Rubin's Pathology:
Clinicopathologic Foundations of Medicine

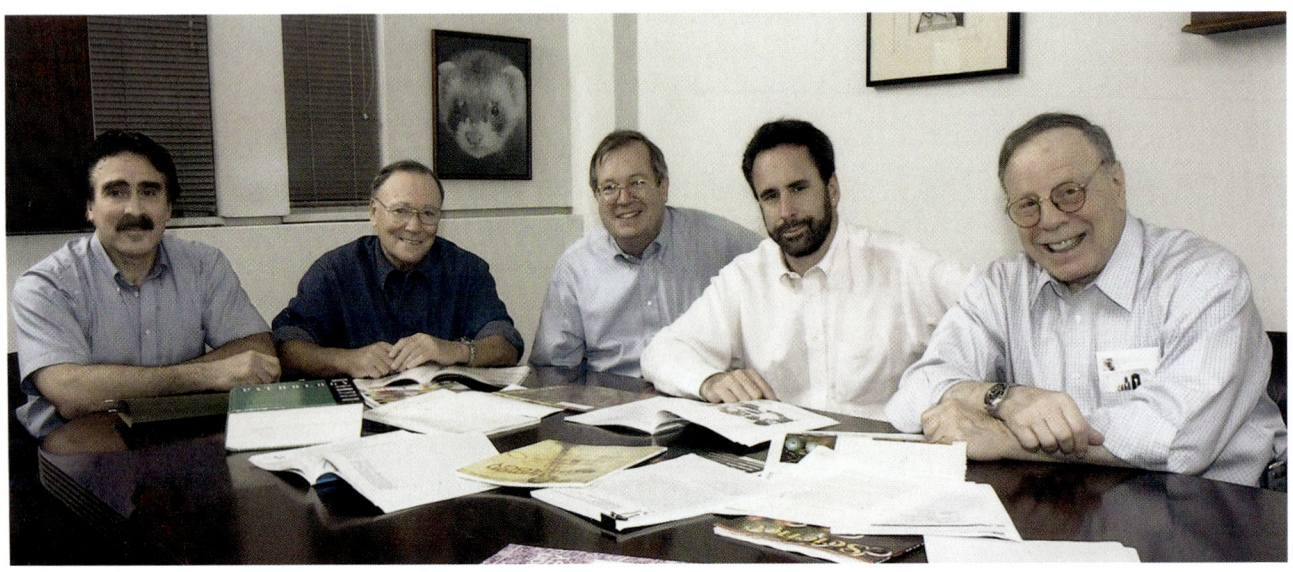

The editorial team at work. From left to right: David Strayer, Emanuel Rubin, Roland Schwarting, Raphael Rubin, Fred Gorstein

Rubin's Pathology:

CLINICOPATHOLOGIC FOUNDATIONS OF MEDICINE, 4TH EDITION

EDITOR-IN-CHIEF:

Emanuel Rubin, MD

Gonzalo E. Aponte
Distinguished Professor of Pathology

ASSOCIATE EDITORS:

Fred Gorstein, MD
Professor of Pathology

Raphael Rubin, MD
Professor of Pathology

Roland Schwarting, MD
Professor of Pathology

David Strayer, M.D., Ph.D.
Professor of Pathology

All are in the Department of Pathology, Anatomy, and Cell Biology
Jefferson Medical College of Thomas Jefferson University
Philadelphia, Pennsylvania

WITH 44 CONTRIBUTORS

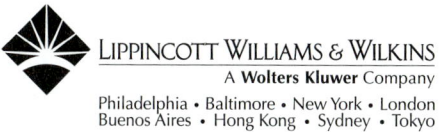

LIPPINCOTT WILLIAMS & WILKINS
A **Wolters Kluwer** Company
Philadelphia • Baltimore • New York • London
Buenos Aires • Hong Kong • Sydney • Tokyo

Dedication:
To my Parents, Jacob and Sophie Rubin and my wife, Linda Anne
Emanuel Rubin

Editor: Betty Sun
Managing Editor: Emilie Linkins
Marketing Manager: Joe Schott
Production Editor: Christina Remsberg
Compositor: Maryland Composition
Printer: RR Donnelley-Willard

Copyright © 2005 Lippincott Williams & Wilkins

351 West Camden Street
Baltimore, Maryland 21201-2436 USA

530 Walnut Street
Philadelphia, PA 19106

All rights reserved. This book is protected by copyright. No part of this book may be reproduced in any form or by any means, including photocopying, or utilized by any information storage and retrieval system without written permission from the copyright owner.

The publisher is not responsible (as a matter of product liability, negligence, or otherwise) for any injury resulting from any material contained herein. This publication contains information relating to general principles of medical care that should not be construed as specific instructions for individual patients. Manufacturers' product information and package inserts should be reviewed for current information, including contraindications, dosages, and precautions.

Printed in the United States of America

First Edition, 1989
Second Edition, 1995
Third Edition, 2001

Library of Congress Cataloging-in-Publication Data

Rubin's pathology: clinicopathologic foundations of medicine/editor-in-chief, Emanuel Rubin; associate editors, Fred Gorstein... [et al.].—4th ed.
  p.; cm.
  Includes index.
  Rev. ed. of: Essential pathology. 3rd ed. c2001.
  ISBN 0-7817-4733-3
  1. Pathology. I. Title: Pathology. II. Rubin, Emanuel, 1928-
III. Gorstein, Fred. IV. Essential pathology.
  [DNLM: 1. Pathology. QZ 4 R896 2004]
  RB111.E856 2004
  616.07—dc22
                                                    2003065889

The publishers have made every effort to trace the copyright holders for borrowed material. If they have inadvertently overlooked any, they will be pleased to make the necessary arrangements at the first opportunity.

To purchase additional copies of this book, call our customer service department at **(800) 638-3030** or fax orders to **(301) 824-7390**. International customers should call **(301) 714-2324**.

Visit Lippincott Williams & Wilkins on the Internet: *http://www.LWW.com*. Lippincott Williams & Wilkins customer service representatives are available from 8:30 am to 6:00 pm, EST.

05 06 07
1 2 3 4 5 6 7 8 9 10

Contributors:

Stuart A. Aaronson, MD
Professor and Director
Derald H. Ruttenberg Cancer Center
Mount Sinai School of Medicine
New York, New York

Michael F. Allard, MD, FRCPC
Associate Professor
Department of Pathology and Laboratory Medicine
University of British Columbia
Scientist and Cardiovascular Pathologist
St. Paul's Hospital—Providence Health Care
Vancouver, British Columbia

Mohammad Alomari
Department of Pathology and Laboratory Medicine
King Faisal Specialist Hospital and Research Center
Riyadh, Saudi Arabia

Karoly Balogh, MD
Associate Professor of Pathology
Harvard Medical School
Boston, Massachusetts

Mary Beth Beasley, MD
Department of Pathology
Providence Portland Medical Center
Portland, Oregon

Marluce Bibbo, MD
Professor
Department of Pathology, Anatomy, and Cell Biology
Jefferson Medical College
Director of Cytopathology
Thomas Jefferson University Hospital
Philadelphia, Pennsylvania

Thomas W. Bouldin, MD
Professor of Pathology and Laboratory Medicine
University of North Carolina School of Medicine
Attending Pathologist
University of North Carolina Hospitals
Chapel Hill, North Carolina

Daniel H. Connor, MD
Visiting Professor of Pathology
Georgetown University School of Medicine
Rockville, Maryland

Mary Cunnane, MD
Clinical Associate Professor
Department of Pathology, Anatomy, and Cell Biology
Jefferson Medical College
Philadelphia, Pennsylvania

Ivan Damjanov, MD, PhD
Professor
Department of Pathology
University of Kansas School of Medicine
Kansas City, Kansas

David Elder, MB, ChB, FRCPA
Professor
Department of Pathology and Laboratory Medicine
University of Pennsylvania
Director of Anatomic Pathology
Hospital of the University of Pennsylvania
Philadelphia, Pennsylvania

Robert M. Genta, MD
Professor and Chairman
Department of Pathology
University of Geneva
Geneva, Switzerland
Adjunct Professor
Department of Pathology and Medicine
Baylor College of Medicine
Houston, Texas

Barry J. Goldstein, MD, PhD
Professor of Medicine, Biochemistry, and Molecular Pharmacology
Director, Division of Endocrinology, Diabetes, and Metabolic Diseases
Jefferson Medical College
Philadelphia, Pennsylvania

Avrum I. Gotlieb, MDCM, FRCP
Professor and Chairman
Department of Laboratory Medicine and Pathobiology
University of Toronto
Toronto, Ontario

J. Charles Jennette, MD
Brinkhous Distinguished Professor and Chairman
Department of Pathology and Laboratory Medicine
University of North Carolina School of Medicine
Chapel Hill, North Carolina

Anthony Alexander Killeen, MB, BCh, PhD, FCAP, FFPath RCPI
Clinical Associate Professor
Department of Pathology
University of Michigan
Ann Arbor, Michigan

Michael J. Klein, MD
Professor of Pathology
Head, Section of Surgical Pathology
University of Alabama at Birmingham
Birmingham, Alabama

Contributors

Gordon K. Klintworth, MD, PhD
Professor
Department of Pathology and Ophthalmology
Duke University Medical Center
Durham, North Carolina

Robert Kisilevsky, MD, PhD, FRCPC
Professor
Department of Pathology and Department of Biochemistry
Queen's University
Kingston, Ontario

William D. Kocher, MD
Clinical Assistant Professor
Department of Pathology
Jefferson Medical College
Philadelphia, Pennsylvania

Robert J. Kurman, MD
Professor of Pathology and Obstetrics and Gynecology
Johns Hopkins University School of Medicine
Director of Gynecologic Pathology
Johns Hopkins Hospital
Baltimore, Maryland

Maria J. Merino, MD
Chief, Surgical Pathology
Laboratory of Pathology
National Cancer Institute
National Institutes of Health
Bethesda, Maryland

Steven McKenzie, MD, PhD
Professor of Medicine and Pediatrics
Jefferson Medical College
Philadelphia, Pennsylvania

Bruce McManus, MD, PhD
Professor
Department of Pathology and Laboratory Medicine
University of British Columbia
Vancouver, British Columbia

Hedwig S. Murphy, MD, PhD
Assistant Professor
Department of Pathology
University of Michigan
Ann Arbor, Michigan

Juan P. Palazzo, MD
Professor of Pathology
Department of Pathology, Anatomy, and Cell Biology
Jefferson Medical College
Philadelphia, Pennsylvania

Stanley J. Robboy, MD
Professor
Department of Pathology, Obstetrics, and Gynecology
Duke University Medical Center
Durham, North Carolina

Emanuel Rubin, MD
Gonzalo E. Aponte Distinguished Professor and Chairman Emeritus
Department of Pathology, Anatomy, and Cell Biology
Jefferson Medical College
Philadelphia, Pennsylvania

Raphael Rubin, MD
Professor
Department of Pathology, Anatomy, and Cell Biology
Jefferson Medical College
Philadelphia, Pennsylvania

Jeffrey E. Saffitz, MD, PhD
Paul E. Lacy and Ellen Lacy Professor of Pathology
Department of Pathology
Washington University School of Medicine
St. Louis, Missouri

Alan Lewis Schiller, MD
Irene Heinz Given and John LaPorte Given Professor and Chairman
Department of Pathology
Mount Sinai School of Medicine
New York, New York

Gregory C. Sephel, PhD
Associate Professor of Pathology
Vanderbilt University School of Medicine
Nashville, Tennessee

Craig A. Storm, MD
Assistant Professor of Pathology
Department of Pathology
Dartmouth Medical School
Hanover, New Hampshire

David Strayer, MD, PhD
Professor
Department of Pathology, Anatomy, and Cell Biology
Jefferson Medical College
Philadelphia, Pennsylvania

Roland Schwarting, MD
Professor
Department of Pathology, Anatomy, and Cell Biology
Jefferson Medical College
Philadelphia, Pennsylvania

Ann D. Thor, MD
Lloyd E. Rader Professor and Chairman
Department of Pathology
University of Oklahoma
Oklahoma City, Oklahoma

William D. Travis, MD
Adjunct Professor of Pathology
Georgetown University
Chairman
Department of Pulmonary and Mediastinal Pathology
Armed Forces Institute of Pathology
Washington, D.C.

John Q. Trojanowski, MD, PhD
Professor
Department of Pathology and Laboratory Medicine
University of Pennsylvania School of Medicine
Center for Neurodegenerative Disease Research
University of Pennsylvania
Philadelphia, Pennsylvania

Beverly Y. Wang, MD
Assistant Professor
Department of Pathology
The Mount Sinai School of Medicine
New York, New York

Jianzhou Wang, MD, PhD
Assistant Professor
Department of Pathology
University of Oklahoma Health Science Center
Oklahoma City, Oklahoma

Peter A. Ward, MD
Godfrey D. Stobbe Professor and Chairman
Department of Pathology
University of Michigan
Ann Arbor, Michigan

Jeffrey S. Warren, MD
Warthin-Weller Professor of Pathology
Department of Pathology
University of Michigan
Ann Arbor, Michigan

Bruce M. Wenig, MD
Professor
Department of Pathology
Albert Einstein College of Medicine
Bronx, New York
Vice Chairman
Department of Pathology
Beth Israel Medical Center
New York, NY.

Stephen C. Woodward, MD
Professor
Department of Pathology
Vanderbilt University
Nashville, Tennessee

Bobby Yanagawa, PhD
Visiting Scientist
Department of Pathology and Laboratory Medicine
University of British Columbia
Vancouver, BC, Canada

Foreword to Rubin's Pathology Fourth Edition

Most medical students seem to approach their pathology course with some degree of trepidation. Gone are the days of sitting for an exam, focusing narrowly on the basic science discipline at hand: anatomy, biochemistry, physiology, etc. Pathology is for most students the first taste of truly synthetic reasoning, the very basis of medicine. Accustomed to the deconstructionist scientific method, the medical student must now master the integration of seemingly disparate disciplines into the Big Picture of pathology.

Such an intellectual paradigm shift is sufficiently difficult in and of itself. Lacking a clear and detailed road map for this journey, many students would find themselves hopelessly lost. For years, Rubin's *Pathology* has served as one of the best guides for students of pathology. With the birth of this Fourth Edition, many welcome changes have now appeared, and medical students have their own colleagues to thank.

Over a year ago, the editors of Rubin's *Pathology* approached me with a proposal to create a formal Student Review Board. For the first time, a major medical student text would be evaluated–page by page–by the end-users themselves. This review board represents some of the best and brightest of our future physicians, balanced by gender, geography, and format of school curriculum. Our goal was to focus the text's content toward that information most relevant for USMLE Step 1 and for clinical rotations.

This Fourth Edition of Rubin's *Pathology* represents the single best source of pathology content for medical students. The revised content, along with substantive improvements in the figures and tables, provides the reader with all the important, high-yield facts necessary for success, and all in a visually engaging manner. Thanks to the expertise and clarity of the chapter authors, along with the critical eye of a dozen student reviewers, medical students have their road map for success in pathology.

Review Board Coordinator: Michael Tomblyn, Rush University Medical School
Nihar Desai, Drexel University School of Medicine
Teresa A. Everson, Medical College of Ohio
Kelly Horton, University of Texas
Jamie Morano, Harvard School of Public Health
Alexa Oster, University of Pennsylvania School of Medicine
James Richter, University of Nevada School of Medicine
Erica Schockett, Brown University School of Medicine
Thomas Semrad, Rush University Medical School
Minesh Shah, University of Illinois Chicago
Sneha Shah, Rush University Medical School

Preface

An honest tale speeds best being plainly told.
(*Shakespeare, Richard III*)

As we stated in the Preface to the previous editions of *Pathology*, this fourth edition continues to view pathology as the medical science that deals with all aspects of disease, but with special reference to the essential nature, the causes, and the development of abnormal conditions. In this sense, literacy in pathology is the bedrock of practice and research for the student of medical science. Thus, wherever possible we have related pathologic changes to clinical manifestations of disease, as reflected in the new subtitle of the book.

As in the earlier editions, *Pathology* maintains the traditional custom of dividing the subject matter into general (Chapters 1–9) and systemic (Chapters 10–30) pathology. General pathology emphasizes the towering achievements in the study of cell and molecular biology, biochemistry, and immunology, all of which are related to the contemporary understanding of the pathogenesis of disease. Although systemic pathology is concerned principally with the description of specific maladies, the concepts detailed in general pathology are utilized to explain their underlying causes. In this approach we are mindful of the admonition of Edmond Halley (1687): "Truth being uniform, and always the same, it is admirable to observe how easily we are enabled to make out very abstruse and difficult matters, when once true and genuine Principles are obtained."

Particular attention continues to be paid throughout to the impact of molecular genetics on our insights into the causes and manifestations of disease, including the correlations between genotype and phenotypic expression. For reference purposes, we have identified many of the relevant gene mutations and their chromosomal locations.

Our original decision to present separate chapters on two systemic diseases, namely diabetes and amyloidosis, has been amply justified by the striking accumulation of new knowledge in these areas. We also recognize the increasing importance of cytopathology as a diagnostic modality by retaining a chapter on this subject.

In his treatise *On the Natural Faculties*, Galen wrote, "the chief merit of language is clearness, and we know that nothing detracts from this as do unfamiliar terms." As in the previous editions, we have always kept this admonition in mind in editing the text and the graphic material. To enhance the clarity of presentation, the fourth edition emphasizes important concepts by incorporating short declarative sentences into secondary headings. We continue with the format of designating for individual diseases separate sections of epidemiology, pathogenesis, pathology, and clinical features, each identified by a unique icon. Attention is often directed to the key points by the use of bulleted lists and boldface type.

To aid the student in understanding and retaining complex and detailed information, we have retained the emphasis on graphic representations of the pathogenesis of disease, the complications of various disorders, and the sequences of pathological alterations. In that context, the initial edition of *Pathology* published in 1988, was the first to utilize line drawings and diagrammatic representations of disease processes for the purpose of teaching pathology to medical students. Because graphic images utilize pattern recognition, one of the most fundamental characteristics of the human brain, they powerfully communicate abstract and complex material, as any lecturer who has referred to a graph will attest. At the same time, we have been guided by Einstein's admonition that "everything should be made as simple as possible, but not simpler." For the fourth edition, we have added numerous new drawings and have revised many of the previous ones. The number of color photographs has also been significantly increased. We welcome the participation of new authors in the large majority of chapters. We are grateful to John Farber for his invaluable contributions to the first three editions and have now assembled a group of expert associate editors to continue this educational project.

Sadly, attempting to edit a comprehensive textbook of pathology without missing any errors is like trying to live without sin—worth the effort, but probably impossible. As Isaac Newton wrote (1703), "To explain all nature is too difficult a task for any one man or even for any one age. Tis much better to do a little with certainty & leave the rest for others that come after you." However, the inevitability of human mistakes has not deterred us from including new and still controversial concepts. Some of these will stand the test of time; the others will be corrected in the next edition.

Emanuel Rubin

Acknowledgments

Much of the material in the fourth edition is derived from chapters in the third edition. The editors acknowledge the fine contributions of the following authors to previous editions.

Adam Bagg
Sue A. Bartow
Hugh Bonner
Stephen W. Chensue
Jeffrey Cossman
John E. Craighead
Maire A. Duggan
Hormoz Ehya
Joseph C. Fantone
John L. Farber
Gregory N. Fuller
Stanley R. Hamilton

Terence J. Harrist
Arthur P. Hays
Robert B. Jennings
Kent J. Johnson
Ernest A. Lack
Antonio Martinez-Hernandez
Wolfgang J. Mergner
Robert O. Peterson
Timothy R. Quinn
Brian Schapiro
Stephen M. Schwartz
Benjamin H. Spargo
Charles Steenbergen, Jr.
Steven L. Teitelbaum
Benjamin F. Trump
F. Stephen Vogel

Table of Contents

Chapter 1:
Cell Injury 2
Emanuel Rubin, David S. Strayer

Chapter 2:
Inflammation 40
Hedwig S. Murphy, Peter A. Ward

Chapter 3:
Repair, Regeneration, and Fibrosis 84
Gregory C. Sephel, Stephen C. Woodward

Chapter 4:
Immunopathology 118
Jeffrey S. Warren, Peter A. Ward

Chapter 5:
Neoplasia 164
Emanuel Rubin, Raphael Rubin, Stuart Aaronson

Chapter 6:
Developmental and Genetic Diseases 214
Emanuel Rubin, Anthony A. Killeen

Chapter 7:
Hemodynamic Disorders 280
Bruce M. McManus, Michael F. Allard, Bobby Yanagawa

Chapter 8:
Environmental and Nutritional Pathology 312
Emanuel Rubin, David S. Strayer

Chapter 9:
Infectious and Parasitic Diseases 356
David Schwartz, Robert M. Genta, Daniel H. Connor

Chapter 10:
Blood Vessels 472
Avrum I. Gotlieb

Chapter 11:
The Heart 520
Jeffrey E. Saffitz

Chapter 12:
The Respiratory System 582
William D. Travis, Mary Beth Beasley

Chapter 13:
The Gastrointestinal Tract 660
Emanuel Rubin, Juan P. Palazzo

Chapter 14:
The Liver and Biliary System 740
Emanuel Rubin, Raphael Rubin

Table of Contents

Chapter 15:
The Pancreas 810

Emanuel Rubin, Raphael Rubin

Chapter 16:
The Kidney 826

J. Charles Jennette

Chapter 17:
The Lower Urinary Tract and Male Reproductive System 886

Ivan Damjanov

Chapter 18:
The Female Reproductive System 926

Stanley J. Robboy, Robert J. Kurman, Maria J. Merino

Chapter 19:
The Breast 996

Ann D. Thor, Jianzhou Wang, Sue A. Bartow

Chapter 20:
Hematopathology 1018

Roland Schwarting, William D. Kocher, Steven McKenzie, Mohammad Alomari

Chapter 21:
The Endocrine System 1124

Emanuel Rubin, Raphael Rubin

Chapter 22:
Diabetes Mellitus 1172

Barry J. Goldstein

Chapter 23:
The Amyloidoses 1186

Robert Kisilevsky

Chapter 24:
The Skin 1202

Craig A. Storm, David E. Elder

Chapter 25:
The Head and Neck 1268

Bruce M. Wenig, Mary Cunnane, Károly Bálogh

Chapter 26:
Bones and Joints 1304

Alan L. Schiller, Beverly Y. Wang, Michael J. Klein

Chapter 27:
Skeletal Muscle 1386

Lawrence C. Kenyon, Mark T. Curtis

Chapter 28:
The Nervous System 1412

John Q. Trojanowski: The Central Nervous System
Thomas W. Bouldin: The Peripheral Nervous System

Chapter 29:
The Eye 1502

Gordon K. Klintworth

Chapter 30:
Cytopathology 1528

Marluce Bibbo

CHAPTER 1

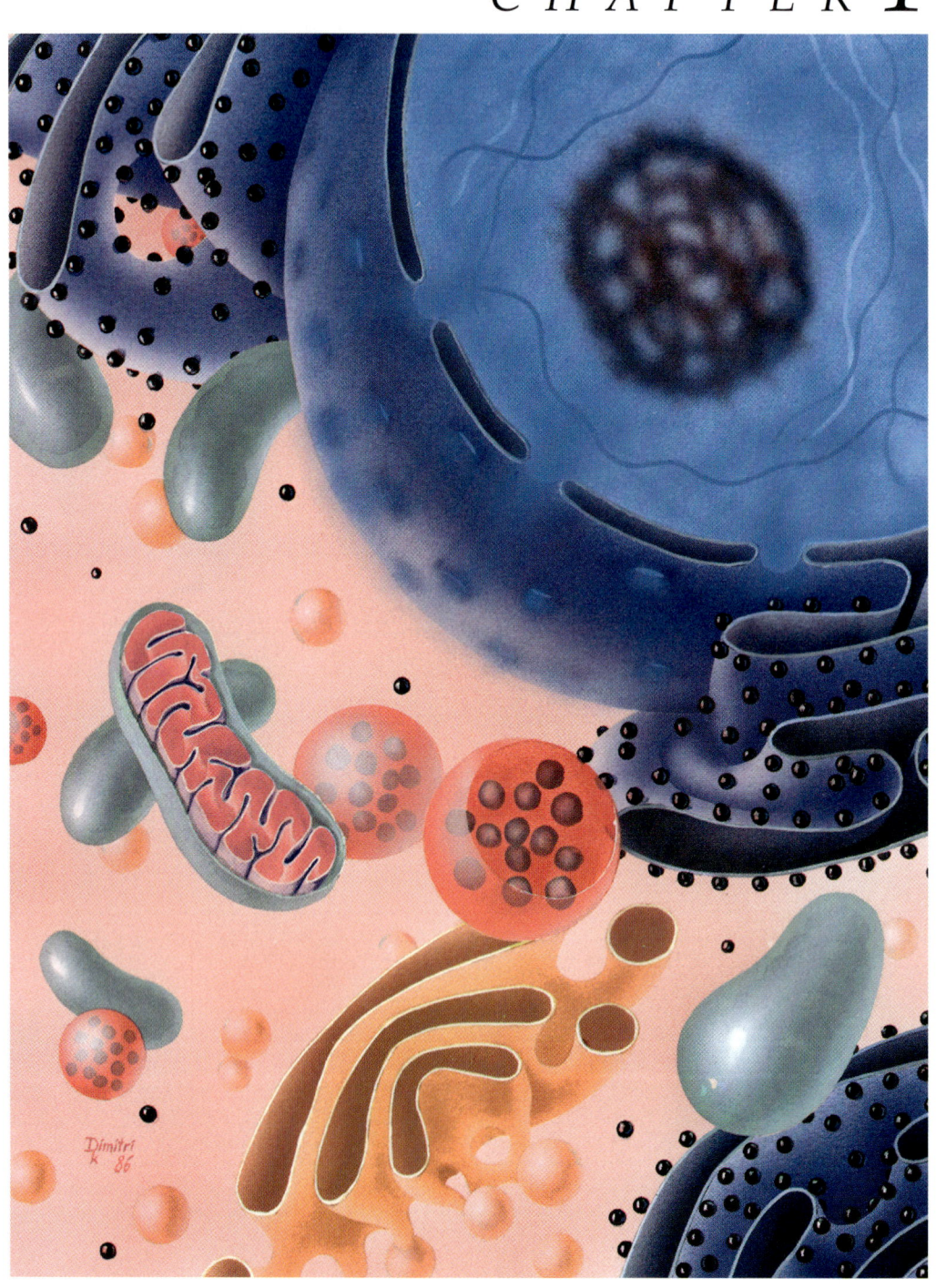

Cell Injury

Emanuel Rubin
David S. Strayer

Reactions to Persistent Stress and Cell Injury
Atrophy
Hypertrophy
Hyperplasia
Metaplasia
Dysplasia
Intracellular Storage
Calcification
Hyaline

Mechanisms and Morphology of Cell Injury
Hydropic Swelling
Subcellular Changes
Ischemic Cell Injury
Oxidative Stress
Ischemia/Reperfusion Injury

Ionizing Radiation
Viral Cytotoxicity
Chemicals
Abnormal G Protein Activity

Cell Death
Necrosis
Apoptosis

Biological Aging
Maximal Life Span
Functional and Structural Changes
The Cellular Basis of Aging
Genetic Factors
Somatic Damage

FIGURE 1-1 *(see opposite page)*
Interior of an idealized cell.

Pathology in its simplest sense is the study of structural and functional abnormalities that are expressed as diseases of organs and systems. Classic theories of disease attributed all disorders to systemic imbalances or to noxious effects of humors on specific organs. In the 19th century, Rudolf Virchow, often referred to as the father of modern pathology, broke sharply with such traditional concepts by proposing that the basis of all disease is injury to the smallest living unit of the body, namely, the cell. A century and a half later, both clinical and experimental pathology remain rooted in Virchow's cellular pathology.

To appreciate the mechanisms of injury to the cell, it is useful to consider its global needs in a philosophical sense. In the reaction against mystical or vitalistic theories of biology, teleology—the study of design or purpose in nature—was discredited as a means of scientific investigation. Nevertheless, although facts can be established only by observations, teleological thinking can be important in framing questions. As an analogy, without an understanding of the goals of chess and prior knowledge that a particular computer is programmed to play it, no analysis of the machine would be likely to uncover its method of operation. Moreover, it would be futile to search for the sources of defects in the specific program or overall operating system while lacking an appreciation of the goals of the device. In this sense, it is helpful to understand the problems with which the cell is confronted and the strategies that have evolved to cope with them.

A living cell must maintain an organization capable of producing energy. Thus, the most pressing need for a free living cell, whether prokaryotic or eukaryotic, is to establish a structural and functional barrier between its internal milieu and a hostile environment. The plasma membrane serves this purpose in several ways:

- It maintains a constant internal ionic composition against very large chemical gradients between the interior and exterior compartments.
- It selectively admits some molecules while excluding or extruding others.
- It provides a structural envelope to contain the informational, synthetic, and catabolic constituents of the cell.
- It provides an environment to house signal transduction molecules that mediate communication between the external and internal milieus.

At the same time, to survive, the cell must be able to adapt to adverse environmental conditions, such as changes in temperature, solute concentrations, or oxygen supply; the presence of noxious agents; and so on. The evolution of multicellular organisms eased the hazardous lot of individual cells by establishing a controlled extracellular environment in which temperature, oxygenation, ionic content, and nutrient supply are relatively constant. It also permitted the luxury of differentiation of cells for such widely divergent functions as nutrient storage (liver cell glycogen and adipocytes), communication (neurons), contractile activity (heart muscle), synthesis of proteins or peptides for export (liver, pancreas, and endocrine cells), absorption (intestine), and defense against foreign invaders (polymorphonuclear leukocytes, lymphocytes, and macrophages).

Cells encounter many stresses as a result of changes in their internal and external environments. **The patterns of response to this stress constitute the cellular bases of disease.** If an injury exceeds the adaptive capacity of the cell, it dies. A cell exposed to persistent sublethal injury has a limited repertoire of responses, the expression of which we interpret as evidence of cell injury. In general, the mammalian cell adapts to injury by conserving its resources; it decreases or ceases its differentiated functions and reverts to its ancestral, unicellular character, which is concerned with functions exclusively dedicated to its own survival. **In this perspective, pathology is the study of cell injury and the expression of a preexisting capacity to adapt to such injury, on the part of either injured or intact cells.** Such an orientation leaves little room for the concept of parallel—normal and pathological—biologies.

REACTIONS TO PERSISTENT STRESS AND CELL INJURY

Persistent stress often leads to chronic cell injury. In general, permanent organ injury is associated with the death of individual cells. By contrast, the cellular response to persistent sublethal injury, whether chemical or physical, reflects adaptation of the cell to a hostile environment. Again, these changes are, for the most part, reversible on discontinuation of the stress. In response to persistent stress, a cell dies or adapts. It is thus our view that at the cellular level it is more appropriate to speak of chronic adaptation than of chronic injury. The major adaptive responses are atrophy, hypertrophy, hyperplasia, metaplasia, dysplasia, and intracellular storage. In addition, certain forms of neoplasia may follow adaptive responses.

Atrophy Is a Decrease in the Size and Function of a Cell

Clinically, atrophy is often recognized as a diminution in the size or function of an organ. Atrophy is often seen in areas of vascular insufficiency or chronic inflammation and may result from disuse of skeletal muscle. Atrophy may be thought of as an adaptive response to stress, in which the cell shrinks and shuts down its differentiated functions, thereby reducing its need for energy to a minimum. In general, the genes expressed in all cells fall into two broad categories, namely, the "housekeeping" genes necessary for the maintenance and survival of any cell and those that determine the differentiated phenotype of any particular cell. With atrophy the expression of differentiation genes is repressed, without significant effects on the expression of housekeeping genes. On restoration of normal conditions, atrophic cells are fully capable of resuming their differentiated functions; size increases to normal, and specialized functions, such as protein synthesis or contractile force, return to their original levels.

One must distinguish atrophy of an organ from cellular atrophy. Reduction in the size of an organ may reflect reversible cell atrophy or may be caused by irreversible loss of cells. For example, atrophy of the brain in Alzheimer disease is secondary to extensive cell death, and the size of the organ cannot be restored (Fig. 1-2). By contrast, atrophy of the ovaries in postmenopausal women is principally due to decreased mass of the ovarian stroma. Atrophy occurs under a variety of conditions outlined below.

Reduced Functional Demand

The most common form of atrophy follows reduced functional demand. For example, after immobilization of a limb in a cast as treatment for a bone fracture or after prolonged bed rest, muscle cells atrophy and muscular strength is reduced. With resumption of normal activity, normal size and function are restored.

Inadequate Supply of Oxygen

Interference with blood supply to tissues is known as ischemia. Total ischemia, with cessation of oxygen perfusion of tissues, results in cell death. Partial ischemia occurs after incomplete occlusion of a blood vessel or in areas of inadequate collateral circulation following a complete vascular occlusion.

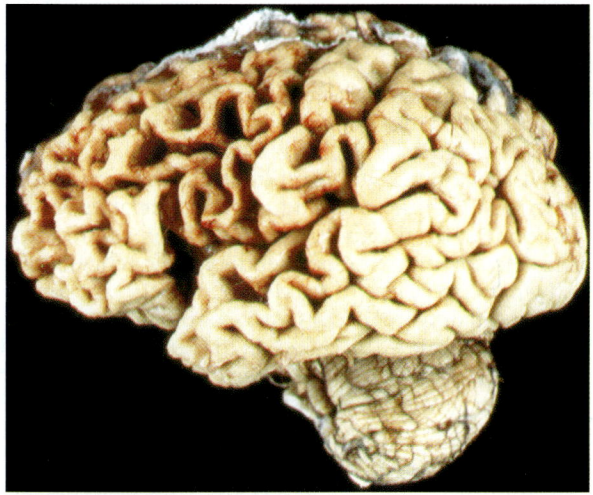

FIGURE 1-2
Atrophy of the brain. Marked atrophy of the frontal lobe is noted in this photograph of the brain. The gyri are thinned and the sulci conspicuously widened.

This results in a chronically reduced oxygen supply, a condition often compatible with cell viability. Under such circumstances, cell atrophy is common. It is frequently seen around the inadequately perfused margins of ischemic necrosis (infarcts) in the heart, brain, and kidneys following vascular occlusion in these organs.

Insufficient Nutrients

Starvation or inadequate nutrition associated with chronic disease leads to cell atrophy, particularly in skeletal muscle. It is striking that reduction in mass is particularly prominent in cells that are not vital to the survival of the organism. One cannot dismiss the possibility that a portion of the cell atrophy attributed to partial ischemia reflects a lack of nutrients.

Interruption of Trophic Signals

The functions of many cells depend on signals transmitted by chemical mediators. The endocrine system and neuromuscular transmission are the best examples. The demands placed on the cell by the actions of hormones or, in the case of skeletal muscle, by synaptic transmission can be eliminated by removing the source of the signal. This can be accomplished through, for example, ablation of an endocrine gland or denervation. If the anterior pituitary is surgically resected, the loss of thyroid-stimulating hormone (TSH), adrenocorticotropic hormone (ACTH, also termed corticotropin), and follicle-stimulating hormone (FSH) results in atrophy of the thyroid, adrenal cortex, and ovaries, respectively. Atrophy secondary to endocrine insufficiency is not restricted to pathological conditions—witness the atrophy of the endometrium caused by decreased estrogen levels following menopause (Fig. 1-3). Moreover, even cancer cells can be induced to undergo atrophy, to some extent, by hormonal deprivation. Androgen-dependent cancer of the prostate partially regresses after the administration of testosterone antagonists. The growth of certain types of thyroid cancer is halted by inhibiting pituitary TSH secretion with thyroxine. Neurological conditions resulting in denervation of muscle, and thus in loss of the neuromuscular transmission necessary for muscle tone, cause atrophy of the affected muscles. The wasting caused by poliomyelitis or traumatic paraplegia falls into this category.

Persistent Cell Injury

Persistent cell injury is most commonly caused by chronic inflammation associated with prolonged viral or bacterial infections. Chronic inflammation may be seen in a variety of other circumstances, including immunological and granulomatous disorders. A good example is the atrophy of the gastric mucosa that occurs in association with chronic gastritis (see Chapter 13). Similarly, villous atrophy of the small intestinal mucosa follows the chronic inflammation characteristic of celiac disease. Even physical injury, such as prolonged pressure in inappropriate locations, produces atrophy. Heart failure leads to increased pressure in sinusoids of the liver because the heart cannot pump the venous return from that organ efficiently. Accordingly, the cells exposed to the greatest pressure—those in the center of the liver lobule—become atrophic.

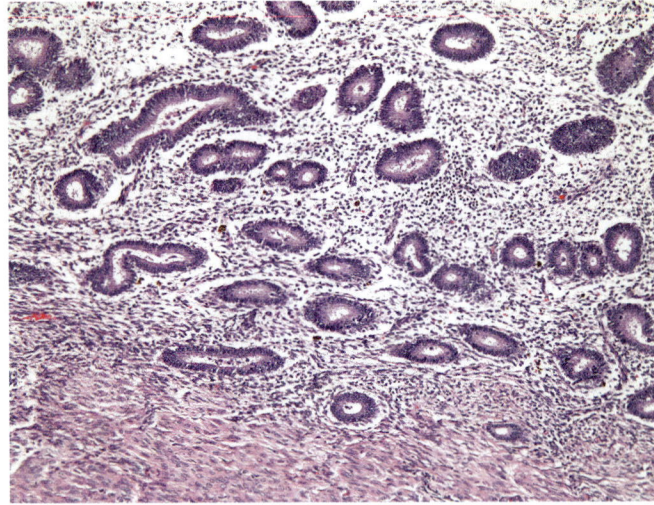
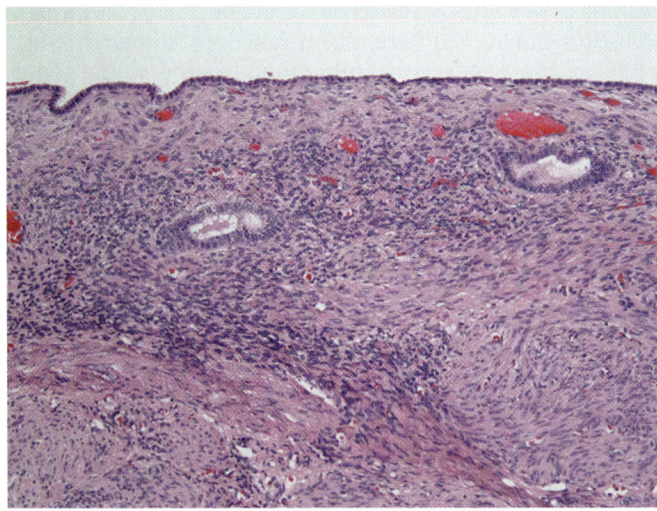

FIGURE 1-3
Proliferative endometrium. A. A section of the uterus from a woman of reproductive age reveals a thick endometrium composed of proliferative glands in an abundant stroma. B. The endometrium of a 75-year-old woman (shown at the same magnification) is thin and contains only a few atrophic and cystic glands.

Aging

One of the hallmarks of aging, particularly in nonreplicating cells such as those of the brain and heart, is cell atrophy. The size of all the parenchymal organs of the body decreases with age. The size of the brain is invariably decreased, and in the very old the size of the heart may be so diminished that the term **senile atrophy** has been used.

Hypertrophy Is an Increase in the Size of a Cell Accompanied by an Augmented Functional Capacity

Hypertrophy is a response to trophic signals or increased functional demands and is commonly a normal process. Hypertrophy can be thought to represent the opposite of atrophy, with increased expression of differentiation genes.

As with atrophy, an increase in size and functional capacity (hypertrophy) of an organ may reflect cellular hypertrophy, an increased number of cells (hyperplasia), or both. In organs composed of nonreplicating cells (i.e., heart and skeletal muscle), organ hypertrophy is invariably secondary to cellular hypertrophy. By contrast, hypertrophy of organs composed of cells that retain the capacity to replicate (e.g., endocrine organs or kidney) involves both cellular hypertrophy and hyperplasia.

Physiological (Hormonal) Hypertrophy

Physiological hypertrophy occurs under the influence of a variety of hormones. Increased production of sex hormones at puberty leads to hypertrophy of the juvenile sex organs and organs associated with secondary sex characteristics. The lactating woman, under the influence of prolactin and estrogen, exhibits hypertrophy of breast tissue.

Although hypertrophy results from certain normal hormonal signals, it is also a response to abnormal levels of hormones. Exogenous anabolic steroids are taken by athletes precisely for their capacity to induce muscle hypertrophy. Endogenous overproduction of TSH by the pituitary is responsible for the thyroid enlargement (goiter) that occurs with nutritional iodine deficiency. In the absence of sufficient iodine, thyroid hormone is not produced. Consequently, there is no feedback inhibition of TSH secretion, and the unopposed TSH, acting as a trophic hormone, induces hypertrophy of thyroid follicular cells. Increased hormone levels can also result from abnormal hormone production by tumors. For example, secretion of ACTH by pituitary tumors results in hypertrophy of the adrenal cortex.

Increased Functional Demand

Hypertrophy caused by increased functional demand is exemplified by greater muscle size and strength following repeated exercise. In an analogous fashion, an exogenous metabolic demand is placed on the liver cell by the administration of drugs that are detoxified by the mixed-function oxidase system. Cytochrome P450 and other enzymes of this drug-metabolizing system reside in the smooth endoplasmic reticulum. The liver cell responds to the metabolic demand of detoxification by increasing the amount of smooth endoplasmic reticulum, with consequent hypertrophy of the cell (Fig. 1-4).

Increased demand occurs under pathological conditions as well. The heart may be called on to increase its contractile force because of mechanical interference with the aortic outflow or because of systemic hypertension, both conditions requiring the heart to eject blood under higher pressure (Fig. 1-5). As in exercise-induced hypertrophy of skeletal muscle, the myocardial cells enlarge, and the heart may more than double in weight. Compensatory enlargement of an organ also results from the loss of functional mass. If one kidney is surgically removed or rendered inoperative because of vascular occlusion, the contralateral kidney hypertrophies to accommodate the increased demand.

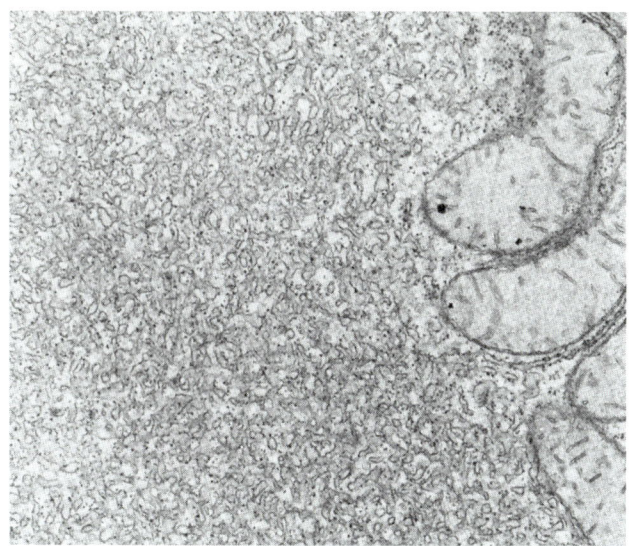

FIGURE 1-4
Proliferation of smooth endoplasmic reticulum in a liver cell in response to phenobarbital administration.

Cellular Mechanisms of Hypertrophy

The elucidation of the cellular and molecular mechanisms underlying the hypertrophic response is still actively pursued, although it is clear that the final steps must include increases in messenger and ribosomal RNA and protein. Thus, cell hypertrophy in some way results from transcriptional regulation. The growth in the size of a cell and DNA replication can be regulated independently by different growth factors. Experimental cardiac hypertrophy is the best-studied model at this time and is discussed in Chapter 11.

The molecular basis of hypertrophy has also been studied in the kidney. After experimental removal of one kidney, the remaining kidney exhibits an increase in both the number and size of the tubular cells. As in the heart, this compensatory hypertrophic response is accompanied by an increased expression of growth-promoting genes (protooncogenes), such as *myc, fos,* and *ras.* When renal tubular cells in culture are exposed to mitogens, they enter into DNA synthesis and divide. However, when the mitogens are added in the presence of inhibitors of DNA synthesis, the cells do not replicate but rather undergo hypertrophy. Thus, the same stimulus can lead to hypertrophy or hyperplasia, depending on the presence of other growth factors or inhibitors.

Hyperplasia Is an Increase in the Number of Cells in an Organ or Tissue

Hypertrophy and hyperplasia are not mutually exclusive and are often seen concurrently.

Hormonal Stimulation

Hormonal signals can induce a physiological hyperplastic effect. For example, the normal increase in estrogen levels at puberty and during the early phase of the menstrual cycle leads to an increased number of both endometrial and uterine stromal cells. A similar hyperplastic response is commonly produced by the administration of exogenous estrogen in postmenopausal women. Estrogens also produce hyperplasia in men. Gynecomastia, an enlargement of the male breast that is characterized by hyperplasia of the epithelial cells lining the ducts, occurs after the treatment of prostatic carcinoma with exogenous estrogens. Similarly, gynecomastia is seen in patients with chronic liver disease, a malady in which circulating estrogen levels are raised because of diminished hepatic inactivation. Hormones produced by tumors can also lead to hyperplasia. For example, secretion of erythropoietin by cancer of the kidney leads to an increase in the number of erythrocyte precursors in the bone marrow.

Increased Functional Demand

Hyperplasia, like hypertrophy, may also follow increased physiological demand. Residence at high altitude, where the oxygen content of the air is relatively low, leads to compensatory hyperplasia of erythrocyte precursors in the bone marrow and an increased number of circulating erythrocytes (secondary polycythemia) (Fig. 1-6). The decrease in the amount of oxygen carried in each erythrocyte is balanced by an increase in the number of cells. On return to sea level, the number of erythrocytes promptly falls to normal. Similarly, chronic blood loss, as in abnormal uterine bleeding, causes hyperplasia of erythrocytic elements.

The immune system's response to many antigens—a vital mechanism for protection from foreign invaders—constitutes another example of demand-induced hyperplasia. Morphologically, lymphocyte hyperplasia is conspicuous in chronic inflammation caused by conditions such as bacterial infection or transplant rejection. An increased demand for parathyroid hormone results in hyperplasia of the parathyroid glands, a sequence found in some cases of chronic renal disease. In such instances, decreased calcium absorption from the small intestine results in mobilization of calcium from the bones to maintain appropriate blood calcium levels. This demand is mediated by parathyroid hormone, and the gland responds with an increase in the number of cells.

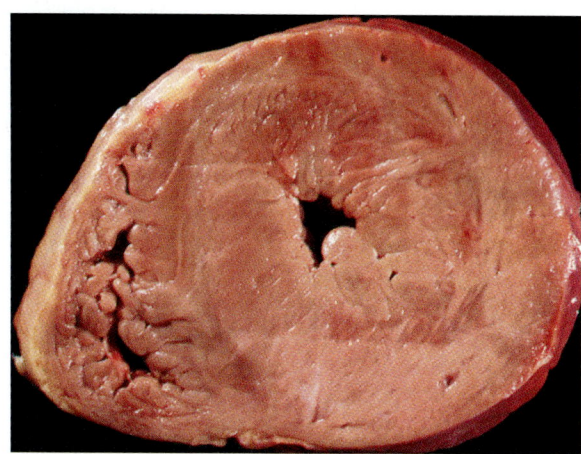

FIGURE 1-5
Myocardial hypertrophy. Cross-section of the heart of a patient with long-standing hypertension shows pronounced, concentric left ventricular hypertrophy.

Chronic Cell Injury

Persistent cell injury may lead to hyperplasia. Chronic inflammation or chronic exposure to physical or chemical injury results in a hyperplastic response. For instance, pressure from ill-fitting shoes causes hyperplasia of the skin of the foot, so-called corns or calluses. It is not too fanciful to consider the primary function of the skin as protection of underlying structures. From this perspective, such hyperplasia, with resultant thickening of the skin, serves to enhance functional capacity. Chronic inflammation of the bladder (chronic cystitis) commonly causes hyperplasia of the bladder epithelium, a condition viewed by endoscopy as whitish plaques of the bladder lining. Inappropriate hyperplasia can itself be harmful—witness the unpleasant consequences of psoriasis, a malady of unknown etiology characterized by conspicuous hyperplasia of the skin (Fig. 1-6).

The cellular and molecular mechanisms that are responsible for the hyperplastic response clearly relate to the control of cell proliferation. These topics are discussed in Chapter 3 and under the heading of liver regeneration in Chapter 14.

Metaplasia Is the Conversion of One Differentiated Cell Type to Another

The most common example of metaplasia is the replacement of a glandular epithelium by a squamous one. It is almost invariably a response to persistent injury and can be thought of as an adaptive mechanism. Columnar or cuboidal lining cells committed to differentiated functions, such as mucus production, assume a simpler form, providing more protection against a pernicious chemical action or the effects of chronic inflammation. Prolonged exposure of the bronchi to tobacco smoke leads to squamous metaplasia of the bronchial epithelium. A comparable response, associated with chronic infection, occurs in the endocervix (Fig. 1-7). In molecular terms, metaplasia represents the substitution of the expression of one set of differentiation genes for another.

Metaplasia is not restricted to squamous differentiation. In cases of chronic reflux of highly acidic gastric contents into the lower esophagus, the squamous epithelium of the esophagus is occasionally replaced by a gastriclike glandular mucosa (Barrett epithelium). This can be thought of as an adap-

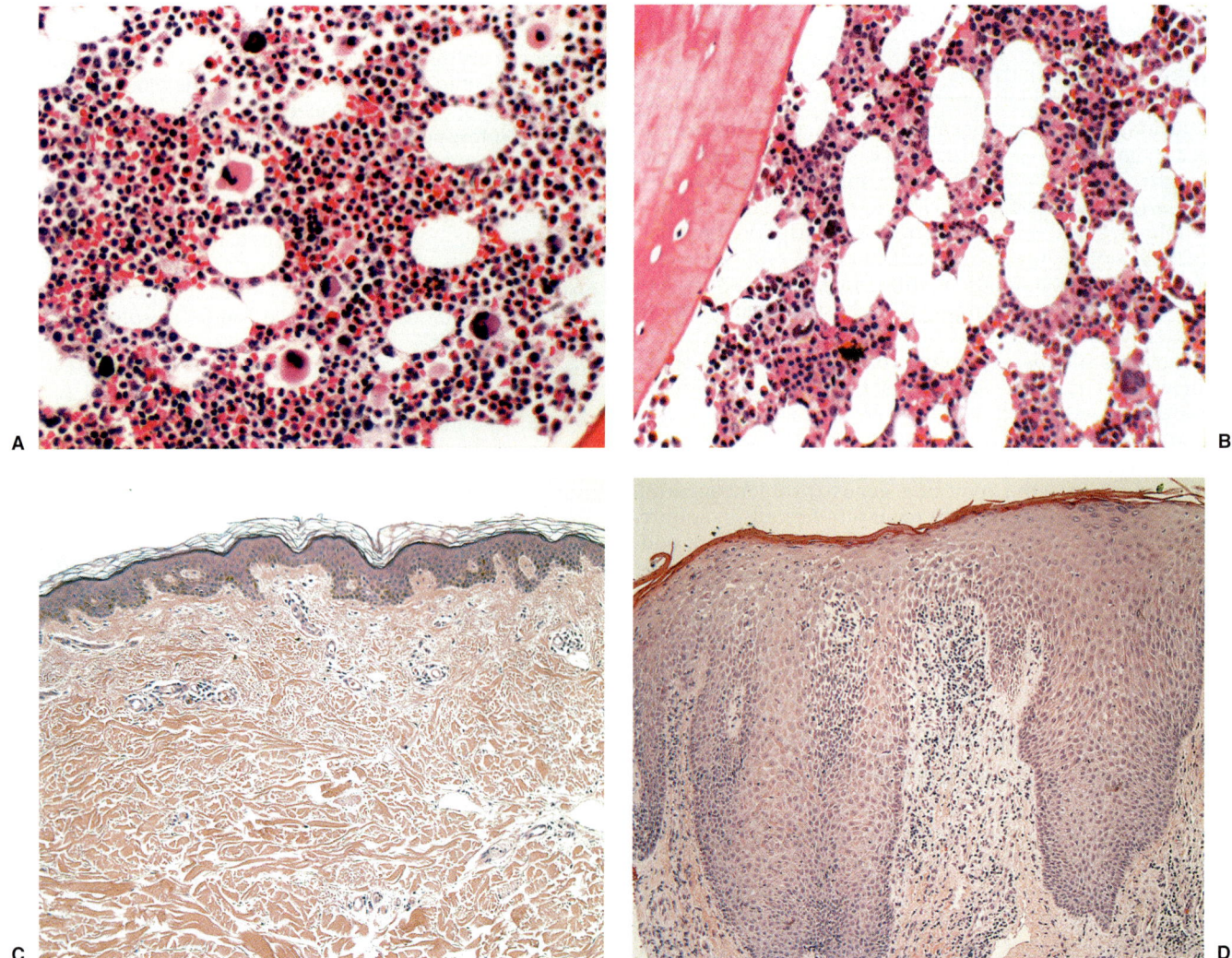

FIGURE 1-6
Hyperplasia. (A) Normal adult bone marrow. (B) Hyperplasia of the bone marrow. (C) Normal epidermis. (D) Epidermal hyperplasia in psoriasis, shown at the same magnification as in C. The epidermis is thickened, owing to an increase in the number of squamous cells.

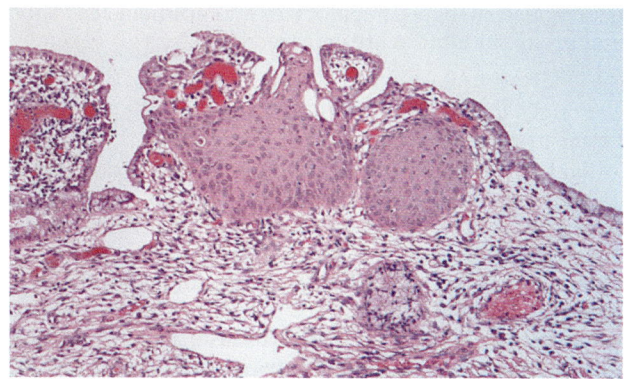

FIGURE 1-7
Squamous metaplasia. A section of endocervix shows the normal columnar epithelium at both margins and a focus of squamous metaplasia in the center.

tive response that protects the esophagus from the injurious effects of gastric acid and pepsin, to which the normal gastric mucosa is resistant. Metaplasia may also consist of replacement of one glandular epithelium by another. In chronic gastritis, a disorder of the stomach characterized by chronic inflammation, atrophic gastric glands are replaced by cells resembling those of the small intestine. The adaptive value of this condition, known as intestinal metaplasia, is not apparent. One also sees metaplasia of transitional epithelium to glandular epithelium in chronic inflammation of the bladder (cystitis glandularis).

Metaplasia is not necessarily a harmless process, even though this response may be thought of as adaptive. For example, in a bronchus, squamous metaplasia may protect against injury produced by tobacco smoke, but it also impairs the production of mucus and ciliary clearance. Furthermore, neoplastic transformation may occur in metaplastic epithelium; cancers of the lung, cervix, stomach, and bladder have their origins in such areas. However, absent continuing injury, there is little stimulus to cell proliferation, and the metaplastic epithelium does not become cancerous.

Metaplasia is usually fully reversible. If the stimulus is removed (e.g., when one stops smoking), the metaplastic epithelium eventually returns to normal.

Dysplasia Refers to Disordered Growth and Maturation of the Cellular Components of a Tissue

The cells that compose an epithelium normally exhibit uniformity of size, shape, and nucleus. Moreover, they are arranged in a regular fashion, as in the progression from plump basal cells to flat superficial cells in a squamous epithelium. When we speak of dysplasia, we mean that this monotonous appearance is disturbed by (1) variations in the size and shape of the cells; (2) enlargement, irregularity, and hyperchromatism of the nuclei; and (3) disorderly arrangement of the cells within the epithelium (Fig. 1-8). Dysplasia occurs most commonly in hyperplastic squamous epithelium, as seen in epidermal actinic keratosis (caused by sunlight) and in areas of squamous metaplasia, such as in the bronchus or the cervix. It is not, however, exclusive to squamous epithelium. Ulcerative colitis, an inflammatory disease of the large intestine, is often complicated by dysplastic changes in the mucosal cells.

Like metaplasia, dysplasia is a response to the persistence of injurious influences and will customarily regress, for example, on cessation of smoking or the disappearance of human papillomavirus from the cervix. However, dysplasia shares many cytological features with cancer, and the line between the two may be very fine indeed. For example, a common diagnostic problem for the pathologist is the distinction between severe dysplasia and early cancer of the cervix. **Dysplasia is a preneoplastic lesion, in the sense that it is a necessary stage in the multistep cellular evolution to cancer.** In fact, dysplasia is today included in the morphological classifications of the stages of intraepithelial neoplasia in a variety of organs (e.g., cervix, prostate, bladder). Accordingly, severe dysplasia is considered an indication for aggressive preventive therapy to cure the underlying cause, eliminate the noxious agent, or surgically remove the offending tissue.

Similar to the development of cancer, dysplasia results from sequential mutations in a proliferating cell population. The fidelity of DNA replication is imperfect, and occasional mutations are inevitable. When a particular mutation confers a growth or survival advantage, the progeny of the affected cell will tend to predominate. In turn, their continued proliferation provides the opportunity for further mutations. The accumulation of such mutations progressively distances the cell from normal regulatory constraints. **Dysplasia is the morphological expression of the disturbance in growth regulation.** However, unlike cancer cells, dysplastic cells are not entirely autonomous, and the histological appearance of the tissue may still revert to normal.

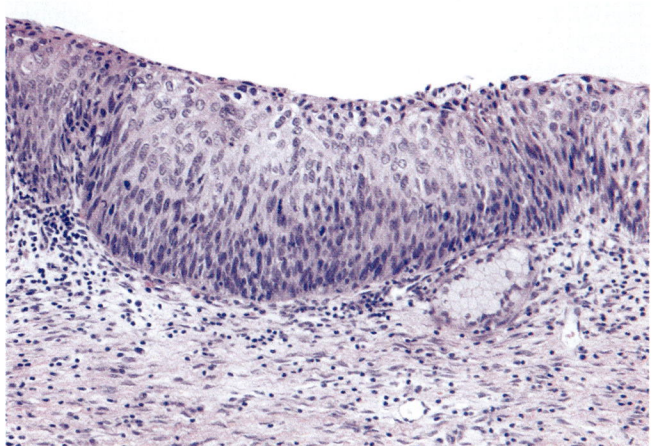

FIGURE 1-8
Dysplasia. The dysplastic epithelium of the uterine cervix lacks the normal polarity, and the individual cells show hyperchromatic nuclei, a larger nucleus-to-cytoplasm ratio, and a disorderly arrangement.

Intracellular Storage Is the Retention of Materials within the Cell

The substance that accumulates may be normal or abnormal, endogenous or exogenous, harmful or innocuous.

- **Nutrients,** such as fat, glycogen, vitamins, and minerals, are stored for later use.
- **Degraded phospholipids,** which result from the turnover of endogenous membranes, are stored in lysosomes and may be recycled.
- **Substances that cannot be metabolized** accumulate in cells. These include (1) endogenous substrates that are not further processed because a key enzyme is missing (hereditary storage diseases), (2) insoluble endogenous pigments (e.g., lipofuscin and melanin), and (3) exogenous particulates, such as inhaled silica and carbon or injected tattoo pigments.
- **Overload of normal body constituents,** including iron, copper, and cholesterol, injures a variety of cells.
- **Abnormal proteins** may be toxic when they are retained within a cell. Examples are Lewy bodies in Parkinson disease and mutant α_1-antitrypsin.

Fat

Bacteria and other unicellular organisms continuously ingest nutrients. By contrast, mammals are freed from the necessity of continuous eating. They can eat periodically and can survive a prolonged fast because they store nutrients in specialized cells for later use—fat in adipocytes and glycogen in the liver, heart, and muscle.

The abnormal accumulation of fat is most conspicuous in the liver, a subject treated in detail in Chapter 14. Briefly, liver cells always contain some fat, because free fatty acids released from adipose tissue are taken up by the liver, where they are either oxidized or converted to triglycerides. Most of the newly synthesized triglycerides are secreted as lipoproteins by the liver. When the delivery of free fatty acids to the liver is increased, as in diabetes, or when the intrahepatic metabolism of lipids is disturbed, as in alcoholism, triglycerides accumulate in the liver cell. Fatty liver is identified morphologically by the presence of lipid globules in the cytoplasm. Other organs, including the heart, kidney, and skeletal muscle, also store fat. One must recognize that fat storage is always reversible, and there is no evidence that the presence of excess fat in the cytoplasm interferes with the function of the cell.

Glycogen

Glycogen is a long-chain polymer of glucose, formed and largely stored in the liver and to a lesser extent in muscles. It is depolymerized to glucose and liberated as needed. Glycogen is degraded in steps by a series of enzymes, each of which may be deficient as a result of an inborn error of metabolism. Regardless of the specific enzyme deficiency, the result is a glycogen storage disease (see Chapter 6). These inherited disorders affect the liver, heart, and skeletal muscle and range from mild and asymptomatic conditions to inexorably progressive and fatal diseases (see Chapters 11, 14, and 27).

The amount of glycogen stored in cells is normally regulated by the blood glucose concentration, and hyperglycemic states are associated with increased glycogen stores. Thus, in uncontrolled diabetes, hepatocytes and epithelial cells of the renal proximal tubules are enlarged by excess glycogen.

Inherited Lysosomal Storage Diseases

Similar to the metabolism of glycogen, the breakdown of certain complex lipids and mucopolysaccharides (glycosaminoglycans) is accomplished by a sequence of enzymatic steps. Since these enzymes are located in the lysosomes, their absence results in the lysosomal storage of incompletely degraded lipids, such as cerebrosides (e.g., Gaucher disease) and gangliosides (e.g., Tay-Sachs disease), or products of the catabolism of mucopolysaccharides (e.g., Hurler and Hunter syndromes). These disorders are all progressive but vary from asymptomatic organomegaly to rapidly fatal brain disease. See Chapter 6 for the metabolic bases of these disorders and Chapters 26 and 28 for specific organ pathology.

Cholesterol

The human body has a love–hate relationship with cholesterol. On the one hand, it is a fundamental component of all plasma membranes. On the other hand, when stored in excess, it is closely associated with atherosclerosis and cardiovascular disease, the leading cause of death in the western world. This subject is discussed in detail in Chapter 10.

Briefly, the initial lesion of atherosclerosis (fatty streak) reflects the accumulation of cholesterol and cholesterol esters in macrophages within the arterial intima. As the disease progresses, smooth muscle cells also store cholesterol. Advanced lesions of atherosclerosis are characterized by the extracellular deposition of cholesterol.

In a number of disorders characterized by elevated blood levels of cholesterol (e.g., familial hypercholesterolemia or primary biliary cirrhosis), macrophages store cholesterol. When clusters of these cells in subcutaneous tissues become grossly visible, they are termed **xanthomas**.

Abnormal Proteins

A number of acquired and inherited diseases are characterized by the intracellular accumulation of abnormal proteins. The deviant tertiary structure of the protein may result from an inherited mutation that alters the normal primary amino acid sequence or may reflect an acquired defect in protein folding. The following are examples:

- α_1-**Antitrypsin deficiency** is a heritable disorder in which mutations in the coding gene for α_1-antitrypsin yield an insoluble protein. This mutant protein is not easily exported by heptocytes, thereby leading to cell injury and cirrhosis (see Chapter 14).
- **Prion diseases** comprise a group of neurodegenerative disorders (spongiform encephalopathies) caused by the accumulation of abnormally folded prion proteins. The anomaly reflects the conversion of the normal α-helical structure to a β-pleated sheet. Abnormal prion proteins may result from an inherited mutation or from exposure to the aberrant form of the protein (see Chapter 28).
- **Lewy bodies** (α-synuclein) are seen in the neurons of the substantia nigra in Parkinson disease (Chapter 28).
- **Neurofibrillary tangles** (tau protein) characterize cortical neurons in Alzheimer disease (Chapter 28).

- **Mallory bodies** (intermediate filaments) are hepatocellular inclusions in alcoholic liver injury (Chapter 14).

Pathogenesis: After nascent polypeptides emerge from the ribosomes, they fold to assume the tertiary configuration of mature proteins. Correct folding requires proteins to assume one particular structure from a constellation of possible but incorrect conformations. Curiously, it is energetically more favorable for the cell to produce a variety of foldings and then edit the protein repertoire than to produce only a single correct conformation. Molecular chaperones associate with polypeptides in the endoplasmic reticulum and promote correct folding, after which they dissociate from those proteins that have assumed the correct conformation (Fig. 1-9). By contrast, incorrectly folded proteins remain bound to their chaperones and are subsequently degraded by a demolition mechanism termed the ubiquitin–proteasome system. Evolutionary preference for energy conservation has dictated that a substantial propor-

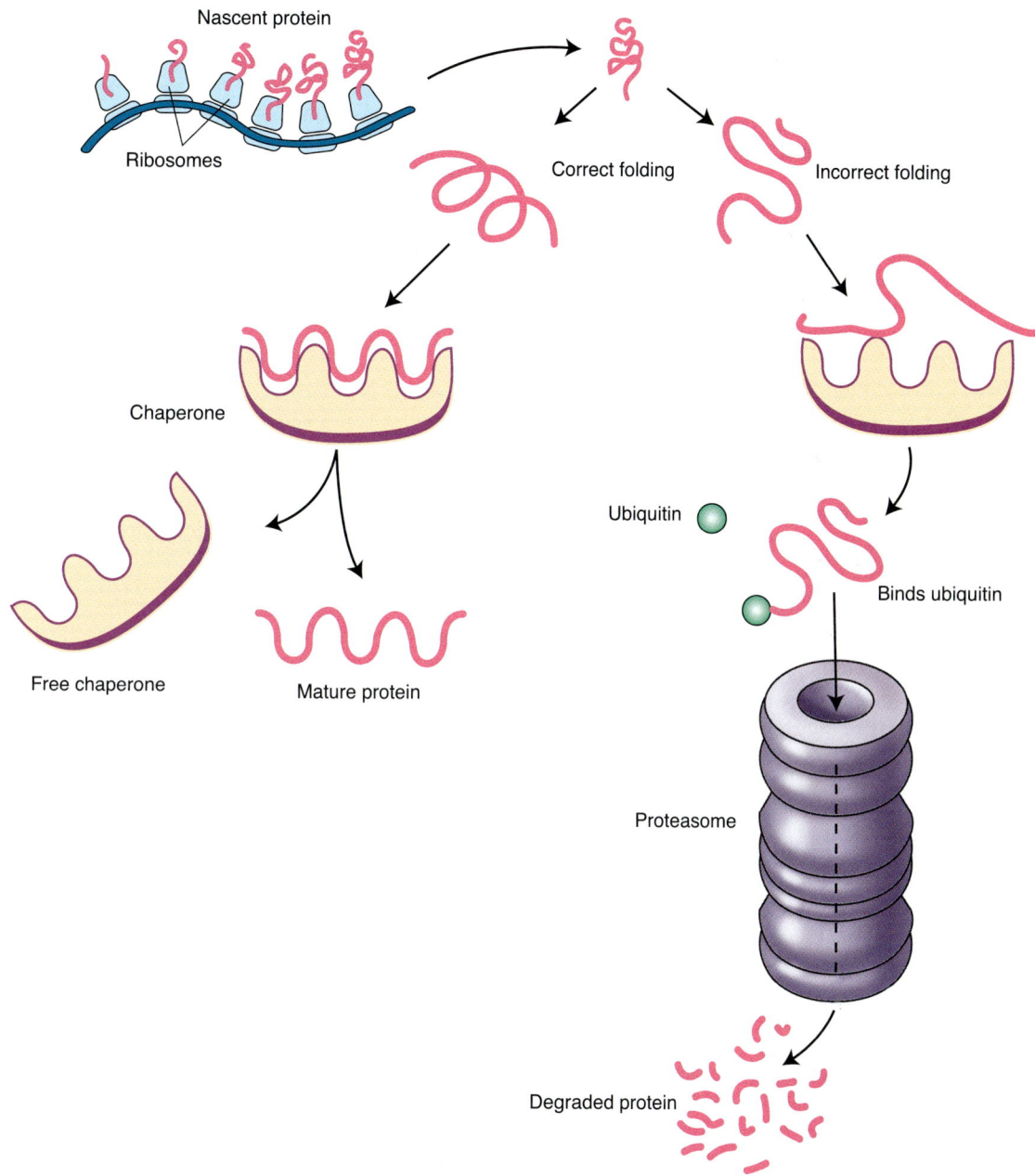

FIGURE 1-9
Differential handling of protein that is correctly folded *(left arrows)* and protein that is incorrectly folded *(right arrows)*. Correctly folded proteins are chaperoned from the ribosomes that produce them to their ultimate cellular destination. Incorrectly folded proteins bind to ubiquitin, an association that directs the protein to proteasomes, where the misfolded protein is degraded.

tion of newly formed proteins are rogues unsuitable for the society of civilized cells.

Numerous hereditary and acquired diseases are caused by evasion of the quality control system designed to promote correct folding and eliminate faulty proteins. Misfolded proteins can injure the cell in a number of ways.

- **Loss of function:** Certain mutations prevent correct folding of crucial proteins, which then do not function properly or cannot be incorporated into the correct site. For example, some mutations that lead to cystic fibrosis cause misfolding of an ion channel protein, which is then sequestered in the endoplasmic reticulum and degraded. Since the protein does not reach its intended destination at the cell membrane, the resulting defect in chloride transport leads to the syndrome termed cystic fibrosis. Other examples of loss of function include mutations of the LDL (low-density lipoprotein) receptor in certain types of hypercholesterolemia and mutations of a copper transport adenosine triphosphatase (ATPase) in Wilson disease.
- **Formation of toxic proteins:** Many of the abnormally folded proteins that accumulate in the cell, either because they form aggregates or because of defects in the system that degrades faulty proteins, are toxic and lead to injury or death of the cell. For the most part, the mechanisms underlying cell injury remain unclear, and the precise targets of the toxic proteins remain to be elucidated. The most prominent examples of the effects of toxic proteins include a number of neurodegenerative diseases, such as Alzheimer disease and Parkinson disease.
- **Retention of secretory proteins:** Many proteins that are destined to be secreted from the cell require a correctly folded conformation to be transported through cellular compartments and released at the cell membrane. Mutations in genes that encode such proteins (e.g., α_1-antitrypsin) lead to cell injury because of massive accumulation of misfolded proteins within the liver cell. Failure to secrete this antiprotease into the circulation also leads to unregulated proteolysis of connective tissue in the lung and loss of pulmonary elasticity (emphysema).
- **Extracellular deposition of aggregated proteins:** Misfolded proteins tend to exhibit a β-pleated conformation in place of random coils or α helices. These abnormal proteins often form insoluble aggregates, which may be visualized as extracellular deposits, the appearance depending upon the specific disease. These accumulations often assume the forms of various types of amyloid and produce cell injury in systemic amyloidoses (see Chapter 23) and a variety of neurodegenerative diseases (see Chapter 28).

Lipofuscin

Lipofuscin, classically known as the "wear-and-tear" pigment, is composed of golden-brown granules found predominantly in cells that either are terminally differentiated (neurons and cardiac myocytes) or cycle only infrequently (hepatocytes) (Fig. 1-10). This material is a normal constituent of many cells and increases with age. It is often more conspicuous in conditions associated with atrophy of an organ.

Lipofuscin derives from the normal turnover of membrane constituents of the cell. Fragments of subcellular organelles are continuously being segregated within autophagic vacuoles in which the lipids and proteins are degraded. Peroxidation of the unsaturated lipids and the formation of heterogeneous lipid–protein complexes render these materials resistant to further digestion. The insoluble products are stored indefinitely as lysosome-derived residual bodies. Despite the occasional prominence of intracellular lipofuscin, there is no reason to believe that this pigment interferes with the function of the cell.

Melanin

Melanin is an insoluble, brown-black pigment found principally in the epidermal cells of the skin, but also in the eye and other organs (Fig. 1-10). It is located in intracellular organelles known as melanosomes and results from the polymerization of certain oxidation products of tyrosine. The amount of melanin is responsible for the differences in skin color among the various races, as well as the color of the eyes. It serves a protective function owing to its ability to absorb ultraviolet light. In white persons, exposure to sunlight increases melanin formation (tanning). The hereditary inability to produce melanin results in the disorder known as *albinism*. The presence of melanin is also a marker of the cancer that arises from melanocytes (melanoma). Melanin is discussed in detail in Chapter 24.

Exogenous Pigments

Anthracosis refers to the storage of carbon particles in the lung and regional lymph nodes (Fig. 1-10). Virtually all urban dwellers inhale particulates of organic carbon generated by the burning of fossil fuels. These particles accumulate in alveolar macrophages and are also transported to hilar and mediastinal lymph nodes, where the indigestible material is stored indefinitely within macrophages. Although the gross appearance of the lungs of persons with anthracosis may be alarming, the condition is innocuous.

Tattoos are the result of the introduction of insoluble metallic and vegetable pigments into the skin, where they are engulfed by dermal macrophages and persist for a lifetime.

Iron and Other Metals

About 25% of the body's total iron content is in an intracellular storage pool composed of the iron-storage proteins **ferritin** and **hemosiderin**. The liver and bone marrow are particularly rich in ferritin, although it is present in virtually all cells. Hemosiderin is a partially denatured form of ferritin that aggregates easily and is recognized microscopically as yellow-brown granules in the cytoplasm. Normally, hemosiderin is found mainly in the spleen, bone marrow, and Kupffer cells of the liver.

Total body iron may be increased by enhanced intestinal iron absorption, as in some anemias, or by parenteral administration of iron-containing erythrocytes in a transfusion. In either case, the excess iron is stored intracellularly as both ferritin and hemosiderin. Increasing the body's total iron content results in a progressive accumulation of hemosiderin, a condition termed **hemosiderosis**. In this condition, iron is present not only in the organs in which it is normally found but also throughout the body, in such places as the skin, pan-

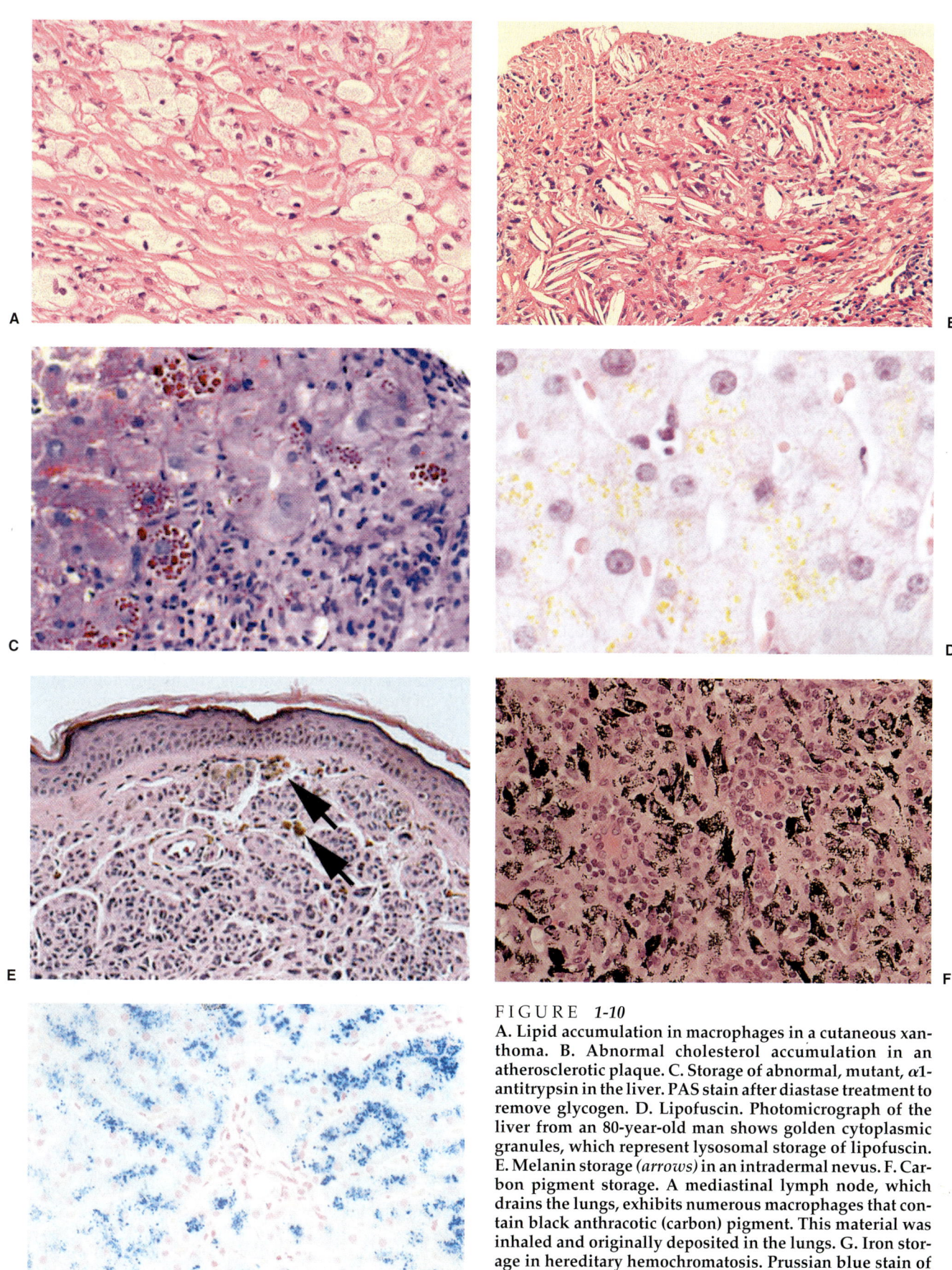

FIGURE 1-10
A. Lipid accumulation in macrophages in a cutaneous xanthoma. B. Abnormal cholesterol accumulation in an atherosclerotic plaque. C. Storage of abnormal, mutant, α1-antitrypsin in the liver. PAS stain after diastase treatment to remove glycogen. D. Lipofuscin. Photomicrograph of the liver from an 80-year-old man shows golden cytoplasmic granules, which represent lysosomal storage of lipofuscin. E. Melanin storage *(arrows)* in an intradermal nevus. F. Carbon pigment storage. A mediastinal lymph node, which drains the lungs, exhibits numerous macrophages that contain black anthracotic (carbon) pigment. This material was inhaled and originally deposited in the lungs. G. Iron storage in hereditary hemochromatosis. Prussian blue stain of the liver reveals large deposits of iron within hepatocellular lysosomes.

creas, heart, kidneys, and endocrine organs. The intracellular accumulation of iron in hemosiderosis does not usually injure the cells. However, there are a number of situations in which the increase in total body iron is extreme; we then speak of **iron overload syndromes** (see Chapter 14), disorders in which iron deposition is so severe that it damages vital organs—the heart, liver, and pancreas. Severe iron overload can result from a genetic abnormality in iron absorption, termed **hereditary hemochromatosis** (Fig. 1-10). Alternatively, severe iron overload may occur after multiple blood transfusions, such as those required in treating hemophilia or certain hereditary anemias.

Excessive iron storage in some organs is also associated with an increased risk of cancer. The pulmonary siderosis encountered among certain metal polishers is accompanied by an increased risk of lung cancer. Hemochromatosis leads to a higher incidence of liver cancer.

Excess accumulation of lead, particularly in children, causes mental retardation and anemia. The storage of other metals also presents dangers. In Wilson disease, a hereditary disorder of copper metabolism, storage of excess copper in the liver and brain leads to severe chronic disease of those organs.

Calcification Is a Normal or Abnormal Process

The deposition of mineral salts of calcium is, of course, a normal process in the formation of bone from cartilage. As we have learned, calcium entry into dead or dying cells is usual, owing to the inability of such cells to maintain a steep calcium gradient. This cellular calcification is not ordinarily visible except as inclusions within mitochondria.

Dystrophic calcification refers to the macroscopic deposition of calcium salts in injured tissues. This type of calcification does not simply reflect an accumulation of calcium derived from the bodies of dead cells but rather represents an extracellular deposition of calcium from the circulation or interstitial fluid. Dystrophic calcification apparently requires the persistence of necrotic tissue; it is often visible to the naked eye and ranges from gritty, sandlike grains to firm, rockhard material. In many locations, such as in cases of tuberculous caseous necrosis in the lung or lymph nodes, calcification has no functional consequences. However, dystrophic calcification may also occur in crucial locations, such as in the mitral or aortic valves (Fig. 1-11). In such instances, calcification leads to impeded blood flow because it produces inflexible valve leaflets and narrowed valve orifices (mitral and aortic stenosis). Dystrophic calcification in atherosclerotic coronary arteries contributes to narrowing of those vessels. Although molecules involved in physiological calcium deposition in bone, e.g., osteopontin, osteonectin, and osteocalcin, are reported in association with dystrophic calcification, the underlying mechanisms of this process remain obscure.

Dystrophic calcification also plays a role in diagnostic radiography. Mammography is based principally on the detection of calcifications in breast cancers; congenital toxoplasmosis, an infection involving the central nervous system, is suggested by the visualization of calcification in the infant brain.

Metastatic calcification reflects deranged calcium metabolism, in contrast to dystrophic calcification, which has its origin in cell injury. Metastatic calcification is associated with an increased serum calcium concentration (hypercalcemia). In general, almost any disorder that increases the serum calcium level can lead to calcification in such inappropriate locations as the alveolar septa of the lung, renal tubules, and blood vessels. Calcification is seen in various disorders, including chronic renal failure, vitamin D intoxication, and hyperparathyroidism.

The formation of stones containing calcium carbonate in sites such as the gallbladder, renal pelvis, bladder, and pancreatic duct is another form of pathological calcification. Under certain circumstances, the mineral salts precipitate from solution and crystallize about foci of organic material. Those who have suffered the agony of gallbladder or renal colic will attest to the unpleasant consequences of this type of calcification.

Hyaline Is a Term That Refers to Any Material That Exhibits a Reddish, Homogeneous Appearance When Stained with Hematoxylin and Eosin

The student will encounter the term *hyaline* in classic descriptions of diverse and unrelated lesions. Standard terminology includes hyaline arteriolosclerosis, alcoholic hyaline in the liver, hyaline membranes in the lung, and hyaline droplets in various cells. The various lesions called hyaline actually have nothing in common. Alcoholic hyaline is composed of cytoskeletal filaments; the hyaline found in arterioles of the kidney is derived from basement membranes; and hyaline membranes consist of plasma proteins deposited in alveoli. The term is anachronistic and of questionable value, although it is still used as a morphological descriptor.

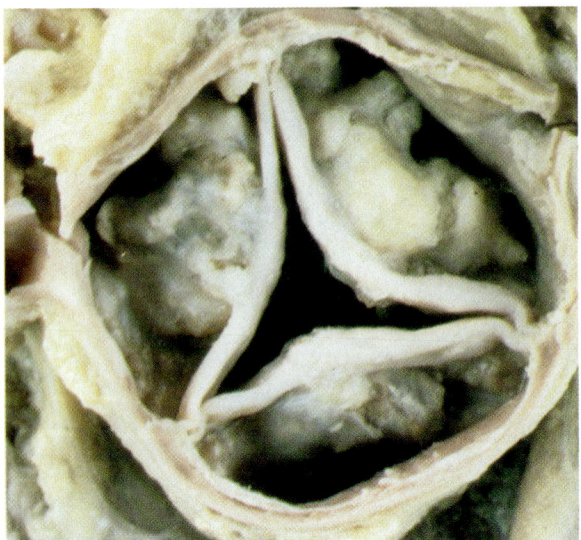

FIGURE 1-11
Calcific aortic stenosis. Large deposits of calcium salts are evident in the cusps and the free margins of the thickened aortic valve, as viewed from above.

MECHANISMS AND MORPHOLOGY OF CELL INJURY

All cells have efficient mechanisms to deal with shifts in environmental conditions. Thus, ion channels open or close; harmful chemicals are detoxified; metabolic stores such as fat or glycogen may be mobilized; and catabolic processes lead to the segregation of internal particulate materials. It is when environmental changes exceed the capacity of the cell to maintain normal homeostasis that we recognize acute cell injury. If the stress is removed in time or if the cell can withstand the assault, cell injury is reversible, and complete structural and functional integrity is restored. For example, when circulation to the heart is interrupted for less than 30 minutes, all structural and functional alterations prove to be reversible. The cell can also be exposed to persistent sublethal stress, as in mechanical irritation of the skin or exposure of the bronchial mucosa to tobacco smoke. In such instances, the cell has time to adapt to reversible injury in a number of ways, each of which has its morphological counterpart. On the other hand, if the stress is severe, irreversible injury leads to death of the cell. The precise moment at which reversible injury gives way to irreversible injury, the "point of no return," cannot be identified at present.

Hydropic Swelling Is a Reversible Increase in Cell Volume

Hydropic swelling is characterized by a large, pale cytoplasm and a normally located nucleus (Fig. 1-12). The greater

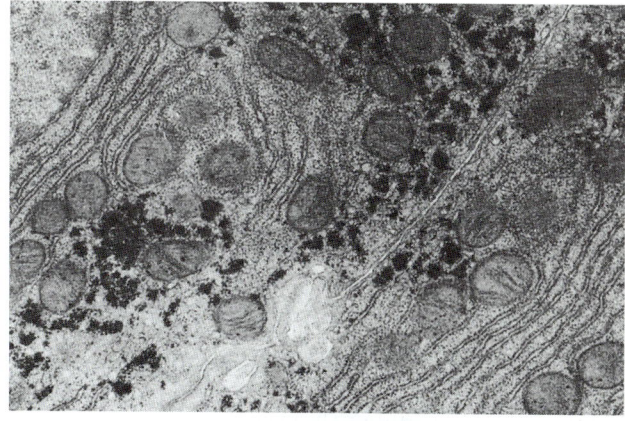
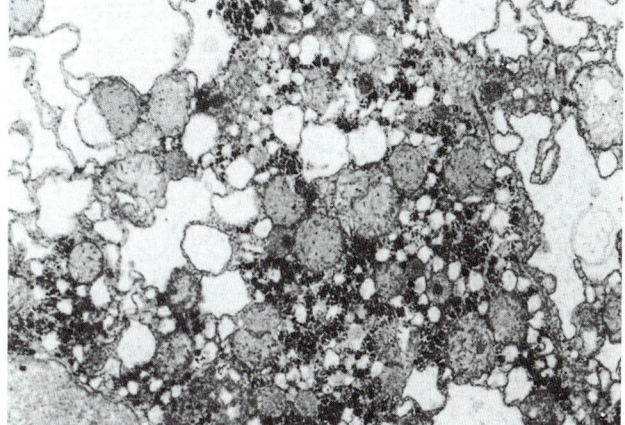

FIGURE 1-13
Ultrastructure of hydropic swelling of a liver cell. A. Two apposed normal hepatocytes with tightly organized, parallel arrays of rough endoplasmic reticulum. B. Swollen hepatocyte in which the cisternae of the endoplasmic reticulum are dilated by excess fluid.

volume reflects an increased water content. Hydropic swelling reflects acute, reversible cell injury and may result from such varied causes as chemical and biological toxins, viral or bacterial infections, ischemia, excessive heat or cold, and so on.

By electron microscopy, the number of organelles is unchanged, although they appear dispersed in a larger volume. The excess fluid accumulates preferentially in the cisternae of the endoplasmic reticulum, which are conspicuously dilated, presumably because of ionic shifts into this compartment (Fig. 1-13). Hydropic swelling is entirely reversible when the cause is removed.

Hydropic swelling results from impairment of cellular volume regulation, a process that controls ionic concentrations in the cytoplasm. This regulation, particularly for sodium, involves three components: (1) the plasma membrane, (2) the plasma membrane sodium pump, and (3) the supply of adenosine triphosphate (ATP). The plasma membrane imposes a barrier to the flow of sodium down a concentration gradient into the cell and prevents a similar efflux of potassium from the cell. The barrier to sodium is imperfect, and the relative leakiness to that ion permits the passive entry of sodium into the cell. To compensate for this intrusion, the energy-dependent plasma membrane sodium pump (Na^+/K^+-ATPase), which is fueled

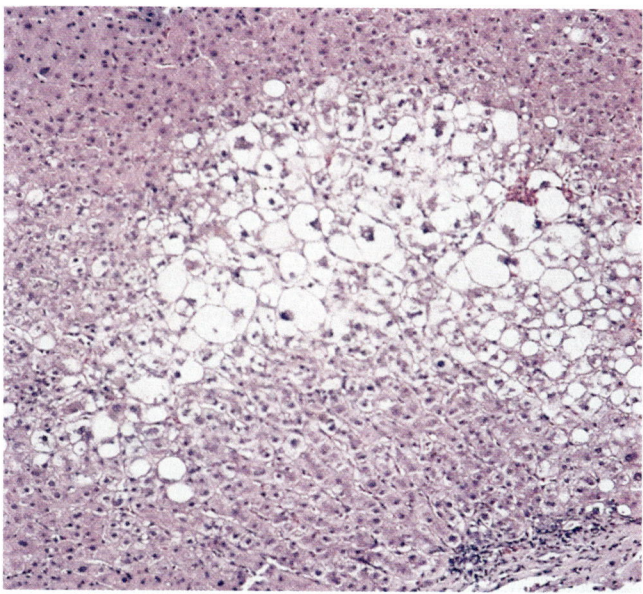

FIGURE 1-12
Hydropic swelling. A needle biopsy of the liver of a patient with toxic hepatic injury shows severe hydropic swelling in the centrilobular zone. The affected hepatocytes exhibit central nuclei and cytoplasm distended (ballooned) by excess fluid.

by ATP, extrudes sodium from the cell. Injurious agents may interfere with this membrane-regulated process by (1) increasing the permeability of the plasma membrane to sodium, thereby exceeding the capacity of the pump to extrude sodium; (2) damaging the pump directly; or (3) interfering with the synthesis of ATP, thereby depriving the pump of its fuel. In any event, the accumulation of sodium in the cell leads to an increase in water content to maintain isosmotic conditions, and the cell then swells.

Subcellular Changes Occur in Reversibly Injured Cells

- **Endoplasmic reticulum:** The cisternae of the endoplasmic reticulum are distended by fluid in hydropic swelling (see Fig. 1-13). In other forms of acute, reversible cell injury, membrane-bound polysomes may undergo disaggregation and detach from the surface of the rough endoplasmic reticulum (Fig. 1-14).
- **Mitochondria:** In some forms of acute injury, particularly ischemia, mitochondria swell (Fig. 1-15). This enlargement reflects the dissipation of the energy gradient and consequent impairment of mitochondrial volume control. Amorphous densities rich in phospholipid may appear, but these effects are fully reversible on recovery.
- **Plasma membrane:** Blebs of the plasma membrane—that is, focal extrusions of the cytoplasm—are occasionally noted. These can detach from the membrane into the external environment without the loss of cell viability.
- **Nucleus:** In the nucleus, reversible injury is reflected principally in nucleolar change. The fibrillar and granular components of the nucleolus may segregate. Alternatively, the granular component may be diminished, leaving only a fibrillar core.

These changes in cell organelles (Fig. 1-16) are reflected in functional derangements (e.g., reduced protein synthesis and impaired energy production). **After withdrawal of an acute stress that has led to reversible cell injury, by definition, the cell returns to its normal state.**

Ischemic Cell Injury Usually Results from Obstruction to the Flow of Blood

When tissues are deprived of oxygen, ATP cannot be produced by aerobic metabolism and is instead generated inefficiently by anaerobic metabolism. Ischemia initiates a series of chemical and pH imbalances, which are accompanied by enhanced generation of injurious free radical species. The damage produced by short periods of ischemia tends to be reversible if the circulation is restored. However, cells subjected to long episodes of ischemia become irreversibly injured and die. The mechanisms of cell damage are discussed below.

Oxidative Stress Leads to Cell Injury in Many Organs

For human life oxygen is both a blessing and a curse. Without it, life is impossible, but its metabolism can produce partially reduced oxygen species that react with virtually any molecule they reach.

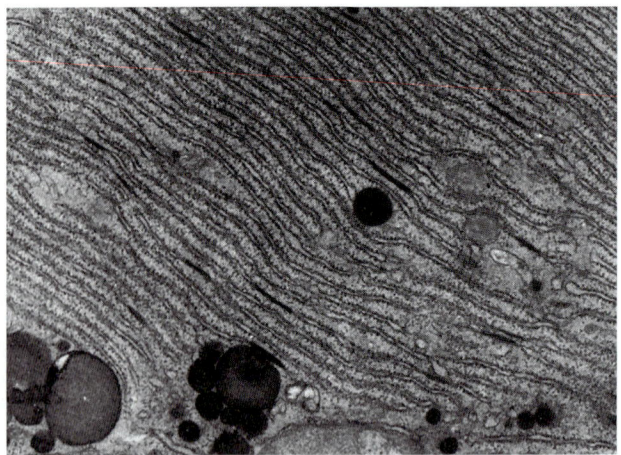
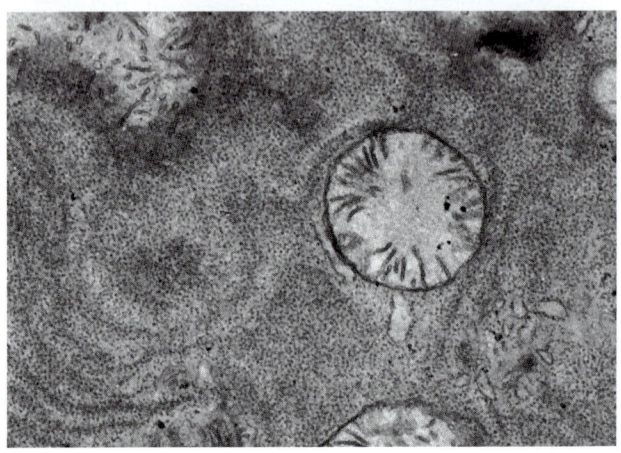

FIGURE 1-14
Disaggregation of membrane-bound polyribosomes in acute, reversible liver injury. A. Normal hepatocyte, in which the profiles of endoplasmic reticulum are studded with ribosomes. B. An injured hepatocyte, showing detachment of ribosomes from the membranes of the endoplasmic reticulum and the accumulation of free ribosomes in the cytoplasm.

Reactive Oxygen Species (ROS)

ROS have been identified as the likely cause of cell injury in many diseases (Fig. 1-17). The inflammatory process, whether acute or chronic, can cause considerable tissue destruction. In such circumstances partially reduced oxygen species produced by phagocytic cells are important mediators of cell injury. Damage to cells resulting from oxygen radicals formed by inflammatory cells has been implicated in diseases of the joints and of many organs, including the kidneys, lungs, and heart. The toxicity of many chemicals may reflect the formation of toxic oxygen species. For example, the killing of cells by ionizing radiation is most likely the result of the direct formation of hydroxyl radicals from the radiolysis of water. There is also evidence of a role for oxygen species in the formation of mutations during chemical carcinogenesis. Finally, oxidative damage has been implicated in biological aging (see below).

Cells also may be injured when oxygen is present at concentrations greater than normal. In the past, this occurred

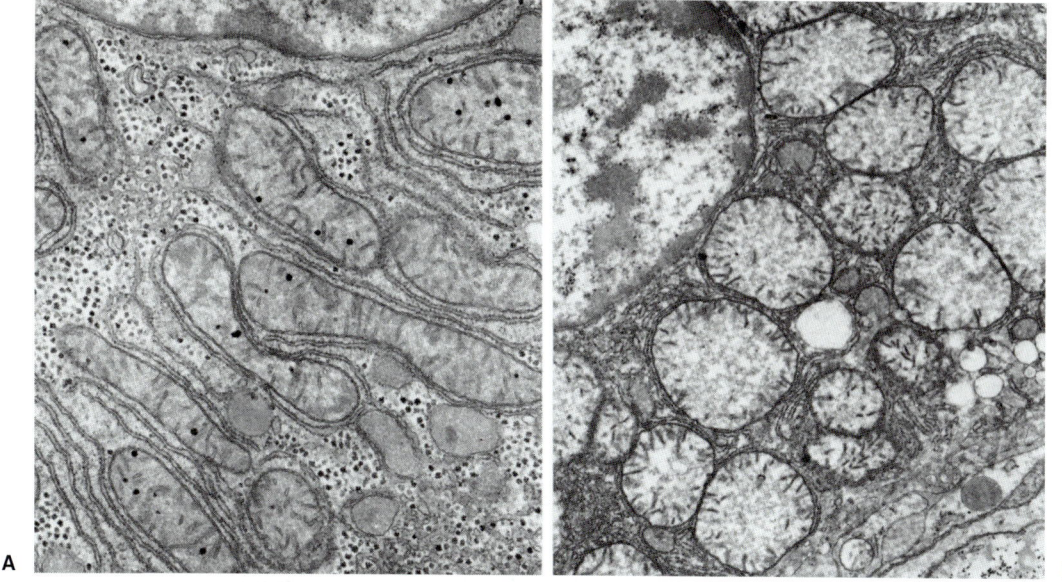

FIGURE 1-15
Mitochondrial swelling in acute ischemic cell injury. A. Normal mitochondria are elongated and display prominent cristae, which traverse the mitochondrial matrix. B. Mitochondria from an ischemic cell are swollen and round and exhibit a decreased matrix density. The cristae are less prominent than in the normal organelle.

largely under therapeutic circumstances in which oxygen was given to patients at concentrations greater than the normal 20% of inspired air. The lungs of adults and the eyes of premature newborns were the major targets of such oxygen toxicity.

Oxygen has a major metabolic role as the terminal acceptor for mitochondrial electron transport. Cytochrome oxidase catalyzes the four-electron reduction of O_2 to water. The resultant energy is harnessed as an electrochemical potential across the mitochondrial inner membrane.

Complete reduction of O_2 to H_2O involves the transfer of four electrons. There are three partially reduced species that are intermediate between O_2 and H_2O, representing transfers of varying numbers of electrons (Fig. 1-18). They are O_2^-, su-

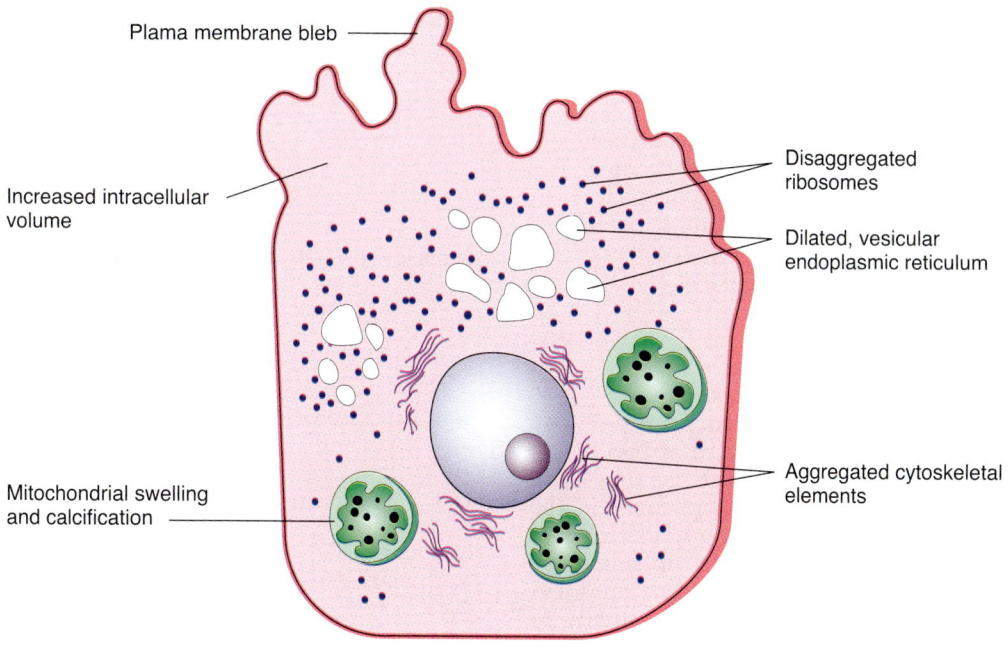

FIGURE 1-16
Ultrastructural features of reversible cell injury.

18 Cell Injury

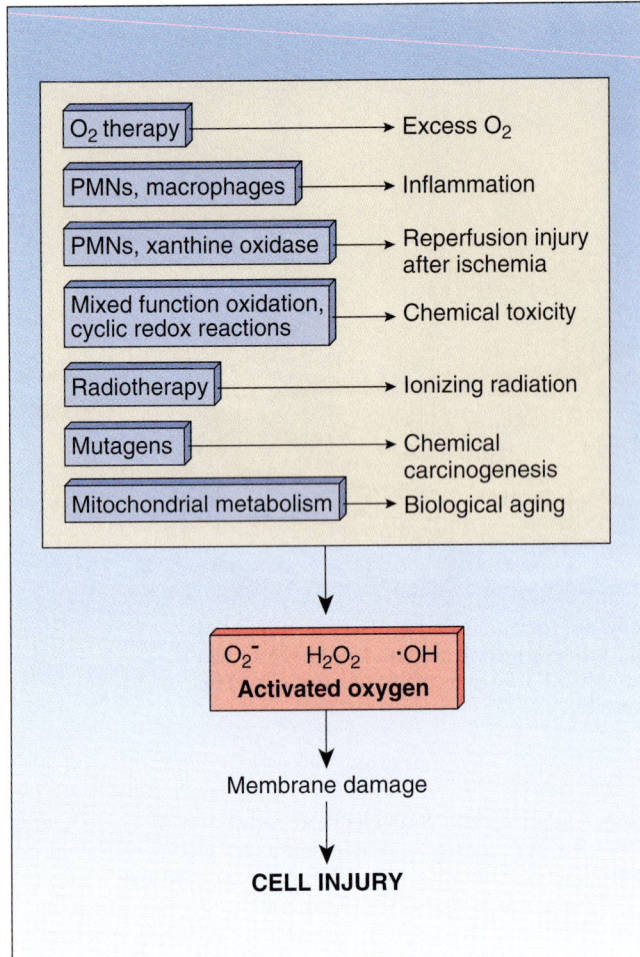

FIGURE 1-17
The role of activated oxygen species in human disease.

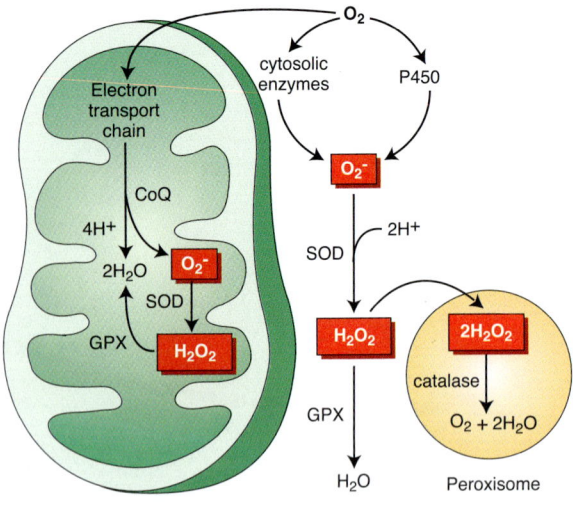

FIGURE 1-18
Mechanisms by which reactive oxygen radicals are generated from molecular oxygen and then detoxified by cellular enzymes. CoQ = coenzyme Q. GPX = glutathione peroxidase. SOD = superoxide dismutase.

Hydrogen Peroxide

O_2^- anions are catabolized by superoxide dismutase to produce H_2O_2. Hydrogen peroxide is also produced directly by a number of oxidases in cytoplasmic peroxisomes (see Fig. 1-18). By itself, H_2O_2 is not particularly injurious, and it is

peroxide (one electron); H_2O_2, hydrogen peroxide (two electrons); and •OH, the hydroxyl radical (three electrons). For the most part these ROS are produced principally by leaks in mitochondrial electron transport, with an additional contribution from the mixed-function oxygenase (P450) system. The major forms of ROS are listed in Table 1-1.

Superoxide

The superoxide anion (O_2^-) is produced principally by leaks in mitochondrial electron transport or as part of the inflammatory response. In the first instance, the promiscuity of coenzyme Q (CoQ) and other imperfections in the electron transport chain allows the transfer of electrons to O_2 to yield O_2^-. In the case of phagocytic inflammatory cells, activation of a plasma membrane oxidase produces O_2^-, which is then converted to H_2O_2 and eventually to other ROS (Fig. 1-19). In turn these ROS attack pathogens, fragments of necrotic cells, or other phagocytosed material (see Chapter 2).

TABLE 1-1 Reactive Oxygen Species (ROS)

Molecule	Attributes
Hydrogen peroxide (H_2O_2)	Forms free radicals via Fe^{2+}-catalyzed Fenton reaction
	Diffuses widely within the cell
Superoxide anion (O_2^-)	Generated by leaks in the electron transport chain and some cytosolic reactions
	Produces other ROS
	Does not readily diffuse far from its origin
Hydroxyl radical (•OH)	Generated from H_2O_2 by Fe^{2+}-catalyzed Fenton reaction
	The intracellular radical most responsible for attack on macromolecules
Peroxynitrite (ONOO•)	Formed from the reaction of nitric oxide (NO) with O_2^- damages macromolecules
Lipid peroxide radicals (RCOO•)	Organic radicals produced during lipid peroxidation
Hypochlorous acid (HOCl)	Produced by macrophages and neutrophils during respiratory burst that accompanies phagocytosis
	Dissociates to yield hypochlorite radical (OCl^-)

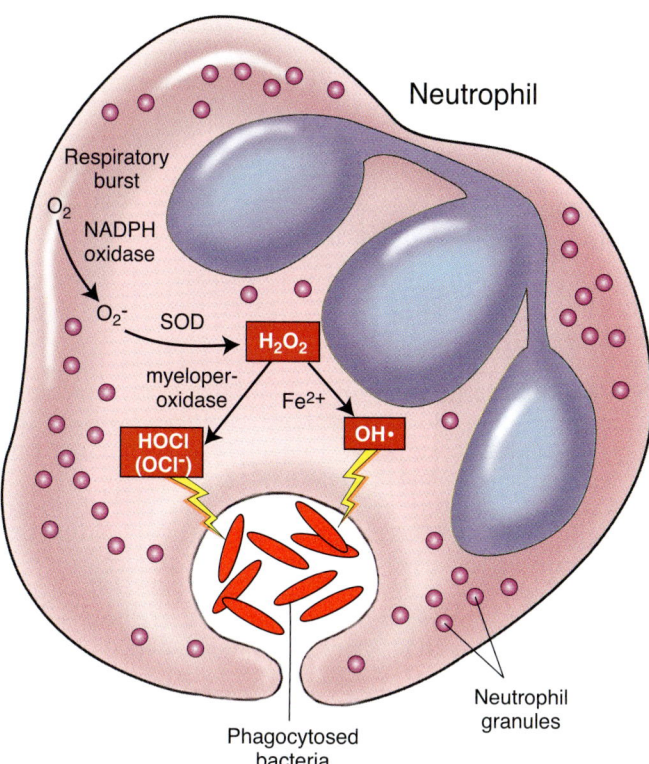

FIGURE 1-19
Generation of reactive oxygen species in neutrophils as a result of phagocytosis of bacteria. SOD = superoxide dismutase.

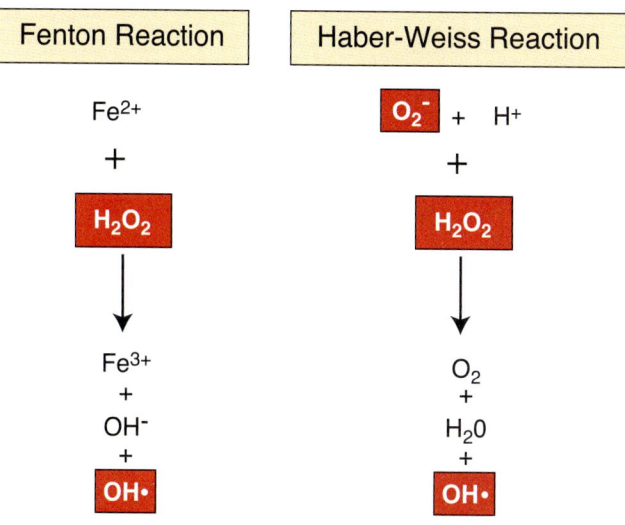

FIGURE 1-20
Fenton and Haber-Weiss reactions to generate the highly reactive hydroxyl radical. Reactive species are shown in red.

largely metabolized to H_2O by catalase. However, when produced in excess, it is converted to highly reactive •OH. In neutrophils, myeloperoxidase transforms H_2O_2 to the potent radical hypochlorite (OCl^-), which is lethal for microorganisms and cells.

Most cells have efficient mechanisms for removing H_2O_2. Two different enzymes reduce H_2O_2 to water: catalase within the peroxisomes and glutathione peroxidase in both the cytosol and the mitochondria (see Fig. 1-18). Glutathione peroxidase uses reduced glutathione (GSH) as a cofactor, producing two molecules of oxidized glutathione (GSSG) for every molecule of H_2O_2 reduced to water. GSSG is re-reduced to GSH by glutathione reductase, with reduced nicotinamide adenine dinucleotide phosphate (NADPH) as the cofactor.

Hydroxyl Radical

Hydroxyl radicals (•OH) are formed by (1) the radiolysis of water, (2) the reaction of H_2O_2 with ferrous iron (the Fenton reaction), and (3) the reaction of O_2^- with H_2O_2 (the Haber-Weiss reaction) (Fig. 1-20). The hydroxyl radical is the most reactive molecule of ROS, and there are several mechanisms by which it can damage macromolecules.

- **Lipid peroxidation:** The hydroxyl radical removes a hydrogen atom from the unsaturated fatty acids of membrane phospholipids, a process that forms a free lipid radical (Fig. 1-21). The lipid radical, in turn, reacts with molecular oxygen and forms a lipid peroxide radical. This peroxide radical can, in turn, function as an initiator, removing another hydrogen atom from a second unsaturated fatty acid. A lipid peroxide and a new lipid radical result, and a chain reaction is initiated. Lipid peroxides are unstable and break down into smaller molecules. The destruction of the unsaturated fatty acids of phospholipids results in a loss of membrane integrity.
- **Protein interactions:** Hydroxyl radicals may also attack proteins. The sulfur-containing amino acids cysteine and methionine, as well as arginine, histidine, and proline, are especially vulnerable to attack by •OH. As a result of oxidative damage, proteins undergo fragmentation, cross-linking, aggregation, and eventually degradation.
- **DNA damage:** DNA is an important target of the hydroxyl radical. A variety of structural alterations include strand breaks, modified bases, and cross-links between strands. In most cases, the integrity of the genome can be reconstituted by the various DNA repair pathways. However, if oxidative damage to DNA is sufficiently extensive, the cell dies.

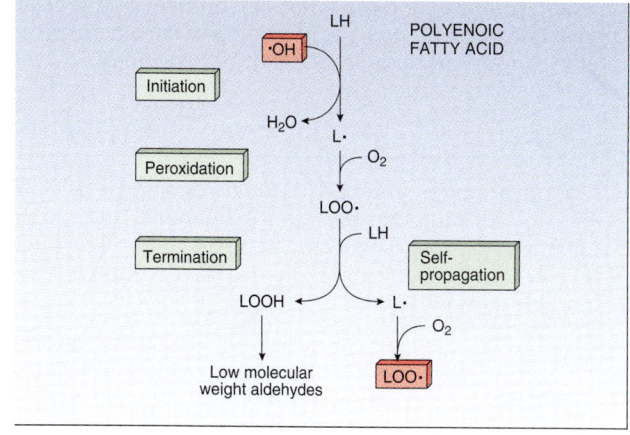

FIGURE 1-21
Lipid peroxidation initiated by the hydroxyl radical.

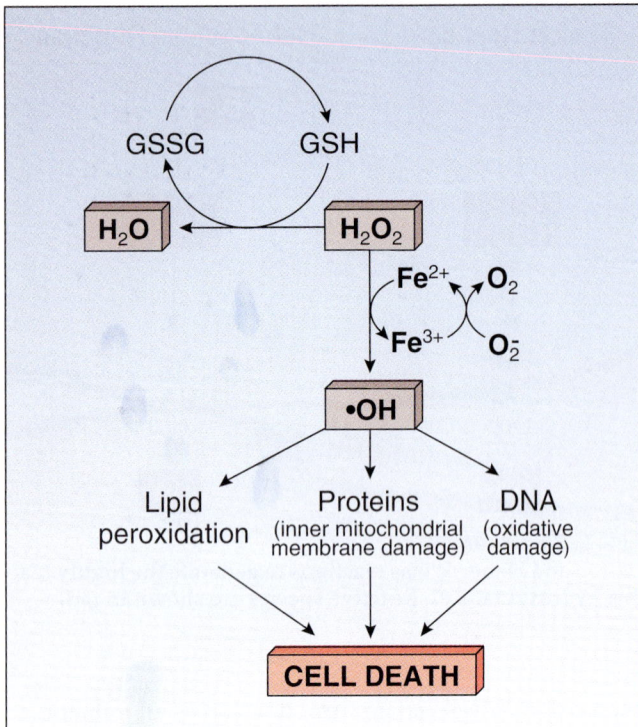

FIGURE 1-22
Mechanisms of cell injury by activated oxygen species.

Figure 1-22 summarizes the mechanisms of cell injury by activated oxygen species.

Peroxynitrite

Peroxynitrite (ONOO$^-$) is formed by the interaction of superoxide (O$_2^-$) with nitric oxide (NO•).

$$NO• + O_2^- \rightarrow ONOO^-$$

The free radical ONOO$^-$ attacks a wide range of biologically important molecules, including lipids, proteins, and DNA. Nitric oxide, a molecule generated in many tissues, is a potent vasodilator and mediator of a number of important biological processes. Thus, the formation of peroxynitrite occupies an important place in free radical toxicology.

Cellular Defenses against Oxygen Free Radicals

Cells manifest potent antioxidant defenses against ROS, including detoxifying enzymes and exogenous free radical scavengers (vitamins). The major enzymes that convert ROS to less reactive molecules are superoxide dismutase, catalase, and glutathione peroxidase.

Detoxifying Enzymes

- **Superoxide dismutase (SOD)** is the first line of defense against O$_2^-$, converting it to H$_2$O$_2$ and O$_2$.

$$2 O_2^- + 2 H^+ \rightarrow O_2 + H_2O_2.$$

- **Catalase**, principally located in peroxisomes, is one of two enzymes that complete the dissolution of O$_2^-$ by eliminating H$_2$O$_2$ and, therefore, its potential conversion to •OH.

$$2 H_2O_2 \rightarrow 2 H_2O + O_2$$

- **Glutathione peroxidase (GPX)** catalyzes the reduction of H$_2$O$_2$ and lipid peroxides in mitochondria and the cytosol.

$$H_2O_2 + 2 GSH \rightarrow 2 H_2O + GSSG$$

Scavengers of ROS

- **Vitamin E (α-tocopherol)** is a terminal electron acceptor and, therefore, blocks free-radical chain reactions. Since it is fat soluble, it exerts its activity in lipid membranes, protecting them against lipid peroxidation.
- **Vitamin C (ascorbate)** is water soluble and reacts directly with O$_2$, •OH, and some products of lipid peroxidation. It also serves to regenerate the reduced form of vitamin E.
- **Retinoids**, the precursors of vitamin A, are lipid soluble and function as chain-breaking antioxidants.

Ischemia/Reperfusion Injury Reflects Oxidative Stress

Ischemia/reperfusion (I/R) injury is a common clinical problem that arises in the setting of occlusive cardiovascular disease, infection, shock, and many other circumstances. The genesis of I/R injury relates to the interplay between transient ischemia and the reestablishment of blood flow (reperfusion). Initially, ischemia produces a type of cellular damage that leads to the generation of free radical species. Subsequently, reperfusion provides abundant molecular oxygen (O$_2$) to combine with free radicals to form reactive oxygen species. The evolution of I/R injury also involves the participation of many other factors. Among these are inflammatory mediators [tumor necrosis factor-α (TNF-α), interleukin-1 (IL-1)], platelet activating factor (PAF), nitric oxide synthase (NOS) and NO•, intercellular adhesion molecules, and many more.

Xanthine Oxidase

Xanthine dehydrogenase may be converted by proteolysis during a period of ischemia into xanthine oxidase. On return of the oxygen supply with reperfusion, the abundant purines derived from the catabolism of ATP during ischemia provide substrates for the activity of xanthine oxidase. This enzyme requires oxygen in catalyzing the formation of uric acid, and activated oxygen species are byproducts of this reaction.

The Role of Neutrophils

An additional source of activated oxygen species during reperfusion is the neutrophil. Alterations in the cell surface that occur during ischemia and on reperfusion induce the adhesion and activation of circulating neutrophils. These cells release large quantities of activated oxygen species and hydrolytic enzymes, both of which may injure the previously ischemic cells.

Reperfusion also prompts endothelial cells to move preformed P-selectin to the cell surface, allowing neutrophils to bind to endothelial membrane intercellular adhesion molecule-1 (ICAM-1) and to roll along endothelial cells (see Chapter 2). The recruitment of these inflammatory cells to the affected area increases the local production of oxygen free radicals.

The Role of Nitric Oxide

There are two major forms of NOS: a constitutive form, which is common to endothelial cells and parenchymal cells (e.g., hepatocytes, neurons), and an inducible form (iNOS), mostly found in inflammatory cells. Nitric oxide dilates the microvasculature by relaxing smooth muscle, inhibits platelet aggregation, and decreases adhesion between leukocytes and the endothelial surface. These activities are all mediated by the ability of NO• to decrease cytosolic Ca^{2+}, both by extrusion of calcium from the cell and by its sequestration within intracellular stores.

NO• also reacts with superoxide (O_2^-) to form the highly reactive species, peroxynitrite ($ONOO^-$). Under normal circumstances, O_2^- is detoxified by SOD, and little $ONOO^-$ is produced. However, I/R disrupts this balance by inactivating SOD and stimulating iNOS, thereby increasing the amount of NO• and favoring the production of peroxynitrite. The free radical gives rise to DNA strand breaks and lipid peroxidation in cell membranes.

Inflammatory Cytokines

I/R injury leads to the release of cytokines that (1) promote vasoconstriction, (2) stimulate the adherence of inflammatory cells and platelets to endothelium, and (3) have effects at sites distant from the ischemic insult itself.

Local release of TNF-α at the site of I/R injury results in chemotaxis and sequestration of neutrophils by upregulating the expression of cell adhesion molecules on both neutrophils and endothelial cells. This cytokine is also responsible for increases in neutrophil trafficking and neutrophil-related damage at locations distant from the site of I/R injury itself, thereby causing systemic effects. By increasing the levels of PAF, I/R injury cripples vascular function both locally and systemically. In addition, augmented release of endothelin during I/R injury promotes the adherence of inflammatory cells and increases vascular tone and permeability.

We can put reperfusion injury in perspective by emphasizing that there are three different degrees of cell injury, depending on the duration of the ischemia:

- With short periods of ischemia, reperfusion (and, therefore, the resupply of oxygen) completely restores the structural and functional integrity of the cell. Cell injury in this case is completely reversible.
- With longer periods of ischemia, reperfusion is not associated with restoration of cell structure and function but rather with deterioration and death of the cells. In this case, lethal cell injury occurs during the period of reperfusion.
- Lethal cell injury may develop during the period of ischemia itself, in which case reperfusion is not a factor. A longer period of ischemia is needed to produce this third type of cell injury. In this case, cell damage does not depend on the formation of activated oxygen species.

Ionizing Radiation Causes Oxidative Stress

The term "ionizing" in reference to electromagnetic radiation connotes an ability to effect the radiolysis of water, thereby directly forming hydroxyl radicals. As noted above, hydroxyl radicals interact with DNA and inhibit DNA replication. For a nonproliferating cell, such as a hepatocyte or a neuron, the inability to divide is of little consequence. For a proliferating cell, however, the prevention of mitosis is a catastrophic loss of function. Once a proliferating cell can no longer divide, it dies by *apoptosis*, which rids the body of those cells that have lost their prime function. Direct mutagenic effects of ionizing radiation on DNA are also important. The cytotoxic effects of ionizing radiation are also dose-dependent. Whereas exposure to significant sources of radiation impairs the replicating capacity of cycling cells, massive doses of radiation may kill both proliferating and quiescent cells directly. Figure 1-23 summarizes the mechanisms of cell killing by ionizing radiation.

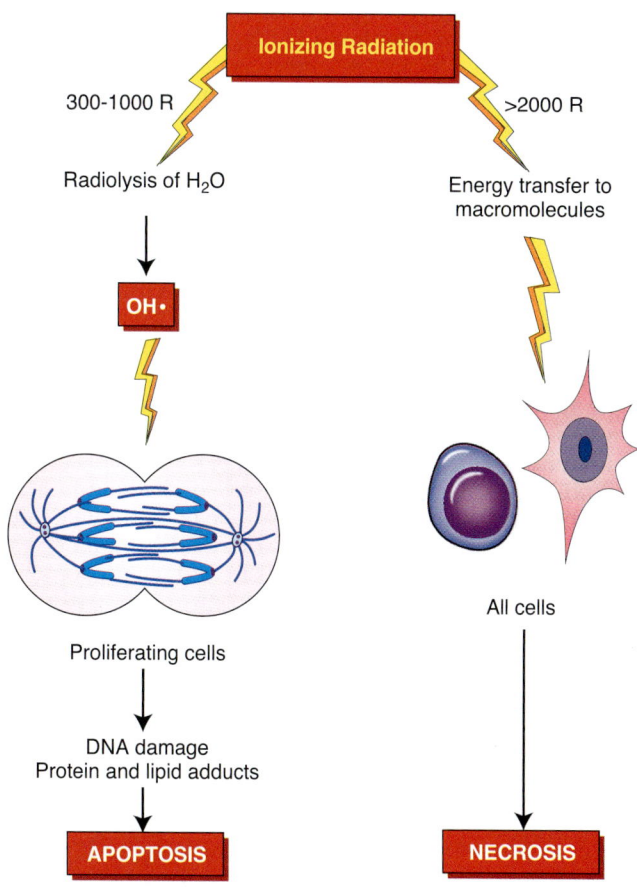

FIGURE 1-23

Mechanisms by which ionizing radiation at low and high doses causes cell death.

Viral Cytotoxicity Is Direct or Immunologically Mediated

The means by which viruses cause cell injury and death are as diverse as the viruses themselves. Unlike bacteria, a virus requires a cellular host to (1) house it; (2) provide the enzymes, substrates, and other resources for viral replication; and (3) serve as a source for dissemination when mature virions are ready to be spread to other cells. Viruses have evolved mechanisms by which they avoid biting the hand that feeds them (at least until they are ready for other hands). The ability of a virus to persist in an infected cell necessitates a parasitic, albeit temporary, relationship with the host cell. During this vulnerable phase, the virus plays a game of cat and mouse with the immune system as a device to evade elimination of the infected cell. This period is followed by a phase in which the virus disseminates, either by budding (which does not necessarily destroy the cell) or by lysis. In some viral infections (e.g., herpes simplex, measles, zoster-varicella), infection of the host cell may last for many years or a lifetime, in which case the cell is not destroyed. There are patterns of cellular injury related to viral infections that deserve a brief mention:

- **Direct toxicity:** Viruses may injure cells directly by subverting cellular enzymes and depleting the cell's nutrients, thereby disrupting the normal homeostatic mechanisms. The mechanisms underlying virus-induced lysis of cells, however, are probably more complex (Fig. 1-24A).
- **Manipulation of apoptosis:** During their replicative cycle, and before virion assembly is complete, there are many viral activities that can elicit apoptosis. For example, apoptosis is activated when the cell detects episomal (extrachromosomal) DNA replication. Since viruses must avoid cell death before they have produced infectious progeny, they have evolved mechanisms to counteract this effect by upregulating antiapoptotic proteins and inhibiting proapoptotic ones. Some viruses also encode proteins that induce apoptosis once daughter virions are mature (Fig. 1-24A).
- **Immunologically mediated cytotoxicity:** Both humoral and cellular arms of the immune system protect against the harmful effects of viral infections by eliminating infected cells. Thus, the presentation of viral proteins to the immune system in the context of a self major histocompatibility complex (MHC) on the cell surface immunizes the body against the invader and elicits both killer cells and antiviral antibodies. These arms of the immune system eliminate virus-infected cells by inducing apoptosis or by lysing the cell with complement (Fig. 1-24B) (see Chapter 4).

Chemicals Injure Cells Directly and Indirectly

Innumerable chemicals can damage almost any cell in the body. The science of toxicology attempts to define the mechanisms that determine both the target cell specificity and the mechanism of action of such chemicals. Toxic chemicals are divided into two general classes: (1) those that interact directly with cellular constituents without requiring metabolic activation and (2) those that are themselves not toxic but are metabolized to yield an ultimate toxin that interacts with the target cell. Whatever the mechanism, the result is usually necrotic cell death (see below).

Liver Necrosis Caused by the Metabolic Products of Chemicals

Studies of a few compounds that produce liver cell injury in rodents have enhanced our understanding of how chemicals injure cells. These studies have focused principally on those compounds that are converted to toxic metabolites. Carbon tetrachloride and acetaminophen are well-studied hepatotoxins. Each is metabolized by the mixed-function oxidase system of the endoplasmic reticulum, and each causes liver cell necrosis. These hepatotoxins are metabolized differently, and it is possible to relate the subsequent evolution of lethal cell injury to the specific features of this metabolism.

Carbon Tetrachloride

The metabolism of carbon tetrachloride (CCl_4) is a model system for toxicological studies. CCl_4 is metabolized via the mixed function oxygenase system (P450) of the liver to a chloride ion and a highly reactive trichloromethyl free radical.

$$CCL_4 + e^- \xrightarrow{P450} CCL_3 \bullet + Cl^-$$

Like the hydroxyl radical, the trichloromethyl radical is a potent initiator of lipid peroxidation, although it may also interact with other macromolecules. However, in view of the rapidity with which CCl_4 kills cells (hours), peroxidative damage to the plasma membrane is the most likely culprit.

Acetaminophen

Acetaminophen, an important constituent of many analgesics, is innocuous in recommended doses, but when consumed to excess it is highly toxic to the liver. Most acetaminophen is enzymatically converted in the liver to nontoxic glucuronide or sulfate metabolites. Less than 5% of acetaminophen is ordinarily metabolized by isoforms of cytochrome P450 to NAPQI (*N*-acetyl-*p*-benzoquinone imine), a highly reactive quinone (Fig. 1-25). However, when large doses of acetaminophen overwhelm the glucuronidation pathway, toxic amounts of NAPQI are formed. NAPQI is responsible for acetaminophen-related toxicity by virtue of its conjugation with either GSH or sulfhydryl groups on liver proteins to form thiol esters. The latter cause extensive cellular dysfunction and lead to injury. At the same time, NAPQI depletes the antioxidant GSH, rendering the cell more susceptible to free radical-induced injury. Thus, conditions that deplete GSH (e.g., starvation) enhance the toxicity of acetaminophen. In addition, the metabolism of acetaminophen is accelerated by chronic alcohol consumption, an effect mediated by an ethanol-induced increase in the 3A4 isoform of P450. As a result, toxic amounts of NAPQI rapidly accumulate and may destroy the liver.

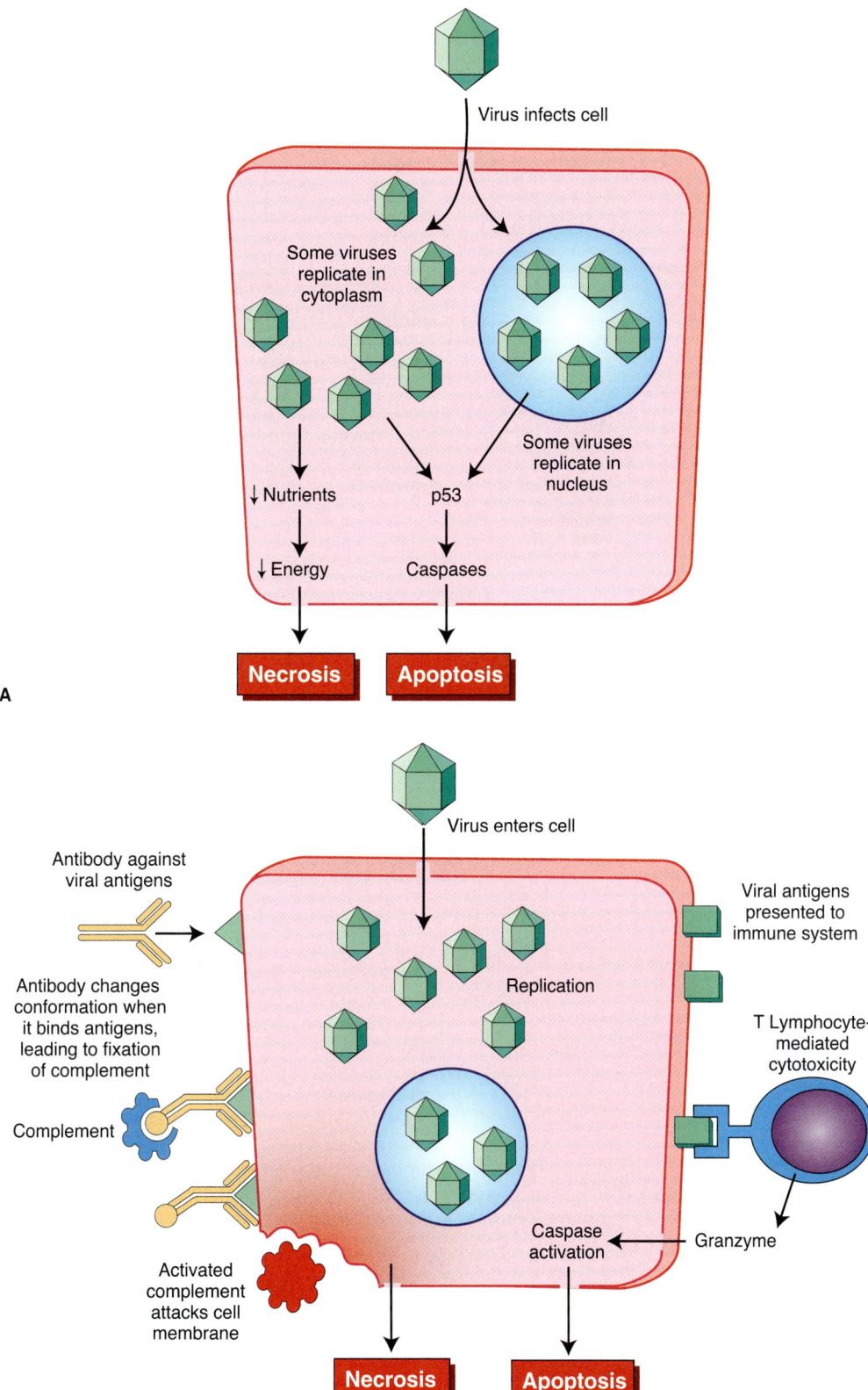

FIGURE 1-24
Cell injury caused by virus infection. A. Direct injury caused by virus infection, involving both depletion of cellular resources and activation of apoptotic signaling mechanisms. B. Mechanisms that lead to immunologically mediated destruction of virus-infected cells.

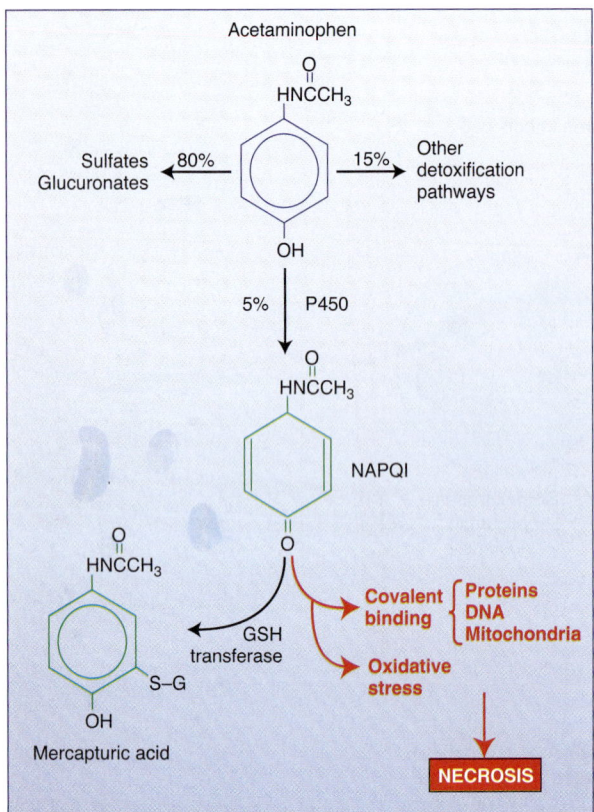

FIGURE 1-25
Chemical reactions involved in acetaminophen hepatotoxicity.

To summarize, the metabolism of hepatotoxic chemicals by mixed-function oxidation leads to cell injury through covalent binding of reactive metabolites and peroxidation of membrane phospholipids. Lipid peroxidation is initiated by (1) a metabolite of the original compound (as with CCl_4) or (2) by activated oxygen species formed during the metabolism of the toxin (as with acetaminophen), the latter augmented by weakened antioxidant defenses.

Chemicals That Are Not Metabolized

Directly cytotoxic chemicals do not have to be metabolized to injure the target cell and interact directly with cellular constituents. The critical cellular targets are diverse and include, for example, mitochondria (heavy metals and cyanide), cytoskeleton (phalloidin, Taxol), and DNA (chemotherapeutic alkylating agents). In addition, the interaction of directly cytotoxic chemicals with glutathione (alkylating agents) weakens the antioxidant defenses of the cell.

Abnormal G Protein Activity Leads to Functional Cell Injury

Normal cell function requires the coordination of numerous activating and regulatory signaling cascades. Hereditary or acquired interference with correct signal transduction can result in significant cellular dysfunction, as illustrated by diseases associated with faulty G proteins **(see Fig. 5-28 and 9-24)**. A variety of membrane receptors (e.g., adrenergic or vasopressin receptors) are linked to intracellular G proteins, which activate downstream signaling. Inherited defects in G protein subunits can lead to constitutive activation of the protein. In one such hereditary syndrome, endocrine manifestations predominate, including multiple tumors in the pituitary and thyroid glands. Another G protein mutation appears to predominate in many cases of essential hypertension, in which exaggerated activation of G protein signaling results in increased vascular responsiveness to stimuli that cause vasoconstriction. Certain microorganisms (e.g., *Vibrio cholerae* and *Escherichia coli*) produce their effects by elaborating toxins that activate G proteins.

Decreased responsiveness of G proteins to ligand–receptor interactions may also be caused by certain mutations in G protein subunits. In addition, G protein activity can be inhibited by certain bacterial products, the most important example being pertussis toxin, the cause of whooping cough.

CELL DEATH

An understanding of the mechanisms underlying cell death is not simply an academic exercise; the manipulation of cell viability by biochemical and pharmacological intervention is currently a major area of research. For example, if we understand the biochemistry of ischemic death of cardiac myocytes, which is responsible for the leading cause of death in the western world, we may be able to prolong their survival after a coronary occlusion until circulation is restored.

Paradoxically, the survival of an organism requires the sacrifice of individual cells. Physiological cell death is integral to the transformation of embryonic anlagen to fully developed organs. It is also crucial for the regulation of cell numbers in a variety of tissues, including the epidermis, the gastrointestinal tract, and the hematopoietic system. Physiological cell death involves the activation of an internal suicide program, which results in cell killing by a process termed **apoptosis.**

By contrast, pathological cell death is not regulated and is invariably injurious to the organism. It may result from a variety of insults to the integrity of the cell (e.g., ischemia, burns, and toxins). When the insult interferes with a vital structure or function of an organelle (plasma membrane, mitochondria, etc.) and does not trigger the preexisting enzymatic cascade of apoptosis, the process is termed **necrosis.** Pathological cell death, however, can also result from apoptosis, as exemplified by viral infections and ionizing radiation.

Necrosis Results from Exogenous Cell Injury and Is Reflected in Geographical Areas of Cell Death

At the cellular level, necrosis is characterized by cell and organelle swelling, ATP depletion, increased permeability of the plasma membrane, release of macromolecules, and eventually inflammation. Although the mechanisms responsible for necrosis depend on the nature of the insult and the organ involved, most instances of necrosis share certain mechanistic similarities. The model of necrotic cell death that has been studied most extensively in mechanistic terms is ischemic injury to cardiac myocytes. The sequence of events is admittedly unique to cardiac myocytes, but most features are pertinent to other cell types and injurious agents.

Necrosis Refers to the Process by Which Exogenous Stress Kills the Cell

Cells exist in a skewed equilibrium with their external environment. The plasma membrane is the barrier that separates the extracellular fluid from the internal milieu. Whatever the nature of the lethal insult, cell necrosis is heralded by disruption of the permeability barrier function of the plasma membrane. In this context, extracellular concentrations of sodium and calcium are orders of magnitude greater than intracellular concentrations, whereas the opposite holds for potassium. The selective ion permeability requires (1) considerable energy, (2) structural integrity of the lipid bilayer, (3) intact ion channel proteins, and (4) a normal association of the membrane with cytoskeletal constituents. When one or more of these elements is severely damaged, the resulting disturbance of the internal ionic balance is thought to represent the "point of no return" for the injured cell.

The role of calcium in the pathogenesis of cell death deserves special mention. The concentration of Ca^{2+} in extracellular fluids is in the millimolar range (10^{-3} M). By contrast, the level in the cytosol is 10,000-fold lower, on the order of 10^{-7} M. Many crucial cellular functions are exquisitely regulated by minute fluctuations in cytosolic free calcium concentration. Thus massive influx of Ca^{2+} through a damaged plasma membrane ensures loss of cell viability.

Coagulative Necrosis

Coagulative necrosis refers to light microscopic alterations in a dead or dying cell (Fig. 1-26). Shortly after the death of a cell, its outline is maintained. When stained with the usual combination of hematoxylin and eosin, the cytoplasm of a necrotic cell is more eosinophilic than usual. The nucleus displays an initial clumping of chromatin followed by its redistribution along the nuclear membrane. Three morphological changes follow:

- **Pyknosis:** The nucleus becomes smaller and stains deeply basophilic as chromatin clumping continues.
- **Karyorrhexis:** The pyknotic nucleus breaks up into many smaller fragments scattered about the cytoplasm.
- **Karyolysis:** The pyknotic nucleus may be extruded from the cell or it may manifest progressive loss of chromatin staining.

Early ultrastructural changes in a dying or dead cell reflect an extension of alterations associated with reversible cell injury (see Figs. 1-14, 1-15). In addition to the nuclear changes described above, the dead cell features dilated endoplasmic reticulum, disaggregated ribosomes, swollen and calcified mitochondria, aggregated cytoskeletal elements, and plasma membrane blebs.

At a variable time after the death of a cell, depending on the tissue and the circumstances, it is subjected to the

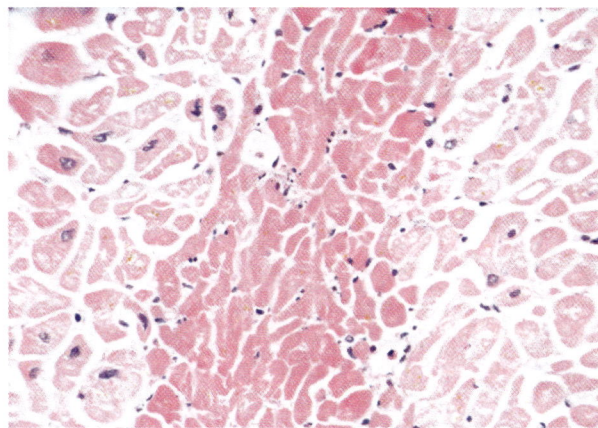

FIGURE 1-26
Coagulative necrosis. Photomicrograph of the heart in a patient with an acute myocardial infarction. In the center, the deeply eosinophilic necrotic cells have lost their nuclei. The necrotic focus is surrounded by paler-staining, viable cardiac myocytes.

lytic activity of intracellular and extracellular enzymes. As a result, the cell disintegrates. This is particularly the case when necrotic cells have elicited an acute inflammatory response.

The morphological appearance of the necrotic cell has traditionally been termed *coagulative necrosis* because of its similarity to the coagulation of proteins that occurs upon heating. However, the usefulness of this historical term today is questionable.

Whereas the morphological features associated with the death of individual cells tend to be uniform across different cell types, the tissue responses are more variable. This diversity is described by a number of terms that reflect specific histological patterns that depend upon the organ and the circumstances.

Liquefactive Necrosis

When the rate of dissolution of the necrotic cells is considerably faster than the rate of repair, the resulting morphological appearance is termed *liquefactive necrosis*. The polymorphonuclear leukocytes of the acute inflammatory reaction are endowed with potent hydrolases capable of digesting dead cells. A sharply localized collection of these acute inflammatory cells, generally in response to a bacterial infection, produces the rapid death and dissolution of tissue. The result is often an **abscess** (Fig. 1-27), defined as a cavity formed by liquefactive necrosis in a solid tissue. Eventually an abscess is walled off by a fibrous capsule that contains its contents.

Coagulative necrosis of the brain as a result of cerebral artery occlusion is frequently followed by rapid dissolution—liquefactive necrosis—of the dead tissue by a mechanism that cannot be attributed to the action of an acute inflammatory response. It is not clear why coagulative necrosis in the brain, and not elsewhere, is followed by the dissolution of the necrotic cells, but the phenomenon may be related

26   Cell Injury

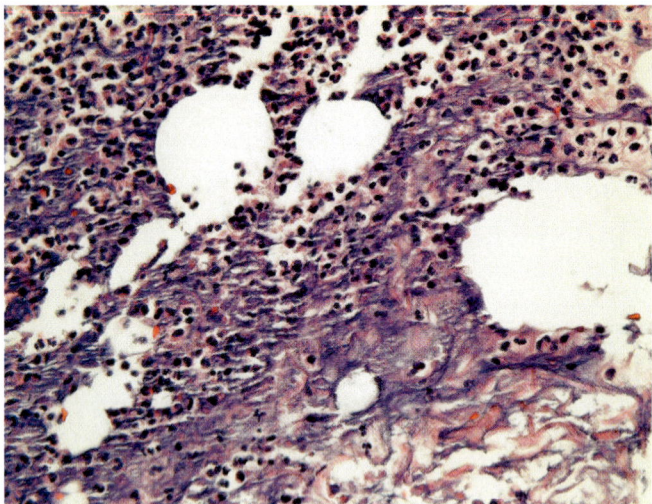

FIGURE 1-27
Liquefactive necrosis in an abscess of the skin. The abscess cavity is filled with polymorphonuclear leukocytes.

to the presence of more abundant lysosomal enzymes or different hydrolases specific to the cells of the central nervous system. Liquefactive necrosis of large areas of the central nervous system can result in the formation of an actual cavity or cyst that will persist for the life of the person.

Fat Necrosis

Fat necrosis specifically affects adipose tissue and most commonly results from pancreatitis or trauma (Fig. 1-28). The unique feature determining this type of necrosis is the presence of triglycerides in adipose tissue. The process begins when digestive enzymes, normally found only in the pancreatic duct and small intestine, are released from injured pancreatic acinar cells and ducts into the extracellular spaces. On extracellular activation, these enzymes digest the pancreas itself as well as the surrounding tissues, including adipose cells, as follows.

1. Phospholipases and proteases attack the plasma membrane of the fat cells, releasing their stored triglycerides.
2. Pancreatic lipase then hydrolyzes the triglycerides, a process that produces free fatty acids.
3. The fatty acids are precipitated as calcium soaps, which accumulate microscopically as amorphous, basophilic deposits at the periphery of the irregular islands of necrotic adipocytes.

On gross examination, fat necrosis appears as an irregular, chalky white area embedded in otherwise normal adipose tissue. In the case of traumatic fat necrosis, we presume that triglycerides and lipases are released from the injured adipocytes. In the breast, fat necrosis secondary to trauma is not uncommon and may mimic a tumor.

Caseous Necrosis

Caseous necrosis is a lesion characteristic of tuberculosis (Fig. 1-29). The lesions of tuberculosis are the tuberculous granulomas, or tubercles. In the center of such a granuloma, the accumulated mononuclear cells mediating the chronic inflammatory reaction to the offending mycobacteria are killed. In caseous necrosis, unlike coagulative necrosis, the necrotic cells fail to retain their cellular outlines. They do not, however, disappear by lysis, as in liquefactive necrosis. Rather, the dead cells persist indefinitely as amorphous, coarsely granular, eosinophilic debris. Grossly, this debris appears grayish white and is soft and friable. It resembles clumpy cheese, hence the name *caseous necrosis*. This distinctive type of necrosis is generally attributed to the toxic effects of the unusual cell wall of the mycobacterium, which contains complex waxes (peptidoglycolipids) that exert potent biological effects.

Fibrinoid Necrosis

Fibrinoid necrosis refers to an alteration of injured blood vessels, in which the insudation and accumulation of plasma proteins cause the wall to stain intensely with eosin (Fig. 1-30). The term is something of a misnomer, however, because the eosinophilia of the accumulated plasma proteins obscures the underlying alterations in the blood vessel, making it difficult, if not impossible, to determine whether there truly is necrosis in the vascular wall.

Necrosis Usually Involves the Accumulation of a Number of Intracellular Insults

The processes by which cells undergo death by necrosis vary according to the cause, the organ, and the cell type. The best

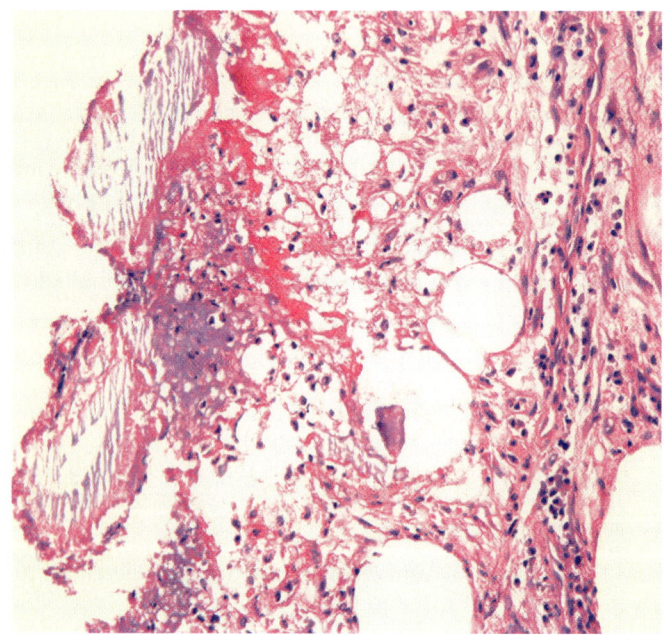

FIGURE 1-28
Fat necrosis. Photomicrograph of peripancreatic adipose tissue from a patient with acute pancreatitis shows an island of necrotic adipocytes adjacent to an acutely inflamed area. Fatty acids are precipitated as calcium soaps, which accumulate as amorphous, basophilic deposits at the periphery of the irregular island of necrotic adipocytes.

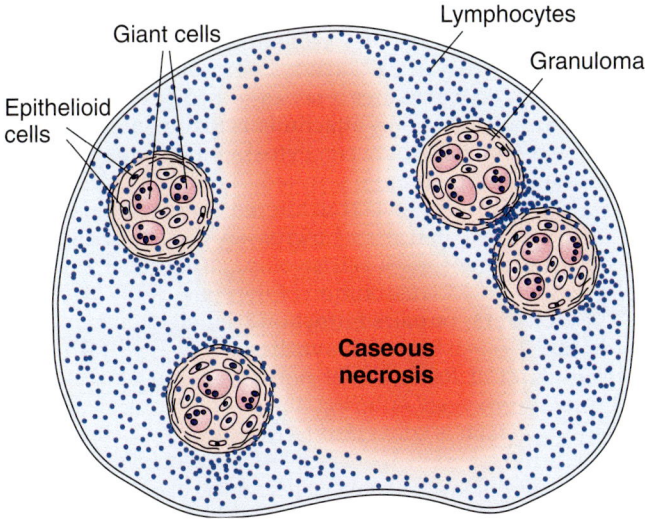

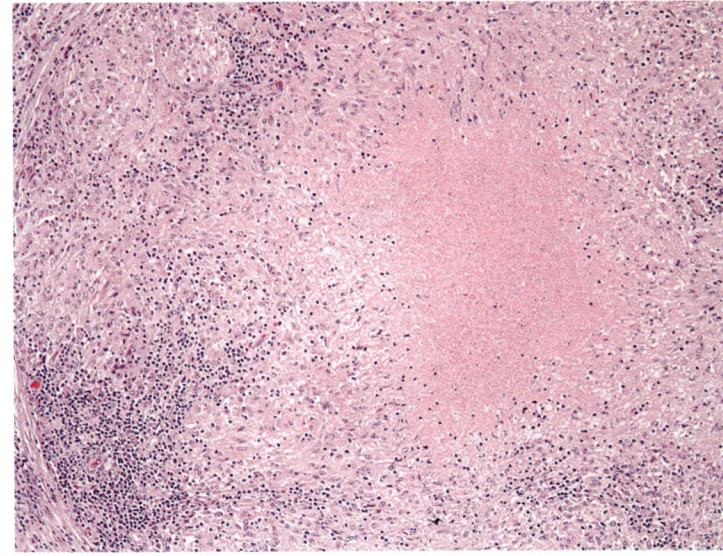

FIGURE 1-29
Caseous necrosis in a tuberculous lymph node. A. The typical amorphous, granular, eosinophilic, necrotic center is surrounded by granulomatous inflammation. B. Photomicrograph showing a tuberculous granuloma with central caseous necrosis.

studied and most clinically important example is ischemic necrosis of cardiac myocytes, the leading cause of death in the western world. The mechanisms underlying the death of cardiac myocytes are in part unique, but the basic processes that are involved are comparable to those in other organs. Some of the unfolding events may occur simultaneously; others may be sequential (Fig. 1-31).

1. **Interruption of blood supply decreases the delivery of O_2 and glucose.** Anoxia, whether it arises from ischemia (e.g., atherosclerosis) or other causes (e.g., blood loss from trauma), decreases the delivery of both oxygen and glucose to the myocyte. For most cells, but especially for cardiac myocytes (which do not store much energy), this combined insult is formidable.
2. **Anaerobic glycolysis leads to overproduction of lactate and a decrease in intracellular pH.** The lack of O_2 during myocardial ischemia not only blocks the production of ATP, but also inhibits the oxidation of pyruvate in the mitochondria. Instead, pyruvate is reduced to lactate in the cytosol, and its accumulation in the cytosol lowers intracellular pH. The acidification of the cytosol then initiates a

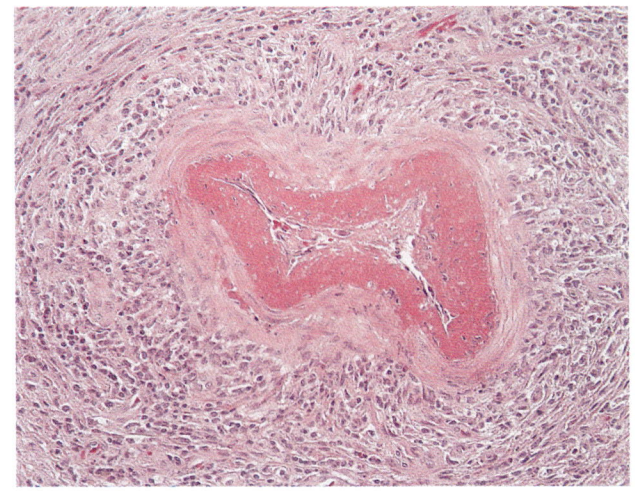

FIGURE 1-30
Fibrinoid necrosis. An inflamed muscular artery in a patient with systemic arteritis shows a sharply demarcated, homogeneous, deeply eosinophilic zone of necrosis.

28 Cell Injury

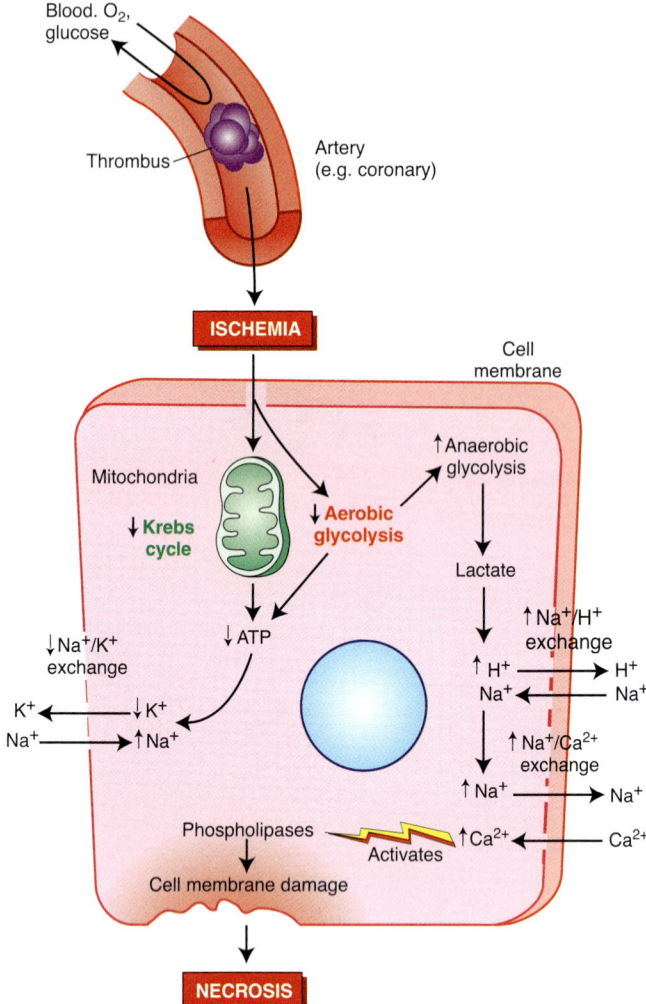

FIGURE 1-31
Mechanisms by which ischemia leads to cell death.

downward spiral of events that propels the cell toward disaster.

3. **Distortion of the activities of pumps in the plasma membrane skews the ionic balance of the cell.** Na^+ accumulates because the lack of ATP renders the Na^+/K^+ ion exchanger inactive, an effect that leads to activation of the Na^+/H^+ ion exchanger. This pump is normally quiescent, but when intracellular acidosis threatens, it pumps H^+ out of the cell in exchange for Na^+ to maintain proper intracellular pH. In turn, the resulting increase in intracellular sodium activates the Na^+/Ca^{2+} ion exchanger, thereby enhancing calcium entry. Ordinarily, excess intracellular Ca^{2+} is extruded by a calcium pump that is ATP dependent. However, ATP is now in very short supply, and Ca^{2+}, therefore, accumulates in the cell.

4. **The activation of phospholipase A_2 and proteases disrupts the plasma membrane and cytoskeleton.** High calcium concentrations in the cytosol of an ischemic cell activate phospholipase A_2 (PLA_2), leading to degradation of membrane phospholipids and the consequent release of free fatty acids and lysophospholipids. The latter act as detergents that solubilize cell membranes. Both fatty acids and lysophospholipids are also potent mediators of inflammation (see Chapter 2), an effect that may further disrupt the integrity of the already compromised cell.

Calcium also activates a series of proteases that attack the cytoskeleton and its attachments to the cell membrane. As the interactions between cytoskeletal proteins and the plasma membrane are disrupted, membrane blebs form, and the shape of the cell is altered. The combination of electrolyte imbalance and increased permeability of the cell membrane causes cell swelling, a frequent morphological prelude to dissolution of the cell.

5. **The lack of O_2 impairs mitochondrial electron transport, thereby decreasing ATP synthesis and facilitating the production of ROS.** Under normal circumstances, about 3% of the oxygen entering the mitochondrial electron transport chain is converted to ROS. During ischemia, the generation of ROS increases because of (1) decreased availability of favored substrates for the electron transport chain, (2) damage to elements of the chain, and (3) reduced activity of mitochondrial SOD. ROS cause peroxidation of cardiolipin, a membrane phospholipid that is unique to mitochondria and is sensitive to oxidative damage by virtue of its high content of unsaturated fatty acids. This attack inhibits the function of the electron transport chain and decreases its ability to produce ATP.

6. **Mitochondrial damage promotes the release of cytochrome c to the cytosol.** In normal cells the mitochondrial permeability transition pore (MPTP) opens and closes sporadically. Ischemic injury to mitochondria causes sustained opening of the MPTP, with resulting loss of cytochrome c from the electron transport chain. This process further diminishes ATP synthesis and may, under some circumstances, also trigger apoptotic cell death (see below).

7. **The cell dies.** When the cell can no longer maintain itself as a metabolic unit, necrotic cell death occurs. The line between reversible and irreversible cell injury (i.e., the "point of no return,") is not precisely defined, but it is probably reached at about the time that the MPTP opens. Although this event by itself is not necessarily lethal, by the time it occurs, disruption of the electron transport chain has become irreparable, and eventually necrotic cell death is inevitable.

Ample evidence from experimental and clinical studies indicates that pharmacological interference with a number of events involved in the pathogenesis of cell necrosis can preserve cell viability after an ischemic insult. The Na^+/H^+ exchanger has become an interesting target for therapeutic intervention to maintain the viability of cardiac myocytes during acute ischemia. Treatments that increase glucose uptake and redress some of the ionic imbalances may preserve myocyte viability under ischemic conditions. Indeed, some success has been reported with the simple administration of a combination of glucose, insulin, and potassium.

Apoptosis, Also Termed Programmed Cell Death, Refers to a Cellular Suicide Mechanism

Apoptosis is a prearranged pathway of cell death, which is triggered by a variety of extracellular and intracellular signals. Apoptosis is part of the balance between the life and death of cells and determines that a cell dies when it is no longer use-

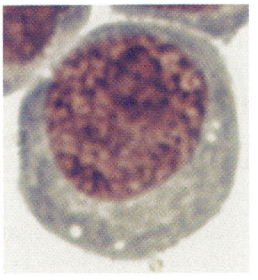 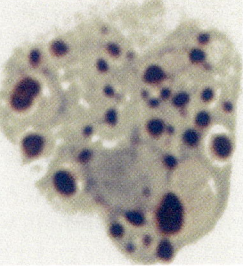

FIGURE 1-32
Apoptosis. A viable leukemic cell *(left)* contrasts with an apoptotic cell *(right)* in which the nucleus has undergone condensation and fragmentation.

ful or when it may be harmful to the larger organism. It is also a self-defense mechanism, destroying cells that have been infected with pathogens or those in which genomic alterations have occurred. In this context, many pathogens have evolved survival mechanisms by which they inactivate key components of the apoptotic signaling cascades. Apoptosis detects and destroys cells that harbor dangerous mutations, thereby maintaining genetic consistency and preventing the development of cancer. By contrast, as in the case of infectious agents, successful clones of tumor cells often devise mechanisms to circumvent apoptosis.

The Morphology of Apoptosis

Apoptotic cells are recognized by nuclear fragmentation and pyknosis, generally against a background of viable cells. Importantly, individual cells or small groups of cells undergo apoptosis, whereas necrosis characteristically involves larger geographical areas of cell death. Ultrastructural features of apoptotic cells include (1) nuclear condensation and fragmentation, (2) segregation of cytoplasmic organelles into distinct regions, (3) blebs of the plasma membrane, and (4) membrane-bound cellular fragments, which often lack nuclei (Fig. 1-32).

Cells that have undergone necrotic cell death tend to elicit strong inflammatory responses. Inflammation, however, is not generally seen in the vicinity of apoptotic cells (Fig. 1-33). Mononuclear phagocytes may contain cellular debris from apoptotic cells, but recruitment of neutrophils or lymphocytes is uncommon (see Chapter 2). In view of the numerous developmental, physiologic and protective functions of apoptosis, the lack of inflammation is clearly beneficial to the organism.

Apoptosis Is Important in Developmental and Physiological Processes

Fetal development involves the sequential appearance and regression of many anatomical structures: some aortic arches do not persist, the mesonephros regresses in favor of the metanephros, interdigital tissues disappear to allow discrete fingers and toes, and excess neurons are pruned from the developing brain. In the generation of immunological diversity, clones of cells that recognize normal self antigens are deleted by apoptosis.

Physiological apoptosis principally involves the progeny of stem cells that are continuously dividing (e.g., stem cells of the hematopoietic system, gastrointestinal mucosa, and epi-

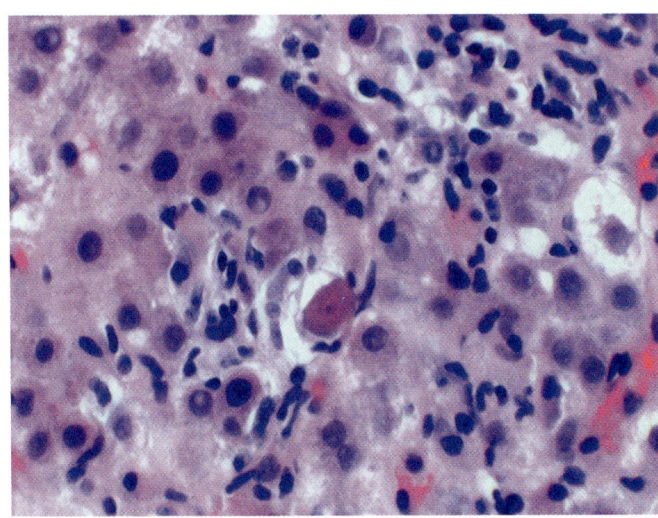 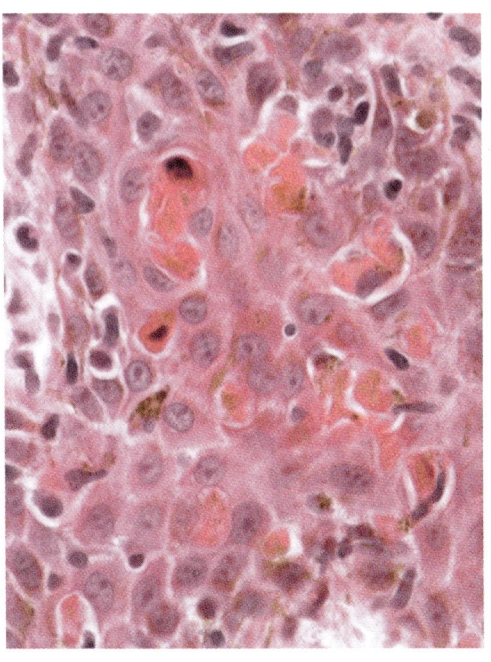

FIGURE 1-33
Histopathologic illustrations of apoptosis in the liver in viral hepatitis (A) and in the skin in erythema multiforme (B).

Apoptosis Eliminates Obsolescent Cells

A normal turnover of cells in many organs is essential to maintain the size and function of that cellular compartment. For example, as cells are continuously supplied to the circulating blood, older and less functional white blood cells must be eliminated to maintain the normal complement of the cells. Indeed, the pathological accumulation of polymorphonuclear leukocytes in chronic myelogenous leukemia results from a mutation that inhibits apoptosis and, therefore, leads to the persistence of these cells. In the mucosa of the small intestine, cells migrate from the depths of the crypts to the tips of the villi, where they undergo apoptosis and are sloughed into the lumen.

Apoptosis also maintains the balance of cellularity in organs that respond to trophic stimuli, such as hormones. An illustration of such an effect is the regression of lactational hyperplasia of the breast in women who have stopped nursing their infants. On the other side of the reproductive divide, postmenopausal women suffer atrophy of the endometrium after hormonal support has withered.

Apoptosis Deletes Mutant Cells

The integrity of an organism requires the recognition of irreparable damage to DNA, after which the damaged cells must be eliminated by apoptosis. There is a finite error rate in DNA replication, owing to the infidelity of DNA polymerases. In addition, environmental stresses such as UV light, ionizing radiation, and DNA-binding chemicals may also alter DNA structure. There are several means, the most important of which is probably p53, by which the cell recognizes genomic abnormalities and "assesses" whether they can be repaired. If the damage to DNA is so severe that it cannot be repaired, the cascade of events leading to apoptosis is activated, and the cell dies. This process protects an organism from the consequences of a nonfunctional cell or one that cannot control its own proliferation (e.g., a cancer cell).

Apoptosis Defends against the Dissemination of Infection

When a cell "detects" episomal (extrachromosomal) DNA replication, as in a viral infection, it tends to initiate apoptosis. This effect can be viewed as a means to eliminate infected cells before they can spread the virus. Many viruses have evolved protective mechanisms to manipulate cellular apoptosis. Viral gene products that inhibit apoptosis have been identified for many viruses, including HIV, human papillomavirus, adenovirus, and many others. In some cases these viral proteins bind and inactivate certain cellular proteins (e.g., p53) that are important in signaling apoptosis. In other instances, they may act at various points in the signaling pathways that activate apoptosis.

Apoptosis Is Signaled by Diverse Stimuli

Apoptosis is a final effector mechanism that can be initiated by many different stimuli, whose signals are propagated by a number of pathways. Unlike necrosis, apoptosis is a process that engages the cell's own signaling cascades. In other words, the cell that undergoes apoptosis is an active participant in its own death (suicide). Most intermediate enzymes that transduce proapoptotic signals belong to a family of cysteine proteases called *caspases*.

Apoptosis Is Initiated by Receptor–Ligand Interactions at the Cell Membrane

The best understood initiators of apoptosis at the cell membrane are the binding of TNF-α to its receptor (TNFR) and that of the Fas ligand to its receptor (Fas, or Fas receptor). TNF-α is most often a free cytokine, whereas Fas ligand is located at the plasma membrane of certain cells, such as cytotoxic effector lymphocytes.

The receptors for TNF-α and Fas ligand become activated upon binding their ligands. These transmembrane proteins posses amino acid sequences in their cytoplasmic tails, termed *death domains,* that serve as docking sites for the death domains of other proteins that participate in the signaling process leading to apoptosis (Fig. 1-34A). After binding to the receptors, the latter proteins activate downstream signaling molecules, especially procaspase-8, which is converted to caspase-8. In turn, caspase-8 initiates an activation cascade of other downstream caspases in the apoptosis pathway. These caspases, (3, 6, and 7) activate a number of nuclear enzymes (e.g., PARP [poly-ADP-ribosyl polymerase]) that mediate the nuclear fragmentation of apoptotic cell death.

Activation of caspase signaling also occurs when killer lymphocytes, principally cytotoxic T cells, recognize a cell as foreign. These lymphocytes then release perforin and granzyme B. Perforin, as its name suggests, punches a hole in the plasma membrane of the target cell, through which granzyme B enters and activates procaspase-8 directly (Fig. 1-34B).

Apoptosis Is Mediated by Mitochondrial Proteins

The mitochondrial membrane is a key regulator of the balance between cell death and cell survival. Proteins of the Bcl-2 family reside in the mitochondrial inner membrane and are either proapoptotic or antiapoptotic (prosurvival). Proapoptotic proteins in this family include Bax, Bak, Bad, and Bik; antiapoptotic proteins are Bcl-2, Bcl-X_L, and A1. These members of the Bcl-2 family form both homo- and heterodimers in the mitochondrial membrane. A preponderance of heterodimers that consist of pro- and antiapoptotic Bcl-2 proteins or homodimers of antiapoptotic proteins promotes cell survival. When the balance shifts to homodimers composed of proapoptotic proteins, the apoptotic cascade is activated (Fig. 1-34C).

ROS (e.g., peroxide) lead to apoptosis by opening the mitochondrial permeability transition pores, resulting in the release of cytochrome c (see below). The formation of the nitric oxide radical (NO•) has similar consequences. ROS also activate neutral sphingomyelinase, a cytosolic enzyme that releases ceramide from sphingomyelin in the plasma membrane. In turn, ceramide stimulates cellular stress responses (stress-activated protein kinases), which then activate procaspase-8.

Activation of p53 by DNA damage or other means also initiates apoptotic signaling through the mitochondria. As a transcription factor, p53 increases the production of the proapoptotic mitochondrial protein Bax and the proapoptotic FasR. Apoptosis is also initiated by p53 through means unrelated to transcriptional activation. The mechanisms by which mitochondria exert such a powerful effect on apoptosis have recently been elucidated (Figure 1-34C). Bcl-2 dimers at the mitochondrial membrane bind the protein Apaf-1. A surfeit of proapoptotic constituents of the Bcl-2 family leads to the release of Apaf-1. At the same time, mitochondrial pores open, and cytochrome c leaks through the mitochondrial membrane. Cytochrome c activates Apaf-1, which in turn converts procaspase-9 to caspase-9. Caspase-9 activates downstream caspases (3, 6, and 7) in the same manner as caspase-8.

Pro- and Antiapoptotic Signals Are in Equilibrium

Apoptosis can be viewed as a default pathway, and the survival of many cells is contingent upon constant antiapoptotic (prosurvival) signals. In other words, the cell must actively choose life rather than succumbing to the despair of apoptosis. The survival signals are transduced through receptors linked to phosphatidylinositol 3-kinase (PI3K), the enzyme that phosphorylates PIP_2 and PIP_3 (phosphatidyl inositol bis-

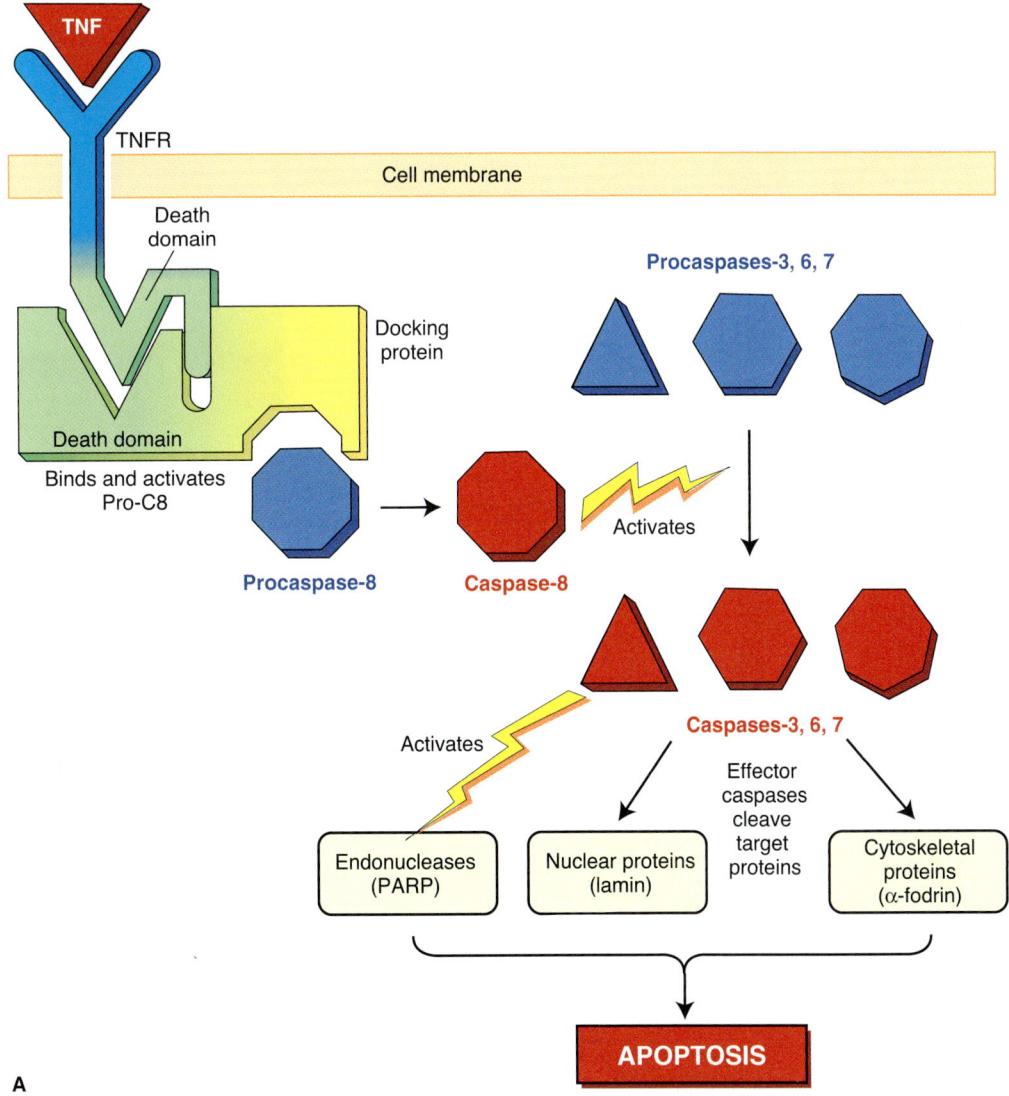

FIGURE 1-34
Mechanisms by which apoptosis may be initiated, signaled, and executed. A. Ligand–receptor interactions that lead to caspase activation.

FIGURE 1-34 (continued)
B. Immunological reactions in which granzyme released by cytotoxic lymphocytes causes apoptosis. C. Opening of the mitochondrial permeability transition pore, leading to Apaf-1 activation thereby triggering the apoptotic cascade.

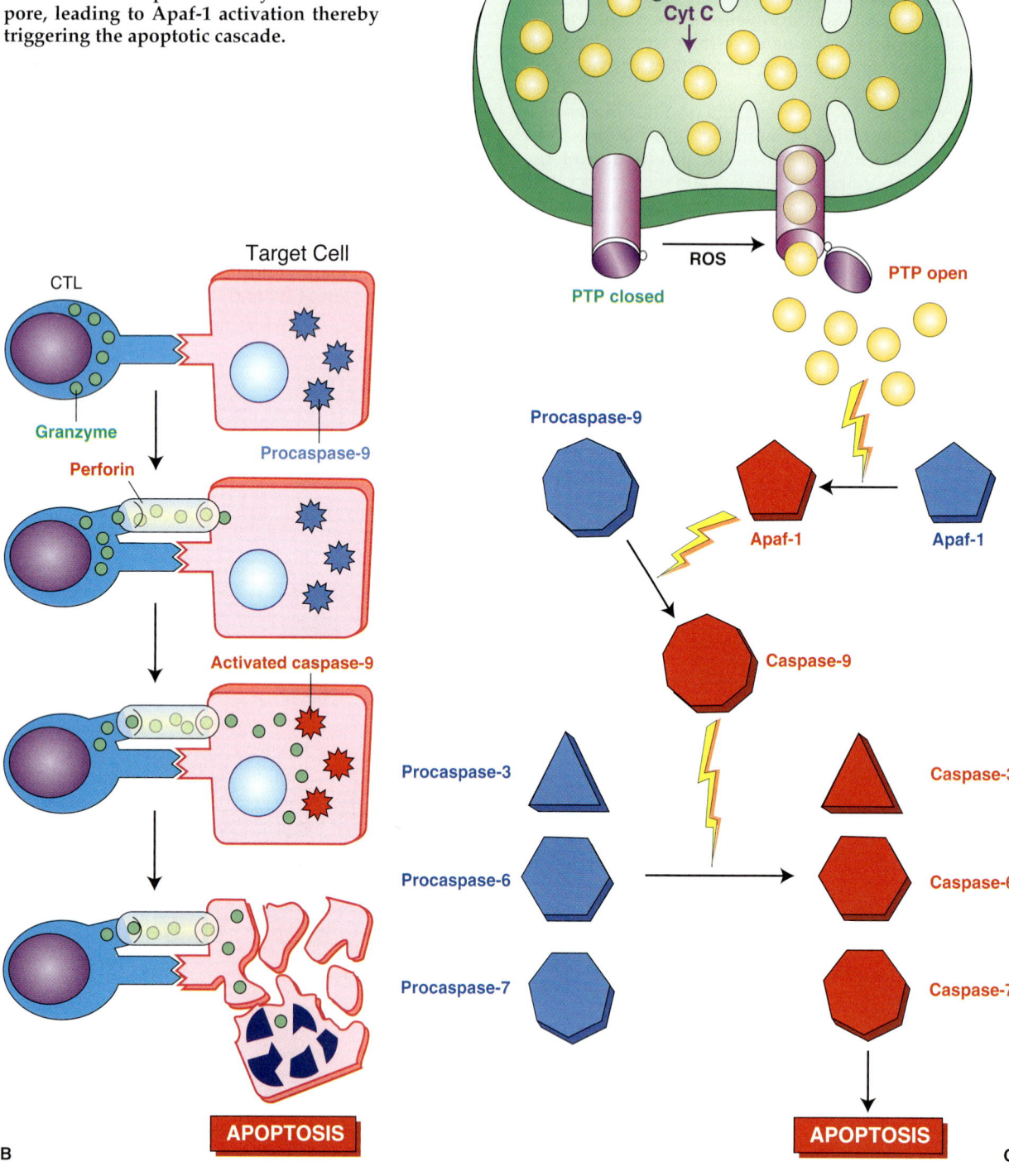

and trisphosphates). By antagonizing apoptosis, PI3K plays a critical role in the vitality of the cell. A prototypical receptor that signals via this mechanism is insulin-like growth factor-1 receptor (IGFR). Paradoxically, PI3K is also activated by TNFR after binding TNF-α. Thus, the same cell membrane receptor that induces apoptosis in some circumstances can also initiate antiapoptotic signaling in other situations.

PI3K exerts antiapoptotic effects through intracellular mediators, which favor survival by activating protein kinase B (PKB), also called Akt. The latter then inactivates several important proapoptotic proteins (e.g., the Bcl-2 family member, Bad). More importantly, PKB activates NFκB (nuclear factor κB), an important transcription factor that promotes the expression of proteins (A1 and Bcl-X_L) that prevent the loss of cytochrome c from mitochondria and promote cell survival. PKB also stimulates signaling mechanisms that activate cell division.

Apoptosis Is Activated by p53

A pivotal molecule in the cell's life-and-death dance is the versatile protein p53, which preserves the viability of an injured cell when DNA damage can be repaired, but propels it toward apoptosis after irreparable harm has occurred (p53 is discussed in greater detail in Chapter 5).

Homeostasis of p53

A delicate balance exists between the stabilization and destruction of p53. Thus, p53 binds to several proteins (e.g., mdm2), which promote its degradation via ubiquitination. The ability of p53 to avoid this pernicious association depends upon certain structural changes in the protein in response to stress, DNA damage, etc. These molecular modifications decrease its interaction with mdm2, thereby enhancing survival of p53 and permitting its accumulation.

Function of p53

After it binds to areas of DNA damage, p53 activates proteins that arrest the cell in G1 of the cell cycle, allowing time for DNA repair to proceed. It also directs DNA repair enzymes to the site of injury. If the DNA damage cannot be repaired, p53 activates mechanisms that terminate in apoptosis.

There are several pathways by which p53 induces apoptosis. This molecule downregulates transcription of the antiapoptotic protein Bcl-2, while it upregulates transcription of the proapoptotic genes *bax* and *bak*. In addition, certain DNA helicases and other enzymes are activated by p53-mediated recognition of DNA damage, an effect that leads to the translocation of a number of proapoptotic proteins (e.g., Fas) from the cell membrane to the cytosol.

Stress also leads to the accumulation of p53. The activation of certain oncogenes, such as *c-myc*, increases the amount of an mdm2-binding protein (p14^{arf}), thereby protecting p53 from mdm2-induced destruction. Additional forms of stress that lead to the accumulation of p53 include hypoxia, depletion of ribonucleotides, and the loss of cell–cell adhesion during oncogenesis.

Inactivation of p53

Proteins of a number of oncogenic viruses inactivate p53 by binding to it. In fact, p53 was first identified as a cellular protein that coprecipitated with certain viral transforming proteins. Inactivating mutations of p53 are the most common DNA alterations in human cancer, which further emphasizes its role as a switch that allows repair of DNA but triggers cellular suicide if that proves to be impossible.

Quantitative Assays for Apoptosis

Apoptotic cells can be detected by demonstrating fragmented DNA. A popular method involves the demonstration of nucleosomal "laddering." This virtually diagnostic pattern of DNA degradation, which is characteristic of apoptotic cell death, results from the cleavage of chromosomal DNA at nucleosomes by activated endonucleases. Since nucleosomes are regularly spaced along the genome, a pattern of regular bands can be seen when fragments of cellular DNA are separated by electrophoresis (Fig. 1-35).

Other assays are also used to detect and quantitate apoptosis. One is the TUNEL assay (terminal deoxyribonucleotidyl transferase [TdT]-mediated dUTP-digoxigenin nick end labeling) in which TdT transfers a fluorescent nucleotide to exposed breakpoints of DNA. Apoptotic cells that have incorporated the labeled nucleotide are then visualized by fluorescence microscopy or flow cytometry. Apoptotic cells that have extruded some of the DNA have less than their normal diploid content. Automated measurement of the amount of DNA in individual cells by flow cytometry thus produces a population distribution according to DNA content (cytofluorograph). Other means of detecting apopto-

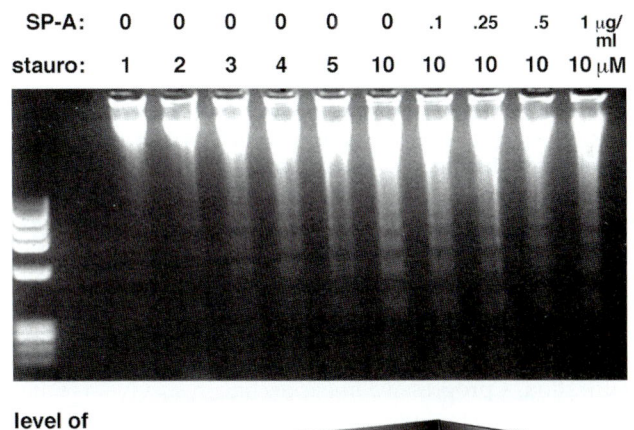

FIGURE 1-35
DNA fragmentation in apoptosis. Agarose gel electrophoresis of DNA isolated from lung epithelial cells treated with different amounts of staurosporine, which induces apoptosis, and with different amounts of surfactant protein-A *(SP-A)*, which protects these cells from apoptosis. The schematic at the bottom illustrates the degree of apoptosis observed in these cells as a function of the concentrations of these two agents. At low concentrations of staurosporine, or at high concentrations of SP-A, genomic DNA is largely unfragmented and thus remains at the top of the gel. By contrast, internucleosomal cleavage of DNA, such as occurs in apoptosis, is reflected in multiple, regularly spaced genomic DNA fragments, resembling a ladder. This phenomenon is called "laddering."

sis depend upon quantitating the activated forms of enzymes that signal apoptosis, including the nuclear proteins PARP and lamin A.

In summary, cells are poised between survival and apoptosis, and their fate rests on a balance of powerful intracellular and extracellular forces, whose signals constantly act upon and counteract each other. In many circumstances, apoptosis is a self-protective programmed mechanism that leads to the suicide of a cell when its survival is deemed detrimental to the organism. In other instances, apoptosis is a pathological process that contributes to many disorders, especially degenerative diseases. Thus, the pharmacological manipulation of apoptosis represents an active frontier of drug development.

BIOLOGICAL AGING

Old age is a consequence of civilization; it is a condition rarely encountered in the animal kingdom or in primitive societies. From an evolutionary perspective, the aging process presents conceptual difficulties. Since animals in the wild do not attain their maximum longevity, how did aging evolve? The consequences of aging arise after the reproductive period and thus should not have an evolutionary impact.

Aging must be distinguished from mortality on the one hand and from disease on the other. Death is a random event; an aged person who does not succumb to the most common cause of death will die from the second, third, or tenth most common cause. Although the increased vulnerability to disease among the elderly is an interesting problem, disease itself is entirely distinct from aging.

Maximal Life Span Has Remained Unchanged

Millennia ago the psalmist, who lived in an era of literate civilization, sang of a natural life span of 70 years, which with vigor may extend to 80. By contrast, it is estimated that the usual age at death of Neolithic humans was 20 to 25 years, and the average life span in some underdeveloped regions today is often barely 10 years more.

The difference between humans in primitive and in civilized environments is analogous to that observed between animals in their natural habitat and those in a zoo (Fig. 1-36). For animals in the wild, after an initial high mortality during maturation, a progressive linear decline in survival is noted, ending at the maximum life span of the species. This steady decrease in the number of mature animals does not reflect aging but rather sporadic events, such as encounters with beasts of prey, accidental trauma, infections, starvation, and so on. On the other hand, survival in the protected environment of a zoo is characterized by slow attrition until old age, at which time the steep decline in numbers is attributable to the aging process. **Interestingly, the maximum life span attained is not significantly altered by a protected environment.** An analogous situation is seen in studies of human mortality (Fig. 1-37). Less than a century ago, the steep linear slope of mortality in human adults principally reflected random accidents and infections. With greater attention to safety and sanitation, the development of antibiotics and other specific drugs, safer blood transfusions, and improved diagnostic and therapeutic methods, the incidence of death through the middle years has substantially decreased. The age-adjusted death rate in the United States has declined by 40% since 1970, and in 2002, life expectancy at birth was 80 years for white females and 75 years for white males. At age 50 years, life expectancy was 32 additional years and 28 additional years, respectively.

Yet the mortality curve during old age remains steep, and the maximum human life span has remained constant at about 110 years. What would happen if diseases associated with old age, such as cardiovascular disease and cancer, were eliminated? Such triumphs would lead to an **ideal survival curve** (see Fig. 1-37) but only a modest increase in average life expectancy. A long period of good health and low mortality rate would inevitably be followed by a precipitously increased mortality owing to aging itself; the life span would, for practical purposes, remain on the lower side of 100 years. Given the current life expectancy, the prevention or cure of the causes of premature death would have little impact on mean longevity.

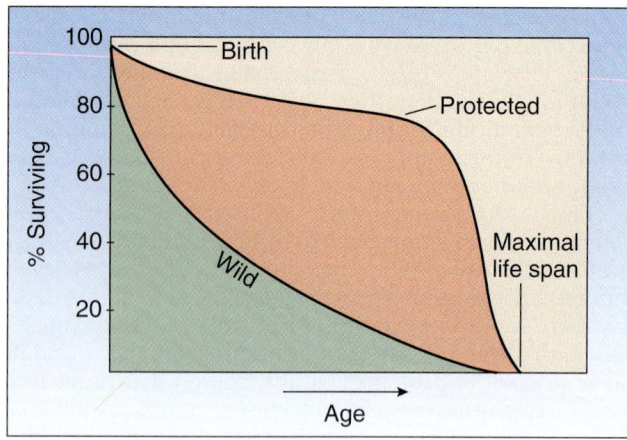

FIGURE 1-36

Life span of animals in their natural environment compared with that in a protected habitat. Note that both curves reach the same maximal life span.

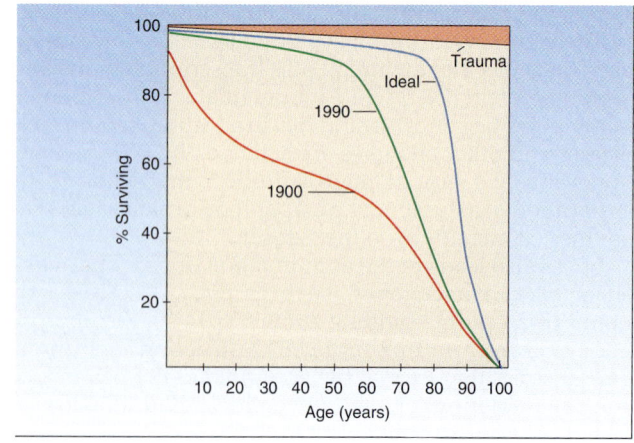

FIGURE 1-37

Ideal human life span contrasted with those seen in 1900 and 1980. Note again that the same maximal life span is reached in all cases.

Why do women live longer than men? The male-to-female ratio is 106:100 at birth, but from that time on, more women than men survive at every age, and at age 75 the male-to-female ratio is 2:3. Interestingly, a greater female longevity is almost universal in the animal kingdom. At the cellular level, somatic cells with the female genotype are no hardier than those with the male pattern. Factors involved in the difference in average human longevity include the greater male mortality rate from violent causes and a greater susceptibility to cardiovascular disease, cancer, respiratory illness, and cirrhosis in middle and old age. The historical differences between the sexes in cigarette smoking and alcohol consumption are also important in the gender gap in longevity. Indeed, smoking alone has been estimated to account for 4 of the 7 years of sex differential in longevity at birth. Thus, if men escape from these hazards, the gap in longevity between the sexes is progressively reduced with advancing age to just over 1 year beyond age 85.

Functional and Structural Changes Accompany Aging

The insidious effects of aging can be detected in otherwise healthy persons. The great leaps of imagination by theoretical physicists and mathematicians are almost exclusively the province of the young, and an athlete in his or her 30s may be referred to as "aged." Even in the absence of specific diseases or vascular abnormalities, beginning in the fourth decade of life there is a progressive decline in many physiological functions (Fig. 1-38), including such easily measurable parameters as muscular strength, cardiac reserve, nerve conduction time, pulmonary vital capacity, glomerular filtration, and vascular elasticity. These functional deteriorations are accompanied by structural changes. Lean body mass decreases, and the proportion of fat rises. Constituents of the connective tissue matrix are progressively crosslinked. Lipofuscin ("wear and tear") pigment accumulates in organs such as the brain, heart, and liver.

The salient characteristic of aging is not so much a decrease in basal functional capacity as it is a reduced ability to adapt to environmental stress. Although the resting pulse is unchanged, the maximal increase with exercise is reduced with age, and the time required for return to a normal heart rate is prolonged. Similarly, the aged show an impaired adaptive response to ingested carbohydrates. The fasting blood sugar level in old age is often normal compared with that of the young, but it rises higher after a carbohydrate meal and declines more slowly.

The Cellular Basis of Aging Is Studied in Culture

Although the biological basis for aging is obscure, there is general agreement that its elucidation, as in all pathological conditions, should be sought at the cellular level. Various theories of cellular aging have been proposed, but the evidence adduced for each is at best indirect and is often derived from data obtained in cultured cells. An adequate theory should be parsimonious, compatible with the species-specific differences in life spans, and consistent with the fact that most non-cycling cells, such as neurons and myocytes, undergo a linear, relatively uniform functional decline with age. In the following discussion, we review the major considerations in this controversial field of investigation.

Support for the concept of a genetically programmed life span comes from studies of replicating cells in tissue culture. Unlike cancer cells, normal cells in tissue culture do not exhibit an unrestrained capacity to replicate. Cultured human fibroblasts undergo about 50 population doublings, after which they are irreversibly arrested in the G1 phase of the cell cycle and no longer divide (Fig. 1-39). If the cells are exposed to an oncogenic virus (e.g., SV40) or a chemical carcinogen, they continue to replicate; in a sense, they become immortal. A rough correlation between the number of population doublings in fibroblasts and life span has been reported in several species. For example, rat fibroblasts exhibit considerably fewer doublings than do human ones. Moreover, cells obtained from persons afflicted with a syndrome of precocious aging, such as progeria (see below), also display a conspicuously reduced number of population doublings in vitro.

There is no demonstrable age-related change in vivo in the replicative capacity of rapidly cycling cells (e.g., epithelial cells of the intestine). One is, therefore, left with the apparent paradox that replicating cells in culture have a limited life span, whereas aging in vivo seems principally to affect the functional capacity of postmitotic cells. In other words, persons do not age because the cells of the intestinal tract or hematopoietic system fail to replicate. However, if one considers that a function of cells in vitro is to proliferate, then they indeed display a major failure in functional capacity, and in many studies cells in culture are used as a model for the study of aging.

Greek mythology postulates that the offspring of unions between immortal gods and mortal humans are mortal, for example, Hercules. Similarly, cellular senescence in vitro is apparently a dominant genetic trait. The evidence for this concept is the demonstration that hybrids between normal human cells in vitro, which exhibit a limited number of cell divisions, and immortalized cells with an indefinite capacity to divide, undergo senescence. This finding shows that senescence is dominant over immortality. Replicative senes-

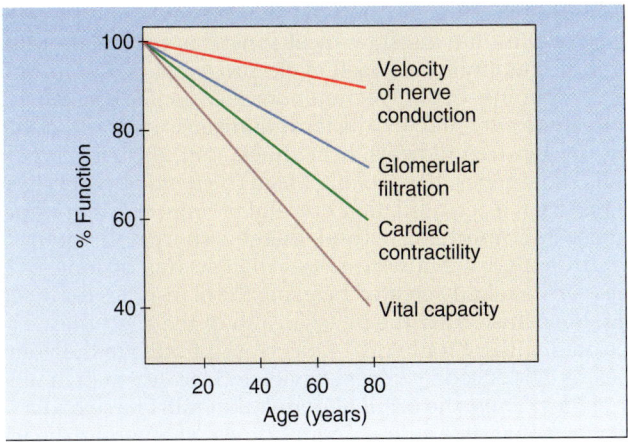

FIGURE 1-38
Decrease in human physiological capacities as a function of age.

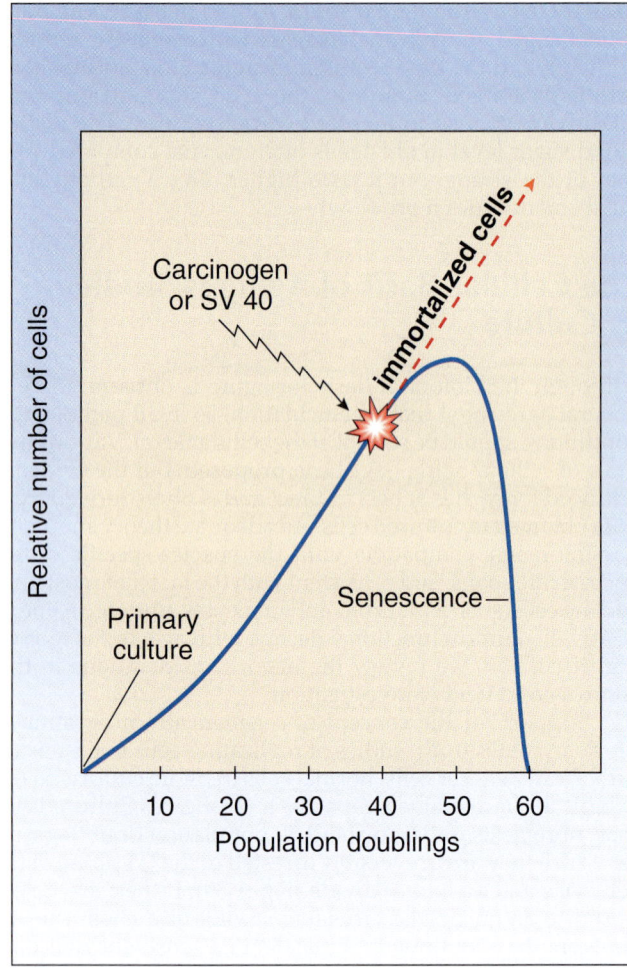

FIGURE 1-39
Cellular senescence in cultured human fibroblasts. The number of cultured cells is a function of the number of population doublings. After about 50 population doublings, the cells no longer divide, and the culture dies out. However, if the cells are transformed with a virus or chemical, cellular senescence is not seen; the cells are "immortalized" and continue to divide indefinitely.

cence–related genes have been identified on a number of human chromosomes, but the precise function(s) encoded by most of them have not been elucidated.

Telomerase and Senescene

An attractive explanation for cell senescence in vitro centers on the genetic elements at the tips of chromosomes, termed *telomeres*. These are composed of short repetitive nucleotide sequences (TTAGGG in vertebrates), which vary in size from 70 in *Tetrahymena* to 2000 in human chromosomes. Since DNA polymerase cannot copy the linear chromosomes all the way to the tip, the telomeres would tend to shorten with each cell division until a critical diminution in size interfered with replication. Moreover, oxidative stress induces single-stranded damage in telomeric DNA, and this defect cannot be repaired in telomeres.

To overcome this "end-replication" problem, most eukaryotic cells use a ribonucleoprotein enzyme termed *telomerase*, which can extend chromosome ends. It has, therefore, been proposed that telomere shortening acts as a molecular clock ("replicometer"), which produces senescence after a defined number of cell divisions in vitro. In this context, ectopic expression of telomerase reverses the senescent phenotype, and after immortalization of cells in vitro, telomerase activity can also be demonstrated.

Senescence also functions as a tumor-suppressing mechanism, limiting the proliferative capacity of cells in vivo. This concept implies that replicative senescence related to telomere shortening did not evolve to cause aging, but is rather an accidental characteristic of a biological device that provides a tumor suppressor function. Thus, the shortening of telomeres to a critical length activates a p53-dependent check point system in the cell cycle. Mice that are mutant for an activated form of p53 display an early onset of phenotypes associated with aging, including a shortened life span, generalized organ atrophy, osteoporosis, and diminished tolerance to a variety of stresses. These data are consistent with the observation that mutant mice that are deficient in telomerase exhibit high levels of activated p53 and also suffer reduced longevity and early senescence-related phenotypes. Other tumor suppressor genes also appear to be activated by telomere shortening, and cyclin-dependent kinase inhibitors (p16, p21, and p27) are regarded as the key effectors of replicative senescence. There is also evidence for a telomere-independent pathway for growth arrest in humans. In view of these data, current concepts hold that growth arrest suppresses tumorigenesis but that the functional changes contribute to aging.

Genetic Factors Influence Aging

Invertebrates, including roundworms and flies, represent a level of biological complexity beyond that afforded by tissue culture. The short generation times of these organisms have been exploited to study genetic influences on aging and longevity.

Caenorhabditis elegans is a worm in which single-gene mutations that extend life span have been identified. A variety of such mutations (*Age* mutations) increase the life span of the nematode up to fivefold, a greater increase than has been reported for any other model. In addition to prolonging the life span, *Age* mutations in *C. elegans* also confer a complex array of other phenotypes. For example, the so-called clock (*clk*) mutations slow most functions that relate to the overall metabolic rate (cell cycle progression, swimming, food pumping, etc.). *Age* mutations also confer resistance to both environmental (extrinsic) and intrinsic stresses, including oxygen free radicals, heat shock, and ultraviolet radiation. Thus, genes that prolong life in *C. elegans* apparently act to reduce the accumulation of cellular "injuries" that impair homeostatic mechanisms and, thereby, shorten life span.

In experiments with *Drosophila*, strains of long-lived flies can be readily created by using the oldest flies for breeding. In such studies, the better health of the aged flies is associated with a "trade-off" of decreased fitness in the young flies, as evidenced by lesser activity and fertility than in wild-type flies. Thus, the original population must have had a set of alleles that determines greater fitness at a young age and decreased fitness at an older one, a phenomenon termed "antagonistic pleiotropy." This doctrine also applies to the protection against cancer by tumor suppressor mechanisms at the price of promoting the aging process.

Diseases of Premature Aging

In humans, the modest correlation in longevity between related persons and the excellent concordance of life span among identical twins lend credence to the concept that aging is influenced by genetic factors. The existence of heritable diseases associated with accelerated aging buttresses this notion. The entire process of aging, including features such as male-pattern baldness, cataracts, and coronary artery disease, is compressed into a span of less than 10 years in a genetic syndrome termed Hutchinson-Guilford **progeria.** The biological basis of this disease is yet to be elucidated.

Werner syndrome (WS) (Fig. 1-40) is a rare autosomal recessive disease characterized by early cataracts, hair loss, atrophy of the skin, osteoporosis, and atherosclerosis. Affected persons are also at increased risk for the development of a variety of cancers. Patients typically die in the fifth decade from either cancer or cardiovascular disease. This phenotype of WS patients gives the impression of premature aging. The gene for WS, located on the short arm of chromosome 8, codes for a DNA helicase, an enzyme that unwinds DNA duplexes to provide access of the template to DNA-binding proteins. Helicases are, thus, crucial for the maintenance of genomic stability. Cells from patients with WS display chromosomal deletions, inversions, and reciprocal translocations (see Chapter 6). It is presumed that the premature aging in this disorder results from the progressive accumulation of genetic damage and consequent functional derangements.

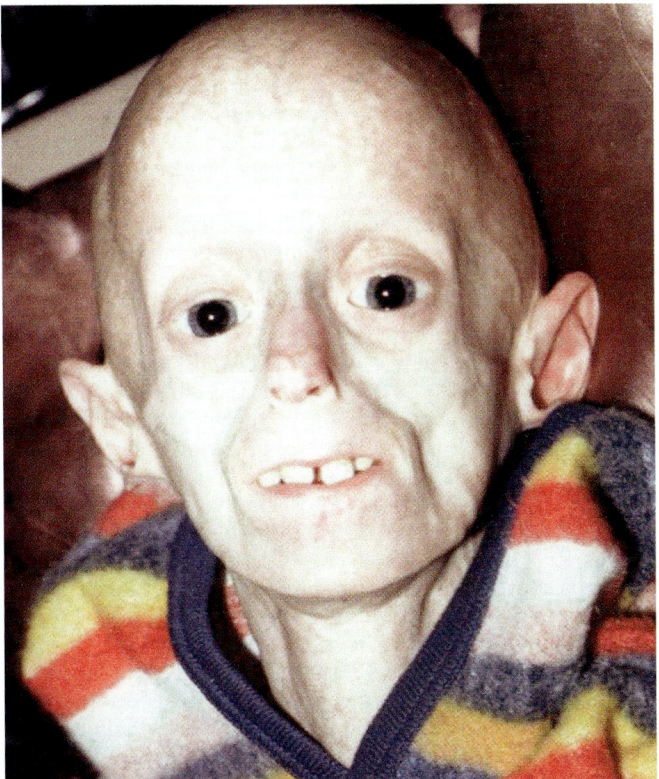

FIGURE 1-40

Progeria. A 10-year old girl shows the typical features of premature aging associated with progeria.

Aging May Reflect Accumulated Somatic Damage

Oxidative stress is an invariable consequence of life in an atmosphere rich in oxygen. An important hypothesis holds that the loss of function characteristic of aging is caused by the progressive and irreversible accrual of molecular oxidative damage. Such lesions would be manifested as (1) peroxidation of membrane lipids, (2) DNA modifications (strand breaks, base alterations, DNA–protein cross-linking), and (3) protein oxidation (loss of sulfhydryl groups, carbonylation). Oxidative stress in normal cells is hardly trivial, with as much as 3% of total oxygen consumption being converted to the generation of superoxide anions and hydrogen peroxide. It has been estimated that a single cell undergoes some 100,000 attacks on DNA a day by oxygen free radicals and that at any one time 10% of protein molecules are modified by carbonyl adducts. Thus, antioxidant defenses are not fully efficient, and progressive oxidative damage to the cell may be responsible, at least in part, for the aging process.

The rate of generation of reactive oxygen species correlates with the overall metabolic rate of an organism. The theory that aging is related to oxidative stress is based on several observations: (1) larger animals usually have longer life spans than smaller ones, (2) the metabolic rate is inversely related to body size (the larger the animal, the lower the metabolic rate), and (3) the generation of activated oxygen species correlates inversely with body size.

The role of oxidative stress in aging has been emphasized by experiments in *Drosophila* in which the overexpression of genes for SOD or catalase significantly prolongs the life span of the fly. Furthermore, as discussed above, virtually all long-lived worms and flies display increased antioxidant defenses. SOD activity in the livers of different primates has also been reported to be proportional to the maximal life span. The correlation of oxidative damage with aging is further exemplified by the demonstration of increased oxidative damage to lipids, proteins, and DNA in aged animals.

Additional evidence for progressive oxidative damage with aging is the deposition of lipofuscin pigment, principally in postmitotic cells of organs such as the brain, heart, and liver. This brown pigment is located in lysosomes and contains products of the peroxidation of unsaturated fatty acids. Although no functional derangements are directly attributed to the accumulation of lipofuscin, it has been proposed that the presence of this pigment reflects continuing lipid peroxidation of cellular membranes as a result of inadequate defenses against the stress of activated oxygen.

Oxidative damage to mitochondria has also been proposed to play a major role in aging. Aerobic respiration in mitochondria is the richest source of reactive oxygen species in the cell. Mitochondrial DNA is extremely sensitive to hydroxyl radical damage and progressively develops more than 100 different DNA deletions over the course of a human life. In turn, these DNA defects may lead to further increases in the mitochondrial generation of toxic oxygen species, thereby establishing a vicious circle.

Caloric restriction in rodents and lower species has been known for more than half a century to increase longevity. However, prolongation of the life span by caloric restriction has not been demonstrated in primates or humans. There is evidence to indicate that the extension of the life span by caloric restriction in rodents is associated with a hypometabolic state, analogous to the effect of the "clock"

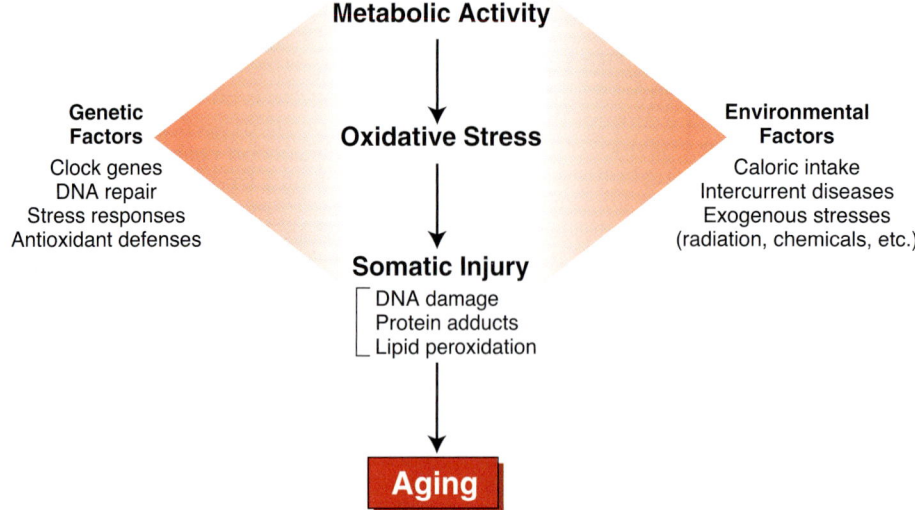

FIGURE 1-41
Factors that influence the development of biological aging.

mutations in *C. elegans*. Animals subjected to caloric restriction show attenuation of age-related increases in the rates of mitochondrial generation of reactive oxygen species, slower accrual of oxidative damage, and decreased evidence of lipid peroxidation and oxidative alterations of proteins.

Summary Hypothesis of Aging

After the reproductive period, evolution loses interest in an individual and abandons the organism to events against which nature confers no protection. As reviewed above, the doctrine of antagonistic pleiotropy posits the existence of genes that are beneficial during development and the reproductive period but exert baleful influences later in life. The alternative hypothesis of mutation accumulation holds that the evolutionary suppression of genes that are harmful to young individuals of a species creates pressure favoring alleles that defer the attainment of a deleterious phenotype until the postreproductive period. Finally, the major nongenetic theories postulate that simple accumulation of various cell injuries eventuates in senescence. Current evidence supports the notion that these hypotheses are not mutually contradictory and that all may contribute to aging (Fig. 1-41). According to this concept, although aging is under some measure of genetic control, **it is unlikely that a predetermined genetic program for aging exists.** It is likely that the combined effects of a number of genes eventually lead to the accumulation of somatic mutations, deficiencies in DNA repair, the accretion of oxidative damage to macromolecules, and a variety of other defects in cell function, all culminating in the progressive failure of homeostatic mechanisms characteristic of aging. As Maimonides said, "The same forces that operate in the birth and temporal existence of man also operate in his destruction and death."

SUGGESTED READING

Baldwin KM, Haddad F: Skeletal muscle plasticity: cellular and molecular responses to altered physical activity paradigms. *American Journal of Physical Medicine & Rehabilitation.* 81:S40–51, 2002.

Bohr VA: Repair of oxidative DNA damage in nuclear and mitochondrial DNA, and some changes with aging in mammalian cells. *Free Radical Biology & Medicine.* 32:804–12, 2002.

Copin MC, Buisine MP, Devisme L, Leroy X, Escande F, Gosselin B, Aubert JP, Porchet N: Normal respiratory mucosa, precursor lesions and lung carcinomas: differential expression of human mucin genes. *Frontiers in Bioscience.* 6:D1264–75, 2001.

Faragher RG: Cell senescence and human aging: where's the link? *Biochemical Society Transactions.* 28:221–6, 2000.

Granger MP, Wright WE, Shay JW: Telomerase in cancer and aging. *Critical Reviews in Oncology-Hematology.* 41:29–40, 2002.

Greider CW: Cellular responses to telomere shortening: cellular senescence as a tumor suppressor mechanism. *Harvey Lectures.* 96:33–50, 2000–2001.

Harkema JR, Wagner JG: Non-allergic models of mucous cell metaplasia and mucus hypersecretion in rat nasal and pulmonary airways. *Novartis Foundation Symposium.* 248:181–97, 2002.

Henry CJ: Mechanisms of changes in basal metabolism during ageing. *European Journal of Clinical Nutrition.* 54 Suppl 3:S77–91, 2000.

Higami Y, Shimokawa I: Apoptosis in the aging process. *Cell & Tissue Research.* 301:125–32, 2000.

Hodes RJ. Hathcock KS. Weng NP. Telomeres in T and B cells. Nature Reviews. *Immunology.* 2:699–706, 2002.

Holleyman CR. Larson DF. Apoptosis in the ischemic reperfused myocardium. *Perfusion.* 16:491–502, 2001.

Hursting SD, Lavigne JA, Berrigan D, Perkins SN, Barrett JC: Calorie restriction, aging, and cancer prevention: mechanisms of action and applicability to humans. *Annual Review of Medicine.* 54:131–52, 2003.

Jaeschke H: Molecular mechanisms of hepatic ischemia-reperfusion injury and preconditioning. *American Journal of Physiology—Gastrointestinal & Liver Physiology.* 284:G15–26, 2003.

Jaeschke H, Knight TR, Bajt ML: The role of oxidant stress and reactive nitrogen species in acetaminophen hepatotoxicity. *Toxicology Letters.* 144:279–88, 2003.

Jassem W, Fuggle SV, Rela M, Koo DD, Heaton ND: The role of mitochondria in ischemia/reperfusion injury. *Transplantation.* 73:493–9, 2002.

Jenkins GJ, Doak SH, Parry JM, D'Souza FR, Griffiths AP, Baxter JN: Genetic pathways involved in the progression of Barrett's metaplasia to adenocarcinoma. *British Journal of Surgery.* 89:824–37, 2002.

Kaminski KA, Bonda TA, Korecki J, Musial WJ: Oxidative stress and neutrophil activation—the two keystones of ischemia/reperfusion injury. *International Journal of Cardiology.* 86:41–59, 2002.

Kolesnick R, Fuks Z: Radiation and ceramide-induced apoptosis. *Oncogene.* 22:5897–906, 2003.

Kowald A: The mitochondrial theory of aging. *Biological Signals & Receptors.* 10:162–75, 2001.

Lalu MM, Wang W, Schulz R: Peroxynitrite in myocardial ischemia-reperfusion injury. *Heart Failure Reviews.* 7:359–69, 2002.

Lawen A: Apoptosis—an introduction. *Bioessays.* 25:888–96, 2003.

Li C, Jackson RM: Reactive species mechanisms of cellular hypoxia-reoxygenation injury. *American Journal of Physiology—Cell Physiology.* 282:C227–41, 2002.

Liaudet L, Szabo G, Szabo C: Oxidative stress and regional ischemia-reperfusion injury: the peroxynitrite-poly-(ADP-ribose) polymerase connection. *Coronary Artery Disease.* 14:115–22, 2003.

McBride WH, Iwamoto KS, Syljuasen R, Pervan M, Pajonk F: The role of the ubiquitin/proteasome system in cellular responses to radiation. *Oncogene.* 22:5755–73, 2003.

Mentzer RM Jr., Lasley RD, Jessel A. Karmazyn M: Intracellular sodium hydrogen exchange inhibition and clinical myocardial protection. *Annals of Thoracic Surgery.* 75:S700–8, 2003.

Murphy E, Cross HR, Steenbergen C: Is Na/Ca exchange during ischemia and reperfusion beneficial or detrimental?. *Annals of the New York Academy of Sciences.* 976:421–30, 2002.

Nieminen AL: Apoptosis and necrosis in health and disease: role of mitochondria. *International Review of Cytology.* 224:29–55, 2003.

Ostler EL, Wallis CV, Sheerin AN, Faragher RG: A model for the phenotypic presentation of Werner's syndrome. *Experimental Gerontology.* 37:285–92, 2002.

Piper HM, Meuter K, Schafer C: Cellular mechanisms of ischemia-reperfusion injury. *Annals of Thoracic Surgery.* 75:S644–8, 2003.

Rensing L, Meyer-Grahle U, Ruoff P: Biological timing and the clock metaphor: oscillatory and hourglass mechanisms. *Chronobiology International.* 18:329–69, 2001.

Ryazanov AG, Nefsky BS: Protein turnover plays a key role in aging: *Mechanisms of Ageing & Development.* 123:207–13, 2002.

Sack MN, Yellon DM: Insulin therapy as an adjunct to reperfusion after acute coronary ischemia: a proposed direct myocardial cell survival effect independent of metabolic modulation. *Journal of the American College of Cardiology.* 41:1404–7, 2003.

Salvemini D, Cuzzocrea S: Superoxide, superoxide dismutase and ischemic injury. *Current Opinion in Investigational Drugs.* 3:886–95, 2002.

Saretzki G, Von Zglinicki T: Replicative aging, telomeres, and oxidative stress. *Annals of the New York Academy of Sciences.* 959:24–9, 2002.

Sax JK, El-Deiry WS: p53 downstream targets and chemosensitivity. *Cell Death & Differentiation.* 10:413–7, 2003.

Schmidt-Ullrich RK, Dent P, Grant S, Mikkelsen RB, Valerie K: Signal transduction and cellular radiation responses. *Radiation Research.* 153:245–57, 2000.

Schultz DR, Harrington WJ Jr.: Apoptosis: programmed cell death at a molecular level. *Seminars in Arthritis & Rheumatism.* 32:345–69, 2003.

Shearer MJ: Role of vitamin K and Gla proteins in the pathophysiology of osteoporosis and vascular calcification. *Current Opinion in Clinical Nutrition & Metabolic Care.* 3:433–8, 2000.

Sohal RS: Role of oxidative stress and protein oxidation in the aging process. *Free Radical Biology & Medicine.* 33:37–44, 2002.

Squier TC: Oxidative stress and protein aggregation during biological aging. *Experimental Gerontology.* 36:1539–50, 2001.

Steensma DP, Timm M, Witzig TE: Flow cytometric methods for detection and quantification of apoptosis. *Methods in Molecular Medicine.* 85:323–32, 2003.

Tatar M, Bartke A, Antebi A: The endocrine regulation of aging by insulin-like signals. *Science.* 299:1346–51, 2003.

Thompson LH, Schild D: Recombinational DNA repair and human disease. *Mutation Research.* 509:49–78, 2002.

Walter L, Miyoshi H, Leverve X, Bernard P, Fontaine E: Regulation of the mitochondrial permeability transition pore by ubiquinone analogs. A progress report. *Free Radical Research.* 36:405–12, 2002.

Wymann MP, Zvelebil M. Laffargue M. Phosphoinositide 3-kinase signalling—which way to target? *Trends in Pharmacological Sciences.* 24:366–76, 2003.

Yoshida H: The role of Apaf-1 in programmed cell death: from worm to tumor. *Cell Structure & Function.* 28:3–9, 2003.

Yu BP, Lim BO, Sugano M: Dietary restriction downregulates free radical and lipid peroxide production: plausible mechanism for elongation of life span. *Journal of Nutritional Science & Vitaminology.* 48:257–64, 2002.

Yuasa Y: DNA methylation in cancer and ageing. *Mechanisms of Ageing & Development.* 123:1649–54, 2002.

CHAPTER 2

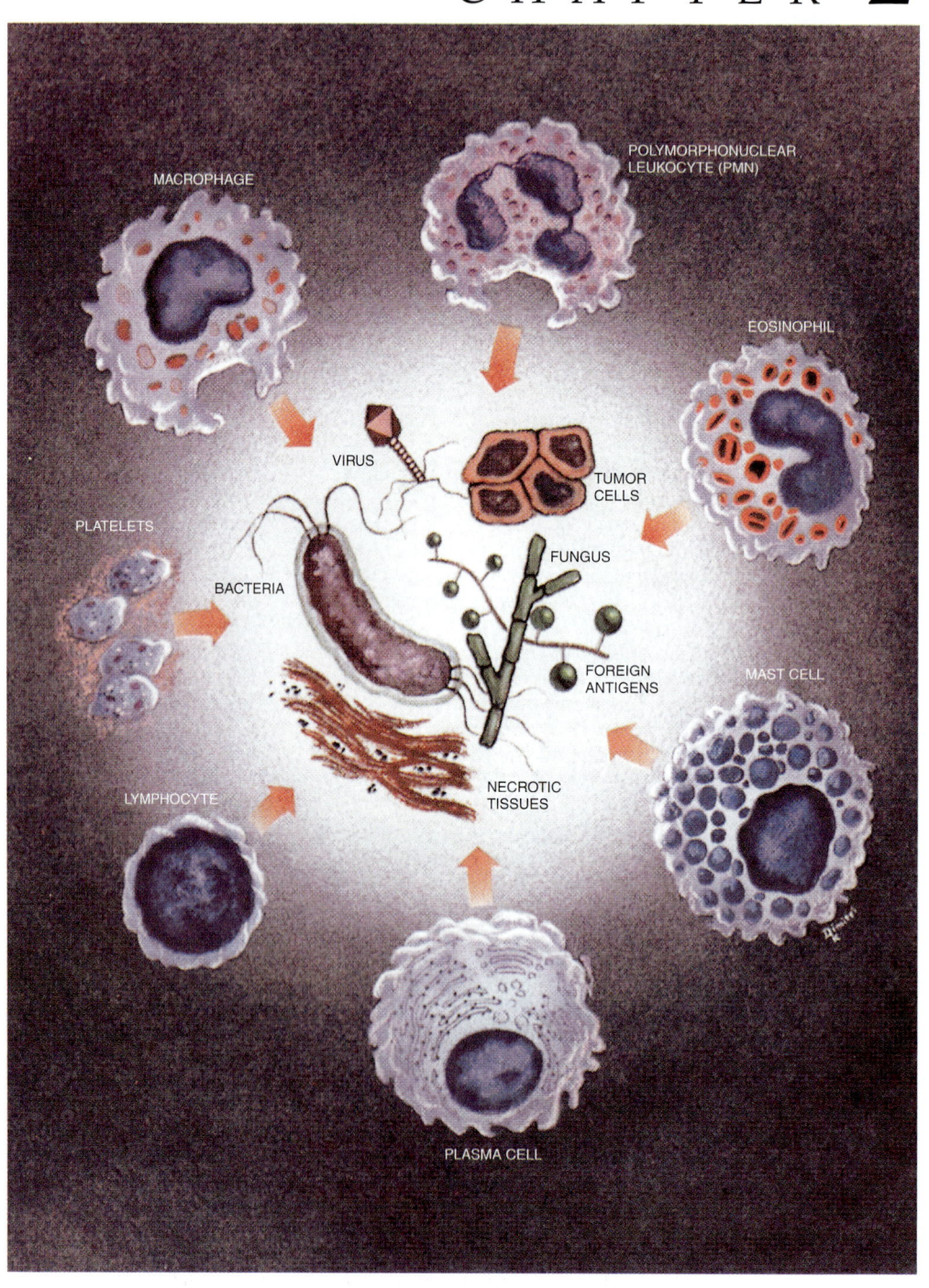

Inflammation

Hedwig S. Murphy
Peter A. Ward

General Considerations

Vascular Events
Vascular and Tissue Fluids

Plasma-Derived Mediators of Inflammation
Hageman Factor
Kinins
Complement

Cell-Derived Mediators of Inflammation
Arachidonic Acid and Platelet-Activating Factor
Prostanoids, Leukotrienes, and Lipoxins
Cytokines
Reactive Oxygen Species
Stress Proteins
Neurokinins

Extracellular Matrix Mediators
Interaction of Cells with the Extracellular Matrix

Cells of Inflammation
Inflammatory Cells and Resident Tissue Cells
Common Intracellular Pathways

Leukocyte Recruitment in Acute Inflammation
Leukocyte Adhesion
Chemotactic Molecules

Leukocyte Functions in Acute Inflammation
Phagocytosis
Neutrophil Enzymes
Oxidative and Nonoxidative Bactericidal Activity

Regulation of Inflammation

Outcomes of Acute Inflammation

Chronic Inflammation

Cells Involved in Chronic Inflammation

Injury and Repair in Chronic Inflammation
Extended Inflammatory Response
Altered Repair Mechanisms

Granulomatous Inflammation

Chronic Inflammation and Malignancy

Systemic Manifestations of Inflammation

FIGURE 2-1 *(see opposite page)*
Participants in acute and chronic inflammatory reactions.

Inflammation is the reaction of a tissue and its microcirculation to a pathogenic insult. It is characterized by the generation of inflammatory mediators and movement of fluid and leukocytes from the blood into extravascular tissues. By this mechanism the host localizes and eliminates metabolically altered cells, foreign particles, microorganisms, or antigens.

The clinical signs of inflammation, termed *phlogosis* by the Greeks and *inflammatio* in Latin, were described in classical times. In the second century AD, the Roman encyclopedist Aulus Celsus described the four cardinal signs of inflammation, namely, **rubor** (redness), **calor** (heat), **tumor** (swelling), and **dolor** (pain). According to medieval concepts, inflammation represented an imbalance of various "humors," including blood, mucus, and bile. The modern understanding of the vascular basis of inflammation began in the 18th century with the observations of John Hunter, who noted dilation of blood vessels and appreciated that pus represented an accumulation of material derived from the blood. That inflammation is usually a reaction to prior tissue injury was described by Rudolf Virchow, whose pupil Julius Cohnheim was the first to associate inflammation with the emigration of leukocytes through the walls of the microvasculature. At the turn of the 19th century, the role of phagocytosis in the inflammatory process was emphasized by the great Russian zoologist Eli Metchnikoff. Finally, the importance of chemical mediators in the inflammatory response was described in 1927 by Thomas Lewis, who demonstrated that histamine and other substances produced an increase in vascular permeability and elicited the migration of leukocytes into the extravascular spaces.

GENERAL CONSIDERATIONS

The primary function of the inflammatory response is the elimination of the pathogenic insult and the removal of injured tissue components. This process of **acute inflammation** accomplishes either regeneration of the normal tissue architecture, with return of physiological function, or the formation of scar tissue to replace what cannot be repaired. Inflammation proceeds as follows:

1. **Initiation** of the mechanisms responsible for the localization and clearance of foreign substances and injured tissues is stimulated by the recognition that injury to tissues has occurred.
2. **Amplification** of the inflammatory response, in which both soluble mediators and cellular inflammatory systems are activated, follows recognition of injury.
3. **Termination** of the inflammatory response, after generation of inflammatory agents and elimination of the foreign agent, is accomplished by specific inhibitors of the mediators.

Under certain conditions, the ability to clear injured tissue and foreign agents is impaired or the regulatory mechanisms of the inflammatory response are altered. In these circumstances, inflammation is harmful to the host and produces excessive tissue destruction and injury, leading to loss of function of the organ or tissue. In other instances, an immune response to residual microbial products or to altered tissue components also triggers a persistent inflammatory reaction, called **chronic inflammation.**

Initiation of the inflammatory response begins as the result of direct injury or stimulation of the cellular or structural components of a tissue, including the following:

- Parenchymal cells
- Microvasculature
- Tissue macrophages and mast cells
- Mesenchymal cells (e.g., fibroblasts)
- Extracellular matrix (ECM)

One of the earliest responses following tissue injury occurs within the microvasculature at the level of the capillary and postcapillary venule. Within this vascular network are the major components of the inflammatory response, including plasma, platelets, erythrocytes, and circulating leukocytes (Figs. 2-1 and 2-2). These components are normally confined to the intravascular compartment by a continuous layer of endothelial cells, which are connected to each other by tight junctions and separated from the tissue by a limiting basement membrane. Following injury to a tissue, changes in the structure of the vascular wall lead to the following:

- Activation of endothelial cells
- Loss of vascular integrity
- Leakage of fluid and plasma components from the intravascular compartment
- Emigration of erythrocytes and leukocytes from the vascular space into the extravascular tissue

Specific inflammatory mediators produced at the sites of injury regulate this response of the vasculature to injury (Fig. 2-3). Among these mediators are vasoactive molecules that act directly on the vasculature to increase vascular permeability. In addition, chemotactic factors are generated and recruit leukocytes from the vascular compartment into the injured tissue. Once present in tissues, these cells secrete additional inflammatory mediators, which either enhance or inhibit the inflammatory response.

Historically, inflammation has been referred to as either acute or chronic, depending on the persistence of the injury, clinical symptoms, and the nature of the inflammatory response. The hallmarks of acute inflammation include (1) accumulation of fluid and plasma components in the affected tissue, (2) intravascular stimulation of platelets, and (3) the

General Considerations

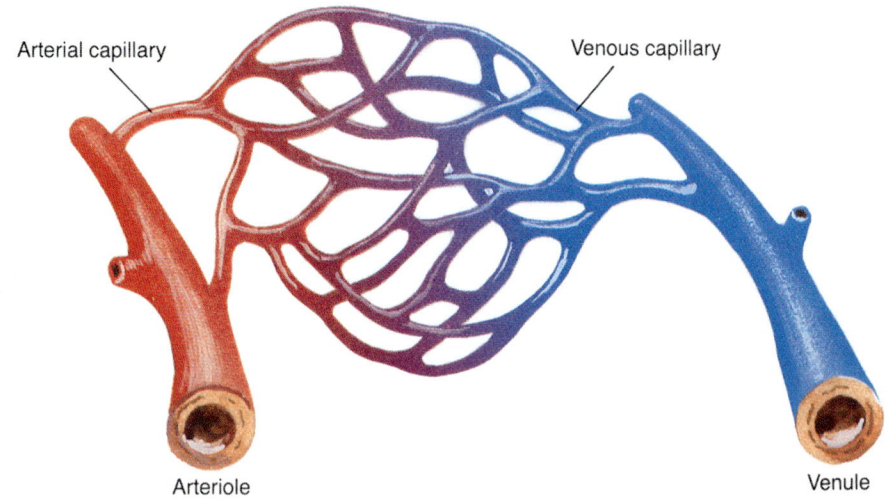

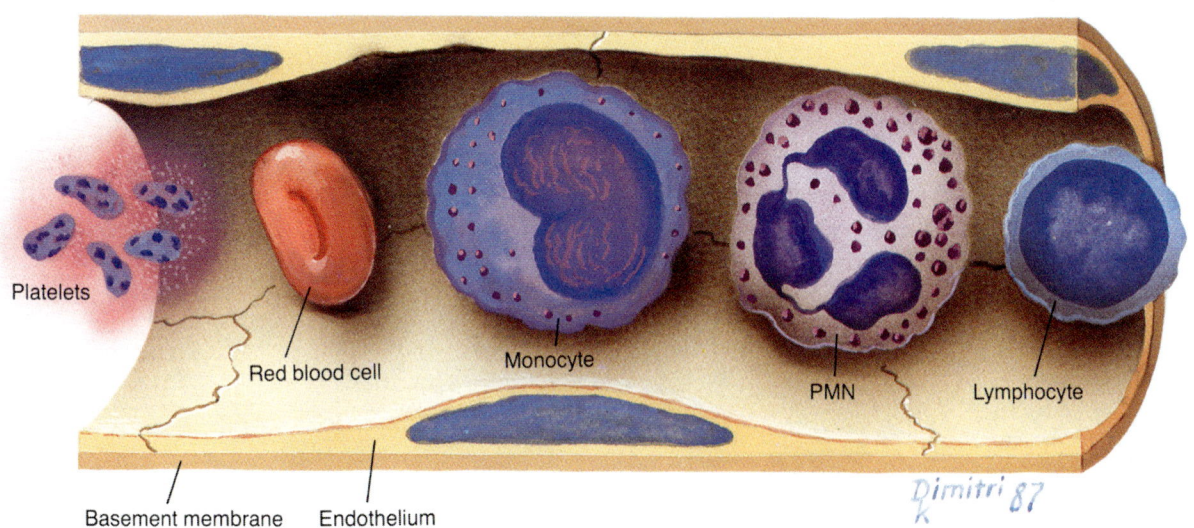

FIGURE 2-2
The microcirculation and cellular components of the blood.

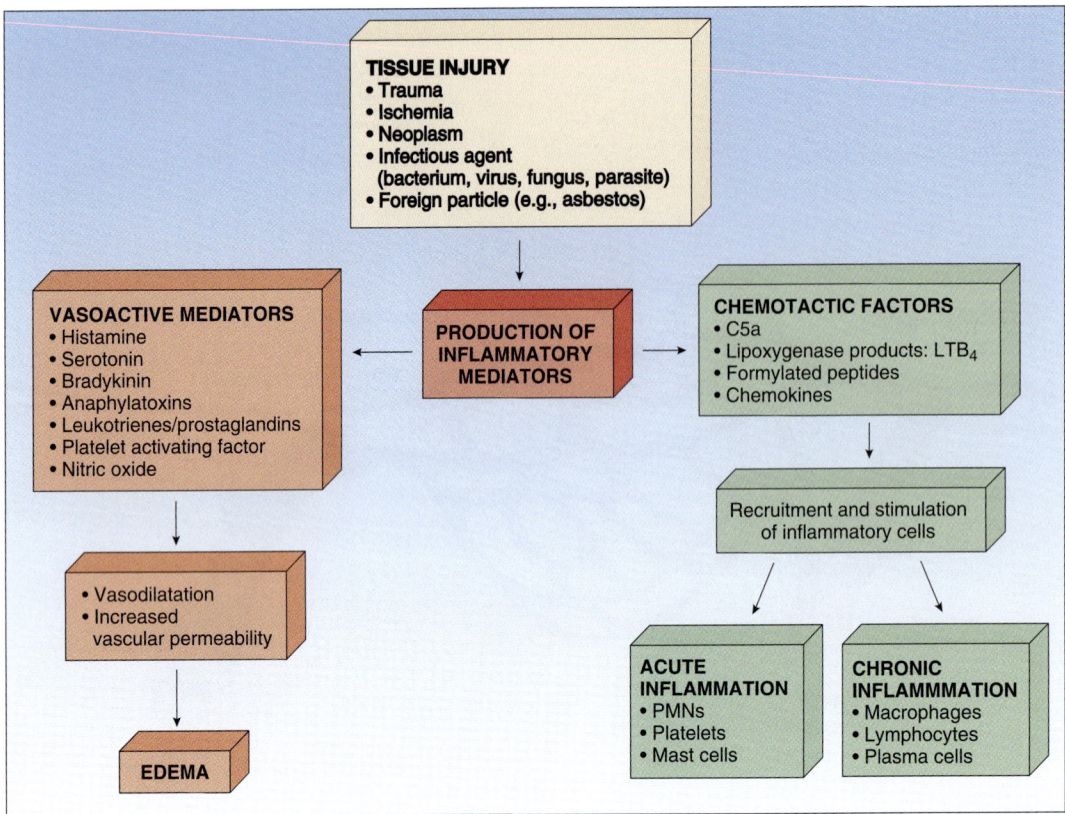

FIGURE 2-3
Mediators of the inflammatory response.

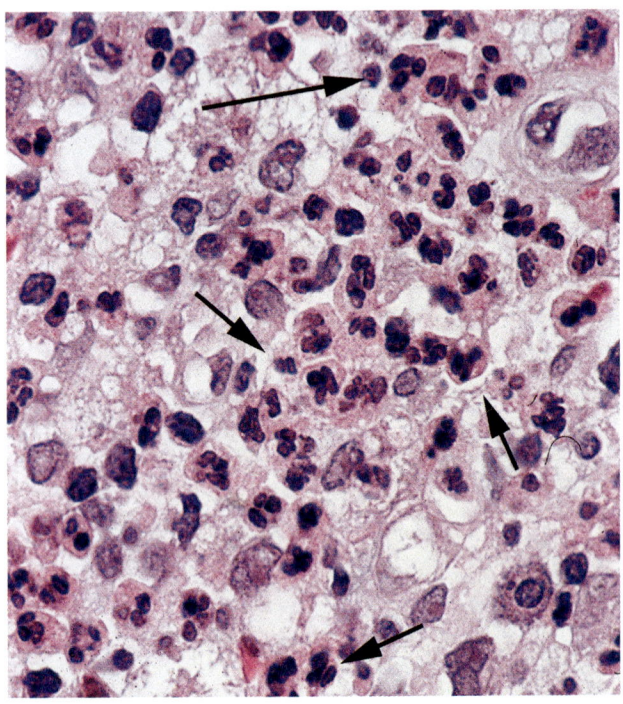

FIGURE 2-4
Acute inflammation with densely packed PMNs with multi-lobed nuclei (*arrows*).

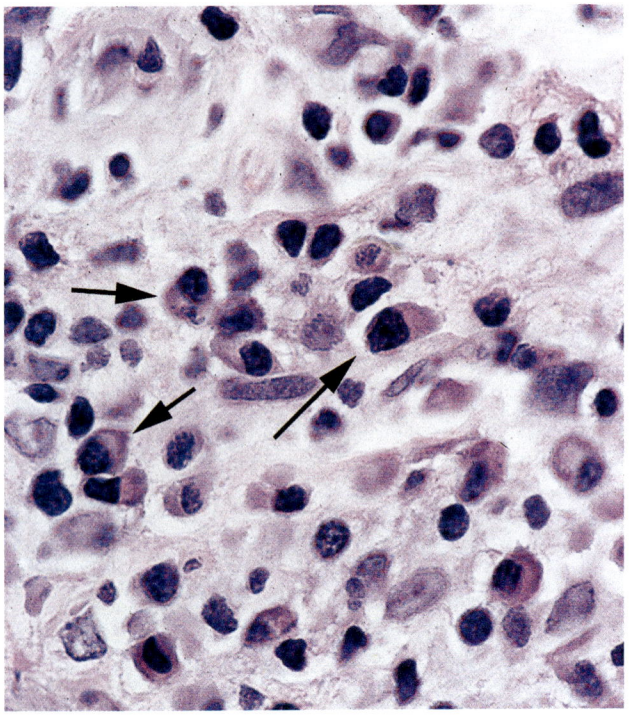

FIGURE 2-5
Chronic inflammation. Lymphocytes, plasma cells (*arrows*), and a few macrophages are present.

presence of polymorphonuclear leukocytes (polymorphonuclear neutrophils, PMNs) (Fig. 2-4). By contrast, the characteristic cell components of chronic inflammation are lymphocytes, plasma cells, and macrophages (Fig. 2-5). The chronic inflammatory response is prolonged, with persistence of inflammatory cells and tissue damage often resulting in aberrant repair.

VASCULAR EVENTS

Fluid exchange occurs normally between intravascular and extravascular spaces, with the endothelium functioning as a permeability barrier. Impairment of this barrier function is a hallmark of acute inflammation. Alterations in vascular permeability may occur transiently in response to chemical mediators, such as histamine and bradykinin. Mechanisms of vascular leakage include endothelial cell contraction, endothelial cell retraction, and alterations in transcytosis. When the endothelial barrier suffers damage, either directly by endothelial injury or indirectly by leukocyte-mediated damage, the loss of the permeability barrier may be extensive and result in edema.

Vascular and Tissue Fluids Are Regulated by a Balance of Forces

Under normal circumstances, there is continual movement of fluid from the intravascular compartment to the extravascular space. Fluid that accumulates in the extravascular space is normally cleared through lymphatics and returned to the circulation. The regulation of the transport of fluid across the vascular wall is described, in part, by the **Starling principle**. According to this law, the interchange of fluid between vascular and extravascular compartments results from a balance of forces that draw fluid into the vascular space or out into tissues (see also Chapter 7). These forces include

- **Hydrostatic pressure** results from blood flow and forces fluid out of the vasculature.
- **Oncotic pressure** reflects the plasma protein concentration, which draws fluid into vessels.
- **Osmotic pressure** is determined by the amounts of sodium and water in vascular and tissue spaces.
- **Lymph flow** (i.e., the passage of fluid through the lymphatic system) continuously drains fluid out of tissues and into lymphatic spaces.

Noninflammatory Edema

When the balance of forces that regulate vascular transport of fluid is altered, flow into the extravascular compartment or clearance through lymphatics is disrupted. The net result is fluid accumulation in the interstitial spaces, termed *edema*. This excess fluid expands the spaces between cells and ECM elements and leads to tissue swelling. A range of clinical conditions, either systemic or organ specific, are associated with edema. Obstruction of venous outflow (thrombosis) or decreased right ventricular function (congestive heart failure) result in a back pressure in the vasculature, thereby increasing hydrostatic pressure. Loss of albumin (kidney disorders) or decreased synthesis of plasma proteins (liver disease, malnutrition) reduce plasma oncotic pressure. Any abnormality of sodium or water retention will alter the osmotic pressure and the balance of fluid forces. Finally, obstruction of lymphatic flow may occur in a number of clinical settings but is most common because of surgical removal of lymph nodes or tumor obstruction. This fluid accumulation is referred to as **lymphedema** (see Chapter 7).

Inflammatory Edema

Among the earliest responses to tissue injury are alterations in the anatomy and function of the microvasculature, which may promote fluid accumulation in tissues (Figs. 2-6 and 2-7). These pathological changes are characteristic of the classic "triple response" first described by Sir Thomas Lewis. In the original experiments, a dull *red line* developed at the site of mild trauma to skin, followed by the development of a *flare* (red halo) and then a *wheal* (swelling). Lewis postulated the presence of a vasoactive mediator that caused vasodilation and increased vascular permeability at the site of injury. The triple response can be explained as follows:

1. **Transient vasoconstriction of arterioles** at the site of injury is the earliest vascular response to mild injury of the skin. This process is mediated by both neurogenic and chemical mediator systems and usually resolves within seconds to minutes.
2. **Vasodilation of precapillary arterioles** then increases blood flow to the tissue, a condition known as *hyperemia*. Vasodilation is caused by the release of specific mediators and is responsible for the redness and warmth at sites of tissue injury.
3. **An increase in the permeability of the endothelial cell barrier** results in *edema*. The loss of fluid from the intravascular compartments as blood passes through the capillary venules leads to local stasis and plugging of dilated small vessels with erythrocytes. These changes are reversible following mild injury, and within several minutes to hours, the extravascular fluid is cleared through lymphatics.

Injury to the vasculature is a dynamic event and frequently involves sequential physiological and pathological changes. **Vasoactive mediators,** originating from both plasma and cellular sources, are generated at sites of tissue injury by a variety of mechanisms. These mediators bind to specific receptors on vascular endothelial and smooth muscle cells, causing vasoconstriction or vasodilation. Vasodilation of arterioles increases blood flow and can exacerbate fluid leakage into the tissue. At the same time, vasoconstriction of postcapillary venules increases the hydrostatic pressure in the capillary bed, potentiating the formation of edema. Vasodilation of venules decreases capillary hydrostatic pressure and inhibits the movement of fluid into the extravascular spaces.

Although the postcapillary venule is the primary site at which vasoactive mediators induce endothelial changes, these molecules affect precapillary vessels as well. Binding of vasoactive mediators to specific receptors on endothelial cells results in their activation, causing endothelial cell reversible contraction and gap formation (Fig. 2-6B). This break in the endothelial barrier leads to the extravasation (leakage) of intravascular fluids into the extravascular space. In contrast to this action of vasoactive mediators, direct injury to the endothelium, such as that caused by burns or caustic chemicals, may result in irreversible damage. In such cases, the endothelium is separated from the basement membrane. This effect leads to cell blebbing (the appearance of blisters or bubbles between the endothelium and the basement membrane) and areas of denuded basement membrane

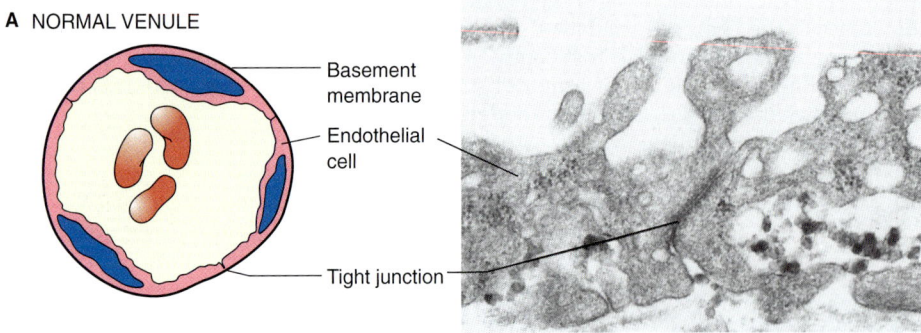
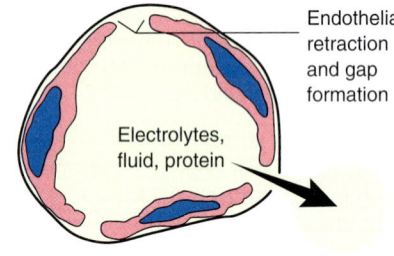 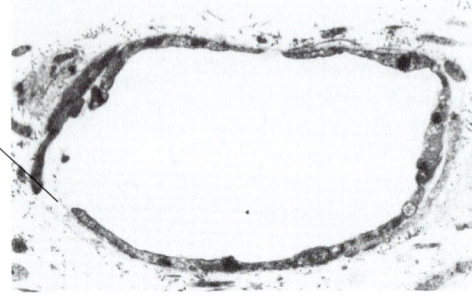 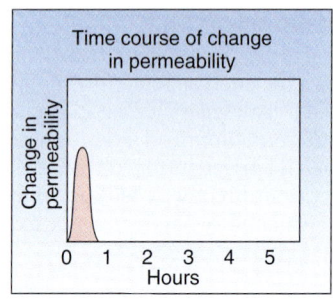
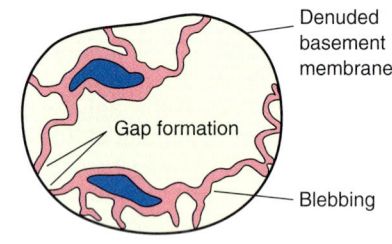 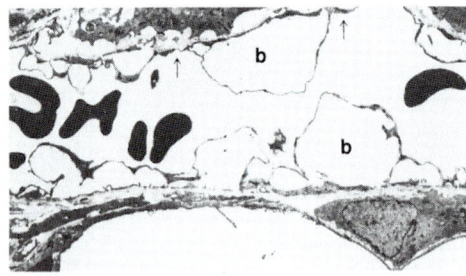 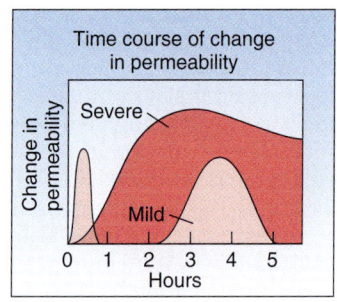

FIGURE 2-6
Responses of the microvasculature to injury. A. The wall of the normal venule is sealed by tight junctions between adjacent endothelial cells. B. During mild vasoactive mediator-induced injury, the endothelial cells separate and permit the passage of the fluid constituents of the blood. C. With severe direct injury, the endothelial cells form blebs (b) and separate from the underlying basement membrane. Areas of denuded basement membrane (arrows) allow a prolonged escape of fluid elements from the microvasculature.

(Fig. 2-6C). Mild direct injury to the endothelium results in a biphasic response: an early change in permeability occurs within 30 minutes after the injury, followed by a second increase in vascular permeability after 3 to 5 hours. When damage is severe, the exudation of intravascular fluid into the extravascular compartment increases progressively, reaching a peak between 3 and 4 hours after injury.

Several definitions are important for understanding the consequences of inflammation:

- **Edema** is the accumulation of fluid within the extravascular compartment and interstitial tissues.
- An **effusion** is excess fluid in the cavities of the body, for instance the peritoneum or pleura.
- A **transudate** is edema fluid with a low protein content (specific gravity < 1.015).
- An **exudate** is edema fluid with a high protein concentration (specific gravity > 1.015), which frequently contains inflammatory cells. Exudates are observed early in acute inflammatory reactions and are produced by mild injuries, such as sunburn or traumatic blisters.
- A **serous exudate,** or **effusion,** is characterized by the absence of a prominent cellular response and has a yellow, strawlike color.
- **Serosanguinous** refers to a serous exudate, or effusion, that contains red blood cells and has a red tinge.
- A **fibrinous exudate** contains large amounts of fibrin as a result of activation of the coagulation system. When a fibrinous exudate occurs on a serosal surface, such as the pleura or pericardium, it is referred to as *fibrinous pleuritis* or *fibrinous pericarditis* (Fig. 2-8).
- A **purulent exudate or effusion** is one that contains prominent cellular components. Purulent exudates and effusions are frequently associated with pathological conditions such as pyogenic bacterial infections, in which the predominant cell type is the PMN (Fig. 2-9).

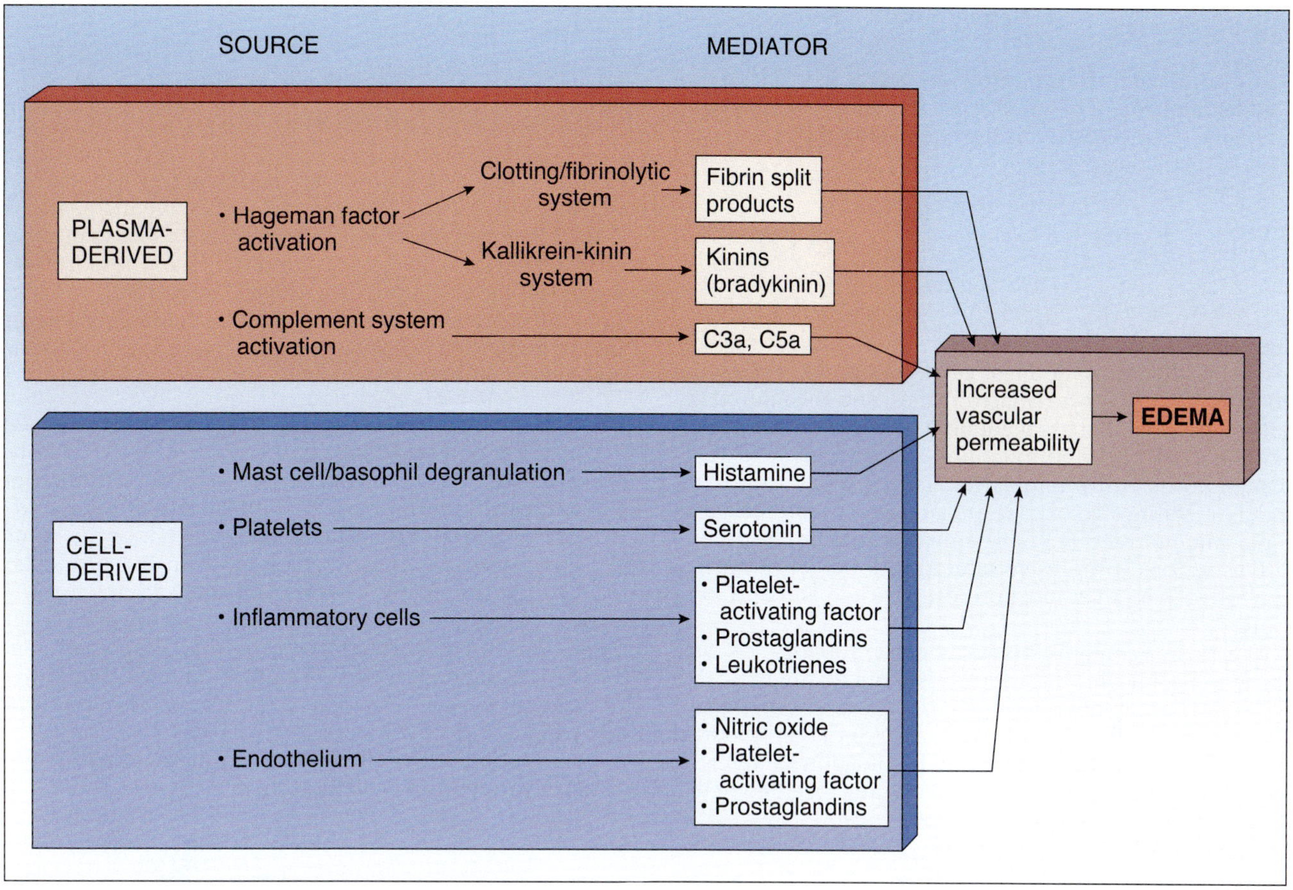

FIGURE 2-7
Vasoactive mediators of increased vascular permeability.

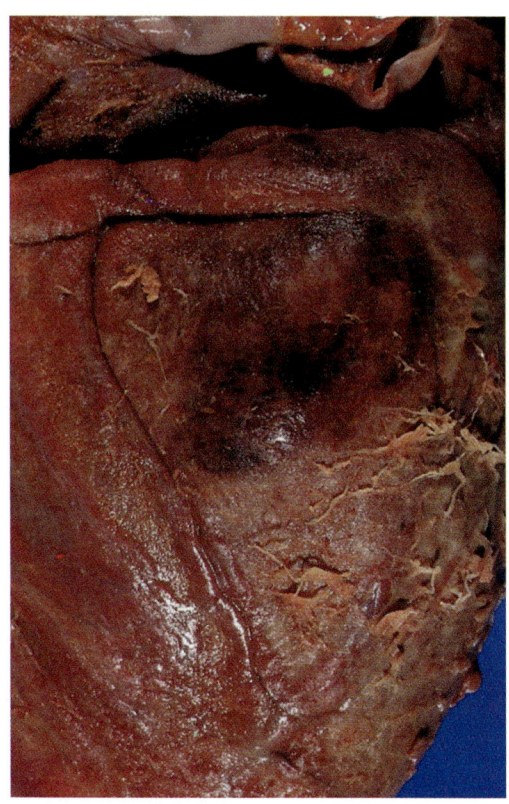

FIGURE 2-8
Fibrinous pericarditis. The heart from a patient who died in renal failure and uremia exhibits a shaggy, fibrinous exudate covering the entire visceral pericardium.

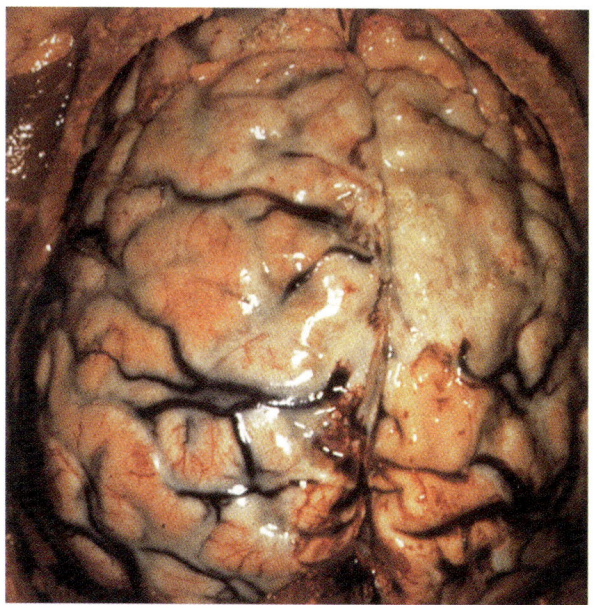

FIGURE 2-9
Purulent exudate. In this patient with bacterial meningitis, a viscid, cream-colored, acute inflammatory exudate is present within the subarachnoid space.

- **Suppurative inflammation** describes a condition in which a purulent exudate is accompanied by significant liquefactive necrosis; it is the equivalent of pus.

PLASMA-DERIVED MEDIATORS OF INFLAMMATION

Potent cellular sources of vasoactive mediators include circulating platelets, tissue mast cells, basophils, PMNs, endothelial cells, monocyte/macrophages, and the injured tissue itself. In general, these mediators (1) are derived from the metabolism of phospholipids and arachidonic acid (e.g., prostaglandins, thromboxanes, leukotrienes, lipoxins, platelet-activating factor), (2) are preformed and stored in cytoplasmic granules (e.g., histamine, serotonin, lysosomal hydrolases), or (3) represent altered production of normal regulators of vascular function (e.g., nitric oxide and neurokinins).

The plasma contains three major enzyme cascades, each of which is composed of a series of sequentially activated proteases. These interrelated systems include (1) the coagulation cascade, (2) kinin generation, and (3) the complement system. The coagulation cascade is discussed in Chapter 10, and the kinin and complement systems are presented here.

Hageman Factor is a Key Source of Vasoactive Mediators

Hageman factor (clotting factor XII), generated within the plasma, provides a key source of vasoactive mediators (Fig. 2-10). Hageman factor is activated by exposure to negatively charged surfaces, such as basement membranes, proteolytic enzymes, bacterial lipopolysaccharide, and foreign materials (including urate crystals in gout). In turn, this process results in the activation of several additional plasma proteases, which lead to the following:

- **Conversion of plasminogen to plasmin:** Plasmin generated by activated Hageman factor induces fibrinolysis. The products of fibrin degradation (fibrin-split products) augment vascular permeability in both the skin and the lung. Plasmin also cleaves components of the complement system, generating biologically active products, including the anaphylatoxins C3a and C5a.
- **Conversion of prekallikrein to kallikrein:** Plasma kallikrein, generated by activated Hageman factor, cleaves high-molecular-weight kininogen, thereby producing several vasoactive peptides of low molecular weight, collectively referred to as *kinins*.
- **Activation of the alternative complement pathway.**
- **Activation of the coagulation system** (see Chapter 10).

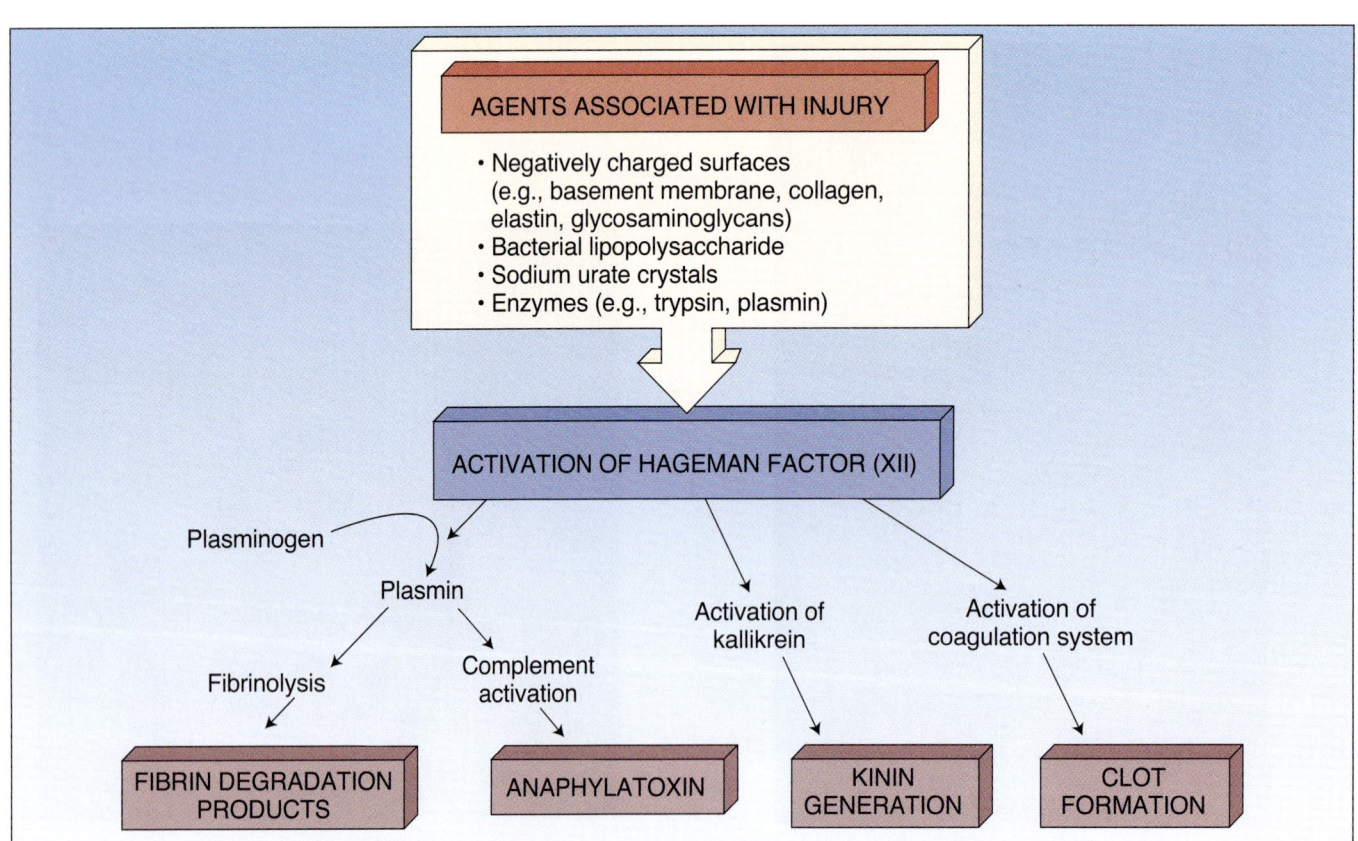

FIGURE 2-10
Hageman factor activation and inflammatory mediator production.

Kinins Amplify the Inflammatory Response

Kinins are formed in plasma and tissue by the action of serine protease kallikreins on the plasma glycoproteins, high-molecular-weight kininogens. These potent inflammatory agents, which include **bradykinin** and related peptides, function in multiple physiological processes including control of blood pressure, contraction and relaxation of smooth muscle, plasma extravasation, cell migration, inflammatory cell activation, and inflammatory mediated pain responses. The immediate effects of kinins are mediated by two receptors: B_1 receptors are induced by inflammatory mediators and are selectively activated by bradykinin metabolites, and B_2 receptors are constitutively and widely expressed. Kinins are rapidly degraded to inactive products by kininases and, therefore, have rapid and short-lived functions. Perhaps the most significant function of kinins is their ability to amplify the inflammatory response by stimulating local tissue cells and inflammatory cells to generate mediators, including prostanoids, cytokines (especially tumor necrosis factor-α [TNF-α] and interleukins), nitric oxide, and tachykinins.

Complement Is Activated through Three Pathways To Form The Membrane Attack Complex

The complement system consists of a group of proteins found in plasma and on cell surfaces, whose primary function is defense against microbes. Complement was first identified as a heat-labile serum factor that killed bacteria and "complemented" antibodies. The complement system is now known to consist of more than 30 proteins, including plasma enzymes, regulatory proteins, and cell lysis proteins, whose principal site of synthesis is the liver. In addition to being a source of vasoactive mediators, components of the complement system are an integral part of the immune system and play an important role in host defense against bacterial infection. The physiological activities of the complement system include (1) defense against pyogenic bacterial infection by opsonization, chemotaxis, activation of leukocytes, and lysis of bacteria and cells; (2) bridging innate and adaptive immunity for defense against microbial agents by augmenting antibody responses and enhancing immunological memory; and (3) disposal of immune products and the products of inflammatory injury by clearance of immune complexes from tissues and removal of apoptotic cells. Complement components also function as vasoactive mediators, termed *anaphylatoxins*. Specific components fix opsonins on cell surfaces and others induce cell lysis by generation of the lytic complex C5b-9 (membrane attack complex [MAC]). The proteins involved in activation of the complement system are themselves activated by three convergent pathways termed *classical, mannose-binding lectin (MBL) and alternative pathways*.

The Classical Pathway

Activators of the classical pathway include antigen-antibody (Ag-Ab) complexes and products of bacteria and viruses, proteases, urate crystals, apoptotic cells, and polyanions (polynucleotides). The proteins of this pathway are designated C1 through C9, and the nomenclature follows the historical order of discovery. The pathway begins when Ag-Ab complexes activate C1 and ends with lysis of the cell. The cascade that leads from complement activation to the formation of the MAC proceeds as follows (Fig. 2-11):

1. **Antibodies bound to antigens on the surface of the bacterial cell bind the C1 complex.** The C1 complex consists of C1q, two molecules of C1r, and two molecules of C1s. Antibodies within the immune complexes bind to C1q, thereby triggering the activation of C1r and C1s.
2. **C1s first cleaves C4, which binds to the bacterial surface and then cleaves C2.** The resulting cleaved molecules form the C4b2a enzyme complex, also called **C3 convertase,** which remains covalently bound to the bacterial surface. This anchors the complement system at specific tissue sites. If a covalent bond is not formed, the complex is inactivated, thereby preventing continuation of the complement cascade in normal host cells or tissues.
3. **C3 convertase cleaves C3 into C3a and C3b.** This is one of the most critical steps in the generation of biologically active complement components. C3a is released as an *anaphylatoxin*, and C3b reacts with cell proteins to localize, or "fix" on the cell surface. C3b and its degradation prod-

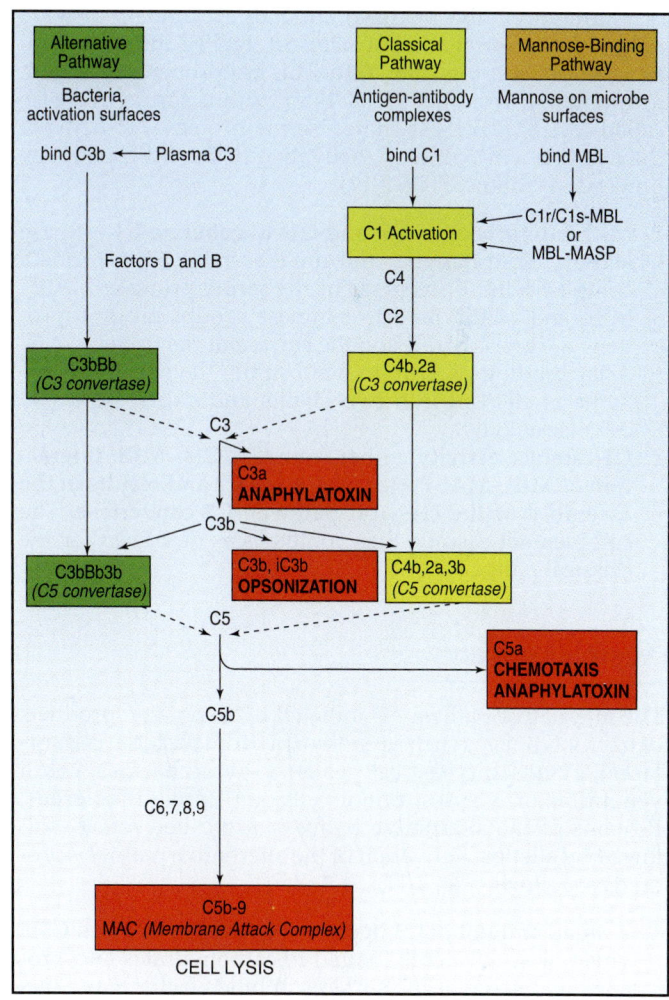

FIGURE 2-11
Complement activation: The alternative, classical and mannose-binding pathways lead to generation of the complement cascade of inflammatory mediators and cell lysis by the MAC.

ucts, especially iC3b, on the surface of pathogens enhance phagocytosis. This process of coating a pathogen with a molecule that enhances phagocytosis is termed *opsonization*, and the molecule is referred to as an *opsonin*.

4. **The complex of C4b, C2a, and C3b (termed C5 convertase) cleaves C5 into C5a and C5b.** C5a functions as an anaphylatoxin, and C5b serves as the nidus for the sequential binding of C6, C7, and C8 to form the MAC.
5. The MAC assembles on target cells, directly inserting into the plasma membrane by hydrophobic binding of C7 to the lipid bilayer. The resulting cylindrical transmembrane channel cripples the barrier function of the plasma membrane and leads to cell lysis.

The Mannose-Binding Pathway

The second complement pathway is the mannose- or lectin-binding pathway, which has some components in common with the classical pathway. This pathway is initiated by binding of microbes bearing terminal mannose groups to *mannose-binding lectin* (MBL), a member of the family of calcium-dependent lectins, termed the *collectins*. This multifunctional acute phase protein has properties similar to those of immunoglobulin M (IgM) antibody (it binds to a wide range of oligosaccharide structures), IgG (it interacts with phagocytic receptors), and C1q. This last property enables it to interact with either C1r-C1s or with a serine protease called MASP (MBL-associated serine protease) to activate the complement pathway. Activation of the MBL pathway proceeds as follows (Fig. 2-11):

1. **MBL interacts with C1r and C1s to generate C1 esterase activity.** Alternatively and preferentially, MBL forms a complex with a precursor of the serine protease MASP. MBL and MASP bind to mannose groups on glycoproteins or carbohydrates on the surface of the bacterial cell. After binding of MBL to a substrate, the MASP proenzyme is cleaved into two chains and expresses a C1-esterase activity.
2. **C1-esterase activity, either from C1r/C1s- MBL interaction or MBL-MASP, cleaves C4 and C2 and results in the assembly of the classical pathway C3 convertase.** The complement cascade then continues as described for the classical pathway.

Alternative Pathway

The alternative pathway is initiated by derivative products of microorganisms such as endotoxin (from bacterial cell surfaces), zymosan (yeast cell walls), polysaccharides, cobra venom factor, viruses, tumor cells, and foreign materials. Proteins of the alternative pathway are called *factors*, followed by a letter. Activation of the alternative pathway proceeds as follows (Fig. 2-11):

1. **A small amount of C3 in plasma cleaves to C3a and C3b.** This C3b is covalently bound to carbohydrates and proteins on microbial cell surfaces. It binds factor B and factor D to form the alternative pathway C3 convertase, C3bBb. This C3 convertase is stabilized by *properdin*.
2. **C3 convertase generates additional C3b and C3a.** The binding of a second C3b molecule to the C3 convertase converts it to a C5 convertase, C3bBb3b.
3. As in the classical pathway, cleavage of C5 by C5 convertase generates C5b and C5a and leads to assembly of the MAC.

The Complement System is Tightly Regulated to Generate Proinflammatory Molecules

Biological Activities of Complement Components

The endpoint of the complement cascade is formation of the MAC and cell lysis. The cleavage products generated at each step in the system not only catalyze the next step in the cascade, but in themselves have additional properties that render them important inflammatory molecules. The following complement components have biological activity (Fig. 2-12):

- **Anaphylatoxins** (C3a, C4a, C5a)
- **Opsonins** (C3b, iC3b)
- **Proinflammatory molecules** (MAC, C5a)

The anaphylatoxins C3a, C4a, and C5a enhance smooth muscle contraction and increase vascular permeability. Both C3a and C5a induce degranulation of mast cells and basophils, and the consequent release of histamine potentiates the increase in vascular permeability. Once the complement system is activated, bacteriolysis may follow, either by means of the assembled MAC or by enhanced bacterial clearance following opsonization. Bacterial *opsonization* is the process by which a specific molecule (e.g., IgG or C3b) binds to the surface of the bacterium. The process enhances phagocytosis by enabling receptors on the phagocytic cell membrane (e.g., the Fc receptor or the C3b receptor) to recognize and bind to the opsonized bacterium. Viruses, parasites, and transformed cells also activate the complement system by similar mechanisms, an effect that leads to their inactivation or death. Receptors for complement components, especially C3b and its degradation products, are crucial not only for bacterial phagocytosis but also for the clearance of soluble Ag-Ab immune complexes (see Chapter 4). Complement receptors on erythrocytes bind and "scavenge" circulating immune complexes that have bound C4b or C3b. In the spleen and liver, mononuclear phagocytic cells bind and degrade the erythrocyte-bound complexes, returning the cells to the circulation.

MAC and C5a activate leukocytes and tissue cells, and MAC activates phagocytic cells to generate oxidants and cytokines. C5a increases vascular permeability and is a potent chemotactic factor, specifically for neutrophils. MAC causes upregulation of the endothelial cell adhesion molecules, ICAM-1, VCAM-1, and E-selectin. MAC, as well as C5a, increases the expression of P-selectin.

Regulation of the Complement System

Proteins in the serum and on cell surfaces protect the host from indiscriminate injury by complement activation products. Deficiencies of several of these regulatory proteins are associated with specific clinical syndromes. Activation of the complement system is regulated primarily by four mechanisms:

- **Spontaneous decay:** The enzymatically active complexes (C4b2a and C3bBb) and their cleavage products

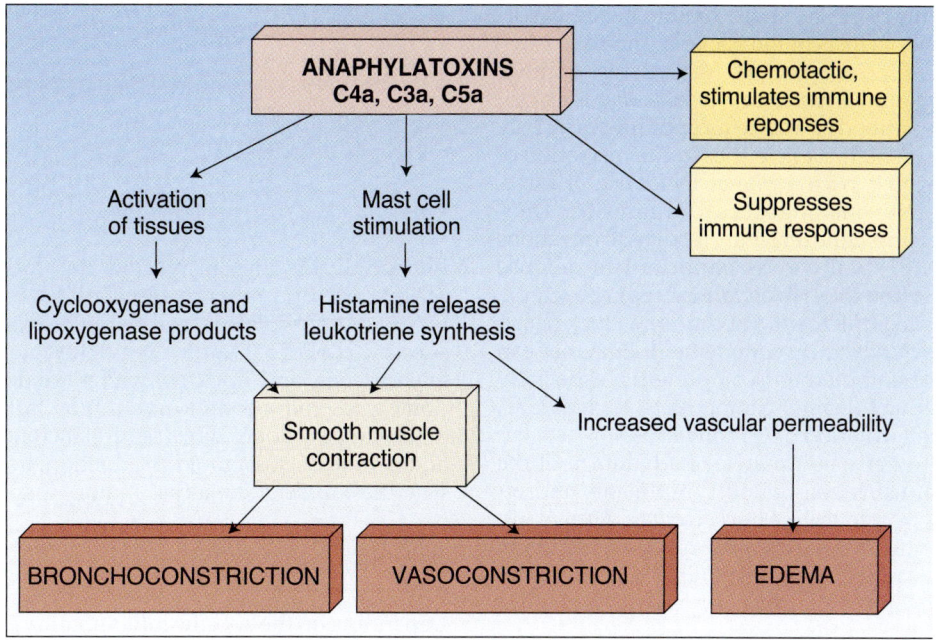

FIGURE 2-12
Biological activity of the anaphylatoxins.

(C3b and C4b) decay, resulting in a decrease in these active byproducts.
- **Proteolytic inactivation:** Specific components are inactivated by interaction with plasma inhibitors. These inhibitors include factor 1 (an inhibitor of C3b and C4b) and serum carboxypeptidase N (SCPN). SCPN cleaves the carboxy-terminal arginine from the anaphylatoxins C4a, C3a, and C5a. Removal of this single amino acid markedly decreases the biological activity of each of these molecules.
- **Binding of active components:** C1 esterase inhibitor (C1 INA) binds C1r and C1s, forming an irreversibly inactive complex. Additional binding proteins in the plasma include factor H and C4b binding protein. These proteins form complexes with C3b and C4b, respectively, and enhance their susceptibility to proteolytic cleavage by factor I.
- **Cell membrane-associated molecules:** Membrane molecules have potent regulatory effects on complement activation. Membrane cofactor protein (protectin, CD59) binds membrane-associated C4b and C3b and promotes its inactivation by factor I. Two proteins that are linked to the cell membrane by glycophosphoinositol (GPI) anchors are decay-accelerating factor (DAF), which breaks down the alternative pathway C3 convertase, and protectin (CD59), which prevents the formation of the MAC.

The Complement System and Disease

The complement system is exquisitely regulated so that activation of complement is focused on the surfaces of microorganisms, whereas deposition on normal cells and tissues is limited. When the mechanisms regulating this balance do not function properly, the complement system can cause tissue injury (Table 2-1).

Immune Complexes

Immune complexes (antigen–antibody complexes) form on bacterial surfaces and associate with the C1q component, thereby triggering activation of the classical pathway. Complement then promotes the physiological clearance of circulating immune complexes. However, when these complexes are formed continuously and in excess (e.g., in chronic immune responses), the relentless activation of complement results in its consumption and, therefore, depletion of complement. Complement inefficiency, whether due to complement depletion, deficient complement binding, or defects in complement activation, results in immune deposition and inflammation, which in turn may trigger autoimmunity.

Infectious Disease

Defense against infection is a key role of complement products, and defective functioning of the complement system leads to increased susceptibility to infection. C3b and iC3b,

TABLE 2-1 Hereditary Complement Deficiencies

Complement Deficiency	Clinical Association
C3b, iC3b, C5, MBL	Pyogenic bacterial infections
	Membranoproliferative glomerulonephritis
C3, properdin, MAC proteins	Neisserial infection
C1 Inhibitor	Hereditary angioedema
CD59	Hemolysis, thrombosis
C1q, C1r and C1s, C4, C2	Systemic lupus erythematosus
Factor H and Factor I	Hemolytic-uremic syndrome
	Membranoproliferative glomerulonephritis

the cleavage fragments of C3, normally bind to bacterial surfaces to promote phagocytosis of the bacteria. Increased susceptibility to pyogenic infection by organisms such as *Haemophilus influenzae* and *Streptococcus pneumoniae* is associated with defects in antibody production, complement proteins, or phagocyte function. Deficiencies in the formation of MAC are also associated with a higher incidence of infections, particularly with meningococcal organisms. Deficiency of MBL in young children with recurrent infections suggests that the MBL pathway is important in defense against bacterial infection in early childhood. Some bacteria, in addition, can resist complement. For example, thick bacterial capsules can prevent lysis by complement. Enzymes can inhibit the effects of complement components, especially C5a, or increase the catabolism of components, such as C3b, thereby reducing the formation of C3 convertase.

Viruses, on the other hand, may take advantage of the complement system, using cell bound components and receptors as an entryway into cells. *Mycobacterium tuberculosis*, Epstein-Barr virus, measles virus, picornaviruses, human immunodeficiency virus (HIV), and flaviviruses use complement components to target inflammatory or epithelial cells.

Inflammation and Necrosis

One of the main functions of the complement system is amplification of the inflammatory response. The anaphylatoxins C5a and C3a activate leukocytes, and C5a and MAC activate endothelial cells, inducing the generation of oxidants and cytokines that are harmful to tissues when in excess. Activation of complement may cause tissue necrosis, after which necrotic tissues are incapable of the normal regulation of complement.

Complement Deficiencies

The importance of an intact and appropriately regulated complement system is exemplified in persons who have deficiencies, either acquired or congenital, of either specific complement components or regulatory proteins (Table 2-1). The most common congenital defect is a C2 deficiency, which is inherited as an autosomal codominant trait, with a gene frequency of approximately 1%. Acquired deficiencies of early complement components occur in patients with some autoimmune diseases, especially those associated with circulating immune complexes. These include certain forms of membranous glomerulonephritis and systemic lupus erythematosus. Congenital deficiencies in the early component of the complement system, including C1q, C1r, C1s, and C4, are strongly associated with susceptibility to systemic lupus erythematosus. Patients with deficiencies of the middle (C3, C5) components have recurrent pyogenic infections, membranoproliferative glomerulonephritis, and rashes, whereas those who lack terminal complement components (C6, C7, or C8) are vulnerable to infections with *Neisseria* species. Such differences in susceptibility further emphasize the importance of individual components of the complement system in host surveillance against bacterial infection. Congenital defects have been reported in regulatory proteins of the complement system, including C1 inhibitor and SCPN. Deficiency of C1 inhibitor, with excessive cleavage of C4 and C2 by C1s, is associated with the syndrome of *hereditary angioedema*, characterized by episodic, painless, nonpitting edema of soft tissues. This disorder is the result of chronic complement activation, with the generation of a vasoactive peptide from C2, and may be life threatening because of the occurrence of laryngeal edema.

CELL-DERIVED MEDIATORS OF INFLAMMATION

Arachidonic Acid and Platelet-Activating Factor Are Derived from Membrane Phospholipids

Phospholipids and fatty acid derivatives released from plasma membranes are metabolized into mediators and homeostatic regulators by inflammatory cells and injured tissues. As part of a complex regulatory network, prostanoids, leukotrienes, and lipoxins, which are derivatives of arachidonic acid, both promote and inhibit inflammation (Table 2-2). The impact depends on several factors, including the level and profile of prostanoid production, both of which change over the course of the inflammatory response (Fig. 2-13).

Arachidonic Acid

Depending on the specific inflammatory cell and the nature of the stimulus, activated cells generate arachidonic acid by one of two pathways (Fig. 2-14). One pathway involves the liberation of arachidonic acid from the glycerol backbone of cell membrane phospholipids (in particular, phosphatidylcholine) by stimulus-induced activation of phospholipase A_2 (PLA_2). The other mechanism for the generation of arachidonic acid is the metabolism of phosphatidylinositol phosphates to diacylglycerol and inositol phosphates by phospholipase C. Diacylglycerol lipase then cleaves arachidonic acid from diacylglycerol. Once generated, arachidonic acid is further metabolized through two pathways: (1) *cyclooxygenation*, with the subsequent production of prostaglandins and thromboxanes, and (2) *lipoxygenation*, to form leukotrienes and lipoxins.

Corticosteroids are widely used to suppress the tissue destruction associated with many inflammatory diseases, including allergic responses, rheumatoid arthritis, and systemic lupus erythematosus. Corticosteroids induce the synthesis of an inhibitor of PLA_2 and block the release of arachidonic acid in inflammatory cells. Although corticosteroids (e.g., prednisone)

TABLE 2-2 **Biological Activities of Arachidonic Acid Metabolites**

Metabolite	Biological Activity
PGE_2, PDG_2	Induce vasodilation, bronchodilation; inhibit inflammatory cell function
PGI_2	Induces vasodilation, bronchodilation; inhibits inflammatory cell function
$PGF_{2\alpha}$	Induces vasodilation, bronchoconstriction
TxA_2	Induces vasoconstriction, bronchoconstriction; enhances inflammatory cell functions (esp. platelets
LTB_4	Chemotactic for phagocytic cells; stimulates phagocytic cell adherence; enhances microvascular permeability
LTC_4, LTD_4, LTE_4,	Induce smooth muscle contraction; constrict pulmonary airways; increase microvascular permeability

Cell-Derived Mediators of Inflammation

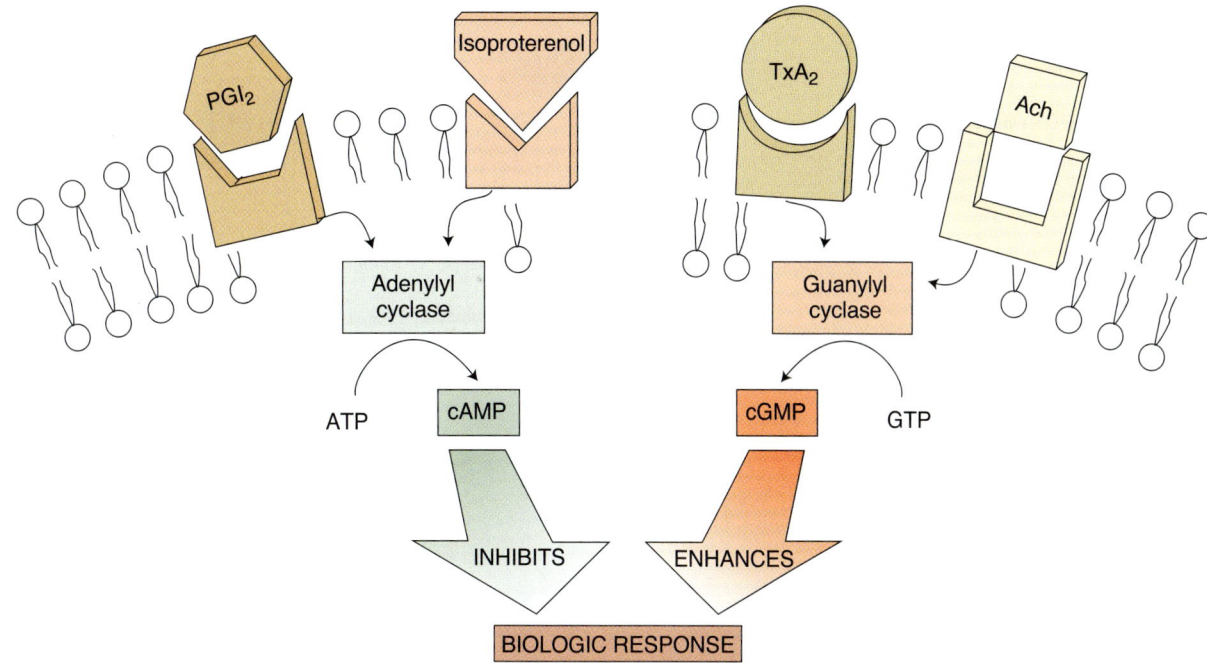

FIGURE 2-13
The biological response of inflammatory cells is modulated by activating and inhibitory cyclic nucleotides. *TxA*, thromboxane A_2; *Ach*, acetylcholine.

are widely used to suppress inflammatory responses, the prolonged administration of these compounds can have significant deleterious effects, including increased risk of infection, damage to connective tissue, and atrophy of the adrenal glands.

Platelet-Activating Factor

Another potent inflammatory mediator derived from membrane phospholipids is platelet-activating factor (PAF), synthesized by virtually all activated inflammatory cells, endothelial cells, and injured tissue cells (Fig. 2-14). During inflammatory and allergic responses, PAF is derived from choline-containing glycerophospholipids in the cell membrane, initially by PLA_2, followed by acetylation by an acetyltransferase. In the plasma, PAF-acetylhydrolase controls PAF activity. Another, de novo, pathway mediates constitutive synthesis of PAF in organs such as brain and kidney and is less important during inflammation.

PAF can function in a *paracrine* (affecting nearby cells), *endocrine* (affecting distant cells), or *juxtacrine* (affecting adjacent cells) manner. In this last function, PAF generated by endothelial cells cooperates with P-selectin. P-selectin lightly tethers a leukocyte to the endothelial cell, allowing PAF from the endothelial cell to bind to its receptor on the leukocyte and inducing intracellular signaling. PAF has a wide range of activities, among which are stimulatory effects on platelets, neutrophils, monocyte/macrophages, endothelial cells, and vascular smooth muscle cells. It induces platelet aggregation and degranulation at sites of tissue injury and enhances the release of serotonin, thereby causing changes in vascular permeability. Because PAF primes leukocytes, it enhances functional responses (e.g., O_2 production, degranulation) to a second stimulus and induces adhesion molecule expression, specifically of integrins. PAF is also an extremely potent vasodilator, augmenting permeability of the microvasculature at sites of tissue injury.

Prostanoids, Leukotrienes, and Lipoxins Are Biologically Active Metabolites Of Arachidonic Acid

Prostanoids

Arachidonic acid is further metabolized by cyclooxygenases 1 and 2 (COX-1, COX-2) to generate prostanoids

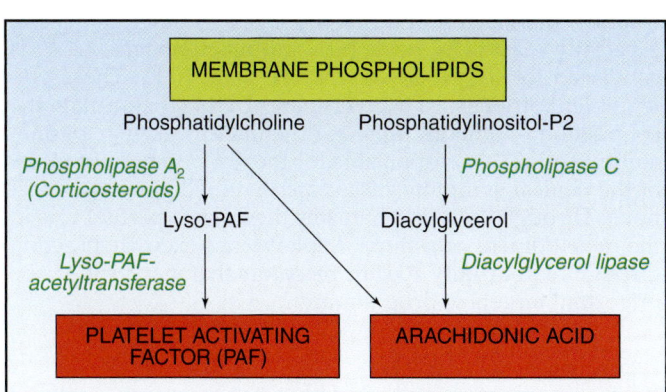

FIGURE 2-14
Membrane-derived mediators. Platelet activating factor and arachidonic acid are derived from membrane phospholipids.

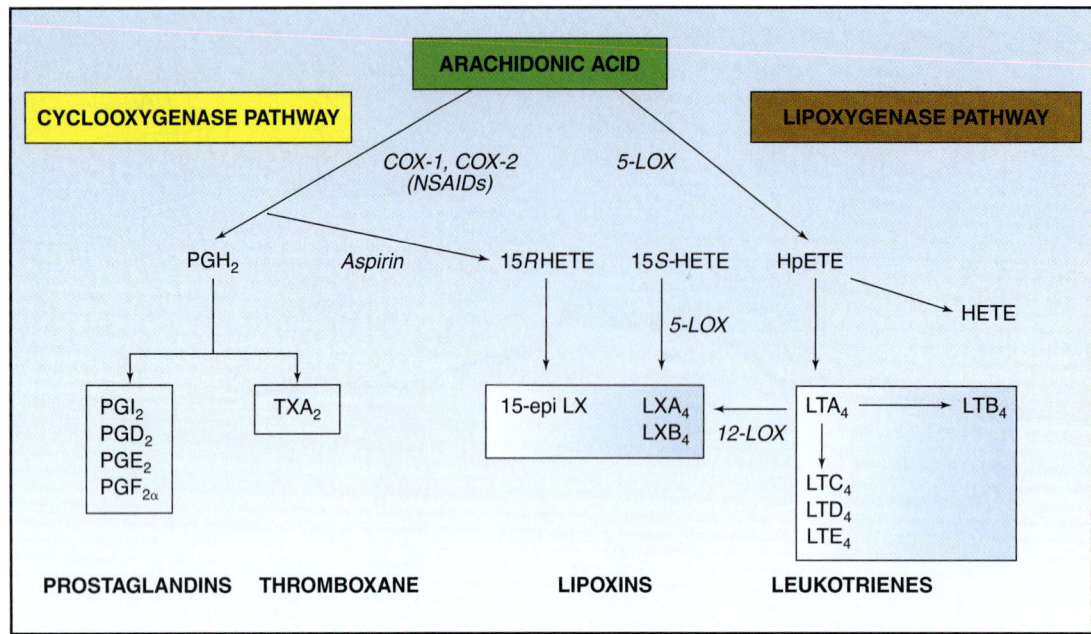

FIGURE 2-15
Arachidonic acid metabolism. The cyclooxygenase pathway of arachidonic acid metabolism generates prostaglandins and thromboxane. The lipoxygenase pathway forms lipoxins and leukotrienes.

(Fig. 2-15). COX-1 is constitutively expressed by most cells, although some studies suggest it may increase upon cell activation. It is a key enzyme in the synthesis of prostaglandins, which (1) protect the gastrointestinal mucosal lining, (2) regulate water/electrolyte balance, (3) stimulate platelet aggregation to maintain normal hemostasis, and (4) maintain resistance to thrombosis on vascular endothelial cell surfaces. COX-2 expression is generally low or undetectable, but increases substantially upon stimulation, generating metabolites important in the induction of pain and inflammation. The early inflammatory prostanoid response is COX-1 dependent; COX-2 becomes the major source of prostanoids as inflammation progresses. Both COX isoforms generate prostaglandin H (PGH_2), which is then the substrate for production of prostacyclin (PGI_2), PGD_2, PGE_2, $PGF_{2\alpha}$, and TXA_2 (thromboxane). The profile of prostaglandin production (i.e., the quantity and variety produced during inflammation) depends in part on the cells present and their activation state. Thus mast cells produce predominantly PGD_2; macrophages generate PGE_2 and TXA_2; platelets are the major source of TXA_2; and endothelial cells produce PGI_2. Prostanoids affect immune cell function by binding to G protein-coupled cell surface receptors, leading to the activation of a range of intracellular signaling pathways in immune cells and resident tissue cells. PGF_2, PGI_2, and TXA_2 bind individual receptors, whereas PGD_2 and PGE_2 bind multiple receptors and receptor subtypes. The repertoire of prostanoid receptors expressed by various immune cells differs, and the functional responses of these cells are, therefore, modified differently according to the prostanoids present.

Inhibition of COX is one mechanism by which *nonsteroidal antiinflammatory drugs* (NSAIDs), including aspirin, indomethacin, and ibuprofen, exert their potent analgesic and antiinflammatory effects. NSAIDS block COX-2 induced formation of prostaglandins, thereby mitigating pain and inflammation. However, they also affect COX-1 and lead to decreased homeostatic functions, resulting in gastric and renal adverse effects. This problem led to the development of COX-2–specific inhibitors.

Leukotrienes

The slow-reacting substance of anaphylaxis (SRS-A) has long been recognized as a smooth muscle stimulant and mediator of hypersensitivity reactions. SRS-A is, in fact, not a single substance but a mixture of leukotrienes, the second major family of derivatives of arachidonic acid (Fig. 2-15). The enzyme 5-lipoxygenase (5-LOX) is responsible for the synthesis of 5-hydroperoxyeicosatetraenoic acid (5-HpETE) and leukotriene A_4 (LTA_4) from arachidonic acid; the latter contains three conjugated double bonds and serves as a precursor for other leukotriene molecules. In the neutrophil and in certain macrophage populations, LTA_4 is metabolized to LTB_4, a compound with potent chemotactic activity for neutrophils, monocytes, and macrophages. In other cell types, especially mast cells, basophils, and macrophages, LTA_4 is converted to LTC_4 followed by LTD_4 and LTE_4. These cysteinyl-leukotrienes, LTC_4, LTD_4, and LTE_4, (1) stimulate the contraction of smooth muscle, (2) enhance vascular permeability, and (3) are responsible for the development of many of the clinical symptoms associated with allergic-type reactions. Through these mechanisms they play a pivotal role in the development of asthma. Leukotrienes exert their action through high-affinity specific receptors that may prove to be important targets of drug therapy.

Lipoxins

The third class of products of arachidonic acid, the lipoxins, is generated within the vascular lumen by cell–cell interactions (Fig. 2-15). Lipoxins are proinflammatory, trihydroxytetraene-containing eicosanoids that are generated during inflammation, atherosclerosis, and thrombosis. Several cell types can synthesize lipoxins from leukotrienes. LTA_4, released by activated leukocytes is available for transcellular enzymatic conversion by neighboring cell types. When platelets are adherent to neutrophils, LTA_4 from neutrophils is converted by platelet 12-lipoxygenase, resulting in the formation of lipoxin A_4 and B_4 (LXA_4 and LXB_4). Monocytes, eosinophils, and airway epithelial cells generate 15S-hydroxyeicosatetraenoic acid (15S-HETE), which is taken up by neutrophils and converted to lipoxins via 5-LOX. Activation of this pathway can also inhibit leukotriene biosynthesis, thereby providing a regulatory pathway.

Aspirin initiates the transcellular biosynthesis of a group of lipoxins termed *aspirin-triggered lipoxins*, or 15-epi-lipoxins (15-epi-LXs). When aspirin is administered in the presence of inflammatory mediators, 15R-HETE is generated by COX-2. Activated neutrophils then convert 15R-HETE to 15 epimeric lipoxins (15-epi-LXs), which are antiinflammatory lipid mediators. This provides another pathway for the beneficial effects of aspirin.

Cytokines Are Cell-Derived Inflammatory Hormones

Cytokines constitute a group of low-molecular-weight proteins secreted by cells. Many of these cytokines are produced at sites of inflammation and include the following:

- Interleukins
- Growth factors and colony-stimulating factors
- Interferons
- Chemokines

Cytokines

The production of cytokines at sites of tissue injury regulates inflammatory responses ranging from initial changes in vascular permeability to resolution and restoration of tissue integrity (Fig. 2-16). These molecules function as inflammatory hormones that exhibit autocrine (affecting themselves), paracrine (affecting nearby cells), and endocrine (affecting cells in other tissues) functions (Fig. 2-17). Most cells can produce cytokines, although cells differ in their cytokine repertoire. Through its production of cytokines, the macrophage is the pivotal cell in the orchestration of the inflammatory response within tissues. *Lipopolysaccharide* (LPS), a molecule derived from the outer cell membrane of gram-negative bacteria, is one of the most potent stimuli of macrophages as well as other cells, including endothelial cells and leukocytes. LPS can activate cells through specific receptors, either directly or after binding with a serum LPS-binding protein (LBP). It is a potent stimulus for the production of TNFα and interleukins (IL-1, IL-6, IL-8, IL-12, and others). Macrophage-derived cytokines modulate endothelial cell–leukocyte adhesion (TNF-α), leukocyte recruitment (IL-8), the acute phase response (IL-6, IL-1), and immune functions (IL-1, IL-6, IL-12).

Interferon-gamma (IFN-γ) is a second potent stimulus for macrophage activation and cytokine production. Although IFN-γ is produced by a subset of T lymphocytes as part of the immune response (see Chapter 4), it is also synthesized by natural killer (NK) cells as a primary host response to intracellular pathogens (e.g., *Listeria monocytogenes*) and certain viral infections. NK cells are lymphocytes that possess large cytoplasmic granules containing cell lysis proteins, which migrate into tissues at sites of injury. When exposed to IL-12 and TNF-α, NK cells are activated to produce IFN-γ. Thus, an amplification pathway exists by which

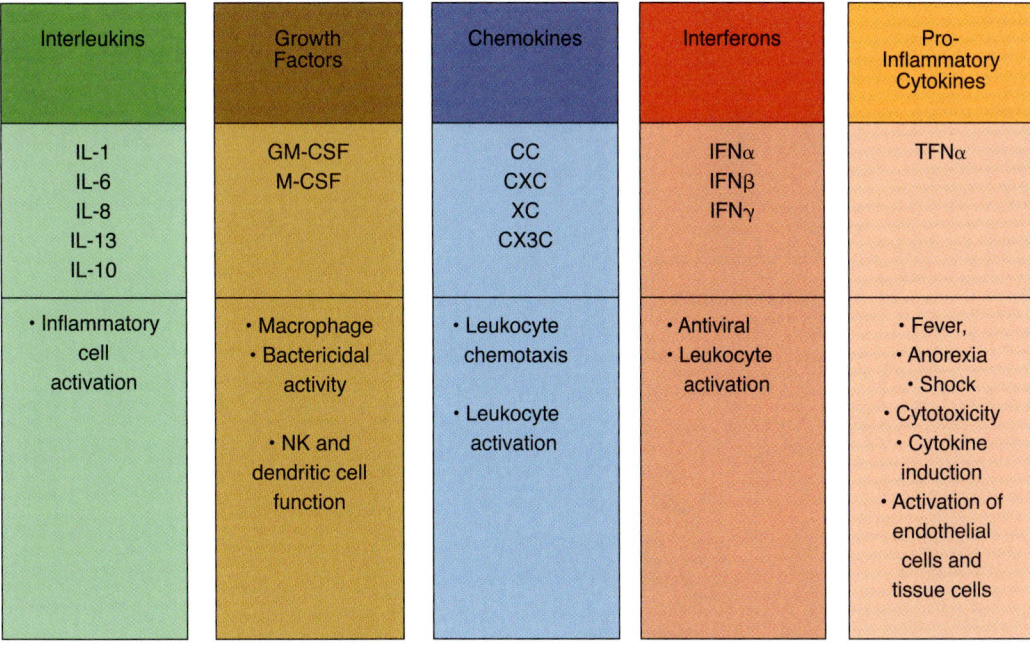

FIGURE 2-16
Cytokines important in inflammation.

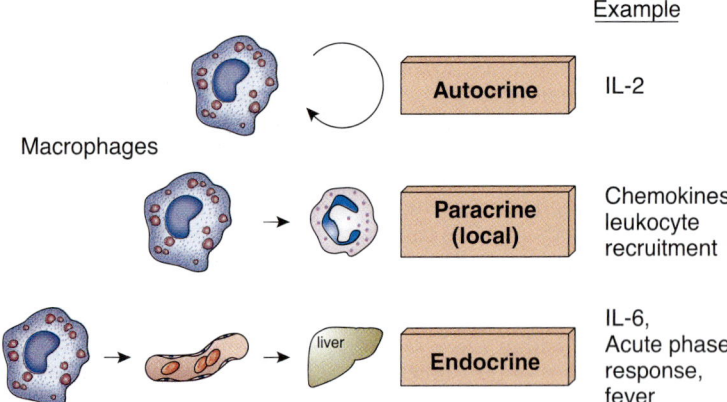

FIGURE 2-17
Functional roles of cytokines.

activated tissue macrophages produce TNF-α and IL-12, thereby stimulating IFN-γ production by NK cells, with subsequent stimulation of additional macrophages (Fig. 2-18).

Chemokines

Chemotactic cytokines, or chemokines, direct the process of cell migration, or chemotaxis, which is a dynamic and energy-dependent activity. Accumulation of inflammatory cells at a site of tissue injury requires the migration of these cells from the vascular space into the extravascular tissue. During migration, the cell extends a pseudopod in the direction of the increasing chemotactic gradient. At the leading front of the pseudopod, marked changes in the levels of intracellular calcium are associated with the assembly and contraction of cytoskeleton proteins. This process results in drawing the remaining tail of the cell along the chemical gradient. The most important chemotactic factors for PMNs are the following:

- C5a, derived from complement
- Bacterial and mitochondrial products, particularly low-molecular-weight N-formylated peptides (such as N-formyl-methionyl-leucyl-phenylalanine [FMLP])
- Products of arachidonic acid metabolism, especially LTB$_4$
- Chemokines

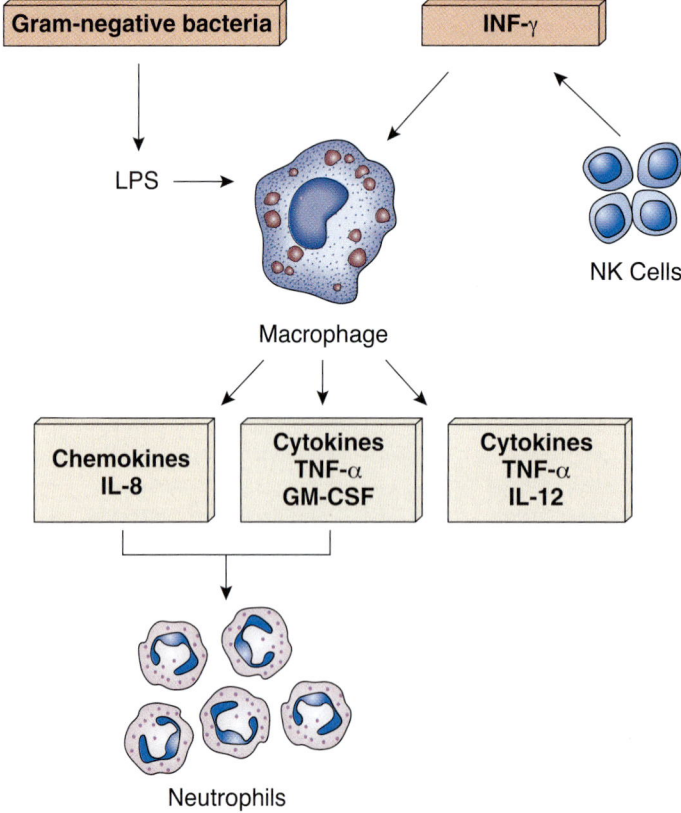

FIGURE 2-18
Cytokine networks: Regulation of macrophage activation.

Chemokines constitute a large class of cytokines (over 50 members) that regulate leukocyte trafficking in inflammation and immunity. In contrast to other cytokines, the chemokines are smaller molecules that interact with G-protein–coupled receptors on target cells. These secretory proteins are produced by a wide variety of cell types, either constitutively or after induction, and differ widely in their biological actions. This diversity may be based on the specific cell types targeted, specific receptor activation, or differences in intracellular signaling.

Two functional classes of chemokines have been distinguished: inflammatory chemokines and homing chemokines. Inflammatory chemokines are produced in response to bacterial toxins and inflammatory cytokines (especially, IL-1, TNF-α and IFN-γ) by a variety of tissue cells as well as leukocytes. These molecules recruit leukocytes during the host inflammatory response. Homing chemokines, which are constitutively expressed and upregulated during disease states, direct the trafficking and homing of lymphocytes and dendritic cells to lymphoid tissues during an immune response. These chemokines are constitutively expressed and upregulated during disease states (see Chapter 4).

Structure and Nomenclature

Chemokines are synthesized as secretory proteins consisting of approximately 70 to 130 amino acids, with four conserved cysteines linked by disulfide bonds. The two major subpopulations, termed *CXC or CC chemokines* (formerly called α and β chemokines) are distinguished by the position of the first two cysteines, which are either separated by one amino acid (CXC) or are adjacent (CC). The disulfide bonds between the two pairs of cysteines determine their three-dimensional rigid loop structure and are essential for receptor recognition and biological activity. The site within the rigid loop acts as a "docking site" and the amino-terminal region binding site is the "triggering domain," which activates the receptor. Two additional classes of chemokines, each with a single member, have been identified. Lymphotactin has two instead of four conserved cysteines (XC), and fractaline (or neurotactin) has three amino acids between the first two cysteines (CX_3C). Chemokines are named according to their structure, followed by "L" and the number of their gene (CCL1, CXCL1, etc.). However, many of the traditional names for chemokines persist in current usage. Chemokine receptors are named according to their structure, "R," and a number (CCR1, CXCR1, etc.). Six receptors for CXC chemokines (CXCRs) and 10 receptors for CC chemokines (CCRs) have been characterized in terms of their function and structure. Most receptors recognize more than one chemokine, and most chemokines recognize more than one receptor. Receptor binding of chemokines to their ligands may result in an agonistic or antagonistic activity, with the same chemokine functioning as an agonist for one receptor and an antagonist for another. Leukocyte recruitment or lymphocyte homing is modulated by a combination of agonistic and antagonistic activities.

Anchoring and Activity

Chemokines function in two ways, as immobilized or as soluble molecules. One of the mechanisms by which chemokines generate a chemotactic gradient is by binding to proteoglycans of the ECM or to cell surfaces. As a result, high concentrations of the chemokines persist at sites of tissue injury. Specific receptors on the surface of the migrating leukocytes bind to the matrix-bound chemokines and associated adhesion molecules, a process that tends to move the cells along the chemotactic gradient to the site of injury. This process of responding to a matrix-bound chemoattractant is termed **haptotaxis.** During leukocyte recruitment to inflamed tissues, chemokines may also be displayed on cytokine-activated vascular endothelial cells. This process can augment very late antigen-4 (VLA-4) integrin- dependent adhesion of leukocytes, resulting in their firm arrest. As soluble molecules, chemokines also control leukocyte motility and localization within the extravascular tissue by establishment of a chemotactic gradient. The multiplicity and combination of chemokine receptors on cells allows an extensive variety in biological function. Neutrophils, monocytes, eosinophils, and basophils share some receptors but express other receptors exclusively. Thus specific chemokine combinations can recruit selective cell populations.

Chemokines in Disease

Chemokines are implicated in a wide variety of acute and chronic diseases. These include disorders with a pronounced inflammatory component, in which case multiple chemokines are expressed in the inflamed tissues. Examples are rheumatoid arthritis, ulcerative colitis, Crohn disease, pulmonary inflammation (chronic bronchitis, asthma), autoimmune diseases (multiple sclerosis, rheumatoid arthritis, systemic lupus erythematosus), and vascular diseases, including atherosclerosis.

Reactive Oxygen Species Function As Signal-Transducing, Bactericidal and Cytotoxic Molecules

Reactive oxygen species (ROS) are chemically reactive molecules derived from oxygen. Under normal circumstances they are rapidly inactivated, but when they are generated inappropriately, they are toxic. ROS activate signal-transduction pathways and combine with proteins, lipids, and DNA, a state termed *oxidative stress*. Sustained oxidative stress leads to loss of cell function and ultimately apoptosis or necrosis. Leukocyte-derived ROS, released within phagosomes, are bactericidal (see below).

The most common ROS important in inflammation include superoxide (O_2^-), nitric oxide (NO•), hydrogen peroxide (H_2O_2), and hydroxyl radical (•OH) (see Chapter 1). The latter two species are primarily involved in tissue injury and antimicrobial defense and are described below.

Superoxide

Molecular oxygen is converted to superoxide anion (O_2^-) by several pathways. Within cells, formation of O_2^- occurs spontaneously near the inner mitochondrial membrane. In vascular endothelial cells, O_2^- is generated by flavoenzymes such as xanthine oxidase, as well as lipoxygenase and cyclooxygenase. Importantly, in the setting of inflammation, leukocytes, as well as endothelial cells, use a reduced nicotinamide adenine dinucleotide phosphate (NADPH) oxidase to produce O_2^-.

The cytosolic purine-metabolizing enzyme, xanthine oxidase, converts xanthine and hypoxanthine to uric acid, thereby generating O_2^-. This pathway is implicated as a major intracellular source of O_2^- in neutrophil-mediated cell injury. Several proinflammatory mediators, including leukocyte elastase and several cytokines, convert xanthine dehydrogenase to the active xanthine oxidase. Intracellular O_2^- interacts with molecules such as NF-κB and AP-1 and activates a number of signal transduction pathways. O_2^- is further metabolized to generate other toxic free radicals, particularly •OH, which participate in inflammatory-mediated cell injury.

The NADPH-oxidase of phagocytic cells, neutrophils, and macrophages, is a multicomponent enzyme complex, by which high concentrations of extracellular and intracellular O_2^- are generated to serve predominantly bactericidal and cytotoxic functions This oxidase uses NADH and NADPH as substrates for electron transfer to molecular oxygen. A similar enzyme complex is present in vascular endothelial cells, where it generates significant, albeit lower, concentrations of O_2^-.

Nitric Oxide

Nitric oxide (NO•) is synthesized by nitric oxide synthase (NOS), which promotes oxidation of the guanidino nitrogen of L-arginine in the presence of molecular oxygen. There are three main isoforms of the enzyme, constitutively expressed neuronal (nNOS) and endothelial (eNOS) nitric oxide synthase and an inducible (iNOS) isoform. Inflammatory cytokines increase expression of the inducible form of NOS, generating intracellular and extracellular NO•. NO•, regardless of the enzyme source, has diverse roles in the physiology and pathophysiology of the vascular system, including the following:

- NO• generated by eNOS functions as *endothelium-derived relaxing factor* (EDRF), which is responsible for mediating vascular smooth muscle relaxation.
- NO• in physiological concentrations, alone and in balance with O_2^-, serves as an intracellular messenger.
- NO• prevents platelet adherence and aggregation at sites of vascular injury, reduces leukocyte recruitment, and scavenges oxygen radicals.
- Excessive production of NO•, especially in parallel with O_2^-, results in the generation of highly cytotoxic molecules.

Stress Proteins Protect against Inflammatory Injury

When cells are subjected to stress conditions, many suffer irreversible injury and die, and others are severely damaged. However, mild heat treatment prior to lethal injury provides tolerance to subsequent injury. This phenomenon is associated with increased expression of the heat shock family of stress proteins (HSPs). Stress proteins belong to multigene families and are named according to molecular size, for example, Hsp27, Hsp70, and Hsp90. These molecules are upregulated by diverse stresses, including oxidative/ischemic stress and inflammation, and are associated with protection during sepsis and metabolic stress. Protein damage and misfolded proteins are common denominators in injury and disease. The protection against nonlethal stress that is mediated by HSPs is attributed to their molecular chaperone function, which increases protein expression by enhanced folding of nascent proteins. Potential functions of stress proteins include suppression of proinflammatory cytokines and NADPH oxidase, increased nitric oxide-mediated cytoprotection, and enhanced collagen synthesis.

Neurokinins Link the Endocrine, Nervous, and Immune Systems

The neurokinin family of peptides includes substance P (SP), neurokinin A (NKA), and neurokinin B (NKB). These peptides are distributed throughout the central and peripheral nervous system and represent a link between the endocrine, nervous, and immune systems. A wide range of biological processes is associated with these peptides, including plasma protein extravasation and edema, vasodilation, smooth-muscle contraction and relaxation, salivary secretion, airway contraction, and transmission of nociceptive responses. As early as 1876, Stricker noted an association between sensory afferent nerves and inflammation. It is now recognized that injury to nerve terminals during inflammation evokes an increase in neurokinins, which in turn influences production of inflammatory mediators, including histamine, nitric oxide, and kinins. The actions of neurokinins are mediated by activation of at least three classes of receptors, NK1, NK2, and NK3, which are distributed in tissues throughout the body. The neurokinin system is linked to inflammation in the following settings:

- **Edema formation:** SP, NKA, and NKB induce edema formation by promoting the release of histamine and serotonin from mast cells.
- **Thermal injury:** SP and NKA are produced after thermal injury and mediate early edema.
- **Arthritis:** SP is widely distributed in nerves in joints and mediates vascular permeability. SP and NKA can modulate the activity of inflammatory and immune cells.
- **Airway inflammation:** SP and NKA have been implicated in bronchoconstriction, mucosal edema, leukocyte adhesion and activation, and increased vascular permeability.

EXTRACELLULAR MATRIX MEDIATORS

Interaction of Cells with the Extracellular Matrix Regulates the Tissue Response to Inflammation

The extracellular environment consists of a macromolecular matrix specific to a given tissue. Resident inflammatory cells interact with this matrix, especially during injury. Collagen, elastic fibers, basement membrane proteins, glycoproteins, and proteoglycans are among the structural macromolecules constituting the ECM (see Chapter 3). Matricellular proteins are secreted macromolecules that serve to link cells to the ECM or to disrupt cell–ECM interactions. Cytokines and growth factors influence the associations among cells, the

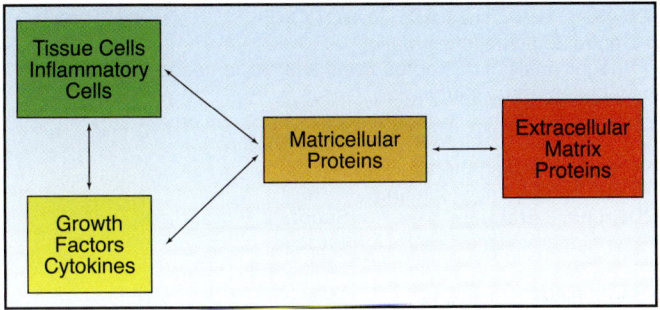

FIGURE 2-19
Extracellular environment contributes to the inflammatory response.

ECM, and matricellular proteins (Fig. 2-19). Matricellular proteins include:

- **SPARC (secreted protein acidic and rich in cysteine)** is a multifunctional glycoprotein that organizes ECM components and modulates growth factor activity. It affects cell proliferation, migration, and differentiation and acts as a counteradhesive protein, especially on endothelial cells.
- **Thrombospondins** are secreted glycoproteins that modulate cell–matrix interactions, influence platelet aggregation, and support neutrophil chemotaxis and adhesion.
- **Tenascins C, X, and R** are counteradhesive proteins expressed during development, tissue injury, and wound healing.
- **Syndecans** are heparan sulfate proteoglycans implicated in the coagulation cascades, growth factor signaling, cell adhesion to the ECM, and tumorigenesis.
- **Osteopontin** is a phosphorylated glycoprotein important in bone mineralization. It also (1) mediates cell–matrix interactions, (2) functions as a cytokine to activate cell signaling pathways (particularly in T cells), (3) is chemotactic for and supports adhesion of leukocytes, and (4) has antiinflammatory effects through its regulation of macrophage function.

CELLS OF INFLAMMATION

Leukocytes are the major cellular components of the inflammatory response and include neutrophils, T and B lymphocytes, monocytes, macrophages, eosinophils, mast cells, and basophils. Although specific functions have been assigned to each of these cell types, they overlap and vary with the phase of inflammation. In addition, local tissue cells interact with one another and with inflammatory cells, in a continuous response to injury and infection.

Inflammatory Cells and Resident Tissue Cells Interact during the Inflammation

Neutrophils

The polymorphonuclear neutrophil, or (PMN), is the hallmark cell of acute inflammation. This cell has a granulated cytoplasm and a nucleus with two to four lobules. PMNs are stored in bone marrow, circulate in the blood, and rapidly accumulate at sites of injury or infection (Fig. 2-20). They are activated in response to phagocytic stimuli, cytokines, chemotactic mediators, or antigen–antibody complexes that bind to specific receptors on their cell membrane. Specifically, neutrophil receptors react with the Fc portion of IgG and IgM molecules; complement system components C5a, C3b, and iC3b; arachidonic acid metabolites (e.g., LTB$_4$), chemotactic factors (e.g., FMLP, IL-8), and cytokines (e.g., TNF-α). In tissues, PMNs phagocytose invading microbes and dead tissue (see below). Once they are recruited into tissue, they do not reenter the circulation.

Endothelial Cells

Endothelial cells are flattened cells that form a monolayer lining the blood vessels. They maintain patency and blood flow through the production of antiplatelet and antithrombotic agents and regulate vascular tone through the production of vasodilators and vasoconstrictors (Fig. 2-21). An intact endothelial cell lining inhibits platelet adhesion and blood clotting, whereas injury to a blood vessel wall alters the endothelial barrier and exposes a local procoagulant signal (Fig. 2-22). The vascular endothelial cell has the capacity either to promote or to inhibit tissue perfusion and inflammatory cell influx through multiple mechanisms, thereby modulating tissue function and the development of the inflammatory response.

Any inflammatory cell circulating through the vascular system must cross the vascular endothelium to extravasate into tissue. Endothelial cells function as gatekeepers in inflammatory cell recruitment, presenting adhesion molecules to anchor flowing leukocytes. They activate leukocytes by these adhesive interactions, as well as by generation of cytokines and presentation of major histocompatibility complex (MHC) class I and II molecules. Endothelial cells respond rapidly to inflammatory agents such as bradykinin and histamine, endotoxin, and cytokines. These substances alter the expression of adhesion molecules required for recruitment of leukocytes and the production of important vasoactive and inflammatory mediators. These mediators include the following:

- **Nitric oxide (NO•):** Originally identified endothelial relaxing factor (EDRF), NO• is a low-molecular-weight vasodilator that inhibits platelet aggregation, regulates vascular tone by stimulating smooth muscle relaxation, and interacts with oxygen radicals to mediate cell injury.
- **Endothelins:** Endothelins-1, -2, and -3 are low-molecular-weight peptides produced by endothelial cells. They are potent vasoconstrictor and pressor agents, which induce prolonged vasoconstriction of vascular smooth muscle.
- **Arachidonic acid-derived contraction factors:** Oxygen radicals generated by the hydroperoxidase activity of cyclooxygenase and prostanoids such as TXA$_2$ and PGH$_2$ induce smooth muscle contraction.
- **Arachidonic acid-derived relaxing factors:** The biological opponent of TXA$_2$, prostacyclin (PGI$_2$) inhibits platelet aggregation and causes vasodilation.
- **Cytokines:** IL-1, IL-6, TNF-α and other inflammatory cytokines are generated by activated endothelial cells.
- **Anticoagulants:** Heparin-like molecules and thrombomodulin inactivate the coagulation cascade (see Chapter 10).

Inflammation

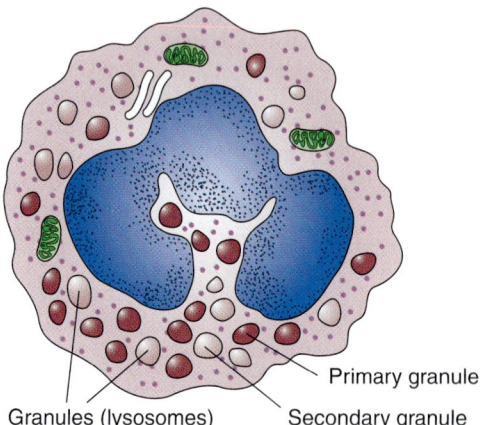

CHARACTERISTICS AND FUNCTIONS
- Central to acute inflammation
- Phagocytosis of microorganisms and tissue debris
- Mediates tissue injury

PRIMARY INFLAMMATORY MEDIATORS
- Reactive oxygen metabolites
- Lysosomal granule contents

Primary granules	Secondary granules
Myeloperoxidase	Lysozyme
Lysozyme	Lactoferrin
Defensins	Collagenase
Bactericidal/permeability increasing protein	Complement activator
	Phospholipase A_2
Elastase	CD11b/CD18
Cathepsins Protease 3	CD11c/CD18
Glucuronidase	Laminin
Mannosidase	
Phospholipase A_2	**Tertiary granules**
	Gelatinase
	Plasminogen activator
	Cathepsins
	Glucuronidase
	Mannosidase

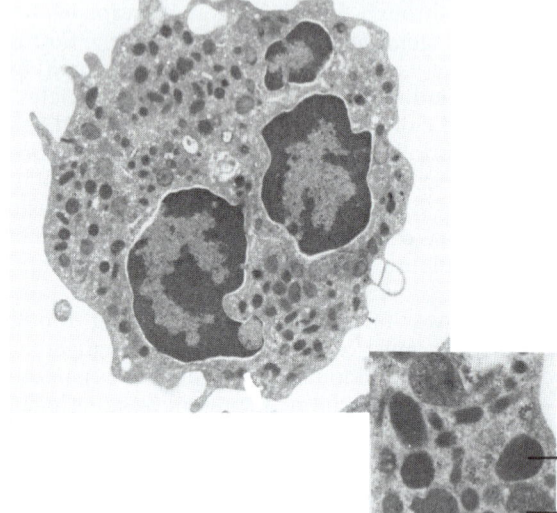

FIGURE 2-20
PMN: Morphology and function.

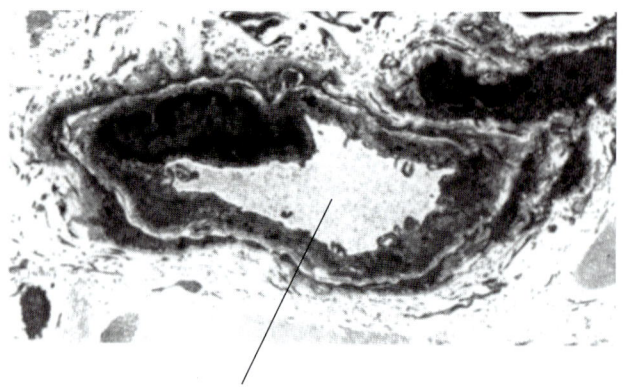

CHARACTERISTICS AND FUNCTIONS
- Maintains vascular integrity
- Regulates platelet aggregation
- Regulates vascular contraction and relaxation
- Mediates leukocyte recruitment in inflammation

PRIMARY INFLAMMATORY MEDIATORS
- von Willebrand factor
- Nitric oxide
- Endothelins
- Prostanoids

FIGURE 2-21
Endothelial cell: Morphology and function

Cells of Inflammation

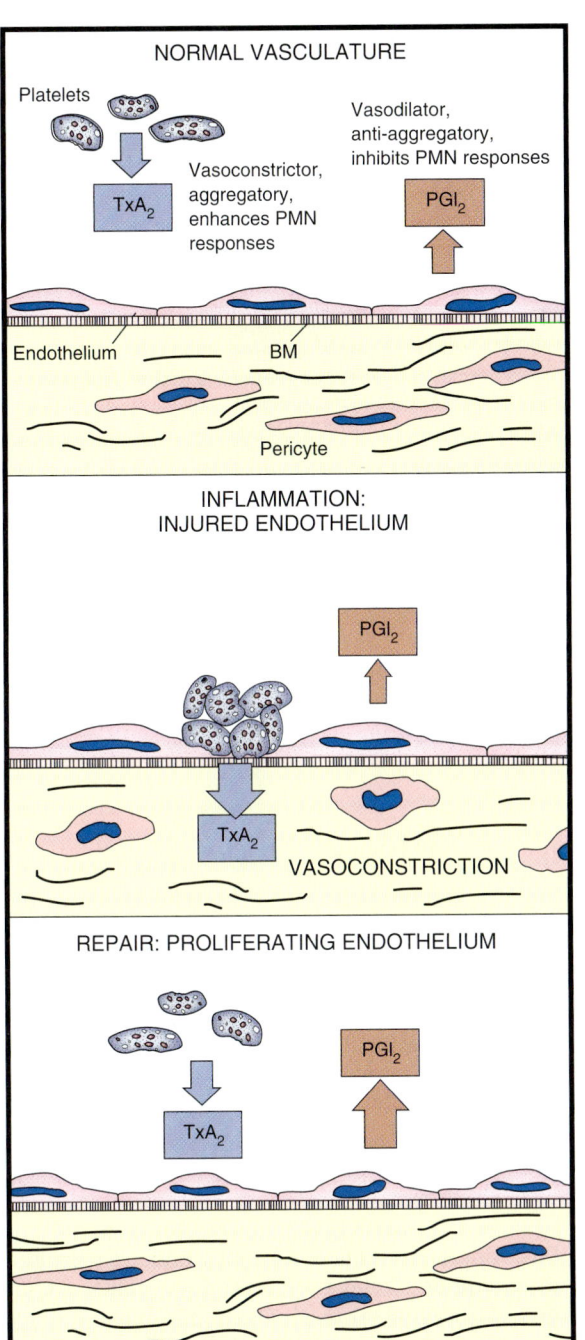
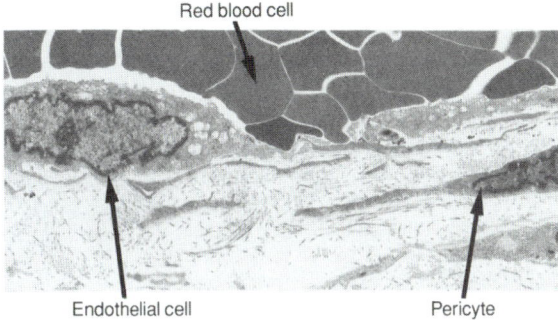
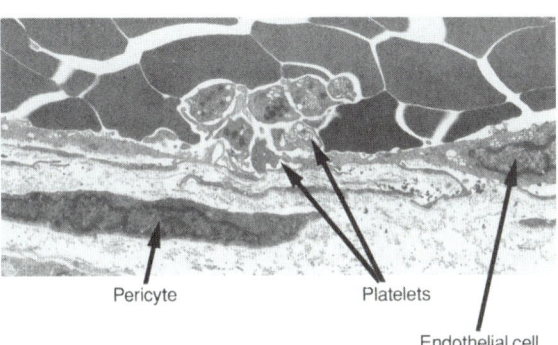

FIGURE 2-22
Regulation of platelet and endothelial cell interactions by thromboxane A_2 (*TXA$_2$*) and prostaglandin I_2 (*PGI$_2$*). During inflammation, the normal balance is shifted to vasoconstriction, platelet aggregation, and PMN responses. During repair, the prostaglandin effects predominate.

- **Fibrinolytic factors:** Tissue-type plasminogen activator (t-PA) promotes fibrinolytic activity.
- **Prothrombotic agents:** von Willebrand factor facilitates adhesion of platelets, and tissue factor activates the extrinsic clotting cascade.

Monocyte/Macrophages

Circulating monocytes (Fig. 2-23) have a single lobed or kidney-shaped nucleus. They are derived from the bone marrow and can exit the circulation to migrate into tissue and become resident macrophages. In response to inflammatory mediators, they accumulate at sites of acute inflammation. Macrophages are phagocytic cells that take up and process microbes and present antigens bound to the **major histocompatibility complex** (MHC) class II to lymphocytes. These cells can also differentiate into dendritic cells, which are highly efficient antigen-presenting cells. Monocyte/macrophages are a source of potent vasoactive mediators, including the products of arachidonic acid metabolism (prostaglandins, leukotrienes), PAF, and inflammatory cy-

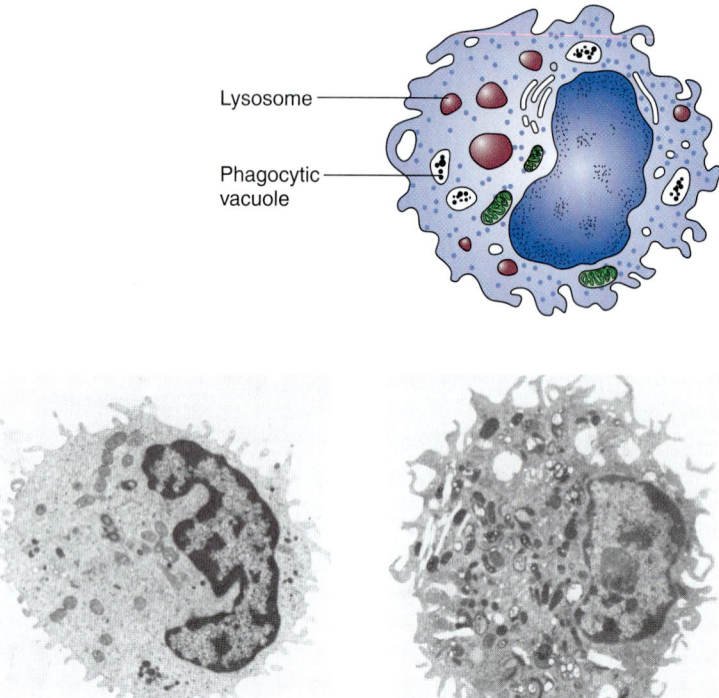

FIGURE 2-23
Monocyte/macrophage: Morphology and function.

tokines. Macrophages are especially important in the maintenance of a chronic inflammatory state.

Mast Cells and Basophils

Mast cells and basophils (Fig. 2-24) are granulated cells that contain receptors for IgE on their cell surface. They are additional cellular sources of vasoactive mediators, particularly in response to allergens. Mast cells are localized within the connective tissue of the body and are especially prevalent along mucosal surfaces of the lung and gastrointestinal tract, the dermis of the skin, and the microvasculature. Basophils are present in low numbers in the circulation and can migrate into tissue.

When IgE-sensitized mast cells or basophils are stimulated by antigen, inflammatory mediators contained in their dense cytoplasmic granules are secreted into extracellular tissues. Degranulation may also be induced by physical agonists, such as cold and trauma, and by cationic proteins derived from platelets and neutrophil lysosomal granules. The granules contain acid mucopolysaccharides (including heparin), serine proteases, chemotactic mediators for neutrophils and eosinophils, and histamine. Histamine is one of the primary mediators of early increased vascular permeability. It acts on the vasculature by binding to specific H_1 receptors in the vascular wall, inducing endothelial cell contraction, gap formation, and edema, an effect that can be inhibited pharmacologically by H_1-receptor antagonists. Stimulation of mast cells and basophils also leads to the release of products of arachidonic acid metabolism, including LTC_4, LTD_4, and LTE_4, and cytokines, such as TNF-α and IL-4. Mast cell products play an important role in the regulation of vascular permeability and bronchial smooth muscle tone, especially in many forms of allergic hypersensitivity reactions (see Chapter 4).

Eosinophils

Eosinophils circulate in the blood and are recruited to tissue in a manner similar to that of PMNs. They are characteristic of IgE-mediated reactions, such as seen in hypersensitivity and allergic and asthmatic responses (Fig. 2-25). Eosinophils contain leukotrienes and PAF, as well as acid phosphatase and peroxidase. They express IgA receptors and contain large granules with eosinophil major basic protein, both of which are involved in defense against parasites.

Platelets

Platelets play a primary role in normal homeostasis and in the initiation and regulation of clot formation. They are sources of inflammatory mediators, including potent vasoactive substances and growth factors that modulate mesenchymal cell proliferation (Fig. 2-26). The platelet is small (2 mm in diameter), lacks a nucleus, and contains three distinct kinds of inclusions: (1) dense granules, rich in serotonin, histamine, calcium, and adenosine diphosphate (ADP); (2) α granules,

Cells of Inflammation

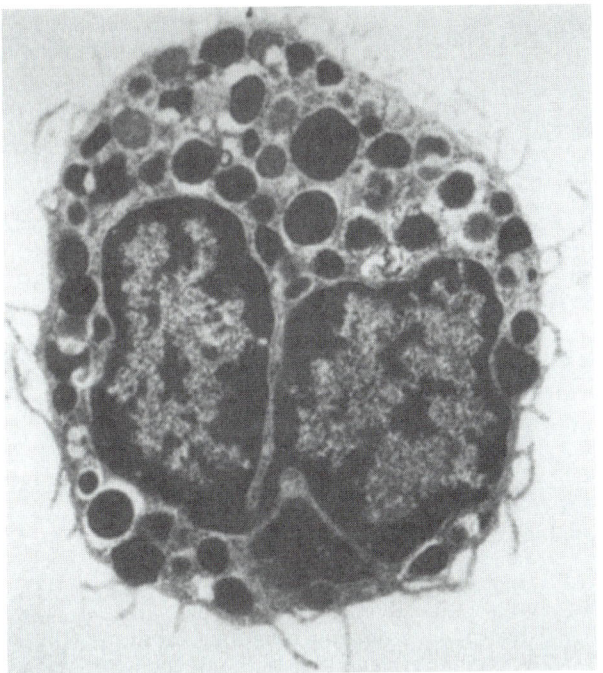

Mast Cell (Basophils)

CHARACTERISTICS AND FUNCTIONS
- Binds IgE molecules
- Contains electron-dense granules

PRIMARY INFLAMMATORY MEDIATORS
- Histamine
- Leukotrienes (LTC, LTD, LTE)
- Platelet activating factor
- Eosinophil chemotactic factors
- Cytokines (e.g., TNF-α IL-4)

FIGURE 2-24
Mast cell: Morphology and functions.

containing fibrinogen, coagulation proteins, platelet-derived growth factor (PDGF), and other peptides and proteins; and (3) lysosomes, which sequester acid hydrolases.

Platelet adherence, aggregation, and degranulation occur when platelets come in contact with fibrillar collagen (following vascular injury that exposes the interstitial matrix proteins) or thrombin (after activation of the coagulation system) (Fig. 2-22). Degranulation is associated with the release of serotonin (5-hydroxytryptamine), which, like histamine, directly increases vascular permeability. In addition, the arachidonic acid metabolite TXA_2, produced by platelets, plays a key role in the second wave of platelet aggregation and mediates smooth muscle constriction. On activation, platelets, as well as phagocytic cells, secrete cationic proteins that neutralize the negative charges on endothelium and promote increased permeability.

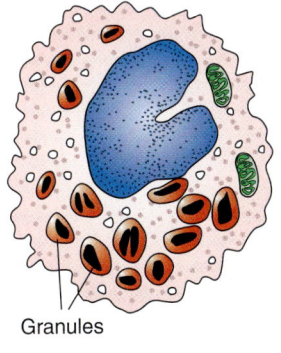
Granules

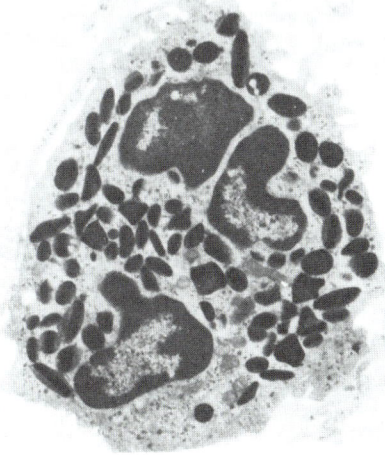

CHARACTERISTICS AND FUNCTIONS
- Associated with:
  - Allergic reactions
  - Parasite-associated inflammatory reactions
  - Chronic inflammation
- Modulates mast cell-mediated reactions

PRIMARY INFLAMMATORY MEDIATORS
- Reactive oxygen metabolites
- Lysosomal granule enzymes
  (primary crystalloid granules)
  - Major basic protein
  - Eosinophil cationic protein
  - Eosinophil peroxidase
  - Acid phosphatase
  - β-glucuronidase
  - Arylsulfatase B
  - Histaminase
- Phospholipase D
- Prostaglandins of E series
- Cytokines

FIGURE 2-25
Eosinophil: Morphology and function.

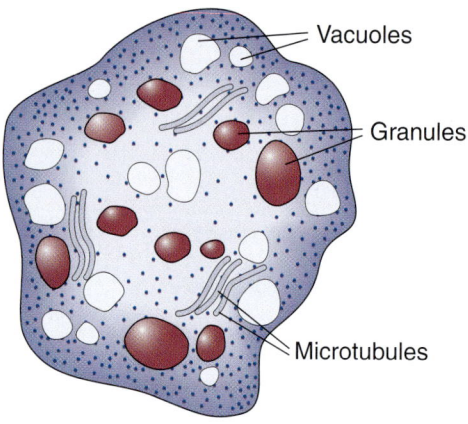 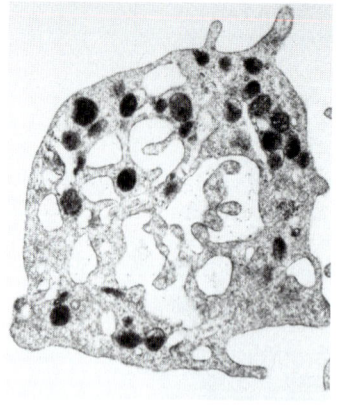

CHARACTERISTICS AND FUNCTIONS
- Thrombosis; promotes clot formation
- Regulates permeability
- Regulates proliferative response of mesenchymal cells

PRIMARY INFLAMMATORY MEDIATORS
- Dense granules
  - Serotonin
  - Ca^{2+}
  - ADP
- α-granules
  - Cationic proteins
  - Fibrinogen and coagulation proteins
  - Platelet-derived growth factor (PDGF)
- Lysosomes
  - Acid hydrolases
- Thromboxane A_2

FIGURE 2-26
Platelet: Morphology and function.

Common Intracellular Pathways Are Associated with Inflammatory Cell Activation

The process by which diverse stimuli lead to the functional responses of inflammatory cells (e.g., degranulation or aggregation) is referred to as *stimulus–response coupling*. Stimuli can include microbial products and the wide array of plasma-derived or cell-derived inflammatory mediators that are described in this chapter. Although intracellular signaling pathways are complex and vary with the cell type and stimulus, some common intracellular pathways are associated with inflammatory cell activation, including G-protein, TNF receptor (TNFR), and JAK-STAT pathways.

G-Protein Pathways

Many chemokines, hormones, and neurotransmitters, as well as other inflammatory mediators, use proteins of the guanine nucleotide-binding family (G proteins) of signal transducers. There are four broad members of this family, which vary in their intracellular connections, but common concepts include the following (Fig. 2-27):

- **Ligand–receptor binding:** The binding of a stimulatory factor to a specific receptor on the cell membrane results in the formation of a ligand–receptor complex. On binding of the stimulus to the receptor, an exchange of GDP for GTP activates the G protein, which dissociates into subunits. These subunits activate phospholipase C and phosphatidylinositol-3-kinase (PI-3-kinase).
- **Phospholipid metabolism of cell membranes:** Phospholipase C hydrolyzes a phosphoinositide in the plasma membrane (phosphatidylinositol bisphosphate [PIP_2]), thereby forming two potent metabolites, diacylglycerol and inositol trisphosphate (IP_3).
- **Elevated cytosolic free calcium:** IP_3 induces the release of stored intracellular calcium. In conjunction with an influx of calcium ions from the extracellular environment, IP_3 increases cytosolic free calcium, a critical event for the activation of most inflammatory cells.
- **Protein phosphorylation and dephosphorylation:** Specific tyrosine kinases bind the ligand–receptor complex and initiate a series of protein phosphorylations.
- **Protein kinase C activation:** Protein kinase C and other protein kinases activate several intracellular signaling pathways, including gene transcription.

TNFR Pathways

TNF is central to the development of inflammation. It also induces apoptosis of tumor cells and regulates immune func-

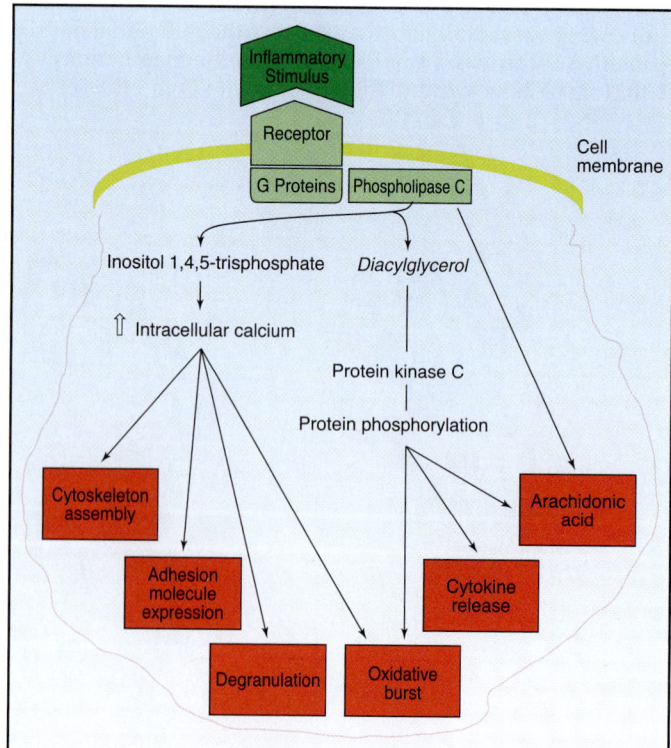

FIGURE 2-27
G-protein–mediated intracellular signal transduction pathway common to many inflammatory stimuli.

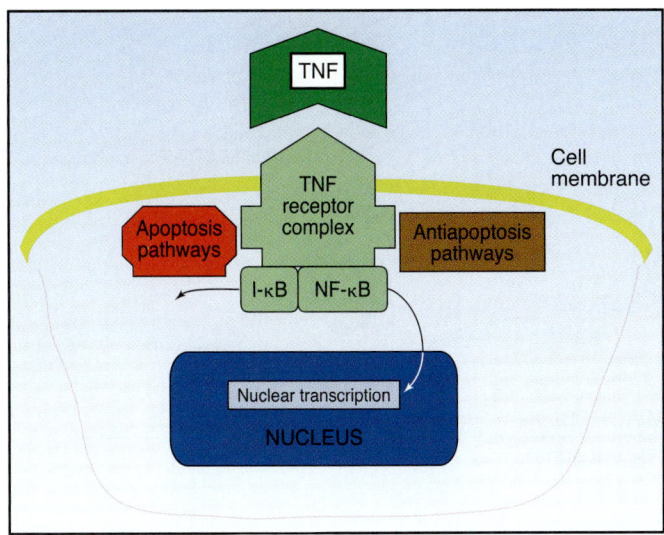

FIGURE 2-28

TNF receptor-mediated intracellular signal transduction pathway.

tions (Fig. 2-28). TNF and related proteins interact with two cell surface receptors, resulting in the formation of a multiprotein signaling complex at the cell membrane. This complex can trigger (1) apoptosis-related enzymes, termed *caspases,* (2) inhibitors of apoptosis, or (3) activation of a nuclear transcription factor called NF-κB, which regulates gene transcription. NF-κB is regulated by its association and disassociation with IκB, an inhibitory component that prevents translocation of NF-κB to the nucleus. This latter pathway is critical to regulation of TNF-mediated events during inflammation.

JAK-STAT Pathways

This pathway provides a direct signaling route from extracellular polypeptides (e.g., growth factors) or cytokines (e.g., interferons or interleukins) through cell receptors to gene promoters in the nucleus. Ligand–receptor interactions generate transcription complexes composed of JAK-STAT (Janus kinase-signal transducer and activator of transcription proteins). STAT proteins translocate to the nucleus, where they interact with gene promoters (Fig. 2-29).

The outcome of these signaling mechanisms involves induction or enhancement of specific functional responses, including phagocytosis, degranulation, cell and platelet aggregation, oxidant production, adhesion molecule expression, cytokine production, and gene transcription. An understanding of inflammatory cell stimulation provides the basis for new strategies for therapeutic modulation of inflammation in human disease.

LEUKOCYTE RECRUITMENT IN ACUTE INFLAMMATION

One of the essential features of inflammation is the accumulation of leukocytes, particularly PMNs, in the affected tissues. Leukocytes adhere to vascular endothelium, becoming activated in the process. They then flatten and migrate from the vasculature, through the endothelial cell layer, and into the surrounding tissue. In the extravascular tissue, PMNs ingest foreign material, microbes, and dead tissue (Fig. 2-30).

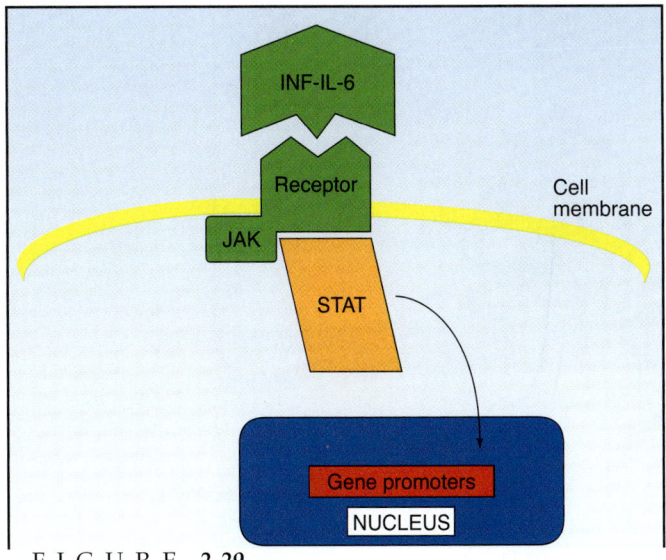

FIGURE 2-29

JAK-STAT–mediated intracellular transduction pathway.

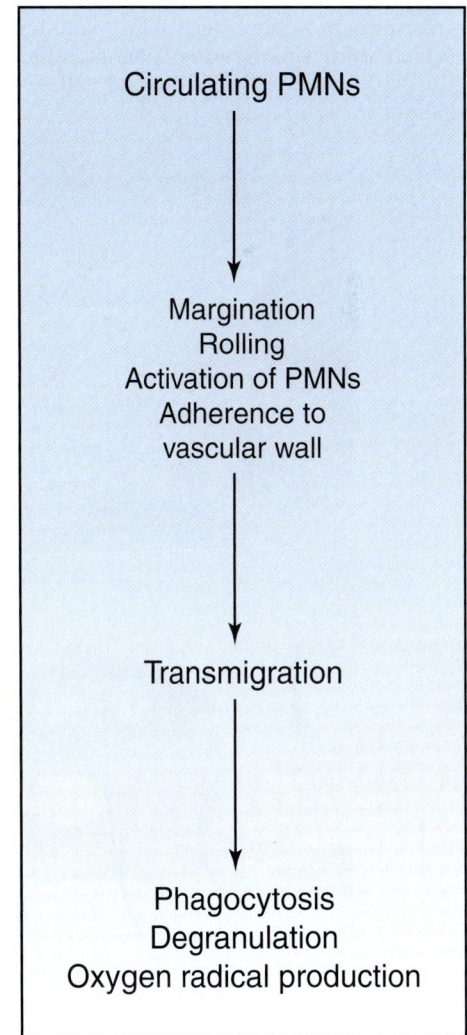

FIGURE 2-30

Leukocyte recruitment and activation.

Inflammation

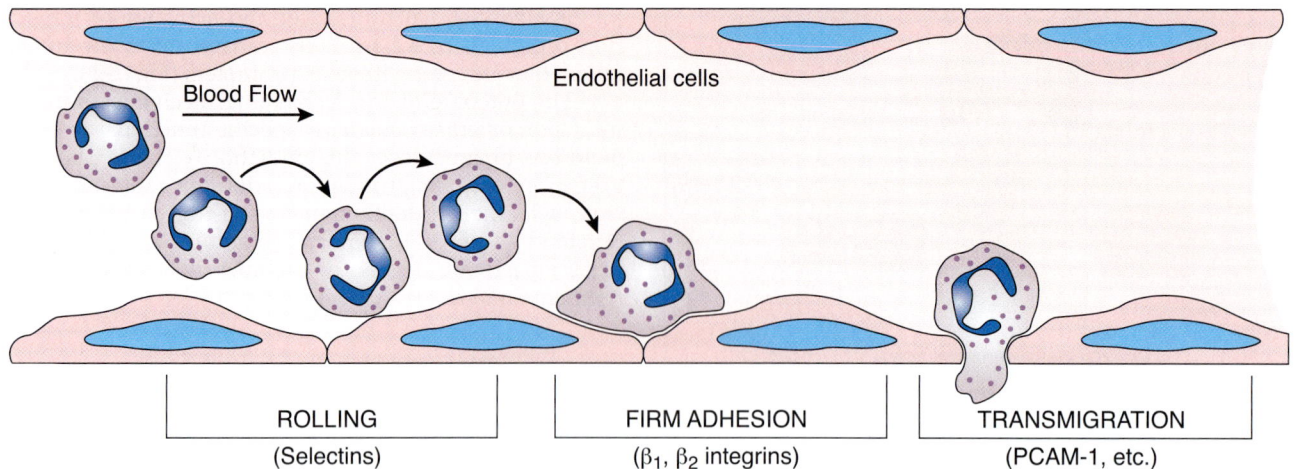

FIGURE 2-31
Mechanisms of leukocyte adherence.

Leukocyte Adhesion to Endothelium Results from Interaction of Complementary Adhesion Molecules

Leukocyte recruitment in the postcapillary venules involves adhesion, which follows a cascade of events initiated by the interaction of leukocytes with endothelial cell selectins, an event referred to as *tethering* (Fig. 2-31). This interaction slows leukocytes in the blood flow, so that they move along the vascular endothelial cell surface with a saltatory movement referred to as *rolling* (Fig. 2-32A). PMNs become activated by proximity to the endothelium and the presence of inflammatory mediators and form strong *adhesion* with the endothelium, resulting in their arrest (Fig. 2-32B). This is followed by *emigration* of leukocytes from the vascular space

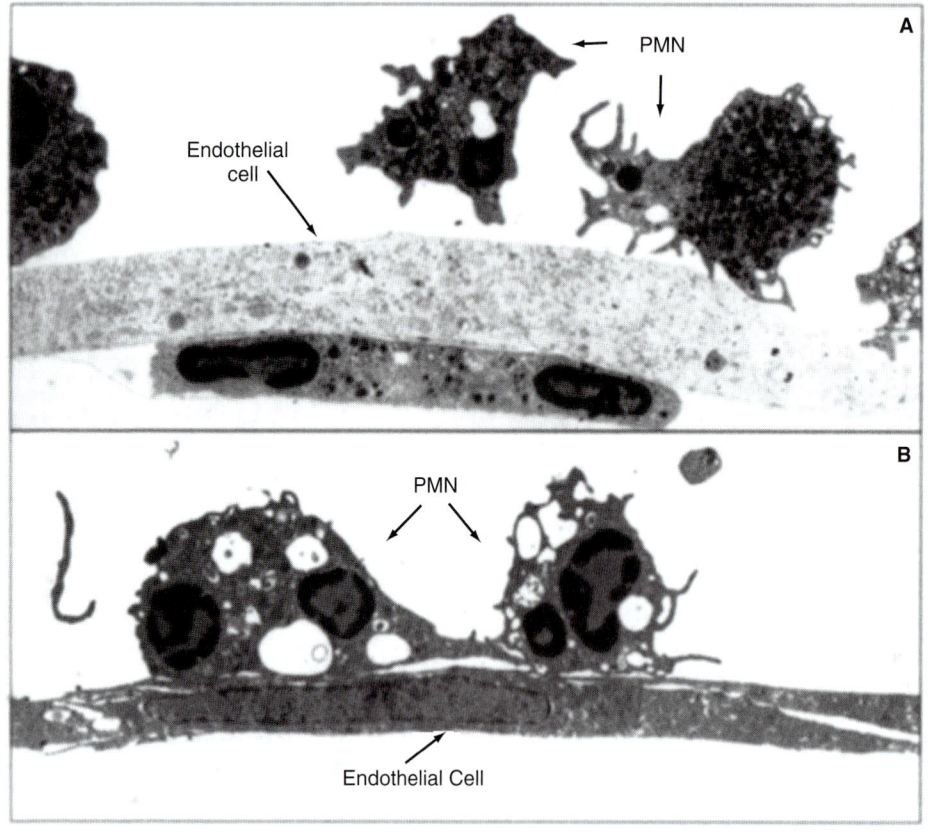

FIGURE 2-32
Leukocyte adhesion to vascular endothelium. A. PMNs roll along the endothelial cell surface. B. Firm adhesion of PMNs to endothelial cell surface.

and migration through extravascular tissue to the site of injury. The events involved in leukocyte recruitment are regulated by (1) expression of adhesion molecules on vascular endothelial cell surfaces, which bind to reciprocal molecules on the surfaces of circulating leukocytes; (2) chemotactic factors, which attract leukocytes along a chemical gradient to the site of injury; and (3) inflammatory mediators, which stimulate resident tissue cells, including vascular endothelial cells.

Adhesion Molecules

Four molecular families of adhesion molecules are involved in leukocyte recruitment (Fig. 2-33).

Selectins

The adhesion molecules in the selectin family include P-selectin, E-selectin, and L-selectin. These are expressed on the surface of platelets, endothelial cells, and leukocytes. The selectins share a similar molecular structure, which includes an extracellular lectin-binding domain. This domain binds to sialylated oligosaccharides, specifically the sialyl-Lewis X moiety on addressins.

P-selectin (CD62P, GMP-140, PADGEM) is preformed and stored within Weibel-Palade bodies of endothelial cells and α-granules of platelets. On stimulation with histamine, thrombin, or specific inflammatory cytokines, P-selectin is rapidly transported to the cell surface, where it binds to sialyl-Lewis X on leukocyte surfaces. Preformed P-selectin can be delivered quickly to the cell surface, allowing rapid adhesive interaction between endothelial cells and leukocytes.

E-selectin (CD62E, ELAM-1) is not normally expressed on endothelial cell surfaces but is induced by inflammatory mediators, such as cytokines or bacterial lipopolysaccharide (LPS). E-selectin mediates adhesion of neutrophils, monocytes, and certain lymphocytes.

L-selectin (CD62L, LAM-1, Leu-8) is expressed on many types of leukocytes and was originally defined as the "homing receptor" for lymphocytes. It serves to bind lymphocytes to high endothelial venules in lymphoid tissue, thereby regulating their trafficking through this tissue.

Addressins

Vascular addressins are mucinlike glycoproteins such as GlyCAM-1, PSGL-1, ESL-1, and CD34. These molecules pos-

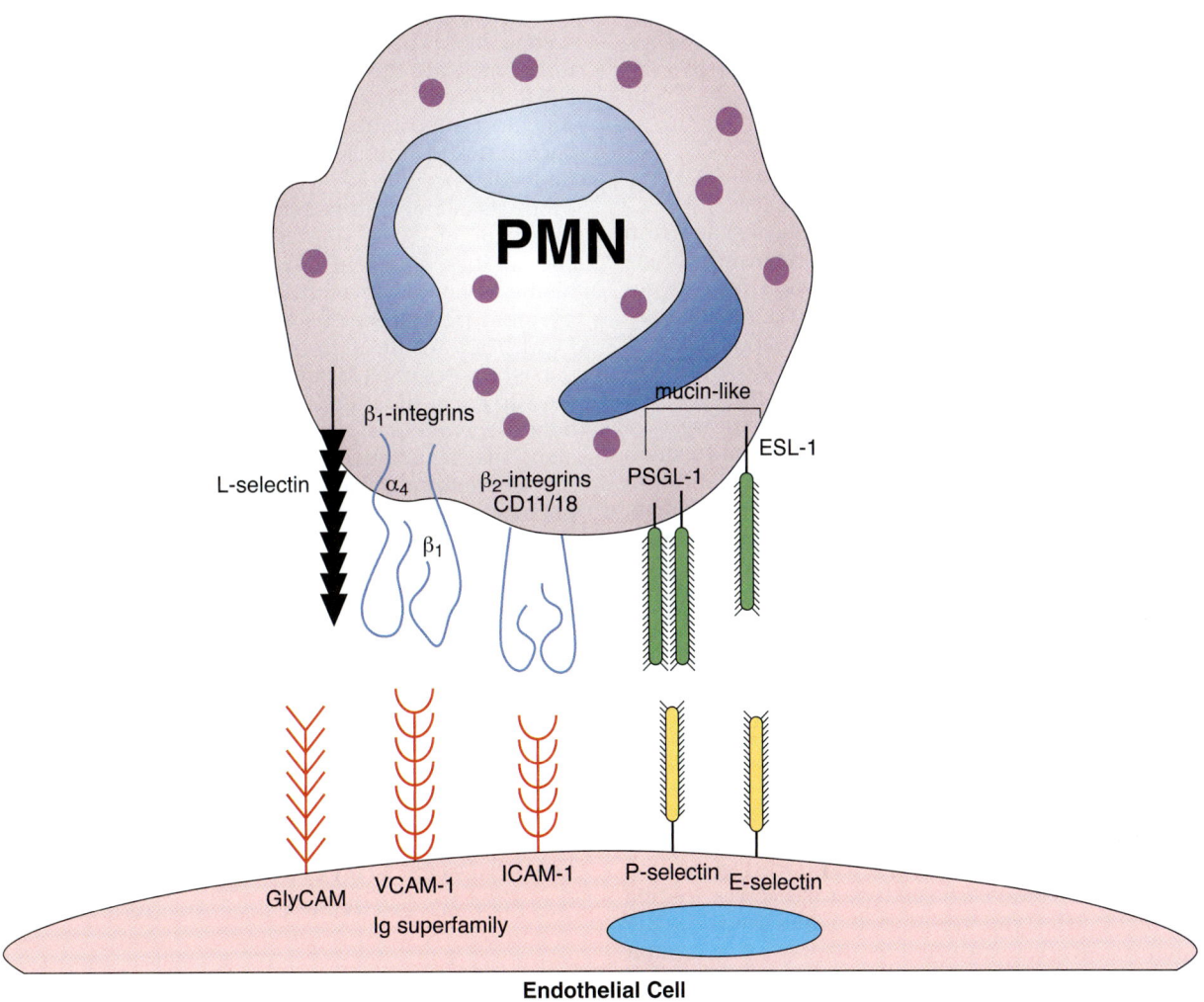

FIGURE 2-33
Leukocyte and endothelial cell adhesion molecules.

sess carbohydrate regions, the sialyl-Lewis X moiety, which binds the lectin domain of selectins. Addressins are expressed on the surface of leukocytes and specific tissue endothelium and regulate the localization of subpopulations of leukocytes. They are also involved in the activation of lymphocytes (see Chapter 4).

Integrins

Chemokines, lipid mediators, and proinflammatory molecules activate a second family of adhesion molecules, the integrins. Integrins consist of transmembrane α and β chains arranged as heterodimers. Molecules in this family participate in cell–cell interactions, as well as cell–ECM binding. The β_1, β_2, and β_7 integrins are involved in leukocyte recruitment. VLA-4 ($\alpha 4\beta 1$) on leukocytes and lymphocytes binds to VCAM-1 on endothelial cells. The $\beta 2$ (CD18) integrins form molecules by association with α integrin chains: $\alpha_1\beta_2$ (also called CD11a/CD18 or LFA-1) and $\alpha_m\beta_2$ (also termed CD11b/CD18 or Mac-1) bind ICAM-1 and ICAM-2.

Immunoglobulins

Adhesion molecules of the immunoglobulin superfamily include ICAM-1, ICAM-2, and VCAM-1, all of which interact with integrins on leukocytes to mediate recruitment. They are expressed on the surfaces of cytokine-stimulated endothelial cells and some leukocytes, as well as certain epithelial cells, such as pulmonary alveolar cells.

Recruitment of Leukocytes

Tethering and rolling, mediated by the selectins, and firm adhesion, involving the integrins, are prerequisites for recruitment of leukocytes from the circulation into tissues and ultimately the inflammatory response. For a rolling cell to adhere, several situations must obtain. First, there must be a reduction in rolling velocity, which may occur by an increase in density of selectins. The early increase in rolling depends on P-selectin, whereas cytokine-induced E-selectin initiates early adhesion. Integrin family members function cooperatively with the selectins to facilitate rolling and firm adhesion of leukocytes, which is crucial for transmigration. Leukocyte integrins bind with the Ig superfamily of ligands expressed on vascular endothelium. These interactions serve further to retard leukocytes, increasing the length of exposure of each leukocyte to the endothelium. The engagement of adhesion molecules also activates intracellular signal transduction pathways by the generation of transmembrane signals. As a result, leukocytes and vascular endothelial cells are further activated, with subsequent upregulation of L-selectin and integrin binding. The net result is firm adhesion.

Recruitment of specific subsets of leukocytes to areas of inflammation may result from unique patterns or relative densities of adhesion molecules on cell surfaces. In the case of subsets of leukocytes, each cell type can express specific adhesion molecules. Cytokines or chemokines specific to the inflammatory process induce the display of adhesion molecules on vascular endothelium and changes in the affinity of these molecules for their ligands (Fig. 2-34). For example, in allergic or asthmatic inflammation, cytokine induction of VCAM-1 on endothelial cells increases the recruitment of the VLA-4–bearing eosinophils in preference to neutrophils, which do not express VLA-4.

Leukocyte recruitment in some tissues may not follow the paradigm just described. In the liver, for example, leukocytes may not need to roll in the narrow sinusoids before adhering to the endothelium. Leukocyte adherence to arterioles and capillaries may also have different requirements, reflecting the different hydrodynamic forces in these vessels.

Chemotactic Molecules Direct Neutrophils to Sites of Injury

Leukocytes must be accurately positioned at the site of inflammatory injury to carry out their biological functions. For specific subsets of leukocytes to present themselves at the site of injury in a timely fashion, they must receive very specific directions. These cells are guided through the vascular and extravascular spaces by a complex interaction of attractants, repellants, and adhesion molecules. *Chemotaxis* refers to the process of directed cell migration, which is a dynamic and energy-dependent activity. Leukocytes recruited from the blood by chemoattractants released by endothelial cells subsequently migrate away from the endothelium toward the target tissue. They travel down a functional gradient of one chemoattractant in response to a second more distal chemoattractant gradient. Neutrophils must integrate the various signals to arrive at the correct site and at the correct time to perform their assigned tasks. The most important chemotactic factors for PMNs are C5a, bacterial and mitochondrial products (particularly low-molecular-weight N-formylated peptides such as FMLP, products of arachidonic acid metabolism, (especially LTB$_4$), products of ECM degradation, and chemokines. The chemokines represent one of the most important mechanisms of leukocyte recruitment because they generate a chemotactic gradient by binding to proteoglycans of the ECM. As a result, high concentrations of the chemokines persist at sites of tissue injury. In turn, specific receptors on the surface of the migrating leukocytes bind to the matrix-bound chemokines, a process that tends to move the cells along the chemotactic gradient to the site of injury.

Chemotactic factors for other cell types, including lymphocytes, basophils, and eosinophils, are also produced at sites of tissue injury and may be secreted by activated endothelial cells, tissue parenchymal cells, or other inflammatory cells. They include PAF, transforming growth factor-β (TGF-β), neutrophilic cationic proteins, and lymphokines. The cocktail of chemokines presented within a tissue largely determines the type of leukocyte attracted to the site. Cells arriving at their destination must then be able to stop in the target tissue. Contact guidance, regulated adhesion, or inhibitory signals may determine the final arrest of specific cells in specific tissue locations.

Leukocytes Traverse the Endothelial Cell Barrier to Gain Access to the Tissue

Diapedesis

Leukocytes adherent to the vascular endothelium emigrate by passing between adjacent endothelial cells, a process

Leukocyte Recruitment in Acute Inflammation

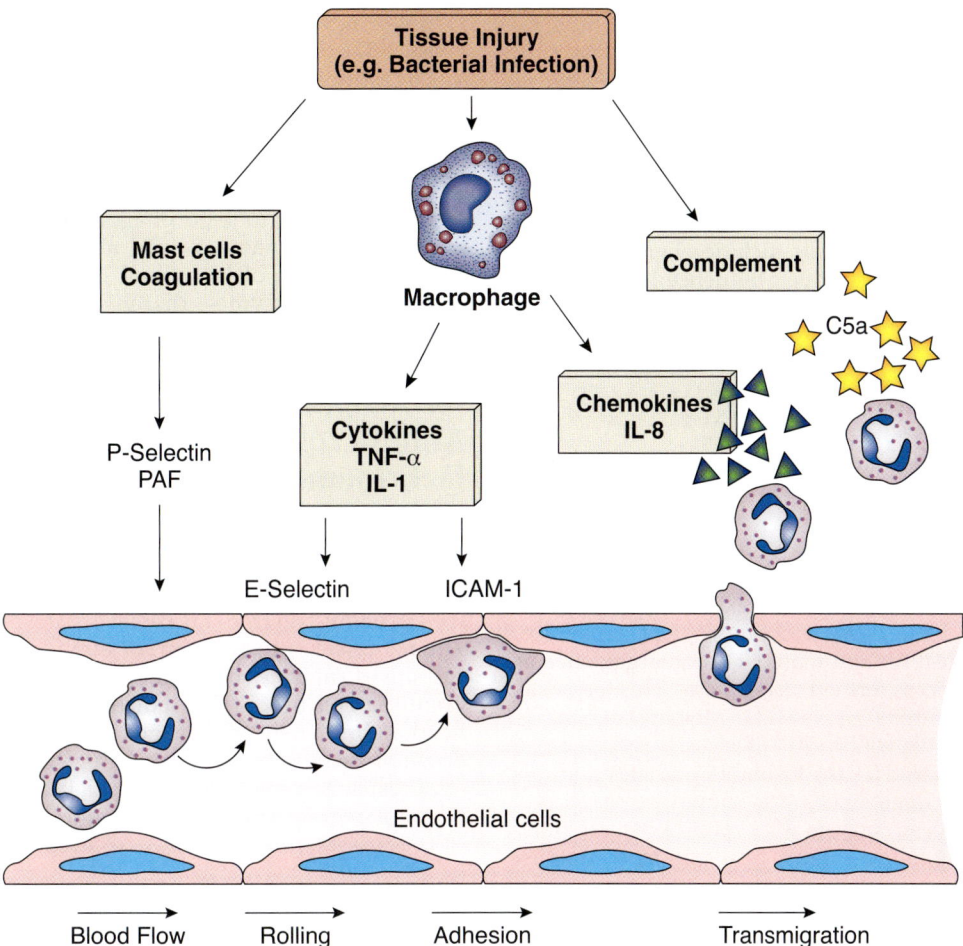

FIGURE 2-34
Regulation of leukocyte recruitment.

called *paracellular diapedesis*. Acting in response to chemokine gradients, neutrophils extend pseudopods and insinuate themselves between the cells and out of the vascular space (Fig. 2-35). Vascular endothelial cells are connected by tight junctions and adherens junctions. Both junctions separate under the influence of inflammatory mediators, intracellular signals generated by adhesion molecule engagement, and signals from the adherent neutrophils. Neutrophils mobilize elastase to their pseudopod membranes, inducing endothelial cell retraction at the advancing portion of the neutrophil. These cells also induce increases in endothelial cell intracellular calcium, to which they respond by pulling apart.

Neutrophils can also migrate through endothelial cells, by *transcellular diapedesis*. PMNs can traverse the endothelial cell cytoplasm, squeezing through small circular pores rather than inducing endothelial cell retraction. In certain tissues, such as gastrointestinal mucosa and secretory glands, which contain fenestrated microvessels, PMNs may traverse thin regions of the endothelium called *fenestrae*, without damaging the endothelial cell. In nonfenestrated microvessels, PMNs may cross the endothelium using endothelial cell caveolae or pinocytotic vesicles, which form small, membrane-bound passageways across the cell.

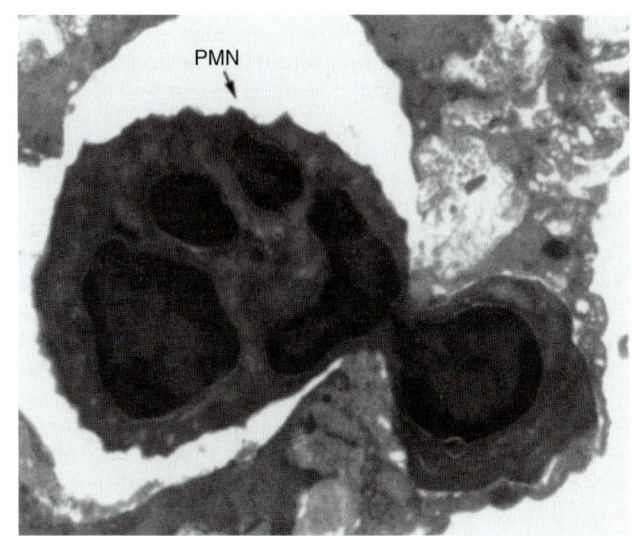

FIGURE 2-35
Leukocyte transmigration. PMN exiting the vascular space by diapedesis across the vascular endothelium.

Tissue Interaction

The selective accumulation of leukocyte subsets at sites of inflammation depends primarily on signals at the blood–endothelial cell interface. Selection also occurs within the tissue stroma itself. After crossing the endothelial cells, leukocytes encounter a stromal microenvironment in which they must interact with cells and the ECM, adhere, and become stationary. Local signals include chemokines, cytokines, and growth factors, which influence leukocytes to anchor within tissue and become further activated.

LEUKOCYTE FUNCTIONS IN ACUTE INFLAMMATION

Leukocytes Phagocytose Microorganisms and Tissue Debris

Many inflammatory cells, including monocytes, tissue macrophages, dendritic cells, and neutrophils, recognize, internalize, and digest foreign material, microorganisms, or cellular debris, a process termed *phagocytosis*. This term was first used over a century ago by Elie Metchnikoff and is now defined as the ingestion by eukaryotic cells of large (generally greater than 0.5 μm) insoluble particles and microorganisms. The effector cells are known as *phagocytes*. The phagocytic process consists of several transmembrane and intracellular signaling events, resulting in a complex sequence.

1. **Recognition:** (Fig. 2-36) Phagocytosis is initiated by the recognition of particles by specific receptors on the surface of the phagocytic cell. The phagocytosis of most biological agents is enhanced by, if not dependent on, their coating (opsonization) with plasma components (opsonins), particularly immunoglobulins or the C3b fragment of complement. Phagocytic cells possess specific opsonic receptors, including those for immunoglobulin Fcγ and complement components. Many pathogens, however, have developed mechanisms to evade phagocytosis by leukocytes. Polysaccharide capsules, protein A, protein M, or peptidoglycans around the bacteria can prevent complement deposition or antigen recognition and receptor binding.
2. **Signaling:** Clustering of opsonins on the bacterial surface results in clustering of the Fcγ receptors in the phagocyte plasma membrane. Subsequent phosphorylation of immunoreceptor tyrosine-based activation motifs (ITAMs), located in the cytosolic domain or γ subunit of the receptor, trigger intracellular signaling events. Tyrosine kinases that associate with the Fcγ receptor are required for signaling during phagocytosis (Fig. 2-37).
3. **Internalization:** In the case of either Fcγ receptor or CR3, actin assembly occurs directly under the phagocytosed target. Polymerized actin filaments push the plasma membrane forward, resulting in formation of a phagocytic cup and engulfment of the foreign agent by the cell membrane. This process involves remodeling of the plasma membrane to increase surface area and to allow the plasma membrane to form pseudopods surrounding the foreign material. "Zippering" of the membrane around the opsonized particle encloses the foreign material in a cytoplasmic vacuole termed a *phagosome* (Figs. 2-36, 2-37).
4. **Digestion:** The phagosome containing the foreign particle or microorganism fuses with cytoplasmic lysosomal granules to form a *phagolysosome*, into which the lysosomal enzymes are released. These hydrolytic enzymes are activated by the acid pH within the phagolysosome, after which they degrade the phagocytosed material. Some microorganisms have evolved mechanisms for preventing degranulation of lysosomal granules or for inhibiting neutrophil enzymes, thereby evading killing by neutrophils.

Neutrophil Enzymes Are Required for Antimicrobial Defense and Debridement.

Although PMNs are critical in the degradation of microbes and cell debris, they also contribute to tissue injury (Fig. 2-38). Cell- and plasma-derived inflammatory mediators, as well as endotoxin from microbial organisms, activate PMNs. The net result is recruitment of these inflammatory cells to the site of injury, where they release the contents of their granules. This process has a dichotomous result. On the one hand, debridement of damaged tissue by proteolytic breakdown of tissue is beneficial. On the other hand, tissue damage is caused by injury to endothelial and epithelial cells and ongoing degradation of connective tissue.

Neutrophil Granules

The armamentarium of enzymes required for the degradation of microbes and tissue is generated and contained within the distinct granules in the cytoplasm of PMNs. These primary, secondary, and tertiary granules are differentiated morphologically and biochemically, each granule displaying a unique spectrum of enzymes (see Fig. 2-20).

- **Primary granules (azurophilic granules):** The constituents of these granules have antimicrobial and proteinase activity and can directly activate other inflammatory cells. Potent acid hydrolases and neutral serine proteases digest a wide variety of macromolecules. Lysozyme and PLA$_2$ are antimicrobial enzymes that degrade bacterial cell walls and biological membranes and are important in killing bacteria. Myeloperoxidase, which is key to the metabolism of hydrogen peroxide, leads to the generation of toxic oxygen radicals.
- **Secondary granules (specific granules):** These structures contain PLA$_2$ and lysozyme. In addition, their contents include the cationic protein, lactoferrin, a vitamin B$_{12}$-binding protein, and a matrix metalloproteinase (collagenase) specific for type IV collagen. Also present in these granules are proteins that initiate the killing of specific cells.
- **Tertiary granules (small storage granules, C granules):** These granules contain the proteinases cathepsin, gelatinase, and urokinase-type plasminogen activator (u-PA). Tertiary granules are released at the leading front of neutrophils during chemotaxis and are the source of enzymes that promote the migration of cells through basement membranes and tissues. Similar granules are present in monocytes and macrophages.

Leukocyte Functions in Acute Inflammation

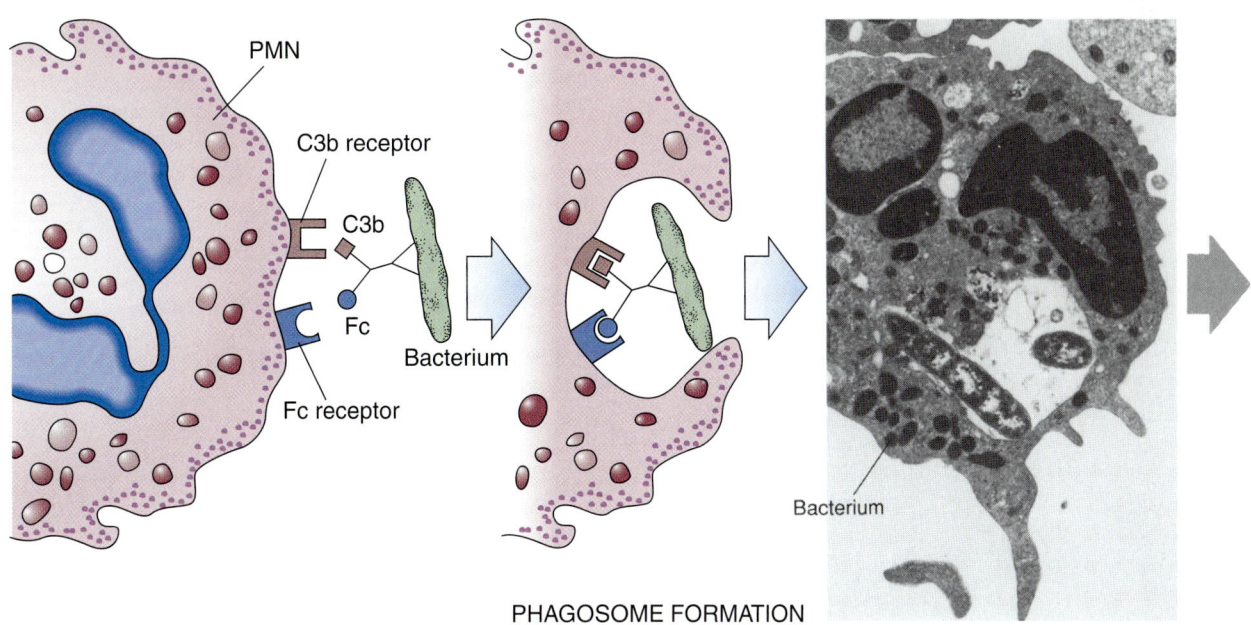

PHAGOSOME FORMATION

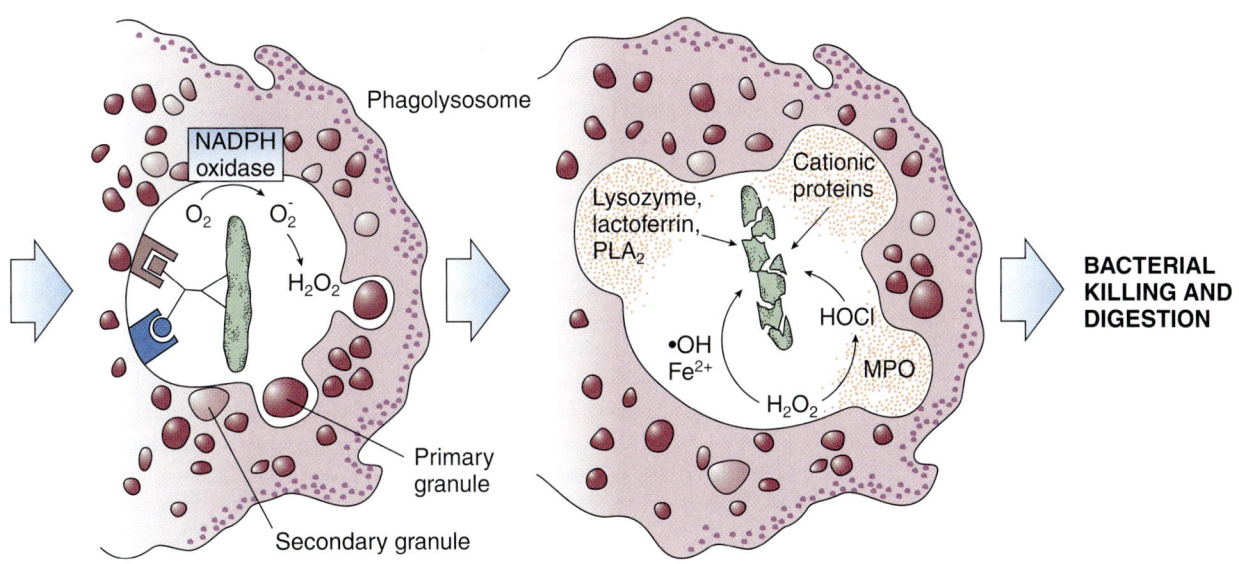

DEGRANULATION AND NADPH OXIDASE ACTIVATION

FIGURE 2-36
Mechanisms of PMN bacterial phagocytosis and cell killing.

Proteinases

Proteolytic enzymes (proteinases) are stored in cytoplasmic granules and secretory vesicles of neutrophils. As these cells emerge from the circulation, released proteinases enable them to penetrate the ECM and migrate to sites of injury. At the site of damaged tissue, they degrade the matrix, cell debris, and pathogens. Neutrophils, however, are not the only source of proteinases. These enzymes are also expressed by most inflammatory cells, including monocytes, eosinophils, basophils, mast cells, and lymphocytes. Moreover, they are produced by tissue cells, including vascular endothelial cells.

Proteinases are enzymes that cleave peptide bonds in polypeptides. They are classified into four groups by their catalytic activity: serine proteinases and metalloproteinases are neutral enzymes capable of activity in extracellular spaces; cysteine proteinases and aspartic proteinases are acidic and function within the acidic environment of lysosomes (Table 2-3).

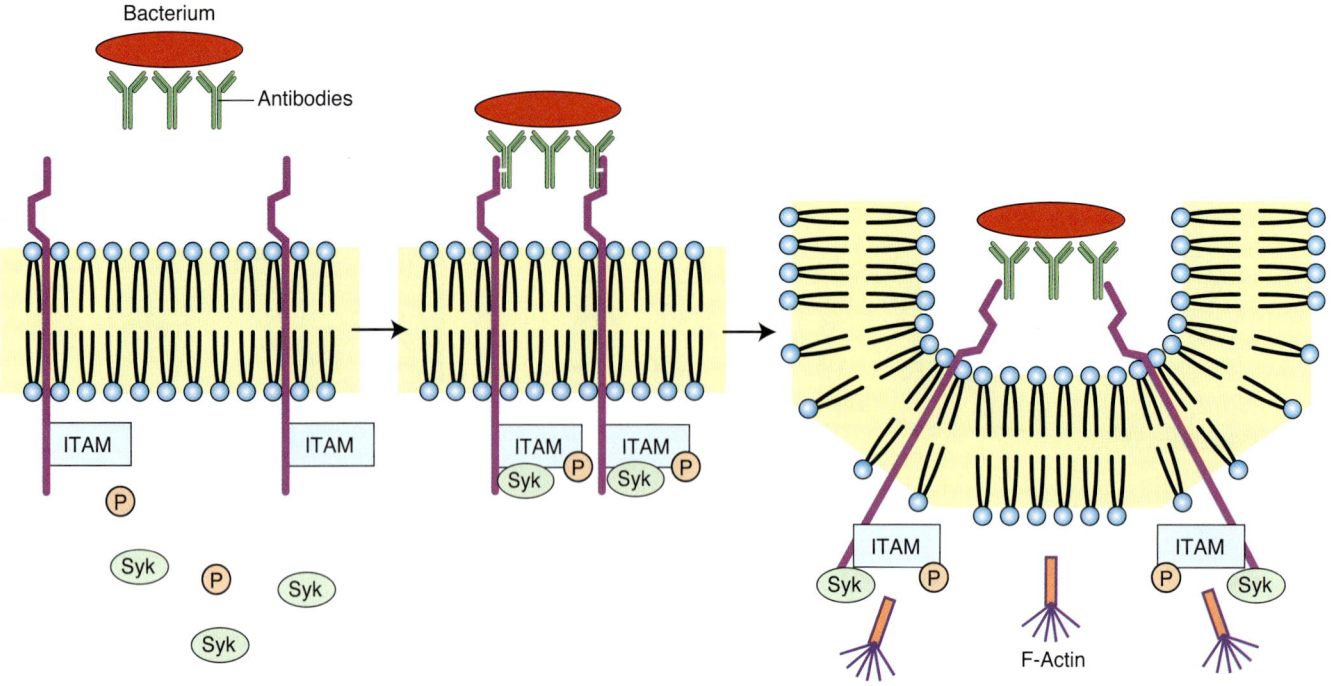

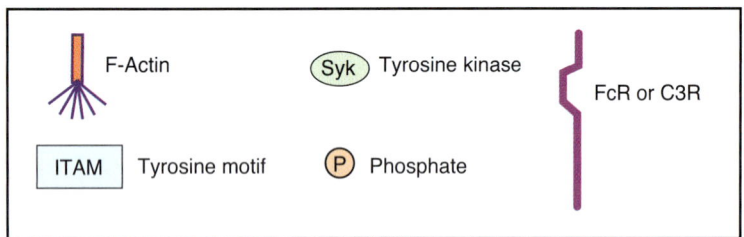

FIGURE 2-37
Intracellular signaling during leukocyte phagocytosis.

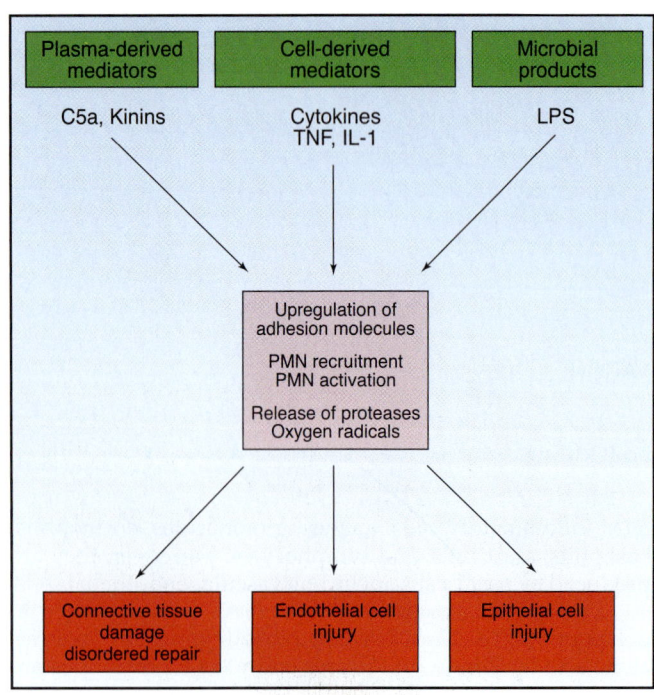

FIGURE 2-38
Leukocyte-mediated inflammatory injury.

TABLE 2-3 Proteinases in Inflammation

Enzyme Class	Examples
Neutral Proteinases	
Serine proteinases	Human leukocyte elastase
	Cathepsin G
	Proteinase 3
	Urokinase-type plasminogen activator
Metalloproteinase	Collagenases (MMP-1, MMP-8, MMP-13)
	Gelatinases (MMP-7, MMP-9)
	Stromelysins (MMP-3, MMP-10, MMP-11)
	Matrilysin (MMP-7)
	Metalloelastase (MMP-12)
	ADAMs-7,-9,-15,-17
Acidic Proteinases	
Cysteine proteinases	Cathepsins, S, L, B, H
Aspartic proteinases	Cathepsin D

MMP: matrix metalloproteinase
ADAM: proteins with *A* Disintegrin and *A* Metalloproteinase domain

These enzymes target a variety of intracellular and extracellular proteins, including:

- Inflammatory products, debris from damaged cells, microbial proteins, and matrix proteins
- Microorganisms
- Plasma proteins, including complement components, clotting factors, immunoglobulins, and cytokines
- Matrix macromolecules (e.g., collagen, elastin, fibronectin, and laminin)
- Lymphocytes and platelets, which are activated by proteinases

Serine Proteinases

Stored as active enzymes within leukocyte granules, serine proteinases degrade a wide variety of extracellular proteins, cell debris and bacteria. Human leukocyte elastase (HLE) is primarily responsible for fibronectin degradation. Cathepsin G (CG) converts angiotensin I to angiotensin II, thereby mediating smooth muscle contraction and vascular permeability. Proteinase 3 (PR3) has antigenic properties related to Wegener granulomatosis. u-PA dissolves fibrin clots, generating plasmin at wound sites. This enzyme plays a key role in leukocyte migration from the vasculature, degrading ECM proteins and activating procollagenases to create a path for leukocytes. Although the serine proteinases are most important for their role in digesting ECM molecules, modification of cytokine activity is an equally significant function. Serine proteases solubilize membrane-bound cytokines and receptors by cleaving active cytokines from their inactive precursors. They also detach cytokine receptors from cell surfaces, thereby regulating cytokine bioactivity.

Metalloproteinases

The metalloproteinase class of enzymes is expanding, with at least 25 members now identified. Matrix metalloproteinases (MMPs, matrixins) degrade all components of the ECM, including basement membranes. They are subclassified according to their substrate specificity into interstitial collagenases, gelatinases, stromelysins, metalloelastases, and matrilysin. Proteins with disintegrin and metalloproteinase domains (ADAMs) regulate neutrophil infiltration by targeting the disintegrins. These molecules are polypeptides that disrupt integrin-mediated binding of cells to each other and to the matrix.

Cysteine Proteinases and Aspartic Proteinases

These acid proteinases function primarily within the lysosomes of leukocytes to degrade intracellular proteins.

Proteinase Inhibitors

The proteolytic environment is regulated by a battery of inhibitors synthesized by inflammatory and tissue cells and present in body fluids and tissue spaces. During wound healing, these antiproteases protect against damage by limiting the activity of proteases. Remodeling of the ECM occurs within the context of the balance between enzymes and inhibitors. In chronic wounds, the continuous influx of neutrophils, with their proteases and reactive oxygen species, overwhelms and inactivates these inhibitors, allowing continuation of proteolysis (see Chapter 3). Known proteinase inhibitors include the following:

- **α_2-Macroglobulin:** nonspecific inhibitor of all classes of proteinases, primarily found in plasma
- **Serpins:** The major inhibitors of serine proteinases
- **α_1-Antiproteases (α_1-antitrypsin, α_1-antichymotrypsin):** Inhibit human leukocyte elastase and cathepsin G
- **Secretory leukocyte proteinase inhibitor (SLPI), Elafin:** Inhibit proteinase 3
- **Plasminogen activator inhibitors (PAIs):** Inhibit u-PA
- **Tissue inhibitors of metalloproteinases (TIMP-1,-2,-3,-4):** Specific for matrix metalloproteinases in tissue

Inflammatory Cells Have Oxidative and Nonoxidative Bactericidal Activity

The bactericidal activity of PMNs and macrophages is mediated in part by the production of reactive oxygen species and in part by oxygen-independent mechanisms.

Bacterial Killing by Oxygen Species

Phagocytosis is accompanied by metabolic reactions within inflammatory cells that lead to the production of a number of oxygen metabolites (see Chapter 1). These products are more reactive than oxygen itself and contribute to the killing of ingested bacteria (Table 2-4).

- **Superoxide anion** (O_2^-): The process of phagocytosis activates a NADPH oxidase in the cell membrane of PMNs. NADPH oxidase is a multicomponent electron transport complex that reduces molecular oxygen to O_2^-. The activation of this enzyme is enhanced by prior exposure of the cells to a chemotactic stimulus or bacterial lipopolysaccharide. NADPH oxidase activation is associated with an increase in oxygen consumption and the stimulation of the hexose monophosphate shunt. Together, these cell responses are referred to as the *respiratory burst*.
- **Hydrogen peroxide** (H_2O_2): O_2^- is rapidly converted to H_2O_2 by superoxide dismutase at the cell surface and within phagolysosomes. H_2O_2 is stable and serves as a substrate for the generation of additional reactive oxidants.
- **Hypochlorous acid:** Myeloperoxidase (MPO), a neutrophil product with a very strong cationic charge, is secreted from granules during exocytosis and catalyzes the conversion of H_2O_2, in the presence of a halide, to form hypochlorous acid. The most prominent halogen in biological systems is chlorine, and thus hypochlorous acid (HOCl) is produced following neutrophil stimulation.

TABLE 2-4 **Reactions Involving Reactive Oxygen Metabolites Produced by Phagocytic Cells**

Reduction of molecular oxygen	
$O_2 + e^- \rightarrow O_2^-$	Superoxide anion
Dismutation of O_2^-	
$O_2^- + O_2^- + 2H^- \rightarrow O_2 + H_2O_2$	Hydrogen peroxide
Haber-Weiss Reaction	
$H_2O_2 + O_2^- + H^+ \rightarrow OH^\cdot + H_2O + O_2$	Hydroxyl radical
Fenton reaction (iron-catalyzed)	
$H_2O_2 + Fe^{2+} \rightarrow Fe^{3+} + OH^- + \cdot OH$	Hydroxyl radical
Myeloperoxidase reaction	
$H_2O_2 + Cl^- + H^- \rightleftharpoons HOCl + H_2O$	Hypochlorous acid

This powerful oxidant is a major bactericidal agent produced by phagocytic cells. In addition, HOCl also participates in the activation of neutrophil-derived collagenase and gelatinase, both of which are secreted as latent enzymes. HOCl also inactivates α_1-antitrypsin.

- **Hydroxyl radical (•OH):** Reduction of H_2O_2 occurs through the Haber-Weiss reaction to form the highly reactive hydroxyl radical (•OH). Although this reaction occurs slowly at physiological pH, in the presence of ferrous iron (Fe^{2+}) the Fenton reaction rapidly converts H_2O_2 to •OH, a radical with potent bactericidal activity. Further reduction of •OH leads to the formation of H_2O.
- **Nitric oxide (NO•):** Phagocytic cells as well as vascular endothelial cells produce nitric oxide (NO•) and its derivatives, which have a remarkable range of physiological and nonphysiological effects. NO• and other oxygen radical species interact with one another to balance their cytotoxic and cytoprotective effects. NO• can react with oxygen radicals to form toxic molecules such as peroxynitrite and *S*-nitrosothiols or it can scavenge O_2^-, thereby reducing the amount of toxic radicals.

Monocytes, macrophages, and eosinophils also produce oxygen radicals, depending on their state of activation and the stimulus to which they are exposed. The production of reactive oxygen metabolites by these cells has been implicated in their bactericidal and fungicidal activity, as well as in their ability to kill certain parasites. The importance of oxygen-dependent mechanisms in the bacterial killing by phagocytic cells is exemplified in chronic granulomatous disease of childhood. Children with this disease suffer from a hereditary deficiency of NADPH oxidase, resulting in a failure to produce superoxide anion and hydrogen peroxide during phagocytosis. Persons with this disorder are susceptible to recurrent infections, especially with gram-positive cocci. Similarly, patients deficient in myeloperoxidase cannot produce HOCl and experience an increased susceptibility to infections with the fungal pathogen *Candida* (Table 2-5).

Nonoxidative Bacterial Killing

Phagocytic cells, particularly PMNs and monocyte/macrophages, exhibit substantial antimicrobial activity that is oxygen independent. This activity relies principally on a number of bactericidal proteins that are preformed constituents of cytoplasmic granules. These include many lysosomal acid hydrolases and specialized noncatalytic proteins with microbicidal activity unique to inflammatory cells.

- **Lysosomal hydrolases:** The primary and secondary granules of neutrophils and the lysosomes of mononuclear phagocytes contain various hydrolases that possess antimicrobial activity, including proteases, lipases, hydrolases active against polysaccharides and DNA, and other enzymes, such as sulfatases and phosphatases.
- **Bactericidal/permeability-increasing protein (BPI):** This cationic protein in the primary granules of PMNs is potently bactericidal toward many gram-negative bacteria but is not toxic to gram-positive bacteria or to eukaryotic cells. BPI inserts into the outer membrane of the bacterial envelope and increases its permeability. Activation of certain phospholipases and enzymes then degrade the bacterial peptidylglycans.
- **Defensins:** Primary granules of PMNs and the lysosomes of some mononuclear phagocytes contain a family of cationic proteins, termed *defensins*, which kill a wide variety of gram-positive and gram-negative bacteria, fungi, and some enveloped viruses. Some of these polypeptides also can kill host cells in a manner that depends on the active metabolism of the target tissue. Defensins are chemotactic for phagocytic leukocytes, immature dendritic cells, and lymphocytes, thereby participating in mobilizing and amplifying antimicrobial immunity.
- **Lactoferrin:** Lactoferrin is an iron-binding glycoprotein contained in the secondary granules of neutrophils. It is also present in most secretory fluids in the body. Its antimicrobial properties are related to its iron-chelating capacity, which allows it to compete with bacteria for iron. In addition, lactoferrin may also participate in oxidative killing of bacteria by enhancing •OH formation.
- **Lysozyme:** This bactericidal enzyme is found in many tissues and fluids in the body and is contained in primary and secondary granules of neutrophils and in the lysosomes of mononuclear phagocytes. The peptidoglycans of gram-positive bacterial cell walls are exquisitely sensitive to degradation by lysozyme; gram-negative bacteria are as a rule resistant to its action.
- **Bactericidal proteins of eosinophils:** Eosinophils contain several granule-bound cationic proteins, the most important of which are major basic protein (MBP) and eosinophilic cationic protein. MBP accounts for about half of the total protein of the eosinophil granule. Both proteins are ineffective against bacteria but are potent cytotoxic agents for many parasites.

TABLE 2-5 Congenital Diseases of Defective Phagocytic Cell Function Characterized by Recurrent Bacterial Infections

Disease	Defect
Leukocyte adhesion deficiency	LAD-1 defective B2-integrin expression or function (CD11/CD18)
	LAD-2 (defective fucosylation, selectin binding)
Hyper-IgE-recurrent infection, (Job) syndrome	Poor chemotaxis
Chediak-Higashi syndrome	Defective lysosomal granules, poor chemotaxis
Neutrophil-specific granule deficiency	Absent neutrophil granules
Chronic granulomatous disease	Deficient NADPH oxidase, with absent H_2O_2 production
Myeloperoxidase deficiency	Deficient HOCl production

Defects in Leukocyte Function

The importance of protection afforded by acute inflammatory cells is emphasized by the frequency and severity of infections in persons with defective phagocytic cells. **The most common defect is actually iatrogenic neutropenia secondary to cancer chemotherapy.** Functional impairment of phagocytic cells may occur almost anywhere in the sequence that includes adherence, emigration, chemotaxis, and phagocytosis. These disorders may be acquired or congenital. Acquired diseases, such as leukemia, diabetes mellitus, malnutrition, viral infections, and sepsis, are often accompanied by defects in inflammatory cell function. Representative examples of congenital diseases linked to defective phagocytic function are shown in Table 2-5.

REGULATION OF INFLAMMATION

The plasma- and cell-derived proinflammatory mediators described above amplify the tissue response and represent a positive feedback loop, with a progressive amplification of the response and subsequent tissue injury. If left unchecked, this intense inflammatory injury leads to organ failure. Complement factors, proinflammatory cytokines, and, in some cases, immune complexes activate signal transduction pathways that control gene expression of proinflammatory mediators, including TNF-α, IL-1, chemokines, and adhesion molecules (Figs. 2-27 to 2-29). Secreted cytokines then propagate the response by activating other cell types, using these and similar pathways.

The response of cells and tissues is primarily in a proinflammatory direction. Endogenous mediators however, control the extent of inflammatory injury by negative feedback inhibition of proinflammatory gene transcription, thereby preventing uncontrolled inflammation. The following are particularly important in the regulation of inflammation:

- **Cytokines:** IL-6, IL-10, IL-11, IL-12, and IL-13 are among the cytokines that limit inflammation by reducing the production of the powerful proinflammatory cytokine, TNF-α. In some instances, this effect occurs because the degradation of the NF-κB inhibitory component IκB is prevented, thereby inhibiting cell activation and the further release of inflammatory mediators.
- **Protease inhibitors:** SLPI and TIMP-2 are particularly important in reducing the responses of a variety of cell types, including macrophages and endothelial cells, and in decreasing connective tissue damage.
- **Lipoxins:** Lipoxins and aspirin-triggered lipoxins are antiinflammatory lipid mediators that inhibit leukotriene biosynthesis.
- **Glucocorticoids:** Stimulation of the hypothalamic-pituitary-adrenal axis results in the release of immunosuppressive glucocorticoids.
- **Kininases:** The potent proinflammatory mediator bradykinin is degraded by kininases in plasma and blood.
- **Phosphatases:** One of the most common mechanisms used by signal transduction pathways that regulate inflammatory cell signaling is rapid and reversible protein phosphorylation (Fig. 2-27). Phosphatases and their associated regulatory proteins provide a balancing dephosphorylating system.

OUTCOMES OF ACUTE INFLAMMATION

As a result of regulatory components and the short life span of neutrophils, acute inflammatory reactions are usually self-limiting and resolve. This resolution involves removal of dead cells, clearance of acute response cells, and regrowth of the stroma. Activation of the inflammatory response results in a number of distinct outcomes:

- **Resolution:** Under ideal conditions the source of the tissue injury is eliminated, the inflammatory response resolves, and normal tissue architecture and physiological function are restored. The progression of inflammation depends on the balance of cell recruitment, cell division, cell emigration, and cell death. For tissue to return to normal, this process must be reversed: the stimulus to injury removed, proinflammatory signals turned off, acute inflammatory cell influx ended, tissue fluid balance restored, cell and tissue debris removed, normal vascular function restored, epithelial barriers repaired, and the ECM regenerated. As the signals for acute inflammation decrease, apoptosis of PMNs limits the immune response and triggers this resolution phase.
- **Abscess:** If the area of acute inflammation is walled off by inflammatory cells and fibrosis, destruction of the tissue by products of PMNs takes place, forming an abscess.
- **Scar:** If the tissue is irreversibly injured, the normal architecture is often replaced by a scar, despite elimination of the initial pathological insult.
- **Lymphadenitis:** Localized acute inflammation and chronic inflammation both lead to a reaction in the lymphatics and lymph nodes that drain the affected tissue. Severe injury causes secondary inflammation of the lymphatic channels (*lymphangitis*) and lymph nodes (*lymphadenitis*). Clinically, the inflamed lymphatic channels in the skin manifest as red streaks, and the lymph nodes themselves are enlarged and painful. Microscopically, the lymph nodes exhibit hyperplasia of the lymphoid follicles and proliferation of mononuclear phagocytes in the sinuses (*sinus histiocytosis*).
- **Persistent inflammation:** Failure to eliminate the pathological insult or inability to trigger resolution results in persistence of the inflammatory reaction. This may be evident as a prolonged acute response, with continued influx of neutrophils and tissue destruction, or more commonly as chronic inflammation.

CHRONIC INFLAMMATION

When the resolution phase of acute inflammation is prevented or becomes disordered, chronic inflammation occurs. In this setting, there is persistence of inflammatory cells, a hyperplastic stromal response, and ultimately tissue destruction and scarring. The end-result is organ dysfunction due to loss of normal tissue integrity.

Acute inflammation and chronic inflammation represent ends of a dynamic continuum, in which the morphological features of these inflammatory responses frequently overlap: (1) inflammation, with recruitment of chronic inflammatory cells is followed by (2) tissue injury due to prolongation of the inflammatory response, and (3) repair, which is often a disordered attempt to restore tissue integrity. The events leading to an amplified inflammatory response resemble those of acute inflammation in a number of aspects:

- **Specific triggers,** microbial products or injury, initiate the response.
- **Chemical mediators** direct recruitment, activation, and interaction of inflammatory cells. Activation of the coag-

ulation and complement cascades generate small peptides that function to prolong the inflammatory response.
- **Inflammatory cells** are recruited from the vascular circulation. Cellular interactions between lymphocytes, macrophages, dendritic cells, and fibroblasts generate antigen-specific responses.
- **Stromal cell activation and extracellular matrix** remodeling occur, both of which affect the cellular immune response. Varying degrees of fibrosis may result, depending on the extent of tissue injury and the persistence of the pathological stimulus and inflammatory response.

Although chronic inflammation is not synonymous with chronic infection, the process may become chronic if the inflammatory response cannot eliminate the injurious agent. It may also be a sequel to acute inflammation or an immune response to a foreign antigen. Signals that result in an extended response include:

- **Parasites, bacteria, and viruses:** These agents can provide the signals for persistence of the inflammatory response, which in this case is directed toward isolating the organism from the host.
- **Trauma:** Extensive tissue damage releases mediators capable of inducing an extended inflammatory response.
- **Cancer:** The presence of chronic inflammatory cells, especially macrophages and T lymphocytes, is the morphological expression of an immune response to malignant cells. Chemotherapy may cause suppression of the normal inflammatory response, resulting in increased susceptibility to infection.
- **Immune factors:** Many autoimmune diseases, including rheumatoid arthritis, chronic thyroiditis, and primary biliary cirrhosis, are characterized by a chronic inflammatory response in the affected tissues. This condition may be associated with the activation of both antibody-dependent and cell-mediated immune mechanisms (see chapter 4). It is thought that the autoimmune response accounts for cellular injury in the affected organs.

CELLS INVOLVED IN CHRONIC INFLAMMATION

The cellular components of the chronic inflammatory response include cells recruited from the circulation (macrophages, plasma cells, lymphocytes, and eosinophils) and tissue cells (fibroblasts and vascular endothelial cells).

Monocyte/Macrophages

Macrophages accumulate through the recruitment of circulating monocytes in response to chemotactic stimuli and their differentiation into tissue macrophages (see Fig. 2-23). The proliferation of resident tissue macrophages also contributes to the local increase in mononuclear phagocytes. The macrophage is the pivotal cell in regulating the reactions that lead to chronic inflammation, since it functions as a source of both inflammatory and immunological mediators. In addition, macrophages regulate lymphocyte responses to antigens and secrete other mediators that modulate the proliferation and function of fibroblasts and endothelial cells (Fig. 2-39).

Within different tissues, resident macrophages differ in their armamentarium of enzymes and can respond to local inflammatory signals. Blood monocytes contain granules with serine proteinases similar to those found in neutrophils. As monocytes circulate in the vascular system, they synthesize additional enzymes, particularly MMPs. When monocytes enter tissue and further differentiate to become macrophages, they acquire the capability of generating additional MMPs and cysteine proteinases but lose their ability to produce serine proteinases. The activity of these enzymes is central to the

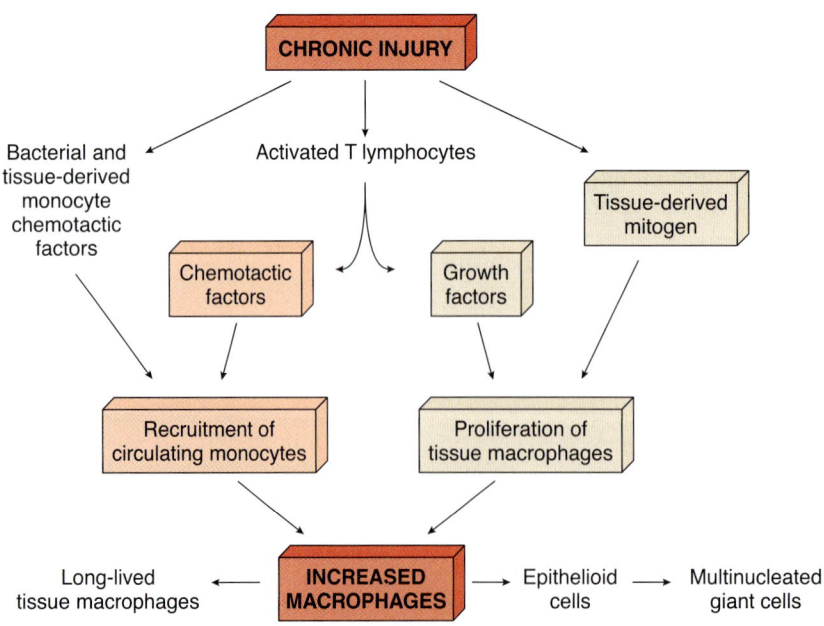

FIGURE 2-39
Accumulation of macrophages in chronic inflammation.

Cells Involved Chronic in Inflammation

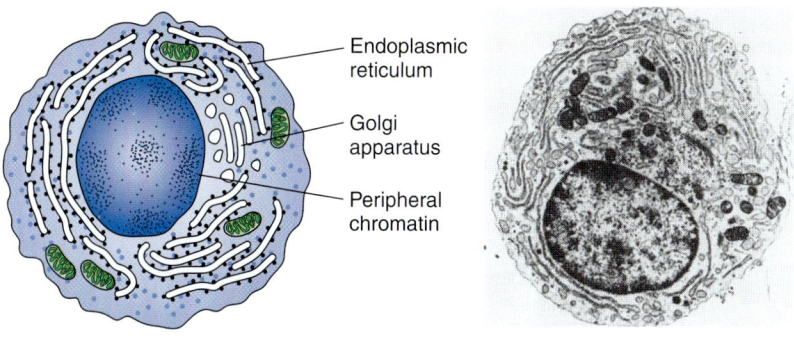

FIGURE 2-40
Plasma cell: Morphology and function.

tissue destruction in chronic inflammation. In emphysema, for example, resident macrophages generate proteinases, particularly MMPs with elastolytic activity, which destroy alveolar walls and recruit blood monocytes into the lung.

Plasma Cells

These lymphoid cells, rich in rough endoplasmic reticulum, are the primary source of antibodies (Fig. 2-40). The production of antibody to specific antigens at sites of chronic inflammation is important in antigen neutralization, clearance of foreign antigens and particles, and antibody-dependent cell-mediated cytotoxicity (see Chapter 4).

Lymphocytes

T and B cells perform vital functions in both humoral and cell-mediated immune responses. T lymphocytes function in the regulation of macrophage activation and recruitment through the secretion of specific mediators (lymphokines), modulate antibody production and cell-mediated cytotoxicity, and maintain an immune memory (Fig. 2-41). NK cells, as well as other lymphocyte subtypes, participate in the defense against viral and bacterial infections.

Naïve lymphocytes home to secondary lymphoid organs, where they encounter antigen-presenting cells. In response to this interaction, they become antigen-specific lymphocytes. Plasma cells and T cells leaving the secondary lymphoid organs circulate in the vascular system and are recruited into peripheral tissues.

Dendritic Cells

Dendritic cells are key to the generation of an immune response to antigen (see Chapter 4). They phagocytose antigen and migrate to lymph nodes, where they present the antigen in the context of a MHC molecule on their cell surfaces. Recognition of antigen and other costimulatory molecules by T cells results in recruitment of specific cell subsets to the inflammatory process. During chronic inflammation, dendritic cells are present in the inflamed tissue, where they help maintain the prolonged response.

Fibroblasts

Fibroblasts are long-lived, ubiquitous cells whose chief function is the generation of ECM elements (Fig. 2-42). They are derived from mesoderm or neural crest tissue and can dif-

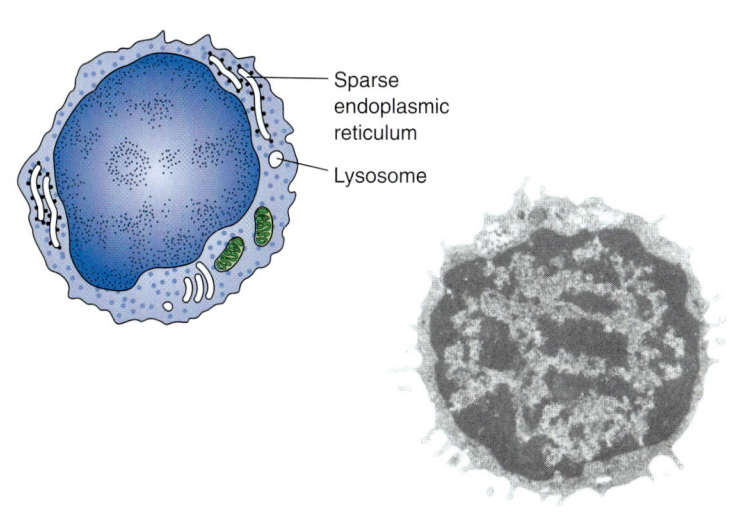

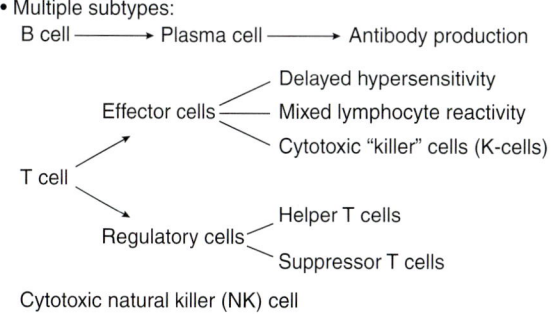

FIGURE 2-41
Lymphocyte: Morphology and function.

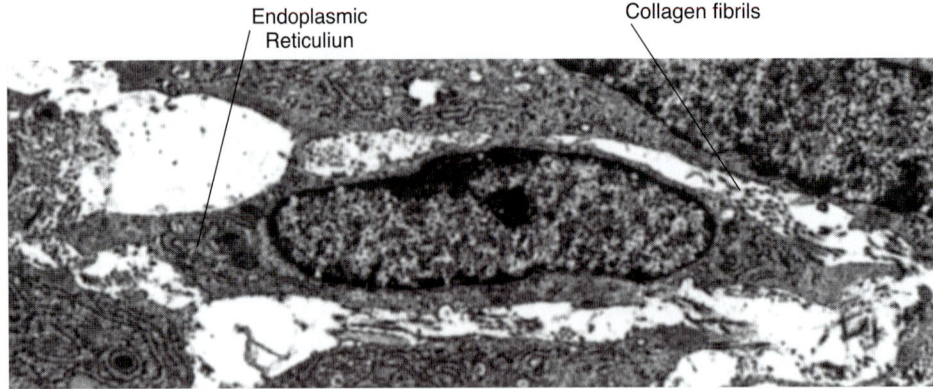

FIGURE 2-42
Fibroblast: Morphology and function.

ferentiate into other connective tissue cells, including chondrocytes, adipocytes, osteocytes, and smooth muscle cells. Fibroblasts are the construction workers of the tissue, rebuilding the scaffolding of ECM upon which tissue is reestablished.

Fibroblasts not only respond to immune signals that induce their proliferation and activation but are also active players in the immune response. These cells interact with inflammatory cells, particularly lymphocytes, via surface molecules and receptors on both cells. For example, CD40 on fibroblasts binds to the ligand on lymphocytes, resulting in activation of both cell types. Activated fibroblasts produce cytokines, chemokines, and prostanoids, creating a tissue microenvironment that further regulates the behavior of inflammatory cells in the damaged tissue. When the mix of immune–regulatory molecules is inappropriate, the transition from acute inflammatory response to restitution of normal tissue does not occur. The fibroblasts maintain a persistent, activated phenotype, resulting in overabundant and often disordered ECM. Fibroblast function is discussed more fully in the context of wound healing in Chapter 3.

Acute Inflammatory Cells

Although neutrophils are generally important in the context of acute inflammation, they may also be present during chronic inflammation, in response to ongoing infection and tissue damage. Eosinophils are conspicuous components of specific types of chronic inflammatory responses. They are particularly evident during allergic-type reactions and parasitic infestations.

INJURY AND REPAIR IN CHRONIC INFLAMMATION

Chronic inflammation is mediated by both immunological and nonimmunological mechanisms and is frequently observed in conjunction with reparative responses, namely, granulation tissue and fibrosis.

An Extended Inflammatory Response Leads to Persistent Injury

The primary role of neutrophils in inflammation is host defense and debridement of damaged tissue. The neutrophil response, however, is a double-edged sword. When the response is appropriate, neutrophil products serve to protect the host by participating in antimicrobial defense and debridement of damaged tissue. When the response is extensive or unregulated, these same products prolong tissue damage and promote chronic inflammation. The same neutrophil enzymes that are beneficial when active intracellularly during phagocytosis can be harmful to the tissues when released to the extracellular environment. During the development of inflammation, neutrophils accumulate in the tissue, and connective tissue is digested by their enzymes.

Persistent tissue injury produced by inflammatory cells is related to the pathogenesis of several diseases, for instance, pulmonary emphysema, rheumatoid arthritis, certain immune complex diseases, gout, and adult respiratory distress syndrome. Phagocytic cell adherence, the escape of reactive oxygen metabolites, and the release of lysosomal enzymes function in a synergistic manner to enhance cytotoxicity and tissue degradation. Proteinase activity is significantly elevated in chronic wounds, creating a proteolytic environment that prevents healing.

Altered Repair Mechanisms Prevent Resolution

Repair processes initiated as part of the inflammatory response can restore normal architecture and function. Early reparative efforts mimic wound healing. However, when the inflammatory response is prolonged, repair processes are incompletely effective and result in altered tissue architecture and tissue dysfunction.

- Ongoing proliferation of epithelial cells can result in *metaplasia*. For example, goblet cell metaplasia characterizes the airways of smokers and asthmatics.

- Fibroblast proliferation and activation results in an increased and abnormal ECM. Since ECM components such as collagen now occupy space that is normally devoted to functioning tissue cells, organ function is altered.
- The ECM may be abnormal. Degradation and production of the matrix change the normal mix of extracellular proteins. For example, elastin degradation plays an important role in the development of emphysema.
- Altered ECM (e.g., fibronectin) can be a chemoattractant for inflammatory cells and present a different scaffolding to cells, resulting in modulation of cell migration.

GRANULOMATOUS INFLAMMATION

Neutrophils ordinarily remove agents that incite an acute inflammatory response. However, there are circumstances in which the substances that provoke the acute inflammatory reaction cannot be digested by the reacting neutrophils. Such a situation is potentially dangerous, because it can lead to a vicious circle of (1) phagocytosis, (2) failure of digestion, (3) death of the neutrophil, and (4) release of the undigested provoking agent. The offending material, once free of the neutrophil, would again be phagocytosed by a newly recruited neutrophil. The result would be persistent and destructive acute inflammation. However, there is a mechanism for dealing with indigestible substances, namely, granulomatous inflammation (Fig. 2-43).

The principal cells involved in granulomatous inflammation are macrophages and lymphocytes. Macrophages are much longer lived than neutrophils. If they are not killed by the noxious agent, they can sequester it in their cytoplasm for indefinite periods, thereby preventing it from continuing to provoke an acute inflammatory reaction. Macrophages are mobile cells that continuously migrate through the extravascular connective tissues of the body. Their recruitment to sites of injury, as well as their activation, is regulated by the local generation of chemotactic factors, particularly bacterial products (e.g., LPS) and cytokines secreted by activated T lymphocytes. Several cytokines stimulate macrophage function (e.g., IFN-γ), whereas others inhibit macrophage activation (e.g., IL-4, IL-10). Thus, lymphocytes are vital for regulating the development and resolution of inflammatory responses. After amassing substances that they cannot digest, the macrophages lose their motility, accumulate at the site of injury, and undergo a characteristic change in their structure that transforms them into pale, epithelioid cells. Nodular collections of these epithelioid cells form *granulomas*, the morphological hallmark of granulomatous inflammation.

Granulomas are small (<2 mm) collections of epithelioid cells (frequently surrounded by a rim of lymphocytes) and multinucleated giant cells, which are formed by the cytoplasmic fusion of macrophages (Fig. 2-44). When the nuclei are arranged around the periphery of the cell in a horseshoe pattern, the cell is termed a *Langhans giant cell* (Fig. 2-45). Frequently, a foreign pathogenic agent (e.g., silica or a *Histoplasma* spore) or other indigestible material is identified within the cytoplasm of a multinucleated giant cell, in which case the term *foreign body giant cell* is used (Fig. 2-46). All the other cell types characteristic of chronic inflammation, including lymphocytes, eosinophils, and fibroblasts, may also be associated with granulomas.

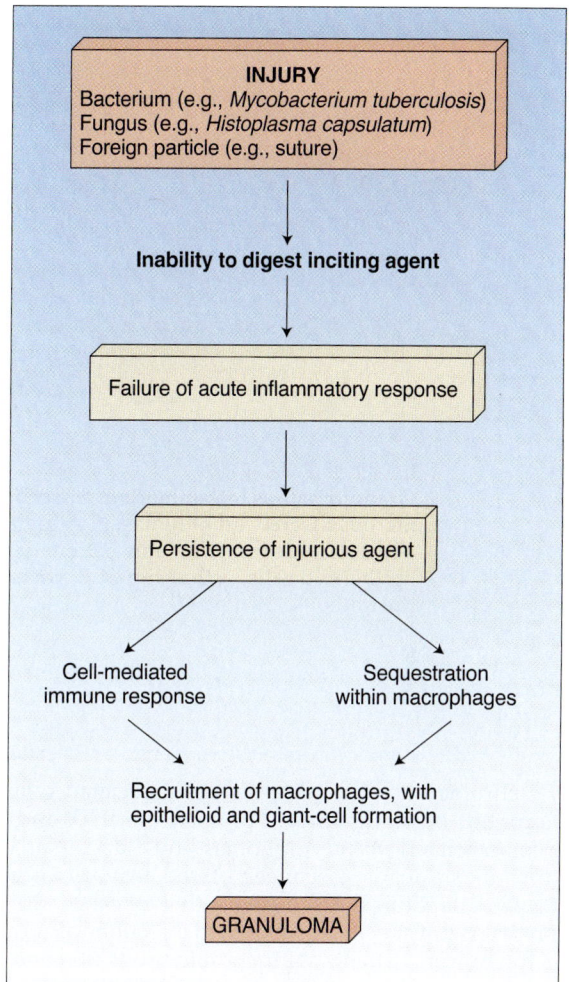

FIGURE 2-43
Mechanism of granuloma formation.

Despite the long life of macrophages in granulomatous reactions, these cells do turn over, albeit slowly. On the death of the macrophage, the offending indigestible agent is released and may continue to provoke an acute inflammatory reaction. Thus, many granulomatous reactions display variable numbers of PMNs. The turnover of epithelioid cells is also influenced by the toxicity of the inciting agent. The more inert the agent, the slower the turnover of the cells. The fate of a granulomatous reaction is influenced not only by the cytotoxicity of the inciting agent but also by its immunogenicity. Immunological sensitivity may develop to a noxious agent that is released slowly from macrophages and epithelioid cells. In particular, cell-mediated immune responses to the inciting agent may modify the granulomatous reaction by recruiting and activating more macrophages and lymphocytes.

Granulomatous inflammation is typical of the tissue response elicited by fungal infections, tuberculosis, leprosy, schistosomiasis, and the presence of foreign material (e.g., suture or talc). It is characteristically associated with areas of caseous necrosis produced by infectious agents, particularly *Mycobacterium tuberculosis*. Some diseases of unknown etiology, especially sarcoidosis, are distinguished by florid granulomatous inflammation, although the inciting agent is not apparent.

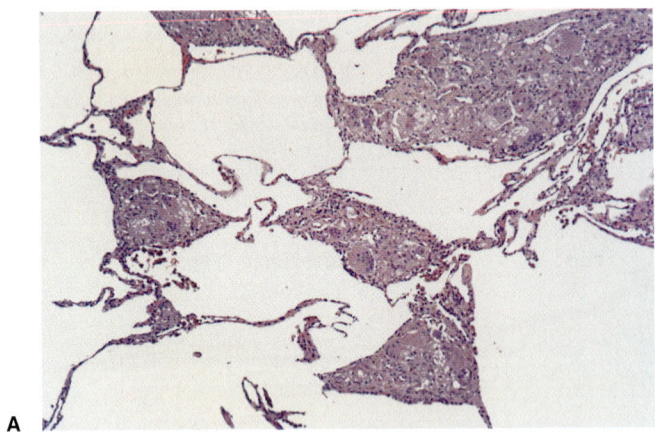 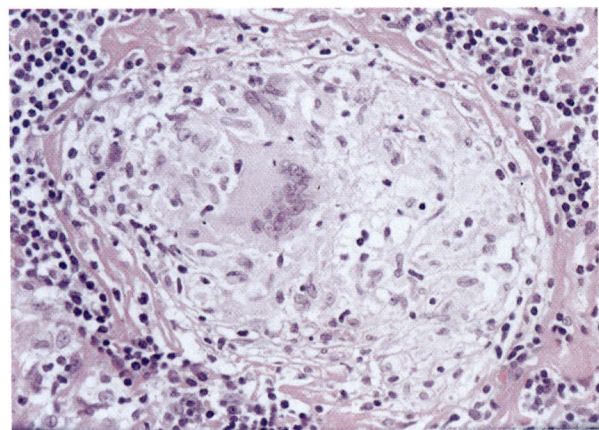

FIGURE 2-44
Granulomatous inflammation. A. Section of lung from a patient with sarcoidosis reveals numerous discrete granulomas. B. A higher-power photomicrograph of a single granuloma in a lymph node from the same patient depicts a multinucleated giant cell amid numerous pale epithelioid cells. A thin rim of fibrosis separates the granuloma from the lymphoid cells of the node.

CHRONIC INFLAMMATION AND MALIGNANCY

Several chronic infectious diseases are associated with the development of malignancy. For example, HIV-induced AIDS is associated with lymphomas and Kaposi sarcoma; schistosomiasis leads to cancer of the urinary bladder; chronic viral hepatitis is associated with liver cancer. Inflammation that is not specifically linked to infection is also a risk factor for cancer. Patients with chronic bronchitis and emphysema, esophagitis, and inflammatory bowel disease have an increased incidence of cancer in those organs. The environment created by chronic inflammation is conducive to the promotion of malignant tumors and may involve a number of mechanisms (see also Chapter 5):

- **Increased cell proliferation:** Mutagenic conditions exist whenever there is increased cell division, such as in inflammatory foci.
- **Oxygen and nitric oxide metabolites:** Inflammatory metabolites, such as nitrosamines, may cause genomic damage.
- **Chronic immune activation:** Chronic antigen exposure induces an altered cytokine profile, leading to suppression of the cell-mediated immune responses and creation of an environment permissive for malignant growth.
- **Angiogenesis:** Growth of new vessels is associated with inflammation and wound healing and is required for maintenance of neoplastic lesions.

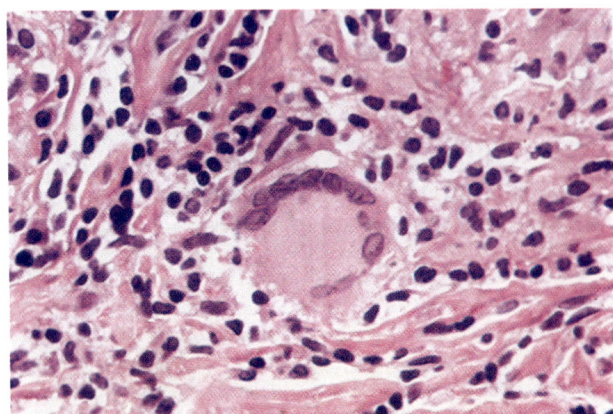

FIGURE 2-45
A Langhans giant cell shows nuclei arranged on the periphery of an abundant cytoplasm.

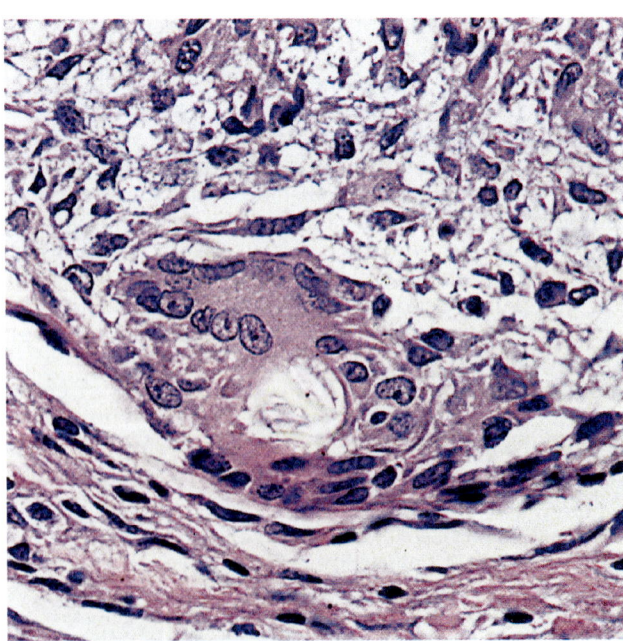

FIGURE 2-46
Foreign body giant cell. The numerous nuclei are randomly arranged in the cytoplasm.

- **Inhibition of apoptosis:** Chronic inflammation suppresses apoptosis. Increased cell division and decreased apoptosis lead to survival and expansion of a mutated cell population.

SYSTEMIC MANIFESTATIONS OF INFLAMMATION

The objective of the inflammatory response is to (1) confine the area of injury, (2) clear the inciting pathological agent and damaged tissue, and (3) restore function to the tissue. However, under certain conditions, local injury may result in prominent systemic effects that can themselves be debilitating. These effects often result from the entry of a pathogen into the bloodstream, a condition known as *sepsis*. This event causes systemic activation of mediator systems in the plasma and inflammatory cells. Alternatively, the local injury may be so severe that it leads to the release of inflammatory mediators, (especially cytokines) into the circulation, thereby causing systemic effects. Cytokines, including IL-1α, IL-1β, TNF-α, IL-6, and interferons, often acting synergistically, are directly or indirectly responsible for both the local and systemic effects of inflammation. The symptoms associated with inflammation, including fever, myalgia, arthralgia, anorexia, and somnolence, are attributable to cytokines. The most prominent systemic manifestations of inflammation, termed the *systemic inflammatory response syndrome* (SIRS), are activation of the hypothalamic-pituitary-adrenal axis, leukocytosis or the acute phase response, fever, and shock.

Hypothalamic-Pituitary-Adrenal Axis

The finding that administration of systemic glucocorticoids have antiinflammatory effects implicated activation of the hypothalamic-pituitary-adrenal axis as a response to chronic inflammation and chronic immune disease. Inflammation results in release of antiinflammatory glucocorticoids from the adrenal cortex, and loss of adrenal function can increase the severity of inflammation. Many of the systemic effects of inflammation are mediated via this axis.

Leukocytosis

Leukocytosis is defined as an increase in the number of circulating leukocytes and commonly accompanies acute inflammation. Neutrophilia is an increase in PMNs, in which immature PMNs ("band" forms) may also be seen in the peripheral blood. It is most common in association with bacterial infections and tissue injury. Leukocytosis is caused by the release of specific mediators by macrophages and perhaps other cells that initially promote an accelerated release of PMNs from the bone marrow. Subsequently, macrophages and T lymphocytes are stimulated to produce a group of proteins (referred to as *colony-stimulating factors*) that induce proliferation of bone marrow hematopoietic precursor cells. On occasion, the circulating levels of leukocytes and their precursors may reach very high levels. Such a situation, referred to as a *leukemoid reaction*, is sometimes difficult to differentiate from leukemia. In contrast to bacterial infections, viral infections (including infectious mononucleosis) are characterized by lymphocytosis, an absolute increase in the number of circulating lymphocytes. Parasitic infestations and certain allergic reactions cause eosinophilia (i.e., an increase in the number of eosinophils in the peripheral blood).

Leukopenia

Leukopenia is defined as an absolute decrease in the circulating white cell count. It is occasionally encountered under conditions of chronic inflammation, especially in patients who are malnourished or who suffer from a chronic debilitating disease such as disseminated cancer. Leukopenia may also be caused by typhoid fever and certain viral and rickettsial infections.

Acute Phase Response

The acute phase response is a regulated physiological reaction that occurs in inflammatory conditions. It is characterized clinically by fever, leukocytosis, decreased appetite, and altered sleep patterns, and chemically by changes in the plasma levels of acute phase proteins. These proteins (Table 2-6) are synthesized primarily by the liver and released in large numbers into the circulation in response to an acute inflammatory challenge. Changes in the plasma levels of acute phase proteins are mediated primarily by IL-1, IL-6, and TNF-α. Increased plasma levels of some acute phase proteins are reflected in an accelerated erythrocyte sedimentation rate, which is a qualitative index used clinically to monitor the activity of many inflammatory diseases.

Fever

Fever is a clinical hallmark of inflammation. Release of exogenous pyrogens (molecules that cause fever) by bacteria, viruses, or injured cells may directly affect the hypothalamic thermoregulatory center. More importantly, they stimulate the production of endogenous pyrogens, namely the cytokines, including IL-1α, IL-1β, and TNF-α as well as the less potent IL-6 and interferons. These cytokines, released primarily from macrophages but from tissue cells as well, have local and systemic effects. IL-1 is a 15-kd protein that stimulates prostaglandin synthesis in the hypothalamic thermoregulatory centers, thereby altering the "thermostat" that controls body temperature. Inhibitors of cyclooxygenase (e.g., aspirin) block the fever response by inhibiting IL-

TABLE 2-6 Acute Phase Proteins

Protein	Function
Mannose binding protein	Opsonization/complement activation
C-reactive protein	Opsonization
α_1-Antitrypsin	Serine protease inhibitor
Haptoglobin	Binds hemoglobin
Ceruloplasmin	Antioxidant, binds copper
Fibrinogen	Coagulation
Serum amyloid A protein	Apolipoprotein
α_2-Macroglobulin	Antiprotease
Cysteine protease inhibitor	Antiprotease

1–stimulated PGE$_2$ synthesis in the hypothalamus. TNF-α and IL-6 also increase body temperature by a direct action on the hypothalamus. Chills (the sensation of cold), rigor (profound chills with shivering and piloerection), and sweats (to allow heat dissipation) are symptoms associated with fever.

Pain

The process of pain is associated with (1) nociception (i.e., the detection of noxious stimuli and transmission of this information to the brain), (2) pain perception, and (3) suffering and pain behavior. Nociception is primarily a neural response initiated in injured tissues by specific nociceptors, which are high-threshold receptors for thermal, chemical, and mechanical stimuli. Most of the chemical mediators of inflammation described in this chapter, including ions, kinins, histamine, nitric oxide, prostanoids, cytokines, and growth factors, either directly or indirectly activate peripheral nociceptors. Kinins, especially bradykinin, are formed following tissue trauma and in inflammation; they activate primary sensory neurons via B$_2$ receptors to mediate pain transmission. Another kinin, des-arg bradykinin, activates B$_1$ receptors to produce pain only during inflammation. Cytokines, particularly TNF-α, IL-1, IL-6, and IL-8, produce pain hypersensitivity to mechanical and thermal stimuli. Prostaglandins and growth factors may directly activate nociceptors but appear to be most important in enhancing nociceptor sensitivity. Pain perception and subsequent behavior arise in response to this enhanced sensitivity to both noxious and normally innocuous stimuli.

Shock

Under conditions of massive tissue injury or infection that spreads to the blood (sepsis), significant quantities of cytokines, especially TNF-α, and the other chemical mediators of inflammation may be generated in the circulation. By their effects on the heart and on the peripheral vascular system, the sustained presence of these mediators induces cardiovascular decompensation. Systemic effects include generalized vasodilation, with increased vascular permeability and intravascular volume loss, and myocardial depression with decreased cardiac output, termed the *systemic inflammatory response syndrome* (see Chapter 6). In severe cases, activation of the coagulation pathways may generate microthrombi throughout the body, with consumption of clotting components and subsequent predisposition to bleeding, a condition defined as *disseminated intravascular coagulation*. The net result is *multisystem organ dysfunction (MODS)* and death (see Chapter 20).

SUGGESTED READING

Books

Collins T: Leukocyte Recruitment, Endothelial Cell Adhesion Molecules, and Transcriptional Control: Insights for Drug Discovery. Kluwer Academic Publishers, Philadelphia, 2001.

Cronstein BN, Weissmann G, Koch A, Serhan CN, Sitkovsky M: Inflammation Kluwer Academic/Plenum Publishers, Philadelphia, 2004.

Gallin JI, Synderman R, Fearon DT, Haynes BF, Nathan C: Inflammation Basic Principles and Clinical Correlates. Lippincott Williams & Wilkins, Philadelphia, 1999.

Gorski A, Krotkiewski H, Zimecki M: Inflammation. Kluwer Academic Publishers, Philadelphia, 2001.

Honn KV, Marnett LJ, Nigam S, Serhan CN, Dennis EA: Eicosanoids and Other Bioactive Lipids In Cancer, Inflammation, and Radiation Injury. Kluwer Academic/Plenum Publishers, Philadelphia, 2003.

Ley K: Physiology of Inflammation. American Physiological Society; 2001.

Pearson JD: Vascular Adhesion Molecules and Inflammation. Springer Verlag, New York, 2002.

Salvemini D, Billiar TM, Vodovotz Y: Nitric Oxide and Inflammation. In Progress in Inflammation Research. Birkhauser Boston, 2001.

Van Eden W: Heat Shock Proteins and Inflammation Research. Birkhauser Boston, 2004.

Whicher JT, Evans SW: Biochemistry of Inflammation. Kluwer Academic/Plenum Publishers, Philadelphia, 1992.

Winyard PD, Blake C. Evans: Free Radicals in Inflammation. In Progress in Inflammation Research. Birkhauser Boston, 2004.

Yazici Z, Folco GC, Drazen JM, Nigam S, Shimizu T, Yazc Z, Yazici Z: Advances in Prostaglandin, Leukotriene and Other Bioactive Lipid Research: Basic Science and Clinical Applications. In Advances in Experimental Medicine and Biology, 525) Kluwer Academic Publishers, 2003.

Review Articles

Baggiolini M: Chemokines in pathology and medicine. *J Intern Med* 250:91, 2001.

Biedermann BC: Vascular endothelium: checkpoint for inflammation and immunity. *News Physiolo Sci* 16:84, 2001.

Booth JW, Trimble WS, and Grinstein S: Membrane dynamics in phagocytosis. *Semin Immunol* 13:357, 2001.

Bornstein P, Sage EH: Matricellular Proteins: extracellular modulators of cell function. *Curr. Opin. Cell Biol.* 14:608, 2002.

Buckley CD, Pilling D, Lord JM, Akbar AN, Scheel-Toellner D, and Salmon M: Fibroblasts regulate the switch from acute resolving to chronic persistent inflammation. *Trends in Immunol* 22:199, 2001.

Fitzgerald GA, Loll P: Cox in a crystal ball: Current status and future premise of Prostaglandin. *J Clin Invest* 107:1335, 2001.

Grisham MB, Jourd'heuil D, and Wink DA: Review article: chronic inflammation and reactive oxygen and nitrogen metabolism—implications in DNA damage and mutagenesis. *Alimentary Pharmacol & Therap* 14:3, 2000.

Ley K: Pathways and Bottlenecks in the Web of Inflammatory Adhesion Molecules and Chemoattractants. *Immunolo Res* 24:87, 2001.

McIntyre TM, Prescott SM, Weyrich AS, Zimmerman GA: Cell-cell interactions: leukocyte-endothelial interactions. *Cur Opin Hematol.* 10:150, 2003.

Nussler AK, Wittel UA, Nussler NC, and Beger HG: Leukocytes, the Janus cells in inflammatory disease. *Langenbecks Arch Surg* 384:222, 1999.

Rossi D, and Zlotnik A: The biology of chemokines and their receptors. *Ann Rev Immunol* 18:217, 2000.

Sears MR: 2000. Consequences of long-term inflammation. The natural history of asthma. *Clin Chest Med* 21:315, 2000.

Steeber DA, and Tedder TF. Adhession molecule cascades direct lymphocyte recirculation and leukocyte migration during inflammation. *Immunolo Res* 22:299, 2001.

Vaday GG, Franitza S, Schor H, Hecht I, Brill A, Cahalon L, Hershkoviz R, and Lider O. Combinatorial signals by inflammatory cytokines and chemokines mediate leukocyte interactions with extracellular matrix. *J Leuk Biology* 69:885, 2001.

Walport MJ: Complement I. *New Eng J Med* 344:1058, 2001.

Walport MJ: Complement II. *New Eng J of Med* 344:1140, 2001.

Watts C, and Amigorena S. Phagocytosis and antigen presentation. *Semin in Immunol* 13:373, 2001.

Willoughby DA, Moore AR, Colville-Nash PR, and Gilroy D. Resolution of inflammation. *Internat J Immunopharmacol* 22:1131, 2000.

Yoshie O: Role of chemokines in trafficking of lymphocytes and dendritic cells. *Internat J Hematol* 72:399, 2000.

CHAPTER 3

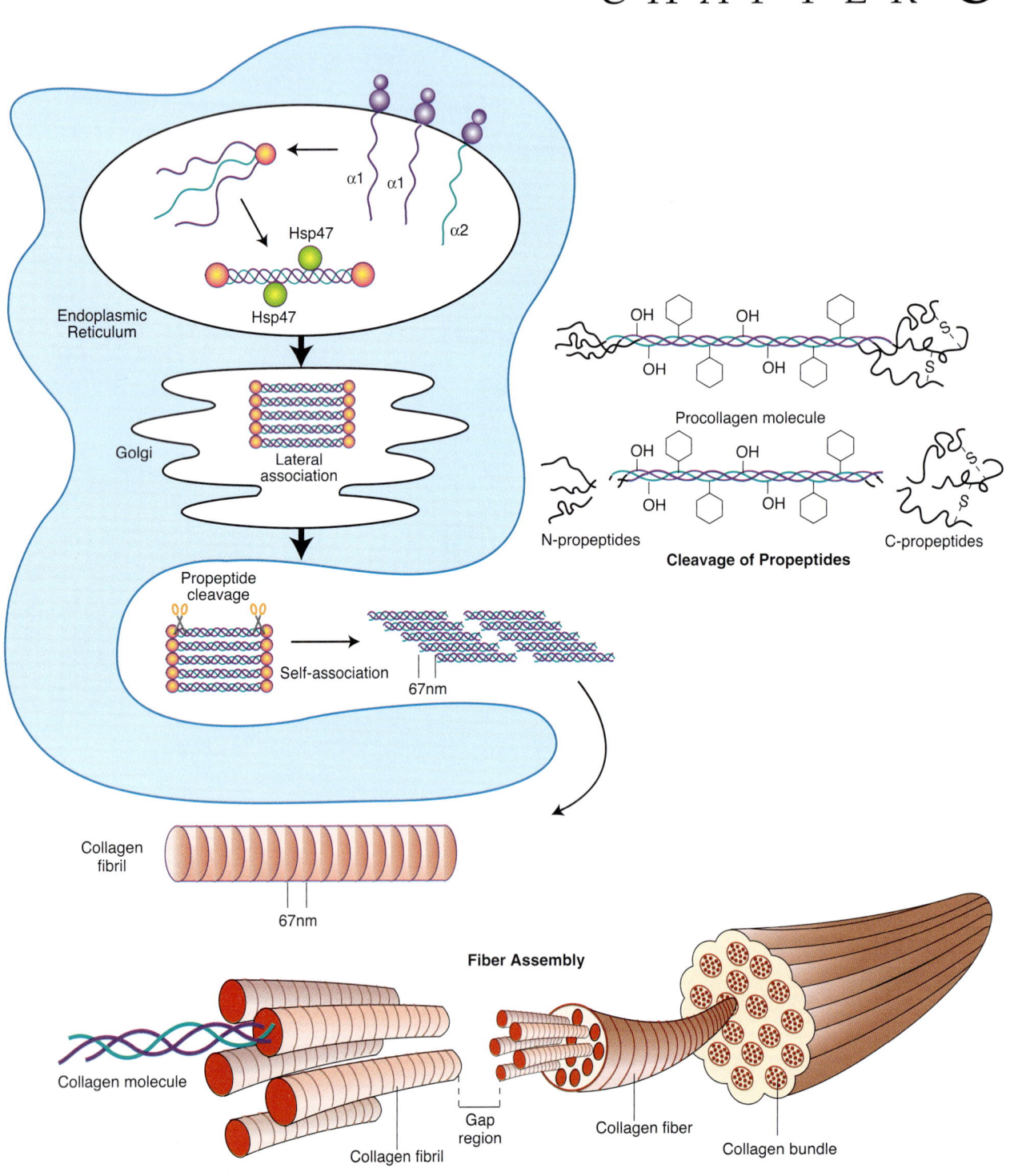

Repair, Regeneration, and Fibrosis

Gregory C. Sephel
Stephen C. Woodward

The Basic Processes of Wound Healing

Migration of Cells

Extracellular Matrix and Repair

Extracellular Matrix Components

Remodeling

Cell Proliferation

Integrated Molecular Signals

Signal Transduction

Repair

Repair and Regeneration

Wound Healing

Regeneration

The Cell Cycle

Cell Proliferation

Regeneration

Conditions That Modify Repair

Local Factors

Repair Patterns

Unsuccessful Wound Repair

FIGURE 3-1 *(see opposite page)*
Collagen synthesis, secretion, and assembly. The steps of collagen synthesis, follow pathways common to all proteins destined for secretion and include a number of posttranslational modifications. Fibrillar collagens are secreted as propeptides, from which the N- and C-terminal noncollagenous domains must be cleaved before fiber assembly can continue. Several collagen molecules associate in a quarter-staggered manner to form collagen fibrils, which associate to form collagen fibers with their characteristic cross-banding (seen by electron microscopy). In turn, collagen fibers associate to form bundles recognizable by light microscopy.

The repair of wounds (i.e., wound healing) was described in the remote past. Physicians in ancient Egypt noted healing in individual cases, and battle surgeons in classic Greece reported injuries produced by swords and other weapons. The clotting of blood to prevent exsanguination was a preoccupation of early writers about wound repair, who recognized hemostasis as the first necessary event in wound healing. At the time of the American Civil War, "laudable pus" was in fashion. Although actually a sign of infection, the development of pus in wounds was thought to be necessary, and its emergence was considered a positive sign in the healing process. Later studies of wound infection led to the discovery that inflammatory cells are primary actors in the repair process. Although scurvy (see Chapter 8) was described in the 16th century British navy, it was not until the 20th century that vitamin C (ascorbic acid) was found to be necessary for the function of prolyl hydroxylase, an enzyme required for proper folding and stabilization of collagen into a triple helix (see Fig. 3-1).

The study of wound healing now encompasses a complex environment containing many matrix proteins, growth factors, and cytokines, which regulate and modulate the repair process. Nearly every stage in the repair process is redundantly controlled, and there is no single rate-limiting step, with the possible exception of the ingress of inflammatory cells.

Successful repair relies upon a crucial balance between the *yin* of matrix deposition and the *yang* of matrix degradation. Thus, wounds that do not heal may reflect excess proteinase activity or decreased matrix accumulation. Conversely, fibrosis and scarring may result from reduced proteinase activity or increased matrix accumulation. Whereas the formation of new collagen during repair is required for increased strength of the healing site, chronic fibrosis is a major component of diseases that involve chronic injury.

THE BASIC PROCESSES OF WOUND HEALING

Many of the basic cellular and molecular mechanisms necessary for wound healing are found in other processes involving dynamic tissue changes, such as development and tumor growth. Three key cellular mechanisms are necessary for wound healing:

- Cellular migration
- Extracellular matrix organization and remodeling
- Cell proliferation

Migration of Cells Initiates Repair

Cells That Migrate to the Wound

The ingress of cells into a wound is initiated by mediators that are either released de novo by resident cells or from reserves stored in the granules of platelets and basophils. The contents of these granules include cytokines, chemoattractants, proteases, and mediators of inflammation. The last (1) control vascular delivery, (2) degrade damaged tissue, and (3) initiate the repair cascade. Platelets are activated when bound to collagen exposed at sites of endothelial damage, and their ensuing aggregation, in combination with fibrin cross-linking, limits blood loss. Activated platelets release platelet-derived growth factor (PDGF) and other molecules that facilitate adhesion, coagulation, vasoconstriction, repair, and clot resorption. Mast cells are bone marrow-derived cells whose granules contain high concentrations of heparin. They reside in connective tissue near small blood vessels and respond to foreign antigens by releasing the contents of their granules, many of which are angiogenic.

Resident macrophages, tissue-fixed mesenchymal cells, and epithelial cells release mediators that not only contribute to the early response, but also perpetuate it. Their numbers are increased through proliferation and recruitment to the site of injury (Fig. 3-2). The following are characteristic of skin wounds:

- **Leukocytes** arrive at the wound site early and migrate rapidly by forming small focal adhesions (focal contacts). A family of small peptide chemoattractants, termed *chemokines,* are capable of restricted or broad recruitment of particular leukocytes (see Chapter 2).
- **Polymorphonuclear leukocytes** are rapidly recruited from the bone marrow and invade the wound site within the first day. They degrade and destroy nonviable tissue by releasing their granular contents.
- **Macrophages** arrive shortly after neutrophils but persist for days or longer. They phagocytose debris and orchestrate the developing granulation tissue by the release of cytokines and chemoattractants.
- **Fibroblasts, myofibroblasts, pericytes, and smooth muscle cells** are recruited by growth factors and matrix degradation products, arriving in a skin wound by day 3 or 4. These cells are responsible for fibroplasia, synthesis of connective tissue matrix, tissue remodeling, wound contraction, and wound strength.
- **Endothelial cells** form nascent capillaries by responding to growth factors and are visible in a skin wound beyond day 3. The development of capillaries is necessary for the exchange of gases, the delivery of nutrients, and the influx of inflammatory cells.

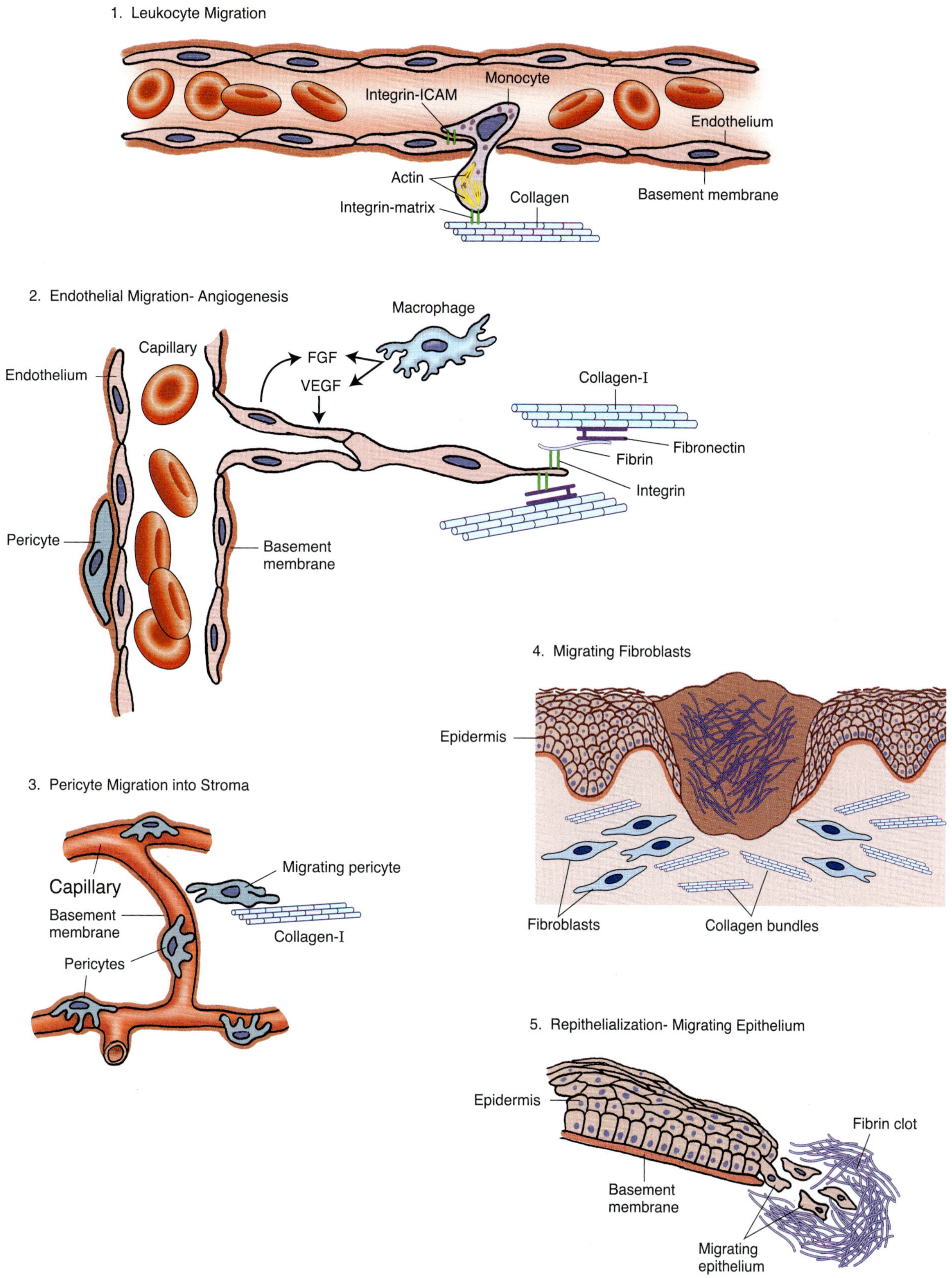

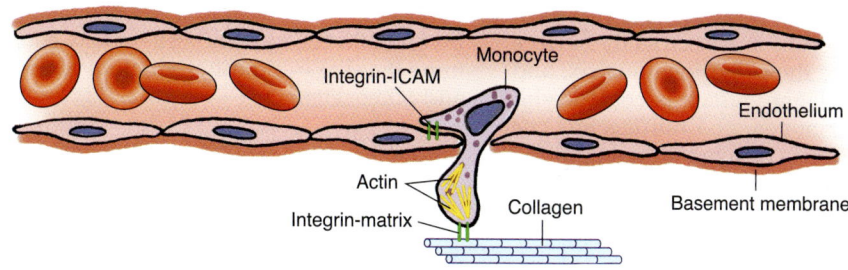

FIGURE 3-2
Cell migrations during repair. *(1)* Leukocytes attach to, and migrate between, capillary endothelial cells, penetrate the basement membrane, and enter the matrix. *(2)* Capillary endothelial cells, released from the basement membrane, migrate through the matrix to form new capillaries. *(3)* Pericytes detach from endothelial cells and their basement membranes to migrate into the matrix. *(4)* Fibroblasts become bipolar and migrate through the matrix to the site of injury. *(5)* Epithelial keratinocytes detach from neighboring cells and basement membranes and migrate between the scab and the wound along the provisional matrix of the dermis.

- **Epithelial cells** in the epidermis move across the surface of a skin wound, penetrate the provisional matrix, and migrate upon stromal collagen, which is coated with plasma glycoproteins, fibrinogen, and fibronectin. The process of reepithelialization is delayed if the migrating epithelial cells must reconstitute a damaged basement membrane. In addition, the phenotype of the epithelial layer is altered in the absence of basement membrane.

Mechanisms of Cell Migration

Cell migration uses the most important mechanism of wound healing, namely, the response of cells to chemical signals (cytokines) and insoluble substrates of the extracellular matrix. Locomotion of the rapidly migrating leukocytes is powered by broad, wavelike, membrane extensions called *lamellipodia*. Slower moving cells, such as fibroblasts, extend narrower, fingerlike membrane protrusions labeled *filopodia*. Cell polarization and membrane extensions are initiated by growth factors or chemokines, which trigger a response by binding to their specific receptors on the cell surface. Actin fibrils polymerize and form a network at the membrane's leading edge, thereby propelling lamellipodia and filopodia forward, with traction provided via attachments to the extracellular matrix substrate. Actin-related proteins (ARPs) stimulate actin assembly, and numerous actin-binding proteins act like molecular tinker toys, rapidly constructing, stabilizing and destabilizing actin networks.

The leading edge of the cell membrane impinges upon the extracellular matrix and adheres to it through transmembrane adhesion receptors termed *integrins* (see Chapter 2). These molecules are highly redundant, and many different heterodimer combinations recognize the same matrix components (Table 3-1). The integrins transmit both mechanical and chemical signals to cells, thereby regulating cellular survival, proliferation, differentiation, and migration. Interestingly, other cell activators, such as cytokines, can "signal" through cytoplasmic tails of integrins from inside the cell to the outside matrix, thereby influencing organization and tension in matrix and tissue. Growth factors and integrins share several common signaling pathways, but integrins are unique in their ability to organize and anchor the cytoskeleton. Cytoskeletal connections are controlled by receptors involved in cell–cell and cell–matrix connections and determine the shape and differentiation of epithelial, endothelial, and other cells.

Focal Adhesions (Focal Contacts)

Focal contacts develop through the adherence of the integrin extracellular domain to the connective tissue matrix. Focal adhesions form under the cell body, whereas smaller focal contacts form at the leading edge of migrating cells. More than 50 proteins have been associated with the formation of adhesion plaques. The Rho-family of GTPases (Rho, Rac, and Cdc42) act as molecular switches that interact with surface receptors to regulate matrix assembly, generate focal adhesions, and organize the actin cytoskeleton. The cytoplasmic domain of integrins is the foundation of a protein cascade that acts to anchor actin stress fibers. So-called adaptor proteins link actin and integrin-binding proteins, thereby providing a connection for actin fibers to interact with the extracellular matrix. Additionally, many of the focal adhesion plaque proteins possess kinase, phosphatase, GTPase, and protease activities, which act upon integrins and enable them to participate in chemical and mechanical signaling. Integrins mechanically sense malleability or resistance in the matrix and respond through focal adhesion complexes to regulate cytoskeletal contractility. This effect controls lamellipodial protrusion and cell migration, differentiation, and growth. The focal contact anchors the actin stress fibers, against which myosins pull to extend or contract the cell body. As the cell moves forward, older adhesions at the rear are weakened or destabilized, allowing the trailing edge to retract.

Extracellular Matrix Sustains the Repair Process

Three types of extracellular matrix contribute to the organization, physical properties, and function of tissue:

- **Basement membrane**
- **Connective tissue (interstitial matrix or stroma)**
- **Provisional matrix**

Basement Membranes

Basement membranes, also called *basal lamina*, are thin, well-defined layers of specialized extracellular matrix that separate the cells that synthesize it from connective tissue (Fig. 3-3). Epithelium, adipocytes, muscle cells, Schwann cells, and capillary endothelium produce basement membranes.

- Basement membranes are constructed from extracellular matrix molecules, including collagen IV, laminin, entactin/nidogen, and perlecan, a heparan sulfate proteoglycan (Table 3-2). They self-assemble into a sandwich-like structure composed of two interacting networks. A network of disulfide-bonded type IV collagen molecules is ionically linked by entactin/nidogen to a planar association of noncovalently bonded laminin molecules (see illustrations in Table 3-2). Network associations are modulated by perlecan, which can interact

TABLE 3-1 **Integrins and Matrix Molecules**

Integrin Ligands in the Extracellular Matrix	Associated Cellular Integrin Receptor Dimers[a]
Collagens	
Stroma or basement membrane	β_1 with α_1 or α_2
Basement membrane	
Laminins	β_1 with $\alpha_{1,2,3,6,\text{ or }7}$
	β_4 with α_6 (hemidesmosome)
Wound (provisional) matrix	
Fibronectins	β_1 with $\alpha_{2,3,4,5,\text{ or }8}$
	α_v with $\beta_{1,3,5,\text{ or }6}$
Fibrinogen	$\alpha_v\beta_3$
Vitronectin	α_v with $\beta_{1,3,\text{ or }5}$
	$\alpha_8\beta_1$
Denatured collagen	$\alpha_3\beta_1$, $\alpha_v\beta_3$

[a] Leukocyte integrins excluded.

The Basic Processes of Wound Healing

TABLE 3-2 Basement Membrane Constituents and Organization

Basement Membrane Components	Chains	Molecular Structure	Molecular Associations	Basement Membrane Aggregate Form
Perlecan (heparan sulfate proteoglycan)	1 protein core; 3 heparan sulfate GAG chains	GAG chains	Laminin, collagen IV, fibronectin, growth factors (VEGF, FGF), chemokines	
Laminin	12-member family; Heterotrimers with α,β,γ chains; 5 α chains, 3 β chains, 3 γ chains	α, β, γ	Integrin and dystroglycan receptors on variety of cells (epithelium, endothelium, muscle, Schwann cells, adipocytes); Forms self-associated noncovalent network assisted by perlecan; Laminin, nidogen/entactin, perlecan, agrin, fibulin	
Nidogen/entactin	2-member family monomeric		Collagen IV, laminin, perlecan, fibulin; Stabilizes basement membrane through association of laminin and collagen IV networks	
Collagen IV	≥3 member family; Heterotrimers; Chains selected from 2 or 3 of 6 unique α chains		Integrin receptors on many cells; Forms covalent self-associated network; Collagen IV, perlecan nidogen/entactin, SPARC	

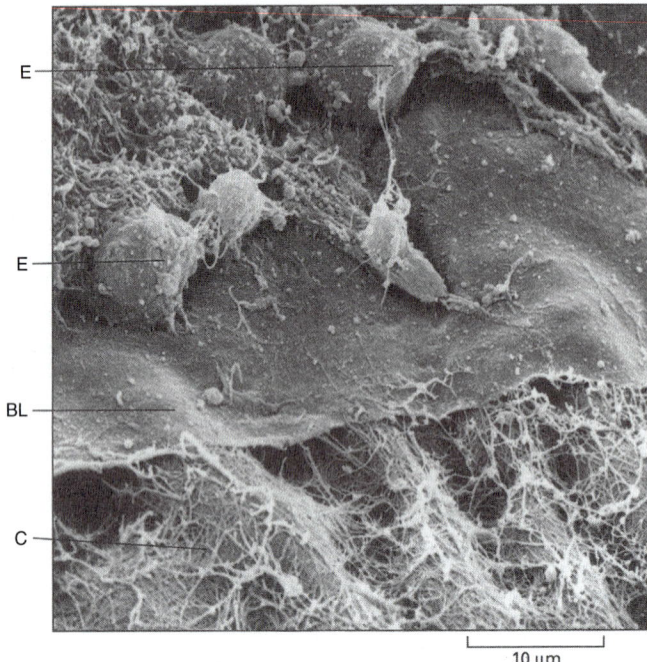
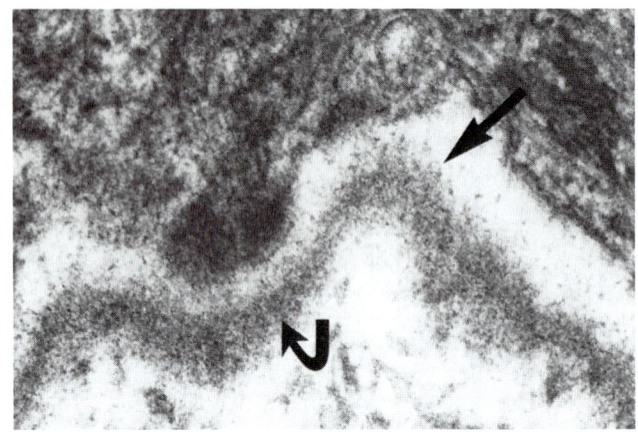

FIGURE 3-3
Scanning electron micrographs of basement membrane. A. Basement membrane (*BL*, basal lamina) separating chick embryo corneal epithelial cells *(E)* from underlying stromal connective tissue with collagen fibrils *(C)*. B. Basement membrane of the epidermis. The layer of lower electron density *(straight arrow)*, the lamina rara, abuts against the plasma membrane of a keratinocyte. The lamina densa *(curved arrow)* is adjacent to the stroma.

with the other three major components. Other minor constituents associate with basement membranes and further define their tissue-specific characteristics. Collagen XVIII, recently reclassified as a heparan sulfate proteoglycan, is associated with basement membranes. A peptide of collagen XVIII, called *endostatin,* was recently demonstrated to be antiangiogenic.

By light microscopy, a basement membrane appears as a thin lamina that is stained by the periodic acid-Schiff stain (PAS). By electron microscopy (Fig. 3-3), it is 40 to 80 nm thick and often appears to contain two layers with different staining densities, possibly an artifact of fixation.

- Within different tissues and during development, the expression of unique members of the collagen IV and laminin families imparts diversity to the basement membrane and the many structures and functions it supports.
- Basement membranes act as filters, cellular anchors, and a surface for migrating epidermal cells after injury. They also serve to reestablish the neuromuscular junction after nerve damage. Basement membranes also determine cell shape, contribute to developmental morphogenesis, and, importantly, provide a repository for growth factors and chemotactic peptides.

Provisional Matrix

Provisional matrix is a term that describes the temporary extracellular organizations of plasma-derived matrix proteins and tissue-derived components that accumulate at sites of injury (e.g. hyaluronan, tenascin, and fibronectin). These molecules associate with the preexisting stromal matrix and serve to stop blood or fluid loss. They also support the migration of monocytes, endothelial cells, epidermal cells, and fibroblasts to the wound site.

Plasma-derived provisional matrix proteins include fibrinogen, fibronectin, and vitronectin. These proteins become insoluble by binding to the stromal matrix and by forming cross-links.

Stromal (Connective Tissue) Matrix

- Connective tissue forms a continuum between tissue elements such as epithelia, nerves, and blood vessels and provides physical protection by conferring resistance to compression or stretching. The connective tissue stroma is also an important medium for the storage and exchange of bioactive proteins.
- Connective tissue contains both extracellular matrix elements and individual cells that synthesize the matrix. The cells are primarily of mesenchymal origin and include fibroblasts, myofibroblasts, adipocytes, chondrocytes, osteocytes, and endothelial cells. Bone marrow-derived cells (e.g., mast cells, macrophages, and transient leukocytes) also populate connective tissue.
- The extracellular matrix of connective tissue, commonly referred to as stroma or interstitium, is defined by fibers formed from a large family of collagen molecules (Table 3-3). Of the fibrillar collagens, type I collagen is the major constituent of bone. Type I and type III collagens are

TABLE 3-3 Collagen Molecular Composition and Structure

Type	Chains (Hetero- or Homo- Trimer)	Macromolecular Association	Aggregate Form
Fibril-forming			
I	α1 and α2(I)		I, II
II	α1(II)		
III	α1(III)		III
V	α1–α4(V)		
Non-fibril-forming (interspersed with non-collagen domains)			
VI	α1–α3(VI)	Dimer, Tetramer	Beaded filament
IX	α1–α3(IX)	IX, GAG	Type II fibril
XII	α1(XII)	XII	Type I fibril
XV / XVIII	α1(XV), α1(XVIII)	XVIII	
Network-forming			
IV	α1–α6(IV)	7S, Tetramer	
VIII	α1 and α2(VIII)	VIII	
X	α1(X)		
Transmembrane and anchoring			
VII	α1(VII)	VII, Dimer	hemidesmosome, Basement membrane, Anchoring fibril, Anchoring plaque in stroma
XVII	α1(XVII)	XVII	

prominent in skin; type II collagen is the predominant form in cartilage. Elastin fibers, which impart elasticity to skin, large blood vessels, and lungs, are decorated by microfibrillar proteins such as fibrillin. The so-called ground substance represents a number of molecules, including glycosaminoglycans (GAGs), proteoglycans, and fibronectin, which provide for many important biological functions of connective tissue in addition to the support and modulation of cell attachment.

Extracellular Matrix Components Are Elaborated and Modified in Repair

Collagens

Collagen is the most abundant protein in the animal kingdom; it is essential for the structural integrity of tissues and organs When collagen synthesis is reduced, delayed, or abnormal, the result is failed wound healing, as seen in scurvy. Excess collagen deposition leads to *fibrosis*. Fibrosis is the basis of connective tissue diseases such as scleroderma and keloids and also accounts for the compromised tissue function that accompanies chronic damage to many organs, including kidney and liver.

The collagen superfamily of insoluble extracellular proteins comprises the constituents of connective tissue in all organs, most notably cornea, arteries, dermis, cartilage, tendons, ligaments, and bone. There are more than 20 collagen proteins, assembled from at least 38 different polypeptide chains. Common to all collagen chains are helical segments, largely composed of glycine, proline, hydroxyproline, and hydroxylysine, in which every third amino acid is glycine (Gly-X-Y). The collagen domain that codes for the glycine repeat is important for the formation of the triple helical structure.

Collagen synthesis is complex and is often used as an example of the complexity of posttranslational protein modification (see Fig. 3-1). Each molecule is made by self-association of three α chains that wind around each other to form a triple helix. The triple helix includes members from an α-chain family that is specific to each collagen type (Table 3-3). The molecule may be a homotrimer, made of three identical α chains, or a heterotrimer, with either two identical α chains and one different α chain or three unique α chains. Collagen chains lose stability when errors occur that change the Gly-X-Y sequence, in which case the molecule is more vulnerable to proteinase activity. In general, successful collagen synthesis results from a series of posttranslational modifications: (1) alignment of the three chains; (2) formation of the triple helix; (3) cleavage of noncollagenous terminal peptides; (4) molecular alignment and association; and (5) covalent cross-linking, which is mediated by the copper-dependent enzyme lysyl oxidase. (see Fig. 3-1).

Fibrillar collagens, namely, types I, II, and III, are the most abundant collagens and appear as long fibrils that are formed from a staggered packing of long, cross-linked collagen molecules, whose triple helix is uninterrupted (Table 3-3). These *fibrillar* collagens turn over slowly and are generally resistant to proteinase digestion, except by specific matrix metalloproteinases. The unique structures of different collagen family members derive from the presence or absence of noncollagenous sequences that interrupt the triple helical regions. Mutations in fibrillar collagens, which do not contain nonhelical interruptions, range from lethal to minor. Type I collagen is the most abundant collagen, and mutations in the gene that encodes this molecule, as seen in osteogenesis imperfecta, result in assembly defects in the triple helix, leading to increased bone fractures, thin dermis, and easy bruising (see Chapter 6).

Molecular diversity in the collagen family supports the variety of forms needed to build tissue structures. Collagens have many biological properties that are important for morphogenesis and wound healing, including cell attachment and migration and the ability to concentrate biologically active glycoproteins in the extracellular matrix. The tensile strength of the collagen fiber enables tissue, and particularly skeletal elements, to resist tremendous pressure and tension. In a wound, collagen synthesis and cross-linking increase the strength of the newly forming tissue until the fully healed wound can resist 70% of the tension of unwounded tissue.

Nonfibrillar collagen family members contain varied numbers of nonhelical domains that interrupt the triple helical segments and confer structural flexibility (Table 3-3). These domains in collagens IV, VIII, and X facilitate the formation of networks, permit unique associations with fibrillar collagens, and modulate collagen-fiber packing. Nonfibrillar collagens V, XII, and XI endow mechanical properties and deformability or support the attachment of epithelial sheets to the dermal matrix. Proteolytic fragments of collagen exhibit a different set of biological properties that are also important in tissue remodeling. For example, fragments of basement membrane collagens IV and XVIII inhibit angiogenesis and tumor growth.

Macromolecular Organization of Collagen

The collagens are called *scleroproteins,* meaning both white and hard; yet in one circumstance, layers of collagen can be translucent, as exemplified by the transparent cornea. The cornea consists of 10 to 20 layers of type I collagen fibers, each layer containing parallel, uniform-sized collagen fibers that are oriented at right angles to the underlying one (Fig. 3-4). In healing, the injured cornea forms disorganized white collagenous scars, which are opaque and interfere with vision.

The structure of the cornea surprises those who have seen only dermal collagen, in a loose, random, basket weave-like network. Yet structured orientation of collagen in human skin has long been known. Plastic surgeons use wrinkle lines to promote inconspicuous healing, the wrinkles indicating the primary direction of the underlying dermal collagen. The tensile strength of skin that is broken parallel to creases and wrinkle lines exceeds that which is broken perpendicular to these lines, further suggesting a structured orientation of dermal collagen.

Elastin and Elastic Fibers

Elastin is a secreted matrix protein that, unlike other stromal proteins, is not glycosylated (Table 3-4). Elastin allows deformable tissues such as skin, uterus, ligament, lung, elastic cartilage, and aorta to stretch and bend and yet recoil. Its lack of carbohydrate and its hydrophobic amino acid sequence make it the most insoluble of all vertebrate proteins. It may

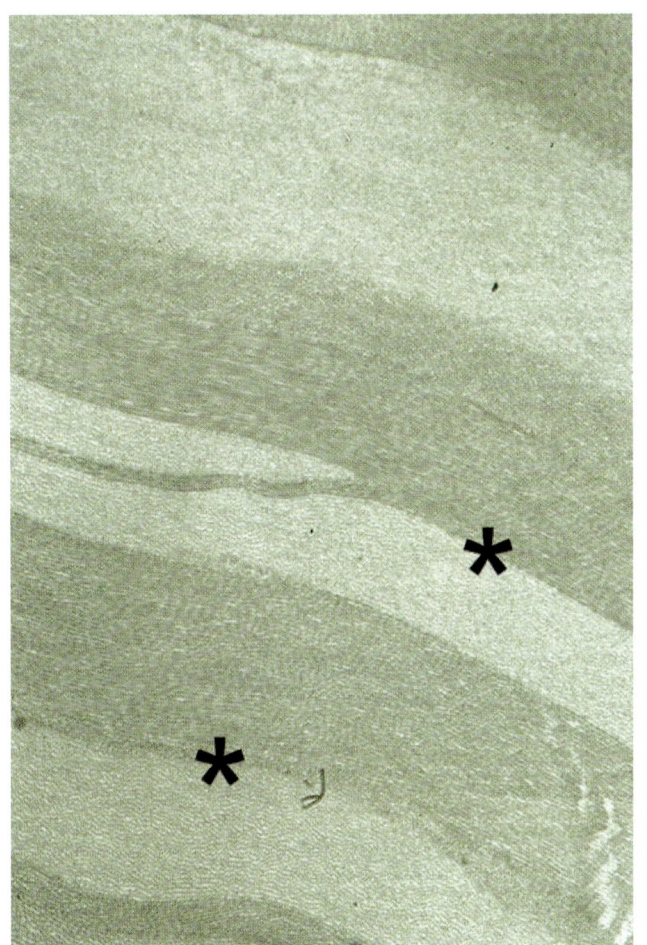 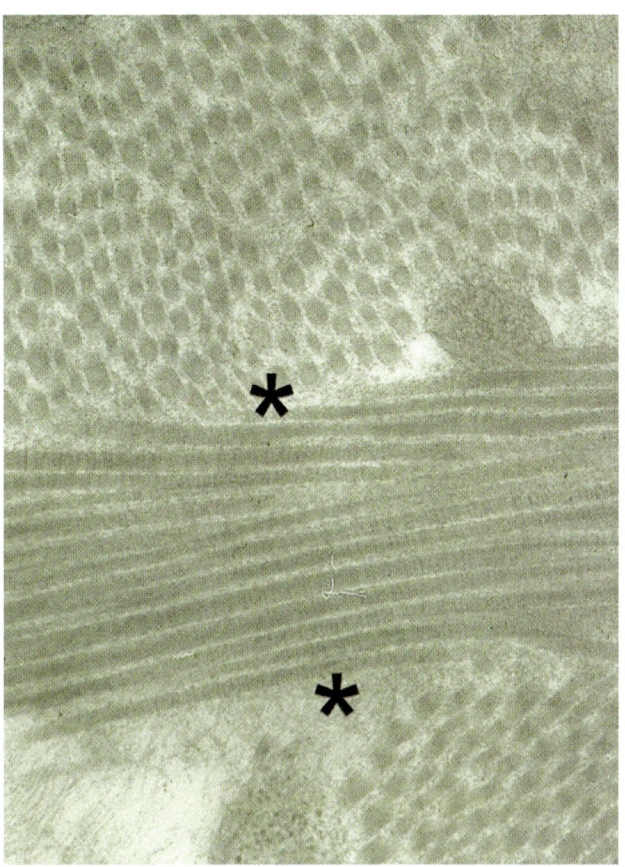

FIGURE 3-4
Human cornea, near center. A. Multiple plywoodlike arrays of collagen fibers are of similar width and are sharply demarcated between asterisks (*). B. The lamellae (*) are at approximately 90° orientation. The central array shows typical cross-banded collagen fibers.

seem surprising, therefore, that elastin fibers are damaged by aging and sun exposure, conditions that lead to age-related loss of dermal suppleness. The elastic fiber is crucial for the function of several vital tissues, yet it is not efficiently replaced during repair of skin and lung. The slow accumulation of functional elastin following damage to skin or lung is offset by the fact that it is degraded with difficulty and turns over slowly. Elastin stability results from its (1) hydrophobicity, (2) extensive covalent cross-linking (mediated by lysyl oxidase, the same enzyme that cross-links collagen), and (3) resistance to most proteolytic enzymes. Arterial wall injury, unlike skin and lung damage, leads to rapid re-formation of the concentric rings of elastic lamellae. This observation illustrates the difference in the elastin synthetic capabilities of the vascular smooth muscle cell and those of dermal or lung fibroblasts.

Elastin is deposited as fibrils, which are complexed with several glycoproteins (microfibrils) that decorate the perimeter of the elastic fiber. The best-characterized microfibrillar protein is *fibrillin* (Table 3-4). When mutated, abnormal fibrillin causes Marfan syndrome, whose pleomorphic manifestations include dissecting aortic aneurysm (see Chapter 6).

Matrix Glycoproteins

The matrix glycoproteins contribute essential biological functions to basement membrane and stromal connective tissue. In general, these molecules are large (150,000 to 1,000,000 kd) multimeric and multidomain proteins, with long arms that bind other matrix molecules and support or modulate cell attachment. Matrix glycoproteins help to (1) organize tissue topography, (2) support cell migration, (3) orient cells, and (4) induce cell behavior. The principal matrix glycoprotein of basement membrane is *laminin*, and that of stromal connective tissue is *fibronectin*.

Laminins

The laminins are a biologically versatile family of basement membrane glycoproteins whose cross-like structure is formed by products of three related gene subfamilies to form α, β, and γ heterotrimers (Table 3-2). There are 12 known laminin isotypes, which are formed from varying combinations of the three chains. The expression of laminin isotypes in specific tissues contributes to the heterogeneity

TABLE 3-4 Noncollagenous Matrix Constituents of Stroma

Stromal Connective Tissue Components	Chains	Molecular Structure	Molecular Associations	Tissue Structures
Fibronectin	Dimeric protein; Chains chosen from ~20 splice variants of one gene	(diagram showing fibrin, collagen, heparin, RGD, heparin cells, fibrin binding regions with N and C termini)	Integrin receptors of many cells (RGD binding site); Plasma fibronectin is soluble; Cellular fibronectin can self-associate into fibrils at cell surface; Collagen, heparin, decorin, fibrin, certain bacteria (opsonin), LTBP (latent transforming growth factor-β binding proteins)	(diagram of CELL with Integrin receptor binding to Collagen or fibrin)
Elastin	Monomer with several splice variants, one gene	Elastin cross-links to form fiber	Self-association to form cross-linked fibers; Formed on scaffold of microfibrils	Elastin fiber decorated with microfibrils
Fibrillin	2 members, 2 genes		Other components of microfibrils (LTBP), fibulin, laminin, versican,	
Versican (hyaluronan-binding proteoglycans)	Family of 4 related genes; 10–30 chondroitin sulfate and dermatan sulfate GAG chains	(diagram with CS)	Linked to hyaluronan via CD-44 (link protein)	(diagram showing Hyaluronan)
Decorin Small leucine-rich proteoglycans	1 protein core, 1 gene; One chondroitin sulfate or dermatan sulfate GAG chain; Biglycan and Fibromodulin structurally related, genetically distinct		Collagen I and II, fibronectin, TGF-β, thrombospondin	Collagen I or II

of tissue morphology and function, in part, by supporting cell attachment. Laminin molecules self-assemble into two-dimensional sheets that associate with type IV collagen sheets and other basement membrane proteins.

The appropriate expression of epidermal laminin is key for both normal epidermal function and reepithelialization of wounds. Epidermal strength is imparted by hemidesmosomes, which develop from the binding of basement membrane laminin to epithelial integrin and collagen VII. The latter is the anchoring fibril that connects the epidermal cell and basement membrane to the dermal connective tissue. Mutations in epidermal laminin, integrin, or collagen VII produce a potentially fatal skin blistering disease, termed *epidermolysis bullosa*.

Fibronectins

Fibronectins are versatile, adhesive glycoproteins widely distributed in stromal connective tissue and deposited in wound provisional matrix (Table 3-4). Fibronectin chains form a V-shaped homo- or heterodimer that is connected at the C terminus by two disulfide bonds. Specific domains within fibronectin bind bacteria, collagen, heparin, fibrin, fibrinogen, and the cell matrix receptor, integrin. Indeed, the integrin receptor family was partly defined by studies demonstrating its specific binding to fibronectin. The multifunctional dimer is designed to link matrix molecules to one another or to cells. Thrombi support cell migration on the fibronectin that links fibrin strands and are stabilized by cross-linking of factor XIII (transglutaminase) to other provisional and dermal matrix components.

Two types of fibronectin are formed from different sources: (1) the less soluble cellular form and (2) a hepatocyte-derived, soluble form in plasma. A plasma-derived thrombus, therefore, contains high concentrations of fibronectin, which is needed for thrombosis and host defense, the latter through opsonization of bacteria. Fibronectin also supports the association of platelets with thrombi and promotes reepithelialization of corneal and cutaneous wounds by promoting keratinocyte attachment and migration. Fibronectin synthesized by mesenchymal cells is polymerized into insoluble fibrils, which are found in granulation tissue and loose connective tissue.

Glycosaminoglycans

GAGs are long, linear polymers of specific repeating disaccharides arranged in sequence. The name of the GAG chain is determined by the disaccharide subunits in the polymer. GAG chains are negatively charged, owing to the presence of carboxylate groups and, with the exception of hyaluronan, the attachment of N- or O-linked sulfate groups to the disaccharide. When the sulfated GAG chains are O-linked to serine residues of protein cores they are called *proteoglycans*.

Hyaluronan

Hyaluronan, the only GAG that is not covalently linked to a protein, exists as a random coil of 2,000 to 25,000 disaccharides. Hyaluronan can associate with proteoglycans (defined below) that contain hyaluronan-binding regions. Certain proteoglycans bind ionically via a linking protein along the hyaluronan backbone to form large, hyaluronan/proteoglycan composites, such as *aggrecan* and *versican* (see Table 3-4), molecules that are found in cartilage and stromal tissues. The negatively charged carboxylate backbone of hyaluronan binds large amounts of water, creating a viscous gel that produces turgor in the matrix. The large size and hydrated viscosity of hyaluronan impart resilience and lubrication to joints and connective tissue, and pericellular accumulation of these molecules enables cell migration through the extracellular matrix.

Proteoglycans

Proteoglycans consist of varying numbers of GAGs, heparan, chondroitin sulfate, and keratan sulfate, linked by O-glycosidic bonds to serines or threonines on specific core proteins. They have a higher carbohydrate content than matrix glycoproteins, and though not branched, demonstrate varied modifications such as sulfation, unique linkages, and varying sequences. Individual proteoglycans differ in size, core proteins, choice of GAG chains, and tissue distribution.

Like the matrix glycoproteins, proteoglycans participate in matrix organization, structural integrity, and cell attachment. Though the protein core of proteoglycans often contains biological activity, the properties of several proteoglycans are largely mediated by the GAG chains themselves. Heparan sulfate GAG chains of basement membrane (perlecan and collagen XVIII) and cell-associated proteoglycans modulate the availability and actions of heparin-binding growth factors, such as vascular endothelial growth factor (VEGF), fibroblast growth factor (FGF), and heparin-binding epidermal growth factor (EGF) (see below). A group of small proteoglycans, which share a core protein domain of leucine-rich repeats, regulates transforming growth factor-β (TGF-β) activity and fibril formation in collagens I and II.

The tissue expressions of extracellular matrix proteins and proteoglycans are summarized in Table 3-5.

Remodeling Is the Long-lasting Phase of Repair

In the later stages of the repair process, inflammatory cells diminish in number, and capillary formation is completed. Remodeling indicates that the equilibrium between collagen deposition and degradation has been restored. The metalloproteinases are the main digestive enzymes in remodeling, but neutrophil protease and serine proteases are also present.

Metalloproteinases and Matrix Degradation

A large family of 25 proteinases, the metalloproteinases (MMPs), are crucial components in wound healing, because they enable cells to migrate through the stroma by degrading matrix proteins. They also activate and inactivate bioactive molecules. The MMPs are synthesized as inactive zymogens and require extracellular activation by already activated MMPs or by serine proteinases. They are classified by the MMP acronym followed by a numerical suffix (e.g., MMP-1) or are called by common names such as collagenase,

TABLE 3-5 Tissue Expression of Extracellular Matrix Molecules

Tissue or Body Fluid	Primary Mesodermal Cell	Prominent Collagen Types	Noncollagenous Matrix Proteins	Glycosaminoglycans Proteoglycans (PGs)
Plasma			Fibronectin, fibrinogen, vitronectin	Hyaluronan
Dermis				
Reticular/papillary	Fibroblast	I, III, V, VI, XII	Fibronectin, elastin, fibrillin	Hyaluronan, decorin, biglycan, versican
Epidermal junction		VII, VXII (BP 180), anchoring fibrils, hemidesmosome		
Muscle	Muscle cell	I, III, V, VI, VIII, XII	Fibronectin, elastin, fibrillin	Aggrecan, biglycan, decorin, fibromodulin
Peri-, epimysium	Fibroblast			
Aortic media/adventitia				
Tendon	Fibroblast	I, III, V, VI, XII	Fibronectin, tensascin (myotendon junction), elastin, fibrillin	Decorin, biglycan, fibromodulin, lumican, versican
Ligament	Fibroblast	I, III, V, VI	Fibronectin, elastin fibrillin	Decorin, biglycan, versican
Cornea	Fibroblast	I, III, V, VI, XII		Lumican, keratocan, Mimecan, biglycan, decorin
Cartilage	Chondrocyte	II, IX, VI, VIII, XI X hypertrophic cartilage	Anchorin CII, fibronectin, tenascin	Hyaluronan, aggrecan, Biglycan, decorin Fibromodulin, lumican, Perlecan (minor)
Bone	Osteocyte	I, V	Osteocalcin, osteopontin, bone sialoprotein, SPARC (osteonectin)	Decorin, fibromodulin, Biglycan
Basement membrane zones	Epithelial, endothelial adipocytes, Schwann cell, muscle cells (endomysium), pericytes	IV, XV, XVIII	Laminin Nidogen/entactin	Heparan sulfate PGs Perlecan Collagen XVIII (vascular) Agrin (neuromuscular junctions)

T A B L E 3-6 Matrix Metalloproteinase Expression in Tissue

Extracellular Matrix Substrate	Matrix Metalloproteinases Shared Substrate Recognition	Matrix Metalloproteinase Partially Shared Substrate Recognition	Included/Excluded
Stromal matrix			
Collagen I			
Collagen III	MMP 1,2,13,14	MMP 3, 10 (not collagen I)	
		MMP 7, 12 (not collagen III)	MMP 9 (excluded)
Fibronectin		MMP 8 (collagens only)	
Elastin	MMP 2		MMP 1, 13, 14 (excluded)
			MMP 9 (included)
Basement membrane			
Laminin			
Entactin/nidogen	MMP 2,3,7,12	MMP 1 (not collagen IV)	MMP 8, 13, 14 (excluded)
Collagen IV		MMP 9 (not entactin)	MMP 7,9,12 (included)
Cartilage			
Collagen II	MMP 1,8,13,14		MMP 2,9 (excluded)
Wound (provisional) matrix			
Fibronectin			
Fibrinogen	MMP 1,2,3,14	MMP 7,12 (not fibrin)	MMP (excluded, other than fibrinogen)
Vitronectin		MMP 9 (not fibronectin)	
Fibrin			

MMP1, collagenase-1; MMP2, gelatinase A; MMP3, stromelysin-1; MMP7, matrilysin; MMP8, collagenase-2; MMP9, gelatinase-B; MMP10, stromelysin-2; MMP12, macrophage elastase; MMP13, collagenase-3; MMP14, MT1-MMP.

stromelysin, and gelatinase. MMPs cleave numerous extracellular substrates, many of which are degraded by more than one MMP (Table 3-6). As with integrins, such redundancy emphasizes the importance of these molecules in regulatory control. The list of molecules needed for wound healing is indistinguishable from the list of MMP substrates. These include

- Clotting factors
- Extracellular matrix proteins
- Latent growth factors and growth factor-binding proteins
- Receptors for matrix molecules and cell–cell adhesion molecules
- Other MMPs, other proteinases, and proteinase inhibitors
- Chemotactic molecules

Most MMPs are closely regulated at the transcriptional level, the exception being MMP-2 (gelatinase A), which is often constitutively expressed. Transcription is regulated by (1) integrin signaling, (2) growth factor signaling, (3) binding to certain matrix proteins, or (4) tensional force on a cell. As would be predicted by the location of their substrates, MMPs are secreted into the extracellular matrix or are membrane bound. Membrane-bound MMPs are either transmembrane molecules or are linked to glycosylphosphatidylinositol (GPI). MMPs 1 and 2 associate with integrins, thereby facilitating cell migration. In addition to enhancing migration and matrix remodeling, MMPs can disrupt cell–cell adhesions and release bioactive molecules stored in the matrix. These include growth factors, chemokines, growth factor-binding proteins, angiogenic/antiangiogenic factors, and bioactive fragments of matrix molecules. Once secreted, MMP activity can be minimized by binding to specific proteinase inhibitors. In addition to the important plasma-derived proteinase inhibitor, α_2-macroglobulin, there is a family of endogenous tissue inhibitors of metalloproteinases (TIMPs).

Cell Proliferation Is Evoked by Cytokines and Matrix

A prominent early feature in injured tissue is a transient increase in cellularity, which serves to initiate and perpetuate granulation tissue and replace damaged cells. Cells of granulation tissue accumulate from labile cell populations (see below), including circulating leukocytes and basal epithelial cells, and from stable cells, such as capillary endothelia and resident mesenchymal cells (fibroblasts, myofibroblasts, pericytes, and smooth muscle cells). Marrow-derived stem cells may also populate wounds, differentiating into endothelial and fibroblast populations. Cells that are terminally differentiated (e.g., cardiac myocytes, neurons) do not contribute to repair or regeneration.

Growth factors and small chemotactic peptides (chemokines) provide soluble autocrine and paracrine signals for cell proliferation, differentiation, and migration. Signals from soluble factors and extracellular matrix also work collectively to influence cell behavior.

Integrated Molecular Signals Mediate Proliferation and Differentiation

The behaviors of cells in healing wounds—proliferation, migration, and altered gene expression—are largely initiated by three receptor systems that share integrated signaling pathways (Fig. 3-5).

- Protein tyrosine kinase receptors for peptide growth factors
- G protein-coupled receptors for chemokines and other factors
- Integrin receptors for extracellular matrix.

Tyrosine kinase receptors, growth factors matrix integrin receptors, and G protein-coupled receptors act in concert to direct cell behavior. These distinct receptor families bind unrelated ligands yet transmit signals within a network of cascading and intersecting pathways that amplify the messages, often activating similar processes. Even different processes, such as proliferation, differentiation, and migration may share signals, such as those that initiate cytoskeletal changes.

Protein Tyrosine Kinase (Growth Factor) Receptors

When bound to growth factors, these receptors dimerize and autophosphorylate, attracting other proteins with Src-homology on the cytoplasmic side of the plasma membrane. Growth factor receptors activate GTPase cascades and PI3K

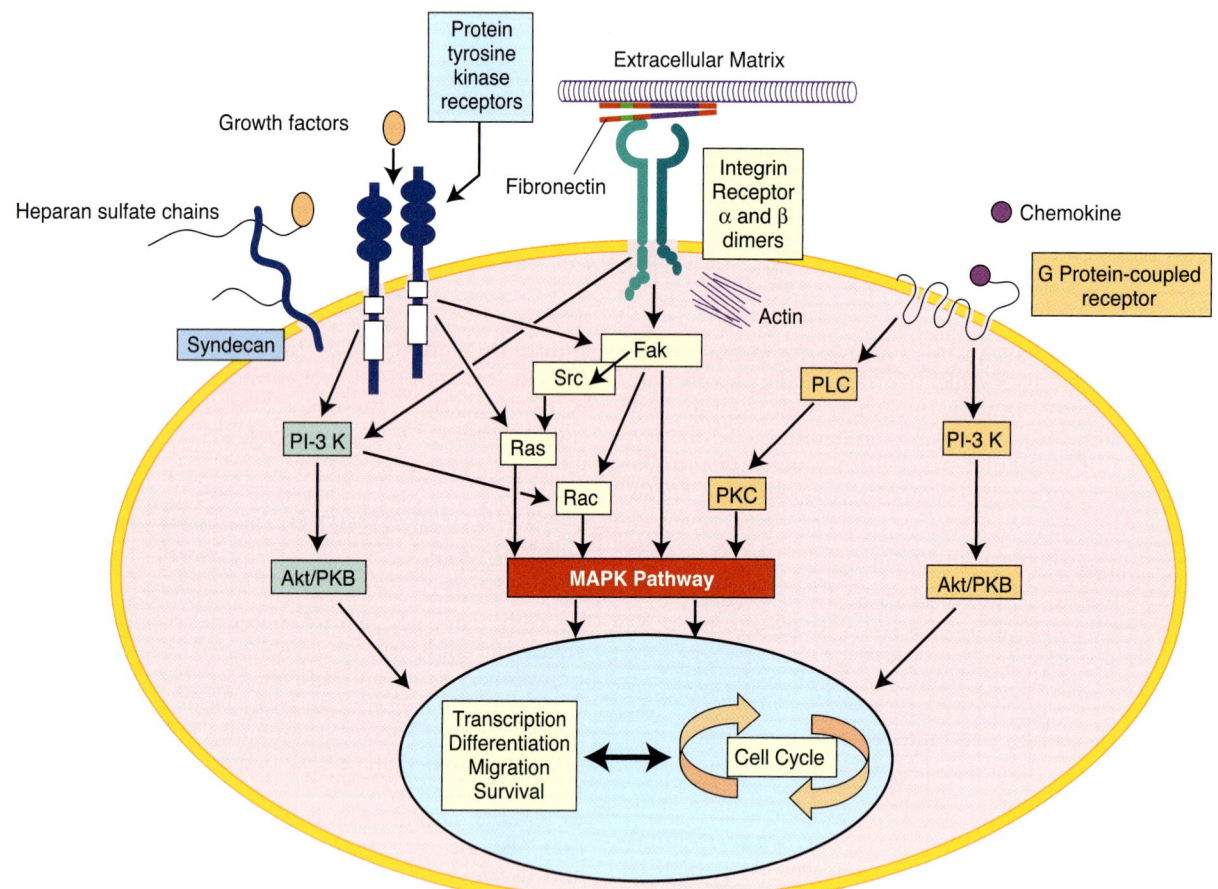

FIGURE 3-5
Summary of shared signaling pathways for integrin, protein tyrosine kinase, and chemokine cell surface receptors. Extracellular matrix is bound by integrin-αβ dimer receptors, which anchor the activated actin cytoskeleton and signal through Src and focal adhesion kinase (FAK) and through the GTPase (Ras, Rac) and PI3K pathways. Growth factors are bound by protein tyrosine kinase receptors, causing them to dimerize, autophosphorylate, and signal through the GTPase and PI3K pathways. VEGF and bFGF signaling is modulated by heparan sulfate proteoglycan (syndecan) receptors, which create a cell-surface reservoir of these growth factors and enable efficient binding to the PTK receptors. Chemokines and certain other cytokines bind the 7-transmembrane G-protein-coupled receptors, which signal through PI3K or the phospholipase C (PLC) and protein kinase C (PKC) pathways. The signals are transduced to Akt/protein kinase B (PKB) or mitogen activated protein kinases (MAP kinases) and into the nucleus, stimulating genes involved in proliferation, differentiation, transcription and migration.

pathways, both of which initiate a cascade of events leading to several signal transduction pathways.

G Protein-Coupled Receptors

These seven-transmembrane receptors for chemokines trigger cyclic AMP, phospholipase C, and JAK-STAT (Janus kinase-signal transducer and activator of transcription) or PI3K pathways, depending on the (1) ligand, (2) specific chemokine receptor, (3) cell type, and (4) particular G protein available.

Integrin Receptors

These cell receptors uniquely function to discern chemical and mechanical information in the extracellular matrix and respond to both by creating attachment sites for the actin cytoskeleton. In this manner they initiate proliferation and differentiation. Accessory proteins help anchor the actin cytoskeleton by attaching protein complexes to the short cytoplasmic tail of integrin and to actin, eventually connecting the actin stress fibers with the extracellular matrix through the integrin receptor (see "Cell Migration"). Two nonreceptor tyrosine kinases, namely, focal adhesion kinase (FAK) and Src, are key signal initiators that interact to trigger early signaling cascades. Autophosphorylation of FAK creates a binding site for Src, which phosphorylates other proteins and builds a protein scaffold that links to actin. Additionally, Src phosphorylates FAK, causing a separate sequence of protein interactions that lead to activation of Ras, a GTPase that activates the mitogen-activated protein (MAP) kinase cascade. Integrin activation also initiates the PI3K pathway.

Three Protein Families Transduce Signals to the Nucleus

The MAP kinase pathway is a series of serine-threonine kinase reactions directed toward the nucleus to initiate transcription that leads to proliferation and differentiation. Signals from these different receptors intersect in commonly used pathways.

GTPases

GTPases such as the Ras- or Rho-type (Rho, Rac, Cdc42) subfamilies are indirectly activated by protein tyrosine kinase receptors and integrin receptors, after which they relay signals to initiate cytoskeletal changes (Rho, Rac). The GTPases initiate a series of serine–threonine kinase reactions in the MAP kinase cascade.

Phosphatidylinositol-3 Kinase (PI3K)

PI3K catalyzes the production of phosphinositide-3,4, 5-trisphosphate (PIP_3) lipids, which accumulate at the cell membrane in response to the activation of tyrosine kinase receptors or G protein-coupled receptors. The serine–threonine kinase Akt (also called protein kinase B) is phosphorylated by phosphoinositide-dependent kinase 1 (PDK1). Akt/PKB then phosphorylates nuclear proteins that affect cell growth and behavior in a cascade distinct from the MAP kinase pathway. The PI3K pathway intersects with growth factor receptor and integrin receptor pathways by PIP_3-derived activation of Rac GTPase, which affects cytoskeletal changes and stimulates the MAP kinase pathway.

Phospholipase C

The $G\alpha_I$ pathway is activated by several chemokine receptors found on endothelial, epithelial, and mast cells, as well as leukocytes. G proteins and protein tyrosine kinase receptors can signal by both the phospholipase C and the PI3K pathways. Phospholipase C hydrolyzes phosphoinositide bisphosphate (PIP_2) into inositol trisphosphate (IP_3) and diacylglycerol (DAG). IP_3 stimulates calcium release, which together with DAG activates protein kinase C (PKC). PKC then activates the MAP kinase pathway.

REPAIR

Outcomes of Injury Include Repair and Regeneration

Repair and regeneration develop following inflammatory responses, inflammation itself being the primary response to tissue injury (see Chapter 2). To understand how inflammation influences repair, it is useful to review the various possible outcomes of acute inflammation. Transient acute inflammation may resolve completely, with locally injured parenchymal elements being regenerated without significant scarring. For example, in recovery from a moderate sunburn, small numbers of acute inflammatory cells temporarily accompany transient vasodilation beneath the solar-injured epidermis. By contrast, progressive acute inflammation, with emergence of macrophage-predominant inflammation, is intrinsic to the sequence of collagen elaboration and repair.

Organization

Organization represents a pathological outcome of an inflammatory response. It occurs in serous cavities such as the pericardium and peritoneal cavities. In pericarditis, fibroblasts secrete and organize collagen within fibrin strands, thereby binding the visceral and parietal pericardium together (Fig. 3-6). This results in constricted ventricular filling of the heart and may require surgical intervention. Fibrin strands sometimes become organized within the peritoneal cavity following intraabdominal surgery. Such adhesions (threads of collagen) can trap loops of bowel and cause intestinal obstruction.

Wound Healing Exhibits a Defined Sequence

Since wounds in the skin and the extremities are easily accessible, they have been extensively used as models. Though more difficult to study, healing within hollow viscera and

Repair, Regeneration, and Fibrosis

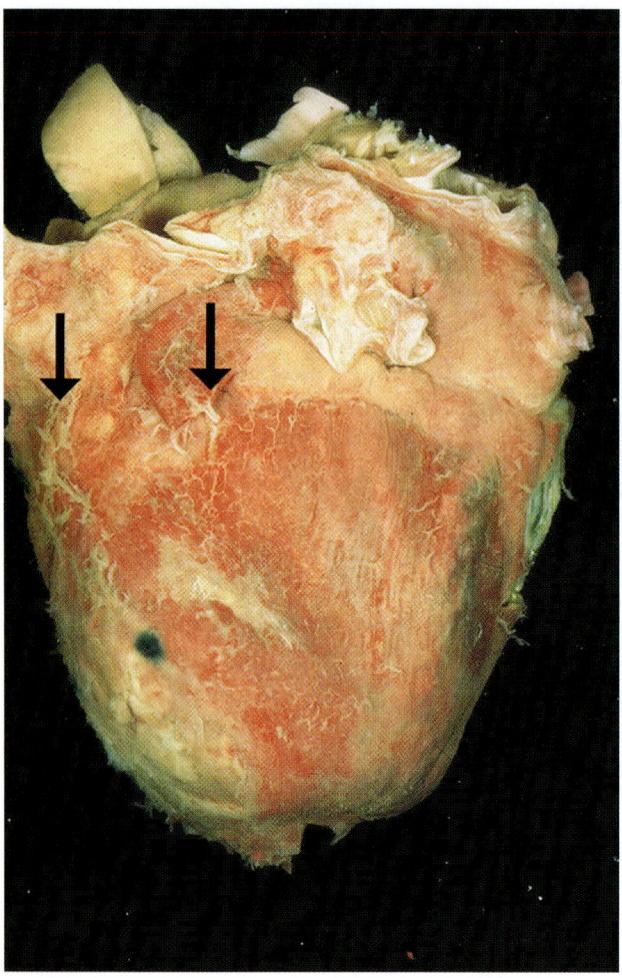

FIGURE 3-6
Organized strands of collagen in constrictive pericarditis *(arrows).*

body cavities generally parallels the repair sequence in skin (Table 3-7 and Fig. 3-7).

Thrombosis

A thrombus (clot), referred to as a *scab*, or *eschar*, after drying out, forms a barrier on the wounded skin to invading surface microorganisms. It also prevents the loss of plasma and tissue fluid. Formed primarily from plasma fibrin, the thrombus is rich in fibronectin. At the site of injury, fibronectin is soon cross-linked by transglutaminase to provide local tensile strength and maintain closure. The thrombus also contains contracting platelets, an initial source of growth factors. Much later, the thrombus undergoes proteolysis, after which it is penetrated by regenerating epithelium. The scab then detaches.

Inflammation

Repair sites vary in the amount of local tissue destruction. For example, the surgical excision of a skin lesion leaves little or no devitalized tissue. Demarcated, localized necrosis accompanies medium-sized myocardial infarcts. By contrast, widespread, irregularly defined necrosis is a feature of a large third-degree burn. Initially, an acute, neutrophil-dominated, inflammatory response liquefies the necrotic tissue. Acute inflammation persists as long as necessary, since repair cannot progress until necrotic structures are liquefied and removed. Subsequently, plasma-derived fibronectin binds to collagen and cell membranes to facilitate phagocytosis. Fibronectin and cellular debris are chemotactic for

TABLE 3-7 Repair in Skin

EARLY	1.	Thrombosis: Formation of a growth factor-rich barrier having significant tensile strength
	2.	Inflammation: Necrotic debris and microorganisms must be removed by neutrophils; the appearance of macrophages signals and initiates repair
	3.	Reepithelialization: Newly formed epithelium establishes a permanent barrier to microorganisms and fluid
MID	4.	Granulation tissue formation and function: This specialized organ of repair is the site of extracellular matrix and collagen secretion; it is vascular, edematous, insensitive, and resistant to infection
	5.	Contraction: Fibroblasts and possibly other cells also transform to actin-containing myofibroblasts, link to each other and collagen, and contract, stimulated by TGF-β_1 or β_2
LATE	6.	Accretion of final tensile strength results primarily from the cross-linking of collagen
	7.	Remodeling: The wound site devascularizes and conforms to stress lines in the skin

FIGURE 3-7
Summary of the healing process. The initial phase of the repair reaction, which typically begins with hemorrhage into the tissues. *(1)* A fibrin clot forms and fills the gap created by the wound. Fibronectin in the extravasated plasma is cross-linked to fibrin, collagen, and other extracellular matrix components by the action of transglutaminases. This cross-linking provides a provisional mechanical stabilization of the wound (0–4 hours). *(2)* Macrophages recruited to the wound area process cell remnants and damaged extracellular matrix. The binding of fibronectin to cell membranes, collagens, proteoglycans, DNA, and bacteria (opsonization) facilitates phagocytosis by these macrophages and contributes to the removal of debris (1–3 days). *(3)* Fibronectin, cell debris, and bacterial products are chemoattractants for a variety of cells that are recruited to the wound site (2–4 days). The intermediate phase of the repair reaction. *(4)* As a new extracellular matrix is deposited at the wound site, the initial fibrin clot is lysed by a combination of extracellular proteolytic enzymes and phagocytosis (2–4 days). *(5)* Concurrent with fibrin removal, there is deposition of a temporary matrix formed by proteoglycans, glycoproteins, and type III collagen (2–5 days). *(6)* Final phase of the repair reaction. Eventually the temporary matrix is removed by a combination of extracellular and intracellular digestion, and the definitive matrix, rich in type I collagen, is deposited (5 days–weeks).

Repair

macrophages and fibroblasts (Fig. 3-7). The appearance of macrophages as the predominant cell at the site of injury signals the onset of the repair process. Macrophages ingest proteolytic products of neutrophils and secrete collagenase, thereby promoting further liquefaction. They also provide growth factors that stimulate fibroblast proliferation, collagen secretion, and neovascularization.

Macrophages

A key step in the development of granulation tissue is the recruitment of monocytes to the site of injury by chemokines and fragments of damaged matrix. The *provisional matrix* is a temporary scaffold of cross-linked plasma glycoproteins, platelets, and other blood-borne cells, which is ultimately replaced by

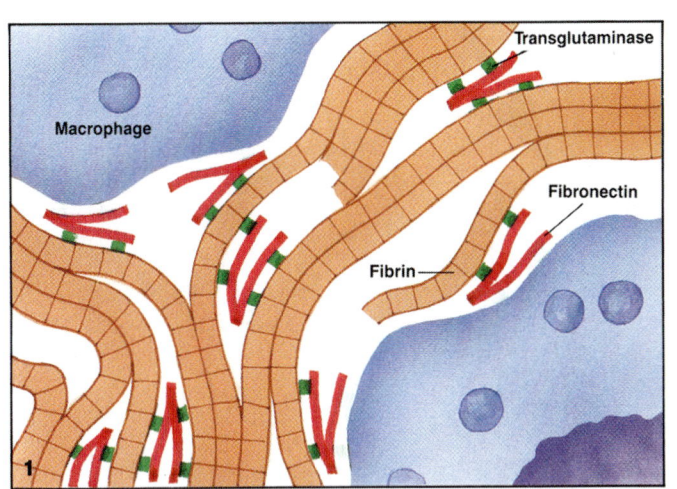
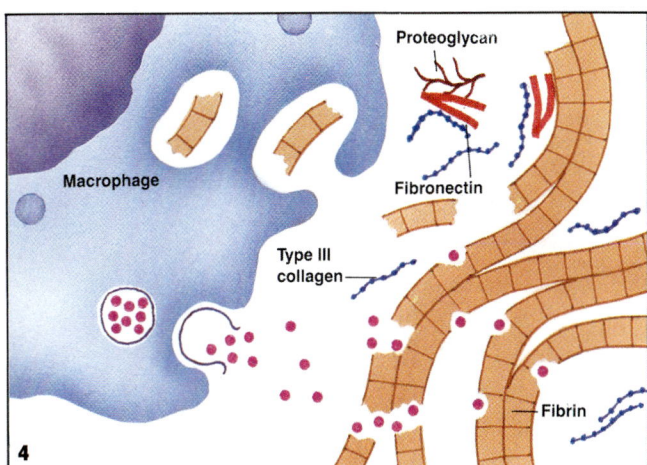
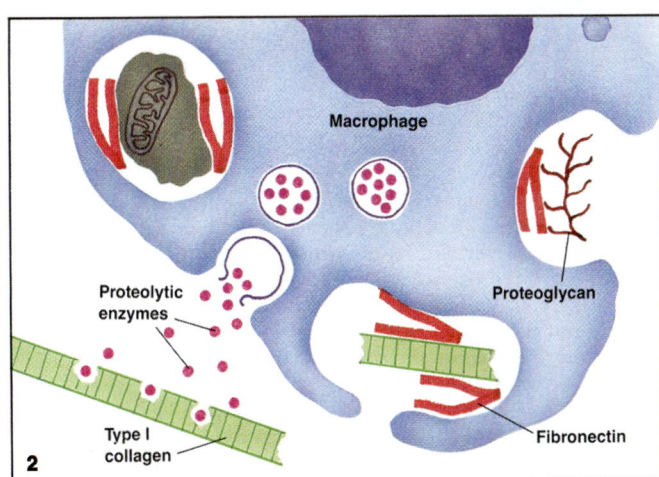
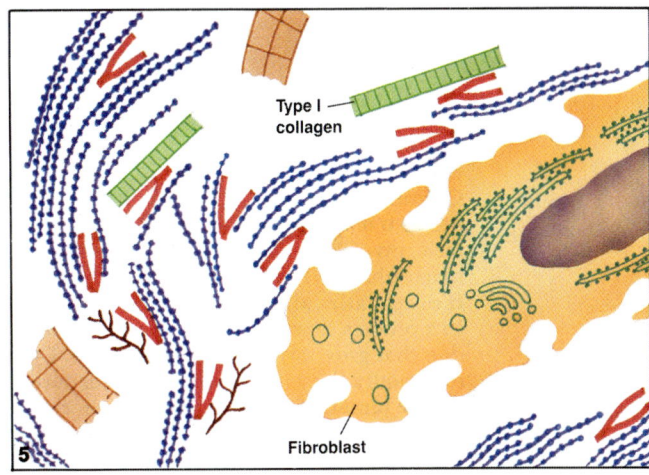
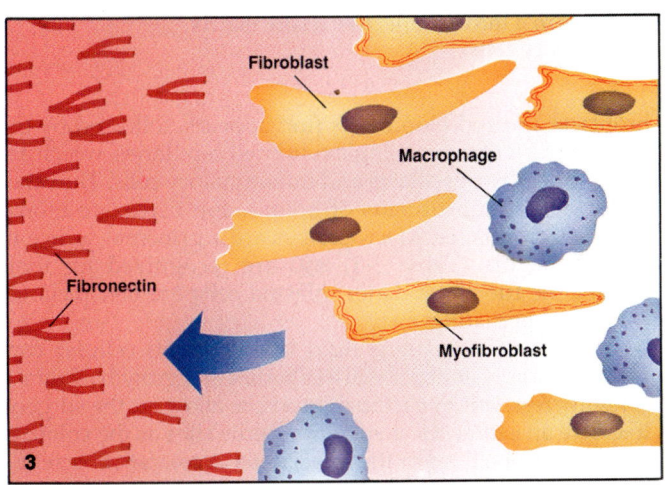
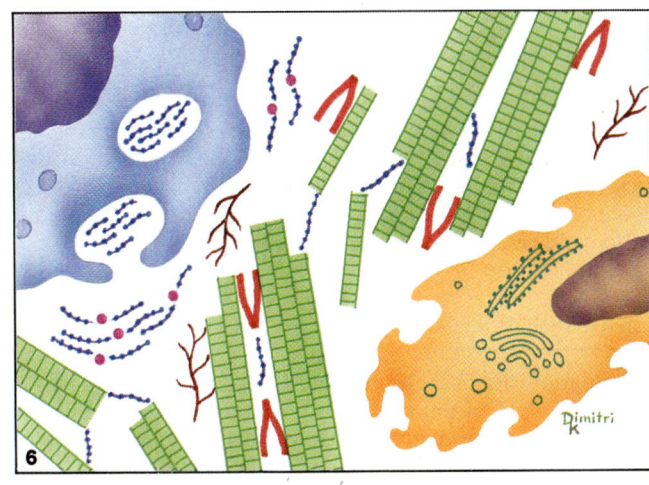

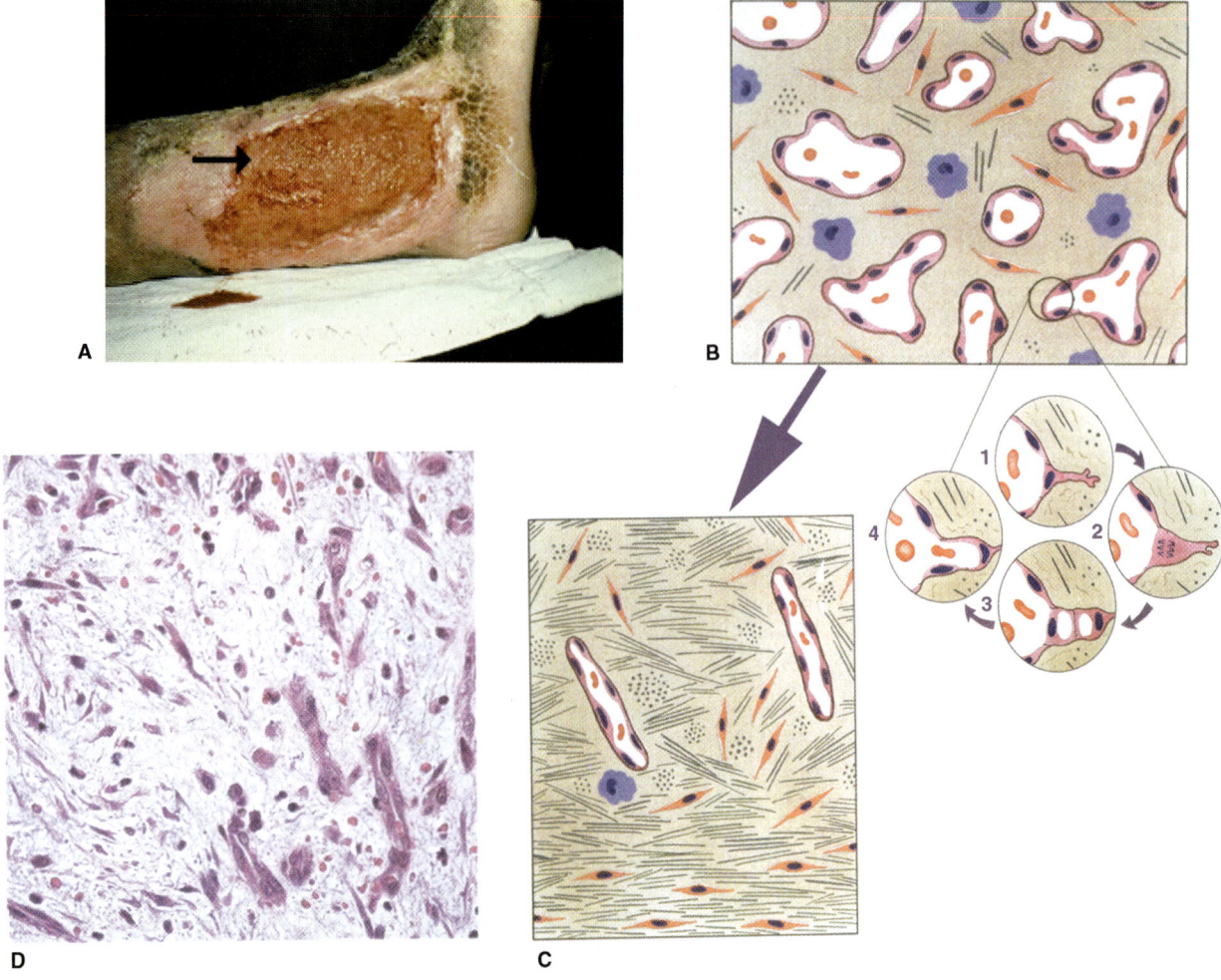

FIGURE 3-8

Granulation tissue. A. A foot ulcer is covered by granulation tissue. B. Granulation tissue has two major components: cells and proliferating capillaries. The cells are mostly fibroblasts, myofibroblasts, and macrophages. The macrophages are derived from monocytes and macrophages. The fibroblasts and myofibroblasts derive from mesenchymal stem cells, and the capillaries arise from adjacent vessels by division of the lining endothelial cells *(detail)*, in a process termed *angiogenesis*. Endothelial cells put out cell extensions, called *pseudopodia*, that grow toward the wound site. Cytoplasmic growth enlarges the pseudopodia, and eventually the cells divide. Vacuoles formed in the daughter cells eventually fuse to create a new lumen. The entire process continues until the sprout encounters another capillary, with which it will connect. At its peak, granulation tissue is the most richly vascularized tissue in the body. C. Once repair has been achieved, most of the newly formed capillaries are obliterated and then reabsorbed, leaving a pale avascular scar. D. A photomicrograph of granulation tissue shows thin-walled vessels embedded in a loose connective tissue matrix containing mesenchymal cells and occasional inflammatory cells.

granulation tissue. Activated macrophages coordinate the development of granulation tissue through the release of growth factors and cytokines. These molecules direct angiogenesis, activate fibroblasts to form new stroma, and continue the degradation and removal of the provisional matrix.

Granulation Tissue

Granulation tissue is the transient, specialized organ of repair. Like the placenta, it is only present where and when needed. It is deceptively simple, with a glistening and pebbled appearance (Fig. 3-8). Microscopically, a mixture of fibroblasts and red blood cells first appears, followed by the development of patent single cell-lined capillaries, which are surrounded by fibroblasts and inflammatory cells. The other early cellular constituents of granulation tissue are monocytes/macrophages. Macrophages are a principal source of growth factors (Table 3-8) and are recognized for their phagocytic functions. Later, plasma cells are conspicuous, even predominating.

Granulation tissue is fluid laden, and its cellular constituents supply antibacterial antibodies and growth factors. It is highly resistant to bacterial infection, allowing the surgeon to create anastomoses at such nonsterile sites as the colon, in which fully one third of the fecal contents consist of bacteria.

TABLE 3-8 Signals in Wound Repair

Phase	Factor(s)	Source	Effects
Coagulation	XIIIA	Plasma	Thrombosis
	TGF-α, TGF-β, PDGF, ECGF	Platelets	Chemoattraction of subsequently involved cells
Inflammation	TGF-β	Neutrophil	Attracts monocytes/macrophages and fibroblasts, differentiates fibroblasts
Granulation tissue formation	Basic FGF, TGF-β	Monocyte/macrophage, then fibroblasts	Various factors are bound to proteoglycan matrix
Angiogenesis	VEGFs	Monocyte/macrophage	Development of blood vessels
Contraction	TGF-β1, β2	Various	Myofibroblasts appear, bind to each other and collagen, and contract
Maturation- arrest of proliferation	TGF-β$_1$	Platelets, monoctyes/macrophages	Accumulation of extracellular matrix
	Heparin sulfate proteoglycan, decorin	Secretory fibroblasts	Capture of TGF-β and basic FGF
	Interferon	Plasma monocytes	Suppresses proliferation of fibroblasts and accumulation of collagen
Remodeling	Increased local oxygen	Repair process	Suppresses release of cytokines
	PDGF-FGF	Platelets, fibroblasts	Induction of MMPs
	Matrix metalloproteinases, t-PAs, u-PAs	Sprouted capillaries, epithelial cells	Remodeling by permitting ingrowth of vessels and restructuring of ECM
	Tissue inhibitors of metalloproteinases	Local, not further defined	Balance the effects of MMPs in the evolving repair site

Fibroblast Proliferation and Matrix Accumulation

The temporary early matrix of granulation tissue contains proteoglycans, glycoproteins, and type III collagen (see Fig. 3-7). The release of cytokines from fixed cells in the damaged tissue causes hemorrhage and attracts inflammatory cells to the site. About 2 to 3 days after injury, activated fibroblasts and capillary sprouts are detected. The shape of fibroblasts in the wound changes from oval to bipolar, as they begin to form collagen (Fig. 3-9) and synthesize other matrix proteins, such as fibronectin. The secretion of type III collagen, initially 20% of the total collagen, is transient and a forerunner

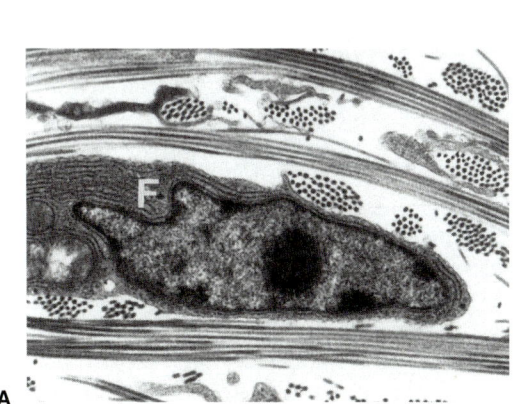
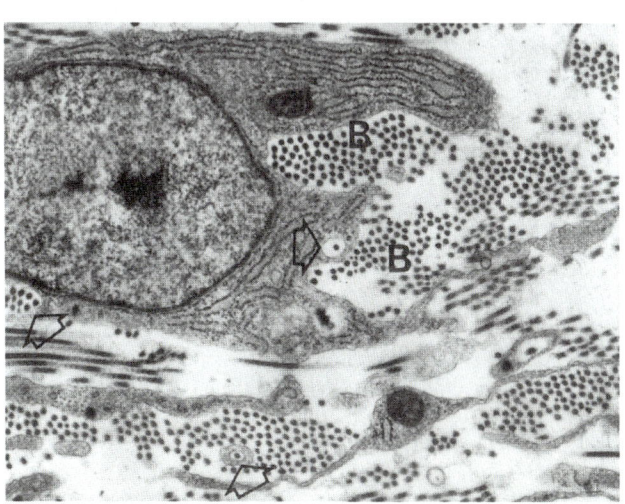

FIGURE 3-9
Fibroblasts and collagen fibers. Electron micrographs. A. Chick embryo fibroblast (F) lying between collagen fibers and an elastin fiber in lower right corner. The collagen fibers are seen as crosswise strands traversing the field and along the long axis, at a right angle, as dots. B. A chick embryo dermal fibroblast with cell surface-associated collagen fibril bundles (B); some bundles are enveloped by fibroblast membrane (arrows). The fibrils are visualized on the long axis as dots.

to the formation of type I collagen, which imparts greater tensile strength. Approaching the peak of matrix accumulation in 5 to 7 days, the release of TGF-β increases the synthesis of collagen and fibronectin and decreases metalloproteinase transcription and matrix degradation. Extracellular cross-linking of newly synthesized collagen progressively increases wound strength.

Growth Factors and Fibroplasia

The initial discovery of EGF and the subsequent identification of at least 20 other growth factors have provided explanations for many of the rapidly changing events in repair and regeneration. Redundancy and interaction among growth factors, other cytokines, and metalloproteinases are illustrated in Figures 3-10, 3-11. The actions of growth factors are not entirely redundant, since each has a predominant function in repair. Specificity derives from (1) temporal expression of different receptors and their isotypes in dissimilar cell populations, (2) variable responses by individual receptors, and (3) latency or activation of growth factors. Tables 3-8, 3-9, and 3-10 show how growth factors control the specific events in repair. Growth factors expressed early (FGF, PDGF, EGF, and keratinocyte growth factor [KGF]) support cell migration and proliferation, whereas those that peak later (TGF-β, and IGF-1) sustain the maturation phase of granulation tissue.

Although the roles of growth factors in the initiation and progression of repair are reasonably well understood, the limiting and terminating events are not well defined. Diminishing anoxia as repair progresses may be key to the arrest of the repair process. Repair may also cease because of reduced turnover of extracellular matrix. Finally, increased storage and decreased availability of growth factors may stabilize the matrix, which may then transmit signals that reduce the effects of growth factors.

Angiogenesis

The Growth of Capillaries

At its peak, granulation tissue has more capillaries per unit volume than any other tissue. New capillary growth is essential for the delivery of oxygen and nutrients to the cells. New capillaries form by angiogenesis (i.e., sprouting of endothelial cells from preexisting capillary venules) (Fig. 3-8) and create the granular appearance for which granulation tissue is named. Less often, new blood vessels form de novo from angioblasts. The latter process is known as *vasculogenesis* and is primarily associated with developmental processes.

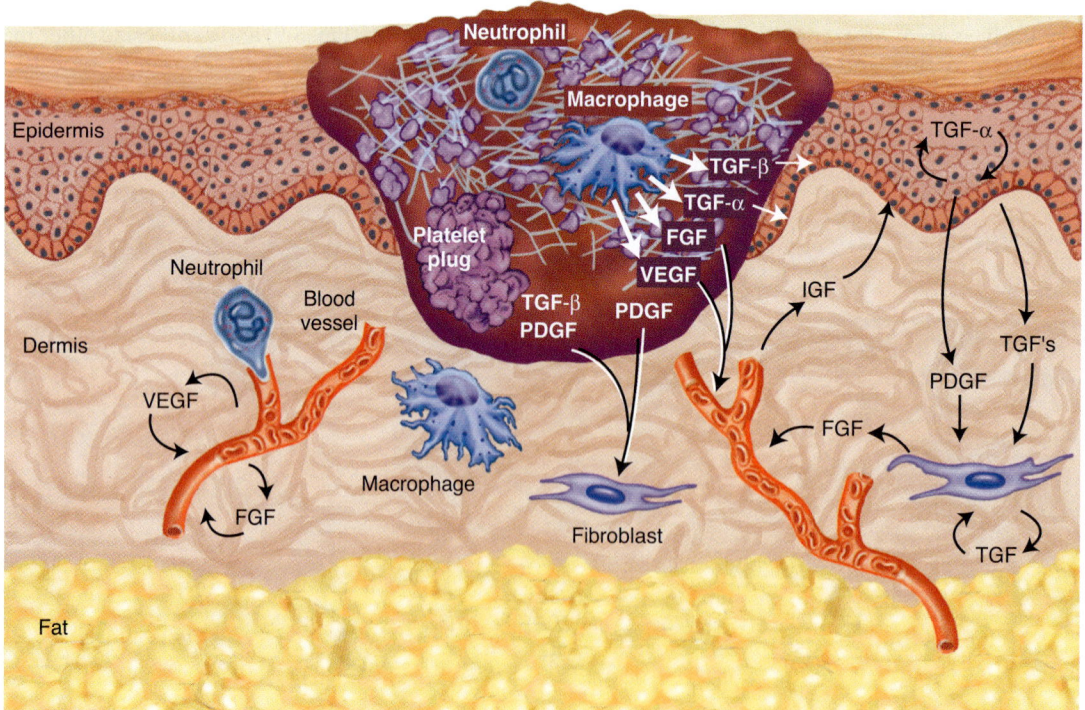

FIGURE 3-10
Cutaneous wound, 2–4 days. Growth factors controlling migration of cells are illustrated. Extensive redundancy is present, and no growth factor is rate limiting. Most factors have multiple effects, as listed in Table 3-10.

Repair 105

4–8 Days

Thrombus

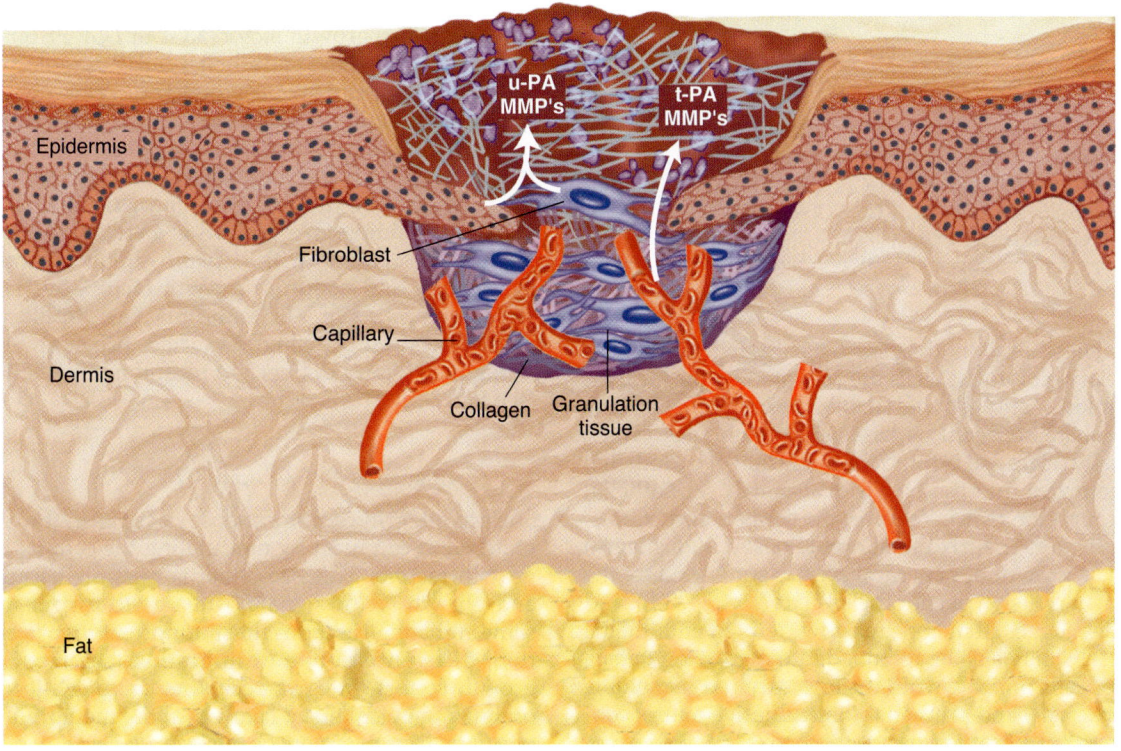

FIGURE 3-11
Cutaneous wound, 4–8 days. Blood vessels are proliferating, and the epidermis is penetrating the thrombus, but not at its surface. The upper portion will become an eschar or scab.

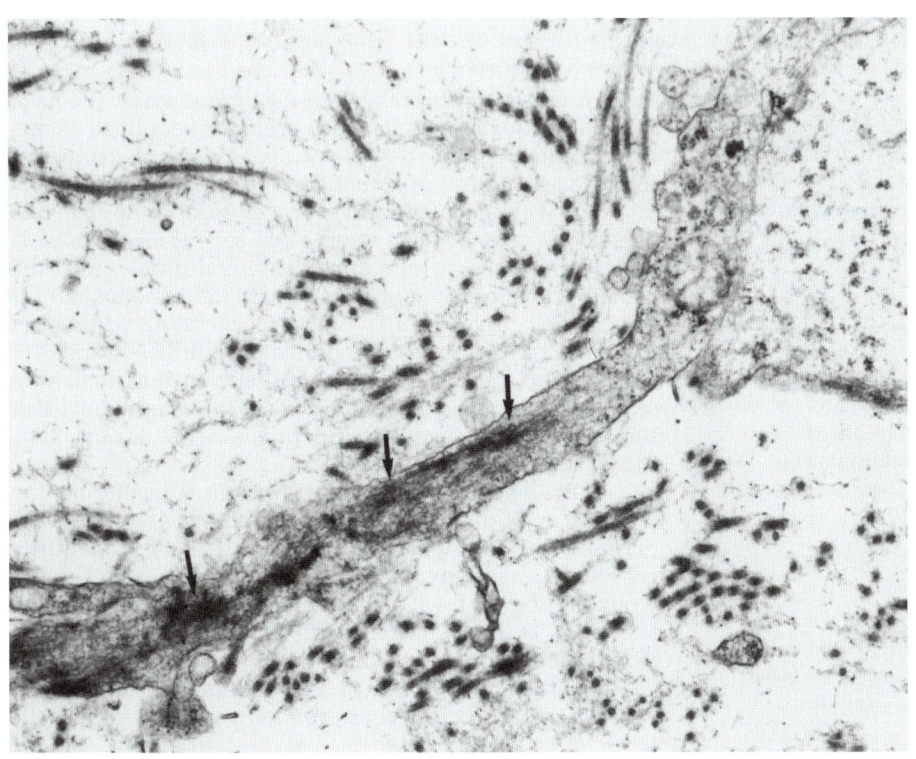

FIGURE 3-12
Myofibroblast viewed by electron microscopy. Myofibroblasts have an important role in the repair reaction. These cells, with features intermediate between those of smooth muscle cells and fibroblasts, are characterized by the presence of discrete bundles of myofilaments in the cytoplasm (arrows).

Repair, Regeneration, and Fibrosis

TABLE 3-9 Growth Factors Control Specific Stages in Repair

Attraction of monoctyes/macrophages	PDGFs, FGFs, TGF-β
Attraction of fibroblasts	PDGFs, FGFs, TGF-β, CTGF, EGFs
Proliferation of fibroblasts	PDGFs, FGFs, EGFs, IGF, CTGF, TNFs
Angiogenesis	VEGFs, FGFs
Collagen synthesis	TGF-β, PDGFs, IGF, CTGF, TNFs
Collagen secretion	PDGFs, FGFs, CTGF, TNFs
Migration and proliferation of epithelium-epidermis	KGF, TGF-α, IGF

Angiogenesis in wound repair is tightly regulated. Quiescent capillary endothelial cells are activated by the local release of cytokines and growth factors. The endothelial cells and pericytes are bordered by basement membranes, which must be locally degraded prior to the migration of endothelial cells and pericytes into the provisional matrix. Endothelial passage through the matrix requires the cooperation of plasminogen activators, matrix metalloproteinases, and integrin receptors. The growth of new capillaries is supported by the proliferation and fusion of endothelial cells (see Fig. 3-8), and recent studies suggest that bone marrow-derived endothelial progenitor cells may also be recruited into a growing vessel. Migration of cells into the wound site is directed by soluble ligands *(chemotaxis)* and proceeds along adhesive matrix substrates *(haptotaxis)*. Once capillary endothelial cells are immobilized, cell–cell contacts form, and an organized basement membrane develops on the exterior of the nascent capillary. Association with pericytes and signals from angiopoietin, TGF-β, and PDGF establish a mature vessel phenotype and help form nonleaky capillaries. New capillaries that have not matured may undergo endothelial apoptosis.

Experimentally, stimulation of angiogenesis in cell culture requires extracellular matrix and growth factors. In vivo angiogenesis is initiated by hypoxia and a redundancy of cytokines, growth factors, and specifically lipids, which enlist angiogenic factors bFGF and VEGF. Activated granulation tissue macrophages and endothelial cells produce bFGF and VEGF, and wound epidermal cells release VEGF in response to keratinocyte growth factor (KGF or FGF-7). Since the chief target of VEGF is the endothelial cell, this molecule is a critical regulator of embryonic vascular development and angiogenesis, regulating endothelial survival, differentiation, and migration. In this context, the loss of one VEGF allele causes lethal defects in the embryonic vasculature.

The binding of angiogenic growth factors to heparan sulfate-containing GAG chains is a crucial feature of angiogenesis. Association with heparan sulfate chains affects the availability and action of growth factors by (1) creating a storage reservoir of VEGF and bFGF in capillary basement membranes and (2) using cell surface proteoglycan receptors to regulate ligand delivery to receptors for VEGF and bFGF (see Fig. 3-5).

Angiogenesis and Receptor Cross-Talk

Surface integrin receptors sense changes in the extracellular matrix and can react by modulating the cellular response to growth factors. This cross-talk is possible because integrin and growth factor signals converge to trigger many of the same signaling cascades that support survival, cell proliferation, differentiation, and migration (see Fig. 3-5). Unlike growth factors, integrin receptors drive cell locomotion by organizing cytoskeletal changes at the membrane. When exposed to growth factors or the loss of an organized basement membrane, quiescent endothelial cells express new integrins that modulate endothelial migration on provisional matrix proteins. Capillary sprouting relies principally on β_1-type integrins, although other integrins are also upregulated during angiogenesis.

Reepithelialization

Epidermis constantly renews itself by mitosis at the basal layer. The squamous cells then cornify or keratinize as they mature and are shed a few days later. Maturation requires an intact layer of basal cells that are in direct contact with one another. If this contact is disrupted, basal epithelial cells reestablish contact with other basal cells through mitosis. The other necessary signal for epidermal differentiation is contact with a basement membrane. In the skin, the hair follicle is the primary source of the regenerating epithelium. Epithelial regeneration is illustrated in Figures 3-10 and 3-11. Once reestablished, the epithelial barrier demarcates the scab from the newly covered wound. When epithelial continuity is reestablished, the epidermis resumes its normal cycle of maturation and shedding.

Epithelialization provides a protective barrier against infection and fluid loss. In addition to epithelial cells, the epidermis includes important immune cells, such as dendritic cells and Langerhans cells. In general, epithelial cells close wounds either by migrating to cover the damaged surface or, less often, by a cinching process called *purse-string closure*. Skin provides the best studied example of epithelial repair.

The basal layer of skin epithelial cells, also called *epidermal cells* or *keratinocytes,* contributes important cytokines (IL-

TABLE 3-10 Growth Factors, Enzymes and Other Factors Regulate Progression of Repair and Fibrosis

Secretion of collagenase	PDGFs EGF, IL-1, TNF, proteases
Movement of surface and stromal cells	t-PA (tissue plasminogen activator)
	u-Pa (urokinase-type plasminogen activator)
	MMPs (matrix metalloproteinase)
	MMP-1 (collagenase 1)
	MMP-2 (gelatinase A)
	MMP-3 (stromelysin 1)
	MMP-13 (collagenase 3)
Maturation or stabilization of blood vessels	Angiopoietins (Ang1, Ang2)
Inhibition of collagen secretion	TGF-β
Reduction in collagen production and turnover	Reduction in anoxia
Collagen cross-linking and maturation	Lysyl oxidase, unknown factor

1, VEGF, TGF-α, PDGF, TGF-β) for the initiation of healing and the immune response. To begin migration, keratinocytes must undergo cellular differentiation before forming a new covering over the wound. Normally, these cells are attached to laminin in the underlying basement membrane by hemidesmosome protein complexes containing $\alpha_6\beta_4$ integrin. The long cytoplasmic tail of the β_4 integrin chain forms a link between the basement membrane and the keratin intermediate filaments of keratinocytes. Among the molecules associated with the hemidesmosome complex are several members of the collagen family, namely, type XVII collagen (BP-180) and collagen type VII, also termed *anchoring fibril* (Table 3-3). The anchoring fibril connects the hemidesmosome–basement membrane complex to the dermal connective tissue collagen fibers.

Epithelial cells are connected at their lateral edges by *adherens junctions* composed of cadherin receptors. Cadherins are calcium-dependent, integral membrane proteins that form extracellular cell–cell connections and anchor intracellular cytoskeletal connections. Cadherins in the adherens junctions bind stable actin bundles to a cytoplasmic complex of α-, β-, and γ-catenins. The layer of actin that encircles the epithelial cytoplasm creates lateral tension and strength and is referred to as the *adhesion belt*. A second epithelial lateral connection that links to the cytoskeleton is the *desmosomal complex*, which is another cadherin-containing receptor complex. This assembly associates intracellularly with γ-catenin but binds keratin filaments rather than actin filaments. The shape and the strength of epithelial sheets result from tension created by cytoskeletal connections to basement membrane and cell to cell connections. Epithelial cells "measure" the presence of cadherin-based lateral attachments by the availability of free β- or γ-catenins. Free catenins are normally degraded, but in the presence of certain growth factors of the TGF-β superfamily, β- and γ-catenins are spared degradation and move to the nucleus, where they act as transcriptional activators. Thus, catenins organize cytoskeleton and perform an important differentiative function.

Cellular migration is the predominant means by which the wound surface is reepithelialized. Migrating epidermal cells originate at the margin of the wound and in hair follicles or sweat glands. If the basement membrane is lost, cells come in contact with unfamiliar stromal components, an effect that stimulates cell locomotion and proteinase expression.

Activation of epithelial motility is driven by the assembly of actin fibers at focal adhesions organized by newly expressed integrin receptors ($\alpha_5\beta_1$, $\alpha v\beta_{5 \text{ or } 6}$ and $\alpha_2\beta_1$). These integrins bind collagen I, fibronectin, vitronectin, and fibrinogen (Table 3-1) and steer the migrating cells along the margin of viable dermis. Movement through cross-linked fibrin apposed to the dermis requires the activation of plasmin from plasminogen to degrade fibrin. Pericellular activation of cell-bound plasminogen is regulated by urokinase-type plasminogen activator (u-PA) and can be localized at the cell surface by the GPI-anchored u-PA receptor (u-PAR). This receptor also interacts with integrin receptors, initiating signaling events for cell migration and proliferation. In addition to degrading fibrinogen and fibrin, plasmin aids in the activation of MMPs. Interstitial collagenase (MMP-1), gelatinase 2 (MMP-2) and stromelysin 1 (MMP-3) are upregulated by keratinocytes migrating on stromal matrix. Proteolytic cleavage of stromal collagens I and III at focal adhesion contacts acts as a release mechanism to allow keratinocyte migration. The epidermal cells resume their normal phenotype after the keratinocytes form a confluent layer over the wound site and attach to the basement membrane.

Wound Contraction

As they heal, open wounds contract and deform. The means by which wounds contract was a mystery until the discovery of a specialized cell of granulation tissue, namely, the *myofibroblast* (Fig. 3-12). This modified fibroblast cannot be distinguished from the collagen-secreting fibroblast by conventional light microscopy. Unlike the fibroblast, the myofibroblast expresses α-smooth muscle actin, desmin, and vimentin, and it responds to pharmacological agents that cause smooth muscle to contract or relax. In short, it is a fibroblast that reacts like a smooth muscle cell. **The myofibroblast is the cell responsible for wound contraction as well as the deforming pathological process termed *wound contracture*.** The appearance of the myofibroblast, usually about the third day of wound healing, is associated with the sudden appearance of contractile forces, which then gradually diminish over the next several weeks. Myofibroblasts exert their contractile effects by forming syncytia in which the myofibroblasts are bound together by tight junctions. By contrast, fibroblasts tend to be solitary cells, surrounded by collagen fibers. The myofibroblast may originate as a pericyte, fibroblast, or stem cell.

Wound Strength

Skin incisions and surgical anastomoses in hollow viscera ultimately develop 75% of the strength of the unwounded site. Despite a rapid increase in tensile strength at 7 to 14 days, by the end of 2 weeks the wound has acquired only about 20% of its ultimate strength. Most of the strength of the healed wound results from intermolecular cross-linking of type I collagen. The 2-month-old incision, although healed, is still visibly obvious. The incision line and suture marks are distinct, vascular, and red. By 1 year, the incision is white and avascular but usually still identifiable. As the scar fades further, it is often slowly deformed into an irregular line by stresses in the skin.

REGENERATION

Regeneration is the renewal of a damaged tissue or a lost appendage that is identical to the original one. An understanding of regeneration requires a discussion of the cell cycle.

The Cell Cycle Leads to Mitosis

The maintenance of the structure of tissues composed of short-lived cells (e.g., gastrointestinal epithelium, epidermis, neutrophils) and the regeneration of injured tissues require rigorously controlled cell proliferation to maintain an appropriate cell number. The cell cycle, (i.e., the period of time between two successive cell divisions) is divided into four phases of unequal duration (Fig. 3-13):

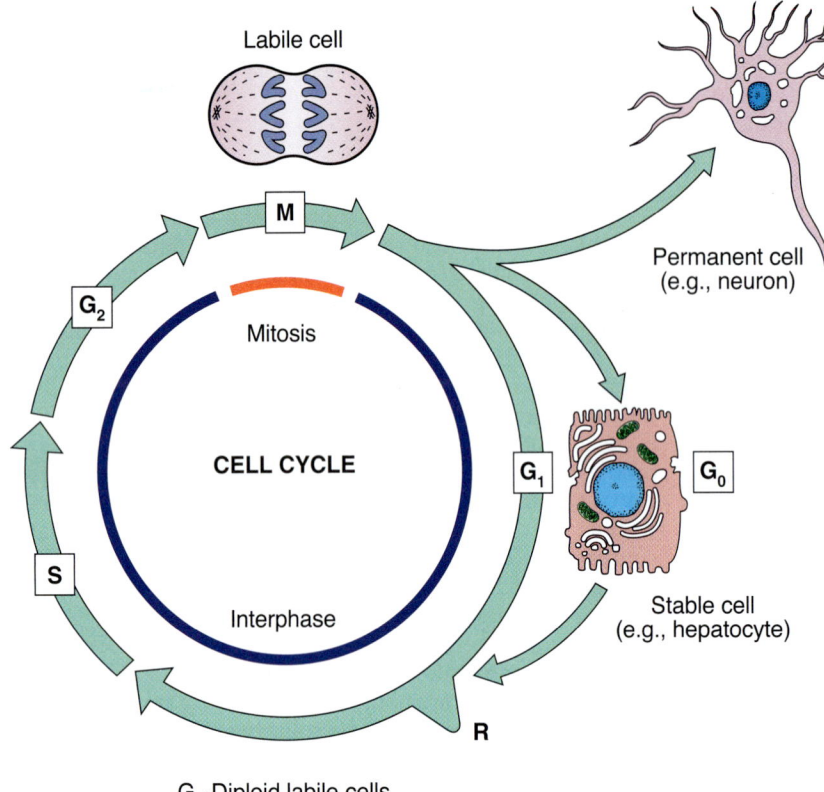

FIGURE 3-13
The cell cycle. Labile cells (e.g., intestinal crypt cells) undergo continuous replication, and the interval between two consecutive mitoses is designated the cell cycle. After division, the cells enter a gap phase (G_1), in which they pursue their own specialized activities. If they continue in the cycle, after passing the restriction point (R) they are committed to a new round of division. The G_1 phase is followed by a period of nuclear DNA synthesis (S) in which all chromosomes are replicated. The S phase is followed by a short gap phase (G_2) and then mitosis. After each cycle, one daughter cell will become committed to differentiation and the other will continue cycling. Other cell types, such as hepatocytes, are stable; that is, after mitosis the cells take up their specialized functions (G_0). They do not reenter the cycle unless stimulated by the loss of other cells. Permanent cells (e.g., neurons) become terminally differentiated after mitosis and cannot reenter the cell cycle.

- **M phase** (M, mitosis): This phase describes the interval between the onset of the mitotic prophase and the conclusion of the telophase, at which time the cell has divided.
- **G_1 phase** (G, gap): Following mitosis, the cell enters the G_1 phase, during which it is devoted to its own specialized activities. The main difference between rapidly dividing and slowly dividing cells is in the length of the G_1 phase.
- **S phase** (S, synthesis): After the G_1 phase, a doubling of DNA takes place in the S phase.
- **G_2 phase:** Upon completion of nuclear DNA duplication, the cells enter the G_2 phase, which is followed by the next mitosis, or M phase. Thus, *interphase* is composed of successive G_1, S, and G_2 phases, which constitute 90% or more of the time required for the total cell cycle.
- **G_0 phase:** Some cells remain quiescent after an M phase and do not divide unless stimulated. After an appropriate stimulus, they may reenter the cycle at G_1 and continue through the cycle to mitosis.

Cells Can Be Classified by Their Proliferative Potential

The cells of the body divide at different rates. Some mature cells do not divide at all, whereas others complete a cycle every 16 to 24 hours.

- **Labile cells** are found in tissues that are in a constant state of renewal, for example, the epithelial lining of the gastrointestinal tract or the hematopoietic system.
- **Stable cells** populate tissues that normally are renewed very slowly but are capable of more rapid renewal after tissue loss. The liver and the proximal renal tubules are examples of stable cell populations.
- **Permanent cells** are terminally differentiated and have lost all capacity for regeneration. Neurons are representative of permanent cells.

Labile Cells

Tissues in which more than 1.5% of the cells are in mitosis at any one time are composed of labile cells. Such tissues include the epidermis; the mucosa of the gastrointestinal, respiratory, urinary, and genital tracts; the bone marrow; and the lymphoid organs. However, not all the cells in these tissues are continuously cycling.

Stem cells are constituents of labile tissues that are programmed to divide continuously. One daughter cell of each division becomes another stem cell, whereas the other follows an irreversible path to terminal differentiation. The basal cells of the epidermis and of the gastrointestinal crypts are examples of stem cells.

Unipotent stem cells give rise to progeny that differentiate into only one type of cell. For instance, the daughter cells of a basal epidermal cell mature only into keratinized cells, which eventually desquamate.

Pluripotent stem cells generate more than one cell type. Hemocytoblasts of the bone marrow yield erythrocytes, neutrophils, eosinophils, basophils, monocytes, lymphocytes, and megakaryocytes.

Tissues composed of labile cells regenerate after injury, provided that enough stem cells remain.

Stable Cells

Stable cells populate tissues in which fewer than 1.5% of the cells are in mitosis. Stable tissues (e.g., endocrine glands, endothelium, and liver) do not have conspicuous stem cells. Rather, their cells require an appropriate stimulus to divide. **It is the potential to replicate and not the actual number of steady state mitoses that determines the ability of an organ to regenerate.** For example, the liver, a stable tissue with less than one mitosis for every 15,000 cells, regenerates rapidly after a loss of as much as 75% of its mass.

Permanent Cells

Permanent cells are terminally differentiated and do not enter the cell cycle. Neurons, cardiac myocytes, and cells of the lens are permanent cells. **If lost, permanent cells cannot be replaced.** Although permanent cells do not divide, most of them do renew their organelles. The extreme example of permanent cells is the lens. Every lens cell generated during embryonic development and postnatal life is preserved in the adult without turnover of its constituents.

Regeneration Is Mediated by Either Stem Cells or Stable Cells

Some regenerative processes may be thought of as a partial recapitulation of embryonic morphogenesis from pluripotent stem cells. Unlike the newt, humans cannot regenerate limbs, but there are notable examples of regenerative processes in bone, skeletal muscle, and liver. As noted above, skin epithelium and hair follicles regenerate from stem cells if the wound does not disrupt the epidermal basement membrane or the hair bulbs. Bone marrow stem cells, which are set aside during embryonic development, replenish the hematopoietic population.

Adult stem cells in the bone marrow and other differentiated tissues differ from embryonic stem cells in that their ability to differentiate into multiple lineages is restricted. Bone marrow also contains mesenchymal and endothelial stem cells, providing a multifaceted regenerative capacity. Bone is a protected storage site with ready accessibility to the circulation. Endothelial stem cells from bone marrow have been implicated in tissue angiogenesis and may supplement endothelial hyperplasia during regeneration of blood vessels. Moreover, bone-marrow derived fibroblasts may populate repairing tissue.

Intestinal epithelium turns over rapidly and is replenished by intestinal stem cells that reside in the crypts of Lieberkuhn. Liver regeneration is partly a misnomer, since the regrowth of liver following partial hepatectomy is a hyperplastic response by mature differentiated hepatocytes and, for the most part, does not involve stem cells. However, there is evidence for stem cell-driven liver regeneration when hepatocytes are damaged by viral hepatitis or toxins. The regenerative potential is thought to arise from "oval cells" in the epithelium of small bile ducts. These putative stem cells have characteristics of both hepatocytes (α-fetoprotein and albumin) and bile duct cells (γ-glutamyl transferase and duct cytokeratins) and may reside in the terminal ductal cells in the canal of Hering.

CONDITIONS THAT MODIFY REPAIR

Local Factors May Retard Healing

Location of the Wound

In addition to the size and shape of the wound, its location also affects healing. Sites in which skin covers bone with little intervening tissue, such as skin over the anterior tibia, are locations where skin cannot contract. Skin lesions in such areas, particularly burns, often require skin grafts because their edges cannot be apposed. Complications or other treatments, such as infection or ionizing radiation, also slow the repair process.

Blood Supply

Lower extremity wounds of diabetics often heal poorly or even require amputation when it otherwise would not be necessary. In such cases, advanced atherosclerosis in the legs compromises blood supply and impedes repair. Varicose veins of the legs slow the venous return and can also cause ulceration and nonhealing. Bed sores (decubitus ulcers) result from prolonged, localized, dependent pressure, which diminishes both arterial and venous blood flow. Joint (articular) cartilage is largely avascular and has limited diffusion capacity; often it cannot mount a vigorous inflammatory response. As a result, articular cartilage repairs poorly, a phenotype that usually worsens with age.

Systemic Factors

No specific effect of age alone on repair has been found. Although the skin of a 90-year-old person, which exhibits reduced collagen and elastin, may heal slowly, the same person's cataract extraction or colon resection heals normally because the bowel and the eye are practically unaffected by age.

Coagulation defects, thrombocytopenia, and anemia impede repair. Local thrombosis decreases platelet activation, thereby reducing the supply of growth factors and limiting the healing cascade. The decrease in tissue oxygen that accompanies severe anemia also interferes with repair. Exogenous corticosteroids retard wound repair by inhibiting collagen and protein synthesis and by exerting antiinflammatory effects.

Specific Sites Exhibit Different Repair Patterns

Skin

Healing in the skin involves both repair, primarily dermal scarring, and regeneration, principally of the epidermis and vasculature. The salient features of primary and secondary healing are provided in Figure 3-14.

Primary healing occurs when the surgeon closely approximates the edges of a wound. The actions of myofibroblasts are minimized, and regeneration of the epidermis is

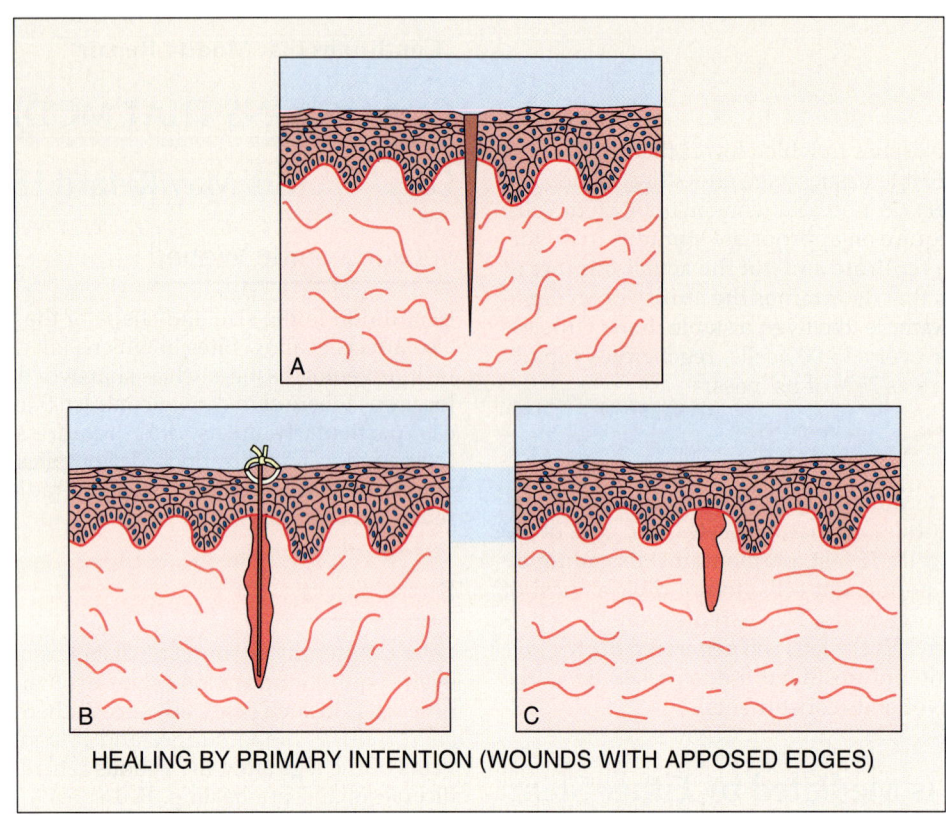

HEALING BY PRIMARY INTENTION (WOUNDS WITH APPOSED EDGES)

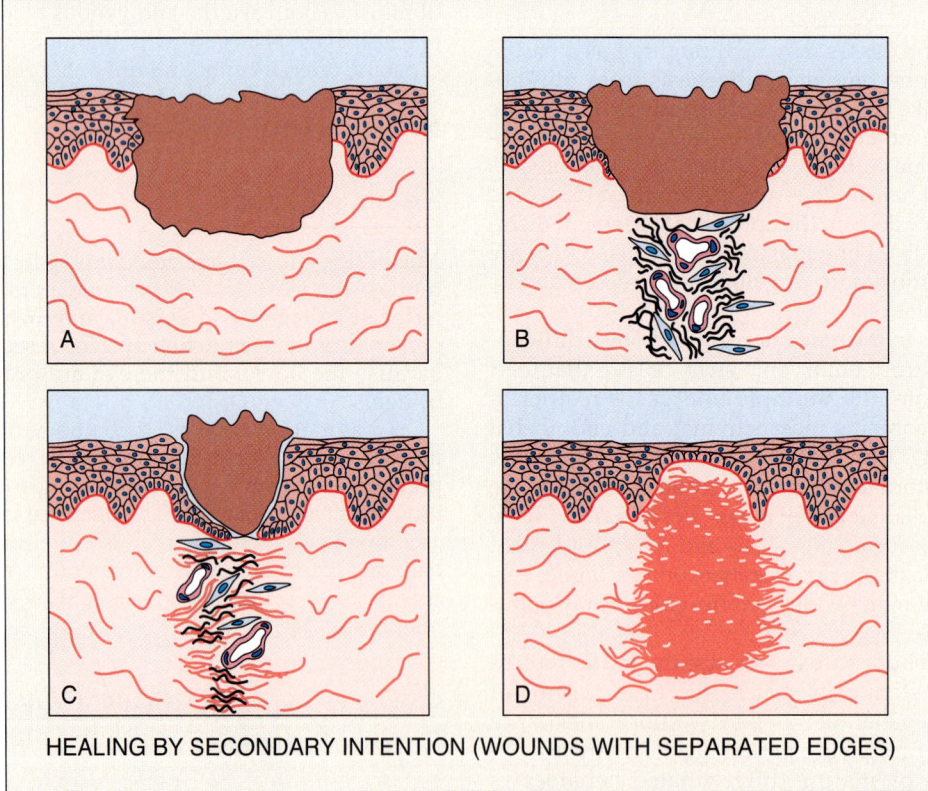

HEALING BY SECONDARY INTENTION (WOUNDS WITH SEPARATED EDGES)

FIGURE 3-14

Healing by primary intention. (*A*) A wound with closely apposed edges and minimal tissue loss. (*B*) Such a wound requires only minimal cell proliferation and neovascularization to heal. (*C*) The result is a small scar. Healing by secondary intention. (*A*) A gouged wound, in which the edges are far apart and in which there is substantial tissue loss. (*B*) This wound requires wound contraction, extensive cell proliferation, and neovascularization (granulation tissue) to heal. (*C*) The wound is reepithelialized from the margins, and collagen fibers are deposited in the granulation tissue. (*D*) Granulation tissue is eventually resorbed and replaced by a large scar that is functionally and esthetically unsatisfactory.

optimal, since epidermal cells need migrate only a minimal distance.

Secondary healing proceeds when a large area of hemorrhage and necrosis cannot be completely corrected surgically. In this situation, myofibroblasts contract the wound, and subsequent scarring repairs the defect.

Liver

Acute chemical injury or fulminant viral hepatitis causes widespread necrosis of hepatocytes. However, if liver failure is not fatal, and if the connective tissue stroma, vasculature, and bile ducts survive, the parenchyma regenerates, and normal form and function are restored. By contrast, chronic injury in viral hepatitis or alcoholism is associated with the development of broad collagenous scars within the hepatic parenchyma, termed *cirrhosis* of the liver (Fig. 3-15). The hepatocytes form regenerative nodules that lack central veins and expand to obstruct blood vessels and bile flow. Portal hypertension and jaundice ensue despite adequate numbers of regenerated but disconnected hepatocytes.

In the Greek myth of Prometheus, a vulture tore out his liver every evening, only to have it grow back by morning. It required more than another two millennia for the demonstration that the liver indeed possesses tremendous regenerative capacity, even though the normal hepatic parenchyma is almost devoid of mitoses and virtually all hepatocytes are in G_0. In the rat, resection of up to 80% of the liver is followed by rapid restoration of a normal-appearing liver. The necessary conditions for hepatic regeneration are complex and beyond the scope of this discussion. Suffice it to say that regeneration is arrested when the normal ratio of liver to total body weight is reestablished; the molecular switch that regulates this ratio is obscure. In human liver transplantation, a partial donation of the right lobe of the liver from a living donor is followed by complete regeneration of the normal liver in both the recipient and the donor.

Kidney

Although kidney has limited regenerative capacity, the removal of one kidney (nephrectomy) is followed by compensatory hypertrophy of the remaining kidney. In the case of renal injury, if it is not extensive and the extracellular matrix framework is not destroyed, the tubular epithelium regenerates. In most renal diseases, however, there is some destruction of the framework. Regeneration is then incomplete, and scar formation is the usual outcome. The regenerative capacity of renal tissue is maximal in cortical tubules, less in medullary tubules, and nonexistent in glomeruli.

Cortical Renal Tubules

Normally, there is some turnover of tubular epithelium, leading to shedding of cells in the urine. No reserve cell has been identified, and simple division accomplishes replacement. The outcome of injury depends on whether the tubular basement membrane is ruptured. If the injury does not produce discontinuities in the basement membrane, the surviving tubular cells in the vicinity of the wound flatten, acquire a squamous appearance, and migrate into the necrotic area along the basement membrane. Mitoses are frequent, and occasional clusters of epithelial cells project into the lumen. Soon, the flattened cells are more cuboidal, and differentiated cytoplasmic elements appear. Tubular morphology and function are normal in 3 to 4 weeks.

Tubulorrhexis

Tubulorrhexis refers to the rupture of the tubular basement membrane. The sequence of events resembles that for tubular damage in which the basement membrane is intact, except that interstitial changes are more prominent. Proliferation of fibroblasts, increased deposition of extracellular matrix, and collapse of the tubular lumen are seen. The final result is regeneration of some tubules and fibrosis of others, usually causing focal losses of functional nephrons.

Medullary Renal Tubules

Medullary diseases of the kidney are often associated with extensive necrosis, which involves tubules, interstitium, and blood vessels. If the lesion is not fatal, the necrotic tissue sloughs into the urine. Healing by fibrosis produces urinary obstruction within the kidney. Although there is some epithelial proliferation, there is no significant regeneration.

Glomeruli

Unlike tubules, glomeruli do not regenerate. Injuries that produce necrosis of glomerular endothelial or epithelial cells, whether focal, segmental, or diffuse, heal by scarring (Fig. 3-16). Mesangial cells are related to smooth muscle cells and seem to have some capacity for regeneration. Following unilateral nephrectomy, the glomeruli in the remaining kid-

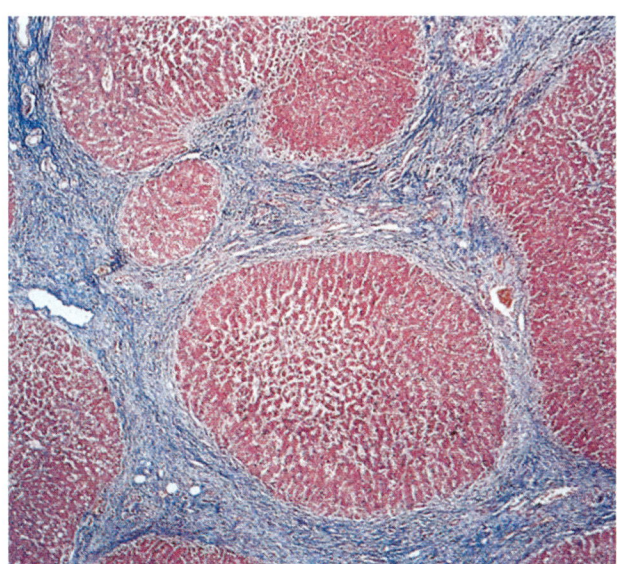

FIGURE 3-15
Cirrhosis of the liver. The consequences of chronic hepatic injury is the formation of regenerating nodules separated by fibrous bands. A microscopic section shows regenerating nodules *(red)* surrounded by bands of connective tissue *(blue)*.

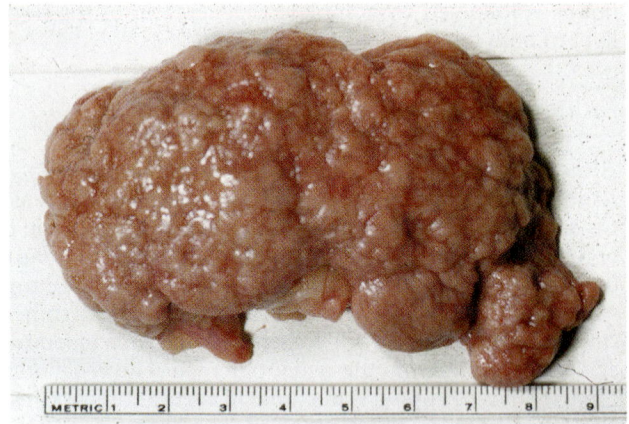 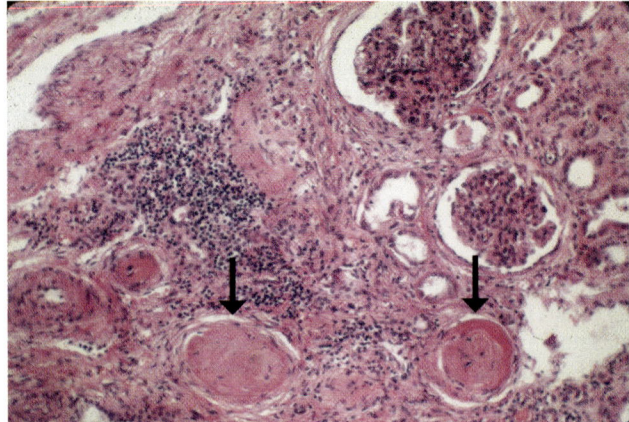

FIGURE 3-16
Obsolescent glomeruli. A. Repeated bacterial urinary tract infections have scarred the kidney. B. Many glomeruli have been destroyed and appear as circular scars *(arrows)*.

ney undergo hypertrophy and hyperplasia to produce greatly enlarged glomeruli.

Lung

The epithelium lining the respiratory tract has an effective regenerative capacity, provided that the underlying extracellular matrix framework is not destroyed. Superficial injuries to tracheal and bronchial epithelia heal by regeneration from the adjacent epithelium. The outcome of alveolar injury ranges from complete regeneration of structure and function to incapacitating fibrosis. As is the case with the liver, the degree of cell necrosis and the extent of the damage to the extracellular matrix framework determine the outcome (Fig. 3-17).

Alveolar Injury with Intact Basement Membranes

Alveolar injury follows a number of insults, for example, infections, shock, and oxygen toxicity. The injury produces a variable degree of alveolar cell necrosis. The alveoli are flooded with an inflammatory exudate particularly rich in plasma proteins. As long as the alveolar basement membrane remains intact, healing is by regeneration, and neutrophils and macrophages clear the alveolar exudate. If these cells fail to liquefy the alveolar exudate, it is organized by granulation tissue, and intraalveolar fibrosis results. Alveolar type II pneumocytes (the alveolar reserve cells) migrate to denuded areas and undergo mitosis to form cells with features intermediate between those of type I and type II pneumocytes. As these cells cover the alveolar surface, they establish contact with other epithelial cells. Mitosis then stops and the cells differentiate into type I pneumocytes.

Alveolar Injury with Disrupted Basement Membranes

Extensive damage to the alveolar basement membrane evokes scarring and fibrosis. Mesenchymal cells from the alveolar septa proliferate and differentiate into fibroblasts and myofibroblasts. The role of macrophage products in inducing fibroblast proliferation in the lung is well documented. The myofibroblasts and fibroblasts migrate into the alveolar spaces, where they secrete extracellular matrix components, mainly type I collagen and proteoglycans, to produce pulmonary fibrosis. The most common chronic pulmonary disease is emphysema, which involves airspace enlargement and the destruction of alveolar walls. Ineffective replacement of elastin is associated with irreversible loss of tissue resiliency and function.

Heart

Cardiac myocytes are permanent, nondividing, terminally differentiated cells. Recent studies, however, have provided evidence for minimal regeneration of cardiac myocytes from previously unrecognized stem or reserve cells. The origin of these cells, whether they reside in the myocardium or migrate there following injury from sites unknown, is not resolved. For practical purposes, myocardial necrosis, from whatever cause, heals by the formation of granulation tissue and eventual scarring (Figs. 3-17, 3-18). Not only does myocardial scarring result in the loss of contractile elements, but the fibrotic tissue also decreases the effectiveness of contraction in the surviving myocardium.

Nervous System

Mature neurons have been described as permanent and postmitotic cells, and recent studies suggesting possible regenerative capacity have not altered well-established observations about injury in the nervous system. Following trauma, only regrowth and reorganization of the surviving neuronal cell processes can reestablish neural connections. Although the peripheral nervous system has the capacity for axonal regeneration, the central nervous system lacks this ability.

Central Nervous System

Any damage to the brain or spinal cord is followed by the growth of capillaries and gliosis (i.e. the proliferation of astrocytes and microglia). Gliosis in the central nervous system

Conditions that Modify Repair 113

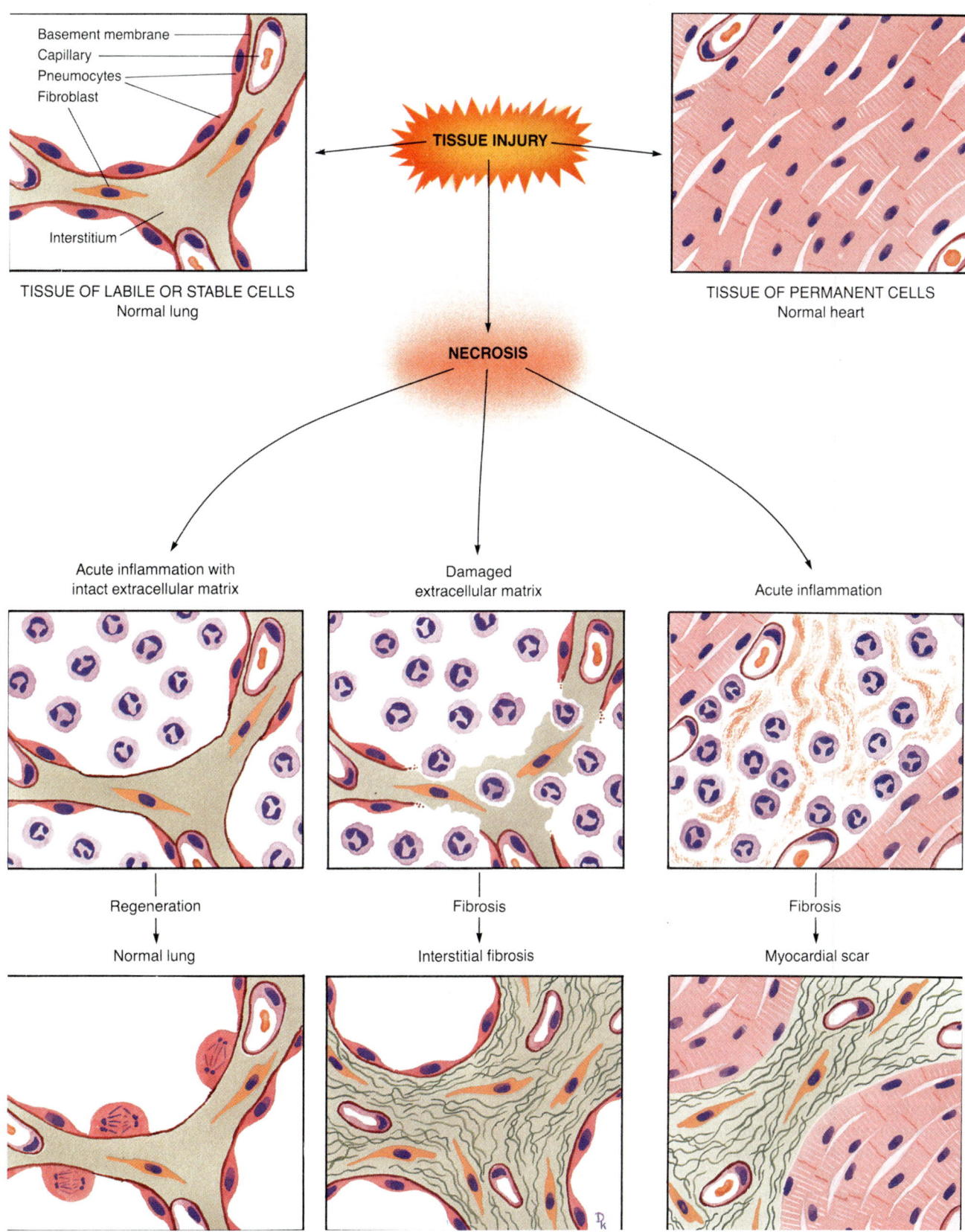

FIGURE 3-17
Overview of repair. This figure provides an overview that interrelates the early dynamic events in repair. The time scale in this figure is not linear; initial tensile strength, the first phase, develops almost immediately. Remodeling is ill defined, extending from its early beginning in repair for weeks or months.

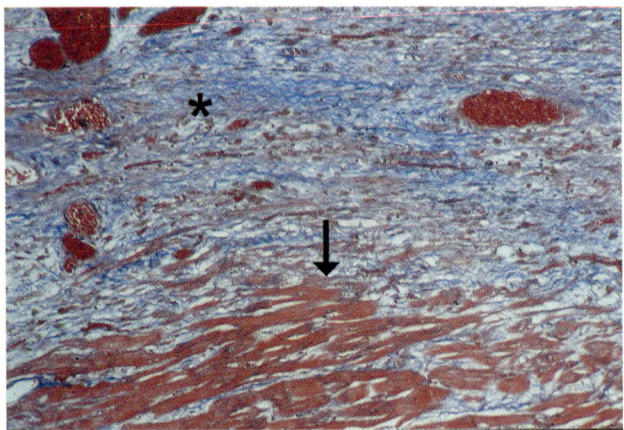

FIGURE 3-18
Myocardial infarction. A section through a healed myocardial infarct shows mature fibrosis (*) and disrupted myocardial fibers (arrow).

is the equivalent of scar formation elsewhere; once established, it remains permanently. In spinal cord injuries, axonal regeneration can be seen up to 2 weeks after injury. After 2 weeks, gliosis has taken place and attempts at axonal regeneration end. In the central nervous system, axonal regeneration occurs only in the hypothalamohypophysial region, where glial and capillary barriers do not interfere with axonal regeneration. Axonal regeneration seems to require contact with extracellular fluid containing plasma proteins.

Peripheral Nervous System

Neurons in the peripheral nervous system can regenerate their axons, and under ideal circumstances, interruption in the continuity of a peripheral nerve results in complete functional recovery. However, if the cut ends are not in perfect alignment or are prevented from establishing continuity by inflammation or a scar, a traumatic neuroma results (Fig. 3-19). This bulbous lesion consists of disorganized axons and proliferating Schwann cells and fibroblasts. The regenerative capacity of the peripheral nervous system can be ascribed to (1) the fact that the blood–nerve barrier, which insulates peripheral axons from extracellular fluids, is not restored for 2 to 3 months and (2) the presence of Schwann cells with basement membranes. Laminin, a basement membrane component, and nerve growth factor (NGF) guide and stimulate neurite growth.

Fetal Wound Repair

Remarkable progress in surgery now permits corrective surgical operations to be performed in utero. Fetal wounds heal without scarring, and at delivery, healed cutaneous incision sites are invisible. The lack of scarring is attributed to the bilayered embryonic epidermis (compared with the adult stratified dermis) and to absence of TGF-β in fetal skin. Fetal skin also contains more MMPs than does adult skin, a circumstance that promotes scarless healing. Reepithelization also differs in fetal skin and postfetal skin. In postfetal skin, epithelial cells creep across the surface of the wound. By contrast, embryonic fetal epithelial cells are pulled forward by the contraction of actin fibers, producing a "purse-string" effect.

Fetal wounds also heal faster than postfetal ones, an effect that may be related to the increased hyaluronic acid content of the extracellular matrix and other factors characteristic of immaturity.

Effects of Scarring

In the absence of the ability to form scars, mammalian life would hardly be possible. Yet scarring in parenchymal organs modifies their complex structure and never improves their function. For example, in the heart, the scar of a myocardial infarction serves to prevent rupture of the heart but reduces the amount of contractile tissue. If extensive enough, it may cause congestive heart failure or the formation of a ventricular aneurysm. Similarly, the aorta that is weakened and scarred by atherosclerosis is prone to dilate as an aneurysm. Scarred mitral and aortic valves following local inflammation caused by rheumatic fever are often stenotic, regurgitant, or both, leading to congestive heart failure. Persistent inflammation within the pericardium produces fibrous adhesions, which result in constrictive pericarditis and heart failure.

Alveolar fibrosis in the lung causes respiratory failure. Infection within the peritoneum or even surgical exploration may lead to adhesions and intestinal obstruction. Immunological injury to the renal glomerulus eventuates in its replacement by a collagenous scar and, if this process is extensive, renal failure. Scarring in the skin following burns or surgical excision of lesions produces unsatisfactory cosmetic results. An important goal of therapeutic intervention is to create optimum conditions for "constructive" scarring and prevent pathological "overshoot" of this process.

Wound Repair Is Often Suboptimal

Abnormalities in any of three healing processes—repair, contraction, and regeneration—result in unsuccessful or prolonged wound healing. The skill of the surgeon is often of critical importance.

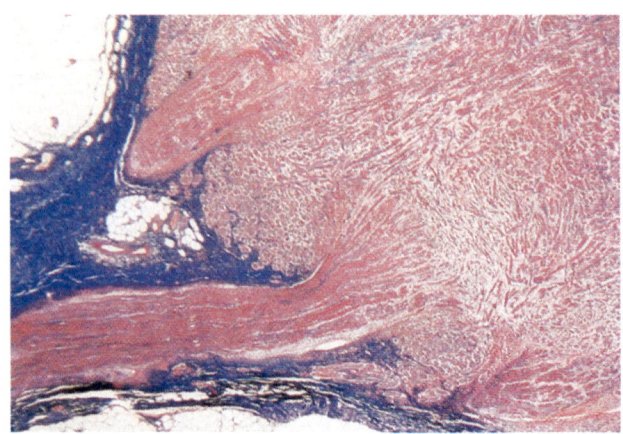

FIGURE 3-19
Traumatic neuroma. In this photomicrograph, the original nerve (lower left) enters the neuroma. The nerve is surrounded by dense collagenous tissue, which appears dark blue with this trichrome stain.

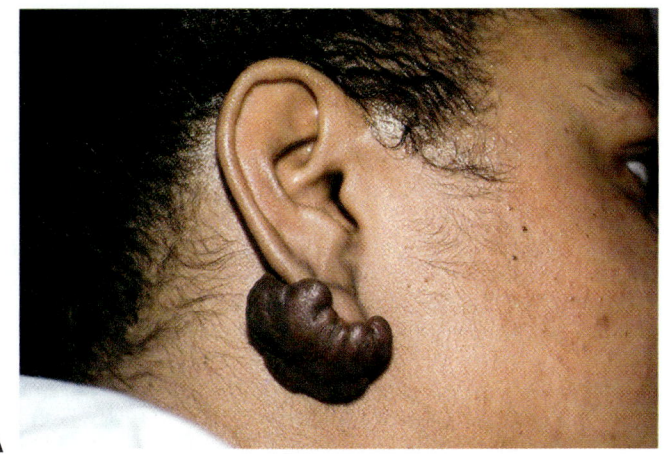
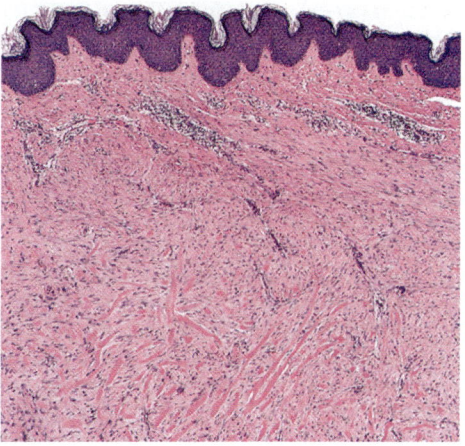

FIGURE 3-20
Keloid. **A.** A light-skinned black woman developed a keloid as a reaction to having her earlobe pierced. **B.** Microscopically, the dermis is markedly thickened by the presence of collagen bundles with random orientation and abundant cells.

Deficient Scar Formation

Inadequate formation of granulation tissue or an inability to form a suitable extracellular matrix leads to deficient scar formation and its complications.

Wound Dehiscence and Incisional Hernias

Dehiscence (the wound splitting open) is most frequent after abdominal surgery and can be a life-threatening complication. Increased mechanical stress on the wound from vomiting, coughing, or bowel obstruction sometimes causes dehiscence of the abdominal wound. Systemic factors predisposing to dehiscence include metabolic deficiency, hypoproteinemia, and the general inanition that often accompanies metastatic cancer. An *incisional hernia* of the abdominal wall refers to a defect caused by prior surgery. Such hernias resulting from weak scars are often the consequence of insufficient deposition of extracellular matrix or inadequate cross-linking in the collagen matrix. Loops of intestine are sometimes trapped within incisional hernias.

Ulceration

Wounds ulcerate because of an inadequate intrinsic blood supply or insufficient vascularization during healing. For example, leg wounds in persons with varicose veins or severe atherosclerosis often ulcerate. Nonhealing wounds also develop in areas devoid of sensation because of persistent trauma. Such *trophic* or *neuropathic* ulcers are commonly seen in diabetic peripheral neuropathy. Occasionally they occur in patients with spinal involvement from tertiary syphilis and leprosy.

Excessive Scar Formation

Excessive deposition of extracellular matrix, mostly excessive collagen, at the wound site results in a hypertrophic scar. *Keloid* is an exuberant scar that tends to progress beyond the site of initial injury and recurs after excision (Fig. 3-20). Histologically, both of these types of scars exhibit broad and irregular collagen bundles, with more capillaries and fibroblasts than expected for a scar of the same age. More clearly defined in keloids than in hypertrophic scars, the rate of collagen synthesis, the ratio of type III to type I collagen, and the number of reducible cross-links, remain high, a situation that indicates a "maturation arrest," or block, in the healing process. Further support for maturation arrest as an explanation for keloid and hypertrophic scars is the overexpression of fibronectin in these lesions. In addition, unlike normal healing tissue, these scar tissues fail to downregulate collagen synthesis when glucocorticoids are administered. Keloids are unsightly, and attempts at surgical repair are always problematic, the outcome likely being a still larger keloid. Dark-skinned persons are more frequently affected by keloids than light-skinned people, and the tendency is sometimes hereditary. By contrast, the occurrence of hypertrophic scars is not associated with skin color or heredity.

Excessive Contraction

A decrease in the size of a wound depends on the presence of myofibroblasts, development of cell–cell contacts, and sustained cell contraction. An exaggeration of these processes is termed *contracture* and results in severe deformity of the wound and surrounding tissues. Interestingly, the regions that normally show minimal wound contraction (e.g., the palms, the soles, and the anterior aspect of the thorax) are the ones prone to contractures. Contractures are particularly conspicuous in the healing of serious burns and can be severe enough to compromise the movement of joints. In the alimentary tract, a contracture (stricture) can result in obstruction to the passage of food in the esophagus or a block in the flow of intestinal contents.

Several diseases are characterized by contracture and irreversible fibrosis of the superficial fascia, including Dupuytren contracture (palmar contracture), Pederhosen disease (plantar contracture), and Peyronie disease (contracture of the cavernous tissues of the penis). In these diseases, there is no known precipitating injury, even though the basic process is similar to contracture in wound healing.

Excessive Regeneration and Repair

In addition to the many responses to injury described thus far, an additional lesion merits consideration, namely *pyogenic granuloma*. This lesion is a localized, persistent, exuberant overgrowth of granulation tissue, most commonly seen in gum tissue in pregnant women. It also develops in the squamocolumnar junction of the uterine cervix and at other sites. An injury preceding the development of pyogenic granuloma cannot usually be found. Like injury-induced granulation tissue, it lacks nerves and can be surgically trimmed without anesthesia. Conceptually, pyogenic granuloma is a transitional lesion, resembling granulation tissue but behaving almost as an autonomous benign neoplasm.

SUGGESTED READING

Books

Alberts B, Johnson A, et al: *Molecular Biology of the Cell*, 4th ed., New York: Garland, 2002.

Falanga, V: *Cutaneous Wound Healing*, first ed., London: Martin Duntiz, Ltd, 2001.

Lodish H, Berk A, et al: *Molecular Cell Biology*, 4th ed., New York: Freeman, 2000.

Royce PM, Steinman B: *Connective Tissue and Its Heritable Disorders: Molecular, Genetic, and Medical Aspects*, 2nd ed., New York: Wiley-Liss, Inc., 2002.

Review Articles

Current Opinion in Cell Biology, Annual October Issue: Cell-to-cell Contact and Extracellular Matrix.

Fine, NA, Mustoe TA: *Wound Healing:* In: *Surgery: Scientific Principles and Practice,* Eds Greenfield LJ, Mulholland MW, Oldham KT, Zelenock GB, and Lillemoe KD, 3rd Ed, Lippincott Williams & Wilkins, Philadelphia, Chap 3 pages 69–85.

Kalluri, R: Basement Membranes: Structure, Assembly and Role in Tumour Angiogenesis. *Nat Rev Cancer* 3(6): 422–433, 2003.

Korbling M and Estrov Z: Adult Stem Cells for Tissue Repair—A new Therapeutic Concept *New Eng J Med* 349: 570–582, 2003.

Pozzi A, Zent R: Integrins: sensors of extracellular matrix and modulators of cell function. *Nephron Exp Nephrol.* 94(3):e77–84, 2003.

Ray LB, Gough NR: Orienteering strategies for a signaling maze. *Science* 296:1633–1657, 2002.

Rosenthal N: Prometheus's Vulture and the Stem-Cell Promise. *New Eng J Med:* 267–274, 2003.

Singer AJ, Clark RAF: Cutaneous wound healing. *New Eng J Med* 341:738–746, 1999.

Steed, DL, Guest Editor: Wound Healing, *Surgical Clinics of North America* 83 (3):entire edition, 2003.

Sternlicht MD and Werb Z: How Matrix Metalloproteinases Regulate Cell Behavior. *Annu Rev Cell Dev Biol* 17: 463–516, 2001.

CHAPTER 4

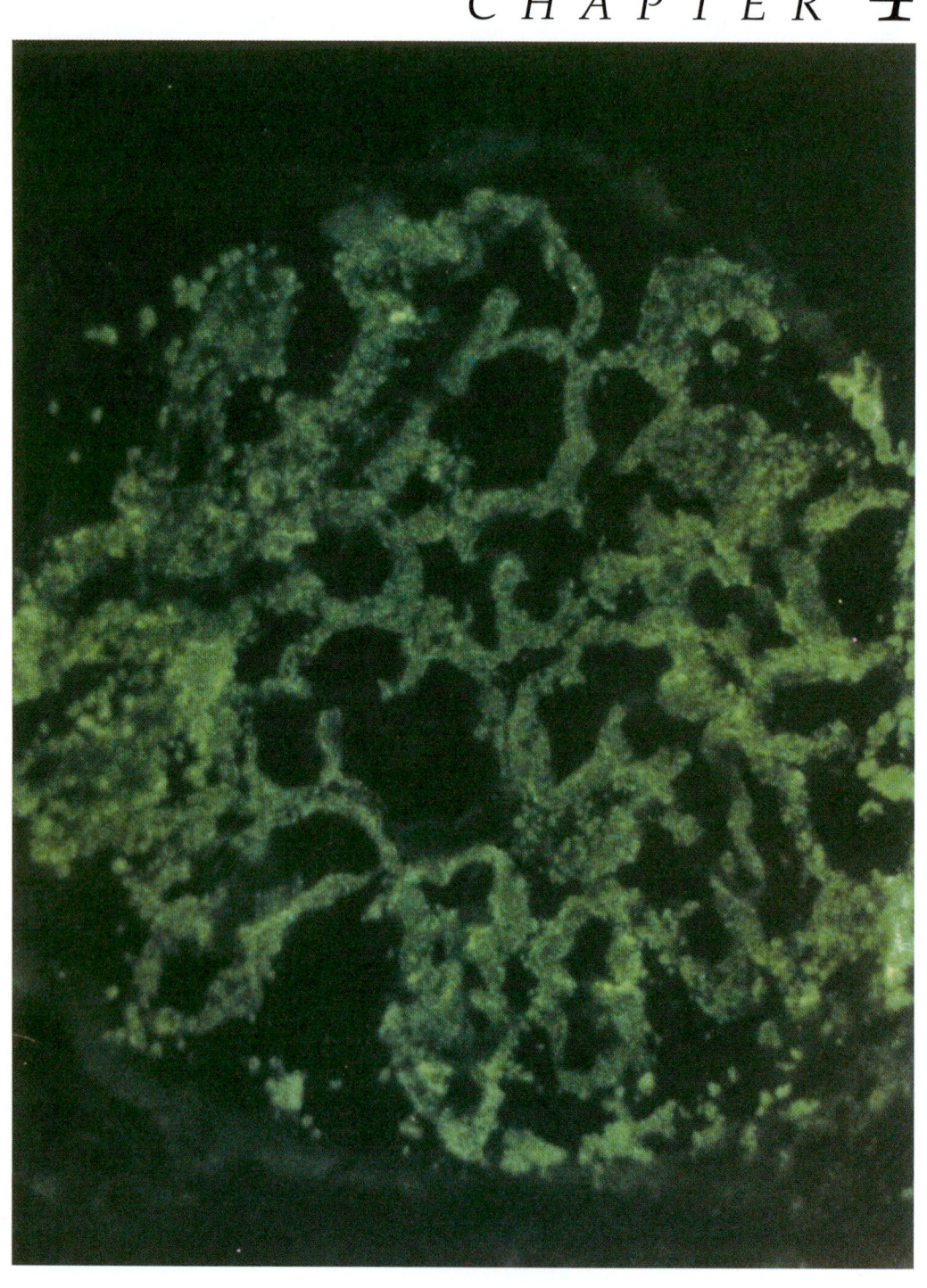

Immunopathology

Jeffrey S. Warren

Biology of the Immune System

Cellular Components of the Immune System

The Major Histocompatibility Complex (MHC)

Integrated Cellular and Humoral Immune Responses

Immunologically Mediated Tissue Injury

Immediate Hypersensitivity Reactions

Non-IgE Antibody–Mediated Hypersensitivity Reactions

Immune Complex Reactions

Cell-Mediated Hypersensitivity Reactions

Immune Reactions to Transplanted Tissues

Hyperacute Rejection

Acute Rejection

Chronic Rejection

Graft-versus-Host Disease

Evaluation of Immune Status

Immunoglobulin Levels

Antibody-Dependent Immunity

Cell-Mediated Immunity

Lymphocyte Populations

Immunodeficiency Diseases

Primary Antibody Deficiency Diseases

Primary T Cell Immunodeficiency Diseases

Combined Immunodeficiency Diseases

Purine Nucleoside Phosphorylase Deficiency

Wiskott-Aldrich Syndrome

Acquired Immunodeficiency Syndrome (AIDS)

Autoimmunity and Autoimmune Diseases

Autoimmune Disease and Immunological Tolerance

Systemic Lupus Erythematosus (SLE)

Lupuslike Diseases

Sjögren Syndrome

Scleroderma (Progressive Systemic Sclerosis)

Polymyositis and Dermatomyositis

FIGURE 4-1 *(see opposite page)*
Direct immunofluorescence reveals glomerular IgG deposition in a renal biopsy from a patient with systemic lupus erythematosus.

The immune system is the major mechanism to protect the host from invasion by foreign agents. An immune response can be elicited by a wide range of agents, including parasites, bacteria, viruses, chemicals, toxins, and drugs. As a component of host defenses, immune responses are (1) characterized by their ability to distinguish self from nonself, (2) by their ability to discriminate among potential invaders (specificity), and (3) by immune memory coupled to the capacity for amplification (i.e., the ability to recall previous exposures and to mount an intensified or anamnestic response).

The hierarchy of complexity of host defense systems within the animal kingdom is exemplified by the following extreme comparison. Protozoans can phagocytize and digest bacteria. Humans possess physical barriers such as regionally adapted epithelia (e.g., thick skin, ciliated respiratory epithelium, and nearly impervious urothelium), chemical–mechanical barriers (e.g., antibacterial lipids and mucus), and indigenous microbial flora that compete with potential pathogens. Patterned hemodynamic responses, soluble and cell surface-associated mediator systems (e.g., complement and coagulation systems), and antigen-nonspecific phagocytes (e.g., resident macrophages, neutrophils) are integral to protective inflammatory responses (see Chapter 2). The host defenses that are not antigen specific are referred to as the "innate" immune system. The antigen-specific or "adaptive" immune system encompasses lymphocytes, plasma cells, antigen-presenting cells (APCs), effector molecules (e.g., immunoglobulins), and a vast array of regulatory mediators. As noted above, the defining features of adaptive immunity include (1) specificity, (2) memory, and (3) the capacity for amplification. Specificity and immunological memory are the direct results of activation by antigens of lymphocyte clones that bear specific receptors. There are many linkages among the various layers of host defense. For example, antibody can specifically bind to an epitope on a bacterium, leading to complement fixation and, in turn, to the generation of chemotactic peptides that attract phagocytic neutrophils.

BIOLOGY OF THE IMMUNE SYSTEM

Cellular Components of the Immune System Develop from Hematopoietic Stem Cells

The cellular components of the immune system are derived from pluripotent hematopoietic stem cells (HSCs). Near the end of the first month of embryogenesis, HSCs appear in the extraembryonic erythropoietic islands adjacent to the yolk sac. At 6 weeks, the primary site of hematopoiesis shifts from the extraembryonic blood islands to the fetal liver to the bone marrow. The process begins at 2 months but by 6 months has completely shifted to the bone marrow. Although there are well-defined sequential changes in the primary site of hematopoiesis, there are periods of overlap. By 8 weeks gestation, lymphoid stem cells derived from HSCs and fated to become T cells circulate to the thymus where they differentiate into mature T lymphocytes. Lymphoid stem cells destined to become B cells differentiate first within the fetal liver (8 weeks) and later within the bone marrow (12 weeks). In the development of both thymic T lymphocytes and bone marrow B lymphocytes, the microenvironments (e.g., thymic epithelium, bone marrow stromal cells, growth factors) are critical. Mature lymphocytes exit the thymus and bone marrow and "home" to peripheral lymphoid tissues (e.g., lymph nodes, spleen, skin, and mucosa). The population of peripheral lymphoid tissues by mature T and B lymphocytes and the rapid deployment and recirculation of mature lymphocytes to different, often remote, parts of the immune system are anatomically specific. "Lymphocyte homing and recirculation" are orchestrated by a series of leukocyte and endothelial surface molecules called *selectins* and *addressins*.

The cells of the immune system express a vast array of surface molecules that are important in cellular differentiation and cell-to-cell communication. These surface molecules serve as useful markers of cellular identity. The International Workshop on Human Leukocyte Differentiation Antigens is responsible for nomenclature of these markers and assigns them so-called cluster of differentiation (CD) numbers. Currently more than 250 different molecules have been assigned CD numbers.

Hematopoietic Stem Cells

The pluripotent HSCs account for 1% of bone marrow mononuclear cells. They exhibit characteristic light-scattering properties as assessed by flow cytometry, usually express a cell surface protein designated CD34, and are generally "lineage negative". Lineage-negative refers to the absence of cell surface molecules that in more mature cells are characteristic of specific lymphocyte subpopulations (e.g., CD2, CD3, CD5, CD7, CD14, CD15, and CD16). Recently, a smaller population of CD34$^-$ HSCs was described. CD34$^+$ HSCs can also be found in the circulation, where they account for 0.01 to 0.1% of mononuclear cells. Bone marrow and peripheral blood HSCs exhibit heterogeneity in terms of their expression of selected lymphocyte markers, myeloid markers, and activation antigens, and they also differ in terms of their capacity to engraft bone marrow. Infusion of peripheral blood HSCs in sufficient numbers into bone marrow transplant recipients leads to faster marrow recovery than that observed in patients who have received marrow-derived HSCs. In clinical stem cell transplantation, it is now common practice for donors to receive recombinant growth factors prior to HSC harvest. This practice has led to higher yields of harvested HSCs and decreased engraftment times. The proportion of bone marrow transplant recipients who receive harvested peripheral blood HSCs rather than marrow-derived HSCs has increased dramatically in recent years.

Lymphopoiesis and Hematopoiesis

All mature lymphoid and hematopoietic cells are derived from a common population of pluripotential HSCs (Fig. 4-2). Each step in lymphopoiesis and hematopoiesis depends on a microenvironment that encompasses specific structural

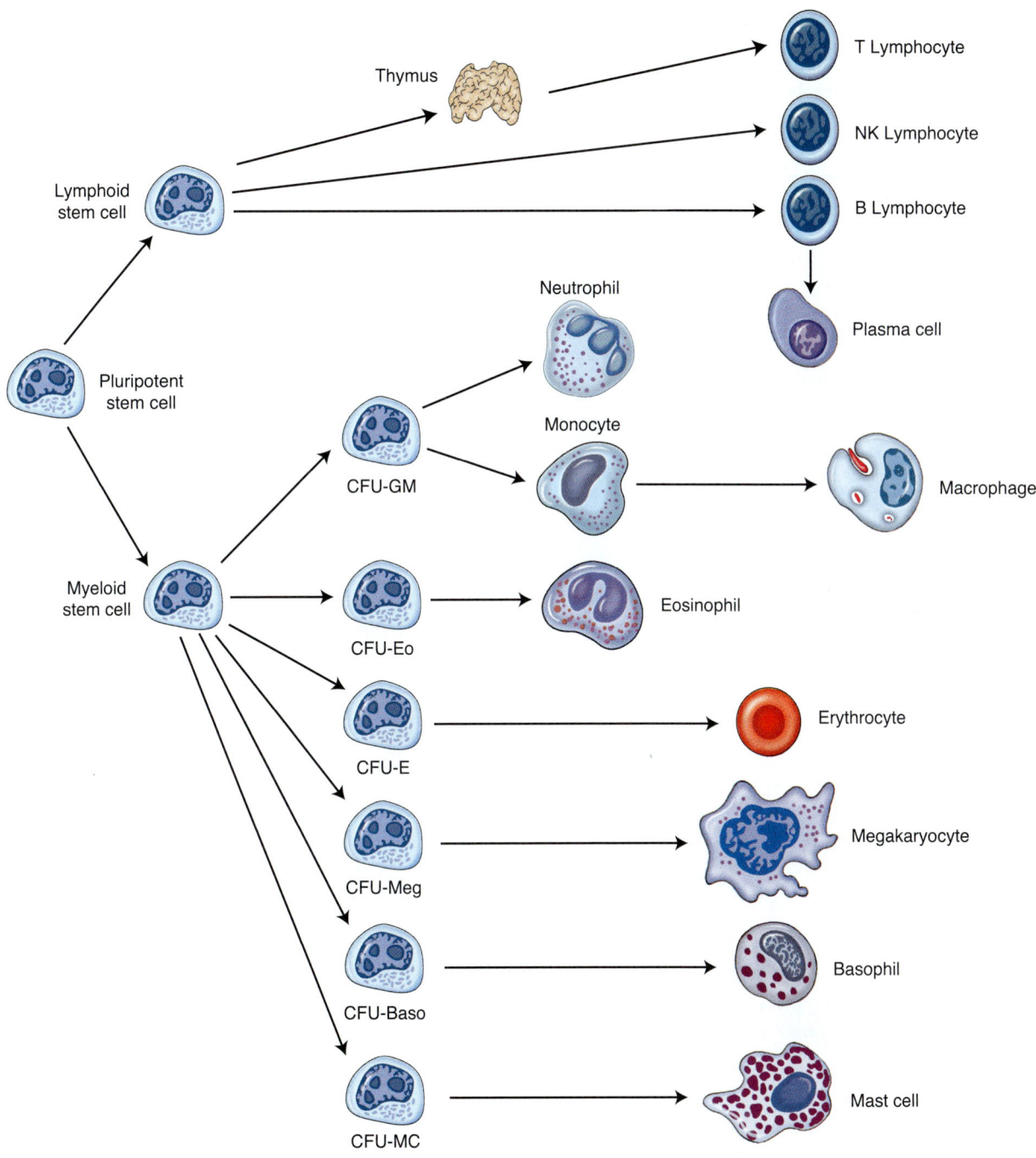

FIGURE 4-2
Pluripotent hematopoietic stem cells differentiate into either lymphoid or myeloid stem cells and, in the case of myeloid stem cells, into lineage-specific colony-forming units (CFUs). Under the influence of an appropriate microenvironment, CFUs give rise to definitive cell types. Lymphoid stem cells are precursors of NK cells, T lymphocytes, and B lymphocytes. B lymphocytes give rise to plasma cells.

features and a complex array of growth factors. The primary branch point in differentiation is between lymphoid progenitors and myeloid progenitors. The former ultimately give rise to T lymphocytes, B lymphocytes, and natural killer (NK) cells, whereas the latter develop into granulocytic, erythroid, monocytic–dendritic, and megakaryocytic colony-forming units (GEMM-CFUs). Downstream, CFUs become more lineage specific. Examples are CFU-GM (granulocyte-monocyte), CFU-Eo (eosinophil), CFU-E (erythrocyte), etc. *CFU* refers to a cell that ultimately gives rise to a specified population of "offspring," such as granulocytes, erythrocytes, monocytes, dendritic cells, and megakaryocytes.

Lymphoid progenitor cells exit the bone marrow and migrate to the thymus, where both alpha/beta (α/β) and gamma/delta (γ/δ) T lymphocytes are formed. "Alpha/beta" and "gamma/delta" refer to the two major classes of heterodimeric T cell receptors (TCRs) that specifically recognize and bind to various antigens. The thymic microenvironment is determined by the epithelial stroma. The early thymus is formed from ectoderm and endoderm derived from the third bronchial cleft and the third and fourth pharyngeal pouches. This thymic anlage is then colonized by HSCs that give rise to T cells, macrophages, and dendritic cells. The thymic cortex is composed of a meshwork of epithelial cell processes that surround groups of immature thymocytes that bear $CD4^+$ and $CD8^+$ surface molecules (Fig. 4-3). As T lymphocytes mature, they percolate into the thymic medulla where, in close proximity to nested groups of epithelial cells,

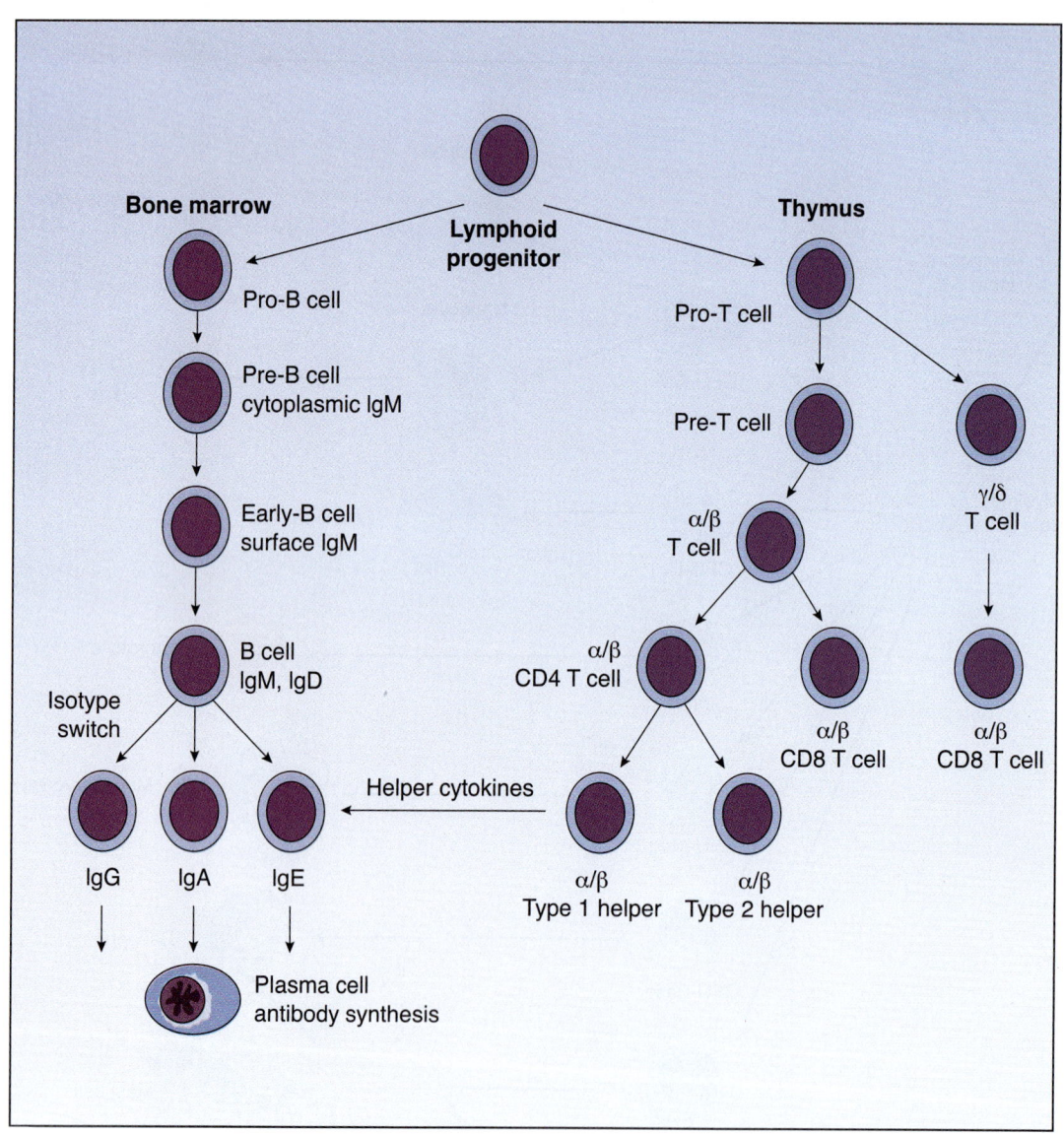

FIGURE 4-3

Lymphoid progenitors (lymphoid stem cells) give rise to mature but naïve T lymphocytes and B lymphocytes. Lymphocytes destined to become T lymphocytes migrate to the thymus where they become either α/β or γ/δ T cells. *Type 1* and *type 2* helper cells refer to functional characteristics of T cells (see text). Other lymphocytes differentiate in the bone marrow and give rise to clonal populations of surface immunoglobulin-producing B cells, which in turn can form plasma cells.

Biology of the Immune System

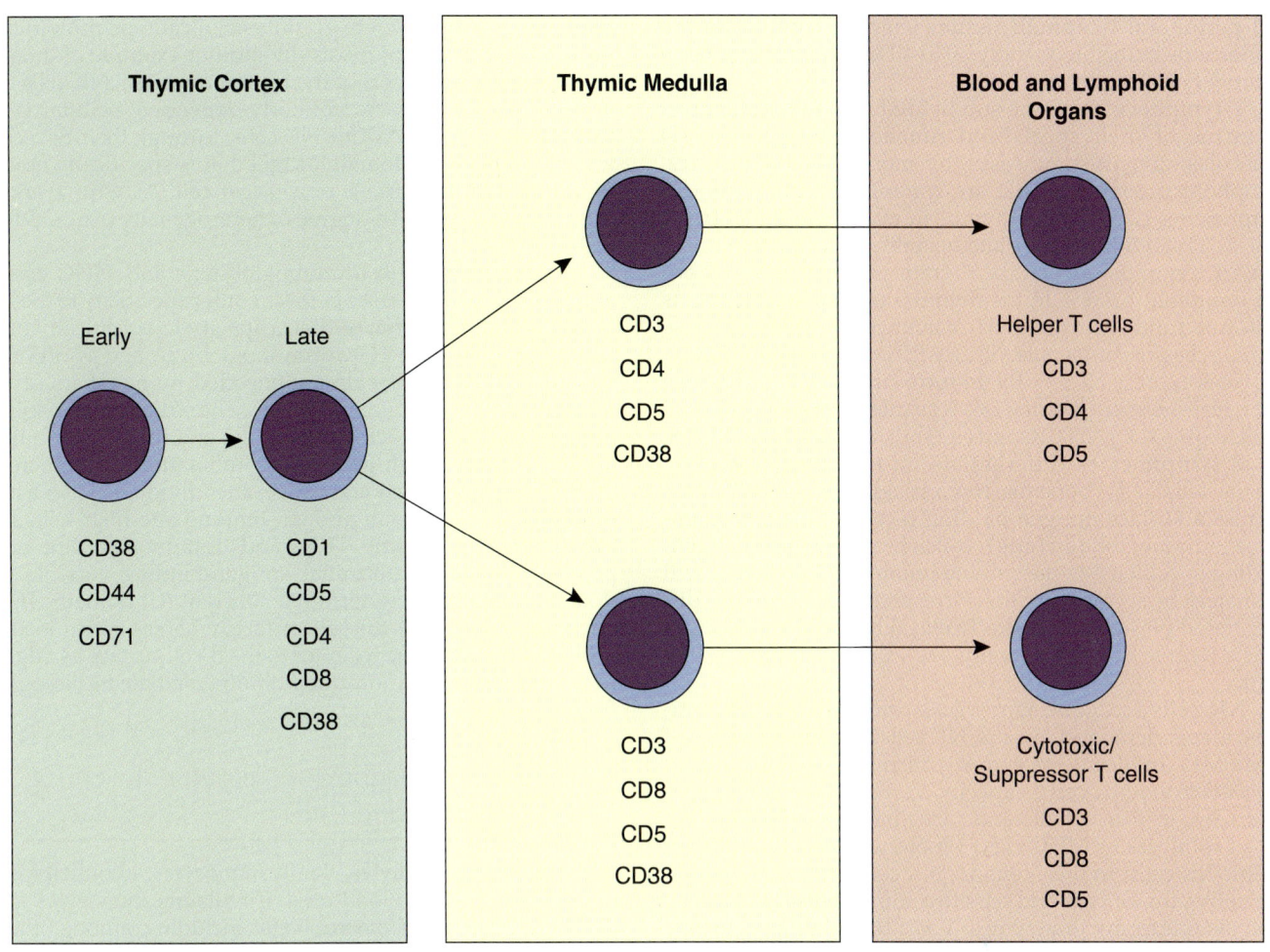

FIGURE 4-4
Lymphoid progenitors that are destined to become mature, but naïve, T cells differentiate as they percolate through the thymus. Peripheral CD4$^+$ and CD8$^+$ T cells are derived from thymic precursor cells that are CD3$^+$, CD4$^+$, and CD8$^+$.

they form more- mature cells that are either CD4$^+$ or CD8$^+$ (Fig. 4-3). The thymic corticomedullary junction contains many bone marrow HSC-derived macrophages and dendritic cells. Much of the process of "positive selection" of thymocytes occurs in the cortex; "negative selection" tends to occur through exposure of developing thymocytes to corticomedullary dendritic cells. *Positive thymic selection* refers to a process in which the transient binding of cell surface TCRs to a person's own MHC class I or II molecules prevents cell death. *Negative thymic selection* is the converse process in which high-affinity TCR-mediated binding to one's own MHC class I or II molecules results in cell death by apoptosis. These complementary thymic selection processes are pivotal to the development of T lymphocytes, which can interact with the host's own cells but not in a manner that results in excessive self-reactivity (see the discussion of tolerance.) Thymic T lymphocyte maturation includes several processes. Developing T cells recombine dispersed genes that encode the heterodimeric α/β or γ/δ TCRs. α/β T lymphocytes progress through stages of development that are characterized as CD4$^-$, CD8$^-$, then CD4$^+$, CD8$^+$, and then either CD4$^+$, CD8$^-$, or CD4$^-$, CD8$^+$ (Fig. 4-4). Most CD4$^+$, CD8$^-$ T cells function as cytotoxic cells.

As noted above, B cell lymphopoiesis in the adult occurs in the bone marrow. Similar to T lymphocyte development, the microenvironment of either the fetal liver or, in adults, the bone marrow, is critical to B lymphocyte development. In both organs, only B lymphocytes that pass through the many stages necessary to produce surface immunoglobulin survive. Conversely, developing B cells in which surface immunoglobulin binds too avidly to self-antigens are negatively selected and eliminated. NK cells are believed to form in both the thymus and bone marrow.

Lymphocytes

There are three major types of lymphocytes—T cells, B cells, and NK cells—which account for 25% of peripheral blood leukocytes. Some 80% of circulating lymphocytes are T cells, 10% B cells, and 10% NK cells. The relative proportions of lymphocytes in the peripheral blood and in the central and peripheral lymphoid tissues vary. In contrast to the proportions in the blood, only 30 to 40% of splenic and bone marrow lymphocytes are T cells.

T lymphocytes can be subdivided into subpopulations by virtue of their specialized functions, by surface CD molecules, and in some cases, by morphological features. Lymphoid progenitors that are committed to becoming T lymphocytes home to the thymus in waves during embryogenesis. Following positive and negative selection or "education," T lymphocytes exit the thymus and populate peripheral lymphoid tissues. In the thymus, antigen-specific TCRs are formed and are expressed in conjunction with CD3, an essential accessory molecule. Nearly 95% of circulating T lymphocytes express α/β TCRs. In turn, circulating α/β T cells also express either CD4 or CD8. A smaller population (5%) of T cells expresses γ/δ TCRs and CD3 but neither CD4 nor CD8.

B lymphocytes differentiate into antibody-secreting plasma cells in the bone marrow. Analogous to T cells, they express a surface antigen-binding receptor, namely membrane immunoglobulin (mIg), which bears the same antigen-binding specificity as the soluble immunoglobulin that will ultimately be secreted by the corresponding terminally differentiated plasma cells. Like T cells, B lymphocytes also exhibit a degree of heterogeneity (e.g., $CD5^+$ [B]) and $CD5^-$ [B2]).

NK cells recognize target cells primarily through antigen-independent mechanisms. NK cells bear several types of class I MHC molecule receptors, which when engaged actually *inhibit* the NK cell's capacity to secrete cytolytic products. Certain tumor cells and virus-infected cells bear reduced numbers of MHC class I molecules and thus do not inhibit NK cells. In this scenario, NK cells engage the virus-infected or tumor cells and secrete complement-like cytolytic proteins (perforin), granzymes A and B, and other lytic factors. NK cells also secrete granulysin, a cationic protein that induces target cell apoptosis. In another example of linkage between different facets of the immune system, NK cells can also lyse target cells via antibody-dependent cellular cytotoxicity (ADCC). In ADCC, NK cells, through their Fc receptors, bind to the Fc domain of IgG that is specifically bound to antigen on the surface of a target cell. As with T and B cells, NK cells exhibit a degree of heterogeneity (e.g., $CD16^+$, $CD16^-$).

TCRs, along with immunoglobulins and MHC class I and class II molecules (see below), confer specificity to the immune system by virtue of their capacity to specifically bind foreign antigens. The TCR, immunoglobulin, and a portion of the MHC class I molecule are encoded by members of the immunoglobulin supergene family. The structural variability and, in turn, high specificity of TCRs and immunoglobulins are achieved through genetic recombination of segmented TCR and Ig genes. As noted above, an individual TCR is a heterodimer that forms an antigen-binding site (Fig. 4-5). The proteins that constitute TCRs and immunoglobulins each possesses an amino-terminal antigen-binding variable (V) domain and a carboxy-terminal constant (C) domain. TCRs anchor the antigen to the cell surface, whereas immunoglobulins either anchor the receptor to the B-cell surface as mIg or, in the case of soluble immunoglobulin, mediate its biological function (Fig. 4-5).

Mononuclear Phagocytes, Antigen-Presenting Cells, and Dendritic Cells

Mononuclear phagocytes, chiefly monocytes, account for 10% of circulating white blood cells. Circulating monocytes give rise to resident tissue macrophages including, among others,

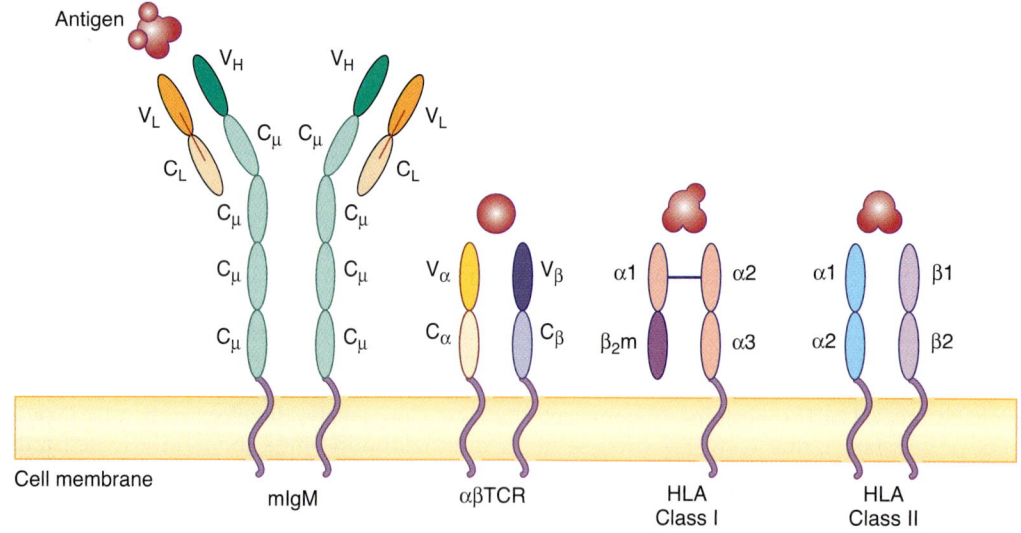

FIGURE 4-5
The antigen-binding sites of TCRs and mIg are formed by the alignment of N-terminal variable domains of two peptide chains. Each variable (V) domain is derived from a transcript that is the product of a random VJ (TCR) or V(D)J (Ig) gene segment rearrangement. The antigen-binding grooves of MHC molecules are formed by the alignment of the $\alpha 1$ and $\alpha 2$ domains of class I and the $\alpha 1$ and $\beta 1$ domains of class II molecules. C indicates a constant domain and $\beta 2m$ represents β_2 microglobulin, which is a component of an intact HLA class I molecule.

Biology of the Immune System

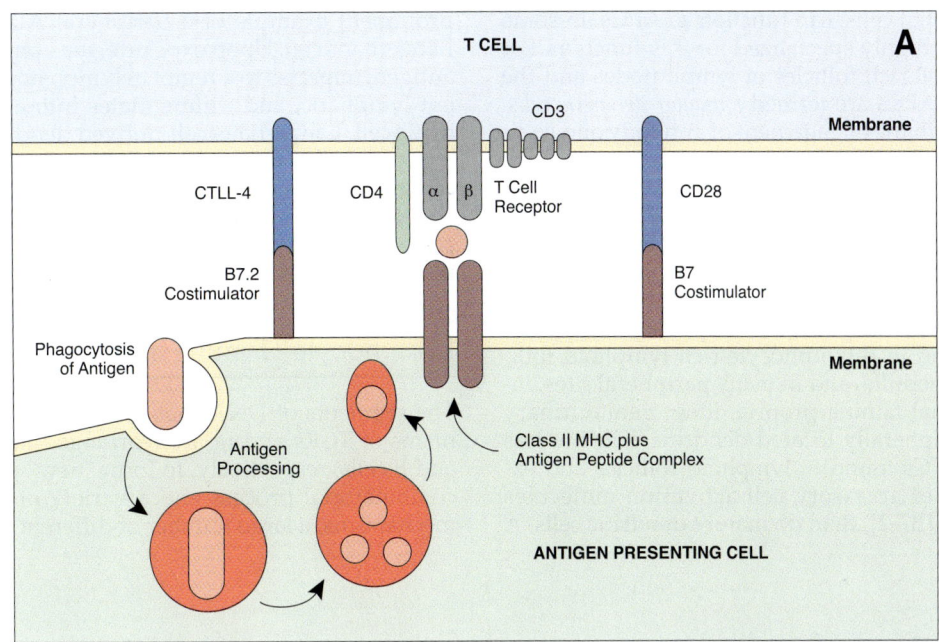

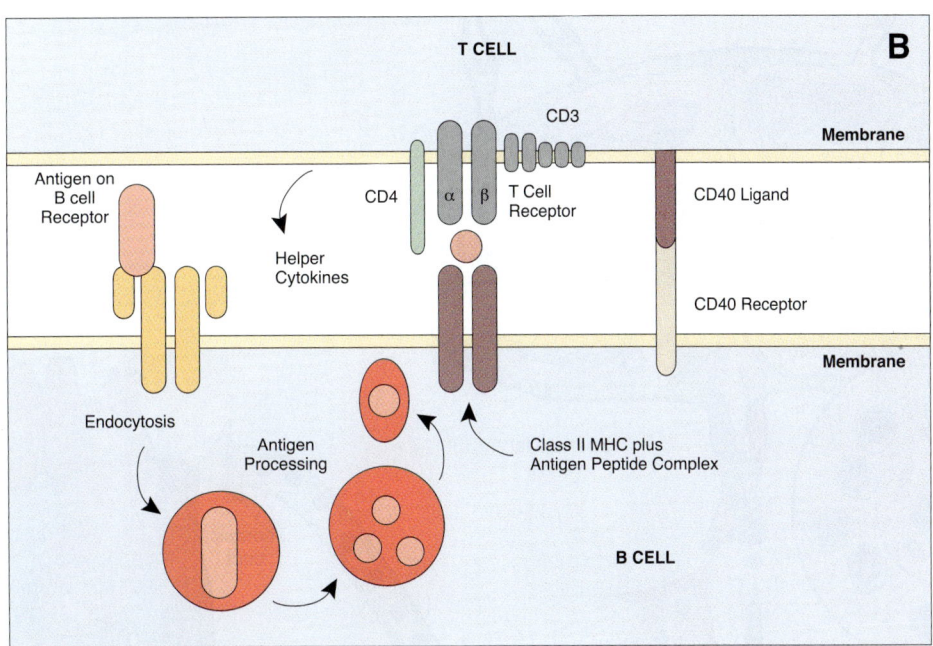

FIGURE 4-6
A. T lymphocyte activation (by the TCR) occurs via peptides cleaved from the phagocytized antigen (antigen processing) and presented to the TCR in the context of a histocompatible class II MHC molecule. T-cell activation also requires accessory or costimulatory signals from CTLL-4 or CD28. B. A similar process applies to B cell–T cell interactions. The B lymphocyte antigen receptor is membrane immunoglobulin.

Kupffer cells, alveolar macrophages, and microglial cells. Monocytes and macrophages express an array of specific cell surface molecules that are important for their host defense functions. These include MHC class II molecules, CD14 (a receptor that binds to bacterial lipopolysaccharide and can trigger cell activation), several types of Fc immunoglobulin receptors, adhesion molecules, and a variety of cytokine receptors that participate in the regulation of monocyte/macrophage function. Activated macrophages produce a variety of cytokines and soluble mediators of host defense (e.g., interferon-γ [IFN-γ], interleukin 1β [IL-1β], tumor necrosis factor-α [TNF-α], and complement components).

Antigen presenting cells (APCs), defined by their function and derived from HSCs, acquire the capacity to present antigen to T lymphocytes in the context of histocompatibility, after the cytokine-driven upregulation of MHC class II molecules (Fig. 4-6). Monocytes, macrophages, dendritic cells, and under certain conditions, B lymphocytes, endothelial cells, and epithelial cells, can function as APCs. In some locations, APCs are highly specialized for this function. For instance, in the B cell-rich follicles of lymph nodes and the spleen, specialized APCs are termed *follicular dendritic cells*. In these sites, through the engagement of antibody and complement via Fc and C3b receptors, APCs trap antigen–antibody complexes. In the case of lymph nodes, such complexes arrive via the afferent lymphatics, and in the spleen, through the blood. Antigen presentation by follicular dendritic cells leads to the generation of memory B lymphocytes.

Dendritic cells are specialized APCs that are termed *dendritic* by virtue of their spiderlike morphological appearance. They are found in B lymphocyte-rich lymphoid follicles, in the thymic medulla, and in many peripheral sites, including the intestinal lamina propria, lung, genitourinary tract, and skin. Peripherally located dendritic cells are less mature than the APCs found in lymphoid follicles and express lower levels of accessory cell activation molecules (CD80 [B7-1], CD86 [B7-2]) than do mature dendritic cells. A prominent example of a peripheral APC is the epidermal Langerhans cell. Upon exposure, the Langerhans cell engulfs antigen, migrates to a regional lymph node through an afferent lymphatic, and differentiates into a more mature dendritic cell. Langerhans cell-derived dendritic cells, which express high densities of MHC class I and II molecules and costimulatory molecules (CD80, CD86), present antigen efficiently to T lymphocytes. Again, antigen presentation to T cells occurs through TCRs in the context of histocompatibility determined by MHC class II molecules.

Lymphocyte Homing and Recirculation

The segments of DNA that encode the antigen-binding domains of TCRs and Ig are rearranged in developing T cells and B cells, respectively, to form "new" genes. Through this combinatorial process and a variety of other contributory mechanisms, a large number of different antigen receptors is

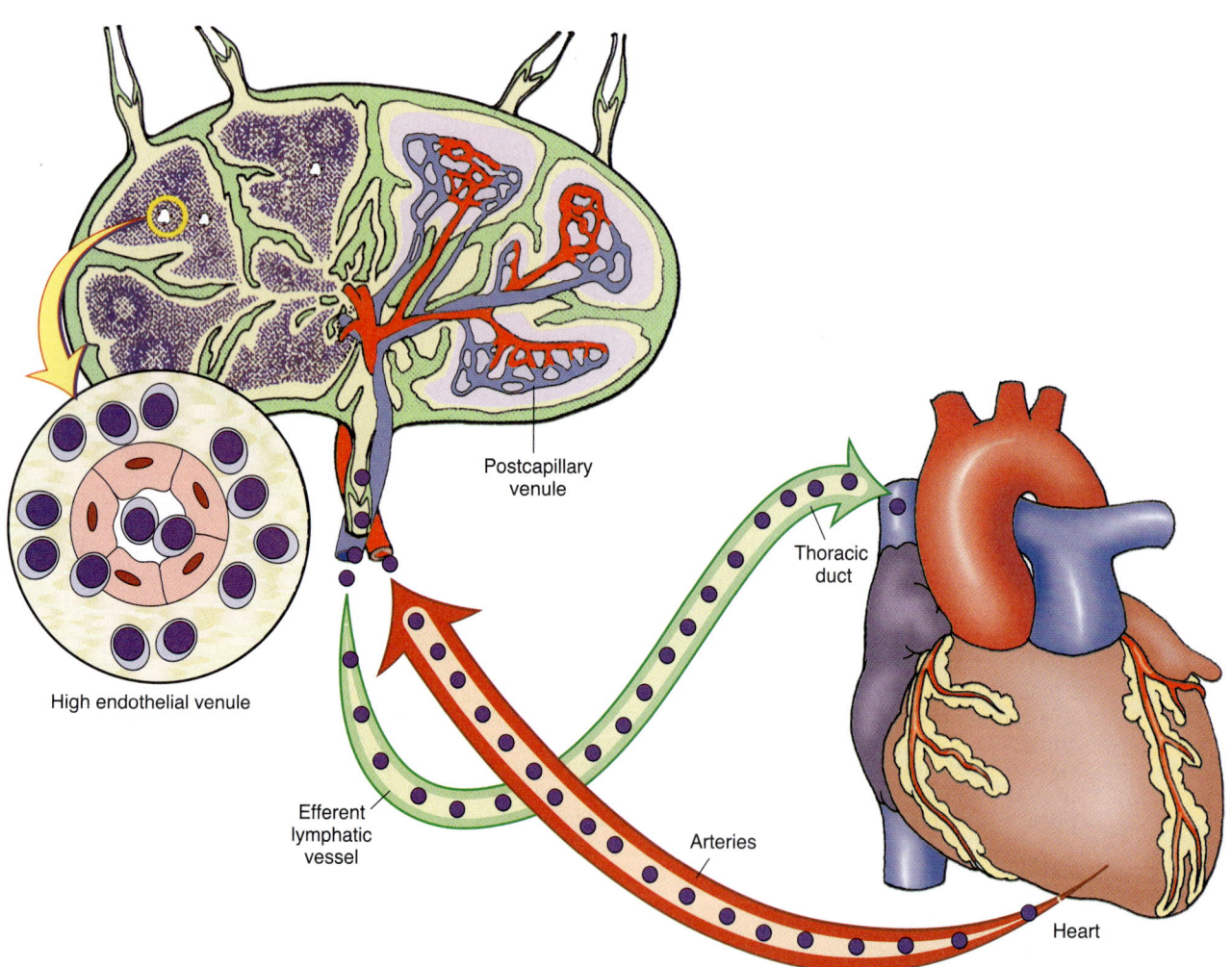

FIGURE 4-7
Blood-borne lymphocytes enter peripheral lymphoid tissues (e.g., lymph nodes) via specialized postcapillary venules referred to as *high endothelial venules* (HEVs). HEVs are lined by specialized high (cuboidal) endothelial cells that express a high density of cell surface CD31 molecules. After extravasation via HEVs, lymphocytes percolate through the lymphoid tissue and reenter the circulation via efferent lymphatics and the thoracic duct.

generated. An adult possesses about 10^{12} lymphocytes, of which only 10% are in the circulation at a given time. Despite the large number of lymphocytes, the number with any specific antigen receptor is relatively small. In addition, the body surfaces that frequently serve as portals of entry for foreign invaders are very large (e.g., skin, 2 m^2; respiratory tract, 100 m^2; gastrointestinal tract, 400 m^2). Lymphocyte trafficking is a necessary aspect of host defense because it allows small numbers of any set of antigen-specific lymphocytes to move to sites of "need." Lymphocyte trafficking, which entails homing and recirculation, has evolved to provide rapid, flexible, and widespread distribution of lymphocytes and a means of focusing specific immunological processes in anatomically discrete sites (e.g., lymph node cortex) (Fig. 4-7).

Following completion of early development, naïve B and T lymphocytes circulate via the vascular system to secondary lymphoid organs and tissues. Included among these tissues are lymph nodes, mucosa-associated lymphoid tissues (e.g., Peyer's patches), and the spleen. In the case of lymph nodes, lymphocyte trafficking occurs through specialized postcapillary venules termed *high endothelial venules (HEVs)* because of the high cuboidal shape of the endothelial cells. HEVs express an array of cellular adhesion molecules (e.g., CD31), which allow lymphocyte binding. The cuboidal shape of HEV cells contributes to a reduction in flow-mediated shear forces, and specialized intercellular connections facilitate the egress of lymphocytes out of the vascular space. Lymphocytes that do not find their cognate antigen as they percolate through secondary lymphoid tissues reenter the circulation through efferent lymphatics and the thoracic duct. By contrast, lymphocytes that have engaged an antigen leave the secondary lymphoid tissue and enter the circulation via lymphatics and the thoracic duct. They then preferentially bind peripheral tissues (e.g., lymph nodes or mucosa-associated lymphoid tissue) from which the activating antigen was introduced. Hence there are at least two major circuits, namely, lymph node and mucosa-associated. Within the mucosa-associated system, nonnaïve lymphocytes can distinguish among the gut, respiratory, and genitourinary tracts. Lymphocyte (and neutrophil) homing into sites of inflammation is mediated by different sets of leukocyte and endothelial cell adhesion molecules (see Chapter 2). The best-understood adhesion molecules involved in lymphocyte–lymphoid tissue trafficking include L-selectins (on lymphocytes) and the peripheral lymph node addressins (PNAd), which serve as attachment sites for lymphocytes. Among others, the addressins include CD34, podocalyxin, mucosal addressin cell adhesion molecule-1 (MadCAM-1), and glycosylation-dependent cell adhesion molecule-1 (GlyCAM-1).

The Major Histocompatibility Complex (MHC) Coordinates Interactions among Immune Cells

The discovery that the sera of multiparous women and multiply transfused patients contain antibodies against foreign blood leukocytes led to the definition of an intricate system of cell surface proteins known as *major histocompatibility antigens*. These antigens are also referred to as *human leukocyte antigens (HLA)* because they were first identified on leukocytes and are expressed in high concentrations on lymphocytes. It has become clear during the last 25 years that HLAs orchestrate many of the cell–cell interactions fundamental to the immune response. Important interactions between cells of the immune system do not occur if there is significant histoincompatibility. Conversely, these antigens are major immunogens and are targets in transplant rejection. The major histocompatibility complex includes class I, II, and III antigens (Fig. 4-8). Class III antigens represent certain complement components and are not histocompatibility antigens.

Class I Histocompatibility Molecules

Class I molecules are encoded by highly polymorphic genes in the A, B, and C regions of the MHC (Fig. 4-8). These loci encode similarly structured molecules that are expressed in virtually all tissues. Class I histocompatibility antigens are heterodimeric structures consisting of two chains, a 44-kd polymorphic transmembrane glycoprotein and a 12-kd nonpolymorphic molecule called β_2-microglobulin. The latter is a superficial surface protein lacking a membrane component and is noncovalently associated with the larger heavy chain. β_2-Microglobulin is encoded by a gene on chromosome 15. Structural polymorphism occurs primarily in the extracellular domains of the α-chain. Since the alleles are expressed codominantly, tissues bear class I antigens inherited from each parent. These antigens are recognized by cytotoxic T cells during graft rejection or during T lymphocyte-mediated killing of virus-infected cells.

Class II Histocompatibility Molecules

Class II molecules are encoded by multiple loci in the D region: DP, DN, DM, DO, DQ, and DR (Fig. 4-8). The D region loci encode structurally similar molecules that are expressed primarily on accessory cells involved in antigen presentation. As noted above, the chief APCs include monocytes, macrophages, dendritic cells, and B lymphocytes. Class II antigens have also been referred to as "Ia" (immunity-associated) antigens. Class II molecules are heterodimers that consist of two noncovalently linked glycoprotein chains. The 34-kd β-chain possesses a single disulfide bond; its extracellular domain is the major site of class II antigenic variability. The 29-kd α-chain exhibits two disulfide bonds. Both chains are transmembrane proteins. As in the case of class I antigens, D alleles are expressed codominantly, and tissues bear antigens from each parent.

Clinical Tissue Typing

Clinical "histocompatibility, HLA, or tissue-typing" laboratories now use several approaches to identify the set of class I and class II antigens expressed by both potential donor tissues and the recipient prior to organ transplantation. For several decades, class I antigens have been serologically defined. Antisera directed against various antigens are tested against donor (or recipient) lymphocytes. The system of nomenclature for class I antigens is based on the locus of origin (A1, A2, A3, B4, B6, C1, C2, etc.). Tissue typing reveals the two different antigens codominantly expressed at each locus; one antigen (double dose) when there is homozygosity. Accordingly, a tissue might express A1, A2, B4, B6, DR3, and DR4 antigens. The products of all loci are not universally typed in clinical laboratories. Increasingly, tissue- typing

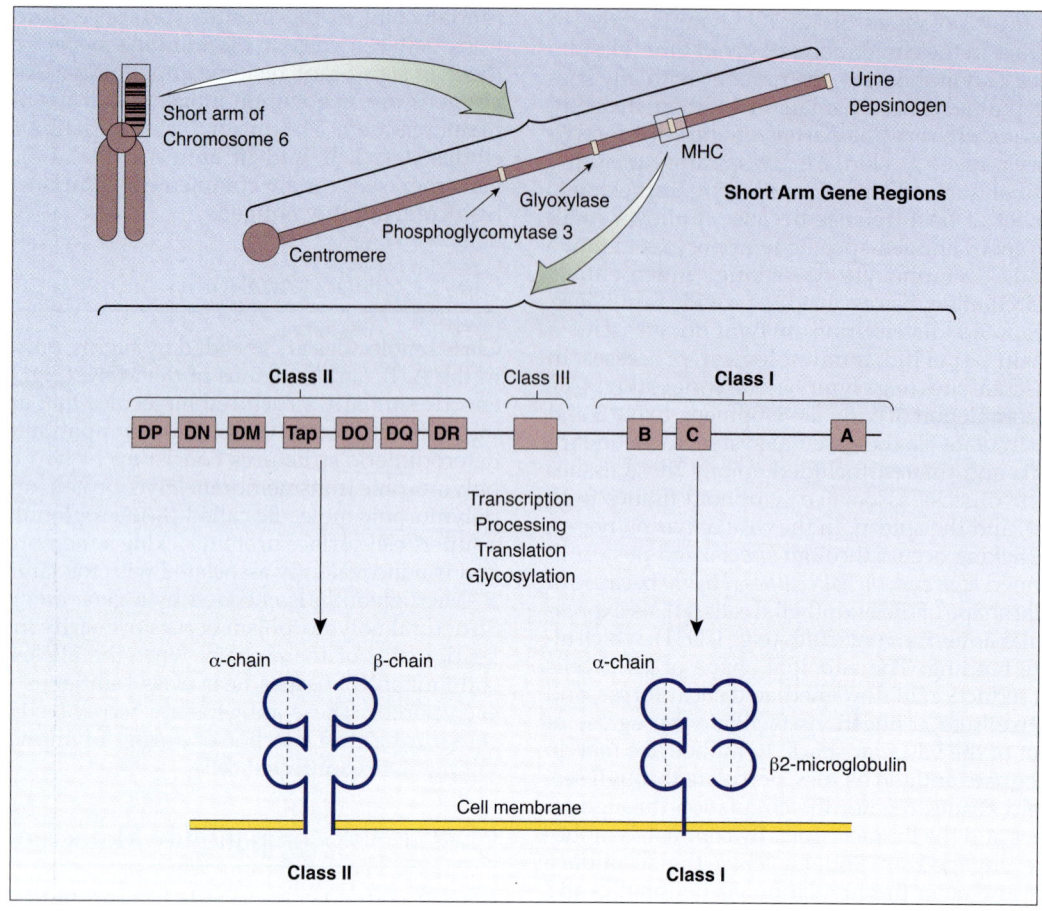

FIGURE 4-8
The highly polymorphic loci that encode major histocompatibility antigens are located on the short arm of chromosome 6. Class I and class II molecules exhibit different structures, but each participates in fundamentally important cell-cell interactions.

laboratories are using molecular methods (see below) to identify class I antigens.

Class II antigens were traditionally defined by serological and functional assay methods, but these have largely been replaced by molecular genetic techniques. It has become clear that there is greater genetic (and structural) variability than previously recognized when the standard for typing was serological. Accordingly, the nomenclature for histocompatibility genes and antigens has become more complex.

Integrated Cellular and Humoral Immune Responses Protect against Invasion by Foreign Agents

T Lymphocyte Interactions

T lymphocytes recognize specific antigens, usually proteins or haptens bound to proteins. They undergo a series of maturational events when engaged via the TCR in the context of a histocompatible (i.e., MHC-matched) APC. Exogenous signals are delivered by cytokines. $CD4^+$ and $CD8^+$ cells are T-cell subsets that possess a variety of effector and regulatory functions. Effector functions include secretion of proinflammatory cytokines and killing of cells that express foreign or altered membrane antigens. Examples of regulatory functions include augmentation and suppression of immune responses, usually by secretion of specific helper or suppressor cytokines.

The $CD4^+$ subset of T cells, and possibly also the $CD8^+$ subset, can be further distinguished by the types of cytokines produced. Helper type 1, or Th1, cells produce interferon-gamma (IFN-γ) and interleukin-2 (IL-2), whereas helper type 2, or Th2, cells secrete IL-4, IL-5, and IL-10. Th1 lymphocytes have been associated with cell-mediated phenomena and Th2 cells with allergic responses. In general, $CD4^+$ T cells promote antibody and inflammatory responses. By contrast, $CD8^+$ cells for the most part exert suppressor and cytotoxic functions. Suppressor cells inhibit the activation phase of immune responses; cytotoxic cells can kill target cells that express specific antigens. However, there is clearly an overlap, since $CD8^+$ cells secrete helper cytokines, and $CD4^+$ Th1 and Th2 cells display cross-regulatory suppressive effects.

An important aspect of T-cell antigen recognition is the requirement for the antigen to be presented on the surface of another cell in association with a histocompatible membrane protein (see Fig. 4-6). As noted above, T cells bear membrane receptor complexes (α/β TCRs plus CD3 accessory molecules) on their surface. For a maximal immune response, the TCR–CD3 complex must interact with the foreign antigen in the context of cell-to-cell histocompatibility. As a consequence, antigens are presented to T cells by accessory cells (APCs) that bear appropriate histocompatibility antigens. Antigens may also be presented to T cells by cells that do not present antigens when they express on their surface a foreign or altered self-protein in association with an appropriate histocompatibility molecule.

CD8$^+$ cells (cytotoxic T cells) recognize antigens in conjunction with class I molecules, whereas CD4$^+$ cells (helper T cells) recognize antigens together with class II molecules. The membrane CD4 and CD8 molecules of α/β T cells help to stabilize binding interactions. γ/δ T cells may also acquire CD8 outside the thymus and thereby use class I antigens for binding target cells. **Remember, foreign class I and class II molecules, which are not histocompatible with the host (e.g., transplanted histocompatibility antigens), are themselves potent immunogens and can be recognized by host T cells.** This is why it is necessary to procure HLA-matched donor tissues for transplant recipients. In addition to the binding of foreign peptides presented by MHC molecules to the TCR complex, a number of other receptor–ligand interactions must occur to maximally activate lymphocytes. Figure 4-6 summarizes some of the key interactions that occur between CD4$^+$ T helper cells and APCs. The CD4$^+$ T cell becomes an activated effector cell when stimulated via the TCR complex and "accessory" receptors (CD28 and CTLL-4), which engage costimulatory molecules (e.g., B7 and B7.2). In turn, the activated T helper cell recognizes an antigen-specific B cell via its receptor. The T helper cell then provides costimulatory and regulatory signals, such as the CD40 ligand and "helper" cytokines (e.g., IL-4 and IL-5).

B Lymphocyte Interactions

Mature B lymphocytes exist primarily in a resting state, awaiting activation by foreign antigens. Activation requires (1) cross-linking of membrane immunoglobulin receptors by antigens presented by accessory cells and (2) interactions with membrane molecules of helper T cells (see Fig. 4-6). The initial stimulus leads to the proliferation and clonal expansion of B cells, a process amplified by cytokines derived from both the accessory cells and T cells. If no additional signal is provided, the proliferating B cells return to the resting state and enter the memory cell pool. These events occur largely in lymphoid tissues and can be seen as germinal centers. Within germinal centers, B cells also undergo further somatic gene rearrangements, leading to the generation of cells that produce the various immunoglobulin isotypes and subclasses.

The term *isotype* refers to the class of the defining heavy chain of an immunoglobulin molecule. In turn, each immunoglobulin subtype exhibits a different array of biological activities. In the absence of antigenic stimulation, different B cell clones express a variety of heavy-chain isotypes and subclasses: IgG ($\gamma1$, $\gamma2$, $\gamma3$, $\gamma4$), IgA ($\alpha1$, $\alpha2$), or IgE (ε). T cells are also involved in the differentiation of B cells. In the presence of antigen, T cells produce helper cytokines that either stimulate B cell isotype switching or induce the proliferation of previously committed isotype populations. For example, IL-4 induces switching to the IgE isotype.

The final stage of B cell differentiation into antibody-synthesizing plasma cells requires exposure to additional products of T lymphocytes (e.g., IL-5, IL-6), especially in the case of protein antigens. However, some polyvalent agents directly induce proliferation of B cells and their differentiation into plasma cells, bypassing the requirements for B-cell growth and differentiation factors. Such agents are called *polyclonal B-cell activators* because they do not interact with antigen-binding sites and hence are not specific antigens. Examples of polyclonal B-cell activators are bacterial products (lipopolysaccharide, staphylococcal protein A) and certain viruses (Epstein-Barr virus, cytomegalovirus).

The predominant type of immunoglobulin produced during an immune response changes with age. Newborns tend to produce predominantly IgM. By contrast, older children and adults initially produce IgM following antigenic challenge but then rapidly shift toward IgG synthesis.

Mononuclear Phagocyte Activities

Mononuclear phagocyte is a general term applied to phagocytic cell populations in virtually all organs and connective tissues. Among these cells are macrophages, monocytes, Kupffer cells of the liver, and alveolar macrophages of the lungs. The older term *histiocyte* is synonymous with *macrophage,* either a circulating or a fixed tissue macrophage. There are subpopulations of macrophages with different functional and phenotypic characteristics. Precursor cells (monoblasts and promonocytes) arise in the bone marrow, enter the circulation as monocytes, and then migrate into tissues, where they take up residence as tissue macrophages. In the lung, liver, and spleen, numerous macrophages populate sinuses and pericapillary zones to form an effective filtering system that removes effete cells and foreign particulate material from the blood. This system was formerly known as the "reticuloendothelial system," but is now termed the "mononuclear phagocyte system." In addition to their "housekeeping" functions, macrophages play a critical role in the induction of immune responses and in both the maintenance and resolution of inflammatory reactions.

Macrophages are important accessory cells by virtue of their expression of class II histocompatibility antigens. They ingest and process antigens for presentation to T cells in conjunction with class II MHC molecules. The subsequent T cell responses are further amplified by macrophage-derived cytokines. One of the best characterized cytokines is IL-1, which, among a pleiotropic set of activities, promotes the expression of the IL-2 receptor on T cells. As a result, T-cell proliferation, which is driven by IL-2, is augmented. Among the broad spectrum of effects of IL-1 on other tissues is preparation of the body to combat infection. For example, IL-1 induces fever and promotes catabolic metabolism.

Macrophages are dominant participants in subacute and chronic inflammatory reactions. During persistent inflammation, increased numbers of monocytes are recruited from the bone marrow. Under chemotactic influences, they migrate into sites of inflammation, where they mature into macrophages. Both recruited and local tissue macrophages proliferate in these foci, where they secrete proteins, lipids, nucleotides, and reactive oxygen metabolites. Functionally, these molecules are digestive, opsonic, cytotoxic, growth promoting, and growth inhibiting.

The functional activities of macrophages and the spectrum of molecules that they produce are regulated by external factors, such as T cell-derived cytokines. Macrophages exposed to such factors become "activated," that is, they acquire a greater capacity to produce reactive oxygen metabolites, kill tumor cells, and eliminate intracellular microorganisms.

If the agent that incites an inflammatory process is poorly digestible, a granulomatous reaction can ensue. Under such conditions, macrophages show additional maturation and become "epithelioid" cells and multinucleated giant cells. Giant cells result from macrophage fusion and appear as syncytia that contain multiple nuclei. Depending upon the inciting agent, different types of giant cells may be formed. For example, granulomas elicited by mycobacteria often contain Langhans-type giant cells, which have a semicircular arrangement of nuclei. Giant cells of foreign body granulomas exhibit a random distribution of nuclei. Both epithelioid cells and giant cells are poorly phagocytic; they mainly sequester and digest foreign material.

IMMUNOLOGICALLY MEDIATED TISSUE INJURY

Immune responses not only protect against invasion by foreign organisms, but they can also lead to tissue damage. Thus, many inflammatory diseases reflect "collateral damage" i.e. they are "byproducts" of immune reactions. A wide variety of foreign substances (e.g., dust, pollen, bacteria, and viruses) can act as antigens and provoke a protective immune response. In certain situations, the protective effects of an immune response give way to deleterious events that may produce a spectrum of lesions. Such lesions can produce manifestations that range from temporary discomfort to substantial injury. For example, in the process of phagocytizing and destroying bacteria, phagocytic cells (neutrophils and macrophages) often cause injury to the surrounding tissue. An immune response that results in tissue injury is broadly referred to as a "hypersensitivity" reaction. A large number of diseases are categorized as immune disorders or immunologically mediated conditions. In these maladies, it is the immune response to a foreign or self-antigen that causes injury. Immune, or hypersensitivity-mediated, diseases are common and include such entities as hives (urticaria), asthma, hay fever, hepatitis, glomerulonephritis, and arthritis.

Hypersensitivity reactions are classified according to the type of immune mechanism (Table 4-1). Type I, II, and III hypersensitivity reactions all require the formation of a specific antibody against an exogenous (foreign) or an endogenous (self) antigen. An exception is a subset of type I reactions. The antibody class is a critical determinant of the mechanism by which tissue injury occurs.

In most type I, or *immediate-type hypersensitivity reactions*, IgE antibody is formed and binds via its Fc domain to high-affinity receptors on mast cells and basophils. The subsequent binding of antigen to the IgE triggers the release of products from these cells and results in the characteristic symptoms of such diseases as urticaria, asthma, and anaphylaxis.

In type II hypersensitivity reactions, IgG or IgM antibody is formed against an antigen, usually a protein on a cell surface. Less commonly, the antigen is an intrinsic structural component of the extracellular matrix (e.g., part of the basement membrane). Such antigen–antibody coupling leads to complement activation, which in turn is responsible for the lysis of the cell (cytotoxicity) or damage to the extracellular matrix. In some type II reactions, other antibody-mediated effects are operative.

In type III hypersensitivity reactions, the antibody responsible for tissue injury is usually IgM or IgG, but the mechanism of tissue injury differs. The antigen is not fixed to the cell surface but rather circulates in the vascular compartment until it is bound by antibody, after which the resulting immune complex is deposited in tissues. Complement activation at sites of antigen–antibody deposition leads to the recruitment of leukocytes, which are responsible for the subsequent tissue injury. In some type III reactions, antigen is bound by antibody in situ.

Type IV reactions, also known as cell-mediated, or delayed-type, hypersensitivity reactions, do not require the formation of an antibody. Rather, antigenic activation of T lymphocytes, usually with the help of macrophages, causes the release of products by these cells, thereby leading to tissue injury.

Many immunological diseases are mediated by more than one type of hypersensitivity reaction. A good example is hypersensitivity pneumonitis, a condition in which lung

TABLE 4-1 Modified Gell and Coombs Classification of Hypersensitivity Reactions

Type	Mechanism	Examples
Type I (anaphylactic type): Immediate hypersensitivity	IgE antibody-mediated mast cell activation and degranulation	Hay fever, asthma, hives, anaphylaxis
	Non-IgE-mediated	Physical urticarias
Type II (cytotoxic type): Cytotoxic antibodies	Cytotoxic (IgG, IgM) antibodies formed against cell surface antigens; complement usually involved	Autoimmune hemolytic anemias, Goodpasture disease
	Noncytotoxic antibodies against cell surface receptors	Graves disease
Type III (immune complex type): Immune complex disease	Antibodies (IgG, IgM, IgA) formed against exogenous or endogenous antigens; complement and leukocytes (neutrophils, macrophages) often involved.	Autoimmune diseases (SLE, rheumatoid arthritis), many types of glomerulonephritis
Type IV (cell-mediated type): Delayed-type hypersensitivity	Mononuclear cells (T lymphocytes, macrophages) with interleukin and lymphokine production	Granulomatous disease (tuberculosis, sarcoidosis)

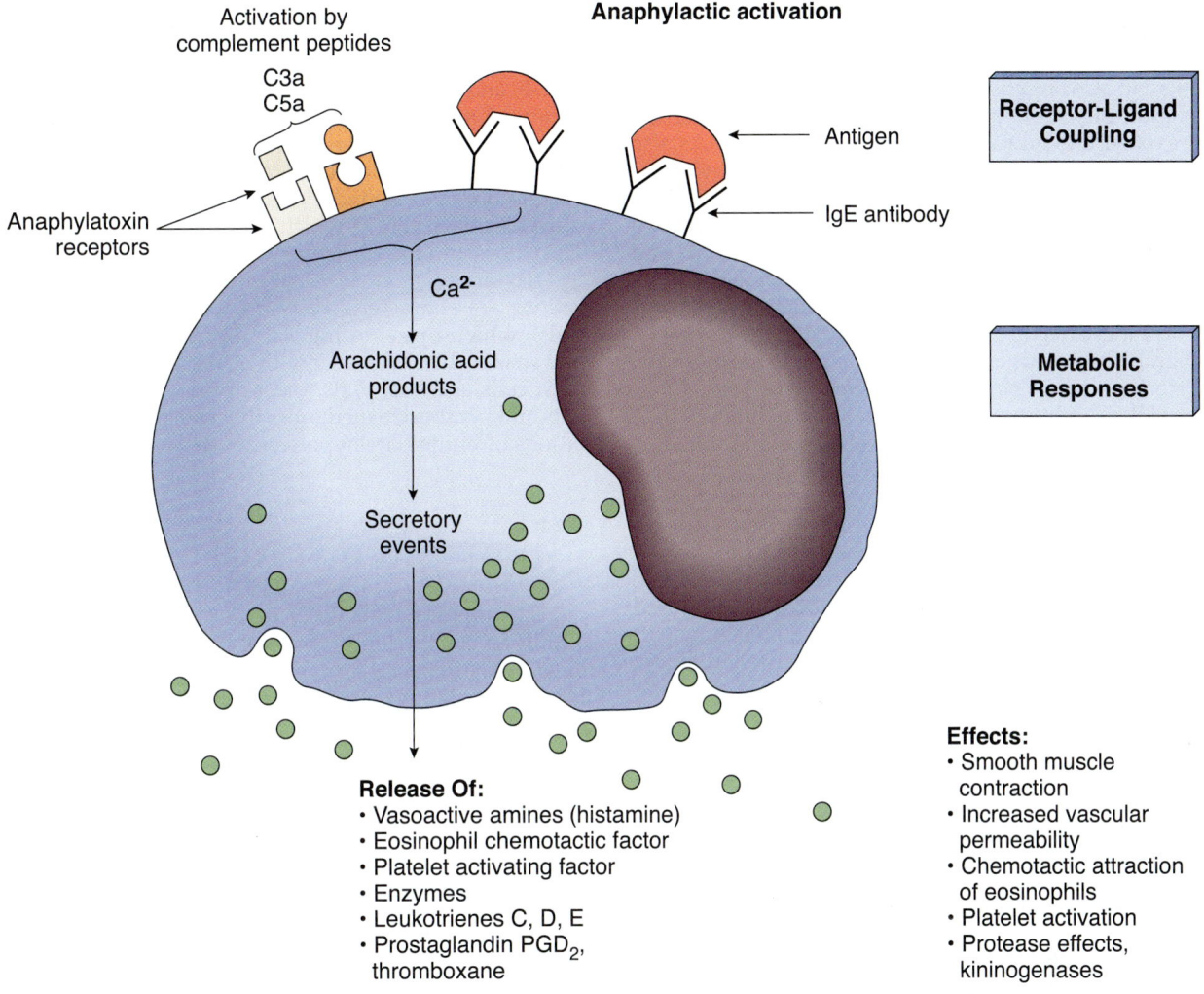

FIGURE 4-9
In a type I hypersensitivity reaction, allergen binds to cytophilic surface IgE antibody on a mast cell or basophil and triggers cell activation and the release of a cascade of proinflammatory mediators. These mediators are responsible for smooth muscle contraction, edema formation, and the recruitment of eosinophils.

injury results from hypersensitivity to inhaled fungal antigens. Types I, III, and IV hypersensitivity reactions all appear to be operative in hypersensitivity pneumonitis.

Type I or Immediate Hypersensitivity Reactions Are Triggered by IgE Bound to Mast Cells

Immediate-type hypersensitivity is manifested by a localized or generalized reaction that occurs immediately (within minutes) after exposure to an antigen or "allergen" to which the person has previously been sensitized. The clinical manifestations of a reaction depend on the site of antigen exposure and extent of sensitization. For example, when a reaction involves the skin, the characteristic local reaction is a "wheal and flare," or *urticaria*. When the localized manifestations of immediate hypersensitivity involve the upper respiratory tract and conjunctiva, causing sneezing and conjunctivitis, we speak of *hay fever* (allergic rhinitis). In its generalized and most severe form, immediate hypersensitivity reactions are associated with bronchoconstriction, airway obstruction, and circulatory collapse, as seen in anaphylactic shock.

Type I hypersensitivity reactions feature the formation of IgE antibody. IgE antibodies are formed by a $CD4^+$, Th2 Tcell–dependent mechanism and bind avidly to Fc-epsilon (Fcε) receptors on mast cells and basophils. The high avidity binding of IgE accounts for the term *cytophilic* antibody. Once exposed to a specific allergen that has resulted in the formation of IgE, a person is sensitized; subsequent responses to the allergen induce an immediate hypersensitivity reaction. After IgE antibody is formed, reexposure to the antigen typically results in the production of additional IgE antibodies, rather than the formation of antibodies of other classes, such as IgM or IgG.

IgE bound to Fcε receptors on mast cells and basophils can persist for a long time, a feature unique to IgE. Upon subsequent reexposure, the soluble antigen or allergen binds to the IgE coupled to its surface Fcε receptor and activates the mast cell or basophil. This event releases the potent inflammatory mediators that are responsible for the manifestations of this type I hypersensitivity reaction. As shown in Figure 4-

9, the antigen (allergen) binds to IgE antibody through its Fab sites. Cross-linking of the antigen to more than one IgE antibody molecule is required to activate the cell. Mast cells and basophils can also be activated by agents other than antibodies. For example, some persons may develop urticaria following exposure to an ice cube (physical urticaria). As also shown in Figure 4-9, the complement-derived anaphylatoxic peptides, C3a and C5a, can directly stimulate mast cells by a different receptor-mediated process. These cell-activating events trigger the release of stored granule constituents and the rapid synthesis and release of other mediators. Some compounds, such as melittin (from bee venom), and some drugs (e.g., morphine) directly activate mast cells and induce the release of granular constituents. Every year many anaphylactic deaths from bee stings occur in the United States.

Regardless of how mast cell activation is initiated, cytosolic calcium influx is required. The rise in cytosolic free calcium is associated with increases in cyclic adenosine 3',5'-monophosphate (cAMP), activation of several metabolic pathways within the mast cell, and the subsequent secretion of both preformed and newly synthesized products.

A number of potent mediators are released from granules within minutes. Because they are preformed and stored in granules, they exert immediate biological effects following their release. Of the granule constituents listed in Figure 4-9, the biogenic amine histamine is perhaps the most important. Histamine induces constriction of vascular and non-vascular smooth muscle, causes microvascular dilation, and increases the permeability of venules. These biological effects are largely mediated through H_1 histamine receptors. Histamine also increases gastric acid secretion through H_2 histamine receptors. In the skin, histamine provokes the wheal- and-flare reaction. In the lung, it is responsible for the early manifestations of immediate hypersensitivity, including bronchospasm, vascular congestion, and edema. Other preformed products released from mast cell granules include heparin, a series of neutral proteases (trypsin, chymotrypsin, carboxypeptidase, and acid hydrolases), and at least two chemotactic factors: a neutrophil chemotactic factor and an eosinophil chemotactic factor. The latter is responsible for the accumulation of eosinophils, a characteristic finding in immediate hypersensitivity.

Activation of mast cells also results in the synthesis of potent inflammatory mediators. Foremost among these molecules are various products of the arachidonic acid pathway that are formed following the activation of phospholipase A_2. Products derived from the activities of cyclooxygenase (prostaglandins D_2, E_2, F_2, and thromboxane) and lipoxygenase (leukotrienes B_4, C_4, D_4, E_4) are formed. Arachidonic acid products, which are also generated by a variety of other cell types, induce smooth muscle contraction, vasodilation, and edema. Leukotrienes C_4, D_4, and E_4, also known as the *slow-reacting substances of anaphylaxis* (SRS-As), are important molecules in the delayed bronchoconstriction phase of anaphylaxis. Leukotriene B_4, a potent chemotactic factor for neutrophils, macrophages, and eosinophils, is formed during anaphylaxis and is involved in attracting inflammatory cells into tissues.

Another inflammatory mediator synthesized by the mast cell is *platelet activating factor* (PAF), a lipid derived from membrane phospholipids. As the name implies, PAF is a potent inducer of platelet aggregation and the release of vasoactive amines from platelets. It has a broad range of biological activities and can activate all types of phagocytic cells.

As mentioned above, activated T cells, specifically Th2 type, produce several cytokines that have important roles in the allergic response. Activated Th2 T-cell subsets produce IL-4, IL-5, and IL-6 in the mouse, leading to IgE production and increased numbers of mast cells and eosinophils. In allergy-prone persons, a similar response occurs via T-cell clones that produce IL-4, IL-6, and IL-2, concentrations of which are also increased in allergic individuals. These persons also have reduced levels of IFN-γ, which suppresses the development of Th2 clones and the subsequent production of IgE.

To summarize, type I (immediate) hypersensitivity reactions are characterized by a specific cytophilic antibody (IgE), which binds to high-affinity receptors on basophils and mast cells and reacts with a specific antigen. Activated mast cells and basophils release preformed (granule) products and synthesize mediators that cause the classic manifestations of immediate hypersensitivity.

Type II or Non-IgE Antibody-Mediated Hypersensitivity Reactions Cause Disease through Several Mechanisms

Type II (or cytotoxic type) hypersensitivity reactions are mediated by antibodies directed against fixed antigens. Type I reactions largely involve IgE, but IgG and IgM mediate type II reactions. The most important characteristic of the latter antibodies is their ability to activate the complement system through the immunoglobulin Fc domain. There are several antibody-dependent mechanisms of cytotoxicity.

The prototypic model of antibody-mediated erythrocyte cytotoxicity is illustrated in Figure 4-10. IgM or IgG antibody binds to an antigen on the surface of the erythrocyte membrane. At sufficient density, bound immunoglobulin leads to complement fixation via C1q and the classic pathway (see Chapter 2).

Once activated, complement can lead to the destruction of the target cell by several distinct mechanisms. Complement products can directly lyse the target cells by the formation of C5b-9 complement complexes (Fig. 4-10). The C5b-9 complex is referred to as the *membrane attack complex* because of its ability to insert like the staves of a barrel into the plasma membrane and form holes or ionic channels, thereby destroying the permeability barrier and inducing cell lysis. This type of complement-mediated cell lysis is exemplified by certain types of autoimmune hemolytic anemias that involve the formation of antibodies against blood group antigens on erythrocytes. In transfusion reactions that result from major blood group incompatibilities, hemolysis occurs through activation of complement.

Complement can indirectly enhance the destruction of a target cell by *opsonization*. Complement activation in proximity to a target cell surface leads to the formation and covalent bonding of C3b (Fig. 4-11). Many phagocytic cells, including neutrophils and macrophages, express C3b receptors on their cell membranes. By binding to its receptor, C3b bridges the target cell and the effector (phagocytic) cell, thereby enhancing phagocytosis and the subsequent intracellular destruction of the complement-coated cell. Certain types of autoimmune hemolytic anemias and some drug reactions are mediated by complement-mediated opsonization.

There is another type of antibody-mediated cytotoxicity that does not require the complement system. **Antibody-dependent cell-mediated cytotoxicity (ADCC)** involves cy-

Immunologically Mediated Tissue Injury

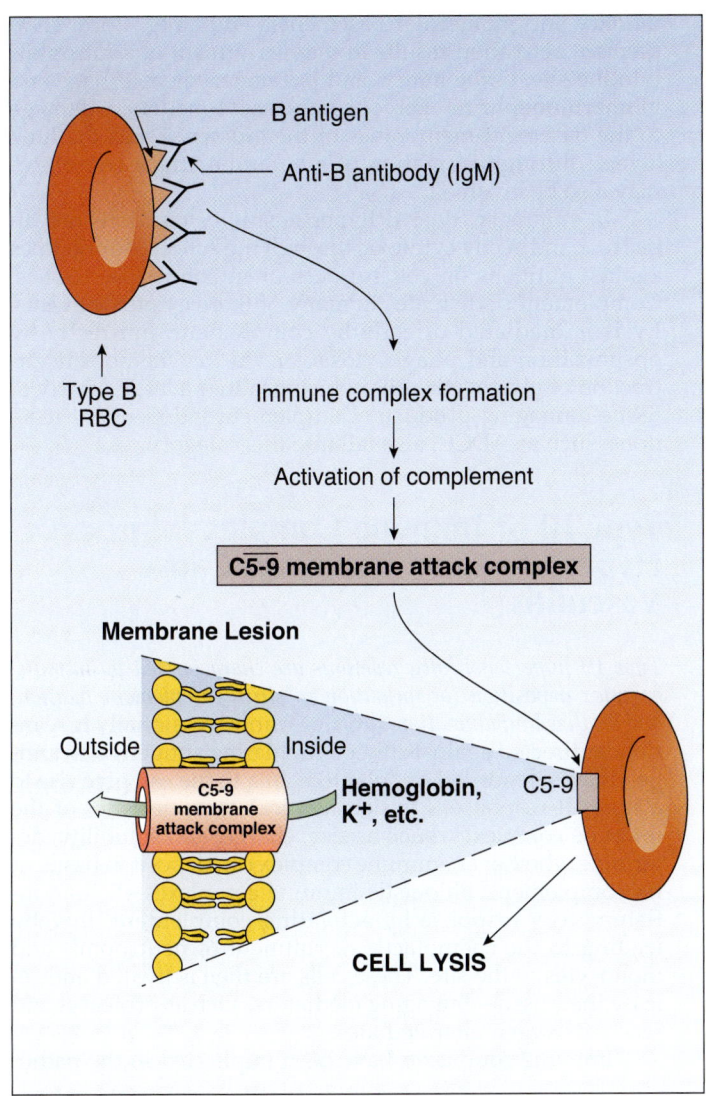

FIGURE 4-10
In a type II hypersensitivity reaction, binding of IgG or IgM antibody to an immobilized antigen promotes complement fixation. Activation of complement leads to amplification of the inflammatory response and membrane attack complex (MAC)-mediated cell lysis.

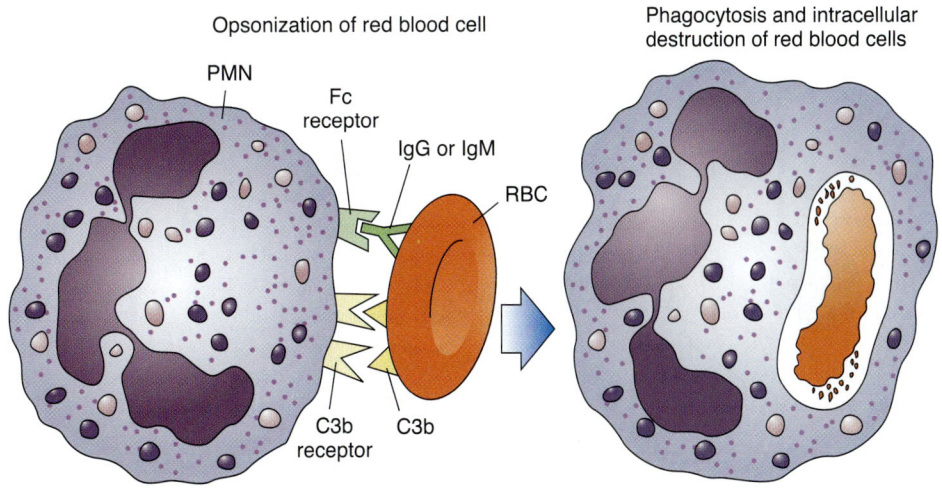

FIGURE 4-11
In a type II hypersensitivity reaction, opsonization by antibody or complement leads to phagocytosis via either Fc or C3b receptors, respectively.

tolytic leukocytes that attack antibody-coated target cells after binding via Fc receptors. Phagocytic cells and NK cells can function as effector cells in ADCC. The mechanisms by which target cells are destroyed in these reactions are not entirely understood. Among an array of mediators, effector cells synthesize homologues of terminal complement proteins (e.g., perforins), which participate in cytotoxic events (see preceding discussion of NK cells). Only rarely is antibody alone directly cytotoxic. In cases involving primarily lymphoid cells, apoptotic mechanisms are activated. ADCC may also be involved in the pathogenesis of some autoimmune diseases (e.g., autoimmune thyroiditis).

In some type II reactions, antibody binding to a specific target cell receptor does not lead to death of the cell but rather to changes in function. Autoimmune diseases such as Graves disease and myasthenia gravis feature autoantibodies against hormone receptors (Fig. 4-12). In Graves disease, autoantibody directed against the thyroid-stimulating hormone (TSH) receptor on thyrocytes mimics the effect of TSH, thereby stimulating thyroxine production and producing hyperthyroidism. By way of contrast, in myasthenia gravis, autoantibodies bind to acetylcholine receptors in the neuromuscular endplate and either block acetylcholine binding or mediate the internalization or destruction of receptors, thereby inhibiting efficient synaptic transmission. Patients with myasthenia gravis thus suffer from muscle weakness. Modulatory autoantibodies against receptors for insulin, prolactin, growth hormone, and other messengers have been described.

Some type II hypersensitivity reactions result from the formation of antibody against a structural connective tissue component. Classic examples are Goodpasture syndrome and the bullous skin diseases, pemphigus and pemphigoid. In these diseases, circulating antibody binds to an intrinsic connective tissue antigen and evokes a local inflammatory response. In the case of Goodpasture syndrome (Fig. 4-13), an autoantibody binds to the noncollagenous domain of type IV collagen, which is a major structural component of pulmonary and glomerular basement membranes. Local complement activation results in the recruitment of neutrophils into the site, tissue injury, and pulmonary hemorrhage and glomerulonephritis. Direct complement-mediated damage to the basement membranes of the glomeruli and the lung alveoli through formation of membrane attack complexes may also be involved.

In summary, type II hypersensitivity reactions are directly or indirectly cytotoxic through the action of antibodies against antigens on cell surfaces or in connective tissues. Complement participates in many of these cytotoxic events. Lysis is mediated directly by complement, indirectly by opsonization and phagocytosis, or via the chemotactic attraction of phagocytic cells, which produce a large variety of tissue-damaging products. Complement-independent reactions, such as ADCC, also fall into this category.

Type III or Immune Complex Hypersensitivity Reactions Cause Vasculitis

Type III hypersensitivity reactions are characterized by immune complex deposition (or formation in situ), complement fixation, and localized inflammation. IgG, IgM, and occasionally IgA antibody directed against either a circulating antigen or an antigen that is deposited or "planted" in a tissue can give rise to a type III response. Physicochemical characteristics of the immune complexes, such as size, charge, and solubility, determine whether an immune complex can deposit in tissue or fix complement. Phlogistic immune complexes elicit an inflammatory response by activating complement, thereby leading to the chemotactic recruitment of neutrophils and monocytes to the site. These cells are then activated and release their tissue-damaging mediators, such as proteases and reactive oxygen intermediates.

Immune complexes have been implicated in the patho-

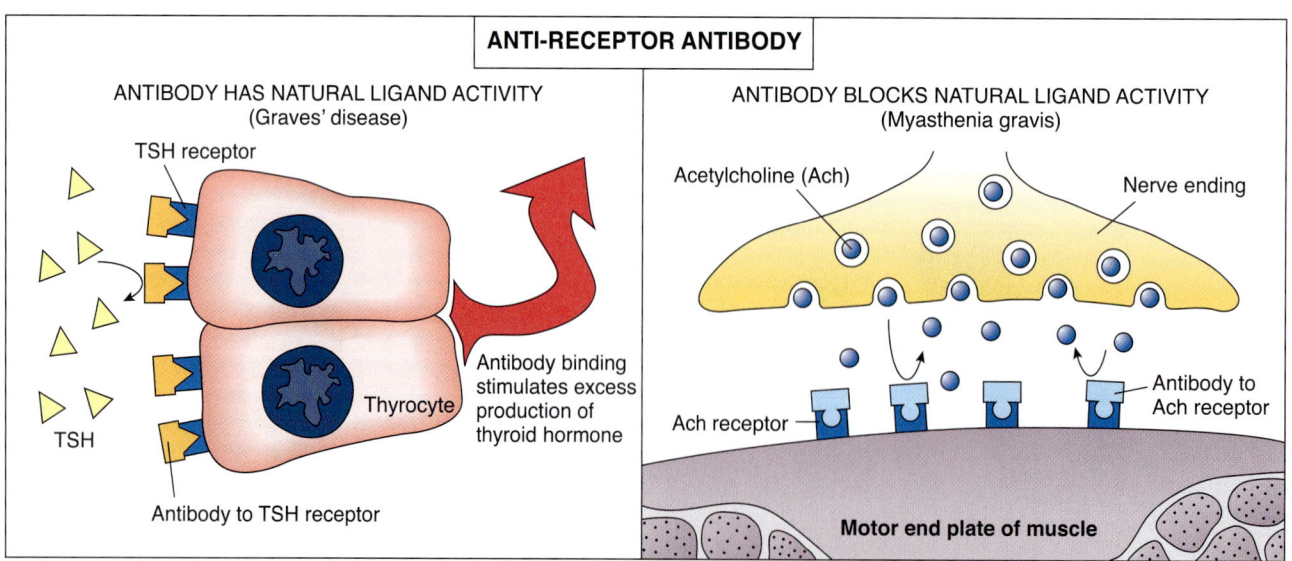

FIGURE 4-12

In a type II hypersensitivity reaction, antibodies bind to a cell surface receptor and induce activation (e.g., TSH receptors in Graves disease) or inhibition/destruction (e.g., acetylcholine receptors in myasthenia gravis).

Immunologically Mediated Tissue Injury

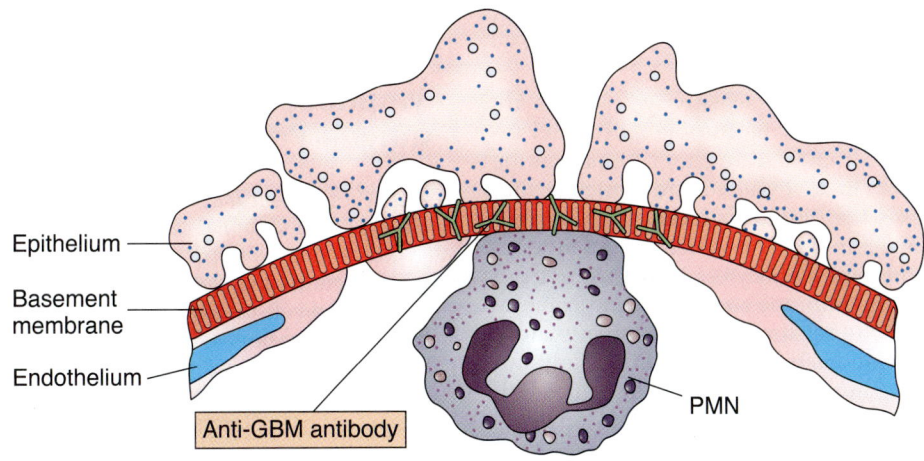

FIGURE 4-13
In a type II hypersensitivity reaction, antibody binds to a surface antigen, activates the complement system, and leads to the recruitment of tissue-damaging inflammatory cells. Several complement-derived peptides (e.g., C5a) are potent chemotactic factors.

genesis of many human diseases. The most compelling cases are those in which the demonstration of immune complexes in the injured tissue correlates with the development of the injury. Convincing examples of this are cryoglobulinemic vasculitis associated with hepatitis C infection, Henoch-Schönlein purpura (in which IgA deposits are found at sites of vasculitis), and systemic lupus erythematosus (anti–double-stranded DNA in vasculitic lesions). In many diseases, immune complexes can be detected in the plasma without concomitant evidence of tissue injury. The physicochemical properties of circulating immune complexes frequently differ from those of complexes deposited in tissues. In some cases, vasopermeability factors may play a role in the localization of circulating immune complexes. The diseases that seem to be most clearly attributable to the deposition of immune complexes are autoimmune diseases of connective tissue, such as systemic lupus erythematosus (SLE) and rheumatoid arthritis, some types of vasculitis, and many varieties of glomerulonephritis.

Serum sickness is an acute, self-limited disease that typically occurs 6 to 8 days after the injection of a foreign protein. Although human serum sickness is uncommon, it does occur in patients who have received foreign proteins as therapeutic agents (e.g., antilymphocyte globulin). Serum sickness is characterized by fever, arthralgias, vasculitis, and acute glomerulonephritis. In experimental acute serum sickness, the levels of exogenously injected antigen in the circulation remain constant until about day 6, after which they fall rapidly (Fig. 4-14). At the same time, immune complexes (containing IgM or IgG bound to antigen) appear in the circulation. Some of these circulating complexes deposit in tissues such as the renal glomeruli and blood vessel walls. They are rendered more soluble by their interaction with the complement system, a process that enhances tissue deposition. The interaction of immune complexes with complement also generates C3a and C5a, which increase vascular permeability by mechanisms described above.

Once phlogistic immune complexes are deposited in tissues, they trigger an inflammatory response. The mechanism of this reaction centers on local activation of the complement system by the complexes and the resulting formation of C5a, which is a potent neutrophil chemoattractant. The recruitment of inflammatory cells is mediated by chemotactic agents such as C5a, leukotriene B$_4$, and IL-8. The adherence and migration of neutrophils into the sites of immune complex deposition are then mediated by a series of cytokine-mediated adhesive interactions (see Chapter 2). A number of cytokines have been implicated in the modulation of this response. The early production of IL-1 and TNF-α mediates the upregulation of adhesion molecules on endothelial cells and the production of other proinflammatory cytokines. These include platelet-derived growth factor (PDGF), transforming growth factor-beta (TGF-β) and the interleukins IL-4, IL-6, and IL-10, which serve to modulate the activation of leukocytes and fibroblasts. Not all cytokines are proinflammatory; IL-10, in particular, downregulates the inflammatory response. Once neutrophils arrive, they are activated through contact with, and ingestion of, immune complexes. Activated leukocytes release many inflammatory mediators, including proteases, reactive oxygen intermediates, and arachidonic acid products, which collectively produce tissue injury. The tissue injury associated with experimental serum sickness mimics that seen in many types of human vasculitis and glomerulonephritis.

The **"Arthus reaction"** has been characterized in an experimental model of vasculitis in which a localized injury is induced by immune complexes (Fig. 4-15). This reaction is classically seen in the dermal blood vessels following the local injection of an antigen to which the individual has been previously sensitized. The circulating antibody and locally injected antigen diffuse toward each other and form immune complex deposits in the walls of small blood vessels. The resulting vascular injury is mediated by complement fixation, followed by the recruitment and activation of neutrophils, which then release their tissue-damaging mediators. Because the injury in the Arthus reaction is caused by recruited neutrophils and their products, 2 to 6 hours are required for evidence of tissue injury. This is in marked contrast to more rapidly evolving type I (immediate) hypersensitivity reactions. Histologically, the walls of affected vessels contain numerous neutrophils and show evidence of damage, with edema and hemorrhage into the surrounding tissue (Fig. 4-15). In addition, the presence of fibrin creates the classic appearance of an immune complex-induced vasculitis, namely, fibrinoid necrosis. This experimental model of localized vasculitis is the prototype for many forms of vasculitis seen in man, for example, the cutaneous vasculitides that characterize certain drug reactions.

To summarize, type III hypersensitivity reactions are the prototypic example of immune complex-mediated injury. Antigen–antibody complexes are either formed in the circulation and deposited in the tissues or are formed in situ. The immune complexes then induce a localized inflammatory response by fixing complement, which leads to the recruitment of neutrophils and monocytes. Activation of these inflammatory cells by the immune complexes and complement, accompanied by the release of potent inflammatory mediators, is directly responsible for the injury. Many human diseases, including autoimmune diseases such as SLE and many types of glomerulonephritis, are mediated by type III hypersensitivity reactions.

Type IV or Cell-Mediated Hypersensitivity Reactions Involve Lymphocytes, Macrophages, and Antigen-Presenting Cells

Type IV or cell-mediated hypersensitivity refers to an antigen-elicited cellular immune reaction that results in tissue damage and does not require the participation of antibodies. Included among these reactions are delayed-type cellular inflammatory responses and cell-mediated cytotoxic effects. These reactions often occur together with superimposed antibody reactions, which often makes it difficult to define these processes. Studies with several experimental models suggest that the type of tissue response is largely determined by the nature of the inciting agent.

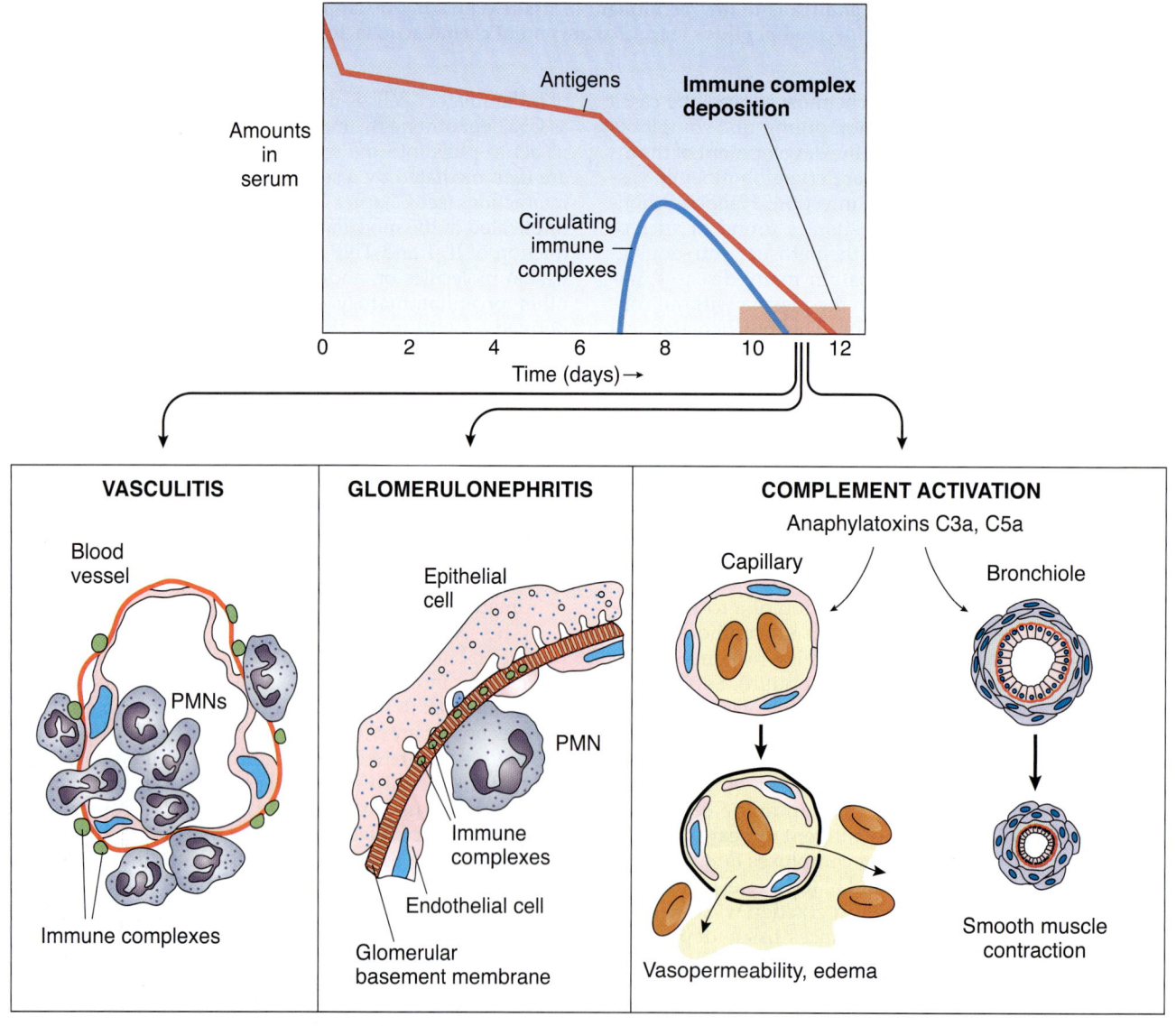

FIGURE 4-14

In type III hypersensitivity, immune complexes are deposited and can lead to complement activation and the recruitment of tissue-damaging inflammatory cells. The ability of immune complexes to mediate tissue injury depends on size, solubility, net charge, and ability to fix complement.

Immunologically Mediated Tissue Injury

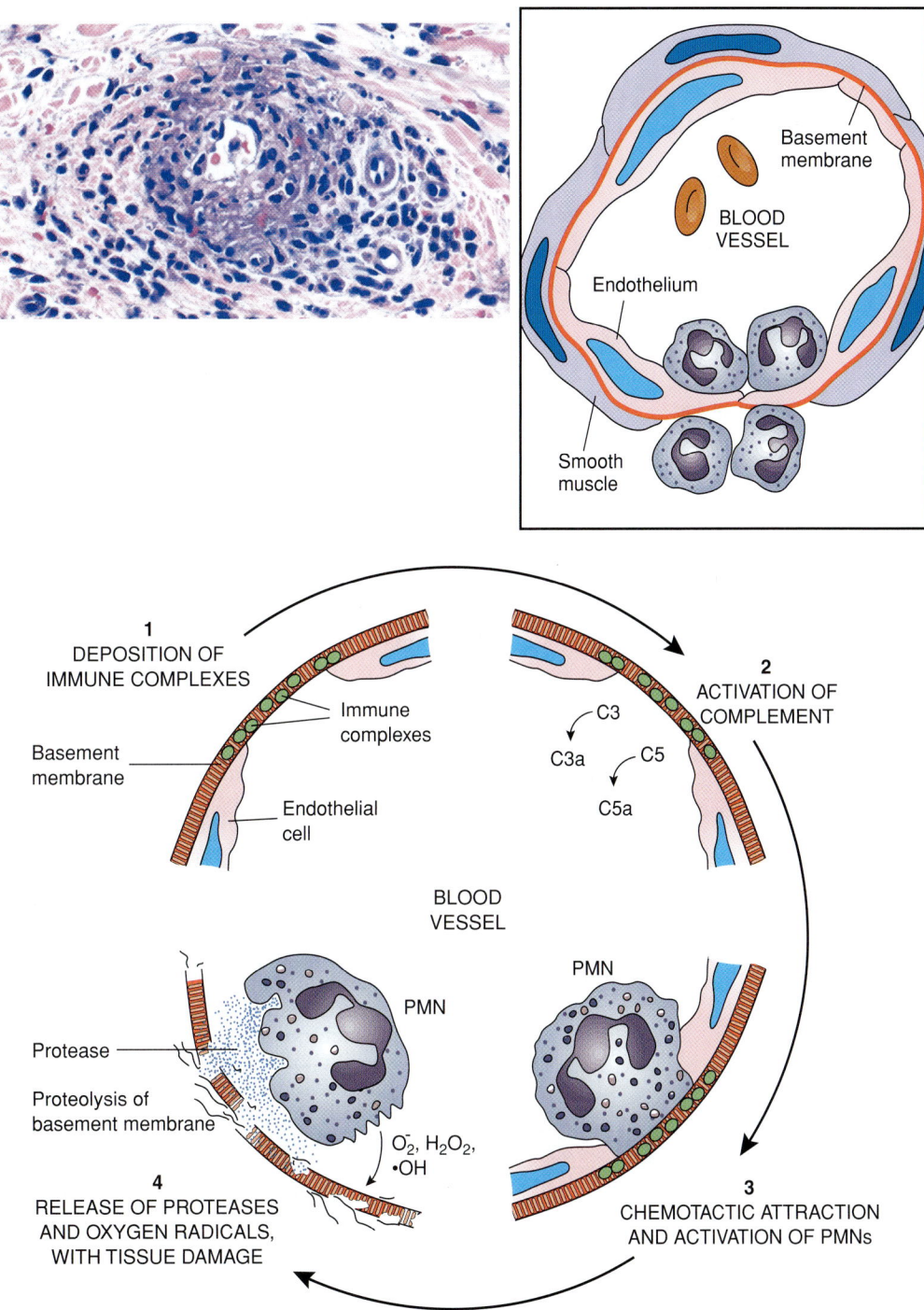

FIGURE 4-15
The Arthus reaction is a type III hypersensitivity reaction characterized by the deposition of immune complexes and the induction of an acute inflammatory response within blood vessel walls. Some vasculitic lesions exhibit fibrinoid necrosis.

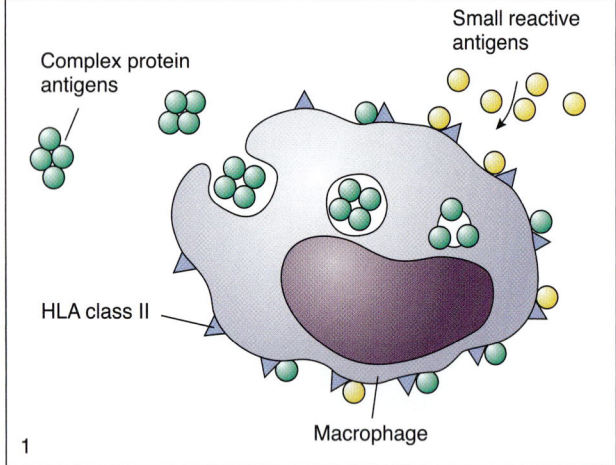
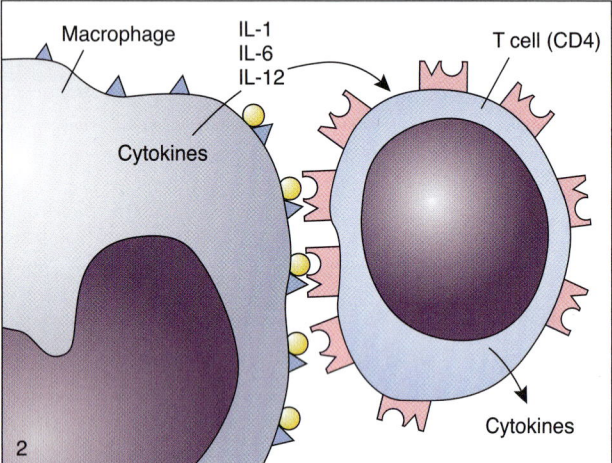
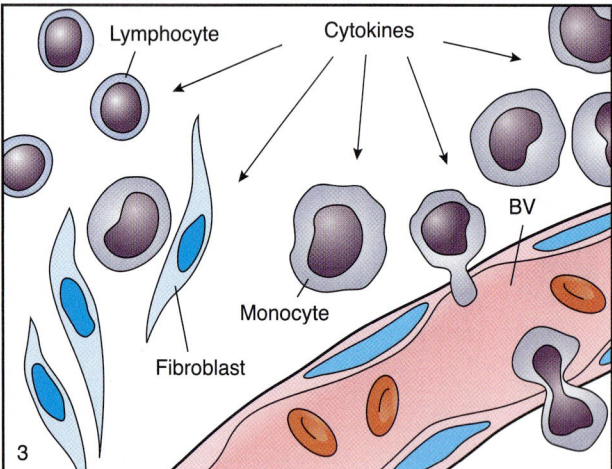

FIGURE 4-16
In a type IV (delayed type) hypersensitivity reaction, complex antigens are phagocytized, processed, and presented on macrophage cell membranes in conjunction with class II MHC antigens. Antigen-specific, histocompatible, cytotoxic T lymphocytes bind the presented antigens and are activated. Activated cytotoxic T cells secrete cytokines that amplify the response.

Classically, delayed-type hypersensitivity is defined as a tissue reaction, primarily involving lymphocytes and mononuclear phagocytes, which occurs in response to a soluble protein antigen and reaches greatest intensity 24 to 48 hours after initiation. An example of a classic type IV reaction is the contact sensitivity response to poison ivy. Although the chemical ligands in poison ivy are not proteins, they bind covalently to cell proteins, after which the compound molecules are recognized by antigen-specific lymphocytes.

Figure 4-16 summarizes the stages of a delayed-type hypersensitivity reaction. In the initial phase, foreign protein antigens or chemical ligands interact with accessory cells (macrophages) bearing class II HLA molecules. The protein antigens are actively processed into short peptides within phagolysosomes of macrophages and then presented on the cell surface in conjunction with the class II HLA molecules. The latter are recognized by CD4$^+$ T cells, which become activated and synthesize an array of cytokines. In turn, the cytokines recruit and activate lymphocytes, monocytes, fibroblasts, and other inflammatory cells. If the antigenic stimulus is eliminated, the reaction spontaneously resolves after about 48 hours. If the stimulus persists, an attempt to sequester the inciting agent may result in a granulomatous reaction.

Another mechanism by which T cells mediate tissue damage is direct cytolysis of target cells. This immune mechanism is important in the destruction and elimination of cells infected by viruses and possibly in tumor cells that express neoantigens. Cytotoxic T cells also play an important role in transplant graft rejection.

Figure 4-17 summarizes the events that occur in T cell–mediated cytotoxicity. In contrast to delayed-type hypersensitivity reactions, cytotoxic CD8$^+$ T cells must simultaneously interact with target antigens joined with class I MHC molecules. In the case of virus-infected cells and tumor cells, foreign antigens are actively presented together with self-MHC antigens. In graft rejection, foreign MHC antigens are themselves potent activators of CD8$^+$ T cells. Once activated by the antigenic stimulus, the proliferation of the cytotoxic cells is promoted by helper cells and is mediated by soluble growth factors such as IL-2. An expanded population of antigen-specific killer cells is thus generated. Actual cell killing involves the binding of the cytotoxic T cell to the target cell, after which the lymphocyte delivers the molecular signals necessary to induce cell lysis.

The defining characteristics of NK cells have been described, but the extent to which such cells participate in tissue-damaging immune reactions is unclear. Mounting evidence indicates that NK cells exert both effector and immunoregulatory functions. Figure 4-18 summarizes target cell killing by NK cells. NK cells can recognize a variety of target cells. Target molecules include membrane glycoproteins that are expressed by certain virus-infected cells and tumor cells. In a series of events similar to those described for cytotoxic T cells, NK cells bind to the target cell through their membrane receptors and then deliver molecular signals that result in lysis. NK cells also express membrane Fc receptors, which can bind antibodies that allow cell killing by ADCC. NK cell activity is influenced by a variety of mediators. For example, NK cell activity is increased by IL-2, IL-12, and IFN-γ and decreased by a variety of prostaglandins.

In summary, type IV hypersensitivity reactions, unlike the other types of hypersensitivity reactions, are not antibody mediated. Rather, antigens are processed by macrophages and presented to antigen-specific T lymphocytes. These lym-

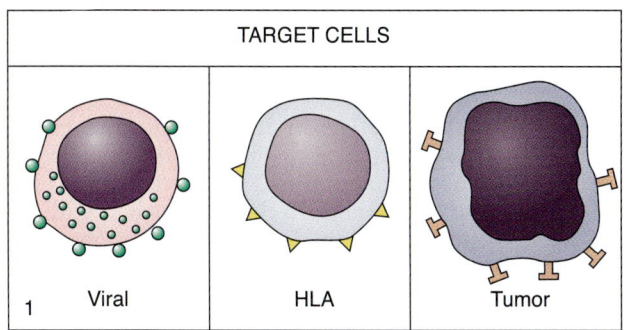

TARGET ANTIGENS
- Virally-coded membrane antigen
- Foreign or modified histocompatibility antigen
- Tumor-specific membrane antigens

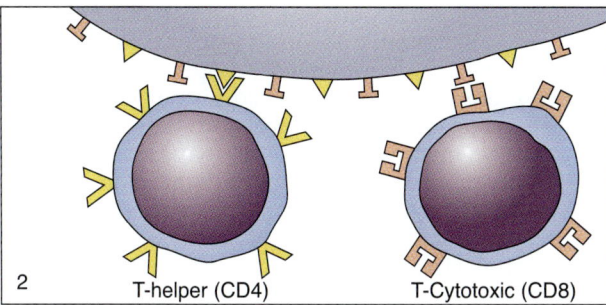

RECOGNITION OF ANTIGEN BY T CELLS
- T-helper cells recognize antigen plus class II molecules
- T-cytotoxic/killer cells recognize antigen plus class I molecules

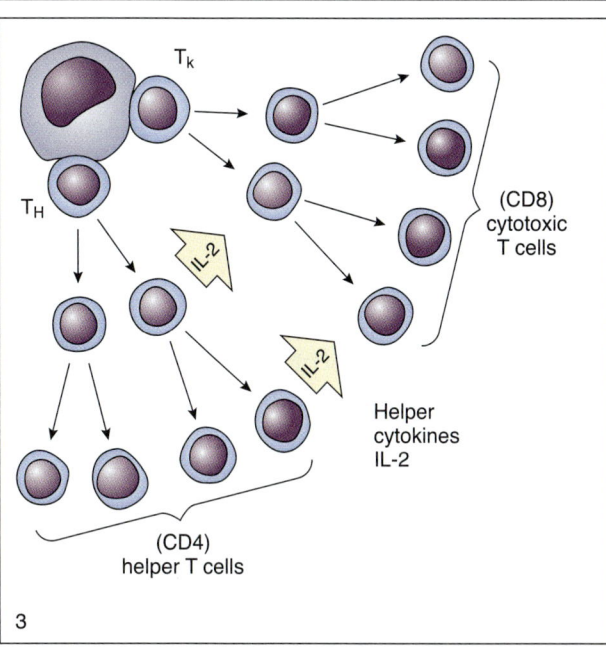

ACTIVATION AND AMPLIFICATION
- T-helper cells activate and proliferate, releasing helper molecules (e.g., IL-2)
- T-cytotoxic/killer cells proliferate in response to helper molecules

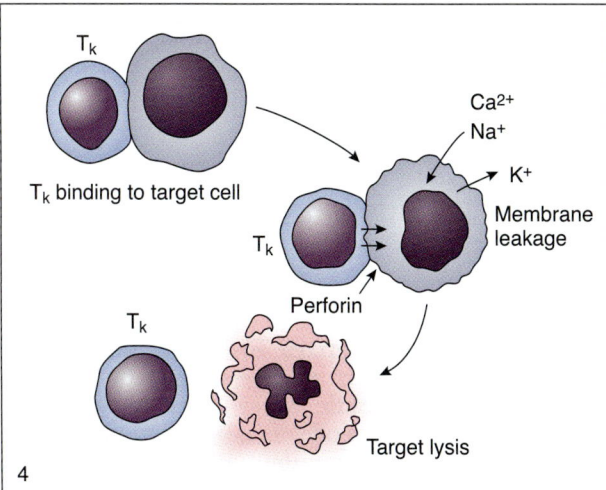

TARGET CELL KILLING
- T-cytotoxic/killer cells bind to target cell
- Killing signals perforin release and target cell loses membrane integrity
- Target cell undergoes lysis

FIGURE 4-17
In T cell-mediated cytotoxicity, potential target cells include virus-infected host cells, malignant host cells, and foreign (histoincompatible transplanted) cells. Cytotoxic T lymphocytes recognize foreign antigens in the context of HLA class I molecules. Activated T cells secrete lytic compounds (e.g., perforin and other mediators) and cytokines that amplify the response.

Immunopathology

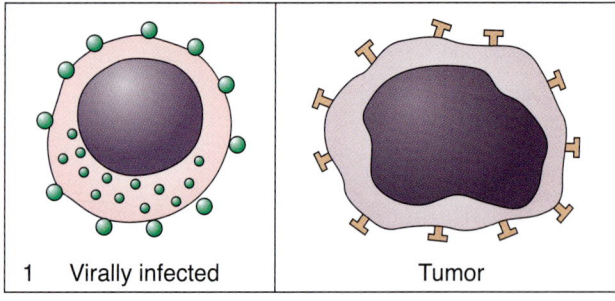
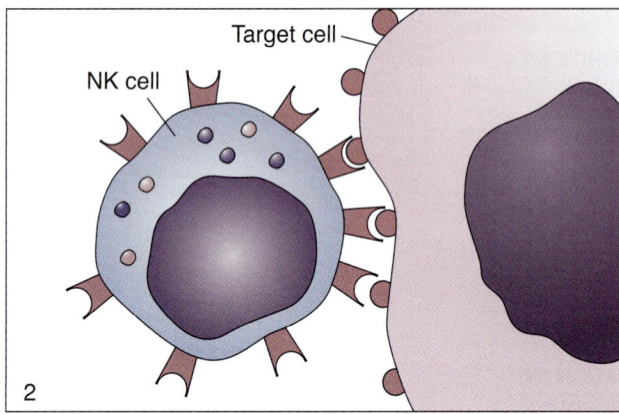
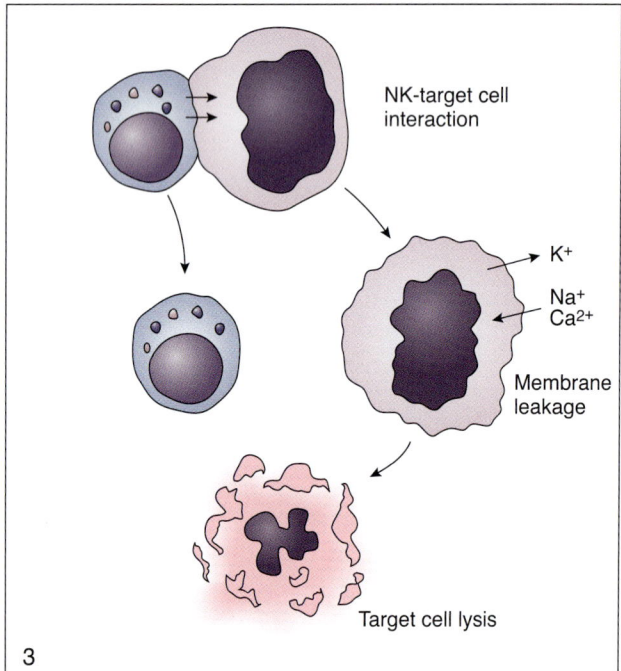

FIGURE 4-18
In NK cell-mediated cytotoxicity, potential target cells include virus-infected and neoplastic cells. NK cells bind target cells, are activated, and secrete lytic compounds.

phocytes become activated and release a variety of mediators that recruit and activate lymphocytes, macrophages, and fibroblasts. The resulting injury is caused by the T lymphocytes themselves, macrophages, or both. The chronic inflammation characteristic of a wide variety of autoimmune diseases including chronic thyroiditis, Sjögren syndrome, and primary biliary cirrhosis, is the result of type IV hypersensitivity.

IMMUNE REACTIONS TO TRANSPLANTED TISSUES

Antigens encoded by the MHC on chromosome 6 are critical immunogenic molecules that can stimulate the rejection of transplanted tissues. Thus, optimal graft survival occurs when the recipient and donor are closely matched with regard to histocompatibility antigens. In practice, an exact HLA match is obtained infrequently, except in the case of transplantation between monozygotic twins. As a result, vigilant monitoring of the functional status of the graft and immunosuppressive therapy are required after transplantation. In recent years, therapeutic advances (e.g., cyclosporine and tacrolimus) have greatly improved transplant success rates, even when there is some documented histoincompatibility. When host-versus-graft immune reactions (rejection) occur, any combination of immune responses may injure the graft. Transplant rejection reactions have been traditionally categorized into "hyperacute, acute, and chronic" rejection, based on the clinical tempo of the response and on the pathophysiological mechanisms involved in each process. However, in practice, there can be overlap of features and ambiguity in diagnosis. The diagnosis of transplant rejection is further complicated by the toxic effects of immunosuppressive drugs and by the potential for either mechanical problems (e.g., vascular thrombosis) or recurrence of original disease (e.g., some types of glomerulonephritis). The following sections describe the types of rejection in the context of renal transplantation (Fig. 4-19). Similar responses occur in other transplanted tissues, although each transplanted tissue type exhibits its own unique problems.

Hyperacute Rejection Occurs within Minutes to Hours after Transplantation

Hyperacute rejection is manifested clinically as a sudden cessation of urine output, along with fever and pain in the area of the graft site. This immediate rejection is catastrophic and necessitates prompt surgical removal of the kidney. The histological features of hyperacute rejection within the transplanted kidney are (1) vascular congestion, (2) fibrin–platelet thrombi within capillaries, (3) neutrophilic vasculitis with fibrinoid necrosis, (4) prominent interstitial edema, and (5) neutrophilic infiltrates (Fig. 4-19). This form of rejection is mediated by preformed antibodies and complement activation products, including chemotactic and other inflammatory mediators. Fortunately, hyperacute rejection is not common when appropriate pretransplantation antibody screening is performed.

Acute Rejection Is Seen within the First Few Weeks or Months after Transplantation

Acute rejection is characterized by an abrupt onset of azotemia and oliguria, which may be associated with fever and graft tenderness. A needle biopsy is often performed to differentiate between an episode of rejection and acute tubular necrosis or toxicity from immunosuppressive agents. The microscopic findings include (1) interstitial infiltrates of lym-

Chronic Rejection Appears Months to Years after Transplantation

In chronic rejection the patient develops progressive azotemia, oliguria, hypertension, and weight gain. The dominant histological features are (1) arterial and arteriolar intimal thickening causing vascular stenosis or obstruction, (2) thickened glomerular capillary walls, (3) tubular atrophy, and (4) interstitial fibrosis (Fig. 4-19). The interstitium often exhibits scattered mononuclear infiltrates, and tubules contain proteinaceous casts. Chronic rejection may be the end-result of repeated episodes of cellular rejection, either asymptomatic or clinically apparent. This advanced state of damage does not respond to therapy. As in the clinical diagnosis, histological features of acute and chronic rejection may overlap and vary in degree, so that a clear distinction is not apparent on renal biopsy.

Graft-versus-Host Disease Occurs When Lymphocytes In the Grafted Tissue Recognize and React to the Recipient

The advent of transplantation of bone marrow into patients whose immune system has been ablated or into otherwise immunodeficient patients has resulted in the complication of graft-versus-host disease. Immunocompetent lymphocytes in the grafted marrow "reject" host tissues. Graft-versus-host disease can also occur when a profoundly immunodeficient patient is transfused with blood products containing HLA-incompatible lymphocytes.

The major organs affected in graft-versus-host disease include the skin, gastrointestinal tract, and liver. The skin and intestine exhibit mononuclear cell infiltrates and epithelial cell necrosis. The liver displays periportal inflammation, damaged bile ducts, and liver cell injury. Clinically, graft-versus-host disease manifests as rash, diarrhea, abdominal cramps, anemia, and liver dysfunction. A chronic form of graft-versus-host disease is characterized by dermal sclerosis, sicca syndrome (dry eyes and dry mouth secondary to chronic inflammation of the lacrimal and salivary glands), and immunodeficiency. Treatment of graft-versus-host disease requires immunosuppressive therapy.

EVALUATION OF IMMUNE STATUS

Clinical suspicion of an immune disorder should trigger testing of immune function. For example, if a patient has chronic, recurrent, or unusual infections, an immune deficiency may be suspected. Alternatively, persons who consistently present with edema and itching following contact with an object in their environment may be suspected of having a hypersensitivity response to an antigen associated with that object. Confirmation of the diagnosis usually requires laboratory studies.

episode will be refractory to therapy. Acute rejection likely involves both cell-mediated and humoral mechanisms of tissue damage. If detected in its early stages, acute rejection can be reversed with immunosuppressive therapy.

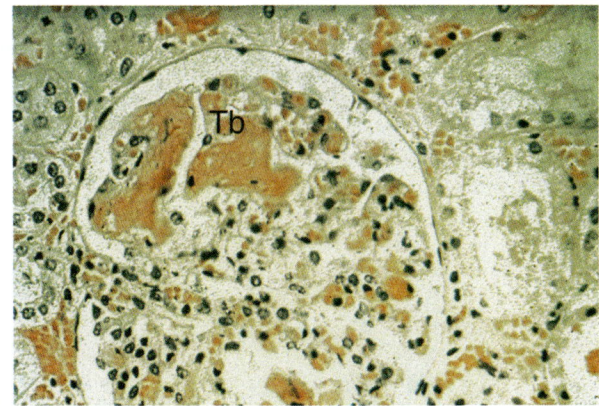
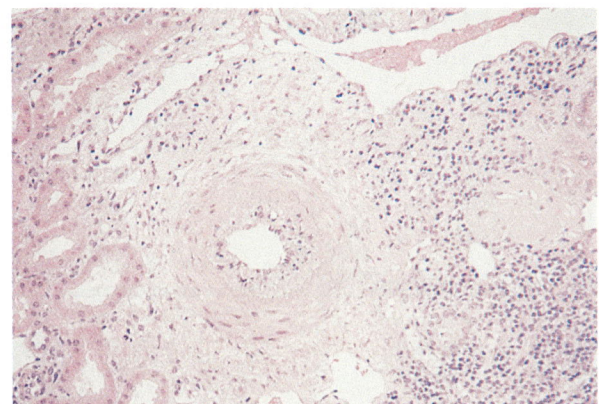
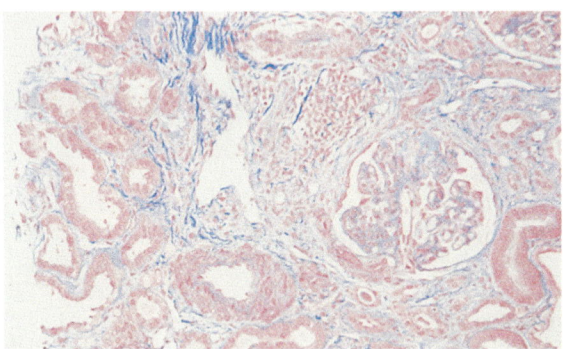

FIGURE 4-19
There are three major forms of renal transplant rejection. A. Hyperacute rejection occurs within minutes to hours after transplantation and is characterized by intravascular fibrin–platelet thrombi. B. Acute cellular rejection occurs within weeks to months after transplantation and is characterized by tubular damage and mononuclear leukocyte infiltration. In this example, the small artery *(in the center of the frame)* exhibits vasculitis. C. Chronic rejection is observed months to years after transplantation and is characterized by tubular atrophy, patchy interstitial mononuclear cell infiltrates, and fibrosis. In this example, glomeruli capillary walls are focally thickened.

phocytes and macrophages, (2) edema, (3) lymphocytic tubulitis, and (4) tubular necrosis (Fig. 4-19). The most severe form also shows vascular damage, manifested as arteritis, fibrinoid necrosis, and thrombosis. Vascular involvement is an ominous sign because it usually means the rejection

Immunoglobulin Levels Are Measured by Electrophoresis

Total concentrations of various immunoglobulins are crudely measured by serum protein electrophoresis. Serum proteins are separated electrophoretically, stained with dyes that bind to proteins, and then quantitated by densitometry. The characteristic electrophoretic pattern of a normal person and that of a person with hypogammaglobulinemia are compared in Fig. 4-20A, along with the densitometric tracings. The immunoglobulins comprise the gamma globulin fraction, which migrates toward the cathode and is reduced in the patient with hypogammaglobulinemia.

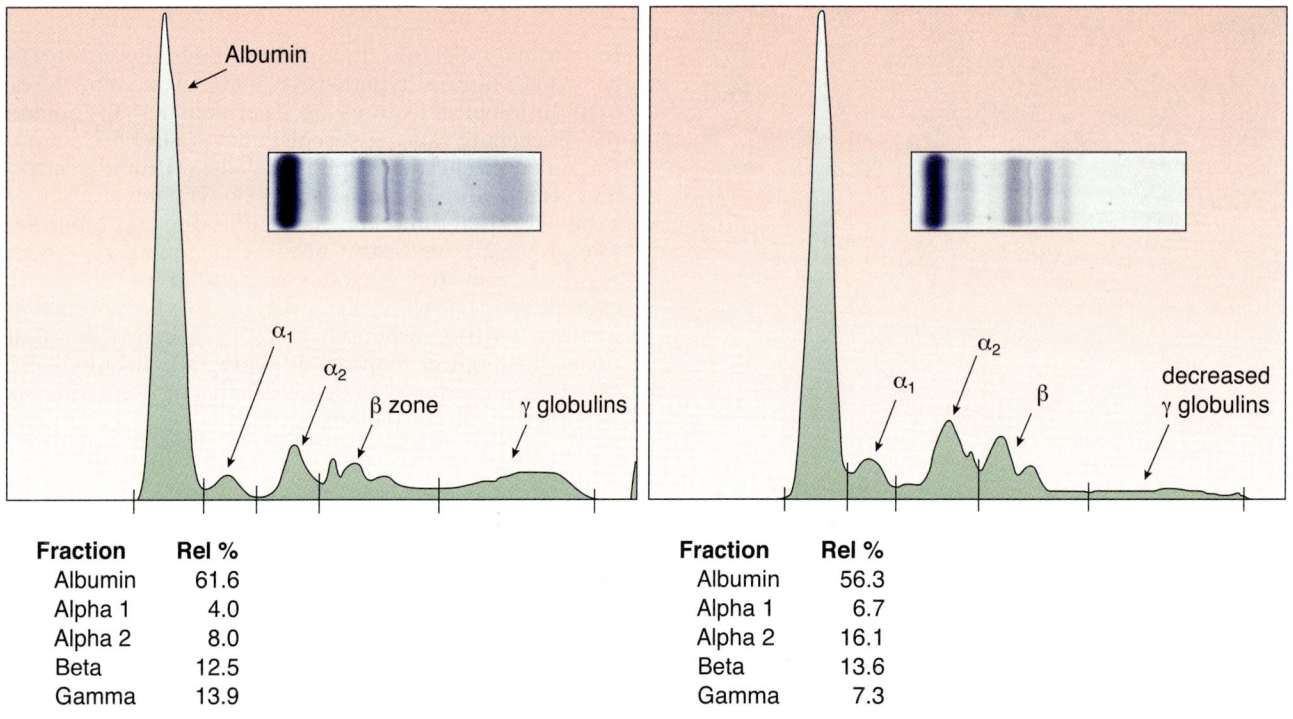

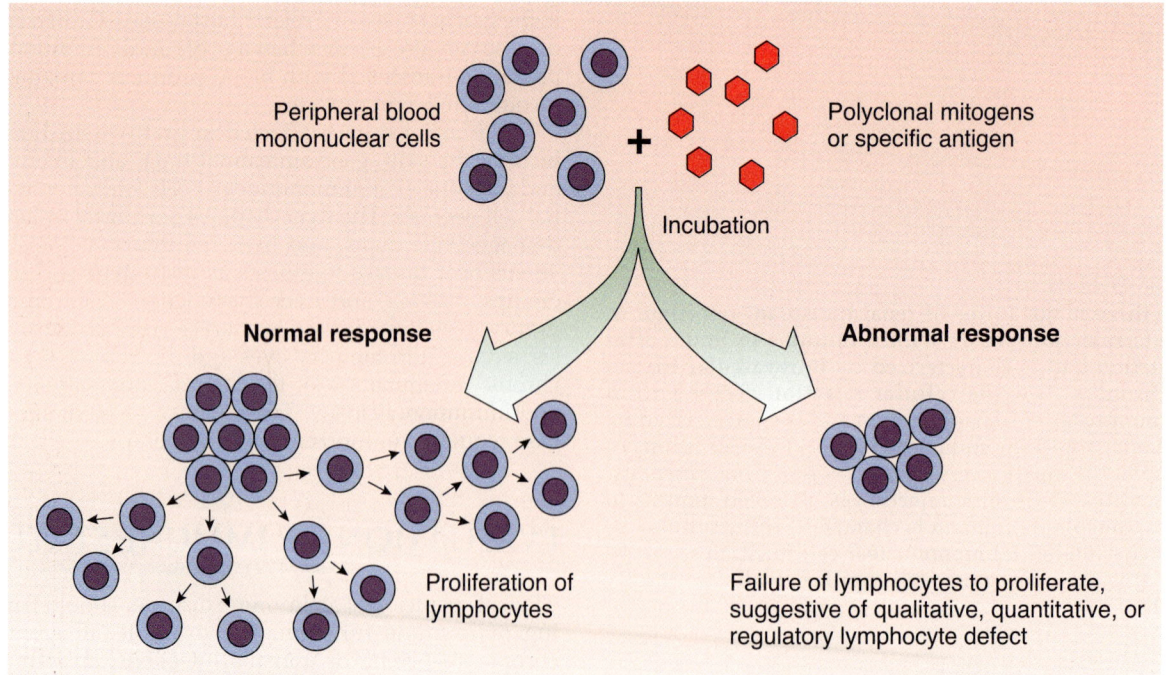

FIGURE 4-20
A. Normal and hypogammaglobulinemic serum protein electrophoresis (SPEP). SPEP provides a rapid means to evaluate the major protein components of serum. B. T-cell mitogenic or blastogenic response assay. This assay tests the capacity of peripheral blood T cells to respond to mitogenic or antigenic stimuli.

Antibody concentrations can be more precisely measured by quantitating individual immunoglobulin isotypes, or classes, with the use of specific antibodies directed against the different heavy chain isotypes. Quantitation allows identification of selective deficiencies of immunoglobulin subclasses and provides a measure of the total serum immunoglobulin concentration. There are numerous conditions that involve selective deficiency of serum IgM, IgG, IgA, or secretory IgA.

Antibody-Dependent Immunity Can Be Assessed by Testing for Antibodies against Specific Antigens

Subtle immune deficiencies can be tested by serological methods that quantitate levels of circulating antibodies to specific antigens to which most people are exposed. Exposure in these cases may be via vaccination or common environmental contact. Examples of such antigens are tetanus toxoid, diphtheria toxoid, and rubella virus. These serological methods may be useful in highlighting deficiencies in specific facets of the B-cell system, in which total serum immunoglobulin levels are not abnormal.

Cell-Mediated Immunity Can Be Measured Using Peripheral Blood T Cells or Skin Sensitivity Testing

Since the large majority of blood lymphocytes are T cells, the total lymphocyte count is a crude index of the ability of the body to generate adequate numbers of T cells. Functional screening of T-cell function can be done by skin testing for delayed-type hypersensitivity to antigens with which most people are assumed to have come into contact. Subjects are given intradermal injections of small amounts of such antigens (e.g., *Candida albicans*). A normal response is swelling and redness of more than 5 mm in diameter at the injection site.

More-sophisticated analyses of T cell function may involve studies in vitro using lymphocyte preparations from the blood. For example, proliferation of T cells in response to specific or nonspecific stimuli can provide an indication of the adequacy of T-lymphocyte function. The basis for these types of studies is shown in Figure 4-20B. Normal T cells proliferate in response to such mitogenic stimuli. T-cell proliferation requires new DNA synthesis, which can be measured by adding labeled nucleotides to the tissue culture medium. For example, a strong proliferative response to the plant lectin phytohemagglutinin (PHA), indicates that the T-cell recognition arm of the immune system is likely to be intact. Weak proliferation in response to PHA suggests either a qualitative or quantitative defect in T cells or a problem in the regulation of T-cell proliferation.

Quantitation of Lymphocyte Populations Is Commonly Done by Flow Cytometry

Another approach to assessing the T- and B-cell arms of the immune system is the quantitation of B and T lymphocytes in the peripheral blood, usually by flow cytometry. Peripheral blood lymphocytes are treated with antibodies directed against B- or T-cell membrane antigens. Many of the plasma membrane antigens used for these analyses have been categorized by the system of "cluster designation," or CD. For example, a B-lymphocyte antigen that may be used for this purpose is CD 20, whereas a commonly used marker of T cells is CD3. T cells are often further subcategorized by their expression of CD4 (helper T cells) or CD8 (effector T cells). CD4 is not unique to T cells; it is also expressed by some mononuclear phagocytes.

Monoclonal antibodies against individual antigens are allowed to bind to the cells in question. These antibodies are conjugated to fluorescent dyes such as fluorescein or rhodamine (fluorophores). A flow cytometer dispenses cells from the whole population in microdroplets, each droplet containing a single cell. As the cell falls, it passes through several lasers designed to excite the common fluorophores. If a cell carries the antigen recognized by the labeled antibody, the fluorophore is excited and emits light of a particular wavelength, which is measured by a detector. The flow cytometer then provides an enumeration of the number of cells that emitted light of the particular wavelength(s) in question, together with the intensity of those emissions. Depending on the number of lasers available in the machine, one or more cell membrane markers can be analyzed simultaneously.

IMMUNODEFICIENCY DISEASES

Immunodeficiency diseases are classified according to whether the defect is acquired or congenital and the type of host defense system that is defective. Disorders of the complement system and primary defects of phagocytes are not discussed here. In stark contrast to the low prevalence of congenital immunodeficiency disorders, HIV-1 infections and AIDS are common, affecting tens of millions of people worldwide. Functional defects in the lymphocytes can be localized to particular maturational stages in the ontogeny of the immune system or to the interruption of discrete immune activation events (Fig. 4-21).

Primary Antibody Deficiency Diseases Are Features of Impaired Production of Specific Antibodies

Primary antibody deficiency diseases are characterized by (1) recurrent bacterial infections, (2) a limited number of specific types of viral infections (e.g., echovirus infections of the central nervous system in patients with Bruton agammaglobulinemia), and (3) subnormal serum concentrations of either all or specific isotypes of immunoglobulin.

Bruton X-Linked Agammaglobulinemia

The congenital disorder Bruton X-linked agammaglobulinemia appears in male infants at 5 to 8 months of age, the period during which maternal antibody levels begin to decline. The infant suffers from recurrent pyogenic infections and severe hypogammaglobulinemia involving all immunoglobulin isotypes. There is an absence of both mature B cells in the

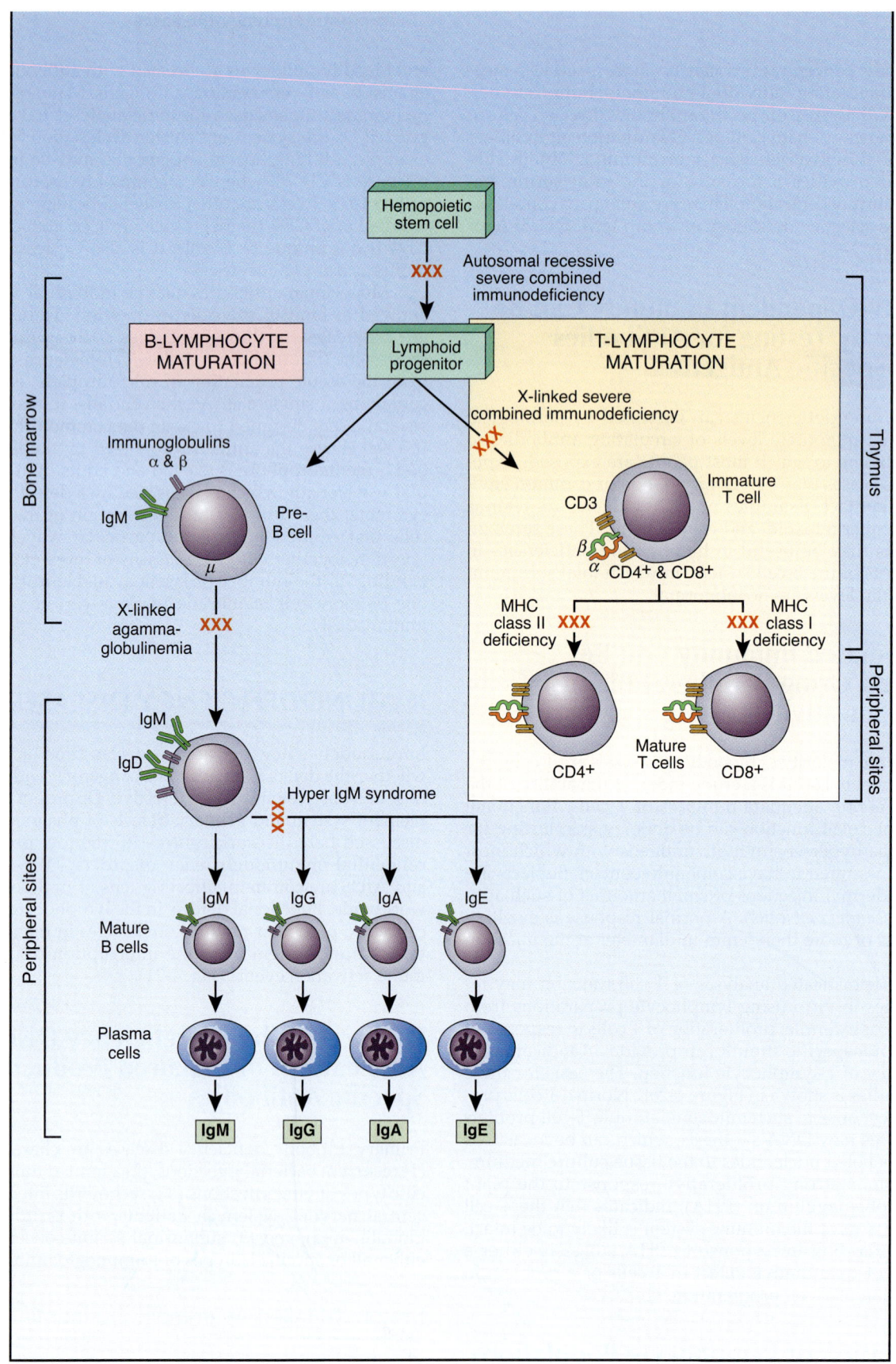

FIGURE 4-21

Hematopoietic stem cells give rise to lymphoid progenitor cells that, in a predetermined manner, populate either the bone marrow or thymus. A number of primary immunodeficiency disorders have been characterized at genetic and molecular mechanistic levels. In a number of immunodeficiency disorders, a discrete molecular defect results in a form of "maturational arrest" in the development of fully differentiated and functional lymphocytes.

TABLE 4-2   Primary Humoral Immunodeficiency Disorders

Disease	Mode of Inheritance[a]	Locus/Gene
Agammaglobulinemia	XL	Xq21.3/*BTK*
Selective antibody class/ subclass deficiencies		
γ1 isotype	AR	14q32.33
γ2 isotype	AR	14q32.33
Partial γ3 isotype	AR	14q32.33
γ4 isotype	AR	14q32.33
IgG subclass ± IgA deficiency	?	—
α1 isotype	AR	14q32.33
α2 isotype	AR	14q32.33
ε isotype	AR	14q32.33
IgA deficiency	Varied	—
Common variable immunodeficiency	Varied	—

[a] XL, X-linked; AR, autosomal recessive.

peripheral blood and plasma cells in the lymphoid tissues. Pre-B cells, however, can be detected. The genetic defect, located on the long arm of the X chromosome, is an inactivating mutation of the gene for B-cell tyrosine kinase (Bruton tyrosine kinase [*BTK*]), an enzyme critical to B-lymphocyte maturation (Table 4-2).

There are a variety of immunoglobulin isotype and subclass deficiency states (Table 4-2). These include selective deletions of immunoglobulin heavy chains and selective loss of light-chain expression. In addition, some patients have normal levels of immunoglobulins but fail to produce antibodies that react with specific antigens, usually polysaccharides. The clinical manifestations of these entities are highly variable; some patients suffer from recurrent mucosal tract infections, whereas others are asymptomatic.

Selective IgA Deficiency

Characterized by low serum concentrations of IgA, selective IgA deficiency is the most common primary immunodeficiency syndrome, with an incidence ranging from 1:700 among Europeans to 1:18,000 in Japanese. Although patients are often asymptomatic, they occasionally present with respiratory or gastrointestinal infections of varying severity. They also display a strong predilection for allergies and collagen vascular diseases. Patients with IgA deficiency have normal numbers of IgA-bearing B cells, and their varied defects result in an inability to synthesize and secrete IgA subclasses (Table 4-2).

Common Variable Immunodeficiency (CVID)

CVID is a heterogenous group of disorders characterized by pronounced hypogammaglobulinemia (Table 4-2). Affected patients present with recurrent severe pyogenic infections, especially pneumonia and diarrhea, the latter often due to infestation with *Giardia lamblia*. Recurrent attacks of herpes simplex are common, and herpes zoster develops in one fifth of patients. The disease appears years to decades after birth, with a mean age at onset of 30 years. The incidence is estimated to be between 1:50,000 and 1:200,000. The inheritance pattern is variable, and the malady features a variety of maturational and regulatory defects of the immune system. A remarkable incidence of malignant disease is seen in CVID, including a 50-fold increase in stomach cancer. Interestingly, lymphoma is 300 times more frequent in women with this immunodeficiency than in affected men. Malabsorption secondary to lymphoid hyperplasia and inflammatory bowel diseases are more frequent. CVID patients are also susceptible to other autoimmune disorders, including hemolytic anemia, neutropenia, thrombocytopenia, and pernicious anemia.

Transient Hypogammaglobulinemia of Infancy

Prolonged hypogammaglobulinemia occurs in transient hypogammaglobulinemia of infancy after maternal antibodies in the infant have reached their nadir. Some affected infants develop recurrent infections and require therapy, but all eventually produce immunoglobulins. Infants with transient hypogammaglobulinemia possess mature B cells that are temporarily unable to produce antibodies. The defect is not well understood but is thought to represent a delay in helper T-cell signal-generating capacity.

Hyper-IgM Syndrome

The hyper-IgM syndrome is often classified as a humoral immunodeficiency because immunoglobulin production is disordered. It could, however, also be classed as a combined humoral and T-lymphocyte defect because the genetic lesion that accounts for the most common X-linked form results in failure to express a T-cell molecule, namely CD40 ligand (Table 4-3). This syndrome actually represents a group of entities, of which 70% are X-linked. Infants with the X-linked form of the disease exhibit pyogenic and opportunistic infections, especially with *Pneumocystis carinii*. They also tend to develop autoimmune diseases involving the formed elements of the blood, especially autoimmune hemolytic anemia, thrombocytopenic purpura, and recurrent, severe neutropenia. Serum levels of IgG and IgA are low, but those of IgM are high normal or conspicuously elevated. Circulating B cells bear only IgM and IgD. The defect appears to be at the level of the "switch" from IgD/IgM to other heavy-chain isotypes. In this context interaction of the CD40 receptor on the surface of the B cell with CD40 ligand is required for isotype switching (see Fig. 4-6).

Primary T Cell Immunodeficiency Diseases Involve Defects in T-Lymphocyte Differentiation or Function

Defects in T-lymphocyte function typically result in recurrent or protracted viral and fungal infections.

DiGeorge Syndrome

In its complete form, the DiGeorge syndrome is one of the most severe T-lymphocyte immunodeficiency disorders. Di-

Immunopathology

TABLE 4-3 Combined Humoral and Cellular Immunodeficiencies

Disease	Locus/Gene	Inheritance[a]
Severe combined immunodeficiency (SCID)		
TB+ SCID		
JAK3 deficiency	19p13.1/*JAK3*	AR
X-linked γc-chain	Xq13.1-q13.3	X
TB- SCID		
Omenn syndrome	11p13/*RAG1, RAG2*	AR
RAG1 deficiency	11p13/*RAG1*	AR
RAG2 deficiency	11p13/*RAG2*	AR
Reticular dysgenesis	—	AR
Abnormal purine metabolism		
Adenosine deaminase (ADA) deficiency	20q13.2-q13.11	AR
Purine nucleoside phosphorylase (PNP) deficiency	14q13.1	AR
Hyper-IgM syndrome		
X-linked (CD40L deficiency)	Xq26.3-q27.1	X
Non-X-linked	—	—
Major histocompatibility complex deficiencies		
MHC class I deficiency	6q21.3/*TAP2*	AR
MHC class II deficiencies	Multiple	AR
Other combined immunodeficiencies		
CD3 deficiencies	11q23/*CD3E, CD3G*	AR
IL-2 receptor α-chain deficiency	10p14-p15/*IL2RA*	AR
ZAP-70 deficiency	2q12/*ZAP70*	AR

[a] XL, X-linked; AR, autosomal recessive.

George syndrome usually appears in an infant with congenital heart defects and severe hypocalcemia (due to hypoparathyroidism) and is recognized shortly after birth. Infants who survive the neonatal period are subject to recurrent or chronic viral, bacterial, fungal, and protozoal infections. DiGeorge syndrome is caused by defective embryological development of the third and fourth pharyngeal pouches, which give rise to the thymus and parathyroid glands. Most patients have a point deletion in the long arm of chromosome 22. In the absence of a thymus, T-cell maturation is interrupted at the pre-T cell stage. The disease has been corrected by transplanting thymic tissue. Most patients have a partial DiGeorge syndrome, in which a small remnant of thymus is present. With time, these persons recover T-cell function without treatment. Some patients with the 22p mutation are not immunodeficient but suffer only from conotruncal cardiac defects.

Chronic Mucocutaneous Candidiasis

The yeast infection chronic mucocutaneous candidiasis is the result of a congenital defect in T-cell function. It is characterized by susceptibility to candidal infections and is associated with an endocrinopathy (hypoparathyroidism, Addison disease, diabetes mellitus). Although most T-cell functions are intact, there is an impaired response to *Candida* antigens. The precise cause of the defect in chronic mucocutaneous candidiasis is unknown, but it could occur at any of several points during T-cell development. Recent studies suggest that persons with this disorder react to *Candida* antigens differently from normal individuals. In particular, they mount a type 2 (IL-4/IL-6) helper T-cell response, which is ineffective in resisting the organism. By contrast, the normal response features type 1 (IL-2/IFN-γ) T cells, which effectively control candidal infections.

Combined Immunodeficiency Diseases Show Reduced Immunoglobulins and Defects in T-Lymphocyte Function

Severe combined immunodeficiencies are conspicuously heterogenous and represent life-threatening disorders (Table 4-3).

Severe Combined Immunodeficiency (SCID)

SCID is a group of disorders of both T and B lymphocytes that are characterized by recurrent viral, bacterial, fungal, and protozoal infections. A virtually complete absence of T cells is associated with severe hypogammaglobulinemia. Many of these infants have severely reduced volumes of lymphoid tissue and an immature thymus that lacks lymphocytes. In some patients, lymphocytes fail to develop beyond pre-B cells and pre-T cells.

SCID occurs in both X-linked and autosomal recessive forms and typically appears before 6 months of age. In some patients with the autosomal recessive form, B lymphocytes are present but do not function, possibly because of a lack of helper cell activity. In the X-linked form, the most common defect is due to a mutation of the γ-chain of the IL-2 receptor, which is also used by receptors for other cytokines, namely IL-4, IL-7, IL-9, and IL-15. Patients with the autosomal recessive form of SCID have demonstrated mutations of the *Jak-3* gene, which encodes a protein kinase that associates with the γ-chain of the cytokine receptors. Thus, abnormalities in the Jak/STAT signaling pathway may account for both of these forms of SCID. Even less common than the so-called T-B positive SCID disorders are the T-B negative SCID diseases, in which neither T nor B lymphocytes are present in appreciable numbers (Table 4-3).

Adenosine Deaminase (ADA) Deficiency

ADA deficiency is an autosomal recessive form of combined immunodeficiency features due to mutations in the adenosine deaminase gene (Table 4-3). Adenosine deaminase participates in the catabolism of purine nucleotides, converting adenosine to inosine or deoxyadenosine to deoxyinosine. If the enzyme is defective or absent, deoxyadenosine and deoxyadenosine triphosphate accumulate. Deoxyadenosine triphosphate inhibits ribonucleotide reductase, thereby causing depletion of deoxyribonucleoside triphosphates and defective lymphocyte function. The clinical manifestations of ADA deficiency range from mild to severe dysfunction of T cells and B cells and include characteristic developmental abnormalities of cartilage.

Purine Nucleoside Phosphorylase Deficiency

Another congenital immunodeficiency syndrome involves an enzyme involved in purine metabolism. This very rare entity is characterized by immune defects attributed to a paucity of circulating T cells, but unlike ADA deficiency, B-cell function is preserved.

Combined immunodeficiencies have been observed in persons with stem cell dysgenesis, impaired expression of MHC class II molecules, defective TCRs (CD3), and mutations in receptor-associated signal transduction enzymes (Table 4-3). All are autosomal recessive conditions and illustrate that appropriate immune function can be undermined at many stages.

WISKOTT-Aldrich Syndrome is an X-Linked Defect in Both B- and T-Cell Function

This rare syndrome is characterized by (1) recurrent infections, (2) hemorrhages secondary to thrombocytopenia, and (3) eczema. It typically manifests in boys within the first few months of life as petechiae and recurrent infections (e.g., diarrhea).

The Wiskott-Aldrich syndrome (WAS) is caused by numerous distinct mutations in a gene on the X chromosome (Xp11.22-11.23) that encodes a protein called WASP (Wiskott-Aldrich syndrome protein), which is expressed at high levels in lymphocytes and megakaryocytes. WASP binds members of the Rho family of GTPases. These enzymes control many cellular processes, including cell morphology and mitogenesis. WASP itself controls the assembly of actin filaments that are required to form microvesicles.

Immunological Abnormalities in WAS

Both cellular and humoral immunities are impaired in WAS. Although the levels of most immunoglobulins are normal or elevated, IgM levels are only about half of normal. Antibody responses to many antigens are normal, but responses to many others may be totally absent. Since many polysaccharide antigens, particularly some bacterial polysaccharides, elicit mainly IgM antibody responses, WAS patients are susceptible to infection with encapsulated organisms such as pneumococci.

Boys with WAS also have selective deficiencies in cell-mediated immunity. Although numbers of $CD4^+$ and $CD8^+$ T cells are normal, these children are largely anergic for cutaneous delayed hypersensitivity. Lymphocytes from WAS patients respond normally to plant lectins that are powerful T-cell mitogens (e.g., PHA), but responses to specific antigens (e.g., *Candida albicans*) are usually meager. In addition, virus-specific cytotoxic T-cell immunity is usually absent, even though virus-specific antibody responses appear to be normal.

Patients with WAS typically have recurrent infections with *Streptococcus pneumoniae, Haemophilus influenzae,* and such opportunistic pathogens as *P. carinii*. They are also prone to viral infections such as cytomegalovirus, and they not infrequently die of disseminated herpes simplex or varicella. Thrombocytopenia may be severe ($<30,000/\mu L$), and the platelets are generally small. One third of these patients typically die of hemorrhage. Rarely, thrombocytopenia alone may be the sole manifestation of mutation in WASP.

A variety of autoimmune diseases may also complicate WAS. These include autoimmune hemolytic anemia and thrombocytopenia, polyarthritis, and vasculitis of coronary and cerebral arteries. These patients also have a high incidence of lymphoproliferative malignancies. The principal form of thrombocytopenia (nonimmune) is almost always cured by splenectomy. Bone marrow transplantation is curative of WAS in more than 90% of cases.

Acquired Immunodeficiency Syndrome (AIDS) Involves Destruction of the Immune System by Human Immunodeficiency Viruses (HIV)

AIDS is a widespread disease that is caused principally by HIV-1, although a small minority of patients are infected with HIV-2. Persons infected with HIV exhibit a variety of immunological defects, the most devastating of which is a complete loss of cellular immunity. As a result, catastrophic opportunistic infections are virtually inevitable. The relentless progression of HIV infection is now recognized as a continuum that extends from an initial asymptomatic state to the immune depletion that characterizes patients with overt AIDS. The fundamental lesion is infection of $CD4^+$ (helper) T lymphocytes by HIV, which leads to the depletion of this cell population and consequent impaired immune function. As a result, rather than dying of HIV infection itself, patients with AIDS usually die of opportunistic infections. There is also a high incidence of malignant tumors, principally B-cell lymphomas and Kaposi sarcoma. Finally, infection of the central nervous system with HIV often leads to a form of encephalopathy termed *AIDS dementia complex*.

 Epidemiology: AIDS was first reported in the United States in 1981 with the recognition of *P. carinii* pneumonia in five homosexual men who had been diagnosed over an 8-month period in Los Angeles. However, antibodies to HIV have been found in stored blood samples from the Congo Republic dating to 1959, although newer polymerase chain reaction (PCR)-based analyses have questioned this finding. In any event, sporadic cases of diseases that can retrospectively be attributed to AIDS certainly occurred in Africa during the 1960s. In the late 1970s, clusters of strange infectious diseases in New York and Miami among homosexual men, intravenous drug users, and Haitians are now recognized as having been secondary to AIDS. By 1982, the unusual infections and the occurrence of Kaposi sarcoma were found to reflect an underlying immune deficiency, and the acronym "AIDS" was coined. At the same time, it became clear that AIDS was spread by contact with the blood of persons suspected of bearing an infectious agent. In addition to homosexual men and intravenous drug users who shared needles, persons at risk were identified among transfusion recipients, heterosexual contacts, and infants born to female drug users. In 1983, the AIDS virus, now termed *HIV-1*, was identified. The development of a serological test for antibodies to HIV-1 in 1985 permitted accurate diagnosis of the infection and allowed much-improved public health surveillance.

Although AIDS is believed to have originated in sub-Saharan Africa, the disease has become a worldwide pandemic. The spread of HIV is attributable to the ease of international travel and enhanced population mobility, which in many societies have coincided with a rapid increase in sexual promiscuity and sexually transmitted diseases. By 1996, the World Health Organization (WHO) estimated that a cumulative total of 6 million cases of AIDS had occurred worldwide. Presently, more than 40 million people are infected with HIV.

By the mid-1990s more than 1 million HIV-positive persons were reported in the United States. Originally, homosexual men represented two thirds of these cases, and 30% were accounted for by intravenous drug users and their sexual partners. However, because of behavioral changes, the prevalence of infection among homosexuals has decreased. Men account for the large majority of AIDS cases in the United States, although the prevalence in women has continued to increase. About 70% of patients with hemophilia A and 35% with hemophilia B who received blood products before 1985 were infected with HIV-1. Fortunately, since that time, donations of blood and plasma have been screened for HIV-1 antibodies, and clotting factor concentrates used in the treatment of hemophilia are treated to inactivate HIV.

Inhabitants of sub-Saharan Africa suffer more from the ravages of AIDS than persons in other regions. Although accurate statistics from this area are not as readily available as in the industrialized countries, in parts of sub-Saharan Africa it is estimated that 25% of the population is HIV-positive. The epidemiological pattern differs from that in the United States, and African patients rarely report homosexuality or intravenous drug use. The sex ratio for AIDS in Africa shows only a slight male predominance, pointing to the predominance of heterosexual spread of the infection.

Many cases of AIDS have been reported in western Europe. As in the United States, most have occurred in homosexual men, intravenous drug users and their sexual partners, and prostitutes. AIDS has been reported increasingly in Asia, and some countries in that region (Thailand, India) have described an exponential increase in the numbers of HIV infections.

Transmission of HIV

It is now clear that with the exception of direct transmission of HIV through blood or blood products, as in intravenous drug users and transfusion recipients, AIDS is transmitted principally as a venereal disease, both homosexually and heterosexually. Significant amounts of HIV have been isolated not only from blood, but also from semen, vaginal secretions, breast milk, and cerebrospinal fluid. Except for cerebrospinal fluid, the occurrence of HIV in these fluids reflects the presence of both lymphocytes and free virus.

Among homosexual men, the receptive partner in anal intercourse is at particularly high risk of becoming infected with HIV. The virus is transmitted from semen through tears in the rectal mucosa and it can infect the epithelial cells of the rectum directly. In heterosexual contact, transmission from male to female is more likely than the reverse, perhaps reflecting the greater concentration of HIV in semen than in vaginal fluids. The risk of infecting a woman with HIV is evidenced by the demonstration that 8 to 50% of women artificially inseminated with semen from donors later shown to be HIV positive became infected with the AIDS virus. Additionally, genital lesions, usually caused by other sexually transmitted diseases, facilitate entry of the virus and lead to a particularly high risk of contracting AIDS.

AIDS is not transmissible by nonsexual, casual exposure to infected persons. A particular concern of health care workers is the possibility of HIV infection from accidental exposure to the virus. In prospective studies of hundreds of health care workers who sustained "needle sticks" or other accidental exposures to blood from AIDS patients, fewer than 1% developed antibodies to HIV. Immediate treatment with antiviral agents is beneficial.

 Pathogenesis: The primary etiologic agent of AIDS is HIV-1, an enveloped RNA retrovirus that contains a reverse transcriptase (RNA-dependent DNA polymerase). HIV-1 is a member of the retrovirus family, specifically the subfamily of lentiviruses. Animal lentiviruses have been recognized for a century, but human lentiviruses have been identified for less than three decades.

The HIV-1 genome consists of two identical 9.7-kd single strands of RNA enclosed within a core of viral proteins. The core is in turn enveloped by a phospholipid bilayer derived from the host cell membrane, in which are found virally encoded glycoproteins (gp120 and gp41). In addition to the *gag, pol,* and *env* genes characteristic of all replication-competent RNA viruses, HIV-1 contains six other genes that code for proteins involved in the regulation of viral replication. The specific target cells for HIV-1 are CD4+ helper T lymphocytes and mononuclear phagocytes, although infection of other cells, such as B lymphocytes, glial cells, and intestinal epithelial cells, occurs.

The replicative life cycle of HIV-1 proceeds as depicted in Figure 4-22.

1. **Binding:** Free HIV or an infected lymphocyte can transmit the virus to an uninfected cell. The HIV envelope glycoprotein gp120, either on the free virus or on the surface of an infected cell, binds to the CD4 molecule on the surface of helper T lymphocytes.

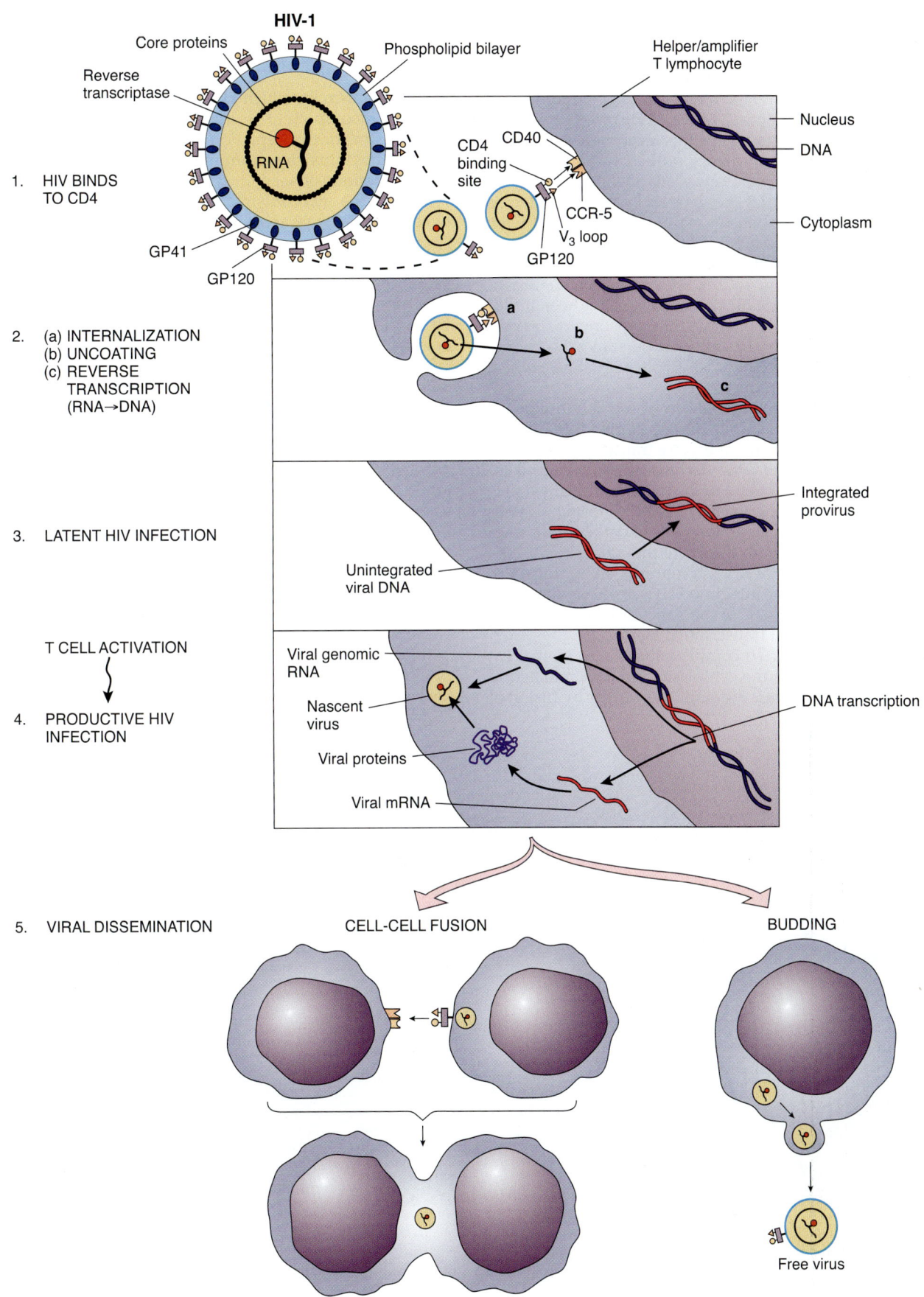

FIGURE 4-22
The life cycle of HIV-1 is a multistep process.

2. **Internalization:** The binding of gp120 to CD4 allows gp41 to insert into the cell membrane of the lymphocyte, thereby promoting fusion of the viral envelope with that of the lymphocyte, with consequent internalization of the virus. The entry of HIV-1 into the target cell in vivo requires viral binding to a coreceptor, β-chemokine receptor 5 (CCR-5). The chemokine ligands for this receptor are RANTES and macrophage inflammatory protien 1α and 1β (MIP-1α, MIP-1β). About 1% of Caucasians are homozygous for major deletions in the CCR-5 gene and remain uninfected with HIV even with extensive exposure to the agent. Even heterozygosity for the mutant CCR-5 allele provides partial protection against HIV infection. Interestingly, the mutant allele is found in up to 20% of Caucasians but is absent in blacks and Asians. Some persons who have been multiply exposed to HIV-1 and who do not seroconvert and possibly some long-term HIV-infected persons who do not progress to AIDS have high levels of chemokines, which may block the coreceptors for HIV.
3. **DNA synthesis:** In the cytoplasm of the T lymphocyte, the virus is uncoated, and its RNA is copied into double-stranded DNA by retroviral reverse transcriptase.
4. **Viral integration:** The DNA derived from the virus is integrated into the host genome by the viral integrase protein, thereby producing the latent proviral form of HIV-1. Viral genes are replicated along with host chromosomes and, therefore, persist for the life of the cell.
5. **Viral replication:** Viral RNA is reproduced by transcriptional activation of the integrated HIV provirus, a process that requires "activation" of the T cell and the presence of certain inducible host transcription factors.
6. **Viral dissemination:** To complete the life cycle, nascent virus is assembled in the cytoplasm and disseminated to other target cells. This is accomplished either by fusion of an infected cell with an uninfected one or by the budding of virions from the plasma membrane of the infected cell (Fig. 4-23).

The mechanism by which HIV kills infected T lymphocytes remains incompletely understood. Among the potential mechanisms for the depletion of CD4$^+$ lymphocytes are direct viral cytotoxicity, immune clearance of infected cells, and the actions of secondary mediators such as cytokines. Whatever the mechanisms, there is a clear association between increasing viral burden and the decline in CD4$^+$ lymphocyte counts.

The long interval between HIV-1 infection and the appearance of the clinical symptoms of AIDS is related to the small number of infected T lymphocytes and the latency of the virus. Only 10^{-5} to 10^{-4} circulating mononuclear cells display detectable viral mRNA, but about 1% of circulating T cells contain proviral DNA. Although many infected cells do not replicate the virus, but rather harbor latent HIV-1, many cells contain actively replicating virus. During latent infection, the virus can exist in three forms: untranscribed viral RNA may exist in the cytoplasm of resting T cells; unintegrated, and thus untranscribed, viral DNA may be present in the cell; in a resting T cell, integrated proviral DNA may remain untranscribed. The mechanisms underlying latency and the conversion to a lytic infection are incompletely understood.

The initiation of viral replication in latent HIV-1 infection critically depends on the induction of host proteins during T-cell activation. The regulation of viral transcription involves the long terminal repeats (LTRs) that flank both ends of the viral genome. The LTRs are activated by many T-cell mitogens and by various cytokines produced by monocyte/macrophages, including TNF-α and IL-1. Moreover, the LTRs can also be activated by proteins produced by other

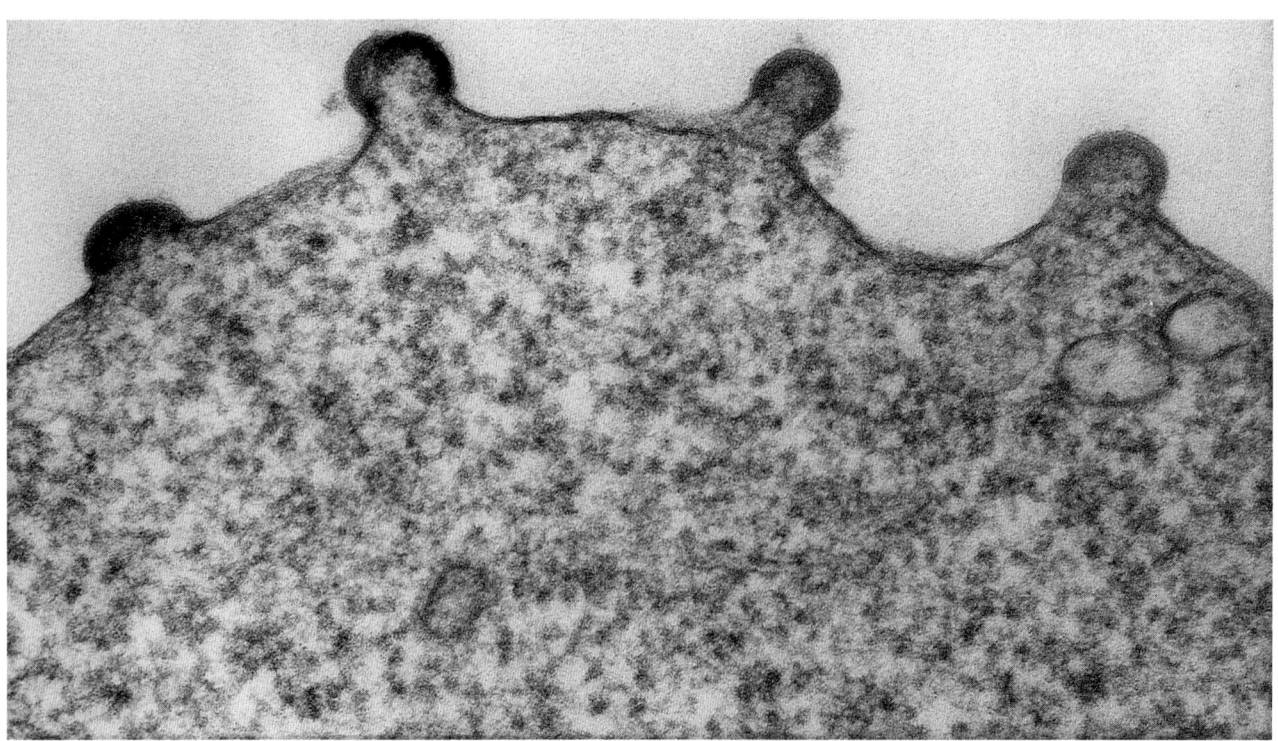

FIGURE 4-23
HIV-1 virions can be seen budding from an infected cells.

viruses known to infect patients with AIDS, such as herpesvirus, Epstein-Barr virus, adenovirus, and cytomegalovirus. Thus, activation of the immune system by a variety of infectious agents may promote HIV replication.

Immunology of AIDS

The destruction of CD4$^+$ T cells by HIV-1 can essentially disable the entire immune system because this subset of lymphocytes exerts critical regulatory and effector functions that involve both cellular and humoral immunity. Thus, in the typical AIDS patient, all elements of the immune system are eventually perturbed, including T cells, B cells, NK cells, and monocyte/macrophages.

CD4$^+$ T lymphocytes include two functional types: helper and amplifier (or inducer) cells. The first population affected in HIV infection is the amplifier subset. Eventually, total CD4$^+$ lymphocyte counts fall to less than 500 cells/μL, and the helper-to-suppressor T-cell ratio declines from a normal of 2.0 to as little as 0.5. The number of CD8$^+$ (cytotoxic/suppressor) cells is variable, although in AIDS, most of these cells seem to be of the cytotoxic variety.

The defects in T-cell function are manifested by defective responses to skin testing with a variety of antigens (delayed hypersensitivity) and by impaired proliferative responses to mitogens and antigens in vitro. Moreover, the deficiency of CD4$^+$ cells reduces the levels of IL-2, the cytokine produced in response to antigens that stimulate cytotoxic T cell killing. Thus, the patient with AIDS cannot generate the antigen-specific cytotoxic T cells that are required for the clearance of viruses and other infectious agents.

In persons infected with HIV, humoral immunity is also abnormal. The production of antibodies in response to specific antigenic stimulation is markedly decreased, often to less than 10% of normal. B cells also demonstrate a decreased proliferative response in vitro to mitogens and antigens. Yet, the serum of patients with AIDS usually shows high levels of polyclonal immunoglobulins, autoantibodies, and immune complexes. This apparent paradox is explained by the fact that concurrent infection with polyclonal B cell-activating viruses (e.g., Epstein-Barr virus or cytomegalovirus) constantly stimulates B cells to produce nonspecific immunoglobulins. The lack of CD4$^+$ lymphocytes impairs the proliferation of cytotoxic T cells that normally would eliminate B cells infected with Epstein-Barr virus.

NK cell activity is severely decreased in AIDS. Since these cells kill both virus-infected cells and tumor cells, this defect may contribute to the appearance of malignant tumors and the viral infections that plague these patients. The suppression of NK cell activity has been related both to a decrease in the number of NK cells and to a reduction in IL-2 levels, owing to the loss of CD4$^+$ cells.

Lentiviruses tend to target monocyte/macrophages, so it is not surprising that macrophages are infected by HIV-1 and may serve as a reservoir for dissemination of the virus. Interestingly, some macrophages express CD4 on their surfaces. Unlike T lymphocytes, which are killed by HIV, infected macrophages exhibit little if any cytotoxicity. Macrophages from patients with AIDS display impaired phagocytosis of immune complexes and opsonized particles, decreased chemotaxis, and impaired responses to antigenic challenges.

Pathology and Clinical Features of AIDS

Untreated AIDS patients exhibit a spectrum of clinical manifestations, beginning with an acute, self-limited illness and ending months to years later in fulminant immunodeficiency and its fatal complications (Fig. 4-24).

Two to 3 weeks after exposure to HIV, before the appearance of antibodies against the virus, infected persons often present with an acute illness that resembles infectious mononucleosis. Less commonly, they manifest neurological symptoms that suggest encephalitis or some form of neuropathy. Fever, myalgia, lymphadenopathy, sore throat, and a macular rash are common. Most of these symptoms resolve within 2 to 3 weeks, although lymphadenopathy, fever, and myalgia may persist for a few months. Seroconversion occurs 1 to 10 weeks after the onset of this acute illness.

Persistent generalized lymphadenopathy is defined as palpable enlargement of lymph nodes at two or more extrainguinal sites, persisting for more than 3 months in a person infected with HIV. The disorder develops either as part of the acute HIV syndrome or within a few months of seroconversion. The most common sites of involvement are the axillary, inguinal, and posterior cervical nodes, although almost any group of lymph nodes can be affected. Many cells within the affected lymph nodes, especially follicular dendritic cells, harbor actively replicating virus. Biopsies of the lymph nodes reveal reactive changes with follicular hyperplasia but are not diagnostic. Persistent generalized lymphadenopathy does not have any prognostic significance with respect to the progression of HIV infection to AIDS.

Most patients infected with HIV express viral antigens and antibodies within 6 months. Viral replication remains at minimal levels for variable times (up to 10 or more years), during which time the infected person is asymptomatic. However, as discussed above, viral replication virtually always resumes at some time, and the number of CD4$^+$ T cells begins to decrease. Patients generally remain asymptomatic until the total number of CD4$^+$ lymphocytes falls below 500/μL. At that time, nonspecific constitutional symptoms may appear, together with opportunistic infections. Below 150 CD4$^+$ cells/μL and CD4:CD8 ratios less than 0.8, the disease progresses rapidly. A wide variety of bacteria, viruses, fungi, and protozoa attack the immunocompromised patient, Kaposi sarcoma and lymphoproliferative disorders may appear, and neurological disease is common.

The diversity of infectious agents that ravage patients with AIDS reads like a textbook of microbiology. It is beyond the scope of this discussion to treat this subject in any detail, and only a few representative examples are mentioned.

The large majority of AIDS patients suffer from opportunistic pulmonary infections. *P. carinii* pneumonia occurs at some time in more than two thirds of patients, and pulmonary infection with cytomegalovirus and *Mycobacterium avium-intracellulare* are common. Patients with AIDS are also susceptible to tuberculosis and *Legionella* infections.

Cryptococcal meningitis is a devastating complication, representing 5 to 8% of all opportunistic infections in patients with AIDS. Toxoplasmosis of the brain is the most common cause of intracerebral mass lesions. Herpes encephalitis occasionally complicates AIDS.

Diarrhea is the single most common gastrointestinal symptom in AIDS, occurring in more than 75% of patients. Simultaneous infections with more than one organism are common. The most frequent pathogens are protozoans, in-

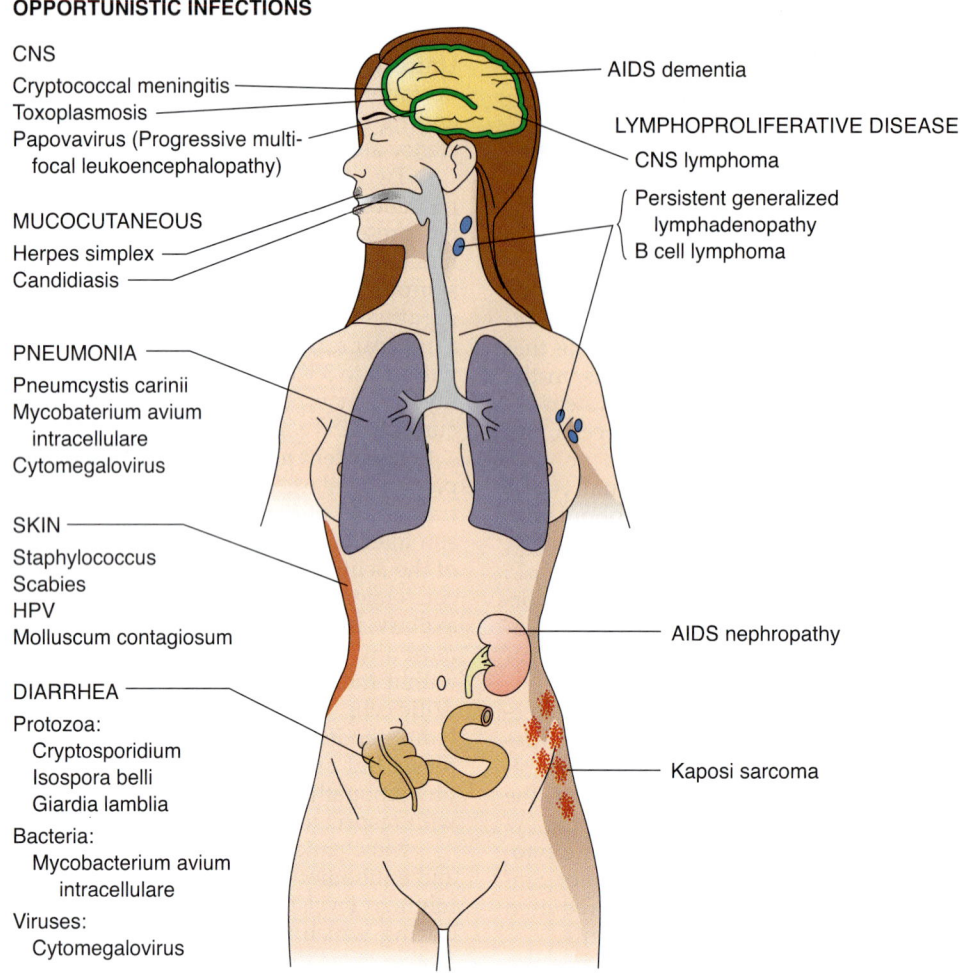

FIGURE 4-24
HIV-1–mediated destruction of the cellular immune system results in AIDS. The infectious and neoplastic complications of AIDS can affect practically every organ system.

cluding *Cryptosporidium, Isospora belli,* and *G. lamblia. M. avium-intracellulare* and *Salmonella* species are the most common bacterial causes of diarrhea in patients with AIDS. Cytomegalovirus infection of the gastrointestinal tract can manifest as a colitis associated with watery diarrhea.

Virtually all patients with AIDS develop some form of skin disease, with infections being prominent causes. *Staphylococcus aureus* is the most common cutaneous bacterial offender, causing bullous impetigo, deeper purulent lesions (ecthyma), and folliculitis. Chronic mucocutaneous herpes simplex infection is so characteristic of AIDS that it is considered an index infection in establishing the diagnosis. Skin lesions produced by *Molluscum contagiosum* and human papillomavirus are common, as are scabies and infections with *Candida* species.

Postmortem studies of patients who have died of AIDS have revealed pathological findings in the central nervous system in more than three fourths of the cases, and neurological symptoms occur in a third of patients. Direct infection of the brain with HIV leads to a subacute encephalopathy, also termed the *AIDS dementia complex.* Progressive multifocal leukoencephalopathy is another lethal complication.

Kaposi sarcoma (KS) is an otherwise rare, multicentric, malignant neoplasm. It is characterized by cutaneous and (less commonly) visceral nodules, in which endothelium-lined channels and vascular spaces are admixed with spindle-shaped cells. The disease was classically described in elderly men but was also associated with immunosuppressive therapy prior to the AIDS pandemic. Treatment with corticosteroids and azathioprine therapy for renal transplantation and autoimmune diseases were found to be associated with some cases of KS. Similarly, patients with AIDS, particularly homosexual men rather than intravenous drug users, are at very high risk of developing KS. In fact, the occurrence of KS in an otherwise healthy person younger than 60 years is considered strong evidence for the diagnosis of AIDS. Unlike the classic indolent variety of KS, the cutaneous tumor in AIDS is commonly aggressive, often involving the gastrointestinal tract or lungs. Lung involvement frequently leads to death.

Recent studies have incriminated a new strain of herpesvirus (HHV8) in all forms of KS, including AIDS-associated KS, the classic European variety in elderly men, and KS in immunosuppressed recipients of organ transplants. HHV8 is also thought to be the cause of a peculiar lymphoma associated with AIDS (*primary effusion lymphoma*) and of *AIDS-associated Castleman disease.* The virus has been detected in both the spindle cells and the flat endothelial cells of KS lesions. The presence of HHV8 in the blood strongly predicts later development of KS. In fact, 75% of HIV-infected persons with HHV8 in the blood developed KS within 5 years. It is thought that HHV8 is sexually transmitted, since almost all homosexual HIV carriers are infected, whereas only a quarter of heterosexual drug users with HIV infection harbor HHV8.

B-cell lymphoproliferative diseases are common in patients with AIDS. Congenital and acquired immunodeficiency states are associated with B-cell hyperplasia, usually manifested as generalized lymphadenopathy. This lymphoproliferative syndrome may be followed by the appearance of high-grade B-cell lymphomas. In fact, patients who have been subjected to immunosuppressive therapy for renal transplants are at a 35-times-greater risk of developing lymphoma, and in one third of these cases, the disease is confined to the central nervous system. The lymphomas in chronically immunodeficient patients may manifest as an invasive polyclonal B-cell proliferation or as a monoclonal B-cell lymphoma. Many of these patients exhibit serological evidence of infection with Epstein-Barr virus, and the genome of this virus has been demonstrated in the neoplastic cells.

B-cell hyperplasia and generalized lymphadenopathy precede the appearance of malignant lymphoproliferative disease. HIV-associated lymphomas usually manifest as the large cell variety, as often noted in other immunodeficient conditions, although a few small cell lymphomas are encountered. A conspicuous feature of lymphomas associated with AIDS is the predilection for extranodal disease, particularly primary lymphomas of the brain. In addition, lymphomas of the gastrointestinal tract, liver, and bone marrow are frequent. The Epstein-Barr virus genome has also been demonstrated in many of the lymphomas occurring with AIDS.

Therapy for HIV Infection

The approaches used to treat HIV infection have focused on targeting HIV proteins that are obligatory for HIV replication and are sufficiently distinct from normal cellular proteins to offer clear targets. Initial agents were designed to inhibit the function of HIV reverse transcriptase (RT), a nonmammalian enzyme. Use of compounds that inhibit RT and, most importantly, the development of drugs that inhibit HIV protease, led to combination chemotherapies to inhibit HIV. These are termed collectively *highly active antiretroviral therapy* (HAART). The introduction of HAART revolutionized the treatment of AIDS, reducing AIDS-related mortality and increasing all indices of health in AIDS patients.

Unlike most retroviral reverse transcriptases, HIV RT lacks an editing function, and HIV mutates much more often than do most other viruses. This high mutation rate not only facilitates its avoidance of the immune system, but also enhances its ability to generate functional mutations that are insensitive to HAART. Although the combination of three or more drugs in most HAART regimens depresses viral replication, HIV mutants resistant to multiple chemotherapeutic agents now represent a significant percentage of HIV isolates. HAART drugs do not cross the blood–brain barrier effectively, and the brain may provide a sanctuary for the virus. Quantitation of HIV^+ cells in the body has led to the conclusion that eradication of the virus from the body is not a realistic expectation using the types of chemotherapy currently available. Finally, even if HAART leads to complete elimination of HIV^+ cells from the blood (as it often does), even temporary cessation of therapy allows reactivation of HIV from reservoirs outside the circulation.

HIV-2

In 1985, otherwise healthy prostitutes in Senegal were discovered to harbor antibodies that cross-reacted with a monkey retrovirus, now termed *simian immunodeficiency virus* (SIV). A year later, a retrovirus similar to HIV-1 was isolated from West African patients with AIDS who were negative for antibodies against HIV-1. Antibodies to this new retrovirus, now termed *HIV-2*, also cross-reacted with SIV antigens. Frozen sera from West Africa dating to the 1960s have been shown to contain antibodies to HIV-2. In Guinea-Bissau, infection with HIV-2 has been shown in 8% of pregnant women, 10% of male blood donors, and more than one third of prostitutes. The infection has now also been reported from other parts of Africa, Europe, and the United States.

HIV-2 is morphologically similar to HIV-1, and the immunodeficiency state associated with HIV-2 infection is indistinguishable from AIDS caused by HIV-1. The risk factors for infection in both diseases seem to be similar. However, HIV-2 is far more difficult to transmit than HIV-1, and persons infected with the former are less likely to progress to AIDS.

AUTOIMMUNITY AND AUTOIMMUNE DISEASES

Autoimmune Disease Occurs after Immunological Tolerance Is Broken

Autoimmunity implies that an immune response has been generated against self-antigens (autoantigens). Central to the concept of autoimmunity is a breakdown in the ability of the immune system to differentiate between self- and non-self-antigens. Autoimmunity was classically interpreted as an abnormal immune response that invariably caused disease. However, it is now clear that autoimmune responses are common and are necessary for the regulation of the immune system. Normally antiidiotype antibodies (antibodies against the antigen-binding site of immunoglobulins), serve as important regulatory proteins for the immune response, and their presence is by definition an autoimmune response. When these regulatory mechanisms are in some way disrupted, the uncontrolled production of autoantibodies, or the appearance of abnormal cell–cell recognition, produces disease. The presence of specific autoantibodies is useful in the diagnosis of autoimmune diseases, but it is not sufficient for a designation of autoimmune disease. It is necessary to demonstrate a cause-and-effect relationship in which the autoimmune reaction (whether cellular or humoral) is directly related to the disease process. At present, only a few diseases (e.g., SLE and thyroiditis) strictly fit this criterion.

An abnormal autoimmune response to self-antigens implies a loss of immune tolerance. The term *tolerance* traditionally denotes a condition in which there is no measurable immune response to specific (usually self) antigens. The reasons for the loss of tolerance in autoimmune diseases are not understood. Experimental studies suggest that normal tolerance to self-antigens is an active process, requiring contact between self-antigens and immune cells. In the fetus, tolerance is readily established to antigens that in the adult cause vigorous immune responses. There is now extensive evidence that induction of tolerance is an active and ongoing set of immune responses that can be produced in a variety of ways. Thus, tolerance is best looked on as an active state in which the immune response is blocked by inhibitory products. Induction of tolerance to an antigen is partly related to the dose of antigen to which cells of the intact organism are exposed. Both T cells and B cells are rendered tolerant—helper T cells after exposure to low doses of the antigen and B cells after large doses.

Theories of Autoimmunity

Inaccessible Self-Antigens

The simplest hypothesis to explain the loss of tolerance in autoimmune disease states that an immune reaction develops to a self-antigen not normally "accessible" to the immune system. Tissue antigens are usually contained within cells and are not exposed or released until some type of tissue injury occurs. When these antigens are released, an immune response develops. Examples of this type of response are antibody formation against spermatozoa, lens tissue, and myelin. Whether these autoantibodies can induce injury directly is another matter. In the case of antisperm antibodies, aside from a localized orchitis, there is no evidence that they induce generalized injury. Thus, although autoantibodies may form against normally "sequestered" antigens, there is only infrequent evidence that they are pathogenic.

Abnormal T-Cell Function

Autoimmune reactions have been claimed to develop as a result of abnormalities in the T-lymphocyte system. Most immune responses require T-cell participation to activate antigen-specific B cells. Thus, alterations in the number or functional activities of helper or suppressor T cells would be expected to influence the ability of the host to mount an immune response. In fact, defects in T cells, particularly suppressor T cells, have been described in many autoimmune diseases. For example, there are reports of defective suppressor cell activity in human and experimental SLE. Lymphocytotropic antibodies have also been described in patients with lupus. Abnormalities in suppressor cell function characterize other autoimmune diseases, including primary biliary cirrhosis, thyroiditis, multiple sclerosis, myasthenia gravis, rheumatoid arthritis, and scleroderma. However, the critical question is whether these alterations in suppressor cell function cause these diseases or whether they merely represent an epiphenomena. Defects in suppressor cell function have also been described in persons with no evidence of autoimmune disease.

There has also been interest in abnormalities in helper T-cell function in autoimmune disease. Helper T cells are defined by their role in antigen-specific B-cell activation. It is believed that these cells maintain the helper T-cell tolerance induced by low doses of antigen. Recent evidence indicates that these cells become autoreactive in many autoimmune diseases. One key mechanism in autoimmunity is DNA hypomethylation caused by drugs and other agents. This effect leads to upregulation of leukocyte function antigen 1 (LFA-1) and B-cell activation independent of antigen. An example of this T-cell autoreactivity and loss of antigen specificity is drug-induced lupus. Experimentally, it is also possible to "break" this type of tolerance by altering the antigen in such a way that the helper cell is activated and triggers the B cells. An example is antigen modification by partial degradation and complexing of the antigen to a carrier protein. Some rheumatic diseases are marked by autoantibodies to partially degraded connective tissue proteins, such as collagen or elastin. In some drug-induced hemolytic anemias, the binding of the drug to the erythrocyte membrane induces hemolysis.

Molecular Mimicry

Another mechanism by which the helper T-cell tolerance is overcome involves antibodies against foreign antigens that cross-react with self-antigens. Here helper T cells function "correctly" and do not induce autoantibody formation. Rather, the efferent limb of the immune response is abnormal. An example is rheumatic heart disease, in which antibodies formed against streptococcal bacterial antigens cross-react with antigens from cardiac muscle—a phenomenon known as *molecular mimicry*.

Polyclonal B-Cell Activation

The loss of tolerance may also involve polyclonal B-cell activation, in which B lymphocytes are directly activated by complex substances that contain many antigenic sites (e.g., bacterial cell walls and viruses). The development of rheumatoid factor in rheumatoid arthritis, anti-DNA antibodies in lupus erythematosus, and other autoantibodies has been described after bacterial, viral, and parasitic infections.

Tissue Injury in Autoimmune Diseases

Autoimmune diseases have traditionally been considered to be prototypic of immune complex disease, which involves complexes that form either in the circulation or in the tissues. Thus, type II (cytotoxic) and type III (immune complex) hypersensitivity reactions are implicated as the cause of tissue injury in most types of autoimmune diseases. Although it is probably true that these hypersensitivity reactions explain most of the autoimmune tissue injury, the story is more complicated. In some types of autoimmune diseases, T cells sensitized to self-antigens (such as thyroglobulin) may directly cause tissue injury (type IV reaction), but it is not clear to what extent.

Another mechanism of tissue injury is antibody-directed cellular cytotoxicity. However, not all autoantibodies cause injury by cytotoxic reactions. In the antireceptor antibody diseases, such as Graves disease and myasthenia gravis, the antibody binds to the receptor but may have no cytotoxic effect itself. In Graves disease, the autoantibody against the TSH receptor acts as an agonist to stimulate the production of thyroid hormone, whereas in myasthenia gravis the autoantibody blocks the binding of acetylcholine to its receptor, thereby impairing neuromuscular synaptic transmission. Anti-insulin receptor antibodies have also been described in diseases such as acanthosis nigricans and ataxia telangiectasia, in which some patients exhibit a form of diabetes characterized by extreme insulin resistance.

Type III hypersensitivity reactions (immune complex disease) explain tissue injury in some types of autoimmune diseases. The prototypical disease in this category is SLE. In this disorder, DNA–anti-DNA complexes are formed in the circulation (or at local sites) and are deposited in tissues, where they induce inflammation and injury, such as occurs in vasculitis and glomerulonephritis. Other examples are rheumatoid arthritis, scleroderma, polymyositis/dermatomyositis, and Sjögren syndrome. All of these disorders are characterized by immune phenomena and are classified under the rubric "collagen vascular" diseases. The clinical manifestations are systemic, and many organs and tissues are typically involved. By contrast, cytotoxic (type II-mediated) autoimmune reactions are, for the most part, organ specific.

Systemic Lupus Erythematosus (SLE) Is a Prototype of Systemic Autoimmune Disease

SLE is a chronic, autoimmune, multisystem, inflammatory disease that may involve almost any organ but characteristically affects the kidneys, joints, serous membranes, and skin. Autoantibodies are formed against a variety of self-antigens, including (1) plasma proteins (complement components and clotting factors), (2) cell surface antigens (lymphocytes, neutrophils, platelets, erythrocytes), (3) intracellular cytoplasmic components (microfilaments, microtubules, lysosomes, ribosomes, RNA), and (4) nuclear DNA, ribonucleoproteins, and histones. The most important diagnostic autoantibodies are those against nuclear antigens—in particular, antibody to double-stranded DNA and to a soluble nuclear antigen complex that is part of the spliceosome and termed Sm (Smith) antigen. High titers of these two autoantibodies (termed *antinuclear antibodies*) are nearly pathognomonic of SLE but are not directly cytotoxic. Antigen–antibody complexes deposit in tissues, leading to the characteristic vasculitis, synovitis, and glomerulonephritis. For this reason, SLE is considered the prototype of type III hypersensitivity reactions. Occasionally, directly cytotoxic antibodies are present, particularly antibodies formed against cell surface antigens of leukocytes and erythrocytes.

The prevalence of SLE varies worldwide and in North America and northern Europe is 40/100,000. In the United States, the disease appears to be more severe in blacks and Hispanics, although socioeconomic factors may in part be responsible. More than 80% of cases are seen in women of childbearing age, and SLE may strike as many as 1 in 1000 women in this age group.

Pathogenesis: The etiology of SLE is unknown. The presence of numerous autoantibodies, particularly antinuclear antibodies, suggests a breakdown in immune surveillance mechanisms that leads to a loss of tolerance. Many of the manifestations of SLE result from the tissue injury caused by immune complex-mediated vasculitis. Other clinical manifestations (e.g., thrombocytopenia or the antiphospholipid syndrome) are caused by autoantibodies directed against serum components or molecules on cell membranes. However, the diagnostic antinuclear antibodies are not incriminated in the pathogenesis of SLE. There appear to be many factors that predispose to the development of SLE (Fig. 4-25).

Although there was at one time interest in C-type viral particles in experimental murine models of SLE, most evidence argues against a viral etiology for human SLE. The clear female predisposition for SLE is true for nearly all autoimmune diseases, and sex hormones may in part be the explanation. The immune response in animals is strongly influenced by sex hormones. In mouse models of SLE, estrogens accelerate the progression of the disease, whereas androgens have a moderating effect. Whether the course of human SLE is influenced in the same manner is controversial. Experimentally, estrogens have been reported to increase the likelihood of overcoming immune tolerance.

Some genetic predisposition to lupus is suggested by a higher prevalence in families, and monozygotic twins exhibit a concordance of 30 to 50%, suggesting that both genetic and environmental factors play a role. The incidence of SLE (and other autoimmune diseases) is higher among persons who express certain MHC class II DR and DQ antigens. These gene products participate in two unlinked functions, namely, immunoregulation and the effector limb of the immune response. Thus, the HLA-B8 haplotype, which is often found in association with autoimmune diseases, is also asso-

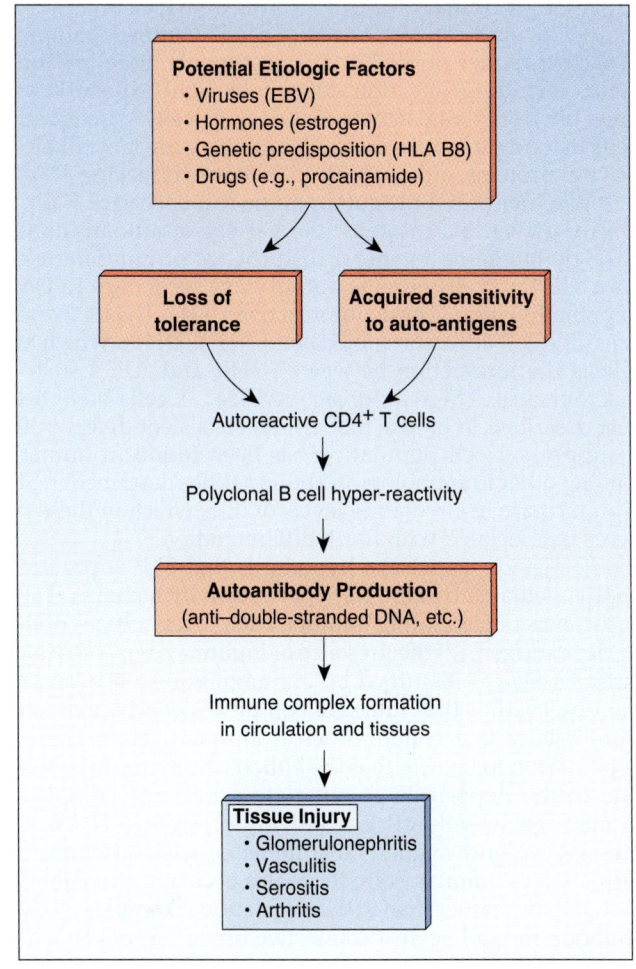

FIGURE 4-25

The pathogenesis of systemic lupus erythematosus is multifactorial.

ciated with the DR antigens in certain immunoregulatory abnormalities. These disorders include abnormal lymphocyte responses to antigens, decreased numbers of circulating suppressor cells, and increased numbers of circulating B cells. Among the effector functions associated with these HLA haplotypes is a decrease in C3b receptors on cells that clear circulating immune complexes. A critical role for the D/DR region in the pathogenesis of SLE is supported by the observation that inherited deficiencies of certain complement components, particularly C2 and C4, are associated with an increased incidence of the disease. The genes that encode these early complement components are within the HLA region, close to the D/DR site.

The production of autoantibodies directed against a large variety of antigens is characteristic of SLE, but the precise mechanisms underlying B-cell hyperreactivity are unknown. Two general hypotheses have been advanced. One attributes the disease to a nonspecific, polyclonal B-cell activation, although the nature of the stimulus is speculative. The second hypothesis holds that the antibodies formed in SLE represent a response to specific antigenic stimulation. Support for the latter supposition comes from the observation that with time the antibodies of SLE demonstrate gene rearrangements and mutations that are typical of an antigen-driven response. Moreover, a patient with SLE often has antibodies to more than one epitope on a single antigen, further suggesting a primary role for an antigen-driven process. Although inciting antigens have not been identified, a number of factors render normal body constituents more immunogenic, including infection, ultraviolet light exposure, and other environmental agents that damage cells. Foreign antigens that might induce molecular mimicry are most likely to be viral proteins, although direct evidence is lacking.

Whether or not the autoimmune response in SLE is primarily driven by antigens, the variety of autoantibodies strongly suggests a general disturbance of immune tolerance. $CD4^+$ T cells become autoreactive secondary to DNA hypomethylation. These autoreactive $CD4^+$ T cells overexpress the cell adhesion molecule LFA-1 (CD11a), which stabilizes the interaction between T cells and APCs such as macrophages. These autoreactive $CD4^+$ T cells have been best described in mouse models; no consistent defect in the T-suppressor cell population has been found in humans. Among other immunological abnormalities described in SLE is an increase in circulating levels of IL-6, which in these patients is associated with B-cell differentiation.

The evidence for the hypothesis that SLE is predominantly mediated by type III hypersensitivity includes (1) the occurrence of circulating immune complexes, which contain nuclear antigen, (2) the presence of immune complexes in injured tissues, as identified by immunofluorescence, and (3) the observation that immune complexes can be extracted from tissues that contain nuclear antigens. Thus, there is good reason to believe that the bulk of the injury in lupus is due to the deposition of circulating immune complexes formed against self-antigens, particularly against DNA. Additional evidence suggests that under certain conditions the formation of immune complexes also occurs in situ—that is, in the tissues rather than in the circulation. Examples include antibody formed against connective tissue components and perhaps the membranous form of lupus glomerulonephritis. Type II hypersensitivity reactions also participate in lupus, since cytotoxic antibodies against leukocytes, erythrocytes, and platelets have been described.

 Pathology and Clinical Features: Because circulating immune complexes deposit in almost all tissues, virtually every organ in the body can be involved.

Skin involvement is common and is manifested by an erythematous rash in sun-exposed sites, a malar "butterfly" rash being the most characteristic. Microscopically, the skin exhibits a perivascular lymphoid infiltrate and liquefactive degeneration of the basal cells. Immunofluorescence studies reveal the deposition of immunoglobulin and complement at the dermal–epidermal junction (*lupus band*).

Joint disease is the most common manifestation of SLE; over 90% of patients have polyarthralgia. An inflammatory synovitis occurs, but unlike rheumatoid arthritis, there is usually no joint destruction.

Renal disease, in particular glomerulonephritis, afflicts three fourths of patients with SLE. IgG antibodies to double-stranded DNA appear to play a prominent role in SLE-induced glomerulonephritis. Four main histological types of glomerulonephritis can be distinguished, as defined in the WHO classification of lupus nephritis.

1. **Mesangial lupus nephritis** is the mildest form of renal involvement. Immune complexes and complement are found almost exclusively in the mesangial regions of the glomeruli, but there are only slight increases in mesangial matrix and the numbers of mesangial cells (Fig. 4-26). These patients have only slight renal dysfunction, typically mild proteinuria and hematuria. The prognosis is excellent.
2. **Focal proliferative lupus nephritis** is characterized by increased cellularity in some but not all (focal) glomeruli (Fig. 4-27). The glomeruli exhibit proliferation of endothelial and mesangial cells and infiltration by neutrophils and monocytes. Necrosis and fibrin deposition are also often present. Immunofluorescence studies and electron microscopy demonstrate the deposition of immunoglobulin and complement, primarily in the mesangial regions of the glomeruli. The prognosis of patients with this form of lupus nephritis is mixed. Some remain with only mild disease; others progress to renal failure.
3. **Diffuse proliferative lupus nephritis** is the most serious type of renal disease. It occurs in as many as half of patients who exhibit clinical renal involvement and is associated with conspicuous increases in glomerular cellularity, fibrin deposition, and necrosis (Fig. 4-28). Epithelial crescents are also commonly seen. Immunofluorescence and electron microscopy disclose widespread deposition of immune complexes throughout the glomeruli, primarily in the mesangium and underneath the glomerular basement membrane (subendothelial). Many patients with this form of lupus nephritis progress to renal failure.
4. **Membranous lupus nephritis** resembles other forms of membranous glomerulonephritis that are associated with massive proteinuria and the nephrotic syndrome. There is often minimal hypercellularity. Instead, the glomeruli display diffusely thickened capillary loops, caused by the deposition of immunoglobulin and complement on the subepithelial surface of the glomerular basement membrane.

Although glomerulonephritis is the most common renal manifestation of SLE, interstitial nephritis or (rarely) a vasculitis can also be seen. In many of these cases, immunoglobulins and complement are present in the intersti-

Autoimmunity and Autoimmune Diseases

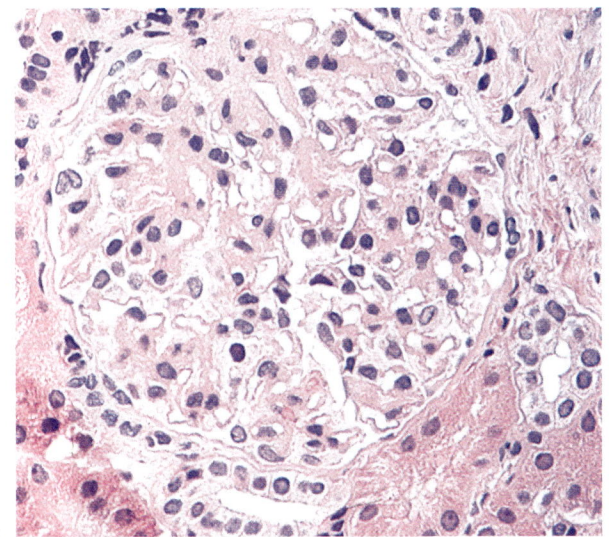
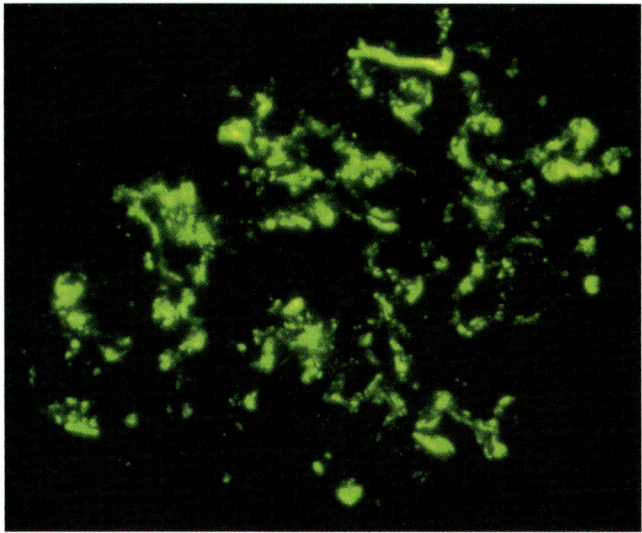

FIGURE 4-26
The mesangial form of lupus glomerulonephritis is characterized by (A) mesangial hypercellularity and (B) the presence of mesangial immunoglobulin (and complement) revealed by direct immunofluorescence.

tium and blood vessels of the kidney. *Involvement of serous membranes* is common in SLE. More than one third of patients have pleuritis and a pleural effusion. Pericarditis and peritonitis occur, but less frequently.

Disorders of the respiratory system in SLE occur frequently. The clinical manifestations are diverse, ranging from pleural disease to upper airway involvement and parenchymal disease of the lungs. Pneumonitis is thought to be caused by the deposition of immune complexes in the alveolar septa and is associated with patchy acute inflammation. Progressive interstitial fibrosis develops in some patients. An increased incidence of pulmonary hypertension has also been reported.

Cardiac involvement is often encountered in SLE, although congestive heart failure is rare and is usually associated with myocarditis. All layers of the heart may be involved, with pericarditis being the most common finding. *Libman-Sacks endocarditis*, which is usually not clinically significant, is characterized by small nonbacterial vegetations on the valve leaflets. These lesions should be differentiated from the larger, bulkier vegetations of bacterial endocarditis or the vegetations of rheumatic endocarditis, which are confined to the lines of valve closure.

Disease of the central nervous system is a life-threatening complication of lupus. Vasculitis is the common underlying lesion leading to hemorrhage and infarction of the brain, which are often lethal.

One third of patients with SLE possess elevated concentrations of **antiphospholipid antibodies.** This autoimmune phenomenon predisposes patients to thromboembolic complications, including stroke, pulmonary embolism, deep venous thrombosis, and portal vein thrombosis.

Other organ involvement occurs less frequently and is often due to *vasculitis*, which is also characteristic of lupus. Lesions in the spleen are characterized by thickening and concentric fibrosis of the penicillary arteries, the so-called onion-skin pattern.

The clinical course of SLE is highly variable and typically exhibits exacerbations and remissions. Before the advent of corticosteroids and other immunosuppressive therapies, SLE was frequently a fatal disease. However, with the recognition of mild forms of the disease, improved antihypertensive medications, and the use of immunosuppressive agents, the overall 10-year survival approaches 90%. The worst prognosis is found in patients with severe disease of the kidneys and brain and those with systolic hypertension.

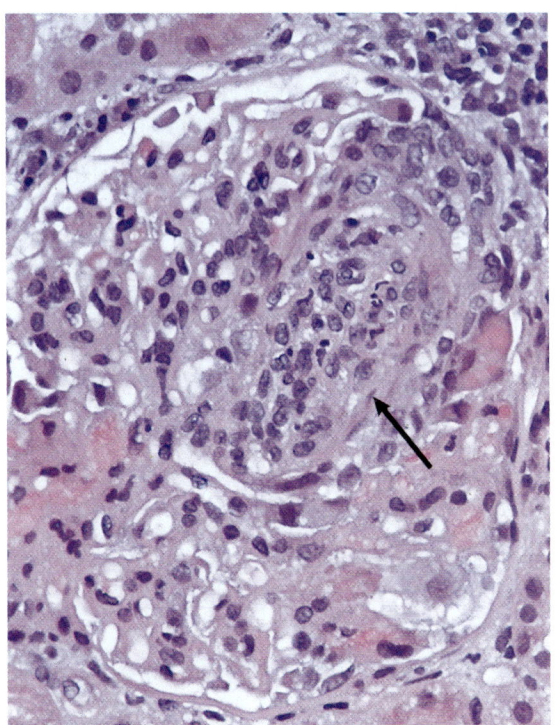

FIGURE 4-27
Focal proliferative lupus glomerulonephritis is characterized by segmental proliferation *(arrow)* in some glomeruli.

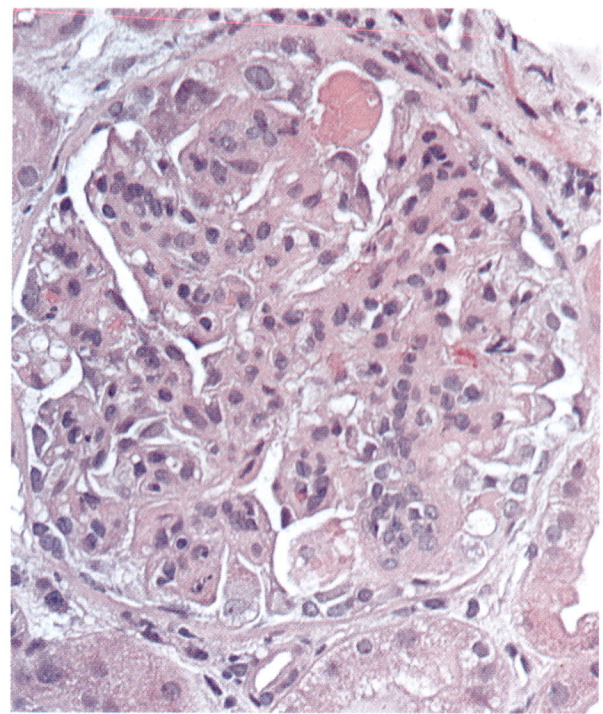
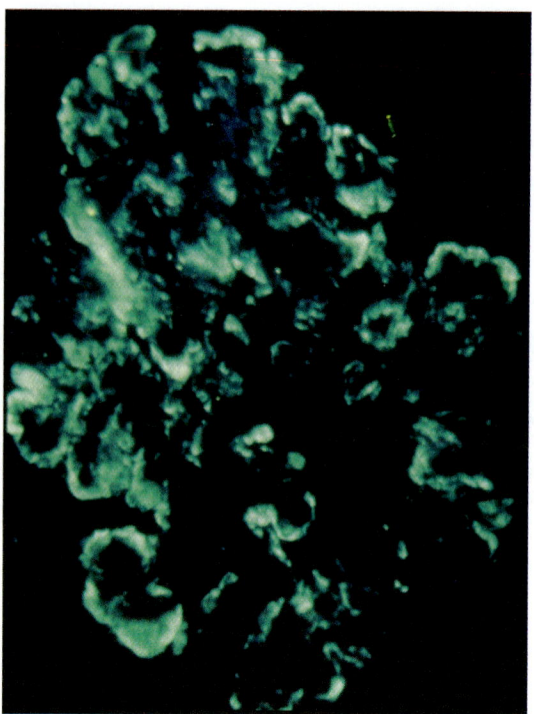

FIGURE 4-28
Diffuse proliferative lupus glomerulonephritis is characterized by (A) a diffuse increase in glomerular cellularity and (B) both mesangial and capillary wall deposition of immunoglobulin (and complement) revealed by direct immunofluorescence.

Lupuslike Diseases Feature Immune Complexes

Drug-Induced Lupus

A syndrome that resembles SLE can occur following the administration of certain drugs, including most notably procainamide (arrhythmias), hydralazine (hypertension), and isoniazid (tuberculosis). Drug-induced lupus ranges from asymptomatic laboratory abnormalities (positive antinuclear antibody [ANA] test result) to the development of a syndrome that is clinically similar to SLE. Unlike SLE, drug-induced lupus shows no sex predominance, and most patients are older than 50 years. Factors that predispose to the development of this syndrome include large daily doses of the offending drug, slow drug-acetylator status, and (in hydralazine-induced lupus) the presence of the HLA-DR4 genotype. As in SLE, the deposition of immune complexes is a feature of drug-induced lupus. Patients with drug-induced lupus typically exhibit constitutional signs, polyarthritis, pleuritis, and a positive ANA test result. In addition, they may develop rheumatoid factor, a false-positive test result for syphilis, and a positive Coombs test result. Unlike in SLE, renal and central nervous system involvement rarely occurs, and it is unusual to find antibodies to double-stranded DNA and Sm antigen. Autoantibodies to histones (which account for the positive ANA test result) are typical of drug-induced lupus. As in idiopathic SLE, autoreactive CD4$^+$ T cells have been implicated in polyclonal B cell activation. Discontinuation of the offending drug is ordinarily curative.

Chronic Discoid Lupus

The most common variety of localized lupus erythematosus is a cutaneous disorder, although identical lesions can occur in some cases of SLE. Erythematous, depigmented, and telangiectatic plaques are found most commonly on the face and scalp. The deposition of immunoglobulins and complement at the dermal–epidermal interface in chronic discoid lupus is similar to that observed in SLE. However, unlike in SLE, the uninvolved skin contains no immune deposits. Although ANAs develop in about one third of patients, antibodies to double-stranded DNA and Sm antigen are not encountered. Most patients with discoid lupus are not otherwise ill, but up to 10% eventually manifest features of SLE.

Subacute Cutaneous Lupus

Subacute cutaneous lupus is characterized by papular and annular lesions, principally on the trunk. The disorder is aggravated by exposure to ultraviolet light (sunlight), although the lesions eventually resolve without scarring. Antibodies to a ribonucleoprotein complex (SS-A or Ro antigen) and an association with HLA-DR3 genotype are characteristic.

Sjögren Syndrome Targets the Salivary and Lacrimal Glands

Sjögren syndrome (SS) is an autoimmune disorder characterized by keratoconjunctivitis sicca (dry eyes) and xerostomia (dry mouth) in the absence of other connective tissue disease. This definition separates primary SS from secondary types that are occasionally associated with other disorders of connective tissue, such as SLE, rheumatoid arthritis, scleroderma, and polymyositis. The primary type is also frequently associated with involvement of other organs, including the thyroid, lung, and kidney.

Primary SS is the second most common connective tissue disorder after SLE and affects up to 3% of the population. Like most autoimmune diseases, it occurs mostly in women (30 to 65 years old). There are strong associations between primary SS and certain MHC types, notably HLA-B8, Dw3, HLA-DR3, DRw-52, HLA-Dw2, and MT2, the last a B-cell alloantigen. Familial clustering occurs, and these families also exhibit a high prevalence of other autoimmune diseases.

The cause of SS is unknown. The production of autoantibodies, particularly ANAs directed against DNA or nonhistone proteins, typically occurs in patients with SS. Autoantibodies to soluble nuclear nonhistone proteins, especially the antigens SS-A a (Ro) and SS-B (La), are found in half of patients with primary SS and are associated with more-severe glandular and extraglandular manifestations. Autoantibodies to DNA or histones are rare, and their presence suggests secondary SS associated with lupus. Organ-specific autoantibodies, such as those directed against salivary gland antigens, are distinctly uncommon. As in SLE, it remains controversial whether the production of autoantibodies in SS primary reflects polyclonal activation of B cells or is essentially antigen driven, although these processes are not mutually exclusive.

SS has become the prototype for the investigation of a viral etiology for autoimmune disease. Particular attention has been paid to the possible roles of Epstein-Barr virus (EBV) and human T cell leukemia virus-1 (HTLV-1). Although it is still difficult to assign a role for EBV in the pathogenesis of SS, there is evidence that reactivation of this virus may be involved in the perpetuation of SS, polyclonal B-cell activation, and the development of lymphoma. In Japan, the seroprevalence of HTLV-1 among patients with SS is 23%, compared with 3.4% among unselected blood donors. Conversely, among HTLV-1 seropositive persons, more than three quarters demonstrated evidence of SS.

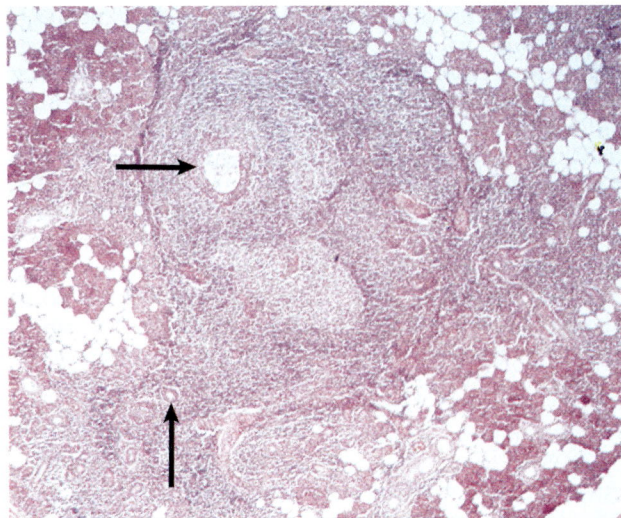

FIGURE 4-29
Minor gland sialadenitis associated with Sjögren syndrome is characterized by an intense lymphoid infiltrate and acinar destruction. The salivary ducts (arrows) are spared.

SS. Pulmonary disease occurs in most patients, particularly bronchial gland atrophy in association with lymphoid infiltration. This effect causes thick tenacious secretions, focal atelectasis, recurrent infections, and bronchiectasis. The gastrointestinal tract is also affected, and many patients have difficulty swallowing (dysphagia). The submucosal glands of the esophagus are infiltrated by lymphocytes. In addition, atrophic gastritis occurs secondary to lymphoid infiltration of the gastric mucosa. Liver disease, especially primary biliary cirrhosis, is present in 5 to 10% of patients with SS and is associated with the destruction of intrahepatic bile ducts and nodular lymphoid infiltrates. Interstitial nephritis and chronic thyroiditis occasionally accompany SS. SS is associated with a 40-fold increased risk of malignant lymphoma, probably through B-cell clonal expansion.

  Pathology and Clinical Features: SS is characterized by an intense lymphocytic infiltrate in the salivary and lacrimal glands (Fig. 4-29). Focal lymphocytic infiltrates in these glands are initially observed in a periductal distribution. Most lobules, especially the centers of the lobules, are affected. Well-defined germinal centers are rare. The lymphoid infiltrates destroy acini and ducts, and the latter often become dilated and filled with cellular debris. The stroma of the gland is preserved, an appearance that helps to differentiate this disorder from lymphoma. The lymphocytic infiltrates in the glands are predominantly CD4+ T cells, but a few B cells are also present. In the late stage of the disease, the glands atrophy and may be replaced by hyalinized tissue and fibrosis. Owing to the absence of tears, the corneas become dry and fissured and may ulcerate. The lack of saliva causes atrophy, inflammation, and cracking of the oral mucosa. The pathology of the salivary and lacrimal glands is described in greater detail in Chapter 25.

Involvement of extraglandular sites is also common in

Scleroderma (Progressive Systemic Sclerosis) Is an Autoimmune Disease of Connective Tissue

 Pathogenesis: Scleroderma is characterized by vasculopathy and excessive collagen deposition in the skin and internal organs, such as the lung, gastrointestinal tract, heart, and kidney. The disease occurs four times as often in women as in men, mostly in persons between 25 and 50 years of age. Familial incidence has been reported. There is an association between HLA-DQB1 and the formation of the autoantibodies characteristic of this disease.

Patients with scleroderma exhibit abnormalities of the humoral and cellular immune systems. The number of circulating B lymphocytes is normal, but there is evidence of hyperactivity, as manifested by hypergammaglobulinemia and cryoglobulinemia. ANAs are common but are usually present in a lower titer than in SLE. Antibodies virtually specific for scleroderma include (1) nucleolar autoantibodies (primarily against RNA polymerase); (2) antibodies to Scl-70, a nonhistone nuclear protein topoisomerase; and (3) anticentromere antibodies, which are associated with the "CREST" variant of the disease (see below). The Scl-70 autoantibody is the most common and specific for the diffuse form of scleroderma and is seen in 70% of these patients. However, there is no correlation between the titer of ANAs and the severity of the disease process. Rheumatoid factor is commonly present in scleroderma, and autoantibodies are occasionally directed against other issues, such as smooth muscle, thyroid gland, and salivary glands. Antibodies against collagen types I and IV have also been described.

Cellular immune derangements are also seen in patients with progressive systemic sclerosis. Reductions in circulating $CD8^+$ T-suppressor cells, evidence of T-cell activation, alterations in functions mediated by IL-1, and elevations in IL-2 and the soluble IL-2 receptor occur in active disease. Increased levels of IL-4 and IL-6 have also been described. The tissues exhibit active mononuclear inflammation, which precedes the development of the vasculopathy and fibrosis characteristic of this disease. In these infiltrates, increased numbers of $CD4^+$ and YS^+ T cells (which adhere to fibroblasts) are present, as well as macrophages. Mast cells (degranulated) are also present in the skin of these patients. The incidence of other autoimmune disorders, such as thyroiditis and primary biliary cirrhosis, is increased in patients with progressive systemic sclerosis. Circulating male fetal cells have been demonstrated in the blood and blood vessel walls of many women with scleroderma who bore male children many years before the onset of the disease. It has been suggested that scleroderma in these patients is similar to graft-versus-host disease.

Progressive systemic sclerosis is characterized by widespread excessive collagen deposition. Although the cause remains unclear, there is emerging evidence that there is expansion and activation of fibrogenic clones of fibroblasts. These clones behave autonomously and display augmented procollagen synthesis, including increased circulating levels of type III collagen aminopropeptide. Several factors may be responsible for this fibroblast activation. The YS^+ T cells adhere to fibroblasts and may induce activation via cytokine generation. Cytokines implicated in this process include TGF-β, which is elevated in the tissues of these patients, as well as IL-1, and IL-4, all of which stimulate fibroblast proliferation and collagen biosynthesis. There is also an increased level of IL-6, which is involved in the upregulation of matrix metalloproteinase and is important in the modulation of collagen metabolism. Activated fibroblasts themselves produce cytokines and growth factors, such as IL-1, prostaglandin E (PGE), TGF-β, and PDGF, which may in turn serve to activate other fibroblasts. Finally, activated fibroblasts also express the adhesion molecule ICAM-1 on their surface, which may be important in the adherence of T cells and macrophages and their subsequent activation.

Pathology: The skin in scleroderma initially displays edema and then induration. The thickened skin shows a striking increase in collagen fibers in the reticular dermis, thinning of the epidermis with loss of rete pegs, atrophy of dermal appendages, hyalinization and obliteration of arterioles, and variable mononuclear infiltrates, consisting primarily of T cells. The stage of induration may progress to atrophy or revert to normal. Increases in collagen deposition can also occur in synovia, lungs, gastrointestinal tract, heart, and kidneys.

Lesions in the arteries, arterioles, and capillaries are typical, and in some cases may be the first demonstrable pathological finding in the disease. Initial subintimal edema with fibrin deposition is followed by thickening and fibrosis of the vessel and reduplication or fraying of the internal elastic lamina. The involved vessels can become severely restricted in terms of blood flow and may become occluded by thrombus.

The kidneys are involved in more than half of patients with scleroderma. They show marked vascular changes, often with focal hemorrhage and cortical infarcts. Among the most severely affected vessels are the interlobular arteries and afferent arterioles. Early fibromuscular thickening of the subintima causes luminal narrowing, which is followed by fibrosis (Fig. 4-30). Fibrinoid necrosis is commonly seen in afferent arterioles. The glomerular alterations are nonspecific, and focal changes range from necrosis extending from the afferent arterioles to fibrosis. There is diffuse deposition of immunoglobulin, complement, and fibrin in affected vessels early in the disease, probably because of increased vascular permeability.

Diffuse interstitial fibrosis is the primary abnormality in the lungs. The disease can progress to end-stage pulmonary fibrosis, so-called honeycomb lung.

Most patients with scleroderma have patchy myocardial fibrosis, and in about one fourth of cases, more than 10% of the myocardium is involved. These lesions result from focal myocardial necrosis, which may reflect focal ischemia secondary to a Raynaud-like reactivity of the coronary microvasculature.

Progressive systemic sclerosis can involve any portion of the gastrointestinal tract. Esophageal dysfunction is the most common and troublesome gastrointestinal complication. Atrophy of the smooth muscle and fibrous replacement are seen

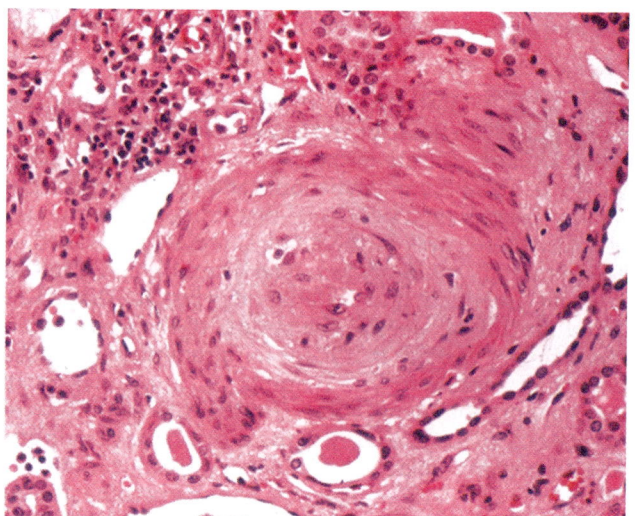

FIGURE 4-30
Scleroderma that affects the kidney is manifested by vascular involvement. Here, the interlobular artery exhibits marked luminal narrowing due to pronounced intimal thickening.

in the lower esophagus. The small bowel is often involved, with patchy fibrosis, principally of the muscular layers.

 Clinical Features: Scleroderma presents as two distinct clinical entities, the generalized (progressive systemic) form and the diffuse cutaneous or the CREST variant. Progressive systemic sclerosis is characterized by severe and progressive disease of the skin and the early onset of all or most of the associated abnormalities of visceral organs. The symptoms usually begin with Raynaud phenomenon, namely, intermittent episodes of ischemia of the fingers, marked by pallor, paresthesias, and pain. These symptoms are accompanied or followed by edema of the fingers and hands, tightening and thickening of the skin, polyarthralgia, and complaints referable to involvement of specific internal organs. The typical patient with generalized scleroderma exhibits "stone facies," owing to tightening of the facial skin and restricted motion of the mouth. The progression of vascular lesions in the fingers is reflected in the appearance of ischemic ulcerations of the fingertips, with subsequent shortening and atrophy of the digits. Many patients suffer from painful tendinitis, and joint pain is common. Involvement of the esophagus leads to hypomotility and dysphagia, and fibrosis in the small bowel interferes with intestinal mobility, with consequent overgrowth of bacteria and secondary malabsorption. Dyspnea on exertion is the initial symptom of pulmonary fibrosis in scleroderma, occurring in more than half of patients. The pulmonary disease progresses to dyspnea at rest and eventually to respiratory failure. Patients with long-standing disease are at risk for the development of pulmonary hypertension and cor pulmonale. Although most patients with scleroderma have some myocardial fibrosis, congestive heart failure is uncommon. However, ventricular arrhythmias can be a cause of sudden death. The vascular involvement of the kidneys in generalized scleroderma is responsible for so-called scleroderma renal crisis, characterized by the sudden onset of malignant hypertension, progressive renal insufficiency, and frequently, microangiopathic hemolytic anemia. The syndrome, which reflects ischemic injury to the kidneys, usually occurs in the first few years of the disease and is marked by conspicuously elevated levels of circulating renin.

The CREST, or diffuse cutaneous, form of scleroderma is a milder disease than generalized scleroderma; it is characterized by *c*alcinosis, *R*aynaud phenomenon, *e*sophageal dysmotility, *s*clerodactyly, and *t*elangiectasia. The diffuse cutaneous variant usually does not exhibit severe systemic involvement early in disease but later can progress, primarily in the form of diffuse interstitial lung fibrosis. Patients with diffuse cutaneous scleroderma often posses circulating anticentromere antibodies.

Polymyositis and Dermatomyositis Are Autoimmune Diseases of Muscle

These chronic inflammatory myopathies together with inclusion body myositis (IBM), comprise a group of rare (1/100,000) autoimmune diseases in children and adults. The most common form is juvenile dermatomyositis. There is an increased incidence in certain families and racial groups; in blacks the incidence is three times that in whites, and women are affected twice as frequently as men A strong association is present with HLA-DR3, HLA-DRw52, and HLA-DQ, as well as with certain alleles of the gene encoding the constant region of the immunoglobulin molecule (the Gm phenotype). In many patients, particularly adult men, there is an association between myositis and cancer. Finally, myositis may also be seen in syndromes that overlap with other autoimmune diseases such as SLE, scleroderma, mixed connective tissue disease, and Sjögren syndrome.

 Pathogenesis: As in other systemic autoimmune diseases, the etiology of these inflammatory myopathies remains to be fully elucidated. Viral agents, such as picornavirus and retroviruses (including HIV), have been suggested as causes, but viral particles have not been detected in human myositis.

In polymyositis and IBM, injury is mediated by activated T cells and macrophages. Muscle damage is associated with $CD8^+$ cytotoxic T cells surrounding muscle fibers that express MHC class I antigens. In vitro, these T cells are directly cytotoxic to autologous muscle fibers. Macrophages are also activated, as assessed by their production of cytokines.

In dermatomyositis, $CD4^+$ T cells are also present in the muscle, but there is evidence that humoral immune mechanisms play the dominant role. B cells occur in the muscle, and the production of antibodies directed against intramuscular capillaries and endothelial cells appears to be important in the disease process. Immunoglobulin and complement are deposited in the walls of the intramuscular capillaries. Complement, in particular C5b-9, has been implicated in the pathogenesis of the vascular injury.

Various autoantibodies are present in 60 to 80% of patients with inflammatory myopathies, including antibodies against muscle antigens such as myosin and various ANAs. The most specific autoantibodies are called *myositis-specific antibodies* (MSAs), a category that includes autoantibodies directed against tRNA synthetases, of which anti-Jo-1 is the most common. These antibodies are found both in polymyositis and dermatomyositis. Other specific but less common MSAs include those directed against a cytoplasmic RNA–protein complex (anti-SRP) found in polymyositis and anti-Mi-2 antibodies directed against nuclear proteins in dermatomyositis. The anti-PM-Scl autoantibody directed against nucleolar proteins is specific for the scleroderma-myositis overlap syndrome. There is no evidence that these specific autoantibodies are directly pathogenic.

 Pathology: The histological features of the various types of myositis are somewhat distinctive, reflecting their different pathogenetic mechanism. Dermatomyositis features a humorally mediated microangiopathy, with early deposition of immune complexes and complement. The inflammatory infiltrate consists primarily of CD41 T cells, B lymphocytes, and macrophages. The end-result of chronic dermatomyositis is a reduction in the number of capillaries in the muscle fibers, with atrophy and fibrosis reflecting secondary ischemia.

Polymyositis and IBM exhibit no evidence of angiopathy. Rather, infiltrates of CD8+ cytotoxic T cells and activated macrophages surround normal-appearing muscle fibers that express MHC class I molecules. Thus, in these diseases, cytotoxic T cells are thought to be primarily responsible for injury to the myocytes. IBM also exhibits pathognomonic vacuolar inclusion bodies in affected myocytes.

In 40% of patients with an inflammatory myopathy, skin involvement is manifested by an erythematous rash on the face (and elsewhere), resembling that seen in SLE. If it involves the eyelids (heliotropic rash), it is considered specific for dermatomyositis. As in SLE, the skin changes are characterized by a perivascular lymphoid infiltrate and liquefactive degeneration of the basal epithelial cells. Immunofluorescence studies of skin are helpful to differentiate between these two entities. In SLE, the deposition of granular immunoglobulin and complement at the dermal–epidermal junction occurs in uninvolved and involved skin and is virtually pathognomonic for that disease. By contrast, dermatomyositis is not associated with the deposition of immune components at the dermal–epidermal junction.

Other organ system, including joints, kidneys, lungs, and the gastrointestinal tract, are also affected. In the childhood form of polymyositis/dermatomyositis, vasculitis may also be present. Renal involvement was initially believed to be rare, but more-recent reports suggest that a small proportion of patients (5–10%) indeed have immune complex-mediated renal disease.

 Clinical Features: The diagnosis of these acquired inflammatory myopathies rests not only on the histological appearance of the involved muscles but also on the location of the involved muscle, electromyographic alterations, and elevated activities of muscle enzymes in the blood, namely, aldolase and the MM isoenzyme of creatine phosphokinase.

The proportion of patients with polymyositis/dermatomyositis who have an associated malignancy is disputed and varies from less than 10% to as many as 50%. In any event, the frequency of cancer is many-fold higher than in the general population. The association with malignancy is particularly evident in men older than 50 years, among whom three fourths have a cancer already diagnosed or will be shown to have cancer within 1 year. Thus, polymyositis/dermatomyositis is often a paraneoplastic syndrome, and a careful search for an underlying malignancy is justified. Most of the cancers are in the lung, colon, and stomach, although in affected women, tumors of the breast, ovaries, and uterus are also encountered.

Dermatomyositis usually responds to treatment with corticosteroids, and the prognosis is generally considered good. Some patients, however, develop classic scleroderma, and others have significant pulmonary and brain involvement.

The inflammatory myopathies are discussed in further detail in Chapter 27.

Mixed Connective Tissue Disease Combines Features of SLE, Scleroderma and Dermatomyositis

The symptoms characteristic of SLE include rash, Raynaud phenomenon, arthritis, and arthralgias, whereas those of scleroderma are swollen hands, esophageal hypomotility, and pulmonary interstitial disease. Some patients also develop symptoms suggestive of rheumatoid arthritis. The incidence of mixed connective tissue disease is unknown. Between 80 and 90% of patients are female, and most are adults (mean age, 37 years). Patients with mixed connective tissue disease have been reported to respond well to corticosteroid therapy, although some studies have challenged this assertion.

The etiology and pathogenesis of mixed connective tissue disease are unknown. Patients often have evidence of B-cell activation with hypergammaglobulinemia and a positive rheumatoid factor assay result. ANAs are present but, unlike in SLE, they are usually not directed against double-stranded DNA. The most distinctive ANA is directed against an extractable nuclear antigen. Specifically, patients with mixed connective tissue disease have high titers of antibody to uridine-rich ribonucleoprotein (anti-U1-RNP) in the absence of other extractable nuclear antigens, including PM-1 and Jo-1. Anti-RNP antibodies are also occasionally seen in SLE but usually in lower titer than in mixed connective tissue disease.

The cause of the formation and maintenance of the high titer of anti-RNP antibody is unclear. However, there is an association with HLA-DR4 and HLA-DR2 genotypes, suggesting a role for T cells in the autoantibody production. There is no direct evidence that these antibodies induce the characteristic involvement of the various organ systems. There is also controversy over whether mixed connective tissue disease is a separate disease entity or represents a heterogeneous collection of patients with SLE, scleroderma, or polymyositis who do not present initially with the classic manifestations of these diseases. For example, in some patients, mixed connective tissue disease seems to have evolved into typical scleroderma. Other patients develop evidence of renal disease, a finding consistent with SLE. Still others differentiate into rheumatoid arthritis. Thus, mixed connective tissue disease in many patients seems to be an intermediate stage in a genetically determined progression to a recognized autoimmune disease. Persons whose disease remains undifferentiated may make up a distinct subset. At this time, whether mixed connective tissue disease represents a distinct entity or simply an overlap of symptoms in patients with other types of collagen vascular diseases remains an open question.

SUGGESTED READING

Books

McClatchey KD: *Clinical laboratory medicine*, 2nd ed. Philadelphia: Lippincott Williams & Wilkins, 2002.

Ochs HL, Smith CIE, Puck JM: *Primary immunodeficiency diseases, a molecular and genetic approach*, 1st ed. New York: Oxford University Press, 1999.

Rich RR, Fleisher TA, Shearer WT, et al.: *Clinical Immunology. Principles and Practice*, 2nd ed. London: Mosby, 2001.

Roitt I, Brosoff J, Male D: *Immunology*, 5th ed. London: Mosby, 1998.

Review Articles

Anderson MK, Rast JP: Evolution of antigen binding receptors. *Annu Rev Immunol* 17:109, 1999.

Arnett FC, Edworthy SM, Block DA, et al.: The American Rheumatism Association 1987 revised criteria for the classification of rheumatoid arthritis. *Arthritis Rheum* 31:315–324, 1988.

Barnaba V: Viruses, hidden self-epitopes and autoimmunity. *Immunol Rev* 152:47–66, 1996.

Boumpas DT, Austin HA, Fessler BJ, Balow JE: Systemic lupus erythematosus: Emerging concepts. Part 1: Renal, neuropsychiatric, cardiovascular, pulmonary, and hematologic disease. *Ann Intern Med* 122:940–950, 1995.

Boumpas DT, Fessler BJ, Austin HA, et al.: Systemic lupus erythematosus: Emerging concepts. Part 2: Dermatologic and joint disease, the antiphospholipid antibody syndrome, pregnancy and hormonal therapy, morbidity and mortality, and pathogenesis. *Ann Intern Med* 123:42–53, 1995.

Butcher EC, Williams M, Youngman K, et al.: Lymphocyte trafficking and regional immunity. *Adv Immunol* 72:209, 1999.

Cantrell D: T cell antigen receptor signal transduction pathways. *Annu Rev Immunol* 15:125, 1997.

Davies JM: Molecular mimicry: Can epitope mimicry induce autoimmune disease? *Immunol Cell Biol* 75:113–126, 1997.

Ebringer A, Wilson C: HLA molecules, bacteria and autoimmunity. *J Med Microbiol* 49:305, 2000.

Fox RI: Sjögren's syndrome: Controversies and progress. *Clin Lab Med* 17:431–444, 1997.

Frederick M, Grimm E, Krohn E, et al.: Cytokine-induced cytotoxic function expressed by lymphocytes of the innate immune system: Distinguishing characteristics of NK and LAK based on functional and molecular markers. *Interferon Cytokine Res* 17:435–447, 1997.

Germain RN: MHC-dependent antigen processing and peptide presentation: providing ligands for T lymphocyte activation. *Cell* 76:287, 1994.

Gianani R, Sarvetnick N: Viruses, cytokines, antigens and autoimmunity. *Proc Natl Acad Sci USA* 93:2257, 1996.

Goodnow CC: Balancing immunity, autoimmunity, and self-tolerance. *N Y Acad Sci* 815:55–66, 1997.

Hayakawa K, Asono M, Shinton SA, et al.: Positive selection of natural autoreactive B cells. *Science* 285:113, 1999.

Hentges F: B lymphocyte ontogeny and immunoglobulin production. *Clin Exp Immunol* 97(suppl 1):3–9, 1994.

Jameson SC, Hogquist KA, Bevan MJ: Positive selection of thymocytes. *Annu Rev Immunol* 13:93, 1995.

Jiminez SA, Hitraya E, Varga J: Pathogenesis of scleroderma: Collagen. *Rheum Dis Clin North Am* 22:647–674, 1996.

Kunkel SL, Lukacs NW, Strieter RM, Chensue SW: Th1 and Th2 responses regulate experimental lung granuloma development. *Sarcoidosis Vasc Diffuse Lung Dis* 13:120–128, 1996.

Lanier LL. NK cell receptors. *Annu Rev Immunol* 16:359, 1998.

Mills JA: Systemic lupus erythematosus. *N Engl J Med* 330:1871–1879, 1994.

Mitchell H, Bolster MB, LeRoy EC: Scleroderma and related conditions. *Med Clin North Am* 81:129–149, 1997.

Nossal GJV. Negative selection of lymphocytes. *Cell* 76:229, 1994.

Oddis CV, Medsger TA Jr: Inflammatory myopathies. *Baillere's Clin Rheumatol* 9:497–514, 1995.

Pantaleo G, Fauci AS: Immunopathogenesis of HIV infection. *Annu Rev Microbiol* 50:825–854, 1996.

Plotz PH: NIH conference. Myositis: Immunologic contributions to understanding cause, pathogenesis, and therapy. *Ann Intern Med* 122:715, 1995.

Romagnani S: Atopic allergy and other hypersensitivities. Interactions between genetic susceptibility, innocuous and/or microbial antigens and the immune system. *Curr Opin Immunol* 9:773, 1997.

Swanson PC, Yung RL, Blatt NB, et al.: New concepts in the pathogenesis of drug-induced lupus. *Lab Invest* 73:746–759, 1995.

White B: Immunologic aspects of scleroderma. *Curr Opin Rheumatol* 7:541–545, 1995.

Yung RL, Johnson KJ, Richardson BC: New concepts in the pathogenesis of drug-induced lupus. *Lab Invest* 73:746–759, 1995.

Zanoyska R: CD4 and CD8: Modulators of T cell receptor recognition of antigen and of immune responses? *Curr Opin Immunol* 10:82, 1998.

CHAPTER 5

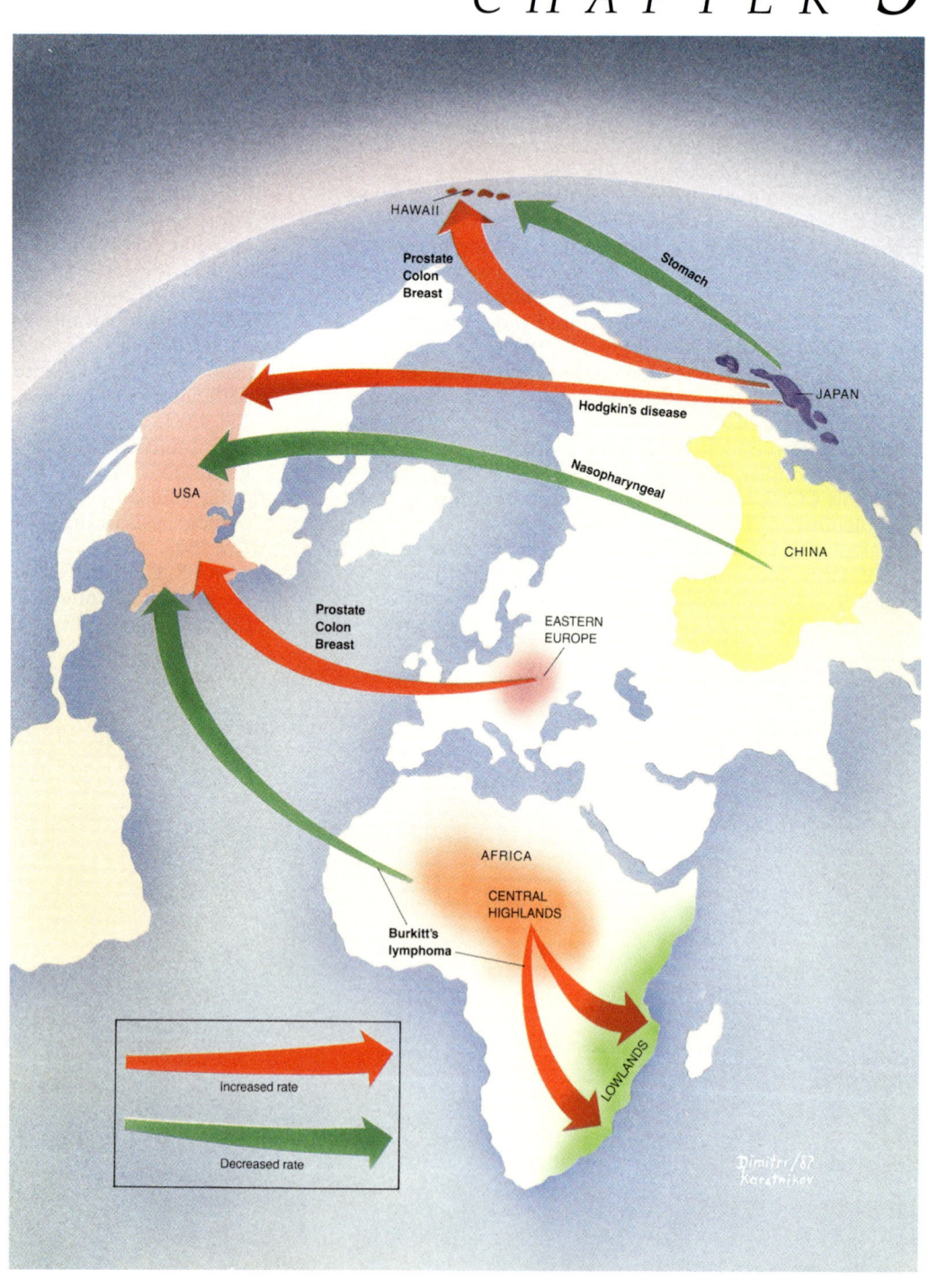

Neoplasia

Emanuel Rubin
Raphael Rubin
Stuart Aaronson

Benign versus Malignant Tumors

Classification of Neoplasms
Benign Tumors
Malignant Tumors

Histological Diagnosis of Malignancy
Benign Tumors
Malignant Tumors
Electron Microscopy of Undifferentiated Tumors
Immunohistochemical Tumor Markers

Invasion and Metastasis
Direct Extension
Metastatic Spread
Invasion and Metastasis

The Grading and Staging of Cancers
Cancer Grading
Cancer Staging

The Biochemistry of the Cancer Cell

The Clonal Origin of Cancer

Cancer As Altered Differentiation

The Growth of Cancers
Tumor Growth Rates
Tumor Angiogenesis
Tumor Dormancy

The Molecular Genetics of Cancer
Transformed Cells
Oncogenes
Tumor Suppressor Genes
DNA Methylation
DNA Repair Genes
Telomerase
Inherited Cancer Syndromes

(continued)

FIGURE 5-1 *(see opposite page)*
Cancer epidemiology. The influence of environmental factors on the incidence of cancer is illustrated by the results of several classic epidemiological studies of migrant populations. Offspring of Japanese immigrants to Hawaii exhibited (1) a decreased incidence of stomach cancer; (2) an increased incidence of cancers of the breast, colon, and prostate; and (3) an increased incidence of Hodgkin disease. The incidence of nasopharyngeal carcinoma decreased in the offspring of immigrants to the United States from China. Eastern Europeans who immigrated to the United States showed an increased incidence of carcinoma of the breast, colon, and prostate. Finally, the incidence of Burkitt lymphoma changed in Africans who immigrated from the central highlands to coastal lowlands or to the United States.

Viruses and Human Cancer

Human T-Cell Leukemia Virus-I (HTLV-I)

DNA Viruses

Chemical Carcinogenesis

Mutagenesis

Multistep Carcinogenesis

Metabolic Activation

Endogenous and Environmental Factors

Physical Carcinogenesis

Ultraviolet Radiation

Asbestos

Foreign Bodies

Tumor Immunology

Immunological Defenses against Cancer

Systemic Effects of Cancer on the Host

Fever

Anorexia and Weight Loss

Endocrine Syndromes

Neurological Syndromes

Skeletal Muscle Syndromes

Hematological Syndromes

The Hypercoagulable State

Gastrointestinal Syndromes

Nephrotic Syndromes

Cutaneous Syndromes

Amyloidosis

The Epidemiology of Cancer

Geographical and Ethnic Differences

Migrant Populations

A neoplasm (Greek, *neo,* new + *plasma,* thing formed) **is the autonomous growth of tissues that have escaped the normal restraints on cell proliferation and exhibit varying degrees of fidelity to their precursors.** However, in some instances, for example follicular lymphoma (see Chapter 20), the accumulation of neoplastic cells reflects an aberration in programmed cell death (apoptosis). The structural resemblance of the neoplastic cell to its cell of origin usually enables specific conclusions about its source and potential behavior. In view of their space-occupying properties, solid neoplasms are termed **tumors** (Gr., *swelling*). Tumors that remain localized are considered *benign,* whereas those that spread to distant sites are termed **malignant, or cancer.** The neoplastic process entails not only cellular proliferation but also a modification of the differentiation of the involved cell types. Thus, in a sense, cancer may be viewed as a burlesque of normal development.

Cancer is actually an ancient disease. Evidence of bone tumors has been found in prehistoric remains, and the disease is mentioned in early writings from India, Egypt, Babylonia, and Greece. Hippocrates is reported to have distinguished benign from malignant growths. He also introduced the term *karkinos,* from which our term *carcinoma* is derived. In particular, Hippocrates described cancer of the breast, and in the second century AD, Paul of Aegina commented on its frequency.

The incidence of neoplastic disease increases with age, and the greater longevity in modern times necessarily enlarges the population at risk. For this reason alone, the overall incidence of cancer is increasing. In previous generations, on average, humans did not live long enough to develop many cancers that are particularly common in middle and old age, such as those of the prostate, colon, pancreas, and kidney. Despite assertions that contemporary society is or will be subject to an "epidemic" of cancer, the epidemiological data do not support such a concept. If all deaths from cancers caused by tobacco smoke are removed from the statistics, there has been no increase in the overall age-adjusted cancer death rate in men in the past half-century, and there has been a continually decreasing rate in women. However, the age-adjusted incidence of specific cancers has fluctuated over this time period.

In general, neoplasms are irreversible, and their growth is, for the most part, autonomous. Several observations are important:

- Neoplasms are derived from cells that normally maintain a proliferative capacity. Thus, mature neurons and cardiac myocytes do not give rise to tumors.
- A tumor may express varying degrees of differentiation, from relatively mature structures that mimic normal tissues to a collection of cells so primitive that the cell of origin cannot be identified.

- The stimulus responsible for the uncontrolled proliferation may not be identifiable; in fact, it is not known for most human neoplasms.
- Neoplasia arises from mutations in genes that regulate cell growth, apoptosis or DNA repair.

BENIGN VERSUS MALIGNANT TUMORS

By definition, benign tumors do not penetrate (invade) adjacent tissue borders, nor do they spread (metastasize) to distant sites. They remain as localized overgrowths in the area in which they arise. As a rule, benign tumors are more differentiated than malignant ones—that is, they more closely resemble their tissue of origin. *By contrast, malignant tumors, or cancers, have the added property of invading contiguous tissues and metastasizing to distant sites, where subpopulations of malignant cells take up residence, grow anew, and again invade.*

In common usage, the terms *benign* and *malignant* refer to the overall biological behavior of a tumor rather than to its morphological characteristics. In most circumstances, malignant tumors kill, whereas benign ones spare the host. However, so-called benign tumors in critical locations can be deadly. For example, a benign intracranial tumor of the meninges (meningioma) can kill by exerting pressure on the brain. A minute benign tumor of the ependymal cells of the third ventricle (ependymoma) can block the circulation of cerebrospinal fluid, and the resulting hydrocephalus is lethal. A benign mesenchymal tumor of the left atrium (myxoma) may kill suddenly by blocking the orifice of the mitral valve. In certain locations, the erosion of a benign tumor of smooth muscle can lead to serious hemorrhage—witness the peptic ulceration of a stromal tumor in the wall of the stomach. On rare occasions, a functioning, benign endocrine adenoma can be life threatening, as in the case of the sudden hypoglycemia associated with an insulinoma of the pancreas or the hypertensive crisis produced by a pheochromocytoma of the adrenal medulla. Conversely, certain types of malignant tumors are so indolent that many are curable by surgical resection. In this category are many cancers of the breast and some malignant tumors of connective tissue, such as fibrosarcoma.

A number of tumors are difficult to classify because they do not fit all the criteria for either benign or malignant neoplasms. The best-known example is basal cell carcinoma of the skin, which is histologically malignant (i.e., it invades aggressively) but only rarely has been reported to metastasize to distant sites. Similarly, the local growth of a pleomorphic adenoma of a salivary gland, which is classified as benign, may be so aggressive that it defies surgical cure.

CLASSIFICATION OF NEOPLASMS

In any language, the classification of objects and concepts is pragmatic and useful only insofar as its general acceptance permits effective communication. Similarly, the nosology of tumors reflects historical concepts, technical jargon, location, origin, descriptive modifiers, and predictors of biological behavior. Although the language of tumor classification is neither rigidly logical nor consistent, it still serves as a reasonable mode of communication.

Benign Tumors Carry the Suffix "oma"

The primary descriptor of any tumor, benign or malignant, is its cell or tissue of origin. The classification of benign tumors is the basis for the names of their malignant variants. **The suffix "oma" for benign tumors is preceded by reference to the cell or tissue of origin.** For example, a benign tumor that resembles chondrocytes is called a *chondroma* (Fig. 5-2). If the tumor resembles the precursor of the chondrocyte, it is labeled *chondroblastoma*. When a chondroma is located entirely within the bone, it is designated *enchondroma*. Tumors of epithelial origin are given a variety of names based on what is believed to be their outstanding characteristic. Thus, a benign tumor of the squamous epithelium may be called simply *epithelioma* or, when branched and exophytic,

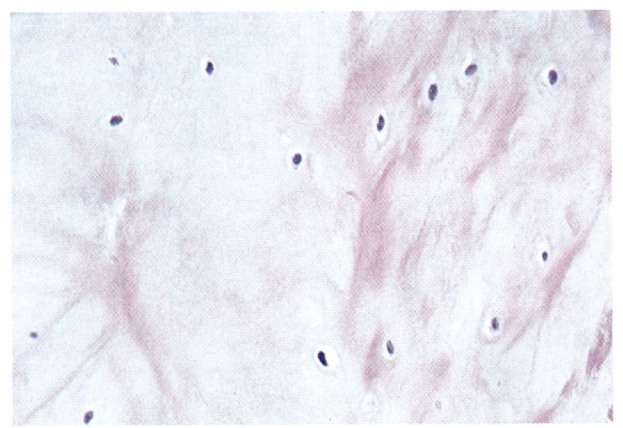
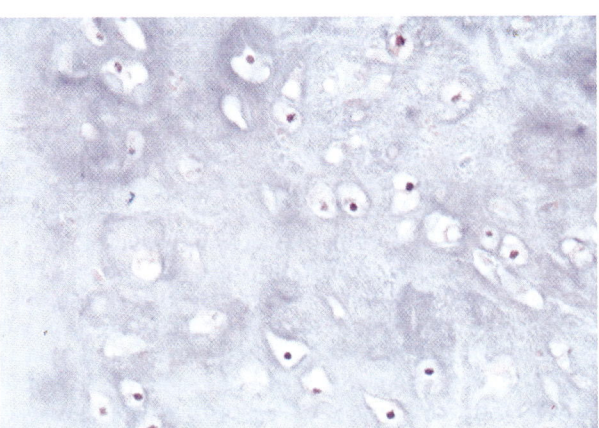

FIGURE 5-2
Benign chondroma. A. Normal cartilage. B. A benign chondroma closely resembles normal cartilage.

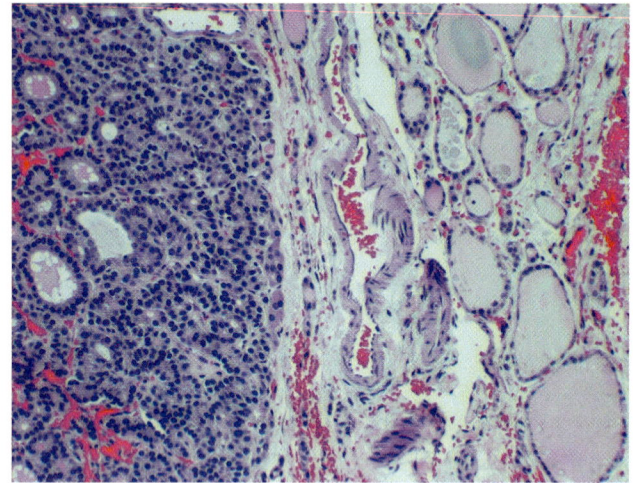

FIGURE 5-3
Benign thyroid adenoma. The follicles of a thyroid adenoma *(left)* contain colloid and resemble those of the normal thyroid tissue *(right)*.

may be termed *papilloma*. Benign tumors arising from glandular epithelium, such as in the colon or the endocrine glands, are named *adenoma*. Accordingly, we refer to a thyroid adenoma (Fig. 5-3) or a pancreatic islet cell adenoma. In some instances, the predominating feature is the gross appearance, in which case we speak, for example, of an *adenomatous polyp* of the colon.

Benign tumors that arise from germ cells and contain derivatives of different germ layers are labeled *teratoma*. These tumors occur principally in the gonads and occasionally in the mediastinum and may contain a variety of structures, such as skin, neurons and glial cells, thyroid, intestinal epithelium, and cartilage. Localized, disordered differentiation during embryonic development results in a *hamartoma*, a disorganized caricature of normal tissue components (Fig. 5-4). Such tumors, which are not strictly neoplasms, contain varying combinations of cartilage, ducts or bronchi, connective tissue, blood vessels, and lymphoid tissue. Ectopic islands of normal tissue, called *choristoma*, may also be mistaken for true neoplasms. These small lesions are represented by pancreatic tissue in the wall of the stomach or intestine, adrenal rests under the renal capsule, and nodules of splenic tissue in the peritoneal cavity. Certain benign growths, recognized clinically as tumors, are not truly neoplastic but rather represent overgrowth of normal tissue elements. Examples are vocal cord polyps, skin tags, and hyperplastic polyps of the colon.

Malignant Tumors Are Mostly Carcinomas or Sarcomas

In general, the malignant counterparts of benign tumors usually carry the same name, except that the suffix "carcinoma" is applied to epithelial cancers and "sarcoma" to those of mesenchymal origin. For instance, a malignant tumor of the stomach is a *gastric adenocarcinoma* or *adenocarcinoma of the stomach* (Fig. 5-5). *Squamous cell carcinoma* is an invasive tumor of the skin or other organs lined by a squamous epithelium (e.g., the esophagus). In addition, squamous cell carcinoma arises in the metaplastic squamous epithelium of the bronchus or endocervix. *Transitional cell carcinoma* is a malignant neoplasm of the bladder or ureters. By contrast, we speak of *chondrosarcoma* (Fig. 5-6) or *fibrosarcoma*. Sometimes the name of the tumor suggests the tissue type of origin, as in *osteogenic sarcoma* or *bronchogenic carcinoma*. Some

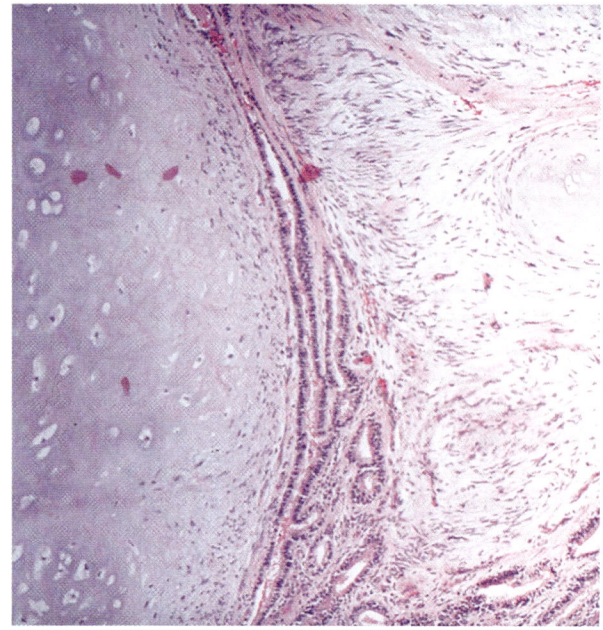

FIGURE 5-4
Hamartoma of the lung. The tumor contains islands of hyaline cartilage and clefts lined by cuboidal epithelium embedded in a fibromuscular stroma.

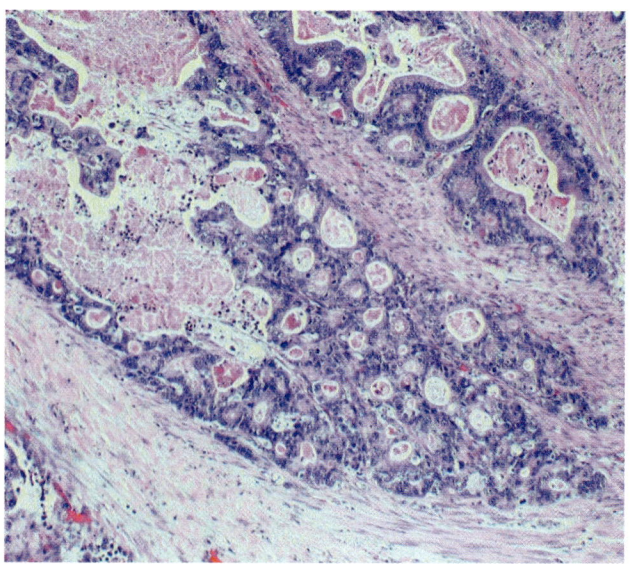

FIGURE 5-5
Adenocarcinoma of the stomach. Irregular neoplastic glands infiltrate the gastric wall.

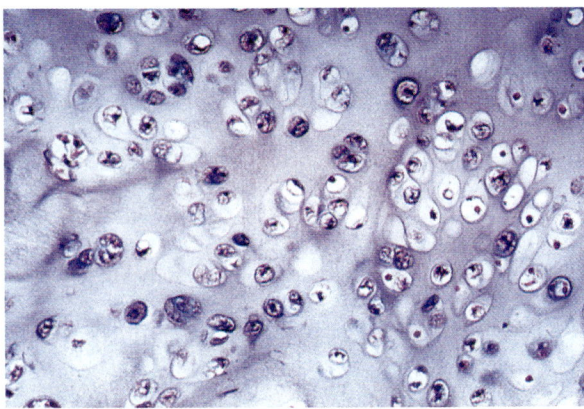

FIGURE 5-6
Chondrosarcoma of bone. The tumor is composed of malignant chondrocytes, which have bizarre shapes and irregular hyperchromatic nuclei, embedded in a cartilaginous matrix. Compare with Figure 5-2.

tumors display neoplastic elements of different cell types but are not germ cell tumors. For example, *fibroadenoma* of the breast, composed of epithelial and stromal elements, is benign, whereas, as the name implies, *adenosquamous carcinoma* of the uterus or the lung is malignant. A rare malignant tumor that contains intermingled carcinomatous and sarcomatous elements is known as *carcinosarcoma*.

The persistence of certain historical terms adds a note of confusion. *Hepatoma* of the liver, *melanoma* of the skin, *seminoma* of the testis, and the lymphoproliferative tumor, *lymphoma*, are all highly malignant. Tumors of the hematopoietic system are a special case in which the relationship to the blood is indicated by the suffix "emia." Thus, *leukemia* refers to a malignant proliferation of leukocytes.

Secondary descriptors (again, with some inconsistencies) refer to a tumor's morphological and functional characteristics. For example, the term *papillary* describes a frond-like structure (Fig. 5-7). *Medullary* signifies a soft, cellular

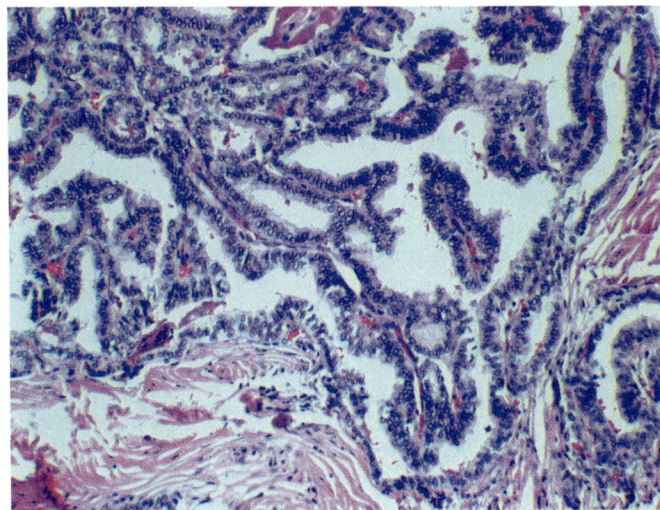

FIGURE 5-7
Papillary adenocarcinoma of the thyroid. The tumor exhibits numerous fronds lined by malignant epithelial cells.

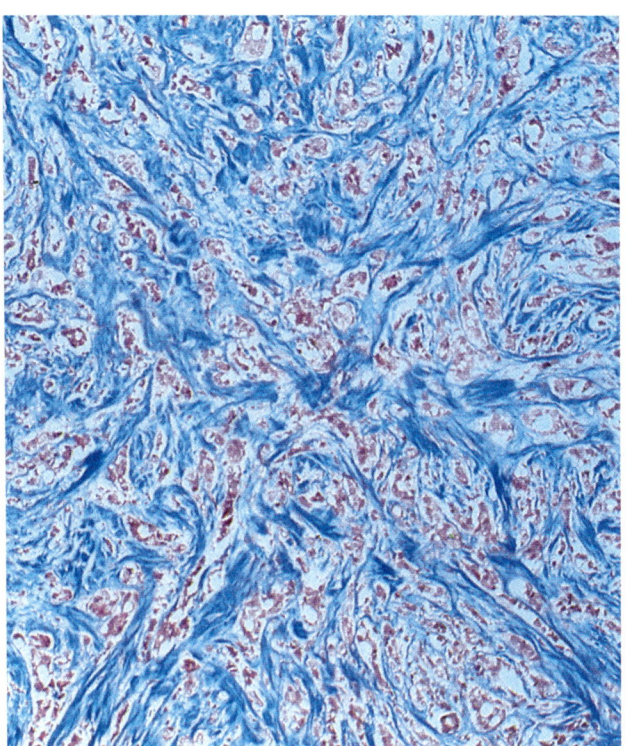

FIGURE 5-8
Scirrhous adenocarcinoma of the breast. A trichrome stain shows nests of cancer cells *(red)* embedded in a dense fibrous stroma *(blue)*.

tumor with little connective tissue stroma, whereas *scirrhous* or *desmoplastic* implies a dense fibrous stroma (Fig. 5-8). *Colloid* carcinomas secrete abundant mucus, in which float islands of tumor cells. *Comedocarcinoma* is an intraductal neoplasm in which necrotic material can be expressed from the ducts. Certain visible secretions of the tumor cells lend their characteristics to the classification—for example, production of mucin or serous fluid. A further designation describes the gross appearance of a cystic mass. From all these considerations we derive such common terms as *papillary serous cystadenocarcinoma* of the ovary, *comedocarcinoma* of the breast, *adenoid cystic carcinoma* of the salivary glands, *polypoid adenocarcinoma* of the stomach, and *medullary carcinoma* of the thyroid. Finally, tumors in which the histogenesis is poorly understood are often given an eponym—for example, Hodgkin disease, Ewing sarcoma of bone, or Brenner tumor of the ovary.

HISTOLOGICAL DIAGNOSIS OF MALIGNANCY

There are no reliable molecular indicators of malignancy, and the "gold standard" for diagnosis of cancer remains routine microscopy. The distinction between benign and malignant tumors is, from a practical point of view, the most important diagnostic challenge faced by the pathologist. In most cases, the differentiation poses few problems; in a few, careful study is required before an accurate diagnosis is secure. However, there remain tumors that defy the diagnostic skills and experience of any pathologist; in these cases, the correct diagnosis must await the clinical outcome. In effect, the criteria used to assess the true biological nature of any tumor are based not on scientific principles but rather on a historical correlation of histological and cytological patterns with clinical outcomes. Although general criteria for malignancy are recognized, they must be used with caution in specific cases. For example, a reactive proliferation of connective cells termed *nodular fasciitis* (Fig. 5-9) has a more alarming histological appearance than many fibrosarcomas, and misdiagnosis can lead to unnecessary surgery. Conversely, many well-differentiated endocrine adenocarcinomas are histologically indistinguishable from benign adenomas.

Benign Tumors Resemble Their Parent Tissue

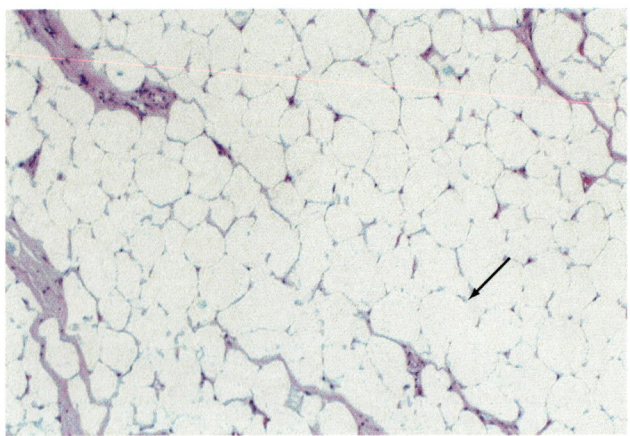

FIGURE 5-10
Lipoma. This subcutaneous, nodular tumor of adipocytes is grossly and microscopically indistinguishable from normal fat.

Benign tumors tend to be histologically and cytologically similar to their tissues of origin. For example, lipomas, despite their often lobulated gross appearance, seem to be composed of normal adipocytes (Fig. 5-10). Fibromas are composed of mature fibroblasts and a collagenous stroma. Chondromas exhibit chondrocytes dispersed in a cartilaginous matrix. Thyroid adenomas form acini and produce thyroglobulin. The gross structure of a benign tumor may depart from the normal and assume papillary or polypoid configurations, as in papillomas of the bladder and skin and adenomatous polyps of the colon. **However, the lining epithelium of a benign tumor resembles that of the normal tissue.** Although many benign tumors are circumscribed by a connective tissue capsule, many equally benign neoplasms are not encapsulated. Unencapsulated benign tumors include papillomas and polyps of the visceral organs, hepatic adenomas, many endocrine adenomas, and hemangiomas. **Remember that the definition of a benign tumor resides above all in its inability to invade adjacent tissue and to metastasize.**

Malignant Tumors Depart from the Parent Tissue Morphologically and Functionally

Despite the histological divergence of malignant tumors from their tissue of origin, an accurate identification of their source depends not only on the location but also on a morphological resemblance to a normal tissue. Some of the histological features that favor malignancy include the following:

- **Anaplasia or cellular atypia:** These terms refer to the lack of differentiated features in a cancer cell. In general, the degree of anaplasia correlates with the aggressiveness of the tumor. Cytological evidence of anaplasia includes (1) variation in the size and shape of cells and cell nuclei *(pleomorphism)*, (2) enlarged and hyperchromatic nuclei with coarsely clumped chromatin and prominent nucleoli, (3) atypical mitoses, and (4) bizarre cells, including tumor giant cells (Fig. 5-11). Many of these features are preceded by a preneoplastic dysplastic epithelium, which may lead to carcinoma in situ (see Chapter 1).
- **Mitotic activity:** Abundant mitoses are characteristic of many malignant tumors but are not a necessary criterion. However, in some cases (e.g., leiomyosarcomas), the diagnosis of malignancy is based on the finding of even a few mitoses.
- **Growth pattern:** In common with many benign tumors, malignant neoplasms often exhibit a disorganized and random growth pattern, which may be expressed as uniform sheets of cells, arrangements around blood vessels, papillary structures, whorls, rosettes, etc. Malignant tumors often outgrow their blood supply and display ischemic necrosis.
- **Invasion:** Malignancy is proved by the demonstration of invasion, particularly of blood vessels and lymphatics.

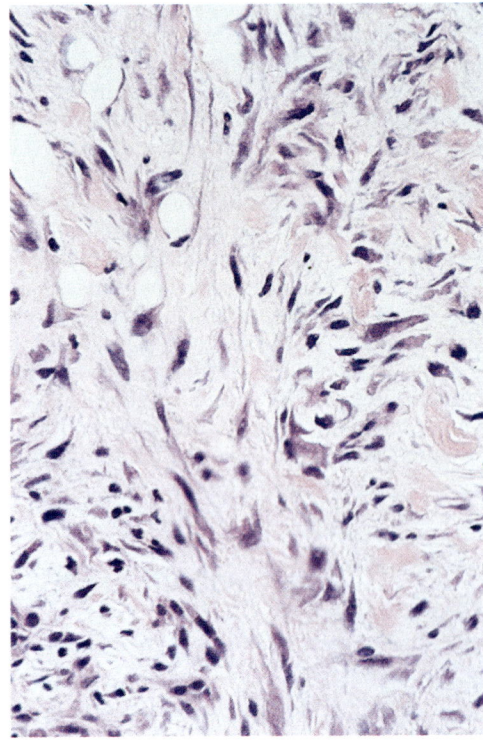

FIGURE 5-9
Nodular fasciitis. This cellular reactive lesion contains atypical and bizarre fibroblasts, which may be mistaken for a fibrosarcoma.

Histological Diagnosis of Malignancy

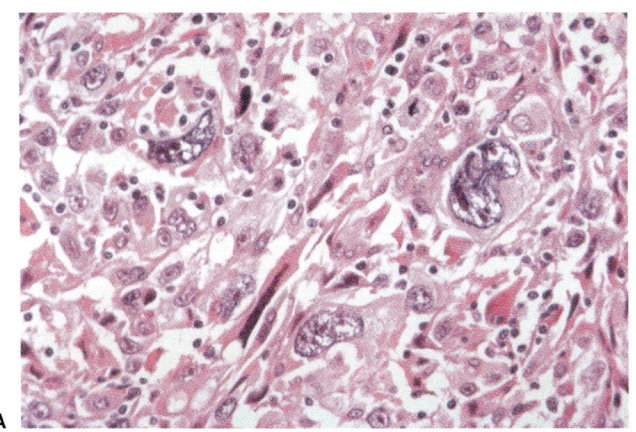
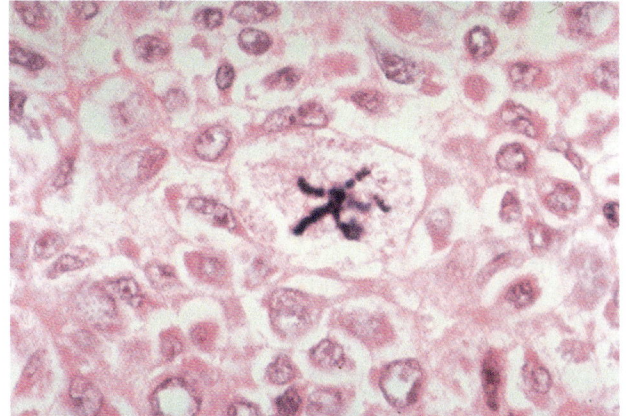
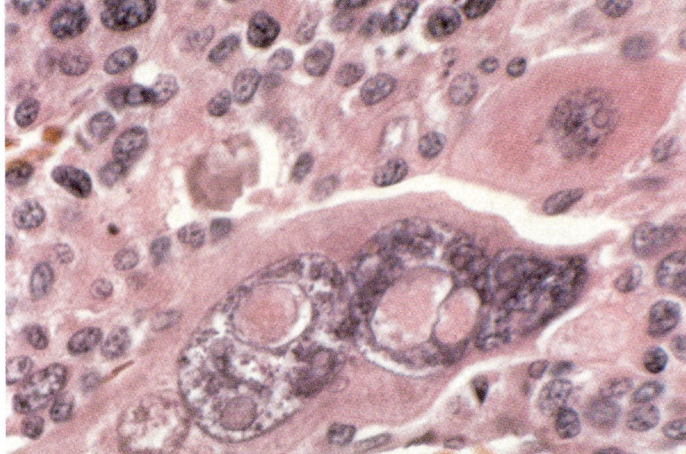

FIGURE 5-11
Anaplastic features of malignant tumors. A. The cells of this anaplastic carcinoma are highly pleomorphic (i.e., they vary in size and shape). The nuclei are hyperchromatic and are large relative to the cytoplasm. B. A malignant cell in metaphase exhibits an abnormal mitotic figure. C. Multinucleated tumor giant cell.

In some circumstances (e.g., squamous carcinoma of the cervix or carcinoma arising in an adenomatous polyp), the diagnosis of malignant transformation is made on the basis of local invasion.

- **Metastases:** The presence of metastases identifies a tumor as malignant. In metastatic disease that was not preceded by a clinically diagnosed primary tumor, the site of origin is often not readily apparent from the morphological characteristics of the tumor. In such cases, electron microscopic examination and the demonstration of specific tumor markers may establish the correct origin.

Electron Microscopy of Undifferentiated Tumors May Identify the Source

There are no specific determinants of malignancy or even of neoplasia itself that can be detected by electron microscopy. On the other hand, this technique may aid in the diagnosis of poorly differentiated cancers, whose classification is problematic by routine light microscopy. For example, carcinomas often exhibit desmosomes and specialized junctional complexes, structures that are not typical of sarcomas or lymphomas. The presence of melanosomes signifies a melanoma, whereas small, membrane-bound granules with a dense core are features of endocrine neoplasms (Fig. 5-12). Another example of a diagnostically useful granule is the characteristic crystal-containing granule of an insulinoma derived from the pancreatic islets.

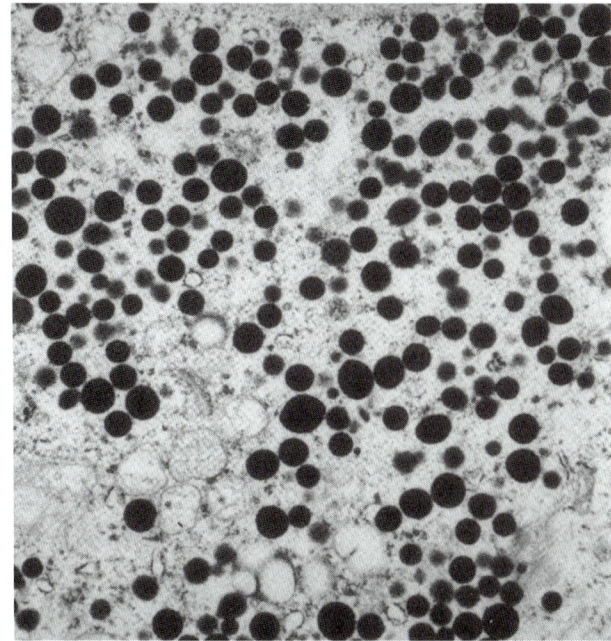

FIGURE 5-12
Electron micrograph of a metastatic cancer of the adrenal medulla (pheochromocytoma). The neuroendocrine origin of this poorly differentiated tumor was identified by the presence of characteristic cytoplasmic secretory granules.

Immunohistochemical Tumor Markers Are Antigens That Point to the Origin of Neoplasms

Tumor markers are products of malignant neoplasms that can be detected in the cells themselves or in body fluids. The ultimate tumor marker would be one that allows the unequivocal distinction between benign and malignant cells, but unfortunately no such marker is in sight. Nevertheless, markers do exist that are often useful in identifying the cell of origin of a metastatic or poorly differentiated primary tumor. Metastatic tumors may be so undifferentiated microscopically as to preclude even the distinction between an epithelial and a mesenchymal origin. Tumor markers rely on the preservation of characteristics of the progenitor cell or the synthesis of specialized proteins by the neoplastic cell to make this distinction. The determination of the cell lineage of undifferentiated tumors is more than an academic exercise, because therapeutic decisions may be based on the appropriate identification. For example, the treatment of carcinomas usually involves surgery, whereas malignant lymphomas are treated with radiation therapy and chemotherapy. Among these diagnostically useful markers are such diverse products as immunoglobulins, fetal proteins, enzymes, hormones, and cytoskeletal and junctional proteins.

Carcinomas uniformly express cytokeratins, which are intermediate filaments belonging to a multigene family of proteins. Lineage-associated markers are often useful in establishing the origin of a poorly differentiated carcinoma. For example, prostatic carcinomas consistently express a glycoprotein named prostate-specific antigen (PSA) and are also positive for prostate-specific acid phosphatase (PSAP). By contrast, colon cancers are consistently negative for these markers, but most of them express carcinoembryonic antigen (CEA). Some thyroid carcinomas demonstrate thyroglobulin, and breast cancers frequently show nuclear receptors for estrogen and progesterone. Expression of the sialated form of the Lewis a antigen (CA 19-9) has been associated with pancreatic and gastrointestinal cancers, whereas CA 125 is a sensitive marker for ovarian cancers.

Neuroendocrine tumors share the positivity for cytok-

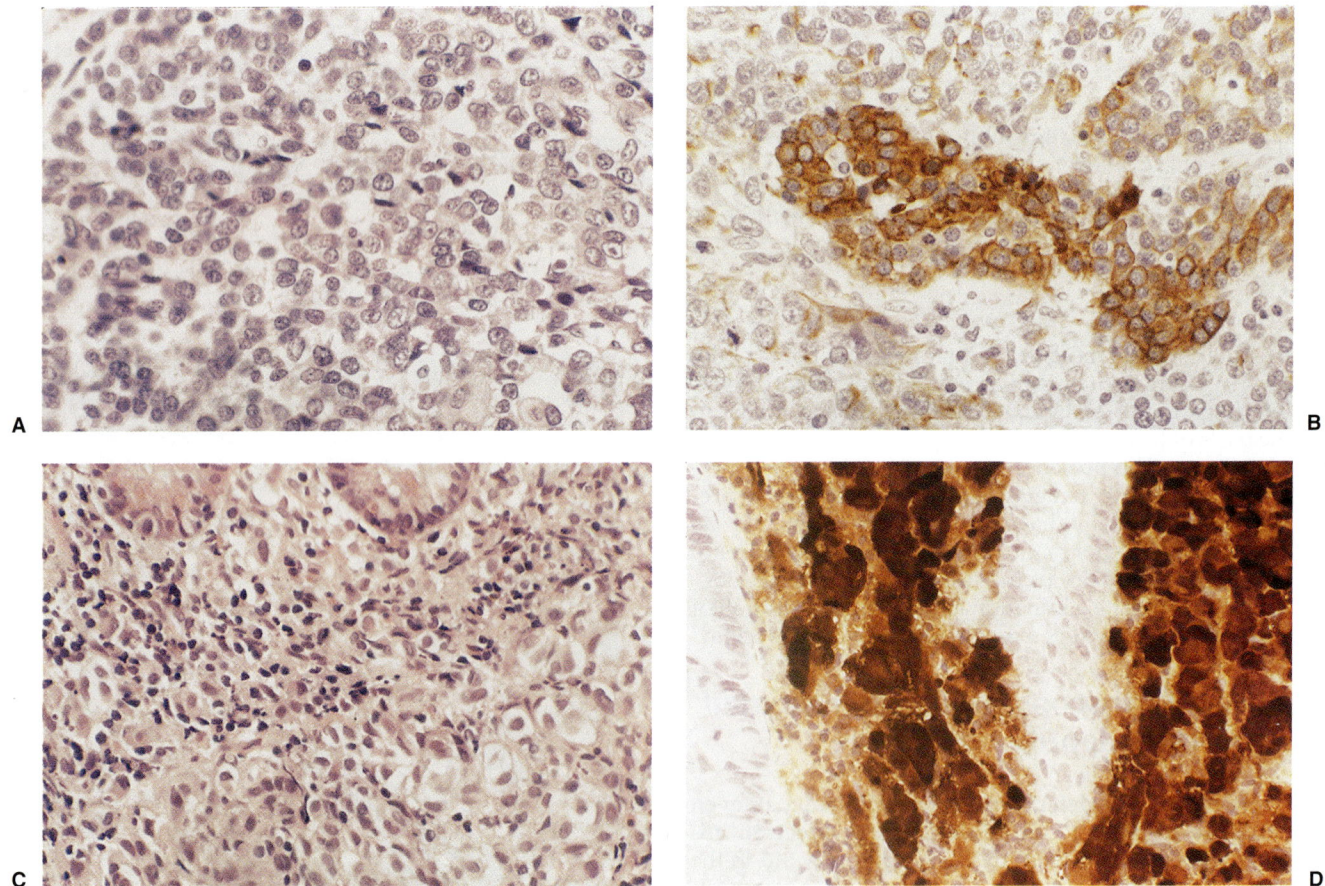

FIGURE 5-13
Tumor markers in the identification of undifferentiated neoplasms. A. A poorly differentiated metastatic bladder cancer is difficult to identify as a carcinoma with the hematoxylin and eosin stain. B. A section of the tumor depicted in A is positive for cytokeratin with an immunoperoxidase stain and is identified as carcinoma. C. A metastasis to the colon of an undifferentiated malignant melanoma is not pigmented, and its origin is unclear. D. An immunoperoxidase stain of the tumor shown in C reveals numerous cells positive for S-100 protein, a commonly used marker for cells of melanocytic origin.

eratins with other carcinomas. However, they can be identified by their content of chromogranins, a family of proteins found in neurosecretory granules. Neuron-specific enolase is another, albeit less specific, marker for neuroendocrine cells. Other markers for neuroendocrine differentiation are synaptophysin and Leu-7 (CD57). Specific antibodies exist for a number of peptide hormones, such as gastrin, bombesin, corticotropic hormone (ACTH), insulin, glucagon, somatostatin, and serotonin.

Malignant melanomas may be unpigmented and appear similar to other poorly differentiated carcinomas. They can be distinguished by immunohistochemical studies (Fig. 5-13). Melanomas express HMB-45 and S-100 protein, but unlike most carcinomas, they are not positive for cytokeratins.

Soft tissue sarcomas express the intermediate filament vimentin. Since this marker is also present in numerous non-mesenchymal tumors, its expression is meaningful only in concert with other markers and morphological criteria. Desmin, another useful intermediate filament, is present in benign and malignant neoplasms originating from either smooth or striated muscle fibers. Muscle-specific actin is another marker for muscle tissue. Neurofilament proteins are excellent markers for tumors originating from neurons, including neuroblastomas and ganglioneuroma. Neuron-specific enolase also shows a strong association with neurogenic tissue and is found in almost all neuroblastomas. Glial fibrillary acidic protein (GFAP), the first intermediate filament discovered, is strongly expressed on astrocytes and in most glial cell neoplasms.

Malignant lymphomas are generally positive for leukocyte common antigen (LCA, CD45). Markers for lymphomas and leukemias are grouped by so-called cluster designations (CD), at present numbering over 200. Markers for CD antigens help to discriminate between T and B lymphocytes, monocytes, and granulocytes and the mature and immature variants of these cells. B-cell malignancies, including plasmacytomas, manifest immunoglobulin light-chain restriction. A single B cell expresses κ or λ light chains. The presence of both κ- and λ-positive B cells argues against malignancy, whereas the demonstration of only one type of light chain on the lymphocytes strongly suggests a monoclonal B-cell lymphoma.

Vascular tumors derived from endothelial cells, including hemangiomas and hemangiosarcomas, are identified by antibodies against factor VIII-related antigen or by the binding of certain lectins.

Proliferating cells display Ki-67 and proliferating cell nuclear antigen (PCNA). Although the presence of proliferating cells alone does not establish a diagnosis of malignancy, the presence of cycling cells at sites in which cell growth is normally absent frequently suggests a cancer.

Serum tumor markers are not disease specific, but they allow monitoring of tumor recurrence after surgery. For example, high serum levels of CEA are associated with carcinomas of the gastrointestinal tract and the breast. Increased levels of serum α-fetoprotein (AFP) suggest liver cancer or a yolk sac tumor. Human chorionic gonadotropin (hCG) is used for monitoring the recurrence of malignant trophoblastic tumors. Elevated CA 19-9 serum titers are found in patients with pancreatic or gastrointestinal cancers, and high CA 125 levels are associated with ovarian carcinomas. Increased serum levels of PSA accompany prostatic cancers.

Elevated titers of human placental alkaline phosphatase (HPAP) occur with seminomas. Table 5-1 lists many of the commonly used tumor markers.

INVASION AND METASTASIS

The two properties that are unique to cancer cells are the ability to invade locally and the capacity to metastasize to distant sites. These characteristics are responsible for the vast majority of deaths from cancer; the primary tumor itself is generally amenable to surgical extirpation.

Direct Extension Damages the Involved Organ and Adjacent Tissues

Most carcinomas begin as localized growths confined to the epithelium in which they arise. As long as these early cancers do not penetrate the basement membrane on which the epithelium rests, such tumors are termed *carcinoma in situ* (Fig. 5-14). In this stage, it is unfortunate that they are asymptomatic, because they are invariably curable. When the in situ tumor acquires invasive potential and extends directly through the underlying basement membrane, it is in a position to compromise neighboring tissues and to metastasize. In situations in which cancer arises from cells that are not confined by a basement membrane, such as connective tissue cells, lymphoid elements, and hepatocytes, an *in situ* stage is not defined.

Malignant tumors characteristically grow within the tissue of origin, where they enlarge and infiltrate normal structures. They may also extend directly beyond the confines of that organ to involve adjacent tissues. In some cases, the growth of the cancer may be so extensive that replacement of the normal tissue results in functional insufficiency of the organ. Such a situation is not uncommon in primary cancer of the liver. Tumors of the brain, such as astrocytomas, infiltrate the brain until they compromise vital regions. The direct extension of malignant tumors within an organ may also be life threatening because of their location. A common example is the intestinal obstruction produced by cancer of the colon (Fig. 5-15).

The invasive growth pattern of malignant tumors often leads to their direct extension outside the tissue of origin, in which case the tumor may secondarily impair the function of an adjacent organ. Squamous carcinoma of the cervix often grows beyond the genital tract to produce vesicovaginal fistulas and obstruct the ureters. Neglected cases of breast cancer are often complicated by extensive ulceration of the skin. Even small tumors can produce severe consequences when they invade vital structures. A small cancer of the lung can cause a bronchopleural fistula when it penetrates the bronchus or exsanguinating hemorrhage when it erodes a blood vessel. The agonizing pain of pancreatic carcinoma results from direct extension of the tumor to the celiac nerve plexus. Tumor cells that reach serous cavities (e.g., those of the peritoneum or pleura) spread easily by direct extension or can be carried by the fluid to new locations on the serous membranes. The most common example is the seeding of the peritoneal cavity by certain types of ovarian cancer (Fig. 5-16).

TABLE 5-1 Frequently Used Markers to Identify Tumors

Marker	Target Cells
Epithelial cells	
Cytokeratins	Carcinomas, mesothelioma
CK7	Many adenocarcinomas
CK20	Gastrointestinal and ovarian carcinomas, bladder transitional cell carcinoma, Merkel cell tumor
Epithelial membrane antigen (EMA)	Carcinomas, mesothelioma, some large cell lymphomas
Ber-Ep4	Most adenocarcinomas, but not in mesothelioma
B72.3 (tumor-associated)	Many adenocarcinomas, but not in mesothelioma
CEA	Many adenocarcinomas, but not in mesothelioma
CD15	Many adenocarcinomas, but not in mesothelioma
Mesothelial cells	
Cytokeratins CK5/6	Mesothelioma
Vimentin	Mesothelioma
HBME	Mesothelioma
Calretinin	Mesothelioma
Melanocytes	
HMB-45	Malignant melanoma
S-100 protein	Malignant melanoma
MART-1	Malignant melanoma
Neuroendocrine and neural cells	
Chromogranins	Neuroendocrine carcinoma, carcinoid tumor
Synaptophysin	Neuroendocrine carcinoma, carcinoid tumor
Neuron-specific enolase	Neuroendocrine carcinoma, carcinoid tumor
CD57	Neuroendocrine carcinoma
Neurofilament proteins	Neuroblastoma
Glial cells	
Glial fibrillary acidic protein (GFAP)	Astrocytoma and other glial tumors
Mesenchymal cells	
Vimentin	Most sarcomas
Desmin	Muscle tumors (myosarcomas)
Muscle-specific actin	Muscle tumors (myosarcomas)
CD99	Ewing sarcoma, peripheral neuroectodermal tumors (PNET)
Specific organs	
Prostate-specific antigen (PSA)	Prostatic cancer
Prostate-specific alkaline phosphatase (PSAP)	Prostatic cancer
Thyroglobulin	Thyroid cancer
α-Fetoprotein (AFP)	Hepatocellular carcinomas, yolk sac tumor
Carcinoembryonic antigen (CEA)	Gastrointestinal cancers
Placental alkaline phosphatase (PLAP)	Seminoma
Human chorionic gonadotropin (hCG)	Trophoblastic tumors
CA19.9	Pancreatic and gastrointestinal carcinomas
CA125	Ovarian carcinoma
Calcitonin	Medullary carcinoma of the thyroid
CD markers	
CD1	Thymocytes, dendritic cells, some T-cell leukemias
CD2	T cells, T-cell malignancies
CD3	T cells, T-cell malignancies
CD4	T-helper cells, T-cell malignancies
CD5	T cells, B-cell chronic lymphocytic leukemia
CD8	Cytotoxic/suppressor T cells
CD10 (common ALL antigen, CALLA)	Some acute lymphoblastic leukemias, follicular lymphoma
	Myeloid leukemias
	Hodgkin lymphoma
CD13	B cells, B-cell malignancies
CD15	B cells, B-cell malignancies
CD19	Large cell lymphomas, Hodgkin lymphoma
CD20	Myeloid leukemias

(continues)

TABLE 5-1 (continued)

Marker	Target Cells
CD30	Leukemias
CD33	Leukemias and lymphomas
CD34	Platelets, acute megakaryoblastic leukemia
CD45 (leucocyte common antigen)	Hairy cell leukemia
Non-CD leukemia/lymphoma markers	
κ-Light chain	B-cell malignancies
λ-Light chain	B-cell malignancies
TdT	Lymphoblastic leukemia
Bcl-1	Mantle cell lymphoma
Bcl-2	Follicular lymphoma
Endothelial markers	
von Willebrand factor (vWF)	Vascular neoplasms
CD31	Vascular neoplasms
CD34	Vascular neoplasms
Lectins	Vascular neoplasms

Metastatic Spread Is the Most Common Cause of Cancer Death

Metastasis refers to the transfer of malignant cells from one site to another not directly connected with it. The invasive properties of malignant tumors bring them into contact with blood and lymphatic vessels. **In the same way that they can invade parenchymal tissue, neoplastic cells can also penetrate vascular and lymphatic channels, through which they are disseminated to distant sites.** In general, metastases resemble the primary tumor histologically, although they are occasionally so anaplastic that their cell of origin is obscure.

Hematogenous Metastases

Cancer cells commonly invade capillaries and venules, whereas the thicker-walled arterioles and arteries are relatively resistant. Before they can form viable metastases, cir-

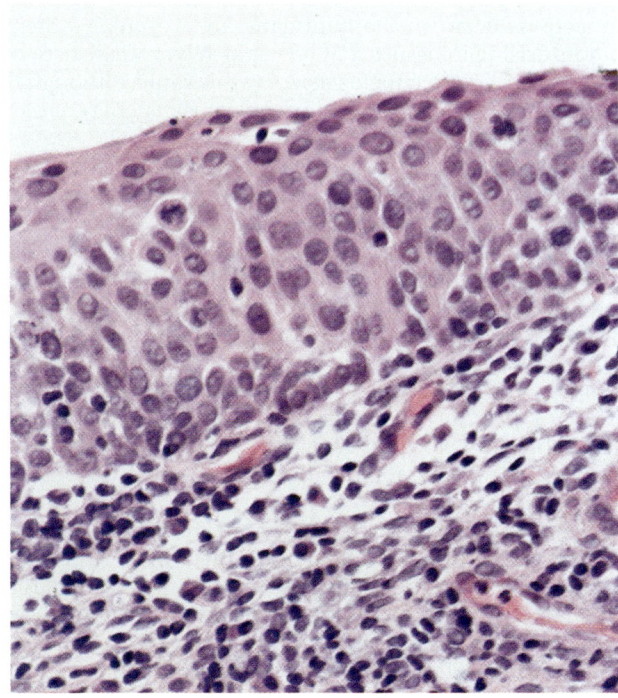

FIGURE 5-14
Carcinoma in situ. A section of the uterine cervix shows neoplastic squamous cells occupying the full thickness of the epithelium and confined to the mucosa by the underlying basement membrane.

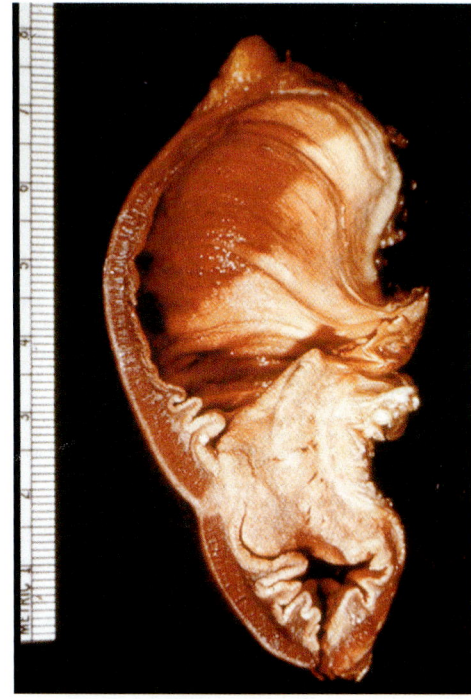

FIGURE 5-15
Adenocarcinoma of the colon with intestinal obstruction. The lumen of the colon at the site of the cancer is narrow. The colon above the obstruction is dilated.

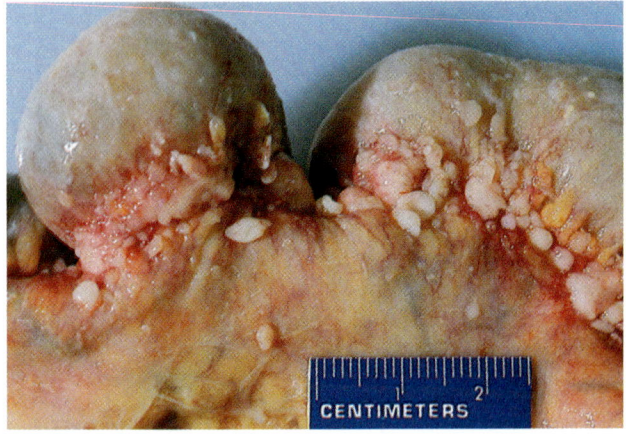

FIGURE 5-16
Peritoneal carcinomatosis. The mesentery attached to a loop of small bowel is studded with small nodules of metastatic ovarian carcinoma.

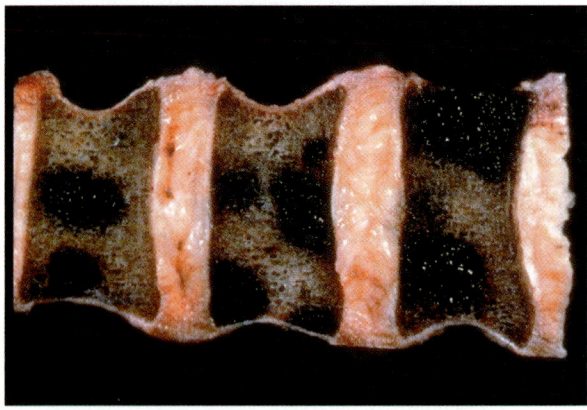

FIGURE 5-18
Multiple pigmented metastases in the vertebral bodies in a patient who died of malignant melanoma.

culating tumor cells must lodge in the vascular bed of the metastatic site (Fig. 5-17). Here they presumably attach to the walls of blood vessels, either to endothelial cells or to naked basement membranes. For many tumors, this sequence of events explains why the liver and the lung are so frequently the sites of metastases. Because abdominal tumors seed the portal system, they lead to hepatic metastases; other tumors penetrate systemic veins that eventually drain into the vena cava and hence to the lungs. In this respect, some tumor cells released into the venous system survive passage through the microcirculation and are thus transported to more distant organs. For instance, tumor cells may traverse the liver and produce pulmonary metastases, and neoplastic cells may also survive passage through the pulmonary microcirculation to reach the brain, bones, (Fig. 5-18), and other organs through arterial dissemination. Neoplastic cells arrested in the microcirculation penetrate the vessel walls at the site of metastasis by use of the same mechanisms by which the primary tumor invades.

Lymphatic Metastases

A historical dogma of metastatic spread held that epithelial tumors (carcinomas) preferentially metastasize through lymphatic channels, whereas mesenchymal neoplasms (sarcomas) are distributed hematogenously. This distinction is no longer considered valid because of clinical observations of metastatic patterns and the demonstration of numerous connections between the lymphatic and vascular systems. Tumors arising in tissues that have a rich lymphatic network (e.g., the breast) often metastasize by this route, although the particular properties of specific neoplasms may play a role in the route of spread.

Basement membranes envelop only the large lymphatic channels; they are lacking in the lymphatic capillaries. Thus, invasive tumor cells may penetrate lymphatic channels more readily than blood vessels. Once in the lymphatic vessels, the cells are carried to the regional draining lymph nodes, where they initially lodge in the marginal sinus and then extend throughout the node. Lymph nodes bearing metastatic deposits may be enlarged to many times their normal size, often exceeding the diameter of the primary lesion. The cut surface of the lymph node usually resembles that of the primary tumor in color and consistency and may also exhibit the necrosis and hemorrhage commonly seen in primary cancers (Fig. 5-19).

The regional lymphatic pattern of metastatic spread is most prominently exemplified by cancer of the breast. In breast cancer, the initial metastases are almost always lymphatic, and these regional lymphatic metastases have considerable prognostic significance. Cancers that arise in the lateral aspect of the breast characteristically spread to the lymph nodes of the axilla; those arising in the medial portion drain to the internal mammary lymph nodes in the thorax.

Lymphatic metastases are occasionally found in lymph nodes distant from the site of the primary tumor; these are termed *skip metastases*. For example, abdominal cancers may initially be signaled by the appearance of an enlarged supra-

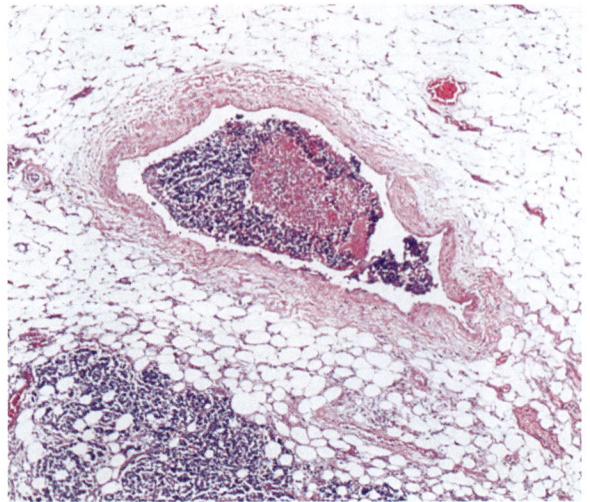

FIGURE 5-17
Hematogenous spread of cancer. A malignant tumor (*bottom*) has invaded adipose tissue and penetrated into a small vein.

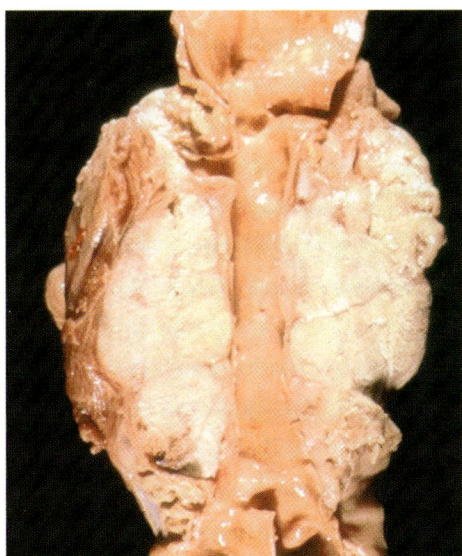

FIGURE 5-19
Metastatic carcinoma in periaortic lymph nodes. The aorta has been opened and the nodes bisected.

clavicular node, the so-called sentinel node. A graphic example of the relationship of lymphatic anatomy to the spread of malignant tumors is afforded by cancers of the testis. Rather than metastasizing to the regional nodes, as do other tumors of the male external genitalia, testicular cancers typically involve the draining abdominal periaortic nodes. The explanation lies in the descent of the testis from an intraabdominal site to the scrotum, during which it is accompanied by its own lymphatic supply.

Seeding of Body Cavities

Malignant tumors that arise in organs adjacent to body cavities (e.g., ovaries, gastrointestinal tract, and lung) may shed malignant cells into these spaces. Such body cavities include principally the peritoneal and pleural cavities, although occasional seeding of the pericardial cavity, joint space, and subarachnoid space, are observed. Similar to tissue culture the tumor in these sites, grows in masses and often produces fluid (e.g., ascites, pleural fluid), sometimes in massive quantities. Mucinous adenocarcinoma may also secrete copious amounts of mucin in these locations.

Invasion and Metastasis Are Multistep Events

A number of steps are required for malignant cells to establish a metastasis (Fig. 5-20):

1. Invasion of the basement membrane underlying the tumor
2. Movement through the extracellular matrix
3. Penetration of vascular or lymphatic channels
4. Survival and arrest within the circulating blood or lymph
5. Exit from the circulation into a new tissue site
6. Survival and growth as a metastasis, a process that involves angiogenesis

Most cancers originate from the malignant transformation of a single cell *(monoclonal origin of tumors)*. Nevertheless, the inherent genetic instability of the malignant phenotype leads to the appearance of subpopulations with diverse biological characteristics and profound variations in their metastatic potential *(tumor heterogeneity)*. The demonstration of tumor heterogeneity has led to the concept that at each step of the metastatic cascade, only the fittest cells survive. Thus, the metastatic process can be viewed as a competition in which a subpopulation of cells within the primary cancer ultimately prevails as a metastasis.

Invasion

Inherent in the definition of a malignant cell is the capacity to invade the surrounding tissue. In epithelial tumors, invasion requires disruption of, and penetration through, the underlying basement membrane and passage through the extracellular matrix. Similarly, circulating cells destined to establish metastases must reproduce these same events to exit from the vascular or lymphatic compartment and establish residence at a distant site.

Adhesion Molecules

The entire metastatic sequence, from the initial binding of the tumor cell to the underlying extracellular matrix to the growth in a distant location, depends on the expression of numerous adhesion molecules by the malignant cells. The display of such surface molecules varies with (1) the type of tumor, (2) the individual clone (tumor heterogeneity), (3) the stage of the malignant progression, and (4) the specific step in the metastatic process.

INTEGRINS: Integrins are transmembrane receptors, each consisting of two α and two β subunits, which together confer substrate specificity on the receptor. These adhesion receptors mediate cell–matrix and cell–cell attachment. The binding of integrins to their ligands also stimulates intracellular signaling and gene expression, which play a role in cell migration, proliferation, differentiation, and survival. In addition, integrins affect the expression, localization, and activation of collagenases (metalloproteinases [MMPs]; see below) and can guide these enzymes to their targets in the extracellular matrix, where they degrade connective tissue and pave the way for the spread of tumor cells.

IMMUNOGLOBULIN SUPERGENE FAMILY: A number of intercellular adhesion molecules belong to this superfamily, including intercellular adhesion molecule-1 (ICAM-1), MUC18, and vascular cell adhesion molecule-1 (VCAM-1). The expression of ICAM-1 correlates positively with the aggressiveness of a variety of tumor cell types.

CADHERINS AND CATENINS: Cadherins are a family of cell–cell adhesion molecules, which are Ca^{2+}-dependent transmembrane glycoproteins. The best-characterized of the cadherins, E-cadherin, is expressed on the surface of all epithelia and mediates cell–cell adhesion by mutual *zipper* interactions. Catenins (α, β, and γ) are proteins that interact with the intracellular domain of E-cadherin and create a me-

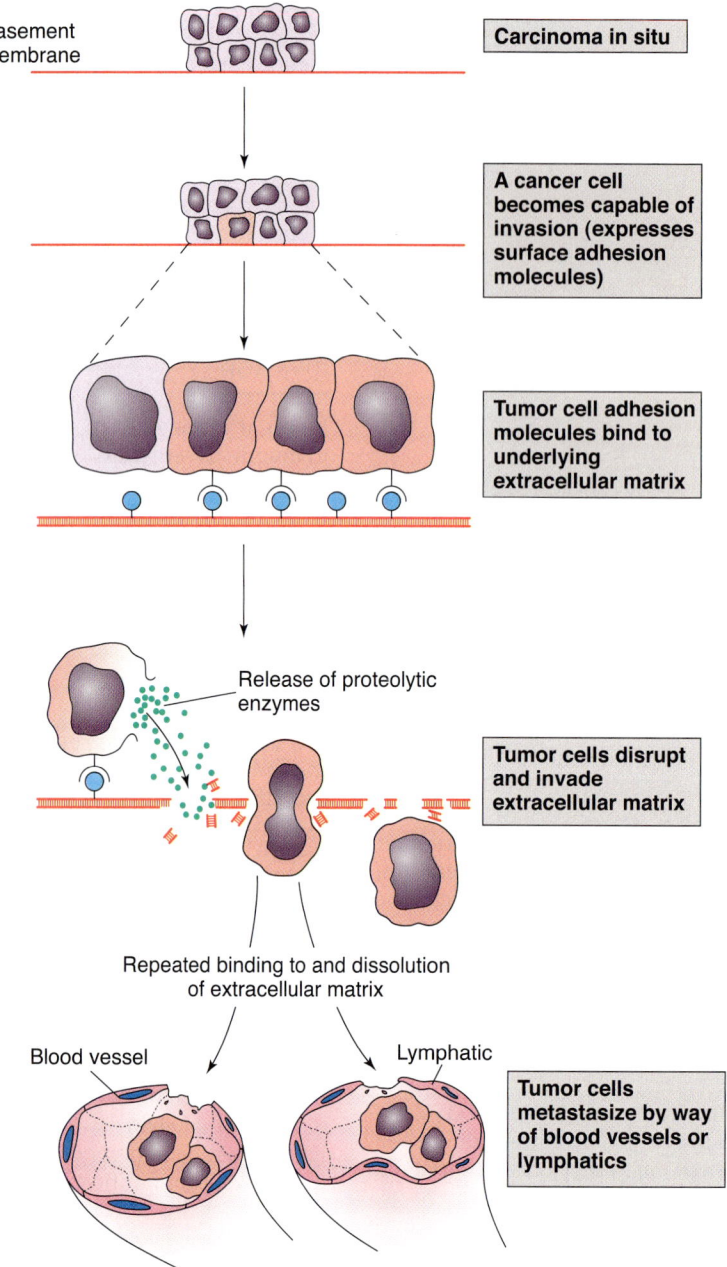

FIGURE 5-20
Mechanisms of tumor invasion and metastasis. The mechanism by which a malignant tumor initially penetrates a confining basement membrane and then invades the surrounding extracellular environment involves several steps. The tumor first acquires the ability to bind components of the extracellular matrix. These interactions are mediated by the expression of a number of adhesion molecules. Proteolytic enzymes are then released from the tumor cells, and the extracellular matrix is degraded. After moving through the extracellular environment, the invading cancer penetrates blood vessels and lymphatics by the same mechanisms.

chanical linkage between the latter and the cytoskeleton, which is essential for effective epithelial cell interactions. Overall, cadherins and catenins suppress invasion and metastasis. The expression of both E-cadherin and catenins is reduced or lost in most carcinomas, an effect that permits individual malignant cells to leave the main tumor mass and metastasize. Interestingly, β-catenin also binds to the adenomatous polyposis coli (APC) gene product, an effect that is independent of its interaction with E-cadherin and α-catenin. Mutations in either the APC or β-catenin gene are implicated in the development of colon cancer (see later and Chapter 13).

Growth Factors and Cytokines

Growth factors and cytokines orchestrate cellular responses during development, differentiation, and repair. Aberrant production of growth factors by tumors contributes to neoangiogenesis and attraction of inflammatory cells and enhances proliferation, migration, and invasive properties of tumor cells. A notable example is *autocrine motility factor* (AMF), a molecule that belongs to a family of tumor cell cytokines that stimulate motility via a receptor-mediated signaling pathway. AMF not only regulates motility but also modulates the expression of cell surface integrins. The expression of the AMF receptor (gp78) in normal cells is regulated by cell contact, whereas in many cancer cells, it is constitutively expressed.

Proteolytic Enzymes

A breach of the basement membrane that separates an epithelium from the underlying mesenchymal compartment is the first event in tumor cell invasion. The basement membrane is composed of a number of extracellular matrix components, including type IV collagen, laminin, and proteoglycans (see Chapter 3). Malignant cells and stromal cells associated with cancers elaborate a variety of proteases that degrade one or more of the basement membrane components. Such enzymes include the urokinase-type plasminogen activator (u-PA) and matrix metalloproteinases (MMPs), including collagenases.

u-PA converts serum plasminogen to plasmin, a serine protease that degrades laminin and activates type IV procollagenase. The activity of u-PA is balanced by plasminogen activator inhibitor (PAI), and changes in the expression of u-PA, the u-PA receptor and PAI have been reported in different cancers.

The MMPs make up a family of zinc-dependent endopeptidases that are susceptible to tissue inhibitors of MMPs (TIMPs). MMPs include interstitial collagenases, stromelysins, gelatinases, and membrane-type MMPs. These enzymes are synthesized and secreted by normal cells under conditions associated with physiological tissue remodeling, such as wound healing and placental implantation. Under these circumstances, a balance between MMPs and TIMPs is strictly regulated. By contrast, the invasive and metastatic phenotypes of cancer cells are characterized by dysregulation of this balance.

A direct correlation between increased expression of MMPs and augmented invasive capacity or metastatic potential of tumor cells has been observed in many cancers. In addition, many of these same tumors exhibit decreased TIMP expression. MMPs are present in either the tumor cells or the surrounding stromal cells or both, depending on the particular neoplasm. In some instances, MMPs secreted by stromal cells are bound to integrins on the surface of the tumor cells, thereby providing a particularly high local concentration of protease activity at the site of tumor invasion. Deregulated MMP activity permits entry of cancer cells into, and their passage through, the extracellular matrix.

Metastasis

Following the invasion of surrounding tissue, malignant cells may spread to distant sites by a process that includes a number of steps:

1. **Invasion of the circulation:** After invading the interstitial tissue, malignant cells penetrate lymphatic or vascular channels. In the lymph nodes, communications between lymphatics and venous tributaries allow the cells access to the systemic circulation. Most tumor cells do not survive their journey in the bloodstream, and less than 0.1% remain to establish a new colony.

2. **Escape from the circulation:** Circulating tumor cells may arrest mechanically in capillaries and venules, where they attach to endothelial cells. This adherence causes retraction of the endothelium, thereby exposing the underlying basement membrane to which the tumor cells now bind. Clumps of tumor cells may also arrest in arterioles, where they grow within the vascular lumen. In both situations, the tumor cells eventually extravasate by mechanisms similar to those responsible for local invasion.

3. **Local growth:** In a hospitable site, the extravasated cancer cells grow in response to autocrine and possibly local growth factors produced by the host tissue. However, a new vascular supply is necessary for the tumor to grow to a diameter greater than 0.5 mm. Thus, many tumors secrete polypeptides (e.g., fibroblast growth factor [FGF], vascular endothelial growth factor [VEGF], transforming growth factor-β [TGF-β], and platelet-derived growth factor [PDGF]), which together trigger and regulate the process of **angiogenesis** (see below). The newly established metastatic colony must also escape detection and destruction by the host immune defenses (see below). The metastasis can metastasize again, either within the same organ or to distant sites.

The establishment of a metastatic colony does not mean that it inevitably enlarges. It is well known clinically that tumors may recur locally or at metastatic sites many years after the primary cancer has been surgically removed. For example, patients treated for breast cancer or malignant melanoma may be apparently cured for 20 or more years, only to have the tumor suddenly recur. The molecular basis for this phenomenon, termed "*tumor dormancy*," is not well understood (see below).

Target Organs in Metastatic Disease

It was recognized more than 100 years ago that the distribution of metastases in breast cancer is not random. In 1889, Paget proposed that the spread of tumor cells to specific secondary sites depends on compatibility between the tumor cells (the seed) and favorable microenvironment factors in the secondary site (the soil). By contrast, others have argued that metastatic spread depends solely on anatomical factors and the blood flow to an organ. Today, there is evidence that both mechanisms operate, depending on the tumor. For example, cancers of the breast, prostate, and thyroid metastasize to bone, a tropism that suggests a favored soil. Conversely, despite their size and abundant blood flow, neither the spleen nor skeletal muscle is a common site of metastases. Yet for many cancers, the vascular anatomy unquestionably influences the pattern of metastatic spread. Malignant tumors of the gastrointestinal tract commonly metastasize to the first capillary bed they encounter, namely the liver. Similarly, lung cancers often spread to the brain. An additional factor that regulates the homing of malignant cells may be the expression of complementary adhesion molecules, either by the cancer cells or those of the organ to which they home.

THE GRADING AND STAGING OF CANCERS

In an attempt to predict the clinical behavior of a malignant tumor and to establish criteria for therapy, many cancers are classified according to cytological and histological grading schemes or by staging protocols that describe the extent of spread.

Cancer Grading Reflects Cellular Characteristics

Low-grade tumors are well differentiated; high-grade ones tend to be anaplastic. Cytological and histological grading, which are necessarily subjective and at best semiquantitative, are based on the degree of anaplasia and on the number of proliferating cells. The degree of anaplasia is determined from the shape and regularity of the cells and from the presence of distinct differentiated features, such as functioning glandlike structures in adenocarcinomas or epithelial pearls in squamous carcinomas. The presence of such characteristics identify a tumor as "well differentiated." By contrast, the cells of "poorly differentiated" malignancies bear little resemblance to their normal counterparts. Evidence of rapid or abnormal growth is provided by (1) large numbers of mitoses, (2) atypical mitoses, (3) nuclear pleomorphism, and (4) tumor giant cells. Most grading schemes classify tumors into three or four grades of increasing malignancy (Fig. 5-21). The general correlation between the cytological grade and the biological behavior of a neoplasm is not invariable: There are many examples of tumors of low cytological grades that exhibit substantial malignant properties.

Cancer Staging Refers to the Extent of Spread

The choice of surgical approach or the selection of treatment modalities is influenced more by the stage of a cancer than by its cytological grade. Moreover, most statistical data related to cancer survival are based on the stage rather than the cytological grade of the tumor. Clinical staging is independent of cytological grading. The significant criteria used for staging vary with different organs. Commonly used criteria include (1) tumor size; (2) the extent of local growth, whether within or without the organ; (3) the presence of lymph node metastases; and (4) the presence of distant metastases. These criteria have been codified in the international **TNM cancer staging system,** in which "T" refers to the size of the primary tumor, "N" to regional node metastases, and "M" to the presence and extent of distant metastases. The definitions of numerical scores for T, N, and M (e.g., T1–T4, N1–N3) vary according to specific tumor types.

In some cases, the distinction between benign and malignant tumors is based solely on size. For example, on the basis of clinical experience with renal cancers, tumors smaller than 2 cm in diameter are generally considered benign adenomas, whereas those of larger size are labeled renal carcinomas. The choice of surgical therapy is often influenced by size alone. For instance, a primary breast cancer smaller than 2 cm in diameter can be treated with local excision and radiation therapy; larger masses often necessitate mastectomy. Local extension can also be used to estimate prognosis, as in the Dukes classification of colorectal cancer. Penetration of the tumor into the muscularis and serosa of the bowel is associated with a poorer prognosis than that of a more superficial tumor. Clearly, the presence of lymph node metastases mandates more-aggressive treatment than

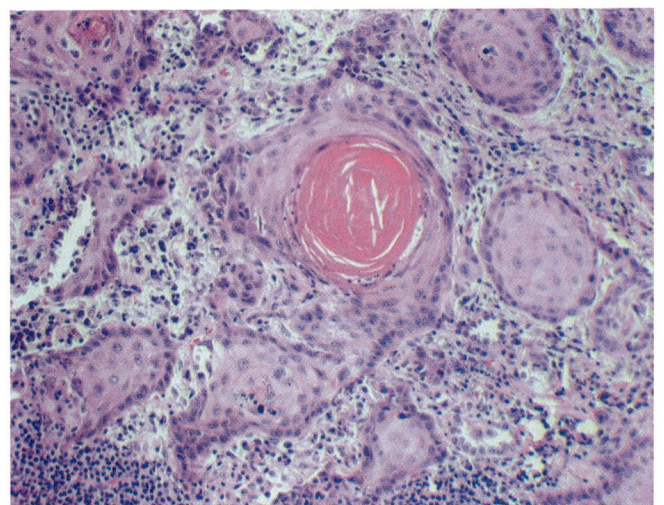
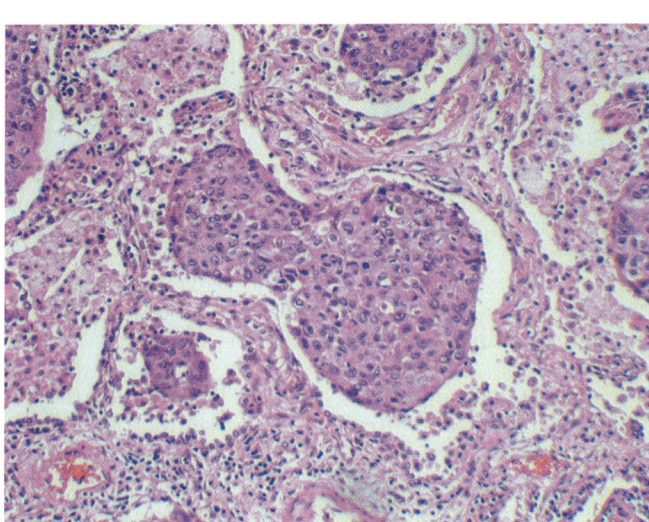

FIGURE 5-21
Cytological grading of squamous cell carcinoma of the lung. A. Well-differentiated (grade 1) squamous cell carcinoma. The tumor cells bear a strong resemblance to normal squamous cells and synthesize keratin, as evidenced by epithelial pearls. B. Poorly differentiated (grade 3) squamous cell carcinoma. The malignant cells are difficult to identify as being of squamous origin.

does their absence, whereas the presence of distant metastases is generally a contraindication to surgical intervention other than for palliation.

THE CLONAL ORIGIN OF CANCER

Studies of human and experimental tumors have provided strong evidence that most cancers arise from a single transformed cell. This theory has been most thoroughly examined in connection with proliferative disorders of the hematopoietic system. The most common piece of clinical evidence in its favor is the production by neoplastic plasma cells of a single immunoglobulin unique to an individual patient with multiple myeloma. Indeed, such a "monoclonal spike" in the serum electrophoresis from a patient with suspected myeloma is regarded as conclusive evidence of the disease. Similarly, cell surface markers have been used to establish a monoclonal origin for many other hematopoietic malignant disorders. For example, B-cell lymphomas are composed of cells that exclusively display either κ or λ light chains on their surface, whereas polyclonal lymphoid proliferations exhibit both types of cells. Monoclonality has also been demonstrated in the individual metastases of a number of solid tumors.

One of the most important observations in regard to the monoclonal origin of cancer was derived from the study of glucose-6-phosphate dehydrogenase in women who were heterozygous for its two isozymes, A and B (Fig. 5-22). These isozymes are encoded by genes located on the X chromosome. Since one X chromosome is randomly inactivated, only one of these genes is expressed in any given cell. Thus, although the genotypes of all cells are the same, their phenotypes vary with regard to the expression of isozyme A or B. An examination of benign uterine smooth muscle tumors (leiomyomas, or "fibroids") revealed that all the cells in an individual tumor expressed either A or B but not both, indicating that each tumor was derived from a single progenitor cell.

CANCER AS ALTERED DIFFERENTIATION

In many cancers, the malignant phenotype reflects, at least in part, defects in the normally strict control of cell proliferation. **However, in some cancers, it is thought that the malignant cells result from a maturation arrest in the sequence of development from a stem cell to a fully differentiated cell.** According to this theory, tumor cells accumulate because the mechanisms that control the total number of cells in the fully differentiated compartment of some tissues do not apply when less-differentiated precursor cells fail to mature.

SQUAMOUS CELL CARCINOMA: In many tumors, most of the neoplastic cells are outside the cell cycle and thus do not contribute to the malignancy of the tumor. For example, as noted above, fewer than 3% of the cells in a squamous carcinoma maintain the malignant potential of the tumor, and most differentiate and die spontaneously. When such terminally differentiated tumor cells are transplanted

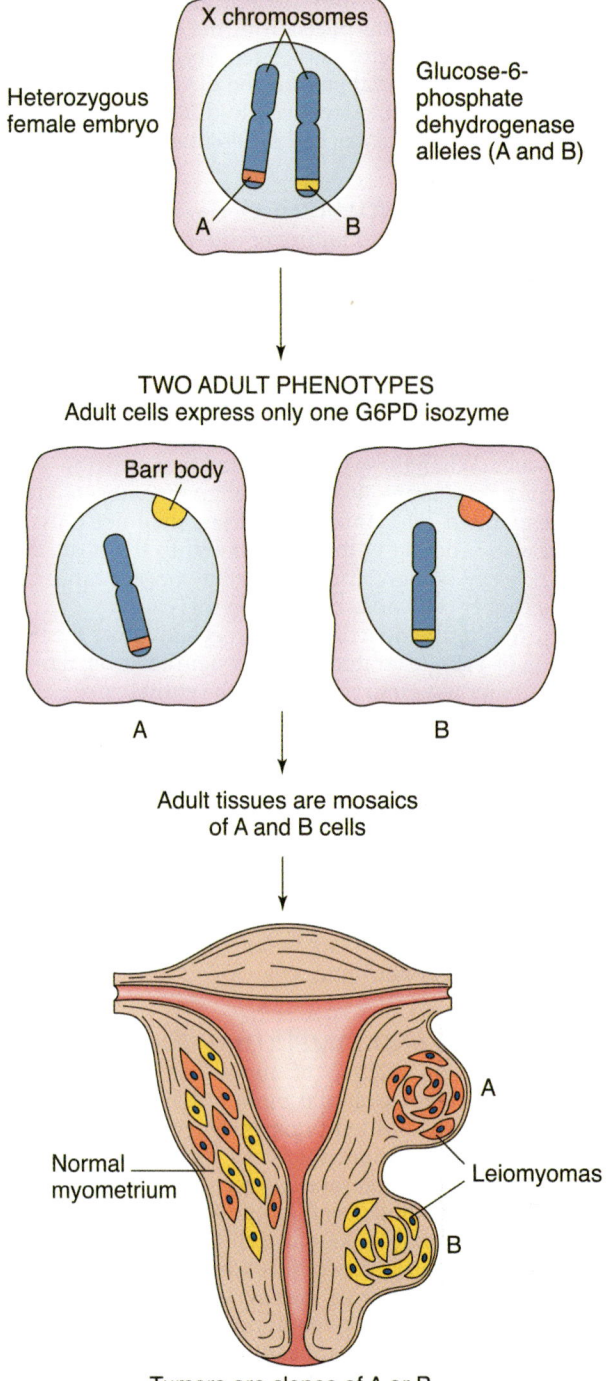

FIGURE 5-22
Monoclonal origin of human tumors. Some females are heterozygous for the two alleles of glucose-6-phosphate dehydrogenase (G6PD) on the long arm of the X chromosome. Early in embryogenesis, one of the X chromosomes is randomly inactivated in every somatic cell and appears cytologically as a Barr body attached to the nuclear membrane. As a result, the tissues are a mosaic of cells that express either the A or the B isozyme of G6PD. Leiomyomas of the uterus have been shown to contain one or the other isozyme (A or B) but not both, a finding that demonstrates the monoclonal origin of the tumors.

into appropriate hosts, they do not grow, whereas their undifferentiated counterparts from the same tumor form typical squamous carcinomas. Such observations support the theory that the initial step in the development of some cancers is a failure of the stem cell to differentiate normally to complete the sequence of cell differentiation.

TERATOCARCINOMA: Further evidence to support the concept of cancer as a failure of differentiation has come from the study of experimental malignant germ cell tumors (teratocarcinomas). A single embryonal carcinoma cell, the stem cell of a teratocarcinoma, when transplanted into a mouse, gives rise to a tumor that contains cells derived from all three germ layers. Clearly, the progeny of the original transplanted tumor cell differentiate into more-mature cells that express recognizable phenotypes of more fully differentiated tissues. When these differentiated tissues of the teratocarcinoma are separated from the malignant embryonal cells and transplanted into compatible hosts, they not only survive but also function with no detriment to the host. These cells are clearly benign, and the dogma "once a cancer cell, always a cancer cell" does not hold in this case.

A further refinement of this approach involves the transplantation of a single teratocarcinoma stem cell from a mouse into an early mouse embryo. At term, the entirely normal pup is a mosaic composed of cells derived from both the embryo proper and the embryonal carcinoma. The progeny of the malignant cell, under the influence of normal developmental controls, has differentiated into mature tissue elements. Thus, the unregulated growth of the cancer cells may be converted into normal patterns of growth and differentiation.

Clinical analogies to the experimental situation do exist. The best known is the rare spontaneous conversion of a malignant neuroblastoma to its better-differentiated, benign counterpart, ganglioneuroma.

LEUKEMIAS AND LYMPHOMAS: The most comprehensive systematic analysis of human neoplasia from the perspective of developmental biology has come from the study of leukemias and lymphomas. During normal B- and T-lymphocyte maturation, there are well-documented sequential changes of membrane antigens and rearrangements of immunoglobulin and T-cell receptor genes. For example, in acute lymphoblastic leukemia of childhood, the neoplastic cells exhibit only partial assembly of the cell surface receptor molecules that characterize mature lymphocytes. In other words, the leukemic cell phenotype bears a strong resemblance to lymphocytes that appear transiently during the developmental sequence of the normal lymphocyte. Thus, the leukemic cells appear to be "frozen" in the act of receptor gene assembly and expression.

Acute myeloid leukemia is similar to acute lymphoblastic leukemia in that the malignant cells express phenotypes of transient, immature myeloid populations. Likewise, studies of chronic lymphocytic leukemias and lymphomas have revealed that these malignant disorders represent clonal expansions of lymphocyte populations corresponding to subsets found in normal lymphoid tissue.

In normal hematopoietic maturation, differentiation is tightly coupled to proliferation—that is, terminally differentiated cells are continually lost, to be replaced by newly proliferated and differentiated cells. By contrast, the data reviewed above suggest that certain leukemias and lymphomas are not truly proliferative disorders but rather reflect an uncoupling of differentiation from proliferation, with resulting accumulation of cells that have not attained terminal differentiation. According to this theory, leukemia and lymphoma may represent the stabilization of a phenotype that is also expressed, though only transiently, in developing normal cells. It has been said that the cell phenotypes in a leukemia or lymphoma can be compared with the phenotype of the ostrich, which is believed to be "primitive and conserved rather than degenerate."

RETINOIDS: The view that certain cancers may reflect impaired differentiation has led to a search for drugs that commit cancer cells to terminal differentiation and, therefore, apoptosis. The interest in the retinoids derives from experiments showing that administration of excess vitamin A or its derivatives inhibits chemically induced carcinogenesis in the skin, lung, bladder, colon, and mammary gland.

A dramatic response to all-*trans*-retinoic acid is generated in acute promyelocytic leukemia, in which the administration of this agent induces a complete remission in most patients. In this disease, the reciprocal translocation between chromosomes 15 and 17 results in a fusion gene consisting of the retinoic acid receptor and the promyelocytic leukemia gene (PML) gene. The chimeric protein blocks myeloid differentiation at the promyelocyte stage, a process that is reversed by retinoic acid. Other forms of retinoic acid have shown limited activity against a variety of tumors. In patients with acute promyelocytic leukemia who are refractory to therapy with retinoic acid, arsenic trioxide, a compound that induces partial nonterminal differentiation of leukemic cells, is surprisingly effective.

THE GROWTH OF CANCERS

Historically, cancer was considered to result from a totally unregulated growth of cells, and a logical corollary was that neoplastic cells divide at a faster rate than normal ones. **It is now clear that tumor cells do not necessarily proliferate more rapidly than their normal counterparts.** Tumor growth depends on other factors, such as the growth fraction (proportion of cycling cells) and the rate of cell death. In normal proliferating tissues (e.g., intestine and bone marrow), an exquisite balance between cell renewal and cell death is maintained. **By contrast, the major determinant of tumor growth is clearly the fact that more cells are produced than die in a given time.** Such an effect can reflect not only an excess of cell proliferation over programmed cell death, but also normal rates of cell renewal in the face of reduced apoptosis.

Tumor Growth Rates May Be Expressed As Doubling Times

Tumor doubling time is the time taken for the number of cells in the mass to double. Internal cancers are not usually detected before they attain a size of about 1 cm^3 (1 g), which corresponds to 10^8 to 10^9 cells. The origin of most tumors from a single cell implies that the mass has doubled at least 30 times to reach this size. If the cancer is neglected and enlarges to the impressive size of 1 kg, it now contains 10^{12} cells. Yet, the growth from 1 g to 1 kg (assuming no cell death) can be achieved by only 10 population doublings. Thus, when cancers are initially detected clinically, they are already far advanced in their natural history. Because of the variable death rate of tumor cells and differences in cell cycle kinetics, the actual doubling time of human tumors is highly unpredictable.

The doubling time is not necessarily correlated with the growth fraction (i.e., the proportion of cells that are within the cell cycle). Since the duration of mitosis in cancer cells is often prolonged, the number of mitoses in a histological section can be misleading as an indicator of overall growth. For example, a doubling in the time required for mitosis results in twice as many visible mitoses without any real increase in the rate of growth. In most cases, the theoretical tumor doubling time, calculated from the growth fraction and the cell cycle time, bears little relation to the actual clinical situation. For example, if a tumor weighing 1 g (often the smallest size clinically detectable) produces 2 new cells per 1000 cells in each mitotic cycle, the theoretical net increase would be a staggering 10^6 cells per hour, a figure totally at variance with the experience with most solid tumors. **Because of this difference between the theoretical and observed growth of tumors, it has been estimated that in human skin tumors, as many as 97% of proliferated cells die spontaneously.** The causes of tumor cell death are not precisely defined but probably include such factors as programmed cell death (apoptosis); inadequate blood supply, with consequent ischemia; a paucity of nutrients; and vulnerability to specific and nonspecific host defenses. From a practical point of view, the duration of a malignant tumor cannot be reasonably estimated from its size when it is first discovered.

Tumor Angiogenesis Refers to the Sprouting of New Capillaries

Angiogenesis is a requirement for the continued growth of cancers, whether primary or metastatic. In the absence of new vessels to supply the nutrients and remove waste products, malignant tumors do not grow larger than 1 to 2 mm in diameter. In this context, the density of capillaries within the primary tumor (e.g., cancers of the breast, prostate, and colon) predicts metastases and decreased survival. Importantly, tumor angiogenesis occurs in nonneoplastic host tissue and is comparable to that in wound healing and other physiological circumstances (see Chapter 3). Neovascularization of the evolving cancer may appear at various stages of tumor development and probably is related to phenotypic and genetic changes in the tumors. However, it is still unclear whether tumor angiogenesis is fundamentally a response to tissue hypoxia or to a distinct angiogenic tumor phenotype by which neoplastic cells secrete angiogenic factors.

A number of factors can stimulate an angiogenic response; some act directly on endothelial cells, whereas others stimulate inflammatory cells to promote the formation of new blood vessels. Among these factors are FGF, TGF-α and TGF-β, tumor necrosis factor-α (TNF-α), VEGF, PDGF, and epidermal growth factor (EGF). VEGF and FGF-2 are thought to be the most important angiogenic factors. The role of such angiogenic factors is underscored by the experimental suppression of tumor growth by both endogenous and synthetic inhibitors of angiogenesis factors. Notably, endogenous inhibitors, angiostatin and endostatin, have been reported to eliminate widespread tumors in mice. Tumor angiogenesis may also be influenced by variations in the production of angiogenic inhibitors, such as thrombospondin, TIMPs, platelet factor 4, and interferons α and β. Other factors that have been documented to influence angiogenesis include adhesion molecules, matrix MMPs, and plasmin. Unfortunately, the clinical effectiveness of angiogenesis inhibitors has yet to be demonstrated.

Tumor Dormancy Accounts for the Interval before the Appearance of Metastases

Often, metastatic disease is not detectable at the time of the removal of a primary cancer. With some tumors, notably breast cancer and melanoma, metastases may remain dormant for many years, only to become apparent without any obvious cause. It is not clear whether tumor dormancy represents a balance between cell growth and cell death or whether the tumor cells are in cell cycle arrest. In the clinical situation, most patients who have undergone a resection for a primary cancer do not evidence any detectable metastases either radiologically or pathologically. Thus, so-called micrometastases consist of single tumor cells or very small clusters. In the case of dormant tumor cells, it is not known whether they remain in G_0 phase of the cell cycle for prolonged periods of time or whether they do not grow because of interference with angiogenesis, unresponsiveness to growth factors, or the presence of immune growth restraints.

THE MOLECULAR GENETICS OF CANCER

The belief that cancer has a genetic basis, embodied in the concept of "cancer genes," has been prevalent for more than half a century and was rooted in the recognition of four factors: (1) hereditary predisposition, (2) the presence of chromosomal abnormalities in neoplastic cells, (3) a correlation between impaired DNA repair and the occurrence of cancer, and (4) the close association between carcinogenesis and mutagenesis. **It is now recognized that the unregulated growth of cancer cells results from the sequential acquisition of somatic mutations in genes that control cell growth, differentiation, and apoptosis or that maintain the integrity of the genome.** Similar mutations may also be present in the germ line of persons with hereditary predispositions to a variety of cancers. Mutations can be produced by environmental mutagens such as chemical carcinogens or radiation (see below). Mutations can also arise during normal cellular metabolism, particularly from the formation of activated oxygen species (see Chapter 1).

It is likely that the most common mechanism of mutagenesis relates to spontaneous errors in DNA replication and repair. Considering that 10^{17} mitoses occur during an average human lifetime, corresponding to incorporation of the more than 10^{26} nucleotides into nascent DNA, it is impossible for this much DNA replication to occur without the introduction of unrepaired errors (mutations). Since the body is composed of some 10^{14} cells and the mutation rate is roughly 10^{-7} per gene per cell division, it is inevitable that everyone is a somatic mosaic at many genetic loci. Most such mutations are of no consequence, because they either do not affect the function of the cell or are lost as a result of the death of the cell. However, if the mutation involves genes that control growth or that protect the stability of the genome, it may give rise to a clone of cells that possess a growth advantage over their normal neighbors. Successive mutations in similar genes result in increasingly aberrant clones until a malignant phenotype eventually emerges. In a sense, the emergence of malignancy may be viewed as an evolutionary process wherein we see only the surviving clones. Moreover, the progression of neoplasms is influenced by selective host pressures.

Transformed Cells Share Common Attributes

The precise definition of cell transformation is difficult, but it is generally accepted that malignant transformation involves somatic mutations that confer a set of common properties. It is estimated that a minimum of 4–7 mutated genes are required for the transformation of a normal cell into a malignant phenotype. This *multistep* process takes place over a period of years, an observation that accounts, at least in part, for the fact that the incidence of cancer increases with age. Although mutations in hundreds of genes have been implicated in the pathogenesis of cancer, individual cancers exhibit unique profiles of genetic alterations. Nevertheless, the disruption of a limited number of regulatory pathways in the cell that leads to deregulation of cell proliferation and suppression of apoptosis confers a neoplastic phenotype to diverse cell types. Metazoans must allow cell proliferation upon demand. Thus, from a teleological perspective, cancer reflects the failure to suppress the deregulated growth of mutated cells.

Cancer cells are remarkably heterogeneous in appearance, growth rate, invasiveness, and metastatic potential, presumably owing to the interplay between diverse acquired mutations and the inherent gene expression of specific cell lineages. Nevertheless, transformed cells share certain biological features:

- Autonomous generation of mitogenic signals
- Insensitivity to exogenous antigrowth signals
- Resistance to apoptosis
- Limitless replicative potential (immortalization)
- Blocked differentiation
- Ability to sustain angiogenesis
- Capacity to invade surrounding tissues
- Potential to metastasize

Normal genes are mutated in various cancers, including cell cycle regulators, signal transduction factors, transcriptional factors, DNA-binding proteins, growth factor receptors, adhesion molecules, effectors of apoptosis, and telomerase. Thus, the concept of specific "cancer genes" is fanciful. The adhesion molecules, transforming genes can be conveniently grouped into three categories:

- **Oncogenes** are altered versions of normal genes, termed *protooncogenes,* that regulate normal cell growth, differentiation, and survival. Gain-of-function (dominant) mutations activate protooncogenes to become oncogenes and are positive effectors of the neoplastic phenotype.
- **Tumor suppressor genes** are normal genes whose products inhibit cellular proliferation. Loss-of-function (recessive) mutations inactivate the inhibitory activities of tumor suppressor genes, thereby permitting unregulated cell growth.
- **Mutator genes (DNA mismatch repair genes)** normally maintain the integrity of the genome and the fidelity of DNA replication. Inactivating mutations of these genes allow the successive accumulation of further mutations.

Oncogenes Are Counterparts of Normal Genes

The concept of oncogenes was originally derived from studies of animal tumor viruses. About three decades ago, research on transforming retroviruses showed that a limited number of viral genes could impart a neoplastic phenotype to virally infected cells. It was subsequently demonstrated that the transfer of specific genes from human tumor cells *(oncogenes)* into rodent cells in vitro could transform the recipient cells. The transforming genes were discovered to be mutant versions of normal genes involved in growth regulation and were termed *protooncogenes*. Transforming viral oncogenes were termed v-*onc* genes, and their cellular counterparts (c-) were individual normal genes (e.g., c-*myc*, c-*jun*, c-*src*).

Mechanisms of Activation of Cellular Oncogenes

There are three general mechanisms by which protooncogene activation is accomplished:

- A mutation of a protooncogene leads to the production of an abnormal protein that is constitutively activated.
- An increase in the expression of the protooncogene causes overproduction of a normal gene product.
- As a general principle, the activation of oncogene proteins is regulated by numerous autoinhibitory mechanisms, which operate as a safeguard against inappropriate activity. Thus, many of the mutations in protooncogenes do not simply "activate" the encoded protein but rather lead to insensitivity to the normal autoinhibitory and regulatory constraints.

Activation by Mutation

Mutations by which protooncogenes are converted to oncogenes may involve point mutations, deletions, or chromosomal translocations. The first oncogene identified in a human tumor was activated c-*ras* from a bladder cancer. This gene was found to have a remarkably subtle alteration, namely, a point mutation in codon 12, a change that results in the substitution of valine for glycine in the ras protein. Subsequent studies of other cancers have revealed point mutations involving other codons of the *ras* gene, suggesting that these positions are critical for the normal function of the ras protein. Since the discovery of mutations in c-*ras*, alterations in other growth-regulatory genes have been described.

Activating, or gain-of-function, mutations in protooncogenes are usually somatic rather than germ line alterations. Germ line mutations in protooncogenes, which are known to be important regulators of growth during development, are ordinarily lethal in utero. There are several exceptions to this rule, including c-*ret,* which is incriminated in the pathogenesis of certain heritable endocrine cancers, and c-*met*, which encodes the receptor for hepatocyte growth factor and is associated with a hereditary form of renal cancer.

Activation by Chromosomal Translocation

Chromosomal translocations (i.e., the transfer of a portion of one chromosome to another) have been implicated in the pathogenesis of several human leukemias and lymphomas. The first and still the best-known example of an acquired chromosomal translocation in a human cancer is the **Philadelphia chromosome,** which is found in 95% of patients with chronic myelogenous leukemia (Fig. 5-23). The c-*abl* protooncogene on chromosome 9 is translocated to chromosome 22, where it is placed in juxtaposition to a site known as the breakpoint cluster region (*bcr*). The c-*abl* gene and *bcr* region unite to produce a hybrid oncogene that codes for an aberrant protein with very high tyrosine kinase activity, which generates mitogenic and antiapoptotic signals. The chromosomal translocation that produces the Philadelphia chromosome is an example of activation of an oncogene by the formation of a chimeric (fusion) protein.

In 75% of patients with Burkitt lymphoma (a type of B-cell lymphoma; see Chapter 20), there is a translocation of c-*myc*, a protooncogene involved in cell cycle progression, from its site on chromosome 8 to a position on chromosome 14 (see Fig. 5-23). This translocation places c-*myc* adjacent to the genes that control the transcription of the immunoglobulin heavy chains. As a result, the c-*myc* protooncogene is activated by the promoter/enhancer sequences of these immunoglobulin genes and is consequently expressed constitutively rather than in a regulated manner. In 25% of patients with Burkitt lymphoma, the c-*myc* protooncogene remains on chromosome 8 but is activated by the translocation of Ig light-chain genes from chromosome 2 or 22 to the 3' end of the c-*myc* gene. In either case, a chromosomal translocation does not create a novel chimeric protein but stimulates the overproduction of a normal gene product. In Burkitt lymphoma, the excessive amount of the normal c-*myc* product, probably in association with other genetic alterations, leads to the emergence of a dominant clone of B cells, driven relentlessly to proliferate as a monoclonal neoplasm. Many other hematopoietic malignancies, lymphomas, and solid tumors reflect activation of oncogenes by chromosomal translocation. Although some malignant conditions are *initiated* by chromosomal translocations, during the *progression* of many cancers, myriad chromosomal abnormalities take place (translocations, breaks, aneuploidy, etc.).

Activation by Gene Amplification

Chromosomal alterations that result in an increased number of copies of a gene (i.e., gene amplification) have been found primarily in human solid tumors. Such aberrations are recognized as (1) **homogeneous staining regions (HSRs)** (Fig. 5-24); (2) **abnormal banding regions** on chromosomes; or (3) **double minutes**, which are visualized as multiple, small, paired, cytoplasmic bodies (Fig. 5-25). In some cases, gene amplification has been shown to involve protooncogenes. For example, HSRs may be seen in neuroblastomas and are all derived from the N-*myc* protooncogene. The presence of N-*myc* HSRs is associated with up to 700-fold amplification of this gene and is a marker of advanced disease with a poor prognosis. Activation of *myc*-family protooncogenes by means of gene amplification has also been demonstrated in small cell carcinoma of the lung, Wilms tumor, and hepatoblastoma.

The *erb B* protooncogene is amplified in up to a third of breast and ovarian cancers. The *erb B* gene (*erb-B2*, also designated *HER2/neu*), codes for a receptor-type tyrosine kinase that shows close structural similarity to the EGF receptor. Amplification of *erb B2* in breast and ovarian cancer may be associated with poor overall survival and decreased time to relapse.

Mechanisms of Oncogene Action

Oncogenes can be classified according to the roles of their normal counterparts (protooncogenes) in the biochemical pathways that regulate growth and differentiation. These include the following (Figs. 5-26 and 5-27):

- Growth factors
- Cell surface receptors
- Intracellular signal transduction pathways
- DNA-binding nuclear proteins (transcription factors)
- Cell cycle proteins (cyclins and cyclin-dependent protein kinases)
- Inhibitors of apoptosis (bcl-2)

Oncogenes and Growth Factors

The binding of soluble extracellular growth factors to their specific surface receptors initiates signaling cascades that eventuate in entry of the cell into the mitotic cycle. A few protooncogenes encode growth factors that stimulate tumor cell growth. In some instances, a growth factor acts upon the same cell that produces it *(autocrine stimulation)*. Other growth factors act upon the receptors of neighboring cells *(paracrine stimulation)*. Examples of growth factors involved in neoplastic transformation include platelet-derived growth factor (PDGF) and fibroblast growth factor (FGF).

PDGF is the protein product of the c-*sis* protooncogene and is a potent mitogen for fibroblasts, smooth muscle cells, and glial cells. Cells derived from human sarcomas and glioblastomas (a malignant glial cell tumor) produce PDGF-like polypeptides; their normal counterparts do not. Transfection of c-*sis* into cultured mouse fibroblasts results in their transformation. Thus, a normal human gene (c-*sis*) that encodes a growth factor (PDGF) acquires transforming capacity when it is constitutively expressed in a cell that responds to this signal.

An oncogene *(HST)* that codes for a protein with homology to FGF has been identified in human stomach cancer and Kaposi sarcoma. Moreover, in rodent models, neoplastic cells often express transforming growth factor (TGF).

Mutational activation of growth factor genes is not well characterized in human cancers. Nevertheless, whether caused by genetic or epigenetic mechanisms, cancer cells generally produce a mixture of growth factors with autocrine or paracrine activity, including insulin-like growth factor-I (IGF-I), PDGF, TGF-α, FGF, colony-stimulating factor-1 (CSF-1), and hepatocyte growth factor (HGF).

Oncogenes and Growth Factor Receptors

Many growth factors stimulate cellular proliferation by interacting with a family of cell surface receptors that are inte-

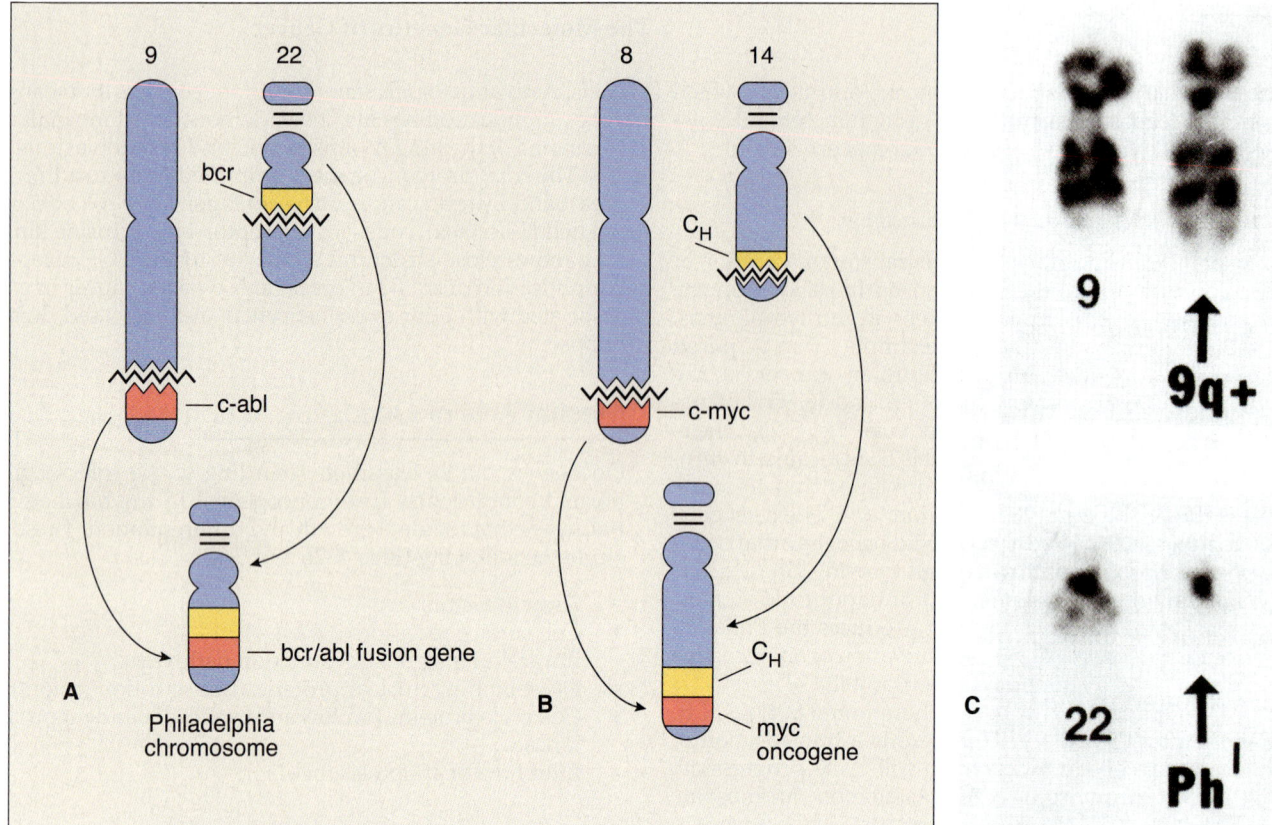

FIGURE 5-23
Oncogene activation by chromosomal translocation. A. Chronic myelogenous leukemia. Breaks at the ends of the long arms of chromosomes 9 and 22 allow reciprocal translocations to occur. The c-*abl* protooncogene on chromosome 9 is translocated to the breakpoint region (*bcr*) of chromosome 22. The result is the Philadelphia chromosome, which contains a new fusion gene coding for a hybrid oncogenic protein (bcr-abl), presumably involved in the pathogenesis of chronic myelogenous leukemia. B. Burkitt lymphoma. In this disorder, chromosomal breaks involve the long arms of chromosomes 8 and 14. The c-*myc* gene on chromosome 8 is translocated to a region on chromosome 14 adjacent to the gene coding for the constant region of an immunoglobulin heavy chain (C_H). The expression of c-*myc* is enhanced by its association with the promoter/enhancer regions of the actively transcribed immunoglobulin genes. C. Karyotypes of a patient with chronic myelogenous leukemia showing the results of reciprocal translocations between chromosomes 9 and 22. The Philadelphia chromosome is recognized by a smaller-than-normal chromosome 22 (22q−). One chromosome 9 (9q+) is larger than its normal counterpart.

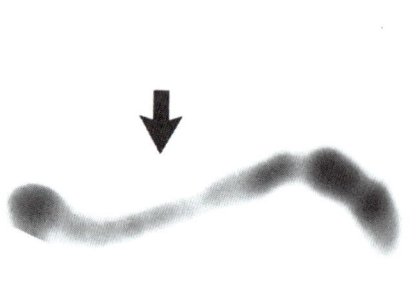

FIGURE 5-24
Homogeneously staining region (HSR; *arrow*) in a chromosome from an ovarian carcinoma.

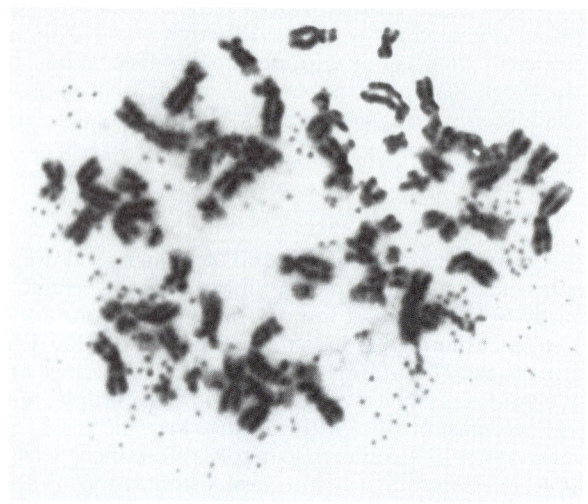

FIGURE 5-25
Double minutes in a karyotype of a soft tissue sarcoma appear as multiple small bodies.

The Molecular Genetics of Cancer

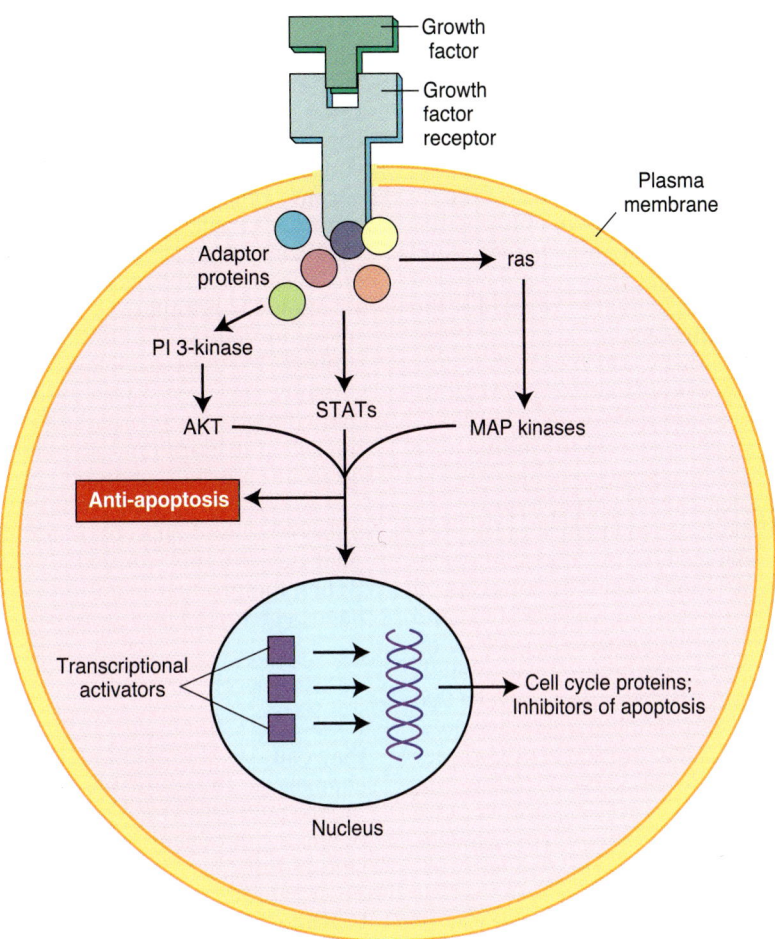

FIGURE 5-26
Signaling pathways controlling proliferation and apoptosis. The activation of growth factor receptors by their ligands causes the binding of adaptor proteins and the activation of a series of intracellular signaling molecules leading to transcriptional activation, the induction of cell cycle proteins, and inhibition of apoptosis. Key targets include *ras*, mitogen activated protein (MAP) kinases, signal transducer and activator transcription factors (STATs), phosphatidylinositol 3-kinase (PI 3-kinase), and the serine/threonine kinase AKT.

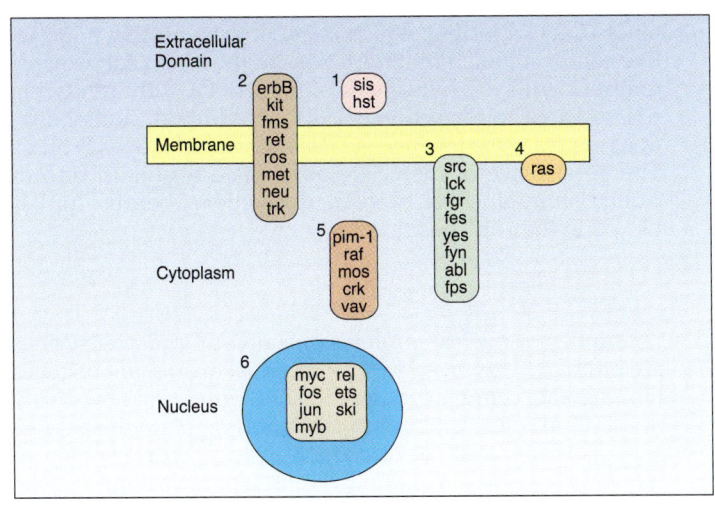

FIGURE 5-27
Cellular compartments in which oncogene or protooncogene products reside. (1) Growth factors, (2) transmembrane growth factor receptors (tyrosine kinase), (3) membrane associated kinases, (4) *ras* GTPase family, (5) cytoplasmic kinases, (6) nuclear transcriptional regulators.

gral membrane proteins with tyrosine kinase activity. In fact, the regulation of the functional responses to growth factors, including cell proliferation, differentiation, and survival, depends principally on the expression of, and relative balance between, various growth factor receptors. Binding of a ligand to the extracellular domain of its receptor stimulates an intrinsic kinase activity in the cytoplasmic domain of the receptor that phosphorylates tyrosine residues on intracellular signaling molecules. **Thus, because growth factor receptors can generate potent mitogenic signals, they harbor a latent oncogenic potential, which when activated overrides the normal controls of signaling pathways.**

The most common mechanism by which growth factors participate in oncogenesis is overexpression of a normal receptor by enhanced activation of promoters or gene amplification. Under normal circumstances, transient binding of a growth factor to its receptor leads to activation of the cytoplasmic tyrosine kinase domain, after which the receptor reverts to its resting state. Certain mutations of growth factor receptors, including truncation of the extracellular or intracellular domains, point mutations, and deletions, result in unrestrained (constitutive) activation of the receptor, independent of ligand binding. For example, the c-*met* protooncogene encodes a receptor for HGF. Point mutations in the intracellular catalytic domain convert the c-*met* protooncogene to an oncogene that is involved in papillary renal cancers. Similarly, germline point mutations in c-*ret* lead to constitutive activation of the receptor and are associated with the multiple endocrine neoplasia syndromes (MEN) and familial medullary thyroid carcinoma (see Chapter 21). Patients with germ line mutations in the catalytic domain of the c-*kit* tyrosine kinase tend to develop gastrointestinal stromal tumors (GIST).

Another abnormality of a growth factor receptor can result from chromosomal translocations that produce hybrid proteins with constitutive tyrosine kinase activity. In the case of the PDGF receptor, a chromosomal translocation [t(5;12)] generates a fusion protein between the cytoplasmic domain of the PDGF receptor and a motif encoded by c-*tel*. The abnormal receptor has been found in patients with myelomonocytic leukemia.

Epigenetic changes that result in increased synthesis of growth factors and their receptors are equally important as mutations and overexpression of growth factor receptors in the pathogenesis of human cancers. In some human malignancies (e.g., breast, ovarian, and stomach cancers), amplification of *her*-2/*neu* results in autocrine activation mediated by overexpression of this growth factor receptor. Of greater importance in human cancers are epigenetic changes that cause increased synthesis of growth factors and receptors.

Oncogenes and Nonreceptor Protein Kinases

A number of proteins that possess tyrosine kinase activity are loosely associated with the inner aspect of the plasma membrane and possess tyrosine kinase activity but are neither integral membrane proteins nor growth factor receptors. The prototype of a viral oncogene that codes for mutant forms of these protein kinases is v-*src* (see Fig. 5-27). A number of other oncogenes (*abl, lck, yes, fgr, fps, fes*) belong to the *src* family. The homologous c-*src* protooncogene product is expressed in most cells, whereas other members of the *src* family are expressed in specialized cell types such as hematopoietic cells and epithelia. The src enzymes are activated by most receptor tyrosine kinases and influence cell proliferation, survival, and invasiveness.

The only member of the *src* family that has been implicated in human tumorigenesis is c-*abl*. As discussed above, in chronic myelogenous leukemia this protooncogene, which codes for a cytoplasmic tyrosine kinase, is translocated from chromosome 9 to the breakpoint cluster region (*bcr*) of chromosome 22. The *bcr-abl* fusion gene encodes a mutant protein with conspicuously elevated tyrosine kinase activity, which is necessary for the oncogenic action of the chimeric protein.

Soluble cytoplasmic oncoproteins (*raf, mos, pim*-1) that phosphorylate serine/threonine residues have also been described. The best-studied of the soluble cytoplasmic oncoproteins, *raf*, plays a role in the signal transduction cascade that converts ligand binding by cell surface receptors into nuclear transcriptional activation. Point mutations in c-*raf* occur in up to 10% of human cancers.

Receptor and nonreceptor tyrosine kinases are dephosphorylated and thereby inactivated by a variety of phosphatases. In this context mutations in the phosphatase PTEN, the product of a tumor suppressor gene (see below), have been linked to a variety of human malignancies.

Ras Oncogenes

Ras is an effector molecule in the signal transduction cascade that couples the activation of growth factor receptors to changes in gene transcription in the nucleus. The *ras* protooncogene codes for a product, p21, that belongs to a family of small cytoplasmic proteins (G proteins) that bind guanosine triphosphate (GTP) and guanosine diphosphate (GDP). The ras protein, p21, is distinct from the integral membrane G proteins that are involved in receptor-mediated signal transduction (Fig. 5-28). The protein p21 is active when it binds GTP and is inactive when it binds GDP. Bound GTP is converted to GDP by the intrinsic GTPase activity of p21. This enzyme activity is normally very low but is stimulated more than 100-fold by a GTPase-activating protein (GAP). Thus, the inactivating switch for the ras protein is the p21 GTPase.

The discovery of an activated version of the *ras* protooncogene in bladder cancer cells was the first demonstration of a human oncogene. The substitution of valine for glycine at position 12 in p21 was the first mutation characterized in a human oncogene. It is now evident that activation of *ras* genes (Ha-*ras*, Ki-*ras*, or N-*ras*) is the most frequent dominant mutation in human cancers.

The mutant forms of p21 are characterized by persistence of GTP binding, which maintains the protein in its active conformation. Point mutations in the *ras* protooncogene interfere with the hydrolysis of GTP to GDP by rendering p21 resistant to the action of GAP. In addition, some mutations decrease the intrinsic ATPase activity of the ras protein. The persistence of the GTP-bound state results in uncontrolled stimulation of *ras*-related functions, because p21 is locked in the "on" position.

Oncogenes and Nuclear Regulatory Proteins

A number of nuclear proteins encoded by protooncogenes are intimately involved in the sequential expression of genes that regulate cellular proliferation and differentiation. Many of these proteins can bind to DNA and regulate the expression of other genes. The transitory expression of several protooncogenes is necessary for the cells to pass through specific

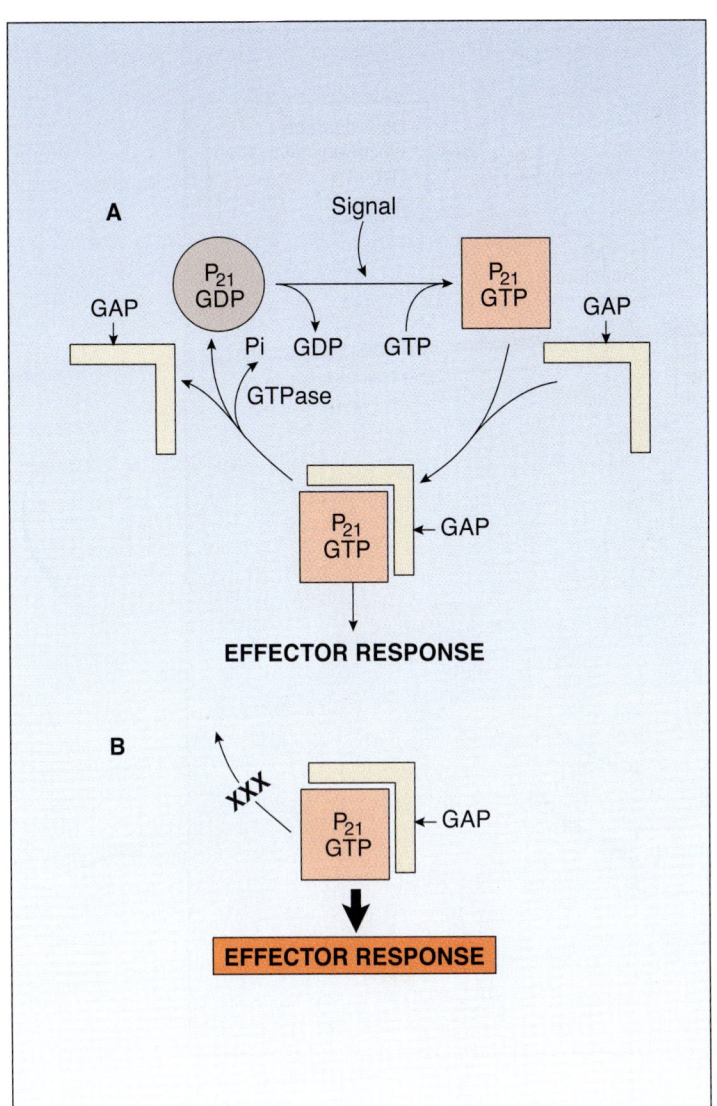

FIGURE 5-28
Mechanism of action of *ras* oncogene. A. Normal. The ras protein p21 exists in two conformational states, determined by the binding of either GDP or GTP. Normally, most of the p21 is in the inactive GDP-bound state. An external stimulus, or signal, triggers the exchange of GTP for GDP, an event that converts p21 to the active state. Activated p21, which is associated with the plasma membrane, binds GTPase-activating protein (GAP) from the cytosol. The binding of GAP has two consequences. In association with other plasma membrane constituents, it initiates the effector response. At the same time, the binding of GAP to p21 GTP stimulates by about 100-fold the intrinsic GTPase activity of p21, thereby promoting the hydrolysis of GTP to GDP and the return of p21 to its inactive state. B. Mutated ras protein is locked into the active GTP-bound state because of an insensitivity of its intrinsic GTPase to GAP or because of a lack of the GTPase activity itself. As a result the effector response is exaggerated, and the cell is transformed.

points in the cell cycle. For example, the binding of PDGF to cultured fibroblasts causes the cells to leave G_0 and enter the G_1 phase of the cell cycle. Shortly thereafter, several genes, including c-*myc*, c-*fos*, and c-*jun*, are expressed. Protooncogenes that are expressed early in the cell cycle, such as *myc* and *fos*, render the cells competent to receive the final signals for mitosis and are, therefore, termed **competence genes**. In general, competence genes play a role in (1) progression from G_1 to S phase in the cell cycle, (2) stability of the genome, (3) apoptosis, and (4) positive or negative effects on cellular maturation. However, the cells are not yet fully programmed to divide by the expression of these genes and will enter S phase and mitosis only after further stimulation by other factors, such as EGF or IGF-I (**progression factors**).

The proteins encoded by c-*fos* and c-*jun* are components of AP-1, a transcription factor that activates the expression of a variety of genes. Mutations of the jun protein eliminate a negative regulatory domain, thereby prolonging its half-life and stimulating progression through G_1. Few mutations of c-*jun* are described in human tumors, but overexpression of the protein has been described in lung and colorectal cancers.

Although nuclear proteins encoded by protooncogenes can promote cellular proliferation, in some circumstances, they stimulate differentiation. A rapid increase in c-*fos* expression follows the induction of differentiation in a variety of cells in vitro, including several hematopoietic cell lines and teratocarcinomas.

c-Myc is a nuclear protein that binds to a variety of other proteins and DNA to regulate gene transcription. Among other proteins, such targets include p53 and ornithine decarboxylase. As discussed above, the translocation characteristic of Burkitt lymphoma (t8:14) constitutively activates *myc* expression, and c-*myc* is also overexpressed in many human malignant tumors (e.g., adenocarcinoma of lung and breast).

Cell Cycle Control

The details of the cell cycle are discussed in Chapter 3. Briefly, cells enter the mitotic cycle by progression from G_0 to G_1 in response to growth factors and cytokines or progress directly from M phase into G_1 in actively dividing cells (Fig. 5-29). During G_1, a commitment to enter the S phase (the phase of DNA replication), is termed the restriction (R) point. The process is regulated by cyclins D and E, which in turn activate members of the cyclin-dependent protein kinases (Cdk) family. The activation of Cdk, which is regulated by specific in-

190   Neoplasia

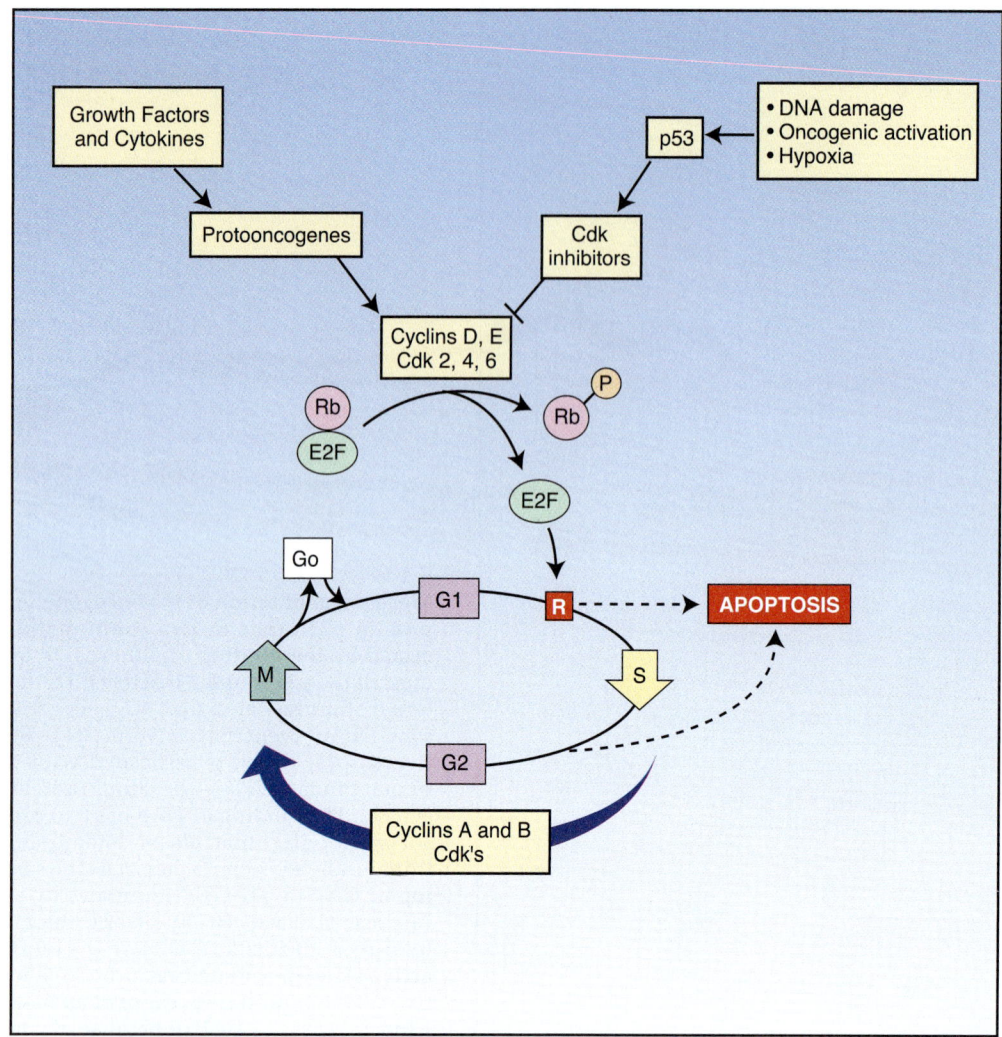

FIGURE 5-29
Regulation of the cell cycle. Cells are stimulated to enter G_1 from G_0 by growth factors and cytokines via protooncogene activation. A critical juncture in the transition of cells from G_1 to S phase is the restriction point (R). A major regulatory event in this process is the phosphorylation of Rb by cyclin-dependent kinases (cdks), which causes the release of the transcriptional activator E2F. Cdks are suppressed by cdk inhibitors that are regulated by p53. Tumor suppressor proteins block cell cycle progression largely within G_1. Interruption of cell cycle progression during G_1 and G_2 may lead to apoptosis as a default pathway. S, G_2, and M phases are also regulated by cyclins, cdks, and cdk inhibitors.

hibitors, leads to the phosphorylation of protein substrates involved in DNA replication. Importantly, Cdk 2, 4, and 6 phosphorylate retinoblastoma protein (pRb), which then unleashes transcription factors of the E2F family. E2F drives the cell past the R point. Other cyclins, Cdks, and their inhibitors regulate S to G_2 and G_2 to M transitions. Cdk inhibitors are regulated by the tumor suppressor protein p53 (see below). Cell cycle progression depends upon regulatory mechanisms that involve "check points," which ensure that the cell does not progress to mitosis until the S phase has been completed and that any DNA damage has been repaired. Blocks in cell cycle progression in G_1 and G_2 often lead to apoptosis as a default pathway. This phenomenon accounts for induction of tumor cell death in response to various chemotherapeutic agents.

Cancer cells often display a loss of R point control through mechanisms such as overexpression of cyclin D1, loss of Cdk inhibitors, or inactivation of the pRb or p53 proteins (see below). A cell in which the R point is no longer controlled tends to display constitutive (rather than regulated) progression through the cell cycle. For example, decreased levels of the Cdk inhibitor P27 are associated with a poor prognosis in adenocarcinoma of the colon and certain cancers of the lung. Conversely, a number of malignant tumors have been shown to overexpress several cyclins and Cdks.

Bcl-2 and Apoptosis

Normal tissue requires an exquisite balance between cell proliferation and cell death (apoptosis, see Chapter 1). Programmed cell death is affected through molecular cascades that reflect two major mechanisms. The **mitochondrial pathway** involves the release of cytochrome c, which serves to trigger caspase activation, thereby leading to cell death. A **death receptor pathway** is unleashed by binding of certain ligands (e.g., Fas, TNF) to cell surface receptors, which results in caspase activation. There is substantial cross-talk between the mitochondrial and the death receptor pathways.

Tumor cells can escape apoptosis by dismantling virtually every aspect of the apoptotic machinery. The most prominent example of suppression of apoptosis in a tumor cell is the upregulation of the antiapoptotic protein bcl-2 in B-cell neoplasia. Bcl-2 and its family regulate permeability of the mitochondrial membranes. Bcl-2 itself exerts an antiapoptotic effect by preventing the release of cytochrome c, thereby protecting the cell from the mitochondrial apoptotic pathway.

Follicular B-cell lymphomas (see Chapter 20) display a characteristic chromosomal translocation, t(14;18), in which the *bcl*-2 gene on chromosome 18 is brought under the transcriptional control of the immunoglobulin light-chain gene promoter, thereby causing overexpression of *bcl*-2. As a result of the antiapoptotic properties of bcl-2, the neoplastic clone accumulates in the affected lymph nodes. Since its demonstration in follicular lymphomas, *bcl*-2 expression has been observed in a variety of other human cancers and non-neoplastic conditions, although the contribution of *bcl*-2 to the disease process in these cases is not defined. Many human cancers show other abnormalities in the apoptotic cascades, including the increased expression of endogenous decoys of the death receptors, overexpression of proteins that block caspase activation, inactivating mutations of proapoptotic proteins, and numerous other mechanisms.

Tumor Suppressor Genes Negatively Regulate Cell Growth

The concept of oncogenes postulates a dominant genetic alteration that results in the overproduction of a normal gene product or the synthesis of an abnormally active mutant protein. A second general mechanism by which a genetic alteration contributes to carcinogenesis is a mutation that creates a deficiency of a normal gene product that exerts a negative regulatory control of cell growth and thereby suppresses tumor formation. Such genes encode negative transcriptional regulators of the cell cycle, signal-transducing molecules, and cell surface receptors. Since both alleles of such tumor suppressor genes ("gatekeeper" genes) must be inactivated to produce the deficit that allows the development of a tumor, it is inferred that the normal suppressor gene is dominant. In this circumstance, the heterozygous state is sufficient to protect against cancer. **The loss of heterozygosity in a tumor suppressor gene by deletion or somatic mutation of the remaining normal allele predisposes to tumor development.**

The Role of Tumor Suppressor Genes in Carcinogenesis

Tumor suppressor genes are increasingly being incriminated in the pathogenesis of both hereditary and spontaneous cancers in humans. Two such genes have been particularly well studied. The retinoblastoma (Rb) and p53 gene products serve to restrain cell division in many tissues, and their absence or inactivation is linked to the development of malignant tumors (see Fig. 5-29). Oncogenic DNA viruses also encode products that interact with these suppressor proteins, thereby inactivating their functions. **Thus, the mechanisms underlying the development of some tumors associated with germ line and somatic mutations and infections with DNA viruses involve the same cellular gene products.**

The Retinoblastoma Gene

Retinoblastoma, a rare childhood cancer, is the prototype of a human tumor whose origin is attributed to the inactivation of a specific tumor suppressor gene. About 40% of cases are associated with a germ line mutation; the remainder are not hereditary. In patients with hereditary retinoblastoma, all somatic cells carry one missing or mutated allele of a gene (the *Rb* gene) located on the long arm of chromosome 13. By contrast, both alleles of the *Rb* gene are inactive in all the retinoblastoma cells. Thus, the *Rb* gene exerts a tumor suppressor function, and the development of hereditary retinoblastoma has been attributed to two genetic events (Knudson's "two-hit" hypothesis) (Fig. 5-30). As mentioned above, the nuclear protein p105Rb is phosphorylated by the activated cyclin/cdk complex, which induces the release of E2F transcription factor, thereby allowing G_1–S phase transition. Additionally, certain products of human DNA viruses (e.g., human papillomavirus) inactivate p105Rb by binding to it. **The function of Rb is the most critical checkpoint in the cell cycle, and inactivating mutations in *Rb* permit unregulated cell proliferation.**

An affected child inherits one defective *Rb* allele together with one normal gene. This heterozygous state is not associated with any observable changes in the retina, presumably because 50% of the *Rb* gene product is sufficient to prevent the development of retinoblastoma. If the remaining normal *Rb* allele is inactivated by deletion or mutation, the loss of its suppressor function leads to the appearance of a retinoblastoma. Thus, the susceptibility to retinoblastoma is inherited in a dominant fashion; that is, the heterozygote develops the disease. Paradoxically, the genetic defect in the tumor itself is recessive. In sporadic cases of retinoblastoma, the child begins life with two normal *Rb* alleles in all somatic cells, but both are inactivated by postzygotic mutations in the retina. Since somatic mutations in the *Rb* gene are uncommon, the incidence of sporadic retinoblastoma is very low (1/30,000).

Children who inherit a mutant *Rb* gene also suffer a 200-fold increased risk of developing mesenchymal tumors in early adult life. More than 20 different cancers have been described, with osteosarcoma being by far the most common. Chromosomal analysis has demonstrated abnormalities of the *Rb* locus in 70% of cases of osteosarcoma and in many instances of small cell lung cancer, carcinomas of the breast, bladder, pancreas, and other human tumors.

The *p53* Gene

The *p53* gene is located on the small arm of chromosome 17, and its protein product is present in virtually all normal tissues. This gene is deleted or mutated in 75% of cases of colorectal cancer and frequently in breast cancer, small cell carcinoma of the lung, hepatocellular carcinoma, astrocytoma,

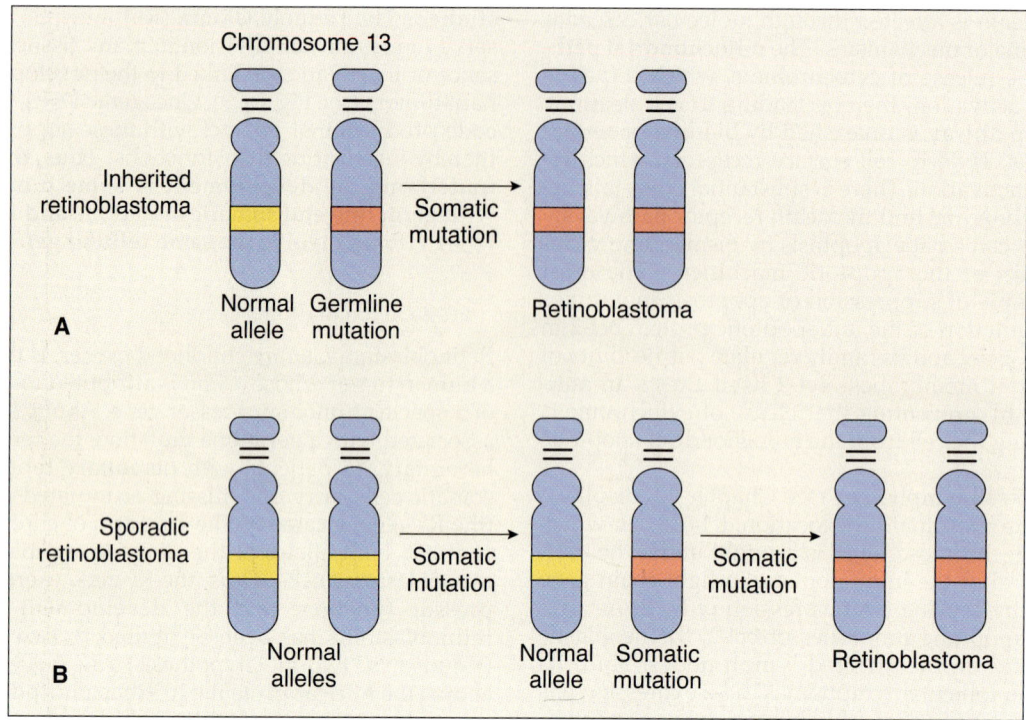

FIGURE 5-30
The "two-hit" origin of retinoblastoma. A. A child with the inherited form of retinoblastoma is born with a germ line mutation in one allele of the retinoblastoma gene located on the long arm of chromosome 13. A second somatic mutation in the retina leads to the inactivation of the functioning *Rb* allele and the subsequent development of a retinoblastoma. B. In sporadic cases of retinoblastoma, the child is born with two normal *Rb* alleles. It requires two independent somatic mutations to inactivate *Rb* gene function and allow the appearance of a neoplastic clone.

and numerous other tumors. **In fact, mutations of *p53* seem to be the most common genetic change in human cancer.**

The p53 molecule is a negative regulator of cell division. In response to DNA damage, oncogenic activation of other proteins, and other stresses (e.g., hypoxia), p53 levels rise and prevent cells from entering the S phase of the cell cycle, thereby allowing time for DNA repair to take place. In this way, p53 acts as a guardian of the genome by restricting uncontrolled cellular proliferation under circumstances in which cells with abnormal DNA might propagate. Inactivating mutations of *p53* allow cells with damaged DNA to progress through the cell cycle.

Many human cancers exhibit deletion of both *p53* alleles, in which case the cell contains no *p53* gene product. By contrast, in some cancers, the malignant cells express one normal *p53* allele and one mutant version. In these cases, the mutant p53 protein forms complexes with the normal p53 protein and thereby inactivates the function of the normal suppressor gene. When a mutant allele inactivates the normal one, the mutant allele is said be a *dominant negative* gene. Theoretically, a cell containing one mutant *p53* allele (i.e., a heterozygote) might have a growth advantage over the normal cells, a situation that would increase the number of cells at risk for a second mutation (loss of heterozygosity) and the development of cancer.

The p53 protein is a transcriptional factor that promotes both the expression of a number of other genes involved in the control of cell cycle progression and apoptosis (see Fig. 5-29). DNA damage and other stresses (e.g., hypoxia) upregulate the expression of *p53*, which in turn enhances the synthesis of CIP1. The latter inactivates cyclin/cdk complexes, thereby leading to cell arrest at the G_1/S checkpoint. Cells arrested at this checkpoint may either repair the DNA damage and then reenter the cycle or they may undergo apoptosis. The stimulation of gene transcription by p53 results in the synthesis of proteins (CIP1, GADD45) that enhance DNA repair by binding to PCNA. In this manner, the upregulation of p53 has two important and related consequences, namely, arresting cell cycle progression and augmenting DNA repair.

Negative regulation of p53 is accomplished by its binding to MDM2 (murine double minute 2) protein. The formation of the MDM2-p53 complex not only inhibits the function of p53 but also targets it for degradation via the ubiquitin pathway. In turn, MDM2 is inhibited by binding to ARF (p14), a protein that is upregulated by any oncogenic stimulus (e.g., *myc*, *ras*, loss of *Rb*) that induces *Rb* phosphorylation and enhances E2F activity. The function of ARF, which maintains the integrity of p53 establishes *ARF* as another tumor suppressor gene. Some cancers in which both *p53* alleles are normal overexpress MDM2, whereas others do not express functional ARF. As in the case of *Rb*, certain DNA tumor viral products, including human papillomavirus E6, promote p53 degradation. Thus, most human cancers display either inactivating mutations of *p53* or abnormalities in the proteins that regulate p53 activity.

Li-Fraumeni syndrome refers to an inherited predisposition to develop cancers in many organs owing to germ line mutations of *p53*. Persons with this condition carry germ line mutations in one *p53* allele, but their tumors display mutations at both alleles. This situation is similar to that determining inherited retinoblastoma and is another example of the two-hit hypothesis.

Other Tumor Suppressor Genes

A number of unrelated syndromes have now been shown to harbor germ line mutations in various tumor suppressor genes.

- *APC* gene: This gene is implicated in the pathogenesis of familial adenomatous polyposis coli and most sporadic colorectal cancers (see Chapter 13). The *APC* gene product binds to, and inhibits, the function of β-catenin, an intracellular protein that transmits signals from E-cadherin cell surface adhesion proteins. β-Catenin activates certain transcription factors (e.g., tcf/crf-1) that activate several genes, including *myc* and cyclin D, which are involved in cell cycle progression. The products of mutant *APC* genes do not bind to β-catenin and are unable to downregulate its activity. As a result, the expression of *myc* and cyclin D1 is not appropriately repressed, thereby promoting cell proliferation. Further evidence for this mechanism of action comes from the observation that many colorectal tumors in which the *APC* gene is intact exhibit activating mutations in the β-catenin gene. Mutations in both *APC* and β-catenin genes have also been described in other malignant tumors, including malignant melanoma and ovarian cancer.
- *WT-1* gene: The tumor suppressor gene *WT-1* is deleted in hereditary Wilms tumor (WT) and is essential for the normal development of the urogenital tract. It encodes a nuclear DNA-binding protein that represses transcription of a variety of genes whose products promote growth and survival, including *PDGF*, *IGF-I*, and *bcl-2*. Loss of *WT-1* gene expression also occurs in many breast cancers and a few other tumors that have been studied.
- *NF-1* gene: Neurofibromatosis (NF) type 1 is related to germ line mutations of the *NF-1* gene, which encodes *neurofibromin*, a negative regulator of *ras*. Inactivation of *NF-1* permits unopposed *ras* function and thereby promotes cell growth. Patients with neurofibromatosis-1 are at a substantial risk for the development of neurogenic sarcomas.
- *VHL* gene: The inactivation of the von Hippel-Lindau (*VHL*) gene causes the VHL syndrome, which is associated with renal cell carcinoma, hemangioblastoma of the brain, and pheochromocytoma. It is also a major gene involved in the pathogenesis of sporadic renal carcinomas. The normal VHL protein complexes with and inhibits elongin, a molecule that promotes transcriptional elongation of growth-promoting genes by RNA polymerases B and C.
- *FHIT* gene: The fragile histidine triad (FHIT) protein is a dinucleoside phosphate hydrolase that is a tumor suppressor. Deletions within the *FHIT* gene, which is found within a fragile chromosome region that is highly susceptible to DNA damage, are associated with cancers of the kidney, lung, digestive tract, and other organs. The mechanism by which loss of FHIT activity contributes to tumorigenesis remains to be elucidated, but the protein has been shown to be proapoptotic and growth suppressive.
- *p15* and *p16* genes: Inactivation of these genes has been identified primarily in breast, pancreas, and prostate tumors, and many other malignancies. The gene products are cdk inhibitors that serve as negative regulators of the cell cycle, and their loss removes a brake on cellular proliferation.
- *DPC4* gene: Some 90% of pancreatic carcinomas feature allelic loss or inactivating mutations in the *DPC4* (deleted in pancreatic cancer) gene. The normal DPC4 product is a transcriptional activator that mediates the growth inhibitory response to TGF-β.
- *BRCA1* and *BRCA2* genes: These breast (BR) cancer (CA) susceptibility genes, which are also incriminated in some ovarian cancers, are tumor suppressors that are involved in checkpoint functions of the cell cycle related to progression of the cell cycle into S phase, particularly by inducing the CDK inhibitor p21. BRAC1 and BRAC2 are also thought to promote DNA repair by binding to RAD51, a molecule that mediates DNA double-strand break repairs, thereby functioning as DNA repair genes (see below).
- *PTEN* gene: Termed the phosphatase and tensin homologue deleted on chromosome 10, this gene is mutated in most prostate cancers and many gliomas and thyroid cancers, as well as other tumors. The gene product suppresses tumor cell growth by antagonizing tyrosine kinases and may also regulate invasion and metastasis through interactions at focal adhesions. Germ line mutations in *PTEN* are responsible for *Cowden syndrome*, a disorder that includes multiple hamartomas and an increased risk of cancers of the breast, thyroid, and endometrium.

Tumor Suppressor Genes and Oncogenic DNA Viruses

Unlike RNA tumor viruses, whose oncogenes have normal cellular counterparts, the transforming genes of DNA viruses are not homologous with any cellular genes. This conundrum was resolved with the discoveries that linked the gene products of oncogenic DNA viruses to the inactivation of tumor suppressor proteins. This phenomenon is analogous to the ability of mutant tumor suppressor proteins to inhibit their normal counterparts. Furthermore, the binding of a human papillomavirus protein to p53 accelerates the degradation of this suppressor protein. It is now recognized that the transforming proteins of polyomaviruses (including SV40), adenoviruses, and human papillomaviruses inactivate both the Rb and p53 proteins by binding to these tumor suppressors. These observations indicate that oncogenic DNA viruses use a common mechanism for altering growth regulation and, thereby, transforming cells.

DNA Methylation Is an Epigenetic Factor in Cancer

DNA methylation represents a regulatory layer for gene transcription. The principal mechanism is the methylation of cytosines within CpG dinucleotides, which occur five times more frequently in so-called CpG islands. These regions span the promoter and the first few exons of more than half of all genes. Methylation of these sequences suppresses gene transcription or maintains prior gene silencing by blocking the binding of transcription factors. Normal methylation of CpG islands is reported in the cases of imprinted genes, inactivated female X chromosomes, germ line genes, and tissue-specific genes. In addition, methylation in the human genome is thought to silence "parasite DNA" such as transposons and endogenous retroviruses, thereby preventing chromosomal instability.

Hypermethylation of many tumor suppressor and DNA repair genes has been demonstrated in human tumors, including the p53 pathway, the APC/β catenin/E-cadherin signaling network, and a number of mismatched DNA repair genes. The pathways controlled by these genes are, therefore, suppressed. For example, about half of human cancers retain unaltered p53. However, the p53 pathway can be inactivated by hypermethylation of *ARF*, thereby preventing inhibition of MDM2 oncogenic protein and the enhancement of p53 degradation. **In this context, aberrant methylation of tumor suppressor genes may be an epigenetic mechanism for a "second hit," thereby leading to loss of heterozygosity.**

The genome of cancer cells also undergoes conspicuous global *hypomethylation*, which may be reflected in up to 60% less DNA methylation than in the normal cell. Gene hypomethylation may lead to chromosomal instability, derepression of growth regulatory genes, and overexpression of antiapoptotic genes. Unlike genetic changes in cancer, epigenetic changes are potentially reversible, and a search for drugs that influence DNA methylation is under way.

Histone acetylation and deacetylation play important roles in transcriptional regulation by modifying chromatin structure. A high degree of histone acetylation is associated with enhanced transcriptional activity, whereas deacetylation is linked to gene silencing. The yin and yang of acetylation and deacetylation of chromatin are fundamental to the process of cell growth. Experimentally, inhibitors of histone deacetylases arrest tumor growth and prevent the progression of metastases. They also promote apoptosis in animal models of leukemia. Although the precise mechanism of action is not clear, such inhibitors have found a role in the treatment of human acute promyelocytic leukemia and lymphoproliferative diseases.

DNA Repair Genes Protect the Integrity of the Genome

The third class of genes in which mutations contribute to the pathogenesis of cancer are genes involved in DNA mismatch repair, or so-called *mutator genes* or *caretaker genes*. The human genome contains roughly 3×10^9 base pairs, distributed evenly among some 10^{14} cells in the body. Considering that DNA is continuously assaulted by mutagenic agents such as radiation, oxidative stress, and chemicals, and that the fidelity of DNA replication is not perfect, it is indeed remarkable that cancer arises in only about one third of the population. In general, the normal versions of the DNA repair genes exercise surveillance over the integrity of genetic information by participating in the cellular response to DNA damage. In this respect, DNA repair genes may be considered "caretaker genes." The loss of these gene functions renders the DNA susceptible to the progressive accumulation of mutations; when these affect protooncogenes or tumor suppressor genes, cancer may result.

HEREDITARY NONPOLYPOSIS COLON CANCER (HNPCC): Also known as Lynch syndrome, HNPCC is a familial predisposition to the development of colorectal cancers in persons who do not suffer from APC (see Chapter 13). It is estimated that some 5% of all colorectal cancers fall into this category. Patients with HNPCC display heterozygous germ line mutations in at least one of five genes involved in the DNA mismatch repair system, whereas the tumors have lost the function of both alleles in the affected gene. After DNA replication is complete, this system leads to the excision and replacement of mismatched nucleotides. Mutations in these error correction genes are associated with up to a 1000-fold general increase in the rate of mutation. Replication errors, termed *microsatellite instability,* are present in the tumor DNA of patients with HNPCC, which arises from uncorrected mispairing of nucleotides and the resulting misalignment of DNA strands. The incidence of cancers of the stomach and small bowel is also increased in patients with HNPCC, and women with this syndrome display an increased risk for endometrial and ovarian cancers.

ATAXIA TELANGIECTASIA: Ataxia telangiectasia (AT) is a rare hereditary syndrome that features cerebellar degeneration, immunological abnormalities, oculocutaneous telangiectasia, and a predisposition to cancer, including lymphomas, leukemias, stomach cancer, and breast cancer. About 15% of patients with this syndrome eventually die from a malignant disease. The gene responsible for AT (AT mutated [*ATM*]), located on chromosome 11q22-q23, codes for a nuclear phosphoprotein that participates in multiple responses to DNA damage, including control of checkpoints in the cell cycle, activation of DNA repair enzymes, and regulation of apoptosis. There is evidence that heterozygous mutations in *ATM* increase the risk of breast cancer in women. In view of a carrier rate of 1% in the general population, it has been suggested that *ATM* mutations may contribute to a significant number of sporadic breast cancers.

XERODERMA PIGMENTOSUM: Xeroderma pigmentosum is an autosomal recessive disease in which increased sensitivity to sunlight is accompanied by a high incidence of skin cancers, including basal cell carcinoma, squamous cell carcinoma, and malignant melanoma. Several xeroderma pigmentosum genes have been identified that are involved in nucleotide excision of UV-damaged DNA.

BLOOM SYNDROME: Bloom syndrome (BS) is an autosomal recessive disorder associated with small size, sun sensitivity, immunodeficiency, and a predisposition to an array of cancers. Cells from BS patients show a high mutation frequency. The BS gene encodes for a protein that has helicase activity involved in repair of DNA damage.

Telomerase Is Activated in Most Cancers

As cells in tissue culture continue to divide, the tips of the chromosomes, termed *telomeres,* progressively shorten (see Chapter 1). These structures are thought to protect the integrity of the DNA at the ends of the chromosomes, possibly by preventing exonuclease attack on these regions. Somatic cells do not normally express telomerase, an enzyme that recognizes the end of a chromosome and adds repetitive telomeric sequences to maintain the length of the telomere. Thus, with each round of cell replication, the telomere progressively shortens. It has been proposed that the length of the telomeres acts as a molecular clock that governs the life span of replicating cells. Since cancer cells have been found to express telomerase, the reactivation of this enzyme is said to be necessary for the immortalization of cancer cells.

Most human cancers show activation of the gene for the catalytic subunit of telomerase, hTERT (human telomerase reverse transcriptase). Although deregulated expression of telomerase might be linked to an increased risk of cancer, telomerase is not classified as an oncogene because it does not lead to growth deregulation. Many immortalized cell lines that express telomerase show no evidence of neoplastic capacity. Thus, despite extensive research in the field, the role of telomerase in oncogenesis remains controversial.

Inherited Cancer Syndromes Encompass a Wide Variety of Tumors

Heritable cancer syndromes attributed to germ line mutations make up only 1% of all cancers. These mutations principally involve tumor suppressor genes and DNA repair genes. As previously discussed for *Rb*, the transmission of a single mutated allele of a tumor suppressor gene results in a heterozygous offspring. Since such persons are at a high risk for loss of heterozygosity (i.e., inactivation of the normal allele), they suffer a conspicuous susceptibility to various types of cancer. Thus, inheritance of cancer susceptibility in such cases is said to be dominant. However, in the tumor cells, both tumor suppressor alleles are inactivated. By contrast, a number of inherited cancer syndromes, mostly involving DNA repair genes, display classical recessive inheritance.

The hereditary tumors can be arbitrarily divided into three categories: (1) inherited malignant tumors (e.g., retinoblastoma, Wilms tumor, and many endocrine tumors), (2) benign inherited tumors that remain benign or have a malignant potential (e.g., APC), and (3) inherited syndromes associated with a high risk of malignant tumors (e.g., Bloom syndrome and AT). Most of these are discussed in detail in the chapters dealing with specific organs, and selected examples are given in Table 5-2. In many cases, the underlying genetic defect responsible for the tumor development has been identified. Some disorders that are difficult to classify, called **phacomatoses** (e.g., tuberous sclerosis, neurofibromatosis), have both developmental and neoplastic features. The tumors associated with these syndromes mostly involve the nervous system.

Although only a small proportion of all cancers show a mendelian pattern of inheritance, certain cancers exhibit an undeniable tendency to run in families. It is estimated that in the case of many tumors, other members of the family of an affected person have a twofold to threefold increase in the risk of developing the same cancer. This predisposition is particularly marked for cancer of the breast and colon. The interplay of heredity and environment is exemplified by the case of lung cancer. Smokers who are closely related to a person with lung cancer have a higher risk of developing lung cancer themselves than smokers without this familial background. **The genomic mechanisms underlying the development of neoplasia are summarized in Figure 5-31.**

VIRUSES AND HUMAN CANCER

Despite the existence of viral oncogenes, the number of human cancers definitely associated with viral infections is limited. Nevertheless, it is estimated that viral infections are responsible for 15% of all human cancers. The strongest associations between the presence of viruses and the development of cancer in humans are (1) the RNA retrovirus human T-cell leukemia virus type I and T-cell leukemia/lymphoma, (2) human papillomavirus (DNA) and carcinoma of the cervix, (3) hepatitis B virus (DNA) and hepatitis C virus (RNA) and primary hepatocellular carcinoma, (4) Epstein-Barr virus and certain forms of lymphoma and nasopharyngeal carcinoma, and (5) human herpesvirus 8 (DNA) and Kaposi sarcoma. Worldwide, infections with hepatitis B virus and human papillomaviruses alone account for 80% of all virus-associated cancers.

Human T-Cell Leukemia Virus-I (HTLV-I) Is a Lymphotropic Agent

The one human cancer that has been firmly linked to infection with an RNA retrovirus is the rare adult T-cell leukemia, which is endemic in southern Japan and the Caribbean basin and occurs sporadically in other parts of the world. The etiological agent, HTLV-I, is tropic for $CD4^+$ T lymphocytes and has also been incriminated in the pathogenesis of a number of neurological disorders. It is estimated that leukemia develops in less than 5% of persons infected with HTLV-I and exhibits a latency period on the order of 40 years for the its development. A closely related virus, HTLV-II, has been associated with only a few cases of lymphoproliferative disorders.

The HTLV-I genome contains no known oncogene and does not integrate at specific sites within the host genome. Oncogenic stimulation by HTLV-I is mediated principally by the viral transcriptional activation protein *tax*. Tax protein not only increases the transcription from its own viral genome, but also promotes the activity of other genes involved in cell proliferation. These include genes that code for IL-2 and its receptor, granulocyte macrophage colony-stimulating factor (GM-CSF), and the protooncogenes c-*fos* and c-*sis*. Lymphocyte transformation in vitro by HTLV-I is initially polyclonal and only later monoclonal. Tax therefore probably initiates transformation, but additional genetic events are required for the appearance of the complete malignant phenotype.

DNA Viruses Encode Proteins That Bind Regulatory Proteins

Four DNA viruses (human papillomavirus, Epstein-Barr virus, hepatitis B virus, and herpesvirus 8) are incriminated in the development of human cancers. The transforming genes of oncogenic DNA viruses exhibit virtually no homology with cellular genes, whereas those of retroviruses (oncogenes) are derived from, and are homologous with, their cellular counterparts (protooncogenes). As discussed above, oncogenic DNA viruses have genes that encode protein products that bind to, and inactivate, specific host proteins (the products of tumor suppressor genes, e.g., *Rb*, *p53*) involved in the regulation of cell proliferation and apoptosis.

Neoplasia

TABLE 5-2 Selected Hereditary Conditions Associated with an Increased Risk of Cancer

Syndrome	Gene	Predominant Malignancies	Gene Function	Inheritance[a]
Chromosomal instablility syndromes				
Bloom syndrome	BLM	Many sites	DNA repair	R
Fanconi anemia	?	Acute myelogenous leukemia	DNA repair	R
Hereditary skin cancer				
Familial melanoma	CDKN2 (p16)	Malignant melanoma	Cell cycle regulation	D
Xeroderma pigmentosum	XP group	Squamous cell carcinoma of skin; malignant melanoma	DNA repair	R
Endocrine system				
Hereditary paraganglioma and pheochromocytoma	SDHD	Paraganglioma; pheochromocytoma	Oxygen sensing and signaling	D
Multiple endocrine neoplasia (MEN) type 1	MEN1	Pancreatic islet cell tumors	Transcriptional regulation	D
Multiple endocrine neoplasia (MEN) type 2	RET	Thyroid medullary carcinoma; Pheochromocytoma (MEN type 2A)	Receptor tyrosine kinase; cell cycle regulation	D
Breast cancer				
Breast/ovary cancer syndrome	BRCA1	Carcinomas of ovary, breat and prostate	DNA repair	D
Site-specific breast cancer	BRCA2	Female and male breast carcinoma; carcinomas of prostate, pancreas and ovary	DNA repair	D
Nervous system				
Retinoblastoma	RB	Retinoblastoma	Cell cycle regulation	D
Phacomatoses				
Neurofibromatosis type 1	NF1	Neurofibrosarcomas; astrocytomas; malignant melanomas	Regulator of *ras*-mediated signaling	D
Neurofibromatosis type 2	NF2	Meningiomas; schwannomas	Regulator of cytoskeleton	D
Tuberous sclerosis	TSC1	Renal cell carcinoma; astrocytoma	Regulator of cytoskeleton	D
Gastrointestinal system				
Familial adenomatous polyposis	APC	Colorectal carcinoma	Cell cycle regulation; migration and adhesion	D
Hereditary nonpolyposis colorectal carcinoma (HNPCC)	hMSH2 hMSH6 hMLH1 hPMS1 hPMS2	Carcinomas of colon, endometrium, ovary, and bladder; malignant melanoma.	DNA repair	D
Juvenile polyposis coli	SMAD4 DPC4	Colorectal carcinoma; endometrial carcinoma	TGFβ signaling	D
Kidney				
Hereditary papillary renal cell carcinoma	MET	Papillary renal cell carcinoma	Receptor tyrosine kinase; cell cycle regulation	D
Wilms tumor	WT	Wilms tumor	Transcriptional regulation	D
Von Hippel-Lindau	VHL	Renal cell carcinoma	Regulator of adhesion	D
Multiple sites				
Carney complex	PRKARIA	Testicular neoplasms; thyroid carcinoma	CAMP signaling	D
Cowden syndrome	PTEN	Colorectal, breast, and thyroid carcinomas	Protein tyrosine phosphatase	D
Li-Fraumeni syndrome	TP53	Breast carcinoma; soft tissue sarcomas; brain tumors; leukemia	Transcriptional regulation	D
Werner syndrome	WRN	Soft tissue sarcomas	DNA repair	R
Ataxia-telangiectasia	ATM	Lymphoma; leukemia	Cell signaling and DNA repair	R

[a] D, autosomal dominant; R, autosomal recessive

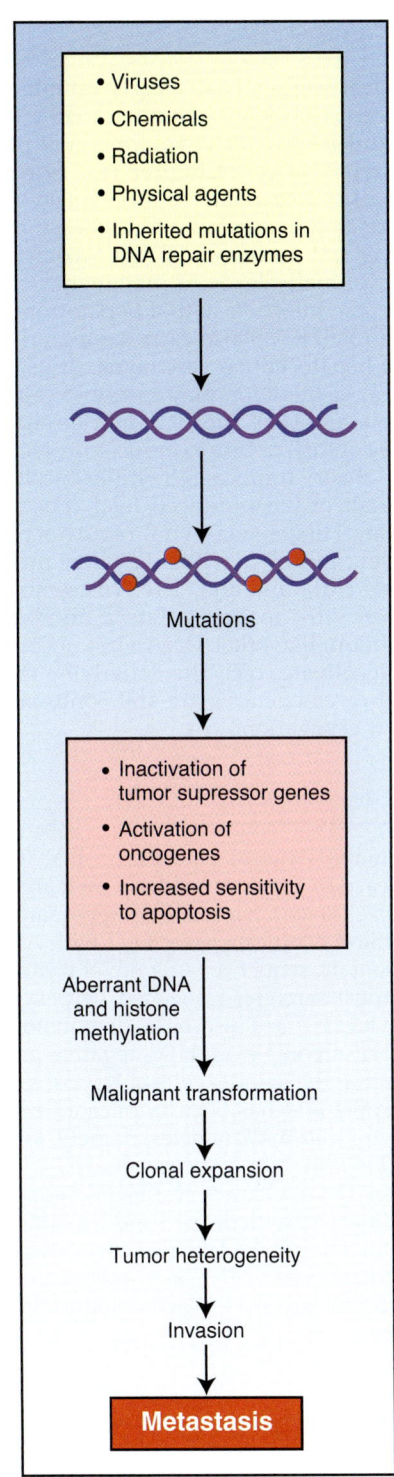

FIGURE 5-31
Summary of the genomic mechanisms of cancer.

Human Papillomaviruses

Human papillomaviruses (HPVs) induce lesions in humans that progress to squamous cell carcinoma. Papillomaviruses manifest a pronounced tropism for epithelial tissues, and their full productive life cycle occurs only in squamous cells. More than 80 distinct HPVs have been identified, and most are associated with benign lesions of squamous epithelium, including warts, laryngeal papillomas, and condylomata acuminata (genital warts) of the vulva, penis, and perianal region. Occasionally, condylomata acuminata and laryngeal papillomas undergo malignant transformation to squamous cell carcinoma. Although warts of the skin invariably remain benign, in a rare hereditary disease termed *epidermodysplasia verruciformis*, HPV produces flat warts that commonly progress to squamous carcinoma. At least 20 HPV types are associated with cancer of the uterine cervix, especially HPV 16 and 18 (see Chapter 18).

The major oncoproteins encoded by HPV are E6 and E7. E6 binds to p53 and targets it for degradation. E7 binds to Rb, thereby releasing its inhibitory effect on cell cycle progression. During the last half century, a cell line derived from cervical cancer, termed *HeLa cells*, has maintained worldwide popularity in the study of cancer. Interestingly, these cells have been found to express HPV-18 E6 and E7, and inactivation of these oncoproteins results in growth arrest. Thus after many years growing in vitro in innumerable laboratories, these cancer cells remain dependent on the expression of HPV proteins.

Epstein-Barr Virus

Epstein-Barr virus (EBV) is a human herpesvirus that is so widely disseminated that 95% of adults in the world have antibodies to it. EBV infects B lymphocytes, transforming them into lymphoblasts with an indefinite life span. In a small proportion of primary infections with EBV, this lymphoblastoid transformation is manifested as infectious mononucleosis (see Chapter 9), a short-lived lymphoproliferative disease. However, EBV is also intimately associated with the development of certain human cancers.

When B lymphocytes are infected with EBV, they acquire the ability to proliferate indefinitely in vitro. A number of EBV genes are implicated in this lymphocyte immortalization, including Epstein-Barr nuclear antigens (EBNAs) and latent-infection-associated membrane proteins (LMPs). The EBNAs maintain the EBV genome in its episomal state and activate the transcription of viral and cellular genes. LMP1 interacts with cellular proteins that normally transduce signals from the TNF receptor, a critical pathway in lymphocyte activation and proliferation. Both EBNAs and LMPs can be demonstrated in most EBV-associated cancers.

BURKITT LYMPHOMA: EBV was the first virus to be unequivocally linked to the development of a human tumor. In 1958, Burkitt described a form of childhood lymphoma in a geographical belt across equatorial Africa, which he suggested might have a viral etiology. A few years later, Epstein and Barr discovered viral particles in cell lines cultured from patients with Burkitt lymphoma.

African Burkitt lymphoma is a B-cell tumor, in which the neoplastic lymphocytes invariably contain EBV in their DNA and manifest EBV-related antigens (see Chapter 20). The tumor has also been recognized in non-African populations, but in those cases, only about 20% contain the EBV genome. The localization of Burkitt lymphoma to equatorial Africa is not understood, but it has been suggested that prolonged stimulation of the immune system by endemic malaria may be important. Under normal circumstances, the EBV-stimulated B-lymphocyte proliferation is controlled by suppressor T cells. The lack of an adequate T-cell response often reported in chronic malarial infections might result in uncontrolled B-cell proliferation, thereby providing the background for further genetic events that lead to the development of lymphoma. As discussed above, one of these is known to be a chromosomal translocation, in which the *c-myc* protooncogene is deregulated by being brought into proximity with an immunoglobulin promoter region. A postulated sequence in the multistep pathogenesis of African Burkitt lymphoma is as follows:

1. Infection and polyclonal lymphoblastoid transformation of B lymphocytes by EBV
2. Proliferation of B cells and inhibition of suppressor T cells induced by malaria
3. Deregulation of the *c-myc* protooncogene by chromosomal translocation in a single transformed B lymphocyte
4. Uncontrolled proliferation of a malignant clone of B lymphocytes

POLYCLONAL LYMPHOPROLIFERATION IN IMMUNODEFICIENT STATES: Congenital or acquired immunodeficiency states can be complicated by the development of EBV-induced B-cell proliferative disorders. These lesions may be clinically and pathologically indistinguishable from true malignant lymphomas, but they differ in that most of them are polyclonal. The incidence of lymphoid neoplasia in immunosuppressed renal transplant recipients is 30 to 50 times that of the general population. In virtually all cases of lymphoproliferations associated with organ transplantation, EBNA or EBV genomic material is present in the neoplastic tissue. Similar B-cell lymphoproliferative disorders are seen in a number of other acquired immunodeficiencies, notably, AIDS. Occasionally, a true monoclonal lymphoma may develop in the background of an EBV-induced lymphoproliferative disorder. As in the case of Burkitt lymphoma, the deficiency of T cells directed against EBV-infected B cells permits the survival of the latter.

Congenital immunodeficiency states, including X-linked lymphoproliferative syndrome (XLP), Wiskott-Aldrich syndrome, and ataxia telangiectasia, are associated with EBV infections and aggressive lymphoproliferations. In the familial disorder XLP, clinical immunodeficiency is commonly inapparent until the onset of a particularly severe, and often fatal, form of infectious mononucleosis. In many of these patients who survive infectious mononucleosis, lymphoproliferative disorders and lymphomas ensue. Patients with XLP lack EBV-specific immune responses, including the formation of cytotoxic T cells that normally eliminate EBV-infected B cells.

NASOPHARYNGEAL CARCINOMA: Nasopharyngeal carcinoma is a variant of squamous cell carcinoma that has a worldwide distribution and is particularly common in certain parts of Africa and Asia. EBV DNA and EBNA are present in virtually all of these cancers. It is thought that epithelial cells are exposed to EBV by lysis of infected lymphocytes traveling through lymphoid-rich epithelium. The pathogenesis of nasopharyngeal carcinoma may be related to infection with EBV in early childhood, with reactivation at 40 to 50 years of age and the appearance of tumors 1 to 2 years thereafter. Fortunately, 70% of patients with this disease are cured by radiation therapy alone.

Hepatitis B Virus

Epidemiological studies have clearly established an association between chronic infection with HBV (chronic hepatitis and cirrhosis) and the development of primary hepatocellular carcinoma (see Chapter 14). Two mechanisms have been invoked to explain the mechanism of carcinogenesis in HBV-related liver cancer. One theory holds that the continued liver cell proliferation that accompanies chronic liver injury eventually leads to malignant transformation. Similarly, chronic infection with a hepatotropic RNA virus (hepatitis C virus [HCV]) also carries a high risk for the development of hepatocellular carcinoma. Thus, chronic liver cell injury and regeneration may suffice to cause hepatocellular carcinoma, and HBV and HCV may be oncogenic in humans by virtue of their ability to induce chronic liver disease.

A second theory implicates a virally encoded protein in the pathogenesis of HBV-induced liver cancer. Transgenic mice expressing HBx, a small viral regulatory protein, also developed liver cancer, but without evident preexisting liver cell injury and inflammation. The *HBx* gene product has been shown in vitro to upregulate a number of cellular genes. In addition, like other DNA viral oncoproteins, HBx binds to and inactivates p53. The underlying mechanisms in HBV-induced carcinogenesis are still controversial and require further investigation.

Human Herpesvirus 8 (HHV 8)

Kaposi sarcoma is a vascular neoplasm that was originally described in eastern European elderly men and later in central African blacks (see Chapter 10). Kaposi sarcoma is today the most common neoplasm associated with AIDS. The neoplastic cells contain sequences of a novel virus HHV 8, also known as Kaposi sarcoma-associated herpesvirus (KSHV). Interestingly, HHV 8 has also been demonstrated in specimens of Kaposi sarcoma from HIV-negative patients. In addition to infecting the spindle cells of Kaposi sarcoma, HHV 8 is lymphotropic and has been implicated in two uncommon B-cell lymphoid malignancies, namely, *primary effusion lymphoma* and *multicentric Castleman disease*.

Like other DNA viruses, the HHV8 genome encodes proteins that interfere with the p53 and RB tumor suppressor pathways. Interestingly, HHV8 also encodes gene products that downregulate class I MHC expression, a mechanism by which the infected cells may evade recognition by cytotoxic T lymphocytes.

CHEMICAL CARCINOGENESIS

The field of chemical carcinogenesis originated some two centuries ago in descriptions of an occupational disease (this was not the first recognition of an occupation-related cancer, since a peculiar predisposition of nuns to breast cancer was appreciated even earlier). The English physician Sir Percival Pott gets credit for relating cancer of the scrotum in chimney sweeps to a specific chemical exposure, namely, soot. Interestingly, the great German pathologist Rudolf Virchow attributed these scrotal tumors to irritation rather than to chemicals. He persisted in this mistaken notion even though at about the same time the high incidence of skin cancer in some German workers had been ascribed to an exposure to coal tar, whose ingredients were known to be remarkably similar to those of soot. Almost a century elapsed between those observations and the realization that other products of the combustion of organic materials are responsible for a man-made epidemic of cancer, namely, cancer of the lung in cigarette smokers.

The experimental production of cancer by chemicals dates to 1915, when Japanese investigators produced skin cancers in rabbits with coal tar. Since that time, the list of organic and inorganic carcinogens has grown exponentially. Yet a curious paradox existed for many years. Many compounds known to be potent carcinogens are relatively inert in terms of chemical reactivity. **The solution to this riddle became apparent in the early 1960s, when it was shown that most, although not all, chemical carcinogens require metabolic activation before they can react with cell constituents.** On the basis of those observations and the close correlation between mutagenicity and carcinogenicity, an in vitro assay using *Salmonella* organisms for screening potential chemical carcinogens—the Ames test—was developed a decade later. Subsequently, a variety of assays for genotoxicity were developed and are still used to screen chemicals and new drugs for potential carcinogenicity.

Chemical Carcinogens Are Mostly Mutagens

Associations between exposure to a specific chemical and human cancers have historically been established on the basis of epidemiological investigations. These studies have numerous inherent disadvantages, including uncertainties in estimated doses, variability of the population, long and variable latency, and dependence on clinical and public health records of questionable accuracy. As an alternative to epidemiological studies, investigators turned to the use of studies involving animals. Indeed, such studies are legally required before the introduction of a new drug. Yet the logarithmic increase in the number of chemicals synthesized every year makes even this method prohibitively cumbersome and expensive. The search for rapid, reproducible, and reliable screening assays for potential carcinogenic activity has centered on the relationship between carcinogenicity and mutagenicity.

A mutagen is an agent that can permanently alter the genetic constitution of a cell. The Ames test uses the appearance of frameshift mutations and base-pair substitutions in a culture of bacteria of a *Salmonella* species. Mutations, unscheduled DNA synthesis, and DNA strand breaks are also detected in rat hepatocytes, mouse lymphoma cells, and Chinese hamster ovary cells. Cultured human cells are now used increasingly for assays of mutagenicity. About 90% of known carcinogens are mutagenic in these systems. Moreover, most, but not all, mutagens are carcinogenic. This close correlation between carcinogenicity and mutagenicity presumably occurs because both reflect damage to DNA. Although not infallible, the in vitro mutagenicity assay has proved to be a valuable tool in screening for the carcinogenic potential of chemicals.

Chemical Carcinogenesis Is a Multistep Process

Studies of chemical carcinogenesis in experimental animals have shed light on the individual stages in the progression of normal cells to cancer. Long before the genetic basis of cancer was appreciated, it was demonstrated that a single application of a carcinogen to the skin of a mouse was not, by itself, sufficient to produce cancer (Fig. 5-32). However, when a proliferative stimulus was then applied locally, in the form of a second, noncarcinogenic, irritating chemical (e.g., a phorbol ester), tumors appeared. The first effect was termed **initiation**. The action of the second, noncarcinogenic chemical was called **promotion**. Subsequently, further experiments in rodent models of a variety of organ-specific cancers (liver, skin, lung, pancreas, colon, etc.) expanded the concept of a two-stage mechanism to our present understanding of carcinogenesis as a multistep process that involves numerous mutations.

From these studies, one can abstract four stages of chemical carcinogenesis:

1. **Initiation** likely represents a mutation in a single cell.
2. **Promotion** follows initiation and reflects the clonal expansion of the initiated cell, in which the mutation has conferred a growth advantage. During promotion, the altered cells remain dependent on the continued presence of the promoting stimulus. This stimulus may be an exogenous chemical or physical agent or may reflect an endogenous mechanism (e.g., hormonal stimulation [breast, prostate] or the effect of bile salts [colon]).
3. **Progression** is the stage in which growth becomes autonomous (i.e., independent of the carcinogen or the promoter). By this time, sufficient mutations have accumulated to immortalize cells.
4. **Cancer,** the end result of the entire sequence, is established when the cells acquire the capacity to invade and metastasize.

The morphological changes that reflect multistep carcinogenesis in humans are best exemplified in epithelia, such as those of the skin, cervix, and colon. Although initiation has no morphological counterpart, promotion and progression are represented by the sequence of hyperplasia, dysplasia, and carcinoma in situ.

Chemical Carcinogens Usually Undergo Metabolic Activation

The International Agency for Research in Cancer (IARC) has listed about 75 chemicals as human carcinogens. Chemicals cause cancer either directly or, more often, after metabolic activation. The direct-acting carcinogens are inherently reactive enough to bind covalently to cellular macromolecules. In addition to a number of organic compounds, such as nitrogen mustard, *bis*(chloromethyl)ether, and benzyl chloride, certain metals are included in this category. Most organic carcinogens, however, require conversion to an ultimate, more reactive compound. This conversion is enzymatic and, for the most part, is effected by the cellular systems involved in drug metabolism and detoxification. Many cells in the body, particularly liver cells, possess enzyme systems that can convert procarcinogens to their active forms. Yet each carcinogen has its own spectrum of target tissues, often limited to a single organ. The basis for organ specificity in chemical carcinogenesis is not well understood.

POLYCYCLIC AROMATIC HYDROCARBONS: The polycyclic aromatic hydrocarbons, originally derived from

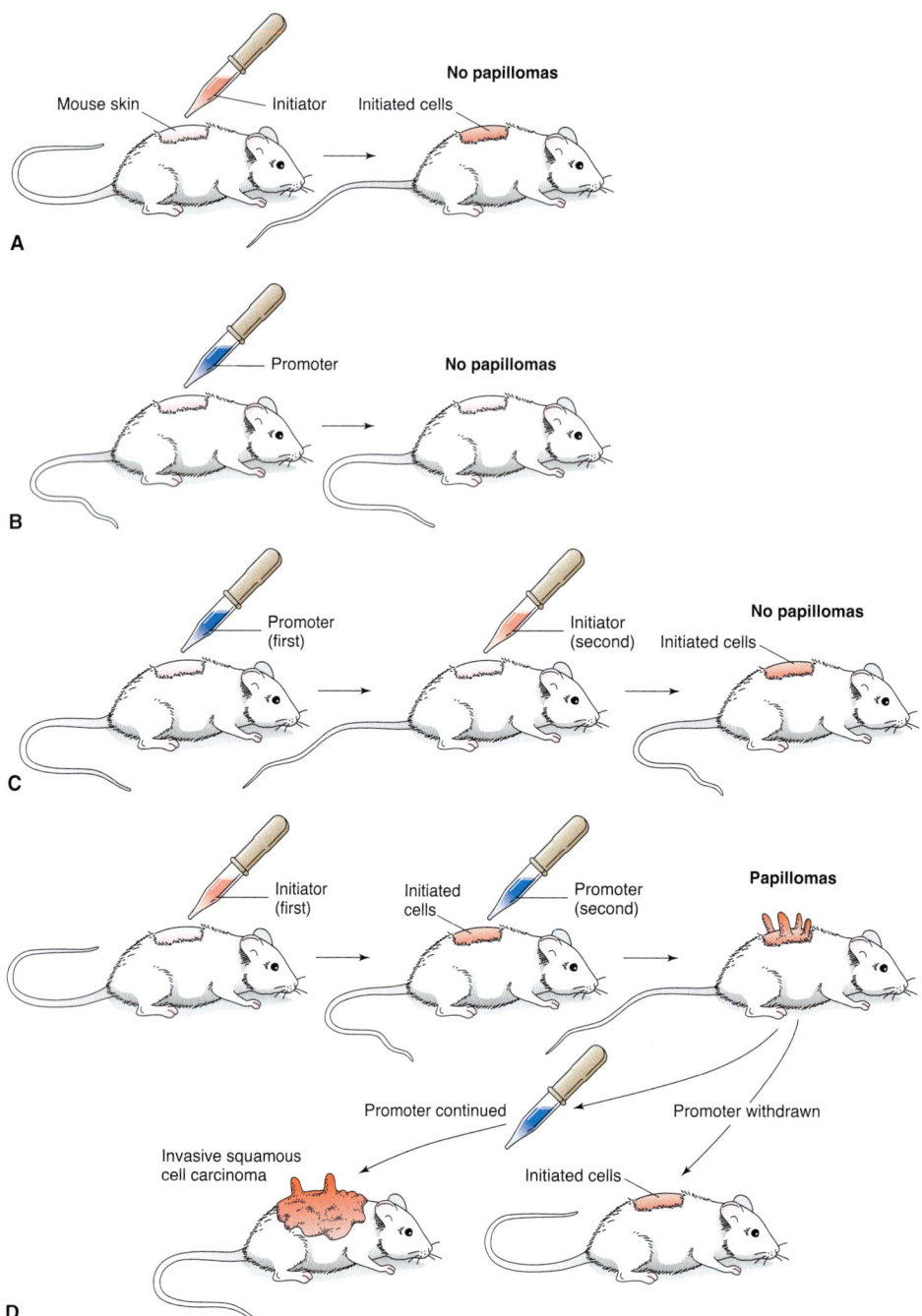

FIGURE 5-32
The concept of initiation and promotion. (A) The single application of an initiator to the skin of a mouse produces initiated cells, but no papillomas form. (B) Likewise, the application of a promoter alone to the skin produces no papillomas. (C) If the promoter is applied to the skin before the application of the initiator, no papillomas form, although initiated cells are present. (D) When the skin is first exposed to the initiator, the subsequent application of the promoter results in papillomas. If the promoter is withdrawn, the papillomas regress, leaving initiated cells in their place. When the promoter is applied to mouse skin bearing papillomas, invasive squamous cell carcinomas are produced.

coal tar, are among the most extensively studied carcinogens. In this class are such model compounds as benzo(a)pyrene, 3-methylcholanthrene, and dibenzanthracene. These compounds have a broad range of target organs and generally produce cancers at the site of application. The specific type of cancer produced varies with the route of administration and includes tumors of the skin, soft tissues, and breast. Since polycyclic hydrocarbons have been identified in cigarette smoke, it has been suggested, but not proved, that they are involved in the production of lung cancer.

Polycyclic hydrocarbons are metabolized by cytochrome P450-dependent mixed-function oxidases to electrophilic epoxides, which in turn react with proteins and nucleic acids. The formation of the epoxide depends on the presence of an unsaturated carbon–carbon bond. For example, vinyl chloride, the simple two-carbon molecule from which the widely used plastic polyvinyl chloride is synthesized, is metabolized to an epoxide, which is responsible for its carcinogenic properties. Workers exposed to the vinyl chloride monomer in the ambient atmosphere later developed angiosarcomas of the liver.

ALKYLATING AGENTS: Many chemotherapeutic drugs (e.g., cyclophosphamide, cisplatin, busulfan) are alkylating agents that transfer alkyl groups (methyl, ethyl, etc.) to macromolecules, including guanines within DNA. Although such drugs destroy cancer cells by damaging DNA, they also lead to a higher risk of a variety of cancers because of similar damage to normal cells. Thus, alkylating chemotherapy carries a significant risk of solid and hematological malignancies at a later time.

AFLATOXIN: In contrast to the polycyclic hydrocarbons, which are for the most part formed either by the combustion of organic material or synthetically, a heterocyclic hydrocarbon, aflatoxin B_1, is a natural product of the fungus *Aspergillus flavus*. Like the polycyclic aromatic hydrocarbons, aflatoxin B_1 is metabolized to an epoxide, which either is detoxified or binds covalently to DNA (Fig. 5-33). Aflatoxin B_1 is among the most potent liver carcinogens recognized, producing tumors in fish, birds, rodents, and primates. Since *Aspergillus* species are ubiquitous, contamination of vegetable foods, particularly peanuts and grains exposed to the warm moist conditions that favor the growth of this mold, may result in the formation of significant amounts of aflatoxin B_1. It has been suggested that in addition to hepatitis B and C, aflatoxin-rich foods may contribute to the high incidence of cancer of the liver in parts of Africa and Asia. In rodents exposed to aflatoxin B_1, the resulting liver tumors exhibit a specific inactivating mutation in the *p53* gene (G:C → T:A transversion at codon 249). Interestingly, human liver cancers in areas of high dietary concentrations of aflatoxin carry the same *p53* mutation.

AROMATIC AMINES AND AZO DYES: Aromatic amines and azo dyes, in contrast to the polycyclic aromatic hydrocarbons, are not ordinarily carcinogenic at the point of application. However, they commonly produce bladder and liver tumors, respectively, when fed to experimental animals. Both aromatic amines and azo dyes are primarily metabolized in the liver. The activation reaction undergone by aromatic amines is N-hydroxylation to form the hydroxylamino derivatives, which are then detoxified by conjugation with glucuronic acid. In the bladder, hydrolysis of the glucuronide releases the reactive hydroxylamine. Occupational exposure to aromatic amines in the form of aniline dyes has resulted in bladder cancer.

Aminoazo dyes are also known to be carcinogenic. At one time, butter yellow (dimethylaminoazobenzene) was used to color margarine or pale winter butter to simulate the richness of summer butter. Maraschino cherries were tinted with scarlet red, a structural component of which is *o*-aminoazotoluene. However, the relationship of these agents to human cancer remains to be elucidated.

NITROSAMINES: Carcinogenic nitrosamines are a subject of considerable study because it is suspected that they may play a role in human gastrointestinal neoplasms and possibly other cancers. The simplest nitrosamine, dimethylnitrosamine, produces kidney and liver tumors in rodents. Nitrosamines are also potent carcinogens in primates, although unambiguous evidence of cancer induction in humans is lacking. However, the extremely high incidence of esophageal carcinoma in the Hunan province of China (100 times higher than in other areas) has been correlated with the high nitrosamine content of the diet. There is concern that nitrosamines may also be implicated in other gastrointestinal cancers because nitrites, commonly added to preserve processed meats and other foods, may react with other dietary components to form nitrosamines. In addition, tobacco-specific nitrosamines have been identified, although a contribution to carcinogenesis has not been proved. Nitrosamines are activated by hydroxylation, followed by formation of a reactive alkyl carbonium ion.

METALS: A number of metals or metal compounds can induce cancer, but the mechanisms by which they do so are unknown. Divalent metal cations, such as Ni^{2+}, Pb^{2+}, Cd^{2+}, Co^{2+}, and Be^{2+}, are electrophilic and can, therefore, react with macromolecules. In addition, metal ions react with guanine and phosphate groups of DNA. A metal ion such as Ni^{2+} can depolymerize polynucleotides. Some metals can bind to purine and pyrimidine bases through covalent bonds or pi electrons of the bases. These reactions all occur in vitro, and the extent to which they occur in vivo is not known. Most metal-induced cancers occur in an occupational setting, and the subject is, therefore, discussed in more detail in Chapter 9, which deals with environmental pathology.

Endogenous and Environmental Factors Influence Chemical Carcinogenesis

Chemical carcinogenesis in experimental animals involves consideration of genetic aspects (species and strain, age and sex of the animal), hormonal status, diet, and the presence or absence of inducers of drug-metabolizing systems and tumor promoters. A similar role for such factors in humans has been postulated on the basis of epidemiological studies.

METABOLISM OF CARCINOGENS: Mixed-function oxidases are enzymes whose activities are genetically determined, and a correlation has been observed between the levels of these enzymes in various strains of mice and their sensitivity to chemical carcinogens. As noted, since most chemical carcinogens require metabolic activation, agents that enhance the activation of procarcinogens to ultimate carcinogens should lead to greater carcinogenicity, whereas those that augment the detoxification pathways should reduce the incidence of cancer. In general, this is the case experimentally. Since humans are exposed to many chemicals in the diet and environment, such interactions are potentially significant.

SEX AND HORMONAL STATUS: These factors are important determinants of susceptibility to chemical carcino-

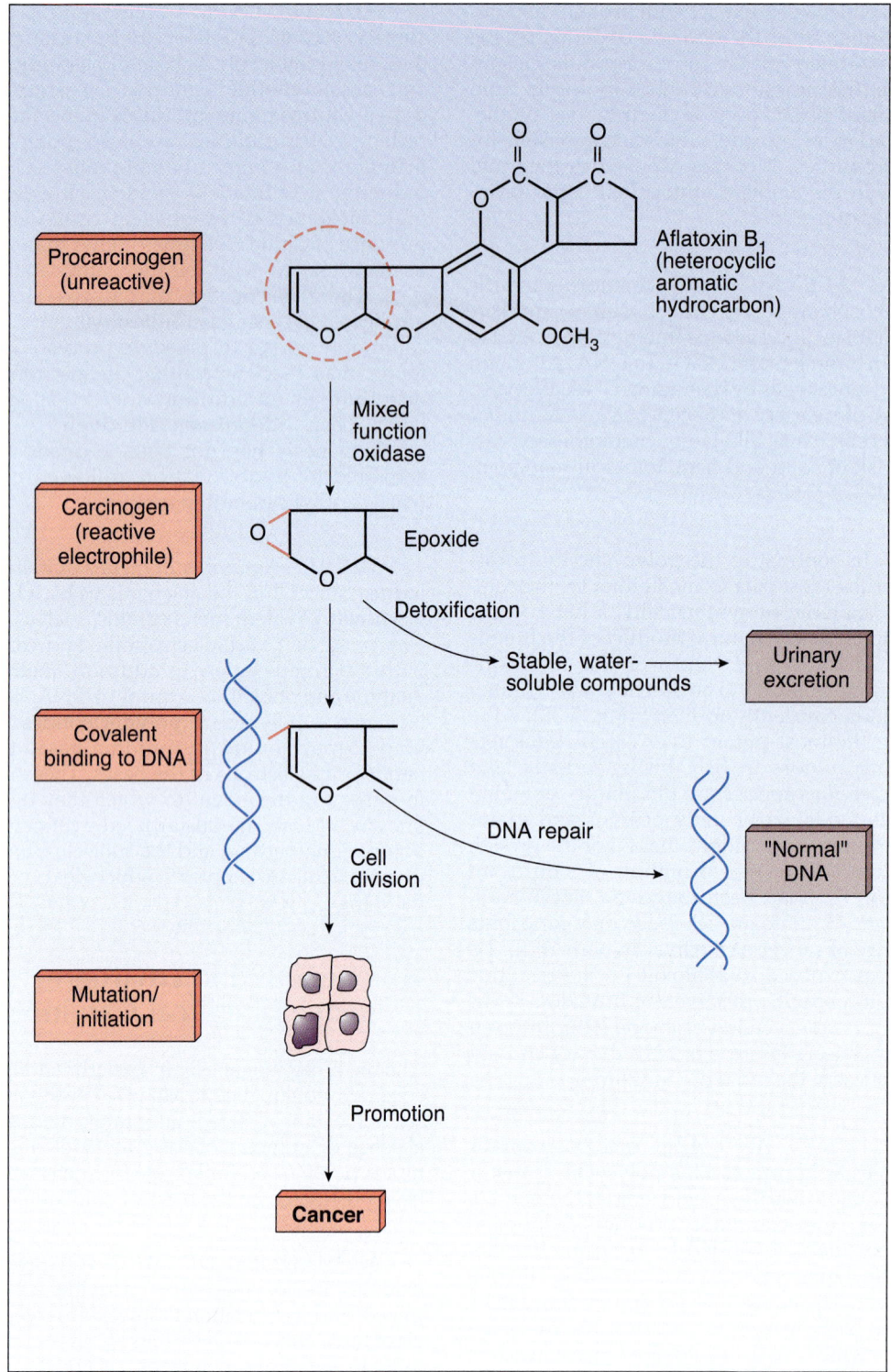

FIGURE 5-33
Metabolic activation of aflatoxin B_1. The unreactive procarcinogen aflatoxin B_1 is metabolized by the mixed-function oxidase of the hepatic endoplasmic reticulum to yield an epoxide. This electrophilic metabolite can be detoxified by conjugation with glutathione (GSH) and excreted in the urine. Alternatively, the epoxide of aflatoxin B_1 can covalently bind to liver cell macromolecules and, in particular, can bind to DNA. The resulting DNA damage can be repaired, a process that restores the integrity of the DNA. If the hepatocyte divides before DNA repair is complete, initiated liver cells result. With the appropriate regimen, these initiated hepatocytes can be promoted to a hepatocellular carcinoma.

gens but are highly variable and in many instances not readily predictable. In most experimental species, male animals are more susceptible to the aromatic amine liver carcinogens than are female animals. By contrast, female mice are more sensitive to the carcinogenic effects of aminoazotoluene and diethylnitrosamine. Moreover, in some instances, when a carcinogen is administered to a sexually immature animal, there is still a sex-linked incidence of cancer in organs that are not primarily responsive to sex hormones, such as the liver. The effects of sex and hormonal status on chemical carcinogenesis in humans are not clear.

DIET: The composition of the diet can affect the level of drug-metabolizing enzymes. A low-protein diet, which reduces the hepatic activity of mixed-function oxidases, is associated with decreased sensitivity to hepatocarcinogens. In the case of dimethylnitrosamine, the decreased incidence of liver tumors is accompanied by an increased incidence of kidney tumors, an observation that emphasizes the fact that the metabolism of carcinogens may be regulated differently in different tissues.

PHYSICAL CARCINOGENESIS

The physical agents of carcinogenesis discussed here are ultraviolet light, asbestos, and foreign bodies. Radiation carcinogenesis is discussed in Chapter 9.

Ultraviolet Radiation Causes Skin Cancers

Among fair-skinned persons, a glowing tan is commonly considered the mark of a successful holiday. However, this overt manifestation of the alleged healthful effects of the sun conceals underlying tissue damage. The harmful effects of solar radiation were recognized by ladies of a bygone era, who shielded themselves from the sun with parasols to maintain a "roses-and-milk" complexion and to prevent wrinkles. The current fad for a tanned complexion has been accompanied not only by cosmetic deterioration of facial skin but also by an increased incidence of the major skin cancers.

Cancers attributed to sun exposure, namely, basal cell carcinoma, squamous carcinoma, and melanoma, occur predominantly in persons of the white race. The skin of persons of the darker races is protected by the increased concentration of melanin pigment, which absorbs ultraviolet radiation. In fair-skinned people, the areas exposed to the sun are most prone to develop skin cancer. Moreover, there is a direct correlation between total exposure to sunlight and the incidence of skin cancer.

Ultraviolet (UV) radiation is the short-wavelength portion of the electromagnetic spectrum adjacent to the violet region of visible light. It appears that only certain portions of the UV spectrum are associated with tissue damage, and a carcinogenic effect occurs at wavelengths between 290 and 320 nm. **The effects of UV radiation on cells include enzyme inactivation, inhibition of cell division, mutagenesis, cell death, and cancer.**

The most important biochemical effect of UV radiation is the formation of *pyrimidine dimers in DNA,* a type of DNA damage that is not seen with any other carcinogen. Pyrimidine dimers may form between thymine and thymine, between thymine and cytosine, or between cytosine pairs alone. Dimer formation leads to a cyclobutane ring, which distorts the phosphodiester backbone of the double helix in the region of each dimer. Unless efficiently eliminated by the nucleotide excision repair pathway, genomic injury produced by UV radiation is mutagenic and carcinogenic.

Xeroderma pigmentosum, an autosomal recessive disease, exemplifies the importance of DNA repair in protecting against the harmful effects of UV radiation. In this rare disorder, a sensitivity to sunlight is accompanied by a high incidence of skin cancers, including basal cell carcinoma, squamous cell carcinoma, and melanoma. Both the neoplastic and nonneoplastic disorders of the skin in xeroderma pigmentosum are attributed to an impairment in the excision of UV-damaged DNA.

Asbestos Causes Mesothelioma

Pulmonary asbestosis and asbestosis-associated neoplasms are discussed in Chapter 12. Here we review possible mechanisms of carcinogenesis attributed to asbestos. In this context, it is not conclusively established whether the cancers related to asbestos exposure should be considered examples of chemical carcinogenesis or of physically induced tumors.

Asbestos, a material widely used in construction, insulation, and manufacturing, is a family of related fibrous silicates, which are classed as "serpentines" or "amphiboles." Serpentines, of which chrysotile is the only example of commercial importance, occur as flexible fibers; the amphiboles, represented principally by crocidolite and amosite, are firm narrow rods.

The characteristic tumor associated with asbestos exposure is malignant mesothelioma of the pleural and peritoneal cavities. This cancer, which is exceedingly rare in the general population, has been reported to occur in 2 to 3% (in some studies even more) of heavily exposed workers. The latent period (i.e., the interval between exposure and the appearance of a tumor) is usually about 20 years but may be twice that figure. It is reasonable to surmise that mesotheliomas of both the pleura and the peritoneum reflect the close contact of these membranes with asbestos fibers transported to them by lymphatic channels.

The pathogenesis of asbestos-associated mesotheliomas is obscure. Thin crocidolite fibers are associated with a considerably greater risk of mesothelioma than the shorter and thicker amosite fibers or the flexible chrysotile fibers. However, the distinction between these fibers in the causation of human disease should not be taken as absolute, particularly since mixtures of these fibers are characteristically found in human lungs. A role for a simian virus, SV40, in the pathogenesis of asbestos-induced mesotheliomas has been postulated, but remains controversial.

An association between cancer of the lung and asbestos exposure is clearly established in smokers. A slight increase in the prevalence of lung cancer has been reported in nonsmokers exposed to asbestos, but the small number of cases renders an association questionable. Claims that exposure to asbestos increases the risk of gastrointestinal cancer have not withstood statistical analysis of the collected data.

Foreign Bodies Produce Experimental Cancer

A number of different sarcomas have been induced in rodents by the implantation of inert materials, such as plastic and metal films, various fibers (including fiberglass), plastic sponges, glass spheres, and dextran polymers. The chemical nature of these implants does not seem to be the critical feature, since disks made of pure carbon also produce sarcomas. Rather, the size, smoothness, and durability of the implanted surface are important. Foreign body carcinogenesis is highly species specific. For example, rats and mice are highly susceptible to foreign body carcinogenesis, but guinea pigs are resistant. **Humans are certainly highly resistant to foreign body carcinogenesis, as evidenced by the lack of cancers following the implantation of prostheses constructed of plastics and metals.** A few reports of cancer developing in the vicinity of foreign bodies in humans probably reflect scar formation, which in some organs seems to be associated with an increased incidence of cancers. Despite numerous contrary claims in lawsuits, there is no evidence that a single traumatic injury can lead to any form of cancer.

TUMOR IMMUNOLOGY

It has long been recognized that malignant tumors elicit a chronic inflammatory response that is unrelated to necrosis or infection of the tumor. This observation led early investigators to postulate a host immune reaction to the neoplastic cells, but a refined understanding awaited the development of modern immunology. The inflammatory reaction is correlated with a better prognosis in some tumors, such as medullary carcinoma of the breast and seminoma, but in general no clear correlation exists. Although the infiltrate is composed principally of T cells and macrophages, suggesting a cell-mediated immune response, the antigens to which the cells respond have not been identified. Despite the paucity of direct evidence in human cancers, it is clear from animal experiments that immune defenses against malignant tumors exist.

Immunological Defenses against Cancer Have Been Demonstrated in Experimental Animals and Man

To invoke a role for an immune defense against cancer, it is necessary to postulate that tumor cells express antigens that differ from those of normal cells and that are recognized as foreign by the host. Such a condition has been indirectly demonstrated in experiments with inbred mice (Fig. 5-34). When cells from a chemically induced or virally induced tumor are transplanted into a syngeneic mouse, the cells form a tumor. When cells from this tumor are passed into a second mouse, they again form a tumor. On the other hand, if the first transplanted tumor is removed before it metastasizes ., the mouse is cured of its tumor), reinjection of the tumor back into the cured mouse will not produce a tumor. ansplanted tumor is rejected because of immunity as a result of the first tumor transplant.** Moreover, tumor cells or preparations of tumor cell membranes, when injected experimentally, augment resistance to tumor growth. Why the original tumor is not destroyed by the immunological reaction remains unexplained.

An important observation is that tumors induced by the same chemical in different mice are antigenically distinct, whereas those induced by the same virus express the same virally determined antigens. Accordingly, mice sensitized to one chemically induced tumor do not reject a second tumor induced by the same chemical. By contrast, mice that have received a virus-induced tumor reject another similar tumor. These experiments provide compelling evidence that immunological mechanisms can play a role in host defenses against tumors, at least against experimental tumors in animals.

Further evidence for the existence of immune mechanisms in the defense against cancer comes from studies in nude mice. These animals are devoid of T cell-mediated immunity and thus accept grafts from different species. Similarly, tumors from different species grow in an unrestrained fashion when transplanted into nude mice.

The effectiveness of immune mechanisms to limit the growth of malignant cells can be demonstrated by mixing mouse tumor cells with immune effector cells from a syngeneic mouse that has been sensitized to the tumor. The mixture is then injected into a normal (unsensitized) syngeneic recipient. In many instances, the growth of the tumor cells in the recipient is inhibited, compared with that of tumor cells mixed with unsensitized lymphoid cells. Similar approaches have been tested in cases of human melanoma. However, it has not proved possible to cure human melanomas by reinjecting tumor-sensitized lymphocytes into the patient.

Tumor Antigens

The immune response to experimental tumors must necessarily be directed against tumor antigens on the surface of the malignant cells. Such antigens can be tumor specific; that is, they are uniquely expressed by the cancer cells but not by their normal cellular counterparts. Alternatively, other tumor antigens represent proteins that are expressed by some normal cells, such as those in developing embryos. Such antigens are tumor associated, rather than tumor specific.

In experimental animals, tumors produced by chemicals and viruses display tumor-specific antigens. As noted above, each chemically induced cancer expresses unique tumor antigens; that is, no two tumors are antigenically alike. The precise nature of these antigens is obscure, although some may be altered histocompatibility antigens. By contrast, all tumors induced by the same virus express the same tumor-specific antigens, presumably because they are products encoded by the viral genome. Interestingly, tumor-specific antigens are expressed weakly or not at all in the neoplasms that appear spontaneously in rodents.

It is much more difficult to document the presence of tumor-specific antigens in human cancers, because patients cannot be subjected to an immunization challenge with tumor cells, as is used in experimental animals (see Fig. 5-34). Yet despite this experimental limitation, candidate human tumor-specific antigens have begun to emerge, for example, virally encoded antigens in tumors whose pathogenesis is linked to viruses (e.g., human papillomavirus). Neoantigens encoded by altered gene sequences have also been detected

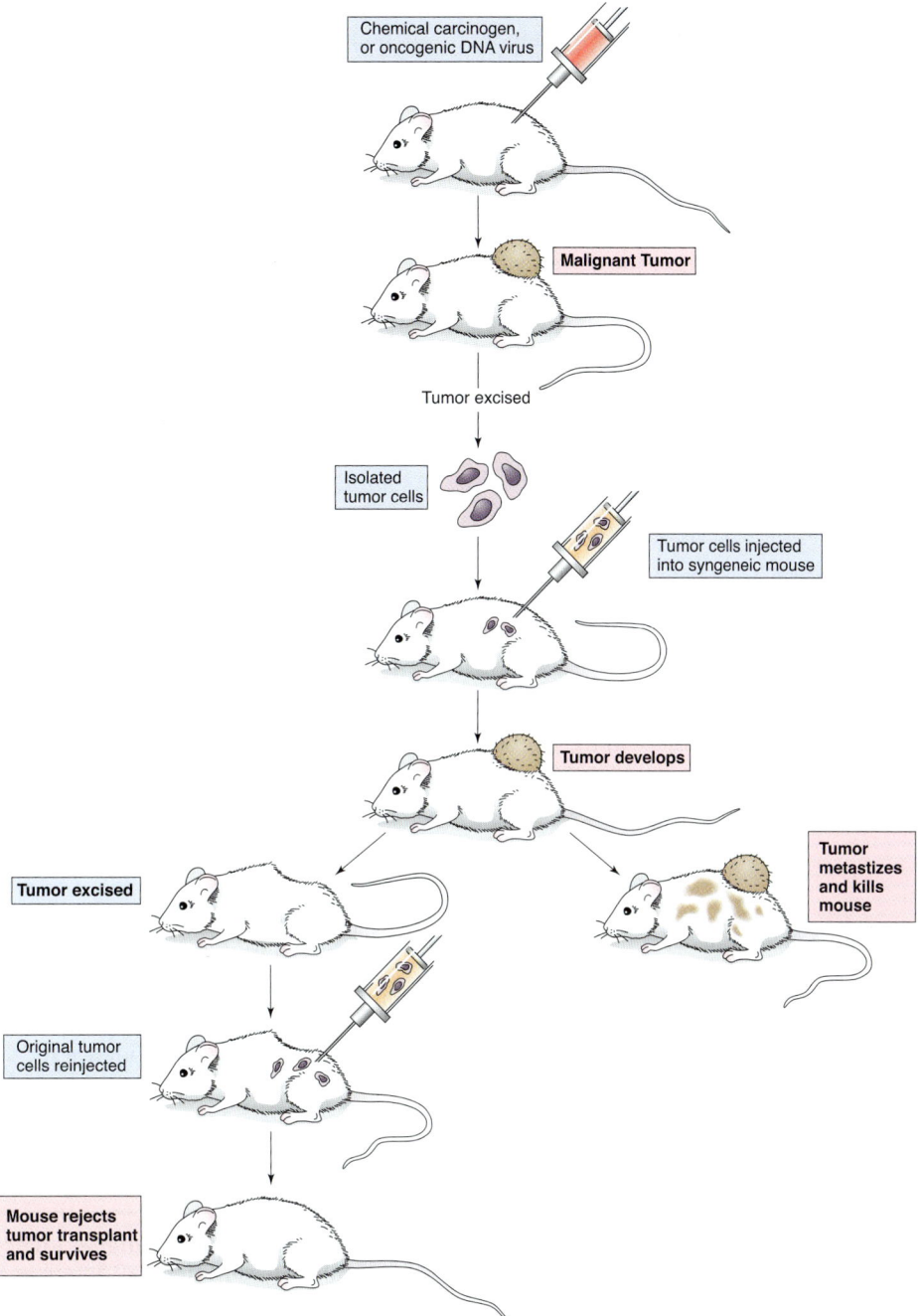

FIGURE 5-34
Immunogenicity of tumors. Cancer cells injected into a syngeneic mouse form tumors, which metastasize and kill the animal. Excision of the tumor before it has metastasized allows the rejection of a second tumor implant, presumably as a consequence of immunity acquired from exposure to the original tumor.

in malignant cells resulting from mutations or translocations. The tumor-specific antigens identified to date are peptides complexed to human leukocyte antigen (HLA) molecules on tumor cell surfaces.

There has been even more progress in identifying tumor-associated antigens for both human and experimental animal tumors. Early studies on melanoma showed that certain HLA-associated peptide antigens correspond to proteins that are present in small amounts in the adult but are abundant during development. Such tumor-associated oncodevelopmental antigens are not specific for a given patient's tumor per se but instead are shared by cancers in different persons and sometimes of varying histological type. Although, there is no reason to believe that immune responses to these fetal antigens play any role in the host defense against cancer, their presence in the blood or the tumor (e.g., carcinoembryonic antigen, α-fetoprotein) is useful in clinical diagnosis and treatment.

Inroads into the identification of tumor antigens have created new opportunities for developing immunotherapies against human cancers, at least in theory. Passive immunotherapies can draw upon tumor-infiltrating lymphocytes with specificity for HLA-associated tumor peptide antigens and antibodies directed against various tumor surface proteins. Alternatively, active immunotherapeutic strategies can invoke tumor antigens as vaccines to elicit systemic antitumor immune responses.

Mechanisms of Immunological Cytotoxicity

The contribution of any specific immunological mechanism to tumor cell destruction in vivo has not been clearly defined. A number of possible mechanisms are recognized (Fig. 5-35):

- **T cell-mediated cytotoxicity:** The capacity of cytotoxic T cells to mediate the specific rejection of transplanted tumors is evidenced by the demonstration that lymphocytes from tumor-bearing hosts can transfer tumor immunity when injected into normal animals. Moreover, the transferred immunity is eliminated by the administration of antibodies directed against T-cell antigens. The mechanisms of T cell-mediated immunological cell killing are discussed in Chapter 4.

- **Natural killer cell-mediated cytotoxicity:** Another set of lymphocytes, the natural killer (NK) cells, have tumoricidal activity that does not depend on prior sensitization. These lymphocytes are generally more effective than untransformed cells in killing tumor cells. Tumor cells that are resistant to the action of NK cells may be lysed by NK cells that have been activated by interleukin (IL)-2. Such activated NK cells are referred to as *lymphokine-activated killer (LAK) cells*.

- **Macrophage-mediated cytotoxicity:** Macrophages are capable of killing tumor cells in a nonspecific manner. However, their role in the control of malignant tumors is far from clear, since under some circumstances in vitro factors derived from macrophages can actually stimulate the proliferation of tumor cells.

- **Antibody-dependent cell-mediated cytotoxicity (ADCC):** Tumor-associated antigens can elicit a humoral antibody response, but these immunoglobulins by themselves do not kill tumor cells. However, as discussed in Chapter 4, such antibodies can participate in ADCC. The antibody binds both to the tumor antigen and to the Fc receptor of the effector cell, thereby bringing the effector cell into direct contact with its target. Depending on the conditions, the effector cells may be a lymphocyte killer cell (null cell), macrophage, or neutrophil.

- **Complement-mediated cytotoxicity:** Tumor cells that have been coated with specific antibodies may be lysed by the activation of complement.

Immune Surveillance

Considering the enormous number of chemical, viral, and physical agents that are carcinogenic, it seems remarkable that the incidence of cancer is not far greater than current statistics indicate. The theory of immune surveillance holds that mutant clones with neoplastic potential frequently arise but are recognized and expunged by cell-mediated immune responses. However, the evidence for this concept is highly controversial, and the subject deserves further study.

Immunological Defenses against Cancer in Humans

Although some circumstantial evidence exists for the participation of immunological defenses in the resistance to cancer in humans, conclusive proof that immunological tumor surveillance is an ongoing process is lacking. Perhaps the strongest argument for immunological tumor rejection in humans is the observation that immunodeficiency, whether acquired or congenital, is associated with an increased incidence of cancers, almost all of which are B-cell lymphomas. Three prominent examples are widely cited: patients with XLP, patients with AIDS, and those who receive immunosuppressive therapy following organ transplantation. In XLP and AIDS, the enormously increased risk can be attributed to a polyclonal lymphoid hyperplasia induced by infection with EBV, coupled with a lack of cytotoxic T cells that normally limit the proliferation of virus-infected B cells. In immunosuppressed transplant patients, who manifest a 75-fold increased incidence of lymphomas, it remains unclear whether a direct effect of immunosuppressive agents on the regulation of lymphocyte proliferation and maturation or a nonspecific depression of immune defenses is responsible.

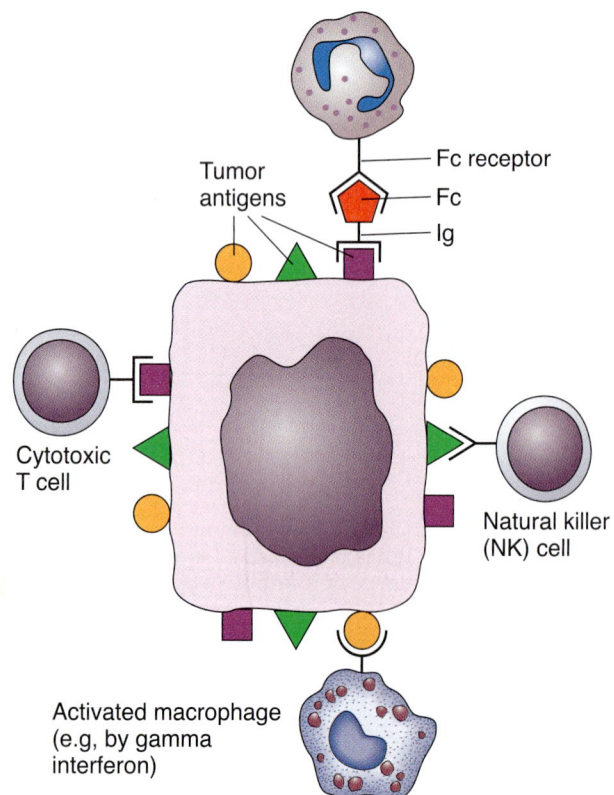

FIGURE 5-35
Possible mechanisms of immunological tumor cytotoxicity in animal studies.

Additional arguments for the effectiveness of immunological defenses against cancer in humans are also far from definitive. Rare instances of the regression of primary and metastatic tumors have been attributed to immunological mechanisms, but many other factors may have been responsible (e.g., hormonal, nutritional, or vascular). Similarly, as noted above, the phenomenon of tumor dormancy may be related to comparable nonimmunological circumstances. The presence of lymphoid cells and macrophages in the stroma of many cancers may represent a reaction to tumor antigens, but their effectiveness in limiting growth is problematic.

Evasion of Immunological Cytotoxicity

The fact that cancer is alive and well despite the presence of potential immunological defenses implies that such mechanisms are either ineffective or that tumor cells can evade immunological cytotoxicity. A number of factors have been proposed to account for the failure of immune responses to limit tumor growth. These explanations remain theoretical and even controversial.

It is intuitively clear that an absence of tumor-specific antigens or a lack of immunogenicity by such antigens will permit unhampered growth of the neoplasm. **In this respect, tumor antigens are sometimes found to be expressed at low levels on human tumors, in conjunction with deficient HLA expression or antigenic peptide processing.** The concept of tumor heterogeneity predicts that even in strongly antigenic tumors, clones will arise that do not express tumor antigens or histocompatibility antigens and thus will be selected for survival. Besides antigenic variation, tumor cells tend to lack surface molecules such as costimulators that are needed for T-cell activation. Additionally, malignant cells can express a variety of immunosuppressive factors that enable them to blunt antitumor immunological responses. Defining and tackling these immune evasion mechanisms will be essential for developing effective immunotherapies for cancer.

SYSTEMIC EFFECTS OF CANCER ON THE HOST

The symptoms of cancer are, for the most part, referable to the local effects of either the primary tumor or its metastases. However, in a minority of patients, cancer produces remote effects that are not attributable to tumor invasion or to metastasis, which are collectively termed *paraneoplastic syndromes*. Although such effects are rarely lethal, in some cases they dominate the clinical course. It is important to recognize these syndromes for several reasons. First, the signs and symptoms of the paraneoplastic syndrome may be the first clinical manifestation of a malignant tumor. When they are recognized, the cancer may be detected early enough to permit a cure. Second, the syndromes may be mistaken for those produced by advanced metastatic disease and may, therefore, lead to inappropriate therapy. Third, when the paraneoplastic syndrome itself is disabling, treatment directed toward alleviating those symptoms may have important palliative effects. Finally, certain tumor products that result in paraneoplastic syndromes provide a means of monitoring recurrence of the cancer in patients who have had surgical resections or are undergoing chemotherapy or radiation therapy.

Fever

It is not uncommon for cancer patients to present initially with fever of unknown origin that cannot be explained by an infectious disease. Fever attributed to cancer correlates with tumor growth, disappears after treatment, and reappears on recurrence. The cancers in which this most commonly occurs are Hodgkin disease, renal cell carcinoma, and osteogenic sarcoma, although many other tumors are occasionally complicated by fever. Tumor cells may themselves release pyrogens or the inflammatory cells in the tumor stroma can produce IL-1.

Anorexia and Weight Loss

A paraneoplastic syndrome of anorexia, weight loss, and cachexia is very common in patients with cancer, often appearing before its malignant cause becomes apparent. For example, a small asymptomatic cancer of the pancreas may be suspected only on the basis of progressive and unexplained weight loss. Although cancer patients often have a decreased caloric intake because of anorexia and abnormalities of taste, restricted food intake does not explain the profound wasting so common among them. The mechanisms responsible for this phenomenon are poorly understood. It is known, however, that unlike starvation, which is associated with a lowered metabolic rate, cancer is often accompanied by an elevated metabolic rate. It has been demonstrated that TNF-α and other cytokines (interferons, IL-6) can produce a wasting syndrome in experimental animals.

Endocrine Syndromes

Malignant tumors may produce a number of peptide hormones whose secretion is not under normal regulatory control. Most of these hormones are normally present in the brain, gastrointestinal tract, or endocrine organs. Their inappropriate secretion can cause a variety of effects.

CUSHING SYNDROME: Ectopic secretion of ACTH by a tumor leads to features of Cushing syndrome, including hypokalemia, hyperglycemia, hypertension, and muscle weakness (see Chapter 21). ACTH production is most commonly seen with cancers of the lung, particularly small cell carcinoma. It also complicates carcinoid tumors and other neuroendocrine tumors, such as pheochromocytoma, neuroblastoma, and medullary carcinoma of the thyroid.

INAPPROPRIATE ANTIDIURESIS: The production of arginine vasopressin (antidiuretic hormone, ADH) by a tumor may cause sodium and water retention to such an extent that it is manifested as water intoxication, resulting in altered mental status, seizures, coma, and sometimes death. The tumor that most often produces this syndrome is small cell carcinoma of the lung. It is also reported with carcinomas of the prostate, gastrointestinal tract, and pancreas and with thymomas, lymphomas, and Hodgkin disease.

HYPERCALCEMIA: A paraneoplastic complication that afflicts 10% of all cancer patients, hypercalcemia, is usually caused by metastatic disease of bone. However, in about one tenth of cases it occurs in the absence of bony metastases. The most common cause of paraneoplastic hypercalcemia is the secretion of a parathormone-like peptide by an epithelial tumor, usually squamous cell carcinoma of the lung or adenocarcinoma of the breast. In multiple myeloma and lymphomas, hypercalcemia is attributed to the secretion of osteoclast activating factor. Other mechanisms of hypercalcemia involve the production of prostaglandins, active metabolites of vitamin D, TGF-α, and TGF-β.

HYPOCALCEMIA: Cancer-induced hypocalcemia is actually more common than hypercalcemia and complicates osteoblastic metastases from cancers of the lung, breast, and prostate. The cause of hypocalcemia is not known. Low calcium levels have been reported in association with calcitonin-secreting medullary carcinoma of the thyroid.

GONADOTROPIC SYNDROMES: Gonadotropins may be secreted by germ cell tumors, gestational trophoblastic tumors (choriocarcinoma, hydatidiform mole), and pituitary tumors. Less commonly, gonadotropin secretion is observed with hepatoblastomas in children and cancers of the lung, colon, breast, and pancreas in adults. High gonadotropin levels lead to precocious puberty in children, gynecomastia in men, and oligomenorrhea in premenopausal women.

HYPOGLYCEMIA: The best-understood cause of hypoglycemia associated with tumors is excessive insulin production by islet cell tumors of the pancreas. Other tumors, especially large mesotheliomas and fibrosarcomas and primary hepatocellular carcinoma, are associated with hypoglycemia. The cause of hypoglycemia in nonendocrine tumors is not established, but the most likely candidate is production of somatomedins (IGFs), a family of peptides normally produced by the liver under regulation by growth hormone.

Neurological Syndromes

Neurological disorders are common in cancer patients, usually resulting from metastases or from endocrine or electrolyte disturbances. Vascular, hemorrhagic, and infectious conditions affecting the nervous system are also common. However, there remains a small group of cancer patients who suffer from a variety of neurological complaints without any demonstrable cause. Most of these cases reflect an autoimmune etiology mediated by circulating antibodies directed against neural antigens or by reactive T cells. Cerebral complications include dementia, subacute cerebellar degeneration, limbic encephalitis, and optic neuritis.

Spinal Cord

Subacute motor neuropathy, a disorder of the spinal cord, is characterized by slowly developing lower motor neuron weakness without sensory changes. It is so strongly associated with cancer that an intensive search for an occult neoplasm, often a lymphoma, should be made in patients who present with these symptoms.

Amyotrophic lateral sclerosis is well described among cancer patients. Conversely, as many as 10% of patients with this disease are found to have cancer.

Peripheral Nerves

Sensorimotor peripheral neuropathy, characterized by distal weakness and wasting and sensory loss, is common in cancer patients and when not associated with an overt neoplasm suggests the possibility of an occult tumor. Interestingly, the removal of the primary tumor usually does not reverse the neuropathy.

Purely sensory neuropathy, resulting from degenerative changes in the dorsal root ganglia, may also develop in persons with cancer.

Autonomic and gastrointestinal neuropathies, manifested as orthostatic hypotension, neurogenic bladder, and intestinal pseudoobstruction, are associated with small cell carcinoma of the lung.

Skeletal Muscle Syndromes

Patients with dermatomyositis or polymyositis have an incidence of cancer five to seven times higher than that in the general population. The association is most conspicuous in affected men older than 50 years; in this group more than 70% have cancer. In most cases, the muscle disorder and cancer present within a year of each other.

Eaton-Lambert syndrome is an uncommon myasthenic disorder that is strongly associated with small cell carcinoma of the lung. Although the symptoms superficially resemble those of true myasthenia gravis, muscle strength improves with exercise, and there is a poor response to an anticholinesterase. Thymoma has a well-recognized association with **myasthenia gravis,** although a wide variety of other tumors have on occasion been linked to this disorder of the neuromuscular junction.

Hematological Syndromes

The most common hematological complications of neoplastic diseases result either from direct infiltration of the marrow or from treatment. However, hematological paraneoplastic syndromes, which antedate the modern era of chemotherapy and radiation therapy, are well described.

Erythrocytosis

Cancer-associated erythrocytosis (polycythemia) is a complication of some tumors, particularly renal cell carcinoma, hepatocellular carcinoma, and cerebellar hemangioblastoma. Interestingly, benign kidney disease, such as cystic disease or hydronephrosis, and uterine myomas can lead to erythrocytosis. Elevated erythropoietin levels are found in the tumor and in the serum in about half of patients with erythrocytosis.

Anemia

One of the most common findings in patients with cancer is anemia, but the mechanism for this disorder is not clear. The anemia is usually normocytic and normochromic, although iron deficiency anemia is common in cancers that bleed into the gastrointestinal tract, such as colorectal cancers. **Pure red cell aplasia,** often associated with thymomas, and megaloblastic anemia are sometimes encountered. **Autoimmune hemolytic anemia** may be associated with B-cell neoplasms and with solid tumors, particularly in the elderly. In fact, autoimmune hemolytic anemia in an older person suggests the possibility of an underlying neoplasm. **Microangiopathic hemolytic anemia** is occasionally seen, often in association with disseminated intravascular coagulation and thrombotic thrombocytopenic purpura.

Leukocytes and Platelets

Paraneoplastic granulocytosis, characterized by a peripheral granulocyte count over 20,000/μL, is a finding that may lead to an erroneous diagnosis of leukemia. This condition is usually caused by the secretion of a colony-stimulating factor by the tumor.

Eosinophilia is occasionally noted in association with cancer, particularly in Hodgkin disease, in which it may occur in one fifth of cases.

Thrombocytosis, with platelet counts above 400,000/μL, occurs in one third of cancer patients. The platelet count usually returns to normal with successful treatment of the malignant disease.

The Hypercoagulable State

The association between cancer and venous thrombosis was noted more than a century ago. Since then, other abnormalities resulting from a hypercoagulable state (e.g., disseminated intravascular coagulation and nonbacterial thrombotic endocarditis) have been recognized. The cause of this hypercoagulable state is still debated.

VENOUS THROMBOSIS: This condition is most distinctly associated with carcinoma of the pancreas, in which there is a 50-fold increased incidence of this complication compared with that in chronic pancreatitis. Venous thrombosis, commonly in the deep veins of the legs, is also particularly frequent in association with other mucin-secreting adenocarcinomas of the gastrointestinal tract and with lung cancer. Tumors of the breast, ovary, prostate, and other organs are occasionally complicated by venous thrombosis.

DISSEMINATED INTRAVASCULAR COAGULATION: The widespread appearance of thrombi in small vessels in association with cancer may come to attention because of the chronic occurrence of thrombotic phenomena or an acute hemorrhagic diathesis. Sometimes a coagulation disorder is detected by laboratory tests alone. This complication is most commonly found with acute promyelocytic leukemia and adenocarcinomas.

NONBACTERIAL THROMBOTIC ENDOCARDITIS: The presence of noninfected verrucous deposits of fibrin and platelets on the left-sided heart valves occurs in cancer patients, particularly in debilitated persons (see Chapter 11). Although the effects on the heart are not of clinical importance, emboli to the brain present a great danger. Paraneoplastic endocarditis may develop early in the course of a cancer and signal its presence long before the tumor would otherwise become symptomatic. This cardiac complication is most common with solid tumors but may occasionally be noted with leukemias and lymphomas.

Gastrointestinal Syndromes

Malabsorption of a variety of dietary components is an occasional paraneoplastic symptom, and half of cancer patients develop some histological abnormalities of the small intestine, even though the tumor may not directly involve the bowel.

Hypoalbuminemia may result from a paraneoplastic depression of albumin synthesis by the liver or, in rare cases, a protein-losing enteropathy.

Nephrotic Syndrome

Nephrotic syndrome, as a consequence of renal vein thrombosis or amyloidosis, is a well-known complication of cancer. The nephrotic syndrome may also represent a paraneoplastic complication in the form of minimal-change disease (lipoid nephrosis) or glomerulonephritis produced by the deposition of immune complexes.

Cutaneous Syndromes

Pigmented lesions and keratoses are well-recognized paraneoplastic effects.

Acanthosis nigricans is a cutaneous disorder marked by hyperkeratosis and pigmentation of the axilla, neck, flexures, and anogenital region. **It is of particular interest because more than half of patients with acanthosis nigricans have cancer.** The development of the disease may precede, accompany, or follow, the detection of the cancer. Over 90% of cases occur in association with gastrointestinal carcinomas, with tumors of the stomach accounting for one half to two thirds.

Exfoliative dermatitis occasionally complicates certain lymphomas and Hodgkin disease, without any cutaneous involvement by tumor.

Erythema gyratum repens is an unusual skin disorder, which presents with scaling and itching and is seen almost exclusively in cancer patients.

Amyloidosis

About 15% of cases of amyloidosis occur in association with cancers, particularly with multiple myeloma and renal cell carcinoma but also with other solid tumors and lymphomas. The presence of amyloidosis implies a poor prognosis; in patients with myeloma, amyloidosis is associated with a median survival of 14 months or less.

THE EPIDEMIOLOGY OF CANCER

The mere compilation of raw epidemiological data is of little use unless they are subjected to careful analysis. In evaluating the relevance of epidemiological observations to cancer causation, the following considerations (Hill criteria) are germane:

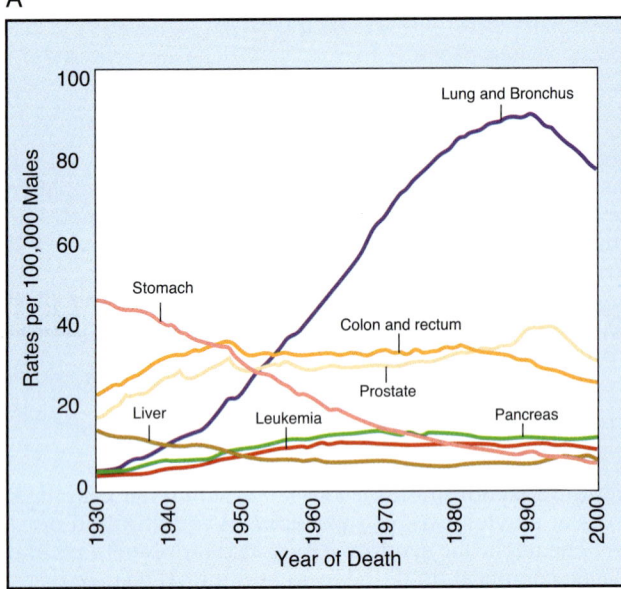

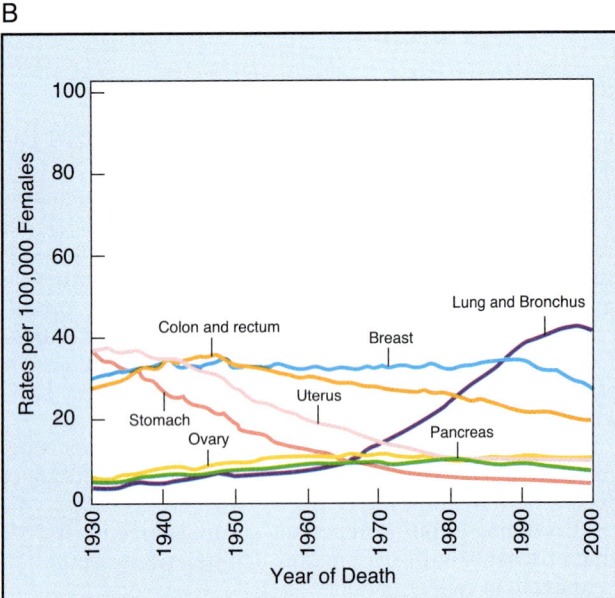

FIGURE 5-36
Cancer death rates in the United States, 1930 to 1999, among men (A) and women (B).

- Strength of the association
- Consistency under different circumstances
- Specificity
- Temporality (i.e., the cause must precede the effect)
- Biological gradient (i.e., there is a dose–response relationship)
- Plausibility
- Coherence (i.e., a cause-and-effect relationship does not violate basic biological principles)
- Analogy to other known associations

It is not mandatory that a valid epidemiological study satisfy all these criteria, nor does adherence to them guarantee that the hypothesis derived from the data is necessarily true. However, as a guideline they remain useful.

Cancer accounts for one fifth of the total mortality in the United States and is the second leading cause of death after cardiovascular diseases and stroke. For most cancers, death rates in the United States have largely remained flat for more than half a century, with some notable exceptions (Fig. 5-36). The death rate from cancer of the lung among men has risen dramatically from 1930, when it was an uncommon tumor, to the present, when it is by far the most common cause of death from cancer in men. As discussed in Chapter 8, the entire epidemic of lung cancer deaths is attributable to smoking. Among women, smoking did not become fashionable until World War II. Considering the time lag needed between starting to smoke and the development of cancer of the lung, it is not surprising that the increased death rate from cancer of the lung in women did not become significant until after 1965. In the United States, the death rate from lung cancer in women now exceeds that for breast cancer, and it is now, as in men, the most common fatal cancer. By contrast, for reasons difficult to fathom, cancer of the stomach, which in 1930 was by far the most common cancer in men and was more common than breast cancer in women, has shown a remarkable and sustained decline in frequency. Similarly, there has been a conspicuous decline in the death rate from cancer of the uterus corpus and cervix, possibly explained by better screening, diagnostic, and therapeutic methods. Overall, after decades of steady increases, the age-adjusted mortality due to all cancers has now reached a plateau. The ranking of the incidence of tumors in men and women in the United States is shown in Table 5-3.

TABLE 5-3 Most Common Tumor Types in Men and Women

Men Tumor Type	%
Prostate	33
Lung and bronchus	14
Colon and rectum	11
Urinary bladder	6
Melanoma	4
Non-Hodgkin lymphoma	4
Kidney	3
Oral cavity	3
Leukemia	3
Pancreas	2
All other sites	17

Women Tumor Type	%
Breast	32
Lung and bronchus	12
Colon and rectum	11
Uterine corpus	6
Ovary	4
Non-Hodgkin lymphoma	4
Melanoma	3
Thyroid	3
Pancreas	2
Urinary bladder	2
All other sites	20

Individual cancers have their own age-related profiles, but for most, increased age is associated with an increased incidence. The most striking example of the dependency on age is carcinoma of the prostate, in which the incidence increases 30-fold between ages 50 and 85 years. Certain neoplastic diseases, such as acute lymphoblastic leukemia in children and testicular cancer in young adults, show different age-related peaks of incidence (Fig. 5-37).

Geographical and Ethnic Differences Influence Cancer Incidence

NASOPHARYNGEAL CANCER: Nasopharyngeal cancer is rare in most of the world except for certain regions of China, Hong Kong, and Singapore.

ESOPHAGEAL CARCINOMA: The range in incidence of esophageal carcinoma varies from extremely low in Mormon women in Utah to a value some 300 times higher in the female population of northern Iran. Particularly high rates of esophageal cancer are noted in a so-called Asian esophageal cancer belt, which includes the great land mass stretching from Turkey to eastern China. Interestingly, throughout this region, as the incidence rises, the proportional excess in males decreases; in some of the areas of highest incidence there is even a female excess. The disease is also more common in certain regions of Africa inhabited predominantly by blacks and among blacks in the United States. The causes of esophageal cancer are obscure, but it is known that it disproportionately affects the poor in many areas of the world, and the combination of alcohol abuse and smoking is associated with a particularly high risk.

STOMACH CANCER: The highest incidence of stomach cancer occurs in Japan, where the disease is almost 10 times as frequent as it is among American whites. A high incidence has also been observed in Latin American countries, particularly Chile. Stomach cancer is also common in Iceland and eastern Europe.

COLORECTAL CANCER: The highest incidence of colorectal cancer is found in the United States, where it is three or four times more common than in Japan, India, Africa, and Latin America. It has been theorized that the high fiber content of the diet in low-risk areas and the high fat content in the United States are related to this difference, although this concept has been seriously questioned.

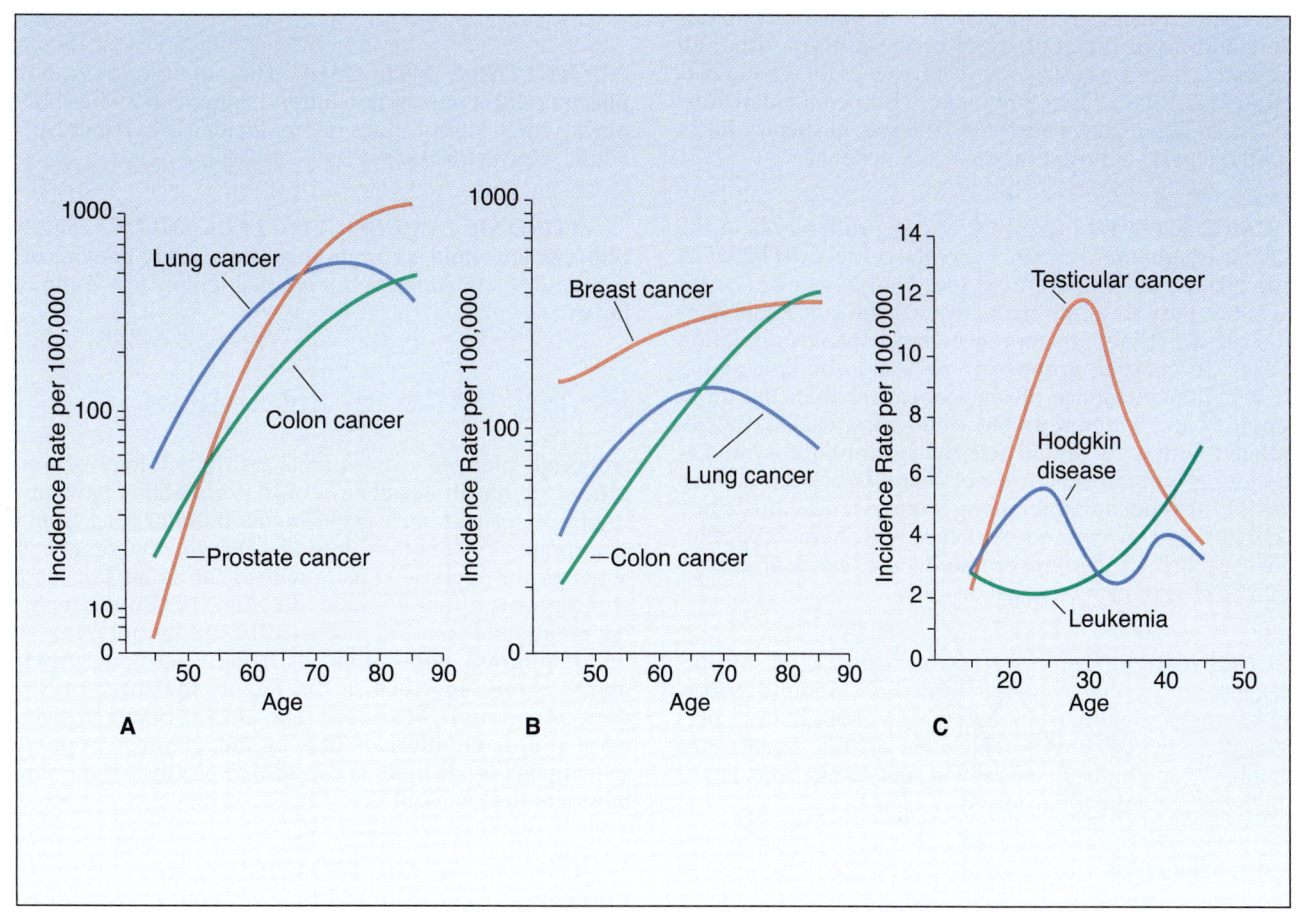

FIGURE 5-37
Incidence of specific cancers as a function of age. (A) Men. (B) Women. (C) Testicular cancer in men and Hodgkin disease and leukemia in both sexes. The incidence of these cancers in C peaks at younger ages than do those in A and B.

LIVER CANCER: There is a strong correlation between the incidence of primary hepatocellular carcinoma and the prevalence of hepatitis B and C. Endemic regions for both diseases include large parts of sub-Saharan Africa and most of the Orient, Indonesia, and the Philippines. It must be remembered that levels of aflatoxin B_1 are high in the staple diets of many of the high-risk areas.

SKIN CANCER: As noted above, the rates for skin cancers vary with skin color and exposure to the sun. Thus, particularly high rates have been reported in northern Australia, where the population is principally of Celtic origin and sun exposure is intense. Increased rates of skin cancer have also been noted among the white population of the American Southwest. The lowest rates are found among persons with pigmented skin (e.g., Japanese, Chinese, and Indians). The rates for African blacks, despite their heavily pigmented skin, are occasionally higher than those for Asians because of the higher incidence of melanomas of the soles and palms in blacks.

BREAST CANCER: Adenocarcinoma of the breast, the most common female cancer in many parts of Europe and North America, shows considerable geographical variation. The rates in African and Asian populations are only one fifth to one sixth of those prevailing in Europe and the United States. Epidemiological studies have contributed little to our understanding of the etiology of breast cancer. Although hormonal factors are clearly involved, except for a good correlation with age at first pregnancy, few confirmed hormonal correlations have surfaced. The role of dietary fat in the pathogenesis of breast cancer is still debated.

CANCER OF THE CERVIX: Striking differences in the incidence of squamous carcinoma of the cervix exist between ethnic groups and different socioeconomic levels. For instance, the very low rate in Ashkenazi Jews of Israel contrasts with a 25 times greater rate in the Hispanic population of Texas. In general, groups of low socioeconomic status have a higher incidence of cervical cancer than the more prosperous and better educated. This cancer is also directly correlated with early sexual activity and multiparity and is rare among women who are not sexually active, such as nuns. It is also uncommon among women whose husbands are circumcised. A strong association with human papillomaviruses has been demonstrated, and cervical cancer should be classed as a venereal disease.

CHORIOCARCINOMA: Choriocarcinoma, an uncommon cancer of trophoblastic differentiation, is found principally in women, following a pregnancy, although it can present as a testicular tumor. The rates of this disease are particularly high in the Pacific rim of Asia (Singapore, Hong Kong, Japan, and the Philippines).

PROSTATIC CANCER: Very low incidences of prostatic cancer are reported for Asian populations, particularly Japanese, whereas the highest rates described are in American blacks, in whom the disease occurs some 25 times more often. The incidence in American and European whites is intermediate.

TESTICULAR CANCER: An unusual aspect of testicular cancer is its universal rarity among black populations. Interestingly, although the rate in American blacks is only about one fourth that in whites, it is still considerably higher than the rate among African blacks.

CANCER OF THE PENIS: This squamous carcinoma is virtually nonexistent among circumcised men of any race but is common in many parts of Africa and Asia.

CANCER OF THE URINARY BLADDER: The rates for transitional cell carcinoma of the bladder are fairly uniform. Squamous carcinoma of the bladder, however, is a special case. Ordinarily far less common than transitional cell carcinoma, it has a high incidence in areas where schistosomal infestation of the bladder (bilharziasis) is endemic.

BURKITT LYMPHOMA: Burkitt lymphoma, a disease of children, was first described in Uganda, where it accounts for half of all childhood tumors. Since then, a high frequency has been observed in other African countries, particularly in hot, humid lowlands. It has been noted that these are areas where malaria is also endemic. High rates have been recorded in other tropical areas, such as Malaysia and New Guinea, but European and American cases are encountered only sporadically.

MULTIPLE MYELOMA: This malignant tumor of plasma cells is uncommon among American whites but displays a three to four times higher incidence in American and South African blacks.

CHRONIC LYMPHOCYTIC LEUKEMIA: Chronic lymphocytic leukemia is common among elderly persons in Europe and North America but is considerably less common in Japan.

Studies of Migrant Populations

Although planned experiments on the etiology of human cancer are hardly feasible, certain populations have unwittingly performed such experiments by migrating from one environment to another. Initially at least, the genetic characteristics of such persons remained the same, but the new environment differed in climate, diet, infectious agents, occupations, and so on. **Consequently, epidemiological studies of migrant populations** (see Fig. 5-1) **have provided many intriguing clues to the factors that may influence the pathogenesis of cancer.** The United States, which has been the destination of one of the greatest population movements of all time, is the source of most of the important data in this field.

CANCER OF THE STOMACH: A study of Japanese residents of Hawaii found that emigrants from Japanese regions with the highest risk of stomach cancer continued to exhibit an excess risk in Hawaii. By contrast, their offspring who were born in Hawaii had the same incidence of this cancer as American whites. Although dietary factors, such as pickled vegetables and salted fish, have been postulated to account for the higher incidence in Japan and the lower incidence in Hawaii, no firm evidence has been adduced to support this contention. More recently it has been shown in Japan that the population in regions at high risk for stomach cancer also display a high prevalence of chronic atrophic gastritis with intestinal metaplasia, lesions that are considered precursors of gastric cancer. Interestingly, when persons from these regions move to low-risk areas, they carry the high prevalence of intestinal metaplasia with them. Thus, the environmental factors associated with stomach cancer may not be directly carcinogenic but rather may be related to atrophic gastritis and intestinal metaplasia.

COLORECTAL, BREAST, ENDOMETRIAL, OVARIAN, AND PROSTATIC CANCERS: Emigrant studies of the incidence of colorectal cancer show opposite trends to those of stomach cancer. Emigrants from low-risk areas in Europe and Japan exhibit an increased risk of colorectal cancer in the United States. Moreover, their offspring continue at higher risk and reach the incidence levels of the general American population. This rule for colorectal cancer also prevails for cancers of the breast, endometrium, ovary, and prostate.

CANCER OF THE LIVER: As noted above, primary hepatocellular carcinoma is common in Asia and Africa, where it has been associated with hepatitis B and C. In American blacks and Asians, however, the neoplasm is no more common than in American whites, a situation that presumably reflects the relatively low prevalence of chronic viral hepatitis in the United States.

BURKITT LYMPHOMA: In Central Africa, emigrants from highland regions to lowland areas, where Burkitt lymphoma is rare, develop tumors at an older age than do those born in endemic areas. This presumably reflects a later age of exposure to EBV or a more potent stimulation of the antigenic response by malaria. Moreover, the incidence of Burkitt lymphoma is higher among emigrants to high-risk areas than among the same group who stay in the low-risk areas. Indeed, the risk of Burkitt lymphoma is higher in emigrants to high-risk areas than among adults who were born in the high-risk area. It is probable that many adults in the high-risk areas who have escaped Burkitt lymphoma in their youth are immune to the disease.

HODGKIN DISEASE: In general, in poorly developed countries the childhood form of Hodgkin disease is the one reported most often. In developed Western countries, by contrast, the disease is most common among young adults. Such a pattern is characteristic of certain viral infections, although there is no evidence for an infectious etiology of Hodgkin disease. An exception to this generalization is noted in Japan, a developed country where young adult disease is distinctly uncommon. Further evidence for an environmental influence is the higher incidence of Hodgkin disease in Americans of Japanese descent than that in Japan.

SUGGESTED READING

Books

Dabbs D: *Diagnostic immunohistochemistry*. New York: Churchill Livingstone, 2002.

Devita VT Jr, Hellman S, Rosenberg A: Cancer: *Principles and practice of oncology*, 6th ed. Philadelphia: Lippincott Williams & Wilkins, 2001.

Souhami RL, Tannock I, Hohenberger P, Horiot, J-C: *Oxford textbook of oncology*. Oxford: Oxford University Press, 2002.

Vogelstein B, Kinzler KW: *The genetic basis of human cancer*. New York: McGraw-Hill, 2002.

Review Articles

Blume-Jensen P, Hunter, T: Oncogenic kinase signaling. *Nature* 411:355–365, 2001.

Brakebusch C, Bouvard D, Stanchi F, et al.: Integrins in invasive growth. *J Clin Invest* 109:999–1006, 2002.

Calvert PM, Frucht H: The genetics of colorectal cancer. *Ann Intern Med* 137:603–612, 2002.

Corn PG, El-Deiry WS: Derangement of growth and differentiation control in oncogenesis. *BioEssays* 24:83–90, 2002.

Evan GI, Vousden KH: Proliferation, cell cycle and apoptosis in cancer. *Nature* 4:342–348, 2001.

Hahn WC, Weinberg RA: Rules for making tumor cells. *N Engl J Med* 347:1593–1603, 2002.

Hickman JA: Apoptosis and tumourigenesis. *Curr Opin Genet Dev*: 12:67–72, 2002.

Jemal A, Murray T, Samuels A, et al.: *CA (Cancer statistics)* 53:5–26, 2003.

Jiang T, Goldberg ID, Shi YE: Complex roles of tissue inhibitors of metalloproteinases in cancer. *Oncogene* 21:2245–2252, 2002.

Marsh DJ, Zori RT: Genetic insights into familial cancers—update and recent discoveries. *Cancer Lett* 181:125–164, 2002.

Munger K: Disruption of oncogene/tumor suppressor networks during human carcinogenesis. *Cancer Invest* 20:71–81, 2002.

Sen F, Vega F, Medeiros J: Molecular methods in the diagnosis of hematologic neoplasms. *Semin Diagn Pathol* 19:72–93, 2002.

White MK, McCubrey JA: Suppression of apoptosis: Role in cell growth and neoplasia. *Leukemia* 15:1011–1021, 2001.

CHAPTER 6

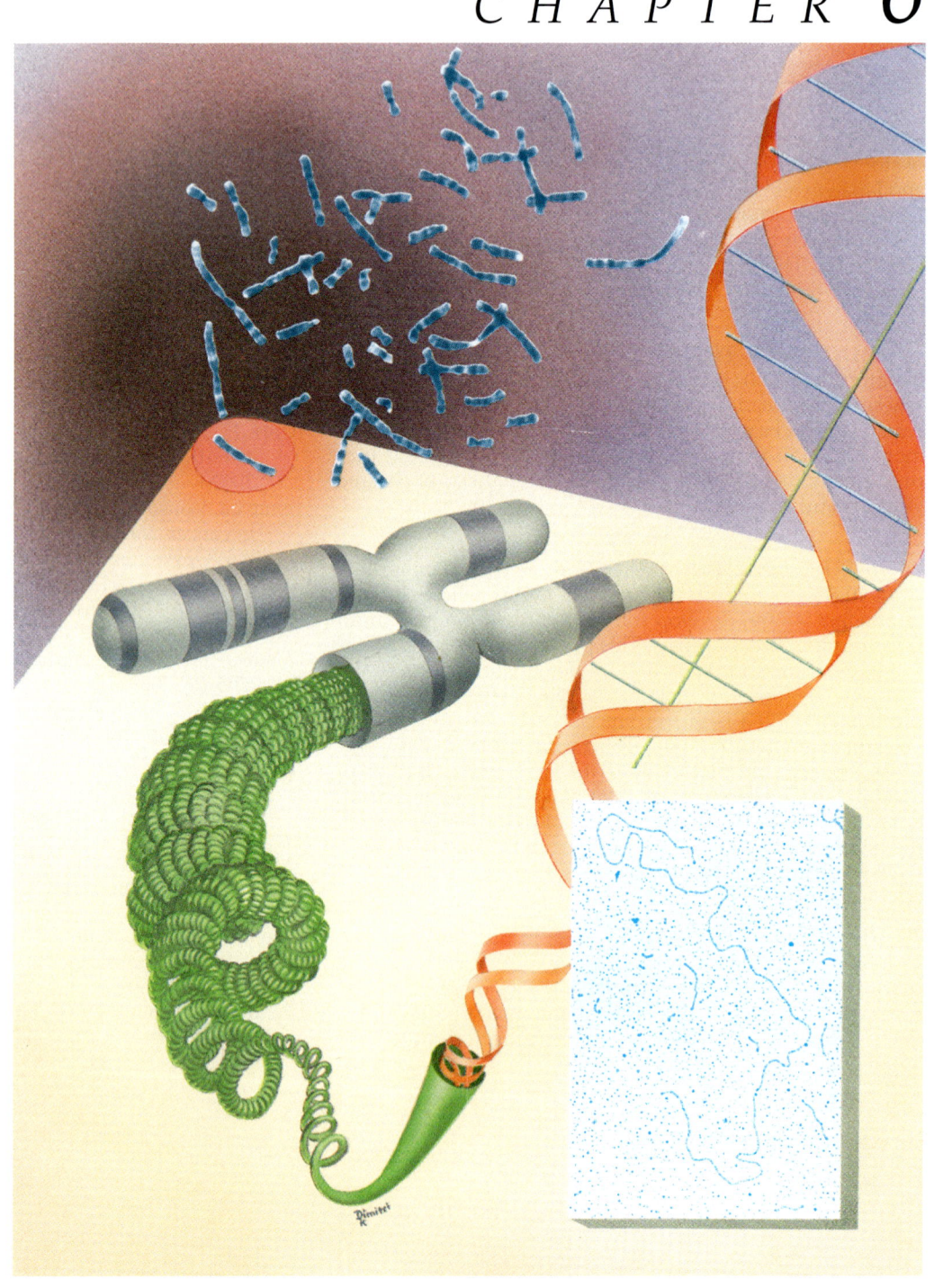

Developmental and Genetic Diseases

Emanuel Rubin
Anthony A. Killeen

Magnitude of the Problem

Principles of Teratology

Errors of Morphogenesis
Clinically Important Malformations

Chromosomal Abnormalities
Normal Chromosomes
Structural Chromosomal Abnormalities
Causes of Abnormal Chromosome Numbers
Syndromes of the Autosomal Chromosomes
Numerical Aberrations of Sex Chromosomes
Single-Gene Abnormalities
Autosomal Dominant Disorders
Heritable Diseases of Connective Tissue
Autosomal Recessive Disorders
Cystic Fibrosis
Lysosomal Storage Diseases
Inborn Errors of Amino Acid Metabolism
X-Linked Disorders

Mitochondrial Diseases

Genetic Imprinting

Multifactorial Inheritance
Cleft Lip and Cleft Palate

Screening for Carriers of Genetic Disorders

Prenatal Diagnosis of Genetic Disorders

Diseases of Infancy and Childhood

Prematurity and Intrauterine Growth Retardation
Organ Immaturity
Respiratory Distress Syndrome (RDS) of the Newborn
Erythroblastosis Fetalis
Birth Injury
Sudden Infant Death Syndrome

Neoplasms of Infancy and Childhood
Benign Tumors and Tumorlike Conditions
Cancers in the Pediatric Age Group

FIGURE 6-1 *(see opposite page)*
Squash preparation of human chromosomes stained by the Giemsa banding technique. The X chromosome is enlarged and depicted schematically.

GLOSSARY

The following terms are used in the text or figures of this chapter:

Allele–An alternative form of a gene.

Alternative splicing–A regulatory mechanism by which variations in the incorporation of a gene's exons, or coding regions, into messenger RNA (mRNA) lead to the production of more than one related protein, or isoform.

Autosomes–All of the nuclear chromosomes except for the sex chromosomes.

Centromere–The constricted region near the center of a chromosome, which has a critical role in cell division.

Codon–A three-base sequence of DNA or RNA that specifies a single amino acid.

Conservative mutation–A change in a DNA or RNA sequence that leads to the replacement of one amino acid with a biochemically similar one.

Epigenetic–A term describing nonmutational phenomena, such as methylation and histone modification, that alter the expression of a gene.

Exon–A region of a gene that codes for a protein.

Frame-shift mutation–The addition or deletion of a number of DNA bases that is not a multiple of three, thus causing a shift in the reading frame of the gene. This shift leads to a change in the reading frame of all parts of the gene that are downstream from the mutation, often creating a premature stop codon and ultimately, a truncated protein.

Gain-of-function mutation–A mutation that produces a protein that takes on a new or enhanced function.

Genomics–The study of the functions and interactions of all the genes in the genome, including their interactions with environmental factors.

Genotype–A person's genetic makeup, as reflected by his or her DNA sequence.

Haplotype–A group of nearby alleles that are inherited together.

Hemizygous–Having a gene on one chromosome for which there is no counterpart on the opposite chromosome.

Heterozygous–Having two different alleles at a specific autosomal (or X chromosomal in a female) gene locus.

Homozygous–Having two identical alleles at a specific autosomal (or X chromosomal in a female) gene locus.

Intron–A region of a gene that does not code for a protein.

Linkage disequilibrium–The nonrandom association in a population of alleles at nearby loci.

Loss-of-function mutation–A mutation that decreases the production or function of a protein (or both).

Missense mutation–A mutation that decreases the production or function of a protein (or both).

Monogenic–Caused by a mutation in a single gene.

Motif–A DNA-sequence pattern within a gene that, because of its similarity to sequences in other known genes, suggests a possible function of the gene, its protein product, or both.

Multifactorial–Caused by the interaction of multiple genetic and environmental factors.

Nonconservative mutation–A change in the DNA or RNA sequence that leads to the replacement of one amino acid with a very dissimilar one.

Nonsense mutation–Substitution of a single DNA base that results in a stop codon, thereby leading to the truncation of a protein.

Penetrance–The likelihood that a person carrying a particular mutant gene will have an altered phenotype.

Phenotype–The clinical presentation or expression of a specific gene or genes, environmental factors, or both.

Point mutation–The substitution of a single DNA base in the normal DNA sequence.

Regulatory mutation–A mutation in a region of the genome in multiple identical or closely related copies.

Repeat sequence–A stretch of bases that occurs in the genome in multiple identical or closely related copies.

Silent mutation–Substitution of single DNA base that produces no change in the amino acid sequence of the encoded protein.

Single-nucleotide polymorphism (SNP)–A common variant in the genome sequence; the human genome contains about 10 million SNPs.

Stop codon–A codon that leads to the termination of a protein rather than the addition of an amino acid. The three stop codons are TGA, TAA, and TAG.

It has been known since biblical times that certain disorders are inherited or related to disturbances in intrauterine development. The earliest sanitary codices contain guidelines on how to choose a healthy spouse, how to conceive healthy children, and what to do or not do during pregnancy. Nevertheless, most of our present scientific knowledge about developmental and genetic disorders has been gathered only within the past three decades, and the exponential growth of molecular genetics has provided the tools for unraveling the etiology and pathogenesis of these disorders. In fact, the molecular basis of most inherited disorders caused by single-gene mutations are either known today or likely to be described within the next few years.

Diseases that originate during prenatal development range from conditions caused solely by factors in the fetal environment to those that are exclusively determined by genomic abnormalities. There are also diseases that exemplify the interaction between genetic defects and environmental influences. An example is phenylketonuria, in which a genetic deficiency of phenylalanine hydroxylase causes mental retardation only if the infant is exposed to dietary phenylalanine.

Developmental and genetic disorders are classified as follows:

- Errors of morphogenesis
- Chromosomal abnormalities
- Single-gene defects
- Polygenic inherited diseases

The fetus may also be injured by adverse transplacental influences or by deformities and injuries caused by intrauterine trauma or during parturition. After birth, acquired diseases of infancy and childhood are also important causes of morbidity and mortality.

MAGNITUDE OF THE PROBLEM

Each year, about one quarter of a million babies are born in the United States with a birth defect. Worldwide, at least 1 in 50 newborns has a major congenital anomaly, 1 in 100 has a single-gene abnormality, and 1 in 200 has a major chromosomal abnormality.

In more than two thirds of all birth defects, the cause is not apparent (Fig. 6-2). No more than 6% of total birth defects can be attributed to uterine factors, maternal disorders such as metabolic imbalances or infections during pregnancy, and other environmental hazards, including exposure to drugs, chemicals, and radiation. Most of the remaining conditions are accounted for by genomic defects, either hereditary traits or spontaneous mutations, and a smaller number by chromosomal abnormalities.

Although chromosomal abnormalities account for only a small fraction of birth defects in newborns, cytogenetic

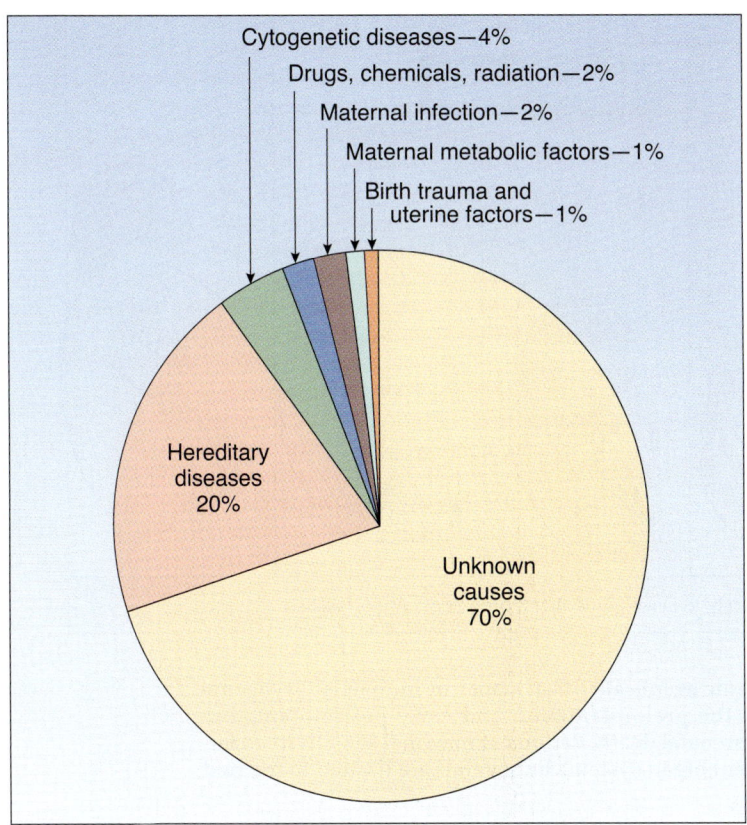

FIGURE 6-2
Causes of birth defects in humans. Most birth defects have unknown causes.

analysis of fetuses spontaneously aborted in early pregnancy indicates that up to 50% have chromosomal abnormalities. **The incidence of specific numerical chromosomal abnormalities in the abortuses is several times higher than in term infants, indicating that most inborn chromosomal defects are lethal.** The conceptus dies in early pregnancy, and only a small number of children with cytogenetic abnormalities are born alive.

In advanced Western countries, developmental and genetic birth defects account for half of the total mortality in infancy and childhood. This contrasts with the situation in less-developed countries, where 95% of infant mortality is attributable to environmental causes such as infectious diseases and malnutrition. In industrialized societies, genetic counseling, early prenatal diagnosis, identification of high-risk pregnancies, and avoidance of possible exogenous teratogens are the only practical approaches that can reduce the incidence of birth anomalies. In this context, prenatal dietary supplementation with folic acid has been shown to reduce the incidence of congenital neural tube defects.

PRINCIPLES OF TERATOLOGY

Teratology is the discipline concerned with the study of developmental anomalies (Gk. *teraton*, monster). **Teratogens** are chemical, physical, and biological agents that cause developmental anomalies. There are few proven teratogens in humans, but many drugs and chemicals are teratogenic in animals and should, therefore, be considered potentially dangerous for humans.

Malformation refers to a morphological defect or abnormality of an organ, part of an organ, or anatomical region that results from perturbed morphogenesis. Exposure to a teratogen may result in a malformation, but this is not invariably the case. Such observations have led to the formulation of general principles of teratology:

- **Susceptibility to teratogens is variable.** Presumably the principal determinants of this variability are the genotypes of the fetus and the mother. Experimental evidence for this concept comes from the demonstration that cer-

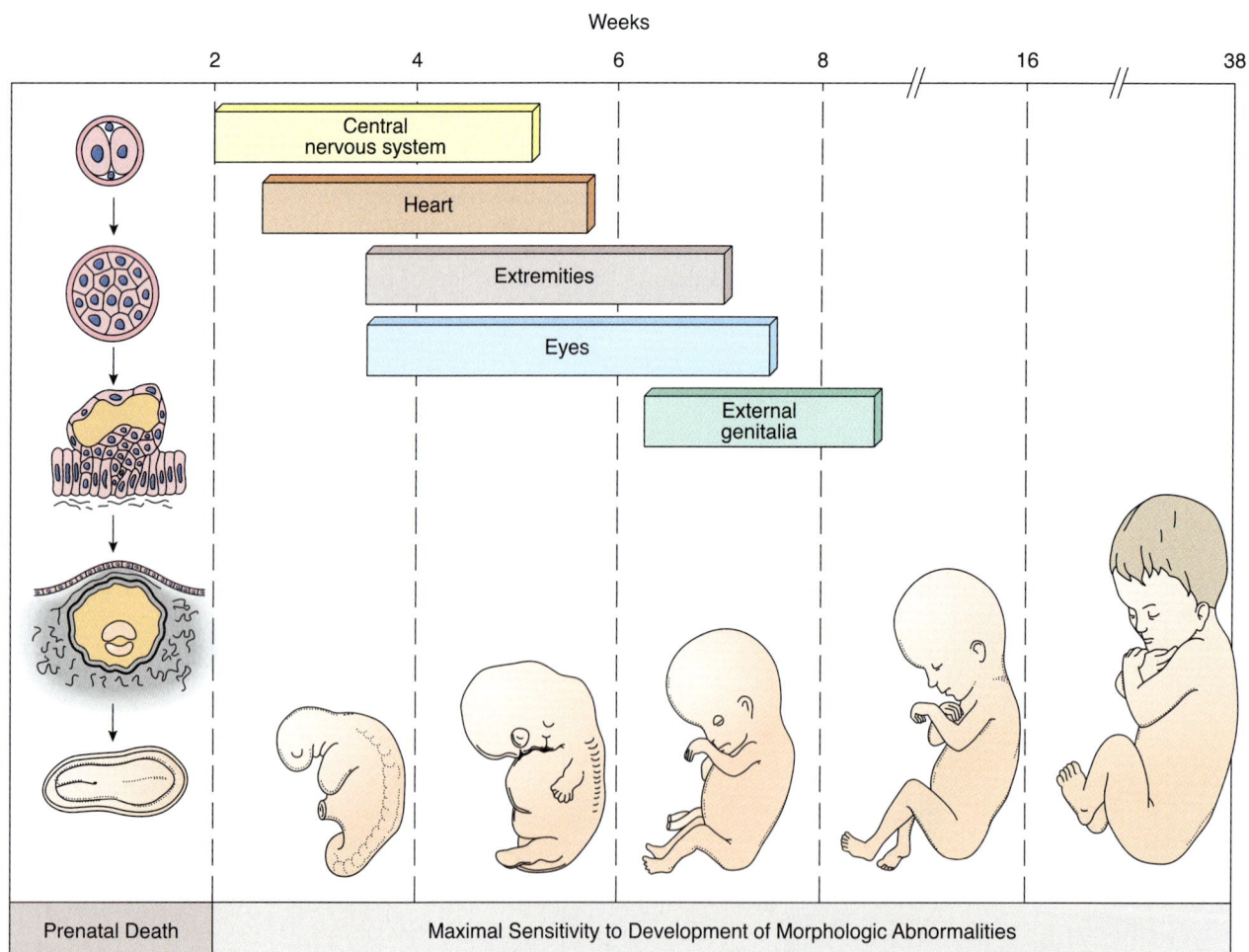

FIGURE 6-3
Sensitivity of specific organs to teratogenic agents at critical stages of human embryogenesis. Exposure to adverse influences in the preimplantation and early postimplantation stages of development (*far left*) **leads to prenatal death. Periods of maximal sensitivity to teratogens** (*horizontal bars*) **vary for different organ systems but overall are limited to the first 8 weeks of pregnancy.**

tain strains of inbred mice are susceptible to some teratogens whereas others are not. An example of human variability in the vulnerability to teratogens is the fetal alcohol syndrome, which affects some children of alcoholic mothers whereas others are resistant.

- **Susceptibility to teratogens is specific for each developmental stage.** Most agents are teratogenic only during critical stages of development (Fig. 6-3). For example, maternal rubella infection causes abnormalities in the fetus only during the first 3 months of pregnancy.
- **The mechanism of teratogenesis is specific for each teratogen.** Teratogenic drugs inhibit the activity of crucial enzymes or receptors, interfere with the formation of the mitotic spindle, or block energy production, thereby inhibiting metabolic steps critical for normal morphogenesis. Many drugs and viruses affect specific tissues (e.g., neurotropism, cardiotropism) and thereby damage some developing organs more than others.
- **Teratogenesis is dose dependent.** Theoretically, this means that each teratogen should have a "safe" dose, below which no teratogenesis occurs. In practice, however, because of the multiple determinants of teratogenesis, all established teratogens should be avoided during pregnancy; an absolutely safe dose cannot be predicted for every woman.
- **Teratogens produce death, growth retardation, malformation, or functional impairment.** The outcome depends on the interaction between the teratogenic influences, the maternal organism, and the fetal–placental unit.

The search for human teratogens requires (1) population surveys, (2) prospective and retrospective studies of single malformations, and (3) the investigation of reported adverse effects of drugs or other chemicals. The list of proven teratogens is long and includes most cytotoxic drugs, alcohol, some antiepileptic drugs, heavy metals, and thalidomide. On the other hand, many drugs and chemicals have been declared safe for use during pregnancy because of negative teratogenic studies in laboratory animals. However, there is species specificity for every drug, and the fact that a drug is not teratogenic for mice and rabbits is not necessarily evidence that it is innocuous for humans. In fact, the best known drug-related teratogenic incident—complex malformations related to the ingestion of the hypnotic drug thalidomide—occurred after the drug was found not to be teratogenic in mice and rats. Interestingly, long after the drug was shown to be teratogenic in humans, its teratogenicity was also demonstrated in rabbits and monkeys.

ERRORS OF MORPHOGENESIS

Normal intrauterine and postnatal development depends on sequential activation and repression of genes inherited from the parents. Although the fertilized ovum (zygote) has all the genes found in the adult organism, most of them are inactive. As the zygote enters cleavage stages of development, individual genes or sets of genes are activated in a stage-specific manner. Initially, activation involves only genes essential for cellular replication and growth, cell-to-cell interaction, and the regulation of important morphogenetic movements. **Abnormally activated or structurally abnormal genes in the zygote and early embryonic cells can result in early death.**

The cells that form the two-cell and four-cell embryos (blastomeres) are developmentally equipotent, and each can give rise to an adult organism. Separation of the embryonic cells at this stage results in identical twins or quadruplets. Since the blastomeres are equipotent and interchangeable, loss of a single blastomere at this stage of development may pass without any serious consequences. On the other hand, since the blastomeres are identical, if one blastomere contains a set of lethal genes, it is likely that other blastomeres contain the same genes. Thus, their activation invariably leads to the death of the conceptus. Furthermore, if the conceptus is exposed to untoward exogenous influences, the noxious agent exerts the same effect on all blastomeres and also causes death. **We conclude that adverse environmental influences on preimplantation-stage embryos exert an all-or-nothing effect: either the conceptus dies or development proceeds uninterrupted, since the interchangeable blastomeres replace the loss.** As a rule, exogenous toxins acting on preimplantation-stage embryos do not produce errors of morphogenesis and do not result in malformations (see Fig. 6-3). **The most common consequence of toxic exposure at the preimplantation stage is embryonic death, which often passes unnoticed or is perceived as heavy, albeit delayed, menstrual bleeding.**

Injury during the first 8 to 10 days after fertilization usually results in an incomplete separation of blastomeres, an effect that leads to the formation of conjoined twins. Symmetric conjoined twins represent incompletely separated twins ("Siamese twins") joined at various anatomical sites, such as the head (craniopagus), thorax (thoracopagus), or rump (ischiopagus). Asymmetric conjoined twins have one well-developed and one rudimentary or hypoplastic twin. The rudimentary twin is always abnormal and is either externally attached to, or internally included in, the body of the better-developed sibling (fetus in fetu). Some of the congenital teratomas, especially those in the sacrococcygeal area, are actually asymmetric monsters.

Most complex developmental abnormalities affecting several organ systems are due to injuries inflicted from the time of implantation of the blastocyst through early organogenesis. In addition to rapid cell division, this period is characterized by differentiation of cells and formation of so-called **developmental fields,** in which cells interact and determine each other's developmental fate. This process leads to irreversible differentiation of groups of cells. Complex morphological movements form organ primordia (anlage), and organs are then interconnected in functionally active systems. **The formation of primordial organ systems is the stage of embryonic development most susceptible to teratogenesis, and many major developmental abnormalities are probably due to faulty gene activity or the deleterious effects of exogenous toxins on the embryo at this time** (see Fig. 6-3). Disorganized or disrupted morphogenesis may have minor or major consequences at the level of (1) cells and tissues, (2) organs or organ systems, and (3) anatomical regions.

Agenesis is the complete absence of an organ primordium. It may manifest as (1) complete absence of an organ, as in unilateral or bilateral agenesis of kidneys; (2) the absence of part of an organ, as in agenesis of the corpus callosum of the brain; or (3) the absence of tissue or cells within an organ, as in the absence of testicular germ cells in congenital infertility ("Sertoli cell only" syndrome).

Aplasia is the absence of an organ coupled with persistence of the organ anlage or a rudiment that never developed completely. Thus, aplasia of the lung refers to a condition in which the main bronchus ends blindly in nondescript tissue composed of rudimentary ducts and connective tissue.

Hypoplasia refers to reduced size owing to the incomplete development of all or part of an organ. Examples include microphthalmia (small eyes), micrognathia (small jaw), and microcephaly (small brain and head).

Dysraphic anomalies are defects caused by the failure of apposed structures to fuse. Spina bifida is an anomaly in which the spinal canal has not closed completely, and the overlying bone and skin have not fused, thus leaving a midline defect.

Involution failures reflect the persistence of embryonic or fetal structures that should involute at certain stages of development. A persistent thyroglossal duct is the result of incomplete involution of the tract that connects the base of the tongue with the developing thyroid.

Division failures are caused by the incomplete cleavage of embryonic tissues, when that process depends on the programmed death of cells. Fingers and toes are formed at the distal end of the limb bud through the loss of cells located between the primordia that contain the cartilage. If these cells do not die in a programmed manner, the fingers will be conjoined or incompletely separated (syndactyly).

Atresia refers to defects caused by the incomplete formation of a lumen. Many hollow organs originate as strands and cords of cells whose centers are programmed to die, thus forming a central cavity or lumen. Atresia of the esophagus is characterized by partial occlusion of the lumen, which was not fully established in embryogenesis.

Dysplasia is caused by abnormal organization of cells into tissues, a situation that results in abnormal histogenesis. (Dysplasia has a different meaning here from that used in characterizing the precancerous lesion epithelial dysplasia [see Chapter 1].) Tuberous sclerosis is a striking example of dysplasia, being characterized by abnormal development of the brain, which contains aggregates of normally developed cells arranged into grossly visible "tubers."

Ectopia, or heterotopia, is an anomaly in which an organ is outside its normal anatomical site. Thus, an ectopic heart is located outside the thorax. Heterotopic parathyroid glands can be located within the thymus in the anterior mediastinum.

Dystopia refers to the retention of an organ at a site where it is located during development. For example, the kidneys are initially in the pelvis and then move into a more craniad lumbar position. Dystopic kidneys are those that remain in the pelvis. Dystopic testes are retained in the inguinal canal, not

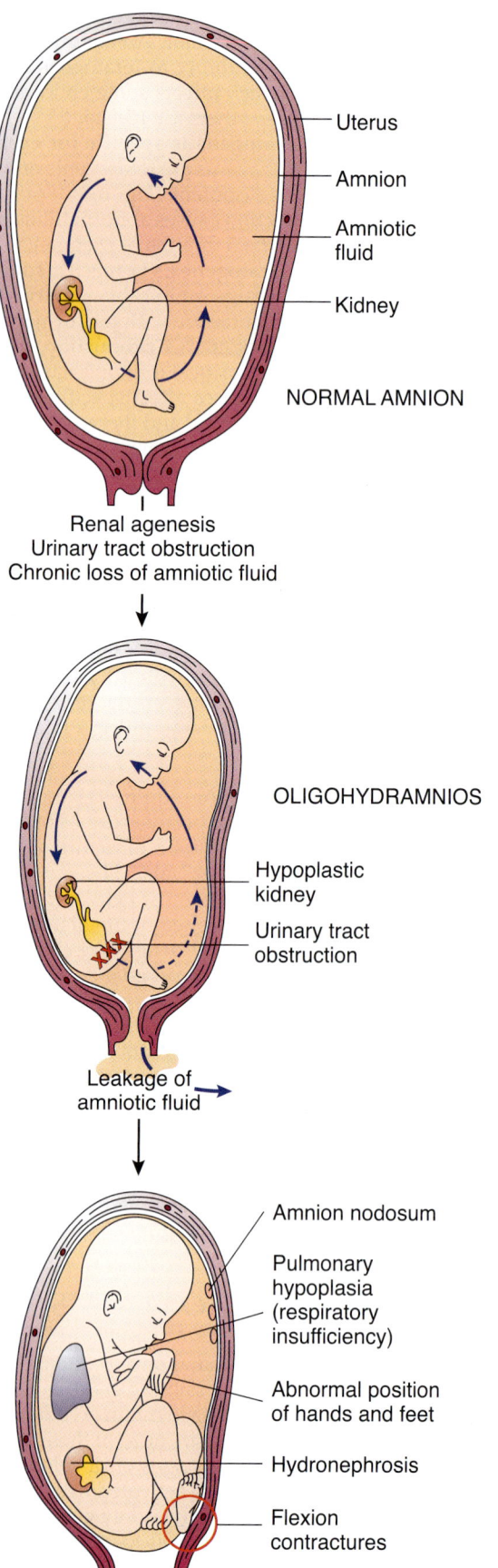

FIGURE 6-4
Potter complex. The fetus normally swallows amniotic fluid and, in turn, excretes urine, thereby maintaining its normal volume of amniotic fluid. In the face of urinary tract disease (e.g., renal agenesis or urinary tract obstruction) or leakage of amniotic fluid, the volume of amniotic fluid decreases, a situation termed *oligohydramnios*. Oligohydramnios results in a number of congenital abnormalities termed *Potter complex*, which includes pulmonary hypoplasia and contractures of the limbs. The amnion has a nodular appearance. In cases of urinary tract obstruction, congenital hydronephrosis is also seen, although this abnormality is not considered part of Potter complex.

having completed their descent into the scrotum (cryptorchidism).

Developmental anomalies caused by interference with morphogenesis are often multiple:

- *A polytopic effect* refers to a situation in which the noxious stimulus affects several organs that are simultaneously in critical stages of development.
- *A monotopic effect* denotes a single localized anomaly that results in a cascade of pathogenetic events.
- *A developmental sequence anomaly* (anomalad or complex anomaly) is a pattern of defects that is related to a single anomaly or pathogenetic mechanism. In a developmental sequence anomaly, different factors lead to the same consequences through a common pathway. Such a situation, which represents the result of a monotopic effect, is well illustrated by Potter complex (Fig. 6-4), in which pulmonary hypoplasia, external signs of intrauterine fetal compression, and morphological changes of the amnion, are all related to oligohydramnios (a severely reduced amount of amniotic fluid). A fetus enclosed in an amniotic sac with insufficient fluid develops the distinctive features of Potter complex irrespective of the cause of the oligohydramnios.

A developmental syndrome refers to multiple anomalies that are pathogenetically related. The term *syndrome* implies a single cause for anomalies in diverse organs that have been damaged by the same polytopic effect during a critical developmental period. Many of the developmental syndromes are related to chromosomal abnormalities or single-gene defects. By contrast, *developmental association, or syntropy,* refers to multiple anomalies that are associated statistically but do not necessarily share the same pathogenetic mechanisms. Many of the anomalies that now seem unrelated may one day prove to have the same cause. However, until such associations are proved, it is important to note that not all multiple congenital defects are interrelated. In practical terms, the birth of a child with multiple anomalies does not prove that the mother was exposed to an exogenous teratogen or that all the diverse anomalies are caused by the same genetic defect. The recognition of specific syndromes, and their distinction from random associations, is essential for the estimation of the risk of recurrence of similar anomalies in subsequent children of the same family.

After the third month of pregnancy, exposure of the human fetus to teratogenic influences rarely results in major errors of morphogenesis. However, morphological and, especially, functional consequences are still found in children exposed to exogenous teratogens during the second and third trimesters. Although organs have already been formed by the end of the third month of pregnancy, most still undergo the restructuring and maturation required for extrauterine life. Functional maturation proceeds at different rates in different organs. For example, the central nervous system does not attain functional maturity until several years after birth and is thus susceptible to adverse exogenous influences not only during pregnancy but for some time after birth.

A deformation is defined as an abnormality of form, shape, or position of a part of the body caused by mechanical forces. Most anatomical defects caused by adverse influences in the latter two trimesters of pregnancy fall into this category. The responsible forces may be external (e.g., amniotic bands in the uterus) or intrinsic (e.g., fetal hypomobility caused by central nervous system injury). Thus, a deformity known as equinovarus foot can be due to the compression of the extremities by the uterine wall in oligohydramnios or to spinal cord abnormalities that lead to defective innervation and movement of the foot.

Clinically Important Malformations Occur in Many Organs and Have Diverse Causes

Anencephaly and Other Neural Tube Defects

Anencephaly

Anencephaly refers to the congenital absence of the cranial vault, with cerebral hemispheres completely missing or reduced to small masses attached to the base of the skull.

Epidemiology: Anencephaly is a typical multifactorial birth defect that exhibits a worldwide geographical variation in incidence. In the United States, the frequency of this anomaly is 0.3 per 1000 live births and stillbirths, whereas in Ireland and Wales, the frequency is 20-fold greater (5 to 6 per 1000 conceptuses). Interestingly, Irish immigrants to North America have the highest incidence of anencephaly on the continent, although it is lower (2 to 3 per 1000) than that in Ireland. A high frequency of anencephaly has also been reported in Iran. The incidence of this disorder is particularly low in blacks.

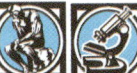

Pathogenesis and Pathology: Anencephaly is a dysraphic defect of neural tube closure. During fetal development the neural plate invaginates and is transformed into the neural tube by fusion of the posterior surfaces (Fig. 6-5). The mesenchymal tissue overlying the primitive neural tube then molds the skull and the vertebral arches posterior to the spinal cord. Failure of the neural tube to close results in the lack of closure of the overlying bony structures of the cranium and an absence of the calvarium, skin, and subcutaneous tissues of this region. The exposed brain is incompletely formed or even entirely absent. In most cases, the base of the skull contains only fragments of neural and ependymal tissue and residues of the meninges. *Acrania* (complete or partial absence of the cranium) results from an injury to the fetus between the 23rd and 26th days of gestation.

Genetic factors seem to play a role in the pathogenesis of anencephaly. The anomaly is twice as common in females as in males, and it occurs with higher frequency in certain families. The risk of a second anencephalic fetus is 2 to 5%, and after two anencephalic fetuses the risk rises to 25% for each subsequent pregnancy.

Folic acid supplied in the periconceptional period lowers the incidence of neural tube defects (NTDs). In 1998, the United States Food and Drug Administration began requiring manufacturers of enriched flour, bread, and some other products to supplement these foods with folate. This mandate has been associated with a significant decrease in the incidence of neural tube defects.

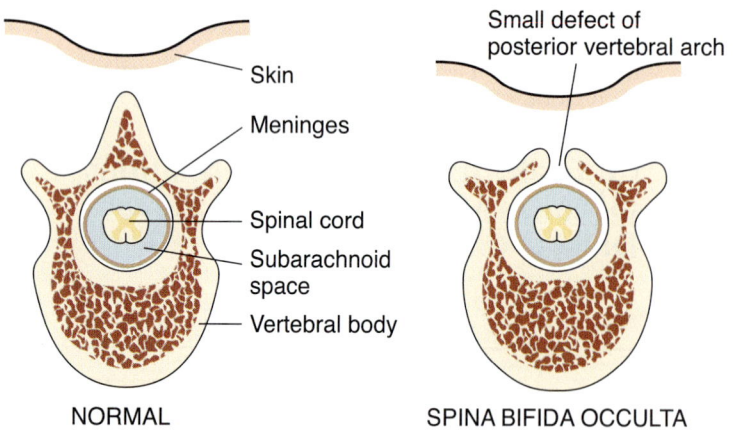
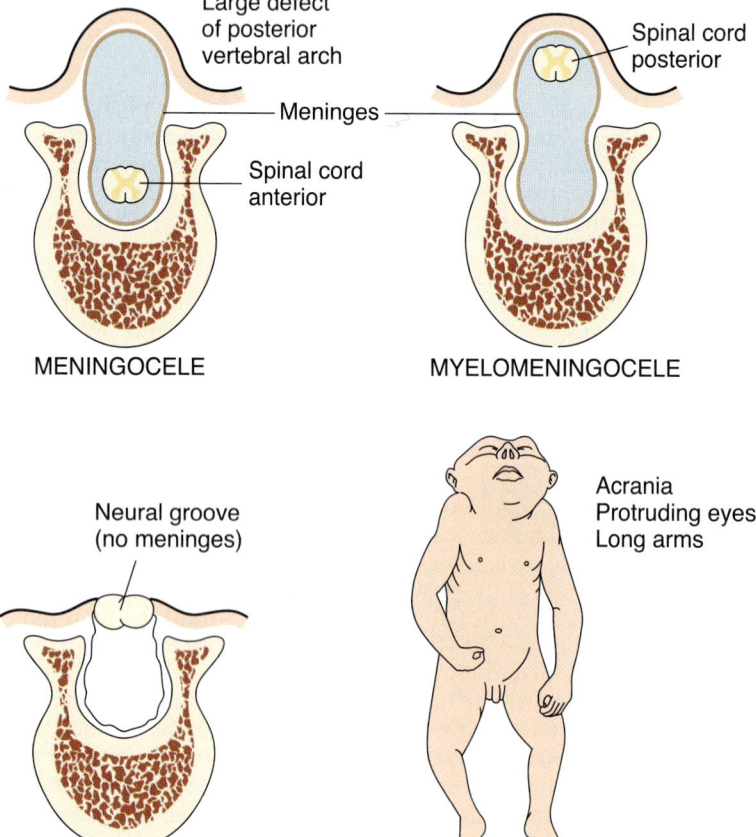

FIGURE 6-5
Dysraphic defects of the neural tube. Incomplete fusion of the neural tube and overlying bone, soft tissues, or skin leads to several defects, varying from mild anomalies (e.g., spina bifida occulta) to severe anomalies (e.g., anencephaly).

Clinical Features: Two thirds of anencephalic fetuses die in utero, and those that are alive at birth rarely survive for more than a week. Screening of pregnant women for serum α-fetoprotein and examination by ultrasonography allow detection of virtually all anencephalic fetuses. The use of organs from anencephalic infants for transplantation remains a thorny ethical problem.

Other Neural Tube Defects

The neural tube closes sequentially in a craniocaudal direction, and a defect in this process results in abnormalities of the vertebral column.

- *Craniorachischisis occurs when defective closure extends from the cranium into the spinal cord and vertebral column.*
- *Spina bifida refers to the incomplete closure of the spinal cord or vertebral column or both.* This anomaly is usually local-

ized to the lumbar region and represents the mildest dysraphic abnormality of the central nervous system. Spina bifida results from an insult between the 25th and 30th days of gestation, reflecting the sequential closure of the neural tube.

- *Meningocele* is a hernial protrusion of the meninges through a defect in the vertebral column.
- *Myelomeningocele* refers to the same condition as meningocele, but it is complicated by hernial protrusion of the spinal cord itself.

Neural tube defects are illustrated in Figure 6-5.

Thalidomide-Induced Malformations

Limb-reduction deformities, involving one or up to all four extremities, are rare congenital defects of mostly obscure origin that affect 1 in 5000 liveborn infants. These defects have been known for ages: a Goya depiction of a typical example is in the Louvre Museum in Paris. In the 1960s, a sudden increase in the incidence of limb-reduction deformities in Germany and England was linked to maternal intake of a sedative during the early stages of pregnancy. Known under the generic name of thalidomide, this derivative of glutamic acid is teratogenic between the 28th and 50th days of pregnancy. Many of the children born to mothers exposed to thalidomide presented with skeletal deformities and pleomorphic defects in other organs, most commonly the ears **(microtia and anotia)** and the heart. Typically, the arms of the affected children were short and malformed (Fig. 6-6) and resembled the flippers of a seal **(phocomelia)**. Sometimes limbs were completely missing **(amelia)**. The central nervous system was not involved, and the children had normal intelligence. After it was recognized that the defects were causally linked to thalidomide, the drug was banned from the market, but not before an estimated 3000 malformed children were born.

Fetal Hydantoin Syndrome

Ten percent of children born to epileptic mothers treated during pregnancy with antiepileptic drugs such as hydantoin show characteristic facial features, hypoplasia of nails and digits, and various congenital heart defects. Since this syndrome occurs only two to three times more often in treated epileptics than in untreated ones, it is uncertain whether the defects are entirely due to the adverse effects of the drug. Nevertheless, it appears that fetal susceptibility to this disorder correlates with the fetal level of the microsomal detoxifying enzyme epoxide hydrolase. Presumably, the accumulation of poorly detoxified reactive intermediates of hydantoin metabolism promotes teratogenesis.

Fetal Alcohol Syndrome

Fetal alcohol syndrome refers to a complex of abnormalities induced by the maternal consumption of alcoholic beverages that includes (1) growth retardation, (2) dysfunction of the central nervous system, and (3) characteristic facial dysmorphology. Since not all children adversely affected by maternal alcohol abuse exhibit the entire spectrum of abnormalities, the term *fetal alcohol effect* is also used.

 Epidemiology and Pathogenesis: An injurious effect of intrauterine exposure to alcohol was noted in biblical times and was reported during the historic London gin epidemic (1720 to 1750). However, it was not until 1968 that a specific syndrome was identified. The prevalence of fetal alcohol syndrome in the United States and Europe is 1 to 3 per 1000 live births. However, in populations with extremely high rates of alcoholism, such as some tribes of Native Americans, the incidence may be astounding (20 to 150 per 1000). **It is thought that abnormalities related to fetal alcohol effect, particularly mild mental deficiency and emotional disorders, are far more common than the full-blown fetal alcohol syndrome.**

The minimum amount of alcohol that results in fetal injury is not well established, but children with the entire spectrum of fetal alcohol syndrome are usually born to mothers who are chronic alcoholics. Heavy alcohol consumption during the first trimester of pregnancy is particularly dangerous. The mechanism by which alcohol damages the developing fetus remains unknown despite a large body of research.

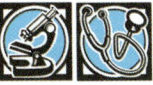 **Pathology and Clinical Features:** Infants born to alcoholic mothers often exhibit prenatal growth retardation, which continues after birth. The facial dysmorphology of fetal alcohol syndrome includes microcephaly, epicanthal folds,

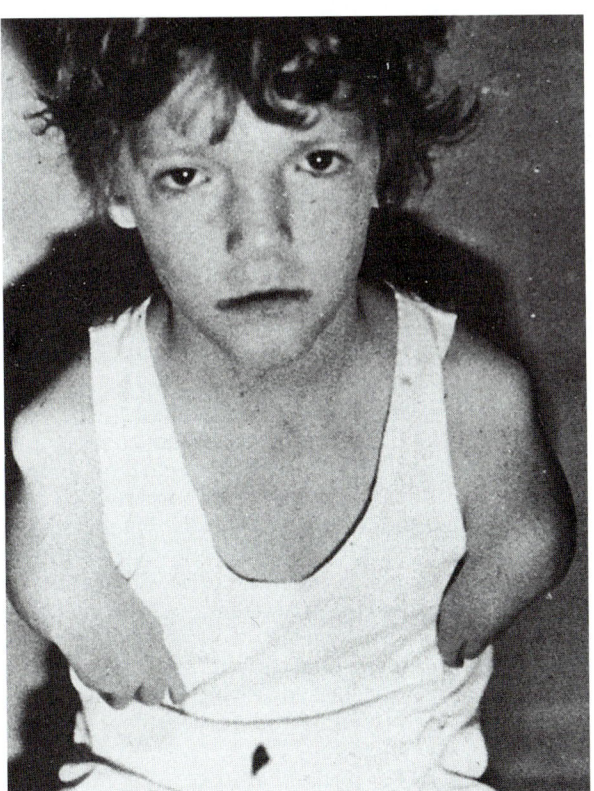

FIGURE 6-6
Thalidomide-induced deformity of the arms.

short palpebral fissures, maxillary hypoplasia, a thin upper lip, a small jaw (micrognathia), and a poorly developed philtrum. Septal defects of the heart are described in as many as one third of patients, although many of these close spontaneously. Minor abnormalities of the joints and limbs may occur.

Fetal alcohol syndrome is a common cause of mental retardation. One fifth of children with fetal alcohol syndrome have IQs below 70, and 40% are between 70 and 85. Even with a normal IQ, these children tend to have short memory spans, impulsiveness, and emotional instability (see Chapter 8).

Torch Complex

The acronym TORCH refers to a complex of similar signs and symptoms produced by fetal or neonatal infection with a variety of microorganisms, including Toxoplasma *(T), rubella (R), cytomegalovirus (C), and herpes simplex virus (H).* In the acronym TORCH, the letter "O" represents "others." The term was coined to alert pediatricians to the fact that infections in the fetus and newborn by TORCH agents are usually indistinguishable from each other and that testing for one of the four major TORCH agents should include testing for the other three and for some possible others as well (Fig. 6-7). "Other" infections include syphilis, tuberculosis, listeriosis, leptospirosis, varicella-zoster virus infection, and Epstein-Barr virus infection. Human immunodeficiency virus (HIV) and human parvovirus (B19) have been suggested as additions to the list.

Infections with TORCH agents occur in 1 to 5% of all liveborn infants in the United States and are among the major causes of neonatal morbidity and mortality. Severe damage inflicted by these organisms is mostly irreparable, and prevention (when possible) is the only alternative. Unfortunately, the titers of serum antibodies against TORCH agents in the newborn or the mother are usually not diagnostic, and the precise cause of the condition often remains obscure.

- **Toxoplasmosis:** Asymptomatic toxoplasmosis is common, and 25% of women in their reproductive years exhibit antibodies to this organism. On the other hand, intrauterine *Toxoplasma* infection occurs in only 0.1% of all pregnancies.
- **Rubella:** The introduction of the rubella vaccine in the United States has virtually eliminated congenital rubella, and fewer than 10 cases are reported each year.
- **Cytomegalovirus:** Two thirds of women of childbearing age test positive for cytomegalovirus immunoglobulin G (IgG), and up to 2% of newborns in the United States are congenitally infected with this virus. Since most normal infants carry maternally transmitted antibodies, the "gold standard" for the diagnosis of cytomegalovirus is a urine culture.
- **Herpesvirus:** Intrauterine infection with herpes simplex virus type 2 (HSV-2) is uncommon, and infection is most often acquired during passage through the birth canal of a mother with active genital herpes. The diagnosis is established by clinical examination of the mother, the appearance of typical skin lesions in the newborn, and serological testing and culture for HSV-2. Congenital herpes infection can be prevented by cesarean section of mothers who exhibit active genital lesions.

The specific organisms of the TORCH complex are discussed in greater detail in Chapter 9.

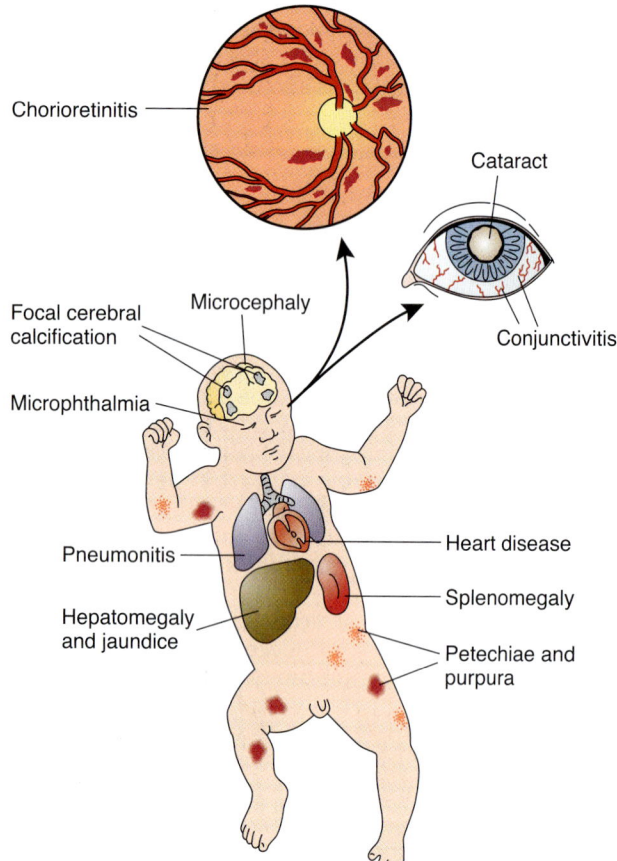

FIGURE 6-7
TORCH complex. Children infected in utero with *Toxoplasma*, rubella virus, cytomegalovirus, or herpes simplex virus show remarkably similar effects.

Pathology: The clinical and pathological findings in the symptomatic newborn vary, and only a minority present with a multisystem disease and the entire spectrum of abnormalities (Table 6-1). Growth retardation and abnormalities of the brain, eyes, liver, hematopoietic system, and heart are common.

Lesions of the brain represent the most serious pathological changes in TORCH-infected children. Acute encephalitis is associated with foci of necrosis, which are initially surrounded by inflammatory cells. Later the lesions become calcified and are visualized radiologically, most prominently in congenital toxoplasmosis. Microcephaly, hydrocephalus, and abnormally shaped gyri and sulci (microgyria) are frequent. Radiologically, defects of cerebral matter (porencephaly), missing olfactory bulbs, and other major brain defects may be identified. Severe brain damage is reflected in psychomotor retardation, neurological defects, and seizures.

Ocular defects are prominent in the TORCH complex, particularly in rubella embryopathy, in which more than two thirds of patients present with cataracts and microphthalmia. Glaucoma and malformations of the retina (coloboma)

TABLE 6-1 **Pathological Findings in the Fetus and Newborn Infected with TORCH Agents**

General	Prematurity, intrauterine retardation	
Central nervous system	Encephalitis	
	Microcephaly	
	Hydrocephaly	
	Intracranial calcifications	
	Psychomotor retardation	
Ear	Inner ear damage with hearing loss	
Eye	Microphthalmia	(R)
	Chorioretinitis	(TCH)
	Pigmented retina	(R)
	Keratoconjunctivitis	(H)
	Cataracts	(RH)
	Glaucoma	(R)
	Visual impairment	(TRCH)
Liver	Hepatomegaly	
	Liver calcifications	(R)
	Jaundice	
Hematopoietic system	Hemolytic and other anemias	
	Thrombocytopenia	
	Splenomegaly	
Skin and mucosae	Vesicular or ulcerative lesions	(H)
	Petechiae and ecchymoses	
Cardiopulmonary system	Pneumonitis	
	Myocarditis	
	Congenital heart disease	
Skeleton	Various bone lesions	

T, Toxoplasma; R, rubella virus; C, cytomegalovirus; H, herpesvirus.

may occur. Choroidoretinitis, which is common in infections with rubella, *Toxoplasma,* and cytomegalovirus, is usually bilateral, and on funduscopy appears as pale, mottled areas surrounded by a pigmented rim. Keratoconjunctivitis is the most common ocular lesion in newborns afflicted with herpes simplex.

Cardiac anomalies occur in many children with the TORCH complex, most commonly in congenital rubella. Patent ductus arteriosus and various septal defects are the most frequent abnormalities, although occasionally stenosis of the pulmonary artery and complex cardiac anomalies are encountered.

Congenital Syphilis

The organism that causes syphilis, *Treponema pallidum,* is transmitted to the fetus by a mother who has acquired syphilis during pregnancy. There is a possibility that the fetus will develop syphilis if the mother became infected in the 2 years preceding the pregnancy, although the actual risk cannot be accurately assessed. It has been estimated that congenital syphilis affects 1 in 2000 liveborn infants in the United States. In pregnant syphilitic women, stillbirth occurs in one third, and of the infants carried to term, two thirds manifest congenital syphilis.

T. pallidum invades the fetus at any point during pregnancy. Early infections most likely induce abortions, and the grossly visible signs of congenital syphilis appear only in fetuses infected after the 16th week of pregnancy. The spirochetes grow in all fetal tissues, and the clinical presentation is thus characterized by protean manifestations.

Children born with congenital syphilis are initially normal or show changes indistinguishable from those of the TORCH complex. The early lesions in various organs teem with spirochetes and are characterized by infiltrates of lymphocytes and plasma cells, particularly around blood vessels and granuloma-like lesions termed **gummas**. Many infants are asymptomatic, only to develop the typical stigmata of congenital syphilis in the first few years of life. Late symptoms of congenital syphilis become apparent many years later and reflect slowly evolving tissue destruction and repair:

- **Rhinitis:** A conspicuous mucopurulent nasal discharge, colloquially known as "snuffles," is almost always present as an early sign of congenital syphilis. The nasal mucosa is edematous and tends to ulcerate, leading to nosebleeds. Destruction of the nasal bridge eventually results in flattening of the nose, so-called *saddle nose*.
- **Skin:** A maculopapular rash is a common early finding in congenital syphilis. The palms and soles are usually affected (similar to secondary syphilis of the adult), although it may involve the entire body or any part. Cracks and fissures *(rhagades)* occur around the mouth, anus, and vulva. Flat raised plaques *(condylomata lata)* around the anus and female genitalia may develop early or after a few years.
- **Visceral organs:** A distinctive pneumonitis, characterized by pale hypocrepitant lungs *(pneumonia alba)*, may develop in the neonatal period. Hepatosplenomegaly, anemia, and lymphadenopathy may also be observed in early congenital syphilis.
- **Teeth:** The buds of the incisor teeth and the 6th-year molars develop early in postnatal life, the time when congenital syphilis is particularly aggressive. Thus, the permanent incisors may be notched *(Hutchinson teeth)* and the molars malformed *(mulberry molars)*.
- **Bones:** The most common osseous lesion is an inflammation of the periosteum together with new bone formation (periostitis). This complication is particularly evident in the anterior tibia, resulting in a distinctive outward curving called *saber shin*.
- **Eye:** A progressive vascularization of the cornea *(interstitial keratitis)* is an especially vexing complication of congenital syphilis, occurring as early as 4 years of age and as late as 20 years. The cornea eventually scars and becomes opaque.
- **Nervous system:** The nervous system is commonly involved in congenital syphilis, with symptoms beginning in infancy or after 1 year of age. **Meningitis** predominates in early congenital syphilis, resulting in convulsions, mild hydrocephalus, and mental retardation. **Meningovascular syphilis** is a common lesion in later syphilis, which may result in deafness, mental retardation, paresis, and other manifestations of neurosyphilis. *Hutchinson triad* refers to the combination of deafness, interstitial keratitis, and notched incisor teeth.

The diagnosis of congenital syphilis is suggested by clinical findings and a history of maternal infection. Serological confirmation of syphilitic infection may be difficult in the newborn because the transplacental transfer of maternal IgG gives false-positive results. Penicillin is still the drug of choice for both intrauterine and postnatal syphilis. If penicillin is given during intrauterine life or during the first 2 years of postnatal life, the prognosis is excellent, and most symptoms of early and late congenital syphilis will be prevented.

CHROMOSOMAL ABNORMALITIES

Cytogenetics is the discipline concerned with the study of chromosomes and chromosomal abnormalities. The classification system now in use is the International System for Human Cytogenetic Nomenclature (ISCN).

The Normal Chromosomal Complement Is 46 Chromosomes: 44 Autosomes and 2 Sex Chromosomes

Cytogenetic analysis can be performed on any spontaneously dividing cell but, in most instances, uses circulating lymphocytes, which are easily stimulated to undergo mitosis. Mitotic cells are treated with colchicine to arrest them in metaphase, after which they are spread on glass slides to disperse the chromosomes. The chromosomes are stained with standard hematological techniques that enable more precise identification of chromosomes on the basis of distinct bands.

Chromosome Structure

Using a stain such as Giemsa, the chromosomes are classified according to their **length** and the positioning of the constriction, or **centromere.** The centromere is the point at which the two identical strand of chromosomal DNA, called *sister chromatids*, attach to each other during mitosis. The location of the centromere is used to classify the chromosomes as *metacentric, submetacentric, or acrocentric. Metacentric chromosomes* (1, 3, 19, and 20) show centromere exactly in the middle. In *submetacentric chromosomes* (2, 4–12, 16–18, and X), the centromere divides the chromosome into a short arm (p, from French, *petit*) and a long arm (q, the next letter in the alphabet). *Acrocentric chromosomes* (13, 14, 15, 21, 22, and Y) display very short arms or stalks and satellites attached to an eccentrically located centromere (see Figs. 6-8 and 6-12).

Hematological stains are used to classify chromosomes into seven groups, conveniently labeled with letters from A to G. Thus, group A contains two large metacentric and a large submetacentric chromosome, group B contains two distinct large submetacentric chromosomes, group C contains six submetacentric chromosomes, and so forth.

Fluorescence In Situ Hybridization (FISH)

FISH uses fluorescently labeled DNA probes to identify individual genes or small regions of chromosomes (Fig. 6-9A). It is also used to demonstrate losses or gains of chromosomal material. By use of probes with different fluorophores, it is possible to demonstrate certain chromosomal translocations. More-recent applications, termed *multicolor FISH*, or *spectral karyotyping,* involve the use of probes that hybridize to entire chromosomes, which facilitates the detection of gross chromosomal abnormalities (Fig. 6-9).

Chromosomal Banding

To identify each chromosome individually, special stains delineate specific bands of different staining intensity on each

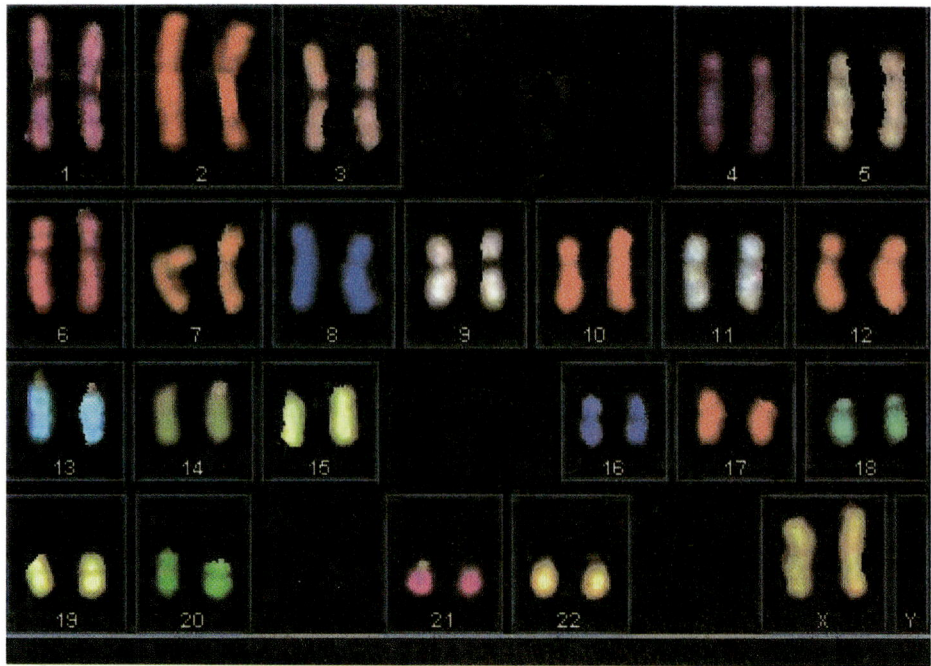

FIGURE 6-8
Spectral karyotype of human chromosomes.

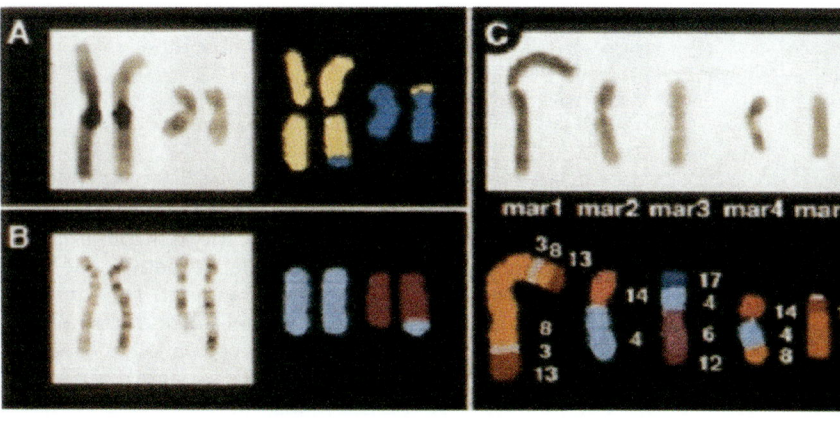

FIGURE 6-9
Translocations in human chromosomes demonstrated by spectral karyotyping. A. Balanced translocation: t (1; 11). B. Unbalanced karyotype: Derivative chromosome 12 with chromosome 4 material attached (partial trisomy for 49 and partial monosomy for 12q). C. Characterization of marker chromosomes from an aneuploid breast cancer showing multiple translocations.

chromosome. **The pattern of bands is unique to each chromosome and makes possible (1) the pairing of two homologous chromosomes, (2) the recognition of each chromosome, and (3) the identification of defects on each segment of a chromosome.**

Chromosome bands are labeled as follows:

- **G bands:** These chromosomal segments stain with Giemsa (hence "G").
- **Q bands:** These bands stain with Giemsa and also fluoresce when stained with quinacrine (hence "Q").
- **R bands:** On appropriate staining, R bands present as the reverse (hence "R") image of G and Q bands; that is, dark G bands are light R bands, and vice versa.
- **C banding:** This is a method for staining centromeres (hence "C") and other portions of chromosomes containing constitutive heterochromatin. By contrast, facultative heterochromatin forms the inactive X chromosome (Barr body).
- **Nucleolar organizing region (NOR) staining:** Secondary constrictions (stalks) of chromosomes with satellites are demonstrated by NOR staining.
- **T banding:** This technique stains the terminal (hence "T") ends of chromosomes.

Structural Chromosomal Abnormalities May Arise during Somatic Cell Division (Mitosis) or during Gametogenesis (Meiosis)

In the case of somatic cell division (most common in rapidly proliferating tissues, e.g., intestines or skin), the structurally abnormal chromosome that arises during mitosis may still code for all of the essential functions of the cell, thereby permitting survival for the normal (usually short) life span of the cell. Alternatively, structural or metabolic deficiencies resulting from a structurally abnormal chromosome may be lethal, in which case only a single cell dies. In both of these instances, structural chromosomal abnormalities that occur during somatic cell division are of no consequence. However, under some circumstances, structural abnormalities may involve protooncogenes and contribute to the pathogenesis of certain cancers (see Chapter 5).

The structural chromosomal abnormalities that origi- nate during gametogenesis are important in a different context, because they are transmitted to all somatic cells of the offspring and may result in heritable diseases. During normal meiosis, homologous chromosomes (e.g., two chromosomes 1) form pairs, termed **bivalents**. By a normal process known as crossing-over, parts of these chromosomes are exchanged, thereby rearranging the genetic constituents of each chromosome. Such an exchange of genetic material may also take place between nonhomologous chromosomes (e.g., between chromosomes 3 and 21), by an abnormal process termed **translocation**. Two major forms of chromosomal translocations are recognized, namely, reciprocal and robertsonian.

Reciprocal Translocations

A reciprocal translocation refers to the exchange of acentric chromosomal segments between two different (nonhomologous) chromosomes (Fig. 6-10). A reciprocal translocation is said to be **balanced** when there is no loss of genetic material, that is, when each chromosomal segment is translocated in its entirety. When such translocations are present in the gametes (sperm or ova), the progeny maintain the abnormal chromosomal structure in all somatic cells. **Since balanced translocations are not associated with the loss of genes or the disruption of vital gene loci, most carriers of such balanced translocations are phenotypically normal.** Balanced reciprocal translocations can be inherited for many generations. Reciprocal translocations are particularly well demonstrated by current banding techniques.

Carriers of balanced translocations, however, are at risk for producing offspring with unbalanced karyotypes and severe phenotypic abnormalities (Fig. 6-11). The abnormal positions of the exchanged chromosomal segments may disturb meiosis and lead to abnormal segregation of chromosomes. In a translocation carrier, the formation of bivalents may be disturbed. To achieve complete pairing of the translocated segments, a complex cross-like structure (quadriradial), which consists of two chromosomes bearing the translocations and their two normal homologues, is formed. Unlike the normal bivalent, which typically resolves by an orderly migration of the two chromosomes to the opposite poles, the quadriradial can divide along several different planes. Some of the resulting gametes carry unbalanced chromosomes and on fertilization result in zygotes

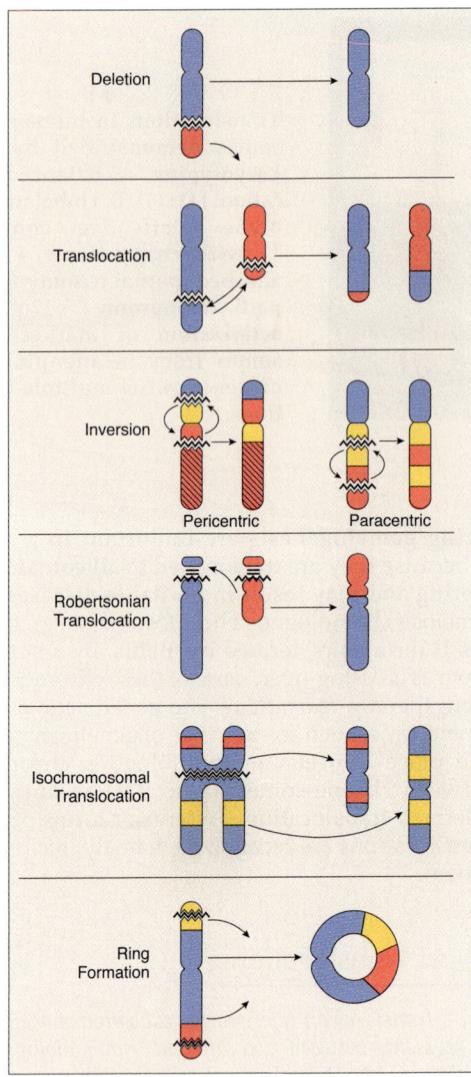

FIGURE 6-10
Structural abnormalities of human chromosomes. The deletion of a portion of a chromosome leads to the loss of genetic material and a shortened chromosome. A reciprocal translocation involves breaks on two nonhomologous chromosomes, with exchange of the acentric segments. An inversion requires two breaks in a single chromosome. If the breaks are on opposite sides of the centromere, the inversion is *pericentric;* it is *paracentric* if the breaks are on the same arm. A robertsonian translocation occurs when two nonhomologous acrocentric chromosomes break near their centromeres, after which the long arms fuse to form one large metacentric chromosome. Isochromosomes arise from faulty centromere division, which leads to duplication of the long arm (iso q) and deletion of the short arm, or the reverse (iso p). Ring chromosomes involve breaks of both telomeric portions of a chromosome, deletion of the acentric fragments, and fusion of the remaining centric portion.

with various combinations of partial trisomy and monosomy for segments of the translocated chromosomes.

Robertsonian Translocations

Robertsonian translocation (centric fusion) involves the centromere of acrocentric chromosomes. When two nonhomologous chromosomes are broken near the centromere, they may exchange two arms to form one large metacentric chromosome and a small chromosomal fragment. The fragment is devoid of a centromere and is usually lost during subsequent divisions. As in a reciprocal translocation, a robertsonian translocation is balanced if there is no significant loss of genetic material. The carrier is also usually phenotypically normal, although he or she may suffer from infertility. **When fertile, however, carriers of balanced robertsonian translocations are at risk of producing unbalanced translocations (see Fig. 6-9) in their gametes, in which case the offspring may be born with congenital malformations.**

Chromosomal Deletions

A deletion is the loss of a portion of a chromosome and involves either a terminal or an intercalary (middle) segment. Disturbances during meiosis in germ cells or breaks of chromatids during mitosis in somatic cells may result in the formation of chromosomal fragments that are not incorporated into any of the chromosomes and are thus lost in subsequent cell divisions.

The shortening of the chromosome because of a deletion may be apparent in routinely stained chromosome preparations. Banding techniques are applied to determine whether the arm of the chromosome is shortened because of a deletion of the terminal portion or because of a double break in the more central portions. The latter event leads to intercalary deletion and subsequent fusion of adjoining residual fragments.

Gametic deletion can be associated with either normal or abnormal development. An example of the latter is the *cri du chat syndrome,* which is associated with the deletion of part of the short arm of chromosome 5. Deletion is related to several cancers in humans, including some hereditary forms of cancer. For example, some familial **retinoblastomas** are associated with deletions in the long arm of chromosome 13. *Wilms tumor aniridia syndrome* is associated with deletions in the short arm of chromosome 11.

Chromosomal Inversions

Chromosomal inversion refers to (1) the break of a chromosome at two points, (2) the inversion of the segment between the breaks,

FIGURE 6-11
Meiotic segregation in a reciprocal balanced translocation involving chromosomes 3 and 6. The pairing of homologous chromosomes 3 and 6 in normal meiosis forms bivalents, which then segregate uniformly to create two gametes, each of which bears a single chromosome 3 and chromosome 6. Here the translocation carrier carries a balanced exchange of portions of the long arms of chromosomes 3 and 6. The chromosomes that carry the translocated genetic material are termed *derivative chromosomes* (der 3 and der 6). Diploid germ cells contain pairs of homologous chromosomes 3 and 6, each of which consists of one normal chromosome and one that carries a translocation. During meiosis, instead of the normal pairing into two bivalents, a quadriradial structure, containing all four chromosomes, is formed. In this circumstance, the chromosomes can segregate along several different planes of cleavage, shown as *X* and *Y*. In addition, the chromosomes can segregate diagonally *(arrows)*. As a result, six different gametes can be produced, four of which are unbalanced and can result in congenital abnormalities.

Chromosomal Abnormalities

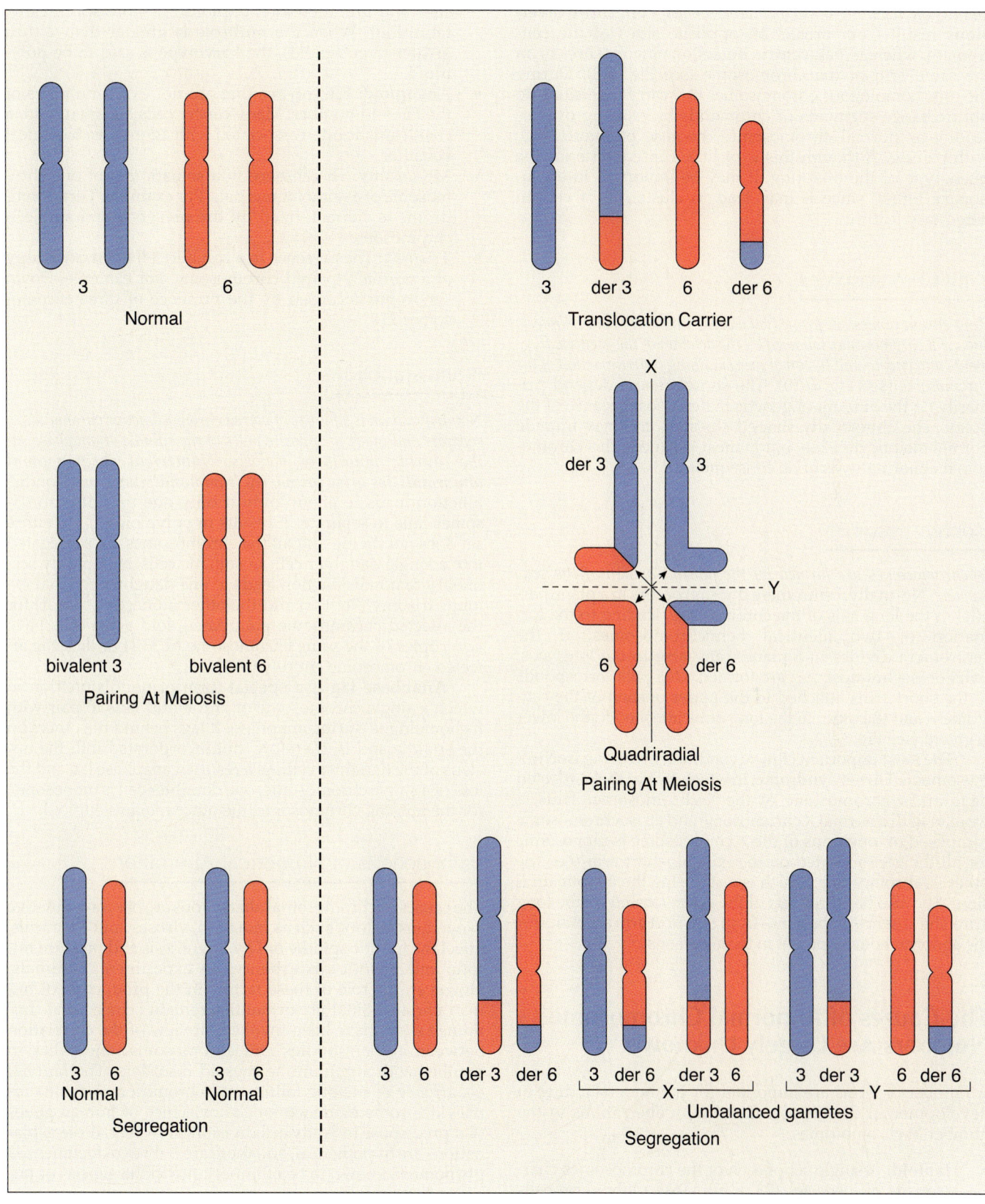

and (3) *the rejoining of the two broken ends.* **Pericentric inversions** result from breaks on opposite sides of the centromere, whereas **paracentric inversions** involve breaks on the same arm of the chromosome (see Fig. 6-8). During meiosis, homologous chromosomes that carry inversions do not exchange segments of chromatids by crossing over as readily as normal chromosomes, because of interference with pairing. Although this is of little consequence for the phenotype of the offspring, it may be important in evolutionary terms, since it may lead to clustering of certain hereditary features.

Ring Chromosomes

Ring chromosomes are formed by a break involving both telomeric ends of a chromosome, followed by the deletion of the acentric fragments and end-to-end fusion of the remaining centric portion of the chromosome (see Fig. 6-10). The consequences depend primarily on the amount of genetic material lost because of the break. The abnormally shaped chromosome may impede normal meiotic division, but in most instances, this chromosomal abnormality is of no consequence.

Isochromosomes

Isochromosomes are formed by the faulty division of the centromere. Normally, centromere division occurs in a plane parallel to the long axis of the chromosome, leading to the formation of two identical hemichromosomes. If the centromere divides in a plane transverse to the long axis, pairs of isochromosomes are formed. One pair corresponds to the short arms attached to the upper portion of the centromere and the other to the long arms attached to the lower segment (see Fig. 6-10).

The most important clinical condition involving isochromosomes is **Turner syndrome,** in which 15% of those affected have an isochromosome of the X chromosome. Thus, a woman with a normal X chromosome and an isochromosome composed of long arms of the X chromosome is monosomic for all the genes located on the missing short arm (i.e., the other isochromosome, which is lost during the meiotic division). She also has three sets of the genes located on the long arm. The absence of the genes from the short arm accounts for the abnormal development in these persons.

The Causes of Abnormal Chromosome Numbers Are Largely Unknown

A number of terms are important for the understanding of developmental defects associated with aberrations in the number of chromosomes.

- **Haploid:** A single set of each of the chromosomes characteristic of a species (23 in humans). Only germ cells have a haploid number (n) of chromosomes.
- **Diploid:** A double set (2n) of each of the chromosomes (46 in humans). Most somatic cells are diploid.
- **Euploid:** Any multiple (from n to 8n) of the haploid number of chromosomes. For example, many normal liver cells contain twice (4n) the DNA of diploid somatic cells and are, therefore, euploid or, more specifically, tetraploid. When the multiple is greater than 2 (i.e., greater than diploid), the karyotype is said to be **polyploid.**
- **Aneuploid:** Karyotypes that are not exact multiples of the haploid number. Many cancer cells are aneuploid, a characteristic often associated with aggressive biological behavior.
- **Monosomy:** The absence in a somatic cell of one chromosome of a homologous pair. For example, Turner syndrome is characterized by the presence of a single X chromosome.
- **Trisomy:** The presence in a somatic cell of an extra copy of a normally paired chromosome. For example, Down syndrome is caused by the presence of three chromosomes 21.

Nondisjunction

Nondisjunction is a failure of paired chromosomes or chromatids to separate and move to opposite poles of the spindle at anaphase, either during mitosis or meiosis. **Numerical chromosomal abnormalities arise primarily from nondisjunction.** Nondisjunction leads to aneuploidy if only one pair of chromosomes fails to separate. It results in polyploidy if the entire set does not divide and all the chromosomes are segregated into a single daughter cell. In somatic cells, aneuploidy secondary to nondisjunction leads to one daughter cell that exhibits trisomy (2n + 1) and the other monosomy (2n–1) for the affected chromosome pair. Aneuploid germ cells have two copies of the same chromosome (n + 1) or lack the affected chromosome entirely (n–1).

Anaphase lag is a special form of nondisjunction in which a single chromosome or chromatid fails to pair with its homologue during anaphase. It lags behind the others on the spindle and is, therefore, not incorporated into the nucleus of the daughter cell. As a result of anaphase lag and the loss of a single chromosome, one daughter cell is monosomic for the missing chromosome; the other remains euploid.

Pathogenesis of Numerical Aberrations

The causes of chromosomal aberrations are obscure. Putative exogenous factors, such as radiation, viruses, and chemicals, affect the mitotic spindle or DNA synthesis and produce mitotic and meiotic disturbances in experimental animals. However, the role of these factors in the production of human chromosomal abnormalities remains conjectural. Immune factors have been invoked, in view of the correlation between autoantibodies and chromosomal anomalies in families with autoimmune thyroid disorders. The familial occurrence of meiotic failure and chromosomal anomalies provides some evidence for the existence of human genes that predispose to faulty cell division. However, these explanations are hypothetical, and there are only two documented phenomena known to be of importance in the genesis of numerical aberrations.

- **Nondisjunction during meiosis occurs more commonly in persons with structurally abnormal chromosomes.** This is probably related to the fact that such chromosomes do not pair or segregate during gametogenesis as readily as do normal ones.

- Children born to older women have more frequent numerical chromosomal abnormalities than those born to younger mothers.

Chromosomal Aberrations at Various Stages of Pregnancy

The chromosomal abnormalities that are found at birth differ from those found in early spontaneous abortions. At birth, the common chromosomal abnormalities are trisomy 21 (most frequent), trisomy 18, trisomy 13, and trisomy of sex chromosomes (47,XXX; 47,XXY; and 47,XYY). Approximately 0.3% of all liveborn infants have a chromosomal abnormality. Among spontaneous abortions, the most commonly observed chromosomal abnormalities are 45,X (most frequent), trisomy 16, trisomy 21, and trisomy 22. However, trisomy of almost any chromosome can be observed in spontaneous abortions. Up to 35% of spontaneous abortions have a chromosomal abnormality, a much higher incidence than is seen in liveborn infants. The reason for these differences is presumably related to survival in utero. Very few fetuses with 45,X survive to term, and trisomy 16 is nearly always lethal in utero; a fetus with trisomy 21 has a better chance of surviving to birth.

Effects of Chromosomal Aberrations

Most major chromosomal abnormalities are incompatible with life. The defects are usually lethal to the developing conceptus, leading to early death and spontaneous abortion. The loss of genetic material (e.g., autosomal monosomies) results in embryos that generally do not survive pregnancy. By contrast, monosomy of the X chromosome (45,X) may be compatible with life, although more than 95% of such embryos are lost during pregnancy. The absence of an X chromosome (i.e., the karyotype 45,Y) invariably results in early abortion.

Autosomal trisomies are associated with several developmental abnormalities, and the affected fetus usually dies during pregnancy or shortly after birth. Trisomy 21, which defines Down syndrome, is an exception, and such persons survive for years. Trisomy of the X chromosome may result in abnormal development but is not lethal.

Mitotic nondisjunction may involve embryonic cells during early stages of development and result in chromosomal aberrations. These are transmitted selectively through some cell lineages but not through others. *The condition in which the body contains two or more karyotypically different cell lines is called* **mosaicism**. Like all chromosomal abnormalities related to nondisjunction, mosaicism may involve autosomes or sex chromosomes. The phenotype of a mosaic person depends on the chromosome involved and the extent of mosaicism. Autosomal mosaicism is rare, most likely because this condition is usually lethal. On the other hand, mosaicism involving sex chromosomes is common and is found in patients with gonadal dysgenesis who present with Turner or Klinefelter syndrome.

Nomenclature of Chromosomal Aberrations

Structural and numerical chromosomal abnormalities are classified according to (1) the total number of chromosomes,

TABLE 6-2 **Chromosomal Nomenclature**

Numerical designation of autosomes	1–22
Sex chromosomes	X, Y
Addition of a whole or part of a chromosome	+
Loss of a whole or part of a chromosome	−
Numerical mosaicism (e.g., 46/47)	/
Short arm of chromosome (petite)	p
Long arm of chromosome	q
Isochromosome	i
Ring chromosome	r
Deletion	del
Insertion	ins
Translocation	t
Derivative chromosome (carrying translocation)	der
Terminal	ter
Representative karyotypes	
Male with trisomy 21 (Down syndrome)	47, XY, +21
Female carrier of fusion-type translocation between chromosomes 14 and 21	45,XX, −14, −21, +t(14q21q)
Cri du chat syndrome (male) with deletion of a portion of the short arm of chromosome 5	46,XY,del(5p)
Male with ring chromosome 19	46,XY,r(19)
Turner syndrome with monosomy X	45,X
Mosaic Klinefelter syndrome	46,XY/47,XXY

(2) the designation (number) of the affected chromosomes, and (3) the nature and location of the defect on the chromosome (Table 6-2). The karyotype is described sequentially in the following order: (1) the total number of chromosomes, (2) the sex chromosome complement, and (3) any abnormality. The short arm of a chromosome is designated **p**, and the long arm is designated **q**. The addition of chromosomal material, whether an entire chromosome or a part of one, is indicated by a plus sign (+) before the number of the affected chromosome, and the loss of chromosomal material by a minus sign (−). Alternatively, the loss (deletion) of part of a chromosome may be designated by the symbol **del** followed by the location of the deleted material on the affected chromosome. A translocation is written as a **t**, followed by brackets containing the involved chromosomes. Structural or numerical chromosomal aberrations are found in 5 to 7 per 1000 liveborn infants, although most are balanced translocations and are asymptomatic.

Syndromes of the Autosomal Chromosomes May Arise from Numerical or Structural Abnormalities

Numerical autosomal aberrations in liveborn infants are virtually all trisomies (Table 6-3). Structural aberrations that may result in clinical disorders include translocations, deletions, and chromosomal breakage.

Trisomy 21 (Down Syndrome)

Trisomy 21 is the single most common cause of mental retardation. Furthermore, liveborn infants represent only a fraction

TABLE 6-3 Clinical Features of the Autosomal Chromosomal Syndromes

Syndromes	Features
Trisomic Syndromes	
Chromosome 21 (Down syndrome 47,XX or XY, +21:1/800)	Epicanthic folds, speckled irides, flat nasal bridge, congenital heart disease, simian crease of palms, Hirschsprung disease, increased risk of leukemia
Chromosome 18 (47,XX or XY, +18: 1/8000)	Female preponderance, micrognathia, congenital heart disease, horseshoe kidney, deformed fingers
Chromosome 13 (47,XX or XY, +13: 1/20,000)	Persistent fetal hemoglobin, microcephaly, congenital heart disease, polycystic kidneys, polydactyly, simian crease
Deletion Syndromes	
5p− syndrome (Cri du chat 46,XX or XY,5p−)	Catlike cry, low birth weight, microcephaly, epicanthic folds, congenital heart disease, short hands and feet, simian crease
11p− syndrome (46,XX or XY, 11p−)	Aniridia, Wilms tumor, gonadoblastoma, male genital ambiguity
13q− syndrome (46,XX or XY,13q−)	Low birth weight, microcephaly, retinoblastoma, congenital heart disease

All of these syndromes are associated with mental retardation.

of all conceptuses with this chromosomal defect. Two thirds are aborted spontaneously or die in utero. Life expectancy is also reduced. Recent advances in the therapy for infections, operations for congenital heart defects, and chemotherapy for leukemia—the leading causes of death in patients with Down syndrome—are increasing life expectancy.

Pathogenesis: There are three mechanisms by which three copies of the genes on chromosome 21 that are responsible for Down syndrome may be present in somatic cells:

- **Nondisjunction** during the first meiotic division of gametogenesis accounts for most (92–95%) patients with Down syndrome that have trisomy 21 (Fig. 6-12). The extra chromosome 21 is of maternal origin in about 95% of Down syndrome children. Interestingly, virtually all maternal nondisjunction seems to result from events occurring in the first meiotic division (meiosis I).
- **Translocation** of an extra long arm of chromosome 21 to another acrocentric chromosome causes about 5% of cases of Down syndrome.
- **Mosaicism** for trisomy 21 is caused by nondisjunction during mitosis of a somatic cell in the early stages of embryogenesis and is responsible for 2% of children born with Down syndrome.

The incidence of trisomy 21 correlates strongly with increasing maternal age; thus, older mothers are at a substantially greater risk of giving birth to an infant with Down syndrome (Fig. 6-13). Up to their mid-30s, women have a constant risk of giving birth to a trisomic child of about 1 per 1000 liveborn infants. The risk then increases dramatically and reaches an incidence of 1 in 30 at age 45 years. The risk of recurrence of Down syndrome in subsequent children born to the same mother is 1%, irrespective of maternal age, unless the syndrome is associated with translocation of chromosome 21.

The mechanism by which increasing maternal age is associated with a greater risk of bearing a child with trisomy 21 is poorly understood. Until recently, alternative hypotheses implicated either an effect caused by aging oocytes or an age-impaired ability of the uterine environment to reject a trisomic conceptus. It is now clear from molecular studies that the maternal age effect is related to maternal nondisjunction events, which implies that the defect lies with the process of meiosis within the oocyte and not with the uterus. Down syndrome associated with a translocation or mosaicism is not related to maternal age.

Down syndrome caused by translocation of an extra portion of chromosome 21 occurs in two situations. Either parent may be a phenotypically normal carrier of a balanced translocation or the translocation may arise de novo during gametogenesis. These translocations are typically robertsonian, tending to involve only acrocentric chromosomes, with short arms consisting of a satellite and stalk (chromosomes 13, 14, 15, 21, and 22). Translocations between these chromosomes are particularly common because they cluster during meiosis and are, therefore, subjected more frequently than other chromosomes to breakage and recombination. The most common translocation in Down syndrome (50%) is fusion of the long arms of chromosomes 21 and 14, t(14q;21q), followed in frequency (40%) by similar fusion involving two chromosomes 21, t(21q;21q).

If the translocation is inherited from a parent, a balanced translocation has been converted to an unbalanced one, as illustrated in Figure 6-9. According to this scheme, one would expect a one in three chance of Down syndrome among the offspring of a carrier of a balanced robertsonian translocation. However, when the mother carries the translocation, the actual incidence is only 10 to 15%, and for unknown reasons, it is less than 5% when the father is the carrier. This reduced incidence probably relates to the early loss of most embryos with trisomy 21.

Molecular Genetics of Down Syndrome

Chromosome 21 is the smallest human autosome, composing less than 2% of the human genome. It has an acrocentric structure, and all genes of known function (other than for ribosomal RNA) are located on the long arm (21q). Based on studies of inherited translocations, in which only a portion of chromosome 21 is duplicated, the region on chromosome 21 responsible for the full Down syndrome phenotype has been restricted to band 21q22.2, a 4-Mb region of DNA termed the **Down syndrome critical region.** The gene(s) responsible for

Chromosomal Abnormalities 233

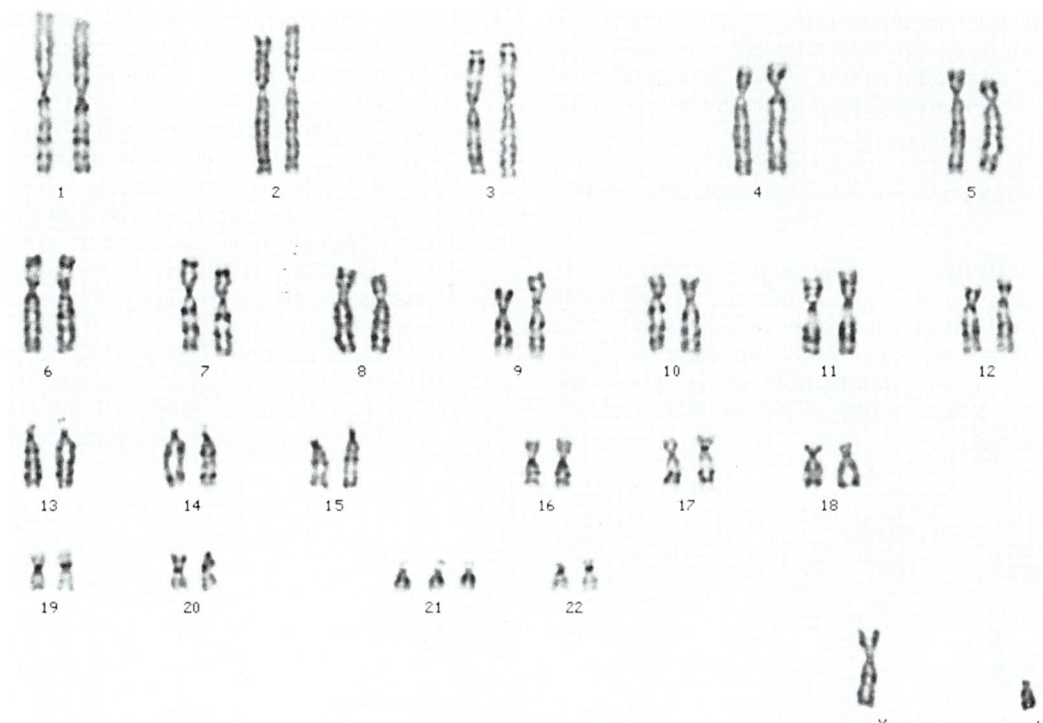

FIGURE 6-12
Trisomy 21 in the karyotype of a child with Down syndrome. All other chromosomes are normal.

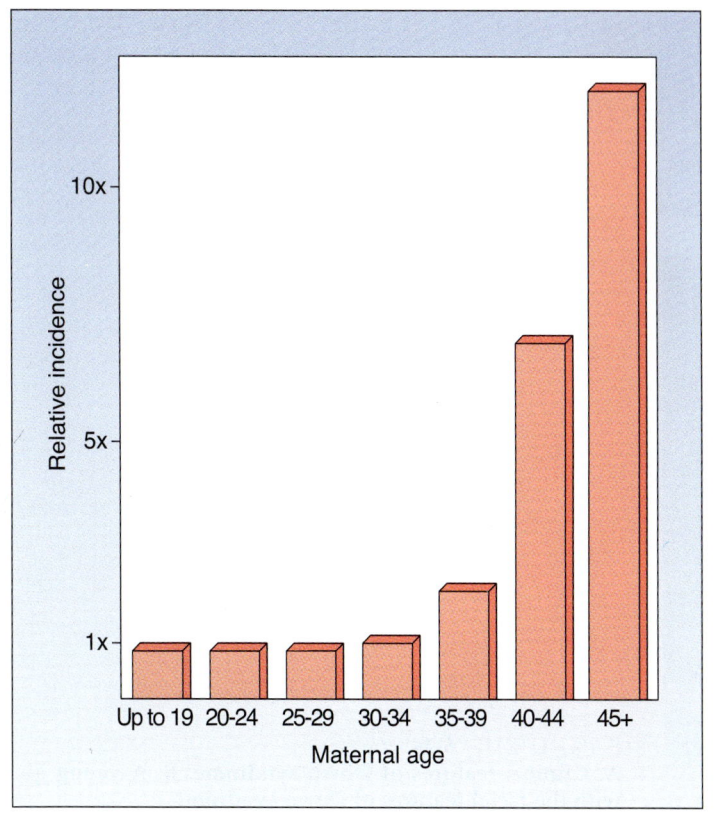

FIGURE 6-13
Incidence of Down syndrome in relation to maternal age. A conspicuous increase in the frequency of this disorder is seen over the age of 35 years.

Down syndrome remains undetermined. Interesting speculation centers on a recently identified homologue of the *Drosophila* gene "minibrain" in this region. Transgenic mice that overexpress the human gene exhibit defects in learning and memory.

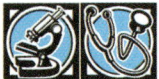

Pathology and Clinical Features: The diagnosis of Down syndrome is ordinarily made at the time of birth by observing the flaccid state and characteristic physical appearance of the infant. The diagnosis is then confirmed by cytogenetic analysis. As the child develops, a typical constellation of abnormalities appears (Fig. 6-14).

- **Mental status:** Children with Down syndrome invariably suffer severe mental retardation, with a relentless and progressive decline in the IQ with age. Beginning with a mean IQ of 70 below the age of 1 year, intelligence deteriorates during the first decade of life to a mean of 30. The major defect seems to be an inability to develop more-advanced cognitive strategies and processes, problems that become more apparent as the child grows older. Although these children have traditionally been described as particularly gentle and affectionate, newer studies have cast serious doubt on the validity of these personality stereotypes.
- **Craniofacial features:** The face and occiput tend to be flat, with a low-bridged nose, reduced interpupillary distance, and oblique palpebral fissures. Epicanthal folds of the eyes impart an Oriental appearance, a feature

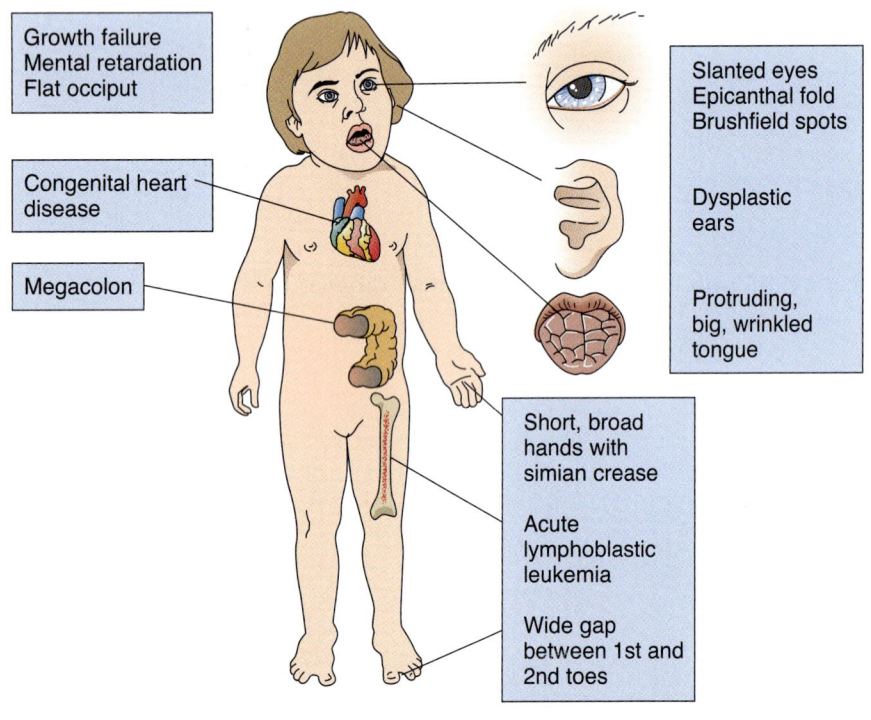

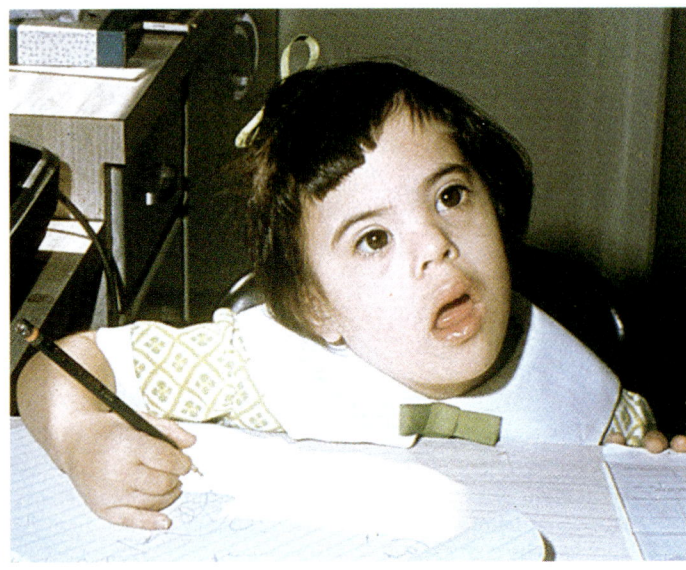

FIGURE 6-14

A. Clinical features of Down syndrome. B. A young girl with the facial features of Down syndrome.

that accounts for the obsolete term *mongolism*. A speckled appearance of the iris is referred to as *Brushfield spots*. The ears are enlarged and malformed. A prominent tongue, which typically lacks a central fissure, protrudes through an open mouth.
- **Heart:** One third of children born with Down syndrome suffer from congenital cardiac disease, and the incidence is even higher in aborted fetuses. The anomalies take the form of atrioventricular canal, ventricular and atrial septal defects, tetralogy of Fallot, and patent ductus arteriosus. Most of the cardiac defects seem to be variations of a common problem in the formation of the venous inflow tract of the heart.
- **Skeleton:** These children tend to be small, owing to shorter than normal bones of the ribs, pelvis, and extremities. The hands are broad and short and exhibit a "simian crease," that is, a single transverse crease across the palm. The middle phalanx of the fifth finger is hypoplastic, an abnormality that leads to inward curvature of this digit.
- **Gastrointestinal tract:** Duodenal stenosis or atresia, imperforate anus, and Hirschsprung disease (megacolon) occur in 2 to 3% of children with Down syndrome.
- **Reproductive system:** Men with trisomy 21 are invariably sterile, owing to arrested spermatogenesis. A few women with Down syndrome have given birth to children, of which 40% had trisomy 21.
- **Immune system:** Although the immune system in Down syndrome has been the subject of numerous studies, no clear pattern of specific defects has emerged. Nevertheless, affected children are unusually susceptible to respiratory and other infections. Prior to the antibiotic era, most of these children died in infancy from infectious diseases.
- **Hematological disorders:** Persons with Down syndrome are at a particularly high risk of developing leukemia at all ages. **The risk of leukemia in Down syndrome children younger than the age of 15 years is about 15-fold greater than normal.** In children younger than the age of 3 years, acute nonlymphocytic leukemia predominates. After that age, when most of the leukemias in Down syndrome occur, most cases are acute lymphoblastic leukemias. The basis for the high incidence of leukemia is unknown, but leukemoid reactions (transient pronounced neutrophilia) are frequent in the newborn with Down syndrome. Interestingly, in mosaic Down syndrome, the proliferating leukocytes are invariably trisomic for chromosome 21.
- **Neurological disorders:** The search for specific neuropathological alterations in the brain associated with Down syndrome has proved futile, and no clear pattern of abnormal "wiring" has emerged. Furthermore, there are no characteristic changes in the electroencephalogram. Nevertheless, it is possible that the nerve cells in trisomy 21 indeed differ from normal. Virtually all electrical parameters and a number of physiological ones are altered in cultured neurons from infants with Down syndrome. One of the most intriguing neurological features of Down syndrome is its association with Alzheimer disease, a relationship that has been appreciated for more than half a century. The morphological lesions characteristic of Alzheimer disease progress in all patients with Down syndrome and are universally demonstrable by age 35. These changes in the brain include (1) granulovacuolar degeneration, (2) neurofibrillary tangles, (3) senile plaques, and (4) loss of neurons (see chapter 28). The senile plaques and cerebral blood vessels of both Alzheimer disease and Down syndrome always contain an amyloid composed of the same fibrillar protein (β-amyloid protein). The similarity between the neuropathological features of Down syndrome and those of Alzheimer disease is also reflected in the appearance of dementia in one fourth to one half of older Down syndrome patients and the progressive loss of many intellectual functions that cannot be attributed to mental retardation alone.
- **Life expectancy:** During the first decade of life, the major determinant of survival in Down syndrome is the presence or absence of congenital heart disease. In those who have a normal heart, only about 5% succumb before age 10, whereas about 25% with heart disease die by that time. After age 10, the estimated life expectancy (the age at death) is 5\5 years, a life span some 20 years or more less than that of the general population. By age 70, only 10% are still alive.

Trisomies of Chromosomes 18, 13, and 22

Trisomy 18 is the second most common autosomal syndrome, occurring about once in 8000 live births, an order of magnitude less frequent than Down syndrome. The disorder results in mental retardation and affects females four times as often as males. Virtually all infants with trisomy 18 suffer from congenital heart disease and succumb within the first 3 months of life.

Trisomies 13 and 22 are rare, and both are associated with mental retardation, congenital heart disease, and other abnormalities. Syndromes associated with trisomies of chromosomes 8 and 9 have also been described.

Translocation Syndromes

The prototypical translocation that results in partial trisomy is Down syndrome. Many other partial trisomies have been documented, the best documented of which is the 9p-trisomy syndrome. In this disorder, the short arm of chromosome 9 may be translocated to a number of different autosomes, and many kindreds in which this syndrome occurs have been described. Importantly, as in Down syndrome, the carriers of a balanced chromosome 9 translocation are asymptomatic but may transmit an unbalanced translocation to their offspring. The clinical disorder is characterized by mental retardation, microcephaly, and other craniofacial abnormalities. A reciprocal translocation between the long arms of chromosomes 22 and 11 is also well known. The children of carriers may have an extra chromosome containing portions of both 11 and 22, in which case they have partial trisomy of both chromosomes, resulting in microcephaly and a variety of other anomalies.

Chromosomal Deletion Syndromes

The deletion of an entire autosomal chromosome (i.e., monosomy) is usually not compatible with life. However, several syndromes arise from the deletions of parts of several chromosomes. In most cases, the congenital syndromes are sporadic, but in a few instances, reciprocal translocations have been demonstrated in the parents. Virtually all of these deletion syndromes are characterized by low birth weight, mental retardation, microcephaly, and craniofacial and skeletal abnormalities. Congenital heart disease and urogenital abnormalities are common.

- **5p–syndrome (cri du chat syndrome):** This is the best-known deletion syndrome, because the high-pitched cry of the infant is similar to that of a kitten and calls attention to the disorder. Most cases are sporadic, but reciprocal translocations have been reported in some parents.
- **11p–syndrome:** Deletion of the short arm of chromosome 11, specifically band 11p13, results in congenital absence of the iris (aniridia) and is often accompanied by Wilms tumor.
- **13q–syndrome:** A deletion of the long arm of chromosome 13 is associated with retinoblastoma, owing to the loss of the *Rb* tumor suppressor gene (see Chapter 5).
- **Other deletion syndromes:** Deletions of both the short and the long arms of chromosome 18 are documented, leading to varying patterns of mental retardation and craniofacial anomalies. The loss of material from chromosomes 19, 20, 21, and 22 is usually associated with the formation of ring chromosomes. Syndromes associated with 21q–and 22q–are the most common and often resemble Down syndrome.
- **Deletions and rearrangements of subtelomeric sequences:** The telomeres are present at the ends of chromosomes and are composed of a repetitive sequence $(TTAGGG)_n$. The subtelomeric regions of chromosomes are rich in genes. Deletions and rearrangements of these regions of the genome have been demonstrated to be a major cause of mild to severe mental retardation and dysmorphic features. These abnormalities generally cannot be demonstrated by conventional cytogenetic stains and require adaptations of FISH for detection.

Chromosomal Breakage Syndromes

A number of recessive syndromes associated with frequent chromosomal breakage and rearrangements are accompanied by a significant risk of leukemia and other cancers. These disorders include xeroderma pigmentosum, Bloom syndrome (congenital telangiectatic erythema with dwarfism), Fanconi anemia (constitutional aplastic pancytopenia), and ataxia telangiectasia. Acquired chromosomal breaks and rearrangements (translocations) are associated with leukemias and lymphomas, the best documented of which are chronic myelogenous leukemia, t(9;22), and Burkitt lymphoma, mostly t(8;14) (see Chapters 5 and 20).

Numerical Aberrations of Sex Chromosomes Are Considerably More Common Than Those of the Autosomes, with the Exception of Trisomy 21

The reasons are not entirely clear, but it is possible that additional sex chromosomes (Fig. 6-15) produce less genetic imbalance than extra autosomes and therefore do not disturb critical stages of development.

The contrast between the X and Y chromosomes is striking. Whereas the X chromosome is one of the larger chromosomes, containing 6% of the total DNA, the Y chromosome is distinctly small. More than 1300 genes in the X chromosome have been identified; whereas the Y chromosome has only about 200 genes, one of which is the testis-determining gene (*SRY*, also known as *TDF*).

The Y Chromosome

Historically, the sex of a person was believed to be determined by the number of X chromosomes, the situation that was observed in genetic studies of *Drosophila*. However, the discoveries that the XXY phenotype (Klinefelter syndrome) is male and that the XO phenotype (Turner syndrome) is female demonstrated the role of the Y chromosome in conferring the male phenotype. The testis-determining gene (*SRY*, sex-determining region, Y) is an intron-less gene near the end of the short arm of the Y chromosome. The *SRY* gene encodes a small nuclear protein with a DNA-binding domain. This protein binds to another protein (SIP-1) to form a complex that functions as a transcriptional activator of autosomal genes whose expression controls the development of the male phenotype. Mutations in this gene are associated with XY females, whereas translocations that introduce this gene into the X chromosome are associated with XX males.

A small proportion of infertile men with azoospermia or severe oligospermia have small deletions in regions of the Y chromosome. However, the size and location of the deletions are variable and do not correlate with the severity of spermatogenic failure.

The X Chromosome

Although males carry only one X chromosome, both males and females produce the same amounts of gene products encoded by the X chromosome. This seeming discrepancy has been explained by the **Lyon effect**, on which the following principles are based:

- In females, one X chromosome is irreversibly inactivated early in embryogenesis. The inactivated X chromosome is detectable in interphase nuclei as a heterochromatic clump of chromatin attached to the inner nuclear membrane, termed the **Barr body**. The inactive X chromosome is extensively methylated at gene control regions and transcriptionally repressed. Nevertheless, a significant minority of X-linked genes escape inactivation and continue to be expressed by both X chromosomes. The probability that an X chromosome is rendered inactive seems to correlate with the level of expression of another X-linked gene, *XIST*, which is expressed only by the inactive partner.
- Either the paternal or maternal X chromosome is inactivated randomly.
- The inactivation of the X chromosome is virtually complete.
- The inactivation of the X chromosome is permanent and transmitted to progeny cells. In other words, paternally or maternally derived X chromosomes are clonally propagated. **Thus, all females are mosaic for paternally and maternally derived X chromosomes.** Mosaicism for glucose-6-phosphate dehydrogenase in females was important in the demonstration of the monoclonal origin of neoplasms (see Chapter 5).

Gametes Sperm / Ovum	X	Y	XY	O
X	46,XX Normal ♀	46,XY Normal ♂	47,XXY Klinefelter ♂	45,X Turner ♀
XX	47,XXX ♀	47,XXY Klinefelter ♂	48,XXXY Klinefelter ♂	46,XX Normal ♀
XXX	48,XXXX ♀	48,XXXY Klinefelter ♂	49,XXXXY Klinefelter ♂	47,XXX Triple X ♀
O	45,X Turner ♀	45,Y LETHAL	46,XY LETHAL	44 LETHAL

● — X chromatin (Barr body)
● — Y chromatin

FIGURE 6-15
Numerical aberrations of sex chromosomes. Nondisjunction in either the male or female gamete is the principal cause of these abnormalities.

The inactivation of the X chromosome poses a problem in understanding the phenotypes of several disorders characterized by an abnormal complement of X chromosomes. If one X chromosome is rendered entirely nonfunctional, persons with XXY (Klinefelter) or XO (Turner) karyotypes should be phenotypically normal. The fact that such persons show a variety of phenotypic abnormalities indicates that the inactivated X chromosome retains some functioning genes. Indeed, a region of the short arm of the X chromosome is known to escape X-inactivation. This region, which can pair with a homologous region on the short arm of the Y chromosome and undergo meiotic recombination between the two, is known as the *pseudoautosomal region*. Genes in this location are present in two functional copies in both males and females. Thus patients with Turner syndrome (45,X) are haploinsufficient for these genes, and patients with more than two X chromosomes (e.g., Klinefelter syndrome) have more than two functional copies. One of the genes in this region, *SHOX*, is associated with height, and its haploinsufficiency in Turner syndrome may explain the short stature associated with this condition. There are also several other genes outside the pseudoautosomal region in the X chromosome that escape X inactivation. **In both phenotypically male and female children with extra X chromosomes, the degree of mental retardation shows a rough correlation with the number of X chromosomes.**

Klinefelter Syndrome (47,XXY)

Klinefelter syndrome, or testicular dysgenesis, is related to the presence of one or more X chromosomes in excess of the normal male XY complement. It is the most important clinical condition associated with trisomy of sex chromosomes (Fig. 6-16). This syndrome is a prominent cause of male hypogonadism and infertility.

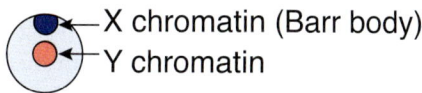Pathogenesis: Most persons with Klinefelter syndrome (80%) have one extra X chromosome, that is, a 47,XXY karyotype. A minority are mosaics (e.g., 46,XY/47,XXY) or have more than two X chromosomes (e.g., 48,XXXY). **Interestingly, regardless of the number of supernumerary X chromosomes (even up to four), the presence of a Y chromosome ensures a male phenotype.** Nevertheless, additional X chromosomes correlate with a more abnormal phenotype, despite the inactivation of the extra X chromosomes. Presumably, the same genes that escape inactivation in the normal female remain functional in Klinefelter syndrome.

Klinefelter syndrome occurs in 1 per 1000 male newborns, roughly comparable to the incidence of Down syn-

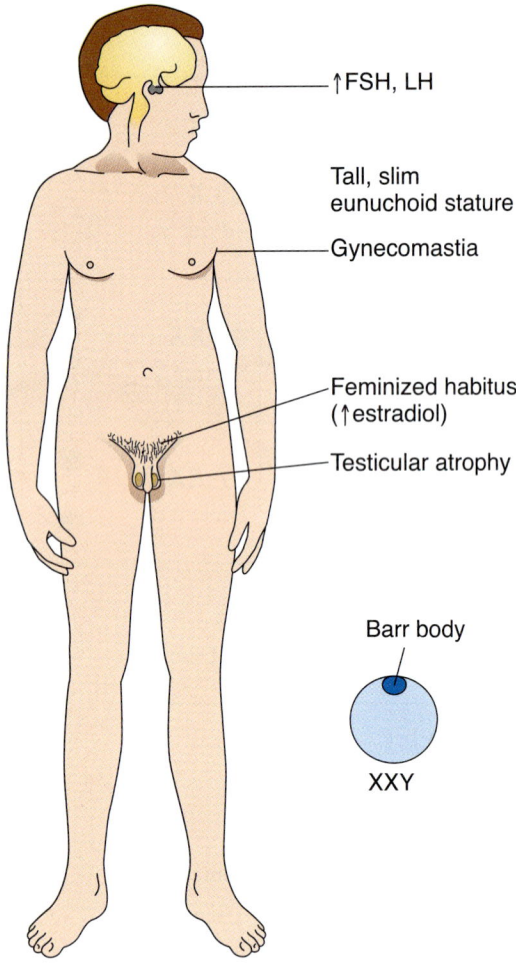

FIGURE 6-16
Clinical features of Klinefelter syndrome.

drome. Interestingly, half of all 47,XXY conceptuses are lost as spontaneous abortions. The additional X chromosome(s) arises as a result of meiotic nondisjunction during gametogenesis. In half of cases, nondisjunction occurs during paternal meiosis I, leading to a sperm containing both an X and a Y chromosome. Fertilization of a normal oocyte by such a sperm gives a zygote with a 47,XXY complement of chromosomes.

 Pathology: After puberty, the intrinsically abnormal testes do not respond to stimulation by gonadotropins and show sequentially regressive alterations. The seminiferous tubules display atrophy, hyalinization, and peritubular fibrosis. Germ cells and Sertoli cells are characteristically absent, and eventually the tubules are represented by dense cords of collagen. Although Leydig cells usually appear to be increased in number, their function is impaired, as evidenced by low testosterone levels in the face of elevated luteinizing hormone (LH) levels.

 Clinical Features: The diagnosis of Klinefelter syndrome is usually not made until after puberty, because the principal manifestations of the disorder during childhood are behavioral and psychiatric. Gross mental retardation is uncommon, although the average IQ is probably somewhat reduced. Since the syndrome is so common, it should be suspected in all boys with some mental deficiency or severe behavioral problems.

Children with Klinefelter syndrome tend to be tall and thin, with relatively long legs (eunuchoid body habitus). Normal testicular growth and masculinization at puberty do not occur, and the testes and penis remain small. Feminine characteristics are manifested as a high-pitched voice, gynecomastia, and a female pattern of pubic hair (female escutcheon). Azoospermia results in infertility. All of these changes are a consequence of hypogonadism and a resulting lack of androgens. Serum testosterone levels are low to normal, whereas those of LH and follicle-stimulating hormone are remarkably high, indicating normal pituitary function. High circulating estradiol levels increase the estradiol-to-testosterone ratio, which determines the degree of feminization. Treatment with testosterone preparations is successful in virilizing these patients but does not restore fertility.

The XYY Male

Interest in the XYY phenotype (1 per 1000 male newborns) derives from studies in penal institutions in which the prevalence of this karyotype was reported to be significantly higher than in the general population. However, the concept that these "supermales" manifest aggressive antisocial behavior as a result of an extra Y chromosome has not been substantiated in other studies, and the topic remains controversial. The only features of the XYY phenotype that are agreed on are tall stature, a tendency toward cystic acne, and some problems in motor and language development. Aneuploidy of the Y chromosome is a consequence of meiotic nondisjunction in the father.

Turner Syndrome (45,X)

Turner syndrome refers to the spectrum of abnormalities that results from the presence of complete or partial monosomy of the X chromosome in a phenotypic female. It is less common than Klinefelter syndrome, occurring in about 1 per 5000 female liveborn infants. In three fourths of cases, the single X chromosome of Turner syndrome is of maternal origin, suggesting that the meiotic error tends to be paternal. The incidence of the syndrome does not correlate with maternal age, and the risk of producing a second affected female infant is not increased.

The 45,X karyotype is actually one of the most common aneuploid abnormalities in human conceptuses, but almost all are aborted spontaneously. In fact, up to 2% of all abortuses manifest this aberration. Since patients with Turner syndrome survive normally after birth, why is the missing X chromosome lethal during fetal development? Moreover, the presence of only one chromosome implies that the inactivated X chromosome in normal females (or the Y chromosome in males) protects against early demise of the embryo. It is believed that homologues of Y genes in the pseudoautosomal region of the X chromosome escape inactivation and are critical to the survival of a female conceptus.

Only about half of women with Turner syndrome lack an entire X chromosome (monosomy X). The remainder are mosaics or display structural aberrations of the X chromosome, such as isochromosome of the long arm, translocations, and deletions. Mosaics characterized by a 45,X/46,XX karyotype (15%) tend to have milder phenotypic manifestations of Turner syndrome and may even be fertile. In about 5% of patients, the mosaic karyotype is 45,X/46,XY, in which case an original male zygote was subsequently modified by a mitotic nondisjunction. Such mosaic persons are at a 20% risk of developing a germ cell cancer and should have prophylactic removal of the abnormal gonads.

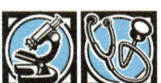 Pathology and Clinical Features: The clinical hallmark of Turner syndrome is sexual infantilism with primary amenorrhea and sterility (Fig. 6-17). In most cases, the disorder is not discovered until the absence of menarche brings the child to medical attention. Virtually all of these women are less than 5 ft (152 cm) tall. Other clinical features include a short, webbed neck (pterygium coli), a low posterior hairline, a wide carrying angle of the arms (cubitus valgus), a broad chest with widely spaced nipples, and hyperconvex fingernails. Half of patients have abnormal urograms, the most common anomalies being horseshoe kidney and malrotation. Many have facial abnormalities, among which are a small mandible, prominent ears, and epicanthal folds. Defective hearing and vision are common, and as many as one fifth are reported to be mentally defective. Pigmented nevi become prominent as the patient ages. For unknown reasons, women with Turner syndrome are at a greater risk for chronic autoimmune thyroiditis and goiter.

Cardiovascular anomalies are common in Turner syndrome, occurring in almost half the patients. Coarctation of the aorta is seen in 15%, and a bicuspid aortic valve is detected by echocardiography in as many as a third. Essential hypertension occurs in some patients, and dissecting aneurysm of the aorta is occasionally a cause of death.

The pathological alterations in the ovary of women with Turner syndrome represent a curious acceleration of the normal aging of this organ. The ovary of a female fetus initially contains 7 million oocytes, of which fewer than half survive to the time of birth. A relentless loss of oocytes continues, so that at menarche only about 5% (400,000) of the original total remain, and at menopause a mere 0.1% have survived. Although the ovaries of fetuses with Turner syndrome initially contain oocytes, they are rapidly degraded, and none remain by 2 years of age. The ovaries are converted to fibrous streaks, whereas the uterus, fallopian tubes, and vagina develop normally. It may be said that the child with Turner syndrome has undergone menopause long before reaching menarche.

Interestingly, families are known in which several women have premature menopause and exhibit deletions of portions of the long arm of one X chromosome. Such data, together with observations of Turner syndrome, further support the concept that the genes controlling ovarian development and function in the inactivated X chromosome continue to be expressed in the normal female.

Children with Turner syndrome are treated with growth hormone and estrogens and enjoy an excellent prognosis for a normal life.

Syndromes in Females with Multiple X Chromosomes

One extra X chromosome in a phenotypic female (i.e., a 47,XXX karyotype) is the most frequent abnormality of sex chromosomes in women, occurring at about the same rate as Klinefelter syndrome. Most of these women are of normal intelligence, although they are reported to display some difficulty in speech, learning, and emotional responses. Minor physical anomalies are encountered, including epicanthal folds and clinodactyly (inward curvature of the fifth finger). Fertility is the rule, but an increased incidence of congenital defects may be found in the children of 47,XXX women.

Women with four and five X chromosomes have been documented, virtually all of whom have been mentally retarded. These women superficially resemble women with Down syndrome and do not mature sexually. Women with supernumerary X chromosomes have additional Barr bodies, indicating inactivation of all but one X chromosome. Clearly, some genes on the inactivated X chromosomes continue to be expressed.

Single Gene Abnormalities Confer Traits That Segregate Sharply within Families

The classic laws of mendelian inheritance, named in honor of Gregor Mendel, are as follows:

- **A mendelian trait** is determined by two copies of the same gene, called alleles, which are located at the same locus on two homologous chromosomes. In the case of the X and Y chromosomes in males, a trait is determined by just one allele.

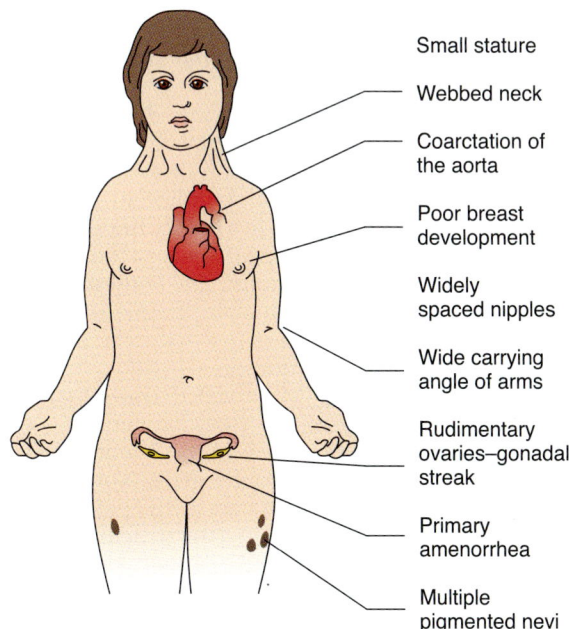

FIGURE 6-17
Clinical features of Turner syndrome.

- **Autosomal genes** refer to those located on one of the 22 autosomes.
- **Sex-linked traits** are encoded by loci on the X chromosome.
- **A dominant phenotypic trait** requires the presence of only one allele of a homologous gene pair. In other words, the dominant phenotype is present whether the allelic genes are homozygous or heterozygous.
- **A recessive phenotypic trait** demands that both alleles be identical, that is homozygous.
- **Codominance** refers to a situation in which both alleles in a heterozygous gene pair are fully expressed (e.g., the AB blood group genes).

Mendelian traits are classified as (1) autosomal dominant, (2) autosomal recessive, (3) sex-linked dominant, or (4) sex-linked recessive. Diseases associated with the expression of sex-linked dominant genes are rare and of little practical significance.

Mutations

The central dogma of molecular biology holds that DNA is transcribed into RNA, which is then processed into mRNA, which in turn is translated into proteins. Thus, a change in DNA can be reflected in either a corresponding change in the amino acid sequence of a specific protein or interference with its synthesis.

A mutation is a stable heritable change in DNA. The consequences of mutations are highly variable. Some have no functional consequences, whereas others are lethal and cannot be transmitted from one generation to another. Between these extremes is a broad range of mutations that account for the profound genetic polymorphisms of any species. **It appears that 1 in 1000 base pairs is polymorphic in the human genome.** Indeed, evolution is based on the occurrence over time of nonlethal mutations that alter the adaptability of a species to its environment. From the viewpoint of human disease, we are interested principally in mutations that result in perceptible alterations in the structure or function of proteins. The major types of mutations encountered in the study of human genetic disorders (Fig. 6-18) are as follows:

- **Point mutations:** The replacement of one base by another is termed a *point mutation*. In the coding region, a point mutation has three consequences.
  A synonymous mutation is one in which the new codon containing the mutation still codes for the same amino acid. For example, UUU and UUC both code for phenylalanine.
  A missense mutation (three fourths of base substitutions in the coding region) refers to a situation in which the new codon codes for a different amino acid. In sickle cell anemia, an adenine to thymine substitution results in the replacement of glutamic acid (GAG) by valine (GUG) in the β-globin chain of hemoglobin.
  A nonsense mutation (4%) is one in which the base substitution changes the normal codon to a termination codon, so that translation is halted at the site of the mutation. For example, UAU codes for tyrosine, but UAA is a stop codon.
- **Frameshift mutations:** The sequence of bases in messenger RNA is read three at a time to determine the amino acid that is to be incorporated in the growing polypeptide. *Insertions or deletions of a number of bases that is not a multiple of 3 into the coding region of DNA changes the reading frame of the message.* In this situation, every codon in the same gene downstream from the mutation has a new sequence and codes for a different amino acid or a termination signal. Frameshift mutations can also alter the transcription, splicing, or processing of mRNA.
- **Large deletions:** When an extensive segment of DNA is deleted, the coding region of a gene may be entirely removed, in which case the protein product is absent. On the other hand, a large deletion may result in the approximation of neighboring genes, thereby producing a fused gene that codes for a hybrid protein, that is, one in which the terminal sequence of one protein is followed by the initial sequence of another.
- **Expansion of unstable trinucleotide repeat sequences:** The human genome contains frequent tandem trinucleotide repeat sequences, some of which are associated with disease. The number of copies of certain repetitive trinucleotide sequences varies among individuals, thereby representing allelic polymorphism of the genes in which they are found. In general, the number of repeats below a particular threshold does not change during mitosis or meiosis, whereas above this threshold, the number of repeats can expand or contract, expansion being far more common. A number of distinct trinucleotide expansions have been identified in human disease (Table 6-4):

Huntington disease (HD): HD is an inherited neurodegenerative disease caused by the expansion of a CAG repeat within the coding sequence of the gene that codes for the protein *huntingtin*. In HD, the stable alleles contain 10 to 30 repeats, whereas persons affected by the disease exhibit 40 to 100 repeats. CAG codes for glutamine, and the abnormal expansion of the polyglutamine tract in HD confers a toxic gain-of-function to huntingtin. Although the precise mechanism by which mutant huntingtin causes selective neuronal loss is not understood, there is evidence to suggest altered protein–protein interactions as the basis for this effect. In addition to HD, expanded CAG repeats have been identified as the cause of a number of other neurodegenerative disorders (see Table 6-4).

Fragile X syndrome: This genetic disorder, the most common cause of inherited mental retardation (see below), is caused by the expansion of a CGG repeat in a noncoding region immediately adjacent to the *FMR1* gene on the X chromosome. In a poorly understood manner, the expanded CGG repeat silences the *FMR1* gene by methylation of its promoter. The abnormal repeat is also associated with an inducible "fragile site" on the X chromosome, which appears in cytogenetic studies as a nonstaining gap or a chromosomal break.

Myotonic dystrophy (MD): MD, the most frequent autosomal muscular dystrophy (see Chapter 27), is caused by expansion of a CTG repeat in the 3′-untranslated region of the myotonic dystrophy gene. Normal persons bear up to 35 CTG repeats, whereas MD patients display up to 2000 repeats. Interestingly, the structure of the protein product of the MD gene, a protein kinase, is unaffected by the mutation. It is suspected that the abnormal expansion renders other nearby genes dysfunctional.

Friedreich ataxia (FA): FA is an autosomal recessive degenerative disease affecting the central nervous

Chromosomal Abnormalities

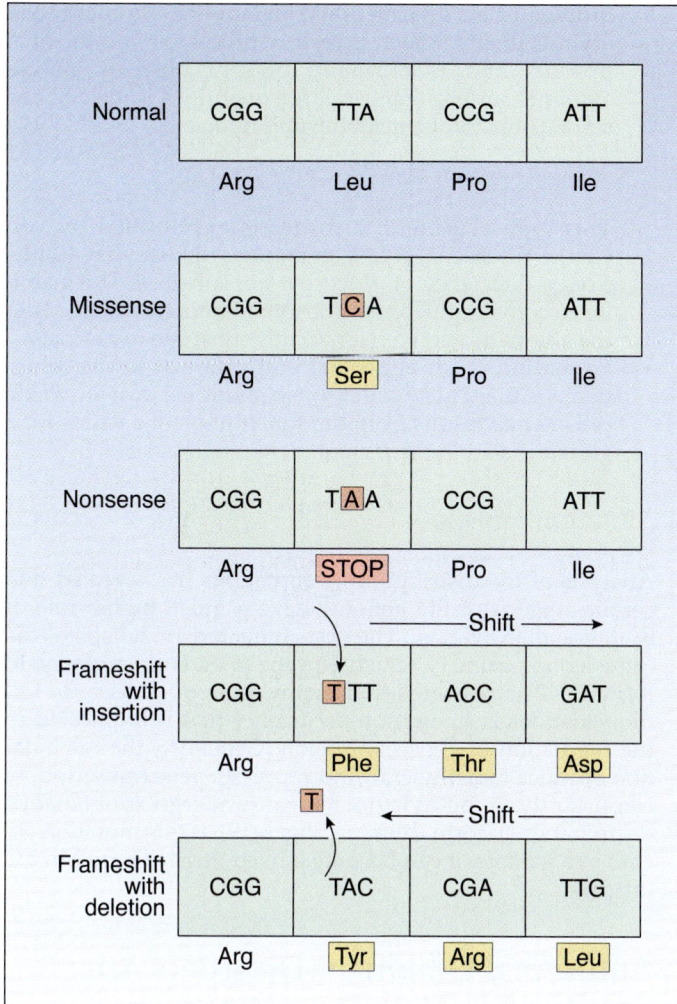

FIGURE 6-18
Point mutations that alter the reading frame of DNA. A variety of mutations in the second codon of a normal sequence of four amino acids is depicted. With a missense mutation, a change from T to C substitutes serine for leucine. With a nonsense mutation, a change from T to A converts the leucine codon to a stop codon. A shift in the reading frame to the right results from insertion of a T, thus changing the sequence of all subsequent amino acids. Conversely, deletion of a T shifts the reading frame one base to the left and also changes the sequence of subsequent amino acids.

system and the heart that is associated with expansion of a GAA repeat in the *frataxin* gene (see Chapter 28), which codes for a mitochondrial protein. Affected persons have 120 to 1700 repeats in the first intron (noncoding) of the frataxin gene.

Functional Consequences of Mutations

A biochemical pathway represents the sequential actions of a series of enzymes, which are coded for by specific genes. A typical pathway can be represented by the conversion of a substrate (A) through intermediate metabolites (B and C) to the final product (D).

$$A \rightarrow B \rightarrow C \rightarrow D$$

initial substrate — intermediary metabolites — end-products

A single gene defect can have several consequences:

- **Failure to complete a metabolic pathway:** In this situation, the end-product (D) is not formed because an en-

TABLE 6-4 Representative Diseases Associated with Trinucleotide Repeats

Disease	Location	Sequence	Normal Length	Premutation	Full Mutation
Huntington disease	4p16.3	CAG	10–35	—	40–100
Kennedy disease	Xq21	CAG	15–25	—	40–55
Spinocerebellar ataxia	6p23	CAG	20–35	—	45–80
Fragile X syndrome	Xq27.3	CGG	5–55	50–200	200–>1000
Myotonic dystrophy	19q13	CTG	5–35	37–50	50–4000
Friedreich ataxia	9q13	GAA	7–30	—	120–1700

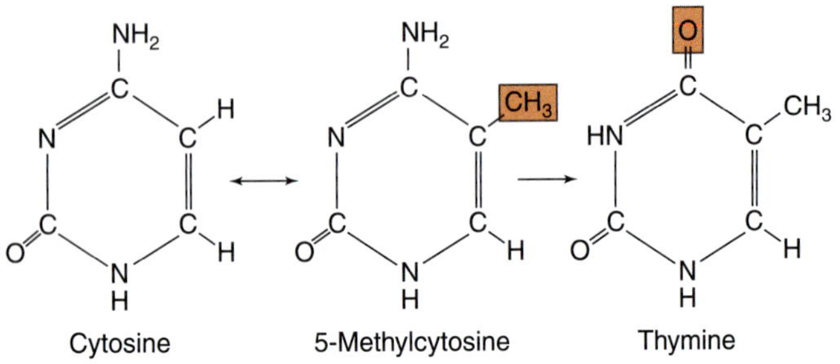

FIGURE 6-19
5-Methylcytosine is formed from cytosine. Spontaneous deamination of 5-methylcytosine produces thymine.

zyme that is essential for the completion of a metabolic sequence is missing:

$$A \rightarrow B \rightarrow C -//\rightarrow (D) (\downarrow)$$

An example of the failure to complete a metabolic pathway is albinism, a pigment disorder caused by a deficiency of tyrosinase. This enzyme catalyzes the conversion of tyrosine to melanin (through the intermediate formation of dihydroxyphenylalanine (DOPA). In the absence of tyrosinase, the end-product, namely melanin, is not formed, and the affected person (an "albino") is devoid of pigment in all organs that normally contain it, primarily the eyes and the skin.

- **Accumulation of unmetabolized substrate:** The enzyme that converts the initial substrate into the first intermediary metabolite may be missing, a situation that results in excessive accumulation of the initial substrate.

$$A (\uparrow) - //\rightarrow B (\downarrow) C (\downarrow) D (\downarrow)$$

An example of this situation is phenylketonuria, a disease in which dietary phenylalanine accumulates owing to an inborn deficiency of phenylalanine hydroxylase. The resulting toxic concentration of phenylalanine interferes with the postnatal development of the brain and causes severe mental retardation.

- **Storage of an intermediary metabolite:** An intermediary metabolite, which is readily processed into the final product and is normally present only in minute amounts, accumulates in large quantities if the enzyme responsible for its metabolism is deficient.

$$A \rightarrow B (\uparrow) - //\rightarrow C (\downarrow) D (\downarrow)$$

This type of genetic disorder is exemplified by von Gierke disease, a glycogen storage disease that results from a deficiency of glucose-6-phosphatase. The inability to convert glucose-6-phosphate into glucose leads to the alternative conversion of this substrate to glycogen.

- **Formation of an abnormal end-product:** In this situation, a mutant gene codes for an abnormal protein. Sickle cell anemia results from the substitution of a valine for a glutamic acid in the β chain of hemoglobin.

Mutation Hotspots

Analysis of the distribution of mutations has revealed that certain regions of the genome have a much higher rate of mutation than average. The best-characterized hotspot is the dinucleotide pair CG, which is prone to undergo mutation to form TG. The reason is that methylation of cytosine in CG dinucleotides is a common occurrence that is implicated in the regulation of gene expression. Generally, the methylation product, 5-methylcytosine, represses gene transcription. Importantly, 5-methylcytosine can undergo spontaneous deamination to form thymine (Fig. 6-19). If this mutation occurs in a gamete, it can become a fixed, heritable trait in the offspring.

Autosomal Dominant Disorders Are Expressed in Heterozygotes

A dominant disease occurs when only one defective gene (i.e., mutant allele) is present, whereas its paired allele on the homologous chromosome is normal. The salient features of autosomal dominant traits are as follows (Fig. 6-20):

- Males and females are equally affected, since by definition, the mutant gene resides on one of the 22 autosomal

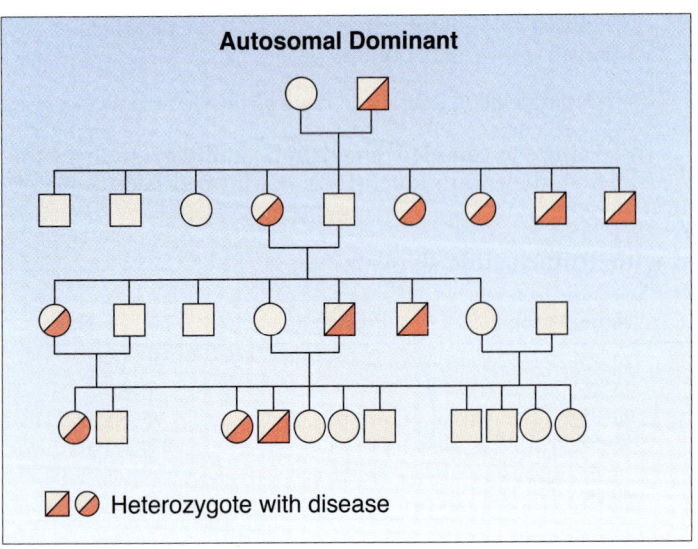

FIGURE 6-20
Autosomal dominant inheritance. Only symptomatic persons transmit the trait to the next generation, and heterozygotes are symptomatic. Both males and females are affected.

chromosomes. As a consequence, there can be father-to-son transmission (which is absent in X-linked dominant disorders).
- The trait encoded by the mutant gene can be transmitted to successive generations (unless the disease interferes with reproductive capacity).
- Unaffected members of the family do not transmit the trait to their offspring. As a corollary, every person with the disease has an affected parent, assuming that the disorder does not represent a new mutation.
- The proportions of normal and diseased offspring of patients with the disorder are on average equal, because most affected persons are heterozygous, whereas their normal mates do not harbor the defective gene.

New Mutations versus Inherited Mutations

As noted above, an autosomal dominant disease may result from a new mutation rather than transmission from an affected parent. Nevertheless, the offspring of persons with a new dominant mutation are at a 50% risk of developing the disease. **The ratio of new mutations to transmitted ones among persons with dominant autosomal disorders varies with the effect of the disease on reproductive capacity.** The greater the impairment of reproductive capacity, the greater the proportion of new mutations. At one end of the spectrum, a dominant mutation that leads to complete infertility would invariably be a new mutation. When reproductive capacity is only partially impaired, the proportion of new mutations is correspondingly lower. Such a situation occurs with tuberous sclerosis, an autosomal dominant condition in which mental retardation limits reproductive potential and in which new mutations account for 80% of cases. However, in a dominant disease that has little effect on reproductive activity (e.g., familial hypercholesterolemia), virtually all affected persons exhibit pedigrees showing classic vertical transmission of the disorder.

Biochemical Basis of Autosomal Dominant Disorders

There are several major mechanisms by which the presence of one mutant allele and one normal allele is responsible for clinical disease.

- When the gene product is a rate-limiting component of a complex metabolic network (e.g., a receptor or an enzyme), half of the normal amount of gene product may be insufficient to maintain the normal state. This is known as *haploinsufficiency*. Examples of this mechanism include β thalassemia and familial hypercholesterolemia.
- In some diseases, the presence of an extra copy of an allele gives rise to a phenotype. An example of this is Charcot-Marie-Tooth disease, type IA, which is caused by a duplication of the peripheral myelin protein-22 gene.
- Constitutive activation of a gene is seen in some familial cancer syndromes. For example, mutations in the *RET* protooncogene are found in families with multiple endocrine neoplasia, type 2. These cause abnormally

TABLE 6-5 **Representative Autosomal Dominant Disorders**

Disease	Frequency	Chromosome
Familial hypercholesterolemia	1/500	19p
von Willebrand disease	1/8000	12p
Hereditary spherocytosis (major forms)	1/5000	14,8
Hereditary elliptocytosis (all forms)	1/2500	1,1p,2q,14
Osteogenesis imperfecta (types I–IV)	1/10,000	17q,7q
Ehlers-Danlos syndrome, type III	1/5000	?
Marfan syndrome	1/10,000	15q
Neurofibromatosis type 1	1/3500	17q
Huntington chorea	1/15,000	4p
Retinoblastoma	1/14,000	13q
Wilms tumor	1/10,000	11p
Familial adenomatous polyposis	1/10,000	5q
Acute intermittent porphyria	1/15,000	11q
Hereditary amyloidosis	1/100,000	18q
Adult polycystic kidney disease	1/1000	16p

increased activity of a tyrosine kinase that stimulates cell proliferation.
- Mutations in genes that encode structural proteins (e.g., collagens and cytoskeletal constituents) result in abnormal molecular interactions and the disruption of normal morphological patterns. Such a situation is exemplified by osteogenesis imperfecta and hereditary spherocytosis.

More than 1000 human diseases are inherited as autosomal dominant traits, although most of them are rare. Examples of human autosomal dominant diseases are given in Table 6-5.

Heritable Diseases of Connective Tissue Are Heterogeneous and Often Inherited As Autosomal Dominant Traits

This discussion is limited to three of the most common and best-studied entities: Marfan syndrome, Ehlers-Danlos syndrome, and osteogenesis imperfecta. Even in these well-delineated disorders, the clinical symptomatology often overlaps. For instance, some patients exhibit the joint dislocations typical of the Ehlers-Danlos syndrome, whereas other members of the same family suffer from multiple fractures characteristic of osteogenesis imperfecta. Yet other persons in the family, with the same genetic defect, may be totally without symptoms. Thus the current classifications, which are based on clinical criteria, will eventually be replaced by references to specific gene defects, in a manner analogous to the hemoglobinopathies.

Marfan Syndrome

Marfan syndrome is an autosomal dominant, inherited disorder of connective tissue characterized by a variety of abnormalities in many organs, including the heart, aorta, skeleton, eyes, and skin. One third of cases represent sporadic mutations. The incidence in the United States is 1 per 10,000.

Pathogenesis: The cause of Marfan syndrome has been established as private missense mutations in the gene coding for *fibrillin-1 (FBN1)*, which has been mapped to the long arm of chromosome 15 (15q21.1). Fibrillin is a family of connective tissue proteins analogous to the collagens, of which there are now about a dozen genetically distinct forms. It is widely distributed in many tissues in the form of a fiber system termed **microfibrils.** By electron microscopy, microfibrils are threadlike filaments that form larger fibers, which are organized into rods, sheets, and interlaced networks. **Microfibrillar fibers** serve as a scaffold for the deposition of elastin during embryonic development, after which they constitute part of elastic tissues. For example, the deposition of elastin on lamellae of microfibrillar fibers produces the concentric rings of elastin in the aortic wall. By use of immunofluorescent microscopy, abnormal microfibrillar fibers have been visualized in all the tissues affected in Marfan syndrome.

Fibrillin-1 is a large, cysteine-rich glycoprotein that forms 10-nm microfibrils in the extracellular matrix of many tissues. Interestingly, the ciliary zonules that suspend the lens of the eye are devoid of elastin but consist almost exclusively of microfibrillar fibers (fibrillin). Dislocation of the lens is a characteristic feature of Marfan syndrome. Deficiencies in the amount and distribution of microfibrillar fibers have been demonstrated in the skin and fibroblast cultures of patients with Marfan syndrome, which renders the elastic fibers incompetent to resist normal stress.

 Pathology and Clinical Features: Persons with Marfan syndrome are usually (but not invariably) tall, and the lower body segment (pubis-to-sole) is longer than the upper body segment. A slender habitus, which reflects a paucity of subcutaneous fat, is complemented by long, thin extremities and fingers, which accounts for the term **arachnodactyly** (spider fingers) (Fig. 6-21). Overall, the affected persons resemble figures in a painting by El Greco.

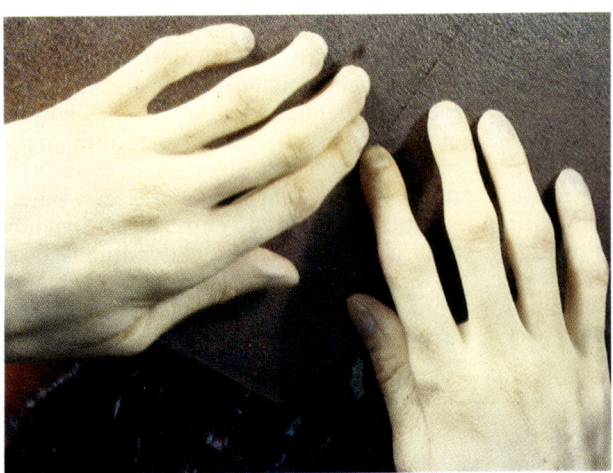

FIGURE 6-21
Long, slender fingers (arachnodactyly) in a patient with Marfan syndrome.

- **Skeletal system:** The skull in Marfan syndrome is characteristically long (dolichocephalic), with prominent frontal eminences. Disorders of the ribs are conspicuous and produce pectus excavatum (concave sternum) and pectus carinatum (pigeon breast). The tendons, ligaments, and joint capsules are weak, a condition that leads to hyperextensibility of the joints (double-jointedness), dislocations, hernias, and kyphoscoliosis; the last is often severe.
- **Cardiovascular system:** The most important cardiovascular defect resides in the aorta, in which the principal lesion is a faulty media. Weakness of the media leads to variable dilation of the ascending aorta and to a high incidence of dissecting aneurysms. The dissecting aneurysm, usually of the ascending aorta, may rupture into the pericardial cavity or make its way down the aorta and rupture into the retroperitoneal space. Dilation of the aortic ring results in aortic regurgitation, which may be severe enough to produce angina pectoris and congestive heart failure. The mitral valve may exhibit redundant valve leaflets and chordae tendineae—changes that result in the mitral valve prolapse syndrome. Cardiovascular disorders are the most common causes of death in Marfan syndrome.

  Microscopic examination of the aorta reveals conspicuous fragmentation and loss of elastic fibers, accompanied by an increase in metachromatic mucopolysaccharide. Focally, the defect in the elastic tissue results in discrete pools of amorphous metachromatic material, reminiscent of that seen in Erdheim (idiopathic) cystic medial necrosis of the aorta. Smooth muscle cells are enlarged and lose their orderly circumferential arrangement.
- **Eyes:** Ocular changes are common in Marfan syndrome and reflect the intrinsic lesion in connective tissue. These include dislocation of the lens (ectopia lentis), severe myopia owing to elongation of the eye, and retinal detachment.

Untreated men with Marfan syndrome usually die in their 30s, and women who are untreated often die in their 40s. However, with the use of drugs that reduce blood pressure and replacement of the aorta with prosthetic grafts, life expectancy approaches normal.

Ehlers-Danlos Syndromes

The Ehlers-Danlos syndromes (EDS) are a group of rare, autosomal dominant, inherited disorders of connective tissue that feature remarkable hyperelasticity and fragility of the skin, joint hypermobility, and often a bleeding diathesis. The disorder is clinically and genetically heterogeneous (Table 6-6). More than 10 varieties of EDS have been distinguished, and the molecular lesions have been identified in several.

 Pathogenesis: The genetic and biochemical lesions in 7 of the 10 types of EDS have been established. **The common feature of all is a generalized defect in collagen, including abnormalities in its molecular structure, synthesis, secretion, and degradation.** In EDS I through IV, VI, and X, electron microscopic studies of the

TABLE 6-6 Ehlers-Danlos Syndromes

Type	Inheritance	Frequency	Biochemical Lesion	Clinical Features
I	AD	1/30,000	Type V collagen	Hyperextensible skin; hypermobile joints
II	AD	1/30,000	Type V collagen	Similar to, but less severe than, type I
III	AD	1/5000	Unknown	Hypermobile joints
IV	AD	1/100,000	Type III collagen	Thin skin, easy bruising, rupture of arteries, intestine and gravid uterus
V	XLR	Rare	Unknown	Similar to type II
VI	AR	Rare	Lysyl hydoxylase	Ocular lesions and blindness, hyperextensible, hypermobile joints
VII	AD	Rare	Type I collagen	Congenital hip dislocation, hypermobile joints
VIII	AD	Rare	Unknown	Periodontal disease, hyperextensible skin
IX	XLR	Rare	Lysyl oxidase (copper metabolism)	Lax skin, bladder diverticula and rupture, skeletal deformities
X	AR	Rare	Fibronectin	Similar to type II

AD, autosomal dominant; AR, autosomal recessive; XLR, X-linked recessive.

skin have shown an increased size of collagen fibrils, with unusually small bundles, features that are consistent with the presence of abnormal collagen. Such changes involve type III collagen in EDS IV and type I collagen in EDS VII. EDS VII arises from mutations that alter the amino-terminal cleavage sites of either the 1 or 2 procollagen chains of type I collagen. Deficiencies of specific collagen- processing enzymes, including lysyl hydroxylase and lysyl oxidase, have been identified in EDS VI and IX, respectively. Whatever the underlying biochemical defect may be, the end result is deficient or defective collagen. Depending on the type of EDS, these molecular lesions are associated with conspicuous weakness of the supporting structures of the skin, joints, arteries, and visceral organs.

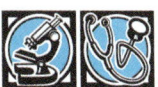

Pathology and Clinical Features: All types of EDS are characterized by soft, fragile, hyperextensible skin. Patients typically can stretch the skin many centimeters, and trivial injuries can lead to serious wounds. Because sutures do not hold well, dehiscence of surgical incisions is common. Hypermobility of the joints allows unusual extension and flexion, a situation that accounted for the "human pretzel" and other contortionists in the freak shows of an earlier age. EDS IV is the most dangerous variety, owing to a tendency to spontaneous rupture of large arteries, the bowel, and the gravid uterus. Death from such complications is common in the third and fourth decades of life.

Ehlers-Danlos syndrome VI also has major complications, including severe kyphoscoliosis, blindness from retinal hemorrhage or rupture of the globe, and death from aortic rupture. Severe periodontal disease, with loss of teeth by the third decade, characterizes EDS VIII. EDS IX features the development of bladder diverticula during childhood, with a danger of bladder rupture, and skeletal deformities.

Many persons who exhibit clinical abnormalities suggesting EDS do not conform to any of the documented types of this disorder. Further genetic and biochemical characterization of such cases is likely to expand the classification of EDS.

Osteogenesis Imperfecta

Osteogenesis imperfecta (OI), or brittle bone disease, is a group of inherited disorders in which a generalized abnormality of connective tissue is expressed principally as fragility of bone. OI is inherited in an autosomal dominant pattern, although there are rare cases that are autosomal recessive.

Pathogenesis: The genetic defects in the four types of OI are heterogeneous, but all affect the synthesis of type I collagen. In 90% of cases, mutations in the pro-α1(I) and pro-α2(I) collagen genes are present, most of them resulting in the substitution of other amino acids for the obligate glycine at every third residue.

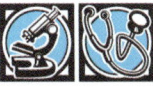

Pathology and Clinical Features: Type I OI is characterized by a normal appearance at birth, but fractures of many bones occur during infancy and at the time the child learns to walk. Such patients have been described as being as "fragile as a china doll." Children with type I OI typically have blue sclerae as a result of the deficiency in collagen fibers, which imparts translucence to the sclera. A high incidence of hearing loss occurs because fractures and fusion of the bones of the middle ear restrict their mobility.

Type II OI is usually fatal in utero or shortly after birth. The infants have a characteristic facial appearance and skeletal abnormalities. Those who are born alive usually die of respiratory failure within the first month of life.

Type III OI is the progressively deforming variant, which is ordinarily detected at birth by the presence of short stature and deformities caused by fractures in utero. Dental defects and hearing loss are common. Unlike the other types of OI, type III is often inherited as an autosomal recessive trait.

Type IV OI is similar to type I, except that the sclerae are normal and the phenotype is more variable.

Osteogenesis imperfecta is discussed in further detail in Chapter 26.

Neurofibromatosis

The neurofibromatoses include two distinct autosomal dominant disorders characterized by the development of multiple neurofibromas, which are benign tumors of peripheral nerves of Schwann cell origin.

Neurofibromatosis Type I (von Recklinghausen Disease)

Neurofibromatosis type I (NF1) is characterized by (1) disfiguring neurofibromas, (2) areas of dark pigmentation of the skin (café au lait spots), and (3) pigmented lesions of the iris (Lisch nodules). It is one of the more common autosomal dominant disorders, affecting 1 in 3500 persons of all races. The *NF1* gene has an unusually high rate of mutation, and half of cases are sporadic rather than familial. The condition was first described in 1882 by von Recklinghausen, but references to this disorder can be found as early as the 13th century. Public interest in the disease was stimulated by the disturbing account in a play and film of a severely disfigured man, the so-called Elephant Man. Interestingly, Joseph Merrick, the original patient, is now thought to have suffered from a different malady, namely, Proteus syndrome.

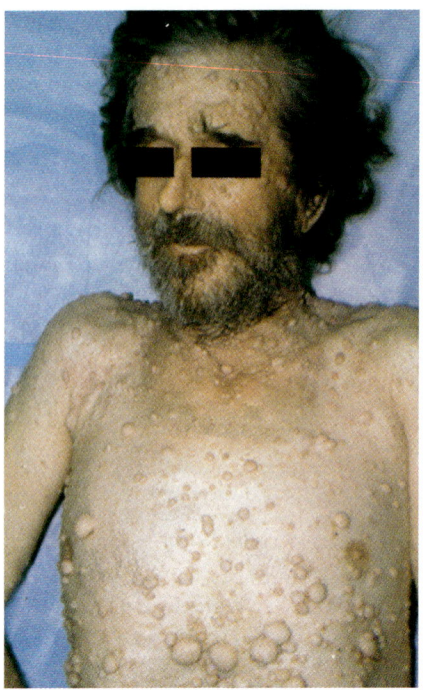

FIGURE 6-22
Neurofibromatosis, type I. Multiple cutaneous neurofibromas are noted on the face and trunk.

 Pathogenesis: Germline mutations in the NF1 gene, located on the long arm of chromosome 17 (17q11.2), include deletions, missense mutations, and nonsense mutations. The protein product of the NF1 gene, termed *neurofibromin*, is expressed in many tissues and belongs to a family of GTPase-activating proteins (GAPs), which inactivate the ras protein (see Chapter 5). In this sense, NF1 is a classic tumor suppressor gene. The loss of GAP activity permits uncontrolled ras activation, an effect that presumably predisposes to the formation of neurofibromas.

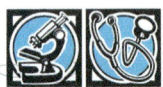 **Pathology and Clinical Features:** The clinical manifestations of NF1 are highly variable and difficult to explain entirely on the basis of a single gene defect. The typical features of NF1 include the following:

- **Neurofibromas:** More than 90% of patients with NF1 develop cutaneous and subcutaneous neurofibromas in late childhood or adolescence. These cutaneous tumors, which may total more than 500, appear as soft, pedunculated masses, usually about 1 cm in diameter (Fig. 6-22). However, on occasion they may reach alarming proportions and dominate the physical appearance of the patient, with lesions up to 25 cm in largest dimension. Subcutaneous neurofibromas present as soft nodules along the course of peripheral nerves. **Plexiform neurofibromas** occur only within the context of NF1 and are diagnostic of that condition. These tumors usually involve the larger peripheral nerves but on occasion may arise from cranial or intraspinal nerves. Plexiform neurofibromas are often large, infiltrative tumors that cause severe disfigurement of the face or an extremity. The microscopic appearance of neurofibromas is discussed in Chapter 28. **One of the major complications of NF1, occurring in 3 to 5% of patients, is the appearance of a neurofibrosarcoma in a neurofibroma, usually a larger one of the plexiform type.** NF1 is also associated with an increased incidence of other neurogenic tumors, including meningioma, optic glioma, and pheochromocytoma.
- **Café au lait spots:** Although normal persons may exhibit occasional light brown patches on the skin, more than 95% of persons affected by NF1 display six or more such lesions. These are over 5 mm before puberty and greater than 1.5 cm thereafter. Café au lait spots tend to be ovoid, with the longer axis oriented in the direction of a cutaneous nerve. Numerous freckles, particularly in the axilla, are also common.
- **Lisch nodules:** More than 90% of persons with NF1 display pigmented nodules of the iris, which consist of masses of melanocytes. These raised lesions are believed to be hamartomas.
- **Skeletal lesions:** A number of bone lesions occur frequently in NF1. These include malformations of the sphenoid bone and thinning of the cortex of the long bones, with bowing and pseudarthrosis of the tibia, bone cysts, and scoliosis.
- **Mental status:** Mild intellectual impairment is frequent in patients with NF1, but severe retardation is not part of the syndrome.
- **Leukemia:** The risk of malignant myeloid disorders in children with NF1 is 200 to 500 times the normal risk. In some patients, both alleles of the NF1 gene are inactivated in the leukemic cells.

Neurofibromatosis Type II (Central Neurofibromatosis)

Neurofibromatosis type II (NF2) refers to a syndrome defined by bilateral tumors of the eighth cranial nerve (acoustic neuromas) and, commonly, by meningiomas and gliomas. The disorder is considerably less common than NF1, occurring in 1 in 50,000 persons. Most patients suffer from bilateral acoustic neuromas, but the condition can be diagnosed in the presence of a unilateral eighth nerve tumor if two of the following are present: neurofibroma, meningioma, glioma, schwannoma, or juvenile posterior lenticular opacity.

Pathogenesis: Despite the superficial similarities between NF1 and NF2, they are not variants of the same disease and, indeed, have separate genetic origins. The *NF2* gene resides in the middle of the long arm of chromosome 22 (22q,11.1-13.1). In contrast to NF1, the tumors in NF2 frequently show deletions or loss of heterozygous DNA markers in the affected chromosome. The *NF2* gene encodes a tumor-suppressor protein termed *merlin*, or *schwannomin*, which is a member of a superfamily of proteins that link the cytoskeleton to the cell membrane. Other members of this family include ezrin, moesin, radixin, talin, and protein 4.1. Merlin is detectable in most differentiated tissues, including Schwann cells.

Achondroplastic Dwarfism

Achondroplastic dwarfism is an autosomal dominant, hereditary disturbance of epiphyseal chondroblastic development that leads to inadequate enchondral bone formation. This abnormality causes a distinctive form of dwarfism characterized by short limbs with a normal head and trunk. The affected person has a small face, a bulging forehead, and a deeply indented bridge of the nose. Achondroplastic dwarfism is not infrequent, occurring in 1 per 3000 live births. Achondroplasia is discussed in Chapter 26.

Familial Hypercholesterolemia

Familial hypercholesterolemia is an autosomal dominant disorder characterized by high levels of low-density lipoproteins (LDLs) in the blood, accompanied by the deposition of cholesterol in arteries, tendons, and skin. It is one of the most common autosomal dominant disorders, and in its heterozygous form, it affects at least one in 500 adults in the United States. Only 1 in 1 million persons is homozygous for the disease. **The interest in this disease stems from the striking acceleration of atherosclerosis and its complications.** This subject is discussed in detail in Chapter 10.

Pathogenesis: Familial hypercholesterolemia results from abnormalities in the gene that codes for the cell surface receptor that removes LDL from the blood. The gene for the LDL receptor is located on the short arm of chromosome 19. More than 150 different mutations in the LDL receptor gene have been described, including insertions, deletions, and nonsense and missense point mutations.

The LDL receptor is (1) synthesized in the endoplasmic reticulum, (2) transferred to the Golgi complex, (3) transported to the cell surface, and (4) internalized by receptor-mediated endocytosis in coated pits after binding LDL. Classes of genetic defects in each of these steps have been described:

- **Class 1:** This is the most common class of defect and leads to failure of the synthesis of nascent LDL-receptor protein in the endoplasmic reticulum. Most class 1 defects reflect large deletions in the gene (null alleles).
- **Class 2:** These mutations prevent the transfer of the nascent receptor from the endoplasmic reticulum to the Golgi apparatus (transport-defective alleles). Thus, the mutant receptor never appears on the cell surface.
- **Class 3:** The LDL receptors of class 3 mutations are expressed on the cell surface but are defective in the ligand-binding domain (binding-defective alleles).
- **Class 4:** In this rare class of mutations, LDL binding to the receptor is normal, but the genetic defect prevents the clustering of the receptors in coated pits, thereby blocking their internalization by endocytosis (internalization-defective alleles).
- **Class 5:** In this situation, the internalized LDL–receptor complex is not discharged from the endosome, and recycling of the receptor to the plasma membrane is defective (recycling-defective alleles).

The LDL receptor resides on the surface of hepatocytes and to some extent on other cells. After binding to the receptor, LDL is internalized and degraded in lysosomes, thereby freeing cholesterol for further metabolism. A deficiency in LDL receptors leads to an increase in plasma LDL because the rate of LDL clearance is inversely proportional to the number of LDL receptors. As a result, LDL cholesterol is taken up by tissue macrophages and accumulates to form occlusive arterial plaques (atheromas) and papules or nodules of lipid-laden macrophages (xanthomas). The central role of the liver in the pathogenesis of familial hypercholesterolemia is confirmed by the successful treatment of this disorder by liver transplantation.

Clinical Features: Heterozygous and homozygous familial hypercholesterolemia constitute two distinct clinical syndromes, reflecting a clear gene-dosage effect. In heterozygotes, elevated blood cholesterol levels (mean, 350 mg/dL; normal, <200 mg/dL) are noted at birth. Tendon xanthomas develop in half the patients before the age of 30 years, and symptoms of coronary heart disease often occur before the age of 40. In homozygotes, the blood cholesterol content reaches astronomic levels (600 to 1200 mg/dL), and virtually all patients exhibit tendon xanthomas and generalized atherosclerosis in childhood. Untreated homozygotes typically die of myocardial infarction before 30 years of age.

Autosomal Recessive Disorders Are Associated with Clinical Symptoms When Both Alleles at a Locus on Homologous Chromosomes Are Defective

In autosomal recessive diseases, the affected person is homozygous for the recessive trait (Fig. 6-23). **Most genetic metabolic diseases exhibit an autosomal recessive mode of inheritance** (Table 6-7). The fact that recessive genes are uncommon and the need for two mutant alleles for the expression of clinical disease determine the important characteristics

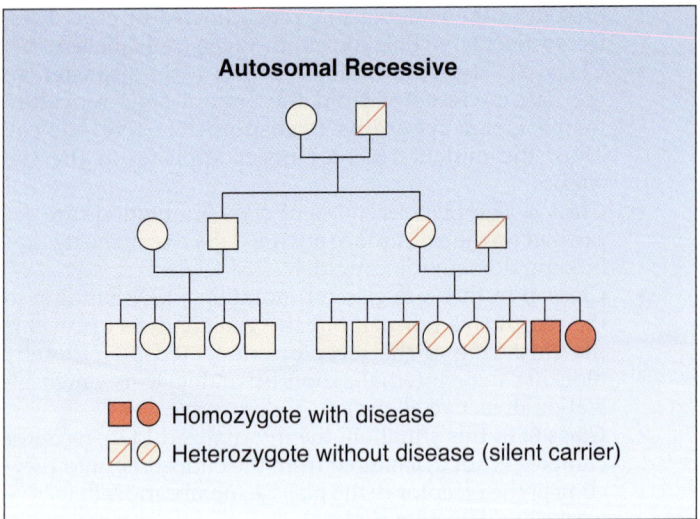

FIGURE 6-23
Autosomal recessive inheritance. Symptoms of the disease appear only in homozygotes, male or female. Heterozygotes are asymptomatic carriers. Symptomatic homozygotes result from the mating of asymptomatic heterozygotes.

of autosomal recessive inheritance. Some of the salient features of autosomal recessive disorders are as follows:

- The more infrequent the mutant gene is in the general population, the lower the probability that unrelated parents carry the trait. **Thus, rare autosomal recessive disorders are often the product of consanguineous marriages.**
- Both parents are usually heterozygous for the trait and are clinically normal.
- Symptoms appear on average in one fourth of the offspring. One half of all offspring are heterozygous for the trait and are therefore asymptomatic.
- As in autosomal dominant disorders, autosomal recessive traits are transmitted equally to males and females, since by definition, the mutant gene resides on one of the 22 different autosomal chromosomes.
- The symptomatology of autosomal recessive disorders is ordinarily less variable than that of dominant diseases. As a result, recessive traits are more commonly evident in childhood, whereas dominant disorders may initially appear in adults.
- The variability in the clinical expression of many autosomal recessive diseases is determined by the residual activity of the affected enzyme. This variability is manifested in (1) different degrees of clinical severity, (2) age at onset, or (3) the existence of acute and chronic forms of the specific disease.

Most mutant genes responsible for autosomal recessive disorders are rare in the general population, because the homozygotes for the trait tend to die before reaching reproductive age. Paradoxically, a few lethal autosomal recessive diseases are common. In the case of sickle cell anemia, it has been suggested that the resistance of the heterozygote to malarial parasitization of the erythrocyte confers a biological advantage that compensates for the loss of homozygotes. Almost all males afflicted with cystic fibrosis are sterile because of congenital bilateral absence of the vas deferens, and females have decreased fertility; any enhanced biological fitness of the heterozygote remains obscure.

New mutations for recessive diseases are difficult to identify clinically because the resulting heterozygotes are asymptomatic. Nonconsanguineous mating of two such heterozygotes would occur by chance only many generations later, if at all.

Biochemical Basis of Autosomal Recessive Disorders

Autosomal recessive diseases characteristically are caused by deficiencies in enzymes rather than abnormalities in structural proteins. A mutation that results in the inactivation of an enzyme does not ordinarily produce an abnormal phenotype, because compensatory mechanisms readily correct the functional defect. For instance, since most cellular enzymes operate at substrate concentrations significantly below saturation, an enzyme deficiency is easily corrected simply by increasing the amount of substrate. By contrast, the loss of both alleles in a homozygote results in the complete loss of enzyme activity, a situation that is not amenable to correction by regulatory mechanisms. It follows that diseases caused by the impairment of catabolic pathways that

TABLE 6-7 **Representative Autosomal Recessive Disorders**

Disease	Frequency	Chromosome
Cystic fibrosis	1/2500	7q
α-Thalassemia	High	16p
β-Thalassemia	High	11p
Sickle cell anemia	High	11p
Myeloperoxidase deficiency	1/2000	17q
Phenylketonuria	1/10,000	12q
Gaucher disease	1/1000	1q
Tay-Sachs disease	1/4000	15q
Hurler syndrome	1/100,000	22p
Glycogen storage disease Ia (von Gierke disease)	1/100,000	17
Wilson disease	1/50,000	13q
Hereditary hemochromatosis	1/1000	6p
α$_1$-Antitrypsin deficiency	1/7000	14q
Oculocutaneous albinism	1/20,000	11q
Alkaptonuria	<1/100,000	3q
Metachromatic leukodystrophy	1/100,000	22q

involve the accumulation of dietary substances (e.g., phenylketonuria, galactosemia) or cellular constituents (e.g., Tay-Sachs, Hurler) are autosomal recessive, since the accumulation of substrate overcomes any partial enzymatic defect in the heterozygote.

Cystic Fibrosis Is the Most Common Lethal Autosomal Recessive Disorder in the White Population

Cystic fibrosis (CF) is an autosomal recessive disorder affecting children, which is characterized by (1) chronic pulmonary disease, (2) deficient exocrine pancreatic function, and (3) other complications of inspissated mucus in a number of organs, including the small intestine, the liver, and the reproductive tract. The disease results from abnormal electrolyte transport caused by impaired function of the chloride channel of epithelial cells.

More than 95% of cases have been reported in whites, and the disease is found only exceptionally in blacks, and almost never in Asians. It is estimated that 1 in 25 whites is a heterozygous carrier of the *CF* gene and the incidence of cystic fibrosis is 1 in 2,500 newborns. The high prevalence of CF mutations in white populations has raised the question of a possible selective advantage for heterozygotes. Although this topic has been a source of lively speculation, a selective advantage for the *CF* gene has yet to be demonstrated.

Pathogenesis: The gene responsible for CF is located on the long arm of chromosome 7 (7q31.2) and encodes a protein of 1480 amino acids termed the *cystic fibrosis transmembrane conductance regulator (CFTR)*. CFTR is a member of the ATP-binding family of membrane transporter proteins that constitutes a chloride channel in most epithelia. The protein has two membrane-spanning domains, two domains that bind ATP, and an "R" domain that contains phosphorylation sites. The activity of the channel is regulated by the balance between kinase and phosphatase activities (i.e., phosphorylation and dephosphorylation). Phosphorylation of the R domain stimulates chloride channel activity by enhancing the binding of ATP. Activation by phosphorylation is principally effected by cAMP-dependent protein kinase A, although other kinases may also contribute. The secretion of chloride anions by mucus-secreting epithelial cells controls the parallel secretion of fluid and, consequently, the viscosity of the mucus. In normal mucus-secreting epithelia, cAMP activates protein kinase A, which in turn phosphorylates the regulatory domain of CFTR and permits channel opening. The binding of ATP to CFTR also contributes to the regulation of channel function.

In CF, the mutations in the gene encoding CFTR that disturb chloride channel function can be classified as follows (Fig. 6-24):

- **Failure of CFTR synthesis:** Mutations of the *CFTR* gene that result in premature termination signals lead to interference with the synthesis of the full-length CFTR protein. As a result there is a complete absence of CFTR-mediated chloride secretion in the involved epithelia.
- **Failure of CFTR transport to the plasma membrane:** Certain mutations prevent the proper folding of the nascent protein, which is then targeted for degradation rather than for transport to the plasma membrane. The mutation responsible for 70% of all cases of CF in the United States, namely the loss of a phenylalanine residue at position 508, (ΔF_{508}), is of this class. However, the contribution of the ΔF_{508} mutation to CF shows significant geographical and ethnic variability. In Denmark, this mutation accounts for almost 90% of all CF cases; among Ashkenazi Jews, the figure is only 30%. An analysis of haplotypes suggested that the ΔF_{508} mutation originated 50,000 years ago in the Middle East, from where it progressively spread throughout the European land mass.
- **Defective ATP binding to CFTR:** Certain mutations allow CFTR proteins to reach the plasma membrane but affect the ATP-binding domains, thereby interfering with the regulation of the channel and decreasing, but not abolishing, chloride secretion.
- **Defective chloride secretion by mutant CFTR:** Mutations in the channel pore inhibit chloride secretion.

The relationship between the these genotypes (more than 1000 mutations are known) and the clinical severity of CF is complicated and not always consistent. The best corre-

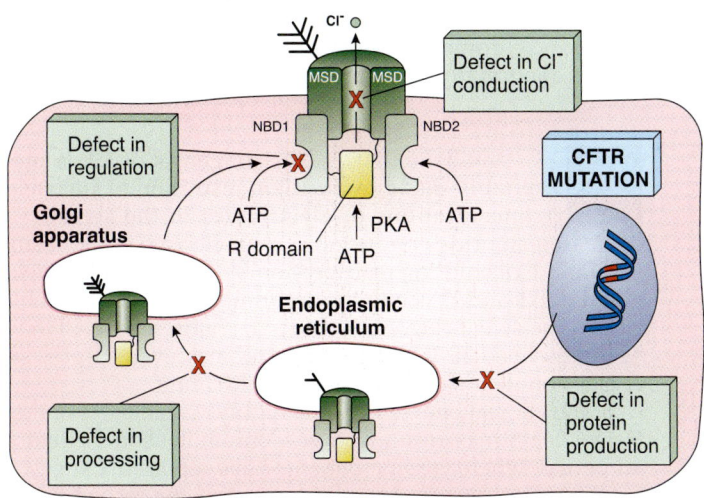

FIGURE 6-24

Cellular sites of the disruptions in the synthesis and function of cystic fibrosis transmembrane conductance regulator (CFTR) in CF.

lation seems to be between children with or without pancreatic insufficiency. Severe symptoms are generally found in those with pancreatic insufficiency (85% of all cases of CF), whereas milder cases are associated with preservation of pancreatic function. Class I and class II mutations are generally found among severely affected patients. By contrast, milder forms of CF feature class III and class IV mutations.

All of the pathological consequences of CF can be attributed to the presence of the abnormally thick mucus, which obstructs the lumina of airways, pancreatic and biliary ducts, and the fetal intestine and impairs mucociliary function in the airways. In fact, an older term for CF was *mucoviscidosis*. The normal CFTR has been shown to correct the deficiency in chloride secretion in cultured cells from patients with CF.

 Pathology: CF affects many organs that produce exocrine secretions.

RESPIRATORY TRACT: **Pulmonary disease is responsible for most of the morbidity and mortality associated with CF.** The earliest lesion is obstruction of bronchioles by mucus, with secondary infection and inflammation of the bronchiolar walls. Recurrent cycles of obstruction and infection result in **chronic bronchiolitis and bronchitis,** which increase in severity as the disease progresses. The mucous glands in the bronchi undergo hypertrophy and hyperplasia, and the airways are distended by thick and tenacious secretions. Widespread **bronchiectasis** becomes apparent by age 10 and often earlier. In the late stages of the disease, large bronchiectatic cysts and lung abscesses are common. Vascular changes of secondary pulmonary hypertension complicate the chronic bronchitis.

PANCREAS: As noted, most (85%) of patients with CF have a form of **chronic pancreatitis,** and in long-standing cases, little or no functional exocrine pancreas remains. The inspissated secretions in the pancreatic ducts produce secondary dilation and cystic change of the distal ducts (Fig. 6-25). Recurrent pancreatitis leads to the loss of acinar cells and extensive fibrosis. At autopsy, the pancreas is often represented simply by cystic fibroadipose tissue containing islets of Langerhans, hence the original designation of this disease as *cystic fibrosis of the pancreas.*

LIVER: Inspissated mucous secretions in the intrahepatic biliary system obstruct the flow of bile in the drainage areas of the affected ducts and are responsible for the development of focal **secondary biliary cirrhosis,** seen in one fourth of patients at autopsy. Microscopically, the liver exhibits inspissated concretions in bile ducts and ductules, chronic portal inflammation, and septal fibrosis. On occasion (2–5%), the hepatic lesions are sufficiently widespread to lead to the clinical manifestations of biliary cirrhosis.

GASTROINTESTINAL TRACT: Shortly after birth, the normal newborn passes the intestinal contents that have accumulated in utero (meconium). The most important lesion of the gastrointestinal tract in CF is small bowel obstruction in the newborn, termed **meconium ileus,** which is caused by the failure to pass meconium in the immediate postpartum

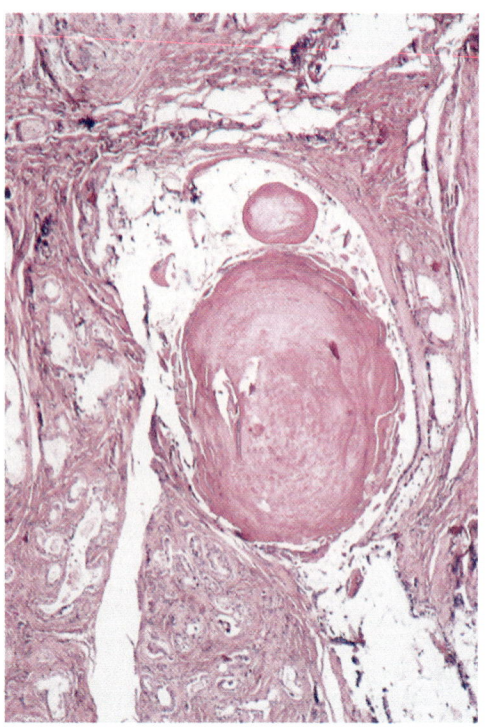

FIGURE 6-25
Intraductal concretion and atrophy of the acini in the pancreas of a patient with cystic fibrosis.

period. This complication, which occurs in 5 to 10% of newborns with CF, has been attributed to the failure of pancreatic secretions to digest meconium, possibly augmented by the greater viscosity of small bowel secretions.

REPRODUCTIVE TRACT: Almost all boys with CF exhibit atrophy or fibrosis of the reproductive duct system, including the vas deferens, epididymis, and seminal vesicles. The pathogenesis of these lesions relates to obstruction of the lumen by inspissated secretions early in life and even in utero. As a result, only 2 to 3% of males become fertile, most demonstrating an absence of spermatozoa in the semen.

Only a minority of women with CF are fertile, and many of them suffer from anovulatory cycles as a result of poor nutrition and chronic infections. Moreover, the cervical mucous plug is abnormally thick and tenacious.

 Clinical Features: **The diagnosis of CF is most reliably made by the demonstration of increased concentrations of electrolytes in the sweat.** The decreased chloride conductance characteristic of CF results in a failure of chloride reabsorption by the cells of the sweat gland ducts and hence to the accumulation of sodium chloride in the sweat (Fig. 6-26). Indeed, children with CF have been described as "tasting salty" and may even display salt crystals on their skin after vigorous sweating.

The clinical course of CF is highly variable. At one extreme, death may result from meconium ileus in the neonatal period, whereas some patients have reportedly survived for 50 years. Improved medical care and the recognition of

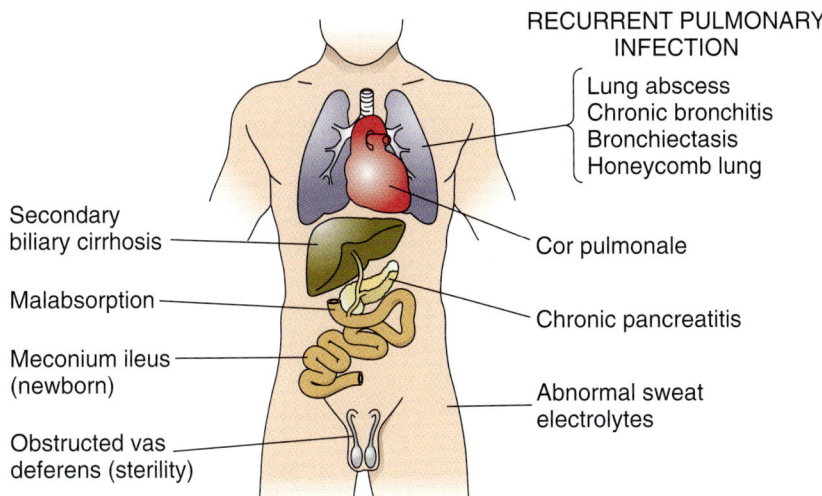

FIGURE 6-26
Clinical features of cystic fibrosis.

milder cases of CF have served to prolong the average life span which is now about 30 years of age.

The pulmonary symptoms of CF begin with cough, which eventually becomes productive of large amounts of tenacious and purulent sputum. Episodes of infectious bronchitis and bronchopneumonia become progressively more frequent, and eventually shortness of breath develops. Respiratory failure and the cardiac complications of pulmonary hypertension (cor pulmonale) are late sequelae.

The most common organisms that infect the respiratory tract in CF are *Staphylococcus* and *Pseudomonas* species. As the disease advances, *Pseudomonas* may be the only organism cultured from the lung. **In fact, the recovery of *Pseudomonas* species, particularly the mucoid variety, from the lungs of a child with chronic pulmonary disease is virtually diagnostic of CF.** Infection with *Burkholderia cepacia* is associated with *cepacia syndrome*, a very severe pulmonary infection that is highly resistant to treatment with antibiotics and is commonly fatal.

The failure of pancreatic exocrine secretion leads to the malabsorption of fat and protein, an effect that is reflected in bulky, foul-smelling stools (steatorrhea), nutritional deficiencies, and growth retardation.

Postural drainage of the airways, antibiotic therapy, and pancreatic enzyme supplementation are the mainstays of the treatment of CF. The molecular prenatal diagnosis of CF in specimens obtained by amniocentesis or chorionic villus sampling is now accurate in 95% of cases.

Lysosomal Storage Diseases Are Characterized by Accumulation of Unmetabolized Normal Substrates in Lysosomes Because of Deficiencies of Specific Acid Hydrolases

Lysosomes are membranous bags of hydrolytic enzymes used for the controlled intracellular digestion of macromolecules. Lysosomal digestive enzymes are referred to as "acid hydrolases" because they function optimally in the acidic range (pH 3.5–5.5), an environment maintained by an ATP-dependent proton pump in the lysosomal membrane. These enzymes degrade virtually all types of biological macromolecules. Extracellular macromolecules that are incorporated by endocytosis or phagocytosis and intracellular constituents that are subjected to autophagy are digested in the lysosomes to their basic components. The end-products may be transported across the lysosomal membrane into the cytosol, where they are reused in the synthesis of new macromolecules.

Virtually all lysosomal storage diseases result from mutations in genes that encode lysosomal hydrolases. A deficiency in one of the more than 40 acid hydrolases can result in an inability to catabolize the normal macromolecular substrate of that enzyme. As a result, the undigested substrate accumulates in the lysosomes, thereby leading to engorgement of these organelles and expansion of the lysosomal compartment of the cell. The resulting distention of the lysosomes is often at the expense of other critical cellular components, particularly in the brain and the heart, and can lead to a failure of cell function.

Lysosomal storage diseases are classified according to the material retained within the lysosomes. Thus, when the substrates that accumulate are sphingolipids, we speak of the *sphingolipidoses*. Similarly, the storage of mucopolysaccharides (glycosaminoglycans) leads to the *mucopolysaccharidoses*. More than 30 distinct lysosomal storage diseases have been described, but we restrict our discussion to the more important examples.

Sphingolipidoses are lysosomal storage diseases characterized by the accumulation of certain lipids derived from the turnover of obsolete cell membranes. Cerebrosides, gangliosides, sphingomyelin, and sulfatides are sphingolipid components of the membranes of a variety of cells. These substances are degraded within lysosomes by complex metabolic pathways to sphingosine and fatty acids (Fig. 6-27). Deficiencies of many of the acid hydrolases that mediate specific steps in these pathways result in the accumulation of undigested intermediate substrates in the lysosomes.

Gaucher Disease

Gaucher disease is characterized by the accumulation of glucosylceramide, primarily in the lysosomes of macrophages. The disor-

252 Developmental and Genetic Diseases

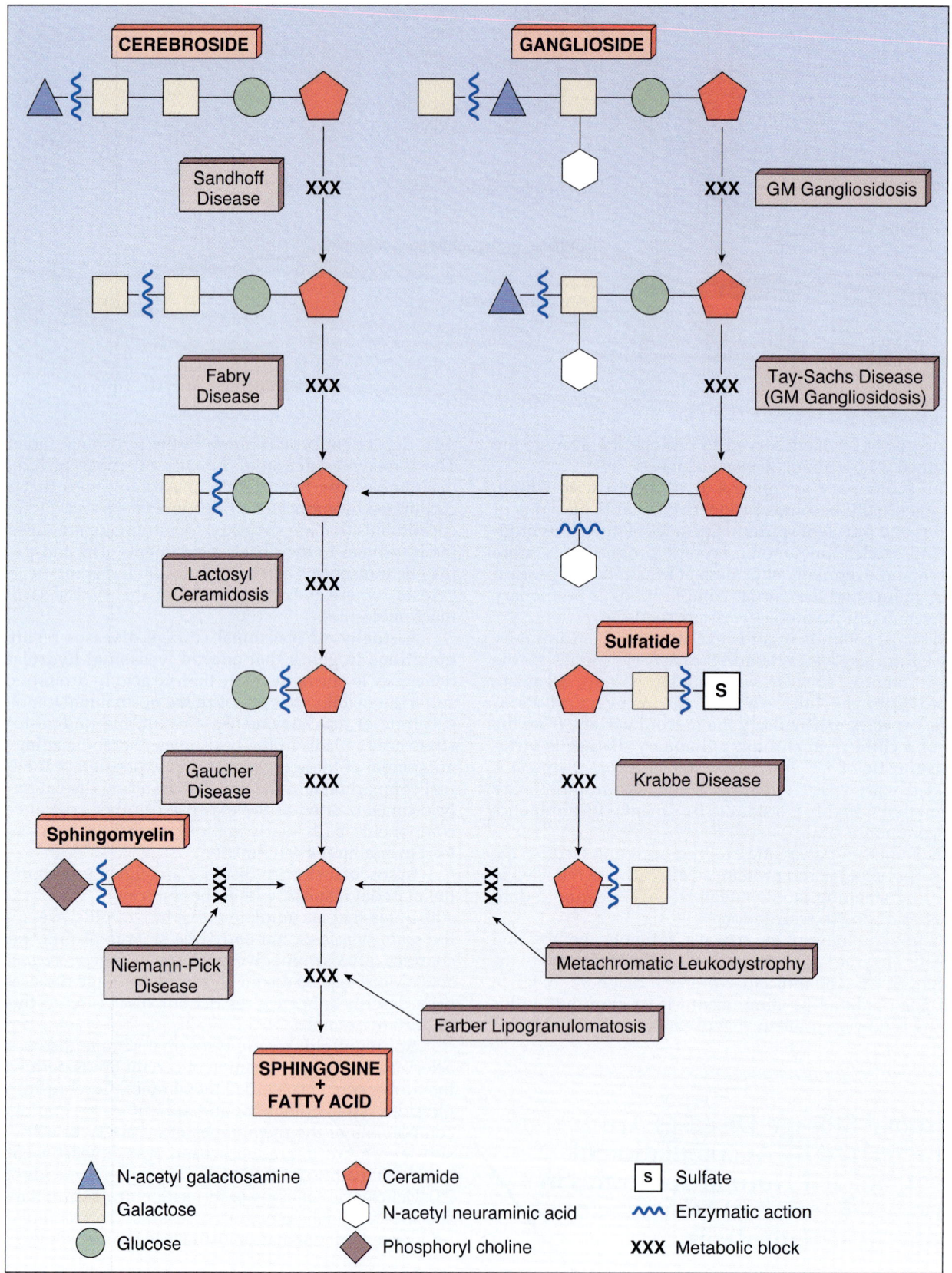

FIGURE 6-27
Disturbances of lipid metabolism in various sphingolipidoses.

der was first described in 1882 in a doctoral thesis by Gaucher, but the familial occurrence was not recognized for some 20 years.

 Pathogenesis: The underlying abnormality in Gaucher disease is a deficiency in glucocerebrosidase, a type of lysosomal acid β-glucosidase. The enzyme deficiency can be traced to a variety of single base mutations in the β-glucosidase gene, which resides on the long arm of chromosome 1 (1q21). Each of the three clinical types of the disease (see below) exhibits heterogeneous mutations in the β-glucosidase gene, although the molecular basis for the phenotypic differences remains to be firmly established.

The glucosylceramide that accumulates in the Gaucher cells in the spleen, liver, bone marrow, and lymph nodes derives principally from the catabolism of senescent leukocytes. The membranes of these cells are rich in the cerebrosides, and when their degradation is blocked by the deficiency of glucocerebrosidase, the intermediate metabolite, glucosylceramide, accumulates. The glucosylceramide of Gaucher cells in the brain is believed to originate from the turnover of plasma membrane gangliosides of cells in the central nervous system.

 Pathology: The hallmark of this disorder is the presence of *Gaucher cells*, which are lipid-laden macrophages that are characteristically present in the red pulp of the spleen, liver sinusoids, lymph nodes, lungs, and bone marrow, although they may be found in virtually any organ of the body. These cells are derived from the resident macrophages in the respective organs, for example, the Kupffer cells in the liver and the alveolar macrophages in the lung. In the uncommon variants of Gaucher disease with involvement of the central nervous system, the Gaucher cells originate from periadventitial cells in the Virchow-Robin spaces.

The Gaucher cell is large (20–100 μm in diameter) and has a clear cytoplasm and an eccentric nucleus (Fig. 6-28). By light microscopy, the cytoplasm has a characteristic fibrillar appearance, which has been likened to "wrinkled tissue paper" and is intensely positive with the periodic acid-Schiff (PAS) stain. By electron microscopy, the storage material is found within enlarged lysosomes and appears as parallel layers of tubular structures.

Enlargement of the spleen is virtually universal in Gaucher disease. In the adult form of the disorder, splenomegaly may be massive, with spleen weights up to 10 kg. The cut surface of the enlarged spleen is firm and pale and often contains sharply demarcated infarcts. Microscopically, the red pulp shows nodular and diffuse infiltrates of Gaucher cells, together with moderate fibrosis.

The liver is usually enlarged by the presence of Gaucher cells within the sinusoids, but the hepatocytes are unaffected. In severe cases, hepatic fibrosis and even cirrhosis may ensue. The extent of bone marrow involvement is variable but leads to some radiological abnormalities in 50 to 75% of cases (see Chapter 26).

Gaucher cells may also be found in many other organs, including the lymph nodes, lungs, endocrine glands, skin, gastrointestinal tract, and kidneys, although symptoms referable to these organs are uncommon.

When the brain is affected, Gaucher cells are present in the Virchow-Robin spaces around blood vessels. In the infantile (neuronopathic) form of Gaucher disease, these cells have also been found in the parenchyma, where they may stimulate gliosis and the formation of microglial nodules.

 Clinical Features: Gaucher disease is classified into three distinct forms, based on the age at onset and degree of neurological involvement.

- **Type 1 (chronic nonneuronopathic):** This variant of Gaucher disease is the most common of all lysosomal storage diseases and is found principally in adult Ashkenazi Jews, among whom the incidence is between 1 in 600 and 1 in 2500. The age at onset is highly variable, with some cases being diagnosed in infants and others in persons 70 years of age. Similarly, the severity of clinical manifestations varies widely. Most cases are not diagnosed until adulthood and present initially as painless splenomegaly and the complications of hypersplenism (i.e., anemia, leukopenia, and thrombocytopenia). Whereas hepatomegaly is common, clinical liver disease is infrequent. Bone involvement, in the form of pain and pathological fractures, is the leading cause of disability and may be severe enough to confine the patient to a wheelchair. The life expectancy of most persons with type 1 Gaucher disease is normal. This type of Gaucher disease is now successfully treated by the intravenous administration of modified acid glucose cerebrosidase, although the extremely high cost limits its use. Marrow transplantation is also effective but is little used because of the risks associated with this therapy. Prenatal diagnosis, based on β-glucosidase activity in amniotic fluid or chorionic villi or on DNA technology, is now routinely available.
- **Type 2 (acute neuronopathic):** Type 2 Gaucher disease is rare and distinctly different from type 1 in the age at onset and the clinical presentation. It usually presents by age 3 months with hepatosplenomegaly and has no ethnic predilection. Within a few months, the infant exhibits neurological signs, with the classic triad of trismus, strabismus, and backward flexion of the neck. Further neu-

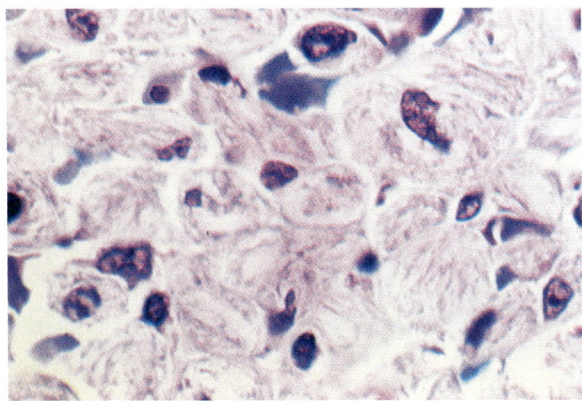

FIGURE 6-28
The spleen in Gaucher disease. Typical Gaucher cells have foamy cytoplasm and eccentrically located nuclei.

rological deterioration rapidly follows, and most patients die before the age of 1 year.
- **Type 3 (subacute neuronopathic):** This form of Gaucher disease is also rare and combines features of type 1 and type 2 disease. Neurological deterioration presents at an older age than in patients with type 2 and is more slowly progressive.

Tay-Sachs Disease (GM$_2$ Gangliosidosis, Type 1)

Tay-Sachs disease is the catastrophic infantile variant of a class of lysosomal storage diseases known as the GM$_2$ gangliosidoses, in which this ganglioside is deposited in neurons of the central nervous system, owing to a failure of lysosomal degradation. The association of a "cherry-red spot" in the retina and profound mental and physical retardation was first pointed out in 1881 by Warren Tay, a British ophthalmologist. Fifteen years later, Bernard Sachs, an American neurologist, described the histological features of the disorder and coined the term "amaurotic (blind) family idiocy." Tay-Sachs disease is inherited as an autosomal recessive trait and is predominantly a disorder of Ashkenazi Jews, in whom the carrier rate is 1 in 30, and the natural incidence of homozygotes is 1 in 4000 live newborns. By contrast, the incidence of Tay-Sachs disease in non-Jewish American populations is less than 1 in 100,000 live births. Screening programs for heterozygotes among Ashkenazi Jews have now reduced the disease incidence by 90%. The other GM$_2$ gangliosidoses are exceedingly rare.

Pathogenesis: Gangliosides are glycosphingolipids consisting of a ceramide and an oligosaccharide chain that contains *N*-acetylneuraminic acid (see Fig. 6-27). They are present in the outer leaflet of the plasma membrane of animal cells, particularly in brain neurons.

The lysosomal catabolism of 1 of the 12 known gangliosides in the brain, namely ganglioside GM$_2$, is accomplished through the activity of the β-hexosaminidases (A and B), which are composed of α and β subunits and require the participation of the GM$_2$-activator protein. A deficiency in any of these components results in clinical disease.

Tay-Sachs disease (also known as hexosaminidase α-subunit deficiency) results from about 50 different mutations in the gene on chromosome 15q23-24 that codes for the α subunit of hexosaminidase A, with a resulting defect in the synthesis of this enzyme. An insertion of four nucleotides in exon 11 is the most common mutation among Ashkenazi Jews, accounting for over two thirds of the carriers, or about 2% of that population. The β subunits are synthesized normally and associate to form the dimer known as hexosaminidase B, the levels of which are normal or even increased in Tay-Sachs disease.

Sandhoff disease is the result of a mutation in the gene on chromosome 5 that encodes the β subunit and leads to deficiencies of both hexosaminidase A and B.

A third, rare variant is the result of a defect in the synthesis of the GM$_2$-activator protein (chromosome 5) in the face of normal activities of the hexosaminidases.

Pathology: GM$_2$ ganglioside accumulates in the lysosomes of all organs in Tay-Sachs disease, but it is most prominent in brain neurons and cells of the retina. The size of the brain varies with the length of survival of the affected infant. Early cases are marked by brain atrophy, whereas the brain may be as much as doubled in weight in those who survive beyond a year. Microscopic examination reveals neurons markedly distended with storage material that stains positively for lipids. By electron microscopy, the neurons are stuffed with "membranous cytoplasmic bodies," which are composed of concentric whorls of lamellar structures (Fig. 6-29). As the disease progresses, neurons are lost, and numerous lipid-laden macrophages are conspicuous in the gray matter of the cerebral cortex. Eventually, gliosis becomes prominent, and myelin and axons in the white matter are lost. The pathological changes in the other forms of GM$_2$ gangliosidosis are similar to those of Tay-Sachs disease, although usually less severe.

Clinical Features: The symptomatology of Tay-Sachs disease appears between 6 and 10 months of age and is characterized by progressive weakness, hypotonia, and decreased attentiveness. Progressive motor and mental deterioration, often with generalized seizures, follow rapidly. Vision is seriously impaired, and blindness (Gk. *amaurosis*) is the feature that was responsible for the original designation of the disease as familial amaurotic idiocy. Involvement of the retinal ganglion cells is detected by ophthalmoscopy as a **cherry-red spot** in the macula. This feature reflects the pallor of the affected cells, which enhances the prominence of the vessels underlying the central fovea. Most children with Tay-Sachs disease die before 4 years of age.

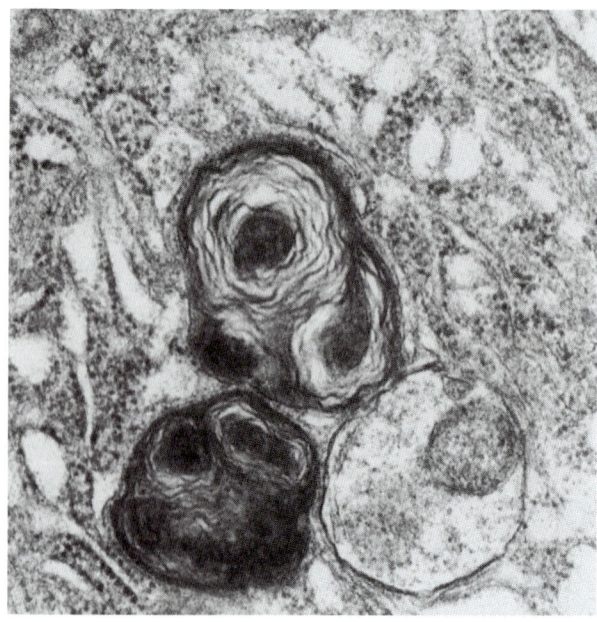

FIGURE 6-29
Tay-Sachs disease. The cytoplasm of the nerve cell contains lysosomes filled with whorled membranes.

Niemann-Pick Disease

Niemann-Pick disease (NPD) refers to lipidoses that are characterized by the lysosomal storage of sphingomyelin in macrophages of many organs, in hepatocytes, and in the brain. These disorders are classified into two categories, termed *types A and B*. Type A NPD appears in infancy and is characterized by hepatosplenomegaly and progressive neurodegeneration, with death occurring by 3 years of age. Type B NPD is more variable and features principally hepatosplenomegaly and minimal neurological symptomatology, with survival to adulthood. A particularly high frequency of NPD is observed among Ashkenazi Jews, but the disorder is present in other ethnic groups. Among the former, the incidence of type A NPD is 1 in 40,000 and of type B 1 in 80,000, with a combined heterozygote prevalence of 1 in 100.

Pathogenesis: Sphingomyelin is a membrane phospholipid composed of phosphorylcholine, sphingosine (a long-chain amino alcohol), and a fatty acid, which accounts for up to 14% of the total phospholipids of the liver, spleen, and brain. The metabolic defect in NPD reflects 12 different mutations in the gene (11p15.1-15.4) that encodes **sphingomyelinase**, the lysosomal enzyme that hydrolyzes sphingomyelin to ceramide and phosphorylcholine. Type A NPD reflects the complete absence of sphingomyelinase activity, whereas in type B patients up to 10% of normal activity can be detected.

Pathology: The characteristic storage cell in NPD is a foam cell, that is, an enlarged (20–90 μm) macrophage in which the cytoplasm is distended by the presence of uniform vacuoles that contain sphingomyelin and cholesterol. By electron microscopy, whorls of concentrically arranged lamellar structures distend the lysosomes.

Foam cells are particularly numerous in the spleen, lymph nodes, and bone marrow but are also found in the liver, lungs, and gastrointestinal tract. The spleen is enlarged, often to massive proportions, and microscopically, foam cells are diffusely distributed throughout the red pulp. Lymph nodes enlarged by foam cells are seen in many locations. The hematopoietic tissues in the bone marrow may be displaced by aggregates of foam cells. The liver is enlarged by the presence of stored sphingomyelin and cholesterol in the lysosomes of both Kupffer cells and hepatocytes.

The brain is the most important organ involved in type A NPD, and neurological damage is the usual cause of death. At autopsy, the brain is atrophic and in severe cases may be reduced to as little as half the normal weight. Neurons are distended by the presence of vacuoles containing the same stored lipids found elsewhere in the body. Advanced cases are characterized by a severe loss of neurons and sometimes by demyelination. Foam cells are noted in many locations. Half of children affected by type A disease demonstrate a cherry-red spot in the retina, similar to that seen in Tay-Sachs disease.

Clinical Features: Type A NPD manifests in early infancy with conspicuous enlargement of the spleen and liver and psychomotor retardation. There is a progressive loss of motor and intellectual function, and the child typically dies between the ages of 2 and 3 years. Most type B patients are identified in childhood because of conspicuous hepatosplenomegaly. Pulmonary infiltration with sphingomyelin-laden macrophages eventually leads to compromised respiratory function in many patients with type B disease. However, these patients have little in the way of neurological symptoms and may survive for many years.

Mucopolysaccharidoses

The mucopolysaccharidoses (MPS) comprise an assortment of lysosomal storage diseases characterized by the accumulation of glycosaminoglycans (mucopolysaccharides) in many organs. All types of MPS are inherited as autosomal recessive traits, with the exception of Hunter syndrome, which is X-linked recessive. These rare diseases are caused by deficiencies in any one of the 10 lysosomal enzymes involved in the sequential degradation of glycosaminoglycans (Fig. 6-30). Six abnormal phenotypes are described, each varying with the specific enzyme deficiency (Table 6-8).

Pathogenesis: Glycosaminoglycans (GAGs) are large polymers composed of repeating disaccharide units containing *N*-acetylhexosamine and a hexose or hexuronic acid. Either of the disaccharide compo-

TABLE 6-8 **Mucopolysaccharidoses**

Type	Eponym	Location of Gene	Clinical Features
I H	Hurler	4p16.3	Organomegaly, cardiac lesions, dysostosis multiplex, corneal clouding, death in childhood
I S	Scheie	4p16.3	Stiff joints, corneal clouding, normal intelligence, longevity
II	Hunter	X	Organomegaly, dysostosis multiplex, mental retardation, death earlier than 15 years of age
III	Sanfillipo	12q14	Mental retardation
IV	Morquio	16q24	Skeletal deformities, corneal clouding
V	Obsolete	—	—
VI	Maroteaux Lamy	5q13–14	Dysostosis multiplex, corneal clouding, death in second decade
VII	Sly	7q21.1–22	Hepatosplenomegaly, dysostosis multiplex

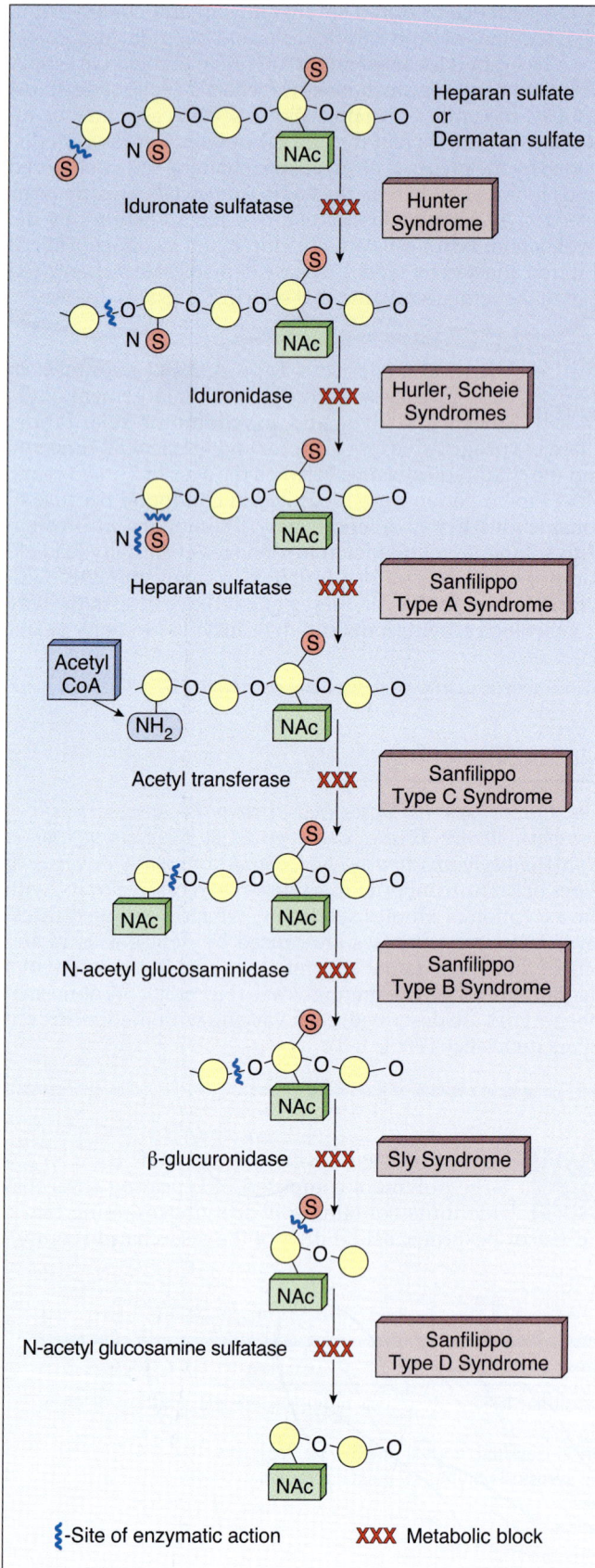

FIGURE 6-30
Metabolic blocks in various mucopolysaccharidoses that affect the degradation of heparan sulfate and dermatan sulfate.

nents may be sulfated. The accumulated GAGs (dermatan sulfate, heparan sulfate, keratan sulfate, and chondroitin sulfates) in MPS are all derived from the cleavage of proteoglycans, which are important constituents of the extracellular matrix. GAGs are degraded in a stepwise fashion by removing sugar residues or sulfate groups. Thus, a deficiency in any one of the glycosidases or sulfatases results in the accumulation of undegraded GAGs. A special case is a deficiency of an N-acetyltransferase, which leads to the deposition of heparan sulfate in Sanfilippo C disease.

 Pathology: Although the severity and location of the lesions in MPS vary with the specific enzyme deficiency, certain features are common to most of these syndromes. The undegraded GAGs tend to accumulate in connective tissue cells, mononuclear phagocytes (including Kupffer cells), endothelial cells, neurons, and hepatocytes. The affected cells are swollen and clear, and stains for metachromasia confirm the presence of GAGs. By electron microscopy, numerous enlarged lysosomes containing granular or striped material are noted.

The most important lesions of the MPS involve the central nervous system, the skeleton, and the heart, although hepatosplenomegaly and corneal clouding are common.

The central nervous system initially demonstrates only the accumulation of GAGs, but with advancing disease, there is an extensive loss of neurons and increasing gliosis, changes that are reflected in cortical atrophy. Communicating hydrocephalus, owing to meningeal involvement, is often reported.

The skeletal deformities are a consequence of the accumulation of GAGs in chondrocytes, a process that eventually interferes with the normal endochondral sequence of ossification. Abnormal foci of osteoid and woven bone are common in the deformed skeleton.

Cardiac lesions are often severe and are characterized by thickening and distortion of the valves, chordae tendineae, and endocardium. The coronary arteries are frequently narrowed by intimal thickening caused by GAG deposits in smooth muscle cells.

Hepatosplenomegaly is secondary to the distention of Kupffer cells and hepatocytes in the liver and the accumulation of macrophages filled with GAGs in the spleen.

 Clinical Features: **Hurler syndrome** (MPS IH), the most severe clinical form of MPS, remains the prototype of these syndromes. The clinical features of the other varieties of MPS are summarized in Table 6-8. The symptoms of Hurler syndrome become apparent between the ages of 6 months and 2 years. These children typically exhibit skeletal deformities, an enlarged liver and spleen, a characteristic facies, and joint stiffness. The combination of coarse facial features and dwarfism is reminiscent of the gargoyle figures decorating Gothic cathedrals and accounts for the term *gargoylism* previously appended to this syndrome.

Children with Hurler syndrome suffer developmental delay, hearing loss, clouding of the cornea, and progressive mental deterioration. Increased intracranial pressure, owing to communicating hydrocephalus, can be troublesome. Most patients die before the age of 10 years from recurrent pulmonary infections and cardiac complications.

The detection of heterozygotes is difficult, because of the overlap in enzyme activity of cultured cells with the normal population. Prenatal diagnosis is possible for all the MPS and is routine for Hurler and Hunter syndromes.

Glycogenoses (Glycogen Storage Diseases)

The glycogenoses are a group at least 10 distinct inherited disorders characterized by the accumulation of glycogen, principally in the liver, skeletal muscle, and heart. Each entity reflects a deficiency of one of the specific enzymes involved in the metabolism of glycogen (Fig. 6-31). With one rare exception (X-linked phosphorylase kinase deficiency), all types of glycogen storage disease represent autosomal recessive traits. The glycogenoses are rare diseases, varying in frequency from 1 in 100,000 to 1 in 1 million.

Glycogen is a large glucose polymer (20,000–30,000 glucose units per molecule), which is stored in most cells to provide a ready source of energy during the fasting state. The liver and muscle are particularly rich in glycogen, although its function is different in each organ. The liver stores glycogen not for its own use but rather for the rapid supply of glucose to the blood, particularly for the benefit of the brain. By contrast, glycogen in skeletal muscle is used as a local fuel when the supply of oxygen or glucose falls. Glycogen is synthesized and degraded sequentially by the action of a number of enzymes, a deficiency in any of which leads to the accumulation of glycogen.

Although each of the glycogen storage diseases involves an accumulation of glycogen, the significant organ involvement varies with the specific enzyme defect. Some predominantly affect the liver, whereas others are principally manifested by cardiac or skeletal muscle dysfunction. **Importantly, the symptoms of a glycogenosis can reflect either the accumulation of glycogen itself (Pompe disease, Andersen disease) or the lack of the glucose that is normally derived from glycogen degradation (von Gierke disease, McArdle disease).** We discuss only several representative examples of the known glycogenoses.

VON GIERKE DISEASE (TYPE IA GLYCOGENOSIS): von Gierke disease is characterized by the accumulation of glycogen in the liver as a result of a deficiency in glucose-6-phosphatase. The symptoms reflect the inability of the liver to convert glycogen to glucose, a defect that results in hepatomegaly and hypo-

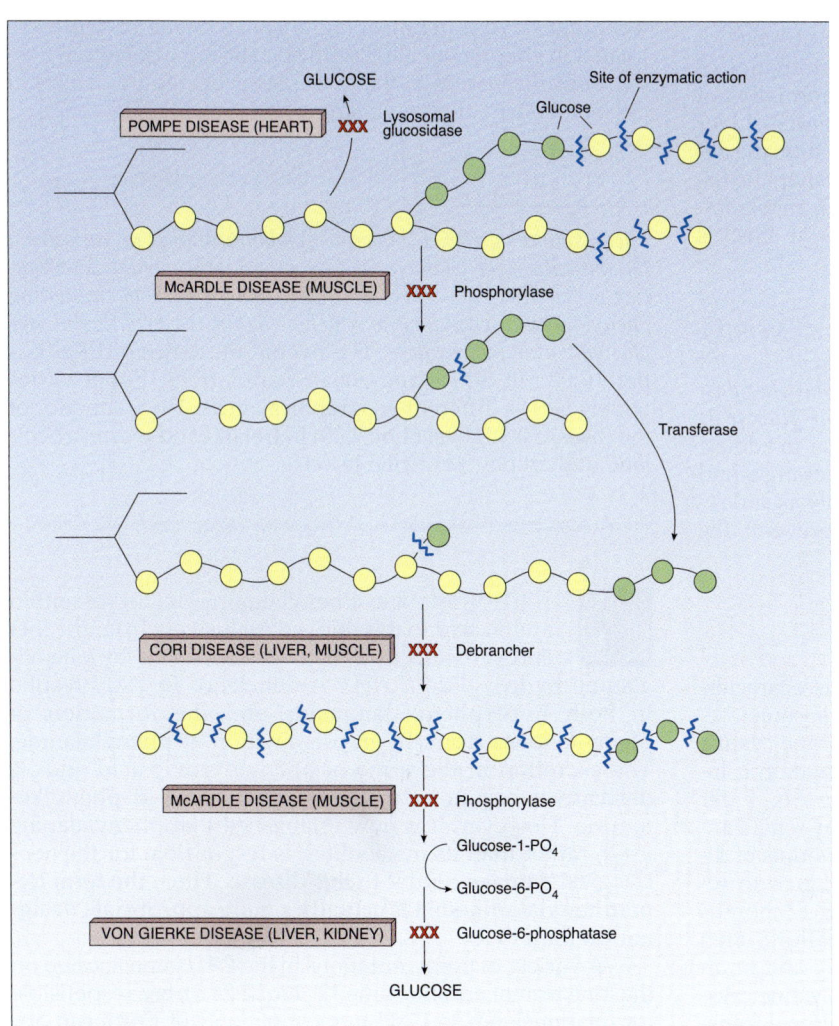

FIGURE 6-31
Sequential catabolism of glycogen and the enzymes that are deficient in various glycogenoses. Glycogen is a long-chain branched polymer of glucose residues, which are connected by α-1,4 linkages, except at branch points, where an α-1,6 linkage is present. Phosphorylase hydrolyzes α-1,4 linkages to a point three glucose residues distal to an α-1,6-linked sugar. These three glucose residues are transferred to the chain linked by α-1,4 bonds, by the bifunctional debrancher enzyme amylo-1,6-glucosidase. Subsequently the same enzyme removes the α-1,6 linked sugar at the original branch point. This creates a linear α-1,4 chain, which is degraded by phosphorylase to glucose-1-phosphate. Following the conversion to glucose-6-phosphate, glucose is released by the action of glucose-6-phosphatase. A small proportion of glycogen is totally degraded within lysosomes by acid α-glucosidase. Red-metabolic block

glycemia. The disorder is usually evident in infancy or early childhood. Although growth is commonly stunted, with modern treatment the prognosis for normal mental development and longevity is generally good.

POMPE DISEASE (TYPE II GLYCOGENOSIS): *Pompe disease is a lysosomal storage disease that involves virtually all organs and results in death from heart failure before the age of 2 years.* The juvenile and adult variants are less common and have a better prognosis. Normally, a small proportion of cytoplasmic glycogen is degraded within lysosomes following an autophagic sequence. Type II glycogenosis is caused by a deficiency in the lysosomal enzyme acid α-glucosidase (17q23), which leads to the inexorable accumulation of undegraded glycogen in the lysosomes of many different cells. Interestingly, the patients do not suffer from hypoglycemia, because the major metabolic pathways of glycogen synthesis and degradation in the cytoplasm remain normal.

ANDERSEN DISEASE (TYPE IV GLYCOGENOSIS): *Andersen disease is a very rare condition in which an abnormal form of glycogen, termed* amylopectin, *is deposited principally in the liver but also in the heart, muscles, and nervous system.* Children with type IV glycogenosis typically die between the ages of 2 and 4 years from **cirrhosis of the liver.** The disorder results from a deficiency in the branching enzyme (amyloglucantransferase) (3p12) responsible for creating the branch points in the normal glycogen molecule. The absence of brancher enzyme leads to the formation and accumulation of an insoluble and toxic form of glycogen that is normally not present in animal cells and resembles plant starch. Liver transplantation cures Andersen disease. Remarkably, the deposits of amylopectin in the heart and other extrahepatic tissues are significantly reduced following liver transplantation, although the mechanism for this paradoxical effect is obscure.

MCARDLE DISEASE (TYPE V GLYCOGENOSIS): *McArdle disease is characterized by the accumulation of glycogen in skeletal muscles, owing to a deficiency of muscle phosphorylase (11q13), the enzyme responsible for the release of glucose-1-phosphate from glycogen.* Symptoms usually appear in adolescence or early adulthood and consist of muscle cramps and spasms during exercise and sometimes myocytolysis and resulting myoglobinuria. Avoidance of exercise prevents the symptoms.

Cystinosis

Cystinosis is a lysosomal storage disease that is characterized by accumulation of crystalline cystine in lysosomes because of the absence of *cystinosin*, a transmembrane cystine transporter. The gene that is affected by this mutation is located at chromosome 17p13. Cystinosis occurs in 1 per 100,000 to 200,000 live births. It is characterized by renal Fanconi syndrome (polydipsia, excretion of large amounts of dilute urine, dehydration, electrolyte imbalances, growth retardation, and rickets) beginning between 6 and 12 months of age. Untreated, cystinosis progresses to renal failure, often before adolescence. Abnormalities in pulmonary and brain function are commonly seen in older patients. Cystine crystals are observed in almost all cells and organs. Renal trans-

T A B L E 6-9 **Representative Inherited Disorders of Amino Acid Metabolism**

Phenylketonuria (hyperphenylalaninemia)
Tyrosinemia
Histidinemia
Ornithine transcarbamylase deficiency (ammonia intoxication)
Carbamyl phosphate synthetase deficiency (ammonia intoxication)
Maple syrup urine disease (branched chain ketoacidemia)
Arginase deficiency
Arginosuccinic acid synthetase deficiency (citrulline accumulation)

plantation can be used to treat the renal failure seen in cystinosis. The use of cysteamine to decrease lysosomal cystine greatly slows the progression of the disease and has resulted in longer survival for patients with cystinosis.

Inborn Errors of Amino Acid Metabolism Manifest with Variably Severe Symptomatology

Heritable disorders involving the metabolism of many amino acids have been described (Table 6-9). Some are lethal in early childhood; others are asymptomatic biochemical defects that have no clinical significance. Some of these are treated in chapters dealing with specific organs. Here we restrict our discussion to the examples provided by defects in the metabolism of phenylalanine and tyrosine (Fig. 6-32).

Phenylketonuria

Phenylketonuria (PKU, hyperphenylalaninemia) is an autosomal recessive disorder characterized by progressive mental deterioration in the first few years of life owing to high levels of circulating phenylalanine secondary to a deficiency of the hepatic enzyme phenylalanine hydroxylase. The overall incidence of PKU is 1 per 10,000 in white and Asian populations, but it varies widely across different geographical areas. The frequency of the disease is highest (1 in 5000) in Ireland and western Scotland and among Yemenite Jews.

Pathogenesis: Phenylalanine is an essential amino acid that is derived exclusively from the diet and is oxidized in the liver to tyrosine by phenylalanine hydroxylase (PAH). A deficiency in PAH results in both hyperphenylalaninemia and the formation of phenylketones from the transamination of phenylalanine. The excretion in the urine of phenylpyruvic acid and its derivatives accounts for the original name of phenylketonuria. However, it is now established that phenylalanine itself, rather than its metabolites, is responsible for the neurological damage central to this disease. **Thus, the term hyperphenylalaninemia is actually a more appropriate designation than PKU.**

A variety of point mutations in the *PAH* gene, located on the long arm of chromosome 12 (12q22-24.1), are responsible for the deficiency in PAH in most patients of European origin. By contrast, PKU among Yemenite Jews has been ascribed to a single deletion in the *PAH* gene. An analysis of family histories of the Yemenite Jewish community has traced the origin of this defect to a common ancestor who lived in Sanà, the capital of Yemen, before the 18th century. A different deletion in the *PAH* gene has been identified in the affected Scottish population.

The mechanism of the neurotoxicity associated with hyperphenylalaninemia during infancy has not been precisely established, but several processes have been implicated: (1) competitive interference with amino acid transport systems in the brain, (2) inhibition of the synthesis of neurotransmitters, and (3) disturbance of other metabolic processes. These effects presumably lead to inadequate development of neurons and defective synthesis of myelin.

The deficiency in PAH activity is not necessarily absolute, and milder hyperphenylalaninemia than occurs in classic PKU is described. In such cases, phenylpyruvic acid is not excreted in the urine. Patients with less than 1% of the normal activity of PAH generally have a PKU phenotype, whereas those with more than 5% are considered to exhibit non-PKU hyperphenylalaninemia. Importantly, the latter do not suffer neurological damage and develop normally. It is presumed that non-PKU hyperphenylalaninemia is caused by mutations different from those in classic PKU.

Malignant hyperphenylalaninemia occurs in a few (<5%) infants with hyperphenylalaninemia. In this condition, dietary restriction of phenylalanine fails to arrest neurological deterioration. These patients have a deficiency in tetrahydrobiopterin (BH_4), a cofactor required for the hydroxylation of phenylalanine by PAH. In some instances, this defect results from a failure to regenerate BH_4, owing to an inherited lack of dihydropteridine reductase (DHPR), the enzyme that reduces dihydrobiopterin (BH_2) to the tetrahydro form (BH_4). The mutant *DHPR* gene is distinct from the *PAH* gene, being located on the short arm of chromosome 4. Alternatively, in some cases the synthesis of BH_4 is impaired. Although these infants with malignant hyperphenylalaninemia are initially indistinguishable phenotypically from those with classic PKU, BH_4 deficiency also interferes with the synthesis of the neurotransmitters dopamine (tyrosine hydroxylase dependent) and serotonin (tryptophan hydroxylase dependent). Thus, the mechanism underlying the brain damage in malignant hyperphenylalaninemia likely involves more than a simple elevation in the levels of phenylalanine.

Clinical Features: Phenylketonuria illustrates the interaction between "nature and nurture" in the pathogenesis of disease. The disorder is based on a genetic defect, but its expression depends on the provision of a dietary constituent. **The affected infant appears normal at birth, but mental retardation is evident within a few months.** By the age of 12 months, the untreated infant has lost about 50 IQ points, which means that a child with nor-

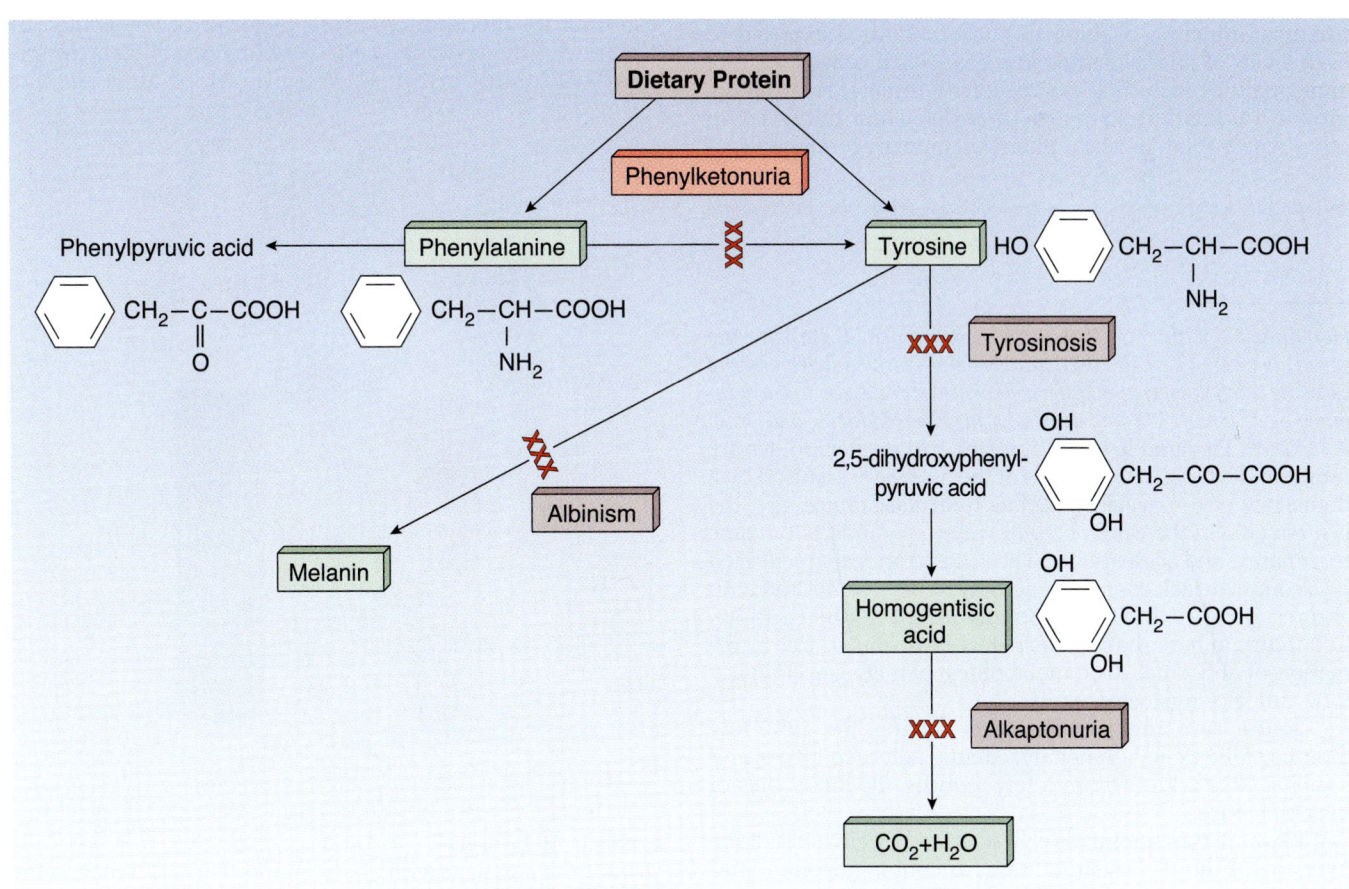

FIGURE 6-32
Diseases caused by disturbances of phenylalanine and tyrosine metabolism.

mal intelligence has been reduced to an imbecile who requires institutionalization. Infants with PKU tend to have fair skin, blond hair, and blue eyes, because the inability to convert phenylalanine to tyrosine leads to reduced melanin synthesis. These patients exude a "mousy" odor, owing to the formation of phenylacetic acid.

The treatment of PKU involves the restriction of phenylalanine in the diet to between 250 and 500 mg/day, which usually requires a semisynthetic formula. The required duration of such dietary therapy is controversial. Although at one time it was believed that the dietary regimen could be relaxed by 6 years of age, that is, after the brain has in large part matured, newer evidence suggests that many older patients suffer some deleterious effect on the reintroduction of phenylalanine into the diet. Thus, it is recommended that some phenylalanine restriction be maintained indefinitely.

In developed countries, the clinical phenotype of classical PKU is now more of historical interest than of significant public health concern. About 10 million newborns worldwide are screened annually for hyperphenylalaninemia by a simple blood test, and most of the estimated 1000 new cases are promptly treated.

The success of newborn screening programs for detection of PKU and prompt institution of a low-phenylalanine diet has offered many PKU homozygotes a normal life and reproductive capacity. With this has come the issue of providing care for expectant mothers who are homozygous for PKU (maternal PKU). Reinstitution of a strictly controlled low-phenylalanine diet is essential during pregnancy if the fetus is to avoid the complications associated with hyperphenylalaninemia of maternal origin. Infants exposed to high levels of phenylalanine in utero have a constellation of abnormalities including microcephaly, mental retardation, growth retardation, and structural defects of the heart. In other words, high levels of phenylalanine are teratogenic.

Tyrosinemia

Hereditary tyrosinemia (hepatorenal tyrosinemia, tyrosinemia type I) is a rare (1 in 100,000) autosomal recessive inborn error of tyrosine catabolism that manifests as acute liver disease in early infancy or as a more chronic disease of the liver, kidneys, and brain in children. Elevated levels of tyrosine and its metabolites are found in the blood. Both forms of the disease are caused by a deficiency of fumarylacetoacetate hydrolase (15q23-25), the last enzyme in the catabolic pathway that converts tyrosine to fumarate and acetoacetate. The acute form is characterized by a complete lack of enzyme activity, whereas children with chronic disease exhibit variable amounts of residual activity. Cell injury in hereditary tyrosinemia is attributed to the formation of abnormal toxic metabolites, namely, succinylacetone and succinylacetoacetate.

Acute tyrosinemia manifests during the first few months of life as hepatomegaly, edema, failure to thrive, and a cabbagelike odor. Within a few months, the infant dies of hepatic failure.

Chronic tyrosinemia is characterized by cirrhosis of the liver, renal tubular dysfunction (Fanconi syndrome), and neurological abnormalities. **Hepatocellular carcinoma supervenes in more than a third of patients.** Most children die before the age of 10 years. Liver transplantation corrects the hepatic metabolic abnormalities and prevents the neurological crises. Combined liver–kidney transplants have also been performed in the treatment of chronic tyrosinemia. Prenatal diagnosis is accomplished by demonstrating succinylacetone in amniotic fluid or fumarylacetoacetate hydrolase deficiency in cells obtained by amniocentesis or chorionic villus sampling.

Alkaptonuria (Ochronosis)

Alkaptonuria is a rare autosomal recessive disease characterized by the excretion of homogentisic acid in the urine, generalized pigmentation, and arthritis. A deficiency in hepatic and renal homogentisic acid oxidase prevents the catabolism of homogentisic acid, an intermediate gene product in the metabolism of phenylalanine and tyrosine. Alkaptonuria is of greater historical significance than of clinical importance. Studies almost a century ago by Garrod and others described the mode of inheritance of alkaptonuria and were among the first to define the concept of hereditary inborn errors of metabolism.

Patients with alkaptonuria excrete urine that darkens rapidly on standing, reflecting the formation of a pigment on the nonenzymatic oxidation of homogentisic acid (Fig. 6-33). In longstanding alkaptonuria, a similar pigment is deposited in numerous tissues, particularly the sclera, cartilage in many areas (ribs, larynx, trachea), tendons, and synovial membranes. Although the pigment appears bluish black on gross examination, it is brown under the microscope, accounting for the term *ochronosis* (color of ocher) coined by Virchow. A degenerative and frequently disabling arthropathy ("ochronotic arthritis") often develops after years of

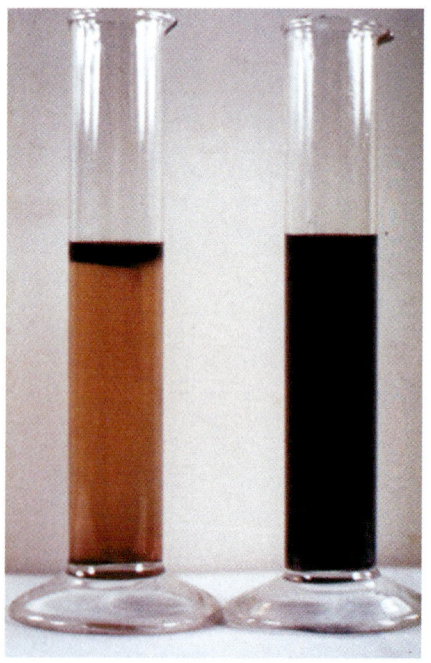

FIGURE 6-33
Urine from a patient with alkaptonuria. The specimen on the left, which has been standing for 15 minutes, shows some darkening at the surface, owing to the oxidation of homogentisic acid. After 2 hours *(right)*, the urine is entirely black.

alkaptonuria. It is tempting to ascribe the joint disease to the pigment deposition, but this has not been proved. Despite the involvement of many organs, alkaptonuria does not reduce the longevity of affected persons.

Albinism

Albinism refers to a heterogeneous group of at least 10 inherited disorders characterized by hypopigmentation as a result of absent or reduced biosynthesis of melanin. This condition is found throughout the animal kingdom (from insects to humans). The most common type is oculocutaneous albinism (OCA), a family of closely related diseases that (with a single rare exception) represent autosomal recessive traits. OCA is characterized by a deficiency or complete absence of melanin pigment in the skin, hair follicles, and eyes. The frequency of OCA in whites varies from 1 per 18,000 in the United States to 1 per 10,000 in Ireland. American blacks have the same high frequency of OCA as the Irish.

The two major forms of OCA are distinguished by the presence or absence of tyrosinase, the first enzyme in the biosynthetic pathway that converts tyrosine to melanin (see fig. 6-32).

Tyrosinase-positive OCA is the most common type of albinism in both whites and blacks. These patients typically begin life with complete albinism, but with age, a small amount of clinically detectable pigment accumulates. The defect responsible for the impairment in melanin synthesis in tyrosinase-positive OCA is attributed to mutations in the *P* gene (15q11.2-13), which is homologous with the mouse pink-eyed *(p)* gene. The *P* gene has been postulated to code for a tyrosine-transport protein.

Tyrosinase-negative OCA is the second most common type of albinism and is characterized by a complete absence of tyrosinase (11q14-21) and melanin, although melanocytes are present and contain unpigmented melanosomes. The affected person has snow-white hair, pale pink skin, blue irides, and prominent red pupils, owing to an absence of retinal pigment. Persons with OCA typically have severe ophthalmic problems, including photophobia, strabismus, nystagmus, and decreased visual acuity. The skin of all types of albinos exhibits a striking sensitivity to sunlight and requires the application of sunscreen lotions to exposed areas. These patients are at a greatly increased risk for the development of squamous cell carcinoma of the skin in sun-exposed sites. In fact, among a group of more than 500 albinos in equatorial Africa, not one survived beyond the age of 40 years, nearly all having succumbed to cancer. Interestingly, albinos seem to have a lower than normal frequency of malignant melanoma.

An X-Linked Disorder Features an Abnormal Gene on the X Chromosome

The expression of an X-linked disorder (Fig. 6-34) is different in males and females. Females, having two X chromosomes, may be homozygous or heterozygous for a given trait. It follows that the clinical expression of the trait in a female is variable, depending on whether it is dominant or recessive. By contrast, males have only one X chromosome and are said to be *hemizygous* for the same trait. **Thus, regardless of whether the trait is dominant or recessive, it is invariably expressed in the male.**

A cardinal attribute of X-linked inheritance, whether dominant or recessive, is the lack of transmission from father to son. This reflects the fact that the symptomatic father donates only his normal Y chromosome to his male offspring. By contrast, he always donates his X chromosome to his daughters, who are therefore obligate carriers of the trait. As a consequence, the disease classically skips a generation in the male, the female carrier transmitting the trait to the grandsons of the original symptomatic male.

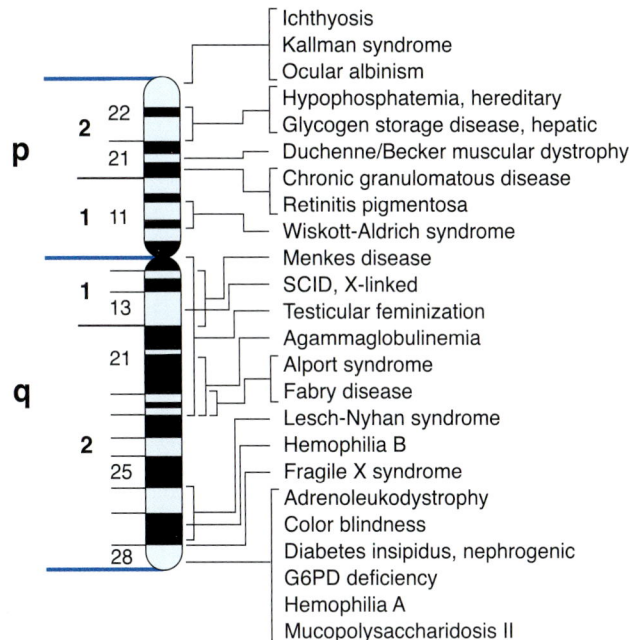

FIGURE 6-34
Localization of representative inherited diseases on the X chromosome.

X-Linked Dominant Traits

X-linked dominance refers to the expression of a trait only in the female, since the hemizygous state in the male precludes a distinction between dominant and recessive inheritance (Fig. 6-35). The distinctive features of X-linked dominant disorders are as follows:

- Females are affected twice as frequently as males.
- A heterozygous woman transmits the disorder to half her children, whether male or female.
- A man with a dominant X-linked disorder transmits the disease only to his daughters.
- The clinical expression of the disease tends to be less severe and more variable in heterozygous females than in hemizygous males.

Only a few X-linked dominant disorders are described, among which are familial hypophosphatemic rickets and ornithine transcarbamylase deficiency. In such diseases, the variations in the phenotypic expression of the trait in the female may be explained, at least in part, by the Lyon effect

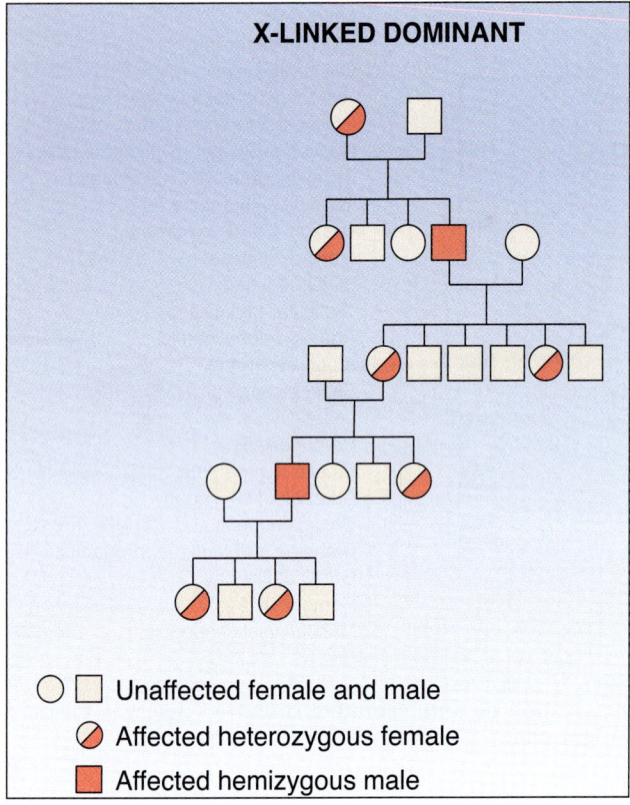

FIGURE 6-35
X-linked dominant inheritance. A heterozygous woman transmits the trait equally to males and females; men transmit the trait only to their daughters. Asymptomatic males and females do not carry the trait.

(i.e., the inactivation of one X chromosome). This random inactivation results in mosaicism for the mutant allele, a condition that may be associated with inconstant expression of the trait.

X-Linked Recessive Traits

Most X-linked traits are recessive; that is, heterozygous females do not exhibit clinical disease (Fig. 6-36). The characteristics of this mode of inheritance are as follows:

- Sons of women who are carriers of the trait have a 50% chance of inheriting the disease; the daughters are not symptomatic.
- All daughters of affected men are asymptomatic carriers, but the sons of these men are free of the trait and, thus, cannot transmit the disease to their children.
- Symptomatic homozygous females result only from the rare mating of an affected man and an asymptomatic, heterozygous woman.
- The trait tends to occur in maternal uncles and in male cousins descended from the mother's sisters.

Table 6-10 presents a list of representative X-linked recessive disorders.

X-Linked Muscular Dystrophies (Duchenne and Becker Muscular Dystrophies)

The muscular dystrophies are a number of devastating muscle diseases, most of which are X-linked, although a few are autosomal recessive. The X-linked muscular dystrophies are among the most frequent human genetic diseases, occurring in 1 per 3500 boys, an incidence approaching that of CF.

Duchenne muscular dystrophy (DMD), the most common variant, is a fatal progressive degeneration of muscle that appears before the age of 4 years (Fig. 6-37).

Becker muscular dystrophy (BMD) is allelic with DMD but is less frequent and milder.

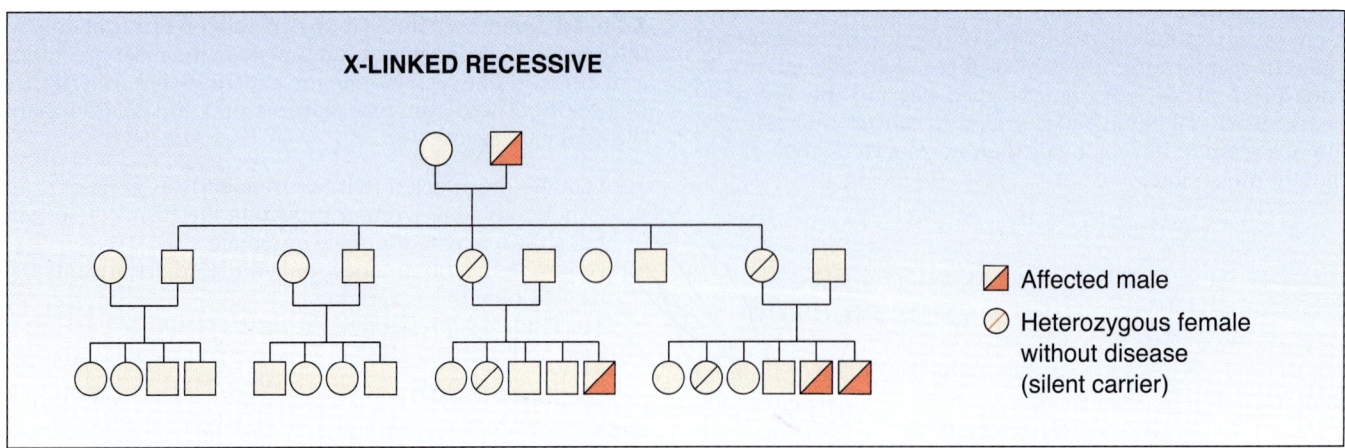

FIGURE 6-36
X-linked recessive inheritance. Only males are affected; daughters of affected men are all asymptomatic carriers. Asymptomatic men do not transmit the trait. Clinical expression of the disease skips a generation.

TABLE 6-10 **Representative X-Linked Recessive Diseases**

Disease	Frequency in Males
Fragile X syndrome	1/2000
Hemophilia A (factor VIII deficiency)	1/10,000
Hemophilia B (factor IX deficiency)	1/70,000
Duchenne-Becker muscular dystrophy	1/3500
Glucose-6-phosphate dehydrogenase deficiency	Up to 30%
Lesch-Nyhan syndrome (HPRT deficiency)	1/10,000
Chronic granulomatous disease	Not rare
X-linked agammaglobulinemia	Not rare
X-linked severe combined immunodeficiency	Rare
Fabry disease	1/40,000
Hunter syndrome	1/70,000
Adrenoleukodystrophy	1/100,000
Menke disease	1/100,000

 Pathogenesis: Both DMD and BMD are caused by a deficiency of *dystrophin*, a member of the family of membrane cytoskeletal proteins, which includes α-actinin and spectrin. The protein is located on the cytoplasmic face of the plasma membrane of muscle cells and is linked to it by integral membrane glycoproteins *(dystrophin-associated glycoprotein complex)*, which in turn are bound to extracellular laminin (Fig. 6-38). Thus, dystrophin molecules form a network connecting actin fibers to the extracellular matrix, a function that probably maintains the mechanical properties of the muscle cell and the flexibility that is needed during the contraction and relaxation of muscle fibers. It has been proposed that the absence of dystrophin leads to a defective membrane that is damaged during contraction, an effect that predisposes to death of the myocyte.

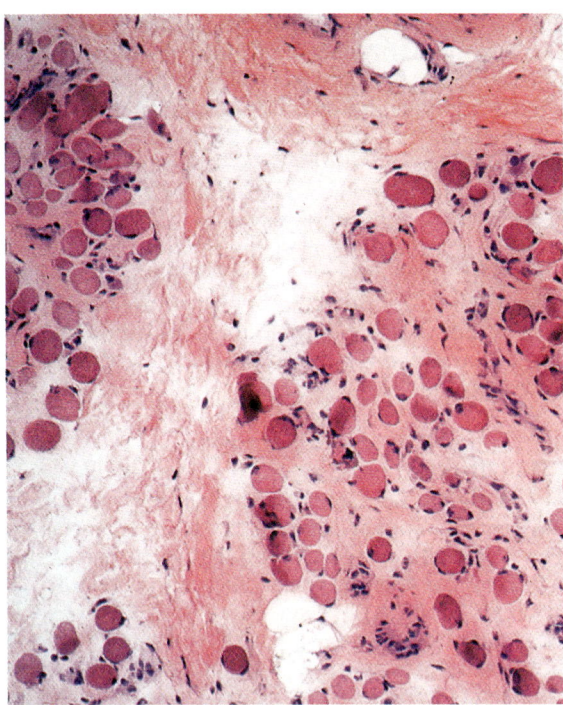

FIGURE 6-37
Dystrophic skeletal muscle in Duchenne muscular dystrophy. The muscle cells are atrophic and embedded in intrafascicular fibrosis. A few inflammatory cells are present.

The *DMD* gene, which encodes dystrophin, is one of the largest known human genes (about 2×10^6 base pairs) and is located on the short arm of the X chromosome (Xp21). Deletions in the *DMD* gene are responsible for the defects in more that 60% of cases of muscular dystrophy, with most of the remaining cases representing point mutations. The more severely affected Duchenne patients have no detectable dys-

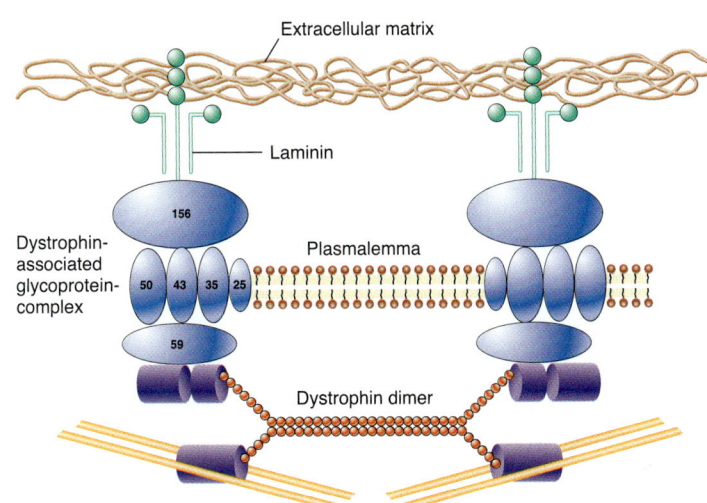

FIGURE 6-38
The correlation of alterations in dystrophin domains with the severity of muscular dystrophy. Small deletions in the N-terminal domain and in both the first 13 and last 8 repeats result in the mild Becker variant. Deletions of the cysteine-rich and adjacent C-terminal domains lead to the severe Duchenne type of muscular dystrophy. Numbers refer to the domains in the dystrophin.

trophin, whereas patients with the Becker variant have a smaller than normal dystrophin molecule. One third of patients with DMD represent new mutations, one third mutations in the mother, and only one third mutations that have been in the family for more than one generation.

In most cases, the differences between DMD and BMD reflect the nature of the mutation in the DMD gene. Almost all (96%) DMD patients have frameshift deletions that result either in the complete absence of detectable dystrophin or in a protein that is reduced in size and exhibits abnormalities or deletions of the C-terminal region. By contrast, 85% of BMD patients harbor in-frame mutations that lead to a truncated version of the protein, but one in which the C-terminal region is conserved.

Clinical Features: The symptoms of DMD progress with age. During the first year of life, the infants appear normal, but more than half fail to walk by 18 months of age. Subsequently, the gait is clumsy. Proximal muscle weakness and pseudohypertrophy of the calf muscles become obvious. More than 90% of afflicted boys are chair-bound by the age of 11 years. In advanced disease, cardiac symptoms are almost universal, and cardiomyopathy is a common cause of death. There is an overall decrease in intelligence, and one fifth of patients are significantly retarded. The presence of dystrophin in the cerebral cortex presumably accounts for this association of DMD with mental deficiency. The mean age at death in boys with DMD is 17 years, a figure that is only 2 years longer than that reported a century ago.

The Becker variant of muscular dystrophy is similar to the Duchenne form but with later onset and milder clinical symptomatology. Virtually all patients are still walking at 12 years of age, and 95% survive beyond the age of 21. Mental retardation is not a feature of the BMD phenotype.

The diagnosis of DMD/BMD in the proper clinical setting is readily made by the demonstration of elevated creatine kinase levels in the blood and characteristic pathological findings in a muscle biopsy (see Chapter 27). Prenatal diagnosis and carrier detection can be accomplished by DNA analysis. Two thirds of carrier women have elevated serum creatine kinase levels.

Hemophilia A (Factor VIII Deficiency)

Hemophilia is an X-linked recessive disorder of blood clotting that results in spontaneous bleeding, particularly into joints, muscles, and internal organs. It is now clear that classic hemophilia is actually two distinct diseases, one resulting from mutations in the gene encoding factor VIII (hemophilia A) and the other caused by defects in the gene for factor IX (hemophilia B). Since hemophilia A is the most frequently encountered sex-linked inherited bleeding disorder (1 per 5000 to 10,000 males), our discussion is limited to that variant.

Hemophilia is one of the oldest human genetic diseases recorded, having been described in the Talmud almost 2000 years ago. Male infants of Jewish families with a history of fatal bleeding after circumcision were accordingly excused from this ritual. The transmission of a bleeding tendency to boys from their unaffected mothers has been known for 200 years. Subsequently, the disorder became a subject of public interest following the dissemination of hemophilia throughout the royal families of Europe by the daughters of Queen Victoria. Finally, the gene for factor VIII was cloned in 1984, allowing investigation of the molecular basis of hemophilia A.

Pathogenesis: The mutations in the very large factor VIII gene at the tip of the long arm of the X chromosome (Xq28) include gene inversions, deletions, point mutations, and insertions. Each family with hemophilia in its history actually harbors a different mutation (private mutant allele). In half of cases of hemophilia A, the disease can be traced through many generations, but in the other half, de novo mutations occurring within two generations are the cause of this bleeding diathesis. In most of these de novo mutations, an origin in the mother, maternal grandfather, or maternal grandmother has been identified.

Pathology and Clinical Features: Patients with hemophilia A exhibit a mild, moderate, or severe bleeding tendency. In most of these patients, the severity of the illness parallels the amount of factor VIII activity in the blood. Half of patients have virtually no factor VIII activity and often suffer spontaneous bleeding. A third of patients, who have up to 10 units of factor VIII per deciliter, have spontaneous bleeding only occasionally, but hemorrhages are common after minor trauma. One fifth of hemophiliacs have more than 10 U/dL and bleed only after significant trauma or surgery.

The most frequent complication of hemophilia A is a deforming arthritis caused by repeated bleeding into many joints. Although uncommon, bleeding into the brain was formerly the most frequent cause of death in hemophiliacs. Hematuria, intestinal obstruction, and respiratory obstruction may all occur with bleeding into the respective organs.

Treatment with factor VIII transfusions to maintain the levels of this clotting factor generally control the bleeding diathesis. Unfortunately, many of these patients developed acquired immunodeficiency syndrome (AIDS) and viral hepatitis as a result of contamination of pooled factor VIII preparations. These complications have been virtually eliminated by screening blood donors and heat treatment to inactivate the HIV in the purified factor VIII product. The availability of human recombinant factor VIII now avoids all infectious complications. Screening of women to detect carriers and prenatal diagnosis of affected fetuses by the use of DNA markers are highly accurate.

Fragile X Syndrome

Fragile X syndrome is the most common form of inherited mental retardation and is caused by expansion of a CGG repeat at the Xq27 fragile site. It is second only to Down syndrome as an identifiable cause of mental retardation. The disease afflicts 1 in 1250 males and 1 in 2500 females.

Pathogenesis: The well-known fact that more males than females are institutionalized for mental retardation was traditionally ascribed to societal factors. However, it was recognized in the early 1970s that X-linked inheritance of mental retardation accounted for most of this excess of males. Whereas fully 20% of all cases of heritable mental retardation are X-linked disorders, one fifth of these are associated with a single genetic defect, namely, an inducible fragile site on the X chromosome (Xq27).

A fragile site represents a specific locus, or band, on a chromosome that breaks easily. It is usually detected in cytogenetic preparations as a nonstaining gap or constriction (Fig. 6-39). Importantly, under the routine conditions of preparing cells for karyotypic analysis, most fragile sites are not detected. However, when the same cells in culture are subjected to treatment that impairs DNA synthesis (e.g., methotrexate, floxuridine), fragile sites are revealed. At least 11, and possibly as many as 50, fragile sites occur in the genomes of most persons, both on autosomes and on the X chromosome. **However, the locus at Xq27 is associated with mental retardation and other clinical findings that characterize fragile X syndrome.** As discussed, the fragile site at the Xq27 locus represents a distinct kind of mutation characterized by amplification of a CGG repeat.

Within fragile X families, the probability of being affected with the disorder is related to the position in the pedigree; that is, later generations are more likely to be affected than earlier ones *(Sherman paradox or genetic anticipation)*. This phenomenon relates to the progressive nature of the triplet repeat expansion. Chromosomes containing more than about 52 repeats can undergo an increase in the number of repeats—so-called expansion. Small expansions can increase, particularly during meiosis in females, leading to larger expansions in successive generations. These are known as *premutations*, and subjects with these small expansions are asymptomatic. Expansions with more than 200 repeats are associated with mental retardation and represent full mutations. Expansion of a premutation to a full mutation during gametogenesis takes place only in females. Thus, the daughters of men with premutations (carriers) are never

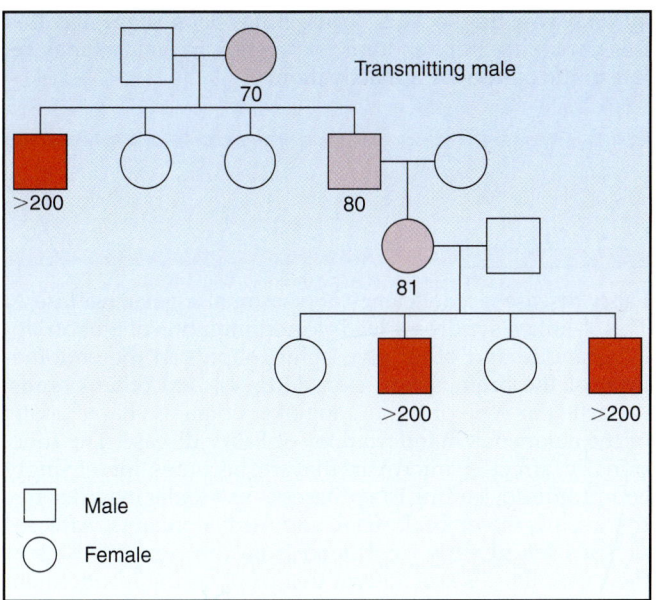

FIGURE 6-40
Inheritance pattern of fragile X syndrome. The number of copies of the trinucleotide repeat (CGG) is shown below selected members in this pedigree. Expansion occurs primarily during meiosis in females. When the number of repeats exceeds ~200, the clinical syndrome is manifested. Individuals shaded pink carry a premutation and are asymptomatic.

clinically symptomatic, whereas the sisters of the transmitting males occasionally produce affected daughters. However, the daughters of carrier males always harbor the premutation. The frequency of conversion of a premutation to a full mutation in such women (i.e., the probability of their sons suffering fragile X syndrome) varies with the length of the expanded tract. Premutations with more than 90 repeats are almost always converted to full mutations. In view of the recessive nature of fragile X syndrome, most of the daughters of carrier males transmit mental retardation to 50% of their sons. These considerations explain the greater risk of the disorder in succeeding generations of fragile X families (Fig. 6-40).

 Clinical Features: The male newborn afflicted with the fragile X syndrome appears normal, but during childhood, characteristic features appear, including an increased head circumference, facial coarsening, joint hyperextensibility, enlarged testes, and abnormalities of the cardiac valves. Mental retardation is profound, with IQ scores varying from 20 to 60. **Interestingly, a significant proportion of autistic male children carry a fragile X chromosome.** Among female carriers who are mentally handicapped, the severity of the impairment varies from a learning disability with normal IQ to serious retardation.

Only 80% of males who exhibit the Xq27 fragile site are mentally retarded; the remaining 20% are clinically normal but can transmit the trait. Among females who are known to bear a fragile X chromosome (obligate carriers), two thirds are intellectually normal, and the fragile site on the X chromosome cannot be demonstrated. By contrast, of the one third of female carriers who are mentally retarded, virtually

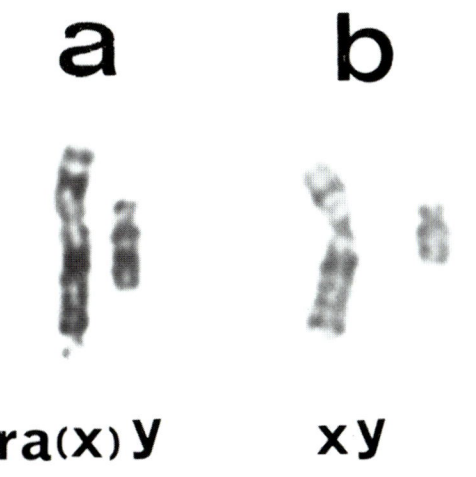

FIGURE 6-39
Fragile X chromosome.

all display a fragile Xq27 locus. It has been suggested that this variability in phenotypic expression in females may relate to the pattern of X inactivation.

Fabry Disease

Fabry disease is a deficiency of lysosomal α-galactosidase A. This X-linked syndrome leads to accumulation of globotriaosylceramide and other glycosphingolipids in the endothelium of the brain, heart, skin, kidneys, and other organs. A particular type of tumor, angiokeratoma, is characteristic of the cutaneous manifestations of Fabry disease. The functionally affected microvasculature becomes increasingly compromised, leading to a progressive vascular insufficiency that results in cerebral, renal, and cardiac infarcts. Affected persons die in early adulthood from the complications of their vascular disease. Recent treatments using recombinant α-D-galactosidase A show promise in arresting the progress of this disease.

MITOCHONDRIAL DISEASES

Mitochondrial proteins are encoded by both the nuclear and mitochondrial genomes. In particular, most respiratory chain proteins are encoded by nuclear genes, whereas several are the products of the mitochondrial genome. A few rare, autosomal recessive (mendelian) disorders that represent defects in nuclear encoded mitochondrial proteins have been described. However, most inherited defects in mitochondrial function result from mutations in the mitochondrial genome itself. An appreciation of these conditions requires an understanding of the unique genetics of the mitochondria. These features include the following:

- **Maternal inheritance:** All vertebrate mitochondria are inherited from the mother via the ovum, which possesses up to 300,000 copies of mitochondrial DNA (mtDNA).
- **Variability of mtDNA copies:** The number of mitochondria and the number of copies of mtDNA per mitochondrion vary in different tissues. Each mitochondrion contains 2 to 10 mtDNA copies, and the need of various cell types for ATP correlates with the DNA content per mitochondrion.
- **Threshold effect:** Since any given cell contains numerous mitochondria and, therefore, hundreds or thousands of mtDNA copies, mutations in mtDNA lead to mixed populations of mutant and normal mitochondrial genomes. This situation is called *heteroplasmy*. The phenotype associated with mtDNA mutations reflects the severity of the mutation, the proportion of mutant genomes, and the demand of the tissue for ATP. In this context, different tissues require different minimum rates (or thresholds) of ATP production to sustain their characteristic metabolic activity; the brain, heart, and skeletal muscle have particularly great energy demands.
- **High mutation rate:** The rate of mutation of mtDNA is considerably higher than that of nuclear DNA, owing (at least in part) to less DNA repair capacity.

Diseases caused by mutations in the mitochondrial genome principally affect the nervous system, heart, and skeletal muscle. The functional deficits in all of these disorders can be traced to inadequate oxidative phosphorylation (OXPHOS). **OXPHOS diseases** have been divided into the following classes: I, nuclear mutations; II, mtDNA point mutations; III, mtDNA deletions; and IV, as yet undefined defects.

All inherited mitochondrial diseases are rare and have variable clinical presentations based on the considerations discussed above. The first human disease caused by an mtDNA point mutation was **Leber hereditary optic neuropathy,** a condition characterized by progressive loss of vision. Since that time, various mitochondrial myopathies and encephalomyopathies have been described; they are discussed in Chapter 27. Hypertrophic cardiomyopathy (see Chapter 11) is also a common manifestation of OXPHOS diseases.

GENETIC IMPRINTING

Genetic imprinting refers to the observation that the phenotype associated with some genes differs depending on whether the allele is inherited from the mother or the father. This phenomenon implies that in the case of imprinted genes, either the maternal or paternal allele is maintained in an inactive state. This normal physiological process results from DNA methylation of cytosine residues in regulatory elements in the imprinted allele. The nonimprinted allele provides the biological function of the genetic locus. If the nonimprinted allele then becomes disrupted through mutation, the imprinted allele cannot compensate for the missing biological function. Imprinting occurs in meiosis during gametogenesis, and the pattern of imprinting is maintained to variable degrees in different tissues. It is reset during meiosis in the next generation, so the selection of a given allele for imprinting can vary from one generation to the next.

In the extreme case, it has been demonstrated experimentally that mammalian embryos in which both sets of chromosomes are derived exclusively from one parent, either the mother or the father, never survive to term. A less severe manifestation of genetic imprinting is seen in *uniparental disomy,* in which both members of a single chromosome pair have been inherited from the same parent. The pair of chromosomes may be copies of one parental chromosome (uniparental isodisomy) or may be the same pair found in one parent (uniparental heterodisomy). Uniparental disomy is a rare anomaly but has been implicated in unexpected patterns of inheritance of genetic traits. For instance, a child with uniparental isodisomy may manifest a recessive disease when only one parent carries the trait, as has been observed in a few cases of cystic fibrosis and hemophilia A. Loss of a chromosome from a trisomy or duplication of a chromosome in the case of a monosomy can lead to uniparental disomy. Interestingly, as many as 1% of viable pregnancies carry uniparental disomy for at least one chromosome.

Genetic imprinting is well illustrated by certain hereditary diseases whose phenotype is determined by the parental source of the mutant allele. Deletion of the 15q11-13 chromosomal locus results in **Prader-Willi syndrome** when the affected chromosome is inherited maternally and in **Angelman syndrome** when it is of paternal origin. The phenotypes of these disorders are remarkably different. Prader-Willi syndrome features hypotonia, obesity, hypogonadism, mental retardation, and a specific facies. By contrast, Angelman syndrome patients are hyperactive, display inappropriate laughter, have a facies different from that of Prader-Willi syndrome, and suffer from seizures. The explanation for Prader-Willi syndrome lies in the imprinting (silencing) of the maternal gene(s) on chromosome 15 and the deletion of the same region on the paternal chromosome. The converse situation obtains in Angelman syndrome, in which the paternal gene is imprinted and the other one is deleted. This pattern is similar to loss of heterozygosity in tumor-suppressor genes by aberrant methylation in some cases of cancer (see Chapter 5). The gene that is responsible for Angelman syndrome appears to be *UBE3A*. The gene(s) responsible for Prader-Willi syndrome have not been definitively identified.

Genetic imprinting is implicated in a number of other situations relevant to human disease. For example, in some childhood cancers, including Wilms tumor, osteosarcoma, bilateral retinoblastoma, and embryonal rhabdomyosarcoma, the maternal allele of a putative tumor-suppressor gene is lost, and the remaining allele is on a chromosome of paternal origin. In the case of familial glomus tumor, an adult neoplasm, both males and females may carry the trait, but it is transmitted only through the male. Thus, the responsible gene is active only when it is located on the paternal autosome. Finally, as noted above, the premutation of fragile X syndrome is expanded to the full mutation only during female gametogenesis, implying that the trinucleotide repeat is treated differently on passage through the female than in the male.

MULTIFACTORIAL INHERITANCE

Multifactorial inheritance is a term that describes a process by which a disease results from the additive effects of a number of abnormal genes and environmental factors. Most normal human traits are inherited neither as dominant nor as recessive mendelian attributes but rather in a more complex manner. For example, multifactorial inheritance determines intelligence, height, skin color, body habitus, and even emotional disposition. Similarly, most of the common chronic disorders of adults represent multifactorial genetic diseases and are well known to "run in families." Such maladies include diabetes, atherosclerosis, and many forms of cancer and arthritis, and hypertension. The inheritance of a number of birth defects is also multifactorial (e.g., cleft lip and palate, pyloric stenosis, and congenital heart disease) (Table 6-11).

The concept of multifactorial inheritance is based on the notion that multiple genes interact with various environmental factors to produce disease in an individual patient. Such inheritance leads to familial aggregation that does not obey simple mendelian rules. As a consequence, the inheritance of polygenic diseases is studied by the methods of population genetics, rather than by the analysis of individual family pedigrees.

The number of involved genes is not known for any polygenic disease. Thus, it is not possible to ascertain accurately the risk of a particular disorder in an individual case. The probability of disease can only be predicted from the number of relatives affected and the severity of their disease, supplemented by statistical projections based on population analyses. Whereas monogenic inheritance implies a specific

TABLE 6-11 Representative Diseases Associated with Multifactorial Inheritance

Adults	Children
Hypertension	Pyloric stenosis
Atherosclerosis	Cleft lip and palate
Diabetes, type II	Congenital heart disease
Allergic diathesis	Meningomyelocele
Psoriasis	Anencephaly
Schizophrenia	Hypospadias
Ankylosing spondylitis	Congenital hip dislocation
Gout	Hirschprung disease

risk of disease (e.g., 25 or 50%), the probability of symptoms in first-degree relatives of a person affected with a polygenic disease is usually on the order of 5 to 10%.

The biological basis of polygenic inheritance rests on the evidence that more than one fourth of all genetic loci in normal humans contain polymorphic alleles. Such genetic heterogeneity provides a background for the wide variability in the susceptibility to many diseases, which is compounded by a multiplicity of interactions with environmental factors.

- **The expression of symptoms is proportional to the number of mutant genes.** Close relatives of an affected person have more mutant genes than the population at large and have a greater chance of expressing clinical disease. The probability of expressing the same number of mutant genes is highest in identical twins.
- **Environmental factors influence the expression of the trait.** Thus, concordance for the disease may occur in only one third of monozygotic twins.
- **The risk in first-degree relatives (parents, siblings, children) is the same (5–10%).** The probability of disease is considerably lower in second-degree relatives.
- **The probability of expression in later offspring is influenced by expression of the trait in earlier siblings.** If one or more children are born with a multifactorial defect, the chance for recurrence in subsequent offspring is doubled. This contrasts with mendelian traits, in which the probability is independent of the number of affected siblings.
- **The more severe the defect, the greater the risk of transmitting it to offspring.** Patients with more-severe polygenic defects presumably have more mutant genes, and their children thus have a greater chance of inheriting the abnormal genes than the offspring of less severely affected persons.
- **Some abnormalities characterized by multifactorial inheritance show a sex predilection.** For example, pyloric stenosis is more common in male infants, whereas congenital dislocation of the hip is more common in females. Such differential susceptibility is believed to represent a difference in the threshold for the expression of mutant genes in the two sexes. For example, if the number of mutant genes required to produce pyloric stenosis in males is A, it may require 4A in the female. In such a circumstance, a woman who had pyloric stenosis as an infant has more mutant genes than a similarly afflicted man to transmit to her children. Indeed, the son of such a woman actually has a 25% chance of being born with

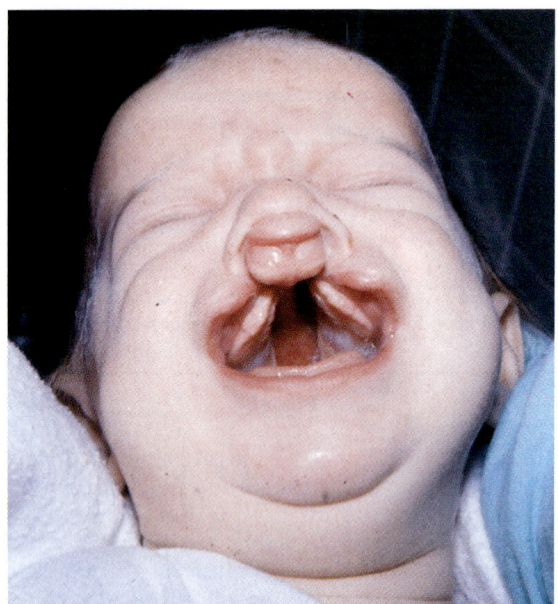

FIGURE 6-41
Cleft lip and palate in an infant.

pyloric stenosis, compared with a 4% risk for the son of an affected man. **As a general rule, if there is an altered sex ratio in the incidence of a polygenic defect, a member of the less commonly affected sex has a much greater probability of transmitting the defect.**

Cleft Lip and Cleft Palate Exemplify Multifactorial Inheritance

At the 35th day of gestation, the frontal prominence fuses with the maxillary process to form the upper lip. This process is under the control of many genes, and disturbances in gene expression (hereditary or environmental) at this time lead to interference with proper fusion and result in cleft lip, with or without cleft palate (Fig. 6-41). This anomaly may also be part of a systemic malformation syndrome caused by teratogens (rubella, anticonvulsants) and is often encountered in children with chromosomal abnormalities.

The incidence of cleft lip, with or without cleft palate, is 1 in 1000, and the incidence of cleft palate alone is 1 in 2500. If one child is born with a cleft lip, the chances are 4% that the second child will exhibit the same defect. If the first two children are affected, the risk of cleft lip increases to 9% for the third child. The more severe the anatomical defect, the greater the probability of transmitting cleft lip will be. Whereas 75% of cases of cleft lip occur in boys, the sons of women with cleft lip have a four times higher risk of acquiring the defect than the sons of affected fathers.

SCREENING FOR CARRIERS OF GENETIC DISORDERS

Until recently, screening for carriers of genetic diseases has not been a common undertaking. Among the Ashkenazi Jewish population, screening to identify carriers of Tay-Sachs disease, an autosomal recessive disease, has been performed because of the relatively high frequency of the disease within that group. A number of other inherited conditions are also included in a so-called "Ashkenazi screen." The objective of such screening is to identify couples in which both members are heterozygous carriers and who therefore have a 25% risk of having an affected offspring with each pregnancy. These couples can be offered prenatal diagnosis to determine the genetic status of the fetus. In vitro fertilization combined with preimplantation genetic diagnosis is available in some centers to ensure that an implanted embryo will not have this disease.

Recently, prenatal screening for carriers of CF has been recommended by national professional organizations. This represents the first large-scale adoption of testing for carriers of genetic diseases. Guidelines recommend that screening for CF be offered to all white and Ashkenazi Jewish women because of the relatively high frequency of CF in these groups. A panel of 25 CF mutations has been chosen for this DNA-based testing. If a woman is a carrier of a CF mutation, then her partner should be tested to determine if the couple is at risk of having an affected offspring. Because of the distribution of CF mutations, the recommended panel will detect only about 80% of known CF mutations in whites, but over 97% among Ashkenazi Jews. Among other ethnic groups, the detection rates are lower.

PRENATAL DIAGNOSIS OF GENETIC DISORDERS

Amniocentesis and chorionic villus biopsy are the most important methods for diagnosis of a developmental or genetic disorder. Both procedures are safe, reliable, and easily performed. The indications for chorionic villus biopsy or amniocentesis in pregnant women are as follows:

- **Age 35 years old and over:** The risk of having a child with Down syndrome is about 1 in 300 for a 40-year-old woman, compared with 1 in 1200 at age 25. This risk rises even higher with advanced maternal age.
- **Previous chromosomal abnormality:** The overall risk of recurrence of Down syndrome in a succeeding child of a woman who has already borne an infant with trisomy 21 is 1%.
- **Translocation carrier:** Estimates of risks to the offspring of translocation carriers vary from 3 to 15%. Carriers of balanced translocations are at increased risk for producing children with unbalanced karyotypes and resulting phenotypic abnormalities.
- **History of familial inborn error of metabolism:** The recessive inborn errors of metabolism have a risk of 25% for each child if each parent is heterozygous for the trait. Prenatal diagnosis can identify disorders for which a definitive biochemical diagnosis can be made.
- **Identified heterozygotes:** Carrier detection programs, such as the Tay-Sachs Disease Prevention Program, identify couples in which both spouses are carriers of the same recessive gene. Each pregnancy in such couples has a 25% risk of an affected child, and prenatal diagnosis can be made routinely.
- **Family history of X-linked disorders:** Fetal sex determination, using amniotic cells, can be offered to women known to be carriers of X-linked disorders. The diagno-

sis of some of these conditions can be established biochemically by amniotic fluid analysis.

New molecular techniques for carrier detection and early prenatal diagnosis are of ever-increasing utility. Gene-specific DNA probes have been developed for many genetic diseases, including hemophilia A and B, the hemoglobinopathies, phenylketonuria, and α_1-antitrypsin deficiency. Most heterozygous carriers for Duchenne and Becker muscular dystrophies, Huntington chorea, and CF can be identified by such techniques.

DISEASES OF INFANCY AND CHILDHOOD

The period from birth to puberty has been traditionally subdivided into several stages.

- Neonatal age (the first 4 weeks)
- Infancy (the first year)
- Early childhood (1 to 4 years)
- Late childhood (5 to 14 years)

Each of these periods has its own distinct anatomical, physiological, and immunological characteristics, which determine the nature and form of various pathological processes. Morbidity and mortality rates in the neonatal period differ considerably from those in infancy and childhood. Infants and children are not simply "small adults," and they may be afflicted by diseases unique to their particular age group.

PREMATURITY AND INTRAUTERINE GROWTH RETARDATION

The duration of human pregnancy is normally 40 ± 2 weeks, and most newborns weigh 3300 ± 600 g. Prematurity has been defined by the World Health Organization as a gestational age of less than 37 weeks (from the first day of the last menstrual period). The traditional definition of prematurity was a birth weight below 2500 g, regardless of gestational age. However, it is now appreciated that full-term infants may weigh less than 2500 g because of intrauterine growth retardation rather than premature birth. **Thus, low-birth-weight infants (>2500 g) are classed as (1) appropriate for gestational age (AGA) or (2) small for gestational age (SGA).**

In the United States, the frequency of low-birth-weight infants is less than 6% among whites, and two thirds of these infants are premature (AGA). By contrast, when the frequency of low-birth-weight infants exceeds 10%, as it does for blacks (>12%), most of these newborns suffer from intrauterine growth retardation and are considered SGA.

About 1% of all infants born in the United States weigh less than 1500 g and are referred to as **very-low-birth-weight infants**. Such babies account for half of all neonatal deaths, and their survival is determined by their birth weight. Historically, newborns weighing more than 1250 g had a 90% survival rate, whereas 2% of those weighing between 500 g and 600 g could be expected to live. Today, in advanced societies in which premature newborns are cared for in neonatal intensive care units, 90% of infants over 750 g survive. Between 500 g and 750 g, 45% survive, of whom more than half develop normally.

- **Etiology:** The factors that predispose to the premature birth of an infant (AGA) are (1) maternal illness, (2) uterine incompetence, (3) fetal disorders, and (4) placental abnormalities. When the life of a fetus is threatened by such conditions, it may be necessary to induce premature delivery to salvage the infant. In a substantial proportion of AGA infants, the cause of premature birth is unknown. Intrauterine growth retardation and the resulting birth of SGA infants are associated with disorders that (1) impair maternal health and nutrition, (2) interfere with placental circulation or function, or (3) disturb the growth or development of the fetus.

 Clinical Features: There is a substantial overlap between the complications of prematurity itself (AGA) and intrauterine growth retardation (SGA). However, certain general principles apply. Prematurity is often associated with severe respiratory distress, metabolic disturbances (e.g., hyperbilirubinemia, hypoglycemia, hypocalcemia), circulatory problems (anemia, hypothermia, hypotension), and bacterial sepsis. By contrast, SGA infants make up a much more heterogeneous group, including many infants with congenital anomalies and infections acquired in utero. Even when these causes of intrauterine growth retardation are excluded, the neonatal complications of SGA infants reflect gestational age more than birth weight. In addition to many of the problems associated with prematurity, SGA infants often suffer from perinatal asphyxia, meconium aspiration, necrotizing enterocolitis, pulmonary hemorrhage, and disorders related to birth defects or inherited metabolic diseases.

Organ Immaturity is a Cause of Neonatal Problems

The maturity of the newborn can be defined in both anatomical and physiological terms. The maturing organs differ morphologically from those in term infants, although complete morphological and physiological maturity of many organs is not achieved for periods varying from days (lungs) to years (brain).

THE LUNGS: Immaturity of the lungs poses one of the most common and immediate threats to the viability of the low-birth-weight infant. The lining cells of the fetal alveoli do not differentiate into type I and type II pneumocytes until late pregnancy. The amniotic fluid, which fills the fetal alveoli, drains from the lungs at birth, after which air expands the respiratory spaces. Often the sluggish respiratory movements of the immature infant do not suffice to evacuate the amniotic fluid from the lungs. As a result, such newborns die of respiratory failure with incompletely expanded lungs. On gross examination, the lungs are not crepitant, and microscopically, the alveoli are variably expanded. The air passages contain desquamated squamous cells *(squames)* and lanugo hair from the fetal skin and protein-rich amniotic fluid (Fig. 6-42). Although this appearance is often termed *amniotic fluid aspiration,* it actually represents retained amniotic fluid.

Alveoli are maintained in the expanded state not only by connective tissue but also by the reduction in surface tension achieved by the presence of **pulmonary surfactant**. This material, which is produced by type II pneumocytes, is a complex mixture of several phospholipids, 75% phosphatidylcholine (lecithin) and 10% phosphatidylglycerol. The composition of lung surfactant changes as the fetus matures: (1) The concentration of lecithin increases rapidly at the beginning of the third trimester and thereafter rises rapidly to reach a peak near term (Fig. 6-43). (2) Whereas most of the lecithin in the mature lung is dipalmitate, in the immature lung it is the less-surface-active α-palmitate, β-myristate species. (3) Phosphatidylglycerol is not present in the lungs before the 36th week of pregnancy. (4) Before the 35th week, the immature surfactant contains a higher proportion of sphingomyelin than adult surfactant.

Pulmonary surfactant is released into the amniotic fluid, which can be sampled by amniocentesis to assess the maturity of the fetal lung. A lecithin-to-sphingomyelin ratio above 2:1 implies that the fetus will survive without developing the respiratory distress syndrome. After the 35th week, the appearance of phosphatidylglycerol in the amniotic fluid is the best proof of the maturity of the fetal lungs.

THE LIVER: The liver of premature infants is morphologically similar to that of the adult organ, with the exception

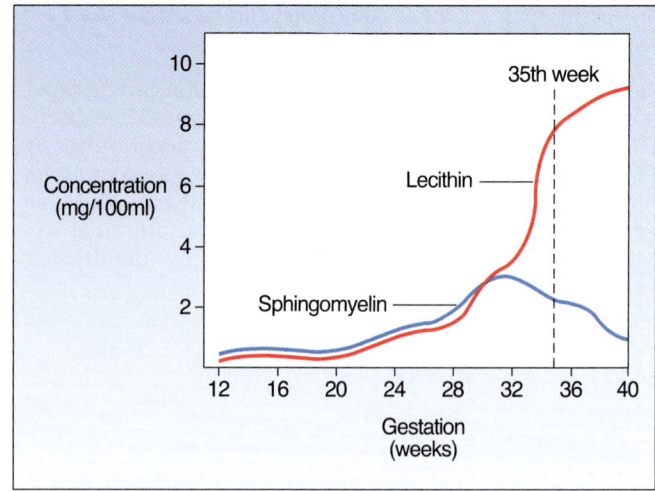

FIGURE 6-43
Changes in amniotic fluid composition during pregnancy.

of conspicuous extramedullary hematopoiesis. However, the hepatocytes tend to be functionally immature. The fetal liver is deficient in glucuronyl transferase and the resulting inability of the organ to conjugate bilirubin often leads to neonatal jaundice. This enzyme deficiency is aggravated by the rapid destruction of fetal erythrocytes, a process that results in an increased supply of bilirubin.

THE BRAIN: Although the brain of the immature newborn differs from that of the adult, both morphologically and functionally, this difference is rarely fatal. On the other hand, the incomplete development of the central nervous system is often reflected in poor vasomotor control, hypothermia, feeding difficulties, and recurrent apnea.

The Apgar Score

Clinical assessments of neonatal maturity are usually performed 1 minute and 5 minutes after delivery, and certain parameters are scored according to the criteria recommended by Virginia Apgar (Table 6-12). In general, the higher the Apgar score, the better the clinical condition of the infant. The score taken at 1 minute is an index of asphyxia and of the need for assisted ventilation. The 5-minute score is a more accurate indication of impending death or the likelihood of persistent neurological damage. For example, in newborns weighing less than 2000 g who have a 5-minute Apgar score of 9 or 10, the mortality during the first month is less than 5%; it is almost 80% when the Apgar score is reduced to 3 or less.

Respiratory Distress Syndrome (RDS) of the Newborn Reflects a Deficiency of Surfactant

RDS is principally associated with prematurity. It is the leading cause of morbidity and mortality among premature in-

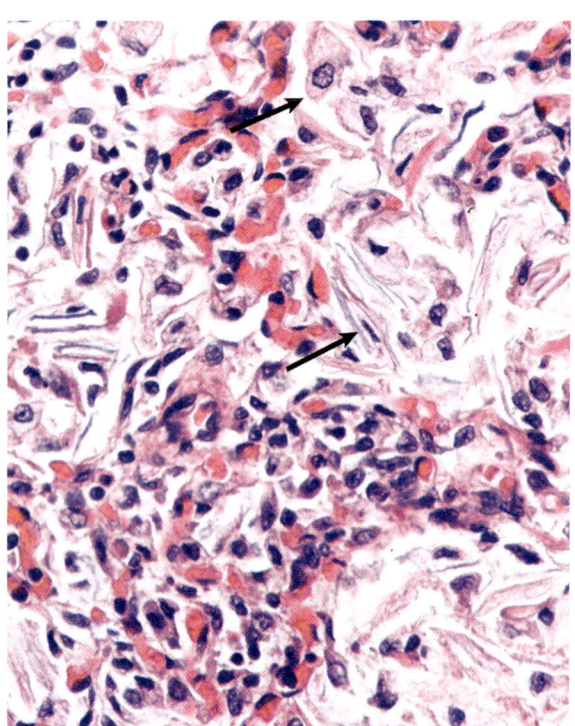

FIGURE 6-42
Retention of amniotic fluid in the lung of a premature newborn. The incompletely expanded lung contains squames *(arrows),* consisting of squamous epithelial cells shed into the amniotic fluid from the fetal skin.

TABLE 6-12 Apgar Score

Sign	0	1	2
Heart rate	Not detectable	Below 100/min	Over 100/min
Respiratory effort	None	Slow, irregular	Good, crying
Muscle tone	Poor	Some flexion of extremities	Active motion
Response to catheter in nostril	No response	Grimace	Cough or sneeze
Color	Blue, pale	Body pink, extremities blue	Completely pink

Sixty seconds after the completion of birth, these five objective signs are evaluated, and each is given a score of 0, 1, or 2. A maximum score of 10 is assigned to infants in the best possible condition.

fants and accounts for half of all neonatal deaths in the United States. The incidence of RDS varies inversely with gestational age and birth weight. Thus, more than half of newborns younger than 28 weeks gestational age are afflicted with RDS, whereas only one fifth of infants between 32 and 36 weeks are affected. In addition to prematurity, other risk factors for RDS include (1) neonatal asphyxia, (2) maternal diabetes, (3) delivery by cesarean section, (4) precipitous delivery, and (5) twin pregnancies.

 Pathogenesis: **The pathogenesis of RDS of the newborn is intimately linked to a deficiency of surfactant** (Fig. 6-44). In the normal newborn, the onset of breathing is associated with a massive release of stored surfactant. This material lowers the surface tension of the alveoli at low lung volumes and thereby prevents collapse (atelectasis) of the alveoli during expiration. As noted above, the immature lung is deficient in both the amount and composition of surfactant. Moreover, any damage to type II pneumocytes (e.g., from asphyxia) will interfere with the synthesis and secretion of surfactant. Atelectasis secondary to surfactant deficiency results in perfused but not ventilated alveoli, a situation that leads to hypoxia and acidosis, with further compromise in the ability of type II pneumocytes to produce surfactant. Moreover, hypoxia produces pulmonary arterial vasoconstriction, thereby increasing right-to-left shunting through the ductus arteriosus and foramen ovale and within the lung itself. The resulting pulmonary ischemia further aggravates alveolar epithelial damage and injures the endothelium of the pulmonary capillaries. The leak of protein-rich fluid into the alveoli from the injured vascular bed contributes to the typical clinical and pathological features of RDS.

 Pathology: On gross examination, the lungs are dark red and airless. Microscopically, the alveoli are collapsed, and the alveolar ducts and respiratory bronchioles are dilated. Within these expanded spaces,

FIGURE 6-44
Pathogenesis of the respiratory distress syndrome of the neonate. Immaturity of the lungs and perinatal asphyxia are the major pathogenetic factors.

Developmental and Genetic Diseases

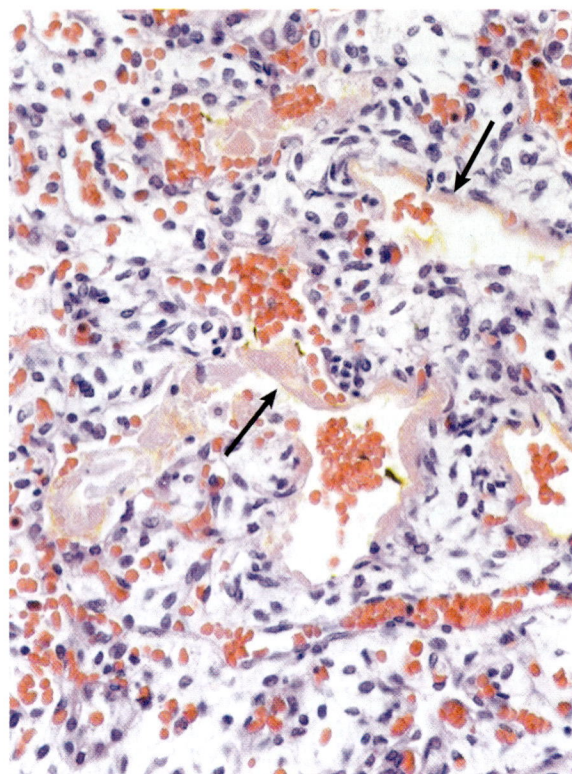

FIGURE 6-45
The lung in respiratory distress syndrome of the neonate. The alveoli are atelectatic, and a dilated alveolar duct is lined by a fibrin-rich hyaline membrane *(arrows)*.

cellular debris, proteinaceous edema fluid, and erythrocytes are evident. The alveolar ducts are lined by conspicuous, eosinophilic, fibrin-rich, amorphous structures, termed *hyaline membranes*, which accounts for the original designation of RDS as *hyaline membrane disease* (Fig. 6-45). The walls of the collapsed alveoli are thick, the capillaries are congested, and the lymphatics are filled with proteinaceous material.

Clinical Features: Most newborns destined to develop RDS appear normal at birth and have high Apgar scores. However, some of these infants have required resuscitation because of intrapartum asphyxia. The first symptom, usually appearing within an hour of birth, is increased respiratory effort, with forceful intercostal retraction and the use of accessory neck muscles. The respiratory rate increases to more than 100 breaths per minute, and cyanosis becomes apparent. The chest radiograph shows a characteristic "ground-glass" granularity, and in terminal stages the fluid-filled alveoli appear as complete "white out" of the lungs. In severe cases, the infant becomes progressively obtunded and flaccid. Long periods of apnea ensue, and the infant eventually dies of asphyxia. Despite advances in neonatal intensive care, the overall mortality of RDS is about 15%, and one third of infants born before 30 weeks of gestational age die of this disorder. In milder cases, the disorder peaks within 3 days, after which gradual improvement takes place.

The major complications of RDS relate to anoxia and acidosis and include the following:

- **Intraventricular cerebral hemorrhage:** The periventricular germinal matrix in the newborn brain is particularly vulnerable to hemorrhage because the dilated, thin-walled veins in this area rupture easily (Fig. 6-46). The pathogenesis of this complication is not fully understood but is believed to reflect anoxic injury to the periventricular capillaries, venous sludging and thrombosis, and impaired vascular autoregulation.
- **Persistence of the patent ductus arteriosus:** In almost one third of newborns who survive RDS, the ductus arteriosus remains patent. With recovery from the pulmonary disease, the pressure in the pulmonary circulation declines, and the higher pressure in the aorta reverses the direction of blood flow in the ductus, thereby creating a persistent left-to-right shunt. Congestive heart failure often ensues and requires correction of the patent ductus.
- **Necrotizing enterocolitis:** This intestinal complication of RDS is the most common acquired gastrointestinal emergency in newborns and is thought to be related to ischemia of the intestinal mucosa. This injury is followed by bacterial colonization, usually with *Clostridium difficile*. The lesions vary from those of typical pseudomembranous enterocolitis to gangrene and perforation of the bowel.
- **Bronchopulmonary dysplasia:** This late complication of RDS usually occurs in infants who weigh less than 1500 g and were maintained on a positive-pressure respirator with high oxygen tensions. It is thought that the disorder results from oxygen toxicity superimposed on RDS. In such patients, respiratory distress persists after the third or fourth day and is reflected in hypoxia, acidosis, oxygen dependency, and the onset of right-sided heart failure. Radiographs of the lungs show a change from almost complete opacification to a spongelike appearance, characterized by small lucent areas alternating with denser foci. Microscopic examination of the lungs reveals hyperplasia of the bronchiolar epithelium and

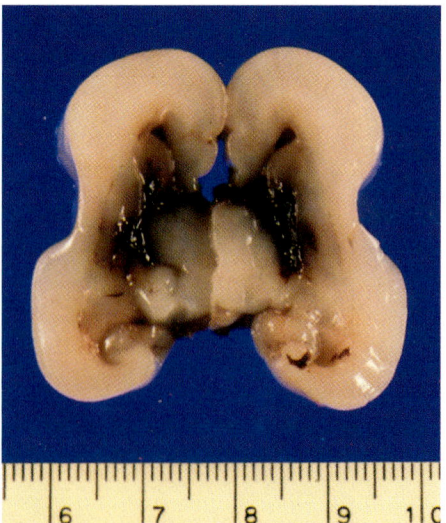

FIGURE 6-46
Intraventricular hemorrhage in a premature infant suffering from respiratory distress syndrome of the neonate.

squamous metaplasia in the bronchi and bronchioles. Atelectasis, interstitial edema, and thickening of the alveolar basement membranes are noted. Most surviving infants eventually recover normal pulmonary function, but right-sided heart failure and viral necrotizing bronchiolitis pose threats to a favorable outcome.

Erythroblastosis Fetalis Is a Hemolytic Disease Caused by Maternal Antibodies against Fetal Erythrocytes

The disorder was first recognized by Hippocrates but was not fully understood until 1940, when the Rh (Rhesus) antigen on erythrocytes was identified. More than 60 antigens on the surface of erythrocytes can elicit an antibody response, but only the D antigen of the Rh group and the ABO system are associated with a significant incidence of hemolytic disease.

Rh Incompatibility

The distribution of Rh antigens among ethnic groups varies. In American whites, 15% are Rh negative (Rh D–), whereas only 8% of blacks are Rh D–. Japanese, Chinese, and Native American Indian populations contain essentially no Rh D–persons. By contrast, in the Basque population, among whom the mutation that causes the Rh D–phenotype may have arisen, the prevalence of Rh D–persons is 35%.

Pathogenesis: The Rh blood group system consists of some 25 components, of which only the alleles cde/CDE need be considered in this discussion. Among infants with erythroblastosis fetalis caused by Rh incompatibility, 90% are due to antibodies against D, with the remaining cases involving C or E. The introduction of Rh-positive fetal erythrocytes (>1 mL) into the circulation of an Rh-negative mother at the time of delivery sensitizes her to the D antigen (Fig. 6-47). Erythroblastosis fetalis does not ordinarily occur during the first pregnancy, because the quantity of fetal blood necessary to sensitize the mother is introduced into her circulation only at the time of delivery, too late to affect the fetus. However, when the sensitized mother again bears an Rh-positive fetus, much smaller quantities of fetal D antigen elicit an increase in antibody titer. In contrast to IgM, IgG antibodies are small enough to cross the placenta and thus produce hemolysis in the fetus. This cycle is exaggerated in multiparous women, and the severity of erythroblastosis tends to increase progressively with each succeeding pregnancy.

Since 15% of white women are Rh D–, and since they have an 85% chance of marrying an Rh D+ man, 13% of all marriages are theoretically at risk for maternal–fetal Rh incompatibility. The actual incidence of erythroblastosis fetalis is, however, much lower. This apparent discrepancy is explained by several factors: (1) More than half of Rh-positive men are heterozygous (D/d), and thus only half of their offspring express the D antigen. (2) Only half of all pregnancies have large enough fetal-to-maternal transfusions to sensitize the mother. (3) Even in those Rh-negative women who are exposed to significant amounts of fetal Rh-positive blood, many do not mount a substantial immune response. Even after multiple pregnancies, only 5% of Rh-negative women are ever delivered of infants with erythroblastosis fetalis.

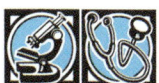

Pathology and Clinical Features: The severity of erythroblastosis fetalis varies from a mild hemolysis to fatal anemia, and the pathological findings are determined by the extent of the hemolytic disease.

- **Death in utero** occurs in the most extreme form of the disease, in which case severe maceration is evident on delivery. Numerous erythroblasts are demonstrable in visceral organs that are not extensively autolyzed.
- **Hydrops fetalis** *refers to the most serious form of erythroblastosis fetalis* (Fig. 6-48) *in liveborn infants and is characterized by severe edema secondary to congestive heart failure caused by the severe anemia.* The infant generally dies, unless adequate exchange transfusions with Rh-negative cells correct the anemia and ameliorate the hemolytic disease. Although the infant is not jaundiced at birth, progressive hyperbilirubinemia develops rapidly. In infants who die, autopsy reveals conspicuous hepatosplenomegaly and bile-stained organs. Microscopically, erythroblastic hyperplasia of the bone marrow and extramedullary hematopoiesis in the liver, spleen, lymph nodes, and other sites are prominent.
- **Kernicterus,** *also termed* **bilirubin encephalopathy,** *is defined as a neurological condition associated with severe jaundice and characterized by bile staining of the brain, particularly of the basal ganglia, pontine nuclei, and dentate nuclei in the cerebellum.* Although brain damage in jaundiced newborns was first mentioned in the 15th century, the association of kernicterus with high levels of unconjugated bilirubin was not appreciated until 1952. Kernicterus (Ger. *kern,* nucleus) is essentially confined to newborns with severe unconjugated hyperbilirubinemia, usually related to erythroblastosis. The bilirubin derived from the destruction of erythrocytes and the catabolism of the released heme is not easily conjugated by the immature liver, which is deficient in glucuronyl transferase.

The development of kernicterus is directly related to the level of unconjugated bilirubin and is rare in term infants when serum bilirubin levels are below 20 mg/dL. Premature infants are more vulnerable to hyperbilirubinemia and may develop kernicterus at levels as low as 12 mg/dL. Bilirubin is thought to injure the cells of the brain by interfering with mitochondrial function. Severe kernicterus leads initially to loss of the startle reflex and athetoid movements, which in 75% progresses to lethargy and death. Most surviving infants have severe choreoathetosis and mental retardation; a minority have varying degrees of intellectual and motor retardation.

PREVENTION AND TREATMENT: Exchange transfusions may keep the maximum serum bilirubin at an acceptable level. However, phototherapy, which converts the toxic

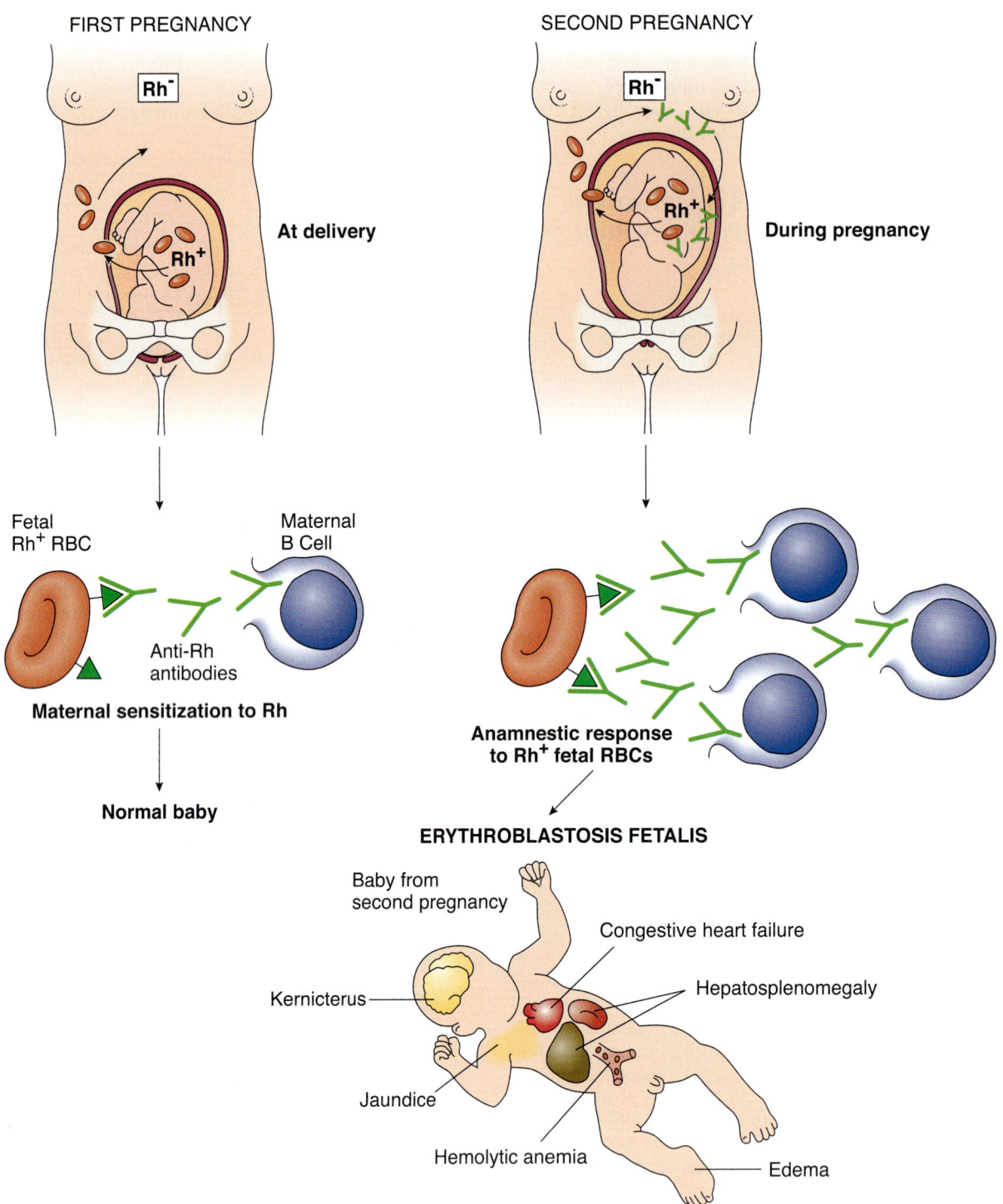

FIGURE 6-47
Pathogenesis of erythroblastosis fetalis due to maternal–fetal Rh incompatibility. Immunization of the Rh-negative mother with Rh-positive erythrocytes in the first pregnancy leads to the formation of anti-Rh antibodies of the IgG type. These antibodies cross the placenta and damage the Rh-positive fetus in subsequent pregnancies.

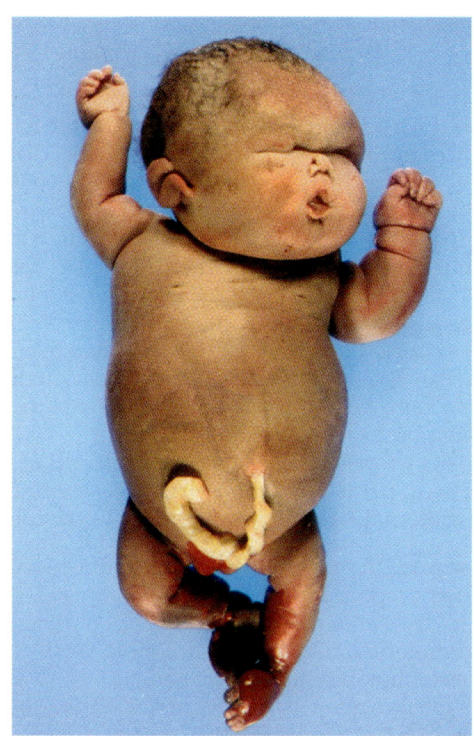

FIGURE 6-48
Hydrops fetalis. The infant shows severe anasarca.

unconjugated bilirubin into isomers that are nontoxic and excreted in the urine, has greatly reduced the need for exchange transfusions.

The incidence of erythroblastosis fetalis secondary to Rh incompatibility has been greatly reduced (to <1% of women at risk) by the use of human anti-D globulin (RhoGAM) within 72 hours of delivery. The quantity of RhoGAM administered to the mother suffices to neutralize 10 mL of antigenic fetal cells that may have entered the maternal circulation during delivery.

ABO Incompatibility

Since the availability of RhoGAM prophylaxis of Rh-negative mothers, the incidence of Rh-incompatible erythroblastosis has drastically decreased, and today ABO incompatibility is the principal cause of hemolytic disease of the newborn. Despite the fact that 25% of pregnancies result in ABO incompatibility between mother and offspring, hemolytic disease develops in only 10% of such children, usually in infants with type A blood. The low antigenicity of the ABO factors in the fetus accounts for the mildness of ABO hemolytic disease. The natural anti-A and anti-B antibodies are IgM, which does not cross the placenta. However, certain incomplete antibodies to A antigen may be IgG, which does cross the placenta. Therefore, ABO isoimmune disease may be seen in firstborn infants. However, most cases of hemolytic anemia from ABO incompatibility are seen after a previous incompatible pregnancy.

Most infants with ABO incompatibility suffer mild disease, and jaundice is the only clinical feature. The complications of erythroblastosis associated with Rh incompatibility are unusual with ABO disease. Nevertheless, kernicterus has occasionally been reported.

Birth Injury Spans the Spectrum from Mechanical Trauma to Anoxic Damage

Some birth injuries relate to poor obstetric manipulation, whereas many are unavoidable sequelae of routine delivery. Birth injuries occur in about 5 per 1000 live births. Factors that predispose to birth injury include cephalopelvic disproportion, dystocia (difficult labor), prematurity, and breech presentation.

Cranial Injury

Caput succedaneum refers to edema of the scalp caused by trauma to the head incurred during the passage through the birth canal. The swelling rapidly disappears and is more a source of parental anxiety than of clinical concern.

Cephalohematoma is defined as a subperiosteal hemorrhage that is confined to a single cranial bone and becomes apparent within the first few hours after birth. It may or may not be associated with a linear fracture of the underlying bone. Most cephalohematomas resolve without complication and require no treatment.

Skull fractures during birth result from the impact of the head on the pelvic bones or pressure from obstetric forceps. Linear fractures, the most common variety, are asymptomatic and do not require any treatment. Depressed fractures are usually caused by trauma from forceps. Although many depressed fractures do not initially produce symptoms, they usually require mechanical elevation because of the risk of underlying cranial trauma from persistent pressure. In contrast to most fractures, those of the occipital bone often extend through the underlying venous sinuses and produce fatal hemorrhage.

Intracranial hemorrhage is one of the most dangerous birth injuries and may be traumatic, secondary to asphyxia, or the result of an underlying bleeding diathesis. Traumatic intracranial hemorrhage occurs in the setting of (1) significant cephalopelvic disproportion, (2) precipitous delivery, (3) breech presentation, (4) prolonged labor, or (5) the inappropriate use of forceps. These traumas can result in **subdural or subarachnoid hemorrhage,** which are commonly secondary to lacerations of the falx cerebri or tentorium cerebelli that involve the vein of Galen or the venous sinuses. As noted above, anoxic injury from asphyxia, particularly in the premature infant, is often associated with intraventricular hemorrhage.

The prognosis for the newborn with intracranial hemorrhage varies with its extent. Massive hemorrhage is often rapidly fatal. If the infant survives, recovery may be complete or the child may be afflicted with chronic neurological residuals, usually in the form of cerebral palsy or hydrocephalus. However, many cases of cerebral palsy have been shown by ultrasound studies to relate to brain damage acquired 2 weeks or more prior to birth rather than from birth trauma.

Peripheral Nerve Injury

Brachial palsy, with varying degrees of paralysis of the upper extremity, is caused by excessive traction on the head and neck or shoulders during delivery. The injury may be permanent if the nerves are severed. Function may return within a few months if the palsy results from edema and hemorrhage.

Phrenic nerve paralysis and associated paralysis of a hemidiaphragm may be associated with brachial palsy and result in breathing difficulties. The condition generally resolves spontaneously within a few months.

Facial nerve palsy usually presents as a unilateral flaccid paralysis of the face caused by injury to the seventh cranial nerve during labor or delivery, especially with forceps. When severe, the entire affected side of the face is paralyzed and even the eyelid cannot be closed. The prognosis again depends on whether the nerve was lacerated or simply injured by pressure.

Fractures

The **clavicle** is more vulnerable to fracture during delivery than any other bone and may be associated with fracture of the **humerus.** Immobilization of the arm and shoulder are almost invariably the only treatment required for complete healing. Fractures of other long bones and the nose occasionally occur during birth but heal easily.

Rupture of the Liver

The only internal organ other than the brain that is injured with any frequency during labor and delivery is the liver. This organ is injured by mechanical pressure during difficult or premature births. Rupture of the liver may lead to the formation of a hematoma large enough to cause a palpable abdominal mass and anemia; surgical repair of the laceration may be required.

Sudden Infant Death Syndrome Does Not Have a Known Cause

The sudden infant death syndrome (SIDS), also known as "crib death," is defined as "the sudden death of an infant or young child which is unexpected by history and in which a thorough postmortem examination fails to demonstrate an adequate cause of death." Although the diagnosis of SIDS is arrived at solely by excluding other specific causes of sudden death, this catastrophe is nevertheless considered a distinct clinicopathological entity. SIDS actually was first described in the American colonies in 1686, but modern attention to the disorder dates only a few decades.

Typically, the victim of SIDS is an apparently healthy young infant who has been asleep without any hint of impending calamity. The infant does not awake spontaneously at the usual time, and when it cannot be aroused, the parent realizes that it has died. Postmortem examination does not disclose a cause of death, such as pneumonia, food aspiration, sepsis, or cerebral hemorrhage. This tragic sequence has aroused great public concern, because it must be separated from homicide, which has been demonstrated in a number of cases to be the true cause of mysterious death in children.

Epidemiology: Beyond the neonatal period, SIDS is the leading cause of death during the first year of life, accounting for more than one third of all deaths in this period. The incidence in the United States is 2 per 1000 live births. Most (90%) cases occur before 6 months of age. Most deaths from SIDS occur during the winter months, but no association between particular respiratory infections and infant death has been established. Most deaths occur at night or during periods associated with sleep. The reported death rates for SIDS have declined dramatically. This has been attributed to the "Back to Sleep" informational campaigns that encourage parents to place infants on their backs for sleeping.

The risk factors for SIDS have been difficult to ascertain and are based principally on retrospective studies. **The strongest maternal risk factors** appear to be the following:

- Low socioeconomic status (limited education, unmarried mother, poor prenatal care)
- Black race
- Age younger than 20 years at first pregnancy
- Cigarette smoking during pregnancy
- Use of illicit drugs during pregnancy

The risk factors for the infant are controversial. The consensus includes the following:

- Low birth weight
- Prematurity
- An illness, often gastrointestinal, within the last 2 weeks before death
- Subsequent siblings of SIDS victims
- Survivors of an apparent life-threatening event, defined as an episode characterized by some combination of apnea, color change, marked alteration in muscle tone, and choking or gagging. A definite cause, such as seizures or aspiration after vomiting, is established in only half the cases of an apparent life-threatening event.

Pathogenesis: The pathogenesis of SIDS remains elusive and controversial, and no clear answers are forthcoming at this time. It is also unclear whether SIDS is a single entity or the common end-point of several different conditions. The most popular hypothesis relates SIDS to a prolonged spell of apnea, followed by cardiac arrhythmia or shock, in sleeping infants who cannot arouse themselves and prevent the process from progressing to a fatal outcome. However, fewer than 10% of parents of SIDS victims report an episode of apnea or an apparent life-threatening event at any time prior to the fatal event. **Thus, while it is possible that sleep apnea contributes to the sequence of events leading to SIDS, available data do not support a strong and predictable relationship between the two conditions.**

Numerous other causes for SIDS have found various champions, but the evidence for any one of these is indeed weak. They include cardiovascular abnormalities triggering fatal arrhythmias, abnormal brainstem sensitivity to respiratory stimuli, gastroesophageal reflux, various types of infections, inborn errors of metabolism, and bronchopulmonary dysplasia.

Pathology: At autopsy, a number of morphological alterations have been described in victims of SIDS, but their relevance to the etiology and pathogenesis of this disorder remains unclear. Chronic hypoxia is said to be evidenced by gliosis of the brainstem, medial hypertrophy of small pulmonary arteries, persistence of extramedullary hematopoiesis in the liver, retention of periadrenal brown fat, and right ventricular hypertrophy. However, with the exception of brainstem gliosis, none of these changes occur with any regularity. Petechiae on the surfaces of the lungs, heart, pleura, and thymus, which have been reported in most infants dying of SIDS, are probably terminal events and have been attributed to negative intrathoracic pressure produced by respiratory efforts.

NEOPLASMS OF INFANCY AND CHILDHOOD

Malignant tumors between the ages of 1 and 15 years are distinctly uncommon, but cancer remains the leading cause of death from disease in this age group. In children, 10% of all deaths are due to malignancies, and only accidental trauma kills a larger number. **Unlike adults, in whom most cancers are of epithelial origin (e.g., carcinomas of the lung, breast, and gastrointestinal tract), most malignant tumors in children arise from hematopoietic, nervous, and soft tissues** (Fig. 6-49). Another feature that distinguishes childhood tumors from those of adults is the fact that many of the former are part of developmental complexes. Examples include Wilms tumor associated with aniridia, genitourinary malformations, and mental retardation (WAGR complex); hemihypertrophy of the body associated with Wilms tumor, hepatoblastoma, and adrenal carcinoma; and tuberous sclerosis in association with renal tumors and rhabdomyomas of the heart. Some neoplasms are apparent at birth and are obviously developmental tumors that have evolved in utero. In addition, abnormally developed organs, persistent organ primordia, and displaced organ rests are all vulnerable to neoplastic transformation.

The individual cancers of childhood, including disorders such as the leukemias, neuroblastoma, Wilms tumor, various sarcomas, and germ cell neoplasms, are discussed in detail in the chapters dealing with the respective organs. The basic principles of neoplasia and carcinogenesis, including those applicable to pediatric cancers, are discussed in Chapter 5.

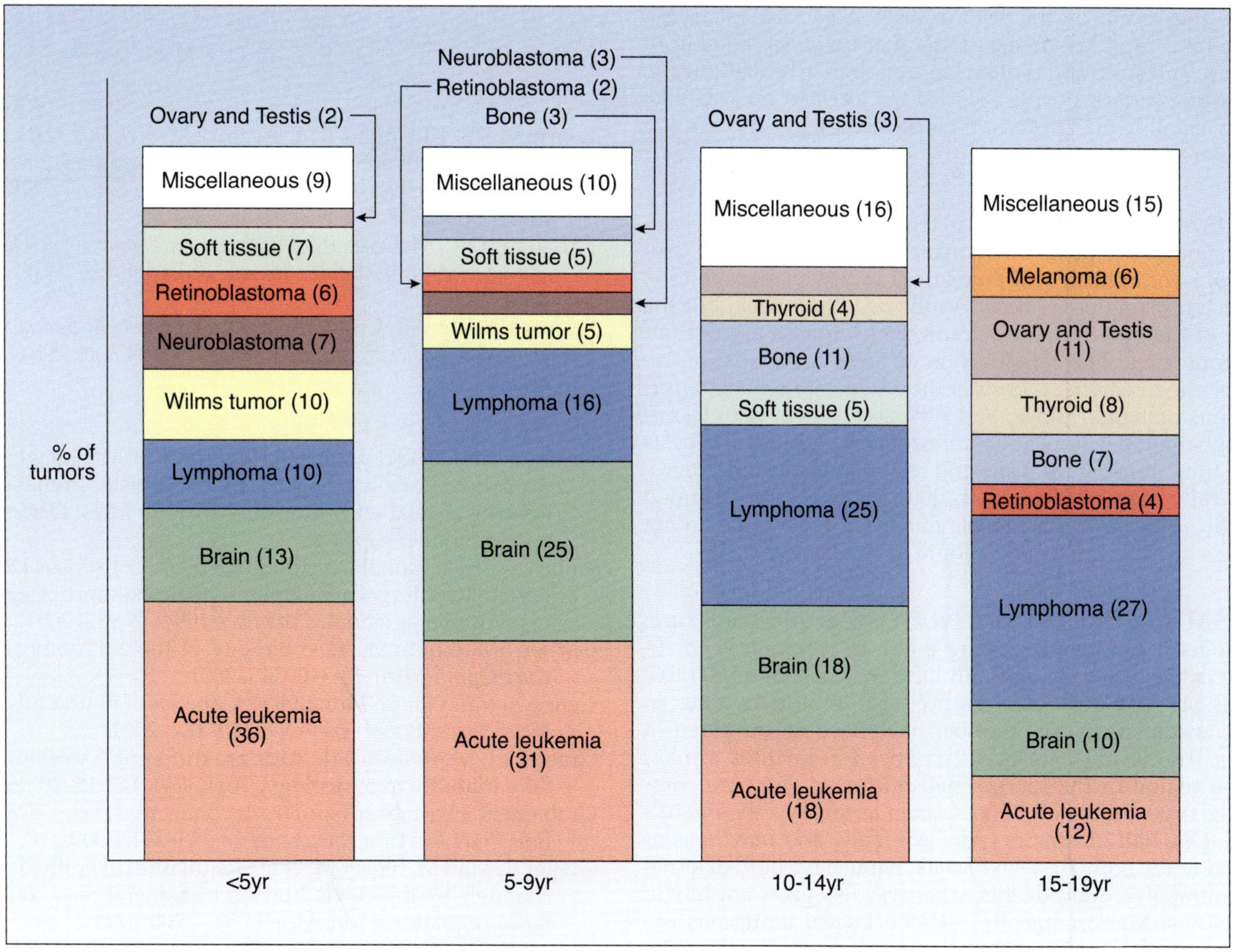

FIGURE 6-49
Distribution of childhood tumors according to age and primary site.

Benign Tumors and Tumorlike Conditions Encompass a Wide Range of Abnormalities

HAMARTOMAS: These lesions represent focal, benign overgrowths of one or more of the mature cellular elements of a normal tissue, often with one element predominating. Although the cells of a hamartoma are often arranged in a highly irregular fashion, the distinction between this developmental abnormality and a true benign neoplasm is often conjectural.

CHORISTOMAS: Also called *heterotopias,* choristomas are similar to hamartomas but are minute or microscopic aggregates of normal tissue components in aberrant locations. Choristomas are represented by rests of pancreatic tissue in the wall of the gastrointestinal tract or of adrenal tissue in the renal cortex.

HEMANGIOMAS: These lesions, of varying size and in diverse locations, are the most frequently encountered tumors in childhood. Whether hemangiomas are true neoplasms or hamartomas is unclear, although half are present at birth and most regress with age. Large, rapidly growing hemangiomas occasionally can be serious lesions, especially when they occur on the head or neck. A *port wine stain* is a congenital capillary hemangioma that involves the skin of the face and scalp and is often large enough to be disfiguring, imparting a dark purple color to the affected area. Unlike many small hemangiomas, they persist for life and are not easily treated.

LYMPHANGIOMAS: Also termed *cystic hygromas,* lymphangiomas are poorly demarcated swellings that are usually present at birth and thereafter rapidly increase in size. Most lymphangiomas occur on the head and neck, but the floor of the mouth, mediastinum, and buttocks are not uncommon sites. The classification of these tumors is imprecise; some researchers consider them developmental malformations or hamartomas, and others call them neoplasms. Lymphangiomas appear as unilocular or multilocular cysts with thin, transparent walls and straw-colored fluid. Microscopically, myriad dilated lymphatic channels are separated by fibrous septa. Unlike hemangiomas, these lesions do not regress spontaneously and should be resected.

SACROCOCCYGEAL TERATOMAS: Although rare, these germ cell neoplasms are the most common solid tumors in the newborn, with an incidence of 1 in 40,000 live births. At least 75% of sacrococcygeal teratomas occur in girls, and a substantial number have been encountered in twins. The tumors are usually noticed at birth as a mass in the region of the sacrum and buttocks. They are commonly large, lobulated masses, often as large as the infant's head. One half of tumors grow externally and may be connected to the body by a small stalk. Some have both external and intrapelvic components, whereas a few grow entirely in the pelvis. Microscopically, sacrococcygeal teratomas are composed of numerous tissues, particularly of neural origin. Most (90%) sacrococcygeal teratomas detected before the age of 2 months are benign, but up to half of those diagnosed later in life are malignant. Associated congenital anomalies of the vertebrae, genitourinary system, and anorectum are common. The lesion should be resected promptly.

Cancers in the Pediatric Age Group Are Uncommon

The incidence of childhood malignancies is 1.3 per 10,000 per year in children under the age of 15 years. The mortality clearly varies with the intrinsic behavior of the tumor and the response to therapy, but as an overall figure, the death rate for childhood cancer is only about one third the incidence. Almost half of all malignant diseases in patients under 15 years of age are acute leukemias and lymphomas. Leukemias alone, particularly acute lymphoblastic leukemia, account for one third of all cases of childhood cancer. Most of the other malignant neoplasms are neuroblastomas, brain tumors, Wilms tumors, retinoblastomas, bone cancers, and various soft tissue sarcomas.

The genetic influences in the development of childhood tumors have been particularly well studied in the case of retinoblastoma, Wilms tumor, and osteosarcoma. The issues relating to the interaction of inherited mutations and environmental influences in the pathogenesis of malignant tumors in both children and adults are discussed in Chapter 5.

SUGGESTED READING

Books

Behrman RE, Kliegman RM, Arvin AM: *Nelson's textbook of pediatrics,* 16th ed. Philadelphia: WB Saunders, 2000.

Killeen AA: *Principles of molecular pathology.* Totowa, NJ: Humana Press, 2003.

Nussbaum RL, McInnes RR, Willard HF: *Thompson & Thompson genetics in medicine,* 6th ed. Philadelphia: WB Saunders, 2001.

Scriver CR, Sly WS, Childs B, et al.: *The metabolic and molecular basis of inherited disease,* 8th ed. New York: McGraw-Hill, 2000.

Review Articles

Anonymous: ACOG practice bulletin. Clinical management guidelines for obstetricians-gynecologists. Prenatal diagnosis of fetal chromosomal abnormalities. *Obstet Gynecol* 97(5 pt 1; suppl 1–12), 2001.

Anonymous: National Institutes of Health Consensus Development Conference Statement: phenylketonuria screening and management. *Pediatrics* 108:972–982, 2001.

Gartler SM, Goldman MA: Biology of the X chromosome. *Curr Opin Pediatr* 13:340–345, 2001.

Gelineau-van Waes J, Finnell RH: Genetics of neural tube defects. *Semin Pediatr Neurol* 8:160–164, 2001.

Graeter LJ, Mortensen ME: Kids are different: Developmental variability in toxicology. *Toxicology* 111:15–20, 1996.

Grahame R. Heritable disorders of connective tissue. *Ballieres Best Pract Res Clin Rheumatol* 14:345–361, 2000.

Greger R, Mall M, Bleich M, et al.: Regulation of epithelial ion channels by the cystic fibrosis transmembrane conductance regulator. *J Mol Med* 74:527–534, 1996.

Gutmann DH: The neurofibromatosis: When less is more. *Hum Mol Genet* 10:747–755, 2001.

Hansis C, Grifo J: Tay-Sachs disease and preimplantation genetic diagnosis. *Adv Genet* 44:311–315, 2001.

Hassold T, Hunt P: To err (meiotically) is human: The genesis of human aneuploidy. *Natl Rev Genet* 2:280–291, 2001.

Hendrickx J, Willems PJ: Genetic deficiencies of the glycogen phosphorylase system. *Hum Genet* 97:551–556, 1996.

Hernandez D, Fisher EM: Down syndrome genetics: Unravelling a multifactorial disorder. *Hum Mol Genet* 5:1411–1416, 1996.

Koch R, Fishler K, Azen C, et al.: The relationship of genotype to phenotype in phenylalanine hydroxylase deficiency. *Biochem Mol Med* 60:92–101, 1997.

Lindblad K, Schalling M: Expanded repeat sequences and disease. *Semin Neurol* 19:289–299, 1999.

Mahenthiralingam E, Baldwin A, Vandamme P: Burkholderia cepacia complex infection in patients with cystic fibrosis. *J Med Microbiol* 51:533–538, 2002.

Mannucci PM, Tuddenham EGD: The hemophilias—from royal genes to gene therapy. *N Engl J Med* 344:1773–1779, 2001.

Nagler J: Sudden infant death syndrome. *Curr Opin Pediatr* 14:247–250, 2002.

Ozawa E, Yoshida M, Suzuki A, et al.: Dystrophin-associated proteins in muscular dystrophy. *Hum Mol Genet* 4(spec. no.):1711–1716, 1995.

Paulsen M, Ferguson-Smith AC: DNA methylation in genomic imprinting, development, and disease. *J Pathol* 195:97–110, 2001.

Polifka JE, Friedman JM: Medical genetics: 1. Clinical teratology in the age of genomics. *Can Med Assoc J* 167:265–273, 2002.

Pope FM, Burrows NP: Ehlers-Danlos syndrome has varied molecular mechanisms. *J Med Genet* 34:400–410, 1997.

Scriver CR: Garrod's foresight; our hindsight. *J Inherit Metab Dis* 24:93–116, 2001.

Thackray H, Tifft C: Fetal alcohol syndrome. *Pediatr Rev* 22:47–55, 2001.

Wraith JE: The mucopolysaccharidoses: A clinical review and guide to management. *Arch Dis Child* 72:263–267, 1995.

CHAPTER 7

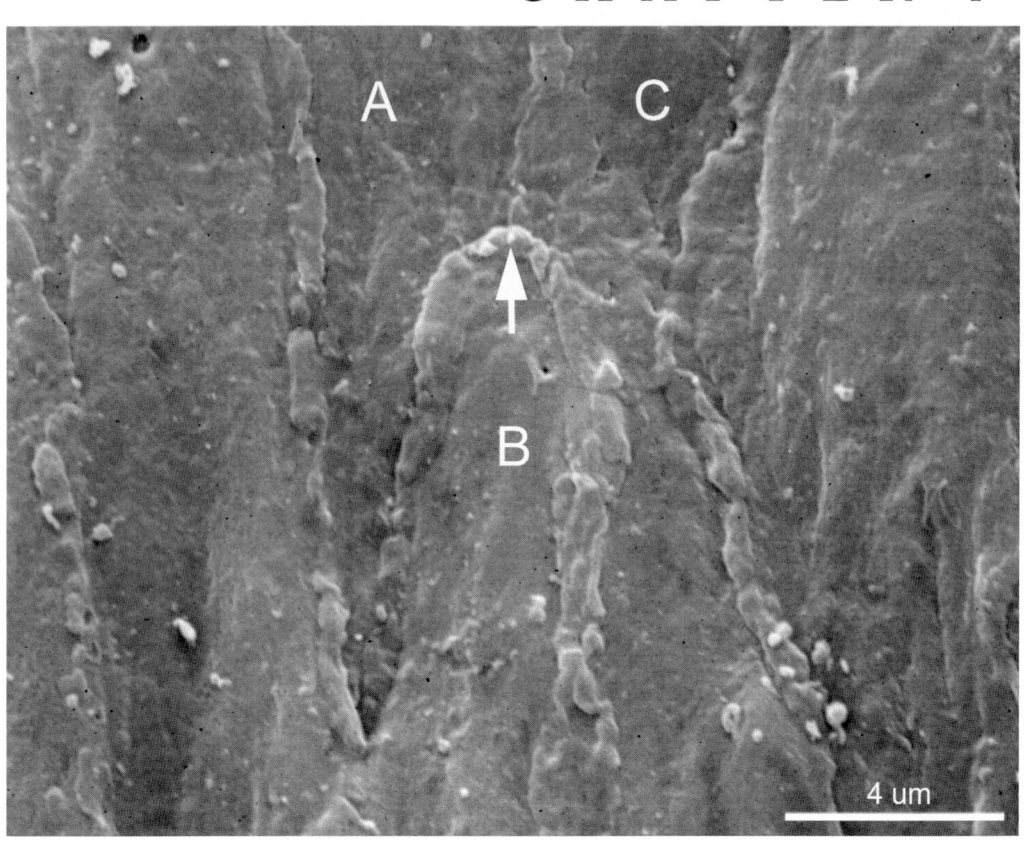

Hemodynamic Disorders

Bruce M. McManus
Michael F. Allard
Bobby Yanagawa

Normal Circulation

The Heart as a Two-Sided Pump

Aorta and Arteries

Microcirculation

Endothelium

Veins and Venules

The Interstitium

Lymphatics

Disorders of Perfusion

Hyperemia

Hemorrhage

Thrombosis

Thrombosis in the Arterial System

Thrombosis in the Heart

Thrombosis in the Venous System

Embolism

Pulmonary Arterial Embolism

Systemic Arterial Embolism

Infarction

Pathology

Infarction in Specific Locations

Edema

Congestive Heart Failure

Pulmonary Edema

Edema in Cirrhosis

Nephrotic Syndrome

Cerebral Edema

Fluid Accumulation in Body Cavities

Fluid Loss and Overload

Dehydration

Overhydration

Shock

Systemic Inflammatory Response Syndrome

Multiple Organ Dysfunction Syndrome (MODS)

FIGURE 7-1 *(see opposite page)*
Scanning electron micrograph of a tricellular corner in the endothelium of a rat coronary artery. The margins of cells *A, B,* and *C* converge to form the tricellular corner at the *arrow*. SEM and freeze-fracture show that tight junctions are discontinuous and form a pore across the endothelium at the tricellular corners through which both molecular species and migrating leukocytes may cross the endothelium. At this corner cell B forms a cytoplasmic extension or flap, *(under the arrow)* that lies over cells A and C.

NORMAL CIRCULATION

Normal function and metabolism of organs and cells depends on an intact circulatory system for the continuous delivery of oxygen, nutrients, hormones, electrolytes, and water and for the removal of metabolic waste and carbon dioxide. The circulatory system is a vascular circuit composed of a muscular pump connected to tubes (or blood vessels) that either deliver blood to the organs and tissues of the body or return blood to the heart to complete the circuit. Delivery and elimination at the cellular level are controlled by exchanges between the intravascular space, interstitial space, cellular space, and lymphatic space, which occur via the smallest-diameter blood vessels in the body (referred to as the microcirculation).

The Heart Is a Two-Sided Pump with Vascular Circuits in Series

The amount of blood pumped by the right ventricle, which pumps blood to the lungs (pulmonary circulation), must, over time, exactly equal the amount of blood pumped by the left ventricle, which distributes blood to the body (systemic circulation). The hemodynamically important parameters are cardiac output, perfusion pressure, and peripheral vascular resistance.

- **Cardiac output** is the volume of blood pumped by each ventricle per minute and represents the total blood flow in the pulmonary and systemic circulations. Cardiac output depends on heart rate and stroke volume. The cardiac output is often indexed to the body surface area (in square meters), termed the *cardiac index*, providing an indication of ventricular function.
- **Perfusion pressure** (also called *driving pressure*) is the difference in dynamic pressure between two points along a blood vessel. Blood flow to any segment of the circulation ultimately depends on the arterial driving pressure. However, each organ can autoregulate flow and, thereby, determine the amount of blood that it receives from the circulation. Such local control of perfusion depends on the continuous modulation of microvascular beds by hormonal, neural, metabolic, and hemodynamic factors.
- **Peripheral vascular resistance** refers to the sum of the factors that determine the regional blood flow in each organ. Two thirds of the resistance in the systemic vasculature is determined by the arterioles.

The sum of all regional flows equals the venous return, which in turn determines the cardiac output. Determination of the cardiac response to inflow (preload) and outflow (afterload) relies on cardiac reflexes as well as cardiac muscle integrity and neurohormonal regulation.

The Aorta and Arteries Are Conducting Vessels

The major functions of the aorta and arteries are the transport of blood to the organs and the conversion of pulsatile flow into sustained regular flow. The latter function derives from the elastic properties of the aorta and the resistance produced by the arteriolar sphincters.

The Microcirculation Includes Arterioles, Capillaries, and Venules

The blood vessels of the microcirculation are less than 100 μM in diameter. Blood from an arteriole enters the capillaries, which freely anastomose with each other (Fig. 7-2A), either directly or through metarterioles. Capillary length, measured from terminal arteriole to collecting venule, ranges from 0.1 to 3 mm, averaging 1 mm. However, the length of the path by which blood cells traverse the capillaries may actually be longer because of their extensive anastomoses. This fact is likely an important factor with respect to microvascular exchange of substances such as oxygen because it will increase the time available for exchange to take place. The large aggregate surface area of capillaries determines that velocity of blood is low, which further enhances microvascular exchange. The density of capillaries in a tissue also influences microvascular exchange by affecting the diffusion distance. For example, in tissues with high oxygen demands, such as the heart, capillary density is very high (Fig. 7-2B). Entry into the capillary system is guarded by precapillary sphincters, except in the case of *thoroughfare channels*, which bypass capillaries and are always open. Since not all capillaries are open at all times, blood flow can be increased by recruitment of additional capillaries. The sum of the flow through the capillary bed, the thoroughfare channels, and the arteriovenous anastomoses determines the regional blood flow. The exact means by which an organ regulates blood flow according to its metabolic needs are still debated, but there is a link between oxygen demand and blood flow. In the heart, blood flow is adjusted on a second-to-second basis. Factors that mediate and link metabolic vasodilation to cellular metabolism include adenosine, other nucleotides, nitric oxide, certain prostaglandins, carbon dioxide, and pH. The microcirculation is an important contributor to all forms of hyperemia and edema and is a target in septic shock (see below). Vasoregulation in conducting arteries, resistance arteries, and veins re-

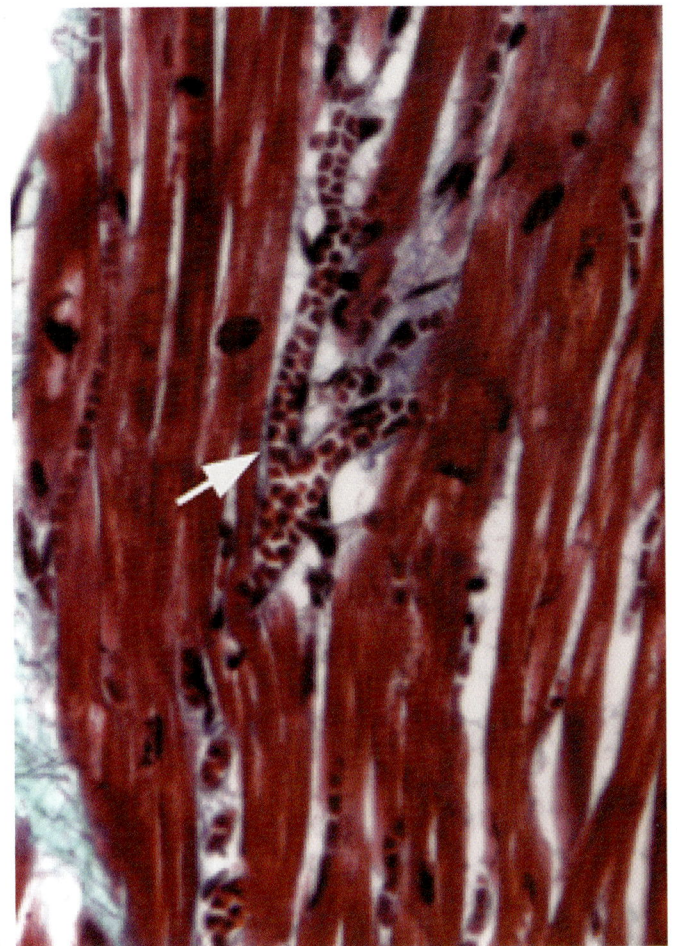
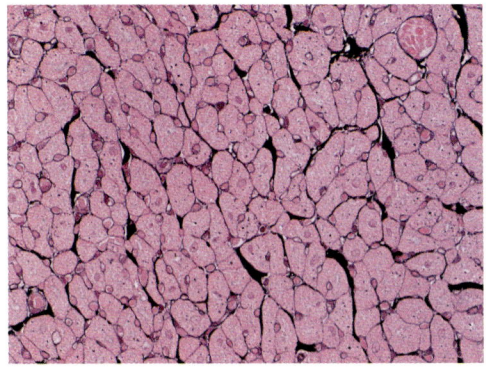

FIGURE 7-2
Microcirculation. Photomicrographs show anastomosing capillaries (arrow) (A) and high capillary density in myocardium (B) (×220).

lies on delicate interactions between blood, endothelium, smooth muscle cells, and surrounding stroma.

The Normal Endothelium Provides a Continuous Partition between Blood and Tissues

Endothelial cells play important physiological roles in anticoagulation, facilitation of migration of substances from blood to tissue and back, regulation of vessel tone (particularly that of resistance arteries), and regulation of vasopermeability.

Veins and Venules Return Blood to the Heart

Blood from the capillaries enters the venules and eventually the veins on its route back to the heart. The veins not only serve as a conduit for blood, but also act as a blood reservoir; 64% of the total blood volume resides in the venous system.

The Interstitium Represents 15% of Total Body Volume

The interstitial fluid between the cells provides a means for the delivery of nutrients and the elimination of waste. Most of the interstitial water is bound to a dense network of glycosaminoglycans.

Lymphatics Reabsorb Interstitial Fluid

Interstitial fluid is reabsorbed into the circulation at the venous end of the capillary, and a small portion is drained through lymphatics. Lymphatic capillaries conduct the lymph from the periphery to the central venous system via the thoracic duct. Normal oscillatory constrictions and relaxations of lymphatic vessels contribute to steady return of lymph fluid to the central circulation. Lymph is a solvent for large molecules that cannot return to the circulation through the blood capillaries.

DISORDERS OF PERFUSION

Hemodynamic disorders are characterized by disturbed perfusion that may result in organ and cellular injury.

Hyperemia Is an Excess of Blood in an Organ

Hyperemia may be caused either by an increased supply of blood from the arterial system (active hyperemia) or by an impediment to the exit of blood through venous pathways (passive hyperemia or congestion).

Active Hyperemia

Active hyperemia is an augmented supply of blood to an organ, usually as a physiological response to an increased functional demand, as in the case of the heart and skeletal muscle during exercise. Neurogenic and hormonal influences play a role in active hyperemia, as exemplified at both extremes of the female reproductive span, namely, the blushing bride and the menopausal flush. Although these examples do not appear to promote any useful function, hyperemia of the skin in febrile states serves to dissipate heat. In addition, skeletal muscle may increase its blood flow (and, thus, oxygen delivery) 20-fold during exercise. The increased blood supply is brought about by arteriolar dilation and recruitment of unperfused capillaries.

The most striking active hyperemia occurs in association with inflammation. Vasoactive materials released by inflammatory cells (see Chapter 2) cause dilation of blood vessels; in the skin this contributes to classic "tumor, rubor, and calor" of inflammation. In pneumonia, for example, the alveolar capillaries are engorged with erythrocytes as a hyperemic response to inflammation. Since inflammation can also damage endothelial cells and increase capillary permeability, inflammatory hyperemia is often accompanied by edema and local extravasation of erythrocytes.

Reactive hyperemia occurs after temporary interruption of blood supply (or ischemia). The release of the obstruction is followed by active hyperemia and is probably due to ischemic tissue injury and release of inflammatory agents such as histamine. **The degree and duration of hyperemia is proportional to the period of occlusion until a plateau of hyperemic response is reached.**

Passive Hyperemia (Congestion)

Passive hyperemia, or congestion, refers to the engorgement of an organ with venous blood. Acute passive congestion is clinically a consequence of acute failure of the left or right ventricle. In the case of acute left ventricular failure, the resultant venous engorgement of the lung leads to the accumulation of a transudate in the alveoli, a condition termed *pulmonary edema*. With acute failure of the right ventricle, the liver can become severely congested.

A generalized increase in venous pressure, typically from chronic heart failure, results in slower blood flow and a consequent increase in the volume of blood in many organs, including the liver, spleen, and kidneys. In the past, heart failure from rheumatic mitral stenosis was a common cause of generalized venous congestion, but with the decline in the prevalence of rheumatic fever and the advent of surgical valve replacement, such cases are unusual. Congestive heart failure secondary to coronary artery disease and hypertension, and right-sided failure because of pulmonary disease, are now more common causes.

Passive congestion may also be confined to a limb or an organ as a result of more-localized obstruction to the venous drainage. Examples include deep venous thrombosis of the leg veins with resulting edema of the lower extremity, and thrombosis of the hepatic veins (Budd-Chiari syndrome) with secondary chronic passive congestion of the liver.

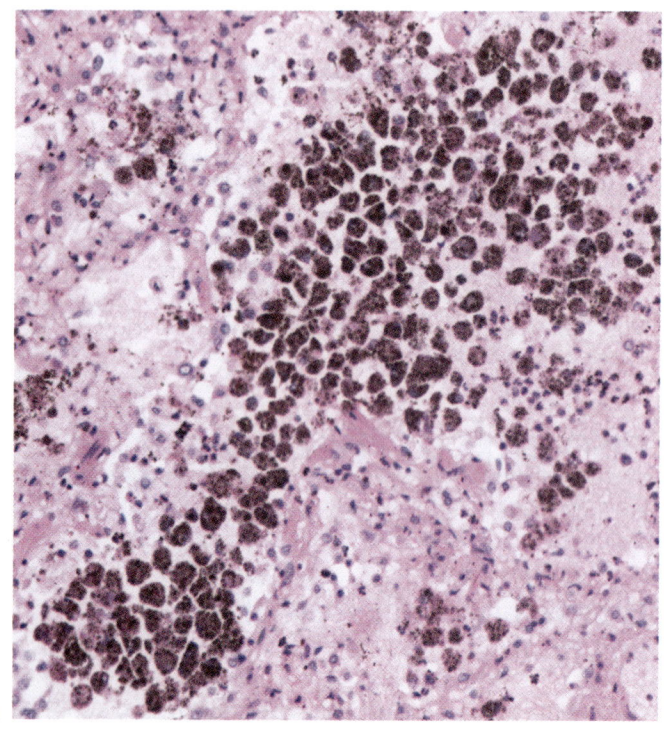
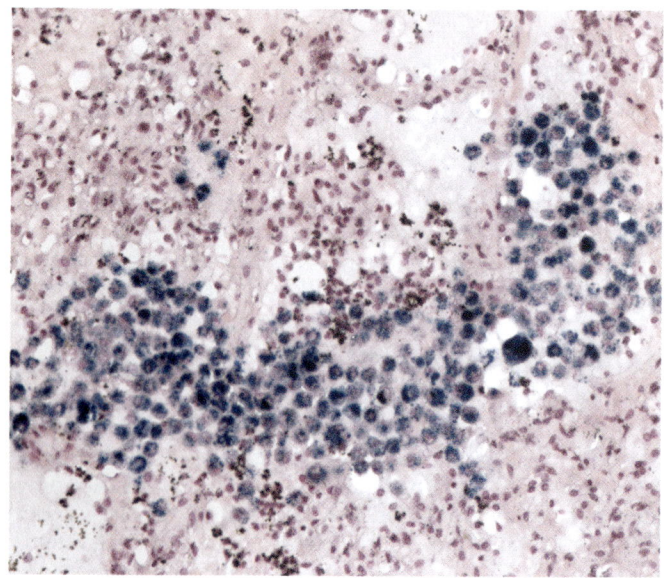

FIGURE 7-3
Passive congestion of lung. A. Hemosiderin-laden macrophages in the lung of a patient with congestive heart failure. B. Macrophages in the lung stain for iron with the Prussian blue stain.

Disorders of Perfusion

THE LUNG: Chronic failure of the left ventricle constitutes an impediment to the exit of blood from the lungs and leads to chronic passive congestion of the lungs. As a result, the pressure in the alveolar capillaries is increased, and these vessels become engorged with blood. The increased pressure in the alveolar capillaries has four major consequences:

- Microhemorrhages release erythrocytes into the alveolar spaces, where they are phagocytosed and degraded by alveolar macrophages. The released iron, in the form of hemosiderin, remains in the macrophages, which are then called "heart failure cells" (Fig. 7-3).
- The increased hydrostatic pressure forces fluid from the blood into the alveolar spaces, resulting in pulmonary edema (Fig. 7-4), a dangerous condition that interferes with gas exchange in the lung.
- The increased pressure, together with other poorly understood factors, stimulates fibrosis in the interstitial spaces of the lung. The presence of fibrosis and iron is viewed grossly as a firm, brown lung *(brown induration)*.
- The increased capillary pressure is transmitted to the pulmonary arterial system, a condition labeled *pulmonary hypertension*. This disorder may lead to right-sided heart failure and consequent generalized systemic venous congestion.

Chapter 12 discusses the morphological changes associated with chronic passive congestion of the lungs.

THE LIVER: The hepatic veins empty into the vena cava immediately inferior to the heart, and the liver is particularly vulnerable to acute or chronic passive congestion. The central veins of the hepatic lobule become dilated. The increased venous pressure is then transferred to the sinusoids, where it leads to dilation of the sinusoids and pressure atrophy of the centrilobular hepatocytes (Fig. 7-5). Grossly, the cut surface of the chronically congested liver exhibits dark foci of centrilobular congestion surrounded by paler zones of unaffected peripheral portions of the lobules. The result is a curious reticulated appearance, that resembles a cross-section of a nutmeg and is appropriately called "nutmeg liver" (Fig. 7-5). In extreme cases associated with acute right ventricular failure, frank hemorrhagic necrosis of the hepatocytes in the centrilobular zones is conspicuous. Prolonged venous congestion of the liver eventually leads to thickening of the central veins and centrilobular fibrosis. Only in the most extreme cases of venous congestion (e.g., constrictive pericarditis or tricuspid stenosis) is the fibrosis sufficiently generalized and severe to justify the label *cardiac cirrhosis*.

THE SPLEEN: Increased pressure in the liver, from cardiac failure or an intrahepatic obstruction to the flow of blood (e.g., cirrhosis), results in higher splenic vein pressure and congestion of the spleen. The organ becomes enlarged and tense, and the cut section oozes dark blood. In long-standing congestion, diffuse fibrosis of the spleen occurs, together with iron-containing, fibrotic, and calcified foci of old hemorrhage (so-called Gamna-Gandy bodies). Fibrocongestive splenomegaly may result in an organ that weighs 250 to 750 g, compared with a normal weight of 150 g. The enlarged spleen sometimes displays excessive functional activity—a condition termed *hypersplenism*—which leads to hematological abnormalities.

EDEMA AND ASCITES: Venous congestion impedes the flow of blood in the capillaries, thereby increasing hydrostatic pressure and promoting edema formation (see below for a discussion of the mechanisms of edema formation). The accumulation of edema fluid in heart failure is particularly noticeable in dependent tissues—the legs and feet in ambulatory patients and the back in bedridden persons. Ascites refers to the accumulation of fluid in the peritoneal space and reflects (among other factors) the lack of tissue rigor, a condition in which there is no countervailing external pressure to oppose hydrostatic pressure within the blood vessels.

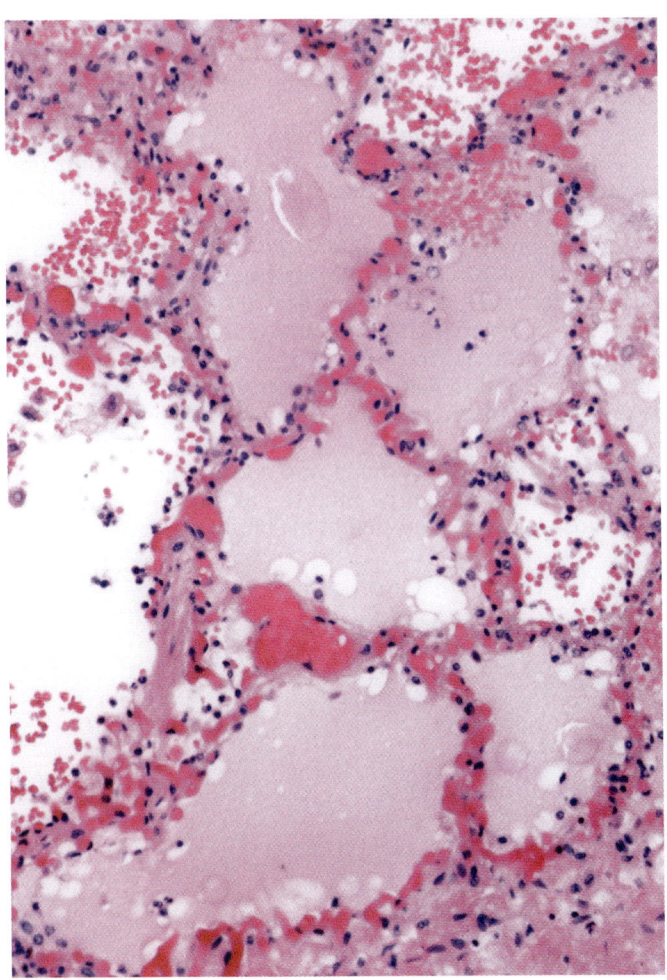

FIGURE 7-4
Pulmonary edema. A patient with congestive heart failure shows pink-staining fluid in the alveoli.

Hemorrhage Is a Discharge of Blood out of the Vascular Compartment

Blood can be released from the circulation to the exterior of the body or into nonvascular body spaces. The most com-

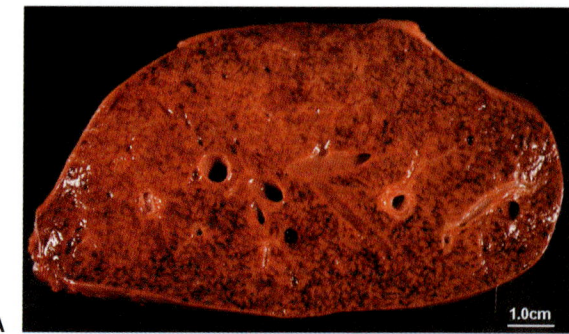
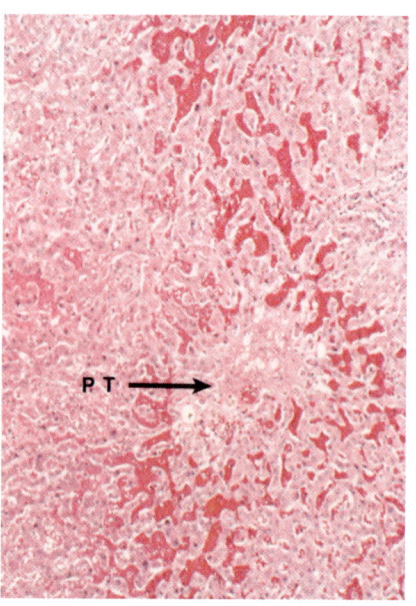

FIGURE 7-5
Passive congestion of liver. A. A gross photograph of liver shows nutmeg appearance, reflecting congestive failure of the right ventricle. B. A photomicrograph of liver shows centrilobular sinusoids dilated with blood. The intervening plates of hepatocytes exhibit pressure atrophy. *PT*, portal tract.

mon and obvious cause is trauma (usually accidental), but bleeding can also occur in association with surgical procedures (e.g., when a blood vessel is lacerated by a scalpel). Severe atherosclerosis may so weaken the wall of the abdominal aorta that it balloons to form an aneurysm, which then may rupture and bleed into the retroperitoneal space. In the same way, an aneurysm may complicate a congenitally weak cerebral artery (berry aneurysm) and lead to subarachnoid hemorrhage. Certain infections (e.g., pulmonary tuberculosis) and invasive neoplasms may erode blood vessels and lead to hemorrhage.

Hemorrhage also results from damage at the level of the capillaries. For instance, rupture of capillaries by blunt trauma is evidenced by the appearance of a bruise. Increased venous pressure also causes extravasation of blood from capillaries in the lung. Vitamin C deficiency, is associated with capillary fragility and bleeding, owing to a defect in the supporting structures. The capillary barrier by itself does not suffice to contain the blood within the intravascular space. The minor trauma imposed on small vessels and capillaries by normal movement requires an intact coagulation system to prevent hemorrhage. Thus, a severe decrease in the number of platelets *(thrombocytopenia)* or a deficiency of a coagulation factor (e.g., factor VIII in hemophilia) is associated with spontaneous hemorrhages unrelated to any apparent trauma (see Chapter 10 for a more detailed discussion of the coagulation system).

A person may exsanguinate into an internal cavity, as in the case of gastrointestinal hemorrhage from a peptic ulcer (arterial hemorrhage) or esophageal varices (venous hemorrhage). In such cases, large amounts of fresh blood fill the entire gastrointestinal tract. Bleeding into a serous cavity can result in the accumulation of a large amount of blood, even to the point of exsanguination. A few definitions are in order:

- **Hematoma:** Hemorrhage into soft tissue. Such collections of blood can be merely painful, as in a muscle bruise, or fatal, if located in the brain.

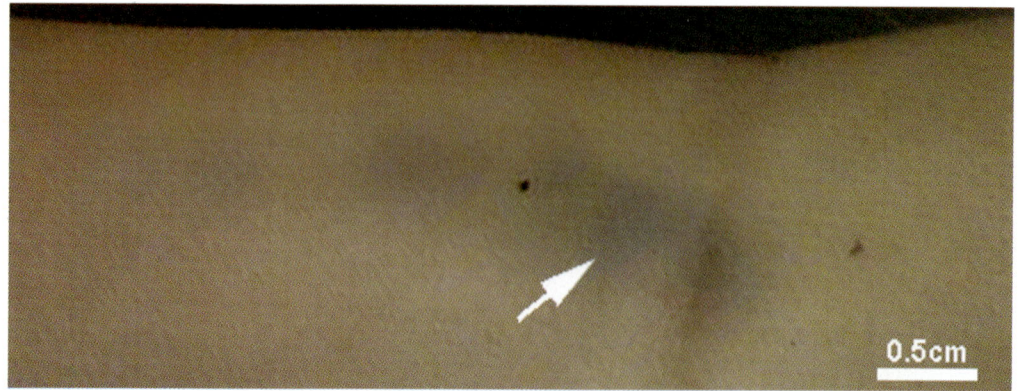

FIGURE 7-6
Ecchymosis *(arrow)* in a forearm caused by a needle puncture.

Thrombosis 287

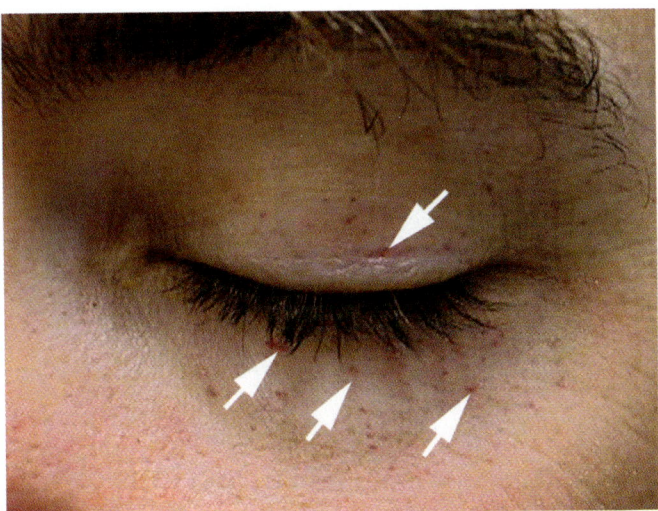

FIGURE 7-7
Petechiae. Periorbital microhemorrhages *(arrows)* appear as red foci.

- **Hemothorax:** Hemorrhage into the pleural cavity.
- **Hemopericardium:** Hemorrhage into the pericardial space.
- **Hemoperitoneum:** Bleeding into the peritoneal cavity.
- **Hemarthrosis:** Bleeding into a joint space.
- **Purpura:** Diffuse superficial hemorrhages in the skin, up to 1 cm in diameter.
- **Ecchymosis:** A larger superficial hemorrhage in the skin (Fig. 7-6). Following such hemorrhage the initially purple discoloration of the skin turns green and then yellow before resolving. This sequence of events reflects the progressive oxidation of bilirubin released from the hemoglobin of degraded erythrocytes. A good example of an ecchymosis is a "black eye."
- **Petechiae:** Pinpoint hemorrhages, usually in the skin or conjunctiva (Fig. 7-7). This lesion represents the rupture of a capillary or arteriole and occurs in conjunction with coagulopathies or vasculitis. Petechiae may also be produced by microemboli from infected heart valves *(bacterial endocarditis)*.

THROMBOSIS

Thrombosis refers to the formation of a thrombus, defined as an aggregate of coagulated blood containing platelets, fibrin, and entrapped cellular elements, within a vascular lumen. A **thrombus** by definition adheres to the vascular endothelium and should be distinguished from a simple blood clot, which reflects only the activation of the coagulation cascade and can form in vitro or in situ in the postmortem state. Similarly, a thrombus differs from a hematoma, which results from hemorrhage and subsequent clotting outside the vascular system. Thrombus formation and the coagulation cascade are discussed in more detail in Chapters 10 and 20. Here we present the causes and consequences of thrombosis in different sites.

Thrombosis in the Arterial System Is Usually due to Atherosclerosis

 Pathogenesis: The most common vessels involved in arterial thrombosis are the coronary, cerebral, mesenteric, and renal arteries and the arteries of the lower extremities. Less commonly, arterial thrombosis occurs in other disorders, including inflammation of the arteries *(arteritis)*, trauma, and diseases of the blood. Thrombi are common in aneurysms (localized dilations of the lumen) of the aorta and its major branches, in which the distortion of blood flow, combined with intrinsic vascular disease, promotes thrombosis.

The pathogenesis of arterial thrombosis involves principally three factors:

- **Damage to the endothelium,** usually by atherosclerosis, disturbs the anticoagulant properties of the vessel wall and serves as the nidus for platelet aggregation and fibrin formation.
- **Alterations in blood flow,** whether from turbulence in an aneurysm or at the sites of arterial bifurcation is conducive to thrombosis. Slowing in narrowed arteries favors thrombosis.
- **Increased coagulability of the blood,** as seen in polycythemia vera or in association with some cancers, leads to an increased risk of thrombosis.

 Pathology: Initially, an arterial thrombus attached to the vessel wall is soft, friable and dark red, with fine alternating bands of yellowish platelets and fibrin, the so-called lines of Zahn (Fig. 7-8). Once formed, arterial thrombi have several possible outcomes.

- **Lysis** of an arterial thrombus may occur, owing to the potent thrombolytic activity of the blood.
- **Propagation** of a thrombus (i.e., an increase in its size) may ensue, because the thrombus serves as the focus for further thrombosis.
- **Organization** refers to the eventual invasion of connective tissue elements, which causes a thrombus to become firm and grayish white.
- **Canalization** is the process by which new lumina lined by endothelial cells form in an organized thrombus (Fig. 7-9). The functional significance of this change is often questionable.
- **Embolization** occurs when a portion or all of the thrombus becomes dislodged and travels through the circulation to become lodged in a blood vessel some distance from the site of thrombus formation (see below for further discussion).

The organized structure of a thrombus reflects a tight interaction between platelets and fibrin and differs in appearance from a postmortem clot or one formed in a test tube. The

288 Hemodynamic Disorders

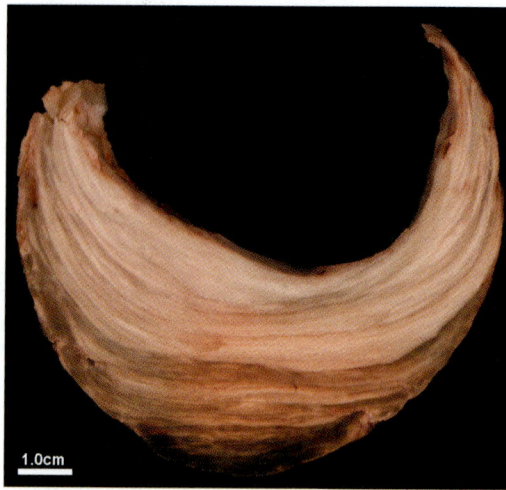

FIGURE 7-8
Arterial thrombus. Gross photograph of a thrombus from an aortic aneurysm shows the laminations of fibrin and platelets known as the lines of Zahn.

lines of Zahn stabilize the thrombus formed during life, whereas the postmortem clot has a more gelatinous structure. Postmortem clots occur in stagnant blood in which gravity fractionates the blood. The part of the clot containing many red blood cells has a reddish, gelatinous appearance, and is referred to as "currant jelly." The overlying clot is firmer and yellow-white, representing coagulated plasma without red blood cells. It is called "chicken fat" because of its color and consistency. Determination of whether or not a clot formed during life (antemortem clot) or after death (postmortem clot) is often important in a medical autopsy and in forensic pathology.

 Clinical Features: **Arterial thrombosis as a consequence of atherosclerosis is the most common cause of death in Western industrialized countries.** Since most arterial thrombi occlude the vessel, they often lead to ischemic necrosis of the tissue supplied by the artery (i.e., an **infarct**). Thus, thrombosis of a coronary or cerebral artery results in a **myocardial infarct** (heart attack) or **cerebral infarct** (stroke), respectively. Other end-arteries that are affected by atherosclerosis and often suffer thrombosis include the mesenteric arteries (intestinal infarction), renal arteries (kidney infarcts), and arteries of the leg (gangrene).

Thrombosis in the Heart Develops on the Endocardium

As in the arterial system, endocardial injury and changes in blood flow in the heart are associated with mural thrombosis, which refers to a thrombus adhering to the underlying wall of the heart. The disorders in which mural thrombosis occurs include the following:

- **Myocardial infarction:** Adherent mural thrombi form in the cavity of the left ventricle over areas of myocardial infarction, owing to damaged endocardium and alterations in blood flow associated with a poorly functional or adynamic segment of the myocardium.
- **Atrial fibrillation:** A disorder of atrial rhythm (atrial fibrillation) leads to slower blood flow and impaired contractility in the left atrium, a situation that predisposes to the formation of mural thrombi in that location.
- **Cardiomyopathy:** Primary diseases of the myocardium are associated with mural thrombi in the left ventricle, presumably because of endocardial injury and altered hemodynamics associated with poor myocardial contractility.
- **Endocarditis:** Small thrombi, termed **vegetations,** may also develop on cardiac valves, usually mitral or aortic, that are damaged by a bacterial infection *(bacterial endocarditis)* (Fig. 7-10). Occasionally, in the absence of valve

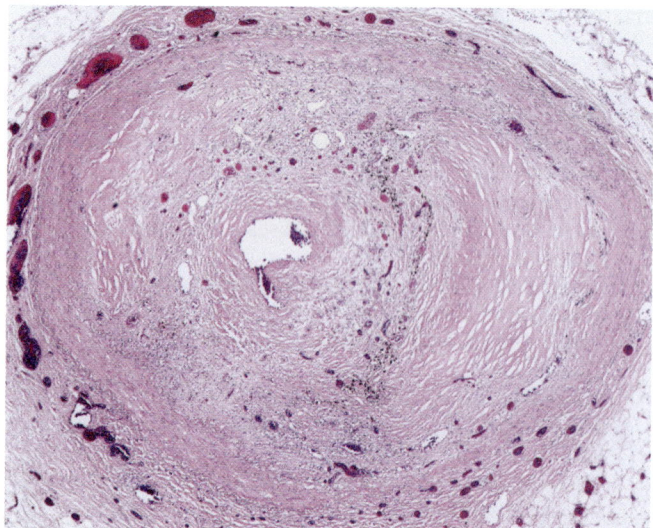

FIGURE 7-9
Canalization of thrombus. Photomicrograph of the left anterior descending coronary artery shows severe atherosclerosis and canalization (×40).

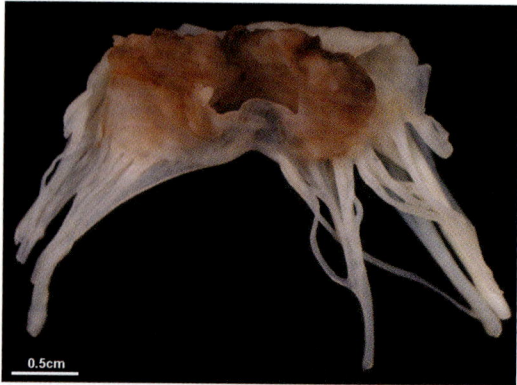

FIGURE 7-10
Endocarditis. The anterior leaflet of the mitral valve is damaged by a friable bacterial vegetation.

infection, vegetations form on a mitral or tricuspid valve injured by systemic lupus erythematosus *(Libman-Sacks endocarditis)*. In chronic wasting states, such as occur with terminal cancer, large, friable vegetations may appear on cardiac valves *(marantic endocarditis)*, possibly reflecting a hypercoagulable state.

The major complication of thrombi in any location in the heart is the detachment of fragments and their transport to distant sites *(embolization)*, where they lodge and occlude arterial vessels.

Thrombosis in the Venous System Is Multifactorial

At one time, venous thrombosis was widely referred to as *thrombophlebitis*, implying that an inflammatory or infectious process had injured the vein, thereby causing thrombosis. However, with recognition that there is no evidence of inflammation in most cases, the term *phlebothrombosis* is more accurate. Nevertheless, both terms have been replaced for the most part by the expression *deep venous thrombosis*. This last term is particularly appropriate for the most common manifestation of the disorder, namely, thrombosis of the deep venous system of the legs.

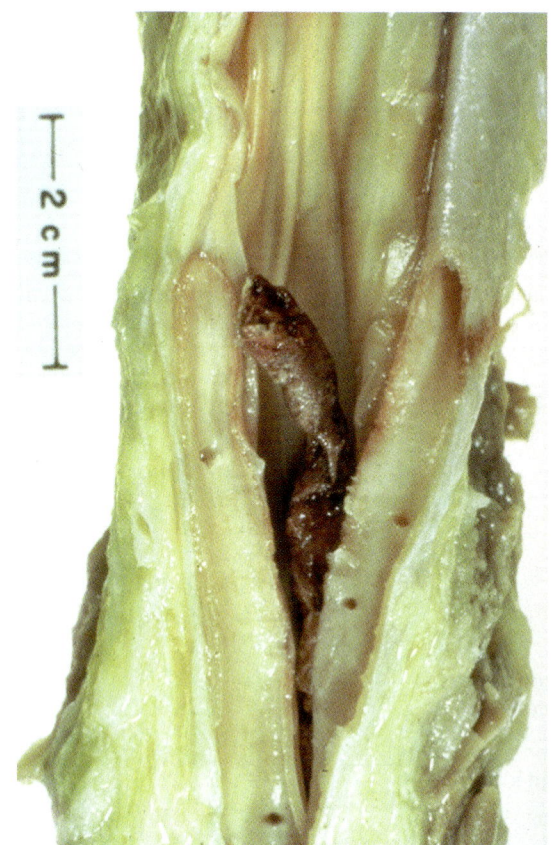

FIGURE 7-11
Venous thrombosis. The femoral vein has been opened to reveal a large thrombus within the lumen.

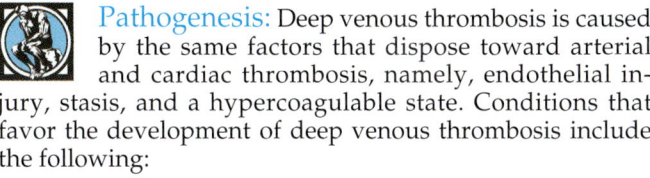 Pathogenesis: Deep venous thrombosis is caused by the same factors that dispose toward arterial and cardiac thrombosis, namely, endothelial injury, stasis, and a hypercoagulable state. Conditions that favor the development of deep venous thrombosis include the following:

- **Stasis** (heart failure, chronic venous insufficiency, postoperative immobilization, prolonged bed rest)
- **Injury** (trauma, surgery, childbirth)
- **Hypercoagulability** (oral contraceptives, late pregnancy, cancer)
- **Advanced age** (venous varicosities, phlebosclerosis)
- **Sickle cell disease** (see Chapter 20 for details)

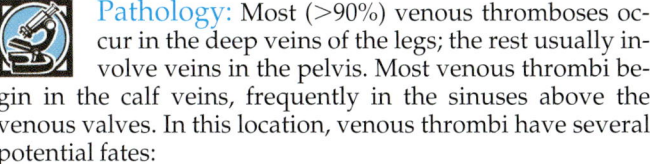 Pathology: Most (>90%) venous thromboses occur in the deep veins of the legs; the rest usually involve veins in the pelvis. Most venous thrombi begin in the calf veins, frequently in the sinuses above the venous valves. In this location, venous thrombi have several potential fates:

- **Lysis:** Venous thrombi generally remain small and are eventually lysed, posing no further threat to health.
- **Organization:** Many thrombi undergo organization similar to those of arterial origin. Small organized venous thrombi may be incorporated into the wall of the vessel; larger ones may undergo canalization, with partial restoration of venous drainage.
- **Propagation:** It is not uncommon for venous thrombi to serve as a nidus for further thrombosis and, thereby, propagate proximally to involve the larger iliofemoral veins (Fig. 7-11).

- **Embolization:** Large venous thrombi or those that have propagated proximally represent a significant hazard to life, since they may dislodge and be carried to the lungs as pulmonary emboli.

Clinical Features: Small thrombi in the calf veins are ordinarily asymptomatic, and even larger thrombi in the iliofemoral system may cause no symptoms. Some patients have tenderness in the calf, often associated with forced dorsiflexion of the foot *(Homans sign)*. Occlusive thrombosis of the femoral or iliac veins leads to severe congestion, edema, and cyanosis of the lower extremity. Symptomatic deep venous thrombosis is treated with systemic anticoagulants, and thrombolytic therapy has been useful in selected cases. In some cases, a filter is inserted into the vena cava to prevent pulmonary embolization.

The function of the venous valves is always impaired in a vein subjected to thrombosis and organization. As a result, chronic deep venous insufficiency (i.e., an impairment of venous drainage) is virtually inevitable. If the lesion is restricted to a small segment of the deep venous system, the condition may remain asymptomatic. However, more extensive involvement results in pigmentation, edema, and induration of the skin of the leg. Ulceration above the medial malleolus can occur in this setting and is often difficult to treat.

Venous thrombi in other locations may also pose severe hazards. Thrombosis of mesenteric veins can cause hemorrhagic infarction of the small bowel; thrombosis of cerebral veins may be fatal; thrombosis of hepatic veins (Budd-Chiari syndrome) may destroy the liver.

EMBOLISM

Embolism is the passage through the venous or arterial circulations of any material capable of lodging in a blood vessel and, thereby, obstructing its lumen. The usual embolus is a thromboembolus—that is, a thrombus formed in one location that detaches from the vessel wall at its point of origin and travels to a distant site.

Pulmonary Arterial Embolism Is Potentially Fatal

For the clinician, pulmonary embolism remains an important diagnostic and therapeutic challenge. In fact, pulmonary thromboemboli are reported in more than half of all autopsies. Furthermore, this complication occurs in 1 to 2% of postoperative patients over the age of 40 years. The risk after surgery increases with advancing age, obesity, length of the operative procedure, postoperative infection, the presence of cancer, and preexisting venous disease.

Most pulmonary emboli (90%) arise from the deep veins of the lower extremities; most of the fatal ones form in the iliofemoral veins (Fig. 7-12). Only half of patients

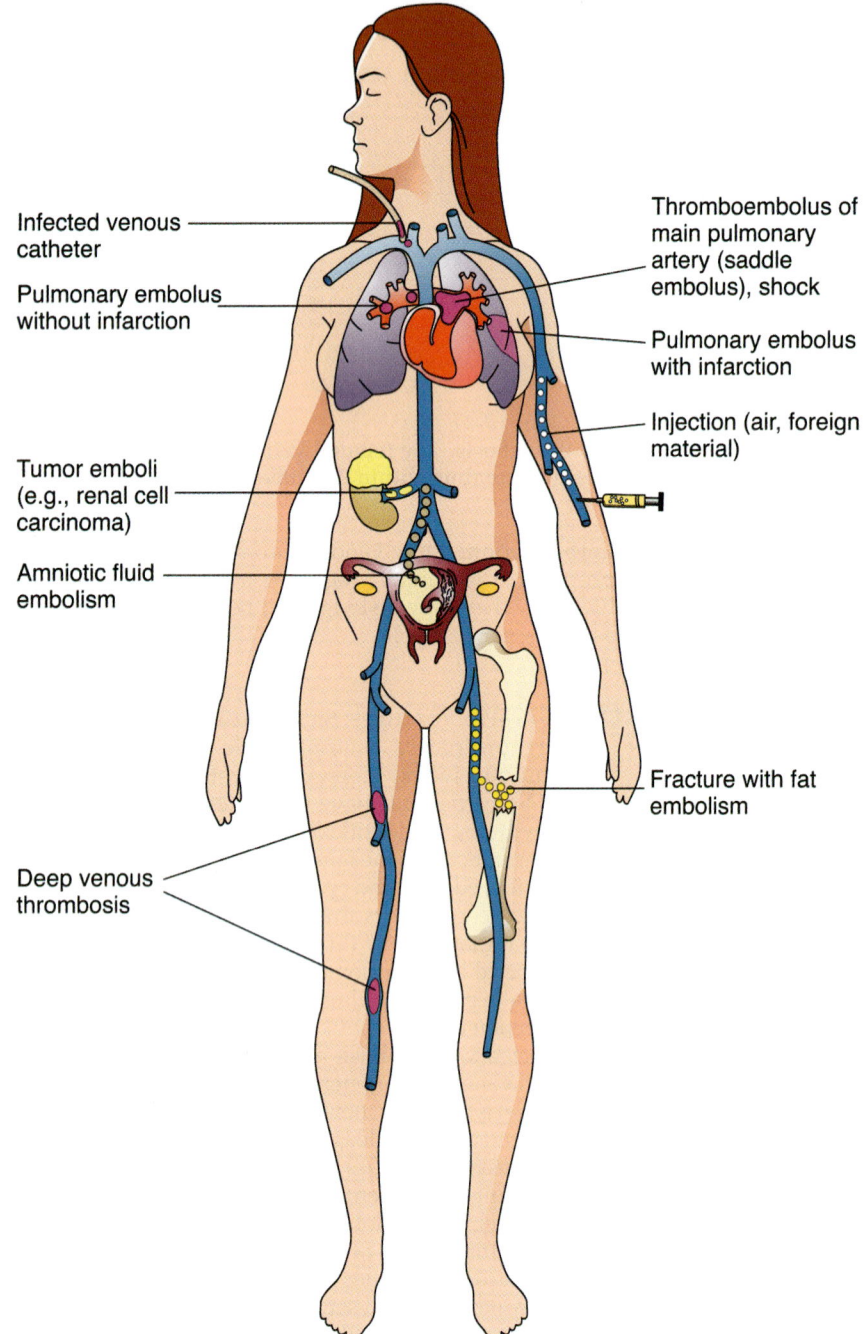

FIGURE *7-12*
Sources and effects of venous emboli.

with pulmonary thromboembolism have signs of deep vein thrombosis. Some thromboemboli arise from the pelvic venous plexus and others from the right side of the heart. Emboli are also derived from thrombi around indwelling lines in the systemic venous system or the pulmonary artery. The upper extremities are a rare source of thromboemboli.

The clinical features of pulmonary embolism are determined by the size of the embolus, the health of the patient, and whether embolization occurs acutely or chronically. Acute pulmonary embolism is divided into the following syndromes:

- Asymptomatic small pulmonary emboli
- Transient dyspnea and tachypnea without other symptoms
- Pulmonary infarction, with pleuritic chest pain, hemoptysis, and pleural effusion
- Cardiovascular collapse with sudden death

Pulmonary embolism that occurs chronically, with numerous (usually asymptomatic) emboli lodged in the small arteries of the lung, can lead to pulmonary hypertension and right-sided heart failure (see below).

Massive Pulmonary Embolism

One of the most dramatic and tragic calamities complicating hospitalization is the sudden collapse and death of a patient who appeared to be well on the way to an uneventful recovery. The cause of this catastrophe is often massive pulmonary embolism as a consequence of the release of a large deep venous thrombus from a lower extremity. Classically, a postoperative patient succumbs immediately on getting out of bed for the first time. The muscular activity dislodges a thrombus that formed as a result of the stasis associated with prolonged bed rest. Excluding deaths related to surgery itself, massive pulmonary embolism is the most common cause of death after major orthopedic surgery and is the most frequent nonobstetric cause of postpartum death. It also is an especially common cause of death in patients who suffer from chronic heart and lung diseases and in those who are subjected to prolonged immobilization for any reason. Prolonged immobilization associated with air travel can also lead to venous thrombosis and, occasionally, sudden death from a pulmonary embolus.

A large pulmonary embolus often lodges at the bifurcation of the main pulmonary artery (*saddle embolus*), thereby obstructing blood flow to both lungs (Fig. 7-13). Large lethal emboli may also be found in the first branching of the right or left pulmonary arteries. Multiple smaller emboli may lodge in secondary branches and prove fatal. With acute obstruction of more than half of the pulmonary arterial tree, the patient often experiences immediate severe hypotension (or shock) and may die within minutes.

The hemodynamic consequences of such massive pulmonary embolism are the result of acute right ventricular failure because of sudden obstruction to outflow and a pronounced reduction in left ventricular cardiac output, secondary to the loss of right ventricular function. The low cardiac output is responsible for the sudden appearance of severe hypotension.

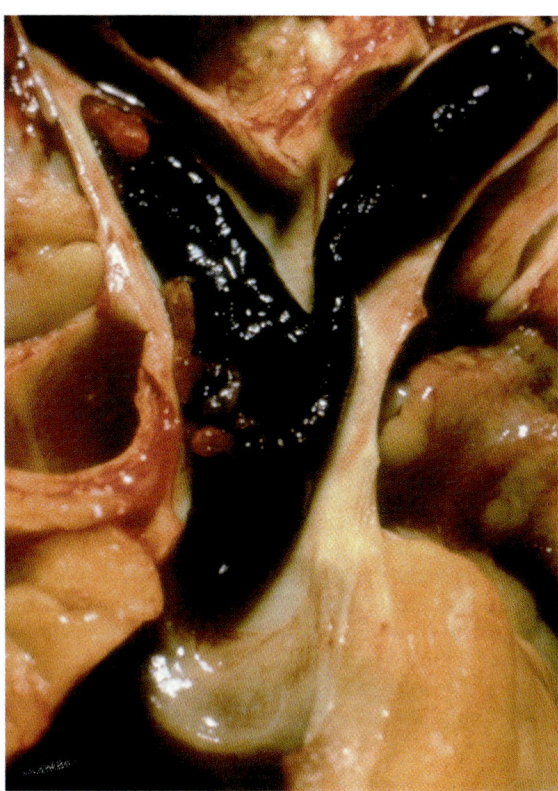

FIGURE 7-13
Pulmonary embolism. The main pulmonary artery and its bifurcation have been opened to reveal a large saddle embolus.

Pulmonary Infarction

Small pulmonary emboli are not ordinarily lethal. They tend to lodge in peripheral pulmonary arteries, and in some patients (15–20% of all pulmonary emboli) they produce infarcts of the lung. Clinically, pulmonary infarction is usually seen in the context of congestive heart failure or chronic lung disease, because the normal dual circulation of the lung ordinarily protects against ischemic necrosis; since the bronchial artery pumps blood into the necrotic area, pulmonary infarcts are typically hemorrhagic. They tend to be pyramidal, with the base of the pyramid on the pleural surface. Patients experience cough, stabbing pleuritic pain, shortness of breath, and occasional hemoptysis. Pleural effusion is common and often bloody. With time, the blood in the infarct is resorbed, and the center of the infarct becomes pale. Granulation tissue forms on the edge of the infarct, after which it is organized to form a fibrous scar.

Pulmonary Embolism without Infarction

Since the lung has a dual circulation, supplied by both the bronchial arteries and the pulmonary artery, most (75%) small pulmonary emboli do not produce infarcts. Although most small emboli do not attract clinical attention, a few lead to a syndrome characterized by dyspnea, cough, chest pain and hypotension. Rarely (3%), recurrent pulmonary emboli produce pulmonary hypertension by mechanical blockage of the arterial bed. In this circumstance, reflex vasoconstriction and bronchial constriction, owing to release of vasoactive substances, may contribute to a reduction in size of the functional pulmonary vascular bed.

In the clinical syndrome of "partial infarction," patients have the clinical and radiological findings of pulmonary infarction due to thromboembolism. However, the lesion resolves instead of contracting to leave a scar. In such cases, hemorrhage and necrosis of the lung tissue in the affected area occur, but the tissue framework remains. Collateral circulation maintains the viability of the tissue and enables its regeneration.

Fate of Pulmonary Thromboemboli

Small pulmonary emboli may completely resolve, depending on (1) the embolic load, (2) the adequacy of the pulmonary vascular reserve, (3) the state of the bronchial collateral circulation, and (4) the activity of the thrombolytic process. Alternatively, thromboemboli may become organized and leave strings of fibrous tissue attached to the vessel wall in the lumen of pulmonary arteries. Radiological studies have indicated that half of all pulmonary thromboemboli are resorbed and organized within 8 weeks, with little narrowing of the vessels involved.

Paradoxical Embolism

Paradoxical embolism refers to emboli that arise in the venous circulation and bypass the lungs by traveling through an incompletely closed foramen ovale, subsequently entering the left side of the heart and blocking flow to the systemic arteries. Since the pressure in the left atrium usually exceeds that in the right, most of these cases occur in the context of a right-to-left shunt (see Chapter 11).

Systemic Arterial Embolism Often Causes Infarcts

Thromboembolism

The heart is the most common source of arterial thromboemboli (Fig. 7-14), which usually arise from mural thrombi (Fig. 7-15) or diseased valves. These emboli tend to lodge at points where the vessel lumen narrows abruptly (e.g., at bifurcations or in the area of an atherosclerotic plaque). The viability of the tissue supplied by the vessel depends on the availability of collateral circulation and on the fate of the embolus itself. The thromboembolus may propagate locally and lead to a more severe obstruction or it may fragment and lyse. Organs that suffer the most from arterial thromboembolism include the following:

- **Brain:** Arterial emboli to the brain cause ischemic necrosis of brain tissue (strokes).
- **Intestine:** In the mesenteric circulation, emboli cause infarction of the bowel, a complication that manifests as an acute abdomen and requires immediate surgery.
- **Lower extremity:** Embolism of an artery of the leg leads to sudden pain, absence of pulses, and a cold limb. In some cases, the limb must be amputated.

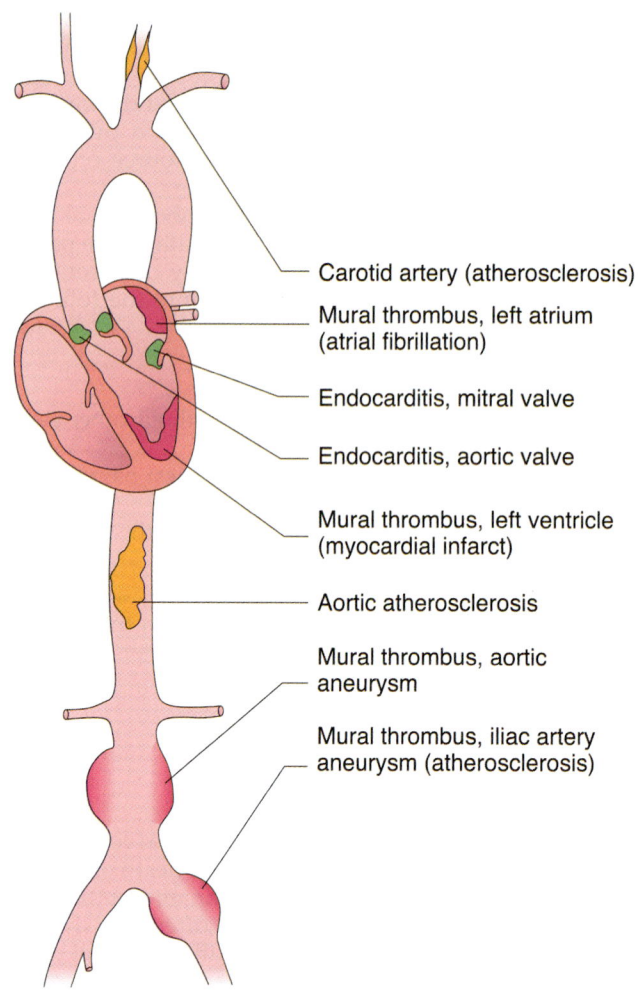

FIGURE 7-14
Sources of arterial emboli.

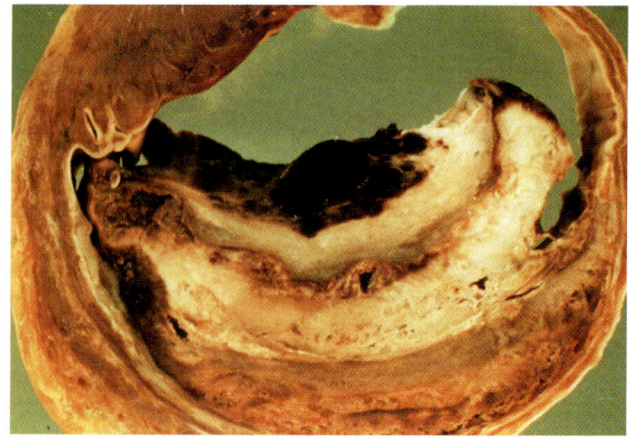

FIGURE 7-15
Mural thrombus of the left ventricle. A laminated thrombus adheres to the endocardium overlying a healed aneurysmal myocardial infarct.

- **Kidney:** Renal artery embolism may infarct the entire kidney but more commonly results in small peripheral infarcts.
- **Heart:** Coronary artery embolism and resulting myocardial infarcts are reported but are rare.

The more common sites of infarction from arterial emboli are summarized in Figure 7-16.

Air Embolism

Air may be introduced into the venous circulation through neck wounds, thoracocentesis, punctures of the great veins during invasive procedures, or hemodialysis. Small amounts of circulating air in the form of bubbles are of little consequence, but quantities of 100 mL or more can lead to sudden death. Air bubbles tend to coalesce and physically obstruct the flow of blood in the right side of the heart, the pulmonary circulation, and the brain. On histological examination, bubbles of air, which appear as empty spaces, can be seen in the capillaries and small vessels of the lung.

Persons exposed to increased atmospheric pressure, such as scuba divers and workers in underwater occupations (e.g., tunnels, drilling platform construction) are subject to *decompression sickness,* a unique form of gas embolism. During descent, large amounts of inert gas (nitrogen or helium) are dissolved in bodily fluids. When the diver ascends, the gas is released from solution and exhaled. However, if the ascent is too rapid, gas bubbles form in the circulation and within tissues, obstructing blood flow and directly injuring cells. Air embolism is the second most common cause of death in sport diving (drowning being the first).

Acute decompression sickness, commonly known as "the bends," is characterized by temporary muscular and joint pain, owing to small vessel obstruction in these tissues. However, involvement of the cerebral blood vessels may be severe enough to cause coma or even death.

Caisson disease refers to decompression sickness in which the vascular obstruction causes multiple foci of ischemic (avascular) necrosis of bone, particularly affecting the head of the femur, tibia, and humerus. This complication was originally described in construction workers in diving bells (or caissons).

Amniotic Fluid Embolism

Amniotic fluid embolism refers to the entry of amniotic fluid containing fetal cells and debris into the maternal circulation through open uterine and cervical veins. It is a rare maternal complication of childbirth, but when it occurs, it is often catastrophic. This disorder usually occurs at the end of labor when the pulmonary emboli are composed of the solid epithelial constituents (squames) contained in the amniotic fluid (Fig. 7-17). Of greater importance is the initiation of a potentially fatal consumptive coagulopathy caused by the high thromboplastin activity of amniotic fluid.

The clinical presentation of amniotic fluid embolism can be dramatic, with the sudden onset of cyanosis and shock, followed by coma and death. If the mother survives this acute episode, she may die of disseminated intravascular coagulation. Should she overcome this complication, she is at substantial risk of developing acute respiratory distress syndrome. Minor amniotic fluid embolism is probably a common asymptomatic event, since autopsies of mothers who have died of other causes in the perinatal period frequently show evidence of this complication.

Fat Embolism

Fat embolism describes the release of emboli of fatty marrow (Fig. 7-18A) *into damaged blood vessels following severe trauma to fat-containing tissue, particularly accompanying bone fractures.* In most instances, fat embolism is clinically inapparent. However, cases of severe fat embolism are marked by the development of a *fat embolism syndrome,* which appears 1 to 3 days after the injury. In its most severe form, which may be fatal,

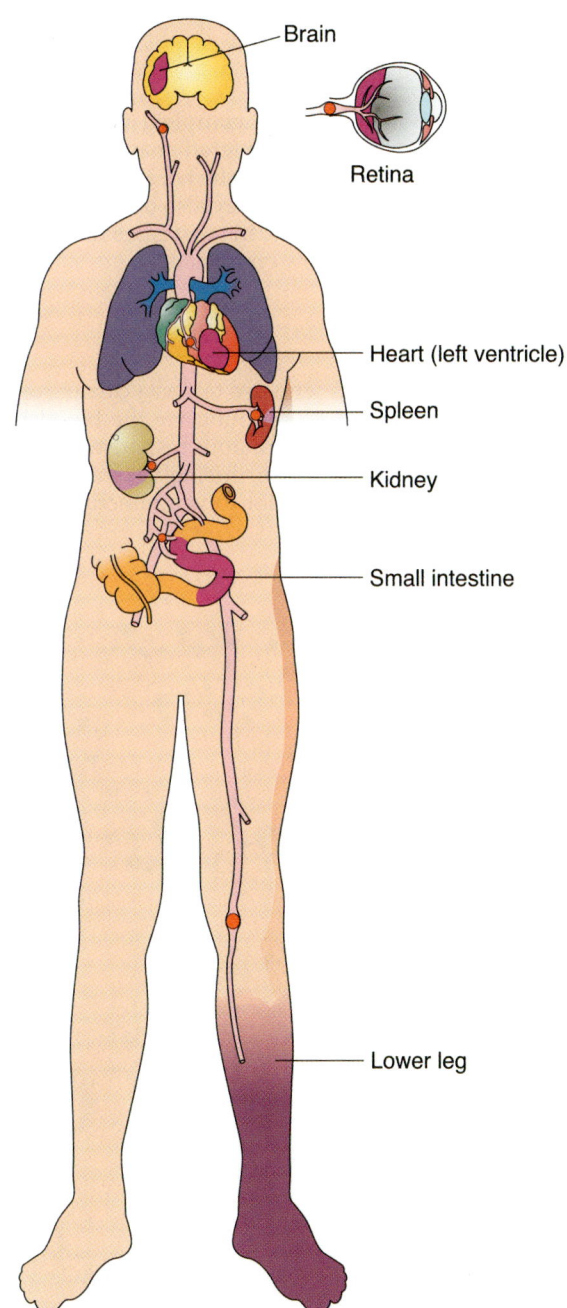

FIGURE 7-16
Common sites of infarction from arterial emboli.

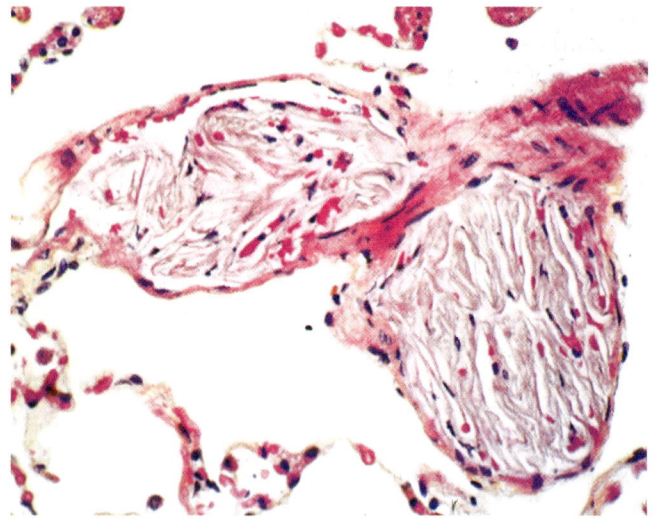

FIGURE 7-17
Amniotic fluid embolism. A section of lung shows pulmonary capillaries distended by epithelial squames.

this syndrome is characterized by respiratory failure, mental changes, thrombocytopenia, and widespread petechiae. A chest radiograph reveals diffuse opacity of the lungs, which may progress to a "whiteout" typical of adult respiratory distress syndrome. At autopsy, innumerable fat globules are seen in the microvasculature of the lungs (Fig. 7-18B) and brain, and sometimes other organs in such cases. The lungs typically exhibit the changes of adult respiratory distress syndrome (see Chapter 12). The lesions in the brain include cerebral edema, small hemorrhages and occasionally microinfarcts.

Fat embolism is usually considered a direct consequence of trauma, with fat entering ruptured capillaries at the site of the fracture. However, this explanation may be too simplistic. It has been suggested that hemorrhage into the marrow cavity and perhaps also into the subcutaneous fat increases the interstitial pressure above capillary pressure, so that fat is forced into the circulation. Moreover, there is more fat in the pulmonary vascular system than can be accounted for by the simple transfer of fat from peripheral depots. In addition, the chemical composition of the fat in the lung differs from that in tissue. Finally, there is a discrepancy between the frequency of fat embolism and bone marrow embolism.

Bone Marrow Embolism

Bone marrow emboli to the lungs, complete with hematopoietic cells and fat, are often encountered at autopsy after cardiac resuscitation, a procedure in which fractures of the sternum and ribs commonly occur. They also occasionally occur after fractures of the long bones. In most cases no symptoms are attributed to bone marrow embolism.

Miscellaneous Pulmonary Emboli

Intravenous drug abusers who use talc as a carrier for illicit drugs may introduce it into the lung via the bloodstream. **Talc emboli** produce a granulomatous response in the lungs (Fig. 7-19). **Cotton emboli** are surprisingly common and are due to cleansing of the skin prior to venipuncture. **Schisto-**

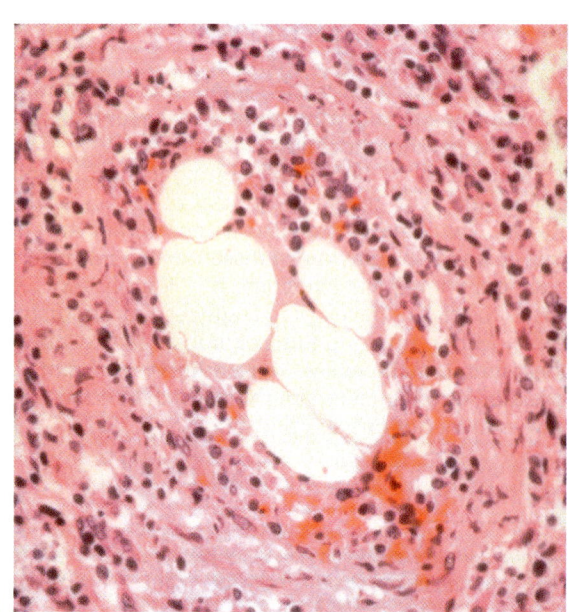
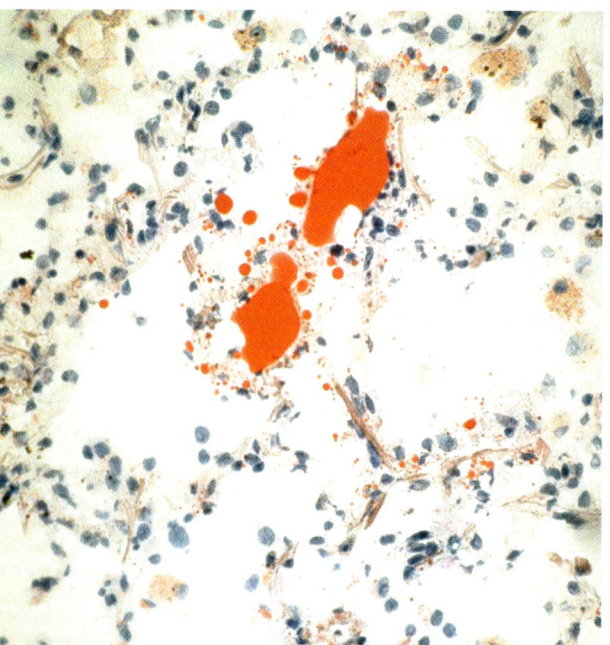

FIGURE 7-18
Fat embolism. A. The lumen of a small pulmonary artery is occluded by a fragment of bone marrow consisting of fat cells and hematopoietic elements. **B.** A frozen section of lung stained with Sudan red shows capillaries occluded by red-staining fat emboli.

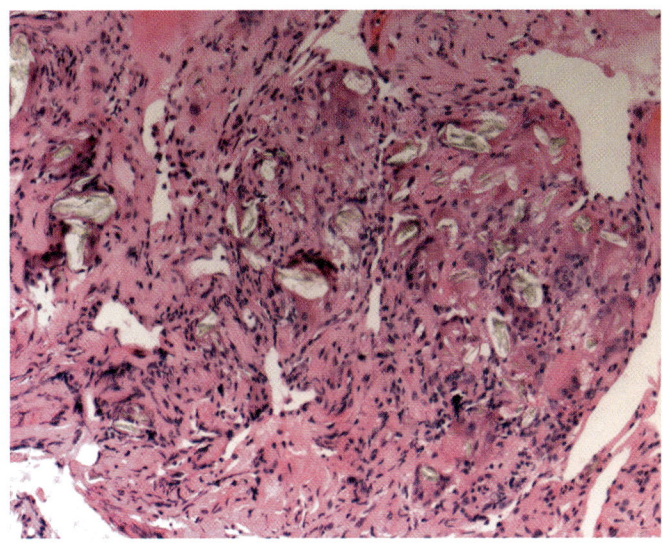 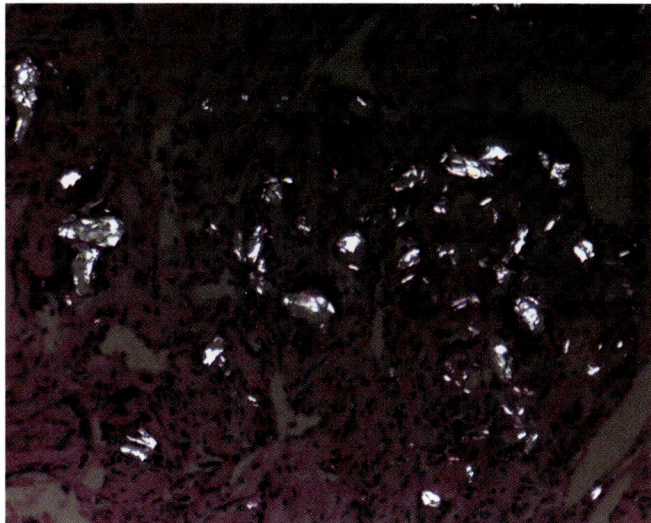

FIGURE 7-19
Talc emboli. A section of lung from an intravenous drug abuser shows talc particles before (A) and after (B) polarization of light (×125).

somiasis may be associated with the embolization of ova to the lungs from the bladder or the gut, in which case they incite a foreign body granulomatous reaction. **Tumor emboli** are occasionally seen in the lung during hematogenous dissemination of cancer.

INFARCTION

Infarction is defined as the process by which coagulative necrosis develops in an area distal to the occlusion of an end-artery. The necrotic zone is termed an *infarct*. Infarcts of vital organs such as the heart, brain, and intestine are serious medical conditions and are major causes of morbidity and mortality. If the victim survives, the infarct heals with a scar. Partial arterial occlusion (i.e., stenosis) occasionally causes necrosis, but more commonly, it results in a variety of atrophic changes associated with chronic ischemia. For example, in the heart these changes include vacuolization of cardiac myocytes, atrophy, loss of muscle cell myofibrils, and interstitial fibrosis.

Pathology: The gross and microscopic appearance of an infarct depends on its location and age. Upon arterial occlusion, the area supplied by the vessel rapidly becomes swollen and deep red. Microscopically, vascular dilation and congestion and occasionally interstitial hemorrhage are noted. Subsequently, several types of infarcts are distinguishable by gross examination.

Pale infarcts are typical in the heart, kidneys, and spleen (Fig. 7-20), although certain infarcts in the kidney may be cystic. *Dry gangrene* of the leg due to arterial occlusion (often noted in diabetes) is actually a large pale infarct. On gross examination, 1 or 2 days after the initial hyperemia, the infarct becomes soft, sharply delineated, and light yellow (Fig. 7-21). The border tends to be dark red, reflecting hemorrhage into the surrounding viable tissue. Microscopically, a pale infarct exhibits uniform coagulative necrosis.

Red infarcts may result from either arterial or venous occlusion and are also characterized by coagulative necrosis. However, they are distinguished by bleeding into the necrotic area from adjacent arteries and veins. Red infarcts occur principally in organs with a dual blood supply, such as the lung, or those with extensive collateral circulation, such as the small intestine and brain. In the heart, a red infarct occurs when the infarcted area is reperfused, as may occur following spontaneous or therapeutically-induced lysis of the occluding thrombus. Grossly, red infarcts are sharply circumscribed, firm, and dark red to purple (Fig. 7-22). Over a period of several days, acute inflammatory cells infiltrate the necrotic area from the viable border. The cellular debris is phagocytosed and digested by polymorphonuclear leukocytes and later by macrophages. Granulation tissue eventu-

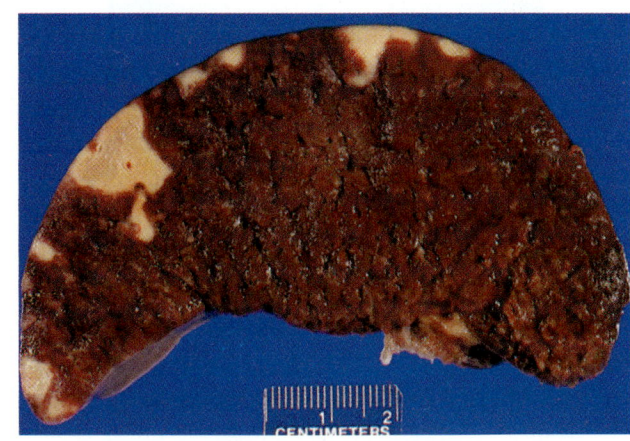

FIGURE 7-20
Spleen infarcts. A cut section of spleen displays multiple pale, wedge-shaped infarcts beneath the capsule.

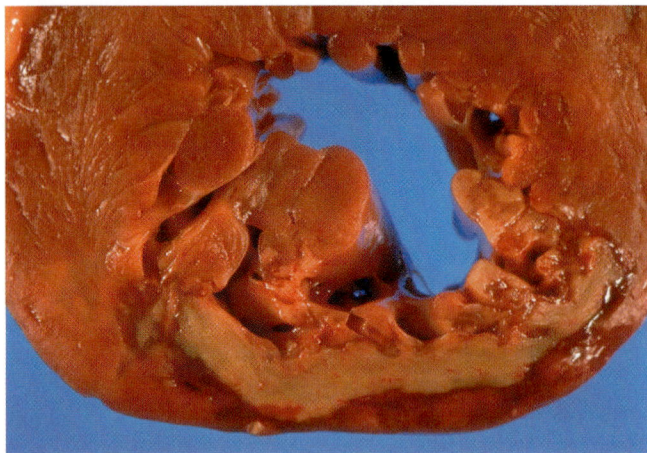

FIGURE 7-21
Acute myocardial infarct. A cross-section of the left ventricle reveals a sharply circumscribed, soft, yellow area of necrosis in the posterior free wall.

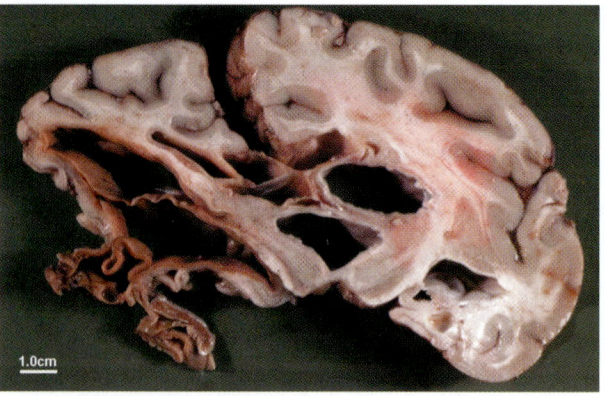

FIGURE 7-23
Cystic infarct. A cross-section of brain in the frontal plane shows a healed cystic infarct.

ally forms, to be replaced ultimately by a scar. In a large infarct of an organ such as the heart or kidney, the necrotic center remains inaccessible to the inflammatory exudate and may persist for months. In the brain, an infarct typically undergoes liquefactive necrosis and may become a fluid-filled cyst, which is (not surprisingly) referred to as a *cystic infarct* (Fig. 7-23).

A *septic infarct* results when the necrotic tissue of an infarct is seeded by pyogenic bacteria and becomes infected. Pulmonary infarcts are not uncommonly infected, presumably because the necrotic tissue offers little resistance to inhaled bacteria. In the case of bacterial endocarditis, the emboli themselves are infected and the resulting infarcts are often septic. A septic infarct may become a frank abscess (Fig. 7-24).

Infarction in Specific Locations Is Often Fatal

Myocardial Infarcts

Myocardial infarcts are transmural (through the entire wall) or subendocardial. A transmural infarct results from complete occlusion of a major extramural coronary artery. Subendocardial infarction reflects prolonged ischemia caused by partially occluding, atherosclerotic, stenotic lesions of the coronary arteries when the requirement for oxygen exceeds the supply. Such a situation prevails in disorders such as shock, anoxia, or severe tachycardia (rapid pulse). A myocardial infarct may be pale or red, depending

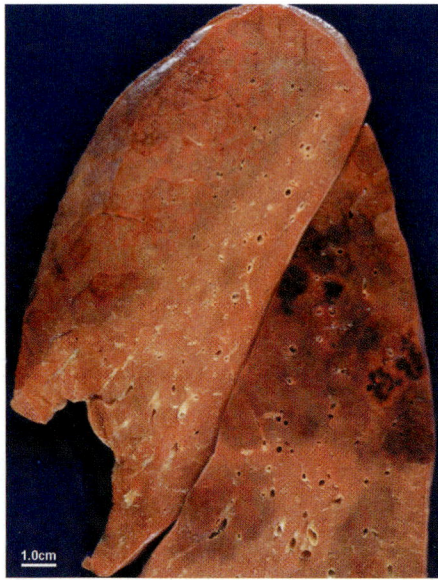

FIGURE 7-22
Red infarct. A sagittal slice of lung shows a hemorrhagic infarct in upper segments of the lower lobe.

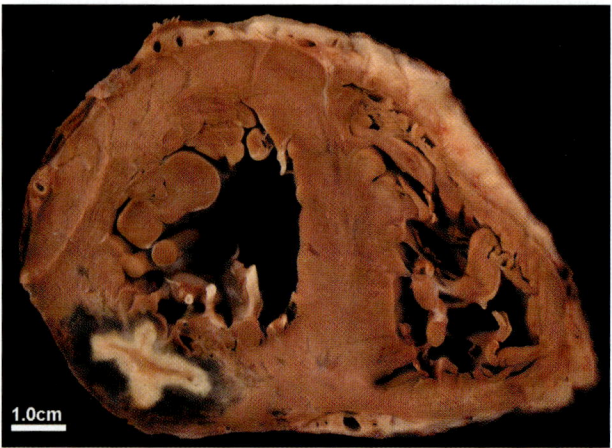

FIGURE 7-24
Septic infarct. A myocardial abscess within the left ventricular free wall was due to infection with *Staphylococcus aureus*.

upon the extent of reflow of blood into the infarcted area (Fig. 7-25).

Pulmonary Infarcts

Only about 10% of pulmonary emboli elicit clinical symptoms referable to pulmonary infarction, usually after occlusion of a middle-sized pulmonary artery. Infarction occurs only if the circulation from the bronchial arteries inadequately compensates for the loss of supply from the pulmonary arteries. This circumstance is often found in congestive heart failure, although stasis in the pulmonary circulation may contribute. Hemorrhage into the alveolar spaces of the necrotic lining tissue occurs within 48 hours.

Cerebral Infarcts

Infarction of the brain may result from local ischemia or a generalized reduction in blood flow. The latter often results from systemic hypotension, as in shock, and produces infarction in the border zones between the distributions of the major cerebral arteries (*watershed infarct*). If prolonged, severe hypotension can cause widespread brain necrosis. The occlusion of a single vessel in the brain (e.g., after an embolus has lodged) causes ischemia and necrosis in a well-defined area. This type of cerebral infarct may be pale or red, the latter being common with embolic occlusions. The occlusion of a large artery produces a wide area of necrosis, which may ultimately resolve as a large fluid-filled cavity in the brain.

Intestinal Infarcts

The earliest tissue changes in intestinal ischemia are necrosis of the tips of the villi in the small intestine and necrosis of the superficial mucosa in the large intestine. In either case, more-severe ischemia leads to hemorrhagic necrosis of the submucosa and muscularis but not the serosa. Small mucosal infarcts heal in a few days, but more severe injury leads to ulceration. These ulcers can eventually reepithelialize. However, if the ulcers are large, they are repaired by scar tissue, a process that may lead to strictures. Severe transmural necrosis is associated with massive bleeding or bowel perforation, complications that often result in irreversible shock, sepsis, and death.

EDEMA

Edema refers to the presence of excess fluid in the interstitial spaces of the body and may be local or generalized. **Local edema** in most instances occurs with inflammation, the "tumor" of "tumor, rubor, and calor." Local edema of a limb, usually the leg, results from venous or lymphatic obstruction. Burns cause prominent local edema by disrupting the permeability of the local vasculature. Local edema may be a prominent component of an immune reaction, for example, urticaria (hives) or edema of the epiglottis or larynx (angioneurotic edema).

Generalized edema, affecting the visceral organs and the skin of the trunk and lower extremities (Fig. 7-26), reflects a global disorder of fluid and electrolyte metabolism, most often occasioned by heart failure. Generalized edema is also seen in certain renal diseases associated with loss of serum proteins to the urine (nephrotic syndrome) and in cirrhosis of the liver. *Anasarca* refers to extreme generalized edema, a condition evidenced by conspicuous fluid accumulation in the subcutaneous tissues, visceral organs, and body cavities. Edema fluid may accumulate in body spaces, such as the pleural cavity (*hydrothorax*), peritoneal cavity (*ascites*), or pericardial cavity (*hydropericardium*).

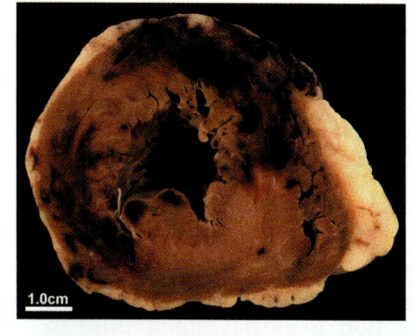
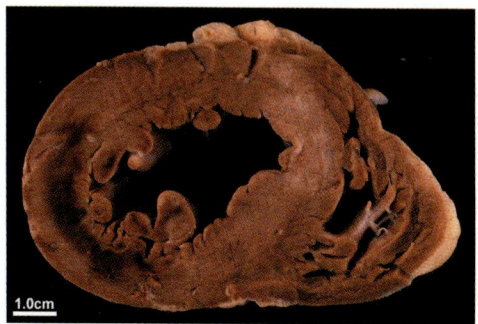

FIGURE 7-25
Myocardial infarction. Transverse sections of ventricular myocardium show reperfused (A), acute and healed together (B), and healed (C) infarction. Reperfusion is typically associated with hemorrhage as in (A) and (B).

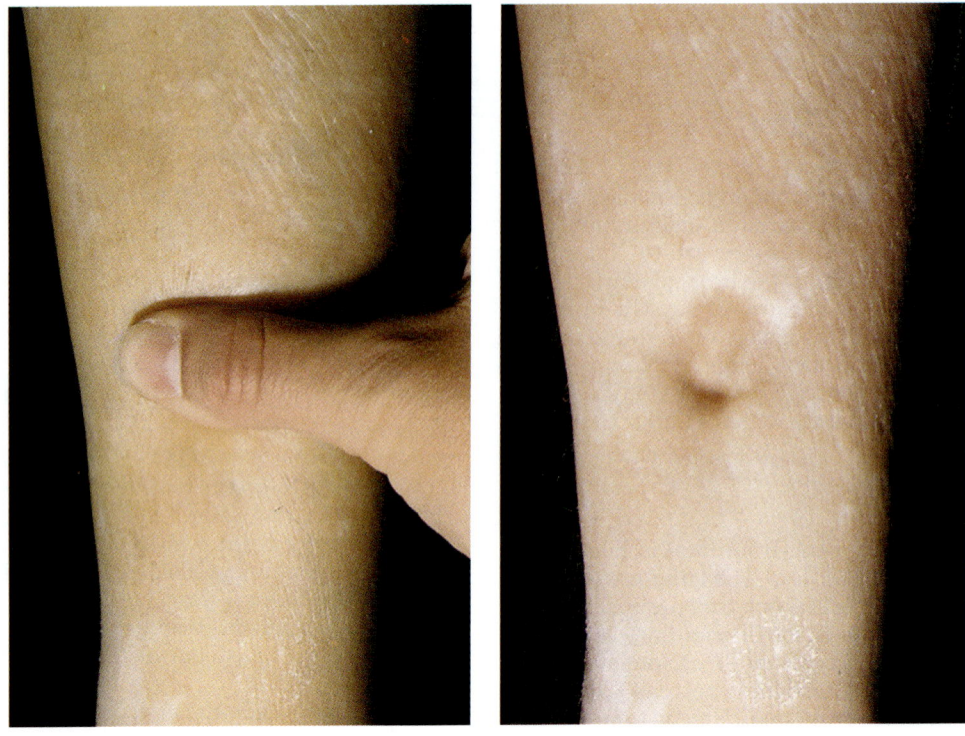

FIGURE 7-26
Pitting edema of the leg. A. In a patient with congestive heart failure, severe edema of the leg is demonstrated by applying pressure with a finger. B, The resulting "pitting" reflects the inelasticity of the fluid-filled tissue.

Normal Capillary Filtration

The normal formation and retention of interstitial fluid depends on filtration and reabsorption at the level of the capillaries (Starling forces). In the arteriolar segment of the capillary, the internal or hydrostatic pressure is 32 mm Hg, and at the middle of the capillary, it is 20 mm. Since the interstitial hydrostatic pressure is only 3 mm Hg, there is an outward fluid filtration of 14 mL/min. The hydrostatic pressure is opposed by the oncotic pressure of the plasma (26 mm Hg), which results in an osmotic reabsorption of 12 mL/min at the venous end of the capillary. Thus, interstitial fluid is formed at the rate of 2 mL/min and is reabsorbed by the lymphatics, so that in equilibrium there is no net fluid gain or loss in the interstitium.

Sodium and Water Metabolism

Water represents 50 to 70% of body weight and comprises two major compartments—the extracellular and the intracellular fluid spaces. Extracellular fluid is further divided into interstitial and vascular compartments. Interstitial fluid constitutes about 75% of the extracellular compartment.

Total body sodium is the principal determinant of extracellular fluid volume because it is the major cation that determines the osmolality of the extracellular fluid. In other words, an increase in total body sodium must be balanced by more extracellular water to maintain constant osmolality. The control of extracellular fluid volume depends to a large extent on the regulation of renal sodium excretion, which is influenced by (1) atrial natriuretic factor, (2) the renin–angiotensin system of the juxtaglomerular apparatus, and (3) sympathetic nervous system activity (see Chapter 10).

Edema Caused by Increased Hydrostatic Pressure

It is intuitively clear that an unopposed increase in hydrostatic pressure will result in greater filtration of fluid into the interstitial space and its retention as edema. Such a situation is particularly prominent in the case of decompensated heart disease, in which back-pressure in the lungs secondary to failure of the left ventricle leads to acute pulmonary edema, and failure of the right side of the heart contributes to systemic edema. Similarly, back-pressure caused by venous obstruction in the lower extremity causes edema of the leg. Obstruction to portal blood flow in cirrhosis of the liver contributes to the formation of abdominal fluid (ascites).

Edema Caused by Decreased Oncotic Pressure

The difference in pressure between the intravascular and interstitial compartments is largely determined by the concentration of plasma proteins, especially that of albumin. Any condition that lowers plasma albumin levels, whether it is albuminuria in the nephrotic syndrome or reduced albumin synthesis in chronic liver disease or severe malnutrition, tends to promote generalized edema.

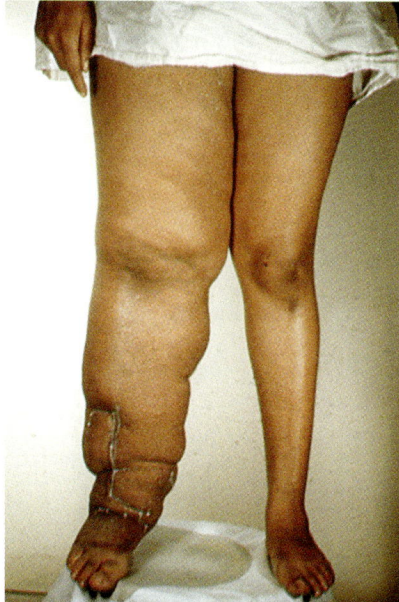

FIGURE 7-27
Edema secondary to lymphatic obstruction. Massive edema of the right lower extremity (elephantiasis) in a patient with obstruction of the lymphatic drainage.

Edema Caused by Lymphatic Obstruction

Under normal circumstances, more fluid is filtered into the interstitial spaces than is reabsorbed into the vascular bed. This excess interstitial fluid is removed by the lymphatics. Thus, obstruction to the lymphatic flow leads to localized edema formation. Lymphatic channels can be obstructed by (1) malignant neoplasms, (2) fibrosis resulting from inflammation or irradiation, and (3) surgical ablation. For instance, the inflammatory response to filarial worms (Bancroftian and Malayan filariasis) can result in lymphatic obstruction that produces massive lymphedema of the scrotum and lower extremities *(elephantiasis)* (Fig. 7-27). Lymphedema of the upper extremity often complicates radical mastectomies for cancer of the breast, owing to the removal of the axillary lymph nodes and lymphatics.

Lymphatic edema differs from other forms of edema in its high protein content, since lymph is the vehicle by which proteins and interstitial cells are returned to the circulation. The increased protein concentration may be a fibrogenic stimulus in the formation of dermal fibrosis in chronic edema (indurated edema).

The Role of Sodium Retention in Edema

Generalized edema and ascites invariably reflect an increased total body sodium content, as a consequence of sodium retention by the kidneys. When peripheral edema is first clinically detectable, the extracellular fluid volume has already expanded by at least 5 L. The most common conditions in which generalized edema is found include congestive heart failure, cirrhosis of the liver, nephrotic syndrome, and some cases of chronic renal insufficiency. The mechanisms of edema formation and representative disorders associated with them are summarized in Figure 7-28 and Table 7-1.

Congestive Heart Failure Is the Consequence of Inadequate Cardiac Output

It is estimated that two to three million people in the United States have congestive heart failure, and 15% die annually. In fact, half of all patients with congestive heart failure who require admission to the hospital will die within 1 year. In the United States, this disorder is most commonly associated with ischemic heart disease, although virtually any chronic cardiac disorder may eventuate in congestive heart failure (see Chapter 11).

 Pathogenesis: The argument regarding the relative contributions of "forward failure" (low cardiac output) versus "backward failure" (venous congestion) in the pathogenesis of the edema of congestive heart failure is no longer a burning issue. It is now recognized that both systolic and diastolic dysfunction contribute to the low cardiac output and high ventricular filling pressure characteristic of congestive heart failure, although systolic dysfunction is more important in most patients.

The inadequacy of the cardiac output in congestive heart failure leads to a decreased glomerular filtration rate and increased secretion of renin. The latter activates angiotensin, leading to the release of aldosterone, subsequent sodium reabsorption, and fluid retention. Furthermore, reduced blood flow to the liver impairs the catabolism of aldosterone, thereby further raising its concentration in the blood. As a compensatory mechanism, increased fluid volume preserves an adequate intracardiac pressure. In addition, increased sympathetic discharge leads to augmented

TABLE 7-1 **Disorders Associated with Edema**

Increased hydrostatic pressure	
Arteriolar dilation	Inflammation
	Heat
Increased venous pressure	Venous thrombosis
	Congestive heart failure
	Cirrhosis (ascites)
	Postural inactivity (e.g., prolonged standing)
Hypervolemia	Sodium retention (e.g., decreased renal function)
Decreased oncotic pressure	
Hypoproteinemia	Nephrotic syndrome
	Cirrhosis
	Protein-losing gastroenteropathy
	Malnutrition
Increased capillary permeability	Inflammation
	Burns
	Adult respiratory distress syndrome
Lymphatic obstruction	Cancer
	Postsurgical lymphedema
	Inflammation

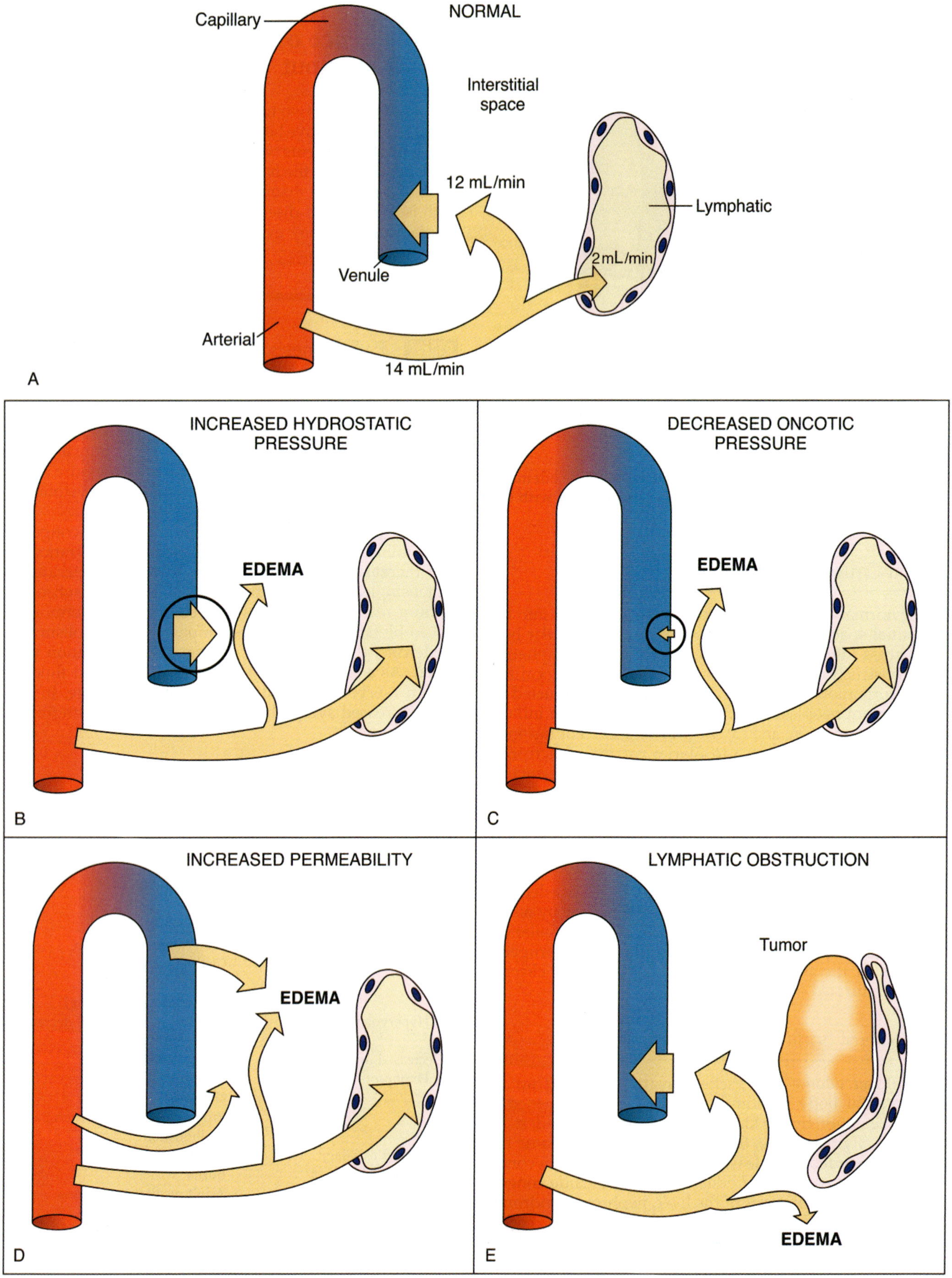

300 Hemodynamic Disorders

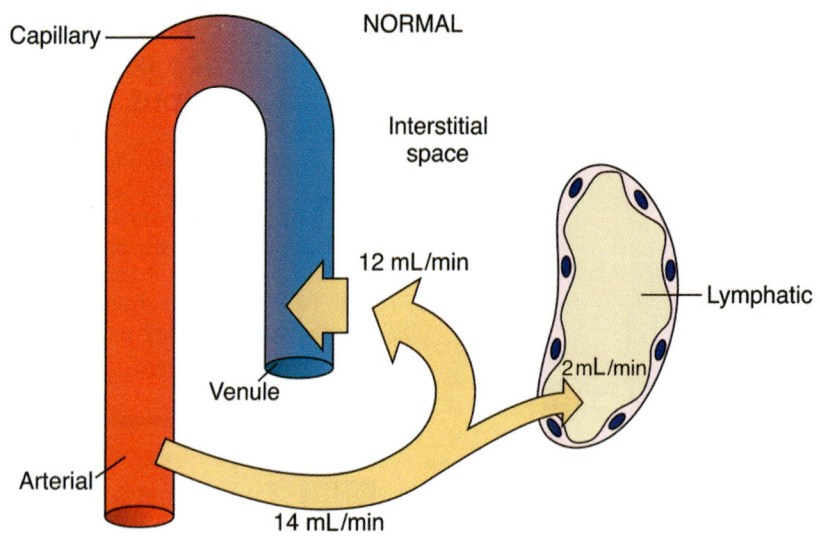

levels of catecholamines, which stimulate cardiac contractility, and further counteract the impairment in cardiac performance. At the same time, distention of the atria by the increased blood volume promotes the release of atrial natriuretic peptide, which stimulates sodium excretion by the kidney.

After long-standing heart failure, these compensatory mechanisms fail, in which case renal sodium retention again becomes important. The further expansion of plasma volume leads to an increase in pulmonary and systemic venous pressure, which produces increased hydrostatic pressure in the respective capillary beds. The increased capillary pressure, together with decreased plasma oncotic pressure, results in the edema of congestive heart failure.

 Pathology: Failure of the left ventricle is associated principally with passive congestion of the lungs and pulmonary edema (Fig. 7-29). When chronic, these conditions lead to pulmonary hypertension and eventual failure of the right ventricle. Right ventricular failure is characterized by generalized subcutaneous edema (most prominent in the dependent portions of the body), ascites, and pleural effusions. The liver, spleen, and other splanchnic organs are typically congested. At autopsy, the heart is enlarged and its chambers dilated (Fig. 7-30).

 Clinical Features: The effects of heart failure depend upon which ventricle is failing, recognizing that both may be in failure simultaneously. Patients in left-sided congestive heart failure complain of shortness of breath *(dyspnea)* on exertion and when recumbent *(orthopnea)*. They may be awakened from sleep by sudden episodes of shortness of breath *(paroxysmal nocturnal dyspnea)*. Physical examination usually reveals distended jugular veins. Persons with right-sided failure have pitting edema of the lower extremities and an enlarged and tender liver. When ascites is present, the abdomen is distended. Patients in congestive heart failure with pulmonary edema have crackling breath sounds *(rales)* caused by the expansion of fluid-filled alveoli.

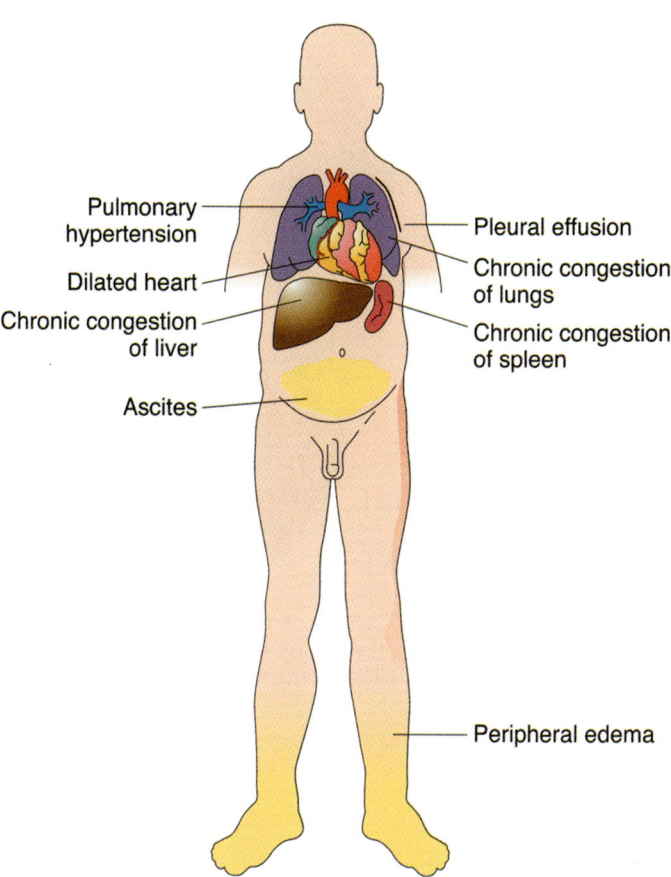

FIGURE 7-29
Pathological consequences of chronic congestive heart failure.

Pulmonary Edema Features Increased Fluid in the Alveolar Spaces and Interstitium of the Lung

This condition leads to decreased gas exchange in the lung, causing hypoxia and retention of carbon dioxide (hypercapnia).

FIGURE 7-28
The capillary system and mechanisms of edema formation. A. Normal. The differential between the hydrostatic and oncotic pressures at the arterial end of the capillary system is responsible for the filtration into the interstitial space of approximately 14 mL of fluid per minute. This fluid is reabsorbed at the venous end at the rate of 12 mL/min. It is also drained through the lymphatic capillaries at a rate of 2 mL/min. Proteins are removed by the lymphatics from the interstitial space. B. Hydrostatic edema. If the hydrostatic pressure at the venous end of the capillary system is elevated, reabsorption decreases. As long as the lymphatics can drain the surplus fluid, no edema results. If their capacity is exceeded, however, edema fluid accumulates. C. Oncotic edema. Edema fluid also accumulates if reabsorption is diminished by decreased oncotic pressure of the vascular bed, owing to a loss of albumin. D. Inflammatory and traumatic edema. Edema, either local or systemic, results if the vascular bed becomes leaky following injury to the endothelium. E. Lymphedema. Lymphatic obstruction causes the accumulation of interstitial fluid because of insufficient reabsorption and deficient removal of proteins, the latter increasing the oncotic pressure of the fluid in the interstitial space.

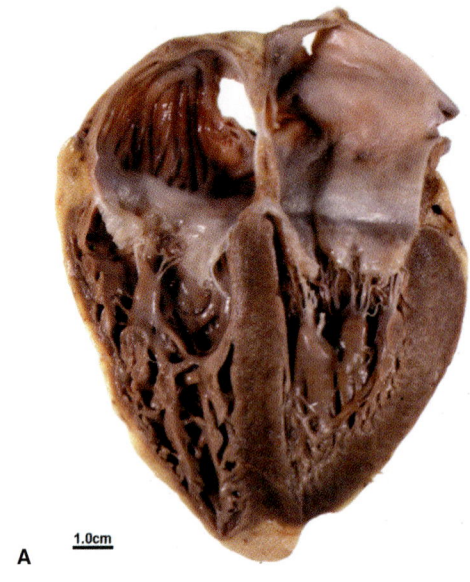
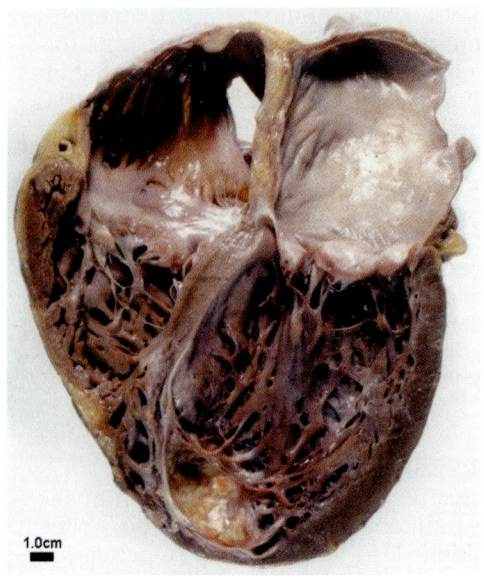

FIGURE 7-30
Congestive heart failure. A normal heart (A) contrasts with a heart dilated because of chronic heart failure secondary to ischemic injury (B).

 Pathogenesis and Pathology: The lung is a loose tissue without much connective tissue support and, therefore, requires certain conditions to prevent the development of edema. Among these protective devices are the following:

- Low perfusion pressure in the lung capillaries, owing to low right ventricular pressure
- Effective drainage of the interstitial space of the lung by lymphatics, which are under a slightly negative pressure and can accommodate up to 10 times the regular lymph flow
- Tight cellular junctions between endothelial cells, which control capillary permeability

If the above-mentioned protective mechanisms are disturbed, pulmonary edema results. The most common causes of pulmonary edema relate to hemodynamic alterations in the heart that increase the perfusion pressure in the pulmonary capillaries and block effective lymphatic drainage. These conditions include left ventricular failure (the most common cause), mitral stenosis, and mitral insufficiency. Disruption of capillary permeability is the cause of pulmonary edema in acute lung injury associated with adult respiratory distress syndrome, inhalation of toxic gases, aspiration of gastric contents, viral infections, and uremia. Acute lung injury is reflected in destruction of endothelial cells or disruption of their tight junctions.

Pulmonary edema may be interstitial or alveolar. Interstitial edema represents the earliest phase and is an exaggeration of the normal process of fluid filtration. Lymphatics become distended, and fluid accumulates in the interstitium of the lobular septa and around veins and bronchovascular bundles. Radiological examination reveals a reticulonodular pattern, more marked in the bases of the lung. Lobular septa become edematous and produce linear shadows (*Kerley B lines*) on the chest radiograph. Edema results in the shunting of blood flow from the bases to the upper lobes of the lungs, and increased airflow resistance occurs because of edema of the bronchovascular tree. Patients are often asymptomatic in this early stage.

When the fluid can no longer be contained in the interstitial space, it spills into the alveoli, a condition termed *alveolar edema*. At this stage, a radiological alveolar pattern is seen, usually worse in the central portions of the lung and in the lower zones. The patient becomes acutely short of breath, and bubbly rales are heard. In extreme cases, frothy fluid is coughed up or wells up out of the trachea.

Microscopic examination of the edematous lung reveals severely congested alveolar capillaries and alveoli filled with a homogeneous, pink-staining fluid permeated by air bubbles (see Fig. 7-4). In cases of pulmonary edema caused by alveolar damage, cell debris, fibrin, and proteins form films of proteinaceous material, called *hyaline membranes,* in the alveoli (Fig. 7-31).

 Clinical Features: Pulmonary fluid accumulation may go unnoticed initially, but eventually dyspnea and coughing become prominent. If the edema is severe, large amounts of frothy, often pink sputum are expectorated. Hypoxemia is manifested as cyanosis.

Pulmonary function is restricted in severe congestion and in interstitial pulmonary edema because the accumulation of fluid in the interstitial space causes reduced compliance (i.e., stiffening of the lung tissue). Thus, increased respiratory work is required to maintain ventilation. Since the alveolar walls are thickened, there is a greater barrier to the exchange of oxygen and carbon dioxide. The exchange of carbon dioxide is less affected than that of oxygen, a situation that results in hypoxia with near-normal carbon

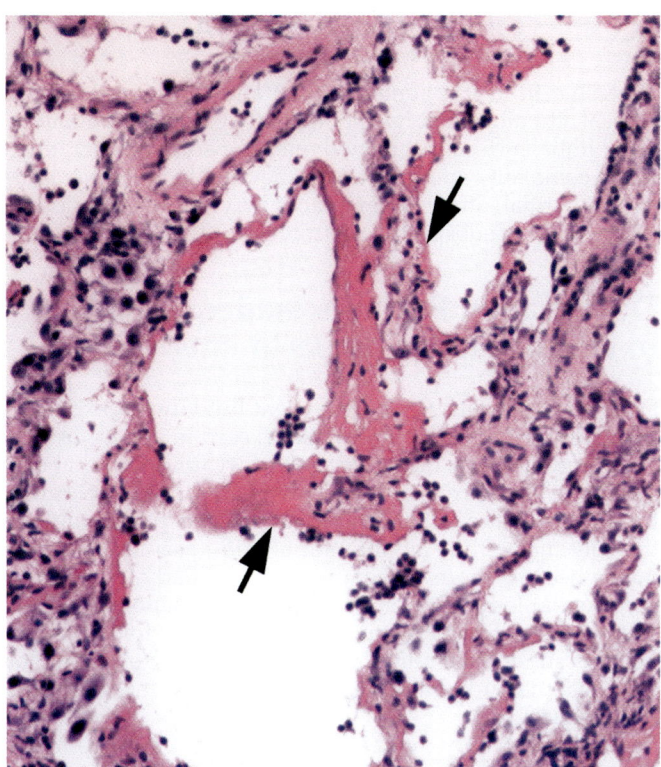

FIGURE 7-31
Pulmonary edema due to diffuse alveolar damage. A section of lung shows hyaline membranes (arrows) in alveoli.

dioxide levels. Mismatch between ventilation (which is reduced) and perfusion (which persists) contributes to the development of hypoxemia in patients with pulmonary edema.

Edema in Cirrhosis of the Liver Is Commonly an End-Stage Condition

Cirrhosis of the liver is often accompanied by ascites and peripheral edema. Scarring of the liver obstructs the portal blood flow and leads to portal hypertension, a condition that increases the hydrostatic pressure in the splanchnic circulation. This situation is compounded by decreased hepatic synthesis of albumin as a result of liver dysfunction. The consequent accumulation of peritoneal fluid leads to a lower effective blood volume, which results in renal retention of sodium by mechanisms similar to those that are operative in congestive heart failure. Alternatively, chronic liver disease itself causes renal retention of sodium. The subsequent expansion of extracellular fluid volume further promotes ascites and edema, thus establishing a vicious circle. In addition, the increased transudation of lymph from the liver capsule adds to the accumulation of fluid in the abdomen.

The Nephrotic Syndrome Reflects Massive Proteinuria

In the nephrotic syndrome, the magnitude of protein loss in the urine exceeds the rate at which it is replaced by the liver. The resulting decline in the concentration of plasma proteins, particularly albumin, reduces the oncotic pressure of the plasma and promotes edema. The ensuing decrease in blood volume stimulates the renin–angiotensin–aldosterone mechanism, leading to sodium retention. The edema is generalized but appears preferentially in soft connective tissues, the eyes, the eyelids, and subcutaneous tissues. Ascites and pleural effusions also occur.

Cerebral Edema Often Causes a Fatal Increase in Intracranial Pressure

Edema of the brain is dangerous because the confined space of the cranium allows little room for expansion. Increased intracranial pressure from edema compromises the blood supply, distorts the gross structure of the brain, and interferes with the function of the central nervous system (see Chapter 28). Cerebral edema is divided into vasogenic, cytotoxic, and interstitial forms.

Vasogenic edema, the most common variety of edema, refers to excess fluid in the extracellular space of the brain. It results from increased vascular permeability, principally in the white matter. The tight endothelial junctions of the blood–brain barrier are disrupted, and fluid filters into the interstitial space. Clinical disorders associated with cerebral vasogenic edema include trauma, neoplasms, encephalitis, abscesses, infarcts, hemorrhage, and toxic brain injury (e.g., lead poisoning).

Cytotoxic edema is equivalent to hydropic cell swelling (i.e., the accumulation of intracellular water). It is usually a response to cell injury, such as that produced by ischemia. Cytotoxic cerebral edema preferentially affects the gray matter.

Interstitial edema is a consequence of hydrocephalus, in which fluid accumulates in the cerebral ventricles and periventricular white matter.

At autopsy, the edematous brain is soft and heavy. The gyri are flattened, and the sulci narrowed. Because of alterations in brain function, patients with cerebral edema suffer vomiting, disorientation, and convulsions. Severe cerebral edema leads to herniation of the cerebral tonsils, ordinarily a lethal event.

Fluid Accumulation in Body Cavities Represents Extensions of the Interstitial Space

The Pleural Space

Pleural effusion (fluid in the pleural space) is a straw-colored transudate of low specific gravity that contains few cells (mainly exfoliated mesothelial cells). Fluid commonly accumulates as an expression of a generalized tendency to form edema in diseases such as the nephrotic syndrome, cirrhosis of the liver, and congestive heart failure. Pleural effusion is also a frequent response to an inflammatory process or tumor in the lung or on the pleural surface.

The Pericardium

Fluid in the pericardial sac may result from either hemorrhage *(hemopericardium)* or injury to the pericardium *(pericardial effusion)*. Pericardial effusions occur with pericardial infections, metastatic neoplasms to the pericardium, uremia, and systemic lupus erythematosus. They are also occasionally encountered after cardiac operations *(postpericardiotomy syndrome)* or radiation therapy for cancer.

Pericardial fluid may accumulate rapidly, particularly with hemorrhage caused by a ruptured myocardial infarct, dissecting aortic aneurysm, or trauma. In this circumstance, the pressure in the pericardial cavity rises to exceed the filling pressure of the heart, a condition termed *cardiac tamponade* (Fig. 7-32). The resulting precipitous decline in cardiac output is often fatal. When fluid in the pericardium accumulates rapidly, the tolerable limit may be only 90 to 120 mL, but a liter or more of fluid can be accommodated when the process is gradual.

Peritoneum

Peritoneal effusion, also called *ascites,* is caused mainly by cirrhosis of the liver, abdominal neoplasms, pancreatitis, cardiac failure, the nephrotic syndrome, and hepatic venous obstruction *(Budd-Chiari syndrome)*. Obstruction of the thoracic duct by cancer may lead to *chylous ascites,* in which the fluid has a milky appearance and a high fat content. The pathogenesis of ascites in cirrhosis of the liver is discussed above.

Patients with severe ascites accumulate many liters of fluid and have a conspicuously distended abdomen. The complications of ascites derive from increased abdominal pressure and include anorexia and vomiting, reflux esophagitis, dyspnea, ventral hernia, and leakage of fluid into the pleural space.

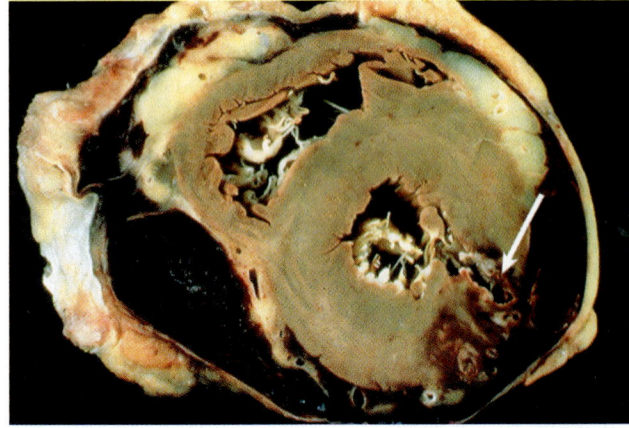

FIGURE 7-32
Cardiac tamponade. A cross-section of the heart shows rupture of a myocardial infarct *(arrow)* with the accumulation of a large quantity of blood in the pericardial cavity.

FLUID LOSS AND OVERLOAD

Excessive fluid loss (dehydration) and fluid overload are clinical situations that have potentially grave consequences. Fluid imbalance causes hemodynamic disorders; alterations in the osmolality and quantity of the fluid in the intravascular, interstitial, and cellular spaces may affect perfusion or the delivery of substrates, electrolytes, or fluids.

Dehydration Features Inadequate Fluid to Fill the Fluid Compartments

Dehydration results from insufficient fluid intake, excessive fluid loss, or both. Water loss may exceed intake in cases of vomiting, diarrhea, burns, excessive sweating, and diabetes insipidus. When excessive fluid loss occurs, fluid is recruited from the interstitial space to the plasma space. The fluids in the cell and within the interstitial and vascular compartments become more concentrated, particularly if there is a preferential loss of water, such as during inappropriate secretion of antidiuretic hormones in diabetes insipidus. When patients suffer from burns, vomiting, excessive sweating, or diarrhea, they not only lose fluid but also suffer electrolyte disturbances.

Clinically, only dryness of the skin and mucous membranes are noted initially, but as dehydration progresses, the turgor of the skin is lost. If dehydration persists, *oliguria* (reduced urine output) occurs as a compensation for the fluid loss. More severe fluid loss is accompanied by a shift of water from the intracellular space to the extracellular space, a process that causes severe cell dysfunction, particularly in the brain. Shrinkage of brain tissue may result in the rupture of small vessels and subsequent bleeding. Systemic blood pressure falls with continuous dehydration, and declining perfusion eventually leads to death.

Overhydration Reflects Fluid Intake That Exceeds the Excretory Capacity of the Kidney

Excessive hydration is ordinarily a rare situation, unless renal injury limits the excretory function of the kidney or the kidney is prevented from proper counterregulation (e.g., through excessive secretion of antidiuretic hormone). Fluid overload today is mostly iatrogenic, caused by the administration of excessive amounts of intravenous fluids. The most serious effect of this type of fluid overload is the induction of cerebral edema or congestive heart failure in patients with cardiac dysfunction.

SHOCK

Shock is a condition of profound hemodynamic and metabolic disturbance characterized by failure of the circulatory system to maintain an appropriate blood supply to the microcirculation, with consequent inadequate perfusion of vital organs. In this often catastrophic circumstance, tissue perfusion and oxygen delivery fall below the levels required to meet normal demands, including a failure to remove metabolites adequately. The term *shock* encompasses all the reactions that occur in response to such disturbances. In the course of uncompensated shock, a rapid circulatory collapse leads to impaired cellular metabolism and death. However, in many cases, compensatory mechanisms sustain the patient, at least for a while. When these adaptations fail, shock becomes irreversible. Shock has been a major cause of morbidity and mortality in intensive care units, and despite endeavors to suppress portions of the immune response, the outcome of shock has been unchanged in the past 50 years.

Shock is not synonymous with low blood pressure, although hypotension is commonly a part of the shock syndrome. Hypotension is actually a late sign in shock and indicates a failure of compensation. At the same time that peripheral blood flow falls below critical levels, extreme vasoconstriction can maintain arterial blood pressure. This distinction between shock and hypotension is important clinically because the rapid restoration of systemic blood flow is the primary goal in treating shock. When blood pressure alone is raised with vasopressive drugs, systemic blood flow may actually be diminished.

Pathogenesis: Decreased perfusion in shock is most commonly the result of a decreased cardiac output, resulting either from the inability of the heart to pump the normal venous return or from a decreased effective blood volume that leads to a decreased venous return. These two mechanisms underlie two of the major types of shock: cardiogenic and hypovolemic shock. Systemic vasodilation, with or without increases in vascular permeability, is responsible for the other categories of shock, namely, septic shock, anaphylactic shock, and neurogenic shock (Fig. 7-33).

Cardiogenic shock is caused by myocardial pump failure. This condition usually arises as a result of a large myocardial infarction, but myocarditis may also be responsible. Conditions that prevent left or right heart filling reduce cardiac output, resulting in "obstructive" shock. Such conditions include pulmonary embolism, cardiac tamponade, and (rarely) atrial myxoma.

Hypovolemic shock is secondary to a pronounced decrease in blood or plasma volume, caused by the loss of fluid from the vascular compartment. Hemorrhage, fluid loss from severe burns, diarrhea, excessive urine formation, perspiration, and trauma are major mechanisms of fluid loss that can lead to hypovolemic shock. In the case of burns or trauma, direct damage to the microcirculation increases vascular permeability.

Septic shock is caused by severe systemic microbial infections. The mechanisms responsible for the development of shock in this setting are complex and are discussed in detail below.

Anaphylactic shock occurs as a consequence of a systemic type I hypersensitivity reaction, which leads to widespread vasodilation and increased vascular permeability.

Neurogenic shock can follow acute injury to the brain or spinal cord, which impairs the neural control of vasomotor tone, thereby leading to generalized vasodilation. In the case of both anaphylactic and neurogenic shock, the subsequent redistribution of blood to the periphery, with or without increased vascular permeability, reduces the effective circulating blood and plasma volume. This effect ultimately leads to the same consequences as observed with hypovolemic shock.

In both hypovolemic and cardiogenic shock, decreased cardiac output and resultant decreased tissue perfusion make up the essential pathogenetic mechanisms in the progression from reversible to irreversible shock. Cellular hypoxia is the common consequence of the initial decrease in tissue perfusion. Although such changes do not result in irreversible injury initially, a vicious circle of decreasing tissue perfusion and further cell injury is perpetuated by several mechanisms:

- Injury to endothelial cells, secondary to the hypoxia caused by decreased tissue perfusion and increased vascular permeability, leads to the escape of fluid from the vascular compartment.
- Increased exudation of fluid from the circulation reduces (1) blood volume, (2) venous return, and (3) cardiac output, thereby aggravating hypoxic cell injury.
- Decreased perfusion of the kidneys and skeletal muscles results in metabolic acidosis, which in turn further decreases cardiac output and tissue perfusion.
- Decreased perfusion of the heart injures the myocardial cells and decreases their ability to pump blood, further reducing cardiac output and tissue perfusion.

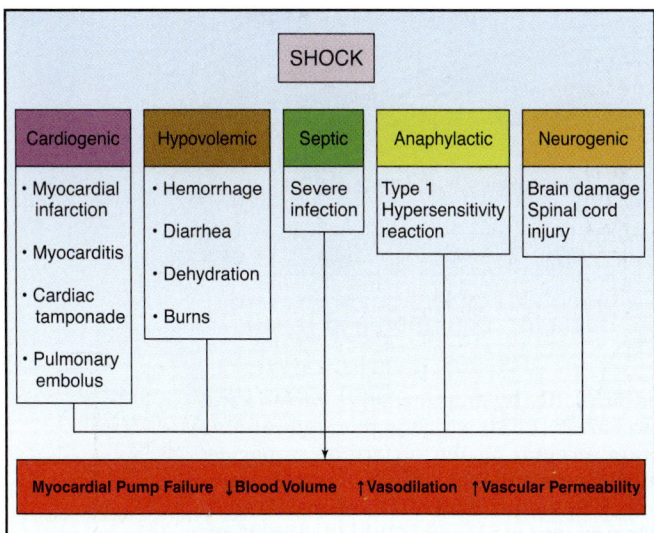

FIGURE 7-33
Classification of shock. Shock results from (1) an inability of the heart to pump adequately (cardiogenic shock) (2) decreased effective blood volume as a consequence of severely reduced blood or plasma volume (hypovolemic shock), or (3) widespread vasodilation (septic, anaphylactic or neurogenic shock). Increased vascular permeability may complicate vasodilation by contributing to reduced effective blood volume.

Systemic Inflammatory Response Syndrome Characterizes Septic Shock

Systemic inflammatory response syndrome (SIRS) is an exaggerated and generalized manifestation of a local immune or inflammatory reaction, and is often fatal. This condition is a hypermetabolic state that features two or more signs of systemic

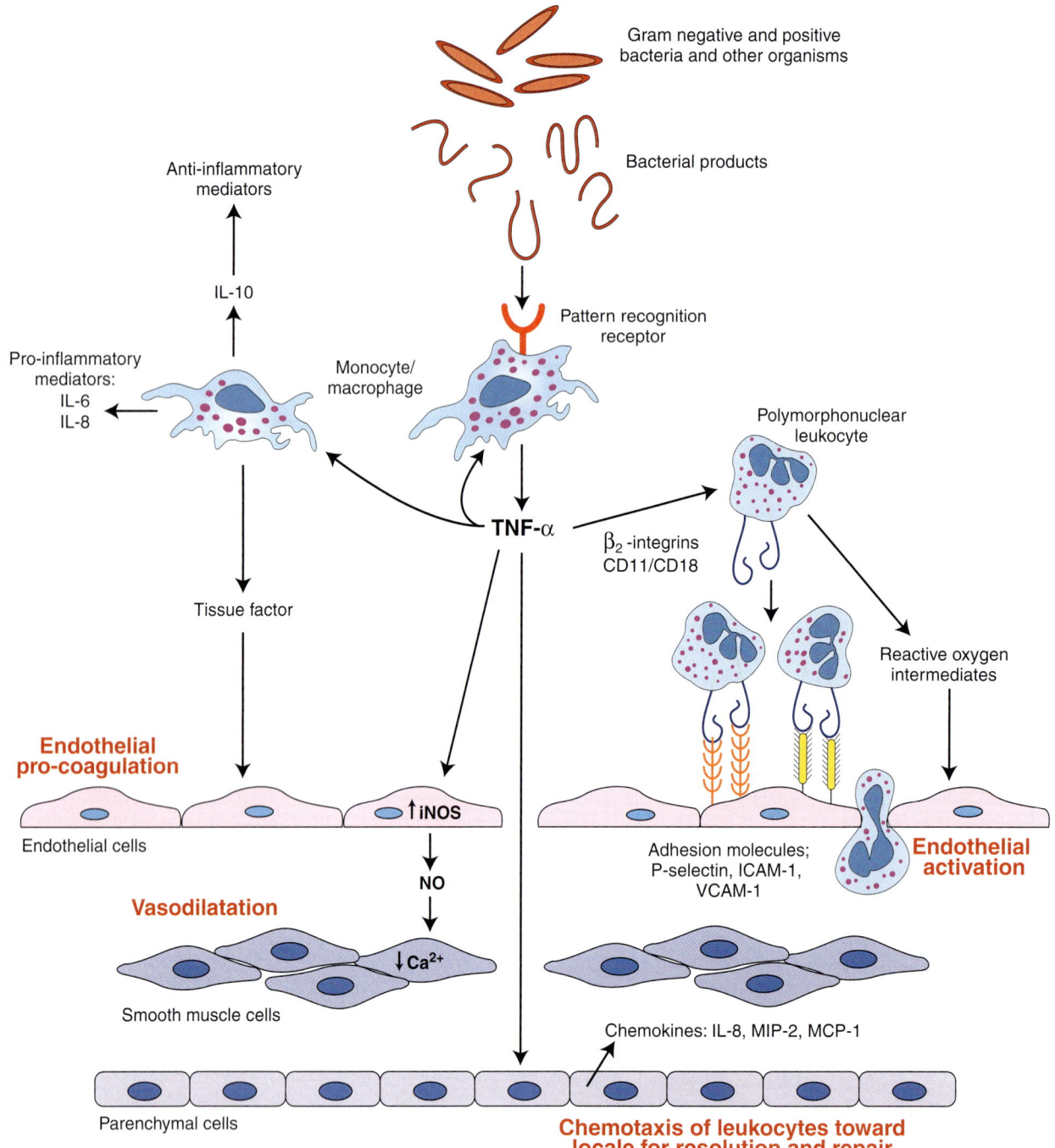

FIGURE 7-34

Pathogenesis of endotoxic shock. Sepsis is caused primarily by gram-negative bacteria and bacterial products such as endotoxin (lipopolysaccharide [LPS]) which is released into the circulation, where it binds to a pattern recognition receptor on the surface of monocyte/macrophages. Such binding stimulates the secretion of substantial quantities of tumor necrosis factor-alpha (TNF-α). TNF-α mediates septic shock by a number of mechanisms: (1) stimulation of the release of various pro- and antiinflammatory mediators; (2) induction of endothelial procoagulation by tissue factor, thereby leading to thrombosis and local ischemia; (3) direct cytotoxic damage to endothelial cells; (4) endothelial activation, which enhances the adherence of polymorphonuclear leukocytes; (5) stimulation of endothelial cell nitric oxide production and vasodilation; and (6) release of chemokines to attract leukocytes for resolution and repair of tissue injury.

inflammation, such as fever, tachycardia, tachypnea, leukocytosis, or leukopenia, in the setting of a known cause of inflammation. *Septic shock* is defined as clinical SIRS so severe that it leads to organ dysfunction and hypotension. The mechanisms responsible for the development of septic shock are illustrated in Figure 7-34. These processes often progress to *multiple organ dysfunction syndrome* (MODS), a term used to describe otherwise unexplained abnormalities of organ function in critically ill patients (see below).

The massive inflammatory reaction defined by SIRS is the consequence of the systemic release of cytokines, the most important being tumor necrosis factor (TNF), interleukin-1 (IL-1), IL-6, and platelet-activating factor (PAF). Actually, over 30 endogenous mediators have been described in this condition, and their collective interactions may be important in the pathogenesis of SIRS.

Septicemia with gram-negative organisms is the most common cause of septic shock. The invading bacteria are responsible for the release of **endotoxin,** a term historically used to describe the cell-associated toxin found in gram-negative bacteria. Endotoxin is a lipopolysaccharide (LPS), whose toxic activity resides in the lipid A component. On entry into the circulation, LPS, via lipid A binds to LPS-binding protein, after which the complex binds to the CD14 receptor on the surface of monocyte/macrophages. The recognition complex resides on the plasma membrane and includes the toll-like receptor (TLR) family of proteins and CD14. TLRs represent the primary sensors of the innate immune system, which collectively recognize bacteria, fungi, and protozoa. They mediate signaling through activation of the transcription factor, nuclear factor-kappaB (NF-κB), and upregulate TNF expression. LPS binding to TLR-4 causes mononuclear phagocytes to secrete large quantities of cytokines, such as TNF, IL-1, IL-6, IL-8, IL-12, and others that mediate a wide variety of responses. The secretion of these cytokines, and the subsequent production of nitric oxide (NO) and procoagulant proteins, ultimately cause the overwhelming cardiovascular collapse characteristic of septic shock. In this context activation of inducible NO synthase (iNOS) by TNF upregulates NO synthesis from L-arginine, an effect that is primarily responsible for the drop in blood pressure during sepsis. TNF is also involved in the pathogenesis of shock unassociated with endotoxemia (e.g., cardiogenic shock). Although LPS is the most potent stimulus for the release of TNF, other antigens also promote its secretion. These include toxin-1 of the toxic shock syndrome; enterotoxin; antigens of mycobacteria, fungi, parasites, and viruses; and products of complement activation.

TNF also exerts beneficial effects by enhancing tissue remodeling, wound healing, and defense against local infections. However, in septic shock this protein is suddenly released in great excess by exposure of macrophages to bacterial endotoxin, resulting in effects that are often lethal. The administration of anti-TNF antibody before exposure of an animal to endotoxin or to gram-negative bacteria completely protects against the development of septic shock. Unfortunately, clinical trials of agents that block TNF or its receptor have thus far not been successful in ameliorating septic shock in humans.

TNF released by monocyte/macrophages exerts a direct toxic effect on endothelial cells by compromising membrane permeability and inducing endothelial cell apoptosis. It also acts indirectly by (1) initiating a cascade of other mediators that amplify its deleterious effects, (2) promoting the adhesion of polymorphonuclear leukocytes to endothelial surfaces, and (3) activating the extrinsic coagulation pathway. The presence of TNF stimulates the release of IL-1 and IL-6, PAF, and other eicosanoids that may mediate tissue injury. Interestingly, nonlethal doses of TNF become fatal when administered together with IL-1. TNF also increases the expression of adhesion molecules, such as intercellular adhesion molecules (ICAMs), vascular cell adhesion molecules (VCAMs), P-selectin, and endothelial-leukocyte adhesion molecules (ELAMs) on endothelial surfaces, thereby promoting leukocyte adhesion and leukostasis. This mechanism presumably plays a role in the respiratory distress syndrome, in which activated neutrophils are sequestered in the pulmonary circulation and damage the alveoli. Other vasoactive peptides include the vasodilatory prostacyclins and endothelin (ET)-1, a potent vasoconstrictor. The pathogenesis of septic shock is summarized in Figure 7-34. Note that the term *septic syndrome* refers to the physiological and metabolic response characteristic of sepsis in the absence of an infection.

Multiple Organ Dysfunction Syndrome (MODS) Is the End-Result of Shock

Improvements in the early treatment of shock and sepsis have allowed patients to survive long enough to manifest a new problem, namely, progressive deterioration of organ function. Almost all septic shock patients suffer from dysfunction of at least one organ, and MODS is seen in one third of cases. MODS also develops in one third of patients afflicted by trauma or burns and in a quarter of those with acute pancreatitis. Whatever the cause, the clinical deterioration of MODS is held to be the result of common mechanisms of tissue injury subsumed under the rubric of SIRS. SIRS/MODS now account for most deaths in noncoronary intensive care units in the United States, with mortality rates well in excess of 50%. In most circumstances an inflammatory reaction reflects a balance between proinflammatory and antiinflammatory factors. Although proinflammatory mediators predominate in SIRS, antiinflammatory factors play an important role in some patients. The result is *compensated antiinflammatory response syndrome (CARS)*, in which paralysis of the immune system leads to a poor outcome. It is now thought that following bacterial infection, there is an initial response of excessive inflammation and septic shock characteristic of SIRS. Such uncontrolled cytokine induction is preceded by a stage of anergy and immune repression, or CARS. Septic patients may cycle between SIRS and CARS, in which case they tend to exhibit increased mortality. Persons with a heterogeneous response are said to have a *"mixed antiinflammatory response syndrome"* (MARS).

An individual genetic background may influence susceptibility to a wide variety of complex illnesses including infections and sepsis. Although determining the genetic background of complex traits is difficult, common single nucleotide polymorphisms such as those for TNF, IL-6 and IL-8, TGF-β, and PDG-F have been shown to affect the severity of disease.

Vascular Compensatory Mechanisms

Compensatory mechanisms in shock maintain blood flow to the heart and the brain, shifting it away from the periphery, skeletal muscle, skin, splanchnic bed, adipose tissue, limbs, and some parenchymal organs. These responses involve the sympathetic nervous system, the release of endogenous vasoconstrictors and hormonal substances, and local vasoregulation. The result is an increased cardiac output achieved by a faster heart rate and augmented myocardial contractility in the presence of enhanced arterial and arteriolar vasoconstriction.

- **Increased sympathetic discharge** augments the release of catecholamines by the adrenal medulla. The skeletal muscle, splanchnic bed, and skin arterioles respond to increased sympathetic discharge; the cardiac and cerebral arterioles are less reactive. In this manner, the increased sympathetic tone tends to shift blood flow from the periphery to the heart and brain. The marked arteriolar vasoconstriction results in reduced capillary hydrostatic pressure and in less fluid shifted into the interstitium, thereby permitting an osmotic fluid shift from the interstitium to the vascular system. The sympathetic–adrenal response can completely compensate for a blood loss of 10% of intravascular volume. With a greater volume deficit, cardiac output and blood pressure are affected, and blood flow to the tissues is reduced.
- **The renin–angiotensin–aldosterone system** also contributes a compensatory mechanism by stimulating sodium and water reabsorption, thereby helping to maintain intravascular volume. A similar water-preserving action is provided by pituitary antidiuretic hormone.
- **Vascular autoregulation** preserves regional blood flow to vital organs, particularly the heart and the brain, by vasodilation of the coronary and cerebral circulations in response to hypoxia and acidosis. Vasoconstriction is mediated largely by the α-adrenergic receptors of the sympathetic nervous system in mesenteric venules and veins, which acts to maintain cardiac filling and arterial pressure. The peripheral circulation of organs such as the skin and skeletal muscles, which are less sensitive to hypoxia, do not display such tightly controlled autoregulation.

 Pathology: Shock is associated with specific changes in a number of organs (Fig. 7-35), including acute tubular necrosis of the kidney, acute respiratory distress syndrome, liver failure, depression of host defense mechanisms, and heart failure.

The Heart

The heart shows petechial hemorrhages of the epicardium and endocardium. Microscopically, necrotic foci in the myocardium range from the loss of single fibers to large areas of necrosis. Prominent contraction bands are visible by light microscopy but are better seen by electron microscopy. Ultrastructurally, flattened areas of the intercalated disk are a sign of cell swelling, and invagination of adjacent cells is considered to be a catecholamine-induced lesion.

The Kidney

Acute tubular necrosis (acute renal failure), a major complication of shock, has been divided into three phases: (1) **the initiation phase**, from the onset of injury to the beginning of renal failure; (2) **the maintenance phase**, from the onset of

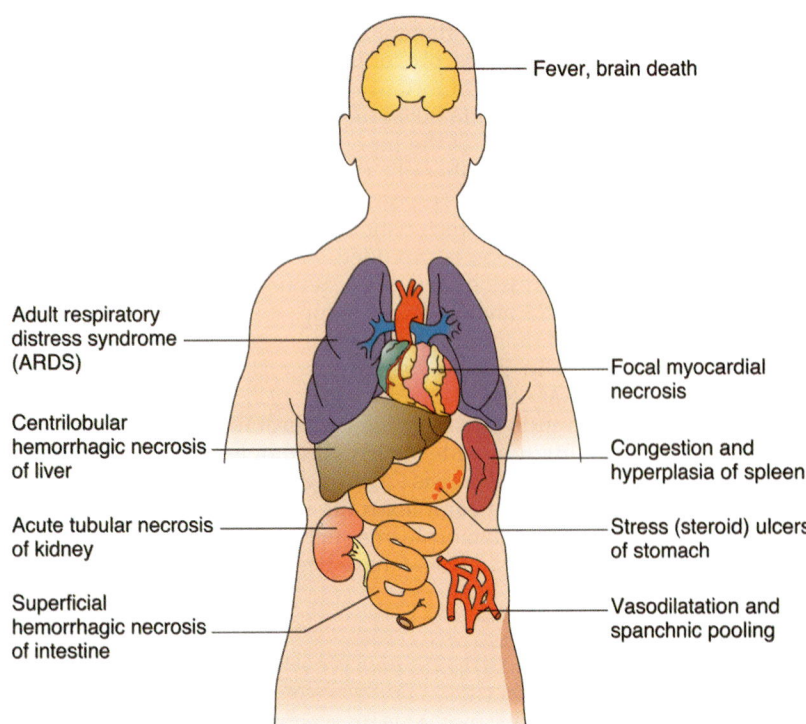

FIGURE 7-35
Complications of shock.

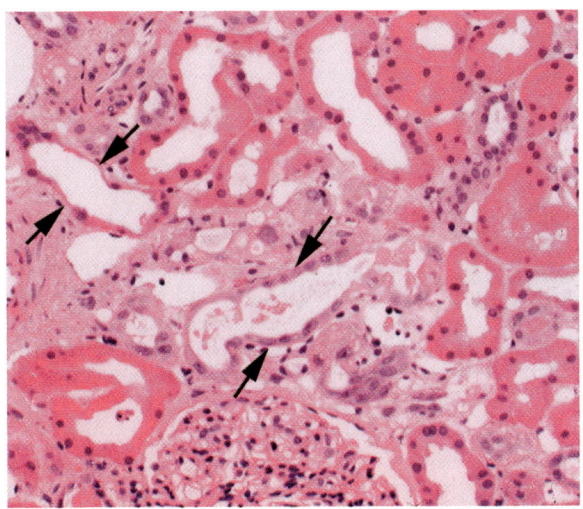

FIGURE 7-36
Acute tubular necrosis. A section of kidney shows swelling and degeneration of tubular epithelium. *Arrows* indicate the thinned epithelium.

renal failure to a stable, reduced renal function; and (3) **the recovery phase**. In those who survive an episode of shock, the recovery phase begins about 10 days after its onset and may last up to 8 weeks.

Renal blood flow is restricted to one third of normal following the acute ischemic phase, an effect that is even more severe in the outer cortex. The constriction of arterioles reduces the filtration pressure, thereby reducing the amount of filtrate and contributing to oliguria. Interstitial edema occurs, possibly through a process termed *backflow*. Excessive vasoconstriction is also related to stimulation of the renin–angiotensin system.

During acute renal failure, the kidney is large, swollen, and congested, although the cortex may be pale. A cross-section reveals blood pooling in the outer stripe of the medulla. Microscopically, fully developed acute tubular necrosis is evidenced by dilation of the proximal tubules and focal necrosis of cells (Fig. 7-36). Frequently, pigmented casts in the tubular lumina indicate leakage of hemoglobin or myoglobin. Coarse, "ropy" casts are seen in the distal nephron and distal convoluted tubules. Interstitial edema is prominent in the cortex, and mononuclear cells accumulate within the tubules and surrounding interstitium. Acute tubular necrosis is discussed in greater detail in Chapter 16.

The Lung

Following the onset of severe and prolonged shock, injury to the alveolar wall can result in *shock lung*, which is a cause of acute respiratory distress syndrome. The sequence of changes is mediated by polymorphonuclear leukocytes and includes interstitial edema, necrosis of endothelial and alveolar epithelial cells, and formation of intravascular microthrombi and hyaline membranes lining the alveolar surface.

Macroscopically, the lung is firm and congested, and a frothy fluid often exudes from the cut surface. Interstitial edema is first seen around the peribronchial connective tissue and lymphatics, subsequently filling the interstitial connective tissue. In this initial period, a large fluid volume drains into the pulmonary lymphatics. If removal of this fluid becomes inadequate, or if the balance of forces that keep the fluid in the interstitial space is disturbed, alveolar edema develops.

Shock-induced lung injury leads to the appearance of hyaline membranes in the alveoli (see Fig. 7-31), which also frequently line the alveolar ducts and terminal bronchioles. These lung changes may heal entirely, but in half of patients, the repair processes cause a thickening of the alveolar wall. Characteristically, type II pneumocytes proliferate to replace the damaged type I pneumocytes and line the alveoli. Fibrous tissue proliferation may lead to organization of the alveolar exudate. These chronic changes may result in persistent respiratory distress and even death. Shock lung and adult respiratory distress syndrome are more fully discussed in Chapter 12.

The Gastrointestinal Tract

Shock often results in diffuse gastrointestinal hemorrhage. Erosions of the gastric mucosa and superficial ischemic necrosis in the intestines are the usual sources of this bleeding. Interruption of the barrier function of the intestine may be related to the development of septicemia. More-severe necrotizing lesions contribute to deterioration in the final phase of shock.

The Liver

In patients who die in shock, the liver is enlarged and has a mottled cut surface that reflects marked centrilobular pooling of blood. The most prominent histological lesion is centrilobular congestion and necrosis. The cells in the center of the lobule are the most distant from the blood supply that comes from the portal tracts and are, therefore, presumably more vulnerable to circulatory disturbances. Hypoxia of the liver leads to the development of cytoplasmic vacuoles, which represent dilated cisternae of the endoplasmic reticulum. An increase in intracellular fat is consistently noted in persons who have survived shock.

The Pancreas

The splanchnic vascular bed, which supplies the pancreas, is particularly affected by impaired circulation during shock. The resulting ischemic damage to the exocrine pancreas unleashes activated catalytic enzymes and causes acute pancreatitis, a complication that further promotes shock.

The Brain

Brain lesions are rare in shock. Occasionally, microscopic hemorrhages are seen, but patients who recover do not ordinarily display neurological deficits. In severe cases, particularly in persons with cerebral atherosclerosis, hemorrhage and necrosis may appear in the overlapping region between the terminal distributions of major arteries, so-called *watershed infarcts*.

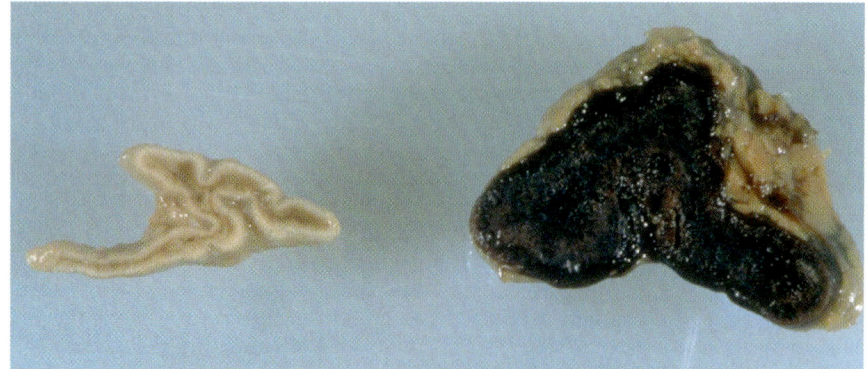

FIGURE 7-37
Waterhouse-Friderichsen syndrome. A normal adrenal gland (left) in contrast to an adrenal gland enlarged by extensive hemorrhage (right), obtained from a patient who died of meningococcemic shock.

The Adrenals

In severe shock, the adrenal glands exhibit conspicuous hemorrhage in the inner cortex. Frequently, this hemorrhage is only focal. However, it can be massive and accompanied by hemorrhagic necrosis of the entire gland, as seen in the *Waterhouse-Friderichsen syndrome* (Fig. 7-37), typically associated with overwhelming meningococcal septicemia.

Host Defenses

The alterations of the immunological system and host defenses in shock are not well defined, although it is common for patients who survive the acute phase to succumb to subsequent overwhelming infection. It may well be that several factors interact, namely, ischemic colitis, tissue trauma, suppression of the immune system, and metabolic suppression of host defenses. Humoral immunity and phagocytic activity by leukocytes and mononuclear macrophages are both depressed, but the mechanisms underlying these effects are not clear.

SUGGESTED READING

Books

Braunwald E: *Heart disease: A textbook of cardiovascular medicine*, 5th ed. Philadelphia: WB Saunders, 1997.

Hall JB, Schmidt GA, Wood LDH: *Principles of critical care*, 2nd ed. New York: McGraw-Hill, 1998.

Kelley WN: *Textbook of internal medicine*, 3rd ed. Philadelphia: Lippincott–Raven, 1997.

Silver, MD, Gotlieb, AI, Schoen, FJ: *Cardiovascular pathology*, 3rd ed. Amsterdam: Churchill Livingstone, 2001.

Virmani R, Burke A, Farb A, Atkinson JB: *Cardiovascular pathology*, Philadelphia: WB Saunders, 2001.

Review Articles

Aird WC: The role of the endothelium in severe sepsis and multiple organ dysfunctional Syndrome. *Blood* 101: 3765–77, 2003.

Aldridge AJ: Role of the neutrophil in septic shock and the adult respiratory distress syndrome. *Europ Surg* 168: 204–14, 2002.

Bateman RM, Sharpe MD, Ellis CG: Bench-to-bedside review: microvascular dysfunction in sepsis—hemodynamics, oxygen transport, and nitric oxide. *Crit Care* 7:359–73, 2003.

Bone RC: Toward a theory regarding the pathogenesis of the systemic inflammatory response syndrome: What we do and do not know about cytokine regulation. *Crit Care Med* 24:163–172, 1996.

Ceppa EP, Fuh KC, Bulkley GB: Mesenteric hemodynamic response to circulatory shock. *Curr Opin Crit Care* 9:127–32, 2003.

Deutschman CS: Acute-phase responses and SIRS/MODS: The good, the bad, and the nebulous. *Crit Care Med* 26: 1630–1631, 1998.

Gando S: Disseminated intravascular coagulation in trauma patients. *Semin Thrombosis Hemostasis* 27:585–92, 2001.

Jacobi J: Pathophysiology of sepsis. *Am J Health Syst Pharm* 59(suppl 1):S3-8, 2002.

Kearon C: Natural history of venous thromboembolism. *Circulation* 107:122–30, 2003.

Knuefermann P, Nemoto S, Baumgarten G, et al.: Cardiac inflammation and innate immunity in septic shock: Is there a role for toll-like receptors? *Chest* 121:1329–1336, 2002.

Kumar A, Haery C, Parrillo JE: Myocardial dysfunction in septic shock. *Crit Care Clin* 16: 251–287, 2000.

Okajima K: Regulation of inflammatory responses by natural anticoagulants. *Immunol Rev* 184:258–274, 2001.

Opal SM, Huber CE: Bench-to-bedside review: Toll-like receptors and their role in septic shock. *Crit Care* 6:125–136, 2002.

Parrillo JE: Pathogenetic mechanisms of septic shock. *N Engl J Med* 3328:1471–1477, 1993.

Strassburg CP: Shock liver. *Best Practice Res Clin Gastroenterol.* 17:369–81, 2003.

Tjardes T, Neugebauer E: Sepsis research in the next millennium: Concentrate on the software rather than the hardware. *Shock* 17:1-8, 2002.

Tracey KJ, Cerami A: Tumor necrosis factor: A pleiotropic cytokine and therapeutic target. *Annu Rev Med* 45:491–503, 1994.

Van Amersfoort ES, Van Berkel TJ, Kuiper J: Receptors, mediators, and mechanisms involved in bacterial sepsis and septic shock. *Clin Microbiol Rev* 16:379–414, 2003.

CHAPTER 8

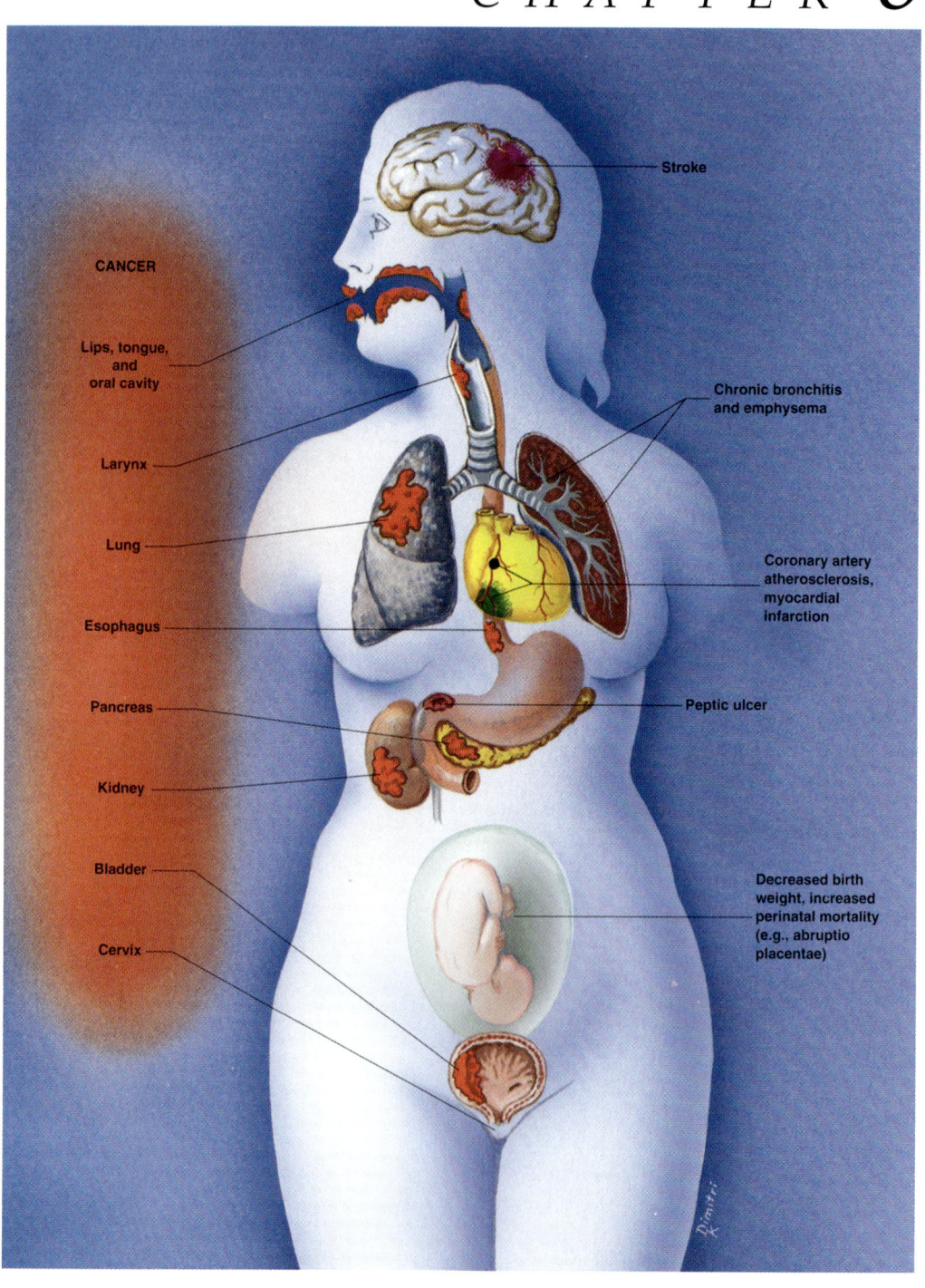

Environmental and Nutritional Pathology

Emanuel Rubin
David Strayer

Smoking

Cardiovascular Disease

Cancer of the Lung

Nonneoplastic Diseases

Female Reproductive Function

Passive Smoking

Alcoholism

Effects of Alcohol on Organs and Tissues

Fetal Alcohol Syndrome

Alcohol and Cancer

Mechanisms of Alcohol-related Injury

Drug Abuse

Heroin

Illicit Stimulants

Intravenous Drug Abuse

Drug Addiction in Pregnant Women

Iatrogenic Drug Injury

Sex Hormones

Oral Contraceptives

Postmenopausal Hormone Replacement Therapy

Environmental Chemicals

Toxic Effects and Hypersensitivity Responses

Occupational Exposure

Thermal Regulatory Dysfunction

Hypothermia

Hyperthermia

Altitude-Related Illnesses

Physical Injuries

Contusions

Abrasions

Lacerations

Wounds

(continued)

FIGURE 8-1 *(see opposite page)*
Diseases associated with cigarette smoking. The cancers whose incidences are known to be increased in cigarette smokers are shown on the *left*. The nonneoplastic diseases associated with cigarette smoking are shown on the *right*.

Radiation

Whole-Body Irradiation

Localized Radiation

Radiation and Cancer

Microwave Radiation, Electromagnetic Fields and Ultrasound

Nutritional Disorders

Obesity

Protein-Calorie Malnutrition

Vitamin Deficiencies

Deficiencies of Essential Trace Minerals

Environmental pathology is the field that deals with the diseases caused by exposure to harmful external agents and deficiencies of vital substances; in a sense it encompasses all nutritional, infectious, chemical, and physical causes of illness. A half century ago, a few physicians cultivated an interest in diseases that seemed to have strict geographical boundaries. "Geographic pathology" was concerned with diseases endemic to certain areas of the world, notably, parasitic and infectious diseases that seemed unique to those locales. A minor component dealt with nutritional disease, and a separate discipline covered forensic medicine. With the discovery that chemical agents mediate a variety of tissue changes and the recognition that many of these causative agents are environmental contaminants, a component called "occupational disease" was added to the roster. In this chapter we concentrate on diseases caused by (1) exposure to toxic agents, (2) physical damage, and (3) nutritional imbalance.

SMOKING

Smoking tobacco is the single largest preventable cause of death in the United States, with direct health costs to the economy of tens of billions of dollars a year. **Over 400,000 deaths a year—about one sixth of the total mortality in the United States—occur prematurely because of smoking.** Estimates have incriminated tobacco in 11 to 30% of cancer deaths (Fig. 8-1), 17 to 30% of cardiovascular deaths, 30% of deaths from lung diseases, and 20 to 30% of the incidence of low-birth-weight infants. Life expectancy is shortened, and overall mortality is proportional to the amount and duration of cigarette smoking, commonly quantitated as "pack-years." (Fig. 8-2). For example, a person who smokes two packs of cigarettes a day at the age of 30 years will live an average of 8 years fewer than a nonsmoker. One of the less desirable fallouts from the feminist movement has been the adoption of the smoking habit by many women. As a result, the epidemic of smoking-related disease that assaulted men more than a generation ago has now reached the female population. Women whose smoking characteristics are similar to those of men exhibit mortality rates similar to those of men. In fact, the mortality from cancer of the lung, almost all of which is related to cigarette smoking, exceeds that from cancers of the breast and prostate, the most common cancers in the United States. The excess mortality associated with cigarette smoking declines after cessation of the habit, and after 15 years of abstinence from cigarettes, the mortality of ex-smokers approaches that of persons who have never smoked at all. Overall mortality among those who smoke only cigars or pipes is only slightly higher than that in the nonsmoking population.

The major diseases responsible for the excess mortality reported in cigarette smokers are, in order of frequency, coronary heart disease, cancer of the lung, and chronic obstructive pulmonary disease (see Fig. 8-1). Smokers also suffer an increased incidence of cancer of the oral cavity, larynx, esophagus, pancreas, bladder, kidney, colon, and cervix. In addition, smokers exhibit excess mortality from atherosclerotic aortic aneurysms and peptic ulcer disease.

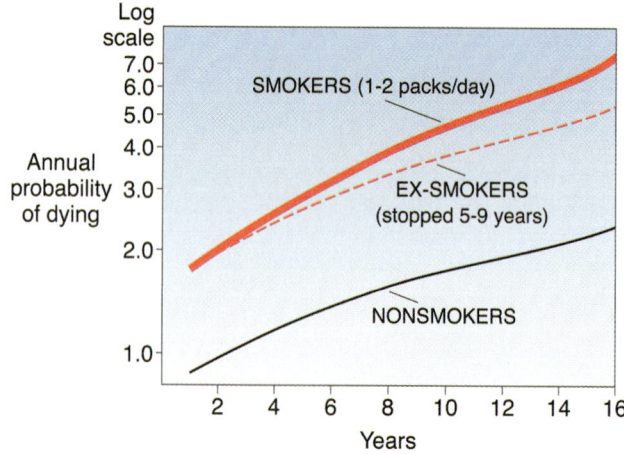

FIGURE 8-2

The risk of dying in smokers and nonsmokers. Note that the annual probability of an individual dying, indicated on the ordinate, is a logarithmic scale. Individuals who have smoked for 1 year have a twofold greater probability of dying than a nonsmoker, whereas those who have smoked for more than 15 years have more than a threefold greater probability of dying.

Cardiovascular Disease Is a Major Complication of Smoking

Cigarette smoking is recognized as a major independent risk factor for myocardial infarction and acts synergistically with other risk factors, such as high blood pressure and elevated blood cholesterol levels (Fig. 8-3). It not only serves to precipitate initial myocardial infarction but also increases the risk for second heart attacks and diminishes survival after a heart attack among those who continue to smoke. Smoking also increases the incidence of sudden cardiac death, possibly by exacerbating regional ischemia, an effect that may promote electrical instability of the heart.

Cigarette smoking is an independent risk factor for ischemic stroke. The risk correlates with the number of cigarettes smoked and is reduced after cessation of smoking. Tobacco use also increases the risk of certain forms of intracranial hemorrhage. The combination of smoking and oral contraceptive use in women older than 35 years of age increases the risk of myocardial infarction. Similarly, the use of cigarettes by women who are using oral contraceptives significantly augments their risk of stroke.

Atherosclerosis of the coronary arteries and the aorta is more severe and extensive among cigarette smokers than among nonsmokers, and the effect is dose related. As a consequence, cigarette smoking is a strong risk factor for atherosclerotic aortic aneurysms. The incidence and severity of atherosclerotic peripheral vascular disease are also remarkably increased by smoking. Smoking is also a major risk factor for coronary vasospasm. It disturbs regional coronary blood flow in patients with coronary artery disease and lowers the threshold for ventricular fibrillation and cardiac arrest in patients with established ischemic heart disease. Other effects of smoking that may predispose to myocardial infarction include pharmacological actions of nicotine itself, inhalation of carbon monoxide, reduction in plasma high-density lipoprotein levels, increased plasma fibrinogen levels, and a higher leukocyte count.

In the earlier part of this century, a peculiar inflammatory and occlusive disease of the vasculature of the lower leg was described in a patient population consisting principally of Eastern European Jews, almost all of whom were heavy smokers. This disorder, termed **Buerger disease,** was characterized by inflammation, fibrosis, and thrombosis of both the artery and its accompanying vein, leading to gangrene and amputation of the lower extremities. Although Buerger disease is unquestionably related to smoking, it is rarely reported today.

Cancer of the Lung Is Largely a Disease of Cigarette Smokers

More than 85% of deaths from cancer of the lung are attributed to cigarette smoking, the single most common cancer death in both men and women in the United States today (Fig. 8-4). Although the precise offenders in cigarette smoke have not been identified, clearly cigarette smoke is toxic and carcinogenic to the bronchial mucosa. When cigarette smoke is passed through a filter, it is separated into gas and particulate phases. Cigarette tar, the material that is deposited on the filter, contains more than 3000 compounds, many of which have been identified as carcinogens, tumor promoters, and ciliotoxic agents. Compounds with similar toxic properties are found in the gas phase, but they are fewer. The risk of developing lung

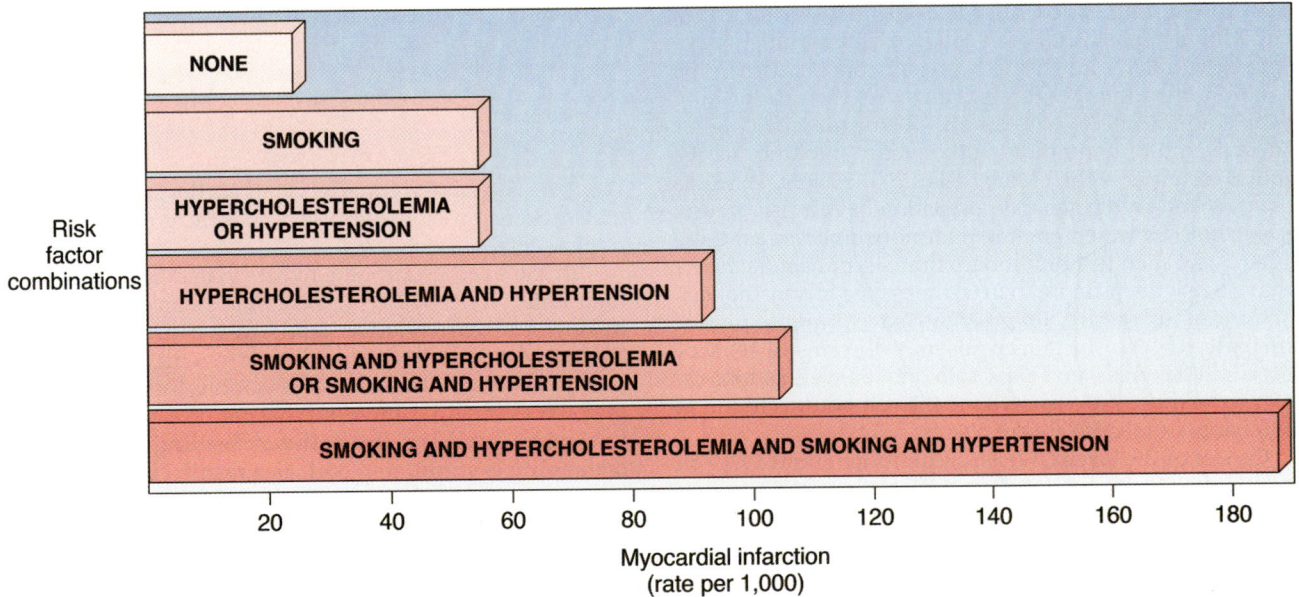

FIGURE 8-3
The risk of myocardial infarction in cigarette smokers. Smoking is an independent risk factor and increases the risk of a myocardial infarction to about the same extent as does hypertension or hypercholesterolemia alone. The effects of smoking are additive to those of these other two risk factors.

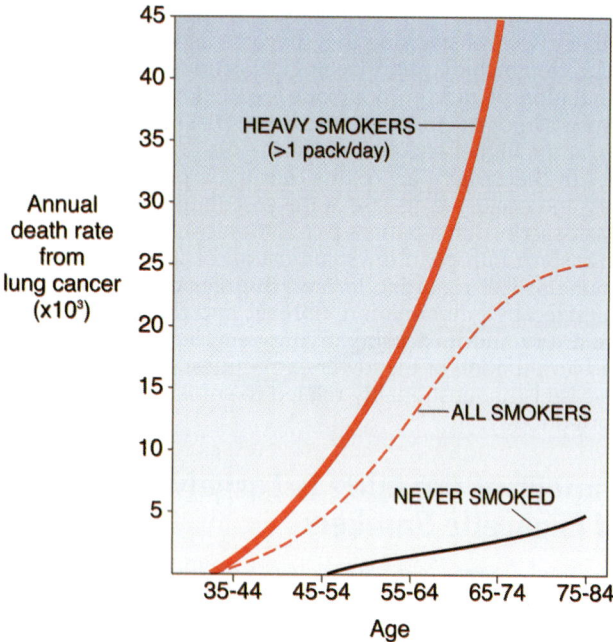

FIGURE 8-4
Death rate from lung cancer among smokers and nonsmokers. Nonsmokers exhibit a small, linear rise in the death rate from lung cancer from the age of 50 onward. By contrast, those who smoke more than one pack per day show an exponential rise in the annual death rate from lung cancer starting at about age 35. By age 70, heavy smokers have about a 20-fold greater death rate from lung cancer than nonsmokers.

cancer is directly related to the number of cigarettes smoked (Fig. 8-5).

Cigarette smoking is also an important factor in the induction of lung cancer that is associated with certain occupational exposures. For instance, uranium miners have an increased rate of lung cancer, presumably because of the inhalation of radon daughters. However, the rate of lung cancer among miners who smoke is considerably higher than that among nonminers with similar smoking habits. Another example is the case of asbestos workers. Whereas heavy smokers in the general population have a risk of lung cancer some 20 times greater than nonsmokers, asbestos workers who manifest pulmonary fibrosis and smoke heavily have a risk that is more than 60 times that of nonsmokers.

Cancers of the lip, tongue, and buccal mucosa occur principally (>90%) in tobacco users. All forms of tobacco use—cigarette, cigar, and pipe smoking, as well as tobacco chewing—expose the oral cavity to the compounds found in raw tobacco or tobacco smoke.

Cancer of the larynx, which accounts for about 1% of all cancer deaths in the United States, involves a similar situation. Among white male smokers the mortality ratio, compared with that in nonsmokers, varies from 6 to 13, and in some large studies, all deaths from cancer of the larynx occurred in smokers.

Cancer of the esophagus in the United States and Great Britain is estimated to result from smoking in 80% of cases.

Cancer of the bladder is twice as frequent a cause of death in cigarette smokers as in nonsmokers. In fact, 30 to 40% of all bladder cancers are attributable to smoking. As with most tobacco-related disorders, there is a clear dose-response relationship between the incidence of bladder cancer, the number of cigarettes smoked per day, and the duration of cigarette smoking.

Adenocarcinoma of the kidney is increased 50 to 100% among smokers. A modest increase in cancer of the renal pelvis has also been documented.

Cancer of the pancreas has shown a steady increase in incidence, which is, at least in part, related to cigarette smoking. The risk ratio in male smokers for adenocarcinoma of the pancreas is 2 to 3, and a dose-response relationship exists (Fig. 8-6). In fact, men who smoke more than two packs a day have a five times greater risk of developing pancreatic cancer than nonsmokers.

Cancer of the uterine cervix is significantly increased in women smokers, and it has been estimated that about 30% of cervical cancer mortality is attributable to this habit.

Acute myelogenous leukemia has been reported by some as associated with smoking, but the issue is controversial.

Smokers Develop Nonneoplastic Diseases

Chronic bronchitis and emphysema are primarily dose-related diseases of smokers (Fig. 8-7) (see Chapter 12).

Peptic ulcer disease has a 70% greater prevalence in male cigarette smokers than in nonsmokers.

Osteoporosis in women is exacerbated by tobacco use. Women who smoke one pack of cigarettes a day during their reproductive period will at the time of menopause exhibit a 5 to 10% deficit in bone density, which is enough to increase the risk of bone fractures.

Thyroid diseases are linked to cigarette smoking. The most conspicuous association is with Graves disease, especially when the hyperthyroidism is complicated by exophthalmos.

Ocular diseases, particularly macular degeneration and cataracts are reportedly more frequent in smokers.

Smoking Impairs Female Reproductive Function

Women who smoke experience an **earlier menopause** than nonsmokers, possibly because of the effects of tobacco on estrogen metabolism.

In the liver, estradiol is hydroxylated to estrone, which then enters one of two irreversible metabolic pathways. In one, 16-hydroxylation leads to the production of estriol, a compound with potent estrogenic activity. In the other, which involves 2-hydroxylation, the end product is methoxyestrone, a compound that has no estrogenic activity. **In women smokers, the pathway leading to the inactive metabolite is stimulated and, as a result, circulating levels of the active estrogen, estriol, are reduced.** As well as earlier menopause, an increased incidence of postmenopausal osteoporosis in smoking women has been attributed to decreased estriol levels.

Fetal Tobacco Syndrome

Fetal tobacco syndrome refers to the deleterious effects of maternal cigarette smoking on the development of the fetus. Infants born to

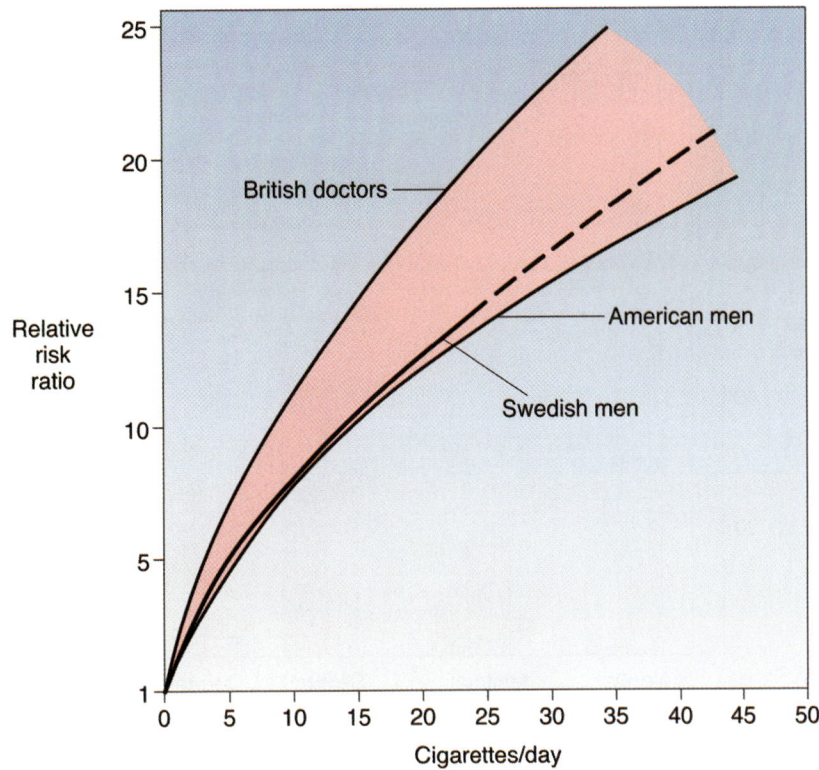

FIGURE 8-5
Dose-dependent relationship between cigarette smoking and the risk of lung cancer. Prospective studies of three different populations of smokers found that the risk of lung cancer depended on the number of cigarettes smoked per day. For example, those who smoke 15 cigarettes a day have about a threefold greater risk of developing lung cancer than those who smoke 5. The *dashed line* is an extrapolation of the data for Swedish men who smoke from 25 to 50 cigarettes a day.

women who smoke during pregnancy are, on average, 200 g lighter than infants born to comparable women who do not smoke. **These infants are not born preterm but rather are small for gestational age at every stage of pregnancy.** The prevalence of newborns weighing less than 2500 g is much greater among mothers who smoke. Among light smokers, there is a 50% increase in the number of newborns weighing less than 2500 g; among heavy smokers, this figure is more than doubled. In fact, 20 to 40% of the incidence of low birth weight can be attributed to maternal cigarette smoking. This decrease in birth weight is independent of other determinants of birth weight, since there is a downward shift of the entire set of weights of smokers' infants (Fig. 8-8). Thus, this effect of smoking is not idiosyncratic but reflects a direct retardation of fetal growth.

The noxious effect of smoking on the fetus is mirrored by its effect on the uteroplacental unit. Every major well-controlled study has shown perinatal mortality to be higher among the offspring of smokers, the increase ranging from 20% among the progeny of women who smoke less than a pack per day to almost 40% among the offspring of those who smoke more than a pack per day. This excess mortality does not reflect specific abnormalities of the fetus but rather problems related to the uteroplacental system. **The incidences of abruptio placentae, placenta previa, uterine bleeding, and premature rupture of the membranes are all increased** (Fig. 8-9). These complications of smoking tend to occur at times when the fetus is not viable or is at great risk, namely, from 20 to 32 weeks of gestation.

Substantial evidence indicates that the injurious effects of maternal cigarette smoking are not limited to the fetus and the newborn but extend to the physical, cognitive, and

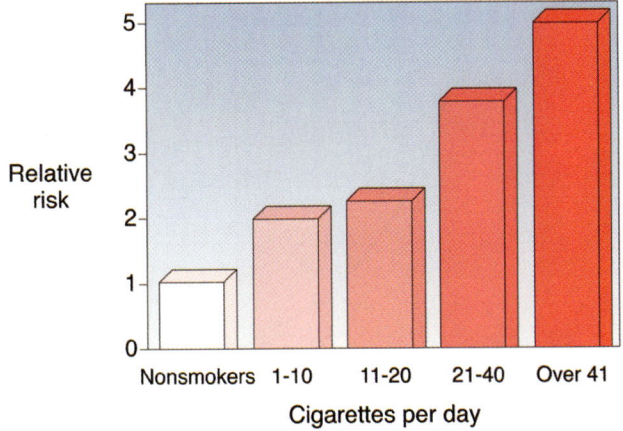

FIGURE 8-6
Dose-dependent relationship between smoking and the risk of pancreatic cancer. The relative risk of pancreatic cancer increases with the number of cigarettes smoked per day.

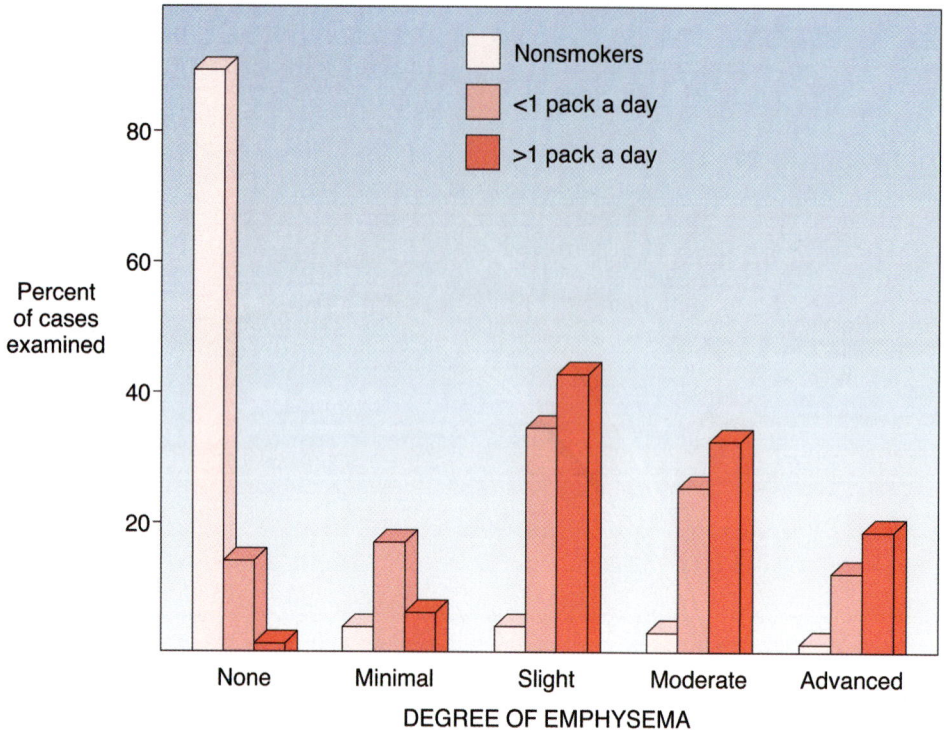

FIGURE 8-7
The association between cigarette smoking and pulmonary emphysema. Some 90% of nonsmokers have no detectable emphysema at autopsy. In contrast, virtually all those who smoke more than one pack per day have morphological evidence of emphysema at autopsy. Emphysema shows a slight dose dependence on the number of cigarettes smoked. Those who smoke less than one pack per day tend to have less-severe emphysema, but 85 to 90% of such smokers have some emphysema at autopsy.

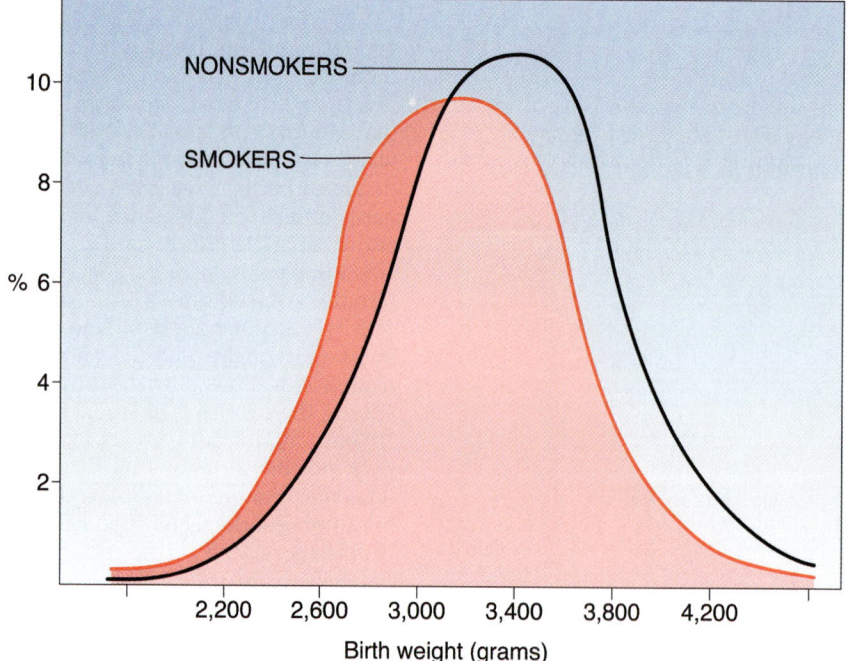

FIGURE 8-8
Effect of smoking on birth weight. Mothers who smoke give birth to smaller infants. In particular, the incidence of babies weighing less than 3000 g is increased significantly by smoking.

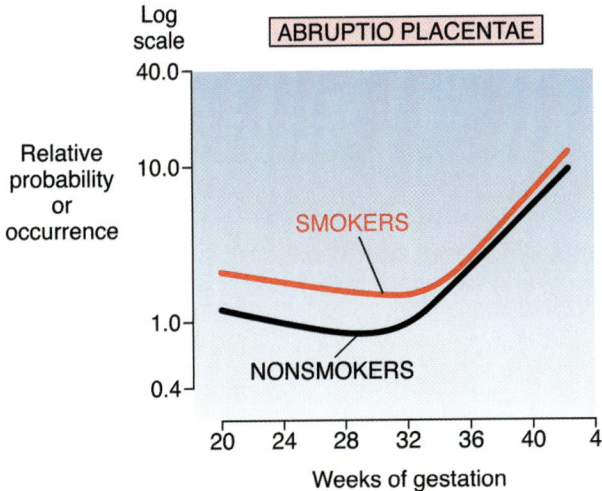
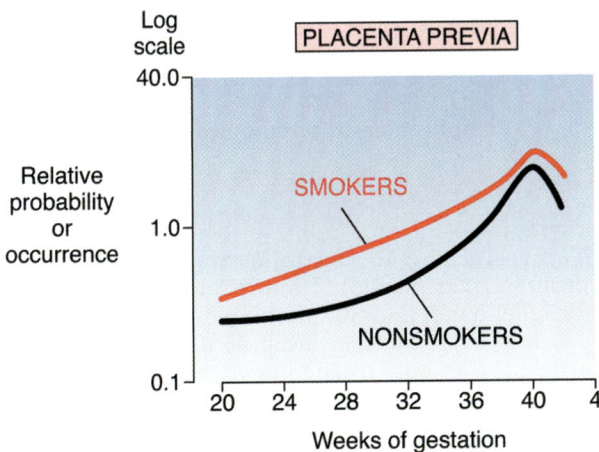
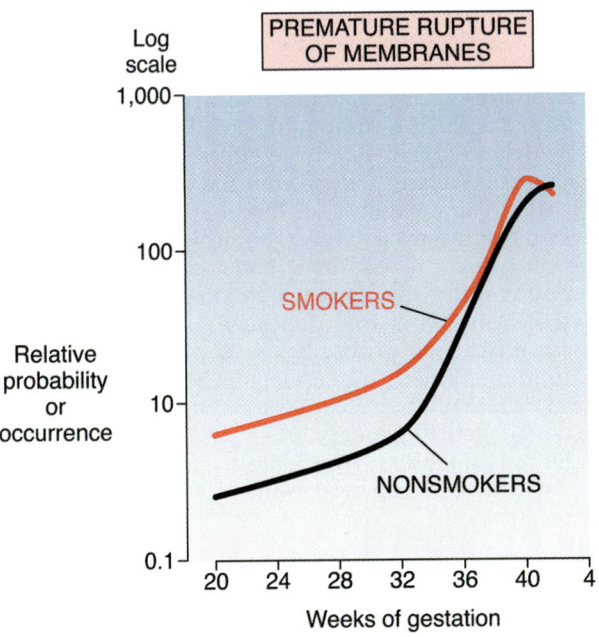

emotional development of the children at older ages. Thus, in a number of studies, the children of mothers who smoke have exhibited measurable deficiencies in physical growth, intellectual maturation, and emotional development that are independent of other known predisposing factors. In the most comprehensive study to date, 17,000 children born during 1 week in Great Britain were studied at ages 7 and 11 years. The children of mothers who smoked 10 or more cigarettes a day during pregnancy were, on average, 1.0 cm shorter than children of nonsmoking mothers and were 3 to 5 months retarded in reading, mathematics, and general intellectual ability. Moreover, the deficits increased with the number of cigarettes smoked during pregnancy.

Passive Smoking Is Defined As Exposure of Nonsmokers to Smoke Produced by Tobacco Smokers

Involuntary exposure to tobacco smoke in the environment has been seriously considered a risk factor for disease in nonsmokers. An increased incidence of respiratory illnesses and hospitalizations has been reported among infants whose parents smoke, and several studies have reported mild impairment of pulmonary function among children of smokers and exacerbation of preexisting asthma. A small increase in the incidence of lung cancer has been attributed to environmental tobacco smoke. However, the relative risks associated with passive smoking are on the order of only about 1.2 (20%), and the subject requires further study.

ALCOHOLISM

Alcoholism is an addiction to ethanol that features dependence and withdrawal symptoms, and results in the acute and chronic toxic effects of alcohol on the body. It is estimated that there are about 12 million alcoholics in the United States, or about one tenth of the population at risk. The proportion may be even higher in other countries, particularly those in which wine is consumed in preference to water. Certain ethnic groups, such as Native Americans and Eskimos, have notoriously high rates of alcoholism. By contrast, other groups, such as Chinese and Jews, experience little alcoholism. Although this addiction is more common in men, the number of female alcoholics has been increasing.

Chronic alcoholism has been defined as the regular intake of a quantity of alcohol that is enough to injure a person

FIGURE 8-9
Effect of smoking on the incidence of abruptio placentae, placenta previa, and the premature rupture of amniotic membranes. In each, the ordinate shows the probability of one of three complications of the third trimester of pregnancy. Note that it is a logarithmic scale. Smoking increases the probability of abruptio placentae and premature rupture of the amniotic membranes prior to 34 weeks of gestation, at which time the fetus is still premature. Smoking increases the risk of placenta previa up to 40 weeks of gestation.

socially, psychologically, or physically. Although there are no firm rules, for most persons, a daily consumption of more than 45 g alcohol should probably be discouraged. Intakes of 100 g or more a day may be dangerous (10 g alcohol = 1 oz, or 30 mL, of 86 proof [43%] spirits).

The short-term effects of alcohol on the brain are familiar to most people, but the mechanism of inebriation is not understood. Like other anesthetic agents, alcohol acts as a central nervous system depressant. However, it is such a weak anesthetic that it must be drunk by the glassful to exert any significant effect. In the normal person, characteristic behavioral changes can be detected at low alcohol concentrations (below 50 mg/dL). Levels above 100 mg/dL are usually associated with gross incoordination, and in American jurisdictions are considered legal evidence of intoxication while driving a motor vehicle. At levels above 300 mg/dL, most people become comatose, and at concentrations above 400 mg/dL, death from respiratory failure is common. In humans, the LD_{50} is about 5 g of alcohol per kilogram of body weight.

The situation is somewhat different in chronic alcoholics, who develop central nervous system tolerance to alcohol. Such persons often easily tolerate blood alcohol levels of 100 to 200 mg/dL, and in fatal automobile accidents, blood levels of 500 to 600 mg/dL or more have been found by medical examiners. The mechanism underlying tolerance has not been established for alcohol or any other drug.

Acute alcohol intoxication is hardly a benign condition. Some 40% of all fatalities from motor vehicle accidents involve alcohol—about 18,000 deaths a year in the United States. Alcoholism is also a major contributor to fatal home accidents, death in fires, and suicide.

Many of the chronic diseases associated with alcoholism were, at one time, attributed to malnutrition, and some alcoholics do suffer from nutritional deficiencies, such as thiamine deficiency (Wernicke encephalopathy) or folic acid deficiency (megaloblastic anemia). **However, most alcoholics have adequate diets, and the great majority of alcohol-related disorders should be attributed to the toxic effects of alcohol.** The diseases associated with alcoholism are discussed in detail in chapters dealing with individual organs, and we restrict this discussion to the spectrum of disease (Fig. 8-10).

Alcohol Ingestion Affects Organs and Tissues

Liver

Liver disease associated with the excess consumption of alcoholic beverages (see Chapter 14) has been recognized for several thousand years, having been implied in the Ayur Veda, the ancient medical text of India. Almost 300 years ago, the noted English clinician Thomas Heberden wrote about the increase in "scirrhous" livers in those who consume large quantities of "spirituous liquors." **Alcoholic liver disease, the most common medical complication of alcoholism, accounts for a large proportion of cases of cirrhosis of the liver** (Fig. 8-11) **in the industrialized countries.** The nature of the alcoholic beverage is largely irrelevant; consumed in excess, beer, wine, whiskey, hard cider, and so on all produce cirrhosis. Only the total daily dose of alcohol itself is relevant.

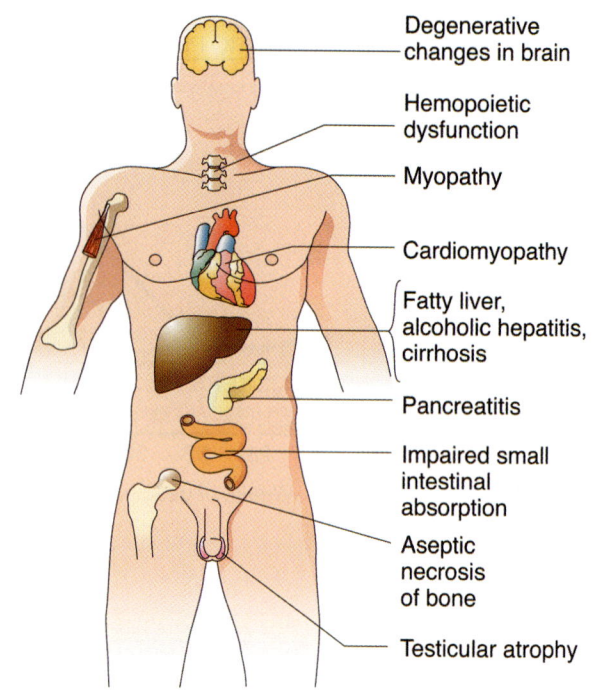

FIGURE 8-10
Complications of chronic alcohol abuse.

Pancreas

Both acute and chronic pancreatitis are complications of alcoholism (see Chapter 15). **Chronic calcifying pancreatitis, on the other hand, is an unquestioned result of alcoholism and an important cause of incapacitating pain, pancreatic insufficiency, and pancreatic stones.**

Heart

Alcohol-related heart disease was recognized over a century ago in Germany, where it was referred to as "beer-drinker's heart." This degenerative disease of the myocardium is a form of dilated cardiomyopathy, termed **alcoholic cardiomyopathy,** and leads to low-output congestive heart failure (see Chapter 11). Although the pathogenesis is obscure, it is widely accepted as a toxic effect of ethanol. This cardiomyopathy clearly differs from the heart disease associated with thiamine deficiency (beri-beri), a disorder characterized by high-output failure. The alcoholic heart seems also to be more susceptible to arrhythmias, and the occurrence of abnormal cardiac rhythms after an alcoholic binge has been called the "holiday heart." Many cases of sudden death in alcoholics are probably caused by sudden, fatal arrhythmias.

In this context, moderate alcohol consumption, or "social drinking" (1 to 2 drinks a day), provides significant protection against coronary artery disease (atherosclerosis) and its consequence, myocardial infarction. Similarly, compared with abstainers, social drinkers have a lower incidence of ischemic stroke.

Skeletal Muscle

Muscle weakness is extremely common in alcoholics and is often attributed to general debility or nutritional deficiency.

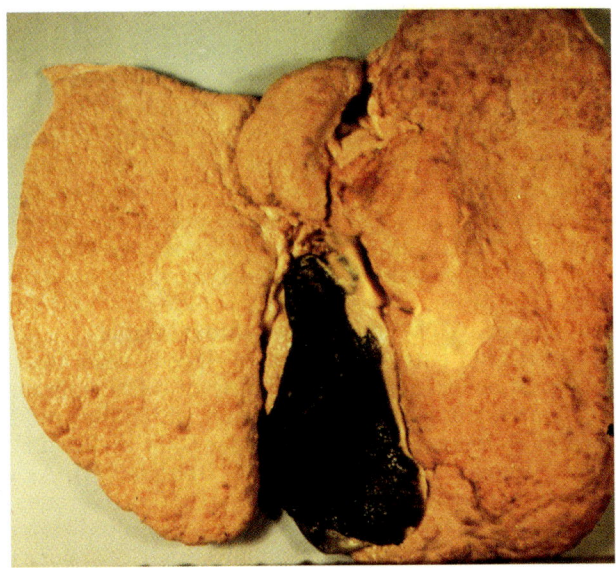

FIGURE 8-11
Cirrhosis of the liver in a chronic alcoholic. The surface displays innumerable small nodules of hepatocytes separated by interconnecting bands of fibrous tissue. The dark structure is the gallbladder.

However, when carefully tested clinically, even well-nourished alcoholics usually show some weakness, particularly of the proximal muscles. A wide range of changes in skeletal muscle occurs in chronic alcoholics, varying from mild alterations in muscle fibers evident only by electron microscopy to a severe, debilitating chronic myopathy, with degeneration of muscle fibers and diffuse fibrosis. On rare occasions, **acute alcoholic rhabdomyolysis**—necrosis of muscle fibers and release of myoglobin to the circulation—occurs. This sudden event can be fatal because of renal failure secondary to myoglobinuria.

Endocrine System

Feminization of male alcoholics, together with loss of libido and potency, is common. The breasts become enlarged (gynecomastia), body hair is lost, and a female distribution of pubic hair (female escutcheon) develops. Some of these changes can be attributed to impaired metabolism of estrogens due to chronic liver disease, but many of the changes—particularly atrophy of the testes—occur in the absence of any liver disease. Chronic alcoholism leads to lower levels of circulating testosterone because of a complex interference with the pituitary–gonadal axis, possibly complicated by accelerated hepatic metabolism of testosterone. Alcohol has been shown to have a direct toxic effect on the testes; thus, sexual impairment in the male is one of the prices exacted by alcoholism.

Gastrointestinal Tract

Since the esophagus and stomach may be exposed to 10 M ethanol, it is not surprising that a direct toxic effect on the mucosa of these organs is common. Injury to the mucosa of both organs is potentiated by the hypersecretion of gastric hydrochloric acid stimulated by ethanol. **Reflux esophagitis** may be particularly painful, and peptic ulcers are also more common in the alcoholic. Violent retching may lead to tears at the esophageal-gastric junction **(Mallory-Weiss syndrome)**, sometimes severe enough to result in exsanguinating hemorrhage (see Chapter 13). The mucosal cells of the small intestine are also exposed to circulating alcohol, and a variety of absorptive abnormalities and ultrastructural changes have been demonstrated. Alcohol inhibits the active transport of amino acids, thiamine, and vitamin B_{12}.

Blood

Megaloblastic anemia secondary to a deficiency of folic acid is not uncommon in malnourished alcoholics. A nutritional deficiency of folic acid is the most important factor, but alcohol is itself considered a weak folic acid antagonist in humans. Moreover, absorption of folate in the small intestine may be decreased in alcoholics. In addition, chronic ethanol intoxication leads directly to an **increase in mean corpuscular volume erythrocytes.** In the presence of alcoholic cirrhosis, the spleen is often enlarged by portal hypertension; in such cases, **hypersplenism** often causes **hemolytic anemia.** Acute transient **thrombocytopenia** is common after acute alcohol intoxication and may result in bleeding. Alcohol also interferes with the aggregation of platelets, thereby contributing to bleeding.

Bone

Chronic alcoholics, particularly postmenopausal women, are at increased risk for **osteoporosis.** Although it is well established that alcohol, at least in vitro, inhibits osteoblast function, the precise mechanism responsible for accelerated bone loss is not understood. Interestingly, moderate alcohol intake seems to exert a protective effect against osteoporosis. Male alcoholics exhibit an unusually high incidence of **aseptic necrosis of the head of the femur.** The mechanism for this complication is also obscure.

Immune System

Alcoholics seem to be prone to many infections (particularly pneumonias) with organisms that are unusual in the general population, such as *Haemophilus influenzae*. Experimentally, a number of alcohol-induced effects on immune function have been reported.

Nervous System

General cortical atrophy of the brain is common in alcoholics and may reflect a toxic effect of alcohol (see Chapter 28). By contrast, most of the characteristic brain diseases in alcoholics are probably a result of nutritional deficiency.

Wernicke encephalopathy is caused by thiamine deficiency and is characterized by mental confusion, ataxia, abnormal ocular motility, and polyneuropathy, reflecting the pathological changes in the diencephalon and brainstem.

Korsakoff psychosis is characterized by retrograde amnesia and confabulatory symptoms. The condition was once believed to be pathognomonic of chronic alcoholism but has now been identified in a number of organic mental syndromes and is considered nonspecific.

Alcoholic cerebellar degeneration is differentiated from other forms of acquired or familial cerebellar degeneration by the uniformity of its manifestations. Progressive unsteadiness of gait, ataxia, incoordination, and reduced deep tendon reflex activity are present.

Central pontine myelinolysis is another characteristic change in the brain of alcoholics, apparently caused by electrolyte imbalance—usually after electrolyte therapy, after an alcoholic binge or during withdrawal. In this complication, a progressive weakness of bulbar muscles terminates in respiratory paralysis.

Amblyopia (impaired vision) is occasionally seen in alcoholics and may result from an alcohol-related decrease in tissue vitamin A, although other vitamin deficiencies may also be involved.

Polyneuropathy is common in chronic alcoholics. This condition is usually associated with deficiencies of thiamine and other B vitamins, but a direct neurotoxic effect of ethanol may play a role. The most common complaints include numbness, paresthesias, pain, weakness, and ataxia.

Fetal Alcohol Syndrome Results from Alcohol Abuse in Pregnancy

Infants born to mothers who consume excess alcohol during pregnancy may show a cluster of abnormalities that together constitute the fetal alcohol syndrome. These include growth retardation, microcephaly, facial dysmorphology, neurological dysfunction, and other congenital anomalies. About 6% of the offspring of alcoholic mothers are afflicted by the full syndrome. More often, the exposure of the fetus to high concentrations of ethanol leads to less severe abnormalities, prominent among which are mental retardation, intrauterine growth retardation, and minor dysmorphic features. The fetal alcohol syndrome is discussed in greater detail in Chapter 6.

Alcohol Increases the Risk of Some Cancers

The incidence of cancer of the oral cavity, larynx, and esophagus is unquestionably higher in alcoholics than in the general population. The precise relationship of cancer to alcohol consumption is confused by the fact that most alcoholics are also smokers. In the case of cancer of the larynx, the combination of excess alcohol intake and smoking may be multiplicative rather than simply additive.

The Mechanisms by Which Alcohol Injures Tissues Are Not Understood

The pathogenesis of ethanol-induced organ damage remains obscure. In the liver, the change in the redox potential occasioned by the metabolism of ethanol has been proposed as a major factor. During the oxidation of ethanol to acetaldehyde, NAD is reduced to NADH, thereby greatly increasing the reducing power of the cell. However, although certain metabolic abnormalities may be attributed to this change in the NAD/NADH ratio, no tissue injury has been directly shown to be caused by it. Moreover, other organs that also exhibit alcohol-induced injury, such as the heart and the pancreas, do not metabolize ethanol to any appreciable extent.

Acetaldehyde is the highly toxic product of alcohol metabolism. In the liver, acetaldehyde is rapidly converted by aldehyde dehydrogenase to acetate, but measurable levels of acetaldehyde can be found in the liver. However, circulating levels of acetaldehyde are extremely low, and it is difficult to attribute all of the changes associated with alcoholism to this metabolite. Other metabolites that have been proposed as causes of tissue injury include fatty acid ethyl esters, phosphatidyl ethanol, and hydroxyethanol.

An effect of ethanol common to all cells, regardless of their origin or location, is disordering of cell membranes. Like all anesthetics, ethanol intercalates within the lipid bilayer and decreases the molecular order of the acyl chains of phospholipids (a process known as fluidization). As an adaptive response, the composition of the membranes is changed, so that they become resistant to this fluidizing effect of ethanol. The relationship of this effect to cell injury requires further study.

DRUG ABUSE

Drug abuse has been defined as "the use of any substance in a manner that deviates from the accepted medical, social, or legal patterns within a given society." For the most part, drug abuse involves agents that are used to alter mood and perception. These chemicals include (1) derivatives of opium (heroin, morphine); (2) depressants (barbiturates, tranquilizers, alcohol); (3) stimulants (cocaine, amphetamines), marijuana, psychedelic drugs (LSD); and (4) inhalants (amyl nitrite, organic solvents such as those in glue). The use of psychotropic chemicals to produce euphoric states has a long history and a worldwide distribution. In addition to alcoholic beverages, examples are hashish in the Middle East, opium in the Far East, coca leaves in South America, and mescaline among Native Americans of the Southwest. However, the current epidemic of drug abuse in western industrialized countries is of recent origin. A notable difference in the pattern of drug intake, namely, the intravenous injection of illicit drugs, reflects the easy availability of syringes and hypodermic needles in industrialized societies. This change in the pattern of drug intake and the development of newer and more-potent drugs have led to a profound change in the nature of the diseases related to drug abuse. The social and emotional consequences of drug abuse are beyond the scope of this chapter, but it should be noted that suicide, homicide, and accidents are responsible for one fourth to one half of deaths related to narcotic abuse. The use of illicit drugs is estimated to cause about 20,000 deaths a year in the United States.

Heroin Is a Potent Diacetyl Derivative of Morphine

Heroin is a commonly used illicit opiate. It is ordinarily administered subcutaneously or intravenously and in the usual dosage is effective for about 5 hours. The drug produces euphoria and drowsiness, but overdoses are characterized by hypothermia, bradycardia, and respiratory depression. Naloxone is a specific opiate antagonist that rapidly reverses the respiratory depression produced by heroin. Withdrawal symptoms are extremely uncomfortable but rarely fatal. Other opiates that are subject to abuse include morphine, Dilaudid, and oxycodone.

Illicit Drugs Are Responsible for Many Pathological Syndromes

Cocaine

Cocaine is an alkaloid derived from South American coca leaves. At one time, it was a drug of the affluent, but its current wide availability has led to an epidemic of use. The traditional route of intake among South American Indians was chewing the raw coca leaves. However, the processing of pure forms of cocaine allowed nasal and intravenous administration. The more potent freebase form of cocaine is hard and is "cracked" into smaller pieces that are smoked ("crack"). The half-life of cocaine in the blood is about 1 hour.

Cocaine users report extreme euphoria and a sense of heightened sensitivity to a variety of stimuli. However, with addiction, paranoid states and conspicuous emotional lability occur. The mechanism of action of cocaine is related to its interference with the reuptake of the neurotransmitter dopamine.

Cocaine overdose leads to anxiety and delirium and occasionally to seizures. Cardiac arrhythmias and other effects on the heart may cause sudden death in otherwise apparently healthy persons. Chronic abuse of cocaine is associated with the occasional development of a characteristic dilated cardiomyopathy, which may be fatal. Abstinence from cocaine does not produce a well-defined withdrawal syndrome.

Amphetamines

Amphetamines were initially used as nasal decongestants, but their ability to disguise fatigue and decrease appetite has led to widespread abuse. These drugs, which are relatively easy to synthesize, are sympathomimetic and resemble cocaine in their effects, although they exhibit a longer duration of action. The most serious complications of the abuse of amphetamines are seizures, cardiac arrhythmias, and hyperthermia. Amphetamine use has been reported to lead to vasculitis of the central nervous system, and both subarachnoid and intracerebral hemorrhages have been described. Physical dependence on amphetamines has not been demonstrated. Numerous analogues of amphetamine have been synthesized, but they differ little in their effects, except that some also have psychedelic properties.

Hallucinogens

Hallucinogens are a group of chemically unrelated drugs that alter perception and sensory experience.

Phencyclidine (PCP) is an anesthetic agent that has psychedelic or hallucinogenic effects. As a recreational drug, it is known as "angel dust" and is taken orally, intranasally, or by smoking. Because the half-life of PCP varies from 12 to 90 hours, its effects are often difficult to control. The anesthetic properties of phencyclidine lead to a diminished capacity to perceive pain and, therefore, to self-injury and trauma. Other than the behavioral effects, PCP commonly produces tachycardia and hypertension, and high doses result in deep coma, seizures, and even decerebrate posturing.

LSD (Lysergic acid diethylamide) is a hallucinogenic drug whose popularity peaked in the late 1960s, and it is little used today. The drug causes perceptual distortion of the senses, interference with logical thought, alteration of time perception, and a sense of depersonalization. "Bad trips" are characterized by anxiety and panic and objectively by sympathomimetic effects that include tachycardia, hypertension, and hyperthermia. Large overdoses cause coma, convulsions, and respiratory arrest.

Organic Solvents

The recreational inhalation of organic solvents is widespread, particularly among adolescents. Various commercial preparations such as fingernail polish, glues, plastic cements, and lighter fluid are all sniffed. Among the active ingredients are benzene, carbon tetrachloride, acetone, and toluene. Acute intoxication with organic solvents is similar to inebriation with alcohol. Large doses produce nausea and vomiting, hallucinations, and eventually coma. Chronic abuse of organic solvents may result in disease of the brain, kidneys, liver, lungs, and hematopoietic system.

Intravenous Drug Abuse Has Many Medical Complications

Apart from reactions related to the pharmacological or physiological effects of substance abuse, the most common complications (15% of directly drug-related deaths) are caused by the introduction of infectious organisms by a parenteral route. The most common infections are local at the site of injection. Among these are cutaneous abscesses, cellulitis, and ulcers (Fig. 8-12). When these heal, "track marks" persist, and these areas may also exhibit hypopigmentation or hyperpigmentation. Thrombophlebitis of the veins draining the sites of injection is common. Self-administration of street drugs can cause tetanus, particularly when the injection is subcutaneous or intramuscular. The intravenous introduction of bacteria also leads to septic complications in many organs. Bacterial endocarditis, often involving *Staphylococcus aureus*, occurs on both sides of the heart (Fig. 8-13). Other complications of bacteremia are pulmonary, renal, and intracranial abscesses; meningitis; osteomyelitis; and mycotic aneurysms (Fig. 8-14).

Perhaps the most feared infectious complications today are of viral etiology. Addicts who exchange needles constitute one of the highest risk groups for acquired immunodeficiency syndrome (AIDS) and viral hepatitis B and C. Addicts also suffer from the complications of viral hepatitis, such as chronic active hepatitis, necrotizing angiitis, and glomerulonephritis. A focal glomerulosclerosis ("heroin nephropathy") is characterized by the presence of immune complexes and has been ascribed to an immune reaction to impurities contaminating illicit drugs.

The intravenous injection of talc, a material used to dilute the pure drug, is associated with the appearance of foreign body granulomas in the lung (Fig. 8-15). These may be severe enough to lead to interstitial pulmonary fibrosis.

324 Environmental and Nutritional Pathology

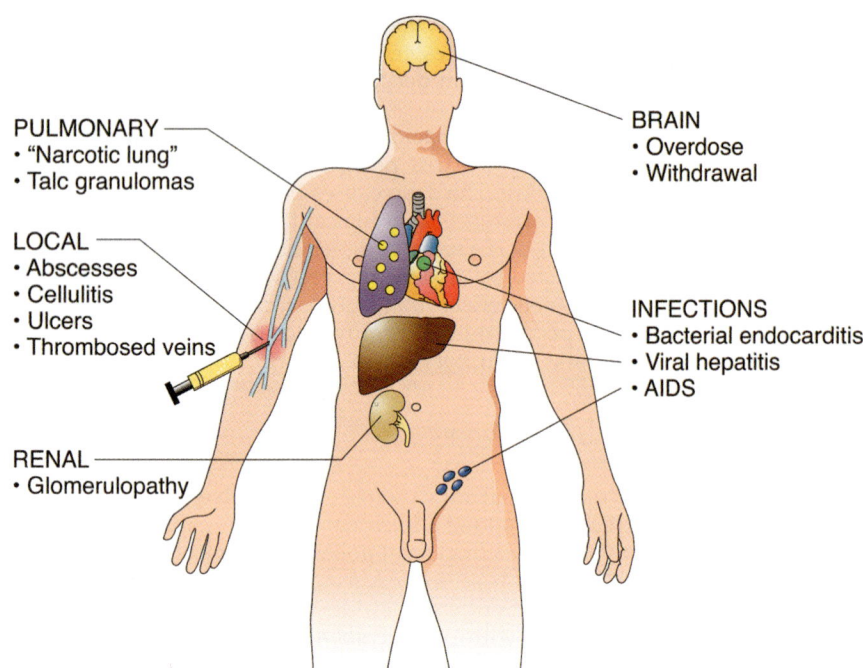

FIGURE 8-12
Complications of intravenous drug abuse.

Drug Addiction in Pregnant Women Poses Risks for the Fetus

Infants of drug-dependent mothers often exhibit a full-blown withdrawal syndrome. Moreover, the appearance of the drug withdrawal syndrome in the fetus during labor may result in excessive fetal movements and increased oxygen demand, a situation that increases the risk of intrapartum hypoxia and meconium aspiration. If labor occurs when maternal drug levels are high, the infant is often born with respiratory depression. Mothers who are addicted to drugs experience higher rates of toxemia of pregnancy and premature labor.

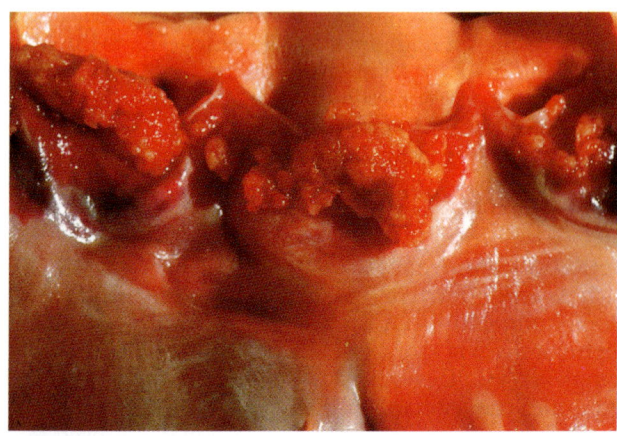

FIGURE 8-13
Bacterial endocarditis. The aortic valve of an intravenous drug abuser displays adherent vegetations.

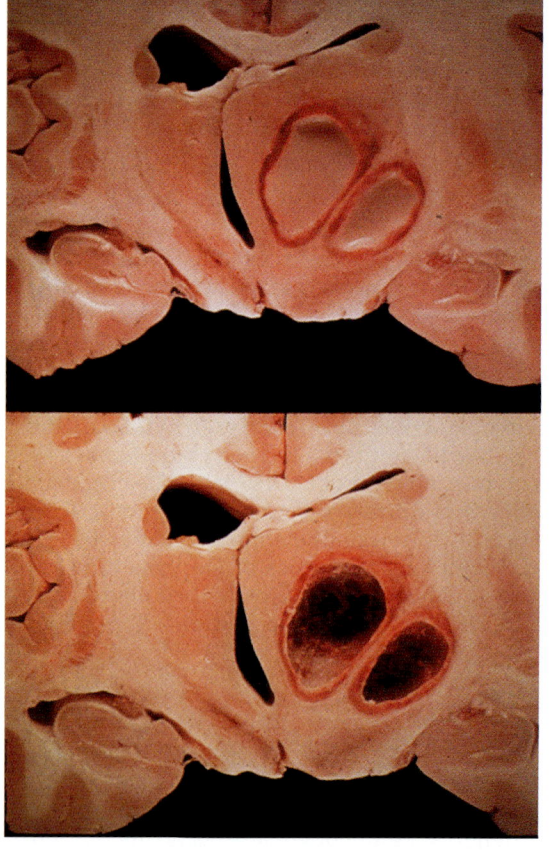

FIGURE 8-14
Brain abscess. *Top,* Cross-section of the brain from an intravenous drug abuser shows two encapsulated cavities containing pus. *Bottom,* The same abscesses after removal of their contents.

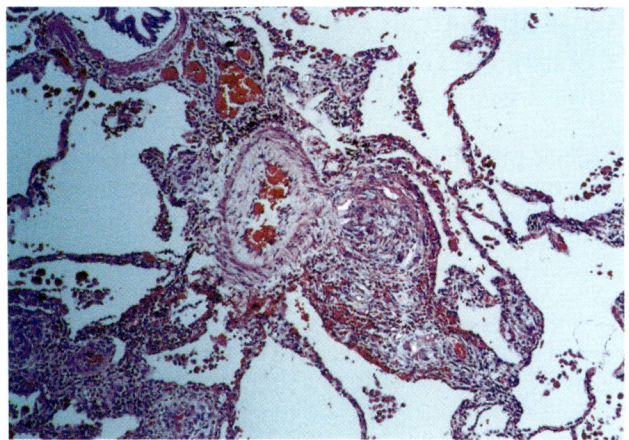

FIGURE 8-15
Talc granulomas in the lung. A section of lung from an intravenous drug abuser viewed under polarized light reveals a granuloma adjacent to a pulmonary artery. The refractile material is talc that was used to dilute the drug prior to its intravenous injection.

IATROGENIC DRUG INJURY

Iatrogenic drug injury refers to the unintended side effects of therapeutic or diagnostic drugs prescribed by physicians. The inadvertent complications of drug administration are so common that they constitute a major public health problem. Although few agents act as specifically and effectively as antibiotics, when properly used, drugs constitute the foundation of patient management. However, the administration of therapeutic agents exacts a price. Adverse reactions are surprisingly common, being found in 2–5% of patients hospitalized on medical services; of these reactions, 2 to 12% are fatal. The typical hospitalized patient is given about 10 different medications, and some receive five times as many. The risk of an adverse reaction increases proportionately with the number of different drugs; for example, the risk of injury is at least 40% when more than 15 drugs are administered. Because they are so ubiquitously prescribed, drugs represent a significant environmental hazard. Untoward effects of drugs result from (1) overdose, (2) an exaggerated physiological response, (3) a genetic predisposition, (4) hypersensitivity mechanisms, (5) interactions with other drugs, and (6) other unknown factors. The characteristic pathological changes associated with drug reactions are treated in chapters dealing with specific organs. An example of a drug reaction is illustrated in Figure 8-16.

SEX HORMONES

Oral Contraceptives Carry a Small Risk of Complications

Hormonal preparations are now the most commonly used contraceptive agents in industrialized countries. Current formulations are combinations of synthetic estrogens and steroids with progesterone-like activity. They act either by inhibiting the surge of gonadotropins at midcycle, thereby preventing ovulation, or by preventing implantation by altering the phase of the endometrium. Most of the complications are produced by the estrogenic component, but some may be related to the progestin component or to a combination of the two (Fig. 8-17).

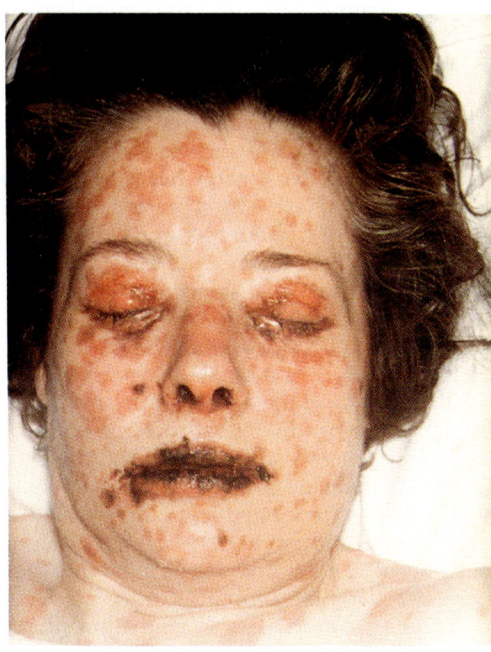

FIGURE 8-16
Erythema multiforme secondary to sulfonamide therapy.

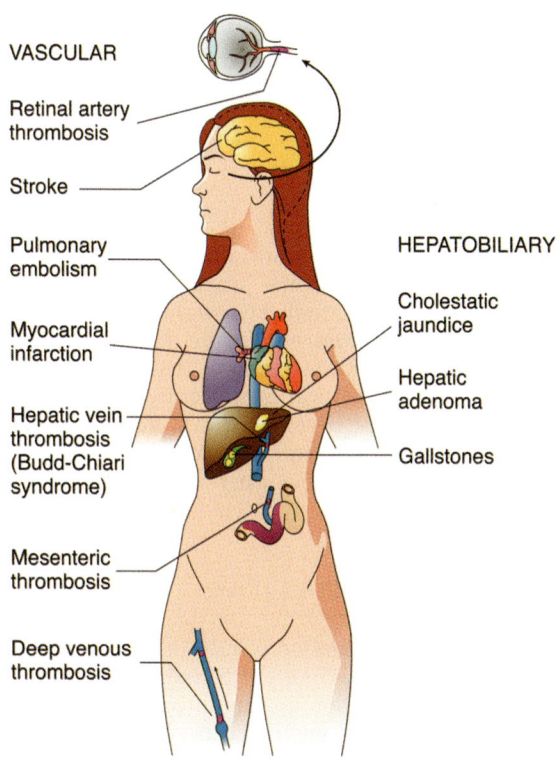

FIGURE 8-17
Complications of oral contraceptives.

Vascular Complications

Deep vein thrombosis is a recognized complication of oral contraceptive use, the risk being increased three to four times. As a consequence, the risk of thromboembolism is correspondingly increased, especially in women who are already at high risk for this condition. Although the incidence of myocardial infarction and stroke is low in women of reproductive age, oral contraceptives slightly increase the risk, particularly in smokers.

Neoplastic Complications

Cancers of the female reproductive organs, namely the ovary, endometrium, and breast, are strongly linked to hormonal influences. The use of an oral contraceptive might increase the risk of such tumors. Fortunately, the available epidemiological data suggest that the use of oral contraceptives actually decreases the risk of ovarian and endometrial cancers by about half, presumably because of suppression of the production of pituitary gonadotropins. With respect to breast cancer, oral contraceptives have not produced an increase in the overall incidence of breast cancer. However, they seem to increase the risk of breast cancer to a small degree in premenopausal women who have used this method of birth control for many years.

Benign liver adenomas are rare hepatic neoplasms that are significantly increased in incidence among women who use oral contraceptives. The risk of these tumors increases conspicuously with the duration of use, particularly after 5 years.

Several small case-control studies in developed countries with low rates of hepatitis B and C infection have suggested an increased risk of **hepatocellular carcinoma** among women using oral contraceptives. Fortunately, this cancer is distinctly uncommon in young women without chronic viral hepatitis, and no more than 1 case in 100,000 long-term users can be expected.

Other Complications

For reasons unknown, oral contraceptives may induce an increased pigmentation of the malar eminences, called **chloasma,** which is accentuated by sunlight and persists for a long time after the contraceptives are discontinued.

Cholelithiasis is more frequent (twofold increase) in women who have used oral contraceptives for 4 years or less, but its incidence becomes lower than normal after that period of time. Thus, oral contraceptives accelerate the process of cholelithiasis but do not increase its overall incidence.

Benefits of Oral Contraceptives

In considering the potential side effects of the use of oral contraceptive agents, it is important to recognize that certain benefits accrue. In addition to a significant reduction in the risk of ovarian and endometrial cancers, the use of these agents decreases the risk of pelvic inflammatory disease, uterine leiomyomas, endometriosis, and fibrocystic disease of the breast.

Postmenopausal Hormone Replacement Therapy Increases the Risk of Some Cancers

Hormone preparations containing combinations of estrogen and progesterone have been given to postmenopausal women in an effort to (1) alleviate menopausal symptoms and (2) decrease the risk of myocardial infarction and osteoporosis. These agents have proved effective in the treatment of postmenopausal symptoms and may mitigate osteoporosis, at least to some extent. However, the incidence of myocardial infarction is unaffected. The frequency of cancers of the breast and endometrium is slightly increased.

ENVIRONMENTAL CHEMICALS

An awareness of the potential hazards posed by the presence of harmful chemicals in the environment is not new. As the following quote from Maimonides shows, concerns about air pollution existed even in the 12th century.

> Comparing the air of cities to the air of deserts is like comparing waters that are befouled and turbid to waters that are fine and pure. In the city, because of the height of its buildings, the narrowness of its streets, and all that pours forth from its inhabitants, the air becomes stagnant, turbid, thick, misty, and foggy. If there is no choice in this matter, if we have grown up in the cities and become accustomed to them, we should endeavor at least to dwell at the outskirts of the city. Wherever the air is altered ever so slightly, you will find men develop dullness of understanding, failure of intelligence, and defects of memory.

Humans inhale, bathe in, and eat a variety of chemical materials that are found as contaminants in foods and in the food chain, the water supply, and the general ecosystem in which they live. However, predictions of widespread destruction of flora and fauna and an epidemic of human cancer have yet to materialize. In fact, efforts to quantitate the potency of environmental contaminants and to estimate past and present human exposure suggest that **naturally occurring chemicals pose a far greater hazard than man-made products**, and the former have been present for eons. Our natural environment is not without risk, and even oxygen can be harmful (see chapter 1).

Several important mechanisms govern the effect of toxic agents, including the toxin's absorption, distribution, metabolism, and excretion. Absorption (whether through pulmonary, gastrointestinal, or dermal routes) depends in part on the chemical structure of the agent. For example, because of their solubility in lipids, the insecticides chlordane and heptachlor are rapidly absorbed and stored in body fat. By contrast, the water-soluble herbicide paraquat is readily eliminated.

The effects of many chemicals are exerted by their metabolic products rather than by the parent compound. The capacity of the xenobiotic systems to modify these materials varies among tissues. Moreover, these detoxifying systems may produce different metabolites in different sites, which may vary in their capacity to produce disease. The cellular content of these enzyme systems varies with age, sex, hormonal and nutritional status, and previous drug intake.

TABLE 8-1 Cancers Associated with Exposure to Occupational Carcinogens

Agent or Occupation	Site of Cancer
Arsenic	Lung cancer
Asbestos	Mesothelioma (pleura and peritoneum)
	Lung cancer (in smokers)
Aromatic amines	Bladder cancer
Benzene	Leukemia, multiple myeloma
bis-(Chloromethyl)ether	Lung cancer
Chromium	Lung cancer
Furniture and shoe manufacturing	Nasal carcinoma
Hematite mining	Lung cancer
Nickel	Lung cancer, paranasal sinus cancer
Tars and oils	Cancers of lung, gastrointestinal tract, bladder, and skin
Vinyl chloride	Angiosarcoma of liver

The storage, distribution, and excretion of these materials control their concentrations in the organism at any given time. It follows that agents stored in adipose tissue exert a prolonged low-level effect, whereas the more water-soluble materials that are easily excreted by the kidney have a shorter duration of action.

The fact that a toxic agent can be detected in the workplace does not mean that it necessarily produces disease. For example, carbon tetrachloride, a recognized species-dependent hepatotoxin, is used frequently in the machining of steel. Yet liver disease derived from this haloalkane is not an occupational hazard in the steel fabricating industry. Thus, although there is little question that chemicals can and do produce human disease, in many cases, our information is far from conclusive.

Among the most important chemical hazards to which humans are exposed are environmental dusts and carcinogens. Inhalation of mineral and organic dusts occurs primarily in occupational settings (e.g., mining, industrial manufacturing, farming) and occasionally as a result of unusual situations (e.g., bird fanciers, pituitary snuff inhalation). The inhalation of mineral dusts leads to the pulmonary diseases known as pneumoconioses, whereas organic dusts produce hypersensitivity pneumonitis. Pneumoconioses were formerly common, but control of dust exposure in the workplace through modification of manufacturing techniques, improvements in air handling, and the use of facial masks has substantially reduced the incidence of these diseases. Because of their importance, pneumoconioses and hypersensitivity pneumonitis are discussed in detail in Chapter 12.

Chemical carcinogens are ubiquitous in the environment, and their potential for causing human disease has elicited widespread concern. In particular, exposure to carcinogens in the workplace has been associated epidemiologically with a number of cancers (Table 8-1). Chemical carcinogenesis is reviewed in Chapter 5.

Toxic Effects Differ from Hypersensitivity Responses

Many substances elicit disease in a variety of animal species in a dose-dependent manner, with a regular time delay and a predictable target organ response. Furthermore, the morphological changes in the injured tissues are constant and reproducible. By contrast, other agents show great variability in the production of disease, an irregular lag before any manifestation of injury, no dose dependency, and a lack of reproducibility. It has been assumed that the predictable dose-response reactions reflect a direct action of the compound or its metabolite on a tissue—that is, a "toxic" effect. The second, unpredictable type of reaction is believed to reflect "hypersensitivity," or an immunological response or idiosyncratic side effect.

Chemical Toxicity May Follow Occupational or Environmental Exposure

Beginning with the industrial revolution, there has been an exponential rise in the number of chemicals manufactured and a corresponding increase in the risk of human exposure. This potential problem has elicited widespread public concern and has particularly attracted the attention of journalists and attorneys. In any consideration of this topic, one must differentiate between the problems of acute poisoning and chronic toxicity. One must also distinguish industrial and accidental exposure from that which is likely to occur in the general environment. The lack of adequate quantitative data in humans and the obvious problems involved in obtaining such information have led to the extrapolation to humans of experimental data derived from animal studies. Such projections can be hazardous because of (1) species differences in sensitivity, (2) differing routes of administration, (3) variations in metabolic pathways, and (4) the use of unrealistically high concentrations of the test agent. Yet the doctrine is enshrined in American law that any agent that produces malignant tumors in any species, and at any dose, is unfit for human use. For example, large doses of the artificial sweeteners saccharin and the cyclamates were reported to be associated with the development of bladder tumors in experimental animals. As a result, the cyclamates have been withdrawn from use and saccharin has been subjected to strong criticism. Yet there are no adequate epidemiological data in humans that suggest a similar harmful effect among those who have regularly consumed these substances.

Except for certain hypersensitivity reactions in susceptible persons, acute poisoning by environmental chemicals does not pose a significant threat to the general population. The concentrations necessary to cause acute functional disorders or structural damage are ordinarily encountered only in the workplace or as a consequence of uncommon accidents. The latter category includes the exposure to the largest amount of tetrachlorodibenzodioxin (TCDD) ever to contaminate the environment, which followed an explosion in a chemical plant in Seveso, Italy, in 1976. This compound, a potent herbicide, is a byproduct of the synthesis of 2,4,5-trichlorphenoxyacetic acid (2,4,5-T), a defoliant used by the U.S. Army in Vietnam under the name "Agent Orange." As expected, some exposed persons developed acute symptoms, although none died. More than 25 years later, with the exception of chloracne, there have been no confirmed chronic effects in the persons exposed at Seveso. Moreover, after 20 years, Air Force veterans exposed to Agent Orange in Vietnam experienced no higher incidence of cancer or other diseases than comparable veterans not so exposed.

Although accidental mass poisonings with the pesticides endrin and parathion have led to as many as 100 deaths in a single event, no chronic sequelae among the survivors have been documented. Despite claims of an association between progressive chronic disease and exposure to pesticides, the small number of cases, coupled with the nonspecific nature of the complaints, does not permit such a conclusion. The action of most environmental toxins is specific, and a causal relationship to disease implies damage to a specific organ or organ system, with specific alterations of these tissues. As a corollary, multisystem involvement, particularly when the symptoms are vague, should be viewed with skepticism. The experimental literature dealing with the short- and long-term toxicity of industrial chemicals is voluminous and complicated and often contradictory. For this reason we largely restrict the following discussion to documented effects in humans.

Volatile Organic Solvents and Vapors

Volatile organic solvents and vapors are widely used in industry to dissolve other compounds (degreasers) and as fuels. With few exceptions, the exposures are industrial or accidental and represent short-term dangers rather than long-term toxicity. An exception is the recreational inhalation of solvents (e.g. "glue sniffing"), typically by adolescents. This activity has acute intoxicating effects on the brain, but no chronic sequelae have been noted. Long-term exposure to organic solvents has, however, been linked to the development of anti–basement membrane glomerulonephritis, with an estimated threefold to ninefold increased risk for this disorder. For the most part, exposure to solvents is by inhalation rather than by ingestion.

- **Chloroform ($CHCl_3$) and carbon tetrachloride (CCl_4):** These solvents exert anesthetic effects on the central nervous system but are better known as hepatotoxins. With both, large doses lead to acute hepatic necrosis, fatty liver, and liver failure. Whereas long-term administration of carbon tetrachloride to rats invariably produces cirrhosis, such a situation does not pertain to humans, because each exposure to the toxin results in recognizable clinical liver injury. Unlike a rat, a person who suffers a bout of jaundice after exposure to carbon tetrachloride will not be permitted another episode of poisoning.
- **Trichloroethylene (C_2HCl_3):** A ubiquitous industrial solvent, trichloroethylene in high concentrations depresses the central nervous system, but hepatotoxicity is minimal. There is no evidence for chronic sequelae in humans following ordinary long-term industrial exposure.
- **Methanol (CH_3OH):** This compound was originally called "wood alcohol" because it was derived from the distillation of wood. The odor and taste of methanol are similar to those of ethanol, and methanol does not carry the burden of a tax. It is, therefore, used by some impoverished chronic alcoholics as a substitute for ethanol or by unscrupulous merchants as an adulterant of alcoholic beverages. In methanol poisoning, inebriation similar to that produced by ethanol is succeeded by gastrointestinal symptoms, visual dysfunction, coma, and death. The major toxicity of methanol is believed to arise from its metabolism to formaldehyde, principally by alcohol dehydrogenase, followed by its oxidation to formic acid by aldehyde dehydrogenase.

  The most characteristic lesion of methanol toxicity is necrosis of retinal ganglion cells and subsequent degeneration of the optic nerve, a process presumably mediated by the metabolites of methanol oxidation. Interestingly, methanol-induced blindness occurs only in primates. It is not clear whether the metabolic acidosis seen in cases of methanol poisoning results from a direct effect of formate or from an inhibition of glucose oxidation.
- **Ethylene glycol ($HOCH_2CH_2OH$):** Commonly used as an antifreeze, ethylene glycol has been ingested by chronic alcoholics as a substitute for ethanol for many years. Poisoning with this compound has come into prominence because it has been used to adulterate wines in Austria and Italy, owing to its sweet taste and solubility. Like methanol, ethylene glycol is much more toxic in humans than in animals. The major toxicity relates to acute tubular necrosis in the kidney. Oxalate crystals in the tubules and oxaluria are often noted.
- **Gasoline and kerosene:** These fuels are mixtures of aliphatic hydrocarbons and branched, unsaturated, and aromatic hydrocarbons. Despite prolonged exposure to gasoline, gas station attendants, auto mechanics, and so on do not manifest any evidence of toxicity. The increased use of kerosene as a home heating fuel has led to accidental poisoning of children.
- **Benzene (C_6H_6):** The prototypic aromatic hydrocarbon is benzene, which must be distinguished from benzine, a mixture of aliphatic hydrocarbons. Benzene is one of the most widely used chemicals in industrial processes, being a starting point for innumerable syntheses and a solvent. It is also a constituent of fuels, accounting for as much as 3% of gasoline. Virtually all cases of acute and chronic benzene toxicity have occurred against the background of industrial exposure. Many instances have been reported in shoemakers and workers in shoe manufacturing, occupations that at one time were associated with heavy exposure to benzene-based glues.

  Acute benzene poisoning primarily affects the central nervous system, and death results from respiratory failure. However, the long-term effects of benzene exposure have attracted the most attention. The bone marrow is the principal target in chronic benzene intoxication. Patients who develop hematological abnormalities characteristically exhibit **hypoplasia or aplasia of the bone marrow and pancytopenia.** Aplastic anemia usually is seen while the workers are still exposed to high concentrations of benzene. In a substantial proportion of cases of benzene-induced anemias, **acute myeloblastic leukemia, erythroleukemia, or multiple myeloma** develops during continuing exposure to benzene, or after a variable latent period following removal of the worker from the hazardous environment. Some cases of acute leukemia have occurred without a prior history of aplastic anemia. Although instances of chronic myeloid and chronic lymphocytic leukemia have been reported, a cause-and-effect relationship with benzene exposure is less convincing than that with cases of acute leukemia. Overall, the risk of leukemia is increased 60-fold in workers exposed to the highest atmospheric concentrations of benzene. The closely related compound toluene, also widely used for its solvent properties, has not been incriminated as a cause of hematological abnormalities.

Agricultural Chemicals

Pesticides, fungicides, herbicides, and organic fertilizers are crucial to the success of modern agriculture. Without the use of pesticides, it is estimated that agricultural production would fall by about half, and it is possible that epidemic and endemic famine would again become commonplace. However, the realization that many of these chemicals persist in soil and water and pose a potential long-term hazard has caused substantial concern. The problem of acute poisoning with very large concentrations of any of these chemicals has already been alluded to, and it is clear that exposure to industrial concentrations or inadvertently contaminated food can cause severe acute illness. A particularly common acute poisoning occurs in children who ingest home gardening preparations.

The symptoms of acute toxicity are often related to the mode of action of the toxin. For example, the organophosphate insecticides exert their effect by inhibiting acetylcholinesterase, and thus acute toxicity in humans is principally reflected in symptoms referable to the nervous system. In the United States, 30 to 40 persons die annually of acute pesticide poisoning. However, in underdeveloped countries, where the use of safety equipment is unusual, many more fatalities occur. If the short-term incident is not fatal, in most cases there are no chronic sequelae. However, delayed neurotoxicity has been reported with a few compounds, the most notorious of which is triorthocresyl phosphate (TOCP). Acute poisoning with this compound leads to a peripheral neuropathy that progresses to motor weakness of limbs, which in some cases is only partially reversible. Contamination of illicit ginger liquor with TOCP in the United States during the 1930s led to an epidemic of "ginger jake paralysis." In Morocco, the adulteration of cooking oil with lubricating oil containing TOCP produced an outbreak of a similar peripheral neuropathy.

The problem of widespread chronic human exposure to low levels of agricultural chemicals has profound health, economic, and legal implications. From a practical point of view, these chemicals cannot be eliminated from our environment, but because they produce a variety of disorders in experimental animals, it is appropriate to search for evidence of disease in humans. Potential effects that have elicited public concern include cancer, chronic degenerative diseases, congenital abnormalities, and a host of nonspecific complaints ranging from asthenia to impotence. However, no persuasive data have emerged to substantiate these fears, with the possible exception of certain types of hematopoietic malignancies in farmers who use large amounts of herbicides, particularly 2,4-dichlorophenoxyacetic acid (2,4-D). In this respect, several studies have linked occupational exposure to herbicides with an increased incidence of soft tissue sarcomas, lymphomas, and Hodgkin disease.

The current state of our knowledge can be summarized with the simple recognition that although chronic toxicity and reproductive failure have been clearly established in predatory birds and fish, there are no reliable data to support a similar link in humans. Until such a connection has been validated, the burden of proof will remain on those who postulate a cause-and-effect relationship.

Aromatic Halogenated Hydrocarbons

The halogenated aromatic hydrocarbons that have received considerable attention include (1) the polychlorinated biphenyls (PCBs), (2) chlorophenols (pentachlorophenol, used as a wood preservative), (3) hexachlorophene, used as an antibacterial agent in soaps), and (4) the dioxin TCDD, a byproduct of the synthesis of herbicides and hexachlorophene and, therefore, a contaminant of these preparations. The lack of chronic effects after acute TCDD poisoning is discussed above. Serious questions have been raised regarding the danger of long-term exposure to dioxin, and there is now a consensus that at the very least this compound is far more carcinogenic in rodents than in humans. The problem of the presence of PCBs in the environment resembles that of agricultural chemicals: long-term animal toxicity is well documented, but no significant increases occur in the incidence of cancer or other diseases in workers exposed to PCBs. The same situation pertains to hexachlorophene and pentachlorophenol.

Cyanide

Prussic acid (HCN) is the classic murderer's tool in detective fiction, where the smell of bitter almonds (*Amygdalus prunus*) betrays the crime. A more contemporary homicidal application of cyanide is its surreptitious addition to a number of commercially available medicinal capsules. Amygdalin, a glycoside found in the pits of several fruits (including apricots, peaches, and wild cherries) and in the seeds of almonds and hydrangeas, is a combination of glucose, benzaldehyde, and cyanide. Although humans do not possess the β-glucosidase needed to liberate the cyanide, intestinal flora can effect this release, thereby leading to cyanide intoxication. Amygdalin is, therefore, far more toxic when ingested than when injected intravenously. These considerations may appear esoteric, except for the fact that extracts of apricot pits were used in the formulation of fraudulent anticancer nostrums and resulted in cases of cyanide poisoning.

Cyanide blocks cellular respiration by reversibly binding to mitochondrial cytochrome oxidase, the terminal acceptor in the electron transport chain, which is responsible for reducing molecular oxygen to water. The pathological consequences are similar to those produced by any acute global anoxia.

Air Pollutants

A precise definition of air pollution is elusive, since the meaning of "pure air" is not established. In the absence of man-made pollutants, the atmosphere has always been dirtied by natural contaminants. These include the products of vegetation (spores, pollens, airborne molds), emissions from decaying plants (carbon dioxide, hydrogen sulfide), volcanic gases and dusts, and aerosolized bacteria and viruses. However, for the purposes of this discussion, the most important pollutants are those generated by the combustion of fossil fuels for the production of heat and energy.

The most important air pollutants that are implicated as factors in human disease are the irritants sulfur dioxide, nitrogen dioxide, and ozone, in addition to suspended particulates and acid aerosols. Particulate air pollution refers to the presence in the atmosphere of solid particles and liquid droplets, which vary in size, composition, and origin. Fine particles (2.5 μm or less in aerodynamic diameter) are a mixture of soot, sulfate and nitrate particles, and acid condensates. Because of their small size, they can be inhaled more deeply into the lungs. Owing to their composition, they are also more toxic than larger particles.

Epidemiological studies of the relationship between urban air pollution and adverse respiratory and cardiovascular effects are difficult to interpret because of the confounding effects of cigarette smoking, social class, occupation, age, and so on. However, it is indisputable that episodes of unusually severe air pollution, such as those that occurred in the Meuse valley in Belgium (1930), Donora, Pennsylvania (1948), and London (1952), were associated with striking increases in mortality. During each of these occurrences, the concentrations of sulfur dioxide and particulates are believed to have been remarkably high.

A substantial body of contemporary epidemiological literature describes adverse health effects from lower levels of particulate air pollution. In studies that adjust for cigarette smoking, the overall mortality in highly polluted cities is still some 25% greater than that in the least polluted areas. The excess mortality is largely attributable to increases in the incidence of lung cancer and cardiopulmonary disease.

Sulfur dioxide results from the combustion of sulfur-containing petroleum and coal in power plants, oil refineries, and industries such as paper mills and smelters. Ozone and nitrogen oxides do not derive principally from industrial activities but rather result from the action of sunlight on the products of vehicular internal combustion engines. Automobiles and trucks emit unburnt hydrocarbons and nitrogen dioxide, after which ultraviolet irradiation leads to complex chemical reactions that produce ozone, various nitrates, and other organic and inorganic compounds in both gas and particulate phases. This mixture of pollutants constitutes the "smog" that is characteristic of areas with numerous vehicles and abundant sunlight. Prolonged exposure to gas-phase pollutants (SO_2, NO_2, and O_3) is associated with an increased frequency of chronic bronchitis and asthmatic attacks and decreased pulmonary function.

A number of studies have established an association between these atmospheric contaminants and both chronic respiratory symptoms and mortality. The adverse effects of this type of air pollution principally involve persons with existing respiratory ailments (asthma, chronic bronchitis, and emphysema) and cardiovascular disease. The evidence to incriminate air pollution in the pathogenesis of chronic respiratory disease in previously healthy persons remains equivocal.

Carbon Monoxide

Carbon monoxide is an odorless and nonirritating gas that results from the incomplete combustion of organic substances. It combines with hemoglobin with an affinity 240 times greater than that of oxygen to form carboxyhemoglobin. The binding of carbon monoxide to hemoglobin also increases the affinity of the remaining heme moieties for oxygen. As a consequence, oxygen does not readily dissociate from such hemoglobin in the tissues and the hypoxia that results from carbon monoxide poisoning is far greater than can be attributed to the loss of oxygen-carrying capacity alone.

Environmental carbon monoxide is derived principally from automobile exhaust emissions, fires, and, in some areas, home heating systems. A concentration of carboxyhemoglobin less than 10% is commonly found in smokers and ordinarily does not produce symptoms. Concentrations up to 30% usually cause only headache and mild exertional dyspnea. Higher levels of carboxyhemoglobin lead to confusion and lethargy; and at concentrations above 50%, coma and convulsions ensue. Levels greater than 60% are usually fatal. In fatal cases of carbon monoxide poisoning, a characteristic cherry-red color is imparted to the skin by the carboxyhemoglobin in the superficial capillaries. Recovery from severe carbon monoxide poisoning may be associated with brain damage, which may be manifested as subtle intellectual deficits, memory loss, or extrapyramidal symptoms (e.g., parkinsonism). Treatment of acute carbon monoxide poisoning, as in persons who attempt suicide or are trapped in fires, consists principally of the administration of 100% oxygen.

Deleterious effects of long-term exposure to low levels of carbon monoxide have been difficult to substantiate. However, concentrations of carboxyhemoglobin below 5 to 8% (often found in smokers) have accelerated the onset of exertional angina and changed the electrocardiograms in patients with ischemic heart disease. Thus, carboxyhemoglobin saturation levels even as low as 2.5% are considered undesirable in such patients.

Metals

Metals are an important group of environmental chemicals that have caused disease in humans from ancient times to the present. Although for centuries lead and mercury were known to cause disease, the industrial revolution was accompanied by a proliferation of occupational exposures to these and other toxic metals. In our own time, attention has increasingly turned to the ominous threat of the pollution of environment by toxic metals.

Lead

Lead is a ubiquitous heavy metal that is common in the environment of industrialized countries. The concentrations of lead in air, water, food, and soil have sharply increased since the onset of the industrial revolution, and a further increase was related to the introduction of leaded gasoline in the earlier part of this century.

Prior to the widespread awareness of chronic exposure to lead in the 1950s and 1960s, the classic symptoms of lead poisoning were commonly encountered in children and adults. In the United States, lead poisoning was primarily a pediatric problem related to pica, the habit of chewing on cribs, toys, furniture, and woodwork and eating painted plaster and fallen paint flakes. Most dwellings built before 1940 were decorated on the interior and exterior with paint that contained lead (up to 40% of dry weight). Children living in dilapidated older homes heavily coated with flaking paint were at significant risk of developing chronic lead poisoning. To these sources of lead was added a heavy burden of atmospheric lead in the form of dust derived from the combustion of lead-containing gasoline. Children and adults living near point sources of environmental lead contamination, such as smelters, were exposed to even higher levels of lead.

In adults, occupational exposure to lead occurred primarily among those engaged in the smelting of lead, a process that releases metal fumes and deposits lead oxide dust in the industrial environment. Lead oxide is a constituent of battery grids, and an occupational exposure to lead is a hazard in the manufacture and recycling of automobile batteries. Accidental poisonings occasionally occurred from the use of pottery that had been improperly fired with a lead glaze, the renovation of an old residence heavily coated with lead paint, the consumption of "moonshine" whiskey made in lead stills, or the "sniffing" of lead-containing gasoline.

METABOLISM: Lead is absorbed through either the lungs or the gastrointestinal tract. Once in the blood, it rapidly equilibrates with the plasma and erythrocytes and is excreted by the kidneys. A portion of blood lead remains freely diffusible and enters either of two types of tissues. Bones, teeth, nails, and hair represent a tightly bound pool of lead that is not generally regarded as harmful. By contrast, the amount of lead in the brain, liver, kidneys, and bone marrow is directly related to its toxic effects. With chronic exposure, 90% of the total body lead burden is in the bones. During metaphyseal bone formation in children, lead and calcium are deposited to produce the increased bone densities ("lead lines") seen radiographically at the metaphysis, thereby providing a simple method of detecting increased body stores of lead in children.

TOXICITY: Classic lead toxicity, which is rarely encountered in the United States today, is manifested in the dysfunction of three important organ systems: (1) the nervous system, (2) the kidneys, and (3) the hematopoietic system (Fig. 8-18).

The brain is the target of lead toxicity in children; adults usually present with manifestation of peripheral neuropathy. Children with lead encephalopathy are typically irritable and ataxic. They may convulse or display altered states of consciousness, from drowsiness to frank coma. Children with blood lead levels above 80 μg/mL, but with concentrations lower than those in children with frank encephalopathy (120 μg/mL), exhibit mild central nervous system symptoms such as clumsiness, irritability, and hyperactivity.

Lead encephalopathy is a condition in which the brain is edematous and displays flattened gyri and compressed ventricles. There may be herniation of the uncus and cerebellar tonsils. Microscopically, congestion, petechial hemorrhages, and foci of neuronal necrosis are seen. A diffuse astrocytic proliferation in both the gray and white matter may accompany these changes. Vascular lesions in the brain are particularly prominent, with dilation and proliferation of capillaries.

Peripheral motor neuropathy is the most common manifestation of lead neurotoxicity in the adult, typically affecting the radial and peroneal nerves and resulting in **wristdrop** and **footdrop**, respectively. Lead-induced neuropathy is probably also the basis of the paroxysms of gastrointestinal pain known as *lead colic*.

Anemia is a cardinal sign of lead intoxication. Lead disrupts heme synthesis in bone marrow erythroblasts through inhibition of δ-aminolevulinic acid dehydratase, the second enzyme in the de novo synthesis of heme. It also inhibits ferrochelatase, the enzyme that catalyzes the incorporation of ferrous iron into the porphyrin ring. The resulting inability to produce heme adequately is expressed as a microcytic and hypochromic anemia resembling that seen in iron deficiency, in which heme synthesis is also impaired. The anemia of lead intoxication is also characterized by prominent basophilic stippling of the erythrocytes, related to the clustering of ribosomes. The life span of the erythrocytes is decreased; thus, the anemia of lead intoxication is due to both ineffective hematopoiesis and accelerated erythrocyte turnover.

Lead nephropathy reflects the toxic effect of the metal on the proximal tubular cells of the kidney. The resulting dysfunction is characterized by aminoaciduria, glycosuria, and hyperphosphaturia (Fanconi syndrome). Such functional alterations are accompanied by the formation of inclusion bodies in the nuclei of the proximal tubular cells. These inclusions are characteristic of lead nephropathy and are composed of a lead–protein complex containing more than 100 times the concentration of lead in the whole kidney.

Lead poisoning is treated with chelating agents such as calcium ethylene diamine tetraacetic acid (EDTA), either alone or in combination with dimercaprol (BAL). Both the hematological and renal manifestations of lead intoxication are usually reversible; the alterations in the central nervous system are generally irreversible.

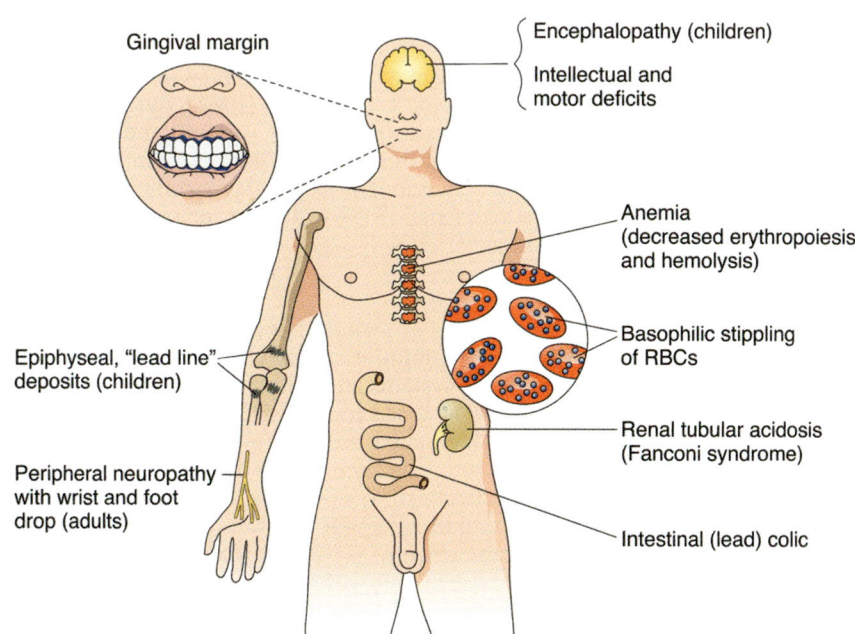

FIGURE 8-18
Complications of lead intoxication.

The laboratory diagnosis of an increased lead burden is made by demonstrating high levels of lead in the blood and increased free erythrocyte protoporphyrin. Elevated urinary excretion of δ-aminolevulinic acid and decreased levels of aminolevulinic acid dehydratase in erythrocytes are confirmatory.

EFFECTS OF CHRONIC EXPOSURE TO LOW LEAD LEVELS: As a result of the increased use of unleaded gasoline, improvements in housing, substitution of titanium for lead in paints, and the control of industrial point sources, ambient levels of lead have fallen significantly in the past three decades. In fact, blood levels in the general population of the United States decreased from an average of 16 μg/dL of blood in 1976 to 1.0 μg/dL in 2000. The dramatic fall in mean blood lead levels has been accompanied by the near elimination of lead-related childhood fatalities and encephalopathy. However, low lead exposure in children, while not producing recognizable symptoms, may permanently decrease cognitive performance. The regulatory safe threshold for blood levels of lead in children has been progressively reduced and is now thought to be below 10 μg/dL.

The evidence is compelling that low lead exposure in children, while not producing recognizable symptoms, creates deficits in intellectual and motor functions that persist into adult life. During the last 15 years, efforts to reduce environmental lead exposure have led to a decrease in the percentage of children in the United States with blood levels of 10 μg of lead or more from 89 to 9%. However, high blood lead concentrations remain a problem among poor, mainly black children, and more vigorous campaigns to ameliorate this situation are justified.

Mercury

Mercury has been used since prehistoric times and has been known to be an occupation-related hazard at least since the Middle Ages. As the use of mercury has changed, so have the populations at risk. At first, mercurialism was mainly a disease of mercury miners. In the 16th and 17th centuries, mercury poisoning was an occupational disease among gilders of gold, silver, or copper, who used mercury in the process of preparing a surface to be decorated. Mercury was subsequently introduced into the manufacture of fur felt, and mercurialism became an occupational hazard of the hatting industry. The neurological syndrome of tremor ("hatter's shakes") and mental symptoms ("mad as a hatter") was well known in the 19th century.

Although mercury poisoning still occurs in some occupations, there has been increasing concern over the potential health hazards brought about by the contamination of many ecosystems following several well-known outbreaks of methylmercury poisoning. The most widely publicized episodes occurred in Japan, first in Minamata Bay in the 1950s and then in Niigata. In both cases, local inhabitants developed severe, chronic organic mercury intoxication. This poisoning was traced to the consumption of fish contaminated with mercury that had been discharged into the environment in the effluents from a fertilizer and a plastics factory. To date, over 1000 cases of methylmercury poisoning have been reported from Japan. In the early 1970s, there was a more extensive outbreak of mercury poisoning in Iraq resulting from the consumption of bread made from cereal grains that had been treated with organic mercury fungicides. Six thousand persons were affected, 500 of whom died. Interestingly, in prenatally exposed children, later studies showed delayed achievement of developmental milestones and abnormal reflexes, despite the fact that fetal exposure was estimated to be 5 to 10 times lower than that for adults.

In the past two decades, it has become ominously clear that mercury released into the environment may be bioconcentrated and enter the food chain. Bacteria in the bottoms of bays and oceans can convert mercury compounds released from industrial wastes into highly neurotoxic organomercurials. These compounds are then transferred up the food chain and are eventually concentrated in the large predatory fish that make up a substantial part of the diet in many countries.

Although inorganic mercury is not efficiently absorbed in the gastrointestinal tract, organic mercurial compounds are readily absorbed because of their lipid solubility. Both inorganic and organic mercury are preferentially concentrated in the kidney, and methylmercury also distributes to the brain. **The kidney is the principal target of the toxicity of inorganic mercury, but the brain is damaged by organic mercurials.**

NEPHROTOXICITY: At one time, mercuric chloride was widely used as an antiseptic, and acute mercuric chloride poisoning was much more common; the compound was ingested by accident or for suicidal purposes. Under such circumstances, **proximal tubular necrosis** was accompanied by oliguric renal failure. Mercurial diuretics were also widely prescribed in the past, and chronic mercury nephrotoxicity was a not uncommon complication of their long-term use. Today, chronic mercurial nephrotoxicity is almost always a consequence of long-term industrial exposure. Proteinuria is common in chronic mercurial nephrotoxicity, and there may be a nephrotic syndrome with more severe intoxication. Pathologically, there is a membranous glomerulonephritis with subepithelial electron-dense deposits, suggesting immune complex deposition.

NEUROTOXICITY: The neurological effects of mercury, now known as **Minamata disease,** are manifested as a constriction of visual fields, paresthesias, ataxia, dysarthria, and hearing loss. Pathologically, there is cerebral and cerebellar atrophy. Microscopically, the cerebellum exhibits atrophy of the granular layer, without loss of Purkinje cells, and spongy softenings in the visual cortex and other cortical regions.

Arsenic

The toxic properties of arsenic have been known for centuries. Arsenic-containing compounds are toxic to a broad spectrum of living systems and, therefore, have been widely used as insecticides, weed killers, and wood preservatives. In the past, the medicinal uses of arsenic ranged from the treatment of a variety of cancers to its use as a "tonic." In the United States, the use of arsenicals in human medicine has declined, although they remain in common use in veterinary medicine and in agriculture. Arsenic compounds contaminate the soil and drinking water as a result of naturally occurring arsenic-rich rock formations or from coal burning and the use of arsenical pesticides. As with mercury, there is evidence for the bioaccumulation of arsenic along the food chain.

Acute arsenic poisoning is almost always the result of accidental or homicidal ingestion, and death is due to **central nervous system toxicity.** For examples, the interested reader is referred to the play "Arsenic and Old Lace" by Joseph Kesselring. Chronic arsenic intoxication is characterized initially by such nonspecific symptoms as malaise and fatigue. Eventually, gastrointestinal disturbances develop, along with changes in the skin and peripheral neuropathy. The latter is characterized by paresthesias, motor palsies, and painful neuritis. On epidemiological grounds, **cancers of the skin and respiratory tract** have been attributed to industrial and agricultural exposure to arsenic. In some parts of the world, exposure of workers in rice paddies to arsenic in the ground water has been associated with skin cancers.

Cadmium

Cadmium is used in the manufacture of alloys, in the production of alkali storage batteries, in electroplating of other metals (e.g., automobile parts and musical instruments), and as a pigment. Fumes of cadmium oxide are released in the course of welding steel parts previously plated with a cadmium anticorrosive.

Short-term cadmium inhalation irritates the respiratory tract, with pulmonary edema the most dangerous result. The lungs and the kidneys are the principal target organs of chronic cadmium intoxication. Emphysema has been the major finding in the fatal cases of chronic cadmium pneumonitis that have been studied. Proteinuria, which reflects tubular rather than glomerular damage, has been the most consistent finding in cadmium workers with renal damage.

Nickel

Nickel is a widely used metal in electronics, coins, steel alloys, batteries, and food processing. Dermatitis ("nickel itch"), the most frequent effect of exposure to nickel, may occur from direct contact with metals containing nickel, such as coins and costume jewelry. The dermatitis is a sensitization reaction; the body reacts to nickel-conjugated proteins formed following the penetration of the epidermis by nickel ions. Exposure to nickel, as to arsenic, increases the risk of development of specific types of cancer. Epidemiological studies have demonstrated that workers who were occupationally exposed to nickel compounds have an increased incidence of **lung cancer and cancer of the nasal cavities**.

Iron

Iron deficiency anemia is a common disease, particularly in women. Oral iron preparations contain largely ferrous sulfate, the form absorbed by the gastrointestinal mucosa and then converted to the trivalent form. Acute poisoning from the accidental ingestion of ferrous sulfate tablets occurs chiefly in children, particularly those between the ages of 1 and 2 years. As little as 1 to 2 g of ferrous sulfate may be lethal, but most fatal cases follow ingestion of 3 to 10 g. Hemorrhagic gastritis and acute liver necrosis have been the most prominent findings at autopsy.

A long-term, excessive dietary intake of iron does not ordinarily lead to abnormal iron accumulation in the body, except in the Bantus of South Africa, among whom it is common. These persons have a high iron content in their diet. Although some of it is derived from iron cooking pots, the major source is the iron drums used for the preparation of fermented alcoholic beverages. The acidic pH of these brews readily solubilizes the iron, and their low alcohol content allows large volumes to be consumed. A large proportion of the excess iron is in the liver, and there is a correlation between the degree of siderosis and the presence of cirrhosis. There is also a high incidence of diabetes and heart disease in this "Bantu siderosis."

Miscellaneous Metals

COBALT: In the 1960s, an epidemic of an unusual cardiomyopathy, clinically characterized by fulminant congestive heart failure, appeared in drinkers of a particular brand of beer, first in the Canadian province of Quebec and subsequently in the United States and Europe. The heart disease was traced to an excessive intake of cobalt, which had been added to the beer to enhance foaming qualities. When the cobalt was removed from the beer, no further cases of heart disease were reported.

ALUMINUM: In 1972, a new syndrome, called "dialysis encephalopathy," was first reported in patients with uremia undergoing chronic renal dialysis. The subsequent finding of high concentrations of aluminum in the gray matter of the brains of patients who died led to the suggestion that the **encephalopathy resulted from aluminum intoxication.** Epidemiological studies implicated the aluminum in the tap water used to prepare the dialysates, and the disease could be eliminated by removing aluminum from the water. Aluminum intoxication with encephalopathy and osteomalacia can occur in patients (generally children) with uremia who are not dialyzed but who are given oral phosphate-binding gels that contain aluminum.

Radioactive Elements

Elements whose radioactive isotopes are potentially hazardous include radium, strontium, uranium, plutonium, thorium, and iodine. The chronic toxicities relate principally to radiation-induced carcinogenesis. The individual tumors reflect the organ localization of the elements and are discussed in the chapters that address specific organ pathology.

THERMAL REGULATORY DYSFUNCTION

Body temperature is regulated by the thermal regulatory center of the hypothalamus, which modifies heat loss from the body, and by heat production, primarily from muscular activity. The hypothalamic center is sensitive to thermal, neural, and humoral stimulation. There is also evidence that it responds to changes in the perfusing blood temperature of as little as 0.5°C. A lowering of skin temperature below 32.8°C (91°F) causes a neural discharge of this center. Fever is produced by a short polypeptide, interleukin-1, which is released from macrophages. There is also a diurnal variation in body temperature of about 0.5°C.

Body heat is produced as a result of cellular metabolic activity and muscular work. Cold stress produces an increase in heat production of 50 to 100% by increasing muscle tone, a modification not associated with significant physical movement. Increased heat production beyond this level requires actual muscular contraction, often in the form of shivering, which can further increase the heat yield considerably.

Heat loss accounts for 50% of the heat produced by the body; the remainder of the heat energy provides for the 37°C ± 1°C body temperature. In large part, heat loss is regulated by the volume of blood. Two major factors are involved in the dermal regulatory system: (1) blood flow to the skin and (2) the use of the thermal energy to warm the portion of the skin surface that is wet with perspiration. Dilation of these arcades to bring the blood nearer the skin surface facilitates the transfer of the heat, a process that underlies the flushed appearance during strenuous exercise or hot weather. The means for heat dissipation from the body are conduction, convection, and radiation of thermal energy, as well as the evaporation of sensible and insensible perspiration from the surface of the skin. Under basal conditions, roughly 5% of the cardiac output goes to the skin, but when vasodilation is called on to increase heat loss, this value may reach roughly half of the normal cardiac output. In the reverse process, environmental cold leads to vasoconstriction and a reduction in blood flow to the skin, an effect seen as blanching.

Although the skin surface is the major avenue of heat loss, smaller quantities of heat energy are lost through the warming of inspired air and through sweating. The skin has abundant sweat glands whose orifices deposit perspiration on the surface. The evaporation of this fluid contributes to the loss of heat energy by extracting the heat of vaporization. At rest, a person normally loses about 1 L of insensible perspiration a day. During strenuous physical activity or in a hot environment, the production of sweat serves as an important additional source of cooling.

The dermis is also provided with a fatty layer that serves as an effective insulator. Humans appear to use body fat as an adaptive device for cold climates. Persons living near and above the Arctic Circle frequently have thicker dermal fat layers than their southern counterparts.

Hypothermia Refers to a Decrease in Body Temperature below 35°C (95°F)

Hypothermia can result in systemic or focal injury, the latter exemplified by **trench foot** or **immersion foot.** In localized hypothermia of these types, actual tissue freezing does not occur. **Frostbite,** by contrast, involves the crystallization of tissue water. Remember that the hospitalized patient, especially if sedated, is often placed in a thermal environment that is cooler than optimal and that can exert a stressful effect. Heat loss during a surgical procedure can be remarkable, and the administration of muscle relaxants further compromises the ability to generate heat.

Generalized Hypothermia

Acute immersion in water at 4°C to 10°C leads to a reduction in central blood flow, coupled with a decreased core body temperature and cooling of the blood perfusing the brain, which results in mental confusion. Muscle tetany makes swimming impossible. Furthermore, an increased vagal discharge leads to premature ventricular contractions, ventricular arrhythmias, and even fibrillation.

In an attempt to increase heat production, the immersed body immediately responds by increasing muscle activity and oxygen consumption. However, there are limits to the sources of energy available for sustained warming. Within 30 minutes, heat loss exceeds heat production because of the combination of high direct conduction of heat from the whole skin surface and the altered muscle tone caused by decreased arterial carbon dioxide and exhaustion. Core temperature then begins to fall. Peripheral vasoconstriction is another response to conserve heat. In addition, there is an increased sympathetic neural discharge, resulting in increased heart and basal metabolic rates and shivering. When the core temperature approaches 35°C, this activity may be three to six times above normal. Below this temperature, declines in respiratory rate, heart rate, and blood pressure ensue because of the reduction in functional reserve.

With prolonged cooling, a "cold-induced" diuresis results in increased blood viscosity. As a result, blood flow decreases and oxygen–hemoglobin association is less effective. Cardiac stroke volume decreases and peripheral vascular resistance increases as a direct result of both blood "sludging" and loss of plasma. The most important factor in causing death is cardiac arrhythmia or sudden cardiac arrest. These observations have been confirmed and extended, largely because of the need to induce hypothermia in some patients undergoing open-heart surgery. In fact, with careful pharmacological control, prolonged periods of lower body temperature can be achieved with no residual harm.

During prolonged hypothermia—for example, after an accident to a mountain climber—several of the consequences of decreased body temperature are related to altered cerebrovascular function. When the body core temperature reaches 32°C (89.6°F), the exposed person becomes lethargic, apathetic, and withdrawn. A characteristic response is inappropriate behavior, including disrobing, even when cold. A further decline in temperature increases the lethargy to intermittent "stupor" and eventually coma. A core temperature below 28°C (82.4°F) results in a weak pulse, feeble respiration, and coma.

Although there are no specific morphological changes in those who have succumbed to hypothermia, the skin exhibits red and purple discolorations, swelling of the ears and hands, and irregular vasoconstriction and vasodilation. Areas of myocytolysis are seen within the heart. The lung may display pulmonary edema and intraalveolar, intrabronchial, and interstitial hemorrhage.

Focal Thermal Alterations

As discussed above, local reduction in tissue temperature, particularly in the skin, is associated with local vasoconstriction. Tissue water crystallizes if blood circulation is insufficient to counter persistent thermal loss. When freezing occurs slowly, ice crystals form within tissue cells and in the interstitial space. Concomitantly, electrolyte-rich gels are excluded. Injury to the cellular organelles reflects the drastic changes in ionic concentrations in the excluded volume. Denaturation of macromolecules follows, as well as physical disruption of cellular membranes by the ice. When freezing is rapid, a gellike structure forms within the cell that lacks the crystalloids of water. This water-solid reduces the extent of mechanical and chemical injury. The most significant cellular damage apparently occurs on thawing, when mechanical disruption of membrane structures occurs. This may be the result of a transformation from the gel to the crystal state.

The most biologically significant cell injury appears in the endothelial lining of the capillaries and venules, an effect that alters small vessel permeability. This injury initiates extravasation of plasma, formation of localized edema and blisters, and an inflammatory reaction. Whereas frostbite results from the actual freezing of water, immersion foot (trench foot) is caused by a prolonged reduction in tissue temperature to a point not low enough to freeze tissue. This cooling causes cellular disruption and vascular changes that resemble those observed during the healing phase of local tissue freezing. The target, again, seems to be the endothelial cell. Local thrombosis and changes caused by altered permeability are prominent. Vascular occlusion often leads to gangrene.

Hyperthermia Means an Increase in Body Temperature

Tissue responses to hyperthermia are similar in some respects to those caused by freezing injuries. In both instances, injury to the vascular endothelium results in altered vascular permeability, edema, and blisters. The degree of injury depends on both the extent of temperature elevation and the rapidity with which it is reached. Clearly, increased temperature of any living system increases its metabolic rate. However, above a certain thermal limit, enzymes denature and other proteins precipitate. In addition, "melting" of the lipid bilayers of cell membranes takes place.

Systemic Hyperthermia

Systemic hyperthermia is an elevation of body core temperature. It occurs because of (1) increased heat production, (2) decreased elimination of heat from the body (reflecting an aberrant response of the thermal regulatory center), or (3) a disturbance of the thermal regulatory center itself. It can also occur because heat is conducted into the body faster than the system can clear the additional "thermal load."

A body temperature above 42.5°C (108.5°F) leads to profound functional disturbances, including general vasodilation, inefficient cardiac function, and altered respiration. Isolated heart–lung preparations fail at about the same temperature, suggesting an inherent temperature limitation in the cardiovascular system and perhaps in the myocardial cells themselves. **In general, systemic temperature elevations above 41 to 42°C are not compatible with life.**

Systemic temperature elevations are commonly designated "fever." During infectious processes and inflammatory responses, interleukin-1 and tumor necrosis factor, derived from macrophages, apparently reset the body's "thermostat" to permit a higher body core temperature. However, this may not be the sole thermal factor.

Few, if any, defined pathological changes are associated with fever alone. Physical findings include increased heart and respiratory rates, peripheral vasodilation, and diaphoresis, all recognized mechanisms for thermal regulation. The central nervous system responds with irritability, restlessness, and (particularly in children) convulsions. Nocturnal temperature elevations with "night sweats" are a feature of pulmonary granulomatous infection (especially tuberculosis) and are also observed in lymphoproliferative diseases. Prolonged temperature elevation can produce wasting, principally because of an increased metabolic rate.

Malignant hyperthermia is a peculiar thermal alteration, accompanied by a hypermetabolic state and often by rhabdomyolysis (muscle necrosis), that occurs after anesthesia in susceptible persons. The cause of this autosomal dominant disorder is associated with mutations in the gene that encodes the ryanodine receptor of the sarcoplasmic reticulum. Muscle damage is caused by an abnormally high calcium concentration produced by accelerated release of Ca^{2+} through the mutant calcium release channel.

Heat stroke is a form of hyperthermia that is not mediated by endogenous pyrogens. It appears under conditions of very high ambient temperatures and reflects impaired cooling responses of the thermal regulatory systems. It characteristically occurs in infants and young children and in the very aged. Often the disorder is associated with an underlying chronic illness and the intake of diuretics, tranquilizers that may affect the hypothalamic thermal regulatory center, or drugs that inhibit perspiration. Another form of heat stroke is seen in healthy men during unusually vigorous exercise. Lactic acidosis, hypocalcemia, and rhabdomyolysis may be severe problems, and almost one third of patients with exertional heat stroke develop myoglobinuric acute renal failure. Heat stroke is not amenable to treatment with standard antipyretics, and only external cooling and fluid and electrolyte replacement are effective therapy.

Cutaneous Burns

Cutaneous burns are the most frequent form of localized hyperthermia. Both the elevated temperature and the rate of temperature change are important in determining the pattern of the tissue response. A temperature of 70°C or higher for several seconds causes necrosis of the entire epidermis, whereas a temperature of 50°C may be sustained for 10 minutes or more without killing the cells.

Cutaneous burns have been separated into three categories of severity: first-, second-, and third-degree burns (Fig. 8-19). A more contemporary classification refers to full-thickness (third-degree) and partial thickness (first- and second-degree) burns.

- **First-degree burns,** such as a mild sunburn, are recognized by congestion and pain but are not associated with necrosis. Mild endothelial injury produces vasodilation, increased vascular permeability, and slight edema.
- **Second-degree burns** cause necrosis of the epithelium but spare the dermis. Clinically, these burns are recognized by blisters, in which the epithelium is separated from the dermis.
- **Third-degree burns** char both the epithelium and the underlying dermis. Histologically, the epidermis and the dermis are carbonized, and the cellular structure is lost.

One of the most serious systemic disturbances caused by extensive cutaneous burns arises from the fact that the de-

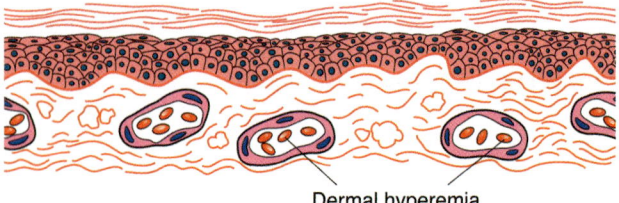
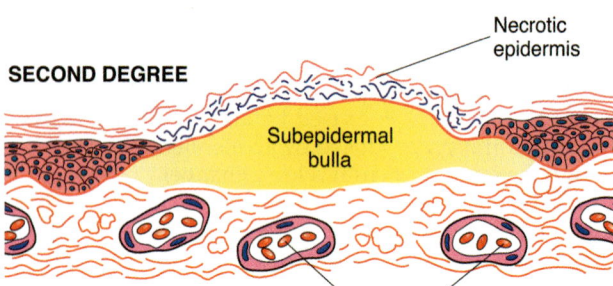
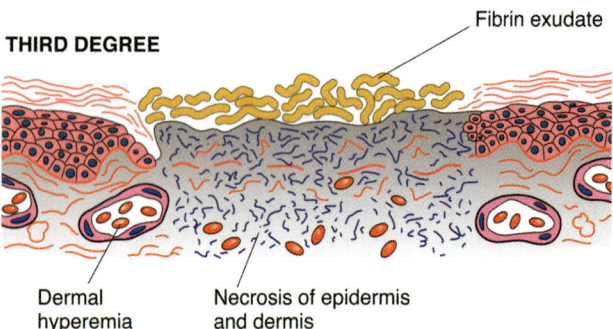

FIGURE 8-19
The pathology of cutaneous burns. A first-degree skin burn exhibits only dilation of the dermal blood vessels. In a second-degree burn, there is necrosis of the epidermis, and subepidermal edema collects under the necrotic epidermis to form a bulla. In a third-degree burn, both the epidermis and dermis are necrotic.

nuded skin surfaces "weep" plasma. Persons with third-degree burns can lose about 0.3 mL of body water per square centimeter of burned area per day. The resulting hemoconcentration and poor vascular perfusion of the skin and other viscera complicate the recovery of these patients. Many severely burned persons, particularly those with more than 70% of their body surface involved with third-degree burns, develop shock and acute tubular necrosis of the kidneys, in which circumstance the mortality is very high. Severely burned patients who survive longer are at great risk of lethal surface infections and sepsis.

The healing of cutaneous burns is related to the extent of the tissue destruction. First-degree burns, by definition, display little if any cell loss, and healing requires only repair or replacement of the injured endothelial cells. Second-degree burns also heal without a scar because the basal cells of the epidermis are not destroyed and serve as a source of regenerating cells for the epithelium. Third-degree burns, in which there is destruction of the entire thickness of the epidermis, pose a separate set of problems. If the destruction spares the skin appendages, reepithelialization can arise from these foci. Initially, islands of proliferation at the orifices of these glands grow and coalesce to cover the surface. Saprophytic infection of the charred tissue is common and poses another difficulty for healing. Deeper burns that destroy the skin appendages require new epidermis to be grafted to the debrided area to establish a functional covering. Burned skin that is not replaced by a graft heals with the formation of a dense scar. Since this connective tissue lacks the elasticity of normal skin, contractures that limit motion may be the eventual result. In severe burns, epithelial layers have been produced in vitro from cultured keratinocytes derived from the patient's own surviving skin. The application of these layers of squamous epithelium to the burned areas has permitted the survival of some severely injured patients who previously would have surely died.

Inhalation Burns

Persons trapped in burning buildings and vehicles are exposed to air and aerosolized flammable materials that have been heated to very high temperatures. The inhalation of these noxious fumes injures or destroys the respiratory tract epithelium from the oral cavity to the alveoli. If the patient survives the acute episode, the end-result of such a burn is the development of adult respiratory distress syndrome (ARDS), which itself may be fatal (see Chapter 12).

Electrical Burns

Electrical injury produces damage through two modalities: (1) an electrical dysfunction of the cardiovascular conduction system and the nervous system and (2) the conversion of electrical energy to heat energy when the current encounters the resistance of the tissues. **Because electrical energy can potentially disrupt the electrical system within the heart, it frequently causes death through ventricular fibrillation.** The amount of current necessary to produce such a disruption depends in part on its pathway through the body and its ease in penetrating the skin. Someone who inadvertently touches a 120-V line in a living room may suffer burns on the hand because of the electrical resistance of the skin that contacts the wire. A person who inadvertently touches the same line in a bathtub may have no cutaneous manifestations but be killed by disordered electrical activity in the heart. In the latter instance, the wet skin provides a low-resistance entry for the current, thereby permitting greater current flow to the entire body.

Electrical burns of the skin reflect the voltage, the area of electrical conductance, and the duration of current flow (Fig. 8-20). Very high-voltage current chars the tissue and produces a third-degree burn. On the other hand, broad, moist surfaces exposed to the same flow exhibit less-severe change. With exposure to very high-voltage currents, the force may be almost "explosive," in which case vaporization of tissue water produces extensive damage.

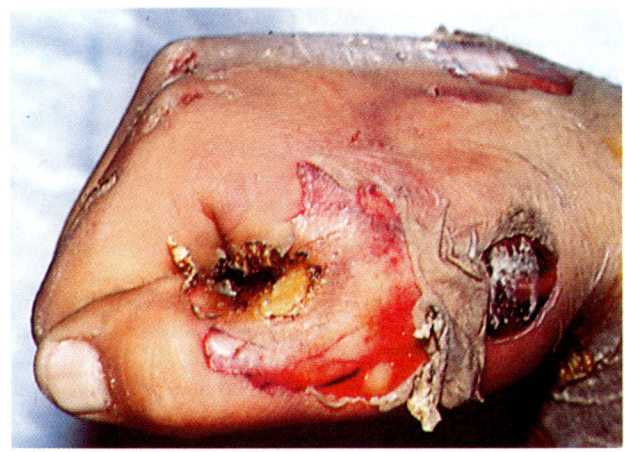

FIGURE 8-20
Electrical burn of the skin. The victim was electrocuted after attempting to stop a fall from a ladder by grasping a high-voltage electrical line.

ALTITUDE-RELATED ILLNESSES

High-altitude illness is rare, in large part because of the acclimation of mountain climbers before extreme altitudes are achieved. However, there is an altitude limit beyond which human life cannot be sustained for prolonged periods. Communities in the Andes succeed at 4000 to 4300 meters. The inhabitants adapt to the decreased pressure and availability of oxygen by developing elevated hematocrits and large "barrel" chests with increased lung volume. Even those who live in this zone do not survive at elevations above 5500 to 6000 meters. Prolonged stays at this altitude result in weight loss, difficulty in sleeping, and lethargy, perhaps because of the redirection of cellular energy simply for survival. For example, 75 to 90% of the oxygen obtained per inspiration at 6000 meters is used for the effort of inspiration alone.

The modifications induced by high altitude are related to decreased atmospheric pressure and, therefore, to decreased oxygen availability. It has been suggested that the decreased oxygen tension and the limited ability of the lungs to extract oxygen at lower pressures produce the hypoxia that is probably the most important factor in causing high-altitude illness. The narrow reserve is illustrated by the observation that physical activity at these elevations leads to a decrease in the partial pressure of arterial oxygen, whereas comparable physical activity at sea level does not change oxygen saturation. At sea level, cardiac output limits exercise; at high altitudes, the diffusing capacity of the lung for oxygen seems to be the determinant.

Acclimation to chronic hypoxia at high altitudes results in a reduced ventilatory drive. Acclimated persons exhibit increases in (1) the number of capillaries per unit of brain, muscle, and myocardium; (2) the amount of myoglobin within tissues; (3) the number of mitochondria per cell; and (4) the hematocrit. An increase in erythrocyte levels of 2'3'-diphosphoglycerate, which enhances oxygen delivery to tissues, occurs within hours, but the induction of polycythemia requires months. Some of the minor effects of high altitude are systemic edema, retinal hemorrhages, and flatus expulsion. The more serious nonfatal diseases are acute and chronic mountain sickness and high-altitude deterioration. Fatal disease can develop in the form of **high-altitude pulmonary edema and high-altitude encephalopathy**.

- **High-altitude systemic edema:** This condition results from an asymptomatic increase in vascular permeability, particularly in the hands, face, and feet, and most often occurs at elevations over 3000 meters. It is reflected only in weight gain; on return to lower altitude, a diuresis causes the edema to disappear. This disorder is twice as common in women as in men. The cause of this peculiar condition is not known, and an endothelial response to hypoxia provides only a partial explanation.
- **High-altitude retinal hemorrhage:** A critical analysis by funduscopic examination revealed that 30 to 60% of those sleeping above 5000 meters had retinal hemorrhages. The initial effect includes retinal vascular engorgement and tortuousness. Optic disc hyperemia is also noted, and multiple flame-shaped hemorrhages subsequently occur. These changes are reversible.
- **High-altitude flatus:** Changes in external pressure and the production of intestinal gas provide for the expansion of the luminal contents of the intestine and increased flatus at altitudes above 3500 meters. No specific physical disease has been associated with these changes, although social problems have been encountered.
- **Acute mountain sickness:** This condition is rare below 2500 meters but is present to some degree in nearly everyone at 3000 to 3600 meters. The initial presentation includes headache, lassitude, anorexia, weakness, and difficulty in sleeping. The pathophysiological mechanism that underlies this disease is in part related to hypoxia and a shift in plasma fluid to the interstitial space. Adaptation through a modification of pulmonary function (increased respiratory rate) causes some amelioration of the disease. Descent to lower altitudes is certainly indicated. Chronic or subacute exacerbation of this disease also occurs, frequently at lower altitudes, and the symptoms may be severe. The basis of the disease is not known.
- **High-altitude deterioration:** Generally occurring at higher elevations (5500 meters or more), high-altitude deterioration presents as a decrease in physical and mental performance. The combination of chronic hypoxia, inadequate fluid intake, and inadequate nutrition, together with decreased plasma volume and hemoconcentration, are aggravating factors.
- **High-altitude pulmonary edema and cerebral edema:** Serious high-altitude problems, including pulmonary edema and cerebral edema, can occur with a rapid ascent to heights over 2500 meters, particularly in susceptible persons who have difficulty tolerating sleeping at higher altitudes. Tachycardia, right ventricular overload, and a marked reduction in arterial oxygen pressure occur, but there is no change in pH or carbon dioxide retention. A characteristic patchy pulmonary infiltrate is noted radiographically. Pulmonary hypertension is common in patients with high-altitude pulmonary edema. Hypoxic vasoconstriction and intravascular thrombosis have been proposed as causes of pulmonary hypertension. Eventually, cardiac output is decreased, and systemic blood pressure falls. The precapillary arterioles become dilated, increasing capillary bed pressure and inducing interstitial and alveolar edema. Autopsy findings in-

clude severe confluent pulmonary edema, proteinaceous alveolar exudates, and hyaline membrane formation. Capillary obstruction by thrombi has been noted. A dilated heart and enlarged pulmonary arteries are commonly found.

- **High-altitude encephalopathy** is characterized by confusion, stupor, and coma. Autopsies have consistently revealed cerebral edema and vascular congestion. A proposed mechanism is severe cerebral hypoxia, with inhibition of the sodium pump and resultant intracellular edema.

PHYSICAL INJURIES

The effect of mechanical trauma is related to the force transmitted to the tissue, the rate at which the transfer occurs, the surface area to which the force is transferred, and the area of the body that is injured. The disruption of the continuity of the tissue results in a wound. However, remember that the transmission of absorbed energy can produce alterations elsewhere in the body.

- **Force expended:** The amount of energy released is related to the velocity and mass of the object that strikes the person or to that of the person who collides with a stationary object. In addition to the lateral displacement, many objects that strike people—from bullets to car wheels—have rotational forces. Prolongation of the period of impact dissipates some of the energy, as when a boxer "rolls with a punch."
- **Transfer area:** The area over which transfer of force occurs is particularly important. The intensity—that is, the force exerted per unit area—decreases with the increasing area. A protective helmet does not lessen the force of a blow or projectile but diffuses it over a larger area.
- **Body area:** The area of the body that is affected by physical trauma plays an important role. The compressibility of the tissue adjacent to the transmitted force in part determines its effect. A blow over a large muscle mass, such as the thigh or upper arm, is often less injurious than a direct blow to a poorly shielded bone, such as the anterior tibia. Furthermore, the distribution of the force is important. Blows over a hollow viscus can rupture the organ because of compression of the fluid or gas it contains; organs nestled beneath the skin, such as the liver, can be easily ruptured. An impact directly over the heart can even disturb its electrical systems.

A Contusion Is a Localized Mechanical Injury with Focal Hemorrhage

A force with sufficient energy may disrupt capillaries and venules within an organ by physical means alone. If this occurs in the skin, a loss of blood into the tissue space occurs, with consequent altered coloration. The change may be so limited that the only histological change is hemorrhage in tissue spaces outside the vascular compartment. The presence of a discrete blood pool within the tissue is termed a *hematoma*. Initially, the deoxygenated blood renders the area blue to blue-black, as in the classic "black eye." Macrophages ingest the erythrocytes and convert the hemoglobin to bilirubin, thereby changing the color from blue to yellow. Both mobilization of the pigment by macrophages and further metabolism of bilirubin cause the yellow to fade to yellowish green and then to disappear.

An Abrasion Is a Skin Defect Caused by Crushes or Scrapes

The disruptive force, which may be direct or tangential, may provide a portal of entry for microorganisms. There may be disruption of the epidermis itself, and there may also be vascular distortion of the cells within the dermis. The impact of the agent and its configuration are frequently seen in these wounds and are of special interest to the forensic pathologist.

A Laceration Is a Split or Tear of the Skin

Lacerations result from an impact stronger than that causing an abrasion and are usually the result of unidirectional displacement. When they have crushed margins, they are termed *abraded lacerations*.

Wounds Are Mechanical Disruptions of Tissue Integrity

An incision is the deliberate opening of the skin by a cutting instrument, usually the surgeon's scalpel. Incisions have particularly sharp edges and, importantly, spare no tissue to the depth of the wound. **Deep penetrating wounds** produced by high-velocity projectiles, such as bullets, are often deceptive, because the energy of the missile as it passes through the body may be released at sites distant from the entrance itself. Bullets, because they rotate, produce a well-defined and usually round entrance wound (Fig. 8-21). Once the projectile enters the flesh, however, it may fragment, tumble, or actually explode, resulting in a remarkable degree of tissue damage and a large, ragged exit wound. The interested student may refer to the reading list at the end of the chapter for further information in this area of forensic pathology.

RADIATION

We can define radiation simply as the emission of energy by one body, its transmission through an intervening medium, and its absorption by another body. By this definition, radiation encompasses the entire electromagnetic spectrum and certain charged particles emitted by radioactive elements. Alpha particles such as the radiation emitted by ^{32}P and the beta particles of elements such as tritium (^3H) and ^{14}C are of immense use scientifically and diagnostically but pose few hazards for humans. High-energy radiation, in the form of gamma or x-rays, mediates most of the biological effects discussed here. We do not consider the effects of ultraviolet radiation here, since they are discussed in Chapters 5 and 24.

Medical practice is inconceivable today without the use of diagnostic and therapeutic radioisotopes, clinical radiographs, and radiation therapy. On the other hand, nuclear explosions and accidental exposure to radiation in nuclear power plants have caused injury and death. Here, we focus

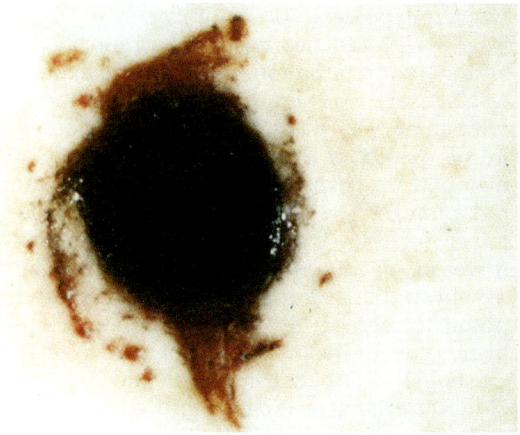
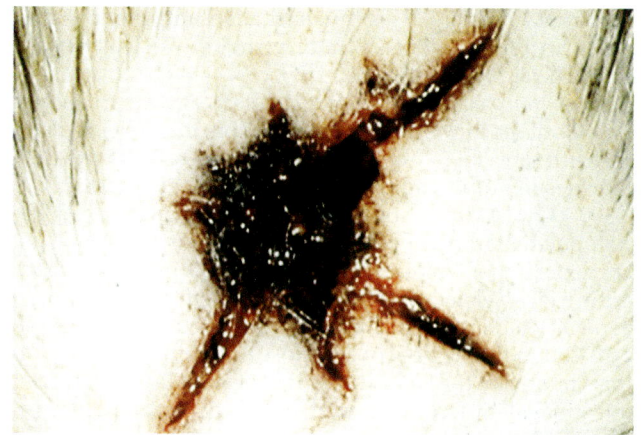

FIGURE 8-21
Bullet wounds. A. The entrance wound is sharply punched out. B. The exit wound is irregular with characteristic stellate lacerations.

on the pathological consequences of radiation exposure. Radiation is quantitated in a number of ways:

- **A roentgen** is a measure of the emission of radiant energy from a source. This unit refers to the amount of ionization produced in air.
- **A rad** measures the absorption of radiant energy, which is biologically the more important parameter. A rad defines the energy, expressed as ergs, absorbed by a tissue. One rad equals 100 ergs per gram of tissue.
- **A gray** (Gy) corresponds to 100 rads (1 joule/kg of tissue), and a centigray (cGy) is equivalent to 1 rad.
- **The rem** unit was introduced to describe the biological effect produced by a rad of high-energy radiation, because low-energy particles produce more biological damage than gamma or x-rays.
- **A sievert** (Sv) is the dose in grays multiplied by an appropriate quality factor Q, so that 1 Sv of radiation is roughly equivalent in biological effectiveness to 1 Gy of gamma rays.

For the purposes of this discussion of radiation-induced pathology, the rad, gray, rem, and sievert are considered comparable. The details of radiation biology are the subject of a voluminous literature, and the student may refer to this chapter's list of suggested reading.

Pathogenesis: At the cellular level, radiation essentially has two effects: (1) a somatic effect, associated with acute cell killing, and (2) the induction of genetic damage. Radiation-induced cell death is believed to be caused by the acute effects of the radiolysis of water (see Chapter 1). The production of activated oxygen species may result in lipid peroxidation, membrane injury, and possibly an interaction with macromolecules of the cell. Genetic damage to the cell, whether caused by direct absorption of energy by DNA (the target theory) or caused indirectly by a reaction of DNA with oxygen radicals, is expressed either as mutation or as reproductive failure. Both mutation and reproductive failure may lead to delayed cell death, and mutation is incriminated in the development of radiation-induced neoplasia.

The differential sensitivity of tissues to radiation has been recognized since the beginning of the century. For example, the intestine and the hematopoietic bone marrow are far more vulnerable to radiation than tissues such as bone and brain. The vulnerability of a tissue to radiation-induced damage depends on its proliferative rate, which in turn correlates with the natural life span of the constituent cells. Damage to the DNA of a long-lived, nonproliferating cell does not necessarily pose a threat to its function or viability because the reproductive and metabolic functions of the cell are separate properties. By contrast, a short-lived, proliferating cell, such as an intestinal crypt cell or a hematopoietic precursor, must be replaced rapidly by the division of stem cells and committed precursors. When radiation-induced DNA damage precludes mitosis of these cells, the mature elements are not replaced, and the tissue can no longer function.

Before discussing the structural and functional injury produced by radiation, it is important to distinguish between whole-body irradiation and localized irradiation. Except for unusual circumstances, as in the high-dose irradiation that precedes bone marrow transplantation, significant levels of whole-body irradiation result only from industrial accidents or from the explosion of nuclear weapons. By contrast, localized irradiation is an inevitable byproduct of any diagnostic radiological procedure, and it is the intended result of radiation therapy. Rapid somatic cell death occurs only with extremely high doses of radiation, well in excess of 1000 rads. It is morphologically indistinguishable from the coagulative necrosis produced by other causes (see Chapter 1). By contrast, irreversible damage to the replicative capacity of cells requires far lower doses, possibly as little as 50 rads.

Whole-Body Irradiation Injures Many Organs

Fortunately, there have been few instances of human disease caused by whole-body irradiation, and most of our information has been derived from studies of Japanese atom bomb survivors. Further information is now available from the study of the survivors of the much smaller sample of persons exposed in the accident at the Chernobyl nuclear power plant in Ukraine in 1986.

Since comparable doses of radiant energy are transmitted to all organs in whole-body irradiation, the development of the different acute radiation syndromes reflects the dissimilarities in vulnerability of the target tissues (Fig. 8-22).

300 cGy: At this dose, a syndrome characterized by **hematopoietic failure** develops within 2 weeks. Following an initial depletion of circulating lymphocytes, a progressive decrease in formed elements of the blood eventually leads to bleeding, anemia, and infection. The last is often the cause of death.

10 Gy: In the vicinity of this dose, the principal cause of death is related to the **gastrointestinal system**. Although gastrointestinal symptoms characterize the entire dose range of whole-body exposure, at higher levels, severe destruction of the entire epithelium of the gastrointestinal tract occurs within 3 days, the time that corresponds to the normal life span of the villous and crypt cells. As a result, the fluid homeostasis of the bowel is disrupted, and severe diarrhea and dehydration ensue. Moreover, the epithelial barrier to intestinal bacteria is breached, and organisms invade and disseminate throughout the body. Septicemia and shock kill the victim.

20 Gy: With exposure to whole-body doses of 20 Gy and above, central nervous system damage causes death within hours. In most cases, cerebral edema and loss of the integrity of the blood–brain barrier, owing to endothelial injury, predominate. With extreme doses, radiation necrosis of neurons can be expected. Convulsions, coma, and death follow.

FETAL EFFECTS: The effects of whole-body irradiation on the human fetus have been documented in studies of the survivors of the atom bomb explosions in Japan. Pregnant women exposed to doses of 25 cGy or above gave birth to infants with reduced head size, diminished overall growth, and mental retardation. (Intrauterine exposure to radiation at Nagasaki was significantly less teratogenic than that at Hiroshima. This disparity has been attributed to a difference in the quality of the radiation in the two cities. The bomb dropped on Hiroshima produced far greater fast-neutron radiation [20% vs. 1% of the total energy released], which is lower in energy than comparable doses of gamma rays and, therefore, produces greater biological damage.)

In studies of the clinical status of children who were exposed to therapeutic doses of radiation in utero, the most likely time for the production of growth retardation and microcephaly was between the 3rd and 20th week of gestation. Other effects of irradiation in utero include hydrocephaly, microphthalmia, chorioretinitis, blindness, spina bifida, cleft palate, clubfeet, and genital abnormalities. Data derived from experimental and human studies strongly support the conclusion that major congenital malformations are highly unlikely with doses below 20 rads after day 14 of pregnancy. However, lower doses may produce more-subtle effects, such as a decrease in mental capacity. **To protect against such a possibility, the established maximum permissible dose to the fetus from exposure of the expectant mother is far below the known teratogenic dose.**

GENETIC EFFECTS: The potential genetic effects of radiation have been the source of considerable public alarm. Again, there is a dearth of evidence, and most of the data on which predictions of human genetic effects are based are derived from experimental data. **After long-term follow-up, even the survivors of Hiroshima and Nagasaki have failed**

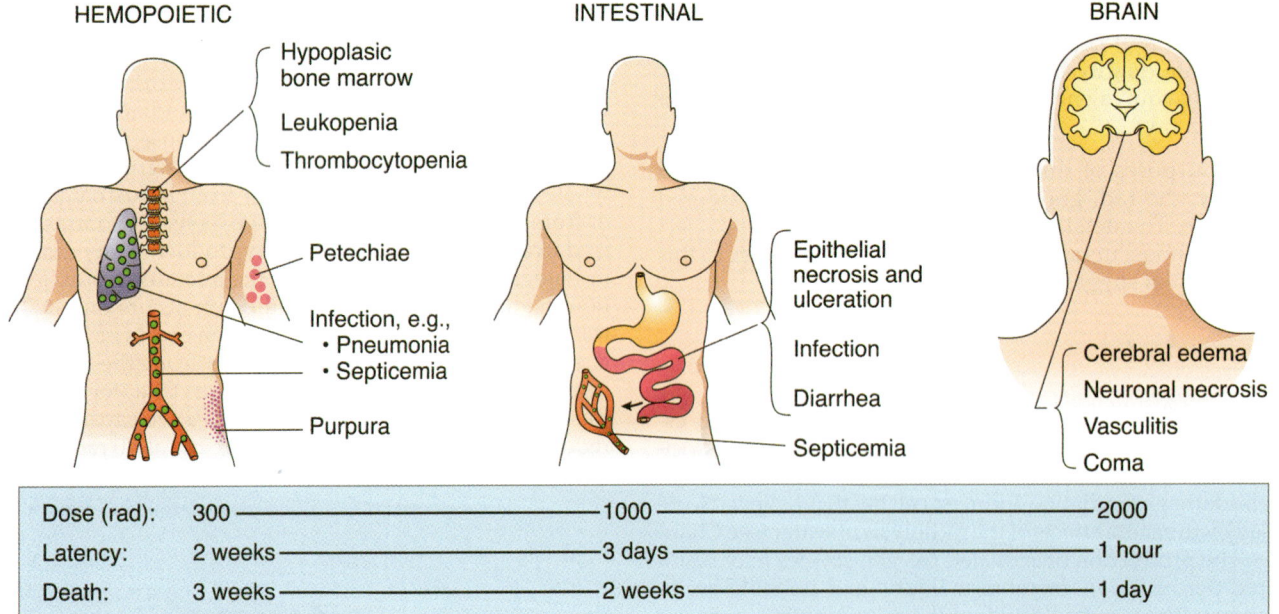

FIGURE 8-22

Acute radiation syndromes. At a dose of approximately 300 rads of whole body radiation, a syndrome characterized by hematopoietic failure develops within 2 weeks. In the vicinity of 1000 rads, a gastrointestinal syndrome with a latency of only 3 days is seen. With doses of 2000 rads or more, disease of the central nervous system appears within 1 hour, and death ensues rapidly.

to manifest evidence of genetic damage in the form of either congenital abnormalities or hereditary diseases in subsequent offspring or their descendants. In experimental animals, the risk of induced mutation per rad is at most only 0.5 to 5% of the risk of spontaneous mutation (estimated to be 10% of live births in humans). In other words, the experimental radiation exposure necessary to double the spontaneous mutation rate is 20 to 200 rads. Thus, even with the most pessimistic estimates, the risk of genetic damage to future generations from radiation appears to be vanishingly small.

AGING: The finding that rodents exposed to whole-body irradiation have a shortened life span has led to the suggestion that radiation accelerates the aging process. A mortality study of the survivors of the atom bomb explosions in Japan has not disclosed any excess mortality not attributable to neoplasia. Nor is there any evidence of acceleration in disease among the survivors in any part of the age range. **Thus, the effects of ionizing radiation on mortality are specific and focal, and there is no reason to believe that premature aging in humans or radiation-induced carcinogenesis is due to a general acceleration of aging.**

Localized Radiation Injury Complicates Radiation Therapy for Tumors

In the course of radiation therapy for malignant neoplasms, some normal tissue is inevitably included in the radiation field. Although almost any organ can be damaged by radiation, the clinically important tissues are the skin, lungs, heart, kidney, bladder, and intestine—organs that are difficult to shield (Fig. 8-23). Localized damage to the bone marrow is clearly of little functional consequence because of the immense reserve capacity of the hematopoietic system.

Pathology: Persistent damage to radiation-exposed tissue can be attributed to two major factors: (1) compromise of the vascular supply and (2) a fibrotic repair reaction to acute necrosis and chronic ischemia. Radiation-induced tissue injury predominantly affects small arteries and arterioles. The endothelial cells are the most sensitive elements in the blood vessels and in the short term exhibit swelling and necrosis. With time, the walls become thickened by endothelial cell proliferation and subintimal deposition of collagen and other connective tissue elements. Striking vacuolization of intimal cells, so-called foam cells, is typical. Fragmentation of the internal elastic lamina, loss of smooth muscle cells, scarring in the media, and fibrosis of the adventitia are seen in the small arteries. Bizarre fibroblasts with large hyperchromatic nuclei are common and probably reflect radiation-induced DNA damage.

Clinical Features: Acute necrosis from radiation is represented by such disorders as **radiation pneumonitis, cystitis, dermatitis,** and diarrhea from **enteritis.** Chronic disease is characterized by **interstitial fibro-**

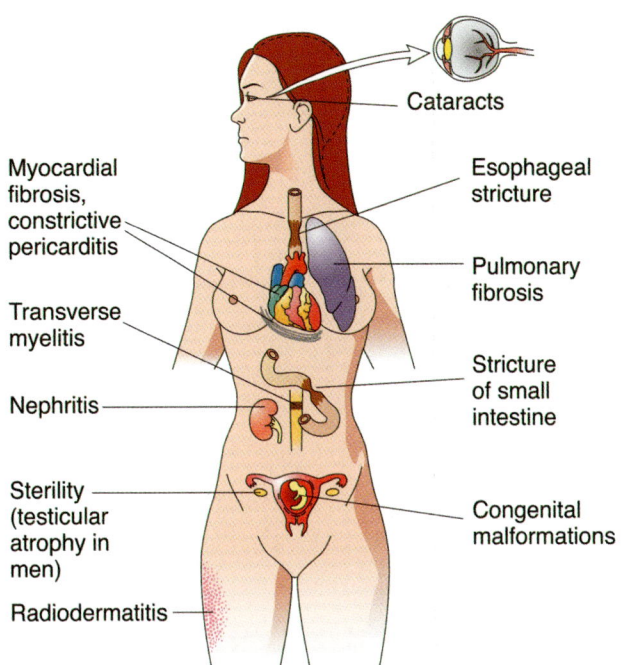

FIGURE 8-23
The nonneoplastic complications of radiation.

sis in the heart and lungs, strictures in the esophagus and small intestine, and **constrictive pericarditis.** Chronic **radiation nephritis,** which simulates malignant nephrosclerosis, is primarily a vascular disease that leads to severe hypertension and progressive renal insufficiency.

Since radiation therapy inevitably traverses the skin, it often causes **radiation dermatitis.** The initial damage is evidenced by dilation of blood vessels, recognized as **erythema.** Necrosis of the skin may follow and linger as **indolent ulcers** that do not heal because the epithelium is unable to regenerate. A further consequence of this poor regenerative capacity is the difficulty faced by the surgeon, for whom the impairment of wound healing in irradiated areas poses a serious problem. **Poorly healed** or **dehisced wounds** or **persistent ulcers** often require full-thickness skin grafts. **Chronic radiation dermatitis** results from the repair and revascularization of the skin and is characterized by atrophy, hyperkeratosis, telangiectasia, and hyperpigmentation (Fig. 8-24).

The gonads, both testes and ovaries, are similar to other tissues in their dependence on continuous cell cycling and are exquisitely radiosensitive. The acute inhibition of mitosis in the testis results in necrosis of the germinal stem cells, the spermatogonia. The combination of radiation-induced vascular injury and direct damage to the germ cells leads to progressive atrophy of the seminiferous tubules, peritubular fibrosis, and loss of reproductive function. However, since the interstitial and Sertoli cells do not cycle rapidly, they are more resistant than the germ cells and so persist, thereby preserving the normal hormonal status. Comparable injury is seen in the irradiated ovary; the follicles become atretic, and the organ eventually becomes fibrous and atrophic.

Cataracts (lenticular opacities) may be produced if the eye lies in the path of the radiation beam. **Transverse myelitis** and paraplegia occur when the spinal cord is unavoidably

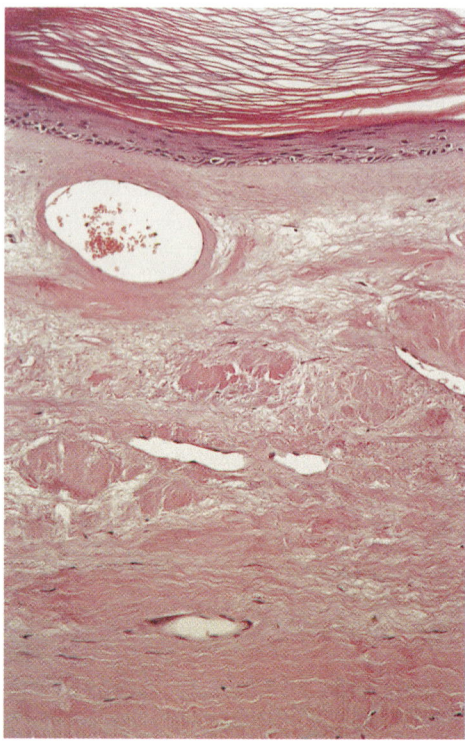

FIGURE 8-24
Chronic radiation dermatitis. The epidermis is atrophic. The dermis is densely fibrotic and contains dilated superficial blood vessels.

irradiated during treatment of certain thoracic or abdominal tumors. **Vascular damage in the cord** may bring about localized ischemia.

High Doses of Radiation Cause Cancer

The evidence that radiation can lead to cancer is incontrovertible and comes from animal experiments and studies of the effects of occupational exposure, radiation therapy for nonneoplastic conditions, the diagnostic use of certain radioisotopes, and the atom bomb explosions (Fig. 8-25). In the early part of this century, scientists and radiologists tested their equipment by placing their hands in the path of the beam. As a result, they developed basal and squamous cell carcinomas of the exposed skin. In addition, early instruments were not properly shielded, and the hazards associated with fluoroscopy were not appreciated. The radiologists of that era suffered an unusually high incidence of leukemia, a situation that has disappeared with the use of modern shielding and protective equipment.

An unusual occupational exposure to radiation occurred among workers who painted radium-containing material onto watches to create luminous dials. These workers were in the habit of licking their paint brushes to produce a point, which led to the ingestion of the radioactive element and its subsequent localization in their bones. As a consequence, they were exposed to a long-lived isotope that persisted in their bones indefinitely. They later experienced a high incidence of cancer of the bone and of the paranasal sinuses. Another example of occupational exposure to a radioactive element is the high rate of lung cancer in uranium miners who have inhaled radioactive dust. Since most of these workers also smoke, it is difficult to distinguish the independent effects from the synergistic effects of radiation in the induction of their cancers, but the evidence strongly favors a synergistic effect.

At one time, thymic irradiation of infants for a mysterious "ailment" known as "status thymicolymphaticus" was popular. The irradiation produced no perceptible improvement in the overall health of these infants, but as adults they developed cancer of the thyroid. An explosive increase in the incidence of thyroid cancer among children in geographical areas contaminated by the nuclear catastrophe at Chernobyl in Ukraine in 1986 has been linked to the release of radioactive iodine isotopes.

The risk of solid tumors, especially breast cancer, is particularly high among adult women who were treated with thoracic radiation for Hodgkin disease as children. Long-term survivors of childhood Hodgkin disease, who were treated with radiation therapy, are at an almost 20-fold increased risk of developing a second neoplasm. Another example of iatrogenic cancer resulted in Great Britain from the widespread use of low-dose spinal irradiation as a treatment for ankylosing spondylitis. A beneficial effect on the course of this disease was claimed, but the penalty was the later development of aplastic anemia, myelogenous leukemia, and other tumors. An increase in brain tumors was found in persons who had received cranial irradiation for tinea capitis infection of the scalp in childhood. Radiation delivered by long-lived radioactive isotopes used for diagnostic purposes was also not without danger. Thorium dioxide (Thorotrast), a material avidly ingested by phagocytic cells, was at one time used for radionuclide imaging. The persistence in the liver of a long-lived radioisotope resulted in the development of a number of tumors, particularly angiosarcomas of the liver.

The survivors of the atom bomb explosions suffered from a number of cancers. These persons exhibited a more than 10-fold increase in the incidence of leukemia, which reached its zenith from 5 to 10 years after exposure and subsequently declined to background rates. (An increased incidence of leukemia was evident in those exposed to doses as low as 50 rads in Hiroshima but required more than 100 rads in Nagasaki. As suggested above, this difference in sensitivity may reflect the greater neutron component of the radiation in Hiroshima.) Two thirds were of cases were acute leukemia; the remainder were of the chronic myelogenous variety. Chronic lymphocytic leukemia, an uncommon disease in Japan, showed no increase in incidence. The risk of multiple myeloma increased fivefold, and there was a small increment in the incidence of lymphoma. The frequency of solid tumors, although not as great as that for leukemia, was clearly increased for the breast, lung, thyroid, gastrointestinal tract, and urinary tract. The development of malignant tumors, including leukemia, showed a dose-response relationship.

LOW-LEVEL RADIATION AND CANCER: Few debates have engendered as much heat and as little light as that concerning the potential carcinogenic effect of low levels of radiation. All assumptions are based on extrapolations to

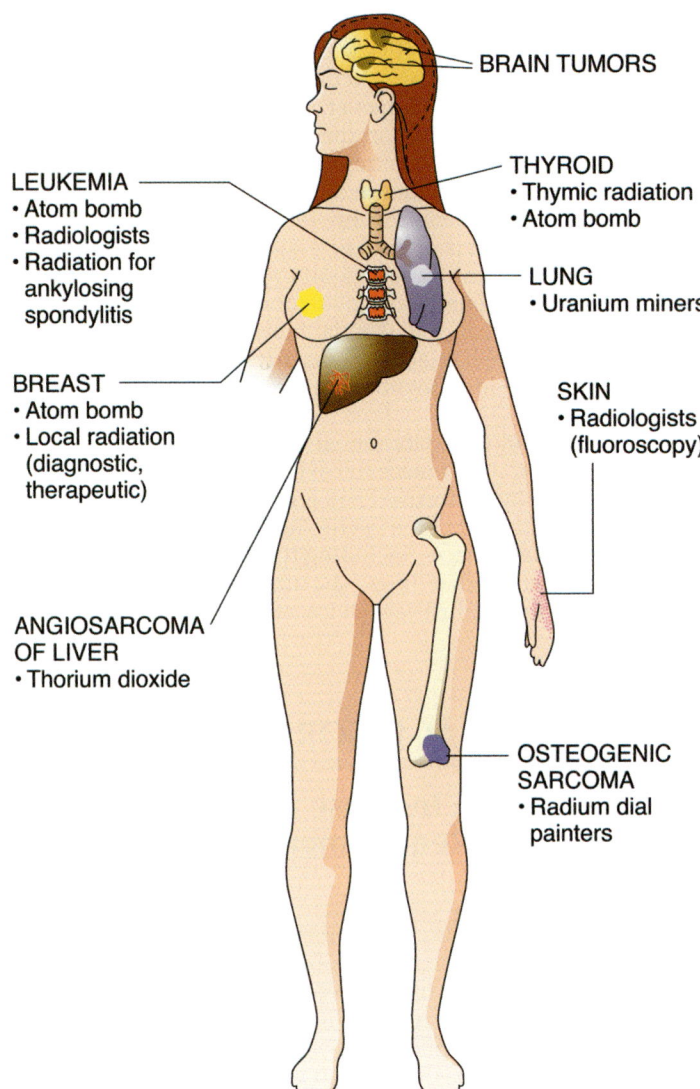

FIGURE 8-25
Radiation-induced cancers.

zero of the risk of cancer at higher doses or from epidemiological studies to which valid exception may be taken. **The key question that needs to be answered is whether there is a threshold dose of radiation below which there is no increase in the incidence of cancer, or whether any exposure carries a significant risk.**

The "linear–no threshold hypothesis"—that is, the theory that postulates no safe dose—is based on a linear (proportional to dose) projection of low doses of radiation to zero. However, as is the case with many drugs, there is no a priori reason to accept such an assumption; an alternative analysis of the same data uses a quadratic (proportional to dose squared) dependence of risk on dose. With this analysis, the proposed "no threshold" curve is steep at higher doses and is appreciably flattened at the lowest ones. A more sophisticated approach is the linear–quadratic analysis, in which the quadratic dependence gives way to a linear dependence at the lowest doses. At low doses, the linear–quadratic model is intermediate between the highest level of risk of radiogenic cancer projected by the linear analysis and the lowest risk indicated by the quadratic projection.

For instance, based on data from the Nagasaki survivors, the risk of leukemia from a 1-cGy dose, expressed as excess cases per million per year, ranges from 2.5 for the linear model to 0.016 for the quadratic model—a 156-fold difference in risk. Comparable differences can be derived from other epidemiological studies of cancer incidence. Thus, the mandated permissible exposures to radiation (which are based on a linear relation) are highly conservative and may exaggerate the risks.

A discussion of the effects of low-level radiation must include consideration of naturally occurring background radiation (i.e., the radiation derived from cosmic and terrestrial radiation and the inhalation and ingestion of natural and man-made radioactive isotopes). This background radiation is estimated to be about 0.1 cGy per year at sea level and somewhat higher at higher altitudes. Since exposure to this radiation is universal, it is clearly impossible to determine directly whether this level of exposure contributes to the spontaneous incidence of cancer in humans. However, using the linear hypothesis to estimate the risk from low levels of background radiation, it has been estimated that the leukemia rate in 20- to 30-year-old women in the United

States that can be attributed to this radiation is between 3 and 4 per million per year. The actual leukemia rate in this group is 18 per million per year; thus, background radiation can only account for about one fifth of cases.

However, other attempts to estimate cancer incidence from the linear hypothesis have yielded conflicting conclusions. For example, a linear extension back from the observed cancer incidence and radiation exposure among uranium miners predicts a cancer rate that is four times higher than the rate actually observed in a population of nonsmokers. Cancer mortality has been recorded in two regions of China that have different levels of background radiation. In the low-background region, persons were exposed to 0.072 cGy per year, while in the high-background region, the exposure was almost three times greater. Despite this difference, no difference in cancer mortality was detected. Moreover, pilots and cabin crews of commercial airlines, who are exposed to significantly higher doses of background radiation at high altitude, have not manifested any increased cancer incidence. These and other studies suggest that the contribution of background radiation to the occurrence of human cancer may not be as significant as many believe.

In summary, the data currently available from radiation studies of cancer induction in animals, chromosomal damage in human cell cultures, malignant transformation of mammalian cells in vitro, and populations exposed to radiation show that the estimates of risk at low doses derived from a linear extrapolation from risk at high doses exaggerate the risk, perhaps by an order of magnitude. On the other hand, the data do not show that the risk of radiogenic cancer from low-level radiation is zero. **When the data from atomic bomb survivors are subjected to a linear–quadratic analysis, the lifetime risk from 1 cGy of whole-body x- or gamma irradiation is 1 excess cancer death per 10,000 persons.**

RADON: The finding that some homes in the United States are contaminated with radon has elicited considerable public concern. Radon is a gas formed as a result of the decay chain of the uranium–radium series of elements. The daughter products of radon emit alpha particles that bind to dust in the home and may be inhaled and deposited in the lungs.

It has been estimated that 4 to 5% of homes in the United States have levels of radon at least five times the average value, and in up to 2%, the concentrations are increased eightfold. Case-control studies of persons living in homes with substantial radon contamination have indicated an excess lifetime risk of lung cancer in nonsmokers of 1 in 200. The risk in smokers seems to be even higher, and the combination of tobacco use and radon exposure may be synergistic. However, more-recent studies in Canada, Finland, Missouri, and China have all found no connection between residential radon exposure and lung cancer risk, and the subject remains controversial.

Microwave Radiation, Electromagnetic Fields and Ultrasound Are Not Ionizing

Microwaves, produced by ovens, radar, and diathermy, are electromagnetic waves that penetrate tissue but do not produce ionization. Unlike x- and gamma radiation, the absorption of microwave energy produces only heat. The activation energy of radiofrequency and microwave radiation is too low to modify chemical bonds or alter DNA below levels that produce thermal effects. Thus, exposure to microwave radiation under ordinary circumstances is highly unlikely to produce any injury. Moreover, an epidemiological study of 20,000 radar technicians in the Navy who were chronically exposed to high levels of microwave radiation failed to detect any increased incidence of cancer.

Considerable controversy also surrounds the possible carcinogenic effects of exposure to nonionizing electromagnetic fields, such as those encountered in the vicinity of high-voltage electric lines. Particular concern has been expressed regarding the risk of leukemia. However, recent epidemiological evidence has led to a consensus that exposure to electromagnetic fields does not raise the incidence of leukemia or other cancers.

Ultrasound, the vibrational waves in air above the audible range, produces mechanical compression but, again, no ionization. Highly focused and energetic ultrasound devices are used to disrupt tissue in vitro for chemical analysis and to clean various surfaces, including teeth. However, there is no reason to believe that diagnostic ultrasound or accidental exposure to any industrial device results in any measurable damage.

NUTRITIONAL DISORDERS

Obesity Is an Increase in Adipose Tissue Beyond the Requirements of the Body

Obesity is the most common nutritional disorder in the industrialized countries, where it is far more common than all the nutritional deficiencies combined. There is no single ratio of increased weight to height or body area at which an increased morbidity and mortality can be said to begin. Thus, as in the case of anemia or hypertension, arbitrary standards are used. Obesity is determined according to body mass index (BMI), calculated as weight (kg)/height (m^2). A BMI of 25 to 30 is classed as overweight, 30 to 40 as obesity, and above 40 as morbid obesity. By these criteria, almost two thirds of American adults and 15% of children are overweight. Genetic factors may play a role in some ethnic and racial groups. For instance, blacks, particularly women, have a considerably higher prevalence of obesity than do whites in the United States.

It is indisputable that obesity results from a chronic excess of caloric intake relative to the expenditure of energy. The ability to store energy in the form of fat during plentiful times clearly confers an evolutionary advantage in an environment in which periods of food scarcity may occur. Presumably, evolution has been unable to anticipate the advances in societal organization and food production that have converted this evolutionary advantage into a leading cause of morbidity and mortality.

Pathogenesis: Whatever the underlying cause of obesity, it clearly results from the excess storage of triglycerides derived from the dietary calories in adipose tissue depots, owing either to excessive caloric intake, insufficient expenditure of energy, or both. The controversies regarding the pathogenesis of obesity are mostly centered on the relative contributions of nature and nurture (i.e., physiological factors as opposed to psychological ones).

The environmental influence on obesity is clearly demonstrated by the conspicuous increase in the prevalence of obesity among Asians and Indians in the United States compared with their counterparts in their native lands. By contrast, studies of identical twins reared apart document a striking concordance in adiposity, indicating a heritability of 80 to 90%. It is fair to say that both genetic and environmental factors are important in the pathogenesis of obesity, but the contributions of each or their interactions vary significantly throughout the population.

Only a minor imbalance between caloric intake and expenditure suffices to produce significant obesity. For example, an excess consumption of only 100 calories per day, the amount contained in a slice of bread, will result in a weight gain of almost 5 kg over the course of a year. The fine balance between caloric intake and energy use necessary to maintain constant body weight implies that each person has an internal set point, or *lipostat,* that regulates these processes.

Excess energy is stored as lipid, largely in the white fatty tissues of the body. Lipid storage, mainly as triglycerides, is achieved by progressive distention of a limited number of adipocytes (beyond childhood, the number of adipocytes in the body does not change appreciably). The size of these cells waxes and wanes in response to imbalances between caloric intake and expenditure.

In modern societies, cycles of feast and famine are no longer a problem, and food is continuously available. However, the mechanisms that regulate appetite and body weight have remained unchanged. There is an equilibrium between anabolic and catabolic neuropeptides. Certain neuropeptides promote food intake, decrease energy expenditure, and enhance fat storage, whereas others have opposite effects. A number of molecules that act as hormones in the regulating of body weight have been described (Fig. 8-26).

Thyroid hormone: Persons with a deficiency of thyroid hormone have lower basal metabolic rates and are heavier than normal, whereas those who produce excess thyroid hormone have higher basal metabolic rates and are thinner. However, although thyroid insufficiency can cause obesity, only a small minority of obese persons lack sufficient thyroid hormone.

Melanocortins: This class of peptides includes adrenocorticotropic hormone (ACTH) and several isotypes of melanocyte-stimulating hormone (MSH). The latter hormones regulate diverse body functions, including energy metabolism, hair color, and maturation of endocrine and other glands. They are different peptide cleavage products of pro-opiomelanocortin and act by binding particular melanocortin receptors (MCRs). MC3R, which is expressed in the hypothalamus and in numerous tissues outside the brain, helps to determine the efficiency with which ingested energy is used. MC4R expression is widespread in the brain and decreases appetite and oxygen consumption.

Leptin: Leptin is the product of the *ob* (obese) gene and is produced by adipose tissue. High levels of blood leptin reflect greater adipocyte mass and lend to a feeling of satiety; low levels, which are seen when body fat is diminished, stimulate appetite. Leptin has an array of other effects on sexual maturation, hematopoiesis, and other systems. Many of these activities can be interpreted as signaling the availability of sufficient energy stores to allow certain physiological processes (e.g., initiation of ovulation) to proceed.

Rare cases of extreme human obesity are caused by genetic deficiencies of either leptin or its receptor. Most obese persons, however, have higher than normal amounts of circulating leptin and are resistant to the effects of leptin on appetite and energy homeostasis seen in normal persons. As a consequence, attempts to "treat" obesity with leptin injections have not been fruitful.

Ghrelin: This 28-amino acid peptide is produced by the endocrine cells of the stomach and, to a lesser extent, the more distal gastrointestinal tract. Ghrelin promotes the release of growth hormone by the hypothalamic–pituitary axis and exerts direct stimulatory effects on cardiovascular, sexual, and other organ function. Its secretion is augmented by fasting and hypoglycemia. Ghrelin, possibly acting through neuropeptide Y-secreting neurons and antagonized by αMSH (see below), provokes appetite powerfully and increases fat storage in adipocytes. It also decreases conversion of stored fat to metabolize energy forms. As a rule, plasma levels of ghrelin are inversely correlated with body weight, but its role in the development or maintenance of obesity remains problematic. Interestingly, gastric stapling, an operation that is effective in treating morbid obesity, results in decreased appetite. This effect has been attributed to decreased ghrelin secretion by the stomach.

Glucagon-like peptide: GLP-1, a protein product of the L cells of the distal gastrointestinal tract, is secreted in response to a glucose load and has numerous effects on the brain and other organs. It stimulates insulin secretion and decreases that of glucagon. GLP-1 increases energy storage as glycogen in liver and muscle and as fat in adipocytes. It also promotes a feeling of satiety, thereby decreasing food

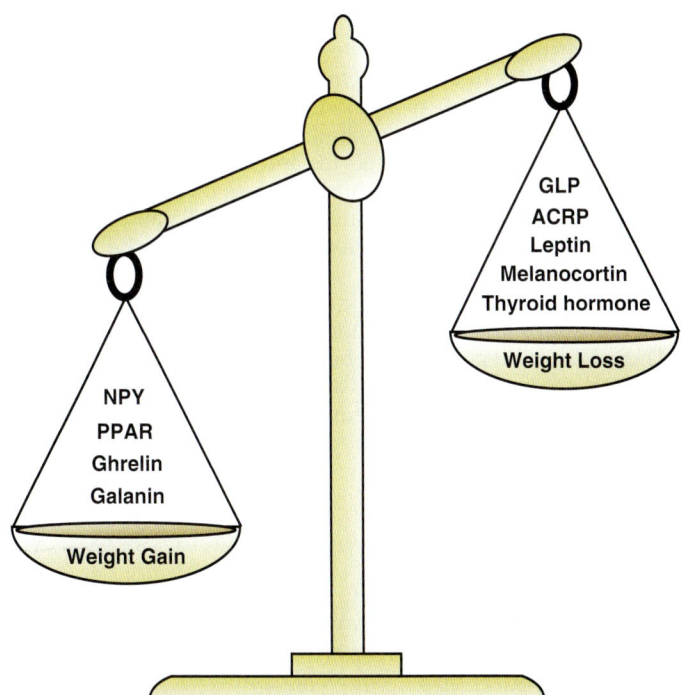

FIGURE 8-26

The balance of chemical mediators that promote fat accumulation (weight gain) and those that promote fat loss (weight loss).

intake. Despite its very short half-life in the blood (2 min), GLP-1 has beneficial effects in type II diabetes, and its repeated administration has led to short-term weight loss. Despite its potential for pharmacological manipulation, there is no defined physiological role for GLP-1 in either weight gain or eating behavior.

Galanin: Galanin and its more recently discovered relative, galanin-like peptide (GALP), are related peptide neurotransmitters that bind to the same neuronal receptors, albeit with different affinities. Galanin stimulates food intake, apparently via central mechanisms, whereas GALP may communicate with LHRH neurons in the hypothalamus. Nevertheless, no clear phenotype linking galanin or GALP to body weight or eating has been identified.

Adipocyte complement-related protein (ACRP30): ACRP30 is a 30-kd peptide made by adipocytes and has been inversely associated with body weight and insulin resistance. ACRP30 levels in the blood are significantly lower in obese than in nonobese persons. Injections of ACRP30 decreased blood glucose independently of insulin and decreased body weight independently of food intake.

Neuropeptide Y: This peptide product of the nucleus solitarius, locus ceruleus, and arcuate nucleus of the hypothalamus is a potent stimulator of appetite. It also decreases the metabolic rate, increases insulin and glucagon secretion, raises the levels of free fatty acids in the blood, and stimulates insulin resistance. Leptin decreases neuropeptide Y secretion, an effect that may be a downstream mediator of leptin's effects. Many of the effects of neuropeptide Y are mediated by two of its several receptors, Y1 and Y5, and development of antagonists to these receptors is an active area of pharmacotherapeutics.

Peroxisome proliferator-activated receptors (PPAR): These proteins are a family of transcription factors; when they bind their ligands, they activate the transcription of targeted genes. PPAR has large ligand-binding pockets, which can combine with a wide variety of compounds (e.g., fatty acids, prostaglandins, and phospholipids). Their "real" ligands in vivo are not known. One isotype, PPARγ, is thought to be most involved in regulating obesity. It is present on adipocytes and, when activated, increases uptake of fatty acids and glucose by adipocytes and their conversion into stored triglycerides. An important class of agents used to treat type II diabetes, the fibrates, binds PPARγ and activates adipocyte glucose uptake, thereby overcoming the insulin resistance of the disease.

In sum, the more that is known about the physiology of energy intake and use, the more its complexity is apparent. There is a striking difference between the effects of these biological mediators in rodents and in humans. Nevertheless, the identification of factors that influence body weight is the basis for a continuing search for pharmacological remedies for obesity.

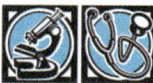 **Pathology and Clinical Features:** The distribution of excess body fat in obesity shows two major patterns. Some overweight persons accumulate fat on the upper trunk, shoulders, and arms, whereas others exhibit pelvic girdle obesity. Persons with upper truncal obesity can usually reduce body fat by diet; those who deposit fat in the buttocks, hip, and lower abdomen retain their obese configuration despite rigorous control of food consumption.

Obesity leads to an increase in overall mortality. **The most important consequence of obesity** (Fig. 8-27) **is maturity-onset (type II) diabetes, which is associated with normal or high levels of circulating insulin and peripheral resistance to insulin's action.** This complication is more frequent in persons with upper truncal obesity than those with pelvic girdle adiposity. In the United States, more than 80% of type II diabetes occurs in obese persons. This subject is more fully discussed in Chapter 22.

Obesity is also linked to atherosclerosis and myocardial infarction. Even mild-to-moderate obesity increases this risk. Obesity is associated with all the major risk factors for myocardial infarction, including hypercholesterolemia, low levels of high-density lipoproteins, diabetes, and hypertension.

Obesity and hypercholesterolemia are also linked to an increased incidence of gallstones, particularly in women. Severe obesity results in the deposition of fat in the liver and minor functional changes, but these are generally of little clinical significance. However, some obese persons display a liver disease termed *nonalcoholic steatohepatitis*, which may have serious consequences (see Chapter 14). Blood uric acid levels are increased in obese persons, as is the incidence of gout.

A number of complications can be traced simply to the physical effect of an increase in body weight and skinfold thickness. Osteoarthritis, or degenerative joint disease, is common in weight-bearing joints such as the hip, knee, and spine. Excessive subcutaneous fat, particularly beneath the breasts and in the crural areas in women, often is responsible for an intertriginous dermatitis, owing to an accumulation of moisture and maceration of the epidermis. The moisture in the intertriginous areas may predispose to fungal infections of the skin. Hernias of the ventral abdominal wall and of the diaphragm are not uncommon. Because the fat deposits place greater pressure on the veins and possibly because tissue turgor is decreased, varicose veins of the lower extremities are more common in obese persons, and the incidence of deep venous thrombosis is increased correspondingly.

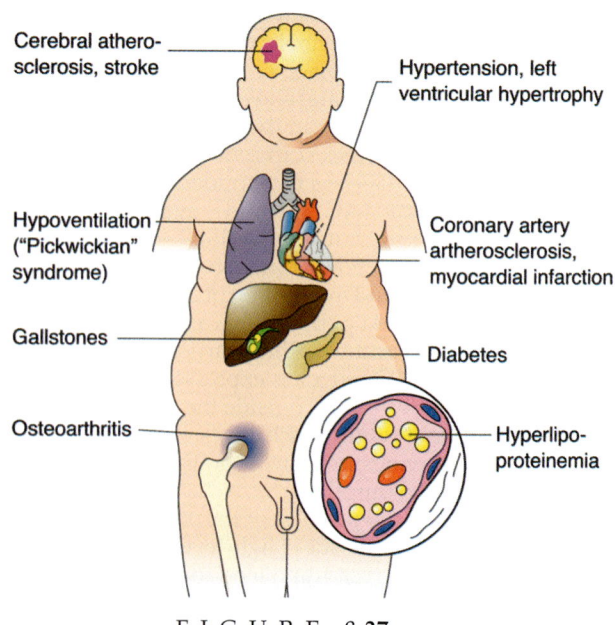

FIGURE 8-27
Complications of obesity.

In morbidly obese persons, the increased abdominal mass hinders chest expansion during inspiration, thereby leading to inadequate respiration. This affliction is referred to as *"Pickwickian syndrome"* after its description by Dickens in the *Pickwick Papers*.

Obesity also poses a physical impediment to surgery, which is made more difficult technically. Because of the longer time needed for surgery, the risks of anesthesia, pulmonary complications, and infection are increased, and the overall surgical mortality for the obese is probably twice as great as that for persons of normal weight.

Obesity also has an important effect on the female reproductive system. **Oligomenorrhea and amenorrhea are common in premenopausal obese women.** Pregnant obese women have a higher incidence of toxemia of pregnancy. Postmenopausal obese women have higher rates of endometrial carcinoma. It has been postulated that the increased body fat provides a larger storage space for estrogens and that the conversion of adrenal androgens to compounds with estrogenic activity is increased. Such mechanisms might lead to greater hormonal stimulation of the endometrium.

The treatment of obesity is difficult, especially in those who have been overweight since childhood. Despite the commercial success of innumerable fad diets that purport to enhance weight loss, there is no evidence that any particular form of caloric restriction is more effective than any other. Simply put, any caloric intake that is less than energy expenditure will result in weight loss. Since some unusual diets (e.g., protein hydrolysates) may actually pose health risks, such as cardiac arrhythmias, the most reasonable regimen for most obese persons is a balanced diet containing less than 1000 calories a day. The use of diuretics to help lose weight borders on the fraudulent, and administration of thyroid hormone has a greater effect on lean body mass than on adipose tissue. Gastric stapling and intestinal bypass operations have been effective in achieving weight loss in morbidly obese persons.

Protein-Calorie Malnutrition Reflects Starvation or Specific Deficiencies

There are two ends of the spectrum of protein-calorie malnutrition, reflecting the relative imbalance between the components of the diet. *Marasmus* refers to a deficiency of calories from all sources. *Kwashiorkor* is a form of malnutrition in children caused by a diet deficient in protein alone. In this discussion we will emphasize childhood nutrition.

Marasmus

Global starvation—that is, a deficiency of all elements of the diet—leads to marasmus. The condition is common throughout the nonindustrialized world, particularly when breast feeding is stopped, and a child must subsist on a calorically inadequate diet. The pathological changes are similar to those in starving adults and consist of decreased body weight, diminished subcutaneous fat, a protuberant abdomen, muscle wasting, and a wrinkled face. In general, the child is a "shrunken old person." Wasting and increased lipofuscin pigment are seen in most visceral organs, especially the heart and the liver. No edema is present. The pulse, blood pressure, and temperature are low, and diarrhea is common. Because immune responses are impaired, the child suffers from numerous infections. An important consequence of marasmus is growth failure. If these children are not provided with an adequate diet during childhood, they will not reach their full potential stature as adults. The effects on ultimate intelligence are controversial.

Kwashiorkor

Kwashiorkor (Fig. 8-28) *is a syndrome that results from a deficiency of protein in a diet relatively high in carbohydrates.* It is one of the most common diseases of infancy and childhood in the nonindustrialized world. Like marasmus, this disorder usually occurs after the infant is weaned, when a protein-poor diet, consisting principally of staple carbohydrates, replaces the mother's milk. Although there is generalized growth failure and muscle wasting, as in marasmus, the subcutaneous fat is normal, owing to an adequate caloric intake. Extreme apathy is a notable feature, in contrast to children with marasmus, who may be alert. Also in contrast to marasmus, severe edema, hepatomegaly, depigmentation of the skin, and dermatoses are usual. "Flaky

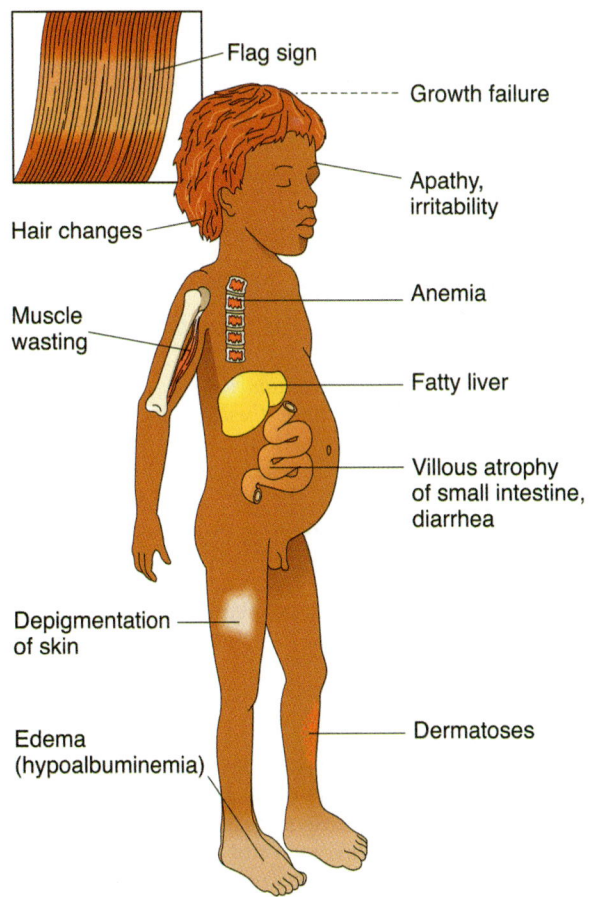

FIGURE 8-28
Complications of kwashiorkor.

paint" lesions of the skin, located on the face, extremities, and perineum, are dry and hyperkeratotic. The hair becomes a sandy or reddish color; a characteristic linear depigmentation of the hair ("flag sign") provides evidence of particularly severe periods of protein deficiency. The abdomen is distended because of flaccid abdominal muscles, hepatomegaly, and ascites due to hypoalbuminemia. Along with generalized atrophy of the viscera, villous atrophy of the intestine may interfere with nutrient absorption, and diarrhea is common. Anemia is a usual feature, although it is not generally life threatening. The nonspecific effects on growth, pulse, temperature, and the immune system are similar to those in marasmus. Although it has been claimed that kwashiorkor not only impairs physical development but also stunts later intellectual growth, the subject requires further study.

Metabolism

β-Carotene is cleaved in the intestinal mucosa to the aldehyde and then reduced to retinoids, which are absorbed with chylomicrons, and stored in the liver, where 90% of the body's vitamin A is located. Usually, rapid transit of food through the small intestine or modification of available lipid by the addition of nonabsorbable lipid carriers (e.g., mineral oil) decreases the absorption of vitamin A.

Vitamin A Deficiency

Although vitamin A deficiency is distinctly uncommon in developed countries, it remains a significant health problem in poorer regions of the world, including much of Africa, China, and Southeast Asia.

Pathology: Microscopically, the liver in kwashiorkor is conspicuously fatty, and the accumulation of lipid within the cytoplasm of the hepatocyte displaces the nucleus to the periphery of the cell. The adequacy of dietary carbohydrate provides the lipid to the hepatocyte, but the inadequate protein stores do not permit the synthesis of enough apoprotein carrier to transport the lipid from the liver cell. The changes, with the possible exception of mental retardation, are fully reversible when sufficient protein is made available. In fact, the fatty liver reverts to normal after early childhood, even when the diet remains deficient in protein. In any event, the hepatic changes are not progressive and are not associated with the development of chronic liver disease.

Pathology: **The lack of vitamin A results principally in squamous metaplasia, especially in glandular epithelium** (Fig. 8-29). As a result, keratin debris blocks sweat and tear glands. Squamous metaplasia is common in the trachea and the bronchi, and bronchopneumonia is a frequent cause of death. The lining epithelia of the renal pelvis, pancreatic ducts, uterus, and salivary glands are also commonly affected. Epithelial changes in the renal pelvis are occasionally associated with kidney stones. With further diminution of vitamin A stores, squamous metaplasia of the epithelial cells of the conjunctiva and tear ducts occurs, which leads to **xerophthalmia**, dryness of the cornea and conjunctiva. The cornea becomes

Vitamins Are Necessary in Trace Amounts for Metabolic Functions

"Vitamin" is a general term for a number of unrelated organic catalysts that are not endogenously synthesized. **The body depends totally on dietary sources for vitamins.** The definition of a vitamin requires demonstration that a lack of this compound results in a clearly definable disease. Thus, vitamins in one species are not necessarily vitamins in another. For example, whereas humans cannot synthesize ascorbic acid (vitamin C) and therefore require dietary ascorbate to prevent scurvy, most lower animals can produce their own ascorbic acid and do not require it as a vitamin.

Vitamin A

Vitamin A, a fat-soluble substance, is important for the maintenance of a number of specialized epithelial linings, skeletal maturation, and the structure of the cell membranes. In addition, it is an important constituent of the photosensitive pigments in the retina. Vitamin A occurs naturally as retinoids or as a precursor, β-carotene. The source of the precursor, carotene, is in plants, principally leafy, green vegetables. Fish livers are a particularly rich source of vitamin A itself.

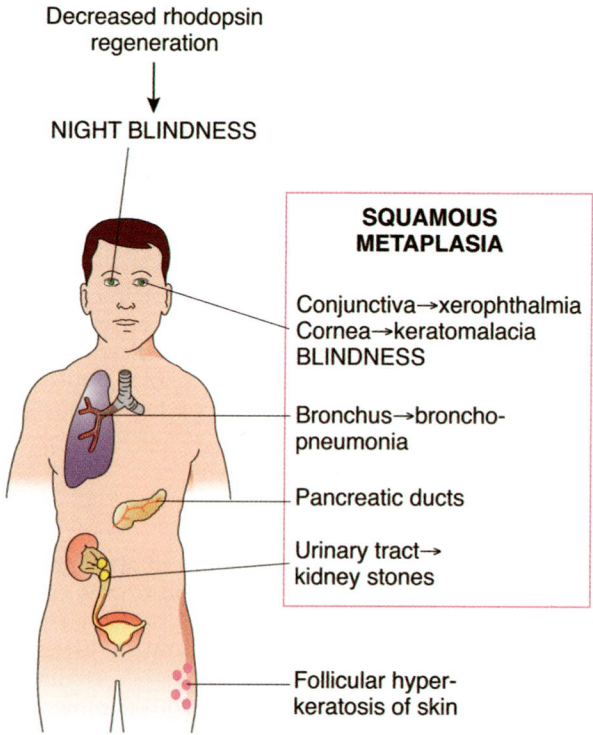

FIGURE 8-29
Complications of vitamin A deficiency.

softened **(keratomalacia)** and is vulnerable to ulceration and bacterial infection, complications that may lead to blindness. **Follicular hyperkeratosis,** a skin disorder that results from occluded sebaceous, is also a feature of this disease.

Clinical Features: The earliest sign of vitamin A deficiency often is diminished vision in dim light. Vitamin A is a necessary component in the pigment of the retinal rods and is active in light transduction. Since the aldehyde of vitamin A, retinal, is constantly being degraded during the generation of the light signal, a continuous supply of vitamin A is necessary for night vision.

Vitamin A Toxicity

Poisoning by excessive doses of vitamin A is usually caused by overenthusiastic administration of vitamin supplements to children. Early Arctic explorers were said to have experienced vitamin A toxicity because they ate polar bear livers, which are particularly rich in the vitamin. Enlargement of the liver and spleen are common; microscopically these organs show lipid-laden macrophages. In the liver, vitamin A is also present in hepatocytes, and prolonged vitamin A toxicity has been incriminated in the production of cirrhosis. Bone pain and neurological symptoms, such as hyperexcitability and headache, may be the presenting symptoms. Discontinuation of excess vitamin A consumption reverses all or most of the lesions. Excessive carotene intake is benign and simply stains the skin yellow, which may be mistaken for jaundice.

Synthetic derivatives of retinoic acid are now increasingly used for their pharmacological effects in alleviating severe acne. Both retinoic acid and a high dietary intake of preformed vitamin A are particularly dangerous in pregnancy because of their potent teratogenic actions.

Vitamin B Complex

Vitamins in the B group of water-soluble vitamins are numbered 1 through 12, but most are not distinct vitamins. The members of the complex currently recognized as true vitamins are vitamins B_1 (thiamine), niacin, B_2 (riboflavin), B_6 (pyridoxine), and B_{12} (cyanocobalamin). With the exception of vitamin B_{12}, which is derived only from animal sources, the vitamins of the B complex are found principally in leafy green vegetables, milk, and liver.

Thiamine

Thiamine was the active ingredient in the original description of vitamin B, which was defined as a water-soluble extract in rice polishings that cured beri-beri (clinical thiamine deficiency). This disease was classically seen in the Orient, where the staple food was polished rice that had been deprived of its thiamine content by processing. With increased awareness of the disease and improved nutrition in some areas, the disorder is less common now than in previous generations. In Western countries, the disease occurs in alcoholics, neglected persons with poor overall nutrition, and food faddists. **The cardinal symptoms of thiamine deficiency are polyneuropathy, edema, and cardiac failure** (Fig. 8-30). The deficiency syndrome is classically divided into **dry beri-beri,** with symptoms referable to the neuromuscular system, and **wet beri-beri,** in which the manifestations of cardiac failure predominate.

Pathogenesis: Patients with dry beri-beri present with paresthesias, depressed reflexes, and weakness and atrophy of the muscles of the extremities. Wet beri-beri is characterized by generalized edema, a reflection of severe congestive failure. The basic lesion is an uncontrolled, generalized vasodilation and significant peripheral arteriovenous shunting. This combination leads to a compensatory increase in cardiac output and eventually to a large dilated heart and congestive heart failure. In the absence of a documented metabolic disease (e.g., hyperthyroidism), high output failure and generalized edema strongly suggest thiamine deficiency.

The biochemical basis for the symptoms of thiamine deficiency is not understood. As a result of the defect in oxida-

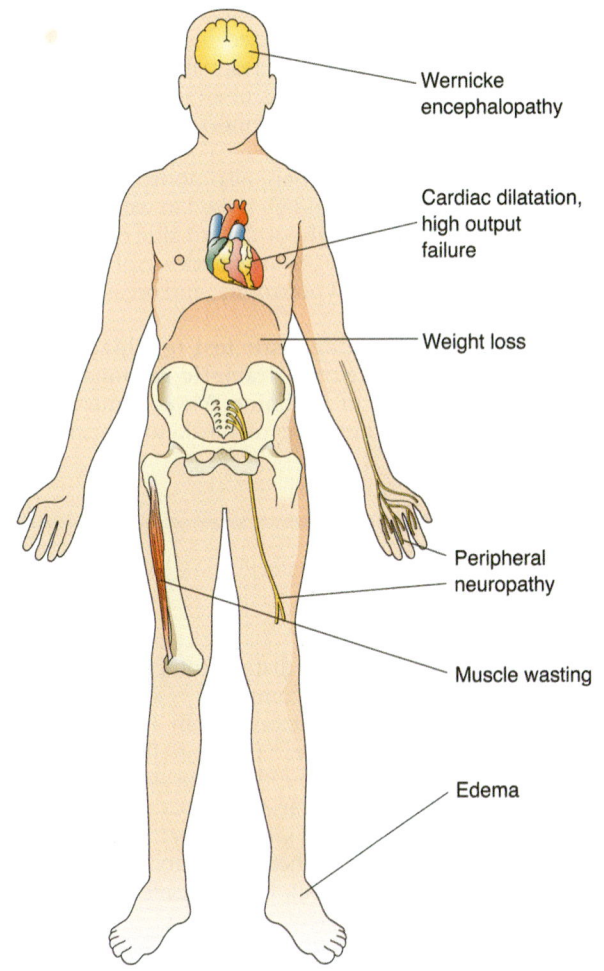

FIGURE 8-30
Complications of thiamine deficiency (beri-beri).

tive decarboxylation, pyruvate accumulates. However, experimental pyruvate administration does not produce the same lesions. Moreover, it is difficult to attribute the symptomatology to a generalized defect in energy metabolism.

 Pathology: Thiamine deficiency in chronic alcoholics may be manifested by involvement of the brain in the form of *Wernicke syndrome,* in which progressive **dementia, ataxia,** and **ophthalmoplegia** (paralysis of the extraocular muscles) are prominent. *Korsakoff syndrome,* in which a thought disorder is conspicuous, at one time was attributed solely to thiamine deficiency, but it now appears to be a finding both in chronic alcoholics and in patients with other organic mental syndromes.

Pathological examination of the nervous system in cases of thiamine deficiency has not defined a pathognomonic change in the peripheral nerves, since similar or identical changes can be seen in a variety of other diseases characterized by peripheral neuropathy. A characteristic alteration is degeneration of myelin sheaths, often beginning in the sciatic nerve and then involving other peripheral nerves and sometimes the spinal cord itself. In the few advanced cases that have been studied, fragmentation of the axons was noted.

In Wernicke encephalopathy, the most striking lesions are found in the mamillary bodies and surrounding areas that abut on the third ventricle. Indeed, atrophy of the mamillary bodies can be visualized in alcoholics by computed tomography and magnetic resonance imaging. Microscopically, degeneration and loss of ganglion cells, rupture of small blood vessels, and ring hemorrhages are seen in the brain.

The changes in the heart are also nonspecific. Grossly, the heart is flabby, dilated, and increased in weight. The process may affect either the right or the left side of the heart or both. The microscopic changes are nondescript and include edema, inconsistent fiber hypertrophy, and occasional foci of fiber degeneration.

The most reliable diagnostic test for thiamine deficiency is an immediate and dramatic response to parenteral administration of thiamine. Measurements of thiamine in the blood and erythrocyte transketolase activity are also useful.

Niacin

Niacin refers to two chemically distinct compounds: nicotinic acid and nicotinamide. These components are derived from dietary niacin or are biosynthesized from available tryptophan. Niacin plays a major role in the formation of NAD and its phosphate (NADP), compounds important in intermediary metabolism and a wide variety of oxidation–reduction reactions. Animal protein, as found in meat, eggs, and milk, is high in tryptophan and is therefore a good source of endogenously synthesized niacin. Niacin itself is available in many types of grain.

PELLAGRA: Pellagra refers to clinical niacin deficiency and is uncommon today.

 Pathogenesis: Pellagra is seen principally in patients who have been weakened by other diseases and in malnourished alcoholics. Food faddists who do not eat sufficient protein may suffer a deficiency of tryptophan, which in combination with a lack of exogenous niacin may result in mild pellagra. Malabsorption of tryptophan, as in *Hartnup disease,* or excessive use of tryptophan for the synthesis of serotonin in the carcinoid syndrome may also lead to mild symptoms of pellagra. Deficiencies of pyridoxine and riboflavin increase the requirement for dietary niacin because both of these cofactors are required for the biosynthesis of niacin from tryptophan. Pellagra is particularly prevalent in areas where corn (maize) is the staple food, because the niacin in corn is chemically bound and thus poorly available. Corn is also a poor source of tryptophan.

 Pathology: Pellagra (Ital., "rough skin") is characterized by the three "Ds" of niacin deficiency: **dermatitis, diarrhea, and dementia** (Fig. 8-31). Areas exposed to light, such as the face and the hands, and those subjected to pressure, such as the knees and the elbows, exhibit a rough, scaly dermatitis. The involvement of the hands leads to so-called glove dermatitis. The lesions are discrete and show areas of pigmentation and of depigmentation. Microscopically, hyperkeratosis, vascularization, and chronic inflammation of the skin are characteristic. Subcutaneous fibrosis and scarring may be seen in late stages. Similar lesions are found in the mucous membranes of the mouth and vagina. In the mouth, inflammation and edema lead to a large, red tongue, which in the chronic stage is fissured and is likened to raw meat. A chronic, watery diarrhea is a typical feature of the disease, presumably caused by mucosal atrophy and ulceration in the entire gastrointestinal tract, particularly in the colon. The dementia, characterized by

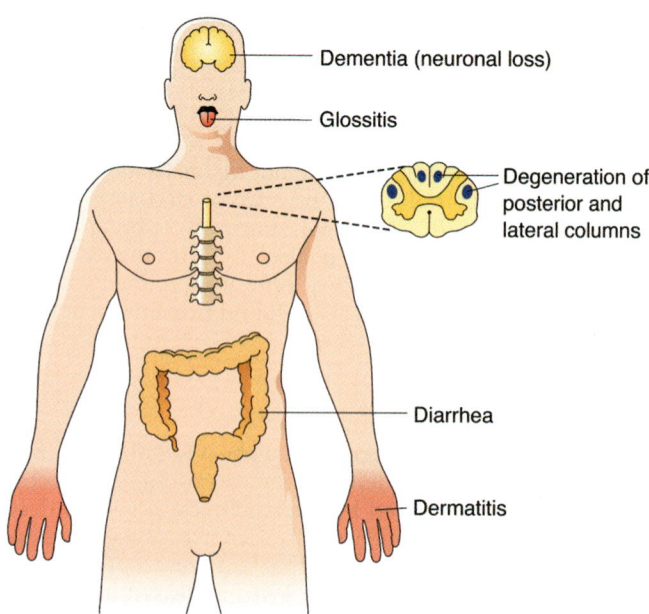

FIGURE 8-31
Complications of niacin deficiency (pellagra).

aberrant ideation bordering on psychosis, is represented in the brain by degeneration of ganglion cells in the cortex. Myelin degeneration of tracts in the spinal cord resembles the subacute combined degeneration of vitamin B_{12} deficiency. Severe long-standing pellagra adds another "D," namely *death*.

Riboflavin

Pathogenesis: Riboflavin, a vitamin derived from many plant and animal sources, is important for the synthesis of flavin nucleotides, which play an important role in electron transport and other reactions in which the transfer of energy is crucial. Riboflavin is converted within the body to flavin mononucleotides and dinucleotides. Clinical symptoms of riboflavin deficiency are uncommon; they are usually seen only in debilitated patients with a variety of diseases and in poorly nourished alcoholics.

Deficiencies of thiamine, riboflavin, and niacin are unusual in industrialized countries because bread and cereals are fortified with these vitamins. Occasionally, a mild deficiency of riboflavin is seen during pregnancy and lactation or during the period of rapid growth of childhood and adolescence, when increased demands are combined with moderate nutritional deprivation.

Pathology: Riboflavin deficiency is manifested principally by lesions of the facial skin and the corneal epithelium. **Cheilosis,** a term used for fissures in the skin at the angles of the mouth, is a characteristic feature (Fig. 8-32). These cracks in the skin may be painful and often become infected. Microscopically, hyperkeratosis and a mild mononuclear infiltrate of the skin are noted. **Seborrheic dermatitis,** an inflammation of the skin that exhibits a greasy, scaling appearance, typically involves the cheeks and the areas behind the ears. The tongue is smooth and purplish (magenta), owing to atrophy of the mucosa. The most troubling lesion may be an **interstitial keratitis of the cornea,** which is followed by opacification of the cornea and eventual ulceration. The localization of the lesions in riboflavin deficiency is not explained biochemically.

Pyridoxine

Vitamin B_6 activity is found in three related, naturally occurring compounds: pyridoxine, pyridoxal, and pyridoxamine. For the sake of convenience, they are all grouped under the heading pyridoxine. These compounds are widely distributed in vegetable and animal foods.

Pathogenesis: Pyridoxine is converted to pyridoxal phosphate, a coenzyme for many enzymes, including transaminases and carboxylases. Pyridoxine deficiency is rarely caused by an inadequate diet, although infants who have been fed a poorly prepared powdered formula in which the pyridoxine has been destroyed during preparation have suffered convulsions. A higher demand for the vitamin, as may occur in pregnancy, may lead to a secondary deficiency state. Of particular concern is the deficiency of pyridoxine that follows prolonged medication with a number of drugs, particularly isoniazid, cycloserine, and penicillamine. A deficiency state is also occasionally reported in alcoholics.

Clinical Features: There are no clinical manifestations of pyridoxine deficiency that can be considered characteristic or pathognomonic. The usual dermatological complications of other B vitamin deficiencies occur with pyridoxine deficiency. **The primary expression of the disease is in the central nervous system, a feature consistent with the role of this vitamin in the formation of pyridoxal-dependent decarboxylase of the neurotransmitter γ-aminobutyric acid (GABA).** In infants and children, diarrhea, anemia, and seizures have occurred.

Conditions are encountered in which there is no clinical or biochemical evidence of pyridoxine deficiency, yet large (pharmacological) doses of the vitamin are useful in treating the disorder. Such diseases are termed *pyridoxine-dependency syndromes* and include anemia, convulsions, and homocystinuria caused by cystathionine synthetase deficiency.

Pyridoxine-responsive anemia is hypochromic and microcytic and therefore can be confused with iron deficiency anemia. Unlike iron deficiency anemia, however, pyridoxine-responsive anemia is characterized by saturation of iron stores and increased saturation of transferrin. Thus, administration of iron may simply make pyridoxine-responsive

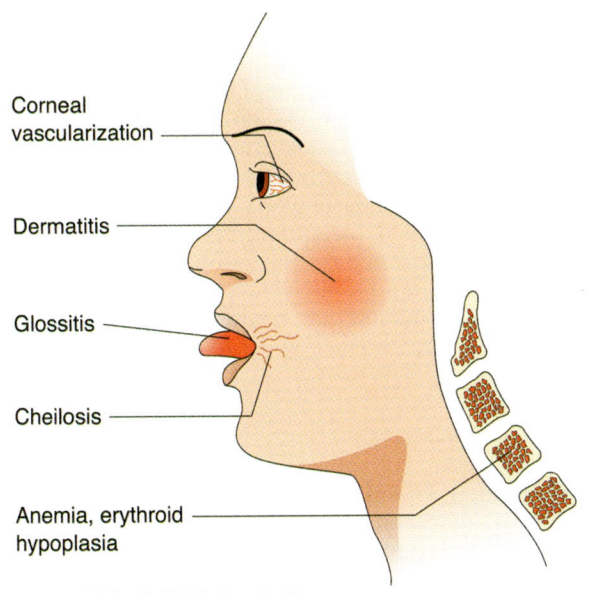

FIGURE 8-32
Complications of riboflavin deficiency.

anemia worse. By definition, the anemia responds well to massive doses of pyridoxine.

Vitamin B₁₂ and Folic Acid Deficiencies

Deficiencies of vitamin B₁₂ are almost always seen in cases of pernicious anemia and result from the lack of secretion of intrinsic factor in the stomach, which prevents absorption of the vitamin in the ileum.

Pathogenesis: Since vitamin B₁₂ is found in almost all animal protein, including meat, milk, and eggs, dietary deficiency is seen only in rare cases of extreme vegetarianism, and that only after many years of a restricted diet. Parasitization of the small intestine by the fish tapeworm *Diphyllobothrium latum* may lead to vitamin B₁₂ deficiency because the parasite absorbs the vitamin in the lumen of the gut.

Deficiency of folic acid is commonly of dietary origin. Leafy vegetables, liver, kidney, and yeast are rich sources of folic acid. However, excessive cooking destroys much of the folic acid in foods. Dietary folic acid deficiency is usually accompanied by multiple vitamin deficiencies. Pregnancy increases the requirement for folic acid 5- to 10-fold. **It has been estimated that two thirds of anemic pregnant women are folate deficient,** although this may be combined with iron deficiency. Folic acid is absorbed principally in the upper third of the small intestine, and thus folate deficiency is common in certain diseases of malabsorption, notably nontropical and tropical sprue. The latter condition responds to treatment with folic acid.

Clinical Features: Deficiencies of both vitamin B₁₂ and folic acid are associated with *megaloblastic anemia*. In addition, pernicious anemia is complicated by a neurological condition called *subacute combined degeneration of the spinal cord*. Comprehensive discussions of vitamin B₁₂ and folic acid deficiencies are found in Chapters 20 and 28. In pregnant women, supplementation of the diet with folic acid prevents spina bifida and other dysraphic anomalies (see Chapter 6).

Vitamin C (Ascorbic Acid)

Pathogenesis: Ascorbic acid is a powerful biological reducing agent that is involved in numerous oxidation–reduction reactions and the transfer of protons. This vitamin is important in the synthesis of chondroitin sulfate and in the hydroxylation of proline to form the hydroxyproline of collagen. It serves many other important functions, such as preventing the oxidation of tetrahydrofolate and augmenting the absorption of iron from the gut. Without vitamin C, the biosynthesis of certain neurotransmitters is impaired because of a reduction in the activity of dopamine β-hydroxylase. Wound healing and immune functions are also under the influence of ascorbic acid. The best dietary sources of vitamin C are citrus fruits, green vegetables, and tomatoes. Humans and the guinea pig cannot make ascorbic acid, an incapacity that can be explained only as an evolutionary quirk.

Scurvy

The term scurvy *refers to the clinical vitamin C deficiency state.* The first demonstration of the need for this vitamin was the remarkable effect of lime in preventing scurvy among 18th century British sailors. The distribution of limes in the British navy led to the name "limey" for the seamen. Scurvy is uncommon in the western world, but is often noted in nonindustrialized countries in which other forms of malnutrition are prevalent. In industrialized countries, scurvy is now a disease of persons afflicted with chronic diseases who do not eat well, the neglected aged and malnourished alcoholics. The stress of cold, heat, fever, or trauma (accidental or surgical) leads to an increased requirement for vitamin C. Children who are fed only milk for the first year of life develop scurvy, as do alcoholics. Mild depression of ascorbic acid levels also occurs in other conditions, including cigarette smoking, tuberculosis, rheumatic fever, and many debilitating disorders. Some women who use oral contraceptives may have a mild decrease in serum vitamin C levels. The rate of catabolism of ascorbic acid is about 3% of the body pool a day, a value that is consistent with the fact that on a diet lacking in vitamin C the symptoms of scurvy take some months to develop.

Pathology: Most of the events associated with vitamin C deficiency are caused by the formation of abnormal collagen that lacks tensile strength (Fig. 8-33). Within 1 to 3 months, subperiosteal hemorrhages lead to pain in the bones and joints. Petechial hemorrhages, ecchymoses, and purpura are common, particularly after mild trauma or at pressure points. Perifollicular hemorrhages in the skin are particularly typical of scurvy. In advanced cases, swollen, bleeding gums are a classic finding. Alveolar bone resorption results in the loss of teeth. Wound healing is poor, and dehiscence of previously healed wounds occurs. Anemia may result from prolonged bleeding, impaired iron absorption, or an associated folic acid deficiency.

In children, vitamin C deficiency leads to growth failure, and collagen-rich structures such as the teeth, bones, and blood vessels develop abnormally. The effects on developing bone are conspicuous and relate principally to impaired function of osteoblasts. The effects of scurvy on bone are discussed in greater detail in Chapter 26. In addi-

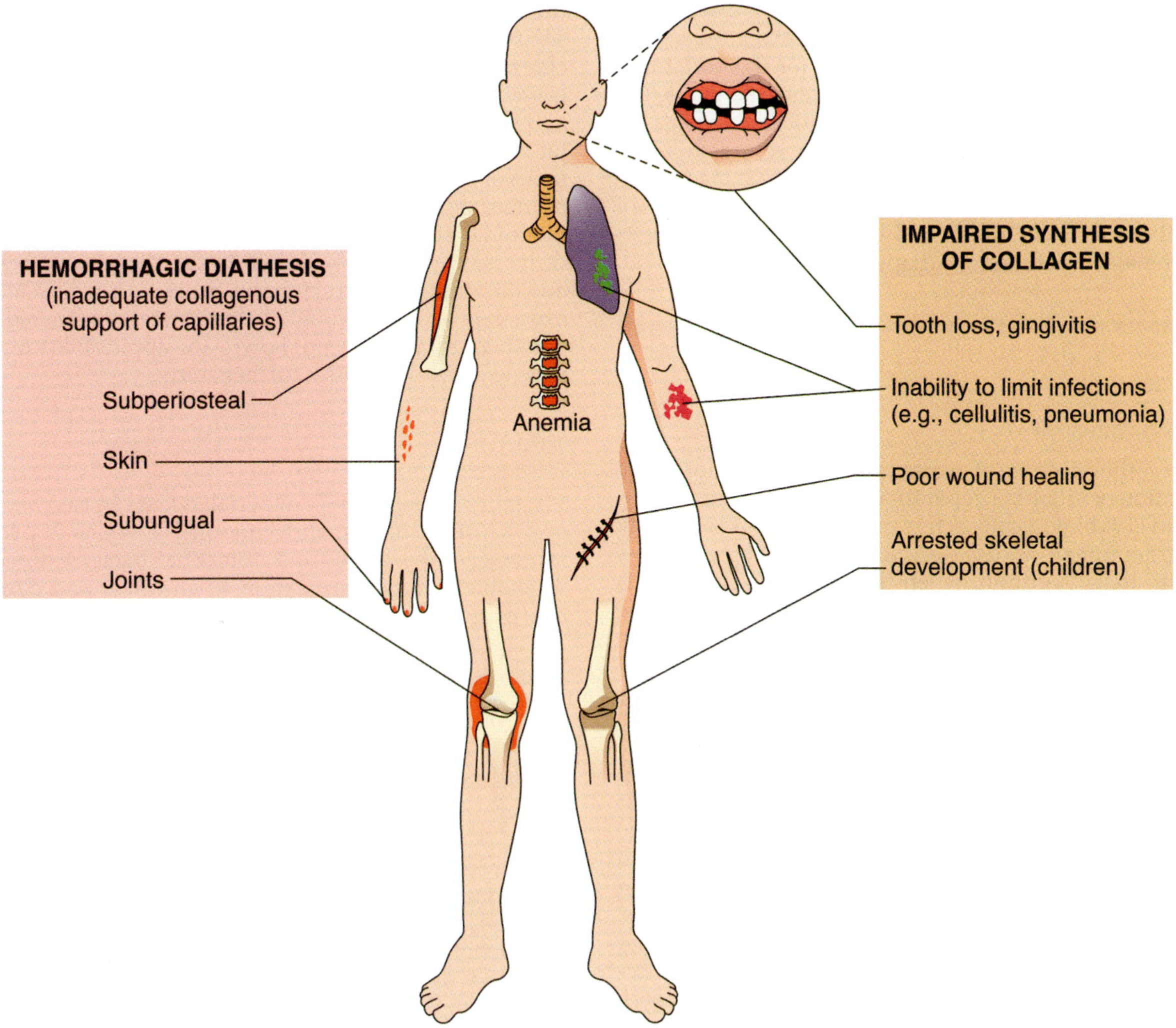

FIGURE 8-33
Complications of vitamin C deficiency (scurvy).

tion to poor wound healing, scorbutic patients have difficulty in walling off an infection to form an abscess, and infections therefore spread more easily. The diagnosis of scurvy is confirmed by finding low levels of ascorbic acid in the serum.

Widespread publicity has attended claims that very large doses of ascorbic acid are useful in the prevention of the common cold and in the treatment of metastatic cancer. There is no credible evidence to support either contention.

Vitamin D

Vitamin D is a fat-soluble steroid hormone found in two forms: vitamin D_3 (cholecalciferol) and vitamin D_2 (ergocalciferol), both of which have equal biological potency in humans. Vitamin D_3 is produced in the skin, and vitamin D_2 is derived from plant ergosterol. The vitamin is absorbed in the jejunum along with fats and is transported in the blood bound to an α-globulin (vitamin D-binding protein). **To achieve biological potency, vitamin D must be hydroxylated to active metabolites in the liver and kidney. The active form of the vitamin promotes calcium and phosphate absorption from the small intestine** and may directly influence mineralization of bone.

Vitamin D Deficiency

 Pathogenesis: Vitamin D deficiency results from (1) insufficient vitamin D in the diet, (2) insufficient production of vitamin D in the skin because of limited sunlight exposure as a result of occupation or dress, (3) inadequate absorption of vitamin D from the diet (as in the fat malabsorption syndromes), or (4) abnormal conversion of vitamin D to its bioactive metabolites. The last occurs in liver disease and chronic renal failure. **In children, vitamin D deficiency causes rickets; in adults, osteomalacia occurs.**

 Clinical Features: The bone lesions of vitamin D deficiency in children (rickets) have been recognized for centuries and were common in the western industrialized world until recently. It was a disease that affected the urban poor to a much greater extent than their rural counterparts. A partial explanation for this difference lies in the greater exposure of rural residents to sunlight. The addition of vitamin D to milk and many processed foods, the administration of vitamin preparations to young children, and generally improved levels of nutrition have made rickets a curiosity in industrialized countries. A full discussion of the metabolism of vitamin D and its relationship to rickets and osteomalacia is found in Chapter 26.

Hypervitaminosis D

The most common cause of excess vitamin D is the inordinate consumption of vitamin preparations. Abnormal conversion of vitamin D to biologically active metabolites is occasionally seen in granulomatous diseases such as sarcoidosis. In cases of calcium malabsorption, when the underlying disease is corrected, the sensitivity of target tissues to vitamin D may be increased.

Pathology: The initial response to excess vitamin D is **hypercalcemia,** which leads to nonspecific symptoms such as weakness and headaches. The increased excretion of calcium by the kidneys results in **nephrolithiasis** or **nephrocalcinosis. Ectopic calcification** in other organs, such as blood vessels, the heart, and lungs, may be seen. Infants are particularly susceptible to excess vitamin D, and if the condition is not corrected, they may develop premature arteriosclerosis, supravalvular aortic stenosis, and renal acidosis.

Vitamin E

Vitamin E is an antioxidant that (experimentally at least) protects membrane phospholipids against lipid peroxidation by free radicals formed by cellular metabolism. The activity of this fat-soluble vitamin is found in a number of dietary constituents, principally in α-tocopherol. Corn and soy beans are particularly rich in vitamin E.

A dietary deficiency of vitamin E is rare, except among patients receiving total parenteral nutrition. Low vitamin E levels have also been found in patients with disorders of fat absorption from the intestine. No clearly definable syndrome associated with vitamin E deficiency has been identified in adults. Inconsistent reports of abnormalities of the posterior columns of the spinal cord, together with functional disturbances of gait, proprioception, and vibration have been recorded. Although the life span of the erythrocyte may be shortened, clinical anemia is not attributable to vitamin E deficiency alone.

In premature infants, hemolytic anemia, thrombocytosis, and edema have been associated with a deficiency of vitamin E. Food faddists and enterprising entrepreneurs have endorsed vitamin E as an antiaging vitamin and an enhancer of sexual potency. There is no objective evidence to support these claims. On the other hand, vitamin E therapy has been reported to improve hemolytic anemia in premature newborns and may reduce the severity but not the incidence of retrolental fibroplasia. Vitamin E is reported to retard the development of cirrhosis in infants with congenital biliary atresia. A number of interesting experimental effects are produced by vitamin E, such as inhibition of (1) platelet aggregation, (2) the conversion of dietary nitrites to carcinogenic nitrosamines, and (3) prostaglandin synthesis. Protection against toxins that exert their activity through the production of free radical oxygen species has also been shown. The applicability of these results to humans requires further study.

Vitamin K

Vitamin K, a fat-soluble material, occurs in two forms: vitamin K_1, from plants, and vitamin K_2, which is principally synthesized by the normal intestinal bacteria. Green leafy vegetables are rich in vitamin K, and liver and dairy products contain smaller amounts.

Pathogenesis: Dietary deficiency is very uncommon in the United States; most cases are associated with other disorders. However, inadequate dietary intake of vitamin K does occasionally occur in conjunction with chronic illness associated with anorexia.

Vitamin K deficiency is common in severe fat malabsorption, as seen in sprue and biliary tract obstruction. The destruction of intestinal flora by antibiotics may also result in vitamin K deficiency. Newborn infants frequently exhibit vitamin K deficiency because the vitamin is not transported well across the placenta, and the sterile gut of the newborn does not have bacteria to produce it. Vitamin K, which confers calcium-binding properties to certain proteins, is important for the activity of four clotting factors: prothrombin, factor VII, factor IX, and factor X. Deficiency of vitamin K can be serious, because it can lead to catastrophic bleeding. Parenteral vitamin K therapy is rapidly effective.

Essential Trace Minerals Are Mostly Components of Enzymes and Cofactors

Essential trace minerals include iron, copper, iodine, zinc, cobalt, selenium, manganese, nickel, chromium, tin, molybdenum, vanadium, silicon, and fluorine. Dietary deficiencies of these minerals are clinically important in the case of iron and iodine, and these are discussed in Chapters 20 and 21, which deal with blood diseases and endocrinological pathology, respectively.

Chronic zinc deficiency has been reported in Iran and Egypt to result in hypogonadal dwarfism in boys. The children usually are those who eat clay, a substance that may bind zinc, but a deficiency in dietary protein is usually also present. An inherited disorder of zinc metabolism, *acrodermatitis en-*

teropathica, which is a chronic form of zinc deficiency, is characterized by diarrhea, rash, hair loss, muscle wasting, and mental irritability. Similar symptoms are seen in acute zinc deficiency associated with total parenteral nutrition. Zinc deficiency is also seen in diseases that cause malabsorption, such as Crohn disease, sprue, cirrhosis, and alcoholism.

Dietary copper deficiency is rare but may occur in certain inherited disorders, in malabsorption syndromes, and during total parenteral nutrition. The most common result is microcytic anemia, although megaloblastic changes have also been described.

Manganese deficiency has been described and causes poor growth, skeletal abnormalities, reproductive impairment, ataxia, and convulsions. **Industrial exposure to manganese** causes symptoms closely related to those of parkinsonism.

CONCLUSION

The dawn of life was marked by an incredibly hostile environment. The earth revolved on its axis more than 10^{12} times before a creature evolved who could consciously manipulate the environment. In the process, the 18-year average life span of Cro-Magnon man has risen for industrialized humans to surpass the biblical 3 score and 10. This remarkable success should not lead us to complacency in our efforts to improve the quality and extent of life, but one must maintain a realistic perspective on the impact of civilization on the environment.

SUGGESTED READING

Books

Amdur MO, Doull J, Klaassen CD: *Casarett and Doull's Toxicology*, 4th ed. New York: Pergamon Press, 1991.

Craighead JE: *Pathology of Environmental and Occupational Disease*. St. Louis: Mosby, 1995.

Di Maio, VJM, Di Maio, D, Di Maio, DJ: *Forensic pathology*, 2nd ed. CRC Press, 2001.

Strickland GT (ed): Nutritional Deficiencies and Heat-associated Illnesses. In: *Hunter's Tropical Medicine*, 6th ed. Philadelphia: WB Saunders, 1984.

Tedeschi CG, Eckert WG, Tedeschi LG: *Forensic Medicine: A Study in Trauma and Environmental Hazards*. Philadelphia: WB Saunders, 1977.

Review Articles

Ames, BB, Gold, LS: The causes and prevention of cancer: the role of the environmnt. *Biotherapy*, 11:205–220(1998).

Baghurst PA, McMichael AJ, Wigg NR: Environmental exposure to lead and children's intelligence at age of seven years. The Port Pirie cohort study. *N Engl J Med* 327:1279–1284, 1992.

Bolger, PM, Schwertz, BA: Mercury and health. *N Engl J Med* 347:1735–1736(2002).

Cohen, BL: Cancer risk from low-level radiation. *Am J Roentgenol* 179:1137–1143(2002).

Craighead JE: *Pathology of environmental and occupational disease*. St. Louis: Mosby, 1995.

Goldfrank LR, Hoffman RS: The cardiovascular effects of cocaine: update 1992. In: *Acute cocaine intoxication: Current methods of treatment*. NIDA Research Monograph No. 123. Rockville, MD: National Institute of Drug Abuse, 1993.

Hacksaw, AK, Law, MR, Wald, NJ: The accumulated evidence on lung cancer and environmental tobacco smoking. *BMJ* 315:980–988(1997).

Hsu, PC Guo, YL: Antioxidant nutrients and lead toxicity. *Toxicol* 180:33–44(2002).

Karch SB: Introduction to the forensic pathology of cocaine. *Am J Forensic Med Pathol* 12:126–131, 1991.

Kjaerheim, K, Gaard, M, Andersen, A: The role of alcohol, tobacco, and dietary factors in upper aerogastric tract cancers: a prospective study of 10,900 Norwegian men. *Cancer Caus & Cont* 9:99–108, 1998.

Krotkiewski, M: Thyroid hormones in the pathogenesis and treatment of obesity. *Eur J Pharmacol* 440:85–98(2002).

La Vecchia, C, Altieri, A, Franceschi, S, Tavani, A: Oral contraceptives and cancer: an update. *Drug Safety* 24:741–754(2001).

Lee, DW, Leinung, MC, Rozhavskaya-Arena, M, Grasso, P: Leptin and the treatment of obesity: its current status. *Eur J Pharmacol* 440:129–139(2002).

Lynge, E, Anttila, A, Hemminki, K: Organic solvents and cancer. *Cancer Causes Control* 8:406–419(1997).

McBride, PE: The health consequences of smoking: cardiovascular disease. *Med Clin N Am* 76:333–353, 1992.

Moysich, KB, Menezes, RJ, Michalek, AM: Chernobyl-related ionizing radiation exposure and cancer risk: an epidemiological review. *Lancet Oncol* 3:269–279(2002).

Muccioli, G, Tschöp, M, Papotti, M, Deghenghi, R, Heiman, M, Ghigo, E: Neuroendocrine and peripheral activities of ghrelin: implication in metabolism and obesity. *Eur J Pharmacol* 440:235–254(2002).

National Council on Radiation Protection and Measurements: The relative biological effectiveness of radiations of different quality. Report No. 104, Bethesda, MD, 1990.

Neuberger, JS, Gesell, TF: Residential radon exposure and lung cancer: risk in nonsmokers. *Health Physics* 83:1–18(2002).

Newcomb, PA, Carbone, PP: The health consequences of smoking. *Med Clin N Am* 76:305–331, 1992.

Raitiola, HS, Pukander, JS: Etiological factors of laryngeal cancer. *Acta Otol-Laryng* 529:S215–S217(1997).

Ravussin, E: Chemical sensors of feast and famine. *J Clin Invest* 109:1537–1540(2002).

Schlecht, NF, Franco, EL, Pintos, J, Kowalski, LP: Effect of smoking cessation and tobacco type on the risk of cancers of the upper aero-digestive tract in Brazil. *Epidemiolo* 10:412–418, 1999.

Shields, PG: Molecular epidemiology of smoking and lung cancer. *Oncogene* 21:6870–6876(2002).

Strickland GT (ed): Nutritional deficiencies and heat-associated illnesses. In: *Hunter's tropical medicine*, 6th ed. Philadelphia: WB Saunders, 1984.

Thackray, H, Tifft, C: Fetal alcohol syndrome. *Pediatr In Rev* 22:47–55(2001).

Tominaga, S: Major avoidable risk factors of cancer. *Cancer Lett* 143:S19–S23(1999).

Vainio, H, Weiderpass, E, Kleihues, P: Smoking cessation in cancer prevention. *Toxicology* 166:47–52(2001).

Webster, EW: Garland lecture: On the question of cancer induction by small x-ray doses. *Am J Roentgenol* 137:647–666, 1981.

Zatonski, W, Becher, H, Lissowska, J, Wahrendorf, J: Tobacco, alcohol, and diet in the etiology of laryngeal cancer: a population-based case-control study. *Canc Caus & Cont* 2:3–10, 1991.

CHAPTER 9

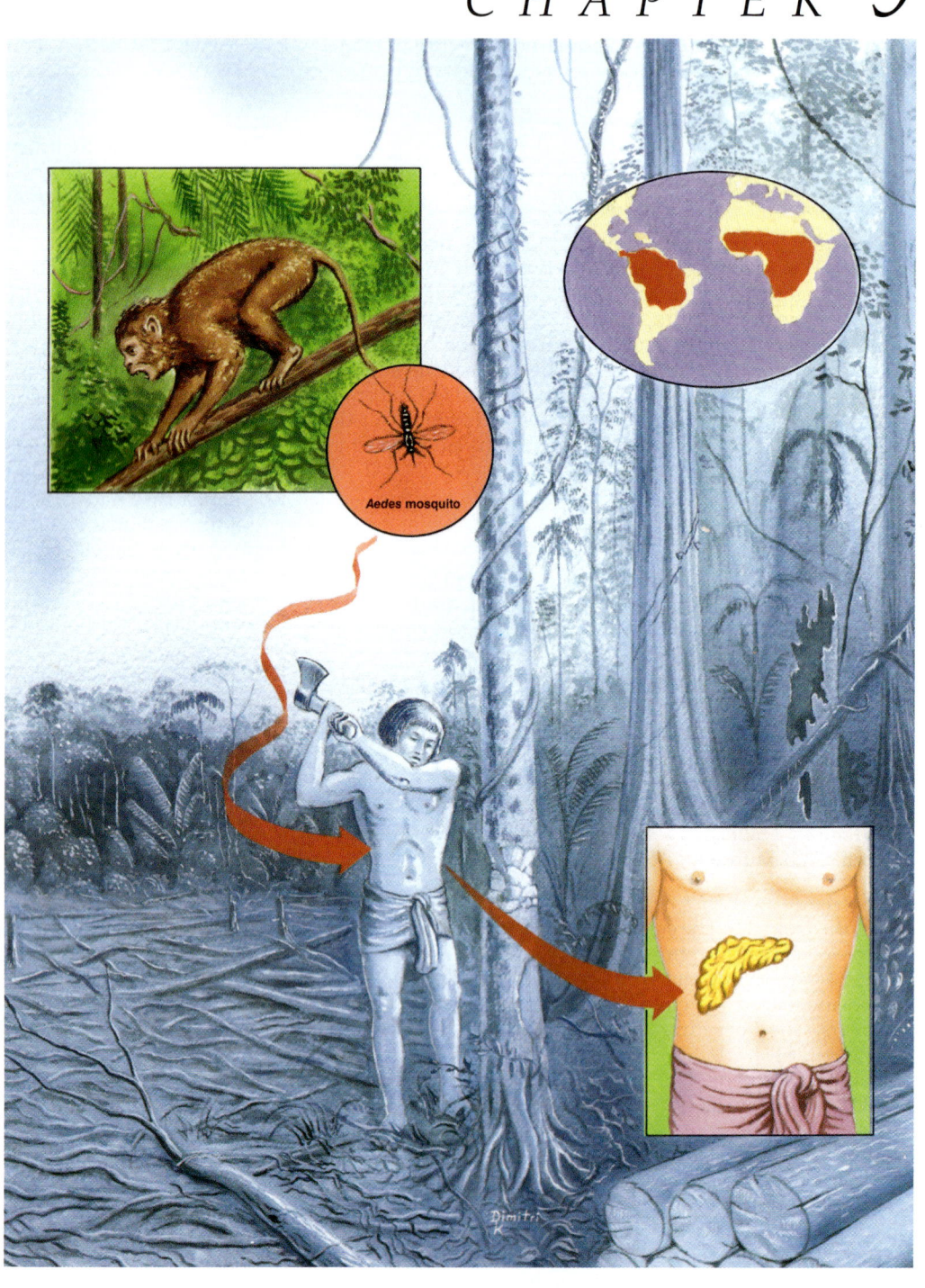

Infectious and Parasitic Diseases

David Schwartz
Robert M. Genta
Daniel H. Connor

Infectivity and Virulence

Host Factors in Infections
Heritable Differences
Age
Behavior
Compromised Host Defenses

Viral Infections

Respiratory Viruses
The Common Cold
Influenza
Parainfluenza Virus
Respiratory Syncytial Virus
Adenovirus
Severe Acute Respiratory Syndrome (SARS)-Associated Coronavirus

Viral Exanthems
Measles (Rubeola)
Rubella
Human Parvovirus B19
Smallpox (Variola)

Mumps

Intestinal Virus Infections
Rotavirus Infection
Norwalk Virus and Other Viral Diarrheas

Viral Hemorrhagic Fevers
Yellow Fever
Ebola Hemorrhagic Fever
West Nile Virus

Herpesvirus
Varicella-Zoster Virus
Herpes Simplex Virus
Epstein-Barr Virus (EBV)
Cytomegalovirus

Human Papillomavirus

(continued)

FIGURE 9-1 *(see opposite page)*
Epidemiology of yellow fever. The usual reservoir for the yellow fever virus is the tree-dwelling monkey. The virus is passed from monkey to monkey in the forest canopy by mosquitoes of the genus *Aedes*. Felling a tree brings mosquitoes down with the tree, increasing the chance of being bitten and inoculated with the virus.

Bacterial Infections

Pyogenic Gram-Positive Cocci

Staphylococcus aureus

Coagulase-Negative Staphylococci

Streptococcus pyogenes

Streptococcus pneumoniae

Group B Streptococci

Bacterial Infections of Childhood

Diphtheria

Pertussis

Haemophilus influenzae

Neisseria meningitides

Sexually Transmitted Bacterial Diseases

Gonorrhea

Chancroid

Granuloma Inguinale

Enteropathogenic Bacterial Infections

Escherichia coli

Salmonella

Shigellosis

Cholera

Campylobacter jejuni

Yersinia

Pulmonary Infections with Gram-Negative Bacteria

Klebsiella and *Enterobacter*

Legionnaires Disease (Legionellosis)

Pseudomonas aeruginosa

Melioidosis

Clostridial Diseases

Clostridial Food Poisoning

Necrotizing Enteritis

Gas Gangrene

Tetanus

Botulism

Clostridium difficile

Bacteria with Animal Reservoirs or Insect Vectors

Brucellosis

Plague

Tularemia

Anthrax

Listeriosis

Cat-Scratch Disease

Glanders

Bartonellosis

Infections Caused by Branching Filamentous Organisms

Actinomycosis

Nocardiosis

Spirochetal Infections

Syphilis

Primary Syphilis

Secondary Syphilis

Tertiary Syphilis

Congenital Syphilis

Nonvenereal Treponematoses

Yaws

Bejel

Pinta

Lyme Disease

Leptospirosis

Relapsing Fever

Fusospirochetal Infections

Tropical Phagedenic Ulcer

Noma

Chlamydial Infections

Chlamydia trachomatis
Genital and Neonatal Infections
Lymphogranuloma Venereum
Trachoma

Psittacosis (Ornithosis)

Chlamydia pneumoniae

Rickettsial Infections

Rocky Mountain Spotted Fever

Epidemic (Louse-Borne) Typhus

Endemic (Murine) Typhus

Scrub Typhus

Q Fever

Mycoplasmal Infections

Mycoplasma pneumoniae

Mycobacteria

Tuberculosis
Primary Tuberculosis
Secondary (Cavitary) Tuberculosis

Leprosy
Tuberculoid Leprosy
Lepromatous Leprosy

***Mycobacterium avium-intracellulare* Complex**
Granulomatous Pulmonary Disease
Disseminated Infection in AIDS

Atypical Mycobacteria

Fungal Infections

Candida

Aspergillosis
Allergic Bronchopulmonary Aspergillosis
Aspergilloma
Invasive Aspergillosis

Mucormycosis (Zygomycosis)

Cryptococcosis

Histoplasmosis

Coccidioidomycosis

Blastomycosis

Paracoccidioidomycosis (South American Blastomycosis)

Sporotrichosis

Chromomycosis

Dermatophyte Infections

Mycetoma

Protozoa

Malaria

Babesiosis

Toxoplasmosis
Toxoplasma Lymphadenopathy Syndrome
Congenital *Toxoplasma* Infections
Toxoplasmosis in Immunocompromised Hosts

***Pneumocystis carinii* Pneumonia**

(continued)

Amebiasis

Intestinal Amebiasis

Amebic Liver Abscess

Cryptosporidiosis

Giardiasis

Leishmaniasis

Localized Cutaneous Leishmaniasis

Mucocutaneous Leishmaniasis

Visceral Leishmaniasis (Kala Azar)

Chagas Disease (American Trypanosomiasis)

Acute Chagas Disease

Chronic Chagas Disease

African Trypanosomiasis

Primary Amebic Meningoencephalitis

Helminthic Infection

Filarial Nematodes

Lymphatic Filariasis

Onchocerciasis

Loiasis

Intestinal Nematodes

Ascariasis

Trichuriasis

Hookworms

Strongyloidiasis

Pinworm Infection (Enterobiasis)

Tissue Nematodes

Trichinosis

Visceral Larva Migrans (Toxocariasis)

Cutaneous Larva Migrans

Dracunculiasis

Trematodes (Flukes)

Schistosomiasis

Clonorchiasis

Paragonimiasis

Fascioliasis

Fasciolopsiasis

Cestodes

Intestinal Tapeworms

Cysticercosis

Echinococcosis

Infectious diseases are the most frequent afflictions of mankind worldwide, the most common reasons that people seek medical care, and the leading causes of death from disease. Bacterial and viral diarrheas, bacterial pneumonias, tuberculosis, measles, malaria, hepatitis B, pertussis, and tetanus kill more people each year than all cancers and cardiovascular diseases (Table 9-1). The impact of infectious diseases is greatest in less-developed countries, where millions of people, mostly children younger than 5 years of age, die of treatable or preventable infectious diseases. Even in the developed countries of Europe and North America, the mortality, morbidity, and loss of economic productivity from infectious diseases is enormous. In the United States each year, infectious diseases cause over 200,000 deaths, more than 50 million days of hospitalization, and almost 2 billion days lost from work or school.

Infectious diseases are disorders in which tissue damage or dysfunction is produced by a microorganism. Many of these diseases, such as influenza, syphilis, and tuberculosis, are contagious, that is, transmissible from person to person. Yet many infectious diseases, such as legionellosis, histoplasmosis, and toxoplasmosis, are not contagious. Humans acquire infecting organisms not only from other humans but also from diverse sources, including animals, insects, soil, air, inanimate objects, and the endogenous microbial flora of the human body.

TABLE 9-1 Sources of Global Deaths

Illness	Annual Deaths
Cardiovascular disease	12×10^6
Diarrheal diseases (Rotavirus, Norwalk-like viruses, *Salmonella, Shigella,* diarrheogenic *E. coli*)	5×10^6
Cancer	4.8×10^6
Pneumonia	4.8×10^6
Tuberculosis	3×10^6
Chronic obstructive lung disease	2.7×10^6
Measles	1.5×10^6
Malaria	$1-2 \times 10^6$
Hepatitis B	$1-2 \times 10^6$
Tetanus (neonatal)	775×10^3
Pertussis (whooping cough)	500×10^3
Maternal mortality	500×10^3
AIDS	200×10^3
Schistosomiasis	200×10^3
Amebiasis	$40-110 \times 10^3$
Hookworm	$50-60 \times 10^3$
Rabies	35×10^3
Typhoid	25×10^3
Yellow fever	25×10^3
African trypanosomiasis (sleeping sickness)	20×10^3
Ascariasis	20×10^3

INFECTIVITY AND VIRULENCE

Virulence refers to the complex of properties that allows an organism to achieve infection and cause disease of different degrees of severity. The organism must (1) gain access to the body, (2) avoid multiple host defenses, (3) accommodate to growth in the human milieu, and (4) parasitize human resources.

HOST FACTORS IN INFECTIONS

The means by which the body prevents or contains infections are known as defense mechanisms (Table 9-2). There are major anatomical barriers to infection—the skin and the aerodynamic filtration system of the upper airway—that prevent most organisms from ever penetrating the body. The mucociliary blanket of the airways is also an essential defense, providing a means of expelling organisms that gain access to the respiratory system. The microbial flora normally resident in the gastrointestinal tract and in various body orifices compete with outside organisms, preventing them from gaining sufficient nutrients or binding sites in the host. The body's orifices are also protected by secretions that possess antimicrobial properties, both nonspecific (e.g., lysozyme and interferon) and specific (usually IgA immunoglobulins). In addition, gastric acid and bile chemically destroy many ingested organisms.

Heritable Differences

The first step in infection is often a highly specific interaction of a binding molecule on the infecting organism with a receptor molecule on the host. If the host lacks the appropriate receptor, then the organism cannot attach to the target. An example is *Plasmodium vivax,* one of the organisms that cause human malaria. It infects human erythrocytes by using the Duffy blood group determinants on the cell surface as receptors. Many persons, particularly blacks, lack these determinants and are not susceptible to infection with *P. vivax.* As a result, *P. vivax* malaria is absent from much of Africa. Similar racial or geographical differences in susceptibility are apparent for many infectious agents, including *Coccidioides immitis,* which is 14 times more common in blacks and 175 times more frequent in persons of Filipino ancestry than in whites.

Age

The effect of age on the outcome of exposure to many infectious agents is well illustrated by fetal infections. Some organisms produce more-severe disease in utero than in children or adults. Infections of the fetus with cytomegalovirus, rubellavirus, parvovirus B19, and *Toxoplasma gondii* interfere with fetal development. Depending on the organism and time of exposure, fetal infection can produce minimal damage, major congenital abnormalities, or death. By contrast, when these organisms infect children or adults, they usually produce asymptomatic or minimally symptomatic diseases.

Age also affects the course of common illnesses, such as the diverse viral and bacterial diarrheas. In older children and adults, these infections cause discomfort and inconvenience, but rarely severe disease. The outcome can be different in children younger than 3 years of age, who cannot compensate for the rapid volume loss resulting from profuse diarrhea.

Other examples include infection with *Mycobacterium tuberculosis,* which produces severe, disseminated tuberculosis in children younger than the age of 3 years, probably because of the immaturity of the cell-mediated immune system. By contrast, older persons fare much better. Maturity, however, is not always an advantage in infections. Epstein-Barr virus is more likely to cause symptomatic infections in adolescents and adults than in younger children. Varicella-zoster virus, the cause of chickenpox, produces more-severe disease in adults, who are more likely to develop viral pneumonia.

The elderly fare more poorly with almost all infections than younger persons. Common respiratory illnesses such as

TABLE 9-2 Host Defenses Against Infection

Skin
Tears
Normal bacterial flora
Gastric acid
Bile
Salivary and pancreatic secretions
Filtration system of nasopharynx
Mucociliary blanket
Bronchial, cervical, urethral, and prostatic secretions
Neutrophils
Monocytes
Complement
Stationary mononuclear phagocyte system
Immunoglobulins
Cell-mediated immunity

influenza and pneumococcal pneumonia are more often fatal in those older than 65 years of age.

Behavior

The link between behavior and infection is probably most obvious for the sexually transmitted diseases. Syphilis, gonorrhea, urogenital chlamydial infections, AIDS, and a number of other infectious diseases are transmitted primarily by sexual contact. The type and number of sexual encounters profoundly influence the risk of acquiring sexually transmitted diseases.

Other aspects of behavior also influence the risk of acquiring infections. Humans contract brucellosis and Q fever, which are primarily bacterial diseases of domesticated farm animals, by close contact with infected animals or their secretions. These infections occur in farmers, herders, meat processors, and, in the case of brucellosis, in persons who drink unpasteurized milk. The transmission of a number of parasitic diseases is strongly affected by behavior. Schistosomiasis, acquired when water-borne infective parasite larvae penetrate the skin of a susceptible host, is primarily a disease of farmers who work in fields irrigated by infected water. In addition, children who swim in lakes and ponds containing these organisms become infected. The larvae of hookworm and *Strongyloides stercoralis* live in humid soil and penetrate the skin of the lower extremities in people who walk barefoot. The introduction of shoes has probably been the single most important factor in reducing the prevalence of infection with soil-transmitted nematodes. Anisakiasis and diphyllobothriasis are helminthic diseases acquired by eating incompletely cooked fish. Toxoplasmosis is a protozoan infection transmitted from animals to humans by ingestion of incompletely cooked, infected meat or by exposure to infected cat feces. Botulism, a food poisoning caused by a bacterial toxin, is contracted by ingestion of improperly canned food.

As humans change their behavior, they open up new possibilities for infectious diseases. Although the agent of Legionnaires disease is common in the environment, aerosols generated by cooling plants, faucets, and humidifiers now have provided the means for causing human infections. Traditional behaviors are not necessarily health promoting. Hundreds of thousands of cases of neonatal tetanus in less-developed countries are linked to coating umbilical stumps with dirt, dung, or even home-made cheese to stop the bleeding. These materials stop the bleeding but often contain the spores of *Clostridium tetani*, which germinate and release the toxin that causes tetanus. In parts of Africa, numerous cases of cysticercosis are caused by the ingestion of locally prepared potions containing, among other ingredients, the stools of persons infected with *Taenia solium*.

Compromised Host Defenses

A disruption or absence of any of the complex host defenses results in increased numbers and severity of infections. Disruption of the skin surface by trauma or burns frequently leads to invasive bacterial or fungal infections. Injury to the mucociliary apparatus of the airways, as occurs in smoking or influenza, impairs the clearing of inhaled microorganisms and results in an increased incidence of bacterial pneumonias. Congenital absence of complement components C5, C6, C7, and C8 prevents formation of a fully functional membrane attack complex and permits disseminated *Neisseria* infections. Diseases and drugs that interfere with neutrophil production or function increase the likelihood of bacterial infection.

The technological capacity to prolong the lives of debilitated persons, the broad use of cytotoxic and immunosuppressive therapies, and the rapid expansion of the AIDS epidemic have led to an exponential increase in the number of patients with severe defects in host defenses. Burn and trauma units, transplantation centers, and medical and surgical intensive care facilities are filled with patients who lack the normal capacity to ward off infections. Many are immunocompromised, meaning that their defects affect their capacity to mount inflammatory or immunological responses. Not only do compromised hosts become infected more easily, but they are often attacked by organisms that are innocuous to normal persons. For example, patients deficient in neutrophils frequently develop life-threatening bloodstream infections with commensal microorganisms that normally populate the skin and gastrointestinal tract.

Organisms that cause disease predominantly in hosts with impaired immunity are known as *opportunistic pathogens*. This term implies that such organisms, many of which are part of the normal endogenous human or environmental microbial flora, take advantage of the host's inadequate defense mechanisms to stage a more violent attack.

Viral Infections

Viruses range in size from 20 to 300 nm and consist of RNA or DNA contained in a protein shell. Some viruses are enveloped in a lipid membrane. **Viruses are incapable of independent metabolism or reproduction and thus are obligate intracellular parasites, requiring living cells in which to replicate.** After invading cells, they divert the cellular biosynthetic and metabolic capacities to the synthesis of viral-encoded nucleic acids and proteins.

Viruses often cause disease by killing the infected cells, but many do not. For example, rotavirus, a common cause of diarrhea, interferes with the function of infected enterocytes without immediately killing them, It prevents enterocytes from synthesizing proteins that transport molecules from the intestinal lumen and thereby causes diarrhea.

Viruses may also promote the release of chemical mediators that elicit inflammatory or immunological responses. The symptoms of the common cold are due to the release of bradykinin from infected cells. Other viruses cause cells to proliferate and form tumors. Human papillomaviruses, for instance, cause squamous cell proliferative lesions, which include common warts and anogenital warts.

Some viruses infect and persist in cells without interfering with cellular functions, a process known as *latency*. Latent viruses can emerge to produce disease long after the primary infection. Opportunistic infections are frequently caused by viruses that have established latent infections. Cytomegalovirus and herpes simplex viruses are among the most frequent opportunistic pathogens because they are commonly present as latent agents and emerge in persons with impaired cell-mediated immunity.

RESPIRATORY VIRUSES

The Common Cold Is the Most Common Viral Disease

The common cold (coryza) is an acute, self-limited disorder of the upper respiratory tract caused by infection with a variety of RNA viruses, including over 100 distinct rhinoviruses and several coronaviruses. Colds are frequent and worldwide in distribution, spreading from person to person by contact with infected secretions. Infection is more likely during the winter months in temperate areas and during the rainy seasons in the tropics, when spread is facilitated by indoor crowding. In the United States, children usually suffer six to eight colds per year and adults two to three.

The viruses infect the nasal respiratory epithelial cells, causing increased mucus production and edema. Rhinoviruses and coronaviruses have a tropism for respiratory epithelium and optimally reproduce at temperatures well below 37°C. Thus, infection remains confined to the cooler passages of the upper airway. Infected cells release chemical mediators, such as bradykinin, which produce most of the symptoms associated with the common cold. Increased mucus production, together with nasal congestion and eustachian tube obstruction, predispose to secondary bacterial infections, resulting in bacterial sinusitis and otitis media. Rhinoviruses and coronaviruses do not destroy the respiratory epithelium and produce no visible alterations. Clinically, the common cold is characterized by rhinorrhea, pharyngitis, cough, and low-grade fever. Symptoms last about a week.

Influenza May Predispose to Bacterial Pneumonia

Influenza is an acute, self-limited, infection of the upper and lower airways, caused by strains of influenza virus. These viruses are enveloped and contain single-stranded RNA.

 Epidemiology: Although three distinct types of influenza virus—types A, B, and C—cause human disease, influenza A is by far the most common pathogen and causes the most-severe disease. Ten to 40 million cases of influenza occur annually in the United States. Influenza is highly contagious, and epidemics often spread around the world. The virus periodically alters its surface antigens, so that the host immunity that develops in one epidemic often does not protect against the next one.

 Pathogenesis: Influenza spreads from person to person by virus-containing respiratory droplets and secretions. Upon reaching the respiratory epithelial cell surface, the virus binds and enters the cell by fusion with the cell membrane, a process mediated by a viral glycoprotein (hemagglutinin) that binds to sialic acid residues on human respiratory epithelium. Once inside the cell, the virus directs it to produce progeny viruses and causes cell death. The infection usually involves both the upper and the lower airways. Destruction of the ciliated epithelium cripples the mucociliary blanket, predisposing to bacterial pneumonia.

 Pathology: In the airways, influenza virus causes necrosis and desquamation of the ciliated respiratory tract epithelium, associated with a predominantly lymphocytic inflammatory infiltrate. Extension of the infection to the lungs leads to necrosis and sloughing of alveolar lining cells and the histological appearance of viral pneumonitis.

 Clinical Features: Clinically, influenza manifests with a rapid onset of fever, chills, myalgia, headaches, weakness, and nonproductive cough. Symptoms may be primarily those of an upper respiratory infection or those of tracheitis, bronchitis, and pneumonia. Epidemics are accompanied by deaths from both the disease and its complications, particularly in the elderly and persons with underlying cardiopulmonary disease. Killed viral vaccines specific to epidemic strains are 75% effective in preventing influenza.

Parainfluenza Virus Is Associated with Croup

The parainfluenza viruses cause acute upper and lower respiratory tract infections, particularly in young children. These enveloped, single-stranded RNA viruses are the most common cause of croup (laryngotracheobronchitis).

 Epidemiology: This condition is common in children younger than the age of 3 years and is characterized by subglottic swelling, airway compression, and respiratory distress. There are four antigenically distinct parainfluenza viruses. These viruses spread from person to person through infectious respiratory aerosols and secretions. Infection is highly contagious, and disease is present worldwide. The parainfluenza viruses are isolated from 10% of young children with acute respiratory tract illnesses.

 Pathogenesis and Pathology: Parainfluenza viruses infect and kill ciliated respiratory epithelial cells and elicit an inflammatory response. In very young children, this process frequently extends into the lower respiratory tract, causing bronchiolitis and pneumonitis. In young children, the trachea is narrow, and the larynx is small. When laryngotracheitis occurs, the local edema compresses the upper airway enough to obstruct breathing and cause croup. Parainfluenza infection is associated with fever, hoarseness, and cough. Croup is evidenced by a characteristic barking cough and inspiratory stridor. In older children and adults symptoms are usually mild.

Respiratory Syncytial Virus Affects Infants

Respiratory syncytial virus (RSV) is an enveloped, single-stranded RNA virus and is the major cause of bronchiolitis and pneumonia in infants.

 Epidemiology: RSV spreads from child to child in respiratory aerosols and secretions. The virus, which is present worldwide, is highly contagious, and most children have been infected with RSV by school age. The spread of RSV is particularly rapid in confined susceptible populations, such as young children on a hospital ward.

  Pathogenesis and Pathology: Viral surface proteins interact with specific receptors on host respiratory epithelium to cause viral binding and fusion. RSV produces necrosis and sloughing of bronchial, bronchiolar, and alveolar epithelium, associated with a predominantly lymphocytic inflammatory infiltrate. Multinucleated syncytial cells are sometimes seen in infected tissues.

 Clinical Features: Infants and young children with RSV bronchiolitis or pneumonitis present with wheezing, cough, and respiratory distress, sometimes accompanied by fever. The illness is usually self-limited, resolving in 1 to 2 weeks. In older children and adults, RSV produces much milder disease. Among otherwise healthy young children, the mortality from RSV infection is very low, but it rises dramatically (to 20–40%) among hospitalized children with congenital heart disease or immunosuppression.

Adenovirus Causes Necrotizing Respiratory Lesions

Adenoviruses are nonenveloped DNA viruses that are isolated from the respiratory and intestinal tract of humans and animals. Certain serotypes are common causes of acute respiratory disease and adenovirus pneumonia in military recruits. Some adenoviruses are important causes of chronic pulmonary disease in infants and young children.

 Pathology: Pathological changes include necrotizing bronchitis and bronchiolitis, in which the sloughed epithelial cells and inflammatory infiltrate may fill the damaged bronchioles. Interstitial pneumonitis is characterized by areas of consolidation with extensive necrosis, hemorrhage, and a mononuclear inflammatory infiltrate. Two distinctive types of intranuclear inclusions—smudge cells and Cowdry type A inclusions—involve bronchiolar epithelial cells and alveolar lining cells.

Adenoviruses types 40 and 41 infect colonic and small intestinal epithelial cells and may cause diarrhea in both immunocompetent and immunocompromised hosts. AIDS patients are particularly susceptible to urinary tract infections caused by adenovirus type 35.

Severe Acute Respiratory Syndrome (SARS)-Associated Coronavirus

In early 1993 an epidemic of severe pneumonia was traced to Guangdong Province of China. The disease then spread by way of travelers to other Asian countries and the United States, Canada, and Europe. The causative agent was quickly identified as a novel coronavirus, which probably mutated from a nonhuman host.

 Pathology: At autopsy, the lungs of patients who died from SARS disclose diffuse alveolar damage. Multinucleated syncytial cells without viral inclusions have also been observed.

 Clinical Features: Clinically, SARS begins with fever and headache, followed shortly by cough and dyspnea. Lymphopenia is common, and the aminotransferase levels are modestly increased. Most patients recover, but the mortality rate is as high as 15% in the elderly and in patients who suffer from other respiratory disorders. No specific treatment is available.

VIRAL EXANTHEMS

Measles (Rubeola) Can Cause a Lethal Respiratory Infection

Measles virus is an enveloped, single-stranded RNA virus that causes an acute, highly contagious, self-limited illness, characterized by upper respiratory tract symptoms, fever, and a rash.

 Epidemiology: The measles virus is transmitted to humans in respiratory aerosols and secretions. In nonimmunized populations, measles is primarily a disease of children. Currently available live, attenuated vaccines are highly effective in preventing measles and in eliminating the spread of the virus. Recent efforts at nationwide immunization have made measles uncommon in the United States. Similar efforts are under way worldwide to immunize all children.

Measles is a particularly severe disease in the very young, the sick, or the malnourished. In impoverished countries, the disease has a high mortality rate (10–25%). In recent years, measles has been estimated to kill 1.5 million children each year and remains a major vaccine-preventable cause of death worldwide. When measles was first introduced to previously unexposed populations (e.g., Native Americans, Pacific Islanders), the resulting widespread infections had devastatingly high mortality rates.

Pathogenesis: The initial site of infection is the mucous membranes of the nasopharynx and bronchi. Two surface glycoproteins, designated the "H" and "F" proteins, mediate viral attachment and fusion with respiratory epithelium. From these cells, the virus extends to the regional lymph nodes and then to the bloodstream, leading to widespread dissemination with prominent involvement of the skin and lymphoid tissues. The rash results from the action of T lymphocytes on virally infected vascular endothelium.

Pathology: Measles virus produces necrosis of infected respiratory epithelium, associated with a predominantly lymphocytic inflammatory infiltrate. In the skin, the virus produces a vasculitis of small blood vessels. Lymphoid hyperplasia is often prominent in the cervical and mesenteric lymph nodes, spleen, and appendix. In lymphoid tissues, the virus sometimes causes fusion of infected cells, producing multinucleated giant cells containing up to 100 nuclei, with both intracytoplasmic and intranuclear inclusions. These cells, named **Warthin-Finkeldey giant cells** (Fig. 9-2), are pathognomonic for measles.

Clinical Features: Measles first manifests with fever, rhinorrhea, cough, and conjunctivitis and progresses to the characteristic mucosal and skin lesions. The mucosal lesions, known as *Koplik spots*, appear on the posterior buccal mucosa and consist of minute gray-white dots on a red base. The skin lesions begin on the face as an erythematous maculopapular rash, which usually spreads to involve the trunk and extremities. The rash fades in 3 to 5 days, and the symptoms gradually resolve. The clinical course of measles may be much more severe in very young children, malnourished persons, or immunocompromised patients. Measles often leads to secondary bacterial infections, especially otitis media and pneumonia.

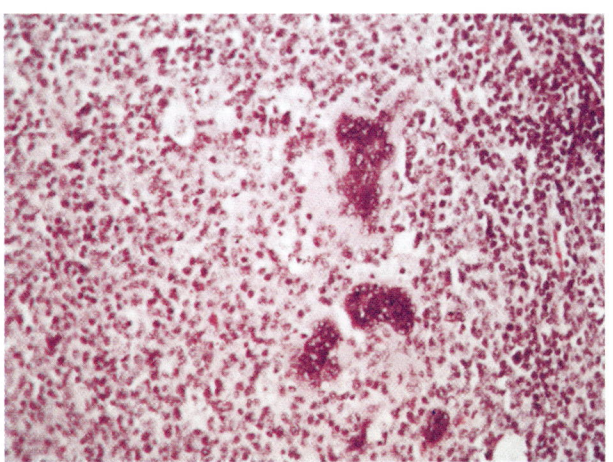

FIGURE 9-2
Warthin-Finkeldey giant cells in measles. A hyperplastic lymph node from a patient with measles shows several multinucleated giant cells.

Rubella Is Associated with Congenital Anomalies

Rubellavirus is an enveloped, single-stranded RNA virus that causes a mild, self-limited systemic disease, usually associated with a rash. Many infections are so mild that they go unnoticed. However, in pregnant women, rubella is a destructive fetal pathogen. Infection early in gestation can produce fetal death, premature delivery, and congenital anomalies, including deafness, cataracts, glaucoma, heart defects, and mental retardation.

Epidemiology: The agent spreads from person to person primarily by the respiratory route. Infection occurs worldwide. Rubella is not highly contagious, and in unvaccinated populations, 10 to 15% of young women remain susceptible to infection into their reproductive years. The live attenuated viral vaccine that is currently available prevents rubella and has largely eliminated the disease from developed countries. This disease is now uncommon in the United States.

Pathogenesis: Rubella infects the respiratory epithelium and then disseminates to various organs through the bloodstream and lymphatics. The rubella rash is believed to result from an immunological response to the disseminated virus. Fetal infection occurs through the placenta during the viremic phase of maternal illness. A congenitally infected fetus remains persistently infected and sheds large amounts of virus in body fluids, even after birth. Maternal infection after 20 weeks' gestation usually does not cause significant fetal disease.

Pathology: In most patients, rubella is a mild, acute febrile illness, with rhinorrhea, conjunctivitis, postauricular lymphadenopathy, and a rash that spreads from face to trunk and extremities. The rash resolves within 3 days, and complications are rare. As many as 30% of infections are completely asymptomatic.

In the fetus, the heart, eye, and brain are the organs most frequently affected. Cardiac lesions include pulmonary valvular stenosis, pulmonary artery hypoplasia, ventricular septal defects, and patent ductus arteriosus. Cataracts, glaucoma, and retinal defects may occur. Deafness is a common complication of fetal rubella. Severe brain involvement can produce microcephaly and mental retardation.

Human Parvovirus B19 Interferes with Erythropoiesis

Human parvovirus B19 is a single-stranded DNA virus that causes systemic infections characterized by rash, arthralgias, and transient interruption in erythrocyte production.

Pathogenesis: Human parvovirus B19 spreads from person to person by the respiratory route. Infection is common and occurs in outbreaks, mostly among children. It is not known which cells, other than erythroid precursors, support parvovirus B19 replication, but replication at some respiratory site prior to dissemination to erythropoietic cells seems likely.

Pathology: Human parvovirus B19 produces characteristic cytopathic effects in erythroid precursor cells. The nucleus of an affected cell is enlarged, and the chromatin is displaced peripherally by central glassy eosinophilic material.

Clinical Features: Most persons suffer a mild exanthematous illness, known as **erythema infectiosum** ("fifth disease"), accompanied by an asymptomatic interruption in erythropoiesis. In persons with chronic hemolytic anemias, however, the interruption in erythrocyte production causes profound, potentially fatal anemia, known as **transient aplastic crisis.** When the fetus is infected by human parvovirus B19, a transient cessation of erythropoiesis can lead to severe anemia, hydrops fetalis, and death in utero, an outcome that occurs in about 10% of maternal infections.

Smallpox (Variola) Is a Dangerous Exanthem That Has Been Eradicated

Smallpox is a highly contagious exanthematous viral infection produced by the variola virus, a member of the family Poxviridae. Related viruses include monkeypox and cowpox.

Epidemiology: Smallpox is evidently an ancient disease. A rash resembling smallpox was found in the mummified remains of the Egyptian pharaoh Ramses V, who died in 1160 BC. The infection was common in Europe and was brought to the New World with the arrival of the Spanish colonists in the 15th and 16th centuries. Jenner performed the first successful vaccination in 1796 when he used cowpox lymph taken from the hand of an infected milkmaid to inoculate a child. In 1967, the World Health Organization (WHO) began its uniquely successful campaign to eradicate smallpox. The last occurrence of endemic smallpox was in Somalia in 1977, and the last reported human cases were laboratory-acquired infections in 1978. On May 8, 1980, the WHO declared the global eradication of smallpox.

Pathogenesis and Pathology: Smallpox was transmitted between smallpox victims and susceptible persons via droplets or aerosol of infected saliva. Viral titers in the saliva were highest during the first week of infection. The virus is highly stable and retains its infectivity for long periods outside its human host. Two distinctive types of smallpox have been recognized. *Variola major* was prevalent in Asia and parts of Africa and represented the prototypical form of the infection. Variola minor (or alastrim) was found in Africa, South America, and Europe and was distinguished by its milder systemic toxicity and smaller pox lesions.

Microscopic features of the skin vesicle of variola show reticular degeneration and scarce areas of ballooning degeneration. The demonstration of eosinophilic, intracytoplasmic inclusion bodies (Guarnieri bodies) has great diagnostic value. Vesicles could also occur in the palate, pharynx, trachea, and esophagus. In severe cases of smallpox there were gastric and intestinal involvement, hepatitis, and interstitial nephritis.

Clinical Features: The incubation period of smallpox is approximately 12 days (range, 7–17 days) following exposure. On exposure to the aerosolized virus, variola travels from the upper and lower respiratory tract to regional lymph nodes, where replication occurs and results in viremia. Clinical manifestations begin abruptly with malaise, fever, vomiting, and headache. The characteristic rash, most prominent on the face but also involving the hands and forearms, follows in 2 to 3 days. Following subsequent eruptions on the lower extremities, the rash spreads centrally during the next week to the trunk. Lesions are more abundant in a centrifugal distribution, that is, on the face and extremities. Lesions progress quickly from macules to papules and then to pustular vesicles (Fig. 9-3). Smallpox lesions generally remain synchronous in their stage of development. In 8 to 14 days after onset, the pustules form scabs, which leave depressed scars on healing after 3 to 4 weeks. The case fatality rate is 30% in unvaccinated persons.

MUMPS

Mumps virus is an enveloped, single-stranded RNA virus that causes an acute, self-limited systemic illness, characterized by parotid gland swelling and meningoencephalitis.

Intestinal Virus Infections

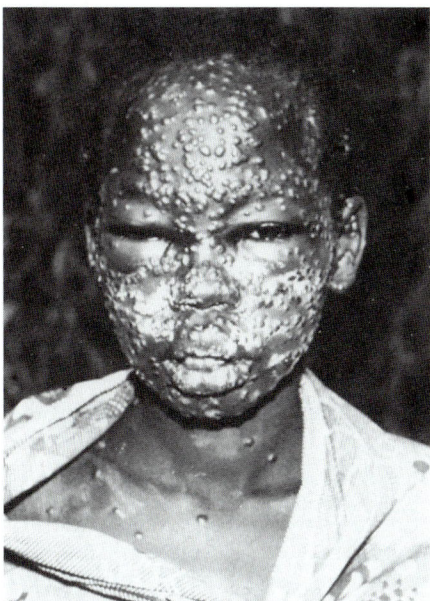

FIGURE 9-3
Smallpox, eastern Congo, 1968.

 Epidemiology: Mumps is present worldwide and is primarily a disease of childhood. The disease spreads from person to person through the respiratory route. Infection is highly contagious, and 90% of exposed, susceptible persons become infected, although only 60 to 70% develop symptoms. A live attenuated mumps vaccine prevents mumps, and the disease has been largely eliminated from most developed countries.

 Pathogenesis: Mumps begins with viral infection of respiratory tract epithelium. The virus then disseminates through the blood and lymphatic systems to infect other sites, most commonly the salivary glands (especially parotids), central nervous system, pancreas, and testes. The central nervous system is involved in more than half of cases, producing symptomatic disease in 10%. Epididymoorchitis occurs in 30% of males infected after puberty.

Pathology: Mumps virus causes necrosis of infected cells, which is associated with a predominantly lymphocytic inflammatory infiltrate. The affected salivary glands are swollen, the ducts lined by necrotic epithelium, and the interstitium infiltrated with lymphocytes. In mumps epididymoorchitis, the testis can be swollen to three times the normal size. The swelling of testicular parenchyma, confined within the tunica albuginea, produces focal infarctions. Mumps orchitis is usually unilateral and, thus, rarely causes sterility.

 Clinical Features: Mumps begins with fever and malaise, followed by painful swelling of the salivary glands, usually one or both parotids. Symptomatic meningeal involvement most often manifests as headache, stiff neck, and vomiting. Prior to widespread vaccination, mumps was a leading cause of viral meningitis and encephalitis in the United States. Although severe disease of the pancreas is rare in mumps, most patients exhibit elevated serum amylase activity.

INTESTINAL VIRUS INFECTIONS

Rotavirus Infection Is the Most Common Cause of Severe Diarrhea Worldwide

Rotavirus produces a profuse watery diarrhea that can lead to dehydration and death if untreated. This double-stranded RNA virus usually infects young children.

 Epidemiology: Rotavirus infection spreads from person to person by the oral–fecal route. Infection is most common among children, who shed huge amounts of virus in the stool. Siblings, playmates, parents, food, water, and environmental surfaces are readily contaminated with the virus. The peak age of infection is 6 months to 2 years, and virtually all children have been infected by the age of 4 years. In the United States, rotavirus causes about 100 deaths in young children and worldwide leads to over 1 million deaths.

 Pathogenesis: Rotavirus infects the enterocytes of the upper small intestine, disrupting the absorption of sugars, fats, and various ions. The resulting osmotic load causes a net loss of fluid into the bowel lumen, producing diarrhea and dehydration. Infected cells are shed from the intestinal villi, and the regenerating epithelium initially lacks full absorptive capabilities.

 Pathology: Pathological changes in rotavirus infection are largely confined to the duodenum and jejunum, where there is shortening of the intestinal villi associated with a mild infiltrate of neutrophils and lymphocytes.

 Clinical Features: Rotavirus infection manifests as vomiting, fever, abdominal pain, and profuse, watery diarrhea. The vomiting usually persists for 2 to 3 days, whereas diarrhea continues for 5 to 8 days. Without adequate fluid replacement, diarrhea can produce fatal dehydration in young children.

Norwalk Virus and Other Viral Diarrheas

In addition to rotavirus, there are numerous other viral causes of diarrhea, including adenoviruses, caliciviruses, and astroviruses. The best understood are the Norwalk family of nonenveloped RNA viruses, a group of caliciviruses that carry a host of individual names (e.g., Norwalk virus, Snow Mountain virus, Sapporo virus) associated with the locations of particular outbreaks. Norwalk viruses are responsible for one third of all outbreaks of diarrheal disease. They produce gastroenteritis in children and adults, with self-limited vomiting and diarrhea, similar to that caused by rotavirus. The Norwalk viruses infect cells of the upper small bowel and produce changes similar to those that occur with rotavirus.

VIRAL HEMORRHAGIC FEVERS

Viral hemorrhagic fevers are a group of at least 20 distinct viral infections that cause varying degrees of hemorrhage and shock and sometimes death. There are many similar viral hemorrhagic fevers in different parts of the world, for the most part named for the area where they were first described. The viral hemorrhagic fevers encompass members of four virus families—the Bunyaviridae, Flaviviridae, Arenaviridae, and Filoviridae. On the basis of differences in routes of transmission, vectors, and other epidemiological characteristics, the viral hemorrhagic fevers have been divided into four groups (Table 9-3): mosquito-borne, tick-borne, zoonotic, and the filoviruses, Marburg and Ebola virus, in which the route of transmission is unknown.

Yellow Fever May Lead to Fulminant Hepatic Failure

Yellow fever is an acute hemorrhagic fever, sometimes associated with extensive hepatic necrosis and jaundice. The illness is caused by an insect-borne flavivirus, an enveloped, single-stranded RNA virus. Other pathogenic flaviviruses cause Omsk hemorrhagic fever and Kyasanur Forest disease.

Epidemiology: Yellow fever was first recognized as a nosological entity in the New World in the 17th century, but its origins probably were in Africa. Today, the virus is restricted to certain regions of Africa and South America, including both jungle and urban settings. The usual reservoir for the virus is tree-dwelling monkeys, the agent being passed among them in the forest canopy by mosquitoes. These monkeys serve as a reservoir because the virus neither kills them nor makes them ill. Humans acquire jungle yellow fever by entering the forest and being bitten by infected *Aedes* mosquitoes (see Fig. 9-1). Felling trees increases the risk of infection, because mosquitoes are brought down with the tree. On returning to the village or city, the human victim becomes the reservoir for epidemic yellow fever in the urban setting, where *Aedes aegyptii* is the vector.

Pathogenesis: On inoculation by the mosquito, the virus multiplies within tissue and vascular endothelium and then disseminates through the bloodstream. The virus has a tropism for liver cells, where it sometimes produces extensive acute hepatocellular destruction. Extensive damage to the endothelium of small blood vessels may lead to the loss of vascular integrity, hemorrhages, and shock.

Pathology: Yellow fever virus causes coagulative necrosis of hepatocytes, which begins among cells in the middle of hepatic lobules and spreads toward the central veins and portal tracts. The infection sometimes produces confluent areas of necrosis in the middle of the hepatic lobules (i.e., midzonal necrosis). In the most severe cases, the entire lobule may be necrotic. Some necrotic hepatocytes lose their nuclei and become intensely eosinophilic. They often dislodge from adjacent hepatocytes, in which case they are known as Councilman bodies (recognized today as apoptotic bodies). Hepatocytes also show microvesicular fatty change.

Clinical Features: Yellow fever is characterized by the abrupt onset of fever, chills, headache, myalgias, nausea, and vomiting. After 3 to 5 days, some patients develop manifestations of hepatic failure, with jaundice (hence the term *yellow fever*), deficiencies of clotting factors, and diffuse hemorrhages. Vomiting of clotted blood ("black vomit") is a classic feature of severe cases of yellow fever. Patients with massive hepatic failure lapse into coma and die, usually within 10 days of onset of illness. The overall mortality of yellow fever is 5%, but among those with jaundice, it rises to 30%.

TABLE 9-3 Viral Hemorrhagic Fevers

Vector	Viral Fever
Mosquitoes	Yellow fever
	Rift valley fever
	Dengue hemorrhagic fever
	Chikungunya hemorrhagic fever
Ticks	Omsk hemorrhagic fever
	Crimean hemorrhagic fever
	Kyasanur forest disease
Rodents	Lassa fever
	Bolivian hemorrhagic fever
	Argentine hemorrhagic fever
	Korean hemorrhagic fever
Undefined	Ebola virus disease
	Marburg virus disease

Ebola Hemorrhagic Fever Is a Fatal African Disease

Ebola hemorrhagic fever is a severe viral disease caused by the Ebola virus, an RNA virus belonging to the Filoviridae. It causes a hemorrhagic disease with a high mortality rate in humans in several regions of Africa. The only other filovirus pathogenic to humans is the Marburg virus, which produces Marburg hemorrhagic fever.

Epidemiology: Ebola virus first emerged in Africa with two major disease outbreaks that occurred almost simultaneously in Zaire and Sudan in 1976. The most recent outbreaks of Ebola hemorrhagic fever occurred in Africa during 2000 to 2001. In Uganda, the virus infected 425 persons with a 53% mortality rate, and in the border area of the Republic of the Congo and Gabon, there were 122 persons infected, with an 80% fatality rate. In the wild, the virus infects humans, gorillas, chimpanzees, and monkeys. The natural reservoir of Ebola virus remains unknown, although it is presumed to have an animal reservoir. Healthcare workers and family members have become infected as a result of viral exposure while treating patients with Ebola hemorrhagic fever or during funerary preparation of the bodies of deceased victims (termed *amplification*). The virus can be transmitted via bodily secretions, blood, and used needles.

 Pathogenesis and Pathology: **Ebola virus results in the most widespread destructive tissue lesions of all viral hemorrhagic fever agents.** The virus undergoes massive replication in endothelial cells, mononuclear phagocytes, and hepatocytes. Necrosis is most severe in the liver, kidneys, gonads, spleen, and lymph nodes. Characteristic findings in the liver include hepatocellular necrosis, Kupffer cell hyperplasia, Councilman bodies, and microsteatosis. The lungs are usually hemorrhagic, and petechial hemorrhages are present in the skin, mucous membranes, and internal organs. Injury to the microvasculature and increased endothelial permeability are important causes of shock.

 Clinical Features: The incubation period varies from 2 to 21 days. The initial symptoms include headache, weakness, and fever followed by diarrhea, nausea, and vomiting. Some patients develop overt hemorrhage including bleeding from injection sites, petechia, gastrointestinal bleeding, and gingival hemorrhage. Pregnant women frequently have spontaneous abortions, and mortality is high among infants born to mothers dying from Ebola hemorrhagic fever.

West Nile Virus

 Epidemiology: The virus is spread between various mosquito vectors and birds, and its increasing geographical distribution is the result of spread by infected migratory birds. West Nile virus (WNV) was isolated in 1937 from the blood of a febrile woman in the West Nile region of Uganda. Since then it has spread rapidly through the Mediterranean and temperate parts of Europe. In 1999, WNV was identified in the Western Hemisphere for the first time when it caused an outbreak of meningoencephalitis in New York City and the surrounding metropolitan area. This outbreak resulted in hospitalization of 59 patients, and caused 7 deaths. By 2003, the infection had been identified in 4000 persons from 40 states and resulted in 263 fatalities.

 Pathogenesis and Pathology: Laboratory findings involve a slightly increased sedimentation rate and a mild leukocytosis; cerebrospinal fluid in patients with central nervous system involvement is clear, with moderate pleiocytosis and elevated protein. The virus can be recovered from blood for up to 10 days in immunocompetent febrile patients, as late as 22 to 28 days after infection in immunocompromised patients; peak viremia occurs 4 to 8 days postinfection. Autopsies of fatal cases from the New York City outbreak revealed mononuclear meningoencephalitis or encephalitis. The inflammation formed microglial nodules and perivascular clusters in the white and gray matter. The brainstem, particularly the medulla, was involved most extensively, and in some cases the cranial nerve roots had endoneural mononuclear inflammation. There were varying degrees of neuronal necrosis in the gray matter, neuronal degeneration, and neuronophagia.

 Clinical Features: Most WNV infections among humans are subclinical, with overt disease occurring in only 1 of 100 infections. The incubation period ranges from 3 to 15 days. When symptoms occur, they usually consist of fever, often accompanied by rash, lymphadenopathy, and polyarthropathy. Patients with severe illness can develop acute aseptic meningitis or encephalitis (associated with neck stiffness, vomiting, confusion, disturbed consciousness, somnolence, tremor of extremities, abnormal reflexes, convulsions, pareses, and coma). Anterior myelitis, hepatosplenomegaly, hepatitis, pancreatitis, and myocarditis occur. The probability of developing severe illness increases with increasing age. Central nervous system infection is associated with a 4 to 13% mortality rate and is highest among elderly persons.

HERPESVIRUS

The virus family Herpesviridae includes a large number of enveloped, DNA viruses, many of which infect humans. Almost all herpesviruses express some common antigenic determinants, and many produce type A nuclear inclusions (acidophilic bodies surrounded by a halo). The most important human pathogens among the herpesviruses are varicella-zoster, herpes simplex, Epstein-Barr virus, human herpesvirus 6 (HHV6, the cause of roseola), and cytomegalovirus. Recently, human herpesvirus 8 (HHV8) was implicated in the pathogenesis of Kaposi sarcoma in HIV-infected patients. Herpesviruses are also distinguished by their capacity to remain latent for long periods of time.

Varicella-Zoster Infection Causes Chickenpox and Herpes Zoster

The first exposure to varicella-zoster virus produces chickenpox, an acute systemic illness whose dominant feature is a generalized vesicular skin eruption (Fig. 9-4). The virus then becomes latent, and its reactivation causes herpes zoster ("shingles"), a localized vesicular skin eruption.

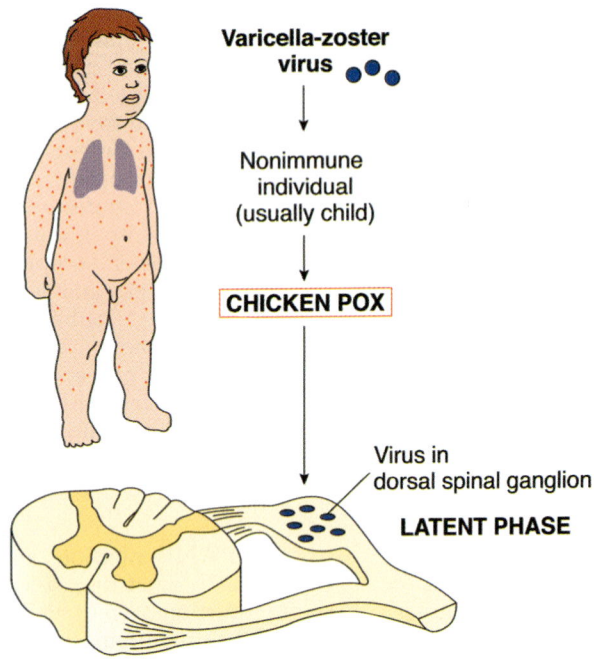

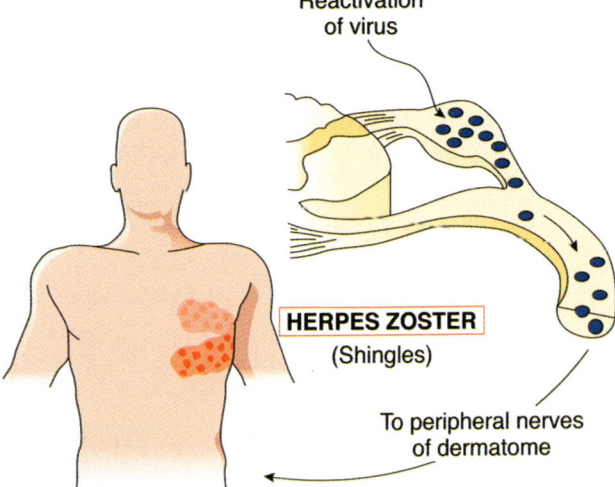

FIGURE 9-4
Varicella (chickenpox) and herpes zoster (shingles). Varicella-zoster virus (VZV) in droplets is inhaled by a nonimmune person (usually a child) and initially causes a "silent" infection of the nasopharynx. This progresses to viremia, seeding of fixed macrophages, and dissemination of VZV to skin (chickenpox) and viscera. VZV resides in a dorsal spinal ganglion, where it remains dormant for many years. Latent VZV is reactivated and spreads from ganglia along the sensory nerves to the peripheral nerves of sensory dermatomes, causing shingles.

 Epidemiology: Varicella-zoster virus is restricted to human hosts and spreads from person to person primarily by the respiratory route. It can also be spread by contact with secretions from the skin lesions. The virus is present worldwide and is highly contagious. Most children in the United States are infected by early school age, but an effective vaccine has reduced this incidence.

 Pathogenesis: Varicella-zoster virus initially infects cells of the respiratory tract or the conjunctival epithelium. There it reproduces and spreads through the bloodstream and lymphatic systems. Many organs are infected during this viremic stage, but skin involvement usually dominates the clinical picture. The virus spreads from the capillary endothelium to the epidermis, where viral replication destroys the basal cells. As a result, the upper layers of the epidermis separate from the basal layer to form vesicles.

During primary infection with varicella-zoster virus, the agent establishes latent infection in perineuronal satellite cells of the dorsal nerve root ganglia. Transcription of viral genes continues during latency, and viral DNA can be demonstrated years after the initial infection.

Shingles occurs when full replication of the virus occurs in ganglion cells, and the agent travels down the sensory nerve serving a single dermatome, where it infects the corresponding epidermis, producing a localized, painful vesicular eruption. The risk of shingles in an infected person increases with age, and most cases occur among the elderly. Impaired cell-mediated immunity also increases the risk of herpes zoster reactivation.

 Pathology: The skin lesions of chickenpox and shingles are indistinguishable from each other and also from the lesions produced by herpes simplex virus (HSV). The vesicle fills with neutrophils and soon erodes to become a shallow ulcer. In infected cells, varicella-zoster virus produces a characteristic cytopathic effect, consisting of nuclear homogenization, intranuclear inclusions (Cowdry type A), and formation of multinucleated cells (Fig. 9-5). The inclusion is large and eosinophilic and is separated from the nuclear membrane by a clear zone (halo). Over several days, the vesicles become pustules, after which they rupture and heal.

 Clinical Features: Chickenpox manifests as fever, malaise, and a distinctive pruritic rash, beginning on the head and spreading to the trunk and extremities. The skin lesions begin as maculopapules that rapidly evolve into vesicles, then pustules that soon ulcerate and crust. Vesicles may also appear on the mucous membranes, especially the mouth. The fever and systemic symptoms resolve in 3 to 5 days; the skin lesions heal in several weeks.

Shingles presents with a unilateral, painful, vesicular eruption, similar in appearance to chickenpox, but in a dermatomal pattern, usually localized to a single dermatome. Pain can persist for months after resolution of the skin lesions.

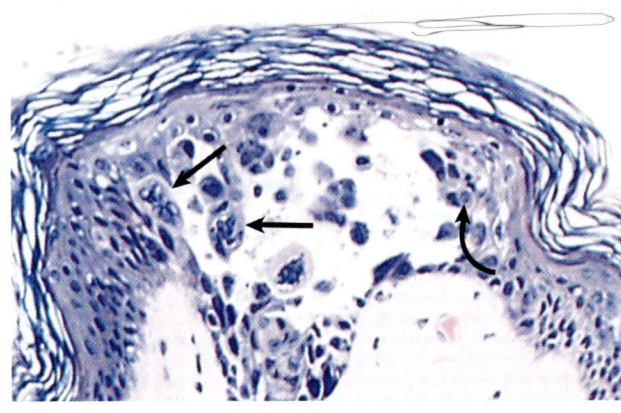

FIGURE 9-5
Varicella. Photomicrograph of the skin from a patient with chickenpox shows an intraepidermal vesicle. Multinucleated giant cells *(straight arrows)* and nuclear inclusions *(curved arrow)* are present.

Herpes Simplex Virus Produces Necrotizing Infections at Diverse Body Sites

Herpes simplex viruses (HSVs) are common human viral pathogens, which most frequently produce recurrent painful vesicular eruptions of the skin and mucous membranes (Table 9-4). Two antigenically and epidemiologically distinct HSVs cause human disease (Fig. 9-6):

- **HSV-1** is transmitted in oral secretions and typically causes disease "above the waist," including oral, facial, and ocular lesions.
- **HSV-2** is transmitted in genital secretions and typically produces disease "below the waist," including genital ulcers and neonatal herpes infection.

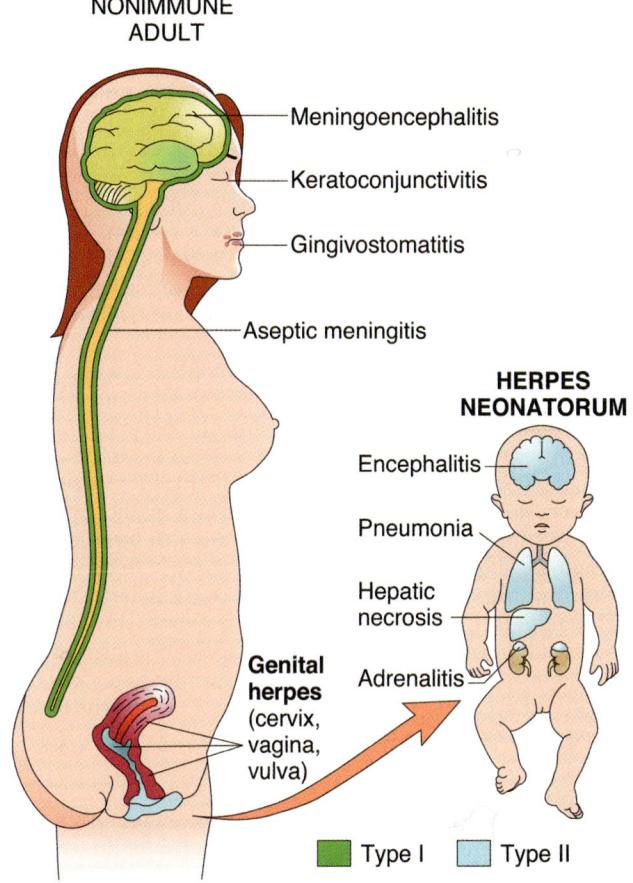

FIGURE 9-6
Herpesvirus infections. HSV-1 infects a nonimmune adult, causing gingivostomatitis ("fever blister" or "cold sore"), keratoconjunctivitis, meningoencephalitis, and aseptic spinal meningitis. HSV-2 infects the genitalia of a nonimmune adult, involving the cervix, vagina, and vulva. HSV-2 infects the fetus as it passes through the birth canal of an infected mother. The infant's lack of a mature immune system results in disseminated infection with HSV-1. The infection is often fatal, involving lung, liver, adrenal glands, and central nervous system.

 Epidemiology: HSV spreads from person to person, primarily through direct contact with infected secretions or open lesions. HSV-1 spreads in oral secretions, and infection frequently occurs in childhood, most persons (50–90%) being infected by adulthood. HSV-2 spreads by contact with genital lesions and is primarily a venereally transmitted pathogen. Neonatal herpes is acquired during passage of the newborn through an infected birth canal.

TABLE 9-4 Herpes Simplex Viral Diseases

Viral Type	Common Presentations	Infrequent Presentations
HSV-1	Oral-labial herpes	Conjunctivitis, keratitis Encephalitis Herpetic whitlow Esophagitis[a] Pneumonia[a] Disseminated infection[a]
HSV-2	Genital herpes	Perinatal infection Disseminated infection[a]

[a] These conditions usually occur in immunocompromised hosts.

 Pathogenesis: Primary HSV disease occurs at a site of initial viral inoculation, such as the oropharynx, genital mucosa, or skin. The virus infects epithelial cells, producing progeny viruses and destroying the basal cells in the squamous epithelium, with resulting formation of vesicles. Cell necrosis also elicits an inflammatory response, initially dominated by neutrophils and then followed by lymphocytes. Primary infection resolves with the development of humoral and cell-mediated immunity to the virus.

Latent infection is established in a manner analogous to that of varicella-zoster virus. The virus invades sensory nerve endings in the oral or genital mucosa, ascends within axons, and establishes a latent infection in sensory neurons within the corresponding ganglia. From time to time, the latent infection is reactivated, and HSV travels back down the nerve to the epithelial site served by the ganglion, where it again infects epithelial cells. Sometimes this secondary infection produces ulcerating vesicular lesions. At other times, the secondary infection does not cause visible tissue destruction, but contagious progeny viruses are shed from the site of infection. Various factors, usually typical for a given person, can induce the reactivation of latent HSV infection. These include intense sunlight, emotional stress, febrile illness, and menstruation. Both HSV-1 and HSV-2 can cause severe protracted and disseminated disease in immunocompromised persons.

Herpes encephalitis is a rare (1 in 100,000 HSV infections), but devastating, manifestation of HSV-1 infection. In some instances, it occurs when the virus, latent in the trigeminal ganglion, is reactivated and travels retrograde to the brain. However, herpes encephalitis also occurs in persons who have no history of "cold sores," and the pathogenesis of the encephalitis in these cases is poorly understood (see Chapter 28). Equally rare is **herpes hepatitis,** which may occur in immunocompromised patients but has been also reported in young, previously healthy pregnant women.

Neonatal herpes is a serious complication of maternal genital herpes. The virus is transmitted to the fetus from the infected birth canal, often the uterine cervix, and readily disseminates in the unprotected newborn child.

Pathology: The skin and mucous membranes are the usual sites of HSV infection, but the disease sometimes involves the brain, eye, liver, lungs, and other organs. In any location, both HSV-1 and HSV-2 cause necrosis of infected cells, which is accompanied by a vigorous inflammatory response. Clusters of painful ulcerating vesicular lesions on the skin or mucous membranes are the most frequent manifestation of HSV infection (Fig. 9-7A). These lesions persist for 1 to 2 weeks and then resolve. The cellular alterations include (1) nuclear homogenization, (2) Cowdry type A intranuclear inclusions, and (3) the formation of multinucleated giant cells (see Fig. 9-7B).

Clinical Features: The clinical features of HSV infections vary according to host susceptibility (e.g., neonate, normal host, compromised host), viral type, and site of infection. A prodromal "tingling" sensation at the site often precedes the appearance of skin lesions. Recurrent lesions appear weeks, months, or years later, at the initial site or at a site subserved by the same nerve ganglion. Recurrent herpetic lesions in the mouth or on the lip are commonly called "cold sores" or "fever blisters" and frequently appear following sun exposure, trauma, or a febrile illness.

Patients with AIDS and other immunocompromised persons are prone to develop herpes esophagitis. Early lesions consist of rounded 1- to 3-mm vesicles located predominantly in the mid to distal esophagus. As the HSV-infected squamous cells slough from the lesions, sharply demarcated ulcers with elevated margins form and coalesce. This process may result in denudation of the esophageal mucosa. Superimposed *Candida* infection is common at this stage. In immunocompromised patients, HSV may also infect the anal mucosa, where it causes painful blisters and ulcers.

Neonatal herpes begins 5 to 7 days after delivery, with irritability, lethargy, and a mucocutaneous vesicular eruption. The infection rapidly spreads to involve multiple organs, including the brain. The infected newborn develops jaundice, bleeding problems, respiratory distress, seizures, and coma. Treatment of severe HSV infections with acyclovir is often effective, but neonatal herpes still carries a high mortality.

Epstein-Barr Virus (EBV) Is the Cause of Infectious Mononucleosis

Infectious mononucleosis is a viral disease characterized by fever, pharyngitis, lymphadenopathy, and increased circulating lymphocytes. By adulthood, most persons have been infected with

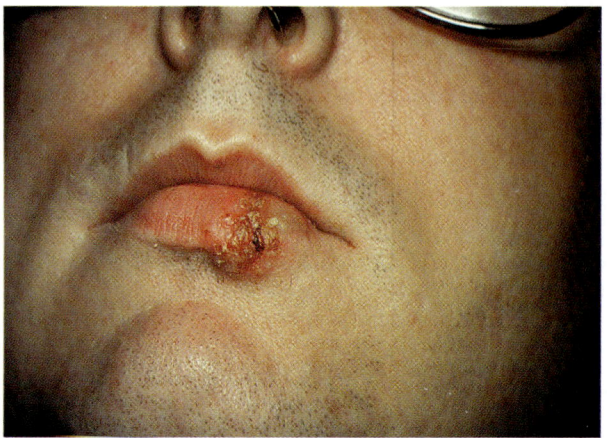
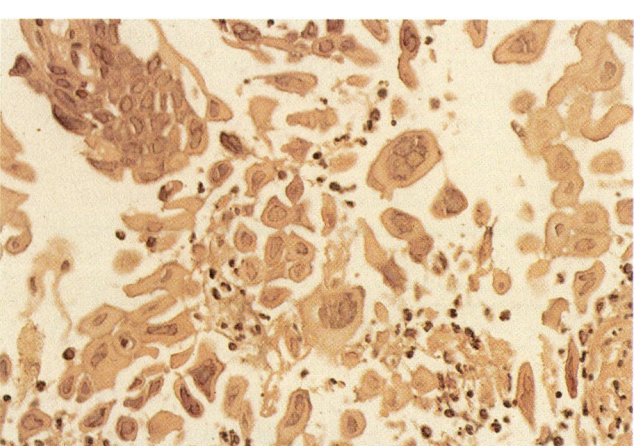

FIGURE 9-7
Herpes simplex, type 1. **A.** Herpetic vesicles are seen on the surface of the lower lip. **B.** Epithelial cells infected with HSV-1 demonstrate Cowdry type A intranuclear inclusions and multinucleated giant cells.

EBV. In most instances, the infection is asymptomatic, but in some persons, EBV causes infectious mononucleosis. EBV infection also has been associated with several cancers, including African Burkitt lymphoma, B-cell lymphoma in immunosuppressed persons, and nasopharyngeal carcinoma. These neoplastic complications are discussed in Chapters 20 and 25.

Epidemiology: In impoverished areas of the world, where children often live in crowded conditions, infection with EBV usually occurs before the age of 3 years, and infectious mononucleosis is not encountered. In developed countries, many persons remain uninfected into adolescence or early adulthood. Two thirds of those newly infected after childhood develop clinically evident infectious mononucleosis.

EBV spreads from person to person primarily through contact with infected oral secretions (Fig. 9-8). Once infected with the virus, persons remain asymptomatically infected for life and a few (10–20%) intermittently shed EBV. This lifelong latent infection with EBV is analogous to latent infections characteristic of the other herpesviruses. Transmission of the virus requires close contact with infected persons. Thus, EBV spreads readily among young children in crowded conditions, where there is considerable "sharing" of oral secretions. Kissing is also an effective mode of transmission.

Pathogenesis: The virus first binds to and infects nasopharyngeal cells and then B lymphocytes, which carry the virus throughout the body, producing a generalized infection of lymphoid tissues.

EBV induces a polyclonal activation of B cells. In turn, the activated B cells stimulate the proliferation of specific killer T lymphocytes and suppressor T cells. The former destroy virally infected B cells, whereas the suppressor cells inhibit the production of immunoglobulins by the B cells. The virus is also implicated in the pathogenesis of Burkitt lymphoma (Fig. 9-9) (see Chapters 5 and 20).

Pathology: The pathological changes of infectious mononucleosis are prominent in the lymph nodes and spleen. In most patients, the lymphadenopathy is symmetric and most striking in the neck. The nodes are movable, discrete, and tender. Microscopically, the general architecture is preserved. The germinal centers are enlarged and have indistinct margins, because of a proliferation of immunoblasts. They contain frequent mitoses and scattered nuclear debris, presumably from degenerated B cells. The nodes contain occasional large hyperchromatic cells with polylobular nuclei that resemble Reed-Sternberg cells. The appearance of the nodes may present diagnostic problems because of the morphological similarity to Hodgkin disease or other lymphomas.

The spleen is large and soft, owing to hyperplasia of the red pulp, and is susceptible to rupture. Many immunoblasts are present throughout the pulp and infiltrate the walls of vessels, the trabeculae, and the capsule. The liver is almost always involved, and the sinusoids and portal tracts contain atypical lymphocytes. One of the features of infectious mononucleosis is a lymphocytosis with atypical lymphocytes, which are activated T lymphocytes with lobulated, eccentric nuclei and vacuolated cytoplasm. They are involved in the suppression and killing of EBV-infected B lymphocytes.

Another distinguishing feature of infectious mononucleosis is the development of a specific heterophile antibody, known as the Paul Bunnell antibody. A heterophile antibody is an immunoglobulin produced in one species that reacts with antigens of another species. Paul Bunnell antibodies are raised in persons with infectious mononucleosis and are recognized by their affinity for sheep erythrocytes. This heterophile reaction is a standard diagnostic test for infectious mononucleosis. Specific serological tests for the presence of antibodies against EBV and for the presence of EBV antigens are also available.

Clinical Features: Infectious mononucleosis manifests as fever, malaise, lymphadenopathy, pharyngitis, and splenomegaly. Patients usually have an elevated leukocyte count, with a predominance of lymphocytes and monocytes. Treatment is supportive, and symptoms usually resolve in 3 to 4 weeks.

Cytomegalovirus Infects Many Persons but Rarely Produces Disease

Cytomegalovirus (CMV) is a congenital and opportunistic pathogen that usually produces an asymptomatic infection. However, the fetus and immunocompromised persons are particularly vulnerable to the destructive effects of the virus. CMV infects 0.5 to 2.0% of all fetuses and injures 10 to 20% of those infected, making it the most common congenital pathogen.

Epidemiology: CMV spreads from person to person by contact with infected secretions and bodily fluids and is transmitted to the fetus across the placenta. Children spread the virus in saliva or urine, whereas among adolescents and adults, transmission occurs primarily through sexual contact.

Pathogenesis: CMV infects various human cells, including epithelial cells, lymphocytes, and monocytes, and establishes latency in white blood cells. The normal immune response rapidly controls CMV infection, and infected persons usually show no ill effects, although they shed virus periodically in body secretions. Like other herpesviruses, CMV can remain latent for life.

When an infected pregnant woman passes the virus to her fetus, the latter is not protected by maternally derived antibodies, and the virus invades fetal cells with little initial immunological response, producing widespread necrosis and inflammation. The virus causes similar lesions in persons with profound suppression of cell-mediated immunity.

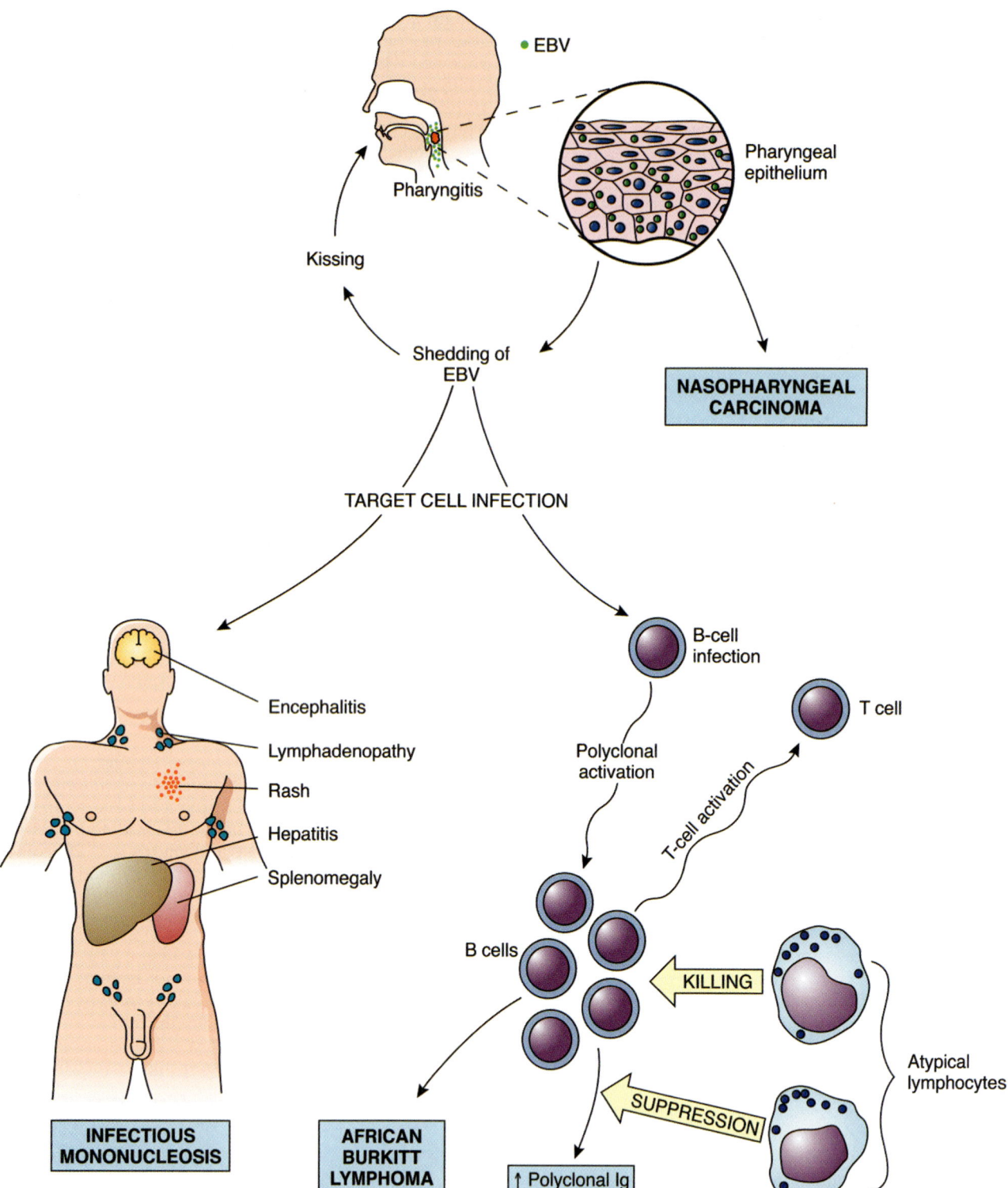

FIGURE 9-8
Role of Epstein-Barr virus (EBV) in infectious mononucleosis, nasopharyngeal carcinoma, and Burkitt lymphoma. EBV invades and replicates within the salivary glands or pharyngeal epithelium and is shed into the saliva and respiratory secretions. In some persons, the virus transforms pharyngeal epithelial cells, leading to nasopharyngeal carcinoma. In persons who are not immune from childhood exposure, EBV causes infectious mononucleosis. EBV infects B lymphocytes, which undergo polyclonal activation. These B cells stimulate the production of atypical lymphocytes, which kill virally infected B cells and suppress the production of immunoglobulins. Some infected B cells are transformed into immature malignant lymphocytes of Burkitt lymphoma.

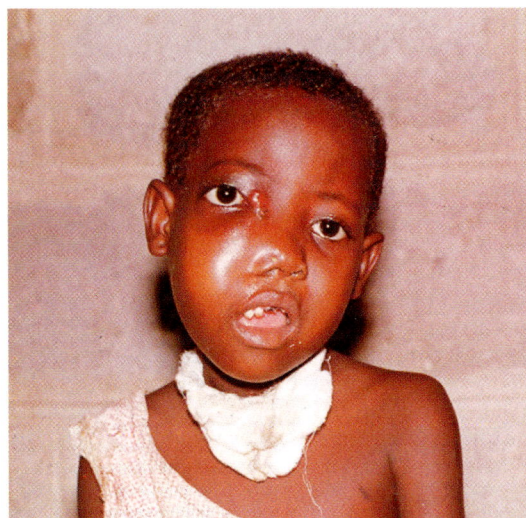

FIGURE 9-9
African Burkitt lymphoma. A tumor of the jaw distorts the child's face.

HUMAN PAPILLOMAVIRUS

Human papillomaviruses (HPVs) cause proliferative lesions of squamous epithelium, including common warts, flat warts, plantar warts, anogenital warts (condyloma acuminatum), and laryngeal papillomatosis. HPV infection also contributes to the development of squamous cell dysplasias and squamous cell carcinomas of the genital tract.

The agents are nonenveloped, double-stranded DNA viruses, which are members of the papovavirus group. Over 60 distinct types of HPV are identified, and different viral types are associated with different lesions. For instance, HPV types 1, 2, and 4 produce common warts and plantar warts. Types 6, 10, 11, and 40 through 45 cause anogenital warts. Types 16, 18, and 31 are associated with squamous cell carcinoma of the female genital tract.

Human papillomavirus infection is widespread and is transmitted from person to person by direct contact. Most children develop common warts. The viruses that cause genital lesions are transmitted sexually.

In most immunosuppressed persons, disseminated CMV infection derives from reactivation of endogenous latent infection, although the virus can also come from exogenous sources.

 Pathology: In the fetus with CMV disease, the most common sites of involvement are the brain, inner ears, eyes, liver, and bone marrow. The most severely affected fetuses may have microcephaly, hydrocephalus, cerebral calcifications, hepatosplenomegaly, and jaundice. Microscopically, the lesions of fetal CMV disease show cellular necrosis and a characteristic cytopathic effect, consisting of marked cellular and nuclear enlargement, with nuclear and cytoplasmic inclusions. The giant nucleus, which is usually solitary, contains a large central inclusion surrounded by a clear zone (Fig. 9-10). The cytoplasmic inclusions are less prominent.

 Clinical Features: Congenitally acquired CMV has a wide range of clinical presentations. Severe disease causes fetal death in utero, conspicuous lesions of the central nervous system, liver disease, and bleeding problems. However, most congenital CMV infections do not produce gross abnormalities, but manifest as subtle neurological or hearing defects, which may not be detected until later in life.

CMV disease in immunosuppressed patients has diverse clinical manifestations. It can manifest as decreased visual acuity (chorioretinitis), diarrhea or gastrointestinal hemorrhage (colonic ulcerations), change in mental status (encephalitis), shortness of breath (pneumonitis), or a wide range of other symptoms. Recently developed antiviral agents, such as ganciclovir, have been effective in arresting some cases of CMV disease in immunosuppressed persons.

 Pathogenesis: HPV infection begins with viral inoculation into a stratified squamous epithelium, where the virus enters the nuclei of basal cells. Infection stimulates the replication of the squamous epithelium, producing the various HPV-associated proliferative lesions. The rapidly growing squamous epithelium replicates innumerable progeny viruses, which are shed in the degenerating superficial cells. Many HPV lesions resolve spontaneously, although depressed cell-mediated immunity is associated with the persistence and spread of HPV lesions. The mechanism by which HPV infections participate in malignant change is discussed in Chapter 5.

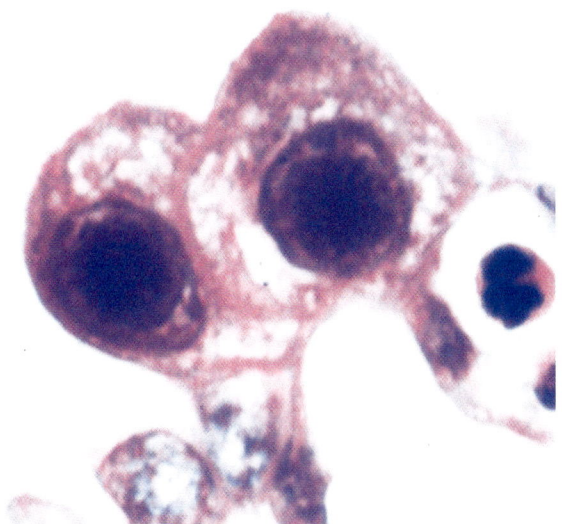

FIGURE 9-10
Cytomegalovirus pneumonitis. Type II pneumocytes display enlarged nuclei containing solitary inclusions surrounded by a clear zone.

Pathology: HPV infection produces squamous proliferative lesions, which vary in appearance and biological behavior. Most lesions show thickening of the affected epithelium, owing to enhanced squamous cell proliferation. Some HPV-infected cells display a characteristic cytopathic effect, termed *koilocytosis*, which features large squamous cells with shrunken nuclei enveloped in large cytoplasmic vacuoles (koilocytes).

 Clinical Features: Common warts (verruca vulgaris) are firm, circumscribed, raised, rough-surfaced lesions, which usually appear on surfaces subject to trauma, especially the hands. **Plantar warts** are similar squamous proliferative lesions on the soles of the feet but are compressed inward by standing and walking.

Anogenital warts (condyloma acuminatum) are soft, raised, fleshy lesions found on the penis, vulva, vaginal wall, cervix, or perianal region. When caused by certain HPV types, flat warts can develop into malignant squamous cell proliferations. The relationship between HPV, cervical intraepithelial neoplasia (CIN), and invasive squamous carcinoma of the cervix is discussed in Chapter 18.

Bacterial Infections

Bacteria are the smallest living cells, ranging in size from 0.1 to 10 μm in greatest dimension. They have three basic structural components: nuclear body, cytosol, and envelope. The nuclear body consists of a single, coiled circular molecule of double-stranded DNA with associated RNA and proteins. The nuclear body is not separated from the cytoplasm by a nuclear membrane, a key feature that distinguishes bacteria, which are prokaryotes, from eukaryotes. The cytosol is densely packed with ribosomes, proteins, and carbohydrates and lacks the structured organelles of eukaryotic cells, such as mitochondria and Golgi apparatus. The nuclear body and cytosol together are surrounded by an envelope, which serves as a permeability barrier but is also actively involved in transport, protein synthesis, energy generation, DNA synthesis, and cell division.

Bacteria are classified according to the structural features of the bacterial envelope. The simplest bacterial envelope consists of only a cell membrane composed of a phospholipid–protein bilayer. For example, the mycoplasmas (discussed below) have such a simple envelope. Most bacteria, however, have a rigid cell wall, which surrounds the cell membrane. Two basic types of bacterial cell walls are identified by their tinctorial properties with the Gram stain.

- **Gram-positive bacteria** retain iodine-crystal violet complexes when decolorized and appear dark blue. Their cell walls contain teichoic acids and a thick peptidoglycan layer.
- **Gram-negative bacteria** lose the iodine-crystal violet stain when decolorized and appear red with a counterstain. The outer membrane of gram-negative bacteria contains a lipopolysaccharide component, known as endotoxin, which is a potent mediator of the shock that complicates infections with these organisms.

Both gram-positive and gram-negative cell walls may be surrounded by an additional layer of polysaccharide or protein gel. When this gel is condensed about the cell wall, it is called a capsule. The capsule aids in bacterial attachment and colonization and may prevent phagocytosis by leukocytes. Bacteria are often described as "encapsulated" or "unencapsulated" because of the importance of the capsule in some infections.

The cell wall confers rigidity to bacteria and allows them to be distinguished on the basis of shape and pattern of growth. Round or oval bacteria are called *cocci*, and those that grow in typical pairs are called *diplococci*. Elongate bacteria are known as *rods* or *bacilli*, and curved ones are termed *vibrios*. Some spiral-shaped bacteria are called *spirochetes*.

Most bacteria can be grown in vitro on artificial media devoid of living cells, and they are frequently described according to their growth requirements on these media. Bacteria that require high levels of oxygen are called *aerobic*, those that grow best in the absence of oxygen are termed *anaerobic*, and those that thrive with limited amounts of oxygen are designated *microaerophilic*. Bacteria that grow well both in the presence and absence of oxygen are referred to as *facultative anaerobes*.

BACTERIAL EXOTOXINS: Many bacteria secrete toxins (exotoxins) that damage human cells either at the site of bacterial growth or at a distant site. These toxins are often named for the site or mechanism of their activity. Thus, those that act on the nervous system are called *neurotoxins* and those that affect intestinal cells are termed *enterotoxins*. Some toxins, such as diphtheria toxin or some of the *Clostridium perfringens* toxins, kill target cells and are referred to as *cytotoxins*. Other toxins, such as the diarrheagenic toxin of *Vibrio cholerae* or the potent neurotoxin of *Clostridium botulinum*, disturb the normal functions of their target cells without causing structural damage or death of these targets. An organism such as *C. perfringens* can produce over 20 different toxins that damage the human body in diverse ways.

BACTERIAL ENDOTOXINS: As mentioned above, gram-negative bacteria contain in their outer membranes a structural element called *lipopolysaccharide*. Also known as *endotoxin*, lipopolysaccharide activates the complement, coagulation, fibrinolysis, and bradykinin systems. It also causes the release of primary mediators of inflammation, including tumor necrosis factor (TNF) and interleukin-1 (IL-1), and various colony-stimulating factors. The actions of endotoxin produce shock, complement depletion, and disseminated intravascular coagulation.

Many bacteria damage tissues through the inflammatory or immune responses that they elicit. *Streptococcus pneumoniae* is an excellent example. It does not produce toxins but possesses a capsule that protects it from phagocytosis while activating the inflammatory response. Within the lung, the encapsulated organism causes an exudation of fluid and cells that fills the alveoli. This inflammatory response impairs breathing but does not, at least initially, limit the proliferation of the organism. *Treponema pallidum*, the spirochete that causes syphilis, persists in the body for years and elicits inflammatory and immune responses that continuously damage host tissues.

Although many common bacterial infections (e.g., *Staphylococcus aureus* skin infections) are characterized by purulent exudates, the tissue response in bacterial disease is highly variable. In some bacterial diseases, such as cholera, botulism, and tetanus, there is no inflammatory response at the critical site of cellular injury. Other bacterial infections, including syphilis and Lyme disease, lead to a predominantly lymphocytic and plasma cellular response. Still others (e.g., brucellosis) are characterized by granuloma formation.

Many bacterial diseases are due to organisms that normally inhabit the human body. There is an extensive endogenous bacterial flora of the gastrointestinal tract, upper respiratory tract, skin, and vagina. Under normal circumstances, these microorganisms are commensal and cause no harm. However, when they gain access to usually sterile sites or when host defenses are impaired, these bacteria can cause extensive destruction. *Staphylococcus aureus, Streptococcus pneumoniae,* and *Escherichia coli* are examples of the normal human flora that are also major human pathogens.

PYOGENIC GRAM-POSITIVE COCCI

Staphylococcus aureus Produces Suppurative Infections

S. aureus is a gram-positive coccus that typically grows in clusters and is one of the most common bacterial pathogens. The organism normally resides on the skin and is readily inoculated into deeper tissues, where it causes suppurative infections. **In fact, it is the most common cause of suppurative infections involving the skin, joints, and bones, and it is a leading cause of infective endocarditis.** S. aureus is commonly distinguished from other, less-virulent staphylococci by the coagulase test. S. aureus is coagulase positive; the other staphylococci are coagulase negative.

S. aureus spreads by direct contact with colonized surfaces or persons. Most children and adults are intermittently colonized with S. aureus, carrying the organism on the skin, in the nares, or on clothing. The organism also survives on inanimate surfaces for long periods.

 Pathogenesis: Many S. aureus infections begin as localized infections of the skin and skin appendages, producing cellulites and abscesses. Equipped with destructive enzymes and toxins, the organism sometimes invades beyond the initial site, spreading by the bloodstream or lymphatic system to almost any location in the body. The bones, joints, and heart valves are the most common sites of metastatic S. aureus infections. S. aureus also causes several distinct diseases by the elaboration of toxins that are carried to distant sites.

 Pathology: When S. aureus is inoculated into a previously sterile site, the infection usually produces suppuration and abscess formation. The abscesses range in size from microscopic foci to lesions several centimeters in diameter and are filled with pus and bacteria.

 Clinical Features: The clinical manifestations of S. aureus disease vary according to the sites and types of infection.

- **Furuncles (boils) and styes:** Deep-seated infections with S. aureus occur in and around hair follicles, often in a nasal carrier. They localize on hairy surfaces, such as the neck, thighs, and buttocks of men and the axillae, pubic area, and eyelids of both sexes. The boil begins as a nodule at the base of a hair follicle, followed by a pimple that remains painful and red for a few days. A yellow apex forms, and the central core becomes necrotic and fluctuant. Rupture or incision of the boil relieves the pain. Styes are boils that involve the sebaceous glands around the eyelid. *Paronychia* refers to staphylococcal infection of the nail bed, and *felons* are the same infections on the palmar side of the fingertips.
- **Carbuncles:** These lesions, mostly on the neck, result from coalescing infections with S. aureus around hair follicles and produce draining sinuses (Fig. 9-11).
- **Scalded skin syndrome:** This disease affects infants and children younger than the age of 3 years who present with a sunburnlike rash, which begins on the face and spreads over the body. Bullae then begin to form, and even gentle rubbing causes the skin to desquamate. The disease begins to resolve in 1 to 2 weeks, as the epithelium regenerates. The desquamation is due to the systemic effects of a specific exotoxin, and the site of S. aureus proliferation is often occult.
- **Osteomyelitis:** Acute staphylococcal osteomyelitis, usually in the bones of the legs, most commonly afflicts boys between 3 and 10 years of age, most of whom have a history of infection or trauma. Osteomyelitis may become chronic if not properly treated. Adults older than 50 years of age are more frequently afflicted with osteomyelitis of the vertebrae, which may follow staphylococcal infections of the skin or urinary tract, prostatic surgery, or pinning of a fracture.

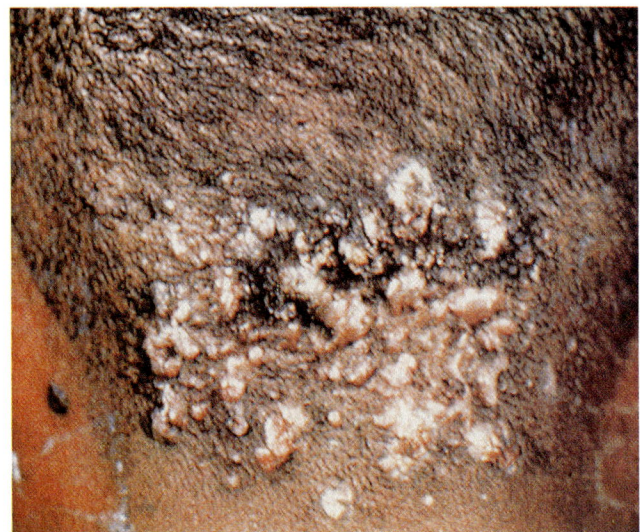

FIGURE *9-11*
Staphylococcal carbuncle. The posterior neck is indurated and shows multiple follicular abscesses discharging purulent material.

- **Infections of burns or surgical wounds:** These sites often become infected with *S. aureus* from the patient's own nasal carriage or from medical personnel. Newborns and elderly, malnourished, diabetic, and obese persons all have increased susceptibility.
- **Respiratory tract infections:** Staphylococcal infections of the respiratory tract are most common in infants younger than 2 years of age, and especially in those younger than 2 months of age. The infection is characterized by ulcers of the upper airway, scattered foci of pneumonia, pleural effusion, empyema, and pneumothorax. In adults, staphylococcal pneumonia may follow viral influenza, a disease that destroys the ciliated surface epithelium and leaves the bronchial surface vulnerable to secondary infections.
- **Bacterial arthritis:** *S. aureus* is the causative organism in half of all cases of septic arthritis, mostly in patients 50 to 70 years old. Rheumatoid arthritis and corticosteroid therapy are common predisposing conditions.
- **Septicemia:** Septicemia with *S. aureus* afflicts patients with lowered resistance who are in the hospital for other diseases. Some have underlying staphylococcal infections (e.g., osteomyelitis, septic arthritis), some have had surgery (e.g., transurethral resection of the prostate), and some have infections from an indwelling intravenous catheter. Miliary abscesses and endocarditis are serious complications.
- **Bacterial endocarditis:** Bacterial endocarditis is a common complication of *S. aureus* septicemia. It may develop spontaneously on normal valves, valves damaged by rheumatic fever, or prosthetic valves. Intravenous drug abuse is a predisposing factor to staphylococcal endocarditis.
- **Toxic shock syndrome:** This disorder most commonly afflicts menstruating women, who present with high fever, nausea, vomiting, diarrhea, and myalgias. Subsequently, they develop shock, and within several days a sunburnlike rash. The disease has been associated with the use of tampons, particularly hyperabsorbent tampons, which provide a site for *S. aureus* replication and toxin elaboration. Toxic shock syndrome occurs rarely in children and men and is then usually associated with an occult *S. aureus* infection.
- **Staphylococcal food poisoning:** Staphylococcal food poisoning typically begins less than 6 hours after a meal. Nausea and vomiting begin abruptly and usually resolve within 12 hours. This disease is caused by preformed toxin, rather than by secretion of toxin by ingested bacteria.

Coagulase-Negative Staphylococci Infect Prosthetic Devices

Coagulase-negative staphylococci are the major cause of infections associated with the introduction of medical devices, including intravenous catheters, prosthetic heart valves, heart pacemakers, orthopedic prostheses, cerebrospinal fluid shunts, and peritoneal catheters.

Disease due to coagulase-negative staphylococci usually derives from the normal bacterial flora. Of the more than 20 known species of coagulase-negative staphylococci, 10 are normal residents of human skin and mucosal surfaces. ***Staphylococcus epidermidis* is the most frequent cause of infections associated with medical devices.** Another species, *S. saprophyticus*, causes 10 to 20% of acute urinary tract infections in young women.

Pathogenesis: Coagulase-negative staphylococci readily contaminate foreign bodies. The organisms slowly proliferate on implanted devices, inducing an inflammatory response that damages adjacent tissue. If the bacteria are present on an intravascular surface, such as the tip of an intravascular catheter, they can spread through the bloodstream to cause metastatic infections. Coagulase-negative staphylococci lack the enzymes and toxins that permit *S. aureus* to cause extensive local tissue destruction. Some strains of coagulase-negative staphylococci produce a polysaccharide gel, called "slime," which enhances adherence of the bacteria to foreign objects and protects them from host antimicrobial defenses.

Pathology: Medical devices infected with coagulase-negative staphylococci are usually thinly coated with tan, fibrinous material. In contrast to infections caused by *S. aureus*, coagulase-negative staphylococcal infections usually do not produce extensive local tissue necrosis or large quantities of pus. Microscopic examination of infected devices shows clusters of gram-positive bacteria embedded in fibrin and cellular debris, with an associated acute inflammatory infiltrate.

Clinical Features: Coagulase-negative staphylococcal infections usually have subtle clinical presentations, and the only symptom of infection may be persistent low-grade fever. Infection of orthopedic prostheses frequently causes progressive loosening and dysfunction of the devices. In most persons, these infections are indolent, but in neutropenic or otherwise severely compromised persons, the infections can be fatal. Treatment usually requires replacement of any infected foreign object and appropriate antibiotic therapy.

Streptococcus pyogenes Causes Suppurative, Toxin-Related and Immunological Reactions

S. pyogenes, also known as group A streptococcus, is one of the most frequent bacterial pathogens of humans, causing many diseases of diverse organ systems, which range from acute self-limited pharyngitis to major illnesses such as rheumatic fever (Fig. 9-12). *S. pyogenes* is a gram-positive coccus that is frequently part of the endogenous flora that colonizes the skin and oropharynx.

The diseases caused by *S. pyogenes* may be considered in two categories: suppurative and nonsuppurative. Suppurative diseases occur at sites where the bacteria invade and cause tissue necrosis, usually inducing an acute inflamma-

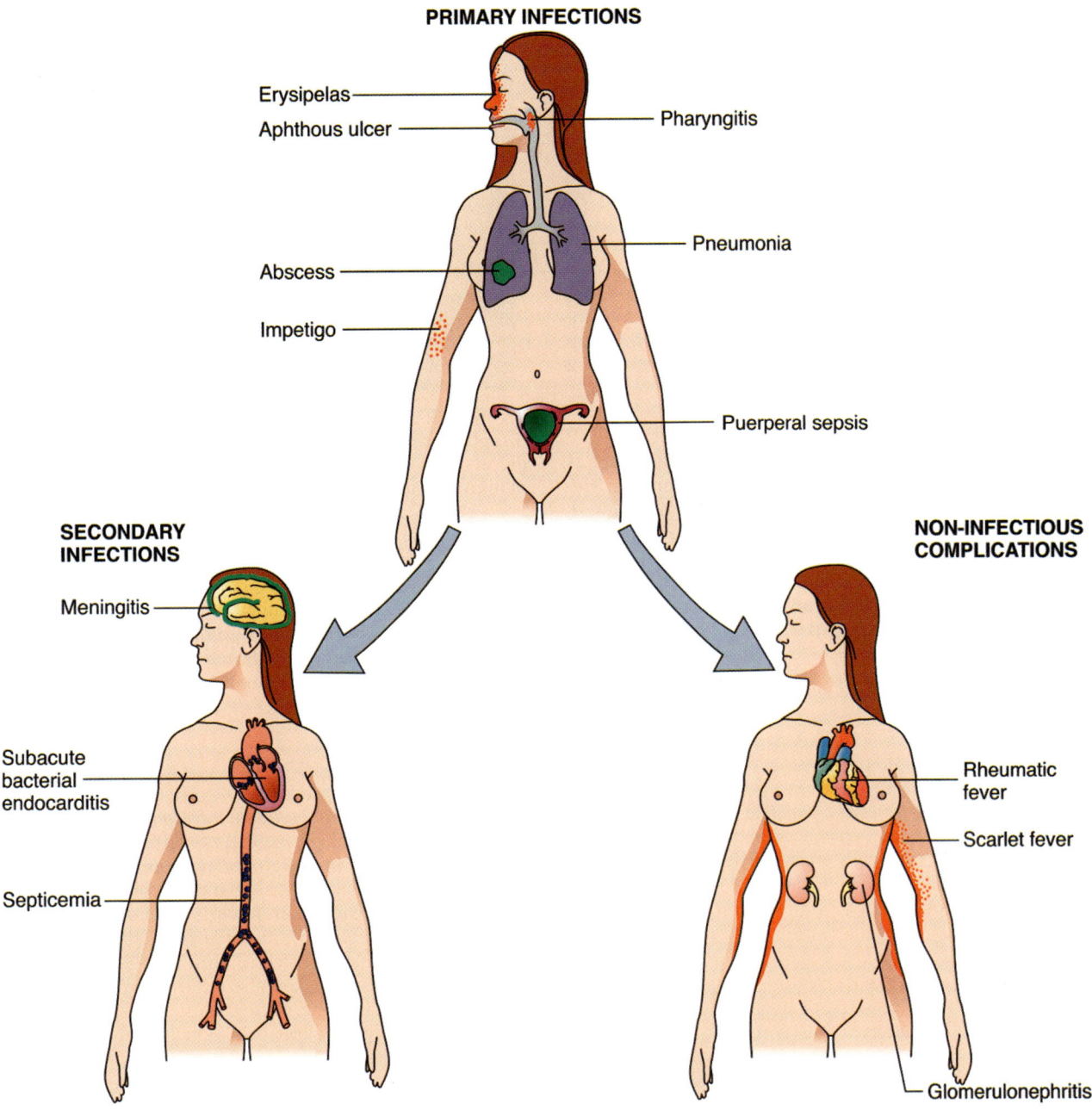

FIGURE 9-12
Streptococcal diseases.

tory response. Suppurative *S. pyogenes* infections include pharyngitis, impetigo, cellulitis, myositis, pneumonia, and puerperal sepsis. By contrast, nonsuppurative diseases occur at sites remote from the site of bacterial invasion. *S. pyogenes* causes two major nonsuppurative complications: rheumatic fever and acute poststreptococcal glomerulonephritis. These (1) involve organ systems far from the sites of streptococcal invasion, (2) usually occur some time after the acute infection, and (3) are probably caused by an immunological response. Rheumatic fever is discussed in Chapter 11, and poststreptococcal glomerulonephritis is described in Chapter 16.

STREPTOCOCCAL EXOTOXINS: *S. pyogenes* elaborates several exotoxins, including erythrogenic toxins and cytolytic toxins (streptolysins S and O). Erythrogenic toxins are responsible for the rash of scarlet fever. Streptolysin S lyses bacterial protoplasts (L forms) and probably destroys neutrophils after they ingest *S. pyogenes*. Streptolysin O induces a persistently high antibody titer, an effect that provides a useful marker for the diagnosis of *S. pyogenes* infections and their nonsuppurative complications.

Streptococcal Pharyngitis ("Strep Throat")

S. pyogenes, the common bacterial cause of pharyngitis, spreads from person to person by direct contact with oral or respiratory secretions. "Strep throat" occurs worldwide, predominantly affecting children and adolescents.

Pathogenesis: *S. pyogenes* attaches to epithelial cells by binding to fibronectin on their surface. The bacterium produces a battery of enzymes, including hemolysins, DNAase, hyaluronidase, and streptokinase, which allow it to damage and invade human tissues. *S. pyogenes* also has cell wall components that protect it from the inflammatory response. One of these, designated *M protein*, protrudes from the cell wall of virulent strains and prevents the deposition of complement, thereby protecting the bacterium from phagocytosis. Another surface protein destroys C5a, blocking the opsonizing effect of complement and inhibiting phagocytosis. The invading organism elicits an acute inflammatory response, often producing an exudate of neutrophils in the tonsillar fossae.

 Clinical Features: "Strep throat" manifests as sore throat, fever, malaise, headache, and an elevated leukocyte count. The disease is self-limited, usually lasting 3 to 5 days. **In a few cases, streptococcal pharyngitis leads to rheumatic fever or acute poststreptococcal glomerulonephritis.** Penicillin treatment shortens the clinical course of "strep throat" and, more importantly, prevents the major nonsuppurative sequelae.

Scarlet Fever

Scarlet fever (scarlatina) describes a punctate red rash that appears on the skin and mucous membranes in some suppurative S. pyogenes *infections, most commonly pharyngitis.* The rash usually begins on the chest and spreads to the extremities. The tongue may develop a yellow-white coating, which sheds to reveal a "beefy-red" surface. Scarlet fever is caused by an erythrogenic toxin.

Erysipelas

Erysipelas is an erythematous swelling of the skin caused chiefly by S. pyogenes (Fig. 9-13). The rash usually begins on the face

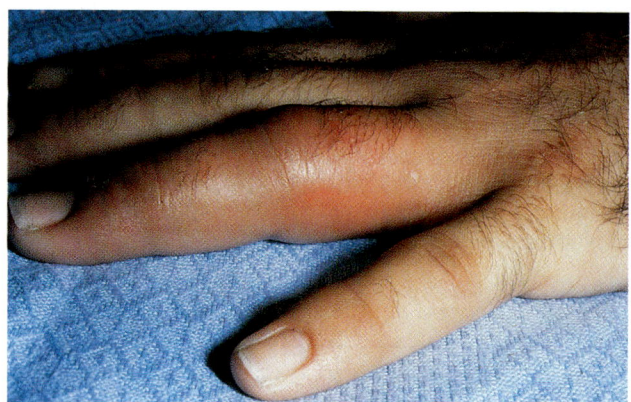

F I G U R E   9-13
Erysipelas. Streptococcal infection of the skin has resulted in an erythematous and swollen finger.

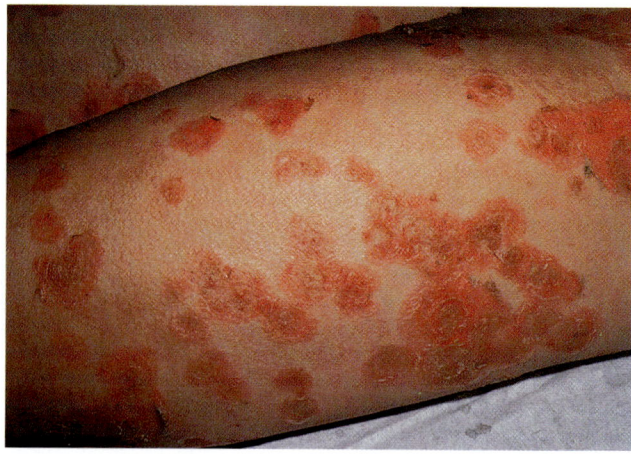

F I G U R E   9-14
Streptococcal impetigo. The lower extremities exhibit numerous erythematous papules, with central ulceration and the formation of crusts.

and spreads rapidly. Erysipelas is common in warm climates but is not often seen before the age of 20 years. A diffuse, edematous, acute inflammatory reaction in the epidermis and dermis extends into the subcutaneous tissues. The inflammatory infiltrate is principally composed of neutrophils and is most intense around vessels and adnexa of the skin. Cutaneous microabscesses and small foci of necrosis are not uncommon.

Impetigo

Impetigo (pyoderma) is a localized, intraepidermal infection of the skin that is caused by S. pyogenes *or* S. aureus. The strains of *S. pyogenes* that cause impetigo are antigenically and epidemiologically distinct from those that cause pharyngitis.

Impetigo spreads from person to person by direct contact. The disease most commonly affects children aged 2 to 5 years. A person, usually a child, first develops skin colonization with the causative organism. Minor trauma or an insect bite then inoculates the bacteria into the skin, where they form an intraepidermal pustule, which ruptures and leaks a purulent exudate.

Lesions begin on exposed body surfaces as localized erythematous papules (Fig. 9-14). These become pustules, which erode within a few days to form a thick honey-colored crust. Impetigo sometimes leads to poststreptococcal glomerulonephritis but not to rheumatic fever.

Streptococcal Cellulitis

S. pyogenes *causes an acute spreading infection of the loose connective tissue of the deeper layers of the dermis.* This suppurative infection results from traumatic inoculation of microorganisms into the skin and frequently occurs on the extremities in the context of impaired lymphatic drainage. Cellulitis usually begins at sites of unnoticed injury and appears as spreading areas of redness, warmth, and swelling.

Puerperal Sepsis

Puerperal sepsis refers to postpartum infection of the uterine cavity by S. pyogenes. The disease was formerly common but is now rare in developed countries. The infection originates from the contaminated hands of attendants at delivery, an association first established by the historic observations of Semmelweiss.

Streptococcus pneumoniae Infection Is a Major Cause of Lobar Pneumonia

Streptococcus pneumoniae, *often simply called pneumococcus, causes pyogenic infections, primarily involving the lungs (pneumonia), middle ear (otitis media), sinuses (sinusitis), and meninges (meningitis).* **It is one of the most common bacterial pathogens of humans, and by age 5, most children in the world have suffered at least one episode of pneumococcal disease (usually otitis media).**

S. pneumoniae is an aerobic, encapsulated, gram-positive diplococcus. There are over 80 antigenically distinct serotypes of pneumococcus; antibody to one serotype does not protect against infection with another. *S. pneumoniae* is a commensal organism in the oropharynx, and virtually all persons are colonized at some time.

  Pathogenesis and Pathology: Pneumococcal disease begins when the organism gains access to sterile sites, usually those in proximity to its normal residence in the oropharynx. Pneumococcal sinusitis and otitis media are usually preceded by a viral illness, such as the common cold, which injures the protective ciliated epithelium and fills the affected air spaces with fluid. Pneumococci then thrive in the nutrient-rich tissue fluid. Infection of the sinuses or middle ear can spread to the adjacent meninges.

Pneumococcal pneumonia arises in a similar fashion. The lower respiratory tract is protected by the mucociliary blanket and cough response, which normally expel organisms that are inhaled into the lower airway. Insults that interfere with respiratory defenses, including influenza, other viral respiratory illness, smoking, and alcoholism, allow access to *S. pneumoniae*. Once in the alveoli, the organisms proliferate and elicit an acute inflammatory response. The polysaccharide capsule of *S. pneumoniae* prevents activation of the alternate complement pathway, thereby blocking the production of the opsonin C3b. Thus, before a specific IgG antibody is produced, the organism can proliferate and spread unimpeded by phagocytes. In the lungs, *S. pneumoniae* spreads rapidly to involve an entire lobe or several lobes (lobar pneumonia). Alveoli fill with proteinaceous fluid, neutrophils, and bacteria. The clinical features of pneumococcal infections are discussed in Chapter 12.

Group B Streptococci Are the Leading Cause of Neonatal Pneumonia, Meningitis, and Sepsis

These organisms are also an infrequent cause of pyogenic infections in adults. Group B streptococci are gram-positive bacteria that grow in short chains. Several thousand neonatal infections with group B streptococci occur in the United States each year, and about 30% of infected infants die. Group B streptococci are part of the normal vaginal flora and are found in 30% of women. Most newborns born to colonized women acquire the organisms as they pass through the birth canal.

  Pathogenesis and Pathology: Particular risk factors associated with the development of neonatal group B streptococcal infections include premature delivery and low levels of maternally derived IgG antibodies against the organism. Newborns have little functional reserve for granulocyte production, and once established, the bacterial infection rapidly overwhelms the body's defense capacity. Group B streptococcal infection may be limited to the lungs or central nervous system or may be widely disseminated. Histopathologically, the involved tissues show a pyogenic response, often with overwhelming numbers of gram-positive cocci.

BACTERIAL INFECTIONS OF CHILDHOOD

Diphtheria Is a Necrotizing Upper Respiratory Tract Infection

Infection with *Corynebacterium diphtheriae*, an aerobic, pleomorphic, gram-positive rod, is sometimes associated with cardiac and neurological disturbances. Diphtheria is preventable by vaccination with inactivated *C. diphtheriae* toxin (toxoid).

 Epidemiology: Humans are the only significant reservoir for *C. diphtheriae*, and most persons are asymptomatic carriers. The organism spreads from person to person in respiratory droplets or oral secretions. At one time, diphtheria was a leading cause of death in children 2 to 15 years of age, but in western countries, immunization programs have largely eliminated the disease. However, diphtheria persists as a major health problem in less-developed countries.

 Pathogenesis: *C. diphtheriae* enters the pharynx, where the organisms proliferate, commonly on the tonsils. Diphtheria toxin is absorbed systemically and acts on tissues throughout the body, with the heart, nerves, and kidneys being most susceptible to damage. Diphtheria toxin is composed of two subunits, designated *A* and *B*. The B subunit binds to glycolipid receptors on target cells, and the A subunit acts within the cytoplasm on elongation factor 2 to interrupt protein synthesis. The toxin is one

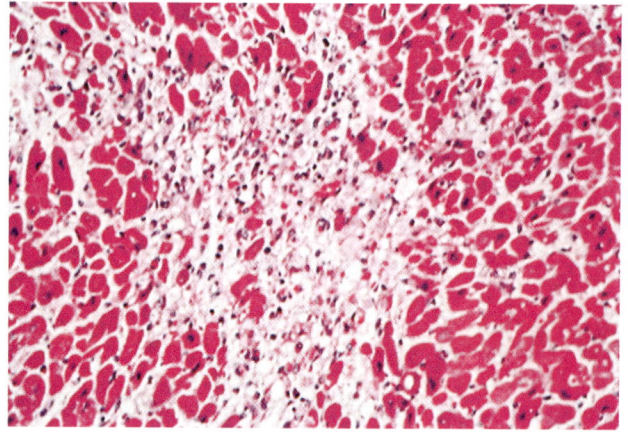

FIGURE 9-15
Diphtheric myocarditis. Focal degeneration of cardiac myocytes is evident.

of the most potent known, and one molecule suffices to kill a cell.

 Pathology: The characteristic lesions of diphtheria are the thick, gray, leathery membranes composed of sloughed epithelium, necrotic debris, neutrophils, fibrin, and bacteria that line the affected respiratory passages (Gk. *diphtheria*, "leather"). The epithelial surface beneath the membranes is denuded, and the submucosa is acutely inflamed and hemorrhagic. The inflammatory process often produces swelling in the surrounding soft tissues, which can be severe enough to cause respiratory compromise. When the heart is affected, the myocardium displays fat droplets in the myocytes and focal necrosis (Fig. 9-15). In the case of neural involvement, the affected peripheral nerves exhibit demyelination.

 Clinical Features: Diphtheria begins with fever, sore throat, and malaise. The dirty gray membrane usually develops first on the tonsils and may spread throughout the posterior oropharynx. The membrane is firmly adherent, and an attempt to strip it from the underlying mucosa produces bleeding. Cardiac and neurological symptoms develop in a minority of infected persons, usually those with the most severe local disease.

Cutaneous diphtheria, which results from inoculation of the organism into a break in the skin, manifests as a pustule or ulcer; it is only rarely associated with cardiac or neurological complications. Diphtheria is treated by prompt administration of antitoxin and antibiotics.

Pertussis Is Commonly Called Whooping Cough

Pertussis is a prolonged upper respiratory tract infection, characterized by debilitating coughing paroxysms. The paroxysm is followed by a long, high-pitched inspiration, the "whoop," which gives the disease its name. The causative organism is *Bordetella pertussis*, a small, gram-negative coccobacillus.

 Epidemiology: *B. pertussis* is highly contagious and spreads from person to person, primarily by infected respiratory aerosols. Humans are the only reservoir of infection. In susceptible populations, pertussis is primarily a disease of children younger than the age of 5 years. Vaccination protects against *B. pertussis*, but worldwide, there are some 50 million cases of pertussis each year, resulting in almost 1 million deaths, particularly in infants.

 Pathogenesis and Pathology: *B. pertussis* initiates infection by attaching to the cilia of respiratory epithelial cells. The organism then elaborates a cytotoxin that kills the ciliated cells. The progressive destruction of ciliated respiratory epithelium and the ensuing inflammatory response cause the local respiratory symptoms. Several other toxins include "pertussis toxin" an agent that causes the pronounced lymphocytosis often associated with whooping cough. Another toxin inhibits adenylyl cyclase, an effect that blocks bacterial phagocytosis.

B. pertussis causes an extensive tracheobronchitis, with necrosis of the ciliated respiratory epithelium and an acute inflammatory response. With the loss of the protective mucociliary blanket, there is an increased risk of pneumonia from aspirated oral bacteria. Coughing paroxysms and vomiting make aspiration likely, and secondary bacterial pneumonia is a common cause of death.

 Clinical Features: Whooping cough is a prolonged upper respiratory tract illness, lasting 4 to 5 weeks and passing through three stages:

- The **catarrhal stage** resembles a common viral upper respiratory tract illness, with low-grade fever, runny nose, conjunctivitis, and cough.
- The **paroxysmal stage** occurs one week into the illness. The cough worsens and becomes paroxysmal, with 5 to 15 consecutive coughs, often followed by an inspiratory whoop. The patient develops a marked lymphocytosis, with the total leukocyte count often exceeding 40,000 cells/μL. The paroxysms persist for 2 to 3 weeks.
- The **convalescent phase** usually lasts for several weeks.

Haemophilus influenzae Causes Pyogenic Infections in Young Children

Haemophilus influenzae infections involve the middle ear, sinuses, facial skin, epiglottis, meninges, lungs, and joints. The organism is a major pediatric bacterial pathogen and the leading cause of bacterial meningitis worldwide. *H. influenzae* is an aerobic, pleomorphic gram-negative coccobacillus that exists in both encapsulated and nonencapsulated strains. Nonencapsulated strains (type a) usually produce localized infections; encapsulated strains, designated type b, are more virulent and cause over 95% of the invasive bacteremic infections.

 Epidemiology: *H. influenzae* is a strict parasite of humans and spreads from person to person, primarily in respiratory droplets and secretions. The organism is normally resident in the human nasopharynx, colonizing 20 to 50% of healthy adults. Most colonizing strains are nonencapsulated, but 3 to 5% are *H. influenzae* type b.

Most severe *H. influenzae* type b infections occur in children younger than the age of 6 years. The incidence of serious disease peaks at 6 to 18 months of age, corresponding to the period between the loss of maternally acquired immunity and the acquisition of native immunity. Complications can be prevented by inoculating infants with *H. influenzae* type b vaccine.

Pathogenesis: Unencapsulated *H. influenzae* strains produce disease by spreading locally from their normal sites of residence to adjoining sterile locations, such as the sinuses or middle ear. This is facilitated by injury to the normal defense mechanisms, as occurs with a viral upper respiratory tract illness. Within these previously sterile sites, unencapsulated organisms proliferate and elicit an acute inflammatory response, which injures the local tissue but eventually contains the infection. Under most circumstances, the unencapsulated strains do not produce bacteremia.

H. influenzae type b is capable of tissue invasion. The capsular polysaccharide of type b organisms allows them to evade phagocytosis, and bacteremic infections are common. Epiglottitis, facial cellulitis, septic arthritis, and meningitis result from invasive bacteremic infections. *H. influenzae* type b also elaborates an IgA protease, which facilitates local survival of the organism in the respiratory tract.

 Pathology: *H. influenzae* elicits a pronounced acute inflammatory response, and specific pathological features vary according to the sites affected. *H. influenzae* meningitis resembles other acute bacterial meningitides, with a predominantly neutrophilic infiltrate in the leptomeninges, sometimes extending into the subarachnoid space.

H. influenzae pneumonia usually complicates chronic lung disease, and in half of patients it follows a viral infection of the respiratory tract. The alveoli are filled with neutrophils, macrophages containing bacilli, and fibrin. The bronchiolar epithelium is necrotic and infiltrated by macrophages.

Epiglottitis consists of swelling and acute inflammation of the epiglottis, aryepiglottic folds, and pyriform sinuses, which sometimes completely obstruct the upper airway. In facial cellulitis, the site of infection and inflammation is the dermis, usually of the cheek or periorbital region.

 Clinical Features: Most bacteremic *H. influenzae* infections afflict young children. **H. influenzae is the most common cause of meningitis in children younger than the age of 2 years.** The onset is insidious and may follow an otherwise unremarkable upper respiratory tract infection or otitis media.

Bronchopneumonia or lobar pneumonia is characterized by fever, cough, purulent sputum, and dyspnea.

Epiglottitis affects primarily children aged 2 to 7 years but also occurs in adults. Death may occur from obstruction of the upper respiratory tract.

Septic arthritis is secondary to bacteremic seeding of large weight-bearing joints. Symptoms include fever, heat, erythema, swelling, and pain on movement.

Facial cellulitis or periorbital cellulitis is another severe bacteremic infection affecting primarily young children. Patients present with fever, profound malaise, and a raised, hot, red-blue discolored area of the face, usually involving the cheek or an area about the eye. There is often concomitant meningitis or septic arthritis.

Neisseria meningitides Causes Pyogenic Meningitis and Overwhelming Shock

Neisseria meningitidis, *commonly termed* meningococcus, *produces disseminated blood-borne infections, often accompanied by shock and profound disturbances in coagulation* (Fig. 9-16). The organism is aerobic and appears as paired, bean-shaped,

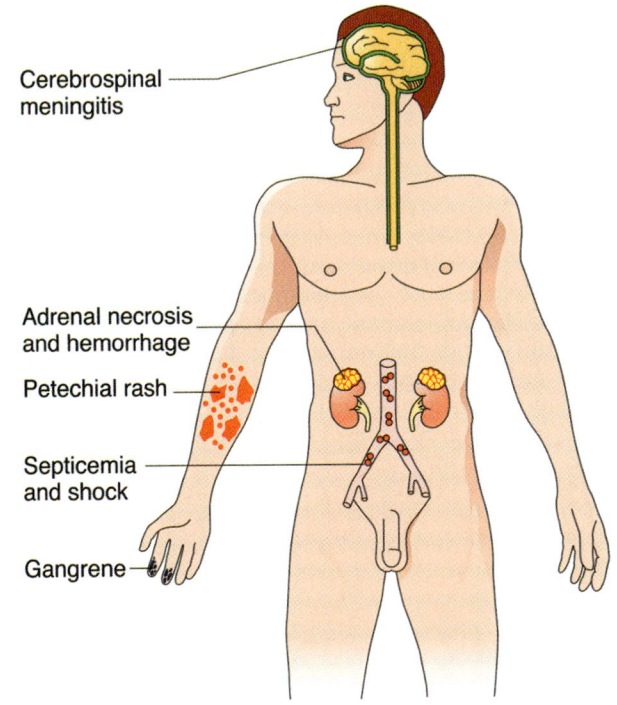

FIGURE 9-16
Meningococcemia. Meningococcal infections have a variety of clinical manifestations including meningitis, septicemia, shock, and associated complications.

gram-negative cocci. There are eight major serogroups, three of which (A, B, C) cause most infections.

Epidemiology: Meningococci spread from person to person, primarily by respiratory droplets. A small proportion (5–15%) of the population carries the organism in the nasopharynx as a commensal. Carriers develop antibodies to the particular colonizing strain of *N. meningitidis* and are immune to meningococcal disease caused by that strain.

Meningococcal diseases appear as sporadic cases, clusters of cases, and epidemics. Most infections in industrialized countries are sporadic and afflict children younger than the age of 5 years. Epidemic disease occurs most frequently in crowded quarters, such as among military recruits in barracks. There are over 6000 cases of meningococcal meningitis each year in the United States, resulting in over 600 deaths. Fatalities from meningococcal disease are more common in less-developed countries.

Pathogenesis: On colonizing the upper respiratory tract, *N. meningitidis* attaches to nonciliated respiratory epithelium by means of its pili. Most exposed persons then develop protective bactericidal antibodies over the following weeks, and some become carriers. If the organism spreads to the bloodstream before the development of protective immunity, it can proliferate rapidly in unprotected human tissue, resulting in fulminant meningococcal disease.

Many of the systemic effects of meningococcal disease are due to the endotoxin of the outer membrane lipopolysaccharide of the bacterium. Endotoxin promotes a conspicuous increase in the production of TNF and the simultaneous activation of the complement and coagulation cascades. Disseminated intravascular coagulation, fibrinolysis, and shock follow.

Pathology: Meningococcal disease can be confined to the central nervous system or may be disseminated throughout the body in the form of septicemia. In the case of meningococcal meningitis, the leptomeninges and subarachnoid space are infiltrated with neutrophils, and the underlying brain parenchyma is swollen and congested. Meningococcal septicemia is characterized by diffuse damage to the endothelium of small blood vessels, resulting in widespread petechiae and purpura in the skin and viscera.

Rarely (3–4% of all cases), vasculitis and thrombosis produce hemorrhagic necrosis of both adrenals, a phenomenon known as the **Waterhouse-Friderichsen syndrome.**

Clinical Features: Meningitis begins with the rapid onset of fever, stiff neck, and headache. In meningococcal sepsis, fever, shock, and mucocutaneous hemorrhages appear abruptly. Patients can progress to shock in minutes, and treatment requires rapid support of blood pressure and antibiotics. In the preantibiotic era, meningococcal disease was almost invariably fatal, but modern treatment has reduced the fatality rate to less than 15%. Some patients who survive the early phase of meningococcemia develop late allergic complications such as polyarthritis, cutaneous vasculitis, and pericarditis. Occasionally, severe vasculitis is associated with extensive cutaneous ulceration and sometimes even gangrene of the distal extremities.

SEXUALLY TRANSMITTED BACTERIAL DISEASES

Gonorrhea Remains a Common Infection That Causes Sterility

Neisseria gonorrhoeae, *also termed* gonococcus, *causes gonorrhea, an acute suppurative infection of the genital tract, which is reflected in urethritis in men and endocervicitis in women. It is one of the oldest and still one of the most common sexually transmitted diseases. N. gonorrhoeae is an aerobic, bean-shaped, gram-negative diplococcus.*

Male homosexuals are at risk for gonococcal pharyngitis and proctitis. In women, infection often ascends the genital tract, producing endometritis, salpingitis, and pelvic inflammatory disease. Ascending spread in men is less common, but when it does occur epididymitis results. Rarely, gonococcal infection becomes bacteremic, in which circumstance septic arthritis and skin lesions develop. Neonatal infections derived from the birth canal of a mother with gonorrhea usually manifest as conjunctivitis, although disseminated infections are occasionally encountered. Neonatal gonococcal conjunctivitis has been largely eliminated in developed countries by the routine instillation of antibiotics into the conjunctiva at birth, but it is still a major cause of blindness in much of Africa and Asia.

Epidemiology: Infection is spread directly from person to person, and except for perinatal transmission, spread is almost always by sexual intercourse. Infected persons who are asymptomatic serve as a significant reservoir of infection. Although effective antibiotic therapy has been available for almost 50 years, the disease remains rampant throughout the world.

Pathogenesis: Gonorrhea begins as an infection of the mucous membranes of the urogenital tract (Fig. 9-17). The bacteria attach to the surface cells, after which they invade superficially and provoke acute inflammation. Gonococcus lacks a true polysaccharide capsule, but hairlike extensions, termed *pili,* project from the cell wall. The pili contain a protease that digests IgA on the mucous membrane, thereby facilitating the attachment of the bacterium to the columnar and transitional epithelium of the urogenital tract.

Sexually Transmitted Bacterial Diseases

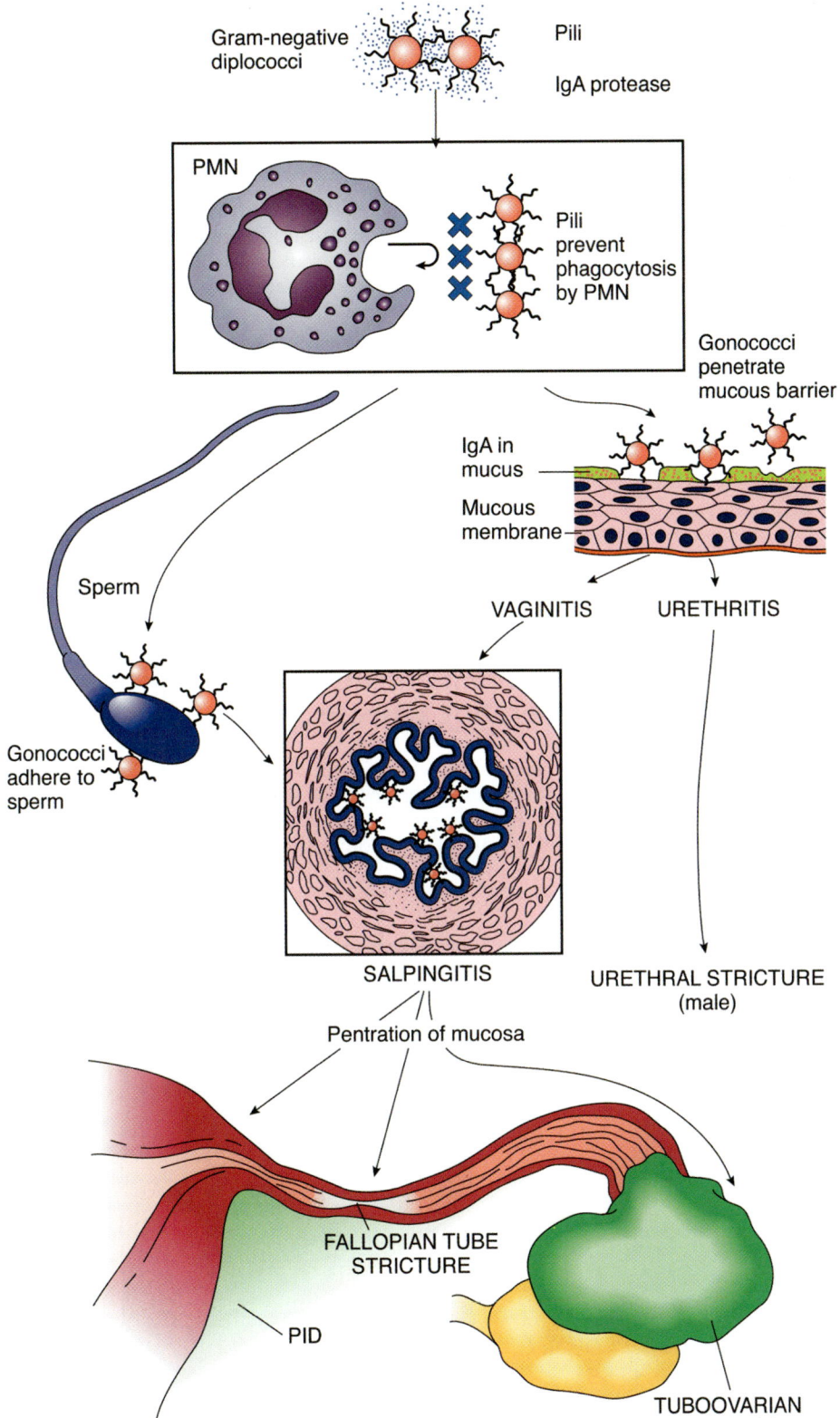

FIGURE 9-17

Pathogenesis of gonococcal infections. *Neisseria gonorrhoeae* is a gram-negative diplococcus whose surface pili form a barrier against phagocytosis by neutrophils. The pili contain an IgA protease that digests IgA on the luminal surface of the mucous membranes of the urethra, endocervix, and fallopian tube, thereby facilitating attachment of gonococci. Gonococci cause endocervicitis, vaginitis, and salpingitis. In men, gonococci attached to the mucous membrane of the urethra cause urethritis and, sometimes, urethral stricture. Gonococci may also attach to sperm heads and be carried into the fallopian tube. Penetration of the mucous membrane by gonococci leads to stricture of the fallopian tube, pelvic inflammatory disease (PID), or tuboovarian abscess.

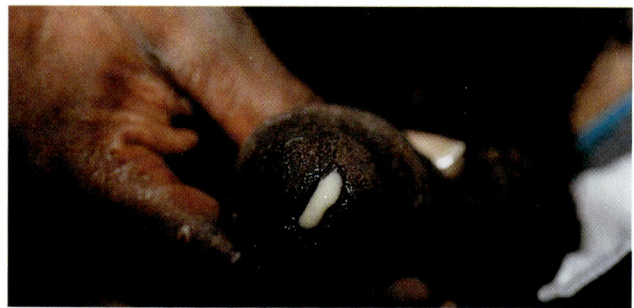

FIGURE 9-18
Acute gonorrhea. A purulent discharge emanates from the penile urethra.

 Pathology: Gonorrhea is a suppurative infection, characterized by a vigorous acute inflammatory response, producing copious pus and often forming submucosal abscesses. Stained smears of pus reveal numerous neutrophils, often containing phagocytosed bacteria. If untreated, the inflammatory response becomes chronic, with macrophages and lymphocytes predominant.

Clinical Features: Men exposed to *N. gonorrhoeae* present with a purulent urethral discharge (Fig. 9-18) and dysuria. If treatment is not instituted promptly, urethral stricture is a common complication. The organisms may also extend to the prostate, epididymis, and accessory glands, where they cause epididymitis and orchitis and may result in infertility.

In about one half of infected women, gonorrhea remains asymptomatic. The other infected women initially exhibit endocervicitis, with a vaginal discharge or bleeding. Urethritis presents as dysuria rather than as a urethral discharge. The infection often extends to the fallopian tubes, where it produces acute and chronic salpingitis and eventually pelvic inflammatory disease. The fallopian tubes swell with pus (Fig. 9-19), causing acute abdominal pain. Infertility occurs when inflammatory adhesions block the tubes.

From the fallopian tubes, gonorrhea spreads to the peritoneum, healing as fine ("violin string") adhesions between the liver and the parietal peritoneum. Chronic endometritis is a persistent complication of gonococcal infection and is usually the consequence of chronic gonococcal salpingitis.

Chancroid Causes Genital Ulcers in Less-Developed Regions

Chancroid, sometimes called "the third venereal disease" (after syphilis and gonorrhea), is an acute sexually transmitted infection caused by Haemophilus ducreyi. The organism is a small, gram-negative bacillus, which appears in tissue as clusters of parallel bacilli and as chains, resembling schools of fish. Chancroid is characterized by painful genital ulcerations and associated lymphadenopathy. The infection is the leading cause of genital ulcers in many less-developed countries, especially in Africa and parts of Asia, and it has been suggested that the genital ulcers facilitate the spread of HIV. The incidence in the United States has risen during the past decade, and there are now about 5000 cases annually.

 Pathology: *H. ducreyi* enters through breaks in the skin, where it multiplies and produces a raised lesion, which then ulcerates. Ulcers vary from 0.1 to 2 cm in diameter. Organisms are carried within macrophages to regional lymph nodes, which may suppurate. Seven to 10 days after the appearance of the primary lesion, half of patients develop unilateral, painful, suppurative, inguinal lymphadenitis (bubo). The overlying skin becomes inflamed, breaks down, and drains pus from the underlying node. The diagnosis is made by identifying the bacillus in tissue sections or gram-stained smears prepared from the ulcers.

Treatment of chancroid with erythromycin is usually effective.

Granuloma Inguinale Is a Tropical Ulcerating Disease

Granuloma inguinale is a sexually transmitted, chronic, superficial ulceration of the genitalia and the inguinal and perianal regions. It is caused by *Calymmatobacterium granulomatis,* a small, encapsulated, nonmotile, gram-negative bacillus.

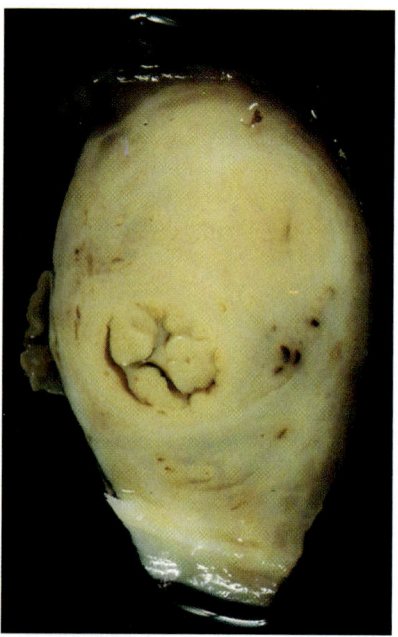

FIGURE 9-19
Gonorrhea of the fallopian tube. Cross-section of a "pus tube" shows thickening of the wall and a lumen swollen with pus.

Epidemiology and Pathogenesis: Humans are the only hosts of *C. granulomatis*. Granuloma inguinale is rare in temperate climates but is common in tropical and subtropical areas. New Guinea, central Australia and India have the highest incidence. Most patients are 15 to 40 years of age, the period of greatest sexual activity. Because male homosexuals who take the passive role have only anal lesions, and because *C. granulomatis* has been isolated from the feces, the organism is believed to inhabit the intestinal tract. It causes granuloma inguinale through autoinoculation, anal intercourse, or vaginal intercourse if the vagina is colonized by the enteric bacteria.

Pathology: The characteristic lesion is a raised, soft, beefy-red, superficial ulcer. The exuberant granulation tissue resembles a fleshy mass herniating through the skin. Microscopically, dermis and subcutis are infiltrated by macrophages and plasma cells and by fewer neutrophils and lymphocytes. Interspersed macrophages contain many bacteria, termed *Donovan bodies* (Fig. 9-20).

Clinical Features: Untreated granuloma inguinale follows an indolent, relapsing course, often healing with an atrophic scar. Secondary fusospirochetal infection may cause ulceration, with mutilation or amputation of the genitalia. Massive scarring of the dermis and subcutis causes genital elephantiasis by lymphatic obstruction. Antibiotic therapy is effective in early cases.

ENTEROPATHOGENIC BACTERIAL INFECTIONS

Escherichia coli is a Frequent Cause of Diarrhea and Urinary Tract Infections

Escherichia coli *is among the most frequent and important bacterial pathogens of humans, causing more than 90% of all urinary tract infections and many cases of diarrheal illness worldwide.* It is also a major opportunistic pathogen, frequently producing pneumonia and sepsis in immunocompromised hosts and meningitis and sepsis in newborns.

E. coli organisms are a group of antigenically and biologically diverse, aerobic (facultatively anaerobic), gram-negative bacteria. Most strains are intestinal commensals, well adapted to growth within the human colon without causing harm to the host. However, *E. coli* can be aggressive when it gains access to usually sterile body sites, such as the urinary tract, meninges, or peritoneum. Strains of *E. coli* that produce diarrhea possess specialized virulence properties, usually plasmid-borne, which confer the capacity to cause intestinal disease.

E. coli Diarrhea

There are four distinct strains of *E. coli* that cause diarrhea.

ENTEROTOXIGENIC E. COLI: *Enterotoxigenic* E. coli *is a major cause of diarrhea in poor tropical areas and probably causes most "traveler's diarrhea" among visitors to such regions.* The organism is acquired from contaminated water and food. Many persons in Latin America, Africa, and Asia carry this strain asymptomatically in their intestine, providing the reservoir.

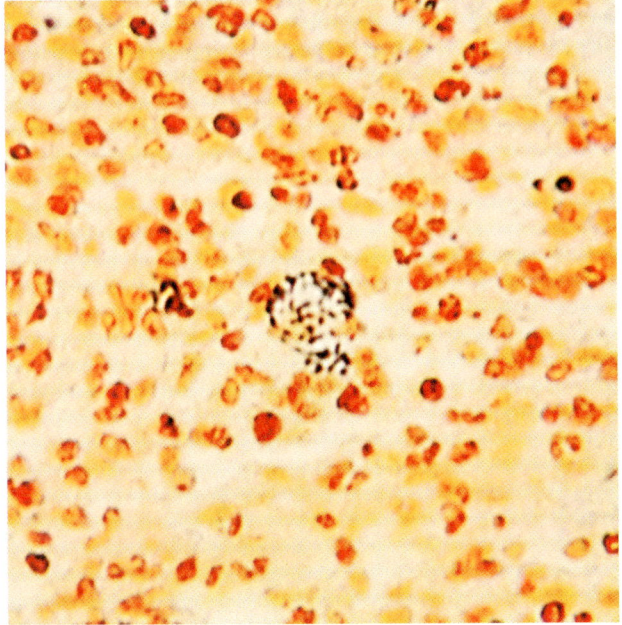

FIGURE 9-20
Granuloma inguinale. A photomicrograph of a skin lesion shows *C. granulomatis* (Donovan bodies) clustered in a large macrophage. Intense silvering by Warthin-Starry technique makes the organisms large, black, and easily seen.

Pathogenesis: Nonimmune persons (local children or travelers from abroad), develop diarrhea when they encounter the organism. Enterotoxigenic strains produce diarrhea by adhering to the intestinal mucosa and elaborating one or more of at least three enterotoxins that cause secretory dysfunction of the small bowel. One of the enterotoxins is structurally and functionally similar to cholera toxin, and another acts on guanylyl cyclase. Enterotoxigenic *E. coli* produces no distinctive macroscopic or light-microscopic alterations in the intestine.

Enterotoxigenic *E. coli* causes an acute, self-limited diarrheal illness with watery stools lacking neutrophils and erythrocytes. In severe cases, the fluid and electrolyte loss can cause extreme dehydration and even death.

ENTEROPATHOGENIC E. COLI: *Historically, enteropathogenic E. coli was the first group of this genus to be identified as a causal agent of diarrhea.* The organism is a major cause of diarrheal illness in poor tropical areas, especially in infants and young children. Although it has virtually disappeared from developed countries, it still causes sporadic outbreaks of diarrhea, particularly among hospitalized infants younger than 2 years of age. Enteropathogenic E. coli is acquired by the ingestion of contaminated food or water. The organism lacks invasive properties and causes disease by adhering to and deforming the microvilli of the intestinal epithelial cells (Fig. 9-21A). Enteropathogenic *E. coli* produces diarrhea, vomiting, fever, and malaise.

ENTEROHEMORRHAGIC E. COLI: *Enterohemorrhagic E. coli (serotype 0157:H7) causes a bloody diarrhea, which occasionally is followed by the hemolytic–uremic syndrome* (see Chapter 16). The source of infection is usually the ingestion of contaminated meat or milk. Enterohemorrhagic *E. coli* adheres to the colonic mucosa and elaborates an enterotoxin, virtually identical to Shiga toxin, that destroys the epithelial cells. Patients infected with *E. coli* 0157:H7 present with cramping abdominal pain, low-grade fever, and sometimes bloody diarrhea. Microscopic examination of the stool shows both leukocytes and erythrocytes.

ENTEROINVASIVE E. COLI: *Enteroinvasive E. coli causes food-borne dysentery which is clinically and pathologically indistinguishable from that caused by* Shigella. The agent shares extensive DNA homology and antigenic and biochemical characteristics with *Shigella*. It invades and destroys mucosal cells of the distal ileum and colon (see Fig. 9-21B). As in shigellosis, the mucosa of the distal ileum and colon are acutely inflamed and focally eroded and are sometimes covered by an inflammatory pseudomembrane. Patients exhibit abdominal pain, fever, tenesmus, and bloody diarrhea. Symptoms persist for about a week. Antibiotic treatment is similar to that for shigellosis.

E. coli Urinary Tract Infection

 Epidemiology: Urinary tract infections with E. coli are most common in sexually active women and in persons of both sexes who have structural or functional abnormalities of the urinary tract. Such infections are extremely common, afflicting more than 10% of the human population, often repeatedly. *E. coli* in the urinary tract usually derives from the resident flora of the perineum and periurethral areas, reflecting fecal contamination of these regions.

 Pathogenesis: *E. coli* gains access to the sterile proximal urinary tract by ascending from the distal urethra. Because the shorter female urethra provides a less effective mechanical barrier to infection, women are much more prone to urinary tract infections. Sexual intercourse can suffice to propel organisms into the female urethra. Uropathogenic *E. coli* organisms have specialized adherence factors (Gal-Gal) on the pili, which enable them to bind to galactopyranosyl-galactopyranoside residues on the uroepithelium. Structural abnormalities of the urinary tract (e.g., congenital deformities, prostatic hyperplasia, strictures) and instrumentation (catheterization) overwhelm normal host defenses and facilitate the establishment of urinary tract infections. These conditions account for most urinary tract infections in men.

 Pathology and Clinical Features: *E. coli* urinary tract infections initially produce an acute inflammatory infiltrate at the site of infection, usually the bladder mucosa. Urinary tract infections involving the bladder or urethra manifest as urinary urgency, burning on urination (dysuria), and leuko-

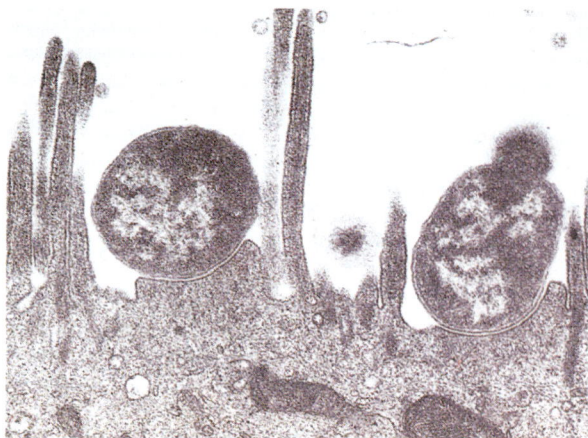
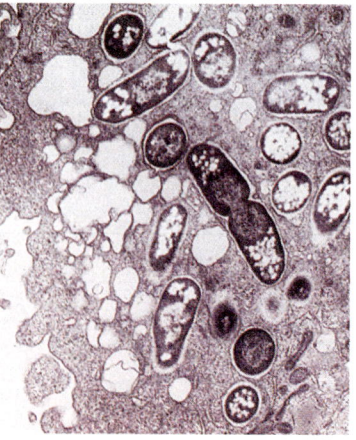

FIGURE 9-21
A. Enteropathogenic *E. coli* infection. An electron micrograph shows adherence of the bacteria to the intestinal mucosal cells and localized destruction of microvilli. B. Enteroinvasive *E. coli* infection. An electron micrograph shows organisms within a cell.

cytes in the urine. If the infection ascends to involve the kidney (pyelonephritis), the patient develops acute flank pain, fever, and an elevated leukocyte count. An infiltrate of neutrophils spills from the mucosa into the urine, and the blood vessels of the submucosa are dilated and congested. Chronic infections exhibit an inflammatory infiltrate of neutrophils and mononuclear cells. Chronic infection of the kidneys may lead to chronic pyelonephritis and renal failure (see Chapter 16).

E. coli Pneumonia

Pneumonias due to enteric gram-negative bacteria are opportunistic infections, mostly occurring in debilitated persons. *E. coli* is the most common cause, but other normal bowel flora, such as *Klebsiella*, *Serratia*, and *Enterobacter* species, produce similar disease. **The following discussion applies to all opportunistic gram-negative pneumonias.**

Pathogenesis and Pathology: Enteric gram-negative bacteria are transiently introduced into the oral cavity of healthy persons, but they cannot compete successfully with the predominant gram-positive flora, which adhere to the fibronectin that coats the surface of mucosal cells. Chronically ill or severely stressed persons elaborate a salivary protease that degrades fibronectin, allowing gram-negative enteric bacteria to overcome the normal gram-positive flora and colonize the oropharynx.

Inevitably, droplets of the resident oral flora are aspirated into the respiratory tract. Debilitated patients often have markedly diminished local defenses and cannot destroy these organisms. Decreased gag and cough reflexes, abnormal neutrophil chemotaxis, injured respiratory epithelium, and the presence of foreign bodies, such as endotracheal tubes, all facilitate entry and survival of the aspirated organisms.

E. coli pneumonia results from the proliferation of aspirated organisms in the terminal airways, usually at multiple sites in the lung. Multifocal areas of consolidation result, and the terminal airways and alveoli are filled with proteinaceous fluid, fibrin, neutrophils, and macrophages.

Clinical Features: Because pneumonia caused by *E. coli* and other enteric gram-negative organisms afflicts patients who are often already severely ill, the symptoms of pneumonia may be less obvious than in healthy persons. Increased malaise, fever, and labored breathing are often the first signs of pneumonia. If *E. coli* pneumonia remains untreated, the organisms may invade the bloodstream to produce a fatal septicemia. Treatment requires parenteral antibiotics.

E. coli Sepsis (Gram-Negative Sepsis)

E. coli is the most common cause of enteric gram-negative sepsis, but various other gram-negative rods, including *Pseudomonas*, *Klebsiella*, and *Enterobacter* species, produce identical disease. **The following discussion pertains to gram-negative sepsis in general.**

Pathogenesis: *E. coli* sepsis is usually an opportunistic infection, occurring in persons with predisposing conditions, such as neutropenia, pyelonephritis, or cirrhosis, and in hospitalized patients. Together with other enteric gram-negative rods that normally reside in the human colon, *E. coli* occasionally seeds the bloodstream. In healthy persons, mononuclear macrophages and circulating neutrophils phagocytose these bacteria. Patients with neutropenia or cirrhosis develop *E. coli* sepsis because of an impaired capacity to eliminate even low-level bacteremias. Persons with ruptured abdominal organs or acute pyelonephritis suffer gram-negative sepsis because the large numbers of organisms that gain access to the circulation overwhelm the normal defenses.

The presence of *E. coli* in the bloodstream causes septic shock through the effects of TNF, whose release from macrophages is stimulated by bacterial endotoxin. Septic shock is discussed in Chapter 7.

Neonatal E. coli Meningitis and Sepsis

E. coli and group B streptococci are the primary causes of meningitis and sepsis in the first month after birth. Both colonize the vagina, and the newborn acquires the organisms on passage through the birth canal. *E. coli* then colonizes the infant's gastrointestinal tract. It is postulated that the organisms spread to the bloodstream from the gastrointestinal tract and then seed the meninges. The pathology of *E. coli* meningitis is identical to that of other bacterial meningitides. Although antibiotic treatment for neonatal *E. coli* meningitis and sepsis is often effective, the mortality rate still ranges from 15 to 50%. Almost half of survivors suffer neurological sequelae.

Salmonella Enterocolitis and Typhoid Fever Are Both Intestinal Infections

The bacterial genus *Salmonella* comprises over 1500 antigenically distinct but biochemically and genetically related gram-negative rods, which cause two important human diseases: *Salmonella* enterocolitis and typhoid fever.

Salmonella Enterocolitis

Salmonella *enterocolitis is an acute self-limited (1 to 3 days) gastrointestinal illness that manifests as nausea, vomiting, diarrhea, and fever.* The infection is typically acquired by ingestion of food contaminated with nontyphoidal *Salmonella* strains and is commonly called Salmonella *food poisoning.*

  Epidemiology: The nontyphoidal *Salmonella* infect diverse animal species, including amphibians, reptiles, birds, and mammals. They also readily contaminate foodstuffs derived from infected animals (e.g., meat, poultry, eggs, or dairy products). If these foods are not cooked, pasteurized, or irradiated, the bacteria persist and proliferate, particularly at warm temperatures. Once a person is infected, the organism can spread from person to person by fecal–oral contamination. Such spread is infrequent among adults but occurs readily among small children in day-care settings or within families. *Salmonella* enterocolitis remains a major cause of childhood mortality in less-developed countries.

Pathogenesis and Pathology: *Salmonella* proliferate in the small intestine and invade enterocytes in the distal small bowel and colon. The nontyphoidal *Salmonella* species elaborate several toxins that contribute to the dysfunction of intestinal cells. The mucosa of the ileum and colon is acutely inflamed and sometimes superficially ulcerated.

 Clinical Features: *Salmonella* enterocolitis characteristically manifests as diarrhea, beginning 12 to 48 hours after the ingestion of contaminated food. This contrasts with staphylococcal food poisoning, which is caused by a preformed toxin and begins 1 to 6 hours after the ingestion of contaminated food. The diarrhea of *Salmonella* food poisoning is self-limited, lasting from 1 to 3 days, and is often accompanied by nausea, vomiting, cramping abdominal pain, and fever. Treatment is supportive, and antibiotics rarely improve the clinical course.

Typhoid Fever

Typhoid fever is an acute systemic illness caused by infection with Salmonella typhi. *Paratyphoid fever is a clinically similar but milder disease that results from infection with other species of* Salmonella, *including* S. paratyphi. *The term* **enteric fever** *includes both typhoid and paratyphoid fever.*

 Epidemiology: Humans are the only natural reservoir for *S. typhi*, and typhoid fever is acquired from convalescing patients or from chronic carriers. The latter tend to be older women with gallstones or biliary scarring, in whom *S. typhi* colonizes the gallbladder or biliary tree. Typhoid fever is spread primarily through the ingestion of contaminated water and food, especially dairy products and shellfish. Less commonly, the organisms are disseminated by direct finger-to-mouth contact with feces, urine, or other secretions. Infected food handlers with poor personal hygiene and urine from patients with typhoidal pyelonephritis can be a significant source of infection. Typhoid fever accounts for over 25,000 annual deaths worldwide but has become uncommon in the United States.

 Pathogenesis: *S. typhi* attaches to and invades the small bowel mucosa without causing clinical enterocolitis. Invasion tends to be most prominent in the ileum in areas overlying Peyer patches, where the organisms are engulfed by macrophages. The organisms block the respiratory burst of the phagocytes and multiply within these cells. They spread first to regional lymph nodes and then throughout the body through the lymphatics and bloodstream, infecting mononuclear macrophages in lymph nodes, bone marrow, liver, and spleen. The infection of macrophages stimulates the production of IL-1 and TNF, thereby causing the prolonged fever, malaise, and wasting characteristic of typhoid fever.

 Pathology: The earliest pathological change in typhoid fever is the degeneration of the brush border of the intestinal epithelium. As bacteria invade, Peyer patches become hypertrophic. In some cases, lymphoid hyperplasia in the intestine progresses to capillary thrombosis, causing necrosis of the overlying mucosa and the characteristic ulcers oriented along the long axis of the bowel (Fig. 9-22). These gastrointestinal ulcerations frequently bleed and occasionally perforate, producing infectious peritonitis. Systemic dissemination of the organisms leads to focal granulomas in the liver, spleen, and other organs, termed **typhoid nodules.** These are composed of aggregates of macrophages ("typhoid cells") containing ingested bacteria, erythrocytes, and degenerated lymphocytes.

 Clinical Features: Prior to the antibiotic era, untreated typhoid fever was classically divided into five stages (Fig. 9-23):

- **Incubation:** (10 to 14 days)
- **Active invasion/bacteremia:** For about a week the patient suffers a variety of nonspecific symptoms, including daily stepwise elevation in temperature (up to 41°C), malaise, headache, arthralgias, and abdominal pain.

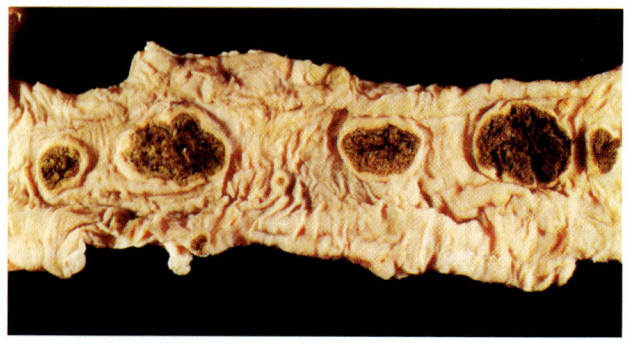

FIGURE 9-22
Ulcers of the terminal ileum in fatal typhoid fever. The ulcers have a longitudinal orientation because they are located over hyperplastic and necrotic Peyer patches.

- **Fastigium:** Fever and malaise increase over several days until the infected person is bedridden. Patients may become toxic as a consequence of the release of endotoxins from dead bacteria. Hepatomegaly is accompanied by derangements in liver function. The spleen is conspicuously enlarged.
- **Lysis:** Patients destined to survive exhibit a gradual reduction in fever, and the toxic symptoms recede. Although gastrointestinal tract bleeding and perforation of the intestine at the site of ulceration may occur in any stage, it is most common during lysis, which commonly lasts a week;
- **Convalescence:** The fever abates, and patients gradually regain strength and recover over a period of several weeks to months. Some patients relapse or have metastatic foci of infection.

The treatment of typhoid fever entails antibiotics and supportive care. Ten to 20% of untreated patients die, usually of secondary complications, such as pneumonia. However, treatment within 3 days of the onset of fever is generally curative.

Shigellosis Is an Acute Bacterial Dysentery

Shigellosis is characterized by a necrotizing infection of the distal small bowel and colon. It is caused by any of four species of *Shigella* (*S. boydii*, *S. dysenteriae*, *S. flexneri*, and *S. sonnei*), which are aerobic, gram-negative rods. Of these species, *S. dysenteriae* is the most virulent. Shigellosis is a self-limited disease that typically presents with abdominal pain and bloody, mucoid stools.

Epidemiology: *Shigella* organisms are spread from person to person by the fecal–oral route. Shigellae have no animal reservoir and do not survive well outside the stool. Therefore, infection usually occurs through ingestion of fecally contaminated food or water, but it can be acquired by oral contact with any contaminated surface (e.g., clothing, towels, or skin surfaces). As a result, endemic shigellosis is more common in populations with poor standards of hygiene and sanitation. Shigellosis is also spread in closed communities, such as hospitals, barracks, and households. In developed countries, *S. flexneri* and *S. sonnei* are more common, and infection tends to be sporadic.

In the United States, there are estimated to be 300,000 cases of shigellosis annually, but the incidence of the disease is much higher in countries lacking sanitary systems for human waste disposal. Like the other diarrheal illnesses, shigellosis is a significant cause of childhood mortality in developing countries.

Pathogenesis: Shigellae are among the most virulent enteropathogens known. Disease is produced by the ingestion of as few as 10 to 100 organisms, and there are few asymptomatic carriers. The agent proliferates rapidly in the small bowel and attaches to enterocytes, where it replicates within the cytoplasm. Endocytosis is essential to the virulence of the organism, and the factor that induces it is encoded on a plasmid. Replicating shigellae kill infected cells and spread to adjacent cells and into the lamina propria.

Shigellae also produce a potent exotoxin, known as *Shiga toxin*. Shiga toxin interferes with the 60S ribosomal subunits and thereby inhibits protein synthesis. It also causes watery diarrhea, probably by inducing a failure of fluid absorption in the colon. Although shigellae extensively damage the epithelium of the ileum and colon, they rarely invade beyond the intestinal lamina propria, and bacteremia is uncommon.

Pathology: The distal colon is almost always affected, although the entire colon and distal ileum can be involved. The affected mucosa is edematous, acutely inflamed, and focally eroded. Ulcers appear first on the edges of mucosal folds, perpendicular to the long axis of the colon. A patchy inflammatory *pseudomembrane*, composed of neutrophils, fibrin, and necrotic epithelium, is commonly found on the most severely affected areas. Regeneration of infected colonic epithelium occurs rapidly, and healing is usually complete within 10 to 14 days.

Clinical Features: Shigellosis often begins with watery diarrhea, which changes in character within 1 to 2 days to the classic dysenteric stools. These are small-volume stools that contain gross blood, sloughed pseudomembranes, and mucus. Cramping abdominal pain, tenesmus, and urgency at stool typically accompany the diarrhea. Symptoms persist for 3 to 8 days, if the disease is untreated. Treatment with antibiotics shortens the course of the illness.

Cholera Is an Epidemic Enteritis Usually Acquired from Contaminated Water

Cholera is a severe diarrheal illness caused by the enterotoxin of Vibrio cholerae, *an aerobic, curved gram-negative rod.* The organism proliferates in the lumen of the small intestine and causes profuse watery diarrhea, rapid dehydration, and (if fluids are not restored) shock and death within 24 hours of the onset of symptoms.

Epidemiology: In the 19th century, cholera was common in most parts of the world, but it periodically "disappeared" spontaneously. A major pandemic occurred between 1961 and 1974, extending throughout Asia, the Middle East, southern Russia, the Mediterranean basin, and parts of Africa. The disease remains endemic in the river deltas of India and Bangladesh, where it may cause up to a half-million deaths annually.

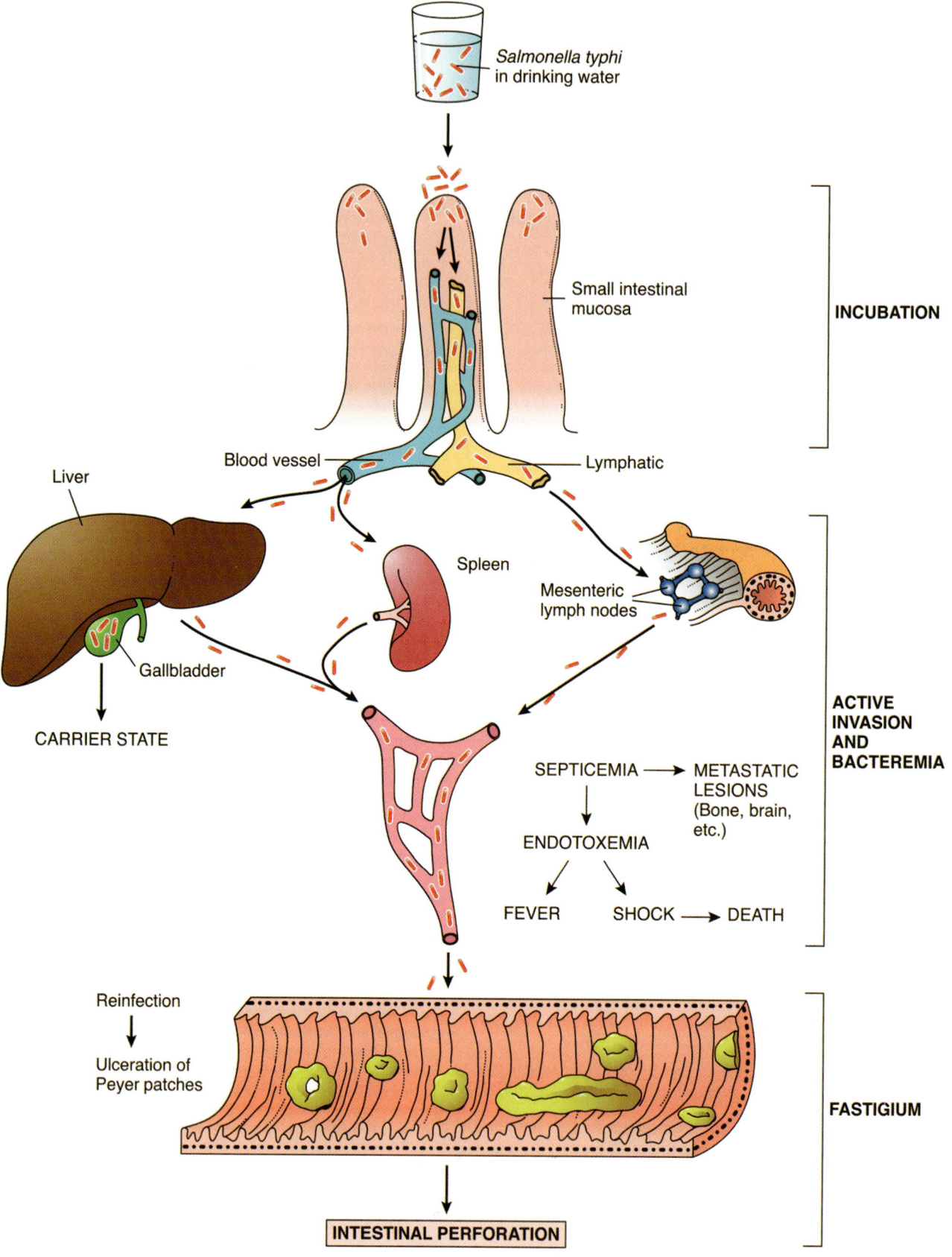

Cholera is acquired by ingesting *V. cholerae*, primarily in contaminated food or water. Epidemics spread readily in areas where human feces pollute the water supply. Shellfish and plankton may serve as a natural reservoir for the organism, and shellfish ingestion accounts for most of the sporadic cases seen in the United States.

Pathogenesis and Pathology: Bacteria that survive passage through the stomach thrive and multiply in the mucous layer of the small bowel. **They do not themselves invade the mucosa but cause diarrhea by the elaboration of a potent exotoxin, known as cholera toxin.** The toxin is composed of A and B subunits. The B subunit binds the toxin to GM$_1$ ganglioside in the cell membrane of the enterocyte. The A subunit then enters the cell, where it activates adenylyl cyclase. The consequent increase in the content of cyclic adenosine monophosphate (cAMP) results in the massive secretion of sodium and water from the enterocyte into the intestinal lumen (Fig. 9-24). The greatest fluid secretion occurs in the small bowel, where there is a net loss of water and electrolytes. *V. cholerae* causes little visible alteration in the affected intestine, which appears grossly normal or only slightly hyperemic. Microscopically, the intestinal epithelium is intact but depleted of mucus.

Clinical Features: Cholera begins with a few loose stools, usually evolving within hours into severe watery diarrhea. The stools are often flecked with mucus, imparting a "rice water" appearance. The volume of diarrhea is highly variable, but the rapidity and volume loss in severe cases can be truly staggering. With adequate volume replacement, infected adults can lose up to 20 L of fluid in a single day. Fluid and electrolyte loss can advance to shock and death within hours if fluid volume is not replaced. Untreated cholera has a 50% mortality rate. Replacement of lost salts and water is a simple, effective treatment, which can often be accomplished by oral rehydration with preparations of salt, glucose, and water. The illness subsides spontaneously in 3 to 6 days. Antibiotic therapy shortens the duration of the illness. Infection with *V. cholerae* confers long-term immunity to the development of recurrent illness, but available vaccines have limited effectiveness.

VIBRIO PARAHAEMOLYTICUS: There are a number of so-called noncholera vibrios, of which *V. parahaemolyticus* is the most common. This organism is a gram-negative bacillus that causes acute gastroenteritis. It is found in marine life and coastal waters around the world in temperate climates, causing outbreaks in the summer. Gastroenteritis is associated with the consumption of inadequately cooked or poorly refrigerated seafood. The clinical syndrome resembles *Salmonella* enteritis, and no deaths have been reported.

Campylobacter jejuni Is the Most Common Cause of Bacterial Diarrhea in the Developed World

C. jejuni is the major human pathogen in the genus Campylobacter *and causes an acute, self-limited inflammatory diarrheal illness.* The organism is distributed worldwide and causes over 2 million cases annually in the United States. *C. jejuni* is a microaerophilic, curved gram-negative rod, morphologically similar to the vibrios.

Epidemiology: *C. jejuni* infection is acquired through contaminated food or water. The bacteria inhabit the gastrointestinal tracts of diverse animal species, including cows, sheep, chickens, and dogs, which constitute a significant animal reservoir for infection. In fact, *Campylobacter* infections cause serious economic losses to farmers because of abortions and infertility of infected cattle and sheep. Raw milk and inadequately cooked poultry and meat are frequent sources of disease. *C. jejuni* can also spread from person to person by fecal–oral contact. The organism is a major cause of childhood mortality in developing countries and is responsible for many cases of "travelers' diarrhea."

FIGURE 9-23
Stages of typhoid fever.
Incubation (10–14 days). Water or food contaminated with *S. typhi* is ingested. Bacilli attach to the villi in the small intestine, invade the mucosa, and pass to the intestinal lymphoid follicles and draining mesenteric lymph nodes. The organisms proliferate further within mononuclear phagocytic cells of the lymphoid follicles, lymph nodes, liver, and spleen. Bacilli are sequestered intracellularly in the intestinal and mesenteric lymphatic system.

Active invasion/bacteremia (1 week). Organisms are released and produce a transient bacteremia. The intestinal mucosa becomes enlarged and necrotic, forming characteristic mucosal lesions. The intestinal lymphoid tissues become hyperplastic and contain "typhoid nodules"—aggregates of macrophages ("typhoid cells") that phagocytose bacteria, erythrocytes, and degenerated lymphocytes. Bacilli proliferate in several organs, reappear in the intestine, are excreted in stool, and may invade through the intestinal wall. **Fastigium (1 week).** Dying bacilli release endotoxins that cause systemic toxemia.

Lysis (1 week). Necrotic intestinal mucosa sloughs, producing ulcers, which hemorrhage or perforate into the peritoneal cavity.

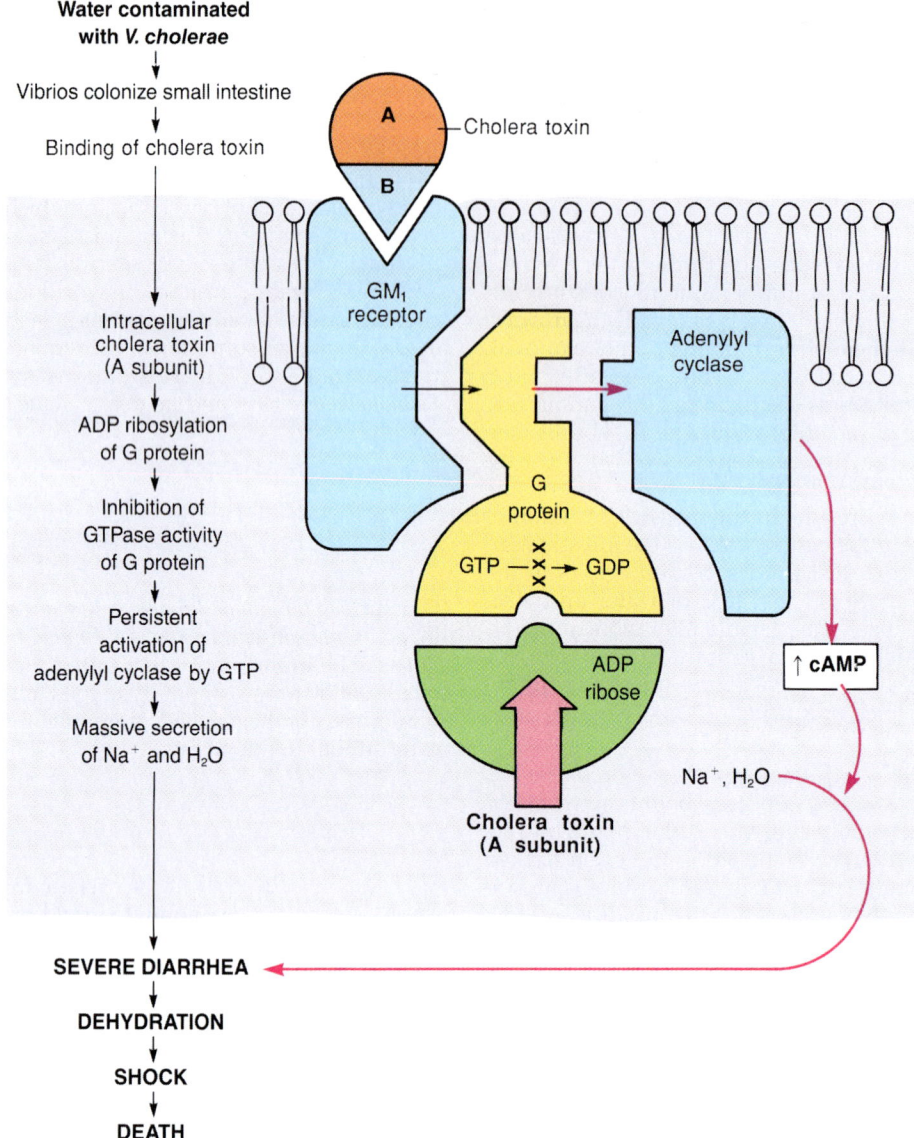

FIGURE 9-24
Cholera. Infection comes from water contaminated with *Vibrio cholerae* or food prepared with contaminated water. Vibrios traverse the stomach, enter the small intestine, and propagate. Although they do not invade the intestinal mucosa, vibrios elaborate a potent toxin that induces a massive outpouring of water and electrolytes. Severe diarrhea ("ricewater stool") leads to dehydration and hypovolemic shock.

Pathogenesis: Ingested *C. jejuni* organisms that survive gastric acidity multiply in the alkaline environment of the upper small intestine. The agent elaborates several toxic proteins that correlate with the severity of the symptoms.

Pathology: *C. jejuni* causes a superficial enterocolitis, primarily involving the terminal ileum and colon, with focal necrosis of the intestinal epithelium, accompanied by an acute inflammatory infiltrate. In severe cases, it progresses to small ulcers and patchy inflammatory exudates (pseudomembranes) composed of necrotic cells, neutrophils, fibrin, and debris. The crypts of the colonic epithelium often fill with neutrophils, forming so-called crypt abscesses. These pathological changes resolve in 7 to 14 days.

Clinical Features: Patients with *C. jejuni* usually produce more than 10 stools per day, varying from profuse watery stools to small-volume stools containing gross blood and mucus. The symptoms resolve in 5 to 7 days. Treatment with antibiotics is probably of marginal benefit. A few patients develop a more severe, protracted illness resembling acute ulcerative colitis.

Yersinia Infections Produce Painful Diarrhea

Y. enterocolitica and *Y. pseudotuberculosis* are gram-negative coccoid or rod-shaped bacteria.

 Epidemiology: These organisms are facultative anaerobes found in the feces of wild and domestic animals, including rodents, sheep, cattle, dogs, cats, and horses. *Y. pseudotuberculosis* is also commonly encountered in domestic birds, including turkeys, ducks, geese, and canaries. Both organisms have been isolated from drinking water and milk. *Y. enterocolitica* is more likely to be acquired from contaminated meat, and *Y. pseudotuberculosis* from contact with infected animals.

 Pathology and Clinical Features: *Y. enterocolitica* proliferates in the ileum, invades the mucosa, produces ulceration and necrosis of Peyer patches, and migrates by way of the lymphatics to the mesenteric lymph nodes. Fever, diarrhea (sometimes bloody), and abdominal pain begin 4 to 10 days after penetration of the mucosa. Abdominal pain in the right lower quadrant has led to an incorrect diagnosis of appendicitis. Arthralgia, arthritis, and erythema nodosum are complications. Septicemia is an uncommon sequel but kills about one half of those affected.

Y. pseudotuberculosis penetrates the ileal mucosa, localizes in ileal–cecal lymph nodes, and produces abscesses and granulomas in the lymph nodes, spleen, and liver. Fever, diarrhea, and abdominal pain may also lead to an erroneous diagnosis of appendicitis.

PULMONARY INFECTIONS WITH GRAM-NEGATIVE BACTERIA

Klebsiella and *Enterobacter* Produce Nosocomial Infections That Cause Necrotizing Lobar Pneumonia

Klebsiella and *Enterobacter* species are short, encapsulated, gram-negative bacilli.

 Epidemiology: These organisms cause 10% of all infections acquired in the hospital, including pneumonia and infections of the urinary tract, biliary tract, and surgical wounds. Person-to-person transmission by hospital personnel is a special hazard. Predisposing factors are obstructive pulmonary disease in endotracheal tubes, indwelling catheters, debilitating conditions, and immunosuppression. Secondary pneumonia caused by these bacteria may complicate influenza or other viral infections of the respiratory tract.

 Pathology: *Klebsiella* and *Enterobacter* species are inhaled and multiply within the alveolar spaces. The pulmonary parenchyma becomes consolidated, and the mucoid exudate that fills the alveoli is dominated by macrophages, fibrin, and edema fluid. As the exudate accumulates, the alveolar walls become compressed and then necrotic. Numerous small abscesses may coalesce and lead to cavitation.

 Clinical Features: The onset of pneumonia is sudden, with fever, pleuritic pain, cough, and a **characteristic thick mucoid sputum.** When infection is severe, these symptoms progress to dyspnea, cyanosis, and death in 2 to 3 days. *Klebsiella* and *Enterobacter* infections may be complicated by a fulminating, often fatal, septicemia, and aggressive antibiotic therapy is required.

Legionnaires Disease (Legionellosis) Is a Noncontagious Environmental Hazard

Legionella species cause pneumonia that ranges from a relatively mild disease to a severe, life-threatening necrotizing pneumonia, known as Legionnaires disease. L. pneumophila is a minute aerobic bacillus that has the cell wall structure of a gram-negative organism but reacts poorly with Gram stains. Six months after an outbreak of a severe respiratory disease of unknown cause at the 1976 state convention of the American Legion in Philadelphia, *L. pneumophila* was first identified by the Centers for Disease Control and Prevention. Subsequently, retrospective studies demonstrated antibodies in sera from previously unexplained epidemics, dating to 1957.

 Epidemiology: *Legionella* is present in small numbers in natural bodies of fresh water. It survives chlorination and proliferates in devices such as cooling towers, water heaters, humidifiers, and evaporative condensers. Infection occurs when persons inhale aerosols from contaminated sources. Legionnaires disease is not contagious, and the organism is not part of the normal human oropharyngeal flora. There are an estimated 75,000 cases of *Legionella* infection in the United States annually.

 Pathogenesis: *Legionella* causes two distinct diseases, namely, pneumonia and *Pontiac fever.* The pathogenesis of *Legionella* pneumonia (Legionnaires disease) is understood in some detail, whereas that of Pontiac fever remains largely a mystery. *Legionella* pneumonia begins with the arrival of the organisms in the terminal bronchioles or alveoli, where they are phagocytosed by alveolar macrophages. The bacteria replicate within the phagosomes and protect themselves by blocking the fusion of lysosomes with the phagosomes. The multiplying *Legionella* are released and infect freshly arriving macrophages. When immunity develops, macrophages are activated and cease to support intracellular growth of the organisms.

The native respiratory tract defenses, such as the mucociliary blanket of the airway, provide a first line of defense against lower respiratory tract *Legionella* infection. Smoking, alcoholism, and chronic lung diseases, which interfere with respiratory defenses, increase the risks of developing *Legionella* pneumonia.

Pathology: Legionnaires disease is an acute bronchopneumonia, usually patchy but sometimes with a lobar pattern of infiltration. Affected alveoli and bronchioles are filled with an exudate composed of proteinaceous fluid, fibrin, macrophages, neutrophils (Fig. 9-25), and microabscesses. The alveolar walls become necrotic and are destroyed. Many macrophages show eccentric nuclei, pushed aside by cytoplasmic vacuoles containing *L. pneumophila*. With resolution of the pneumonia, the lungs heal with little permanent damage.

Clinical Features: After an incubation of 2 to 10 days, the clinical onset is characterized by a rapidly progressive pneumonia, accompanied by fever, a nonproductive cough, and myalgia. Chest radiographs reveal unilateral, diffuse, patchy consolidation, progressing to widespread nodular consolidation. Toxic symptoms, hypoxia, and obtundation may be prominent, and death may follow within a few days. In those who survive, convalescence is prolonged. The mortality rate among hospitalized patients averages 15%, although there is a much greater risk of death among persons with serious underlying illness. Erythromycin is the antibiotic of choice.

Pontiac fever is a self-limited, flulike illness with fever, malaise, myalgias, and headache. It differs from Legionnaires disease in showing no evidence of pulmonary consolidation. The disease resolves spontaneously in 3 to 5 days.

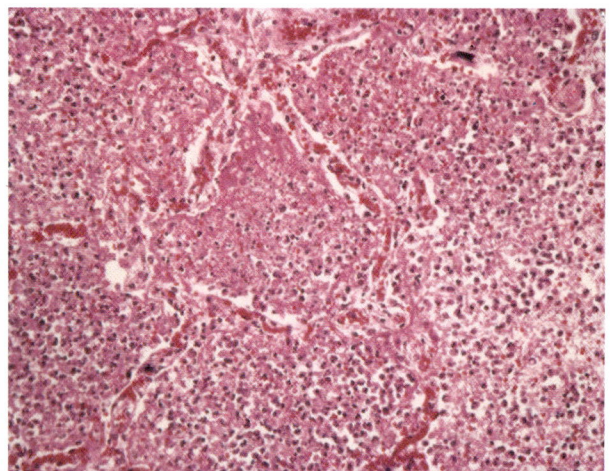

FIGURE 9-25
Legionnaires pneumonia. The alveoli are packed with an exudate composed of fibrin, macrophages, and neutrophils.

Pseudomonas aeruginosa, a Hospital-Acquired Pathogen, Is Among the Most Antibiotic-Resistant Bacteria

Pseudomonas aeruginosa is a major opportunistic pathogen. The organism only infrequently infects humans. However, it can cause disease, particularly in the hospital environment, where it is associated with pneumonia, wound infections, urinary tract disease, and sepsis in debilitated persons. Burns, urinary catheterization, cystic fibrosis, diabetes, and neutropenia all predispose to infection with *P. aeruginosa*.

P. aeruginosa is a ubiquitous aerobic, gram-negative rod that requires moisture and only minimal nutrients. It thrives in soil and water, on animals, and on moist environmental surfaces. **Antibiotic use tends to select for *P. aeruginosa* infection, since the organism is resistant to most antibiotics.**

Pathogenesis: *P. aeruginosa* elaborates an array of proteins that allow it to attach to, invade, and destroy host tissues, while avoiding host inflammatory and immune defenses. Injury to epithelial cells uncovers surface molecules that serve as binding sites for the pili of *P. aeruginosa*. Many strains of *P. aeruginosa* produce a proteoglycan that surrounds the bacteria and protects them from mucociliary action, complement, and phagocytes. The organism releases extracellular enzymes, including an elastase, an alkaline protease, and a cytotoxin, which facilitate tissue invasion and are partially responsible for the necrotizing lesions of *Pseudomonas* infections. The elastase is probably responsible for the distinctive ability of *P. aeruginosa* to invade blood vessel walls. The organism also produces systemic pathological effects through endotoxin and several systemically active exotoxins.

Pathology: *Pseudomonas* infection produces an acute inflammatory response. The organism often invades small arteries and veins, producing vascular thrombosis and hemorrhagic necrosis, particularly in the lungs and skin. Blood vessel invasion predisposes to dissemination and sepsis and leads to the development of multiple nodular lesions in the lungs. Gram stains of necrotic tissue infected with *Pseudomonas* commonly show blood vessel walls densely infiltrated with organisms. Sometimes disseminated infections are marked by the development of typical skin lesions called **ecthyma gangrenosum.** These nodular, necrotic lesions represent sites where the organism has disseminated to the skin, invaded blood vessels, and produced localized hemorrhagic infarctions.

Clinical Features: *Pseudomonas* infections are among the most aggressive human bacterial diseases, often progressing rapidly to sepsis. They require immediate medical intervention and are associated with high mortality.

Melioidosis Features Abscesses in Many Organs

Melioidosis (Rangoon beggars disease) is an uncommon disease caused by Pseudomonas pseudomallei, *a small gram-negative bacillus in the soil and surface water of Southeast Asia and other tropical areas.* During the conflict in Vietnam, several hundred servicemen acquired melioidosis. The organism flourishes in wet environments, such as rice paddies and marshes. The skin is the usual portal of entry, and organisms enter through preexisting lesions, including penetrating wounds and burns. Humans may also be infected by inhaling contaminated dust or aerosolized droplets. The incubation period may last months to years, and the clinical course is variable.

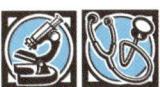

Pathology and Clinical Features: *Acute melioidosis is a pulmonary infection, ranging from a mild tracheobronchitis to an overwhelming cavitary pneumonia* (Fig. 9-26). Patients with severe cases present with the sudden onset of high fever, constitutional symptoms, and a cough that may produce blood-stained sputum. Splenomegaly, hepatomegaly, and jaundice are sometimes present. Diarrhea may be as severe as that in cholera. Fulminating septicemia, shock, coma, and death may develop in spite of antibiotic therapy. Acute septicemic melioidosis causes discrete abscesses throughout the body, especially in the lungs, liver, spleen, and lymph nodes.

Chronic melioidosis is a persistent localized infection involving the lungs, skin, bones, or other organs. The lesions are suppurative or granulomatous abscesses and in the lung may be mistaken for tuberculosis. Chronic melioidosis may lie dormant for months or years, only to appear suddenly—hence the colloquial name "Vietnamese time bomb."

CLOSTRIDIAL DISEASES

Clostridia are gram-positive, spore-forming bacilli that are obligate anaerobes. The vegetative bacilli are found in the gastrointestinal tract of herbivorous animals and humans.

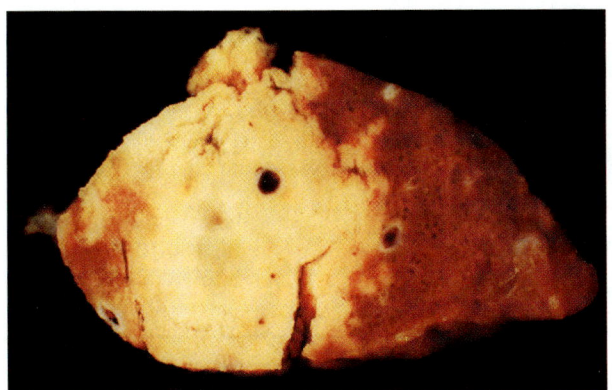

FIGURE 9-26
Acute melioidosis. The lung is consolidated and necrotic.

Anaerobic conditions promote vegetative division, whereas aerobic ones lead to sporulation. Spores pass in animal feces and contaminate soil and plants, where they survive unfavorable environmental circumstances. Under anaerobic conditions, the spores revert to vegetative cells, thereby completing the cycle. During sporulation, vegetative cells degenerate and their plasmids produce a variety of specific toxins that cause widely differing diseases, depending on the species (Fig. 9-27).

- **Food poisoning and necrotizing enteritis (pigbel)** are caused by the enterotoxins of *Clostridium perfringens*.
- **Gas gangrene** is produced by the myotoxins of *C. perfringens*, *C. novyi*, *C. septicum*, and other species.
- **Tetanus** is related to the neurotoxin of *C. tetani*.
- **Botulism** results from the action of the neurotoxin of *C. botulinum*.
- **Pseudomembranous enterocolitis** reflects the action of the exotoxins of *C. difficile*.

Clostridial Food Poisoning Is Self-Limited

Clostridium perfringens is one of the most common causes of bacterial food poisoning in the world, characterized by an acute, generally benign, diarrheal disease, usually lasting less than 24 hours. It is omnipresent in the environment, contaminating soil, water, air samples, clothing, dust, and meat.

Spores of *C. perfringens* survive cooking temperatures and germinate to yield vegetative forms, which proliferate when food is allowed to stand without refrigeration. Cooking drives out enough air to make the food anaerobic, a condition that is conducive to growth but not to sporulation. As a result, the contaminated food contains the vegetative clostridia but little preformed enterotoxin. The vegetative bacteria sporulate in the small bowel, where they elaborate a variety of exotoxins, which are cytotoxic to enterocytes and cause the loss of intracellular ions and fluid. Certain types of food, including meats, gravies, and sauces, are ideal substrates for *C. perfringens*. Clostridial food poisoning presents as abdominal cramping and watery diarrhea. Symptoms begin 8 to 24 hours after the ingestion of contaminated food and usually resolve within 24 hours.

Necrotizing Enteritis Is a Catastrophic Childhood Infection in New Guinea

Clostridium perfringens type C also produces an enterotoxin that causes a necrotizing enterocolitis. The illness is seldom encountered in the industrialized world but is still endemic in the highlands of New Guinea, especially in children who have participated in pig feasts (hence the pidgin term *pigbel*).

Pathogenesis: Spit roasting of pig carcasses encourages the growth of *C. perfringens*. Adults tend not to develop pigbel, because they have circulating antibodies. The normal diet of the children is derived principally from sweet potatoes. The combination of protein malnutrition and the presence of a trypsin inhibitor in sweet potatoes renders the children deficient in intestinal

398 Infectious and Parasitic Diseases

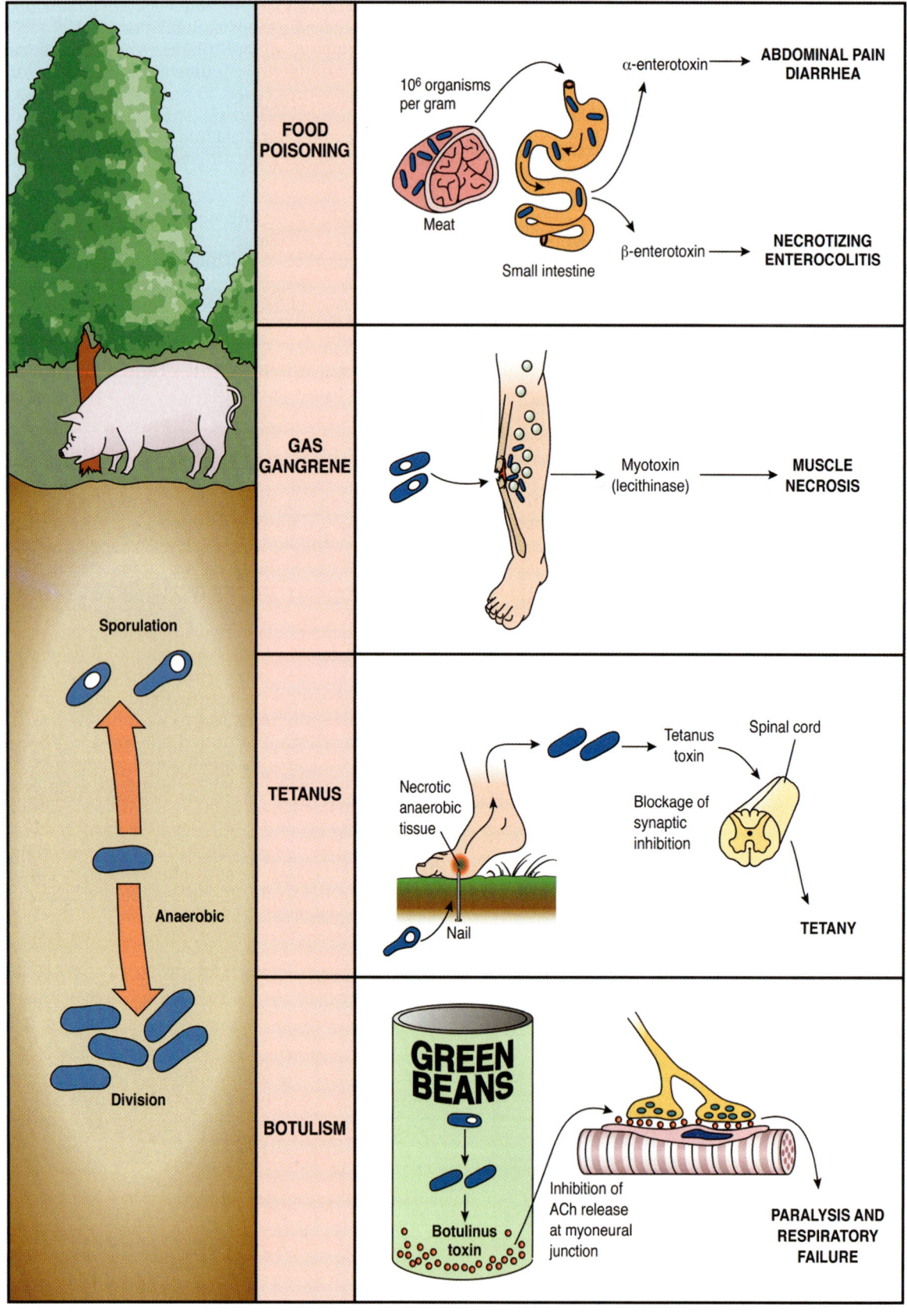

proteases, to which the enterotoxin of *C. perfringens* is very sensitive.

 Pathology: Necrotizing enteritis is a segmental disease that may be restricted to a few centimeters or may involve the entire small intestine. Green, necrotic pseudomembranes are seen in segmental areas of necrosis and peritonitis. More-advanced lesions perforate the bowel wall. Histological sections reveal infarction of the intestinal mucosa, with edema, hemorrhage, and a suppurative transmural infiltrate.

 Clinical Features: About 48 hours after the ingestion of contaminated meat, children exhibit severe abdominal pain and distention, vomiting, and passage of bloody or black stools. Some patients die within 24 hours of onset; others have mild gastroenteritis. Half of patients require segmental resection of the bowel. Passive immunization with specific antitoxin and active immunization with a pigbel toxoid vaccine reduce morbidity and mortality.

Gas Gangrene May Complicate Penetrating Wounds

Gas gangrene (clostridial myonecrosis) is a necrotizing, gas-forming infection that begins in contaminated wounds and spreads rapidly to adjacent tissues. The disease can be fatal within hours of onset. *C. perfringens* is the most common cause of gas gangrene, but other clostridial species occasionally produce the disease.

 Pathogenesis: Gas gangrene follows the deposition of *C. perfringens* into tissue under anaerobic conditions. The anaerobic conditions necessary to foster clostridial growth obtain only in the presence of extensive devitalized tissue, such as occurs with severe trauma, wartime injuries, and septic abortions. Clostridial myonecrosis is rare when wounds are subjected to prompt and thorough debridement of traumatized tissue.

The necrosis of previously healthy muscle is caused by myotoxins elaborated by a few species of clostridia. *C. perfringens* type A is the most common source of myotoxin (80–90% of cases), but myotoxin may also be produced by *C. novyi* and *C. septicum*. Clostridial myotoxin is a phospholipase that destroys the membranes of muscle cells, leukocytes, and erythrocytes.

 Pathology: Affected tissues rapidly become mottled and then frankly necrotic. Tissues such as muscle may even liquefy. The overlying skin becomes tense, as edema and gas expand the underlying soft tissues. Microscopic examination shows extensive tissue necrosis with dissolution of the normal cellular architecture. A striking feature is the paucity of neutrophils, which are apparently destroyed by the myotoxin. Gram stain of affected tissues often shows typical, lozenge-shaped, gram-positive rods.

 Clinical Features: The incubation period of gas gangrene is commonly 2 to 4 days after injury. Sudden, severe pain occurs at the site of the wound, which is tender and edematous. The skin darkens, because of hemorrhage and cutaneous necrosis. The lesion develops a

FIGURE 9-27

Clostridial diseases. Clostridia in the vegetative form (bacilli) inhabit the gastrointestinal tract of humans and animals. Spores pass in the feces, contaminate soil and plant materials, and are ingested or enter sites of penetrating wounds. Under anaerobic conditions they revert to vegetative forms. Plasmids in the vegetative forms elaborate toxins that cause several clostridial diseases.

Food poisoning and necrotizing enteritis. Meat dishes left to cool at room temperature grow large numbers of clostridia (>10^6 organisms per gram). When contaminated meat is ingested, *C. perfringens* types A and C produce α enterotoxin in the small intestine during sporulation, causing abdominal pain and diarrhea. Type C also produces β enterotoxin.

Gas gangrene. Clostridia are widespread and may contaminate a traumatic wound or surgical operation. *C. perfringens* type A elaborates a myotoxin (α toxin), a lecithinase that destroys cell membranes, alters capillary permeability, and causes severe hemolysis following intravenous injection. The toxin causes necrosis of previously healthy skeletal muscle.

Tetanus. Spores of *C. tetani* are in soil and enter the site of an accidental wound. Necrotic tissue at the wound site causes spores to revert to the vegetative form (bacilli). Autolysis of vegetative forms releases tetanus toxin. The toxin is transported in peripheral nerves and (retrograde) through axons to the anterior horn cells of the spinal cord. The toxin blocks synaptic inhibition, and the accumulation of acetylcholine in damaged synapses leads to rigidity and spasms of the skeletal musculature (tetany).

Botulism. Improperly canned food is contaminated by the vegetative form of *C. botulinum*, which proliferates under aerobic conditions and elaborates a neurotoxin. After the food is ingested, the neurotoxin is absorbed from the small intestine and eventually reaches the myoneural junction, where it inhibits the release of acetylcholine. The result is a symmetric descending paralysis of cranial nerves, trunk, and limbs, with eventual respiratory paralysis and death.

thick, serosanguineous discharge, which has a fragrant odor and may contain gas bubbles. Hemolytic anemia, hypotension, and renal failure may develop, and in the terminal stages, coma, jaundice, and shock supervene.

Tetanus Reflects the Release of a Bacterial Neurotoxin

Tetanus is a severe, acute neurological syndrome of humans and other mammals caused by tetanus toxin, an extremely potent neurotoxin elaborated by plasmids of C. tetani. *The disease is characterized by spastic contractions of skeletal muscles. It is also known as "lockjaw" because of early involvement of the muscles of mastication.*

 Epidemiology: C. tetani is present in the soil and the lower intestine of many animals. Tetanus occurs when the organism contaminates wounds and proliferates in tissue, releasing its exotoxin. Using a vaccine composed of inactivated tetanus toxin, immunization programs have largely eliminated the disease from developed countries. Nonetheless, tetanus remains a frequent and lethal disease in developing countries. Many deaths occur in newborns in primitive societies, owing to the custom of coating the umbilical stump with dirt or dung to prevent bleeding.

 Pathogenesis: At the site of injury, necrotic tissue and suppuration contribute to creating an anaerobic environment, a condition that causes spores to revert to vegetative cells. Tetanus toxin is released from autolyzed vegetative cells. Although the clostridial infection remains localized, the potent neurotoxin *(tetanospasmin)* undergoes retrograde transport through the ventral roots of peripheral nerves to the anterior horn cells of the spinal cord. The toxin crosses the synapse and binds to ganglioside receptors on presynaptic terminals of motor neurons in the ventral horns. Following internalization, the endopeptidase activity of the toxin selectively cleaves a protein responsible for the exocytosis of synaptic vesicles. As a result, the release of inhibitory neurotransmitters is blocked, thereby permitting unopposed neural stimulation and sustained contraction of skeletal muscles (tetany). The block to the release of inhibitory neurotransmitters also induces heart rate acceleration, hypertension, and cardiovascular instability.

 Clinical Features: The incubation period of tetanus is 1 to 3 weeks. The disease begins subtly with fatigue, weakness, and muscle cramping that progresses to muscle rigidity. Spastic rigidity often begins in the muscles of the face, giving rise to lockjaw, which extends to several facial muscles, causing a fixed grin *(risus sardonicus)*. Rigidity of the muscles of the back produces a backward arching *(opisthotonos)* (Fig. 9-28). Abrupt stimuli, including noise, light, or touch, can precipitate painful generalized muscle spasms. Prolonged spasm of the respiratory and laryngeal musculature may lead to death. Infants

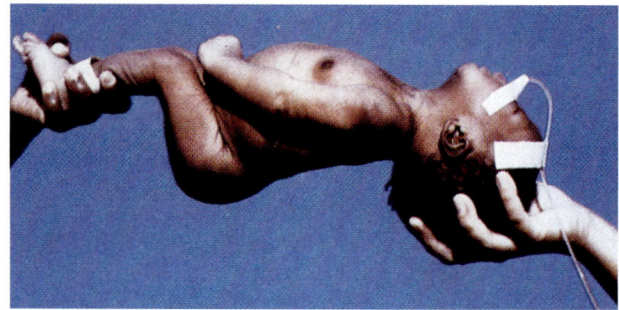

FIGURE 9-28
Tetanus. Opisthotonus (backward arching) in an infant due to intense contraction of the paravertebral muscles.

and persons older than 50 years of age have the highest mortality.

Botulism Follows the Ingestion of Food Containing Preformed Neurotoxins

Botulism is a paralyzing illness that involves C. botulinum. *The disease is characterized by a symmetric descending paralysis of cranial nerves, limbs, and trunk.*

 Epidemiology: The spores of *C. botulinum* are widely distributed and are especially resistant to drying and boiling. **In the United States, the toxin is most commonly present in vegetables or other foods that have been improperly home canned and stored without refrigeration. These circumstances provide suitable anaerobic conditions for the growth of the vegetative cells that elaborate the neurotoxins (A–G).** Botulism can also be contracted from home-cured ham and other meats that have been left unrefrigerated for several days and from raw, smoked, and fermented fish products. The disease is also caused by the absorption of toxin from organisms proliferating in the intestine of infants *(infantile botulism)* or rarely by the absorption of toxin from organisms growing in contaminated wounds *(wound botulism)*.

 Pathogenesis: After food containing botulinum neurotoxin is ingested, the toxin resists gastric digestion and is readily absorbed into the blood from the proximal small intestine. Circulating toxin reaches the cholinergic nerve endings at the myoneural junction and binds to gangliosides of the presynaptic nerve terminals. In this location, it inhibits the release of acetylcholine to produce a flaccid paralysis.

 Clinical Features: Botulism is characterized by a descending paralysis, first affecting the cranial nerves and beginning with blurred vision, photophobia, dry mouth, and dysarthria. Weakness progresses to involve the neck muscles, extremities, diaphragm, and accessory muscles of breathing. Respiratory weakness can progress rapidly to complete respiratory arrest and death. Untreated botulism is usually lethal, but treatment with antitoxin reduces the mortality to 25%.

Clostridium difficile Colitis Follows Antibiotic Treatment

C. difficile colitis is an acute necrotizing infection of the terminal small bowel and colon. It is responsible for a large fraction (25–50%) of the antibiotic-associated diarrheas and is potentially lethal.

Epidemiology: *C. difficile* resides in the colon in some healthy persons. A change in intestinal flora, usually precipitated by antibiotic administration, allows the organism to flourish, produce toxin, and damage the colonic mucosa. Such colitis can also be precipitated by other insults to the colonic flora, such as bowel surgery, dietary changes, and antineoplastic chemotherapeutic agents. In hospitals where many patients receive antibiotics, fecal shedding of the organism results in person-to-person spread.

Pathogenesis: As mentioned above, the colonic bacteria ordinarily prevent the pathogenic action of *C. difficile*, but alterations in the normal flora permit the organism to proliferate, elaborate toxins, and destroy mucosal cells. The bacterium does not invade the colonic mucosa but rather produces two exotoxins. Toxin A causes fluid secretion; toxin B is directly cytopathic.

Pathology: *C. difficile* destroys colonic mucosal cells and incites an acute inflammatory infiltrate. Lesions range from focal colitis limited to a few crypts and only detectable on biopsy, to massive confluent mucosal ulceration. The inflammatory infiltrate initially involves only the mucosa, but if the disease progresses, it can extend into the submucosa and muscularis propria. An inflammatory exudate, called a "pseudomembrane," often forms over affected areas of the colon. This membrane is composed of cellular debris, neutrophils, and fibrin. *C. difficile* colitis is often called *pseudomembranous colitis,* even though this organism is only one of several causes of this condition.

Clinical Features: *C. difficile* colitis may present with very mild symptoms or with diarrhea, fever, and abdominal pain. Stools may be profuse and often contain neutrophils. The symptoms and signs are not specific and do not distinguish *C. difficile* colitis from other acute inflammatory diarrheal illnesses. Mild cases of *C. difficile* diarrhea can often be treated simply by discontinuing the precipitating antibiotic. More-severe cases require treatment with an antibiotic effective against *C. difficile*.

BACTERIA WITH ANIMAL RESERVOIRS OR INSECT VECTORS

Brucellosis Is a Chronic Febrile Disease Acquired from Domestic Animals

Brucellosis is a zoonotic disease caused by one of four Brucella *species. Human brucellosis may manifest as an acute systemic disease or as a chronic infection characterized by waxing and waning febrile episodes, weight loss, and fatigue.* Brucella *species are small, aerobic, gram-negative rods that in humans primarily infect monocytes/macrophages.*

Epidemiology: Each species of *Brucella* has its own animal reservoir:

- *B. melitensis:* sheep and goats
- *B. abortus:* cattle
- *B. suis:* swine
- *B. canis:* dogs

Brucellosis is encountered worldwide, and virtually every type of domesticated animal and many wild ones are affected. The organisms reside in the genitourinary systems of animals, and infection is often endemic in animal herds. Humans acquire the bacteria by several mechanisms, including (1) contact with infected blood or tissue, (2) ingestion of contaminated meat or milk, or (3) inhalation of contaminated aerosols. Brucellosis is an occupational hazard among ranchers, herders, veterinarians, and slaughterhouse workers.

Elimination of infected animals and vaccination of herds have reduced the incidence of brucellosis in many countries, including the United States, where only about 200 cases are reported annually. Yet, the disease remains prevalent throughout Central and South America, Africa, Asia, and Southern Europe. Unpasteurized milk and cheese remain a major source of infection in these areas. In the arctic and subarctic regions, humans acquire brucellosis by eating raw bone marrow of infected reindeer.

Pathology: Bacteria enter the circulation through skin abrasions, the conjunctiva, oropharynx, or lungs. They then spread in the bloodstream to the liver, spleen, lymph nodes, and bone marrow, where they multiply in macrophages. Generalized hyperplasia of these cells may ensue, causing lymphadenopathy and hepatosplenomegaly in 15% of patients infected with *B. melitensis* and in 40% of those infected with *B. abortus*. Patients infected with *B. abortus* develop conspicuous noncaseating granulomas in the liver, spleen, lymph nodes, and bone marrow. By contrast, classic granulomas are not present in patients infected with *B. melitensis*, who may have only small aggregates of mononuclear inflammatory cells scattered throughout the liver. *B. suis* infection may cause suppurative liver abscesses rather than granulomas. The organisms usually cannot be demonstrated histologically. Periodic release of organisms from infected phagocytic cells may be responsible for the febrile episodes of the illness.

Clinical Features: Brucellosis is a systemic infection that can involve any organ or organ system of the body, with an insidious onset in half of cases. The disease is characterized by a multitude of somatic complaints, such as fever, sweats, anorexia, fatigue, weight loss, and depression. Fever occurs in all patients at some time during the illness, but it can wax and wane (hence the term *undulant fever*) over a period of weeks to months when untreated. The mortality rate from brucellosis is less than 1%; death is usually caused by endocarditis.

The most common complications of brucellosis involve the bones and joints and include spondylitis of the lumbar spine and suppuration in large joints. Peripheral neuritis, meningitis, orchitis, endocarditis, myocarditis, and pulmonary lesions are described. Prolonged treatment with tetracycline is usually effective; the relapse rate is dramatically reduced if rifampin or an aminoglycoside is added.

Plague Was Responsible for Devastating Epidemics of the "Black Death"

Yersinia pestis *causes plague, a bacteremic infection that is usually accompanied by enlarged, painful regional lymph nodes (buboes) and is often fatal.* Historically, the disease was the scourge of the civilized world. *Y. pestis* is a short gram-negative rod that tends to stain more heavily at the ends (i.e., bipolar staining), particularly with Giemsa stains.

Epidemiology: *Y. pestis* infection is an endemic zoonosis in many parts of the world, including the Americas, Africa, and Asia. The organisms are found in wild rodents, such as rats, squirrels, and prairie dogs. Fleas transmit the bacterium from animal to animal, and most human infections result from the bites of infected fleas. Some infected humans develop plague pneumonia, shedding large numbers of organisms in aerosolized respiratory secretions. Infection can be transmitted from person to person in these respiratory aerosols.

Major plague epidemics have occurred when *Y. pestis* was introduced into large urban rat populations in crowded, squalid cities. Infection spreads first among the rats; as the rats die, large numbers of infected fleas begin feeding on the human population, causing widespread disease. Spread from rats to persons, the "black death" of the mid-14th century killed over one fourth of the European population.

Plague still occurs as sporadic cases throughout endemic areas. In the United States, 30 to 40 cases of plague occur annually, most in the desert southwest.

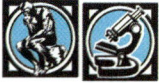

Pathogenesis and Pathology: After inoculation into the skin, *Y. pestis* is phagocytosed by neutrophils and macrophages. Organisms ingested by neutrophils are killed, but those engulfed by macrophages survive and replicate intracellularly. The bacteria are carried to regional lymph nodes, where they continue to multiply, producing extensive hemorrhagic necrosis. From the regional lymph nodes, they disseminate throughout the body through the bloodstream and lymphatics. In the lungs, *Y. pestis* produces a necrotizing pneumonitis that releases organisms into the alveoli and airways. These are expelled by coughing, enabling pneumonic spread of the disease.

Affected lymph nodes, known as "buboes," are frequently enlarged and fluctuant, owing to extensive hemorrhagic necrosis. Microscopic examination shows irregular zones of cytolysis with large numbers of bacteria in cellular debris. In plague pneumonia, the consolidation can be patchy or diffuse. Microscopically, the affected portions of the lung show hemorrhagic necrosis of alveolar walls, and large numbers of bacteria are apparent within the alveoli. Infected patients often develop necrotic, hemorrhagic skin lesions, hence the name "black death" for this disease.

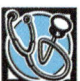

Clinical Features: There are three clinical presentations of *Y. pestis* infection, although they often overlap.

Bubonic plague begins within 2 to 8 days of the flea bite, with headache, fever, and myalgias, accompanied by painful enlargement of regional lymph nodes, most commonly those of the groin, because flea bites usually occur in the lower extremities. The disease progresses to septic shock within hours to days after the appearance of the bubo.

Septicemic plague (10% of cases) occurs when bacteria are inoculated directly into the blood and do not produce buboes. Patients die of the overwhelming growth of the bacteria in the bloodstream. Fever, prostration, and meningitis occur suddenly, and death ensues within 48 hours. All blood vessels contain bacilli, and fibrin casts surround the organisms in renal glomeruli and dermal vessels.

Pneumonic plague results from the inhalation of airborne particles from the carcasses of animals or the cough of infected persons. Within 2 to 5 days after infection, there is a sudden onset of high fever, cough, and dyspnea. The sputum teems with bacilli. Respiratory insufficiency and endotoxic shock kill the patient within 1 to 2 days.

All types of plague carry a high mortality rate (50–75%) if untreated. Tetracycline combined with streptomycin is the recommended therapy.

Tularemia Is an Acute Febrile, Granulomatous Disease Acquired from Rabbits

Tularemia is caused by Francisella tularensis, *a small, gram-negative coccobacillus.*

Epidemiology: Tularemia is a zoonosis whose most important reservoirs are rabbits and rodents, although other wild and domestic animals may harbor the organisms. Human infection with *F. tularensis* results from contact with infected animals or from the bites of infected insects, including ticks, deerflies, and mosquitoes.

Ticks and rabbits are responsible for most human infections. The blood-sucking insect inoculates the organism into the skin on feeding. The bacteria may also be inoculated into unnoticed breaks in the skin by direct contact with an infected animal. In addition, tularemia can result from the inhalation of infected aerosols, ingestion of contaminated food and water, or inoculation into the eye. Tularemia is found in temperate zones of the Northern Hemisphere. The incidence of the infection has fallen dramatically in the United States in the past five decades, to about 250 cases annually, presumably related to a decline in hunting and trapping.

 Pathogenesis: *F. tularensis* multiplies at the site of inoculation, where it produces a focal ulceration. The bacteria then spread to regional lymph nodes. Dissemination in the bloodstream leads to metastatic infections that involve the monocyte/macrophage system and sometimes the lungs, heart, and kidneys. *F. tularensis* survives within macrophages until these cells are activated by a cell-mediated immune response to the infection.

 Pathology: Lesions of tularemia occur at the inoculation site and in lymph nodes, spleen, liver, bone marrow, lungs (Fig. 9-29), heart, and kidneys. The initial skin lesion is an exudative, pyogenic ulcer. Later, disseminated lesions undergo central necrosis and are surrounded by a perimeter of granulomatous reaction resembling the lesions of tuberculosis. Hyperemia and the presence of numerous macrophages in the sinuses make lymph nodes large and firm; they subsequently soften as necrosis and suppuration develop. The spleen tends to be enlarged but shows only nonspecific changes. The pulmonary lesions resemble those of primary tuberculosis.

Clinical Features: The incubation period of tularemia ranges from 1 to 14 days, depending on the dose and route of transmission, with a mean of 3 to 4 days. There are four distinct clinical presentations.

- **Ulceroglandular tularemia** is the most common form of the disease (80–90% of cases) and begins as a tender, erythematous papule at the site of inoculation, usually on a limb. This develops into a pustule, which then ulcerates. The regional lymph nodes become large and tender and may suppurate and drain through sinus tracts. In some instances, generalized lymphadenopathy (glandular tularemia) is the first manifestation of the infection.

The initial bacteremia is accompanied by fever, headache, myalgias, and occasionally prostration. Within a week, generalized lymphadenopathy and splenomegaly become evident. The most serious infections are complicated by secondary pneumonia and endotoxic shock, in which case the prognosis is grave. Some patients develop meningitis, endocarditis, pericarditis, or osteomyelitis.

- **Oculoglandular tularemia** is rare (<2% of cases) and is characterized by a primary papule in the conjunctiva, which forms a pustule and ulcerates. Lymphadenopathy of the head and neck become prominent. Severe ulceration may cause blindness, owing to penetration of the sclera and infection of the optic nerve.
- **Typhoidal tularemia** is diagnosed when fever, hepatosplenomegaly, and toxemia are the presenting signs and symptoms.
- **Pneumonic tularemia**, in which pneumonia is a major feature, may complicate any of the other types.

The duration of illness is 1 week to 3 months, but this may be shortened by prompt treatment with streptomycin.

Anthrax Is Rapidly Fatal When It Disseminates

Anthrax is a necrotizing disease caused by Bacillus anthracis, *which is a large spore-forming, gram-positive rod.*

 Epidemiology: Anthrax has been recognized for centuries, and descriptions of disease consistent with anthrax were reported in early Hebrew, Roman, and Greek records. The major reservoirs are goats, sheep, cattle, horses, pigs, and dogs. Spores form in the soil and dead animals, resisting heat, desiccation, and chemical disinfection for years. Humans are infected when spores enter the body through breaks in the skin, by inhalation, or by ingestion. Human disease may also result from exposure to contaminated animal byproducts, such as hides, wool, brushes, or bone meal.

Anthrax has been a persistent problem in Iran, Turkey, Pakistan, and Sudan. One of the largest recorded naturally occurring outbreaks of anthrax occurred in Zimbabwe, when an estimated 10,000 persons became infected in 1978 to 1980. In North America, human infection is extremely rare (one case per year for the past few years) and usually results from exposure to imported animal products.

 Pathogenesis: The spores of *B. anthracis* germinate in the human body to yield vegetative bacteria that multiply and release a potent necrotizing

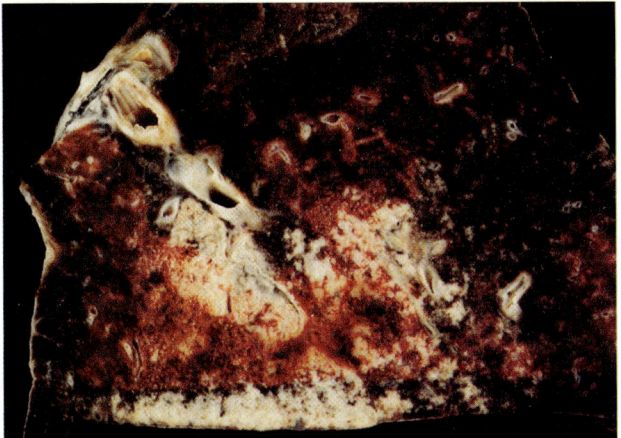

FIGURE 9-29
Tularemia. The lung shows firm, consolidated, and necrotic areas.

toxin. In 80% of cases of cutaneous anthrax, the infection remains localized, and the host immunological response eventually eliminates the organism. If the infection disseminates, as occurs when the organisms are inhaled or ingested, the resulting widespread tissue destruction is usually fatal.

 Pathology: *B. anthracis* produces extensive tissue necrosis at the sites of infection, associated with only a mild infiltrate of neutrophils. Cutaneous lesions are ulcerated, contain numerous organisms, and are covered by a black scab. Pulmonary infection produces a necrotizing, hemorrhagic pneumonia, associated with hemorrhagic necrosis of mediastinal lymph nodes and widespread dissemination of the organism.

 Clinical Features: There are four presentations of anthrax, depending on the site of inoculation.

- **Malignant pustule** accounts for 95% of all anthrax and is the cutaneous form of the disease. The infected person presents with an elevated cutaneous papule that enlarges and erodes into an ulcer. Bloody purulent exudate accumulates and gradually darkens to purple or black. The ulcer is often surrounded by a zone of brawny edema, which seems disproportionately large relative to the size of the ulcer. Regional lymphadenitis portends a poor prognosis, because invasion of lymphatics precedes septicemia. If the infection does not disseminate, the cutaneous lesions heal without sequelae.
- **Pulmonary, or inhalational, anthrax,** sometimes called "woolsorters' disease," is a hazard of handling raw wool and develops after the inhalation of the spores of *B. anthracis*. Pulmonary anthrax presents as a flulike illness that rapidly progresses to respiratory failure and shock. Death often ensues within 24 to 48 hours of onset. Only 18 cases of inhalational anthrax were reported in the United States from 1900 to 1980. As a result of the anthrax bioterror attack in the United States in 2001, 11 cases of inhalational anthrax occurred. The only hope is early antibiotic therapy.
- **Septicemic anthrax** more commonly follows pulmonary anthrax than malignant pustule. Disseminated intravascular coagulation is a common complication. Moreover, a bacterial toxin depresses the respiratory center, which explains why death can occur even when antibiotic therapy has cured the infection.
- **Gastrointestinal anthrax** is rare and is acquired by eating contaminated meat. Ulceration of the stomach or bowel and invasion of the regional lymphatics are common. Death is caused by fulminant diarrhea and massive ascites.

Listeriosis Is a Systemic Multiorgan Infection That Carries a High Mortality

Listeriosis is caused by Listeria monocytogenes, *a small, motile, gram-positive coccobacillus.*

 Epidemiology: Listeriosis is usually sporadic but may also be epidemic. The organism has been isolated worldwide from surface water, soil, vegetation, the feces of healthy persons, many species of wild and domestic mammals, and several species of birds. However, the spread of infection from animals to humans is rare. Most human infections are in urban rather than rural environments and, in the Northern Hemisphere, occur during July and August. *L. monocytogenes* grows at refrigerator temperatures, and outbreaks of listeriosis have been traced to unpasteurized milk, contaminated cheese, and other dairy products.

 Pathogenesis: *L. monocytogenes* has an unusual life cycle, which accounts for its ability to evade intracellular and extracellular antibacterial defense mechanisms. After phagocytosis by host cells, the organism enters a phagolysosome, where the acidic pH activates *listeriolysin O,* an exotoxin that disrupts the vesicular membrane and permits escape of the bacterium into the cytoplasm. After replicating, the bacteria usurp the contractile elements of the host cytoskeleton to form elongated protrusions that are engulfed by adjacent cells. Thus, *Listeria* spread from one cell to another without exposure to the extracellular environment.

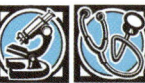 **Pathology and Clinical Features:** Most *Listeria* infections fall into one of two groups. **Listeriosis of pregnancy includes prenatal and postnatal infections.** Listeriosis of the adult population is most commonly characterized by **meningoencephalitis and septicemia,** but may be localized to skin, eyes, lymph nodes, endocardium, or bones.

Maternal infection early in pregnancy leads to abortion or premature delivery. Infected infants rapidly develop respiratory distress, hepatosplenomegaly, cutaneous and mucosal papules, leukopenia, and thrombocytopenia. Intrauterine infections involve many organs and tissues, including the amniotic fluid, placenta, and the umbilical cord. Widespread abscesses are found in many organs. Microscopically, foci of necrosis and suppuration contain many bacteria. Older lesions tend to be granulomatous. Neurological sequelae are common, and the mortality is high even with prompt antibiotic therapy. Neonatal listeriosis may also be acquired during delivery, in which case the onset of clinical disease is 3 days to 2 weeks after birth.

Chronic alcoholics, patients with cancer, those receiving immunosuppressive therapy, and patients with AIDS are far more susceptible to infection than is the general population. Meningitis is the most common form of the disease in adults and resembles other bacterial meningitides.

Septicemic listeriosis is a severe febrile illness most common in immunodeficient patients. It may lead to shock and disseminated intravascular coagulation, a situation that may be erroneously diagnosed as gram-negative sepsis. Prolonged treatment with antimicrobials is usually required because patients tend to experience relapse if therapy is administered for less than 3 weeks. The mortality from systemic listeriosis remains at 25%.

Cat-Scratch Disease Is a Self-Limited Granulomatous Lymphadenitis

Cat-scratch disease is a self-limited infection usually caused by Bartonella henselae, *and more rarely by* B. quintana. The bacteria are small (0.2–0.6 µm) gram-negative rods. These organisms are difficult to culture but are easily seen in tissue sections of the skin, lymph nodes, and conjunctiva, when stained with a silver impregnation technique (Fig. 9-30).

 Epidemiology: The reservoir is thought to be cats; various surveys have shown that up to 30% of cats are bacteremic. Infection begins when the bacillus is inoculated into the skin by the claws of cats (and rarely, other animals) or by thorns or splinters. Sometimes the conjunctiva is contaminated by close contact with a cat, possibly by licking around the eye. Infections are more common in children (80%) than in adults, and there may be clustering of cases when a stray cat joins a family.

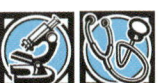 Pathology and Clinical Features: Bacteria multiply in the walls of small vessels and about collagen fibers at the site of inoculation. The organisms are then carried to regional lymph nodes, where they produce a suppurative and granulomatous lymphadenitis. In early lesions, clusters of bacteria fill and expand the lumina of small blood vessels, but they are rare in late lesions. After a papule develops at the site of inoculation, tenderness and enlargement of regional lymph nodes ensue. The nodes remain enlarged for 3 to 4 months and may drain through the skin. About half of patients have other symptoms, including fever and malaise, rash, a brief encephalitis, and erythema nodosum. *Parinaud oculoglandular syndrome* (preauricular adenopathy secondary to conjunctival infection) is common. No antibiotic has been accepted as beneficial.

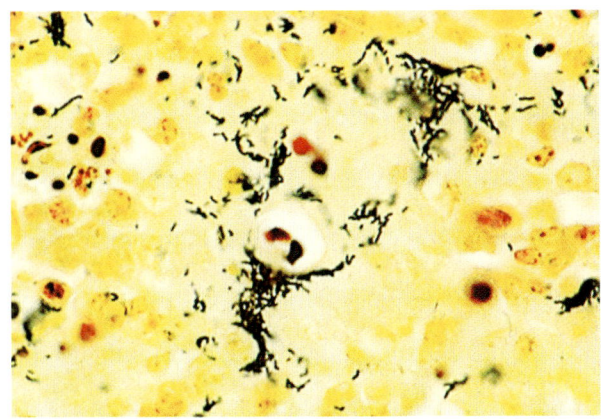

FIGURE 9-30
Cat-scratch disease. Section of a lymph node shows the bacilli, which are gram-negative but difficult to visualize with tissue gram stains. They are blackened by the Warthin-Starry silver impregnation technique.

Glanders Is a Granulomatous Infection Acquired from Horses

Glanders is an infection of equine species (horses, mules, donkeys) that is only rarely transmitted to humans, in whom it causes acute or chronic granulomatous disease. The cause is *Pseudomonas mallei,* a small gram-negative, nonmotile bacillus. Although uncommon, the infection remains endemic in South America, Asia, and Africa. Humans acquire the disease by contact with infected equines through broken skin or by inhalation of contaminated aerosols.

Acute glanders is characterized by bacteremia, with severe prostration and fever. Granulomatous abscesses may form in subcutaneous tissues and many other organs, including the lung, liver, spleen, muscles, and joints. Acute glanders is almost always fatal.

Chronic glanders features low-grade fever, draining abscesses of the skin, lymphadenopathy, and hepatosplenomegaly. Granulomas in many organs mimic tuberculosis. The mortality in chronic glanders exceeds 50%.

Bartonellosis Causes Acute Anemia and Chronic Skin Disease

Bartonellosis is an infection by Bartonella bacilliformis, *a small, multiflagellated, gram- negative coccobacillus (Oroya fever) (verruga peruana).*

 Epidemiology: Bartonellosis occurs only in Peru, Ecuador, and Colombia in river valleys of the Andes and is transmitted by sandflies. Humans provide the only reservoir and acquire the infection at sunrise and sunset, when sandflies are most active. In endemic areas, 10 to 15% of the population have latent infections. Newcomers are susceptible, whereas the indigenous population tends to be resistant.

 Pathology and Clinical Features: Bartonellosis presents a biphasic pattern, with acute hemolytic anemia (Oroya fever) first, followed some months later by a chronic dermal phase (verruga peruana). Either phase may occur by itself.

The most severe consequence of bartonellosis is hemolytic anemia. After *B. bacilliformis* has been inoculated into the skin by a sandfly, the bacteria proliferate in the vascular endothelium and then invade erythrocytes, thereby producing profound hemolysis.

The **acute anemic phase** follows an incubation period of 3 weeks and is characterized by abrupt onset of fever, skeletal pains, and a severe, hemolytic anemia. In untreated bartonellosis, 40% of patients in the anemic phase die. Secondary *Salmonella* sepsis is frequent and contributes to the high mortality.

The **dermal eruptive phase** of bartonellosis may coexist with the anemic phase but is usually separated by an interval of 3 to 6 months. Many small hemangioma-like lesions stud the dermis, and bacteria may be identified in endothelial cells. Nodular lesions may be prominent on the extensor surfaces of the arms and legs. Large deep-seated lesions, which tend to ulcerate, develop near joints and limit motion. The dermal eruptive phase is often prolonged but eventually heals spontaneously. The mortality in this phase is less than 5%.

INFECTIONS CAUSED BY BRANCHING FILAMENTOUS ORGANISMS

Actinomycosis Is Characterized by Abscesses and Sinus Tracts

Actinomycosis is a slowly progressive, suppurative, fibrosing infection involving the jaw, thorax, or abdomen. The disease is caused by a number of anaerobic and microaerophilic bacteria termed *Actinomyces*. These organisms are branching, filamentous, gram-positive rods that normally reside in the human oropharynx, gastrointestinal tract, and vagina. Although *Actinomyces* organisms are now recognized as bacteria, they were long considered fungi because of their filamentous morphology. Several *Actinomyces* species cause human disease, the most common being *Actinomyces israelii*.

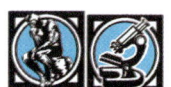 Pathogenesis and Pathology: *Actinomyces* is not ordinarily virulent, and the organisms reside as saprophytes in the body without producing disease. Two uncommon conditions must occur for *Actinomyces* to establish disease. First, the organism must be inoculated into deeper tissues, since it cannot invade. Second, an anaerobic atmosphere is necessary for the bacteria to proliferate. Trauma can produce tissue necrosis, providing an excellent anaerobic medium for growth of *Actinomyces*, and can inoculate the organism into normally sterile tissue. Actinomycosis occurs at four distinct sites:

- **Cervicofacial actinomycosis** results from jaw injury, dental extraction, or dental manipulation.
- **Thoracic actinomycosis** is caused by the aspiration of organisms contaminating dental debris.
- **Abdominal actinomycosis** follows traumatic or surgical disruption of the bowel, especially the appendix.
- **Pelvic actinomycosis** is associated with the prolonged use of intrauterine devices (IUDs).

Actinomycosis begins as a nidus of proliferating organisms that attracts an acute inflammatory infiltrate. The small abscess grows slowly, becoming a series of abscesses connected by sinus tracts. Tracts burrow across normal tissue boundaries and into adjacent organs. Eventually, a tract may penetrate onto an external surface or mucosal membrane, producing a draining sinus. The walls of the abscess and tracts are composed of granulation tissue, often thick, densely fibrotic, and chronically inflamed. Within the abscesses and sinuses are pus and colonies of organisms.

The colonies of *Actinomyces* within these lesions can grow to several millimeters in diameter and be visible to the naked eye. They appear as hard, yellow grains known as *sulfur granules*, because of their resemblance to elemental sulfur. Sulfur granules consist of tangled masses of narrow, branching filaments, embedded in a polysaccharide–protein matrix *(Splendore-Hoeppli material).* Histologically, the colonies appear as rounded, basophilic grains with scalloped eosinophilic borders (Fig. 9-31A). The individual filaments of *Actinomyces* cannot be discerned with the hematoxylin and eosin stain but are readily visible on Gram staining or silver impregnation (see Fig. 9-31B).

 Clinical Features: The signs and symptoms of actinomycosis vary according to the site of infection. Actinomycosis originating in a tooth socket or the tonsils is characterized by swelling of the jaw ("lumpy jaw"), face, and neck, at first painless and fluctuant but later painful. In pulmonary infections, sinus tracts may penetrate from lobe to lobe, through the pleura, and into ribs and vertebrae. Abdominal or pelvic disease may be encountered as an expanding mass, suggesting a locally spreading tumor. Actinomycosis responds to prolonged antibiotic therapy, and penicillin is highly effective.

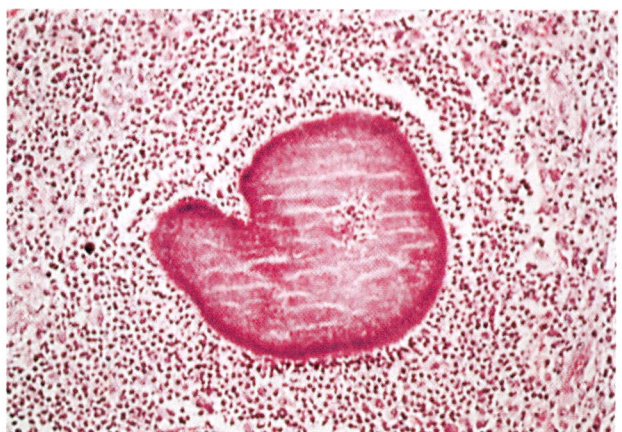
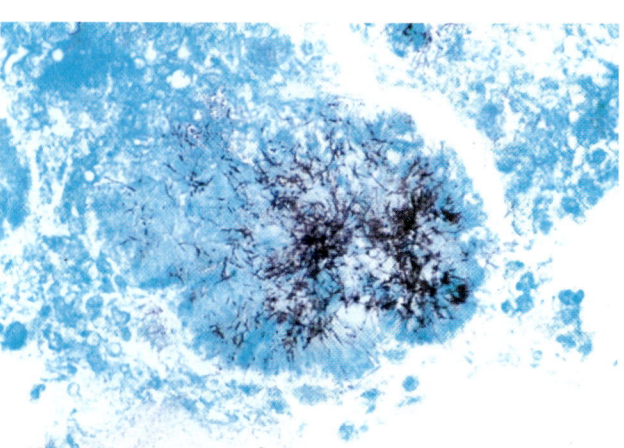

FIGURE *9-31*

Actinomycosis. A. A typical sulfur granule lies within an abscess. **B.** The individual filaments of *A. israeli* are readily visible with the silver impregnation technique.

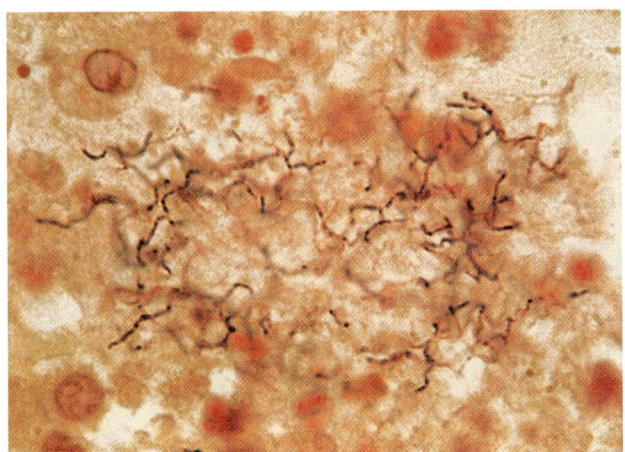

FIGURE 9-32
Nocardiosis. A silver stain of a necrotic exudate reveals the branching, filamentous rods of *N. asteroides*.

Nocardiosis Is a Respiratory Infection in Immunocompromised Persons

Nocardiosis is a suppurative infection of the lung that often spreads to the brain and skin. Nocardia are aerobic, gram-positive filamentous, branching bacteria. They are weakly acid-fast, a characteristic used to distinguish them from the morphologically similar actinomycetes.

 Epidemiology: *Nocardia* species are widely distributed in soil, and human disease is caused by inhalation or inoculation of soil-borne organisms. The infection is not transmitted from person to person. *Nocardia asteroides* is the species that most frequently produces human disease. Nocardiosis is most common in persons with impaired immunity, particularly cell-mediated immunity. Organ transplantation, long-term corticosteroid therapy, lymphomas, leukemias, and various other debilitating diseases predispose to *Nocardia* infections.

Two other pathogenic species of *Nocardia*, namely *N. brasiliensis* and *N. caviae*, may cause pulmonary nocardiosis resembling that produced by *N. asteroides*. However, they are usually encountered in underdeveloped countries as a cause of mycetomas.

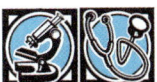 **Pathology and Clinical Features:** The respiratory tract is the usual portal of entry for *Nocardia*. The organism elicits a brisk infiltrate of neutrophils, and disease begins as a slowly progressive, pyogenic pneumonia. If the infected person mounts a vigorous cell-mediated immune response, the infection may be eliminated. In immunocompromised persons, however, *Nocardia* produces pulmonary abscesses, which are frequently multiple and confluent. Direct extension to the pleura, trachea, and heart and metastases to the brain or skin through the circulation carry a grave prognosis. Nocardial abscesses are filled with neutrophils, necrotic debris, and scattered organisms. Bacteria can be demonstrated by silver impregnation (Fig. 9-32). With the Gram stain, they appear as beaded, filamentous, gram-positive rods. Untreated nocardiosis is usually fatal. Sulfonamides or related antibiotics for several months are often effective therapy.

Spirochetal Infections

Spirochetes are long, slender, helical bacteria with specialized cell envelopes that permit them to move by flexion and rotation. The thinner organisms are below the resolving power of routine light microscopy, and specialized techniques, such as darkfield microscopy or silver impregnation, are needed for their demonstration. Although spirochetes have the basic cell wall structure of gram-negative bacteria, they stain poorly with the Gram stain.

Three genera of spirochetes, *Treponema*, *Borrelia*, and *Leptospira*, cause human disease (Table 9-5). Spirochetes are adept at evading host inflammatory and immunological de-

TABLE 9-5 Spirochete Infections

Disease	Organism	Clinical Manifestation	Distribution	Mode of Transmission
	Treponemes			
Syphilis	*T. pallidum*	See text	Common worldwide	Sexual contact, congenital
Bejel	*T. endenicum (T. Pallidum, subspecies endenicum)*	Mucosal, skin, and bone lesions	Middle East	Mouth-to-mouth contact
Yaws	*T. pertenue (T. pallidum subspecies pertenue)*	Skin and bone	Tropics	Skin-to-skin contact
Pinta	*T. carateum*	Skin lesions	Latin America	Skin-to-skin contact
	Borrelia			
Lyme disease	*B. burgdorferi*	See text	North America, Europe, Russia, Asia, Africa, Australia	Tick bite
Relapsing fever	*B. recurrentis* and related species	Relapsing flulike illness	Worldwide	Tick bite, louse bite
	Leptospira			
Leptospirosis	*L. interrogans*	Flulike illness, meningitis	Worldwide	Contact with animal urine

408 Infectious and Parasitic Diseases

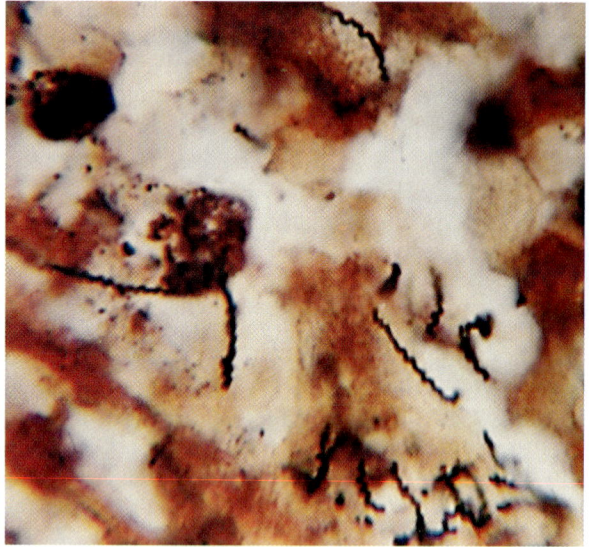

FIGURE 9-33
Syphilis. Spirochetes of *T. pallidum*, visualized by silver impregnation, in the eye of a child with congenital syphilis.

fenses, and diseases caused by these organisms are all chronic or relapsing.

SYPHILIS

Syphilis (lues) is a chronic, sexually transmitted, systemic infection caused by Treponema pallidum. *T. pallidum* is a thin, long spirochete (Fig. 9-33) that cannot be grown in artificial media. The disease was first recognized in Europe in the 1490s and has been related to the return of Christopher Columbus and his seamen from the New World. Urbanization and mass movements of people caused by war contributed to its rapid spread. Originally, syphilis was an acute disease that caused destructive skin lesions and early death, but it has become milder, with a more protracted and insidious clinical course.

 Epidemiology: Syphilis is a worldwide disease that is transmitted almost exclusively by sexual contact. The infection is also spread from an infected mother to her fetus *(congenital syphilis)*. In the United States, the incidence of primary and secondary syphilis declined after the introduction of penicillin therapy at the end of World War II.

 Pathogenesis: *T. pallidum* is very fragile and is killed by soap, antiseptics, drying, and cold. Person-to-person transmission requires direct contact between a rich source of spirochetes (e.g., an open lesion) and mucous membranes or abraded skin of the genital organs, rectum, mouth, fingers, or nipples. The organisms reproduce at the site of inoculation, pass to regional lymph nodes, gain access to the systemic circulation, and are disseminated throughout the body. Although *T. pallidum* induces an inflammatory response and is taken up by phagocytic cells, it persists and proliferates. Chronic infection and inflammation cause tissue destruction, sometimes for decades. The course of syphilis is classically divided into three stages (Fig. 9-34).

Primary Syphilis Features a Chancre

The classic lesion of primary syphilis is the chancre (Fig. 9-35), a characteristic ulcer located at the site of *T. pallidum* inocula-

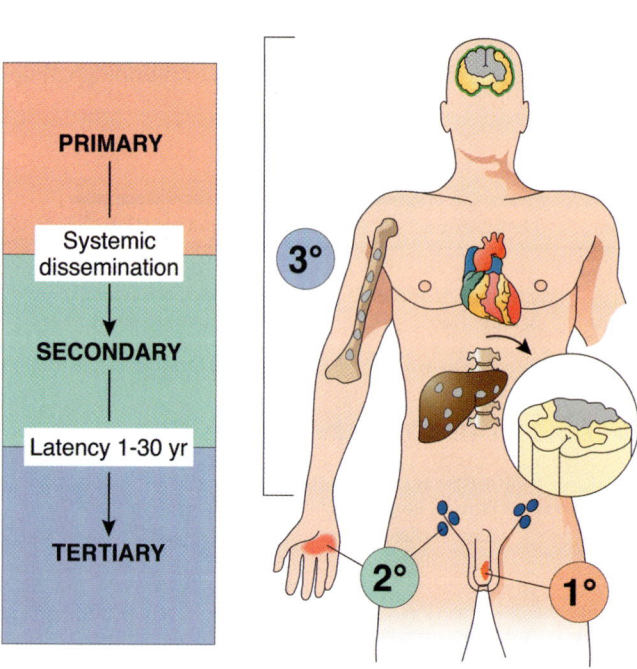

FIGURE 9-34
Clinical characteristics of the various stages of syphilis.

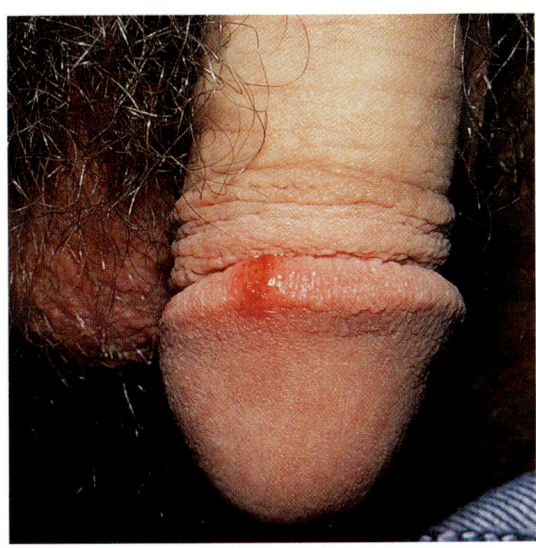

FIGURE 9-35
Syphilitic chancre. A patient with primary syphilis displays a raised, erythematous penile lesion.

tion, usually the penis, vulva, anus, or mouth. It appears 1 week to 3 months after exposure, with an average incubation period of 3 weeks. The chancre tends to be solitary and has a firm, raised border. Spirochetes tend to be concentrated in the walls of vessels and in the epidermis around the ulcer. **Chancres, as well as the lesions of the other stages of syphilis, display a characteristic "luetic vasculitis," in which endothelial cells proliferate and swell, and the walls of the vessels become thickened by lymphocytes and fibrous tissue.**

The chancre quickly erodes to a characteristic ulcer. Chancres are painless and can go unnoticed in some locations, such as the uterine cervix, anal canal, and mouth. The chancre lasts from 3 to 12 weeks and is frequently accompanied by inguinal lymphadenopathy. It heals without scarring.

Secondary Syphilis Reflects Dissemination of Spirochetes

Secondary syphilis features systemic dissemination and proliferation of *T. pallidum* and is characterized by lesions in the skin, mucous membranes, lymph nodes, meninges, stomach, and liver. The lesions show a perivascular lymphocytic infiltrate and endarteritis obliterans.

- **Skin:** The most common presentation of secondary syphilis is an erythematous and maculopapular rash, involving the trunk and extremities and often including the palms (Fig. 9-36) and soles. The rash appears 2 weeks to 3 months after the chancre heals. A variety of other skin lesions in secondary syphilis includes **condylomata lata** (exudative plaques in the perineum, vulva, or scrotum, which abound in spirochetes) (Fig. 9-37), **follicular syphilids** (small papular lesions around hair follicles that cause loss of hair), and **nummular syphilids** (coinlike lesions involving the face and perineum).
- **Mucous membranes:** Lesions on mucosal surfaces of the mouth and genital organs, called *mucous patches*, teem with organisms and are highly infectious.
- **Lymph nodes:** Characteristic changes in lymph nodes, especially epitrochlear nodes, include a thickened capsule, follicular hyperplasia, increased numbers of plasma cells and macrophages, and luetic vasculitis. Numerous spirochetes are present in the lymph nodes of secondary syphilis.
- **Meninges:** Although the meninges are commonly seeded with *T. pallidum*, this involvement is frequently asymptomatic.

Tertiary Syphilis Causes Neurological and Vascular Diseases

After the lesions of secondary syphilis have subsided, an asymptomatic period lasts for years or decades. However, spirochetes continue to multiply, and the deep-seated lesions of tertiary syphilis gradually develop in one third of untreated patients. Focal ischemic necrosis secondary to obliterative endarteritis is the underlying mechanism for many of the processes associated with tertiary syphilis. *T. pallidum* induces a mononuclear inflammatory infiltrate predominantly composed of lymphocytes and plasma cells. These cells infiltrate small arteries and arterioles, producing a characteristic obstructive vascular lesion *(endarteritis obliterans)*. The small arteries are inflamed, and their endothelial cells are swollen. They are surrounded by concentric layers of proliferating fibroblasts, which confer an "onion skin" appearance to the vascular lesions.

- **Syphilitic aortitis:** This lesion results from a slowly progressive endarteritis obliterans of the vasa vasorum that eventually leads to necrosis of the aortic media, a grad-

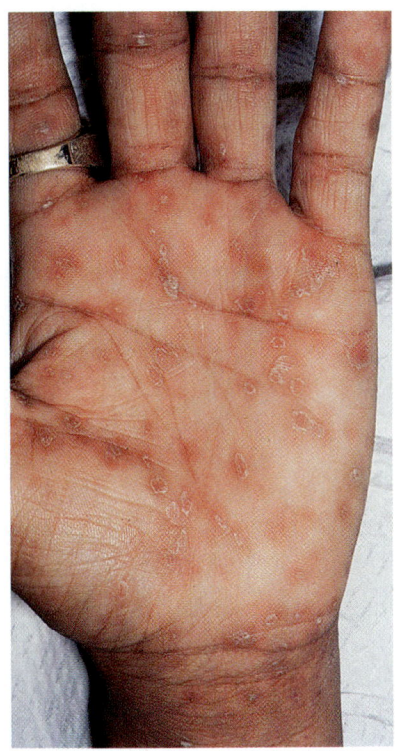

FIGURE 9-36
Secondary syphilis. A maculopapular rash is present on the palm.

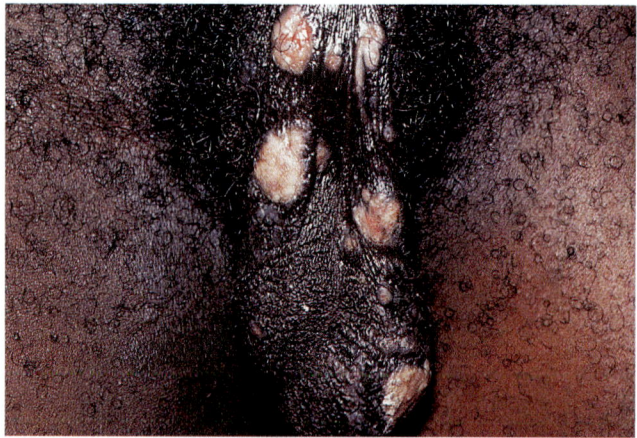
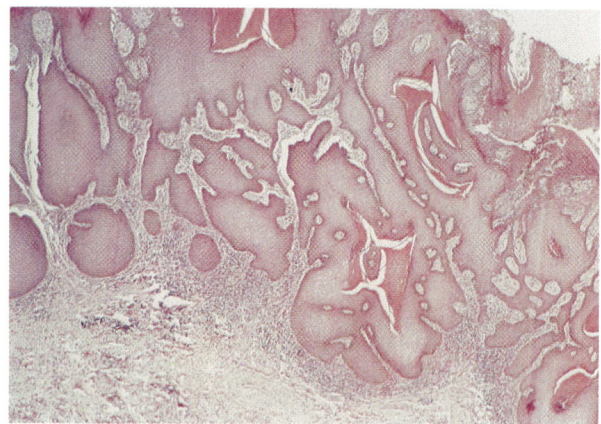

FIGURE 9-37
Condylomata lata in secondary syphillis. A. Whitish plaques are seen on the vulva and perineum. B. A photomicrograph shows papillomatous hyperplasia of the epidermis with underlying chronic inflammation.

ual weakening and stretching of the aortic wall, and the formation of an aortic aneurysm. The syphilitic aneurysm is saccular and involves the ascending aorta, an unusual site for the much more common atherosclerotic aneurysms. On gross examination, the intima of the aorta appears rough and pitted *(tree-bark appearance)* (Fig. 9-38). The aortic media is gradually replaced by scar tissue, after which the aorta loses its strength and resilience. The aorta gradually stretches, becoming progressively thinner to the point of rupture, massive hemorrhage, and sudden death. **Damage to, and scarring of, the ascending aorta also commonly lead to dilation of the aortic ring, separation of the valve cusps, and regurgitation of blood through the aortic valve (aortic insufficiency).** Luetic vasculitis of the coronary arteries may narrow or occlude these vessels and cause myocardial infarction.

- **Neurosyphilis:** The slowly progressive infection damages the meninges, cerebral cortex, spinal cord, cranial nerves, or eyes. Tertiary syphilis involving the central nervous system is subclassified according to the predominant tissue affected. Thus, there are references to **meningovascular syphilis** (meninges), **tabes dorsalis** (spinal cord), and **general paresis** (cerebral cortex). The lesions of neurosyphilis are discussed in Chapter 28.
- **Benign tertiary syphilis:** The appearance of a gumma (Fig. 9-39) in any organ or tissue is the hallmark of benign tertiary syphilis. Gummas are most commonly found in the skin, bone, and joints, although lesions can occur at any body site. These granulomatous lesions are composed of a central area of coagulative necrosis, epithelioid macrophages, occasional giant cells, and peripheral fibrous tissue. Gummas are usually localized lesions that do not significantly damage the patient.

Congenital Syphilis Is Acquired in Utero

When *T. pallidum* is transmitted from an infected mother to the fetus, the organism disseminates in fetal tissues, which are injured by the proliferating organisms and accompanying inflammatory response. Fetal infection produces still-

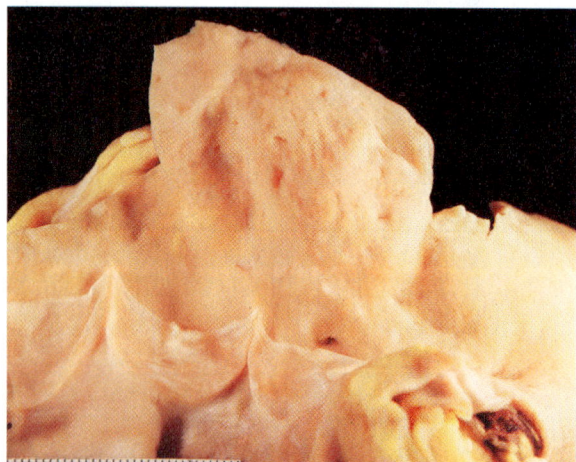

FIGURE 9-38
Syphilitic aortitis. The ascending aorta exhibits a roughened intima ("tree bark" appearance), owing to destruction of the media.

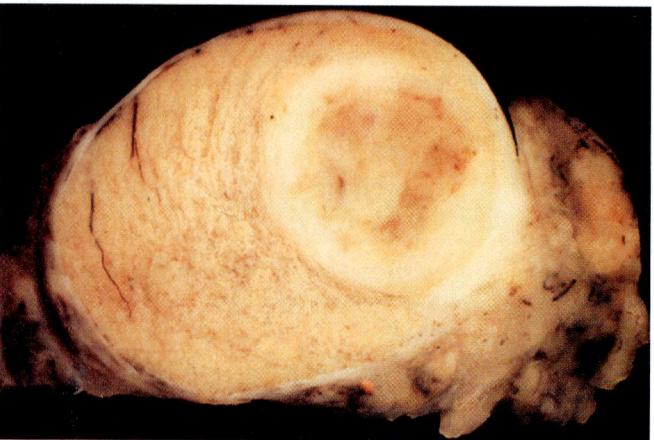

FIGURE 9-39
Syphilitic gumma. A patient with tertiary syphilis shows a sharply circumscribed gumma in the testis, characterized by a fibrogranulomatous wall and a necrotic center.

birth, neonatal illness or death, or progressive postnatal disease.

Pathology: Histopathologically, the lesions of congenital syphilis are identical to those of adult disease. Infected tissues show a chronic inflammatory infiltrate, composed of lymphocytes and plasma cells, and endarteritis obliterans. Virtually any tissue can be affected, but skin, bones, teeth, joints, liver, and central nervous systems are characteristically involved (see Chapter 6).

Clinical Features: The presentation of congenital syphilis is variable, and infected newborns are often asymptomatic. Early signs of infection include a rhinitis **(snuffles)** and a desquamative rash. Infection of periosteum, bone, cartilage, and dental pulp produce deformities of bones and teeth, including **saddle nose,** anterior bowing of the legs **(saber shins),** and peg-shaped upper incisor teeth **(Hutchinson teeth).** Progression of congenital syphilis can be arrested by penicillin.

NONVENEREAL TREPONEMATOSES

In tropical and subtropical countries, there is a group of nonvenereal, chronic diseases that are caused by treponemes indistinguishable from *T. pallidum*. Like syphilis, they result from the inoculation of the organism into mucocutaneous surfaces. They also pass through clearly defined clinical and pathological stages, including a primary lesion at the site of inoculation, secondary skin eruptions, a latent period, and a tertiary, late stage.

Yaws is a Tropical Disease that Affects Many Organs

Yaws is caused by *T. pertenue* and occurs among poor rural populations in warm, humid areas of tropical Africa, South America, Southeast Asia, and Oceania. Children and adolescents living in deprived tropical regions are at risk. Transmission is by skin-to-skin contact and is facilitated by breaks or abrasions. Two to 5 weeks after exposure, a single "mother yaw" appears at the site of inoculation, usually on an exposed part. The lesion begins as a papule and becomes a 2- to 5-cm "raspberry-like" papilloma. The secondary or disseminated stage begins with the eruption of similar, but smaller, yaws on other parts of the skin. Microscopically, the mother yaw and the disseminated lesions show hyperkeratosis, papillary acanthosis, and an intense neutrophilic infiltrate of the epidermis. The epidermis at the apex of the papilloma lyses to form a shallow ulcer, and plasma cells invade the upper dermis. Spirochetes are numerous in the dermal papillae.

Painful papillomas on the soles of the feet lead patients to walk on the side of their feet like a crab, a condition called *"crab yaw."* The treponemes are borne by the blood to bones, lymph nodes, and skin. There they grow during a latent period of 5 or more years. The lesions in the late stage include gummas of the skin, which are destructive to the face and upper airway. Periostitis of the tibia causes "saber shins" or "boomerang legs." A single dose of long-acting penicillin cures yaws.

Bejel Is Characterized by Gummas of the Skin, Airways, and Bone

Bejel (also known as "endemic syphilis") has a focal distribution in Africa, western Asia, and Australia. Bejel is transmitted by nonvenereal routes, such as from an infected infant to the breast of the mother, from mouth to mouth, or from utensils to the mouth, and is caused by *T. pallidum* subspecies *endemicum*. Other than on the nursing breast, primary lesions are rare. Secondary lesions in the mouth are identical to the mucosal lesions of syphilis and may spread from the upper airway to the larynx. Lesions of the perineum and bone are encountered, and gummas of the breast occur.

Pinta Is a Tropical Skin Disease

Pinta (Sp., "painted" or "blemish") is a treponematosis characterized by variably colored spots on the skin. It is caused by *T. carateum* and prevails in remote, arid, inland regions and river valleys of the American tropics. The lesions of the three stages of pinta are limited to the skin and tend to merge. Transmission is by skin-to-skin inoculation, usually after long intimate contact with an infected person.

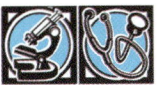

Pathology and Clinical Features: Ten days after inoculation, a small papule appears, most often on the leg. The lesion enlarges and in 1 to 3 months may involve a 10-cm patch of skin. The papule flattens and displays irregular margins and a scaly and pigmented surface. The lesion initially appears slate blue in dark-skinned persons, but after several years it leaves an area of hypopigmentation. In secondary pinta (5–18 months later), generalized pale, pink macules *(pintids)* appear on exposed surfaces. These lesions later become depigmented and hyperkeratotic. Treponemes abound in the primary and secondary lesions but not in the late ones. The latter are characterized by acanthosis and hyperkeratosis of the epidermis, follicular plugging, elongation of rete ridges, intraepidermal microabscesses, and an absence of pigment in the basal layer. The inflammatory infiltrate is diminished in the tertiary stage. A single dose of long-acting penicillin is curative.

LYME DISEASE

Lyme disease is a chronic systemic infection, which begins with a characteristic skin lesion and later manifests as cardiac, neurological, or joint disturbances. The causative agent is *Borrelia burgdorferi*, a large, microaerophilic spirochete.

Epidemiology: Lyme disease was first described in patients from Lyme, Connecticut, but was later recognized in many other areas. *B. burgdorferi* is transmitted from its animal reservoir to humans by the bite of the minute *Ixodes* tick. The insect is found in wooded areas, where it usually feeds on mice and deer. Transmission to humans is most likely to occur from May through July, when nymph forms of the tick feed.

Lyme disease is a growing problem in the United States, where the disease has become the most common tick-borne illness, causing an estimated 15,000 to 20,000 cases annually. Disease is concentrated mainly in three areas, along the eastern seaboard from Maryland to Massachusetts, in the Midwest in Minnesota and Wisconsin, and in the West in California and Oregon. The disease is also present in Europe, Australia, countries of the former Soviet Union, Japan, and China.

Pathology and Clinical Features: *B. burgdorferi* reproduces locally at the site of inoculation, spreads to regional lymph nodes, and is disseminated throughout the body in the bloodstream. Like other spirochetal diseases, Lyme disease is chronic, occurring in stages, with remissions and exacerbations. Studies of skin and synovium have shown that *B. burgdorferi* elicits a chronic inflammatory infiltrate, composed of lymphocytes and plasma cells. In patients who died of the disease, organisms have been seen at autopsy in virtually every organ affected, including skin, myocardium, liver, central nervous system, and the musculoskeletal system.

Lyme disease is a prolonged illness in which three clinical stages are described.

- **Stage 1:** A distinctive feature of the first stage of Lyme disease is the characteristic skin lesion, *erythema chronicum migrans*, which appears at the site of the tick bite. This begins 3 to 35 days after the bite as an erythematous macule or papule, which grows to become an erythematous patch 3 to 7 cm in diameter. It often is intensely red at its periphery and shows some central clearing, imparting an annular appearance to the lesion. Erythema chronicum migrans is accompanied by fever, fatigue, headache, arthralgias, and regional lymphadenopathy. Secondary annular skin lesions develop in about half of patients and in some cases persist for long periods. During this phase, patients experience constant malaise and fatigue, headache, and fever. Intermittent manifestations may also include meningeal irritation, migratory myalgia, cough, generalized lymphadenopathy, and testicular swelling.
- **Stage 2:** The second stage, which begins within several weeks to months of the appearance of the skin lesion, is characterized by exacerbation of migratory musculoskeletal pains and the development of cardiac and neurological abnormalities. In 10% of infected persons, conduction abnormalities, particularly atrioventricular block, result from myocarditis. Neurological abnormalities, most commonly meningitis and facial nerve palsies, occur in 15% of patients.
- **Stage 3:** The third stage of Lyme disease begins months to years after the tick bite and is manifested by joint, skin, and neurological abnormalities. Joint abnormalities develop in over half of infected persons and include severe arthritis of the large joints, especially the knee. The histopathological changes in affected joints are virtually indistinguishable from those of rheumatoid arthritis, with villous hypertrophy and a conspicuous mononuclear infiltrate in the subsynovial lining area.

It is now recognized that neurological manifestations may begin months to years after the onset of the disease. They range from intermittent tingling paresthesias without demonstrable neurological deficits to slowly progressive encephalomyelitis, transverse myelitis, organic brain syndromes, and dementia. There is a distinctive late skin manifestation of Lyme disease, *acrodermatitis chronica atrophicans*, which occurs years after erythema chronicum migrans and presents as patchy atrophy and sclerosis of the skin.

The diagnosis of Lyme disease is established by culturing *B. burgdorferi* from infected patients, but the yield is low. Therefore, the determination of antibody titers (initially IgM and later IgG) against the organism remains the most practical way to establish the diagnosis. Treatment with tetracycline or erythromycin is effective in eliminating early Lyme disease. In later stages and when there are extensive extracutaneous manifestations, high doses of intravenous penicillin G and other combinations of antibiotic regimens for long periods are necessary.

LEPTOSPIROSIS

Leptospirosis is an infection with spirochetes of the genus Leptospira, *which is for the most part (90% of patients) a mild, self-limited, febrile disease. In persons with more-severe infections, hepatic and renal failure may prove fatal.*

Epidemiology: Leptospirosis is a zoonosis of worldwide distribution. Leptospires penetrate abraded skin or mucous membranes following contact with infected rats, contaminated water, or mud. Since warm, moist environments favor survival of the spirochetes, the incidence is higher in the tropics. Between 30 and 100 cases of leptospirosis are reported annually in the United States, some of them in slaughterhouse workers and trappers, but recently some cases were reported among destitute persons in urban areas. Soldiers engaged in jungle warfare during the Vietnam War were at particular risk.

Pathology and Clinical Features: The symptoms of leptospirosis begin 4 days to 3 weeks after exposure to *L. interrogans*. In most cases, the disease resolves within a week without sequelae. In more severe infections, leptospirosis is a biphasic disease.

- The **leptospiremic phase** is characterized by the presence of leptospires in the blood and cerebrospinal fluid. There is an abrupt onset of fever, shaking chills, headache, and

myalgias. After 1 to 2 weeks, the symptoms abate as the leptospires disappear from the blood and bodily fluids.
- The **immune phase,** which begins within 3 days of the end of the leptospiremic phase, is accompanied by the production of IgM antibodies. The earlier symptoms recur, and signs of meningeal irritation become apparent. At this time, the cerebrospinal fluid shows a prominent pleiocytosis. In severe cases, jaundice appears and may be followed by hepatic and renal failure and the appearance of widespread hemorrhages and shock. This severe form of leptospirosis has historically been referred to as *Weil disease.*

Untreated Weil disease carries a mortality rate of 5 to 30%. At autopsy the tissues in Weil disease are bile stained, and hemorrhages are observed in many organs. Microscopically, the principal lesion is a diffuse vasculitis with capillary injury. The liver shows dissociation of the liver cell plates, erythrophagocytosis by Kupffer cells, minimal necrosis of hepatocytes, neutrophils in the sinusoids, and a mixed inflammatory cell infiltrate in the portal tracts. The kidneys display swollen and necrotic tubules. Spirochetes are numerous in the lumina of the tubules and particularly in bile-stained casts (Fig. 9-40).

RELAPSING FEVER

Relapsing fever is an acute, febrile, septicemic illness caused by spirochetes of the genus Borrelia. There are two main types of relapsing fever:

- **Epidemic relapsing fever** is caused by *B. recurrentis* and is transmitted by the bite of an infected louse. Humans are the only reservoir.
- **Endemic relapsing fever** is produced by a number of *Borrelia* species and is transmitted from rodents and other animals by the bite of an infected tick.

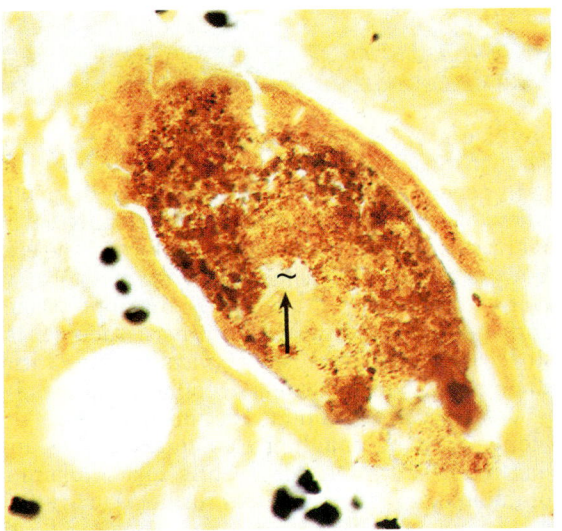

FIGURE 9-40
Leptospirosis. A distal renal tubule is obstructed by a bile-stained mass of hemoglobin and cellular debris. A leptospire *(arrow)* is in the center of this mass.

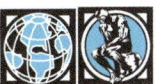 Epidemiology and Pathogenesis: The human body louse, *Pediculus humanus humanus*, becomes infected with *B. recurrentis* when it feeds on an infected person. The spirochetes cross the gut wall of the louse into the hemolymph, where they multiply. Here they remain, unless the louse is crushed when feeding. If this occurs, the borrelliae escape and penetrate at the site of the bite or even through the intact skin. War, crowded migrant worker camps, and heavy clothing during cold weather all favor mobilization of lice and the spread of relapsing fever. Furthermore, lice dislike the higher temperatures of the feverish victims and seek new hosts, another factor in the rapid spread of relapsing fever during epidemics. Louse-borne relapsing fever is currently encountered in a number of African countries, especially Ethiopia and Sudan, and is also seen in the South American Andes.

In endemic, tick-borne relapsing fever, ticks are infected while biting rats and other hosts. The borrelliae grow in the hemocoelom of the tick and invade other tissues, including the salivary glands. Humans are infected by the saliva or coxal fluid of the tick. Ticks have a considerably longer life span than lice and may harbor spirochetes for 12 to 15 years without a blood meal. Tick-borne relapsing fever occurs sporadically worldwide.

 Pathology: In fatal infections, the spleen is enlarged and contains miliary microabscesses. Spirochetes form tangled aggregates around the necrotic centers. Lymphocytes and neutrophils infiltrate central and midzonal areas of the liver, where spirochetes lie free in the sinusoids. Focal hemorrhages involve many organs.

 Clinical Features: Following the bite of an infected arthropod, fever, headache, myalgias, arthralgias, and lethargy appear within 1 to 2 weeks. The liver and spleen enlarge, and there are petechiae of the skin, conjunctival hemorrhages, and abdominal tenderness. Within 3 to 9 days after the onset of symptoms, the fever ends abruptly, only to begin 7 to 10 days later. During the afebrile period, the spirochetes disappear from the blood and change their antigenic coats. With each relapse, the symptoms are milder and the duration of illness is shorter. In severe cases, the initial episode may be characterized by a rash, meningitis, myocarditis, liver failure, and coma. Tetracycline is an effective treatment for both types of relapsing fever.

FUSOSPIROCHETAL INFECTIONS

Tropical Phagedenic Ulcer Is a Painful Lesion of the Leg

Tropical phagedenic (rapid spreading and sloughing) ulcer, also known as *tropical foot,* is a painful, necrotizing lesion of the skin and subcutaneous tissues of the leg that afflicts persons in tropical climates. Although the flora in the ulcers are often mixed, bacteriological studies indicate *Bacillus fusiformis* and *Treponema vincentii* to be causal. Malnutrition may predispose the patient to infection.

 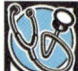 **Pathology and Clinical Features:** The lesion usually starts on the skin at a point of trauma and develops rapidly. The surface sloughs to form an ulcer with raised borders and a cup-shaped crater, which contains a gray, putrid exudates (Fig. 9-41). The ulcer may be so deep that the underlying bone and tendons are exposed. The margin becomes fibrotic, but complete healing may be delayed for years. In addition to secondary infection, tibial osteomyelitis and squamous cell carcinoma may be late complications. Antibiotics may be effective, but reconstructive plastic surgery is often necessary to close the defect.

Noma Is a Destructive Lesion of the Face

Noma (gangrenous stomatitis, cancrum oris) is a rapidly progressive necrosis of soft tissues and bones of the mouth and face and, less commonly, of such other sites as the chest, limbs, and genitalia. It afflicts malnourished children in the tropics, many of whom are further debilitated by recent infections (e.g., measles, malaria, leishmaniasis). A variety of bacteria may be recovered from these lesions, but *Treponema vincentii*, *Bacillus fusiformis*, *Bacteroides* spp., and *Corynebacterium* spp. tend to predominate.

  Pathology and Clinical Features: The ulceration is destructive and disfiguring and usually unilateral (Fig. 9-42). The initial lesion is a small papule, often on the cheek opposite the

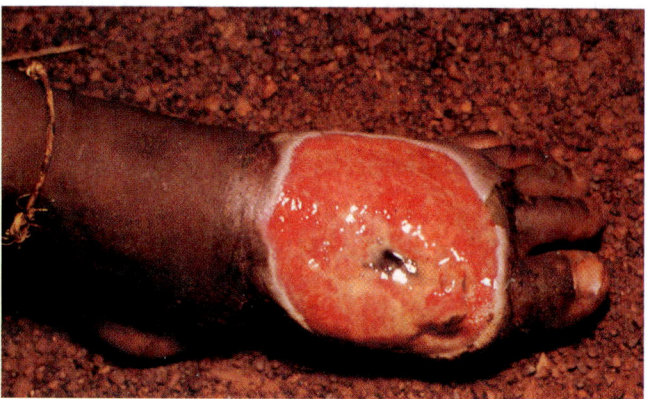

FIGURE 9-41
Tropical phagedenic ulcer caused by infection by fusospirochetal organisms, following penetrating trauma.

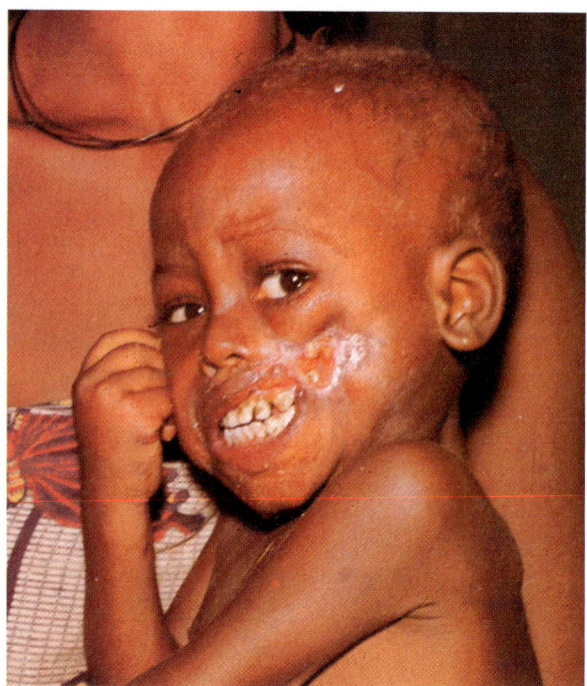

FIGURE 9-42
Noma. There is massive destruction of the soft tissues and bones of the mouth and cheek.

molars or premolars. From this early lesion, large malodorous defects quickly develop. The lesions are painful, and advanced lesions reveal necrosis of the skin, muscle, and adipose tissue, with exposure of underlying bone. In the absence of treatment, patients usually die. Antibiotics are helpful, but reconstructive surgery is often required to correct the deformity.

Chlamydial Infections

Chlamydiae are obligate intracellular parasites that are smaller than most other bacteria. They lack the enzymatic capacity to generate ATP and must parasitize the metabolic machinery of a host cell to reproduce. The chlamydial life cycle involves two distinct morphological forms. The **elementary body** is the smaller, metabolically inactive form, which survives extracellularly. It attaches to the appropriate host cell and induces endocytosis, forming a vacuole. It then transforms into the larger, metabolically active form, the **reticulate body,** which commandeers host cell metabolism to fuel chlamydial replication. The reticulate body divides repeatedly, forming daughter elementary bodies and destroying the host cell. Necrotic debris elicits inflammatory and immunological responses that further damage infected tissue.

Chlamydial infections are widespread among birds and mammals, and as many as 20% of humans are infected. Three species of chlamydiae (*C. trachomatis*, *C. psittaci*, and *C. pneumoniae*) cause human infection.

CHLAMYDIA TRACHOMATIS INFECTION

The species *C. trachomatis* contains a variety of strains (serovars), which cause three distinct types of disease: (1) genital and neonatal disease, (2) lymphogranuloma venereum, and (3) trachoma.

Genital and Neonatal Infections with *C. trachomatis* Are among the Most Common Sexually Transmitted Diseases

C. trachomatis serovars D through K cause a genital epithelial infection that has surpassed gonorrhea as the leading cause of sexually contracted disease in North America. In men, this infection produces urethritis and sometimes epididymitis or proctitis. In women, the infection usually begins with cervicitis, which can progress to endometritis, salpingitis, and generalized infection of the pelvic adnexal organs (pelvic inflammatory disease). Repeated infections of the fallopian tubes are particularly associated with scarring, which may interfere with passage of sperm or fertilized ova and result in infertility or ectopic pregnancy. Perinatal transmission of *C. trachomatis* causes neonatal conjunctivitis and pneumonia.

Epidemiology: The organism spreads from person to person in infected genital secretions. Infection is chronic and frequently asymptomatic, providing an enormous reservoir for transmission. As with all sexually transmitted diseases, persons with the largest number of sexual partners are at greatest risk of infection. Newborns acquire the organism by contact with infected endocervical secretions on passage through an infected birth canal. Two thirds of exposed newborns develop *C. trachomatis* conjunctivitis.

Pathology: Chlamydial infection elicits an inflammatory infiltrate of neutrophils and lymphocytes. Lymphoid aggregates, with or without germinal centers, may appear at the site of infection. In newborns, the conjunctival epithelium often contains characteristic vacuolar cytoplasmic inclusions, and the disease is frequently called *inclusion conjunctivitis*. Most genital infections are asymptomatic. In men, clinically apparent infection presents as a purulent penile discharge, associated with dysuria and urinary urgency. Chlamydial cervicitis causes a mucopurulent drainage from the cervical os.

Clinical Features: Chlamydial disease in the newborn presents as reddened conjunctivae with a watery or purulent discharge. Untreated neonatal conjunctivitis is potentially serious, although it may resolve without sequelae. Chlamydial pneumonia manifests in the second or third month with tachypnea and paroxysmal cough, usually without fever. Inclusion conjunctivitis is treated with systemic or topical antibiotics.

Lymphogranuloma Venereum Involves Lymph Nodes and May Result in Scarring

Lymphogranuloma venereum is a sexually transmitted disease that begins as a genital ulcer, progresses to a local necrotizing lymphadenitis (Fig. 9-43A), *and may eventuate in local scarring.* The disease is caused by *C. trachomatis* serovars L1 through L3.

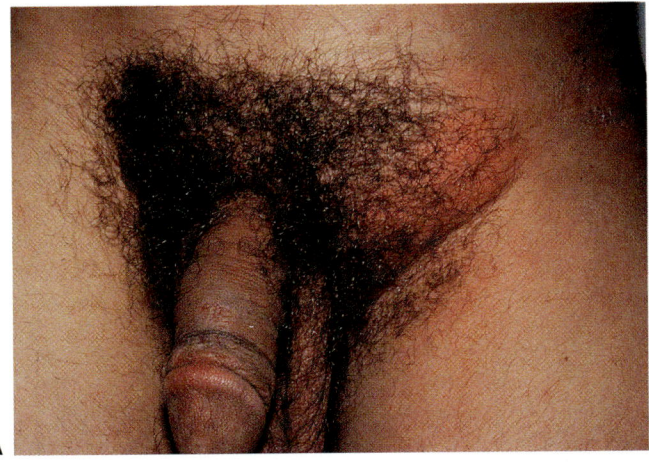
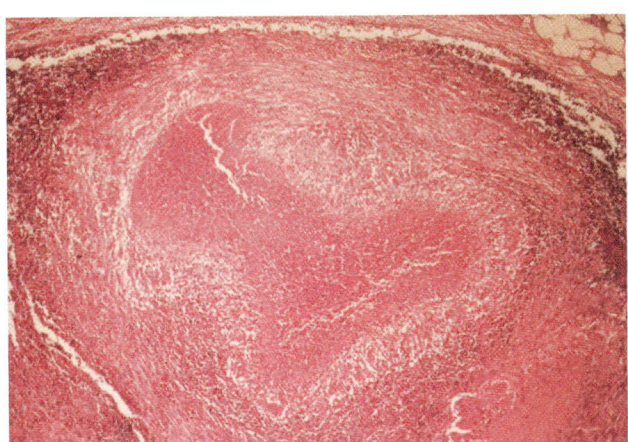

FIGURE 9-43
Lymphogranuloma venereum. A. Painful inguinal lymphadenopathy in a man infected with *C. trachomatis*. B. Microscopic section of a lymph node shows a necrotic central area surrounded by a granulomatous zone.

Epidemiology: Lymphogranuloma venereum is uncommon in developed countries, but it is endemic in the tropics and subtropics. It accounts for 5% of sexually transmitted disease in Africa, India, parts of southeast Asia, South America, and the Caribbean. In North America and Europe, lymphogranuloma venereum is now primarily a disease of homosexual men.

 Pathology: The organism is introduced through a break in the skin. After an incubation period of 4 to 21 days, an ulcer appears, usually on the penis, vagina, or cervix, although lips, tongue, and fingers may also be primary sites. The organisms are transported by lymphatics to regional lymph nodes, where a necrotizing lymphadenitis erupts 1 to 3 weeks after the primary lesion. Abscesses develop within involved lymph nodes, often extending to adjacent lymph nodes. Over the next few weeks, the nodes become tender and fluctuant and frequently ulcerate and discharge pus. The intense inflammatory process can result in severe scarring, which may produce chronic lymphatic obstruction, ischemic necrosis of overlying structures, or strictures and adhesions. The necrotizing process produces enlarged and matted lymph nodes, containing multiple, coalescing abscesses, which often develop a stellate shape (see Fig. 9-43B). The abscesses have a granulomatous appearance, containing neutrophils and necrotic debris in the center, surrounded by palisading epithelioid cells, macrophages, and occasional giant cells. The abscesses are rimmed by lymphocytes, plasma cells, and fibrous tissue. The nodal architecture is eventually effaced by fibrosis.

 Clinical Features: Patients with lymphogranuloma venereum present with lymphadenopathy. Most infections resolve completely, even without antimicrobial therapy. However, progressive ulceration of the penis, urethra, or scrotum, with fistulas and urethral stricture, develop in 5% of men. Women and homosexual men often present with hemorrhagic proctitis, and most late complications, such as rectal stricture, rectovaginal fistulas, and genital elephantiasis, occur in women.

Trachoma Is a Leading Cause of Blindness in Many Developing Countries

Trachoma is a chronic infection of the conjunctiva that progressively scars the conjunctiva and cornea. C. trachomatis serovars A, B, Ba, and C cause the disease.

 Epidemiology: Trachoma is worldwide, associated with poverty, and most prevalent in dry or sandy regions. Only humans are naturally infected, and poor personal hygiene and inadequate public sanitation are common factors. Trachoma remains a major problem in parts of Africa, India, and the Middle East. The infection is spread mostly by direct contact, but it may also be transmitted by fomites, contaminated water, and probably flies. Subclinical infections are an important reservoir. In endemic areas, infection is acquired early in childhood, becomes chronic, and eventually progresses to blindness.

 Pathology: When C. trachomatis is inoculated into the eye, it reproduces within the conjunctival epithelium, thereby inciting a mixed acute and chronic inflammatory infiltrate. Histological examination of the early lesions shows chronic inflammation, lymphoid aggregates, focal degeneration of the conjunctiva, and chlamydial inclusions within the conjunctival epithelium. As trachoma progresses, the lymphoid aggregates enlarge, and the conjunctiva becomes scarred and focally hypertrophic. The cornea is invaded by blood vessels and fibroblasts, forming a scar reminiscent of a cloth ("pannus" in Latin), and is eventually opacified.

 Clinical Features: Early trachoma is characterized by the abrupt onset of palpebral and conjunctival inflammation, which leads to tearing, purulent conjunctivitis, and photophobia. The lymphoid aggregates can be seen as small yellow grains beneath the palpebral conjunctivae within 3 to 4 weeks of infection. After months or years, deformities of the eyelids eventually interfere with normal ocular function, and secondary bacterial infections and corneal ulcerations are common. Blindness is a common end point.

PSITTACOSIS (ORNITHOSIS)

Psittacosis is a self-limited pneumonia transmitted to humans from birds. The causative agent, *Chlamydia psittaci,* is spread by infected birds, and the resulting disease is known as both psittacosis (association with parrots) or ornithosis (association with birds in general).

 Epidemiology: C. psittaci is present in the blood, tissues, excreta, and feathers of infected birds. Humans inhale infectious excreta or dust from feathers. Although infection is endemic in tropical birds, C. psittaci can infect almost any species. Human disease has resulted from exposure to various bird species, including parrots, parakeets, canaries, pigeons, sea gulls, ducks, chickens, and turkeys. Use of tetracycline-containing bird feeds and quarantine of imported tropical birds limits the spread of disease, and fewer than 50 cases of psittacosis are reported annually in the United States.

 Pathology: C. psittaci first infects pulmonary macrophages, which carry the organism to the phagocytic cells of the liver and spleen, where it reproduces. The organism is then distributed by the blood-

TABLE 9-6 Rickettsial Infections

Disease	Organism	Distribution	Transmission
	Spotted-fever group		
Rocky Mountain spotted fever	R. rickettsii	Americas	Ticks
Queensland tick fever	R. australis	Australia	Ticks
Boutonneuse fever, Kenya tick fever	R. conorii	Mediterranean, Africa, India	Ticks
Siberian tick fever	R. sibirica	Siberia, Mongolia	Ticks
Rickettsialpox	R. akari	United States, Russia, Central Asia, Korea, Africa	Mites
	Typhus group		
Louse-borne typhus (epidemic typhus)	R. prowazekii	Latin America, Africa, Asia	Lice
Murine typhus (endemic typhus)	R. typhi	Worldwide	Fleas
Scrub typhus	R. tsutsugamushi	South Pacific, Asia	Mites
Q fever	Coxiella burnetti	Worldwide	Inhalation

stream, producing systemic infection, particularly diffuse involvement of the lungs. *C. psittaci* reproduces in alveolar lining cells, whose destruction elicits an inflammatory response.

The pneumonia is predominantly interstitial, and the inflammatory infiltrate within alveolar septa is composed largely of lymphocytes. Type II pneumocytes are hyperplastic and may show characteristic chlamydial cytoplasmic inclusions. In severe pulmonary disease, hemorrhage and fibrin fill the alveoli, and bacterial superinfection may produce multiple abscesses. Dissemination of the infection is characterized by foci of necrosis in the liver and spleen and diffuse mononuclear cell infiltrates in the heart, kidneys, and brain.

Clinical Features: The spectrum of clinical illness varies widely. There is usually a persistent dry cough, accompanied by constitutional symptoms of high fever, headache, malaise, myalgias, and arthralgias. If untreated, the fever persists for 2 to 3 weeks and then subsides as the pulmonary disease regresses. The mortality rate in the preantibiotic era exceeded 20%, but with tetracycline therapy, the disease is only rarely fatal.

CHLAMYDIA PNEUMONIAE

Chlamydia pneumoniae is a chlamydial pathogen that causes acute, self-limited, usually mild respiratory tract infections, including pneumonia. C. pneumoniae is transmitted from person to person, and infection appears to be very common. In the developed world, half of all adults show evidence of past exposure, but only 10% of infections result in clinically apparent pneumonia. Symptomatic persons complain of fever, sore throat, and cough. Severe pneumonia occurs only in those with an underlying pulmonary condition. In most cases, untreated disease resolves in 2 to 4 weeks.

Rickettsial Infections

The rickettsiae are small, gram-negative coccobacillary bacteria that are obligate intracellular pathogens and cannot replicate outside a host. Rickettsiae can synthesize their own ATP via a proton-translocating ATPase and can also obtain ATP from the host through the ATP/ADP translocase. The organisms induce endocytosis by target cells and replicate within the cytoplasm of the host cell. They have the cell wall structure of gram-negative bacteria but, unlike chlamydiae, replicate by binary fission. Although structurally gram-negative, the rickettsiae do not stain well with the Gram stain and are best demonstrated by the Gimenez method or with acridine orange.

Humans are accidental hosts for most species of *Rickettsia*. The organisms reside in animals and insects and do not require humans for perpetuation. Human rickettsial infection results from insect bites. Several species of *Rickettsia* cause different human diseases (Table 9-6), but rickettsial infections have many features in common. **The human target cell for all rickettsiae is the endothelial cell of capillaries and other small blood vessels.** The organisms reproduce within these cells, killing them in the process and producing a necrotizing vasculitis. Human rickettsial infections are traditionally divided into the "spotted fever group" and the "typhus group."

ROCKY MOUNTAIN SPOTTED FEVER

Rocky Mountain spotted fever is an acute, potentially fatal, systemic vasculitis, usually manifested by headache, fever and rash. The causative organism, Rickettsia rickettsii, is transmitted to humans by tick bites.

Epidemiology: Rocky Mountain spotted fever is acquired by bites of infected ticks, which are the vectors for *R. rickettsii*. The organism passes from mother to progeny ticks without killing them, thereby maintaining a natural reservoir for human infection. Rocky Mountain spotted fever occurs in various areas throughout North, Central, and South America. In the United States, most cases occur in a large cluster of states extending from the eastern seaboard (Georgia to New York) westward to Texas, Oklahoma, and Kansas. Cases in the Rocky Mountain region are uncommon. The name of the disease is misleading, deriving from its discovery in Idaho, rather than its area of greatest prevalence. Some 500 cases occur annually in the United States.

Pathogenesis: *R. rickettsii* in the salivary glands of the tick is introduced into the skin while the tick is feeding. The organisms spread via lymphatics and small blood vessels to the systemic and pulmonary circulation. Here they attach to vascular endothelial cells, are engulfed, and reproduce within the cytoplasm. They are then shed into the vascular and lymphatic systems. Further infection and destruction of vascular endothelium causes a systemic vasculitis. The rash, produced by inflammatory damage to cutaneous vessels, is the most visible manifestation of the generalized phenomenon of vascular injury. Whereas other rickettsiae infect only capillary endothelial cells, *R. rickettsii* spreads to vascular smooth muscle and endothelium of larger vessels. Extensive damage to blood vessel walls causes loss of vascular integrity, exudation of fluid, and disseminated intravascular coagulation. Fluid loss can be so extensive that it leads to shock. Damage to pulmonary capillaries can produce pulmonary edema and acute alveolar injury.

Pathology: The vascular lesions of Rocky Mountain spotted fever are found throughout the body, affecting capillaries, venules, arterioles, and sometimes larger vessels. Necrosis and reactive hyperplasia of vascular endothelium are often associated with thrombosis of the smaller-caliber vessels. Vessel walls are infiltrated, initially with neutrophils and macrophages and later with lymphocytes and plasma cells. Microscopic infarctions and extravasation of blood into surrounding tissues are common. The orientation of the intracellular bacilli in parallel rows and in an end-to-end pattern gives them the appearance of a "flotilla at anchor facing the wind."

Clinical Features: Rocky Mountain spotted fever manifests with fever, headache, and myalgias, followed by a rash. The skin lesions begin as a maculopapular eruption but rapidly become petechial, spreading centripetally from the distal extremities to the trunk (Fig. 9-44). Cutaneous lesions usually appear on the palms and soles, a distinctive feature of the disease. If untreated, more than 20 to 50% of infected persons die within 8 to 15 days. Prompt diagnosis and antibiotic treatment (chloramphenicol and tetracycline) is life saving, and in the United States, mortality has been reduced to less than 5%.

EPIDEMIC (LOUSE-BORNE) TYPHUS

Epidemic typhus is a severe systemic vasculitis transmitted by the bite of infected lice. The disease is caused by *Rickettsia prowazekii*, an organism that has a human-louse-human life cycle (Fig. 9-45).

Epidemiology: *R. prowazekii* is transmitted from one infected person to another by the bite of an infected body louse. The disease is widely distributed in some regions of Africa, Asia, Europe, and the Western Hemisphere. Devastating epidemics of typhus were associated with cold climates, poor sanitation, and crowding during natural disasters, famine or war. Infrequent bathing and lack of changes of clothing lead to louse infestation of human populations and consequently epidemics of typhus. With the mass displacements of populations in Eastern Europe in World War I, epidemic typhus affected over 30 million persons, killing over 3 million. Epidemic louse-borne typhus last occurred in the United States in 1921.

Pathogenesis: After a louse takes a blood meal from a person infected with *R. prowazekii*, the organisms enter the epithelial cells of the midgut, multiply, and rupture the cells within 3 to 5 days. Large numbers of rickettsiae are released into the lumen of the louse intestine. The louse deposits its contaminated feces on the skin or clothing of a second host, where they may remain infectious for more than 3 months. A person becomes infected when the contaminated louse feces penetrate an abrasion or scratch or when the person inhales airborne rickettsiae from clothing containing louse feces. Epidemic typhus begins with localized infection of capillary endothelium and progresses to a systemic vasculitis. Louse-borne typhus differs from the other rickettsial diseases in that *R. prowazekii* can establish la-

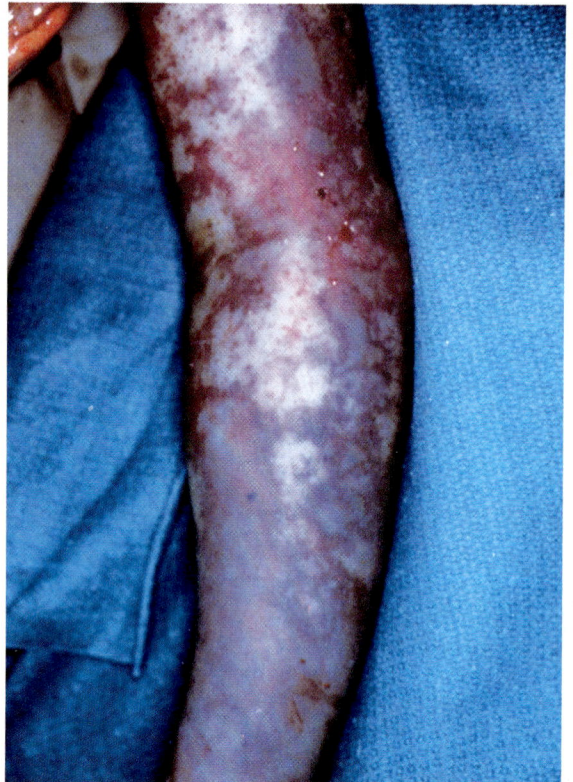

FIGURE 9-44
Rocky mountain spotted fever. A severe petechial and purpuric eruption is noted on the arm in this fatal case.

Scrub Typhus

tent infection and produce recrudescent disease *(Brill-Zinsser disease)* many years after primary infection.

 Pathology: The pathological changes produced by *R. prowazekii* are similar to those of Rocky Mountain spotted fever and the other rickettsial diseases. At autopsy, there are few gross findings except for splenomegaly and occasional areas of necrosis. Microscopically, collections of mononuclear cells are found in various organs (e.g., skin, brain, and heart). The infiltrate includes mast cells, lymphocytes, plasma cells, and macrophages, which are frequently arranged as *typhus nodules* around arterioles and capillaries. Throughout the body, the endothelium of small blood vessels is focally necrotic and hyperplastic, and the walls contain inflammatory cells. Rickettsiae can be demonstrated within the endothelial cells.

 Clinical Features: Louse-borne typhus is characterized by fever, headache, and myalgias, followed by a rash. Macular lesions, which become petechial, appear on the upper trunk and axillary folds and spread centrifugally to the extremities. In fatal cases, the rash commonly becomes confluent and purpuric. Mild rickettsial pneumonia is followed by a superimposed bacterial pneumonia. Dying patients may exhibit the symptoms of encephalitis, myocarditis, interstitial pneumonia, interstitial nephritis, and shock. Fatalities usually occur during the second or third week of illness. In patients who recover, the symptoms abate after about 3 weeks.

Epidemic typhus can be controlled by large-scale delousing of the population, by steam sterilization of clothing, and the use of insecticides.

ENDEMIC (MURINE) TYPHUS

Endemic typhus is similar to epidemic typhus but tends to be a milder disease. Humans are infected with *R. typhi* by interrupting the rat-flea-rat cycle of transmission. When the flea defecates on the surface of the skin, the feces contaminate the small wound made by the bite. The rickettsiae also contaminate clothes and become airborne. When they are inhaled, they cause pulmonary infection. Outbreaks of murine typhus are associated with an exploding population of rats, although sporadic infections occur in the southwestern United States. These are associated with rat-infested dwellings and with occupations that bring humans into contact with rats, such as the handling and storage of grain.

SCRUB TYPHUS

Scrub typhus **(Tsutsugamushi fever)** *is an acute, febrile illness of humans that is caused by* Rickettsia tsutsugamushi. Rodents are the natural mammalian reservoir. From rats, the organism is passed to trombiculid mites known as chiggers. These insects transmit the infection to their larvae, which crawl to the tips of vegetation and attach to passers-by. While feeding, mites inoculate the organisms into the skin. Rickettsemia and lymphadenopathy follow shortly. Scrub ty-

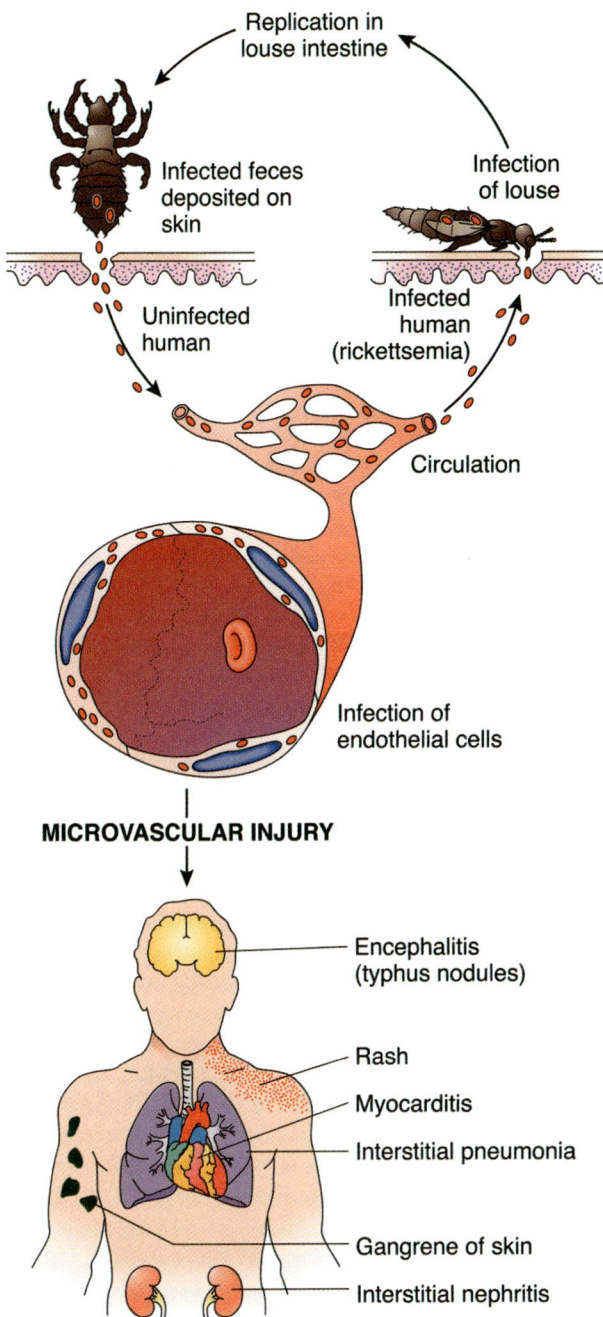

FIGURE 9-45
Epidemic typhus (louse-borne typhus). *R. prowazekii* has a man-louse-man life cycle. The organism multiplies in endothelial cells, which detach, rupture, and release organisms into the circulation (rickettsemia). A louse taking a blood meal becomes infected with rickettsiae, which enter the epithelial cells of its midgut, multiply, and rupture the cells, thereby releasing rickettsiae into the lumen of the louse intestine. Contaminated feces are deposited on the skin or clothing of a second host, penetrate an abrasion or are inhaled. The rickettsiae then enter endothelial cells, multiply, and rupture the cells, thus completing the cycle.

phus is widely distributed in eastern and southern Asia, and the islands of the southern and western Pacific, including Japan. Endemic infection is unknown in the western world.

A multiloculated vesicle forms at the inoculation site and ulcerates, after which an eschar forms. As the lesion heals, there is a sudden onset of headache and fever, followed by pneumonia, a macular rash, lymphadenopathy, and hepatosplenomegaly. Severe infections are complicated by meningoencephalitis, myocarditis, and shock. The mortality rates in untreated patients have ranged up to 30%.

Q FEVER

Q fever is a self-limited, systemic infection, usually manifesting as headache, fever, and myalgias. The disease is caused by *Coxiella burnetii,* a small pleomorphic coccobacillus with a gram-negative cell wall. Unlike true rickettsiae, *C. burnetii* enters cells by a passive mechanism, being phagocytized by macrophages. *C. burnetii* infection does not produce a vasculitis, and thus there is no associated rash.

Epidemiology: Humans acquire Q fever by exposure to infected animals or animal products. Infection is endemic in many wild and domesticated animals, but cattle, sheep, and goats are the usual sources of human infection. These animals shed large numbers of organisms in urine, feces, milk, bodily fluids, and birth products. Q fever is most often seen in herders, slaughterhouse workers, veterinarians, dairy workers, and other persons with occupational exposure to infected domesticated animals. Aerosol droplets may spread the infection from person to person. Q fever is rare in the United States.

Pathology: Q fever begins with the inhalation of organisms, after which they are phagocytosed by alveolar macrophages and replicate in phagolysosomes. Recruitment of neutrophils and macrophages produces a focal bronchopneumonia. The nonactivated phagocytes fail to kill *C. burnetii,* and the organism disseminates through the body, primarily infecting cells of the monocyte/macrophage system. Most infections resolve with the onset of specific cell-mediated immunity, but occasional cases persist as chronic infections.

The lungs and liver are the organs most prominently involved in Q fever. The lungs demonstrate single or multiple irregular areas of consolidation, in which the pulmonary parenchyma is infiltrated by neutrophils and macrophages. Organisms may be demonstrated in macrophages by the Giemsa stain. Hepatic involvement in Q fever is usually characterized by multiple microscopic granulomas, which have a distinctive "fibrin ring" or "doughnut ring" configuration. In these granulomas, epithelioid macrophages encircle a ring of fibrin, sometimes containing a lipid vacuole.

Clinical Features: In most cases in endemic areas, Q fever is a self-limited mildly symptomatic febrile disease. More-severe cases typically present as headache, fever, fatigue, and myalgias, with no rash. Pulmonary infection is virtually always present, but it may appear as an atypical pneumonia with dry cough, a rapidly

TABLE 9-7 **Mycoplasmal Infections**

Organism	Disease
Mycoplasma pneumoniae	Tracheobronchitis
	Pneumonia
	Pharyngitis
	Otitis media
Ureaplasma urealyticum	Urethritis
	Chorioamnionitis
	Postpartum fever
Mycoplasma hominis	Postpartum fever

progressive pneumonia, or chest roentgenographic abnormalities without significant respiratory symptoms. Many patients have some hepatosplenomegaly. The disease resolves spontaneously in 2 to 14 days.

Mycoplasmal Infections

The mycoplasmas, formerly known as pleuropneumonia-like organisms, are the smallest free-living prokaryotes, measuring less than 0.3 μm in greatest dimension. They lack the rigid cell walls of the more complex bacteria. Mycoplasmas are widespread, both geographically and ecologically, as saprophytes and as parasites of a broad range of animals and plants. Numerous *Mycoplasma* species are known to inhabit the human body, but only three are pathogenic: *M. pneumoniae, M. hominis,* and *Ureaplasma urealyticum.* The diseases associated with these organisms are shown in Table 9-7.

MYCOPLASMA PNEUMONIAE

M. pneumoniae produces acute, self-limited lower respiratory tract infections, affecting mostly children and young adults. M. pneumoniae can also cause pharyngitis and otitis media.

Epidemiology: Most infections occur in small groups of persons who have frequent close contact (e.g., families, college fraternities, military units, and residents of closed institutions). The organism is spread by aerosol transmission from person to person over a period of several months, with an attack rate exceeding 50% within the group. *M. pneumoniae* infection occurs worldwide, and in developed countries, the organism causes 15 to 20% of all pneumonias.

Pathogenesis: *M. pneumoniae* initiates infection by attaching to a glycolipid on the surface of the respiratory epithelium. The organism remains outside the cells, where it reproduces and causes progressive dysfunction and eventual death of the host cells. Because *M. pneumoniae* infection rarely produces symptomatic disease in children younger than the age of 5 years, it is thought that the host immune response plays a role in tissue injury.

Pathology: Pneumonia caused by *M. pneumoniae* usually shows patchy consolidation of a single segment of a lower lung lobe, although the process can be more widespread. The mucosa of the affected airways is edematous and infiltrated by a predominantly mononuclear inflammatory infiltrate. The alveoli display a largely interstitial process, with reactive alveolar lining cells and infiltration by mononuclear cells. The pulmonary changes are often complicated by bacterial superinfection. The organism itself is too small to be detected in infected tissue by routine light microscopy.

Clinical Features: Mycoplasma pneumonia tends to be milder than other bacterial pneumonias, which has earned the disease the appellation "walking pneumonia." Fever ordinarily persists for no more than 2 weeks, although the cough may linger for 6 weeks or more. Death from *M. pneumoniae* infection is rare.

Mycobacteria

The mycobacteria are distinctive organisms, 2 to 10 μm in length, which share the cell wall architecture of gram-positive bacteria but also contain large amounts of lipid. The high lipid content interferes with staining by aniline dyes, including crystal violet used in the Gram stain. Thus, although the mycobacteria are gram-positive on a structural basis, this property is difficult to demonstrate by routine staining. The waxy lipids of the cell wall make the mycobacteria "acid fast" (i.e., they retain carbolfuchsin after rinsing with acid alcohol).

The mycobacteria grow more slowly than other pathogenic bacteria, and mycobacterial diseases are all chronic, slowly progressive illnesses. The organisms produce no known toxins, and they damage human tissues by inducing inflammatory and immunological responses. Most mycobacterial pathogens can replicate within cells of the monocyte/macrophage lineage and elicit granulomatous inflammation. The outcome of mycobacterial infection is largely determined by the host's capacity to contain the organism through delayed-type hypersensitivity mechanisms and cell-mediated immune responses.

The two primary mycobacterial pathogens, *Mycobacterium tuberculosis* and *M. leprae*, exclusively infect humans and enjoy no environmental reservoir. The remaining pathogenic mycobacteria are environmental organisms, which only occasionally cause human disease.

TUBERCULOSIS

Tuberculosis is a chronic, communicable disease in which the lungs are the prime target, although any organ may be infected. The disease is caused principally by M. tuberculosis hominis *(Koch bacillus) but also occasionally by* M. tuberculosis bovis. **The characteristic lesion is a spherical granuloma with central caseous necrosis.**

M. tuberculosis is a slender, beaded, nonmotile, acid-fast bacillus (Fig. 9-46) that is an obligate aerobe. The organism grows slowly in culture, with a doubling time of 24 hours, and 3 to 6 weeks are commonly required to produce visible growth in culture.

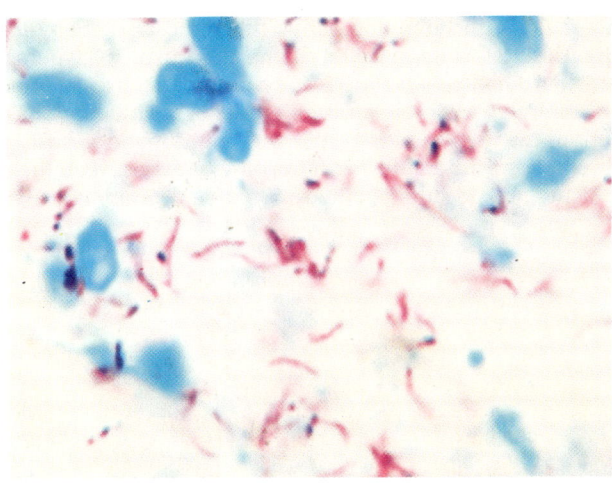
FIGURE 9-46
Mycobacterium tuberculosis. **A smear of a pulmonary lesion shows slender, beaded, acid-fast bacilli.**

Epidemiology: Distributed throughout the world, tuberculosis is clearly one of the most important bacterial diseases in humans. Although the risk of infection has been significantly reduced in developed countries, it remains high for HIV-infected persons; homeless, and malnourished persons in impoverished areas; and immigrants from regions where the disease is endemic. In the United States, for example, the annual incidence of tuberculosis is 12 per 100,000, and the mortality is 1 to 2 per 100,000. By contrast, in some developing countries, the incidence reaches 450 per 100,000, and many of these persons die of the disease. There are also racial and ethnic differences—Africans, Native Americans, and Eskimos being the most susceptible. In the United States, tuberculosis is highest among the elderly, possibly reflecting reactivation of infections acquired earlier in life before the decline in the prevalence of the disease.

M. tuberculosis is transmitted from person to person by aerosolized droplets. Coughing, sneezing, and talking all create aerosolized respiratory droplets; usually, the droplets evaporate, leaving an organism *(droplet nucleus)* that is readily carried in the air. Tuberculosis can also be caused by *M. tuberculosis bovis*, an animal pathogen closely related to *M. tuberculosis hominis*, which is acquired by the ingestion of infected milk. It has ceased to be a significant public health problem in countries where milk is pasteurized or milk-producing animals are inspected.

Pathogenesis: Depending on the age and immunological status of the infected person as well as the total burden of organisms, tuberculosis can pursue radically different courses. Some patients exhibit only an indolent, completely asymptomatic infection; in others, tuberculosis progresses to disseminated destructive disease. Many more persons are infected with *M. tuberculosis* than develop clinical symptoms, and a distinction is made between tuberculous infection and active tuberculosis. **Tuberculous infection** refers to growth of the organism in a person, whether the infection produces symptomatic disease or not. *Active tuberculosis* is the term for the subset of tuberculous infections manifested by destructive, symptomatic disease.

Primary tuberculosis occurs on first exposure to the organism and can pursue either an indolent or an aggressive course (Fig. 9-47). **Secondary tuberculosis** refers to disease that develops long after the primary infection, most commonly as a result of the reactivation of the primary infection. Secondary tuberculosis can also be produced by exposure to exogenous organisms and is always an active disease.

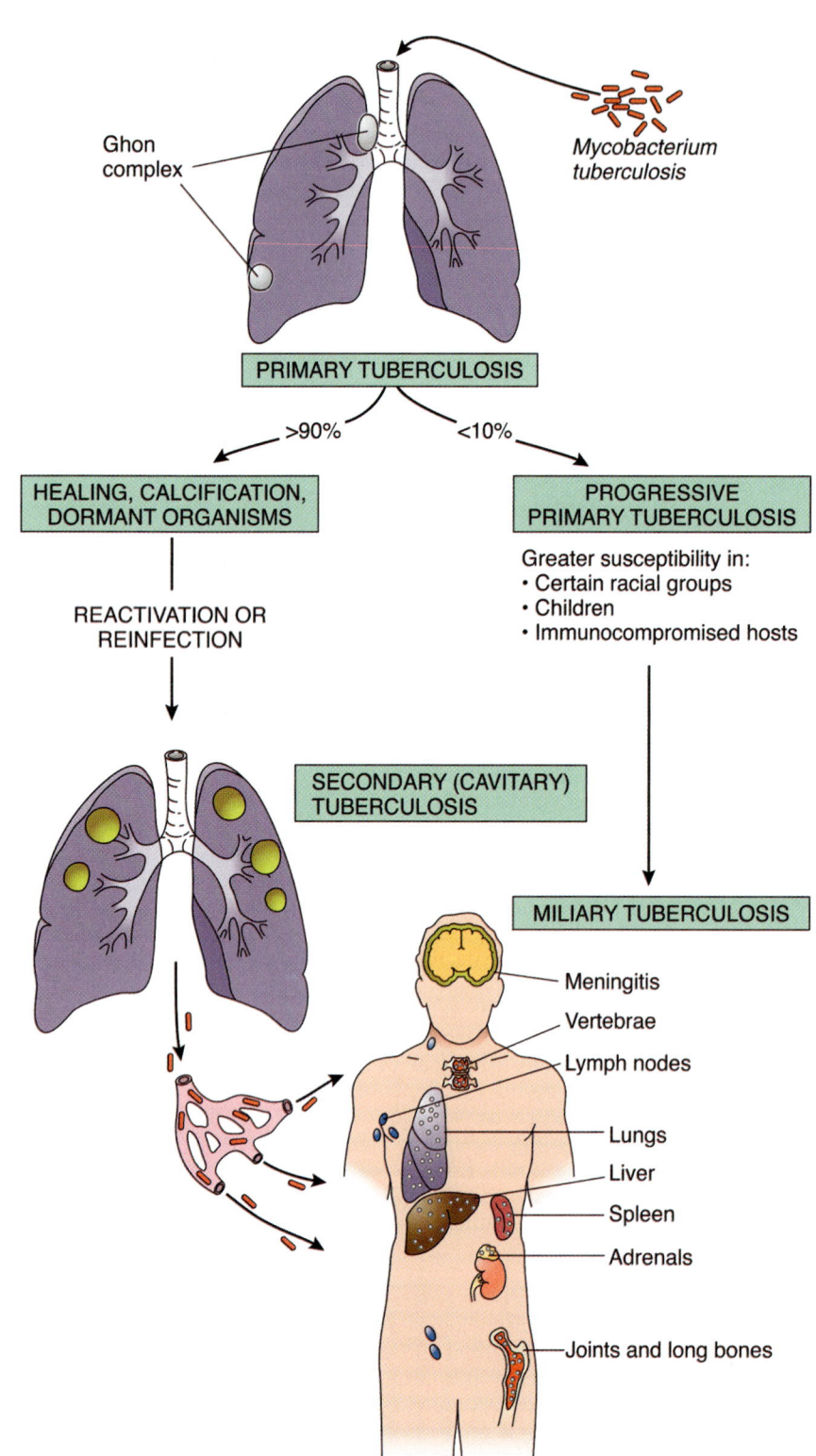

FIGURE 9-47
Stages of the tuberculosis. Primary tuberculosis (in a person lacking previous contact or immune responsiveness). Progressive primary tuberculosis develops in less than 10% of infected normal adults, but more frequently in children and immunosuppressed patients.

Secondary (cavitary) tuberculosis results from reactivation of dormant endogenous bacilli or reinfection with exogenous bacilli. Miliary tuberculosis is caused by dissemination of tubercle bacilli to produce numerous, minute, yellow-white lesions (resembling millet seeds) in distant organs.

Primary Tuberculosis Is an Infection of Persons Who Have Not Had Prior Contact with the Tubercle Bacillus

Pathogenesis: Inhaled *M. tuberculosis* is deposited in the alveoli, usually in the lower segments of the lower and middle lobes and anterior segments of the upper lobes. The organisms are phagocytosed by alveolar macrophages but resist killing; the cell wall lipids of *M. tuberculosis* apparently block the fusion of phagosomes and lysosomes and allow the bacilli to proliferate within the macrophages. As the tubercle bacilli multiply, macrophages degrade some mycobacteria and present antigen to T lymphocytes. Some macrophages carry organisms from the lung to regional (hilar and mediastinal) lymph nodes, from which they may be disseminated by the bloodstream to other areas in the body. The bacilli continue to proliferate at the primary site of deposition in the lungs, as well as at other hospitable sites, including lymph nodes, kidneys, meninges, epiphyseal plates of long bones and vertebrae, and apical areas of the lungs.

Although the macrophages that first ingest *M. tuberculosis* cannot kill these organisms, they initiate hypersensitivity and cell-mediated immunological responses that eventually contain the infection. Infected macrophages present tuberculous antigens to T lymphocytes. A clone of sensitized cells proliferates, produces interferon γ, and activates macrophages, thereby increasing their concentrations of lytic enzymes and augmenting their capacity to kill mycobacteria. When released, the lytic enzymes in these activated macrophages, which include epithelioid macrophages and Langhans giant cells, also damage host tissues.

The development of a population of activated lymphocytes responsive to *M. tuberculosis* antigen constitutes the hypersensitivity response to the organism. The related development of activated macrophages capable of ingesting and destroying the bacilli comprises the cell-mediated immune response. These responses work in concert to combat the proliferating organisms, a process that requires 3 to 6 weeks to come into play.

If the infected person is immunologically competent and the burden of organisms is small, a vigorous granulomatous reaction is produced. Tubercle bacilli are ingested and killed by activated macrophages, surrounded by fibrous tissue, and successfully contained. When the number of organisms is high, the hypersensitivity reaction produces significant tissue necrosis, which has a characteristic cheeselike (caseous) consistency. Although not invariably caused by *M. tuberculosis*, caseous necrosis is so strongly associated with tuberculosis, that its discovery in tissue must raise a suspicion of this disease.

In immunologically immature subjects (a young child or immunosuppressed patient) granulomas are poorly formed or not formed at all, and infection progresses at the primary site in the lung, in the regional lymph nodes, or in multiple sites of dissemination. This process produces *progressive primary tuberculosis*.

 Pathology: The lung lesion of primary tuberculous infection is known as the *Ghon focus*. It is located in the subpleural area of the upper segments of the lower lobes or in the lower segments of the upper lobes. Initially, the Ghon focus is a small, ill-defined area of inflammatory consolidation. The infection then drains to the hilar lymph nodes. The combination of the peripheral Ghon focus and the involved mediastinal or hilar lymph nodes is called the *Ghon complex*.

Microscopically, the classic lesion of tuberculosis is a caseous granuloma (Fig. 9-48), which has a soft, semisolid core surrounded by epithelioid macrophages, Langhans giant cells, lymphocytes, and peripheral fibrous tissue. If the infected person lacks an appropriate immunological response, the granuloma formed in response to *M. tuberculosis* is less organized and may consist of only an aggregate of macrophages, lacking the architecture and Langhans giant cells of the classic granuloma.

In over 90% of normal adults, tuberculous infection follows a self-limited course. In both the lungs and the lymph nodes, the lesions of the Ghon complex heal, undergoing shrinkage, fibrous scarring, and calcification, the last visible radiographically. A small proportion of the organisms may remain viable for years. Later, if immune mechanisms wane or fail, the resting bacilli may proliferate and break out, causing serious secondary tuberculosis.

Progressive primary tuberculosis is an alternative course in which the immune response fails to control the multiplication of the tubercle bacilli. Infection takes this course in less than 10% of normal adults, but it is common in children younger than 5 years of age and in patients with suppressed or defective immunity. The Ghon focus in the lung enlarges and may even erode into the bronchial tree. The affected hilar and mediastinal lymph nodes also enlarge, sometimes compressing the bronchi to produce atelectasis of the distal lung; collapse of the middle lobe *(middle lobe syndrome)* is a common result of this compression. In some instances, the infected lymph nodes erode into an airway to spread organisms throughout the lungs.

Miliary tuberculosis refers to infection at disseminated sites that produces multiple, small, yellow, nodular lesions in several organs (Fig. 9-49). The term *miliary* was coined to emphasize the resemblance of the disseminated lesions to millet seeds. The lungs, lymph nodes, kidneys, adrenals, bone marrow, spleen, and liver are common sites of miliary lesions. Pro-

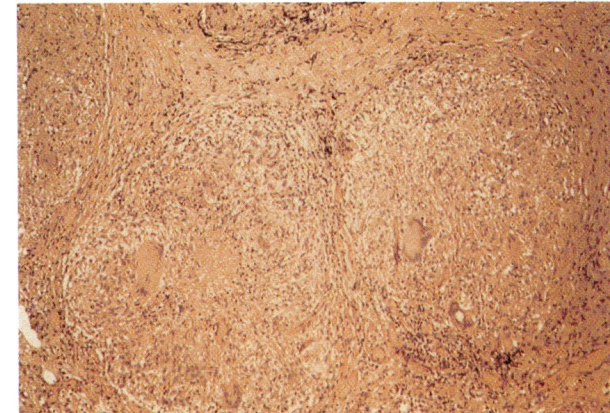

FIGURE 9-48
Primary tuberculosis. Photomicrograph of a hilar lymph node shows a tuberculous granuloma with central caseation.

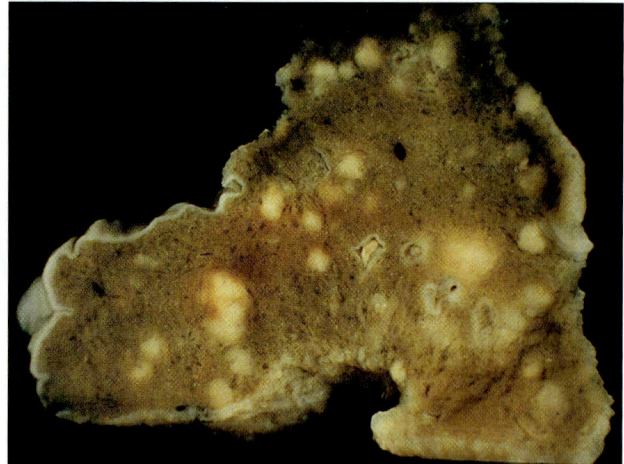
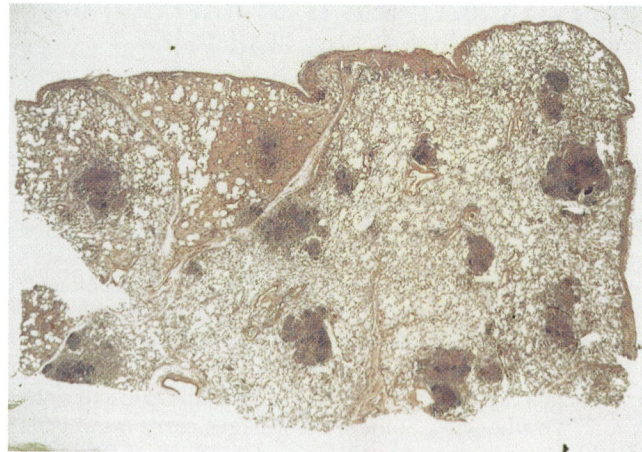

FIGURE 9-49
Miliary tuberculosis. A. The cut surface of the lung reveals numerous uniform, white nodules. B. A low-power photomicrograph discloses many foci of granulomatous inflammation.

gressive disease may involve the meninges and cause tuberculous meningitis.

Clinical Features: Most persons successfully contain the primary infection, and primary tuberculosis is generally asymptomatic. In those who develop progressive primary disease, the symptoms are usually insidious and nonspecific, with fever, weight loss, fatigue, and night sweats. Sometimes the onset of symptoms is abrupt, and the disease manifests as high fever, pleurisy, a pleural effusion, and lymphadenitis. Cough and hemoptysis develop only when active pulmonary disease is well established. With disseminated (miliary) tuberculosis, symptoms vary according to the organs affected and tend to occur late in the course of disease.

Secondary (Cavitary) Tuberculosis Occurs in Previously Infected Persons

Secondary tuberculosis results from the proliferation of M. tuberculosis *in a person who has been previously infected and has mounted an immunological response.* The source of the bacteria in secondary tuberculosis may be either dormant organisms from old granulomas (which is usually the case) or newly acquired bacilli. Various conditions predispose to the reemergence of endogenous (dormant) *M. tuberculosis,* including cancer, antineoplastic chemotherapy, immunosuppressive therapy, AIDS, and old age. Secondary tuberculosis may develop even decades after the primary infection.

Pathology: The lungs are by far the most common site for secondary tuberculosis, although any locale may manifest secondary disease. In the lungs, secondary tuberculosis usually begins in the apical–posterior segments of the upper lobes, where organisms are commonly seeded during the primary infection. The bacilli proliferate at these sites and elicit an inflammatory response, which results in a localized area of consolidation. **The ensuing T cell-mediated immune responses to the now familiar tuberculous antigens lead to tissue necrosis and the production of tuberculous cavities** (Fig. 9-50). Apical cavities are optimal sites for the multiplication of *M. tuberculosis,* and large numbers of organisms are produced in this environment. Cavities are typically 2 to 4 cm in diameter when first detected clinically but can range to well over 10 cm. Tuberculous cavities contain caseous material teeming with mycobacteria and are surrounded by a granulomatous response.

The pulmonary lesions of secondary tuberculosis may be complicated by a variety of secondary effects. These include (1) scarring and calcification; (2) spread to other areas; (3) pleural fibrosis and adhesions; (4) rupture of a caseous lesion, spilling bacilli into the pleural cavity; (5) erosion into a

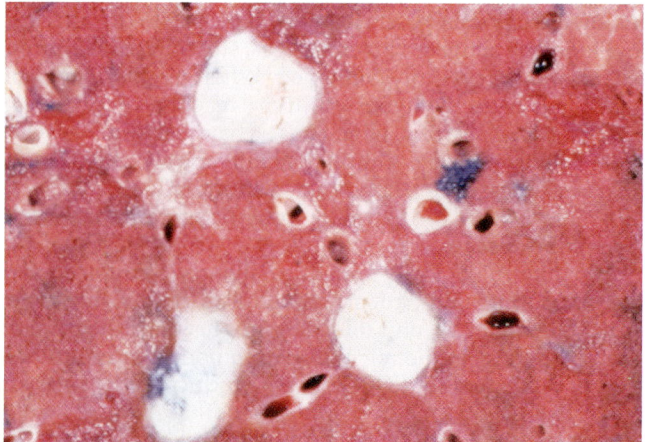

FIGURE 9-50
Secondary pulmonary tuberculosis. A cross-section of lung shows several tuberculous cavities filled with necrotic, caseous material.

bronchus, which seeds the bronchioles, bronchi, and trachea; and (6) implantation of bacilli in the larynx, causing hoarseness and pain on swallowing. Tubercle bacilli may also spread throughout the body through the lymphatics and bloodstream to cause miliary tuberculosis.

Clinical Features: Cough (which may be erroneously attributed to smoking or to a cold), low-grade fever, general malaise, fatigue, anorexia, weight loss, and often night sweats are the usual manifestations. Cavitary disease may be accompanied by hemoptysis, on occasion severe enough to cause exsanguination. Chest radiographs showing unilateral or bilateral apical cavities suggest the diagnosis of secondary tuberculosis. If the disease is disseminated, the signs and symptoms reflect the particular organs involved.

Untreated secondary tuberculosis is a wasting disease that is eventually fatal. Prior to the antibiotic era, chronic cavitary tuberculosis was one of the most common causes of secondary amyloidosis. Tuberculosis is treated with prolonged courses of antituberculous antibiotics, including isoniazid, pyrazinamide, rifampin, and ethambutol. Strains of *M. tuberculosis* that are resistant to these antibiotics have recently emerged, usually as a result of failure to take prescribed medications consistently and for the full time.

LEPROSY

Leprosy (Hansen disease) is a chronic, slowly progressive, destructive process involving peripheral nerves, skin, and mucous membranes, caused by Mycobacterium leprae. This agent is a slender, weakly acid-fast rod, which cannot be cultured on artificial media or in cell culture.

Epidemiology: Leprosy is one of the oldest recognized human diseases. Lepers were isolated from the community in the Old Testament, although some of those segregated persons may have suffered from psoriasis and other skin conditions. For centuries, leprosy was widespread in Europe, including England. In 1873, Hansen documented the first human bacterial pathogen when he described the lepra bacillus in fresh mounts of scrapings from a skin lesion of a Norwegian patient.

Lepra bacilli multiply in experimental animals at sites with temperatures below that of the internal organs, such as the foot pads of mice and the ear lobes of hamsters, rats, and other rodents. Naturally acquired leprosy has been recognized in armadillos in Louisiana and Texas. Lepra bacilli have been experimentally transmitted to armadillos, whose susceptibility is related, at least in part, to their low body temperature (32–35°C).

Leprosy is transmitted from person to person, usually as a result of years of intimate contact. *M. leprae* is shed in nasal secretions or from ulcerated lesions of an infected person. The mode of infection is unclear, but it probably involves inoculation of bacilli into the respiratory tract or into open wounds. Although leprosy is now rare in developed countries, 15 million persons are infected worldwide, primarily in tropical areas, including India, Papua-New Guinea, Southeast Asia, and tropical Africa. Fewer than 400 cases are diagnosed annually in the United States; most in immigrants from endemic areas.

Pathogenesis: *M. leprae* multiplies best at temperatures below core human body temperature, and lesions tend to occur in cooler parts of the body (e.g., the hands and face). Leprosy exhibits a bewildering variety of clinical and pathological features. The lesions vary from the small, insignificant, and self-healing macules of tuberculoid leprosy to the diffuse, disfiguring, and sometimes fatal lesions of lepromatous leprosy (Fig. 9-51). This extreme variation in the presentation of the disease is probably related to differences in immune reactivity.

Most (95%) persons have a natural protective immunity to *M. leprae* and are not infected, even through intimate and prolonged exposure. In the susceptible population (5%) who may develop symptomatic infections, a broad immunological spectrum ranges from anergy to hyperergy. **Anergic patients (i.e., those with little or no resistance) have lepromatous leprosy, whereas hyperergic patients (i.e., those with high resistance) develop tuberculoid leprosy.** *Borderline leprosy* is the term applied to the broad middle ground into which most symptomatic patients fall.

Tuberculoid Leprosy Occurs in Infected Persons Who Mount an Effective Granulomatous Response

Pathology: Tuberculoid leprosy is characterized by a single lesion or very few lesions of the skin, which usually appear on the face, extremities, or trunk. Microscopically the lesions show well-formed, circumscribed dermal granulomas, composed of epithelioid macrophages, Langhans giant cells, and lymphocytes. Nerve fibers are almost invariably swollen and infiltrated with lymphocytes. The destruction of small dermal nerve twigs accounts for the sensory deficit associated with tuberculoid leprosy. Bacilli are rare and often not found with acid-fast stains. The condition is termed *tuberculoid leprosy* because the granulomas vaguely resemble the lesions of tuberculosis. However, the granulomas of leprosy lack caseous necrosis.

Clinical Features: The skin lesions of tuberculoid leprosy appear as well-demarcated, hypopigmented or erythematous, dry, hairless patches, with raised outer edges. Nerve involvement causes diminished sensation or numbness within the patch. As the lesion expands at its periphery, it often heals centrally. In contrast to lepromatous leprosy, the lesions of tuberculoid leprosy cause minimal disfigurement and are not infectious.

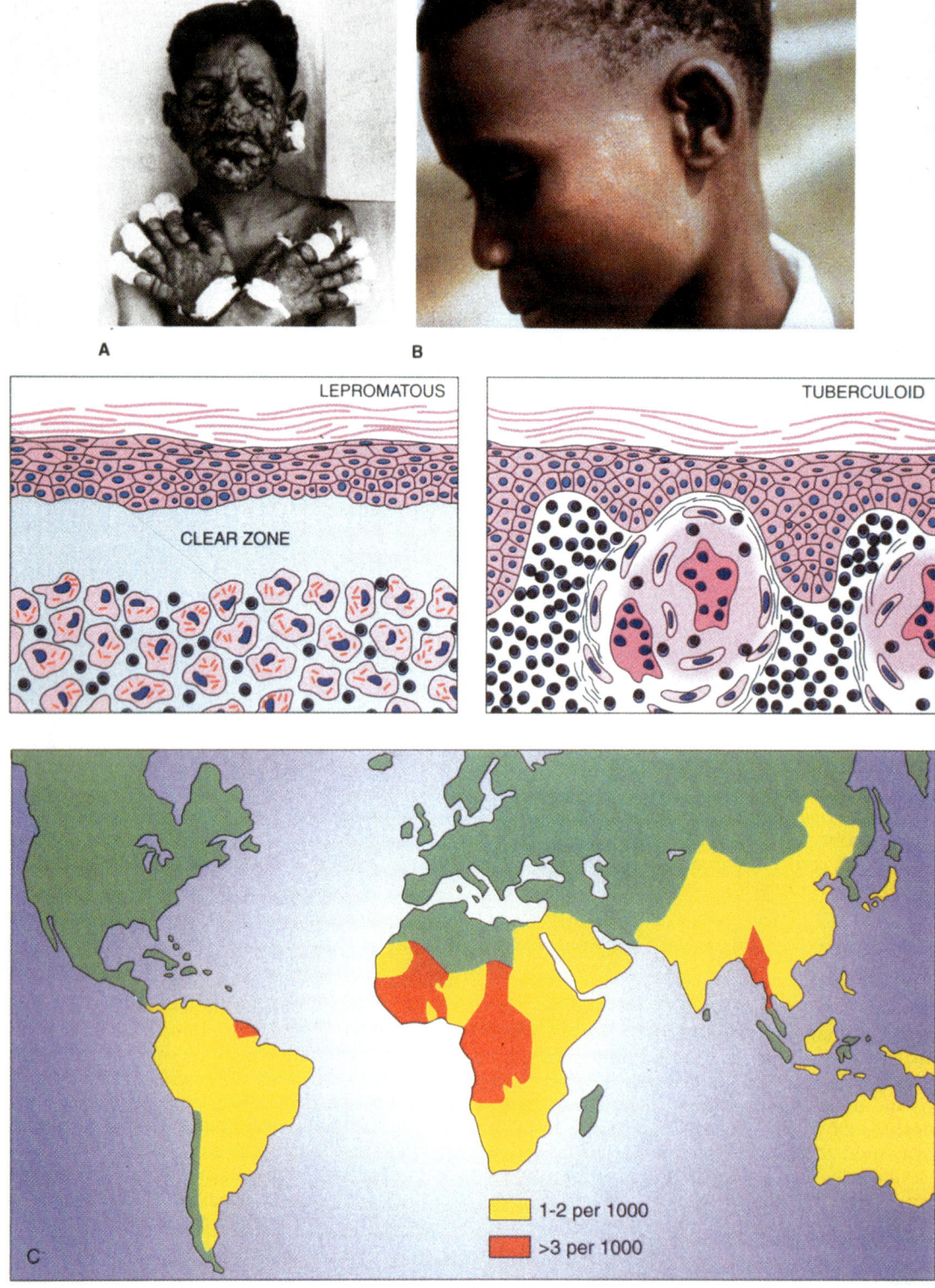

FIGURE 9-51

A. *(Top)* Lepromatous leprosy. There is diffuse involvement, including a leonine face, loss of eyebrows and eyelashes, and nodular distortions, especially on the face, ears, forearms, and hands—the exposed (cool) parts of the body. *(Bottom)* The nodular skin lesions of advanced lepromatous leprosy. Swelling has flattened the epidermis (loss of Rete ridges). A characteristic "clear zone" of uninvolved dermis separates the epidermis from tumorlike accumulations of macrophages, each containing numerous lepra bacilli *(M. leprae)*. B. *(Top)* Tuberculoid leprosy on the cheek, showing a hypopigmented macule with a raised, infiltrated border. The central portion may be hypesthetic or anesthetic. *(Bottom)* Macular skin lesion of tuberculoid leprosy. Skin from the raised "infiltrated" margin of the plaque contains discrete granulomas that extend to the basal layer of the epidermis (without a clear zone). The granulomas are composed of epithelioid cells and Langhans giant cells, and are associated with lymphocytes and plasma cells. Lepra bacilli are rare. C. Distribution of leprosy. Prevalence is greatest in tropical regions of Africa, Asia, and Latin America.

Lepromatous Leprosy Reflects an Inadequate Immune Response to the Lepra Bacillus

Pathology: Lepromatous leprosy exhibits multiple, tumorlike lesions of the skin, eyes, testes, nerves, lymph nodes, and spleen. Nodular or diffuse infiltrates of foamy macrophages contain myriad bacilli (Fig. 9-52). The epidermis is stretched thinly over the nodules, and beneath it is a narrow, uninvolved "clear zone" of the dermis. Rather than destroying the bacilli, the macrophages appear to act as microincubators. When subjected to acid-fast stains, the numerous organisms within the foamy macrophages appear as aggregates of acid-fast material, called *globi*. The dermal infiltrates expand slowly to distort and disfigure the face, ears, and upper airway and to destroy the eyes, eyebrows and eyelashes, nerves, and testes.

Clinical Features: The nodular skin lesions of lepromatous leprosy sometimes ulcerate. Claw-shaped hands, hammertoes, saddle nose, and pendulous ear lobes are common deformities. Nodular lesions of the face may coalesce to produce a lionlike appearance *(leonine facies)*. Involvement of the upper respiratory tract leads to a chronic nasal discharge and voice change, and infection of the eyes may cause blindness.

The most commonly used drug, dapsone, effectively eliminates the lepra bacilli in 4 to 5 years, but it must be continued indefinitely. Dapsone-resistant strains of *M. leprae* have appeared, and multidrug regimens are often used.

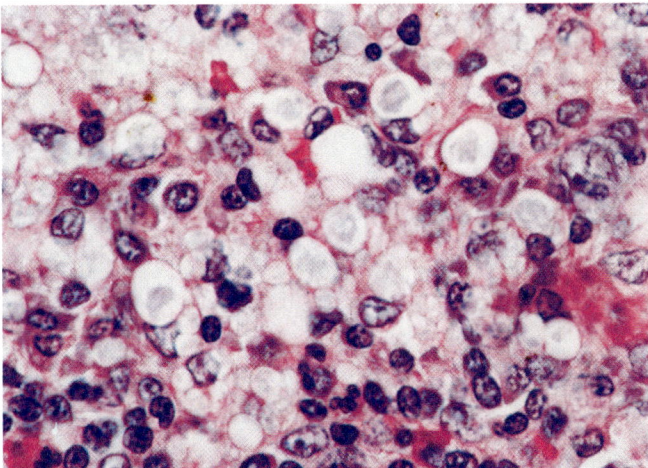

FIGURE 9-52
Lepromatous leprosy. A section of skin shows a tumorlike mass of foamy macrophages. The faint masses within the vacuolated macrophages are enormous numbers of lepra bacilli.

MYCOBACTERIUM AVIUM-INTRACELLULARE COMPLEX

Mycobacterium avium and *Mycobacterium intracellulare* are similar mycobacterial species, which cause identical diseases and are classed together as *M. avium-intracellulare* (MAI) complex, or simply MAI. MAI causes two types of disease: (1) a rare, slowly progressive granulomatous pulmonary disease in immunocompetent persons and (2) a progressive systemic disease in patients with AIDS. Prior to the AIDS epidemic, infection with MAI was a medical curiosity, but today it is the third most common opportunistic infection in AIDS patients in the United States.

MAI is found in soil, water, and foodstuffs worldwide. Humans probably acquire MAI from the environment by inhalation of aerosols from infected water sources, and colonization by the organisms is common. As many as 70% of healthy persons show immunological responsiveness to MAI, indicating prior exposure.

MAI Granulomatous Pulmonary Disease Occurs in Immunocompetent Persons

Most immunocompetent persons with granulomatous pulmonary disease caused by MAI are older (aged 50–70 years), and many suffer from preexisting pulmonary disease. The disease is clinically and pathologically similar to tuberculosis but progresses much more slowly. Both infections produce pulmonary nodules and cavities, and microscopically both show similar caseating granulomas.

Clinical Features: The most common antecedent illnesses predisposing to pulmonary infection with MAI are chronic obstructive pulmonary disease, treated tuberculosis, pneumoconioses, and bronchiectasis. Cough is a frequent symptom, but the disease lacks the fever, night sweats, fatigue, and weight loss that characterize tuberculosis. MAI pulmonary disease is indolent or only slowly progressive, producing a gradual decline in pulmonary function over years or decades. The organism is invariably resistant in vitro to all first-line antituberculous drugs. Combinations of these drugs are used in treatment, but the results are often disappointing.

M. avium-intracellulare Causes Disseminated Infection in AIDS

One third of AIDS patients in the United States develop overt MAI infections, and as many as one half have evidence of infection at autopsy.

Pathogenesis: In AIDS patients, progressive depletion of helper T cells cripples the immune responses that normally prevent MAI disease. Al-

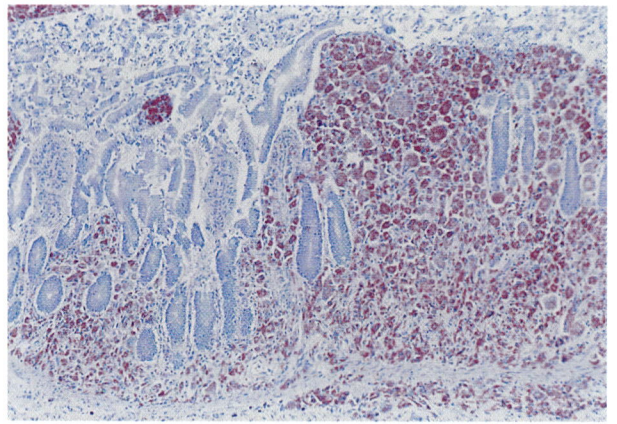

FIGURE 9-53
Mycobacterium avium-intracellulare (MAI). A section of small bowel from a patient with AIDS reveals the presence of numerous macrophages stuffed with acid-fast bacilli in the lamina propria.

though macrophages phagocytose the organisms, they are unable to kill them. The bacilli replicate, fill the cells, spread to other macrophages, and are disseminated throughout the body by the lymphatics and bloodstream.

 Pathology: Infected macrophages are found in various organs, particularly the bowel, lymph nodes, spleen, liver, bone marrow, and lungs. Proliferation of organisms and recruitment of additional macrophages produce expanding nodular lesions, ranging from structured epithelioid granulomas containing few organisms to loose aggregates of foamy macrophages packed with acid-fast bacilli (Fig. 9-53). Eventually, lymph nodes, spleen, and bone marrow may be almost completely replaced by aggregates of macrophages, and lesions in the bowel erode into the lumen of the gut.

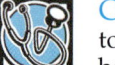 **Clinical Features:** The early, constitutional symptoms of MAI disease in AIDS resemble those of tuberculosis and include fever, night sweats, fatigue, and weight loss. Progressive involvement of the small bowel produces malabsorption and diarrhea, often accompanied by abdominal pain. Although the lungs are commonly involved, pulmonary disease is usually clinically insignificant. Combinations of as many as five or more different antibiotics, usually including clarithromycin, may control, but rarely cure, disseminated MAI infection in AIDS patients.

ATYPICAL MYCOBACTERIA

Several other species of environmental mycobacteria occasionally produce human disease. These organisms are also present in surface waters, dust, and dirt, and people acquire infection by inhalation, inoculation, or ingestion of environmental material.

These bacteria, including MAI, are often lumped together as the "atypical mycobacteria" (in contrast to *M. tuberculosis*, regarded as the "typical" mycobacterium). The atypical mycobacteria are biologically diverse, and the uncommon diseases that they produce in humans differ in circumstances of acquisition, pathology, clinical presentations, and therapies. The features of these diseases are compared in Table 9-8.

M. kansasii causes a chronic, slowly progressive granulomatous pulmonary disease in older persons (over age 50 years), similar to that produced by MAI in immunocompetent patients.

M. scrofulaceum, a common soil inhabitant, causes a draining, granulomatous, cervical lymphadenitis in young children (aged 1–5 years). The infection affects the submandibular lymph nodes and probably results from inoculation or ingestion of organisms by toddlers playing in soil. The disease is localized, and surgical excision of the affected lymph nodes is curative.

TABLE 9-8 Atypical Mycobacterial Infections

Organism	Disease	Ages Affected	Pathology	Source	Distribution
M. kansasii	Chronic granulomatous pulmonary disease (similar to that caused by *M. avium-intracellulare*)	50–70	Granulomatous inflammation	Inhaled organisms from soil, dust, or water	Worldwide
M. scrofulaceum	Cervical lymphadenitis	1–5	Granulomatous inflammation	Probably ingested organisms from soil or dust	Worldwide
M. marinum	Localized skin lesions	All	Granulomatous inflammation	Direct inoculation of organisms from fish or underwater surfaces (swimming pools, fish tanks)	Worldwide
M. ulcerans	Large, solitary, severe ulcer of skin and subcutaneous tissue	Usually 5–25	Coagulative necrosis	Probably inoculation of environmental organisms	Australia, Africa
M. fortuitum-chelonei	Infections associated with traumatic or iatrogenic inoculations	All	Pyogenic inflammation	Inoculation of environmental organisms	Worldwide

M. marinum, commonly found on underwater surfaces, produces a localized nodular skin lesion ("swimming pool granuloma"), sometimes with lymphatic involvement. Infection is acquired by traumatic inoculation, such as abrading an elbow on a swimming pool ladder or cutting a finger on a fish spine. The tissue reaction can be pyogenic or granulomatous.

M. ulcerans leads to a severe ulcerating skin disease in Australia, Africa, and New Guinea. The infection presents as a solitary, undermining, deep ulcer of the skin and subcutaneous fat of the extremities.

M. chelonae and *M. fortuitum* are closely related organisms that are present throughout the environment. Infection is associated with traumatic or iatrogenic inoculation of material contaminated with organisms. Painless, fluctuant abscesses appear at the site of inoculation, ulcerate, and gradually heal spontaneously. The tissue reaction can be pyogenic or granulomatous.

Fungal Infections

Of more than 100,000 known fungi, only a few invade and destroy human tissue. Of these, most are "opportunists"—that is, they infect only persons with impaired immune mechanisms. **Thus, corticosteroid administration, antineoplastic therapy, and congenital or acquired T-cell deficiencies all predispose to mycotic infections.**

Fungi are larger and more complex organisms than bacteria, ranging in size from 2 to 100 μm. They are eukaryotes, having nuclear membranes and cytoplasmic organelles, such as mitochondria and endoplasmic reticulum.

There are two basic morphological types of fungi: yeasts and molds.

- **Yeasts** are the unicellular form of fungi. They are round or oval cells that reproduce by budding, a process in which the daughter organism pinches off from the parent. Some yeasts produce buds that do not detach but instead produce a chain of elongated yeast cells that resemble hyphae and are termed *pseudohyphae*.
- **Molds** are multicellular filamentous fungal colonies that consist of branching tubules, 2 to 10 μm in diameter, termed *hyphae*. The mass of tangled hyphae in the mold form is called a *mycelium*. Some hyphae are separated by septa that are located at regular intervals; others are nonseptate.
- **Dimorphic fungi** can grow as either yeasts or molds, depending on the environmental circumstances.

Most fungi are visible on tissue sections stained with hematoxylin and eosin. The periodic acid–Schiff (PAS) reaction and Gomori methenamine silver (GMS) stain outline fungal cell walls and are commonly used to detect fungal infection in tissues.

CANDIDA

The genus *Candida*, comprising over 20 species of yeasts, includes the most common opportunistic pathogens. Many *Candida* species are endogenous human flora, well adapted to life on or in the human body. However, they can cause disease when host defenses are compromised. Although the various forms of candidiasis vary in clinical severity, most are localized, superficial diseases, limited to a particular mucocutaneous site, including the following:

- **Intertrigo:** infection of opposed skin surfaces
- **Paronychia:** infection of the nail bed
- **Diaper rash**
- **Vulvovaginitis**
- **Thrush:** oral infection
- **Esophagitis**

Candidal infections of deep tissues are much less common than superficial infections but can be life threatening. The most common deep sites affected are the brain, eye, kidney, and heart. Deep infections, with candidal sepsis and disseminated candidiasis, occur only in immunologically compromised persons and are often fatal.

Most candidal infections derive from endogenous flora. *C. albicans* resides in small numbers in the oropharynx, gastrointestinal tract, and vagina and is the most frequent candidal pathogen, being responsible for more than 95% of these infections.

Pathogenesis: Mechanical barriers, inflammatory cells, humoral immunity, and cell-mediated immunity relegate *Candida* to superficial, nonsterile sites. In turn, the resident bacterial flora normally limits the number of fungal organisms. Bacteria (1) block candidal attachment to epithelial cells, (2) compete with the organisms for nutrients, and (3) prevent conversion of the fungus to its tissue-invasive forms. When any of the above defenses is compromised, candidal infections can occur (Table 9-9). **Antibiotic use results in the suppression of the competing bacterial flora and is the most common precipitating factor for candidiasis.** Under conditions of unopposed growth, the yeast converts to its invasive form (hyphae or pseudohyphae), invades superficially, and elicits an inflammatory or immunological response.

Even though Candida inhabits the skin surface, it does not produce cutaneous disease without some predisposing skin lesion. The most common precipitating factor is maceration, a softening and destruction of the skin. Chronically warm and moist areas, such as those between fingers and toes, between skinfolds, and under diapers, are prone to maceration and thus superficial candidal disease.

TABLE 9-9 **Candidal Infections**

Disease	Predisposing Conditions
Superficial Infections	
Intertrigo (opposed skin surfaces)	Maceration
Paronychia (nail beds)	Maceration
Diaper rash	Maceration
Vulvovaginitis	Alteration in normal flora
Thrush (oral)	Decreased cell-mediated immunity
Esophagitis	Decreased cell-mediated immunity
Deep Infections	
Urinary tract infections	Indwelling urinary catheters
Sepsis and disseminated infection	Neutropenia, indwelling vascular catheters, and change in normal flora

The incidence of severe candidal infections has increased in recent years, in part owing to increased numbers of neutropenic and immunodeficient patients. Frequent use of potent broad-spectrum antibiotics leads to extensive candidal colonization in debilitated patients. Expanded use of medical devices, such as intravascular catheters, monitoring devices, endotracheal tubes, and urinary catheters, provides access to sterile sites. Intravenous drug users also develop deep candidal infections because of inoculation of the fungi into the bloodstream.

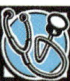 **Pathology and Clinical Features:** Superficial infections of the skin, oropharynx (Fig. 9-54A), and esophagus show invasive organisms in the most superficial layers of the epithelium and are associated with acute inflammatory infiltrates. Yeasts, pseudohyphae, and hyphae are present (see Fig. 9-54B). The yeast cells are round and 3 to 4 μm in diameter, and the hyphae are septate. Candidal vaginitis is characterized by superficial invasion of the squamous epithelium, but the inflammatory infiltrate is usually sparse. Deep candidal infections consist of multiple microscopic abscesses composed of yeasts and hyphae, necrotic debris, and neutrophils. Rarely, a granulomatous response to the organism occurs.

The various superficial cutaneous infections manifest as tender, erythematous papules, which expand to form confluent erythematous areas.

- **Thrush:** This lesion involves the tongue and mucous membranes of the mouth. Early in life, oral thrush is the most common form of mucocutaneous candidiasis, and candidal vaginitis during pregnancy predisposes the newborn to infection. Thrush consists of friable, white, curdlike membranes adherent to the affected surfaces. These patches are composed of fungi, necrotic debris, neutrophils, and bacteria and can be dislodged by scraping. Removal of the membranes leaves a painful, bleeding surface.

- **Candidal vulvovaginitis:** This condition appears as vaginal and vulvar itching, associated with a thick, white vaginal discharge. Involved areas of the vulva are erythematous and tender. Candidal vaginitis is most intense when the vaginal pH is low. Antibacterial antibiotics, pregnancy, diabetes, and corticosteroids predispose to the development of this common form of vaginitis.

- **Candidal sepsis and disseminated candidiasis:** Systemic candidiasis is rare, and it is ordinarily a terminal event of an underlying disorder associated with an altered immune system. In addition to C. albicans, other candidal species can produce invasive candidiasis. The organisms may enter through an ulcerative lesion of the skin or mucous membrane, or may be introduced by iatrogenic means (e.g., peritoneal dialysis, intravenous lines, or urinary catheters). The urinary tract is most commonly involved, and the incidence in women is four times that in men. Renal lesions may be blood-borne or may arise from an ascending pyelonephritis.

- **Candidal endocarditis:** This infection is characterized by large vegetations on the valves and a high incidence of embolization to large arteries. In most patients with candidal endocarditis, the cause is not immunosuppression but unusual vulnerability. Drug addicts who use unsterilized needles and persons with preexisting valvular disease who have had prolonged antibacterial therapy or indwelling vascular catheters are at risk for endocarditis. One of the most serious complications of invasive candidiasis is septic embolism to the brain.

ASPERGILLOSIS

Aspergillus species are common environmental fungi that produce opportunistic infections, usually involving the

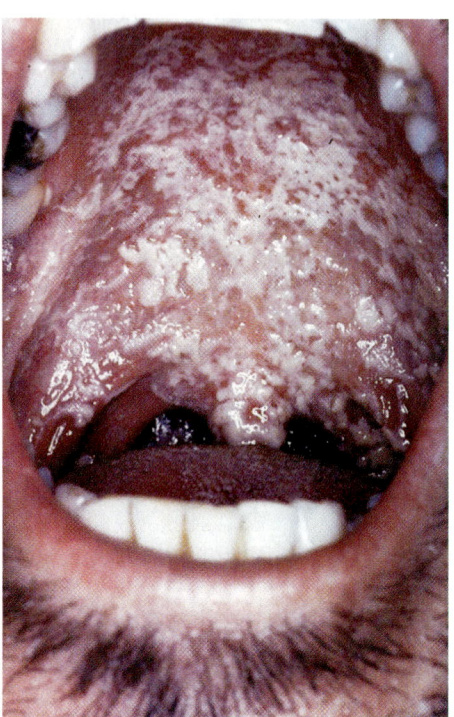
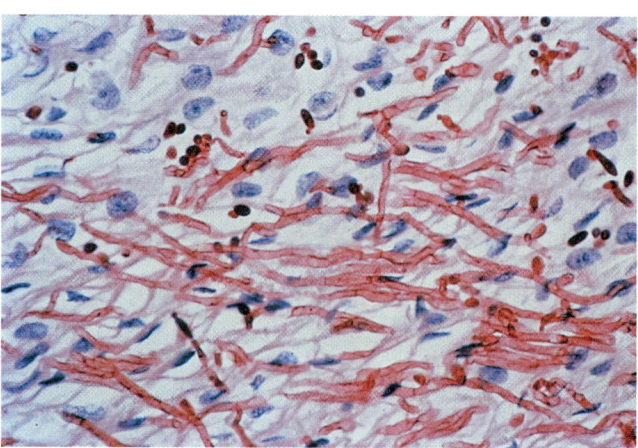

FIGURE 9-54

Candidiasis. A. The oral cavity of a patient with AIDS is covered by a white, curdlike exudate containing numerous fungal organisms. **B.** A PAS stain shows numerous septate hyphae and yeast forms.

lungs. There are three distinct types of pulmonary aspergillosis: (1) allergic bronchopulmonary aspergillosis, (2) colonization of a preexisting pulmonary cavity (aspergilloma or fungus ball), and (3) invasive aspergillosis. Of the over 200 identified species of *Aspergillus,* approximately 20 have been associated with human disease. One species, *A. fumigatus,* is by far the most frequent human pathogen.

Epidemiology: *Aspergillus* is present throughout the world, growing as saprophytes in soil, decaying plant matter, and dung. Pulmonary aspergillosis is acquired by inhalation of environmental organisms. The fungus reproduces by releasing numerous small (2–3 μm) spores, known as *conidia,* which are carried in the air into almost every human environment. The spores are small enough to reach the alveoli when inhaled. Exposure to *Aspergillus* is greatest when its native habitat is disturbed, as during soil excavations or handling of decaying organic matter.

Aspergillus has a characteristic appearance in tissue. Septate hyphae, 2 to 7 μm in diameter and branching progressively at acute angles, are seen. The multiple dichotomous branching is responsible for the name *Aspergillus* (from the Latin *aspergere,* "to sprinkle"). It derived from a fancied resemblance to the aspergillum, a device used to sprinkle holy water during religious ceremonies of the Catholic church.

Allergic Bronchopulmonary Aspergillosis Complicates Asthma

The inhalation of *Aspergillus* spores exposes the airways and the alveoli to *Aspergillus* antigens; subsequent contact initiates an allergic response in susceptible persons. The situation is aggravated if the spores germinate and grow in the airways, thereby producing long-term exposure to the antigen. Allergic bronchopulmonary aspergillosis is virtually restricted to asthmatics, 20% of whom eventually develop this disorder.

Bronchi and bronchioles in allergic bronchopulmonary aspergillosis are inflamed, with an infiltrate of lymphocytes, plasma cells, and variable numbers of eosinophils. Sometimes the airways are impacted with mucus and fungal hyphae. Patients experience exacerbations of asthma, often accompanied by pulmonary infiltrates and eosinophilia.

Aspergilloma Occurs in Persons with Pulmonary Cavities or Bronchiectasis

Inhaled spores germinate in the warm humid atmosphere provided by these hollows and fill them with masses of hyphae. The organisms do not invade, being confined to the air spaces by neutrophils and macrophages.

Pathology: An aspergilloma, also termed *fungus ball,* consists of a dense, round or lobulated mass of tangled hyphae, 1 to 7 cm in diameter, within a fibrous cavity. The wall of the cavity is composed of collagenous connective tissue, infiltrated by lymphocytes and plasma cells. The hyphae do not invade the adjacent pulmonary parenchyma.

Clinical Features: Aspergillomas occur in persons with underlying lung disease, most commonly old cavitary tuberculosis, and the symptoms correspond to the underlying disease. The radiological appearance of a dense round ball in a cavity is characteristic. For the most part, aspergillomas are best left untreated, but surgical excision may be indicated in some cases.

Invasive Aspergillosis Afflicts Neutropenic Patients

Any condition that profoundly diminishes the number or activity of neutrophils predisposes to invasive aspergillosis. The most common circumstances are acute leukemia and high-dose cytotoxic therapy, both of which are accompanied by depletion of bone marrow elements. In profoundly neutropenic patients, inhaled spores germinate to produce hyphae, which invade through the bronchi into the pulmonary parenchyma, from where the fungi may spread widely.

Pathology: *Aspergillus* readily invades blood vessels and produces thrombosis (Fig. 9-55). As a result, multiple nodular infarcts are found throughout both lungs. Involvement of larger pulmonary arteries results in large, wedge-shaped, pleural-based infarcts. Vascular invasion by the fungi also leads to widespread dissemination of the infection to the brain, heart, kidney, and other organs. Microscopically, *Aspergillus* hyphae are arranged radially around blood vessels and extend through their walls from the surrounding pulmonary parenchyma. Acute aspergillosis may also start in a nasal sinus and spread to the face, orbit, and brain.

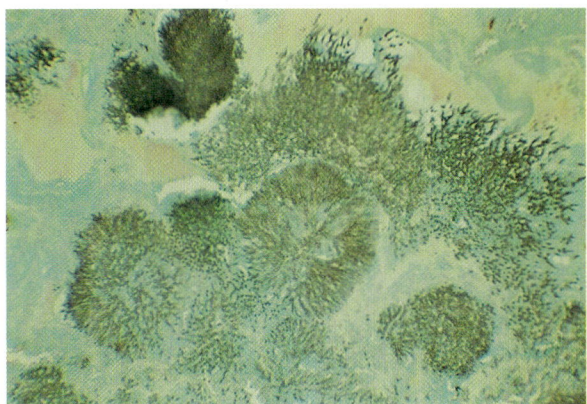

FIGURE 9-55

Invasive aspergillosis. A section of lung impregnated with silver shows branching fungal hyphae surrounding blood vessels and invading the adjacent parenchyma.

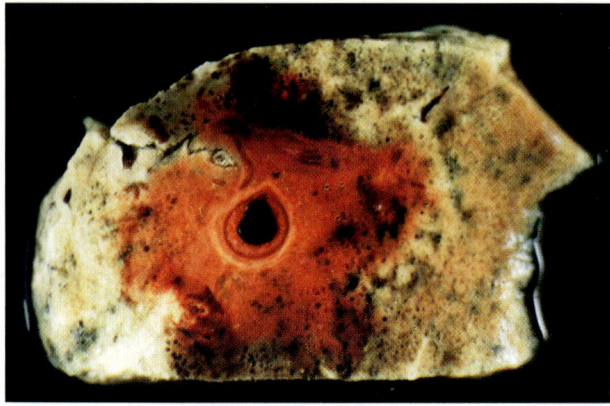

FIGURE 9-56
Pulmonary mucormycosis. A cross-section of the lung shows the vessel in the center of the field to be invaded by mucormycetes and occluded by a septic thrombus. The surrounding tissue is infarcted.

Clinical Features: Invasive aspergillosis manifests as fever and multifocal pulmonary infiltrates in a patient with profound neutropenia. Because of the frequent thrombosis and bloodstream dissemination, invasive aspergillosis is often fatal. Antifungal therapy with amphotericin B may be successful but must be initiated early and given in high doses.

MUCORMYCOSIS (ZYGOMYCOSIS)

Several related environmental fungi, namely, *Rhizopus, Mucor, Rhizomucor,* and *Absidia* species, produce severe, necrotizing, invasive, opportunistic infections that begin in the nasal sinuses or lungs. These organisms are members of the class Zygomycetes, order Mucorales, and the infections that they produce are usually called mucormycoses or zygomycoses.

Zygomycetes have a characteristic appearance in tissue sections and can usually be distinguished from other pathogenic fungi. They are large (8–15 μm across), branch at right angles, have thin walls, and lack septa. In sections, they appear as hollow tubes. Lacking cross walls, their liquid contents flow, leaving long empty segments. Zygomycetes also may resemble "twisted ribbons," which represent collapsed hyphae.

Epidemiology: *Rhizopus, Rhizomucor, Mucor,* and *Absidia* are ubiquitous in the environment, inhabiting soil, food, and decaying vegetable matter. The spores are inhaled, and in susceptible persons, disease begins in the lungs. Mucormycosis occurs almost exclusively in the context of an underlying illness, particularly, severe diabetes, underlying pulmonary disease, cancer, or profound neutropenia.

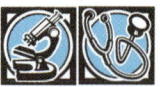

Pathology and Clinical Features: The three predominant forms of mucormycosis are rhinocerebral, pulmonary, and subcutaneous.

- **Rhinocerebral mucormycosis:** In this disease, fungi proliferate in the nasal sinuses and invade surrounding tissues, extending into the facial soft tissues, nerves, blood vessels, and brain. The palate or nasal turbinates are covered by a black crust, and the underlying tissue is friable and hemorrhagic. The fungal hyphae grow into the arteries and cause a devastating, rapidly progressive, septic infarction of the affected tissues. Extension into the brain leads to a fatal, necrotizing, hemorrhagic encephalitis. Therapy requires surgical excision of involved tissues, administration of amphotericin B, and correction of the predisposing abnormality.
- **Pulmonary mucormycosis:** This infection resembles invasive pulmonary aspergillosis, including vascular invasion and multiple areas of septic infarction throughout the lungs (Fig. 9-56). Both rhinocerebral and pulmonary mucormycosis are usually fatal.
- **Subcutaneous zygomycosis:** This infection is limited to the tropics and is caused by *Basidiobolus haptosporus*. The fungus grows slowly in the panniculus, producing a gradually enlarging, hard inflammatory mass, usually on the shoulder, trunk, buttock, or thigh.

CRYPTOCOCCOSIS

Cryptococcosis is a systemic mycosis caused by Cryptococcus neoformans, *which principally affects the meninges and the lungs* (Fig. 9-57). *C. neoformans* has a worldwide distribution. The main reservoir for the fungus is pigeon droppings, which are

FIGURE 9-57
Pulmonary and disseminated fungal infection. Fungi grow in soil, air, and the feces of birds and bats and produce spores, some of which are infectious. When inhaled, spores cause primary pulmonary infection. In a few patients, the infection disseminates.
   Histoplasmosis. Primary infection is in the lung. In susceptible patients, the fungus disseminates to target organs, namely, the monocyte/macrophage system (liver, spleen, lymph nodes, and bone marrow), and the tongue, mucous membranes of mouth, and the adrenals.
   Cryptococcosis. Primary infection of the lung disseminates to the meninges.
   Blastomycosis. Primary infection of the lung disseminates widely. The principal targets are the brain, meninges, skin, spleen, bone, and kidney.
   Coccidioidomycosis. Primary infection of the lung may disseminate widely. The skin, meninges, and bone are common targets.

Cryptococcosis

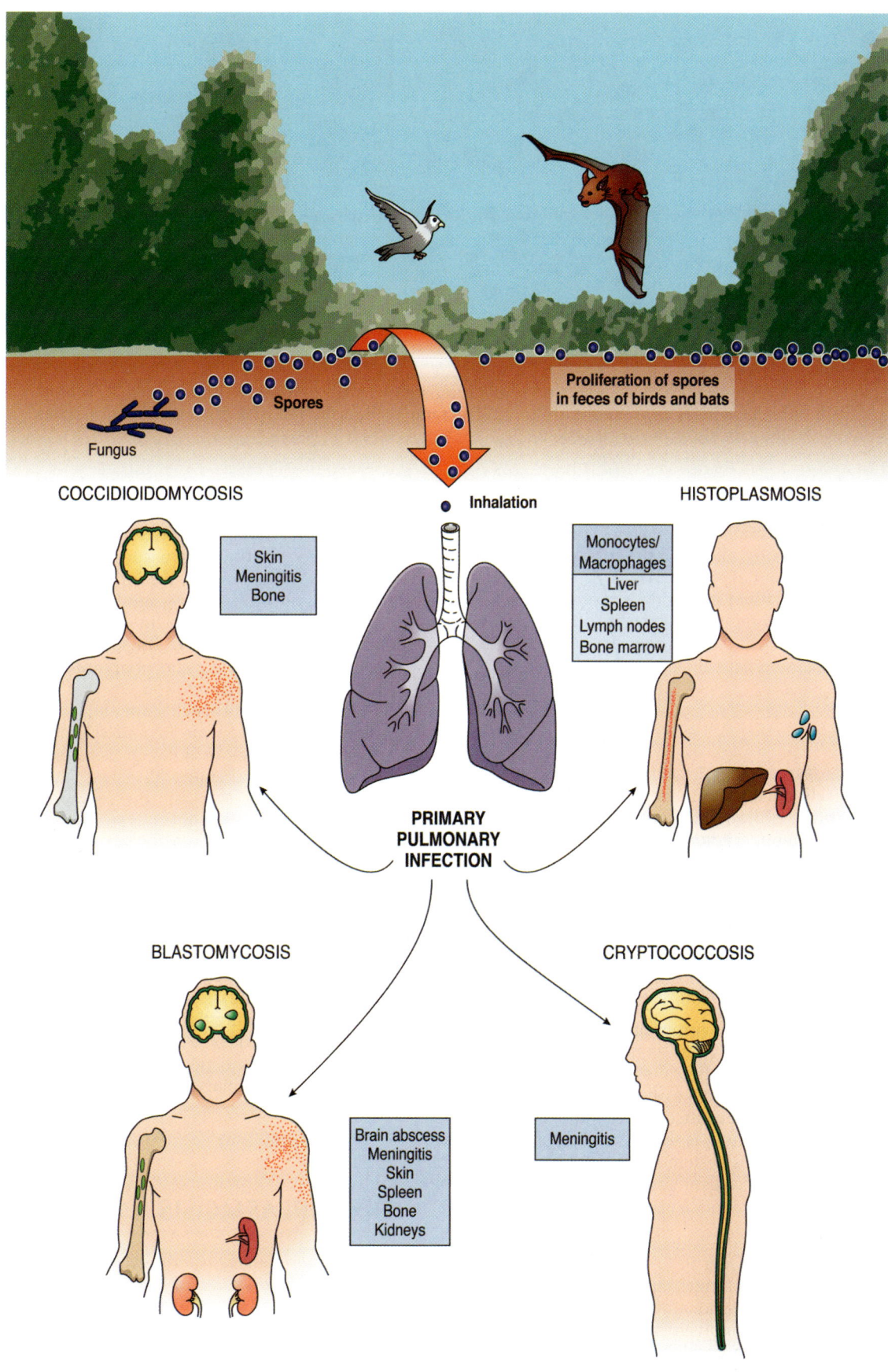

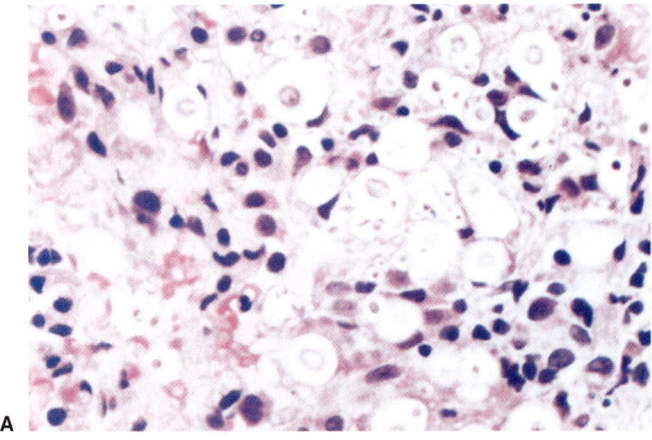 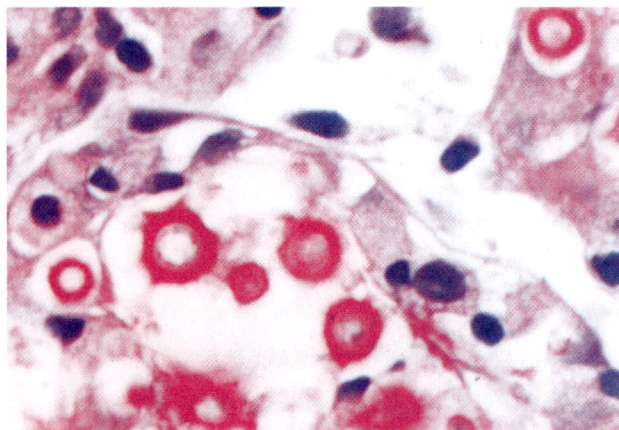

FIGURE 9-58
Cryptococcosis. A. In a section of the lung stained with hematoxylin and eosin, *C. neoformans* appears as holes or bubbles. B. The same section stained with mucicarmine illustrates the capsule of the organism.

alkaline and hyperosmolar. These conditions keep the cryptococci small, thereby allowing the inhaled organisms to penetrate to the terminal bronchioles. *C. neoformans* is unique among pathogenic fungi in having a proteoglycan capsule, which is essential for their pathogenicity. The organisms appear as faintly stained, basophilic yeasts with a clear 3- to 5-μm thick mucinous capsule.

 Epidemiology: *Cryptococcus* almost exclusively affects persons with impaired cell-mediated immunity. Although the organism is ubiquitous, and exposure is common, cryptococcosis remains a rare disease in the absence of a predisposing illness. Disease is uncommon even among persons such as pigeon fanciers, who are exposed to large inocula of the organism. Cryptococcosis occurs in patients with AIDS, lymphomas (particularly Hodgkin disease), leukemias, and sarcoidosis and in those treated with high doses of corticosteroids.

 Pathogenesis: In immunologically intact persons, neutrophils and alveolar macrophages kill *C. neoformans*, and no clinical disease develops. By contrast, in a patient with defective cell-mediated immunity, the cryptococci survive, reproduce locally, and then disseminate. Even though the lung is the site of entry of the organism, the central nervous system is the most common site of disease, owing to the excellent environment provided by the cerebrospinal fluid.

 Pathology: Over 95% of cryptococcal infections involve the meninges and the brain. Lesions in the lungs can be demonstrated in half of patients, and a small minority have involvement of the skin, liver, spleen, adrenals, and bones. In cryptococcal meningoencephalitis, the entire brain is swollen and soft, and the leptomeninges are thickened and gelatinous, owing to infiltration by the thickly encapsulated organisms. The inflammatory response is highly variable but is often minimal, with large numbers of cryptococci infiltrating tissue that is devoid of inflammatory cells. When present, the inflammatory response is neutrophilic, lymphocytic, or granulomatous.

Cryptococcosis in the lung may appear as diffuse disease or as isolated areas of consolidation. The affected alveoli are distended by clusters of organisms, usually with minimal associated inflammation.

Because of its thick capsule, C. neoformans stains poorly with the routine hematoxylin and eosin stain and appears as bubbles or holes in tissue sections (Fig. 9-58A). The routine fungal stains (PAS and GMS) demonstrate the yeasts well but fail to stain the polysaccharide capsule. As a result, the organism appears to be surrounded by a halo. The capsule can be demonstrated with a mucicarmine stain (see Fig. 9-58B).

 Clinical Features: Cryptococcal disease of the central nervous system often begins insidiously with nonfocal symptoms, including headache, dizziness, sleepiness, and loss of coordination. Untreated cryptococcal meningitis is invariably fatal, and therapy requires prolonged systemic administration of antifungal medication. Cryptococcal pneumonia presents as diffuse progressive pulmonary disease.

HISTOPLASMOSIS

Histoplasmosis is a mycosis caused by Histoplasma capsulatum, *which is usually self-limited but may lead to a systemic granulomatous disease.* Although most cases of histoplasmosis are asymptomatic, progressive disseminated infections occur in persons with impaired cell-mediated immunity. *H. capsulatum* is a dimorphic fungus of worldwide distribution that grows as a mold at ambient temperatures and always as a yeast in the body (37°C). The yeast cell is round and has a central basophilic body surrounded by a clear zone or halo, which in turn is encircled by a rigid cell wall 2 to 4 μm in diameter. In caseous lesions, where the yeasts are degenerating, silver impregnation identifies the remains of the yeasts.

Epidemiology: Histoplasmosis is acquired by the inhalation of infectious spores of *H. capsulatum* (see Fig. 9-57). The reservoir for the fungus is in bird droppings and in the soil. In the Americas, hyperendemic areas are in the eastern and central United States, western Mexico, Central America, the northern countries of South America, and Argentina. In the tropics, bat nests, caves, and soil beneath trees are foci of exposure.

Pathogenesis: Histoplasmosis resembles tuberculosis in many ways. Primary infection begins with phagocytosis of microconidia by alveolar macrophages. Like *M. tuberculosis*, *H. capsulatum* reproduces in immunologically naïve macrophages. As the organisms grow, additional macrophages are recruited to the site of infection, producing an area of pulmonary consolidation. A few macrophages carry organisms first to hilar and mediastinal lymph nodes, and then throughout the body, where the fungi further infect cells of the monocyte/macrophage system. The organisms proliferate within parasitized macrophages until the host mounts hypersensitivity and cell-mediated immune responses, usually within 1 to 3 weeks. The normal immunological response contains the organisms in most infected persons. Activated macrophages destroy the phagocytosed yeasts, forming necrotizing granulomas at the sites of infection.

The course of the infection varies with the size of the infecting inoculum and the immunological competence of the host. Most infections (95%) involve small inocula of organisms in immunologically competent persons. They affect small areas of the lung and regional lymph nodes and remain unnoticed. On the other hand, inhalation of a large inoculum, as occurs in an excavated bird roost, may lead to rapidly evolving pulmonary histoplasmosis, with large areas of consolidation, prominent mediastinal and hilar nodal involvement, and extension of the infection to the liver, spleen, and bone marrow.

Disseminated histoplasmosis develops in persons who fail to mount an effective immune response to *H. capsulatum*. Infants, persons with AIDS, and patients treated with corticosteroids are at particular risk. In addition, some persons with no known underlying illness also develop disseminated histoplasmosis.

Pathology: **Acute self-limited histoplasmosis** is characterized by the development of necrotizing, caseous granulomas in the lung, mediastinal and hilar lymph nodes, spleen, and liver. Early in the course of infection, the caseous material is surrounded by macrophages, Langhans giant cells, lymphocytes, and plasma cells. Yeast forms of *H. capsulatum* can be demonstrated both within macrophages and in the caseous material. Eventually, the cellular components of the granuloma largely disappear, and the caseous material calcifies, forming a "fibrocaseous nodule" (Fig. 9-59A).

Disseminated histoplasmosis is characterized by progressive organ infiltration with macrophages containing *H. capsulatum* (see Fig. 9-59B). In mild cases, the immunological response is sufficient to inhibit, but not eliminate, the infection. For long periods, the disease remains largely confined to the macrophages in the infected organs. In cases of profound immunodeficiency, large clusters of macrophages filled with *H. capsulatum* infiltrate the liver, spleen, lungs, intestine, adrenals, and meninges.

Clinical Features: Most infections are asymptomatic, but with extensive disease, patients present with fever, headache, and cough. The symptoms persist for a few days to a few weeks, but the disease requires no therapy.

Disseminated histoplasmosis features weight loss, intermittent fever, and weakness. In cases of subtle immunodeficiency, the disease may persist and progress for years, even

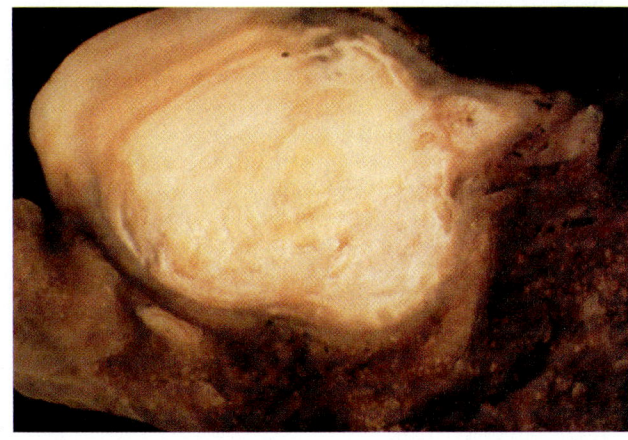
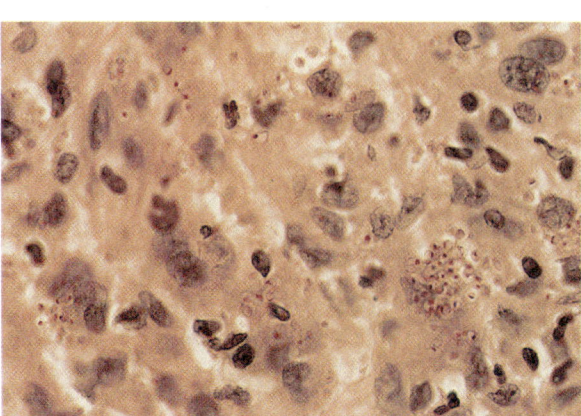

FIGURE 9-59
Histoplasmosis. **A.** A section of lung shows an encapsulated, subpleural, fibrocaseous nodule. **B.** A section of liver from a patient with disseminated histoplasmosis reveals Kupffer cells containing numerous yeasts of *H. capsulatum* (PAS stain).

decades. With more-profound immunodeficiency, disseminated histoplasmosis progresses rapidly, often causing high fever, cough, pancytopenia, and changes in mental status. Disseminated histoplasmosis is treated with systemic antifungal agents.

COCCIDIOIDOMYCOSIS

Coccidioidomycosis is a chronic, necrotizing mycotic infection that clinically and pathologically resembles tuberculosis. The disease, caused by *Coccidioides immitis*, includes a spectrum of infections that begin as focal pneumonitis. Most are mild and asymptomatic and are limited to the lungs and regional lymph nodes. Occasionally, *C. immitis* infections spread outside the lungs to produce life-threatening disease.

Epidemiology: *C. immitis* is a dimorphic fungus that grows as a mold in the soil, where it forms spores. The spores are inhaled into the alveoli and terminal bronchioles (see Fig. 9-57), enlarge into spherules, and then mature to form sporangia, which are structures that are 30 to 60 μm across. The sporangia gradually fill with endospores, 1 to 5 μm across, which accumulate by endosporulation, a process unique among the pathogenic fungi. The sporangia eventually rupture and release endospores, which then repeat the cycle.

C. immitis is present in the soil in restricted climatic regions, particularly the Lower Sonoran life zones of the Western hemisphere. These are areas with sparse rainfall, hot summers, and mild winters. In the United States, large portions of California, Arizona, New Mexico, and Texas are a natural habitat for *C. immitis*. The disease is particularly common in the San Joaquin Valley of California, where it is called "valley fever." Coccidioidomycosis also occurs in Mexico and parts of South America.

Long-term residents of endemic regions are almost invariably infected with *C. immitis*, and even brief visits to these areas can produce infection (usually asymptomatic). Dry, windy weather, which lifts spores into the air, favors infection. Coccidioidomycosis is not contagious.

Pathogenesis: Coccidioidomycosis begins with focal bronchopneumonia at the site where the spores are deposited. These elicit a mixed inflammatory infiltrate composed of neutrophils and macrophages, but the spores survive the onslaught of the immunologically naïve inflammatory cells. The host cannot control the infection until inflammatory cells become activated. With the onset of specific hypersensitivity and cell-mediated immune responses, necrotizing granulomas form, killing or containing the fungi.

Like those of tuberculosis and histoplasmosis, the course of coccidioidomycosis varies according to the size of the infecting inoculum and the immunological status of the host. A broad spectrum of illness ranges from acute self-limited disease to disseminated infections. Coccidioidomycosis begins with focal bronchopneumonia. **Most infections are produced by small inocula of organisms in immunologically competent hosts and are acute and self-limited.** Extensive pulmonary involvement and fulminant disease may occur in persons from a nonendemic region exposed to large numbers of organisms (e.g., New Yorkers who participate in an archaeological dig in southern Arizona).

Disseminated coccidioidomycosis occurs in immunocompromised persons, either from a primary infection or from reactivation of old disease. Patients with lymphoma, leukemia, or AIDS and those receiving immunosuppressive therapy are at risk of dissemination. Certain racial groups, including Filipinos, other Asians, and blacks, are particularly susceptible to dissemination of coccidioidomycosis, probably because of a specific immunological defect. The risk of dissemination in Filipinos is actually 175 times that in whites. Pregnant women are also unusually susceptible to spread of the disease if they develop primary infection during the latter half of pregnancy.

Pathology: Acute self-limited coccidioidomycosis produces a solitary lesion or patchy areas of pulmonary consolidation, in which the affected alveoli are infiltrated by neutrophils and macrophages (Fig. 9-60). *C. immitis* spherules elicit an infiltrate of macrophages, whereas the endospores attract predominantly neutrophils. With the onset of an immune reaction, a necrotizing, caseous granuloma develops. A successful immunological response causes the granuloma to heal, sometimes leaving a fibrocaseous nodule composed of caseous material and rimmed by residual macrophages and a thin capsule. In contrast to histoplasmosis, the old granulomas of coccidioidomycosis rarely calcify.

The spherules and endospores of *C. immitis* both stain with hematoxylin and eosin. Spherules in various stages of development appear as basophilic rings. Mature spherules (sporangia) contain endospores that appear as smaller basophilic rings. As in other fungal infections, PAS and GMS stains can be used to enhance the staining of *C. immitis*.

Disseminated coccidioidomycosis may involve almost any body site and may manifest as a single extrathoracic site

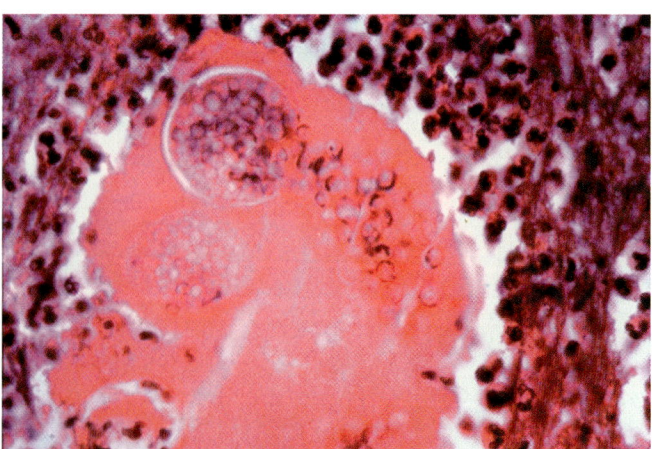

FIGURE 9-60
Coccidioidomycosis. A photomicrograph of the lung from a patient with acute coccidioidal pneumonia shows an acute inflammatory infiltrate surrounding spherules and endospores of *C. immitis*.

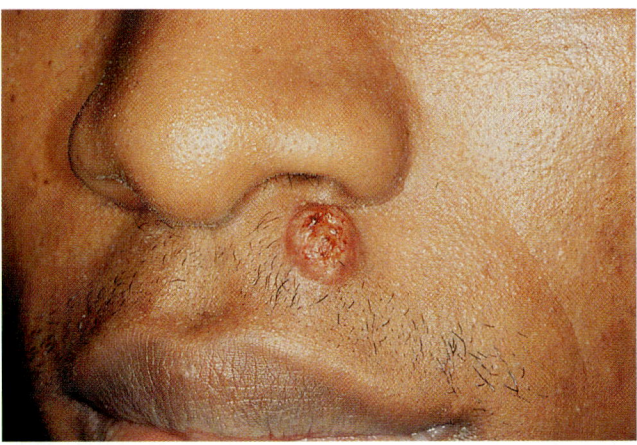

FIGURE 9-61
Disseminated coccidioidomycosis. A single raised, central ulcerated lesion is present on the face.

or as widespread disease, including lesions of the skin (Fig. 9-61), bones, meninges, liver, spleen, and genitourinary tract. The inflammatory response at the sites of dissemination is highly variable, ranging from an infiltrate of neutrophils to a granulomatous response.

Clinical Features: Coccidioidomycosis is a disease of protean manifestations, which vary from a subclinical respiratory infection to one that disseminates and is rapidly fatal. Physicians in endemic areas who are most experienced in diagnosing coccidioidomycosis state that almost any complaint or syndrome may be a manifestation of this infection. It thus joins syphilis and typhoid fever as a "great imitator."

Most persons with coccidioidomycosis (>60%) are asymptomatic. The others develop a flulike syndrome, characterized by fever, cough, chest pain, and malaise. Infection usually resolves spontaneously. Cavitation is the most frequent complication of pulmonary coccidioidomycosis, although it fortunately occurs in only few patients (<5%). The cavity, which may be mistaken for tuberculosis, is usually solitary and may persist for years. Progression or reactivation may lead to destructive lesions in the lungs, or more seriously, to disseminated lesions.

The signs and symptoms of disseminated coccidioidomycosis vary according to the site affected. Coccidioidal meningitis manifests with headache, fever, alteration in mental statis, or seizures and is fatal if untreated. Skin lesions of disseminated coccidioidomycosis frequently have a warty appearance (see Fig. 9-61). Even with prolonged amphotericin B therapy, the prognosis is poor in acute disseminated coccidioidomycosis.

BLASTOMYCOSIS

Blastomycosis is a chronic granulomatous and suppurative disease of the lungs, which is often followed by dissemination to other body sites, principally the skin and bone. The causative organism is *Blastomyces dermatitidis,* a dimorphic fungus that grows as a mold in warm moist soil, rich in decaying vegetable matter.

 Epidemiology: Blastomycosis is acquired by the inhalation of infectious spores from the soil (see Fig. 9-57). The infection occurs within restricted geographical regions of North America, Central and South America, Africa, and possibly the Middle East. In North America, the fungus is endemic along the distributions of the Mississippi and Ohio Rivers, the Great Lakes, and the St. Lawrence River. Disturbance of the soil, either by construction or by leisure activities such as hunting or camping, leads to the formation of aerosols containing fungal spores.

 Pathogenesis: The inhaled spores of *B. dermatitidis* germinate to form yeasts, which reproduce by budding. The host responds to the proliferating organisms with neutrophils and macrophages, producing a focal bronchopneumonia. Despite the inflammatory response, the organisms persist until the onset of specific hypersensitivity and cell-mediated immunity, when activated neutrophils and macrophages kill them.

 Pathology: Blastomycosis is usually confined to the lungs, where the infection most frequently produces small areas of pulmonary consolidation. *B. dermatitidis* incites a mixed suppurative and granulomatous inflammatory response, and even in the same patient, lesions may range from neutrophilic abscesses to epithelioid granulomas. Although the pulmonary disease usually resolves by scarring, some patients develop progressive miliary lesions or cavities. When the infection spreads outside the lungs, the skin (>50%) and bones (>10%), are common sites of involvement. Skin infection often elicits a marked pseudoepitheliomatous hyperplasia, imparting a warty appearance to the lesions.

The infected areas contain numerous yeasts of *B. dermatitidis,* which are spherical and 8 to 14 μm across, with broad-based buds and multiple nuclei in a central body (Fig. 9-62). With the hematoxylin and eosin stain, the yeasts appear as rings with thick, sharply defined cell walls. The yeasts may be found in epithelioid cells, macrophages, or giant cells or they may lie free in microabscesses.

 Clinical Features: Pulmonary blastomycosis is self-limited in one third of cases. Symptomatic acute infection presents as a flulike illness, with fever, arthralgias, and myalgias. Progressive pulmonary disease is characterized by low-grade fever, weight loss, cough, and predominantly upper lobe infiltrates on the chest radiograph. Skin lesions, which often resemble squamous cell carcinomas of the skin, are the most common manifestation of extrapulmonary dissemination. Although the pulmonary infection may apparently resolve completely, in some patients, blastomycosis may appear at distant sites months to years later.

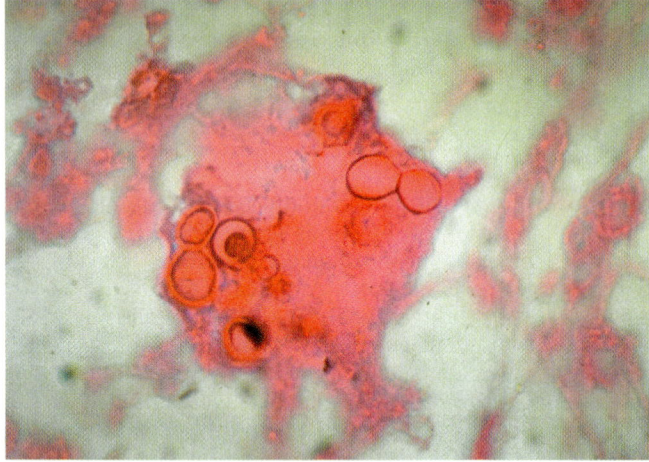

FIGURE 9-62
Blastomycosis. The yeasts of *B. dermatitidis* have a doubly contoured wall and nuclei in the central body. The buds have broad-based attachments.

PARACOCCIDIOIDOMYCOSIS (SOUTH AMERICAN BLASTOMYCOSIS)

Paracoccidioidomycosis is a chronic granulomatous infection that begins with pulmonary involvement and disseminates to involve the skin, oropharynx, adrenals, and the macrophages of the liver, spleen, and lymph nodes. The causative organism is *Paracoccidioides brasiliensis*, a dimorphic fungus, whose mold form is thought to reside in the soil.

 Epidemiology: Paracoccidioidomycosis is acquired by the inhalation of spores from the environment in restricted regions of Central and South America. Most infections are asymptomatic. Reactivation of latent infection occurs, and persons can develop active disease many years after moving from an endemic region. Interestingly, men develop symptomatic infections 15 times more often than women, presumably because of hormonal influences on the conversion of the organism to its yeast phase.

 Pathology: Paracoccidioidomycosis can involve the lungs alone (Fig. 9-63) or multiple extrapulmonary sites, most commonly skin, mucosal surfaces, and lymph nodes. *P. brasiliensis* elicits a mixed suppurative and granulomatous response, producing lesions similar to those seen in blastomycosis and coccidioidomycosis.

Clinical Features: Paracoccidioidomycosis is usually an acute, self-limited, and minimally symptomatic disease. The symptoms of progressive pulmonary involvement resemble those of tuberculosis. Chronic mucocutaneous ulcers are a frequent manifestation of extrapulmonary disease.

SPOROTRICHOSIS

Sporotrichosis is a chronic infection of the skin, subcutaneous tissues, and regional lymph nodes caused by Sporothrix schenckii. This dimorphic fungus grows as a mold in soil and decaying plant matter and as yeast in the body.

Epidemiology: Sporotrichosis is endemic in parts of the Americas and southern Africa. Most cases are cutaneous, resulting from the accidental inoculation of the fungus from thorns or splinters or by handling reeds or grasses. Cutaneous sporotrichosis is particularly common among gardeners (especially rose gardeners), nursery workers, and other persons who suffer abrasions while working with soil, moss, hay, or timbers. However, infected animals, particularly cats, can also transmit the disease.

Pathology: On inoculation into the skin, *S. schenckii* proliferates locally, inducing an inflammatory response that produces an ulceronodular lesion. The infection frequently spreads along subcutaneous lymphatic channels, resulting in a chain of similar nodular skin lesions (Fig. 9-64A). Extracutaneous disease is much less common than skin disease. Joint and bone involvement is the most frequent form of extracutaneous disease, and infections of the wrist, elbow, ankle, or knee account for most (80%) of the cases.

The lesions of cutaneous sporotrichosis are usually centered in the dermis or subcutaneous tissue. The periphery of

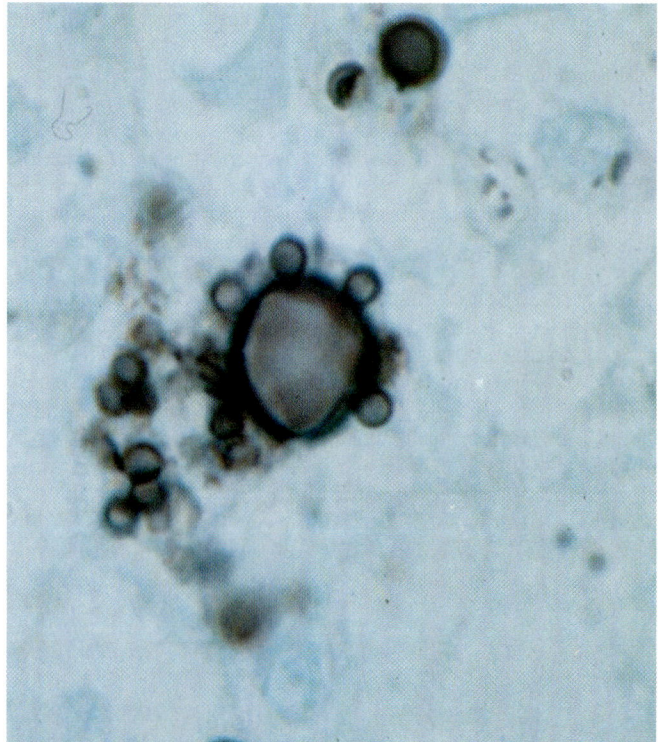

FIGURE 9-63
Paracoccidioidomycosis. The lung contains *P. braziliensis*, which displays many external buds arising circumferentially from the mother organism.

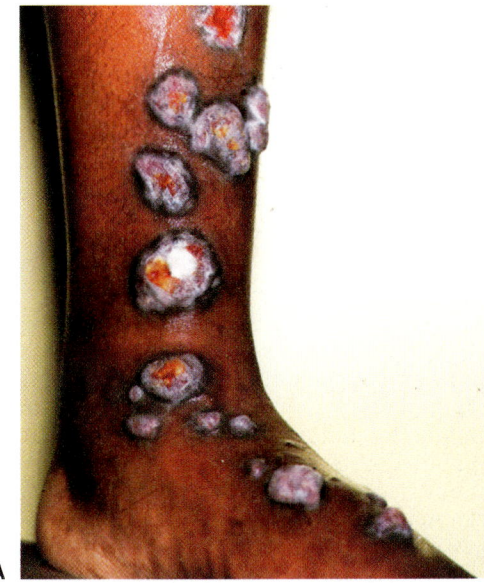
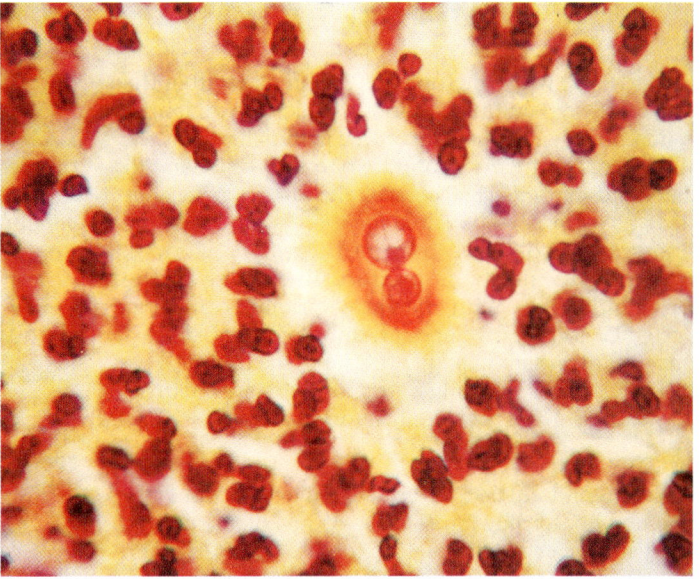

FIGURE 9-64
Sporotrichosis. A. The leg shows typical lymphocutaneous spread. B. A section of the lesion in (A) shows an asteroid body, composed of a pair of budding yeasts of *S. schenckii* surrounded by a layer of Splendore-Hoeppli substance, with radiating projections.

the nodules is granulomatous, and the center is suppurative. The surrounding skin displays exuberant pseudoepitheliomatous hyperplasia. Some of the yeasts are surrounded by an eosinophilic, spiculated zone and are termed *asteroid bodies* (see Fig. 9-64B). The material surrounding the yeasts (*Splendore-Hoeppli substance*) probably consists of antigen–antibody complexes.

Clinical Features: Cutaneous sporotrichosis begins as a solitary nodular lesion at the site of inoculation, typically on a hand, arm, or leg. Weeks after the appearance of the first lesion, additional nodules may appear along the lymphatic drainage of the primary lesion. The nodules frequently ulcerate and drain serosanguineous fluid. Joint involvement appears as pain and swelling of the affected joint, without involvement of the overlying skin. If untreated, cutaneous sporotrichosis continues to spread along the skin. The skin infection responds to systemic iodine therapy, but extracutaneous sporotrichosis requires systemic antifungal therapy.

CHROMOMYCOSIS

Chromomycosis is a chronic infection of the skin caused by several species of fungi that live as saprophytes in soil and decaying vegetable matter. The fungi are brown, round, thick walled, and 8 μm across and have been likened to "copper pennies" (Fig. 9-65). The infection is most common in barefooted agricultural workers in the tropics, in whom the fungus is implanted by trauma, usually below the knee. The lesions begin as papules and over the years become verrucous, crusted, and sometimes ulcerated. The infection spreads by contiguous growth and through lymphatics and eventually may involve an entire limb.

DERMATOPHYTE INFECTIONS

Dermatophytes are fungi that cause localized superficial infections of keratinized tissues, including skin, hair, and nails. There are about 40 species of dermatophytes within three genera: *Trichophyton*, *Microsporum*, and *Epidermophyton*. Although dermatophyte infections are minor illnesses, they are among the most common skin diseases for which persons seek medical care. Dermatophytes are resident in the soil, on animals, and on other humans. Most dermatophyte infections in temperate countries are acquired by direct contact with persons who have infected hairs or skin scales.

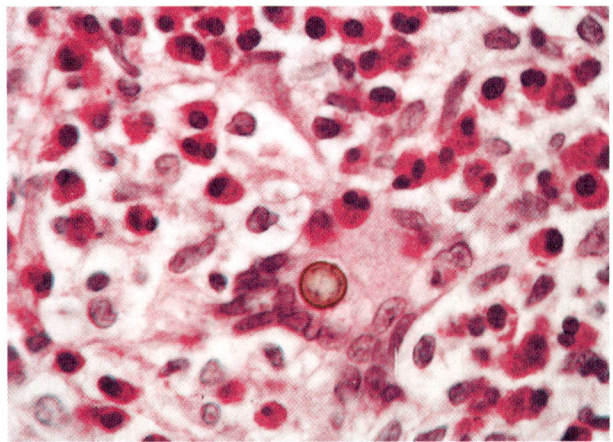

FIGURE 9-65
Chromomycosis. A section of skin shows a giant cell in the center, which contains a thick-walled, brown, sclerotic body (copper penny), representing the fungus.

Pathology: Dermatophytes proliferate within the superficial keratinized tissues, which are no longer viable. In skin, they spread centrifugally from the inoculation site, producing round, expanding lesions with sharply defined margins. The clinical appearance once suggested that a worm is responsible for the disease, thus the names "ringworm" and "tinea" (from the Latin *tinea*, "worm").

Dermatophyte infections produce thickening of the squamous epithelium, with increased numbers of keratinized cells. Lesions severe enough to be biopsied show a mild lymphocytic inflammatory infiltrate in the dermis. Hyphae and spores of the infecting dermatophytes are confined to the nonviable portions of skin, hair, and nails.

Clinical Features: Dermatophyte infections are named according to the sites of involvement (e.g., scalp, tinea capitis; feet, tinea pedis, "athlete's foot"; nails, tinea unguium; and intertriginous areas of the groin, tinea cruris, "jock itch"). These infections range from asymptomatic disease to chronic, fiercely pruritic eruptions. Dermatophyte infections are treated with topical antifungal agents.

MYCETOMA

A mycetoma is a slowly progressive, localized, and often disfiguring infection of the skin, soft tissues, and bone produced by inoculation of various soil-dwelling fungi and filamentous bacteria. The foot is the most common site of infection, and the disease is also known as Madura foot. Responsible organisms include *Madurella mycetomatis, Petrilidium boydii, Actinomadura madurae,* and *Nocardia brasiliensis.*

Epidemiology: Mycetoma usually occurs in the tropics among farmers and outdoor laborers whose skin is exposed to trauma. The foot is a common site of infection in locales where persons walk barefoot on soggy ground. Frequent immersion of the foot macerates the skin, facilitating deep inoculation with soil organisms.

Pathology: Within the subcutaneous tissue, the inoculated organisms proliferate and spread to adjacent tissues, including bone. The infection incites a mixed suppurative and granulomatous inflammatory infiltrate, which fails to eliminate the infecting organism. Surrounding granulation tissue and scarring produce progressive disfigurement of the affected sites.

A mycetoma begins as a solitary subcutaneous abscess, which slowly expands to form multiple abscesses interconnected by sinus tracts (Fig. 9-66A). The sinus tracts eventually drain to the skin surface. The abscesses contain colonies of compact bacteria or fungi surrounded by neutrophils and an outer layer of granulomatous inflammation. The colonies of organisms, called "grains," resemble the "sulfur granules" of actinomycosis (see Fig. 9-66B).

Clinical Features: A mycetoma initially manifests as a painless, localized swelling at the site of a penetrating injury. The lesion slowly expands, eventually producing sinus tracts, which tend to follow fascial planes in their lateral and deep spread through connective tissue, muscle, and bone. The treatment is usually radical excision of the affected area.

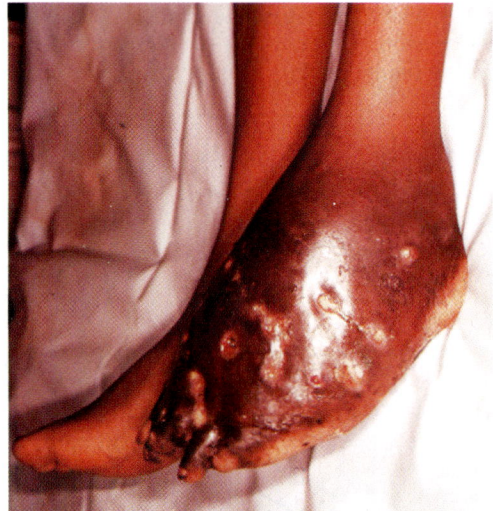
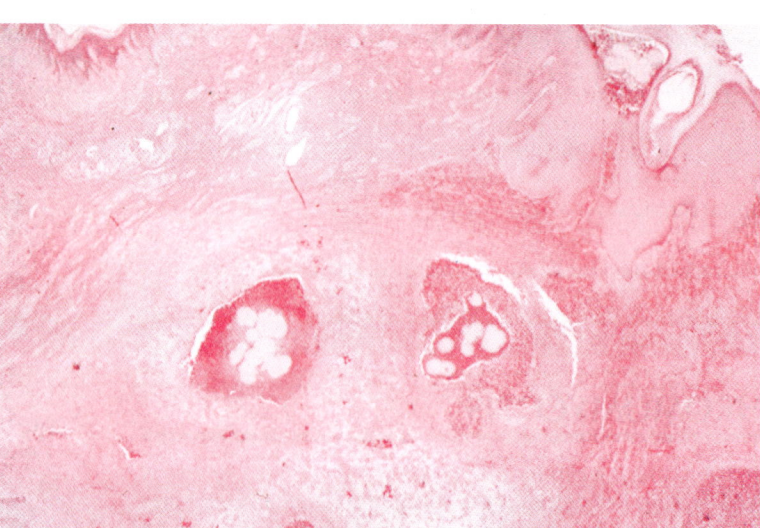

FIGURE 9-66

Mycetoma of the foot. A. The foot is swollen and painful and drains through the skin. The extremity was amputated. **B.** A photomicrograph of (A) demonstrates mycotic grains in the dermis. Fungal clusters *(P. boydii)* are surrounded by an abscess with a granulomatous perimeter. The grains are erupting through the surface and are in a tunnel of keratin.

Protozoa

The protozoa are single-celled eukaryotes that fall into three general classes: amebae, flagellates, and sporozoites. Amebae move by projection of cytoplasmic extensions termed *pseudopods*. Flagellates move through threadlike structures, known as flagella, which extend out from the cell membrane. Sporozoites do not possess organelles of locomotion and also differ from the amebae and flagellates in their mode of replication.

Protozoa cause human disease by diverse mechanisms. Some, such as *Entamoeba histolytica*, are extracellular parasites capable of digesting and invading human tissues. Others, such as the plasmodia, are obligate intracellular parasites, which replicate within human cells, thereby killing them. Still others, such as the trypanosomes, damage human tissue largely through the inflammatory and immunological responses that they elicit. Some of the protozoa (e.g., *Toxoplasma gondii*) can establish latent infections and produce reactivation disease in immunocompromised hosts.

MALARIA

Malaria is a mosquito-borne, hemolytic, febrile illness. Malaria infects over 200 million persons and yearly kills more than 1 million. Four species of *Plasmodium* cause malaria: *P. falciparum*, *P. vivax*, *P. ovale*, and *P. malariae*. All of these plasmodia infect and destroy human erythrocytes, producing chills, fever, anemia, and splenomegaly. *P. falciparum* causes more- severe disease than the other plasmodial species and accounts for most malarial deaths.

Epidemiology: Malaria has been eradicated in developed countries but continues to be a scourge in tropical and subtropical areas, especially Africa, parts of South and Central America, India, and Southeast Asia (Fig. 9-67). The rural poor, infants, children, malnourished persons, and pregnant women are all especially susceptible to infection.

Malaria is transmitted from person to person by the bite of the female *Anopheles* mosquito. *P. falciparum* and *P. vivax* are the most common pathogens, but there is considerable geographical variation in species distribution. *P. vivax* is rare in Africa, where much of the black population lacks the erythrocyte cell surface receptors required for infection. *P. falciparum* and *P. ovale* are the predominant species in Africa. *P. malariae* is the least common and mildest form of malaria, although it enjoys a broad geographical distribution.

Pathogenesis: The life cycle of the *Plasmodium* species responsible for human malaria requires both human and mosquito hosts (Fig. 9-68). Infected humans produce forms of the organism (gametocytes) that mosquitoes acquire on feeding. Within these insects, the organism reproduces sexually, producing plasmodial forms (*sporozoites*), which the mosquito transmits to humans when it feeds.

The anopheline mosquito inoculates malarial sporozoites into the human bloodstream, where they undergo asexual division (*schizogony*). Circulating sporozoites rapidly invade hepatocytes and reproduce in the liver, yielding numerous daughter organisms, known as *merozoites* (exoerythrocytic phase). Within 2 to 3 weeks of hepatic infec-

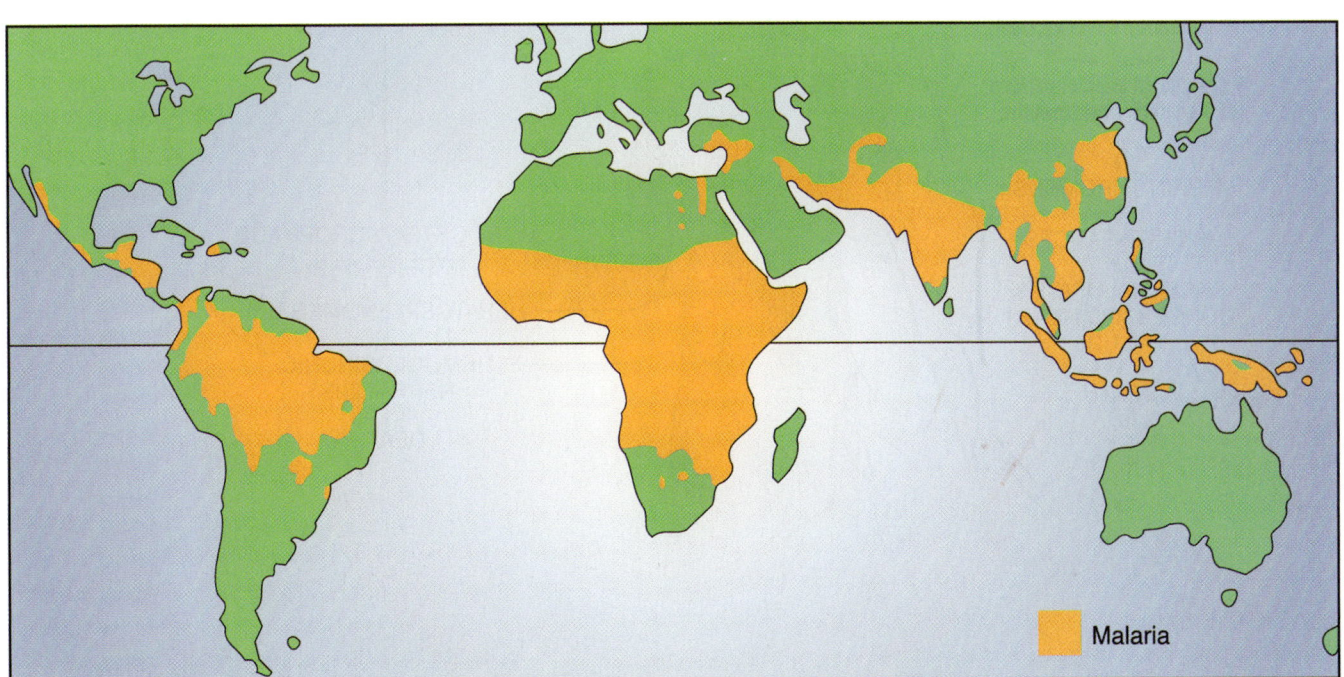

FIGURE 9-67
The geographical distribution of malaria.

442 Infectious and Parasitic Diseases

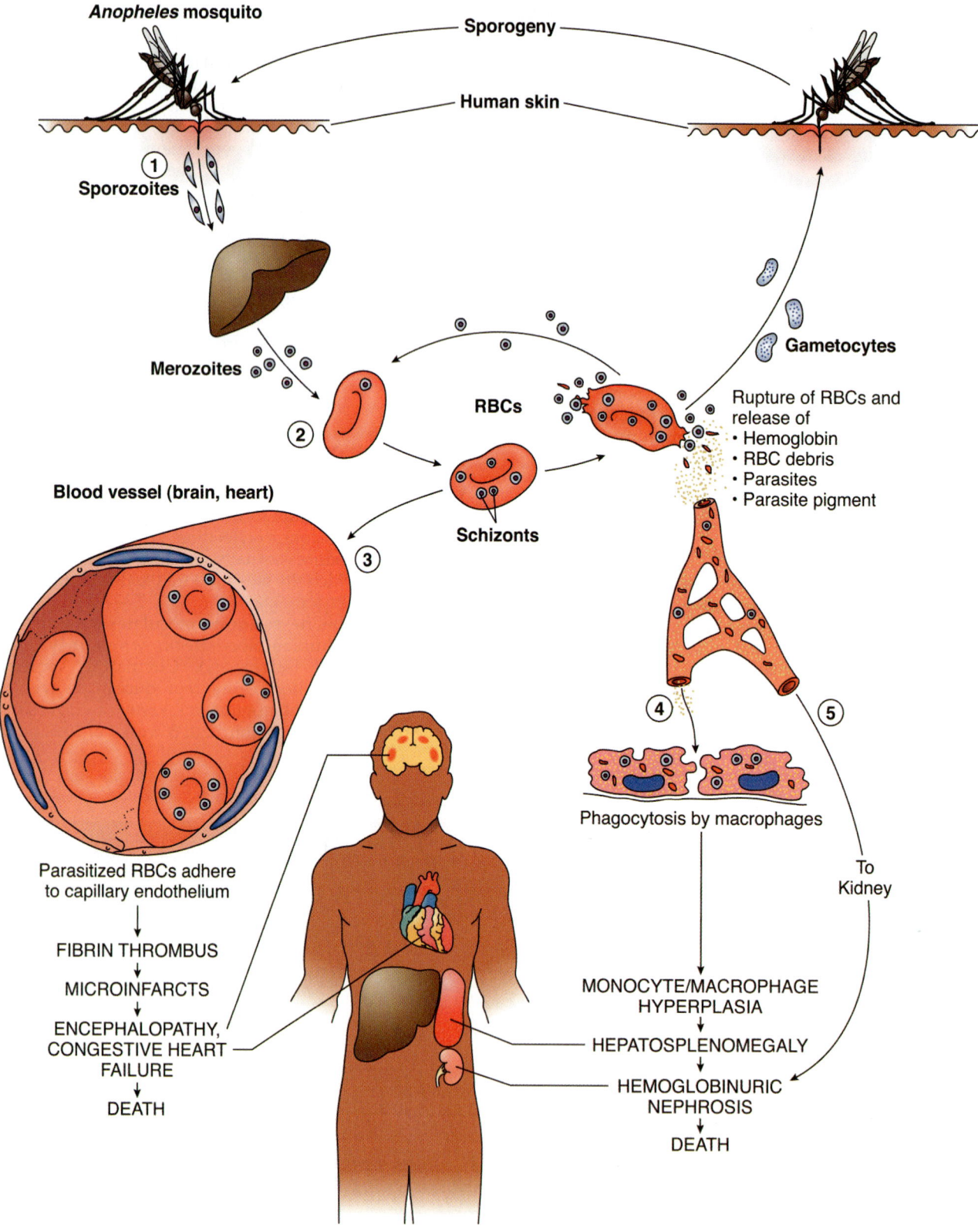

tion, merozoites exit into the bloodstream by rupturing host hepatocytes and invade erythrocytes, establishing the erythrocytic phase of malarial infection.

The merozoites feed on hemoglobin, grow, and reproduce within the erythrocytes. Within 2 to 4 days, mature progeny merozoites are produced. These burst from infected erythrocytes and invade previously uninfected red cells, initiating another cycle of erythrocytic parasitism. The erythrocytic cycle is repeated many times. Eventually, subpopulations of merozoites differentiate into sexual forms known as gametocytes. A mosquito feeding on an infected host ingests gametocytes, thereby completing the life cycle of the malarial parasite.

The rupture of infected erythrocytes causes the chills and fever of malaria through the release of pyrogenic material. Anemia results both from the rupture of circulating infected erythrocytes and from sequestration of cells in the enlarging spleen. Hepatosplenomegaly reflects the response of the fixed mononuclear phagocytes of the liver and spleen to the parasitism and destruction of red cells.

P. falciparum, the cause of malignant malaria, produces much more aggressive disease than the other plasmodia. This organism is distinguished from other malarial parasites in four respects:

- It has no secondary exoerythrocytic (hepatic) stage.
- It parasitizes erythrocytes of any age, causing marked parasitemia and anemia. In other types of malaria, only subpopulations of erythrocytes (e.g., only young or old forms) are parasitized, and thus low-level parasitemias and more modest anemias occur.
- There may be several parasites in a single red cell.
- *P. falciparum* alters the flow characteristics and adhesive properties of infected erythrocytes, so that they adhere to the endothelial cells of small blood vessels. The obstruction of small blood vessels frequently produces severe tissue ischemia, which is probably the most important factor in the virulence of *P. falciparum*.

Pathology: In all forms of malaria, the spleen and liver enlarge as erythrocytes are sequestered by the fixed mononuclear phagocyte system. The organs of this system (liver, spleen, lymph nodes) are darkened ("slate gray") by macrophages filled with hemosiderin and malarial pigment, the end-product of parasitic digestion of hemoglobin.

The adherence of infected red cells to the microvascular endothelium in falciparum malaria has two consequences. First, parasitized erythrocytes attached to endothelial cells do not circulate, so patients with severe falciparum malaria have few circulating parasites. Second, capillaries of deep organs, especially the brain, become obstructed, leading to ischemia of the brain, kidneys, and lungs. The brains of persons who die of cerebral malaria show congestion and thrombosis of small blood vessels in the white matter, which are rimmed with edema and hemorrhage ("ring hemorrhages") (Fig. 9-69). Obstruction of blood flow in the kidney produces acute renal failure, whereas intravascular hemolysis leads to hemoglobinuric nephrosis (*blackwater fever*). In the lung, damage to alveolar capillaries produces pulmonary edema and acute alveolar damage.

Clinical Features: Recurrent bouts of chills and high fever, known as *paroxysms*, are characteristic of malaria. The paroxysm begins with chills and sometimes headache. This "cold phase" of the paroxysm is then followed by a "hot phase" of high, spiking fever and tachycardia, often accompanied by nausea, vomiting, and abdominal pain. The high fever produces marked vasodilation and often associated orthostatic hypotension. When the fever defervesces after several hours, the patient is usually exhausted and drenched in sweat, the "wet phase" of the paroxysm.

A period of 2 to 3 days then follows during which the patient feels well, only to be followed by a new paroxysm. The paroxysms recur for weeks, eventually subsiding as the infected person mounts an immunological response. Each paroxysm corresponds to the rupture of infected erythrocytes and the release of daughter merozoites. As the mononuclear macrophage system responds to the infection, patients develop hepatosplenomegaly. Splenic enlargement can be dramatic (some of the largest spleens on record represent the effects of chronic malaria). Hypersplenism can exacerbate the anemia of malarial infection. *P. falciparum* infection produces a graver disease than the other forms of malaria. As the level of parasitemia grows, fever can become virtually continuous. Ischemic injury to the brain causes symptoms ranging from somnolence, hallucinations, and behavioral changes to

---

FIGURE 9-68
Life cycle of malaria. An *Anopheles* mosquito bites an infected person, taking blood that contains micro- and macrogametocytes (sexual forms). In the mosquito, sexual multiplication (sporogony) produces infective sporozoites in the salivary glands. *(1)* During the mosquito bite, sporozoites are inoculated into the bloodstream of the vertebrate host. Some sporozoites leave the blood and enter the hepatocytes, where they multiply asexually (exoerythrocytic schizogony), and form thousands of uninucleated merozoites. *(2)* Rupture of hepatocytes releases merozoites, which penetrate erythrocytes and become trophozoites, which then divide to form numerous schizonts (intraerythrocytic schizogony). Schizonts divide to form more merozoites, which are released on the rupture of erythrocytes and reenter other erythrocytes to begin a new cycle. After several cycles, subpopulations of merozoites develop into micro- and macrogametocytes, which are taken up by another mosquito to complete the cycle. *(3)* Parasitized erythrocytes obstruct capillaries of the brain, heart, kidney, and other deep organs. Adherence of parasitized erythrocytes to capillary endothelial cells causes fibrin thrombi, which produce microinfarcts. These result in encephalopathy, congestive heart failure, pulmonary edema, and frequently death. Ruptured erythrocytes release hemoglobin, erythrocyte debris, and malarial pigment. *(4)* Phagocytosis leads to monocyte/macrophage hyperplasia and hepatosplenomegaly. *(5)* Released hemoglobin produces hemoglobinuric nephrosis, which may be fatal.

444 Infectious and Parasitic Diseases

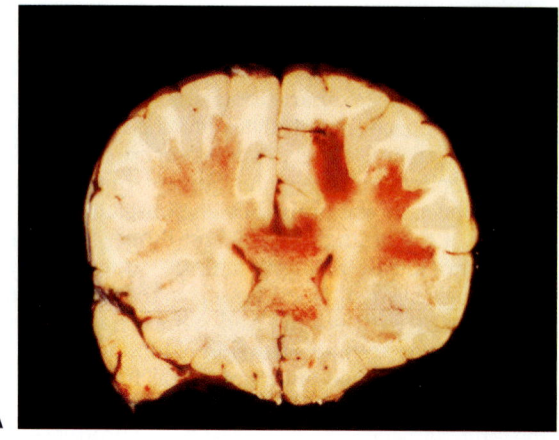
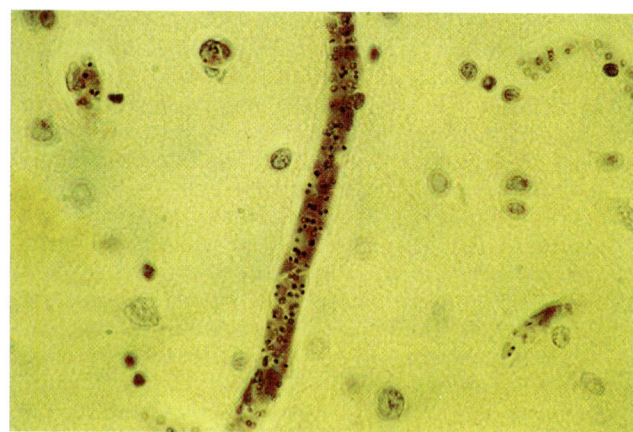
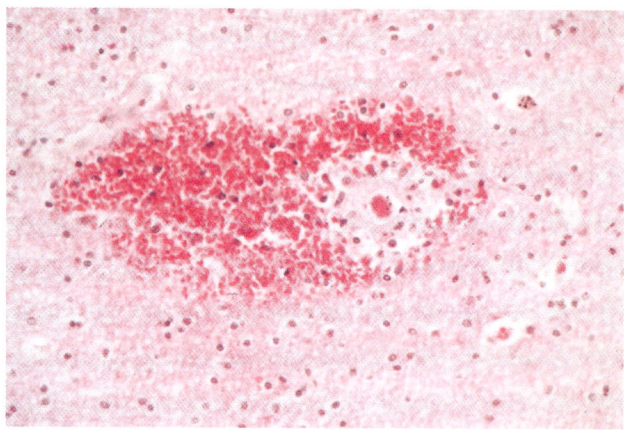

FIGURE 9-69
Acute falciparum malaria of the brain. A. There is severe diffuse congestion of the white matter and focal hemorrhages. B. A section of (A) shows a capillary packed with parasitized erythrocytes. C. Another section of (A) displays a ring hemorrhage around a thrombosed capillary, which contains parasitized erythrocytes in a fibrin thrombus.

seizures and coma. Central nervous system disease has a mortality of 20 to 50%.

Malaria is diagnosed by the demonstration of the organisms on Giemsa-stained smears of peripheral blood, and the different species of Plasmodium are distinguished by their appearance in infected erythrocytes. Malarias other than falciparum malaria are treated with oral chloroquine, sometimes with the addition of primaquine. Therapy for falciparum malaria varies, as new treatments are constantly being developed to meet the challenge of widespread chloroquine resistance.

BABESIOSIS

Babesiosis is a malaria-like infection caused by protozoa of the genus Babesia, *which is transmitted by hard-bodied ticks.*

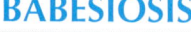 Epidemiology: *Babesia* infections are common in animals and in some locations are responsible for serious economic losses to the livestock industry. By contrast, human babesiosis is almost a medical curiosity, with the parasites infecting humans only when they intrude into the zoonotic cycle between the tick vector and its vertebrate host. Human babesiosis has been reported only in Europe and North America. Infections in the United States have been concentrated in islands off the New England coast.

 Pathogenesis and Pathology: The causative organisms, which resemble those of malaria, invade and destroy erythrocytes. However, they differ from malarial parasites in several important ways: they (1) are transmitted by ticks, (2) make no pigment, (3) produce no sexual forms, and (4) have no exoerythrocytic stage. *Babesia* spp. infect a variety of mammals, including cattle, horses, and dogs. The parasites are ingested by ticks when they feed on infected animals, after which the organisms are transmitted in the saliva when the tick feeds again. *Babesia* spp. invade red cells, where the organisms assume an ameboid, round, rod-shaped, or irregular appearance. They are 1 to 5 μm in diameter; with the Giemsa stain, they have a blue cytoplasm and a mass of red chromatin.

 Clinical Features: Splenectomy and diabetes are predisposing factors for babesiosis. After an incubation period of 2 to 6 weeks, the patient experiences the sudden onset of chills and fever, sometimes with muscle aches and pains, prostration, jaundice, dark urine, and diarrhea. The progressive invasion and destruction of erythrocytes causes hemoglobinemia, hemoglobinuria, and renal failure. The disease is usually self-limited, but uncontrolled infections can be fatal. *Babesia* spp. are resistant to most antiprotozoal drugs used in human medicine.

TOXOPLASMOSIS

Toxoplasmosis is a worldwide infectious disease caused by the protozoan Toxoplasma gondii. *Most infections are asymptomatic, but when they occur in the fetus or an immunocompromised host, devastating necrotizing disease may result.*

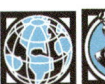 **Epidemiology and Pathogenesis:** In some areas (e.g., France), the prevalence of *T. gondii* infection exceeds 80% of adults; in other regions (e.g., the southwestern part of the United States), only few people are infected. *T. gondii* infects a wide variety of mammals and birds as intermediate hosts. The only final host is the cat, which becomes infected by ingesting cysts of the organism in the tissues of an infected mouse or other intermediate host. Within the cat's intestinal epithelium, five multiplicative stages end with the shedding of oocysts. The oocysts sporulate in feces and soil and differentiate into sporocysts, which contain sporozoites. The sporocysts are ingested by intermediate hosts, such as birds, mice, or humans. The sporozoites develop in the intermediate host to complete the life cycle. *T. gondii* has two stages in tissue, tachyzoites and bradyzoites, both crescent-shaped and measuring 2 × 6 μm. During acute infection, tachyzoites multiply rapidly to form "groups" within intracellular vacuoles of the parasitized cells, a process that eventually causes the rupture of the cells. Tachyzoites spread from the gut through the lymphatics to regional lymph nodes and through the blood to the liver, lungs, heart, brain, and other organs. During chronic infection, the organisms, now called *bradyzoites*, multiply slowly. The bradyzoites store PAS-positive material, and hundreds of organisms are tightly packed in "cysts." The cysts originate in intracellular vacuoles, enlarge beyond the usual size of the cell, and push the nucleus to the periphery.

Except for congenital infection, toxoplasmosis is acquired by the ingestion of infectious forms of the organism. In the tropics, where infection is generally acquired in childhood, oocysts in contaminated soil are the principal source of infection. In developed countries, the ingestion of incompletely cooked meat (lamb and pork) that contains *Toxoplasma* tissue cysts is the major mechanism of infection. Another source of infection is cat feces. The oocysts contaminate the hands and food of persons who live in close association with cats. Congenital infection is acquired by transplacental transmission of infectious forms from an acutely infected (usually asymptomatic) mother to the fetus.

The active infection is usually terminated by cell-mediated immunological responses. **In most *T. gondii* infections, little significant tissue destruction occurs before the immunological response brings the active phase of the infection under control, and infected persons suffer few clinical effects.** *T. gondii* establishes latent infection, however, by forming the dormant tissue cysts in some infected cells. These survive for decades in host cells. If the infected person loses cell-mediated immunity, the organism can emerge from its encysted form and reestablish a destructive infection.

Toxoplasma Lymphadenopathy Syndrome Occurs in Immunocompetent Persons

 Pathology: The most frequent manifestation of *T. gondii* infection in the immunocompetent host is lymphadenopathy. Virtually any lymph node group may be involved, but enlarged cervical nodes are most readily apparent. The histological appearance of affected lymph nodes is distinctive, with numerous epithelioid macrophages surrounding and encroaching on reactive germinal centers.

 Clinical Features: In *Toxoplasma* lymphadenitis (Fig. 9-70A), patients present with nontender regional lymph node enlargement, sometimes accompanied by fever, sore throat, hepatosplenomegaly, and circu-

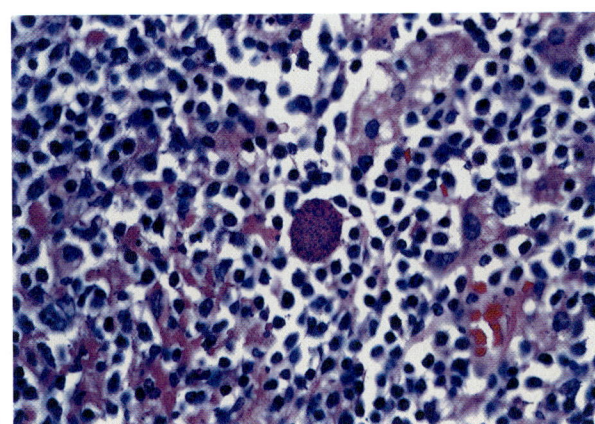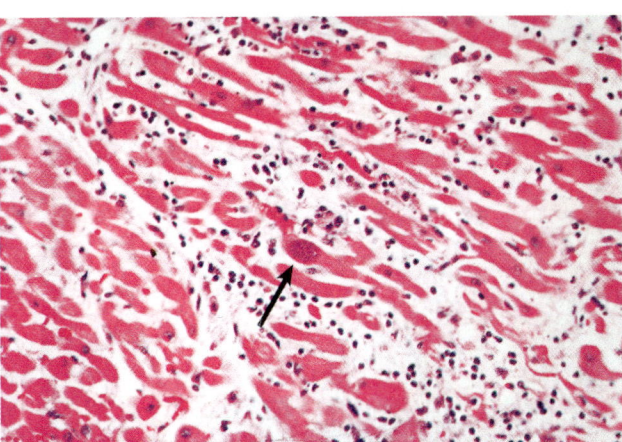

FIGURE 9-70
Toxoplasmosis. A. A photomicrograph of an enlarged lymph node reveals bradyzoites of *T. gondii* within a cyst. **B.** A section of heart shows a cyst of bradyzoites of *T. gondii* within a myofiber *(arrow)*, with edema and inflammatory cells in the adjacent tissue.

lating atypical lymphocytes. Hepatitis, myocarditis (see Fig. 9-70B), and myositis have been documented. Lymphadenopathy usually resolves spontaneously in several weeks to several months, and therapy is seldom required.

Congenital *Toxoplasma* Infections Principally Affect the Brain

T. gondii infection in the fetus is much more destructive than in the child or adult (see Chapter 6).

Pathology: The developing brain and eye are readily infected, and the fetus lacks the immunological capacity to contain the infection. Central nervous system infection produces a necrotizing meningoencephalitis, which in the most severe cases results in the loss of brain parenchyma, cerebral calcifications, and marked hydrocephalus (Fig. 9-71). Ocular infection causes chorioretinitis (i.e., necrosis and inflammation of the choroid and retina).

Clinical Features: The most severe fetal disease is produced by infection early in pregnancy and often terminates in spontaneous abortion. In infants born with congenital toxoplasmosis, the effects of brain involvement range from severe mental retardation and seizures to subtle psychomotor defects. Ocular involvement may cause congenital visual impairment. Latent ocular infection established in utero may also recrudesce later in life to produce visual loss. Some newborns have *Toxoplasma* hepatitis, with large areas of necrosis and giant cells. Adrenal necrosis is also occasionally observed. Congenital toxoplasmosis requires therapy with antiprotozoal agents.

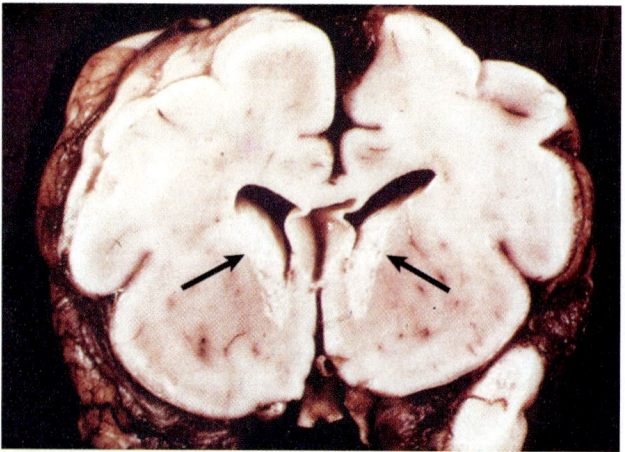

FIGURE 9-71
Congenital toxoplasmosis. The brain of a premature infant reveals subependymal necrosis with calcification appearing as bilaterally symmetric areas of whitish discoloration (*arrows*).

Toxoplasmosis in Immunocompromised Hosts Produces Encephalitis

Devastating *T. gondii* infections occur in persons with decreased cell-mediated immunity (e.g., patients with AIDS or those receiving immunosuppressive therapy for transplantation). In most cases, the disease represents reactivation of a latent infection. The brain is the most commonly affected organ, where infection with *T. gondii* produces a multifocal necrotizing encephalitis. Patients with encephalitis present with paresis, seizures, alterations in visual acuity, and changes in mentation. *Toxoplasma* encephalitis in the immunocompromised patient is fatal if not treated with effective antiprotozoal agents.

PNEUMOCYSTIS CARINII PNEUMONIA

Pneumocystis carinii causes progressive, often fatal, pneumonia in persons with severely impaired cell-mediated immunity and is the one of the most common opportunistic pathogens in persons with AIDS. The organism is now tentatively classified with the fungi, although it lacks the ergosterol characteristic of most fungi.

Epidemiology: *P. carinii* is distributed worldwide, and since 75% of the population have acquired antibodies by 5 years of age, it is believed that the organisms are inhaled by all. In persons with intact cell-mediated immunity, *P. carinii* infection is rapidly contained without producing symptoms.

In the 1960s and 1970s, 100 to 200 cases of active *Pneumocystis* disease were reported annually in the United States, primarily among persons with hematological malignancies, transplant recipients, or patients treated with corticosteroids or cytotoxic therapy. The situation changed dramatically in the 1980s with the AIDS pandemic. Before the new protease inhibitors became available, **80% of all AIDS patients developed *Pneumocystis carinii* pneumonia during the course of their illness.**

Pathogenesis: *P. carinii* reproduces in association with alveolar type 1 lining cells, and active disease is confined to the lungs. Infection begins with the attachment of the *Pneumocystis* trophozoite to the alveolar lining cell. The trophozoite feeds on the host cell, enlarges, and transforms into the cyst form, which contains daughter organisms. The cyst ruptures to release new trophozoites, which attach to additional alveolar lining cells. If the process is not checked by the host immune system or antibiotic therapy, the infected alveoli eventually fill with organisms and proteinaceous fluid. The progressive filling of alveoli prevents adequate gas exchange, and the patient slowly suffocates.

It is assumed, but not proven, that most cases of pneumocystosis derive from latent endogenous infection. Outbreaks of *Pneumocystis* pneumonia have also occurred among severely malnourished (and thus immunosuppressed) infants in nurseries; these uncommon cases are believed to represent primary infection with the organism.

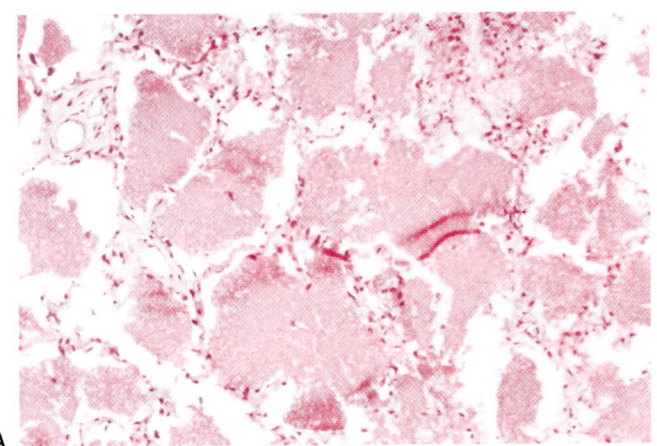
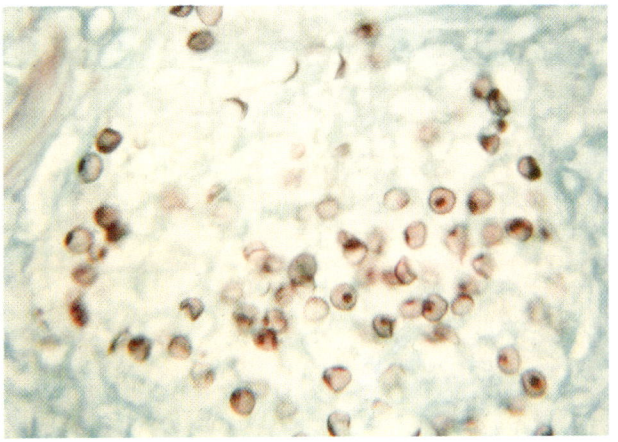

FIGURE 9-72
Pneumocystis carinii pneumonia. **A.** The alveoli contain a frothy eosinophilic material that is composed of alveolar macrophages and cysts and trophozoites of *P. carinii*. **B.** A silver stain shows crescent-shaped organisms, which are collapsed and degenerated. Some have a characteristic dark spot in their walls.

Pathology: *P. carinii* causes progressive consolidation of the lungs. Microscopically, the alveoli contain a frothy eosinophilic material, which is composed of alveolar macrophages and cysts and trophozoites of *P. carinii* (Fig. 9-72). There are hyaline membranes and prominent type 2 pneumocytes. In newborns, alveolar septa are thickened by lymphoid cells and macrophages. The prominence of plasma cells in the infantile disease led to the now obsolete term *plasma cell pneumonia*.

The various forms of *P. carinii* are best visualized with methenamine silver stains. The cyst form measures about 60 μm in diameter (see Fig. 9-72B); extracellular trophozoites and intracystic forms of the organism appear as irregularly shaped cells, 1 to 3 μm across, with punctate violet nuclei by Giemsa staining.

Clinical Features: *P. carinii* pneumonia features fever and progressive shortness of breath, often exacerbated by exertion and accompanied by a nonproductive cough. The dyspnea may be subtle in onset and slowly progressive over many weeks. Chest radiographs show a diffuse pulmonary process. The diagnosis requires recovery of alveolar material (by bronchoscopy, endobronchial washing, or sputum induction) for staining. *P. carinii* pneumonia is fatal if untreated. Therapy consists of the administration of trimethoprim-sulfamethoxazole or pentamidine.

AMEBIASIS

Amebiasis refers to an infection with Entamoeba histolytica, *which principally involves the colon and occasionally the liver*. *E. histolytica* is named for its lytic actions on tissue. Intestinal infection ranges from asymptomatic colonization to severe invasive infections with bloody diarrhea. On occasion, the parasites spread beyond the colon to involve other organs. The most common site of extraintestinal disease is the liver, where *E. histolytica* causes slowly expanding, necrotizing abscesses.

Epidemiology: Humans are the only known reservoir for *E. histolytica*, which reproduces in the colon and passes in the feces. Although amebiasis is worldwide, it is more common and more severe in tropical and subtropical areas, where poor sanitation prevails. **Amebiasis is acquired by ingestion of materials contaminated with human feces.**

Pathogenesis: *E. histolytica* has three distinct stages: the trophozoite, the precyst, and the cyst.

Amebic trophozoites, 15 to 20 μm across, are found in the stools of patients with acute symptoms. They are spherical or oval and have a thin cell membrane, a single nucleus, condensed chromatin on the interior of the nuclear membrane, and a central karyosome. The trophozoites sometimes contain phagocytosed erythrocytes. PAS stains the cytoplasm of the trophozoites and makes them stand out in tissue sections.

Amebic cysts are the infecting stage and are found only in the stools, since they do not invade tissue. They are spherical, have thick walls, measure 5 to 25 μm across, and usually have four nuclei. From the stools, they contaminate water, food, or fingers. (Fig. 9-73). On ingestion, the cysts traverse the stomach and excyst in the lower ileum. A metacystic ameba containing four nuclei divides to form four small, immature trophozoites, which then grow to full size. The trophozoites thrive in the colon and feed on bacteria and human cells. Trophozoites may colonize any portion of the large bowel, but the area of maximum disease is usually the cecum. Patients with symptomatic amebic colitis pass both cysts and trophozoites, but the latter survive only briefly outside the body and are also destroyed by gastric secretions. Host factors, such as nutritional status, coexistent colonic flora, and immunological status, also contribute to

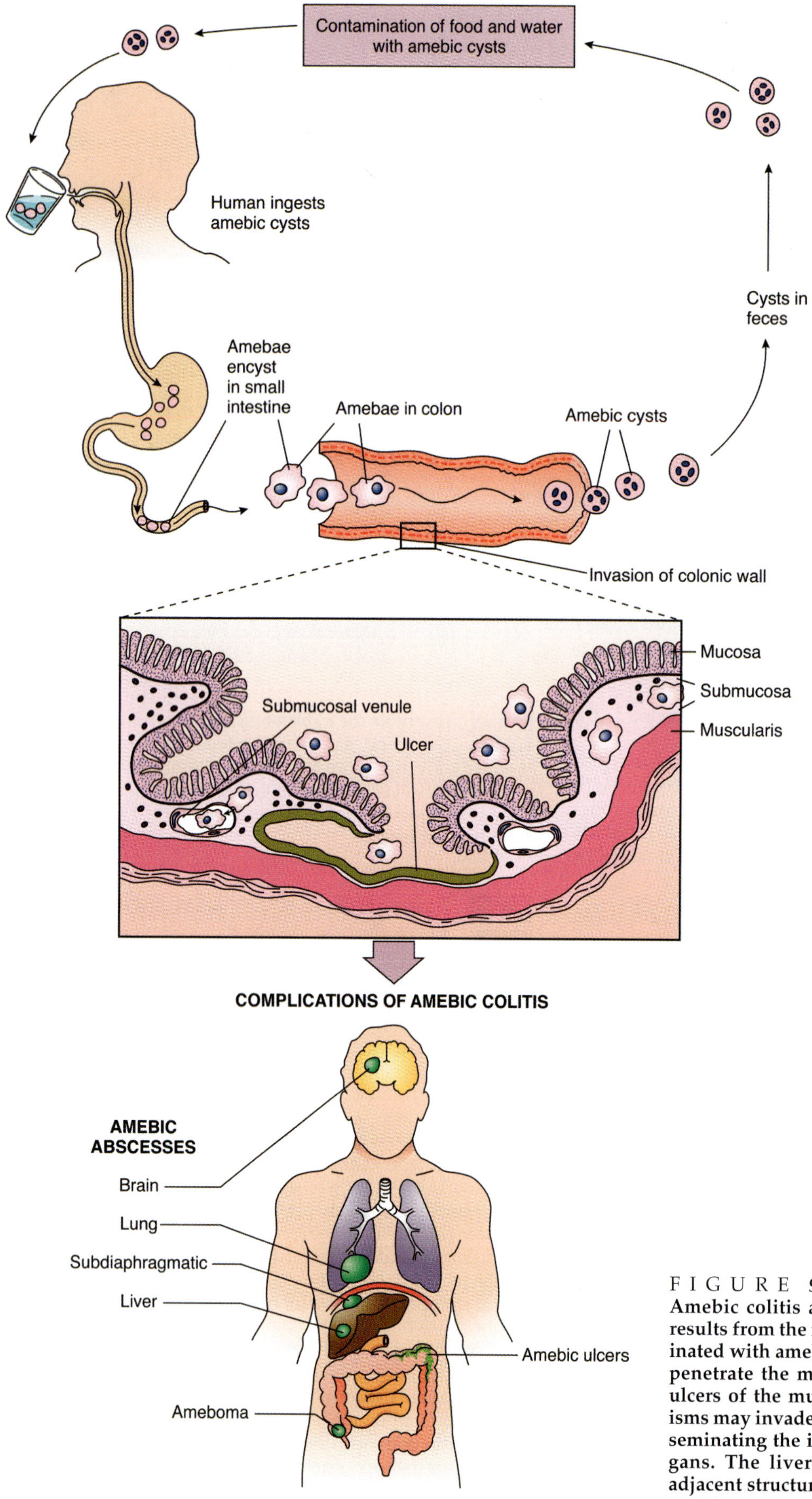

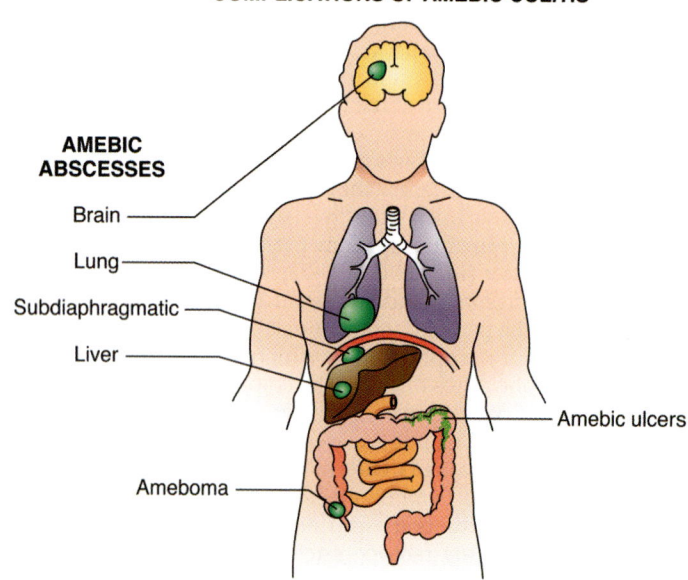

FIGURE 9-73
Amebic colitis and its complications. Amebiasis results from the ingestion of food or water contaminated with amebic cysts. In the colon, the amebae penetrate the mucosa and produce flask-shaped ulcers of the mucosa and submucosa. The organisms may invade submucosal venules, thereby disseminating the infection to the liver and other organs. The liver abscess can expand to involve adjacent structures.

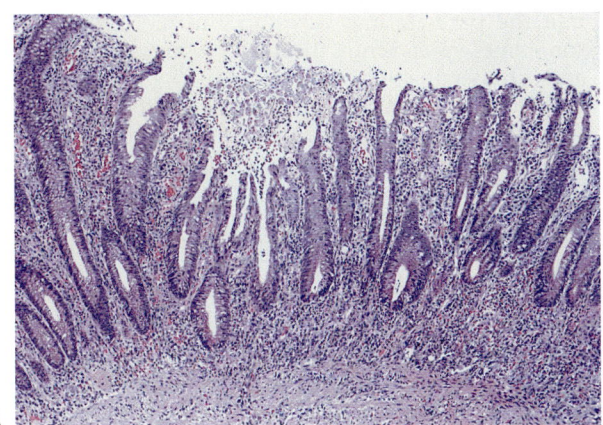 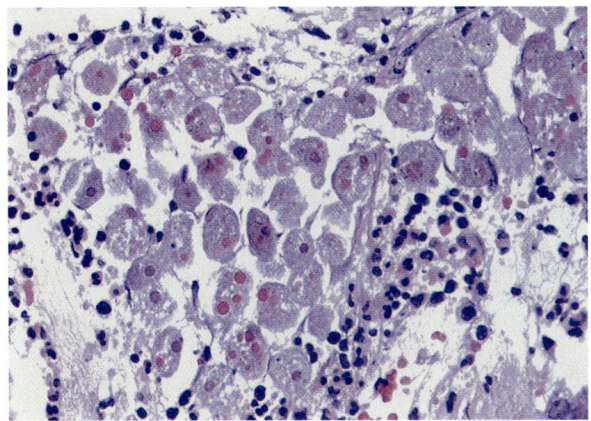

FIGURE 9-74

Intestinal amebiasis. **A.** The colonic mucosa shows superficial ulceration beneath a cluster of trophozoites of *E. histolytica*. The lamina propria contains excess acute and chronic inflammatory cells, including eosinophils. **B.** Higher-power view shows numerous trophozoites in the luminal exudate.

the course of *E. histolytica* infection. Invasion begins with the attachment of a trophozoite to a colonic epithelial cell. The organism kills the target cell by elaborating a lytic protein that breaches the cell membrane. Progressive death of mucosal cells produces a superficial ulcer.

Intestinal Amebiasis Is an Ulcerating Disease of the Colon

 Pathology: Amebic lesions begin as small foci of necrosis that progress to ulcers (Fig. 9-74A). Undermining of the ulcer margin and confluence of the expanding ulcers lead to sloughing of the mucosa in irregular, geographical patterns. The bed of the ulcer is gray and necrotic, being composed of fibrin and cellular debris. The exudate raises the undermined mucosa, producing chronic amebic ulcers whose shape has been described as resembling a flask or a bottle neck.

Trophozoites are found on the surface of the ulcer, in the exudate, and in the crater (see Fig. 9-74B). They are also frequent in the submucosa, muscularis propria, serosa, and small veins of the submucosa. There is little inflammatory response in early amebic ulcers. However, as the ulcer enlarges, acute and chronic inflammatory cells accumulate.

An **ameboma** is an infrequent complication of amebiasis, occurring when amebae invade through the intestinal wall. The lesion consists of an inflammatory thickening of the wall of the bowel that resembles colon cancer and tends to form a "napkin-ring constriction." It consists of granulation tissue, fibrosis, and clusters of trophozoites.

 Clinical Features: Intestinal amebiasis ranges from a completely asymptomatic infection to a severe dysenteric disease. The incubation period for acute amebic colitis is 8 to 10 days. Gradually increasing abdominal discomfort, tenderness, and cramps are accompanied by chills and fever. Nausea, vomiting, malodorous flatus, and intermittent constipation are typical features. Liquid stools (up to 25 a day) contain bloody mucus, but the diarrhea is rarely prolonged enough to result in dehydration. Amebic colitis often persists for months or years, and patients may become emaciated and anemic. The clinical features are occasionally bizarre and sometimes must be differentiated from those of appendicitis, cholecystitis, intestinal obstruction, or diverticulitis. In severe amebic colitis, massive destruction of the colonic mucosa may lead to fatal hemorrhage, perforation, or peritonitis. Therapy for intestinal amebiasis includes metronidazole, which acts against trophozoites, and diloxanide, which is effective against cysts.

Amebic Liver Abscess Is a Major Complication of Intestinal Amebiasis

 Pathology: *E. histolytica* trophozoites that have invaded into submucosal veins of the colon enter the portal circulation and reach the liver. Here the organisms kill hepatocytes, producing a slowly expanding necrotic cavity, filled with a dark brown, odorless semisolid material, reported to resemble "anchovy paste" in color and consistency (Fig. 9-75). Neutrophils are rare within the cavity, and trophozoites are found along the edges adjacent to hepatocytes.

An amebic liver abscess may expand and rupture through the capsule, extending into the peritoneum, diaphragm, pleural cavity, lungs, or pericardium. Rarely, a liver abscess, or even a lesion in the colon, may spread amebae to the brain by a hematogenous route to form large necrotic lesions.

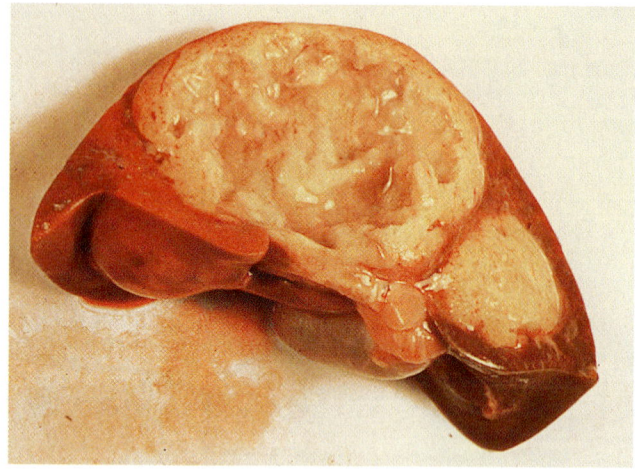

FIGURE 9-75
Amebic abscesses of the liver. The cut surface of the liver shows multiple abscesses containing "anchovy paste" material.

 Clinical Features: Patients with amebic liver abscess present with severe right upper quadrant pain, low-grade fever, and weight loss. Only a minority of patients give a history of an antecedent diarrheal illness, and *E. histolytica* is demonstrated in the feces of less than one third of patients with extraintestinal disease. The diagnosis is usually made by radiological or ultrasound demonstration of the abscess, in conjunction with serological testing for antibodies to *E. histolytica*. Amebic abscess is treated by percutaneous or surgical drainage and antiamebic drugs.

CRYPTOSPORIDIOSIS

Cryptosporidiosis refers to an enteric infection with a protozoan of the genus Cryptosporidium *that causes diarrheal disease in persons with compromised immunity.* The infection varies from a self-limited gastrointestinal infection to a potentially life-threatening diarrheal illness. Cryptosporidiosis is acquired by the ingestion of *Cryptosporidium* oocysts, which are shed in the feces of infected humans and animals. Most infections probably result from person-to-person transmission, but many domesticated animals harbor the parasite, providing a large reservoir for human infection.

 Pathogenesis and Pathology: The *Cryptosporidium* oocyst survives passage through the stomach and releases forms that attach to the microvillous surface of the small bowel. Unlike *Toxoplasma* and other coccidia, *Cryptosporidium* remains an extracellular parasite. The organisms reproduce on the luminal surface of the gastrointestinal tract, from the stomach to the rectum, forming progeny that also attach to the epithelium.

In immunologically competent persons, the infection is terminated by unknown immune responses. Patients with AIDS and some congenital immunodeficiencies cannot contain the parasite and develop chronic infections, which sometimes spread from the bowel to involve the gallbladder and intrahepatic bile ducts.

Cryptosporidiosis produces no grossly visible alterations. The organisms are visible microscopically as round, 2- to 4-μm blebs attached to the luminal surface of the epithelium. In the small intestine, there may be moderate or severe chronic inflammation in the lamina propria and some villous atrophy that is directly related to the density of the parasites. The colon exhibits a chronic active colitis, with minimal architectural disruption.

 Clinical Features: Cryptosporidiosis presents as a profuse, watery diarrhea, sometimes accompanied by cramping abdominal pain or low-grade fever. Extraordinary volumes of fluid can be lost as diarrhea, and intensive fluid replacement is required. In immunologically competent persons, the diarrheal illness resolves spontaneously in 1 to 2 weeks. In the immunocompromised patient, diarrhea persists indefinitely and may contribute to death.

GIARDIASIS

Giardiasis is an infection of the small intestine caused by the flagellated protozoan Giardia lamblia *and characterized by abdominal cramping and diarrhea.*

 Epidemiology: *G. lamblia* has a worldwide distribution, with a prevalence of infection from less than 1% to more than 25% in some areas with warmer climates and crowded, unsanitary environments. Children are more susceptible than adults. Giardiasis is acquired by the ingestion of infectious cyst forms of the organism, which are shed in the feces of infected humans and animals. Infection spreads directly from person to person and also in contaminated water or food. *Giardia* can be acquired from wilderness water sources, where infected animals, such as beavers and bears, serve as the reservoir of infection. The infection may be epidemic, and outbreaks have occurred in orphanages and institutions.

 Pathogenesis and Pathology: *G. lamblia* has two stages: trophozoites and cysts. The trophozoites are flat, pear-shaped, binucleate organisms, with four pairs of flagella. They are most numerous in the duodenum and proximal small intestine. A curved, disklike "sucker plate" on the ventral surface aids mucosal attachment. The ingested cysts contain two or four nuclei and revert to trophozoites on reaching the intestine. The stools usually contain only cysts, but trophozoites may also be present in patients with diarrhea.

Giardia cysts survive gastric acidity and rupture within the duodenum and jejunum to release trophozoites. The latter attach to the microvilli of the small bowel epithelium and reproduce. Giardiasis produces no grossly visible alterations. Microscopic examination shows *Giardia* trophozoites on the surface of villi and within crypts, with minimal associated mucosal changes.

 Clinical Features: Although *G. lamblia* is a harmless commensal in most persons, it can cause acute or chronic symptoms. Acute giardiasis manifests with the abrupt onset of abdominal cramping and frequent, foul-smelling stools. The course of infection is highly variable. In some patients, the symptoms resolve spontaneously in 1 to 4 weeks. Others complain of persistent abdominal cramping and poorly formed stools for months. In children, chronic giardiasis may cause malabsorption, weight loss and retarded growth. The infection is treated effectively with various antibiotics, including metronidazole.

LEISHMANIASIS

Leishmaniae are protozoans that are transmitted to humans by insect bites and cause a spectrum of clinical syndromes, ranging from indolent, self-resolving cutaneous ulcers to fatal disseminated disease. There are numerous species of *Leishmania*, which differ in their natural habitats and the types of disease that they produce.

 Epidemiology: Leishmaniasis is transmitted by the bites of *Phlebotomus* sandflies, which acquire infection from feeding on infected animals. In many subtropical and tropical areas, leishmanial infection is endemic in animal populations; thus, gerbils, dogs, ground squirrels, foxes, and jackals serve as reservoirs and potential sources for transmission to humans. Leishmaniasis is primarily a disease of less-developed countries where humans live in close proximity to animal hosts and the fly vector. There are estimated to be 20 million persons infected worldwide.

 Pathogenesis: Infection begins when the organisms are inoculated into human skin by the bite of the sandfly. Shortly thereafter, leishmaniae are phagocytosed by mononuclear phagocytes and transformed into amastigotes, which reproduce within the macrophage. Daughter amastigotes eventually rupture from the cell and spread to other macrophages. Reproduction continues in this way, and eventually a cluster of infected macrophages forms at the site of inoculation.

From this initial local infection, the disease may take widely divergent courses depending on two factors: the immunological capabilities of the host and the infecting species of *Leishmania*. Three distinct clinical entities are recognized: (1) localized cutaneous leishmaniasis, (2) mucocutaneous leishmaniasis, and (3) visceral leishmaniasis.

Localized Cutaneous Leishmaniasis Is an Ulcerating Disorder

Several *Leishmania* species in Central and South America, Northern Africa, the Middle East, India, and China produce localized cutaneous disease, also known as "oriental sore" or "tropical sore."

 Pathology: Localized cutaneous leishmaniasis begins as a collection of amastigote-filled macrophages that ulcerates the overlying epidermis. In tissue sections, the oval amastigotes measure 2 μm and contain two internal structures, a nucleus and a kinetoplast. When examined under low power, the amastigotes in macrophages appear as multiple regular cytoplasmic dots, known as *Leishman-Donovan bodies*. With the progressive development of cell-mediated immunity to the parasite, macrophages become activated and kill the intracellular parasites. The lesion slowly assumes a more mature granulomatous appearance, with epithelioid macrophages, Langhans giant cells, plasma cells, and lymphocytes. Over the course of months, the cutaneous ulcer heals spontaneously.

 Clinical Features: Cutaneous leishmaniasis begins as an itching, solitary papule, which erodes to form a shallow ulcer with a sharp, raised border. This ulcer can grow to 6 to 8 cm in diameter. Satellite lesions develop along draining lymphatics. The ulcers begin to resolve at 3 to 6 months, but healing may take a year or longer.

Diffuse cutaneous leishmaniasis develops in some patients who lack specific cell-mediated immune responses to leishmaniae. The disease begins as a single nodule, but adjacent satellite nodules slowly form, eventually involving much of the skin. These lesions so closely resemble lepromatous leprosy that some patients have been cared for in leprosaria. The nodule of anergic leishmaniasis is caused by enormous numbers of macrophages replete with leishmaniae.

Mucocutaneous Leishmaniasis Is a Late Complication of Cutaneous Leishmaniasis

Mucocutaneous leishmaniasis is caused by infection with *L. braziliensis*. Most cases occur in Central and South America, where rodents and sloths are reservoirs for the organism.

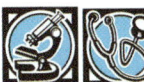 **Pathology and Clinical Features:** The early course and pathological changes of mucocutaneous leishmaniasis are similar to those of localized cutaneous leishmaniasis. A solitary ulcer appears, expands, and resolves spontaneously. Years after the primary lesion has healed, an ulcer develops at a

mucocutaneous junction, such as the larynx, nasal septum, anus, or vulva. The mucosal lesion is slowly progressive, highly destructive, and disfiguring, eroding mucosal surfaces and cartilage. Destruction of the nasal septum sometimes produces a "tapir nose" deformity. The ulcers may also kill the patient by obstructing the airways. Mucocutaneous leishmaniasis requires treatment with systemic antiprotozoal agents.

Visceral Leishmaniasis (Kala Azar) Is a Potentially Fatal Infection of the Monocyte/Macrophage System

Epidemiology: Kala azar is produced by several subspecies of L. donovani. The reservoirs of the agent and the susceptible age groups vary in different parts of the world. Humans are the reservoir in India, and foxes in southern France, central Italy, and some parts of South America. Jackals are the source of infection for sporadic cases in rural areas of the Middle East and Central Asia. Dogs harbor the organism in the Mediterranean basin, China, and some parts of South America. The reservoirs in Africa are incompletely known but may include humans, domestic dogs, rats, and other rodents.

Pathology: Infection with L. donovani begins with a localized collection of infected macrophages at the site of a sandfly bite (Fig. 9-76); which spread the organisms throughout the mononuclear phagocyte system. Most infected persons destroy L. donovani by a cell-mediated immune response, but 5% cannot contain the organisms and develop disseminated disease. Young children and malnourished persons are especially prone to develop visceral leishmaniasis. The liver (Fig. 9-77A), spleen, and lymph nodes become massively enlarged, as the macrophages in these organs fill with proliferating leishmanial amastigotes. The normal architecture of these organs and the bone marrow is progressively supplanted by sheets of parasitized macrophages (see Fig. 9-77B). Eventually, these cells accumulate in other organs, including the heart and kidney.

Clinical Features: Patients with visceral leishmaniasis suffer persistent fever, with progressive weight loss, hepatosplenomegaly, anemia, thrombocytopenia, and leukopenia. Light-skinned persons develop darkening of the skin; the Hindi name for leishmaniasis, *kala azar,* means "black sickness." Over the course of months, the patient with visceral leishmaniasis becomes profoundly cachectic, and the spleen enlarges massively. If untreated, the disease is invariably fatal. Treatment entails systemic antiprotozoal therapy.

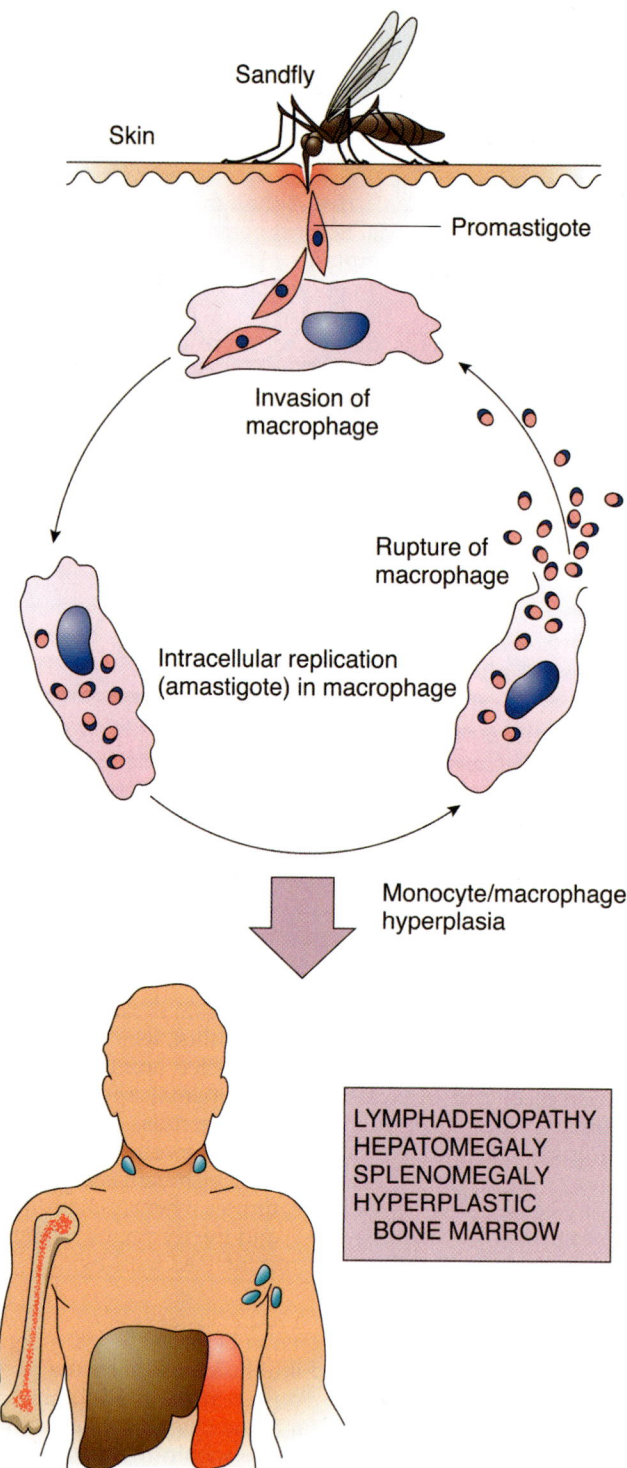

FIGURE 9-76
Leishmaniasis. Blood-sucking sandflies ingest amastigotes from an infected host. These are transformed in the sandfly gut into promastigotes, which multiply and are injected into the next vertebrate host. There they invade macrophages, revert to the amastigote form, and multiply, eventually rupturing the cell. They then invade other macrophages, thus completing the cycle.

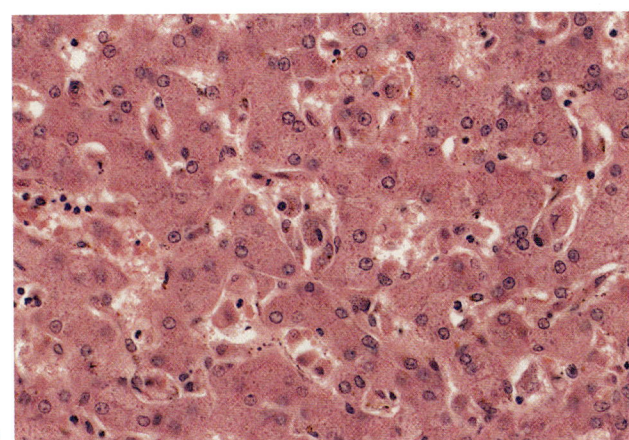

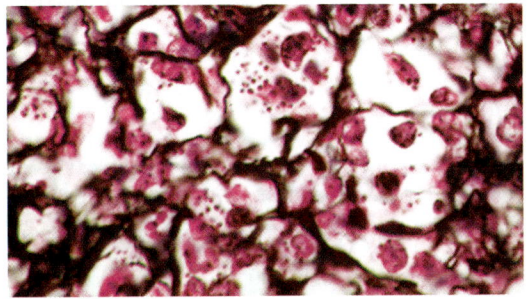

FIGURE 9-77
Visceral leishmaniasis. A. A photomicrograph of an enlarged liver shows prominent Kupffer cells distended by leishmanial amastigotes. B. A section of bone marrow subjected to silver impregnation shows macrophages filled with proliferating leishmanial amastigotes.

CHAGAS DISEASE (AMERICAN TRYPANOSOMIASIS)

Chagas disease is an insect-borne, zoonotic infection by the protozoan Trypanosoma cruzi, *which causes a systemic infection of humans. Acute manifestations and long-term sequelae occur in the heart and gastrointestinal tract.*

 Epidemiology: *T. cruzi* infection is endemic in wild and domesticated animals (e.g., rats, dogs, goats, cats, armadillos) in Central and South America, where the parasite is transmitted by the reduviid ("kissing") bug. Infection with *T. cruzi* is promoted by contact between humans and infected bugs, usually in mud or thatched dwellings of the rural and suburban poor. The bugs hide in cracks of rickety houses and in vegetal roofing, emerge at night, and feed on sleeping victims. Congenital infection occurs upon passage of the parasite from mother to fetus. It is estimated that some 20 million persons in Latin America are infected with *T. cruzi*, more than half of whom live in Brazil. An annual total of 50,000 deaths are attributable to Chagas disease.

Pathogenesis: The infective forms of *T. cruzi* are discharged in the feces of the reduviid bug while it takes its blood meal. Itching and scratching promote contamination of the wound by the insect feces. The trypomastigotes penetrate through the site of the bite or other abrasions or may penetrate the mucosa of the eyes or lips. Once in the body, they lose their flagella and undulating membranes, round up to become amastigotes, and enter macrophages, where they undergo repeated divisions. Amastigotes also invade other sites, including cardiac myofibers and brain. Within the host cells, amastigotes differentiate into trypomastigotes, which break out and enter the bloodstream (Fig. 9-78). Ingested in a subsequent bite of a reduviid bug, trypomastigotes multiply in the alimentary tract of the insect and differentiate into metacyclic trypomastigotes, which congregate in the rectum of the bug and are discharged in the feces.

T. cruzi infects cells at the site of inoculation, reproducing within them to form a localized nodular inflammatory lesion, known as a *chagoma*. The organism then disseminates in the bloodstream, infecting cells throughout the body. Strains of *T. cruzi* differ in their predominant target cells; infections of cardiac myocytes, gastrointestinal ganglion cells, and meninges produce the most significant disease. The parasitemia and widespread cellular infection are responsible for the systemic symptoms of acute Chagas disease. The onset of cell-mediated immunity eliminates the acute manifestations, but chronic tissue damage may continue. The progressive destruction of cells at sites of *T. cruzi* infection, particularly the heart, esophagus, and colon, causes dysfunction of these organs, manifested decades after the acute infection.

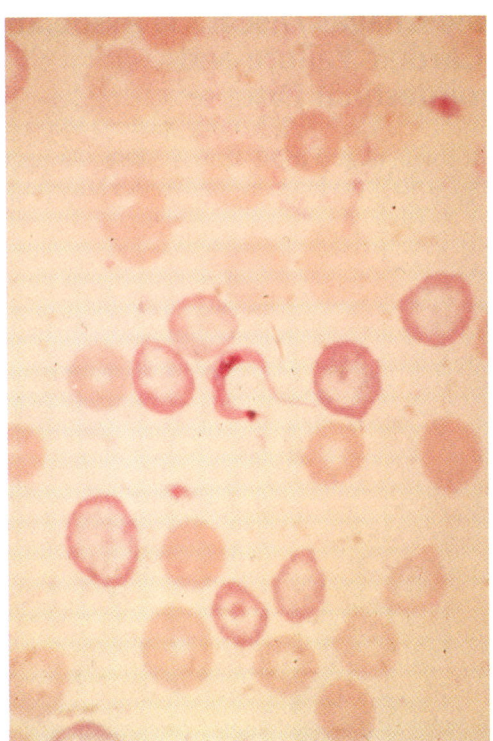

FIGURE 9-78
Chagas disease. A blood smear demonstrates a trypomastigote of *T. cruzi* with its characteristic "C" shape, flagellum, nucleus, and terminal kinetoplast.

Acute Chagas Disease May Cause Fatal Myocarditis

 Pathology: *T. cruzi* circulates in the blood as a 20-μm long, curved, flagellate that is easily recognized on blood films. Within infected cells, it reproduces as a nonflagellated amastigote, 2 to 4 μm in diameter. In fatal cases, the heart is enlarged and dilated, with a pale, focally hemorrhagic myocardium. Microscopically, numerous parasites are seen in the heart, and amastigotes are evident within pseudocysts in myofibers (Fig. 9-79). There is extensive chronic inflammation, and phagocytosis of parasites is conspicuous.

Clinical Features: Acute symptoms develop after an incubation period of 1 to 2 weeks following inoculation with *T. cruzi*. A subcutaneous, inflammatory nodule, the chagoma, develops at the site. Parasitemia appears 2 to 3 weeks after inoculation and is usually associated with a mild illness characterized by fever, malaise, lymphadenopathy, and hepatosplenomegaly. However, the disease can be lethal when there is extensive myocardial or meningeal involvement.

Chronic Chagas Disease Is Associated with Cardiac Failure and Gastrointestinal Disease

The most frequent and most serious consequences of infection with *T. cruzi* develop years or decades after the acute infection. It is estimated that 10 to 40% of acutely infected persons eventually develop chronic disease. In this phase of the illness, *T. cruzi* is no longer present in the blood or tissue. Infected organs have been damaged, however, by a chronic, progressive inflammatory process.

 Pathology and Clinical Features: Chronic myocarditis is characterized by a dilated heart, prominent right ventricular outflow tract, and dilation of the valve rings. The interventricular septum is often deviated to the right and may immobilize the adjacent tricuspid leaflet. Microscopically, there is extensive interstitial fibrosis, hypertrophied myofibers, and focal lymphocytic inflammation, often involving the cardiac conduction system. Progressive cardiac fibrosis causes dysrhythmia or congestive heart failure. In endemic regions, chronic Chagas disease is a leading cause of heart failure in young adults.

Megaesophagus, that is, dilation of the esophagus caused by failure of the lower esophageal sphincter (achalasia), is a common complication of chronic Chagas disease. It results from the destruction of parasympathetic ganglion cells in the wall of the lower esophagus and leads to difficulty in swallowing, which may be so severe that the patient can consume only liquids.

Megacolon, massive dilation of the large bowel, is similar to megaesophagus in that the myenteric plexus of the colon is destroyed. The progressive aganglionosis of the colon causes severe constipation.

Congenital Chagas disease occurs in some pregnant women with parasitemia. Infection of the placenta and fetus leads to spontaneous abortion. In the infrequent live births, the infants die of encephalitis within a few days or weeks.

Antiprotozoal chemotherapy is effective for acute Chagas disease but is of no value for its chronic sequelae. Cardiac transplantation has been effective in a number of patients.

AFRICAN TRYPANOSOMIASIS

African trypanosomiasis, popularly termed sleeping sickness, *is an infection with* Trypanosoma brucei gambiense *or* T. brucei rhodesiense, *which produces a life-threatening meningoencephalitis.* Gambian trypanosomiasis is a chronic infection often lasting more than a year. By contrast, East African (Rhodesian) trypanosomiasis is a rapidly progressive infection that kills the patient in 3 to 6 months. The organisms are curved flagellates, 15 to 30 μm in length. Although they can be demonstrated in blood or cerebrospinal fluid, they are difficult to find in infected tissues.

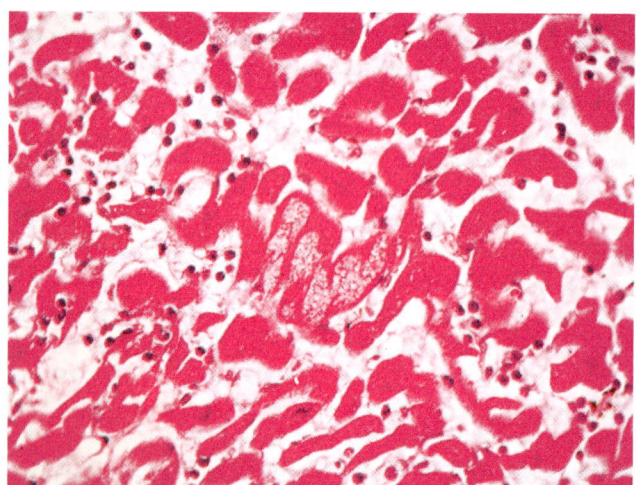

FIGURE 9-79
Acute Chagas myocarditis. The myofibers in the center contain numerous amastigotes of *T. cruzi* and are surrounded by edema and chronic inflammation.

 Epidemiology: *T. brucei gambiense* and *T. brucei rhodesiense* are hemoflagellate protozoa that are transmitted by several species of blood-sucking tsetse flies of the genus *Glossina*. The patchy distribution of African trypanosomiasis is related to the habitats of the tsetse flies. In Gambian trypanosomiasis, *T. brucei gambiense*

is transmitted by tsetse flies of the riverine bush, mainly in endemic pockets of West and Central Africa. **Humans are the only important reservoir for this trypanosome.**

In East African trypanosomiasis, *T. brucei rhodesiense* is spread by tsetse flies of the woodland savanna of East Africa. Antelope, other game animals, and domestic cattle are natural reservoirs of *T. brucei rhodesiense*. **Infection of humans is an occupational hazard of game wardens, fishermen, and cattle herders.**

 Pathogenesis: While biting an infected animal or human, the tsetse fly ingests trypomastigotes with the blood (Fig. 9-80). These forms (1) lose their coat of surface antigen, (2) multiply in the midgut of the fly, (3) migrate to the salivary gland, (4) develop over a 3-week period through the epimastigote stage, and (5) multiply in the fly's saliva as infective metacyclic trypomastigotes. During another bite, the metacyclic trypomastigotes are injected into the lymphatics and blood vessels of a new host. The organisms disseminate to the bone marrow and tissue fluids, and some eventually invade the central nervous system. After replicating by binary fission in blood, lymph, and spinal fluid, trypomastigotes are ingested by another fly to complete the cycle.

The pathogenesis of African trypanosomiasis involves the formation of immune complexes by variable trypanosomal antigens and antibodies. In addition, the production of autoantibodies to antigenic components of erythrocytes, brain, and heart may participate in the production of disease. The trypanosome evades immune attack in the mammalian host by periodically altering its glycoprotein antigenic coat. The alterations take place in a genetically determined pattern, not by mutation. Thus, each wave of circulating trypomastigotes includes immunologically distinct antigenic variants that are a step ahead of the immune response.

 Pathology: *T. brucei* multiplies at the site of inoculation, occasionally producing a localized nodular lesion termed a *primary chancre*. Early in the course of the disease, there is prominent generalized involvement of lymph nodes and spleen. Microscopic changes in the affected nodes and spleen include foci of lymphocyte and macrophage hyperplasia. Infection eventually localizes to

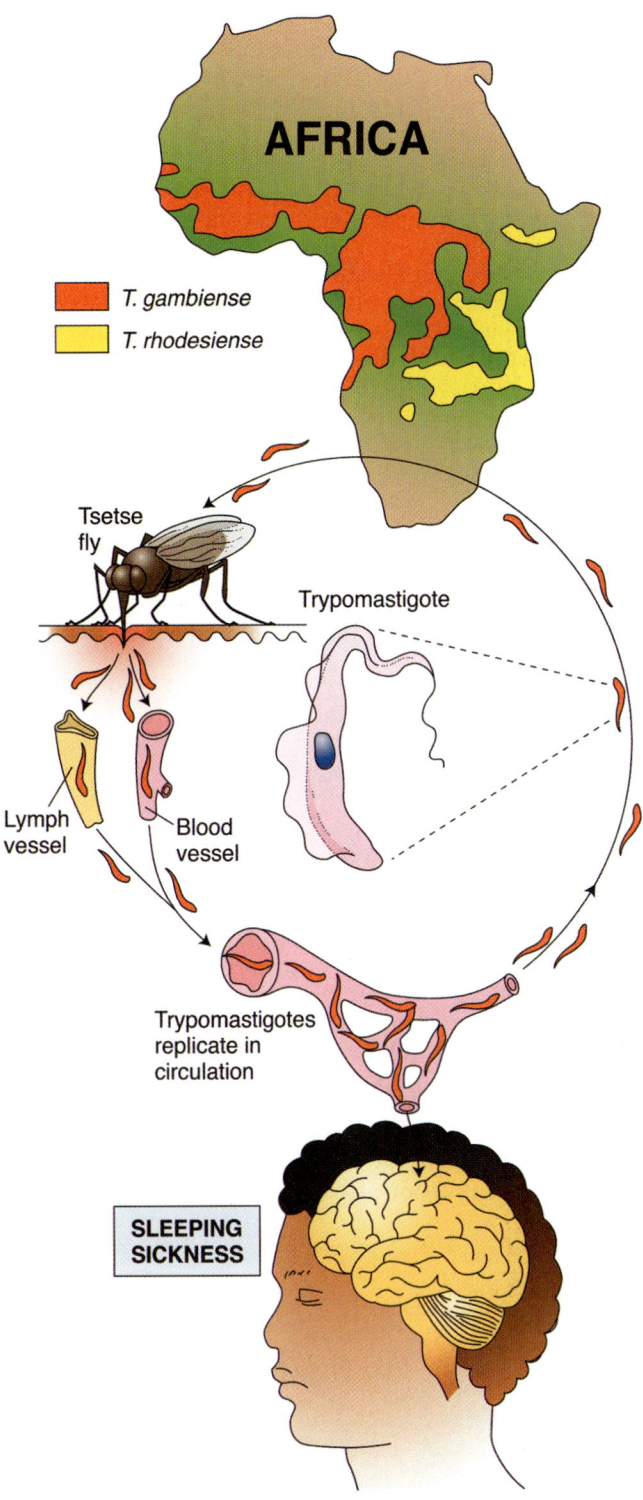

FIGURE 9-80

African trypanosomiasis (sleeping sickness). The distribution of Gambian and Rhodesian trypanosomiasis is related to the habitats of the vector tsetse flies (*Glossina* spp.). A tsetse fly bites an infected animal or human and ingests trypomastigotes, which multiply into infective, metacyclic trypomastigotes. During another fly bite, these are injected into lymphatic and blood vessels of a new host. A primary chancre develops at the site of the bite (stage 1a). Trypomastigotes replicate further in the blood and lymph, causing a systemic infection (stage 1b). Another fly ingests hypomastigotes to complete the cycle. In stage 2, invasion of the central nervous system by trypomastigotes leads to meningoencephalomyelitis and associated symptoms, including lethargy and daytime somnolence. Patients with Rhodesian trypanosomiasis may die within a few months.

the small blood vessels of the central nervous system, where the replicating organisms elicit a destructive vasculitis, producing the progressive decrease in mentation characteristic of sleeping sickness. In *T. brucei rhodesiense* infection, the organisms also localize to blood vessels in the heart, sometimes causing a fulminant myocarditis.

Lesions in the lymph nodes, brain, heart, and various other sites (including the inoculation site) show vasculitis of small blood vessels, with endothelial cell hyperplasia and dense perivascular infiltrates of lymphocytes, macrophages, and plasma cells. Vasculitis of the meninges and brain causes destruction of neurons, demyelination, and gliosis. The perivascular infiltrate thickens the leptomeninges and involves the Virchow-Robin spaces (Fig. 9-81).

 Clinical Features: African trypanosomiasis is divided into three clinical stages:

1. **Primary chancre:** After an incubation period of 5 to 15 days, a 3- to 4-cm papillary swelling topped by a central red spot appears at the dermal inoculation site. The chancre subsides spontaneously within 3 weeks.
2. **Systemic infection:** Shortly after the appearance of the chancre (if any) and within 3 weeks of the bite, invasion of the bloodstream is marked by intermittent fever, which lasts up to a week and is often accompanied by splenomegaly and local and generalized lymphadenopathy. *Winterbottom sign* refers to enlargement of the posterior cervical lymph nodes and is characteristic of Gambian trypanosomiasis. The evolving illness is marked by remitting irregular fevers, headache, joint pains, lethargy, and muscle wasting. Myocarditis may be a complication and is more common and severe in Rhodesian trypanosomiasis. Dysfunction of the lungs, kidneys, liver, and endocrine system is frequently observed in both forms of the disease.
3. **Brain invasion:** Differences between the forms of sleeping sickness are primarily a matter of time scale, especially with regard to invasion of the brain. This feature develops early (weeks or months) in Rhodesian trypanosomiasis and late (months or years) in the Gambian form. Brain invasion is marked by apathy, daytime somnolence, and sometimes coma. A diffuse meningoencephalitis is characterized by tremors of the tongue and fingers; fasciculations of the muscles of the limbs, face, lips, and tongue; oscillatory movements of the arms, head, neck, and trunk; indistinct speech; and cerebellar ataxia, leading to problems in walking.

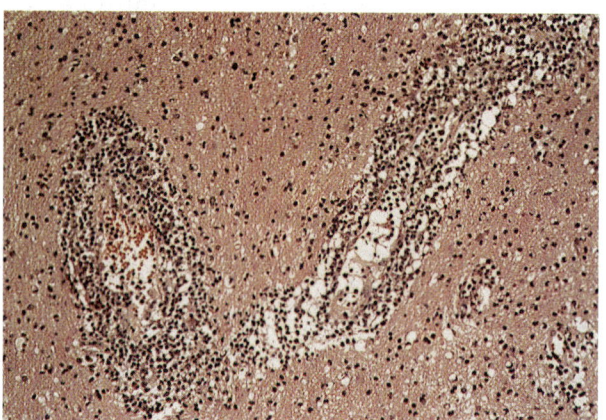

FIGURE 9-81
African trypanosomiasis. A section of brain from a patient who died from infection with *T. brucei rhodesiense* shows a perivascular mononuclear cell infiltrate.

PRIMARY AMEBIC MENINGOENCEPHALITIS

Amebic meningoencephalitis, caused by Naegleria fowleri, *is a fatal, suppurative inflammation of the brain and meninges.*

 Epidemiology: *N. fowleri* is a free-living, soil ameba that inhabits ponds and lakes throughout tropical and subtropical regions but has occasionally been found in temperate areas. Primary amebic meningoencephalitis is a rare disease (fewer than 300 reported cases) affecting persons who swim or bathe in these waters. The disease has been recognized in many parts of the world, including the United States, Europe, Australia, New Zealand, South America, and Africa.

 Pathogenesis and Pathology: *N. fowleri* is inoculated into the nasal mucosa near the cribriform plate when a person swims in or dives into water containing high concentrations of the organism. The amebae subsequently invade the olfactory nerves, migrate through the cribriform plate to the olfactory bulbs, and then proliferate in the meninges and brain.

In tissue sections, trophozoites of *Naegleria* measure 8 to 15 μm across. The nuclei are sharply outlined and stain deeply with hematoxylin. On gross examination, the brain is swollen and soft, with vascular congestion and a purulent exudate on the meningeal surface, most prominent over the lateral and basal areas. There is massive destruction of the brain by amebae, which invade the brain along the Virchow-Robin spaces. Thrombosis and destruction of blood vessels are associated with extensive hemorrhage. The olfactory tract and bulbs are enveloped and destroyed, and there is an exudate between the bulb and the inferior surface of the temporal lobe. Extensive proliferation of *Naegleria* in the brain often leads to the formation of solid masses of amebae (amebomas). Meningitis can extend the full length of the cord.

 Clinical Features: Primary amebic meningoencephalitis due to *N. fowleri* begins suddenly with fever, nausea, vomiting, and headache. The disease progresses rapidly, and within hours the patient suffers profound deterioration in mental status. The cerebrospinal fluid contains numerous neutrophils, blood, and amebae. The disease is rapidly fatal.

Helminthic Infection

Helminths, or worms, are among the most common human pathogens. At any given time, 25 to 50% of the world's population is infected with at least one helminth species. Although most helminthic infections cause little harm, some produce significant disease. Schistosomiasis, for instance, ranks among the leading global causes of morbidity and mortality.

Helminths are the largest and most complex organisms capable of living within the human body. Their adult forms range from 0.5 mm more than 1 m in length, and most are readily visible to the naked eye. Helminths are multicellular animals with differentiated tissues, including specialized nervous tissues, digestive tissues, and reproductive systems. Their maturation from eggs or larvae to adult worms is complex, often involving multiple morphological transformations (molts). Some helminths undergo these metamorphoses in different hosts before attaining adulthood, and the human host may be only one in a series that supports this maturation process. Within the human body, the helminths frequently migrate from the port of entry through several organs to a site of final infection.

Most helminths that infect humans are well adapted to human parasitism, producing limited or no damage to host tissues. Helminth infections are acquired by ingestion, direct skin penetration, or insect bites. Unlike viruses, bacteria, and fungi, the helminths (with two exceptions) cannot multiply within the human body; thus the inoculation of a single organism cannot be amplified into an overwhelming infection. The exceptions are *Strongyloides stercoralis* and *Capillaria philippinensis*, which can complete their life cycle and multiply within the human body.

Helminths cause disease in various ways. A few compete with their human host for certain nutrients. Some grow to block vital structures, producing disease by mass effect. Most, however, cause dysfunction through the destructive inflammatory and immunological responses that they elicit. For example, morbidity in schistosomiasis, the most destructive helminthic infection, results from the granulomatous response to the schistosome eggs deposited in tissue.

Eosinophils contain basic proteins toxic to some helminths and are a major component of the inflammatory responses to these organisms. Parasitic helminths are divided into three broad categories based on overall morphology and the structure of digestive tissues.

- **Roundworms (nematodes)** are elongate cylindrical organisms with tubular digestive tracts.
- **Flatworms (trematodes)** are dorsoventrally flattened organisms with digestive tracts that end in blind loops.
- **Tapeworms (cestodes)** are segmented organisms with separate head and body parts; they lack a digestive tract and absorb nutrients through their outer walls.

FILARIAL NEMATODES

Lymphatic Filariasis Results in Massive Lymphedema (Elephantiasis)

Lymphatic filariasis (bancroftian and Malayan filariasis) is an inflammatory parasitic infection of lymphatic vessels caused by the filarial roundworms *Wuchereria bancrofti* and *Brugia malayi*. The adult worms inhabit the lymphatics, most frequently those in the inguinal, epitrochlear, and axillary lymph nodes, testis, and epididymis. There they cause acute lymphangitis and, in a minority of infected subjects, eventual lymphatic obstruction, leading to severe lymphedema (Fig. 9-82). These and similar organisms are known as filarial worms, because of their threadlike appearance (from the Latin *filum*, meaning thread).

Epidemiology: The elephantiasis characteristic of lymphatic filariasis was familiar to Hindi and Persian physicians as early as 600 BC. Humans, the only definitive host of these filarial nematodes, acquire infection from the bites of at least 80 species of mosquitoes of the genera *Culex, Aedes, Anopheles,* and *Mansonia*. *W. bancrofti* infection is widespread in southern Asia, the Pacific, Africa, and portions of South America. *B. malayi* is localized to coastal southern Asia and western Pacific islands. Worldwide, between 100 and 200 million persons are estimated to be infected.

Pathogenesis: Mosquito bites transmit infectious larvae that migrate to lymphatics and lymph nodes. After maturing into adult forms over several months, the worms mate and the female releases microfilariae into lymphatics and the bloodstream. The manifestations of filariasis result from the inflammatory response to degenerating adult worms in the lymphatics. Repeated filarial infections are common in endemic regions and produce numerous bouts of lymphangitis *(filarial fevers),* which eventually (over years) cause extensive scarring and obstruction of lymphatics. The lymphatic obstruction produces localized dependent edema, most commonly affecting the legs, arms, genitalia, and breasts. In its most severe form (less than 5% of the infected population), this edematous distortion of body parts is known as *elephantiasis*.

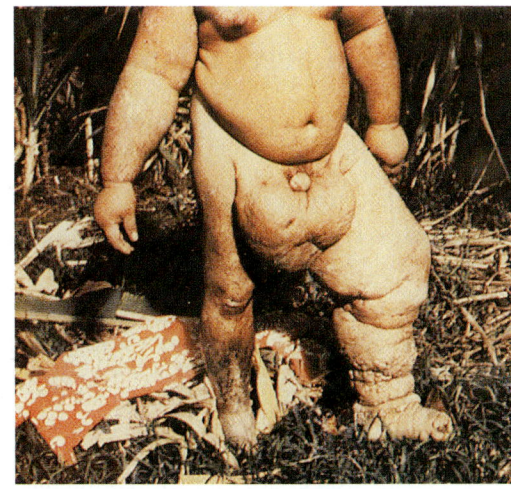

FIGURE 9-82
Bancroftian filariasis. Massive lymphedema (elephantiasis) of the scrotum and left lower extremity are present.

Pathology: The adult nematode is a white, threadlike worm that is much convoluted within the lymph nodes. The female is twice the size of the male and measures 80 to 100 mm in length and 0.20 to 0.3 mm in width. In blood films stained with Giemsa, the microfilariae appear as gracefully curved worms, measuring about 300 μm in length.

The lymphatic vessels harboring the adult worms are dilated, and the endothelial lining is thickened. In the adjacent tissue, a chronic inflammatory infiltrate, including eosinophils, surrounds the worms. A granulomatous reaction may develop, and degenerating worms can provoke acute inflammation. Microfilariae are seen in blood vessels and lymphatics, and degenerating microfilariae also provoke a chronic inflammatory reaction. After repeated bouts of lymphangitis, the lymph nodes and lymphatics become densely fibrotic, often containing calcified remnants of the worms.

 Clinical Features: In endemic areas, most of the infected population displays either antifilarial antibodies with no detectable infection or asymptomatic microfilaremia. A smaller number of the infected persons develop recurrent episodes of filarial fevers, with malaise, lymphadenopathy, and lymphangitis, which persist for 1 to 2 weeks and then resolve spontaneously. In a small subset of these patients, the late manifestations of disease appear after two to three decades of recurrent bouts of filarial fevers. Lymphatic obstruction produces chronic edema of dependent tissues, and the overlying skin becomes thickened and warty. The diagnosis is made by identifying the microfilariae in blood samples. Diethylcarbamazine and ivermectin are the agents effective against lymphatic filariasis.

Occult filariasis, a condition characterized by indirect evidence of filarial infection (circulating antifilarial antibodies), is the cause of *tropical pulmonary eosinophilia*. This condition is virtually restricted to southern India and some Pacific Islands. Patients present with cough, wheezing diffuse pulmonary infiltrates, and peripheral eosinophilia. The severity ranges from mild asthma to fatal pneumonia.

Onchocerciasis Causes Blindness

Onchocerciasis ("river blindness") is a chronic inflammatory disease of the skin, eyes, and lymphatics caused by the filarial nematode *Onchocerca volvulus*.

 Epidemiology: Onchocerciasis is one of the world's major endemic diseases, afflicting an estimated 40 million persons, of whom 2 million are blind. Humans are the only definitive host. On biting, *Simulium damnosum* blackflies transmit infectious larvae to humans. These insects require rapidly running water for breeding, and onchocerciasis is therefore endemic along rivers and streams (hence the name "*river blindness*") in parts of tropical Africa, southern Mexico, Central America, and South America.

 Pathogenesis: Adult worms live as coiled tangled masses in the deep fasciae and subcutaneous tissues. They do not cause tissue damage and do not elicit inflammatory responses, but the gravid females release millions of microfilariae, which migrate into the skin, eyes, lymph nodes, and deep organs, thereby producing corresponding onchocercal lesions. Ocular onchocerciasis results from the migration of microfilariae into all regions of the eye, from the cornea to the optic nerve head.

When microfilariae die, they incite a vigorous inflammatory and immunological response. Inflammatory damage to the cornea, choroids, or retina leads to partial or total loss of vision. The inflammatory response in the skin results in microabscess formation and chronic degenerative changes in the epidermis and dermis. In the lymph nodes and lymphatics, the response to dying microfilariae causes chronic lymphatic obstruction and localized dependent edema.

 Pathology: *Onchocerca volvulus* is a thin, very long nematode, the female measuring 400 × 0.3 mm and the male 30 × 0.2 mm. Masses of adult worms become encapsulated by a fibrous scar, forming discrete, 1- to 3-cm, *onchocercal nodules* in the deep dermis and subcutaneous tissues. Nodules form over bony prominences of the skull, scapula, ribs, iliac crest, trochanter, sacrum, and knee. Microscopically, the subcutaneous nodules have an outer fibrous layer and a central inflammatory infiltrate, which varies from suppurative to granulomatous. The active lesions in the eyes and lymphatics all show degenerating microfilariae surrounded by chronic inflammation, including eosinophils. Involvement of the eye leads to sclerosing keratitis, iridocyclitis, chorioretinitis, and optic atrophy. The femoral inguinal nodes become enlarged and then fibrotic.

 Clinical Features: Symptoms of onchocerciasis result from the inflammatory response to degenerating microfilariae. Skin manifestations begin with generalized pruritus that becomes so intense that it often interferes with sleeping. Continuing damage produces areas of depigmentation, hypertrophy, or atrophy of the skin. Progressive destruction of the cornea, choroids, or uvea leads to loss of vision. Chronic lymphadenitis results in localized edema that may cause chronic swelling (elephantiasis) of the legs, scrotum, or other dependent portions of the body. Systemic antihelminthic therapy, particularly with ivermectin, is effective in treating onchocerciasis.

Loiasis Principally Affects the Eyes and Skin

Loiasis is infection by the filarial nematode Loa loa, *the African "eyeworm."*

  Epidemiology and Pathogenesis: The infestation is prevalent in the rain forests of Central and West Africa. Humans and ba-

Intestinal Nematodes

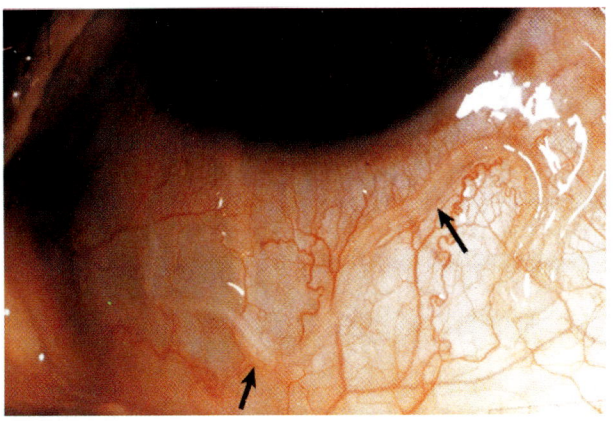

FIGURE 9-83
Loiasis. A threadlike *L. loa (arrows)* is migrating in the subconjunctival tissues.

boons are the definitive hosts, and infection is transmitted by mango flies. Adult worms (4 cm long) migrate in the skin and occasionally cross the eye beneath the conjunctiva, making the patient acutely aware of this infection (Fig. 9-83). Gravid worms discharge microfilariae, which circulate in the bloodstream during the day but reside in capillaries of the skin, lungs, and other organs at night.

 Pathology: Migrating worms cause no inflammation, but static ones are surrounded by eosinophils, other inflammatory cells, and a foreign body giant cell reaction. Rarely, infected subjects may develop acute generalized loiasis. At autopsy, these patients have obstructive fibrin thrombi in small vessels of most organs, which contain degenerating microfilariae. When the brain is involved, obstruction of vessels by filarial thrombi kills the patient through sudden and diffuse ischemia.

 Clinical Features: Most infections are asymptomatic but persist for years. Some patients have pruritic, red, subcutaneous "Calabar" swellings, which may be a reaction to migrating adult worms or to microfilariae in the skin. Ocular symptoms include swelling of the eyelids, itching, and pain. Worms may be extracted during their migration beneath the conjunctiva. Systemic reactions include fever, pain, itching, urticaria, and eosinophilia. Dead worms in or near major nerves may cause paresthesia or paralysis. Treatment with microfilariacides may cause massive death of microfilariae and provoke fever, meningoencephalitis, and death.

INTESTINAL NEMATODES

The adult forms of a number of nematode species (Table 9-10) reside in the human bowel but rarely cause symptomatic disease. In fact, clinical symptoms occur almost exclusively in persons who are infected with large numbers of worms or in those who are immunocompromised. Humans are the exclusive or primary host for all of the intestinal nematodes, and infection spreads from person to person through eggs or larvae passed in the stool or deposited in the perianal region. Infection is most prevalent in locations where hand washing and hygienic disposal of human feces are lacking (e.g., less-developed countries, day-care centers). Warm, moist climates are required for environmental survival of the infectious forms of many of the intestinal nematodes, and these worms are, therefore, endemic in tropical and subtropical environments.

Ascariasis Is Usually an Asymptomatic Infestation of the Small Bowel

Ascariasis refers to infection by the large roundworm Ascaris lumbricoides. It is the most common helminth infection of humans, affecting at least one billion people, usually without causing symptoms. Ascariasis is found worldwide, but infection is most common in areas with warm climates and poor sanitation.

 Pathogenesis: Adult worms live in the small intestine, where gravid females discharge eggs that pass in the feces. The eggs hatch when ingested, and the *Ascaris* larvae emerge in the small intestine, penetrate the bowel wall, and reach the lungs through the venous circulation. From the pulmonary capillaries they enter the

TABLE 9-10 Intestinal Nematodes

Species	Common Name	Site of Adult Worm	Clinical Manifestations
Ascaris lumbricoides	Roundworm	Small bowel	Allergic reactions to lung migration; intestinal obstruction
Ancylostoma duodenale	Hookworm	Small bowel	Allergic reactions to cutaneous inoculation and lung migration; intestinal blood loss
Necator americanus	Hookworm	Small bowel	Allergic reactions to cutaneous inoculation and lung migration; intestinal blood loss
Trichuris trichiura	Whipworm	Large bowel	Abdominal pain and diarrhea; rectal prolapse (rare)
Strongyloides stercoralis	Threadworm	Small bowel	Abdominal pain and diarrhea; dissemination to extraintestinal sites in immunocompromised persons
Enterobius vermicularis	Pinworm	Cecum, appendix	Perianal and perineal itching

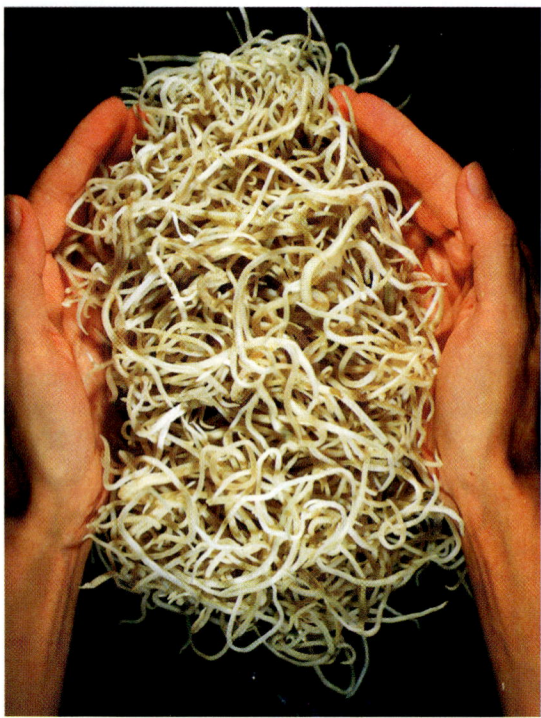

FIGURE 9-84
Ascariasis. This mass of over 800 worms of *A. lumbricoides* obstructed and infarcted the ileum of a 2-year-old girl in South Africa.

alveolar spaces and migrate up the trachea to the glottis, where they are swallowed and again reach the small bowel. They mature in the small bowel and live as adult worms within the lumen for 1 to 2 years.

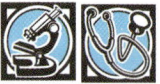 **Pathology and Clinical Features:** Adult worms (15–35 cm long) usually cause no pathological changes. Heavy infections may cause vomiting, malnutrition and sometimes intestinal obstruction (Fig. 9-84). On rare occasions, worms migrate into the ampulla of Vater or the pancreatic or biliary ducts, where they may cause biliary obstruction, acute pancreatitis, suppurative cholangitis, and liver abscesses. Eggs deposited in the liver or other tissues may produce necrosis, granulomatous inflammation, and fibrosis. *Ascaris* pneumonia, which may be fatal, develops when large numbers of larvae migrate within the air spaces.

The diagnosis of ascariasis is made by identifying eggs in the feces. Occasionally, adult worms may pass with the stools or even emerge from the nose or mouth. Ascaricidal drugs are effective.

Trichuriasis Is a Superficially Invasive Infection of the Large Bowel

Trichuriasis is caused by the intestinal nematode Trichuris trichiura *("whipworm").*

 Epidemiology: Whipworm infection is found worldwide, with over 800 million persons infected. Although parasitism is most common in areas with warm, moist climates and poor sanitation, it is estimated that over 2 million persons in the United States are infected. Children are especially susceptible. Adult worms live in the cecum and upper colon, where female worms produce eggs that pass in the feces. Eggs embryonate in moist soil and become infective in 3 weeks. Humans are infected by ingesting eggs in contaminated soil, food, or drink.

  Pathogenesis and Pathology: Larvae emerge from the ingested eggs in the small bowel and migrate to the cecum and colon, where the adult worms burrow their anterior portions into the superficial mucosa (Fig. 9-85). This invasion causes small erosions, focal active inflammation, and continuous loss of small quantities of blood. *T. trichiura* measures 3 to 5 cm in length, with a long, slender anterior portion and a short, blunt posterior.

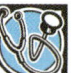 **Clinical Features:** Most *T. trichiura* infections are asymptomatic. Heavy infestation of worms may produce cramping abdominal pain, bloody diarrhea, weight loss, and anemia. The diagnosis is made by finding the characteristic eggs in the stool. Mebendazole is effective therapy.

Hookworms Cause Intestinal Blood Loss and Anemia

Necator americanus and Ancylostoma duodenale ("hookworms") are intestinal nematodes that infect the human small bowel. These worms lacerate the bowel mucosa, causing intestinal blood loss, which can produce symptomatic disease in heavy infestations.

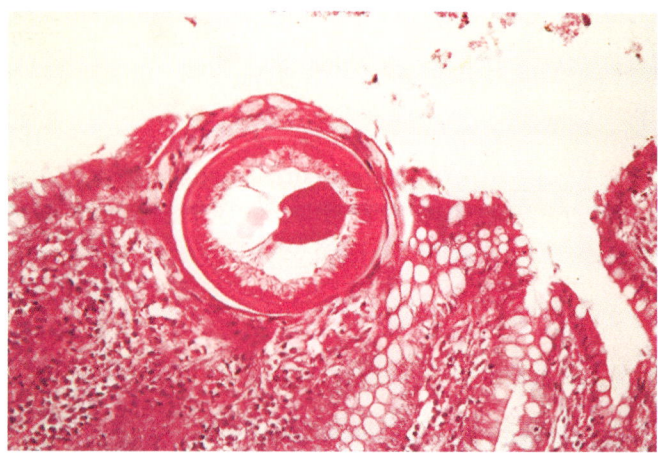

FIGURE 9-85
Trichuriasis. The anterior "whip" end of *T. trichiura* is threaded into the mucosa of the colon.

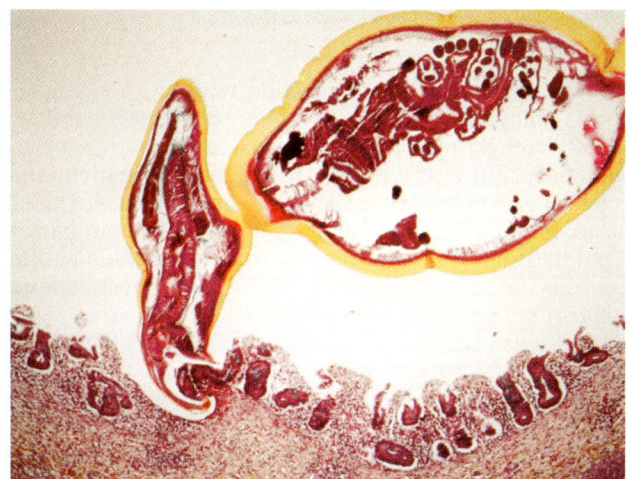

FIGURE 9-86
Ancylostomiasis. Section of the ileum shows two portions of a single adult worm, *A. duodenale*. A plug of mucosa is in the buccal cavity of the hookworm.

 Epidemiology: Hookworm infections are encountered in moist, warm, temperate and tropical areas and cause serious public health problems across large areas of the globe. In fact, both *A. duodenale* ("Old World" hookworm) and *N. americanus* ("American" hookworm) prevail on most continents and have overlapping epidemiological boundaries. Worldwide, more than 700 million persons are infected with hookworms, and it is estimated that a half-million persons in the United States harbor the parasite.

  Pathogenesis and Pathology: On contact with human skin, filariform larvae directly penetrate the epidermis and enter the venous circulation. They travel to the lungs, where they lodge in alveolar capillaries. After rupturing into the alveoli, the larvae migrate up the trachea to the glottis and are then swallowed. They molt in the duodenum, attach to the mucosal wall with toothlike buckle plates, clamp off a section of the villus, and ingest it (Fig. 9-86). With extensive worm infections, particularly with *A. duodenale*, the blood loss can be considerable and result in anemia. Hookworms measure about 1 cm in length. The worms are grossly visible attached to the mucosal surface of the small bowel, alongside punctate areas of hemorrhages. There is no associated inflammation.

 Clinical Features: Although most persons with hookworm infection are not symptomatic, infection with this parasite is the most important cause of chronic anemia worldwide. In persons with heavy worm burdens (particularly women who consume a diet low in iron) and in populations with inadequate iron intake, chronic intestinal blood loss can produce severe iron deficiency anemia. Skin penetration is sometimes associated with a pruritic eruption ("ground itch"), and the phase of larval migration through the lungs occasionally causes asthma-like symptoms.

Strongyloidiasis Is Disseminated in Immunocompromised Hosts

Strongyloidiasis refers to a small intestinal infection with the nematode Strongyloides stercoralis *("threadworm"). Although most cases of strongyloidiasis are asymptomatic, the infection can progress to lethal disseminated disease in immunocompromised persons.* Infection is most frequent in areas with warm, moist climates and poor sanitation. However, endemic pockets of strongyloidiasis still exist in the United States, particularly in the Appalachian region and in institutions where personal hygiene is poor, such as hospitals for the mentally ill.

  Pathogenesis and Pathology: *S. stercoralis* is the smallest of the intestinal nematodes, measuring 0.2 to 0.3 cm in length. The adult females are buried in the crypts of the duodenum or jejunum but produce no visible alterations. Microscopic examination shows the coiled females, along with eggs and developing larvae, within the mucosa, usually with no associated inflammation (Fig. 9-87).

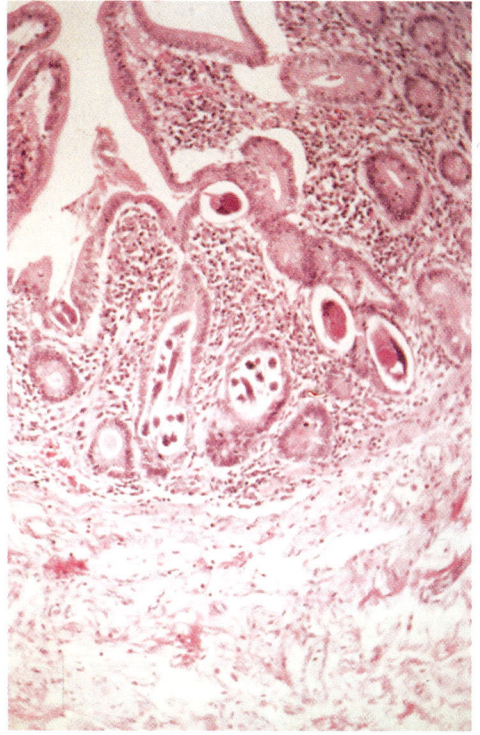

FIGURE 9-87
Strongyloidiasis. A section of jejunum shows adult worms, larvae, and eggs of *S. stercoralis* in the mucosal crypts. The lamina propria is infiltrated with lymphocytes, plasma cells, and eosinophils. The patient had a hyperinfected syndrome and presented with malabsorption.

Parasitic females live within the mucosa of the small intestine, where they lay eggs that hatch quickly and release rhabditiform larvae. The larvae are passed in the feces, and in the soil become filariform, the infective stage that penetrates human skin. On entering the skin, *S. stercoralis* larvae pass in the bloodstream to the lungs and then to the small bowel, in a manner similar to that of hookworms. The worms mature in the small bowel. In contrast to other intestinal nematodes, *S. stercoralis* may reproduce within the human host by a mechanism known as *autoinfection*. This process occurs when rhabditiform larvae become infective (filariform) within the host's intestine and repenetrate either the intestinal wall or the perianal skin, thereby starting a new parasitic cycle within a single host.

Clinical Features: Most infected persons are completely asymptomatic, but moderate eosinophilia is common. **Disseminated strongyloidiasis or hyperinfection syndrome** occurs in patients with suppressed immunity, particularly those receiving corticosteroids. In such patients, the rate of internal autoinfection is greatly increased, and extraordinary numbers of filariform larvae penetrate the intestinal walls and disseminate to distant organs. In disseminated strongyloidiasis, the gut may exhibit ulceration, edema, and severe inflammation. Sepsis, usually with gram-negative organisms, and infection of parenchymal organs occur almost invariably. If untreated, disseminated strongyloidiasis is fatal; even with prompt treatment with thiabendazole or ivermectin, only a third of patients survive.

Pinworm Infection (Enterobiasis) Leads to Perianal Itching

Enterobius vermicularis ("*pinworm*") *is an intestinal nematode that is encountered worldwide but is more frequent in temperate zones.* Although people can be infected at any age, parasitism is most common among young children. It is estimated that more than 200 million persons are infected with *E. vermicularis* worldwide; some 5 million school-age children harbor the worm in the United States.

The adult female worm resides in the cecum and appendix but migrates to the perianal and perineal skin to deposit eggs. The eggs stick to fingers, bed linens, towels, and clothing and are readily transmitted from person to person. Ingested eggs hatch in the small bowel to yield larvae that mature into adult worms. Some infected persons are asymptomatic, but most complain of perineal pruritus, caused by the migrating worms depositing eggs. Several agents, including mebendazole, are effective against pinworms.

TISSUE NEMATODES

Trichinosis Is Myositis Acquired by Eating Pork

Trichinosis is produced by the roundworm Trichinella spiralis.

Epidemiology: Infection with *T. spiralis* is cosmopolitan but is most common in eastern and central Europe, North America, and South America. Humans acquire trichinosis by ingesting inadequately cooked meat containing encysted *T. spiralis* larvae. The larvae are found in the skeletal muscles of various carnivorous or omnivorous wild and domesticated animals, including pigs, rats, bears, and walruses. Pork is the most common source of human trichinosis (Fig. 9-88).

Animals acquire trichinosis by feeding on the flesh of other infected animals. Infection is common among some wild animal populations and can be readily introduced into domesticated animals, such as pigs, when they feed on garbage or uncooked meat. Meat inspection programs and restriction of feeding practices have largely eliminated *T. spiralis* from domesticated pigs in many developed countries. Although only about 100 cases of trichinosis are reported in the United States annually, these represent only the most severely symptomatic cases, and infection is probably much more common.

Pathogenesis: Within the small bowel, *T. spiralis* larvae emerge from the ingested tissue cysts and burrow into the intestinal mucosa, where they develop into adult worms. The adults mate, and the female worm liberates larvae that invade the intestinal wall and enter the circulation. Production of larvae may continue for 1 to 4 months, until the worms are finally expelled from the intestine. The larvae can invade nearly any tissue but can survive only in striated skeletal muscle, where they encyst and remain viable for years. The resulting myositis is especially prominent in the diaphragm, extrinsic ocular muscles, tongue, intercostal muscles, gastrocnemius, and deltoids. Sometimes the central nervous system or heart is also involved in the inflammatory response, producing a meningoencephalitis or myocarditis.

Pathology: The skeletal muscles are the major sites of tissue damage in trichinosis. When a larva infects a myocyte, the cell undergoes basophilic degeneration and swelling. Early myocyte infection elicits an intense inflammatory infiltrate rich in eosinophils and macrophages. The larva grows to 10 times its initial size, folds on itself, and develops a capsule. With encapsulation, the inflammatory infiltrate subsides. Several years later, the larva dies and the cyst calcifies. In *T. spiralis* infections, the small bowel is grossly unremarkable. In heavy infestations, adult worms may be found on microscopic examination at the base of villi and may be associated with an inflammatory infiltrate.

Clinical Features: Most human infections with *T. spiralis* involve small numbers of cysts and are totally asymptomatic. Symptomatic trichinosis is usually a self-limited disease from which patients recover in a few months. When large numbers of cysts are eaten, abdominal pain and diarrhea may result from small bowel

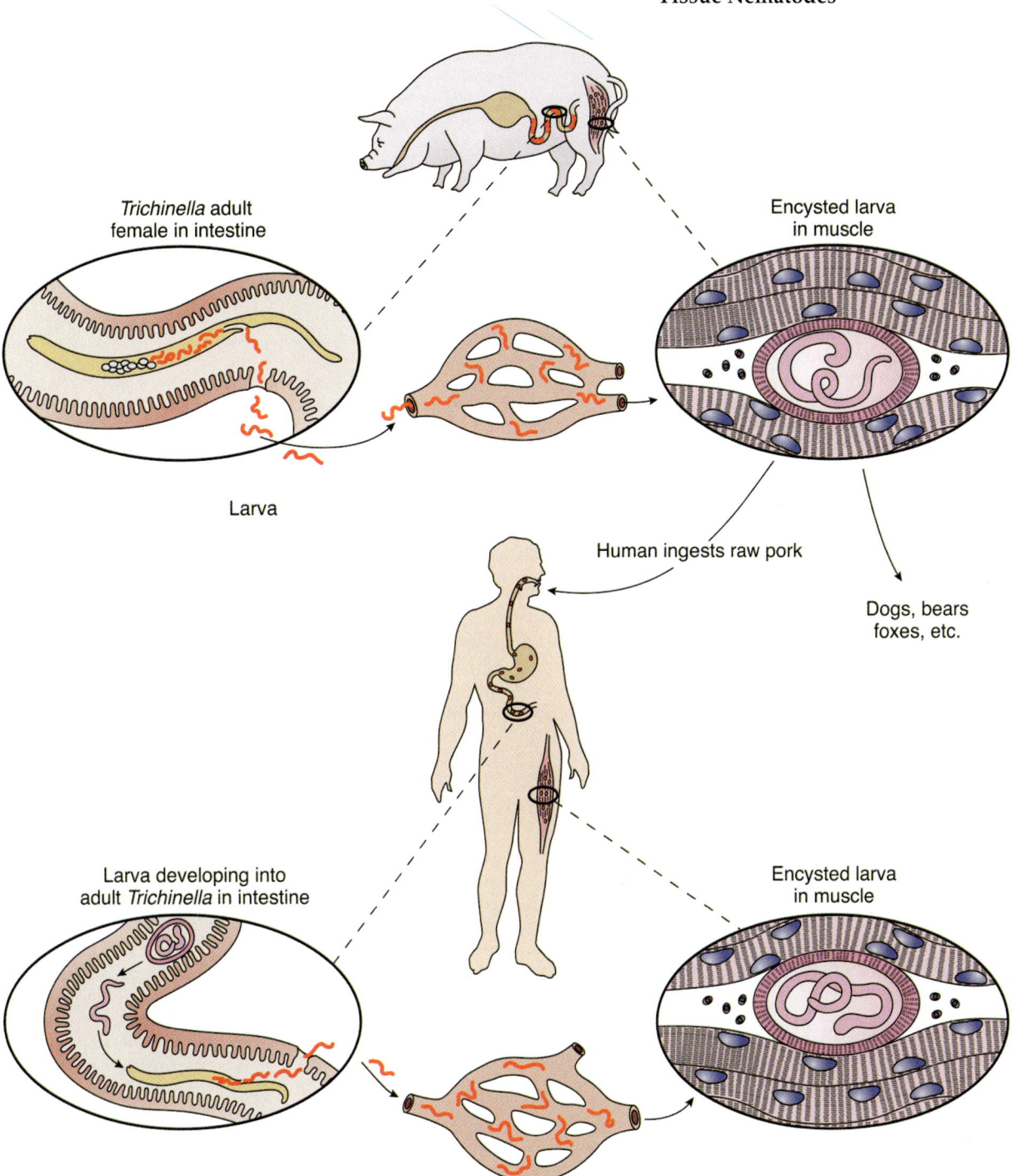

FIGURE 9-88
Trichinosis. After being ingested by the pig, cysts of *Trichinella* are digested in the gastrointestinal tract, liberating larvae that mature to adult worms. Female worms release larvae that penetrate the intestinal wall, enter the circulation, and lodge in striated muscle, where they encyst. When humans ingest inadequately cooked pork, the cycle is repeated, resulting in the muscle disease characteristic of trichinosis.

invasion by the worms. The major clinical manifestations develop several days later with the onset of skeletal muscle invasion. Patients suffer severe pain and tenderness of affected skeletal muscles, together with fever and weakness. Eosinophilia may be extreme (over 50% of all leukocytes). Involvement of the extraocular muscles produces periorbital edema. Infection of the brain or myocardium can be fatal. Severe cases of trichinosis are treated with corticosteroids to attenuate the inflammatory response. Antihelminthic drugs are required to remove adult worms from the intestine.

Visceral Larva Migrans (Toxocariasis) Is Transmitted by Cats and Dogs

Visceral larva migrans is an infection of deep organs by helminthic larvae migrating in aberrant hosts.

 Pathogenesis and Pathology: The infestation is a sporadic disease, primarily of young children, which characteristically occurs in areas where there are overcrowded dwellings, dogs, and cats. The most common causes of visceral larva migrans are *Toxocara* species, especially *T. canis* and *T. cati*. These roundworms live in the intestines of dogs and cats, and infection is transmitted to humans by the ingestion of embryonated ova. Ingested eggs hatch, and the larvae invade the intestinal wall. They are carried to the liver, from where a few emerge to reach the systemic circulation and may be carried to any part of the body. In tissues, larvae die and stimulate the formation of small granulomas, which eventually heal by scarring.

 Clinical Features: Many cases of visceral larva migrans are asymptomatic, but any infection can potentially cause severe disease. The typical symptomatic patient is a child with hypereosinophilia, pneumonitis, and hypergammaglobulinemia. In these patients, ocular manifestations are common, and the chief complaint is often the loss of vision in one eye. In fact, eyes with toxocaral endophthalmitis have been enucleated on the supposition that the lesion was a retinoblastoma. The infection is generally self-limited, and symptoms disappear within a year. The disease is treated with diethylcarbamazine and thiabendazole.

Cutaneous Larva Migrans Is a Pruritic Eruption

Cutaneous larva migrans is caused by the migration of a variety of larval nematodes through the skin. The migrating worms provoke severe inflammation, which appears as serpiginous urticarial trails (Fig. 9-89). The names applied to cutaneous larva migrans are as varied as the organisms that cause it and include creeping eruptions, sand worm, plumber's itch, duck hunter's itch, and epidermis linearis migrans. The more common larval nematodes include *S. stercoralis, Ancylostoma braziliensis,* and *Necator americanus*. Dogs and cats infected with hookworms are the major source of the disease. Outbreaks of cutaneous larva migrans occur at subtropical and tropical beaches. Plumbers who crawl under houses and animal caretakers are frequently infected. Thiabendazole is the treatment of choice.

Dracunculiasis Features Long Adult Worms beneath the Skin

Dracunculiasis is an infection of the connective and subcutaneous tissues with the guinea worm, **Dracunculus medinensis.**

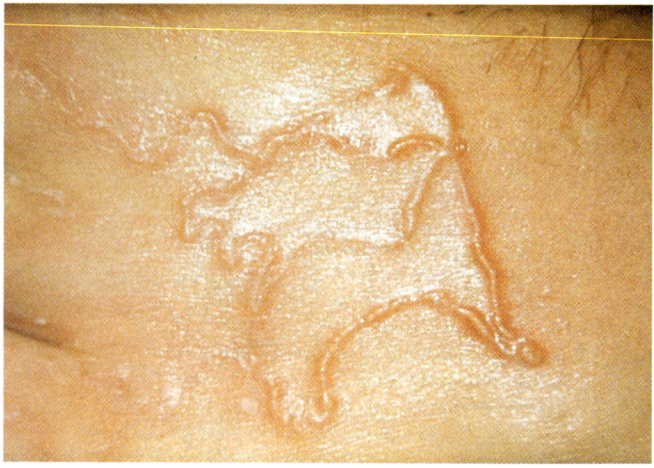

FIGURE 9-89
Cutaneous larva migrans. The skin shows a creeping eruption with the characteristic serpiginous, raised lesion.

 Epidemiology: Dracunculiasis is common in rural areas of sub-Saharan Africa, the Middle East, India, and Pakistan, where it is estimated that 10 million persons are infected. The disease is transmitted in drinking water contaminated with the intermediate host, a microscopic aquatic crustacean of the genus *Cyclops*.

 Pathogenesis and Pathology: The adult female nematode resides in subcutaneous tissues and releases numerous larvae through an ulcerated blister. When the infected part is immersed in water, the larvae are ingested by the *Cyclops* crustaceans, which are in turn ingested by humans.

About a year after ingestion of infected crustaceans, systemic allergic symptoms, including a pruritic urticarial rash, appear. A reddish papule, often around the ankles, develops and vesiculates. Beneath this sterile blister is the anterior end of the female worm. The blister bursts when it comes into contact with water, and the female worm, now measuring up to 120 cm in length and containing 3 million larvae, partially emerges (Fig. 9-90). The worm then spews myriad larvae into the water. Secondary infection of the blister, often with spreading cellulitis, is common. Dead worms provoke an intense inflammatory response, accounting for the debilitation seen in many patients with dracunculosis. The worm is often extracted by local practitioners by progressively twisting it onto a small stick. Treatment also includes anthelminthic drugs.

TREMATODES (FLUKES)

Schistosomiasis Produces Diseases of the Liver and Bladder

Schistosomiasis (bilharziasis) is the most important helminthic disease of humans, in which intense inflammatory and immunological responses damage the liver, intestine, or urinary bladder.

Trematodes (Flukes)

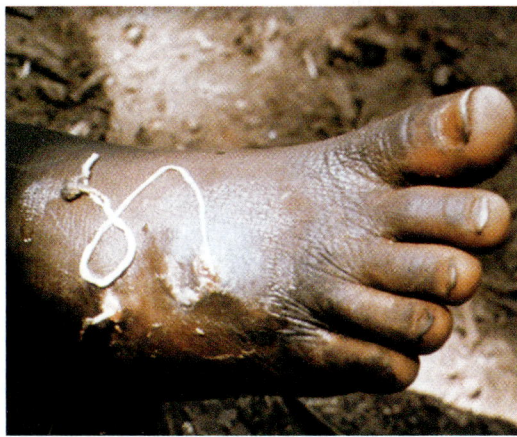

FIGURE 9-90
Dracunculiasis. A female guinea worm is seen emerging from the foot, which is swollen because of secondary bacterial infection.

Three species of schistosomes, namely, *Schistosoma mansoni, S. haematobium,* and *S. japonicum,* are responsible for the disease.

 Epidemiology: Schistosomiasis causes greater morbidity and mortality than all other worm infections. The disease affects about 10% of the world's population and ranks second only to malaria as a cause of disabling disease. The three schistosomal pathogens inhabit distinct geographical regions, dictated by the distribution of their specific host snail species (Fig. 9-91). *S. mansoni* is found in much of tropical Africa, parts of southwest Asia, South America, and the Caribbean islands. *S. haematobium* is endemic in large regions of tropical Africa and parts of the Middle East. *S. japonicum* occurs in parts of China, the Philippines, Southeast Asia, and India.

Pathogenesis: The schistosomes have complicated life cycles, alternating between asexual generations in the invertebrate host (snail) and sexual generations in the vertebrate host (Fig. 9-92). A schistosome egg hatches in fresh water, liberating a motile form (*miracidium*) that penetrates a snail, where it develops into the final larval stage, the cercaria. The cercaria escapes from the snail into the water and penetrates the skin of the human host, during which process it loses its forked tail and becomes a *schistosomulum.* The schistosomula migrate through tissues, penetrate blood vessels, and are carried to the lung and subsequently to the liver. In the intestinal venules of the portal drainage, the schistosomula mature, forming pairs of male and female worms. The female worms of *S. mansoni* and *S. japonicum* deposit eggs in the intestinal venules, whereas *S. haematobium* lays eggs in those of the urinary bladder. Embryos develop during the passage of eggs through the tissues, and the larvae are mature when the eggs pass through the wall of the intestine or the urinary bladder and are discharged in the feces or urine. The eggs hatch in fresh water, liberating miracidia and completing the life cycle.

 Pathology: **The basic lesion is a circumscribed granuloma or a cellular infiltrate of eosinophils and neutrophils around an egg.** Adult schisto-

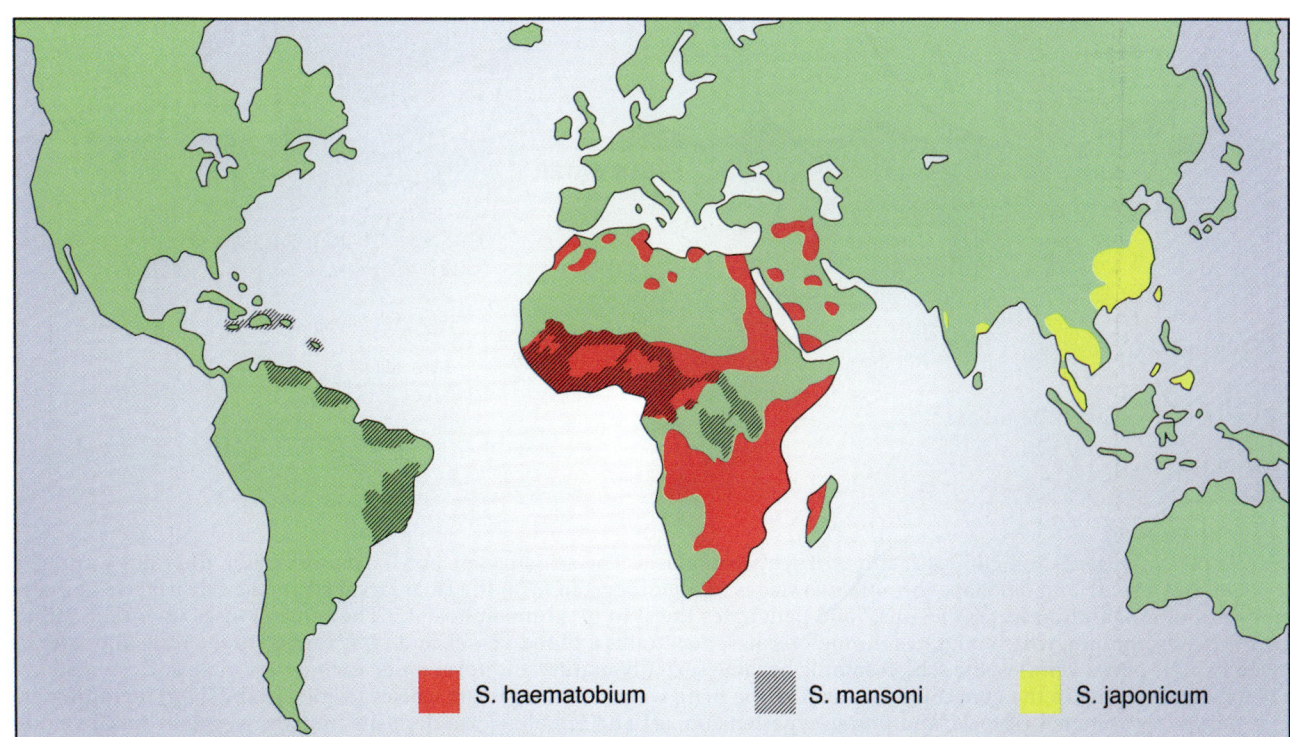

FIGURE 9-91
Distribution of schistosomiasis caused by *S. mansoni, S. haematobium,* and *S. japonicum.*

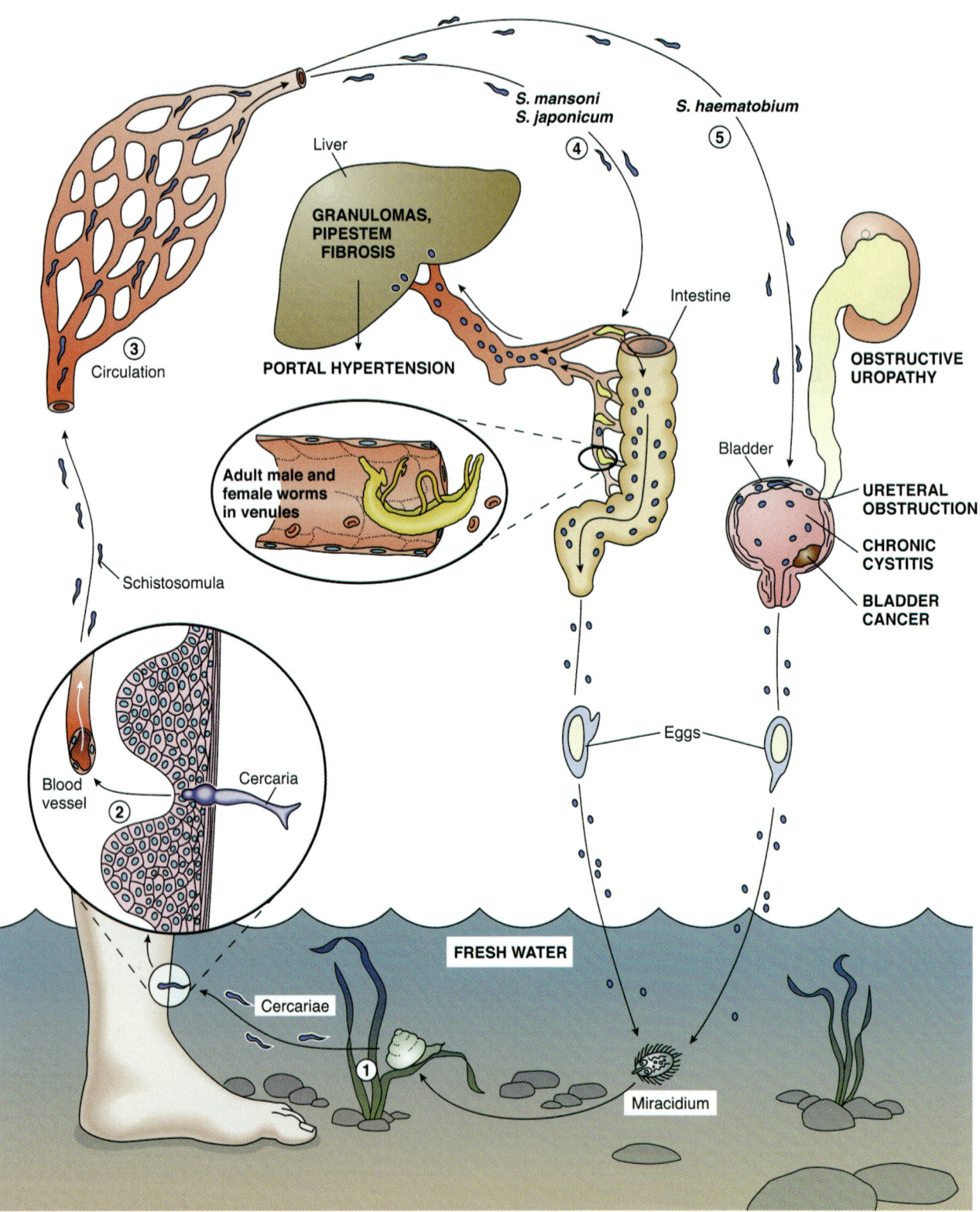

FIGURE 9-92

Life cycle of *Schistosoma* and clinical features of schistosomiasis. The schistosome egg hatches in water, liberates a miracidium that penetrates a snail, and develops through two stages to a sporocyst to form the final larval stage, the cercaria. *(1)* The cercaria escapes from the snail into water, "swims," and penetrates the skin of a human host. *(2)* The cercaria loses its forked tail to become a schistosomulum, which migrates through tissues, penetrates a blood vessel, and *(3)* is carried to the lung and later to the liver. In hepatic portal venules, the schistosomula become sexually mature and form pairs, each with a male and a female worm, the female worm lying in the gynecophoral canal of the male worm. The organism causes lesions in the liver, including granulomas, portal ("pipestem") fibrosis, and portal hypertension. *(4)* The female worm deposits immature eggs in small venules of the intestine and rectum (*S. mansoni* and *S. japonicum*) or *(5)* of the urinary bladder (*S. haematobium*). The bladder infestation leads to obstructive uropathy, ureteral obstruction, chronic cystitis, and bladder cancer. Embryos develop during passage of the eggs through tissues, and larvae are mature when eggs pass through the wall of the intestine or urinary bladder. Eggs hatch in water and liberate miracidia to complete the cycle.

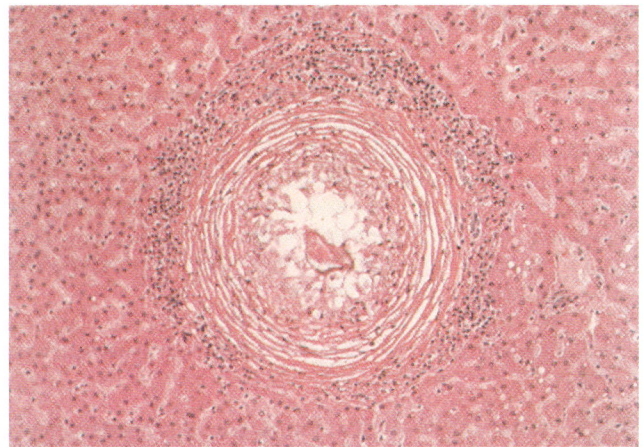

FIGURE 9-93
Hepatic schistosomiasis. A hepatic granuloma surrounds a degenerating egg of *S. mansoni*.

somes provoke no inflammation while alive in the veins. Granulomas that form about the eggs also obstruct the microvascular blood supply and produce ischemic damage to adjacent tissue. The result is progressive scarring and dysfunction in the affected organs.

The female worm deposits hundreds or thousands of eggs daily for 5 to 35 years. Most infected persons harbor fewer than 10 adult females. However, when the worm burden is large, the granulomatous response to the enormous number of eggs poses significant problems. The site of involvement is determined by the tropism of the particular schistosome species.

- *S. mansoni* inhabits the branches of the inferior mesenteric vein, thereby affecting the distal colon and liver.
- *S. haematobium* winds its way to the veins serving the rectum, bladder, and pelvic organs.
- *S. japonicum* deposits eggs predominantly in the branches of the superior mesenteric vein, thereby damaging the small bowel, ascending colon, and liver.

Liver disease caused by *S. mansoni* or *S. japonicum* begins as periportal granulomatous inflammation (Fig. 9-93) and progresses to dense periportal fibrosis *(pipestem fibrosis)* (Fig. 9-94).

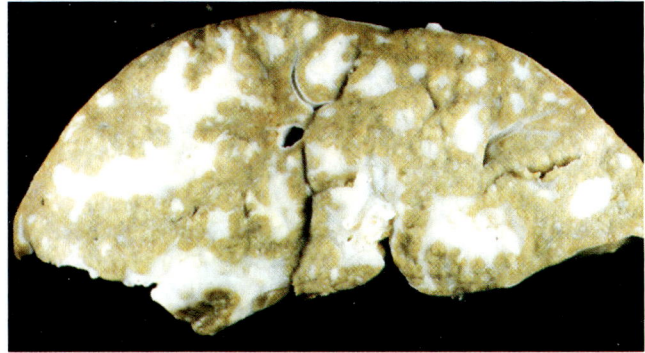

FIGURE 9-94
Hepatic schistosomiasis. Chronic infection of the liver with *S. japonicum* has led to the characteristic "pipestem" fibrosis.

In severe cases of hepatic schistosomiasis, this effect results in obstruction of portal blood flow and portal hypertension. *S. mansoni* and *S. japonicum* also damage the intestine, where the granulomatous response produces inflammatory polyps and foci of mucosal and submucosal fibrosis.

Urogenital schistosomiasis, caused by *S. haematobium*, features eggs that are most numerous in the bladder, ureter, and seminal vesicles, although they may also reach lungs, colon, and appendix. Eggs in the urinary bladder and ureters lead to a granulomatous reaction, inflammatory protuberances, and patches of mucosal and mural fibrosis. These can obstruct urine flow, producing secondary inflammatory damage to the bladder, ureters, and kidneys. **The bladder disease produced by *S. haematobium* is related to the development of squamous cell carcinoma of the bladder.**

The granulomas of schistosomiasis surround schistosome eggs. Eosinophils often predominate in early granulomas. In older granulomas, epithelioid macrophages and giant cells are conspicuous, and the oldest granulomas are densely fibrotic. The eggs of the various schistosomal species are identified on the basis of their size and shape.

 Clinical Features: Skin penetration by the schistosome larvae is sometimes associated with a self-limited, intensely pruritic rash. Most cases are dominated by the manifestations of chronic granulomatous tissue damage. Hepatic involvement leads to portal hypertension, with splenomegaly, ascites, and bleeding esophageal varices. Although intestinal disease is usually only minimally symptomatic, some patients experience abdominal pain and blood in the stools. Schistosomiasis of the bladder causes hematuria, recurrent urinary tract infections, and sometimes progressive obstruction leading to renal failure. The diagnosis is made by identifying schistosome eggs in the urine or feces. Although schistosomes are effectively killed by systemic antihelminthic agents, the structural changes resulting from extensive fibrosis and scarring are irreversible.

Clonorchiasis Leads To Biliary Obstruction

Clonorchiasis is an infection of the hepatic biliary system by the Chinese liver fluke, Clonorchis sinensis. *Although the presence of the fluke usually causes only mild symptoms, it is sometimes associated with bile duct stones, cholangitis, and bile duct cancer.*

 Epidemiology: Clonorchiasis is endemic in east Asia, from Vietnam to Korea, where uncooked freshwater fish is common fare. In parts of Vietnam, China, and Japan, over 50% of the adult population is infected. Human infection is acquired by the ingestion of inadequately cooked freshwater fish containing *C. sinensis* larvae.

Adult worms are flat and transparent, live in human bile ducts, and pass eggs to the intestine and feces. After ingestion by a specific snail, the egg hatches into a miracidium.

Cercariae escape from the snail and seek out certain fish, which they penetrate and in which they encyst. When humans eat the fish, the cercariae emerge in the duodenum, enter the common bile duct through the ampulla of Vater, and mature in the distal bile ducts to an adult fluke.

 Pathogenesis and Pathology: The presence of *Clonorchis* in the bile ducts elicits an inflammatory response, which fails to eliminate the worm but which causes dilation and fibrosis of the ducts. Sometimes the worms cause calculus formation within the hepatic bile ducts, leading to ductal obstruction. The adult *Clonorchis* persists in the ducts for decades, and long-standing infection is associated with an increased incidence of carcinoma of the bile duct epithelium (cholangiocarcinoma).

In heavy *Clonorchis* infections, the liver may be up to three times the normal size. Dilated bile ducts are seen through the capsule, and the cut surface is punctuated with thick-walled dilated bile ducts (Fig. 9-95). The flukes (up to 2.5 cm in length), sometimes in the thousands, can be expressed from the bile ducts. Microscopically, the epithelial lining of the ducts is initially hyperplastic and then becomes metaplastic. The surrounding stroma is fibrotic. Secondary bacterial infection is common and may be associated with suppurative cholangitis. Eggs deposited in the hepatic parenchyma are surrounded by a fibrous and granulomatous reaction. Masses of eggs may become lodged in the bile ducts and cause cholangitis. The pancreatic ducts may also be invaded and become dilated, thickened, lined by metaplastic epithelium, and eventually surrounded by scar tissue.

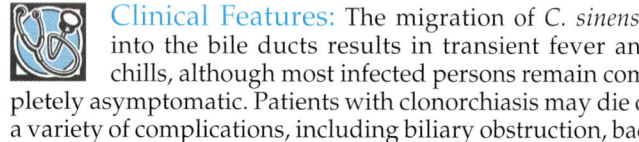 Clinical Features: The migration of *C. sinensis* into the bile ducts results in transient fever and chills, although most infected persons remain completely asymptomatic. Patients with clonorchiasis may die of a variety of complications, including biliary obstruction, bacterial cholangitis, pancreatitis, and cholangiocarcinoma. The diagnosis of clonorchiasis is made by identifying the eggs of *C. sinensis* in stools or duodenal aspirates. The infestation is treated effectively with systemic antihelminthic agents.

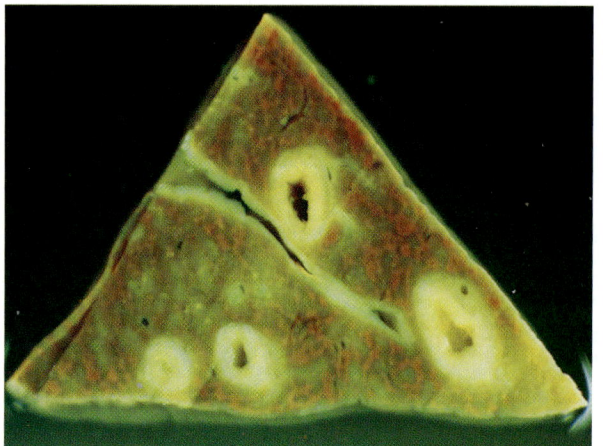

FIGURE 9-95
Clonorchiasis of the liver. The bile ducts are greatly thickened and dilated because of the presence of adult flukes *(C. sinensis).*

Paragonimiasis Is a Lung Disease

Paragonimiasis refers to a pulmonary infection by several species of the genus *Paragonimus,* the oriental lung fluke. The most common human pathogen is *P. westermani.* The infestation is common in Asian countries (Korea, the Philippines, Taiwan, and China), where uncooked, lightly salted, or wine-soaked fresh crabs are considered delicacies. The use of raw crab juices as medicinal beverages or seasonings also has been associated with the infection.

 Clinical Features: Pulmonary paragonimiasis is frequently misdiagnosed as tuberculosis. The disease manifests as fever, malaise, night sweats, chest pain, and cough. However, unlike tuberculosis, peripheral eosinophilia is common. The sputum is sometimes blood tinged, and chest radiographs reveal transient diffuse pulmonary infiltrates. The prognosis in pulmonary paragonimiasis is good, but ectopic lesions of the brain may be fatal. Eggs in the sputum or stools provide the definitive diagnosis.

Fascioliasis Is a Biliary Disease Acquired from Sheep

Fascioliasis is an infection of the liver by the sheep liver fluke, Fasciola hepatica. Humans may acquire the infection wherever sheep are raised. They become infected by eating vegetation, such as watercress, that is contaminated with the cysts passed by sheep.

 Pathogenesis: After reaching the duodenum, cysts liberate metacercariae that pass into the peritoneal cavity, penetrate the liver, and migrate through the hepatic parenchyma into the bile ducts. The larvae mature to adults and live in both the intrahepatic and extrahepatic bile ducts. Later, the adult flukes penetrate the wall of the bile ducts and wander back into the liver parenchyma, where they feed on liver cells and deposit their eggs.

 Pathology and Clinical Features: The eggs of *F. hepatica* lead to hepatic abscesses and granulomas. The worms induce hyperplasia of the lining epithelium of the bile ducts, portal and periductal fibrosis, proliferation of bile ductules, and varying degrees of biliary obstruction. Eosinophilia, vomiting, and acute gastric pain are characteristic features. Severe untreated infections may be fatal. The diagnosis is made by recovering eggs from the stools or biliary tract.

Fasciolopsiasis Is an Infestation of the Small Intestine

Fasciolopsiasis is caused by the giant intestinal fluke, Fasciolopsis buski. The disease prevails throughout most of the Orient. Humans acquire the infection by eating aquatic vegetables contaminated with the encysted cercariae. The worm is large (3 × 7 cm) and attaches to the duodenal or jejunal wall. The point of attachment may ulcerate and become infected, causing pain similar to that of a peptic ulcer. Acute symptoms may also be caused by intestinal obstruction or by toxins released by large numbers of worms. The diagnosis is made by identifying the eggs of *F. buski* in the stool. Treatment is with systemic antihelminthic agents.

CESTODES INTESTINAL TAPEWORMS

Taenia saginata, Taenia solium, and *Diphyllobothrium latum* are tapeworms that infect humans, growing to their adult forms within the intestine (Table 9-11). The presence of these adult worms rarely damages the human host.

Epidemiology: The intestinal tapeworm infections are acquired by eating inadequately cooked beef *(T. saginata)*, pork *(T. solium)*, or fish *(D. latum)* that contain the larval forms of the organisms. The life cycles of these tapeworms involve cystic larval stages in animals and worm stages in the human. The life cycles of the beef and pork tapeworms require that the animals ingest material tainted with infected human feces. The cystic larval forms of the worms develop in the muscles of the animals. Modern cattle and pig farming practices, together with meat inspection, have largely eliminated beef and pork tapeworms in industrialized countries, but infection remains common throughout the underdeveloped world. Fish tapeworm infection is prevalent in regions where raw, pickled, or partly cooked freshwater fish are common fare. Tapeworm infections are usually asymptomatic. Often the most significant concern is the distress produced when the infected person passes portions of the worm in the stool. The fish tapeworm *(D. latum)* competes for vitamin B_{12}, and a small number (<2%) of infected persons develop a deficiency of this nutrient.

TABLE 9-11 Tapeworm Infections

Species	Human Disease	Source of Human Infection
Taenia saginata	Adult tapeworm in intestine	Beef
Taenia solium	Adult tapeworm in intestine; cysticercosis	Pork; human feces
Diphyllobothrium latum	Adult tapeworm in intestine	Fish
Echinococcus granulosus	Hydatid cyst disease	Dog feces

Cysticercosis Is a Systemic Infection by the Larvae of the Pork Tapeworm

The adult *T. solium* is acquired by eating undercooked pork infected with cysticerci (measly pork).

Pathogenesis: Pigs acquire cysticerci by ingesting eggs of *T. solium* shed in human feces. This cycle, although a public health concern, is essentially benign for both humans and pigs. **However, when humans accidentally ingest the eggs from human feces and become infected with cysticerci, the consequences may be catastrophic.** The eggs release oncospheres, which penetrate the wall of the gut, enter the bloodstream, lodge in tissue, encyst, and differentiate to cysticerci.

Pathology: The cysticercus is a spherical, milky white cyst about 1 cm in diameter that contains fluid and an invaginated scolex (head of the worm) with birefringent hooklets. Viable cysts can be shelled out from the infected tissue. The cysticerci remain viable for an indefinite period and provoke no inflammation; rather, as they grow they compress adjacent tissues. Degenerating cysts, the ones usually responsible for symptoms, are attached to the tissue and are densely inflamed with eosinophils, neutrophils, lymphocytes, and plasma cells. Multiple cysticerci in the brain sometimes impart a "Swiss cheese" appearance to the tissue (Fig. 9-96).

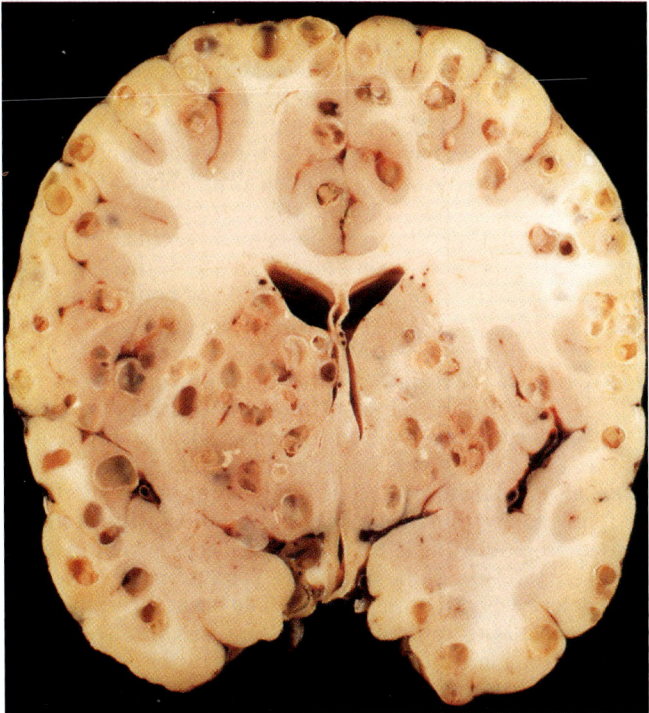

FIGURE 9-96
Cysticercosis. A cross-section of the brain from a patient infected with the larvae of *T. solium* shows many cysticerci in the gray matter, imparting a "Swiss cheese" appearance.

Clinical Features: Cysticercosis of the brain manifests as headaches or seizures, and symptoms vary according to the sites affected. Massive cysticercosis of the brain causes convulsions and death. Cysticerci in the retina blind the patient. In the heart, cysticerci may cause arrhythmias and sudden death. Depending on the site of involvement, cysticercosis is treated with surgery or antihelminthic therapy.

Echinococcosis Features Cysts of the Liver and Lungs

Echinococcosis (hydatid disease) is a zoonotic infection caused by larval cestodes of the genus *Echinococcus*. The most common offender is *E. granulosus*, which causes cystic hydatid disease. Rarely, *E. multilocularis* and *E. vogeli* infect humans.

 Epidemiology: Infestation with the tapeworm *E. granulosus* is endemic in sheep, goats, and cattle and their attendant dogs. Dogs contaminate their habitats (and their human keepers) with infectious eggs. Humans become infected when they inadvertently ingest the tapeworm eggs. The resulting hydatid disease is present worldwide among herding populations who live in close proximity to dogs and herd animals, especially in Australia, New Zealand, Argentina, Greece, and herding countries of Africa and the Middle East. In the United States, hydatid cyst disease is seen among immigrants and among the indigenous sheep-herding populations of the southwest.

E. multilocularis causes the alveolar hydatid disease in humans. Dogs and cats are domestic definitive hosts, and the domestic intermediate host is the house mouse. Rare infections by *E. multilocularis* have been reported in Germany, Switzerland, China, and the republics of the former Soviet Union.

Dogs are definitive hosts for *E. vogeli*. Humans may become accidental intermediate hosts for *E. vogeli* by ingesting eggs shed by domestic dogs. Polycystic hydatid disease caused by *E. vogeli* has been reported in Central and South America.

 Pathogenesis: The adult tapeworms (2–6 mm long) live in the small intestine of a carnivorous host, such as the wolf, fox, coyote, jackal, or dog (Fig. 9-97). *E. granulosus* has a scolex with suckers and numerous hooklets for attachment to the intestinal mucosa. A short neck is followed by three segments (proglottids). The terminal gravid proglottid breaks off and releases eggs, which are eliminated in the feces of the carnivore. Contaminated herbage is then eaten by herbivorous intermediate hosts, including deer, moose, antelopes, cattle, and sheep. Humans are also infected by ingesting plant material contaminated by the cestode eggs. Larvae released from the eggs penetrate the wall of the gut, enter the bloodstream, and disseminate to deep organs, where they grow to form large cysts containing brood capsules and scolices. When the flesh of the herbivore is eaten by a carnivore, the scolices develop into sexually mature worms in the latter, thereby completing the cycle.

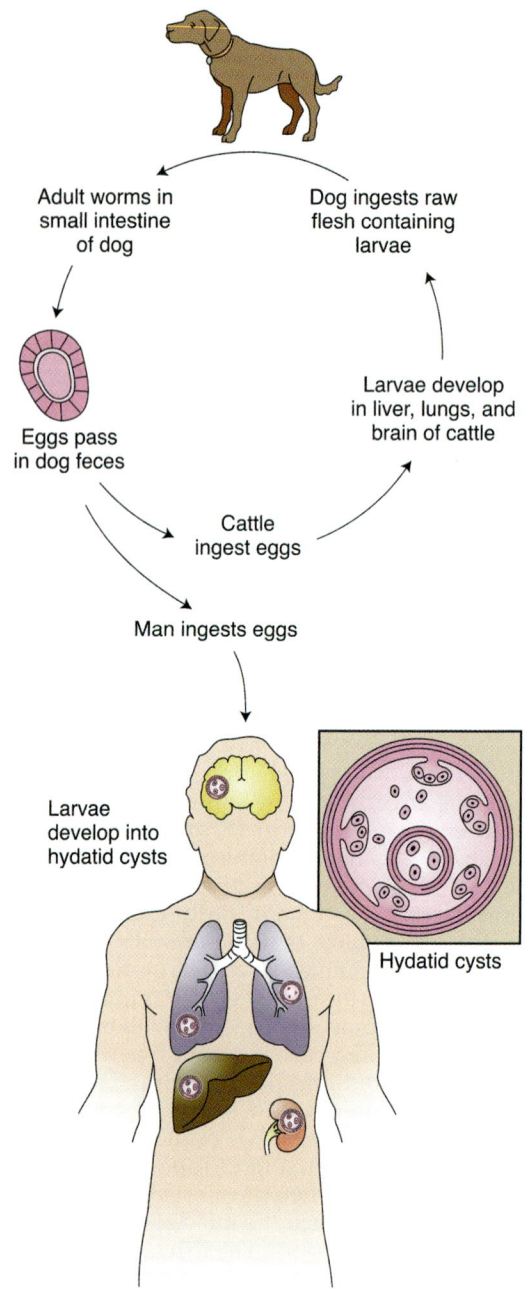

FIGURE 9-97

Life cycle of *Echinococcus granulosus* and cystic hydatid disease. The adult cestode lives in the small intestine of a dog (the definitive host). A gravid proglottid ruptures, releasing cestode eggs into the dog's feces. Cestode eggs are ingested by cattle or sheep (the intermediate hosts), hatch in the intestine, and release oncospheres that penetrate the wall of the gut, enter the bloodstream, disseminate to various deep organs, and grow to form hydatid cysts, containing brood capsules and scolices. When another dog ingests raw flesh from the cattle or sheep, the scolices are ingested and develop into mature worms in the dog's intestine to complete the cycle. A person who ingests cestode eggs in contaminated plant material becomes an accidental intermediate host. The larvae increase in size, but the parasite reaches a "dead end" without developing into an adult tapeworm. Hydatid cysts in humans occur predominantly in the liver but may also involve lung, kidney, brain, and other organs.

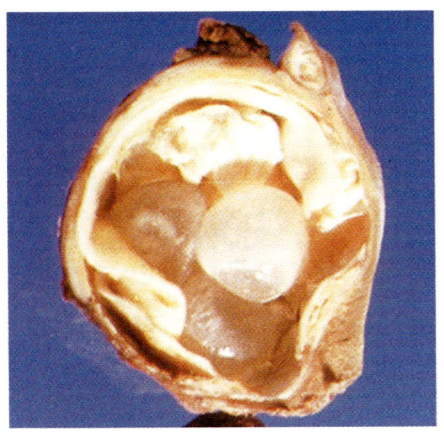 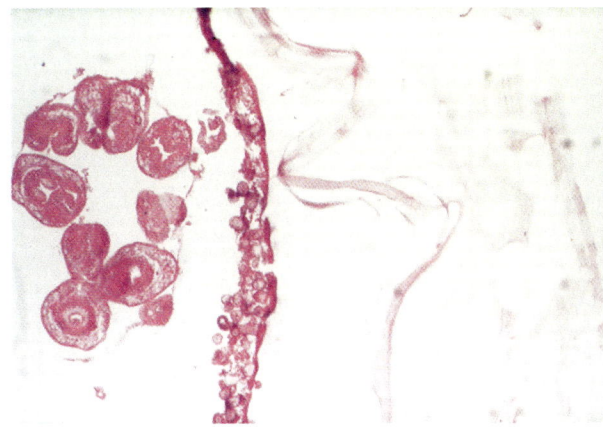

FIGURE 9-98
Echinococcal cyst. **A.** An echinococcal cyst showing daughter cysts was resected from the liver of a patient infected with *E. granulosus*. **B.** A photomicrograph of the cyst wall shows *(from right to left)* a laminated, non nuclear layer, a nucleated germinal layer with brood capsules attached, and numerous scolices in the cyst cavity.

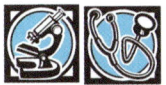 **Pathology and Clinical Features:** The slowly growing hydatid cyst is found by chance or becomes obvious when its size and position interferes with normal bodily functions. A hepatic cyst often manifests as a palpable mass in the right upper quadrant. Compression of intrahepatic bile ducts by the cyst may lead to obstructive jaundice. Pulmonary cysts (Fig. 9-98) are often asymptomatic and discovered incidentally on a chest radiograph.

A major complication of cyst rupture is the seeding of adjacent tissues with brood capsules and scolices. When these "seeds" germinate, they produce many additional cysts, each with the growth potential of the original cyst. Traumatic rupture of a hydatid cyst of the liver or other abdominal organ results in severe diffuse pain, resembling that of peritonitis. The rupture of a cyst in the lung may cause pneumothorax and empyema. Moreover, when a hydatid cyst ruptures into a body cavity, the release of cyst contents can cause fatal allergic reactions. Treatment of echinococcal cysts frequently requires careful surgical removal. Cysts must be sterilized with formalin before drainage or extirpation to prevent intraoperative anaphylactic shock.

SUGGESTED READING

Books

Baron S (ed): *Medical microbiology*, 4th ed. New York: Churchill Livingstone, 1996.

Connor DH, Chandler FW, Schwartz DA, et al. (eds): *Pathology of infectious diseases*, vol I and II. Stamford, CT: Appleton & Lange, 1997.

Cook M: *Manson's tropical disease*, 20th ed. Philadelphia: WB Saunders, 1995.

Gorbach SL, Bartlett JG, Blacklow NR (eds): *Infectious diseases in medicine and surgery*, 2nd ed. Philadelphia: WB Saunders, 1997.

Gutierrez Y: *Diagnostic pathology of parasitic infections with clinical correlations*. Philadelphia: Lea & Febiger, 1990.

Holmes KK, Mardh P, Sparling PF, et al. (eds): *Sexually transmitted diseases*, 3rd ed. New York: McGraw-Hill, 1997.

Mandell GL, Bennett JE, Dolin E (eds): *Principles and practice of infectious diseases*, 3rd ed. New York: Churchill Livingstone, 1995.

Murray PR (ed): *Manual of clinical microbiology*, 6th ed. Washington, DC: ASM Press, 1995.

Remington JS, Klein JO (eds): *Infectious diseases of the fetus and newborn infant*, 4th ed. Philadelphia: WB Saunders, 1994.

Rippon JW: *Medical mycology: the pathogenic fungi and the pathogenic actinomycetes*, 3rd ed. Philadelphia: WB Saunders, 1988.

Rom WN, Garay SM (eds): *Tuberculosis*. Boston: Little Brown, 1996.

Reviews

Genta RM: Diarrhea in helminthic infections. *Clin Infect Dis* 19:S122–S129, 1993.

Meslin FX: Surveillance and control of emerging zoonoses. *World Health Stat Q* 45:200–207, 1992.

Steere AC: Lyme disease. *N Engl J Med* 321:586–596, 1989.

Walker DH, Barbour AG, Olivier JH, et al.: Emerging bacterial zoonotic and vector-borne diseases. Ecological and epidemiological factors. *JAMA* 275:463–469, 1996.

Walker DH, Yamolska O, Grinberg LM: Death at Sverdlovsk: What have we learned? *Am J Pathol* 144:1135–1141, 1994.

CHAPTER 10

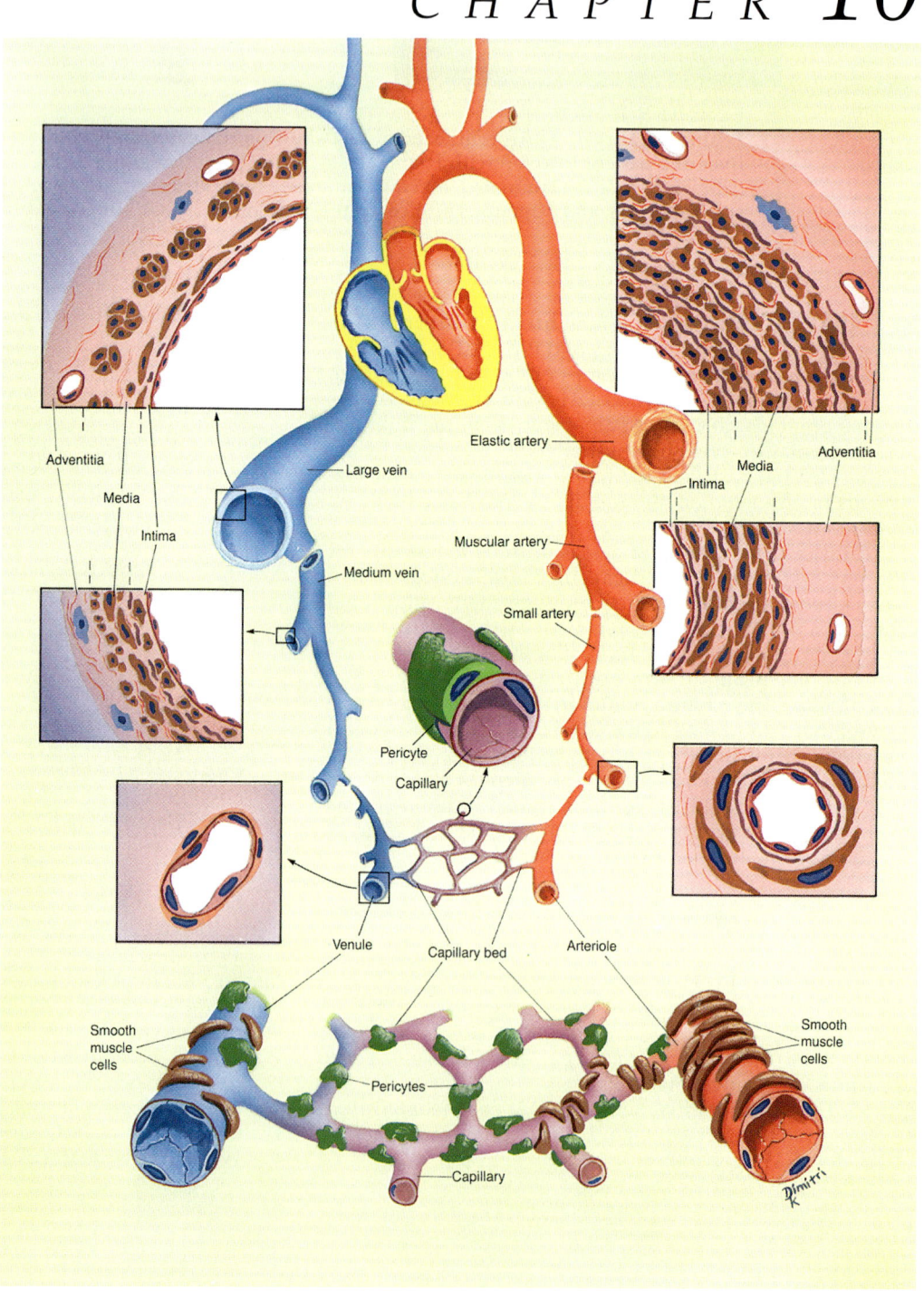

Blood Vessels

Avrum I. Gotlieb

Embryonic Development and Structure of Blood Vessels

The Vessel Wall

Arteries

Capillaries

Veins

Lymphatics

Hemostasis and Thrombosis

Blood Coagulation

Platelet Adhesion and Aggregation

Endothelial Factors

Clot Lysis

Atherosclerosis

Restenosis

Risk Factors

Lipid Metabolism

Hypertensive Vascular Disease

Mönckeberg Medial Sclerosis

Raynaud Phenomenon

Fibromuscular Dysplasia

Vasculitis

Polyarteritis Nodosa

Hypersensitivity Angiitis

Allergic Granulomatosis and Angiitis (Churg-Strauss Syndrome)

Giant Cell Arteritis (Temporal Arteritis, Granulomatous Arteritis)

Wegener Granulomatosis

Takayasu Arteritis

Kawasaki Disease (Mucocutaneous Lymph Node Syndrome)

Thromboangiitis Obliterans (Buerger Disease)

Behçet Disease

Radiation Vasculitis

Rickettsial Vasculitis

Aneurysms

Abdominal Aortic Aneurysms

Aneurysms of Cerebral Arteries

Dissecting Aneurysm

Syphilitic Aneurysms

Mycotic (Infectious) Aneurysms

(continued)

FIGURE 10-1 *(see opposite page)*
Subdivisions and histological structure of the vascular system. Each subdivision is subject to a set of pathological changes conditioned by the structure–function relationship of that part of the system. For example, the aorta, an elastic artery subject to great pressure, frequently shows a pathological dilation (aneurysm) if the supporting elastic media is damaged. Muscular arteries are the most significant sites of atherosclerosis. Small arteries, particularly arterioles, are sites of hypertensive changes. Capillary beds, venules, and veins each display their own types of pathological changes.

Veins

Varicose Veins

Deep Venous Thrombosis

Lymphatic Vessels

Lymphangitis

Lymphatic Obstruction

Benign Tumors of Blood Vessels

Hemangiomas

Glomus Tumor (Glomangioma)

Hemangioendothelioma

Malignant Tumors of Blood Vessels

Angiosarcoma

Hemangiopericytoma

Kaposi Sarcoma

Tumors of the Lymphatic System

Capillary Lymphangioma

Cystic Lymphangioma (Cystic Hygroma, Cavernous Lymphangioma)

Lymphangiosarcoma

EMBRYONIC DEVELOPMENT AND STRUCTURE OF BLOOD VESSELS

Vascular smooth muscle cells are derived from the local mesoderm after the endothelial tubes are formed. The smooth muscle cells that populate the major arteries in the upper part of the body represent "mesectoderm," derived from neural crest cells (Fig. 10-2). Thus, although smooth muscle cells of the media appear uniform, they exhibit significant heterogeneity. This has important implications for the development of pathological lesions in the vascular system. The contractile properties of smooth muscle cells also vary according to the location of the blood vessel, some being more reactive to various stimuli than others.

The Vessel Wall Comprises Endothelial Cells and Smooth Muscle Cells

Most vascular diseases result from the dysfunction of endothelial and smooth cells.

Endothelial Cells

The endothelium is (1) a macromolecular barrier, (2) a thromboresistant surface, (3) a modulator of vascular smooth muscle cell function, and (4) a highly metabolic cell intimately involved in several biological functions, including coagulation, inflammation, and repair.

A single row of endothelium lines the tunica intima, the innermost layer of the vessel wall (Fig. 10-3). The integrity of the endothelial cells depends on several types of adhesion complexes. These junctions are essential for the maintenance of proper endothelial function and the permeation of solutes across this barrier. Moreover, the interaction of endothelial cells with circulating white blood cells is also governed, in part, by the expression of adhesive molecules (see Chapter 2). The receptors for adhesion molecules and their ligands fall into three functional categories:

- **Cell-substrate adhesion molecules** provide for the attachment of endothelial cells to their substrate (e.g., basal lamina) and also regulate signal transduction pathways. For example, integrins are receptors for the binding of endothelial cells to adhesive glycoproteins, including laminin, fibronectin, and thrombospondin. Integrins are transmembrane proteins that bind to the complex of proteins that regulate adhesion at focal contact sites and are associated with the cell cytoskeleton (Fig. 10-4).
- **Cell–cell adhesion molecules** attach one endothelial cell to another. For instance, cadherin is located at intercellular adhesion junctions, and occludin at intercellular tight junctions. The cadherins are linked to the actin cytoskeleton by catenins.
- **Leukocyte adhesion molecules** are located at the endothelial cell surface and are available after activation of endothelial cells. Different types of leukocytes adhere to endothelial cells through adhesion molecules. For example E-selectin and P-selectin are present on the endothelial surface and bind ligands on leukocytes. P-selectin binds to counterreceptors such as P-selectin glycoprotein ligand-1 (PSGL-1). Vascular cell adhesion molecule 1 (VCAM-1) and intercellular adhesion molecule 1 (ICAM-1) on the endothelial surface bind to very late antigen 4 (VLA-4) and leukocyte function antigen-1 (LFA-1) on leukocytes.

A layer of connective tissue is interposed between the endothelium and the underlying smooth muscle of the tunica media. At one time the endothelium was considered to be an uncomplicated structural barrier that simply modulated permeation through the vessel wall by providing pores of appropriate size. The endothelial cells do not normally proliferate, but in the face of vascular injury and loss of endothelium, they spread, migrate, and proliferate rapidly to reestablish the integrity of the endothelium (Fig. 10-5). We now recognize that endothelial cells actually accomplish a large variety of metabolic functions (Table 10-1) and that endothelial dysfunction is important in the pathogenesis of vascular disease. In some diseases, endothelial dysfunction is associated with the subendothelial accumulation of blood-borne materials. For example, the accretion of lipid beneath the endothelium in atherosclerotic lesions reflects the failure of the endothelium to serve as an effective barrier between tissue and plasma.

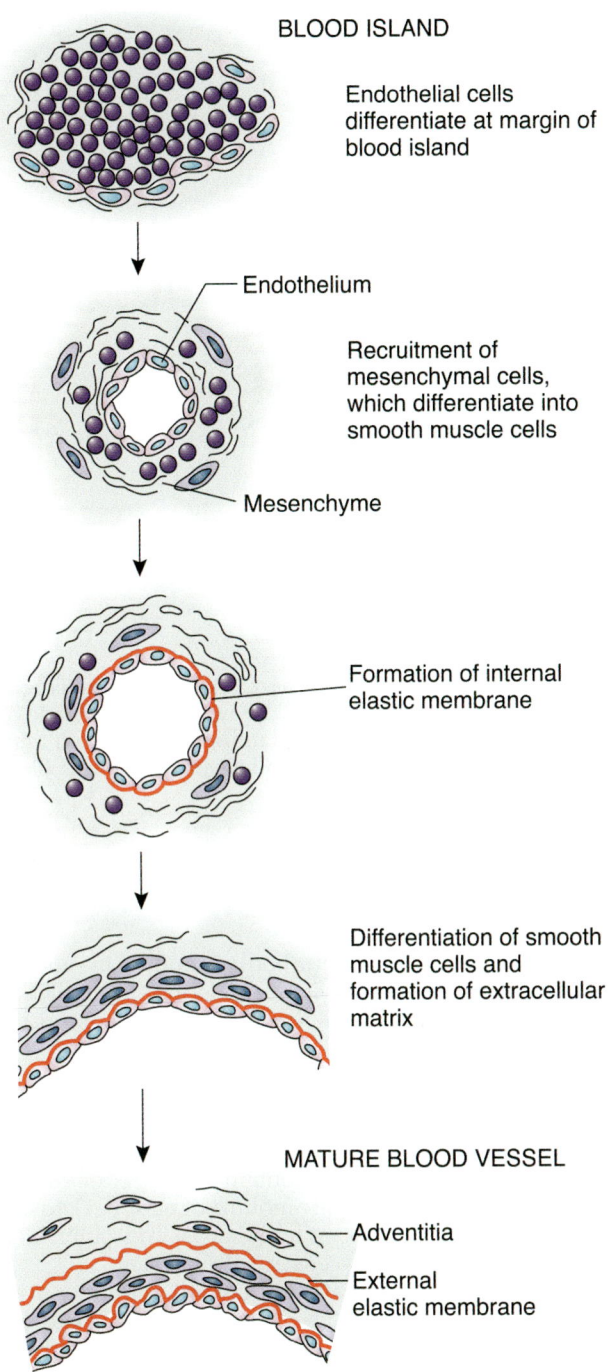

FIGURE 10-2
Differentiation of vessels in early embryos. The course of events from the development of blood islands on the chorioallantoic membrane starts with differentiation of endothelium and proceeds to fully developed arteries and veins.

synthase (NOS), which produces nitric oxide from arginine, is constitutively expressed, it can be regulated. NO inhibits the adhesion and aggregation of platelets by attenuating the rise in intracellular free calcium induced by a variety of agonists. NO modulates vascular tone as well as the proliferation of vascular smooth muscle cells by increasing cyclic guanosine monophosphate (cGMP) formation, with subsequent activation of cGMP-dependent protein kinase. NO likely plays a physiological role in the control of the vascular tone of large arteries and resistance vessels. Both prostacyclin and NO are released following stimulation of endothelial receptors by agonists, and they act together to inhibit platelet aggregation. Compounds that promote the release of NO include acetylcholine, bradykinin, and ADP. NO is more labile than even prostacyclin, with a half-life of 6 seconds.

Vascular tone is also affected by a number of bioactive peptides. The endothelins are a family of potent vasoconstrictive proteins synthesized by the endothelium. Their functional effects are mediated by two distinct receptor subtypes; both are found on smooth muscle cells, but only one on endothelial cells. Angiotensin II, which is also a potent vasoconstrictor, is derived from angiotensin I through the action of angiotensin-converting enzyme (ACE), which is located in the endothelium.

Endothelial cell-derived factors are also important in the control of the immune response. Like macrophages, endothelial cells express class II histocompatibility antigens when they are stimulated. In this way, they can participate with monocytes—or even replace them—in activating lymphocytes. Immune responses to endothelial cells are a major part of organ rejection following transplantation.

Smooth Muscle Cells

Smooth muscle cells maintain the integrity of the vessel and provide support for the endothelium. They control blood flow by contracting or dilating in response to specific stimuli. Smooth muscle cells synthesize the connective tissue matrix of the vessel wall, which includes elastin, collagen, and proteoglycans. Like endothelial cells, smooth muscle cells show very low levels of proliferation in the normal artery but proliferate in response to vessel injury.

Leukocytes that enter the vessel wall, especially macrophages and lymphocytes, also promote vascular disease. In acute vasculitis, polymorphonuclear leukocytes are also important. The cells surrounding the vessel wall, including fibroblasts in the connective tissue of the adventitia and pericytes of capillaries and venules, may also contribute to the pathogenesis of vascular diseases. Pericytes influence endothelial cell function, and the fibroblasts of the adventitia proliferate and migrate in reaction to medial disruption, as occurs in severe vasculitis and following angioplasty.

Arteries Include Conducting and Resistance Vessels

The simple two-cell structure of blood vessels is made more complex by the organization of the wall into layers called "tunicae" (see Fig. 10-1).

Endothelial cells synthesize a number of biologically active factors. Some factors are potent bioactive molecules that are released locally, act at short distances, and are rapidly inactivated. Endothelial cells release autocoids, thereby exerting effects on vascular tone and platelet activity. For example, prostacyclin relaxes smooth muscle and inhibits the aggregation of platelets. Although endothelial nitric oxide

476 Blood Vessels

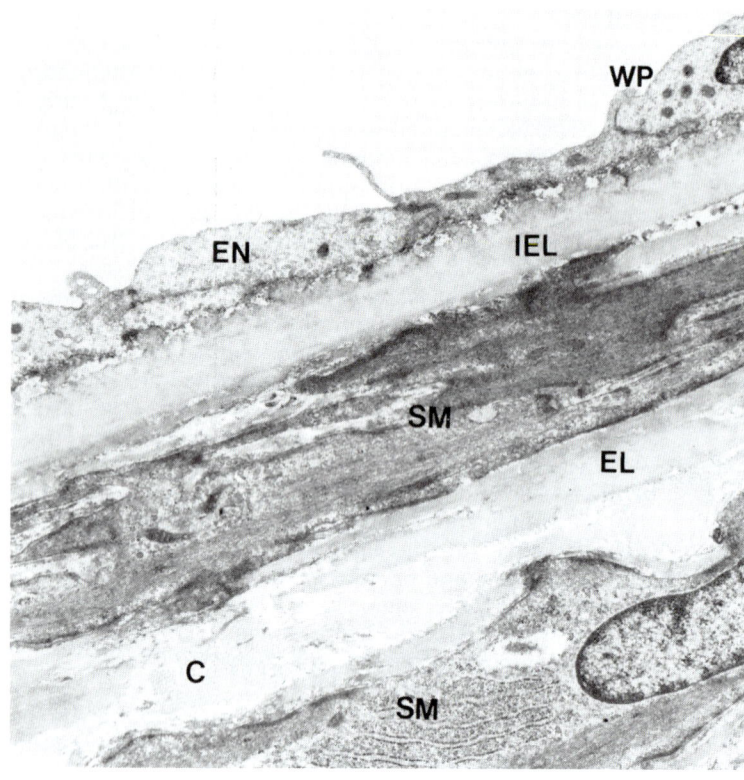

FIGURE 10-3
Luminal side of the rat aorta. An electron micrograph shows endothelial cells *(EN)* with Weibel-Palade bodies *(WP)*, internal elastic lamina *(IEL)*, smooth muscle cells *(SM)*, collagen *(C)*, and elastic lamellae *(EL)*.

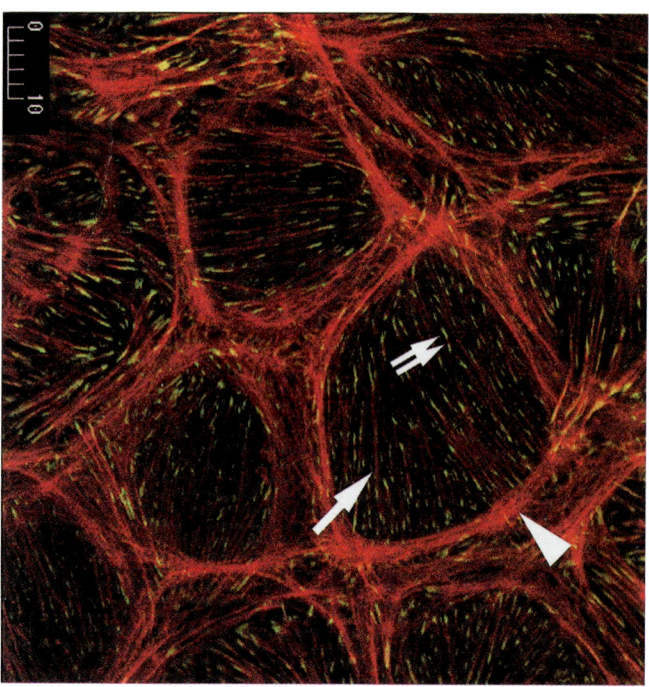

FIGURE 10-4
Focal adhesion protein, vinculin. Porcine aortic endothelial cells were grown to confluency and double-stained for actin/vinculin. Endothelial cells in confluent monolayers contain a *dense peripheral band* (DPB) of actin microfilament bundles *(arrow head)* and central microfilament or "stress fibers" *(single arrow)*. Vinculin in confluent monolayer localizes to the tips of stress fibers *(double arrow)*.

Elastic Arteries

The largest blood vessels in the body, including the aorta, are the elastic arteries. They function as conduits to smaller arterial branches for blood from the heart and are composed of three layers:

- **Tunica intima:** This layer consists of the endothelium, a few smooth muscle cells, and the connective tissue on the luminal side of the internal elastic lamina. The intima of the aorta is thick and contains a matrix of collagen, proteoglycans, and small amounts of elastin. Occasional resident lymphocytes, macrophages, and other blood-derived inflammatory cells are also present.
- **Tunica media:** The next layer outward, the tunica media, displays layers of smooth muscle cells. In the elastic arteries, elastic fibers are interposed between smooth muscle cells and minimize energy loss during the pressure changes between systole and diastole. A breakdown of the media, particularly of its elastic layers, leads to dilation of the artery, called an *aneurysm*. Much of the disease that occurs in arteries (e.g., atherosclerosis) involves proliferation of medial smooth muscle cells. Alternatively, during normal aging and in hypertension, smooth muscle cells replicate their DNA without cell division. As a result, they become tetraploid, octaploid, or of even higher ploidy.

Medial smooth muscle cells may also undergo atrophy or cell death because they do not receive adequate nutrients or cannot effectively exchange wastes with the circulating blood. In smaller vessels, particularly those with fewer than 30 layers of smooth muscle cells, nutrition for the media is provided only from the lumen

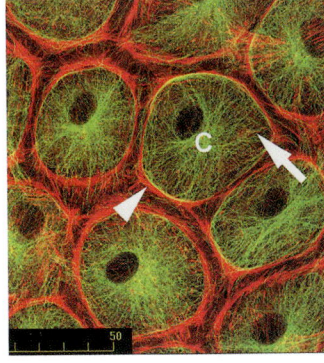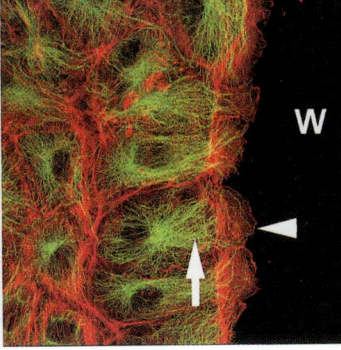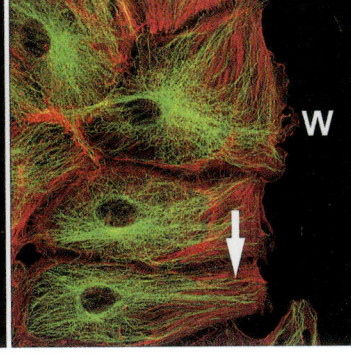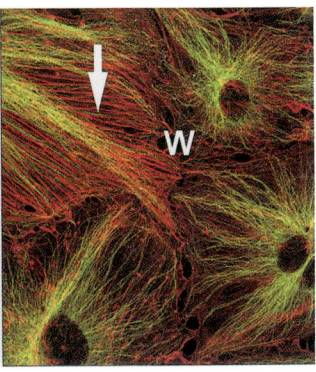

FIGURE 10-5
Remodeling in response to loss of endothelial integrity. Porcine aortic endothelial cells were grown to confluency, and a 1-mm wound was created using a scraper. Cells were fixed and double-stained for actin/tublin at 2, 6, and 24 hours after wounding. A. Endothelial cells in confluent monolayers contain a dense peripheral band (DPB) of actin microfilament bundles (*arrow head*) and centrosomes (*c*) toward the cell periphery. B. 2 hours after wounding, there is formation of lamellipodia (*arrow head*), and stress fibers (*arrow*) rearrange to become parallel to the wound edge (*w*). Centrosomes migrate around the nucleus toward the wound edge, and the microtubules begin emanating toward the wound (*w*). C. By 6 hours, changes in microtubules and microfilaments are more prominent, the microtubule/microfilaments are more prominent, and the microtubule–microfilament networks (*arrow*) begin to reorganize perpendicular to the wound edge (*w*) as the cells begin to spread. D. 24 hours after wounding, the microtubule–microfilament networks (*arrow*) are aligned perpendicular to the wound edge (*w*) as the cells migrate into the wound.

of the blood vessel, from which it permeates through the endothelium and the layers of smooth muscle. However, in larger blood vessels such as the aorta, this pathway is inadequate. Blood vessels that have more than 28 layers of smooth muscle cells display a vasculature of their own, namely the *vasa vasorum*.

TABLE 10-1 Functions of Endothelial Cells of the Blood Vessels

---

Permeability barrier
Vasoactive factors: Nitric oxide (EDRF), endothelin
Antithrombotic agent production: Prostacyclin (PGI$_2$), adenine metabolites
Prothrombotic agent production: Factor VIIIa (von Willebrand factor)
Anticoagulant production: Thrombomodulin, other proteins
Fibrinolytic agent production: Tissue plasminogen activator, urokinase-like factor
Procoagulant production: Tissue factor, plasminogen activator/inhibitor, factor V
Inflammatory mediator production: Interleukin-1, cell adhesion molecules
Receptors for factor IX, factor X, low-density lipoproteins, modified low-density lipoproteins, thrombin
Growth factor production: Blood cell colony-stimulating factors, insulin-like growth factors, fibroblast growth factor, platelet-derived growth factor
Growth inhibitor: Heparin
Replication

These small vessels penetrate the exterior of the artery and provide blood for the tunica media. The rich blood supply that develops in atherosclerotic plaques is derived from the vasa vasorum. The tunica media also contains autonomic nerve fibers that influence vascular contractility.

- **Tunica adventitia**: The most external layer of the vessel wall is composed of fibroblasts, connective tissue, small vessels that give rise to the vasa vasorum, and nerves. Occasional inflammatory cells may also be present in the adventitia.

Muscular Arteries

The blood conducted by the elastic arteries is distributed to individual organs through large muscular arteries (Fig. 10-6). The tunica media of a muscular artery consists of layers of smooth muscle cells without prominent bands of elastin, although a prominent internal elastic lamina and usually an external elastic lamina are seen. The continuity of the internal elastic lamina is interrupted by fenestrae, which permit the migration of smooth muscle cells from the media into the intima. The absence of the heavy elastin layers allows more-efficient contraction of the muscular arteries. The intima of the muscular arteries, like that of the aorta, also contains smooth muscle cells, connective tissue, and occasional inflammatory cells. Vasa vasorum penetrate the walls of the thicker muscular arteries but are not seen in the smaller ones. As the vascular tree branches further, the tunica media becomes thinner. Except for the endothelium, the tunica intima disappears.

478   Blood Vessels

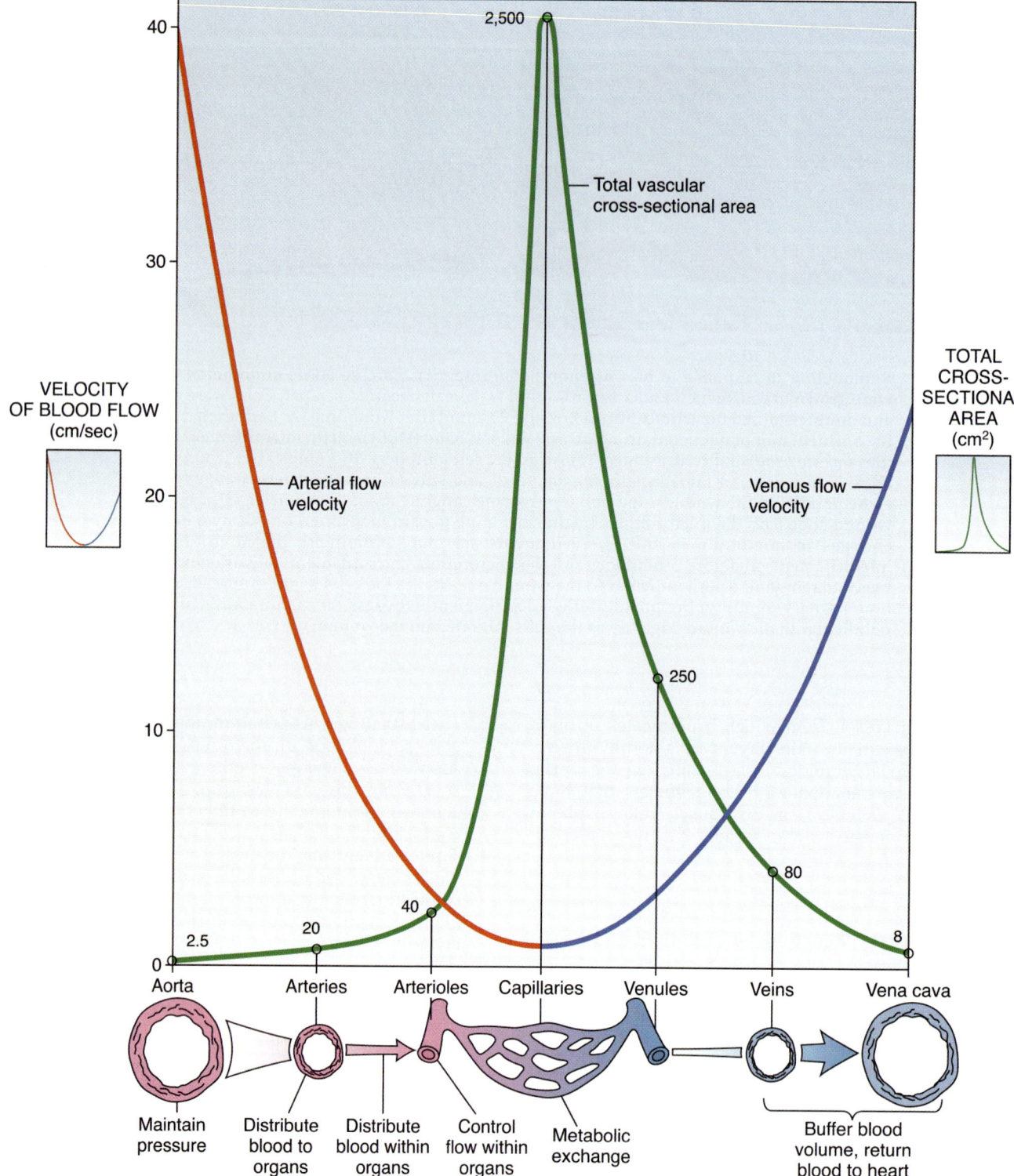

FIGURE 10-6
Relationship between velocity of blood flow and cross-sectional area in the vasculature. The vascular tree is a circuit that conducts blood from the heart through large-diameter, low-resistance conducting vessels to small arteries and arterioles, which lower blood pressure and protect the capillaries. The capillaries are thin-walled and allow the exchange of nutrients and waste products between tissue and blood, a process that requires a very large surface area. The circuit back to the heart is completed by the veins, which are distensible and provide a volume buffer that acts as a capacitance for the vascular circuit.

The small muscular arteries play an important role in the regulation of blood flow. The narrow lumen of these vessels produces increased resistance, thereby reducing blood pressure to levels appropriate for the exchange of water and plasma constituents across the thin-walled capillaries. The small muscular arteries, sometimes called *resistance vessels*, also maintain systemic pressure by regulating total peripheral resistance.

Arterioles

The arterioles are the smallest elements of the arterial vascular tree and consist of an endothelial lining surrounded by one or two layers of smooth muscle cells. No elastic layers are evident. The smallest arterioles provide dynamic regulation of blood flow by controlling the distribution of blood in the capillary tree.

Capillaries Permit Transport from the Blood to the Interstitium

In the smallest blood vessels, namely the capillaries, the endothelium is supported only by sparse smooth muscle cells. The capillary endothelium provides for the interchange of solutes and cells between the blood and the extracellular fluid. A necessary feature of this exchange is a marked lowering of pressure, which prevents the vascular fluid from shifting into the extracellular space.

The capillary endothelium acts as a semipermeable membrane, in which the exchange of plasma solutes with extracellular fluid is controlled by molecular size and charge. It also synthesizes factors that influence the surrounding cells, modifies molecules in transit across the endothelium, and synthesizes inflammatory mediators.

Pericytes are modified smooth muscle cells that surround the capillaries. They share a basement membrane with the endothelial cell, thereby bringing the two cells into close contact (see Fig. 10-1). The functions of pericytes are largely unknown. They may have a contractile function and may regulate the function of adjacent endothelial cells, especially their proliferation. The adventitia of the capillary merges with the surrounding connective tissue and cannot be distinguished from it.

The permeability of capillaries depends on the ultrastructure of their endothelial cells. Brain capillaries are highly impermeable because the endothelium has tightly sealed junctions between individual cells, which prevent the exchange of proteins across the vessel wall. Transport in other capillary beds is mediated either by the passage of molecules through incomplete cell junctions or by pinocytosis, a process by which molecules traverse the cytoplasm through vesicular transport. Some investigators hold that little transport occurs by way of micropinocytosis. Rather, they contend that vesicles are connected with each other, to provide a channel for direct transport of plasma proteins across the cytoplasm. In some locations, the capillary endothelium itself may be fenestrated. It may have permanent channels across the endothelium or it may exhibit discontinuous gaps between endothelial cells. Fenestrated capillaries in the renal glomerulus are specifically adapted to filter plasma. The liver sinusoids, which are not true capillaries, also show a fenestrated endothelium, which permits free access of the plasma to the liver cell.

Veins Return Blood to the Heart

The venules are the first vessels that collect blood from the capillaries. The thin media of the venule is appropriate for a vessel that is not required to withstand a high luminal pressure. Venules merge into small and medium-sized veins, which in turn converge into large veins. The walls of large veins do not display the characteristic elastic lamellae of elastic arteries, and even the internal elastic lamina is well developed only in the largest veins. The media is thin and is virtually absent in the smaller tributaries. Many veins, particularly those in the extremities, have valves formed by endothelial-lined folds of the tunica intima. These structures prevent backflow and assist in the transport of blood under the low-pressure conditions of the venous circulation. The postcapillary venules are the site of leukocyte transmigration into tissue in inflammatory reactions.

Lymphatics Drain Interstitial Fluid

The lymphatic vessels are composed essentially of endothelium. The filtrate from capillaries and venules enters the lymphatics, which act as a pathway to the regional lymph nodes for cells, foreign material, and microorganisms.

HEMOSTASIS AND THROMBOSIS

Hemostasis is defined as the arrest of hemorrhage and is a response to vascular injury. This process involves vasoconstriction, tissue swelling, coagulation, platelet aggregation, and thrombosis.

The hemostatic system is an exquisitely controlled mechanism that prevents blood loss following injury. The complex system comprises (1) a network of activating and inactivating enzymes and (2) cofactors derived from different cells and tissues, some circulating and some locally produced (Table 10-2). The disorders of hemostasis are discussed in detail in Chapter 20.

The hemostatic complex can be divided into several functional areas that combine coagulation of blood proteins and aggregation of platelets to form a hemostatic "plug." *Thrombosis refers to the formation of a blood clot in the circulation.* A thrombus is an aggregate of coagulated blood that contains platelets, fibrin, leukocytes, and red blood cells. The formation of a thrombus involves a "tug of war" between factors that promote thrombosis and those that inhibit it. Thrombosis occurs when antithrombotic systems fail to balance prothrombotic processes.

One must understand the difference between coagulation and thrombosis. Coagulation can occur in vitro as a result of the activation of the clotting cascade. By contrast, thrombosis is the formation of a blood clot in situ. Thrombosis also involves (1) the adherence and aggregation of platelets, (2) the participation of cellular elements of the monocyte/macrophage system, and (3) active participation of endothelial cells.

TABLE 10-2 Coagulation Factor Designations

Factor	Standard Name	Alternative Designations
I	Fibrinogen	
II	Prothrombin	
III	Tissue factor	Thromboplastin
IV	Calcium ions	
V	Proaccelerin	Labile factor, accelerator globulin (AcG), thrombogen
(VI)		No longer considered in the scheme of hemostasis
VII	Proconvertin	Stable factor, serum prothrombin conversion accelerator (SPCA)
VIII	Antihemophilic factor (AHF)	Antihemophilic globulin (AHG), antihemophilic factor A, platelet co-factor 1, thromboplastinogen
IX	Plasma thromboplastin (PTC)	Christmas factor, antihemophilic factor B, autoprothrombin II, platelet co-factor 2
X	Stuart factor	Prower factor, autoprothrombin III, thrombokinase
XI	Plasma thromboplastin antecedent (PTA)	Antihemophilic factor C
XII	Hageman factor	Glass factor, contact factor
XIII	Fibrin stabilizing factor (FSF)	Laki-Lorand factor (LLF), fibrinase, plasma transglutaminase, fibrinoligase
—	Prekallikrein	Fletcher factor
—	HMW kininogen	High-molecular-weight kininogen, contact activation cofactor, Fitzgerald factor, Williams factor, Flaujeac factor, Reid factor, Washington factor

Blood Coagulation Occurs When Fibrinogen Is Converted to Fibrin

Coagulation of blood entails the conversion of soluble plasma fibrinogen to an insoluble fibrillar polymer, fibrin, a reaction catalyzed by the proteolytic enzyme thrombin. This event cannot represent a sudden process, since the entire circulation might be converted into a massive clot. Instead, a series of finely tuned steps is mediated by a number of coagulation factors (Table 10-2), many of which are restricted by specific inhibitors This coagulation cascade amplifies the initial signal into the eventual generation of thrombin. The production of thrombin is probably the most important factor in the progression and stabilization of the thrombus.

Historically, the coagulation cascade was divided into two arms, termed the "intrinsic" and "extrinsic" pathways. The intrinsic pathway was so-named because blood clotting could be initiated without the addition of an extrinsic trigger and required only contact of factor XII with a thrombogenic surface. By contrast, the extrinsic pathway depended on the fact that in vivo coagulation requires the exposure of blood to an extravascular tissue factor. However, today we recognize that this partition of the coagulation cascade into two distinct arms is arbitrary and does not accurately reflect the underlying mechanisms of clotting.

The current view of the coagulation cascade (Fig. 10-7) highlights the importance of *tissue factor* (TF), a membrane-bound glycoprotein. The dynamic association of factor VIIa–TF complexes with TF pathway inhibitor (TFPI) is crucial to the generation of a thrombus. TFPI inhibits the initiation of the coagulation cascade by binding to the TF–Fxa–FVIIa complex. A major pool of TFPI located on the surface of endothelial cells likely regulates coagulation. The initiation of hemostasis takes place when activated factor VII (VIIa) encounters TF at the site of injury. As a result, small amounts of factors X and IX are activated to form Xa and IXa. The activation of larger amounts of X to Xa is promoted by factors VIIIa and IXa. Traces of thrombin catalyze the activation of factor XI, which in turn augments the conversion of factor IX to IXa. The complex of IXa and VIII converts larger amounts of factor X to Xa, which then binds Va to form the *prothrombinase complex*. This complex then converts prothrombin to thrombin, which functions as a serine protease.

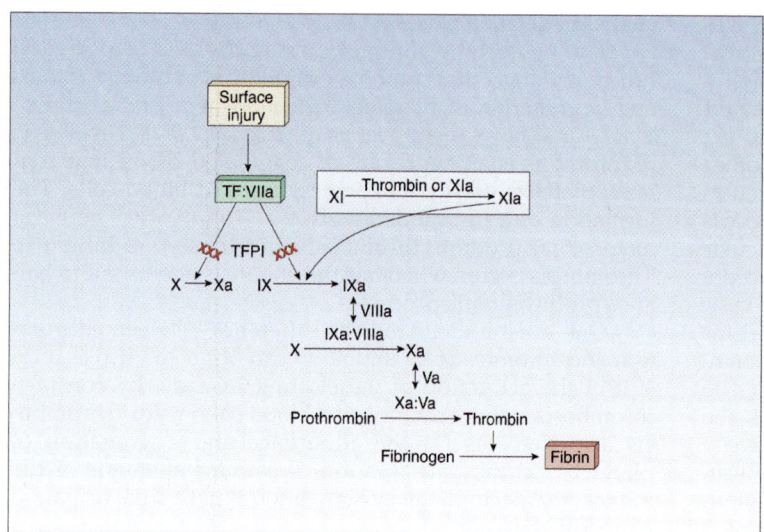

FIGURE 10-7

Coagulation cascade. The coagulation cascade is initiated by endothelial injury, which releases tissue factor. The latter combines with activated factor VII (VIIa) to form a complex that activates small amounts of X to Xa and IX to IXa. The complex of IXa with VIIIa further activates X. The complex of Xa with Va then catalyzes the conversion of prothrombin to thrombin, after which fibrin is formed from fibrinogen.

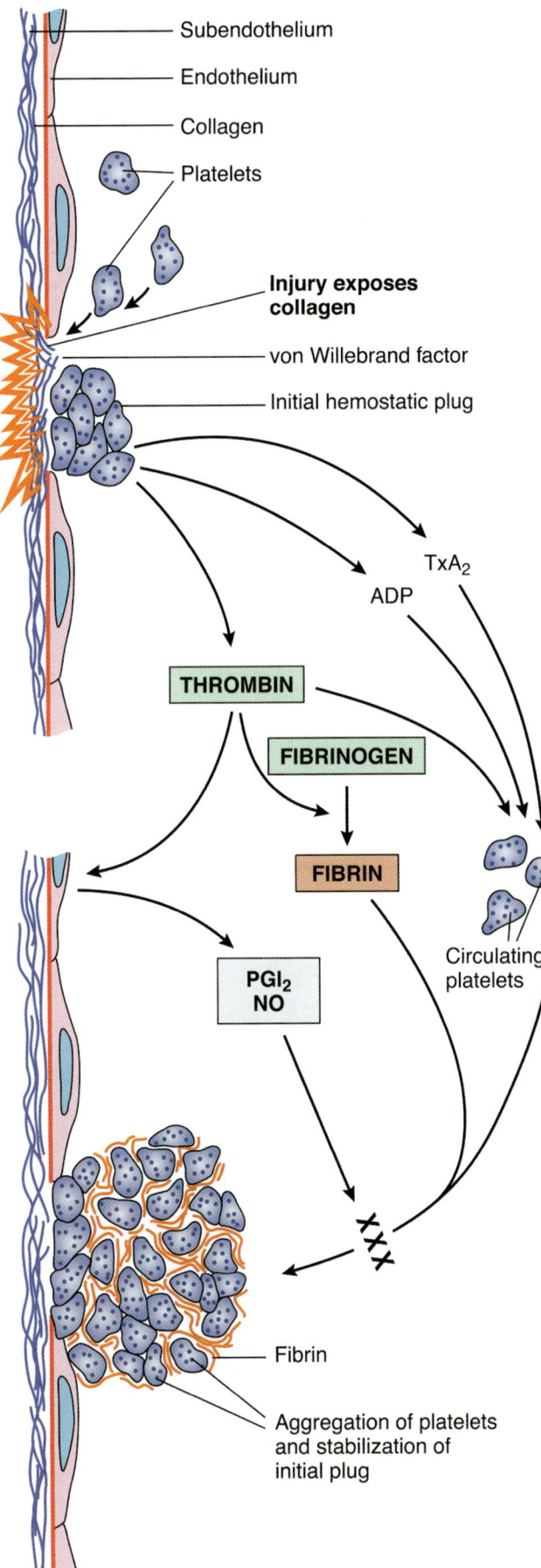

Hemostasis and Thrombosis

Besides its important role in the coagulation cascade and in platelet aggregation, thrombin modulates numerous endothelial cell functions. Thrombin participates in the production of fibrinolytic molecules and the regulation of growth factors and leukocyte adhesion molecules. It also mediates the protein C anticoagulant pathway by binding to thrombomodulin on the surface of endothelial cells. Factor V, an essential coagulation factor, also exhibits anticoagulant activity by exerting a cofactor function in the activated protein C system, which then downregulates factor VIIIa activity. Thrombin also increases endothelial permeability by promoting alterations in endothelial cell shape and disruption of cell–cell adhesion junctions.

Platelet Adhesion and Aggregation Occur after Injury to a Blood Vessel

Under normal circumstances circulating platelets are in a nonadherent state. However, injury upregulates platelet adhesiveness, after which platelets interact with one another to form a platelet thrombus, that is, an aggregate of activated platelets (Fig. 10-8). Changes in platelet shape that reflect reorganization of actin microfilaments are essential for platelet aggregation. Platelet aggregates occlude injured small vessels and prevent the leakage of blood.

Once platelets are stimulated to adhere to the vessel wall, their granular contents are released, in part by contraction of the platelet cytoskeleton. In turn, these granules promote aggregation with new platelets. Platelet adhesion is enhanced by the release of subendothelial von Willebrand factor, which is adhesive for Gp1b platelet membrane protein and for fibrinogen. Activated platelets also release ADP and thromboxane A_2, which recruit additional platelets to the process The platelet membrane protein complex GpIIb–IIIa adheres to fibrinogen, thereby forming bridges between platelets, an effect that enhances aggregation and stabilizes the forming thrombus. Activated platelets, in turn, release factors that initiate clotting, resulting in the formation of a complex thrombus on the vessel wall. Thrombin itself suffices to stimulate further release of platelet granules and subsequent recruitment of new platelets.

Endothelial Factors Regulate Both Anticoagulant and Procoagulant Processes

The endothelium is intimately involved in the initiation and propagation of thrombosis. The major initiating event that

---

FIGURE 10-8
The role of platelets in thrombosis. Following vessel wall injury and alteration in flow, platelets adhere and then aggregate. ADP and thromboxane A_2 are released and, along with locally generated thrombin, recruit additional platelets, causing the mass to enlarge. The growing platelet thrombus is stabilized by fibrin. Other elements, including leukocytes and red blood cells, are also incorporated into the thrombus. The release of prostacyclin *(PGI$_2$)* and nitric oxide *(NO)* by endothelial cells regulates the process by inhibiting platelet aggregation.

triggers most thrombosis is injury to the endothelium (see Fig. 10-8). Thrombus formation is normally prevented by blood flow and the antithrombotic properties of the endothelium. Thrombi may form when endothelial function is altered, when endothelial continuity is lost, or when flow in a blood vessel becomes turbulent or static. Simple loss of endothelial cells or injury to a vessel with good flow produces platelet pavementing but not thrombosis (Fig. 10-9).

For thrombosis to occur, either endothelial continuity must be disrupted or the endothelial cell surface must change from an anticoagulant surface to a procoagulant one. The most common denuding injury is the progressive disruption of endothelium by an atherosclerotic plaque. Denuding endothelial injury has also been described in other conditions, including homocystinuria, hypoxia, and endotoxemia. Endothelial injury and denudation also occur during interventional therapies for atherosclerotic disease, including the construction of saphenous vein bypass grafts, angioplasty, insertion of intravascular stents, and atherectomy. In addition, the interactions of a thrombus with underlying endothelial cells may further disturb endothelial integrity. For example, both fibrin and thrombin initiate endothelial shape changes and promote disruption of endothelial integrity.

Endothelial cells can also repair areas of endothelial loss by spreading and migrating into the area of denudation. This is followed by endothelial cell proliferation to restore normal cell density. However, these mechanisms become dysfunctional at sites of persistent damage to endothelium.

The endothelium plays an active role in the control of thrombosis (Table 10-3). The major antithrombotic mechanism of the endothelium seems to be the secretion of prostaglandin I_2 (prostacyclin), which inhibits platelet aggregation. Endothelial NO is also a potent inhibitor of platelet aggregation and adhesion to the vessel wall, although it may play only a minor role. Several other features of the endothelium support its antithrombotic activity. Endothelial cells metabolize ADP, a strong promoter of thrombogenesis, to metabolites that are antithrombogenic. The lu-

TABLE 10-3 Regulation of Coagulation at the Endothelial Cell Surface

Down-Regulation
1. Thrombin inactivators
   a. Antithrombin III
   b. Thrombomodulin
2. Activated protein C pathway
   a. Synthesis and expression of thrombomodulin
   b. Synthesis and expression of protein S
   c. Thrombomodulin-mediated activation of protein C
   d. Inactivation of factor V_a and factor VIII_a by APC-protein S complex
3. Tissue factor pathway inhibition
4. Fibrinolysis
   a. Synthesis of tissue plasminogen activator, urokinase plasminogen activator, and plasminogen activator inhibitor 1
   b. Conversion of GLU-plasminogen to LYS-plasminogen
   c. APC-mediated potentiation
5. Synthesis of unsaturated fatty acid metabolites
   a. Lipoxygenase metabolites-13-HODE
   b. Cyclooxygenase metabolites-PGI_2 and PGE_2

Procoagulant Pathways
1. Synthesis and expression of:
   a. Tissue factor (thromboplastin)
   b. Factor V
   c. Platelet activating factor (PAF)
2. Binding of clotting factors IX/IX_a, X (prothrombinase complex)
3. Down-regulation of APC pathway
4. Increased synthesis of plasminogen activator inhibitor
5. Synthesis of 15-HPETE

minal surface of the endothelium is coated with heparan sulfate, a molecule that binds a number of clotting factors, including the antiprotease α_2-macroglobulin. Endothelial cells may also lyse some clots as they form. In addition, they take up vasoactive amines released from adherent platelets and may limit coagulation by consuming thrombin.

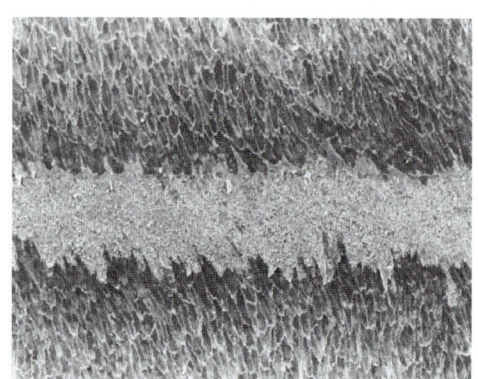
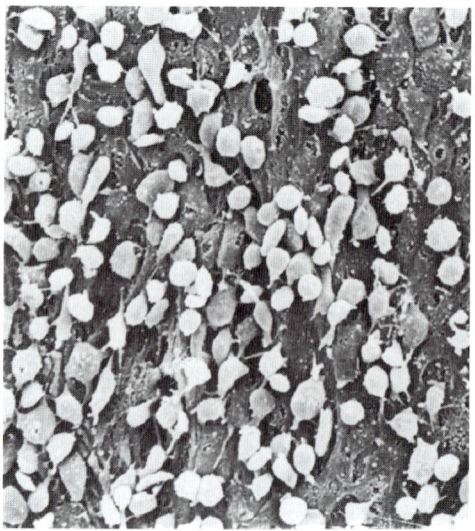

FIGURE 10-9
Scanning electron micrograph of the endothelial surface of a rat aorta 1 hour after the endothelial cells were removed by scraping with a nylon filament. A. Intact endothelium and scratched portion. B. Higher-power view of the scratched area shows a pavement of intact platelets that adheres to the underlying connective tissue in the high-velocity arterial stream.

There are several more mechanisms by which endothelial cells express anticoagulant mechanisms. A cofactor on the endothelial cell surface inactivates thrombin by forming a complex with it and antithrombin 3 (a plasma antiprotease). Thrombin itself activates protein C through an interaction with its receptor, termed *thrombomodulin*, which is located on the surface of endothelial cells. Both protein C and thrombomodulin are synthesized by endothelial cells. Activated protein C destroys coagulation factors V and VIII. TFPI generated during coagulation is bound to endothelium, where it inhibits the TF–VIIa complex. TF and TFPI are synthesized and secreted by endothelial cells as well as other vascular cells.

The presence of these thrombotic and antithrombotic mechanisms on the endothelial surface has raised the intriguing possibility that endothelial dysfunction alone might lead to thrombosis. There is also evidence that endothelial cells have prothrombotic functions. At least in culture, endothelial cells synthesize von Willebrand factor, which promotes platelet adherence and activates clotting factor V. Cultured endothelial cells also bind factors IX and X, a process that favors coagulation on the endothelial surface in vivo. Finally, inflammatory agents, including cytokines released from monocytes, activate procoagulant activities on the surface of an intact endothelium. Endothelial cells treated with interleukin-1 or tumor necrosis factor present thromboplastin to the plasma, thereby potentially initiating coagulation through the extrinsic pathway. Thus, one can envision that procoagulant injuries at the surface of blood vessels are produced either by the loss of a normal endothelial function or by the stimulation of an abnormal one.

Clot Lysis Is a Regulatory Mechanism

A thrombus may undergo several fates, including (1) lysis, (2) growth and propagation, (3) embolization, or (4) organization and canalization. The combination of aggregated platelets and clotted blood is made unstable by the activation of the fibrinolytic enzyme plasmin (Fig. 10-10). During clot formation, plasminogen is bound to fibrin and, therefore, is an integral part of the forming platelet mass. Endothelial cells synthesize plasminogen activator, but in larger thrombi, circulating plasminogen may also be converted to plasmin by products of the coagulation cascade. Plasminogen activator bound to fibrin activates plasmin. In turn, by digesting fibrin, plasmin lyses the clots and disrupts the thrombus. The clearance of fibrin also prevents its accumulation in the atherosclerotic plaque, where it tends to promote plaque growth and attract inflammatory cells. Endothelial cells also synthesize plasminogen activator inhibitor-1 (PAI-1), and plasmin is inhibited by α_2 antiplasmin. Thus, the regional fibrinolytic balance depends on the balance between plasminogen activation and inhibition.

ATHEROSCLEROSIS

Atherosclerosis is a disease of large and medium-sized elastic and muscular arteries that results in the progressive accumulation within the intima of inflammatory cells, smooth muscle cells, lipid, and connective tissue. The classical atherosclerotic lesion is best described as a fibroinflammatory lipid plaque *(atheroma)*. The

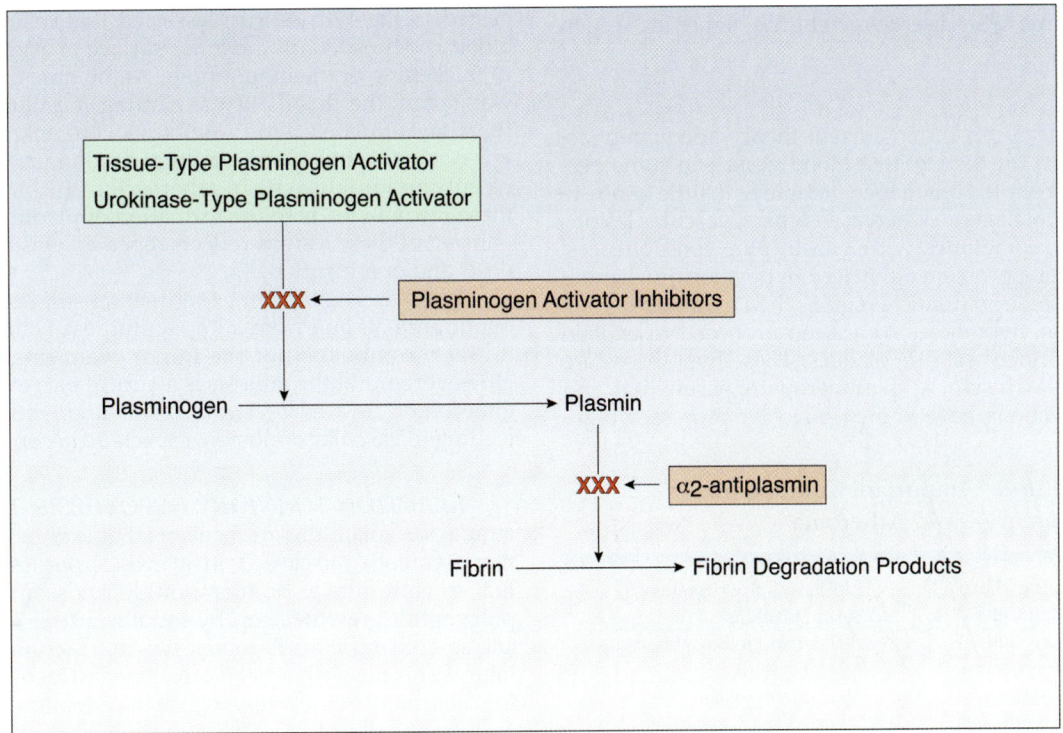

FIGURE *10-10*
Mechanisms of fibrinolysis. Plasmin formed from plasminogen lyses fibrin. The conversion of plasminogen to plasmin and the activity of plasmin itself are suppressed by specific inhibitors.

TABLE 10-4 Atherogenesis

- Initiation and growth of fibro-inflammatory lipid atheroma is a slowly evolving dynamic process with superimposed acute events
- Risk factors accelerate progression
- The pathogenesis is multifactorial and thus the relative importance of specific genetic and environmental factors may vary in individuals.
- Interactions between cellular and matrix components of the vessel wall, and serum constituents, leukocytes, platelets, and physical forces regulate the formation of the fibro-inflammatory lipid atheroma.

pathogenesis of the atherosclerotic plaque is a dynamic process that usually occurs over several decades (Table 10-4, Table 10-5). The continued growth of the lesions encroaches on other layers of the arterial wall and narrows the lumen of the vessel. Atherosclerotic lesions are also referred to as atherosclerotic plaques, atheromas, fibrous plaques, or fibro-fatty lesions.

Epidemiology: The major complications of atherosclerosis, including ischemic heart disease, myocardial infarction, stroke, and gangrene of the extremities, account for more than half of the annual mortality in the United States. In fact, ischemic heart disease is by itself the leading cause of death. The incidence of ischemic heart disease in the United States and other western countries rose progressively from the turn of the century to a peak in the late 1960s. Subsequently it has fallen by more than 30%. There are wide geographical and racial variations in the incidence of ischemic heart disease. For example, the mortality from ischemic heart disease is eightfold higher in Sweden than it is in Japan.

Pathogenesis: No current theory adequately accounts for the fact that blood vessels in some persons conduct blood for a lifetime with little or no evidence of arterial disease, whereas in others, vascular lesions develop early, sometimes with catastrophic consequences. Another puzzling problem is that lesions develop much more frequently in some anatomical regions than in others.

At least six hypotheses have been proposed to explain the origins of atherosclerotic plaques. These hypotheses are not mutually exclusive, and numerous experimental and clinical observations have shown how the processes highlighted in one theory are linked to those of another. Viewed in this light, most of the controversies lie in opinions about which process is most important in the initiation of the lesions or their progression to clinically significant disease.

INSUDATION HYPOTHESIS: Conventional wisdom has for some years held that the critical events in atherosclerosis center on the focal accumulation of fat in the vessel wall. The insudation hypothesis states that the lipid in these lesions is derived from plasma lipoproteins, a view consistent with the role of blood lipids as risk factors for myocardial infarction. Although there is still controversy over how the lipid enters the vessel wall, the insudation hypothesis is now widely accepted. Whereas this hypothesis explains the source of plaque lipid, it does not provide a complete explanation for the pathogenesis of the atherosclerotic lesion. Many other clinically important features of the plaque, such as smooth muscle proliferation and thrombosis, remain unexplained. Thus lipid deposition appears to be a necessary but not sufficient condition to explain atherosclerosis.

Low-density lipoprotein (LDL) is the form of lipid in the plasma that has been most closely associated with accelerated atherosclerosis. The LDL particle is far too large (20 nm in diameter) to penetrate the tightly closed endothelial cell junctions. However, endothelial cells have receptors for both LDL and modified forms of LDL. Transport can occur across an intact endothelium either by receptor-mediated uptake of lipoprotein or by nonspecific uptake into micropinocytic channels. Alternatively, lipid may be engulfed by macrophages in the blood and then transported into the vascular wall inside these cells as they transmigrate between endothelial cells.

ENCRUSTATION HYPOTHESIS: A theory first suggested in the 19th century asserted that material from the blood is deposited on the inner surface of arteries and leads to thickening of the inner lining. At the time this suggestion was made, the details of the clotting mechanisms and the functions of platelets in thrombosis were unknown. A modern version of this idea holds that small mural thrombi represent the initial event in atherosclerosis. Organization of these thrombi leads to the formation of plaques, and the expansion of these lesions reflects repeated episodes of thrombosis and organization.

We now know from experimental studies of hyperlipidemic animals and from autopsy studies of children that the mural thrombus is not the initial event in atherogenesis. However, mural thrombosis is a critical part of the later progression of the atherosclerotic lesion and is the major event leading to vascular occlusion, especially in coronary arteries.

REACTION TO INJURY HYPOTHESIS: This theory attempts to explain the mechanisms that lead to the accumulation of smooth muscle cells in atherosclerotic lesions. It is held that smooth muscle proliferation depends on the release of polypeptide growth factors by endothelial cells, macrophages, and smooth muscle cells themselves that accumulate at sites of injury. This theory has been broadened to focus on the role of the cells found in the artery wall in the initiation and growth of an atherosclerotic lesion. It has recently been modified to suggest that the cellular responses that occur during the pathogenesis of the atherosclerotic lesion constitute an inflammatory and fibroproliferative response to injury. In this theory, endothelial dysfunction compromises the integrity of the en-

TABLE 10-5 Important Components of Fibroinflammatory Lipid Atheroma

Cells	- Endothelial Cells	Lipids and lipoproteins
	- Foam Cells	Serum proteins
	- Giant Cells	Platelet and leukocyte products
	- Lymphocytes	Necrotic debris
	- Mast Cells	New microvessels
	- Macrophages	Hydroxyapatite crystals
Matrix	- Collagen	Growth factors
	- Elastin	Oxidants/Antioxidants
	- Glycoproteins	Proteolytic enzymes
	- Proteoglycans	Procoagulant factors

dothelial barrier to macromolecules and activates leukocyte adhesion molecules to promote the infiltration of macrophages in the subendothelium.

The "reaction to injury" hypothesis evolved from the discovery that the growth of smooth muscle cells in culture requires one or more platelet-derived polypeptides. The best known of these is platelet-derived growth factor (PDGF), which is secreted by both macrophages and vascular wall cells. PDGF is not only mitogenic for smooth muscle cells in vitro, but is also chemotactic for them. Thus, in addition to stimulating the proliferation of cells already located in the intima, PDGF may recruit smooth muscle cells from the media. The number of growth factors that can potentially induce proliferation of cells in culture has multiplied and now include fibroblast growth factor (FGF), PDGF, transforming growth factor-β (TGF-β), thrombin, LDL, endothelin, and others. There are also growth inhibitors, such as heparin and NO.

MONOCLONAL HYPOTHESIS: The monoclonal concept is focused on smooth muscle proliferation and was originally derived from the observation that the fibrous caps of atherosclerotic plaques (see below) are composed of smooth muscle cells. Furthermore, these cells appear to migrate from the underlying media and then proliferate. Can the lesion, therefore, arise as an aberration of growth control in one, or at most a few cells, in a manner analogous to the process in a benign smooth muscle tumor such as a leiomyoma? On the other hand, might it not arise from the polyclonal proliferation of many cells, as would be expected in a healing wound?

Based on studies of women who are mosaic for X-linked markers, it has been established that many plaques are monoclonal; that is, they originate from one or very few smooth muscle cells. The monoclonality of the fibrous cap suggests that some unknown etiological factor, perhaps circulating mutagens or viruses, might induce cap formation by altering growth control in the smooth muscle cells of the arterial wall. Although research has been done on the possible role of viruses in the pathogenesis of atherosclerosis, particularly herpesvirus and cytomegalovirus, a cause-and-effect relationship has not been established.

INTIMAL CELL MASS AND NEOINTIMA FORMATION HYPOTHESIS: The location of atherosclerotic lesions has been related to the focal accumulation of smooth muscle cells in the normal intima at branch points and other sites in certain vessels, particularly the coronary arteries. Intimal cell masses or neointimal thickening are found in infancy (more pronounced in males), and their distribution resembles that of intimal cell masses in children and atherosclerotic lesions in adults. Intimal cell masses in animals fed high-fat diets develop into lesions that display many of the characteristics of fully developed human atherosclerotic plaques. These observations suggest that the intimal cell mass may be either the early lesion of atherosclerosis or a precursor of it.

Little is known about the development of the intimal cell mass, its growth potential, or its clonality. If the intimal cell mass is indeed the precursor of atherosclerosis, it is probable that all humans are susceptible to this disease. In that case other factors, such as hyperlipidemia or hypertension, are critical for the progression of the disease to a clinically significant state.

HEMODYNAMIC HYPOTHESIS: The role of hemodynamics in the origin of atherosclerosis is frequently mentioned, and certain observations are compatible with the concept that elevated blood pressure enhances the process. The distribution of atherosclerotic lesions in large vessels, and the differences in location and frequency of lesions in different vascular beds, has encouraged a belief in the role of hemodynamic factors. In humans, atherosclerotic lesions tend to occur at sites where shear stresses are low but fluctuate rapidly, whereas in rabbit models of hypercholesterolemia, atherosclerotic lesions form in areas exposed to high shear. The fact that hypertension enhances the severity of atherosclerotic lesions in various systems, further promotes the idea that hemodynamic factors are somehow involved in the development of atherosclerosis.

An example of the role of hypertension in large arteries is seen in the pulmonary artery, which rarely exhibits atherosclerosis. In cases of pulmonary hypertension, typical fibrous atheromatous plaques can be found in the pulmonary artery and its major branches. There is reason to believe that shear stress may aggravate endothelial cell dysfunction and accelerate the development of atherosclerotic lesions. For example, hemodynamic forces induce gene expression of several factors in endothelial cells that are likely to promote atherosclerosis, including FGF-2, TF, plasminogen activator, and endothelin. However, shear stress also induces gene expression of agents that may be antiatherogenic, including NOS and PAI-1.

A Unifying Hypothesis

The sequence of events in the development of atherosclerosis (Figs. 10-11 to 10-14) may begin as early as the fetal stage, with the formation of intimal cell masses, or perhaps shortly after birth, when fatty streaks begin to evolve. However, the characteristic lesion, which is not initially clinically significant, requires as long as 20 to 30 years to form. Once formed, serious acute complications may occur or complicated lesions may emerge after several more years of development.

To tie the foregoing concepts together, we can construct a hypothetical sequence divided into three stages: an initiation and formation stage, an adaptation stage, and a clinical stage. Biologically active molecules regulate a number of cellular functions that are atherogenic. The role of modifier genes in the atherogenic phenotype must also be considered.

Initiation and Formation Stage

1. The intimal lesion initially occurs at sites that are predisposed to lesion formation, owing to endothelial dysfunction or the accumulation of subendothelial smooth muscle cells, as occurs in an intimal cell mass at branch points. In persons at increased risk of atherosclerosis, lesions also occur in areas that are not predisposed to the disease.
2. Lipid accumulation in these foci depends on disruption of the integrity of the endothelial barrier or the properties of intimal smooth muscle cells. The types of connective tissue synthesized by the cells in the intima also render these sites prone to lipid accumulation. Oxidative stress in endothelial cells and macrophages leads to cell-

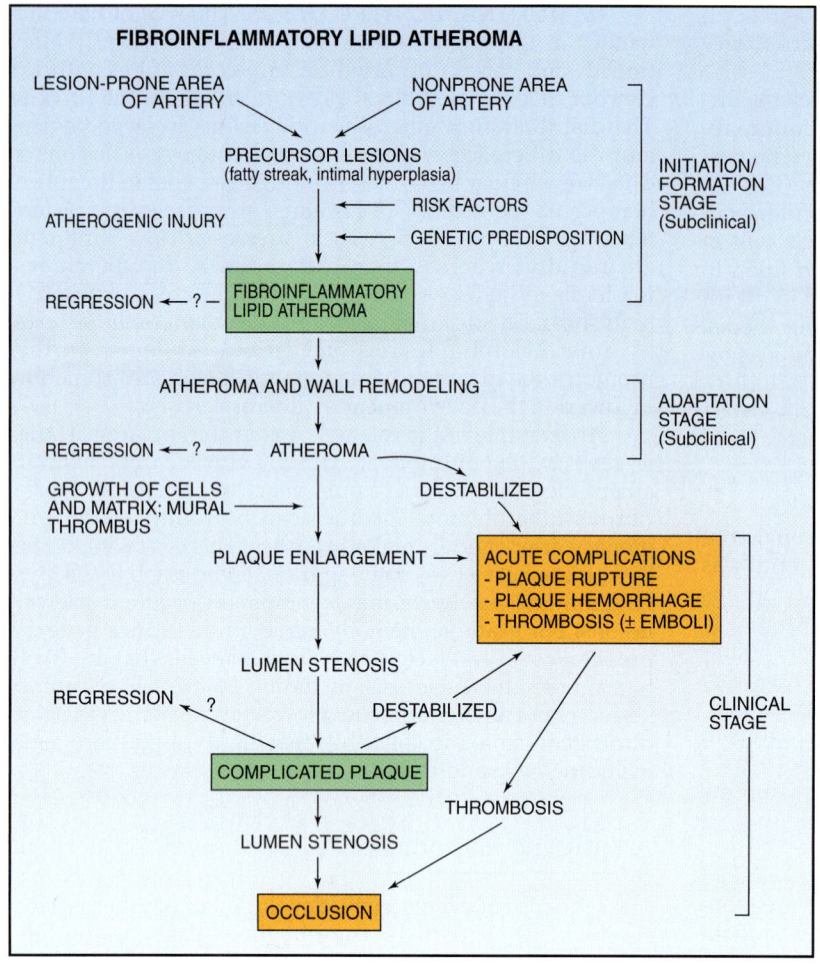

FIGURE 10-11
A unifying hypothesis for the pathogenesis of atherosclerosis.

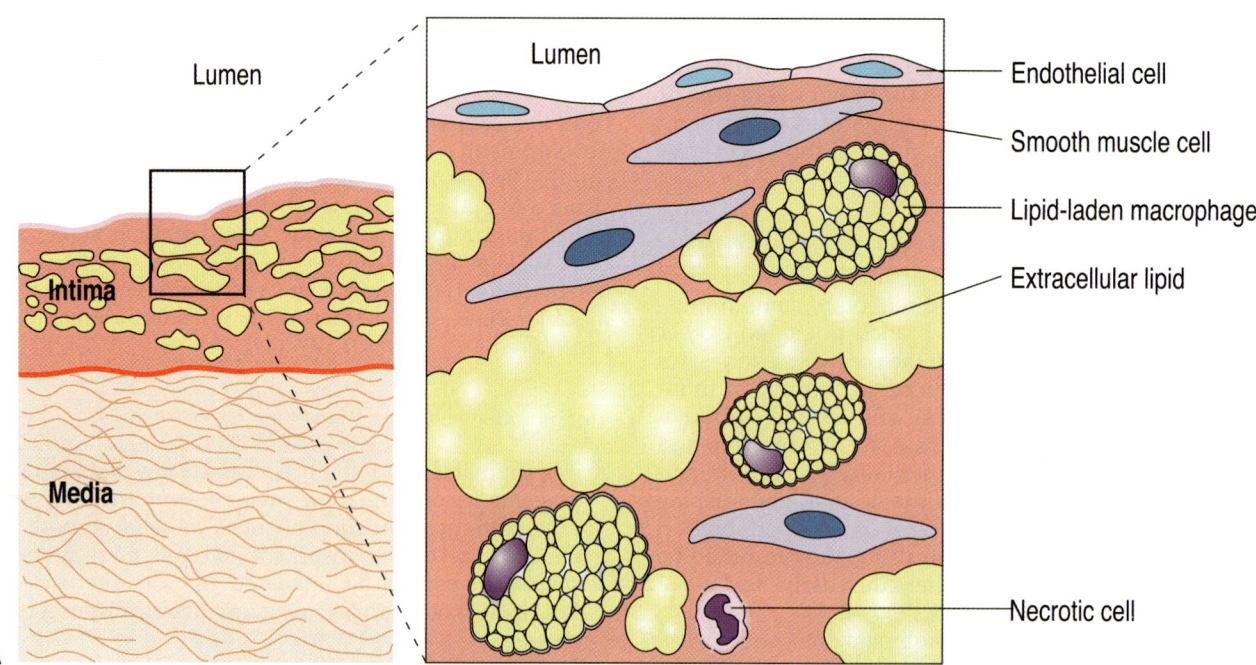

FIGURE 10-12
Fatty streak of atherosclerosis. A. The fatty streak, composed largely of foamy macrophages, is presumed to be an early stage in the formation of atherosclerotic lesions. Note the intimal thickening in the *left panel* and the infiltrating cells in the enlargement on the *right*. B. The aorta of a young man shows numerous fatty streaks on the luminal surface when stained with Sudan red. The unstained specimen is shown on the *right*.

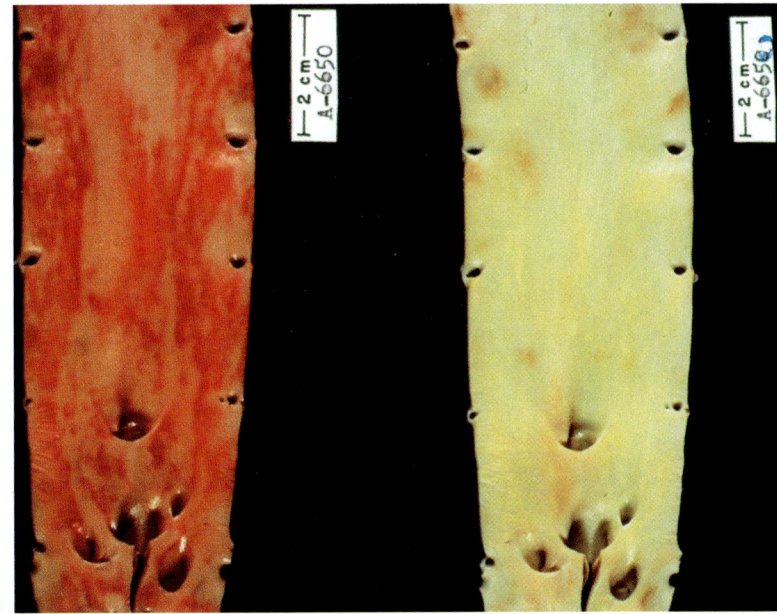

FIGURE 10-12 (continued)

ular dysfunction and damage is produced by vascular bioactive proteins and lipids, especially LDLs. Cell injury, promotes the accumulation of macrophages and a few lymphocytes.
3. As proposed in the "reaction to injury" hypothesis, mononuclear macrophages may play a central role by participating in lipid accumulation and releasing growth factors, thereby stimulating further accumulation of smooth muscle cells. *Oxidized lipoproteins* induce tissue damage and further macrophage accumulation. Monocyte/macrophages synthesize PDGF, FGF, TNF, IL-1, interferon-α (IFN-α), and TGF-β, each of which can modu-

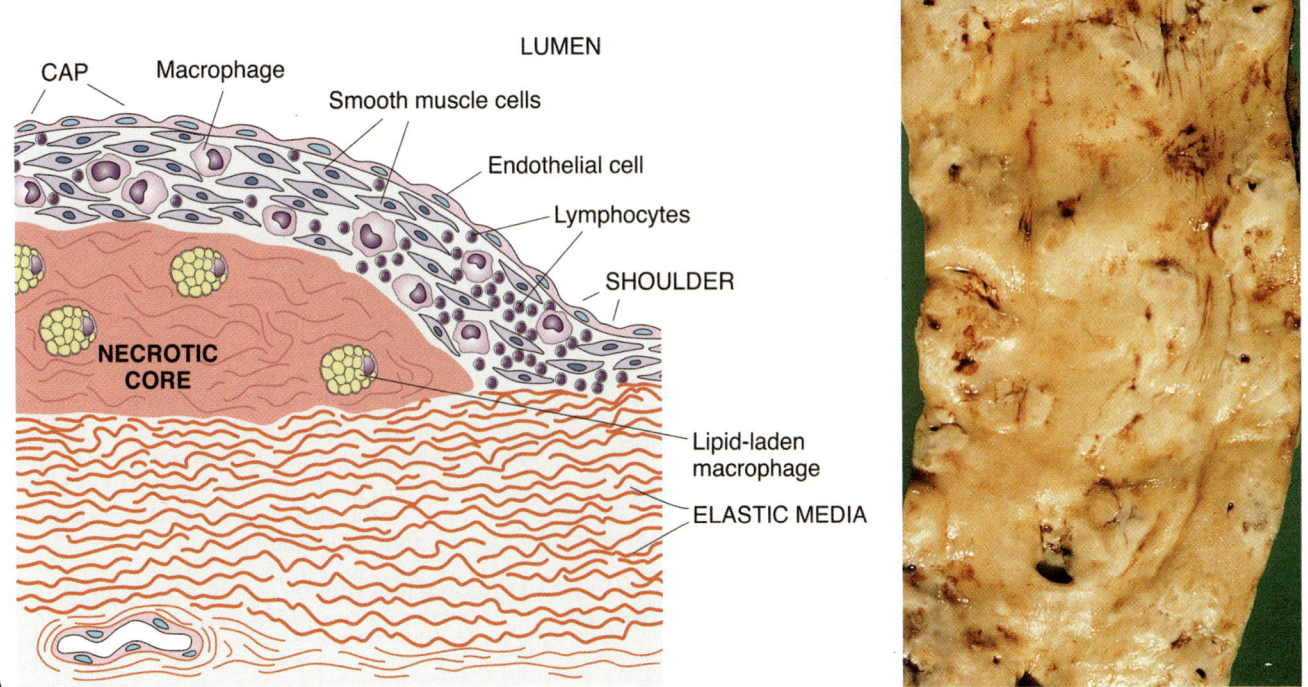

FIGURE 10-13
Fibrofatty plaque of atherosclerosis. (*A*) In this fully developed fibrous plaque, the core contains lipid-filled macrophages and necrotic smooth muscle cell debris. The "fibrous" cap is composed largely of smooth muscle cells, which produce collagen, small amounts of elastin, and glycosaminoglycans. Also shown are infiltrating macrophages and lymphocytes. Note that the endothelium over the surface of the fibrous cap frequently appears intact. (*B*) The aorta shows discrete, raised, tan plaques. Focal plaque ulcerations are also evident.

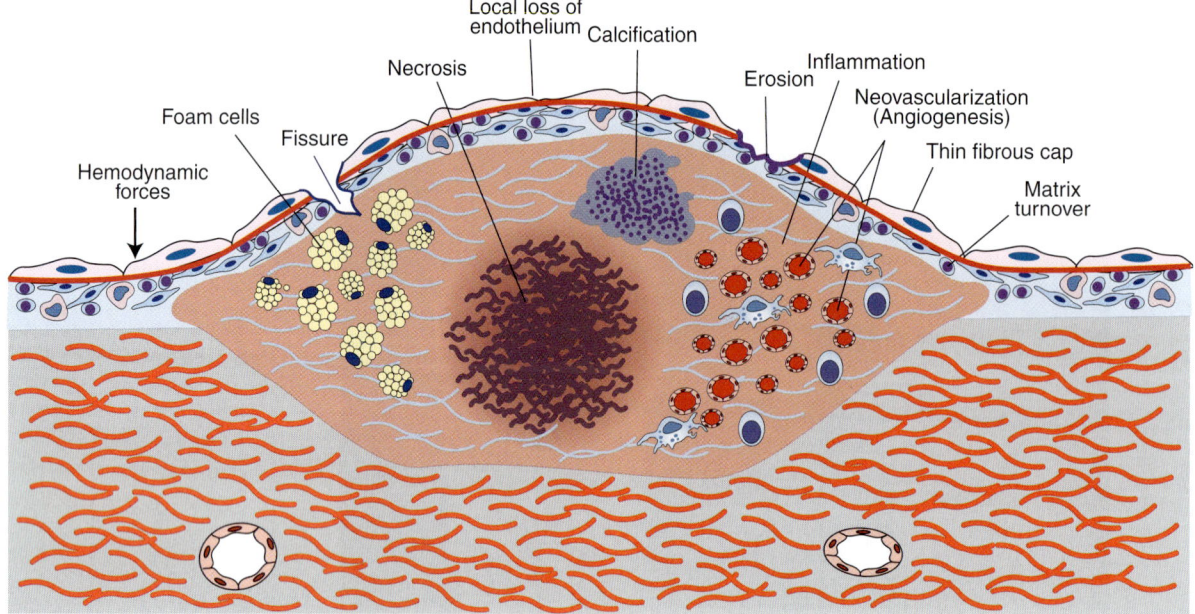

FIGURE 10-14
Factors involved in the pathogenesis of complicated atherosclerotic plaques.

late the growth of smooth muscle or endothelial cells, either positively or negatively. For example, IFN-α and TGF-β inhibit cell proliferation and could account for the failure of endothelial cells to maintain continuity over the lesion. Alternatively, such molecules could inhibit growth-stimulatory peptides. Of particular interest is the discovery that IL-1 and TNF stimulate endothelial cells to produce platelet-activating factor (PAF), TF, and PAI. Thus, the combination of macrophages and endothelial cells may transform the normal anticoagulant vascular surface to a procoagulant one.

4. As the lesion progresses, mural thrombosis on the damaged intima stimulates the release of PDGF, which accelerates smooth muscle proliferation and the secretion of matrix components. The thrombus becomes organized and is incorporated into the plaque.
5. The deeper parts of the thickened intima are poorly nourished and undergo necrosis, an event augmented by proteolytic enzymes released by macrophages and tissue damage caused by oxidized LDL and other agents.
6. The fibroinflammatory lipid plaque is formed, angiogenesis promotes its vascularization, and the plaque becomes heterogeneous with respect to inflammatory cell infiltration and matrix organization.

Adaptation Stage

7. As the lumen is encroached upon by the plaque (e.g., in coronary arteries), the wall of the artery undergoes remodeling to maintain the lumen size. Once a plaque encroaches upon half the lumen, compensatory remodeling can no longer maintain normal patency, and the artery becomes narrowed (stenosis). Hemodynamic shear stress is an important regulator of vessel wall remodeling. It is likely that cell proliferation, apoptosis, and matrix synthesis and degradation modulate remodeling of the vessel and the plaque in the face of atherosclerosis.

Clinical Stage

8. Plaque progression continues as the plaque encroaches on the lumen. Hemorrhage into a plaque without rupture may increase its size. The expression of HLA-DR antigens on both endothelial cells and smooth muscle cells in plaques implies that these cells have undergone some type of immunological activation, perhaps in response to IFN-γ released by activated T cells in the plaque. In this scenario, the presence of T cells reflects an autoimmune response that is important for the progression of atherosclerotic lesions.
9. Complications develop in the plaque, including surface ulceration, fissure formation, calcification, and aneurysm formation. Activated mast cells are found at sites of erosion and may release proinflammatory mediators and cytokines. Continued plaque growth leads to severe stenosis or occlusion of the lumen. Plaque rupture and ensuing thrombosis and occlusion may precipitate acute catastrophic events in these advanced plaques. Recent angiographic studies suggest that plaques causing less than 50% stenosis may also rupture. Factors that promote rupture of a plaque include (1) hemodynamic shear stress on the shoulder of the plaque, (2) inflammatory activity at the interface between an area of lipid deposition and fibrous tissue, and (3) the presence of metalloproteinases that digest connective tissue matrix.

Figure 10-11 shows how these hypothetical mechanisms may operate in the pathogenesis of atherosclerosis.

 ## Pathology:

The Initial Lesion of Atherosclerosis

Two distinct lesions have been proposed as the initial structural abnormality of atherosclerosis.

FATTY STREAK: Fatty streaks are flat or slightly elevated lesions that contain accumulations of intracellular and extracellular lipid in the intima. They are found in young children as well as in adults. In these simple focal lesions, cells filled with lipid droplets ("foam cells") accumulate (see Figs. 10-11 and 10-12). Cells with the greatest amount of lipid are indeed macrophages, but smooth muscle cells also contain fat.

In children who die accidentally, significant numbers of fatty streaks may be evident in many parts of the arterial tree. However, they do not correspond to the distribution of atherosclerotic lesions in adults. For example, fatty spots are common in the thoracic aorta in children, but atherosclerosis in adults is typically prominent in the abdominal aorta. Nonetheless, many believe that fatty infiltration represents the initial lesion of atherosclerosis and that other factors control the distribution of the later and more clinically significant lesions.

INTIMAL CELL MASS: As we have already proposed, the intimal cell mass is an alternative candidate for the initial lesion of atherosclerosis. Intimal cell masses are white, thickened areas at branch points in the arterial tree. Microscopically, they contain smooth muscle cells and connective tissue but no lipid. The location of these lesions, also known as "cushions," at arterial branch sites correlates well with the location of later atherosclerotic lesions.

The concept of the intimal cell mass as the initial lesion is controversial. First, if it is indeed the initial lesion of atherosclerosis, then the very early stages of lesion development should be common to everyone, regardless of age. However, a gradual increase in the thickness of the intima occurs diffusely throughout large arteries as a normal part of aging. For this reason many prefer to distinguish intimal thickening from atherosclerosis.

The Characteristic Lesion of Atherosclerosis

The characteristic lesion of atherosclerosis is the fibroinflammatory lipid plaque. On gross examination, simple plaques are elevated, pale yellow, smooth-surfaced lesions. They are focal in distribution and irregular in shape but have well-defined borders. Fibrofatty plaques (see Fig. 10-13), which represent more-advanced lesions, tend to be oval, with a larger diameter of 8 to 12 cm. In smaller vessels, such as the coronary or cerebral arteries, a plaque is often eccentric; that is, it occupies only part of the circumference of the lumen. In later stages, the fusion of plaques in muscular arteries can give rise to larger lesions, which occupy several square centimeters.

Microscopically, the atherosclerotic plaque is initially covered by endothelium and tends to involve the intima and only very little of the upper media (see Fig. 10-13). The area between the lumen and the necrotic core, termed the *fibrous cap*, contains smooth muscle cells, macrophages, lymphocytes, lipid-laden cells (foam cells) and connective tissue components. The central core contains necrotic debris. Cholesterol crystals and foreign body giant cells may be present within the fibrous tissue and the necrotic areas. Foam cells represent both macrophages and smooth muscle cells that have taken up lipids. Numerous inflammatory and immune cells, especially T cells, are present within a plaque.

Neovascularization is an important contributor to plaque growth and its subsequent complication (see Fig. 10-14). It is postulated that vessels grow in from the vasa vasorum. They are rare in healthy coronary arteries but plentiful in atherosclerotic plaques. Newly formed vessels are fragile and may rupture, resulting in acute expansion of the plaque from intraplaque hemorrhage. Foci of hemosiderin-laden macrophages are often present in the plaque, indicating a remote plaque hemorrhage.

Complicated Atherosclerotic Plaques

The term *complicated* plaque describes several conditions: erosion, ulceration or fissuring of the surface of the plaque; plaque hemorrhage; mural thrombosis; calcification; and aneurysm (Figs. 10-14 and 10-15). Progression from a simple fibrofatty atherosclerotic plaque to a complicated lesion may occur in some persons while they are still in their 20s, but in most affected people by 50 or 60 years of age (Fig. 10-16). Cellular interactions involved in the progression of atherosclerotic lesions are summarized in Fig. 10-17.

Calcification occurs in areas of necrosis and elsewhere in the plaque. Calcification in the artery is thought to depend on mineral deposition and resorption, which are regulated by osteoblast-like and osteoclast-like cells in the vessel wall.

Mural thrombosis results from turbulent blood flow around the plaque, at the site of its protrusion into the lu-

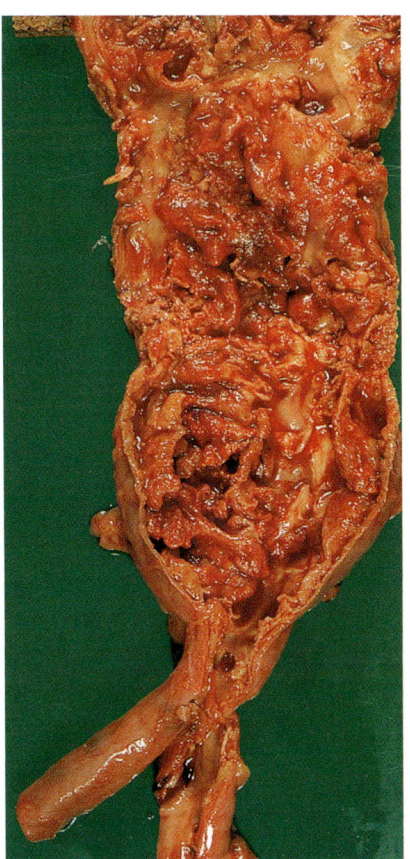

FIGURE *10-15*
Complicated lesions of atherosclerosis. The luminal surface of the abdominal aorta and the common iliac arteries shows numerous fibrous plaques and raised, ulcerated lesions containing friable, atheromatous debris. The distal portion of the aorta displays a small aneurysmal dilation.

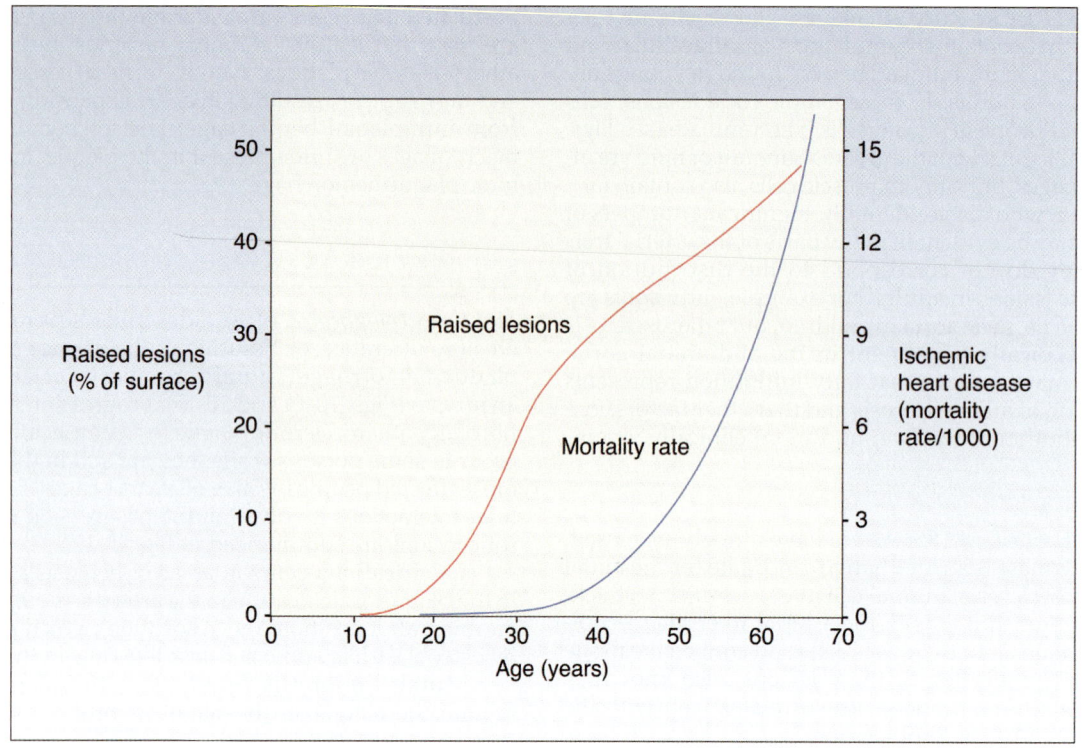

FIGURE 10-16
Raised lesions in coronary arteries and the mortality rate from ischemic heart disease as a function of age. There is a protracted incubation period of about 25 years between the appearance of raised lesions in the coronary vessels and their lethal complications.

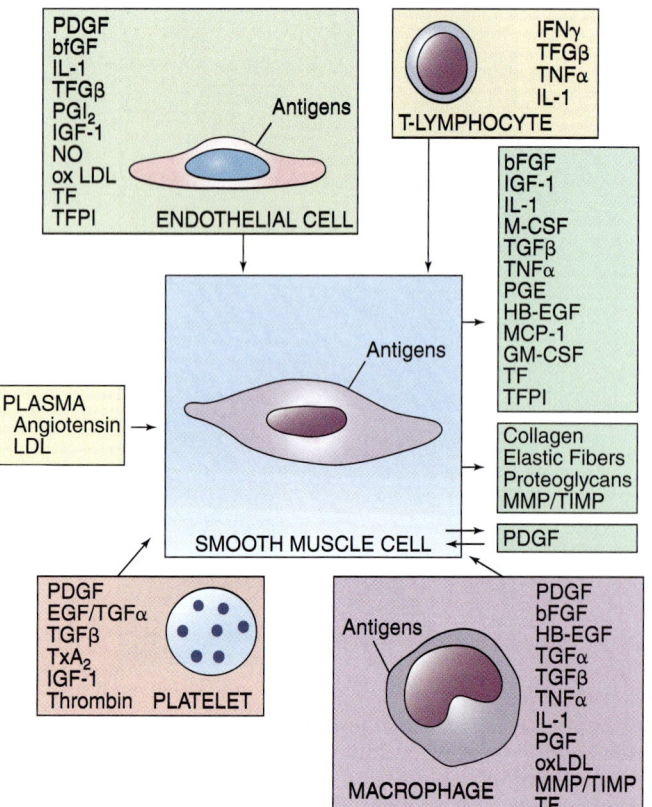

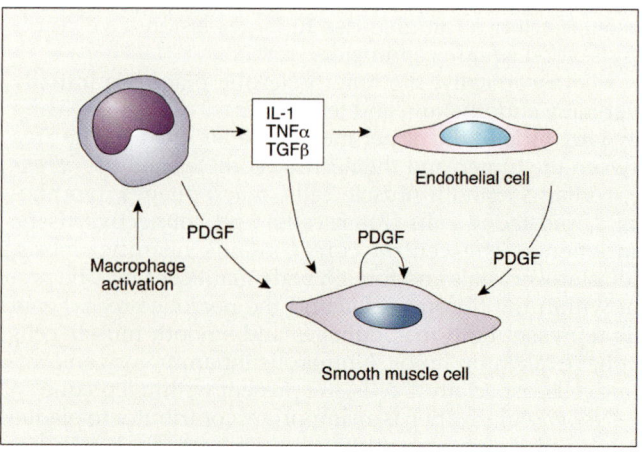

FIGURE 10-17
Cellular interactions in the progression of the atherosclerotic plaque. A. Endothelium, platelets, macrophages, T lymphocytes, and smooth muscle cells elaborate a variety of cytokines, growth factors, and other substances. The scheme illustrated here emphasizes their influence on smooth muscle cells. B. The cellular interactions that promote the proliferation of smooth cells.

men. The disturbance in flow also causes damage to the endothelial lining, which may become locally denuded and no longer present a thromboresistant surface. Thrombi often form at sites of erosion and fissuring on the surface of the fibrous cap of the plaque. Mural thrombi in the proximal region of a coronary artery may embolize to more distal sites.

The vulnerable atheroma has structural and functional alterations that predispose the patient to acute ischemic syndromes.

Atheroma destabilization may occur at any time when the dynamic balance of opposing biological and physical processes is disrupted, leading to mural thrombosis, fibrous cap rupture, or intraplaque hemorrhage. Clinically silent ruptures have been demonstrated, indicating that they can heal.

Thrombosis may occur on the surface of a plaque at the site of an ulceration or even when the surface appears to be intact. As noted above, endothelial dysfunction results in a prothombotic phenotype.

Sequelae to Plaque Rupture

In a ruptured plaque, the necrotic material that comes in contact with the blood contains TF and is very thrombogenic. The adjacent endothelium displays reduced TFPI levels (tipping the balance to coagulation) and reduced antiplatelet and fibrinolytic activities. The presence of circulating markers of inflammation suggests that procoagulant inflammatory mediators may also be operative.

Once the plaque ruptures, the thrombogenic material in the plaque promotes thrombosis in the lumen, resulting in the formation of an occlusive thrombus. Plaque rupture may also heal without clinical complications. Plaque hemorrhage due to rupture of thin, newly formed vessels within the plaque, may occur within the plaque with or without a subsequent rupture of the fibrous cap. In the latter case the hemorrhage may result in expansion of the size of the plaque, thus narrowing the lumen further. The hemorrhage will be resorbed over time within the plaque, and residual hemosiderin-laden macrophages persist as evidence of a previous hemorrhage.

Most plaques that rupture show less than 50% luminal stenosis, and over 95% display less than 70% stenosis. Plaque rupture often occurs at the shoulder of the plaque, suggesting that hemodynamic shear stress plays a role in weakening and tearing the fibrous cap. If not repaired, endothelial loss leads to erosion of the plaque, thereby weakening the fibrous cap and exposing the plaque to blood constituents. Plaque rupture has been associated with (1) areas of inflammation, (2) large lipid core size, (3) thin fibrous cap (<65 μM), (4) reduced number of smooth muscle cells owing to apoptosis, and (5) the balance of proteolytic enzymes and their inhibitors in the fibrous cap. Calcification of a plaque has also been associated with rupture.

Several circulating markers have been associated with plaque burden, including C-reactive protein, fibrinogen, soluble VCAM, IL-1, IL-6, and TNF.

Complications of Atherosclerosis

The complications of atherosclerosis vary with the location and the size of the affected vessel and the chronicity of the process (Fig. 10-18).

- **Acute occlusion:** Thrombosis on an atherosclerotic plaque, may abruptly occlude the lumen of a muscular

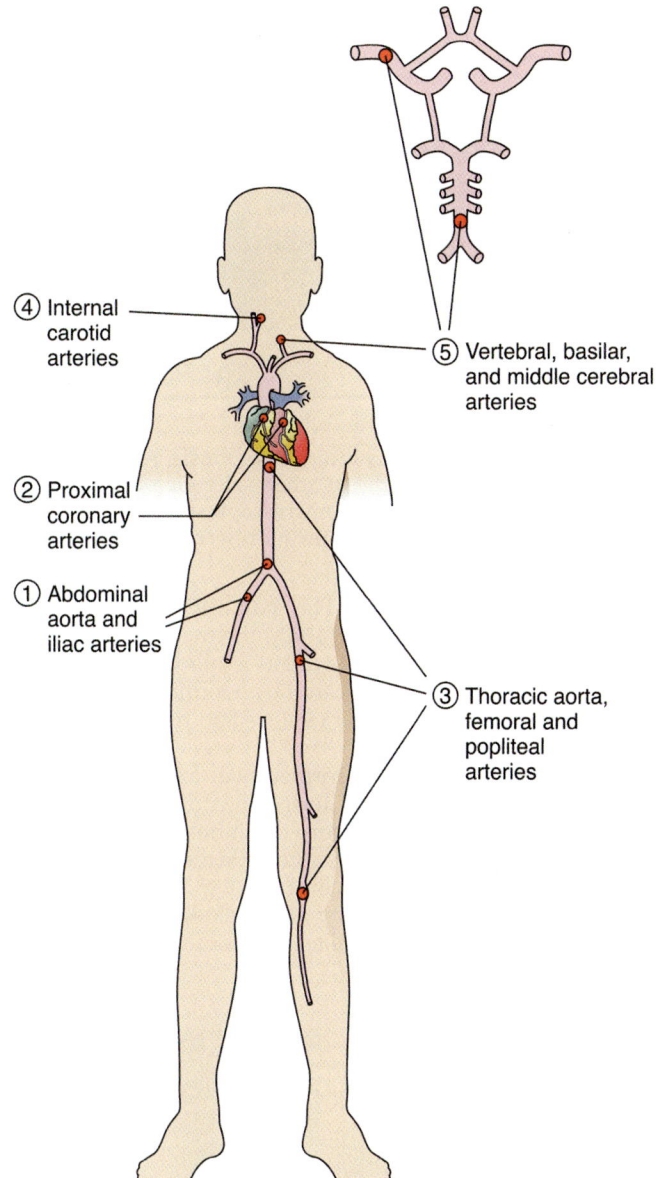

FIGURE 10-18
Sites of severe atherosclerosis in order of frequency.

artery (Fig. 10-19). The result is ischemic necrosis (infarction) of the tissue supplied by that vessel, manifested clinically as myocardial infarction, stroke, or gangrene of the intestine or lower extremities. Some occlusive thrombi can be dissolved by enzymes that activate plasma fibrinolytic activity, including streptokinase and tissue plasminogen activator (Fig. 10-20).

- **Chronic narrowing of the vessel lumen:** As an atherosclerotic plaque grows, it often impinges on the lumen, thereby progressively reducing the blood flow to the distribution of the artery. Chronic ischemia of the affected tissue is evidenced by atrophy of the organ, as exemplified by (1) unilateral renal artery stenosis with atrophy of a kidney, (2) intestinal stricture in mesenteric artery atherosclerosis, or (3) ischemic atrophy of the skin in a diabetic with severe peripheral vascular disease.

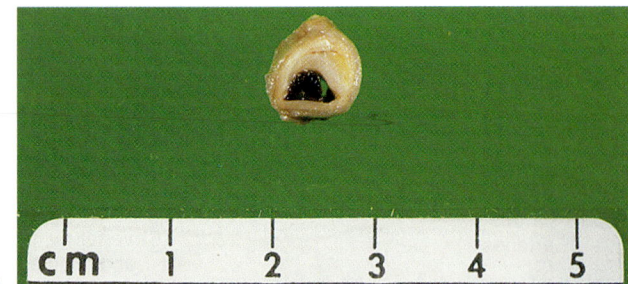

FIGURE 10-19
Coronary artery thrombosis. A. A cross-section of a coronary artery shows a fresh thrombus overlying an atherosclerotic plaque and occluding the lumen. B. Atherosclerotic coronary occlusion. A microscopic section of a coronary artery shows severe atherosclerosis and a recent thrombus in the narrowed lumen.

- **Aneurysm formation:** The complicated lesions of atherosclerosis may extend into the media of an elastic artery and so weaken the wall as to allow the formation of an aneurysm, typically in the abdominal aorta. These aneurysms may suddenly rupture and precipitate a vascular catastrophe.
- **Embolism:** A thrombus formed over an atherosclerotic plaque may detach and lodge in a distal vessel. For example, embolization from a thrombus in an abdominal aortic aneurysm may acutely occlude the popliteal artery, with subsequent gangrene of the leg. Ulceration of an atherosclerotic plaque may also dislodge atheromatous debris and produce so-called cholesterol crystal emboli,

which appear as needle-shaped spaces in affected tissues (Fig. 10-21), most commonly in the kidney.

Restenosis Occurs after Interventional Therapy

Angioplasty is an important form of interventional therapy for occlusive atherosclerotic vascular disease, especially that of the epicardial coronary arteries. A balloon catheter is inserted into the coronary arteries, where it is inflated to dilate the stenotic artery. The balloon causes endothelial damage and tears in the atherosclerotic plaque and the media. In 30 to 40% of cases in which the vessel lumen is satisfactorily dilated, restenosis of the vessel takes place over a period of 3 to 6 months.

Intimal hyperplasia due to smooth muscle proliferation and matrix deposition, with or without an organized mural thrombus on the luminal surface, leads to restenosis. In ad-

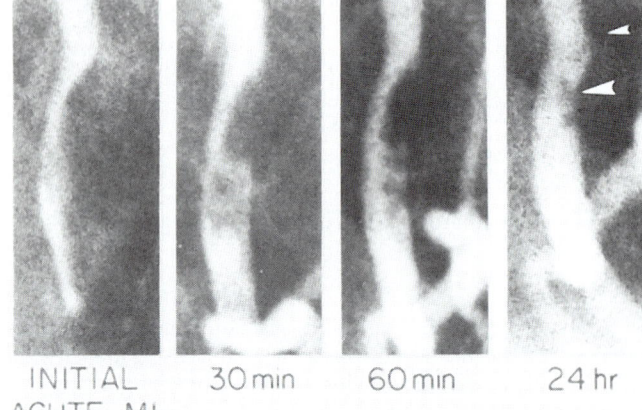

FIGURE 10-20
Dissolution of coronary artery thrombus. These coronary angiograms show a thrombus (initial) in the coronary artery of a 48-year-old man, 3 hours after the onset of the symptoms of acute myocardial infarction. He was immediately infused with recombinant human tissue plasminogen activator. Successive frames show stages of dissolution of the thrombus. By 60 minutes after the beginning of infusion, the thrombus is distinctly smaller. The infusion was continued for 6 hours, and at 24 hours the thrombus is almost completely lysed. The lower arrow indicates a small remaining portion of plaque or thrombus; the apparent bulge indicated by the upper arrow is interpreted as an ulceration of the plaque.

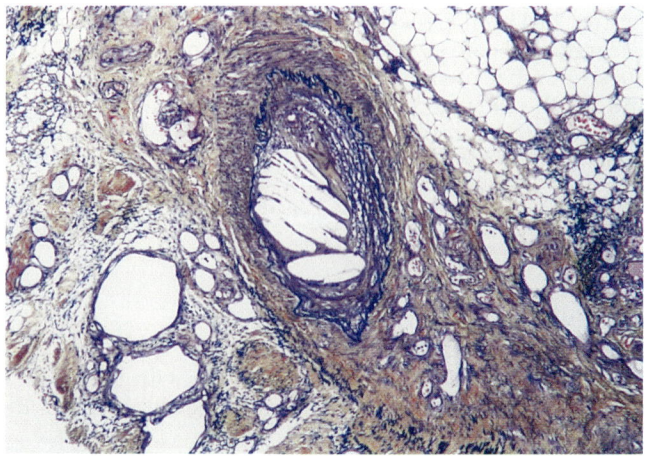

FIGURE 10-21
Cholesterol crystal embolus. Needle-shaped clefts are seen in an atherosclerotic embolus that has occluded a small artery.

dition, the dynamic process of vascular wall remodeling, induced in part by the trauma to the vessel wall and involving the adventitia, also results in luminal narrowing through contraction of the vessel wall. The use of stents coated with biologically active agents has resulted in less restenosis.

Transplanted saphenous veins are used as autografts in coronary artery bypass operations and undergo a series of adaptive and reparative changes. These include (1) intimal thickening associated with phlebosclerosis, (2) occasional foci of medial calcification, (3) focal muscle cell hypertrophy, and eventually (4) scarring of the adventitia. Venous grafts in place for a few years have atherosclerotic plaques indistinguishable from those found in native coronary arteries. Half of grafts occlude within 5 to 10 years, owing to neointimal hyperplasia and atherosclerosis.

Risk Factors for Atherosclerosis Are Predictors of Ischemic Events

Any factor associated with a doubling in the incidence of ischemic heart disease has been defined as a "risk factor."

- **Hypertension:** An increase in blood pressure is consistently associated with an augmented risk of myocardial infarction. Although the incidence of complications of hypertension was previously attributed to the diastolic component, there is increasing evidence that the systolic pressure is equally important. In fact, men with systolic blood pressures over 160 mm Hg have almost three times the incidence of myocardial infarction as those with blood pressures under 120 mm Hg. Control of hypertension has resulted in a significant decrease in the incidence of myocardial infarction and stroke.
- **Blood cholesterol level:** The levels of serum cholesterol have been directly correlated with the incidence of ischemic heart disease. Indeed, of all the known risk factors, serum cholesterol seems to be the most important determinant of the geographical differences in the incidence of atherosclerotic coronary artery disease. In the absence of genetic disorders of lipid metabolism (see below), the amount of cholesterol in the blood is strongly related to the dietary intake of saturated fat. A number of studies have demonstrated a reduction in the incidence of myocardial infarction following treatment with potent cholesterol-lowering drugs, so-called *statins*.
- **Cigarette smoking:** Atherosclerosis of the coronary arteries and the aorta is more severe and extensive among cigarette smokers than among nonsmokers, and the effect is dose-related (see Chapter 8). As a result, the incidence of myocardial infarction, ischemic stroke, and abdominal aortic aneurysms is markedly increased among smokers.
- **Diabetes:** Diabetics have a substantially greater risk of occlusive atherosclerotic vascular disease in many organs, but the relative contributions of carbohydrate intolerance itself, advanced glycation end-products, and secondary changes in blood lipids are not well defined.
- **Increasing age and male sex:** These factors are strong determinants of the risk for myocardial infarction, but both are probably secondary to the accumulated effects of other risk factors.
- **Physical inactivity and stressful life patterns:** Both of these factors have been correlated with an increased risk of ischemic heart disease, although their precise relationship to the evolution of atherosclerosis is not established.
- **Homocysteine:** Homocystinuria is a rare autosomal recessive disease caused by mutations in the gene encoding cystathionine synthase. The disorder results in premature and severe atherosclerosis. Mild elevations of plasma homocysteine are common and represent an independent risk factor for atherosclerosis of the coronary arteries and other large vessels. The increased risk of vascular disease associated with high levels of plasma homocysteine is comparable to that of smoking or hyperlipidemia. Homocysteine is toxic to endothelial cells and inhibits several anticoagulant mechanisms in endothelial cells. It inhibits thrombomodulin on the endothelial cell surface, the antithrombin III binding activity of heparan sulfate proteoglycan, the binding of tissue plasminogen activator, and the ecto-ADPase activity on the endothelial cell surface, which promotes the aggregation of platelets. In addition, oxidative interactions between homocysteine, lipoproteins, and cholesterol have been shown.

A low dietary intake of folic acid may aggravate an underlying genetic predisposition to hyperhomocysteinemia, but it has not been established that treatment with folic acid actually protects against atherosclerotic vascular disease.

TABLE 10-6 The Apolipoproteins

Apolipoprotein	Approximate Molecular Weight	Major Density Class	Major Sites of Synthesis in Humans	Major Function in Lipoprotein Metabolism
AI	28,000	HDL	Liver, intestine	Activates lecithin: cholesterol acyltransferase
AII	18,000	HDL	Liver, intestine	
AIV	45,000	Chylomicrons	Intestine	
B-100	250,000	VLDL IDL LDL	Liver	Binds to LDL receptor
B-48	125,000	Chylomicrons VLDL IDL	Intestine	
CI	6500	Chylomicrons VLDL HDL	Liver	Activates lecithin: cholesterol acyltransferase
CII	10,000	Chylomicrons VLDL HDL	Liver	Activates lipoprotein lipase
CIII	10,000	Chylomicrons	Liver	Inhibits lipoprotein uptake by the liver
D	20,000	HDL		Cholesteryl ester exchange protein
E	40,000	Chylomicrons VLDL HDL	Liver, macrophage	Binds to E receptor system

- **C-Reactive Protein**: Elevated concentrations of C-reactive protein, an acute phase reactant that is a marker for systemic inflammation, have been linked to an increased risk of myocardial infarction and ischemic stroke. This finding suggests that systemic inflammation may indeed contribute to atherogenesis.

Infection and Atherosclerosis

Seroepidemiologic studies have implicated infection as a possible contributing factor in the pathogenesis of atherosclerosis. *Chlamydia pneumoniae* and cytomegalovirus have been the most studied, although there is also interest in *Helicobacter pylori*, herpesvirus, and other organisms. Genomic sequences of these agents have been found in human atherosclerotic lesions, but whether they are causally associated or simply enter the diseased artery wall is not known. Viral infection is compatible with the importance of cell proliferation in the formation of atheromatous plaques.

Lipid Metabolism Is the Major Factor in Atherosclerosis

Since Virchow in the 19th century, first identified cholesterol crystals in atherosclerotic lesions, a large body of information on lipoproteins and their role in lipid transport and metabolism and atherosclerosis has evolved. The insolubility of cholesterol and other lipids (mainly triglycerides) necessitates a special transport system. This function is subserved by a system of lipoprotein particles (Table 10-6; Fig. 10-22), which have been divided into classes according to their density. The major classes of particles are as follows:

- Chylomicrons
- Very-low-density lipoproteins (VLDLs)
- Low-density lipoproteins (LDLs)
- High-density lipoproteins (HDLs)

Each of these particles consists of a lipid core with associated proteins (apolipoproteins), as indicated in Table 10-6. The metabolic pathways for lipoproteins containing the B apolipoproteins (apoB) are two major lipoprotein cascades, one originating from the intestine and the other from the liver (Fig. 10-23).

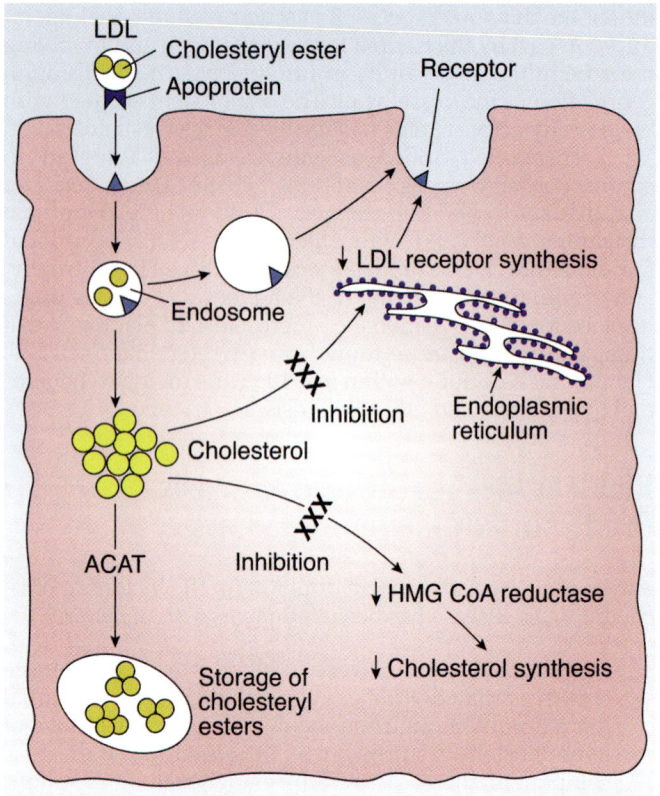

FIGURE 10-22
The relationship between circulating low-density lipoprotein *(LDL)*-cholesterol, LDL receptors, and the synthesis of cholesterol. LDL, which contains cholesteryl esters, is taken up by cells into vesicles by a receptor-mediated pathway to form an endosome. The receptor and lipids are dissociated, and the receptor is returned to the cell surface. The exogenous cholesterol, now in the cytoplasm, causes a reduction in receptor synthesis in the endoplasmic reticulum and inhibits the activity of HMG–CoA reductase in the cholesterol synthesizing pathway. Excess cholesterol in the cell is esterified to cholesteryl esters and stored in vacuoles.

FIGURE 10-23
Exogenous and endogenous cholesterol transport pathway. In the exogenous pathway, cholesterol and fatty acids from food are absorbed through the intestinal mucosa. Fatty acid chains are linked to glycerol to form triglycerides. Triglycerides and cholesterol are packaged into chylomicrons that are returned via the lymph to the blood. The lipids are coupled to proteins by enzymes such as the microsomal transfer protein complex. In the capillaries (mainly of fat tissue and muscle, but also other tissues), the ester bonds holding the fatty acids in triglycerides are split by lipoprotein lipase. Fatty acids are removed, leaving cholesterol-rich lipoprotein remnants. These bind to special remnant receptors and are taken up by liver cells. The cholesterol of the remnant is either secreted into the intestine, largely as bile acids, or packaged as VLDL particles, which are then secreted into the circulation. This is the first step in the endogenous cycle. In fat or muscle tissue the triglyceride is removed from the VLDL with the aid of lipoprotein lipase. The IDL particles (not shown) remain in the circulation. Some IDL is immediately taken up by the liver via the mediation of LDL receptors for ApoB/E. The remaining IDL in the circulation is either taken up by nonliver cells or converted to LDL. Most of the LDL in the circulation binds to hepatocytes or other cells and is removed from the circulation. HDLs take up cholesterol from cells. This cholesterol is esterified by the enzyme lecithin: cholesterol acyltransferase *(LCAT)*, after which the esters are transferred to LDL and taken up by cells.

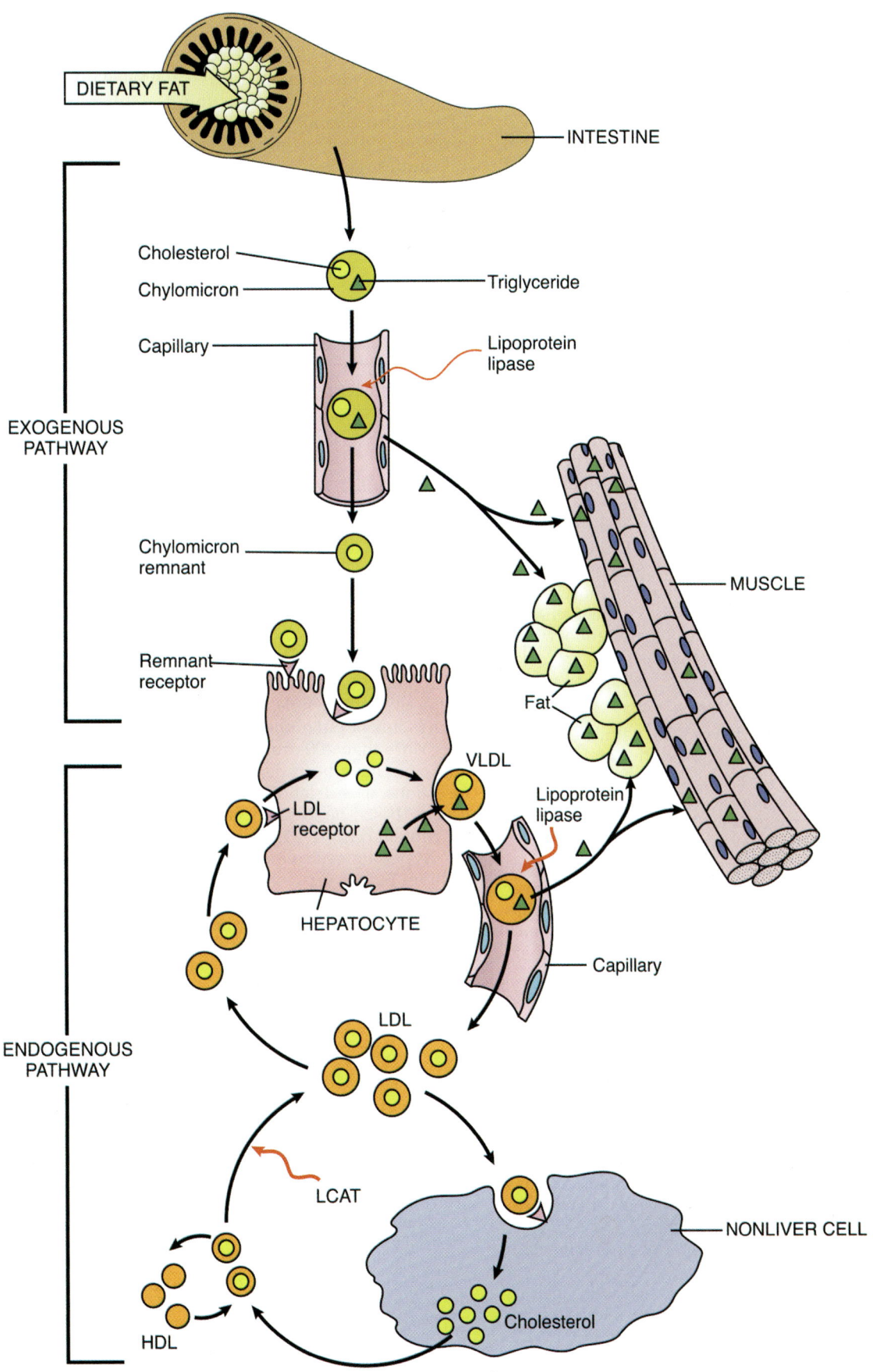

EXOGENOUS PATHWAY: This metabolic route involves chylomicrons containing apoB-48 secreted by the intestine. Following secretion, chylomicrons rapidly acquire apoCII and apoE from HDL. These triglyceride-rich lipoproteins primarily transport lipid from the intestine to the liver. The triglycerides in chylomicrons are hydrolyzed by lipoprotein lipase, which is attached to the surface of capillary endothelial cells. ApoCII activates lipoprotein lipase and causes removal of triglycerides. Thus, chylomicrons are converted to "remnants" and finally to intermediate-density lipoproteins (IDLs). The chylomicron remnants are removed by the hepatocytes through an apoE-mediated (remnant) receptor process.

ENDOGENOUS PATHWAY: This network of reactions involves triglyceride-rich lipoproteins containing apoB-100 secreted by the liver. As with the chylomicrons, the liver VLDL particles acquire apoCII and apoE from HDL shortly after their secretion. The triglycerides on VLDL undergo hydrolysis by lipoprotein lipase. The lipoproteins containing apoB-100 are initially converted to IDLs and finally to LDLs. With the conversion of IDL to LDL, most apoCII and apoE dissociates from the particles and reassociates with HDL. The conversion of IDL to LDL may, in part, be mediated by hepatic lipase. This enzyme functions both as a triglyceride hydrolase and, more importantly, as a phospholipase. LDL, which contains apoB-100, interacts with high-affinity receptors on hepatocytes and on peripheral cells, including smooth muscle cells, fibroblasts, and adrenal cells (see Fig. 10-21). The interaction of LDL with its receptor initiates receptor-mediated endocytosis, which is followed by the catabolism of LDL.

HIGH-DENSITY LIPOPROTEIN: HDL containing apoAI and apoAII is synthesized by several pathways. These include direct secretion of HDL by the intestine and liver and transfer of the lipid and apolipoprotein constituents released during the lipolysis of lipoproteins that contain apoB. Two major functions have been proposed for HDL: (1) a reservoir for apolipoproteins, particularly apoCII and apoE, and (2) an interaction with cells in the transport system to carry extrahepatic cholesterol, including that in the arterial wall, to the liver for ultimate removal from the body. The latter function has been termed *reverse cholesterol transport.* The cholesterol removed from the cells is principally free cholesterol, which rapidly undergoes esterification to cholesteryl esters. Cholesteryl esters are transferred to the core of the lipoprotein particle or are exchanged to VLDL and LDL. The transfer of cholesteryl esters between lipoprotein particles is mediated by specific transfer proteins such as cholesterol ester transfer protein. Defects in cholesteryl ester transfer and exchange lead to dyslipoproteinemia, increased intracellular cholesteryl ester concentrations, and premature atherosclerosis.

LOW-DENSITY LIPOPROTEIN: LDL cholesterol has numerous effects on the function of endothelial cells, smooth muscle cells, and monocyte/macrophages. For example, LDL regulates cyclooxygenase-2–dependent prostacyclin formation in vitro.

Each of the cell types in atherosclerotic lesions (macrophages, endothelial cells, smooth muscle cells) can oxidize LDL, a change that facilitates its recognition by the macrophage scavenger receptor and results in massive uptake of cholesterol by macrophages. Oxidized lipoproteins also affect other processes that may contribute to atherogenesis, including the regulation of vascular tone, the activation of inflammatory and immune responses, and coagulation (Table 10-7). Oxidized LDL is toxic to cells of the vascular wall and may lead to disrupted endothelial integrity and accumulation of cell debris within the atheroma. Oxidized LDL is also chemotactic for macrophages, thereby further promoting their accumulation in atheromas. Epidemiological studies suggest that the dietary intake of antioxidants is inversely associated with the risk of atherosclerosis, implying that oxidized LDL may be an important mediator of vascular disease. Further investigation is, however, necessary to establish this point.

Hereditary Disorders of Lipid Metabolism and Atherosclerosis

Familial clustering of ischemic heart disease has been recognized for decades, and a number of heritable dyslipoproteinemias are now recognized (Table 10-8).

FAMILIAL HYPERCHOLESTEROLEMIA: The LDL receptor is a cell surface glycoprotein that regulates plasma cholesterol by mediating the endocytosis and recycling of apoE, the major cholesterol transport protein in human plasma. Mutations in the LDL receptor gene, located on the short arm of chromosome 19, are responsible for familial hypercholesterolemia, an autosomal dominant disease in which the prevalence of heterozygotes is about 1 in 500 persons. However, among persons who have had myocardial infarctions associated with hyperlipidemia, the prevalence of familial hypercholesterolemia is much higher, reaching 6% in some populations.

More than 400 mutant alleles for familial hypercholesterolemia have been described, including point mutations, insertions, and deletions. The mutations fall into five main classes, based on their effects on the functions of the receptor protein (Fig. 10-24). The genetic considerations of familial hypercholesterolemia are discussed more fully in Chapter 6.

The early onset and malignant course of ischemic heart disease in patients with homozygous familial hypercholesterolemia may be the most compelling argument for a relationship between circulating cholesterol and the development of atherosclerosis. Homozygotes exhibit plasma

TABLE 10-7 **Important Cellular Processes in Atherogenesis**

Angiogenesis	Cell-physical forces interactions
Cell adhesion	Cell proliferation
Cell-cell communication	Inflammatory and immune
-soluble factors	reactions
-cell junctions	Matrix synthesis and
Cell contractility	degradation
Cell death; necrosis and	Mineralization
apoptosis	Phenotypic modulation
Cell injury, reactive oxygen	Thrombosis and modulation
species	of coagulation, fibrinolysis and
Cell-matrix interactions	platelet activation
Cell migration and chemotaxis	Vasomotor regulation

TABLE 10-8 Molecular Defects in Dyslipoproteinemias

Disease	Genetic Defect	Clinical Features
Apolipoprotein Defects		
ApoA1 deficiency	ApoA1 truncations or rearrangements (11q23)	Absent HDL, severe atherosclerosis
ApoA1 variants	ApoA1 point mutations (11q23)	Reduced HDL, variable atherosclerosis
Abetalipoproteinemia (absence of both ApoB-100 and ApoB-48)	Microsomal triglyceride protein mutations (4q22–24)	Ataxia, malabsorption, hemolytic anemia, visual defects, absence of atherosclerosis
ApoB-100 absence	Unknown (2p24)	Mild ataxia, malabsorption, absence of atherosclerosis
ApoCII deficiency	ApoCII mutations (19q13.2)	Type I hyperlipidemia: severe hypertriglyceridemia, variable atherosclerosis
ApoE variants	ApoE mutations (19q13.2)	Type III hyperlipidemia: elevated triglycerides, premature atherosclerosis
Enzyme Defects		
Lipoprotein lipase deficiency	Lipoprotein lipase mutations (8p22)	Type I hyperlipidemia: hypertriglyceridemia; minimal atherosclerosis
Hepatic lipase deficiency	Hepatic lipase mutations (15q21–23)	Elevations of IDL and HDL; severe atherosclerosis
Lecithin:cholesterol acyltransferase deficiency	LCAT mutations (16q22.1)	Mild hypertriglyceridemia; reduced HDL; corneal opacities; variable atherosclerosis
Receptor Defect		
Familial hypercholesterolemia	LDL receptor mutations (19p13.2)	Type II hyperlipidemia: severe elevation of LDL; premature atherosclerosis

cholesterol levels between 600 and 1000 mg/dL, a value fourfold to sixfold higher than the mean value in most whites. Most untreated homozygotes die from coronary artery disease before the age of 20 years. In heterozygotes, LDL cholesterol levels vary from 250 to 500 mg/dL, roughly twice the normal range. These patients also suffer from premature myocardial infarction but at a later age than do the homozygotes (40–45 years in men).

In addition to the accelerated accumulation of cholesterol in the arteries (premature atherosclerosis), LDL cholesterol also deposits in skin and tendons to form xanthomas (Fig. 10-25). In some cases (before age 10 in homozygotes), an arcus lipoides is present in the cornea.

APOLIPOPROTEIN E (APOE): Genetic variations in various apoproteins are also known to be accompanied by alterations in LDL levels. Polymorphisms are present in apoE, and variants of apolipoprotein AI and AII have also been observed. Apolipoprotein E is one of the main protein constituents of VLDL and of a subclass of HDL. The gene locus that codes for apoE is polymorphic; three common alleles, E2, E3, and E4, code for three major apoE isoforms, respectively, and determine the six apoE phenotypes. Some 20% of the variability in serum cholesterol has been attributed to apoE polymorphism. In men, the apoE 3/2 phenotype is associated with a 20% lower LDL level than the most common phenotype, apoE 3/3. By contrast, the E4 allele is associated with elevated serum cholesterol. Interestingly, there is an increased frequency of the E2 allele and a decreased frequency of E4 among male octogenarians.

HIGH-DENSITY LIPOPROTEIN: An inverse correlation between ischemic heart disease and HDL cholesterol levels has been established. The genes for apolipoproteins AI and CIII reside on chromosome 11 and are physically linked, whereas the gene for A-II is on chromosome 1. Polymorphisms of apoAI are associated with premature atherosclerosis, as are rare cases of hereditary apoAI deficiency. Factors that increase HDL levels include female gender, estrogens, vigorous exercise, and moderate alcohol consumption. Decreased HDL occurs with low-fat diets and diets high in polyunsaturated fats, truncal obesity, diabetes, smoking, and androgen administration. Hypertriglyceridemia is one of the most frequent metabolic abnormalities observed in association with low HDL cholesterol.

LIPOPROTEIN (a) (Lp[a]): High circulating levels of Lp(a) are associated with an augmented risk of atherosclerotic disease of the coronary arteries and larger cerebral vessels. The plasma level of this cholesterol-rich lipoprotein varies over a wide range (<1 to >140 mg/dL) and appears to be independent of LDL levels. The Lp(a)-specific protein, apo(a), has been detected in atherosclerotic lesions, and high Lp(a) levels have been correlated with target organ damage in hypertensive patients.

Lp(a) is an LDL-like particle to which the glycoprotein apo(a) is attached through a disulfide bridge with apoB-100. Apo(a) is coded for by a gene on chromosome 6 (6q2.7), close to the gene for plasminogen, with which apo(a) is highly homologous. Both apo(a) and plasminogen display similar domains that mediate an interaction with fibrin and cell surface

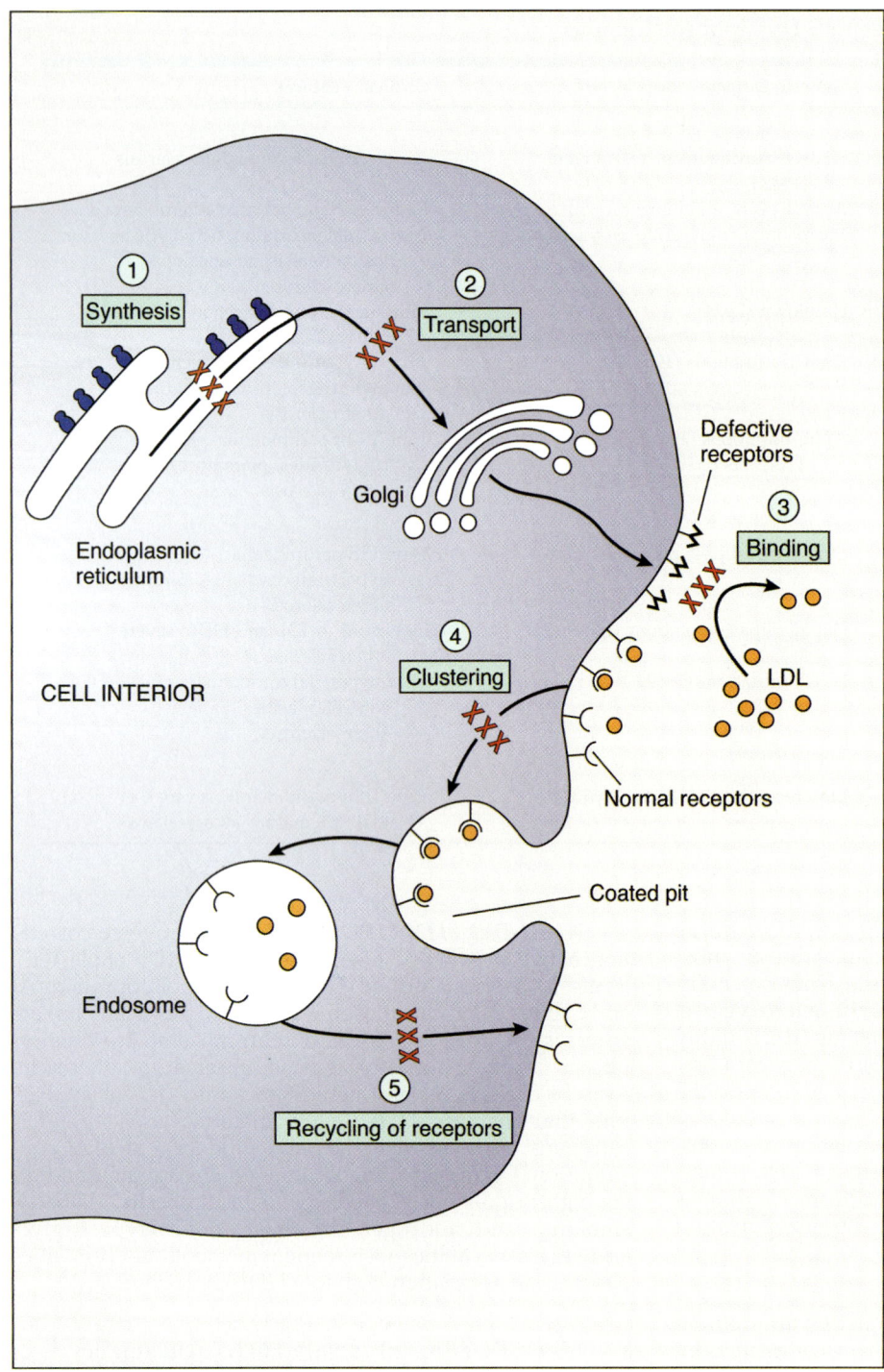

FIGURE 10-24
Mutations of the LDL receptor in familial hypercholesterolemia.

receptors. Lp(a) enhances the delivery of cholesterol to injured blood vessels, suppresses the generation of plasmin, and promotes the proliferation of smooth muscle cells. Thus, it may be an important link between atherosclerosis and thrombosis.

Lp(a) plasma levels are heritable and not altered by the usual cholesterol-lowering drugs, although they are reduced by nicotinic acid therapy. Taken together, this information distinguishes a risk factor that appears superficially to be related to serum cholesterol, but the effect of which may actually be linked to an alteration in clot lysis.

HYPERTENSIVE VASCULAR DISEASE

Hypertension affects up to 20% of the population in industrial countries and is present in more than half of cases of myocardial infarction, stroke, and chronic renal disease. Blacks are particularly prone to the ravages of hypertension and are more likely than whites to experience severe complications. Three fourths of patients with dissecting aortic aneurysm, intracerebral hemorrhage, or rupture of the myocardial wall also have elevated blood pressure. The etiology

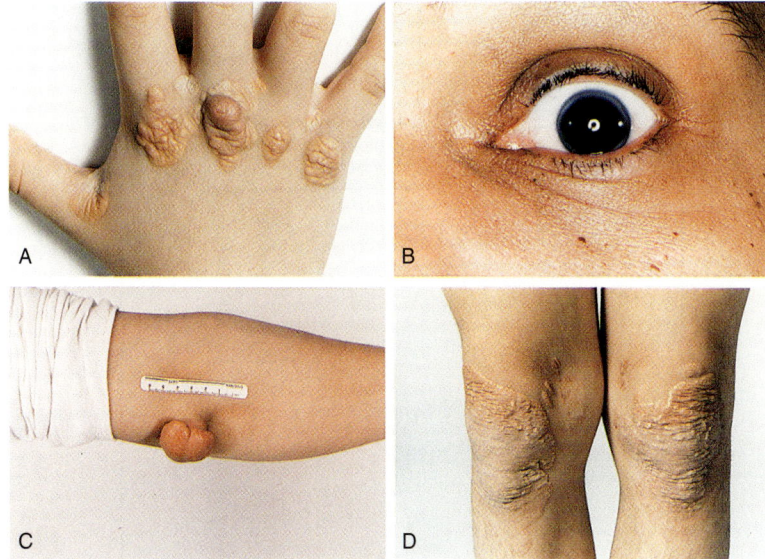

FIGURE 10-25
Xanthomas in familial hypercholesterolemia. Arcus lipoides represents the deposition of lipids in the peripheral cornea.

of most hypertension remains obscure; 95% of patients have no clearly identifiable cause. Thus, most hypertensive persons are described as having "essential" or "primary" hypertension. Whatever the etiology, it has become clear that the treatment of hypertension prolongs life.

The definition of hypertension depends on a statistical estimate of the distribution of systolic and diastolic blood pressures in the general population. Over the course of the day, blood pressure varies widely, depending on exertion, emotional state, and other poorly understood factors. Blood pressure also varies with age. The mean systolic blood pressure in 20-year-old men is about 130 mm Hg, but the 95% confidence limits range from 105 to 150 mm Hg. With age, the average systolic blood pressure increases, so that in 80-year-olds, it reaches 170 mm Hg, with the 95% confidence limits extending from 125 to 220. The World Health Organization has defined hypertension as a systolic pressure above 160 mm Hg and a diastolic pressure above 90, or both.

 Pathogenesis: Blood pressure is simply the product of cardiac output and the systemic vascular resistance to blood flow. However, both of these functions are critically influenced by renal function and sodium homeostasis. The most widespread hypothesis holds that primary hypertension results from an imbalance in the interactions between these mechanisms (Fig. 10-26).

A complex endocrine axis centers on the renin–angiotensin system. Renal artery occlusion or dietary salt restriction leads to increased secretion of renin by the kidney. Renin is a protease that splits angiotensinogen to a decapeptide, termed *angiotensin I*. In turn, angiotensin I is converted to angiotensin II by ACE, a protein found on surface of the endothelial cells. Angiotensin II is a vasoconstrictor that also affects centers in the central nervous system that control sympathetic outflow and stimulate aldosterone release from the adrenal gland. Aldosterone acts on renal tubules to increase sodium reabsorption. The net effect of all these actions is an increase in total body fluid volume. Thus,

the *renin–angiotensin* system elevates blood pressure by three mechanisms:

- Increased sympathetic output
- Increased mineralocorticoid secretion
- Direct vasoconstriction

The renin–angiotensin–aldosterone axis is antagonized by atrial natriuretic factor (ANF), a hormone secreted by specialized cells in the cardiac atria. ANF binds to specific receptors in the kidney and increases the urinary excretion of sodium, thereby opposing the vasoconstrictor effects of angiotensin II. Secretion of ANF may be controlled by atrial distention, a consequence of increased volume, or by as-yet undefined endocrine interactions.

The importance of this axis of hormones in regulating blood pressure in hypertension is demonstrated by the therapeutic success of sympathetic antagonists (β-adrenergic blockers), diuretics, and inhibitors of ACE. Nonetheless, it has proved difficult to identify a central defect in the rennin–angiotensin axis, because the vasculature responds quickly to hemodynamic changes in the tissues by autoregulation (Fig. 10-27).

In the case of hypertension, the end-result of autoregulation is always increased peripheral resistance. For example, hypertension can be induced experimentally by surgical resection of large amounts of renal tissue, followed by the administration of excess sodium and water. Cardiac output, and therefore blood pressure, is rapidly increased as a result of the rapid change in blood volume. However, within a few days, pressure-induced diuresis results in a return to near-normal cardiac output and plasma volume. At this point, blood pressure is maintained by increased peripheral resistance. Even though the elevation in blood pressure was initially due to increased volume, compensatory mechanisms have successfully masked the volume changes and caused apparent essential hypertension. It is possible that many cases of human hypertension also represent the end-stage of a process that begins with alterations in cardiac output, salt metabolism, or ANF release.

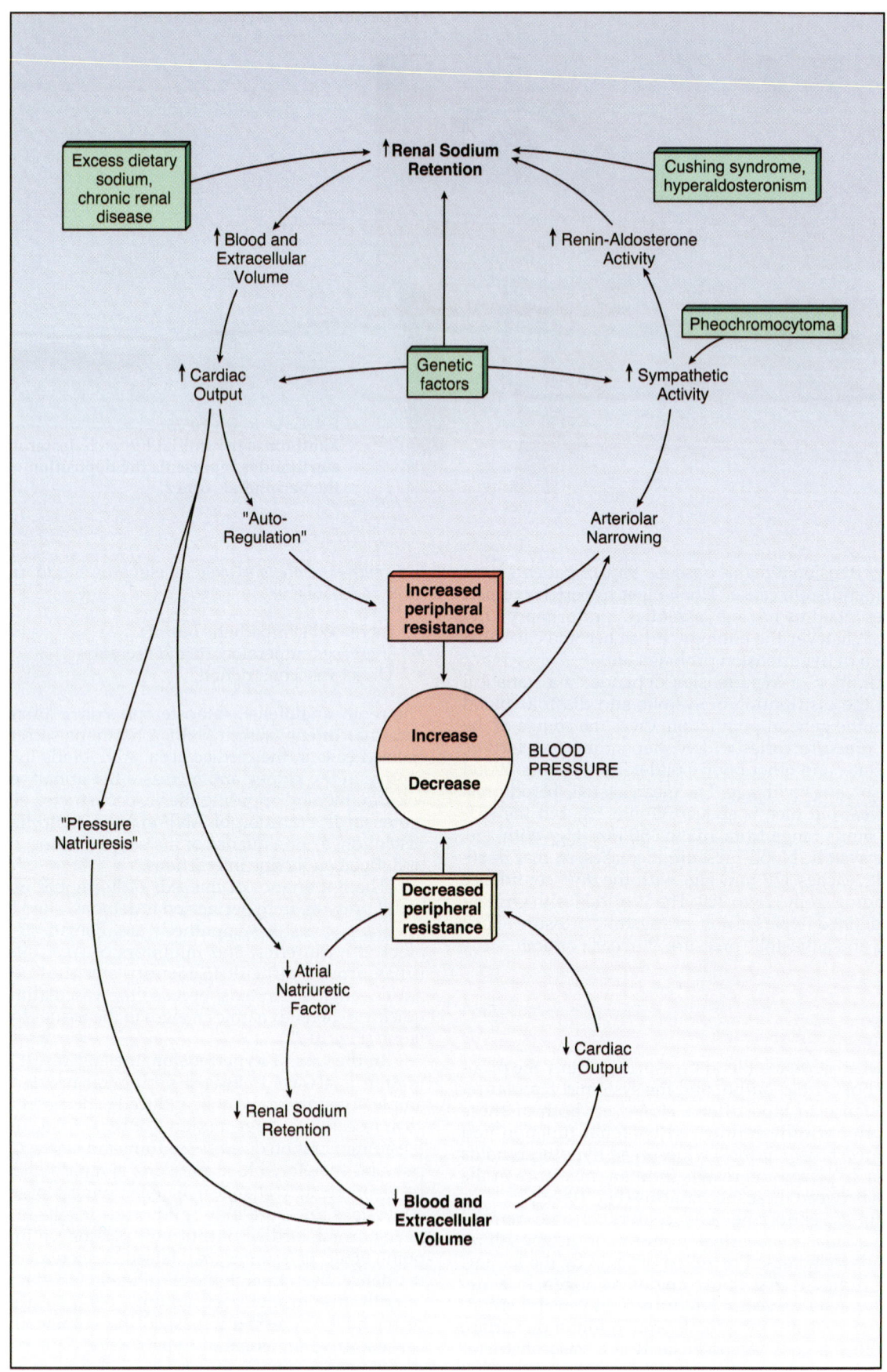

FIGURE 10-26
Factors contributing to hypertension and the counterregulatory factors that lower blood pressure. An imbalance in these factors results in the increased peripheral resistance that is responsible for most cases of essential (primary) hypertension. Note the central role of peripheral resistance.

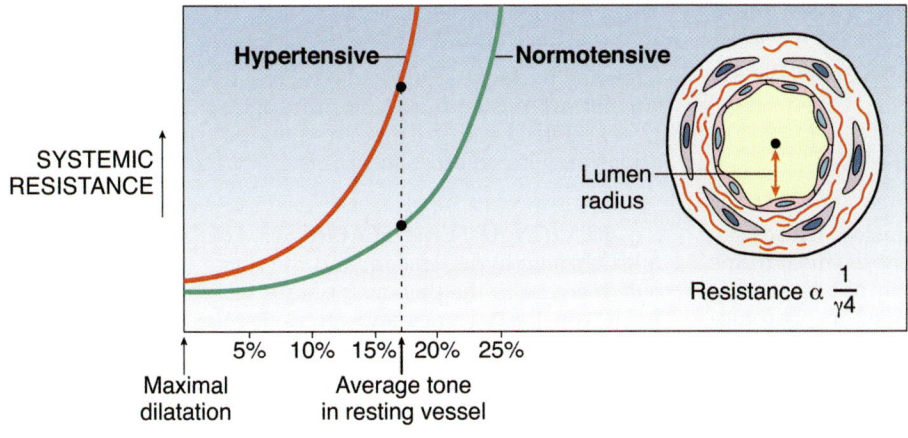

FIGURE 10-27
Structural autoregulation of blood pressure. Hypertension, regardless of its primary cause, increases the ability of the resistance vessel walls to respond to vasoactive stimuli. Resistance is increased even in maximally dilated vessels because the lumen size is decreased in the hypertensive vascular bed. As the smooth muscle cells contract, the increase in vessel wall thickness increases the resistance, which is inversely proportional to the fourth power of the radius of the lumen. Note that at the average resting muscular tone, the resistance in hypertensive persons is considerably higher than normal.

Molecular Genetics of Hypertension

We know from family and twin studies that genetic factors are likely to be important in the pathogenesis of essential hypertension. For example, there is a familial association of hypertension with alterations in the membrane transport of sodium (measured as lithium transport). Interestingly, spontaneous hypertension can be produced in rats in as few as six generations of inbreeding for elevated blood pressure. However, no specific genetic defect has been shown to be causal in rats or humans. The inheritance of essential hypertension is most likely polygenic and not due to single-gene conditions.

Although essential hypertension likely involves the interactions of a number of gene products, the study of rare mendelian forms of hypertension has provided a novel opportunity to identify candidate genes that may contribute to the control of blood pressure. Three hereditary forms of human hypertension have been defined in which a single gene mutation results in high blood pressure:

- **Glucocorticoid-remediable aldosteronism (GRA):** GRA is an autosomal dominant trait in which congenital hypertension is mediated by the mineralocorticoid receptor in the kidney. In this condition, the excess production of aldosterone is prompted by corticotropin (ACTH) rather than by the normal secretagogue for aldosterone, angiotensin II. The aldosterone synthase gene on chromosome 8 is normally expressed in the adrenal glomerulosa, where its product catalyzes the biosynthesis of aldosterone. This gene is 95% homologous with the steroid 11β-hydroxylase gene, which regulates the biosynthesis of cortisol in the adrenal fasciculata. Located in close proximity on the same chromosome, mutations in the aldosterone synthase and 11β-hydroxylase genes create a hybrid gene, with ectopic production of aldosterone in the zona fasciculata under the control of ACTH. In turn, the unrestrained secretion of mineralocorticoids leads to prolonged volume expansion and hypertension.
- **Syndrome of apparent mineralocorticoid excess (AME):** In this autosomal recessive form of early-onset hypertension, stimulation of the mineralocorticoid receptor is present in the face of very low levels of aldosterone. Under normal circumstances, the mineralocorticoid receptor responds not only to aldosterone but also to cortisol, albeit much more weakly. The aldosterone-like activity of cortisol is suppressed through its conversion to cortisone by 11β-hydroxysteroid dehydrogenase in the renal tubular epithelial cells. In AME, inactivating mutations in the gene for this enzyme allow cortisol to accumulate and constitutively stimulate the mineralocorticoid receptor. Interestingly, the consumption of large quantities of licorice can produce a syndrome similar to AME, and a substance in licorice (glycyrrhetinic acid) inhibits 11β-hydroxysteroid dehydrogenase.
- **Liddle syndrome:** Patients with this autosomal dominant form of hypertension exhibit low levels of mineralocorticoids but have a constitutively activated sodium channel in the renal tubule. The defect represents a "gain-of-function" mutation in the gene on chromosome 16 that codes for the amiloride-sensitive epithelial sodium channel. Sustained activation of the channel results in excessive renal reabsorption of salt and water independent of the action of mineralocorticoids, thereby leading to volume expansion and hypertension.

The mutations that cause hereditary hypertension all result in constitutively increased renal sodium reabsorption. Conversely, mutations that result in sodium wastage (pseudohypoaldosteronism type I and Gitelman syndrome) are associated with profound hypotension. Thus, these mendelian disorders illustrate the central role for sodium homeostasis in the control of blood pressure. It has been speculated that the sensitivity of human blood pressure to salt reflects the evolution of man in the salt-poor environment of sub-Saharan Africa. According to this scenario, mechanisms evolved to conserve total body sodium. However, with the salt-rich diet prevalent in industrialized countries, these adaptive mechanisms have become a liability and have led to an epidemic of hypertension.

Increasing evidence indicates that common polymorphisms of the angiotensinogen gene contribute to essential hypertension. Three findings buttress the potential importance of angiotensinogen variants: (1) the angiotensinogen locus shows linkage to elevated blood pressure in sibling pairs; (2) specific angiotensinogen variants have been linked to hypertension in case-control studies; and (3) the same variants are associated with increased levels of plasma angiotensinogen.

Acquired Causes of Hypertension

In a small proportion of cases of hypertension, causes are identifiable. These include renal artery stenosis, most forms of chronic renal disease, primary elevation of aldosterone levels (Conn syndrome), Cushing syndrome, pheochromocytoma, hyperthyroidism, coarctation of the aorta, and renin-secreting tumors. In addition, persons with severe atherosclerosis may have a high systolic pressure, because the sclerotic aorta cannot properly absorb the kinetic energy of the pulse wave.

Pathology: The central lesion in most cases of hypertension is a decrease in the caliber of the lumen of small muscular arteries and arterioles (Fig. 10-27). These resistance vessels control the flow of blood through the capillary bed. The lumen may be restricted by active contraction of the vessel wall, an increase in the structural mass of the vessel wall, or both. Structural changes in hypertension have been demonstrated by morphometric analysis of the arterial walls. Constriction of a structurally thicker vessel wall would be expected to produce an even more marked narrowing of the lumen than would occur with a normal thinner wall. The rapid drop in blood pressure after the treatment of hypertensive animals or persons with smooth muscle relaxants suggests that active constriction is very important.

Arteriosclerosis

Chronic hypertension leads to reactive changes in the smaller arteries and arterioles throughout the body, collectively referred to as *arteriosclerosis*. In the arterioles, the alterations are termed *arteriolosclerosis*.

BENIGN ARTERIOSCLEROSIS: This condition reflects mild chronic hypertension, and the major change is a variable increase in the thickness of arterial walls (Fig. 10-28A). In the smallest arteries and arterioles, these lesions are referred to as *hyaline arteriosclerosis and arteriolosclerosis*. "Hyaline" refers to the glassy, scarred appearance of the blood vessel walls as seen by light microscopy. The wall of the arteriole is thickened by the deposition of basement membrane material and by the accumulation of plasma proteins (Fig. 10-28B). The small muscular arteries display new layers of elastin, manifesting as reduplication of the intimal elastic lamina, and increased connective tissue. The vascular lesions of benign arteriosclerosis are particularly evident in the kidney, where they result in loss of renal parenchyma, termed *benign nephrosclerosis* (see Chapter 17).

The finding of benign arteriosclerosis is not diagnostic of hypertension, since comparable morphological alterations commonly occur as part of the aging process. However, hyaline arteriosclerosis is accelerated in diabetes and in hypertension, diseases that are also associated with accelerated atherosclerosis.

MALIGNANT (ACCELERATED) HYPERTENSION: This term refers to a situation in which elevated blood pressure results in rapidly progressive vascular compromise, with the onset of symptomatic disease of the brain, heart, or kidney. Although malignant hypertension cannot be defined strictly by the degree of blood pressure elevation, it is ordinarily not evident with pressures below 160/110 mm Hg.

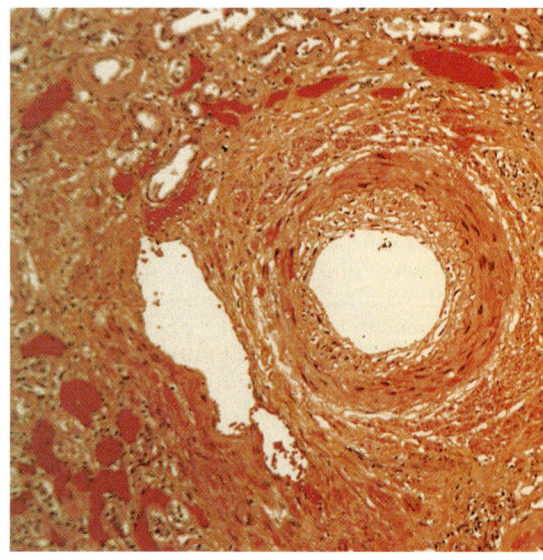
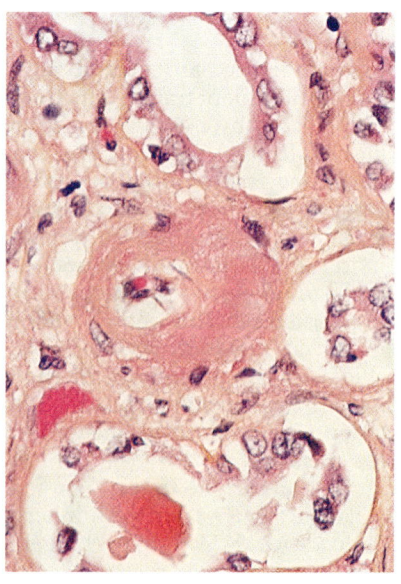

FIGURE *10-28*
Benign arteriosclerosis. A. A cross-section of a renal intralobular shows irregular thickening of the intima. B. A renal arteriole exhibits hyalin arteriolosclerosis.

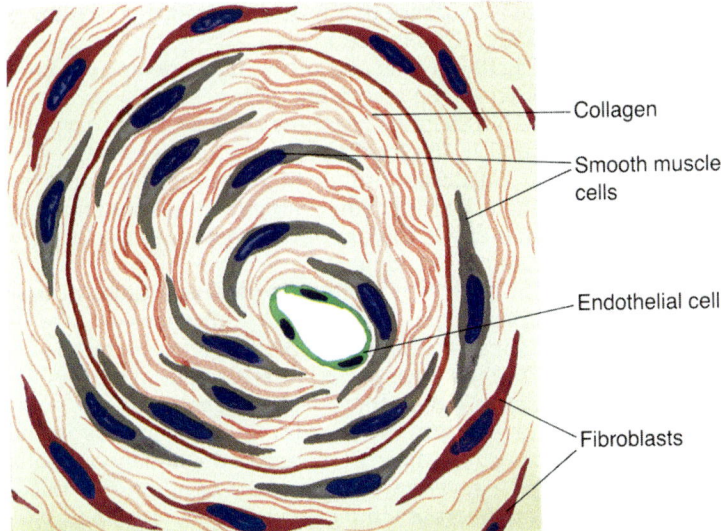

FIGURE 10-29
Arteriolosclerosis. In cases of hypertension, the arterioles exhibit smooth muscle cell proliferation and increased amounts of intercellular collagen and glycosaminoglycans, resulting in an "onion-skin" appearance. The mass of smooth muscle and associated elements tends to fix the size of the lumen and restrict the arteriole's capacity to dilate.

Modern antihypertensive therapy has made malignant hypertension a rare disorder.

The morphological changes associated with moderate elevations of blood pressure are often too subtle to be detected by simple histological studies. On the other hand, severe or malignant hypertension produces dramatic changes, particularly at the microvascular level. Segmental constriction and dilation of the retinal arterioles in severely hypertensive persons are sufficiently prominent to allow the diagnosis of hypertension by ophthalmoscopy. If the blood pressure rises rapidly, the retinal arterioles cannot resist the increased pressure, and microaneurysms, focal hemorrhages, and scarring of the retina result. Ischemic necrosis and edema of the retina are visible with the ophthalmoscope as "cotton wool spots" (see Chapter 29). These retinal changes are typical of those in other resistance vessels when the pressure rises rapidly.

In malignant hypertension, small muscular arteries show segmental dilation as a result of necrosis of smooth muscle cells. Endothelial integrity is lost in these regions, and the increase in vascular permeability leads to the entry of plasma proteins into the vessel wall, the deposition of fibrin, and an appearance termed *fibrinoid necrosis*. The period of acute injury is rapidly followed by smooth muscle proliferation and a striking concentric increase in the number of layers of smooth muscle cells, which yields the so-called onion-skin appearance (Fig. 10-29). This form of smooth muscle proliferation may be a response to the release of growth factors derived from platelets and other cells at the sites of vascular injury. Taken together, these changes are labeled *malignant arteriosclerosis or arteriolosclerosis*, depending on the size of the vessels affected. In the kidney, the lesions of malignant hypertension are known as *malignant nephrosclerosis*.

MONCKEBERG MEDIAL SCLEROSIS

Mönckeberg medial sclerosis refers to degenerative calcification of the media of large and medium-sized muscular arteries. The disorder occurs principally in older persons and most often involve the arteries of the upper and lower extremities.

 Pathology: On gross examination, the involved arteries are hard and dilated. Microscopically, the smooth muscle of the media is focally replaced by pale-staining, acellular, hyalinized fibrous tissue, which exhibits concentric dystrophic calcification. Osseous metaplasia in calcified areas is occasionally observed. Mönckeberg medial sclerosis is distinct from atherosclerosis and ordinarily does not lead to any clinical disorder.

RAYNAUD PHENOMENON

Raynaud phenomenon refers to intermittent, bilateral attacks of ischemia of the fingers or toes and sometimes of the ears or nose. It is characterized by severe pallor (Fig. 10-30) and is often accompanied by paresthesias and pain. The symptoms are precipitated by cold or emotional stimuli and relieved by heat.

Raynaud phenomenon may occur as an isolated disorder or as a prominent feature of a number of systemic diseases of connective tissue (collagen vascular disorders), particularly scleroderma and systemic lupus erythematosus. The entity includes primary and secondary cold sensitivity, livedo reticularis, and acrocyanosis. Whatever the cause, Raynaud phenomenon represents arterial vasospasm in the skin.

Primary cold sensitivity of the Raynaud type is more common in women, often starting in the late teens. It is bilateral and symmetric and, on rare occasions, may lead to ulcers or gangrene of the tips of the digits. The hands are more commonly affected than the feet.

FIBROMUSCULAR DYSPLASIA

Fibromuscular dysplasia is a rare, noninflammatory thickening of large and medium-sized muscular arteries, which is distinct from atherosclerosis and arteriosclerosis. The cause is unknown. In the

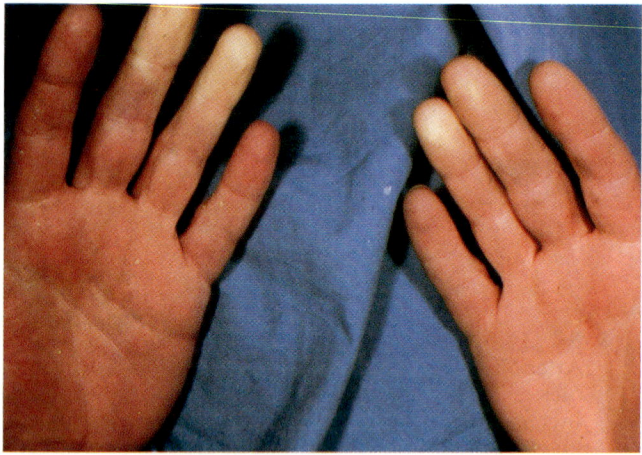

FIGURE 10-30
Raynaud phenomenon. The tips of the fingers show marked pallor.

renal arteries, the stenosis produced by this condition is an important cause of renovascular hypertension, although the disorder may affect almost any other vessel, including the carotid, vertebral, and splanchnic arteries. Fibromuscular dysplasia is typically a disease of women during their reproductive years, but it can appear at any age, even in childhood.

Pathology: In most cases, the distal two thirds of the renal artery and its primary branches display several segmental stenoses, which represent fibrous and muscular ridges that project into the lumen. Microscopically, these segments exhibit a disorderly arrangement and proliferation of the cellular elements of the vessel wall, without necrosis or inflammation. Smooth muscle is replaced by fibrous tissue and myofibroblasts. In some cases, intimal fibroplasia predominates, and in unusual instances, connective tissue encircles the adventitia. Other than renal hypertension, the major complication of fibromuscular dysplasia is dissecting aneurysm of the affected arteries.

VASCULITIS

Vasculitis refers to inflammation and necrosis of blood vessels, including arteries, veins, and capillaries (Table 10-9). Arteries or veins may be damaged by immune mechanisms, infectious agents, mechanical trauma, radiation, or toxins. However, in many cases of vasculitis, no specific cause is determined.

Pathogenesis: Vasculitic syndromes are thought to involve immune mechanisms, including (1) the deposition of immune complexes, (2) a direct attack on the vessels by circulating antibodies, and (3) various forms of cell-mediated immunity. Although the agents responsible for inciting the immune reaction are largely unknown, there is evidence that in some instances vasculitis is associated with a viral infection.

Serum sickness was one of the first human immunological disorders to be associated with vasculitis. In animal models of serum sickness, immune complexes and complement are found in the local tissue reaction (see Chapter 4). However, in most cases of human vasculitis, the search for immune complexes has yielded variable results, and firm evidence for immune complexes in the pathogenesis of most cases of vasculitis is lacking.

Viral antigens have been suspected as a cause of vasculitis in experimental animals and in humans. A case in point is chronic infection with hepatitis B virus, which is associated with some cases of polyarteritis nodosa. In this circumstance, both circulating viral antigen–antibody complexes and deposition of these immune complexes in the vascular lesions have been demonstrated. Human vasculitis has also been associated with a variety of other viral infections, including herpes simplex, cytomegalovirus, and parvovirus. In addition, several bacterial antigens have been identified in the lesions of some patients with vasculitis.

Small vessel vasculitides (e.g., Wegener granulomatosis and microscopic polyarteritis; see below) are associated with antineutrophil cytoplasmic antibodies (ANCA), but the contribution of these autoantibodies to the pathogenesis of the vasculitis is not understood. ANCA may cause endothelial damage by activating neutrophils, and antibody titers correlate with disease activity in some cases. ANCA is detected by indirect immunofluorescence assays using the patient's serum and ethanol-fixed neutrophils. Common patterns include a perinuclear immunofluorescence (P-ANCA, mainly against myeloperoxidase) and a more general cytoplasmic immunofluorescence (C-ANCA, mainly against proteinase 3). Although the significance of ANCA requires further study, myeloperoxidase and proteinase 3 are expressed on the surface of neutrophils activated by cytokines in vitro, which then leads to degranulation.

TABLE 10-9 **Inflammatory Disorders of Blood Vessels**

Polyarteritis nodosa group of systemic necrotizing vasculitis
   Classic polyarteritis nodosa
     Allergic angiitis and granulomatosis (Churg-Strauss variant)
     "Overlap syndrome" of systemic angiitis
Hypersensitivity vasculitis
   Serum sickness and similar reactions
   Henoch-Schönlein purpura
   Vasculitis associated with connective tissue disorders
   Vasculitis in cases of essential mixed cryoglobulinemia
   Vasculitis associated with other primary disorders
Wegener granulomatosis
Lymphomatoid granulomatosis
Giant cell arteritis
   Temporal arteritis
   Takayasu arteritis
Central nervous system vasculitis
Vasculitis associated with cancer
Mucocutaneous lymph node syndrome (Kawasaki disease)
Thromboangiitis obliterans (Buerger disease)
Behçet disease
Miscellaneous vasculitis syndromes

Polyarteritis Nodosa Is an Acute, Necrotizing Vasculitis

Polyarteritis nodosa affects medium-sized and smaller muscular arteries, and occasionally larger arteries. It is somewhat more common in men than in women. The disease was regarded as a rarity until the 1940s, when there was a striking rise in its incidence. The increased frequency of polyarteritis nodosa at that time seemed to be associated with the widespread use of antisera to bacteria and toxins produced in animals and with the administration of sulfonamides. The incidence of polyarteritis nodosa now seems to be subsiding.

 Pathology: The characteristic lesions of polyarteritis nodosa are found in small to medium-sized muscular arteries and are distributed in a patchy manner. However, on occasion they extend into larger arteries, such as the renal, splenic, or coronary arteries. Each lesion is no more than a millimeter long and may involve the entire circumference of the vessel or only a part of it. The most prominent morphological feature of the affected artery is an area of fibrinoid necrosis, in which the medial muscle and adjacent tissues are fused into a structureless eosinophilic mass that stains for fibrin. A vigorous acute inflammatory response envelops the area of necrosis, usually involving the entire adventitia (periarteritis), and extends through the other coats of the vessel (Fig. 10-31). Neutrophils, lymphocytes, plasma cells, and macrophages are present in varying proportions, and eosinophils are often conspicuous. Polyarteritis nodosa affecting small vessels is frequently associated with the presence of P-ANCA (see below).

As a result of thrombosis in the affected segment of an artery, infarcts are commonly found in the involved organs. Injury to larger arteries results in the formation of small aneurysms (<0.5 cm in diameter), particularly in branches of the renal, coronary, and cerebral arteries. An aneurysm may rupture and, if located in a critical area, may be the source of fatal hemorrhage.

If the patient survives for some months, many of the vascular lesions will show evidence of healing, especially if corticosteroids have been administered. The necrotic tissue and inflammatory exudate are resorbed, and the vessel is left with fibrosis of the media and conspicuous gaps in the elastic laminae.

Clinical Features: The clinical manifestations of polyarteritis nodosa are highly variable, depending on the chance occurrence of lesions in different organs. The kidneys, heart, skeletal muscle, skin, and mesentery are most frequently involved, but lesions may occur in almost any organ of the body, including the bowel, pancreas, lungs, liver, and brain. Constitutional symptoms such as fever and weight loss are common.

Without treatment, polyarteritis nodosa is usually fatal, but antiinflammatory and immunosuppressive therapy, in the form of corticosteroids and cyclophosphamide, leads to remissions or cures in most patients.

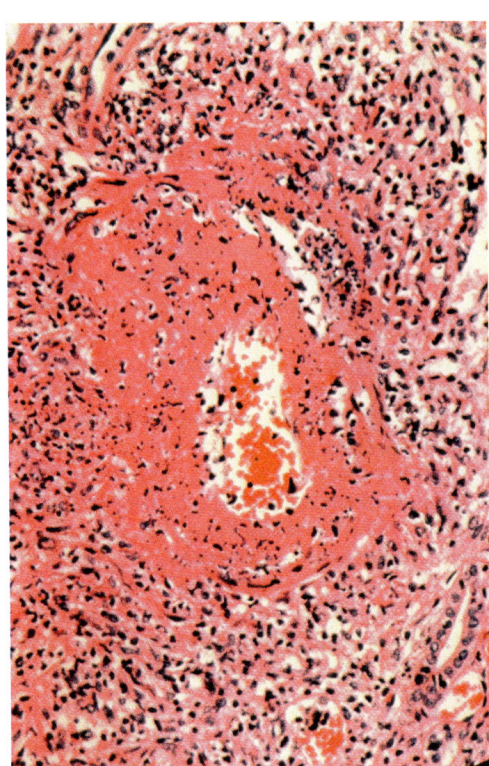

FIGURE 10-31
Polyarteritis nodosa. The intense inflammatory cell infiltrate in the arterial wall and surrounding connective tissue is associated with fibrinoid necrosis and disruption of the vessel wall.

Hypersensitivity Angiitis Is a Response to Exogenous Substances

Hypersensitivity angiitis refers to a broad category of inflammatory vascular lesions that are thought to represent a reaction to foreign materials (e.g. bacterial products or drugs). In the case of vascular lesions confined predominantly to the skin, the terms *leukocytoclastic vasculitis* (referring to the nuclear debris from disintegrating neutrophils), *cutaneous vasculitis*, or *cutaneous necrotizing venulitis* (emphasizing the predominant involvement of the venules) are applied. *Systemic hypersensitivity angiitis*, also referred to as *microscopic polyarteritis*, affects many of the same organs as polyarteritis nodosa but is restricted to the smallest arteries and arterioles.

 Clinical Features: Cutaneous vasculitis may follow the administration of a wide variety of drugs, including aspirin, penicillin, and thiazide diuretics. It is also commonly related to disparate infections such as streptococcal and staphylococcal illnesses, viral hepatitis, tuberculosis, and bacterial endocarditis. The disease typically presents as palpable purpura, principally on the lower extremities. Microscopically, the superficial cutaneous venules display fibrinoid necrosis and an acute inflammatory reaction. Cutaneous vasculitis is generally self-limited. A detailed description of cutaneous necrotizing venulitis is found in Chapter 24.

Systemic hypersensitivity angiitis may be an isolated entity or a feature of other conditions, including collagen vascular diseases (lupus erythematosus, rheumatoid arthritis, Sjögren syndrome), Henoch-Schönlein purpura, dysproteinemias, and a variety of malignant neoplasms. Patients with systemic hypersensitivity angiitis may also exhibit purpuric lesions in the skin. The most feared complication of microscopic polyarteritis is renal involvement, characterized by rapidly progressive glomerulonephritis and renal failure (see Chapter 16). Microscopic polyarteritis is strongly associated with the presence of ANCA (60% P-ANCA and 40% C-ANCA).

Allergic Granulomatosis and Angiitis (Churg-Strauss Syndrome) Features Eosinophilia

Churg-Strauss syndrome is a systemic vasculitis that occurs in young persons with asthma. Two thirds of patients exhibit C-ANCA or P-ANCA.

Pathology: Widespread necrotizing vascular lesions of the small and medium-sized arteries (Fig. 10-32), arterioles, and veins are found in the lungs, spleen, kidney, heart, liver, central nervous system, and other organs. The lesions are characterized by granulomas and an intense eosinophilic infiltrate in and around blood vessels. The resulting fibrinoid necrosis, thrombosis, and aneurysm formation may simulate polyarteritis nodosa, although Churg-Strauss syndrome seems to be a distinct entity. The disease must also be distinguished from other eosinophilic syndromes, such as parasitic and fungal infestations, Wegener granulomatosis, eosinophilic pneumonia (Loeffler syndrome), and drug vasculitis.

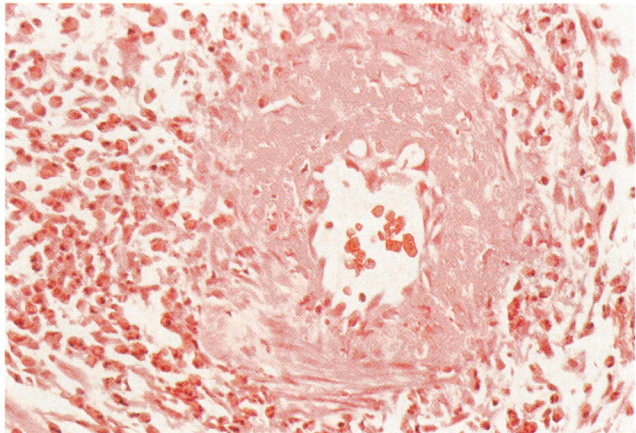

FIGURE 10-32
Churg-Strauss syndrome. A medium-sized artery shows fibrinoid necrosis and a surrounding eosinophilic infiltrate.

Untreated persons with allergic granulomatosis and angiitis have a poor prognosis, but corticosteroids are now almost always successful in the treatment of the disease.

Giant Cell Arteritis (Temporal Arteritis, Granulomatous Arteritis) Is the Most Common Vasculitis

Giant cell arteritis describes a focal, chronic, granulomatous inflammation of the temporal arteries. Although the disease most often affects the temporal artery, it can also involve additional cranial arteries, the aorta (giant cell aortitis) and its branches, and occasionally other arteries. The average age at onset is 70 years, and the disease rarely occurs in those younger than age 50. The incidence rises with age and may reach 1% by 80 years of age. Women are affected slightly more often than men. The age at onset helps differentiate this entity from other vasculitides that may affect the same vessels, such as Takayasu disease, which occurs in much younger persons.

Pathogenesis: The etiology of giant cell arteritis is obscure. The association of this disease with HLA-DR4 and its occurrence in first-degree relatives support a genetic component in its pathogenesis. The morphological alterations, including the presence of activated $CD4^+$ T-helper cells and association with a specific polymorphism of the leukocyte adhesion molecule ICAM-1, suggest an immunological reaction. The generalized muscle aching and widespread distribution of its manifestations are consistent with a relationship to rheumatoid diseases.

Pathology: In giant cell arteritis, the affected vessel is cordlike and exhibits nodular thickening. The lumen is reduced to a slit or may be obliterated by a thrombus. Microscopic examination reveals granulomatous inflammation of the media and intima, consisting of aggregates of macrophages, lymphocytes and plasma cells, with varying admixtures of eosinophils and neutrophils (Fig. 10-33A). Giant cells tend to be distributed at the site of the internal elastic lamina (Fig. 10-33B) but vary widely in number. Both foreign-body giant cells and Langhans giant cells may be found. Foci of necrosis are characterized by changes in the internal elastica, which becomes swollen, irregular, and fragmented, and in advanced lesions may completely disappear. Fragments of the elastica occasionally appear in the giant cells. In the late stages, the intima is conspicuously thickened, and the media is fibrotic. Thrombosis may obliterate the lumen, after which organization and canalization occur.

Clinical Features: Giant cell arteritis tends to be benign and self-limited, with the symptoms subsiding in 6 to 12 months. Patients present with headache and throbbing temporal pain. In some instances, there are early constitutional symptoms, including malaise, fever, and weight loss, accompanied by generalized muscular aching or stiffness in the shoulders and hips. The throb-

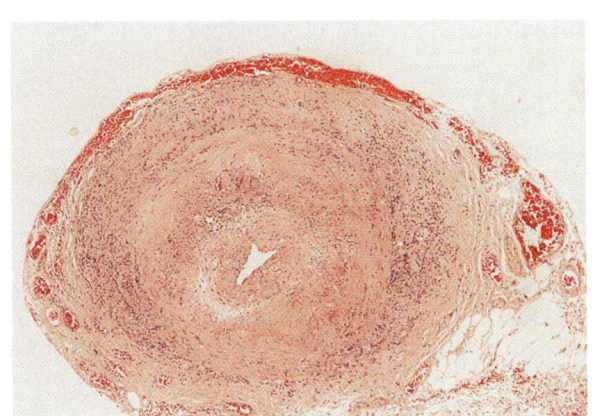
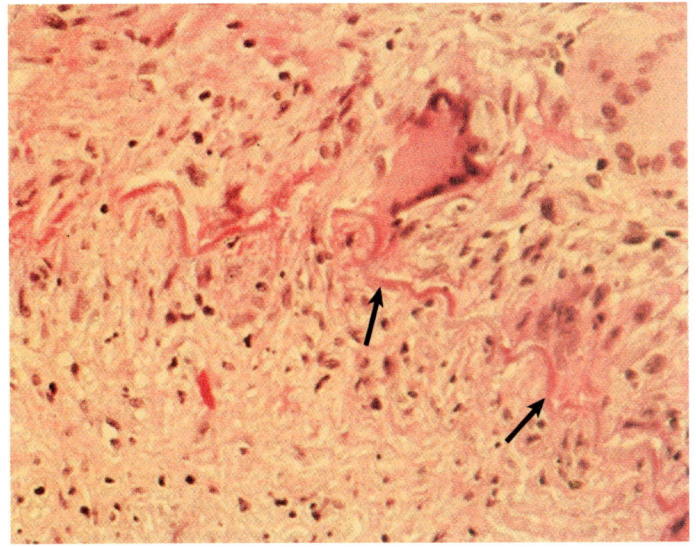

FIGURE 10-33
Temporal arteritis. A. A photomicrograph of a temporal artery shows chronic inflammation throughout the wall, giant cells, and a lumen severely narrowed by intimal thickening. B. A high-power view shows giant cells adjacent to the fragmented internal elastic lamina *(arrows)*.

bing and pain over the temporal artery are accompanied by swelling, tenderness, and redness in the skin overlying the vessel. Visual symptoms occur in almost half of patients and may proceed from transient to permanent blindness in one or both eyes. In an occasional patient, the disease gives rise to infarcts in the myocardium, brain, or gastrointestinal tract, which may be fatal. Biopsy of the temporal artery may not disclose the disease in as many as 40% of patients with otherwise classic manifestations. The response to corticosteroid therapy is usually dramatic, with symptoms subsiding in a matter of days.

Wegener Granulomatosis Is a Vasculitis of the Respiratory Tract and Kidney

Wegener granulomatosis is a systemic necrotizing vasculitis of unknown etiology characterized by granulomatous lesions of the nose, sinuses, and lungs and renal glomerular disease. Men are affected more often than women, usually in the fifth and sixth decades of life. The etiology of the disease is unknown, and no infectious agent has been uncovered. More than 90% of patients with Wegener granulomatosis exhibit ANCA in the blood, of whom 75% have C-ANCA. It has been suggested that these antibodies activate circulating neutrophils to attack blood vessels. The response to immunosuppressive therapy supports an immunological basis for the disease.

Pathology: The lesions of Wegener granulomatosis feature parenchymal necrosis, vasculitis, and a granulomatous inflammation composed of neutrophils, lymphocytes, plasma cells, macrophages, and eosinophils. The individual lesions in the lung may be as large as 5 cm across and must be distinguished from those of tuberculosis. Vasculitis involving small arteries and veins may be found anywhere but occurs most frequently in the respiratory tract (Fig. 10-34), kidney, and spleen. The arteritis is char-

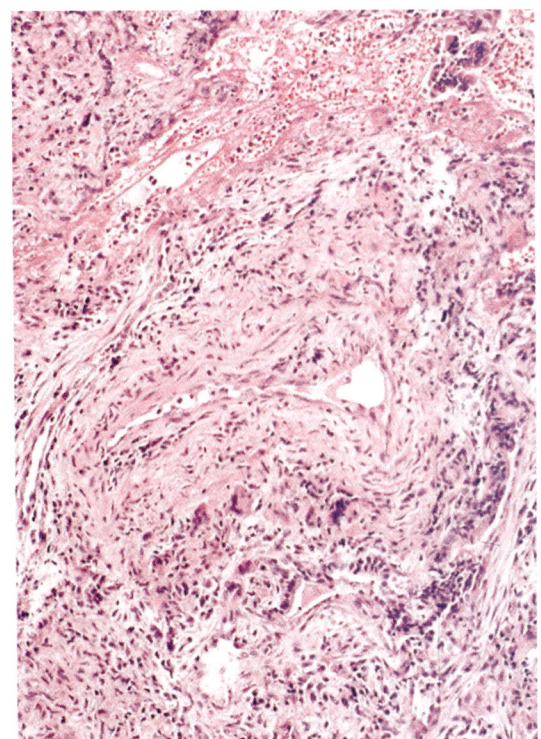

FIGURE 10-34
Wegener granulomatosis. A photomicrograph of the lung shows vasculitis of a pulmonary artery. There are chronic inflammatory cells and Langhans giant cells in the wall, together with thickening of the intima.

acterized principally by chronic inflammation, although acute inflammation, necrotizing and nonnecrotizing granulomatous inflammation, and fibrinoid necrosis are frequently present. Medial thickening and intimal proliferation are common and often result in narrowing or obliteration of the lumen.

The most prominent pulmonary feature is a persistent bilateral pneumonitis, with nodular infiltrates that undergo cavitation in a manner similar to that of tuberculous lesions (although the mechanisms are clearly different). Chronic sinusitis and ulcerations of the nasopharyngeal mucosa are common. The kidney initially exhibits focal necrotizing glomerulonephritis, which progresses to crescentic glomerulonephritis (see Chapter 17).

Clinical Features: Most patients with Wegener granulomatosis present with symptoms referable to the respiratory tract, particularly pneumonitis and sinusitis. In fact, the lung is eventually involved in over 90% of patients. Radiologically, multiple pulmonary infiltrates, which are often cavitary, are prominent. Hematuria and proteinuria are common, and the glomerular disease can progress to renal failure. Rash, muscular pains, joint involvement, and neurological symptoms occur. In untreated Wegener granulomatosis, most persons (80%) die within a year of onset, with a mean survival of 5 to 6 months. Treatment with cyclophosphamide produces a striking improvement in the prognosis, and both complete remissions and substantial disease-free intervals are induced in most patients. Interestingly, the administration of antimicrobial sulfa drugs significantly reduces the incidence of relapses, suggesting a relationship of the disease to bacterial infections.

Takayasu Arteritis Affects the Aorta

Takayasu arteritis refers to an inflammatory disorder of large arteries, classically the aortic arch and its major branches. The malady has a worldwide distribution and primarily affects young women (90%), most of whom are younger than 30 years of age. The cause of Takayasu arteritis is unknown, but an autoimmune basis has been proposed.

Pathology: Takayasu arteritis is classified according to the extent of aortic involvement: (1) disease restricted to the aortic arch and its branches, (2) arteritis involving only the descending thoracic and abdominal aorta and its branches, and (3) combined involvement of the arch and descending aorta. The pulmonary artery is also occasionally affected, and involvement of the retinal vasculature is often a prominent feature.

On gross examination, the aorta is thickened, and the intima exhibits focal, raised plaques. The branches of the aorta often display localized stenosis or occlusion, which interferes with blood flow and accounts for the synonym *"pulseless disease"* when the subclavian arteries are affected. The aorta, particularly the distal thoracic and abdominal segments, commonly shows variably sized aneurysms. The early lesions of the aorta and its main branches consist of an acute panarteritis, with infiltrates of neutrophils, mononuclear cells, and occasional Langhans giant cells. Inflammation of the vasa vasorum in Takayasu arteritis requires differentiation from syphilitic aortitis. Late lesions display fibrosis and severe intimal proliferation, and secondary atherosclerotic changes may obscure the basic disease.

Clinical Features: Patients with early Takayasu arteritis complain of constitutional symptoms, dizziness, visual disturbances, dyspnea, and occasionally syncope. As the disease progresses, cardiac symptoms become more severe, and intermittent claudication of the arms or legs appears. Asymmetric differences in blood pressure may develop, and the pulse in one extremity may actually disappear. Hypertension may reflect coarctation of the aorta or renal artery stenosis. Most patients eventually manifest congestive heart failure or loss of visual acuity, ranging from field defects to total blindness. Early Takayasu arteritis responds to corticosteroids, but the later lesions require surgical reconstruction.

Kawasaki Disease (Mucocutaneous Lymph Node Syndrome) Is a Childhood Vasculitis That Targets Coronary Arteries

Kawasaki disease is an acute necrotizing vasculitis of infancy and early childhood characterized by high fever, rash, conjunctival and oral lesions, and lymphadenitis. In 70% of patients, the vasculitis affects the coronary arteries and leads to the formation of coronary artery aneurysms (Fig. 10-35). Such lesions are the cause of death in 1 to 2% of cases.

Pathogenesis: Kawasaki disease is usually self-limited, and although an infectious cause has been sought, none has been conclusively proved. Infection with parvovirus B19 has been implicated in some cases, and there is evidence for various bacterial infections in others. The common theme seems to be viral or bacterial production of superantigens, molecules that bind to MHC class II receptors and the V-beta region of the T-cell receptor, thereby overstimulating the immune system. Autoantibodies to both endothelial and smooth muscle cells have been identified in some patients.

Thromboangiitis Obliterans (Buerger Disease) Features Peripheral Vascular Disease in Smokers

Thromboangiitis obliterans defines an occlusive inflammatory disease of the medium and small arteries in the distal arms and legs. At one time Buerger disease occurred almost exclusively in

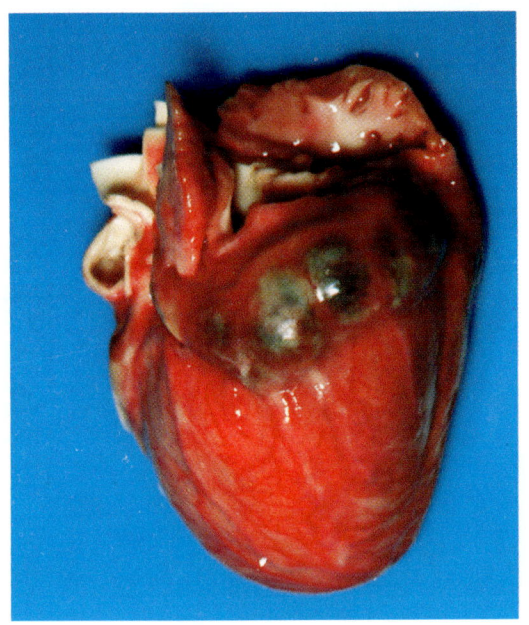
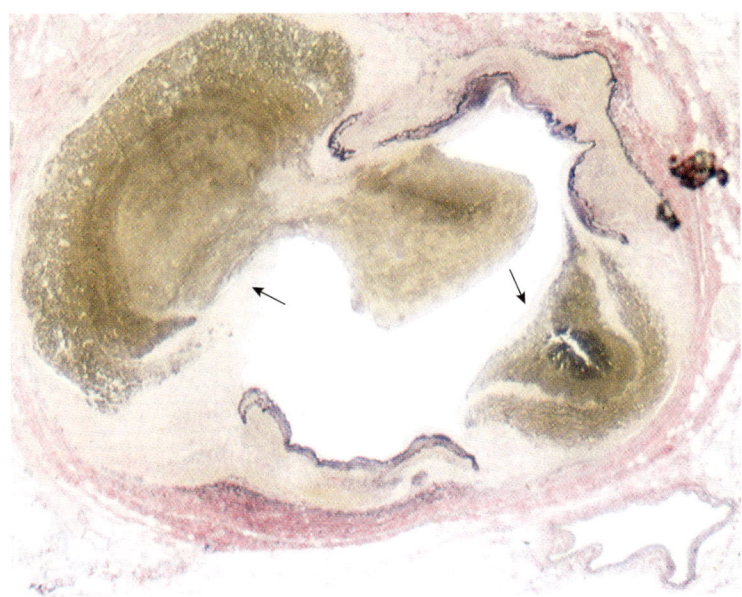

FIGURE 10-35
Kawasaki disease. A. The heart of a child who died from Kawasaki disease shows conspicuous coronary artery aneurysms. B. A microscopic section of a coronary artery from the same patient shows two large defects *(arrows)* in the internal elastic lamina, with two small aneurysms filled with thrombus.

young and middle-aged men who smoked heavily, but it is now described in women as well.

 Pathogenesis: The etiological role of smoking in Buerger disease is emphasized by the observation that cessation of smoking can be followed by a remission, and resumption of smoking by an exacerbation. Yet the mechanism of action of tobacco smoke is obscure. Interestingly, certain polyphenols from tobacco elicit antibodies and can induce inflammation. Smokers show a higher incidence of such sensitivity to tobacco than do nonsmokers. Cell-mediated hypersensitivity to collagen types II and III has also been observed. Endothelium-dependent vasodilatory responses in nondiseased blood vessels are dysfunctional in some patients, suggesting that there may be a generalized impairment of endothelial function.

Although at one time the disorder was common in Jewish men in Eastern Europe and their immigrant counterparts in the United States, Buerger disease is now rare in both locations. Its greater frequency in Japan, Israel, and India suggests possible predisposing genetic factors. An increased prevalence of HLA-A9 and HLA-B5 haplotypes among patients with the disease lends further credence to the idea that a genetically controlled hypersensitivity to tobacco is involved in the pathogenesis of disease.

 Pathology: The earliest change in Buerger disease is an acute inflammation of medium-sized and small arteries. The neutrophilic infiltrate extends to involve neighboring veins and nerves. The involvement of the endothelium in the inflamed areas leads to thrombosis and obliteration of the lumen (Fig. 10-36A). Small microabscesses of the vessel wall, featuring a central area of neutrophils surrounded by fibroblasts and Langhans giant cells, distinguish the process from thrombosis associated with atherosclerosis. The early lesions often become severe enough to result in gangrene of the extremity, for which the only treatment is amputation. Late in the course of the disease, the thrombi are completely organized and partly canalized.

 Clinical Features: The symptoms of Buerger disease usually start between the ages of 25 and 40 years and take the form of intermittent claudication (cramping pains in muscles following exercise, which are quickly relieved by rest). Patients often present with painful ulceration of a digit, which can progresses to destruction of the tips of the involved digits (Fig. 10-36B). Persons with Buerger disease who continue to smoke may slowly lose both hands and feet.

Behçet Disease Is a Widespread Vasculitis of Many Organs

Behçet disease is a systemic vasculitis characterized by oral aphthous ulcers, genital ulceration, and ocular inflammation and occasionally lesions in the central nervous system, the gastrointestinal tract, and the cardiovascular system. Both large and small vessels display vasculitis. The mucocutaneous lesions show a nonspecific vasculitis of arterioles, capillaries, and venules,

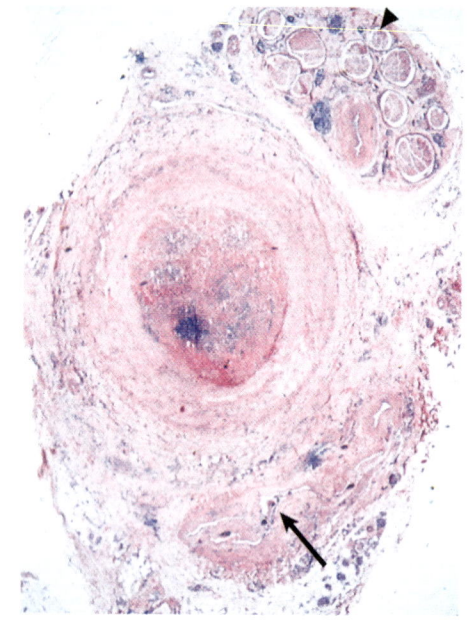
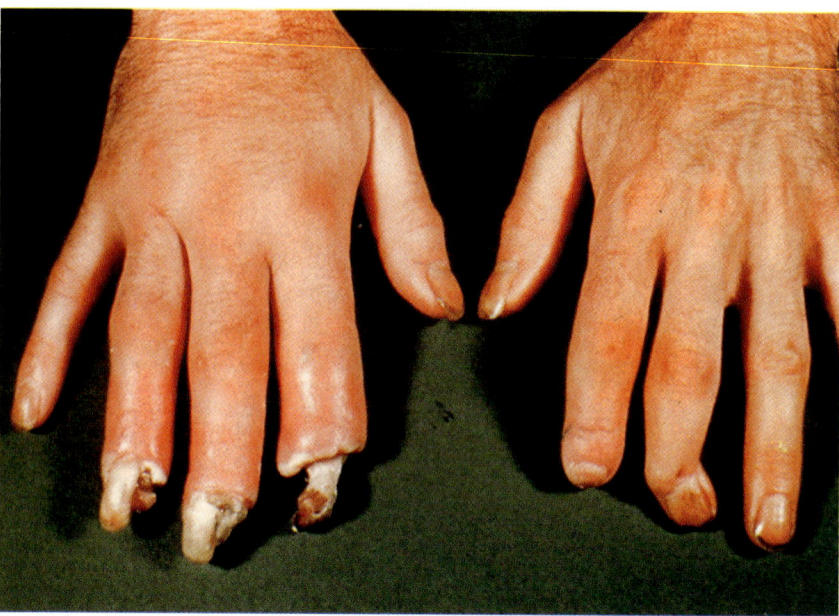

FIGURE 10-36
Buerger disease. A. Section of the upper extremity shows an organized arterial thrombus that has occluded the lumen. Some inflammatory cells are evident in the adventitial fat. In this instance, the vein *(arrow)* and the adjacent nerve *(arrowhead)* show foci of chronic inflammation. B. The hand shows necrosis of the tips of the fingers.

characterized by infiltration of the walls and perivascular tissue by lymphocytes and plasma cells. Occasional endothelial cells are proliferated and swollen. Medium- sized and large arteries disclose destructive arteritis, with fibrinoid necrosis, mononuclear infiltration, thrombosis, aneurysms, and hemorrhage. The cause of Behçet syndrome is unknown, but an association with specific HLA subtypes suggests an immune basis. The disease often responds to corticosteroids.

Radiation Vasculitis Presents an Acute and a Chronic Phase

The acute phase of radiation vasculitis shows endothelial injury and denudation, ballooning degeneration of intimal smooth muscle cells and macrophages, and medial smooth muscle cell necrosis, which may be fibrinoid. Thrombosis may be present in small arteries and arterioles. In the chronic phase, intimal hyperplasia and fibrosis of the vessel wall are noted. Occasionally the vessel shows complete fibrous occlusion. Radiation damage predisposes to accelerated atherosclerosis.

Rickettsial Vasculitis Is Caused by Intracellular Parasites

Rickettsiae are obligate intracellular parasites that produce a characteristic vasculitis. The vasculitis in each of the different rickettsial diseases affects different types of small vessels, and its extent and severity varies. In general, the organisms disseminate from the entry site into the bloodstream and invade endothelial cells, smooth muscle cells of the media of small vessels, and capillaries. These infections are discussed in detail in Chapter 9.

ANEURYSMS

Arterial aneurysms are localized dilations of blood vessels caused by a congenital or acquired weakness in the media. They are not rare, and their incidence tends to rise with age. Aneurysms of the aorta and other arteries are found in as many as 10% of autopsies. The wall of an aneurysm is formed by the stretched remnants of the arterial wall.

Aneurysms are classified by location, configuration, and etiology (Fig. 10-37). The location refers to the type of vessel involved—artery or vein—and the specific vessel affected, such as the aorta or popliteal artery. The gross morphology of aneurysms reveals several different pathological features.

- **A fusiform aneurysm** is an ovoid swelling parallel to the long axis of the vessel.
- **A saccular aneurysm** is a bubblelike outpouching of the arterial wall at the site of a weakened media.
- **A dissecting aneurysm** is actually a dissecting hematoma, in which hemorrhage into the media separates the layers of the vascular wall by a column of blood.
- **An arteriovenous aneurysm** is a direct communication between an artery and a vein.

Abdominal Aortic Aneurysms Are Complications of Atherosclerosis

An aneurysm of the abdominal aorta is defined as a dilation of the vessel in which its diameter is increased at least 50%. They are the most frequent aneurysms, usually developing after the age of 50 years, and are associated with severe atherosclerosis of the artery, with a prevalence rising to 6% after the age of 80 years. Aortic aneurysms occur much more often in men than in women, and half of patients are hypertensive. Occasion-

Aneurysms

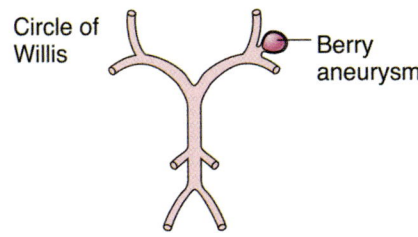

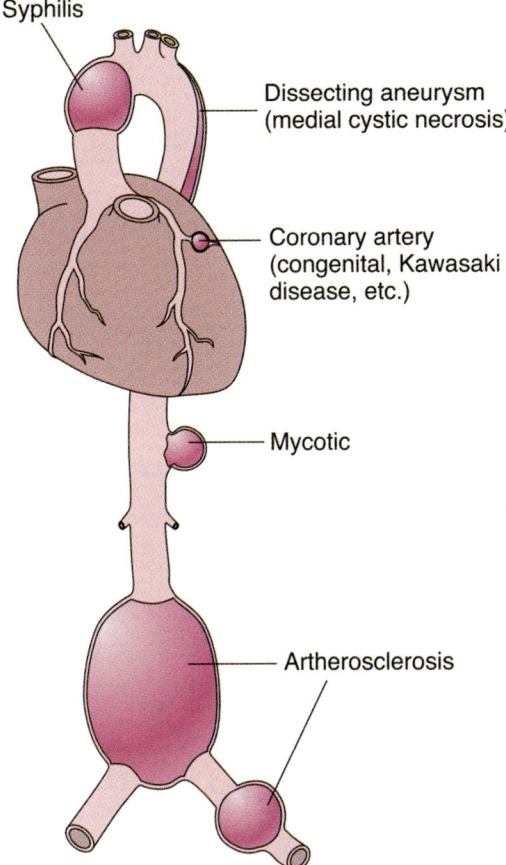

FIGURE 10-37
The locations of aneurysms. Syphilitic aneurysms are the common variety in the ascending aorta, which is usually spared by the atherosclerotic process. Atherosclerotic aneurysms can occur in the abdominal aorta or muscular arteries, including the coronary and popliteal arteries and other vessels. Berry aneurysms are seen in the circle of Willis, mainly at branch points; their rupture leads to subarachnoid hemorrhage. Mycotic aneurysms occur almost anywhere that bacteria can deposit on vessel walls.

ally, aneurysms are found in the ascending arch and descending parts of the thoracic aorta, and they also can occur in the iliac and popliteal arteries.

Although abdominal aortic aneurysms invariably occur in the context of atherosclerosis, it is thought that the disease is actually multifactorial. Familial clustering suggests a role for genetic predisposition. A variety of changes in the extracellular matrix of the aortic wall has been described, and hemodynamic factors have also been implicated, particularly with regard to hypertension.

 Pathology: Most abdominal aneurysms of the aorta are distal to the renal arteries and proximal to the bifurcation (Fig. 10-38). The aneurysms are usually fusiform, although saccular varieties are occasionally encountered. The lesions may be of almost any size, but most of the symptomatic ones are more than 5 to 6 cm in diameter. Some of these aneurysms extend into the iliac arteries, which occasionally exhibit distinct aneurysms distal to the one in the aorta. Aneurysms that extend above the renal arteries may occlude the origin of the superior mesenteric artery and the celiac axis.

Most abdominal aortic aneurysms are lined by raised, ulcerated, and calcified (complicated) atherosclerotic lesions. Most contain a mural thrombus of varying degrees of organization. Portions of the thrombus may dislodge and be carried in the bloodstream as emboli to peripheral arteries. Infrequently, the thrombus itself may enlarge enough to compromise the lumen of the aorta.

Microscopic examination reveals complicated atherosclerotic lesions, with destruction of the normal arterial wall and its replacement by fibrous tissue. Remnants of normal media are seen focally, and atheromatous lesions extend to variable depths. The adventitia is thickened and focally inflamed, as a response to severe atherosclerosis.

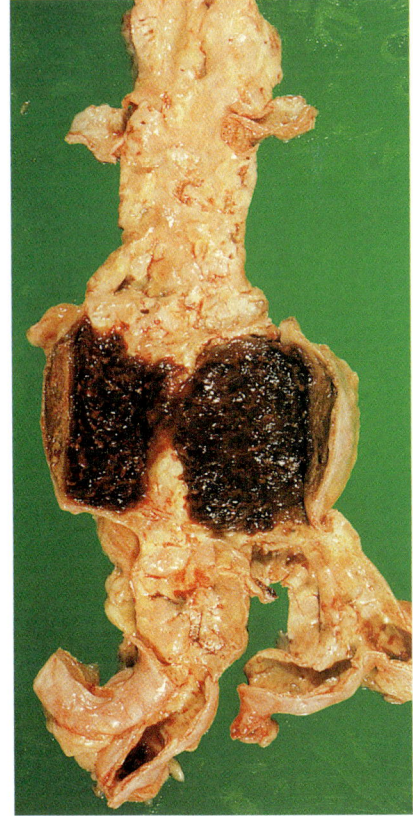

FIGURE 10-38
Atherosclerotic aneurysm of the abdominal aorta. The aneurysm has been opened longitudinally to reveal a large mural thrombus in the lumen. The aorta and common iliac arteries display complicated lesions of atherosclerosis.

Clinical Features: Many abdominal aortic aneurysms are asymptomatic and are discovered only by the palpation of a mass in the abdomen or during radiological examination for some other reason. In some cases the condition is brought to medical attention by the onset of abdominal pain, which often reflects the expansion of the aneurysm. Abrupt occlusion of a peripheral artery by an embolus from the mural thrombus presents as sudden ischemia of a lower limb. The most dreaded complication of aortic aneurysms is rupture and exsanguinating retroperitoneal (or thoracic) hemorrhage, in which case the patient presents with pain, shock, and a pulsatile mass in the abdomen. Such a situation is an acute emergency, and even with prompt surgical intervention, half of patients die. Therefore, large aneurysms, even if entirely asymptomatic, are often replaced by or bypassed with prosthetic grafts.

The risk of rupture of an abdominal aortic aneurysm relates to the size of the lesion. Aneurysms less than 4 cm in diameter rarely rupture (2%), whereas 25 to 40% of those larger than 5 cm in diameter rupture within 5 years of their discovery.

Aneurysms of Cerebral Arteries Lead to Subarachnoid Hemorrhage

The most common type of cerebral aneurysm is saccular and is called a *berry aneurysm*, because it resembles a berry attached to a twig of the arterial tree. The aneurysm results from a congenital defect in a branch point of the arterial wall. Berry aneurysms tend to arise at one of the branching angles of the circle of Willis or in one of the arterial branches. The most common sites are (1) between the anterior cerebral artery and the anterior communicating artery, (2) between the internal carotid artery and the posterior communicating artery, and (3) between the first main divisions of the middle cerebral artery and the bifurcation of the internal carotid artery. Berry aneurysms are discussed in detail in Chapter 28.

Dissecting Aneurysm Is a Hematoma of the Aortic Wall

Dissecting aneurysm refers to the entry of blood into the arterial wall and its extension along the length of the vessel (Fig. 10-39).

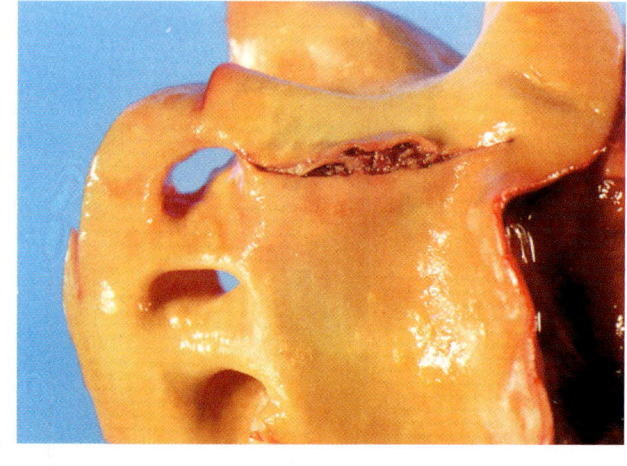
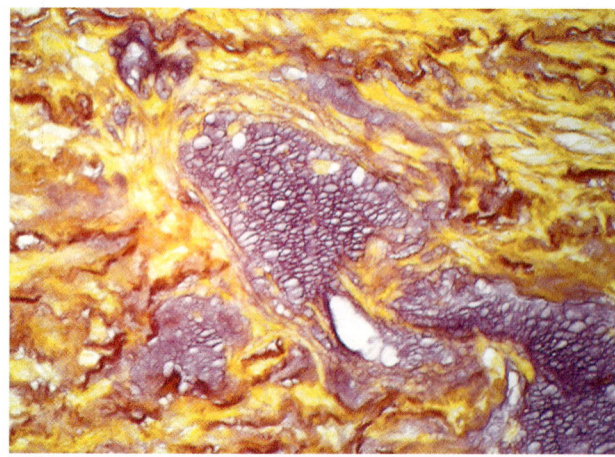
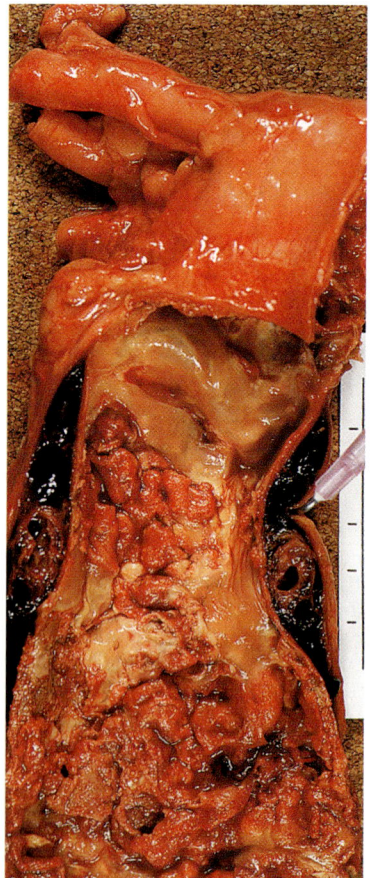

FIGURE 10-39
Dissecting aneurysm of the aorta. A. A transverse tear is present in the aortic arch. The orifices of the great vessels are on the *left*. B. The thoracic aorta has been open longitudinally and reveals clotted blood dissecting the media of the vessel. The luminal surface shows extensive complicated lesions of atherosclerosis. C. A section of the aortic wall stained with aldehyde fuchsin shows pools of metachromatic material characteristic of the degenerative process known as cystic medial necrosis.

In effect, the blood is encompassed by a false lumen within the wall of the artery. Although this lesion is conventionally termed an aneurysm, it is actually a form of hematoma. Dissecting aneurysm most often affects the aorta and its major branches. The frequency of occurrence has been estimated to be as high as 1 in 400 autopsies, with men being affected three times as frequently as women. A dissecting aneurysm may occur at almost any age, but is most common in the sixth and seventh decades of life. Most patients have a history of hypertension.

Pathogenesis: The pathogenesis of dissecting aneurysm in most instances can be traced to a weakening of the aortic media. The changes were originally described as *cystic medial necrosis (of Erdheim)*, because focal loss of elastic and muscle fibers in the media leads to "cystic" spaces filled with a metachromatic myxoid material. These spaces are not true cysts but are rather pools of matrix collected between the cells and tissues of the media. The cause of the medial degeneration is not known. Some cases of dissecting aneurysm represent a complication of Marfan syndrome (see Chapter 6). Aging also results in mild degenerative changes in the aorta, characterized by focal elastin loss and medial fibrosis. In animals, defective cross-linking of collagen induced by a copper-deficient diet (lysyl oxidase is a copper-dependent enzyme) causes dissecting aneurysm of the aorta. The same lesion is produced by feeding β-aminopropionitrile, an inhibitor of lysyl oxidase. Persons with Wilson disease who are treated with penicillamine, a copper chelator, also may develop medial necrosis of the aorta. Taken together, these data suggest that the common factor in these several situations is a defect that leads to weakness of the connective tissue of the aorta.

The initial event that triggers medial dissection is controversial. More than 95% of cases of dissecting aneurysm show a transverse tear in the intima and internal media, and many investigators hold that spontaneous laceration of the intima allows blood from the lumen to enter and dissect the media. Alternatively, it has been proposed that hemorrhage from the vasa vasorum into the media weakened by cystic medial necrosis initiates stress on the intima, which in turn leads to the ubiquitous intimal tear.

Pathology: Most intimal tears are found in the ascending aorta, 1 or 2 cm above the aortic ring. The dissection in the media, which occurs within seconds, separates the inner two thirds of the aorta from the outer third. It can also involve the coronary arteries, great vessels of the neck, or the renal, mesenteric, or iliac arteries. Since the outer wall of the false channel of the dissecting aneurysm is thin, hemorrhage into the extravascular space, including the pericardium, mediastinum, pleural space, and retroperitoneum, is a frequent cause of death. In 5 to 10% of cases, the blood within the dissecting aneurysm reenters the lumen through a second distal tear to form a "*double-barreled aorta.*" In a comparable proportion, a reentry site leads to communication of the aorta with a major artery, most often the iliac artery.

Clinical Features: The typical patient with an aortic dissection presents with the acute onset of severe, "tearing" pain in the anterior chest, which is sometimes misdiagnosed as myocardial infarction. A loss of one or more arterial pulses is common, and a murmur of aortic regurgitation is often present. Whereas hypertension is a frequent finding, hypotension is an ominous sign, suggesting aortic rupture. Cardiac tamponade or congestive heart failure is diagnosed by the usual criteria.

Before antihypertensive and surgical treatment became available, more than a third of patients with aortic dissection died within 24 hours, and 80% succumbed by 2 weeks. Of the survivors, half died within 3 months. Surgical intervention and control of hypertension have now reduced the overall mortality to less than 20%.

Syphilitic Aneurysms Reflect an Aortitis

Syphilitic (luetic) aneurysms were once the most common form of aortic aneurysm, but the decline in the prevalence of syphilis has led to a marked decrease in syphilitic vascular disease, including aortitis and aneurysms. These aneurysms preferentially affect the ascending aorta, where microscopic examination shows endarteritis and periarteritis of the vasa vasorum. These vessels ramify in the adventitia and penetrate the outer and middle thirds of the aorta, where they become encircled by lymphocytes, plasma cells, and macrophages. Obliterative changes in the vasa vasorum cause focal necrosis and scarring of the media, with disruption and disorganization of the elastic lamellae. The depressed medial scars lead to a roughened intimal surface, which imparts a "tree bark" appearance (Fig. 10-40). The weakened wall of the ascending aorta and aortic arch eventually yields to the relentless pressure of the blood and balloons to form a fusiform aneurysm.

Mycotic (Infectious) Aneurysms

Mycotic aneurysms result from the weakening of the vessel wall by a microbial infection and have a tendency to rupture

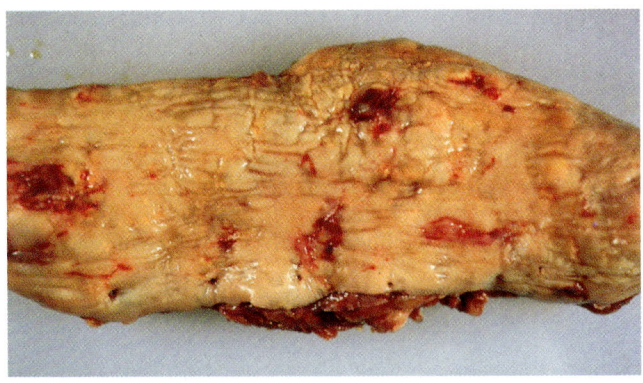

FIGURE *10-40*

Syphilitic aortitis. The thoracic aorta is dilated, and its inner surface shows the typical "tree bark" appearance.

and hemorrhage. They may develop in the aortic wall or in cerebral vessels during the course of a septicemia, most commonly secondary to bacterial endocarditis. Mesenteric, splenic, or renal arteries are also common sites of involvement. In addition, mycotic aneurysms may occur adjacent to a tuberculous infection or a bacterial abscess.

VEINS

Varicose Veins of the Legs Involve the Superficial Saphenous System

A varicose vein is an enlarged and tortuous blood vessel. Superficial varicosities of the leg veins, usually in the saphenous system, are among the most common ailments of humans. They vary from a trivial knot of dilated veins to disabling distention of the whole venous system of the leg, with secondary trophic disturbances. It has been estimated that as much as 10 to 20% of the population have some varicosities in the leg veins, but only a fraction of these persons develop symptoms.

Pathogenesis: There are a number of risk factor for varicose veins:

- **Age:** The incidence of varicose veins rises with age and may reach 50% in persons older than the age of 50 years. The increase in the frequency of varicose veins with age may reflect degenerative changes of the connective tissues in the vein walls, together with loss of the supporting fat and connective tissues, a more flaccid muscle tone, and inactivity.
- **Sex:** In the 30- to 50-year-old age group, women are affected by varicose veins more often than men, particularly women who have experienced the increased venous pressure associated with the weight of the pregnant uterus on the iliac veins.
- **Heredity:** There is a strong familial predisposition to varicose veins, possibly owing to inherited configurations or structural weaknesses of the walls or valves of the veins.
- **Posture:** Since four-legged animals do not develop varicose veins, this abnormality may be regarded as a price exacted by the erect posture. The pressure in the leg veins is 5 to 10 times greater in the erect position than in the recumbent one. As a result, the incidence of varicose veins is increased among persons whose occupations require them to stand in one place for long periods, such as dentists and sales clerks.
- **Obesity:** Excessive body weight increases the incidence of varicose veins, possibly because of an increase in intraabdominal pressure or the poor support offered by subcutaneous fat to the vessel walls.

Other factors that augment venous pressure in the legs can cause varicose veins. These include pelvic tumors, congestive heart failure, and thrombotic obstruction of the main venous trunks of the thigh or pelvis.

In the pathogenesis of varicose veins, it is not clear whether incompetence of the valves or dilation of the vessels comes first. Whatever the case, the two reinforce each other. The vein increases both in length and diameter, so that tortuousities develop. Once the process has begun, the varicosity extends progressively throughout the length of the affected vein. As each valve becomes incompetent, a progressively increasing strain is thrown on the vessel and valve below.

Pathology: Microscopically, varicose veins exhibit variations in the thickness of the wall. Thinning due to dilation is present in some areas, whereas others are thickened by smooth muscle hypertrophy, subintimal fibrosis, and the incorporation of mural thrombi into the wall. Patchy calcification is frequently seen. Valvular deformities consist of thickening, shortening, and rolling of the cusps.

Clinical Features: The diagnosis of varicose veins of the leg is easily made by inspection. Except for their cosmetic impact, most varicose veins are without clinical effects and require no treatment. The principal symptoms are aching in the legs, aggravated by standing and relieved by elevation. Severe varicosities (Fig. 10-41) may lead to trophic alterations in the skin drained by the affected veins, termed *stasis dermatitis*. Surgical intervention is mandated in the presence of ulceration of the overlying skin, spontaneous bleeding, or extensive thrombosis (which may lead to pulmonary embolism).

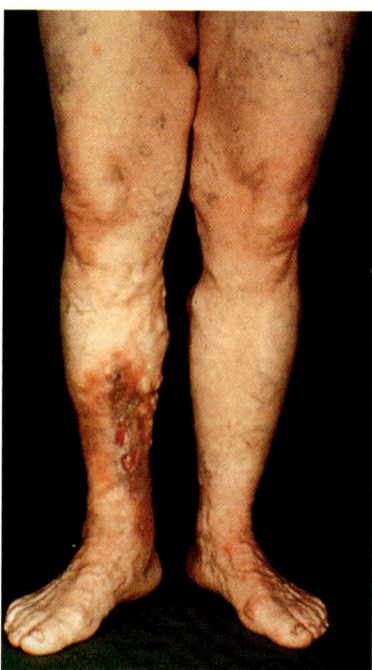

FIGURE *10-41*
Varicose veins of the legs. Severe varicosities of the superficial leg veins have led to stasis dermatitis and secondary ulcerations.

Varicose Veins at Other Sites

HEMORRHOIDS: These dilations of the veins of the rectum and anal canal may occur inside or outside the anal sphincter (see Chapter 13). Although there may be a hereditary predisposition, the condition is aggravated by constipation and pregnancy. It may also result from venous obstruction by rectal tumors. Hemorrhoids often bleed, a sign that can cause confusion with bleeding rectal cancers. Thrombosed hemorrhoids are exquisitely painful.

ESOPHAGEAL VARICES: This complication of portal hypertension is caused mainly by cirrhosis of the liver (see Chapter 14). High portal pressure leads to distention of the anastomoses between the portal system and the systemic veins at the lower end of the esophagus. Although they may be prominent radiologically, esophageal varices are usually unimpressive at autopsy. After their collapse at death, often all that is evident on gross examination are bluish streaks in the esophageal mucosa. Hemorrhage from esophageal varices is one of the most common causes of death in cirrhosis.

VARICOCELE: This palpable mass in the scrotum is formed by varicosities of the pampiniform plexus (see Chapter 17).

Deep Venous Thrombosis Principally Affects Leg Veins

- **Thrombophlebitis** describes inflammation and secondary thrombosis of small veins and sometimes larger ones, commonly as part of a local reaction to bacterial infection.
- **Phlebothrombosis** is the term for venous thrombosis that occurs in the absence of an initiating infection or inflammation.
- **Deep venous thrombosis** now refers to both phlebothrombosis and thrombophlebitis. Since most cases of venous thrombosis are not associated with inflammation or infection, the condition is currently associated with prolonged bed rest or reduced cardiac output. It is most frequent in the deep leg veins and can be a major threat to life because of embolization to the lung (witness the well-known phenomenon of sudden death occurring on ambulation after surgery). Deficiencies of anticoagulants, such as protein C and antithrombin, result in an increased incidence of venous thromboembolism. Deep venous thrombosis is discussed more fully in Chapter 7.

LYMPHATIC VESSELS

The lymphatic vessels are thin-walled low-pressure channels that provide drainage of plasma filtrates, cells, and foreign material from the interstitial spaces. The lymphatic vessels show greater permeability than blood vessels, in part because of the presence of fewer tight junctions in the former. In this way, they serve as pathways for the spread of two major pathological processes, namely, inflammation and neoplasia.

Lymphangitis Reflects the Entrance of Bacteria and Inflammatory Cells into the Lymphatic Drainage

The transport of infectious material to the regional lymph nodes incites *lymphadenitis*. The periphery of a focus of inflammation reveals dilated lymphatics filled with fluid exudate, cells, cellular debris, and bacteria. When the tissues are expanded by exudate, there is a comparable distention of the lymphatic channels and an opening of intercellular channels between endothelial cells.

Almost any virulent pathogen can cause acute lymphangitis, but β-hemolytic streptococci (pyogenes) are particularly notorious offenders. The process may extend beyond the lymphatic channels into the surrounding tissues. The draining lymph nodes are regularly enlarged and inflamed. Painful subcutaneous red streaks, often accompanied by painful regional lymph nodes, characterize acute lymphangitis.

Lymphatic Obstruction Causes Lymphedema

Lymphatics may be obstructed by scar tissue, intraluminal tumor cells, pressure from surrounding tumor tissue, or plugging with parasites. Since collateral lymphatic routes are abundant, lymphedema (distention of tissue by lymph) usually occurs only when major trunks are obstructed, especially in the axilla or groin. For example, when radical mastectomy for breast cancer was routine, dissection of the axillary lymph nodes frequently disrupted lymphatic channels and led to lymphedema of the arm. Prolonged lymphatic obstruction causes progressive dilation of lymphatic vessels, called *lymphangiectasia*, and overgrowth of fibrous tissue. The term *elephantiasis* describes a lymphedematous limb that has become grossly enlarged. An important cause of elephantiasis in the tropics is filariasis, in which a parasitic worm invades the lymphatics (see Chapter 9).

Milroy disease is *an inherited type of lymphedema that is present at birth.* It usually affects only one limb, but it may be more extensive and involve the eyelids and lips. The affected tissues show enormously dilated lymphatic channels, and the entire area appears honeycombed or spongy. This lesion is more properly considered lymphangiectasia rather than simply lymphedema.

BENIGN TUMORS OF BLOOD VESSELS

Tumors of the vascular system are common, and many are not true neoplasms but rather hamartomas, that is, masses of mature but disorganized cells and tissues characteristic of the particular organ.

Hemangiomas Are Common Benign Tumors Composed of Vascular Channels

Hemangiomas usually occur in the skin but may also be found in internal organs.

Pathogenesis: Although they are clearly benign, the origin of hemangiomas is uncertain; they represent either true neoplasms or hamartomas. The evidence in favor of a hamartoma (i.e., a malformation) includes the following: (1) the lesion is present at birth; (2) it grows only with the growth of the rest of the body and remains limited in size; and (3) following cessation of growth, it usually remains unchanged indefinitely, unless accidents such as trauma, thrombosis, or hemorrhage supervene.

The development of these vascular malformations recalls the embryology of the vascular system. A network of endothelial channels undergoes remodeling, acquiring a muscular coat and adventitia. In this view, vascular malformations reflect the persistence of the original or modified channels and mixtures of connective tissue elements derived from the mesenchyme. Hemangiomas are classified by histological type and location.

 Pathology:

CAPILLARY HEMANGIOMA: This lesion is composed of vascular channels that have the size and structure of normal capillaries. Capillary hemangiomas may be located in any tissue. The most common sites are the skin, subcutaneous tissues, mucous membranes of the lips and the mouth, and internal viscera, including the spleen, kidneys, and liver. Capillary hemangiomas vary from a few millimeters to several centimeters in diameter. They are bright red to blue, depending on the degree of oxygenation of the blood. In the skin, capillary hemangiomas are known as "*birthmarks*" or "*ruby spots.*" The only disability is cosmetic disfiguration.

JUVENILE HEMANGIOMA: Also called *strawberry hemangiomas,* these lesions are found on the skin of newborns. They grow rapidly in the first few months of life, begin to fade at 1 to 3 years of age, and completely regress in most (80%) cases by 5 years of age. Histologically, juvenile hemangioma is composed of packed masses of capillaries separated by a connective tissue stroma. The endothelium-lined channels are usually filled with blood. Thromboses, sometimes organized, are often seen. Occasionally, the vascular channels rupture, causing scarring and the accumulation of hemosiderin pigment. Juvenile hemangiomas are usually well demarcated despite the lack of a capsule, although fingerlike projections of the vascular tissue may give the impression of invasion. However, the growths are not malignant, and they do not invade or metastasize.

CAVERNOUS HEMANGIOMA: This designation is reserved for lesions consisting of large vascular channels, frequently interspersed with small, capillary-type vessels. Cavernous hemangiomas occur in the skin (Fig. 10-42), where they are termed *port wine stains*. They also appear on mucosal surfaces and visceral organs, including the spleen, liver, and pancreas. Occasionally, they are found in the brain, where after long quiescent periods they may slowly enlarge and cause neurological symptoms.

A cavernous hemangioma appears as a red-blue, soft, spongy mass, with a diameter of up to several centimeters.

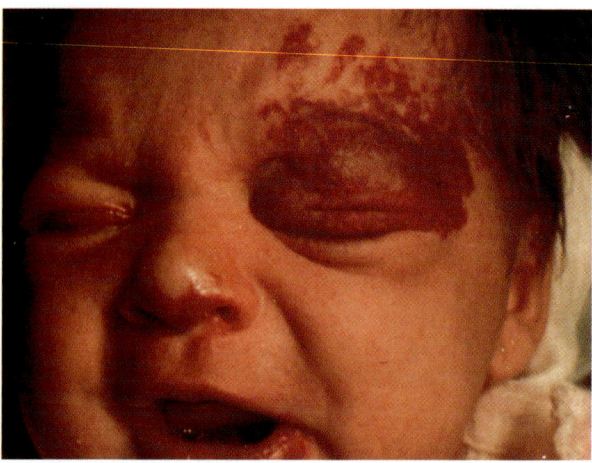

FIGURE 10-42
Congenital cavernous hemangioma of the skin.

Unlike the capillary hemangioma, a cavernous hemangioma does not regress spontaneously. Although the lesion is demarcated by a sharp border, it is not encapsulated. Large endothelial lined, blood-containing spaces are separated by sparse connective tissue. Cavernous hemangiomas can undergo a variety of changes, including thrombosis and fibrosis, cystic cavitation, and intracystic hemorrhage.

MULTIPLE HEMANGIOMATOUS SYNDROMES: A number of hemangiomas may be found in a single tissue. Two or more tissues may be involved, such as the skin and the nervous system or the spleen and the liver. Eponym enthusiasts have defined various combinations of sites. For example, *von Hippel-Lindau syndrome* is a rare entity in which cavernous hemangiomas occur within the cerebellum or brainstem and the retina. *Sturge-Weber syndrome* is characterized by a developmental disturbance of blood vessels in the brain and skin. Other closely related lesions are plexiform or racemose angiomas, cirsoid aneurysms, and angiomatous dilation of vessels of the brain and elsewhere.

Glomus Tumor (Glomangioma) Is a Painful Arteriolar–Venous Anastomosis

A glomus tumor is a benign neoplasm of the glomus body. Glomus bodies are normal neuromyoarterial receptors that are sensitive to temperature and regulate arteriolar flow. They are widely distributed in the skin but are most frequent in the distal regions of the fingers and toes. This pattern is reflected in the location of glomus tumors at these sites, typically in a subungual location.

 Pathology: The lesions are small, usually less than 1 cm in diameter, and many are smaller than a few millimeters. In the skin, they are slightly elevated, rounded, red-blue, and firm (Fig. 10-43). The two

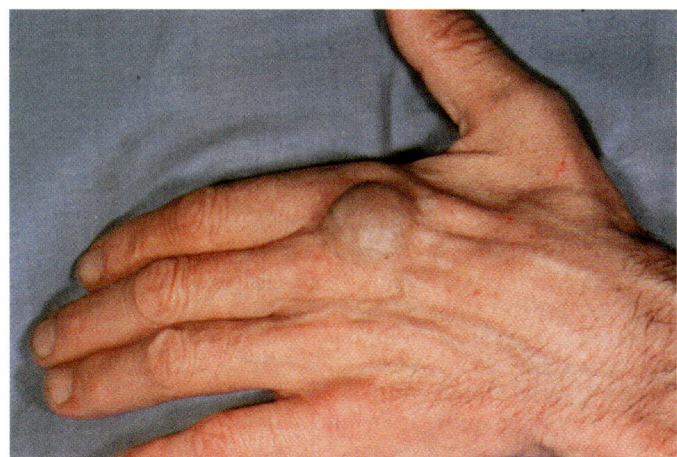
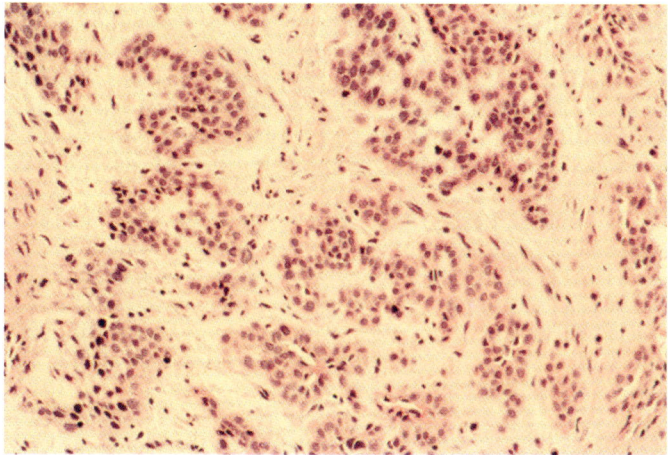

FIGURE 10-43
Glomus tumor. (A) The dorsal surface of the hand displays a prominent tumor nodule on the proximal third finger. (B) A photomicrograph of A reveals nests of glomus tumor cells embedded in a fibrovascular stroma.

main histological components are branching vascular channels in a connective tissue stroma and aggregates or nests of the specialized glomus cells. The latter are regular, round to cuboidal cells that reveal typical smooth muscle cell features by electron microscopy.

Hemangioendothelioma May Metastasize to Distant Sites

Hemangioendothelioma refers to a vascular tumor of endothelial cells that is intermediate between benign hemangiomas and frankly malignant angiosarcomas. The epithelioid, or histiocytoid, variant displays endothelial cells with considerable eosinophilic, often vacuolated, cytoplasm. Vascular lumina are evident, and there is a paucity of mitoses. These tumors occur in almost all locations. Surgical removal is generally curative, but about one fifth of patients develop metastases.

Spindle cell hemangioendothelioma occurs principally in males of any age, usually in the dermis and subcutaneous tissue of the distal extremities. The tumor features vascular, endothelial lined spaces into which papillary projections extend. Although the lesion may recur locally after excision, this variant of hemangioendothelioma rarely metastasizes.

MALIGNANT TUMORS OF BLOOD VESSELS

Malignant vascular neoplasms are rare, and only a few arise in preexisting benign tumors.

Angiosarcoma Features Neoplastic Endothelial Cells

Angiosarcoma is a rare, highly malignant tumor composed of single or multiple masses of malignant endothelial cells. The lesions occur in either sex and at any age and begin as small, painless, sharply demarcated, red nodules. The most common locations are skin, soft tissue, breast, bone, liver, and spleen. Eventually, most angiosarcomas enlarge to become pale gray, fleshy masses without a capsule. Often these tumors undergo central necrosis, with softening and hemorrhage.

 Pathology: Angiosarcomas exhibit varying degrees of differentiation, ranging from those composed mainly of distinct vascular elements to undifferentiated tumors with few recognizable blood channels. The latter display frequent mitoses, pleomorphism, and giant cells and tend to be more malignant. Almost half of patients with angiosarcoma die of the disease.

Angiosarcoma of the liver is of special interest because of its association with environmental carcinogens, particularly arsenic (a component of pesticides) and vinyl chloride (used in the production of plastics). Hepatic angiosarcoma has also been associated with the administration of thorium dioxide (Thorotrast), a material used by radiologists prior to 1950. This radioactive contrast medium is engulfed by the macrophages of the liver sinusoids, where it remains for life.

There is a long latent period between exposure to the chemicals or radionuclide and the development of angiosarcoma of the liver. The earliest detectable changes are atypism and diffuse hyperplasia of the cells lining the hepatic sinusoids. The tumors are frequently multicentric and may arise in the spleen as well as the liver. Hepatic angiosarcomas are highly malignant and exhibit both local invasion and metastatic spread.

Hemangiopericytoma

Hemangiopericytoma is a rare malignant neoplasm that presumably arises from pericytes, the modified smooth muscle cells that are external to the walls of capillaries and arterioles. These tumors present as small masses and consist of capillary-like channels surrounded by, and frequently enclosed within, nests and masses of round to spindle-shaped cells. The tumor cell type is identified by a characteristic investment of basement membrane, similar to that of its normal counterpart.

Hemangiopericytomas can occur anywhere, but are most frequently encountered in the retroperitoneum and lower extremities. Most hemangiopericytomas are removed surgically without having invaded or metastasized. The reported metastatic rate varies from 10 to 50%, depending on the series. Malignant hemangiopericytomas metastasize to lungs, bone, liver, and lymph nodes.

Kaposi Sarcoma Is a Complication of AIDS

Kaposi sarcoma is a malignant tumor derived from endothelial cells.

Epidemiology: Kaposi sarcoma was originally described in the 19th century by Moritz Kaposi (née Kohn) as a sporadic tumor in the sixth and seventh decades of life, with an incidence 10 times higher in men than in women. However, this picture has changed dramatically, and Kaposi sarcoma has now appeared in epidemic form in association with AIDS. For some years before AIDS appeared, Kaposi sarcoma was known to be common in parts of Central Africa (where AIDS is now rampant) and to afflict younger men. The etiology of this formerly rare disease is now clearer. Its association with the current AIDS epidemic as a widespread, multifocal lesion suggests that it is related to the loss of immunity. A virus of the herpes family (HHV8) has been detected in endothelial and spindle cells of Kaposi sarcoma and is thought to contribute to the genesis of the tumor (see Chapter 4).

Pathology: Kaposi sarcoma begins as painful purple or brown nodules in the skin, varying from 1 mm to 1 cm in diameter. They occur most often on the hands or feet but may appear anywhere in the body. The histological appearance of Kaposi sarcoma is highly variable. One form resembles a simple hemangioma and is characterized by tightly packed clusters of capillaries and scattered hemosiderin-laden macrophages. In other forms of the tumor, the lesions are highly cellular and the vascular spaces are less prominent (Fig. 10-44). These lesions may be difficult to distinguish from fibrosarcomas, but the characteristic features of endothelial cells can be demonstrated immunochemically and by electron microscopy. Although Kaposi sarcoma is considered a malignant lesion and may be widely disseminated in the body, it is only exceptionally a cause of death.

TUMORS OF THE LYMPHATIC SYSTEM

Many histological and clinical variants of local enlargements of the lymphatics have been described, and it is difficult to distinguish among anomalies, proliferations due to stasis, and true neoplasms. In general, lymphatic tumors are distinguished by their size and location. The spaces may be small, as in capillary lymphangiomas, or large and dilated, as in cystic or cavernous lesions. Lymphangiomatous lesions can arise at almost any site, including the skin, mediastinum, retroperitoneum, spleen, and other locations.

Capillary Lymphangioma

Sometimes called "simple lymphangiomas," these benign tumors are small, circumscribed, grayish pink, fleshy nodules, which can be single or multiple. They are subcutaneous and found in the skin of the face, lips, chest, genitalia, or extremities. Capillary lymphangiomas are composed of variably sized, thin-walled spaces that are lined by endothelial cells and contain lymph and occasional leukocytes.

Cystic Lymphangioma (Cystic Hygroma, Cavernous Lymphangioma)

These benign lesions occur most often in the neck and axilla, less commonly in the mediastinum, and occasionally in the retroperitoneum. They may reach a size of 10 to 15 cm in diameter or more and fill the axilla or distort structures of the neck.

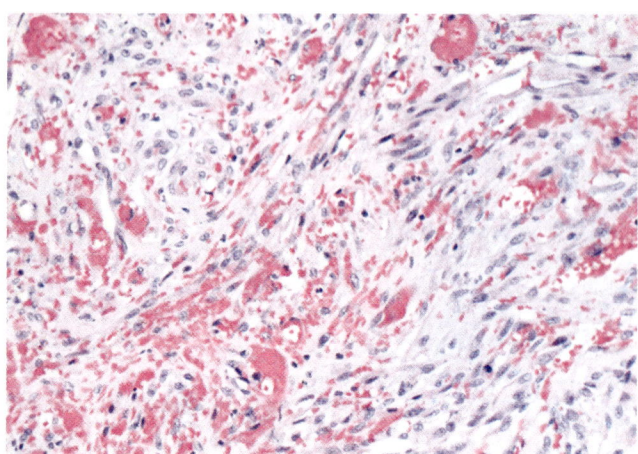

FIGURE 10-44
Kaposi sarcoma. A photomicrograph of a vascular lesion from a patient with acquired immune deficiency syndrome shows numerous poorly differentiated, spindle-shape neoplastic cells and a vascular lesion filled with red blood cells.

Pathology: Cystic lymphangiomas are soft, spongy, and pink, and watery fluid exudes from their cut surface. Microscopically, they are composed of endothelial lined spaces that contain a protein-rich fluid. These spaces are distinguished from blood vessels by their lack of erythrocytes and leukocytes. An abundance of irregularly distributed smooth muscle and connective tissue cells may be present.

Lymphangiosarcoma May Follow Lymphedema or Radiation

A rare malignant tumor develops in 0.1 to 0.5% of patients with lymphedema of the arm following radical mastectomy. A distinction between this tumor and angiosarcoma is difficult, and some authors equate the two cancers. Lymphangiosarcoma may also occur in other regions, for example, in the leg following radiation therapy for uterine cervical carcinoma.

 Pathology: Lymphangiosarcomas present as purplish, frequently multiple nodules in the edematous skin. Histologically, the nodules are composed of cells that resemble capillary endothelial cells and display zonulae adherentes between the cells. The walls of the tumor vessels have a rudimentary form of basal basement membrane. Lymphangiosarcomas are highly malignant and, despite radical surgery, carry a poor prognosis.

SUGGESTED READING

Books

Gotlieb AI, Silver MD: Atherosclerosis: Pathogenesis and pathology. In: Silver MD, Gotlieb AI, Schoen FJ (eds): *Cardiovascular pathology*. New York: Churchill Livingstone, 2001:68–106.

McManus BM, Braunwald E: *Atlas of cardiovascular pathology*. Philadelphia: Current Medicine Inc, 2000.

Virmani R, Burke A, Farb A. *Atlas of cardiovascular pathology*. Philadelphia: WB Saunders, 1996.

Review Articles

Davies MJ, Bland JM, Hangartner JR, et al.: Factors influencing the presence or absence of acute coronary artery thrombi in sudden ischemic death. *Eur Heart J* 10:203–208, 1989.

Frank H: Characterization of atherosclerotic plaque by magnetic resonance imaging. *Am Heart J* 141:S45-48, 2001.

Libby P: Coronary artery injury and the biology of atherosclerosis: Inflammation, thrombosis, and stabilization. *Am J Cardiol* 86:3J–9J, 2000.

Nicholson AC, Hajjar DP: Herpesviruses in atherosclerosis and thrombosis: Etiologic agents or ubiquitous bystanders? *Arterioscler Thromb Vasc Biol* 18:339–348, 1998.

Orlic D, Kajstura J, Chimenti S, et al.: Transplanted adult bone marrow cells repair myocardial infarcts in mice. *Ann NY Acad Sci* 938:221–229, 2001.

Schoen FJ, Libby P: Cardiac transplant graft arteriosclerosis. *Trends Cardiovasc Med* 1:216–223, 1991.

Stary HC, Blankenhorn DH, Chandler AB, et al.: A definition of the intima of human arteries and of its atherosclerosis-prone regions: A report from the Committee on Vascular Lesions of the Council on Arteriosclerosis, American Heart Association. *Circulation* 85:391–405, 1992.

Stary HC, Chandler AB, Dinsmore RE, et al.: A definition of advanced types of atherosclerotic lesions and a histological classification of atherosclerosis: A report from the Committee on Vascular Lesions of the Council on Arteriosclerosis, American Heart Association. *Arterioscler Thromb Vas Biol* 15:1512–1531, 1995.

Stary HC, Chandler AB, Glagov S, et al.: A definition of initial, fatty streak, and intermediate lesions of atherosclerosis: A report from the Committee on Vascular Lesions of the Council on Arteriosclerosis, American Heart Association. *Arterioscler Thromb* 14:840–856, 1994.

Van der Wal AC, Becker AE: Atherosclerotic plaque rupture—pathologic basis of plaque stability and instability. *Cardiovasc Res* 41:334–344, 1999.

Virmani R, Burke AP, Farb A: Sudden cardiac death. *Cardiovasc Pathol* 10:275–282, 2001.

Virmani R, Kolodogie FD, Burke AP, et al.: Lessons from sudden coronary death. A comprehensive morphological classification scheme for atherosclerotic lesions. *Arterioscler Thromb Vasc Biol* 20:1262–1275, 2000.

Vyalov S, Langille BL, Gotlieb AI: Low shear stress disrupts repair processes and slows in vivo reendothelialization. *Am J Pathol* 149:2107–2118, 1996.

Waller BF, Orr CM, Pinkerton CA, et al.: Morphologic observations late after coronary balloon angioplasty: Mechanisms of acute injury and relationship to restenosis. *Radiology* 174:961–967, 1990.

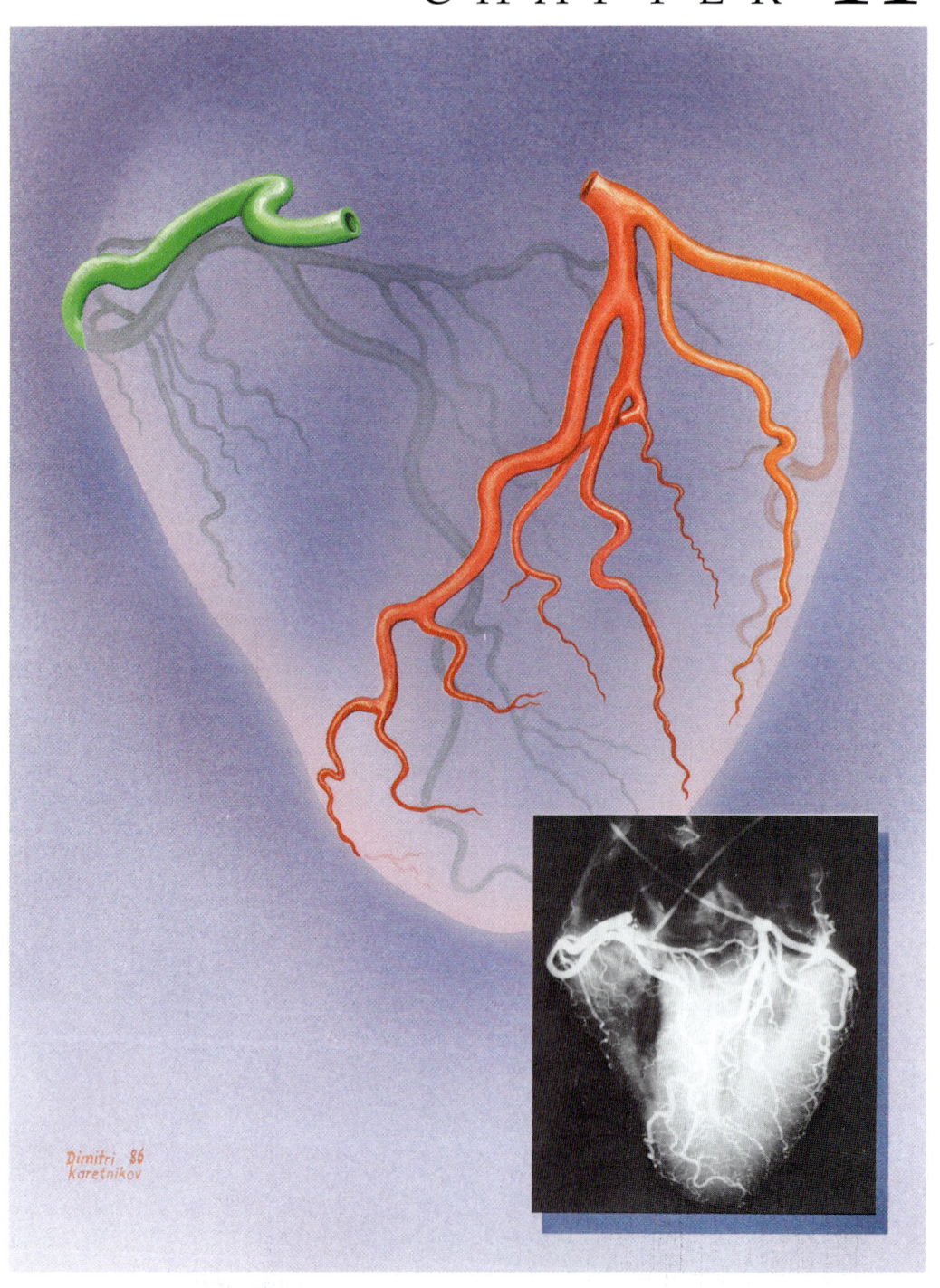

CHAPTER 11

The Heart

Jeffrey E. Saffitz

Anatomy of the Heart

The Cardiac Myocyte

The Conduction System

The Coronary Arteries

Myocardial Hypertrophy and Heart Failure

Congenital Heart Disease

Classification of Congenital Heart Disease

Initial Left-to-Right Shunt

Tetralogy of Fallot (Dominant Right-to-Left Shunt)

Congenital Heart Diseases without Shunts

Ischemic Heart Disease

Conditions That Limit the Supply of Blood to the Heart

Conditions That Limit Oxygen Availability

Increased Oxygen Demand

Clinical Diagnosis of Acute Myocardial Infarction

Complications of Myocardial Infarction

Therapeutic Interventions that Limit Infarct Size

Chronic Ischemic Heart Disease

Hypertensive Heart Disease

Effects of Hypertension on the Heart

Cause of Death in Patients with Hypertension

Cor Pulmonale

Acquired Valvular and Endocardial Diseases

Rheumatic Heart Disease

Collagen Vascular Diseases

Bacterial Endocarditis

Nonbacterial Thrombotic Endocarditis

Calcific Aortic Stenosis

Calcification of the Mitral Valve Annulus

Mitral Valve Prolapse

Papillary Muscle Dysfunction

Carcinoid Heart Disease

Primary Myocardial Diseases

Myocarditis

Metabolic Diseases of the Heart

Hyperthyroid Heart Disease

Hypothyroid Heart Disease

Thiamine Deficiency (Beriberi) Heart Disease

(continued)

FIGURE 11-1 *(see opposite page)*
The coronary circulation. The right coronary artery *(green)* supplies the back of the left ventricle and gives rise to the posterior descending artery. The left main coronary artery *(red)* divides into the anterior descending and the circumflex branches. *(Inset)* Postmortem coronary arteriogram.

Cardiomyopathy

Idiopathic Dilated Cardiomyopathy

Secondary Dilated Cardiomyopathy

Hypertrophic Cardiomyopathy

Restrictive Cardiomyopathy

Cardiac Tumors

Cardiac Myxoma

Rhabdomyoma

Papillary Fibroelastoma

Other Tumors

Diseases of the Pericardium

Pericardial Effusion

Acute Pericarditis

Constrictive Pericarditis

Pathology of Interventional Therapies

Coronary Angioplasty and Stenting

Coronary Bypass Grafts

Prosthetic Valves

Heart Transplantation

The heart is a fist-sized muscular pump that has a remarkable capacity to work unceasingly for the 80 or more years of a human lifetime. As demand requires, it can increase its output manyfold, in part because the coronary circulation can augment its blood flow to a rate more than 10 times normal. The ventricles also respond to a short-term increase in their workload by dilating, in accordance with Starling law of the heart. When an increased workload is imposed for a longer period (e.g., in cases of essential hypertension) the left ventricle hypertrophies, an adaptation that increases its work capacity. However, when this compensatory mechanism reaches its limits, the heart no longer provides an adequate supply of blood to the peripheral tissues, and the result is congestive heart failure. Damage to the myocardium, caused mostly by ischemic heart disease, also limits the capacity of the left ventricle to pump blood and similarly results in heart failure.

ANATOMY OF THE HEART

The heart of an adult man weighs 280 to 340 g, and that of a woman, 230 to 280 g. The organ is a two-sided pump, with blood entering each side through a thin-walled atrium, from which it is propelled forward by thicker muscular ventricles. Owing to the low venous pressure and the relatively low afterload on the right side, the right ventricle is considerably thinner (<0.5 cm) than the left ventricle (1.3–1.5 cm). Blood enters the ventricles across the atrioventricular valves, the mitral valve on the left and the tricuspid valve on the right. The leaflets of these valves are held in place by the chordae tendineae, which are strong fibrous cords attached via papillary muscles to the inner surface of the ventricular wall. The aorta and pulmonary arteries are guarded by the aortic and pulmonary valves, respectively, each consisting of three semilunar cusps. The wall of the heart is composed of three layers: an outer epicardium, a middle myocardium, and an inner endocardium. The heart is surrounded and enclosed by the visceral and parietal pericardia, which are separated by the pericardial cavity.

The Cardiac Myocyte

The myocardium is composed of a syncytial network of myocytes, each of which has a single nucleus and is separated from adjacent cells by intercalated disks, which contain cell–cell mechanical and electrical junctions. Electron microscopy reveals the structure and distribution of the sarcolemma, the sarcoplasmic reticulum (SR), the T system of tubules, the nucleus and numerous mitochondria (Fig. 11-2). The contractile elements of the myocyte, the myofilaments, are arranged in bundles, referred to as myofibrils, which are separated by mitochondria and SR. The myofibrils are organized into repeating units termed *sarcomeres*.

The sarcomere is the basic functional unit of the contractile apparatus. It consists of a Z line on each end and interdigitated thick and thin filaments, which are oriented perpendicular to the Z line (see Fig. 11-2). The thick filaments contain myosin heavy chains, myosin binding protein C, and myosin light chains. The thick filaments, which are limited to the A band, interact with the giant sarcomeric protein, *titin* (~27,000 amino acids long), which spans from the Z line to the M line, thereby forming a third filament system of the sarcomere. Titin helps maintain precise assembly of myofibrillar proteins and contributes to the viscoelastic properties of cardiac muscle. The thin filaments contain actin and regulatory proteins, including tropomyosin and the troponin complex (troponins I, C and T), and extend from the Z line through the I band and into the A band. The interaction of these myofilaments generates the force for contraction. The amount of force that can be generated is proportional to the extent of overlap between adjoining thick and thin filaments and is at a maximum when the sarcomeres are 2.0 to 2.2 μm in length.

When the sarcomere length is less than 2 μm, the thin filaments slide across each other and overlap, decreasing the potential for force-generating cross-links. When the sarcomere is stretched beyond 2.2 μm, there is a decrease in force that is proportional to the widening of the H zone. **This mechanism is the basis for Starling law of the heart, which states that the contractile force of the heart is a function of diastolic fiber length.** The average sarcomere length is

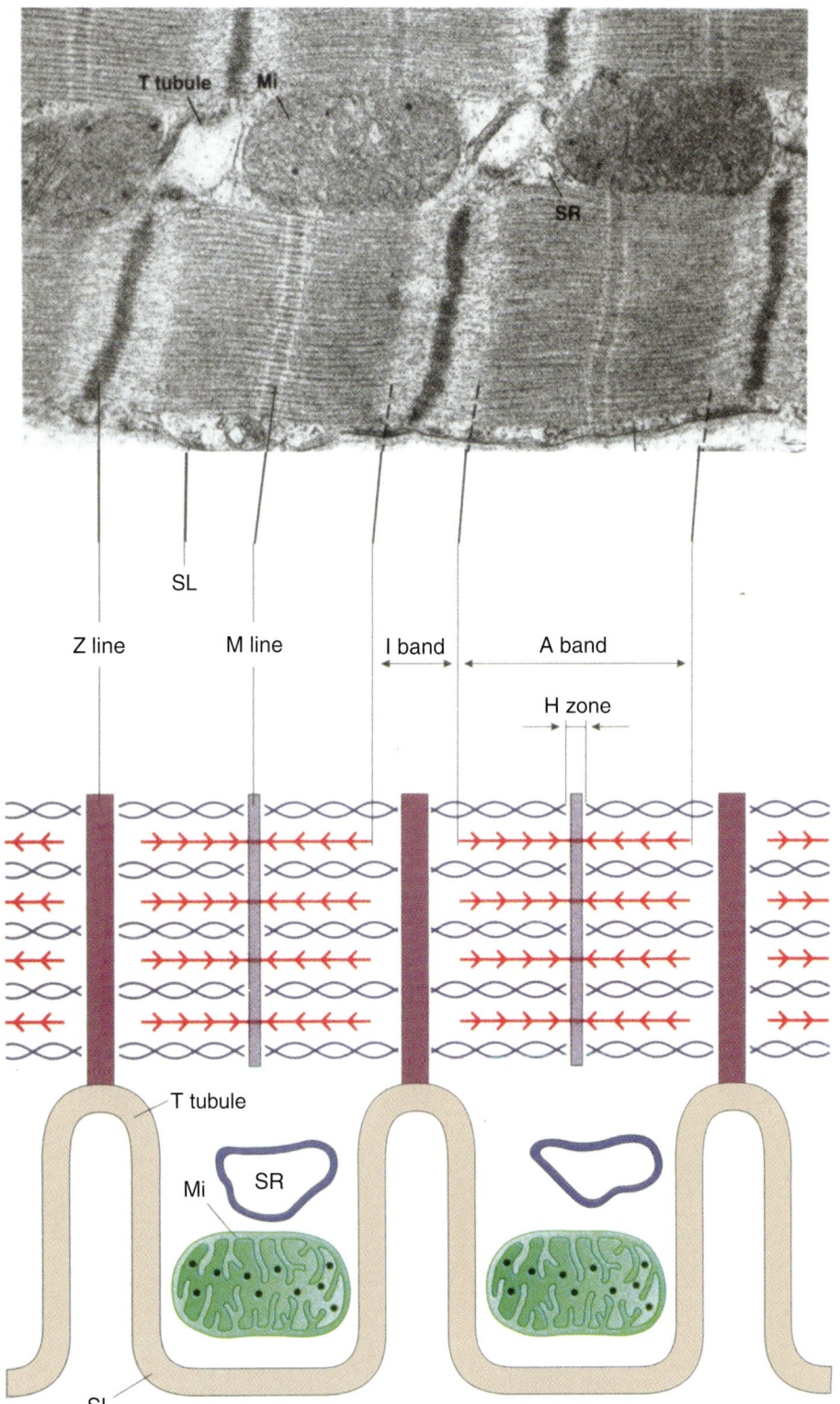

FIGURE 11-2
Ultrastructure of the myocardium. *(Top)* Electron micrograph of left ventricle in the longitudinal plane, showing the sarcolemma *(SL)*; the sarcomeres of the myofibrils, delimited by Z lines; A bands; I bands; H zones; and M lines. Also present are mitochondria *(Mi)*, sarcoplasmic reticulum *(SR)*, and T tubules. The I bands and H zones are absent when the myofibrils are shortened. *(Bottom)* The structural basis for the banding shown in the electron micrograph. The fine threads that extend at right angles to the thick (myosin) filaments are the cross bridges that form the force-generating cross-links with actin. The amount of force that can be generated is proportional to the length of the adjoining myofilaments and is at a maximum when the sarcomeres are between 2 and 2.2 μm in length. When the sarcomeres are less than 2 μm in length, the thin filaments slide across each other and overlap, decreasing the potential for force-generating cross-links; similarly, when the sarcomeres are stretched beyond 2.2 μm, there is a decrease in force that is proportional to the widening of the H zone. This mechanism can be invoked as the basis for Starling law of the heart.

about 2.2 μm when the end-diastolic pressure in the left ventricle is at the upper limit of normal.

The contraction of cardiac muscle is initiated by an increase in cytosolic free calcium. In the normal myocyte, the action potential triggers the entry of calcium into the myocyte through voltage-gated L-type calcium channels in the sarcolemma. In turn, calcium penetrating into the cell stimulates the release, via the cardiac ryanodine receptor (RyR2), of calcium sequestered in the SR (Ca^{2+}-induced Ca^{2+} release). The increase in cytosolic free calcium produces a conformational change in the regulatory proteins of the myofilaments, in particular troponin, which permits the cross-bridges between actin and myosin to break and reform repetitively. As a result, the filaments slide over one another,

524   The Heart

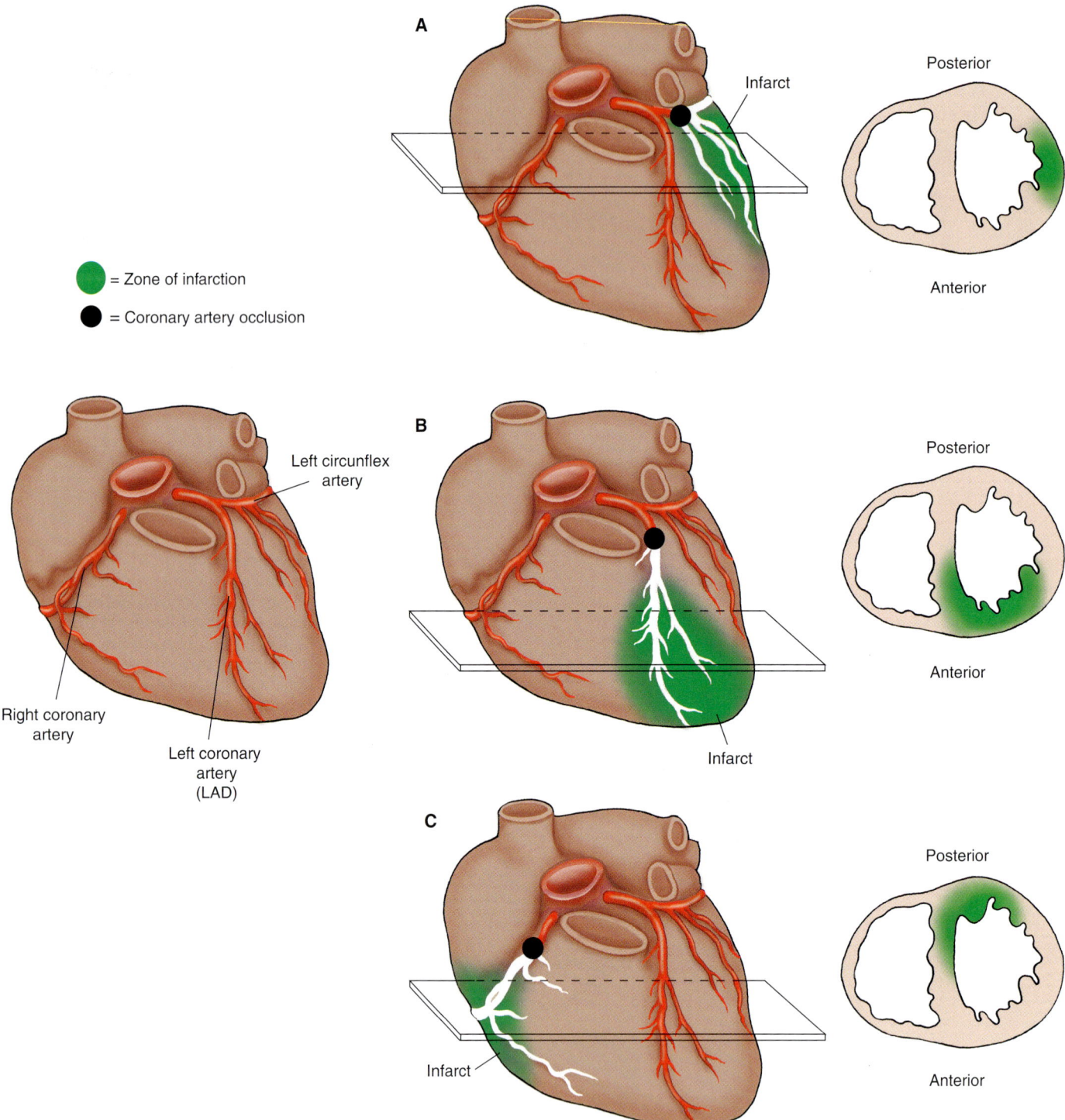

FIGURE 11-3
Position of left ventricular infarcts resulting from occlusion of each of the three main coronary arteries. A. Posterolateral infarct, which follows occlusion of the left circumflex artery and is present in the posterolateral wall. B. Anterior infarct, which follows occlusion of the anterior descending branch *(LAD)* of the left coronary artery. The infarct is located in the anterior wall and adjacent two thirds of the septum. It involves the entire circumference of the wall near the apex. C. A posterior ("inferior" or "diaphragmatic") infarct results from occlusion of the right coronary artery and involves the posterior wall, including the posterior third of the interventricular septum and the posterior papillary muscle in the basal half of the ventricle.

causing contraction of the myocardium. **The number of contractile sites activated and the resulting force that is generated are directly proportional to the concentration of calcium in the vicinity of the myofibrils.**

The myocardium relaxes when the cytosolic calcium returns to its normal low concentration of 10^{-7} M. This process depends on the calcium ATPase of the SR, which pumps Ca^{2+} from the cytosol into the SR. Cytosolic Ca^{2+} also is lowered by its outward transport through sodium–calcium exchange and the sarcolemmal calcium pumps. **Thus, myocardial relaxation is an active, energy-requiring event.**

The Conduction System

The cardiac conduction system consists of specialized myocytes that have two major functions: (1) they initiate the heartbeat by generating electric current through their automatic rhythmicity, which is more rapid in the sinoatrial node than in the more distal parts of the system; and (2) they distribute electric current to activate atrial and ventricular myocardium in an appropriate temporal–spatial pattern. Generally, fibers of the atrioventricular conduction system conduct impulses at a faster rate (~1–2 m/sec) than do the working (contractile) atrial and ventricular fibers (~0.5–1 m/sec). By contrast, conduction through the atrioventricular node is exceptionally slow (~0.1 m/sec). Slow conduction through the atrioventricular junction delays activation of the ventricles, and thereby facilitates their filling.

The heartbeat normally originates in the sinoatrial node. If the sinoatrial node is diseased or otherwise prevented from functioning as the pacemaker, more-distal components of the conduction system or even the ventricular muscle itself assume the role of pacemaker. As a rule, the more distal the pacemaker site, the slower the heart rate. On leaving the sinoatrial node, the electrical impulse activates the atria. Atrial wavefronts converge on the atrioventricular node, which conducts the impulse through the common bundle (bundle of His) to the left and right bundle branches of the Purkinje system. Purkinje fibers run within the endocardium on either side of the interventricular septum and distribute current to the overlying ventricular muscle. During each cycle, ventricular contraction begins along the interventricular septum and at the apex. It progresses from apex to base, resulting in smooth and efficient ejection of blood into the great vessels.

In the normal adult heart, the His bundle is the only electrical connection between the atria and the ventricles. Occasionally, however, additional abnormal connections may arise as small bundles or tracts of cardiac myocytes. Such "bypass tracts" can activate ventricular muscle before the normal impulse arrives via the conduction system and are found in patients with the *Wolff-Parkinson-White syndrome* and in various forms of supraventricular tachycardia. Congenital discontinuities in the conduction system may be caused by placentally transmitted autoantibodies in mothers with connective tissue disease such as systemic lupus erythematosus. Acquired defects may arise as a result of infarction, inflammatory or infiltrative disease, cardiac surgery, or cardiac catheterization.

The Coronary Arteries

The right and left main coronary arteries originate in, or immediately above, the sinuses of Valsalva of the aortic valve (see Fig. 11-1). The left main coronary artery bifurcates within 1 cm of its origin into the left anterior descending (LAD) and left circumflex coronary arteries. The left circumflex coronary artery rests in the left atrioventricular groove and supplies the lateral wall of the left ventricle (Fig. 11-3). The LAD coronary artery lies in the anterior interventricular groove and provides blood to (1) the anterior left ventricle, (2) the adjacent anterior right ventricle, and (3) the anterior half-to-two thirds of the interventricular septum. In the apical region, the LAD coronary artery supplies the ventricles circumferentially (see Fig. 11-3).

The right coronary artery travels along the right atrioventricular groove and nourishes the bulk of the right ventricle and the posteroseptal region of the left ventricle (see Fig. 11-3), including the posterior third-to-half of the interventricular septum at the base of the heart (also referred to as the "inferior" or "diaphragmatic" wall). From these distributions, one can predict the location of infarcts that result from occlusion of any of the three major epicardial coronary arteries (see Fig. 11-3).

The epicardial coronary arteries are usually arranged in a so-called right coronary-dominant distribution. The pattern of dominance is determined by the coronary artery that contributes most of the blood to the posterior descending coronary artery (see Fig. 11-1). Ten percent of human hearts display a left-dominant pattern, with the left circumflex coronary artery supplying the posterior descending coronary artery.

Blood flow in the myocardium occurs inward from epicardium to endocardium. Thus, as a general rule, **the endocardium is most vulnerable to ischemia** when flow through a major epicardial coronary artery is compromised. Some of the small intramyocardial coronary arteries branch as they course through the ventricular wall; others maintain a large diameter and pass to the endocardial surface without branching (Fig. 11-4). Because the capillary networks arising from these penetrating arteries do not interconnect, the borders between viable and infarcted myocardium after coronary artery occlusion are distinct.

The epicardial portion of each coronary artery fills and expands during systole and empties and narrows during diastole. The intramyocardial arteries have the opposite action and are narrowed by the systolic muscular pressure. As a result, blood flow within the myocardium, especially in the subendocardial regions of the ventricle, is decreased or absent during systole. Nevertheless, because of autoregulation, blood flow is roughly equal throughout the myocardium.

MYOCARDIAL HYPERTROPHY AND HEART FAILURE

In the normal heart the ventricles are compliant, and diastolic filling occurs at low atrial pressures. During systole, the ventricles contract vigorously and eject about 60% of the blood present in the ventricle at the end of diastole (ejection fraction). When the heart is injured, regardless of the cause of cardiac dysfunction, the clinical consequences are similar. **If the initial impairment is severe, cardiac output is not maintained despite compensatory changes, and the result is acute, life-threatening, cardiogenic shock.** When the functional impairment is less extensive, compensatory mecha-

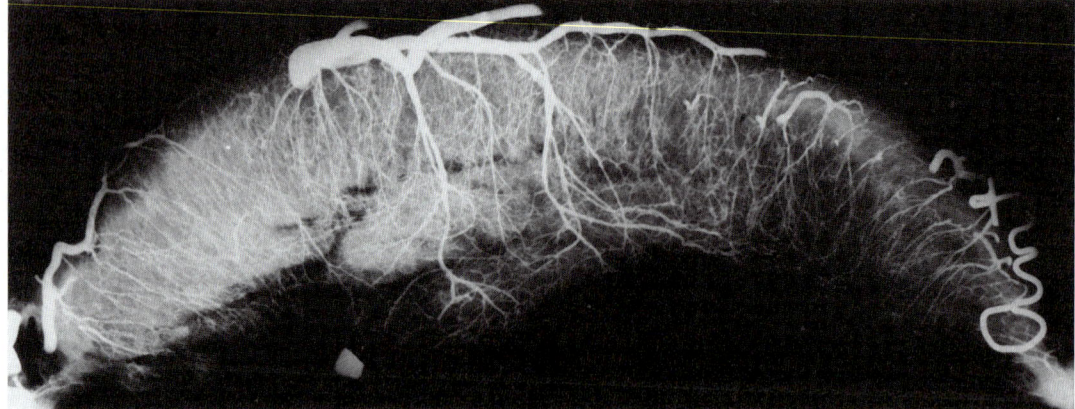

FIGURE 11-4
Arteriogram of a longitudinal segment of the posterior wall of the left ventricle including the posterior papillary muscle. Note the two types of branches passing into the myocardium at right angles to the epicardial artery *(top)*: class A, which quickly divide into a fine network, and class B, which maintain a large diameter and pass with little branching into the subendocardial region and the papillary muscle.

nisms (see below) allow the cardiac output to be maintained by increasing diastolic ventricular filling pressure and end-diastolic volume. This situation results in the characteristic signs and symptoms of congestive heart failure. Because of the heart's capacity to compensate, congestive heart failure is often tolerated for many years.

The ability of the heart to compensate after cardiac injury is based on the same mechanisms that allow cardiac output to increase in response to stress. **The fundamental compensatory mechanism is based on the Frank-Starling mechanism, which states that the stroke volume of the heart is a function of diastolic fiber length and that, within certain limits, the normal heart will pump whatever volume is brought to it by the venous circulation** (Fig. 11-5). Stroke volume is a measure of ventricular function. It is enhanced by increasing ventricular end-diastolic volume secondary to an increase in atrial filling pressure.

The increase in contractile force that occurs in response to ventricular dilation is a consequence of myofibrillar organization, in which stretching of the sarcomeres results in a greater potential for overlap of thick and thin filaments during contraction. This effect allows enhanced force generation, provided that the sarcomere is not stretched beyond 2.2 µm. When there is a sudden need to increase cardiac output in a normal heart, such as during exercise, catecholamine stimulation causes an increase in both heart rate and contractility. The latter is mediated primarily through modulation of the activities of key proteins that regulate calcium transients during excitation–contraction coupling. As a result, the normal relationship between end-diastolic volume and stroke volume is shifted upward (from curve A to curve X in Fig. 11-5). End-diastolic volume may also increase, resulting in a large increase in cardiac output.

In the presence of cardiac injury, overall cardiac function tends to be depressed in the basal state. Under these circumstances, higher than normal filling pressures are required to maintain cardiac output (curve Y in Fig. 11-5). Moreover, during cardiac failure, catecholamine stimulation is often present in the basal state, so that a comparable increase in cardiac output requires a larger increase in atrial pressure in the failing heart than in the normal one. **The most prominent feature of heart failure is the abnormally high atrial filling pressure relative to stroke volume.** However, the absolute values of stroke volume and cardiac output are generally well maintained.

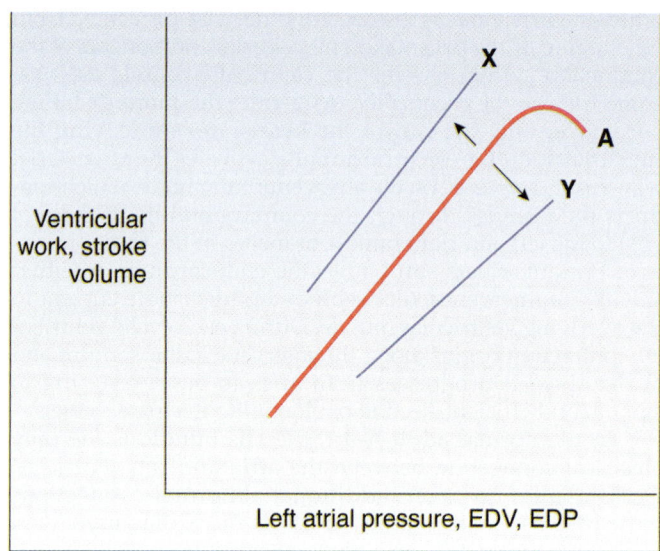

FIGURE 11-5
Relation between the work of the heart (or stroke volume) and the level of venous inflow, as measured by atrial pressure, ventricular end-diastolic volume, or end-diastolic pressure. *Curve A* indicates that as ventricular end-diastolic volume (EDV), end-diastolic pressure (EDP), or left atrial pressure increases, the amount of work done by the heart increases linearly up to a point. Beyond this point, the work done decreases, and the heart fails. However, the downslope of this curve is reached only at very high left atrial pressures. The curve may shift upward to position *X* or downward to position *Y*, depending on whether contractility has increased (e.g., because of the action of norepinephrine) or decreased (i.e., in failure), respectively. The failing heart usually functions on the ascending limb of a depressed curve.

Pathogenesis: Myocardial hypertrophy is an adaptive response that augments the contractile strength of the myocytes. It develops as a compensatory response to hemodynamic overload, which occurs in association with chronic hypertension or valvular stenosis (pressure overload), myocardial injury, valvular insufficiency (volume overload), and other stresses that increase the workload of the heart. The importance of this adaptive mechanism was noted more than a century ago by Austin Flint, who suggested that like the enlargement of skeletal muscle in athletes, cardiac hypertrophy compensates for hemodynamic overloading of the heart. A distinction must be made, however, between *physiological* hypertrophy of the heart, which develops in highly trained athletes, and *pathological* hypertrophy, which occurs in response to injury or overload. The hypertrophic response features enlargement of cardiac myocytes and accumulation of sarcomeric proteins, without an increase in the number of cardiac myocytes. Initially, hypertrophy reflects a compensatory and potentially reversible mechanism, but with persistent stress on the heart, the myocardium becomes irreversibly enlarged and dilated (Fig. 11-6).

Receptor-mediated events that are triggered by a stimulus act by autocrine and paracrine mechanisms to promote the hypertrophic response. Contractile cells respond to mechanical stimuli, such as stretching in response to an external load, by activating receptor-mediated signaling pathways that produce the hypertrophic response. Among the most important ligands that activate hypertrophy pathways are (1) angiotensin II, (2) endothelin-1, and (3) various growth factors, including insulin-like growth factor-1 (IGF-1) and transforming growth factor-β (TGF-β). Some of these mediators may also act on interstitial fibroblasts in the heart to promote synthesis and deposition of extracellular matrix. The most important signaling cascades involve (1) mitogen-activated protein kinase (MAPK) and protein kinase C (PKC) pathways, which are activated by G protein-coupled receptors, and (2) calcineurin A and calcium/calmodulin- dependent protein kinase (CamK) pathways, which are regulated by calcium. Events mediated by the adrenergic receptor have been implicated in the transition from compensatory hypertrophy to heart failure.

ANGIOTENSIN II (ANG II): All components of the renin–angiotensin system (renin, angiotensinogen, angiotensin-converting enzyme [ACE], and Ang II receptors)

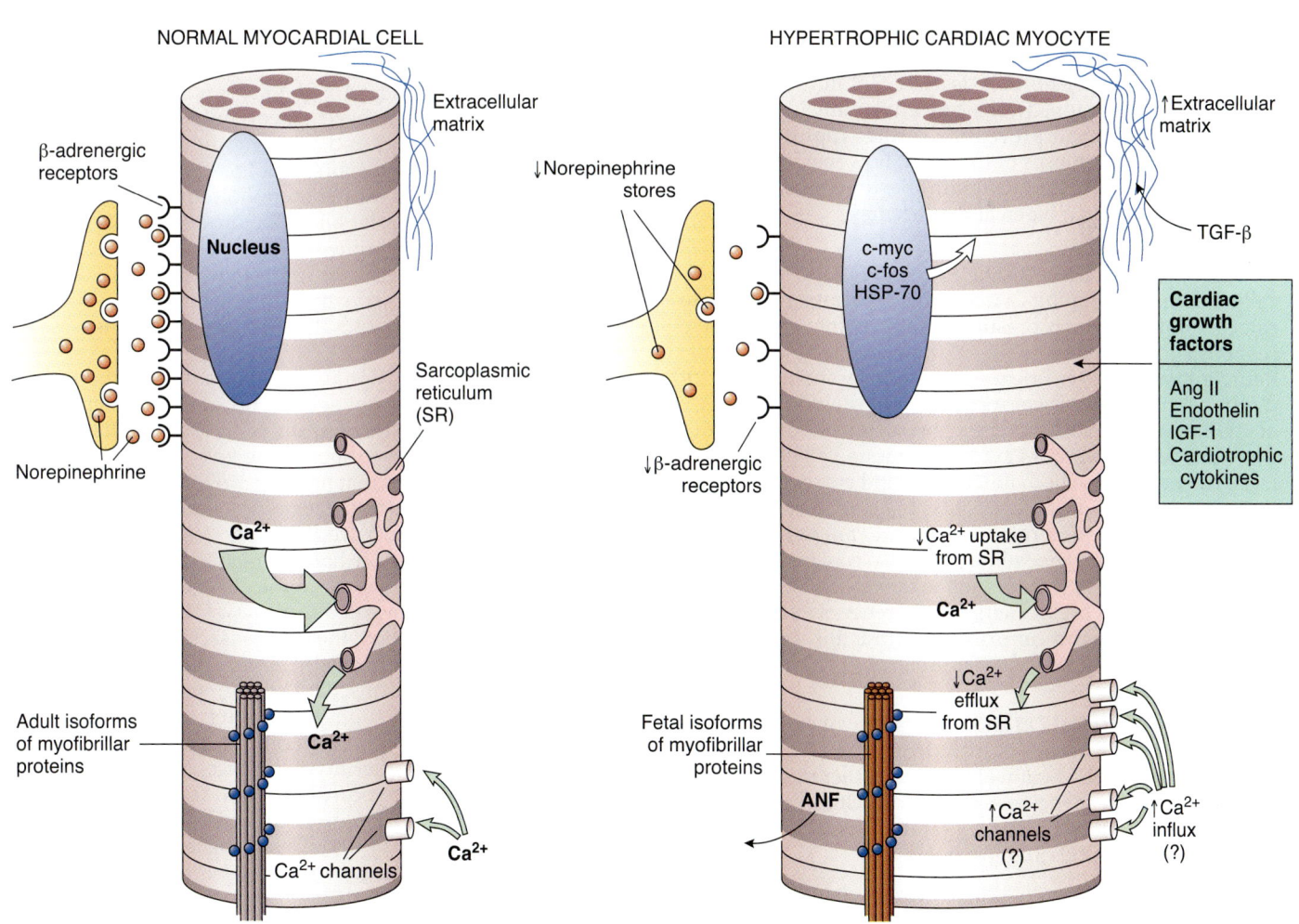

FIGURE 11-6
Biochemical characteristics of myocardial hypertrophy and congestive heart failure.

are present in both cardiac myocytes and interstitial fibroblasts of the myocardium. Ang II is released locally in response to load or stress stimuli and acts by autocrine and paracrine mechanisms to promote myocyte hypertrophy and the production of extracellular matrix. In this context, treatment with an ACE inhibitor tends to reverse cardiac hypertrophy and normalize heart size. ACE inhibitors also prevent cardiac hypertrophy induced by experimental hypertension, without reducing the elevated arterial pressure.

ENDOTHELIN-1 (ET-1): ET-1 is a powerful vasoconstrictor produced by a variety of cells, including endothelial cells and cardiac myocytes. This peptide is also a potent growth factor for cardiac myocytes. Like Ang II, ET-1 activates MAPK cascades on binding to its receptor to promote cardiac hypertrophy.

INSULIN-LIKE GROWTH FACTOR-1: IGF-1 is a growth-promoting peptide that is synthesized locally in most tissues. As a growth factor for cardiac myocytes, substantial evidence exists in experimental models that IGF-1 participates in the pathogenesis of cardiac hypertrophy.

EXTRACELLULAR MATRIX: Short-term overload of the heart leads to a prompt increase in collagen synthesis. Interstitial fibrosis, which occurs in virtually all forms of heart failure, is an obligatory feature of the hypertrophic response. Deposition of matrix proteins results, at least in part, from stimulation of cardiac fibroblasts by TGF-β and Ang II. After myocardial infarction, fibrosis is important in replacing necrotic myocytes and preventing cardiac rupture. As with many adaptive responses of the heart, however, myocardial fibrosis eventually interferes with diastolic relaxation and impairs diffusion of oxygen and nutrients.

β-ADRENERGIC DESENSITIZATION: The chronically failing heart exhibits a markedly depressed response to catecholamines, which presumably represents an adaptive response to the elevated circulating levels of autonomic neurotransmitters in heart failure. Desensitization of β-adrenergic receptors contributes to the sluggish response of the failing heart to exercise. Chronic overstimulation of these myocyte receptors by endogenous catecholamines leads to a decrease in both the number and responsiveness of receptors. In addition, there appears to be a defect in the coupling of the β-adrenergic receptor to adenylyl cyclase through G proteins. The failing heart also contains less norepinephrine stored in the autonomic nerve endings. Interestingly, treatment with blockers of β-adrenergic receptors reduces mortality and improves contractile function in patients with advanced heart failure.

CALCIUM HOMEOSTASIS: A variety of defects in calcium homeostasis occurs in hypertrophy and heart failure. The expression and function of important calcium-regulating proteins in cardiac myocytes are altered, including (1) the cardiac ryanodine receptor (RyR2), (2) the SR Ca^{2+}-dependent ATPase (SERCA), and (3) phospholamban.

- **RyR2,** the major calcium release channel in the SR, is activated during the action potential by the influx of extracellular Ca^{2+} through voltage-gated calcium channels in the sarcolemma. A decrease in the number of RyR2 channels impairs contractile function by reducing the rate of Ca^{2+} release from the SR.
- **SERCA** is the pump responsible for reuptake of Ca^{2+} back into SR once contraction has occurred. Decreased Ca^{2+} uptake by the SR is mediated by a reduced amount and abnormal regulation of SERCA. As a result, interference with Ca^{2+} sequestration during diastole leads to impaired relaxation.
- **Phospholamban** is a key regulator of cardiac contractility that inhibits SERCA. Enhanced phospholamban–SERCA interactions lead to chronically elevated Ca^{2+} levels during diastole and have been implicated in chronic heart failure.
- **Calcineurin A and CamK pathways,** both of which are regulated by Ca^{2+}, have also been implicated in the hypertrophic response.

The hypertrophic response involves changes in gene expression in cardiac myocytes, including activation of protooncogenes and reexpression of "fetal" genes.

PROTOONCOGENES AND MYOCARDIAL HYPERTROPHY: Within an hour of the stress produced by acute pressure overload, myocardial cells respond by expressing the protooncogenes c-*jun* and c-*fos* and heat shock protein 70 (HSP 70). It is likely that transcription of protooncogenes helps orchestrate the reexpression of fetal protein isoforms in the hypertrophic heart.

EXPRESSION OF FETAL GENES: A number of protein isoforms are expressed in the fetal heart but not after birth. In cardiac hypertrophy induced by hemodynamic overload, many of these genes are reexpressed. For example, atrial natriuretic factor (ANF) is expressed in both the ventricle and atrium in the fetus, but after birth, the production of ANF is restricted to the atrium. In the hypertrophic ventricle, however, ANF and brain natriuretic protein (BNP) are abundantly reexpressed and serve to reduce hemodynamic overload through their effects on salt and water metabolism (see Chapter 7).

Cardiac hypertrophy is also accompanied by the reexpression of fetal isoforms of several contractile proteins. In the rat, the normal adult isoform is β-myosin that has high ATPase activity and a rapid shortening velocity. By contrast, the fetal type is β-myosin that has lower ATPase activity and a slower shortening velocity. In experimental cardiac hypertrophy, "fast" β-myosin is replaced by "slow" β-myosin, leading to impaired myocardial contractility. However, this change in myosin gene expression is also adaptive, since it increases the tension generated during systole and improves the efficiency of contraction, thereby conserving energy. Hypertrophied human hearts exhibit similar, but not identical, changes in myosin isoforms. The human ventricle contains only slow myosin, and the hypertrophic heart exhibits a change from fast to slow myosin only in the atrium. However, fetal isoforms of other myofibrillar proteins appear in the human ventricular myocardium, including fetal forms of actin and tropomyosin. The hypertrophied heart also contains abnormal varieties of lactic dehydrogenase (LDH), creatine kinase (CK), and the sarcolemmal sodium pump.

Another adaptive gene switch occurs in expression of proteins involved in energy metabolism. The fetal heart relies primarily on maternally-derived glucose for ATP production. After birth, however, the heart downregulates genes encoding glycolytic enzymes and increases the expression of genes that encode proteins involved in β-oxidation of fatty acids. The failing heart reverts to using glucose by re-expressing the fetal pattern of genes regulating energy metabolism. Although a mole of glucose yields less ATP than a mole of fatty acid, glycolytic metabolism requires less oxygen. In the case of the failing heart, this switch is, therefore, advantageous.

Apoptosis of cardiac myocytes may play an important role in heart failure. A 5-fold increase in the number of cardiac myocytes undergoing apoptosis has been observed in animal models of heart disease, and senescent rats have 30% fewer cardiac myocytes than young ones.

 Pathology: Anything that increases the workload of the heart for a prolonged period or produces structural damage may eventuate in myocardial failure. **Ischemic heart disease is by far the most common condition responsible for cardiac failure, accounting for more than 80% of deaths from heart disease.** Most of the remaining deaths are caused by nonischemic forms of heart muscle disease (cardiomyopathies) and congenital heart disease. Virtually all of the organs of the body suffer the effects of heart failure. The subject is discussed in detail in Chapter 7, and only the salient features are reviewed here.

Other than the changes characteristic of specific disease entities (e.g., ischemic heart disease or cardiac amyloidosis) the morphological changes in the failing heart are nonspecific. **Ventricular hypertrophy is observed in virtually all conditions associated with chronic heart failure.** Initially, only the left ventricle may become hypertrophied, as in the case of compensated hypertensive heart disease. But when the left ventricle fails, some right ventricular hypertrophy usually follows, owing to the increased work load imposed on the right ventricle by the failing left ventricle. **In most cases of clinically apparent heart failure, the ventricles are conspicuously dilated.** The distribution of end-organ involvement depends on whether the heart failure is predominantly left-sided or right-sided.

Left-sided heart failure is the more common type of heart failure, because the most frequent causes of cardiac injury (e.g., ischemic heart disease and hypertension) primarily affect the left ventricle. In a compensatory response to left ventricular failure, left atrial and pulmonary venous pressures increase, resulting in passive pulmonary congestion. The capillaries in the alveolar septa fill with blood, and small ruptures allow the escape of erythrocytes. As a result, the alveoli contain many hemosiderin-laden macrophages (so-called heart failure cells). Moreover, if capillary hydrostatic pressure exceeds plasma osmotic pressure, fluid leaks from the capillaries into the alveoli. The resultant *pulmonary edema* may be massive, with alveoli being "drowned" in a transudate. Interstitial pulmonary fibrosis results when congestion is present over an extended period.

Right-sided heart failure commonly complicates left-sided failure, or it can develop independently secondary to intrinsic pulmonary disease or pulmonary hypertension, which create resistance to blood flow through the lungs. As a consequence, right atrial pressure and systemic venous pressure both increase, resulting in jugular venous distention, edema of the lower extremities, and congestion of the liver and spleen. Hepatic congestion in heart failure is characterized by distended central veins, which stand out on the cut surface of the liver as dark red foci against the yellow of the

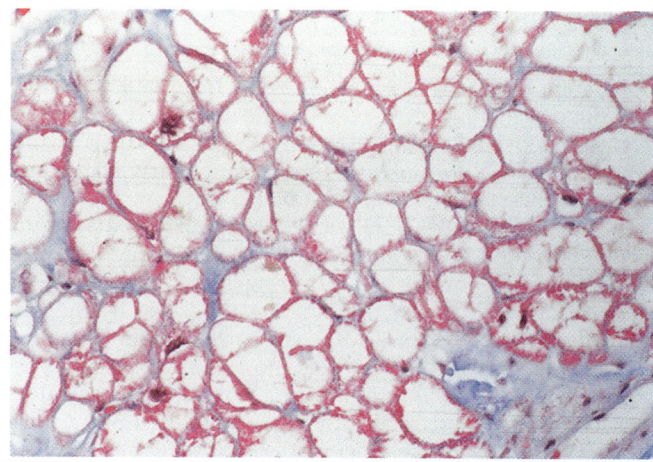

FIGURE 11-7
Severe myocytolysis in a patient with end-stage heart failure. Chronically injured myocytes show dramatic loss of myofibrils, giving the cells a marked vacuolated appearance. Only a thin rim of contractile cytoplasm is present, immediately beneath the sarcolemma.

cells in the periphery of the lobule. This gives the liver a gross appearance that has been compared to the cut surface of a nutmeg (hence the term **nutmeg liver;** see Chapter 14).

Chronically injured cardiac myocytes exhibit degenerative changes characterized by loss of myofibrils. Regardless of the type of injury, dysfunctional myocytes lose sarcomeres and show a corresponding increase in cytosol and glycogen, which causes the cells to appear vacuolated (myocytolysis) (Fig. 11-7). These changes are apparently reversible and likely result from perturbations in myocyte metabolism. Myofibrillar loss may be an adaptive response designed to enhance myocyte survival in the face of chronic injury. This histopathological appearance is especially prominent in "*hibernating myocardium,*" a condition in which contractile function is impaired at rest in the setting of reduced coronary blood flow.

 Clinical Features: The clinical symptoms of left-sided failure include dyspnea on exertion, orthopnea (dyspnea when lying down), and paroxysmal nocturnal dyspnea. Dyspnea on exertion reflects the increasing pulmonary congestion that accompanies a higher end-diastolic pressure in the left atrium and ventricle. Orthopnea and paroxysmal nocturnal dyspnea result when thoracic blood volume increases, owing to reduced blood volume in the lower extremities when the patient is recumbent.

Although much of the clinical presentation of heart failure can be explained by venous congestion (backward failure), two aspects of congestive failure involve inadequate arterial perfusion of vital organs (forward failure). Most patients with left-sided heart failure retain sodium and water (edema), owing to decreased renal perfusion, a decreased glomerular filtration rate, and activation of the renin–angiotensin–aldosterone system (see Chapter 7). Inadequate cerebral perfusion can result in confusion, memory loss, and disorientation, and reduced perfusion of skeletal muscle leads to fatigue and weakness.

CONGENITAL HEART DISEASE

Congenital heart disease (CHD) results from faulty embryonic development, expressed either as misplaced structures (e.g., transposition of the great vessels) or an arrest in the progression of a normal structure from an early stage to a more advanced one (e.g., atrial septal defect).

The incidence of CHD is cited as almost 1% of all live births. This figure does not include certain common defects that are not functionally significant, such as an anatomically patent foramen ovale that is functionally closed by the left atrial flap that covers it. In this circumstance, the foramen ovale remains closed as long as the left atrial pressure is higher than that in the right atrium. A bicuspid aortic valve is also common and is usually asymptomatic until adulthood. The figures for the incidence of particular cardiovascular anomalies vary, depending on many factors, and a range derived from several sources is shown in Table 11-1.

Pathogenesis: The cause of CHD is usually not ascertained. However, it is worthwhile to determine whether the defect in any one case can be recognized as being mainly of genetic origin or primarily acquired, because this consideration is important to parents with respect to planning future pregnancies. Most congenital defects of the heart reflect a combination of multifactorial genetic and environmental influences. As in other diseases with multifactorial inheritance (see Chapter 6), the risk of recurrence increases among the siblings of an affected child. Whereas the incidence of CHD in the general population is 1%, it increases to 2 to 15% for a second pregnancy after the birth of a child with a heart defect. The risk for a third affected child may be as high as 30%. Moreover, an infant born to a mother with CHD also has an increased risk of cardiac defects.

Single-gene syndromes are only rare causes of CHD. A number of chromosomal abnormalities are associated with an increased incidence of congenital anomalies of the heart, most prominently Down syndrome (trisomy 21), but also other trisomies, Turner syndrome, and DiGeorge syndrome. However, these account for no more than 5% of all cases of CHD.

The best evidence for an intrauterine influence on the occurrence of congenital cardiac defects relates to maternal infection with rubellavirus during the first trimester, especially during the first 4 weeks of gestation. An association with other viral infections is suspected but is not as well documented. The maternal use of certain drugs in early pregnancy is also associated with an increased number of cardiac defects in the offspring. For example, the thalidomide syndrome (phocomelia) was associated with a 10% incidence of CHD. Other drugs implicated in the pathogenesis of CHD include alcohol, phenytoin, amphetamines, lithium, and estrogenic steroids. Maternal diabetes is also associated with an increased incidence of CHD.

Classification of Congenital Heart Disease

There are several ways to categorize hearts with congenital defects. One of the earliest clinically useful schemes was proposed by Maude Abbott, who grouped cases in three categories according to the presence or absence of cyanosis, as follows:

- **The acyanotic group** does not have an abnormal communication between the two circulations. Examples of the acyanotic group described by Abbott include coarctation of the aorta, right-sided aortic arch, and Ebstein malformation.
- **The cyanose tardive** group is defined as an initial left-to-right shunt with late reversal of flow. Abbott illustrated this group with cases of patent ductus arteriosus (PDA), patent foramen ovale, and ventricular septal defect. In patients with these anomalies, cyanosis supervenes later (i.e., tardive). Although the shunt is initially from left to right, it later becomes a right-to-left shunt (Eisenmenger complex) because progressive changes in pulmonary vessels increase vascular resistance in the lungs to the point where right ventricular pressure exceeds left ventricular pressure.
- **The cyanotic group** describes a permanent right-to-left shunt. This category of CHD includes tetralogy of Fallot, truncus arteriosus, tricuspid atresia, and complete transposition of the great vessels.

Since Abbott's grouping, numerous classification schemes have been developed to provide the detail necessary to meet clinical requirements, especially those of the cardiac surgeon. A more contemporary classification divides the cases into the groups shown in Table 11-2.

Initial Left-to-Right Shunt Reflects Higher Left-Sided Pressure

Ventricular Septal Defect

Ventricular septal defects are the most common of all congenital heart lesions (see Table 11-2) and occur as isolated lesions or in combination with other malformations.

Pathogenesis: The fetal heart consists of a single chamber until the fifth week of gestation, after which it is divided by the development of the interatrial and interventricular septa and by the formation of

TABLE 11-1 Relative Incidence of Specific Anomalies in Patients with Congenital Heart Disease

Ventricular septal defects—25 to 30%
Atrial septal defects—10 to 15%
Patent ductus arteriosus—10 to 20%
Tetralogy of Fallot—4 to 9%
Pulmonary stenosis—5 to 7%
Coarctation of the aorta—5 to 7%
Aortic stenosis—4 to 6%
Complete transposition of the great arteries—4 to 10%
Truncus arteriosus—2%
Tricuspid atresia—1%

T A B L E *11-2* **Classification of Congenital Heart Disease**

Initial left-to-right shunt
  Ventricular septal defect
  Atrial septal defect
  Patent ductus arteriosus
  Persistent truncus arteriosus
  Anomalous pulmonary venous drainage
  Hypoplastic left heart syndrome

Right-to-left shunt
  Tetralogy of Fallot
  Tricuspid atresia

No shunt
  Complete transposition of the great vessels
  Coarctation of the aorta
  Pulmonary stenosis
  Aortic stenosis
  Coronary artery origin from pulmonary artery
  Ebstein malformation
  Complete heart block
  Endocardial fibroelastosis

the atrioventricular valves from the endocardial cushions. A muscular interventricular septum grows upward from the apex toward the base of the heart (Fig. 11-8). The muscular septum is joined by the down-growing membranous septum, thereby separating the right and left ventricles. **The most common ventricular septal defect is related to the failure of the membranous portion of the septum to form in whole or in part.**

Pathology: Ventricular septal defects vary in size. They occur as (1) a small hole in the membranous septum, (2) a large defect involving more than the membranous region (perimembranous defects), (3) defects in the muscular portion, which are more common anteriorly but can occur anywhere in the muscular septum, or (4) complete absence of the muscular septum (leaving a single ventricle).

Ventricular septal defects occur most commonly in the superior portion of the septum below the outflow tract of the pulmonary artery (below the crista supraventricularis, i.e., infracristal), and behind the septal leaflet of the tricuspid valve. The common bundle (bundle of His) is located immediately below the defect (inlet type). Less commonly, the defect occurs above the crista supraventricularis (supracristal) and just below the pulmonary valve (infraarterial). The supracristal variety of septal defect is often associated with other defects, such as an overriding pulmonary artery (the *Taussig-Bing* type of double-outlet right ventricle), transposition of the great vessels, or persistent truncus arteriosus.

Clinical Features: A small septal defect may have little functional significance and may actually close spontaneously as the child matures. Closure is accomplished by either hypertrophy of the adjacent muscle or adherence of the tricuspid valve leaflets to the margins of the defect. In infants with large septal defects, the higher pressure in the left ventricle creates initially a left-to-right shunt. Left ventricular dilation and congestive heart failure are common complications of such shunts. If the defect is small enough to permit prolonged survival, the augmented pulmonary blood flow caused by shunting of blood into the right ventricle eventually results in thickening of the pulmonary arteries and increased pulmonary vascular resistance. This increased vascular resistance may be so great that the direction of the shunt is reversed and goes from right to left *(Eisenmenger complex)*. A patient with this condition displays late onset of cyanosis (i.e., tardive cyanosis). These children develop right ventricular hypertrophy and right-sided congestive heart failure.

Additional complications of ventricular septal defects include (1) infective endocarditis at the site of the lesion, (2) paradoxical emboli, and (3) prolapse of an aortic valve cusp (with resulting aortic valve insufficiency). Large ventricular septal defects are repaired surgically, usually in infancy.

Atrial Septal Defects

Atrial septal defects range in severity from clinically insignificant and asymptomatic anomalies to chronic, life-threatening conditions.

Pathogenesis: The embryological development of the atrial septum occurs in a sequence that permits the continued passage of oxygenated placental blood from the right to the left atrium through the patent foramen. The developing atrial septum is programmed to permit this right-to-left shunt to continue until birth. Beginning at the fifth week of intrauterine life, the septum primum extends downward from the roof of the atrium to join with the endocardial cushions, thereby closing the incomplete segment, or "ostium primum" (see Fig. 11-8). Before this closure is complete, the midportion of the septum primum develops a defect, or "ostium secundum," so that right-to-left flow continues. During the sixth week, a second septum (septum secundum) develops to the right of the septum primum, passing from the roof of the atrium toward the endocardial cushions. This process leaves a patent foramen at about the midpoint of the septum, known as the *foramen ovale*. The defect persists after birth until it is sealed off by the fusion of the septum primum and septum secundum, after which it is termed the *fossa ovalis*.

Pathology: The atrial septum may be defective at a number of sites (see Fig 11-8).

- **Patent foramen ovale:** Tissue derived from the septum primum situated on the left side of the foramen ovale functions as a flap valve that normally fuses with the margins of the foramen ovale, thereby sealing the opening. An incomplete seal of the foramen ovale, which

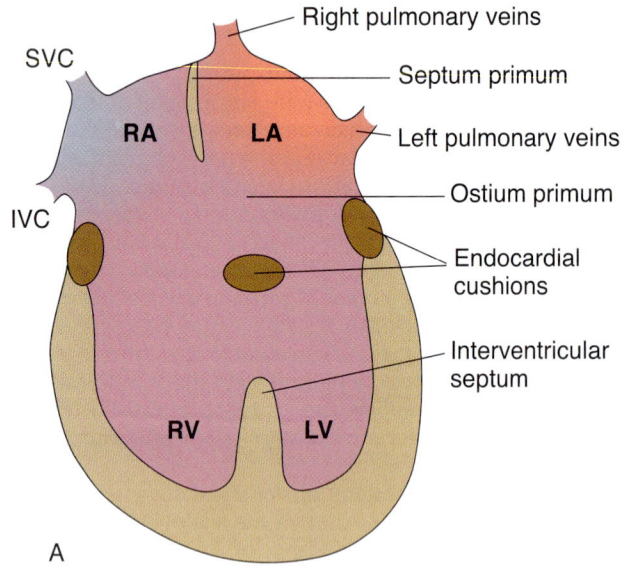
A

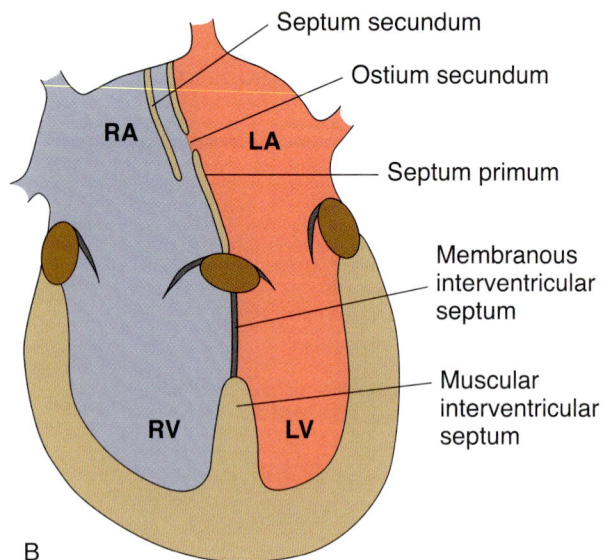
B

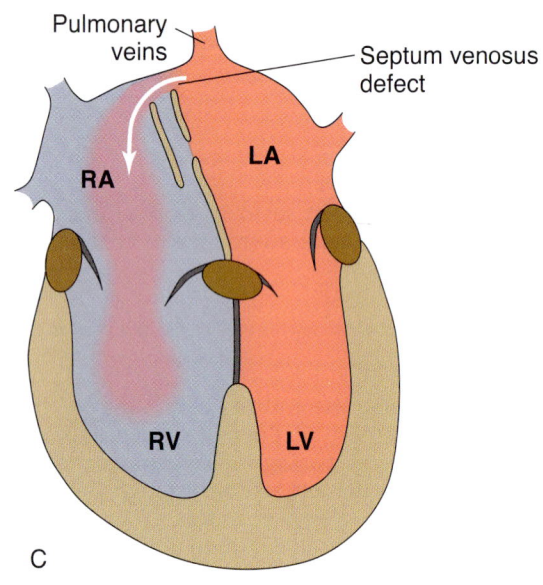
C

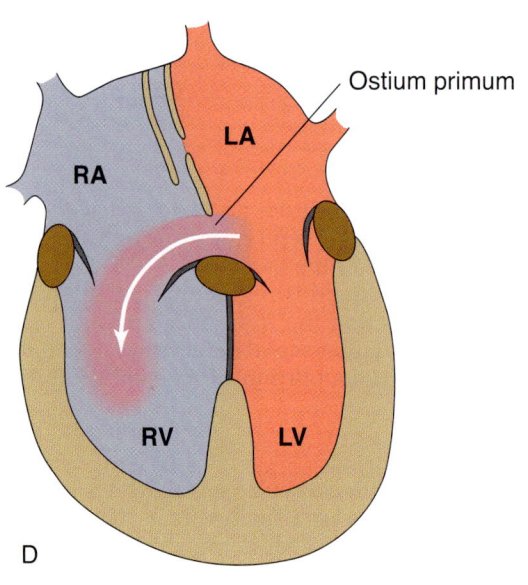
D

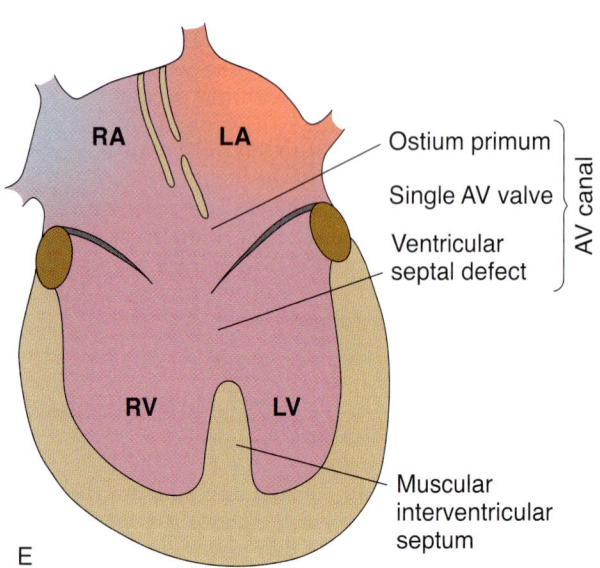
E

can be detected with a probe *(probe patent foramen ovale)*, is found in 25% of normal adults and is not normally functional. However, it may become a true shunt if circumstances increase the right atrial pressure, as can occur with recurrent pulmonary thromboemboli. If this situation develops, a right-to-left shunt will be produced, and thromboemboli from the right-sided circulation will pass directly into the systemic circulation. These paradoxical emboli can produce infarcts in many parts of the arterial circulation, most commonly in the brain, heart, spleen, intestines, kidneys, and lower extremities. A widely patent foramen ovale is occasionally encountered and is actually an acquired atrial septal defect caused by a disproportion between the size of the foramen ovale and the length of the valve covering it.

- **Atrial septal defect, ostium secundum type:** This lesion is by far the most common of the atrial septal defects, accounting for 90% of all cases. It reflects a true deficiency of the atrial septum and should not be confused with a patent foramen ovale. An ostium secundum defect occurs in the middle portion of the septum and varies in size, ranging from a trivial opening to a large defect of the entire fossa ovalis region. A small defect is usually not functional, but if it is larger, it may allow shunting of sufficient blood from the left to the right side of the heart to produce dilation and hypertrophy of the right atrium and right ventricle. Under these circumstances, the diameter of the pulmonary artery may exceed that of the aorta.

  Lutembacher syndrome, a variant of the ostium secundum type of atrial septal defect, is defined as the combination of mitral stenosis and an ostium secundum type of atrial septal defect. Mitral stenosis may be due to either a congenital malformation or rheumatic fever. It is thought that increased left atrial pressure secondary to mitral valve obstruction influences the continued patency of the atrial septum.

- **Sinus venosus defect:** This anomaly occurs in the upper portion of the atrial septum, above the fossa ovalis, near the entry of the superior vena cava. It is usually accompanied by drainage of the right pulmonary veins into the right atrium or superior vena cava. This uncommon defect occurs in only 5% of atrial septal defects.

- **Atrial septal defect, ostium primum type:** This condition involves the region adjacent to the endocardial cushion and is also rare, making up 7% of all atrial septal defects. There are usually clefts in the anterior leaflet of the mitral valve and the septal leaflet of the tricuspid valve, which may be accompanied by an associated defect in the adjacent interventricular septum.

- **Atrioventricular canal:**

  Persistent common atrioventricular canal represents fully developed combined atrial and ventricular septal defects. Although ordinarily rare, this defect is common in patients with Down syndrome.

  Complete atrioventricular canal is the consequence of a failure of the atrioventricular endocardial cushions to fuse. As a result, the defect includes (1) an enlarged ostium primum atrial septal defect, (2) an inlet ventricular septal defect, and (3) clefts in the septal leaflets of the tricuspid and mitral valves.

  Incomplete (partial) atrioventricular canal is a situation in which an ostium primum atrial septal defect is adjacent to the atrioventricular valves, which are often abnormal.

- **Coronary sinus atrial septal defect:** This abnormality is the rarest of the atrial septal defects. It is situated in the posteroinferior part of the interatrial septum at the site of the coronary sinus ostium and is associated with a persistent left superior vena cava, which drains into the roof of the left atrium.

 Clinical Features: Young children with atrial septal defects are ordinarily asymptomatic, although they may complain of easy fatigability and dyspnea on exertion. Later in life, usually in adulthood, changes in the pulmonary vasculature may reverse the flow of blood through the defect and create a right-to-left shunt. In such cases, cyanosis and clubbing of the fingers ensue. Complications of atrial septal defects include atrial arrhythmias, pulmonary hypertension, right ventricular hypertrophy, heart failure, paradoxical emboli, and bacterial endocarditis. Symptomatic cases are treated surgically.

FIGURE 11-8
Pathogenesis of ventricular and atrial septal defects. **A.** The common atrial chamber is being separated into the right and left atria (*RA* and *LA*) by the septum primum. Because the septum primum has not yet joined the endocardial cushions, there is an open ostium primum. The ventricular cavity is being divided by a muscular interventricular septum into right and left chambers (*RV* and *LV*). *SVC*, superior vena cava; *IVC*, inferior vena cava. **B.** The septum primum has joined the endocardial cushions but at the same time has developed an opening in its midportion (the ostium secundum). This opening is partly overlaid by the septum secundum, which has grown down to cover, in part, the foramen ovale. Simultaneously, the membranous septum joins the muscular interventricular septum to the base of the heart, completely separating the ventricles. **C.** The sinus venosus type of atrial septal defect is located in the most cephalad region and is adjacent to the inflow of the right pulmonary veins, which thus tend to open into the right atrium. **D.** The ostium primum defect occurs just above the atrioventricular valve ring, sometimes in the presence of an intact valve ring. It may also, in conjunction with a defect of the valve ring and ventricular septum, form an atrioventricular canal, as shown in (**E**). This common opening allows free communication between the atria and the ventricles.

Patent Ductus Arteriosus

Early in its development, the embryo supposedly recapitulates an ancestral evolutionary stage, with six aortic arches connecting the ventral and dorsal aortas as part of the branchial cleft system (Fig. 11-9). The left sixth aortic arch is partly preserved as the pulmonary arteries, and the arterial continuation on the left to the descending thoracic aorta is retained as the *ductus arteriosus*. The ductus conveys most of the pulmonary outflow into the aorta. After birth, the ductus contracts in response to the increased arterial oxygen content and becomes occluded by fibrosis (ligamentum arteriosus).

Pathogenesis: Persistent PDA is one of the most common congenital cardiac defects and is especially frequent in infants whose mothers were infected with rubellavirus early in pregnancy. It is also common in premature infants, in whom this structure is anatomically normal but in whom prematurity precluded closure. In these patients, the ductus usually closes spontaneously. In full-term infants with PDA, however, the ductus has an abnormal endothelium and media and only rarely closes spontaneously.

Clinical Features: The lumen of a PDA varies greatly. A small shunt has little effect on the heart, whereas a large one leads to considerable diversion of blood from the aorta to the low-pressure pulmonary artery. In severe cases, more than half of the left ventricular output may be shunted into the pulmonary circulation. As a result of the increased demand for cardiac output, left ventricular hypertrophy and heart failure ensue. In patients with a large PDA, the increased volume and pressure of blood in the pulmonary circulation eventually lead to pulmonary hypertension and its cardiac complications. Infective endarteritis is a frequent complication in untreated patients with PDA.

Patent ductus arteriosus can be corrected surgically or by cardiac catheterization. The PDA can be caused to contract and then close by the instillation of inhibitors of prostaglandin synthesis (e.g., indomethacin). Conversely, the ductus arteriosus can be kept open after birth by the administration of prostaglandins (PGE_2). This effect is used in treating patients born with a cardiac defect whose survival requires the presence of a left-to-right or right-to-left shunt. Examples include patients with isolated pulmonary stenosis, complete transposition of the great vessels, or hypoplastic left heart syndrome.

Aortopulmonary window is a defect between the base of the aorta and the pulmonary artery. It is a rare condition that is functionally similar to PDA and is clinically difficult to differentiate from it.

Other abnormalities of the aortic arch system can be predicted by visualizing the variations that could occur in the de-

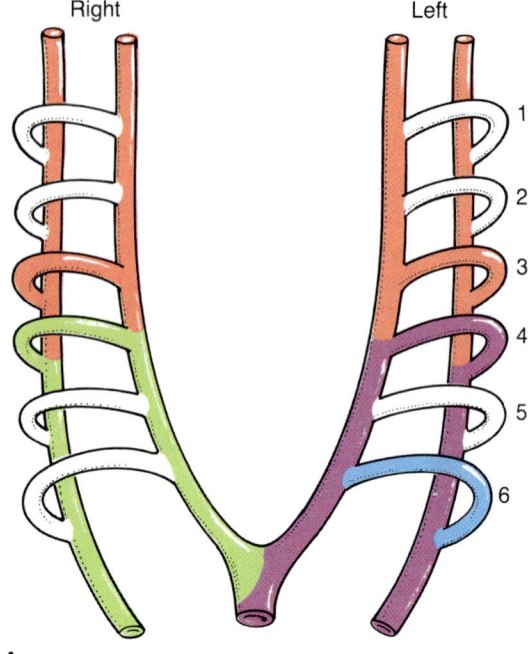

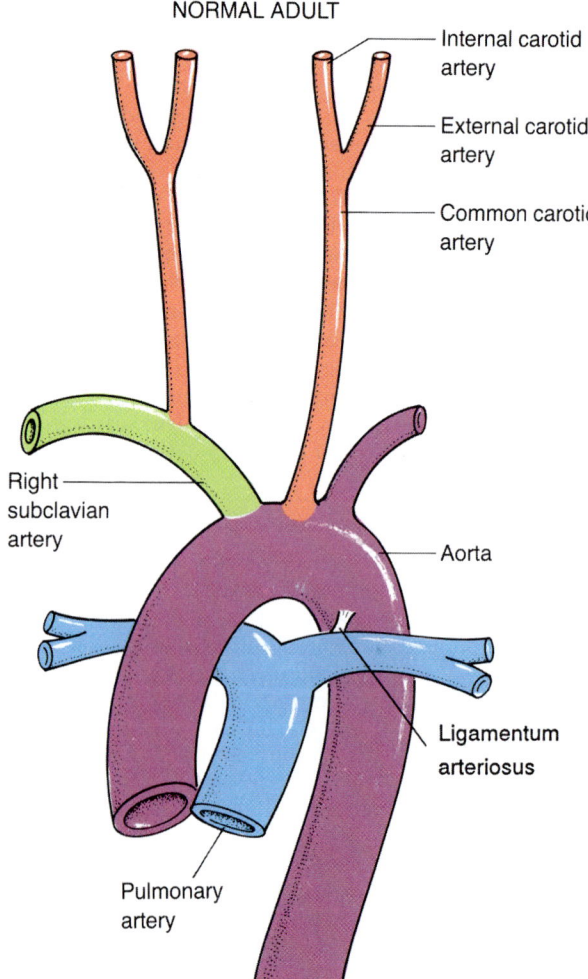

FIGURE 11-9
Derivatives of the aortic arches. **A.** Complete primitive aortic arch system. **B.** In the normal adult, the left fourth aortic arch is preserved as the arch of the adult aorta, and the left sixth arch gives rise to the pulmonary artery and ligamentum arteriosus (closed ductus arteriosus).

velopment of the complete aortic arch system (see Fig. 11-9). For example, the right side of the aortic arch system rather than the left may be retained, resulting in the condition known as a *right aortic arch*. This variant is seen in about 25% of patients with tetralogy of Fallot and in 50% of patients with truncus arteriosus. A right aortic arch is innocuous unless it creates a vascular ring that compresses the esophagus and trachea.

Truncus Arteriosus

Persistent truncus arteriosus refers to a common trunk for the origin of the aorta, pulmonary arteries, and coronary arteries. It results from absent or incomplete partitioning of the truncus arteriosus by the spiral septum.

Pathology: There are several variants of truncus arteriosus:

- **Type 1** is the most common variant and consists of a single trunk that gives rise to a common pulmonary artery and ascending aorta.
- **Type 2** displays right and left pulmonary arteries that originate from a common site in the posterior midline of the truncus.
- **Type 3** has separate pulmonary arteries that originate laterally from a common trunk.
- **Type 4** consists of other rare variants in which there is no pulmonary trunk at all and in which the pulmonary circulation is supplied from the aorta by enlarged bronchial arteries. This type is difficult to differentiate from tetralogy of Fallot with pulmonary artery atresia.

Truncus arteriosus always overrides a ventricular septal defect and receives blood from both ventricles. The valve of the truncus usually has three semilunar cusps but may have as few as two or as many as six. The coronary arteries arise from the base of the valve.

Clinical Features: Most infants with truncus arteriosus have torrential pulmonary blood flow, causing heart failure, recurrent respiratory tract infections, and often early death. In children with prolonged survival, pulmonary vascular disease develops, in which case cyanosis, polycythemia, and clubbing of the fingers appear. Open-heart surgery is an effective treatment.

Hypoplastic Left Heart Syndrome

Pathology: This usually profound malformation is characterized by hypoplasia of the left ventricle and ascending aorta and hypoplasia or atresia of the left-sided valves. Severe aortic valvular stenosis or aortic atresia is often the main defect. Some mitral valve structures are usually present, although the mitral valve may also be atretic. If the mitral valve is atretic rather than hypoplastic, the left ventricle may consist of only a thin slit lined by endocardium.

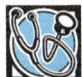

Clinical Features: Atresia of the aortic valve precludes left ventricular outflow into the aorta. There is an obligate left-to-right shunt through the patent foramen ovale, and cardiac output occurs entirely via the right ventricle and pulmonary artery. Systemic blood flow depends on flow from the pulmonary trunk to the aorta through the patent ductus arteriosus. Coronary blood flow depends on retrograde flow from a hypoplastic ascending aorta to the sinuses of Valsalva. Because pulmonary vascular resistance is high at birth, and both the foramen ovale and the ductus arteriosus are patent, newborns with hypoplastic left heart syndrome may appear well initially. However, as pulmonary vascular resistance falls, systemic blood flow (and especially coronary blood flow) decreases, and the infants become symptomatic. More than 95% of these infants will die within the first month of life without surgical intervention. Treatment includes surgical approaches or cardiac transplantation.

Anomalous Pulmonary Vein Drainage

The pulmonary veins form a network in the dorsal mesoderm. A bud from the region of the atrium joins the pulmonary venous confluence, and eventually all four pulmonary veins drain into the left atrium. Failure of these tissues to join correctly results in various venous anomalies.

Pathology: **Total anomalous pulmonary vein drainage** may occur as an isolated defect, or it may be part of the asplenia syndrome (splenic agenesis, congenital heart defects, and situs inversus of abdominal organs). Most commonly, the pulmonary veins drain into a common pulmonary venous chamber, and then through a persistent left superior vena cava (the persistent left pericardial vein) into the innominate vein or into the right superior vena cava. A second route for the common pulmonary vein drainage leads into the coronary sinus. A third drainage route consists of persistent posterior and subcardinal veins, which form a middorsal trunk that crosses the diaphragm and enters the portal vein or the ductus venosus. The third type of drainage is often associated with some pulmonary venous obstruction.

Clinical Features: In total anomalous pulmonary drainage, there is no direct venous return to the left side of the heart, and life is sustained only in the presence of an atrial septal defect or a patent foramen ovale. Heart failure, severe hypoxemia, and pulmonary venous obstruction result from total anomalous pulmonary vein drainage. Good results have been obtained with surgical correction.

Partial anomalous pulmonary venous drainage may result from less severe circulatory impairment. This anomaly may involve one or two pulmonary veins, especially in association with a sinus venosus type of atrial septal defect. The prognosis is excellent, similar to that for atrial septal defects.

Tetralogy of Fallot (Dominant Right-to-Left Shunt) Is the Most Common Cyanotic CHD

Tetralogy of Fallot represents 10% of all cases of CHD.

Pathology

The four anatomical changes that define the tetralogy of Fallot are as follows (Fig. 11-10):

- **Pulmonary stenosis**
- **Ventricular septal defect**
- **Dextroposition of the aorta so that it overrides the ventricular septal defect**
- **Right ventricular hypertrophy**

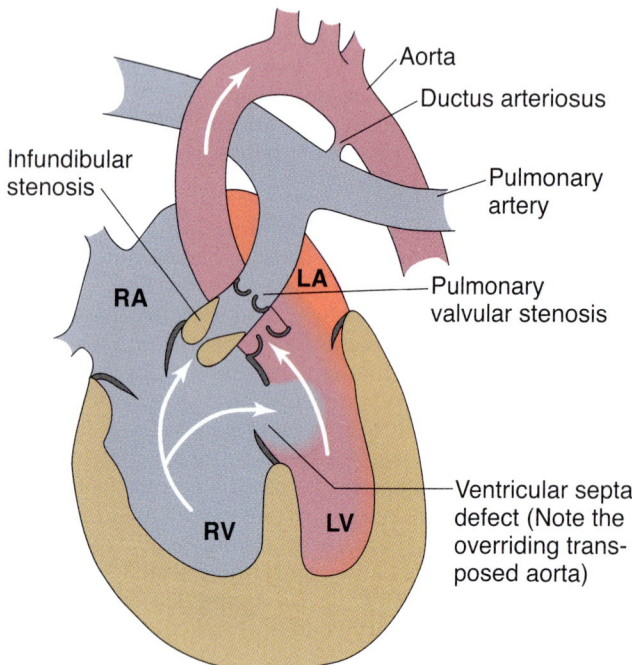

FIGURE 11-10
Tetralogy of Fallot. Note the pulmonary stenosis, which is due to infundibular hypertrophy as well as pulmonary valvular stenosis. The ventricular septal defect involves the membranous septum region. Dextroposition of the aorta and right ventricular hypertrophy are shown. Because of the pulmonary obstruction, the shunt is from right to left, and the patient is cyanotic.

The ventricular septal defect, which may be as large as the aortic orifice, is the result of incomplete closure of the membranous septum and involves both the muscular septum and the endocardial cushions. In addition, the development of the spiral septum, which normally divides the common truncus region into an aorta and pulmonary artery, is abnormal. As a result, the aorta is displaced into a more dextral position overlying the septal defect. The ventricular septal defect is immediately below the overriding aorta. Pulmonary stenosis is due to subpulmonary muscular hypertrophy, with an enlarged infundibular muscle obstructing blood flow into the pulmonary artery. In about one third of these hearts, the valve itself is the main cause of the stenosis; in such cases, the valve is usually funnel shaped, with the narrow part more distal.

The heart is hypertrophied in such a way as to give it a boot shape. Almost half of patients with tetralogy of Fallot display other cardiac anomalies, including ostium secundum atrial septal defects, PDA, left superior vena cava, and endocardial cushion defects. The aortic arch is on the right side in about 25% of cases of tetralogy of Fallot. The surgeon must remember that a large branch of the right coronary artery may cross the pulmonary conus region, which is the site of the cardiotomy made to enlarge the outflow tract. Patency of the ductus arteriosus is actually protective, because it provides a source of blood to the otherwise deprived pulmonary vascular bed.

Clinical Features: In the face of severe pulmonary stenosis, right ventricular blood is shunted through the ventricular septal defect into the aorta, resulting in arterial desaturation and cyanosis. Surgical correction is typically performed in the first 2 years of life. In children who are unrepaired, dyspnea on exertion is particularly noticeable, and the affected child often assumes a squatting position to relieve the shortness of breath. Physical development is characteristically retarded. Owing to marked polycythemia, cerebral thromboses may complicate the course of the disease. The patients are also at risk for bacterial endocarditis and brain abscesses. Increasing cyanosis and shortness of breath may indicate that a beneficial PDA has closed spontaneously. Left-sided heart failure is not a common complication.

In the absence of surgical intervention, tetralogy of Fallot carries a dismal prognosis. However, total correction is now possible with open-heart surgery, which carries less than 10% mortality. After successful surgery, the patients are asymptomatic and have an excellent long-term prognosis.

Tricuspid Atresia

Pathology: *Tricuspid atresia, or congenital absence of the tricuspid valve, results in an obligate right-to-left shunt through the patent foramen ovale.* This defect usually occurs with a ventricular septal defect through which blood gains access to the pulmonary artery. Type I tricuspid atresia, (75% of patients with tricuspid atresia) is associated with normally related great arteries. Type II is associated with D-transposition of the great arteries, and type III (rare) features L-malposition.

 Clinical Features: Infants with tricuspid atresia present with cyanosis due to right-to-left shunt at the atrial level. If the ventricular septal defect is small, limitation of pulmonary blood flow can result in even more significant cyanosis. In this scenario, a prominent cardiac murmur is typically noted. Surgical intervention is aimed at bypassing the atretic tricuspid valve and small right ventricle. Staged surgical palliation is the goal of current therapy.

Congenital Heart Diseases without Shunts Involve Various Cardiovascular Sites

Transposition of the Great Arteries

Transposition of the great arteries (TGA) refers to a situation in which the aorta arises from the right ventricle and the pulmonary artery from the left ventricle. The condition shows a male predominance and is more common in the offspring of mothers with diabetes. TGA is responsible for more than half of deaths in infants with cyanotic heart disease younger than 1 year.

 Pathogenesis: The normal division of the embryonic truncus arteriosus into the aorta and pulmonary artery depends on the spiral septum. Its abnormal development can produce aberrant positioning of the great arteries, such that the aorta is anterior to the pulmonary artery and connects with the right ventricle. In this circumstance, the pulmonary artery receives the outflow of the left ventricle (Fig. 11-11). Because the venous blood from the right side of the heart flows to the aorta, and the oxygenated blood from the lungs returns to the pulmonary artery, there are in effect two independent and parallel blood circuits for the systemic and pulmonary circulations. Thus, survival is possible only in the presence of a communication between the circuits. Virtually all infants with TGA have an atrial septal defect. One half of patients exhibit a ventricular septal defect, and two thirds have a PDA.

 Pathology: The aorta normally arises posterior to the pulmonary artery and to the left of it. In its ascending portion, it courses behind and to the right of the pulmonary artery. In TGA, the aorta is anterior to the pulmonary artery and to its right ("D" or dextrotransposition) all the way from its origin.

 Clinical Features: Before the advent of cardiac surgery, the outlook for infants born with TGA was hopeless, with 90% dying within the first year.

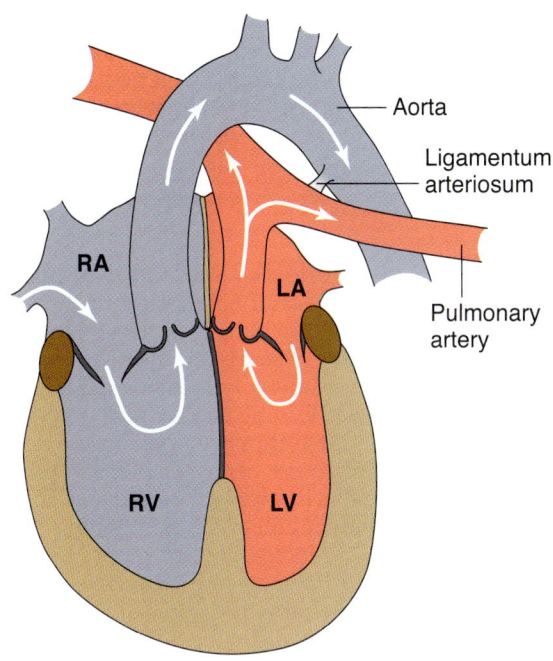

FIGURE 11-11
Complete transposition of great arteries, regular type. The aorta is anterior to, and to the right of, the pulmonary artery ("D-transposition") and arises from the right ventricle. In the absence of interatrial or interventricular connections or patent ductus arteriosus, this anomaly is incompatible with life.

However, it is now possible to correct the malformation within the first 2 weeks of life by means of an arterial-switch operation, with an overall survival rate of 90%.

Congenitally corrected transposition is a condition in which the aorta is anterior to, but passes to the left of, the pulmonary artery ("L" transposition). Although the great arteries are thus abnormally related to each other and arise from discordant ventricles, the circulatory pattern is functionally corrected because of coexistent atrioventricular discordance. Patients in whom corrected TGA is the only malformation are clinically entirely normal. Unfortunately, many cases are complicated by other cardiac anomalies, which require their own specific interventions.

The *Taussig-Bing malformation* is a double-outlet right ventricle (both great vessels arise from the right ventricle) in which a ventricular septal defect is above the crista supraventricularis and directly beneath an overriding pulmonary artery. This condition is functionally and clinically similar to TGA with a ventricular septal defect and pulmonary hypertension.

Coarctation of the Aorta

Coarctation of the aorta is a local constriction of the aorta that almost always occurs immediately below the origin of the left subclavian artery at the site of the ductus arteriosus. Rare coarctations can occur at any point from the aortic arch to the abdominal bifurcation. The condition is two to five times more frequent in males than females and is associated with a bicuspid aortic valve in two thirds of cases. Malformations of the mitral valve, ventricular septal defects, and subaortic stenosis may also accompany coarctation of the aorta. There is a particular association of coarctation with Turner syndrome. An increased incidence of berry aneurysms in the brain is also observed.

 **Pathogenesis and Pathology:** The pathogenesis of coarctation of the aorta is related to the pattern of flow in the ductus arteriosus during fetal life (Fig. 11-12). In utero blood flow through the ductus is considerably greater than that across the aortic valve. The blood leaving the ductus is diverted into two streams by a posterior aortic shelf opposite the orifice of the ductus. One stream passes cephalad into the relatively hypoplastic aortic isthmus to supply the head and upper extremities; the other stream enters the descending thoracic aorta. In late fetal life, the increasing left ventricular output dilates the isthmus, and the increased blood flow bypasses the obstruction (represented by the posterior shelf) through the wide ductal orifice. After birth, the ductal orifice is obliterated, and the posterior shelf normally involutes, thereby removing the obstruction. The shelf may not involute because of inadequate antegrade flow in the aortic arch in utero due to anomalies that limit left ventricular output (e.g., bicuspid aortic valve). Alternatively, in many instances the obstructing shelf fails to involute for unknown reasons. In any event, the result is the most common type of coarctation of the aorta, a *juxtaductal constriction*.

The *infantile (preductal) type of coarctation* results when the aortic isthmus remains narrow (hypoplastic) into late fetal life and after birth. This lesion is usually accompanied by a patent ductus arteriosus and a right-to-left shunt through a ventricular septal defect.

 Clinical Features: The clinical hallmark of coarctation of the aorta is a discrepancy in blood pressure in the upper and lower extremities. The pressure gradient produced by the coarctation causes hypertension proximal to the narrowed segment and, occasionally, dilation of that portion of the aorta.

Hypertension in the upper part of the body results in left ventricular hypertrophy and may produce dizziness, headaches, and nosebleeds. The increased pressure may also increase the risk of rupture of a berry aneurysm and conse-

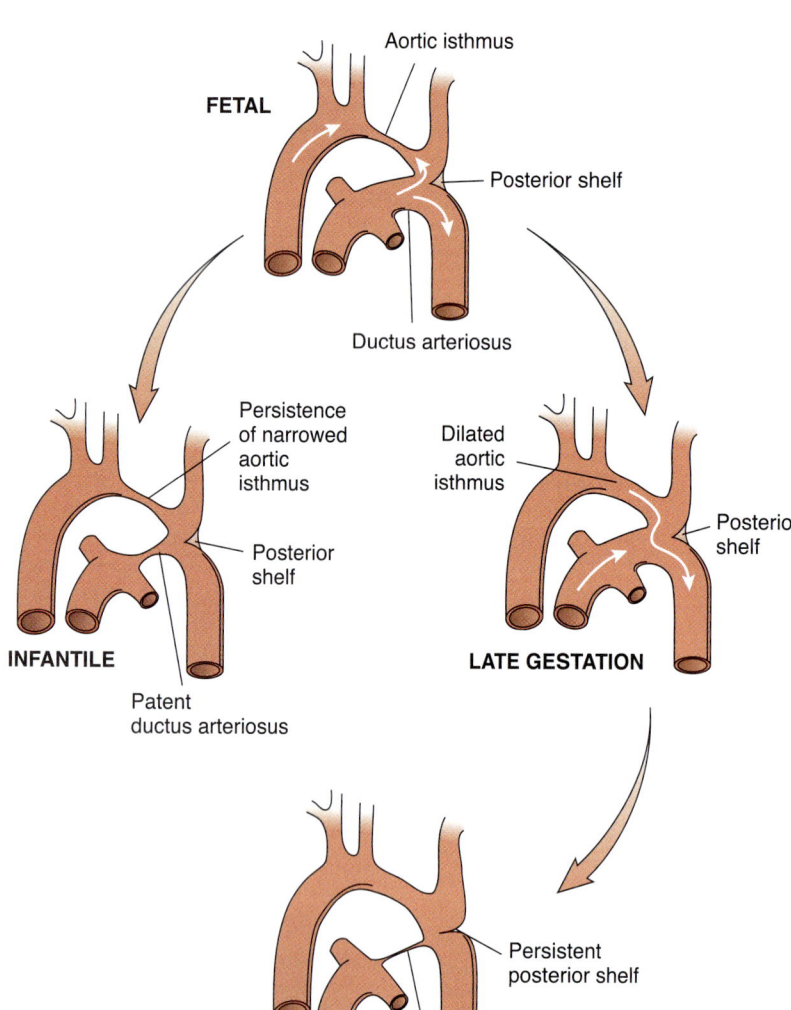

FIGURE 11-12
Pathogenesis of coarctation of the aorta. In the fetus, ductal blood is diverted into cephalad and descending streams by the posterior aortic shelf. In late fetal life, the isthmus dilates and the increased descending blood flow is accommodated by the ductal orifice. After birth, if the shelf does not undergo the normal involution, obliteration of the ductal orifice does not permit free flow around the persistent posterior shelf, thereby creating a juxtaductal obstruction of blood flow to the distal aorta. If the aortic isthmus does not dilate during late fetal life, it remains narrow, resulting in an infantile or preductal coarctation. In this circumstance, the ductus arteriosus usually remains patent.

quent subarachnoid hemorrhage. Hypotension below the coarctation leads to weakness, pallor, and coldness of the lower extremities. In an attempt to bridge the obstruction between the upper and lower aortic segments, collateral vessels enlarge. Radiological examination of the chest shows **notching of the inner surfaces of the ribs**, produced by increased pressure in the markedly dilated intercostal arteries.

Most patients with coarctation of the aorta who remain untreated die by age 40 years. Complications include (1) heart failure, (2) rupture of a dissecting aneurysm (secondary to cystic medial necrosis of the aorta), (3) infective endarteritis at the point of narrowing or at the site of jet-stream impingement on the wall immediately distal to the coarctation, (4) cerebral hemorrhage, and (5) stenosis or infective endocarditis of a bicuspid aortic valve. Coarctation of the aorta is successfully treated by surgical excision of the narrowed segment, preferably between 1 and 2 years of age for asymptomatic patients. Balloon dilation of the narrowed area by cardiac catheterization has also been performed.

Pulmonary Stenosis

Pulmonary stenosis results from (1) developmental deformities arising from the endocardial cushion region of the heart (with involvement of the pulmonary valves), (2) an abnormality of the right ventricular infundibular muscle (subvalvular or infundibular stenosis, especially as part of tetralogy of Fallot), or (3) abnormal development of the more distal parts of the pulmonary artery tree (peripheral pulmonary stenosis). Peripheral pulmonary stenosis, which is a much less common condition than the other two, may produce "coarctation" of the pulmonary arteries at one or several sites. This anomaly is more frequent in newborn infants with *Williams syndrome,* a disorder often associated with deletion mutations in the gene encoding elastin.

Isolated pulmonary stenosis ordinarily involves the valve cusps, which are fused to form an inverted cone or funnel type of constriction. The artery distal to the valve may develop poststenotic dilation after several years. In severe cases, infants exhibit hypertrophy of the right ventricle and atrium. In the presence of a patent foramen ovale, there is a right-to-left shunt with cyanosis, secondary polycythemia, and clubbing of the fingers. Good results have been obtained with balloon dilation of the stenotic valve by cardiac catheterization.

Congenital Aortic Stenosis

Three types of congenital aortic stenosis are recognized: valvular, subvalvular, and supravalvular.

VALVULAR AORTIC STENOSIS: The most common type of congenital aortic stenosis arises through abnormal development of the endocardial cushions and usually produces a bicuspid valve. A congenitally bicuspid aortic valve is considerably more frequent (4:1) in males than in females and is associated with other cardiac anomalies (e.g., coarctation of the aorta) in 20% of cases. The bicuspid valve typically features fusion of two of the three semilunar cusps (the right coronary cusp with one of the adjacent two cusps).

 Clinical Features: Many children with bicuspid aortic stenosis are asymptomatic. Over the years, the resulting bicuspid valve tends to become thickened and calcified, generally leading to symptoms in adulthood. More severe forms of congenital aortic stenosis result in a unicommissural valve or one without any commissures. These malformations cause symptoms in early life. Exertional dyspnea and angina pectoris may be prominent features. Sudden death poses a distinct threat to patients with severe obstruction, principally owing to ventricular arrhythmias. Bacterial endocarditis sometimes complicates the course of the disease. In symptomatic cases, aortic valvulotomy has had a high degree of success, although valve replacement is occasionally indicated.

SUBVALVULAR AORTIC STENOSIS: This defect accounts for 10% of all cases of congenital aortic stenosis and is caused by the abnormal development of a band of subvalvular fibroelastic tissue or a muscular ridge. The stenosis results from a membranous diaphragm or fibrous ring that surrounds the left ventricular outflow tract immediately below the aortic valve. It is twice as common in males as in females.

In many persons with subvalvular aortic stenosis, thickening and immobility of the aortic cusps develops, with mild aortic regurgitation. Bacterial endocarditis carries its own risks and may also aggravate the regurgitation. Surgical treatment of subvalvular aortic stenosis is accomplished by excising the membrane or fibrous ridge.

SUPRAVALVULAR AORTIC STENOSIS: This type of stenosis is much less common than the other two forms and is often associated with idiopathic infantile hypercalcemia (*Williams syndrome*), characterized by mental retardation and multiple system disorders.

Origin of a Coronary Artery from the Pulmonary Artery

A single coronary artery or, rarely, both may originate from the pulmonary artery rather than the aorta. When one coronary artery has an anomalous origin (most commonly the left coronary), anastomoses develop between the right and left coronary arteries. This produces an arteriovenous shunt through which blood flows from the artery originating from the aorta to that arising from the pulmonary artery. As a result, the myocardium supplied by the anomalous artery is vulnerable to episodes of ischemia. The result may be myocardial infarction, fibrosis and calcification, and endocardial fibroelastosis.

Ebstein Malformation

Ebstein malformation results from downward displacement of an abnormal tricuspid valve into an underdeveloped right ventricle. One or more of the tricuspid valve leaflets is plastered to the right ventricular wall for a variable distance below the right atrioventricular annulus.

Pathology: The septal and posterior leaflets of the tricuspid valve are usually involved in Ebstein malformation. They are irregularly elongated and adherent to the right ventricular wall, so that the upper part of the right ventricular cavity (inflow region) functions separately from the distal chamber. The anterior leaflet is usually the least involved of the three and may be normal. The valve ring may or may not be displaced downward from its usual position. In any event, the effective tricuspid valve orifice is displaced downward into the ventricle, thereby dividing it into two separate parts: the "atrialized" ventricle (proximal ventricle) and the functional right ventricle (distal ventricle). In two thirds of cases, conspicuous dilation of the functional ventricle hinders its ability to pump blood efficiently through the pulmonary arteries. The degree of insufficiency of the tricuspid valve depends on the severity and configuration of the defect in the leaflets.

 Clinical Features: Ebstein malformation leads to heart failure, massive right atrial dilation, arrhythmias with palpitations and tachycardia, and sudden death. Surgical treatment of Ebstein malformation has met with variable success.

Congenital Heart Block

 Pathogenesis: Congenital complete heart block usually occurs in association with other cardiac anomalies. In such cases, disruption in the continuity of the conduction system is probably caused by the accompanying cardiac abnormality. However, in cases of isolated complete heart block, failure of the atrioventricular conduction system is believed to result from the lack of regression of the sulcus tissue, which entirely encloses the conducting tissue during early development. Congenital heart block in the absence of structural heart disease has been linked to maternal connective tissue disease, especially systemic lupus erythematosus. In the presence of maternal SS-A/Ro or SS-B/La autoantibodies that are placentally transmitted to the fetus, the incidence of congenital complete heart block approaches 100%.

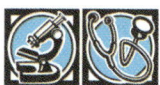 **Pathology and Clinical Features:** The hearts of patients with congenital heart block tend to show a lack of continuity between the atrial myocardium and the atrioventricular node. Alternatively, the defect may consist of a fibrous separation of the atrioventricular node from the ventricular conducting tissue. Although the heart rate is abnormally slow, patients with isolated heart block often have little functional difficulty. Later in life, cardiac hypertrophy, attacks of Stokes–Adams syncope (dizziness and unexpected fainting), arrhythmias, and heart failure may develop.

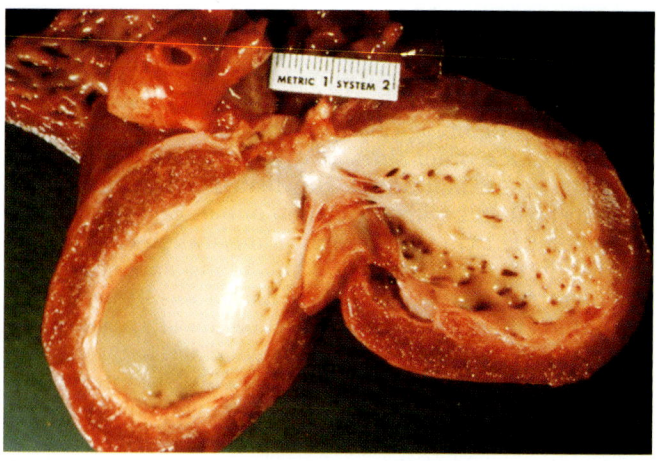

FIGURE 11-13

Endocardial fibroelastosis. The left ventricle of an infant who died of endocardial fibroelastosis has been opened to reveal a thickened endocardium lining most of the cavity and virtually obliterating the trabeculae carneae.

Endocardial Fibroelastosis

Endocardial fibroelastosis (EFE) is characterized by fibroelastic thickening of the endocardium of the left ventricle, which may also affect the valves. The disorder is classified as primary or secondary, the latter being far more common.

SECONDARY ENDOCARDIAL FIBROELASTOSIS: This disorder occurs in association with underlying cardiovascular anomalies that lead to left ventricular hypertrophy in the face of an inability to meet the increased oxygen demands of the myocardium. Thus secondary EFE is a frequent complication of congenital aortic stenosis (including hypoplastic left ventricle syndrome) and coarctation of the aorta. Presumably, some type of endocardial injury is involved in its pathogenesis.

 Pathology: On gross examination, the endocardium of the left ventricle displays irregular, opaque, grey-white patches, which also may be present on the cardiac valves. Microscopically, these plaques are areas of endocardial fibroelastotic thickening, frequently accompanied by degeneration of adjacent subendocardial myocytes. The valves may show collagenous thickening.

PRIMARY ENDOCARDIAL FIBROELASTOSIS: Defined as fibroelastosis in the absence of any associated lesion, this disorder is now quite rare. It afflicts infants, usually between 4 and 10 months of age. Although the disease has occurred in siblings, no specific mode of inheritance has been established. Recent evidence has linked primary endocardial fibroelastosis to mumps infection, which may explain why this condition is now so rarely encountered.

Pathology: The left ventricle is usually conspicuously dilated but occasionally contracted and hypertrophic. Diffuse endocardial thickening involves most of the left ventricle (Fig. 11-13) and the aortic and mitral valve leaflets. The thickened endocardium tends to obscure the trabecular pattern of the underlying myocardium, and the papillary muscles and chordae tendineae are thick and short. Mural thrombi may complicate the situation.

Infants with primary EFE develop progressive heart failure. The prognosis is dismal, and cardiac transplantation offers the only hope for a cure.

Dextrocardia

Dextrocardia refers to a rightward orientation of the base–apex axis of the heart, and is often associated with a mirror image of the normal left-sided location and configuration. The position of the ventricles is determined by the direction of the embryonic cardiac loop. If the loop protrudes to the right, the future right ventricle develops on the right and the left ventricle comes to occupy its proper position. If the loop protrudes to the left, the opposite occurs.

Pathology: When dextrocardia occurs without abnormal positioning of the visceral organs (situs inversus), the condition is invariably associated with severe cardiovascular anomalies. These include transposition of the great arteries, a variety of atrial and ventricular septal defects, anomalous pulmonary venous drainage, and many others. In dextrocardia that occurs in combination with situs inversus, the heart is functionally normal, although minor anomalies are not uncommon.

ISCHEMIC HEART DISEASE

Ischemic heart disease is, in most cases, a consequence of atherosclerosis of the coronary arteries. It develops when blood flow is inadequate to meet the oxygen demands of the heart. **Ischemic heart disease is by far the most common type of heart disease in the United States and other industrialized nations, where it remains the leading cause of death. It is responsible for at least 80% of all deaths attributable to heart disease.** By contrast, atherosclerotic heart disease is far less frequent in underdeveloped countries, such as those of Africa and many parts of Asia. The principal effects of ischemic heart disease are angina pectoris, myocardial infarction, chronic congestive heart failure, and sudden death.

ANGINA PECTORIS: *This term refers to the pain of myocardial ischemia. It typically occurs in the substernal portion of the chest and may radiate into the left arm, the jaw, and the epigastrium. It is the single most common symptom of ischemic heart disease.* Coronary atherosclerosis usually becomes symptomatic only when the luminal cross-sectional area of the affected vessel is reduced by more than 75%. A patient with typical angina pectoris exhibits recurrent episodes of chest pain, usually brought on by increased physical activity or emotional excitement. The pain is of limited duration (1–15 minutes) and is relieved by reducing physical activity or by treatment with sublingual nitroglycerin (a potent vasodilator).

Although the most common cause of angina pectoris is severe coronary atherosclerosis, decreased coronary blood flow can result from other conditions, including coronary vasospasm, aortic stenosis, or aortic insufficiency. Angina pectoris is not associated with any characteristic anatomical change in the myocardium as long as the duration and severity of the ischemic episode are insufficient to cause myocardial necrosis.

Prinzmetal angina (variant angina) *is an atypical form of angina that occurs at rest and is caused by coronary artery spasm.* The responsible mechanisms are not fully understood. Spasm can occur in structurally normal coronary arteries and may be part of a systemic syndrome of abnormal arterial vasomotor reactivity, which includes migraine headache and Raynaud phenomenon. Usually, however, it develops in atherosclerotic coronary arteries, often in a portion of the vessel adjacent to an atherosclerotic plaque. Whereas coronary artery spasm may contribute to the pathogenesis of an acute myocardial infarction or to the size of the infarct, it is generally not the principal cause of infarction.

Unstable angina, *a variety of chest pain that has a less predictable relationship to exercise than does stable angina and may occur during rest or sleep, is associated with the development of nonocclusive thrombi over atherosclerotic plaques.* In some cases of unstable angina, episodes of chest pain become progressively more frequent and of longer duration over a 3- to 4-day period. The electrocardiographic changes are not characteristic of infarction, and the serum levels of cardiac-specific intracellular proteins, such as MB-CK or cardiac troponins T or I, (evidence of myocardial necrosis), do not become elevated. Unstable angina is also termed *preinfarction angina*, *accelerated angina*, or "*crescendo*" *angina*. Without pharmacological or mechanical intervention to "open up" the coronary narrowing, many patients with unstable angina progress to myocardial infarction.

MYOCARDIAL INFARCT: *Myocardial infarct refers to a discrete focus of ischemic necrosis in the heart.* This definition excludes patchy foci of necrosis caused by drugs, toxins, or viruses. The development of an infarct is related to the duration of ischemia and the metabolic rate of the ischemic tissue. In experimental coronary artery ligation, foci of necrosis form after 20 minutes of ischemia and become more extensive as the period of ischemia lengthens.

CHRONIC CONGESTIVE HEART FAILURE: Because early mortality associated with acute myocardial infarction has fallen to less than 5%, many patients with ischemic heart disease survive longer and eventually develop chronic congestive heart failure. More than 75% of all heart failure patients have coronary artery disease as the major cause of their heart failure. Contractile impairment in these patients is due to irreversible loss of myocardium (previous infarcts) and hypoperfusion of surviving muscle, which leads to chronic ventricular dysfunction ("hibernating" myocardium). Many of these patients die suddenly, especially those in whom contractile impairment is not severe. Others develop progressive pump failure and die of multi-organ failure. Because coronary artery disease is often so extensive in these patients, and many have already undergone coronary artery bypass surgery, the only treatments available are cardiac transplantation or the use of artificial pumps (ventricular assist devices).

SUDDEN DEATH: In some patients, the first and only clinical manifestation of ischemic heart disease is sudden death due to spontaneous ventricular fibrillation. Some authorities consider death to be sudden only if it occurs within 1 hour of the onset of symptoms. Others regard death within 24 hours after the onset of symptoms to be sudden or require that sudden death be diagnosed only if it is unexpected. **In any event, coronary atherosclerosis underlies most cases of cardiac death occurring during the first hour after the onset of symptoms.**

Experimental animals subjected to acute coronary occlusion show a high incidence of ventricular fibrillation during the first hour of ischemia. Sudden cardiac death due to ventricular fibrillation also occurs in humans as a result of acute thrombosis of a coronary artery. On the other hand, such an arrhythmia also appears in patients with marked coronary artery disease and no detectable thrombosis. Clinical studies of patients who have been defibrillated and survived an arrhythmia have shown that most have not had acute myocardial infarction. No serum markers of myocardial necrosis can be found, and electrocardiographic changes indicating infarction do not develop. Thus, it appears that in many cases, a lethal arrhythmia is triggered by acute ischemia without overt myocardial infarction. The presence of a healed infarct or ventricular hypertrophy increases the risk that an episode of acute ischemia will initiate a life-threatening ventricular arrhythmia.

Epidemiology: **The major risk factors that predispose a person to coronary artery disease are (1) systemic hypertension, (2) cigarette smoking, (3) diabetes mellitus, and (4) elevated blood cholesterol level.** Any one of these factors significantly increases the risk of myocardial infarction, but the combination of multiple factors augments the risk more than sevenfold (see Chapter 8).

During the 20th century, the United States experienced first a dramatic increase and then a dramatic reversal in mortality from ischemic heart disease. In 1950, the age-adjusted death rate from myocardial infarction was 226 per 100,000 cases; 40 years later it was only 108. This shift is due to many factors, including reduction in smoking, consumption of less saturated fat in the diet, and the development of new drugs to control hypertension, reduce cholesterol, and dissolve coronary thrombi. Important advances in medical technology include the construction of coronary care units, coronary revascularization procedures, and the use of defibrillators and ventricular assist devices. During the second half of the 20th century, much attention was focused on the role of hyperlipidemia in the pathogenesis of coronary artery atherosclerosis. This was driven initially by epidemiological evidence showing that populations in which men have high mean serum cholesterol values exhibit a high rate of coronary artery disease. Since then, multiple studies have established that elevated serum low-density lipoproteins (LDLs) increase risk, whereas high levels of high-density lipoproteins (HDLs) decrease the risk of myocardial infarction. The total cholesterol/HDL cholesterol ratio appears to be a better predictor of coronary artery disease than the serum cholesterol level alone.

Although the blood lipid profile is an important determinant for the risk of atherogenesis, the other major risk factors exert powerful independent effects. A person with a blood pressure of 160/95 mm Hg has twice the risk of ischemic heart disease as one whose blood pressure is 140/75 mm Hg or less. Cigarette smoking is another major preventible cause of coronary artery disease, and the risk of ischemic heart disease is increased in proportion to the number of cigarettes smoked. Serum factors involved in thrombosis or thrombolysis or which contribute to endothelial injury have also been implicated in atherogenesis. For example, the level of plasma fibrinogen directly correlates with the risk of ischemic heart disease, presumably because of the role of fibrinogen in atherogenesis and coronary artery thrombosis. Other factors reported to contribute to an increased risk of myocardial infarction include factor VII, plasminogen activator inhibitor-1 (PAI-1), homocysteine, and decreased fibrinolytic activity. Levels of selected serum markers of inflammation such as C-reactive protein are predictors of ischemic heart disease risk.

During the past several years, there has been a remarkable increase in the incidence of type II diabetes in the United States, which has mirrored a similar increase in obesity. Ischemic heart disease is a major consequence of both type I and type II diabetes, the risk being twofold to threefold greater than that in the nondiabetic population. Conversely, atherosclerotic cardiovascular disease (myocardial infarction, stroke, peripheral vascular disease) accounts for 80% of all deaths in patients with diabetes.

Other risk factors for ischemic heart disease include the following:

- **Obesity:** In a major, longitudinal study of one population (Framingham Heart Study), obesity was an independent risk factor for cardiovascular disease, with an increased risk for obese persons over lean ones of 2 to 2.5.
- **Age:** The risk of infarction is greater with increasing age, up to age 80 years.
- **Sex:** Men remain at increased risk of ischemic heart disease, with 60% of coronary events occurring in men. Angina pectoris is considerably more frequent in men than in women; the ratio at ages younger than 50 years is 4:1 and that at age 60 years is 2:1.
- **Family history:** In one study that controlled for other risk factors, relatives of patients with ischemic heart disease had a twofold to fourfold increased risk for coronary artery disease. The genetic basis for this familial risk may interact with the other risk factors.
- **Use of oral contraceptives:** Women older than 35 years who smoke cigarettes and use oral contraceptives have a modestly increased incidence of myocardial infarction.
- **Sedentary life habits:** Regular exercise seems to reduce the risk of myocardial infarction, perhaps by increasing HDL levels. In one study, the least fit quartile of persons

subjected to exercise testing had a risk of myocardial infarction 6 times greater than that of persons in the fittest quartile.
- **Personality features:** Early studies suggested that aggressive, time-conscious, executive-type individuals ("type A" personality) have a higher incidence of heart disease than more easygoing, relaxed persons ("type B" personality). "Coronary-prone" subjects, those of the type A behavior pattern, tend to differ from type B individuals by having higher plasma triglyceride and cholesterol levels and greater urinary catecholamine excretion. However, the relationship between coronary artery disease and type A personality is controversial, and recent studies have failed to show the strong association previously reported.

Many Conditions Limit the Supply of Blood to the Heart

The heart is an aerobic organ, requiring oxidative phosphorylation to provide energy for contraction. The anaerobic glycolysis used by skeletal muscle under conditions of extreme physical exertion is an insufficient source of energy for cardiac contraction. Ischemic heart disease is caused by an imbalance between the oxygen demands of the myocardium and the supply of oxygenated blood (Table 11-3).

Atherosclerosis and Thrombosis

The pathogenesis of atherosclerosis is described in detail in Chapter 10. Here we only briefly discuss the features that are of special importance in relation to ischemic heart disease. The coronary arteries are conductance vessels, small muscu-

TABLE 11-3 **Causes of Ischemic Heart Disease**

Decreased supply of oxygen
  Conditions that influence the supply of blood
   Atherosclerosis and thrombosis
   Thromboemboli
   Coronary artery spasm
   Collateral blood vessels
   Blood pressure, cardiac output, and heart rate
   Miscellaneous: arteritis (e.g., periarteritis nodosa), dissecting aneurysm, luetic aortitis, anomalous origin of coronary artery, muscular bridging of coronary artery
  Conditions that influence the availability of oxygen in the blood
   Anemia
   Shift in the hemoglobin-oxygen dissociation curve
   Carbon monoxide
   Cyanide

Increased oxygen demand (i.e., increased cardiac work)
   Hypertension
   Valvular stenosis or insufficiency
   Hyperthyroidism
   Fever
   Thiamine deficiency
   Catecholamines

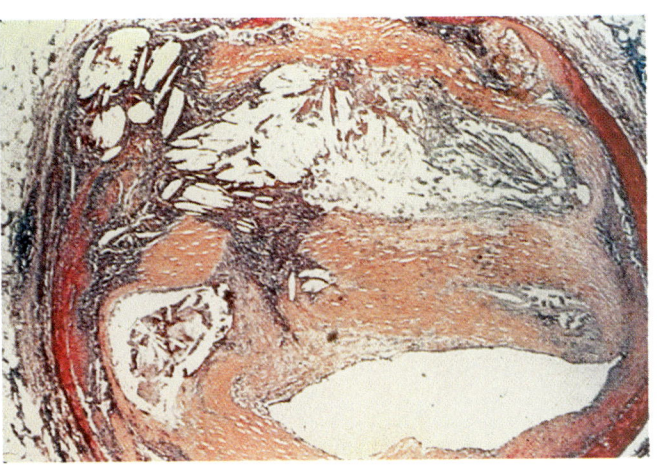

FIGURE **11-14**
Coronary atherosclerosis. Cross-section of an epicardial coronary artery shows severe atherosclerosis. The wall is thickened, and the lumen is reduced to a small slit by accumulation of atheromatous debris, including cholesterol crystals (needle-like spaces).

lar arteries with a prominent internal elastic lamina. Their principal role is to deliver blood to the regulatory vasculature (small intramural arteries and arterioles), which controls nutritive myocardial blood flow. A healthy person has substantial coronary flow reserve, and myocardial perfusion can be increased to 4 to 8 times the resting blood flow. In the normal heart, the large coronary arteries provide almost no resistance to blood flow; and the myocardial circulation is controlled mainly by constriction and dilation of small, intramyocardial branches less than 400 μm in diameter. In advanced atherosclerosis of the main epicardial coronary arteries (Fig. 11-14), luminal stenosis causes a decrease in blood pressure distal to the narrowed zone. To compensate for the reduced perfusion pressure, the microvessels dilate, thereby maintaining normal resting blood flow. As a result, most patients with coronary atherosclerosis do not have ischemia or angina at rest. However, with exercise, the capacity of the microcirculation to dilate further becomes limiting, and the demand for oxygen by the myocardium exceeds the blood supply. The result is ischemia and angina.

Maximal blood flow to the myocardium is not impaired until about 75% of the cross-sectional area of coronary artery (~50% of the diameter as assessed during coronary angiography) is compromised by atherosclerosis. However, resting blood flow is not reduced until more than 90% of the lumen is occluded. In patients with long-standing angina pectoris, the extent and distribution of collateral circulation exerts an important influence on the risk of acute myocardial infarction. There are conditions (e.g., hypotension or tachycardia) in which the demand for oxygen and the perfusion pressure may be in such imbalance that myocardial infarction ensues even when the narrowing of a coronary artery is not ordinarily sufficient to produce ischemia.

Although myocardial infarction often occurs during physically demanding activities such as running or shoveling snow, many infarcts occur at rest or even during sleep. Thus, for most persons, conversion of the clinically silent disease of coronary atherosclerosis to the catastrophic event of myocardial infarction involves a sudden, marked decrease in myocardial blood flow, with or without an increase in myo-

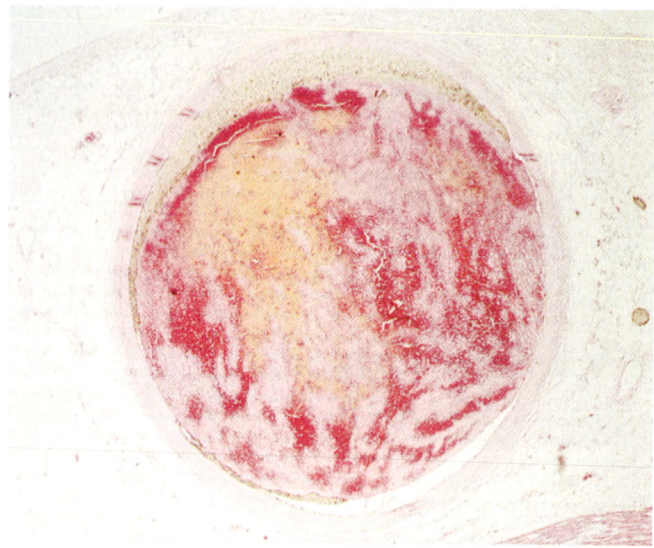

FIGURE 11-15
Thromboembolus in the left anterior descending coronary artery of a man who had old rheumatic heart disease, mitral stenosis, and a mural thrombus in the left atrial appendage.

cardial oxygen demand. **It is now well established that coronary artery thrombosis is the event that usually precipitates an acute myocardial infarction. Thrombosis typically results from spontaneous rupture of an atherosclerotic plaque, usually in a region that contains numerous inflammatory cells and a thin fibrous cap.** The initiating event may be hemorrhage into or beneath the plaque.

Thromboemboli

Thromboembolism is a rare cause of myocardial infarction, and the coronary embolus is usually traced to the heart itself. The most common source is valvular vegetations, caused either by infective or nonbacterial endocarditis. Coronary emboli occur in patients with atrial fibrillation and mitral valve disease who have mural thrombi in the left atrial appendage (Fig. 11-15). Thromboembolic occlusion of a coronary artery is also seen in patients with mural thrombi in the left ventricle secondary to infarction, aneurysm, or dilated cardiomyopathy.

Coronary Collateral Circulation

Normal coronary arteries function as end-arteries. Although most normal hearts have anastomoses 20 to 200 μm in diameter between coronary vessels, these collateral vessels do not function under normal circumstances because there is no pressure gradient between the arteries that they connect. However, after abrupt occlusion of a coronary artery, the resulting pressure differential allows blood to flow from the patent coronary artery to the ischemic area. Extensive collateral connections develop in hearts with severe coronary atherosclerosis. These collaterals may actually provide enough arterial flow to prevent infarction completely or to limit its size when a major epicardial coronary artery undergoes acute thrombotic occlusion

Well-developed coronary collaterals can explain certain unusual situations, such as anterior infarction after recent thrombotic occlusion of the right coronary artery (so-called infarction at a distance). This circumstance reflects the presence of coronary collaterals between the LAD and right coronary arteries that formed in response to gradual atherosclerotic narrowing of the LAD. As a result, myocardium normally supplied by the LAD coronary artery distal to the occlusion now depends on blood flow from the right coronary artery through the collaterals. Under these conditions, acute thrombosis of the right coronary artery results in paradoxical infarction of the anterior left ventricle.

Other Conditions That Limit Coronary Blood Flow

- **Coronary arteritis** is caused by various vasculitides such as polyarteritis nodosa or Kawasaki disease. It may produce luminal narrowing due to thickening of the vessel wall. It can also create local aneurysms that become occluded by thrombus.
- **Dissecting aneurysm of the aorta** occasionally extends into and obstructs the coronary arteries. Occasionally, medial necrosis and dissecting aneurysms are confined to the coronary artery.
- **Syphilitic aortitis** characteristically involves the ascending aorta, where it may obliterate a coronary artery orifice.
- **Congenital anomalous origin of a coronary artery** (origin of a coronary artery from the pulmonary trunk or passage of an anomalous coronary artery between the aorta and pulmonary artery) has been associated with sudden death.
- **An intramural course of the LAD coronary artery** may cause myocardial ischemia and sudden death. This artery normally runs in the epicardial fat, but in some hearts, it dips into the myocardium for a short distance. The muscular bridge over the LAD coronary artery may compress the vessel during systole or predispose to coronary spasm.

Many Situations Limit Oxygen Availability

Anemia is a common cause of decreased oxygen supply to the myocardium. Although a heart with normal circulation can survive severe anemia, the presence of coronary atherosclerosis may limit the capacity to increase coronary blood flow to such an extent that cardiac necrosis results. Furthermore, anemia increases the workload of the heart because increased cardiac output is required to oxygenate vital organs adequately.

Carbon monoxide poisoning decreases oxygen delivery to the tissues. The high affinity of hemoglobin for carbon monoxide displaces oxygen, thereby causing oxygen deprivation of the tissues. In this respect cigarette smoking produces significant levels of carboxyhemoglobin (a measure of CO) in the blood.

Increased Oxygen Demand May Cause Cardiac Ischemia

Any increase in the workload of the heart augments its need for oxygen. Conditions that increase blood pressure or cardiac output, such as exercise or pregnancy, result in increased oxygen demand by the myocardium, which may contribute to angina pectoris or myocardial infarction. Disorders in this category include valvular disease (mitral or aortic insufficiency, aortic stenosis), infection, and conditions such as hypertension, coarctation of the aorta, and hypertrophic cardiomyopathy. The increased metabolic rate and tachycardia in patients with hyperthyroidism is accompanied by an increase in oxygen demand as well as an increase in the workload of the heart. In fact, treatment of the underlying thyroid disease is the most effective therapy for a hyperthyroid patient with symptoms of ischemic heart disease. Fever also increases the basal metabolic rate, cardiac output, and heart rate.

Myocardial Infarcts Display Specific Locations and Microscopic Features

Pathology

Location of Infarcts

Infarcts may involve predominantly the subendocardial portion of the myocardium or they may be transmural. There are important differences between these two types of infarctions (Table 11-4).

A subendocardial infarct affects the inner one third to one half of the left ventricle. It may arise within the territory of one of the major epicardial coronary arteries or it may be circumferential, involving the subendocardial territories of multiple coronary arteries. Subendocardial infarction generally occurs as a consequence of hypoperfusion of the heart. It may result from atherosclerosis in a specific coronary artery or develop in disorders that limit myocardial blood flow globally, such as aortic stenosis, hemorrhagic shock, or hypoperfusion during the course of cardiopulmonary bypass. Most subendocardial infarcts occur in the absence of occlusive coronary thrombi, although small particles of platelet–fibrin thrombus may be seen in the epicardial coronary artery that supplies the region of infarction. In the case of circumferential subendocardial infarction caused by global hypoperfusion of the myocardium, coronary artery stenosis need not be present. Because necrosis is limited to the inner layers of the heart, complications arising in transmural infarcts (e.g., pericarditis and ventricular rupture) are not seen in subendocardial infarcts.

A transmural infarct involves the full thickness of the left ventricular wall and most often follows occlusion of a coronary artery. As a result, transmural infarcts typically conform to the distribution of one of the three major coronary arteries (see Fig. 11-3).

- **Right coronary artery:** Occlusion of the proximal portion of this vessel results in an infarct of the posterior basal region of the left ventricle and the posterior third to half of the interventricular septum ("inferior" infarct).
- **LAD coronary artery:** Blockage of this artery produces an infarct of the apical, anterior, and anteroseptal walls of the left ventricle.
- **Left circumflex coronary artery:** Obstruction of this vessel is the least common cause of myocardial infarction and leads to an infarct of the lateral wall of the left ventricle.

Myocardial infarction does not occur instantaneously. Rather, it first develops in the subendocardium and progresses as a wave front of necrosis from subendocardium to subepicardium over the course of several hours. Transient coronary occlusion may result in only subendocardial necrosis, whereas persistent occlusion leads eventually to transmural necrosis. The goal of acute coronary interventions (pharmacological or mechanical thrombolysis) is the interruption of this wave front and limitation of myocardial necrosis.

The volume of arterial collateral flow is the chief factor in the transmural progression of an infarct. With chronic cardiac ischemia, the presence of extensive collateral vessels, which preferentially supply the outer or subepicardial layer, often limits the infarct to the subendocardial portion of the myocardium. However, in fatal cases of acute myocardial infarction, transmural infarcts are more common than those restricted to the subendocardium.

Infarcts involve the left ventricle much more commonly and extensively than the right ventricle. This difference may be partly explained by the greater workload imposed on the left ventricle by systemic vascular resistance and the greater thickness of the left ventricular wall. Right ventricular hypertrophy (e.g., in cases of pulmonary hypertension) increases the incidence of right ventricular infarction. Infarction of the posterior right ventricle occurs in about a third of left ventricular posteroseptal infarcts (right coronary artery territory), but infarcts limited to the right ventricle are rare.

Macroscopic Characteristics of Myocardial Infarcts

The early stages in the evolution of a myocardial infarct have been characterized most thoroughly in experimental animals. About 10 seconds after ligation of a coronary artery, the affected myocardium becomes cyanotic and, rather than contracting, bulges outward during systole. If the obstruction is promptly relieved, myocardial contractions resume,

TABLE 11-4 Differences between Subendocardial and Transmural Infarcts

Subendocardial Infarcts	Transmural Infarcts
Multifocal	Unifocal
Patchy	Solid
Circumferential	In distribution of a specific coronary artery
Coronary thrombosis rare	Coronary thrombosis common
Often result from hypotension or shock	Often causes shock
No epicarditis	Epicarditis common
Do not form aneurysms	May result in aneurysm

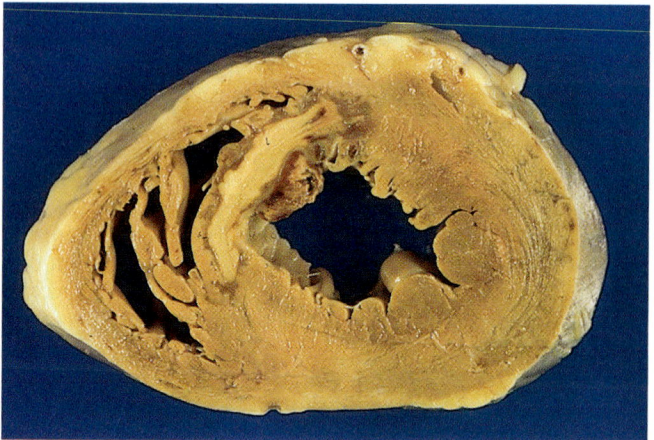

FIGURE 11-16
Acute myocardial infarct. A transverse section of the heart of a patient who died a few days after the onset of severe chest pain shows a transmural infarct in the anteroseptal region of the left ventricle (LAD coronary artery territory). The necrotic myocardium is soft, yellowish, and sharply demarcated.

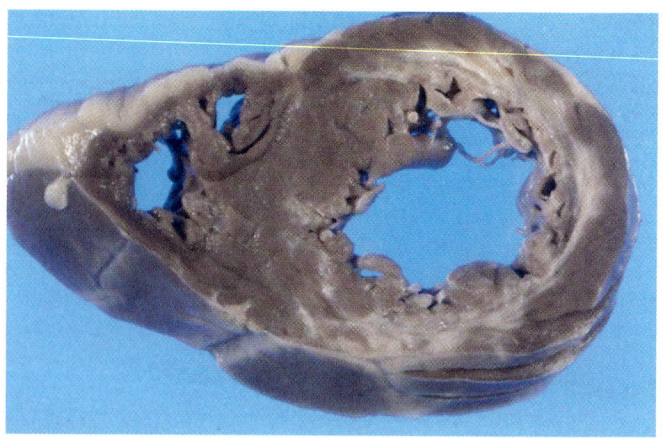

FIGURE 11-17
Healed myocardial infarct. A cross-section of the heart from a man who died after a long history of angina pectoris and several myocardial infarctions shows circumferential scarring of the left ventricle.

and no anatomical damage ensues, although contractility may be depressed in the postischemic tissue for many hours *(stunned myocardium)*. This reversible stage continues for 20 to 30 minutes of total ischemia, beyond which time damaged myocytes progressively die.

On gross examination, an acute myocardial infarct is not identifiable within the first 12 hours after the onset. By 24 hours, the infarct can be recognized on the cut surface of the involved ventricle by its pallor. After 3 to 5 days, the infarct becomes mottled and more sharply outlined, with a central pale, yellowish, necrotic region bordered by a hyperemic zone (Fig. 11-16). By 2 to 3 weeks, the infarcted region is depressed and soft, with a refractile, gelatinous appearance. Older, healed infarcts are firm and contracted and have the pale gray appearance of scar tissue (Fig. 11-17).

Microscopic Characteristics of Myocardial Infarcts

THE FIRST 24 HOURS: Electron microscopy is required to discern the earliest morphological features of ischemic injury (Fig. 11-18). Reversibly injured myocytes show subtle changes of sarcoplasmic edema, mild mitochondrial

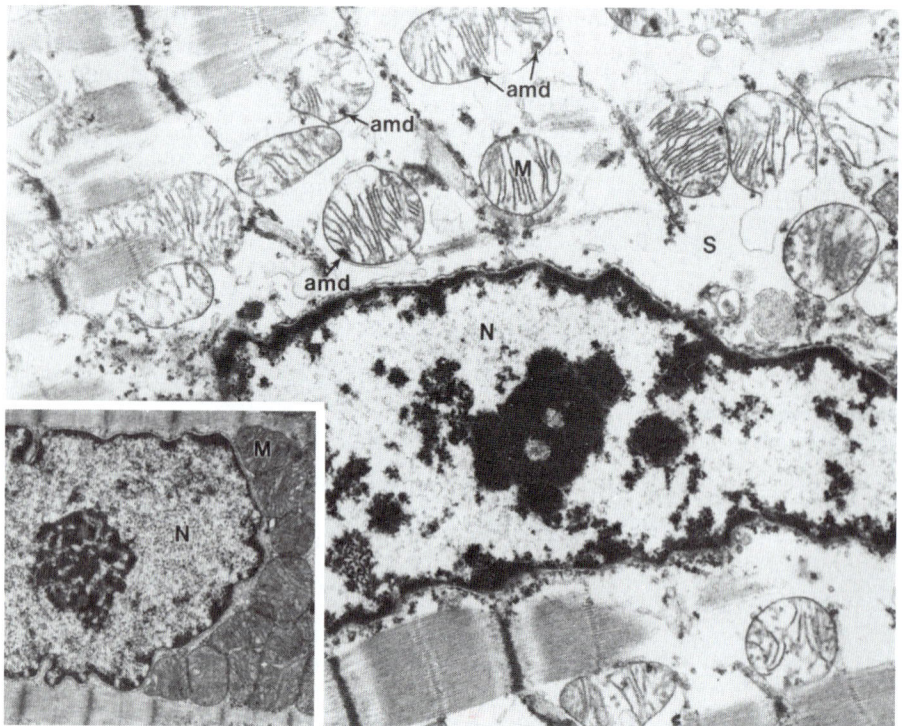

FIGURE 11-18
Ultrastructure of myocardial ischemia. Electron micrograph of an irreversibly injured myocyte from a canine heart subjected to 40 minutes of low-flow ischemia induced by proximal occlusion of the circumflex branch of the left coronary artery. (*Inset* shows a nonischemic control myocyte from the same heart, N-nucleus.) The affected myocyte is swollen and has abundant clear sarcoplasm (*S*). The mitochondria (*M*) are also swollen and contain amorphous matrix densities (*amd*), which are characteristic of lethal cell injury. The sarcolemma of this myocyte (*not shown*) exhibited small areas of disruption. The chromatin of the nucleus (*N*) is aggregated peripherally, in contrast to the uniformly distributed chromatin in normal tissue.

swelling, and loss of glycogen. After 30 to 60 minutes of ischemia, when myocyte injury has become irreversible, the mitochondria are greatly swollen and exhibit disorganized cristae and amorphous matrix densities. The nucleus shows clumping and margination of chromatin, and the sarcolemma is focally disrupted.

The loss of sarcolemmal integrity leads to the release of intracellular proteins, such as myoglobin, lactic dehydrogenase (LDH), CK, and troponins I and T. Ion gradients are also dissipated, and tissue potassium decreases as sodium and chloride increase.

The noncontractile ischemic myocytes are stretched with each systole and become *"wavy fibers."* By 24 hours, the myocytes are deeply eosinophilic (Fig. 11-19) and show the characteristic changes of coagulation necrosis. However, it takes several days for the myocyte nucleus to disappear totally.

TWO TO 3 DAYS: Polymorphonuclear leukocytes are attracted to the necrotic myocytes, but they gain access only at the periphery of the infarct, where blood flow is maintained. Hence they accumulate at the infarct border and reach a maximal concentration after 2 to 3 days (Figs. 11-19 and 11-20). Interstitial edema and microscopic areas of hemorrhage may also appear. By 2 to 3 days, the muscle cells are more clearly necrotic, nuclei disappear, and striations become less prominent. Some of the polymorphonuclear leukocytes that were attracted to the area begin to undergo karyorrhexis.

FIVE TO 7 DAYS: By this time, the acute inflammatory leukocytic response has abated, so that few, if any, polymorphonuclear leukocytes remain. The periphery of the infarcted region shows phagocytosis of the dead muscle by

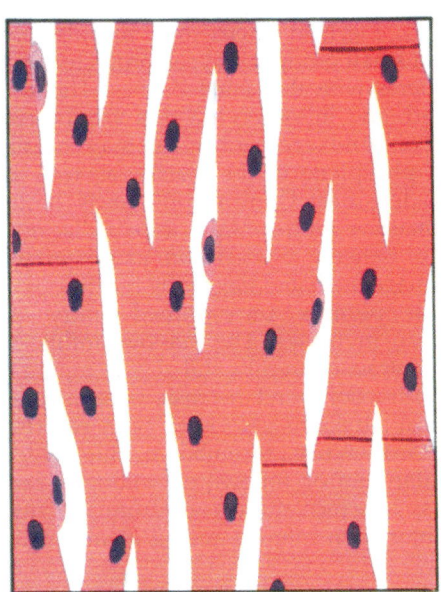
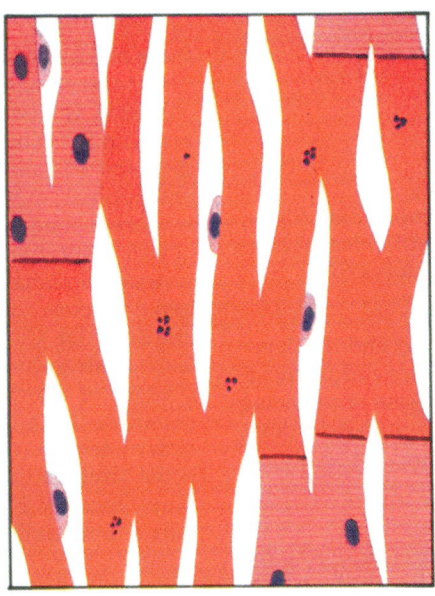
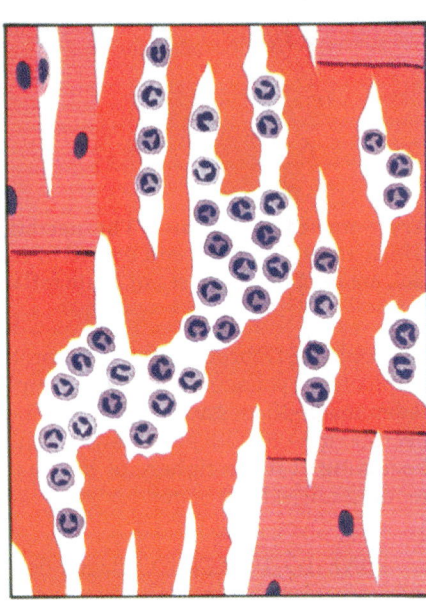

A,B,C Normal 12-18 hours 1 day

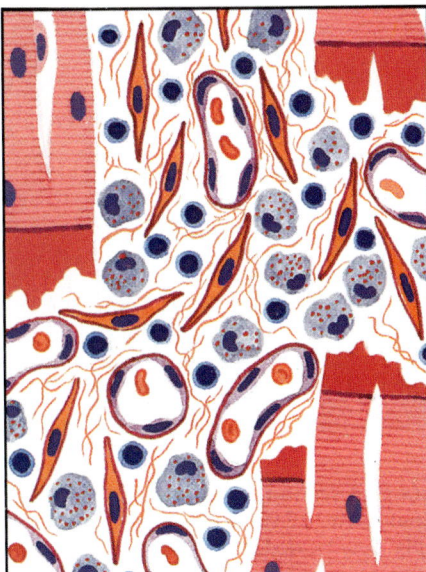
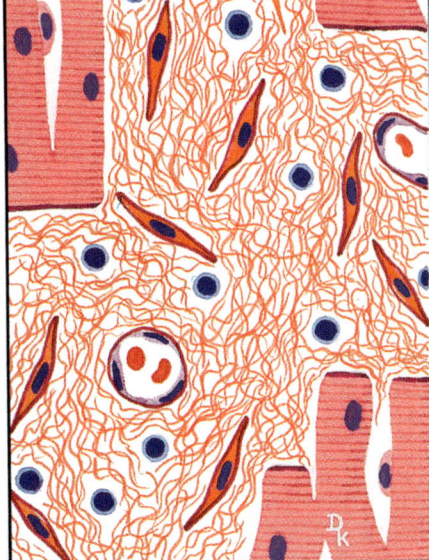

D,E

FIGURE 11-19
Development of a myocardial infarct. A. Normal myocardium. B. After about 12 to 18 hours, the infarcted myocardium shows eosinophilia *(red staining)* in sections of the heart stained with hematoxylin and eosin. C. About 24 hours after the onset of infarction, polymorphonuclear neutrophils infiltrate necrotic myocytes at the periphery of the infarct. D. After about 3 weeks, peripheral portions of the infarct are composed of granulation tissue with prominent capillaries, fibroblasts, lymphoid cells, and macrophages. The necrotic debris has been largely removed from this area, and a small amount of collagen has been laid down. E. After 3 months or more, the infarcted region has been replaced by scar tissue.

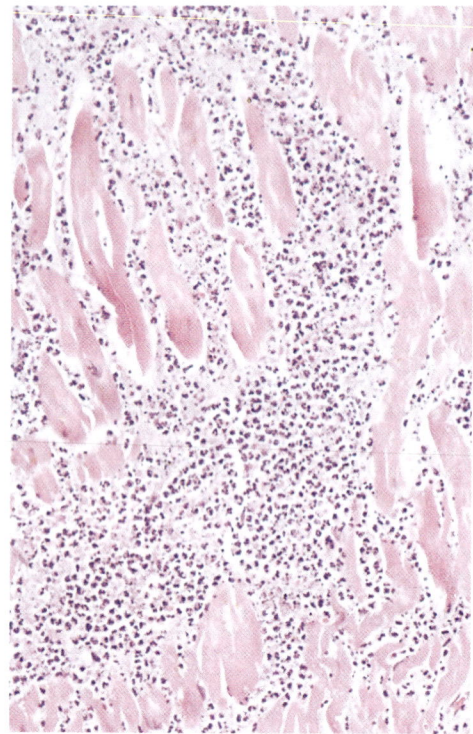

FIGURE 11-20
Acute myocardial infarct. The necrotic myocardial fibers, which are eosinophilic and devoid of cross striations and nuclei, are immersed in a sea of acute inflammatory cells.

macrophages. Fibroblasts begin to proliferate, and the deposition of new collagen is evident. Lymphocytes and pigment-laden macrophages are prominent. The process of replacing necrotic muscle with scar tissue is initiated at about 5 days, beginning at the periphery of the infarct and gradually extending toward the center.

ONE TO 3 WEEKS: Collagen deposition proceeds, the inflammatory infiltrate gradually recedes, and the newly sprouted capillaries are progressively obliterated.

MORE THAN 4 WEEKS: Considerable dense fibrous tissue is present. The debris is progressively removed, and the scar becomes more solid and less cellular as it matures (Fig. 11-21).

This sequence of inflammatory and reparative events can be altered by local or systemic factors. For example, the immediate extension of an infarct into a region that previously displayed patchy necrosis may not show the expected changes. A large infarct tends not to mature in its center as rapidly as a smaller infarct. In estimating the age of a large infarct, it is more accurate to base the interpretation on the outer border where repair begins, rather than on changes in the central region. In fact, in some large infarcts, rather than being removed, the dead myocytes remain indefinitely in a "mummified" form.

Reperfusion of Ischemic Myocardium

The foregoing descriptions pertain to healing of infarcts caused by persistent coronary occlusion, such as those arising from thrombotic occlusion of an epicardial coronary artery. However, blood flow may be restored to regions of evolving infarcts either because of spontaneous thrombolysis or in response to pharmacological or mechanical means of opening up occluded coronary arteries. Under these circumstances, the gross and microscopic pathology of infarct healing becomes altered. Reperfused infarcts are typically hemorrhagic, the result of blood flow through a damaged microvasculature. Thus, whereas infarcts following persistent occlusion become grossly apparent only after about 12 hours and appear pale, reperfused infarcts can be identified immediately by the presence of hemorrhage. Reperfusion also accelerates the acute inflammatory response. Neutrophils can gain access throughout the infarct rather than only at the periphery. They accumulate more rapidly but also disappear more rapidly. In general, replacement of necrotic muscle by fibrous scar also proceeds more quickly, at least in areas of the infarct in which perfusion persists.

One of the most characteristic features of reperfused infarcts is **contraction band necrosis.** Contraction bands are thick, irregular, transverse eosinophilic bands in necrotic myocytes (Fig. 11-22). Electron microscopy reveals that these bands consist of small groups of hypercontracted and disorganized sarcomeres with thickened Z lines. The sarcolemma is disrupted, and mitochondria that are located between the contraction bands are swollen and may contain deposits of calcium phosphate in the matrix, as well as amorphous matrix densities. Contraction bands occur whenever there is a massive influx of Ca^{2+} into cardiac myocytes. Reperfusion of ischemic myocardium causes extensive sarcolemmal damage mediated largely by reactive oxygen species, which permits unrestrained entry of extracellular Ca^{2+} into myocytes. The massive influx of Ca^{2+} leads to hypercontraction in cells still able to mount a contractile effort. Contraction band necrosis is seen most prominently in clinical situations associated with reperfusion of necrotic myocardium (e.g., thrombolytic therapy for acute myocardial infarction or following prolonged cardiopulmonary bypass in which the myocardium has sustained irreversible injury). In infarcts arising from persis-

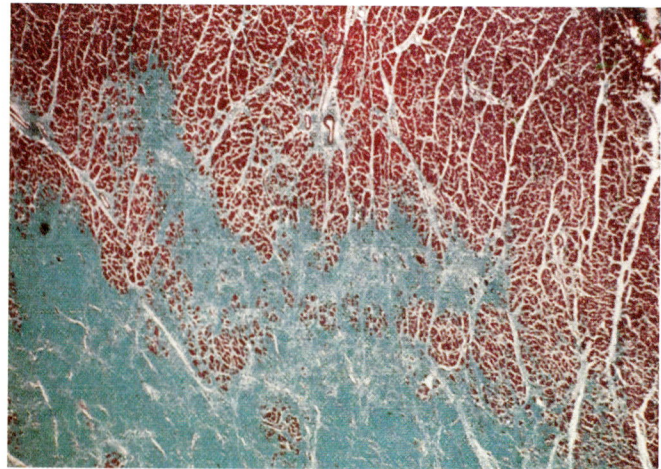

FIGURE 11-21
Healed myocardial infarct. A section at the edge of a healed infarct stained for collagen shows dense, acellular regions of collagenous matrix sharply demarcated from the adjacent viable myocardium.

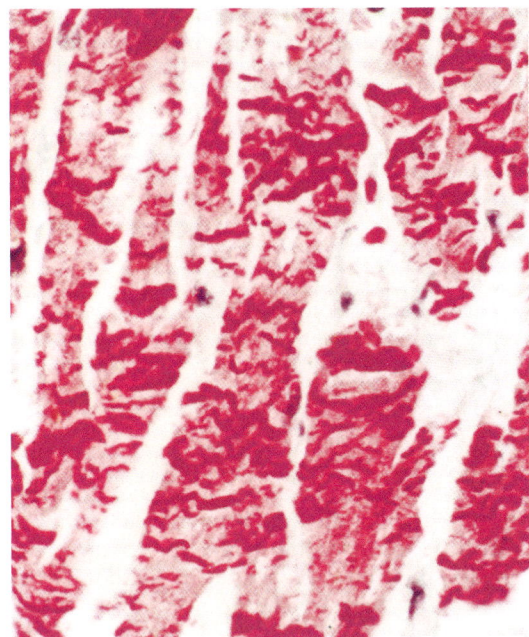

FIGURE 11-22
Contraction band necrosis. A section of infarcted myocardium shows prominent, thick, wavy, transverse bands in myofibers.

tent coronary occlusion, microscopic foci of contraction band necrosis are often seen at the margins, where dynamic ebb and flow of blood creates conditions that favor Ca^{2+} influx. Other conditions associated with contraction band injury include massive catecholamine release in patients with pheochromocytoma or head injuries, or patients in shock treated with large doses of pressors.

 Clinical Features:

Diagnosis

The onset of acute myocardial infarction is often sudden and associated with severe substernal or precordial crushing pain. The pain may be experienced as epigastric burning (simulating indigestion) or may extend into the jaw or down the inside of either arm. It is often accompanied by sweating, nausea, vomiting, and shortness of breath. In some cases, an acute myocardial infarction is preceded by unstable angina of several days duration. **One fourth to one half of all nonfatal myocardial infarctions occur without any symptoms, and the infarcts are identified only later by electrocardiographic changes or at autopsy.** These "clinically silent" infarcts are particularly common among diabetic patients with autonomic dysfunction and are also seen in cardiac transplant patients whose hearts are denervated.

The diagnosis of acute myocardial infarction is confirmed by electrocardiography and the appearance of increased levels of certain enzymes or proteins in the serum. The electrocardiogram exhibits new Q waves and changes in the ST segment and the conformation of the T wave. Identification in serum of cardiac proteins such as the MB isoform of CK or cardiac troponins T and I is evidence of myocardial necrosis.

Complications of Myocardial Infarction

Early mortality in acute myocardial infarction (within 30 days) has dropped from 30% in the 1950s to less than 5% today. Nevertheless, the clinical course following acute infarction may be dominated by a variety of functional or mechanical complications of the infarct.

ARRHYTHMIAS: Virtually all patients who have a myocardial infarct have an abnormality of cardiac rhythm at some time during the course of their illness. Arrhythmias still account for half of all deaths caused by ischemic heart disease, although the advent of coronary care units and defibrillators has greatly reduced early mortality. Acute infarction is often associated with premature ventricular beats, sinus bradycardia, ventricular tachycardia, ventricular fibrillation, and paroxysmal atrial tachycardia. Partial or complete heart block can also occur. The causes of these arrhythmias are often multifactorial. Acute ischemia alters conduction, increases automaticity, and promotes triggered activity related to afterdepolarizations. Enhanced sympathetic activity mediated by increased levels of local or circulating catecholamines plays an important role.

LEFT VENTRICULAR FAILURE AND CARDIOGENIC SHOCK: Development of left ventricular failure soon after myocardial infarction is an ominous sign that generally indicates massive loss of muscle. Fortunately, the incidence of cardiogenic shock is now less than 5%, owing to the development of techniques that limit the extent of infarction (thrombolytic therapy, angioplasty) or assist the damaged myocardium (intraaortic balloon pump). Cardiogenic shock tends to develop early after infarction when 40% or more of the left ventricle has been lost; mortality is as high as 90%.

EXTENSION OF THE INFARCT: Clinically recognizable extension of an acute myocardial infarct occurs in the first 1 to 2 weeks in up to 10% of patients. In careful echocardiographic studies, half of all patients with anterior myocardial infarction showed some extension of the infarct during the first 2 weeks, indicating that many episodes of infarct extension are not recognized. Clinically significant infarct extension is associated with a doubling of mortality.

RUPTURE OF THE FREE WALL OF THE MYOCARDIUM: Myocardial rupture (Fig. 11-23) may occur at almost any time during the first 3 weeks following acute myocardial infarction but is most common between the first and fourth days, when the infarcted wall is weakest. During this vulnerable period, the infarct is composed of soft, necrotic tissue in which the extracellular matrix has been degraded by proteases released by inflammatory cells before deposition of new matrix has taken place. Once scar tissue begins to form, rupture becomes less likely. Rupture of the free wall is

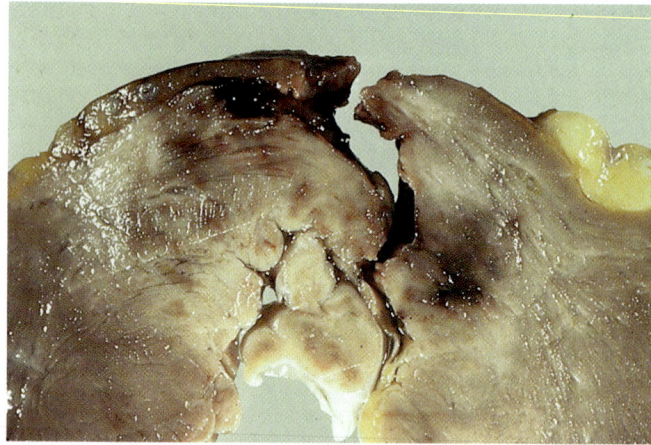

FIGURE 11-23
Rupture of an acute myocardial infarct. An elderly woman with a recent myocardial infarct died of cardiac tamponade. The pericardium was filled with blood, and the cut surface of the left ventricle shows a linear rupture of the necrotic myocardium.

a complication of transmural infarcts; surviving muscle overlying subendocardial infarcts prevents rupture. However, rupture usually occurs in relatively small transmural infarcts. The remaining viable, contractile myocardium produces mechanical forces that can initiate and propagate tearing along the lateral border of the infarct where neutrophils have accumulated.

Rupture of the free wall of the left ventricle most often results in hemopericardium and death due to pericardial tamponade. Myocardial rupture accounts for 10% of deaths after acute myocardial infarction in hospitalized patients. This complication is more common in elderly patients who have sustained a first infarct (most of whom are women). In rare instances, a ruptured ventricle may become walled off, and the patient survives with a false aneurysm (Fig. 11-24).

OTHER FORMS OF MYOCARDIAL RUPTURE: A few patients in whom a myocardial infarct involves the interventricular septum develop **septal perforation,** varying in length from 1 cm or more. The magnitude of the resulting left-to-right shunt and, therefore, the prognosis vary with the size of the rupture.

Rupture of a portion of a papillary muscle results in mitral regurgitation. In some cases, an entire papillary muscle is transected, in which case, massive mitral valve incompetence may be fatal.

ANEURYSMS: Left ventricular aneurysms complicate 10 to 15% of transmural myocardial infarcts. After acute transmural infarction, the affected ventricular wall tends to bulge outward during systole in one third of patients. As the infarct heals, the newly deposited collagenous matrix is susceptible to further stretching, although eventually the scar tissue becomes nondistensible. Localized thinning and stretching of the ventricular wall in the region of a healing myocardial infarct has been termed *infarct expansion* but is actually an early aneurysm. Such an aneurysm is composed of a thin layer of necrotic myocardium and collagenous tissue, which expands with each contraction of the heart. As the evolving aneurysm becomes more fibrotic, its tensile strength increases. However, the aneurysm continues to dilate with each beat, thereby "stealing" some of the left ventricular output and contributing to the workload of the heart. Patients with left ventricular aneurysms are at increased risk of developing ventricular tachycardia, owing to increased opportunities for reentry along the periphery of the aneurysm. Mural thrombi often develop within aneurysms and are a source of systemic emboli.

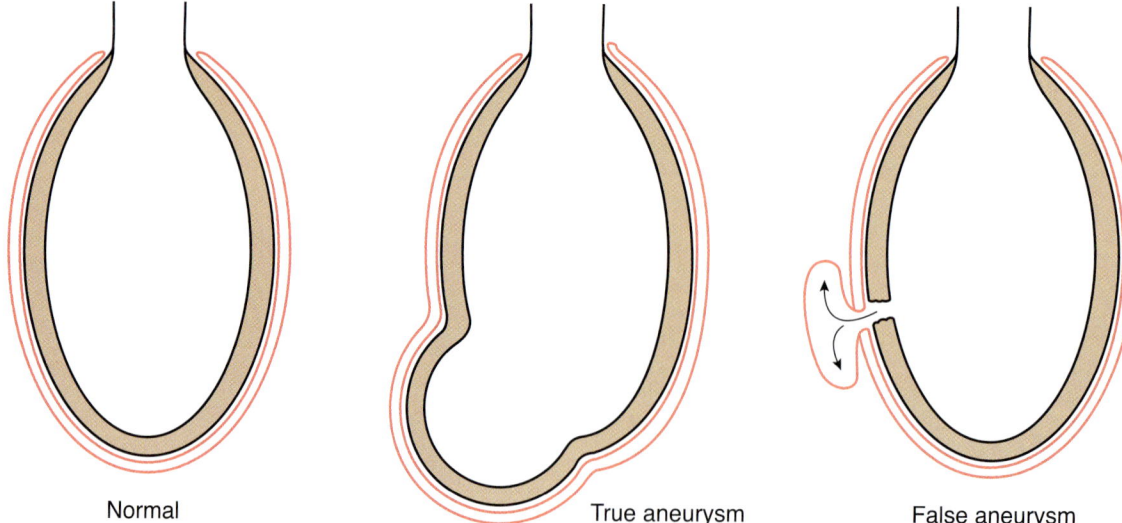

FIGURE 11-24
True and false aneurysms of the left ventricle. *(Left)* Normal heart. The left ventricular wall *(shaded)* is enclosed by the pericardial sac. *(Center)* True aneurysm shows an intact wall *(black),* which bulges outward. *(Right)* False aneurysm shows a ruptured infarct that is walled off externally by adherent pericardium. Note that the mouth of the true aneurysm is wider than that of the false aneurysm.

A distinction should be made between "true" and "false" aneurysms (see Fig. 11-24). True aneurysms are much more common than false aneurysms and are caused by bulging of the weakened, but intact, left ventricular wall (Fig. 11-25). By contrast, false aneurysms result from the rupture of a portion of the left ventricle that has been walled off by pericardial scar tissue. Thus, the wall of a false aneurysm is composed of pericardium and scar tissue but not left ventricular myocardium.

MURAL THROMBOSIS AND EMBOLISM: Half of all patients who die after myocardial infarction are discovered at autopsy to have mural thrombi overlying the infarct (Fig. 11-26). This finding is particularly frequent when the infarct involves the apex of the heart. In turn, half of these patients have some evidence of systemic embolization. Inflammation of the endocardium lining an infarct promotes platelet adhesion and fibrin deposition. Moreover, the poor contractile function of the underlying myocardium allows the fibrin–platelet mural thrombus to grow. Particles of thrombus can detach and be swept along with the arterial blood, potentially causing strokes or myocardial or visceral infarcts. Documented mural thrombosis justifies anticoagulant therapy and antiplatelet medications.

PERICARDITIS: A transmural myocardial infarct involves the epicardium and leads to inflammation of the pericardium in 10 to 20% of patients. Pericarditis is manifested clinically as chest pain and may produce a pericardial friction rub. A fourth of patients with acute myocardial infarction,

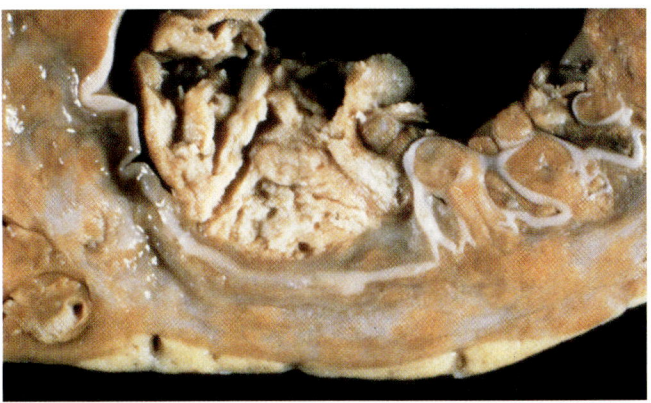

FIGURE 11-26
Mural thrombus overlying a healed myocardial infarct. In this cross-section of a fixed heart, an organized, friable, grayish white mural thrombus overlies a thickened endocardium situated over a scarred myocardium.

particularly those with larger infarcts and congestive heart failure, develop a pericardial effusion, with or without pericarditis. Less frequently, anticoagulant therapy has been associated with the appearance of a hemorrhagic pericardial effusion and even with cardiac tamponade.

Postmyocardial infarction syndrome *(Dressler syndrome)* refers to a delayed form of pericarditis that develops 2 to 10 weeks after infarction. A similar disorder may occur after cardiac surgery. The fact that antibodies to heart muscle appear in patients with Dressler syndrome and the observation that the condition is ameliorated by corticosteroid therapy suggest that this condition has an immunological basis.

Therapeutic Interventions that Limit Infarct Size

Because the amount of myocardium that undergoes necrosis is an important predictor of morbidity and mortality, any therapy that limits infarct size should be beneficial. By definition, such therapy is directed at preventing the death of reversibly injured, ischemic myocytes and limiting infarct extension. Damaged myocytes can be salvaged for some time after the onset of ischemia if the tissue can be reperfused with arterial blood.

Restoration of arterial blood flow remains the only way to salvage ischemic myocytes permanently, although a number of interventions can delay ischemic injury. The most notable is hypothermia, which is used during cardiac surgery to minimize myocardial injury during cardiopulmonary bypass. Several methods have been developed to restore blood flow to the area of myocardium supplied by an obstructed coronary artery.

Thrombolytic enzymes such as tissue plasminogen activator or streptokinase can be infused intravenously to dissolve the clot causing the obstruction.

Percutaneous transluminal coronary angioplasty (PTCA) refers to dilation of a narrowed coronary artery by the inflation of a balloon catheter. This can be performed as a primary procedure immediately after the onset of ischemia or as a rescue procedure when thrombolytic agents fail to restore arterial blood flow. PTCA also allows the placement of a stent in the coronary artery to maintain the patency of the lumen.

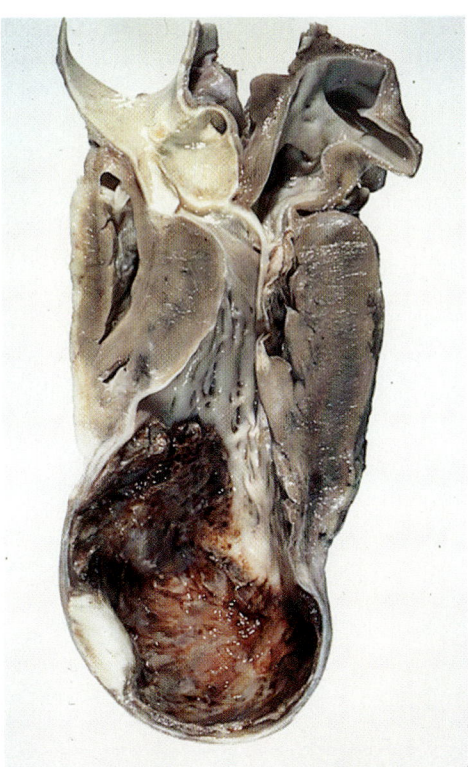

FIGURE 11-25
Ventricular aneurysm. The heart of a patient with a history of an anteroapical myocardial infarct who developed a massive ventricular aneurysm. The apex of the heart shows marked thinning and aneurysmal dilation.

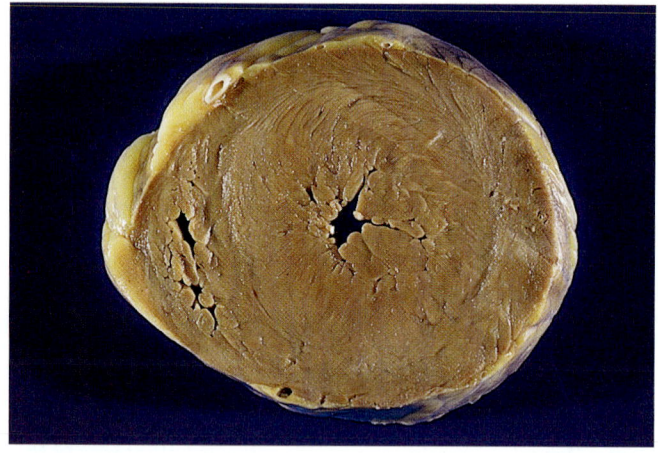

FIGURE 11-27
Hypertensive heart disease. A transverse section of the heart shows marked hypertrophy of the left ventricular myocardium without dilation of the chamber. The right ventricle is of normal dimensions.

Coronary artery bypass grafting can restore blood flow to the distal segment of a coronary artery with a proximal occlusion.

Procedures that restore blood flow must be performed as quickly as possible, preferably in the first few hours after the onset of symptoms. Beyond 6 hours, it is unlikely that much salvageable ischemic myocardium remains.

Chronic Ischemic Heart Disease Can Lead to Cardiomyopathy

In a minority of patients with severe coronary atherosclerosis, myocardial contractility is impaired globally in the absence of discrete infarcts, a situation that mimics dilated cardiomyopathy. This situation usually reflects a combination of ischemic myocardial dysfunction, diffuse fibrosis, and multiple small healed infarcts. However, there remains a group of patients with left ventricular failure in whom cardiac dysfunction occurs without obvious infarction. These patients are said to have *ischemic cardiomyopathy*. In some patients, the dysfunctional myocardium has been subjected to repetitive episodes of ischemic injury, which causes degenerative changes in myocytes, characterized principally by loss of myofibrils (hibernating myocardium) (see Fig. 11-7). The contractile function of hibernating myocardium is restored when the affected tissue is revascularized. Thus, to the extent that hibernation plays a role in ischemic cardiomyopathy, surgical revascularization is potentially beneficial.

HYPERTENSIVE HEART DISEASE

Hypertension has been defined by the World Health Organization as a persistent increase of systemic blood pressure to levels above 140 mm Hg systolic or 90 mm Hg diastolic, or both (see Chapter 10). Systemic hypertension is one of the most prevalent and serious causes of coronary artery and myocardial disease in the United States. Chronic hypertension leads to pressure overload resulting first in compensatory left ventricular hypertrophy and, eventually, cardiac failure. The term *hypertensive heart disease* is used when the heart is enlarged in the absence of a cause other than hypertension.

 Pathology: Hypertension causes compensatory left ventricular hypertrophy as a result of the increased workload imposed on the heart. The left ventricular free walls and interventricular septum become thickened uniformly and concentrically (Fig. 11-27), and the overall weight of the heart increases, exceeding 375 g in men and 350 g in women. Microscopically, the hypertrophic myocardial cells have an increased diameter, with enlarged, hyperchromatic, and rectangular ("boxcar") nuclei (Fig. 11-28).

 Clinical Features: Myocardial hypertrophy clearly adds to the ability of the heart to handle an increased workload. However, there is a limit beyond which additional hypertrophy is no longer compensatory. This upper limit to useful hypertrophy may reflect the increasing diffusion distance between the interstitium and the center of each myofiber; if the distance becomes too great, the supply of oxygen to the myofiber will be deficient.

Diastolic dysfunction is the most common functional abnormality caused by hypertension and by itself can lead to congestive heart failure. Some interstitial fibrosis typically develops as part of the hypertrophic response, which further contributes to left ventricular stiffness. **Hypertension also is associated with increased severity of atherosclerosis of the**

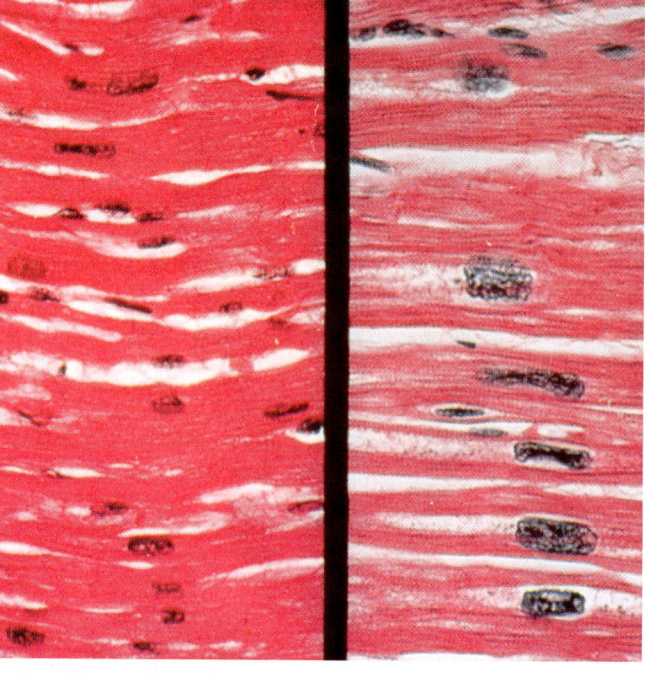

FIGURE 11-28
Hypertensive heart disease with myocardial hypertrophy. (*Left*) Normal myocardium. (*Right*) Hypertrophic myocardium shows thicker fibers and enlarged, hyperchromatic, rectangular nuclei.

TABLE 11-5   Causes of Cor Pulmonale

Parenchymal diseases of the lung
   Chronic bronchitis and emphysema
   Pulmonary fibrosis (from any cause)
   Cystic fibrosis

Pulmonary Vascular Diseases
   Recurrent pulmonary emboli
   Primary pulmonary hypertension
   Peripheral pulmonary stenosis
   Intravenous drug abuse
   Residence at high altitude
   Schistosomiasis

Congenital heart diseases

Impaired movement of the thoracic cage
   Kyphoscoliosis
   Pickwickian syndrome
   Pleural fibrosis
   Neuromuscular disorders
   Idiopathic hypoventilation

coronary arteries. The combination of increased cardiac workload (systolic dysfunction), diastolic dysfunction, and narrowed coronary arteries leads to a greater risk of myocardial ischemia, infarction, and heart failure.

Congestive heart failure is the most common cause of death in untreated hypertensive patients. Intracerebral hemorrhage is also a frequent fatal complication. In addition, death may result from coronary atherosclerosis and myocardial infarction, dissecting aneurysm of the aorta, or ruptured berry aneurysm of the cerebral circulation. Renal failure may supervene when nephrosclerosis induced by hypertension becomes severe.

COR PULMONALE

Cor pulmonale is defined as right ventricular hypertrophy and dilation secondary to pulmonary hypertension. Increased pressure in the pulmonary circulation may reflect a disorder of the pulmonary parenchyma or, more rarely, a primary disease of the vasculature (e.g., primary pulmonary hypertension, recurrent small pulmonary emboli).

Acute cor pulmonale refers to the sudden occurrence of pulmonary hypertension, most commonly as a result of sudden, massive pulmonary embolization. This condition causes acute right-sided heart failure and is a medical emergency. At autopsy, the only cardiac findings are severe dilation of the right ventricle and sometimes of the right atrium.

Chronic cor pulmonale is a common heart disease, accounting for 30 to 40% of all cases of heart failure in an English study and 10 to 30% in a series in the United States. This frequency reflects the prevalence of chronic pulmonary disease in these countries, especially chronic bronchitis and emphysema. In many cases of chronic disease of the lung, the severity of pulmonary hypertension correlates more closely with survival than any other variable. In fact, fewer than 10% of patients with a pulmonary artery pressure greater than 45 mm Hg survive 5 years.

 Pathogenesis: Chronic cor pulmonale may be caused by any pulmonary disease that interferes with ventilatory mechanics or gas exchange or obstructs the pulmonary vasculature (Table 11-5). **The most common causes of chronic cor pulmonale are chronic obstructive pulmonary disease and pulmonary fibrosis.** Severe kyphoscoliosis may deform the chest wall and interfere with its function as a bellows, resulting in hypoxemia and pulmonary vasoconstriction. A few cases of cor pulmonale are attributed to *primary pulmonary hypertension,* a disorder of unknown etiology. As discussed above, some congenital heart diseases associated with increased pulmonary blood flow are complicated by pulmonary hypertension and cor pulmonale.

The pathogenesis of pulmonary hypertension secondary to recurrent pulmonary emboli is related clearly to progressive mechanical obstruction of blood flow. However, mechanisms of pulmonary hypertension in chronic parenchymal diseases of the lungs are more complicated. In addition to the obliteration of blood vessels in the lung, these disorders also lead to pulmonary arteriolar vasoconstriction, which reduces the effective cross-sectional area of the pulmonary vascular bed without destroying the vessels. Hypoxia, acidosis, and hypercapnia directly cause pulmonary vasoconstriction. Hypoxia also increases pulmonary vascular resistance indirectly by leading to polycythemia, which causes hyperviscosity of the blood. Persons living at very high altitude, for instance, natives of the South American Andes mountain range, often develop cor pulmonale secondary to the effects of chronic hypoxemia.

 Pathology: Chronic cor pulmonale is characterized by conspicuous hypertrophy of the right ventricle (Fig. 11-29), which can measure more than 1.0 cm in thickness (normal range, 0.3–0.5 cm). Dilation of the right ventricle and right atrium are often present. Normally,

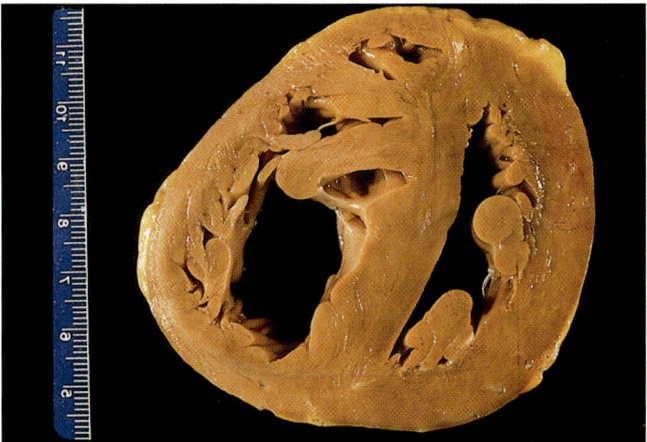

FIGURE 11-29
Cor pulmonale. A transverse section of the heart from a patient with primary (idiopathic) pulmonary hypertension shows a markedly hypertrophied right ventricle (on the left). The right ventricular free wall has a thickness equal to the left ventricular wall. The right ventricle is dilated. The straightened interventricular septum has lost its normal curvature toward the left ventricle as part of the remodeling process in cor pulmonale.

the interventricular septum is concave to the left (i.e., it is part of the left ventricle). With development of severe right ventricular hypertrophy, the interventricular septum remodels by straightening or even becoming concave to the right.

ACQUIRED VALVULAR AND ENDOCARDIAL DISEASES

A variety of inflammatory, infectious, and degenerative diseases damage the cardiac valves and impair their function. The valves normally consist of thin flexible membranes, which close tightly to prevent backward blood flow. When the valves become damaged, the leaflets or cusps may be thickened and fused enough to narrow the aperture and obstruct blood flow, a condition labeled *valvular stenosis*. Diseases that destroy valve tissue may also allow retrograde blood flow, termed *valvular regurgitation or insufficiency*. In many instances, diseases involving the cardiac valves produce both stenosis and insufficiency, but generally one or the other predominates.

Stenosis of a cardiac valve results in hypertrophy of the myocardium proximal (in terms of blood flow) to the obstruction. **Pressure overload** eventually causes myocardial dilation and failure of the chamber proximal to the valve, once compensatory mechanisms have been exhausted. Thus, mitral stenosis leads to left atrial hypertrophy and dilation. As the left atrium decompensates and can no longer force the venous return through the stenotic mitral valve, signs of pulmonary congestion develop and are followed by right ventricular hypertrophy and even cor pulmonale. Similarly, aortic stenosis causes left ventricular hypertrophy and eventually left heart failure.

Valvular regurgitation or insufficiency also results in hypertrophy and dilation of the cardiac chamber proximal to the valve, owing to **volume overload**. In aortic insufficiency, the left ventricle first hypertrophies and then dilates when it can no longer accommodate the regurgitant volume and provide adequate cardiac output. On the other hand, an incompetent mitral valve leads to hypertrophy and dilation of both the left atrium and left ventricle, because both are subjected to volume overload. Marked left ventricular dilation from any condition in which cardiac contractility is inadequate (e.g., congestive failure after a large myocardial infarct) also may widen the mitral valve ring. This effect may be so severe that the valve leaflets cannot close properly, thereby causing mitral regurgitation.

The semilunar valves are structurally and functionally simple compared with the atrioventricular valves, which consist not only of the valve leaflets but also muscular valve annuli and the subvalvular apparatus (the chordae tendineae and papillary muscles). In general, valvular stenosis involves pathological changes of the leaflets themselves, but regurgitation can be caused by abnormalities of the valve leaflets, annulus, or subvalvular apparatus.

Rheumatic Heart Disease Encompasses Acute Myocarditis and Residual Valvular Deformities

Acute Rheumatic Fever

Rheumatic fever (RF) is a multisystem childhood disease that follows a streptococcal infection and is characterized by an inflammatory reaction involving the heart, joints, and central nervous system.

 Epidemiology: RF is a complication of an acute streptococcal infection, almost always pharyngitis (i.e., "strep" throat) (see Chapter 9). The offending agent is *Streptococcus pyogenes*, also known as group A, β-hemolytic *Streptococcus*. In some epidemics of streptococcal pharyngitis, the incidence of RF has been as high as 3%. RF is principally a disease of childhood, the median age being 9 to 11 years, although it can occur in adults.

In the first half of the 20th century, RF reached almost epidemic proportions in the United States, but the incidence of this disease has decreased dramatically. In the period from 1950 to 1972, the death rate fell from 14.5 to 6.8 per 100,000, and it has decreased further since that time. Although this decline may have been partly the result of widespread antibiotic treatment, such therapy cannot account for the entire reduction, because the death rate had begun to decrease well before antibiotics were generally available. It is probable that improved socioeconomic conditions, in particular less crowded living circumstances, contributed to the decrease. **Despite its declining importance in the industrialized countries, RF remains a leading cause of death of heart disease in persons between the ages of 5 and 25 years in less-developed regions.**

 Pathogenesis: The pathogenesis of RF remains unclear, and with the exception of the link to streptococcal infection, no theory has been proven unequivocally. Most hypotheses relate rheumatic carditis to immunological phenomena. It has been proposed that antibodies raised against streptococcal antigens cross-react with heart antigens, an observation that raises the possibility of an autoimmune etiology related to so-called molecular mimicry (Fig. 11-30).

FIGURE 11-30

Biological factors in rheumatic heart disease. The upper portion illustrates the initiating β-hemolytic streptococcal infection of the throat, which introduces the streptococcal antigens into the body and may also activate cytotoxic T cells. These antigens lead to the production of antibodies against various antigenic components of the streptococcus, which can cross-react with certain cardiac antigens, including those from the myocyte sarcolemma and glycoproteins of the valves. This may be the mechanism for inflammation of the heart in acute rheumatic fever, which involves all cardiac layers (endocarditis, myocarditis, and pericarditis). This inflammation becomes apparent after a latent period of 2 to 3 weeks. Active inflammation of the valves may eventually lead to chronic valvular stenosis or insufficiency. These lesions involve the mitral, aortic, tricuspid, and pulmonary valves, in that order of frequency.

Acquired Valvular and Endocardial Diseases

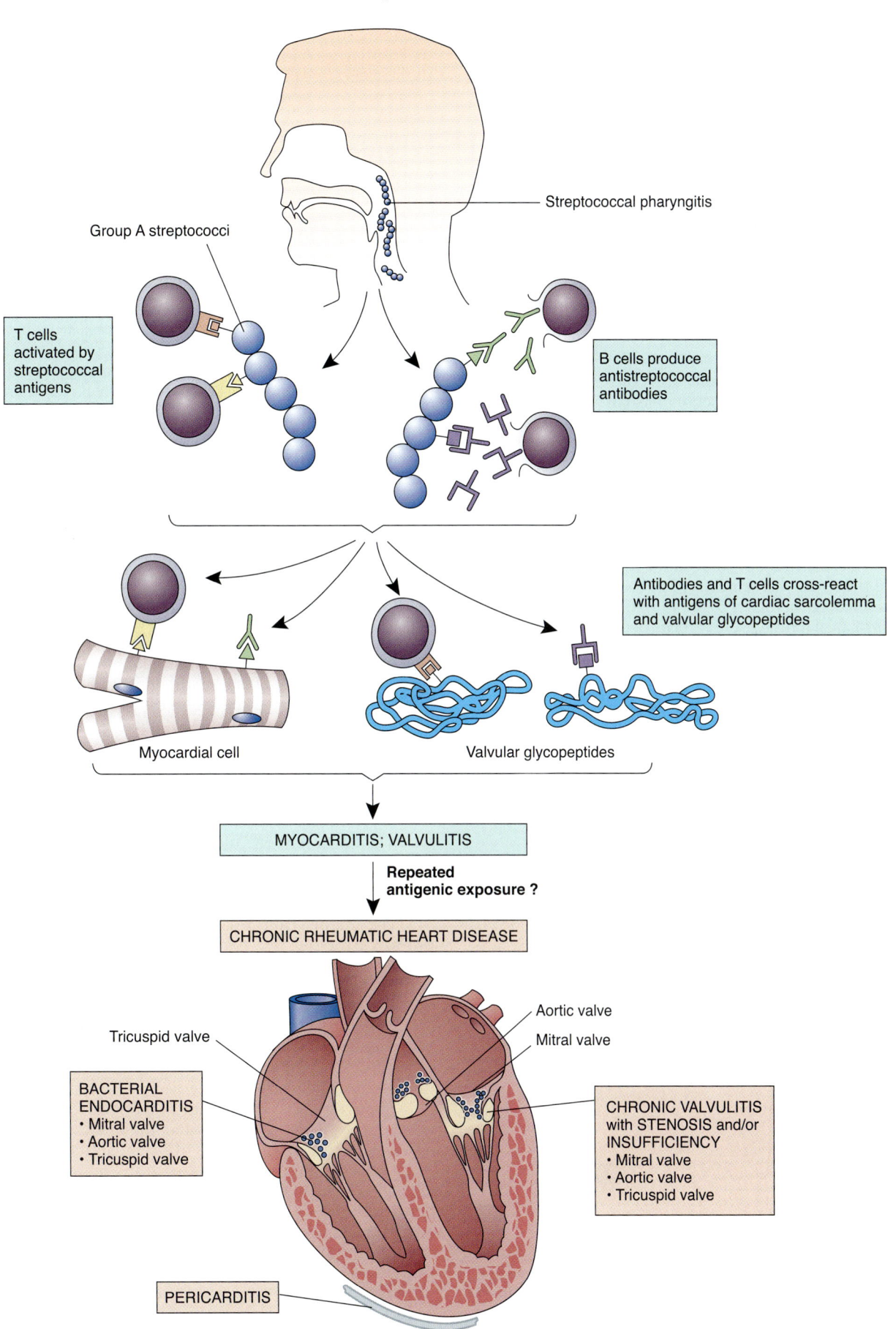

Streptococcal antigens structurally similar to those in the heart include hyaluronate in the bacterial capsule, cell wall polysaccharides similar to the carbohydrate moiety of heart valve glycoproteins, and bacterial membrane antigens that share epitopes with sarcolemma and smooth muscle constituents. Although antibodies to these antigens are found in patients with RF, it has not been proved that they are cytotoxic or that they are directly involved in the pathogenesis of the disease. A direct toxic effect of some streptococcal product on the myocardium has not yet been excluded.

 Pathology: Acute rheumatic heart disease is a pancarditis, involving all three layers (endocardium, myocardium, and pericardium) of the heart.

MYOCARDITIS: In severe cases of RF, a few patients may die during the earliest acute phase of the illness before the characteristic granulomatous inflammation has developed. At this early stage, the heart tends to be dilated and exhibits a nonspecific myocarditis, in which lymphocytes and macrophages predominate, although a few neutrophils and eosinophils may be evident. Fibrinoid degeneration of collagen, in which the fibers become swollen, fragmented, and eosinophilic, is characteristic of this early phase.

The *Aschoff body* is the characteristic granulomatous lesion of rheumatic myocarditis (Fig. 11-31), developing several weeks after the onset of symptoms. This structure initially consists of a perivascular focus of swollen eosinophilic collagen surrounded by lymphocytes, plasma cells, and macrophages. With time, the Aschoff body assumes a granulomatous appearance, with a central fibrinoid focus associated with a perimeter of lymphocytes, plasma cells, macrophages, and giant cells. Eventually, the Aschoff body is replaced by a nodule of scar tissue.

Anitschkow cells are unusual cells within the Aschoff body, whose nuclei contain a central band of chromatin. In cross-section, these nuclei have an "owl eye" appearance, and when cut longitudinally, they resemble a caterpillar. These cells are cardiac macrophages that are normally present in small numbers but accumulate and become prominent in certain types of inflammatory diseases of the heart. Anitschkow cells may become multinucleated, in which case they are termed *Aschoff giant cells*.

PERICARDITIS: Tenacious irregular deposits of fibrin are found on both the visceral and parietal surfaces of the pericardium during the acute inflammatory phase of RF. These deposits resemble the shaggy surfaces of two slices of buttered bread that have been pulled apart (*bread-and-butter pericarditis*). The pericarditis may be recognized clinically by hearing a friction rub, but it has little functional effect and ordinarily does not lead to constrictive pericarditis.

ENDOCARDITIS: During the acute stage of rheumatic carditis, the valve leaflets become inflamed and edematous. Although all four valves are affected, the left-sided valves develop the most injury because they close under greater pressures than do the right-sided valves. The result is damage and focal loss of endothelium along the lines of closure of the valve leaflets. This leads to deposition of tiny nodules of fibrin which can be recognized grossly as "verrucae" along the leaflets (so-called verrucous endocarditis of acute RF).

 Clinical Features: There is no specific test for RF, and the clinical diagnosis is made when two major—or one major and two minor—criteria (the Jones criteria) are met. If the diagnosis is supported by evidence of a recent streptococcal infection, the probability of RF is high.

The **major criteria** of acute RF include carditis (murmurs, cardiomegaly, pericarditis, and congestive heart failure), polyarthritis, chorea, erythema marginatum, and subcutaneous nodules.

The minor criteria are a previous history of RF, arthralgia, fever, certain laboratory tests indicating an inflammatory process (e.g., increased sedimentation rate, positive test result for C-reactive protein, leukocytosis), and electrocardiographic changes.

The symptoms of RF occur 2 to 3 weeks after an infection with *S. pyogenes*. By this time, the throat culture is usually negative. Increasing titers of serum antibodies to group A streptococcal antigens, such as antistreptolysin O, anti-DNAase B, and antihyaluronidase, provide concrete evidence of a recent infection with group A *Streptococcus*. The acute symptoms of RF usually subside within 3 months, but in the presence of severe carditis, clinical activity may continue for 6 months or more. The mortality from acute rheumatic carditis is low, and the main cause of death is heart failure caused by myocarditis, although valvular dysfunction may also play a role.

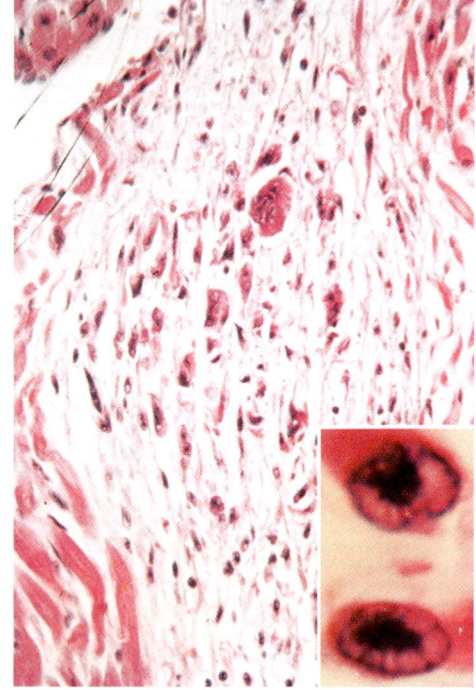

FIGURE 11-31
Acute rheumatic heart disease. An Aschoff body is located interstitially in the myocardium. Note collagen degeneration, lymphocytes, and a multinucleated Aschoff giant cell. (Inset) Nuclei of Anitschkow myocytes, showing "owl-eye" appearance in cross-section and "caterpillar" shape longitudinally.

Chronic Rheumatic Heart Disease

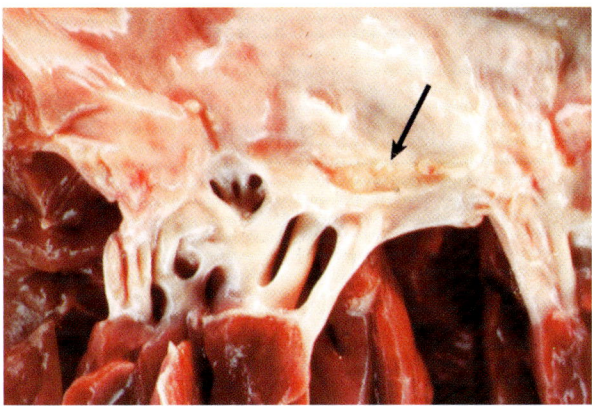

FIGURE 11-32
Chronic rheumatic valvulitis. The mitral valve leaflets are thickened and focally calcified *(arrow)*, and the commissures are partially fused. The chordae tendineae are also short, thick, and fused.

Pathology: The myocardial and pericardial components of rheumatic pancarditis typically resolve without permanent sequelae. By contrast, the acute valvulitis of RF often results in long-term structural and functional alterations. During the healing phase, the valve leaflets develop diffuse fibrosis, causing them to become thickened, shrunken, and less pliable. At the same time, healing of the verrucous lesions along the lines of closure often leads to formation of fibrous "adhesions" between the leaflets, especially at the commissures (commissural fusion). The result is a stenotic valve that does not open freely because the leaflets are rigid and partially fused. Blood flow across such a valve is turbulent, which can cause even more scarring and deformation of the leaflets because of chronic "wear and tear" on the valve. Severe valvular scarring may develop months or years after a single bout of acute RF. On the other hand, recurrent episodes of acute RF are common and result in repeated and progressively increasing damage to the heart valves.

The mitral valve is the most commonly and severely affected valve in chronic rheumatic disease. The mitral valve snaps shut under systolic pressure and, thus, bears the greatest mechanical burden of all cardiac valves. Chronic mitral valvulitis is characterized by conspicuous, irregular thickening and calcification of the leaflets, often with fusion of the commissures and the chordae tendineae (Fig. 11-32). In severe chronic rheumatic mitral valve disease, the valve orifice becomes reduced to a fixed narrow opening that has the appearance of a "fish mouth" when viewed from the ventricular aspect (Fig. 11-33). Mitral stenosis is the predominant functional lesion, but such a valve is also regurgitant. The chronic regurgitation produces a "jet" of blood directed

Recurrent attacks of RF are associated with types of group A β-hemolytic streptococci to which the patient has not been previously exposed and, therefore, to which immunity has not developed. The rate of recurrence of RF is related to the elapsed interval between the initial episode and a subsequent streptococcal infection. In patients with a history of a recent attack of RF, the recurrence rate is as high as 65%, whereas after 10 years, a streptococcal infection is followed by an acute relapse in only 5%.

Prompt treatment of streptococcal pharyngitis with antibiotics prevents an initial attack of RF and, less often, a recurrence of the disease. There is no specific treatment for acute RF, but corticosteroids and salicylates are helpful in managing the symptoms.

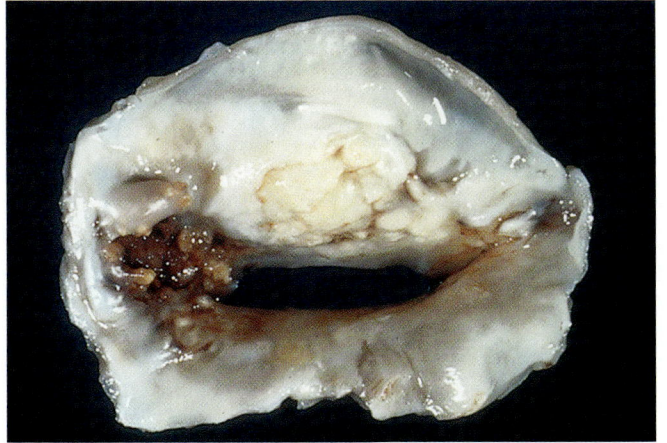
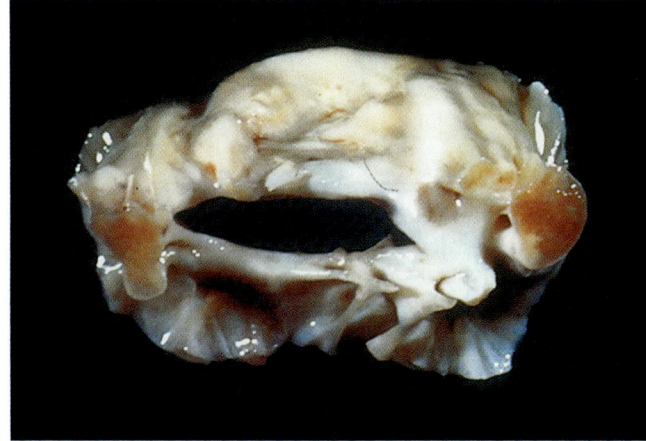

A   B

FIGURE 11-33
Chronic rheumatic valvulitis. A view of a surgically excised rheumatic mitral valve from the left atrium (A) and left ventricle (B) shows rigid, thickened, and fused leaflets with a narrow orifice, creating the characteristic "fish mouth" appearance of rheumatic mitral stenosis. Note that the tips of the papillary muscles *(shown in B)* are directly attached to the underside of the valve leaflets, reflecting marked shortening and fusion of the chordae tendineae.

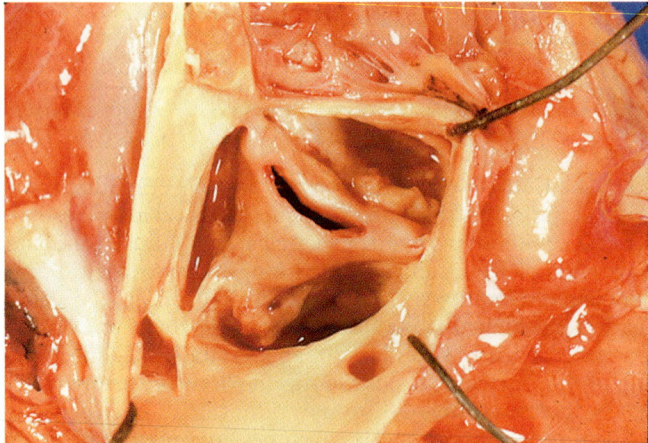

FIGURE 11-34
Chronic rheumatic valvulitis. An example of severe rheumatic aortic stenosis. Three sinuses of Valsalva are recognizable, but the cusps are rigidly fibrotic and calcified, and extensive fusion of the commissures has narrowed the orifice into a fixed slitlike configuration that does not change during the cardiac cycle.

at the posterior aspect of the left atrium, which damages the atrial endocardium and produces a discrete focus of rough, wrinkled endocardium referred to as a *MacCallum patch*.

The aortic valve, which snaps shut under diastolic pressure, is the second most commonly involved valve in rheumatic heart disease. Diffuse fibrous thickening of the cusps and fusion of the commissures cause aortic stenosis, which may be mild initially but which progresses because of the chronic effects of turbulent blood flow across the valve. Often, the cusps become rigidly calcified as the patient ages, resulting in stenosis and insufficiency, although either lesion may predominate (Fig. 11-34). The lower pressures experienced by the right-sided valves are usually protective. In cases of recurrent RF, however, the tricuspid valve may become deformed, virtually always in association with mitral and aortic lesions. The pulmonic valve is rarely affected.

Complications of Chronic Rheumatic Heart Disease

- **Bacterial endocarditis** follows episodes of bacteremia, such as those that occur during dental procedures. The scarred valves of rheumatic heart disease provide an attractive environment for bacteria that would bypass a normal valve.
- **Mural thrombi** form in the atrial or ventricular chambers in 40% of patients with rheumatic valvular disease. They give rise to thromboemboli, which can produce infarcts in various organs. Rarely, a large thrombus in the left atrial appendage develops a stalk and acts as a ball valve that obstructs the mitral valve orifice.
- **Congestive heart failure** is associated with rheumatic disease of both the mitral and aortic valves.
- **Adhesive pericarditis** commonly follows the fibrinous pericarditis of the acute attack, but almost never results in constrictive pericarditis.

Collagen Vascular Diseases Affect Valves and Myocardium

Systemic Lupus Erythematosus

The heart is often involved in systemic lupus erythematosus (SLE), but the cardiac symptoms are usually less prominent than other manifestations of the disease.

 Pathology: The most common cardiac lesion is fibrinous pericarditis, usually with an effusion. Myocarditis in SLE, at least in the form of subclinical left ventricular dysfunction, is also common and reflects the severity of the disease in other organs. Microscopically, fibrinoid necrosis of small vessels and focal degeneration of interstitial tissue are seen.

Endocarditis is the most striking cardiac lesion of SLE. Verrucous vegetations, measuring up to 4 mm across, occur on the endocardial surfaces and are termed *Libman-Sacks endocarditis*. They are most common on the surfaces of the mitral valve (Fig. 11-35), characteristically the undersurface, close to the origin of the leaflets from the valve ring. Rare aortic valve involvement has been described, and the verrucae may extend onto the chordae tendineae and the papillary muscles. Ordinarily, Libman-Sacks endocarditis heals without scarring and does not produce a functional deficit.

Rheumatoid Arthritis

On rare occasions, the heart is involved in patients with rheumatoid arthritis. Characteristic rheumatoid granulomatous inflammation, with fibrinoid necrosis and palisaded lymphocytes and macrophages, may occur in the pericardium, myocardium, or valves. Involvement of the heart in rheumatoid arthritis does not compromise function.

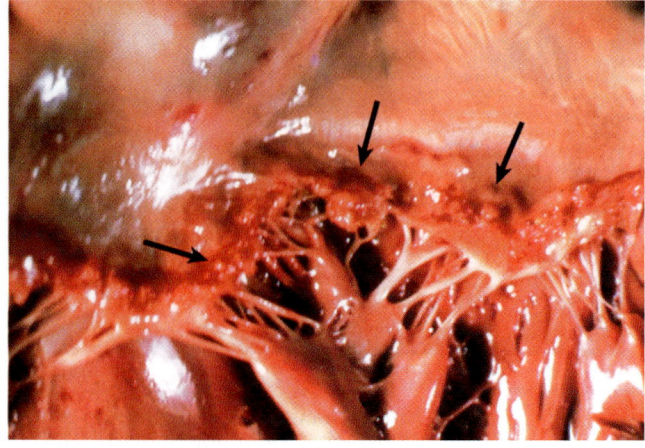

FIGURE 11-35
Libman-Sacks endocarditis. The heart of a patient who died of complications of systemic lupus erythematosus displays verrucous vegetations on the leaflets of the mitral valve.

TABLE 11-6 Etiological Factors in Bacterial Endocarditis

	Children (%)		Adults (%)	
	Newborns	<15 years	15–60 years	>60 years
Underlying disease				
Congenital heart disease	30	80	10	2
Rheumatic heart disease	—	5	25	8
Mitral valve prolapse	—	10	10	10
Valvular calcification	—	—	5	30
Intravenous drug abuse	—	—	15	10
Other	—	—	10	10
None	70	5	25	30
Microorganisms[a]				
Staphylococcus aureus	45	25	35	30
Coagulase-negative staphylococci	10	5	5	10
Streptococci	15	45	45	35
Enterococci	—	5	5	15
Gram-negative bacteria	10	5	5	5
Fungi	10	Rare	Rare	Rare
Negative culture	5	10	5	5

[a] 5% of neonatal infections are polymicrobial

Ankylosing Spondylitis

A characteristic aortic valve lesion develops in as many as 10% of patients with long-standing ankylosing spondylitis. The aortic valve ring is dilated, and the valve cusps are scarred and shortened. Focal inflammatory lesions occur in all layers of the aortic wall, particularly near the valve ring. The principal functional consequence is aortic regurgitation.

Scleroderma (Progressive Systemic Sclerosis)

Involvement of the heart in patients with scleroderma is second only to renal disease as a cause of death in this illness. The myocardium exhibits intimal sclerosis of small arteries, which leads to small infarcts and patchy fibrosis. As a result, congestive heart failure and arrhythmias are common. In fact, electrocardiographic studies have revealed ventricular ectopy in two thirds of patients with scleroderma and serious arrhythmias in one fourth. Cor pulmonale secondary to interstitial fibrosis of the lungs and hypertensive heart disease (caused by renal involvement) are also seen.

Polyarteritis Nodosa

The heart is involved in up to 75% of cases of polyarteritis nodosa. The necrotizing lesions in branches of the coronary arteries result in myocardial infarction, arrhythmias, or heart block. Cardiac hypertrophy and failure secondary to renal vascular hypertension often occur.

Bacterial Endocarditis Refers to Infection of the Cardiac Valves

Fungi, chlamydia, and rickettsiae may also produce an infective endocarditis, but such cases are distinctly uncommon. Before the antibiotic era, bacterial endocarditis was untreatable and almost invariably fatal. The infection was classified according to its clinical course as either acute or subacute endocarditis.

Acute bacterial endocarditis was described as an infection of a normal cardiac valve by highly virulent suppurative organisms, typically *Staphylococcus aureus* and *S. pyogenes*. The affected valve was rapidly destroyed, and the patient died within 6 weeks in acute heart failure or of overwhelming sepsis.

Subacute bacterial endocarditis was a less fulminant disease in which less-virulent organisms (e.g., *Staphylococcus viridans* or *Staphylococcus epidermidis*) infected a structurally abnormal valve, which typically had been deformed by rheumatic heart disease. In these cases, patients typically survived for 6 months or more, and infectious complications were uncommon.

The development of antimicrobial therapy changed the clinical patterns of bacterial endocarditis, and the classical presentations described earlier are today unusual. The disease is now classified according to the anatomical location and the offending organism (Table 11-6).

 Epidemiology: Most children with bacterial endocarditis have an underlying cardiac lesion. In the past, rheumatic heart disease accounted for a third of such cases. However, with the declining incidence of RF, fewer than 10% of cases of bacterial endocarditis in children are today attributable to this disease. **The most common predisposing condition for bacterial endocarditis in children is now congenital heart disease.**

The epidemiology of bacterial endocarditis has also changed in adults. Whereas rheumatic heart disease comprised three fourths of the cases in the past, it now underlies only a few. More than half of adults with bacterial endocarditis have no predisposing cardiac lesion. **Mitral valve prolapse and congenital heart disease are today the most frequent bases for bacterial endocarditis in adults.**

In **rheumatic heart disease,** the mitral valve is affected in more than 85% of cases of bacterial endocarditis, and the aortic valve is involved in 50%. Involvement of a single valve occurs more often in women (2:1) in the case of mitral valve disease, whereas the male-to-female ratio in isolated aortic endocarditis is 4:1.

Intravenous drug abusers inject pathogenic organisms along with their illicit drugs, and bacterial endocarditis is a notorious complication. In such patients, 80% have no underlying cardiac lesion, and the tricuspid valve is infected in fully half of cases. The most common source of bacteria in intravenous drug abusers is the skin, with *S. aureus* causing more than half of the infections.

Prosthetic valves are the site of infection in 15% of all cases of endocarditis in adults, and 4% of patients with prosthetic valves have this complication. Staphylococci are again responsible for half of these infections, with most of the remainder being caused by gram-negative aerobic organisms, streptococci and enterococci, and fungi. Another iatrogenic form of endocarditis originates from the bacterial colonization of indwelling vascular catheters.

Transient bacteremia from any procedure may lead to infective endocarditis. Examples include dental procedures, urinary catheterization, gastrointestinal endoscopy, and obstetric procedures. Antibiotic prophylaxis is recommended during such maneuvers for patients at increased risk for bacterial endocarditis (e.g., those with a history of rheumatic fever or the presence of a cardiac murmur).

The elderly also show an increasing tendency to develop endocarditis. A number of degenerative changes in the cardiac valves predispose to endocarditis, including calcific aortic stenosis and calcification of the mitral annulus. Diabetes and pregnancy are also associated with an increased incidence of bacterial endocarditis.

 Pathogenesis: Virulent organisms, such as *S. aureus*, can infect apparently normal valves, but the mechanism of such bacterial colonization is poorly understood. The pathogenesis of the infection of a damaged valve by less-virulent organisms has been related to (1) hemodynamic factors, (2) the formation of an initially sterile platelet–fibrin thrombus, and (3) the adherence properties of the microorganisms.

A key feature is abnormal blood flow across a damaged valve. The pressure gradient formed across a narrow orifice (valve or congenital defect) produces turbulent flow at the periphery and a high-velocity jet stream at the center, both of which tend to denude endothelial surfaces of valves on the low-pressure side of the orifice. This leads to focal deposition of platelets and fibrin, creating small sterile vegetations that are hospitable sites for bacterial colonization and growth. Microorganisms that gain access to the circulation, as a result of a dental procedure for example, can be deposited within the vegetations. In this protected environment, colony counts upon culture may reach 10^{10} organisms per gram of tissue.

Factors that promote adherence of bacteria to the sterile vegetations are believed to be important in the pathogenesis of endocarditis. Cell-associated and circulating fibronectin both bind to surface molecules of the bacteria, thereby facilitating adhesion of fibrin, collagen, and cells. Some microorganisms produce extracellular polysaccharides, which also function as adhesion factors.

 Pathology: Bacterial endocarditis most commonly involves the left-sided heart valves (mitral or aortic valves or both).

The most frequent congenital heart lesions that underlie bacterial endocarditis are patent ductus arteriosus, tetralogy of Fallot, ventricular septal defect, and bicuspid aortic valve, which is an increasingly recognized risk factor, especially in men older than 60 years. **As a rule, vegetations in bacterial endocarditis form on the atrial side of the atrioventricular valves and the ventricular side of the semilunar valves,** often at points of closure of the leaflets or cusps (Fig. 11-36). They are composed of platelets, fibrin, cell debris, and masses of organisms. The underlying valve tissue is edematous and inflamed and may eventually become so damaged that the leaflet perforates, causing regurgitation. The lesions vary in size from a small, superficial deposit to bulky, exuberant vegetations. The infective process may spread locally to involve the valve ring or the adjacent mural endocardium and chordae tendineae.

Infected thromboemboli travel to multiple systemic sites, causing infarcts or abscesses in many organs, including the brain, kidneys, intestine, and spleen.

Focal segmental glomerulonephritis is another complication of infective endocarditis (see Chapter 16). The disease is the result of immune-complex deposition in glomeruli, producing a patchy hemorrhagic appearance of the kidneys referred to as *flea-bitten kidneys.*

Clinical Features: Many patients manifest the early symptoms of bacterial endocarditis within a week of the bacteremic episode, and almost all are symptomatic within 2 weeks. The disease begins with nonspecific symptoms of low-grade fever, fatigue, anorexia, and weight loss. Heart murmurs develop almost invariably, often with a changing pattern, during the course of the disease. In cases of more than 6 weeks duration, splenomegaly, pe-

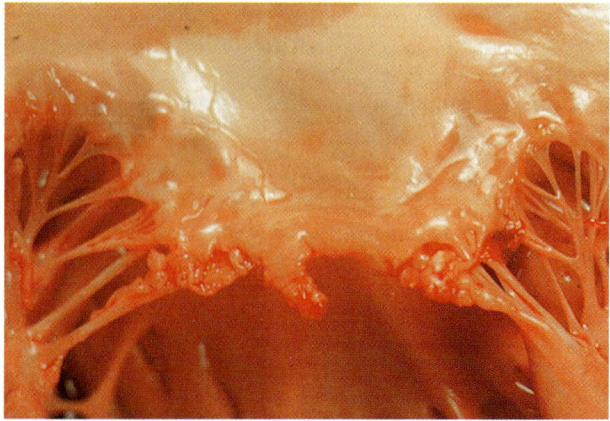

FIGURE 11-36

Bacterial endocarditis. The mitral valve shows destructive vegetations, which have eroded through the free margins of the valve leaflets.

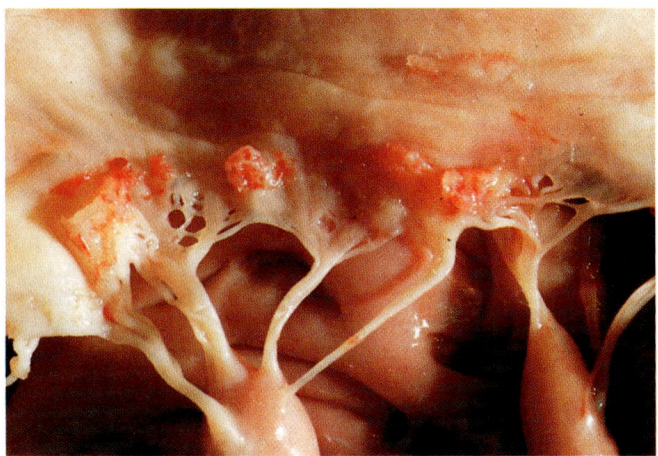

FIGURE 11-37
Marantic endocarditis. Sterile platelet–fibrin vegetations are seen on the leaflets of a structurally normal mitral valve.

techiae, and clubbing of the fingers are frequent. In a third of patients, systemic emboli are recognized at some time during the illness. Pulmonary emboli characterize tricuspid valve endocarditis in drug addicts. One third of the victims of bacterial endocarditis manifest some evidence of neurological dysfunction, owing to the frequency of embolization to the brain. Mycotic aneurysms of cerebral vessels, brain abscesses, and intracerebral bleeding are observed.

Antibacterial therapy is effective in limiting the morbidity and mortality of bacterial endocarditis, and most patients defervesce within a week of instituting such therapy. However, the prognosis depends to some extent on the offending organism and the stage at which the infection is treated. **A third of cases of endocarditis caused by S. aureus are still fatal.** Surgical replacement of a valve destroyed by endocarditis is a risky procedure that carries high surgical mortality unless the infection has been fully cleared. **The most common serious complication of bacterial endocarditis is congestive heart failure, usually as a result of the destruction of a valve.** Myocardial abscesses and infarction secondary to coronary artery emboli occasionally contribute to heart failure. At this stage the prognosis is grim.

Nonbacterial Thrombotic Endocarditis Is a Complication of Wasting Diseases

Nonbacterial thrombotic endocarditis (NBTE), also known as marantic endocarditis, refers to the presence of sterile vegetations on apparently normal cardiac valves, almost always in association with cancer or some other wasting disease. NBTE affects the mitral (Fig. 11-37) and aortic valves with equal frequency. Its gross appearance is similar to that of infective endocarditis, but it does not destroy the affected valve, and on microscopic examination, neither inflammation nor microorganisms can be demonstrated.

The cause of NBTE is poorly understood. It has been attributed to increased blood coagulability or immune-complex deposition. It is seen commonly as a paraneoplastic condition, usually complicating adenocarcinomas (particularly of the pancreas and lung) and hematological malignancies. It may also be part of the disseminated intravascular coagulation syndrome or accompany a variety of debilitating nonneoplastic diseases, thus accounting for the synonym "marantic endocarditis" (Gr., *marantikos*, "wasting away"). The principal danger posed by NBTE is embolization to distant organs, clinically manifested as infarcts of many organs.

Calcific Aortic Stenosis Reflects Chronic Damage to the Valve

Calcific aortic stenosis refers to a narrowing of the aortic valve orifice as a result of the deposition of calcium in the cusps and valve ring.

 **Pathogenesis and Pathology:** Calcific aortic stenosis has three main causes.

- **Rheumatic aortic valve disease** is characterized by diffuse fibrous thickening and scarring of the cusps, commissural fusion, and deposition of calcium, all of which reduce the valve orifice and limit mobility of the valve (see Fig. 11-34). Rheumatic aortic stenosis virtually never occurs in isolation; there is nearly always evidence of rheumatic mitral valve disease as well. Now that acute rheumatic fever has become so rare in the United States and most elderly patients with rheumatic valve disease have either undergone valve replacement or died, calcific aortic stenosis is usually attributed to other major cause.
- **Senile calcific stenosis** develops in elderly patients as a degenerative process involving a symmetric tricuspid aortic valve. The valve cusps become rigidly calcified, but there is no commissural fusion (Fig. 11-38), which is

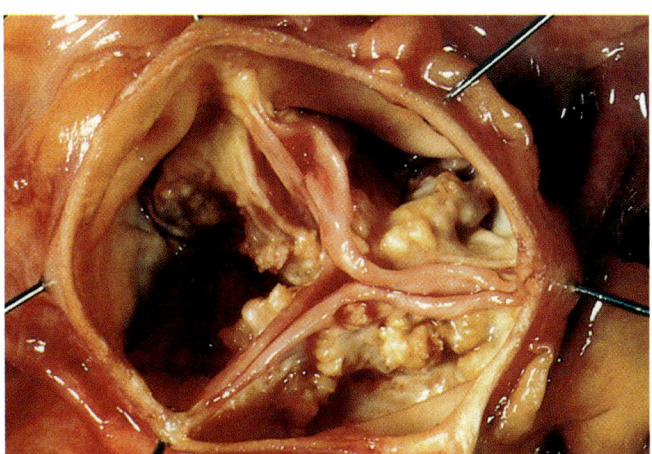

FIGURE 11-38
Calcific aortic stenosis in a three-cuspid aortic valve in an elderly person. The leaflets are heavily calcified, but there is no commissural fusion (compare with Fig. 11-34).

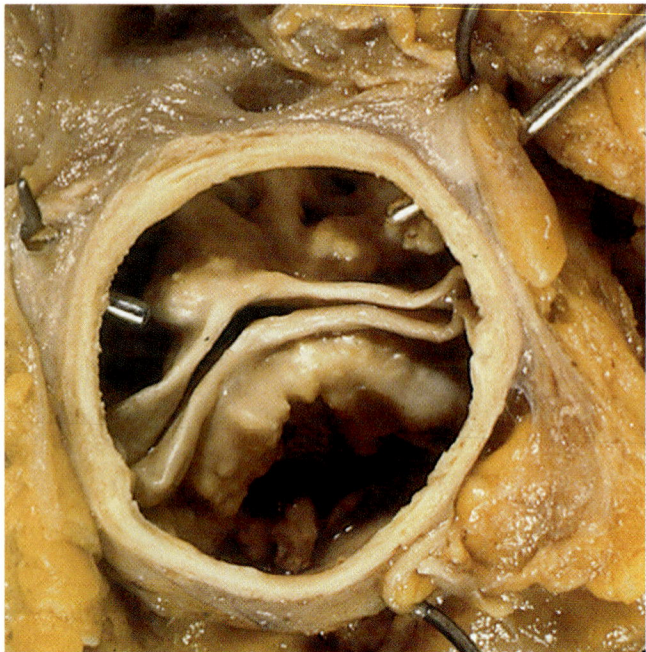

FIGURE 11-39
Calcific aortic stenosis of a congenitally bicuspid aortic valve. The two leaflets are heavily calcified, but there is no commissural fusion.

a hallmark of the rheumatic aortic valve. The mitral valve is usually normal in patients with senile calcific aortic stenosis.

- **Congenital bicuspid aortic stenosis** often develops with age (Fig. 11-39).

Calcific aortic stenosis in both congenitally malformed valves and normal ones is probably related to the cumulative effect of years of trauma, owing to turbulent blood flow around the valve. For example, although the bicuspid valve is not inherently stenotic, its orifice is elliptical rather than round, and flow across the valve is somewhat turbulent. Increasing rigidity of the cusps eventually produces functional derangements, typically in patients beyond the age of 60. In any of the forms of calcific aortic stenosis, dystrophic calcification produces nodules restricted to the base and lower half of the cusps, rarely involving the free margins. In the absence of rheumatic scarring, the commissures are not fused, and three distinct cusps are evident.

Clinical Features: Severe aortic stenosis results in striking concentric left ventricular hypertrophy. Eventually, the heart dilates and fails. The disease is treated with great success (5-year survival rate of 85%) with surgical valve replacement, provided that the operation is performed before ventricular dysfunction becomes irreversible. The hypertrophic left ventricle is then restored to normal size.

Calcification of the Mitral Valve Annulus Is Usually Asymptomatic

Calcification of the mitral valve annulus occurs commonly in the elderly and is usually without functional significance, although it often produces a murmur. However, if it is severe enough to interfere with closure of the mitral leaflets during systole, mitral regurgitation occurs. Calcification of the mitral valve annulus in the elderly differs from the calcification that occurs in rheumatic mitral valve disease. The former features little or no deformation of the valve leaflets, and the calcification is most prominent in the annulus rather than the leaflets. About 40% of women older than 90 years exhibit this lesion, whereas in men the incidence is only 15%. Calcification of the mitral valve annulus is aggravated by the presence of aortic stenosis, hypertension, and diabetes.

Calcific deposits transform the mitral ring into a rigid, curved bar up to 2 cm in diameter, which may be evident radiologically. The posterior mitral leaflet is often distorted and displaced upward. Amorphous masses of calcified material first develop in the connective tissue of the valve ring. However, with time, the calcification extends into the base of the leaflets and eventually to the ventricular septum.

Mitral Valve Prolapse Is the Most Common Indication for Valve Replacement

Mitral valve prolapse (MVP) refers to a condition in which the mitral valve leaflets become enlarged and redundant, and the chordae tendineae become thinned and elongated such that the billowed leaflets prolapse into the left atrium during systole. (Fig. 11-40A). Also referred to as "floppy mitral valve syndrome," MVP is the most frequent cause of mitral regurgitation that requires surgical replacement of the valve. As much as 5% of the adult population may show echocardiographic evidence of MVP, although most will not have regurgitation severe enough to warrant surgical intervention.

Pathogenesis: MVP has an important hereditary component, and many cases appear to be transmitted as an autosomal dominant trait. Patients with primary MVP exhibit a striking accumulation of myxomatous connective tissue in the center of the valve leaflet (Fig. 11-40B). This abnormality is believed to be related to an undefined defect in the metabolism of the extracellular matrix. The amount of proteoglycans in the mitral valve is increased, and by electron microscopy, collagen fibrils are fragmented. Presumably, the defect in the extracellular matrix allows the leaflets and chordae to enlarge and stretch under the high-pressure conditions they experience during the cardiac cycle. MVP is usually an isolated finding, although it may occur in the context of a variety of other conditions, including Marfan syndrome, inherited disorders of collagen metabolism, and myotonic muscular dystrophy. It is also seen in association with hyperthyroidism, certain congenital heart lesions, and von Willebrand disease. There seems to be an unusually high incidence of MVP in persons with an asthenic habitus and a number of congenital thoracic deformities.

Pathology: On gross examination, the mitral valve leaflets are redundant and deformed (see Fig. 11-40A), and on cross-section, they have a gelatinous appearance and a slippery texture, owing to accumulation of acid mucopolysaccharides (proteoglycans). The myxomatous degenerative process affects not only the mitral valve leaflets but also the annulus and the chordae tendineae, which increases the degree of prolapse and regurgitation. Damage to the chordae may be so severe that chordal rupture occurs, producing a flail mitral valve that is totally incompetent. Although the mitral valve is usually the only valve affected, myxomatous degeneration can develop in the other cardiac valves, especially in patients with Marfan syndrome, 90% of whom have some clinical evidence of MVP.

 Clinical Features: Most patients with MVP are asymptomatic. Clinical recognition of the abnormality is based on recognition of the classical auscultatory findings of a mid-to-late systolic click, caused by the snap of the redundant leaflets as they prolapse into the left atrium. A late systolic murmur is present if mitral regurgitation is significant. Endocarditis, both infective and nonbacterial, is sometimes a serious complication, and cerebral emboli are common. Significant mitral regurgitation develops in 15% of patients after 10 to 15 years of MVP, after which mitral valve replacement is indicated.

Papillary Muscle Dysfunction Produces Mitral Regurgitation

Dysfunction of the left ventricular papillary muscles is most often caused by ischemia. The papillary muscles are especially vulnerable to ischemic injury because they are supplied by the terminal branches of the intramyocardial coronary arteries. Thus, any reduction in coronary blood flow may preferentially interfere with the function of the papillary muscles. Brief periods of ischemia (e.g., during episodes of angina pectoris) can result in transient papillary muscle dysfunction (stunning) and temporary mitral regurgitation. By contrast, severe myocardial infarction and subsequent scarring of the papillary muscles can lead to permanent mitral regurgitation. In fact, one third of all patients being evaluated for coronary artery bypass surgery have some evidence of "ischemic mitral regurgitation." Papillary muscle dysfunction may also be associated with a healed myocardial infarct, in which impaired contractility of the myocardium at the base of the papillary muscle interferes with its function. Rarely, patients may suddenly develop life-threatening mitral regurgitation after rupture of an acutely infarcted papillary muscle.

Carcinoid Heart Disease Involves the Right-Sided Valves

Carcinoid heart disease is an unusual condition that uniquely affects the right side of the heart and produces tricuspid regurgitation and pulmonary stenosis. It arises in patients with carcinoid tumors, usually of the small intestine, that have metastasized to the liver.

 Pathogenesis: The pathogenesis of carcinoid heart disease is not fully understood. The valvular and endocardial lesions are thought to be caused by high concentrations of serotonin or other vasoactive amines and peptides produced by the tumor in the liver. Because these moieties are metabolized in the lung, carcinoid heart disease affects the right side of the heart almost exclusively. There are rare reports of left-sided involvement in patients with atrial or ventricular septal defects.

During the 1990s, reports surfaced of mitral and aortic valve disease in patients taking the appetite-suppressing

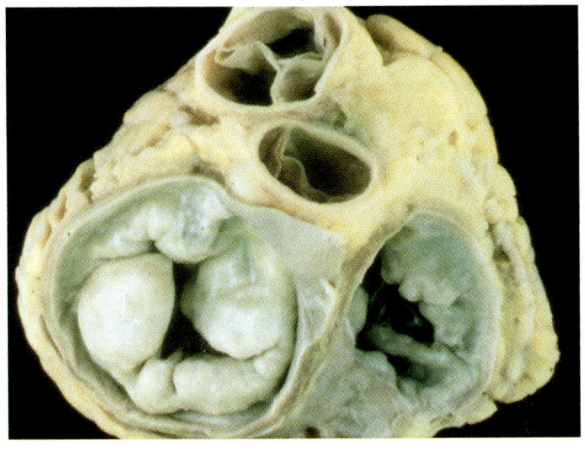
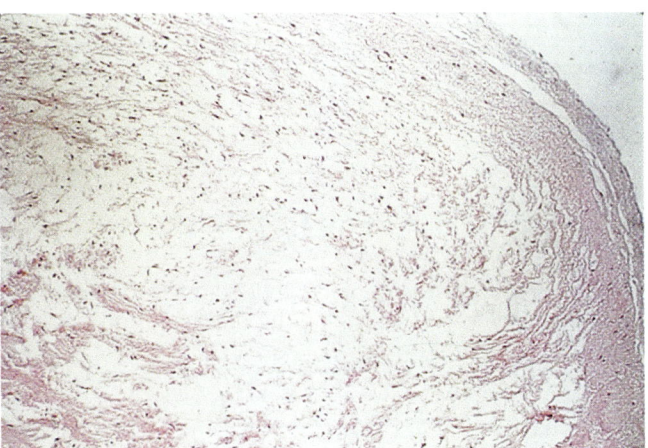

FIGURE 11-40
Mitral valve prolapse. A. A view of the mitral valve *(left)* from the left atrium shows redundant and deformed leaflets, which billow into the left atrial cavity. **B.** A microscopic section of one of the mitral valve leaflets reveals conspicuous myxomatous connective tissue in the center of the leaflet.

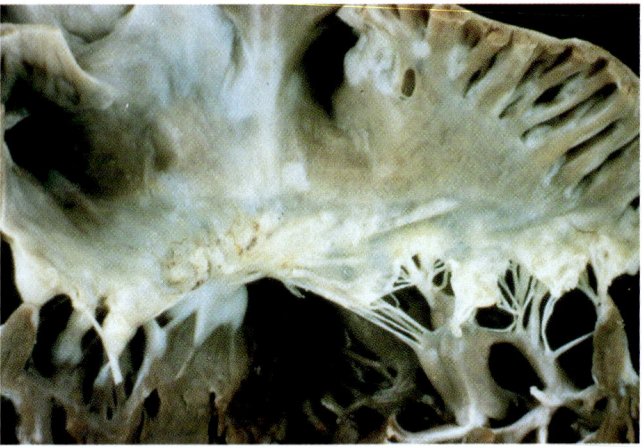

FIGURE 11-41
Carcinoid heart disease. Pearly white deposits are seen on the tricuspid valve leaflets and adjacent endocardium. Although the valve leaflets have not been destroyed, they have become deformed and "stuck down" on the ventricular endocardium, which usually produces tricuspid regurgitation.

drugs fenfluramine–phentermine ("fen-phen"). The gross and microscopic features of the valve lesions are strikingly similar to that seen in carcinoid heart disease, except that they develop on the left-sided valves. Because these drugs interfere with serotonin metabolism and signaling, it has been suggested that the pathogenesis of fen-phen and carcinoid valve disease is similar.

 Pathology: The cardiac lesions consist of plaque-like deposits of dense, pearly gray, fibrous tissue on the tricuspid (Fig. 11-41) and pulmonary valves and on the endocardial surface of the right ventricle. Microscopically, these patches of fibrous tissue appear "tacked on" to the valve leaflets and are not associated with inflammation or apparent damage to the underlying valve structures. However, the leaflets become deformed, and their surface area, reduced. As a result, the tricuspid leaflets become "stuck down" on the adjacent right ventricular mural endocardium, resulting in tricuspid insufficiency or stenosis. Shrinkage of the pulmonary valve and its annulus leads to pulmonary stenosis.

PRIMARY MYOCARDIAL DISEASES

Primary myocardial diseases can be divided into inflammatory diseases (myocarditis), metabolic diseases, and cardiomyopathies.

Myocarditis Can Be Caused by Infections, Toxins, and Immune Reactions

Myocarditis refers to inflammation of the myocardium associated with necrosis and degeneration of myocytes. This definition specifically excludes ischemic heart disease. The true incidence of myocarditis is difficult to establish because many cases are asymptomatic. Myocarditis can occur at any age but is most common in children between the ages of 1 and 10. It is one of the few heart diseases that can produce acute heart failure in previously healthy children, adolescents, or young adults. Severe myocarditis can cause arrhythmias and even sudden cardiac death.

Viral Myocarditis

Most cases of myocarditis in North America occur without an easily demonstrable cause. The large majority are believed to be viral, although the evidence is usually circumstantial unless polymerase chain reaction (PCR) studies are performed to identify viral nucleic acids in heart biopsies. The most common viruses that cause myocarditis are listed in Table 11-7.

 Pathogenesis: The pathogenesis of viral myocarditis is believed to involve direct viral cytotoxicity or cell-mediated immune reactions directed against infected myocytes. There is substantial evidence for both mechanisms. In animal models, inoculation of a cardiotropic virus is followed shortly by replication of the virus in the myocardium. Microscopically, only small isolated foci of acute myocyte necrosis with little if any inflammatory cell infiltration are seen, and there is little evidence of functional impairment. Over the next few days, mononuclear cells, principally T lymphocytes and macrophages, infiltrate the myocardium extensively. At the point of maximum inflammation, the animals show signs of heart failure, although viral cultures of both blood and myocardium are negative. This finding is consistent with the observation that patients with symptomatic myocarditis generally have negative viral cultures. Nevertheless, it may still be possible to identify viral nucleic acid sequences by PCR. Furthermore, viral proteins may degrade some components of the myocyte cytoskeleton and thereby contribute to contractile dysfunc-

TABLE 11-7 **Causes of Myocarditis**

Idiopathic

Infectious

- Viral: Coxsackievirus, echovirus, influenza virus, human immunodeficiency virus, and many others
- Rickettsial: Typhus, Rocky Mountain spotted fever
- Bacterial: Diphtheria, staphylococcal, streptococcal, meningococcal, borrelial (Lyme disease) and leptospiral infection
- Fungi and protozoan parasites: Chagas disease, toxoplasmosis, aspergillosis, cryptococcal, and candidal infection
- Metazoan parasites: *Echinococcus, Trichina*

Noninfectious

- Hypersensitivity and immunologically related diseases: Rheumatic fever, systemic lupus erythematosus, scleroderma, drug reaction (e.g., to penicillin or sulfonamide), and rheumatoid arthritis
- Radiation
- Miscellaneous: Sarcoidosis, uremia

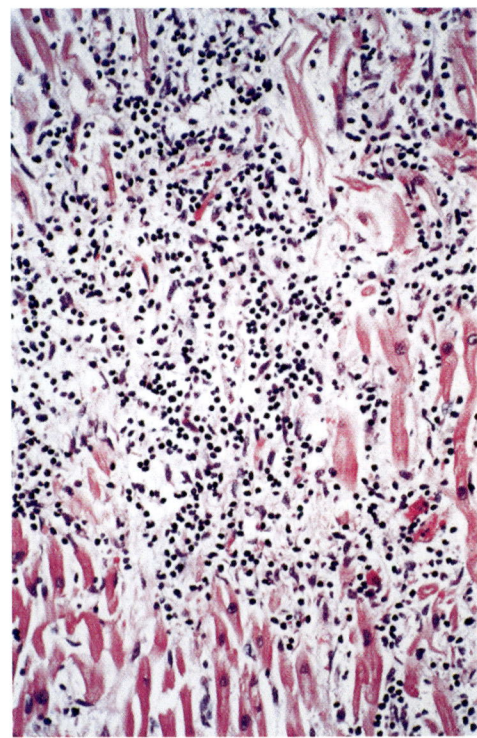

FIGURE 11-42
Viral myocarditis. The myocardial fibers are disrupted by a prominent interstitial infiltrate of lymphocytes and macrophages.

tion. In some models of experimental viral myocarditis, it is clear that T lymphocytes cause much or all of the myocyte injury. The stimulus for the immune attack on the myocyte has not been established but appears to involve the major histocompatibility antigens.

 Pathology: The hearts of patients with myocarditis who develop clinical heart failure during the active inflammatory phase show biventricular dilation and generalized hypokinesis of the myocardium. At autopsy, the heart of a patient dying of acute illness is flabby and dilated. The histological changes of viral myocarditis vary with the clinical severity of the disease, but with few exceptions, the microscopic features are nonspecific and indistinguishable from toxic myocarditis. Most cases show a patchy or diffuse interstitial, predominantly mononuclear, inflammatory infiltrate composed principally of T lymphocytes and macrophages (Fig. 11-42). Multinucleated giant cells may also be present. The inflammatory cells often surround individual myocytes, and focal myocyte necrosis is seen. During the resolving phase, fibroblast proliferation and interstitial collagen deposition predominate. Ordinarily, neutrophils are not seen in viral myocarditis. However, when necrosis is extensive, the histological features may be reminiscent of those seen in an infarct, namely a neutrophilic infiltrate followed by organization and repair. Most viruses that cause myocarditis also cause pericarditis.

 Clinical Features: Many persons who develop viral myocarditis may be asymptomatic. When symptoms do occur, they usually begin a few weeks after infection. Most patients recover from acute myocarditis, although a few die of congestive heart failure or arrhythmias. The disease may be unusually severe in infants and pregnant women. Despite resolution of the active inflammatory phase of viral myocarditis, subtle functional impairment may persist for years, and progression to overt cardiomyopathy is well documented. There is no specific treatment for viral myocarditis, and supportive measures are the rule.

MYOCARDITIS IN AIDS: A significant proportion of symptomatic AIDS patients have some clinical or pathological evidence of cardiac disease (pericardial effusions, myocarditis, endocarditis, or cardiomyopathy). An unusually high incidence of viral myocarditis due to cardiotropic viruses, such as Coxsackie B and adenovirus, has been documented in this population. HIV infection of cardiac myocytes appears to play a minor role.

Other Forms of Infectious Myocarditis

In addition to viruses, other microorganisms that gain access to the bloodstream can infect the heart. For example, brucellosis, meningococcemia, and psittacosis are often associated with an infectious myocarditis. Moreover, some bacteria (e.g., diphtheria organisms) produce cardiotoxins, which may produce a fatal myocarditis. The most common cause of myocarditis in South America is infection with the protozoan *Trypanosoma cruzi,* the agent of Chagas disease (see Chapter 9).

Bacterial infection of the myocardium is characterized by multiple foci of a mixed inflammatory cell infiltrate, with neutrophils as the major component. Microabscesses can occur when septic emboli lodge in the coronary circulation, often as a consequence of infective endocarditis.

Rickettsial diseases commonly cause widespread vasculitis, which affects small coronary blood vessels.

Fungal infection of the myocardium typically occurs in immunocompromised patients, although the heart is relatively resistant to fungal infection.

Toxoplasmosis can involve the myocardium in immunosuppressed patients; the intracellular parasites proliferate within cardiac myocytes and elicit a focal mixed inflammatory response, with neutrophils and eosinophils.

Chagas disease is associated with the proliferation of parasites within cardiac myocytes and a mixed inflammatory cell infiltrate, composed principally of lymphocytes, plasma cells, and macrophages.

Hypersensitivity Myocarditis

Hypersensitivity reactions to many drugs can affect the heart.

 Pathology: The inflammation consists of an interstitial and perivascular infiltrate, which is often confined to the myocardium and does not affect other organs. The inflammatory infiltrate in hypersensitivity myocarditis resembles that seen in viral myocarditis, but the former displays numerous eosinophils, as well as lymphocytes and plasma cells. Another typical feature is the virtual absence of myocyte necrosis, even when the infiltrate is intense.

 Clinical Features: Hypersensitivity myocarditis is usually clinically silent, and the diagnosis is often made as an incidental finding at autopsy. However, it may produce chest pain and electrocardiographic changes that resemble acute myocardial ischemia. Occasionally, it can be responsible for fatal ventricular arrhythmias. When the disease causes symptoms, treatment consists of discontinuing the offending drug and administering corticosteroids or immunosuppressive agents.

Giant Cell Myocarditis

Giant cell myocarditis is a rare, highly aggressive disease of the heart characterized by intense inflammation, extensive areas of myocyte necrosis, and numerous multinucleated giant cells. The cause of the disorder is unknown, but it is sometimes encountered in association with systemic lupus erythematosus, hyperthyroidism, and thymoma. Although an autoimmune cause has been suggested, no persuasive evidence for this theory has been presented.

Giant cell myocarditis is usually a rapidly fatal disease of adults in the third to fifth decades of life, although it can also occur in adolescents. Patients die of congestive heart failure or sudden death from arrhythmias. At autopsy, the heart is flabby and dilated and may contain mural thrombi. Microscopically, prominent giant cells, together with lymphoid cells and macrophages, are seen at the margins of serpiginous areas of myocardial necrosis. The only effective treatment for giant cell myocarditis is cardiac transplantation. However, the disease recurs in the transplanted heart in one fourth of cases. Aside from cardiac transplantation, there is no effective therapy.

METABOLIC DISEASES OF THE HEART

Hyperthyroidism Causes High-Output Failure

Hyperthyroidism causes conspicuous tachycardia and an increased cardiac workload, owing to decreased peripheral resistance and increased cardiac output. The disorder may eventually lead to angina pectoris and high-output failure. In addition to its multiple effects in the body, thyroid hormone has direct inotropic and chronotropic effects on the heart. Thyroid hormone (1) increases the activity of the sarcolemmal sodium pump, (2) enhances the synthesis of a myosin isoform with rapid ATPase activity and reduces production of a slower isoform, and (3) upregulates expression of slow calcium channels in the sarcolemma, thereby facilitating contractility.

Hypothyroid Heart Disease Diminishes Cardiac Output

Patients with severe hypothyroidism (myxedema) have decreased cardiac output, reduced heart rate, and impaired myocardial contractility, changes that are the reverse of those seen in hyperthyroidism. There may be a pericardial effusion created by increased capillary permeability and leakage of fluid and protein into the pericardial cavity. The pulse pressure is decreased because of increased peripheral resistance and decreased blood volume.

The hearts of patients with myxedema are flabby and dilated, and the myocardium exhibits myofiber swelling. Basophilic (mucinous) degeneration is common. Interstitial fibrosis may also be present. Despite these changes, myxedema does not produce congestive heart failure in the absence of other cardiac disorders.

Thiamine Deficiency (Beriberi) Heart Disease is Similar to Hyperthyroidism

Beriberi heart disease develops in patients who consume a diet inadequate in vitamin B_1 (thiamine) for at least 3 months (see Chapter 8). It is seen in parts of Asia in which the diet consists largely of shelled rice. In the United States, thiamine deficiency is seen occasionally in alcoholics or neglected persons. Beriberi heart disease results in decreased peripheral vascular resistance and increased cardiac output, a combination similar to that produced by hyperthyroidism. The result is high-output failure. Interestingly, heart failure may develop so suddenly that the patient dies within 2 days of the onset of symptoms. At autopsy, the heart is dilated and shows only nonspecific microscopic changes.

CARDIOMYOPATHY

Cardiomyopathy refers to a primary disease of the myocardium and excludes damage caused by extrinsic factors Dilated cardiomyopathy (DCM) is the most common type of cardiomyopathy and is characterized by biventricular dilation, impaired contractility, and eventually congestive heart failure. DCM can develop in response to a large number of known insults that directly injure cardiac myocytes ("secondary DCM"), or it may be idiopathic (primary).

Idiopathic Dilated Cardiomyopathy Is Characterized by Impaired Contractility

 Pathogenesis: Numerous theories regarding the cause of idiopathic DCM have been proposed, but none has been established.

Genetic factors now appear to be more important than previously believed. Among patients with idiopathic DCM, a third have a familial disease. The proportion may be even greater because incomplete penetrance often makes it difficult to identify early or latent disease in family members. Most familial cases seem to be transmitted as an autosomal dominant trait, but autosomal recessive, X-linked recessive, and mitochondrial inheritance pattern have all been described.

Mutations in several known genes including those encoding dystrophin, δ-sarcoglycan, troponin T, β-myosin heavy chain, actin, lamin A/C, and desmin have been identified as a cause of a phenotype (Table 11-8). A current hypothesis holds that **defects in force transmission lead to development of a dilated, poorly contracting heart** (Fig 11-43). Stabilization of sarcomeres by attachments of the actin cytoskeleton to the extracellular matrix via dystrophin and δ-sarcoglycan may be perturbed by mutations in genes encoding these proteins. Mutations in the cytoskeletal protein desmin may act similarly. Interestingly, mutations in proteins such as actin, troponin T and β-myosin heavy chain may produce either dilated or hypertrophic cardiomyopathy phenotypes, perhaps depending on whether they produce a defect in force generation (hypertrophic cardiomyopathy) or force transmission. For example, actin mutations associated with hypertrophic cardiomyopathy have been localized to a portion of the molecule near a myosin-binding site, which could impair sarcomeric function. By contrast, DCM-associated mutations in actin are located within the region that binds to the dystrophin–sarcoglycan complex (Fig. 11-43). It has been suggested that defects in lamin A/C, filamentous proteins associated with the inner surface of the nuclear envelope could make the nucleus more vulnerable to mechanical stress and, thereby, cause myocyte death.

Viral myocarditis may eventually lead to DCM, but the responsible mechanism(s) are not well understood. Interestingly, a protease expressed by cardiotropic enteroviruses, has been shown to cleave dystrophin, thus providing a potential mechanistic link between viral infection and development of a dilated cardiomyopathy phenotype. As noted above, in some instances the acute inflammatory phase of viral myocarditis may be followed by an autoimmune attack on the myocardium, which injures cardiac myocytes and eventually causes DCM.

Immunological abnormalities involving both cellular and humoral effects have been recognized in both myocarditis and idiopathic DCM. Autoantibodies to cardiac antigens that have been identified include those directed against a variety of mitochondrial antigens, cardiac myosin, and β-adrenergic receptors. However, as in many cases of autoimmune disease, a pathogenic role for immune mechanisms remains to be proved, and circulating autoantibodies may simply result from rather than cause long-standing myocardial injury.

Pathology: The pathological changes in patients with DCM are generally nonspecific and are similar whether the disorder is idiopathic or secondary to a known injurious agent. At autopsy, the heart is invariably enlarged, reflecting conspicuous left and right ventricular hypertrophy. The weight of the heart may be as much as tripled (>900 g). As a rule, all chambers of the heart are dilated, although the ventricles are more severely affected than the atria (Fig. 11-44). At end-stage, left ventricular dilation is usually so severe that the left ventricular wall appears to be of normal thickness or even thinned. The myocardium is flabby and pale, and small subendocardial scars are occasionally evident. The endocardium of the left ventricle, espe-

TABLE 11-8 **Gene Defects Associated with Dilated Cardiomyopathy (DCM)**

Gene Product	Chromosome and Inheritance[a]		Skeletal Involvement	High Risk of SD or HF[b]	Remarks	Mutations in the Same Gene Can Cause MD or HCM[c]
Dystrophin	Xp21	X	Mild	HF	Rapid progression to end-stage heart failure	Becker and Duchenne MD
Troponin T	1q3	AD	Not reported	SD, HF	Early-onset ventricular dilation	HCM
δ-Sarcoglycan	5q33–q34	AD	None to subclinical	SD, HF	Early-onset ventricular dilation	Limb girdle MD
β-Myosin heavy chain	14q11.2–12	AD	None	HF	Early-onset ventricular dilation	HCM
Actin	15q14	AD	Not reported		Defect located in dystrophin-binding region	HCM
Lamin A/C	1q21.3	AD	None to mild	SD	Occurs in DCM associated with conduction abnormalities	Emerey-Dreifuss MD, Limb girdle MD
Desmin	2q35	AD	None to severe		Can develop severe skeletal weakness	Desmin skeletal myopathy
Titin	2q31	AD	None		Two mutations in Z-line binding domain	HCM in one case

[a] X, X-linked; AD, autosomal dominant.
[b] SD, sudden death; HF, rapid progression to heart failure.
[c] MD, primary muscular dystrophy; HCM, hypertrophic cardiomyopathy.

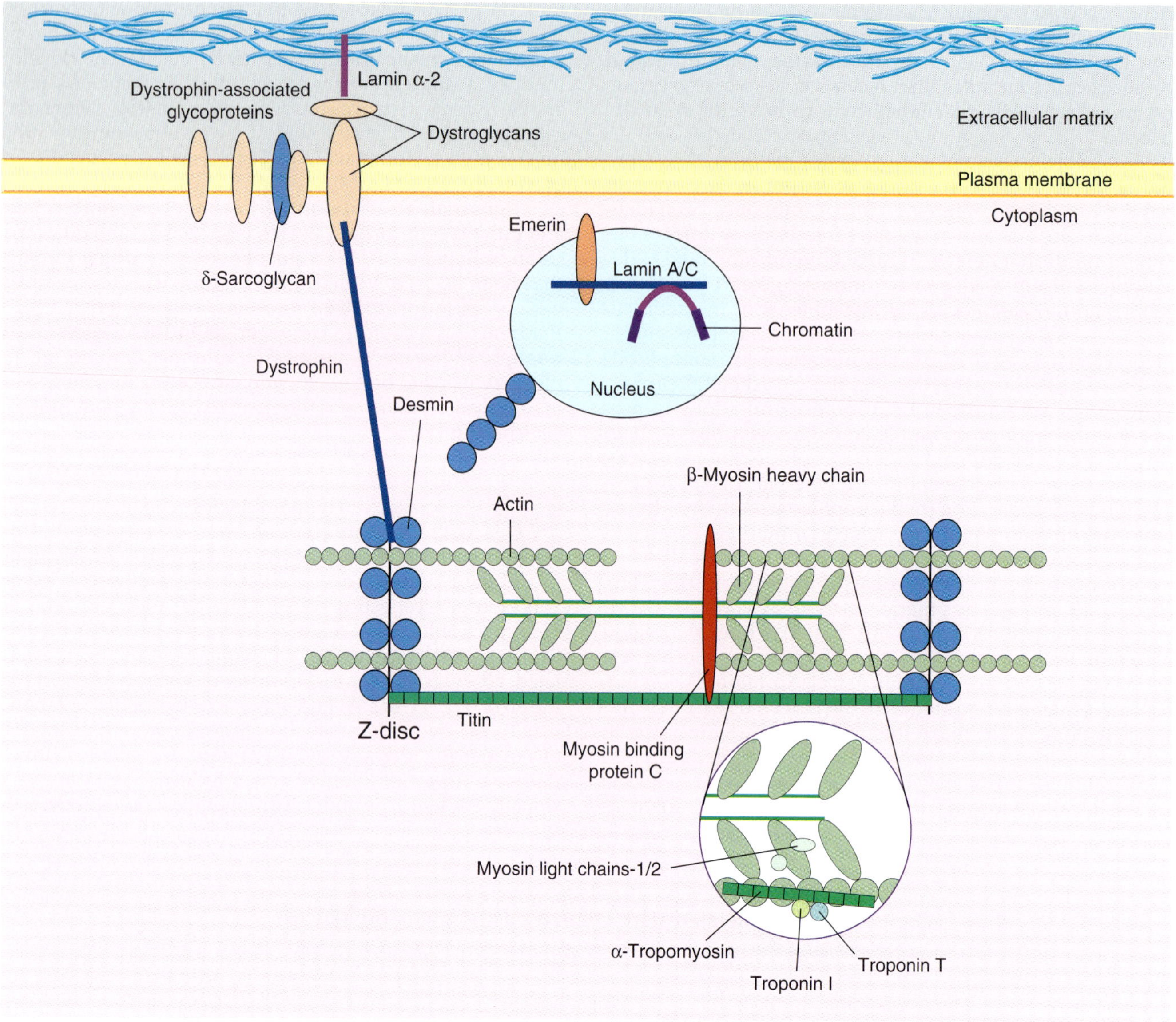

FIGURE 11-43
Subcellular distribution and molecular interactions of mutant proteins implicated in the pathogenesis of dilated and hypertrophic cardiomyopathy. The specific mutations responsible for each type are provided in Tables 11-8 and 11-9.

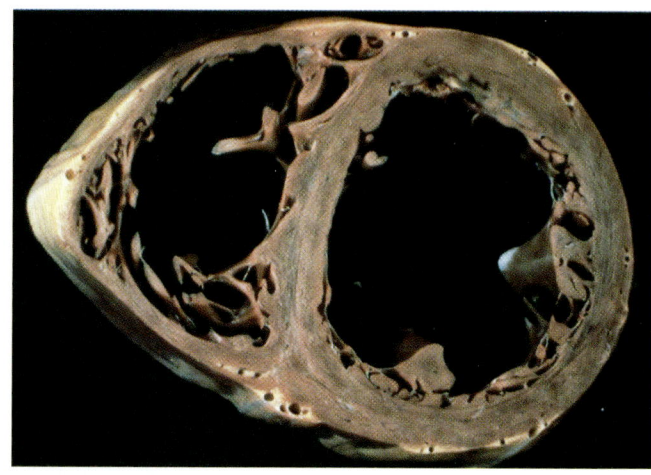

FIGURE 11-44
Idiopathic dilated cardiomyopathy. A transverse section of the enlarged heart reveals conspicuous dilation of both ventricles. Although the ventricular wall appears thinned, the increased mass of the heart indicates considerable hypertrophy.

cially at the apex, tends to be thickened. Adherent mural thrombi are often present in this area.

Microscopically, DCM is characterized by both atrophic and hypertrophic myocardial fibers. Cardiac myocytes, especially in the subendocardium, often show advanced degenerative changes characterized by myofibrillar loss, an effect that gives the cells a vacant, vacuolated appearance. Interstitial and perivascular fibrosis of the myocardium is evident, also most prominently in the subendocardial zone. Scattered chronic inflammatory cells may be present, but they are not conspicuous. Electron microscopy typically shows loss of sarcomeres and an apparent increase in the number of mitochondria.

 Clinical Features: The clinical courses of idiopathic and secondary DCM are comparable. The disease begins insidiously with compensatory ventricular hypertrophy and asymptomatic left ventricular dilation. Commonly, exercise intolerance progresses relentlessly to frank congestive heart failure, and 75% of patients die within 5 years of the onset of symptoms. Half of all deaths in DCM patients are sudden and are attributed to ventricular arrhythmias Abnormalities in intracellular Ca^{2+} handling and certain repolarizing currents are common features in all forms of heart failure. They tend to prolong the QT interval and increase the likelihood of arrhythmias initiated by triggered activity. Although supportive treatment is useful, cardiac transplantation or use of a ventricular assist device eventually becomes the only option.

Secondary Dilated Cardiomyopathy Has Varied Causes

Almost 100 distinct myocardial diseases can result in the clinical features of DCM. Thus, secondary DCM is best viewed as a final common pathway for the effects of virtually any toxic, metabolic, or infectious disorder that directly injures cardiac myocytes. In this context, alcohol abuse, hypertension, pregnancy, and viral myocarditis predispose to secondary DCM. Diabetes mellitus and cigarette smoking have also been linked to an increased incidence of this disorder.

Toxic Cardiomyopathy

Numerous chemicals and drugs cause myocardial injury, but only a few of the more important chemicals are discussed here.

ETHANOL: Alcoholic cardiomyopathy is the single most common identifiable cause of DCM in the United States and Europe. Ethanol abuse can lead to chronic, progressive cardiac dysfunction, which may be fatal. The disorder is more common in men, because alcoholism is more frequent in men than in women. The typical patient is between 30 and 55 years of age and has been drinking heavily for at least 10 years.

 Pathogenesis: The mechanism by which alcohol injures the heart remains obscure, but the degree of myocardial damage has been correlated with the total lifetime dose of ethanol. It is clear that ethanol exerts an immediate negative inotropic effect. Furthermore, metabolism of ethyl alcohol by the myocardium produces ethyl esters of fatty acids, which are believed to interfere with fatty acid oxidation, the principal metabolic pathway used by the heart to generate ATP. Although the immediate action of alcohol on the cardiac myocyte is entirely reversible, the injury eventually becomes irreversible. Abstinence ameliorates or even reverses the early stages of alcoholic cardiomyopathy but may be too late in advanced stages.

COBALT: Cobalt cardiomyopathy was originally misdiagnosed as alcoholic cardiomyopathy in the mid-1960s, because persons who drank large amounts of a certain type of beer developed DCM. It was subsequently shown that the cardiac manifestations were actually caused by the toxic effects of cobalt, which had been added as a foam stabilizer. Interestingly, cobalt cardiomyopathy was reported almost exclusively in alcohol abusers rather than in moderate drinkers.

CATECHOLAMINES: In high concentrations, catecholamines can cause focal myocyte necrosis. Toxic myocarditis may occur in patients with pheochromocytomas, in persons who require high doses of inotropic drugs to maintain blood pressure, and in accident victims who sustain massive head trauma. Multiple mechanisms contribute to myocardial injury, but the most important is enhanced calcium flux into myocytes. Focal ischemia caused by platelet aggregation and microvascular constriction may also contribute.

ANTHRACYCLINES: Doxorubicin (adriamycin) and other anthracycline drugs are potent chemotherapeutic agents whose usefulness is limited by a cumulative, dose-dependent, cardiac toxicity. The major effect is a chronic, irreversible degeneration of cardiac myocytes, characterized pathologically by vacuolization and loss of myofibrils and functionally by depressed contractility. Myocyte necrosis is rare, but once severe degeneration occurs, intractable congestive heart failure develops, and the prognosis is grim.

 Pathogenesis: Dilated cardiomyopathy begins to appear in patients who receive a cumulative dose of more than 500 mg doxorubicin per m^2, and those who are treated with more than 550 mg/m^2 have a 35% incidence of cardiomyopathy. The mechanism by which anthracyclines damage the heart appears related to a diminished capacity to handle reactive oxygen species. Although the heart is relatively resistant to radiation injury, anthracyclines and radiation act synergistically. Thus, a patient who has re-

CEIVED radiotherapy to the mediastinum is at risk of developing anthracycline cardiac toxicity at a lower dose than one who was not irradiated.

CYCLOPHOSPHAMIDE: This potent chemotherapeutic drug is often used in high doses before bone marrow transplantation. Although it is not responsible for classical DCM, it can cause pericarditis and occasionally massive hemorrhagic myocarditis. The latter is thought to be secondary to endothelial injury and thrombocytopenia.

COCAINE: The use of this illicit drug is frequently associated with chest pain and palpitations. Although true DCM is not a usual complication of cocaine abuse, myocarditis, focal necrosis, and thickening of intramyocardial coronary arteries have been reported. Myocardial ischemia or infarction associated with cocaine use has been attributed to coronary vasoconstriction in the presence of increased myocardial oxygen demand. Sudden death due to spontaneous ventricular tachyarrhythmias is well documented. The mechanisms underlying the arrhythmogenic effects of cocaine include vasoconstriction, sympathomimetic activity, hypersensitivity responses, and direct toxicity.

Cardiomyopathy of Pregnancy

A unique form of DCM develops during the last trimester of pregnancy or during the first 6 months after delivery. The disorder is relatively uncommon in the United States, but in some regions of Africa, it is encountered in as many as 1% of pregnant women. The risk of cardiomyopathy of pregnancy is greatest in black, multiparous women older than 30 years. The cause of this form of DCM is unknown. Some patients exhibit inflammatory cells in heart biopsies taken during the symptomatic phase of the illness, consistent with the hypothesis that disordered immunity may underlie development of DCM in this setting.

Unlike most other varieties of DCM, half of women with cardiomyopathy of pregnancy spontaneously recover normal cardiac function. The other half is left with persistent left ventricular dysfunction or proceed to overt congestive heart failure and early death. In patients who survive, subsequent pregnancies pose a high risk of recurrence and maternal mortality.

Hypertrophic Cardiomyopathy Is a Genetic Disease

Hypertrophic cardiomyopathy (HCM) refers to a condition in which cardiac hypertrophy develops for no apparent reason and is out of proportion to the hemodynamic load on the heart. The disorder is probably genetically determined in most patients and is identified as an autosomal dominant trait in half of patients. Many patients without a family history probably have spontaneous mutations or a mild form of disease that is difficult to detect. HCM is now recognized to be far more frequent than previously appreciated, with a prevalence in the United States of about 1 in 500.

Pathogenesis: The clinical picture of HCM is caused by more than 100 mutations in at least nine genes encoding proteins of the sarcomere (Table 11-9 and Fig.11-43). The mutated genes most commonly involved are those encoding (1) β-myosin heavy chain (35%), (2) myosin-binding protein C (20%), and (3) troponin T (15%). Mutations in other genes such as titin and myosin light chains are rare. The mutant protein is incorporated into the sarcomere, where it acts in a dominant-negative fashion to alter sarcomeric function. This proposed mechanism has led to the hypothesis that **development of HCM is related to defects in force generation owing to altered sarcomeric function.** In turn, hypertrophy develops as a compensatory response. Other mutations, such as those involving myosin light chain and α-tropomyosin genes, may actually enhance contractility and, thereby, lead to hypertrophy. Still others (e.g., mutations in the myosin-binding protein C gene) may produce proteins

TABLE 11-9 Gene Defects Associated with Hypertrophic Cardiomyopathy (HCM)

Gene product	Chromosome	Risk of Sudden Death	Mutations	Remarks
β-Myosin heavy chain	14q11-2-12	High[a]	Missense	Degree of hypertrophy correlates with risk of sudden death
Myosin-binding protein C	11p11.2	Low	Missense, deletions, splice defects	Benign clinical course, progressive hypertrophy with late onset
Troponin T	1q3	High	Missense, deletions, splice defects	High risk of sudden death; mild or absent hypertrophy
Troponin I	19q13.4	High	Missense	Apical variant of HCM, occasionally DCM-like features in elderly patients
α-Tropomyosin	15q22	High	Missense	Usually favorable prognosis, high phenotypic variability
Myosin light chain-1	3p21	Low	Missense	Papillary muscle thickening, only rare cases
Myosin light chain-2	12q23–24.3	Low	Missense	Papillary muscle thickening, only rare cases
Actin	15q14	Low	Missense	Some mutations also cause DCM
α-Myosin heavy chain	Spontaneous	Low	Missense	Late onset; rare
Titin	Spontaneous	—	Missense	Only one patient reported

[a] For selected mutations.

that do not become incorporated into sarcomeres. These might lead to hypertrophy through a lack of the functional protein, rather than by a dominant-negative effect.

It is possible to relate specific mutations to certain clinical features of HCM (see Table 11-9). For example, selected mutations in β-myosin heavy chain and troponin T genes are associated with a high risk of sudden death. In the case of the β-myosin heavy chain mutations, the risk of sudden death correlates with the amount of hypertrophy, whereas the troponin T mutations, which are also linked to sudden death, produce minimal or no hypertrophy. HCM in patients with myosin-binding protein C mutations is usually clinically benign and associated with slowly progressive hypertrophy developing late in life.

Pathology: The heart in HCM is always enlarged, but the degree of hypertrophy is variable in different genetic forms. The wall of the left ventricle is thick, and its cavity is small, sometimes being reduced to a slit. The papillary muscles and trabeculae carneae are prominent and encroach on the ventricular lumen. More than half of cases exhibit asymmetric hypertrophy of the interventricular septum, with a ratio of the thickness of the septum to that of the left ventricular free wall greater than 1.5 (Fig. 11-45A). There are some rare genetic forms of HCM in which only the apical portion of the left ventricle or the papillary muscles are selectively hypertrophied. Often, the thickened, hypertrophied interventricular septum bulges into the left ventricular outflow tract during the early phase of ventricular systole, causing subvalvular obstruction of the aortic outflow tract. In this situation, an endocardial mural plaque is typically seen in the outflow tract, corresponding to the contact point where the anterior mitral valve leaflet impinges on the septal wall of the outflow tract during systole. Both atria are commonly dilated.

The most notable histological feature of HCM is myofiber disarray, which is most extensive in the interventricular septum. Instead of the usual parallel arrangement of myocytes into muscle bundles, myofiber disarray is characterized by an oblique and often perpendicular orientation of adjacent hypertrophic myocytes (see Fig. 11-45B). By electron microscopy, the myofibrils and myofilaments within the individual myocytes are also disorganized. Such structural derangements are also frequently present in infants with congenital heart defects and can be observed under a wide variety of circumstances. However, they are always extensive in HCM and are not as widespread in other situations. There is usually hyperplasia of interstitial cells, and intramural coronary arteries may become thick and cellular (Fig. 11-45C).

Clinical Features: Most patients with HCM have few if any symptoms, and the diagnosis is commonly made during screening of the family with an affected member. Despite the absence of symptoms, such persons may be at risk for sudden death, particularly during severe exertion. In fact, unsuspected HCM is a common abnormality found at autopsy in young competitive athletes who die suddenly. Clinical recognition of HCM can occur at any age, often in the third, fourth, or fifth decade of life, but the disorder also is encountered in the elderly. Some patients with HCM become incapacitated by cardiac symptoms, of which dyspnea, angina pectoris, and syncope are the most common. The clinical course tends to remain stable for many years, although eventually the disease can progress to congestive heart failure. In 10% of patients, DCM supervenes.

Despite the fact that mutant proteins impair the sarcomere, contractile function in HCM tends to be hyperdynamic. Ejection fractions are typically very high, and most of the stroke volume is ejected during early systole. The most prominent dysfunctional aspect of HCM is decreased left ventricular compliance (diastolic dysfunction), which results in increased end-diastolic pressure. Mitral regurgitation is also seen in many HCM patients. These features contribute to the atrial dilation commonly seen in HCM. In one fourth of patients, functional obstruction of the left ventricular outflow tract occurs near the end of systole, resulting in a pressure gradient between the apex and the subvalvular region of the left ventricle.

Hypertrophic cardiomyopathy responds paradoxically to pharmacological interventions. Heart failure from other causes is typically treated with cardiac glycosides to increase myocardial contractility and with diuretics to reduce intravascular volume. In HCM, these drugs aggravate symptoms. The most efficacious drugs for the treatment of HCM are β-adrenergic blockers and calcium channel blockers. These agents reduce contractility, decrease outflow-tract obstruction, and may improve left ventricular relaxation during diastole. Surgical removal of a portion of the hypertrophic septum or injection of ethanol into a septal artery to cause localized infarction has been successful in relieving symptoms of obstruction but seems to have no impact on the risk of sudden death.

Restrictive Cardiomyopathy Impairs Diastolic Function

Restrictive cardiomyopathy refers to a group of diseases in which myocardial or endocardial abnormalities limit diastolic filling, while allowing contractile function to remain normal. It is the least common category of cardiomyopathy in western countries, although in some less-developed regions (e.g., parts of equatorial Africa, South America, and Asia), endomyocardial disease related to parasitic infections leads to many cases of restrictive cardiomyopathy.

Pathogenesis and Pathology: Restrictive cardiomyopathy is caused by (1) interstitial infiltration of amyloid, metastatic carcinoma, or sarcoid granulomas; (2) endomyocardial disease characterized by marked fibrotic thickening of the endocardium; (3) storage diseases, including hemochromatosis; and (4) a marked increase in interstitial fibrous tissue. The pathophysiological consequence is a pre-load-dependent state, characterized by defective diastolic compliance, restricted ventricular filling, increased end-diastolic pressure, atrial dilation, and venous congestion. In many respects, these hemodynamic changes are similar to the consequences of constrictive pericarditis. Many cases of restrictive car-

572   The Heart

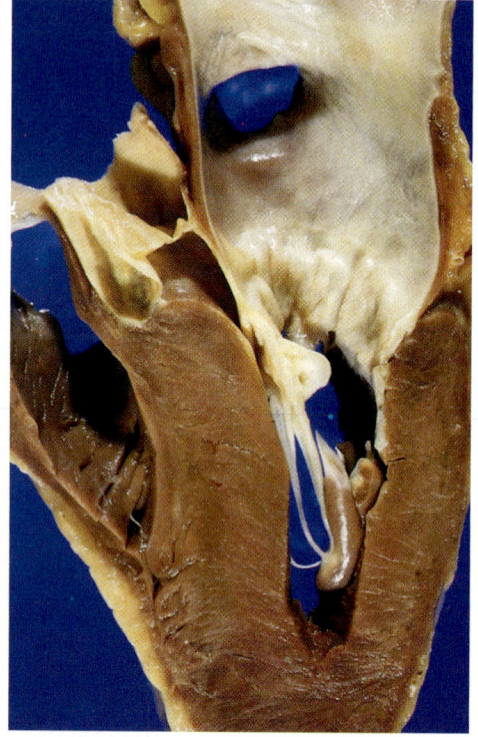
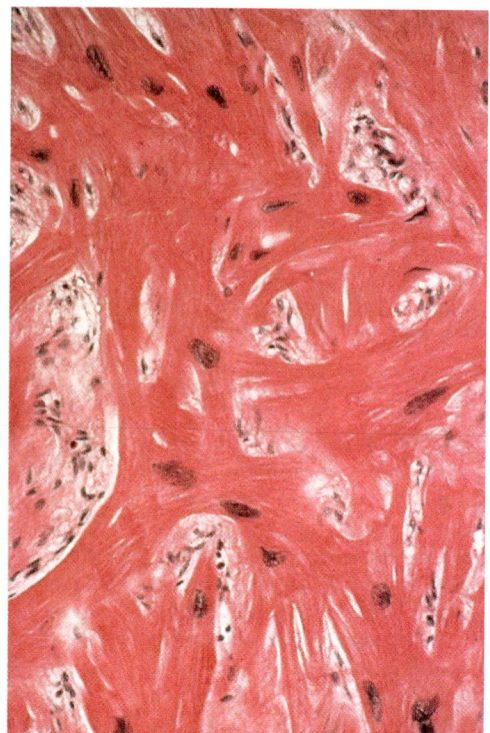
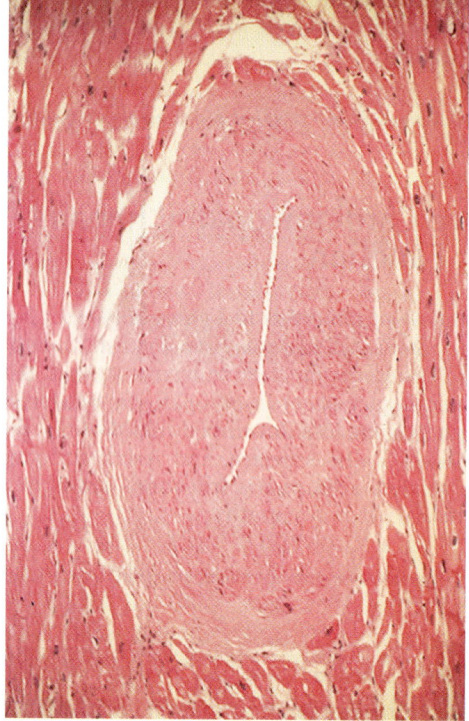

FIGURE 11-45
Hypertrophic cardiomyopathy. A. The heart has been opened to show striking asymmetric left ventricular hypertrophy. The interventricular septum is thicker than the free wall of the left ventricle and impinges on the outflow tract such that it contacts the underside of the anterior mitral valve leaflet. B. A section of the myocardium shows the characteristic myofiber disarray and hyperplasia of interstitial cells. C. A small intramural coronary artery shows a thickened, hypercellular media. This type of remodeling of coronary vessels could contribute to development of angina-like symptoms in some patients with HCM.

diomyopathy are classified as idiopathic, with interstitial fibrosis as the only histological abnormality.

The disease almost invariably progresses to congestive heart failure, and only 10% of the patients survive for 10 years.

Amyloidosis

The heart is affected in most of the generalized forms of amyloidosis (see Chapter 23). In fact, restrictive cardiomyopathy is the most common cause of death in AL amyloidosis of plasma cell dyscrasias.

Pathology: Amyloid infiltration of the heart results in cardiac enlargement without ventricular dilation, and the gross appearance of the heart may resemble that of hypertrophic cardiomyopathy. The ventricular walls are typically thickened, firm, and rubbery. Microscopically, amyloid accumulation is most prominent in interstitial, perivascular, and endocardial regions (Fig. 11-46). Endocardial involvement is particularly common in the atria, where nodular endocardial deposits often impart a granular appearance and gritty texture to the endocardial surface. Amyloid deposits also can cause thickening of cardiac valves. In rare cases, amyloid deposition within the walls of intramural coronary arteries narrows the lumens and causes ischemic injury.

 Clinical Features: Cardiac amyloidosis is most often seen as a restrictive cardiomyopathy, with symptoms predominantly referable to right-sided heart failure. Infiltration of the conduction system can result in arrhythmias, and sudden cardiac death is not unusual. Cardiomegaly is characteristically prominent. Echocardiography shows marked wall thickening and decreased wall motion. Low voltage of the QRS complex is a characteristic feature of the electrocardiogram.

Some patients with cardiac amyloidosis initially present with congestive heart failure secondary to impaired systolic or contractile function. In these patients, the diastolic dysfunction is often inconspicuous. As in patients with a restrictive presentation, the prognosis is grim. Survival for more than 1 year once the disease becomes symptomatic is unusual.

SENILE CARDIAC AMYLOIDOSIS: *Senile cardiac amyloidosis refers to the deposition of a protein closely related to prealbumin (transthyretin) in the hearts of elderly persons (see* Chapter 23). The disorder may be present to some extent in up to 25% of patients who are 80 years old or older. It not only involves the heart (atria and ventricles) but, in many cases, the lungs and rectum as well. Amyloid deposits also may be found in blood vessel walls in many organs, but virtually never in the renal glomeruli. The functional significance of senile cardiac amyloidosis is often minimal, and most of the time, it is identified as an incidental finding at autopsy. Even when the amyloid deposition is extensive and is associated with symptoms of congestive heart failure, the progression of the disease is much slower than that in AL amyloidosis.

Two additional forms of isolated cardiovascular amyloidosis are common in the elderly: senile aortic amyloidosis and isolated atrial amyloidosis. Neither of these forms of amyloid contains prealbumin or closely related proteins.

Endomyocardial Disease

Endomyocardial disease (EMD) comprises two geographically separate disorders.

ENDOMYOCARDIAL FIBROSIS: This disorder is particularly common in equatorial Africa, where it accounts for 10 to 20% of all deaths attributed to heart disease. The malady is also occasionally encountered in other tropical and subtropical regions of the world. It is most common is children and young adults but has been reported to occur in persons up to age 70 years. Endomyocardial fibrosis leads to progressive myocardial failure and has a poor prognosis, although survival for as long as 12 years has been reported.

EOSINOPHILIC ENDOMYOCARDIAL DISEASE (LOFFLER ENDOCARDITIS): This is a cardiac disorder of temperate regions characterized by hypereosinophilia (as high as $50,000/\mu L$). The disease is usually encountered in men in the fifth decade and is often accompanied by rash. Löffler endocarditis typically progresses to congestive heart failure and death, although corticosteroids may improve the survival rate.

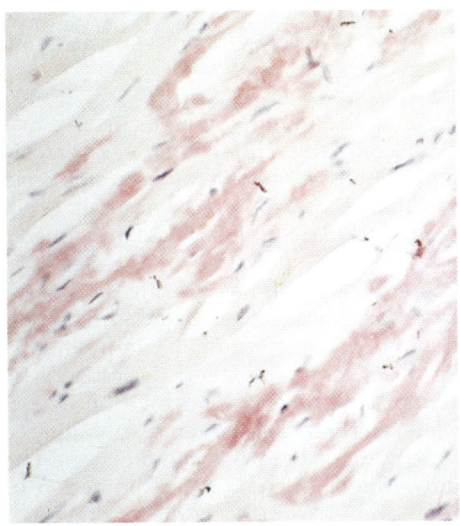
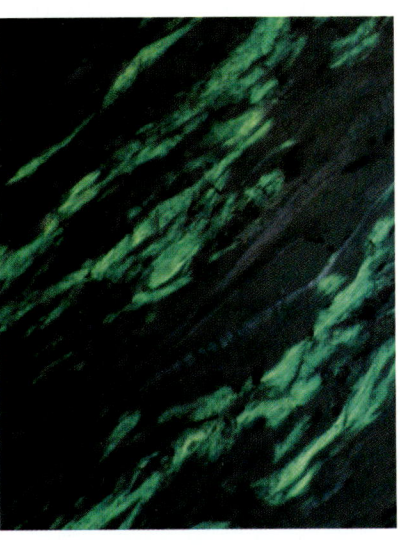

FIGURE 11-46
Cardiac amyloidosis. A. A section of myocardium stained with Congo red shows interstitial, pink-staining deposits of amyloid. B. Under polarized light, the same section displays the characteristic green birefringence of amyloid fibrils.

Pathogenesis: In the past, endomyocardial fibrosis and Löffler endocarditis were considered distinct entities, but there is a growing consensus that they represent variants of the same underlying disease. EMD is suspected to result from myocardial injury produced by eosinophils, possibly mediated by cardiotoxic constituents of the granules. In the tropics, transient high blood eosinophil counts often result from parasitic infestations; in temperate climates, idiopathic hypereosinophilia is often persistent.

EMD can be divided into three stages:

1. The necrotic stage occurs within the first few months of the illness and is characterized by an intense eosinophilic infiltrate involving the inner layers of the myocardium, usually of both ventricles. The infiltrate is perivascular and interstitial, and there is evidence of vascular injury and myocyte necrosis. The necrotic stage lasts for several months, but significant functional impairment is rare.
2. The thrombotic stage develops about a year later and features mural thrombi attached to the injured and slightly thickened endocardium. At this time, the myocardium is no longer inflamed but shows early hypertrophy. Embolization is a common complication.
3. The fibrotic stage is the chronic phase of EMD and features conspicuous fibrotic thickening of the endocardium. Marked endocardial fibrosis results in decreased compliance and abnormal diastolic function. Adherence of the posterior mitral valve leaflet to the endocardium results in mitral regurgitation or, in the case of the right side, tricuspid regurgitation.

 Pathology: At autopsy, a grayish white layer of thickened endocardium extends from the apex of the left ventricle over the posterior papillary muscle to the posterior leaflet of the mitral valve and for a short distance into the left outflow tract. On cut section of the ventricle, endocardial fibrosis spreads into the inner one third to one half of the wall. Mural thrombi in various stages of organization may be present. When the right ventricle is involved, the entire cavity may exhibit endocardial thickening, which may penetrate as far as the epicardium. Microscopically, the fibrotic endocardium contains only a few elastic fibers. Myofibers trapped within the collagenous tissue display nonspecific degenerative changes.

Storage Diseases

The various lysosomal storage diseases are discussed in detail in Chapter 6, and only the cardiac manifestations are reviewed here.

GLYCOGEN STORAGE DISEASES: Of the various forms of glycogen storage disease, types II (Pompe disease), III (Cori disease), and IV (Andersen disease) affect the heart. The most common and severe cardiac involvement occurs with type II glycogen storage disease. In infants with this condition, the heart is markedly enlarged (up to seven times normal), and endocardial fibroelastosis is seen in 20% of patients. The myocytes are vacuolated as a result of the large amounts of stored glycogen. The functional changes are those of a restrictive type of cardiomyopathy, and the usual cause of death is cardiac failure.

MUCOPOLYSACCHARIDOSES: Several of the mucopolysaccharidoses involve the heart. Cardiac disease results from lysosomal accumulation of mucopolysaccharides (glycosaminoglycans) in various cells. In general, pseudohypertrophy of the ventricles develops, and contractility gradually diminishes. The coronary arteries may be narrowed by thickening of the intima and media, and in Hurler and Hunter syndromes, myocardial infarction is common. The valve leaflets may be thickened, thereby producing progressive valvular dysfunction, manifested as aortic stenosis (Scheie syndrome) or mitral regurgitation (Hurler and Morquio syndromes). Cor pulmonale may result from pulmonary hypertension related to narrowing of the airways.

SPHINGOLIPIDOSES: *Fabry disease* may result in accumulation of glycosphingolipids in the heart, with functional and pathological changes similar to those that complicate the mucopolysaccharidoses. *Gaucher disease,* which only rarely involves the heart, may feature interstitial infiltration of the left ventricle by cerebroside-laden macrophages, leading to impairment of left ventricular compliance and cardiac output.

HEMOCHROMATOSIS: This multiorgan disease is associated with excessive iron deposition in many tissues (see Chapter 14). The degree of iron deposition in the heart varies and only roughly correlates with that in other organs. Involvement of the heart creates features of both dilated and restrictive cardiomyopathy, with systolic and diastolic impairment. **Congestive heart failure occurs in as many as one third of patients with hemochromatosis.**

At autopsy, the heart is dilated, and the ventricular walls are thickened. The brown color seen on gross examination correlates with the deposition of iron in cardiac myocytes. Interstitial fibrosis is invariable, but its extent does not correlate well with the degree of iron accumulation. The severity of myocardial dysfunction seems to be proportional to the quantity of iron deposited.

Sarcoidosis

Sarcoidosis is a generalized granulomatous disease that can involve the heart (see Chapter 12). A quarter of sarcoidosis cases that come to autopsy show some granulomas in the heart, but fewer than 5% of patients with this condition have clinical symptoms. Sarcoid heart disease is seen clinically as a mixed pattern of dilated and restrictive cardiomyopathy. Sarcoid granulomas are highly necrotizing and often produce large areas of myocardial damage. The base of the interventricular septum is preferentially involved. Because this region contains major components of the atrioventricular conduction system, bundle branch blocks or complete heart block are often seen. More serious life-threatening arrhythmias are also common, and the rate of sudden death is high. Microscopic examination of the heart in severe cases of sarcoid heart disease reveals infil-

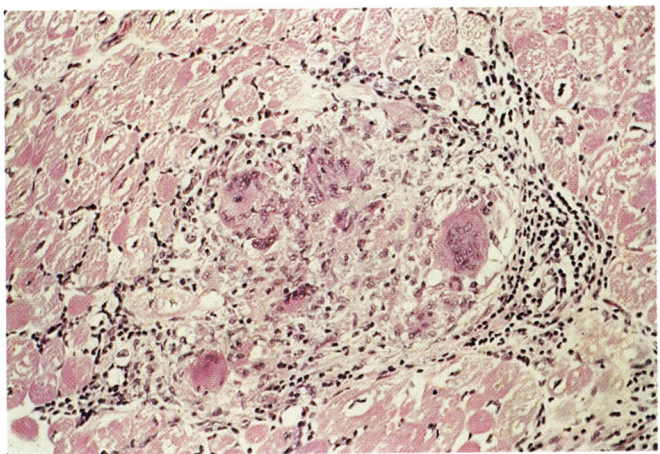

FIGURE 11-47
Cardiac sarcoidosis. The myocardium is infiltrated by non-caseating granulomas, with prominent giant cells. There is considerable destruction of cardiac myocytes with fibrosis.

tration of the myocardium by noncaseating granulomas, massive destruction of myocytes, and replacement by interstitial fibrosis (Fig. 11-47).

CARDIAC TUMORS

Primary cardiac tumors are rare, but when they occur, they can result in serious problems.

Cardiac Myxoma Is the Most Common Primary Tumor of the Heart

Cardiac myxoma accounts for 35 to 50% of all primary cardiac tumors. The tumor is usually sporadic, but it is occasionally associated with familial autosomal dominant syndromes.

 Pathology: Most myxomas (75%) arise in the left atrium, although they can occur in any cardiac chamber or on a valve. The tumor appears as a glistening, gelatinous, polypoid mass, usually 5 to 6 cm in diameter, with a short stalk (Fig. 11-48). It may be sufficiently mobile to obstruct the mitral valve orifice. Microscopically, cardiac myxoma has a loose myxoid stroma containing abundant proteoglycans. Polygonal stellate cells are found within the matrix, occurring singly or in small clusters.

 Clinical Features: More than half of patients with left atrial myxoma have clinical evidence of mitral valve dysfunction. Although the tumor does not metastasize in the usual sense, it often embolizes. A third of patients with a myxoma of the left atrium or left ventricle die from embolization of the tumor to the brain. Surgical removal of the tumor is successful in most cases.

Rhabdomyoma Is a Childhood Tumor

Rhabdomyoma is the most common primary cardiac tumor in infants and children and forms nodular masses in the myocardium. Cardiac rhabdomyoma may actually be a hamartoma rather than a true neoplasm, although the issue is still debated. Almost all rhabdomyomas are multiple and involve both the left and right ventricles and, in one third of cases, the atria as well. In half of cases, the tumor mass projects into the cardiac chamber and obstructs the lumen or the valve orifices.

 Pathology: On gross examination, cardiac rhabdomyomas are pale masses, varying from 1 mm to several centimeters in diameter. Microscopically, tumor cells show small central nuclei and abundant glycogen-rich clear cytoplasm, in which fibrillar processes containing sarcomeres radiate to the margin of the cell ("spider cell"). Rhabdomyomas often occur in association with tuberous sclerosis (one third to one half of cases). A few cardiac rhabdomyomas have been successfully excised.

Papillary Fibroelastoma Involves the Valves

Papillary fronds resembling a sea anemone and measuring up to 3 to 4 cm in diameter may grow on the heart valves. These tumors are not neoplasms and are more appropriately

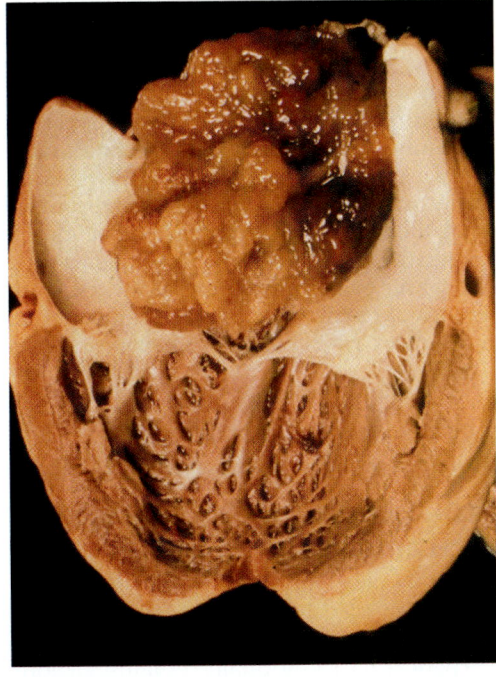

FIGURE 11-48
Cardiac myxoma. The left atrium contains a large, polypoid tumor that protrudes into the mitral valve orifice.

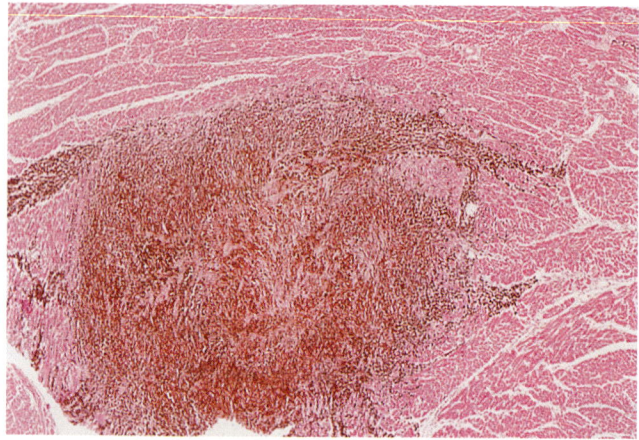

FIGURE 11-49
Malignant melanoma metastatic to the heart. The myocardium contains a heavily pigmented tumor metastasis.

termed *hamartomas*. The fronds have a central dense core of collagen and elastic fibers surrounded by looser connective tissue. They are covered by a continuation of the endothelial cells of the valve on which the tumor originates. In most instances, papillary fibroelastomas pose no clinical problem, but they have the potential to fragment and embolize to other organs, or they may occlude a coronary artery orifice and produce myocardial ischemia.

Other Tumors

Other primary tumors of the heart are even rarer than those described above. These include angiomas, fibromas, lymphangiomas, neurofibromas, and the sarcomatous counterparts of these tumors. Lipomatous hypertrophy of the interatrial septum and encapsulated lipomas have been reported.

Metastatic tumors of the heart are seen most frequently in patients with the most prevalent forms of carcinomas—those of the lung, breast, and gastrointestinal tract. Nevertheless, only a minority of patients with these tumors will show cardiac metastases. Lymphomas and leukemia also may involve the heart. Of all tumors, the one most likely to metastasize to the heart is malignant melanoma (Fig. 11-49). Metastatic cancer of the myocardium can result in clinical manifestations of restrictive cardiomyopathy, particularly if the cardiac tumors are associated with extensive fibrosis.

DISEASES OF THE PERICARDIUM

Pericardial Effusion Can Cause Cardiac Tamponade

Pericardial effusion refers to the accumulation of excess fluid, in the form of either a transudate or an exudate, within the pericardial cavity. The pericardial sac normally contains no more than 50 mL of lubricating fluid. If the pericardium is slowly distended, it can stretch to accommodate as much as 2 L of fluid without notable hemodynamic consequences. However, rapid accumulation of as little as 150 to 200 mL of pericardial fluid or blood may significantly increase intrapericardial pressure and thereby restrict diastolic filling, especially of the right ventricle.

Serous pericardial effusion is often a complication of an increase in extracellular fluid volume, as occurs in congestive heart failure or the nephrotic syndrome. The fluid has a low protein content and few cellular elements.

Chylous effusion (fluid containing chylomicrons) results from a communication of the thoracic duct with the pericardial space secondary to lymphatic obstruction by tumor or infection.

Serosanguineous pericardial effusion may develop after chest trauma, either accidentally or caused by cardiopulmonary resuscitation.

Hemopericardium refers to bleeding directly into the pericardial cavity (Fig. 11-50). The most common cause is ventricular free wall rupture at a myocardial infarct. Less frequent causes are penetrating cardiac trauma, rupture of a dissecting aneurysm of the aorta, infiltration of a vessel by tumor, or a bleeding diathesis.

Cardiac tamponade is the syndrome produced by the rapid accumulation of pericardial fluid, which restricts the filling of the heart. The hemodynamic consequences range from a minimally symptomatic condition to abrupt cardiovascular collapse and death. As the pericardial pressure increases, it reaches and then exceeds the central venous pressure, thereby limiting the return of blood to the heart. Cardiac output and blood pressure decrease, and *pulsus paradoxus* (an abnormal decrease in systolic pressure with inspiration) occurs in almost all patients. Acute cardiac tamponade is almost invariably fatal unless the pressure is relieved by

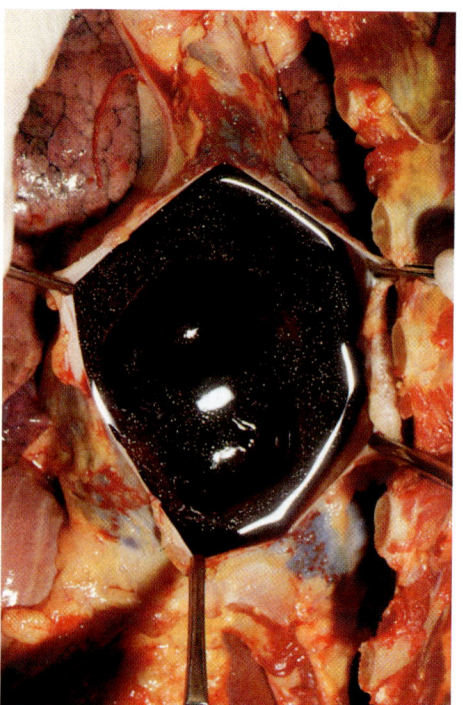

FIGURE 11-50
Hemopericardium. The parietal pericardium has been opened to reveal the pericardial cavity distended with fresh blood. The patient sustained a rupture of a myocardial infarct.

removal of the pericardial fluid, by either needle pericardiocentesis or surgical procedures.

Acute Pericarditis May Follow Viral Infections

Pericarditis refers to inflammation of the visceral or parietal pericardium.

Pathogenesis: The causes of pericarditis are similar to those for myocarditis (see Table 11-7). In most cases, the cause of acute pericarditis is obscure and (as in myocarditis) is attributed to undiagnosed viral infection. At one time, pneumococcal pericarditis secondary to lobar pneumonia was not uncommon, but today all forms of bacterial pericarditis are unusual. Metastatic neoplasms may induce a serofibrinous or hemorrhagic exudate and inflammatory reaction when they involve the pericardium. The most common tumors to involve the pericardium and cause a malignant pericardial effusion are breast and lung carcinomas. Pericarditis associated with myocardial infarction and rheumatic fever is discussed above.

Pathology: Acute pericarditis can be classified as **fibrinous, purulent,** or **hemorrhagic,** depending on the gross and microscopic characteristics of the pericardial surfaces and fluid. The most common form is fibrinous pericarditis, in which the normal smooth, glistening appearance of the pericardial surfaces becomes replaced by a dull, granular fibrin-rich exudate (Fig. 11-51). The rough texture of the inflamed pericardial surfaces produces the characteristic friction rub heard by auscultation. The effusion fluid in fibrinous pericarditis is usually rich in protein, and the pericardium contains primarily mononuclear inflammatory cells. Uremia can cause fibrinous pericarditis (Fig. 11-52), although with the widespread availability of renal dialysis, uremic pericarditis is now unusual in the United States. The most common causes are viral infection and pericarditis following myocardial infarcts.

Bacterial infection leads to a purulent pericarditis, in which the pericardial exudate resembles pus and contains many neutrophils. Bleeding into the pericardial space caused by aggressive infectious or neoplastic processes or coagulation defects leads to hemorrhagic pericarditis.

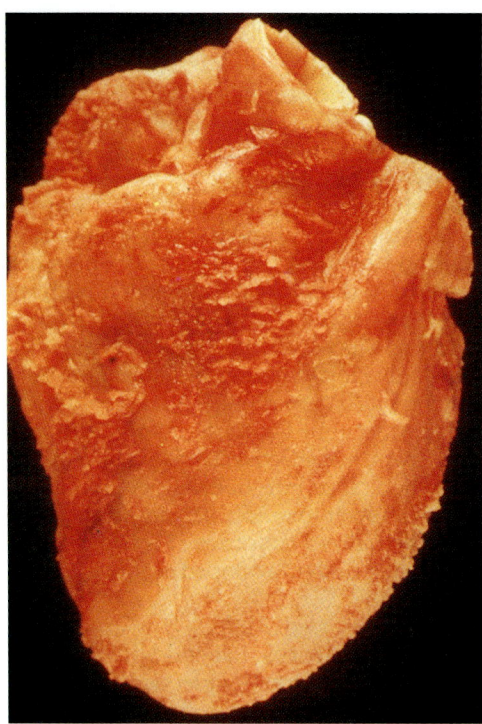

FIGURE *11-52*
Fibrinous pericarditis. The heart of a patient who died in uremia displays a shaggy, fibrinous exudate covering the visceral pericardium.

Clinical Features: The initial manifestation of acute pericarditis is sudden, severe, substernal chest pain, sometimes referred to the back, shoulder, or neck. It is distinguished from the pain of angina pectoris or myocardial infarction by its failure to radiate down the left arm. A characteristic pericardial friction rub is easily heard. Electrocardiographic changes reflect repolarization abnormalities of the myocardium.

Idiopathic or viral pericarditis is a self-limited disorder, although it may infrequently lead to constrictive pericarditis. Corticosteroids are the treatment of choice. The therapy for other specific forms of acute pericarditis varies with the cause.

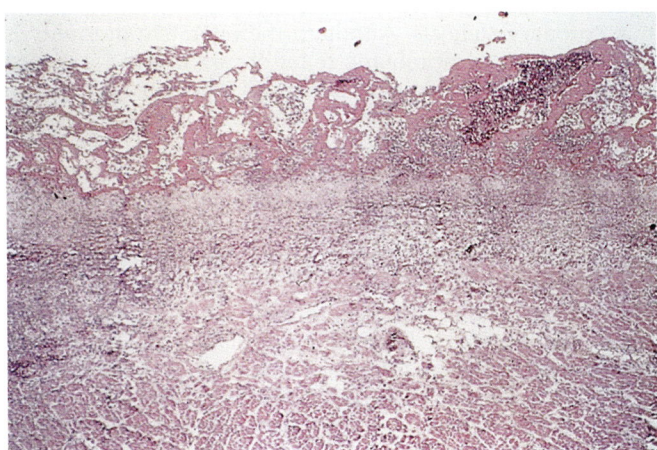

FIGURE *11-51*
Fibrinous pericardial exudate. The epicardial surface is edematous, inflamed, and covered with tentacles of fibrin.

Constrictive Pericarditis May Mimic Right Heart Failure

Constrictive pericarditis is a chronic fibrosing disease of the pericardium that compresses the heart and restricts inflow.

Pathogenesis and Pathology: A misnomer, constrictive pericarditis is not an active inflammatory condition. Rather, it results from an exuberant healing response following acute pericardial injury in which the pericardial space becomes obliterated and the visceral and parietal layers become fused in a dense, rigid mass of fibrous tissue. The scarred pericardium may be so thick (up to 3 cm) that it narrows the orifices of the venae cavae (Fig. 11-53). The fibrous envelope may contain deposits of calcium. The condition is infrequent today and, in developed countries, is predominantly idiopathic. Previous radiation therapy to the mediastinum and cardiac surgery account for more than one third of cases, whereas in others, constrictive pericarditis evolves from a purulent or tuberculous infection. Although tuberculosis today accounts for fewer than 15% of cases of constrictive pericarditis in industrialized countries, it is still the major cause of this condition in underdeveloped regions.

 Clinical Features: Patients with constrictive pericarditis have a small, quiet heart in which venous inflow is restricted, and the rigid pericardium determines the diastolic volume of the heart. These patients have high venous pressure, low cardiac output, small pulse pressure, and fluid retention with ascites and peripheral edema. Total pericardiectomy is the treatment of choice.

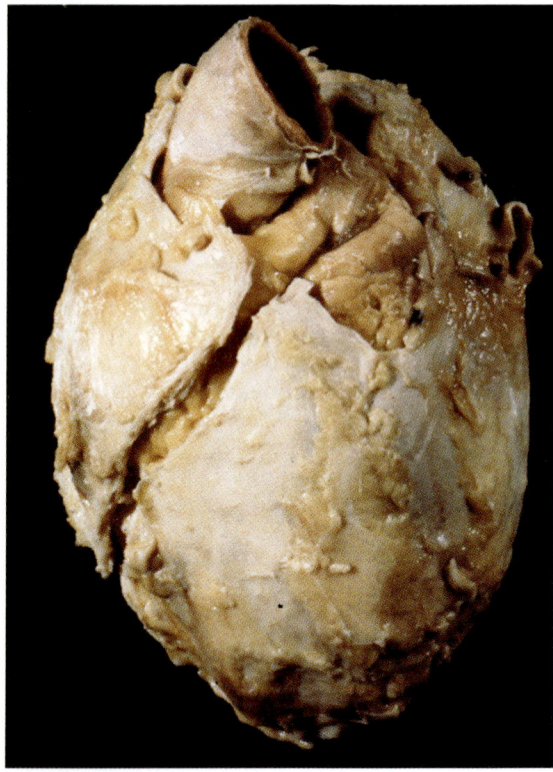

FIGURE 11-53
Constrictive pericarditis. The pericardial space has been obliterated, and the heart is encased in a fibrotic, thickened pericardium.

Adhesive pericarditis is a much milder form of healing of an inflamed pericardium. Commonly seen as an incidental finding at autopsy, it is the outcome of many different types of pericarditis that have healed and left only minor fibrous adhesions between the visceral and parietal surfaces.

PATHOLOGY OF INTERVENTIONAL THERAPIES

Coronary Angioplasty and Stenting Treat Atherosclerotic Coronary Disease

PTCA and stenting are used to mechanically dilate an artery narrowed by an atherosclerotic plaque and maintain the lumen in an open configuration. A catheter containing a deflated balloon covered by a collapsed cylindrical metallic mesh (referred to as a *stent*) is advanced through the stenotic segment. Inflation of the balloon fractures the plaque and stretches the underlying vessel wall. As the stent deploys, it holds the fragmented wall open and keeps the lumen patent. Acute complications of PTCA are uncommon and include coronary artery dissection, acute thrombotic occlusion, and perforation. Progressive restenosis of the lumen develops after PTCA in up to 40% of patients within 4 to 6 months, but the use of stents has reduced this incidence. This complication is the result of a fibroproliferative response of intimal smooth muscle cells to injury sustained during the procedure, resulting in variable amounts of intimal thickening and hyperplasia. Administration of antiplatelet drugs, use of drug-coated stents, and localized irradiation at the site of angioplasty have been successful in limiting the proliferative response of the vessel wall to injury.

Coronary Bypass Grafts Circumvent Obstructed Segments

Coronary bypass grafting, using either a saphenous vein or the left internal mammary artery as a bypass conduit, is a commonly performed procedure for the treatment of proximal coronary stenosis. Although the operative mortality is low and early symptomatic relief occurs in most patients, improvement in myocardial perfusion is not permanent, owing to several complications in the grafts. These include (1) early thrombosis, (2) intimal hyperplasia, and (3) atherosclerosis of vein grafts. Moreover, progressive atherosclerosis of the native coronary arteries is not affected by the grafting procedure.

Internal mammary artery grafts develop fewer pathological changes and, therefore, last longer than vein grafts. Excised saphenous vein segments used as grafts are subjected to unavoidable surgical manipulation and experience an interval of ischemia during harvesting, which results in endothelial cell injury. Once the vein is grafted and arterial blood begins to flow, the vein is exposed to much higher blood pressures than those in its previous location. Finally, the diameter of the vein, which is expanded by arterial blood pressure, is usually much greater than the diameter of the distal coronary artery at the graft anastomosis, a mismatch that promotes blood stasis. In the immediate postoperative period, these factors enhance the probability of thrombosis and probably play a role in the eventual development of intimal hyperplasia. Intimal hyperplasia is characterized by a concentric proliferation of smooth muscle cells and fibroblasts and the deposition of collagen in the intima of the vein. After several years, lipid deposition and atherosclerotic plaque formation can occur in the thickened intima of vein grafts, a process that is accelerated in patients with hyperlipidemia. Atherosclerosis is the most frequent cause of vein graft failure in patients who have had good graft function for several years after surgery.

Because arteries are better suited than veins to serve as aortocoronary bypass conduits, some surgeons have developed total arterial bypass procedures that use the internal mammary, radial, and selected abdominal arteries, which can be harvested without causing significant end-organ damage.

Prosthetic Valves

In most patients with severe valve dysfunction, the best prospect for long-term symptomatic improvement is valve replacement. Operative mortality is low, especially for patients with good preoperative myocardial function. Half of all patients with prosthetic valves are free of complications after 10 years. Heart-valve prostheses can be divided into two categories: those with tissue components and those that are composed entirely of synthetic materials (mechanical valves).

Tissue valves: The most commonly used tissue-valve prostheses are fabricated by using a mechanical frame to which glutaraldehyde-fixed porcine aortic valve cusps or pieces of bovine pericardium are attached. These valves have good hemodynamic characteristics, cause little obstruction, and resist thromboembolic complications. Unfortunately, they are not very durable. The most common cause of failure of tissue-valve prostheses is tissue degeneration with severe calcification and fragmentation of the prosthetic valve cusps. This complication affects virtually all porcine aortic valves within 5 years after implantation and is responsible for valve failure in 20 to 30% of patients within 10 years.

Mechanical valves: The most widely used mechanical prostheses involve single or bileaflet tilting disk designs that do not obstruct blood flow across the valve and have excellent durability. However, the risk of thromboembolism makes long-term anticoagulant therapy imperative.

Heart Transplantation Cures End-Stage Heart Disease

Development of effective immunosuppressive drugs and institution of surveillance endomyocardial biopsy protocols has made cardiac transplantation an effective treatment for end-stage heart disease.

Allograft rejection, however, is a major complication of cardiac transplantation.

Hyperacute rejection occurs in the presence of blood-group incompatibility or major histocompatibility differences. In these situations, preformed antibodies initiate immediate vascular injury in the donor heart, with diffuse hemorrhage, edema, intracapillary platelet–fibrin thrombi, vascular necrosis and infiltration of neutrophils. Screening for blood-group incompatibility has rendered this complication rare.

Acute humoral rejection is another unusual form of allograft rejection, characterized by vascular deposition of immunoglobulin and complement, endothelial cell swelling, and edema. This form of rejection has a worse prognosis than acute cellular rejection.

Acute cellular rejection, the most common form of allograft rejection, occurs in most transplant patients during the first few months after transplantation. Mild cellular rejection begins as perivascular T-cell infiltration, which is focal and is not associated with acute myocyte necrosis. This reaction often resolves spontaneously and, therefore, does not necessitate a change in the immunosuppressive regimen. Moderate cellular rejection is characterized by T-cell infiltration into adjacent interstitial spaces, where lymphocytes surround individual myocytes and expand the interstitium (Fig. 11-54). In this instance, focal acute myocyte necrosis is also present. Moderate cellular rejection usually does not produce detectable functional impairment and tends to resolve within a few days to a week after treatment. However, additional immunosuppressive therapy is instituted because moderate cellular rejection can progress to severe rejection. The latter is characterized by vascular damage, widespread myocyte necrosis, neutrophil infiltration, interstitial hemorrhage, and functional impairment, which is difficult to reverse.

The early stage of significant cellular allograft rejection typically produces no symptoms. Once symptoms develop, rejection is usually much more advanced and has caused irrecoverable loss of cardiac myocytes. The most reliable screening procedure is endomyocardial biopsy of the right side of the interventricular septum, performed by cardiac catheterization.

Chronic vascular rejection, also referred to as *accelerated coronary artery disease,* **is the most common cause of death in heart transplant patients after the first year following transplantation.** It affects the proximal and distal epicardial coronary arteries, the penetrating coronary artery branches, and even the arterioles. Microscopically, accelerated coronary artery disease is characterized by concentric intimal proliferation (Fig. 11-55), which can lead to coronary occlusion and myocardial infarction. This complication is

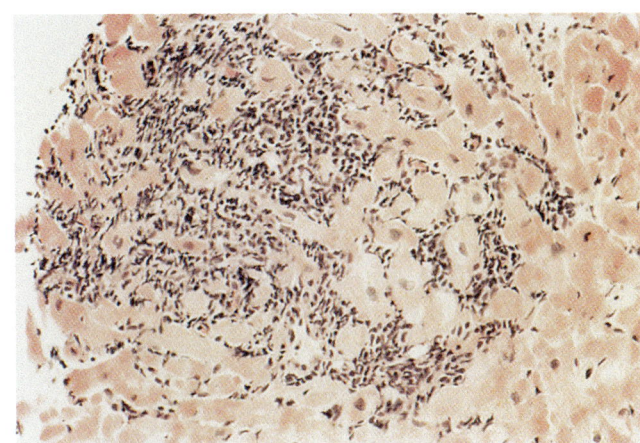

FIGURE 11-54
Cardiac transplant rejection. An endomyocardial biopsy shows lymphocytes surrounding individual myocytes and expanding the interstitium.

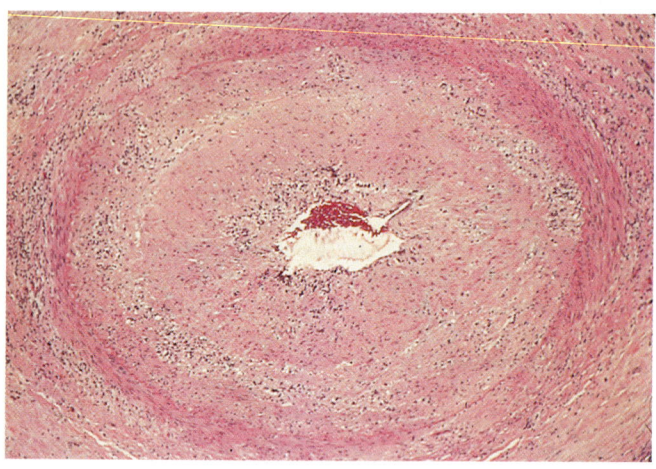

FIGURE 11-55
Chronic cardiac transplant rejection. An intramyocardial branch of a coronary artery shows prominent intimal proliferation and inflammation with narrowing of the lumen.

silent because the transplanted heart is denervated. Thus extensive myocardial damage can develop before the transplant patient is aware that ischemic injury has occurred.

SUGGESTED READING

Books

Braunwald E (ed): *Essential atlas of heart disease,* 2nd ed. Philadelphia: Current Medicine, 2001.

Braunwald E, Zipes DP, Libby P (eds): *Heart disease: A textbook of cardiovascular medicine,* 6th ed. Philadelphia: WB Saunders, 2001.

Fozzard HA, Haber E, Jennings RB, et al. (eds.): *The heart and cardiovascular system: Scientific foundations.* New York: Raven Press, 1991.

Lilly LS (ed): *Pathophysiology of heart disease,* 2nd ed. Philadelphia: Lippincott Williams & Wilkins, 1997.

Perloff JK: *The clinical recognition of congenital heart disease,* 4th ed. Philadelphia: WB Saunders, 1994.

Perloff JK, Child JS: *Congenital heart disease in adults,* 2nd ed. Philadelphia: WB Saunders, 1998.

Schoen FJ: *Interventional and surgical cardiovascular pathology.* Philadelphia: WB Saunders, 1989.

Silver MD, Gotlieb AI, Schoen FJ (eds): *Cardiovascular pathology,* 2nd ed. New York: Churchill Livingstone, 2001.

Review Articles

Aretz HT, Billingham ME, Edwards WD, et al.: Myocarditis. *Am J Cardiovasc Pathol* 1:3–14, 1987.

Armoundas AA, Wu R, Juang G, et al.: Electrical and structural remodeling of the failing ventricle. *Pharmacol Ther* 92:213–230, 2001.

Dare AJ, Veinot JP, Edwards WD, et al.: New observations on the etiology of aortic valve disease. *Hum Pathol* 24: 1330–1338, 1993.

Devereux RB: Recent developments in the diagnosis and management of mitral prolapse. *Curr Opin Cardiol* 10: 107–116, 1995.

Hunter JJ, Chien KR: Signaling pathways for cardiac hypertrophy and failure. *N Engl J Med* 341:1276–1283, 1999.

Kim KS, Hufnagel G, Chapman NM, Tracy S: The group B coxsackieviruses and myocarditis. *Rev Med Virol* 6:355–368, 2001.

Kloner RA, Bolli R, Marban E, et al.: Medical and cellular implications of stunning, hibernation, and preconditioning: An NHLBI workshop. *Circulation* 18:1848–1867, 1998.

Marian AJ: Pathogenesis of diverse clinical and pathological phenotypes in hypertrophic cardiomyopathy. *Lancet* 355:58–60, 2000.

Mylonakis E, Calderwood SB: Infective endocarditis in adults. *N Engl J Med* 18:1318–1330, 2001.

Roberts R, Sigwart U: New concepts in hypertrophic cardiomyopathies, Part I. *Circulation* 104:2113–2116, 2001.

Roberts R, Sigwart U: New concepts in hypertrophic cardiomyopathies, Part II. *Circulation* 104:2249–2252, 2001.

Seidman JG, Seidman C: The genetic basis for cardiomyopathy: from mutation identification to mechanistic paradigms. *Cell* 104:557–567, 2001.

Towbin JA: The role of cytoskeletal proteins in cardiomyopathies. *Current Opin Cell Biol* 10:131–139, 1998.

Virmani R, Burke AP, Farb A: Sudden cardiac death. *Cardiovasc Pathol* 10:211–218, 2001.

CHAPTER 12

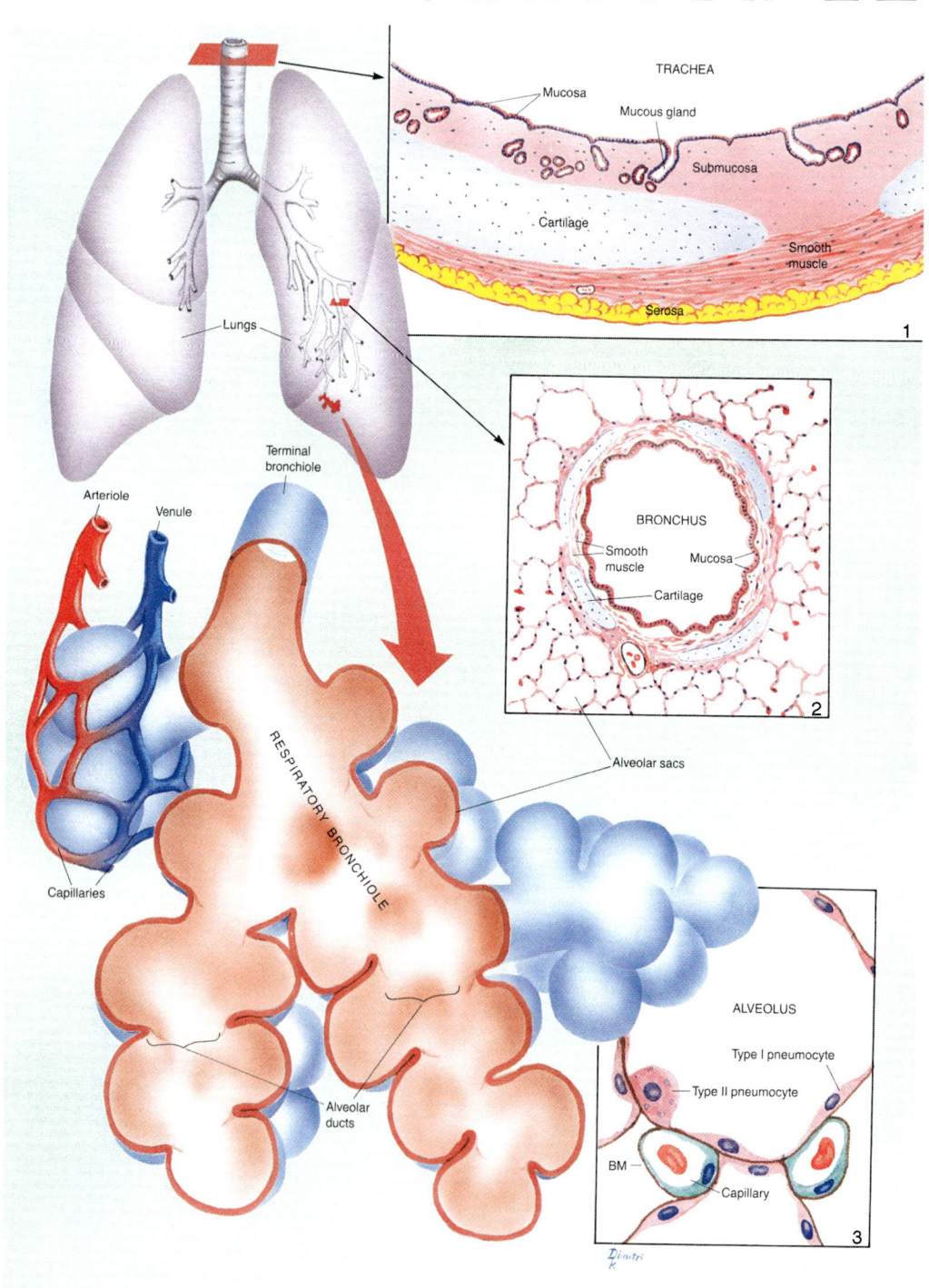

The Respiratory System

William D. Travis
Mary Beth Beasley
Emanuel Rubin

Embryology

Anatomy

Defense Mechanisms

The Lungs

Congenital Anomalies of the Lungs

Diseases of the Bronchi and Bronchioles
Infections
Irritant Gases
Bronchocentric Granulomatosis
Constrictive Bronchiolitis
Bronchial Obstruction
Bronchiectasis

Infections
Bacterial Pneumonia
Mycoplasma
Tuberculosis
Actinomycosis
Nocardia
Fungal Infections
Viral Pneumonia
Lung Abscess

Diffuse Alveolar Damage (Acute Respiratory Distress Syndrome)

Rare Alveolar Diseases
Alveolar Proteinosis
Diffuse Pulmonary Hemorrhage Syndromes
Eosinophilic Pneumonia
Endogenous Lipid Pneumonia
Exogenous Lipid Pneumonia

Obstructive Pulmonary Diseases
Chronic Bronchitis
Emphysema
Asthma

Pneumoconioses
Silicosis
Coal Workers' Pneumoconiosis
Asbestos-Related Diseases
Berylliosis
Talcosis

(continued)

FIGURE 12-1 *(see opposite page)*
Anatomy of the lung. The conducting structures of the lung include (1) the trachea, which has horseshoe-shaped cartilages; (2) the bronchi, which have plates of cartilage in their walls (both the trachea and bronchi have mucus-secreting glands in their walls); and (3) the bronchioles, which do not have cartilage in their walls and terminate in the terminal bronchioles. The gas-exchanging components compose the unit distal to the terminal bronchiole, namely, the acinus. Alveoli are lined by type I cells, which are large, flat cells that cover most of the alveolar wall, and by type II cells, which secrete surfactant and are the progenitor cells of the alveolar epithelium. Gas exchange occurs at the level of the alveolar wall.

Interstitial Lung Disease

Hypersensitivity Pneumonitis (Extrinsic Allergic Alveolitis)

Sarcoidosis

Interstitial Pneumonia

Desquamative Interstitial Pneumonia

Respiratory Bronchiolitis–Interstitial Lung Disease

Organizing Pneumonia Pattern (Cryptogenic Organizing Pneumonia)

Lymphoid Interstitial Pneumonia

Langerhans Cell Histiocytosis (Histiocytosis X)

Lymphangioleiomyomatosis

Lung Transplantation

Vasculitis and Granulomatosis

Wegener Granulomatosis

Churg-Strauss Syndrome (Allergic Angiitis and Granulomatosis)

Necrotizing Sarcoid Granulomatosis

Pulmonary Hypertension

Precapillary versus Postcapillary Pulmonary Hypertension

Functional Resistance to Arterial Flow (Vasoconstriction)

Cardiac Causes of Pulmonary Hypertension

Pulmonary Venoocclusive Disease

Pulmonary Hamartoma

Carcinoma of the Lung

General Features

Pulmonary Metastases

The Pleura

Pneumothorax

Pleural Effusion

Pleuritis

Tumors of the Pleura

Localized (Solitary) Fibrous Tumor of the Pleura

Malignant Mesothelioma

EMBRYOLOGY

The respiratory system comprises the larynx, trachea, bronchi, bronchioles, and alveoli. During the fourth week of gestation, the laryngotracheal groove develops as a ventral outpouching of the foregut.

The embryonic period of lung development occurs between 4 and 6 weeks' gestation. During this period, the tracheobronchial bud divides to form the proximal airways complete to the segmental level.

The pseudoglandular period occupies weeks 6 to 16 of gestation, after which time the distal airways are formed up to the level of the terminal bronchioles.

The acinar or canalicular period encompasses weeks 17 to 28 of gestation. This is the time when (1) the framework of the gas-exchanging unit of the lung develops, (2) the acinus is formed, (3) the vascular system develops, (4) capillaries reach the epithelium, and (5) gas exchange becomes possible. At this point extrauterine life becomes possible.

The saccular period extends from 28 to 34 weeks of gestation. The primary saccules become subdivided by secondary crests, a process that results in greater complexity of the gas-exchanging surface and thinning of air-space walls.

The alveolar period corresponds to 34 to 36 weeks of gestation and is the last step in lung development when alveoli begin developing. At birth, the number of alveoli is highly variable, ranging from 20–150 million. Most alveoli develop in the first 2 years of life.

ANATOMY

TRACHEA AND BRONCHI: The trachea is a hollow tube measuring up to 25 cm in length and up to 2.5 cm in diameter. The right bronchus diverges at a lesser angle from the trachea than does the left, which is why foreign material is more frequently aspirated on the right side (Fig. 12-1). On entering the lung, the bronchi divide into lobar bronchi and then into segmental bronchi, which supply the 19 segments of the lung. Because the segments are individual units with their own bronchovascular supply, they can be resected individually.

The tracheobronchial tree contains cartilage and submucosal mucous glands in the wall. The latter are compound tubular glands that display both mucous cells (pale) and serous cells (granular, more basophilic). The tracheobronchial tree is lined by a pseudostratified epithelium, which appears as layers, although all cells reach the basement membrane. Most of the cells are ciliated, but mucus-secreting (goblet) cells also exist, as well as basal cells that do not reach the surface. The basal cells are thought to be precursor cells that differentiate to form the more specialized cells of the tracheobronchial epithelium. In addition, there are nonciliated columnar cells, or *Clara cells,* which accumulate and detoxify many inhaled toxic agents (e.g., nitrogen dioxide). Scattered in the tracheobronchial mucosa are *Kulchitsky cells,* which are neuroendocrine cells that contain a variety of hormonally active polypeptides and vasoactive amines.

BRONCHIOLES: Distal to the bronchi are bronchioles, which differ from the bronchi by the absence of cartilage and mucus-secreting glands (Fig. 12-1). The epithelium of the bronchioles becomes thinner with progressive branchings, until only one cell layer is present. The last purely conducting structure free of alveoli is the *terminal bronchiole,* which has a circumferential layer of pseudostratified ciliated respiratory epithelium and a smooth muscle wall. Mucous cells gradually disappear from the lining of the bronchioles until they are entirely replaced in the small bronchioles by the nonciliated, columnar Clara cells. The terminal bronchioles divide into the *respiratory bronchioles,* which merge into *alveolar ducts* and *alveoli.* The *acinus,* which is the unit of gas exchange in the lung, consists of respiratory bronchioles, alveolar ducts, and alveoli.

ALVEOLI: The alveoli are lined by two types of epithelium (Fig. 12-1). **Type I cells cover 95% of the alveolar surface, although they comprise only 40% of all the epithelial cells of the alveolus.** They are thin and have a large surface area, a combination that facilitates gas exchange. **Type II cells produce surfactant and account for 60% of the alveolar lining cells.** However, because they are more cuboidal, they contribute only 5% of the alveolar surface. Type I cells are particularly vulnerable to injury. When they are lost, type II pneumocytes multiply and differentiate to form new type I cells, thereby reconstituting the alveolar surface.

The alveolar epithelial and endothelial cells are arranged ideally for gas exchange. The cytoplasm of the epithelial and endothelial cells is spread very thinly on either side of a fused basement membrane, allowing efficient exchange of oxygen and carbon dioxide. An abundant capillary network covers 85 to 95% of the alveolar surface. Away from the site of gas exchange, there is more abundant interstitial connective tissue consisting of collagen, elastin, and proteoglycans. In addition, fibroblasts and myofibroblasts may be present. This expanded region forms the interstitial space of the alveolar wall, where significant fluid and molecular exchange occurs.

PULMONARY VASCULATURE: The lung has a dual blood supply, composed of the pulmonary circulation and the bronchial system. The pulmonary arteries accompany the airways in a sheath of connective tissue, termed the *bronchovascular bundle.* The more proximal arteries are elastic. They are succeeded by muscular arteries, the pulmonary arterioles, and eventually the pulmonary capillaries.

The smallest veins, which resemble the smallest arteries, join with other veins and drain into the lobular septa, connective tissue partitions that subdivide the lung into small respiratory units. The veins then continue in the lobular septa, joining other veins to form a network that is separate from the bronchovascular bundles.

The bronchial arteries arise from the thoracic aorta and nourish the bronchial tree as far as the respiratory bronchioles. These arteries are accompanied by their respective veins, which drain into the azygous or hemiazygous veins.

There are no lymphatics in most alveolar walls. The lymphatics commence in alveoli at the periphery of the acinus, which lies along a lobular septum, a bronchovascular bundle, or the pleura. The lymphatics of the lobular septa and bronchovascular bundle accompany these structures, and the pleural lymphatics drain toward the hilus through the bronchovascular lymphatics.

DEFENSE MECHANISMS

The respiratory system has effective defense mechanisms to cope with the numerous particulates and infectious agents inhaled on inspiration.

The **nose and trachea** warm and humidify the air entering the lung. The nose traps almost all particles more than 10 μm in diameter and about half of all particles with an aerodynamic diameter of 3 μm (Fig. 12-2). (Aerodynamic diameter refers to the way particles behave in air rather than to their actual size.)

The **mucociliary blanket** of the airway epithelium disposes of particles 2 to 10 μm in diameter. The ciliary beat drives the mucous blanket toward the trachea, and particles that land on it are thus removed from the lungs and swallowed or coughed up.

Alveolar macrophages protect the alveolar space. These cells are derived from the bone marrow, probably undergo a maturation division in the interstitium of the lung, and then enter the alveolar space. They are particularly effective in dealing with particles whose aerodynamic diameter is less than 2 μm. Very small particles are not phagocytosed and are exhaled.

The Lungs

CONGENITAL ANOMALIES

BRONCHIAL ATRESIA: This abnormality most often involves the bronchus to the apical posterior segment of the left upper lobe. In infants, the lesion may result in an overexpanded part of the lung. In later life, the overexpanded lobe may also be emphysematous. Bronchial mucus accumulating distal to the atretic region may appear on radiological examination as a mass.

PULMONARY HYPOPLASIA: This condition reflects incomplete or defective development of the lung. The lung is smaller than normal, owing to fewer acini or a decrease in their size. Pulmonary hypoplasia is the most common congenital lesion of the lung, being found in 10% of neonatal autopsies. In most cases (90%), it occurs in association with other congenital anomalies, most of which impinge on the thorax. The lesion may be accompanied by hypoplasia of the bronchi and pulmonary vessels if the insult occurs early in gestation, as in congenital diaphragmatic hernia. Pulmonary hypoplasia also is seen in trisomies 13, 18, and 21.

Pathogenesis: Three major factors have been implicated as causes of pulmonary hypoplasia:

- **Compression of the lung** is usually caused by a congenital diaphragmatic hernia, typically on the left side, owing to failure of the pleuroperitoneal canal to close. Varying degrees of herniation of abdominal viscera are present in the affected hemithorax, and the degree of hypoplasia is variable. At one extreme, the lung on the affected side is reduced to a small nubbin of tissue, and the lung on the opposite side is severely hypoplastic. At the other extreme, the hypoplasia is so slight that the infant has no symptoms, and the abnormalities are noted incidentally on a routine chest radiograph. Other causes of hypoplasia include abnormalities of the chest wall, pleural effusions, and ascites, as in hydrops fetalis.
- **Oligohydramnios** (an inadequate volume of amniotic fluid) is usually due to genitourinary anomalies and is an important cause of pulmonary hypoplasia.
- **Decreased respiration** has been shown experimentally to produce hypoplastic lungs, which may be caused by a lack of repetitive stretching of the lung.

CONGENITAL CYSTIC ADENOMATOID MALFORMATION: This common anomaly consists of abnormal bronchiolar structures of varying sizes or distribution. Most cases are encountered in the first 2 years of life. The lesion usually affects one lobe of the lung and histologically consists of multiple cystlike spaces lined by bronchiolar epithelium and separated by loose fibrous tissue (Fig. 12-3). Some patients with congenital cystic adenomatoid malformation have other congenital anomalies. The most common presenting symptom is respiratory distress and cyanosis. Surgical resection is the treatment of choice.

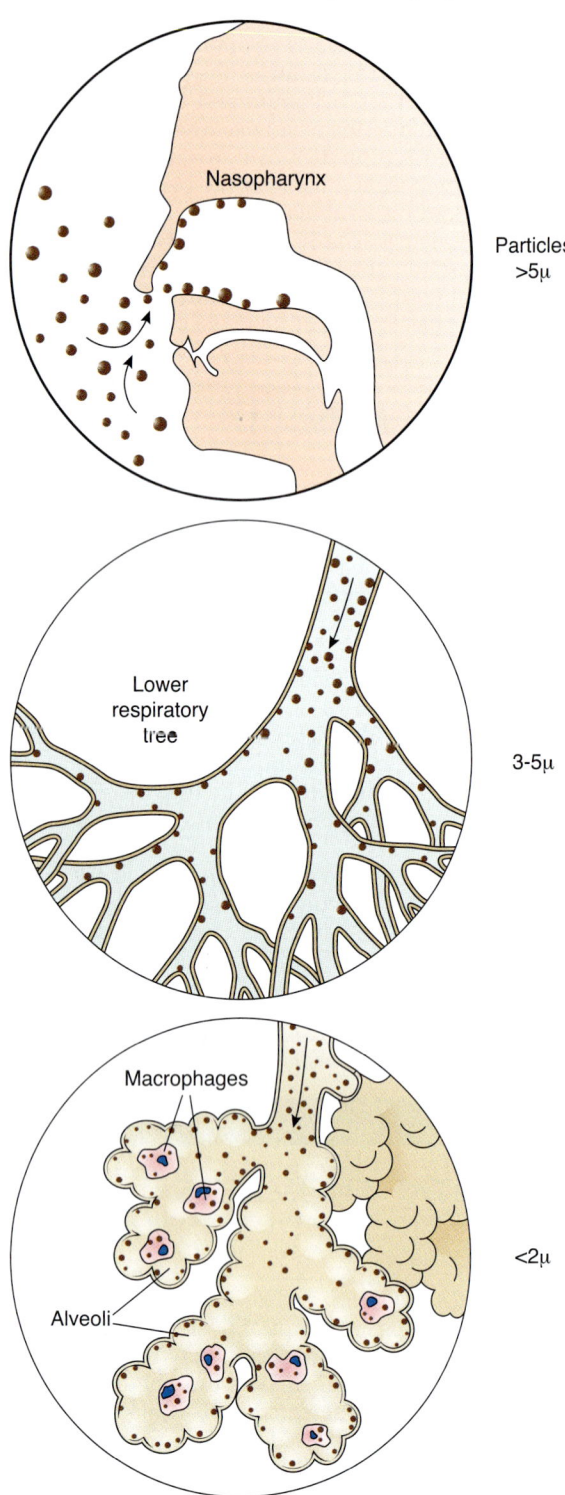

FIGURE 12-2
Deposition of particles in the respiratory tract. Large particles are trapped in the nose. Intermediate-sized particles deposit on the bronchi and bronchioles and are removed by the mucociliary blanket. Smaller particles terminate in the air spaces and are removed by macrophages. Very small particles behave as a gas and are breathed out.

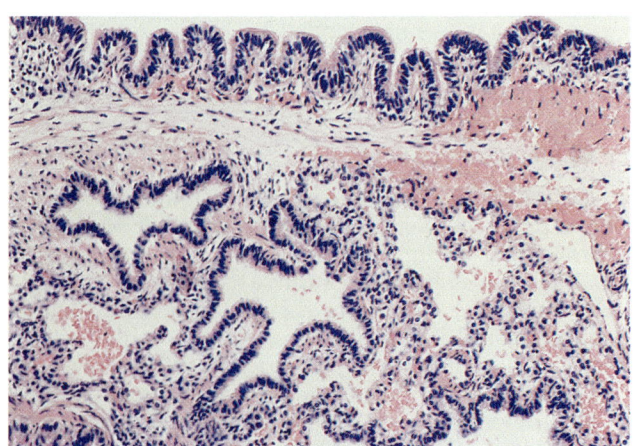

FIGURE 12-3
Congenital cystic adenomatoid malformation. Multiple glandlike spaces are lined by bronchiolar epithelium.

BRONCHOGENIC CYST: *This lesion is a discrete, extrapulmonary, fluid-filled mass that is lined by respiratory epithelium and limited by walls that contain muscle and cartilage.* It is most commonly found in the middle mediastinum. In the newborn, a bronchogenic cyst may compress a major airway and cause respiratory distress. Secondary infection of the cyst in older patients may lead to hemorrhage and perforation. Many bronchogenic cysts are asymptomatic and are found on routine chest radiographs.

EXTRALOBAR SEQUESTRATION: *Extralobar sequestration is a mass of lung tissue that is not connected to the bronchial tree and is located outside the visceral pleura.* An abnormal artery, usually arising from the aorta, supplies the sequestered tissue (Fig. 12-4).

 Pathogenesis: This lesion is thought to originate from an outpouching of the foregut, which is separate from the pulmonary anlage but later becomes detached from the original foregut. The lesion occurs 3 to 4 times as often in male as in female infants, and in two thirds of patients, it is associated with other anomalies.

 Pathology: On gross examination, extralobar sequestration appears as a pyramidal or round mass covered by pleura, ranging from 1 to 15 cm in greatest dimension. Microscopically, dilated bronchioles, alveolar ducts, and alveoli are noted. Infection or infarction may alter the histological appearance.

 Clinical Features: In half of cases, extralobar sequestration is recognized in the first month of life, and by age 2 years, the diagnosis has been made in 75% of patients. In the neonatal period, often during the first

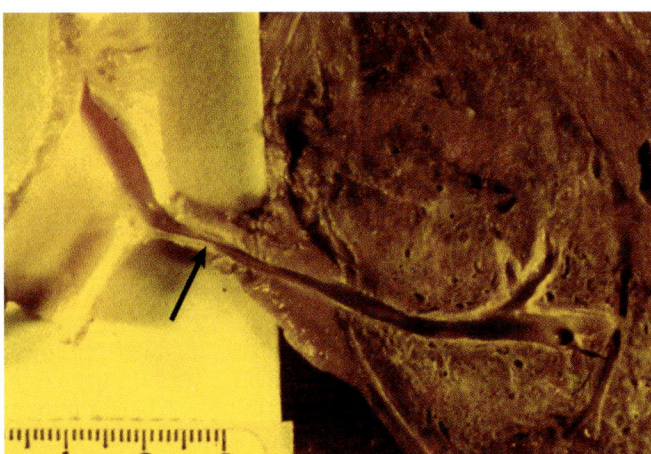

FIGURE 12-4
Extralobar sequestration. The sequestered pulmonary tissue is situated outside the lung parenchyma. It is supplied by an aberrant artery *(arrow)* **from the aorta and is not connected to the bronchial tree.**

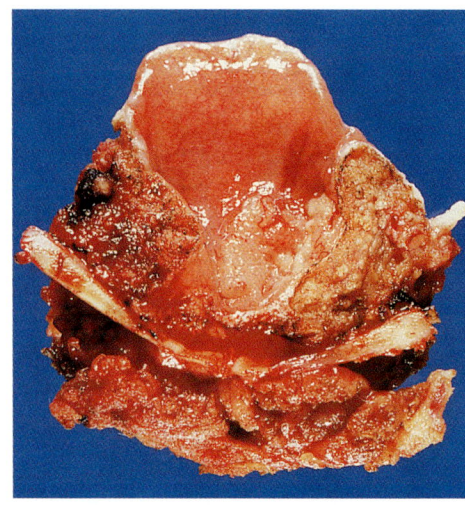

FIGURE 12-5
Intralobar sequestration. The sequestered tissue lies within the visceral pleura and exhibits cystic change and dense fibrosis. An aberrant arterial supply to this lesion was identified (not shown).

day of life, the disorder may manifest as dyspnea and cyanosis. In older children, the lesion frequently comes to medical attention because of recurrent bronchopulmonary infections. Surgical excision is curative.

INTRALOBAR SEQUESTRATION: *Intralobar sequestration is a mass of lung tissue within the visceral pleura that is isolated from the tracheobronchial tree and is supplied by a systemic artery* (Fig. 12-5). For many years, this lesion was considered a congenital malformation, but it is now thought to be acquired.

 Pathology: Intralobar sequestration is found in a lower lobe in almost all (98%) cases, and bilateral involvement is distinctly unusual. On gross examination, the sequestered pulmonary tissue shows the result of chronic recurrent pneumonia, with end-stage fibrosis and honeycomb cystic changes. The cysts range up to 5 cm in diameter and lie in a dense fibrous stroma. Microscopically, the cystic spaces are mostly lined by cuboidal or columnar epithelium, and the lumen contains foamy macrophages and eosinophilic material. Interstitial chronic inflammation and hyperplasia of lymphoid follicles is often prominent. Acute and organizing pneumonia may be seen.

 Clinical Features: Symptoms of cough, sputum production, and recurrent pneumonia are noted in almost all patients. Most cases are discovered in adolescents or young adults. Only one fourth of patients are in the first decade of life, and the lesion is only rarely identified in infants. Surgical resection is often indicated.

DISEASES OF THE BRONCHI AND BRONCHIOLES

Most of the entities subsumed under bronchial and bronchiolar diseases deal with acute conditions and their sequelae. We reserve the discussion of chronic bronchitis for the section devoted to chronic obstructive pulmonary disease.

Airway Infections Occur Principally in Children

In this section, we distinguish between infections of the airways and parenchyma for reasons of classification and convenience, but this division should not be thought of as rigid. The agents causing these infections are discussed in detail in Chapter 9.

Many infectious agents that involve the intrapulmonary airways tend to affect the more peripheral airways *(bronchiolitis)*. The classic examples are adenovirus, measles, and respiratory syncytial virus. All appear to be more serious in malnourished children and populations not ordinarily exposed to these agents. Severe symptomatic illnesses are mostly confined to infants and children, and recovery is the rule. Symptoms include cough, a feeling of tightness in the chest, and, in extreme cases, shortness of breath and even cyanosis.

INFLUENZA: This is a characteristic example of tracheobronchitis, and in the occasional patient who dies with this infection, the appearance of the bronchi is dramatic. The surface of the airway is fiery red, reflecting acute inflammation and congestion of the mucosa.

ADENOVIRUS: Infection with this virus produces the most serious sequelae, including extensive inflammation of bronchioles (Fig. 12-6) and subsequent healing by fibrosis. Bronchioles may become obliterated or occluded by loose fibrous tissue *(obliterative bronchiolitis)*.

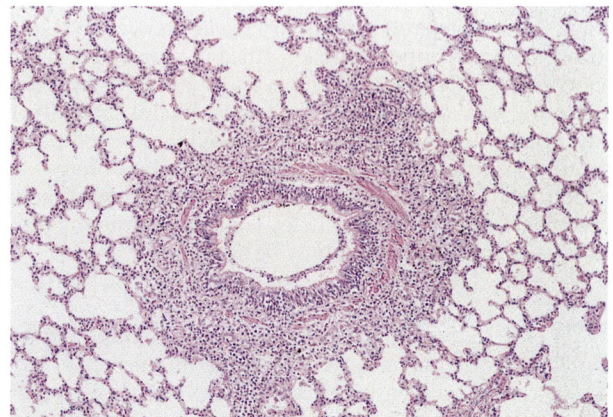

FIGURE 12-6
Bronchiolitis due to adenovirus. The wall of this bronchiole shows an intense chronic inflammatory infiltrate with local extension into the surrounding peribronchial tissue.

RESPIRATORY SYNCYTIAL VIRUS: Infection with this agent tends to occur in epidemics in nurseries. It is usually a self-limited illness, but rare fatal cases occur. It can cause nosocomial infection in children and (rarely) in adults. Histologically, one encounters peribronchiolar inflammation and disorganization of the epithelium. Severe overdistention of the lung parenchyma may be found without obvious bronchiolar obstruction, possibly because of displacement of surfactant from the bronchiolar surface.

MEASLES: At one time a major cause of bronchiolitis, measles is no longer a problem in developed countries because of the advent of the measles vaccine. However, measles-induced bronchiolitis still remains a serious problem elsewhere, particularly in populations seldom exposed to the virus. Similar to adenovirus, it may result in bronchiolar obliteration and bronchiectasis.

BORDETELLA PERTUSSIS: This bacterium commonly infects the airways and is the cause of **whooping cough**. After the introduction of a pertussis vaccine, the disease became rare in the United States, but it has become increasingly common in England, where vaccination is no longer compulsory. Clinically, whooping cough is typified by fever and severe prolonged bouts of coughing, followed by a characteristic deep whooping inspiration. Severe bronchial and bronchiolar inflammation has been found in fatal cases. Whooping cough commonly preceded the development of bronchiectasis in the past, but this is no longer the case in areas where children are routinely immunized.

HAEMOPHILUS INFLUENZAE AND STREPTOCOCCUS PNEUMONIAE: These organisms have been implicated in exacerbations of chronic bronchitis. Such episodes contribute to the morbidity of chronic bronchitis and are treated with antibiotics.

CANDIDA ALBICANS: This fungus is a normal commensal organism in the oral cavity, gut, and vagina and is best known for its infection of those regions. *Candida* may also affect the lungs, usually as a noninvasive growth on the surface epithelium of the airways, where it may produce mucosal ulceration. Predisposing factors for invasive growth include trauma, burns, gastrointestinal surgery, and indwelling catheters, as well as neutropenia associated with a history of acute leukemia and cytotoxic chemotherapy.

Irritant Gases Involve Air Pollution or Accidents

Of the irritant gases in the atmosphere, the important ones are oxidants (ozone, oxides of nitrogen) and sulfur dioxide. Oxidants are particularly related to the action of sunlight on automobile exhaust fumes and are important in major urban areas that have temperature inversions. Sulfur dioxide is derived mainly from the burning of fossil fuels. Although the precise effects of these agents in low concentration is not certain, and although they clearly have a high nuisance value, it seems unlikely that they are a major cause of serious respiratory disease. However, they may compound the adverse effects of tobacco smoke. Indeed, persons living in urban and more polluted areas have worse pulmonary function, as expressed by reduced expiratory flow rates, than do those who reside in cleaner environments. Respiratory infections are also more common in young children in regions of high pollution. However, the decrement in function and increase in symptoms is small in the healthy population.

In persons with chronic pulmonary disease, the situation is different. Of particular relevance is the experimental observation that ozone makes the airways more reactive, an effect related to airway inflammation. Thus, air pollution may exacerbate the symptoms of asthmatic persons and those with established respiratory disease. In high concentrations, irritant gases produce serious morphological and functional effects.

NITROGEN DIOXIDE (NO₂): Exposure to NO₂ is often encountered in industrial settings, including welding, electroplating, metal cleaning, and blasting. The gas is also produced by decaying grain stored in silos. Because NO₂ is heavier than air, it accumulates immediately above the surface of the grain. A worker entering the silo inhales high concentrations of the gas, with resulting injury to the lung, a condition known as *silo-filler disease*. The onset of respiratory symptoms is delayed for up to 30 hours, after which time the patient is seen with cough and dyspnea. Although most patients recover, some have developed progressive bronchiolitis obliterans and have died in respiratory failure.

SULFUR DIOXIDE (SO₂): This highly soluble gas, when inhaled over the long term by experimental animals, produces lesions in the more central airways that resemble chronic bronchitis and that may progress to squamous metaplasia. In humans, exposure to very high concentrations of SO₂ has been associated with severe inflammation and bronchiolitis.

CHLORINE AND AMMONIA: These gases are released in high concentrations in industrial accidents. On inhalation, they produce extensive bronchial and bronchiolar mucosal injury. Secondary inflammation may culminate in extensive bronchiectasis, in part from bronchiolar obliteration and in part from direct damage to the bronchi.

Bronchocentric Granulomatosis Usually Reflects Allergic Responses to Infection

Bronchocentric granulomatosis refers to nonspecific granulomatous inflammation centered on bronchi or bronchioles (Fig. 12-7). The histological pattern can be seen in a wide variety of clinical settings and is not a distinct clinical entity. Bronchocentric granulomatosis can be the predominant pulmonary pathological finding in two groups of patients, asthmatics and nonasthmatics.

Asthmatic patients, for the most part, have allergic bronchopulmonary aspergillosis (see below). In addition to the lesion of bronchocentric granulomatosis, such patients demonstrate bronchial mucous plugs, bronchiectasis and bronchiolectasis, and eosinophilic pneumonia. Irregular, fragmented *Aspergillus* hyphae may be seen in the mucous

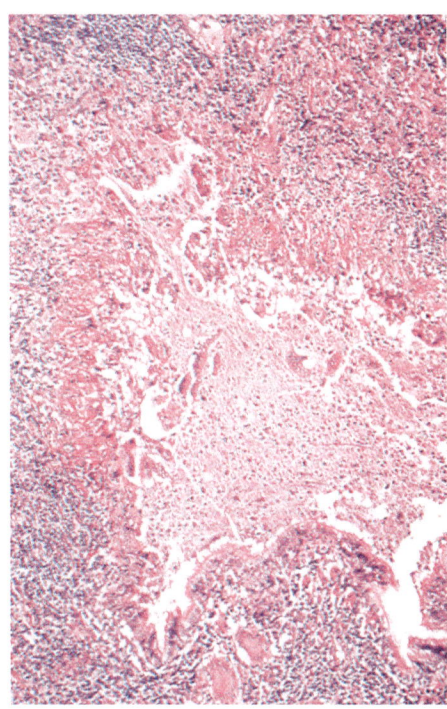

FIGURE 12-7
Bronchocentric granulomatosis. The wall of a bronchiole is destroyed by necrotizing granulomatous inflammation. The lumen is filled with necrotic debris.

plugs. A nonspecific secondary vasculitis is centered on the airways rather than the vessels.

Nonasthmatic patients with bronchocentric granulomatosis are likely to have an infection, especially tuberculosis or fungal organisms such as *Histoplasma capsulatum*. Bronchocentric granulomatosis can also be a manifestation of rheumatoid arthritis, ankylosing spondylitis, and Wegener granulomatosis. In the absence of any of these potential causes, bronchocentric granulomatosis is regarded as *idiopathic*. Patients with *idiopathic* bronchocentric granulomatosis may respond well to corticosteroid therapy.

Constrictive Bronchiolitis May Obliterate the Airway

Constrictive bronchiolitis is an uncommon disorder in which an initial inflammatory bronchiolitis is followed by bronchiolar scarring and fibrosis, resulting in constrictive narrowing and eventually complete obliteration of the airway lumen (Fig. 12-8). *Obliterative bronchiolitis* is a synonym.

 Pathology: Bronchioles show chronic mural inflammation and varying amounts of submucosal fibrosis. These lesions are often focal and may be difficult to identify. Elastic stains may assist in recognizing the scarred bronchioles. Bronchiolectasis and mucous plugs may be seen in adjacent airways. The surrounding lung is usually normal.

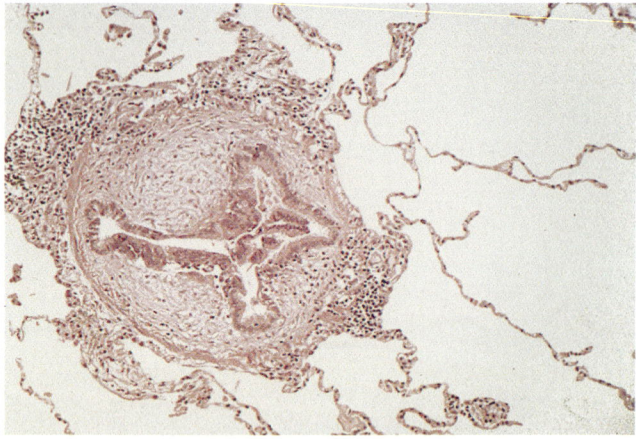

FIGURE 12-8
Constrictive bronchiolitis. The lumen of a bronchiole is markedly narrowed, owing to marked submucosal fibrosis.

Clinical Features: Patients may have dyspnea and wheezing owing to severe obstructive pulmonary function. The chest radiograph and computed tomography (CT) scan may be normal, or they may show overinflation, caused by air trapping distal to the obliterated bronchioles. This pattern of fibrosis is seen in a number of situations, including: (1) bone marrow transplantation (graft-versus-host disease), (2) lung transplantation (chronic rejection), (3) collagen vascular diseases (especially rheumatoid arthritis), (4) postinfectious disorders (especially viral infections), (5) after inhalation of toxins (sulfur dioxide, ammonia, phosgene), and (6) intake of certain drugs (penicillamine). It also may occur as an idiopathic entity. Most patients have a relentless progressive clinical course. Although many are treated with steroids, there is no known effective therapy for this disease.

Bronchial Obstruction Leads to Atelectasis

Bronchial obstruction in adults is most often the consequence of the endobronchial extension of primary lung tumors, although mucous plugs from aspirated gastric contents or foreign bodies may be responsible, especially in children. In the case of partial obstruction, the trapped air may lead to overdistention of the distal affected segment; complete obstruction results in atelectasis. Areas distal to the obstruction are also susceptible to pneumonia, pulmonary abscess, and bronchiectasis (see below).

Atelectasis

Atelectasis refers to the collapse of expanded lung tissue (Fig. 12-9). If the supply of air is obstructed, the loss of gas from the alveoli to the blood causes collapse of the affected region. Atelectasis is an important postoperative complication of abdominal surgery, occurring because of (1) mucous obstruction of a bronchus and (2) diminished respiratory movement resulting from postoperative pain. It is often asymptomatic, but when severe, it results in hypoxemia and a shift of the mediastinum *toward* the affected side.

Although atelectasis is usually caused by bronchial obstruction, it may also result from direct compression of the lung (e.g., hydrothorax or pneumothorax). Such compression, if severe enough, seriously compromises the function of the affected lung and causes a mediastinal shift *away* from the affected side.

In long-standing atelectasis, the collapsed lung becomes fibrotic and the bronchi dilate, in part because of infection distal to the obstructed bronchus. Permanent bronchial dilation (bronchiectasis) results.

Right middle lobe syndrome refers to atelectasis secondary to obstruction of the bronchus to the right middle lobe. The bronchial obstruction is usually due to external compression by hilar lymph nodes. This bronchus is particularly susceptible to external compression because it is long and slender and surrounded by lymph nodes. Histologically, the lung shows bronchiectasis, chronic bronchitis and bronchiolitis, lymphoid hyperplasia, abscess formation, and dense fibrosis. Both acute and organizing pneumonia may be present. The lymph node enlargement can be due to tuberculous lymphadenitis or metastatic lung cancer. In a substantial proportion of cases, the cause of the bronchial obstruction remains undetermined.

Bronchiectasis Is the Irreversible Dilation of Bronchi

Bronchiectasis is caused by the destruction of the muscular and elastic elements of their the bronchial walls.

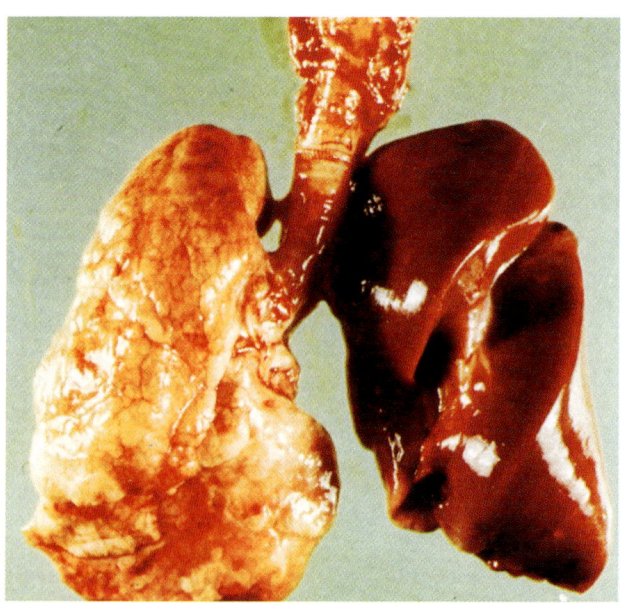

FIGURE 12-9
Atelectasis. The right lung of an infant is pale and expanded by air; the left lung is collapsed.

Pathogenesis: Bronchiectasis is either obstructive or nonobstructive.

Obstructive bronchiectasis is localized to a segment of the lung distal to a mechanical obstruction of a central bronchus by a variety of lesions, including tumors, inhaled foreign bodies, mucous plugs in asthma, and compressive lymphadenopathy. **Nonobstructive bronchiectasis** is usually a complication of respiratory infections or defects in the defense mechanisms that protect the airways from infection. It may be localized or generalized.

Localized nonobstructive bronchiectasis was once a common disease, usually resulting from childhood bronchopulmonary infections such as measles, pertussis, or other bacterial infections. Although vaccines and antibiotics have reduced the frequency of bronchiectasis, one half to two thirds of all cases still follow a bronchopulmonary infection. At present, adenovirus and respiratory syncytial virus infections are frequent causes of bronchiectasis in children. Childhood respiratory infections remain important causes of bronchiectasis in less-developed parts of the world.

Generalized bronchiectasis is, for the most part, secondary to inherited impairment in host defense mechanisms or acquired conditions that permit the introduction of infectious organisms into the airways. The acquired disorders that predispose to bronchiectasis include (1) neurological diseases that impair consciousness, swallowing, respiratory excursions, and the cough reflex; (2) incompetence of the lower esophageal sphincter; (3) nasogastric intubation; and (4) chronic bronchitis. The principal inherited conditions associated with generalized bronchiectasis are cystic fibrosis, the dyskinetic ciliary syndromes, hypogammaglobulinemias, and deficiencies of specific IgG subclasses.

Kartagener syndrome is one of the immotile cilia (ciliary dyskinesia) syndromes and comprises the triad of dextrocardia (with or without situs inversus), bronchiectasis, and sinusitis. This disorder is associated with a defect in the structure of cilia, characterized by an absence of inner or outer dynein arms. Other dyskinetic ciliary syndromes include radial spoke deficiency *(Sturgess syndrome)* and an absence of the central doublet of the cilium. Cilia are deficient throughout the body in immotile cilia syndromes. As a result, sterility in both men and women is usual, because of impaired ciliary mobility in the vas deferens and the fallopian tube. In the respiratory tract, ciliary defects lead to repeated upper and lower respiratory tract infections in the lung and, thus, to bronchiectasis.

Immunodeficiency diseases similarly predispose to repeated pulmonary infections and are associated with bronchiectasis. Hypogammaglobulinemia can result in recurrent pulmonary infections owing to the absence of IgA or IgG antibodies that protect against viruses or bacteria. Acquired and inherited disorders of neutrophils also lead to a greater risk of respiratory infections and bronchiectasis.

 Pathology: On gross examination, bronchial dilation is classified as saccular, varicose, or cylindrical.

- **Saccular bronchiectasis** affects the proximal third to fourth branches of the bronchi (Fig. 12-10). These bronchi

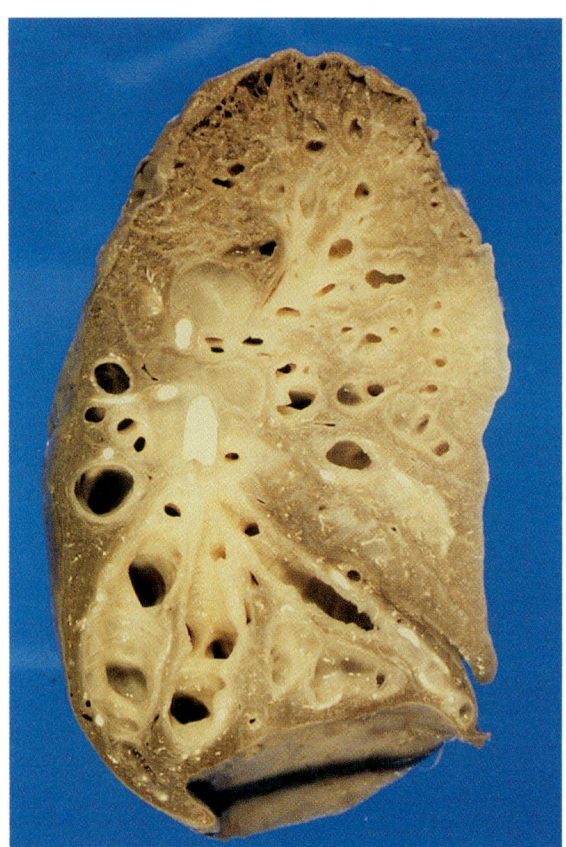

FIGURE 12-10
Bronchiectasis. The resected upper lobe shows widely dilated bronchi, with thickening of the bronchial walls and collapse and fibrosis of the pulmonary parenchyma.

are severely dilated and end blindly in dilated sacs, with collapse and fibrosis of the distal lung parenchyma.
- **Cylindrical bronchiectasis** involves the sixth to eighth bronchial branchings, which show uniform, moderate dilation. It is a milder disease than saccular bronchiectasis and leads to fewer clinical symptoms.
- **Varicose bronchiectasis** results in bronchi that resemble varicose veins when visualized by radiological bronchography, with irregular dilations and constrictions. Two to eight branchings of bronchi are recognized grossly. Bronchiolar obliteration is not as severe, and parenchymal abnormalities are variable.

Generalized bronchiectasis is usually bilateral and is most common in the lower lobes, the left more commonly involved than the right. Localized bronchiectasis may be situated wherever the obstruction or infection occurred. The bronchi are dilated and have white or yellow thickened walls. The bronchial lumen frequently contains thick, mucopurulent secretions. Microscopically, severe inflammation of bronchi and bronchioles results in destruction of all components of the bronchial wall. With the consequent collapse of distal lung parenchyma, the damaged bronchi dilate. Inflammation of the central airways leads to hypersecretion of mucus and abnormalities of the surface epithelium, including an increase in number of goblet cells and squamous metaplasia of the epithelium. Lymphoid follicles are often seen in the bronchial walls. The distal bronchi and bronchioles are scarred and often obliterated. The bronchial arteries increase in size to supply the inflamed bronchial wall and fibrous tissue. A vicious circle may be established, because a pool of mucus is liable to further infection, which leads to progressive destruction of the bronchial walls.

Clinical Features: Patients with bronchiectasis are seen with chronic productive cough, often with several hundred milliliters of mucopurulent sputum a day. Hemoptysis is a common symptom, owing to erosion by the bronchial inflammation through the wall of the adjacent bronchial arteries. Dyspnea and wheezing are variable, depending on the extent of the disease. Pneumonia is a common complication, and patients with long-standing cases are at risk of chronic hypoxia and pulmonary hypertension. Radiologically, the bronchi appear dilated and have thickened walls. Today the definitive diagnosis is made by CT scans of the lung. Surgical treatment of localized bronchiectasis may be necessary, especially if complications such as severe hemoptysis or pneumonia arise. However, in the generalized disease, surgical resection is more palliative than curative.

Acute, reversible dilation of bronchi may occur as a consequence of bacterial or viral bronchopulmonary infection, and it may take months before the bronchi return to normal size.

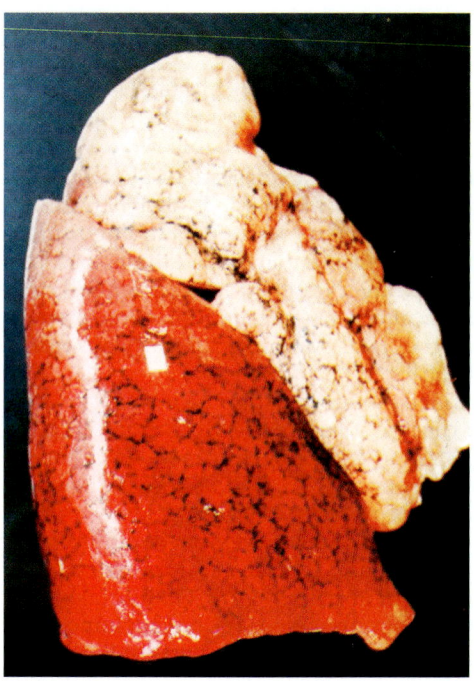

FIGURE *12-11*
Lobar pneumonia. The entire left lower lobe is consolidated and in the stage of red hepatization. The upper lobe is normally expanded.

INFECTIONS

Pulmonary infections are discussed in detail in Chapter 9. The major pulmonary entities are described below, with particular emphasis on pathological features.

Bacterial Pneumonia Remains an Important Cause of Death

Pneumonia *is a generic term that refers to inflammation and consolidation (solidification) of the pulmonary parenchyma.* Traditionally, bacterial pneumonias were classified as either lobar pneumonia or bronchopneumonia, but these terms have little clinical relevance today. In general, the term *lobar pneumonia* refers to consolidation of an entire lobe (Fig. 12-11); *bronchopneumonia* signifies scattered solid foci in the same or several lobes (Fig. 12-12).

Pneumococcal pneumonia was the classic example of lobar pneumonia, but today the involvement of a lobe tends to be incomplete, and more than one lobe is usually affected. By contrast, bronchopneumonia remains a common cause of death and is often found at autopsy. It typically develops in terminally ill patients, usually in the dependent and posterior portions of the lung. Scattered irregular foci of pneumonia are centered on terminal bronchioles and respiratory bronchioles. Bronchiolitis is present, with exudation of polymorphonuclear leukocytes into the adjacent alveoli. Large continuous areas of alveolar involvement do not occur in bronchopneumonia.

Bacterial pneumonias occur in three settings:

- **Community-acquired pneumonia** arises outside the hospital in persons with no primary disorder of the immune system.
- **Nosocomial pneumonia** represents an infection spread by organisms in the hospital environment to particularly susceptible patients.
- **Opportunistic pneumonia** afflicts persons whose immune status is compromised.

Pathogenesis: Most bacteria that cause pneumonia are normal inhabitants of the oropharynx and nasopharynx and reach the alveoli by aspiration of secretions. Other routes of infection include inhalation of microorganisms from the environment, hematogenous dissemination from an infectious focus elsewhere, and (rarely) spread of bacteria from an adjacent site. A change in the oropharyngeal flora from the normal commensals to a virulent organism often precedes the development of pneumonia. A number of conditions predispose to infection by depressing the host defenses, including cigarette smoking, chronic bronchitis, alcoholism, severe malnutrition, wasting diseases, and poorly controlled diabetes. Alterations in oropharyngeal flora commonly occur in debilitated or immunosuppressed patients in the hospital, in whom nosocomial pneumonia can occur in as many as 25%.

Infections

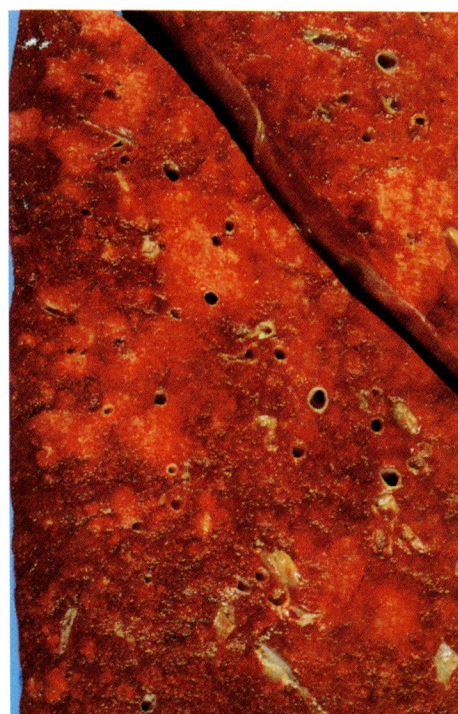

FIGURE 12-12
Bronchopneumonia. Scattered foci of consolidation are centered on bronchi and bronchioles.

Bacterial pneumonias should be classified on the basis of the etiological agent, because the clinical and morphological features, and thus the therapeutic implications, often vary with the causative organism.

Pneumococcal Pneumonia

Despite the impact of antibiotic therapy, pneumonia caused by *Streptococcus pneumoniae* (pneumococcus) remains a significant problem. Pneumococcal pneumonia is principally a disease of young to middle-aged adults. It is rare in infants, less common in the elderly, and considerably more frequent in men than in women.

 Pathogenesis: Pneumococcal pneumonia is mostly a consequence of altered defense barriers in the respiratory tract. Frequently this pneumonia follows a viral infection of the upper respiratory tract (e.g., influenza). The bronchial secretions stimulated by a viral infection provide a hospitable environment for the proliferation of *S. pneumoniae* organisms, which are normal flora of the nasopharynx. The thin, watery secretions carry the organisms into the alveoli, thereby initiating an inflammatory response. The remarkably severe acute inflammation with spreading edema suggests that immunological mechanisms may be involved. The aspiration of pneumococci is also promoted by factors that impair the epiglottic reflex, including exposure to cold, anesthesia, and alcohol intoxication. Injury to the lung caused by factors such as congestive heart failure and irritant gases also renders the lung more susceptible to pneumococcal pneumonia.

The capsule of the pneumococcus provides a defense against phagocytosis by the alveolar macrophages, and the organisms must, therefore, be opsonized before they can be ingested and killed. In an immune-competent person, antipneumococcal antibodies function as opsonins, but a host that has not been exposed to the specific infecting strain of *S. pneumoniae* can achieve opsonization only through the alternative complement pathway.

 Pathology: In the earliest stage of pneumococcal pneumonia, protein-rich edema fluid containing numerous organisms fills the alveoli (Fig. 12-13). Marked congestion of the capillaries is followed by a massive outpouring of polymorphonuclear leukocytes, accompanied by intraalveolar hemorrhage (Fig. 12-14). Because the firm consistency of the affected lung is reminiscent of the liver, this stage has been aptly named *red hepatization*.

The next phase, occurring after 2 or more days, depending on the success of treatment, involves the lysis of polymorphonuclear leukocytes and the appearance of macrophages. The latter phagocytose the fragmented polymorphonuclear leukocytes and other inflammatory debris. At this stage, the congestion has diminished, but the lung still remains firm (*grey hepatization*). The alveolar exudate is then removed, and the lung gradually returns to normal.

A number of complications may follow pneumococcal pneumonia:

- **Pleuritis,** often painful, is common, because the pneumonia readily extends to the pleura.
- **Pleural effusion** occurs frequently, but usually resolves.
- **Pyothorax** results from an infection of a pleural effusion and may heal with extensive fibrosis.
- **Empyema** (a loculated collection of pus with fibrous walls) results from the persistence of pyothorax.
- **Bacteremia** is present in more than 25% of patients in the early stages of pneumococcal pneumonia and may lead to endocarditis or meningitis. Patients whose spleens have been removed often die of this bacteremia.
- **Pulmonary fibrosis** is a rare complication in which the intraalveolar exudate becomes organized and forms intraalveolar plugs of granulation tissue, also known as *organizing pneumonia*. Gradually, increasing alveolar fibrosis leads to a shrunken and firm lobe, a rare complication known as *carnification*.
- **Lung abscess** is an unusual complication of pneumococcal pneumonia.

 Clinical Features: The onset of pneumococcal pneumonia is acute, with fever and chills. Chest pain secondary to pleural involvement is common. Hemoptysis is frequent and is characteristically "rusty," because it is derived from altered blood in alveolar spaces. Radiological examination shows alveolar filling in large areas of lung, producing a solid appearance that extends to

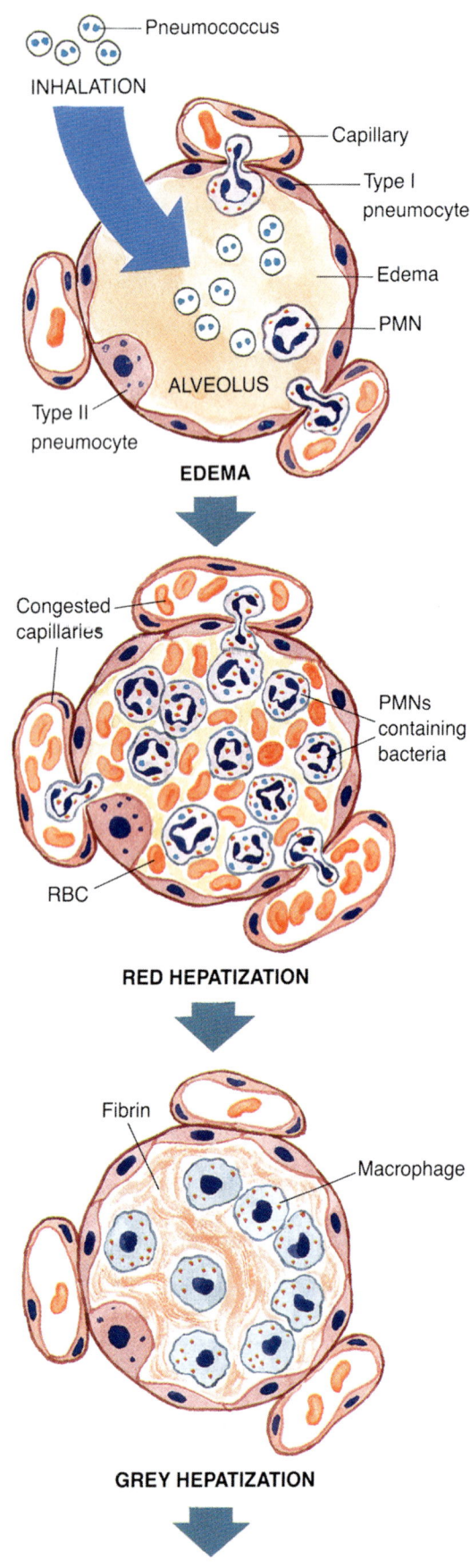

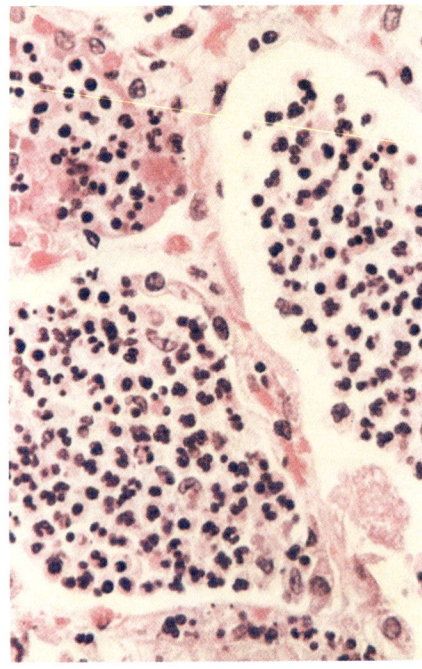

FIGURE 12-14
Pneumococcal pneumonia. The alveoli are packed with an exudate composed of polymorphonuclear leukocytes and occasional macrophages.

entire lobes or segments. Before antibiotic therapy, the clinical course was characterized by severe fever, dyspnea, debility, and even loss of consciousness. The dramatic event was the *crisis*, occurring 5 to 10 days after the onset of respiratory symptoms, when the moribund patient would suddenly become afebrile and return from death's door. The satisfactory resolution of the crisis was the result of the immune response to the infection. Unfortunately, all too often the outcome was not favorable, and in one third of cases, the patient died. However, in the modern era, pneumococcal pneumonia is treated effectively with antibiotics. Although the symptoms of pneumonia respond rapidly to antibiotic therapy, radiologically, the lesion still takes several days to resolve.

Klebsiella Pneumonia

Other than *S. pneumoniae*, *Klebsiella pneumoniae* is the only organism that causes lobar pneumonia with any frequency.

FIGURE 12-13
Pathogenesis of pneumococcal lobar pneumonia. Pneumococci, characteristically in pairs (diplococci), multiply rapidly in the alveolar spaces and produce extensive edema. They incite an acute inflammatory response in which polymorphonuclear leukocytes and congestion are prominent (red hepatization). As the inflammatory process progresses, macrophages replace the polymorphonuclear leukocytes and ingest debris (grey hepatization). The process usually resolves, but complications may ensue.

However, it accounts for no more than 1% of all cases of community-acquired pneumonia. The disease is commonly associated with alcoholism and is seen most frequently in middle-aged men, although persons with diabetes and chronic pulmonary disease are also at risk.

Pathology: The stages in *Klebsiella* pneumonia are not so well described as those in pneumococcal pneumonia, but the congestion and hemorrhage in the acute phase are less pronounced. *K. pneumoniae* has a thick, gelatinous capsule, a feature that is responsible for the characteristic mucoid appearance of the cut surface of the lung. Another distinctive feature of *Klebsiella* pneumonia is an increase in the size of the affected lobe, so that the fissure "bulges" toward the unaffected region. There is a tendency toward necrosis of tissue and abscess formation. A serious complication is *bronchopleural fistula*, (i.e., a communication between the bronchial airway and the pleural space).

The onset of *Klebsiella* pneumonia is less dramatic than that of pneumococcal pneumonia, but the disease may be more dangerous. Before the antibiotic era, mortality rates in *Klebsiella* pneumonia ranged from 50 to 80%. Even with prompt antibiotic treatment, the mortality is still considerable.

Staphylococcal Pneumonia

Staphylococcal pneumonia is an uncommon community-acquired disease, accounting for only 1% of these bacterial pneumonias. However, pulmonary infection with *S. aureus* is common as a superinfection after influenza and other viral respiratory tract infections. In the 1918 influenza pandemic, it was a major cause of death. Repeated episodes of staphylococcal pneumonia are encountered in patients with cystic fibrosis, owing to colonization of the bronchiectatic airways. Nosocomial staphylococcal pneumonia typically occurs in weakened, chronically ill patients, who are prone to aspiration, and in intubated persons.

Pathology: Like staphylococcal infection elsewhere, staphylococcal pneumonia is characterized by the development of abscesses. In contrast to the classic solitary lung abscess, the multiple foci of staphylococcal pneumonia produce many small abscesses. In infants and, to a lesser extent, in adults, these may lead to *pneumatoceles*, thin-walled cystic spaces lined primarily by respiratory tissue. Pneumatoceles may expand rapidly and compress the surrounding lung or they may rupture into the pleural cavity and cause a tension pneumothorax. A pneumatocele develops when an abscess breaks into an airway, thereby allowing the expansion of the former by the pressure of inspired air. Cavitation and pleural effusions are common complications of staphylococcal pneumonia, but empyema is infrequent.

Staphylococcal pneumonia requires aggressive antibiotic treatment, particularly in view of the numerous antibiotic-resistant strains of *S. aureus*.

Streptococcal Pneumonia

Pulmonary infection with group A *Streptococcus pyogenes* was identified among soldiers as early as the 19th century, and its pathological features were described during World War I. Streptococcal pneumonia typically follows viral respiratory tract infections and is thought to have been the common superinfection in the 1918–1919 influenza pandemic. It is distinctly unusual in a community setting but is occasionally encountered in debilitated persons.

Pathology: On gross examination, the lungs of patients who die of streptococcal pneumonia are heavy and display bloody edema. Dry consolidation (hepatization) is not a feature of the disease. Microscopically, the alveoli are filled with fibrin-containing fluid, but neutrophils are few. After prolonged pneumonia, alveolar necrosis may be encountered. Empyema is a common complication.

Clinical Features: Patients with streptococcal pneumonia have abrupt fever, dyspnea, cough, chest pain, hemoptysis, and often cyanosis. Radiologically, a pattern of bronchopneumonia is observed, and lobar consolidation is not seen. Intensive antibiotic therapy is indicated.

Streptococcal pneumonia in the newborn is usually caused by group B streptococci (*S. agalactiae*), a normal resident of the female genital tract. The symptoms are similar to those of the infantile respiratory distress syndrome. The infants, however, are often full term, have severe toxemia, and may die within a few hours.

Legionella Pneumonia

In 1976, a mysterious respiratory ailment that carried a high mortality broke out at an American Legion convention in Philadelphia. The responsible organism, *Legionella pneumophila*, was soon identified as a fastidious bacterium, with special requirements to grow in culture. Serological and histological studies revealed that several previously unrecognized epidemics of the same disease had occurred.

Legionella organisms thrive in aquatic environments, and outbreaks of pneumonia have been traced to contaminated water in air-conditioning cooling towers, evaporative condensers, and construction sites. Person-to-person spread does not occur, and there is no animal or human reservoir.

Pathology: In fatal cases of *Legionella* pneumonia, multiple lobes exhibit a bronchopneumonia, with large confluent areas. Microscopically, the alveoli contain fibrin and inflammatory cells, with either neutrophils or macrophages predominating. Necrosis of inflammatory cells (leukocytoclasis) may be extensive. If the patient survives for several weeks, the exudate may show fibrous organization. One third of cases have been complicated by empyema. The *Legionella* organisms are usually abundant within and without the phagocytic cells. They are difficult to visualize with conventional stains and are gram negative with the Brown and Hopp's stain. Silver impregnation methods and immunofluorescent stains highlight the bacteria.

 Clinical Features: The onset of *Legionella* pneumonia tends to be abrupt, with malaise, fever, muscle aches and pains, and, curiously, abdominal pain. A productive cough is usual, and chest pain due to pleuritis occasionally occurs. The chest radiograph is variable, but the most common pattern is the presence of focal alveolar infiltrates, which may be bilateral. The symptoms are usually less severe than the chest radiographs suggest. Mortality has been high (10–20%), especially in immunocompromised patients. Erythromycin is the antibiotic of choice.

Pontiac fever, also caused by *Legionella* species, is mainly a febrile illness with slight respiratory symptoms, radiological abnormalities, and a good prognosis. It has occurred in epidemics in office buildings and affects apparently healthy persons.

Opportunistic Pneumonia Caused by Gram-Negative Bacteria

Pneumonias caused by gram-negative organisms have become more common with the advent of immunosuppressive and cytotoxic therapies, treatment with broad-spectrum antibiotics, and the epidemic of AIDS. The most common bacteria are *Escherichia coli* and *Pseudomonas aeruginosa*.

ESCHERICHIA COLI: Pneumonia caused by *E. coli* is a recognized complication of bacteremia after gastrointestinal and urogenital surgery, even in patients who are not immunosuppressed. It also is encountered in cancer patients given chemotherapy and in persons with chronic lung or heart disease. It occurs as a bronchopneumonia and responds poorly to treatment.

PSEUDOMONAS AERUGINOSA: *Pseudomonas* pneumonia is most often seen in immunocompromised persons, in patients with burns, and in those with cystic fibrosis. A history of antibiotic treatment of another infection is common. Often an infectious vasculitis, in which large numbers of organisms can be seen in the wall of a blood vessel, results in pulmonary infarction. *Pseudomonas* infection is common in cystic fibrosis, probably because of the favorable environment provided by the abnormal bronchial secretions. Antibiotic treatment of *Pseudomonas* pneumonia is often unsatisfactory.

Pneumonia Caused by Anaerobic Organisms

Many anaerobic organisms are normal commensals of the oral cavity, especially in patients with poor dental hygiene. These include certain streptococci, fusobacteria, and *Bacteroides* species. Aspiration of these organisms commonly occurs with swallowing disorders, as seen in stuporous alcoholics, anesthetized patients, and persons subject to seizures. Pulmonary infection with anaerobic organisms leads to necrotizing pneumonias, which are frequently complicated by lung abscesses. The most dramatic complication is gangrene of the lung, a result of thrombosis of a branch of the pulmonary artery and consequent infarction. This is regarded as a medical emergency and requires resection of the affected lung.

Psittacosis

Psittacosis is a pulmonary infection that results from the inhalation of **Chlamydia psittaci** *in dust contaminated with excreta from birds, usually pets and often parrots.* It is characterized by severe systemic symptoms, with fever, malaise, and muscle aches, but surprisingly few respiratory symptoms other than cough. Chest radiographs may be negative, and when abnormal, they show irregular consolidation and an interstitial pattern. The morphological patterns in most cases are unknown, but the disease is likely to be an interstitial pneumonia. In fatal cases, varying degrees of diffuse alveolar damage are present, together with edema, intraalveolar pneumonia, and necrosis.

Anthrax Pneumonia and Pneumonic Plague

Recent world events have refocused a great deal of attention toward infectious agents that may be used as potential weapons of bioterrorism. Chief among these are *Bacillus anthracis* and *Yersinia pestis*.

Bacillus anthracis, the causative agent of anthrax, is a gram-positive spore-forming bacillus. Anthrax occurs in many species of domestic animals, and infection of humans is seen infrequently or in sporadic outbreaks. Transmission is via direct contact with the spores, and person-to-person transmission is uncommon. Cutaneous anthrax is rarely fatal, whereas inhalational anthrax has a high mortality. Anthrax spores are highly resistant to drying, and when inhaled they are transported to the mediastinal lymph nodes. From there, the bacilli emerge and are rapidly transmitted through the bloodstream to other organs, including the lungs. Hemorrhagic necrosis of the infected organs ensues, the most pronounced of which is a hemorrhagic mediastinal mass. In the lungs, the disease is manifested by hemorrhagic bronchitis and confluent areas of hemorrhagic pneumonia.

Yersinia pestis, the causative agent of *plague,* produces two forms of infection, a bubonic form and a pneumonic form. In pneumonic plague the organisms are inhaled directly without transmission by an arthropod vector, and the disease may be spread from person to person,. The lungs typically show extensive hemorrhagic bronchopneumonia, pleuritis, and enlargement of mediastinal lymph nodes. The untreated disease progresses rapidly and is highly fatal.

Mycoplasma Pneumoniae Causes Atypical Pneumonia

In contrast to lobar pneumonia, the onset of atypical pneumonia is insidious, leukocytosis is absent or slight, and the course is prolonged. Respiratory symptoms may be minimal or severe, and the chest radiograph shows a patchy intraalveolar pneumonia or an interstitial infiltrate. The infection characteristically causes a bronchiolitis with a neutrophilic intraluminal exudate and an intense lymphoplasmacytic infiltrate in the bronchiolar wall (Fig. 12-15). Mycoplasma lack the rigid cell wall characteristic of most bacteria and are thus slow growing and often difficult to isolate by traditional culture methods. The diagnosis is often established clinically on the basis of serological studies detecting *M. pneumoniae* antibodies or cold agglutinins. Erythromycin is an effective antibiotic, and the infection is only rarely fatal.

Tuberculosis Is the Classic Granulomatous Infection

No chest disease has had as dramatic a history as tuberculosis. Known since ancient Egypt, it became the scourge of 19th century Europe and North America. There was an exponential decline in the prevalence of tuberculosis in the 20th century, and the advent of antituberculosis drugs has further diminished the impact of the disease. However, the recent resurgence of tuberculosis and the emergence of drug-resistant strains, particularly among patients with AIDS, has rekindled interest in this disease. The infection is discussed in detail in Chapter 9, and here we consider only the pulmonary pathology.

Tuberculosis represents infection with *Mycobacterium tuberculosis*, although atypical mycobacterial infections may mimic tuberculosis. The disease is divided into primary and secondary (or reactivation) tuberculosis.

PRIMARY TUBERCULOSIS: The disease is acquired from the initial exposure to *M. tuberculosis*, most commonly as a result of inhaling infected aerosols produced by coughing by a person with cavitary tuberculosis. The inhaled organisms multiply in the alveoli because the alveolar macrophages cannot readily kill the bacteria.

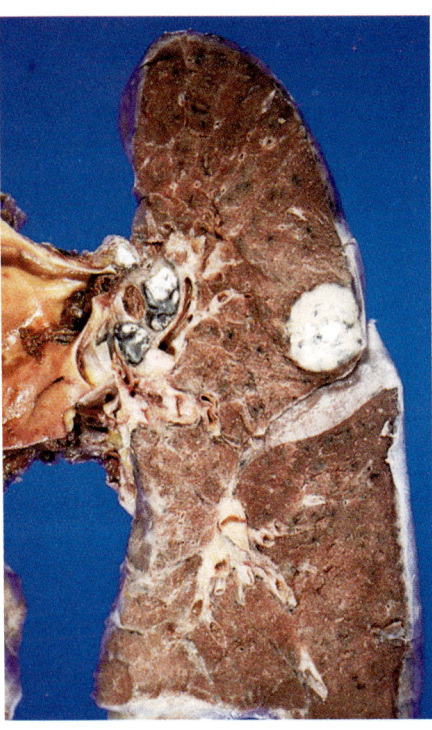

FIGURE 12-16
Primary tuberculosis. A healed Ranke complex is represented by a subpleural nodule and involved hilar lymph nodes.

 Pathology: The **Ghon complex** is the first lesion of primary tuberculosis and consists of a peripheral parenchymal granuloma, often in the upper lobes. When it is associated with an enlarged mediastinal lymph node a *Ranke complex* is formed (Fig. 12-16). On gross examination, the healed, subpleural Ghon nodule is 1 to 2 cm in diameter, well circumscribed, and centrally necrotic. In later stages, the lesion is fibrotic and calcified. Microscopically, a granuloma with central caseous necrosis (Fig. 12-17) shows varying degrees of fibrosis. The microscopic features of the draining hilar lymph nodes are similar to those of the peripheral parenchymal lesion.

Most (90% or more) primary infections are asymptomatic, and the lesions remain localized and heal. In some instances, self-limited extension to the pleura, with secondary

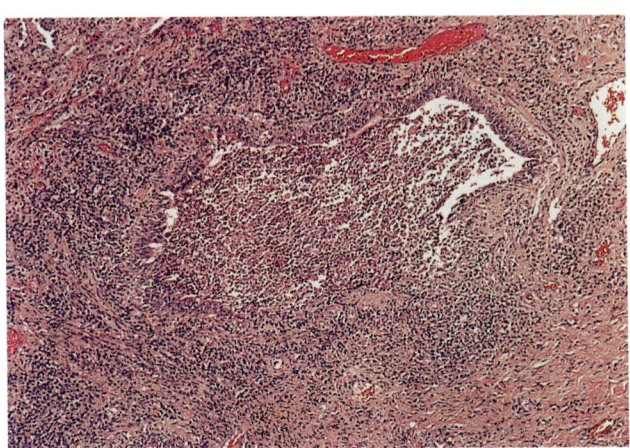

FIGURE 12-15
Mycoplasma pneumonia. Chronic bronchiolitis with a neutrophilic luminal exudate.

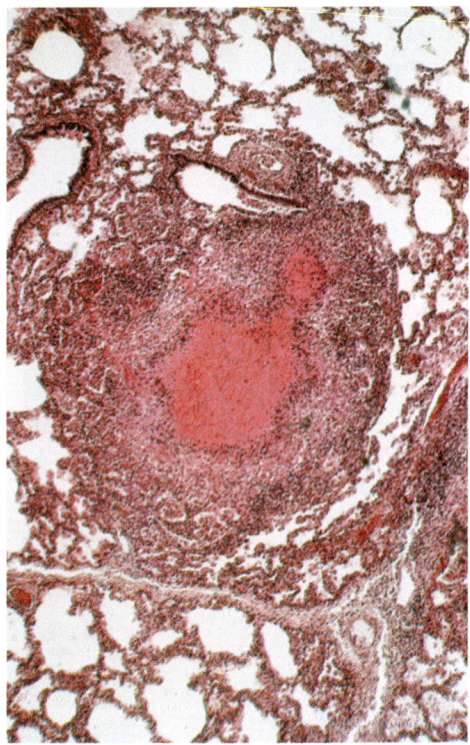

FIGURE 12-17
Necrotizing granuloma due to *M. tuberculosis*. A small tuberculous granuloma with conspicuous central caseation is present in the pulmonary parenchyma. The necrotic center is surrounded by histiocytes, giant cells, and fibrous tissue.

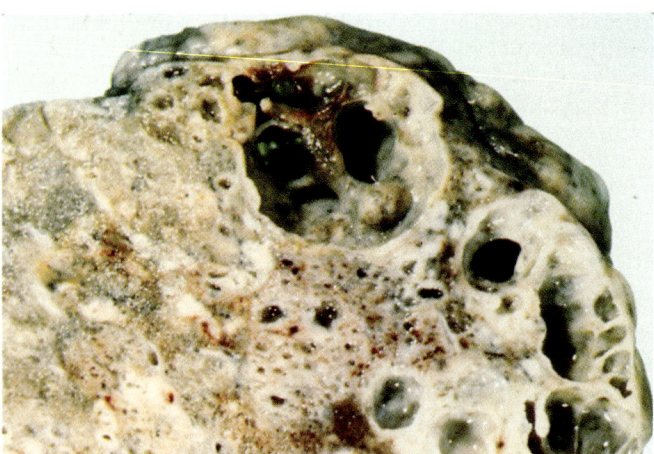

FIGURE 12-18
Cavitary tuberculosis. The apex of the left upper lobe shows tuberculous cavities surrounded by consolidated and fibrotic pulmonary parenchyma that contains small tubercles.

pleural effusion, occurs. Less commonly, primary tuberculosis does not remain limited but spreads to other parts of the lung *(progressive primary tuberculosis)*. This condition is usually seen in early childhood or in immunosuppressed adults. The initial lesion enlarges, producing necrotic areas up to 6 cm or more in greatest dimension. Central liquefaction results in cavities, which may expand to occupy most of the lower lobe. At the same time, the draining lymph nodes display similar histological changes. Erosion of a bronchus by the necrotizing process leads to further pulmonary dissemination of the disease.

SECONDARY TUBERCULOSIS: This stage represents either the reactivation of primary pulmonary tuberculosis or a new infection in a host previously sensitized by primary tuberculosis.

 Pathology: The initial reaction to *M. tuberculosis* is different in secondary tuberculosis. A cellular immune response occurs after a latent interval and leads to the formation of many granulomas and extensive tissue necrosis. The apical and posterior segments of the upper lobes are most commonly involved, but the superior segment of the lower lobe is also often affected, and no part of the lung can be excluded. A diffuse, fibrotic, poorly defined lesion develops, which displays focal areas of caseous necrosis. Often these foci heal and calcify, but some erode into a bronchus, after which drainage of infectious material creates a tuberculous cavity.

Tuberculous cavities range in size from less than 1 cm in diameter to large, cystic areas that occupy almost the entire lung. Most cavities measure 3 to 10 cm in diameter and tend to be situated in the apices of the upper lobes (Fig. 12-18), although they may occur anywhere in the lung. The wall of the cavity is composed of an inner, thin, gray membrane encompassing soft necrotic nodules; a middle zone of granulation tissue; and an outer collagenous border. The lumen is filled with caseous material containing acid-fast bacilli. The tuberculous cavity often communicates freely with a bronchus, and release of the infectious material into the airways serves to disseminate the infection within the lung. The walls of healed tuberculous cavities eventually become fibrotic and calcified.

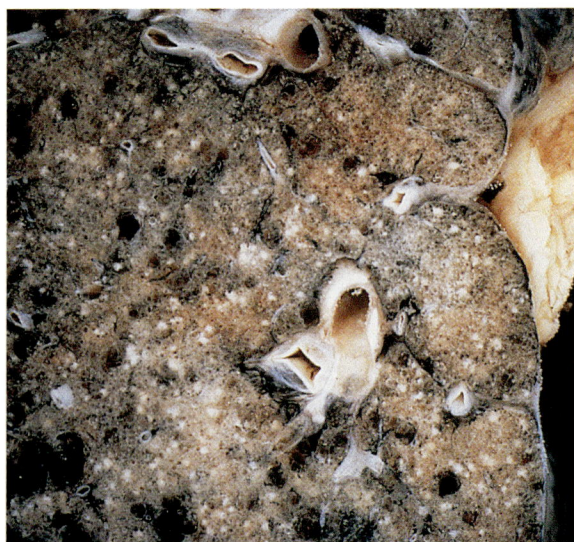

FIGURE 12-19
Miliary tuberculosis. Multiple millimeter-sized nodules are scattered throughout the lung parenchyma.

Secondary tuberculosis is associated with a number of complications:

- **Miliary tuberculosis** refers to the presence of multiple, small (size of millet seeds) tuberculous granulomas (Fig. 12-19) in many organs. It results from the hematogenous dissemination of the organisms, usually from secondary pulmonary tuberculosis, but occasionally from primary pulmonary tuberculosis or from other sites.
- **Hemoptysis** is caused by the erosion of small pulmonary arteries in the wall of a cavity. It may be severe enough to drown patients in their own blood.
- **Bronchopleural fistula** occurs when a subpleural cavity ruptures into the pleural space. In turn, tuberculous empyema and pneumothorax result.
- **Tuberculous laryngitis** is a consequence of coughing up infectious material.
- **Intestinal tuberculosis** may follow the swallowing of the same tuberculous material.
- **Aspergilloma** is a fungal mass that follows superinfection of a persistent open cavity with *Aspergillus*; it may fill the entire cavity.

MYCOBACTERIUM AVIUM-INTRACELLULARE (MAI): In AIDS patients, the ability to form a granulomatous reaction may be impaired, and MAI pneumonia is characterized by an extensive infiltrate of macrophages and innumerable acid-fast organisms (Fig. 12-20).

Actinomycosis Features Multiple Lung Abscesses

Actinomycosis is caused by infection with actinomycetes, and the usual pulmonary organism is *Actinomyces israelii*. Although actinomycetes resemble fungi in appearance, they are more closely related to bacteria. These gram-positive organisms, which normally inhabit the mouth and nose, infect the lung either by aspiration of oropharyngeal contents or by extension from an actinomycotic subdiaphragmatic abscess or liver abscess.

Pathology: The lung lesions consist of multiple, interconnecting, small lung abscesses. The margin of an abscess is granulomatous, but the central necrotic area is purulent and contains colonies of organisms, which form "sulfur granules." The colonies consist of thin, branching, filamentous gram-positive bacteria. Clubbed basophilic filaments are noted at the margins of the colonies, which are visible to the naked eye as small yellow particles (sulfur granules). The abscesses invade the pleura and produce bronchopulmonary fistulas and empyema. They may also invade the chest wall.

Nocardia Is Usually an Opportunistic Organism

Nocardia is a gram-positive bacillus that causes an acute progressive or chronic bacterial pneumonia. It is frequently encountered in immunocompromised persons, particularly patients with lymphomas, neutropenia, chronic granulomatous disease of childhood, and pulmonary alveolar proteinosis. *N. asteroides* is the most common species to cause pneumonia.

Pathology: Histologically, the lungs show abscesses (Fig. 12-21A), which may have granulomatous features in chronic infections. The organisms are delicate, beaded, thin filaments, which branch mostly at

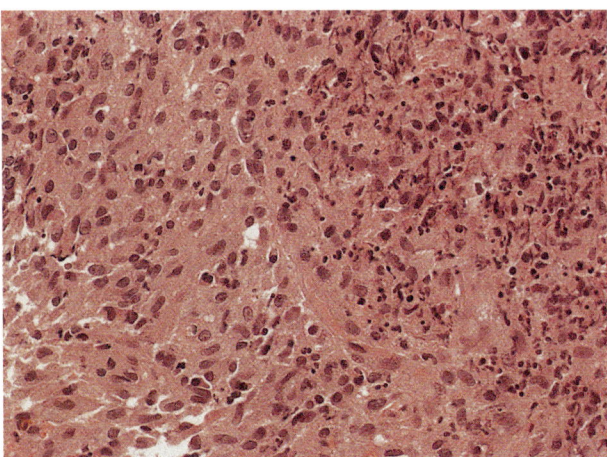
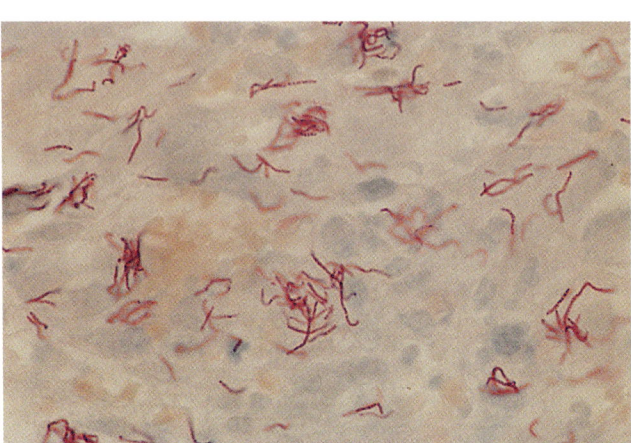

FIGURE 12-20
Mycobacterium avium-intracellulare pneumonia in AIDS. A. The pneumonia is characterized by an extensive infiltrate of macrophages. B. The Ziehl-Neelsen stain shows numerous acid-fast organisms.

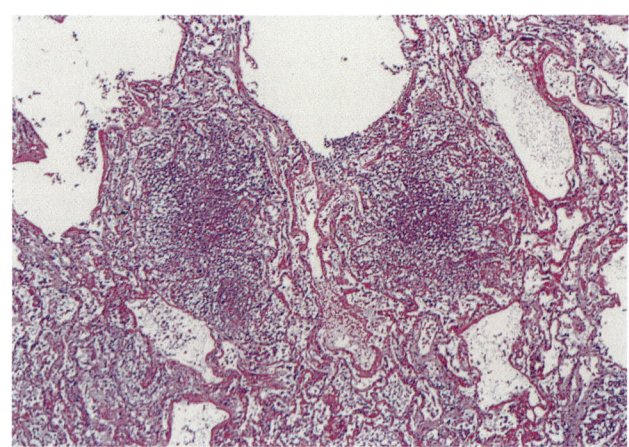
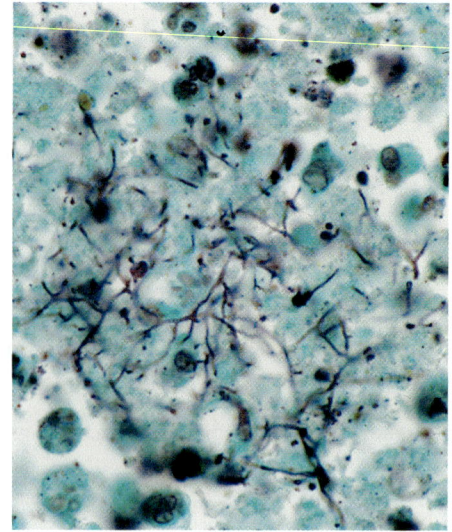

FIGURE 12-21
Nocardiosis. A. This lung shows abscesses consisting of focal collections of acute inflammation. B. The organisms are thin, filamentous, branching bacteria (Gomori methenamine silver).

right angles (see Fig. 12-21B). The highly branching pattern may resemble "Chinese characters." In tissue sections, the organisms are best seen with the Gomori methenamine silver stain (see Fig. 12-21B) or a gram stain. They are also weakly acid fast.

Fungal Infections are Geographic or Opportunistic

Histoplasmosis

Histoplasmosis is a disease of the midwestern and southeastern regions of the United States, particularly the Mississippi and Ohio valleys. The disease is caused by inhalation of *Histoplasma capsulatum* in infected dust, commonly from bird droppings.

 Pathology: Histoplasmosis has many clinical and pathological similarities to tuberculosis. Most infections are asymptomatic and result in lesions comparable to the Ghon complex, including a parenchymal granuloma and similar lesions in the draining lymph nodes. The granulomas are particularly prone to calcify, often with a concentric laminar pattern. The acute phase, in which numerous organisms are seen within macrophages, is followed by granulomatous inflammation, with central areas of necrosis in the lesions. The granulomas heal by fibrosis and calcification, although the central necrotic areas may persist.

In a few cases, the pulmonary lesion progresses or reactivates, which leads to a progressive fibrotic and necrotic lesion that closely resembles reactivation tuberculosis. However, the lesion of histoplasmosis has a more fibrotic appearance than that of tuberculosis, and cavitation is less common. The reason for progression is not known, although a large infective dose and a poor host response are usually considered to be responsible. Immunocompromised persons are at particular risk for dissemination of *Histoplasma* within the lungs and spread to other organs.

Coccidioidomycosis

Coccidioidomycosis, caused by the inhalation of spores of *Coccidioides immitis,* was originally known as San Joaquin Valley fever, after the location where the disease has been endemic for many years. However, the infection is widely spread throughout the southwestern part of the United States and shares many of the clinical and pathological features of histoplasmosis and tuberculosis.

 Pathology: In most instances, the lesions are limited to a peripheral parenchymal granuloma, with or without lymph node granulomas. In a few instances, the lesion is progressive, although the rate of progression is slow. Immunocompromised persons may experience rapid progression of the disease, with release of endospores into the lung, in which case the tissue reaction may be purulent as well as granulomatous.

Cryptococcosis

Cryptococcosis results from the inhalation of spores of *Cryptococcus neoformans,* an organism frequently encountered in pigeon droppings. The pulmonary lesions range from small parenchymal granulomas to several large granulomatous nodules, pneumonic consolidation, and even cavitation. Most serious cases of pulmonary cryptococcosis occur in immunocompromised persons, in whom the organisms proliferate extensively within alveolar spaces, with little tissue reaction.

North American Blastomycosis

Blastomycosis is an uncommon condition caused by *Blastomyces dermatitidis*. It is concentrated in the basins of the Missouri, Mississippi, and Ohio rivers in the United States and in southern Manitoba and northwestern Ontario in Canada. The clinical and pathological features resemble those associated with the fungi mentioned earlier. The infection manifests as a lesion resembling a Ghon complex or as a progressive pneumonitis. Unlike the tuberculous Ghon complex, the focal lesion of blastomycosis exhibits central necrosis with a purulent reaction, surrounded by granulomatous inflammation.

Aspergillosis

Infection of the lungs by *Aspergillus* species, usually *A. niger* or *A. fumigatus,* can occur under a number of circumstances.

- **Invasive aspergillosis:** This is the most serious manifestation of *Aspergillus* infection, occurring almost exclusively as an opportunistic infection in persons with compromised immunity, usually because of cytotoxic therapy or AIDS. The lungs exhibit patchy, multifocal areas of consolidation and occasionally cavities. Extensive blood vessel invasion (usually arterial [Fig. 12-22]) results in occlusion, thrombosis, and infarction of lung tissue. Invasive aspergillosis is a fulminant pulmonary infection that is not amenable to therapy.
- **Aspergilloma ("fungus ball" or mycetoma):** *Aspergillus* species may grow in preexisting cavities, such as those caused by tuberculosis or bronchiectasis. They proliferate to form a fungus ball within the cavities (Fig. 12-23).

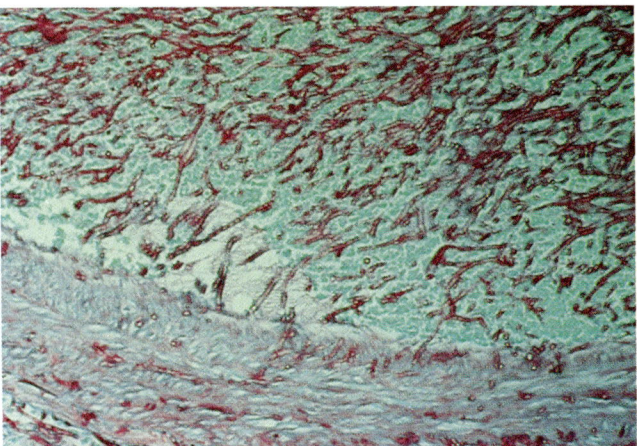

FIGURE 12-22
Invasive pulmonary aspergillosis. A branch of the pulmonary artery shows fungal hyphae in the wall and within the lumen.

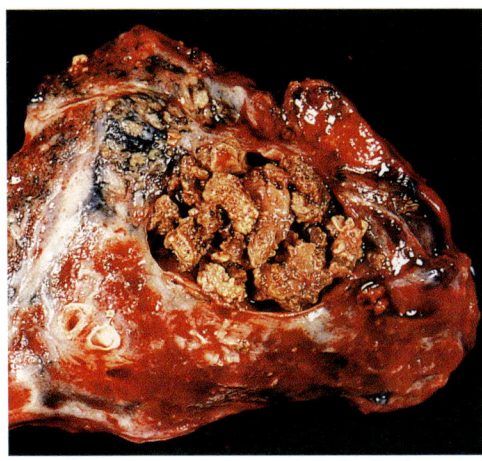

FIGURE 12-23
***Aspergillus* fungus ball. The lung contains a cavity filled with a fungus ball.**

Radiological examination shows a large mass within a cavity that is separated from the wall by air. In most instances, the fungus ball is clinically unrecognized and represents merely an interesting radiological finding. However, sometimes it becomes clinically evident, the most important symptom being hemoptysis, owing either to the underlying condition, or less commonly, to fungal infection of the cavity wall.

- **Allergic bronchopulmonary aspergillosis (ABPA):** Certain asthmatic persons demonstrate an unusual immunological reaction to *Aspergillus* characterized by (1) transient pulmonary infiltrates on chest radiographs, (2) eosinophilia of blood and sputum, (3) skin sensitivity and serum precipitins to *A. fumigatus*, and (4) increased levels of serum IgE. Radiologically, thickened bronchial walls and mucous plugs in the bronchi are visualized

 Pathology: Morphologically, proximal (central) bronchiectasis, involving segmental bronchi and the next two to four orders of subsegmental bronchi, is almost invariable. Histologically, the lungs show bronchial and bronchiolar mucous plugs, with infiltrates of eosinophils (Fig. 12-24A,B). Bronchocentric granulomatosis and eosinophilic pneumonia may be present. The bronchial mucus may contain septate, branching fungal hyphae, with 45° branching. Interestingly, the peripheral bronchial tree is spared.

Clinically, patients with ABPA have wheezing, chest pain, and cough, commonly producing thick mucous plugs. The administration of systemic corticosteroids usually controls the acute episode.

Pneumocystis carinii

First described as "plasma cell pneumonia," pulmonary infection with *Pneumocystis carinii* was identified in malnourished infants at the end of World War II. The disease came into prominence in North America with the advent of

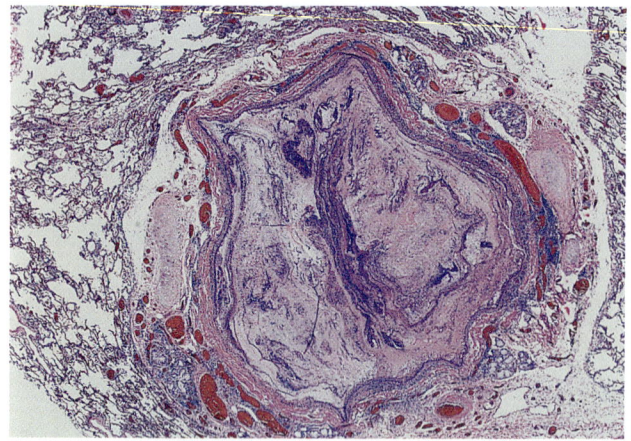
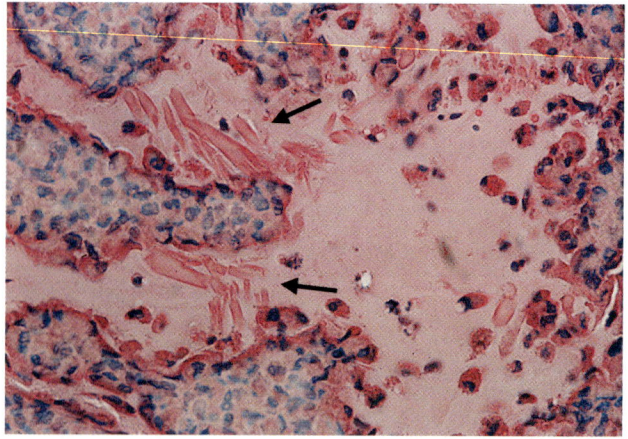

FIGURE 12-24
Allergic bronchopulmonary aspergillosis. A. A dilated bronchus is filled with a mucous plug that has dense layers of eosinophilic infiltrates. B. Higher magnification shows numerous eosinophils and Charcot-Leyden crystals *(arrows)*.

renal transplantation and immunosuppression. Since then, it has been recognized as a major pulmonary complication of chemotherapy for malignant disease. **It is also the most frequent cause of infectious pneumonia in patients with AIDS.** Once considered a protozoan, *Pneumocystis* has been reclassified as a fungus.

Pathology: The classic lesion of *Pneumocystis* pneumonia comprises an interstitial infiltrate of plasma cells and lymphocytes, diffuse alveolar damage (see below), and hyperplasia of type II pneumocytes. The alveoli are filled with a characteristic foamy exudate, the organisms appearing as small bubbles in a background of proteinaceous exudate (Fig. 12-25A). With silver impregnation, the cysts appear as round or indented ("crescent moon") bodies, 5 μm in diameter (see Fig. 12-25B). A darkly stained focus represents focal thickening of the capsule. After sporozoites develop within the cyst, it ruptures and assumes an indented shape. The sporozoites develop into trophozoites, which may be recognized with stains such as Giemsa in cytological specimens; they are very difficult to see in routine histological sections. Granulomatous inflammation in *Pneumocystis* pneumonia is rare but may be seen in up to 5% of lung biopsies from HIV-infected patients.

Clinical Features: Clinically and radiologically, the presentation of *Pneumocystis* pneumonia is variable. At one extreme, the symptoms are minimal; at the other, there is rapidly progressive respiratory failure. In HIV-infected patients, thin-walled cysts may develop and predispose to pneumothorax. The diagnosis is made by identifying the organism with a variety of procedures including sputum examination, bronchoalveolar lavage, transbronchial biopsy, needle aspiration of the lung, and open-lung biopsy. Treatment is with trimethoprim–sulfamethoxazole or pentamidine.

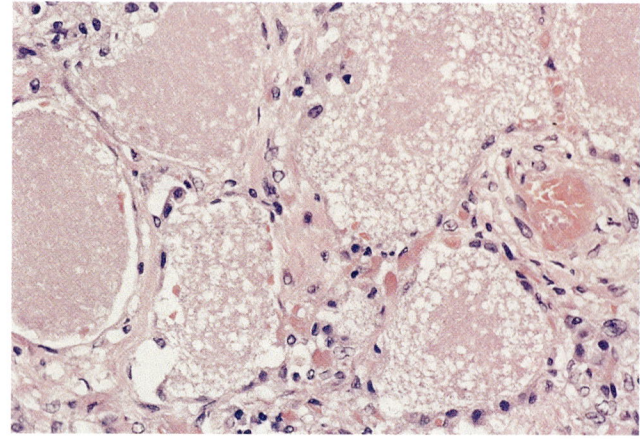
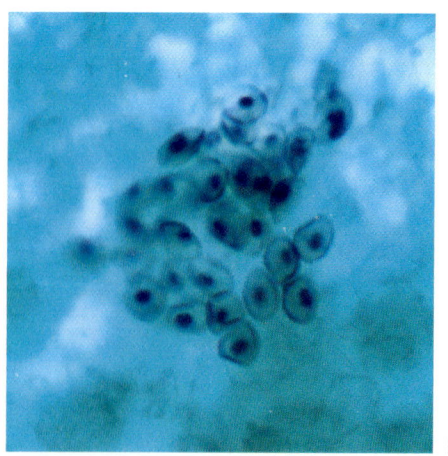

FIGURE 12-25
Pneumocystis carinii pneumonia. A. The alveoli are filled with a foamy exudate, and the interstitium is thickened and contains a chronic inflammatory infiltrate. B. A centrifuged bronchoalveolar lavage specimen impregnated with silver shows a cluster of *Pneumocystis* cysts.

Viral Pneumonia Features Interstitial Inflammation

Viral infections of the pulmonary parenchyma produce diffuse alveolar damage and interstitial (rather than alveolar) pneumonia.

Pathology: Initially, viral infections affect the alveolar epithelium and result in a mononuclear infiltrate in the interstitium of the lung (Fig. 12-26). Necrosis of type I epithelial cells and the formation of hyaline membranes result in an appearance that is indistinguishable from diffuse alveolar damage from other causes. In some instances, the alveolar damage may be indolent, in which case the disease is characterized by hyperplasia of type II pneumocytes and interstitial inflammation. This appearance contrasts with that of most bacterial infections, in which an intraalveolar exudate predominates and in which the interstitium is only incidentally involved (Fig. 12-27).

Cytomegalovirus produces a characteristic interstitial pneumonia. Initially described in infants, it is now well recognized in immunocompromised persons. This viral pneumonia features an intense interstitial infiltrate of lymphocytes. The alveoli are lined by type II cells that have regenerated to cover the epithelial defect left by necrosis of type I cells. The infected alveolar cells are very large (cytomegaly) and display a single, dark, basophilic nuclear inclusion with a peripheral halo and multiple indistinct cytoplasmic, basophilic inclusions (Fig. 12-28).

Measles infection, which involves both the airways and the parenchyma, is characterized by the presence of very large (100 μm across) multinucleated giant cells that have nuclear inclusions and large eosinophilic cytoplasmic inclusions (Fig. 12-29). Although interstitial pneumonia is a well-characterized complication of measles, it is rarely fatal, except in immunocompromised, previously unexposed persons.

Varicella infection (both chickenpox and herpes zoster) produces disseminated, focally necrotic lesions in the lung, as well as interstitial pneumonia. Pulmonary involvement is usually asymptomatic, except in immunocompromised hosts, in whom it may be fatal. The viral inclusions are nuclear, eosinophilic, and refractile and are surrounded by a clear halo. Multinucleation can occur.

Herpes simplex can cause a necrotizing tracheobronchitis as well as diffuse alveolar damage. The viral inclusions are identical to those seen in varicella infection.

Adenovirus pneumonia results in a necrotizing bronchiolitis and bronchopneumonia. It can cause two types of nuclear inclusions: eosinophilic nuclear inclusions surrounded by a clear halo and "smudge cells" with indistinct, basophilic, nuclear inclusions that fill the entire nucleus and are surrounded by only a thin rim of chromatin. (Fig. 12-30).

Lung Abscess Is Usually Caused By Aspiration

Lung abscess, recognized since the time of Hippocrates, is a localized accumulation of pus accompanied by the destruction of pulmonary parenchyma, including alveoli, airways, and blood vessels.

Pathogenesis: The most common cause of pulmonary abscess is aspiration, often in the setting of depressed consciousness. Most (>90%) cases of lung abscess reflect the aspiration of anaerobic bacteria from the oropharynx. The infections are typically polymicrobial, with fusiform bacteria and *Bacteroides* species often isolated. Other organisms encountered in lung abscesses caused by aspiration include *S. aureus, K. pneumoniae, S. pneumoniae,* and *Nocardia.*

The deposition of enough bacteria to produce a lung abscess requires two conditions. A large number of anaerobic bacteria must be present in the oral flora, a situation encountered in persons with poor oral hygiene or periodontal disease. In addition, the cough reflex or tracheobronchial clearance must be impaired. Not surprisingly, alcoholism is the single most common condition predisposing to lung abscess. Persons with drug overdose, epileptics, and neurologically impaired patients are also at risk. Other causes of lung abscess include necrotizing pneumonias, bronchial obstruction, infected pulmonary emboli, penetrating trauma, and extension of infection from tissues adjacent to the lung.

Pathology: Lung abscesses mostly range from 2 to 6 cm in diameter, and 10 to 20% have multiple cavities, usually after a necrotizing pneumonia or a shower of septic pulmonary emboli. The right side of the lung is more prone than is the left to the development of a lung abscess, because the right main bronchus follows the direction of the trachea more closely at its bifurcation. Acute lung abscesses are not well separated from the surrounding pulmonary parenchyma. They exhibit abundant polymorphonuclear leukocytes and, depending on the age of the lesion, variable numbers of macrophages. Debris derived from necrotic tissue may be evident. The abscess is surrounded by hemorrhage, fibrin, and inflammatory cells. As the abscess ages, a fibrous wall forms around the margin. Lung abscesses differ from those elsewhere in their capacity for spontaneous drainage. The cavity thus formed contains air, necrotic debris, and inflammatory exudate (Fig. 12-31), creating a fluid level that is easily visualized radiographically. The lining of the cavity becomes covered with regenerating squamous epithelium. In an old abscess, the wall may become lined by ciliated respiratory epithelium, making the cavity difficult to distinguish from bronchiectasis.

Clinical Features: Almost all patients with lung abscess are first seen with cough and fever. One of the most characteristic symptoms is the production of large amounts of foul-smelling sputum. Many patients complain of pleuritic chest pain, and 20% develop hemoptysis.

The differential diagnosis of lung abscess includes cancer of the lung and cavitary tuberculosis. Indeed, cancer

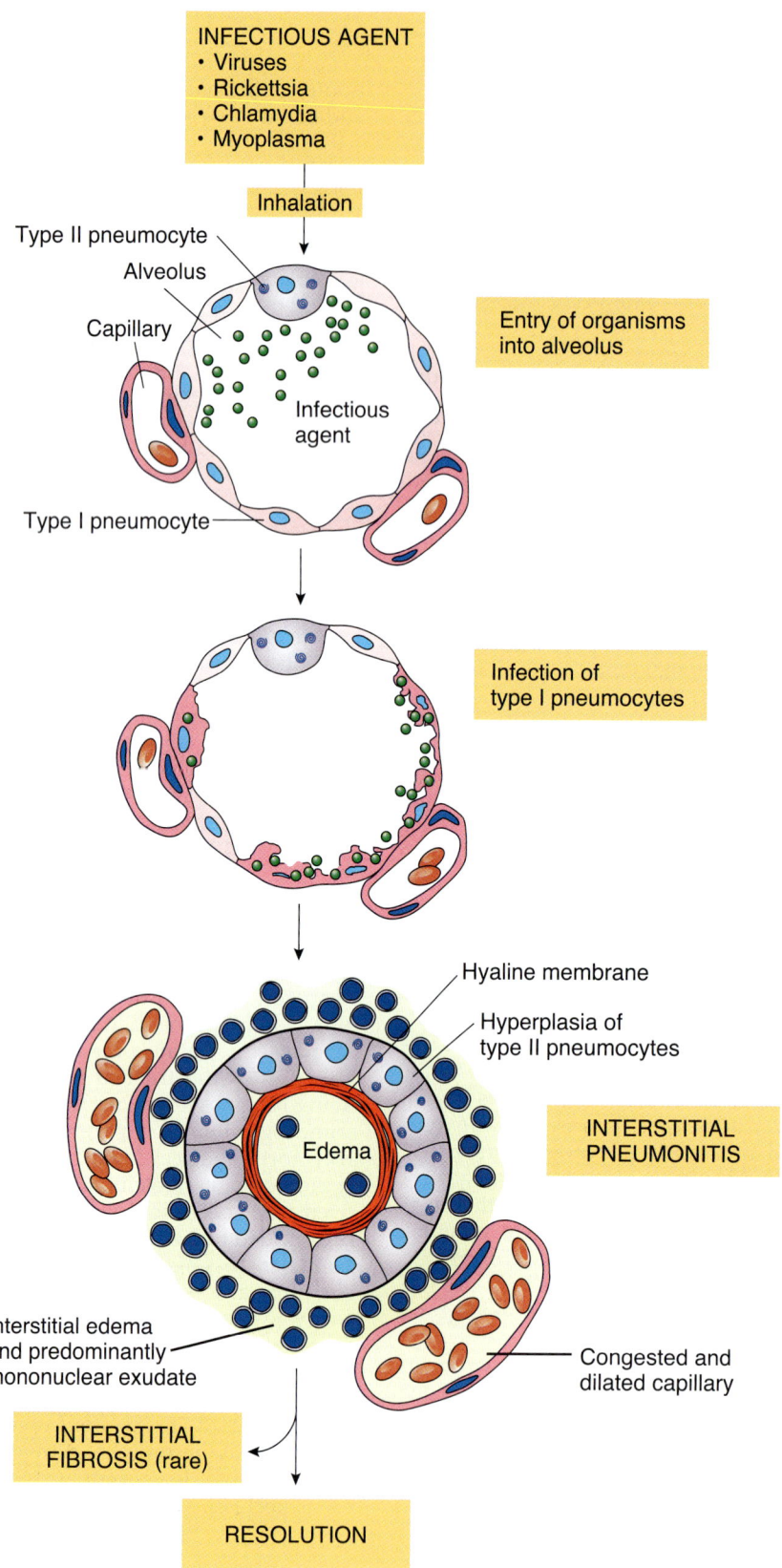

FIGURE 12-26
Pathogenesis of interstitial pneumonia. Although interstitial pneumonia is most commonly caused by viruses, other organisms also may cause significant interstitial inflammation. Type I cells are the most sensitive to damage, and loss of their integrity leads to intraalveolar edema. The proteinaceous exudate and cell debris form hyaline membranes, and type II cells multiply to line the alveoli. Interstitial inflammation is characterized mainly by mononuclear cells. The disease generally resolves completely but occasionally progresses to interstitial fibrosis.

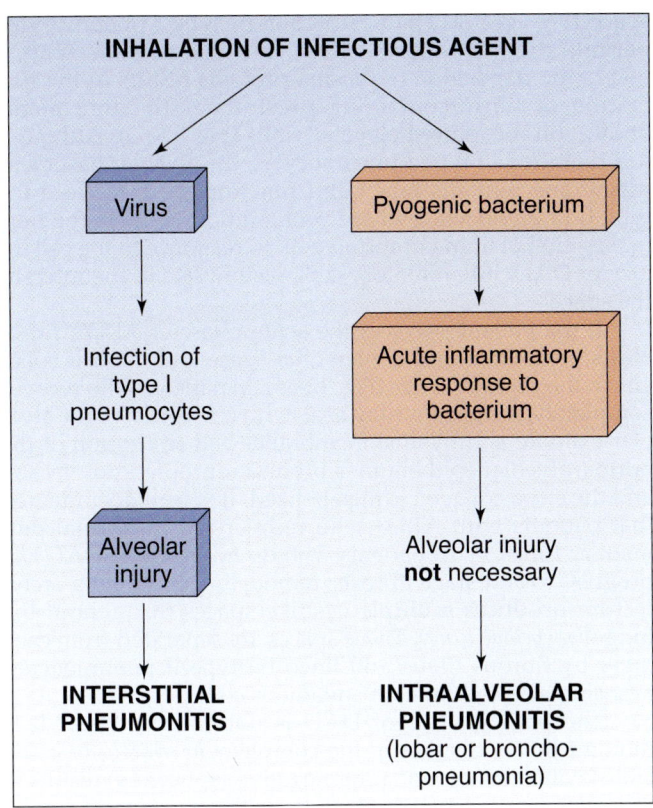

FIGURE 12-27
Pathogenesis of interstitial and intraalveolar pneumonitis.

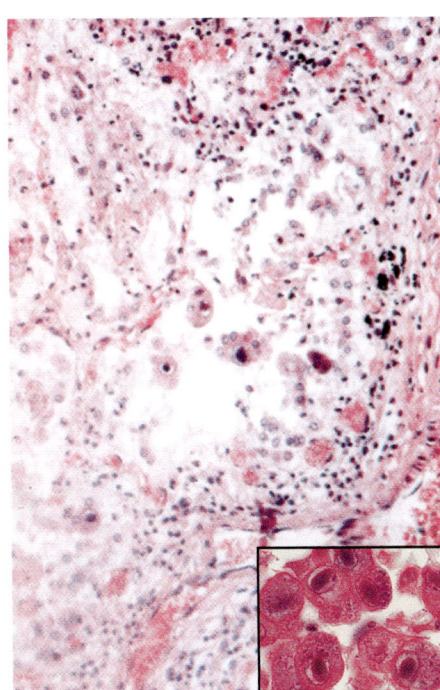

FIGURE 12-28
Cytomegalovirus pneumonitis. The infected alveolar cells are enlarged and display the typical dark-blue nuclear inclusions. *Inset:* A higher-power view shows infected alveolar cells that display a single basophilic nuclear inclusion with a perinuclear halo and multiple, indistinct, basophilic, cytoplasmic inclusions.

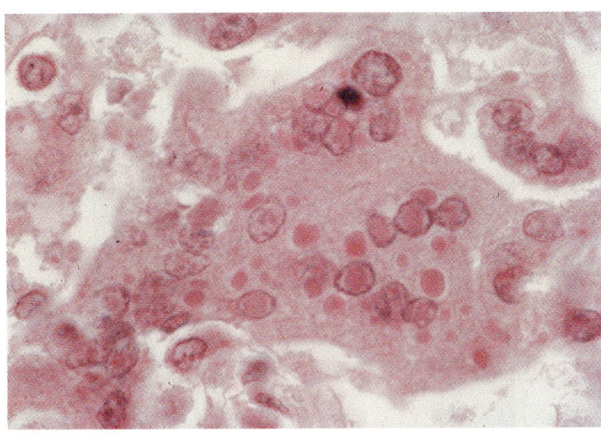

FIGURE 12-29
Measles pneumonitis. This multinucleated giant cell shows single, eosinophilic, refractile inclusions within each of the nuclei, as well as multiple, irregular, eosinophilic, cytoplasmic inclusions.

is now a more common cause of cavitation than is lung abscess. About half of all cases of cavitation due to cancer reflect necrosis of the tumor; the others follow obstruction of the bronchi and subsequent infection. A tuberculous cavity only rarely displays the air–fluid level characteristic of a lung abscess.

Complications of lung abscess include rupture into the pleural space, with resulting empyema and severe hemoptysis. The abscess may drain into a bronchus, with subsequent dissemination of the infection to other parts of the lung. Despite vigorous antimicrobial therapy, principally directed against anaerobic bacteria, the mortality of lung abscess remains in the range of 5 to 10%.

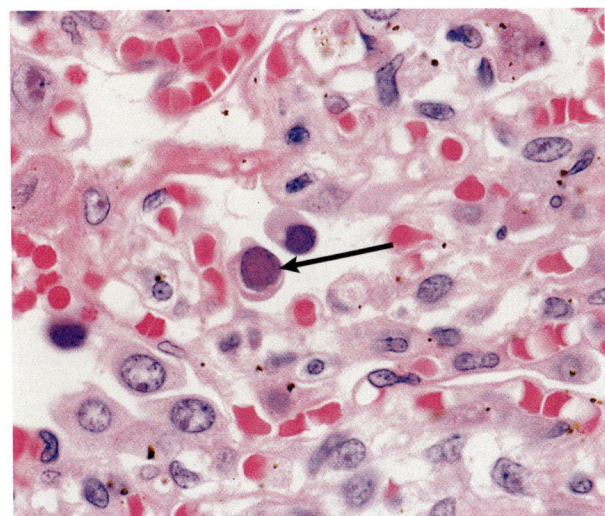

FIGURE 12-30
Adenovirus pneumonia. The "smudge" cell in the center consists of a smudgy basophilic nuclear inclusion.

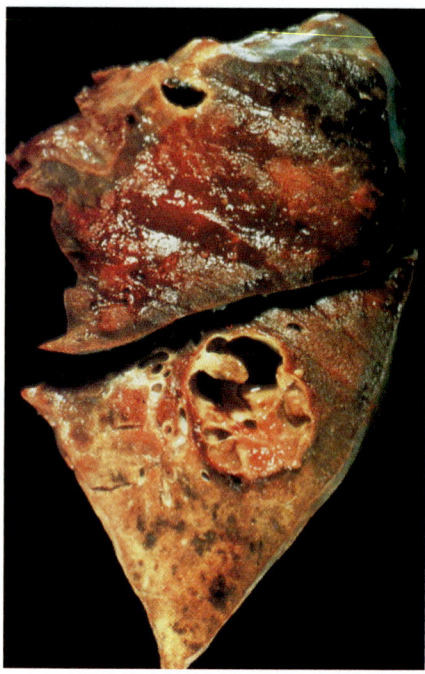

FIGURE 12-31
Pulmonary abscess. A large, cystic abscess contains a purulent exudate and is contained by a fibrous wall. Pneumonia is present in the surrounding pulmonary parenchyma.

DIFFUSE ALVEOLAR DAMAGE (ACUTE RESPIRATORY DISTRESS SYNDROME)

Diffuse alveolar damage (DAD) refers to a nonspecific pattern of reaction to injury of alveolar epithelial and endothelial cells from a variety of acute insults (Table 12-1). The clinical counterpart of severe DAD is the acute respiratory distress syndrome (ARDS). In this disorder, a patient with apparently normal lungs sustains pulmonary damage and then develops rapidly progressive respiratory failure. The condition reflects decreased lung compliance (usually requiring mechanical ventilation) and hypoxemia and features extensive radiological opacities in both lungs ("white-out"). The overall mortality of ARDS is more than 50%, and in patients older than 60 years, it is as high as 90%.

 Pathogenesis: DAD is a final common pathway of pathological changes caused by a large variety of insults (see Table 12-1). These include respiratory tract infections, sepsis, shock, aspiration of gastric contents, inhalation of toxic gases, near-drowning, radiation pneumonitis, and a large assortment of drugs and other chemicals. Some patients have an idiopathic form of DAD in which no cause can be found. Although these conditions are quite diverse, they can all injure the epithelial and endothelial cells of the alveoli, thereby producing DAD. **Importantly, the precise cause of DAD cannot be determined from the morphological appearance of the lung alone, unless a specific infectious agent is identified.**

Injury to endothelial cells allows the leakage of protein-rich fluid from the alveolar capillaries into the interstitial space (Fig. 12-32). The destruction of type I pneumocytes permits the exudation of fluid into the alveolar spaces, where the deposition of plasma proteins results in the formation of fibrin-containing precipitates (hyaline membranes) on the injured alveolar walls (Fig. 12-33). Although it is denuded of type I pneumocytes, the alveolar basement membrane remains intact and functions as a scaffold for type II pneumocytes, whose proliferation replaces the normal epithelial lining of the alveoli. In response to the cell injury of DAD, inflammatory cells accumulate in the interstitial space.

If the patient survives the acute phase of ARDS, fibroblasts proliferate in the interstitial space and deposit collagen in the alveolar walls (Fig. 12-34). In patients who recover completely, the lesions may heal, with resorption of the alveolar exudate and hyaline membranes and restitution of the normal alveolar epithelium. Fibroblastic proliferation ceases, and the extra collagen is metabolized. It is well documented that patients with ARDS who recover regain normal pulmonary function. In patients who do not recover, DAD can progress to end-stage fibrosis; remodeling of the lung architecture produces multiple cystlike spaces throughout the lung *(honeycomb lung)*. These spaces are separated from each other by fibrous tissue and lined by type II pneumocytes, bronchiolar epithelium, or squamous cells.

The pathogenesis of DAD is not entirely clear. It is thought that activation of the complement system (e.g., by endotoxin in the case of gram-negative septicemia) results in the sequestration of neutrophils in the marginating pool. Only a small proportion, perhaps one third, of neutrophils actively circulate in the blood; most of the remainder are found in the lung. Normally, the neutrophils cause no damage, but after activation by complement, they release oxygen radicals and hydrolytic enzymes, which damage the capillary endothelium of the lung. The role of polymorphonuclear leukocytes in the pathogenesis of DAD is still debated because ARDS has been reported in severely neutropenic patients.

In DAD produced by inhalation of toxic gases or near-drowning, the damage occurs primarily at the alveolar epithelial surface. The alveolar epithelial junctions are usually very tight; damage to the epithelium disrupts these junctions, permitting exudation of fluid and proteins from the interstitium into the alveolar spaces.

 Pathology: The evolution of DAD can be divided into two periods: the initial exudative phase, followed by an organizing phase.

TABLE 12-1 Important Causes of the Adult Respiratory Distress Syndrome

Nonthoracic trauma	Drugs and therapeutic agents
Shock due to any cause	Heroin
Fat embolism	Oxygen
	Radiation
Infection	Paraquat
Gram-negative septicemia	Cytotoxic drugs
Other bacterial infections	
Viral infections	
Aspiration	
Near-drowning	
Aspiration of gastric contents	

Diffuse Alveolar Damage (Acute Respiratory Distress Syndrome)

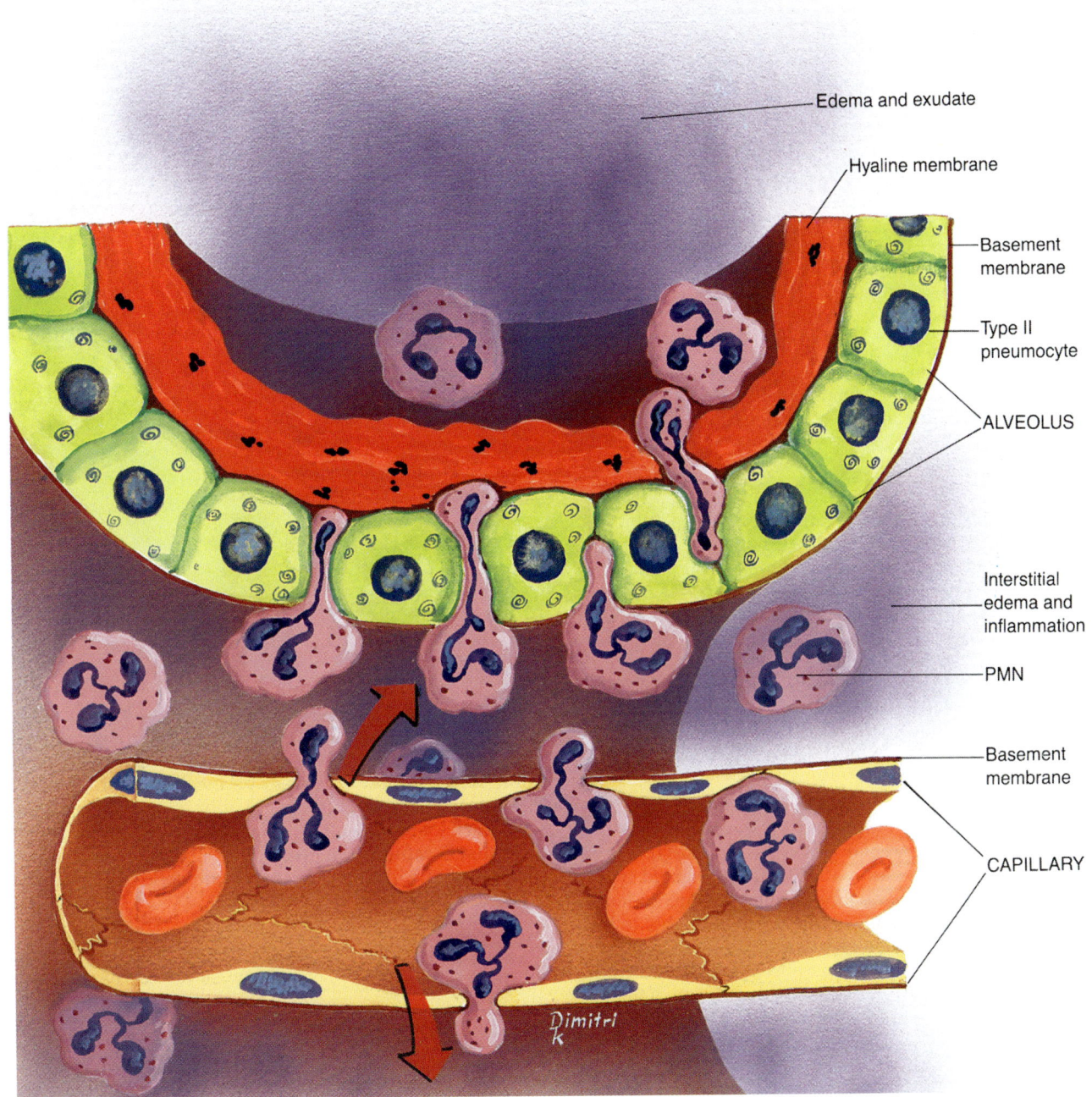

FIGURE 12-32
Diffuse alveolar damage (adult respiratory distress syndrome, ARDS). In ARDS, type I cells die as a result of diffuse alveolar damage. Intraalveolar edema follows, after which there is formation of hyaline membranes composed of proteinaceous exudate and cell debris. In the acute phase, the lungs are markedly congested and heavy. Type II cells multiply to line the alveolar surface. Interstitial inflammation is characteristic. The lesion may heal completely or progress to interstitial fibrosis.

The exudative phase of DAD develops during the first week after the pulmonary insult and features edema, exudation of plasma proteins, accumulation of inflammatory cells, and hyaline membranes (see Fig. 12-33). The earliest manifestation of alveolar injury is evidenced by electron microscopy, which reveals degenerative changes in both endothelial cells and type I pneumocytes. This is followed by the sloughing of type I cells and the appearance of denuded basement membranes. Interstitial and alveolar edema is prominent by the first day but soon recedes. Hyaline membranes begin to appear by the second day and are the most conspicuous morphological feature of the exudative phase

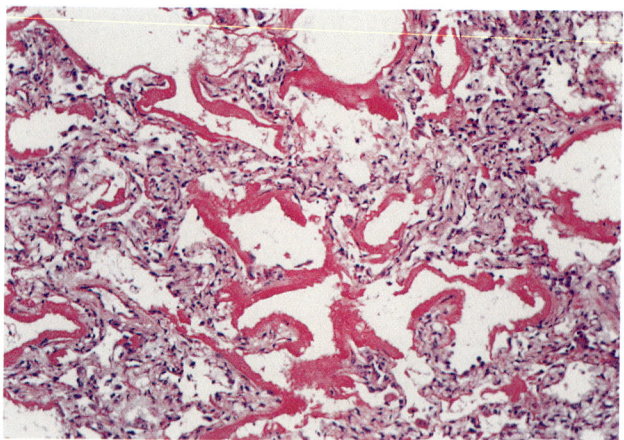

FIGURE 12-33
Diffuse alveolar damage, acute (exudative) phase. The alveolar septa are thickened by edema and a sparse inflammatory infiltrate. The alveoli are lined by eosinophilic hyaline membranes.

after 4 to 5 days. These eosinophilic, glassy "membranes" consist of precipitated plasma proteins and the cytoplasmic and nuclear debris from sloughed epithelial cells. Interstitial inflammation, consisting of lymphocytes, plasma cells and macrophages, is apparent early and reaches its maximum in about a week. Toward the end of the first week and persisting during the subsequent organizing stage, regularly spaced, cuboidal type II pneumocytes become arrayed along the denuded alveolar septa. The alveolar capillaries and pulmonary arterioles may exhibit fibrin thrombi. In fatal cases of DAD, the lungs are heavy, edematous, and virtually airless.

The organizing phase of DAD, beginning about a week after the initial injury, is marked by the proliferation of fibroblasts within the alveolar walls (see Fig. 12-34). During this phase interstitial inflammation and proliferated type II pneumocytes persist, but hyaline membranes are no longer formed. Alveolar macrophages digest the remnants of hyaline membranes and other cellular debris. Loose fibrosis thickens the alveolar septa. This fibrosis resolves in mild cases; in severe ones, it progresses to restructuring of the pulmonary parenchyma and cyst formation.

 Clinical Features: Patients destined to develop ARDS have a symptom-free interval for a few hours after the initial insult, after which tachypnea and dyspnea mark the onset of the syndrome. At this time, arterial hypoxemia and decreased P_{CO_2} are evident on measurement of blood gases. As ARDS progresses, the dyspnea worsens, and the patient becomes cyanotic. Diffuse, bilateral interstitial and alveolar infiltrates are noted radiologically. The arterial hypoxemia at this stage cannot be reversed simply by increasing the oxygen tension of inspired air, and mechanical ventilation becomes necessary. In fatal cases the combination of increasing tachypnea and decreasing tidal volume eventuates in alveolar hypoventilation, progressive hypoxemia, and increasing P_{CO_2}.

Patients who survive ARDS may recover normal pulmonary function but, in severe cases, are left with scarred lungs, respiratory dysfunction, and, in some instances, pulmonary hypertension.

Diffuse Alveolar Damage May Have Specific Causes

Oxygen

During World War II, aviators were required to breathe increased concentrations of oxygen at high altitude. To study possible pulmonary damage, animal experiments were carried out and demonstrated harmful effects of oxygen on the lung. Later observations with patients who were administered high levels of oxygen for respiratory problems documented the development of DAD. Pulmonary lesions have developed in patients with long-term exposure to as little as 28% oxygen, but it is usually safe to breathe 40 to 60% oxygen for long periods. The mechanism of oxygen toxicity is thought to be related to increased production of activated oxygen species in the lung.

Shock

ARDS often follows shock from any cause, including gram-negative sepsis, trauma, or blood loss, in which case the pulmonary condition is colloquially referred to as "shock lung." Although the pathogenesis of DAD associated with shock is poorly understood, it is likely multifactorial. Tissue necrosis in organs damaged by trauma or by ischemia may lead to the release of vasoactive peptides into the circulation, which enhance vascular permeability in the lung. Disseminated intravascular coagulation may damage alveolar capillaries, and fat emboli from bone fractures may obstruct the distal capillary bed of the lung. The pathogenesis of endothelial cell injury in endotoxic shock is discussed in Chapter 7.

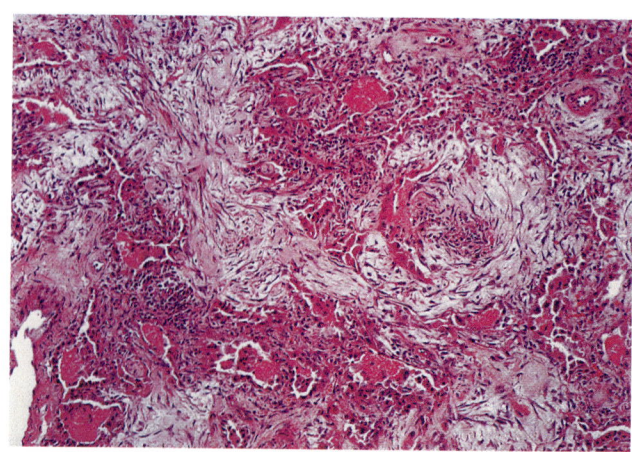

FIGURE 12-34
Diffuse alveolar damage, acute and organizing phase. In addition to hyaline membranes, the alveolar walls are thickened by fibroblasts and loose connective tissue.

Aspiration

The aspiration of gastric contents introduces acid with a pH less than 3.0 into the alveoli. DAD develops as a result of the severe chemical injury to the alveolar lining cells. In near-drowning, the aspiration of water leads to pulmonary injury and the clinical picture of ARDS.

Drug-Induced Diffuse Alveolar Damage

The long list of drugs that cause DAD includes most chemotherapeutic agents. The best known is bleomycin, but other frequently used agents, such as 1,3-bis-(2-chloroethyl)-1-nitrosourea (BCNU), methotrexate, 5-fluorouracil, busulfan, and cyclophosphamide, are known causes. Thus, as a general rule, all cytotoxic agents should be suspected as a cause of DAD. With bleomycin, an imprecise dose-dependent relation has been demonstrated, but such an effect is not apparent with most other drugs.

Bizarre, atypical, hyperchromatic nuclei in type II cells are particularly common in cases of alveolar damage from chemotherapeutic agents (Fig. 12-35). The damage progresses despite discontinuation of the offending agent, although it may be modified by the administration of corticosteroids. Progressive interstitial fibrosis occurs, usually with retention of the lung structure. Methotrexate differs from the other chemotherapeutic agents in that it may sometimes cause a hypersensitivity reaction in the lung. Under these circumstances, DAD is reversible after the drug is discontinued. The lesions that reflect hypersensitivity are characterized by granulomatous inflammation and occasionally vasculitis.

Drugs other than chemotherapeutic agents also cause DAD. Examples are nitrofurantoin, amiodarone, and penicillamine.

Radiation Pneumonitis

Radiation pneumonitis occurs in two forms, acute DAD and chronic pulmonary fibrosis. Alveolar injury is believed to be caused by the generation of oxygen radicals through the radiolysis of water.

Acute radiation pneumonitis occurs in as many as 10% of patients irradiated for cancer of the lung or breast or for mediastinal lymphoma. DAD caused by radiation is, for the most part, dose related and appears 1 to 6 months after radiation therapy. Patients have fever, cough, and dyspnea. Microscopic examination of the lungs reveals atypical alveolar lining cells, with enlarged hyperchromatic nuclei and multinucleated cells. Most patients recover from acute radiation pneumonitis.

Chronic radiation pneumonitis is characterized by interstitial fibrosis and may follow acute DAD or may develop insidiously. Lung biopsy demonstrates interstitial fibrosis, radiation-induced vascular changes, and atypical type II pneumocytes. The disease remains asymptomatic unless a substantial volume of the lung is affected.

Paraquat

The inhalation of the widely used herbicide paraquat is associated with DAD. Pulmonary disease becomes apparent 4 to 7 days after ingestion, as ARDS develops. Patients rarely recover once pulmonary complications have evolved. A curious intraalveolar exudate and organization occur, as well as the more usual interstitial fibrosis. The intraalveolar exudate organizes in such a way that the alveolar framework persists and the airspaces are filled with loose granulation tissue.

Respiratory Distress Syndrome of the Newborn

The counterpart of ARDS in newborns is termed respiratory distress syndrome (RDS) of the newborn. The disease also is associated with DAD, which is known as **hyaline membrane disease** in this circumstance. Prior to the use of exogenous surfactant treatment of RDS, oxygen tensions greater than 80% and mechanical ventilation were associated with the development of **bronchopulmonary dysplasia**. This infantile disorder was caused initially by damage to the pulmonary acini and later by repair, which led to atelectasis, fibrosis, and the destruction of clusters of acini. Since the advent of surfactant replacement therapy, the necrotizing bronchiolitis and alveolar septal fibrosis of bronchopulmonary dysplasia have largely disappeared, and the major change now encountered is one of decreased alveolarization in infants following birth. RDS of the newborn and bronchopulmonary dysplasia are discussed in further detail in Chapter 6.

RARE ALVEOLAR DISEASES

Alveolar Proteinosis Features Excess Intraalveolar Surfactant

Alveolar proteinosis, also termed lipoproteinosis, *is a rare condition in which the alveoli are filled with a granular eosinophilic material, which is periodic acid–Schiff (PAS)-positive, diastase resistant, and rich in lipids.* The disease was initially described as idiopathic, but recent studies have associated alveolar proteinosis with (1) compromised immunity; (2) a number of cancers, particularly leukemia and lymphoma; (3) res-

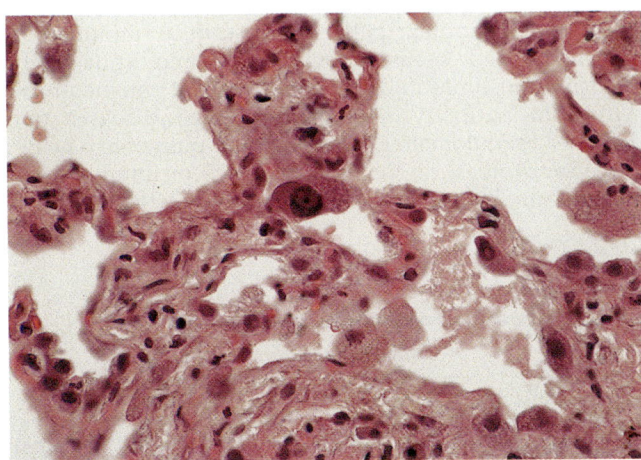

FIGURE 12-35
Diffuse alveolar damage associated with busulfan treatment. An atypical pneumocyte was encountered in a case of organizing diffuse alveolar damage (DAD) associated with busulfan therapy.

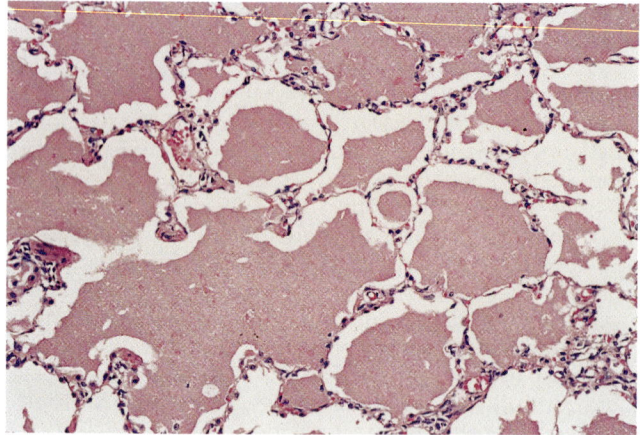

FIGURE 12-36
Alveolar proteinosis. The alveoli and alveolar ducts contain a granular, eosinophilic material.

debris, foamy macrophages, ghosts of degenerated cells, and detached type II pneumocytes. Importantly, the interstitial architecture of the lung is intact, and little inflammation is present.

Clinical Features: Alveolar proteinosis is a disease of adults, although a few cases have been reported in infants and children. Patients have fever, a productive cough, and dyspnea. The most common finding on the chest radiograph is diffuse, bilateral, symmetric, alveolar infiltrates, which may radiate from the hilar regions. Repeated respiratory tract infections, often with fungi or *Nocardia,* are a common complication. Before treatment became available, alveolar proteinosis gradually progressed to respiratory failure in one third of patients. Today, bronchoalveolar lavage is used to remove the alveolar material, and repeated lavage (sometimes for years) cures or halts the progress of the disease.

piratory infections; and (4) exposure to environmental inorganic dusts.

Pathogenesis: The origin of alveolar proteinosis is obscure, but it is suspected that impaired activity of alveolar macrophages and overproduction of lipid (surfactant) by type II pneumocytes may be responsible. However, the large amount of protein in the material indicates an additional (although unknown) mechanism. In most cases, no etiological agent is identifiable.

Pathology: On gross examination, the lungs in alveolar proteinosis are very heavy and viscid, and yellow fluid leaks from the cut surface. Scattered, firm, yellow-white nodules vary in size from a few millimeters to 2 cm in diameter. On microscopic examination, the granular material is noted not only in the alveoli, but also in the respiratory bronchioles and alveolar ducts (Fig. 12-36). The intraalveolar material often stains with an antibody to surfactant apoprotein, and electron microscopy reveals concentrically laminated myelin figures and lamellar bodies identical to the cytoplasmic inclusions of type II pneumocytes. Within the eosinophilic material may be found cellular

Diffuse Pulmonary Hemorrhage Syndromes Are Mainly Immune Disorders

Diffuse alveolar hemorrhage can occur in a wide variety of clinical settings (Table 12-2). Histologically, the diseases are characterized by acute hemorrhage (numerous intraalveolar red blood cells) or chronic hemorrhage (hemosiderosis). In virtually all of these disorders, a neutrophilic infiltrate of the alveolar wall *(neutrophilic capillaritis)* is present and is reminiscent of leukocytoclastic vasculitis seen in other organs such as the skin. This lesion tends to be most prominent in hemorrhagic syndromes associated with Wegener granulomatosis or systemic lupus erythematosus.

Diffuse pulmonary hemorrhage syndromes can be classified according to the associated immunofluorescence patterns. A linear pattern of fluorescence is seen in anti–basement membrane antibody disease or Goodpasture syndrome. A granular pattern is present in immune complex–associated diseases, such as systemic lupus erythematosus. Pauciimmune disorders consist of anti–neutrophil cytoplasm antibody (ANCA)-associated diseases (e.g., Wegener granulomatosis or idiopathic pulmonary hemorrhage syndromes), in which no etiology or immunological mechanism can be determined (see Table 12-2).

TABLE 12-2 Conditions of Pulmonary Hemorrhage

Disease	Immunological Mechanism	Immunofluorescence Pattern
Goodpasture syndrome	Anti-basement membrane antibody	Linear
Systemic lupus erythematosus	Immune complexes	Granular
Mixed cryoglobulinemia		
Henoch-Schönlein purpura		
IgA disease		
Wegener granulomatosis	Antineutrophil cytoplasmic antibody (ANCA)	Negative or pauciimmune
Idiopathic glomerulonephritis		
Idiopathic pulmonary hemorrhage	No immunological marker	

Goodpasture Syndrome

Goodpasture syndrome refers to a triad of diffuse alveolar hemorrhage, glomerulonephritis, and a circulating cytotoxic autoantibody to a component of basement membranes. The cross-reactivity between the basement membrane of the alveolus and the glomerulus accounts for the simultaneous attack on the lung and kidney. The pathogenesis of Goodpasture syndrome is discussed in greater detail in Chapter 16.

Pathology: Patients with Goodpasture syndrome suffer extensive intraalveolar hemorrhage (Fig. 12-37A). On gross examination, the lungs are dark red and heavy in the acute phase and rusty brown later, when the erythrocytes have been phagocytosed. Histologically, erythrocytes and hemosiderin-laden macrophages fill the airspaces. There is suggestive evidence of an "alveolitis" in the form of neutrophils in and around alveolar capillaries, although this reaction may be transient. The alveolar septa are mildly thickened by interstitial fibrosis and hyperplasia of type II pneumocytes. By immunofluorescence, linear deposition of IgG and complement is demonstrated in the basement membranes of the alveoli and glomeruli (see Fig. 12-37B).

Clinical Features: Patients with Goodpasture syndrome are typically young men, although the disease may affect adults of either sex and of any age. Most (95%) patients are seen initially with hemoptysis, often accompanied by dyspnea, weakness, and mild anemia. Evidence of glomerulonephritis follows the pulmonary manifestations in about 3 months (1 week to 1 year), although some patients do not develop renal disease. Radiographic examination reveals diffuse, bilateral alveolar infiltrates, which may resolve rapidly in a matter of days as the erythrocytes lyse and are phagocytosed. Hypoxemia and respiratory alkalosis are common, but respiratory function returns to normal as the hemorrhage resolves. The diagnosis is made on the basis of a renal or pulmonary biopsy.

Goodpasture syndrome is treated by the administration of corticosteroids and cytotoxic drugs and by plasmapheresis. Before such aggressive treatment was instituted, the mortality of Goodpasture syndrome was 80%, but even with current treatment, the 2-year survival is only 50%, and the outlook is worse when renal failure is present.

Idiopathic Pulmonary Hemorrhage

Idiopathic pulmonary hemorrhage (also known as idiopathic pulmonary hemosiderosis) is a rare disease characterized by diffuse alveolar bleeding similar to that of Goodpasture syndrome but without renal involvement or the presence of anti–basement membrane antibodies. Microscopically, idiopathic pulmonary hemorrhage is indistinguishable from the lung of Goodpasture syndrome.

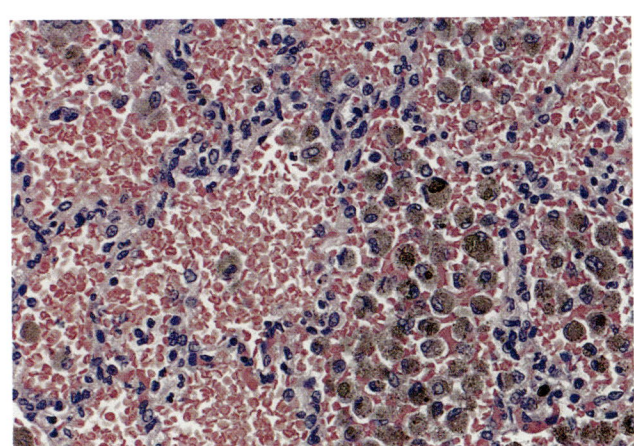
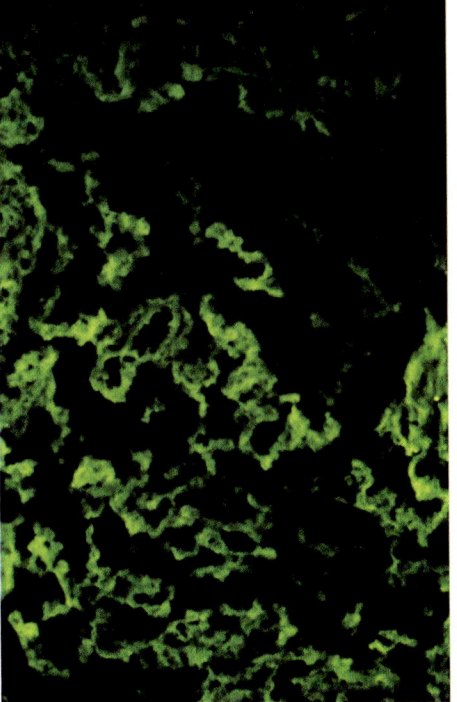

FIGURE 12-37
Goodpasture syndrome. **A.** A section of lung shows extensive intraalveolar hemorrhage. The alveolar septa are thickened, and the alveoli are lined by hyperplastic type II pneumocytes. **B.** Linear deposition of IgG within the alveolar septa is demonstrated by immunofluorescence.

Clinical Features: The malady primarily affects children, but 20% of patients are adults, usually younger than 30 years. There is a 2:1 male predominance in adults, but an equal sex distribution in children. The patients are first seen with cough (with or without hemoptysis), dyspnea, substernal chest pain, fatigue, and iron-deficiency anemia. Pulmonary hemorrhages are recurrent and intermittent, and the course is more protracted than that of Goodpasture syndrome.

The response to corticosteroids is variable, and the mean survival is 3 to 5 years. One fourth of patients die rapidly of massive hemorrhage. Another fourth have persistent, active disease; repeated episodes of hemoptysis result in interstitial fibrosis and cor pulmonale. In another fourth of patients, the disease remains inactive, but persistent dyspnea and anemia are troublesome. The remaining patients recover completely without recurrence.

Hypersensitivity to cow's milk in infants and children generally younger than 2 years can result in diffuse pulmonary hemorrhage similar to that seen in idiopathic pulmonary hemorrhage. Removal of milk from the diet ameliorates the condition.

Eosinophilic Pneumonia Is Principally an Allergic Disorder

Eosinophilic pneumonia refers to the accumulation of eosinophils in alveolar spaces. Eosinophilic pneumonia is classified as idiopathic or secondary to an underlying illness (Table 12-3).

TABLE 12-3 Types of Eosinophilic Pneumonia

Idiopathic
  Chronic eosinophilic pneumonia
  Acute eosinophilic pneumonia
  Simple eosinophilic pneumonia (Löffler syndrome)

Secondary eosinophilic pneumonia
  Infection
    Parasitic
      Tropical eosinophilic pneumonia
        Ascaris lumbricoides, Toxocara canis, filaria
      Dirofilaria
    Fungal
      Aspergillus
  Drug-induced
    Antibiotics
    Cytotoxic drugs
    Antiinflammatory agents
    Antihypertensive drugs
    L-Tryptophan (eosinophilic fasciitis)
  Immunological or systemic diseases
    Allergic bronchopulmonary aspergillosis
    Churg-Strauss syndrome
    Hypereosinophilic syndrome

Idiopathic Eosinophilic Pneumonia

SIMPLE EOSINOPHILIC PNEUMONIA: Simple eosinophilic pneumonia (Löffler syndrome) is a mild condition characterized by fleeting pulmonary infiltrates, which usually resolve within a month. Patients typically have peripheral blood eosinophilia but are often asymptomatic. Histologically, the lung shows eosinophilic pneumonia, but the diagnosis is usually established clinically, and lung biopsy is rarely performed.

ACUTE EOSINOPHILIC PNEUMONIA: In this disorder, patients are first seen with fewer than 7 days of symptoms, which include fever, hypoxemia, and diffuse interstitial and alveolar infiltrates on chest radiograph. The etiology of acute eosinophilic pneumonia is not known, but it is thought to be a type of hypersensitivity reaction. Although peripheral blood eosinophilia is frequently absent, bronchoalveolar lavage consistently demonstrates increased eosinophils. Leukocytosis is usually present. Histologically, the lung shows eosinophilic pneumonia accompanied by features of diffuse alveolar damage (i.e., hyaline membranes). Patients respond dramatically to corticosteroids, and in contrast to chronic eosinophilic pneumonia, acute eosinophilic pneumonia does not recur.

CHRONIC EOSINOPHILIC PNEUMONIA: The etiology of chronic eosinophilic pneumonia is unknown, but an allergic diathesis is noted in some patients.

Pathology: The alveolar spaces are flooded with eosinophils, alveolar macrophages, and a proteinaceous exudate (Fig. 12-38). In some cases, there is also an eosinophilic interstitial pneumonia, and hyperplasia of type II pneumocytes may be prominent. Eosinophilic ab-

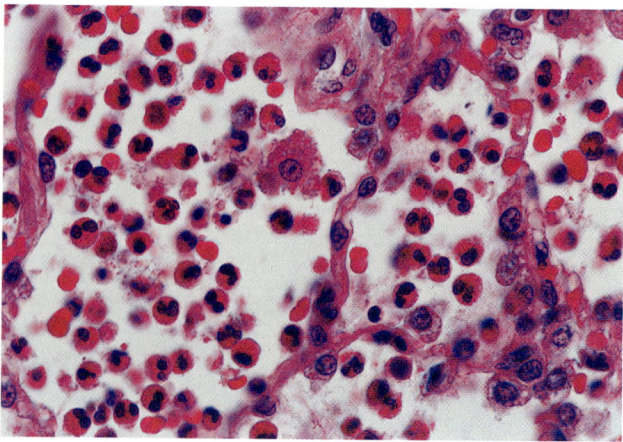
FIGURE 12-38
Eosinophilic pneumonia. The alveolar spaces are filled with an inflammatory exudate composed of eosinophils and macrophages. The alveolar septa are thickened by the presence of numerous eosinophils.

scesses, formed by a central mass of necrotic eosinophils surrounded by palisaded macrophages, are sometimes encountered. A mild eosinophilic vasculitis may be seen. Bronchiolitis obliterans and organizing pneumonia are also occasionally described.

Clinical Features: Patients have fever, night sweats, weight loss, cough productive of eosinophils, and dyspnea. Asthma is present in many patients, and circulating eosinophilia may be conspicuous. The chest radiograph is diagnostic and has been described as "the photographic negative of pulmonary edema," characterized by peripheral alveolar infiltrates with sparing of the hilum. The response to corticosteroids is dramatic and helps to confirm the diagnosis.

Secondary Eosinophilic Pneumonia

Eosinophilic pneumonia can occur in a variety of known clinical settings, including parasitic or fungal infection, drug toxicity, and systemic disorders such as Churg-Strauss syndrome. In industrialized countries, the most frequent cause of eosinophilic pneumonia is drug hypersensitivity, including reactions to antibiotics, antiinflammatory agents, cytotoxic drugs, and antihypertensive agents. The pulmonary disease resolves without long-term sequelae. The clinical presentations and histological findings are the same as described above.

INFECTIOUS EOSINOPHILIC PNEUMONIA: The classic form of eosinophilic pneumonia associated with parasitic infection is *tropical eosinophilic pneumonia*. The migration of parasites through the lung is often accompanied by an acute, self-limited, respiratory illness, characterized clinically by (1) fever, (2) a cough productive of sputum containing eosinophils, and (3) transient pulmonary infiltrates.

In temperate zones, *Ascaris lumbricoides* is the usual inciting organism. Hypersensitivity to *Toxocara canis* is also occasionally encountered. However, the most distinctive infection associated with eosinophilic pneumonia is allergic bronchopulmonary aspergillosis (see discussion above on aspergillosis).

In tropical regions, eosinophilic pneumonia is most commonly a response to infestation with the filarial nematodes *Wuchereria bancrofti* and *Brugia malayi*, although other parasites may also produce this syndrome.

Endogenous Lipid Pneumonia Reflects Bronchial Obstruction

Endogenous lipid pneumonia, also termed golden pneumonia, *is a localized condition distal to an obstructed airway, characterized by lipid-laden macrophages in the alveolar spaces.* The size of the affected area corresponds to the caliber of the involved bronchus. Bronchial obstruction results in the retention of secretions and breakdown products of inflammatory and epithelial cells. Whereas the protein component is readily digested, lipids are phagocytosed by macrophages, which fill the alveoli distal to the obstruction.

Pathology: On gross examination, endogenous lipid pneumonia has a characteristic golden-yellow color that reflects the accumulation of fine lipid droplets within alveolar macrophages. Microscopically, alveoli are flooded by foamy macrophages, with needle-shaped clefts characteristic of cholesterol crystals. The alveolar walls typically remain intact. The pneumonia is accompanied by mild chronic inflammation and fibrosis. If the obstruction is relieved, the affected parenchyma can return to its normal state, unless bronchiectasis and chronic recurrent bronchopneumonia have led to irreversible parenchymal changes.

Exogenous Lipid Pneumonia Is a Response to Aspirated Oils

Causes of exogenous pneumonia include mineral oil (a laxative and a carrier for medications in nose drops), vegetable oils used in cooking, and animal oils ingested in the form of cod-liver oil and other vitamin preparations. Oil-based contrast media used for radiological bronchography has also been associated with the disorder. Exogenous lipid pneumonia is most common in older persons who take nose drops or laxatives at bedtime and aspirate during sleep. Children may aspirate oily medications while vigorously resisting the dosing.

Pathology: On gross examination, exogenous lipid pneumonia appears as a gray, poorly demarcated, greasy lesion. Microscopically, foamy macrophages are seen in the alveolar and interstitial spaces (Fig. 12-39). Large oil droplets in both locations are sur-

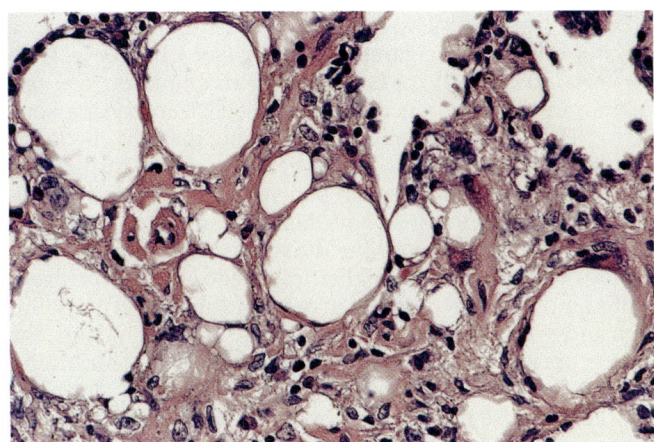

FIGURE 12-39
Exogenous lipid pneumonia (mineral oil aspiration). The cystic spaces are empty because the lipid was washed out during paraffin processing. A giant-cell reaction is also present.

rounded by a foreign-body granulomatous response. Because most of the oil washes out in paraffin processing, empty vacuolar spaces are noted in histological sections. In chronic cases, the affected areas may become densely fibrotic.

Patients with exogenous lipid pneumonia are usually asymptomatic, and the condition is brought to medical attention when a mass simulating an infectious process or a tumor is noted on a chest radiograph.

OBSTRUCTIVE PULMONARY DISEASES

Several different diseases, including chronic bronchitis, emphysema, asthma, and in some classifications, bronchiectasis and cystic fibrosis, are grouped together because they have in common an obstruction to air flow in the lungs.

Chronic obstructive pulmonary disease (COPD) is a nonspecific term that describes patients with chronic bronchitis or emphysema who evidence a decrease in forced expiratory volume, measured by spirometric pulmonary function tests.

Air flow has a hydraulic basis and can be reduced in two ways: by increasing the resistance to air flow or by reducing the outflow pressure. In the lung, narrowed airways produce increased resistance, whereas loss of elastic recoil results in diminished pressure. Airway narrowing occurs in chronic bronchitis or asthma, and emphysema causes loss of recoil.

Chronic Bronchitis Is a Malady of Smokers

Chronic bronchitis is defined clinically as the presence of a chronic productive cough without a discernible cause for more than half the time over a period of 2 years. The pathological definition of the disease is less satisfactory, because the morphological alterations represent a continuum; in milder chronic bronchitis, they overlap with those seen in ostensibly normal persons.

 Pathogenesis: Chronic bronchitis is primarily a disease of cigarette smoking (see Chapter 8), with **90% of all cases occurring in smokers.** The frequency of chronic bronchitis is less than 5% in nonsmokers, 10 to 15% in moderate smokers, and more than 25% in heavy smokers. The frequency and severity of acute respiratory tract infections is increased in patients with chronic bronchitis; conversely, infections have been incriminated in the etiology and progression of the disease. Although population studies demonstrated a higher prevalence of chronic bronchitis among urban dwellers in areas of substantial air pollution and in workers exposed to toxic industrial inhalants, the effects of cigarette smoking far outweigh other contributing factors.

The precise mechanisms by which cigarette smoke and other pollutants produce bronchial injury are poorly understood. Experimentally, rodents subjected to the inhalation of cigarette smoke or sulfur dioxide, or to the instillation of dilute acids, exhibit squamous metaplasia of the bronchial epithelium. A similar change is produced by the introduction of certain proteases into the bronchi, an effect that is pre-

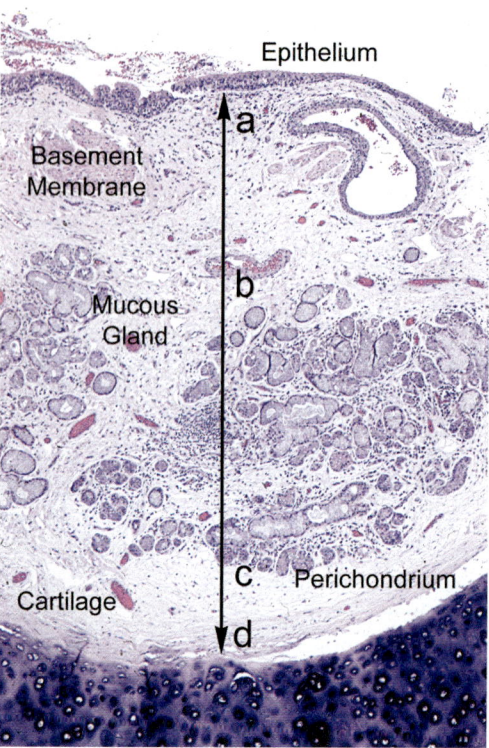

FIGURE 12-40
Chronic bronchitis. The bronchial submucosa is greatly expanded by hyperplastic submucosal glands that compose well over 50% of the thickness of the bronchial wall. The Reid index equals the maximum thickness of the bronchial mucous glands internal to the cartilage (*b to c*) divided by the bronchial wall thickness (*a to d*).

vented by pretreatment with antiproteases. Metaplasia of the bronchial epithelium can also be induced in rodents by adrenergic and cholinergic agonists, suggesting that autonomic stimulation may play a role in the pathogenesis of chronic bronchitis.

 Pathology: The principal morphological finding in chronic bronchitis is an increase in the size of the bronchial mucus-secreting apparatus (Fig. 12-40). Two types of cells line the mucous glands: pale mucous cells, which are the most common, and serous cells, which are more basophilic and contain granules. **Chronic bronchitis is characterized by hyperplasia and hypertrophy of the mucous cells and an increased proportion of mucous to serous cells.** As a result, both the individual acini and the glands become larger (Fig. 12-41).

The Reid index is a measure of the increase in the size of the mucous glands (Fig. 12-40). The area occupied by the glands in the plane vertical to the cartilage and epithelium is expressed as a proportion of the thickness of the entire bronchial wall (basement membrane to inner perichondrium). The normal value of the Reid index is 0.4 or less; it is more than 0.5 in chronic bronchitis.

Other morphological changes in chronic bronchitis are variable and include the following:

- Excess mucus in the central and peripheral airways
- "Pits" on the surface of the bronchial epithelium, which

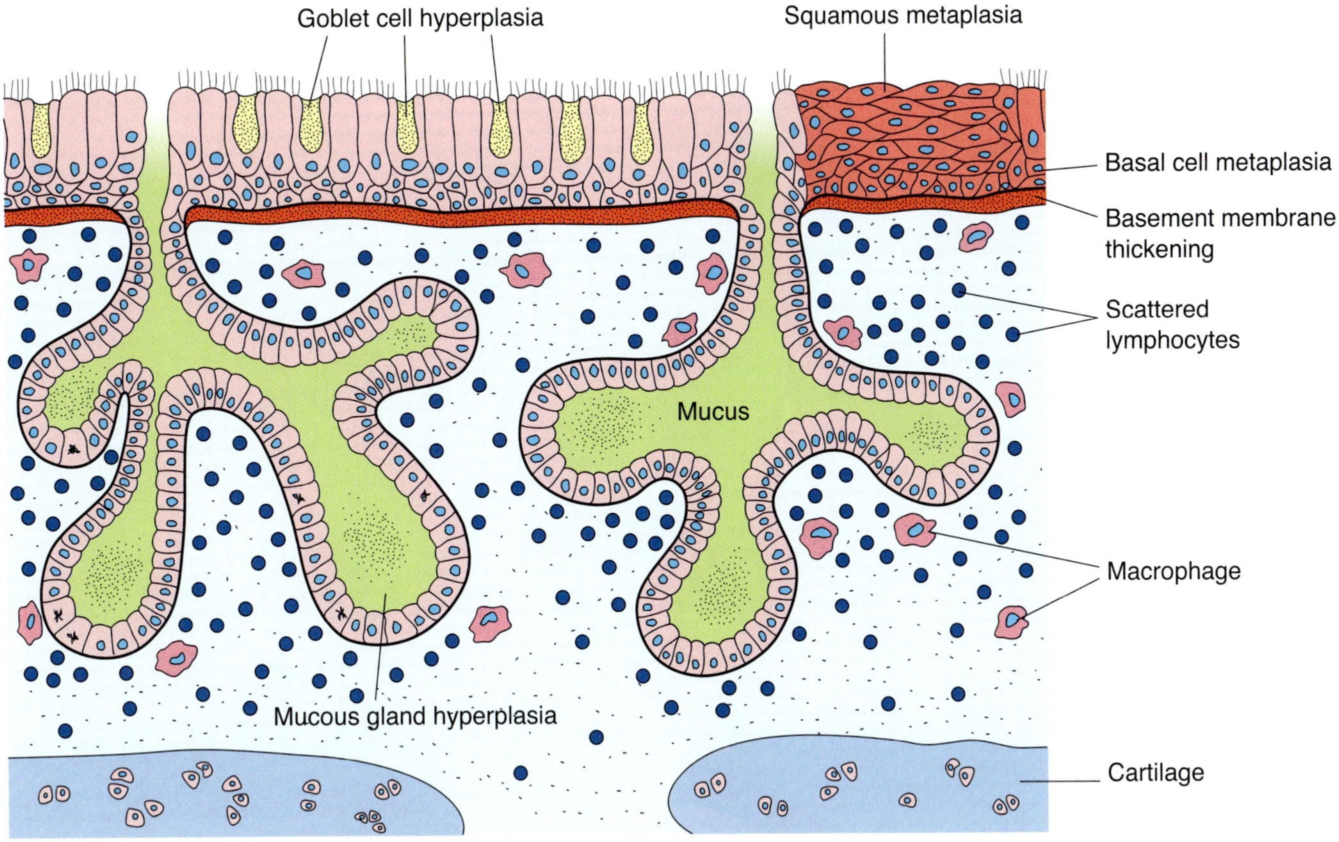

Obstructive Pulmonary Disease

Goblet cell hyperplasia

Squamous metaplasia

Basal cell metaplasia

Basement membrane thickening

Scattered lymphocytes

Mucus

Macrophage

Mucous gland hyperplasia

Cartilage

FIGURE 12-41
Chronic bronchitis. Morphological changes in chronic bronchitis.

represent dilated bronchial gland ducts into which open several glands
- Thickening of the bronchial wall by mucous gland enlargement and edema, which leads to encroachment on the bronchial lumen
- An increase in the number of goblet cells (hyperplasia)
- Increased amounts of smooth muscle, which may indicate bronchial hyperreactivity
- Squamous metaplasia of the bronchial epithelium in chronic bronchitis reflecting epithelial damage from tobacco smoke, an effect that is probably independent of the other morphological features of chronic bronchitis

 Clinical Features: Chronic bronchitis is often accompanied by emphysema (see below); it is often difficult to separate the relative contribution of each disease to the clinical presentation. In general, patients with predominantly chronic bronchitis have had a productive cough for many years. Cough and sputum production are initially more severe in the winter months, but as the malady becomes more chronic, it progresses from hibernal to perennial. Exertional dyspnea and cyanosis supervene, and cor pulmonale may ensue. The combination of cyanosis and edema secondary to cor pulmonale has led to the label "blue bloater" for such patients.

Acute respiratory failure in patients with advanced chronic bronchitis, consisting of progressive hypoxemia and hypercapnia, may be precipitated by pulmonary infections, thromboembolism, and left ventricular failure and by major episodes of air pollution. Because of retained mucous secretions, patients with chronic bronchitis are at an increased risk of bacterial infections of the lung, particularly with *H. influenzae* and *S. pneumoniae*.

Persons with chronic bronchitis must be admonished to stop smoking. Prompt antibiotic treatment of pulmonary infections, administration of bronchodilator drugs, and occasionally bronchopulmonary drainage are the mainstays of treatment.

Emphysema Causes Overinflation of the Lungs in Smokers

Emphysema is a chronic lung disease characterized as enlargement of the airspaces distal to the terminal bronchioles, with destruction of their walls but without fibrosis. Emphysema is classified in anatomical terms, but the classification should not obscure the fact that **the severity of emphysema is more important than the type.** In practical terms, as emphysema becomes

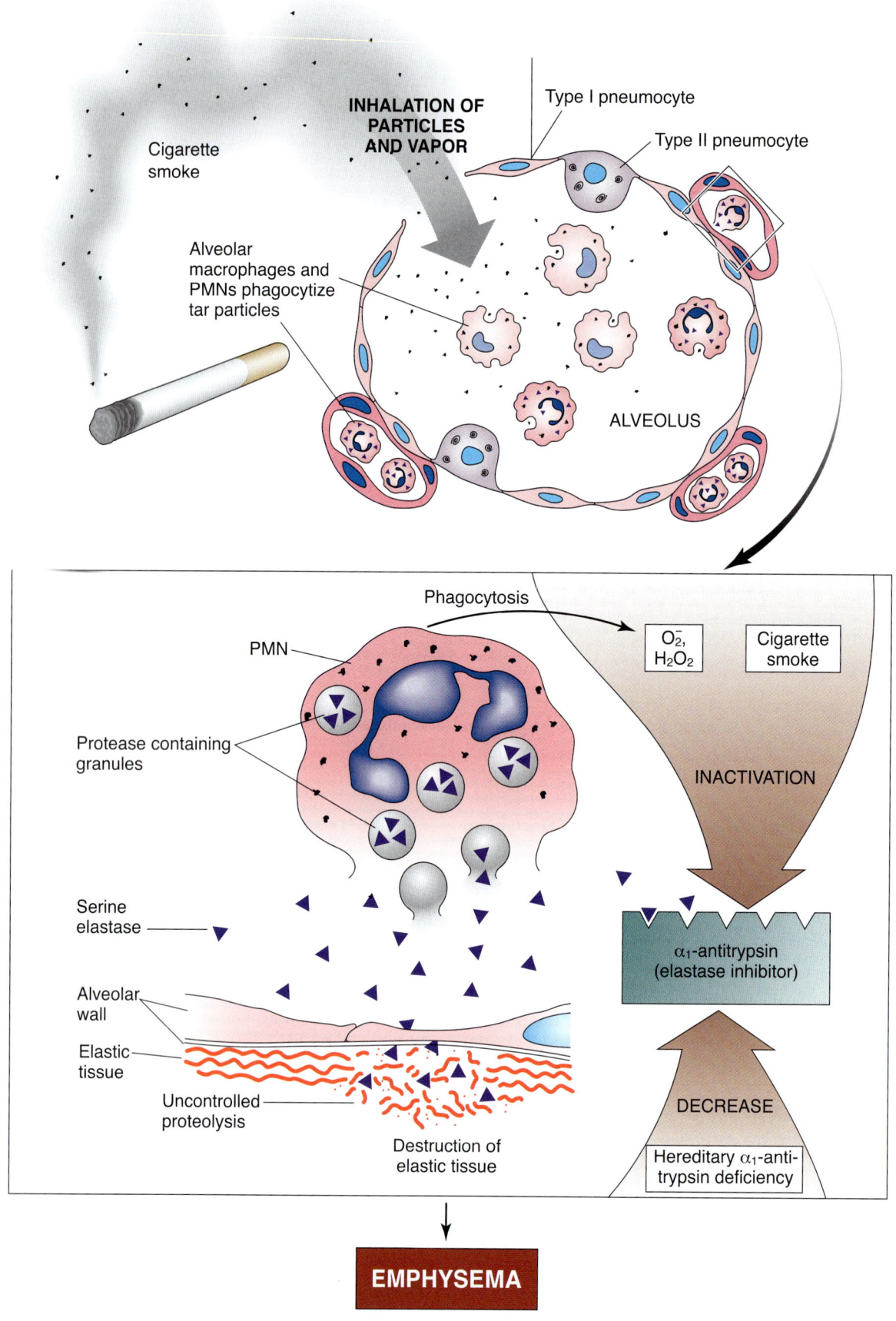

FIGURE 12-42
The proteolysis–antiproteolysis theory of the pathogenesis of emphysema. Cigarette (tobacco) smoking is closely related to the development of emphysema. Some product in tobacco smoke induces an inflammatory reaction. The serine elastase in polymorphonuclear leukocytes, which is a particularly potent elastolytic agent, injures the elastic tissue of the lung. Normally, this enzyme activity is inhibited by α_1-antitrypsin, but tobacco smoke, directly or through the generation of free radicals, inactivates α_1-antitrypsin (protease inhibitor).

more severe, it becomes more difficult to classify, a situation similar to that of end-stage renal disease or cirrhosis of the liver. Moreover, several anatomical patterns may be present in the same lung.

Pathogenesis: **The major cause of emphysema is cigarette smoking, and moderate-to-severe emphysema is rare in nonsmokers (see Chapter 8).** The dominant hypothesis concerning the pathogenesis of emphysema is the proteolysis–antiproteolysis theory (Fig. 12-42). It is thought that a balance exists between elastin synthesis and catabolism in the lung. In other words, emphysema results when elastolytic activity increases or antielastolytic activity is reduced.

Increased numbers of neutrophils, which contain serine elastase and other proteases, are found in the bronchoalveolar lavage fluid of smokers. Smoking also reduces α_1-antitrypsin activity, owing to the oxidation of methionine residues in the enzyme. In this way, unopposed and increased elastolytic activity leads to the destruction of elastic tissue in the walls of the distal airspaces, thereby impairing elastic recoil. At the same time, other cellular proteases may be involved in injury to the airspace walls. Although the proteolysis–antiproteolysis theory is attractive as an explanation for smokers' emphysema, it awaits further confirmation.

α_1-*ANTITRYPSIN DEFICIENCY:* A hereditary deficiency in α_1-antitrypsin (α_1-AT) accounts for about 1% of all patients with a clinical diagnosis of COPD and is considerably more common in young persons with severe emphysema. α_1-AT, a circulating glycoprotein produced in the liver, is a major inhibitor of a variety of proteases, including elastase, trypsin, chymotrypsin, thrombin, and bacterial proteases. In fact, it accounts for 90% of antiproteinase activity in the blood. In the lung, the most important action of α_1-AT is its inhibition of neutrophil elastase, an enzyme that digests elastin and other structural components of the alveolar septa.

The amount and type of α_1-AT is determined by a pair of codominant alleles, referred to as *Pi* (protease inhibitor). The most common genotype, *PiM*, and some 75 variants are now recognized. The most serious abnormality is associated with the *PiZ* allele, which occurs in some 5% of the population. It is more common in persons of Scandinavian origin and is rare in Jews, blacks, and Japanese. *PiZZ* homozygotes have only 15 to 20% of the normal plasma concentration of α_1-AT because the abnormal protein is poorly secreted by the liver. These persons are at risk for the development of both cirrhosis of the liver (see Chapter 14) and emphysema. **In fact, most patients with clinically diagnosed emphysema younger than age 40 years have α_1-AT deficiency (PiZ).** *PiZZ* homozygotes who do not smoke show a mean age at onset of emphysema between ages 45 and 50 years; those who smoke develop emphysema at about age 35 years. However, two thirds of nonsmoking *PiZZ* homozygotes show no evidence of emphysema. The association of α_1-AT deficiency with emphysema supports the concept that cigarette smoking by itself causes emphysema by altering the balance of the protease–antiprotease system in the lung.

Pathology: Emphysema is morphologically classified according to the location of the lesions within the pulmonary acinus (Fig. 12-43). Only the proximal part of the acinus (respiratory bronchiole) is selectively involved in centrilobular emphysema, whereas the entire acinus is destroyed in panacinar emphysema.

CENTRILOBULAR EMPHYSEMA: This form of emphysema is the most frequently encountered variant and the one usually associated with cigarette smoking and with clinical symptoms. Centrilobular emphysema is characterized by destruction of the cluster of terminal bronchioles near the end of the bronchiolar tree in the central part of the pulmonary lobule (Fig. 12-44A). The lobule is the smallest portion of the lung bounded by septa and includes several acini. The dilated respiratory bronchioles form enlarged airspaces that are separated from each other and from the lobular septa by normal alveolar ducts and alveoli. As centrilobular emphysema progresses, these distal structures also may be involved (see Fig. 12-44B). The bronchioles proximal to the emphysematous spaces are inflamed and narrowed. Centrilobular emphysema is most severe in the upper zones of the lung, the upper lobe and the superior segment of the lower lobe.

Focal dust emphysema, a disease of coal miners, resembles centrilobular emphysema but differs in that the enlarged spaces are smaller and more regular and inflammation of the bronchioles is not apparent. Importantly, the lesion is primarily distensive rather than destructive. Focal dust emphysema is discussed below in the section on coal worker's pneumoconiosis.

PANACINAR EMPHYSEMA: In this type of emphysema, the acinus is uniformly involved, with destruction of the alveolar septa from the center to the periphery of the acinus (Fig. 12-45A,B). The loss of alveolar septa is illustrated in the histological comparison of lung affected by α_1-AT deficiency with normal lung at the same magnification (Fig. 12-46). In the final stage, panacinar emphysema leaves behind a lacy network of supporting tissue *(cotton-candy lung)*. This variant occurs in several different situations. Diffuse panacinar emphysema is the typical lesion associated with α_1-AT deficiency. It is also often found in cigarette smokers in association with centrilobular emphysema. In such cases, the panacinar pattern tends to occur in the lower zones of the lung, whereas centrilobular emphysema is seen in the upper regions.

LOCALIZED EMPHYSEMA: This condition, previously known as "paraseptal emphysema," is characterized by the destruction of alveoli and resulting emphysema in only one or at most a few locations. The remainder of the lungs is normal. The lesion is usually found at the apex of an upper lobe, although it may occur anywhere in the pulmonary parenchyma, such as in a subpleural location (Fig. 12-47). Although it is of no clinical significance itself, rupture of an area of localized emphysema produces spontaneous pneumothorax (see below). Progression of localized emphysema can result in a large area of destruction, termed a *bulla,* which ranges in size from as small as 2 cm to a large lesion that occupies an entire hemothorax.

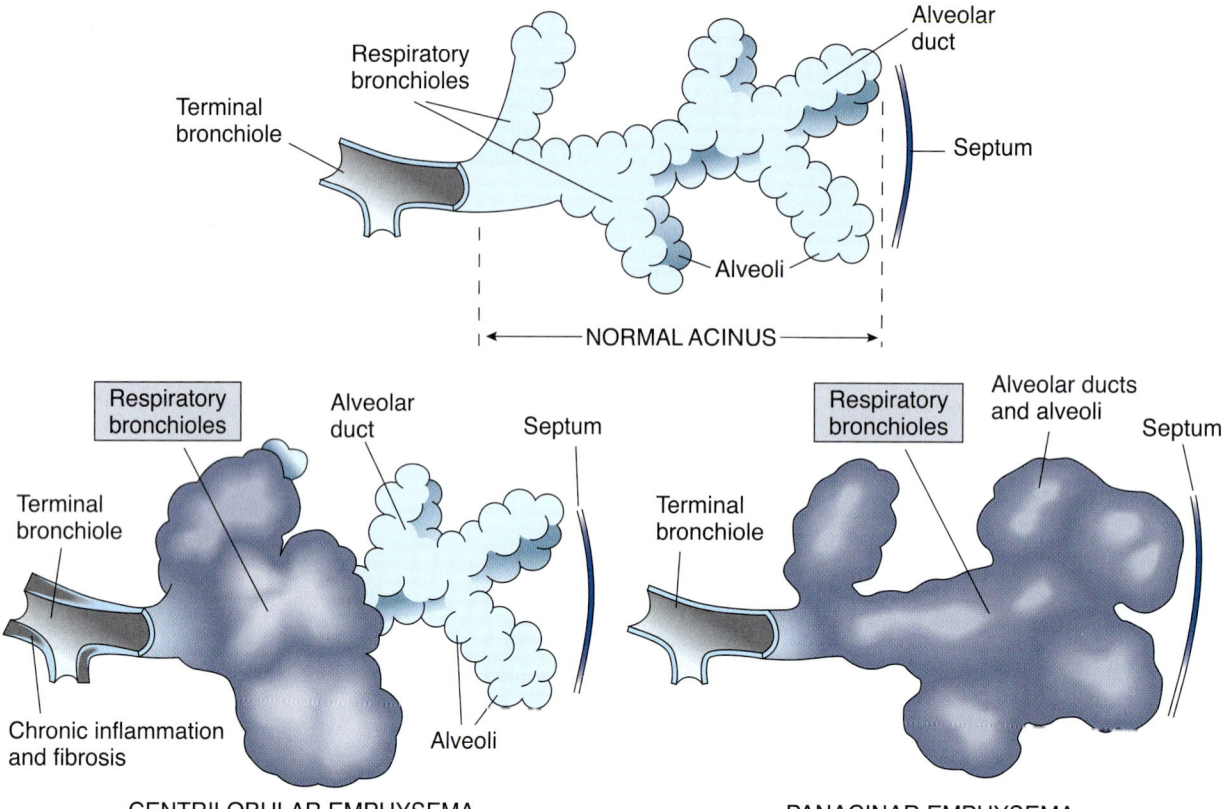

FIGURE 12-43
Types of emphysema. The acinus is the unit gas-exchanging structure of the lung distal to the terminal bronchiole. It consists of (in order) respiratory bronchioles, alveolar ducts, alveolar sacs, and alveoli. In centrilobular (proximal acinar) emphysema, the respiratory bronchioles are predominantly involved. In paraseptal (distal acinar) emphysema, the alveolar ducts are particularly affected. In panacinar (panlobular) emphysema, the acinus is uniformly damaged.

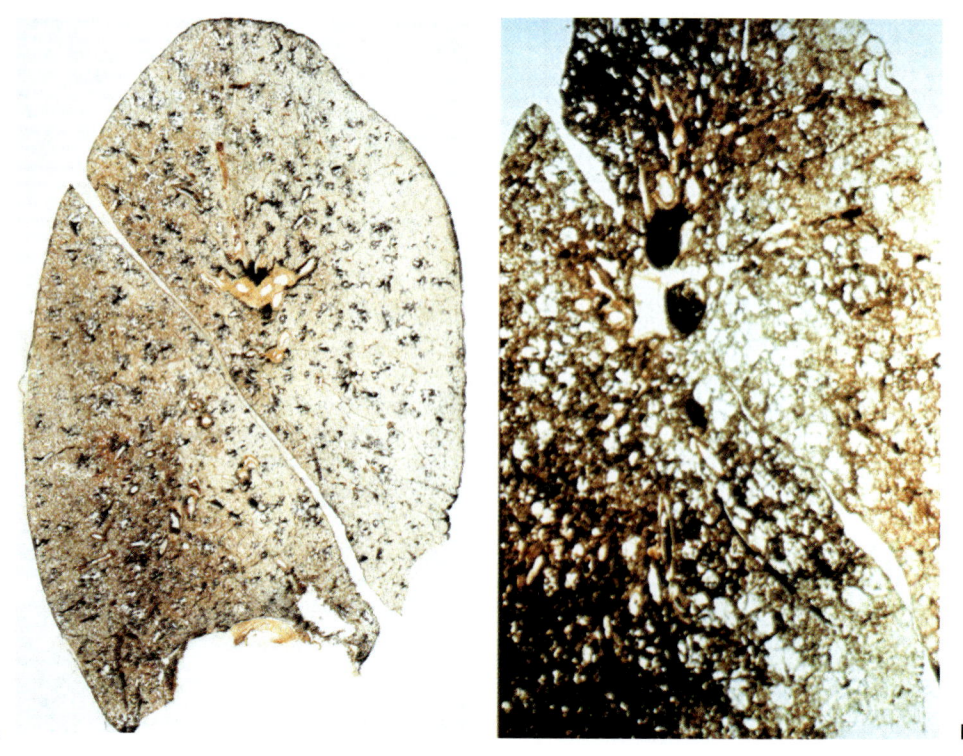

Obstructive Pulmonary Disease

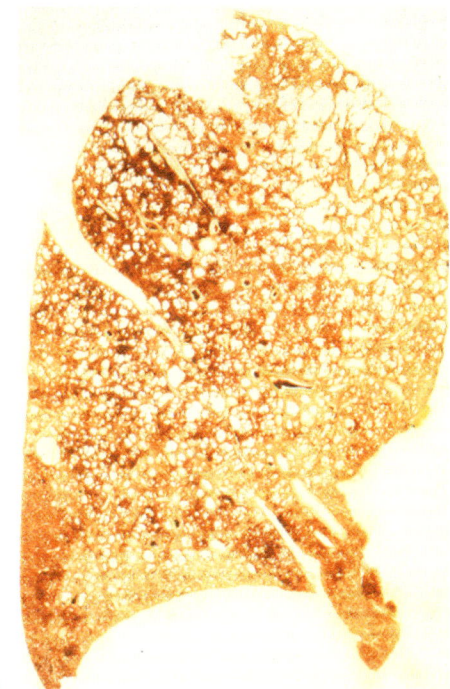

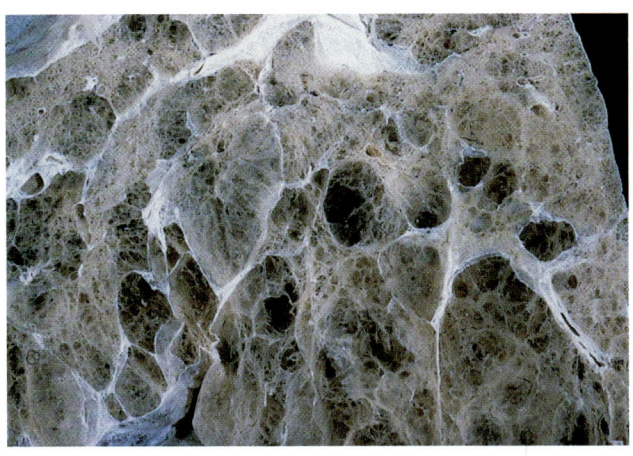

FIGURE 12-45
Panacinar emphysema. A. A whole mount of the left lung from a patient with severe emphysema reveals widespread destruction of the pulmonary parenchyma, which in some areas leaves behind only a lacy network of supporting tissue. B. The lung from this patient with α_1-antitrypsin deficiency shows a panacinar pattern of emphysema. The loss of alveolar walls has resulted in markedly enlarged air spaces.

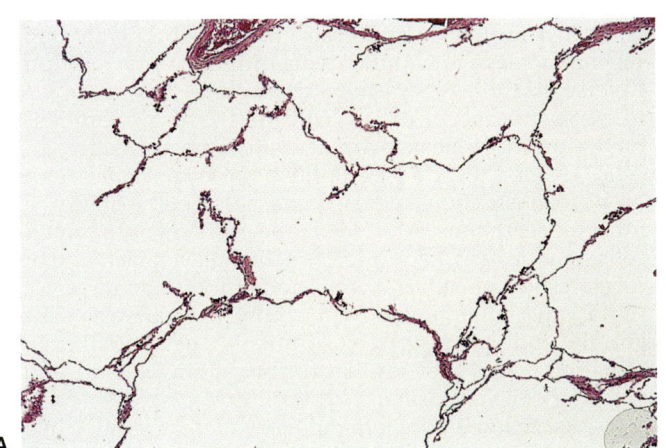

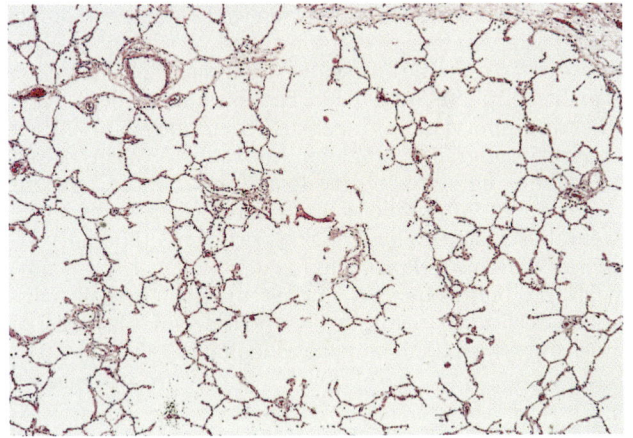

FIGURE 12-46
Panacinar emphysema. A. This lung, from a patient with α_1-antitrypsin deficiency, shows large, irregular air spaces and a markedly reduced number of alveolar walls. B. The extensive loss of alveolar walls in A is emphasized by comparison with this section of normal lung at the same magnification.

FIGURE 12-44
Centrilobular emphysema. A. A whole mount of the left lung of a smoker with mild emphysema shows enlarged air spaces scattered throughout both lobes, which represent destruction of the terminal bronchioles in the central part of the pulmonary lobule. These abnormal spaces are surrounded by intact pulmonary parenchyma. B. In a more advanced case of centrilobular emphysema, the destruction of the lung has progressed to produce large, irregular air spaces.

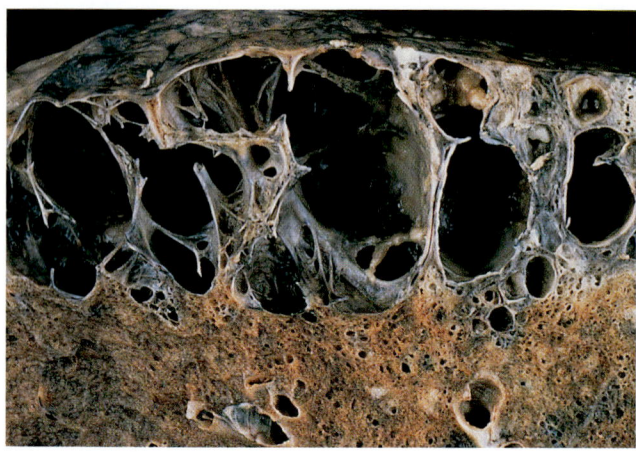

FIGURE 12-47
Localized emphysema. The subpleural parenchyma shows markedly enlarged air spaces owing to the loss of alveolar tissue.

Clinical Features: Most patients with symptomatic emphysema are seen at age 60 years or older with a prolonged history of exertional dyspnea but a minimal, nonproductive cough. They have lost weight and use the accessory muscles of respiration to breathe. Weight loss is probably due less to the lack of calories than to the increased work of breathing. Tachypnea and a prolonged expiratory phase are typical. The most prominent radiological abnormality is overinflation of the lung, as evidenced by enlarged lungs, depressed diaphragms, and an increased posteroanterior diameter *(barrel chest)*. The bronchovascular markings do not extend to the peripheral lung fields. Because these patients have a higher respiratory rate and an increased minute volume, they can maintain arterial hemoglobin saturation at near-normal levels and are therefore referred to as "pink puffers." In contrast to patients with predominantly chronic bronchitis, those with emphysema are at lower risk of recurrent pulmonary infections and are not so prone to the development of cor pulmonale. The clinical course of emphysema is marked by an inexorable decline in respiratory function and progressive dyspnea, for which no treatment is adequate.

Asthma Is Characterized by Episodic Air-Flow Obstruction

Asthma is a chronic lung disease caused by increased responsiveness of the airways to a variety of stimuli. Patients typically have paroxysms of wheezing, dyspnea, and cough. Acute episodes of asthma may alternate with asymptomatic periods or they may be superimposed on a background of chronic airway obstruction. When severe acute asthma is unresponsive to therapy, it is referred to as *status asthmaticus*. Most asthmatic patients, even when apparently well, have some persistent airflow obstruction and morphological lesions.

In the United States, bronchial asthma is a common disorder, affecting up to 10% of children and 5% of adults. For reasons unknown, since 1980, the prevalence of asthma in the United States has doubled. Although the initial attack of the disease can occur at any age, half of cases appear in patients younger than 10 years, and the incidence is twice as high in boys as in girls. By age 30 years, both sexes are affected equally.

 Pathogenesis: Asthma was classically divided into two major categories depending on the inciting factors. Extrinsic (allergic) asthma referred to a condition in which bronchospasm is induced by inhaled antigens, usually in children with a personal or family history of allergic disease (e.g., eczema, urticaria, or hay fever). By contrast, intrinsic (idiosyncratic) asthma was a disease of adults in which bronchial hyperreactivity was produced in persons who had no apparent allergic diathesis by a variety of factors unrelated to immune mechanisms. These distinctions implied rigid differences in pathogenetic mechanisms, but as greater knowledge of asthma has been obtained, such distinctions have been blurred. At this time, it seems more appropriate simply to discuss asthma in terms of the different inciting factors and the common effector pathways.

The consensus hypothesis attributes bronchial hyperresponsiveness in asthma to an inflammatory reaction to diverse stimuli. As a result of exposure to an inciting factor (e.g., allergens, drugs, cold, exercise), inflammatory mediators are released by activated macrophages, mast cells, eosinophils, and basophils. These molecules induce bronchoconstriction, increased vascular permeability, and mucous secretions. Moreover, the resident inflammatory cells may be activated to release chemotactic factors that in turn recruit more effector cells and amplify the response of the airways. Inflammation of the bronchial walls also may injure the epithelium, thereby stimulating nerve endings and initiating neural reflexes that further aggravate and propagate the bronchospasm.

A large number of inflammatory mediators and chemotactic factors have been implicated in the production of the bronchospasm and mucous hypersecretion of asthma. The relative contributions of the different substances probably vary with the inciting stimulus. The best-studied situation associated with the induction of asthma is the inhalation of allergens.

In a sensitized person, an inhaled allergen interacts with T_H2 cells and IgE antibody bound to the surface of mast cells that are interspersed among the epithelial cells of the bronchial mucosa (Fig. 12-48). As a result, T_H2 cells and

FIGURE 12-48
Pathogenesis of asthma. A. Immunologically mediated asthma. Allergens interact with immunoglobulin E (IgE) on mast cells, either on the surface of the epithelium or, when there is abnormal permeability of the epithelium, in the submucosa. Mediators are released and may react locally or by reflexes mediated through the vagus. B. The discharge of eosinophilic granules further impairs mucociliary function and damages epithelial cells. Epithelial cell injury stimulates nerve endings in the mucosa, thereby initiating an autonomic discharge that contributes to airway narrowing and mucous secretion.

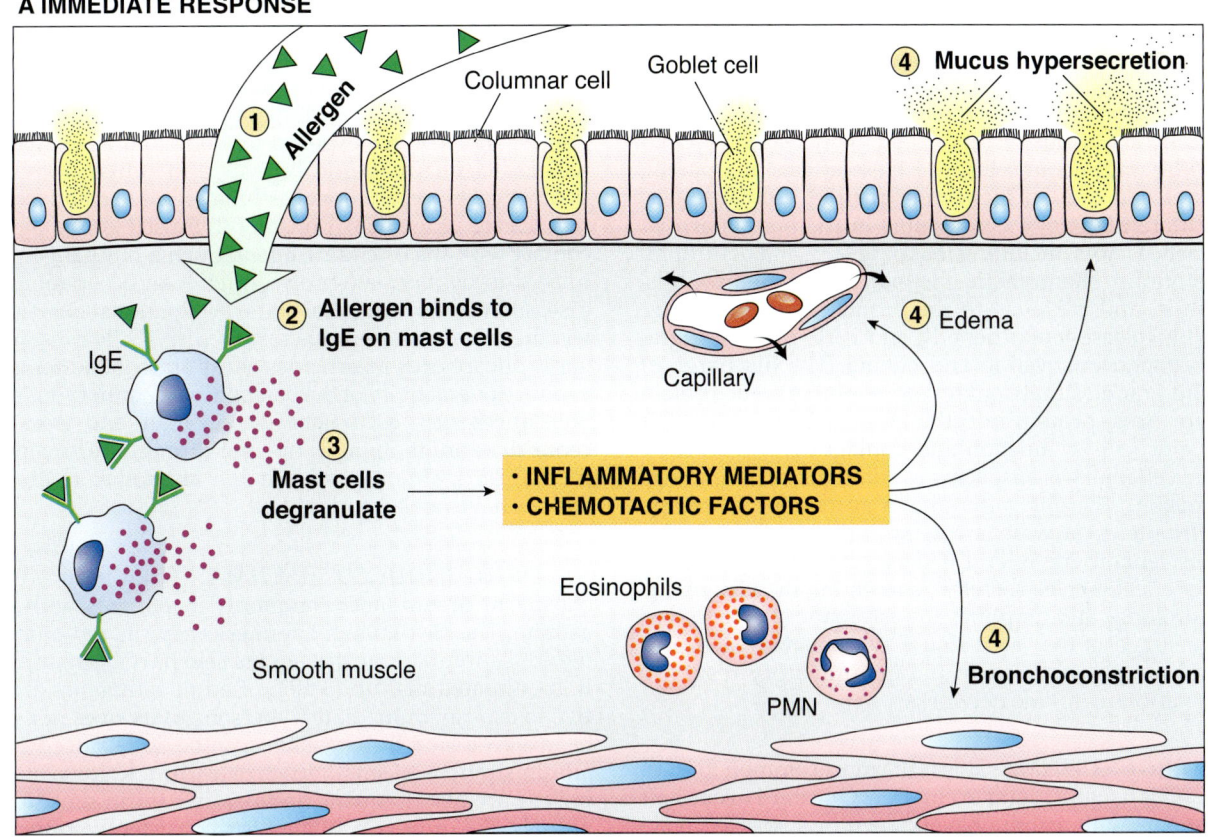
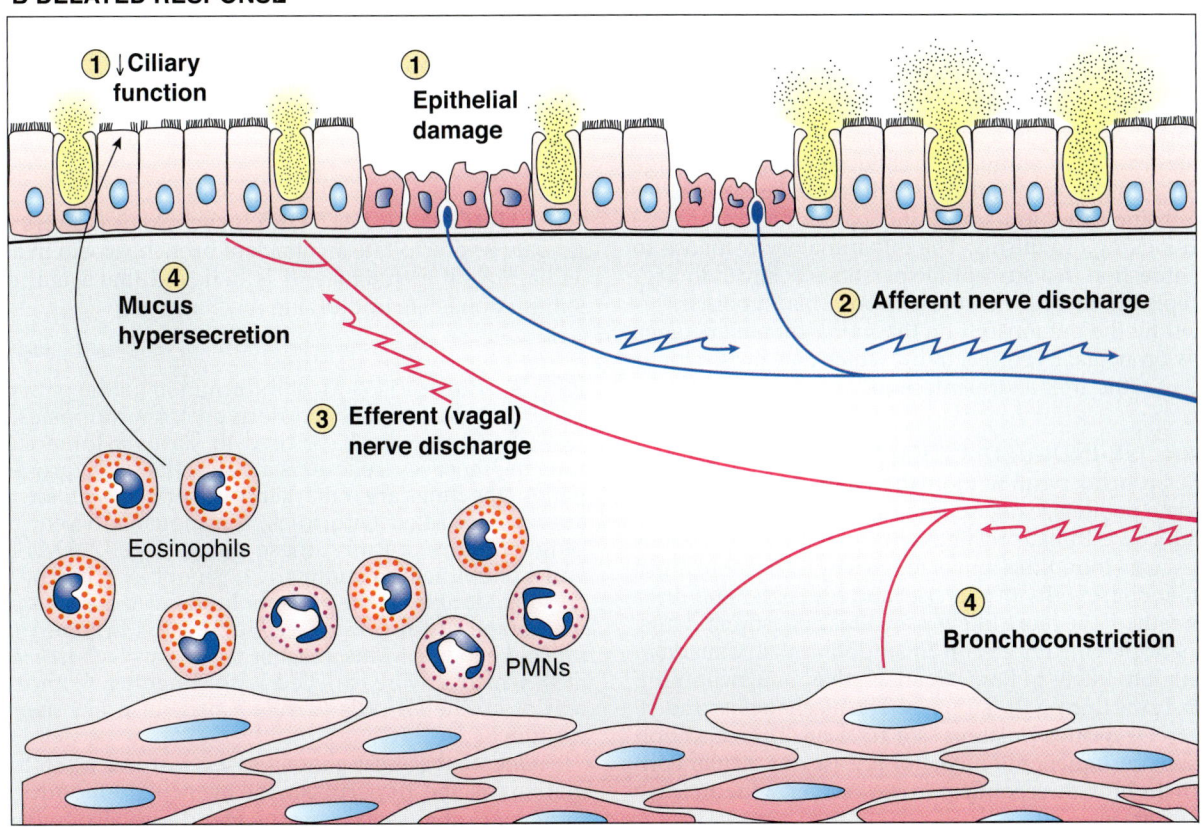

mast cells release mediators of type I (immediate) hypersensitivity, including histamine, bradykinin, leukotrienes, prostaglandins, thromboxane A_2 and platelet-activating factor (PAF), as well as cytokines such as interleukin (IL)-4 and IL-5. The inflammatory mediators lead to (1) smooth muscle contraction, (2) mucous secretion, and (3) increased vascular permeability and edema. Each of these effects is a potent, albeit reversible, cause of airway obstruction. IL-5 causes terminal differentiation of eosinophils in the bone marrow. Chemotactic factors, including leukotriene B_4 and neutrophil and eosinophil chemotactic factors, attract neutrophils, eosinophils, and platelets to the bronchial wall. In turn, eosinophils release leukotriene B_4 and PAF, thereby aggravating bronchoconstriction and edema. The discharge of eosinophil granules that contain eosinophil cationic protein and major basic protein into the bronchial lumen further impairs mucociliary function and damages epithelial cells. Epithelial cell injury is suspected to stimulate nerve endings in the mucosa, thereby initiating an autonomic discharge that contributes to airway narrowing and mucous secretion. Moreover, leukotriene B_4 and PAF recruit more eosinophils and other effector cells, thereby augmenting the vicious circle that prolongs and amplifies the asthmatic attack. Recent evidence suggests that activated T lymphocytes also contribute to the propagation of the inflammatory response through various cytokine networks.

ALLERGIC ASTHMA: This is the most common form of asthma and is usually found in children. One third to one half of all patients with asthma have known or suspected reactions to airborne allergens. Common allergens include pollens, animal hair or fur, and contamination of house dust with mites. Allergic asthma is strongly correlated with skin-test reactivity. Half of all children with asthma have a substantial or complete remission of symptoms by age 20 years, but a considerable number have a recurrence after age 30 years.

INFECTIOUS ASTHMA: A common precipitating factor in childhood asthma is a viral respiratory tract infection rather than an allergic stimulus. In children younger than age 2 years, respiratory syncytial virus is the usual agent; in older children, rhinovirus, influenza, and parainfluenza are the common inciting organisms. The inflammatory response to the viral infection in a susceptible person is believed to trigger the episode of bronchoconstriction. This hypothesis is supported by the demonstration that nonasthmatic persons also show bronchial hyperreactivity, which may persist for as long as 2 months after a viral infection.

EXERCISE-INDUCED ASTHMA: Exercise can precipitate some bronchospasm in more than half of all asthmatics, and in some patients, exercise is the only inciting factor. Exercise-induced asthma is related to the magnitude of heat or water loss from the epithelium of the airways. The more rapid the ventilation (severity of exercise) and the colder and drier the air breathed, the more likely is an attack of asthma. Thus, an asthmatic playing hockey on an outdoor rink in Canada in winter is more likely to have an attack than one swimming slowly in Texas during the summer. The mechanisms underlying exercise-induced asthma are unclear. The condition may be the consequence of mediator release or vascular congestion in the bronchi secondary to rewarming of the airways after the exertion.

OCCUPATIONAL ASTHMA: More than 80 different occupational exposures have been linked to the development of asthma. In some instances, these substances provoke allergic asthma by IgE-related hypersensitivity mechanisms. Examples of those affected by this malady include animal handlers, bakers, and workers exposed to wood and vegetable dusts, metal salts, pharmaceutical agents, and industrial chemicals. In other cases, occupational asthma seems to result from a direct release of mediators of smooth muscle contraction after contact with the offending agent. Such a mechanism is postulated in byssinosis ("brown lung"), an occupational lung disease in cotton workers. Some occupational exposures affect the autonomic nervous system directly. For instance, organic phosphorus insecticides act as anticholinesterases and produce overactivity of the parasympathetic nervous system. Substances such as toluene diisocyanate and western red cedar dust are thought to operate through hypersensitivity mechanisms, although specific IgE antibodies to these substances have not been identified.

DRUG-INDUCED ASTHMA: Drug-induced bronchospasm occurs most commonly in patients with known asthma. The best-known offender is aspirin, but other nonsteroidal antiinflammatory agents also have been implicated. It is estimated that up to 10% of adult asthmatics are sensitive to aspirin. Immediate hypersensitivity does not seem to be involved, and these patients can be desensitized by daily administrations of small doses of aspirin. Rhinitis and nasal polyps are also frequent findings in aspirin-sensitive individuals. β-Adrenergic antagonists consistently induce bronchoconstriction in asthmatics and are contraindicated in such patients.

AIR POLLUTION: Massive air pollution, usually in episodes associated with temperature inversions, is associated with bronchospasm in patients with asthma and other preexisting lung diseases. Sulfur dioxide, oxides of nitrogen, and ozone are the commonly implicated environmental pollutants.

EMOTIONAL FACTORS: Psychological stress can aggravate or precipitate an attack of bronchospasm in as many as half of all asthmatics. It is believed that vagal efferent stimulation is the underlying mechanism.

Pathology: Most information on the pathology of asthma has been derived from autopsies on patients who have died in status asthmaticus, and thus the most severe lesions are described. On gross examination, the lungs are remarkably distended with air, and the airways are filled with thick, tenacious, adherent mucous plugs. Microscopically, these plugs (Fig. 12-49A) contain strips of epithelium and many eosinophils. Charcot-Leyden crystals, derived from phospholipids of the eosinophil cell membrane, are also seen (see Fig. 12-24B). In some cases, the mucoid exudate forms a cast of the airways *(Curschmann spirals),* which may be expelled with coughing. Compact clusters of epithelial cells *(Creola bodies)* also are seen in the sputum.

One of the most characteristic features of status asthmaticus is the hyperplasia of bronchial smooth muscle. Bronchial submucosal mucous glands are also hyperplastic

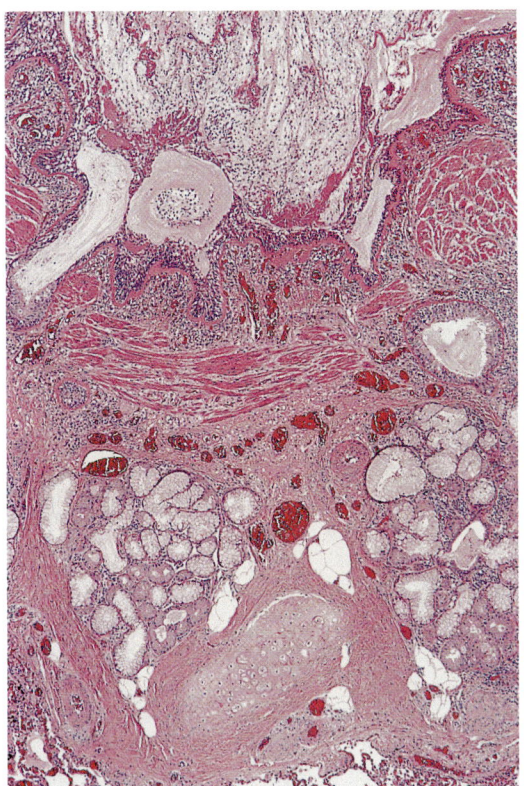
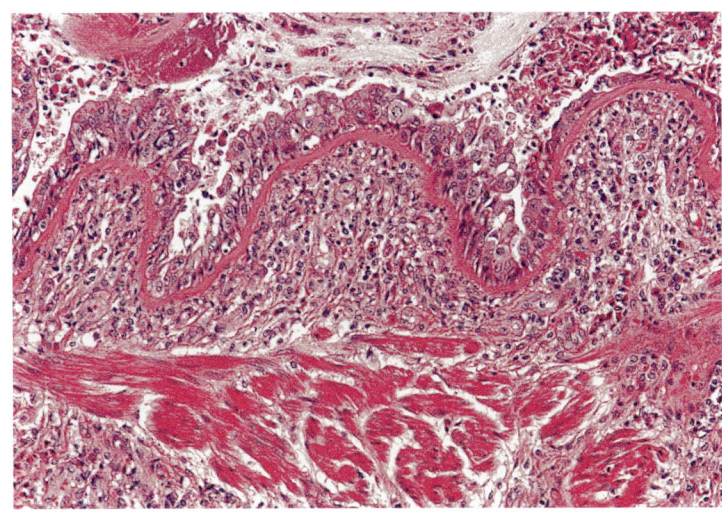

FIGURE 12-49

Asthma. **A.** A section of lung from a patient who died in status asthmaticus reveals a bronchus containing a luminal mucous plug, submucosal gland hyperplasia, and smooth muscle hyperplasia. **B.** Higher magnification shows hyaline thickening of the subepithelial basement membrane and marked inflammation of the bronchiolar wall, with numerous eosinophils. The mucosa exhibits an inflamed and metaplastic epithelium.

(see Fig. 12-49A). The submucosa is edematous and contains a mixed inflammatory infiltrate, including variable numbers of eosinophils. The epithelium does not display the normal pseudostratified appearance and may be denuded, with only the basal cells remaining (see Fig. 12-49B). The basal cells are hyperplastic, and squamous metaplasia is seen. An increase in goblet cells (goblet cell hyperplasia) is also apparent. Characteristically, the epithelial basement membrane appears thickened, owing to an increase in collagen deep to the true basal lamina.

Clinical Features: A typical attack of asthma begins with a feeling of tightness in the chest and a nonproductive cough. Both inspiratory and expiratory wheezes appear, the respiratory rate increases, and the patient becomes dyspneic. Characteristically, the expiratory phase is particularly prolonged. The end of the attack is often heralded by severe coughing and the expectoration of thick, mucus-containing Curschmann spirals, eosinophils, and Charcot–Leyden crystals.

Status asthmaticus refers to increasingly severe bronchoconstriction that does not respond to the drugs that usually abort the acute attack. This situation is potentially serious and requires hospitalization. Patients in status asthmaticus have hypoxemia and often hypercapnia, and in particularly severe episodes, they may die. They require oxygen and other pharmacological interventions.

The cornerstone of treatment in asthma is pharmacological and includes the administration of β-adrenergic agonists, inhaled corticosteroids, cromolyn sodium, methylxanthines, and anticholinergic agents. Systemic corticosteroids are reserved for status asthmaticus or resistant chronic asthma. The inhalation of bronchodilators often provides dramatic relief.

PNEUMOCONIOSES

The pneumoconioses are pulmonary diseases caused by the inhalation of inorganic dusts. More than 40 inhaled minerals cause lung lesions and radiographic abnormalities. Most, such as tin, barium, and iron, are innocuous and simply accumulate in the lung. However, some lead to crippling pulmonary diseases. The specific types of pneumoconioses are named according to the substance inhaled (e.g., silicosis, asbestosis, talcosis). In certain instances, the offending agent is uncertain, and often the occupation is simply cited (e.g., *arc welder's lung*). Historically, occupations were recognized as predisposing to lung disease before an etiological agent was recognized. Thus, *knife grinder's lung* was used before this malady was recognized as silicosis.

The most important factor in the production of symptomatic pneumoconioses is the capacity of inhaled dusts to stimulate fibrosis (Fig. 12-50). Thus, small amounts of silica or asbestos may produce extensive fibrosis, whereas coal and iron are only weakly fibrogenic.

In general, lung lesions produced by inorganic dusts reflect the dose and size of the particles delivered to the lung. The dose is a function of the amount of dust in the ambient

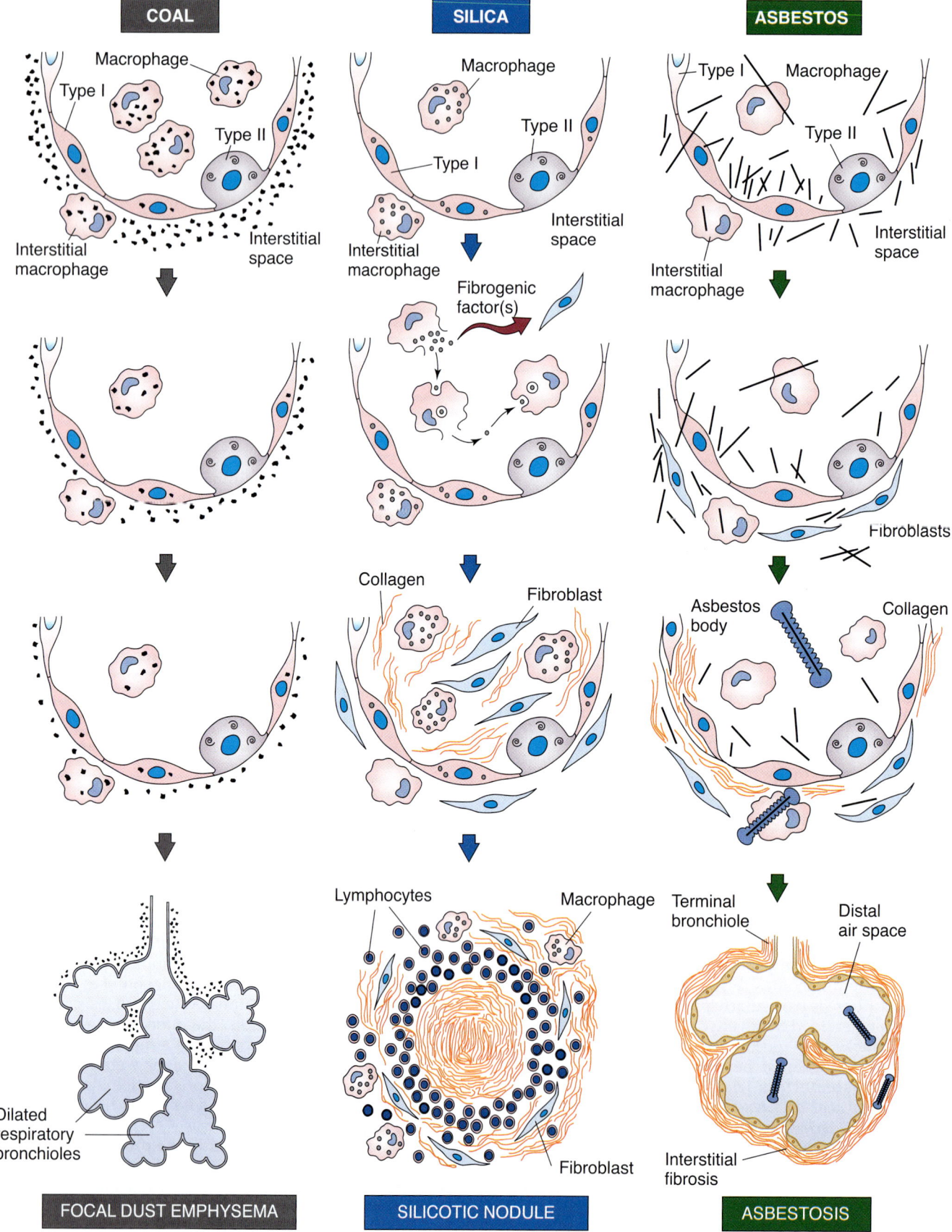

air and the time spent working in the environment. Because the inhaled particles are often irregular, it is important to express their size as aerodynamic particle diameter, a parameter that describes the motion of the particle in inspired air. The aerodynamic particle diameter determines where the inhaled dusts deposit in the lung (see Fig. 12-2). The most dangerous particles are those that reach the peripheral zones (i.e., the smallest bronchioles and the acini). Most large particles (>10 µm in diameter) deposit on the bronchi and bronchioles and are removed by the mucociliary escalator. The smaller particles terminate in the acinus, and the smallest ones behave as a gas and are exhaled.

The alveolar macrophages ingest the inhaled particles and constitute the primary defense mechanism of the alveolar space. Most of the phagocytosed particles ascend to the mucociliary carpet and are expectorated or swallowed. Others migrate into the interstitium of the lung and then into the lymphatics. A significant number of ingested particles accumulate in and about respiratory bronchioles and terminal bronchioles. Other particles are not phagocytosed but migrate through epithelial cells into the interstitium.

Silicosis Is Caused by the Inhalation of Silicon Dioxide (Silica)

The earth's crust is composed largely of silicon and its oxides, and silicosis is one of the oldest recorded diseases, possibly having begun in the Paleolithic period when humans began to fashion flint instruments. Dyspnea in metal diggers was reported by Hippocrates, and early Dutch pathologists wrote that the lungs of stone cutters sectioned like a mass of sand. The 19th-century English literature provided numerous descriptions of silicosis, and the disease remained the major cause of death in workers exposed to silica dust for the first half of the 20th century.

Silicosis was described historically as a disease of sandblasters. Mining also involves exposure to silica, as do numerous other occupations, including stone cutting, polishing and sharpening of metals, ceramic manufacturing, foundry work, and the cleaning of boilers. The use of air-handling equipment and masks has substantially reduced the incidence of silicosis.

Pathogenesis: The biological effects of silica particles depend on a number of factors, some involving the particle itself and others related to the host response. Crystalline silica (quartz) is more toxic than amorphous forms, and its biological activity is related to its surface properties. Particles of 0.2 to 2.0 µm are the most dangerous. Removal of the soluble surface layer by acid washing or the creation of new surfaces by sandblasting enhances the biological activity of silica particles.

After their inhalation, silica particles are ingested by alveolar macrophages. Silicon hydroxide groups on the surface of the particles form hydrogen bonds with phospholipids and proteins, an interaction that is presumed to damage cellular membranes and thereby kill the macrophages. The dead cells release free silica particles and fibrogenic factors. The released silica is then reingested by macrophages, and the process is amplified.

 Pathology:

SIMPLE NODULAR SILICOSIS: This is the most common form of silicosis and is almost inevitable in any worker with long-term exposure to silica. Twenty to 40 years after the initial exposure to silica (but sometimes after only 10 years), the lungs contain silicotic nodules. These characteristic lesions are less than 1 cm in diameter, usually 2 to 4 mm. On histological examination, they have a characteristic whorled appearance, with concentrically arranged collagen that forms the largest part of the nodule (Fig. 12-51). At the periphery, there are aggregates of mononuclear cells, mostly lymphocytes and fibroblasts. Polarized light reveals doubly refractile needle-shaped silicates within the nodule.

The hilar nodes may become enlarged and calcified, often at the periphery of the node *(eggshell calcification)*. Simple silicosis is not ordinarily associated with significant respiratory dysfunction.

PROGRESSIVE MASSIVE FIBROSIS: Progressive massive fibrosis is defined radiologically as nodular masses of more than 2 cm diameter in a background of simple silicosis. These larger lesions represent the coalescence of smaller nodules. Most of these lesions are 5 to 10 cm across and are usually located in the upper zones of the lungs bilaterally (Fig. 12-52). Morphologically, the lesions often exhibit central cavitation. Progressive massive fibrosis is related to the amount of silica in the lung. Disability is caused by the destruction of lung tissue that has been incorporated into the nodules.

ACUTE SILICOSIS: Now uncommon, acute silicosis results from heavy exposure to finely particulate silica during sandblasting or boiler scaling. It is associated with diffuse fibrosis of the lung, but silicotic nodules are not found. Dense eosinophilic material accumulates in alveolar spaces to pro-

FIGURE 12-50
Pathogenesis of pneumoconioses. The three most important pneumoconioses are illustrated. In simple coal workers' pneumoconiosis, massive amounts of dust are inhaled and engulfed by macrophages. The macrophages pass into the interstitium of the lung and aggregate around the respiratory bronchioles. Subsequently, the bronchioles dilate. In silicosis, the silica particles are toxic to macrophages, which die and release a fibrogenic factor. In turn the released silica is again phagocytosed by other macrophages. The result is a dense fibrotic nodule, the silicotic nodule. Asbestosis is characterized by little dust and much interstitial fibrosis. Asbestos bodies are the classic features.

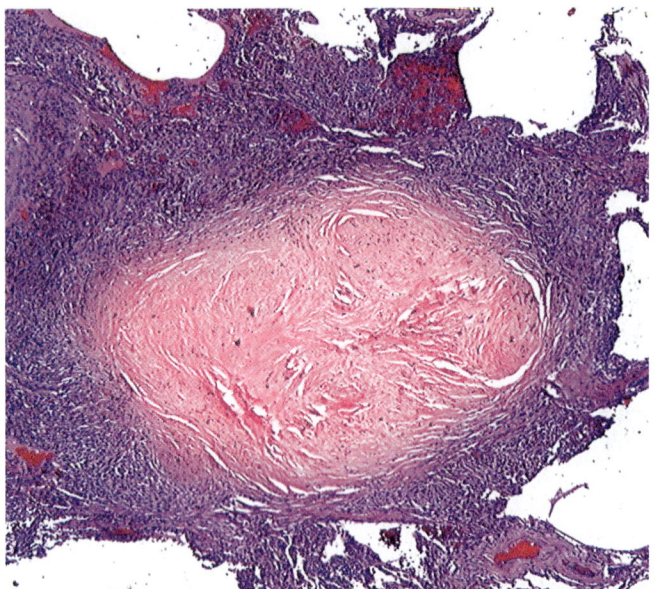

FIGURE 12-51
Silicosis. A silicotic nodule is composed of concentric whorls of dense, sparsely cellular collagen. At the edge of the nodule are dust deposits that contain carbon pigment and silica particles.

duce an appearance that resembles alveolar lipoproteinosis (*silicoproteinosis*). The disease progresses rapidly over a few years, in contrast to other forms of silicosis in which progression is measured in decades. On radiological examination, acute silicosis shows diffuse linear fibrosis and reduced lung volume. Clinically, there is a severe restrictive defect.

Clinical Features: Simple silicosis is usually a radiological diagnosis without significant symptoms. Dyspnea on exertion and later at rest suggests progressive massive fibrosis or other complications of silicosis. In acute silicosis, dyspnea may become rapidly disabling, after which respiratory failure ensues.

It is well recognized that tuberculosis is much more common in patients with silicosis than in the general population. The incidence of tuberculosis in patients with silicosis is higher in acute silicosis and among populations with a high prevalence of tuberculosis. Despite a decline in the incidence of tuberculosis in the general population, the association with silicosis has persisted. Silicosis does not predispose to lung cancers.

Coal Workers' Pneumoconiosis Reflects Inhalation of Carbon Particles

Pathogenesis: Coal dust is composed of amorphous carbon and other constituents of the earth's surface, including variable amounts of silica. Anthracite (hard) coal contains significantly more quartz than does the bituminous variety (soft coal). Workers in certain occupations, such as those who work within mines, inhale more quartz particles than those working above ground or loading coal for transport. In this context, one must recognize that amorphous carbon by itself is not fibrogenic, owing to its inability to kill alveolar macrophages. It is simply a nuisance dust that causes an innocuous anthracosis. By contrast, silica is highly fibrogenic, and the inhalation of anthracotic particles may therefore lead to the lesions of *anthracosilicosis*.

Pathology: Coal worker's pneumoconiosis (CWP) is typically divided into the categories of *simple CWP* and *complicated CWP* (a.k.a. progressive massive fibrosis). The characteristic pulmonary lesions of **simple CWP** include the nonpalpable coal-dust *macules* and the palpable coal-dust *nodule,* both of which are typically multiple and scattered throughout the lung as 1- to 4-mm black foci. Microscopically, the coal-dust **macule** exhibits numerous carbon-laden macrophages, which surround the distal respiratory bronchioles, extend to fill adjacent alveolar spaces, and infiltrate the peribronchiolar interstitial space. There is an accompanying mild dilation of respiratory bronchioles *(focal dust emphysema),* which probably results from atrophy of smooth muscle. **Nodules** consist of dust-laden macrophages associated with a fibrotic stroma. Nodules are round or irregular in outline and may or may not be associ-

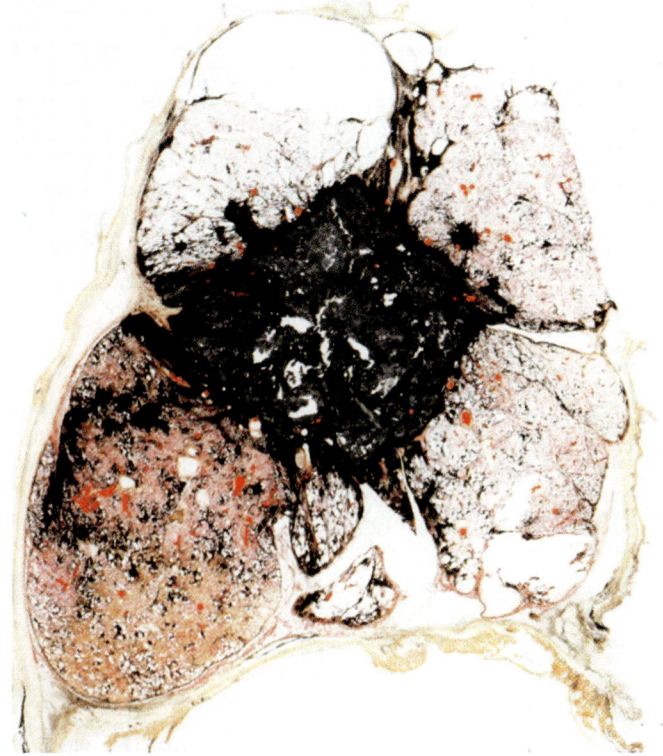

FIGURE 12-52
Progressive massive fibrosis. A whole mount of a silicotic lung from a coal miner shows a large area of dense fibrosis containing entrapped carbon particles.

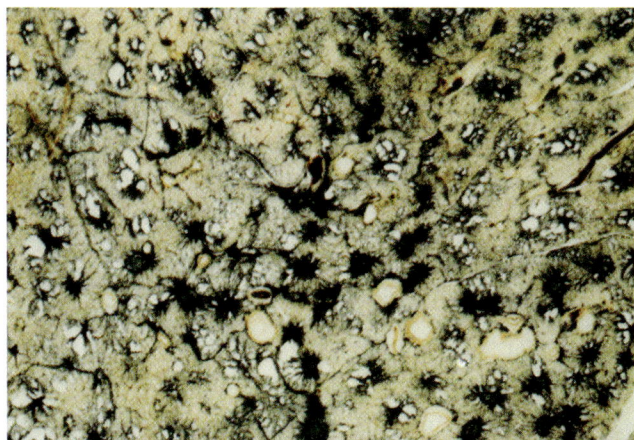

FIGURE 12-53
Anthracosilicosis. A whole mount of the lung of a coal miner demonstrates scattered, irregular, pigmented nodules throughout the parenchyma.

ated with bronchioles. They occur when coal is admixed with fibrogenic dusts such as silica and are more properly classified as anthracosilicosis (Fig. 12-53). Coal-dust macules and nodules appear on a chest radiograph as small nodular densities. Although simple coal workers' pneumoconiosis was once thought to cause severe disability, it is now clear that it causes at worst a minor impairment of pulmonary function. When coal miners have severe air-flow obstruction, it is usually due to smoking. **Complicated CWP** occurs on a background of simple CWP and is defined as a lesion 2.0 cm or greater in size. Patients with complicated CWP may have significant respiratory impairment.

Caplan syndrome was originally described as the presence of rheumatoid nodules (*Caplan nodules*) in the lungs of coal miners with rheumatoid arthritis. However, the term *Caplan syndrome* is now also used for the association of pulmonary rheumatoid nodules with other pneumoconioses, such as silicosis or asbestosis. These nodular lesions are large (1–10 cm in diameter), multiple, bilateral, and usually peripheral. Microscopically, a Caplan nodule has the appearance of a rheumatoid nodule associated with inhaled dust deposits. Rheumatoid nodules consist of large, central, necrotic areas surrounded by a border of chronic inflammation and palisading macrophages. Caplan nodules are similar but not identical to rheumatoid nodules and may represent a combination of silicotic and rheumatoid nodules.

Asbestos-Related Diseases Are Reactive or Neoplastic

Asbestos (Greek, *unquenchable*) is a generic term that embraces a group of fibrous silicate minerals that occur as long, thin fibers. This mineral has been used for a variety of purposes for more than 4000 years, since early Finns fashioned pottery from the material. The Roman vestal virgins used asbestos in the manufacture of oil-lamp wicks, and Marco Polo remarked on the asbestos-containing Chinese cloth that resisted fire. In the modern era, asbestos has been used in a variety of products including insulation, construction materials, and brake linings. Asbestos mining proceeded exponentially in the 20th century until its deleterious effects eventually elicited alarm.

Asbestos occurs in six natural types, which can be broadly divided into two mineralogical groups. *Chrysotile*, which accounts for the bulk of commercially used asbestos, and the *amphiboles*, which include amosite, crocidolite, tremolite, actinolite, and anthophyllite. Of the amphiboles, only amosite and crocidolite have been used commercially to any extent. If coal is the classic example of much dust and little fibrosis, asbestos is the prototype of little dust and much fibrosis (see Fig. 12-50). Exposure to asbestos can result in a number of thoracic complications including asbestosis, benign pleural effusion, diffuse pleural fibrosis, pleural plaques, rounded atelectasis, and mesothelioma (Table 12-4). All of the commercially used forms of asbestos have been associated with the asbestos-related lung diseases. However, owing to differing properties, the amphiboles, and crocidolite in particular, have a much greater propensity to produce disease than does chrysotile.

ASBESTOSIS: *Asbestosis refers to the diffuse interstitial fibrosis that results from the inhalation of asbestos fibers.* The disease occurs as a result of the processing and handling of asbestos, rather than mining, which is a surface operation. Exposure starts with the baggers who package asbestos and continues with those who modify or use it, such as workers who make asbestos products (tiles, cement, insulation material) and those in the construction and shipbuilding industries.

 Pathogenesis: Asbestos fibers are long (up to 100 μm) but thin (0.5–1 μm), so their aerodynamic particle diameter is small. They deposit in the distal airways and alveoli, particularly at the bifurcations of alveolar ducts. The smallest particles are engulfed by macrophages, but many of the larger fibers penetrate into the interstitial space. The first lesion is an alveolitis that is directly related to asbestos exposure. Release of inflammatory mediators by activated macrophages and the fibrogenic character of the free asbestos fibers in the interstitium promote interstitial pulmonary fibrosis.

 Pathology: Asbestosis is characterized by bilateral, diffuse interstitial fibrosis and asbestos bodies in the lung (Fig. 12-54). In the early stages, fibrosis

TABLE 12-4 **Asbestos-Related Lung Disease**

Pleural lesions	Interstitial lung disease
Benign pleural effusion	Asbestosis
Parietal pleural plaques	
Diffuse pleural fibrosis	**Malignant mesothelioma**
Rounded atelectasis	**Carcinoma of the lung (in smokers)**

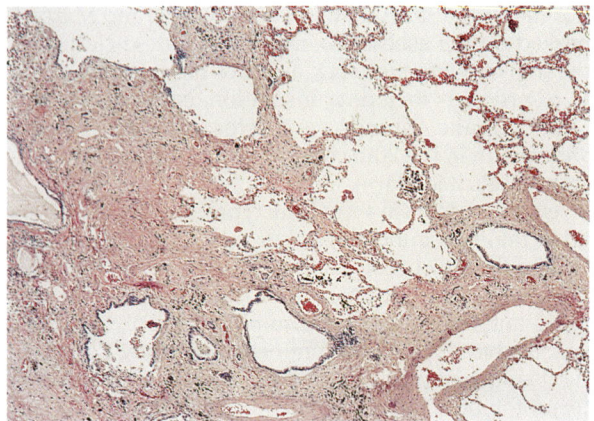

FIGURE 12-54
Asbestosis. The lung shows patchy, dense, interstitial fibrosis.

occurs in and around alveolar ducts and respiratory bronchioles, as well as in the periphery of the acinus. Asbestos fibers that deposit in the bronchioles and respiratory bronchioles incite a fibrogenic response in these locations that leads to mild chronic air-flow obstruction. Thus, asbestos may produce an obstructive as well as a restrictive defect. As the disease becomes more advanced, fibrosis spreads beyond the peribronchiolar location and eventually results in an end-stage or ("honeycomb") lung. Asbestosis is usually more severe in the lower zones of the lung.

Asbestos bodies are found in the walls of the bronchioles or within alveolar spaces, often engulfed by alveolar macrophages. The particle has distinctive morphological features, consisting of a clear, thin asbestos fiber (10–50 μm long) surrounded by a beaded iron–protein coat. By light microscopy, it is golden brown (Fig. 12-55) and stains strongly with the Prussian blue stain for iron. The fibers are only partly engulfed by macrophages because they are too large for a single cell. The macrophages coat the asbestos fiber with protein, proteoglycans, and ferritin.

The incidental finding of asbestos bodies in autopsies does not warrant a diagnosis of asbestosis; the lungs must show diffuse interstitial fibrosis as well as asbestos bodies. Digests and concentrates of lung tissue show that asbestos bodies occur to varying degrees in the lungs of virtually all patients who come to autopsy.

BENIGN PLEURAL EFFUSION: Benign pleural effusion associated with the inhalation of asbestos is diagnosed by four criteria: (1) a history of asbestos exposure, (2) identification of a pleural effusion with radiographs or thoracentesis, (3) absence of other diseases that could cause effusion, and (4) no malignant tumor after 3 years of follow-up. Pleural effusions often occur within 10 years of initial exposure and have been observed in about 3% of workers exposed to asbestos.

PLEURAL PLAQUES: Pleural plaques typically occur on the parietal and diaphragmatic pleura, often 10 to 20 years after exposure to asbestos. Plaques may be found in up to 15% of the general population, and half of all patients with plaques at autopsy may not have a history of asbestos exposure. Plaques are found most often on the parietal pleura, in the posterolateral regions of the lower thorax, and on the domes of the diaphragm.

On gross examination, pleural plaques are pearly white and have a smooth or nodular surface (Fig. 12-56). They are usually bilateral, although not necessarily symmetric. Plaques may become quite large, measuring more than 10 cm in diameter, and may become calcified. Histologically, they consist of acellular, dense, hyalinized fibrous tissue, with numerous slitlike spaces in a parallel fashion *(basket-weave pattern)*. Pleural plaques are not a predictor of asbestosis.

DIFFUSE PLEURAL FIBROSIS: Fibrosis limited to the pleura is usually detected at least 10 years after initial exposure to asbestos. It must be distinguished from asbestosis, in which fibrosis diffusely affects the interstitium of the underlying lung parenchyma. Plaques and pleural fibrosis can occur in association with all types of asbestos.

ROUNDED ATELECTASIS: Asbestosis exposure occasionally leads to a condition in which pleural fibrosis and ad-

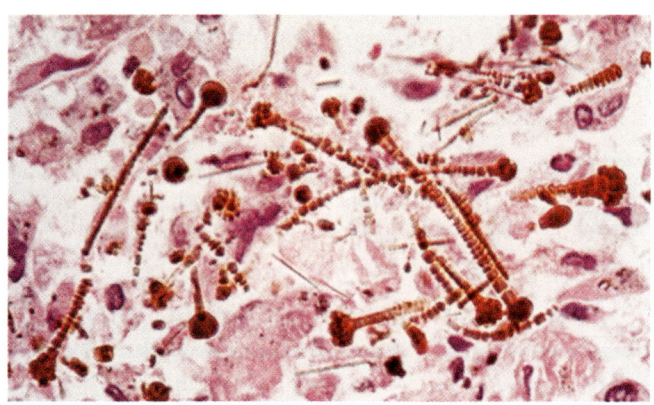

FIGURE 12-55
Asbestos bodies. These ferruginous bodies are golden brown and beaded, with a central, colorless, nonbirefringent core fiber. Asbestos bodies are encrusted with protein and iron.

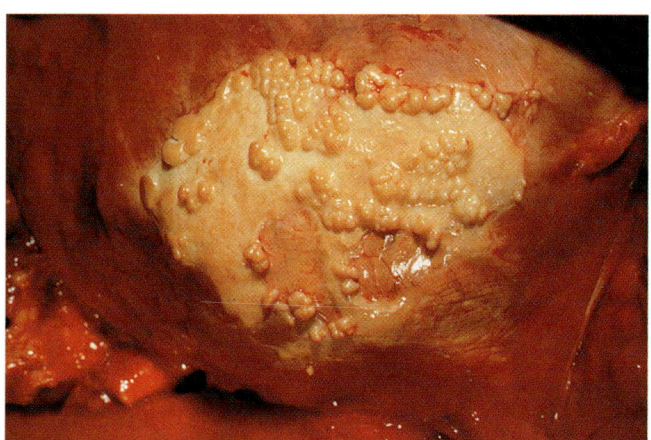

FIGURE 12-56
Pleural plaque. The dome of the diaphragm is covered by a smooth, pearly white, nodular plaque.

hesions are associated with atelectasis, which has a rounded appearance on chest radiograph. Radiographically, rounded atelectasis is characterized by a pleural-based, rounded or oval, 2.5- to 5.0-cm shadow, which usually lies along the posterior surface of a lower lobe. Pathologically, the lung shows pleural fibrosis or plaques, with curved pleural invaginations extending several centimeters into the underlying parenchyma. The condition is entirely benign.

MESOTHELIOMA: **A clear-cut relation between asbestos exposure and malignant mesothelioma is firmly established.** Sometimes the exposure is slight, as in the wives of asbestos workers who wash their husbands' clothes. More often mesothelioma is found in workers heavily exposed to asbestos, predominantly of the crocidolite variety. The clinical and pathological features of this disease are discussed below with diseases of the pleura.

CARCINOMA OF THE LUNG: Although lung cancer has been reported to be three to five times more common in nonsmoking asbestos workers than in similar workers not exposed to asbestos, this figure is based on small numbers and remains to be firmly established. However, in asbestos workers who smoke, the incidence of carcinoma of the lung is vastly increased; the reported risk for the incidence of carcinoma of the lung is increased up to 60 times that of the general population. The link between asbestos and lung cancer is most convincingly supported in the presence of asbestosis (diffuse interstitial fibrosis).

Berylliosis Displays Noncaseating Granulomas

Berylliosis refers to the pulmonary disease that follows the inhalation of beryllium. Today this metal is used principally in structural materials in aerospace industries, in the manufacture of industrial ceramics, and in atomic reactors. Exposure to beryllium also may occur during the mining and extraction of beryllium ores.

Pathology: Berylliosis occurs as an acute chemical pneumonitis or a chronic pneumoconiosis. In the acute form, symptoms begin within hours or days after inhalation of metal particles and are reflected pathologically in diffuse alveolar damage. Of all persons with acute beryllium pneumonitis, 10% progress to chronic disease, although chronic berylliosis is often encountered in workers without any history of an acute illness.

Chronic berylliosis differs from other pneumoconioses in that the amount and duration of exposure may be small, and the lesion is suspected to be a hypersensitivity phenomenon. Pathologically, the pulmonary lesions are indistinguishable from those of sarcoidosis (see below). Multiple noncaseating granulomas are distributed along the pleura, septa, and bronchovascular bundles (Fig. 12-57). The beryllium lymphocyte proliferation test may aid in separating these two entities. Progression of the disease can result in end-stage fibrosis and *honeycomb lung*. Patients with chronic berylliosis have an insidious onset of dyspnea 15 or more years after the initial exposure. The disease appears to be associated with an increased risk of lung cancer.

Talcosis Results From Prolonged and Heavy Exposure to Talc Dust

Talc consists of magnesium silicates that are used in a number of industries for their lubricant properties and in cosmetics and pharmaceuticals. Occupational exposure to talc occurs among workers engaged in the mining and milling of the mineral and in the leather, rubber, paper, and textile industries. Industrial talc is usually mixed with other minerals such as asbestos or silica. Cosmetic talc is more than 90% pure and rarely causes lung disease.

Pathology: On gross examination, the lesions of talcosis vary from minute nodules to severe fibrosis. Microscopically, foreign-body granulomas associated with birefringent platelike talc particles are scattered throughout the parenchyma, which displays fibrotic nodules and interstitial fibrosis. The associated minerals, such as silica or asbestos, may contribute to the fibrotic changes.

Intravenous drug abusers who use talc as the carrier material for illicit drugs develop vascular and interstitial granulomas in the lung, together with variable degrees of fibrosis. Arterial changes of pulmonary hypertension are common, and persons with these changes may initially be seen with cor pulmonale.

INTERSTITIAL LUNG DISEASE

A large number of pulmonary disorders are grouped as interstitial, infiltrative, or restrictive diseases because they are characterized by inflammatory infiltrates in the interstitial

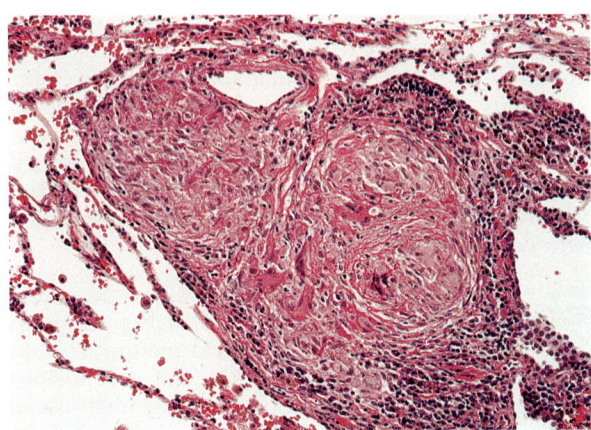

FIGURE 12-57

Berylliosis. A noncaseating granuloma consists of a nodular collection of epithelioid macrophages and multinucleated giant cells.

space and have similar clinical and radiological presentations. These diverse maladies (1) are acute or chronic, (2) are of known or unknown etiology, and (3) vary from minimally symptomatic conditions to severely incapacitating and lethal interstitial fibrosis. Restrictive lung diseases are typically characterized by decreased lung volume and decreased oxygen-diffusing capacity on pulmonary function studies.

Hypersensitivity Pneumonitis (Extrinsic Allergic Alveolitis) Is a Response to Inhaled Antigens

Pathogenesis: A wide variety of antigens is known to cause hypersensitivity pneumonitis. The inhalation of these antigens leads to acute or chronic interstitial inflammation in the lung. Most of the responsible antigens are encountered in occupational settings, and the diseases are often labeled according to the specific vocation. For example, *farmer's lung* occurs in farmers exposed to *Micropolyspora faeni* from moldy hay, *bagassosis* results from exposure to *Thermoactinomyces sacchari* in moldy sugar cane, *maple bark–stripper's disease* is seen in persons exposed to the fungus *Cryptostroma corticale* from moldy maple bark, and *bird fancier's lung* affects bird keepers with long-term exposure to proteins from bird feathers, blood, and excrement. Other causes of hypersensitivity pneumonitis include the inhalation of pituitary snuff (*pituitary snuff taker's disease*), moldy cork (*suberosis*), and moldy compost (*mushroom worker's disease*). Hypersensitivity pneumonitis may also be caused by fungi growing in stagnant water in air conditioners, swimming pools, hot tubs, and central heating units. Skin tests and serum precipitating antibodies are often used to confirm the diagnosis. In many cases, especially in the chronic form of hypersensitivity pneumonitis, the inciting antigen is never identified.

Acute hypersensitivity pneumonitis is characterized by a neutrophilic infiltrate in the alveoli and respiratory bronchioles; chronic lesions display mononuclear cells and granulomas, typical of delayed hypersensitivity. In most cases, precipitating IgG antibodies against the offending agent are demonstrated in the serum. Hypersensitivity pneumonitis represents a combination of immune complex-mediated (type III) and cell-mediated (type IV) hypersensitivity reactions, although the precise contribution of each is still debated (Fig. 12-58). Importantly, most persons with serum precipitins to inhaled antigens do not develop hypersensitivity pneumonitis on exposure, a fact that suggests a genetic component in host susceptibility.

Pathology: In florid cases of hypersensitivity pneumonitis, the histological picture is strongly suggestive; in subtle cases, the diagnosis may require careful clinical correlation, and even then the diagnosis may remain tentative. The main microscopic features of chronic hypersensitivity pneumonitis include a bronchiolocentric cellular interstitial pneumonia, noncaseating granulomas, and organizing pneumonia (Fig. 12-59A,B). The bronchiolocentric cellular interstitial infiltrate varies from severe to subtle and consists of lymphocytes, plasma cells, and macrophages; eosinophils are distinctly uncommon. Poorly formed noncaseating granulomas are present in two thirds of cases (see Fig. 12-59B). Organizing pneumonia is found in two thirds of cases and may form the lesion of bronchiolitis obliterans (see Fig. 12-59A). In the end stage, the interstitial inflammation recedes, leaving pulmonary fibrosis, which may resemble usual interstitial pneumonia.

Clinical Features: Hypersensitivity pneumonitis may be first seen as acute, subacute, or chronic pulmonary disease, depending on the frequency and intensity of exposure to the offending antigen. The prototype of hypersensitivity pneumonitis is "farmer's lung," caused by the inhalation of thermophilic actinomycetes that grow in moldy hay. Typically, a farm worker enters a barn where hay has been stored for winter feeding. After a lag period of 4 to 6 hours, the worker rapidly develops dyspnea, cough, and mild fever. The symptoms remit within 24 to 48 hours but return on reexposure; with time, they become chronic. Patients with the chronic form of hypersensitivity pneumonitis have a more nonspecific presentation, with the indolent onset of dyspnea and cor pulmonale.

Pulmonary-function studies show a restrictive pattern, characterized by decreased compliance, reduced diffusion capacity, and hypoxemia. In the chronic stage of hypersensitivity pneumonitis, airway obstruction may become troublesome. Bronchoalveolar lavage shows a T lymphocytosis, with a predominance of $CD8^+$ suppressor/cytotoxic cells. Removal of the environmental antigen is the only adequate treatment for hypersensitivity pneumonitis. Steroid therapy may be effective in acute forms and for some chronically affected patients.

Sarcoidosis Is a Granulomatous Disease of Unknown Etiology

In sarcoidosis the lung is the most frequently involved organ, but the lymph nodes, skin, and eye are also common targets (Fig. 12-60).

Epidemiology: Sarcoidosis is a worldwide disease, affecting all races and both sexes. The differences in the prevalence of the disease among racial and ethnic groups are remarkable. In North America, sarcoidosis occurs much more frequently in blacks than in whites, the ratio being about 15:1. Whereas sarcoidosis is frequent among blacks in South Africa, it is reported to be uncommon in tropical Africa. The disease is often encountered in Scandinavian countries, where the prevalence is 64/100,000, compared with 10/100,000 in France and 3/100,000 in Poland. The reported prevalence of sarcoidosis in Irish women in London is an astonishing 200/100,000. The illness is distinctly uncommon in China.

Pathogenesis: Although the exact pathogenesis of sarcoidosis remains obscure, there is a consensus that it represents an exaggerated cellular immune response on the part of helper/inducer T lymphocytes to ex-

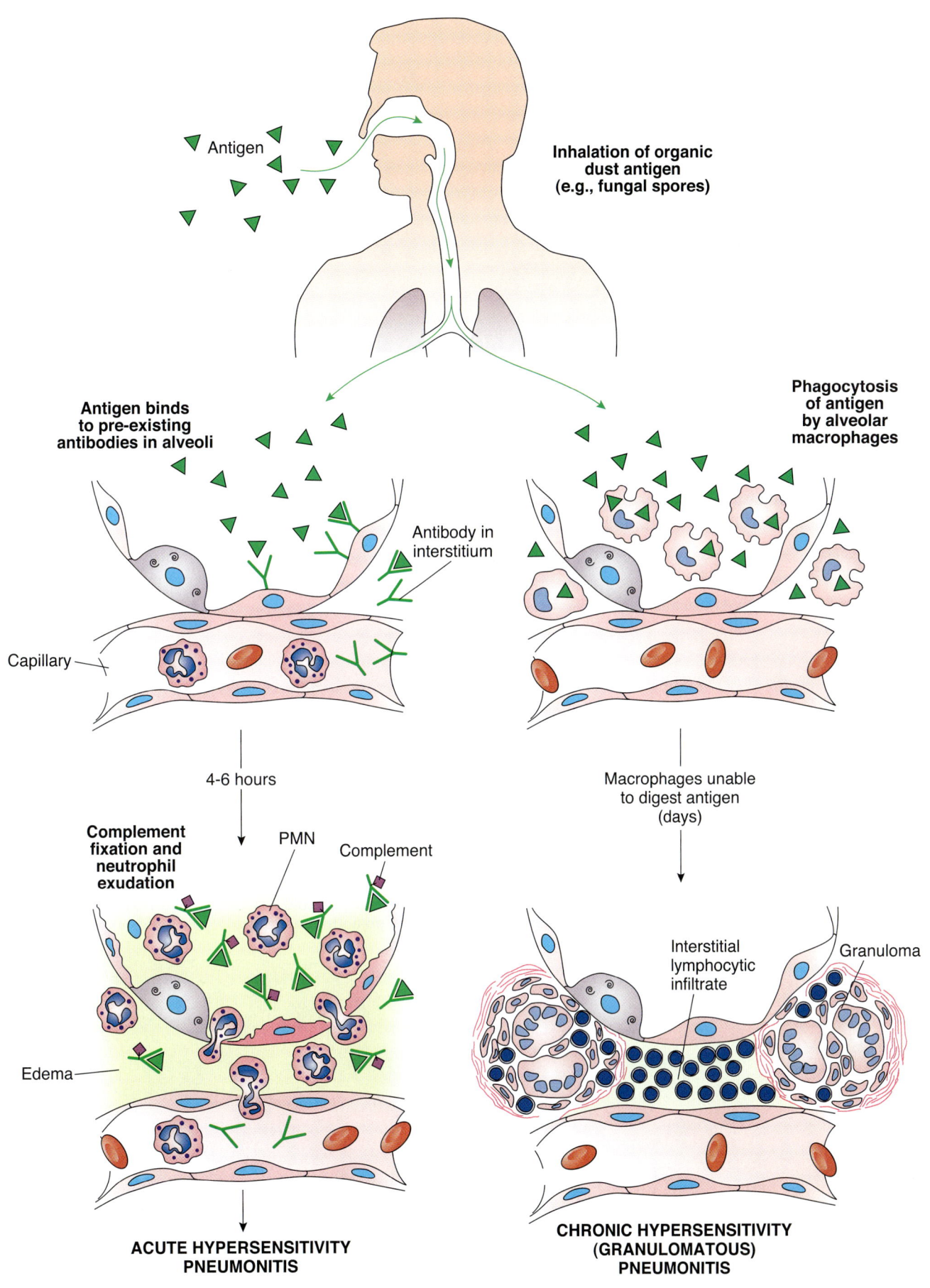

FIGURE 12-58
Hypersensitivity pneumonitis. An antigen–antibody reaction occurs in the acute phase and leads to acute hypersensitivity pneumonitis. If exposure is continued, this is followed by a cellular or subacute phase, with the formation of granulomas and chronic interstitial pneumonitis.

632 The Respiratory System

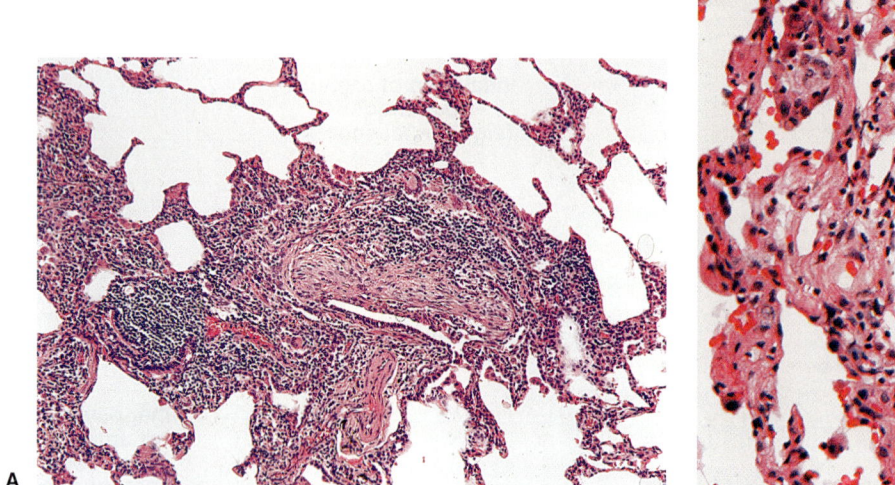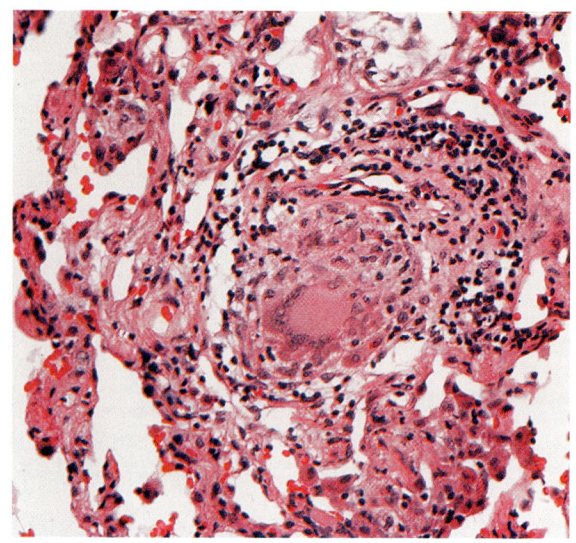

FIGURE *12-59*
Hypersensitivity pneumonitis. A. A lung biopsy specimen shows a mild peribronchiolar chronic inflammatory interstitial infiltrate, with a focus of intraluminal organizing fibrosis. B. Focal poorly formed granulomas were scattered in the lung biopsy specimen.

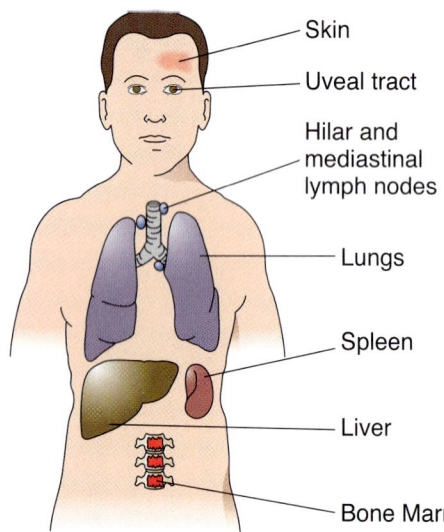

FIGURE *12-60*
Organs commonly affected by sarcoidosis. Sarcoidosis involves many organs, most commonly the lymph nodes and lung.

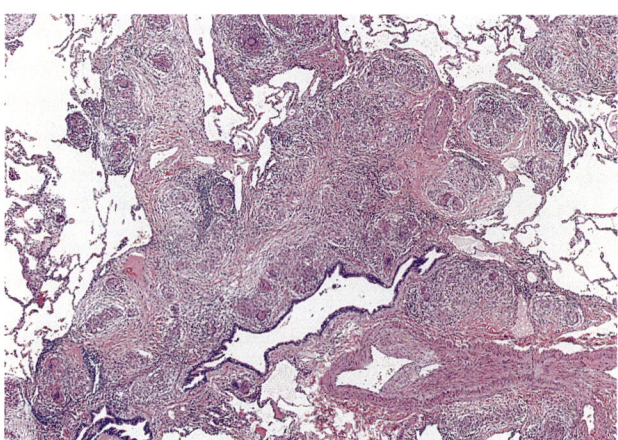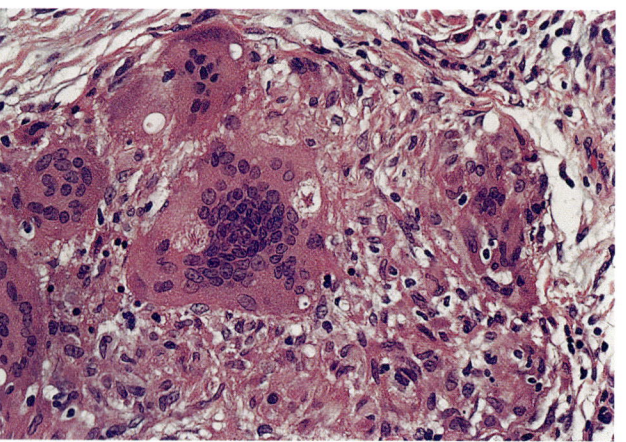

FIGURE *12-61*
Sarcoidosis. A. Multiple noncaseating granulomas are present along the bronchovascular interstitium. B. Noncaseating granulomas consist of tight clusters of epithelioid macrophages and multinucleated giant cells. Several asteroid bodies are present.

ogenous antigens or autoantigens. These cells accumulate in the affected organs, where they secrete lymphokines and recruit macrophages, which participate in the formation of noncaseating granulomas. The organs that contain sarcoid granulomas exhibit a $CD4^+$ to $CD8^+$ T-cell ratio of 10:1, compared with a ratio of 2:1 in uninvolved tissues. The basis for this abnormal accumulation of helper/inducer T lymphocytes is unclear. Perhaps a defect in suppressor-cell function permits unopposed helper-cell proliferation. In addition, inherited or acquired differences in immune-response genes may favor the response of one type of T cell over another. Nonspecific polyclonal activation of B cells by T-helper cells leads to hyperglobulinemia, a characteristic feature of active sarcoidosis.

Pathology: Pulmonary sarcoidosis most commonly affects the lung and hilar lymph nodes, although either involvement may occur separately. Radiologically, a diffuse reticulonodular infiltrate is typical, but in occasional cases, larger nodules are present. Histologically, multiple sarcoid granulomas are scattered in the interstitium of the lung (Fig. 12-61). The distribution is distinctive—along the pleura and interlobular septa and around the bronchovascular bundles (see Fig. 12-61A). Frequent bronchial or bronchiolar submucosal infiltration by sarcoid granulomas accounts for the high diagnostic yield (>90%) on bronchoscopic biopsy. Granulomas in the airways may occasionally be so prominent as to lead to airway obstruction (endobronchial sarcoid).

The cellular granulomatous phase of sarcoidosis can progress to a fibrotic phase. Fibrosis often begins at the periphery of the granuloma and may show an onion-skin pattern of lamellar fibrosis around the giant cells. Although significant necrosis is usually absent, small foci of necrosis are seen in one third of open lung biopsies. Interstitial chronic inflammation tends to be inconspicuous. Vasculitis can be demonstrated in two thirds of open lung biopsy specimens from patients with sarcoidosis. Asteroid bodies (star-shaped crystals) may be seen in the granulomas (see Fig. 12-61B). Schaumann bodies (small calcifications with a lamellar structure) may also be present.

In most cases of pulmonary sarcoidosis, interstitial fibrosis is not a prominent feature. However, in rare instances, progressive pulmonary fibrosis leads to a honeycomb lung and resulting respiratory insufficiency and cor pulmonale.

Clinical Features: Sarcoidosis most commonly occurs in young adults of both sexes. **Acute sarcoidosis** has an abrupt onset, usually followed by spontaneous remission within 2 years and an excellent response to steroids. **Chronic sarcoidosis** has an insidious onset, and patients are more likely to have persistent or progressive disease. Sarcoidosis causes several chest radiographic patterns, the most classic of which is bilateral hilar adenopathy, with or without interstitial pulmonary infiltrates. The malady may also affect the skin (erythema nodosum and lupus pernio), more commonly in women. Black patients tend to have more severe uveitis, skin disease, and lacrimal gland involvement. Cough and dyspnea are the major respiratory complaints. However, the disease can be mild, and the diagnosis may be discovered as an incidental finding on a chest radiograph in an asymptomatic patient.

No laboratory test is specific for the diagnosis of sarcoidosis. Transbronchial lung biopsy, by means of a fiberoptic bronchoscope often reveals granulomas. Occasionally, the diagnosis is based on finding multiple noncaseating granulomas in the biopsy of a mediastinal lymph node by mediastinoscopy. Bronchoalveolar lavage often demonstrates an increase in the proportion of T lymphocytes that show a predominance of $CD4^+$ cells. Increased uptake of gallium-67, a material phagocytosed by activated macrophages, can demonstrate granulomatous areas. The serum level of angiotensin-converting enzyme (ACE) is elevated in two thirds of patients with active sarcoidosis, and the 24-hour urine calcium excretion is frequently increased. The laboratory data, together with the clinical and radiological findings, allow the diagnosis of sarcoidosis to be established with a high probability.

The other organs commonly involved by sarcoidosis include the skin, eye, heart, central nervous system, extrathoracic lymph nodes, spleen, and liver. These are discussed separately in individual chapters.

The prognosis in pulmonary sarcoidosis is favorable, and most patients do not manifest clinically significant sequelae. Resolution occurs in 60% of patients with pulmonary sarcoidosis but is less likely in older patients and those with extrathoracic lesions, particularly in the bone and skin. In up to 20% of cases, the disorder does not remit or recurs at intervals, but it directly accounts for the death of the patient in only 10% of cases. Corticosteroid therapy is effective for active sarcoidosis.

Usual Interstitial Pneumonia Refers Clinically to Idiopathic Pulmonary Fibrosis

Usual interstitial pneumonia (UIP) demonstrates a histological pattern that occurs in a variety of clinical settings, including collagen vascular disease, chronic hypersensitivity pneumonitis, drug toxicity, and asbestosis. Most commonly it has no known cause. In the latter setting, the clinical terms idiopathic pulmonary fibrosis (IPF) or cryptogenic fibrosing alveolitis (CFA), are appropriate. UIP is one of the most common types of interstitial pneumonia, with an annual incidence of 6 to 14.6 cases per 100,000 persons. It has a slight male predominance and has a mean age at onset of 50 to 60 years.

Pathogenesis: The etiology of UIP is unknown, but viral, genetic, and immunological factors are thought to play a role. A viral etiology is favored by the history of a flulike illness in some patients. A genetic role is suggested by cases of familial UIP and the association of UIP-like diseases in patients with inherited disorders such as neurofibromatosis and Hermansky-Pudlak syndrome. An immunological component has been proposed because of the presence of an associated collagen vascular disease in about 20% of cases, including rheumatoid arthritis, systemic lupus erythematosus, and progressive systemic sclerosis. UIP also occurs in the context of other autoimmune disorders (e.g., Hashimoto thyroiditis, primary biliary cirrhosis, chronic

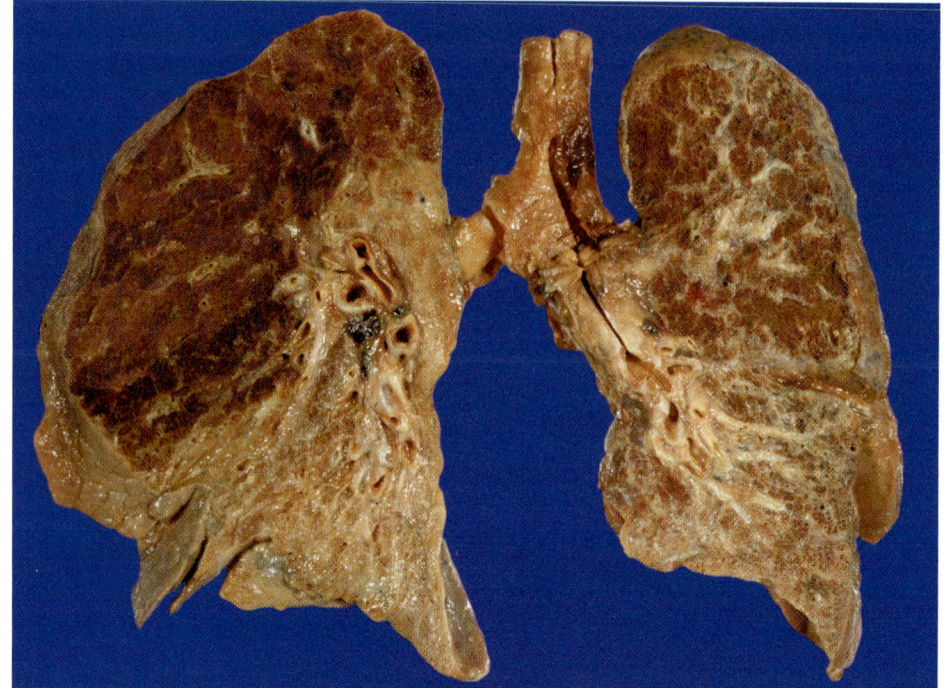
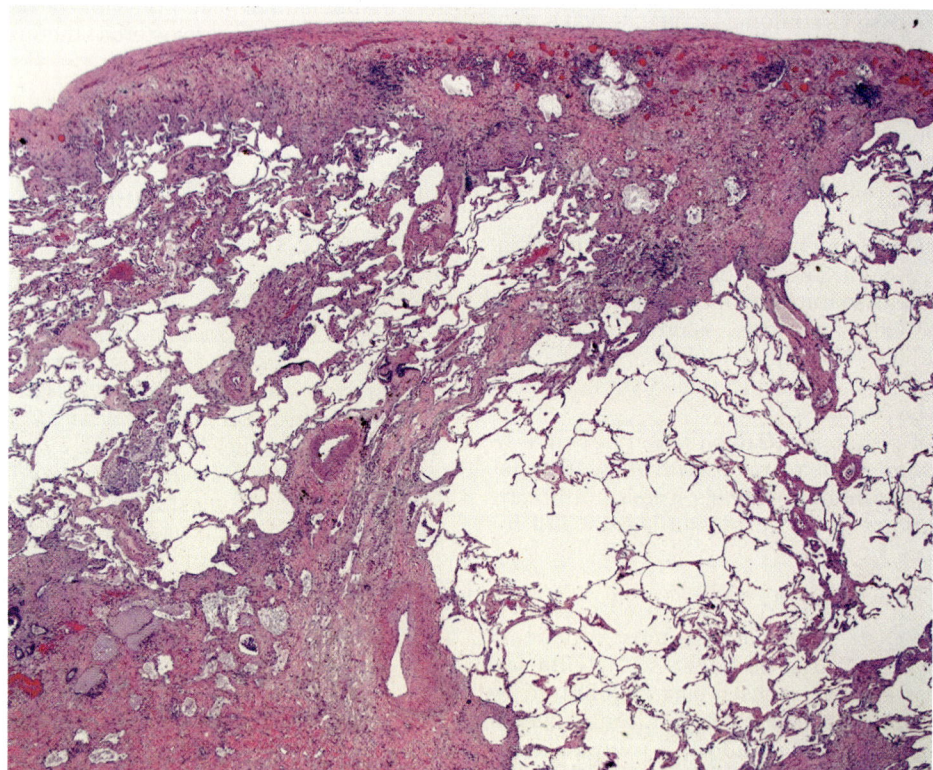

FIGURE 12-62
Usual interstitial pneumonitis. A. A gross specimen of the lung shows patchy dense scarring with extensive areas of honeycomb cystic change, predominantly affecting the lower lobes. This patient also had polymyositis. B. A microscopic view shows patchy subpleural fibrosis with microscopic honeycomb fibrosis. The areas of dense fibrosis display remodeling, with loss of the normal lung architecture.

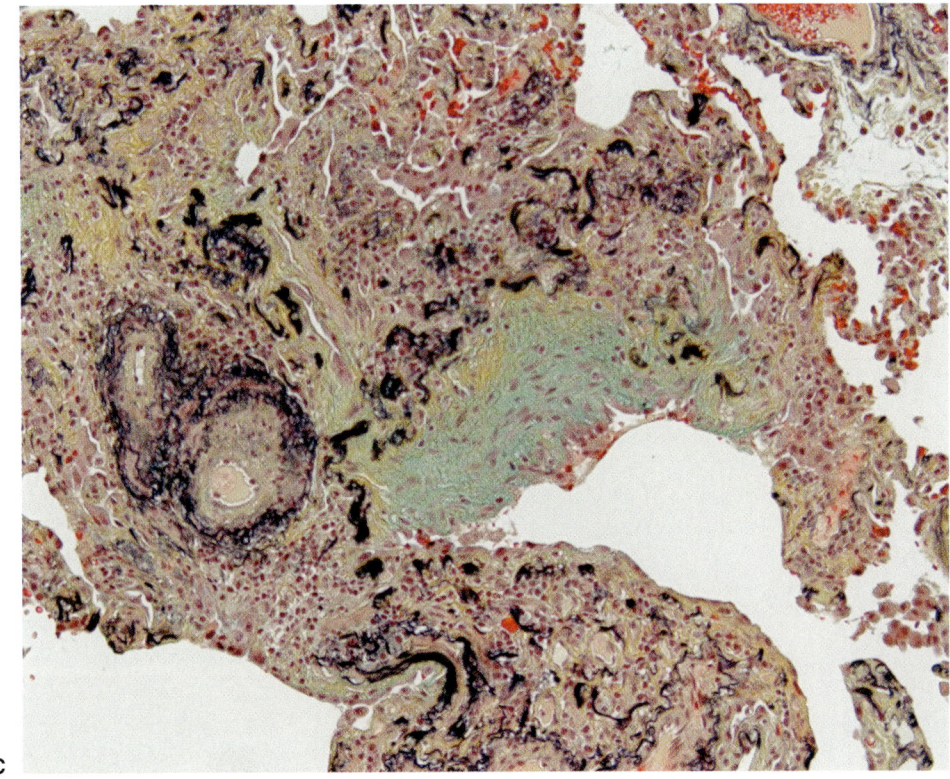

FIGURE 12-62 (continued)
C. Movat stain highlights the fibroblastic focus in green, which contrasts with the adjacent area of yellow staining of dense collagen and black staining of collapsed elastic fibers.

hepatitis, idiopathic thrombocytopenic purpura, and myasthenia gravis.) In addition, patients with UIP frequently exhibit circulating autoantibodies (e.g., antinuclear antibodies and rheumatoid factor). Immune complexes have been demonstrated in the circulation, the inflamed alveolar walls, and bronchoalveolar-lavage specimens, although the antigen has not been identified. It has been postulated that alveolar macrophages become activated on phagocytosis of immune complexes, after which they release cytokines that recruit neutrophils. In turn, polymorphonuclear leukocytes damage the alveolar walls, setting in motion a series of events that culminates in interstitial fibrosis.

Variants of UIP include *nonspecifc interstitial pneumonia* and *acute interstial pneumonia,* but it is not clear whether they are distict entities or points on the spectrum of UIP.

 Pathology: The lungs are small in UIP, and the fibrosis tends to be worse in the lower lobes, in the subpleural regions, and along the interlobular septa. Retraction of the scars, especially of lobular septa, gives the external surface of the lung a hobnail appearance, reminiscent of cirrhosis of the liver. Grossly, fibrosis is often patchy, with areas of dense scarring and honeycomb cystic change (Fig. 12-62A).

The histological hallmark of UIP is patchy chronic inflammation and interstitial fibrosis, with areas of normal lung adjacent to fibrotic areas (see Fig. 12-62B). The fibrosis itself exhibits what has been termed "temporal heterogeneity," meaning that the fibrosis is of different ages. Areas of loose fibroblastic tissue (fibroblast foci) are found adjacent to dense collagen (Fig. 12-62C). The fibrosis is most pronounced beneath the pleura and adjacent to the interlobular septa (Fig. 12-62B). Because of alveolitis and subsequent fibrosis, the distal part of the acinus shrinks, and the proximal bronchioles dilate. The bronchiolar epithelium grows into the dilated air spaces, which may represent damaged proximal respiratory bronchioles but are no longer recognized as such (Fig. 12-63). The areas of dense scarring fibrosis cause remodeling of the lung architecture, resulting in collapse of alveolar walls and formation of cystic spaces (see Fig. 12-62A). The cystic spaces are typically lined by bronchiolar or cuboidal epithelium and contain mucus, macrophages, or neutrophils. Interstitial chronic inflammation is mild or moderate. Lymphoid aggregates, sometimes containing germinal centers, are occasionally noted, particularly in UIP associated with rheumatoid arthritis. Extensive vascular changes, particularly intimal fibrosis and thickening of the media, may be associated with pulmonary hypertension.

Clinical Features: UIP begins insidiously, with the gradual onset of dyspnea on exertion and dry cough, usually over a period of 5 to 10 years. Clinically, patients have restrictive lung disease. Chest radiographs show diffuse bilateral infiltrates, predominantly in the lower lobes, and a reticular pattern. Clubbing of the fingers is common, especially late in the course of disease. In

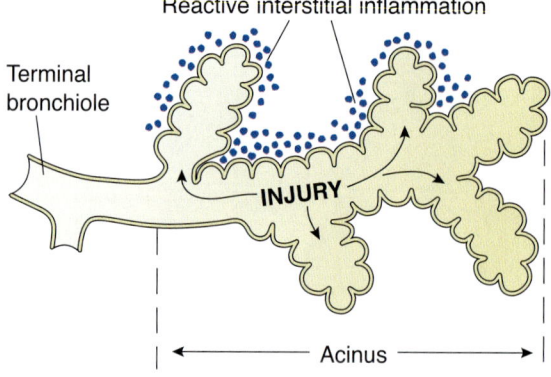

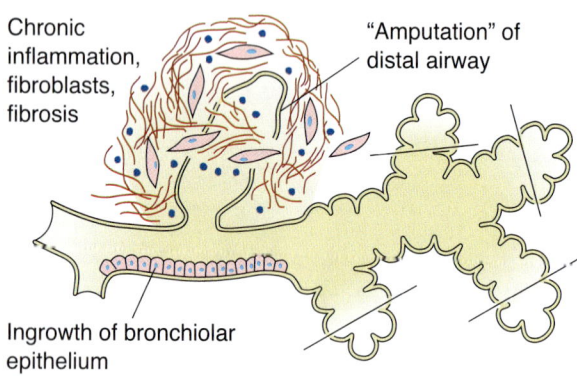

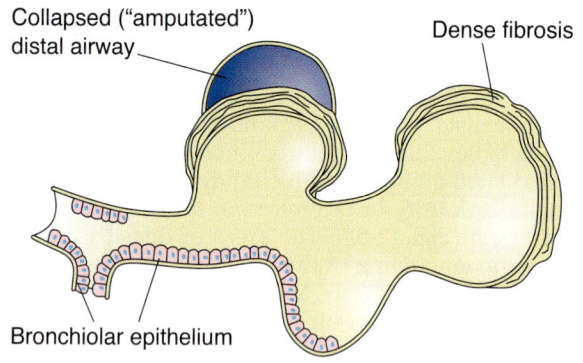

FIGURE 12-63
Pathogenesis of honeycomb lung. Honeycomb lung is the result of a variety of injuries. Interstitial and alveolar inflammation destroys ("amputates") the distal part of the acinus. The proximal parts dilate and become lined by bronchiolar epithelium.

approximately 50% of patients, high resolution CT shows distinctive findings, consisting of peripheral, subpleural reticular opacities and honeycombing, predominantly in the posterior aspects of the lower lobes.

The classic auscultatory finding consists of late inspiratory crackles and fine ("Velcro") rales at the lung bases. Tachypnea at rest, cyanosis, and cor pulmonale eventually ensue. The prognosis is bleak, with a mean survival of 4 to 6 years. Patients are treated with corticosteroids and sometimes cyclophosphamide, but lung transplantation generally offers the only hope of a cure.

Desquamative Interstitial Pneumonia Features Intraalveolar Macrophage Accumulation

Desquamative interstitial pneumonia (DIP) is a chronic, fibrosing, interstitial pneumonitis of unknown etiology (Fig. 12-64A,B). The term *desquamative* is actually a misnomer that originated from the belief that the intraalveolar cells were desquamated epithelial cells, whereas they are now recognized as macrophages. DIP is distinguished from UIP by the preservation of alveolar architecture in the former and the lack of patchy scarring and remodeling of lung parenchyma characteristic of UIP. The macrophages contain a fine golden-

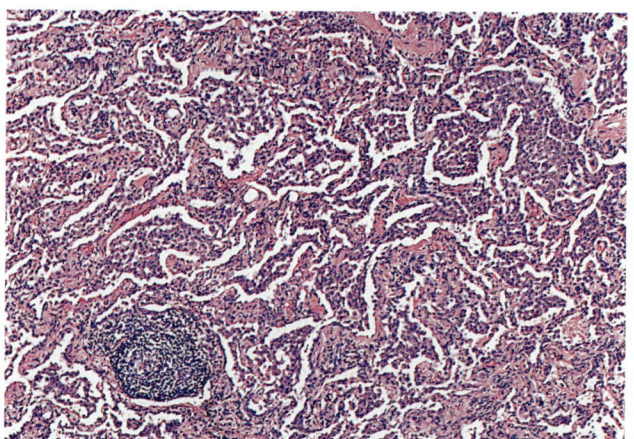

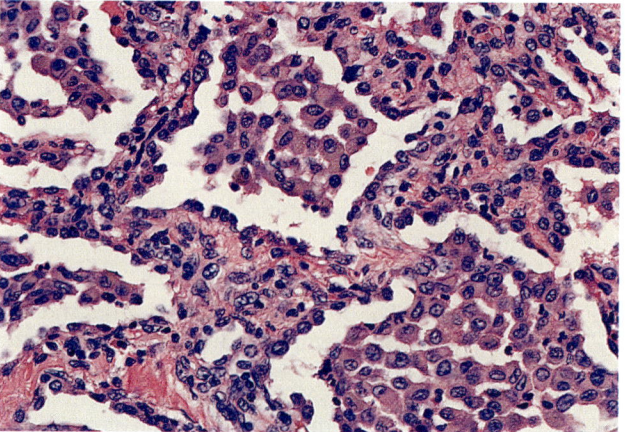

FIGURE 12-64
Desquamative interstitial pneumonia (DIP). A. A diffuse process in the lungs is characterized by the accumulation of alveolar macrophages, preservation of the alveolar architecture, and a lymphoid aggregate. B. In addition to alveolar macrophage accumulation, there is mild alveolar septal fibrosis, type II pneumocyte hyperplasia, and mild interstitial chronic inflammation.

brown pigment. Alveolar walls in DIP may, however, show mild thickening by chronic inflammation and interstitial fibrosis (see Fig. 12-64B). Scattered lymphoid aggregates also may be present. Hyperplasia of type II pneumocytes is often prominent.

DIP is seen almost exclusively in cigarette smokers, typically in the fourth or fifth decade, and occurs in males twice as often as females. The prevailing opinion is that DIP and respiratory bronchiolitis–interstitial lung disease (RB-ILD; below) represent a spectrum of disease related to cigarette smoking, although the mechanism is unclear. The radiographic picture of DIP is not specific but is most frequently described as bilateral ground glass infiltrates with a lower lobe predominance. DIP has a much better prognosis than UIP, with an overall 10-year survival between 70 and 100%. Most patients respond well to steroid therapy and smoking cessation.

Respiratory Bronchiolitis–Interstitial Lung Disease Demonstrates Bronchiolocentric Macrophages

Respiratory bronchiolitis (RB) is a histological lesion that occurs in cigarette smokers. It is encountered most often as an incidental histological finding, but rarely it may be the sole cause of interstitial lung disease, and the clinical term *respiratory bronchiolitis–interstitial lung disease (RB-ILD)* is appropriate.

 Pathology: Histologically, the process is patchy and consists of prominent accumulation of pigmented macrophages in the air spaces, centered on bronchioles (Fig. 12-65). The macrophages are present within the lumina of bronchioles and the adjacent alveolar spaces. The bronchiolar walls show mild chronic inflammation and fibrosis. However, interstitial fibrosis does not extend into the surrounding lung. The pigment within the macrophages is usually brown and finely granular. In contrast to DIP, in which the process is diffuse, in RB the lesion is bronchiolocentric and patchy.

 Clinical Features: Clinically, patients have mild respiratory dysfunction. Radiographically, there is an upper lobe predominance, with thickening of the peripheral bronchioles. Patients with RB–ILD have an excellent prognosis, and the symptoms usually resolve after cessation of smoking.

Organizing Pneumonia Pattern (Cryptogenic Organizing Pneumonia) Displays Fibroblastic Plugs in Alveoli and Bronchioles

Organizing pneumonia pattern was previously referred to as *bronchiolitis obliterans–organizing pneumonia (BOOP)*. This disorder features polypoid plugs of tissue that fill the bronchiolar lumen, whereas respiratory bronchiolitis (described above) demonstrates fibrosis of the bronchiolar wall and luminal narrowing. Organizing pneumonia pattern is not specific for any particular etiological agent, and the cause cannot be determined from the morphological appearance. It is observed in many settings, including respiratory tract infections (particularly viral bronchiolitis), inhalation of toxic materials, administration of a number of drugs, and several inflammatory processes (e.g., collagen vascular diseases). Importantly, a substantial number of cases remain idiopathic and are referred to as cryptogenic organizing pneumonia (or idiopathic BOOP).

 Pathology: Histologically, organizing pneumonia pattern features patchy areas of loose organizing fibrosis and chronic inflammatory cells in the distal airways adjacent to normal lung. Plugs of organizing fibrosis occlude bronchioles (bronchiolitis obliterans), alveolar ducts, and surrounding alveoli (organizing pneumonia; Fig. 12-66), but there is little connective tissue within bronchioles. Thus the pattern is more an organizing pneumonia than a bronchiolitis obliterans. The architecture of the lung is preserved, with none of the remodeling or honeycomb changes seen in UIP. Owing to the occlusion of the distal airways, an obstructive or endogenous lipid pneumonia may develop. The alveolar septa are only slightly thickened with chronic inflammatory cells, and there is only mild hyperplasia of type II pneumocytes.

 Clinical Features: Organizing pneumonia pattern has a mean age of presentation of 55 years and is first seen with the acute onset of fever, cough, and dyspnea. Many patients have a history of a flulike illness 4 to 6 weeks before the onset of symptoms. As noted above, some may have predisposing conditions. Chest radiographs reveal localized opacities or bilateral interstitial infiltrates,

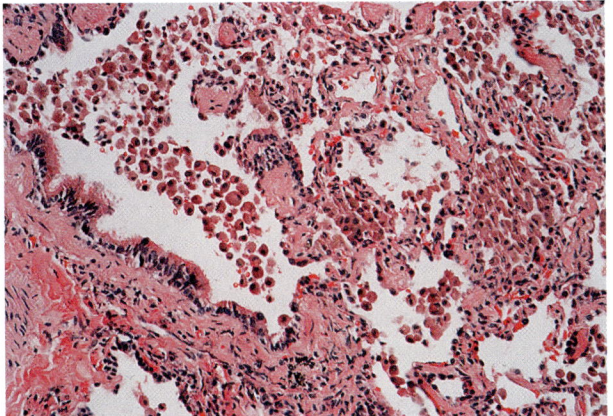

FIGURE 12-65
Respiratory bronchiolitis. There is marked accumulation of macrophages within the bronchioles and surrounding air spaces. Mild fibrotic thickening and chronic inflammation of the bronchiolar wall are present.

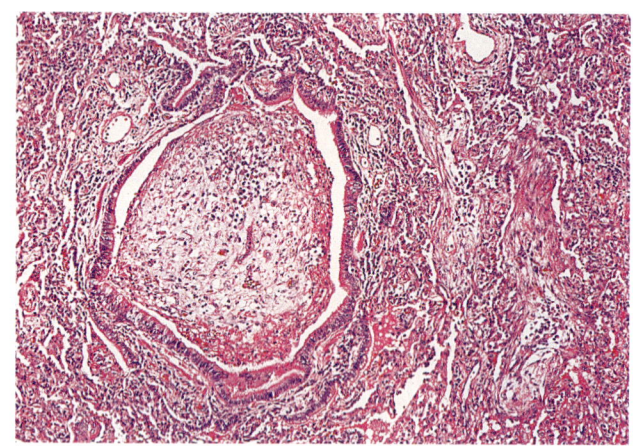
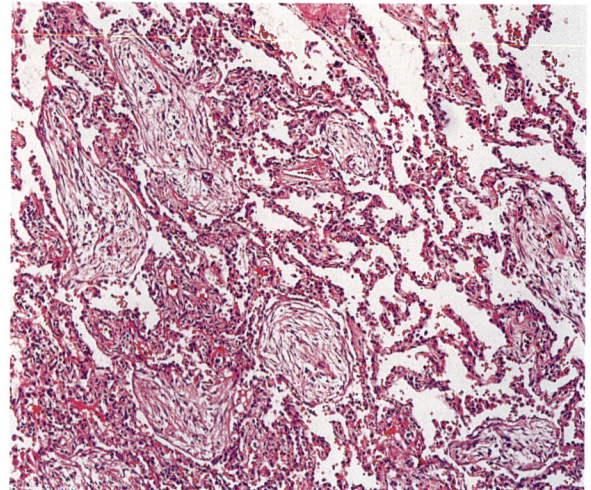

FIGURE 12-66
Organizing pneumonia pattern. **A.** Polypoid plugs of loose fibrous tissue are present in a bronchiole and the adjacent alveolar ducts and alveoli. **B.** The alveolar spaces contain similar plugs of loose organizing connective tissue.

which may migrate over time. Pulmonary function studies demonstrate a restrictive ventilatory pattern. Corticosteroid therapy is effective, and some patients recover within weeks to months even without therapy.

Lymphoid Interstitial Pneumonia Occurs in the Setting of Autoimmune Diseases

Lymphoid interstitial pneumonia (LIP) is a rare pneumonitis in which lymphoid infiltrates are distributed diffusely in the interstitial spaces of the lung.

Pathology: The hallmark of LIP is diffuse infiltration of alveolar septa and peribronchiolar spaces by lymphocytes, plasma cells, and macrophages (Fig. 12-67). The alveolar architecture is preserved without scarring or remodeling of the lung architecture. Hyperplasia of type II pneumocytes may be conspicuous, and inconspicuous foci of organizing interstitial fibrosis are occasionally present. Sarcoidlike, noncaseating granulomas are often seen. The alveolar spaces tend to contain a proteinaceous exudate. Occasionally, scattered lymphoid aggregates are present, some containing germinal centers. Hyperplasia of the peribronchiolar lymphoid tissue may be prominent.

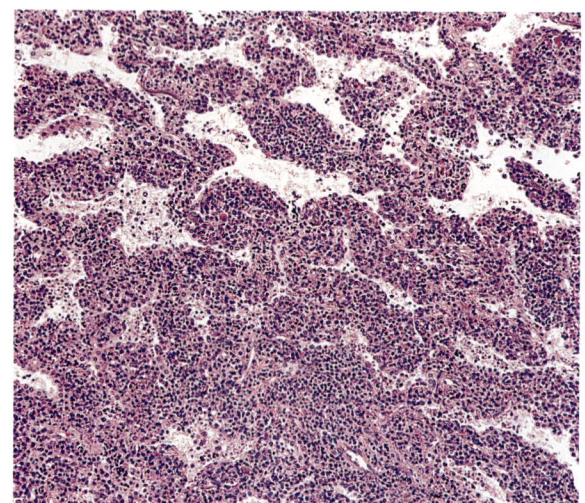
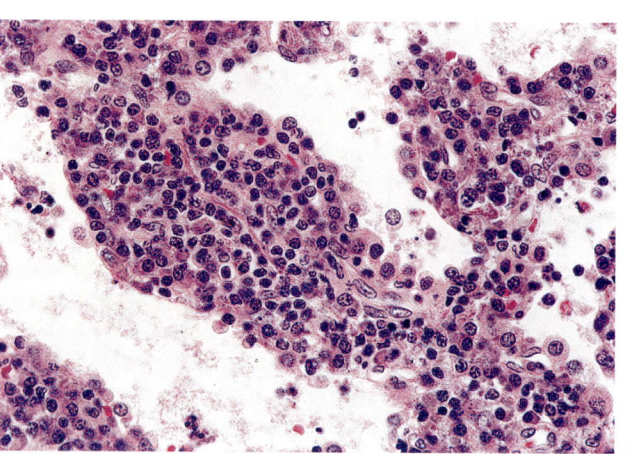

FIGURE 12-67
Lymphocytic interstitial pneumonia (LIP). **A.** The walls of the alveolar septa are diffusely infiltrated by chronic inflammation. **B.** The inflammatory infiltrate is composed of lymphocytes and plasma cells.

TABLE 12-5 **Conditions Associated with Lymphocytic Interstitial Pneumonia (LIP)**

Idiopathic	Immunodeficiency
Dysproteinemia	HIV infection
Polyclonal gammopathy	Severe combined immunodeficiency syndrome
Macroglobulinemia	
Hypogammaglobulinemia	**Infection**
Pernicious anemia	*Pneumocystis carinii* pneumonia
Collagen vascular disease	Epstein-Barr virus (lymphoproliferative disorder)
Sjögren syndrome	Chronic active hepatitis
Systemic lupus erythematosus	**Iatrogenic**
Rheumatoid arthritis	Bone marrow transplantation
	Phenytoin (Dilantin)

 Clinical Features: Although LIP may be idiopathic, it often occurs in a variety of clinical settings (Table 12-5), particularly in patients with dysproteinemia, collagen vascular disease (especially Sjögren syndrome), and HIV infection. It is principally encountered in adults, but cases in children are recorded. In children, LIP is one of the defining criteria for the diagnosis of AIDS. Associated autoimmune manifestations include increased or reduced serum gamma globulins, a variety of dysproteinemias, and increased circulating autoantibodies, such as rheumatoid factor and antinuclear antibodies. Rarely, lymphoma can develop in patients with LIP, particularly in those with Sjögren syndrome and AIDS.

Patients with LIP have cough and progressive dyspnea. The course of the disease varies from an indolent condition to one that progresses to end-stage lung and respiratory failure. Corticosteroids and cytotoxic agents have been of some benefit.

Langerhans Cell Histiocytosis (Histiocytosis X) Encompasses a Spectrum of Localized and Systemic Cell Proliferations

Different presentations of Langerhans cell histiocytosis (LCH) have been called eosinophilic granuloma, Hand-Schüller-Christian disease, and Letterer-Siwe disease. LCH can affect the lung as a distinctive form of interstitial lung disease. In adults, the disorder occurs most often as an isolated form (also known as *pulmonary eosinophilic granuloma*), with extrapulmonary manifestations such as bone lesions or diabetes insipidus occurring in 10 to 15% of cases. **Virtually all of these patients are cigarette smokers.** In children, lung involvement may occur in association with Letterer-Siwe disease or Hand-Schüller-Christian disease.

 Pathology: Histologically, pulmonary LCH appears as scattered nodular infiltrates with a stellate border extending into the surrounding interstitium (Fig. 12-68A). These lesions are frequently centered on bronchioles or in a subpleural location. The cellular lesions consist of varying proportions of Langerhans cells admixed with

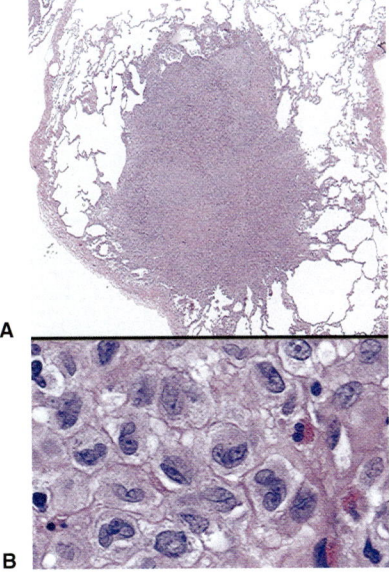
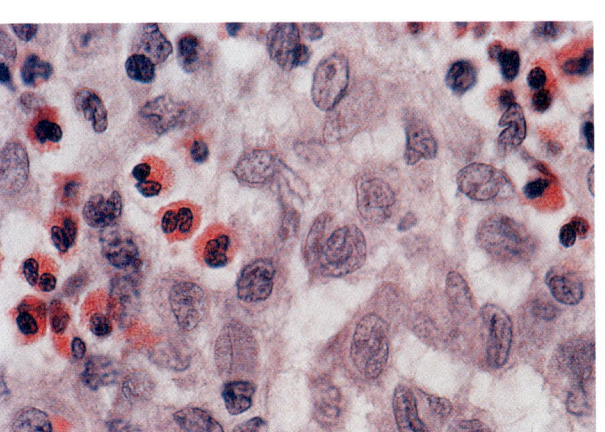

FIGURE 12-68
Langerhans cell histiocytosis. A. The interstitial nodular infiltrate has a stellate shape, with extension of the cells into the adjacent alveolar septa. B. The infiltrate has numerous Langerhans cells that have a moderate amount of eosinophilic cytoplasm and prominently grooved nuclei. Several eosinophils are also present. C. A higher power view shows Langerhans cells and eosinophils.

lymphocytes, eosinophils, and macrophages. Langerhans cells are round to oval, with a moderate amount of eosinophilic cytoplasm and prominently grooved nuclei that contain small inconspicuous nucleoli (see Fig. 12-68B and C). As the disease progresses, the lesions cavitate and become fibrotic. Eventually, honeycomb fibrosis can result. The lung parenchyma adjacent to the nodular lesions may show marked accumulation of intraalveolar macrophages, owing to respiratory bronchiolitis induced by smoking.

Langerhans cells have distinctive characteristics, including (1) cytoplasmic Birbeck granules (detected by electron microscopy), (2) C3, IgG-F_c receptors, CD1 and HLA-DR, and (3) S-100 protein expression. Whether pulmonary LCH represents a neoplastic proliferation or an abnormal immunological response to antigens within cigarette smoke remains to be determined.

Clinical Features: Pulmonary LCH usually affects patients in the third and fourth decades of life. The most common presenting manifestations are a nonproductive cough, dyspnea on exertion, and spontaneous pneumothorax. Some 25% of patients are asymptomatic at the time of diagnosis. Chest radiographs show diffuse bilateral reticulonodular lesions, usually in the upper lobes. The lesions frequently undergo cavitation. Although most patients have a good prognosis, some develop chronic pulmonary dysfunction. In a small subset of cases, progressive pulmonary fibrosis can lead to death. Cessation of smoking is beneficial in the early stages of the disease.

Lymphangioleiomyomatosis Features Smooth Muscle in the Lung and Lymphatics

Lymphangioleiomyomatosis (LAM) is a rare interstitial lung disease that occurs in women of childbearing age and is characterized by the widespread abnormal proliferation of smooth muscle in the lung, mediastinal and retroperitoneal lymph nodes, and the major lymphatic ducts. The etiology of LAM is unknown, but clinical responses to oophorectomy and progesterone therapy suggest that the smooth muscle proliferation is under hormonal control. The occurrence of LAM in patients with tuberous sclerosis and the association of LAM with renal angiomyolipomas have led to speculation that LAM may represent a *forme fruste* of tuberous sclerosis.

Pathology: On gross examination, the lungs show bilateral, diffuse enlargement, with extensive cystic changes resembling those of emphysema (Fig. 12-69A). Histologically, numerous cystic spaces are lined by focal nodules or bundles of abnormal smooth muscle cells. These round or spindle-shaped cells (LAM cells) resemble immature smooth muscle cells but lack the parallel orientation of the normal smooth muscle surrounding airways and blood vessels (see Fig. 12-69B). The smooth muscle proliferation typically follows a lymphatic distribution in the lung, around blood vessels and bronchioles, and along the pleura and interlobular septa. Blood vessel walls, especially in small pulmonary veins, also may be infiltrated, resulting in micro-

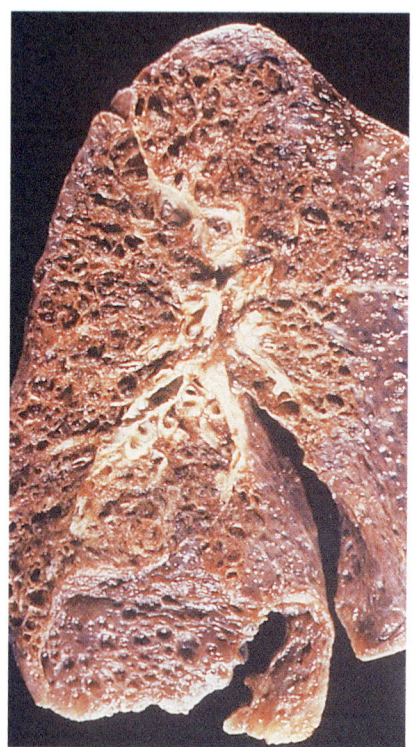
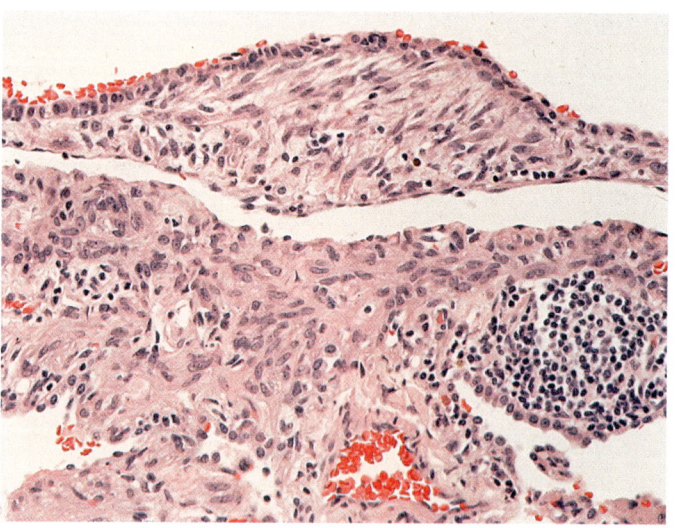

FIGURE 12-69
Lymphangioleiomyomatosis. A. The cut surface of the lung displays extensive cystic change, which resembles emphysema. B. An abnormal cystic space is lined by smooth muscle bundles in which the myocytes are haphazardly arranged.

scopic hemorrhage and hemosiderin accumulation in alveolar macrophages. Immunohistochemical staining for HMB-45 (a melanoma antigen) specifically decorates the LAM cells but not other smooth muscle cells in the lung. Estrogen or progesterone receptors are occasionally demonstrated in LAM cells.

 Clinical Features: Patients with LAM have shortness of breath, spontaneous pneumothorax, hemoptysis, cough, and chylous effusions. In early stages, the chest radiograph may appear normal. However, as the disease progresses, a diffuse interstitial reticular or cystic pattern may appear on the radiograph. Pleural effusions, marked hyperinflation of the lungs, and pneumothorax may ensue. Pulmonary function tests show markedly increased total lung capacity, decreased diffusing capacity, and obstructive or restrictive features. Although some patients have an indolent clinical course, many die of progressive respiratory failure. Hormonal ablation through oophorectomy, as well as antiestrogen (tamoxifen) and progesterone therapy, have shown some promise.

LUNG TRANSPLANTATION

Patients who undergo lung transplantation manifest acute and chronic rejection and infection. Histological clues to acute rejection include perivascular infiltrates of small round lymphocytes, plasmacytoid lymphocytes, macrophages, and eosinophils. In severe cases, the inflammation may spill over into adjacent alveoli, and hyaline membranes may be seen. In chronic rejection, the major pattern of injury is bronchiolitis obliterans, characterized by bronchiolar inflammation and varying degrees of fibrosis. The latter can take the form of polypoid plugs of intraluminal granulation tissue or concentric mural fibrosis, with the pattern of obliterative bronchiolitis (Fig. 12-70). Bronchiectasis is common in long-term survivors of lung transplants, an outcome that may be due to poor perfusion of the airways, denervation, and recurrent airway infection.

A spectrum of opportunistic infections, including bacteria, fungi, viral agents, and *P. carinii*, can be seen in transplant patients. The most common fungal pneumonias are due to *Candida* and *Aspergillus* species. Cytomegalovirus is the most common cause of viral pneumonia. **Lymphoproliferative disorders** occur in 3 to 8% of lung-transplant patients who survive more than 30 days. These neoplasms are secondary to uncontrolled proliferation of B lymphocytes infected with the Epstein-Barr virus (EBV) as a result of immunosuppression by cyclosporine.

VASCULITIS AND GRANULOMATOSIS

Many pulmonary conditions result in vasculitis, most of which are secondary to other inflammatory processes, such as necrotizing granulomatous infections. Only a few primary idiopathic vasculitis syndromes affect the lung, the most important of which are Wegener granulomatosis, Churg-Strauss granulomatosis, and necrotizing sarcoid granulomatosis.

Wegener Granulomatosis Affects the Respiratory Tract and Kidneys

Wegener granulomatosis (WG) is a disease of unknown cause that is characterized by aseptic, necrotizing, granulomatous inflammation and vasculitis that affect the upper and lower respiratory tracts and the kidneys. The disease is described in Chapter 10. The glomerulonephritis associated with WG is discussed in Chapter 16, and the lesions of the upper respiratory tract are described in Chapter 25. In this section, we deal only with the pulmonary manifestations of WG.

Pathology: The pulmonary features of WG include necrotizing granulomatous inflammation, parenchymal necrosis, and vasculitis. In most cases of pulmonary WG, multiple bilateral nodules, averaging 2 to 3 cm in diameter, are seen in the lungs. The nodules have an irregular edge, a tan-brown or hemorrhagic cut surface, and frequent central cavitation.

Nodules of parenchymal consolidation consist of (1) tissue necrosis; (2) granulomatous inflammation with a mixed inflammatory infiltrate composed of lymphocytes, plasma cells, neutrophils, eosinophils, macrophages, and giant cells; and (3) fibrosis. Necrosis can take the form of neutrophilic microabscesses or large basophilic zones of "geographical" necrosis with irregular serpiginous borders (Fig. 12-71A). The granulomas may show several patterns, including palisading macrophages along the border of the large necrotic zones, loosely clustered multinucleated giant cells, and scattered giant cells. Vasculitis may affect arteries (see Fig. 12-71B), veins, or capillaries, and the vascular lesions may show acute, chronic, or granulomatous inflammation. The most common pattern of fibrosis consists of a nonspecific organizing pneumonia at the edges of the nodules of inflammatory

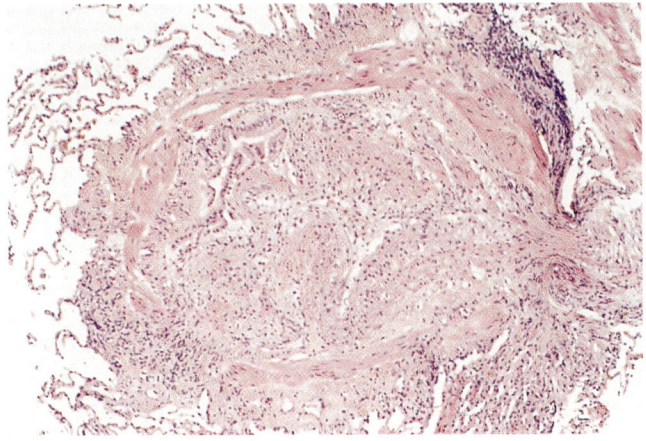

FIGURE 12-70
Obliterative bronchiolitis, chronic rejection in lung transplantation. The lumen of this bronchiole is virtually entirely obliterated by concentric fibrosis.

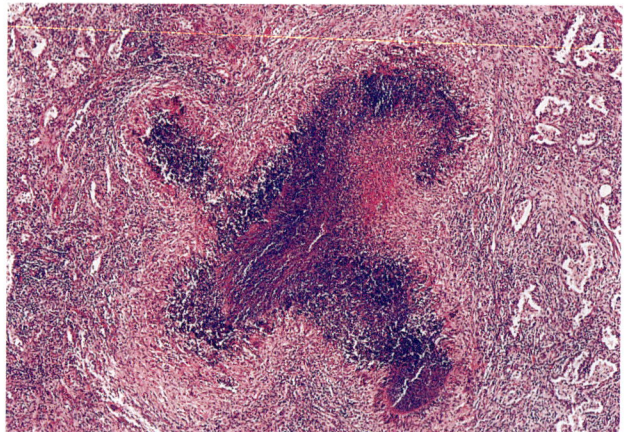 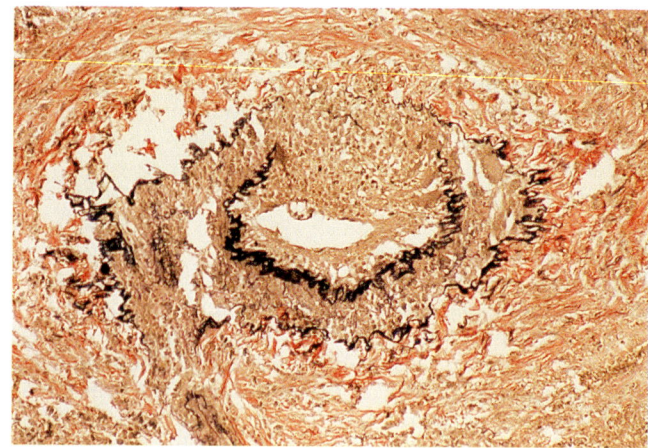

FIGURE 12-71
A. Wegener granulomatosis. This large area of necrosis has a "geographical" pattern with serpiginous borders and a basophilic center. B. Vasculitis in this artery is characterized by a focal, eccentric, transmural chronic inflammatory infiltrate that destroys the inner and outer elastic laminae (elastic stain).

consolidation. The lungs often show acute or chronic intraalveolar hemorrhage. "Neutrophilic capillaritis," consisting of neutrophilic infiltration of alveolar walls, is often present.

Clinical Features: WG most commonly affects the head and neck, followed by the lung, kidney, and eye. Respiratory manifestations include cough, hemoptysis, and pleuritis. Chest radiographs commonly show multiple intrapulmonary nodules, although single nodules may also be encountered. Head and neck manifestations consist of sinusitis, nasal disease, otitis media, hearing loss, subglottic stenosis, ear pain, cough, and oral lesions. Other systemic manifestations are arthralgias, fever, skin lesions, weight loss, peripheral neuropathy, central nervous system abnormalities, and pericarditis.

Diffuse pulmonary hemorrhage is an important complication of WG, seen as a fulminant life-threatening crisis characterized by severe respiratory failure. It is usually accompanied by acute renal failure.

The serum anti-neutrophil cytoplasm antibody (ANCA) test is a useful marker for WG and other vasculitis syndromes. When these antibodies react with ethanol-fixed neutrophils, there are two major immunofluorescence patterns: cytoplasmic or classical (C-ANCA) and perinuclear (P-ANCA). C-ANCAs react with proteinase 3 and occur in more than 85% of patients with active generalized WG. Most P-ANCAs have a specificity for myeloperoxidase and are encountered in patients with idiopathic necrotizing and crescentic glomerulonephritis and in patients with polyarteritis nodosa and Churg-Strauss syndrome.

Most patients with WG are treated effectively with corticosteroids and cyclophosphamide. Some patients respond to therapy with trimethoprim-sulfamethoxazole, suggesting the possibility of a bacterial infection.

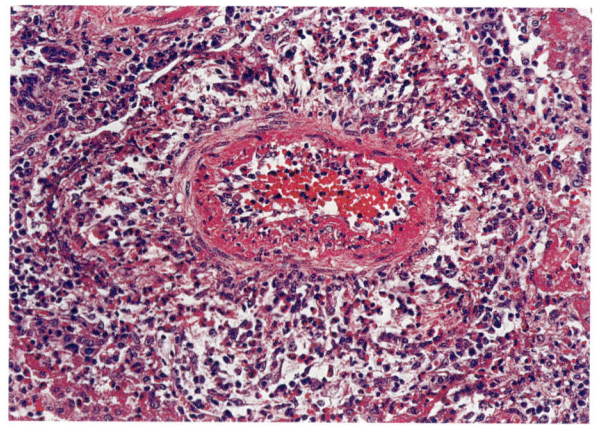 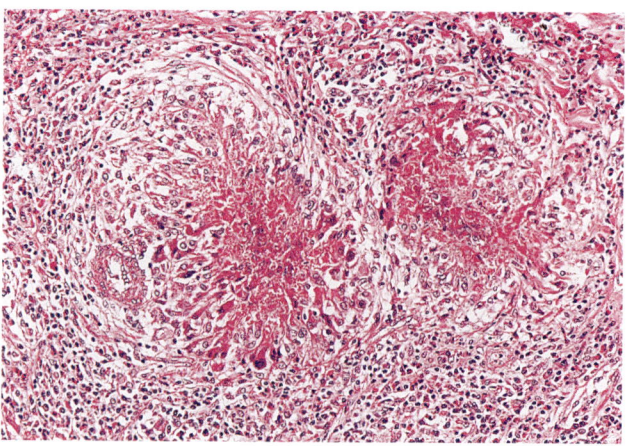

FIGURE 12-72
Churg-Strauss syndrome. A. An artery shows severe vasculitis consisting of a dense infiltrate of chronic inflammatory cells and eosinophils. B. A necrotic ("allergic") granuloma has a central eosinophilic area of necrosis surrounded by palisading macrophages and giant cells.

Churg-Strauss Syndrome (Allergic Angiitis and Granulomatosis) Is Defined by Asthma, Eosinophilia, and Vasculitis

Churg-Strauss syndrome is a disorder of unknown etiology.

Pathology: The lungs of patients with Churg-Strauss syndrome show changes of asthmatic bronchitis or bronchiolitis (see above discussion of asthma). Histological features include eosinophilic pneumonia, vasculitis (Fig. 12-72A), parenchymal necrosis (see Fig. 12-72B), and granulomatous inflammation. Infiltrates of eosinophils may be seen in any anatomical compartment of the lung. Involvement of blood vessel walls causes vasculitis and damage to airway walls and results in bronchitis or bronchiolitis. The vasculitis exhibits varying types of inflammatory cells, including eosinophils, lymphocytes, plasma cells, macrophages, giant cells, and neutrophils (see Fig. 12-72A). Necrotic foci have eosinophilic centers owing to the accumulation of dead eosinophils (see Fig. 12-72B).

Clinical Features: Churg-Strauss syndrome passes through three clinical phases.

Prodrome: Patients have one or more of the following: allergic rhinitis, asthma, peripheral eosinophilia, and eosinophilic infiltrative disease (eosinophilic pneumonia or eosinophilic enteritis).

Systemic vasculitic phase: Extrapulmonary vasculitic manifestations are present, such as cutaneous leukocytoclastic vasculitis, or peripheral neuropathy.

Postvasculitic phase: Patients may continue to have asthma and allergic rhinitis, and complications of neuropathy and hypertension may persist. Cardiovascular manifestations are common and often consist of pericarditis, hypertension, and cardiac failure. Renal disease and sinus involvement are usually less severe than those in WG.

Churg-Strauss patients usually are positive for P-ANCA during the vasculitic phase. Most patients respond to corticosteroid therapy, but cyclophosphamide may be needed in severe cases.

Necrotizing Sarcoid Granulomatosis Demonstrates Large Zones of Necrosis and Vasculitis

Necrotizing sarcoid granulomatosis is a rare condition that features nodular confluent sarcoidal granulomas (Fig. 12-73). This disorder is not a systemic vasculitis, but a disorder usually limited to the lung. The vasculitis displays giant cells, necrotizing granulomas (see Fig. 12-73B), and chronic inflammation consisting of lymphocytes and plasma cells. Most patients are asymptomatic, and chest radiographs typically show multiple, well-circumscribed, pulmonary nodules. Extrapulmonary disease is uncommon, and localized lesions may be treated effectively by surgical removal. Corticosteroids are usually effective for patients with multiple lesions. The prognosis is excellent.

PULMONARY HYPERTENSION

In fetal life, the pulmonary arterial walls are thick, and pulmonary arterial pressure is correspondingly high. Blood is oxygenated through the placenta rather than through the lungs. Thus, the high fetal pulmonary arterial pressure serves to shunt the output of the right ventricle through the ductus arteriosus into the systemic circulation, effectively bypassing the lungs.

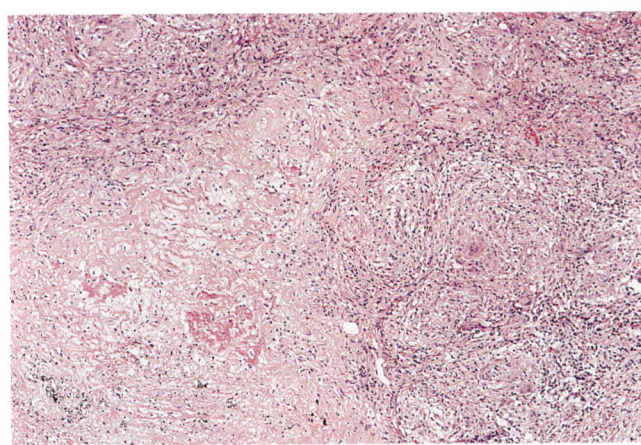
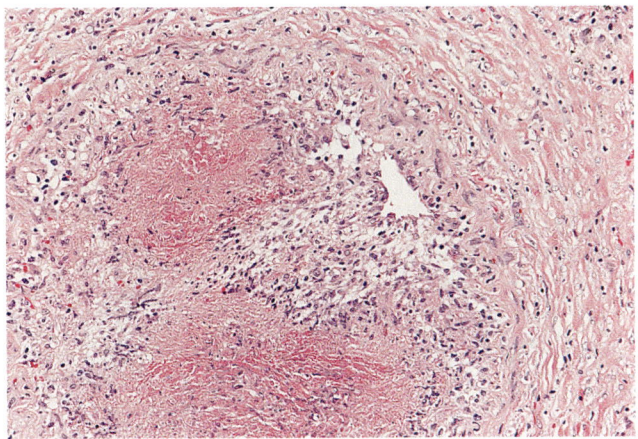

FIGURE 12-73
Necrotizing sarcoid granulomatosis. A. A large area of necrosis is surrounded by confluent sarcoidal granulomas. B. The vasculitis consists of a necrotizing granuloma in the wall of an artery.

After birth, the lungs assume the obligation of oxygenating the venous blood, and the ductus arteriosus closes. Under these circumstances, the lungs must adapt to accept the entire cardiac output, a situation that demands the high-volume and low-pressure system of the mature lung. Accordingly, by the third day of life, the pulmonary arteries dilate, their walls become thin, and pulmonary arterial pressure correspondingly declines. Increased pulmonary arterial pressure is defined as a mean pressure exceeding 25 mm Hg at rest.

In the child or the adult, the pressure within the pulmonary arterial system may be increased either by augmented flow or by increased vascular resistance. Whatever the cause, characteristic morphological abnormalities result from increased pulmonary artery pressure (Fig. 12-74). The grading system for the arterial changes of pulmonary hypertension were originally designed to assess the severity of pulmonary hypertension in patients with congenital heart disease. The system was devised to determine if corrective cardiac surgery would reverse the hypertensive changes. Grades 1, 2, and 3 are generally reversible; grades 4 and above are generally not.

Grade 1: Medial hypertrophy of muscular pulmonary arteries and the appearance of smooth muscle in the pulmonary arterioles
Grade 2: Intimal proliferation with increasing medial hypertrophy
Grade 3: Intimal fibrosis of muscular pulmonary arteries and arterioles, which may be occlusive (Fig. 12-75A)
Grade 4: Formation of plexiform lesions together with dilation and thinning of pulmonary arteries. These nodular lesions are composed of irregular interlacing blood channels and impose a further obstruction in the pulmonary circulation (see Fig. 12-75B).
Grade 5: Plexiform lesions in combination with dilation or angiomatoid lesions. Rupture of dilated thin walled vessel, with parenchymal hemorrhage and hemosiderosis, is also present.
Grade 6: Fibrinoid necrosis of the arteries and arterioles

With all grades of pulmonary hypertension, atherosclerosis is seen in the largest pulmonary arteries. In this respect, even mild atherosclerosis is uncommon when pulmonary arterial pressure is normal. As a result of the increased pressure in the lesser circulation, hypertrophy of the right ventricle occurs (cor pulmonale).

Precapillary versus Postcapillary Pulmonary Hypertension

Conceptually, it is helpful to consider pulmonary hypertension in terms of precapillary versus postcapillary origins, indicating that the primary source of increased flow or resistance is proximal or distal to the pulmonary capillary bed, respectively. Precapillary hypertension includes left-to-right cardiac shunts as well as primary pulmonary hypertension, thromboembolic pulmonary hypertension, and hypertension secondary to fibrotic lung disease and hypoxia. Postcapillary hypertension includes pulmonary venoocclusive disease as well as hypertension secondary to left-sided cardiac disorders such as mitral stenosis and aortic coarctation.

Left-to-Right Shunts

A shunt from the systemic circulation to the pulmonary circulation results in increased flow through the lungs. Most cases represent congenital left-to-right shunts (see Chapter 11). An additional lesion is present when hypertension exists from birth. At this time, the pulmonary artery and the aorta have about the same number of elastic lamellae in their media. In normal infants, there is a loss of elastic lamellae in the pulmonary artery after birth, but when pulmonary hypertension is present, the fetal pattern persists.

Primary Pulmonary Hypertension

Primary pulmonary hypertension is a rare condition caused by increased tone within the pulmonary arteries. It occurs at all ages, but is most common in young women in their 20s

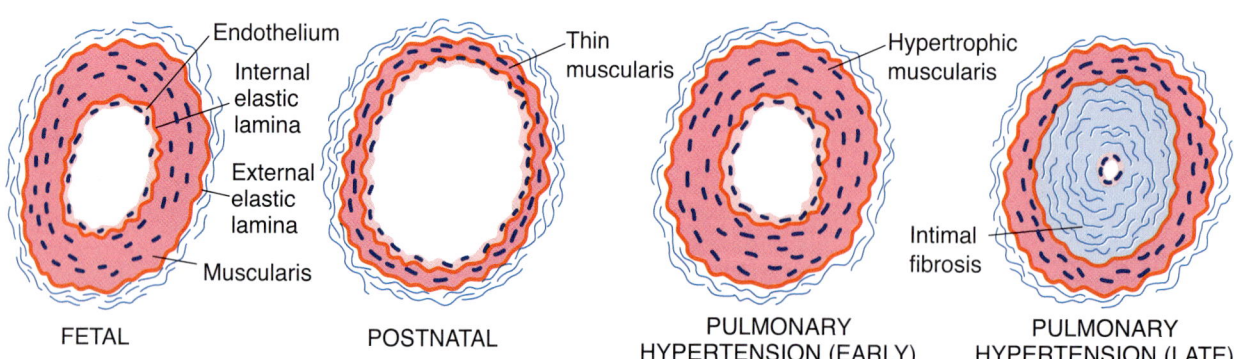

FIGURE 12-74
Histopathology of pulmonary hypertension. In late gestation, the pulmonary arteries have thick walls. After birth, the vessels dilate, and the walls become thin. Mild pulmonary hypertension is characterized by thickening of the media. As pulmonary hypertension becomes more severe, there is extensive intimal fibrosis and muscle thickening.

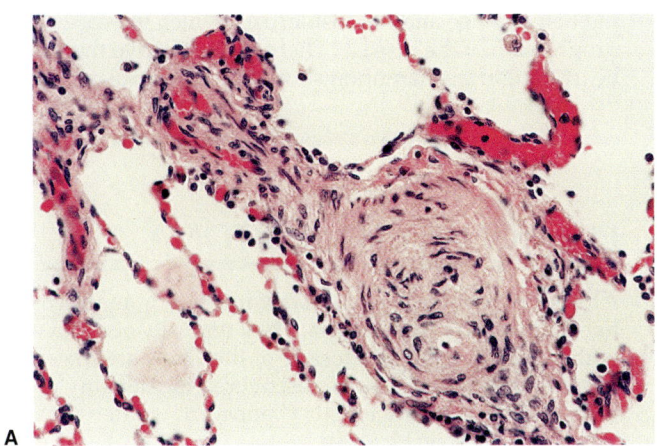
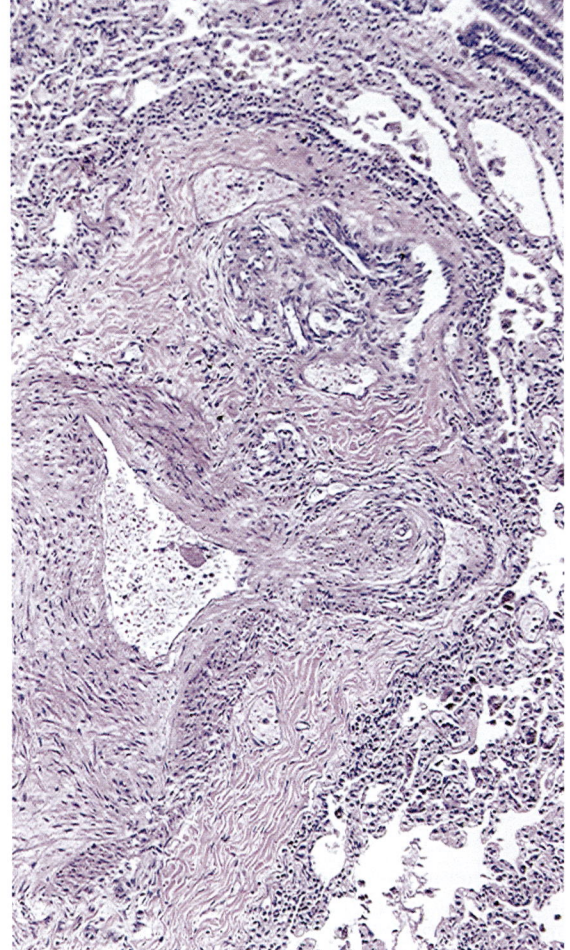

FIGURE 12-75
Pulmonary arterial hypertension. A. A small pulmonary artery is virtually occluded by concentric intimal fibrosis and thickening of the media. B. A plexiform lesion is characterized by a glomeruloid proliferation of thin-walled vessels adjacent to a parent artery, which shows marked hypertensive changes of intimal fibrosis and medial thickening.

and 30s. The disorder is seen as an insidious onset of dyspnea. Physical signs and radiological abnormalities are initially slight, but with time they become more apparent. Severe morphological changes of pulmonary hypertension (i.e., plexiform lesions) eventually ensue, and the patients die of cor pulmonale. Medical treatment is ineffective, and the disease is an indication for heart–lung transplantation. Although primary pulmonary hypertension is typically an idiopathic disorder, some patients with collagen vascular diseases have identical clinical and morphological findings.

Recurrent Pulmonary Emboli

Multiple thromboemboli in the smaller pulmonary vessels often result from asymptomatic, episodic showers of small emboli from the periphery. Gradually restricting the pulmonary circulation, they eventuate in pulmonary hypertension. Some patients have evidence of peripheral venous thrombosis, usually in the leg veins, or a history of circumstances predisposing to venous thrombosis. In addition to the vascular lesions of pulmonary hypertension, organized thromboemboli are evidenced by fibrous bands ("webs") that extend across the lumina of small pulmonary arteries. If the condition is diagnosed during life, placement of a filter in the inferior vena cava prevents further embolization.

Functional Resistance to Arterial Flow (Vasoconstriction)

Any disorder that produces hypoxemia can result in constriction of small pulmonary arteries and pulmonary hypertension. Predisposing conditions include chronic airflow obstruction (chronic bronchitis), interstitial lung disease, and living at high altitude. Severe kyphoscoliosis or extreme obesity *(Pickwickian syndrome)* may interfere with the mechanics of ventilation and can cause hypoxemia and pulmonary hypertension.

Cardiac Causes of Pulmonary Hypertension

Left ventricular failure from any cause increases pulmonary venous pressure and, to some extent, pulmonary arterial pressure. By contrast, mitral stenosis produces severe venous hy-

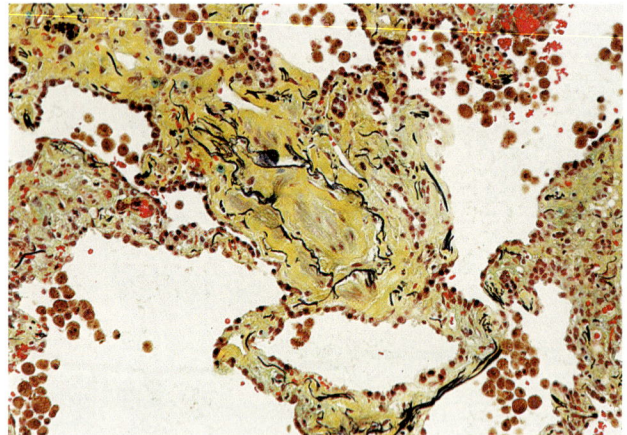

FIGURE 12-76
Venoocclusive disease of the lung. This pulmonary vein is occluded by intimal fibrosis (Movat stain).

pertension and significant pulmonary artery hypertension. In such cases, the lungs exhibit lesions of both pulmonary hypertension and chronic passive congestion (see Chapter 7).

Pulmonary Venoocclusive Disease Involves Fibrotic Obstruction of Small Veins

Pulmonary veno-occlusive disease is a rare condition of uncertain etiology characterized by extensive occlusion of small pulmonary veins and venules by loose, sparsely cellular, intimal fibrosis (Fig. 12-76). Some large veins may also be involved, and in half of cases, similar but less severe lesions involve the pulmonary arteries. Canalization of the obstructive lesions suggests that they represent organized thrombi. The disease has been reported to follow viral infections, exposure to toxic agents, and chemotherapy. More than half of cases are encountered in the first 3 decades of life. In children, girls and boys are affected similarly, but after age 15 years, pulmonary venoocclusive disease is more common in men.

 Pathology: Pulmonary venoocclusive disease produces severe pulmonary hypertension. Gross examination reveals brown induration of the lung and atherosclerosis of large pulmonary arteries. Microscopic examination shows partial or total occlusion of small veins and venules and eccentric intimal thickening of larger veins. Moderate fibrosis of the alveolar walls is usually noted, and foci of hemosiderosis are common. The pulmonary arterial tree exhibits severe lesions of pulmonary hypertension. Recent thrombi are regularly observed.

 Clinical Features: The clinical presentation of progressive dyspnea is similar to that of primary pulmonary hypertension, but pulmonary venoocclusive disease has a more fulminant course. Radiological examination reveals scattered infiltrates in the lung, representing hemorrhage and hemosiderosis, which increase with the progression of the disease. There is no effective therapy, and heart–lung transplantation should be contemplated.

PULMONARY HAMARTOMA

Although the term *hamartoma* implies a malformation, **hamartomas are true tumors.** They typically occur in adults, with a peak in the sixth decade of life. They are the cause of some 10% of "coin" lesions discovered incidentally on chest radiographs. A characteristic ("popcorn") pattern of calcification is often seen by x-ray.

 Pathology: Grossly, pulmonary hamartomas appear as solitary, circumscribed, lobulated masses, averaging 2 cm in diameter, with a white or gray, cartilaginous cut surface (Fig. 12-77A). The tumor consists of elements usually present in the lung, including cartilage, fibromyxoid connective tissue, fat, bone, and occasionally smooth muscle (see Fig. 12-77B). These components are interspersed with clefts lined by respiratory epithelium. The tumor is benign and well circumscribed and shells out from the surrounding lung parenchyma. Most hamartomas occur in the peripheral parenchyma, but 10% occur in a central endobronchial location. The latter may be seen with symptoms due to bronchial obstruction.

CARCINOMA OF THE LUNG

 Epidemiology: Carcinoma of the lung is the most common cause of cancer death worldwide, including the United States. Regarded as a rare tumor as late as 1945, it now occurs in epidemic proportions. In the United States, it is the most common cause of cancer death in both men and women. Some 85% of lung cancers occur in cigarette smokers (see Chapter 8). Most types are linked to cigarette smoking, but the strongest association is with squamous cell carcinoma and small cell carcinoma. The nonsmoker who develops cancer of the lung usually has an adenocarcinoma. The peak age for lung cancer is between age 60 and 70 years, and most patients are between 50 and 80 years old. There is a male predominance, but the male-to-female ratio is decreasing, owing to the increase in smoking among women.

 Pathogenesis: Mutations in the K-*ras* oncogene, particularly in codons 12 and 13, are found in 25% of adenocarcinomas, 20% of large cell carcinomas, and 5% of squamous cell carcinomas but only rarely in small cell lung carcinoma. Mutations in K-*ras* are correlated with

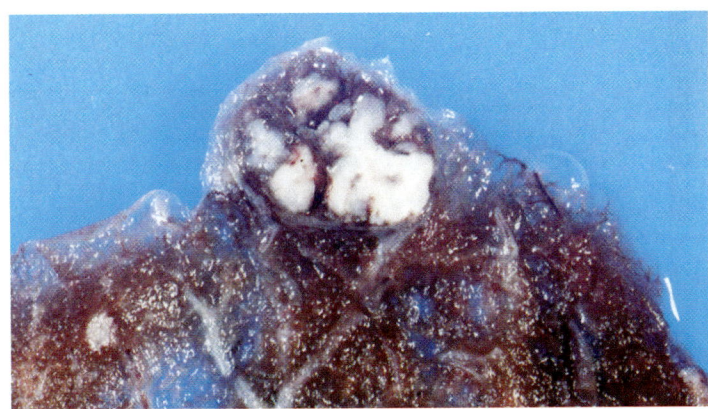
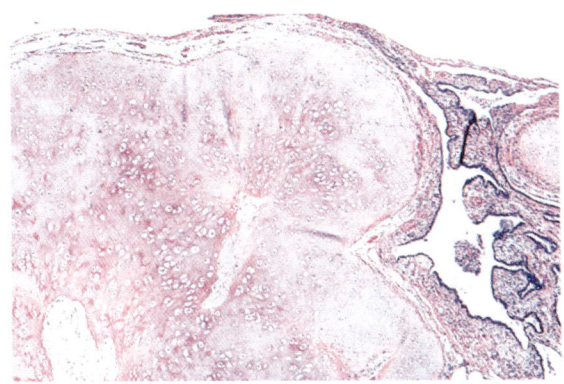

FIGURE 12-77
Pulmonary hamartoma. **A.** The cut surface of a sharply circumscribed, peripheral pulmonary nodule shows a lobulated structure. **B.** A photomicrograph reveals nodules of hyaline cartilage separated by connective tissue lined by respiratory epithelium.

cigarette smoking and have been reported to be associated with a poor prognosis in patients with adenocarcinoma. *Myc* oncogene overexpression occurs in 10 to 40% of small cell carcinomas but is rare in other types. Two important tumor-suppressor genes in lung cancer are the *p53* and retinoblastoma *(Rb)* genes. Mutations in the *p53* gene are found in more than 80% of small cell carcinomas and 50% of non-small cell tumors. *Rb* mutations occur in more than 80% of small cell carcinomas and 25% of non-small cell cancers. Deletions in the short arm of chromosome 3 (3p) are frequently found in all types of lung cancers. The protooncogene *bcl-2*, which encodes a protein that inhibits programmed cell death (apoptosis), is expressed in 25% of squamous cell carcinomas and 10% of adenocarcinomas.

 Pathology: In the past, the term *bronchogenic* carcinoma was often used for primary lung cancer, but it is perhaps too specific, implying an origin from the bronchi. A substantial proportion, perhaps one fourth, of primary lung cancers do not have an obvious bronchial origin. The most important issue in the histological subclassification of lung cancer is the separation of small cell carcinoma from the other types (non-small cell carcinoma), because small cell carcinoma responds to chemotherapy, whereas other histological types do not.

Histological subtyping of lung cancer is based on the best-differentiated component, unless an area of small cell carcinoma is present. However, the differentiation of tumors is *graded* according to the worst-differentiated component. For example, if a tumor consists mostly of poorly differentiated large cells but has foci of squamous cells or adenocarcinoma, it is classified as a poorly differentiated squamous cell carcinoma or adenocarcinoma, respectively. Any cancer with a component of small cell carcinoma is regarded as a subtype of that tumor (see below).

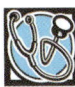 Clinical Features: The overall 5-year survival for all lung cancer patients has remained at 15% over the past 2 decades. The 5-year survival at all stages is 42% for bronchioloalveolar carcinoma, 17% for adenocarcinoma, 15% for squamous cell carcinoma, 11% for large cell carcinoma, and 5% for small cell carcinoma. Tumor stage remains the single most important predictor of prognosis.

General Features Common to All Subtypes

LOCAL EFFECTS: Lung cancer can produce cough, dyspnea, hemoptysis, chest pain, obstructive pneumonia, and pleural effusion. Growth of a lung cancer (usually squamous) in the apex of the lung *(Pancoast tumor)* may extend to involve the eighth cervical and first and second thoracic nerves, which results in shoulder pain radiating in an ulnar distribution down the arm *(Pancoast syndrome)*. A Pancoast tumor also may paralyze the cervical sympathetic nerves and cause *Horner syndrome,* characterized on the affected side by (1) depression of the eyeball (enophthalmos), (2) ptosis of the upper eyelid, (3) constriction of the pupil (miosis), and (4) absence of sweating (anhidrosis).

Most central endobronchial tumors produce symptoms related to bronchial obstruction: persistent cough, hemoptysis, and obstructive pneumonia or atelectasis. Effusions can result from extension of the tumor into the pleura or pericardium. Lymphangitic spread of the tumor within the lung may interfere with oxygenation. Tumors that arise in the periphery of the lung are more likely to be discovered either on routine chest radiographs or after they have become advanced. The latter circumstance features invasion of the chest wall with resulting chest pain, the superior vena cava syndrome, and nerve-entrapment syndromes.

MEDIASTINAL SPREAD: Growth of the tumor within the mediastinum can cause the superior vena cava syndrome (owing to tumorous obstruction of this vein) and nerve-entrapment syndromes.

METASTASES: Carcinomas of the lung metastasize most frequently to the regional lymph nodes, particularly the hilar and mediastinal nodes, but also to the brain, bone, and liver. The most frequent site of extranodal metastases is

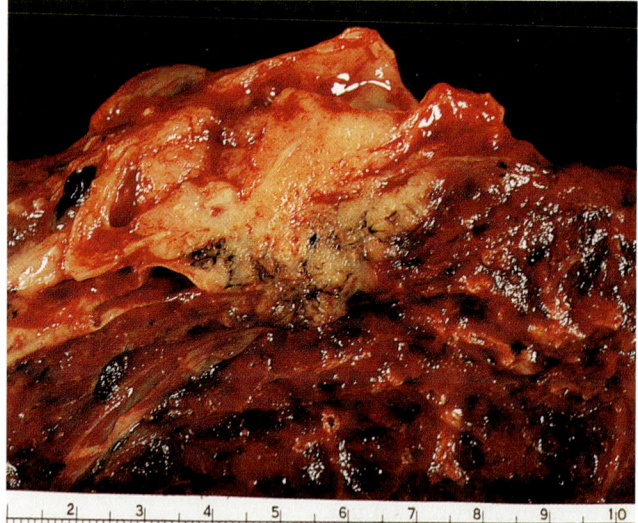
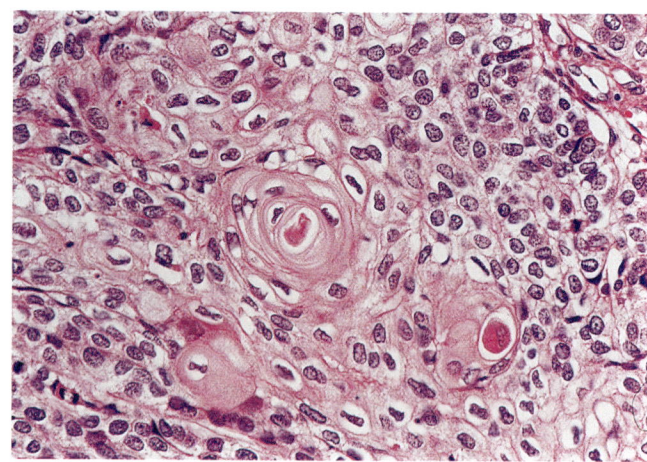

FIGURE 12-78
Squamous cell carcinoma of the lung. A. The tumor grows within the lumen of a bronchus and invades the adjacent intrapulmonary lymph node. B. A photomicrograph shows well-differentiated squamous cell carcinoma with a keratin pearl composed of cells with brightly eosinophilic cytoplasm.

the adrenal gland, although adrenal insufficiency is distinctly uncommon.

PARANEOPLASTIC SYNDROMES: Disorders associated with lung cancer include acanthosis nigricans, dermatomyositis/polymyositis, clubbing of the fingers, and myasthenic syndromes, such as Eaton-Lambert syndrome and progressive multifocal encephalopathy. Endocrine syndromes are also encountered, for example, Cushing syndrome or inappropriate release of antidiuretic hormone by small cell carcinoma, and hypercalcemia (secretion of a parathormone-like substance by squamous cell carcinoma).

Squamous Cell Carcinoma

Squamous cell carcinoma accounts for 30% of all invasive lung cancers in the United States. After injury to the bronchial epithelium, such as occurs with cigarette smoking, regeneration from the pluripotent basal layer commonly occurs in the form of squamous metaplasia. The metaplastic mucosa follows the same sequence of dysplasia, carcinoma in situ, and invasive tumor as that observed in sites that are normally lined by squamous epithelium, such as the cervix or skin.

Pathology: Most squamous cell carcinomas arise in the central portion of the lung from the major or segmental bronchi, although 10% arise in the periphery. On gross examination, they tend to be firm, grey-white, 3- to 5-cm ulcerated lesions that extend through the bronchial wall into the adjacent parenchyma (Fig. 12-78A). The appearance of the cut surface is variable, depending on the degree of necrosis and hemorrhage. Central cavitation is frequent. On occasion, a central squamous carcinoma occurs as an endobronchial tumor.

The microscopic appearance of squamous cell carcinoma is highly variable. Well-differentiated squamous cell carcinomas display keratin "pearls," which appear as small round nests of brightly eosinophilic aggregates of keratin surrounded by concentric ("onion skin") layers of squamous cells (see Fig. 12-78B). Individual cell keratinization also occurs, in which the cytoplasm of the cell assumes a glassy, intensely eosinophilic appearance. Intercellular bridges are identified in some well-differentiated squamous cancers as slender gaps between adjacent cells, which are traversed by fine strands of cytoplasm. By contrast, some squamous tumors are so poorly differentiated that they do not exhibit even small foci of keratinization and are difficult to distinguish from large cell, small cell, or spindle cell carcinomas. Tumor cells may be readily found in the sputum, in which case the diagnosis is made by exfoliative cytology.

Adenocarcinoma

Adenocarcinoma of the lung comprises for a third of all invasive lung cancers. In the United States it has overtaken squamous cell carcinoma as the most common subtype of lung cancer and is the most common type in women. It tends to arise in the periphery and is often associated with pleural fibrosis and subpleural scars, which can result in pleural puckering (Fig. 12-79). In the past, these cancers were thought to arise in scars secondary to old tuberculosis or healed infarcts but it is now recognized that most of these scars represent a desmoplastic response to the tumor.

Carcinoma of the Lung

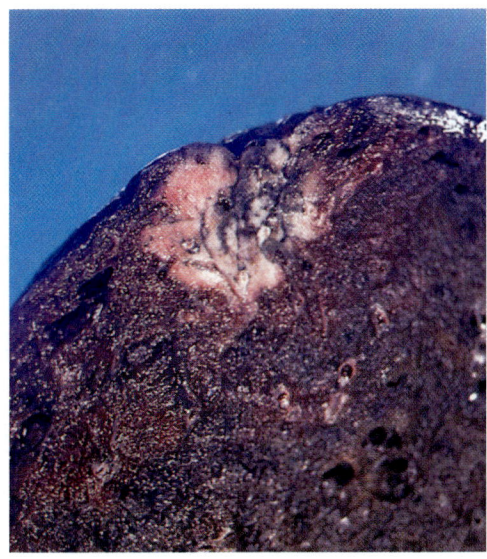

FIGURE 12-79
Adenocarcinoma of the lung. A peripheral tumor of the right upper lobe has an irregular border and a tan or grey cut surface and causes puckering of the overlying pleura.

 Pathology: At initial presentation, adenocarcinomas of the lung most often appear as irregular masses 2 to 5 cm in diameter, although they may be so large that they completely replace an entire lobe of the lung. On cut section, the tumor is grayish white and often glistening, depending on the amount of mucus production. Central adenocarcinomas may have predominantly endobronchial growth and invade bronchial cartilage.

There are four major subtypes of adenocarcinoma, as defined by the World Health Organization (Figs 12-80, 12-81, and 12-82): (1) acinar, (2) papillary, (3) solid with mucus formation, and (4) bronchioloalveolar. Although some adenocarcinomas consist purely of one of these patterns, it is common to encounter a mixture of these histological subtypes. Bronchioloalveolar carcinoma is distinctive enough to merit special attention (see below).

Pulmonary adenocarcinoma may reflect the architecture and cell population of any part of the respiratory mucosa, from the large bronchi to the smallest bronchioles. The neoplastic cells may resemble ciliated or nonciliated columnar epithelial cells, goblet cells, cells of bronchial glands, or Clara cells. The most common histological type of adenocarcinoma features the acinar pattern, which is distinguished by regular glands lined by cuboidal or columnar cells, (see Fig. 12-80A). Papillary adenocarcinomas exhibit a single cell layer on a core of fibrovascular connective tissue (see Fig. 12-80B). Solid adenocarcinomas with mucus formation are poorly differentiated tumors, which are distinguished from large cell carcino-

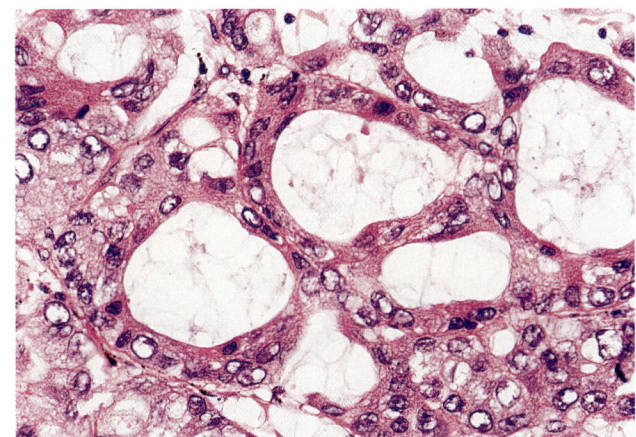

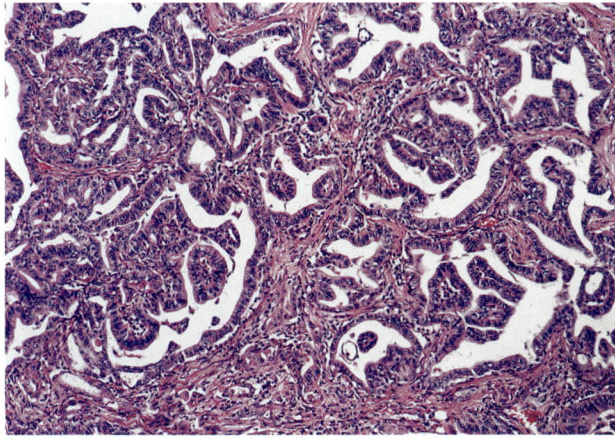

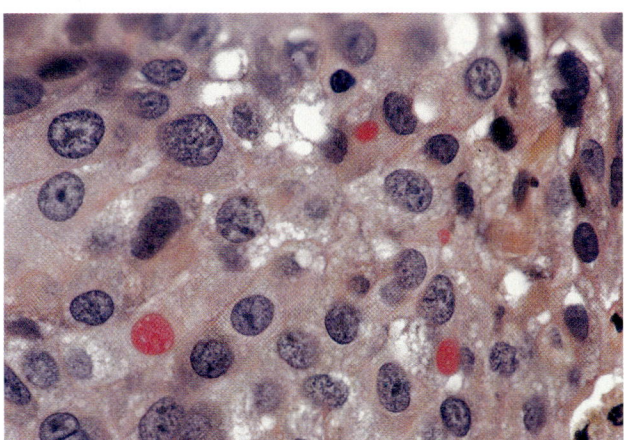

FIGURE 12-80
Adenocarcinoma of the lung. A. The malignant epithelial cells of an acinar adenocarcinoma form glands. B. A papillary adenocarcinoma consists of malignant epithelial cells growing along thin fibrovascular cores. C. A tumor grows in the pattern of solid adenocarcinoma with mucin formation. Several intracytoplasmic mucin droplets stain positively with the mucicarmine stain.

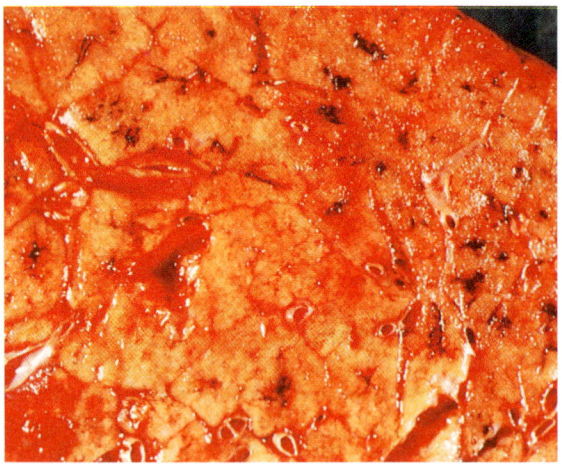

FIGURE 12-81
Bronchioloalveolar carcinoma. The cut surface of the lung is solid, glistening, and mucoid, an appearance that reflects a diffusely infiltrating tumor.

mas by the demonstration of mucin with the mucicarmine stain or PAS reaction (see Fig. 12-80C).

Patients with stage I adenocarcinomas (localized to the lung) who undergo complete surgical removal have a 5-year survival of 50 to 80%.

Bronchioloalveolar Carcinoma

Bronchioloalveolar carcinoma is a distinctive subtype of adenocarcinoma that grows along preexisting alveolar walls and accounts for 1 to 5% of all invasive lung tumors. It has not been definitively linked to smoking. Copious mucin in the sputum *(bronchorrhea)* is a distinctive sign of bronchioloalveolar carcinoma but is seen in fewer than 10% of patients.

On gross examination, bronchioloalveolar carcinoma may appear as a single peripheral nodule or coin lesion (>50% of cases), multiple nodules, or a diffuse infiltrate indistinguishable from lobar pneumonia (Fig. 12-81). Two thirds of tumors are nonmucinous, consisting of Clara cells and type II pneumocytes (Fig. 12-82A); the remaining third are mucinous tumors featuring goblet cells (see Fig. 12-82B). The nonmucinous tumors exhibit cuboidal cells growing along the alveolar walls. The mucinous tumors are composed of columnar cells with abundant apical cytoplasm filled with mucus. It is important to exclude the possibility that the tumor is actually a pulmonary metastasis, particularly for mucinous tumors.

Patients with stage I bronchioloalveolar carcinomas have a good prognosis; those who have multiple nodules or diffuse lung involvement are more likely to have a poor outcome.

Small Cell Carcinoma

Small cell carcinoma (previously "oat cell" carcinoma) is a highly malignant epithelial tumor of the lung that exhibits neuroendocrine features. It accounts for 20% of all lung cancers and is strongly associated with cigarette smoking. In the past, the male-to-female ratio was 10:1, but it is now 2:1. The tumor grows and metastasizes rapidly, and 70% of patients are first seen in an advanced stage. A variety of paraneoplastic syndromes are distinctive for small cell carcinoma, including diabetes insipidus, ectopic ACTH (corticotropin) syndrome, and the Eaton-Lambert syndrome.

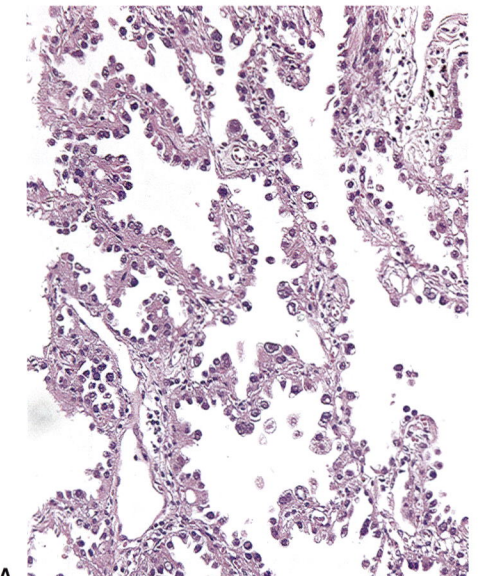
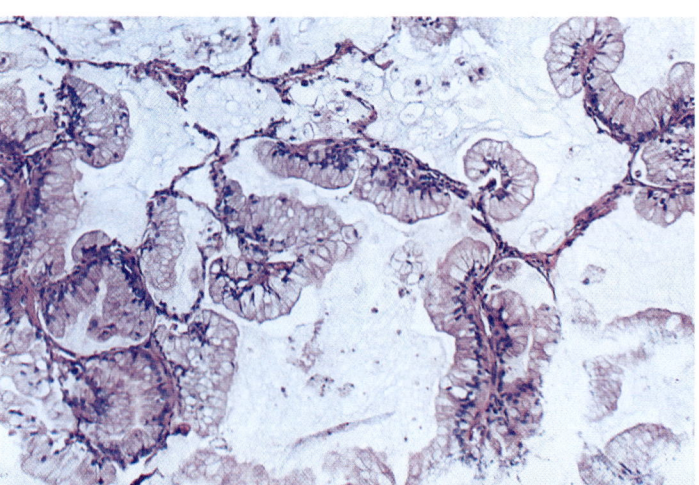

FIGURE 12-82
Bronchioloalveolar carcinoma. **A.** Nonmucinous bronchioloalveolar carcinomas consist of atypical cuboidal to low columnar cells proliferating along the existing alveolar walls. **B.** Mucinous bronchioloalveolar carcinoma consists of tall columnar cells filled with apical cytoplasmic mucin that grow along the existing alveolar walls.

Pathology: Small cell carcinoma usually appears as a perihilar mass, frequently with extensive lymph node metastases. On cut section, it is soft and white but often shows extensive hemorrhage and necrosis. The tumor typically spreads along the bronchi in a submucosal and circumferential fashion.

Histologically, small cell carcinoma consists of sheets of small, round, oval or spindle-shaped cells. The tumor cells display scant cytoplasm and distinctive nuclear characteristics, which include finely granular nuclear chromatin and absent or inconspicuous nucleoli (Fig. 12-83). By electron microscopy, many of the cells contain secretory neuroendocrine granules. A high mitotic rate is characteristic, with an average of 60 to 70 mitoses per 10 high-power fields. Necrosis is frequent and extensive. Basophilic nuclear staining of vascular walls by DNA from necrotic tumor cells *(the Azzopardi effect)* is common in necrotic areas. Although there is no absolute measure for the size of the tumor cells, a useful rule of thumb in small cell carcinoma is the diameter of three small lymphocytes.

The important difference between small cell carcinoma and other lung cancers is its more marked sensitivity to chemotherapy. From an oncologist's standpoint, therefore, all other lung cancers are grouped together under the term "non-small cell carcinoma."

Large Cell Carcinoma

Large cell carcinoma is a diagnosis of exclusion in a poorly differentiated tumor that does not show features of squamous or glandular differentiation and has been shown not to be a small cell carcinoma (Fig. 12-84). This tumor type accounts for 10% of all invasive lung tumors. The cells are large and exhibit ample cytoplasm. The nuclei frequently show prominent nucleoli and vesicular chromatin. Some large cell carcinomas exhibit pleomorphic giant cells or spindle cells.

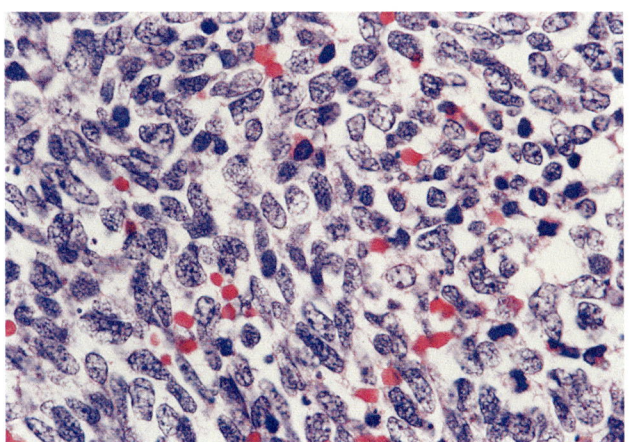

FIGURE 12-83
Small cell carcinoma of the lung. This tumor consists of small oval to spindle-shaped cells with scant cytoplasm, finely granular nuclear chromatin, and conspicuous mitoses.

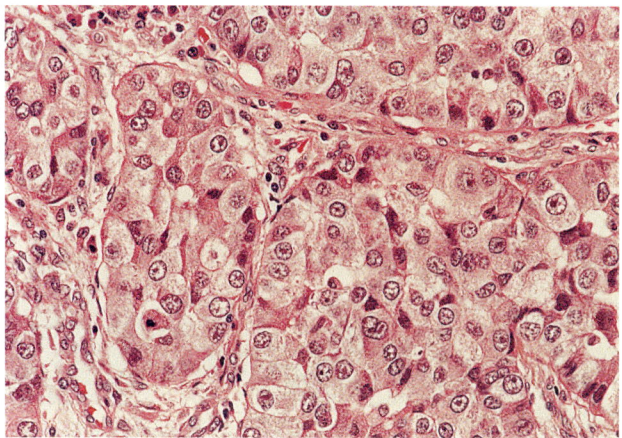

FIGURE 12-84
Large cell carcinoma of the lung. This poorly differentiated tumor is growing in sheets. The tumor cells are large and contain ample cytoplasm and prominent nucleoli.

Carcinoid Tumors

Carcinoid tumors of the lung comprise a group of neuroendocrine neoplasms derived from the pluripotential basal layer of the respiratory epithelium. They exhibit a neuroendocrine differentiation similar to that of the resident Kulchitsky cells. In this respect, carcinoid tumors bear a resemblance to small cell carcinomas. These neoplasms account for 2% of all primary lung cancers, show no sex predilection, and are not related to cigarette smoking. Although neuropeptides are readily demonstrated in the tumor cells, most are endocrinologically silent. A small subset of cases is associated with an endocrinopathy, such as Cushing syndrome with ectopic ACTH production by tumor cells. The carcinoid syndrome (see Chapter 13) occurs in 1% of cases, usually in the setting of hepatic metastases.

 Pathology: One third of carcinoid tumors are central, one third are peripheral (subpleural), and one third are situated in the midportion of the lung. Central carcinoid tumors tend to have a large endobronchial component, with a fleshy, smooth, polypoid mass protruding into the bronchial lumen (Fig. 12-85A). The tumors average 3.0 cm in diameter, but range from 0.5 to 10 cm.

Carcinoid tumors are characterized histologically by an organoid growth pattern and uniform cytological features, consisting of an eosinophilic, finely granular cytoplasm and nuclei that display a finely granular chromatin pattern (see Fig. 12-85B). A variety of neuroendocrine patterns may be seen, including trabecular growth, peripheral palisading, and rosettes.

Atypical carcinoid tumors are distinguished from typical carcinoids by the following criteria: (1) increased mitotic activity, with 2 to 10 mitotic figures per 10 high-power fields; (2) tumor necrosis (Fig. 12-86); (3) areas of increased cellularity and disorganization of the architecture; and (4) nuclear pleomorphism, hyperchromatism, and a high nuclear/cytoplasmic ratio.

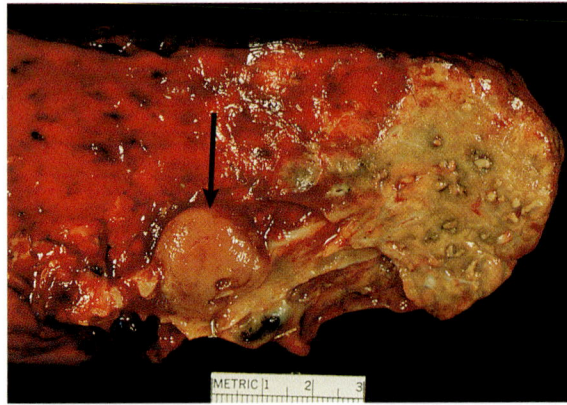
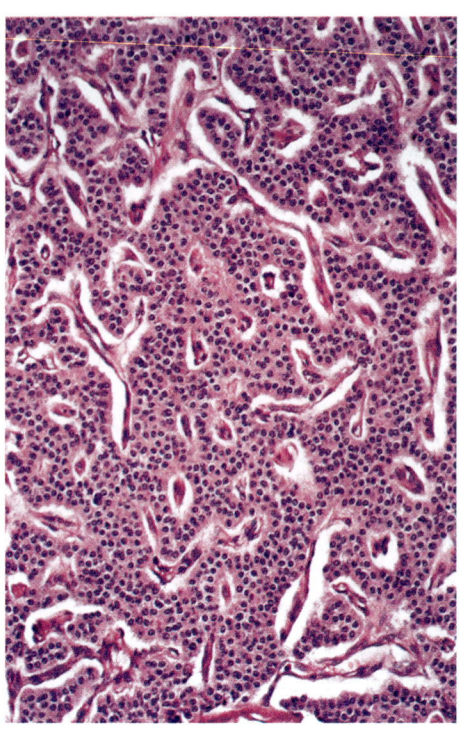

FIGURE 12-85
Carcinoid tumor of the lung. A. A central carcinoid tumor (arrow) is circumscribed and protrudes into the lumen of the main bronchus. The compression of the bronchus by the tumor caused the postobstructive pneumonia seen in the distal lung parenchyma *(right)*. B. A microscopic view shows ribbons of tumor cells embedded in a vascular stroma.

Clinical Features: The indolent nature of carcinoid tumors is reflected in the finding that half the patients are asymptomatic at presentation. The tumors are usually discovered because of a mass in a chest radiograph. In symptomatic patients, the most common pulmonary manifestations include hemoptysis, postobstructive pneumonitis, and dyspnea. There is a slight female predominance. The mean age at the time of diagnosis is 55 years, but carcinoid tumors can occur at any age. In fact, bronchial carcinoids are the most common lung tumor in childhood. Atypical carcinoid tumors tend to be more aggressive than typical ones. Regional lymph node metastases are found in 20% of patients with typical carcinoids and in 50% of those with atypical carcinoids. Patients with typical carcinoids have an excellent prognosis, with a 90% 5-year survival after surgery, compared with 60% for patients with atypical carcinoids.

Rare Pulmonary Tumors

INFLAMMATORY PSEUDOTUMOR: Inflammatory pseudotumor of the lung is an uncommon lesion that consists of nodular masses of inflammatory cells and fibroblasts. Most of these masses are contained within the lung, although the pleura may be involved. In 5% of cases, the tumor invades structures outside the lung, such as the esophagus, mediastinum, chest wall, diaphragm, or pericardium.

Inflammatory pseudotumor is regarded as an inflammatory, nonneoplastic process, despite the occasional case that recurs and behaves in a locally aggressive fashion. A previous history of a pulmonary infection can be elicited in one third of patients. Some fibrohistiocytic variants exhibit clonality by cytogenetic studies, suggesting that occasional tumors may actually be neoplastic.

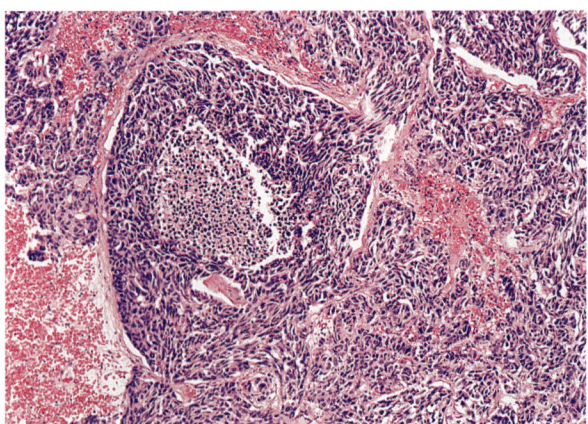

FIGURE 12-86
Atypical carcinoid tumor of the lung. A cellular tumor shows central necrosis and a disorganized architecture.

Pathology: The tumors are solitary circumscribed, with a mean size of 4 cm. Virtually any inflammatory cells may be present, including lymphocytes, plasma cells, macrophages, giant cells, mast cells, and eosinophils. Inflammatory pseudotumor causes consolidation of the lung parenchyma and loss of architecture. Two major histological patterns are fibrohistiocytic (Fig. 12-87) and plasma cell granuloma, depending on the predominant component. In some cases, foamy macrophages impart a xanthomatous pattern.

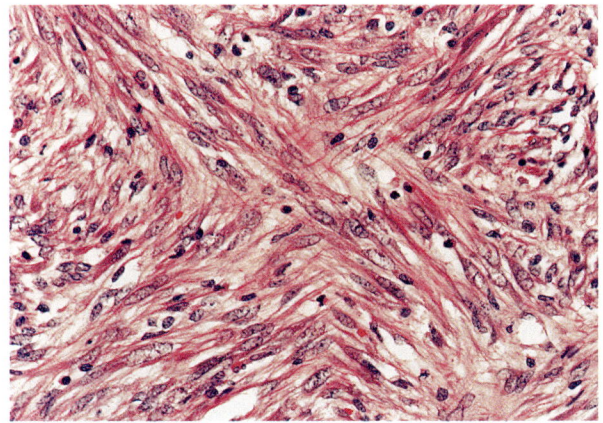

FIGURE 12-87
Inflammatory pseudotumor. A photomicrograph shows intersecting spindle cells and scattered lymphocytes and macrophages.

 Clinical Features: Most patients are younger than 40 years, although inflammatory pseudotumor can occur at any age and is one of the most common lung tumors of childhood. Half of patients are asymptomatic at presentation. Most inflammatory pseudotumors are cured by surgical excision, but 5% recur within the chest.

PULMONARY EPITHELIOID HEMANGIOEN-DOTHELIOMA: Pulmonary epithelioid hemangioendotheliomas are rare tumors that represent low-grade vascular sarcomas. Most patients are young adults, and 80% are women. The course tends to be indolent, and half of the patients are asymptomatic.

Pathology: Most patients are first seen with multiple pulmonary nodules. Histologically, the tumor consists of oval-shaped nodules that have a central, sclerotic, hypocellular zone and a cellular peripheral zone. The tumor spreads within alveolar spaces (Fig. 12-88). The tumor cells have abundant cytoplasm, with frequent intracytoplasmic vascular lumina, which may contain red blood cells. The intercellular stroma consists of an abundant eosinophilic matrix. The tumors express vascular markers, such as factor VIII. Epithelioid hemangioendotheliomas with a histological pattern similar to that seen in the lung may occur in the liver, bone, and soft tissue. Pulmonary epithelioid hemangioendothelioma is a slow-growing tumor, with a mean survival of 5 years.

CARCINOSARCOMA: Occasionally, cancers of the lung have the appearance of both a carcinoma and a sarcoma in different parts of the tumor, and the two are usually intimately mingled. In most cases, the epithelial component is a squamous carcinoma, and the sarcomatous one is composed of spindle cells. The sarcomatous portion may also exhibit heterologous elements, such as osteosarcoma, chondrosarcoma, and rhabdomyosarcoma. Metastases can contain both histological components of the primary tumor. The primary approach to therapy for carcinosarcoma is surgery, but the prognosis is poor, with a median survival of 9 to 12 months.

PULMONARY BLASTOMA: This malignant tumor resembles embryonal lung, with a glandular component consisting of poorly differentiated columnar cells arranged in tubules, without mucous secretion. The intervening tumor is formed by spindle cells that resemble embryonal mesoderm. There is a histological overlap between pulmonary blastoma and carcinosarcoma, including heterologous elements, and the clinical features are similar.

Despite the embryonal appearance of pulmonary blastoma, the tumor occurs primarily in adults (median age range, 35–43 years), and most patients are cigarette smokers. The prognosis for patients with biphasic tumors is poor and comparable to that for carcinoma of the lung.

MUCOEPIDERMOID CARCINOMA AND ADENOID CYSTIC CARCINOMA: These neoplasms resemble their namesakes in the salivary glands. They are derived from the tracheobronchial mucous glands and are seen in the trachea or proximal bronchus as a luminal mass, often associated with obstructive symptoms. Adenoid cystic carcinomas are difficult to resect locally and often metastasize.

PULMONARY ARTERY SARCOMA: Pulmonary artery sarcoma is a rare tumor of connective tissue (Fig. 12-89), which has a histological spectrum, including fibrosarcoma, leiomyosarcoma, osteosarcoma, rhabdomyosarcoma, angiosarcoma, or unclassifiable sarcoma. These tumors are rarely diagnosed during life and may be discovered because of pulmonary hypertension. The tumor often grows in an intraluminal fashion within proximal arteries and may extend in a wormlike fashion to peripheral pulmonary artery branches, resulting in peripheral infarcts.

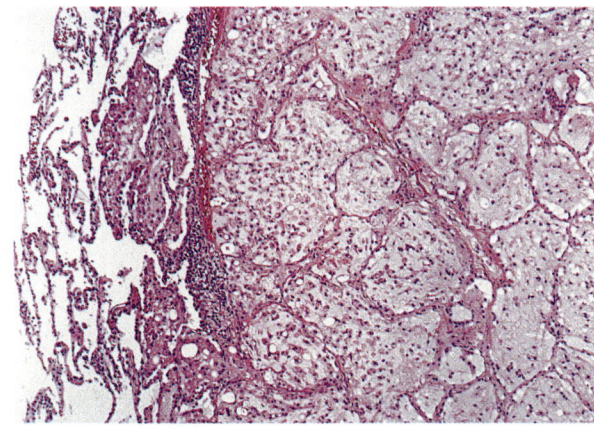

FIGURE 12-88
Epithelioid hemangioendothelioma. A nodule of tumor has spread within alveolar spaces.

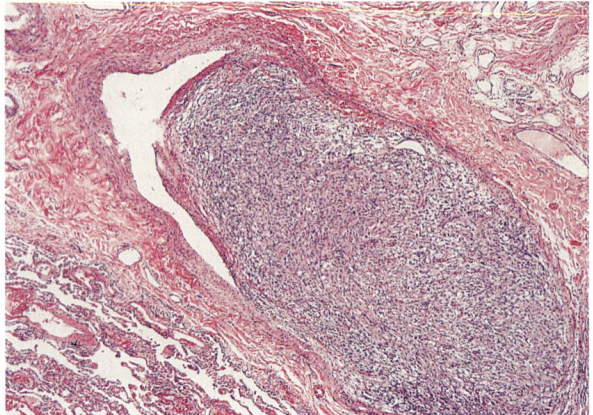

FIGURE 12-89
Pulmonary artery sarcoma. A polypoid mass of malignant spindle cells is spreading within the lumen of this pulmonary artery.

Lymphomatoid Granulomatosis

Lymphomatoid granulomatosis is a lymphoproliferative disorder characterized by pulmonary nodular lymphoid infiltrates with frequent central necrosis and vascular permeation (Fig. 12-90). It is a disease of middle-aged persons. The lung is the major location, but the kidney, skin, and upper respiratory tract also may be involved. The lymphoid infiltrate is angiocentric and angioinvasive and consists of polymorphous, small to medium-sized lymphocytes. Scattered, large, atypical, immunoblast-like cells represent B cells infected with Epstein-Barr virus. The smaller cells are T lymphocytes.

Despite remissions induced by chemotherapy, half of all patients eventually develop large cell lymphoma. Even with aggressive treatment, the overall prognosis of lymphomatoid granulomatosis is poor.

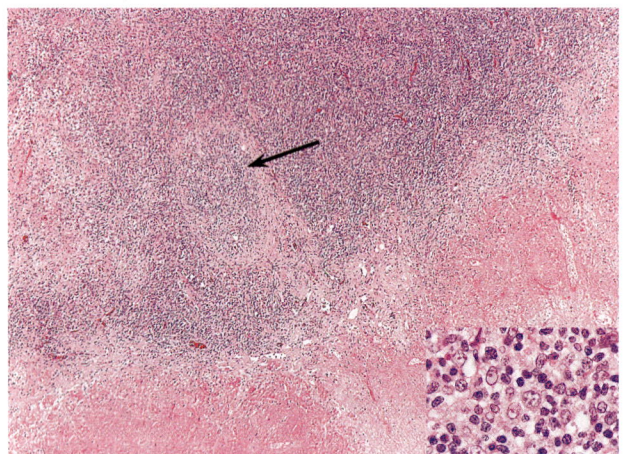

FIGURE 12-90
Lymphomatoid granulomatosis. This extensively necrotic nodular mass consists of a cellular lymphoid infiltrate that penetrates a blood vessel *(arrow)* at the edge of the lesion. *Inset:* The lymphoid infiltrate is composed of a polymorphous population of small, medium-sized, and large atypical lymphoid cells.

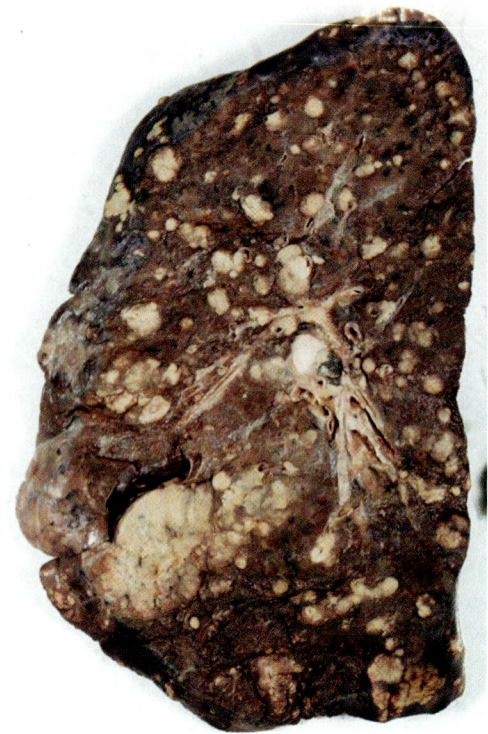

FIGURE 12-91
Metastatic carcinoma of the lung. A section through the lung shows numerous nodules of metastatic carcinoma corresponding to "cannon ball" metastases seen radiologically.

Pulmonary Metastases Represent the Most Common Neoplasm of the Lung

In one third of all fatal cancers, pulmonary metastases are evident at autopsy. Metastatic tumors in the lung are typically multiple and circumscribed. When large nodules are seen in the lungs radiologically, they are called "cannon ball" metastases (Fig. 12-91). The histological appearance of most metastases resembles that of the primary tumor. Uncommonly, metastatic tumors mimic widespread bronchioloalveolar carcinoma, the usual primary site being the pancreas or stomach.

Lymphangitic carcinoma is a condition in which the metastatic tumor spreads widely through the pulmonary lymphatic channels to form a sheath of tumor around the bronchovascular tree and the veins. Clinically, patients suffer from cough and shortness of breath and display a diffuse reticulonodular pattern on the chest radiograph. The common primary sites are the breast, stomach, pancreas, and colon.

The Pleura

PNEUMOTHORAX

Pneumothorax is defined as the presence of air in the pleural cavity. It may be due to traumatic perforation of the pleura or may be "spontaneous." Traumatic causes include penetrating wounds of the chest wall (e.g., a stab wound or a rib fracture). Traumatic pneumothorax is most commonly iatrogenic and is seen after aspiration of fluid from the pleura (thoracentesis), pleural or lung biopsies, transbronchial biopsies, and positive pressure-assisted ventilation.

Spontaneous pneumothorax is typically encountered in young adults. For example, while exercising vigorously, a tall young man develops acute chest pain and shortness of breath. A chest radiograph reveals collapse of the lung on the side of the pain and a large collection of air in the pleural space. The condition is due to the rupture of an emphysematous lesion, usually a subpleural emphysematous bleb. In most cases, spontaneous pneumothorax subsides by itself, but some patients required withdrawal of the air.

Tension pneumothorax refers to unilateral pneumothorax extensive enough to shift the mediastinum to the opposite side, with compression of the opposite lung. The condition may be life threatening and must be relieved by immediate drainage.

Bronchopleural fistula is a serious condition in which there is free communication between the airway and the pleura. It is usually iatrogenic, caused by the interruption of bronchial continuity by biopsy or surgery. It may also be due to extensive infection and necrosis of lung tissue, in which case the infection is more important than the air.

PLEURAL EFFUSION

Pleural effusion is the accumulation of excess fluid in the pleural cavity. Only a small amount of fluid in the pleural cavity lubricates the space between the lung and the chest wall. Fluid is secreted into the pleural space from the parietal pleura and absorbed by the visceral pleura. The severity of a pleural effusion varies from a few milliliters of fluid, which is detected only radiologically as obliteration of the costophrenic angle, to a massive accumulation that shifts the mediastinum and the trachea to the opposite side.

HYDROTHORAX: *This term refers to an effusion that resembles water and would be regarded as edema elsewhere.* It may be due to increased hydrostatic pressure within the capillaries, as occurs in patients with heart failure or in any condition that produces systemic or pulmonary edema. Hydrothorax also occurs in patients with low serum osmotic pressure, as in nephrotic syndrome, cirrhosis of the liver, or severe starvation. Other important causes of hydrothorax are the collagen vascular diseases (notably systemic lupus erythematosus and rheumatoid arthritis) and asbestos exposure.

PYOTHORAX: *A turbid effusion containing many polymorphonuclear leukocytes (pyothorax) results from infections of the pleura.* This condition may occasionally be caused by an external penetrating wound that brings pyogenic organisms into the pleural space. More commonly, it is a complication of bacterial pneumonia that extends to the pleural surface, the classic example of which is pneumococcal pneumonia. Pyothorax is a rare complication of medical procedures involving the pleural cavity.

EMPYEMA: *This disorder is a variant of pyothorax in which thick pus accumulates within the pleural cavity, often with loculation and fibrosis.*

HEMOTHORAX: *This term refers to blood in the pleural cavity as a result of trauma or rupture of a vessel (e.g., dissecting aneurysm of the aorta).* A pleural effusion may be blood-stained in tuberculosis, cancers involving the pleura, and pulmonary infarction.

CHYLOTHORAX: *This condition is defined as the accumulation in the pleural cavity of a milky, lipid-rich fluid (chyle) as a result of lymphatic obstruction.* It has an ominous portent, because obstruction of the lymphatics suggests disease of the lymph nodes in the posterior mediastinum. Chylothorax is thus found as a rare complication of malignant tumors in the mediastinum, such as lymphoma. In tropical countries, chylothorax results from nematode infestations. Chylothorax can also be seen in pulmonary lymphangioleiomyomatosis.

PLEURITIS

Pleuritis, or inflammation of the pleura, may result from the extension of any pulmonary infection to the visceral pleura, bacterial infections within the pleural cavity, viral infections, collagen vascular disease, or pulmonary infarction that involves the surface of the lung. The most striking symptom is sharp, stabbing chest pain on inspiration. It is frequently associated with a pleural effusion.

TUMORS OF THE PLEURA

Localized (Solitary) Fibrous Tumor of the Pleura Is Often Malignant

Solitary fibrous tumor of the pleura is an uncommon localized neoplasm arising in association with the pleura. Most are benign, but one third are malignant. Some 80% of the tumors arise on the visceral pleura, with the remainder originating in the parietal pleura. Similar tumors can develop in any location associated with a mesothelial surface, including the mediastinum, peritoneum, pericardium, liver, and tunica vaginalis. In the past, these tumors were thought to be derived from mesothelium, but they actually arise from the submesothelial connective tissue. The lesion has not been linked to asbestos exposure.

 Pathology: Of fibrous tumors of the pleura that are attached to the visceral pleura, more than half have a pedicle, often measuring 1 cm in length. The tumors range up to 40 cm, and more than 60% exceed 10 cm in size. Weights up to 3800 g are recorded. The cut surface is grey-white, with a nodular, whorled, or lobulated appearance (Fig. 12-92A). Cysts are occasionally present, especially at the base near the pleural attachment.

The most common histological feature is the "patternless pattern," followed by hemangiopericytoma-like, storiform, herringbone, leiomyoma-like, or neurofibroma-like arrangements (Fig. 12-92B). The patternless pattern consists of fibroblast-like cells and connective tissue arranged in a random or disorderly pattern. The tumor cells are spindle- to oval-shaped, often with a fibroblast-like appearance. The collagen is compressed between the cells in a lacy network or it may form dense, wirelike bands. Histological features in favor of malignancy include increased cellularity, pleomorphism, necrosis, and more than four mitoses per 10 high-power fields.

Clinical Features: The median age of patients diagnosed with localized fibrous tumor of the pleura is 55 years (range, 9–86 years) without any sex predominance. The most common presenting symptom is chest pain, followed by shortness of breath, cough, hypoglycemia, weight loss, hemoptysis, fever, and night sweats. Patients with benign fibrous tumors of pleura have an excellent prognosis. Half of histologically malignant tumors are cured if completely resected.

Malignant Mesothelioma is the Major Complication of Asbestos Exposure

Malignant mesothelioma is a neoplasm of mesothelial cells that is most common in the pleura but also occurs in the peritoneum, pericardium, and the tunica vaginalis of the testis.

Epidemiology: The tumor affects some 2000 new persons a year in the United States. **In the United States, Great Britain, and South Africa, some 80% of patients report exposure to asbestos.** The latency period between asbestos exposure and the appearance of malignant mesothelioma is usually to 40 years, with a range of 12 to 60 years.

Pathology: On gross examination, pleural mesothelioma characteristically encases and compresses the lung, extending into fissures and interlobar septa. This distribution of tumor is often referred to as a "pleural rind." (Fig. 12-93A). Invasion of the pulmonary parenchyma is generally limited to the periphery adjacent to the tumor, and lymph nodes tend to be spared. Microscopically, classic mesothelioma exhibits a biphasic appearance, with epithelial and sarcomatous patterns (see Fig. 12-93B). Glands and tubules that resemble adenocarcinoma are admixed with sheets of spindle cells that are similar to a fibrosarcoma. In some instances, only the epithelial component is apparent, in which case, it is difficult to distinguish mesothelioma from adenocarcinoma. Less commonly, only the sarcomatous component is present. Useful criteria for the diagnosis of mesothelioma include the absence of mucin, the presence of hyaluronic

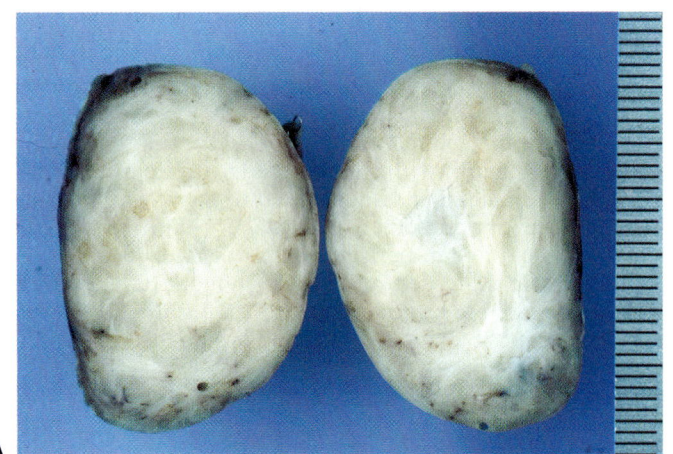

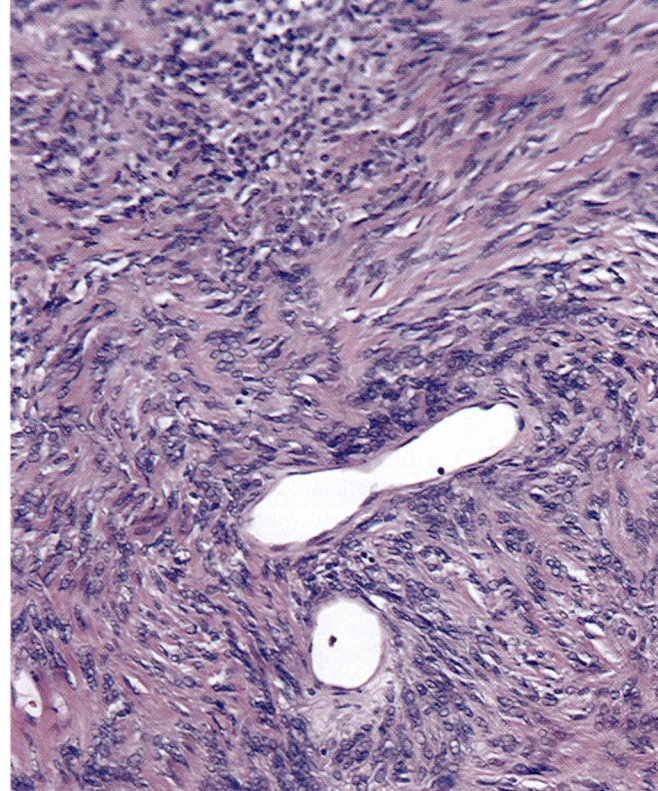

FIGURE 12-92
Pleural localized fibrous tumor. A. The tumor is circumscribed with a whorled, tan, cut surface. **B.** The tumor cells are round to oval and spindle shaped, with a dense eosinophilic or "ropy" collagen stroma and slitlike blood vessels.

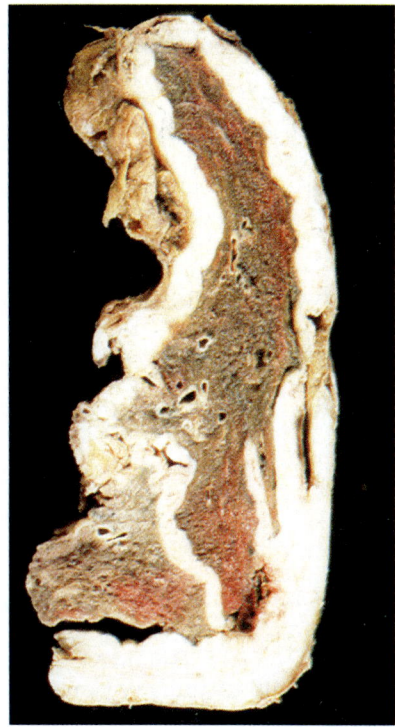 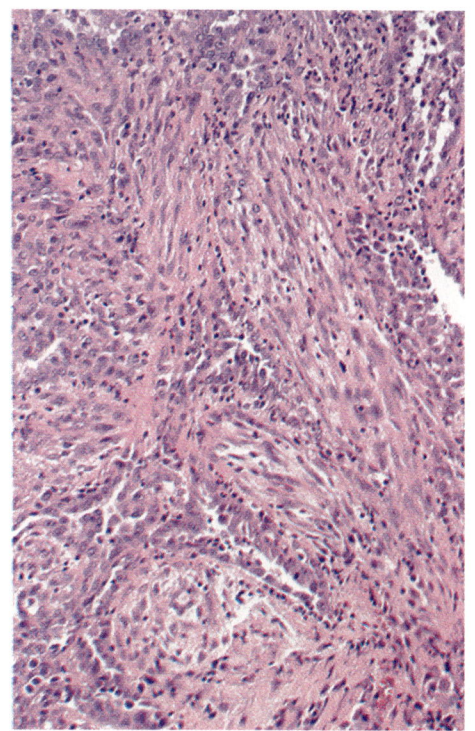

FIGURE 12-93
Pleural malignant mesothelioma. A. The lung is encased by a dense pleural tumor that extends along the interlobar fissures but does not involve the underlying lung parenchyma. B. This mesothelioma is composed of a biphasic pattern of epithelial and sarcomatous elements.

acid (positive Alcian blue staining), and the demonstration of long, slender microvilli by electron microscopy.

The application of immunohistochemistry provides more-refined criteria for differentiating mesothelioma from adenocarcinoma. Adenocarcinomas are often, but not invariably, positive for carcinoembryonic antigen, Leu-M1, B72.3, and BER-EP4. Mesotheliomas are negative for these markers. Both mesothelioma and adenocarcinoma are positive for cytokeratins. Calretinin, a recently developed marker, usually stains mesotheliomas, whereas adenocarcinoma is typically negative. WT-1 (Wilms Tumor-1) is another marker often found in mesotheliomas.

Clinical Features: The average age of patients with mesothelioma is 60 years. Patients are first seen with a pleural effusion or a pleural mass, chest pain, and nonspecific symptoms, such as weight loss and malaise. Pleural mesotheliomas tend to spread locally within the chest cavity, invading and compressing major structures. Metastases can occur to the lung parenchyma and mediastinal lymph nodes, as well as to extrathoracic sites such as the liver, bones, peritoneum, and adrenals. Treatment is ineffective, and the prognosis is hopeless.

SUGGESTED READING

Books

Churg A, Green FHY: *Pathology of occupational lung disease.* Baltimore: Williams & Wilkins, 1998.

Colby TV: *Atlas of pulmonary surgical pathology.* Philadelphia: WB Saunders, 1991.

Colby TV, Koss MN, Travis WD: *Tumors of the lower respiratory tract.* Armed Forces Institute of Pathology Fascicle, Third series. Washington, DC: Armed Forces Institute of Pathology, 1995.

Dail DH, Hammar SP: *Pulmonary pathology.* New York: Springer-Verlag, 1994.

Fishman AP, Elias JA: *Pulmonary diseases and disorders.* New York: McGraw-Hill, Health Professions Division, 1998.

Katzenstein AL: *Surgical pathology of non-neoplastic lung disease.* Philadelphia: WB Saunders, 1997.

Murray JF, Nadel JA, Mason RJ, Boushey HA Jr: *Textbook of respiratory medicine.* Philadelphia: WB Saunders, 2000.

Pass HI, Mitchell JB, Johnson DH, et al. (eds): *Lung cancer: Principles and practice.* Philadelphia: Lippincott–Raven, 2000.

Roggli VL, Greenberg SD, Pratt PC: *Pathology of asbestos-associated diseases.* Boston: Little, Brown, 1992.

Schwartz MI, King TE (eds): *Interstitial lung disease.* Hamilton, BC: Decker, 1998.

Spencer H, Hasleton PS: *Spencer's pathology of the lung.* New York: McGraw-Hill, Health Professions Division, 1996.

Thurlbeck WM, Churg A: *Pathology of the lung.* New York: Thieme Medical Publishers, 1995.

Travis WD, Colby TV, Corrin B, et al. in collaboration with Sobin LH, and pathologists from 14 Countries. *Histological typing of lung and pleural tumors.* Berlin: Springer, 1999.

Travis WD, Colby TV, Koss MN, et al.: *Non-neoplastic disorders of the lower respiratory tract.* Washington, DC: American Registry of Pathology, 2002.

Review Articles

Statement on sarcoidosis. Joint Statement of the American Thoracic Society (ATS), the European Respiratory Society (ERS) and the World Association of Sarcoidosis and Other Granulomatous Disorders (WASOG) adopted by the ATS Board of Directors and by the ERS Executive Committee, February 1999. *Am J Respir Crit Care Med* 160(2):736–755, 1999.

Agostini C, Semenzato G: Immunology of idiopathic pulmonary fibrosis. *Curr Opin Pulm Med* 2:364–369, 1996.

Bjoraker JA, Ryu JH, Edwin MK, et al.: Prognostic significance of histopathologic subsets in idiopathic pulmonary fibrosis. *J Respir Crit Care Med* 157:199–203, 1998.

Busse WW, Lemanske RF: Review articles: Advances in immunology: Asthma. *N Engl J Med* 344:350–362, 2001.

Epler GR: Bronchiolitis obliterans organizing pneumonia. *Arch Intern Med* 161(2):158–164, 2001.

Evans MD, Pryor WA: Cigarette smoking, emphysema, and damage to alpha 1-proteinase inhibitor. *Am J Physiol* 266:493–611, 1994.

Guthrie R: Community-acquired lower respiratory tract infections: etiology and treatment. Chest 120:2021–2034, 2001.

King TE Jr, Costabel U, Cordier J-F, et al.: Idiopathic pulmonary fibrosis: Diagnosis and treatment. *Am J Respir Crit Care Med* 161:646–664, 2000.

Knight KR, Burdeon JG, Cook L, et al.: The proteinase-antiproteinase theory of emphysema: A speculative analysis of recent advances into the pathogenesis of emphysema. *Respirology* 2:91–95, 1997.

Katzenstein AL, Myers JL: Idiopathic pulmonary fibrosis: Clinical relevance of pathologic classification. *Am J Respir Crit Care Med* 157(4 Pt 1):1301–1315, 1998.

Lynch JP 3rd, Kazerooni EA, Gay SE: Pulmonary sarcoidosis. *Clin Chest Med* 18:755–785, 1997.

Martinez FJ: Diagnosing chronic obstructive pulmonary disease. The importance of differentiating asthma, emphysema, and chronic bronchitis. *Postgrad Med* 103(4):112–125, 1998.

Nicotra MB: Bronchiectasis. *Semin Respir Infect* 9:31–40, 1994.

Otto WR: Lung stem cells. *Int J Exp Pathol* 78:291–310, 1997.

Peak JK: The epidemiology of asthma: *Curr Opin Pulm Med* 2:7–15, 1996.

Ross JA, Rosen GD: The molecular biology of lung cancer. *Curr Opin Pulm Med* 8(4):265–269, 2002.

Salvaggio JE: Extrinsic allergic alveolitis (hypersensitivity pneumonitis): Past, present, and future. *Clin Exp Allergy* 27(suppl 1):18–25, 1997.

Schulger NW, Rom WN: The host immune response to tuberculosis. *Am J Respir Crit Care Med* 157:679–691, 1998.

Travis WD, King TE, Bateman ED, et al.: ATS/ERS International Multidisciplinary Consensus Classification of Idiopathic Interstitial Pneumonia. *Am J Respir Crit Care Med* 165:277–304, 2002.

CHAPTER 13

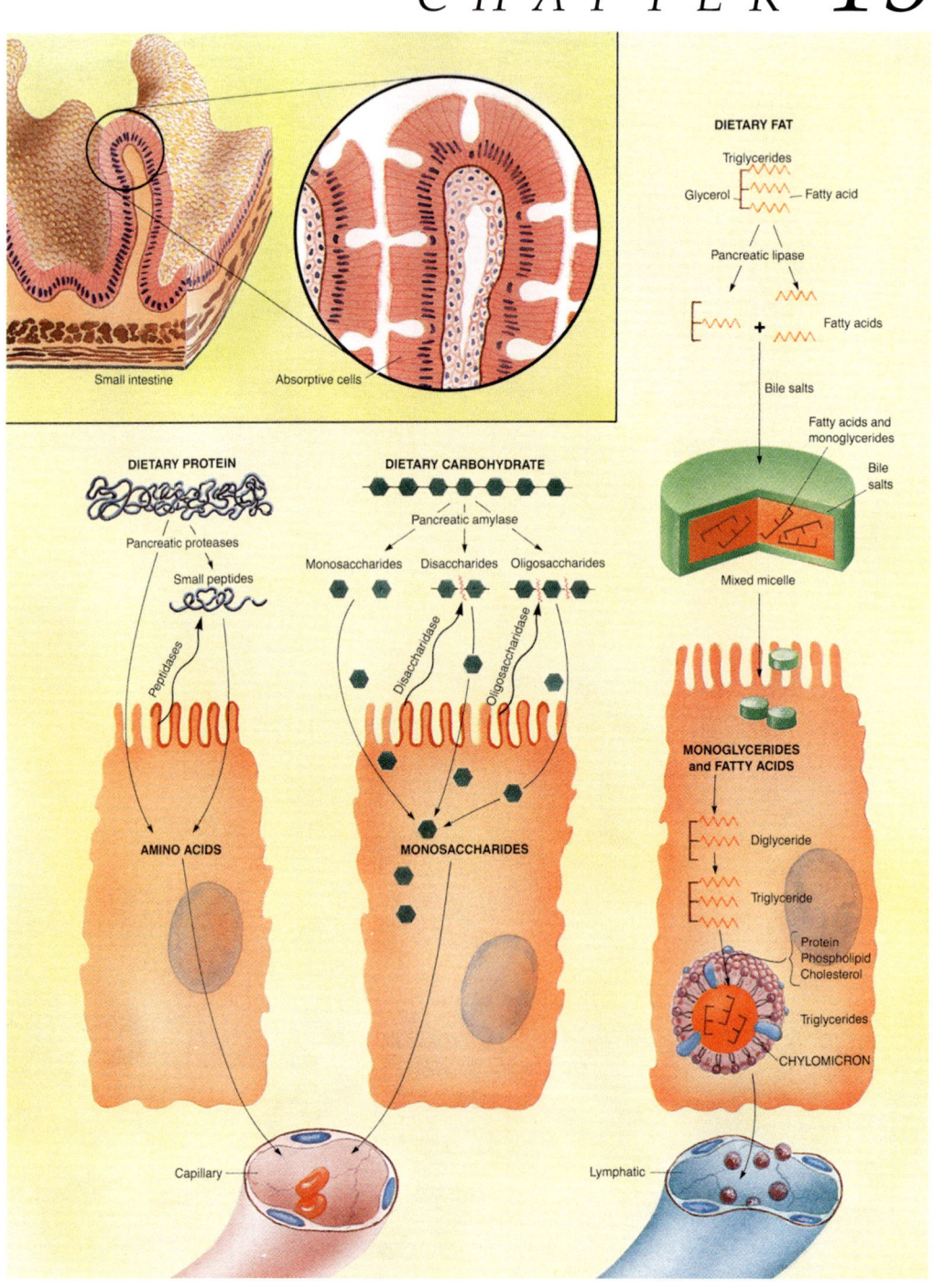

The Gastrointestinal Tract

Emanuel Rubin
Juan P. Palazzo

The Esophagus

Anatomy

Congenital Disorders

Tracheoesophageal Fistula

Rings and Webs

Esophageal Diverticula

Motor Disorders

Achalasia

Scleroderma

Hiatal Hernia

Esophagitis

Reflux Esophagitis

Barrett Esophagus

Infective Esophagitis

Esophagitis of Systemic Illness

Esophagitis Produced by Physical Agents

Esophageal Varices

Lacerations and Perforations

Neoplasms

The Stomach

Anatomy

Congenital Disorders

Pyloric Stenosis

Diaphragmatic Hernia

Rare Abnormalities

Gastritis

Acute Hemorrhagic Gastritis

Chronic Gastritis

Menetrier Disease

Peptic Ulcer Disease

Benign Neoplasms

Stromal Tumors

Epithelial Polyps

Malignant Tumors

Carcinoma of the Stomach

Carcinoid Tumors

Gastric Lymphoma

Gastrointestinal Stromal Tumor

Mechanical Disorders

Bezoars

(continued)

FIGURE 13-1 *(see opposite page)*
Mechanisms of nutrient absorption in the small intestine.

The Small Intestine

Anatomy

Congenital Disorders
Atresia and Stenosis
Duplications
Meckel Diverticulum
Malrotation
Meconium Ileus

Infections
Bacterial Diarrhea
Viral Gastroenteritis
Intestinal Tuberculosis
Intestinal Fungi
Parasites

Vascular Diseases
Acute Intestinal Ischemia
Chronic Intestinal Ischemia

Crohn Disease

Malabsorption
Luminal-Phase Malabsorption
Intestinal-Phase Malabsorption
Laboratory Evaluation
Lactase Deficiency
Celiac Disease
Whipple Disease
Hypogammaglobulinemia
Congenital Lymphangiectasia
Tropical Sprue

Neoplasms
Benign Tumors
Malignant Tumors

Pneumatosis Cystoides Intestinalis

The Large Intestine

Anatomy

Congenital Disorders
Congenital Megacolon (Hirschsprung Disease)
Acquired Megacolon
Anorectal Malformations

Infections
Pseudomembranous Colitis
Neonatal Necrotizing Enterocolitis

Diverticular Disease
Diverticulosis
Diverticulitis

Idiopathic Inflammatory Bowel Disease
Crohn Disease
Ulcerative Colitis
Collagenous Colitis and Lymphocytic Colitis

Vascular Diseases
Ischemic Colitis
Angiodysplasia (Vascular Ectasia)
Hemorrhoids

Radiation Enterocolitis

Solitary Rectal Ulcer Syndrome

Polyps of the Colorectum
Adenomatous Polyps
Serrated Adenoma
Familial Adenomatous Polyposis
Nonneoplastic Polyps

Malignant Tumors
Adenocarcinoma of the Colon and Rectum
Carcinoid Tumors (Neuroendocrine Tumors)
Large Bowel Lymphoma
Cancers of the Anal Canal

Miscellaneous Disorders

Endometriosis

Melanosis Coli

Stercoral Ulcers

The Appendix

Anatomy

Appendicitis

Mucocele

Neoplasms

The Peritoneum

Peritonitis

Bacterial Peritonitis

Chemical Peritonitis

Familial Paroxysmal Polyserositis (Familial Mediterranean Fever)

Retroperitoneal Fibrosis

Neoplasms

The Esophagus

ANATOMY

Embryologically, the gut and the respiratory tract arise from the same anlage and constitute a single tube. This structure divides into two separate tubes, the esophagus being dorsal and the future respiratory tract, ventral. Initially, columnar epithelium lines the esophagus in its early embryonic development, but it is replaced by a stratified squamous epithelium.

The adult esophagus is a 25-cm tube that serves as a conduit for the passage of food and liquid into the stomach. It contains both striated and smooth muscle in its upper portion and smooth muscle alone in its lower portion. The organ is fixed superiorly at the cricopharyngeus muscle, which is considered the upper esophageal sphincter. It courses inferiorly through the posterior mediastinum behind the trachea and the heart and exits the thorax through the hiatus of the diaphragm. Tonic muscular contraction at the lower end of the esophagus creates an action similar to that of a one-way flutter valve. The so-called *lower esophageal sphincter* is not a true anatomical sphincter but rather a functional one.

The esophagus has a mucosa, submucosa, muscularis propria, and adventitia. The transition from the squamous mucosa of the esophagus to the gastric mucosa at the esophagogastric junction occurs abruptly at the level of the diaphragm. The esophageal submucosa contains mucous glands and a rich lymphatic plexus. The lymphatics of the upper third of the esophagus drain to the cervical lymph nodes, those of the middle third to the mediastinal nodes, and those of the lower third to the celiac and gastric lymph nodes. These anatomical features are significant in the spread of esophageal cancer.

The venous drainage of the esophagus is important in portal hypertension, in which esophageal varices occur. These varices are invariably found in the lower third of the esophagus, because the veins of the upper third drain into the superior vena cava, and those of the middle third drain into the azygous system. Only the veins of the lower third of the esophagus drain into the portal vein by way of the gastric veins.

CONGENITAL DISORDERS

Tracheoesophageal Fistula Leads to Aspiration Pneumonia

The most common esophageal anomaly is tracheoesophageal fistula (Fig. 13-2). It is frequently combined with some form of **esophageal atresia.** In some cases, it has been associated with a complex of anomalies identified by the acronym Vater syndrome (*v*ertebral defects, *a*nal atresia, *tr*acheo*e*sophageal fistula, and *r*enal dysplasia). Maternal hydramnios has been recorded in some cases of esophageal atresia and, less commonly, in cases of tracheoesophageal fistula. Esophageal atresia and fistulas are often associated with congenital heart disease.

Pathology: In 90% of tracheoesophageal fistulas, the upper portion of the esophagus ends in a blind pouch, and the superior end of the lower segment communicates with the trachea. **In this type of atresia, the upper blind sac soon fills with mucus, which the infant then aspirates.** Surgical correction is feasible albeit difficult.

Among the remaining 10% of cases, the most common fistula involves a communication between the proximal esophagus and the trachea; the lower esophageal pouch

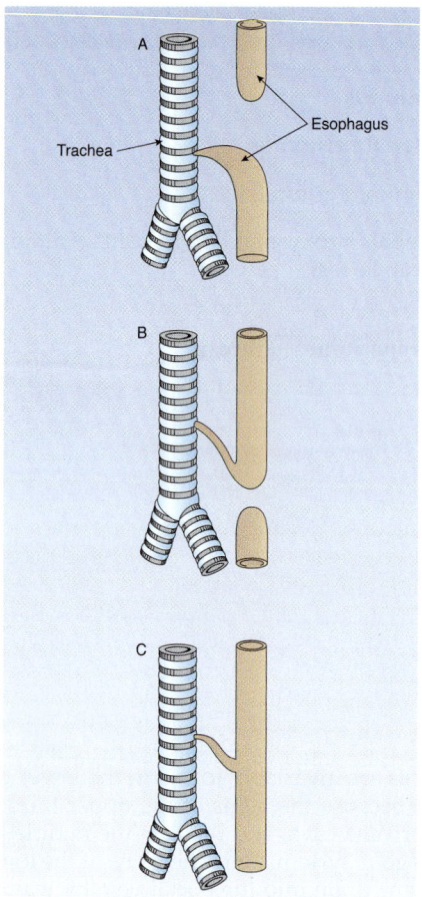

FIGURE 13-2
Congenital tracheoesophageal fistulas. *(A)* The most common type is a communication between the trachea and the lower portion of the esophagus. The upper segment of the esophagus ends in a blind sac. *(B)* In a few cases, the proximal esophagus communicates with the trachea. *(C)* The least common anomaly, the H type, is a fistula between a continuous esophagus and the trachea.

communicates with the stomach. **Infants with this condition develop aspiration immediately after birth.** In another variant, termed an *H-type fistula*, a communication exists between an intact esophagus and an intact trachea. In some cases, the lesion becomes symptomatic only in adulthood, when repeated pulmonary infections call attention to it.

CONGENITAL ESOPHAGEAL STENOSIS: This condition is surprisingly resistant to mechanical dilation. In some instances, pulmonary tissue is found in the stenotic region.

BRONCHOPULMONARY FOREGUT MALFORMATION: This uncommon tracheoesophageal developmental anomaly consists of a mass of abnormal pulmonary tissue within the lung. Such tissue is invested by its own separate pleural lining and communicates with the lower esophagus. Passage of esophageal contents into the lung leads to repeated pulmonary infections or an enlarging mediastinal mass.

Rings and Webs Cause Dysphagia

ESOPHAGEAL WEBS: Occasionally, a thin mucosal membrane projects into the lumen of the esophagus. Usually single, the webs are sometimes multiple and can be found anywhere in the esophagus. Esophageal webs are often successfully treated by dilation with large rubber bougies; occasionally, they can be excised with biopsy forceps during endoscopy.

PLUMMER-VINSON (PATERSON-KELLY) SYNDROME: This disorder is characterized by *(1) a cervical esophageal web, (2) mucosal lesions of the mouth and pharynx, and (3) iron-deficiency anemia.* Dysphagia, often associated with aspiration of swallowed food, is the most common clinical manifestation. Ninety percent of cases occur in women. **Carcinoma of the oropharynx and upper esophagus is a recognized complication of the Plummer-Vinson syndrome.**

SCHATZKI RING: This lower esophageal narrowing is usually seen at the gastroesophageal junction (Fig. 13-3). The upper surface of the mucosal ring exhibits stratified squamous epithelium; the lower is lined by columnar epithelium. Although it has been noted in as many as 14% of barium meal examinations, Schatzki ring is usually asymptomatic. Patients with narrow Schatzki rings however, may complain of intermittent dysphagia.

Esophageal Diverticula Often Reflect Motor Dysfunction

A *true* esophageal diverticulum is an outpouching of the wall that contains all layers of the esophagus. When the sac lacks a muscular layer, it is known as a *false* diverticulum. Esophageal diverticula occur in the hypopharyngeal area above the upper esophageal sphincter, in the middle esophagus, and immediately proximal to the lower esophageal sphincter.

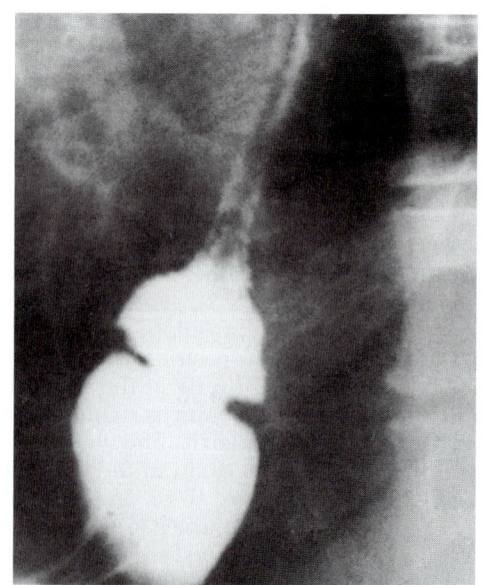

FIGURE 13-3
Schatzki mucosal ring. A contrast radiograph illustrates the lower esophageal narrowing.

ZENKER DIVERTICULUM: *Zenker diverticulum is an uncommon lesion that appears high in the esophagus and affects men more than women.* It was once believed to result from luminal pressure exerted in a structurally weak area and was therefore classed as a *pulsion diverticulum*. The cause is probably more complicated, but disordered function of the cricopharyngeal musculature is still generally thought to be involved in the pathogenesis of this false diverticulum. Most affected persons who come to medical attention are older than 60 years, an observation that supports the belief that this diverticulum is acquired.

Zenker diverticula can enlarge conspicuously and accumulate a large amount of food. The typical symptom is regurgitation of food eaten some time previously (occasionally days), in the absence of dysphagia. Recurrent aspiration pneumonia may be a serious complication. When symptoms are severe, surgical intervention is the rule.

TRACTION DIVERTICULA: *Traction diverticula are outpouchings that occur principally in the midportion of the esophagus.* They were so named because of their attachment to adjacent mediastinal lymph nodes, usually associated with tuberculous lymphadenitis. However, such adhesions are today uncommon, and it is believed that these pouches often reflect a disturbance in the motor function of the esophagus. A diverticulum in the midesophagus ordinarily has a wide stoma, and the pouch is usually higher than its orifice. Thus, it does not retain food or secretions and remains asymptomatic, with only rare complications.

EPIPHRENIC DIVERTICULA: *These diverticula are located immediately above the diaphragm.* Motor disturbances of the esophagus (e.g., achalasia, diffuse esophageal spasm) are found in two thirds of patients with this true diverticulum. In addition, reflux esophagitis may play a role in the pathogenesis of epiphrenic diverticula.

Unlike other diverticula, epiphrenic diverticula are encountered in young persons. Nocturnal regurgitation of large amounts of fluid stored in the diverticulum during the day is typical. When symptoms are severe, surgical intervention directed toward correcting the motor abnormality (e.g., myotomy) is appropriate.

INTRAMURAL PSEUDODIVERTICULOSIS: *This rare disorder is characterized by numerous small (1- to 3-mm) diverticula in the wall of the esophagus.* The lesions are not true diverticula but rather dilated ducts of the submucosal glands. The principal symptom is dysphagia.

MOTOR DISORDERS

The automatic coordination of muscular movement during swallowing is termed a *motor function* and results in the free passage of food through the esophagus. The hallmark of motor disorders is difficulty in swallowing, termed *dysphagia*. Dysphagia is often manifested by an awareness of the lack of progression of a bolus of food and in itself is not painful. Pain on swallowing is called *odynophagia*. Motor disorders can be caused by the following:

- **Dysfunction of striated muscle** in the upper esophagus
- **Systemic diseases of skeletal muscle** such as myasthenia gravis, dermatomyositis, amyloidosis, hyperthyroidism, and myxedema
- **Neurological diseases** that affect nerves to skeletal muscle (e.g., cerebrovascular accidents, amyotrophic lateral sclerosis)
- **Peripheral neuropathy** associated with diabetes or alcoholism

Achalasia Features Impaired Function of the Lower Esophageal Sphincter

Achalasia, at one time termed cardiospasm, *is characterized by failure of the lower esophageal sphincter to relax in response to swallowing and the absence of peristalsis in the body of the esophagus.* As a result of these defects in both the outflow tract and the pumping mechanisms of the esophagus, food is retained within the esophagus, and the organ hypertrophies and dilates conspicuously (Fig. 13-4).

Achalasia is associated with a loss or absence of ganglion cells in the myenteric plexus of the esophagus. Degenerative changes in the dorsal motor nucleus of the vagus and the extraesophageal vagus nerves have also been described. The loss of ganglion cells is occasionally accompanied by chronic inflammation. In Latin America, achalasia is a common complication of **Chagas disease**, in which the ganglion cells are destroyed by *Trypanosoma cruzi*.

Dysphagia, occasionally odynophagia, and regurgitation of material retained in the esophagus are common symptoms of achalasia. Squamous carcinoma is also a complication. Treatment is by dilation or surgical myotomy, which can lead to gastroesophageal reflux.

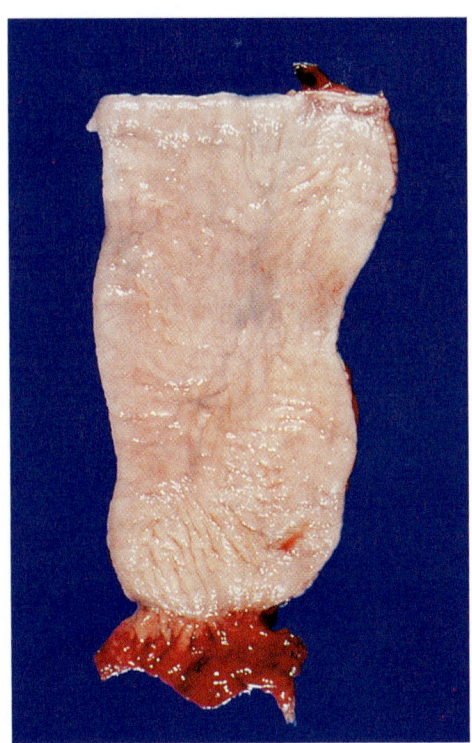

FIGURE *13-4*
Esophagus and upper stomach of a patient with advanced achalasia. The esophagus is markedly dilated above the esophagogastric junction, where the lower esophageal sphincter is located. The esophageal mucosa is redundant and has hyperplastic squamous epithelium.

666   The Gastrointestinal Tract

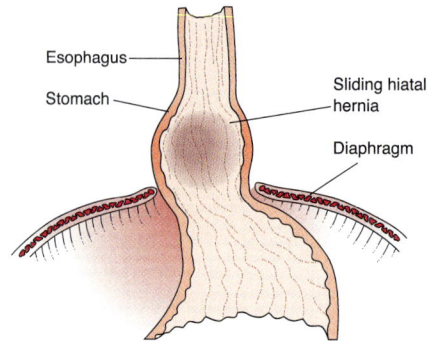
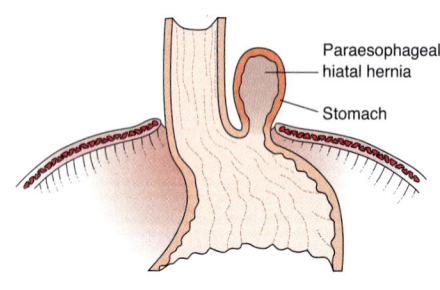
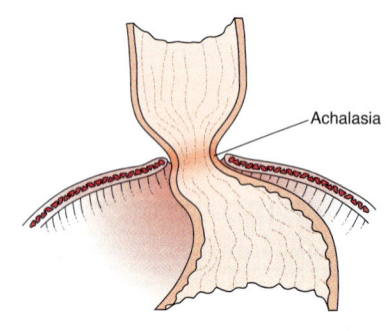
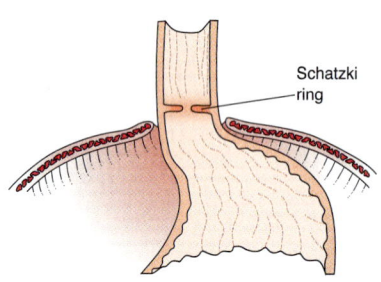

FIGURE 13-5
Disorders of the esophageal outlet.

Microscopically, fibrosis of the esophageal smooth muscle (especially the inner layer of the muscularis propria) and nonspecific inflammatory changes are seen. Intimal fibrosis of the small arteries and arterioles is common and may play a role in the pathogenesis of the fibrosis. Clinically, patients have dysphagia and heartburn caused by peptic esophagitis, owing to reflux of acid from the stomach.

HIATAL HERNIA

Hiatal hernia is a herniation of the stomach through an enlarged esophageal hiatus in the diaphragm. Two basic types of hiatal hernia are observed (Fig. 13-5).

SLIDING HERNIA: *An enlargement of the diaphragmatic hiatus and laxity of the circumferential connective tissue allows a cap of gastric mucosa to move upward to a position above the diaphragm.* This condition is common. Sliding hiatal hernia is asymptomatic in most patients, and only 5% of patients diagnosed radiologically complain of symptoms referable to gastroesophageal reflux.

PARAESOPHAGEAL HERNIA: *This form of hiatal hernia is characterized by herniation of a portion of the gastric fundus alongside the esophagus through a defect in the diaphragmatic connective tissue membrane that defines the esophageal hiatus.* The hernia progressively enlarges, and the hiatus grows increasingly wide. In extreme cases, most of the stomach herniates into the thorax.

 Clinical Features: Symptoms of hiatal hernia, particularly heartburn and regurgitation, are attributed to gastroesophageal reflux of gastric contents, which is primarily related to incompetence of the lower esophageal sphincter. Classically, the symptoms are exacerbated when the affected person is recumbent, which facilitates acid reflux. Dysphagia, painful swallowing, and occasionally bleeding may also be troublesome. Large herniations carry a risk of gastric volvulus or intrathoracic gastric dilation.

Sliding hiatal hernias generally do not require surgical repair; symptoms are often treated medically. By contrast, an enlarging paraesophageal hernia should be surgically treated, even in the absence of symptoms.

Scleroderma Causes Fibrosis of the Esophageal Wall

Scleroderma (progressive systemic sclerosis) causes fibrosis in many organs and produces a severe abnormality of esophageal muscle function. The disease affects principally the lower esophageal sphincter, which may become so impaired that the lower esophagus and upper stomach are no longer distinct functional entities and are visualized as a common cavity. In addition, there may be a lack of peristalsis in the entire esophagus.

ESOPHAGITIS

Reflux Esophagitis Is Caused by Regurgitation of Gastric Contents

By far the most common type of esophagitis, reflux esophagitis is often found in conjunction with a sliding hiatal hernia, although it may occur through an incompetent lower esophageal sphincter without any demonstrable anatomical lesion.

Esophagitis

 Pathogenesis: The principal barrier to the reflux of gastric contents into the esophagus is the lower esophageal sphincter. Transient reflux is a normal event, particularly after a meal. When these episodes become more frequent and are prolonged, esophagitis results. Agents that cause a decrease in the pressure of the lower esophageal sphincter (e.g., alcohol, chocolate, fatty foods, cigarette smoking) are also associated with reflux. Certain central nervous system depressants (e.g., morphine, diazepam), pregnancy, estrogen therapy, and the presence of a nasogastric tube may lead to reflux esophagitis. Although acid is damaging to the esophageal mucosa, the combination of acid and pepsin may be particularly injurious. Moreover, gastric fluid often contains refluxed bile from the duodenum, which is harmful to the esophageal mucosa. Alcohol, hot beverages, and spicy foods also may damage the mucosa directly.

Pathology: The earliest grossly evident alteration produced by gastroesophageal reflux is hyperemia. When reflux is chronic, reactive thickening of the squamous epithelium, traditionally termed *leukoplakia*, is occasionally seen as irregular grayish white patches. Areas affected by reflux are susceptible to superficial mucosal erosions and ulcers, which often appear as vertical linear streaks. Microscopically, mild injury to the squamous epithelium is manifested by balloon cells (enlarged cells with clear cytoplasm due to intracellular edema and influx of plasma proteins). The basal region of the epithelium is thickened, and the papillae of the lamina propria are elongated and extend toward the surface because of reactive proliferation. Capillary vessels within the papillae are often dilated. An increase in lymphocytes is seen in the squamous epithelium, and eosinophils and neutrophils may be present.

Esophageal stricture may eventuate in those patients in whom the ulcer persists and damages the esophageal wall deep to the lamina propria. In this circumstance, reactive fibrosis can narrow the esophageal lumen. Such a stricture is usually sharply localized and situated near the lower esophageal sphincter, although it may extend considerably higher. If an esophageal stricture seriously interferes with the passage of food, the esophagus becomes dilated above the narrowing. The most common clinical complaint is progressive dysphagia.

Barrett Esophagus Is a Precancerous Lesion

Barrett epithelium is defined as replacement of the squamous epithelium of the esophagus by columnar epithelium as a result of chronic gastroesophageal reflux. The incidence of Barrett esophagus has been increasing in recent years, particularly among white men. This disorder occurs in the lower third of the esophagus but may extend higher.

There is a slight male predominance and a more than twofold increased risk for Barrett esophagus among smokers. Patients with Barrett esophagus are placed in a regular surveillance program to detect early microscopic evidence of dysplastic mucosa.

 Pathology: The metaplastic Barrett epithelium may partially involve the circumference of short segments or may line the entire lower esophagus (Fig. 13-6A). Histologically, the lesion is characterized by a distinctive intestine-like epithelium composed of goblet cells and surface cells similar to those of incompletely intestinalized gastric mucosa (see Fig. 13-6B). Complete intestinal metaplasia, with Paneth cells and absorptive cells, occurs occasionally in Barrett epithelium. Inflammatory changes are usually superimposed on the epithelial alterations. **Barrett esophagus carries a serious risk of malignant transformation to adenocarcinoma,** and the risk correlates with the length of the involved esophagus and the degree of dysplasia (see below).1

Infective Esophagitis Is Associated with Immunosuppression

CANDIDA ESOPHAGITIS: This fungal infection has become commonplace because of an increasing number of immunocompromised persons who (1) receive chemotherapy for malignant disease, (2) are treated with immunosuppressive drugs after organ transplantation, or (3) have contracted AIDS. Esophageal candidiasis also occurs in patients with diabetes, those receiving antibiotic therapy, and uncommonly in persons with no known predisposing factors. Dysphagia and severe pain on swallowing are usual.

 Pathology: In mild cases of candidiasis, a few small, elevated white plaques surrounded by a hyperemic zone are present on the mucosa of the middle or lower third of the esophagus. In severe cases, confluent pseudomembranes lie on a hyperemic and edematous mucosa. Microscopically, *Candida* sometimes involves only the superficial layers of the squamous epithelium. The candidal pseudomembrane contains fungal mycelia, necrotic debris, and fibrin. Involvement of the deeper layers of the esophageal wall can lead to disseminated candidiasis or fibrosis, sometimes severe enough to create a stricture.

HERPETIC ESOPHAGITIS: Esophageal infection with herpesvirus type I is most frequently associated with lymphomas and leukemias and is often manifested by odynophagia.

 Pathology: The well-developed lesions of herpetic esophagitis are grossly similar to those of candidiasis. In early cases, vesicles, small erosions, or plaques are noted; as the infection progresses, these may coalesce to form larger lesions. Microscopically, the lesions are superficial, and the epithelial cells exhibit typical herpetic in-

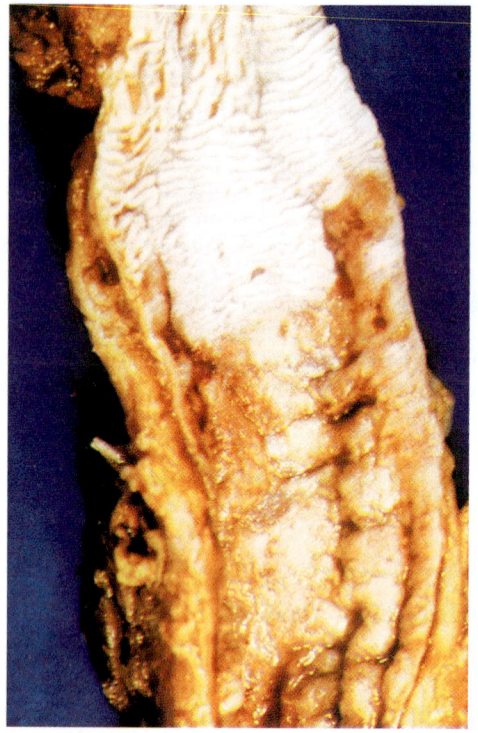
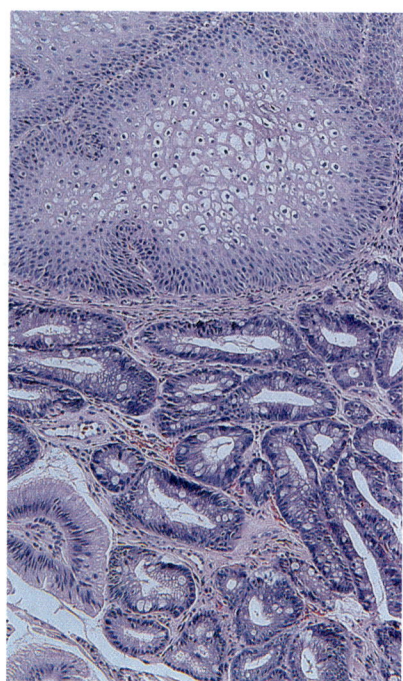

FIGURE 13-6
Barrett esophagus. A. The white squamous mucosa of the proximal esophagus (*top*) is contrasted with the columnar lining of the distal Barrett esophagus (*bottom*). B. Gastroesophageal junction showing metaplastic mucosa with numerous goblet cells.

clusions in their nuclei (Fig. 13-7). Multinucleated epithelial cells are occasionally encountered, but stromal cells are spared. Necrosis of infected cells leads to ulceration, and candidal and bacterial superinfection results in the formation of pseudomembranes.

CYTOMEGALOVIRUS ESOPHAGITIS: Esophageal involvement with cytomegalovirus usually reflects systemic viral disease in patients with AIDS. Ulceration of the mucosa, similar to that seen in herpetic esophagitis, is common. Characteristic inclusion bodies of cytomegalovirus are present in the endothelial cells and fibroblasts of the granulation tissue, but the epithelium is spared.

Chemical Esophagitis Results from the Ingestion of Corrosive Agents

Chemical injury to the esophagus usually reflects accidental poisoning in children, attempted suicide in adults, or contact with medication. Ingestion of strong alkaline agents (e.g., lye) or strong acids (e.g., sulfuric or hydrochloric acid), both of which are used in various cleaning solutions, can produce chemical esophagitis. The alkaline solutions are particularly insidious, because they are generally odorless and tasteless and therefore easily swallowed before protective reflexes come into play.

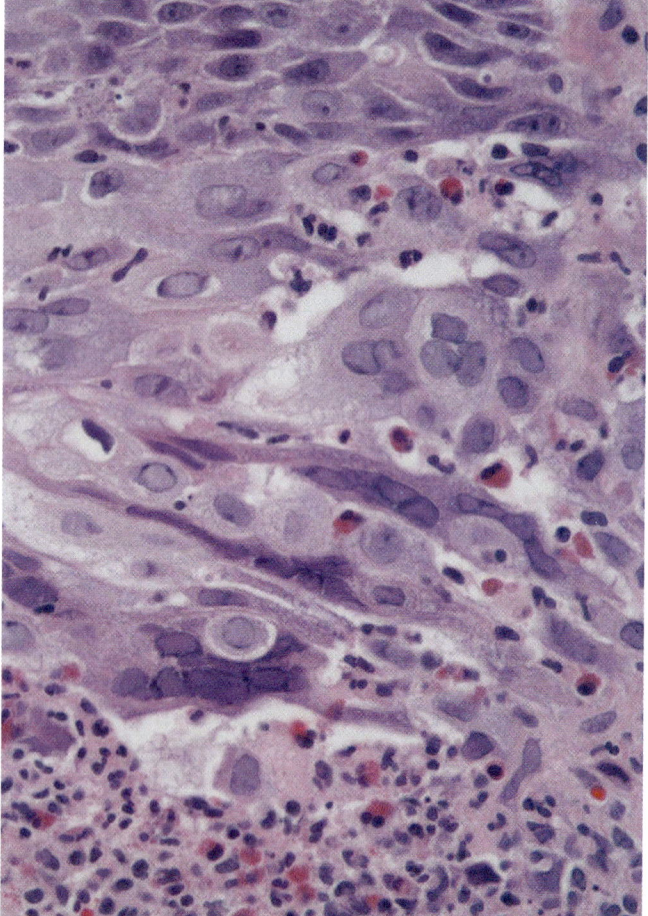

FIGURE 13-7
Herpetic esophagitis. Multinucleated giant cells with nuclear inclusions are seen in the squamous mucosa.

Pathology: Histologically, alkali-induced liquefactive necrosis is accompanied by conspicuous inflammation and saponification of the membrane lipids in the epithelium, submucosa, and muscularis propria of the esophagus and stomach. Thrombosis of small vessels adds ischemic necrosis to the injury. Severe injury is the rule with liquid alkali, but less than 25% of those who ingest granular preparations have severe complications.

Strong acids produce immediate coagulation necrosis, which results in a protective eschar that limits injury and penetration. Nevertheless, half of patients who ingest concentrated hydrochloric or sulfuric acid have severe esophageal injury.

Drug-related esophagitis is most often caused by direct chemical effects on the squamous-lined mucosa, especially with capsules; esophageal dysmotility and cardiac enlargement (which impinges on the esophagus) may be contributing factors. Allergic reactions to drugs may cause esophagitis reflected by an increased number of eosinophils in the esophageal mucosa.

Esophagitis May Complicate Systemic Illnesses

The squamous mucosa of the esophagus is similar to that of the skin and shares some reactions with that organ.

The dystrophic form of epidermolysis bullosa involves all organs that are lined by, or derived from, squamous epithelium, including the skin, nails, teeth, and esophagus. The bullae, which occur episodically, evolve from fluid-filled vesicles to weeping ulcers. Dysphagia and painful swallowing are the rule. Severe cases result in stricture, usually in the upper esophagus.

Pemphigoid produces subepithelial bullae in the skin and esophagus, but the disease does not lead to scarring. Other dermatological disorders associated with esophagitis include pemphigus, dermatitis herpetiformis, Behçet syndrome, and erythema multiforme.

Graft-versus-host disease in recipients of bone marrow transplants can cause esophageal lesions and dysphagia, odynophagia, and gastroesophageal reflux. The upper and middle thirds of the esophageal mucosa appear friable, and motor function of the esophagus is impaired.

Esophagitis Is Produced by Physical Agents

External irradiation for the treatment of thoracic cancers may include portions of the esophagus and lead to esophagitis and even stricture. **Nasogastric tubes** produce pressure ulcers of the esophageal mucosa in patients who have them in place for prolonged periods, although acid reflux also plays a role in these cases.

ESOPHAGEAL VARICES

Esophageal varices are dilated veins immediately beneath the mucosa (Fig. 13-8) *that are prone to rupture and hemorrhage* (see Chapter 14). They arise in the lower third of the esophagus, virtually always in the setting of portal hypertension resulting from cirrhosis of the liver. The lower esophageal veins are linked to the portal system through gastroesophageal anastomoses. If the portal pressure exceeds a critical level, these anastomoses become prominent in the upper stomach and lower esophagus. When the varices are greater than 5 mm in diameter, they are likely to rupture, in which case, life-threatening hemorrhage ensues. Reflux injury or infective esophagitis can contribute to variceal bleeding.

LACERATIONS AND PERFORATIONS

Lacerations of the esophagus result from external trauma, such as automobile accidents and falls from great heights, and from medical instrumentation. However, the most common cause is severe vomiting, during which the intra-

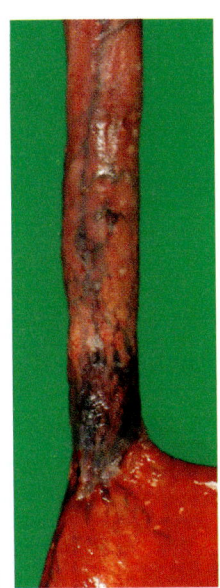
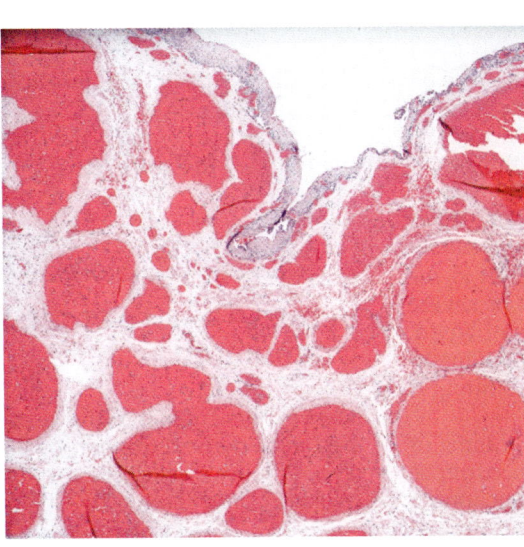

FIGURE 13-8
Esophageal varices. A. Numerous prominent blue venous channels are seen beneath the mucosa of the everted esophagus, particularly above the gastroesophageal junction. **B.** Section of the esophagus reveals numerous dilated submucosal veins.

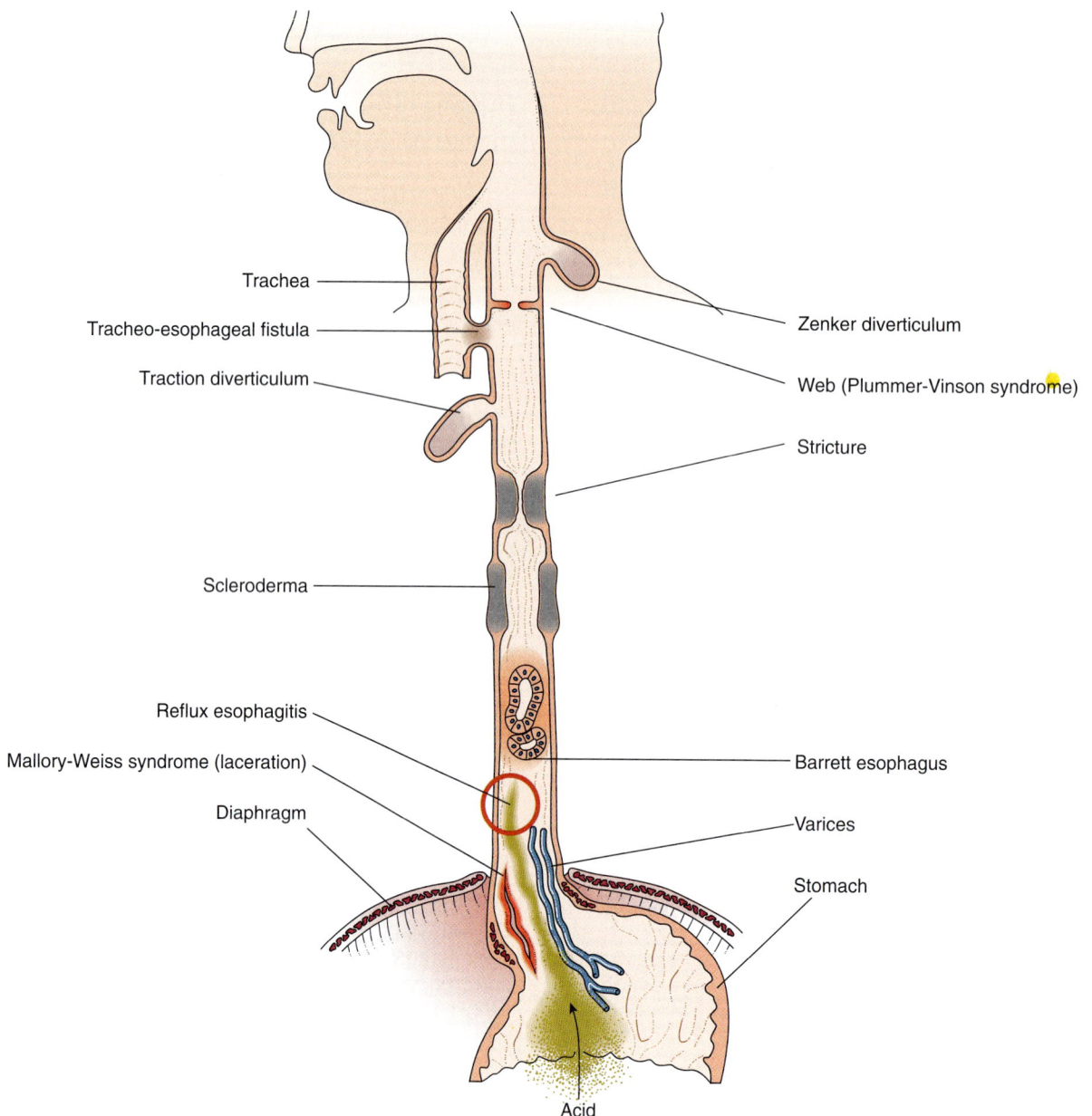

FIGURE 13-9
Nonneoplastic disorders of the esophagus.

esophageal pressure may rise as high as 300 mm Hg. The diaphragm descends rapidly, and a portion of the upper stomach is forced up through the hiatus. As a result, forceful retching may cause mucosal tears, beginning in the gastric epithelium and extending into the esophagus.

Mallory-Weiss syndrome refers to severe retching, often associated with alcoholism, that leads to mucosal lacerations of the upper stomach and lower esophagus. These tears result in the vomiting of bright red blood, and bleeding may be severe enough to require the transfusion of many units of blood. The lacerations may also cause perforation into the mediastinum. Rupture of the esophagus as a result of vomiting is known as *Boerhaave syndrome*.

Perforation of the esophagus, whether from trauma or vomiting, can be catastrophic. It is a well-known occurrence in newborns, in whom it is caused occasionally by suctioning or feeding with a nasogastric tube. However, it may also occur spontaneously.

The major nonneoplastic disorders of the esophagus are summarized in Figure 13-9.

NEOPLASMS

Benign Tumors of the Esophagus are Uncommon

Most benign tumors of the gastrointestinal tract are considered to be derived from either the pacemaker cell of Cajal or smooth muscle cells. The former are referred to as *gastrointestinal stromal tumors,* or GIST, and most of them express

CD117 (c-*kit* gene). A higher percentage of benign tumors of the esophagus display smooth muscle markers and are considered leiomyomas. Macroscopically, the normal mucosa is elevated over an intramural mass, which on microscopic examination is composed of spindle cells.

Carcinoma of the Esophagus Varies Geographically and Histologically

Epidemiology: Most cancers of the esophagus worldwide are squamous cell carcinomas (Fig. 13-10) but adenocarcinoma is now more common in the United States (see below). The incidence of this tumor in the United States is low, however, and esophageal cancer accounts for only about 2% of all cancer deaths.

Worldwide geographical variations in the incidence of carcinoma of the esophagus are striking, and areas of high incidence are located adjacent to areas of low incidence. There is an esophageal cancer belt extending across Asia from the Caspian Sea region of northern Iran and the former Soviet Union through Central Asia and Mongolia to northern China. In parts of China, the mortality rate from esophageal cancer in men is reported to be some 70 times that in the United States. American blacks have a considerably higher incidence than do whites, and in the United States, urban dwellers are at greater risk than those in rural areas. Cancer of the esophagus is also common in certain regions of France, Finland, Switzerland, Chile, Japan, India, and Africa.

Pathogenesis: The geographical variations in esophageal cancer, even in relatively homogeneous populations, suggest that environmental factors contribute strongly to the development of this disease. However, no single factor has been incriminated as the cause of esophageal cancer.

- **Excessive consumption of alcohol** is a major risk factor in the United States, even when cigarette smoking is taken into account.
- **Cigarette smoking** is associated with a 5- to 10-fold increased risk of esophageal cancer, and the number of cigarettes smoked correlates with the presence of dysplasia in the esophageal epithelium.
- **Nitrosamines** and aniline dyes produce esophageal cancer in animals. Although high levels of nitrosamines and other potentially carcinogenic compounds have been found in the diets of persons living in high-incidence areas, direct evidence for their contribution to esophageal cancer is lacking. Moreover, such chemical agents have not been detected in many high-risk areas, such as northern Iran.
- **Diets lacking in fresh fruits, vegetables, animal protein, and trace metals** have been described in areas with endemic esophageal cancer, and in some hyperendemic areas, deficiencies of various vitamins and minerals have

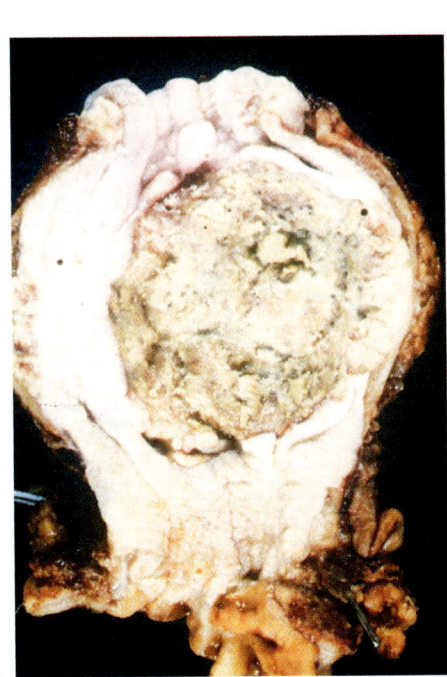
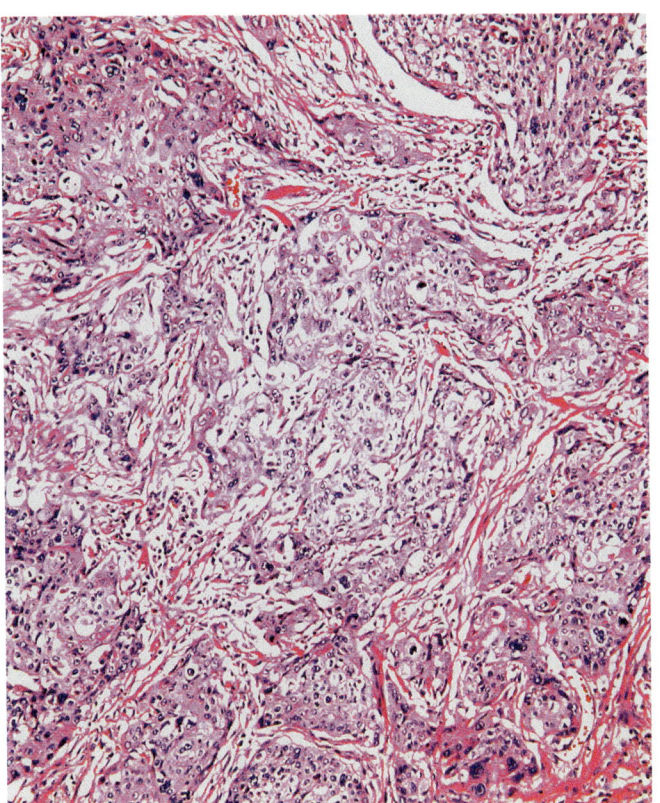

FIGURE 13-10
A. Carcinoma of the esophagus. A large, fungating, ulcerated squamous carcinoma of the esophagus is surrounded by apparently normal mucosa. **B.** Invasive carcinoma with keratin formation infiltrating the wall of the esophagus.

been claimed. However, the close proximity of endemic and nonendemic areas renders a causative role for these dietary factors unlikely.

- **Plummer-Vinson syndrome, celiac sprue, and achalasia** are associated with an increased incidence of esophageal cancer, but the cause for this risk has not been explained.
- **Chronic esophagitis** has been related to esophageal cancer in areas in which this tumor is endemic.
- **Chemical injury with esophageal stricture** is a risk factor. Five percent of persons who have an esophageal stricture after ingestion of lye develop cancer 20 to 40 years later.
- **Webs, rings, and diverticula** are sometimes associated with esophageal cancer.

 Pathology: About half the cases of esophageal cancer involve the lower third of the esophagus; the middle and upper thirds account for the remainder. Grossly, the tumors are of three types: (1) polypoid, which projects into the lumen (see Fig. 13-10); (2) ulcerating, which is usually smaller than polypoid; and (3) infiltrating, in which the principal plane of growth is in the wall. The bulky polypoid tumors tend to obstruct early, whereas the ulcerated ones are more likely to bleed. The infiltrating tumors gradually narrow the lumen by circumferential compression. Local extension of the tumor into adjoining mediastinal structures is commonly a major problem.

Microscopically, in squamous carcinoma the neoplastic squamous cells range from well differentiated, with epithelial "pearls" (see Fig. 13-10), to poorly differentiated tumors that lack evidence of squamous differentiation. Occasional tumors have a predominant spindle cell population of tumors cells (metaplastic carcinoma).

The rich lymphatic drainage of the esophagus provides a route for most metastases. Accordingly, tumors of the upper third metastasize to the cervical, internal jugular, and supraclavicular nodes. Cancer of the middle third metastasizes to the paratracheal and hilar lymph nodes and to nodes in the aortic, cardiac, and paraesophageal regions. Because the lower third of the esophagus is fed by the left gastric artery, which is accomplished by lymphatics, tumors in this portion of the esophagus spread to retroperitoneal, celiac, and left gastric nodes. Visceral metastases to the liver and lung are common, and almost any organ may be involved.

 Clinical Features: The most common presenting complaint is dysphagia, but by this time most tumors are unresectable. Patients with esophageal cancer are almost invariably cachectic, owing to anorexia, difficulty in swallowing, and the remote effects of a malignant tumor. Odynophagia occurs in half of patients, and persistent pain suggests mediastinal extension of the tumor or involvement of spinal nerves. Compression of the recurrent laryngeal nerve produces hoarseness, and tracheoesophageal fistula is manifested clinically by a chronic cough.

Surgery and radiation therapy are useful for palliation, but the prognosis remains dismal. Many patients are inoperable, and of those who undergo surgery, only 20% survive for 5 years.

Adenocarcinoma of the Esophagus

Adenocarcinoma of the esophagus is now more common (60%) in the United States than is squamous carcinoma, because the incidence has increased in recent years. **Virtually all adenocarcinomas arise in the background of Barrett esophagus,** although a rare case originates in submucosal mucous glands of the esophagus. The symptoms and clinical course of adenocarcinoma of the esophagus are similar to those of squamous cell carcinoma.

The Stomach

ANATOMY

The stomach, a J-shaped saccular organ with a volume of 1200 to 1500 mL, arises as a dilation of the primitive foregut. It is continuous with the esophagus superiorly and the duodenum inferiorly. Situated in the upper abdomen, the stomach extends from the left hypochondrium across the epigastrium. The convexity of the stomach, extending leftward from the gastroesophageal junction, is termed the **greater curvature**. The concavity of the right side of the stomach, called the **lesser curvature,** is only about one fourth as long as the greater curvature. The entire stomach is invested in peritoneum, which descends from the greater curvature as the **greater omentum**.

The interior of the stomach has been divided into five regions, from superior to inferior (Fig. 13-11):

1. The **cardia** is a small, grossly indistinct zone that extends a short distance from the gastroesophageal junction.
2. The **fundus** is the dome-shaped part of the stomach that is located to the left of the cardia and extends superiorly above a line drawn horizontally through the gastroesophageal junction.

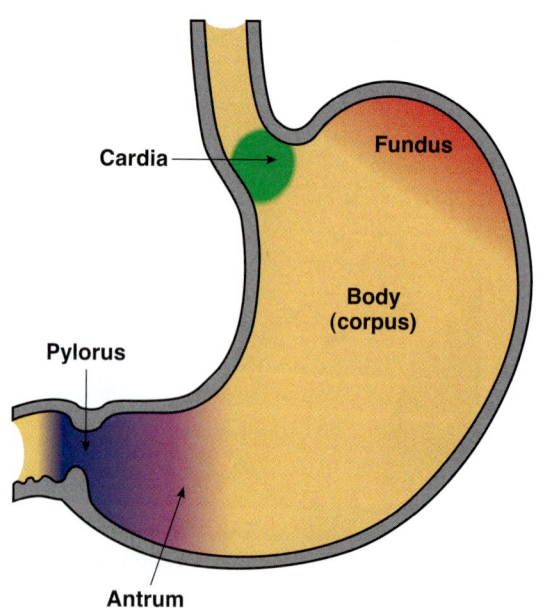

FIGURE 13-11
Anatomical regions of the stomach.

3. **The body, or corpus,** constitutes two thirds of the entire stomach and descends from the fundus to the most inferior region, where the organ turns right to form the bottom of the J.
4. **The antrum** is the distal third of the stomach. It is positioned horizontally and extends from the body to the pyloric sphincter.
5. **The pyloric sphincter** is the most distal tubular segment of the stomach, which is entirely surrounded by the thick muscular layer that governs the passage of food into the duodenum.

The wall of the stomach is composed of a mucosa, submucosa, muscularis, and serosa. The lining of the fundus and body of the stomach has prominent folds, the gastric rugae.

Branches of the celiac, hepatic, and splenic arteries supply blood to the stomach. The gastric veins drain either directly into the portal system or indirectly through the splenic and superior mesenteric veins. A rich plexus of lymphatic channels empties into the gastric and other regional lymph nodes. Both vagal nerves supply parasympathetic innervation to the stomach, and the celiac plexus provides sympathetic innervation.

The histological appearance of the gastric mucosa varies according to the anatomical region. The surface has a mucus-secreting, columnar epithelium that extends into numerous foveolae, or pits. These represent the orifices of millions of branched, tubular glands. There are three types of glands:

- **The cardiac glands** are located in the cardia.
- **The parietal (oxyntic) glands** are found in the body and fundus of the stomach.
- **The pyloric glands** are situated in the antrum and the pyloric canal.

The gastric glands, the principal secretory elements of the stomach, are densely arranged perpendicular to the mucosa and enter the base of the foveola through a narrowed segment called *the neck of the gland*. The gastric glands contain five cell types:

- **Zymogen, or chief, cells:** These cells reside primarily in the lower half of the gastric gland. They are pyramidal, basophilic cells filled with zymogen granules that contain pepsinogen.
- **Parietal, or oxyntic, cells:** These cells occupy the upper half of the gastric gland. They are oval or pyramidal eosinophilic cells that secrete hydrochloric acid. They contain numerous mitochondria that provide energy for the ion transport necessary for acid secretion. Ultrastructurally, parietal cells exhibit numerous invaginations of the surface membrane, **secretory canaliculi,** which vastly expand the surface area for acid secretion. The parietal cells are also the source of intrinsic factor, which is necessary for the intestinal absorption of vitamin B_{12}.
- **Mucous neck cells:** These mucus-secreting, basophilic components are interspersed among the parietal cells in the neck of the gastric gland.
- **Endocrine cells:** These cells are scattered in the gastric glands, mostly between the zymogen cells and the basement membrane. They are small, round, or pyramidal cells filled with granules that are stained with silver salts. Those that reduce silver without prior treatment are termed *argentaffin cells*. These cells also reduce chromium salts and are therefore included in the designation *enterochromaffin cells*. In other endocrine cells, termed *argyrophil cells,* prior reaction with a reducing substance is necessary before the granules stain with silver. Endocrine cells are scattered among the pyloric glands and contain biogenic amines such as serotonin and polypeptide hormones (e.g., gastrin and somatostatin). The endocrine cells include G cells, which secrete gastrin. Vasoactive intestinal peptide (VIP) is found in neural elements of the mucosa but not within endocrine cells.
- **Pyloric glands** are branched and conspicuously coiled structures, emptying into foveolae that are substantially deeper than those in other portions of the stomach. The glands are lined by pale cells similar in appearance to mucous neck cells and cells of Brunner glands in the duodenum. The endocrine cells include G cells, which secrete gastrin.
- **Cardiac glands** are lined by cells that are similar to mucous neck cells and those of the pyloric glands but lack G cells.

CONGENITAL DISORDERS

Congenital Pyloric Stenosis Causes Projectile Vomiting in Infancy

Congenital pyloric stenosis is a concentric enlargement of the pyloric sphincter and narrowing of the pyloric canal that obstructs the outlet of the stomach. This disorder is the most common indication for abdominal surgery in the initial 6 months of life. It is four times more common in boys than in girls and affects first-born children more often than subsequent ones. Congenital pyloric stenosis occurs in 1 in 250 white infants but is rare in blacks and Asians.

Pathogenesis: Congenital pyloric stenosis may have a genetic basis; there is a familial tendency, and the condition is more common in identical twins than in fraternal ones. Pyloric stenosis also has been recorded in the context of other developmental abnormalities, such as Turner syndrome, trisomy 18, and esophageal atresia. Embryopathies associated with rubella infection and maternal intake of thalidomide have also been associated with congenital pyloric stenosis. In some cases, congenital pyloric stenosis is associated with a deficiency of nitric oxide synthase in the nerves of pyloric smooth muscle (nitric oxide mediates relaxation of smooth muscle).

Pathology: Gross examination of the stomach shows concentric enlargement of the pylorus and narrowing of the pyloric canal. The only consistent microscopic abnormality is extreme hypertrophy of the circular muscle coat. After pyloromyotomy, the lesion disappears, although occasionally a small mass remains.

Clinical Features: The symptoms of pyloric stenosis usually become apparent within the first month of life, when the infant manifests projectile vomiting. The consequent loss of hydrochloric acid results in hypochloremic alkalosis in one third of infants. A palpable pyloric lesion and visible peristalsis are characteristic of the disorder. Surgical incision of the hypertrophied pyloric muscle is curative.

Congenital Diaphragmatic Hernia

Congenital diaphragmatic hernias of variable size and location are associated with defective closure of embryological foramina or abnormalities of the esophageal hiatus. These hernias are often associated with congenital malrotations of the intestine. The stomach, together with other abdominal organs, may eventrate into the thoracic cavity.

Rare Congenital Abnormalities

DUPLICATIONS, DIVERTICULA, AND CYSTS: These lesions are usually lined by normal gastric mucosa and are distinctly uncommon. Whereas all layers of the stomach wall tend to be present in congenital duplications, muscle coats are often deficient in diverticula and cysts. Patients with these disorders are generally asymptomatic.

SITUS INVERSUS: This causes the stomach to be located to the right of the midline, as is the esophageal hiatus. Correspondingly, the duodenum is on the left.

ECTOPIC PANCREATIC TISSUE: Nodules of pancreatic tissue are common in the wall of the antrum and pylorus. Histologically, these embryonic rests are identical to normal pancreatic tissue, except that islets are rare. Heterotopic pancreatic tissue is usually asymptomatic, but pyloric obstruction and epigastric pain have been reported.

PARTIAL GASTRIC ATRESIAS: Lack of development of the body, antrum, and pylorus have been described, as have cases in which the stomach ends blindly.

CONGENITAL PYLORIC AND ANTRAL MEMBRANES: These lesions are presumably caused by failure of the stomach to canalize during embryogenesis. They may cause symptoms of obstruction in the neonatal period but more commonly become symptomatic in adults.

GASTRITIS

Acute Hemorrhagic Gastritis Is Associated with Drugs and Stress

Acute hemorrhagic erosive gastritis is characterized by necrosis of the mucosa. Erosion of the mucosa may extend into the deeper tissues to form an ulcer. The necrosis is accompanied by an acute inflammatory response and hemorrhage, which may be severe enough to result in exsanguination.

 Pathogenesis: Acute hemorrhagic gastritis is most commonly associated with the intake of aspirin, other nonsteroidal antiinflammatory agents, or excess alcohol, or with ischemic injury. These agents are directly injurious to the gastric mucosa and exert their effects topically. The oral administration of corticosteroids is also occasionally complicated by acute hemorrhagic gastritis. Uncommonly, the accidental or suicidal ingestion of corrosive substances, such as those that produce erosive esophagitis, produces acute gastric injury. Any serious illness that is accompanied by profound physiological alterations that require substantial medical or surgical intervention renders the gastric mucosa more vulnerable to acute hemorrhagic gastritis because of mucosal ischemia. The factor common to all forms of acute hemorrhagic gastritis is thought to be the breakdown of the mucosal barrier, permitting acid-induced injury.

Stress ulcers and erosions are long known to occur in severely burned persons *(Curling ulcer)* and commonly result in bleeding. The ulceration may be deep enough to cause perforation of the stomach. Patients occasionally exhibit both gastric and duodenal ulcers.

Trauma to the central nervous system, either accidental or surgical *(Cushing ulcer),* is another cause of stress ulcers. These ulcers, which also may occur in the esophagus or duodenum, are characteristically deep and carry a substantial risk of perforation. Injury to the brain, particularly if it results in a decerebrate state, often leads to increased acid secretion in the stomach, presumably as a result of increased vagal tone. **Severe trauma,** especially if accompanied by **shock, prolonged sepsis,** and **incapacitation** from many debilitating chronic diseases also predispose to the development of acute hemorrhagic gastritis.

Hypersecretion of gastric acid has been incriminated in the pathogenesis of acute hemorrhagic gastritis, but its role is not clear. Acid secretion is often increased in some circumstances, such as neurological trauma, but the development of stress ulcers is not generally accompanied by any such increase. Nevertheless, gastric acid plays a permissive role, because inhibition of gastric acid secretion (e.g., with histamine-receptor antagonists) protects against the development of stress ulcers.

Microcirculatory changes in the stomach induced by shock or sepsis suggest that ischemic injury may contribute to the development of acute hemorrhagic gastritis.

Each of these defensive factors of the gastric mucosa has been individually investigated as follows:

- **Corticosteroids and aspirin** lead to decreased mucus production and gastric ulcers after experimental administration.
- **Prostaglandin deficiency,** caused by nonsteroidal antiinflammatory agents that inhibit prostaglandin synthesis, has been postulated to decrease the mucosal resistance to the contents of the stomach. By contrast, certain prostaglandins that stimulate mucus secretion also protect against gastric erosions.
- **Renewal of gastric epithelial cells** is clearly necessary for healing erosions of any etiology.

- **Decreased intramural pH of the gastric mucosa** has been demonstrated to protect against gastric erosions in hemorrhagic shock. Thus, acid-induced damage to the gastric mucosa is important in the pathogenesis of certain erosions.

 Pathology: Acute hemorrhagic gastritis is characterized grossly by widespread petechial hemorrhages in any portion of the stomach or regions of confluent mucosal or submucosal bleeding (Fig. 13-12). These lesions vary in size from 1 to 25 mm across and appear occasionally as sharply punched-out ulcers. Microscopically, patchy mucosal necrosis, which can extend to the submucosa, is visualized adjacent to normal mucosa. Fibrinous exudate, edema, and hemorrhage in the lamina propria are present in early lesions. The necrotic epithelium is eventually sloughed, but deeper erosions and hemorrhage may be present. In extreme cases, penetrating ulcers are associated with necrosis extending through to the serosa.

 Clinical Features: The symptoms of acute hemorrhagic gastritis range from vague abdominal discomfort to massive, life-threatening hemorrhage or the clinical manifestations of gastric perforation. Patients with gastritis induced by aspirin and other nonsteroidal antiinflammatory agents may be seen with hypochromic, microcytic anemia caused by undetected chronic bleeding. However, in patients with a severe underlying illness, the first sign of stress ulcers may be exsanguinating hemorrhage. Treatment with antacids and histamine-receptor antagonists has proved useful.

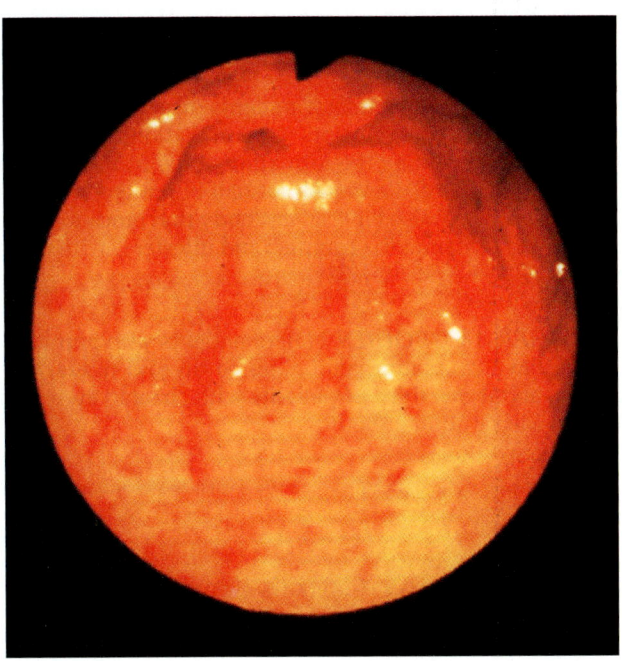

FIGURE 13-12
Erosive gastritis. This endoscopic view of the stomach in a patient who was ingesting aspirin reveals acute hemorrhagic lesions.

Chronic Gastritis is Autoimmune or Environmental

Chronic gastritis refers to chronic inflammatory diseases of the stomach, which range from mild superficial involvement of the gastric mucosa to severe atrophy. It actually comprises a heterogeneous group of disorders that have distinct anatomical distributions within the stomach, varying etiologies, and characteristic complications. The predominant symptom that has been ascribed to chronic gastritis has been dyspepsia. The diseases are also commonly discovered in asymptomatic persons undergoing routine endoscopic screening.

Autoimmune Atrophic Gastritis and Pernicious Anemia

Autoimmune atrophic gastritis refers to a chronic, diffuse inflammatory disease of the stomach that is restricted to the body and fundus and is associated with autoimmune phenomena. This disorder typically exhibits the following:

- Diffuse atrophic gastritis in the body and fundus of the stomach, with lack of, or minimal involvement of, the antrum
- Antibodies to parietal cells and intrinsic factor
- Significant reduction in or absence of gastric secretion, including acid
- Increased serum gastrin, owing to G-cell hyperplasia of the antral mucosa
- Enterochromaffin-like (ECL) cell hyperplasia in atrophic oxyntic mucosa, secondary to gastrin stimulation

Pernicious anemia is a megaloblastic anemia that is caused by malabsorption of vitamin B_{12}, occasioned by a deficiency of intrinsic factor. **In most cases, pernicious anemia is a complication of autoimmune gastritis.** The latter disorder is also associated with extragastric autoimmune diseases such as chronic thyroiditis, Graves disease, Addison disease, vitiligo, diabetes mellitus type I, and myasthenia gravis.

 Pathogenesis: Autoimmune gastritis is so named because of the presence of autoantibodies and the association with other diseases that have a similar pathogenesis.

CYTOTOXIC ANTIBODIES: Circulating antibodies to parietal cells, some of which are cytotoxic in the presence of complement, occur in 90% of patients with pernicious anemia. Parietal cell autoantibodies react with the α and β subunits of the proton pump (H^+/K^+ ATPase). This enzyme, which is the major protein of the secretory canaliculi of parietal cells, mediates the secretion of H^+ in exchange for K^+. Importantly, some 20% of persons older than 60 years exhibit parietal cell antibodies, but few have pernicious anemia.

INTRINSIC FACTOR ANTIBODIES: In addition to the postulated immunological destruction of parietal cells, two types of autoantibodies to intrinsic factor are common in pernicious anemia. Two thirds of patients display an antibody to intrinsic factor that prevents its combination with vitamin B_{12}, thereby preventing the formation of the complex that is later absorbed in the ileum. About half of patients with this blocking antibody also have an antibody that binds to the intrinsic factor–vitamin B_{12} complex and interferes with its absorption.

OTHER ANTIBODIES: Half of patients with pernicious anemia have circulating antibodies to thyroid tissue. Conversely, about one third of patients with chronic thyroiditis possess gastric autoantibodies.

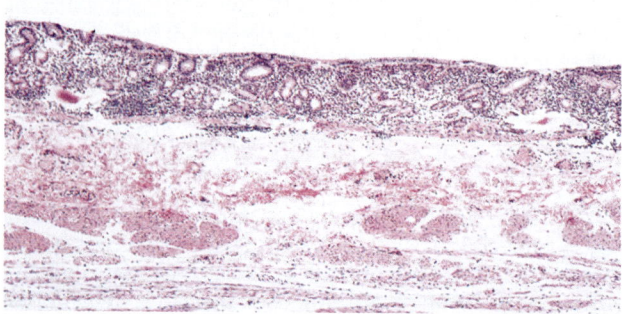

FIGURE 13-13

Atrophic gastritis. The gastric mucosa is thinned and displays a conspicuous chronic inflammatory infiltrate that separates the atrophic glands.

Multifocal Atrophic Gastritis (Environmental Metaplastic Atrophic Gastritis)

Multifocal atrophic gastritis is a disease of uncertain etiology that typically involves the antrum and adjacent areas of the body. This form of chronic gastritis has the following features:

- It is considerably more common than the autoimmune variety of atrophic gastritis and is four times as frequent among whites as in other races.
- It is not linked to autoimmune phenomena.
- Like autoimmune gastritis, it is often associated with reduced acid secretion (hypochlorhydria).
- Complete absence of gastric secretion (achlorhydria) and pernicious anemia are uncommon.

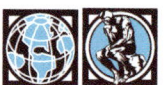 **Epidemiology and Pathogenesis:** The age and geographical distribution of environmental metaplastic atrophic gastritis parallel those of carcinoma of the stomach, and this type of gastritis seems to be a precursor of this cancer. The disease exhibits a striking localization to certain populations, being particularly common in Asia, Scandinavia, and parts of Europe and Latin America. It also demonstrates an increasing incidence with age in all populations in which it is prevalent. The offspring of emigrants from areas of high risk for stomach cancer to those of low risk lose their predisposition to this tumor. The environmental factors in its etiology include *Helicobacter pylori* infection (see below) and diet.

 Pathology of Autoimmune and Multifocal Atrophic Gastritis: The pathological features of autoimmune and multifocal atrophic gastritis are similar, except for the localization of the autoimmune type to the fundus and body and the multifocal variety mainly to the antrum.

ATROPHIC GASTRITIS: This condition is characterized by prominent chronic inflammation in the lamina propria. Occasionally, lymphoid cells are arranged as follicles, an appearance that has led to an erroneous diagnosis of lymphoma, especially in patients with *H. pylori* infection (see below). Involvement of the gastric glands leads to degenerative changes in their epithelial cells and ultimately to a conspicuous reduction in the number of glands (thus the name *atrophic gastritis*; Fig. 13-13). Eventually, the inflammatory process may abate, leaving only a thin atrophic mucosa, in which case the term *gastric atrophy* is applied.

INTESTINAL METAPLASIA: This lesion is a common and important histopathological feature of both the autoimmune and multifocal types of atrophic gastritis. In response to injury of the gastric mucosa, the normal epithelium is replaced by one composed of cells of the intestinal type (Fig. 13-14). Numerous mucin-containing goblet cells and enterocytes line cryptlike glands. Paneth cells, which are not normal inhabitants of the gastric mucosa, are present. Intestinal-type villi may occasionally form. The various endocrine

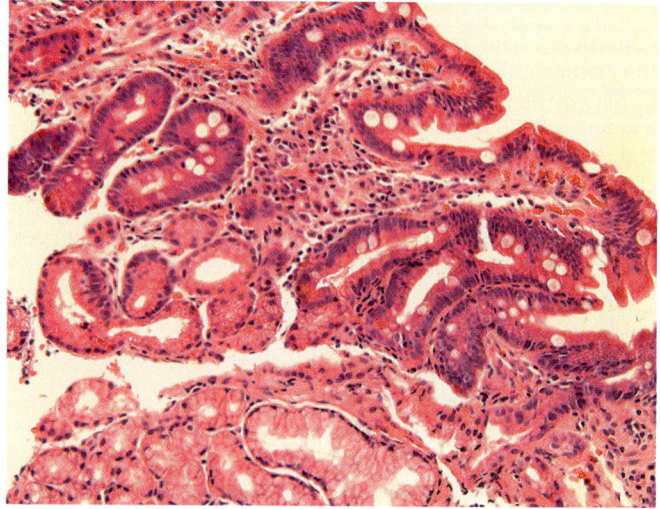

FIGURE 13-14

Chronic gastritis with intestinal metaplasia. The atrophic glands show goblet cells, and there is chronic inflammation in the lamina propria.

cells, normally situated near the basement membrane of the gastric glands, are clustered at the base of the crypts, similar to their location in the intestine. Mitoses are more numerous than in the normal gastric mucosa. In most cases of intestinal metaplasia, islands of metaplastic epithelium alternate with atrophic gastric glands, but in severe cases, large areas of the mucosa may resemble colon or small intestine, complete with villi and Paneth cells. The metaplastic cells also contain enzymes characteristic of the intestine but not of the stomach (e.g., alkaline phosphatase, aminopeptidase). Moreover, whereas gastric secretions contain principally neutral mucins, the goblet cells of the metaplastic epithelium produce the typical intestinal acid mucins.

In the fundus of the stomach with autoimmune atrophic gastritis, the normal parietal and zymogen cells may be replaced by clear mucous glands similar to those of the cardia or antrum, a change termed *pseudopyloric metaplasia*. Therefore, the pathologist must know the precise location from which a biopsy specimen was taken, because fundal pseudopyloric metaplasia may be mistaken for gastritis of the antrum. Immunohistochemical analysis for gastrin-containing cells is helpful in determining the anatomical localization of the biopsy.

Atrophic Gastritis and Stomach Cancer

Persons with atrophic gastritis of the autoimmune or multifocal type have an increased incidence of carcinoma of the stomach. Reliable statistics about this relation are difficult to obtain, because atrophic gastritis is usually asymptomatic and therefore does not ordinarily come under medical scrutiny. However, patients with pernicious anemia, who invariably have atrophic gastritis, have a 3-fold increased risk of developing gastric adenocarcinoma and a 13-fold increased risk for carcinoid (neuroendocrine) tumors.

Cancer arises in the antrum several times more frequently than in the body of the stomach, suggesting that antral gastritis is related to the development of carcinoma of the stomach.

Intestinal metaplasia of the stomach has been particularly identified as a preneoplastic lesion for several reasons: (1) gastric cancer arises in areas of metaplastic epithelium; (2) half of all cancers of the stomach are of the intestinal cell type; and (3) many cancers of the stomach show aminopeptidase activity similar to that seen in areas of intestinal metaplasia. Moreover, all grades of epithelial dysplasia, from low grade dysplasia to carcinoma in situ, have been observed in the metaplastic intestinal epithelium and are considered to be the precursors of invasive gastric cancer.

Helicobacter pylori Gastritis

H. pylori gastritis is a chronic inflammatory disease of the antrum and body of the stomach caused by H. pylori and occasionally by H. heilmannii. It is the most common type of chronic gastritis in the United States, and the organism causes one of the most frequent chronic infections. *H. pylori* infection is also strongly associated with peptic ulcer disease of the stomach and the duodenum (see below).

 Pathogenesis: *Helicobacter* species are small, curved, gram-negative rods (Proteobacteria) that bear polar flagella and display a corkscrew-like motion. *H. pylori* has been isolated from diverse populations throughout the world. The prevalence of infection with this organism increases with age, and by age 60 years, half the population has serological evidence of infection. Twin studies have shown genetic influences in susceptibility to infection with *H. pylori*. Intrafamilial clustering of *H. pylori* infection suggests that there may be person-to-person spread of these bacteria. Two thirds of those who have been infected with *H. pylori* manifest histopathological evidence of chronic gastritis.

The reasons for accepting *H. pylori* as the pathogen responsible for chronic antral gastritis rather than as a commensal that colonizes injured gastric mucosa are as follows: (1) Gastritis develops in healthy persons after ingestion of the organism; (2) *H. pylori* is attached to the epithelium in areas of chronic gastritis and is absent from uninvolved areas of the gastric mucosa; (3) eradication of the infection with bismuth or antibiotics cures gastritis; (4) antibodies against *H. pylori* are routinely found in persons with chronic gastritis; and (5) the increasing prevalence of *H. pylori* infection with age parallels that of chronic gastritis.

H. pylori is found only on the epithelial surface and does not invade the gastric mucosa. The pathogenicity of the agent is related to the *cag* pathogenicity island in its genome—a horizontally acquired locus of 40 kb that contains 31 genes. This virulence marker is putatively associated with duodenal ulcer and gastric cancer. A separate region of the genome contains the gene for vacuolating cytotoxin (*vac A*), which is also associated with duodenal ulcer disease. Chronic infection with *H. pylori* also predisposes to the development of MALT, (mucosa-associated lymphoid tissue) lymphoma of the stomach.

 Pathology: The curved rods of *H. pylori* are found in the surface mucus of the epithelial cells and in the gastric foveolae (Fig. 13-15). The uncommon bacterium *H. heilmannii* is long and has tight spirals, an appearance similar to that of spirochetes. Active gastritis features polymorphonuclear leukocytes in glands and their lumina and increased numbers of plasma cells and lymphocytes in the lamina propria. Lymphoid hyperplasia with germinal centers is frequent.

Reactive (Chemical) Gastropathy

Reflux gastropathy refers to chronic gastric injury (chemical gastropathy) that results from the reflux of alkaline duodenal contents, pancreatic secretions, and bile into the stomach. Whereas conspicuous reflux gastropathy is most common after gastroduodenostomy or gastrojejunostomy, a milder form is often identified in intact stomachs from patients with gastric ulcer, gallstone dyspepsia, postcholecystectomy syndrome, and various motor disturbances of the distal stomach.

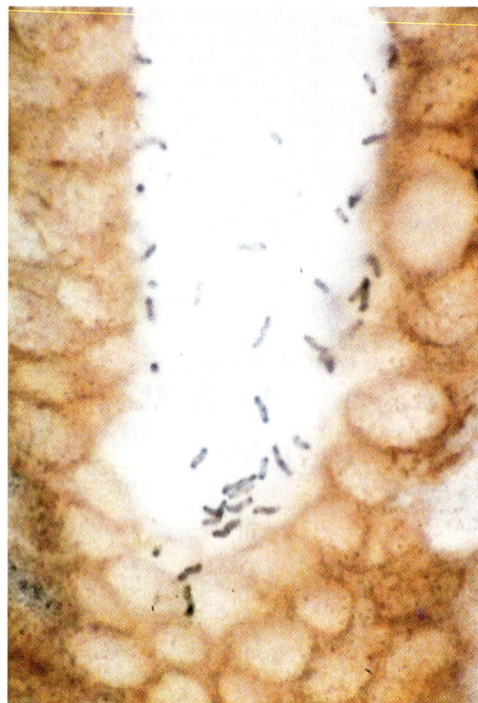

FIGURE 13-15
Helicobacter pylori- associated gastritis. The microorganisms appear on silver staining as small, curved rods on the surface of the gastric mucosa.

The histopathological appearance is dominated by foveolar hyperplasia, edema, congestion, and fibromuscular proliferation in the lamina propria. There is a paucity of inflammatory cells, although eosinophils may be prominent. Long-term exposure to nonsteroidal antiinflammatory drugs also results in reactive gastropathy.

Idiopathic Granulomatous Gastritis

Idiopathic granulomatous gastritis is defined as the presence of epithelioid granulomas in the gastric mucosa when specific granulomatous diseases have been excluded. Occasionally, the granulomas are found in association with atrophic gastritis. The condition is benign and ordinarily asymptomatic.

Eosinophilic Gastritis

Eosinophilic gastritis, often in association with eosinophilic enteritis, is disease in which eosinophils involve all layers of the stomach wall or are selectively localized in a single layer. In classic cases, the disease affects principally the antrum and pylorus, where a diffuse thickening of the wall, presumably by muscular hypertrophy, may narrow the pylorus and cause symptoms of obstruction. These are occasionally severe enough to require surgical relief. In some cases, ulceration in the affected area leads to chronic blood loss and anemia. Peripheral eosinophilia and a history of food allergies are common, but many patients have neither. Treatment with corticosteroids is often effective.

Allergic gastroenteritis occurs in young children with a conspicuous allergic diathesis, who are seen with anemia, edema, and protein-losing enteropathy. Gastric biopsy reveals an eosinophilic infiltrate limited to the mucosa.

Menetrier Disease Causes Protein Loss

Menetrier disease (hyperplastic hypersecretory gastropathy) is an uncommon disorder of the stomach characterized by enlarged rugae. It is often accompanied by a severe loss of plasma proteins (including albumin) from the altered gastric mucosa. The disease occurs in two forms, a childhood form due to cytomegalovirus infection and an adult form attributed to overexpression of TGF-α.

 Pathology: The stomach is increased in weight by as much as 900 to 1200 g. The folds of the greater curvature in the fundus and body of the stomach and occasionally in the antrum are increased in height and thickness, forming a convoluted brainlike surface (Fig. 13-16). Microscopically, Menetrier disease is restricted to the oxyntic mucosa. Hyperplasia of the gastric pits results in a conspicuous increase in their depth and a tortuous (corkscrew) structure. Mucus-secreting cells of the surface or neck type line the foveolae. The glands are elongated, and many appear cystic. These dilated glands, which are lined by superficial-type, mucus-secreting epithelial cells rather than parietal and chief cells, may penetrate the muscularis mucosae, in which case they resemble the sinuses of

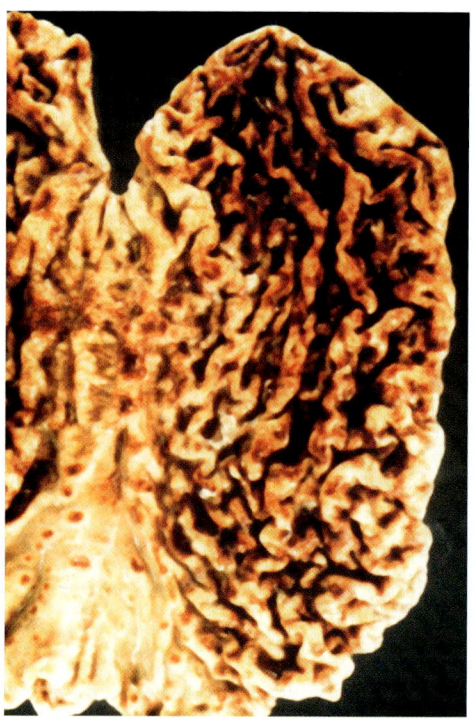

FIGURE 13-16
Menetrier disease. The folds of the stomach are increased in height and thickness, forming a convoluted surface.

Rokitansky-Aschoff in the gallbladder. Pseudopyloric metaplasia is occasionally noted, but intestinal metaplasia does not occur. Lymphocytes, plasma cells, and occasional neutrophils are seen in the lamina propria.

Clinical Features: Menetrier disease is four times more common in men than in women and affects persons of all ages. The presenting symptom is usually postprandial pain, relieved by antacids. Weight loss, sometimes of rapid onset, occasionally occurs. Peripheral edema is common, and in some cases, ascites and cachexia simulate the presence of cancer. These manifestations of the disease are related to a loss of plasma proteins from the gastric mucosa. The cause of the enormous protein loss into the lumen of the stomach is obscure, but amelioration has been reported after treatment with anticholinergic agents or an inhibitor of acid secretion. Although gastric acidity is usually low, severe peptic ulceration associated with hyperacidity has occasionally been observed.

Menetrier disease does not usually resolve spontaneously in adults, and in intractable cases, partial gastrectomy is necessary. **The disorder is considered a precancerous condition, and periodic endoscopic surveillance is recommended.** Cytomegalovirus-associated Menetrier disease in children is often self-limited.

PEPTIC ULCER DISEASE

"Peptic ulcer disease" refers to breaks in the mucosa of the stomach and small intestine, principally the proximal duodenum, that are produced by the action of gastric secretions. Peptic ulcers of the stomach and duodenum are estimated to afflict 10% of the population of Western industrialized countries at some time during their lives. Although peptic ulceration can occur as high as Barrett esophagus and as low as Meckel diverticulum with gastric heterotopia, **for practical purposes, peptic ulcer disease affects the distal stomach and proximal duodenum.** Many clinical and epidemiological features distinguish gastric from duodenal ulcers; the common factor that unites them is the gastric secretion of hydrochloric acid.

 Epidemiology: Both the incidence and the prevalence of duodenal ulcers have declined substantially during the past 30 years.

The age profile of peptic ulcer disease has progressively increased in the past 50 years. The peak incidence of duodenal ulcer disease is now between the ages of 30 and 60 years, although the disorder may occur in persons of any age, and even in infants. Gastric ulcers afflict the middle-aged and elderly more than the young.

The sex distribution of duodenal ulcers has shown a striking change, from a marked female predilection in the 19th century to a current male predominance. By contrast, the incidence of gastric ulcers is similar in men and women.

Racial differences in the incidence of peptic ulcers have been observed, but the studies of different ethnic populations are confounded by variations in many other environmental factors. For example, in Africa, duodenal ulcers are rare among blacks, whereas in the United States, the incidence is the same in blacks and whites. The preponderance of evidence suggests that in an urban Western setting, all ethnic groups are susceptible.

Surveys in the United States and Great Britain have suggested an inverse relation between duodenal ulcers and socioeconomic status and education, although the trends are not marked.

 Pathogenesis: Numerous etiological factors have been implicated in the pathogenesis of peptic ulcers, but no single agent seems to be responsible.

Environmental Factors

DIET: Despite the folk wisdom that holds that spicy food and caffeine are ulcerogenic, the evidence to support the contention that the consumption of any food or beverage, including coffee and alcohol, contributes to the development or persistence of peptic ulcers is surprisingly meager. However, cirrhosis from any cause is associated with an increased incidence of peptic ulcers.

DRUGS: **Aspirin** is an important contributing factor in the genesis of duodenal and especially gastric ulcers. **Other nonsteroidal antiinflammatory agents and analgesics** have been incriminated in the production of peptic ulcers. Prolonged treatment with high doses of corticosteroids has been claimed to increase slightly the risk of peptic ulceration.

CIGARETTE SMOKING: Smoking is a definite risk factor for duodenal and gastric ulcers, particularly gastric ulcers.

Genetic Factors

First-degree relatives of patients with duodenal ulcers have a threefold increased risk of developing a duodenal ulcer but do not have a similar increase for gastric ulcer. Patients with gastric ulcers similarly breed true. These data are confirmed by a considerably higher concordance for these ulcers in monozygotic than in dizygotic twins. The fact that identical twins show only a 50% concordance indicates that genetic factors alone do not suffice to produce an ulcer; environmental factors must also be involved.

Blood-group antigens provide further evidence for the role of genetic factors. The risk of duodenal ulcer is 30% higher in persons with type O blood than in those with types A, B, and AB. Interestingly, patients with gastric ulcers do not exhibit a greater frequency of blood group O. The fourth of the population who do not secrete blood-group antigens in the saliva and gastric juice are at a 50% increased risk of developing a duodenal ulcer. The risk of duodenal ulceration is increased (2.5:1) when nonsecretory status is combined with blood group O, a combination that occurs in 10% of the white population.

Pepsinogen I is secreted by the chief and mucous neck cells of the gastric mucosa and appears in the gastric juice, blood, and urine. Serum levels of this proenzyme correlate with the gastric capacity for acid secretion and are considered a measure of parietal cell mass. **A person with a high circulating level of pepsinogen I is at five times the normal risk of developing a duodenal ulcer.** Hyperpepsinogenemia I is present in half of children of ulcer patients with hyperpepsinogenemia and has been attributed to autosomal dominant inheritance. Thus, hyperpepsinogenemia is thought to indicate a genetically predetermined increase in parietal cell mass.

Familial tendencies for other features are reported in ulcer patients. Many patients with peptic ulcer have normal pepsinogen I secretion, and familial aggregation has also been demonstrated among such persons. Familial clustering of duodenal ulcers and rapid gastric emptying have been demonstrated, and familial hyperfunction of gastrin-secreting cells (G cells) in the antrum is also reported. Patients with a childhood duodenal ulcer are considerably more likely to have a family history of an ulcer diathesis than are persons in whom the disease begins when they are adults.

Hydrochloric Acid

The formation and persistence of peptic ulcers in both the stomach and duodenum require the gastric secretion of acid. This is evidenced principally by the following: (1) all patients with duodenal ulcers and almost all with gastric ulcers are gastric acid secretors; (2) the experimental production of ulcers in animals requires the production of acid; (3) hypersecretion of acid is present in many, but not all, patients with duodenal ulcers (there is no evidence that overproduction of acid by itself is necessary or sufficient to explain duodenal ulceration); and (4) surgical or medical treatment that reduces acid production results in the healing of peptic ulcers. The gastric secretion of pepsin, which may also play a role in the production of peptic ulcers, parallels that of hydrochloric acid.

Physiological Factors in Duodenal Ulcers

The maximal capacity for acid production by the stomach reflects total parietal cell mass. Both parietal cell mass and maximal acid secretion are increased up to twofold in patients with duodenal ulcers. However, there is a large overlap with normal values, and **only one third of these patients secrete excess acid.** The increase in parietal cells is paralleled by a comparable increase in chief cells, a situation that is consistent with the increased prevalence of hyperpepsinogenemia in patients with ulcers.

The gastric secretion of acid stimulated by food is increased in magnitude and duration in patients with duodenal ulcer, although here, too, there is significant overlap with normal values. In a few patients, this may involve, at least in part, an altered response of the G cells to meals. Such persons exhibit postprandial hypergastrinemia and an increase in the number of G cells in the antrum. Most patients with duodenal ulcers, however, show no evidence of G-cell hyperfunction.

Acid secretion in patients with duodenal ulcers may also be more sensitive than normal to gastric secretagogues such as gastrin, possibly as a result of increased vagal tone or a greater than normal affinity of the parietal cells for gastrin. It is further possible that the brisk secretion of acid after a meal is stimulated by increased vagal tone.

Accelerated gastric emptying, a condition that might lead to excessive acidification of the duodenum, has been noted in patients with duodenal ulcers. However, as with other factors, there is substantial overlap with normal rates. Normally, acidification of the duodenal bulb inhibits further gastric emptying. In most patients with duodenal ulcer, this feedback inhibitory mechanism is absent, and duodenal acidification results in continued, rather than delayed, gastric emptying. Rapid gastric emptying may in some cases be an inherited abnormality.

The pH of the duodenal bulb reflects the balance between the delivery of gastric juice and its neutralization by biliary, pancreatic, and duodenal secretions. The production of duodenal ulcers requires an acidic pH in the bulb, that is, an excess of acid over neutralizing secretions. In ulcer patients, the duodenal pH after a meal decreases to a lower level and remains depressed for a longer time than that in normal persons. This duodenal hyperacidity certainly reflects the gastric factors discussed above. The role of neutralizing factors, particularly secretin-stimulated bicarbonate secretion by the pancreas and production of bicarbonate by the duodenal mucosa, is uncertain.

Impaired mucosal defenses have been invoked as contributing to peptic ulceration. The mucosal factors, including the function of prostaglandins, may or may not be similar to those protecting the gastric mucosa (see above).

Physiological Factors in Gastric Ulcers

Gastric ulcers almost invariably arise in the setting of *H. pylori* gastritis or chemical gastritis that results in injury to the epithelium. The mechanisms by which chronic gastritis predisposes to the development of stomach ulcers remain obscure. **Most patients with gastric ulcers secrete less acid than do those with duodenal ulcers and even less than normal persons.** The factors implicated include (1) back-diffusion of acid into the mucosa, (2) decreased parietal cell mass, and (3) abnormalities of the parietal cells themselves. A minority of patients with gastric ulcers exhibit acid hypersecretion. In these persons, the ulcers are usually near the pylorus and are considered variants of duodenal ulcers. Interestingly, the intense gastric hypersecretion that occurs in the Zollinger-Ellison syndrome is associated with severe ulceration of the duodenum and even the jejunum but rarely with gastric ulcers.

The occurrence of gastric ulcers in the presence of gastric hyposecretion implies the following possibilities: (1) the gastric mucosa is in some way particularly sensitive to low concentrations of acid; (2) some material other than acid damages the mucosa, especially nonsteroidal antiinflammatory drugs; or (3) the gastric mucosa is exposed to potentially injurious agents for an unusually long period. As discussed above, the mucosal barrier to the action of acid, and perhaps to other contents of the stomach, may be impaired in some patients with gastric ulcers, although the evidence is far from conclusive. Reflux of bile (particularly deoxycholic acid and lysolecithin) and pancreatic secretions have been suggested as causes of gastric ulcers.

The Role of *Helicobacter pylori*

***Helicobacter pylori* has been isolated from the gastric antrum of virtually all patients with duodenal ulcers.** The converse is not true; that is, only a small minority of persons infected with *H. pylori* have duodenal ulcer disease. Thus, *H. pylori* infection may be accepted as a necessary, but not sufficient, condition for the development of peptic ulcer disease of the duodenum.

The mechanisms by which *H. pylori* infection predisposes to duodenal ulcers are not completely known, but a few possible mechanisms have been proposed. Cytokines produced by the inflammatory cells that respond to *H. pylori* infection stimulate gastrin release and suppress somatostatin secretion. Interleukin (IL)-1β, an acid inhibitor, has also emerged as an important mediator of inflammation in *H. pylori*-infected gastric mucosa. These effects, together with the release of histamine metabolites from the organism itself, may stimulate basal gastric acid secretion. In addition, luminal cytokines from the stomach may enter and injure the duodenal epithelium. There is some evidence that *H. pylori* infection blocks inhibitory signals from the antrum to both the G cells and the parietal cell region, resulting in increased gastrin release and impaired inhibition of gastric acid secretion. Such an effect might lead to an increased load of acid in the duodenum, thereby contributing to the development of duodenal ulcers. Owing to acidification of the duodenal bulb, islands of metaplastic gastric mucosa in the duodenum occur in many patients with peptic ulcers. This gastric epithelium in the duodenum sometimes shows the same colonization with *H. pylori* as does the gastric mucosa. It has been postulated that infection of the metaplastic epithelium by *H. pylori* might render the mucosa more susceptible to peptic injury (Fig. 13-17).

Infection with *H. pylori* is probably also important in the pathogenesis of gastric ulcers, because this organism is responsible for most cases of the chronic gastritis that underlies this disease. It is estimated that about 75% of patients with gastric ulcers harbor *H. pylori*. The remaining 25% of cases may represent an association with other types of chronic gastritis. The various gastric and duodenal factors

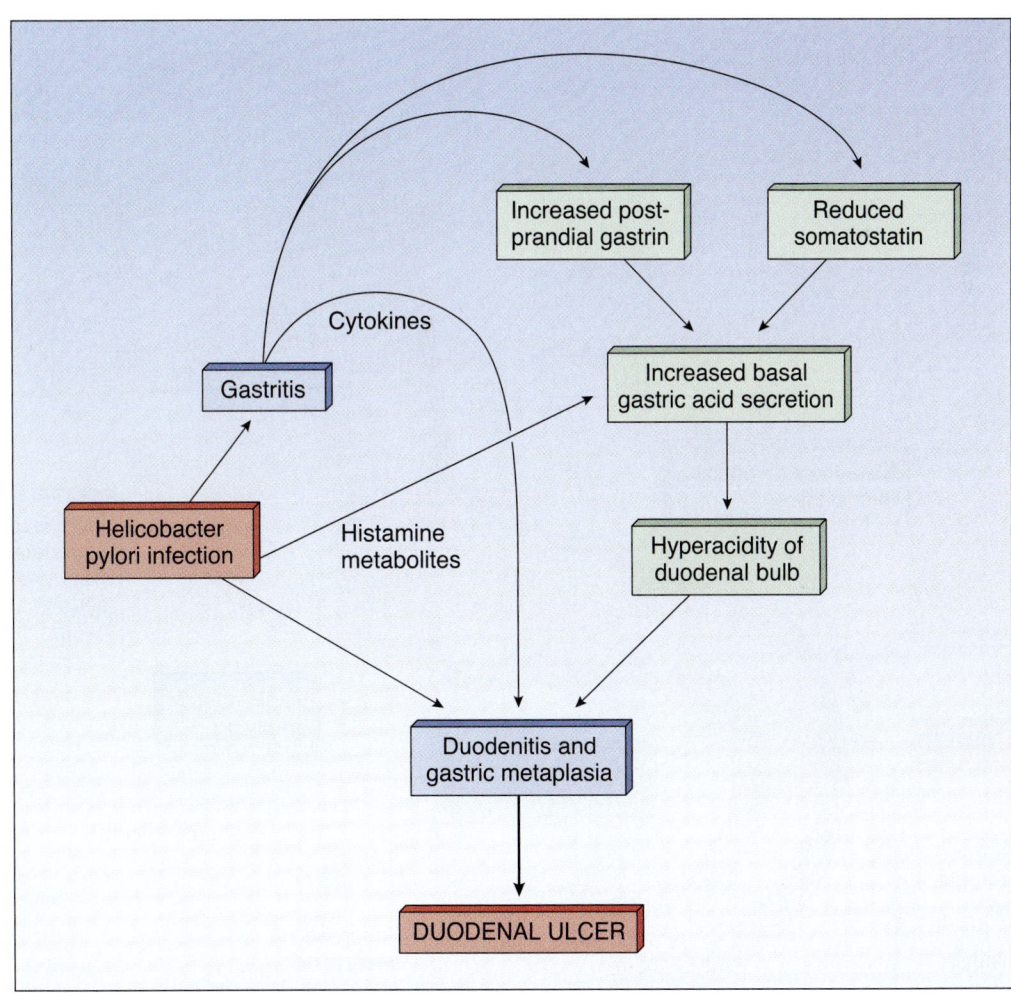

FIGURE 13-17
Possible mechanisms in the pathogenesis of duodenal ulcer disease associated with *Helicobacter pylori* infection.

that have been implicated as possible mechanisms in the pathogenesis of duodenal ulceration are summarized in Figure 13-18.

Diseases Associated with Peptic Ulcers

CIRRHOSIS: The incidence of duodenal ulcers in patients with cirrhosis is 10 times that in normal persons.

CHRONIC RENAL FAILURE: End-stage renal disease with hemodialysis results in a greater than normal risk for the development of peptic ulcers. Patients subjected to renal transplantation also show a substantially increased incidence of peptic ulceration and its complications, such as bleeding and perforation.

HEREDITARY ENDOCRINE SYNDROMES: There is an increased incidence of peptic ulcers in persons with **multiple endocrine neoplasia, type I** (see Chapter 21). Zollinger-Ellison syndrome, a cause of severe peptic ulceration, is characterized by gastric hypersecretion caused by a gastrin-producing islet cell adenoma of the pancreas.

α_1-ANTITRYPSIN DEFICIENCY: This hereditary disorder is associated with peptic ulcers in almost one third of patients, and this incidence is even higher in patients who have pulmonary disease as well. Moreover, the number of heterozygotes for α_1-antitrypsin deficiency among relatives of patients with peptic ulcer is increased.

CHRONIC PULMONARY DISEASE: Long-standing pulmonary dysfunction significantly increases the risk of ulcers, and it is estimated that fully one fourth of patients with such disorders have peptic ulcer disease. Conversely, chronic lung disease is increased twofold to threefold in persons who have peptic ulcers.

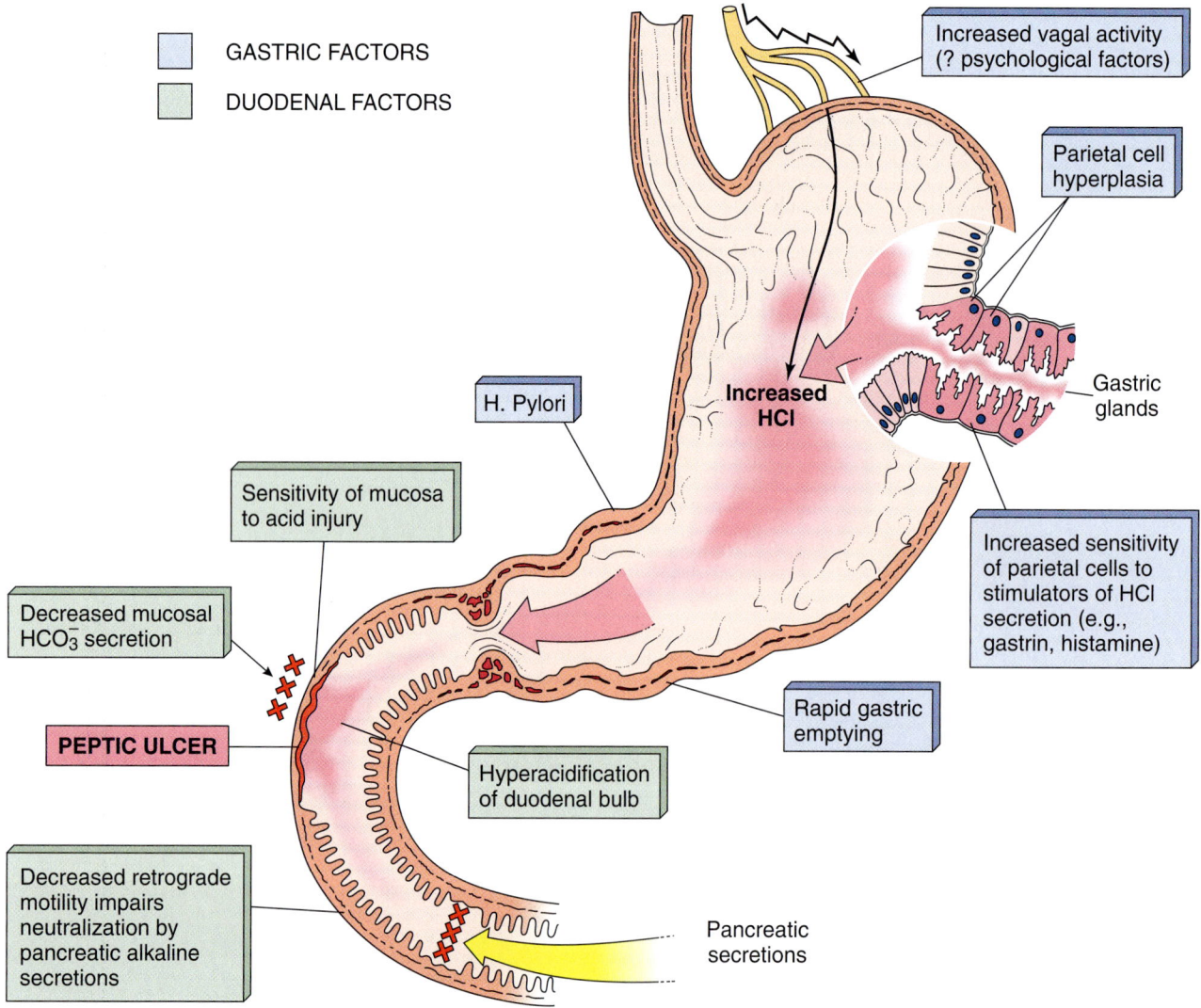

FIGURE 13-18

Gastric and duodenal factors in the pathogenesis of duodenal peptic ulcers.

Pathology: Most peptic ulcers arise in the lesser curvature of the stomach, in the antral and prepyloric regions, and in the first part of the duodenum.

Gastric ulcers (Fig. 13-19) are usually single and less than 2 cm in diameter. Ulcers on the lesser curvature are commonly associated with chronic gastritis, whereas those on the greater curvature are often related to nonsteroidal antiinflammatory drugs. The edges tend to be sharply punched out, with overhanging margins. Deeply penetrating ulcers produce a serosal exudate that may cause adherence of the stomach to the surrounding structures. Scarring of ulcers in the prepyloric region may be severe enough to produce pyloric stenosis. **On gross examination, it may be exceedingly difficult to distinguish chronic peptic ulcer from an ulcerated gastric carcinoma.** Thus, when examining the stomach, the endoscopist is required to take multiple biopsy specimens from the edges and bed of any gastric ulcer.

Duodenal ulcers (Fig. 13-20) are ordinarily located on the anterior or posterior wall of the first part of the duodenum, within a short distance of the pylorus. The lesion is usually solitary, but it is not uncommon to find paired ulcers on both walls, so-called kissing ulcers.

Microscopically, gastric and duodenal ulcers have a similar appearance (Fig. 13-21). From the lumen outward, the following are noted: (1) a superficial zone of fibrinopurulent exudate; (2) necrotic tissue; (3) granulation tissue; and (4) fibrotic tissue at the base of the ulcer, which exhibits variable degrees of chronic inflammation. The ulceration sometimes penetrates the muscle layers, thereby causing them to be interrupted by scar tissue after healing. Blood vessels on

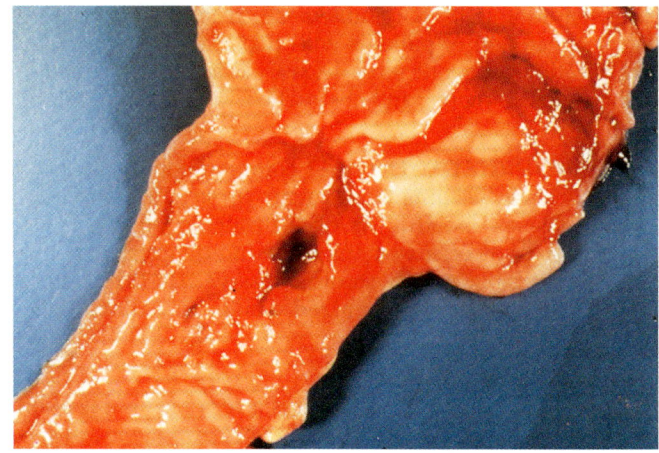

FIGURE 13-20
Duodenal ulcer. A sharply punched-out peptic ulcer of the duodenum is situated immediately below the pylorus.

the margins of the ulcer are often thrombosed. The mucosa at the margins of the ulcer tends to be hyperplastic and with healing grows over the ulcerated area as a single layer of epithelium. Duodenal ulcers are usually accompanied by peptic duodenitis, with Brunner gland hyperplasia and gastric mucin cell metaplasia.

Clinical Features: The symptoms of gastric and duodenal ulcers are sufficiently similar that the two conditions are generally not distinguishable by history or physical examination. The classic case of duodenal ulcer is characterized by epigastric pain that is experienced 1–3 hours after a meal or that awakens the patient at night. Both alkali and food are said to relieve the symptoms. Dyspeptic symptoms commonly associated with gallbladder dis-

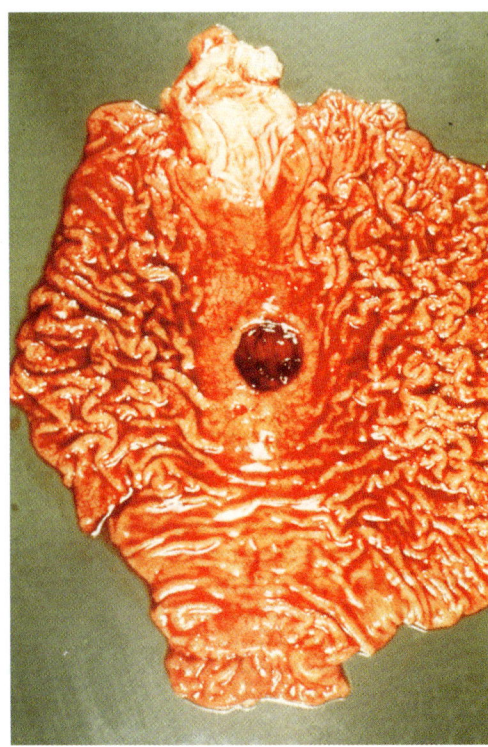

FIGURE 13-19
Gastric ulcer. The stomach has been opened to reveal a sharply demarcated, deep peptic ulcer on the lesser curvature.

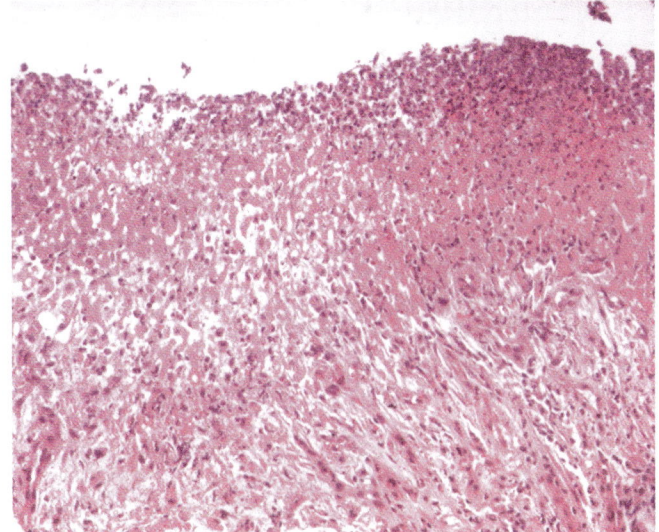

FIGURE 13-21
Peptic ulcer of the stomach. A photomicrograph of the ulcer shows the mucosa to be denuded. The surface is covered with a fibrinous exudate containing neutrophils, with inflamed granulation tissue below.

ease, including fatty food intolerance, distention, and belching, occur in half of patients with peptic ulcers. The major complications of peptic ulcer disease are hemorrhage, perforation with peritonitis, and obstruction.

HEMORRHAGE: The most common complication of peptic ulcers is bleeding, occurring in up to 20% of patients. In many cases, bleeding is occult and, in an otherwise asymptomatic ulcer, may manifest as iron-deficiency anemia or as occult blood in the stools. **Massive life-threatening hemorrhage is a well-recognized danger in patients with active peptic ulcers.**

PERFORATION: Perforation is a serious complication of peptic ulcer disease that occurs in 5% of patients; in one third of cases, there are no antecedent symptoms referable to peptic ulcer. Perforations are seen more commonly with duodenal than with gastric ulcers, most occurring on the anterior wall of the duodenum. Because the anterior walls of the stomach and duodenum are undefended by contiguous tissue, ulcers in these locations are more likely to be complicated by free perforation, which leads to generalized peritonitis and the accumulation of air in the abdominal cavity, called *pneumoperitoneum*. Posterior gastric ulcers perforate into the lesser peritoneal sac, where the inflammatory reaction may be contained. When ulcers penetrate into the pancreas, liver, or greater omentum, they cause intractable symptoms. They may also penetrate the biliary tract and fill it with air.

Perforated ulcers continue to be associated with a high mortality. The overall mortality for perforated gastric ulcers is 10 to 40%, two to three times more than that for duodenal ulcers (~10%). Perforations are occasionally complicated by hemorrhage. Although shock, abdominal distention, and pain are common symptoms, perforations are occasionally diagnosed for the first time at autopsy, particularly in institutionalized, elderly patients.

PYLORIC OBSTRUCTION (GASTRIC OUTLET OBSTRUCTION): Pyloric obstruction occurs in up to 10% of ulcer patients, and peptic ulcer disease is its most common cause in adults. Narrowing of the pyloric lumen by an adjacent peptic ulcer may be caused by muscular spasm, edema, muscular hypertrophy, or contraction of scar tissue; most commonly it is due to a combination of these. Eventually obstruction may ensue.

DEVELOPMENT OF COMBINED ULCERS: The simultaneous occurrence of gastric and duodenal ulcers in the same patient is far greater than can be accounted for by chance alone. Patients with gastric ulcers have a substantially increased risk of developing a subsequent duodenal ulcer, and vice versa.

MALIGNANT TRANSFORMATION OF A BENIGN GASTRIC ULCER: It is extremely difficult to distinguish a cancer arising in a preexisting gastric ulcer from an ulcerated primary carcinoma. This difficulty does not complicate the study of duodenal ulcers, because **malignant transformation of a duodenal ulcer is very uncommon.** However, although cancers originating in benign peptic ulcers probably account for fewer than 1% of all malignant tumors in the stomach, such tumors have been well documented.

BENIGN NEOPLASMS

Stromal Tumors in the Stomach Tend to Be Benign

All gastrointestinal stromal tumors (GISTs) are derived from the pacemaker cells of Cajal and include the vast majority of mesenchymal derived stromal tumors of the entire gastrointestinal tract. The pacemaker cells and the tumor cells express the *c-kit* oncogene (CD117) that encodes a tyrosine kinase that regulates cell proliferation and apoptosis. The criteria to evaluate malignancy in all GISTs include size, necrosis, and the number of mitotic figures. Interestingly, many of the gastric GISTs, independently of their size, tend to behave in a benign fashion, as opposed to small and large bowel tumors, which are more commonly malignant.

Gastric GISTs are usually submucosal (Fig. 13-22) and covered by intact mucosa or, when they project externally, by peritoneum. The cut surface has a whorled appearance. Microscopically, the tumors show variable cellularity and are composed of spindle-shaped cells with cytoplasmic vacuoles embedded in a collagenous stroma. The cells are disposed in whorls and interlacing bundles. The presence of bizarre and giant nuclei is not necessarily a sign of malignancy.

GISTs can also appear more epithelioid, with cells that are polygonal and have eosinophilic cytoplasm. With very few exceptions, stromal tumors of the gastrointestinal tract are considered tumors of low malignant potential. Treatment of GISTs consists mainly of surgical resection.

Epithelial Polyps May Be Precancerous

HYPERPLASTIC POLYPS: These lesions represent most gastric polyps. They may be single or multiple and are seen as pedunculated or sessile lesions of variable sizes. Hyperplastic polyps are common in the atrophic oxyntic mucosa of the body and fundus of patients with autoimmune metaplastic atrophic gastritis, but they also occur in the antrum of patients with *H. pylori* gastritis. Microscopically, the polyps consist of elongated, branched crypts lined by foveolar epithelium, beneath which pyloric or gastric glands are present. **Hyperplastic polyps have no malignant potential.**

TUBULAR ADENOMAS (ADENOMATOUS POLYPS): These are true neoplasms that occur most commonly in the antrum. The polyps range from less than 1 cm in diameter to a considerable size, the average being about 4 cm. Most adenomatous polyps are sessile and more often single than multiple. Microscopically, adenomas are composed of tubular structures or a combination of tubular and villous structures. The glands are usually lined by dysplastic epithelium, which is sometimes intestinalized. **Adenomatous polyps manifest a malignant potential, variably reported at 5 to 75%.** This risk increases with the size of the polyp and is greatest for lesions larger than 2 cm in diameter. Dysplasia can also occur in flat gastric mucosa. The presence of multiple tubular adenomas in patients with familial adenomatous polyposis greatly increases the risk of developing adenocarcinoma.

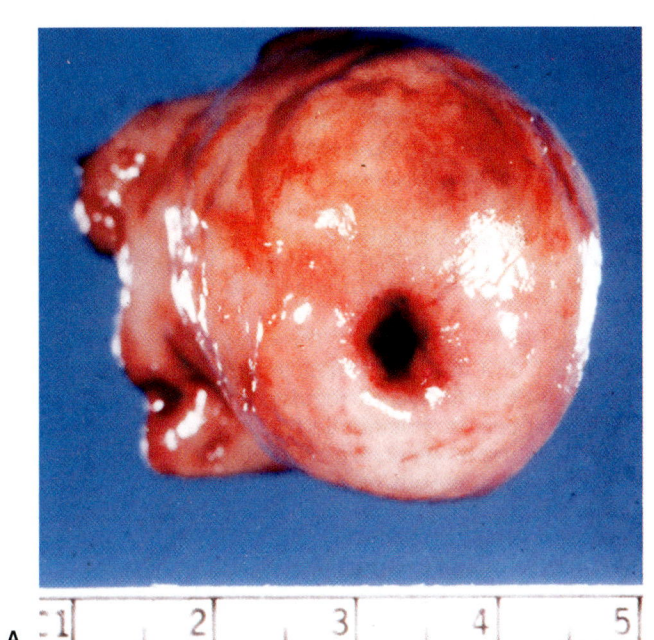
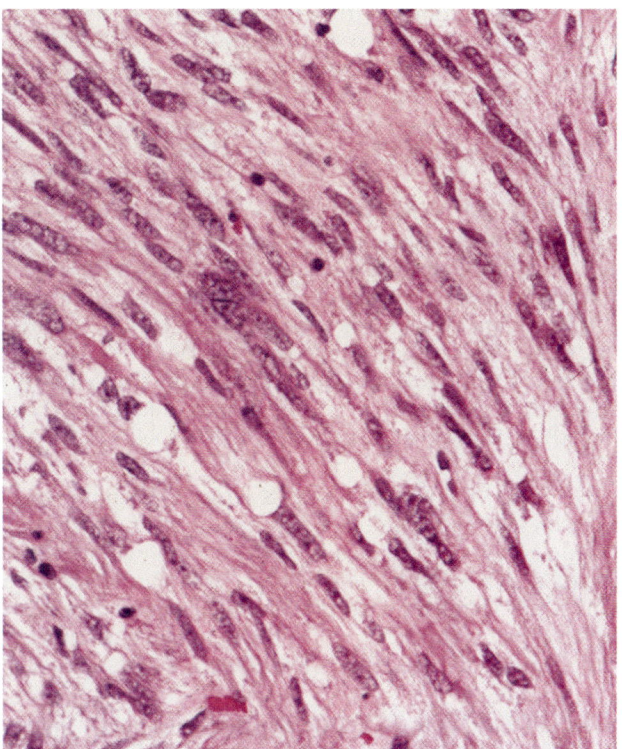

FIGURE 13-22
A. Gastrointestinal stromal tumor of the stomach. The resected tumor is submucosal and covered by a focally ulcerated mucosa. B. Microscopic examination of the tumor shows spindle cells with vacuolated cytoplasms.

TREATMENT: In the past, patients with peptic ulcers were subjected to subtotal gastrectomy. However, the disease is now cured by the administration of antibiotics to eliminate H. pylori and the use of inhibitors of acid secretion, including histamine receptor blockers and proton pump inhibitors.

FUNDIC GLAND POLYPS: Fundic gland polyps are characterized by dilated oxyntic glands lined by parietal and chief cells and by mucous cell metaplasia. They are common in patients with familial adenomatous polyposis and patients treated with proton pump inhibitors. These polyps are not considered preneoplastic, and patients do not have an increased risk of developing gastric carcinoma.

MALIGNANT TUMORS

Carcinoma of the Stomach Relates to Many Environmental Factors

Epidemiology: As recently as the mid-20th century, carcinoma of the stomach was the most common cause of death from cancer among men in the United States. For reasons that have not been explained, the incidence of gastric carcinoma has steadily decreased and now accounts for only about 3% of cancer deaths in the United States. The incidence of stomach cancer remains exceedingly high in such countries as Japan and Chile, where the rates are seven to eight times that in the United States. Although the cause of gastric cancer is unknown, emigrants from high-risk to low-risk areas show a decline in the incidence of cancer of the stomach (see Chapter 5), an observation that strongly implicates environmental factors in its pathogenesis.

 Pathogenesis: Although correlations have been demonstrated with a number of factors, the cause of gastric cancer remains elusive.

DIETARY FACTORS: Ingredients in the diet have been invoked to account for geographical variations in the incidence of gastric cancer. Carcinoma of the stomach is more common among persons who eat large amounts of starch, smoked fish and meat, and pickled vegetables. Benzpyrene, a potent carcinogen, has been detected in smoked foods.

NITROSAMINES: Attention has been focused on the possible role of nitrosamines, which are powerful animal carcinogens, in the pathogenesis of cancer of the stomach. Secondary amines are converted nonenzymatically to nitrosamines in the presence of nitrates or nitrites. High nitrate concentrations have been found in the soil and water in certain areas where the incidence of gastric cancer is high, and processed meats and vegetables are high in nitrates and nitrites.

The decreased incidence of gastric cancer in the United States has been paralleled by an increased use of refrigeration, a practice that inhibits the conversion of nitrates to nitrites and also obviates the need to add such compounds for food preservation. The consumption of whole milk and fresh vegetables rich in vitamin C is inversely related to the occurrence of stomach cancer. Vitamin C has been shown to inhibit the nitrosation of secondary amines in vivo.

GENETIC FACTORS: Hereditary traits have not been identified in most cases of carcinoma of the stomach, although a few familial clusters and several cases in twins have been reported. Gastric cancer occurs in higher frequency in hereditary nonpolyposis colorectal cancer (HNPCC) syndrome, a disorder caused by germline mutations of genes responsible for DNA nucleotide mismatch repair. Blood type A is found in 38% of the general population, whereas half of patients with gastric cancer display this blood type.

AGE AND SEX: Gastric cancer is uncommon in persons younger than 30 years and shows a sharp peak in incidence in persons older than 50 years. However, the age at onset seems to be somewhat lower in Japan, where the disease is endemic. In the United States, there is only a slight male predominance, but in countries with a high incidence of this tumor, the male-to-female ratio is about 2:1.

HELICOBACTER PYLORI: **Serological studies have demonstrated a high prevalence of gastric infection with *H. pylori* many years before the appearance of stomach cancer.** Persons seropositive for *H. pylori* were three times more likely than seronegative persons to develop gastric adenocarcinoma in the ensuing 1 to 24 years of follow-up. In view of the observation that the risk of stomach cancer is determined largely by environmental factors in the first decades of life, it is noteworthy that populations at high risk for this tumor exhibit a high prevalence of infection with *H. pylori* in children, whereas those at low risk do not. Since gastric adenocarcinoma develops in only a small proportion of persons infected with *H. pylori,* and since some stomach cancers are found in noninfected persons, this infection alone is neither sufficient nor necessary for gastric carcinogenesis.

LOW-SOCIOECONOMIC SETTINGS: These situations pose an increased risk of gastric cancer, an observation that has been used to explain the higher frequency of the tumor among American blacks and the fact that the incidence of the disease in that population has not declined as rapidly as it has among whites.

Atrophic gastritis, pernicious anemia, subtotal gastrectomy, and gastric adenomatous polyps are discussed above as factors associated with a high risk of stomach cancer.

Pathology: Adenocarcinoma of the stomach accounts for more than 95% of all malignant gastric tumors. It occurs in two major but overlapping types: diffuse and intestinal. Cancers are most common in the distal stomach, on the lesser curvature of the antrum, and in the prepyloric region. Adenocarcinoma is rare in the fundus but may occur in any location.

ADVANCED GASTRIC CANCER: By the time most gastric cancers in the Western world are detected, they are advanced; that is, they have penetrated beyond the submucosa into the muscularis propria and may extend through the serosa. The macroscopic appearance of these advanced cancers is of great importance not only to the pathologist but also to the radiologist and the endoscopist, who may be called on to distinguish carcinomas from benign lesions and to assess the degree of spread.

Advanced gastric cancers are divided into three major macroscopic types:

- **Polypoid (fungating) adenocarcinoma** accounts for one third of advanced cancers. It is a solid mass, often several centimeters in diameter, that projects into the lumen of the stomach. The surface may be partly ulcerated, and the deeper tissues may or may not be infiltrated.
- **Ulcerating adenocarcinoma** constitutes another third of all gastric cancers. It is visualized as a shallow ulcer of variable size (Fig. 13-23). The surrounding tissue is firm, raised, and nodular. Characteristically, the lateral margins of the ulcer are irregular, and the base is ragged. This appearance stands in contrast to that of the usual benign peptic ulcer, which exhibits punched-out margins and a smooth base. Despite these differences, the radiological differentiation of ulcerating cancer from peptic ulcer is occasionally difficult.
- **Diffuse or infiltrating adenocarcinoma** composes one tenth of all stomach cancers. No true tumor mass is seen macroscopically; instead, the wall of the stomach is conspicuously thickened and firm (Fig. 13-24). When the entire stomach is involved, the term *linitis plastica* is applied. In the diffuse type of gastric carcinoma, the invading tumor cells induce extensive fibrosis in the submucosa and muscularis. As a result, the wall is stiff and may be more than 2 cm thick.

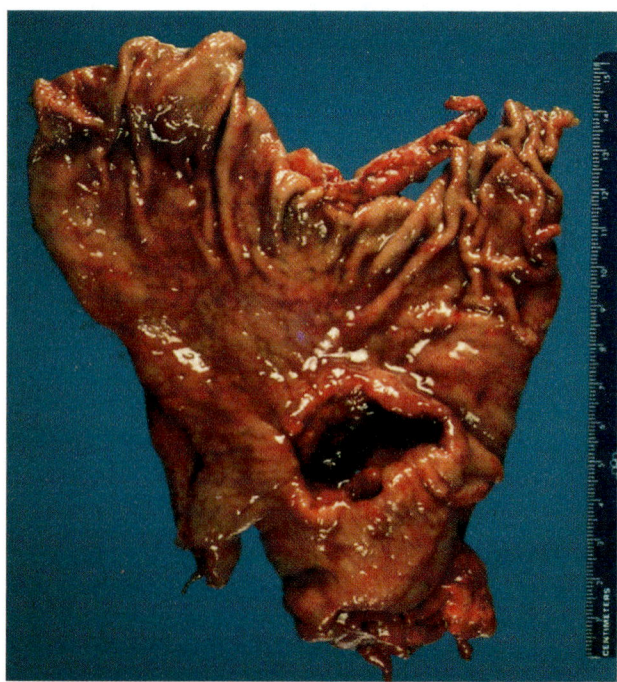

FIGURE 13-23
Ulcerating carcinoma of the stomach. The stomach has been opened along the greater curvature to reveal a large, centrally ulcerated adenocarcinoma in the antrum, characterized by raised, indurated margins.

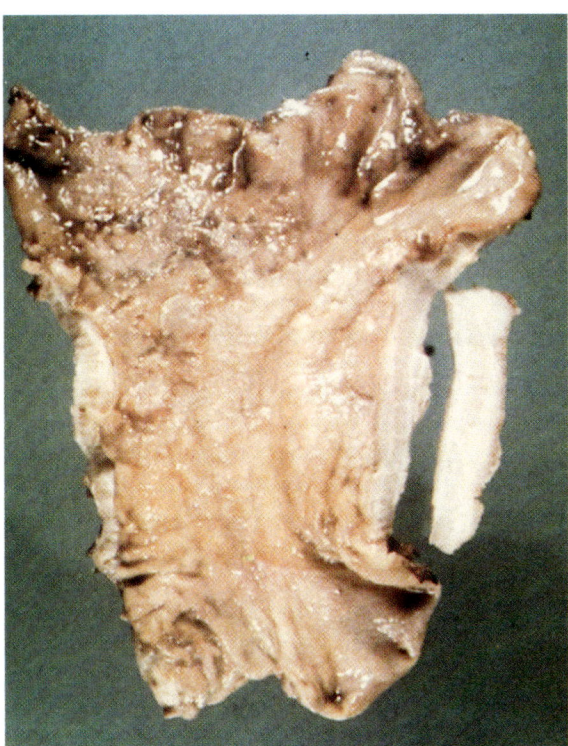

FIGURE 13-24
Infiltrating gastric carcinoma (linitis plastica). The wall of the stomach is thickened and indurated by a diffusely infiltrating cancer.

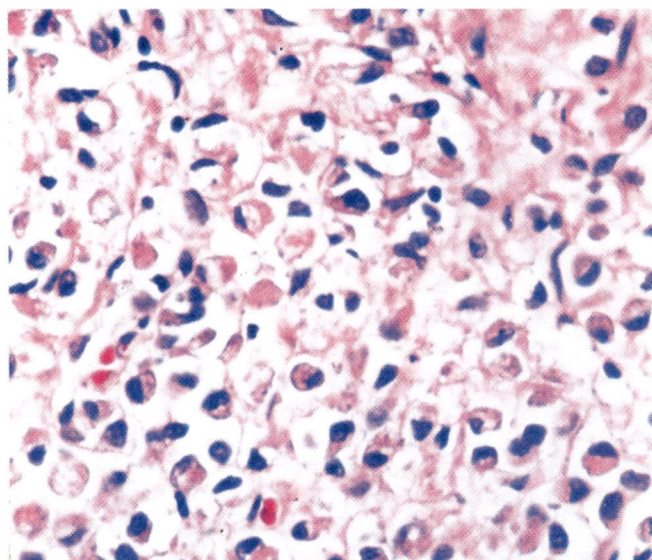

FIGURE 13-25
Poorly differentiated gastric adenocarcinoma with signet ring cells. The intracellular mucin displaces the nuclei to the periphery of the tumor cells

Microscopically, the histological pattern of advanced gastric cancer varies from a well-differentiated adenocarcinoma with gland formation (intestinal type) to a poorly differentiated carcinoma without gland formation. The polypoid variant typically contains well-differentiated glands, whereas linitis plastica is characteristically poorly differentiated. Particularly in the ulcerated type of cancer, the tumor cells may be arranged in cords or small foci. Tumor cells may contain cytoplasmic mucin that displaces the nucleus to the periphery of the cell, resulting in the so-called signet ring cell (Fig. 13-25). Extracellular mucinous material may be so prominent that the malignant cells seem to float in a gelatinous matrix, in which case it is called a *mucinous (colloid) carcinoma.* Cancers that display papillary infoldings are termed *papillary adenocarcinomas,* and those that form solid tumor masses are referred to as *medullary carcinomas.*

EARLY GASTRIC CANCER: Early gastric cancer is defined as a tumor that is confined to the mucosa or submucosa (Fig. 13-26). An earlier term, *superficial spreading carcinoma,* is synonymous with early gastric cancer. In Japan, early gastric cancer accounts for fully one third of all stomach cancers, whereas in the United States and Europe, it constitutes only about 5%.

Early gastric cancer is strictly a pathological diagnosis based on depth of invasion; the term does not refer to the duration of the disease, its size, the presence of symptoms, the absence of metastases, or the curability. In fact, up to 20% of early gastric cancers are already metastatic to lymph nodes at the time of detection.

Like advanced cancer, most early gastric cancers are found in the distal stomach and have been classified by Japanese investigators according to their macroscopic appearance. Three major types are recognized:

- **Type I** protrudes into the lumen as a polypoid or nodular mass.
- **Type II** is a superficial, flat lesion that may be slightly elevated or depressed.
- **Type III** is an excavated malignant ulcer that does not ordinarily occur alone but rather represents ulceration of type I or type II tumors.

The polypoid and the superficial elevated varieties of early gastric cancer are typically well-differentiated intestinal-

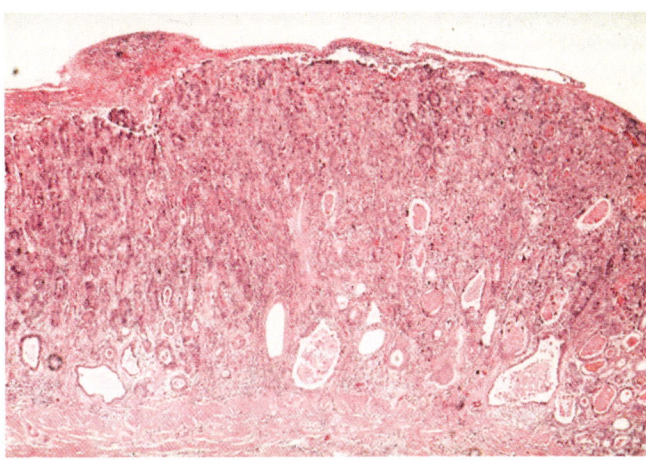

FIGURE 13-26
Early gastric cancer. Gastric adenocarcinoma showing malignant glands infiltrating into the submucosa.

type adenocarcinomas. In the flattened or depressed superficial early cancers, the pattern ranges from well differentiated to poorly differentiated. The excavated lesions have the highest proportion of undifferentiated tumors.

Most gastric cancers of the intestinal type originate from epithelium that has undergone intestinal metaplasia. By contrast, less-differentiated and anaplastic tumors of the diffuse type are more likely to originate from the necks of gastric glands without intestinal metaplasia.

Intuitively, one would suppose that early gastric cancer would be the precursor of advanced gastric cancer. However, this is not always the case, and early gastric cancer may sometimes be a different disease from advanced cancer. It may exhibit a more benign course and greater curability because of an inherently lower biological potential for invasion, possibly related to the differences between the intestinal and gastric cell types. For example, even in the presence of lymph node metastases, early gastric cancer has a considerably better prognosis than advanced cancer. The 10-year survival rate for surgically treated advanced gastric cancer is about 20%, compared with 95% for early gastric cancer. Moreover, the mean age at onset of early gastric cancer is uniformly younger than that of advanced cancer, and the early variety shows a striking geographical distribution.

Gastric cancer metastasizes principally by the lymphatic route to regional lymph nodes of the lesser and greater curvature, the porta hepatis, and the subpyloric region. Distant lymphatic metastases also occur, the most common being an enlarged supraclavicular node, called *Virchow node*. Hematogenous spread may seed any organ, including the liver, lung, or brain. Direct extension to nearby organs is often encountered. Carcinoma of the stomach can also spread to the ovary, where it commonly elicits a desmoplastic response, in which case it is termed a *Krukenberg tumor*. Figure 13-27 schematically depicts the major types of gastric cancer.

 Clinical Features: In the United States and Europe, most patients with gastric cancer have metastases by the time they are seen for examination. Thus, the symptoms and course are usually those of advanced cancer. The most frequent initial symptom is weight loss, usually associated with anorexia and nausea. Most patients complain of epigastric or back pain, a symptom that mimics benign gastric ulcer and is often relieved by antacids or H_2-receptor antagonists. However, as the disease advances, symptomatic amelioration with medical therapy disappears.

Obstruction of the gastric outlet may occur with large tumors of the antrum or prepyloric region. Massive bleeding is uncommon, but chronic bleeding is often reflected in the finding of occult blood in the stools and anemia. Tumors that involve the esophagogastric junction result in dysphagia and occasionally mimic achalasia and esophageal adenocarcinoma.

Patients with early gastric cancer may be asymptomatic but usually complain of dyspepsia or epigastric pain. Weight loss, melena, and anemia are present in a minority of patients.

Carcinoembryonic antigen is increased in the blood of one fourth of patients with advanced gastric cancer. This test has little value in the diagnosis of stomach cancer, but it may be helpful in monitoring the course of metastatic disease or of postoperative recurrence.

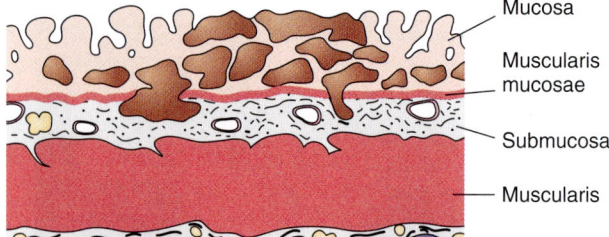
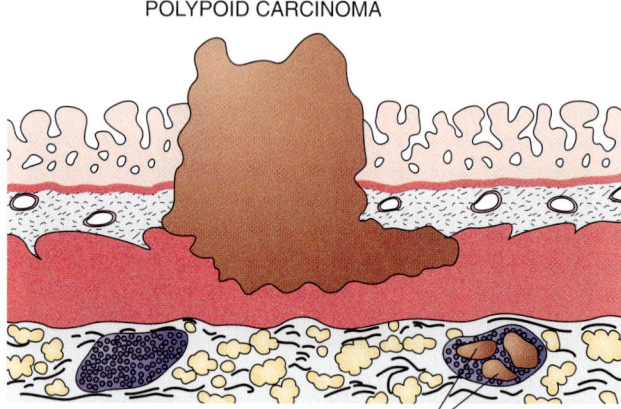
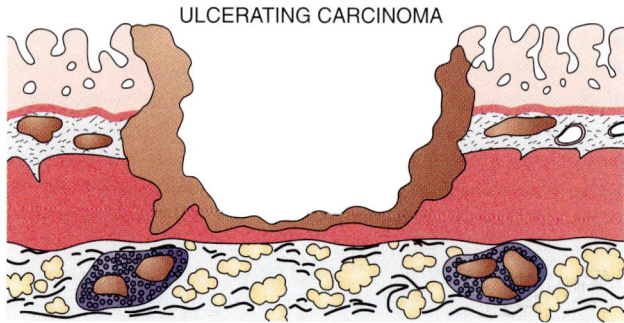
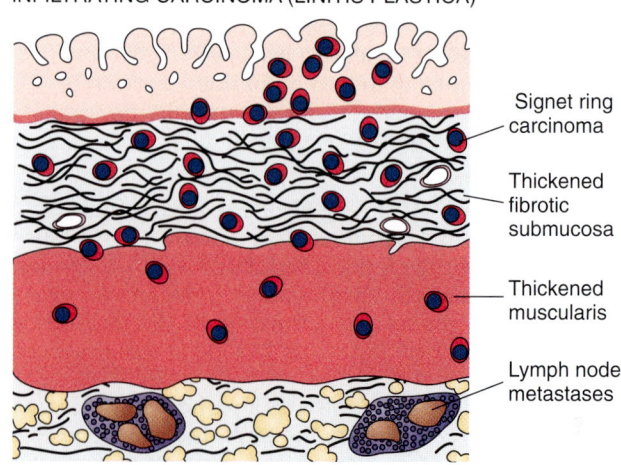

FIGURE 13-27
The major types of gastric cancer.

Carcinoid Tumors Are of Low-Grade Malignancy

Various endocrine cells in the normal gastric mucosa may give rise to neoplasms, collectively termed *carcinoid tumor (neuroendocrine tumors)*. All the carcinoid tumors of the gastrointestinal tract have a potential for local recurrence and metastasis. The probability of metastases depends more on the size than on the histopathological characteristics. Most of the gastric carcinoids do not display hormonal function, although an occasional one secretes serotonin, and their metastases can cause the carcinoid syndrome. Many gastric microcarcinoids occur in the setting of autoimmune metaplastic atrophic gastritis and pernicious anemia.

Gastric Lymphoma Is the Most Common Extranodal Lymphoma

Primary lymphoma of the stomach accounts for about 5% of all malignant stomach tumors and comprises 20% of all extranodal lymphomas. **Clinically and radiologically, gastric lymphoma mimics gastric adenocarcinoma.** The presenting symptoms of gastric lymphoma are weight loss, dyspepsia, and abdominal pain, which are similar to symptoms of gastric adenocarcinoma. The age at diagnosis is usually 40 to 65 years, and there is no sex predominance. The tumors often cannot be differentiated from carcinoma, because they may be polypoid, ulcerating, or diffuse. Most gastric lymphomas are low-grade B-cell neoplasms of the MALToma type (**mu**cosa-**a**ssociated **l**ymphoid **t**issue) and arise in the setting of chronic *H. pylori* gastritis with lymphoid hyperplasia. Some of these lymphomas regress after eradication of the *H. pylori* infection. Other histopathological varieties are similar to those in primary nodal lymphomas.

Malignant Gastrointestinal Stromal Tumor (GIST)

Malignant GISTs constitute about 1% of gastric cancers. They are seen as palpable masses in up to half of patients with this tumor. It is often difficult to predict the biological behavior of a GIST from its morphological appearance in the absence of infiltration or metastases. Macroscopically malignant GISTs are larger than their benign counterparts. Cellular pleomorphism and hyperchromasia may be present in both benign and malignant tumors, but the size and number of mitoses are greater in malignant GISTs. In some cases, the true biology of the tumor becomes apparent only after long-term follow-up. Metastases are usually to the liver and the peritoneal surfaces, and direct spread to adjacent tissues may occur. The treatment is surgical excision. Recently, a drug that specifically inhibits the kit-signal transduction pathway (imatinib) offers promising results in the treatment of patients with advanced metastatic GISTs.

MECHANICAL DISORDERS

RUPTURE OF THE STOMACH: This event is most commonly associated with blunt abdominal trauma from automobile accidents. **Spontaneous gastric perforation** typically occurs in middle-aged women and follows gastric overdistention, severe vomiting, labor and delivery, or the production of excess carbon dioxide after ingestion of sodium bicarbonate. Distention of the stomach during cardiopulmonary resuscitation has resulted in rupture of the stomach. The consequences of rupture and spontaneous perforation are disastrous, and early surgical repair is crucial for survival.

VOLVULUS OF THE STOMACH: This rare condition refers to torsion of the stomach upon itself. Severe abdominal pain, upper gastrointestinal obstruction, and shock accompany interruption of blood flow and blockage of the lumen. A gastric tumor or pressure from an extragastric mass may warp the anatomy of the stomach and allow it to twist. Nasogastric decompression and surgical repair are the usual treatment.

DIVERTICULA OF THE STOMACH: These outpouchings of the gastric wall are rare, developing after prolonged stress from tumors, ulcers, gastritis, and surgery. Diverticula in the cardia are not associated with such conditions; they presumably result from congenital weakness of the wall or perhaps unusual intraluminal pressure at this site. Patients are either asymptomatic or complain of nonspecific symptoms. Hemorrhage and perforation are uncommon complications.

BEZOARS

Bezoars are foreign bodies in the stomach of animals and humans that are composed of food or hair that has been altered by the digestive process.

PHYTOBEZOAR: These vegetable concretions are unusual in the normal stomach, except in persons who eat many persimmons or swallow unchewed bubble gum. Phytobezoars are usually found in persons with conditions that cause delayed gastric emptying, such as peripheral neuropathy of diabetes or gastric cancer, and in persons undergoing therapy with anticholinergic agents.

In the past few decades, phytobezoars have been found principally in patients who display delayed gastric emptying and hypochlorhydria after partial gastrectomy, particularly when the surgery has included vagotomy. Plant bezoars contain vegetable or fruit fibers. Most patients with persimmon bezoars have bleeding from an associated gastric ulcer.

The preferred treatment of phytobezoars is chemical attack with cellulase; in some cases, manual disruption by endoscopic techniques, including jets of water, has been successful. However, enzymatic therapy is usually not effective for persimmon bezoars, and surgery is required.

TRICHOBEZOAR: This mass is a hairball within a gelatinous matrix; it is usually seen in long-haired girls or young women who eat their own hair as a nervous habit. Such a bezoar may grow by accretion to form a complete cast of the stomach, reaching a size of up to 3 kg (Fig. 13-28). Strands of hair may extend into the bowel as far as the transverse colon, the so-called *Rapunzel syndrome*.

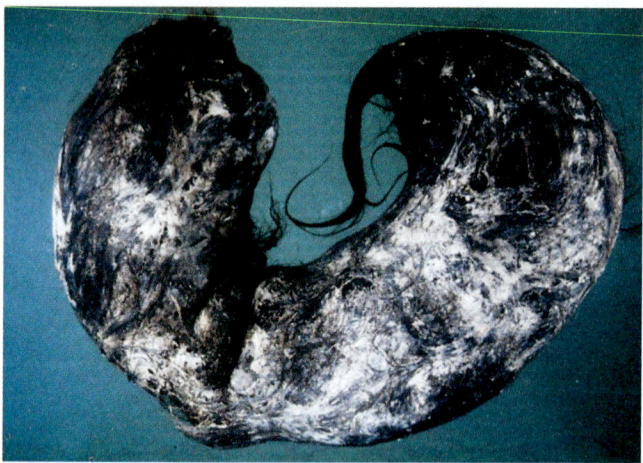

FIGURE 13-28
Trichobezoar (hairball). A mass of hair in a gelatinous matrix forms a cast of the stomach.

The Small Intestine

ANATOMY

Early in development, the intestinal tract begins as a tube that joins the stomach to the cloaca. This tube progressively elongates, and its cephalic portion becomes the segment that extends from the distal duodenum to the proximal ileum. The more caudal portion develops into the distal ileum and the proximal two thirds of the transverse colon. The vitelline duct, which connects the primitive duct with the yolk sac, may persist as a Meckel diverticulum. To achieve the final position of the intestine, the fetal gut undergoes a complex series of rotations.

The small intestine extends from the pylorus to the ileocecal valve and, depending on the tone of its muscle, measures from 3.5 to 6.5 m in length. It is divided into three regions:

1. **The duodenum** extends to the ligament of Treitz.
2. **The jejunum** is the proximal 40% of the remainder of the small intestine.
3. **The ileum** is the distal 60%.

The entire length of the small intestine, which is disposed in redundant loops, is movable, except for the duodenum, which is almost entirely retroperitoneal and therefore fixed.

The C-shaped duodenum surrounds the head of the pancreas and receives the biliary drainage of the liver and the pancreatic secretions through the common bile duct at the ampulla of Vater. The distal duodenum becomes invested by mesentery and merges with the jejunum at the ligament of Treitz. The proximity of the duodenum to its neighbors means that it may be affected by disorders such as cancer of the pancreas and cholecystoduodenal fistulas. Conversely, duodenal ulcers may penetrate into the pancreas or liver. There is no demarcation between the jejunum and ileum, which merge gradually. The wall of the jejunum is thicker and its lumen wider than that of the ileum.

The plicae circularis, the spiral folds that consist of mucosa and submucosa, are most prominent in the distal duodenum and proximal jejunum, usually disappearing in the terminal ileum. **Peyer patches** are lymphoid aggregates in the submucosa measuring up to 3 cm in diameter. They are located in the antimesenteric aspect of the distal half of the ileum. The ileocecal valve is not a true valve but rather a muscular sphincter that regulates the flow of intestinal contents into the cecum.

The duodenum is served by the pancreaticoduodenal branch of the hepatic artery, which arises from the celiac artery. The jejunum and ileum are supplied by the superior mesenteric artery (a branch of the aorta), which is arranged in arcades in the mesentery, thereby providing abundant collateral circulation in its distal reaches. The veins draining the small intestine empty into the portal venous system. The lymphatic channels of the duodenum drain to the portal and pyloric lymph nodes; those of the jejunum and ileum communicate with the mesenteric lymph nodes. The lymphatics of the terminal ileum empty into the ileocolic nodes. The small intestine is innervated by sympathetic fibers from the celiac plexus and ganglia and by parasympathetic fibers from the vagus nerve. The wall of the small intestine is composed of four layers: the mucosa, the submucosa, the muscularis, and the serosa. In the retroperitoneal duodenum, however, only the anterior wall is covered by a serosa.

SEROSA AND MUSCULARIS PROPRIA: The serosa consists of loose connective tissue bounded by a single layer of mesothelial cells. The muscularis propria has an outer longitudinal layer and an inner circular layer, both of which function in a coordinated manner to propel the intestinal contents by peristalsis.

SUBMUCOSA: This region consists of vascularized connective tissue and a few scattered lymphocytes, plasma cells, and macrophages, with an occasional mast cell and eosinophil. In the duodenum, the submucosa is occupied by the Brunner glands, branched structures that contain mucous and serous cells. These secrete mucus and bicarbonate, which protect the duodenal mucosa from peptic ulceration. The lymphatic and venous capillaries of the mucosa drain into a highly developed system of lymphatic and venous plexuses in the submucosa. *The myenteric nerve plexus of Auerbach,* which lies between the two layers of the muscularis, and *Meissner plexus* in the submucosa are interconnected.

MUCOSA: The distinctive feature of the intestinal mucosa is its arrangement in villi, fingerlike projections 0.5 to 1 mm in length that expand the absorptive area enormously. The macroscopic structure of the villi varies in different regions of the small intestine. In the proximal duodenum, the villi tend to be broad and blunted, whereas in the distal duodenum and proximal jejunum, they have a more slender, leaf-shaped appearance. Shorter, finger-shaped villi are the rule in the distal jejunum and ileum.

The villi are composed of a columnar epithelium resting on a basement membrane, a lamina propria, and a muscularis mucosae, which separates the mucosa from the submucosa. The connective tissue of the lamina propria forms the core of the villus and surrounds the crypts of Lieberkuhn at the base of the villi. The normal lamina propria is home to a variety of mesenchymal cells, including lymphocytes, plasma cells, and macrophages. Plasma cells in this location principally secrete immunoglobulin A (IgA) into the intestinal lumen or the lamina propria itself. Occasional eosinophils and mast cells are scattered throughout. A few smooth muscle cells and fibroblasts are also present. The cellular composition of the lamina propria reflects its role in protecting against invasion by bacteria that may penetrate the mucosa and segregating foreign material that breaches the mucosa.

Some IgA is produced by plasma cells in the lamina propria as a dimer that diffuses through the basement membrane of the crypt. IgA then reaches the basal or lateral surface of the epithelial cell, where it combines with the secretory component produced by that cell. The resulting *secretory IgA* molecule is taken up by the epithelial cell and secreted into the lumen. Secretory IgA, which is more resistant to proteolysis than is serum IgA, binds food antigens and prevents bacterial adherence to the intestinal epithelial cells. Moreover, IgA can neutralize bacterial toxins and inhibit the replication and mucosal penetration of viruses.

Lymphoid nodules (MALT) are scattered throughout the mucosa and aggregate into visible Peyer patches. The columnar epithelial cells of the villi are principally absorptive, whereas those lining the crypts are the source of cell renewal and secretion.

Absorptive cells, or enterocytes (see Fig. 13-1), are the principal lining cells of the intestinal villi. The villi also exhibit a few goblet and endocrine cells. Enterocytes are tall and display basally situated nuclei. Numerous microvilli extend from the surface of these cells into the lumen, thereby hugely increasing the absorptive surface. The plasma membrane of the microvilli is covered by a glycocalyx (fuzzy coat) produced by the absorptive cell. Disaccharidases and peptidases reside in this glycocalyx. Certain receptors, such as that for the intrinsic factor–vitamin B_{12} complex in the ileum, are also present in the membrane–glycocalyx complex. The cytoplasm immediately beneath the microvilli contains a network of actin microfilaments, termed the *terminal web*. These filaments, which are also associated with myosin and other contractile proteins, insert into the core of the microvilli and presumably serve as a contractile apparatus. The lateral borders of adjacent plasma membranes form tight junctions that are impermeable to macromolecules but permit passive transport of small molecules by the paracellular route. Absorbed material is transported from the epithelial cell into the intercellular space between absorptive cells through the lateral or basal plasma membranes. It then penetrates the basement membrane, traverses the lamina propria, and enters a capillary or a lymphatic channel.

Four cell types are recognized in the crypts:

- **Paneth cells** at the base of the crypts are similar to the zymogen cells of the pancreas and salivary glands that are actively engaged in exocrine secretion. Within Paneth cells, eosinophilic secretory granules fill a basophilic cytoplasm. These cells play a role in mucosal defense, as evidenced by the presence of lysozyme, anti-microbial products, including peptides called *crypt defensins* (cryptdins), and CD95 ligand, which is a member of the tumor necrosis factor (TNF) family of cytokines.
- **Goblet cells** of the lateral walls of the crypts are flask shaped and filled with mucus granules. They are similar in structure and function to goblet cells elsewhere and contain neutral and acid mucins.
- **Endocrine cells,** both argentaffin and argyrophilic, appear inverted, with an apical nucleus and basal granules. The basal location of the granules implies that they are secreted into the lamina propria rather than the lumen. These cells produce numerous gastrointestinal hormones and peptides, including gastrin, secretin, cholecystokinin, glucagon, VIP, and serotonin. The secretion of such hormones in response to appropriate stimuli is presumed to regulate many gastrointestinal functions. As in other tissues, primary tumors derived from these cells often exhibit striking hormone secretion.
- **Undifferentiated cells** are located in the lateral walls of the crypts and are interspersed between the Paneth cells at their bases. They are the most numerous cells of the crypts. Small glycoprotein secretory granules are grouped in the apical cytoplasm of some of the undifferentiated cells. These cells function as the reserve cells from which all the other mucosal cells are renewed, and thus mitoses are numerous among them.

Cell renewal in the small intestine is limited to the crypts, where undifferentiated cells divide. The newly formed cells migrate up the villus, where they terminally differentiate into absorptive cells and goblet cells and eventually undergo apoptosis or slough into the lumen at the tip of the villus. Their absorptive capacity is maximal when the cells reach the upper third of the villus. The mucosal epithelium of the small intestine is replaced within a period of 4 to 7 days. This rapid cell proliferation explains why the intestinal epithelium is particularly sensitive to radiation and chemotherapeutic agents.

CONGENITAL DISORDERS

Atresia and Stenosis Cause Neonatal Intestinal Obstruction

ATRESIA: Atresia is defined as a complete occlusion of the intestinal lumen, which may be manifested as (1) a thin intraluminal diaphragm, (2) blind proximal and distal sacs joined by a cord, or (3) disconnected blind ends. One fourth of atresias are associated with meconium ileus, and cystic fibrosis is discovered in one tenth of the cases.

STENOSIS: This abnormality is an incomplete stricture of the small intestine, which narrows but does not occlude, the lumen. Stenosis may also be caused by an incomplete diaphragm. Although the condition is usually symptomatic in infancy, cases in middle-aged adults have been recorded.

One fourth of mothers of fetuses with high intestinal atresia develop polyhydramnios during the last trimester, presumably because the fetus does not swallow amniotic fluid. Intestinal atresia or stenosis is diagnosed on the basis of persistent vomiting of bile-containing fluid within the first day of life. Meconium is not passed. The obstructed fetal intestine is dilated and filled with fluid, a condition detectable with imaging techniques. Surgical correction is usually successful, but coexistent anomalies often complicate the course.

Duplications

Gastrointestinal duplications (enteric cysts), which may occur from the esophagus to the anus, are spherical or tubular structures attached to the alimentary tract. They may be seen as cystic structures or may communicate with the lumen of the gastrointestinal tract. Intestinal duplications are most common in the ileum and less so in the jejunum. The duplications have a smooth muscle wall and an epithelium of the gastrointestinal type. Communicating duplications are often lined by gastric mucosa, a situation that may lead to peptic ulceration, bleeding, or perforation.

Meckel Diverticulum Causes Bleeding, Obstruction, and Perforation

Meckel diverticulum, caused by persistence of the vitelline duct, is an outpouching of the gut on the antimesenteric border of the ileum, 60 to 100 cm from the ileocecal valve in adults. It is the most common and the most clinically significant congenital anomaly of the small intestine (Fig. 13-29). Two thirds of patients are younger than 2 years.

Pathology: Meckel diverticulum is about 5 cm in length, with a diameter slightly less than that of the ileum but considerably larger than that of the appendix. A fibrous cord may hang freely from the apex of the diverticulum or may be attached to the umbilicus, and fistulas between Meckel diverticulum and the umbilicus have been described.

Meckel diverticulum is a true diverticulum in that it possesses all the coats of the normal intestine, and the mucosa is similar to that of the adjoining ileum. Most Meckel diverticula are asymptomatic and discovered only as incidental findings at laparotomy for other causes or at autopsy. Of the minority that becomes symptomatic, about half contain ectopic gastric, duodenal, pancreatic, biliary, or colonic tissue.

Clinical Features: Meckel diverticulum may lead to a number of complications.

- **Hemorrhage:** The most common complication is bleeding, which is responsible for half of all lower gastrointestinal hemorrhage in children. Bleeding results from **peptic ulceration** of the ileum adjacent to the ectopic gastric mucosa.
- **Intestinal obstruction:** The diverticulum may act as a lead point for **intussusception** and thereby cause intestinal obstruction. Obstruction can also be caused by **volvulus** around the fibrotic remnant of the vitelline duct.
- **Diverticulitis:** Inflammation of a Meckel diverticulum (i.e., diverticulitis) leads to symptoms indistinguishable from those of appendicitis. Thus, the surgeon who operates for acute appendicitis, but encounters a normal appendix, is well advised to search for a Meckel diverticulum.
- **Perforation:** Peptic ulceration, either in the diverticulum or in the ileum, may cause perforation, and lead to rapidly spreading peritonitis.
- **Fistula:** A fecal discharge from the umbilicus may be observed.

Malrotation

Defective intestinal rotation in fetal life leads to abnormal positions of the small intestine and colon, anomalous attachments, and bands. The clinical importance of such rotational anomalies lies in their propensity to cause catastrophic volvulus of the small and large intestine and incarceration of the bowel in an internal hernia.

Meconium Ileus Complicates Cystic Fibrosis

Cystic fibrosis often has as its earliest manifestation neonatal intestinal obstruction, caused by the accumulation of tenacious meconium in the small intestine. The abnormal consistency of the meconium reflects a deficiency in pancreatic enzymes and high viscosity of the intestinal mucus. Usually the distal ileum is contracted beyond the obstruction, whereas the midileum proximal to the inspissated meconium is dilated. In half of affected infants, meconium ileus is complicated by (1) volvulus, (2) perforation with meconium peritonitis, or (3) intestinal atresia. Meconium ileus must be differentiated from the distal intestinal obstruction syndrome associated with cystic fibrosis, in which a small plug of meconium in the distal colon may eventually be passed, thereby relieving the obstruction.

Successful treatment of meconium ileus may be accomplished by means of a hypertonic enema containing a detergent. Complicated meconium ileus always requires surgical intervention.

INFECTIONS

Bacterial Diarrhea Remains a Cause of Death Worldwide

Despite advances in the identification of organisms, antibiotic therapy, and fluid and electrolyte replacement, infec-

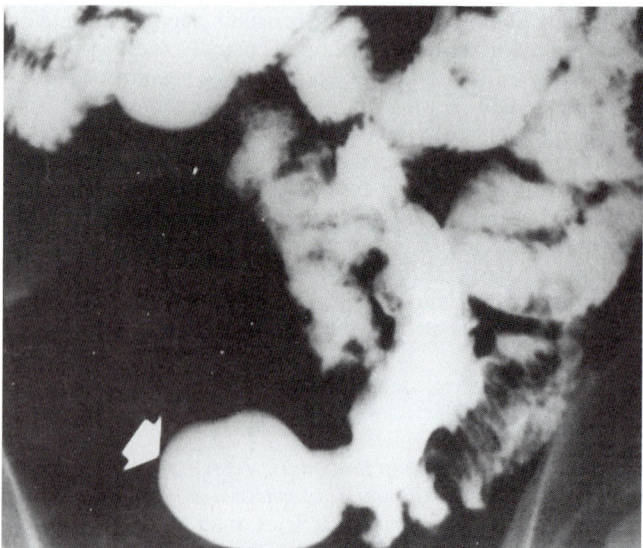

FIGURE 13-29
Meckel diverticulum. A contrast radiograph of the small intestine shows a barium-filled diverticulum of the ileum *(arrow)*.

tious diarrhea still causes many deaths worldwide. This is particularly true in underdeveloped countries and in infants. The normal small bowel has few microorganisms (usually <10^4/mL), mostly aerobic bacilli such as lactobacilli. These organisms travel in the food stream and ordinarily do not colonize the small intestine. Infectious diarrheal states are caused by colonization with bacteria such as toxigenic strains of *Escherichia coli* and *Vibrio cholerae*.

The most significant factor in infectious diarrhea is increased intestinal secretion, stimulated by bacterial toxins and enteric hormones. Decreased absorption and increased peristaltic activity contribute less to the diarrhea.

The colon harbors an abundant bacterial flora, with a concentration seven orders of magnitude greater than that of the small intestine. In the colon, anaerobic bacteria (e.g., *Bacteroides* and *Clostridium* species) outnumber aerobic organisms by a factor of 1000. With the more rapid transit of intestinal contents during a diarrheal episode, the flora is shifted to a more aerobic population, including *E. coli*, *Klebsiella*, and *Proteus*. Moreover, the offending organisms themselves become conspicuous, and pathogens of the small intestine such as *V. cholerae* may be the major isolate in the stools.

The paucity of bacteria in the stomach and small intestine is accounted for by a number of protective mechanisms: (1) gastric acid production is inimical to bacterial growth, which explains the overgrowth of bacteria in the stomach in the presence of achlorhydria; (2) bile has antimicrobial activity; (3) the peristaltic propulsion of intestinal contents limits the time available for bacterial accumulation; (4) the normal flora secrete their own antimicrobial substances to maintain an ecological balance (indeed, treatment with broad-spectrum antibiotics alters the natural flora and allows overgrowth of ordinarily harmless organisms); and (5) the plasma cells of the lamina propria secrete IgA into the intestinal lumen.

The individual agents responsible for infectious diarrhea are discussed in Chapter 9. Here we only briefly review the major entities. The agents of infectious diarrhea are conveniently classified into toxigenic organisms, which produce diarrhea by elaborating toxins, adherent bacteria, and invasive bacteria.

Toxigenic Diarrhea

The prototypic organisms that produce diarrhea by secreting toxins are V. cholerae and toxigenic strains of E. coli. Toxigenic diarrhea is characterized by the following:

- Damage to the intestinal mucosa is minimal or absent.
- The organism remains on the mucosal surface, where it secretes its toxin.
- Fluid secreted into the small intestine causes watery diarrhea, which can lead to dehydration, particularly in the case of cholera.

Although many organisms have been isolated in so-called travelers' diarrhea, the most common pathogen in almost all studies is toxigenic *E. coli*.

Diarrhea Caused by Invasive Bacteria

Invasive bacteria, as their name implies, cause diarrhea by directly injuring the intestinal mucosa. Among these organisms, *Shigella*, *Salmonella*, and certain strains of *E. coli*, *Yersinia*, and *Campylobacter* are the most widely recognized. Invasive organisms tend to infect the distal ileum and colon, whereas toxigenic bacteria mainly involve the upper intestinal tract. The mechanism by which they produce diarrhea has not been clarified. Enterotoxins have been identified, but their role in causing diarrhea has not been established. Invasion of the mucosa by bacteria increases the synthesis of prostaglandins in the affected tissue, and inhibitors of prostaglandin synthesis seem to block fluid secretion. It is also possible that the damaged mucosa is unable to resorb fluid from the lumen.

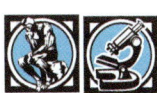 Pathogenesis and Pathology:

SHIGELLOSIS: Shigellosis principally affects the colon, although the terminal ileum is occasionally involved. Microscopically, a granular and hemorrhagic mucosa exhibits numerous shallow serpiginous ulcers. The inflammation, which is especially severe in the sigmoid colon and rectum, is usually superficial. In the early stage, the accumulation of neutrophils in damaged crypts (crypt abscesses) is similar to that in ulcerative colitis, and the lymphoid follicles of the mucosa break down to form ulcers. As the infection recedes, the ulcers heal and the mucosa returns to normal.

TYPHOID FEVER: Typhoid fever (*Salmonella* enteritis) is today uncommon in the industrialized world but still presents a problem in underdeveloped countries. Necrosis of lymphoid tissue, principally in the terminal ileum, leads to scattered ulcers. Infection of Peyer patches results in oval ulcers, in which the longer dimension is in the long axis of the intestine. Occasionally, lymphoid follicles in the large bowel or the appendix are ulcerated. The base of the ulcer is composed of black necrotic tissue mixed with fibrin.

Microscopically, the early lesions of typhoid fever contain large basophilic macrophages filled with typhoid bacilli, erythrocytes, and necrotic debris. Necrosis of lymphoid follicles becomes confluent, and mucosal ulceration follows. Similar lymphoid hyperplasia and necrosis are seen in the regional lymph nodes. Healing of the ulcers is complete within a week of the acute symptoms and leaves little fibrosis or other sequelae. **Intestinal hemorrhage and perforation,** principally in the ileum, are the most feared complications of typhoid fever and tend to occur in the third week and during convalescence.

NONTYPHOIDAL SALMONELLOSIS: Formerly known as *paratyphoid fever*, this enteritis is caused by *Salmonella* strains other than *S. typhi* and is generally a far less serious illness than typhoid fever. The principal target is the ileum, although minor involvement of the colon may also take place. The organisms invade the mucosa, which shows mild ulceration, edema, and infiltration with neutrophils. Hematogenous dissemination from the intestine may carry the infection to bones, joints, and meninges. Interestingly, there seems to be a relation between sickle cell anemia and *Salmonella* osteomyelitis, presumably because phagocytosis of the products of hemolysis prevents further cellular ingestion of the *Salmonella* organisms and allows their dissemination through the bloodstream.

ENTEROINVASIVE AND ENTEROHEMORRHAGIC STRAINS OF *E. COLI*: These organisms are uncommon causes of a bloody diarrhea that resemble shigellosis. Certain strains of *E. coli*, particularly serotype 0157:H7, produce *Shigella*-like toxins, but the role of these proteins in the pathogenesis of the enterocolitis is not understood. Serotype 0157:H7 has also been implicated in the pathogenesis of the hemolytic–uremic syndrome in children.

YERSINIA ENTEROCOLITIS: *Yersinia enterocolitica* and *Y. pseudotuberculosis* are transmitted by pets or contaminated food, and infection is most common in young children. *Yersinia* infection causes diarrhea, cramps, and fever and lasts 1 to 3 weeks. The disease is characterized by hyperplasia of Peyer patches, with acute ulceration of the overlying mucosa. The fibrinopurulent exudate that covers the ulcers often contains many organisms.

In addition to causing enterocolitis, *Yersinia* causes acute mesenteric adenitis and pain in the right lower quadrant. Infected children have undergone laparotomy because of a mistaken diagnosis of appendicitis. Microscopically the lymph nodes show epithelioid granulomas with central necrotic zones in the case of infection with *Y. pseudotuberculosis*. The ileum and appendix may contain similar granulomas, causing an appearance that has been mistaken for Crohn disease.

Adults, who are less susceptible to infection with *Yersinia* than are children, have an acute diarrhea, often followed within a few weeks by erythema nodosum, erythema multiforme, or polyarthritis. Patients with chronic debilitating diseases may develop a fatal *Yersinia* bacteremia that is resistant to antibiotic treatment. Interestingly, persons with thalassemia have a propensity for *Y. enterocolitica* infection.

CAMPYLOBACTER JEJUNI: Infection with *C. jejuni* is now recognized as one of the most important causes of bacterial diarrhea. Some investigators have reported a higher incidence of *Campylobacter* than of nontyphoidal *Salmonella* and *Shigella* infections in the United States, and in one survey from Great Britain, half of all bacterial diarrhea was caused by *Campylobacter*. Humans are involved mainly by contact with infected domestic animals or through ingestion of poorly cooked or contaminated food. Adults usually recover from the diarrheal illness in less than 1 week.

Food Poisoning

Infectious agents can produce diarrhea by elaborating enterotoxins in contaminated food that is then ingested.

STAPHYLOCOCCUS AUREUS: This widespread bacterium is a common cause of food poisoning. Symptoms result from the ingestion of food contaminated with strains of *Staphylococcus* that produce an exotoxin that damages the epithelium of the gastrointestinal tract. Within 6 hours of the ingestion of tainted food, severe vomiting and abdominal cramps occur, often followed by diarrhea. Most patients recover in 1 to 2 days.

CLOSTRIDIUM PERFRINGENS: This bacterium elaborates an enterotoxin that causes vomiting and diarrhea. Although the organism is anaerobic, it can tolerate exposure to air for as long as 3 days. Maximal activity of the clostridial enterotoxin is in the ileum. In most cases, watery diarrhea and severe abdominal pain that begin 8 to 24 hours after ingestion of the contaminated food last only about 1 day.

Viral Gastroenteritis Is Caused by Diverse Agents

ROTAVIRUS: Infection with this virus is a common cause of infantile diarrhea and accounts for about half of the cases of acute diarrhea in hospitalized children younger than 2 years. Rotavirus has been demonstrated in duodenal biopsy specimens and is associated with injury to the surface epithelium and impaired intestinal absorption for periods of up to 2 months.

NORWALK VIRUSES: These agents account for one third of the epidemics of viral gastroenteritis in the United States. The virus targets the upper small intestine, where it causes patchy mucosal lesions and malabsorption. Vomiting and diarrhea are usual, but the symptoms resolve within 2 days.

Other viruses that have been implicated as etiological agents of infective diarrhea include echovirus, coxsackievirus, cytomegalovirus, adenovirus, and coronavirus.

Intestinal Tuberculosis Occurs after Ingesting the Bacillus

Historically an important disease, gastrointestinal tuberculosis is now uncommon in industrialized countries, although it is still a problem in underdeveloped areas of the world. At one time, a large proportion of intestinal tuberculosis involved infection with *Mycobacterium bovis*, which was principally transmitted by contaminated milk. However, the control of tuberculosis in dairy herds and the pasteurization of milk have made infection with this organism a curiosity.

Most cases of intestinal tuberculosis are caused either by the ingestion of bacteria in food or by the swallowing of infectious sputum. After it is ingested, the tubercle bacillus, protected from digestion by its waxy capsule, passes into the small bowel. The bacterium then establishes a locus of infection, usually (90% of patients) in the ileocecal region, where lymphoid tissue is abundant. Infection also occurs in the colon, jejunum, appendix, rectum, and duodenum, in that order of frequency.

 Pathology: The macroscopic presentation of intestinal tuberculosis is divided into three categories:

- **Ulcerative intestinal tuberculosis:** This type is seen in more than half of patients and is characterized by one or more circular ulcers of varying size in the transverse

plane of the bowel. As the ulcers heal, reactive fibrosis may cause a circumferential ("napkin ring") stricture of the bowel lumen. Mesenteric lymph nodes are typically enlarged and display caseous necrosis.
- **Hypertrophic intestinal tuberculosis:** In pure form, this variety is uncommon (10% of patients). It affects the ileocecal region or the colon, which exhibits an exuberant inflammatory and fibroblastic reaction throughout the thickness of the wall. Protrusion of the hypertrophic lesion into the bowel lumen may mimic carcinoma.
- **Ulcerohypertrophic intestinal tuberculosis:** This variant is seen in about one third of patients and combines the features of the ulcerative and hypertrophic forms. Microscopically, typical tuberculous granulomas are found in all layers of the bowel wall, particularly in Peyer patches and lymphoid follicles, and in the mesenteric lymph nodes. Seen at autopsy or in surgical specimens, old tuberculous strictures are difficult to distinguish from other causes of stricture, such as ischemic enterocolitis or Crohn disease.

 Clinical Features: Almost all patients with intestinal tuberculosis complain of chronic abdominal pain, and about two thirds have a palpable abdominal mass, usually in the right lower quadrant. Malnutrition, weight loss, fever, and weakness are common. Complications of intestinal tuberculosis include obstruction, fistulas, perforation, and abscess.

Intestinal Fungi Produce Opportunistic Infections

The gastrointestinal tract is not normally a hospitable environment for fungi. The number of commensal organisms is miniscule, and such agents are restricted to yeasts and anaerobic actinomycetes. **Therefore, fungal infection of the gastrointestinal tract occurs almost exclusively in immunocompromised persons.** Suppression of the normal bacterial flora by antibiotics also favors fungal growth. Under these circumstances, the most common mycosis is caused by *Candida*. Other fungi, including *Histoplasma* and *Mucor,* are occasionally found.

 Pathology: Candidiasis and mucormycosis typically cause mucosal erosions; these may progress to larger ulcers that are surrounded by hemorrhage and necrosis. The inflammation is characteristically neutrophilic, and there may be remarkably little reaction to the fungi because of immunosuppression. Mucormycosis often exhibits invasion of blood vessels with thrombosis and infarction, but hematogenous dissemination from the intestine is rare. Disseminated histoplasmosis may involve the bowel, where it causes elevated plaques that ulcerate and may even perforate.

Parasites of the Small Intestine

Parasitic diseases of the small bowel are discussed in detail in Chapter 9 and summarized in Figure 13-30. These parasites include (1) **protozoa,** such as *Giardia lamblia, Coccidia* species, and cryptosporidia; (2) **nematodes (roundworms)** such as *Ascaris, Strongyloides,* and hookworms; and (3) **flatworms.** The flatworms are divided into tapeworms (cestodes), which include *Diphyllobothrium latum, Taenia solium, Taenia saginata,* and *Hymenolepis nana.* Flukes (trematodes) include various schistosomes and the giant intestinal fluke *Fasciolopsis buski.* In addition, trichinosis has an intestinal phase during which vomiting, diarrhea, and colic mimic acute food poisoning or bacterial enteritis.

VASCULAR DISEASES

Decreased blood flow to the intestines from any cause can lead to ischemic bowel disease. Analogous to coronary heart disease, there is a spectrum of manifestations. The most common type of ischemic bowel disease is acute intestinal ischemia, which is associated with injury ranging from mucosal necrosis to transmural infarction of the bowel. Chronic intestinal ischemic syndromes are less common and generally require the severe compromise of two or more major arteries, usually by atherosclerosis.

Acute Intestinal Ischemia Mostly Involves the Superior Mesenteric Artery

 Pathogenesis:

ARTERIAL OCCLUSION: The sudden occlusion of a large artery by thrombosis or embolization leads to infarction of the small bowel before collateral circulation comes into play. Depending on the size of the artery, infarction may be segmental or may lead to gangrene of virtually the entire small bowel (Fig. 13-31). Occlusive intestinal infarction is most often caused by embolic or thrombotic occlusion of the superior mesenteric artery. A lesser number are the result of vasculitis, which often involves small arteries. In addition to intrinsic vascular lesions, volvulus, intussusception, and incarceration of the intestine in a hernial sac may all lead to arterial as well as venous occlusion.

NONOCCLUSIVE INTESTINAL ISCHEMIA: Intestinal ischemic necrosis in which no acute vascular occlusion is evident is today more common than the occlusive type. Nonocclusive intestinal infarction may be extensive and is seen in hypoxic patients with reduced cardiac output from shock of a variety of causes including hemorrhage, sepsis, and acute myocardial infarction. Shock leads to redistribution of blood flow to the brain and other vital organs. In addition, patients in shock often receive α-adrenergic agents, which may fur-

CATEGORY	ORGANISMS	TRANSMISSION
PROTOZOON	Giardia	Fecal-oral
ROUND WORMS (NEMATODES)	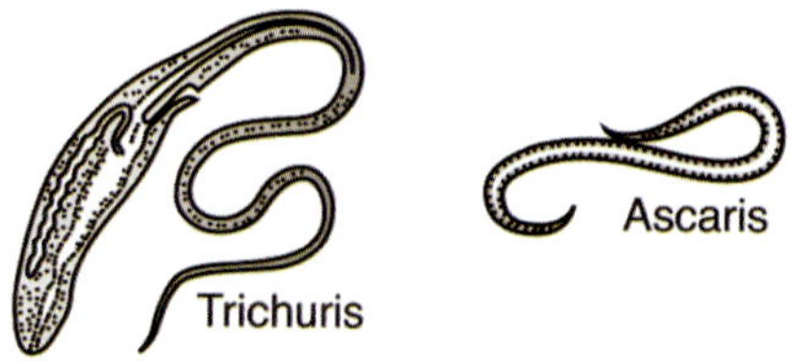 Trichuris, Ascaris	Fecal-oral
ROUND WORMS (NEMATODES)	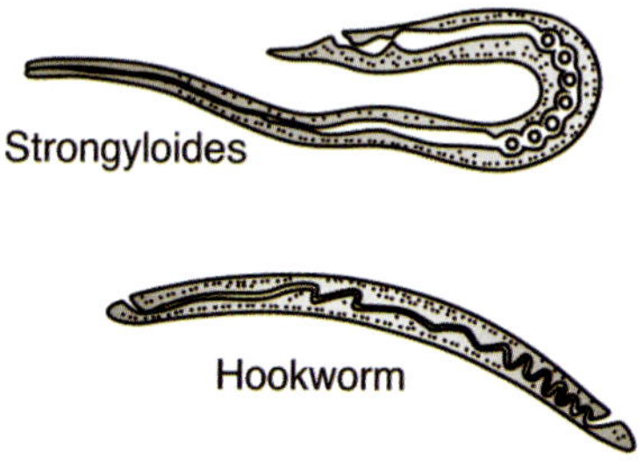 Strongyloides, Hookworm	Free living larvae in soil penetrate skin
TAPEWORMS (CESTODES)	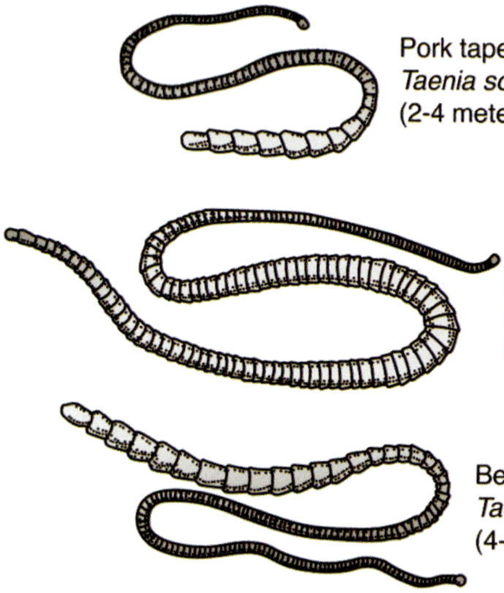 Pork tapeworm *Taenia solium* (2-4 meters); Fish tapeworm *Diphyllobothrium latum* (3-10 meters); Beef tapeworm *Taenia saginata* (4-8 meters)	Undercooked or raw flesh containing cysts
TAPEWORMS (CESTODES)	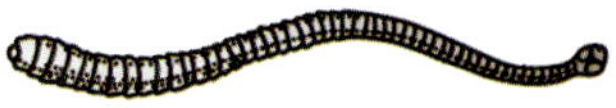 Human tapeworm *Hymenolepis nana* (0.5-5 meters)	Fecal-oral
FLUKE (TREMATODE)	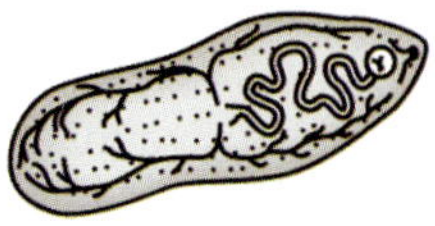 *Fasciolopsis buski*	Fecal-oral (with intermediate host)

FIGURE 13-30
Parasites of the small bowel.

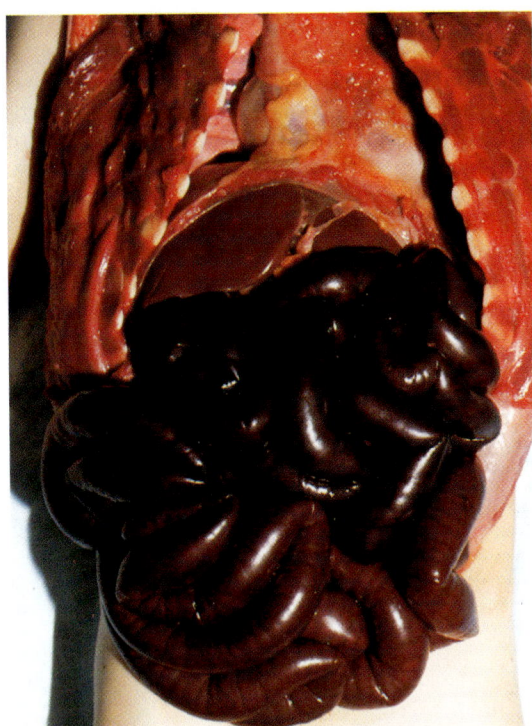

FIGURE 13-31
Infarct of the small bowel. This infant died after an episode of intense abdominal pain and shock. Autopsy demonstrated volvulus of the small bowel that had occluded the superior mesenteric artery. The entire small bowel is dilated, gangrenous, and hemorrhagic.

ther shunt blood away from the intestine. The drastically lowered perfusion pressure in the arterioles leads to their collapse, thereby aggravating the ischemia.

THROMBOSIS OF THE MESENTERIC VEINS: This cause of intestinal ischemia occurs under a variety of conditions, including hypercoagulable states, stasis, and inflammation (pylephlebitis). Almost all thromboses affect the superior mesenteric vein, and only 5% of cases involve the inferior mesenteric vein. The collateral flow in the distribution of the superior mesenteric vein usually suffices to preclude infarction of the intestine.

 Pathology: Infarcted bowel is edematous and diffusely purple. The demarcation between infarcted bowel and normal tissue is usually sharp, although venous occlusion may lead to a more diffuse appearance. Extensive hemorrhage is seen in the mucosa and submucosa. Hemorrhage is prominent especially in the case of venous occlusion (e.g., mesenteric vein thrombosis). The mucosal surface shows irregular white sloughs, the wall becomes thin and distended, and bubbles of gas (pneumatosis) may be present in the bowel wall and mesenteric veins. The serosal surface is cloudy and covered by an inflammatory exudate.

The dysfunction of smooth muscle interferes with peristalsis and leads to *adynamic ileus*, a condition in which the bowel proximal to the lesion is dilated and filled with fluid. Intestinal organisms may pass through the damaged wall and cause **peritonitis** or **septicemia**.

In nonocclusive intestinal ischemia, the principal lesion is restricted initially to the mucosa. Mucosal changes range from foci of dilated capillaries with a few extravasated erythrocytes to severe hemorrhagic necrosis and bleeding into the lumen. If the patient survives the episode of hypoperfusion, the bowel may be completely repaired, or it may heal with granulation tissue and fibrosis, with eventual **stricture formation.**

 Clinical Features: In mesenteric artery occlusion, the abrupt onset of abdominal pain is virtually invariable. Bloody diarrhea, hematemesis, and shock are common, and in untreated cases, perforation is frequent. **As the infarction progresses, systemic manifestations become more severe (multiple organ dysfunction syndrome).** In extensive infarction, as a result of occlusion in the proximal portion of the superior mesenteric artery, almost the entire small bowel must be resected, a situation that is not compatible with ultimate survival.

Chronic Intestinal Ischemia Leads to Recurrent Abdominal Pain

Atherosclerotic narrowing of the major splanchnic arteries results in chronic intestinal ischemia. As in the heart, it causes intermittent abdominal pain, termed *intestinal (abdominal) angina*. Characteristically, the pain begins within a half hour of eating and lasts for a few hours. Many cases of frank infarction of the intestine are preceded by abdominal angina. Recurrent abdominal pain has also been ascribed to pressure on the celiac axis from surrounding structures and has been labeled the *celiac compression syndrome*.

 Pathology: Chronic ischemia of the small bowel may lead to fibrosis and the formation of a stricture. Ischemic strictures of the small bowel, which may be single or multiple, produce intestinal obstruction or, occasionally, malabsorption resulting from stasis and bacterial overgrowth. These strictures are concentric, and the mucosa of this region is atrophic and often exhibits one or more small ulcers. The submucosa is thickened and fibrotic and displays granulation tissue, which may extend into the muscular layers.

CROHN DISEASE

Crohn disease, a chronic inflammatory disorder of the bowel wall, can affect any region of the upper and lower gastrointestinal tract, but the right colon and ileocecal regions are the most commonly affected. Crohn disease is discussed below in the section on inflammatory bowel disease.

MALABSORPTION

Malabsorption is a general term used to describe a number of clinical conditions in which important nutrients are inadequately absorbed by the gastrointestinal tract. Although some nutrient absorption occurs in the stomach and colon, only absorption from the small intestine, mainly in the proximal portion, is clinically important. The two substances that are preferentially absorbed by the distal small intestine are bile salts and vitamin B_{12}.

Normal intestinal absorption is characterized by a luminal phase and an intestinal phase (Fig. 13-32). The **luminal phase,** consisting of those processes that occur within the lumen of the small intestine, alters the physicochemical state of the various nutrients such that they can be taken up by the absorptive cells in the small bowel epithelium. The **intestinal phase** includes those processes that occur in the cells and transport channels of the intestinal wall. Each phase includes several critical components, and derangement of one or more leads to impaired absorption.

In the luminal phase of intestinal absorption, **pancreatic enzymes** and **bile acids** must be secreted into the duodenal lumen in adequate amounts and in a normal physicochemical condition. Two additional factors are important for optimal activity of both pancreatic enzymes and bile salts: a normal and regulated flow of gastric contents into the duodenum and an appropriately high pH of the duodenal contents. Normal pancreatic enzyme excretion into the duodenum requires adequate pancreatic exocrine function and an unobstructed flow of pancreatic juice.

The supply of a normal quantity and quality of bile to the duodenum requires (1) adequate hepatocellular function, (2) unobstructed flow of bile, and (3) an intact enterohepatic circulation of bile salts. The enterohepatic circulation of bile begins with absorption of most of the intestinal bile salts from the distal ileum and ends with their excretion into the duodenum through the bile ducts. Normally, 95% of intestinal bile salts are recycled through the enterohepatic circulation, with the remaining 5% being excreted in the stools. The essential conditions for the normal functioning of the enterohepatic circulation are (1) normal intestinal microflora,

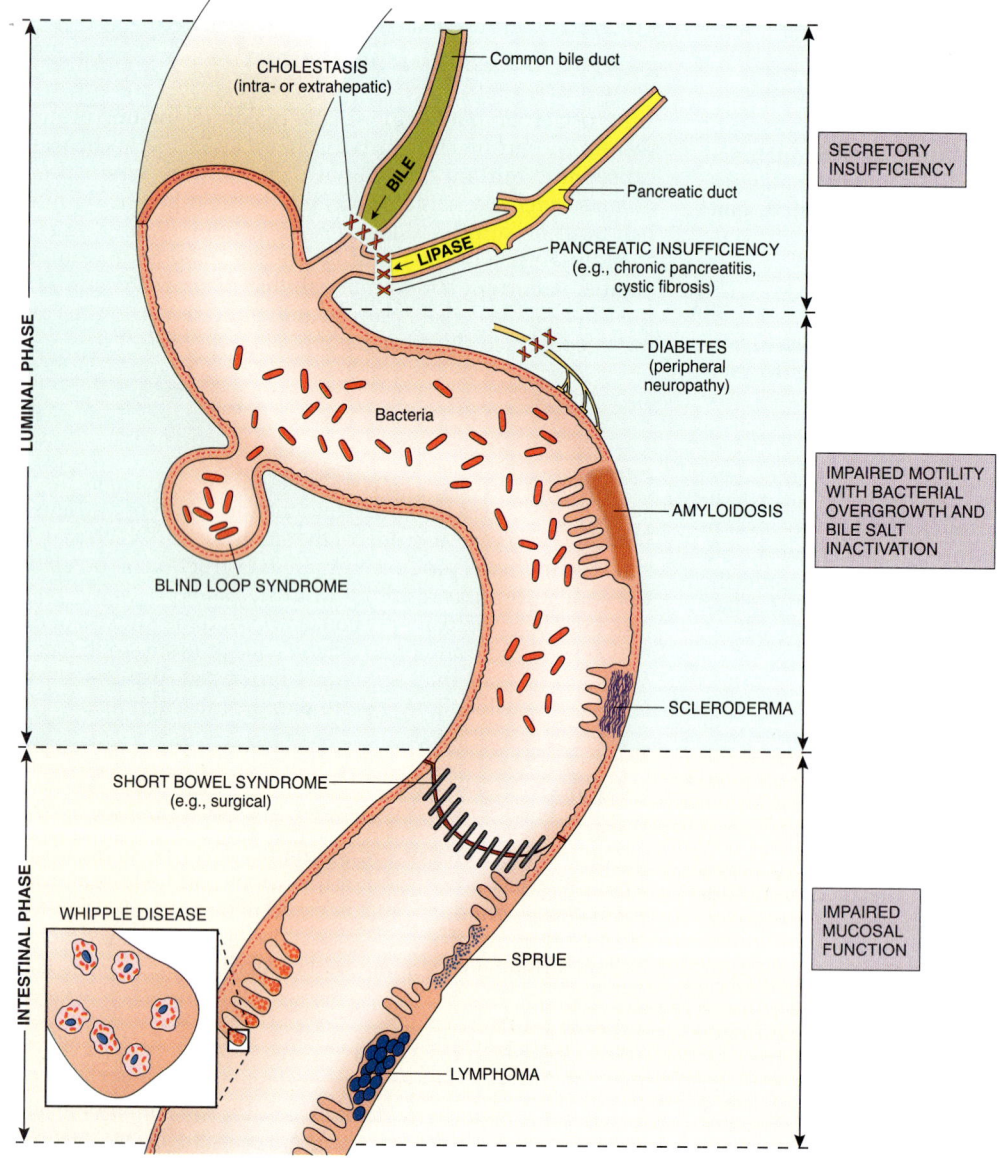

FIGURE 13-32
Causes of malabsorption

(2) normal ileal absorptive function, and (3) an unobstructed biliary system.

Luminal-Phase Malabsorption Often Reflects Insufficient Bile Acids

Interruption of the normal continuity of the distal stomach and duodenum occurs after gastroduodenal surgery (gastrectomy, antrectomy, pyloroplasty).

Pancreatic dysfunction can occur as a result of chronic pancreatitis, pancreatic carcinoma, or cystic fibrosis.

Deficient or ineffective bile salts may result from three possible causes:

- **Impaired excretion of bile** resulting from liver disease.
- **Bacterial overgrowth** from a disturbance in the motility of the gut. This condition is seen in such conditions as blind-loop syndrome, multiple diverticula of the small bowel, and muscular or neurogenic defects of the intestinal wall (e.g., amyloidosis, scleroderma, diabetic enteropathy). When gastrointestinal motility is defective, bile salts are deconjugated by the excess bacterial flora, after which they are ineffective in the process of micelle formation, which is essential for the normal absorption of monoglycerides and free fatty acids.
- **Deficient bile salts** as a consequence of the absence or bypass of the distal ileum caused by surgical excision, surgical anastomoses, fistulas, or ileal disease (e.g., Crohn disease, lymphoma).

Intestinal-Phase Malabsorption Frequently Reflects Specific Enzyme Defects or Impaired Transport

Although abnormalities in any one of the four components of the intestinal phase may cause malabsorption, some diseases affect more than one of these components. Figure 13-32 summarizes the major causes of malabsorption.

 Pathogenesis:

MICROVILLI: The intestinal disaccharidases and oligopeptidases are integrally bound to the microvillous membranes. Disaccharidases are essential for sugar absorption, because only monosaccharides can be absorbed by the intestinal epithelial cells. Oligopeptides and dipeptides may be absorbed by alternate mechanisms that do not require peptidases. Abnormal function of the microvilli may be primary, as in the primary disaccharidase deficiencies, or secondary, when there is damage to the villi, as in celiac disease (sprue). The various enzyme deficiencies (e.g., of lactase) are characterized by intolerance for the corresponding disaccharides.

ABSORPTIVE AREA: The considerable length of the small bowel and the amplification of its surface wall by the intestinal folds (valves of Kerkring) provide a large absorptive surface. If sufficiently severe, a diminution in this area results in malabsorption. The surface area may be diminished by (1) small bowel resection (short bowel syndrome), (2) gastrocolic fistula (bypassing the small intestine), or (3) mucosal damage due to a number of small intestinal diseases (celiac disease, tropical sprue, and Whipple disease).

METABOLIC FUNCTION OF THE ABSORPTIVE CELLS: For their subsequent transport to the circulation, nutrients within the absorptive cells depend on their metabolism within these cells. There, monoglycerides and free fatty acids are reassembled into triglycerides and coated with proteins (apoproteins) to form chylomicrons and lipoprotein particles. Specific metabolic dysfunction is seen in abetalipoproteinemia (associated with erythrocyte acanthocytosis), a disorder in which the absorptive cells cannot synthesize the apoprotein required for the assembly of lipoproteins and chylomicrons. Nonspecific damage to small intestinal epithelial cells occurs in celiac disease, tropical sprue, Whipple disease, and hyperacidity due to gastrinoma.

TRANSPORT: Nutrients are transported from the intestinal epithelium through the intestinal wall by way of blood capillaries and lymphatic vessels. Impaired transport of nutrients through these conduits is probably an important factor in the malabsorption associated with Whipple disease, intestinal lymphoma, and congenital lymphangiectasia.

 Clinical Features: Malabsorption may be either specific or generalized.

- *Specific or isolated malabsorption* refers to an identifiable molecular defect that causes malabsorption of a single nutrient. Examples of this group are the disaccharidase deficiencies (notably lactase deficiency) and deficiency of gastric intrinsic factor, which causes malabsorption of vitamin B_{12} and consequently pernicious anemia. Specific deficiency states may be manifested by anemia resulting from a deficiency of iron, folic acid, or vitamin B_{12} or a combination of these three. Patients may have a bleeding diathesis due to vitamin K deficiency, or malabsorption of vitamin D and calcium may lead to tetany, osteomalacia (in adults), or rickets (in children). In some persons, a deficiency of water-soluble vitamins of the B group may occur.
- *Generalized malabsorption* describes a condition in which the absorption of several or all major nutrient classes is impaired. This condition leads to generalized malnutrition. In adults, this is manifested by weight loss and sometimes cachexia; in children, it is expressed as "failure to thrive" with poor growth and weight gain.

Secondary effects of nonabsorbed or partially absorbed substances may lead to diarrhea. In disaccharidase deficiency, the unhydrolyzed sugars in the gut are metabolized by colonic bacteria to lactic acid, carbon dioxide, and water, a process that results in explosive fermentative diarrhea. In patients with ileal dysfunction, bile salts that are not absorbed pass into the colon and cause choleretic diarrhea because of the stimulation of colonic secretion.

Laboratory Evaluation Detects Specific Forms of Malabsorption

Laboratory tests are available to examine absorptive capacity. For example, disaccharidase deficiency is diagnosed by measurement of blood sugar after the oral administration of a standard amount of disaccharide, as in the **lactose-tolerance test,** or by measurement of the activity of disaccharidase in a small bowel biopsy specimen. Vitamin B_{12} absorption is assessed by the **Schilling test,** in which isotopically labeled vitamin B_{12} is administered orally and its blood level then determined. This test also helps to distinguish between malabsorption resulting from intrinsic-factor deficiency and other causes of vitamin B_{12} malabsorption.

In generalized malabsorption, there is almost always impaired absorption of dietary fat. Quantitative fecal fat analysis is the most reliable and sensitive test of overall digestive and absorptive function and serves as a standard for all other tests for malabsorption. Steatorrhea (fat in the stools) is the hallmark of generalized malabsorption, and the two terms are often used interchangeably.

A few of the tests currently in use for the evaluation of various causes of malabsorption merit mention.

- **D-Xylose Absorption:** Xylose is a 5-carbon sugar whose absorption does not require any of the components of the luminal phase. Blood levels and urinary excretion of this compound after ingestion of a defined amount thus serve as useful tests for the intestinal phase of absorption.
- **$^{14}CO_2$-cholyl-glycine breath test:** Measurement of $^{14}CO_2$ in exhaled air after oral administration of $^{14}CO_2$-cholylglycine is a test of bile salt absorption by the ileum. It is used in the diagnosis of the blind- or stagnant-loop syndrome (caused by bacterial overgrowth) and of ileal absorptive function. A newer test to detect bacterial overgrowth is the ^{14}C-xylose breath test.
- **Schilling test:** Originally devised for the diagnosis of pernicious anemia, the Schilling test has been modified for additional use as a test of ileal absorptive function, bacterial overgrowth, and pancreatic function.

Lactase Deficiency Causes Intolerance to Milk Products

The intestinal brush border contains disaccharidases that are important for the absorption of carbohydrates. As a prominent constituent of milk and many other dairy products, lactose is one of the most common disaccharides in the diet. Acquired lactase deficiency is a widespread disorder of carbohydrate absorption. Typically, symptoms of the disease begin in adolescence. Patients complain of abdominal distention, flatulence, and diarrhea after the ingestion of dairy products. Eliminating milk and its products from the diet relieves these symptoms. Diseases that injure the intestinal mucosa (e.g., celiac disease or radiation enteritis) may also lead to acquired lactase deficiency. Congenital lactase deficiency is rare but may be lethal if not recognized.

Celiac Disease Reflects an Immune Response to Gluten in Cereals

Celiac disease (celiac sprue, gluten-sensitive enteropathy) is a syndrome characterized by (1) generalized malabsorption; (2) small intestinal mucosal lesions; and (3) a prompt clinical and histopathological response to the withdrawal of gluten-containing foods from the diet.

Epidemiology: The disorder is worldwide and affects all ethnic groups. There is a slight female predominance, the sex ratio being 1.3:1. The malady may be seen at any time after the introduction of cereals into the diet. Most cases are diagnosed during childhood, although the disease may become clinically apparent for the first time as late as the seventh decade of life.

Pathogenesis: Genetic predisposition and gliadin exposure are crucial factors in the development of celiac disease.

ROLE OF CEREAL PROTEINS: Experiments on successfully treated, asymptomatic patients with celiac disease have shown that the ingestion or instillation of wheat, barley, or rye flour into the small intestine is followed by the clinical features and histopathological changes typical of celiac sprue. Other grains, such as rice and corn flour, do not have such an effect. Both the water-insoluble portion of wheat flour, **gluten,** and an alcoholic extract called **gliadin** have the same effect.

GENETIC FACTORS: The pathogenesis of celiac sprue involves the interplay of complex genetic factors and an abnormal immunological response to ingested cereal antigens. Overt celiac sprue and latent disease are frequent among family members. Concordance for celiac disease in first-degree relatives ranges between 8 and 18% and reaches 70% in monozygotic twins. About 90% of patients with celiac disease carry the class I histocompatibility antigen HLA-B8, and a comparable frequency has been reported for the class II HLA antigens DR8 and DQ2.

IMMUNOLOGICAL FACTORS: The intestinal lesion in celiac disease is characterized by damage to the epithelial cells and a marked increase in the number of T lymphocytes within the epithelium and of plasma cells in the lamina propria. Gliadin challenge of persons with treated celiac sprue stimulates local immunoglobulin synthesis.

A region of amino acid sequence homology has been found between α-gliadin and a protein of an adenovirus (serotype 12) that infects the human gastrointestinal tract. Most (90%) untreated patients with celiac disease have serological evidence of prior infection with this virus. Subsequent exposure of a genetically susceptible person to gluten-containing cereals might then stimulate an immunological reaction to gliadin bound to the surface of intestinal epithelial cells.

Antigliadin and antiendomysial antibodies in the serum are present in almost all patients with celiac disease, but their role in the pathogenesis of the disease remains to be established.

ASSOCIATION WITH DERMATITIS HERPETI-FORMIS: Celiac disease is occasionally associated with dermatitis herpetiformis, a vesicular skin disease that typically affects the extensor surfaces and the exposed parts of the body. In this disorder, subepidermal neutrophilic infiltration leads to local edema and blister formation. Deposits of IgA are detected in the region of the basement membrane. Almost all patients with dermatitis herpetiformis have a small bowel mucosal lesion similar to that of celiac disease, although only 10% have overt malabsorption. Treatment with a strict gluten-free diet is followed by improvement in both the gastrointestinal symptoms and the skin lesions. The histocompatibility antigen HLA-B8 is much more frequent in patients with dermatitis herpetiformis than in normal persons.

Malabsorption in celiac disease probably results from multiple factors, including reduced surface area of the intestinal mucosa (due to the blunting of villi and microvilli) and impaired intracellular metabolism within the damaged epithelial cells. A probable aggravating factor is secondary disaccharidase deficiency, related to damage to the microvilli. A hypothetical mechanism for the pathogenesis of celiac disease is presented in Figure 13-33.

 Pathology: A microscopic finding in small bowel biopsies that can precede the more characteristic findings is a lymphocytic infiltrate involving the crypts and surface epithelium within normal appearing villi. The hallmark of celiac disease is a flat mucosa, with (1) blunting or total disappearance of villi, (2) damaged epithelial cells on the mucosal surface with numerous intraepithelial lymphocytes (T cells), and (3) increased plasma cells in the lamina propria but not in the deeper layers (Fig. 13-34). The most severe histological abnormalities in untreated celiac disease usually occur in the duodenum and proximal jejunum. There is a progressive decrease in severity distally, and in some cases the ileal mucosa appears virtually normal. The clinical severity of the disease is related to the length of the affected intestine.

The total thickness of the mucosa may not be decreased, because lengthening of the crypts compensates for shortening of the villi. The absorptive cells are flattened and more basophilic than normal, and the basal polarity of their nuclei is lost. The numbers of lymphocytes and plasma cells in the lamina propria is markedly increased. Most of the plasma cells produce IgA (as in the normal small bowel). The numbers of polymorphonuclear leukocytes and eosinophils may also be increased in the epithelium and lamina propria.

 Clinical Features: **Celiac disease is characterized by generalized malabsorption.** Not infrequently, overt signs of malabsorption in children are lacking, and the disease is suspected only because of growth retardation. Often the symptoms and signs of generalized malabsorption are initially manifested in older children, adolescents, and adults. With the application of Ig A antiendomysium and IgA anti-tissue transglutaminase antibodies, it has become evident that celiac disease is a more common disorder than previously thought.

The systemic manifestations of celiac disease are related to the various deficiency states that result from generalized malabsorption. Late complications in some cases include ulcerative jejunitis and T-cell lymphoma of the small bowel. Adenocarcinoma of the small bowel and carcinoma of the oropharynx and esophagus also occur and an increased risk for colorectal carcinoma has been reported. Other extraintestinal manifestations include follicular keratosis, peripheral

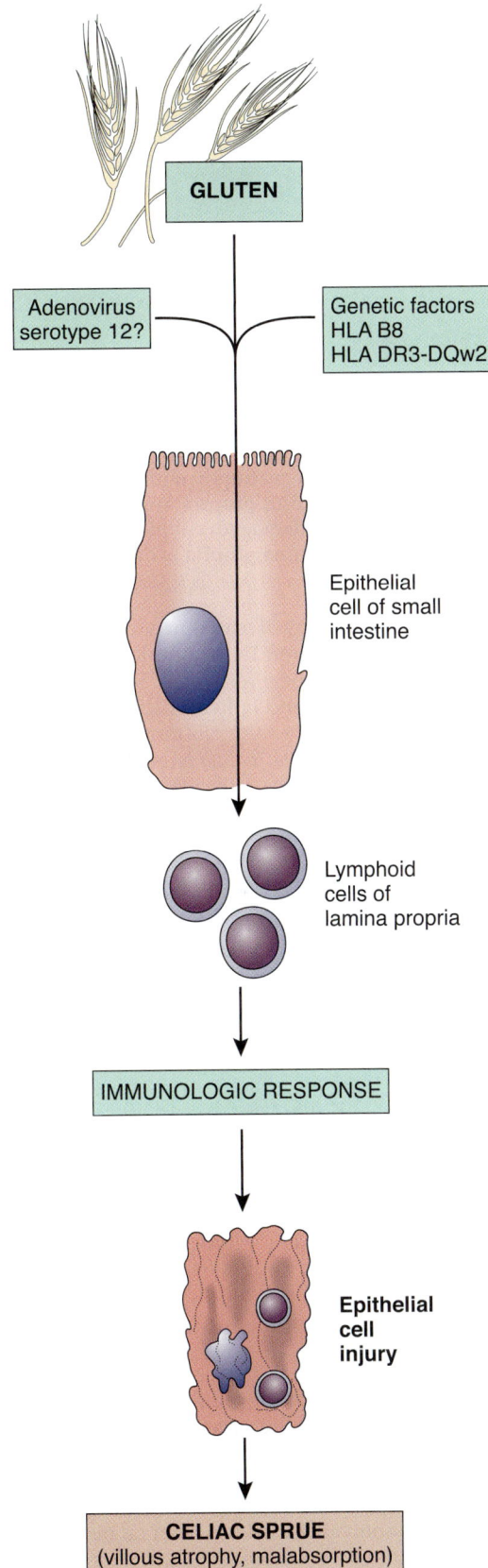

FIGURE 13-33
Hypothetical mechanisms in the pathogenesis of celiac disease.

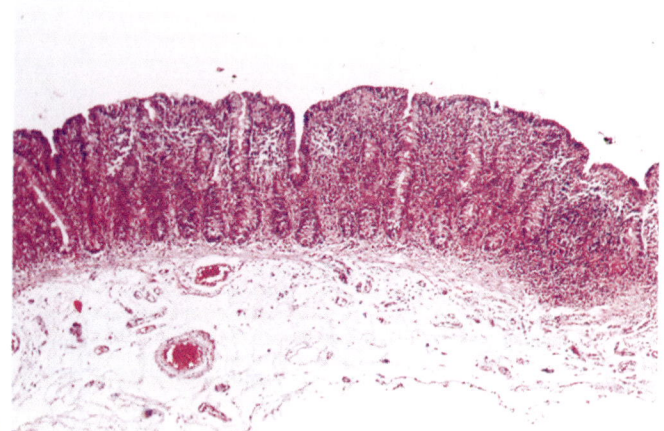
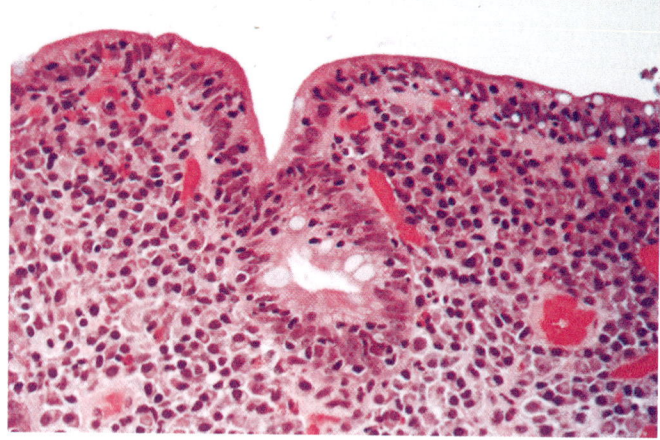

FIGURE 13-34
A. Villous atrophy with a flat surface, elongation of the crypts, and chronic inflammation of the lamina propria are characteristic of long-standing disease. B. A higher-power view shows damaged, cuboidal surface epithelium with numerous intraepithelial lymphocytes. The lamina propria is densely infiltrated by lymphocytes and plasma cells.

neuropathy, and infertility. Treatment with a strict gluten-free diet is usually followed by a complete and prolonged clinical and histopathological remission. Some patients have refractory sprue and respond only to corticosteroids.

Collagenous sprue refers to a rare disorder characterized by the deposition of collagen in the lamina propria of the small bowel. The disorder initially mimics celiac disease but does not respond to the removal of gluten from the diet. The prognosis in collagenous sprue is grave, and all reported patients have died of the disease.

Whipple Disease Is an Infection of the Small Bowel

Whipple disease is a rare, infectious disorder of the small intestine in which malabsorption is the most prominent feature. It most commonly affects white men in their 30s and 40s. The disease is systemic, and other clinical findings include fever, increased skin pigmentation, anemia, lymphadenopathy, arthritis, pericarditis, pleurisy, endocarditis, and central nervous system involvement.

Pathogenesis: **Whipple disease typically shows infiltration of the small bowel mucosa by macrophages that are packed with small, rod-shaped bacilli.** Dramatic clinical remissions occur with antibiotic therapy. The causative organism has been identified as one of the actinomycetes and has been named *Tropheryma whippelii*. Interestingly, *T. whippelii* is distantly related to mycobacteria such as *M. avium-intracellulare* and *M. paratuberculosis*, both of which have been associated with illnesses resembling Whipple disease. The results of several studies suggest that host susceptibility factors, possibly defective T-lymphocyte function, may be important in predisposing toward the disease. Macrophages from patients with Whipple disease exhibit decreased ability to degrade intracellular microorganisms. Patients have reduced numbers of circulating cells expressing CD11b, a cell-adhesion and complement-receptor molecule on macrophages, which is involved in the activation of intracellular killing of pathogens.

Pathology: The bowel wall is thickened and edematous, and the mesenteric lymph nodes are usually enlarged. Histological examination of the small intestine reveals flat, thickened villi and extensive infiltration of the lamina propria with large foamy macrophages (Fig. 13-35A). **The cytoplasm of these macrophages is filled with large glycoprotein granules that stain strongly with PAS** (Fig. 13-35B). Importantly, the other normal cellular components of the lamina propria (i.e., plasma cells and lymphocytes) are depleted. The lymphatic vessels in the mucosa and submucosa are dilated, and large lipid droplets abound within lymphatics and in extracellular spaces, a finding that suggests obstruction of the lymphatics. In contrast to the striking distortion of the villous architecture, the epithelial cells show only patchy abnormalities, including attenuation of the microvilli and accumulation of lipid droplets within the cytoplasm.

Electron-microscopic examination reveals numerous small bacilli within macrophages and free in the lamina propria (see Fig. 13-35C). The PAS-positive granules seen by light microscopy correspond to lysosomes engorged with bacilli in various stages of degeneration. Many bacilli cluster immediately beneath the epithelial basement membrane.

The mesenteric lymph nodes draining the affected segments of small bowel reveal similar microscopic changes. A characteristic infiltration by macrophages containing bacilli may also be found in most other organs. Heart lesions may include vegetations on the heart valves, which contain bacilli-laden macrophages, sometimes with superimposed streptococcal endocarditis. Treatment of Whipple disease is with appropriate antibiotics.

Abetalipoproteinemia Results from a Metabolic Defect in Absorptive Cells

Abetalipoproteinemia is an autosomal recessive inherited disease characterized by a failure to synthesize apoprotein B, a constituent of the membrane coat of low-density lipoproteins. Small intestinal absorptive cells that lack apoprotein B fail to assemble chylomicrons, an essential component of lipid transport out of the cell. These are manifested in erythrocytes as acanthocytosis and in the central nervous system as selective demyelinization, particularly of the posterior columns. Typical neurological manifestations are loss of deep tendon reflexes, sensory ataxia, and a mild form of retinitis pigmentosa. The serum shows a total absence of chylomicrons, very-low-density lipoproteins, and low-density lipoproteins. In addition, serum levels of cholesterol and triglycerides are low, and the bulk of serum lipids is carried within high-density lipoprotein particles.

Histologically, the villi, lamina propria, and submucosa appear normal. The epithelial cells contain lipid vacuoles, but no lipid is seen in the intestinal lymphatics. This lipid probably represents triglyceride that has been assembled within the cell but cannot be transported into the basolateral intercellular space because of the lack of apoprotein B.

Malabsorption in abetalipoproteinemia is partially reversed by ingestion of medium-chain (rather than the usual long-chain) triglycerides; these lipids are transported through the absorptive cells without an apoprotein coat.

Hypogammaglobulinemia May Interfere with Absorption

Malabsorption occurs frequently in patients with acquired hypogammaglobulinemia. The histopathological appearance of the small intestine includes a paucity or lack of

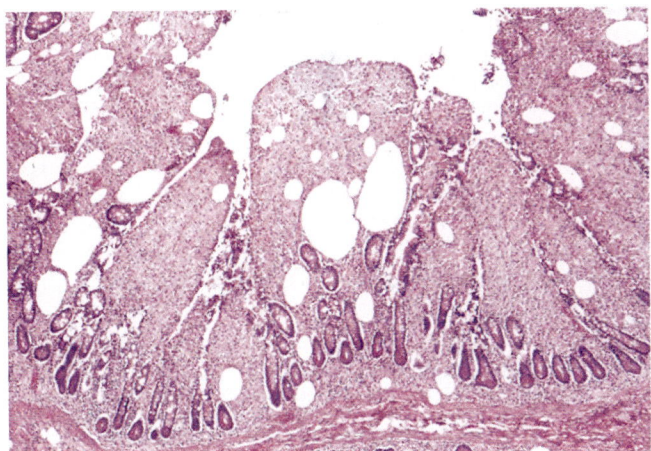
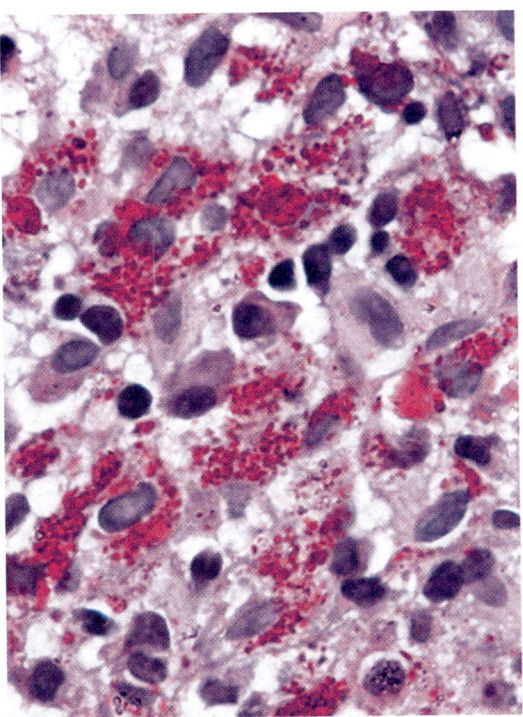
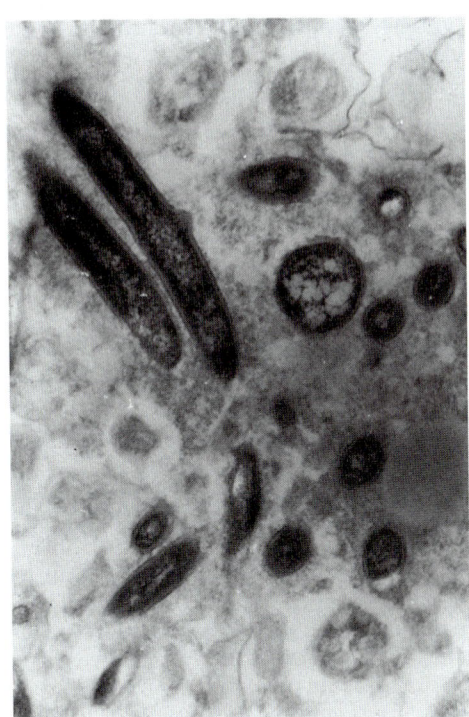

FIGURE 13-35

Whipple disease. A. A photomicrograph of a section of jejunal mucosa shows distortion of the villi. The lamina propria is packed with large, pale-staining macrophages. Dilated mucosal lymphatics are prominent. **B.** A periodic acid–Schiff (PAS) reaction shows numerous macrophages filled with cytoplasmic granular material. **C.** An electron micrograph shows small bacilli in a macrophage.

plasma cells in the lamina propria and often nodular lymphoid hyperplasia. Occasionally, there is a flat mucosa, similar to the lesion of celiac sprue; in this case, the disorder is termed *hypogammaglobulinemic sprue.*

Most hypogammaglobulinemic patients with malabsorption are infected in the small intestine with *Giardia lamblia.* Appropriate treatment with metronidazole is followed by improved intestinal absorption.

Congenital Lymphangiectasia Is a Generalized Malformation That Causes Malabsorption

Congenital lymphangiectasia is a poorly understood disease that usually begins in childhood. A syndrome of intestinal lymphangiectasia and peripheral lymphedema is known as *Milroy disease.* In addition to steatorrhea caused by impaired transport of chylomicrons by intestinal lymphatics, patients with congenital lymphangiectasia have *protein-losing enteropathy,* a condition characterized by excessive loss of plasma proteins into the gut.

Other important features of congenital lymphangiectasia are lymphopenia and impaired cell-mediated immunity, caused by the loss of small lymphocytes into the bowel lumen. Chylous ascites (milky, lipid-containing peritoneal fluid) occurs in some patients as a result of leakage of lymph from the mesenteric or serosal lymphatic vessels into the peritoneal cavity.

The lesions of congenital lymphangiectasia are recognized macroscopically as opalescent white spots and microscopically as **dilated lymphatics (lacteals)** in the lamina propria. The submucosal lymphatics also tend to be dilated. The epithelium is normal, but the villi may be blunted or even absent in areas overlying severe lymphatic dilation.

Acquired intestinal lymphangiectasia, with all or some of the associated clinical features described above, also occurs as a secondary manifestation of small intestinal or retroperitoneal lymphoma, other retroperitoneal tumors, tuberculosis, sarcoidosis, chronic pancreatitis, and retroperitoneal fibrosis.

Tropical Sprue Is Linked to Folate Deficiency

Tropical sprue is a poorly understood disease of obscure cause that is endemic in certain tropical areas and is characterized by progressively severe malabsorption and nutritional deficiency. Cure, or at least amelioration of the symptoms, usually follows treatment with oral tetracycline and folic acid. The cause of tropical sprue is not known. Some studies suggest that **long-standing contamination of the bowel with bacteria,** perhaps toxigenic strains of *E. coli,* may be important and that the resultant **folate deficiency** may play a role in perpetuating the intestinal lesion.

The histological findings are variable, ranging from mild widening and blunting of villi to a completely flat mucosa similar to that seen in celiac sprue. The morphological injury in the epithelium and the inflammation of the lamina propria usually parallel the severity of the alterations in the villi.

Typically, steatorrhea, anemia, and weight loss are followed by progressively severe manifestations of folic acid and vitamin B_{12} deficiencies and hypoalbuminemia. Laboratory findings include increased fecal fat, impaired D-xylose absorption, megaloblastic anemia, and decreased disaccharidase activity in the intestinal mucosa.

Radiation Enteritis Results from Radiotherapy

Abdominal irradiation may cause transient damage to the small intestinal mucosa. Anorexia, abdominal cramps, and changes in bowel habits occur frequently during the course of abdominal radiation therapy, and laboratory studies in such patients indicate malabsorption of bile salts and disaccharides. Transient histological changes in the small bowel include shortening of the villi, increased cellularity in the lamina propria, and submucosal edema.

Occasionally, subacute or chronic radiation damage does occur, especially when (1) the radiation dose is very high, (2) segments of small bowel become fixed as a result of postoperative or inflammatory adhesions, (3) the blood supply to the bowel is impaired, or (4) radiation is combined with chemotherapeutic agents that may augment radiation damage.

The major histological features of subacute and chronic radiation damage to the small intestine are similar to those seen elsewhere in the gastrointestinal tract and include (1) mucosal ulceration, (2) swelling and detachment of endothelial cells of the small arterioles in the submucosa, (3) obliteration by fibrin plugs of the lumina of the arterioles, and (4) the presence of large foam cells beneath the intima. Thickening and fibrosis of the submucosa ensue, together with signs of progressive ischemia, to produce stricture.

MECHANICAL OBSTRUCTION

Mechanical obstruction to the passage of intestinal contents can be caused by (1) a luminal mass, (2) an intrinsic lesion of the bowel wall, or (3) extrinsic compression.

INTUSSUSCEPTION: This is a form of intraluminal small bowel obstruction in which a segment of bowel (intussusceptum) protrudes distally into a surrounding outer portion (intussuscipiens). This condition is usually a disorder of infants or young children, in whom it occurs without a known cause. In adults, the leading point of an intussusception is usually a lesion in the bowel wall, such as Meckel diverticulum or a tumor. Once the leading point is entrapped in the intussuscipiens, peristalsis drives the intussusceptum forward. In addition to acute intestinal obstruction, intussusception compresses the blood supply to the intussusceptum, which may become infarcted. If the obstruction is not relieved spontaneously, treatment requires surgery.

VOLVULUS: This is a cause of an acute abdomen and is an example of intestinal obstruction in which a segment of gut twists on its mesentery, thereby kinking the bowel and usually interrupting the blood supply. Volvulus is virtually always a consequence of an underlying congenital abnormality. Malrotation of the bowel permits undue mobility of the bowel loops and predisposes to **midgut volvulus.** When the cecum or right colon is invested with a mesentery rather than being retroperitoneal, the result may be **cecal volvulus.** An unusually long sigmoid colon, which occurs sometimes in patients with idiopathic chronic constipation, permits the development of **sigmoid volvulus.**

ADHESIONS: Fibrous scars caused by previous surgery or peritonitis cause obstruction by kinking or angulating the bowel or directly compressing the lumen.

HERNIAS: Loops of small bowel may be incarcerated in an inguinal or femoral hernia, in which case, the lumen may become obstructed, and the vascular supply compromised. Similarly, portions of the bowel may be trapped internally by hernias that represent congenital or surgically acquired defects in the mesentery.

NEOPLASMS

Tumors of the small intestine constitute fewer than 5% of all gastrointestinal tumors.

Benign Tumors

Adenomas

Adenomas of the small intestine resemble those of the colon. According to the predominant component, adenomatous polyps of the small intestine may be tubular, villous, or tubulovillous. Villous adenoma is rare in the small intestine, usually occurring in the duodenum, especially the periampullary region. Although most adenomas remain benign, some, especially the villous type, undergo malignant transformation. Benign adenomas are frequently asymptomatic, but bleeding and intussusception are occasional complications.

Peutz–Jeghers Syndrome

Peutz–Jeghers syndrome is an autosomal dominant hereditary disorder characterized by intestinal hamartomatous polyps and mucocutaneous melanin pigmentation, which is particularly evident on the face, buccal mucosa, hands, feet, and perianal and genital areas. Except for the buccal pigmentation, the frecklelike macular lesions usually fade at puberty. The polyps occur most commonly in the proximal regions of the small intestine but are sometimes seen in the stomach and the colon. Patients usually have symptoms of obstruction or intussusception; in as many as one fourth of cases, however, the diagnosis is suggested by pigmentation in an otherwise asymptomatic person.

Peutz-Jeghers syndrome is associated with inactivating mutations of a gene *(LKB1)* on chromosome 19p that encodes a protein kinase. Carriers of the defective gene are also at increased risk for cancers of the breast, pancreas, testis, and ovary.

The polyps in Peutz-Jeghers syndrome are hamartomas. Histologically, a branching network of smooth muscle fibers continuous with the muscularis mucosae supports the glandular epithelium of the polyp (Fig. 13-36). Peutz-Jeghers polyps are generally considered benign, but 3% of patients develop adenocarcinoma, although not necessarily in the hamartomatous polyps.

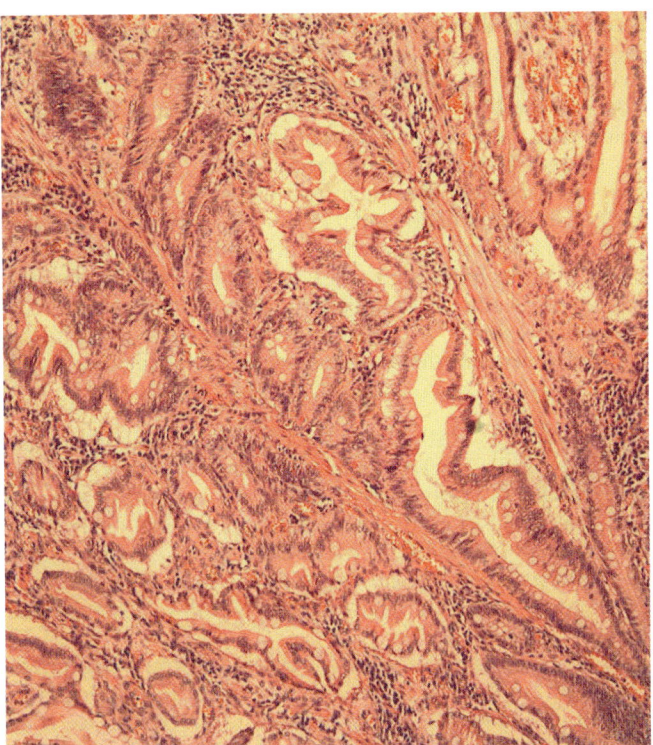

FIGURE *13-36*
Peutz-Jeghers polyp. In this hamartomatous polyp, the glandular epithelium, composed of both goblet cells and absorptive cells, is supported by a network of smooth muscle.

Gastrointestinal Stromal Tumors

GISTs occur at all levels of the small intestine but are most common in the jejunum. They grow as intramural masses covered by intact mucosa and are similar to those in other locations. Intestinal obstruction is uncommon, but volvulus may be a complication.

Lipomas

Lipomas occur throughout the length of the small intestine but are most common in the distal ileum. Although for the most part asymptomatic, these submucosal tumors may become large and produce intestinal obstruction, usually as a result of intussusception. The overlying mucosa may become ulcerated and bleed.

Malignant Tumors of the Small Bowel are Uncommon

Adenocarcinoma

 Epidemiology: Although adenocarcinoma of the small intestine accounts for a minute proportion of all gastrointestinal tumors, it constitutes half of all malignant small bowel tumors. Most adenocarcinomas are located in the duodenum and jejunum. The majority occur in middle-aged persons, and there is a moderate male predominance. Interestingly, the geographical variation in the incidence of small bowel adenocarcinoma correlates with that of colon cancer but not with that of stomach cancer.

A risk factor for adenocarcinoma is Crohn disease of the small bowel. The mean age for the appearance of an adenocarcinoma of the small intestine is 10 years younger than average in patients with Crohn disease, and the cancer tends to occur in the same area as the inflammatory lesions, namely the ileum. Familial adenomatous polyposis, hereditary nonpolyposis colorectal cancer syndrome (Lynch syndrome), and celiac disease are additional risk factors.

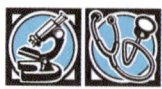 **Pathology and Clinical Features:** Adenocarcinoma of the small intestine may be polypoid or ulcerative or simply annular and stenosing. In addition to causing intestinal obstruction directly, a polypoid tumor may be the lead point of an intussusception. Adenocarcinomas originate from the epithelium of the crypts rather than the villi and, therefore, resemble colorectal cancers.

The symptoms of adenocarcinoma of the small bowel are commonly those of progressive intestinal obstruction. Occult bleeding is common and often leads to iron-deficiency anemia. Adenocarcinoma of the duodenum may involve the papilla of Vater, in which case it is termed *ampullary carcinoma*. This tumor causes obstructive jaundice or pancreatitis. By the time the patient becomes symptomatic, most adenocarcinomas have metastasized to local lymph nodes, and overall 5-year survival is less than 20%. This neoplasm is the second most common cause of death in patients with familial adenomatous polyposis.

Primary Intestinal Lymphoma

Primary lymphoma originates in nodules of lymphoid tissue normally present in the mucosa and superficial submucosa, termed mucosa-associated lymphoid tissue (MALT). Lymphoma represents the second most common malignant tumor of the small intestine in industrialized countries, where it accounts for about 15% of small bowel cancers. By contrast, another type of primary lymphoma comprises more than two thirds of all cancers of the small intestine in underdeveloped countries. The latter variety of intestinal lymphoma was originally described in Mediterranean populations, but it is now clear that it is distributed throughout the poorer parts of the world. Because these two types of lymphoma have distinct epidemiological, clinical, and pathological features, they are labeled, respectively, the Western type and the Mediterranean variety.

The cause of primary lymphoma of the small bowel is unknown, but an association with celiac disease is well documented, occurring in as many as one tenth of patients with primary lymphoma. It is assumed that the persistent activation of lymphocytes in the bowel is related to the subsequent development of T-cell lymphoma. However, although a gluten-free diet usually improves the inflammatory component of the enteropathy, T-cell lymphoma can still occur.

The risk of intestinal lymphoma is also increased in conditions that favor the development of nodal lymphoma, particularly immunodeficiency following treatment with immunosuppressive drugs.

MEDITERRANEAN LYMPHOMA: Mediterranean lymphoma typically occurs in poor countries in young men of low socioeconomic status; it is therefore thought by some to have an environmental cause. **This neoplasm has been associated with a proliferative disorder of intestinal B lymphocytes that secrete the heavy chain of immunoglobulin A without light chains, termed *α-heavy chain disease*.** Mediterranean lymphoma and α-chain disease are believed to be the same disorder, termed *immunoproliferative small intestinal disease*.

Mediterranean intestinal lymphoma predominantly involves the duodenum and proximal jejunum. A long segment of small intestine, or even the entire small bowel, is characteristically affected. The lymphoma typically is seen as a diffuse infiltration of the mucosa and submucosa by plasmacytoid lymphocytes or plasma cells (Fig. 13-37). Lymphomatous infiltration of the mucosa leads to mucosal atrophy and severe malabsorption.

WESTERN-TYPE INTESTINAL LYMPHOMA: This disorder usually affects adults older than 40 years and children younger than 10 years. It is most common in the ileum, where it is seen as (1) a fungating mass that projects into the lumen, (2) an elevated ulcerated lesion, (3) a diffuse segmental thickening of the bowel wall, or (4) plaquelike mucosal nodules. As a result, intestinal obstruction, intussusception, and perforation are important complications. Occult bleeding is common, although massive acute hemorrhage may also occur. Microscopically, all varieties of malignant lymphoma are encountered. When extraintestinal spread is present, the 5-year survival rate is less than 10%.

Chronic abdominal pain, diarrhea, and clubbing of the fingers are the most frequent clinical signs of intestinal lymphoma. Diarrhea and weight loss reflect the underlying malabsorption. Patients with Mediterranean lymphoma tend to survive longer than those with the Western type of lymphoma.

Carcinoid Tumor (Neuroendocrine Tumors)

Carcinoid tumors of the gastrointestinal tract can secrete all the peptides and amines produced by their normal counterparts, the most common being serotonin. **Carcinoid tumors account for about 20% of all malignant tumors of the small intestine.** Most carcinoid tumors are found incidentally in the appendix, and most of the remainder occur in the ileum. Interestingly, 2% of carcinoid tumors of the small bowel arise in a Meckel diverticulum.

All carcinoid tumors are considered tumors with low malignant potential. In general, the malignant potential of intestinal carcinoid tumors appears to be related to their size. Those smaller than 1 cm in diameter are rarely malignant, 50% of those between 1 and 2 cm in diameter metastasize, and 80% of those larger than 2 cm in diameter metastasize.

Carcinoid tumors of the gastrointestinal tract, especially those of the small intestine, are often multicentric; that is, multiple primary tumors arise, either simultaneously or at different times. They are also seen in association with the multiple endocrine neoplasia (MEN) syndromes, most commonly with type I. Because neuroendocrine cells are

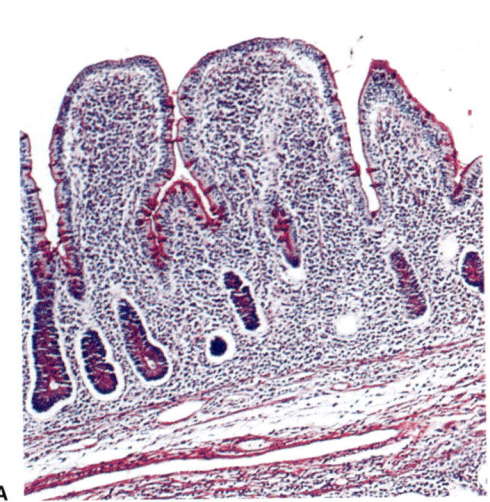
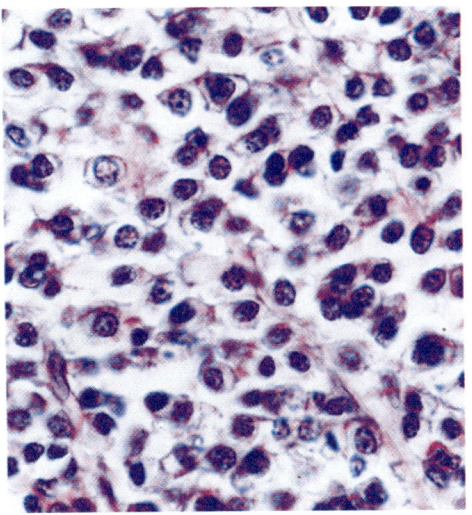

FIGURE 13-37
Mediterranean intestinal lymphoma. A. The villi are short and blunted, and the lamina propria is filled with lymphoid cells. The goblet cells are red with this periodic acid–Schiff stain. B. A high-power view of A shows neoplastic plasmacytoid lymphocytes.

widespread, carcinoid tumors are found in a variety of other locations, including the pancreas, bronchus, ovary, and testis.

Pathology: Macroscopically, small carcinoid tumors present as submucosal nodules covered by intact mucosa. Large carcinoids may grow in a polypoid, intramural, or annular pattern (Fig. 13-38A) and often undergo secondary ulceration. The cut surface is firm and white to yellow. As they enlarge, carcinoid tumors invade the muscular coat and penetrate the serosa, often causing a conspicuous desmoplastic reaction. This fibrosis is responsible for peritoneal adhesions and kinking of the bowel, which may lead to intestinal obstruction.

Microscopically, the neoplasms appear as nests, cords, and rosettes of uniform small, round cells (see Fig. 13-38B). Occasional glandlike structures are also encountered. The nuclei exhibit a remarkable regularity, and mitoses are rare.

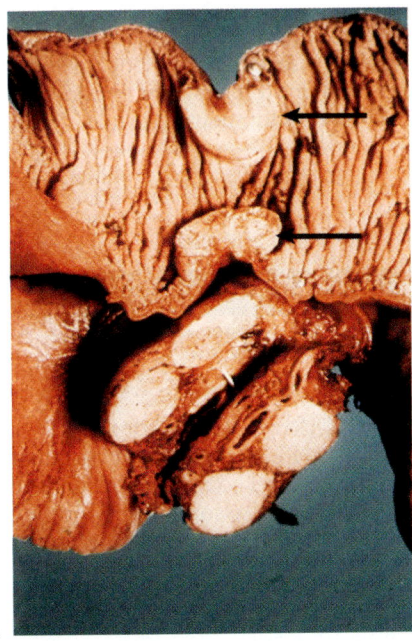
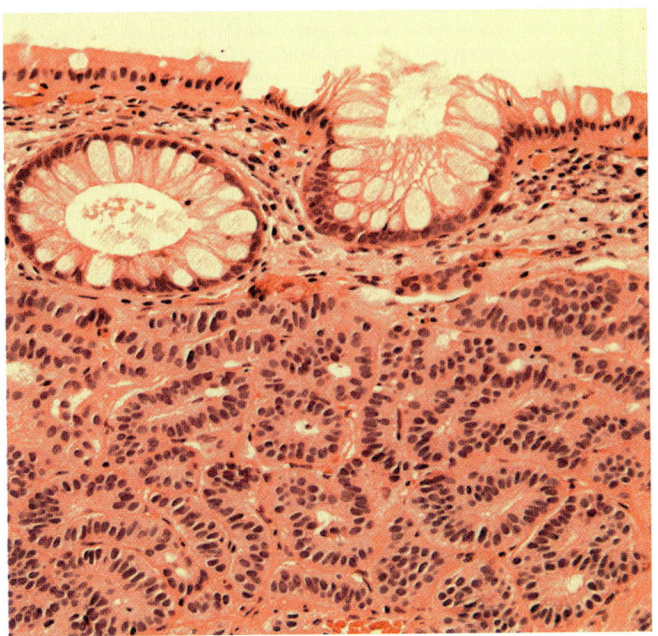

FIGURE 13-38
Carcinoid tumor of the small intestine. A. A bisected annular carcinoid tumor (arrows) constricts the lumen of the small intestine. Lymph node metastases are evident. B. A photomicrograph of the lesion in A demonstrates cords of uniform small, round cells.

An abundant eosinophilic cytoplasm contains cytoplasmic granules, which by electron microscopy are typically of the neurosecretory type. Goblet cell carcinoids or adenocarcinoid tumors have glandular differentiation. These tumors have a higher rate of aggressive behavior than do typical carcinoids.

Carcinoid tumors metastasize first to regional lymph nodes. Subsequently, hematogenous spread produces metastases at distant sites, particularly the liver.

 Clinical Features: **Carcinoid syndrome** is a unique clinical condition that marks carcinoid tumors. The disorder is caused by the release of a variety of active tumor products. Although most carcinoids are to some extent functional, this syndrome ordinarily occurs only in patients with extensive hepatic metastases. **The classic symptoms of the carcinoid syndrome include diarrhea (often the most distressing symptom), episodic flushing, bronchospasm, cyanosis, telangiectasia, and skin lesions.** Half of patients also have right-sided cardiac valvular disease. Diarrhea is thought to be caused by serotonin.

After its release into the blood, serotonin is metabolized to 5-hydroxyindoleacetic acid (5-HIAA) by monoamine oxidase either in the tumor or in other tissues. The presence of 5-HIAA in the urine is a diagnostic test for the carcinoid syndrome. Whereas the liver, lung, and brain all have high levels of activity of monoamine oxidase and (presumably) of enzymes that inactivate other tumor secretions, the right side of the heart is exposed to the full effects of tumor products that have been released into the vena cava from hepatic metastases. As a result, endocardial fibrosis occurs, probably as a reaction to endothelial damage. Fibrous plaques form on the tricuspid and pulmonic valves, the endocardium of the right-sided cardiac chambers, the vena cava, the coronary sinus, and the pulmonary artery. **Distortion of the valves leads to pulmonic stenosis and tricuspid regurgitation.**

Malignant Gastrointestinal Stromal Tumors

The diagnostic criteria applied to GISTs of the small bowel are the same as those tumors in other locations of the gastrointestinal tract.

Metastatic Tumors

The most common malignant tumors that involve the small intestine are metastatic. Cancer of adjacent organs (e.g., stomach, pancreas, or colon) may spread to the small intestine by direct extension. Cancers of the lung and female genital organs and melanomas are the most frequent primary sites of small-intestinal metastases. Secondary involvement of the small intestine with systemic lymphoma may simulate metastatic carcinoma. Solitary, submucosal metastatic tumors may easily be mistaken for a primary cancer, and the symptoms may be indistinguishable.

PNEUMATOSIS CYSTOIDES INTESTINALIS

Pneumatosis cystoides intestinalis is an uncommon disorder in which numerous pockets of gas are found in the wall of the gut anywhere in the gastrointestinal tract. Most cases are associated with an underlying gastrointestinal disease, including intestinal obstruction, peptic ulcer, Crohn disease, mesenteric ischemia, volvulus, and neonatal necrotizing enterocolitis. Some are associated with chronic obstructive pulmonary disease or mechanical ventilation. Pneumatosis in adults is ordinarily benign, depending on the underlying disease. However, intestinal pneumatosis associated with neonatal necrotizing enteritis has a high mortality.

The cause of intestinal pneumatosis depends on the associated conditions. A mechanical break in the continuity of the mucosa allows the entry of air from the lumen to the submucosa. Alternatively, the gas can be a product of bacterial action, particularly in neonatal necrotizing enterocolitis. Dissection of air bubbles along the mesentery is common in patients with obstructive pulmonary disease or ventilation.

 Pathology: Macroscopically, the cysts appear as bubbles under the serosa of the intestine, and the bowel wall feels spongy. In some cases, the air cysts are located principally in the submucosa, in which case, the cut surface of the bowel wall appears to be honeycombed. The cysts vary from a few millimeters to several centimeters in diameter. Cysts may also occur in the stomach and the mesentery. Microscopic examination reveals cystic spaces in the submucosa or beneath the serosa, which are often lined by large macrophages and multinucleated giant cells.

 Clinical Features: Many cases are found during investigation of symptoms unrelated to the pneumatosis. Some patients have episodic diarrhea. There is often blood in the stools, and rectal bleeding may be brisk. When intestinal pneumatosis is a complication of neonatal necrotizing enterocolitis, bowel perforation and peritonitis are frequent, but these complications are rare in adults.

Gas cysts may disappear spontaneously or may persist for years. Relief of symptoms may be obtained by oxygen inhalation or treatment with metronidazole.

The Large Intestine

ANATOMY

The large intestine, defined as the portion of the gastrointestinal tract from the ileocecal valve to the anus, is 90 to 125 cm in length in adults and comprises the colon and rectum. The proximal part shares a common embryological origin with the small intestine, both being derived from the embryonic midgut and supplied by the superior mesenteric artery. The distal half of the large intestine is embryologically distinct. It is derived from the embryonic hindgut, is supplied by the inferior mesenteric artery, and serves principally as a storage organ.

MACROSCOPIC FEATURES: The large intestine is traditionally divided into six regions in a sequence that proceeds from the ileocecal valve distally: (1) cecum, (2) ascending colon, (3) transverse colon, (4) descending colon, (5) sigmoid colon, and (6) rectum. The bend between the ascending and transverse colon in the right upper quadrant is called the *hepatic flexure* and that between the transverse and descending segments in the left upper quadrant is termed the *splenic flexure*. The caliber of the lumen progressively diminishes from the cecum to the sigmoid colon.

Like the small intestine, the colon is endowed with outer longitudinal and inner circular muscle coats. However, in the colon, the longitudinal muscle has three separate bundles, termed the *taeniae coli*. Evaginations of the colonic wall between the taeniae, called the *haustra*, appear as external sacculations. The appendices epiploicae are small serosal masses of fat, invested by peritoneum. The vermiform appendix arises at the apex of the cecum and terminates as a blind tube; it averages about 8 cm in length but occasionally measures up to 20 cm.

The ileocecal valve functions as a sphincter to regulate the flow of intestinal contents into the cecum. However, it is an incompetent sphincter, and reflux of cecal contents into the ileum is usual. The internal sphincter of the anal canal is continuous with colonic smooth muscle. The external anal sphincter, the major mechanism by which continence of the bowel is maintained, surrounds the anal canal with a layer of skeletal muscle. The mucosal surface of the large bowel has prominent folds, which are less pronounced in the rectum.

MICROSCOPIC FEATURES: Histologically, the surface of the colonic mucosa is flat and punctuated by numerous pits, termed *crypts of Lieberkuhn*. The mucosa of the surface and crypts is lined by a tall columnar epithelium. The surface epithelium consists primarily of simple columnar cells and occasional goblet cells. The crypts are lined mostly by goblet cells, except at their basFs, where a few undifferentiated cells and a variety of neuroendocrine cells are located. The basal undifferentiated cells constitute the reserve cell population of the colonic mucosa and exhibit numerous mitoses. Mucosal cells migrate from the bases of the crypts toward the luminal surface. Programmed cell death (apoptosis) and sloughing of the mucosal cells balance proliferation in maintaining the crypt epithelial cell population.

The lamina propria of the colonic mucosa contains lymphocytes, plasma cells, macrophages, and fibroblasts. Eosinophils may be encountered. Lymphoid aggregates interrupt the continuity of the muscularis mucosae and extend into the submucosa. The submucosa is similar to that in the small intestine, but lymphatic channels are far less prominent. The lymphatics drain into paracolic nodes in the serosal fat, intermediate nodes located along the course of the colic blood vessels, and central nodes clustered near the aorta. Parasympathetic and sympathetic innervations terminate in Meissner submucosal and Auerbach myenteric plexuses.

CONGENITAL DISORDERS

Congenital Megacolon (Hirschsprung Disease) Reflects a Segmental Absence of Ganglion Cells

Hirschsprung disease is a disorder in which colonic dilation (Fig. 13-39) *results from a defect in the innervation of the colorectum.*

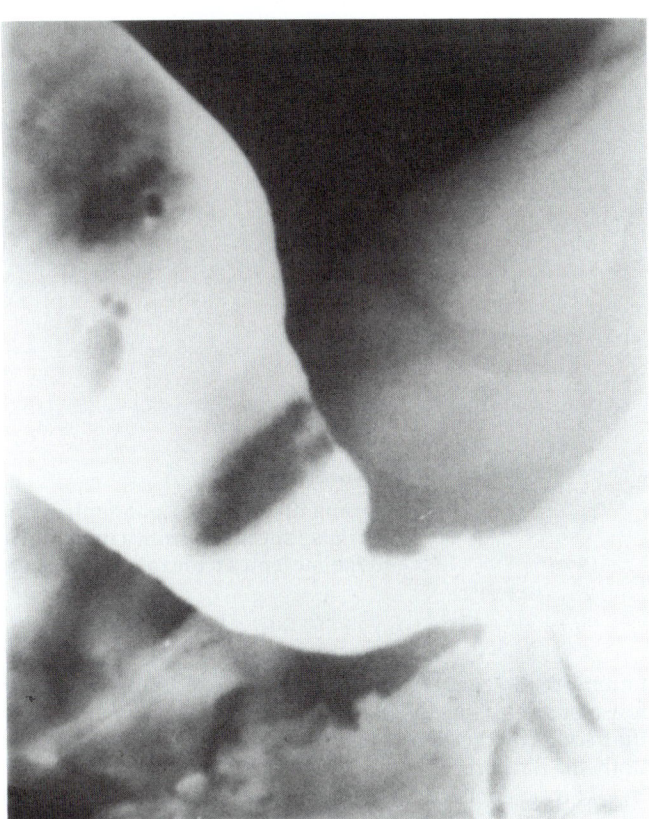

FIGURE 13-39
Hirschsprung disease. A contrast radiograph shows marked dilation of the rectosigmoid colon proximal to the narrowed rectum.

The lesion is a congenital absence of ganglion cells, in most cases in the wall of the rectum (Fig. 13-40). In one fourth of cases, ganglion cells are deficient in more-proximal portions of the colon, and in unusual instances, the lesion may extend as far as the small intestine. The incidence of the disorder is estimated to be 1 in 5000 live births, and 80% of patients are male.

 Pathogenesis: The pathogenesis of Hirschsprung disease can be traced to an interruption of the developmental sequence that leads to innervation of the colon. The normal caudal migration of cells from the neural crest that eventually gives rise to the intramural ganglion cells is interrupted. Because the internal anal sphincter marks the terminus of this migration, the aganglionic segment always includes the rectum and may extend for variable distances proximally, depending on the point at which the primitive neuroblasts are halted. Given that the aganglionic rectum and occasionally the adjacent colon are permanently contracted because of the absence of relaxation stimuli, the fecal contents do not readily enter this stenotic area. The proximal bowel becomes dilated because of functional distal obstruction.

Most cases of Hirschsprung disease are sporadic, but 10% of cases are familial. Half of the familial cases and 15% of sporadic ones are associated with inactivating gene mutations of the RET receptor tyrosine kinase on chromosome 10q (see MEN2 syndrome, Chapter 21). Some cases involve mu-

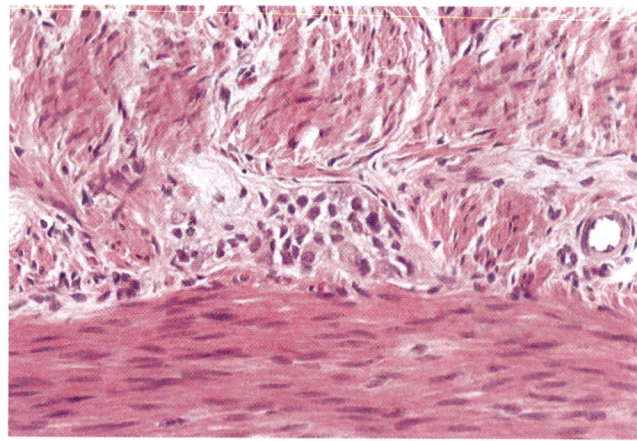
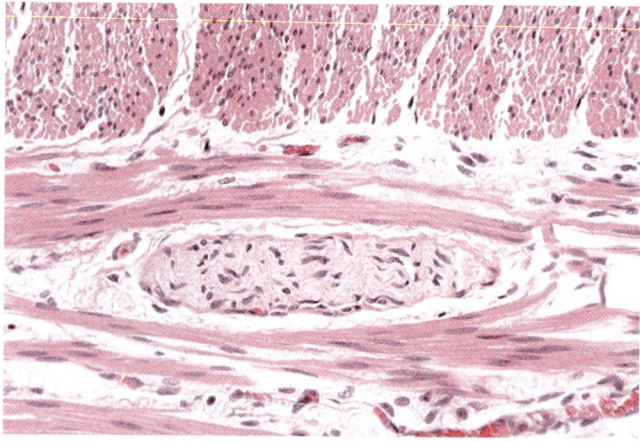

FIGURE 13-40
Hirschsprung disease. A. A photomicrograph of ganglion cells in the wall of the rectum. B. A rectal biopsy specimen from a patient with Hirschsprung disease shows a nonmyelinated nerve in the mesenteric plexus and an absence of ganglion cells.

tations of the gene for the endothelin-B receptor. Finally, a few instances of the disease are due to mutations in the genes that code for the ligands of the RET receptor and the endothelin-B receptor.

The incidence of congenital megacolon is 10 times higher than normal in infants with **Down syndrome,** and 2% of patients with Down syndrome are born with Hirschsprung disease. Although most cases of aganglionosis of the colon are uncomplicated by other lesions, the disorder also has been reported in conjunction with a number of other congenital abnormalities, including anomalies of the kidneys and lower urinary tract, imperforate anus, and ventricular septal defect.

Pathology: The colon and rectum in Hirschsprung disease reveal a constricted and spastic segment that corresponds to the aganglionic zone. Proximal to this area, the bowel is conspicuously dilated. The definitive diagnosis of Hirschsprung disease is made on the basis of absence of ganglion cells in a rectal biopsy specimen. Additionally, there is a striking increase in nonmyelinated cholinergic nerve fibers in the submucosa and between the muscle coats (neural hyperplasia). The absence of ganglion cells leads to accumulation of the enzyme acetylcholinesterase and acetylcholine. The histochemical demonstration of this enzyme, which is not visualized in the normal rectal mucosa, enhances the reliability of the diagnosis based on rectal biopsy. Neuronal dysplasia has features of Hirschsprung disease, but ganglion cells, albeit histopathologically abnormal, are present. Interestingly, like achalasia, which is caused by the destruction of esophageal ganglion cells, Chagas disease may cause aganglionic megacolon.

Clinical Features: Hirschsprung disease is the most common cause of congenital intestinal obstruction. The clinical signs are delayed passage of meconium by the newborn and the development of vomiting in the first few days of life. In some cases, complete intestinal obstruction requires immediate surgical relief. In children who have short rectal segments lacking ganglion cells and who have only partial obstruction, constipation, abdominal distention, and recurrent fecal impactions characterize the clinical course.

The most serious complication of congenital megacolon is an enterocolitis, in which necrosis and ulceration affect the dilated proximal segment of the colon and may extend into the small intestine. The treatment for Hirschsprung disease is surgical removal of the aganglionic segment and reconstruction.

Acquired Megacolon Often Reflects Laxative Use

Acquired megacolon sometimes occurs in children and often has a psychogenic background. It is also frequently associated with chronic constipation and the prolonged use of laxatives ("cathartic colon"). However, some cases in which ganglion cells are demonstrated by rectal biopsy begin in infancy and are associated with fecal incontinence. The cause of this apparently organic disturbance is not well understood, but the disorder is believed to represent a functional abnormality of colonic motility. Acquired megacolon in adults can result from disorders that interfere with the innervation of the bowel or smooth muscle function. Examples include diabetic neuropathy, parkinsonism, myotonic dystrophy, scleroderma, amyloidosis, and hypothyroidism.

Anorectal Malformations Are Developmental Defects

Anorectal malformations are among the most common anomalies and vary from minor narrowing to serious and complex defects. These lesions result from arrested development of the caudal region of the gut in the first 6 months of fetal life. The classification of these anomalies is based on the relation of the terminal bowel to the levator ani muscle. The classes are (1) high or supralevator deformities, in which the bowel ends above the pelvic floor; (2) intermediate deformities; and (3) low or translevator deformities, in which the bowel ends below the pelvic floor.

- **Anorectal agenesis and rectal atresia** are supralevator deformities.
- **Anal agenesis and anorectal stenosis** are classified as intermediate deformities.
- **Imperforate anus** is a low or translevator deformity in which the opening is covered by a cutaneous membrane behind which meconium is visible. **Anal stenosis** is a variant of imperforate anus.
- **Fistulas** between the malformation and the bladder, urethra, vagina, or skin may occur in all types of anorectal anomalies.

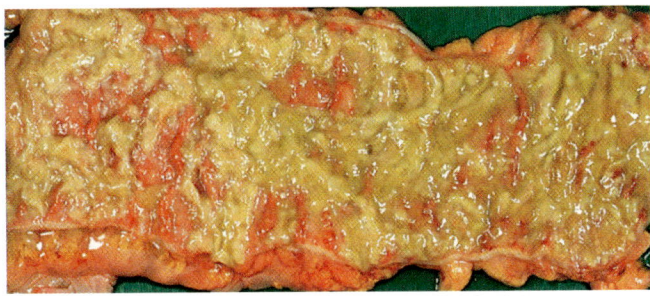

FIGURE 13-41
Pseudomembranous colitis. The mucosal surface of the colon is covered by raised, irregular plaques composed of necrotic debris and an acute inflammatory exudate.

INFECTIONS

Many of the principal bacterial and parasitic infections that affect the colon, including tuberculosis and amebiasis, are discussed either in Chapter 9 or above in the context of infectious diarrhea in the section on the small intestine. Most of the remaining infectious diseases are transmitted sexually and involve the anorectal region, often in male homosexuals. They include gonorrhea, syphilis, lymphogranuloma venereum, anorectal herpes, and venereal warts (condylomata acuminata). There is also a high incidence of colonic infections (e.g., amebiasis and shigellosis) among immunosuppressed patients. Within this last group and in patients with bone marrow transplants there is a high incidence of cytomegalovirus and herpes infection of the gastrointestinal tract.

Pseudomembranous Colitis Follows Antibiotic Treatment

Pseudomembranous colitis is a generic term for an inflammatory disease of the colon that is characterized by exudative plaques on the mucosa.

 Pathogenesis: After the introduction of antibiotics in the early 1950s, the administration of these drugs, principally tetracycline and chloramphenicol, was recognized to predispose to pseudomembranous colitis. *Clostridium difficile*, which has also been implicated in neonatal necrotizing enterocolitis, is the offending organism. The organism is not invasive, but it produces toxins that damage the colonic mucosa.

Other predisposing conditions include various diseases of the colon, shock, burns, uremia, and chemotherapy.

The mechanism by which *C. difficile* becomes pathogenic is not entirely clear. Alteration of fecal flora by antibiotics contributes. Only 2 to 3% of healthy adults harbor the organism, whereas 10 to 20% of persons who have recently been treated with antibiotics are infected. However, the microbe can be isolated from the stools of 95% of patients with antibiotic-associated pseudomembranous colitis.

 Pathology: Macroscopically, the colon, particularly the rectosigmoid region, exhibits raised yellowish plaques up to 2 cm in diameter that adhere to the underlying mucosa (Fig. 13-41). The intervening mucosa appears congested and edematous but is not ulcerated. In severe cases, the plaques coalesce to form extensive pseudomembranes. Microscopic examination of the lesions discloses necrosis of the superficial epithelium, which is believed to be the initial pathological event. Subsequently, the crypts become disrupted and are expanded by mucin and neutrophils. The pseudomembrane consists of the debris of necrotic epithelial cells, mucus, fibrin, and neutrophils.

When both the small and the large bowel are involved, the condition is referred to as *pseudomembranous enterocolitis*. Pseudomembranes are occasionally encountered in other enteric infections, such as those involving *S. aureus*, *Candida*, invasive bacteria, and verotoxin-producing *E. coli*. Ischemic bowel disease may also show pseudomembranes.

 Clinical Features: Antibiotic-associated infections with *C. difficile* are virtually always accompanied by diarrhea, but in most cases, the disorder does not progress to colitis. In patients who develop pseudomembranous colitis, fever, leukocytosis, and abdominal cramps are superimposed on the diarrhea. In the preantibiotic era, this form of colitis was a catastrophic event, and many patients died within hours or days from ileus and irreversible shock. Today, pseudomembranous colitis, although still a serious disease, is usually controlled with antibiotics and supportive fluid and electrolyte therapy.

Neonatal Necrotizing Enterocolitis Complicates Prematurity

Necrotizing enterocolitis is one of the most common acquired surgical emergencies in newborns. It is particularly common in premature infants after oral feeding and is believed to be related principally to an ischemic event involving the intestinal mucosa, which is followed by bacterial colonization, usually with *C. difficile*. The lesions vary from those of typical pseudomembranous enterocolitis to gangrene and perforation of the bowel.

DIVERTICULAR DISEASE

Diverticular disease refers to two entities: a condition termed *diverticulosis* and an inflammatory complication called *diverticulitis*.

Diverticulosis Reflects Environmental and Structural Factors

Diverticulosis is an acquired herniation (diverticulum) of the mucosa and submucosa through the muscular layers of the colon.

 Epidemiology: Diverticulosis shows a striking geographical variation, being common in Western societies and infrequent in Asia, Africa, and underdeveloped countries. Diverticulosis increases in frequency with age. Some 10% of persons in Western countries are afflicted.

 Pathogenesis: The striking variation in the prevalence of diverticulosis implies that environmental factors are primarily responsible for the disease. Western populations consume a diet in which refined carbohydrates and meat have replaced crude cereal grains, and it is widely assumed that the lack of indigestible fibers in some way predisposes to the formation of diverticula in susceptible persons. In this respect, the larger fecal mass in those who ingest a high-fiber diet diminishes spontaneous motility and intraluminal pressure in the colon.

INCREASED INTRALUMINAL PRESSURE: According to the fiber hypothesis, a lack of dietary residue in the Western diet leads to sustained bowel contractions and a consequent increase in intraluminal pressure. Such prolonged increased pressure is believed to lead to herniation of the superficial coats of the colon through the muscular layers into the serosa.

DEFECTS IN THE WALL OF THE COLON: In addition to pressure, defects in the wall of the colon are required for the formation of a diverticulum. The circular muscle of the colon is interrupted by connective tissue clefts at the sites of penetration by the nutrient vessels that supply the submucosa and mucosa. In persons of advancing age, this connective tissue loses its resilience and, therefore, its resistance to the effects of increased intraluminal pressure. This concept is supported by the observation that persons with heritable disorders of connective tissue (e.g., Marfan syndrome, Ehlers-Danlos syndrome) acquire precocious diverticulosis, primarily of the small bowel.

 Pathology: The abnormal structures that characterize diverticulosis are not true diverticula, which contain all layers of the intestinal wall, but rather pseudodiverticula, in which only the mucosa and submucosa are herniated through the muscle layers. The sigmoid colon is affected in 95% of cases, but diverticulosis can affect any segment of the colon, including the cecum. Diverticula vary in number from a few to several hundred. Most appear in parallel rows between the mesenteric and lateral taeniae. The diverticula, which measure up to 1 cm in greatest dimension, are connected to the intestinal lumen by necks of varying length and caliber. The muscular wall of the affected colon is consistently thickened.

Microscopically, a diverticulum characteristically is seen as a flasklike structure that extends from the lumen through the muscle layers (Fig. 13-42). The wall of the diverticulum is in continuity with the surface mucosa and therefore displays an epithelium and a submucosa. The base of the diverticulum is formed by serosal connective tissue.

 Clinical Features: **Diverticulosis is generally asymptomatic, and 80% of affected persons remain symptom free.** Many patients with diverticulosis complain of episodic colicky abdominal pain. Both constipation and diarrhea, sometimes alternating, may occur, and flatulence is common. **Sudden, painless, and severe bleeding from colonic diverticula** is a cause of serious lower gastrointestinal hemorrhage in the elderly, occurring in as many as 5% of persons with diverticulosis. Chronic blood loss may lead to anemia.

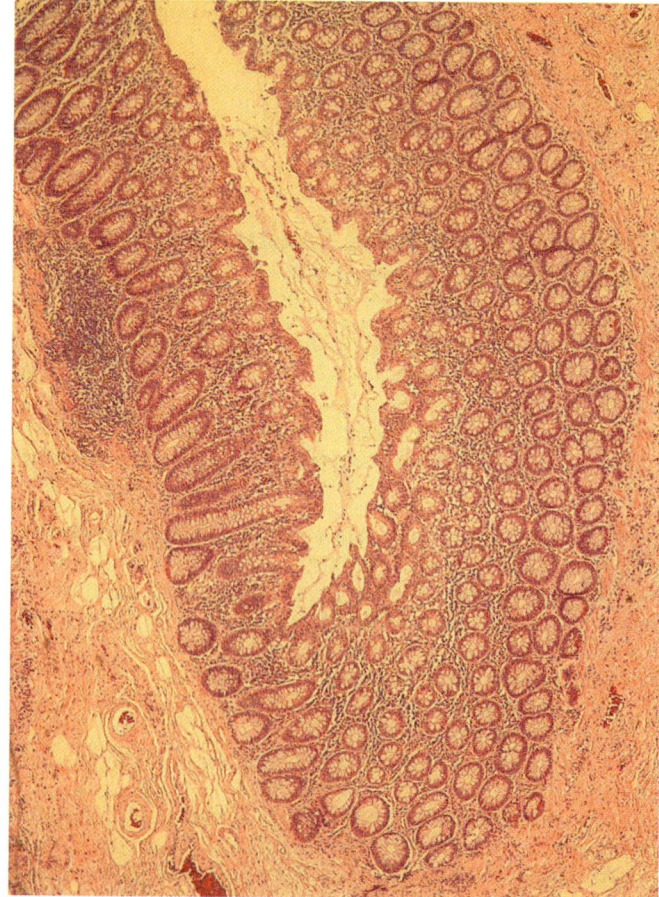

FIGURE 13-42
Diverticulosis of the colon. The herniated mucosa extends through the muscular layers of the wall.

Diverticulitis Refers to Inflammation at the Base of a Diverticulum

Diverticulitis presumably results from the irritation caused by retained fecal material. Although most persons with diverticulosis remain asymptomatic, in 10 to 20%, diverticulitis supervenes at some time in their lives.

Pathology: Diverticulitis produces inflammation of the wall of the diverticulum, an event that may result in perforation and the release of fecal bacteria into the peridiverticular tissues. The resulting abscess is usually contained by the appendices epiploicae and the pericolonic tissue, but infrequently, free perforation leads to generalized peritonitis. Fibrosis in response to repeated episodes of diverticulitis may constrict the lumen of the bowel, thereby causing colonic obstruction. Fistulas may form between the colon and adjacent organs, including the bladder, vagina, small intestine, and skin of the abdomen. Additional complications include pylephlebitis and liver abscesses.

Clinical Features: The most common symptoms of diverticulitis, usually following microscopic or gross perforation of the diverticulum, are persistent lower abdominal pain and fever. Changes in bowel habits, ranging from diarrhea to constipation, are frequent, and dysuria indicates irritation of the bladder. Most patients exhibit tenderness in the left lower quadrant, and a mass in that area is not infrequently palpated. Leukocytosis is the rule. Antibiotic treatment and supportive measures usually succeed in alleviating acute diverticulitis, but about 20% of patients eventually require surgical intervention.

INFLAMMATORY BOWEL DISEASE

Inflammatory bowel disease is a term that describes two diseases: Crohn disease and ulcerative colitis. Although these two disorders usually differ enough to be clearly distinguishable, they have certain common features. Yet similarities apart, Crohn disease and ulcerative colitis have different clinical courses and natural histories.

Crohn Disease Is a Segmental Transmural Inflammation of the Intestine

Crohn disease is a transmural, chronic inflammatory disease that may affect any part of the digestive tract but occurs principally in the distal small intestine and occasionally the right colon. It has variously been referred to as *terminal ileitis* and *regional ileitis* when it involves mainly the ileum, and *granulomatous colitis* and *transmural colitis* when it principally affects the colon. **Crohn disease may involve any part of the gastrointestinal tract and even extraintestinal tissues.**

Epidemiology: Crohn disease occurs throughout the world, with an annual incidence of 0.5 to 5 per 100,000. Reports from various countries indicate that the incidence has increased dramatically over the past 30 years. The disease usually appears in adolescents or young adults and is most common among persons of European origin, with a considerably higher frequency among Jews. There is a slight female predominance (1.6:1).

Pathogenesis: Epidemiological studies, particularly concordance rates in twin pairs and siblings, strongly implicate genetic susceptibility in the pathogenesis of Crohn disease. A family history of inflammatory bowel disease is more common in Crohn disease than in ulcerative colitis. A putative susceptibility locus for Crohn disease has been assigned to the centromeric region of chromosome 16, at least in non-Jewish patients. Other susceptibility loci may reside on chromosomes 3, 7, and 12. *NOD2* and *CARD15* mutations determine ileal disease, and the clinical pattern of Crohn disease has been linked to specific genotypes. Crohn disease has only rarely been described in both a husband and a wife, a fact that suggests that environmental factors alone do not suffice to cause the disease. Interestingly, smoking has been associated with Crohn disease, whereas ulcerative colitis distinctly uncommon in smokers. Several infectious agents have been suggested as possible causative agents. Bacteria that have been cultured from tissue involved with Crohn disease include a variant of *Pseudomonas* and atypical mycobacteria. The bacterial flora that may play a role in Crohn disease do not seem to be involved in ulcerative colitis.

Several studies have shown impairment of cell-mediated immunity in patients with Crohn disease. Some investigators have suggested increased suppressor T-cell activity, and others have claimed depressed phagocytic function.

The possibility that Crohn disease might be caused by immune-mediated damage to the intestine is suggested by the chronic and recurrent nature of the inflammation and by the occurrence of systemic manifestations that are frequently associated with autoimmune diseases. In recent years, most immunological studies have been concerned with the possible role of cell-mediated cytotoxicity. Some studies support the hypothesis that cytotoxic T cells sensitized to bacterial or other antigens damage the intestinal wall. In this respect, cyclosporine, a potent inhibitor of cell-mediated immunity that is widely used to prevent rejection of transplanted organs, has been reported to ameliorate the symptoms of Crohn disease.

The production of TNF-α is increased in vitro in mucosal cells derived from patients with Crohn disease. Moreover, in these patients, a shift in the mucosal balance of T-cell mediated cytokine production toward TNF-α was observed. Importantly, the administration of anti–TNF-α antibodies to patients with Crohn disease provides effective short-term symptom remission.

The fecal stream appears to be of prime importance in the pathogenesis of Crohn disease, as evidenced by (1) the beneficial effects of surgical bypass, (2) the pattern of preanastomotic recurrence in patients with side-to-end anastomotic sites, and (3) the frequency of early inflammatory lesions (aphthoid erosions) in the epithelium in association with mucosal lymphoid tissue.

Pathology: Two major features characterize the pathology of Crohn disease and serve to differentiate it from other inflammatory diseases of the gastrointestinal tract. First, the inflammation usually involves all layers of the bowel wall and is, therefore, referred to as *transmural inflammatory disease*. Second, the inflammation of the intestine is discontinuous; that is, segments of inflamed tissue are separated by apparently normal intestine.

It is convenient to classify Crohn disease into four broad macroscopic patterns, although many patients do not fit precisely into any one of them. The disease involves (1) mainly the ileum and cecum in about 50% of cases, (2) only the small intestine in 15%, (3) only the colon in 20%, and (4) principally the anorectal region in 15%. Disease of the ileum and cecum is more frequent in young persons; colitis is common in older patients. Crohn disease is occasionally observed in the duodenum and stomach as a focal acute inflammatory process with or without granulomas. More rarely, it occurs in the esophagus and oral cavity, almost always in association with small intestinal Crohn disease. In women with anorectal Crohn disease, the inflammation may spread to involve the external genitalia.

The macroscopic and microscopic pathology of Crohn disease is variable and may comprise almost any combination of features considered characteristic of the disease. On gross examination, the bowel appears thickened and edematous, as does the adjacent mesentery. Mesenteric fat often wraps around the bowel ("creeping fat"). Mesenteric lymph nodes are frequently enlarged, firm, and matted together. The intestinal lumen is narrowed by edema in early cases and by a combination of edema and fibrosis in long-standing disease. Nodular swelling, fibrosis, and ulceration of the mucosa lead to a "cobblestone" appearance (Fig. 13-43). In early cases, the ulcers have either an aphthous or a serpiginous appearance; later they become deeper and appear as linear clefts or fissures.

The cut surface of the bowel wall shows the transmural nature of the disease, with thickening, edema, and fibrosis of all layers. Involved loops of bowel often become adherent, and fistulas between such segments are frequent. These fistulas, presumably a late result of the deep mural ulcers, may also penetrate from the bowel into other organs, including the bladder, uterus, vagina, and skin. Most fistulas end blindly, forming abscess cavities within the peritoneal cavity, in the mesentery, or in retroperitoneal structures. Lesions in the distal rectum and anus may create perianal fistulas, a well-known presenting feature of Crohn disease.

Microscopically, Crohn disease appears as a chronic inflammatory process. During early phases of the disease, the inflammation may be confined to the mucosa and submucosa. Small, superficial mucosal ulcerations (aphthous ulcers) are seen, together with mucosal and submucosal edema and an increase in the number of lymphocytes, plasma cells, and macrophages. Destruction of the mucosal architecture, with regenerative changes in the crypts and villous distortion, are frequent. Pyloric metaplasia and Paneth cell hyperplasia is common in the small intestine and the colorectum. Later, long, deep, fissurelike ulcers are seen, and vascular hyalinization and fibrosis become apparent.

The microscopic hallmark of Crohn disease is transmural nodular lymphoid aggregates, accompanied by proliferative changes of the muscularis mucosae and nerves of the submucosal and myenteric plexuses (Fig. 13-44). **Discrete, noncaseating granulomas, mostly in the submucosa, may be present.** Indistinguishable from those of sarcoidosis, these granulomas consist of focal aggregates of epithelioid cells, vaguely limited by a rim of lymphocytes. Multinucleated giant cells may be present, and the center of the granulomas usually displays hyaline material and only very rarely necrosis.

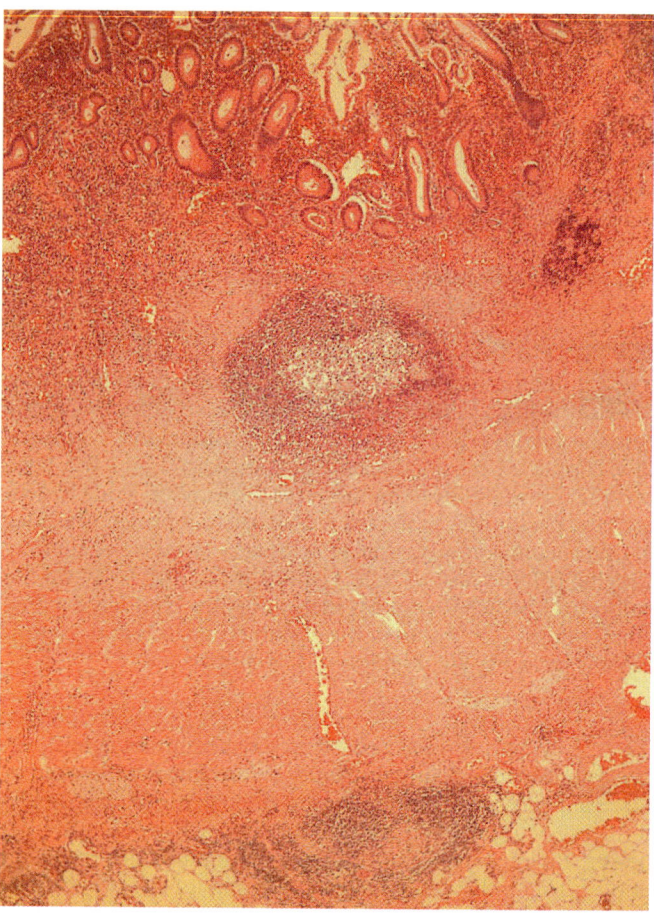
FIGURE 13-44
Crohn disease. A section of the colon shows transmural inflammation with germinal centers and granulomas.

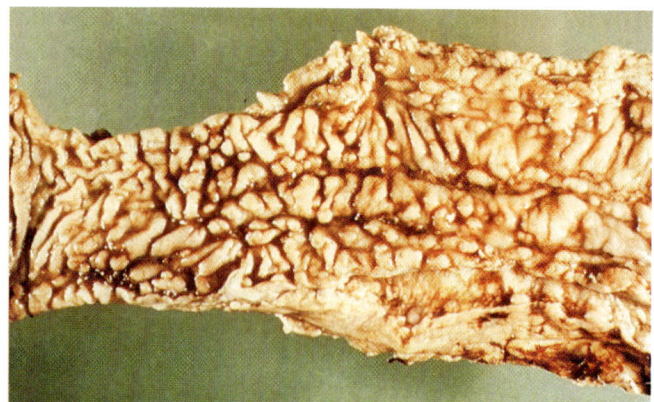
FIGURE 13-43
Crohn disease. The mucosal surface of the colon displays a "cobblestone" appearance owing to the presence of linear ulcerations and edema and inflammation of the intervening tissue.

Although the presence of discrete granulomas is strong evidence in favor of Crohn disease, the absence of granulomas by no means excludes the diagnosis, since less than half the cases show the typical granulomas.

The pathological features of Crohn disease are summarized in Figure 13-45.

Clinical Features: The clinical manifestations and the natural history of Crohn disease are highly variable and are related to the anatomical localization of the disease. The most frequent symptoms are **abdominal pain and diarrhea,** which occur in more than 75% of patients, and recurrent **fever,** evident in 50%. When the disease involves mainly the ileum and cecum, the sudden onset may mimic appendicitis, and the diagnosis of Crohn disease is occasionally made first at the time of abdominal surgery. If the disease predominantly involves the ileum, the major clinical features are right lower quadrant pain, intermittent diarrhea and fever, and frequently a tender mass in the right lower quadrant of the abdomen. In cases of diffuse small intestinal involvement, **malabsorption** and malnutrition may be the major features. Lipid malabsorption may also result from interruption of the enterohepatic cycle of bile salts because of ileal disease. Crohn disease of the colon leads to **diarrhea** and sometimes **colonic bleeding.** In a few patients, the major site of involvement is the anorectal region, and recurrent anorectal fistulas are the presenting sign.

Intestinal obstruction and fistulas are the most common intestinal complications of Crohn disease. Occasionally, free perforation of the bowel occurs. **The risk of small bowel cancer is increased at least threefold in patients with Crohn disease, and the disease also predisposes to colorectal cancer.** When Crohn disease begins in childhood, its major man-

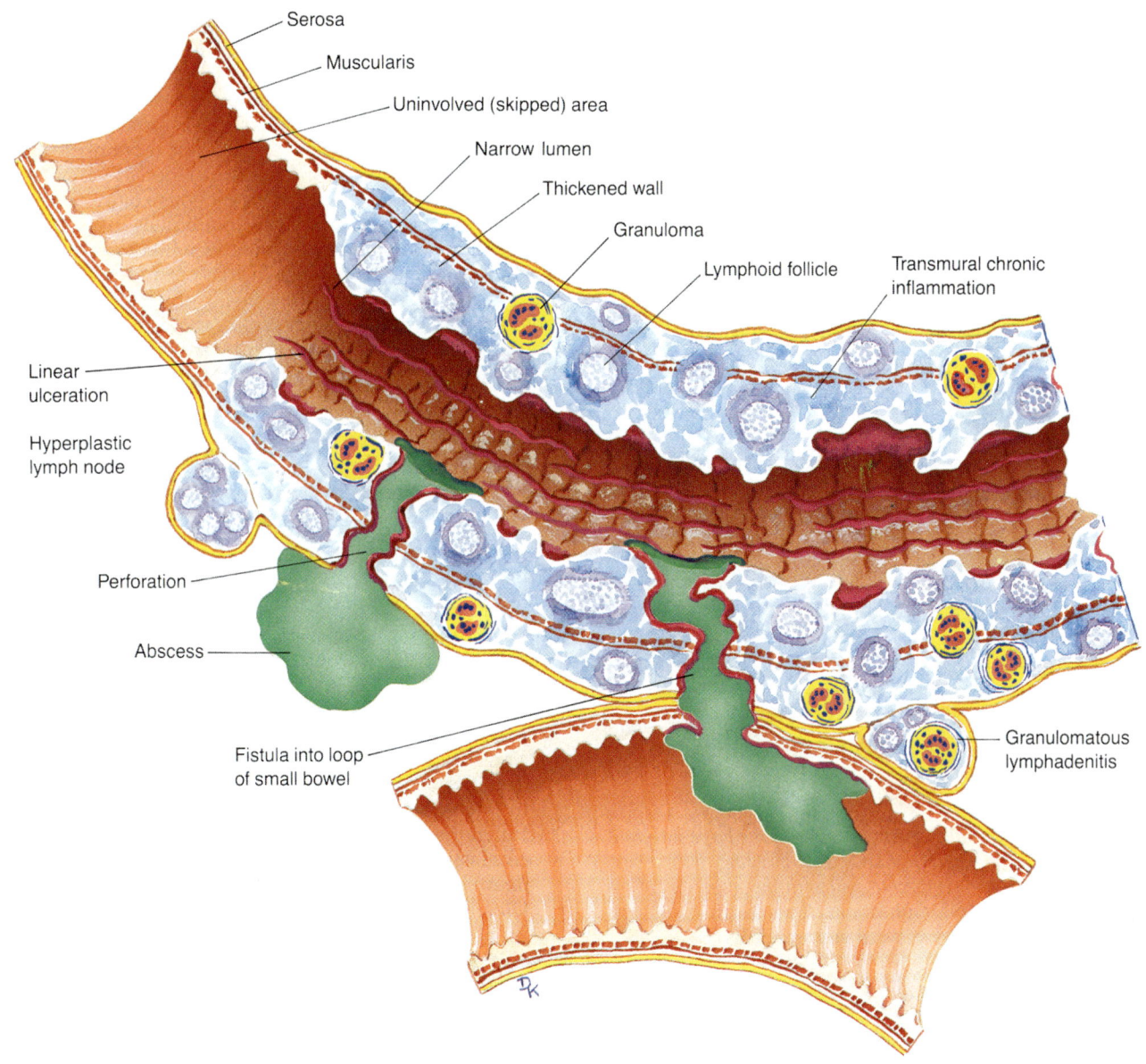

FIGURE 13-45
Crohn disease. A schematic representation of the major features of Crohn disease in the small intestine.

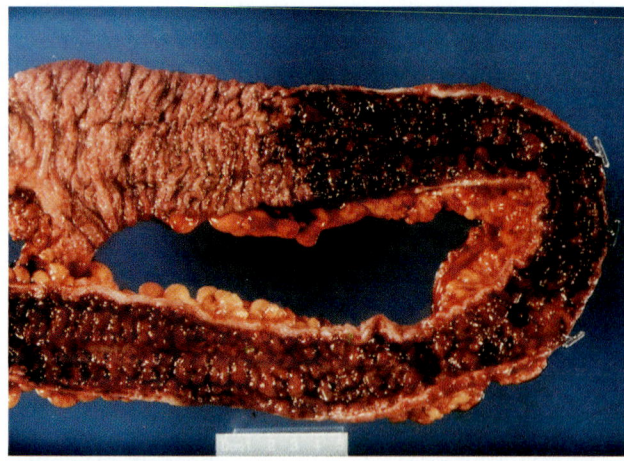

FIGURE 13-46
Ulcerative colitis. Prominent erythema and ulceration of the colon begin in the ascending colon and are most severe in the rectosigmoid area.

ifestation may be retardation of growth and physical development. Systemic complications also include liver disease (pericholangitis, sclerosing cholangitis), cholelithiasis, oxalate stones in the kidneys, and amyloidosis. The most frequent extraintestinal inflammatory features are in the eye (episcleritis or uveitis), the medium-sized joints (arthritis), and the skin (erythema nodosum).

No curative treatment is available for Crohn disease. Several medications are effective in suppressing the inflammatory reaction, including corticosteroids, sulfasalazine, metronidazole, 6-mercaptopurine, cyclosporine and anti-TNF antibodies. Surgical resection of obstructed areas or of severely involved portions of intestine and drainage of abscesses caused by fistulas are required in some cases. Preanastomotic or prestomal recurrence of the disease after construction of an enterostomy is a hallmark of Crohn disease, a feature that makes clinical management difficult. The need for repeated resections can lead to short-bowel syndrome in some patients.

Ulcerative Colitis Is a Chronic Superficial Inflammation of the Colon and Rectum

Ulcerative colitis is an inflammatory disease of the large intestine characterized by chronic diarrhea and rectal bleeding, with a pattern of exacerbations and remissions and with the possibility of serious local and systemic complications. The disorder occurs principally, but not exclusively, in young adults.

 Epidemiology: In Europe and North America, ulcerative colitis has an annual incidence of 4 to 7 per 100,000 population and a prevalence of 40 to 80 per 100,000. The disease usually begins in early adult life, with a peak incidence in the third decade of life. However, it also occurs in childhood and in old age. In the United States, whites are affected more commonly than blacks.

 Pathogenesis: The cause of ulcerative colitis is not known. Attempts to implicate a viral or bacterial agent have given only inconsistent results. In some families, as many as six patients with this disease have been described, and concordance has been reported in monozygotic twins. However, available family studies do not suggest any distinct mode of genetic transmission, and studies of HLA distribution in patients with ulcerative colitis have not demonstrated a consistent pattern.

The possibility that an abnormal immune response may play a role in the pathogenesis of ulcerative colitis has been studied extensively. The presence of abundant lymphoid tissue throughout the colon has made such a possibility attractive, as has the documented association of this disorder with immunorelated features, such as uveitis, erythema nodosum, and vasculitis. Several studies have demonstrated an increased frequency of circulating antibodies against antigens in colonic epithelial cells and against cross-reacting antigens in enterobacteria. Furthermore, in vitro studies of cell-mediated immune function have shown that mononuclear cells from the colonic mucosa and from the blood of patients with ulcerative colitis are toxic for autologous colonic epithelial cells. Antineutrophil cytoplasmic antibodies (ANCAs) have been demonstrated in 80% of patients with ulcerative colitis. However, these abnormalities are not found exclusively in patients with ulcerative colitis, nor are any of these changes a prerequisite for the development of the disease. It is, therefore, possible that all of these immune features are, the result, rather than the cause, of the mucosal damage.

 Pathology: Three major pathological features characterize ulcerative colitis and help to differentiate it from other inflammatory conditions:

- **Ulcerative colitis is a diffuse disease.** It usually extends from the most distal part of the rectum for a variable distance proximally (Fig. 13-46). When the disease involves the rectum alone, it is referred to as *ulcerative proctitis*. When the inflammatory process extends toward the splenic flexure, the terms *proctosigmoiditis* and *left-sided colitis* are applied. Sparing of the rectum or involvement of the right side of the colon alone is rare and suggests the possibility of another disorder, such as Crohn disease.
- **The inflammatory process of ulcerative colitis is predominantly limited to the colon and rectum.** It rarely involves the small intestine, stomach, or esophagus. When the cecum is affected, the disease ends at the ileocecal valve, although minor inflammation of the adjacent ileum is sometimes noted (backwash ileitis).
- **Ulcerative colitis is essentially a disease of the mucosa.** Involvement of deeper layers is uncommon, occurring only in fulminant cases, usually in association with toxic megacolon.

The following morphological sequence may develop rapidly or over a course of years.

EARLY COLITIS: Early in the evolution of the disease, the mucosal surface appears raw, red, and granular. It is frequently covered with a yellowish exudate and bleeds easily. Later small, superficial erosions or ulcers may appear. These occasionally coalesce to form irregular, shallow, ulcerated areas that appear to surround islands of intact mucosa.

The microscopic features of early ulcerative colitis correlate well with the colonoscopic appearances and include (1) mucosal congestion, edema, and microscopic hemorrhages; (2) a diffuse chronic inflammatory infiltrate in the lamina propria; and (3) damage and distortion of the colorectal crypts, which are often surrounded and infiltrated by neutrophils. Suppurative necrosis of the crypt epithelium gives rise to the characteristic *crypt abscess*, which appears as a dilated crypt filled with neutrophils (Fig. 13-47).

PROGRESSIVE COLITIS: As the disease continues, mucosal folds are lost (atrophy). Lateral extension and coalescence of crypt abscesses can undermine the mucosa, leaving areas of ulceration adjacent to hanging fragments of mucosa. Such mucosal excrescences are termed *inflammatory polyps* (Fig. 13-48). Tissue destruction is accompanied by manifestations of tissue repair. Granulation tissue develops in denuded areas. Importantly, the strictures characteristic of Crohn disease are absent. Microscopically, the colorectal crypts may appear tortuous, branched, and shortened in the late stages, and the mucosa may be diffusely atrophic.

ADVANCED COLITIS: In long-standing cases, the large bowel is often shortened, especially in the left side. The mucosal folds are indistinct and are replaced by a granular or smooth mucosal pattern. Microscopically, advanced ulcerative colitis is characterized by mucosal atrophy and a chronic inflammatory infiltrate in the mucosa and superficial submucosa. Paneth metaplasia is common.

 Clinical Features: The clinical course and manifestations of ulcerative colitis are highly variable. Most patients (70%) have intermittent attacks, with partial or complete remission between attacks. A small number (<10%) have a very long remission (several years) after their first attack. The remaining 20% have continuous symptoms without remission.

MILD COLITIS: Half of patients with ulcerative colitis have mild disease. Their major symptom is rectal bleeding, sometimes accompanied by tenesmus (rectal pressure and discomfort). The disease in these patients is usually limited to the rectum but may extend to the distal sigmoid colon. Extraintestinal complications are uncommon, and in most patients in this category, the disease remains mild throughout their lives.

MODERATE COLITIS: About 40% of patients are categorized as having moderate ulcerative colitis. They usually have recurrent episodes of loose bloody stools, crampy abdominal pain, and frequently low-grade fever, lasting days or weeks. Moderate anemia is a common result of chronic fecal blood loss.

SEVERE COLITIS: A small minority (10%) of patients have severe or fulminant ulcerative colitis, sometimes from its onset but often during a flare of activity. They have more than 6, and sometimes more than 20, bloody bowel movements daily, frequently accompanied by fever and other systemic manifestations. The loss of blood and fluids rapidly leads to anemia, dehydration, and electrolyte depletion. Massive hemorrhage is occasionally life threatening. A particularly dangerous complication of fulminant colitis is *toxic megacolon*, which is characterized by extreme dilation of the colon. Patients with this condition are at high risk for perforation of the colon. Fulminant ulcerative colitis is a medical emergency requiring immediate, intensive medical therapy and, in some cases, prompt colectomy. About 15% of patients with fulminant ulcerative colitis die of the disease.

The medical treatment of ulcerative colitis is governed by the sites involved and the severity of the inflammation. The 5-aminosalicylate–based compounds are the mainstays for the treatment of patients with mild-to-moderate ulcerative colitis. Corticosteroids and immunosuppressive and im-

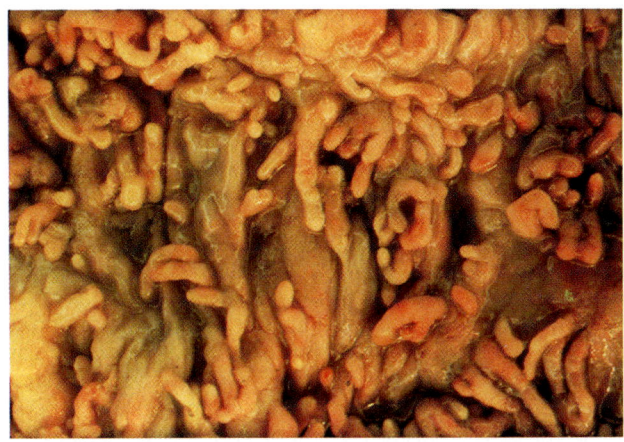

FIGURE 13-48
Inflammatory polyps of the colon in ulcerative colitis. Nodules of regenerative mucosa and inflammation surrounded by denuded areas provide a diffuse polypoid appearance of the mucosa.

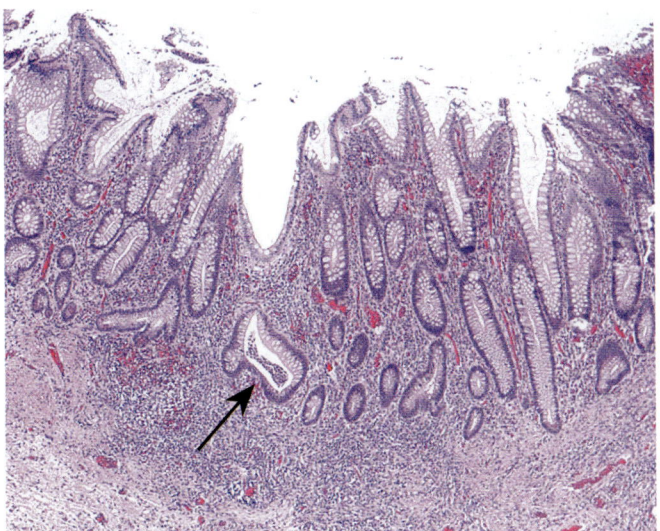

FIGURE 13-47
Ulcerative colitis. A section of the colonic mucosa shows gland distortion, crypt abscess (arrow), and basal lymphoplasmacytosis.

munoregulatory agents (azathioprine or mercaptopurine) are used in patients who have severe and refractory disease.

Extraintestinal Manifestations

Arthritis is seen in 25% of patients with ulcerative colitis. Eye inflammation (mostly **uveitis**) develops in about 10%, and skin lesions occur in about the same number. The most common cutaneous lesions are **erythema nodosum** and **pyoderma gangrenosum**, the latter a serious, noninfective disorder characterized by deep, purulent, necrotic ulcers in the skin.

Liver disease occurs in 3% of patients, the most common pathological findings being pericholangitis and fatty liver. Sclerosing cholangitis and carcinoma of the bile ducts are both associated with ulcerative colitis. Chronic active hepatitis is occasionally encountered. Thromboembolic phenomena, mostly deep vein thromboses of the lower extremities, occur in 6% of ulcerative colitis patients.

The various complications of ulcerative colitis are shown in Figure 13-49.

Differential Diagnosis

The most important conditions to be distinguished from ulcerative colitis are other forms of chronic colitis due to specifically treatable causes and Crohn disease. Other conditions that should be considered in the differential diagnosis of ulcerative colitis are bacterial infections and amebic colitis, especially in areas where it is endemic. When the inflammation is limited to the rectum, other infectious agents, including viruses, *Chlamydia,* fungi, and other parasites merit consideration. Proctitis due to these agents is common in male homosexuals, and a variety of opportunistic infections of the bowel are encountered in patients with AIDS. Other conditions that may mimic ulcerative colitis are ischemic colitis, antibiotic-associated colitis, radiation injury, and the solitary rectal ulcer syndrome.

The distinction between ulcerative colitis and Crohn colitis is based on the difference in anatomical localization

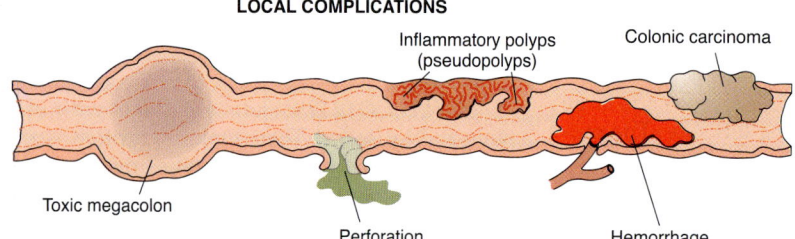
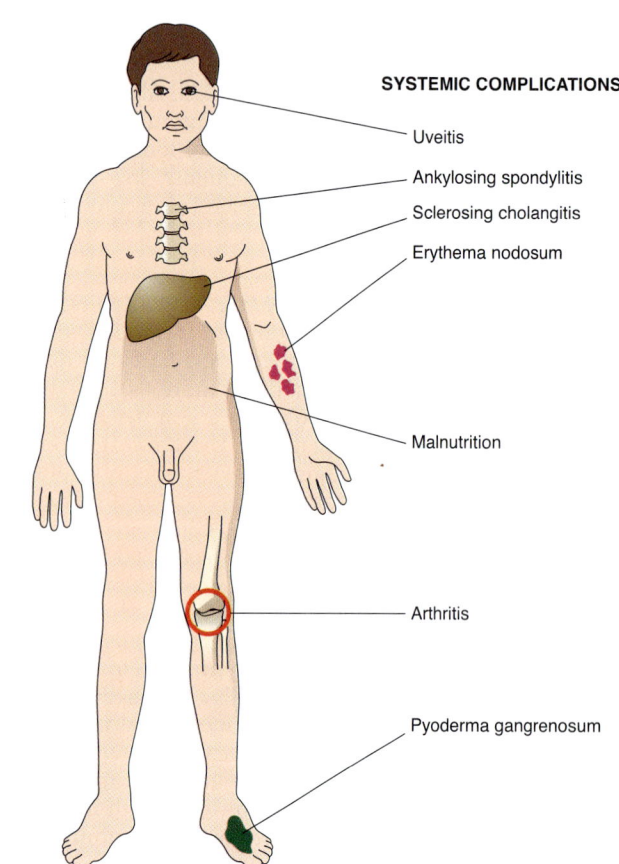

FIGURE 13-49
Complications of ulcerative colitis.

TABLE 13-1 **Comparison of the Pathological Features in the Colon of Crohn Disease and Ulcerative Colitis**

Lesion	Crohn Disease	Ulcerative Colitis
Macroscopic		
Thickened bowel wall	Typical	Uncommon
Luminal narrowing	Typical	Uncommon
"Skip" lesions	Common	Absent
Right colon predominance	Typical	Absent
Fissures and fistulas	Common	Absent
Circumscribed ulcers	Common	Absent
Confluent linear ulcers	Common	Absent
Pseudopolyps	Absent	Common
Microscopic		
Transmural inflammation	Typical	Uncommon
Submucosal fibrosis	Typical	Absent
Fissures	Typical	Rare
Granulomas	Common	Absent
Crypt abscesses	Uncommon	Typical

and histopathological appearance (Table 13-1). Ulcerative colitis is a diffuse process, usually more severe distally. By contrast, Crohn colitis is a patchy or segmental disease, with frequent sparing of the rectum. The inflammation in ulcerative colitis is superficial (i.e., usually limited to the mucosa) and is characterized by an acute inflammatory infiltrate, with neutrophils and crypt abscesses. By contrast, Crohn colitis is transmural and involves all layers, with granulomas in some of the specimens.

Demarcation of the disease at the ileocecal valve or in the colon distal to it favors ulcerative colitis. Involvement of the terminal ileum suggests Crohn colitis.

In 10% of cases, a precise diagnosis of ulcerative colitis versus Crohn colitis cannot be made, and the inflammatory bowel disease is termed *indeterminate colitis*. The distinction between ulcerative colitis and Crohn colitis is important because of (1) different surgical therapy (Crohn disease often has recurrences, so that continent ileostomy and ileoanal pouch procedures may be contraindicated), (2) a higher risk of cancer in ulcerative colitis, and (3) different medical therapy.

Ulcerative Colitis and Colorectal Cancer

Persons with long-standing ulcerative colitis have a higher risk of colorectal cancer than the general population. The risk is related to the extent of colorectal involvement and the duration of the inflammatory disease. Thus, persons with involvement of the entire colon are at the greatest risk of developing colorectal cancer. In patients with inflammatory disease limited to the rectum, colorectal cancer is no more common than in the general population. An incidence of colorectal cancer in the range of 5 to 10% for each decade of pancolitis is seen in the United States. Young age at the onset of colitis does not seem to be an independent risk factor, but because patients in whom ulcerative colitis develops at a young age have a longer duration of disease, they also have a high cumulative incidence of cancer.

EPITHELIAL DYSPLASIA: Colorectal epithelial dysplasia is a neoplastic epithelial proliferation and the precursor to colorectal carcinoma in patients with long-standing ulcerative colitis (Fig. 13-50). The histopathological criteria include (1) alteration of mucosal architecture, (2) epithelial abnormalities (hypercellularity and stratification of nuclei), and (3) epithelial dysplasia (variation in the size, shape, and staining qualities of nuclei). Dysplasia is divided into low-grade and high-grade dysplasia. High-grade epithelial dysplasia reflects a high risk for the development of colorectal cancer, and when identified in a biopsy, it is a strong indication for colectomy. Routine surveillance by colonoscopic biopsy of all patients with ulcerative colitis is, therefore, recommended.

Collagenous Colitis and Lymphocytic Colitis Cause Chronic Diarrhea

Collagenous colitis is a rare, inflammatory disorder of the colon characterized clinically by chronic watery diarrhea and pathologically by a thickened subepithelial collagen band. The disorder mainly afflicts middle-aged and elderly women.

The colonic mucosa appears grossly normal. The histopathological diagnosis of collagenous colitis is made by the demonstration of a chronic inflammatory cell infiltrate in the mucosa and a band of collagen immediately beneath the surface epithelium that measures up to 80 μm versus 5 to 7 μm in normal persons (Fig. 13-51). The surface epithelium displays flattened or cuboidal cells and even separation of the epithelial cells from the underlying structures. Intraepithelial lymphocytes are common. The lamina propria contains increased numbers of chronic inflammatory cells, and neutrophils are also found in some patients. *Lymphocytic colitis* also features prominent infiltration of the damaged colonic epithelium by lymphocytes but lacks the collagen table and has an equal sex distribution. Patients with lymphocytic colitis have more than 10 lymphocytes for every 100 epithelial cells.

The etiologies of collagenous colitis and lymphocytic colitis are unknown. It has been postulated that the fibrosis of collagenous colitis may result from persistent inflammation. Although the diseases have not been consistently linked

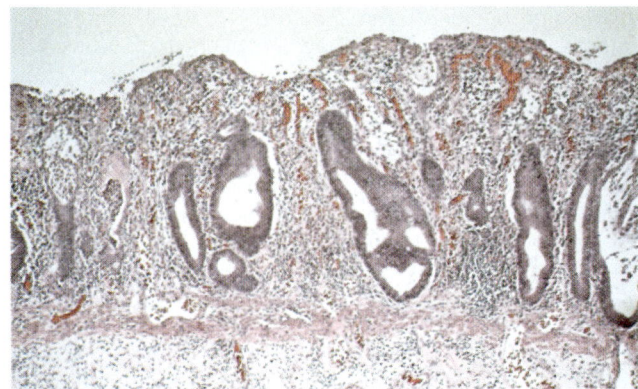

FIGURE 13-50
Epithelial dysplasia in ulcerative colitis. The colonic mucosa exhibits severe inflammation and irregular crypts lined by dysplastic epithelial cells. The epithelial cells exhibit hyperchromatic nuclei and stratification.

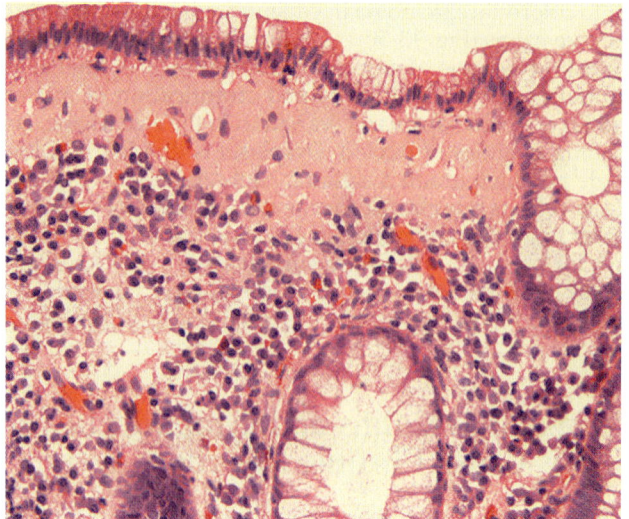

FIGURE 13-51
Collagenous colitis. A thickened band of collagen is evident beneath the surface epithelium. The lamina propria shows an increased number of chronic inflammatory cells.

to other systemic disorders, an autoimmune etiology also has been suggested, based on a putative association with rheumatoid arthritis and thyroid dysfunction. Compared with patients with collagenous colitis, those with lymphocytic colitis have an increased frequency of HLA-A1 and a decreased frequency of A3. Many patients with these diseases have taken nonsteroidal antiinflammatory drugs. Lymphocytic colitis is common in patients with celiac disease.

VASCULAR DISEASES

Ischemic Colitis

The colon is subject to the same types of ischemic injury as is the small intestine. Unlike the small bowel, extensive infarction of the colon is uncommon and chronic segmental disease is the rule. The most vulnerable areas are those between adjacent arterial distributions, so-called watershed areas. For example, the splenic flexure lies between the regions supplied by the superior and inferior mesenteric arteries, and the rectosigmoid area shares the blood from the inferior mesenteric and internal iliac arteries. However, the rectum itself is usually spared in ischemic colitis. Because most cases of ischemic colitis are caused by atherosclerotic narrowing of major intestinal arteries, intestinal disease usually occurs in persons over the age of 50 years.

Pathology: Some patients are seen with the symptoms and complications of bowel infarction and require immediate surgical intervention. However, in most patients, the acute signs stabilize, and radiographic examination shows only the pattern associated with intramural hemorrhage and edema. On endoscopy, multiple ulcers, hemorrhagic nodular lesions, or a pseudomembrane is seen. Biopsy reveals the characteristic changes of ischemic necrosis of the bowel: mucosal ulcerations, crypt abscesses, edema, and hemorrhage (Figure 13-52). Such patients may recover completely or may develop a colonic stricture, in which case, surgical removal of the obstructing segment becomes necessary. Segments of ischemic stricture show variable mucosal ulceration and inflammation, as well as widening of the submucosa by granulation tissue and fibrosis. Hemosiderin-laden macrophages may be noted, and patchy fibrosis of the muscular coats also may be present.

 Clinical Features: Ischemic disease of the rectosigmoid area typically manifests as abdominal pain, rectal bleeding, and a change in bowel habits. On clinical grounds alone, ischemic colitis often cannot be distinguished from certain forms of infective colitis, ulcerative colitis, and Crohn disease of the colon. The prognosis and treatment of patients with ischemic colitis depends on the primary cause and the extent of involvement. The goal is to improve the blood supply to the colon by treating the overall cardiovascular status of the patients. Acute interruption of blood supply to the colon can be fatal in neonates and elderly persons.

Angiodysplasia (Vascular Ectasia) Is a Cause of Intestinal Bleeding

Angiodysplasia (vascular ectasia) refers to localized arteriovenous malformations, predominantly in the cecum and ascending colon, which produce lower intestinal bleeding. The mean age at presentation is 60 years. Younger persons preferentially exhibit lesions at other sites, including the rectum, stomach, and small bowel. Interestingly, angiodysplasia is associated with aortic valve disease in some patients. It has been suggested that the disorder may be the result of chronic circulatory in-

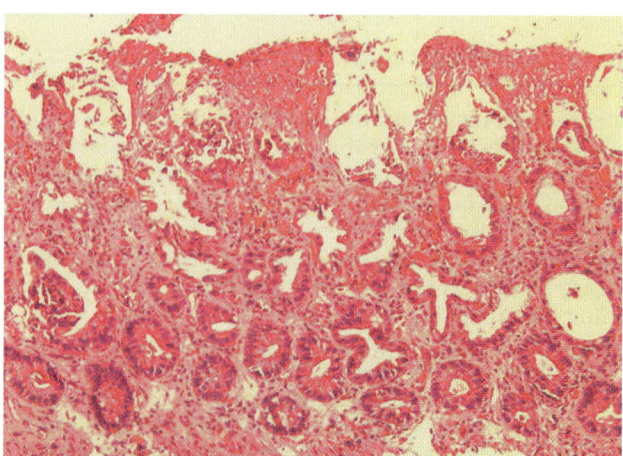

FIGURE 13-52
Ischemic colitis. Colonic mucosa with marked mucin depletion, surface ulceration, and fibrosis of the lamina propria.

sufficiency of the intestine, intestinal muscle hypertrophy, and resulting venous obstruction. Patients typically complain of multiple bleeding episodes, although the lesions also may cause chronic occult bleeding. Radiological studies and examination at laparotomy are usually negative. Thus, the diagnosis is difficult and often requires selective mesenteric arteriography or colonoscopy. Surgical removal of the affected segment is curative.

Pathology: The resected specimen displays small, often multiple hemangiomatous lesions, usually less than 0.5 cm in diameter. Microscopically, the veins and capillaries of the submucosa are tortuous, thin walled, and dilated. The attenuated walls of these vessels are presumably responsible for their propensity to bleed.

Hemorrhoids

Hemorrhoids are dilated venous channels of the hemorrhoidal plexuses that result from the downward displacement of the anal cushions. Internal hemorrhoids arise from the superior hemorrhoidal plexus above the pectinate line, whereas external hemorrhoids originate from the inferior hemorrhoidal plexus below that line. **Hemorrhoids are common in Western countries, to some degree afflicting at least half the population older than 50 years.** Hemorrhoids are common in pregnancy, presumably because of the increased abdominal pressure.

Pathology: Microscopic examination of hemorrhoidectomy specimens discloses dilated vascular spaces with excess smooth muscle in their walls. Hemorrhage and thrombosis of varying severity are common.

Clinical Features: The salient clinical feature of hemorrhoids is bleeding, and chronic blood loss may lead to **iron-deficiency anemia. Rectal prolapse** often develops in patients with hemorrhoids. Prolapsed hemorrhoids may become irreducible, a situation that leads to painful strangulated hemorrhoids. **Thrombosis** of external hemorrhoids is exquisitely painful and requires evacuation of the intravascular clot.

RADIATION ENTEROCOLITIS

Radiation therapy for malignant disease of the pelvis or abdomen may be complicated by injury to the small intestine and colon.

Pathology: Clinically significant radiation colitis is most common in the rectum. The lesions produced by radiation therapy range from a reversible injury of the intestinal mucosa to chronic inflammation, ulceration, and fibrosis of the intestine. In the short term, radiation results in epithelial and endothelial damage, including decreased mitoses and, in the small bowel, shortening of the villi. Mucosal inflammation is conspicuous, and in the colorectal crypts, abscesses may be seen. Failure of epithelial renewal may lead to ulceration. Subacute changes, occurring 2 to 12 months after radiation therapy, are noted after the mucosa has healed. Damage to submucosal vessels leads to thrombosis. The submucosa becomes fibrotic and often contains bizarre fibroblasts. As a result of radiation vascular injury, progressive ischemia further damages the bowel.

Complications of radiation enterocolitis include perforation and the subsequent development of internal fistulas, hemorrhage, and stricture, occasionally severe enough to lead to intestinal obstruction.

SOLITARY RECTAL ULCER SYNDROME

Internal mucosal prolapse of the rectum can produce mucosal changes that can be mistaken clinically and pathologically for chronic inflammatory disease or a neoplasm. The hallmark of solitary rectal ulcer syndrome is smooth muscle proliferation from the muscularis mucosae into the lamina propria. Despite the name, some patients have no ulcers, whereas others display multiple erosions or ulcers. Mucosal abnormalities often appear as a mass that can simulate a neoplasm. Dilated glands can be entrapped in the rectal wall, a condition termed *colitis cystica profunda*.

POLYPS OF THE COLON AND RECTUM

A gastrointestinal polyp is defined as a mass that protrudes into the lumen of the gut. Polyps are subdivided according to their attachment to the bowel wall (e.g., sessile or pedunculated, with a discrete stalk), their histopathological appearance (e.g., hyperplastic, serrated, or adenomatous), and their neoplastic potential (i.e., benign or malignant). By themselves, polyps are only infrequently symptomatic, and their clinical importance lies in their potential for malignant transformation.

Adenomatous Polyps Are Premalignant Lesions

Adenomatous polyps (tubular adenomas) are neoplasms that arise from the mucosal epithelium. They are composed of neoplastic epithelial cells that have migrated to the surface and have accumulated beyond the needs for replacement of the cells sloughed into the lumen.

Epidemiology: The prevalence of adenomatous polyps of the colon is highest in industrialized countries. As in diverticular disease, the diet is the only consistent environmental difference between high-risk and low-risk populations that has been identified. In the United States, it appears that at least one adenomatous polyp is present in half of the adult population, a figure that increases to more than two thirds among persons older than 65 years. There is a modest male predominance (1.4:1), and blacks have a higher proportion of right-sided adenomas and cancers. In one fourth of those who have at least one adenoma, two or more are present.

Pathology: Almost half of all adenomatous polyps of the colon in the United States are located in the rectosigmoid region and can, therefore, be detected by digital examination or by sigmoidoscopy. The remaining half are evenly distributed throughout the rest of the colon. The macroscopic appearance of an adenoma varies from a barely visible nodule or small, pedunculated adenoma to a large, sessile (flat) adenoma. Adenomas are classified by their architecture into tubular, villous, and tubulovillous types.

TUBULAR ADENOMAS: These polyps constitute two thirds of the benign large bowel adenomas. Tubular adenomas are typically smooth-surfaced lesions, usually less than 2 cm in diameter, which often have a stalk (Fig. 13-53A). Some tubular adenomas, particularly the smaller ones, are sessile.

Microscopically, tubular adenoma exhibits closely packed epithelial tubules, which may be uniform or may be irregular and excessively branched (see Fig. 13-53B). The tubules are embedded in a fibrovascular stroma similar to the normal lamina propria. Although most tubular adenomas display little epithelial dysplasia, one fifth (particularly larger tumors) show a range of more pronounced dysplastic features, which vary from mild nuclear pleomorphism to frank invasive carcinoma (Fig. 13-54). In high-grade dysplasia, the glands become crowded and highly irregular in size and shape. Papillary or cribriform (sievelike or perforated) growth patterns are common. **As long as the dysplastic focus remains confined to the mucosa, the lesion is invariably cured by resection of the polyp.**

The risk of invasive carcinoma correlates with the size of the tubular adenoma. Only 1% of tubular adenomas smaller than 1 cm across display invasive cancer at the time of resection; among those between 1 and 2 cm, 10% are found to harbor malignancy, and among those greater than 2 cm, 35% are cancerous. Small flat adenomas may be missed during conventional endoscopy and have a high malignant potential.

VILLOUS ADENOMAS: These polyps constitute one tenth of colonic adenomas and are found predominantly in the rectosigmoid region. They are typically large, broad-based, elevated lesions that grossly display a shaggy, cauliflower-like surface (Fig. 13-55A) but can be small and pedunculated. More than half are larger than 2 cm in diameter, and on occasion, they reach a size of 10 to 15 cm across. Microscopically, villous adenomas are composed of thin, tall, fingerlike processes that superficially resemble the villi of the small intestine. They are lined externally by neoplastic epithelial cells and are supported by a core of fibrovascular

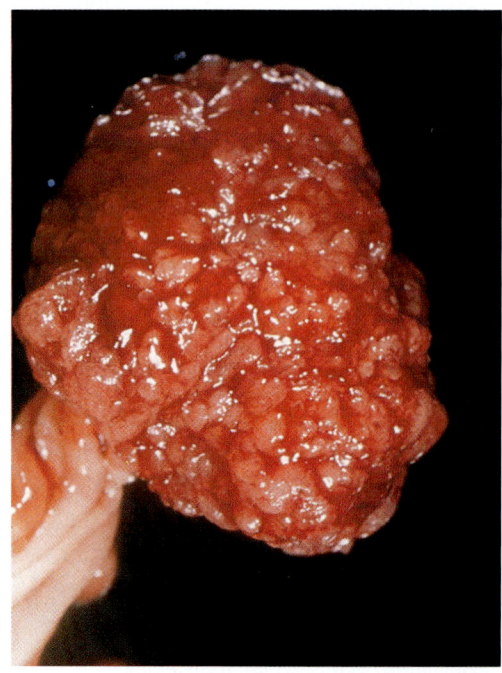
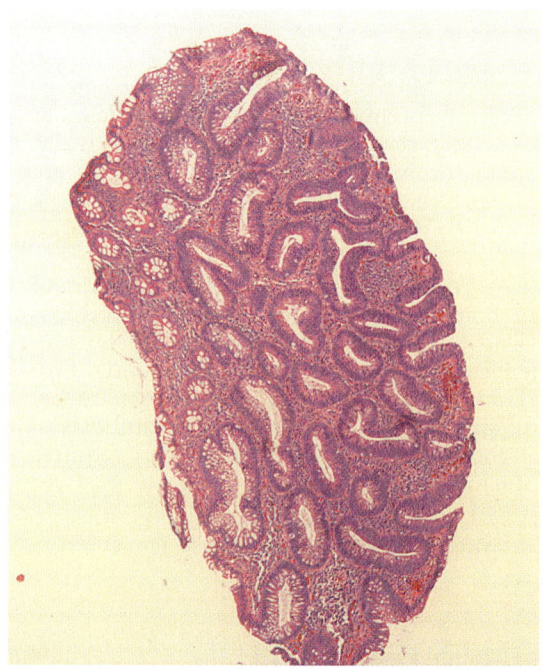

FIGURE 13-53
Tubular adenoma of the colon. A. A pedunculated tubular adenoma. B. A low-power photomicrograph of a tubular adenoma of the colon shows irregular crypts lined by pseudostratified epithelium with hyperchromatic nuclei.

Polyps of the Colon and Rectum

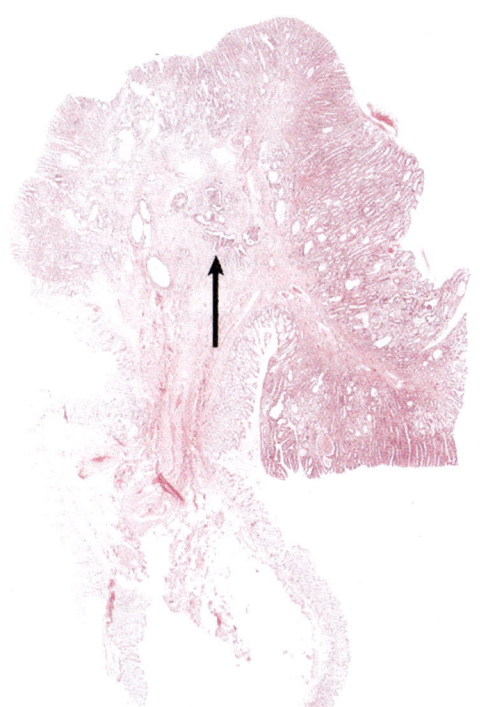

FIGURE 13-54
Adenocarcinoma arising in a pedunculated adenomatous polyp. A low-power photomicrograph shows irregular neoplastic glands *(arrow)* invading the stalk.

connective tissue corresponding to the normal lamina propria (see Fig. 13-55B).

The histopathology of dysplasia in villous adenomas is comparable to that in tubular adenomas. **However, in contrast to tubular adenomas, villous adenomas more frequently contain foci of carcinoma.** In polyps less than 1 cm across, the risk is 10 times higher than that for comparably sized tubular adenomas. Of greater importance is the fact that villous adenomas greater than 2 cm in size have a 50% prevalence of invasive carcinoma at the time of resection. **Given that most villous adenomas measure more than 2 cm in greatest dimension, more than one third of all resected villous adenomas contain invasive cancer.**

TUBULOVILLOUS ADENOMAS: Many adenomatous polyps manifest both tubular and villous features. Polyps with more than 25% and less than 75% villous architecture are termed tubulovillous. These adenomas tend to be intermediate in distribution and size between the tubular and villous forms, one fourth to one third being larger than 2 cm across. Tubulovillous polyps are also intermediate between tubular and villous adenomas in the risk of invasive carcinoma.

 Pathogenesis: The precursor to colorectal carcinoma is dysplasia, usually in the form of an adenoma. The pathogenesis of adenomas of the colon and rectum involves a neoplastic alteration of crypt epithelial homeostasis characterized by (1) diminished apoptosis, (2) persistence of cell replication, and (3) failure of maturation and differentiation in the epithelial cells that migrate to-

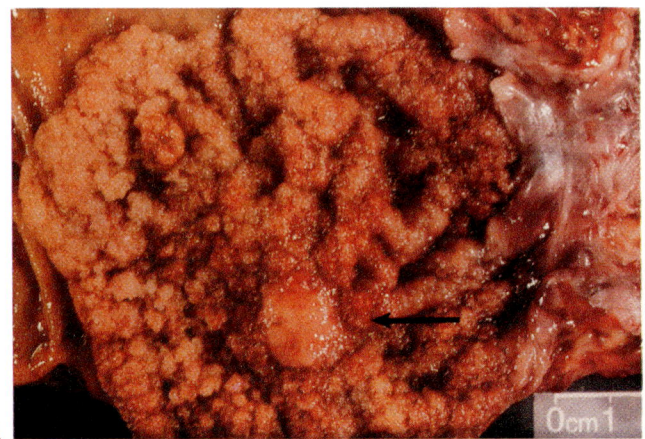
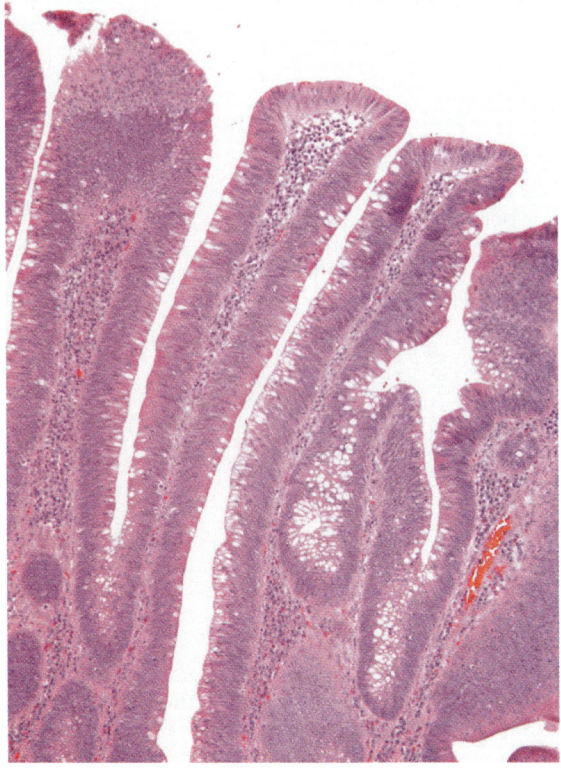

FIGURE 13-55
Villous adenoma of the colon. A. The colon contains a large, broad-based, elevated lesion that has a cauliflower-like surface. A firm area near the center of the lesion proved on histological examination to be an adenocarcinoma. B. Microscopic examination shows fingerlike processes with fibrovascular cores line by hyperchromatic nuclei.

ward the surface of the crypts (Fig. 13-56). Normally, DNA synthesis ceases when the cells reach the upper third of the crypts, after which they mature, migrate to the surface, and become senescent. They then undergo apoptosis or are sloughed into the lumen. Adenomas arise from a focal disruption of this orderly sequence, such that the epithelial cells maintain their proliferative capacity throughout the entire depth of the crypt. Thus, mitotic figures are initially visualized not only along the entire length of the crypt but also on the mucosal surface. As the lesion evolves, cell proliferation exceeds the rate of apoptosis and sloughing, and the cells begin to accumulate in the upper crypts and on the surface. Eventually, the accumulated cells on the surface of the mucosa form tubules or villous structures, in concert with stromal elements.

ADENOMATOUS POLYPS AND COLORECTAL CANCER: The origin of colon cancer in adenomatous polyps is supported by the following:

- **The geographical coincidence** in the frequencies of adenomatous polyps and colorectal cancer suggests a causal relation. In geographical regions in which there is a high risk of colorectal cancer, adenomatous polyps tend to be larger, are more often villous, and display more high-grade dysplasia than those in low-risk areas. The anatomical distribution of adenomas and carcinomas is similar, both being most frequent in the sigmoid colon in Western countries.
- **The average age at onset** of adenomatous polyps is earlier than that of colorectal cancer, suggesting that the latter follows the former. Adenomatous polyps tend to antedate colon cancer by 10 to 15 years.
- **Carcinomas are found in adenomas,** and some carcinomas have adenomatous remnants at their periphery.
- **An associated carcinoma** is commonly found in colons that harbor adenomas. Conversely, one third of colons resected for cancer contain an adenomatous polyp. Moreover, the presence of an adenomatous polyp in the same colon specimen resected for cancer doubles the risk that another carcinoma will develop in the remaining colon.
- **In familial adenomatosis polyposis** (see below), the innumerable adenomatous polyps are initially benign, but cancer of the colorectum invariably develops at a later age.

Prophylactic polypectomies have significantly reduced the risk of subsequent cancer development, a finding that provides powerful support for the concept that most colorectal cancers arise in adenomatous polyps.

Serrated Adenoma

Serrated adenomas show the sawtoothlike architecture seen in hyperplastic polyps, but the cytological features resemble those of adenomatous polyps and display nuclear elongation and pseudostratification. The cytoplasm is abundant and eosinophilic and contains mucin droplets. These polyps occur with higher frequency in the proximal colon. Serrated adenomas can progress to cancer.

Familial Adenomatous Polyposis Invariably Leads to Cancer

Familial adenomatous polyposis (FAP), also termed *adenomatous polyposis coli* (APC), a rare, autosomal dominant inherited trait with almost complete penetrance, accounts for less than 1% of colorectal cancers. It is characterized by the progressive development of innumerable adenomatous polyps of the colorectum, particularly in the rectosigmoid re-

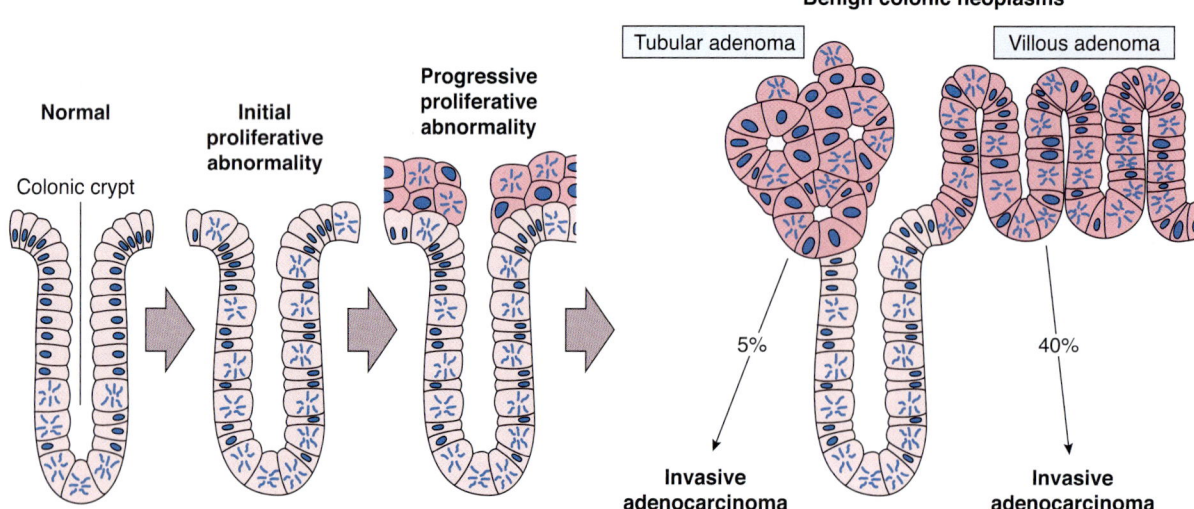

FIGURE 13-56
The histogenesis of adenomatous polyps of the colon. The initial proliferative abnormality of the colonic mucosa, the extension of the mitotic zone in the crypts, leads to the accumulation of mucosal cells. The formation of adenomas may reflect epithelial–mesenchymal interactions.

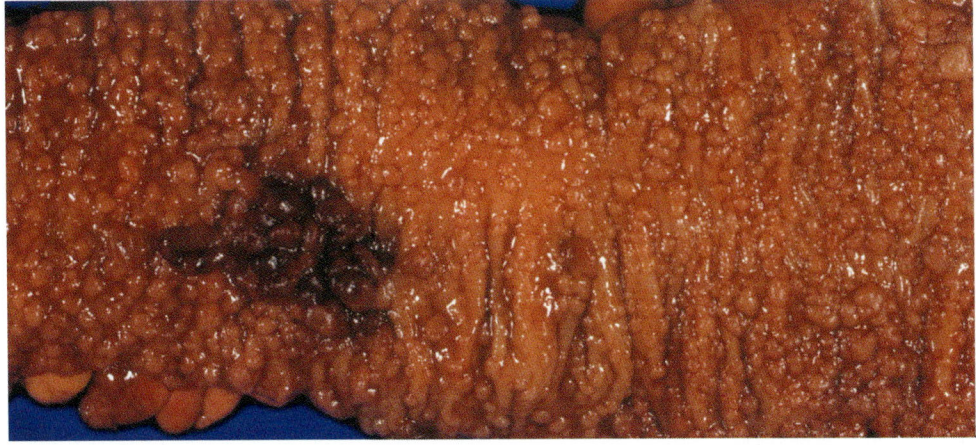

FIGURE 13-57
Familial polyposis. The mucosal surface of the colon is covered by numerous tubular adenomas.

gion. The disorder is caused by a germline mutation of the *APC* gene on the long arm of chromosome 5 (5q21-22) (see below). Most cases are familial, but 30 to 50% are due to new mutations. FAP is characterized by hundreds to thousands of adenomas carpeting the colorectal mucosa, sometimes throughout its length (Fig. 13-57). The adenomas are mostly of the tubular variety, although tubulovillous and villous adenomas are also present. Microscopic adenomas, sometimes involving a single crypt, are numerous. Although a few polyps are usually present by age 10, the mean age for the occurrence of symptoms is 36 years, by which time cancer is already present in many patients. **Carcinoma of the colon and rectum is inevitable, the mean age of onset being 40 years.** Total colectomy before the onset of cancer is curative. However, some patients also manifest tubular adenomas in the small intestine and stomach that have the same malignant potential as those in the colon.

Genetic testing for FAP is available, but mutations are found in only 75% of familial cases. Subtypes of FAP include the following:

Attenuated FAP: In this condition adenomas in the colon number less than 100.

Gardner syndrome: This variant features extracolonic lesions including osteomas of the skull, mandible, and long bones; epidermoid cysts; desmoid tumors; and congenital hypertrophy of the retinal pigment epithelium. *APC* gene mutations do not predict this phenotype.

Turcot syndrome: This rare disorder combines FAP with malignant tumors of the central nervous system. Many cases, especially those with medulloblastoma, are due to germline mutation of the *APC* gene. Some cases, especially those with glioblastoma multiforme, are part of the spectrum of the hereditary nonpolyposis colorectal cancer syndrome (see below).

Nonneoplastic Polyps Are Acquired Lesions

The nonneoplastic polyps are entirely different entities and are grouped together solely because of their gross appearance as raised lesions of the colonic mucosa.

Hyperplastic Polyps (Metaplastic Polyps)

Hyperplastic polyps are small, sessile mucosal excrescences that display exaggerated crypt architecture. They are the most common polypoid lesions of the colon and are particularly frequent in the rectum. Hyperplastic polyps present in 40% of rectal specimens in persons younger than 40 years and in 75% of older persons. These polyps are more common than usual in colons that contain adenomatous polyps and in populations with higher rates of colorectal cancer. Thus, these asymptomatic lesions reflect an increased risk of colorectal cancer. *Ras* mutations and overexpression of *Bcl-2* have been found in a number of hyperplastic polyps. Patients with hyperplastic polyposis (multiple hyperplastic polyps of the colon) have frequent allelic loss of chromosome 1p. Those with large hyperplastic polyps of the right colon have an increased risk of right-sided adenocarcinoma.

Pathogenesis: The pathogenesis of the hyperplastic polyp is believed to involve a defect in the proliferation and maturation of the normal mucosal epithelium. In a hyperplastic polyp, proliferation occurs at the base of the crypt, and the upward migration of the cells is slowed. Thus, the epithelial cells differentiate and acquire absorptive characteristics lower in the crypts. Moreover, the cells persist on the surface mucosa longer do than normal cells.

Pathology: Hyperplastic polyps are seen macroscopically as small, sessile, raised mucosal nodules, which measure up to 0.5 cm in diameter but occasionally can be larger. They are almost always multiple and have even been mistaken for FAP. Histologically, the crypts of the hyperplastic polyp are elongated and may exhibit cystic dilation (Fig. 13-58). The epithelium is composed of goblet cells and absorptive cells, without any dysplasia.

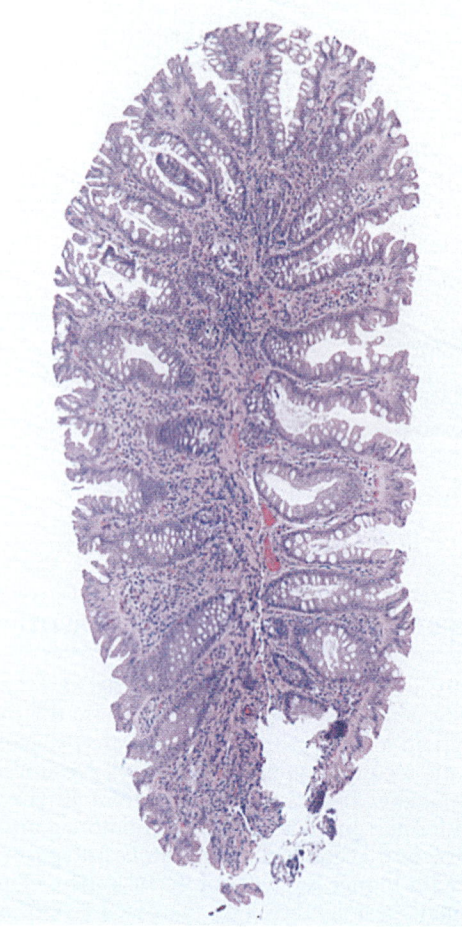

FIGURE 13-58
Hyperplastic polyp. A low-power photomicrograph shows elongated crypts with a sawtooth appearance lined by goblet cells.

Inflammatory Polyps

Inflammatory polyps are not true neoplasms but rather elevated nodules of inflamed and regenerating epithelium. Such polyps are commonly found in association with ulcerative colitis and Crohn disease; they are also encountered in cases of amebic colitis and bacterial dysentery. Microscopically, inflammatory polyps are composed of a variable component of distorted and inflamed mucosal glands, often intermixed with granulation tissue (Fig. 13-59).

As healing proceeds, epithelial regeneration characterized by large, basophilic epithelial cells restores the mucosal architecture. Although these lesions are themselves not precancerous, they occur in chronic inflammatory diseases that are associated with a high incidence of cancer (e.g., ulcerative colitis) and must therefore be distinguished from adenomatous polyps.

Lymphoid Polyps

Lymphoid polyps are submucosal accumulations of lymphoid tissue, almost invariably in the rectum, which are seen as single, sessile nodules measuring from pinpoint size to as large as 5 cm in diameter. On occasion, multiple lesions impart a cobblestone appearance to the mucosa. Microscopically, these polyps are covered by intact mucosa and are composed of prominent lymphoid follicles with germinal centers. In this context, lymphoid tissue is normally present in the colorectal mucosa. Lymphoid polyps are more common in women than in men and occur at any age, including childhood. The lesions are benign and usually asymptomatic.

Nodular lymphoid hyperplasia, *a condition seen primarily in children or with common variable immunodeficiency syndrome, features an excessive accumulation of the normal follicular lymphoid tissue of the colon.* Macroscopically, the mucosa exhibits numerous small sessile or polypoid nodules up to 0.5 cm in diameter. The microscopic appearance is similar to that of

Juvenile Polyps (Retention Polyps)

Juvenile polyps are classified as hamartomatous proliferations of the colonic mucosa. They are most common in children younger than 10 years, although one third occur in adults.

Pathology: Juvenile polyps are single or (rarely) multiple and occur most commonly in the rectum, although they may be seen anywhere in the small or large bowel. Grossly, most polyps are pedunculated lesions up to 2 cm in diameter. They have a smooth, rounded surface, in contrast to the fissured surface of an adenomatous polyp. Histologically, dilated and cystic epithelial tubules filled with mucus (hence the name "retention polyp") are embedded in a fibrovascular lamina propria. Surface epithelial erosion is common, and reactive epithelial proliferation is evident, but the epithelium usually lacks dysplasia.

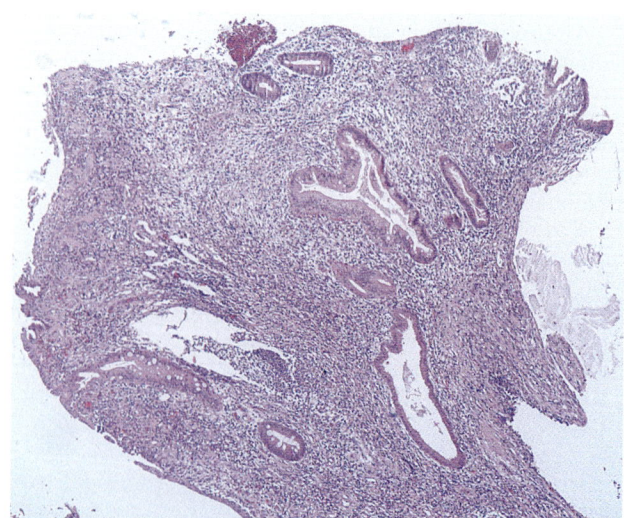

FIGURE 13-59
Inflammatory polyp. A low-power photomicrograph shows dilated glands embedded in an edematous and inflamed lamina propria.

lymphoid polyps. The condition is only rarely related to malignant lymphoma, but the radiological appearance can be mistaken for FAP.

MALIGNANT TUMORS

Adenocarcinoma of the Colon and Rectum Is an Example of Multistep Carcinogenesis

In Western industrialized societies, colorectal cancer is the most common cause of cancer deaths that are not directly attributable to tobacco use. Some 5% of Americans develop this cancer during their lifetime. Although the widely used term *colorectal* implies a common biology, the differences between cancers of the colon and rectum seem to be more fundamental than simple location. For instance, whereas colon cancer is much more common in the United States than in Japan, the incidence of rectal cancer in the two populations is nearly the same. In general, rectosigmoid carcinoma accounts for a considerably higher proportion of all large bowel cancers in populations at high risk for this tumor (including the United States) than in low-risk populations. Moreover, cancer of the colon shows a slight female preponderance, whereas cancer of the rectum is somewhat more common in men. The proportion of cancers in the distal colorectum has been declining in recent decades.

Pathogenesis: Most cancers of the colon and rectum arise in adenomatous polyps, and therefore factors associated with the development of such polyps are relevant to the genesis of colorectal cancer. The importance of environmental factors in the pathogenesis of colorectal cancer is emphasized by the high incidence of the disease in industrialized countries and among emigrants from low-risk to high-risk regions.

DIETARY FIBER: The major environmental risk factor for colorectal cancer has been suggested to be the diet, specifically **a diet low in indigestible fiber and high in animal fat.** As discussed above, such a diet also has been implicated in the etiology of other colonic diseases, including diverticulosis and appendicitis. A number of studies have reported that compared with a high-fiber diet a low-fiber one is associated with slower transit of fecal contents through the colon, thereby permitting longer exposure of the mucosa to substances in the stools. It has been suggested that fiber may bind potential mutagens and, by increasing the bulk of the stools, dilute their concentration. Newer analyses of the epidemiological data have, however, weakened the case for an association between the fiber content of the diet and the incidence of colorectal cancer. Moreover, in clinical trials dietary fiber exerted little protective effect against colorectal adenomas.

DIETARY FAT: The consumption of animal fats is paralleled by an increased incidence of colorectal cancer. Moreover, a lower content of animal fat in the diet of certain ethnic groups in the United States is accompanied by a lower incidence of colorectal cancer. The ingestion of fat elicits the secretion of bile into the intestine, and some bile acids have been said to enhance the tumorigenicity of experimental intestinal carcinogens. In this context, cholecystectomy, a procedure that increases the colonic content of secondary bile acids, has been claimed in some studies (although not in others) to be associated with an increased risk of right-sided colon cancer.

ANAEROBIC BACTERIA: The feces of persons in high-risk populations have a higher content of anaerobic bacteria than do those in low-risk populations. Such microorganisms, particularly *Bacteroides* species, can convert bile salts into compounds that are potentially mutagenic. Repopulation of the colon with *Lactobacillus* protects experimental animals against chemically induced colon cancer.

OTHER DIETARY FACTORS: A low prevalence of colorectal cancer has been correlated with **high levels of selenium** in the soil and plants of certain geographical areas. In this context, the endogenous antioxidant glutathione peroxidase is a selenium-containing enzyme. **Exogenous antioxidants** (e.g., butylated hydroxytoluene and vitamin E) and a reducing agent such as ascorbic acid have protected animals against the experimental production of colonic cancer. **Diets rich in cruciferous vegetables** (e.g., cauliflower, Brussels sprouts, and cabbage) and those that provide vitamin A are said to be associated with a lower incidence of colorectal cancer.

Molecular Genetics of Colorectal Cancer

In 85% of cases of colorectal carcinoma, it has been estimated that a minimum of 8 to 10 mutational events must accumulate before the development of an invasive cancer with metastatic potential. This process is initiated in histologically normal mucosa, proceeds through an adenomatous precursor stage, and terminates as invasive adenocarcinoma.

The most important events are illustrated in Figure 13-60 and involve the following genes:

- *APC* **gene**: As discussed above, germline mutations in the *APC* (adenomatous polyposis coli) gene, a putative tumor-suppressor gene, are responsible for familial adenomatous polyposis. Importantly, most sporadic colorectal cancers harbor a mutation in the same gene. Some of the tumors that lack an *APC* defect display mutations in the β-catenin gene, whose product binds to the *APC* protein. A specific *APC* mutation (T→A, 1307) is found in 6% of Ashkenazi Jews and seems to render surrounding regions of the gene susceptible to inactivating frameshift mutations. Mutations of the *APC* gene have been demonstrated in the normal colonic mucosa preceding the development of sporadic adenomas. These data suggest an important role for the *APC* gene in the early development of most colorectal neoplasms.
- *Ras* **oncogene**: Activating mutations of the *ras* protooncogene occur early in tubular adenomas of the colon.
- *DCC* **gene**: A putative tumor-suppressor gene, labeled "deleted in colon cancer" (*DCC*) and located on chromosome 18, is often missing in colorectal cancers.

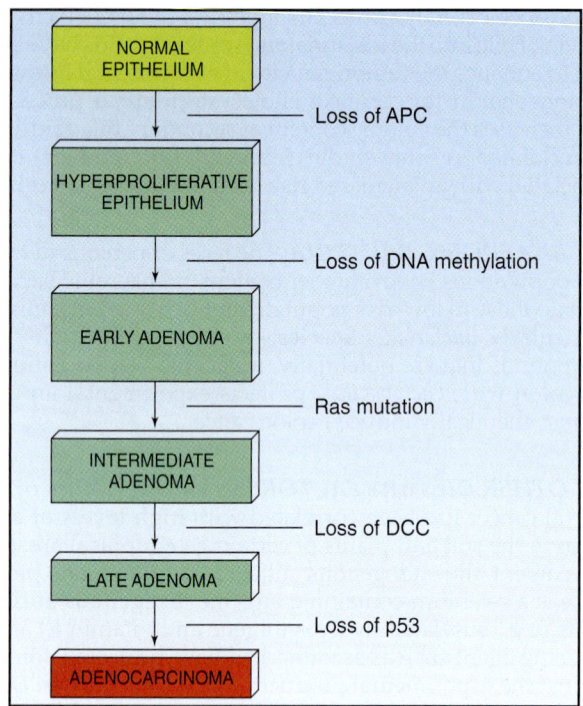

FIGURE 13-60
Model of some of the genetic alterations involved in colonic carcinogenesis following the tumor suppressor pathway.

- **p53 tumor-suppressor gene:** In the most common type of adenocarcinoma of the colon, mutation of *p53* participates in the transition from adenoma to carcinoma and is a late event in the carcinogenic pathway.

In 15% of colorectal cancers, DNA mismatch repair (MMR) is impaired, resulting in deficient repair of spontaneous replication errors, particularly in simple repetitive sequences (microsatellites).

MMR deficiencies can occur through two mechanisms in a hereditary form (hereditary nonpolyposis colorectal carcinoma, HNPCC, Lynch syndrome), a germline mutation in one of the MMR genes is followed by a somatic mutation of the other allele ("second hit") later in life. In a sporadic form, hypermethylation of the promoter of the MMR gene, *MLH1*, inactivates transcription of the gene.

Risk Factors

AGE: Increasing age is probably the single most important risk factor for colorectal cancer in the general population. The risk is low before age 40 years and increases steadily to age 50 years, after which it doubles with each decade.

PRIOR COLORECTAL CANCER: Patients who have previously suffered colorectal cancer have an increased risk of a subsequent tumor. In fact, 5 to 10% of patients treated for colorectal cancer subsequently develop a second malignant lesion of the colorectum. Moreover, 2 to 5% of patients in whom a colorectal cancer is discovered harbor a second primary (synchronous) cancer of the colorectum.

ULCERATIVE COLITIS AND CROHN DISEASE: These chronic inflammatory diseases increase the risk of colorectal cancer in proportion to their duration and extent of involvement within the large bowel.

GENETIC FACTORS: Colorectal cancer is increased in frequency among relatives of patients with the disease, a finding that suggests a genetic contribution to the development of the tumor. Persons who have two or more first- or second-degree relatives with colorectal cancer constitute 20% of all patients with this tumor. Some 5 to 10% of all colorectal cancers are inherited as autosomal dominant traits. A history of cancer at other sites, particularly breast or genital cancer in women, is associated with a higher than normal frequency of colorectal cancer.

DIET: As previously noted, prospective studies involving large populations in various countries have reported that the daily consumption of red meat and animal fat leads to a higher risk of colorectal cancer than that in persons who eat little or no meat.

 Pathology: The gross appearance of colorectal cancers is similar to that of adenocarcinomas elsewhere in the gastrointestinal tract. They tend to be **polypoid and ulcerating or infiltrative and may be annular and constrictive** (Fig. 13-61A). Polypoid cancers are more common on the right side of the colon, particularly in the cecum, where the large caliber of the colon allows unimpeded intraluminal growth. Annular constricting tumors occur more often in the distal portions of the colon. Ulceration of tumors, irrespective of the growth pattern, is common.

The vast majority of colorectal cancers are adenocarcinomas (see Fig. 13-61B) that are microscopically similar to their counterparts in other portions of the gastrointestinal tract. Some 10 to 15% secrete considerable quantities of mucin; these are classed as *mucinous* adenocarcinomas. The degree of differentiation influences the prognosis; better-differentiated tumors tend to have a more favorable outlook.

Colorectal cancer spreads by direct extension or invasion of vessels. **Direct spread of colorectal cancer** is commonly observed in resected specimens. The connective tissues of the serosa offer little resistance to the spread of the tumor, and cancer cells are often found in the fat and serosa at some distance from the primary tumor. The peritoneum is occasionally involved, in which case, there may be multiple deposits throughout the abdomen.

Colorectal cancer invades lymphatic channels and initially involves the lymph nodes immediately underlying the tumor. Venous invasion leads to blood-borne metastases, which involve the liver in most patients with metastatic disease. The prognosis of colorectal cancer is more closely related to the extension of the tumor through the wall of the large bowel than to its size or histopathological characteristics. Colorectal cancers are often staged according to the Astler and Coller modified classification of the Dukes system using the following criteria (Figure 13-62):

- **Stage A:** Tumor confined to the mucosa
- **Stage B₁:** Tumor invading the muscularis propria, but not penetrating to the serosa

- **Stage B₂:** Tumor invading to the serosa without lymph node metastases
- **Stage C₁:** B₁ tumors with metastases to regional lymph nodes
- **Stage C₂:** B₂ tumors with metastases to regional lymph nodes
- **Stage D:** Distant metastases

In the widely used TNM classification (tumor, lymph nodes, metastasis), T1 tumor invades the submucosa; T2 tumor infiltrates into, but not through, the muscularis propria; T3 tumor invades into the subserosal tissue; and T4 tumors penetrate the serosa or involves adjacent organs.

 Clinical Features: In its initial stages, colorectal cancer is clinically silent. As the tumor grows, the most common sign is **occult blood in the feces** when the tumor is in the proximal portions of the colon. Both occult blood and **bright red blood** may occur in the feces when the lesion is in the distal colorectum. In the right side of the colon, particularly in the cecum, where the diameter of the lumen is large and the fecal contents liquid, tumors can grow to large size without causing symptoms of obstruction. In this situation, chronic asymptomatic bleeding typically causes **iron-deficiency anemia,** which is often the first indication of colorectal cancer. By contrast, cancers on the left side of the colon, where the caliber of the lumen is small and the fecal contents more solid, often constrict the lumen, producing **obstructive symptoms.** These are manifested as changes in bowel habits and abdominal pain. Occasionally, colorectal cancer **perforates** early and induces peritonitis. When the tumor has extended beyond the confines of the colorectum, it may produce enterocutaneous and rectovaginal **fistulas,** tumor masses in the abdominal wall, bladder symptoms, and sciatic nerve pain. Intraabdominal spread may cause **small intestinal obstruction** and **ascites** with malignant cells.

A positive test result for occult blood in the feces with reagent-impregnated paper predicts the presence of a cancer or an adenoma in 50% of cases. Periodic fiberoptic colonoscopy and testing for occult blood in the feces improves the prognosis of colorectal cancer, because these methods can often detect the disease at an early stage.

The only curative treatment for colorectal cancer is surgery. Small polyps are easily removed endoscopically; large lesions require segmental resection. Tumors close to the anal verge often necessitate abdominal–perineal resection and colostomy, although newer surgical techniques frequently allow sphincter preservation. In rectal cancers, the combination of adjuvant chemotherapy and radiotherapy before surgery improves the prognosis. Among newer methods, the detection of guanylyl cyclase C mRNA in regional lymph nodes can be used as a biomarker to detect recurrences.

Hereditary Nonpolyposis Colorectal Cancer Syndrome

Hereditary nonpolyposis colorectal cancer (HNPCC) syndrome (Warthin-Lynch syndrome) is an autosomal dominant inherited disease that accounts for 3 to 5% of all colorectal cancers. The syndrome is characterized by (1) the onset of colorectal cancer at a young age (Table 13-2); (2) few adenomas (hence "nonpolyposis"); (3) a high frequency of carcinomas proximal to the splenic flexure (70%); (4) multiple synchronous or metachronous colorectal cancers; and (5) extracolonic cancers, including endometrial and ovarian cancers, adenocarcinomas

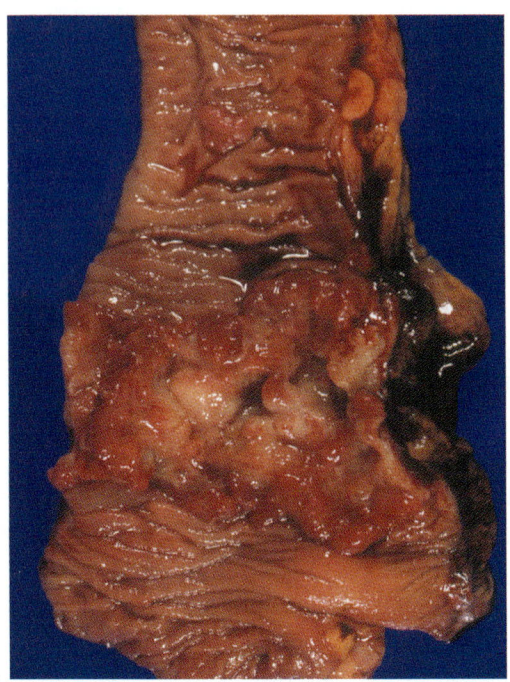
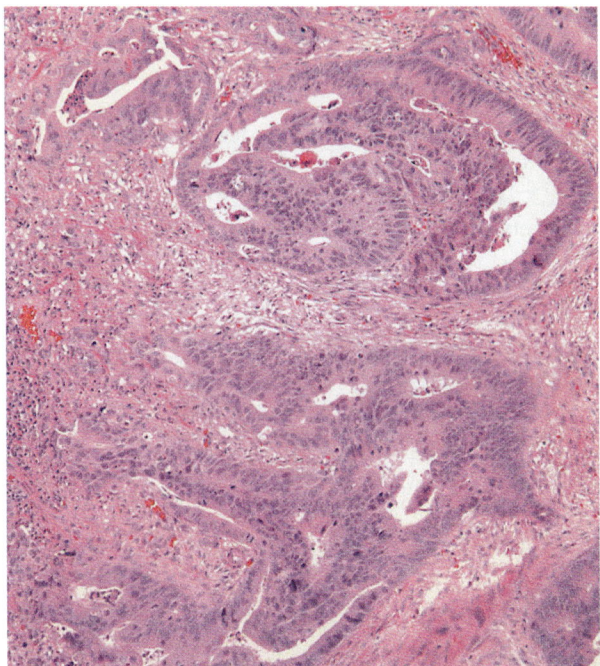

FIGURE 13-61
Adenocarcinoma of the colon. A. The opened colon contains an elevated, centrally ulcerated, infiltrating mass. B. A section taken from the tumor shows infiltrating malignant glands.

730 The Gastrointestinal Tract

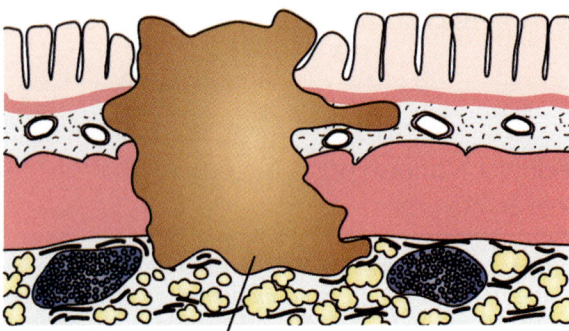

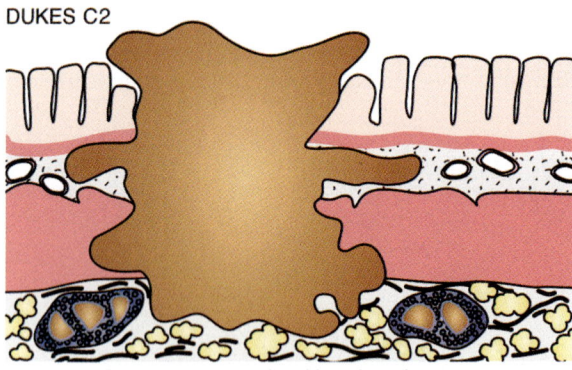

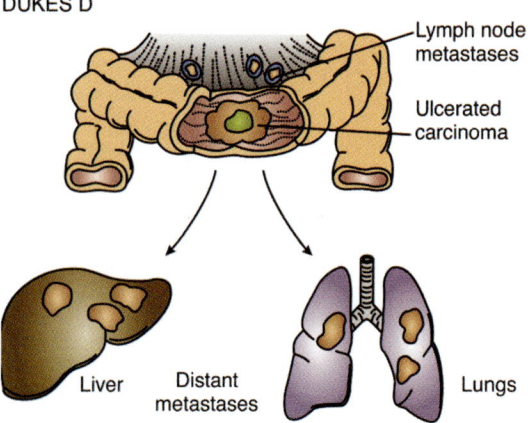

FIGURE 13-62
Astler and Coller-modified classification of the Dukes system of stages of the colon cancer.

TABLE 13-2 **Hereditary Nonpolyposis Colorectal Cancer**

Amsterdam criteria
  At least three relatives must have histologically verified colorectal cancer:
  One must be a first-degree relative of the other two
  At least two successive generations must be affected
  At least one of the relatives with colorectal cancer must have received the diagnosis before the age of 50 years
  Familial adenomatous polyposis must have been excluded

Bethesda guidelines
  Amsterdam I criteria met
  Individuals with more than one HNPCC
  Colorectal cancer (CRC) and first-degree relative with CRC/HNPCC, one cancer younger than 45 years or one adenoma younger than 40
  CRC/endometrial cancer younger than age 45
  Rigt-sided CRC, undifferentiated, younger than 45
  Signet-ring CRC younger than 45
  Adenomas younger than 40 years

of the stomach, small intestine, and hepatobiliary tract and transitional cell carcinomas of the renal pelvis and ureter. (Fig. 13-63). Patients with HNPCC may also have sebaceous adenomas, sebaceous carcinomas, and multiple keratoacanthomas. Histologically, HNPCC-related colorectal cancers are characterized by a high frequency of mucinous, signet ring cell, and solid (medullary) carcinomas and frequent intratumoral lymphocytes.

 Pathogenesis: HNPCC is caused by germline mutations in one of the DNA mismatch repair genes. In most cases, *hMSH2* (human MutS homolog 2) on chromosome 2p and *hMLH1* (human MutL homolog 1) on chromosome 3p are affected. A smaller number of cases are caused by mutations in *hMSH6* (human MutS homolog 6) and *hPMS2* (human postmeiotic segregation 2) on chromosomes 2p and 7p, respectively. In patients with HNPCC there is a germline mutation in one allele of one of the mismatch repair genes, and the second allele is deleted in a somatic "second hit." The resulting DNA mismatch repair deficiency prevents spontaneous replication errors from being repaired. This leads to widespread genomic instability, particularly in simple repetitive sequences (microsatellites), which are particularly prone to replication errors. Thus, genes for growth control and differentiation and other mismatch repair genes are disabled when they are affected by the genomic instability.

Mismatch repair deficiencies can be screened for by looking for microsatellite instability and loss of immunohistochemical expression of mismatch repair proteins in the tumor. If suspicion of HNPCC persists, mutation analysis of the mismatch repair genes is available.

Carcinoid Tumors (Neuroendocrine Tumors)

Carcinoid tumors of the colorectum behave like similar tumors of the small intestine. Half of carcinoid tumors of the colorectum have metastasized by the time they are discovered.

Large Bowel Lymphoma

Primary lymphoma of the colorectum is uncommon. The neoplasm may be seen as (1) segmental involvement of the mucosa, (2) diffuse polypoid lesions, or (3) a mass extending beyond the confines of the colorectum. The presenting symptoms are similar to those of other primary intestinal cancers, but the diffuse polypoid form may resemble inflammatory polyps or adenomatous polyps. Most large bowel lymphomas are derived from B cells.

Cancers of the Anal Canal Are Epidermoid Carcinomas

Carcinomas of the anal canal, which constitute 2% of cancers of the large bowel, may arise at or above the dentate line. These tumors occur in both sexes, but are more common in women and in blacks.

Pathology: Although anal cancers have various histological patterns, such as squamous, basaloid (cloacogenic), or mucoepidermoid, there are few clinical differences in behavior among the different tumor types, and they can be conveniently classed as *epidermoid carcinoma*. *Bowen disease of the anus* represents squamous carcinoma in situ, whereas *extramammary Paget disease* at this site reflects intraepithelial adenocarcinoma (either primary of the mucosa or metastatic). Carcinoma of the anus penetrates directly into the surrounding tissues, including the internal and external sphincters, perianal soft tissues, prostate, and vagina.

Clinical Features: Infection with human papilloma virus (HPV) and chronic inflammatory disease of the anus (e.g., venereal disease), fissures, and trauma predispose to anal cancer. Factors associated with genital carcinoma (cancer of the penis, scrotum, cervix, or vulva), poor hygiene, indiscriminate sexual practices, and genital warts also contribute to the development of anal cancer.

The usual symptoms of anal cancers include bleeding, pain, and an anal or rectal mass. Often the tumor is not clinically recognized as a malignant lesion and may be discovered only in a hemorrhoidectomy specimen. Combined chemotherapy and radiation therapy is the customary treatment, although abdominal–perineal resection is sometimes carried out. More than half of patients survive for at least 5 years.

MISCELLANEOUS DISORDERS

Endometriosis May Lead to Obstructive Symptoms

Endometriosis involves the colon and rectum in 15 to 20% of cases but is ordinarily asymptomatic and discovered only incidentally during laparotomy for other reasons. When symptoms do occur (abdominal pain, constipation, and even intestinal obstruction), they may be mistaken for those of colorectal cancer. *Endometriomas* are seen as indurated tumors of up to 5 cm in diameter in the serosa and muscularis propria of the bowel, although they may penetrate the submucosa. As a result of repeated hemorrhage, the lesions are surrounded by reactive fibrosis.

Melanosis Coli Refers to Pigment in the Colonic Mucosa

Despite the name, the pigment is not melanin, but rather, lipofuscin. Persons with melanosis coli are chronic users of anthracene-type cathartics, including cascara sagrada, rhubarb, senna, and aloe, and the finding can indicate surreptitious laxative abuse.

Melanosis coli imparts a dark brown color to the mucosa. Microscopically, macrophages in the lamina propria contain brown pigment granules. The pigment is lysosomal and is derived from the breakdown of cellular membranes.

Stercoral Ulcers

Incomplete evacuation of the feces, usually in association with debilitating disease or old age, may lead to the formation of a large mass of stool that cannot be passed, termed *fecal impaction*. Stercoral ulcers result from pressure necrosis of the mucosa caused by the fecal mass. Although such ulcers are most common in the rectosigmoid region, they have also been reported as proximally as the transverse colon. The most feared complications are severe rectal bleeding and perforation.

Gastrointestinal Diseases Are Common Complications of AIDS

The epidemic of AIDS due to infection with the human immunodeficiency virus (HIV) has resulted in numerous gastrointestinal infections previously considered rare. Most patients with AIDS (50–90%) have chronic diarrhea. Virtually all forms of infectious agents, including bacteria, fungi, protozoa, and viruses afflict patients with AIDS (Table 13-3).

Kaposi sarcoma of the gastrointestinal tract is found almost exclusively in patients with AIDS. One third to one half of AIDS patients with cutaneous Kaposi sarcoma exhibit involvement of the gastrointestinal tract. In most patients, intestinal Kaposi sarcoma does not lead to symptoms, although gastrointestinal bleeding, obstruction, and malabsorption have been reported.

A common presentation of lymphoma complicating AIDS is involvement of the gastrointestinal tract. Any portion may be affected. The histological appearance and prog-

TABLE 13-3 Gastrointestinal Pathogens Associated with AIDS

Bacteria	Protozoa
Mycobacterium avium-intracellulare	*Cryptosporidium*
Shigella	*Toxoplasma*
Salmonella	*Giardia*
Clostridium difficile	*Entameba histolytica*
	Microsporidia
Viruses	*Isospora belli*
Cytomegalovirus	
Herpes simplex	**Helminths**
	Strongyloides
Fungi	*Enterobius*
Candida	
Aspergillus	

nosis of these tumors in AIDS patients are similar to those elsewhere.

The Appendix

ANATOMY

The vermiform appendix, which is usually 8 to 10 cm in length, typically has a retrocecal attachment to the cecum, but its tip is generally not fixed and can therefore move freely. The appendix is invested with a mesentery called the *mesoappendix*. The wall of the appendix is composed of the same layers as the rest of the intestine. The most prominent microscopic feature is the predominance of submucosal lymphoid tissue, which develops in early infancy, reaches its largest size during adolescence, and then progressively atrophies.

APPENDICITIS

Acute appendicitis is an inflammatory disease of the wall of the vermiform appendix that leads to transmural inflammation and perforation and peritonitis. This condition is by far the most common disease of the appendix and is the most frequent cause of an abdominal emergency. Although the incidence peaks in the second and third decades, acute appendicitis may occur in persons of any age.

 Pathogenesis: **Acute appendicitis relates to obstruction of its orifice, with secondary distention of the lumen and bacterial invasion of the wall.** Mechanical obstruction by fecaliths or solid fecal material in the cecum is demonstrated in one third of cases. Occasionally tumors, parasites such as *Enterobius vermicularis*, or foreign bodies are incriminated. Lymphoid hyperplasia as a result of bacterial or viral infection (e.g., by *Salmonella* or measles) may obstruct the lumen and lead to appendicitis. **However, no obstruction is demonstrated in up to half of patients with appendicitis,** and the factor that precipitates the disease in these patients is unknown.

As secretions distend the obstructed appendix, the intraluminal pressure increases and eventually exceeds the venous pressure, thereby causing venous stasis and ischemia. As a result, the mucosa ulcerates and permits invasion by intestinal bacteria. The accumulation of neutrophils produces microabscesses. Interestingly, appendectomy protects against the development of ulcerative colitis but not Crohn disease.

 Pathology: Macroscopically, the appendix is congested, tense, and covered by a fibrinous exudate. The lumen often contains purulent material, and a fecalith may be evident (Fig. 13-63). Microscopically, early cases show mucosal microabscesses and a purulent exudate in the lumen. As the infection progresses, the entire wall becomes infiltrated with neutrophils, which eventually reach the serosa. Perforation of the wall releases the luminal contents into the peritoneal cavity.

The complications of appendicitis are principally related to perforation, which occurs in one third of children and young adults. Almost all children younger than 2 years have a perforated appendix at the time of operation, as do three fourths of patients older than 60 years.

- **Periappendiceal abscesses** are common, although abscesses may develop anywhere in the abdominal cavity.
- **Fistulous tracts** may appear between the perforated appendix and adjacent structures, including the small and large bowel, bladder, vagina, or abdominal wall.
- **Pylephlebitis** (thrombophlebitis of the intrahepatic portal vein radicals) and **secondary hepatic abscesses** may occur, because venous blood from the appendix drains into the superior mesenteric vein.
- **Diffuse peritonitis and septicemia** are dangerous sequelae.
- **Wound infection** is the most common complication of acute appendicitis after surgery; it occurs in one fourth of patients with perforation and in one third of those who develop a periappendiceal abscess.

 Clinical Features: Acute appendicitis is typically manifested as epigastric or periumbilical cramping pain, but the pain may be diffuse or initially restricted to the right lower quadrant. Shortly thereafter, nau-

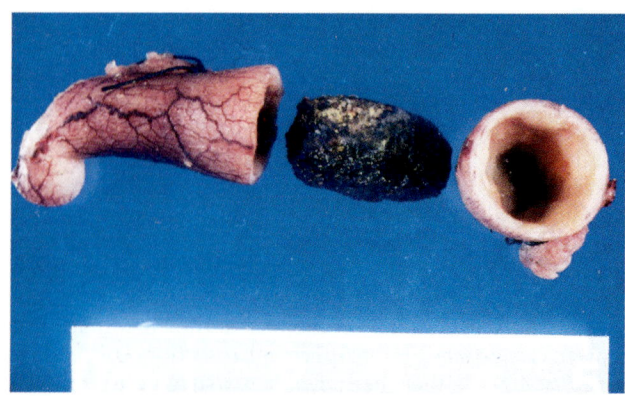

FIGURE 13-63
Acute appendicitis. The lumen of this acutely inflamed appendix is dilated and contains a large fecalith.

sea and vomiting occur, and the patient develops a low-grade fever and moderate leukocytosis. The pain shifts to the right lower quadrant, where point tenderness is the rule. A diseased retrocecal appendix is shielded from the anterior abdominal wall by the cecum and ileum; atypical symptoms are therefore easily misinterpreted because of their poor localization. In the elderly, appendicitis may produce only vague symptoms, and the diagnosis is often not made until perforation occurs. A number of conditions that do not require surgery are not infrequently misdiagnosed as appendicitis, especially mesenteric adenitis in children, Meckel diverticulitis, rupture of an ovarian follicle during ovulation, and acute salpingitis.

The treatment of acute appendicitis is surgical in the vast majority of cases. Because perforation carries a much higher risk of death than does laparoscopic surgery, early surgical intervention is warranted, even when the diagnosis of acute appendicitis is not entirely secure.

Other Causes of Appendicitis

Yersinia infection of the ileum may also involve the appendix.

Tuberculous appendicitis is usually found in association with tuberculous enteritis, and rare cases of **actinomycotic infections** are recorded.

Crohn disease of the terminal ileum involves the appendix in one fourth of cases and may affect it even when the inflammatory lesions are localized to distant sites in the small intestine or colon. Ulcerative colitis may also affect the mucosa of the appendix.

MUCOCELE

Mucocele refers to a dilated mucus-filled appendix. The pathogenesis may be neoplastic or nonneoplastic. In the nonneoplastic variety chronic obstruction leads to the retention of mucus in the appendiceal lumen.

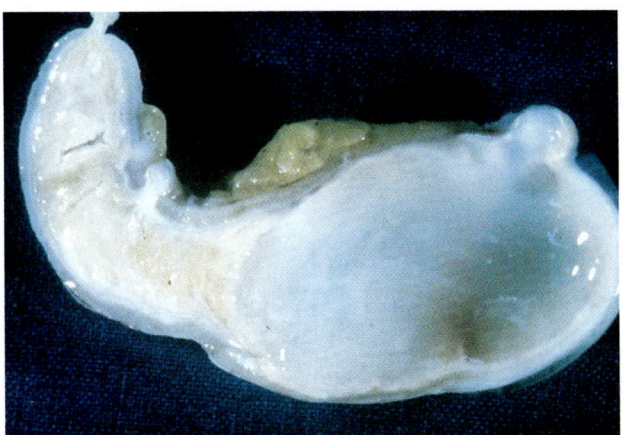

FIGURE 13-64
Mucocele of the appendix. The appendix is conspicuously dilated by mucinous material secreted by a cystadenoma.

In the presence of a mucinous cystadenoma (Fig. 13-64) or a mucinous cystadenocarcinoma, the dilated appendix is lined by a villous adenomatous mucosa. Cystadenocarcinoma exhibits infiltrating neoplastic glands into the wall of the appendix.

A mucocele may become secondarily infected and rupture, thereby discharging mucin and debris into the peritoneal cavity. This material may be mistaken at laparotomy for tumor implants on the peritoneum. However, when the mucocele results from mucus secretion by a cystadenoma or cystadenocarcinoma of the appendix, perforation may lead to seeding of the peritoneum by mucus-secreting tumor cells, a condition known as *pseudomyxoma peritonei*. In less than one third of cases, pseudomyxoma peritonei is caused by disease of the appendix; in half, it originates from ovarian mucinous cystadenocarcinoma.

NEOPLASMS

Carcinoid tumors of the appendix are common, and in this location are unlikely to metastasize.

Figures 13-65 through 13-68 summarize the causes of gastrointestinal bleeding and obstruction and the major benign and malignant tumors of the gastrointestinal tract.

The Peritoneum

The peritoneum is the mesothelial lining of the abdominal cavity and its viscera. The visceral peritoneum invests the gastrointestinal tract from the stomach to the rectum and encircles the liver. The parietal peritoneum lines the abdominal wall and the retroperitoneal space. The omentum, which has a double layer of peritoneum, encloses blood vessels and a variable amount of fat.

PERITONITIS

Bacterial Peritonitis Is Usually Caused by Intestinal Organisms

 Pathogenesis

PERFORATION: A number of situations are associated with the introduction of microorganisms into the peritoneal cavity. **The most common cause of bacterial peritonitis is perforation of an abdominal viscus,** as in an inflamed appendix, peptic ulcer, or colonic diverticulum. Peritonitis results in an acute abdomen, in which severe abdominal pain and tenderness predominate. Nausea, vomiting, and a high fever are usual, and in severe cases, generalized peritonitis, paralytic ileus, and septic shock ensue. Often the perforation becomes "walled off," in which case, a peritoneal abscess results.

The bacteria released into the peritoneal cavity from the gastrointestinal tract vary according to the site of perforation

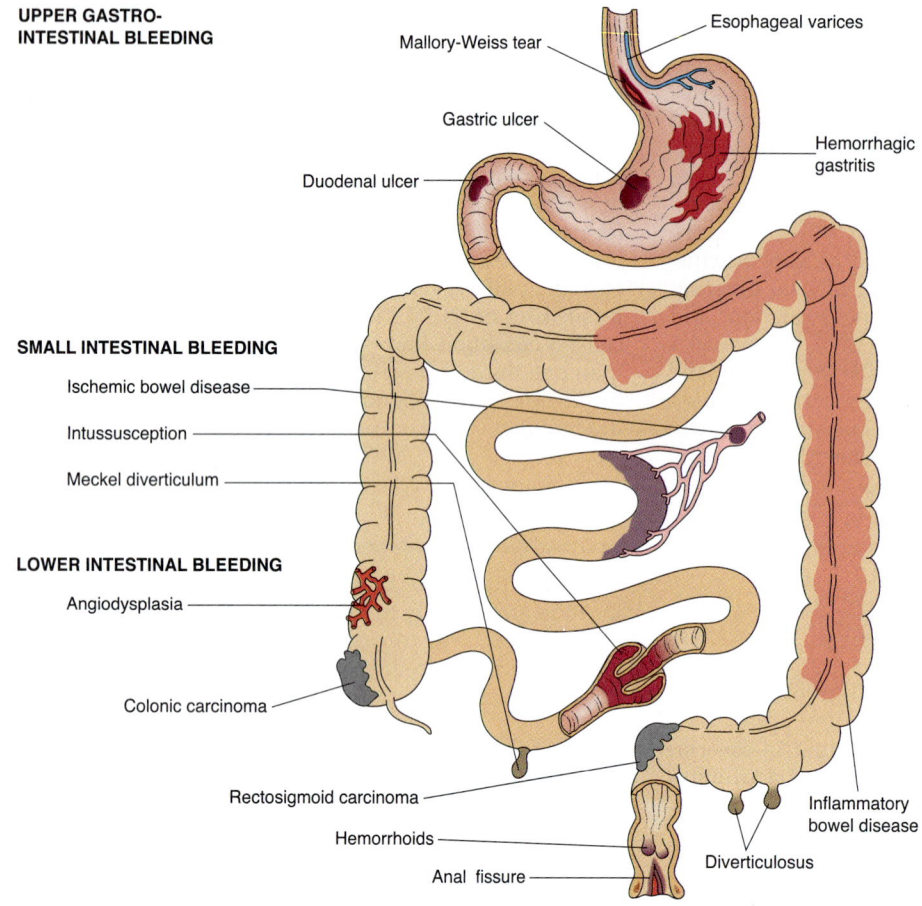

FIGURE 13-65
Causes of gastrointestinal bleeding.

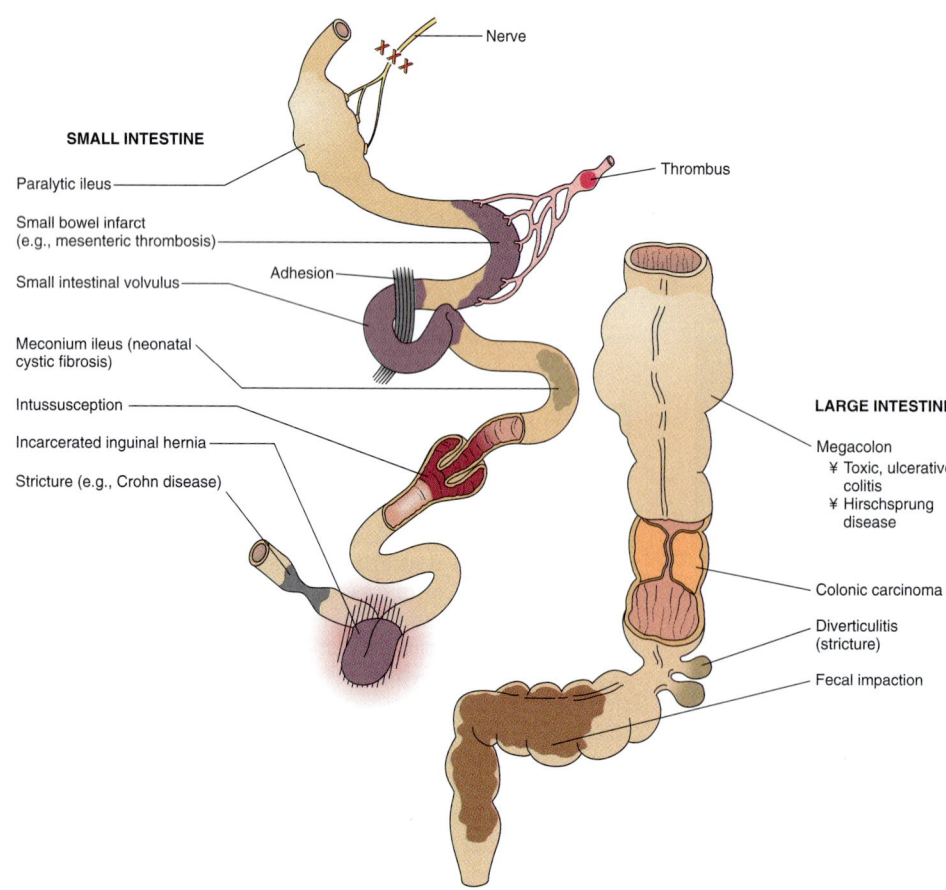

FIGURE 13-66
Causes of gastrointestinal obstruction.

Peritonitis 735

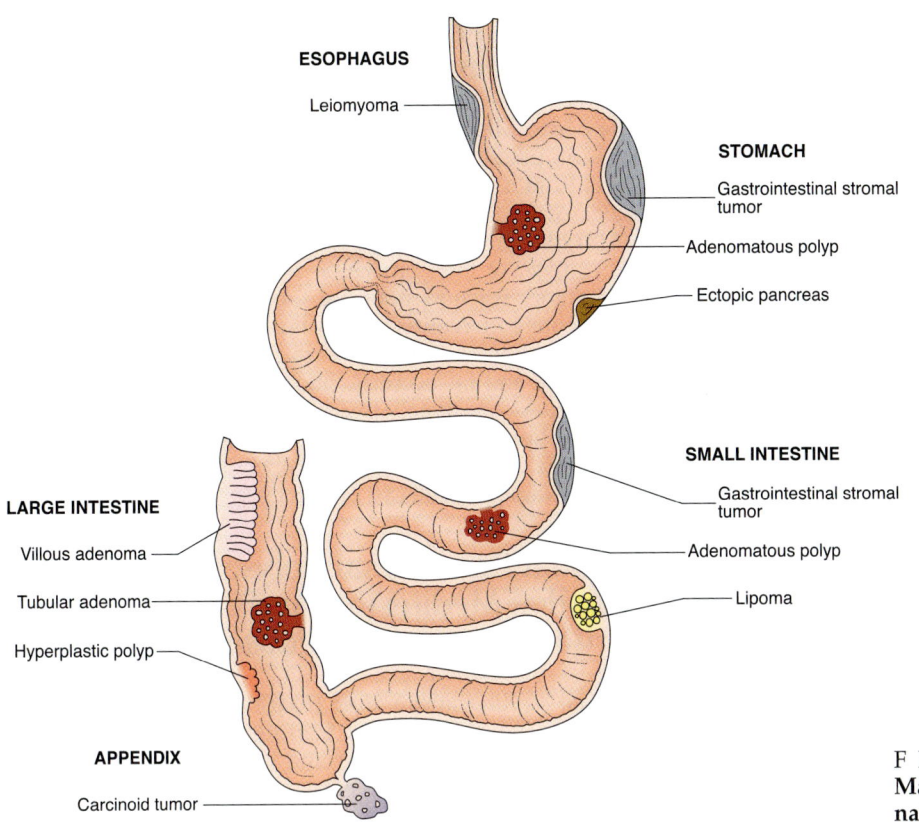

FIGURE 13-67
Major benign tumors of the gastrointestinal tract.

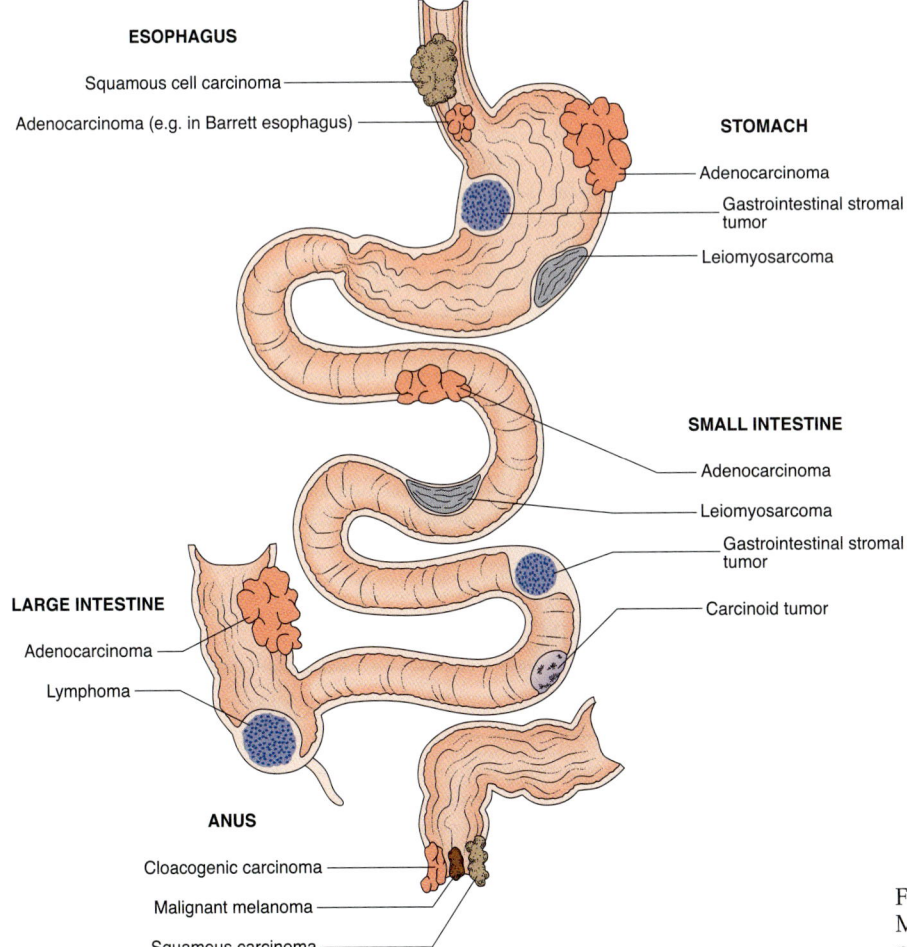

FIGURE 13-68
Major malignant tumors of the gastrointestinal tract.

and the duration of the peritonitis. Commonly, several aerobic and anaerobic species are cultured, including *E. coli, Bacteroides* species, various *Streptococcus* species, and *Clostridium*. Despite treatment with antibiotics, surgical drainage and debridement, and supportive measures, generalized peritonitis is still associated with substantial mortality and is especially dangerous in the elderly.

PERITONEAL DIALYSIS: Chronic peritoneal dialysis is today a frequent cause of bacterial peritonitis, owing to contamination of instruments or dialysate. The clinical course is usually milder than that noted with a perforated viscus, and the offending organisms are mostly *Staphylococcus* and *Streptococcus* species. One fourth of cases of peritonitis associated with chronic dialysis are aseptic; they are presumably caused by some chemical in the dialysate to which the peritoneum is sensitive.

SPONTANEOUS BACTERIAL PERITONITIS: This term refers to a peritoneal infection in the absence of a clear precipitating circumstance, such as a perforated viscus. **The most common cause of spontaneous bacterial peritonitis in adults is cirrhosis complicated by portal hypertension and ascites.** The pathogenesis appears to involve translocation of enteric organisms, mainly gram-negative bacilli, from the gut to mesenteric lymph nodes. Seeding of ascitic fluid then ensues, with depressed phagocytic activity and low antibacterial activity in ascitic fluid.

Spontaneous bacterial peritonitis in children can be a complication of the **nephrotic syndrome,** in part because ascites is more common in nephrotic children than in adults. Since the advent of the antibiotic era, most cases of spontaneous peritonitis in children are caused by gram-negative organisms, usually derived from urinary tract infections. The disease causes symptoms of an acute abdomen and ordinarily leads to surgical intervention, unless the child is known to have the nephrotic syndrome. Even with antibiotic treatment, the mortality remains at 5 to 10%.

TUBERCULOUS PERITONITIS: This infection is an unusual form of bacterial peritonitis. It is rarely seen in industrialized countries today, but occasionally complicates tuberculosis in developing countries. Many patients with tuberculous peritonitis do not have apparent pulmonary or miliary tuberculosis, an observation that suggests the activation of latent tuberculous foci in the peritoneum derived from previous hematogenous dissemination.

Pathology: The macroscopic appearance of bacterial peritonitis is like that of purulent infection elsewhere. A fibrinopurulent exudate covers the surface of the intestines, and on organization, fibrinous and fibrous adhesions form between loops of bowel, which become joined to each other. Such adhesions may eventually be lysed, or they may lead to **volvulus** and **intestinal obstruction.** Bacterial salpingitis, usually gonococcal, may lead to pelvic peritonitis and adhesions, which define **pelvic inflammatory disease.**

Chemical Peritonitis Results from Endogenous Sources

Bile peritonitis results from the escape of bile into the peritoneum, usually from a perforated gallbladder but sometimes from a needle biopsy of the liver. This abrupt insult may lead to shock.

Hydrochloric acid or hemorrhage from a perforated peptic ulcer of the stomach or duodenum may elicit an inflammatory reaction in the peritoneum.

Acute pancreatitis causes the release and activation of potent lipolytic and proteolytic enzymes that produce severe peritonitis and fat necrosis. Shock is common and may be lethal unless adequately treated.

Foreign materials introduced by surgery (e.g., talc) or by trauma are unusual causes of chemical peritonitis.

Leakage of urine can produce ascites.

Familial Paroxysmal Polyserositis (Familial Mediterranean Fever) Leads to Peritonitis and Amyloidosis

Familial Mediterranean fever (FMF) is an inherited autosomal recessive disorder that features recurrent episodes of aseptic peritonitis with fever and abdominal pain. The disease reflects mutations in a gene on the short arm of chromosome 16. FMF initially is seen as peritonitis in half of cases and as arthritis in one fourth. Pleuritis is the first complaint in only 5% of patients. However, almost all affected persons eventually manifest peritonitis, and more than half develop arthritis and pleuritis at some time. The disease predominates in Sephardic Jews and other Mediterranean populations, such as Armenians, Turks, and Arabs. The pathogenesis of FMF remains obscure, but in the absence of complications, the prognosis is good. Unfortunately, **amyloidosis** is a frequent complication (see Chapter 23).

RETROPERITONEAL FIBROSIS

Idiopathic retroperitoneal fibrosis, an uncommon fibrosing condition of the abdomen, becomes symptomatic when it causes obstruction of the ureters. Although no cause is discernible in most cases, the disorder has been linked to treatment of migraine headaches with methysergide. A similar idiopathic fibrosis also has been described in the mediastinum and may affect the mesentery, causing secondary intestinal obstruction.

NEOPLASMS

Mesenteric and Omental Cysts

Mesenteric and omental cysts are generally of lymphatic origin but may derive from other embryonic tissues. Usually a slowly enlarging, painless mass is discovered in a child older than 10 years. The cyst may come to medical attention because of rupture, bleeding, torsion, or intestinal obstruction. Surgical excision is curative.

Mesothelioma

One fourth of all mesotheliomas arise in the peritoneum, and mesotheliomas are the most common primary tumor of that tissue. **Like pleural mesotheliomas, most of these malignant tumors are associated with exposure to asbestos.** The pathological characteristics of peritoneal mesotheliomas are identical to those of their pleural counterparts (see - Chapter 12).

Primary Peritoneal Carcinoma

Primary peritoneal carcinoma presents as tumor masses involving the omentum and peritoneum. It is morphologically identical to ovarian serous carcinoma of the ovary, except that the ovaries are normal.

Metastatic Carcinoma

Metastatic carcinoma is by far the most common malignant disorder of the peritoneum. Ovarian, gastric, and pancreatic carcinomas are particularly likely to seed the peritoneum, but any intraabdominal carcinoma can spread to the peritoneum.

SUGGESTED READING

Books

Fenoglio-Preiser CM, Noffsinger AE, Stemmermann GN, et al.: *Gastrointestinal pathology: An atlas and text.* Lippincott Williams & Wilkins, 1999.

Lewin K, Riddell RH, Weinstein WM: *Gastrointestinal pathology and its clinical implications.* New York: Igaku-Shoin, 1992.

Morson BC, Dawson IMP, Day DW, et al.: *Morson and Dawson's gastrointestinal pathology*, 3rd ed. Oxford: Blackwell Scientific, 1990.

Sleisenger MH, Fordtran JS (eds): *Gastrointestinal disease,* 5th ed. Philadelphia: WB Saunders, 1993.

Yamada T (ed): *Textbook of gastroenterology,* 2nd ed. Philadelphia: JB Lippincott, 1995.

Review Articles

Ahmad T, Armuzzi A, Bunce M, et al.: The molecular classification of the clinical manifestations of Crohn's disease. *Gastroenterology* 122:854–866, 2002.

Bocker-Edmonston T, Cuesta KH, Burkholder S, et al.: Colorectal carcinomas with high microsatellite instability: defining a distinct immunologic and molecular entity with respect to prognostic markers. *Hum Pathol* 31: 1506–1514, 2000

Bond JH, for the practice parameters committee of the American College of Gastroenterology: Polyp guideline: Diagnosis, treatment, and surveillance for patients with colorectal polyps. *Am J Gastroenterol* 95:3053–3063, 2000.

Brandtzaeg P, Haraldsen G, Rugtveit J: Immunopathology of human inflammatory bowel disease. *Semin Immunopathol* 18:555–589, 1997.

Cagir B, Gelman A, Park J, et al.: Guanylyl cyclase C messenger RNA is a biomarker for recurrent stage II colorectal cancer. *Ann Intern Med* 131:805–812, 1999.

Carter PS: Anal cancer: Current perspectives. *Dig Dis* 11: 239–251, 1993.

Cave DR: Transmission and epidemiology of *Helicobacter pylori. Am J Med* 100:12S–17S, 1996.

Czinn SJ, Nedrud JG: Immunopathology of *Helicobacter pylori* infection and disease. *Semin Immunopathol* 18:495–514, 1997.

Dieterich W, Ehnis T, Bauer M: Identification of tissue transglutaminase as the autoantigen of celiac disease. *Nat Med* 3:P797–801, 1997

Dixon MF, Genta RM, Yardley JH, Correa P: Classification and grading of gastritis: The updated Sydney System. International Workshop on the Histopathology of Gastritis, Houston 1994. *Am J Surg Pathol* 20:1161–1181, 1996.

Eaden JA, Mayberry JF: Colorectal cancer complicating ulcerative colitis: A review. *Am J Gastrointest* 95:2710–2719, 2000.

Falk GW: Barrett's esophagus. *Gastroenterology* 122:1569–1591, 2002.

Farrell RJ, Kelly CP: Diagnosis of celiac sprue. *Am J Gastroenterol* 96:3237–3246, 2001

Fiocchi C: Inflammatory bowel disease: Etiology and pathogenesis. *Gastroenterology* 115:182–205, 1998.

Fletcher CDM, Berman JJ, Corless C, et al.: Diagnosis of gastrointestinal stromal tumors: A consensus approach. *Hum Pathol* 33:459–465, 2002.

Fodde R, Smits R, Clevers H: APC, signal transduction and genetic instability in colorectal cancer. *Nat Rev* 1:55–67, 2001.

Foulkes WD: A tale of four syndromes: Familial adenomatous polyposis, Gardner syndrome, attenuated APC and Turcot syndrome. *Q J Med* 88:853–863, 1995.

Giardiello FM, Lazenby AJ, Bayless TM: The new colitides, collagenous, lymphocytic and diversion colitis. *Gastroenterol Clin North Am* 24:717–729, 1995.

Gretz JE, Achem SR: The watermelon stomach: Clinical presentation, diagnosis and treatment. *Am J Gastrointest* 93: 890–895, 1998.

Gryfe R, Kim H, Hsieh ETK: Tumor microsatellite instability and clinical outcome in young patients with colorectal cancer. *N Engl J Med* 342:69–77, 2000.

Howden CW: Clinical expressions of *Helicobacter pylori* infection. *Am J Med* 100:27S–32S, 1996.

Huntsman DG, Carneiro F, Lewis FR: Early gastric cancer in young, asymptomatic carriers of germ-line E-cadherin mutations. *N Engl J Med* 344:1904–1909, 2001.

Jass JR: Serrated route to colorectal cancer: Back street or super highway? *J Pathol* 193:283–285, 2001.

Kinzler KW, Vogelstein B: Lessons from hereditary colorectal cancer. *Cell* 87:159–170, 1996.

Kozol RA, Dekhne N: *Helicobacter pylori* and the pathogenesis of duodenal ulcer. *J Lab Clin Med* 124:623–626, 1994.

Kulke MH, Mayer RJ: Carcinoid tumors. *N Engl J Med* 340: 858–868, 1999.

Mittal RK, Balaban DH: The esophagogastric junction. *N Engl J Med* 336:924–932, 1997.

Quellette AJ, Selsted ME: Paneth cell defensins: Endogenous peptide components of intestinal host defense. *FASEB J* 10:1280–1289, 1996.

Pardi DS, Smyrk TC, Tremaine WJ, Sandborn WJ: Microscopic colitis: A review. *Am J Gastrointest* 97:794–802, 2002.

Peek RM, Blaser MJ: Helicobacter pylori and gastrointestinal tract adenocarcinomas. *Nat Rev* 2:28–37, 2002.

Podolsky, D: Inflammatory bowel disease. *N Engl J Med* 347:417–429, 2002.

Raoult D, Birg ML, La Scola B et al.: Cultivation of the Bacillus of Whipple's disease. *N Engl J Med* 342:620–625, 2000.

Sampliner RE, and the practice parameters committee of the American College of Gastroenterology: Updated guidelines for the diagnosis, surveillance, and therapy of Barrett's esophagus. *Am J Gastroenterol* 97:1888–1895, 2002.

Savarino SJ: Diarrhoeal disease: Current concepts and future challenges: Enteroadherent *Escherichia coli:* a heterogeneous group of E. coli implicated as diarrhoeal pathogens. *Trans R Soc Trop Med Hyg* 87(suppl 3):49–53, 1993.

Schatzkin A, Lanza E, Corle D, et al.: Lack of effect of a low-fat, high-fiber diet on the recurrence of colorectal adenomas. *N Engl J Med* 3421149–1155, 2000.

Schlemper RJ, Riddell RH, Kato Y, et al.: The Viena classification of gastrointestinal epithelial neoplasia. *Gut* 47:251–255, 2000.

Schneider T, Ullrich R, Zeitz M: Immunopathology of human immunodeficiency virus infection in the gastrointestinal tract. *Semin Immunopathol* 18:515–534, 1997.

Schuppan D: Current concepts of celiac disease pathogenesis. *Gastroenterology* 119:234–242, 2000.

Scott H, Nilsen E, Sollid LM, et al.: Immunopathology of gluten-sensitive enteropathy. *Semin Immunopathol* 18:535–554, 1997.

Spechler SJ: Barrett's esophagus. *N Engl J Med* 346:836–842, 2002.

Spigelman AD, Arese P, Phillips RK: Polyposis: The Peutz-Jeghers syndrome. *Br J Surg* 82:1311–1314, 1995.

Suerbaum S, Michetti P: Helicobacter Pylori infection. *N Engl J Med* 347:1175–1186, 2002.

Voutilainen M, Farkkila M, Mecklin JP, et al. and The Central Finland Endoscopy Study Group. *Am J Gastroenterol* 94:3175–3180, 1999.

Voutilainen M, Farkkila M, Pekka Mecklin J, et al.: Chronic inflammation at the gastroesophageal junction (carditis) appears to be a specific finding related to Helicobacter pylori infection and gastroesophageal reflux disease. *Am J Gastroenterol* 94:3175–3180, 1999.

Wheeler JMD: DNA mismatch repair genes and colorectal cancer. *Gut* 47:148–153, 2000.

CHAPTER 14

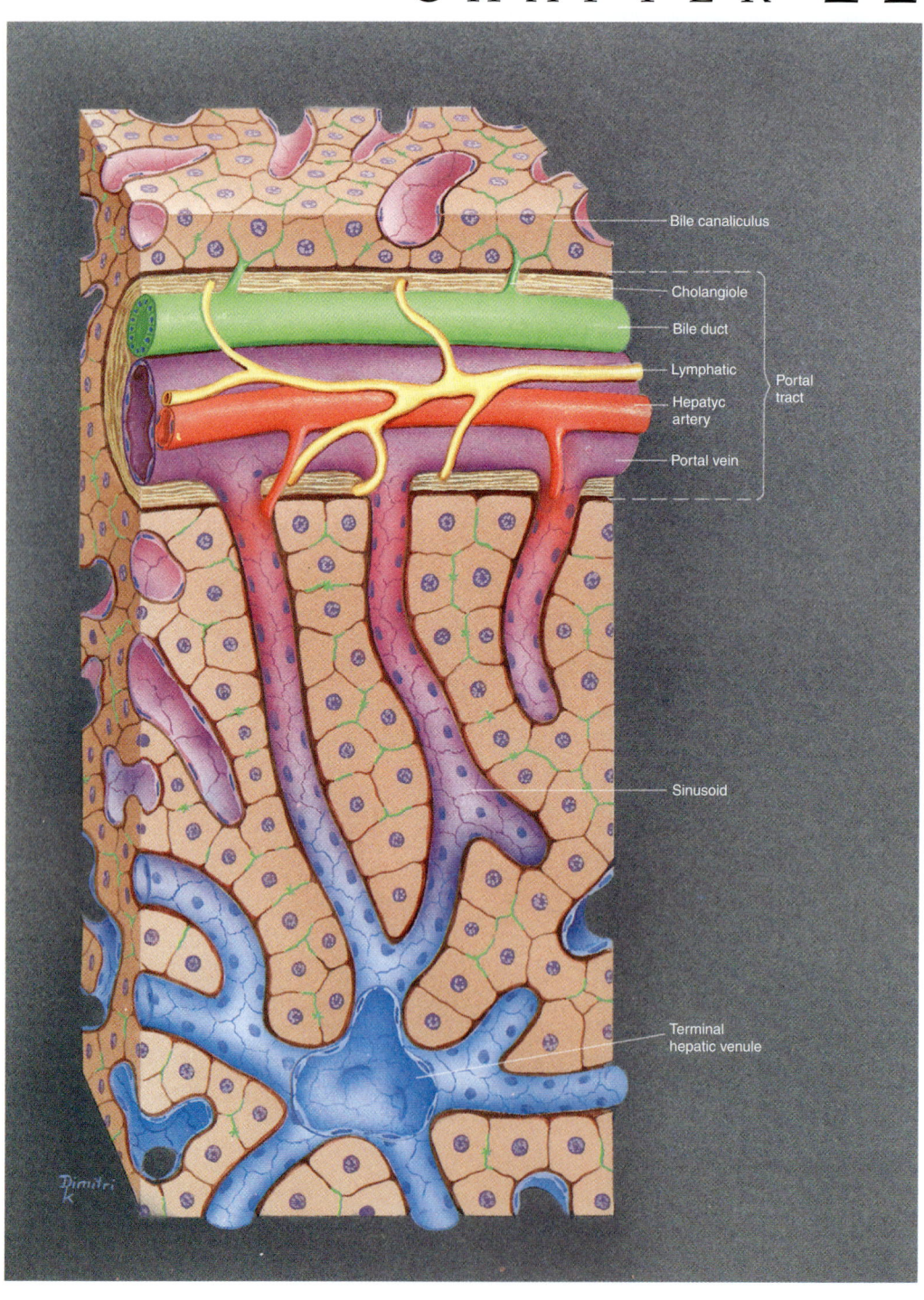

The Liver and Biliary System

Emanuel Rubin
Raphael Rubin

The Liver

Anatomy
The Liver Lobule
The Liver Acinus
The Hepatocyte
The Hepatic Sinusoid

Functions of the Liver
Regeneration

Bilirubin Metabolism and the Mechanisms of Jaundice
Heme Catabolism
Overproduction of Bilirubin
Decreased Hepatic Uptake of Bilirubin
Decreased Bilirubin Conjugation
Decreased Transport of Conjugated Bilirubin
Sepsis
Neonatal (Physiological) Jaundice
Impaired Canalicular Bile Flow

Cirrhosis

Hepatic Failure
Inadequate Hepatic Clearance of Bilirubin
Hepatic Encephalopathy

Defects Of Coagulation
Hypoalbuminemia
Hepatorenal Syndrome
Pulmonary Complications
Endocrine Complications

Portal Hypertension
Intrahepatic Portal Hypertension
Prehepatic Portal Hypertension
Posthepatic Portal Hypertension
Complications of Portal Hypertension

Viral Hepatitis
Hepatitis A
Hepatitis B
Hepatitis D
Hepatitis C
Hepatitis E

Pathology of Viral Hepatitis
Acute Hepatitis
Chronic Hepatitis

Autoimmune Hepatitis

Alcoholic Liver Disease
Metabolism of Ethanol
Liver Diseases and Alcohol Consumption

(continued)

FIGURE 14-1 *(see opposite page)*
Microanatomy of the liver.

Nonalcoholic Fatty Liver Disease

Primary Biliary Cirrhosis

Primary Sclerosing Cholangitis

Extrahepatic Biliary Obstruction

Iron-Overload Syndromes
Hereditary Hemochromatosis
Secondary Iron Overload Syndromes

Heritable Disorders Associated with Cirrhosis
Wilson Disease
Cystic Fibrosis
Inborn Errors of Carbohydrate Metabolism

Indian Childhood Cirrhosis

Toxic Liver Injury
Zonal Hepatocellular Necrosis
Fatty Liver
Intrahepatic Cholestasis
Lesions Resembling Viral Hepatitis
Chronic Hepatitis
Granulomatous Hepatitis
Vascular Lesions
Neoplastic Lesions

The Porphyrias

Vascular Disorders
Congestive Heart Failure
Shock
Infarction

Bacterial Infections

Parasitic Infestations
Protozoal Diseases
Helminthic Diseases
Leptospirosis (Weil Disease)

Syphilis

Cholestatic Syndromes of Infancy
Neonatal Hepatitis
Biliary Atresia

Benign Tumors and Tumor-like Lesions
Adenomas
Focal Nodular Hyperplasia
Nodular Regenerative Hyperplasia
Hemangiomas
Cystic Diseases

Malignant Tumors of the Liver
Hepatocellular Carcinoma
Cholangiocarcinoma
Hepatoblastoma
Hemangiosarcoma
Metastatic Cancer

Liver Transplantation

The Gallbladder and Extrahepatic Bile Ducts

Anatomy

Congenital Anomalies

Cholelithiasis
Cholesterol Stones
Pigment Stones

Acute Cholecystitis

Chronic Cholecystitis

Cholesterolosis

Tumors
Benign Tumors
Carcinoma of the Bile Duct and the Ampulla of Vater

The Liver

ANATOMY

The liver arises from the embryonic foregut as an entodermal bud that differentiates into the hepatic diverticulum. Strands of entodermal cells mingle with proliferating mesenchymal cells to form all the structures of the adult liver, the gallbladder, and the extrahepatic biliary ducts.

The liver is the largest visceral organ in the body; in the average adult man it weighs about 1500 g. Situated in the right upper quadrant of the abdomen immediately below the diaphragm, it consists of two lobes, a larger **right lobe** and a smaller **left lobe**, which meet at the level of the gallbladder bed. Inferiorly, the right lobe exhibits lesser segments, the **caudate** and **quadrate lobes**. The **gallbladder** is located inferiorly in a fossa of the right hepatic lobe and normally extends slightly beyond the inferior margin of the liver.

The liver has a dual blood supply consisting of (1) **the hepatic artery,** a branch of the celiac axis, and (2) **the portal vein,** formed by the convergence of the splenic and superior mesenteric veins. **The hepatic veins** drain into the inferior vena cava, which is partly surrounded by the posterior surface of the liver. The hepatic lymphatics drain principally into lymph nodes of the porta hepatis and the celiac axis.

The common hepatic duct, formed by the union of the right and left hepatic ducts, receives the cystic duct from the gallbladder to form the common bile duct. The common bile duct joins with the pancreatic duct just before emptying into the duodenum. It terminates in the ampulla of Vater, where its lumen is guarded by the sphincter of Oddi.

The Liver Lobule Is the Basic Unit of the Liver

The liver lobule is a polyhedral structure (Figs. 14-1 through 14-3), classically depicted as a hexagon. **Portal triads** (or portal tracts), found peripherally at the angles of the polygon, are so named because they contain intrahepatic branches of the (1) **bile ducts,** (2) **hepatic artery,** and (3) **portal vein.** The collagenous portal tracts are surrounded by an adjacent circumferential layer of hepatocytes called *the limiting plate*. As its name implies, the **central vein** (also known as the *terminal hepatic venule*) resides in the center of the lobule. Radiating from it are **one-cell-thick plates of hepatocytes,** which extend to the perimeter of the lobule, where they are continuous with the plates of other lobules. Between the plates of hepatocytes are the **hepatic sinusoids,** which are lined by endothelial cells, Kupffer cells, and stellate cells.

The large blood vessels that enter the liver at the porta hepatis eventually divide into the small interlobular branches of the hepatic artery and portal vein in the portal triads. From the portal triads, the interlobular vessels distribute blood to the hepatic sinusoids, where it flows centripetally into the central vein. The central veins coalesce to form sublobular veins, which eventually merge into the hepatic veins.

Bile flows in a direction opposite to that of the blood. Bile is secreted by hepatocytes into the bile canaliculi, formed by the apposed lateral surfaces of contiguous hepatocytes. Contraction of the bile canaliculus, mediated by the pericanalicular cytoskeleton of the hepatocytes, propels the bile toward the portal tract.

From the canaliculi, the bile flows into the bile ductules (canals of Hering or cholangioles) at the border of the portal tract and then enters a branch of the intrahepatic bile ducts. Within each lobe of the liver, smaller bile ducts progressively merge, eventually forming the right and left hepatic ducts.

The Liver Acinus Is the Functional Interpretation of the Lobule

The classic lobule described above is depicted as arranged around the central vein simply because of the histological appearance of the liver. **However, from a functional point of view, the lobule can be thought of as an acinus with its center in the portal tract** (see Fig. 14-2). Such a concept takes into account the functional gradients that exist within the lobule. Concentrations of oxygen, nutrients, and hormones in the blood are highest at the portal tracts and decline progressively as the blood courses through the sinusoids to the central vein. This functional heterogeneity of the liver lobule can be expressed in terms of concentric functional zones around portal tracts. **Zone 1,** the most highly oxygenated zone, encircles the portal tracts, whereas **zone 3,** which surrounds the central veins, is oxygen poor. The intermediate or midlobular area is referred to as **zone 2.** Differences in hepatocytes are not restricted to blood flow. The acinus is also heterogeneous with respect to metabolism, independent of oxygenation. In particular, toxic injury is often prominent in zone 3 owing to enrichment in hepatocyte enzymes involved in drug detoxification and biotransformation. For convenience, pathological changes in the liver are usually designated in relation to the classic histological lobule. For example, centrilobular necrosis refers to a lesion around the central veins, whereas periportal fibrosis is seen at the periphery of the classic lobule.

The Hepatocyte Performs the Major Functions of the Liver

About 60% of the total cell population of the liver consists of hepatocytes, although these cells account for 90% of the vol-

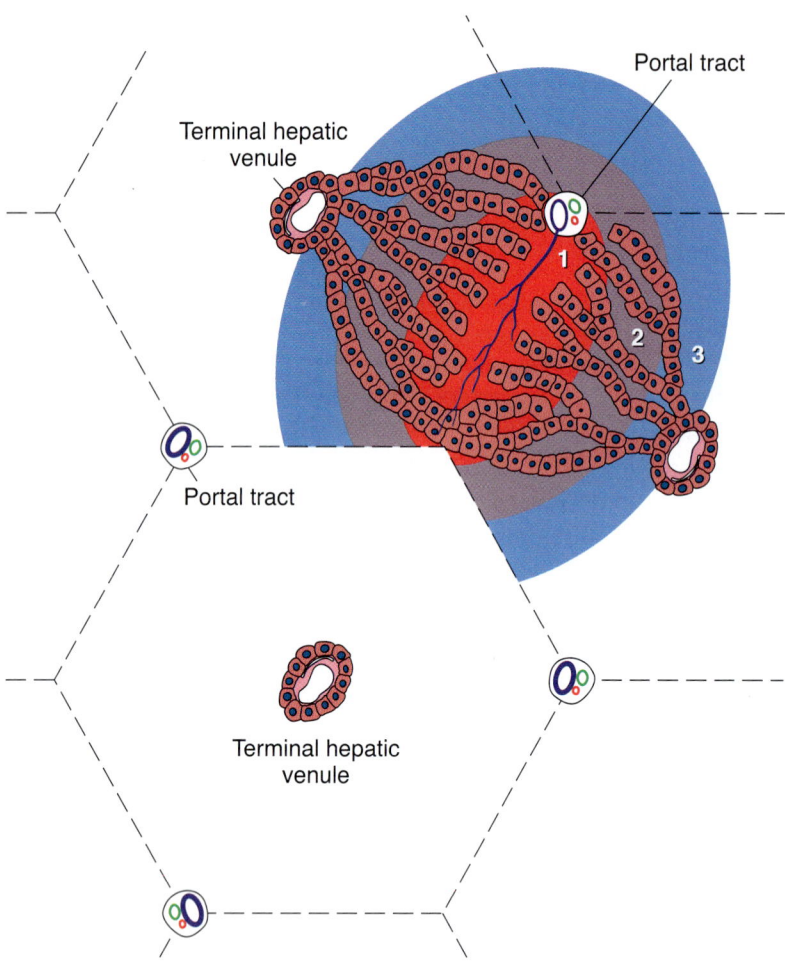

FIGURE 14-2
Morphological and functional concepts of the liver lobule. In the classic, morphological liver lobule, the periphery of the hexagonal lobule is anchored in the portal tracts, and the terminal hepatic venule is in the center. The functional liver lobule is an acinus derived from the gradients of oxygen and nutrients in the sinusoidal blood. In this scheme, the portal tract, with the richest content of oxygen and nutrients, is in the center (zone 1). The region most distant from the portal tract (zone 3) is poor in oxygen and nutrients and surrounds the terminal hepatic venule.

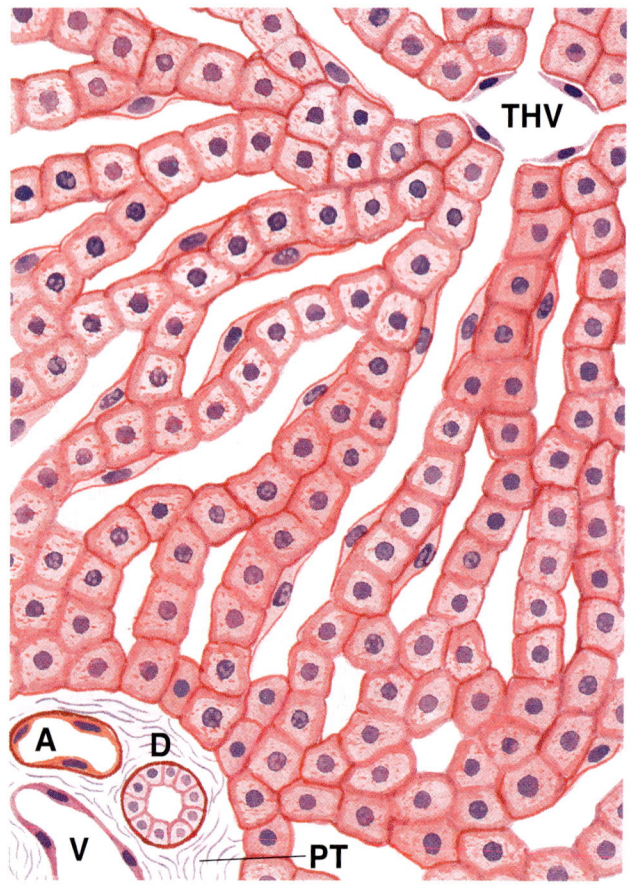

FIGURE 14-3
Schematic representation of the normal liver lobule. The portal tract *(PT)* contains branches of the hepatic artery *(A)*, portal vein *(V)*, and interlobular bile duct *(D)*. The liver cell plates converge to the terminal hepatic venule *(THV)*.

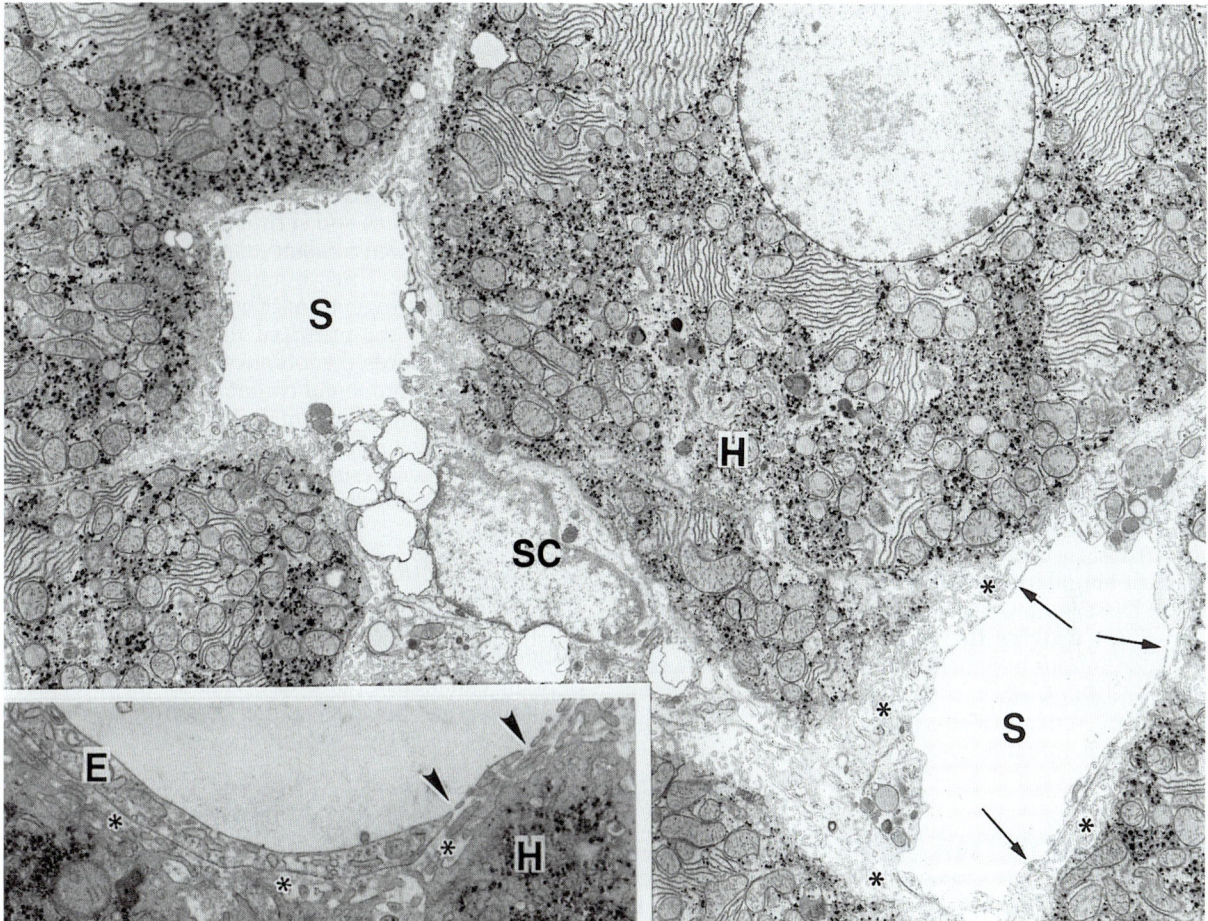

FIGURE 14-4
Hepatic sinusoids and space of Disse. An electron micrograph illustrates the relationship between hepatocytes, sinusoids, the space of Disse, and hepatic stellate cells (Ito cells, fat-storing cells). *H*, hepatocyte; *S*, sinusoid; *SC*, stellate cell; *arrow*, endothelial cell; *asterisk*, space of Disse. The *inset* illustrates the relationship between hepatocytes (*H*) and endothelial cells (*E*). The *arrowheads* indicate fenestrae in the endothelial cells; the *asterisks* are in the space of Disse.

ume of the liver. The hepatocyte, roughly 30 μm across, has three specialized surfaces: sinusoidal, lateral, and canalicular. Each cell has two sinusoidal surfaces, which exhibit numerous slender microvilli. The sinusoidal surface is separated from the endothelial cells that line the sinusoids by the **space of Disse** (Fig. 14-4). The canalicular surfaces of adjacent hepatocytes form the **bile canaliculus,** a collecting structure that is actually an intercellular space without a separate and distinct wall. The canalicular surface displays microvilli extending into the lumen. A tight junctional complex between adjacent hepatocytes prevents leakage of bile from the canaliculus. The lateral, or intercellular, surfaces of adjacent hepatocytes are in close contact and contain gap junctions.

The centrally placed, spherical nucleus of the hepatocyte exhibits one or more nucleoli. The nuclei vary in size in ratios of 2 (diploid), 4 (tetraploid), and 8 (octaploid), with most being diploid. The cytoplasm is rich in organelles and shows prominent rough and smooth endoplasmic reticulum, Golgi complexes, mitochondria, lysosomes, and peroxisomes. In addition, in the fed state, abundant glycogen and occasional fat droplets are evident.

The Hepatic Sinusoid Is the Channel through Which Blood Traverses the Liver

The sinusoids contain three cell types: endothelial, Kupffer, and stellate cells.

ENDOTHELIAL CELLS: The hepatic sinusoid is lined by a sheet of endothelial cells, which are penetrated by numerous holes called **fenestrae.** Unlike their counterparts in other tissues, adjacent endothelial cells do not form junctions, and there are many gaps between them. The result is a sievelike structure that affords free communication between the sinusoidal lumen and the space of Disse. Free access of sinusoidal plasma to the hepatocyte is further facilitated by the absence of a basement membrane between the endothelial cells and liver cells.

KUPFFER CELLS: The phagocytic Kupffer cells are located either in the gaps between adjacent endothelial cells or on their surfaces. Kupffer cells belong to the monocyte/macrophage system derived from the bone marrow. For that reason, after liver transplantation, the Kupffer cell population eventually originates from the recipient rather than the donor. Like other macrophages, they provide a first line of defense against infection and circulating toxic molecules (e.g., endotoxin). Activated Kupffer cells also release a variety of cytokines, including tumor necrosis factor (TNF), interleukins, interferons, and transforming growth factors (TGFs) α and β.

STELLATE CELLS: Beneath the endothelial cells in the space of Disse are found occasional stellate cells (also known as Ito cells), which have specialized storage capacities. These cells contain fat, vitamin A, and other lipid-soluble vitamins. The stellate cell also secretes extracellular matrix components, including various collagens, laminin, and proteoglycans. In a number of pathological states, these matrix constituents are formed in great excess, leading to the hepatic fibrosis characteristic of cirrhosis.

The most abundant extracellular matrix component in the space of Disse is fibronectin. Occasional bundles of type I collagen fibers provide the scaffold of the liver lobule. There is no continuous basement membrane barrier between the plasma and the surface of the hepatocyte, although by light microscopy, reticulin stains impart the false impression of a continuous membrane.

FUNCTIONS OF THE LIVER

The hepatocyte subserves a wide variety of functions, which can be broadly categorized as metabolic, synthetic, storage, catabolic, and excretory.

METABOLIC FUNCTIONS: The liver is the central organ of **glucose homeostasis** and responds rapidly to fluctuations in the concentration of blood glucose. In the fed state, excess blood glucose is shunted to the liver to be stored as glycogen; in the fasting state, the liver maintains blood glucose levels by glycogenolysis and gluconeogenesis. For **gluconeogenesis,** the liver uses amino acids, lactate, and glycerol. The nitrogenous portion of amino acids is converted to urea. Free fatty acids are taken up by the liver, where they are oxidized to produce energy. Alternatively, they are converted to triglycerides, and secreted in the form of **lipoproteins** to be used elsewhere.

SYNTHETIC FUNCTIONS: Most serum proteins, with the major exception of the immunoglobulins, are synthesized in the liver. **Albumin** is the principal source of plasma oncotic pressure, and its decrease in chronic liver disease contributes to the development of edema and ascites. Blood coagulation depends on the continuous production of **clotting factors,** most of which, including prothrombin and fibrinogen, are synthesized by hepatocytes. Liver failure is thus characterized by a severe and often life-threatening bleeding diathesis. Endothelial cells of the liver manufacture **factor VIII,** and hemophilia is ameliorated by liver transplantation. **Complement** and other acute-phase reactants are also secreted by the liver, as are numerous specific binding proteins—for example, the **binding proteins** for iron, copper, and vitamin A.

STORAGE FUNCTIONS: The liver is an important storage site for glycogen, triglycerides, iron, copper, and lipid-soluble vitamins. Severe liver disease can result from excessive storage—for instance, abnormal glycogen in type IV glycogenosis and excess iron in hemochromatosis.

CATABOLIC FUNCTIONS: Endogenous substances, including hormones and serum proteins, are catabolized by the liver to maintain a balance between their production and their elimination. Thus, in chronic liver disease, impaired catabolism of estrogens contributes to feminization in men. The liver is also the principal site for the **detoxification of foreign compounds** (xenobiotics), such as drugs, industrial chemicals, environmental contaminants, and perhaps products of bacterial metabolism in the intestine. Removal of ammonia, a product of amino acid metabolism, occurs principally in the liver. Serum ammonia increases in liver failure and is used as a marker for this condition.

EXCRETORY FUNCTIONS: The principal excretory product of the liver is **bile,** an aqueous mixture of conjugated bilirubin, bile acids, phospholipids, cholesterol, and electrolytes. Bile not only provides a repository for the products of heme catabolism but is also vital for fat absorption in the small intestine. Bile also contains immunoglobulin A (IgA), which is involved in an enterohepatic circulation.

Regeneration Is a Unique Characteristic of the Liver

Liver size is normally maintained within narrow limits relative to body size. When liver tissue is damaged (e.g., after a mechanical, toxic, or viral challenge that has caused a substantial loss of functional tissue), recovery occurs by regrowth of the undamaged tissue in a process called *liver regeneration*. The parenchymal cells in the liver, which normally are in a fully differentiated, quiescent state (G_0), reenter the cell cycle and go through one or more synchronized rounds of replication to recover the original size of the tissue. Uniquely, this process takes place while maintaining the differentiated functions of the liver. Several phases can be distinguished in liver regeneration:

Priming: The tissue has to recognize that damage has occurred and that the remaining functional parenchymal cells have to make the transition from the quiescent G0 state to the G1 phase of the cell cycle. This phase is often referred to as "priming." It is associated with the expression of a large number of immediate-early genes, many of which are transcription factors required for the expression of cell cycle proteins. The priming phase depends on the release of different cytokines, notably TNF-α and interleukin-6 (IL-6).

Progression to mitosis: The second phase involves progression through the G1 phase of the cell cycle and transition into S phase, where DNA synthesis occurs. This sequence is followed by the G2 phase and M phase, where cell division takes place. A number of growth factors promote this part of the process, including hepatocyte growth factor, also known as scatter factor (HGF/SF), epidermal growth factor (EGF), TGF-α, and several others. The intracellular signaling events that are involved in the progression through the cell cycle remain largely unknown. After completion of one or two rounds of cell division (depending on need), the cells revert to the quiescent state and resume normal function.

Nonparenchymal cells: The third phase of liver regeneration involves the replication of nonparenchymal cells (sinusoidal endothelial cells, Kupffer cells, stellate cells, and biliary epithelial cells) and the remodeling of the tissue architecture, with recovery of the original structure of liver cell plates. Little is known about the factors that guide this part of the process or how the liver recognizes the recovery of its normal size and architecture.

Conditions that interfere with the regenerative process may result in permanent liver dysfunction and lead to fibrosis and cirrhosis.

BILIRUBIN METABOLISM AND THE MECHANISMS OF JAUNDICE

Bilirubin Is the End Product of Heme Catabolism

Bilirubin has no known physiological function, although a role as an antioxidant has been suggested. **Up to 85% of bilirubin is derived from senescent erythrocytes,** which are removed from the circulation by mononuclear phagocytes of the spleen, bone marrow, and liver. The remaining bilirubin arises from the degradation of heme produced from other sources, the most important of which is the premature breakdown of hemoglobin in developing erythroid cells in the bone marrow.

Bilirubin is released from phagocytes and other cells into the circulation, where it is bound to albumin for transport to the liver. Albumin in the circulation and the extracellular space constitutes a large binding reservoir for bilirubin and ensures a low extracellular concentration of free (unbound) bilirubin. Free bilirubin, unlike that bound to albumin or conjugated with glucuronic acid, is toxic to the brain in newborns and in high concentrations causes irreversible brain injury termed **kernicterus.** In this respect, certain drugs that compete with bilirubin for binding sites on albumin (e.g., sulfonamides and salicylates) tend to shift bilirubin from the plasma into tissues and thereby increase its cytotoxicity.

The transfer of bilirubin from the blood to the bile involves four steps:

1. **Uptake:** On reaching the sinusoidal plasma membrane of the hepatocyte, the albumin–bilirubin complex is dissociated, and bilirubin is transported across the plasma membrane. This transport system has the characteristics of a carrier-mediated process and likely involves specific recognition of bilirubin by a plasma membrane receptor.
2. **Binding:** Within the hepatocyte, bilirubin is bound to cytosolic proteins, in this case a group of proteins known collectively as glutathione-S-transferases (also termed *ligandin*). Ligandin binds bilirubin and prevents its reflux into the circulation and its nonspecific diffusion into inappropriate compartments of the hepatocyte.
3. **Conjugation:** For its excretion, bilirubin must be converted to a water-soluble compound by complexing with glucuronic acid. Bilirubin is transferred to the endoplasmic reticulum, which contains the uridine diphosphate-glucuronyl transferase (UGT) system responsible for the conjugation of bilirubin with glucuronic acid. This reaction forms water-soluble bilirubin diglucuronide and a small amount (<10%) of the monoglucuronide.
4. **Excretion:** Conjugated bilirubin diffuses through the cytosol to the bile canaliculus, where it is excreted into the bile by an energy-dependent carrier-mediated process that is the rate-limiting step for overall transhepatic transport of bilirubin.

After its excretion into the small intestine in bile, conjugated bilirubin is not absorbed and remains intact until it reaches the distal small bowel and colon, where it is hydrolyzed by the bacterial flora to free bilirubin. In turn, free bilirubin (now unconjugated) is reduced to a mixture of pyrroles, known collectively as *urobilinogen*. Most of the urobilinogen is excreted in the feces, but a small proportion is absorbed in the terminal ileum and colon, returned to the liver, and reexcreted into the bile. Bile acids are also reabsorbed in the terminal ileum and salvaged by the liver. Collectively, the reabsorption of bile constituents is referred to as the *enterohepatic circulation of bile*. Some urobilinogen escapes reabsorption by the liver and reaches the systemic circulation, after which it is excreted in the urine.

- **Hyperbilirubinemia** refers to an increased concentration of bilirubin in the blood (>1.0 mg/dL).
- **Jaundice** or **icterus** describes yellow skin and sclerae (Fig. 14-5), whose color becomes apparent when the circulating bilirubin concentration exceeds 2.0 to 2.5 mg/dL.
- **Cholestasis** is the presence of plugs of inspissated bile in dilated bile canaliculi and visible bile pigment in hepatocytes.
- **Cholestatic jaundice** is characterized by histological cholestasis and hyperbilirubinemia.

As shown in Figure 14-6, many conditions are associated with hyperbilirubinemia. Overproduction of bilirubin, interference with hepatic uptake or intracellular metabolism of bilirubin, and impairment of bile excretion are all causes of jaundice.

Overproduction of Bilirubin Can Lead to Unconjugated Hyperbilirubinemia

An increased production of bilirubin results from increased destruction of erythrocytes (i.e., hemolytic anemia) or ineffective erythropoiesis (dyserythropoiesis). In unusual circumstances, the breakdown of erythrocytes in a large hematoma (e.g., after trauma) may also provide excess bilirubin.

In the adult, even severe hemolytic anemia does not produce a sustained rise in serum bilirubin concentration beyond

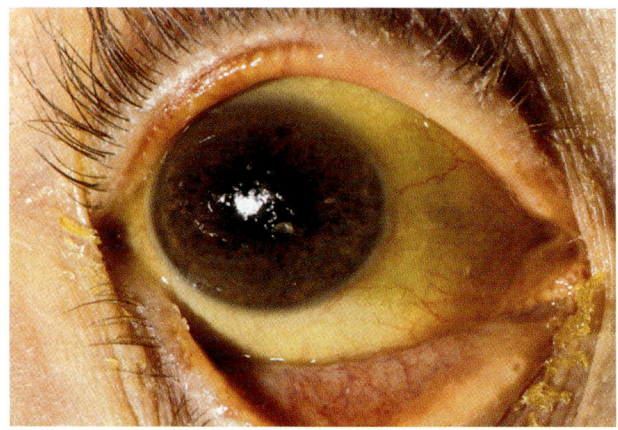

FIGURE *14-5*

Jaundice. A patient in hepatic failure displays a yellow sclera.

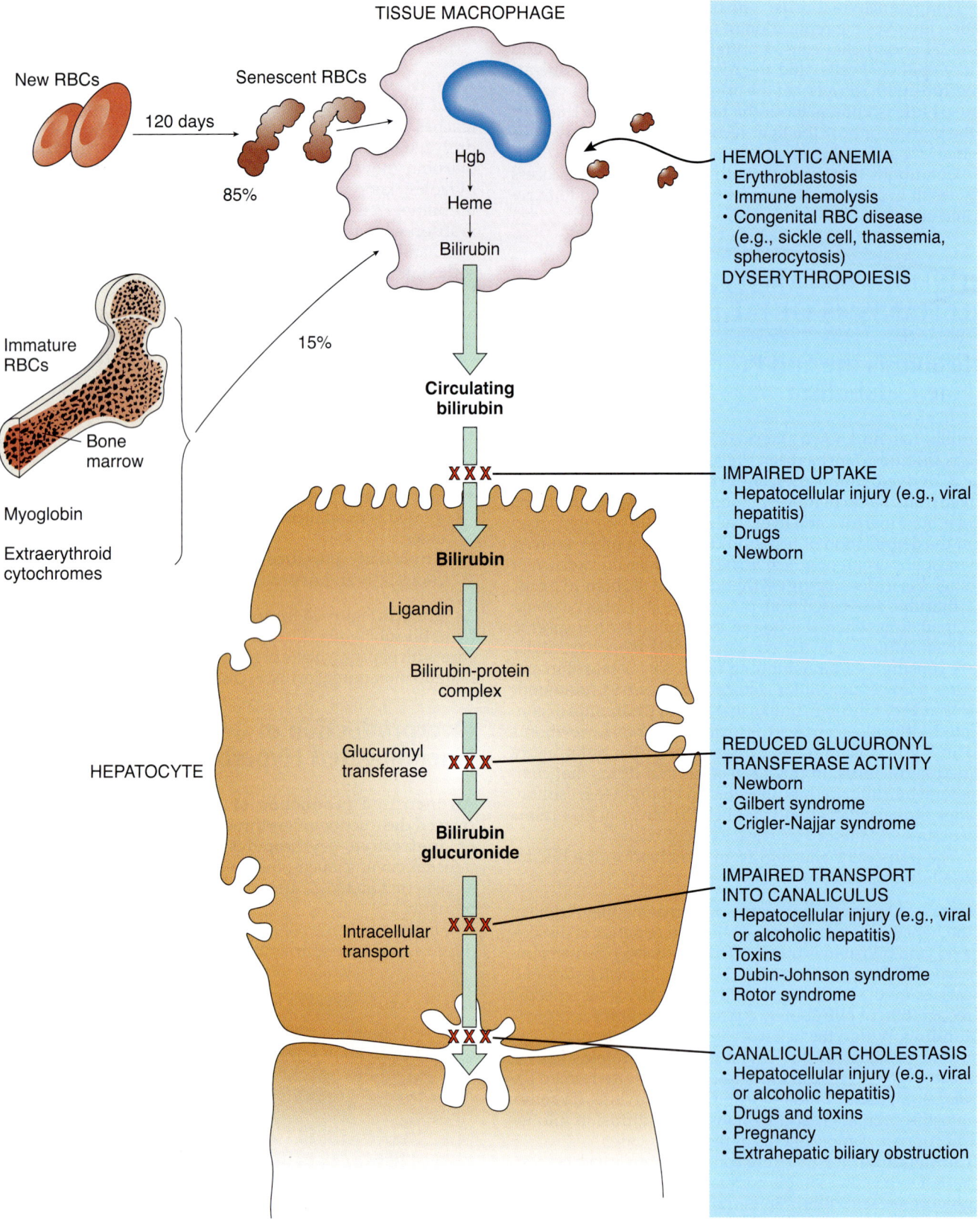

FIGURE 14-6
Mechanisms of jaundice at the level of the hepatocyte. Bilirubin is derived principally from the senescence of circulating red blood cells, with a smaller contribution from the degradation of erythropoietic elements in the bone marrow, myoglobin, and extraerythroid cytochromes. Jaundice results from overproduction of bilirubin (hemolytic anemia), dyserythropoiesis, or defects in its hepatic metabolism. The locations of specific blocks in the metabolic pathway of bilirubin in the hepatocyte are illustrated.

4.0 mg/dL, provided that hepatic bilirubin clearance remains normal. However, the combination of prolonged hemolysis, as in sickle cell anemia, and intrinsic liver disease, such as viral hepatitis, leads to extraordinarily high levels of circulating bilirubin (up to 100 mg/dL) and pronounced jaundice.

The hyperbilirubinemia of uncomplicated hemolytic disease principally involves unconjugated bilirubin, whereas in parenchymal liver disease, both conjugated and unconjugated bilirubin participate. Although the unconjugated hyperbilirubinemia of hemolytic disease is of little clinical significance in the adult, in the newborn it may be catastrophic. Hemolytic disease of the newborn may result in concentrations of unconjugated bilirubin high enough to cause kernicterus (see Chapter 6). Kernicterus has generally been associated with bilirubin concentrations over 20 mg/dL, but subtle psychomotor retardation may follow considerably lower bilirubin concentrations.

In disorders characterized by ineffective erythropoiesis (e.g., megaloblastic and sideroblastic anemias), the fraction of bilirubin derived from the bone marrow may be increased to the point that hyperbilirubinemia develops. A rare hereditary disease of unknown etiology, *primary shunt hyperbilirubinemia* or *idiopathic dyserythropoietic jaundice*, is characterized by massive overproduction of bilirubin in the bone marrow and is associated with chronic unconjugated hyperbilirubinemia.

Decreased Hepatic Uptake of Bilirubin Is a Common Cause of Jaundice

Hyperbilirubinemia can result from impaired hepatic uptake of unconjugated bilirubin. Such a situation occurs in generalized liver cell injury, exemplified by viral hepatitis. Certain drugs (e.g., rifampin and probenecid) interfere with the net uptake of bilirubin by the liver cell and may produce a mild unconjugated hyperbilirubinemia.

Decreased Bilirubin Conjugation Occurs in a Number of Hereditary Syndromes

Crigler-Najjar Syndrome

Crigler-Najjar syndrome type I is a rare recessively inherited malady characterized by chronic, severe unconjugated hyperbilirubinemia, owing to the complete absence of hepatic UGT activity. A variety of mutations in the *UGT* gene lead to the synthesis of a completely inactive enzyme. As a result, treatment with phenobarbital, an inducer of microsomal enzymes (including UGT), is without effect.

The bile in this condition is colorless and contains no conjugated bilirubin and no more than trace amounts of unconjugated bilirubin. **The morphological appearance of the liver is normal.** In the era before liver transplantation, infants with Crigler-Najjar syndrome type I invariably developed bilirubin encephalopathy and usually died in the first year of life.

Crigler-Najjar syndrome type II is similar to but less severe than type I and manifests only a partial decrease in the activity of UGT. Both autosomal recessive and dominant mutations in the *UGT* gene (the latter having incomplete penetrance) result in partial inactivation of the enzyme, and treatment with phenobarbital induces a decrease in unconjugated hyperbilirubinemia. This feature is the most reliable criterion for distinguishing type II from type I Crigler-Najjar syndrome. Almost all patients with type II syndrome develop normally, but neurological changes resembling kernicterus are observed in some.

Gilbert Syndrome

Gilbert syndrome is an inherited, mild, chronic unconjugated hyperbilirubinemia (<6 mg/dL) that is caused by impaired clearance of bilirubin in the absence of any detectable functional or structural liver disease. The syndrome runs in families, and both autosomal dominant and recessive patterns of inheritance have been suggested, although the latter is favored today. Mutations of the *UGT* gene in the promotor region lead to reduced transcription of the gene and, consequently, inadequate synthesis of the enzyme. In a few patients with a normal *UGT* gene promotor region, missense mutations of the coding region have been described. It has long been known that factors that increase serum bilirubin concentrations in normal persons, such as fasting or an intercurrent illness, produce an exaggerated increase in serum bilirubin levels in persons with Gilbert syndrome. Mild hemolysis, which also tends to increase bilirubin levels, is believed to occur in more than half of persons with Gilbert syndrome, but the mechanism is unclear.

Gilbert syndrome is exceptionally common, occurring in 3 to 7% of the population. It is seen more often in men than in women and is usually recognized after puberty. The sex differences and the age at onset suggest that hormones influence the modulation of bilirubin metabolism in the liver. Gilbert syndrome is harmless and, for the most part, without symptoms.

Decreased Transport of Conjugated Bilirubin Often Involves Mutations in the Multidrug Resistance Protein (MRP) Family

MRPs mediate organic ion transport across membranes, including conjugated bilirubin, bile acids, and phospholipids. Mutations in these proteins impair hepatocellular secretion of bilirubin glucuronides and other organic anions into the canalicular lumen. The diseases vary in severity from innocuous to lethal, owing to the heterogeneity of the mutations.

Dubin-Johnson Syndrome

Dubin-Johnson syndrome is a benign autosomal recessive disease characterized by chronic conjugated hyperbilirubinemia and conspicuous melanin-like pigment deposition in the liver. The disease is linked to mutations that result in the complete absence of MRP2 protein in hepatocytes. In addition to impaired secretion of bilirubin glucuronides, there is an accompanying defect in the hepatic excretion of coproporphyrins and a consequent alteration in urinary coproporphyrin excretion. The syndrome is rare among most populations, but certain groups that tend to have high rates of intermarriage, such as Iranian Jews and Japanese in remote areas, have a considerably higher incidence.

Dubin-Johnson syndrome can be distinguished from other conditions associated with conjugated hyperbilirubinemia by studies of **urinary coproporphyrin excretion.** There are two forms of human coproporphyrins, termed **iso-**

mer I and **isomer III**. Normally, isomer I constitutes 25% of urinary coproporphyrins. In Dubin-Johnson syndrome, although total urinary coproporphyrin excretion is normal, this isomer accounts for fully 80%. By contrast, in most hepatic disorders associated with jaundice, total urinary coproporphyrin excretion is increased, but coproporphyrin I constitutes less than 65%. Thus, a finding of normal excretion of total urinary coproporphyrins combined with more than 80% as isomer I is diagnostic of Dubin-Johnson syndrome

Pathology: The microscopic appearance of the liver is entirely normal in Dubin-Johnson syndrome, except for the accumulation of coarse, iron-free, **dark-brown granules** in hepatocytes and Kupffer cells, primarily in the centrilobular zone (Fig. 14-7). By electron microscopy, the pigment is seen in enlarged lysosomes. Since hepatocytes do not synthesize melanin, it has been suggested that the pigment reflects the autooxidation of anionic metabolites (e.g., tyrosine, phenylalanine, tryptophan) and possibly of epinephrine. The accumulation of this intracellular pigment is reflected in a grossly pigmented, or "black," liver.

Clinical Features: Except for mild intermittent jaundice, most patients with Dubin-Johnson syndrome do not complain of any symptoms. As in Gilbert syndrome, vague nonspecific complaints are common. Half of those affected have dark urine. In women, the disease may be discovered when jaundice appears during pregnancy or as a result of the use of oral contraceptives. The serum bilirubin value varies from 2 to 5 mg/dL, although it may be much higher transiently. About 60% of the increased bilirubin in the serum is conjugated.

Rotor Syndrome

Rotor syndrome is a familial conjugated hyperbilirubinemia that is clinically similar to Dubin-Johnson syndrome but without the associated pigmentation of the liver. The disease is inherited as an autosomal recessive trait. Although the disorder clinically resembles Dubin-Johnson syndrome, it is a distinct entity. A defect in hepatic uptake or intracellular binding of organic ions has been postulated as the basis of Rotor syndrome. In addition, the pattern of urinary coproporphyrin excretion is similar to that of most hepatobiliary disorders accompanied by conjugated hyperbilirubinemia (i.e., increased total urinary coproporphyrins with 65% of isomer I). As in the Dubin-Johnson syndrome, patients with Rotor syndrome have few symptoms and lead normal lives.

Benign Recurrent Intrahepatic Cholestasis

Benign recurrent intrahepatic cholestasis is characterized by self-limited, periodic episodes of intrahepatic cholestasis preceded by malaise and itching. The occurrence of familial cases suggests a genetic origin. Symptoms tend to last from several weeks to several months. The mean number of attacks in a lifetime is 3 to 5, but some affected persons have as many as 10 attacks. Recurrences have been noted at intervals of weeks to years. Serum bilirubin levels during the acute episodes are in the range of 10 to 20 mg/dL, and most of the bilirubin is conjugated.

The liver shows centrilobular cholestasis (bile plugs in bile canaliculi) and a few mononuclear inflammatory cells in the portal tracts. All the structural and functional alterations disappear during remissions, and no permanent sequelae have been reported.

Intrahepatic Cholestasis of Pregnancy

Intrahepatic cholestasis of pregnancy is a disorder characterized by pruritus and cholestatic jaundice that usually occurs in the last trimester of each pregnancy and promptly disappears after delivery. Half of patients with intrahepatic cholestasis of pregnancy have other family members who have experienced jaundice during pregnancy or after the use of oral contraceptives; the remainder are sporadic. In some familial cases, mutations in the MRP protein genes have been described. The increase in gonadal and placental hormones during pregnancy is likely responsible for the cholestasis in susceptible women. Maternal health is unaffected by this disease, but the effects on the fetus are often grave and include fetal distress, stillbirth, prematurity, and increased risk of intracranial hemorrhage during delivery. The liver of the mother exhibits no specific changes other than centrilobular cholestasis.

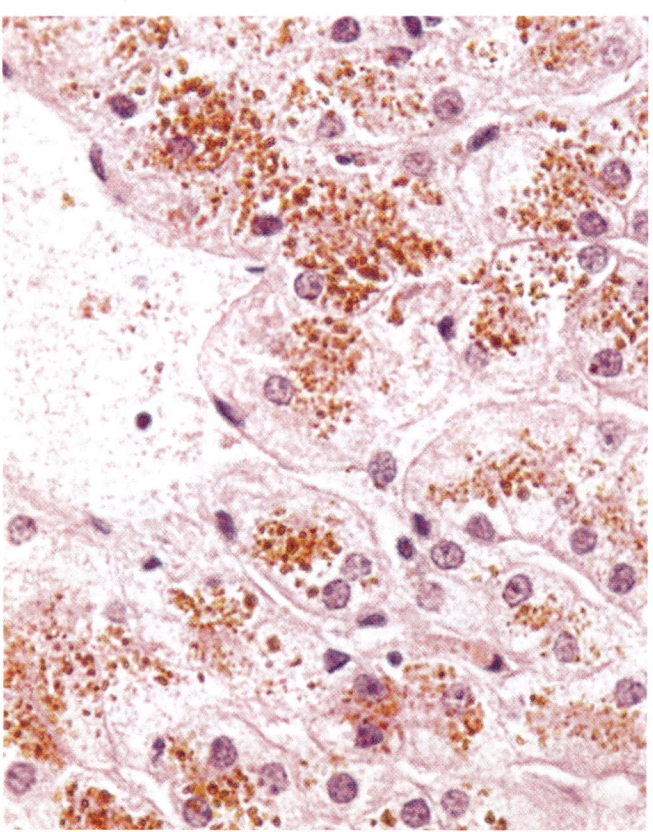

FIGURE 14-7
Dubin-Johnson syndrome. The hepatocytes contain coarse, iron-free, dark-brown granules.

Familial Intrahepatic Cholestasis (Byler Syndrome)

Byler syndrome is a heterogeneous group of uncommon, inherited, autosomal recessive disorders of infancy or early childhood in which intrahepatic cholestasis progresses relentlessly to cirrhosis. Although Byler syndrome was originally described in several Amish families, all of whom were named Byler, it is not limited to that ethnic group. These disorders have been linked to mutations in genes involved in hepatocellular bile transport systems, including MPRs. There is an associated high incidence of retinitis pigmentosa, and the children are often mentally retarded. Most affected children die within the first 2 years of life.

Sepsis Can Cause Jaundice

Severe conjugated hyperbilirubinemia may be associated with septicemia involving both gram-positive and gram-negative bacteria, although the latter infection is more common. In these situations, the serum alkaline phosphatase activity and cholesterol levels are usually low, suggesting the possibility of an isolated defect in the excretion of conjugated bilirubin. In jaundice associated with sepsis, the histological changes in the liver are nonspecific and include mild canalicular cholestasis and slight fat accumulation. The portal tracts may contain excess inflammatory cells, and varying degrees of proliferation of bile ductules may be seen. Occasionally, dilated ductules are filled with inspissated bile.

Neonatal (Physiological) Jaundice Occurs in Most Newborns

Infants who exhibit hyperbilirubinemia in the absence of any specific disorder are said to suffer from physiological jaundice.

Pathogenesis: In the fetus, the transhepatic clearance of bilirubin is negligible; hepatic uptake, conjugation, and biliary excretion are all much lower than in children and adults. Hepatic UGT activity is less than 1% of that in adults, and ligandin levels are low. Nevertheless, fetal bilirubin levels remain low because bilirubin traverses the placenta, after which it is conjugated and excreted by the maternal liver.

The liver of the newborn assumes the responsibility for bilirubin clearance before its conjugating and excretory capacities are fully developed. Moreover, the demands on the liver in the newborn are actually increased because of augmented destruction of circulating erythrocytes during this period. **As a consequence, 70% of normal newborns exhibit transient unconjugated hyperbilirubinemia.** This physiological jaundice is more pronounced in premature infants, both because the hepatic clearance of bilirubin is less developed and because the turnover of erythrocytes is more pronounced than in the term infant. The hepatic bilirubin-conjugating capacity reaches adult levels about 2 weeks after birth; the ligandin level takes somewhat longer to reach adult values. As a result of this hepatic maturation, serum bilirubin levels rapidly decline to adult values shortly after birth. Absorption of light by unconjugated bilirubin generates water-soluble bilirubin isomers. Thus, phototherapy is now routinely used in cases of neonatal jaundice.

In cases of maternal–fetal blood group incompatibilities that lead to erythroblastosis fetalis (see Chapter 6), a striking overproduction of bilirubin in the fetus results from immune-mediated hemolysis. However, although newborns with erythroblastosis fetalis display increased bilirubin levels in cord blood, jaundice becomes severe only after birth, because maternal metabolism of bilirubin no longer compensates for the immaturity of the neonatal liver.

Impaired Canalicular Bile Flow Accompanied by Visible Biliary Pigment (Cholestasis) Reflects either Extrahepatic or Intrahepatic Biliary Obstruction

Functionally, cholestasis represents decreased bile flow through the canaliculus and reduced secretion of water, bilirubin, and bile acids by the hepatocyte. The clinical diagnosis is based on the accumulation in the blood of materials normally transferred to the bile, including bilirubin, cholesterol, and bile acids, and the presence in the blood of elevated activities of certain enzymes, typically alkaline phosphatase. Cholestasis may be produced by intrinsic liver disease, in which case the term *intrahepatic cholestasis* is used, or by obstruction of the large bile ducts, a condition known as *extrahepatic cholestasis*. In any event, cholestasis is caused by a defect in the transport of bile across the canalicular membrane.

The secretion of bile into the canaliculus and its passage into the biliary collecting system are active processes that depend on a number of factors, including (1) the functional and structural characteristics of the canalicular microvilli, (2) the permeability of the canalicular plasma membrane, (3) the intracellular contractile system surrounding the canaliculus (microfilaments, microtubules), and (4) the interaction of bile acids with the secretory apparatus.

Pathogenesis: The biochemical basis of cholestasis is not entirely clear, but a number of abnormalities in the formation and movement of bile have been described. In the case of extrahepatic biliary obstruction, the effects clearly begin with increased pressure in the bile ducts. However, in the early stages, the biochemical and morphological events at the canalicular level are similar to those that occur with intrahepatic cholestasis, including **a centrilobular predilection for the appearance of canalicular bile plugs** (Fig. 14-8).

The invariable presence of bile constituents in the blood of persons with cholestasis implies regurgitation of conjugated bilirubin from the hepatocyte into the bloodstream. The hepatic clearance of unconjugated bilirubin in cholestasis is normal. Even in the presence of complete bile duct obstruction, the serum bilirubin level rises only as high as 30 to 35 mg/dL because renal excretion of bilirubin prevents further accumulation.

Both intrahepatic and extrahepatic cholestasis are characterized initially by a preferential localization of visible bile

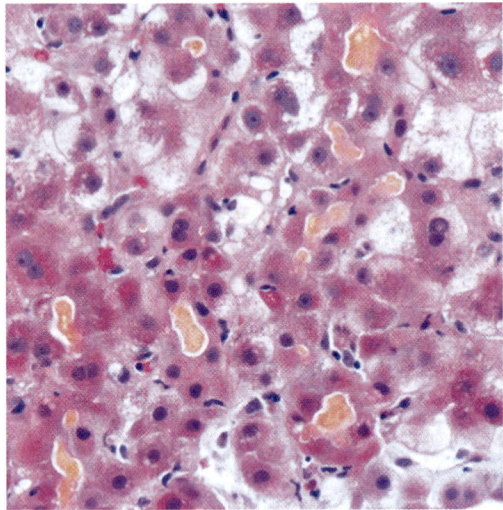

FIGURE 14-8
Bile stasis. A photomicrograph of the liver shows prominent bile plugs in dilated bile canaliculi.

pigment in the centrilobular zone. Fluid secretion into the canalicular bile is divided into two components: one dependent on the secretion of bile acids and the other independent of bile acid secretion. Since the periportal hepatocytes secrete most of the bile acids, the fluid content in the periportal zone of the canaliculus exceeds that in the central zone, a condition that tends to keep bilirubin in solution. Moreover, the bile acids themselves, which act as detergents in the intestine, also solubilize aggregates of bilirubin in the periportal areas. To the above factors is added the higher activity of microsomal mixed-function oxidases in the central zone, which predisposes central hepatocytes to injury by a variety of drugs and toxins. Such an effect may favor the deposition of bile in the centrilobular areas in cholestatic disorders.

DAMAGE TO THE CANALICULAR PLASMA MEMBRANE: The canalicular plasma membrane is the site of sodium (and therefore fluid) secretion into the bile. In addition, this membrane participates in the secretion of bile acids and bilirubin. The secretion of fluid is under the control of the Na^+/K^+-ATPase of the canalicular membrane. Alterations in the canalicular membrane by agents capable of perturbing its lipid structure (e.g., chlorpromazine) inhibit Na^+/K^+-ATPase and decrease bile flow. Similarly, ethinyl estradiol increases the cholesterol content of the canalicular membrane, inhibits ATPase, and interferes with bile flow. Morphological alterations in the canalicular membrane (e.g., those associated with the infusion of certain monohydroxy bile acids, such as taurolithocholate) are also accompanied by a decreased bile flow.

ALTERATION IN THE CONTRACTILE PROPERTIES OF THE CANALICULUS: Cinematography has shown that bile is propelled along the canaliculus by a **peristalsis-like contractile activity of the hepatocytes.** Agents that interact with the pericanalicular actin microfilaments (e.g., cytochalasin, phalloidin, and possibly chlorpromazine) inhibit this peristalsis and may cause cholestasis.

ALTERATIONS IN THE PERMEABILITY OF THE CANALICULAR MEMBRANE: It has been suggested that certain agents that produce cholestasis, including estrogens and taurolithocholate, permit back-diffusion of bile components by making the canalicular membrane more permeable, or "leaky."

 Pathology: **The morphological hallmark of cholestasis is the presence of brownish bile pigment within dilated canaliculi and in hepatocytes.** By electron microscopy, the canaliculus is enlarged, and the microvilli are blunted and fewer in number or even absent (Fig. 14-9). Bile stasis in the hepatocyte is reflected in the presence of large, inhomogeneous, bile-laden lysosomes.

When cholestasis persists, secondary morphological abnormalities develop. Scattered necrotic hepatocytes probably reflect a toxic effect of excess intracellular bile. Within the sinusoid, the macrophages and resident Kupffer cells contain bile pigment and cellular debris. **Whereas early cholestasis is restricted almost exclusively to the central zone, chronic cholestasis is also marked by the appearance of bile plugs in the periphery of the lobule.**

In long-standing cholestasis (usually the result of extrahepatic biliary obstruction), groups of hepatocytes manifest (1) hydropic swelling, (2) diffuse impregnation with bile pigment, and (3) a reticulated appearance. This triad is termed *feathery degeneration.* The necrosis of such cells, together with

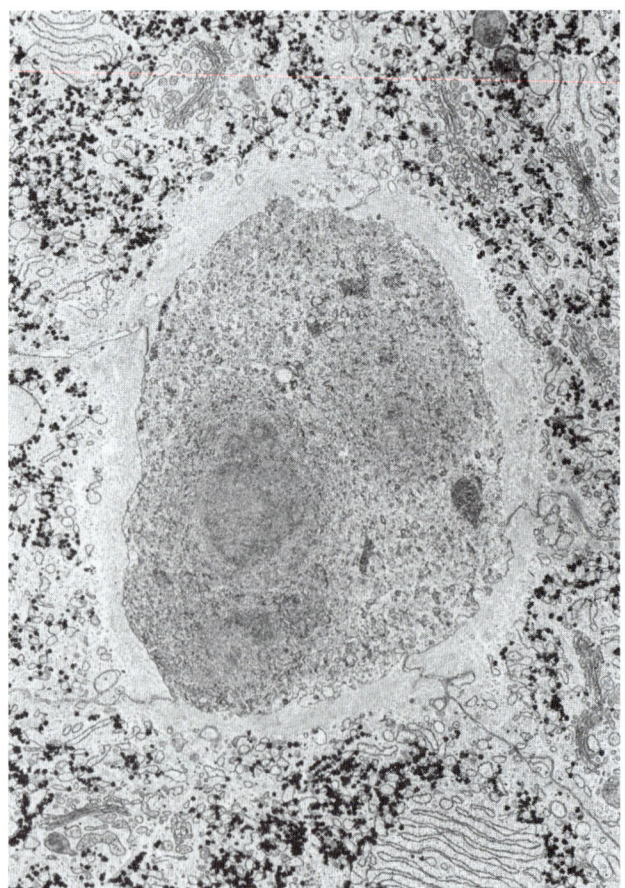

FIGURE 14-9
Cholestasis. An electron micrograph reveals a distended bile canaliculus that has a thickened, filamentous ectoplasmic zone and encloses a granular bile plug.

the accumulation of extravasated bile in the area, results in a golden-yellow focus of extracellular pigment and debris known as a *bile infarct or bile lake* (Fig. 14-10).

The sites of obstruction to the flow of bile in the liver are depicted in Figure 14-11.

CIRRHOSIS

Cirrhosis, the end stage of chronic liver disease, is defined as the destruction of the normal hepatic architecture by fibrous septa that encompass regenerative nodules of hepatocytes. This morphological pattern invariably results from persistent liver cell necrosis. Advanced cases of cirrhosis all tend to have a similar appearance, and often the cause can no longer be ascertained by morphological examination alone. During earlier stages, on the other hand, the characteristic features of the inciting pathogenic insult may be evident. For example, fat and Mallory bodies are typical of alcoholic liver injury, whereas chronic inflammation and periportal necrosis define chronic hepatitis.

The number of terms applied to the different forms of cirrhosis rivals the number of causative agents incriminated in chronic liver disease. Out of this apparent complexity, we

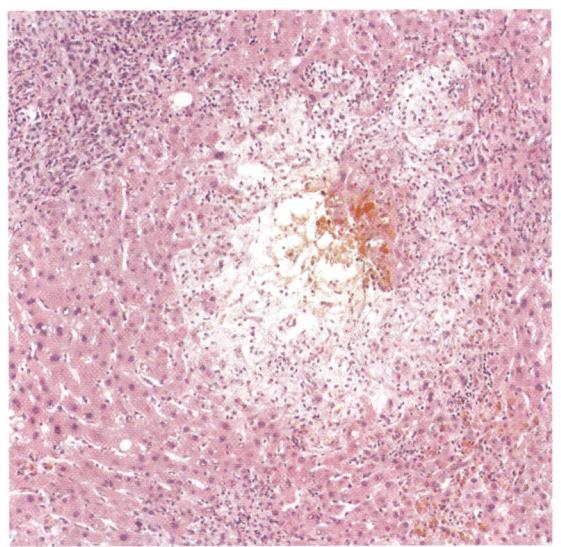

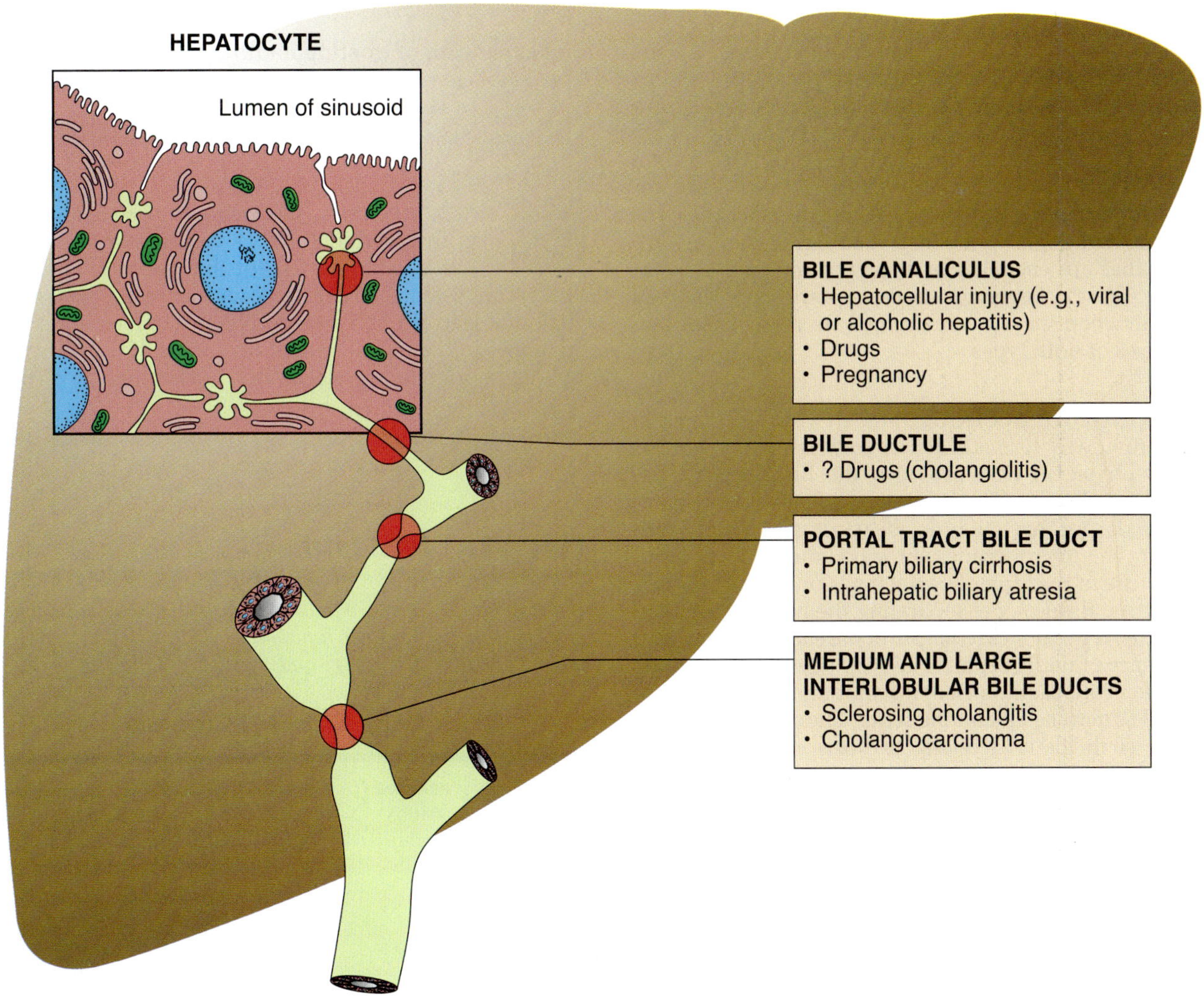

FIGURE 14-10
Bile infarct (bile lake). A photomicrograph of the liver in a patient with extrahepatic biliary obstruction shows an area of necrosis and the accumulation of extravasated bile.

FIGURE 14-11
Sites of cholestasis.

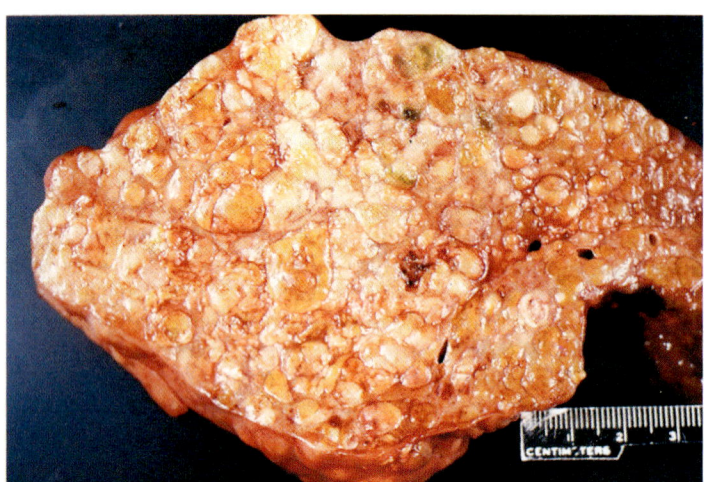
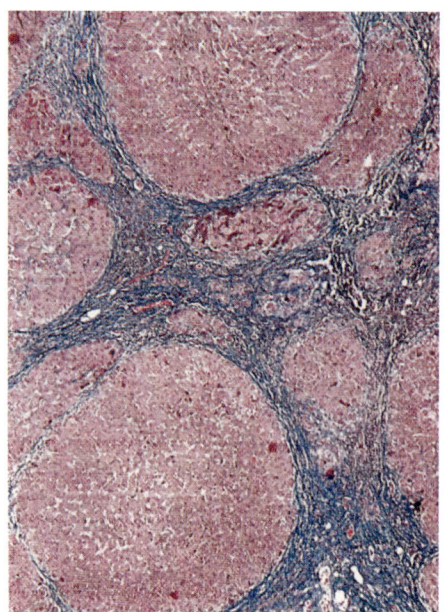

FIGURE *14-12*
Macronodular cirrhosis. A. The liver is misshapen, and the cut surface reveals irregular nodules and connective tissue septa of varying width. **B.** A photomicrograph shows nodules of varying size and irregular fibrous septa.

can extract a simple spectrum of nodular patterns. At one end of this spectrum, usually in the early evolution of cirrhosis, is the *micronodular* type, characterized by small, uniform nodules separated by thin fibrous septa (see Fig. 14-40, below). At the other end of the spectrum, ordinarily late in the course of the disease, is *macronodular cirrhosis*. This pattern consists of grossly visible, coarse, irregular nodules that are mirrored histologically by large nodules of varying size and shape that are encircled by bands of connective tissue (Fig. 14-12). These collagenous septa also vary conspicuously in width. Between these two extremes are many cases that show features of both types.

MICRONODULAR CIRRHOSIS: This form of liver disease was previously termed *Laennec cirrhosis*, which honors the French physician who provided the first accurate description of this disease. Micronodular cirrhosis exhibits nodules scarcely larger than a lobule, measuring less than 3 mm in diameter. The micronodules show no landmarks of lobular architecture in the form of portal tracts or central venules. The connective tissue septa separating the nodules are usually thin, but irregular focal collapse of parenchyma may lead to the presence of wider septa. In active stages of the cirrhotic process, numerous mononuclear inflammatory cells and proliferated bile ductules inhabit the septa. The prototype of micronodular cirrhosis is alcoholic cirrhosis, but this pattern may also be observed in cirrhosis of many other causes.

MACRONODULAR CIRRHOSIS: Macronodular cirrhosis is classically associated with chronic hepatitis. It also occasionally results from submassive confluent necrosis (see below), in which case the liver may be grossly misshapen. The connective tissue septa in macronodular cirrhosis are characteristically broad and contain elements of preexisting portal tracts, mononuclear inflammatory cells, and proliferated bile ductules. **Micronodular cirrhosis can be converted into a macronodular pattern by continued regeneration and expansion of existing nodules.** This is particularly true of alcoholics who are persuaded to abstain from drinking.

 Pathogenesis: The diseases associated with cirrhosis are listed in Table 14-1. It is clear that they have little in common except that they are all accompanied by persistent liver cell necrosis. Most cases of cirrhosis are attributable to alcoholism and chronic viral hepatitis. Despite advances in diagnostic modalities, some 15% of cases are of unknown origin and are classified as **cryptogenic cirrhosis**.

HEPATIC FAILURE

Hepatic failure is the clinical syndrome that occurs when the mass of liver cells or their function is inadequate to sustain the vital metabolic, detoxifying, and synthetic activities of the liver.

TABLE *14-1* **Causes of Cirrhosis**

Alcoholic liver disease	Glycogen storage disease, types III and IV
Chronic viral hepatitis	
Primary biliary cirrhosis	Galactosemia
Autoimmune hepatitis	Hereditary fructose intolerance
Extrahepatic biliary obstruction	Tyrosinemia
	Hereditary storage diseases:
Sclerosing cholangitis	Gaucher, Niemann-Pick,
Hemochromatosis	Wolman, mucopoly-
Wilson disease	saccharidoses
Cystic fibrosis	Zellweger syndrome
α_1-Antitrypsin deficiency	Indian childhood cirrhosis

Hepatic Failure

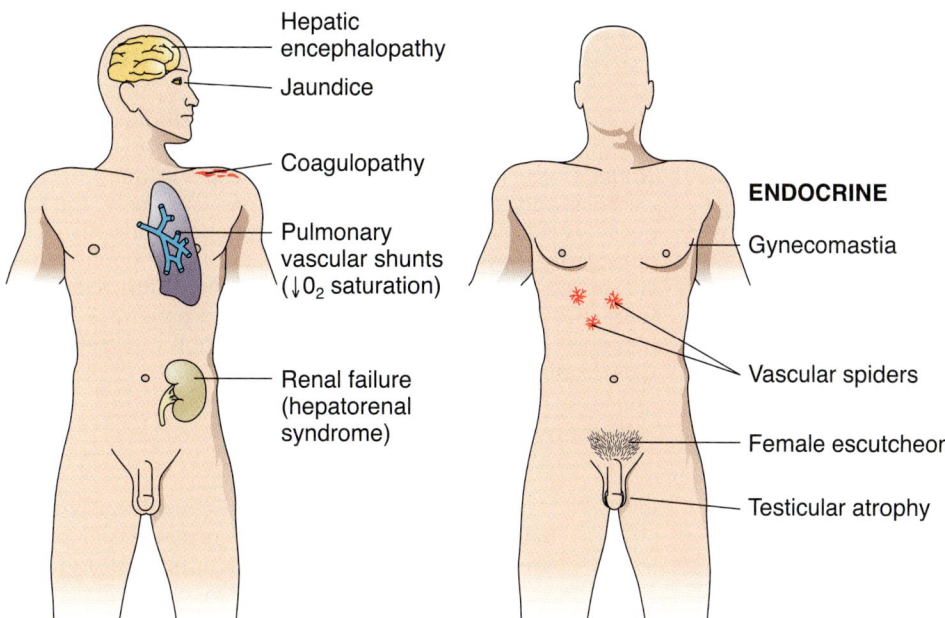

FIGURE 14-13
Complications of hepatic failure.

Liver failure may develop acutely, most commonly as a result of viral hepatitis or toxic liver injury. By contrast, chronic liver diseases, such as chronic viral hepatitis or cirrhosis, may lead to an insidious onset of hepatic failure. The consequences of acute and chronic hepatic failure are depicted in Figure 14-13, which deals with the complications of cirrhosis, the most common cause of hepatic failure. Although advances in supportive care have improved survival in acute hepatic failure, the mortality rate for this condition remains above 50%.

Inadequate Clearance of Bilirubin by the Liver Causes Jaundice

Hyperbilirubinemia associated with hepatic failure is for the most part conjugated, but the level of unconjugated bilirubin also tends to increase. On occasion, increased erythrocyte turnover may add to unconjugated hyperbilirubinemia, thereby aggravating the jaundice.

Hepatic Encephalopathy Refers to Neurological Signs and Symptoms of Liver Failure

Hepatic encephalopathy progresses according to the following stages:

Stage I: Sleep disturbance, irritability, and personality changes
Stage II: Lethargy and disorientation
Stage III: Deep somnolence
Stage IV: Coma

This sequence may occur over a period of many months or may evolve rapidly in days or weeks in cases of fulminant hepatic failure. Associated neurological symptoms include (1) a flapping tremor of the hands, called *asterixis*, and hyperactive reflexes in the earlier stages; (2) extensor toe responses later; and (3) a decerebrate posture in the terminal stages. Whereas intensive supportive measures may be adequate therapy in the early stages of hepatic encephalopathy, patients with stages III and IV encephalopathy are usually salvaged only by liver transplantation.

 Pathogenesis: The pathogenesis of hepatic encephalopathy remains elusive, and no single factor has been proved to account for the clinical syndrome. It is probable that encephalopathy is caused in part by toxic compounds absorbed from the intestine that have escaped hepatic detoxification, because of either hepatocyte dysfunction or the existence of structural or functional vascular shunts. The latter mechanism is particularly evident after the surgical construction of a portal–systemic anastomosis (portal vein to inferior vena cava or its equivalent) for the relief of portal hypertension (see below), which accounts for the synonym *portasystemic encephalopathy*.

AMMONIA: Levels of ammonia are usually increased in the blood and brain of patients with hepatic encephalopathy. Most of the body's ammonia is of dietary origin and is derived from ingestion of ammonia in foods, digestion of proteins in the small intestine, and bacterial catabolism of dietary protein and urea secreted into the intestine. The brain detoxifies ammonia by synthesizing glutamate and glutamine, and excess levels of these molecules may alter neurotransmission and brain osmolality. However, the correlation between the increased concentration of blood ammonia and the severity of hepatic encephalopathy is inexact, and the neurotoxic effect of ammonia remains unexplained.

GABA: Neural inhibition, mediated by the γ-aminobutyric acid (GABA)–benzodiazepine receptor complex, is accentuated in hepatic encephalopathy by increased levels of benzodiazepine-like molecules.

OTHER SUBSTANCES: A number of other compounds have been suggested as contributing to the pathogenesis of hepatic encephalopathy. Among these are **mercaptans**, which result from the breakdown of sulfur-containing amino acids in the colon. The characteristic breath odor of patients with hepatic failure, termed *fetor hepaticus*, reflects the presence of mercaptans in saliva. Another hypothesis for the pathogenesis of hepatic encephalopathy holds that increased blood levels of aromatic amino acids, typical of hepatic failure, lead to decreased synthesis of normal neurotransmitters such as norepinephrine and augmented production of **false neurotransmitters** (e.g., octopamine). A toxic effect of **phenols** and **short-chain fatty acids** on the brain has also been postulated. Finally, there is experimental evidence for a disturbance in the blood–brain barrier in hepatic failure.

Pathology: In patients who have died with chronic liver disease and hepatic coma, the most striking changes are found in the astrocytes, termed *Alzheimer type II astrocytes*. These brain cells are increased in number and size and show swelling, nuclear enlargement, and nuclear inclusions. The deep layers of the cerebral cortex and subcortical white matter, the basal ganglia, and the cerebellum exhibit laminar necrosis and a spongiform appearance.

In patients with acute hepatic failure, **cerebral edema** is the major cause of death, occurring in more than half the cases, often in conjunction with uncal and cerebellar herniation. This edema is not simply a terminal event but is rather a specific lesion associated with hepatic coma, although the precise mechanism is obscure.

Defects Of Coagulation Often Cause Bleeding

Reduced hepatic synthesis of coagulation factors and thrombocytopenia are the principal causes for the impaired hemostasis in liver failure. Decreased production of clotting factors (fibrinogen, prothrombin, and factors V, VII, IX, and X) reflects the generalized impairment of protein synthesis by the liver.

A low platelet count ($<80,000/\mu L$) occurs commonly in hepatic failure and is accompanied by qualitative abnormalities in platelet function. Thrombocytopenia may result from (1) hypersplenism, (2) bone marrow depression, or (3) the consumption of circulating platelets by intravascular coagulation.

Disseminated intravascular coagulation (DIC) occurs frequently in liver failure. Intravascular coagulation may be stimulated by necrosis of liver cells, activation of factor XII (Hageman factor) by endotoxin, or inadequate hepatic clearance of activated clotting factors from the circulation.

Hypoalbuminemia Complicates Hepatic Failure

A decreased level of circulating albumin is secondary to impaired hepatic synthesis of albumin and is an important factor in the pathogenesis of the edema that often complicates chronic liver disease.

Hepatorenal Syndrome Refers to Renal Failure Secondary to Hepatic Failure

Hepatorenal syndrome is characterized by the features of renal hypoperfusion, namely, oliguria, azotemia, and increased plasma creatinine levels. The syndrome usually occurs in the setting of cirrhosis and indicates a poor prognosis. Curiously, the kidneys clearly maintain the ability to function normally. Kidneys from patients who have died of the hepatorenal syndrome function well when transplanted into recipients with chronic renal failure. Conversely, in patients with the hepatorenal syndrome, liver transplantation can restore renal function.

Pathogenesis: **The major determinant of the hepatorenal syndrome is decreased renal blood flow and a consequent reduction in glomerular filtration rate.** A reduction in the effective circulating blood volume leads to compensatory renal vasoconstriction. The resulting decrease in renal perfusion and the shunting of blood from the cortex to the medulla cause reduced glomerular filtration. Vasoactive substances produced by the failing liver or inadequately cleared by it seem to contribute to the renal hemodynamic changes. In any event, the hepatorenal syndrome is caused by inadequate perfusion of the kidneys when local vasodilation can no longer counteract the effects of vasoconstriction.

Pathology: At autopsy, jaundiced patients with the hepatorenal syndrome show bile staining of renal tubular cells and bile casts in the lumina, so-called *biliary nephrosis*. However, these morphological alterations are not believed to contribute to the renal dysfunction.

Pulmonary Complications Are Frequent in Cirrhosis

Decreased arterial oxygen saturation may be severe enough to result in cyanosis. Arteriovenous shunts in the lungs of patients with cirrhosis shift the hemoglobin dissociation curve to the right (reduced affinity for oxygen). In addition, ventilatory and perfusion deficits may play a role. Arterial desaturation is responsible for the clubbing of the fingers occasionally encountered in chronic liver disease.

Endocrine Complications Are Associated with Cirrhosis

It is important to distinguish between the direct effects of alcohol abuse, a common cause of liver disease, and changes that are better attributed to hepatic dysfunction. Chronic liver failure in men leads to feminization, characterized by gynecomastia, a female body habitus, and a female distribution of pubic hair (female escutcheon). In addition, vascular manifestations of hyperestrogenism are common and include **spider angiomas** in the territory drained by the superior vena cava (upper trunk and face) and **palmar erythema. Feminization** is attributed to reduced hepatic catabolism of estrogens and weak androgens. The weak androgens (androstenedione and dehydroepiandrosterone) are converted to estrogenic compounds in peripheral tissues, thereby adding to the burden of circulating estrogens. Moreover, extrahepatic portal–systemic shunts secondary to portal hypertension in cirrhosis permit these hormones to bypass the liver.

Men who suffer from alcoholic liver disease are more likely to be feminized than those with liver disease from other causes, and the feminization is usually more severe. In addition, chronic alcoholics also suffer hypogonadism, manifested by testicular atrophy, impotence, and loss of libido. Alcoholic women also exhibit gonadal failure, presenting as oligomenorrhea, amenorrhea, infertility, ovarian atrophy, and loss of secondary sex characteristics. These effects on gonadal function in both sexes reflect a direct toxic action of alcohol independent of chronic liver disease.

PORTAL HYPERTENSION

Portal hypertension is defined as a sustained increase in portal venous pressure and results from obstruction to blood flow somewhere in the portal circuit. Arising at the junction of the superior mesenteric vein with the splenic vein, the portal vein carries the major venous drainage from the gastrointestinal tract, the pancreas, and the spleen into the liver. It delivers two thirds of the hepatic blood flow but accounts for less than half of the total oxygen supply, the remainder being supplied by the hepatic artery. Normally, the pressure in the portal vein is only 7 to 14 cm H_2O (5–10 mm Hg). A pressure greater than 30 cm H_2O is considered evidence of portal hypertension. **The major complications of increased portal pressure and the opening of collateral channels are bleeding from gastroesophageal varices, ascites, and splenomegaly.**

For the sake of convenience, obstruction to the flow of portal blood can be pictured as (1) prehepatic, occurring before the blood enters the liver; (2) intrahepatic, occurring during transit through the portal tracts and lobules; and (3) posthepatic, occurring after exit of the blood from the lobules (Fig. 14-14).

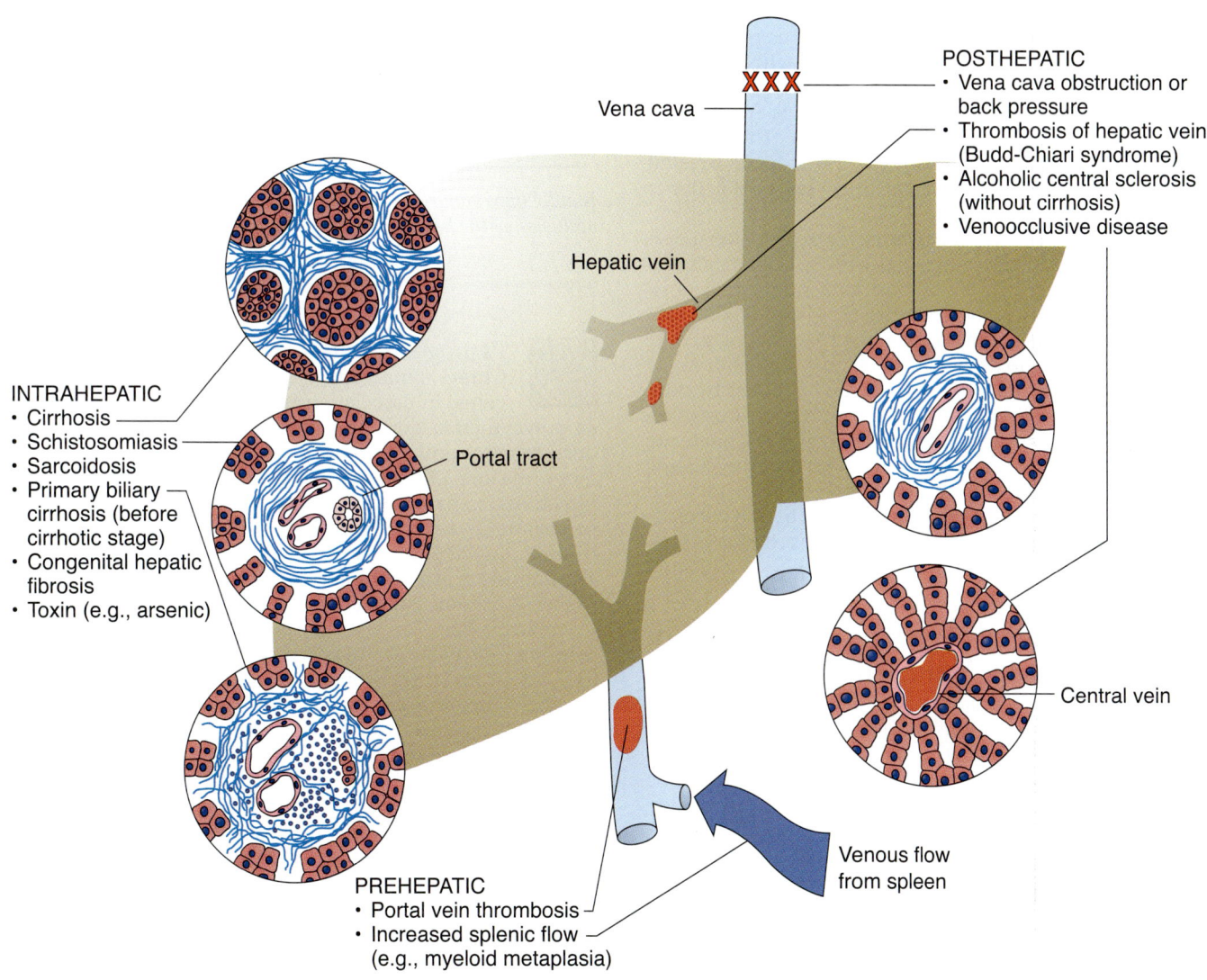

FIGURE 14-14
Causes of portal hypertension.

Intrahepatic Portal Hypertension Is Usually Caused by Cirrhosis

Regenerative nodules in the cirrhotic liver impinge on the hepatic veins, thereby obstructing blood flow distal to the lobules. The small portal veins and venules are trapped, narrowed, and often obliterated by scarring of the portal tracts. Moreover, blood flow through the hepatic artery is increased and small arteriovenous communications become functional. In this way, portal hypertension due to obstruction of blood flow distal to the sinusoid is augmented by increased arterial blood flow. In addition, increased splanchnic arterial blood flow, whose cause is unclear, is an important factor in the maintenance of portal hypertension. Central vein sclerosis and sinusoidal fibrosis also contribute to the development of portal hypertension in alcoholic liver disease. In fact, portal hypertension can result from alcoholic central sclerosis, even in cases that do not progress to cirrhosis.

Worldwide, hepatic schistosomiasis (*S. mansoni* and *S. japonicum*) is a major cause of intrahepatic portal hypertension. The ova released from the intestinal veins traverse the portal system and lodge in the intrahepatic portal venules, where they elicit a granulomatous reaction that heals by scarring. Because the obstruction within the liver occurs predominantly before the portal blood enters the hepatic sinusoids, **hepatic schistosomiasis is functionally similar to prehepatic portal hypertension.** Thus, hepatic function is well maintained, but the intrahepatic presinusoidal vascular obstruction leads to severe portal hypertension.

Idiopathic portal hypertension refers to occasional cases of intrahepatic portal hypertension with splenomegaly that occur in the absence of any demonstrable intrahepatic or extrahepatic disease. In some countries (England, Japan), idiopathic portal hypertension accounts for 15 to 35% of all cases that require surgery to decompress the portal circulation.

Intrahepatic portal hypertension can be caused by other conditions that interfere with the flow of blood through the liver, including (1) cystic disease of the liver (see Chapter 16, which includes a discussion of cystic disease of the kidney), (2) partial nodular transformation of the liver in the region of the porta hepatis, and (3) nodular regenerative hyperplasia (small regenerative nodules without fibrosis that compress the intervening hepatic parenchyma).

Prehepatic Portal Hypertension Is Often Caused by Portal Vein Thrombosis

Portal vein thrombosis occurs most commonly in the setting of cirrhosis. Other causes of portal vein thrombosis include tumors, infections, hypercoagulability states, pancreatitis, and surgical trauma. Some cases are of unknown etiology. Primary hepatocellular carcinoma characteristically invades branches of the portal vein and occasionally occludes the main portal vein. When the portal vein is obstructed by a septic thrombus, bacteria may seed the intrahepatic branches of the portal vein *(suppurative pylephlebitis)* and cause multiple hepatic abscesses.

Occlusion of the portal vein may be manifested in the neonatal period or in early childhood. In some cases, umbilical sepsis is an important cause, but other local and systemic infections may also play a role. Sometimes the thrombosed portal or splenic vein is replaced by a fibrous cord or interlacing vascular channels, a condition termed *cavernous transformation*.

The liver normally offers little resistance to the outflow of blood through the sinusoids and can, therefore, accommodate substantial increases in blood flow without a secondary increase in pressure. However, under some uncommon circumstances, increased portal venous blood flow can result in prehepatic portal hypertension. An arteriovenous fistula (i.e., an abnormal communication between an artery and the portal vein) may lead to prehepatic portal hypertension. It generally arises from trauma or rupture of an aneurysm of the splenic or hepatic artery. Such a fistula may also be found in association with hereditary hemorrhagic telangiectasia (Osler-Weber-Rendu syndrome). Portal hypertension also occasionally occurs in patients with splenomegaly from a variety of causes, including polycythemia vera, myeloid metaplasia, and chronic myelogenous leukemia. In cirrhosis, the accompanying splenomegaly may further aggravate portal hypertension.

Posthepatic Portal Hypertension Refers to Obstruction to Blood Flow beyond the Liver Lobules

Budd-Chiari Syndrome

Budd-Chiari syndrome is a congestive disease of the liver caused by occlusion of the hepatic veins and their tributaries.

Pathogenesis: The principal cause of the Budd-Chiari syndrome is thrombosis of the hepatic veins, in association with such diverse conditions as polycythemia vera and other myeloproliferative disorders, hypercoagulable states associated with malignant tumors, the use of oral contraceptives, pregnancy, bacterial infections, paroxysmal nocturnal hemoglobinuria, metastatic and primary tumors in the liver, and surgical trauma. In 20% of cases, no specific cause is evident. Thrombosis is most common in the large hepatic veins close to their exit from the liver and in the intrahepatic portion of the inferior vena cava. In parts of Africa and the Orient, membranous webs of unknown cause, presumably congenital, compromise the vena cava above the orifices of the hepatic veins and commonly cause the Budd-Chiari syndrome. Increased back-pressure in the venous system caused by severe congestive heart failure, tricuspid stenosis or regurgitation, or constrictive pericarditis may mimic the Budd-Chiari syndrome.

Hepatic venoocclusive disease is a variant of the Budd-Chiari syndrome and is caused by occlusion of the central venules and small branches of the hepatic veins. Most commonly, this disorder is traced to the ingestion of toxic pyrrolizidine alkaloids present in plants of the *Crotalaria* and *Senecio* families, which are used in the formulation of "bush teas" in primitive societies. It is also seen in patients treated with certain antineoplastic chemotherapeutic agents, and after hepatic irradiation. Venoocclusive disease also occurs in association with bone marrow transplantation, possibly as a manifestation of graft-versus-host disease.

 Pathology: In the acute stage of **hepatic vein thrombosis**, the liver is swollen and tense, and the cut surface exhibits a mottled appearance and oozes blood (Fig. 14-15A). In the chronic stage, the cut surface is paler, and the liver is firm, owing to an increase in connective tissue. Microscopically, the hepatic veins display thrombi in varying stages of evolution, from recent clots to well-organized thrombi that have been canalized.

In the acute stage of both the Budd-Chiari syndrome and venoocclusive disease, the sinusoids of the central zone are dilated and packed with erythrocytes. The liver cell plates are compressed, and there is necrosis of centrilobular hepatocytes (see Fig. 14-15B). In long-standing venous congestion, fibrosis of the central zone radiating into the more peripheral portions of the lobules is conspicuous. The sinusoids are dilated, and the central to midzonal hepatocytes show pressure atrophy. Eventually, connective tissue septa link adjacent central zones to form nodules with a single portal tract in the center, a process known as *reverse lobulation*. The fibrosis is usually not severe enough to justify a label of cirrhosis.

 Clinical Features: **Complete thrombosis of the hepatic veins presents as an acute illness characterized by abdominal pain, enlargement of the liver, ascites, and mild jaundice.** Acute hepatic failure and death often occur rapidly. The more usual course, in which the obstruction of the hepatic venous circulation is incomplete, is marked by similar symptoms but may pursue a protracted course over periods ranging from a month to a few years. More than 90% of patients with Budd-Chiari syndrome develop ascites, usually severe, and splenomegaly is seen in over 30%. Typically, the serum bilirubin and aminotransferase activities increase only modestly. Most patients eventually die in hepatic failure or from the complications of portal hypertension. Liver transplantation has been successful in curing the disease.

Portal Hypertension Leads to Systemic Complications

Esophageal Varices

Esophageal varices represent the most important complication of portal hypertension and arise from the opening of portal–systemic collaterals as an adaptation to decompress the portal venous system. One of the most common causes of death in patients with cirrhosis and other disorders associated with portal hypertension is exsanguinating upper gastrointestinal tract hemorrhage from **bleeding esophageal varices.**

 Pathogenesis: The collaterals of most clinical significance are located in the submucosa of the lower esophagus and upper stomach and are the result of communications between the portal vein and the gastric coronary vein. Because of the increased blood flow and higher pressure that follow the opening of these collaterals, the submucosal veins in the vicinity of the esophagogastric junction become dilated and protrude into the lumen (See chapter 13). There is no simple correlation between portal venous pressure and the risk of variceal bleeding, although the risk does rise with increasing size of the varices.

 Clinical Features: The prognosis in patients with bleeding esophageal varices is poor, and the acute mortality may be as high as 40%. In patients with cir-

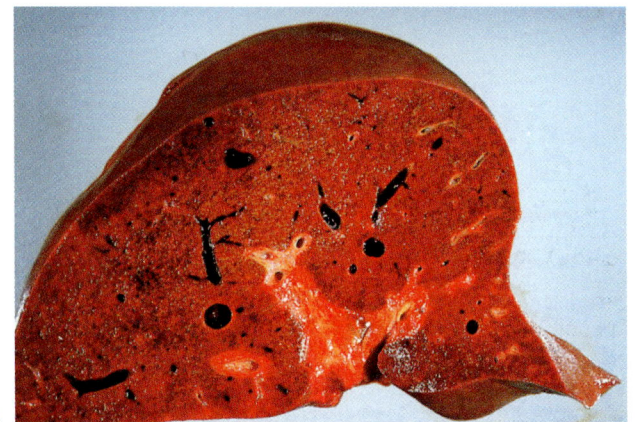
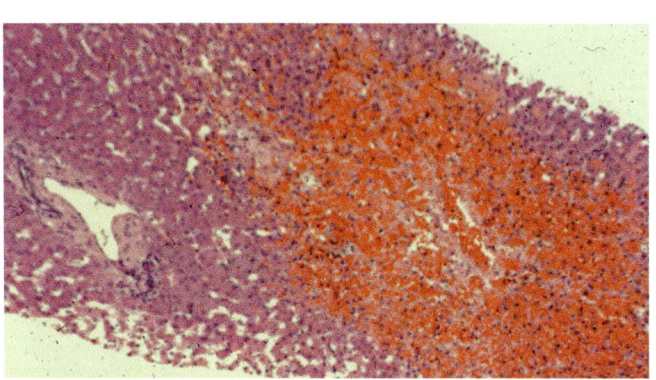

FIGURE 14-15
Budd-Chiari syndrome. A. The cut surface of the liver from a patient who died from Budd-Chiari syndrome shows thrombosis of the hepatic veins and diffuse congestion of the parenchyma. B. A needle biopsy of the liver from a patient with acute Budd-Chiari syndrome reveals centrilobular necrosis and hemorrhage.

rhosis who survive an initial episode of variceal bleeding, long-term survival is unlikely because of a high risk of rebleeding or worsening liver failure. By contrast, patients in whom the portal hypertension is caused by a presinusoidal block, such as hepatic schistosomiasis, have a much better prognosis than those with cirrhosis because of the absence of underlying liver dysfunction. Importantly, death associated with bleeding esophageal varices is frequently not attributable directly to exsanguination and shock. Rather it is the result of hepatic failure precipitated by stress, ischemic necrosis of the liver, and the encephalopathy caused by the acute nitrogenous load imposed by blood in the intestinal tract.

Acute variceal hemorrhage may be treated by direct tamponade with an inflatable balloon, injection of varices with sclerosing agents through an endoscope, endoscopic variceal ligation, or intravenous administration of vasopressin to reduce splanchnic blood flow and portal venous pressure. For patients with repeated episodes of variceal bleeding in whom sclerotherapy has failed, permanent decompression of the portal circulation can be achieved by surgically constructed portasystemic shunts. These procedures divert blood from the high-pressure portal circulation to the lower-pressure systemic venous circulation. Intrahepatic portasystemic shunts can also be constructed by invasive angiography, in which a catheter in a hepatic vein is thrust through hepatic parenchyma into a dilated branch of the portal vein (transjugular intrahepatic portasystemic shunt [TIPS]). In some cases, liver transplantation is an alternative to shunt surgery.

The back-pressure in the portal vein is also transmitted to its tributaries, including the inferior hemorrhoidal veins, which become dilated and tortuous (*anorectal varices*). Collateral veins radiating about the umbilicus produce a pattern known as *caput medusae*.

Splenomegaly

The spleen in portal hypertension enlarges progressively and often gives rise to the syndrome of *hypersplenism*—that is, a decrease in the life span of all of the formed elements of

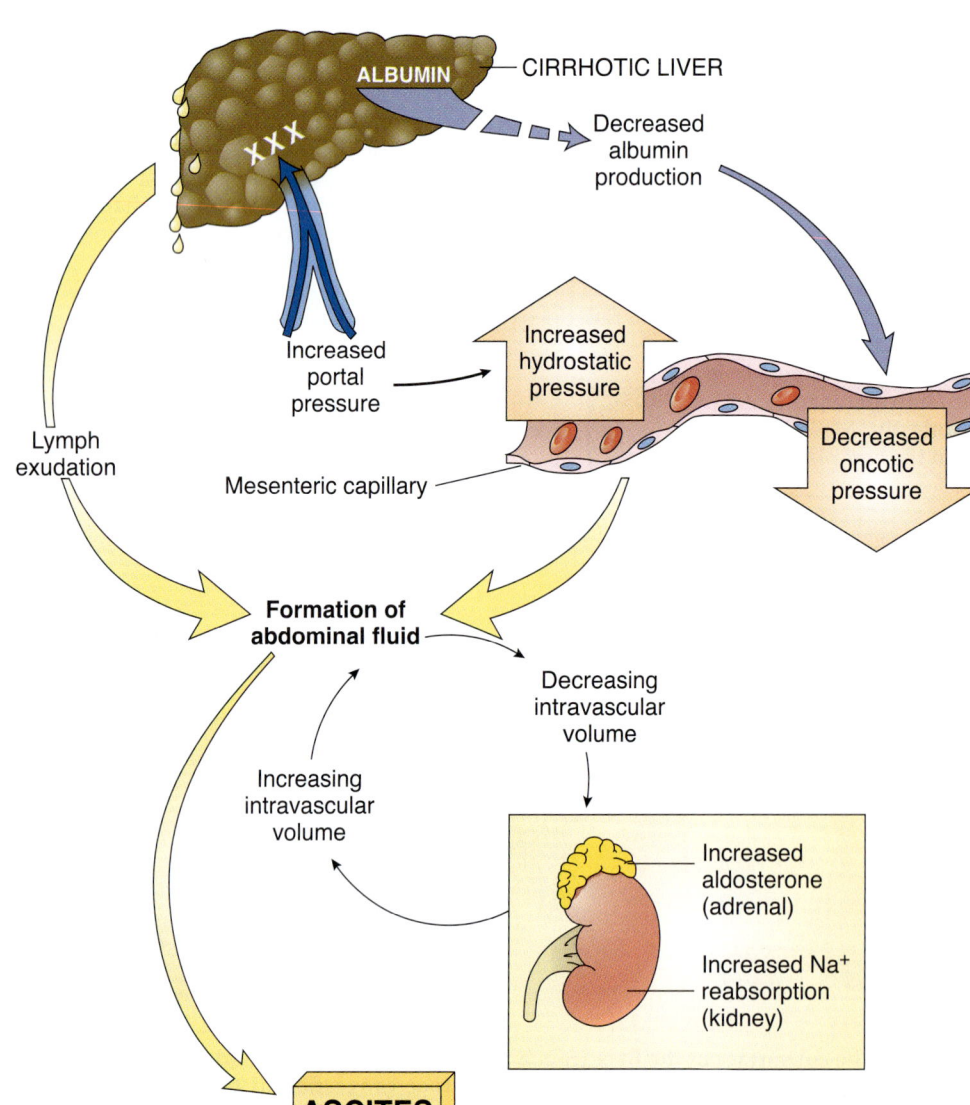

FIGURE *14-16*
Pathogenesis of ascites. In addition to the other factors depicted, the traditional concept holds that renal retention of sodium is a response to a decreased "effective" blood volume. An alternative view (overflow hypothesis) considers the increased renal reabsorption of sodium to be a primary effect of cirrhosis that precedes the formation of ascites. Peripheral vasodilation should also considered.

the blood and, therefore, a reduction in their circulating numbers (pancytopenia). Hypersplenism is attributed to an increased rate of removal of erythrocytes, leukocytes, and platelets because of the prolonged transit time through the hyperplastic spleen.

On gross examination, the spleen is firm and enlarged, up to 1000 g, and its cut surface is uniformly deep red, with an inapparent white pulp. Microscopically, the splenic sinusoids are dilated, and their walls are thickened by fibrous tissue and lined by hyperplastic endothelial cells and macrophages. Focal hemorrhages lead to the formation of fibrotic, iron-laden nodules, known as *Gamna-Gandy bodies*.

Ascites

Ascites refers to the accumulation of fluid in the peritoneal cavity. It often accompanies portal hypertension, and the amount of fluid may be so great (frequently many liters) that it not only distends the abdomen but also interferes with breathing. The onset of ascites in cirrhosis is associated with a poor prognosis.

 Pathogenesis: The retention of sodium and water in cirrhosis is clearly important in the pathogenesis of ascites. The mechanisms for altered sodium and water homeostasis in cirrhosis remain controversial, but three major hypotheses can be considered:

- **Hypovolemia:** It was initially held that increased pressure in the portal system caused sodium and water transudation into the abdominal cavity. The resulting hypovolemia was postulated to stimulate increased renal sodium and water retention (Fig. 14-16).
- **Overflow:** Subsequently, it was shown that the total blood volume in cirrhotic patients with ascites actually increases rather than decreases. In fact, blood volume expansion and sodium and water retention by the kidney precede the formation of ascites. These findings suggest that renal sodium and water retention in decompensated cirrhosis results from an alteration in volume regulation that is not secondary to decreased intravascular volume.
- **Vasodilation:** It has been proposed that peripheral arterial vasodilation is an initiating event in the renal retention of sodium and water in cirrhosis. This vasodilation results in a decreased effective arterial blood volume, owing to the diversion of blood to the periphery. This process serves as a potent stimulus for the renal retention of sodium and water.

Other factors contribute to the formation of ascites in cirrhosis. Portal hypertension increases the hydrostatic pressure in the mesenteric capillaries. At the same time, the low serum albumin characteristic of cirrhosis is associated with decreased plasma oncotic pressure. As in the formation of peripheral edema (see Chapter 7), the resulting imbalance in Starling forces leads to transudation of fluid into the peritoneal cavity. Finally, the rate of formation of hepatic lymph exceeds the capacity of the lymphatics to remove it, and the liver "weeps" lymph into the abdomen.

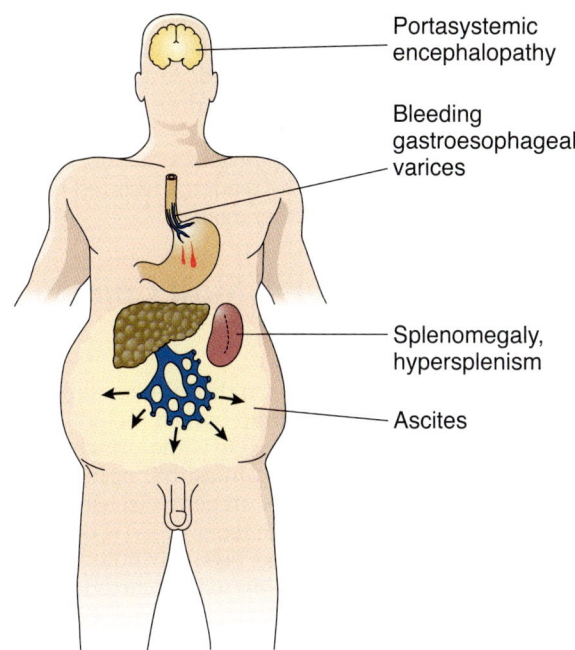

FIGURE *14-17*
Complications of portal hypertension.

Spontaneous Bacterial Peritonitis

Spontaneous bacterial peritonitis is an important complication in patients with both cirrhosis and ascites. The infection is extremely dangerous and carries a very high mortality, even when treated with antibiotics. Presumably, the ascitic fluid is seeded with bacteria from the blood or lymph or by the passage of bacteria through the bowel wall. Typically, the leukocyte count in the ascitic fluid of spontaneous bacterial peritonitis is greater than $500/\mu L$, and more than half are neutrophils.

The complications of portal hypertension are summarized in Figure 14-17.

VIRAL HEPATITIS

Viral hepatitis is an infection of hepatocytes that produces necrosis and inflammation of the liver. The disease has been recognized as "epidemic jaundice" for millennia. Many viruses and other infectious agents can produce hepatitis and jaundice (Table 14-2), but in the industrialized world, more than 95%

TABLE *14-2* **Infectious Agents That Cause Hepatitis**

Hepatitis A virus	Herpes simplex virus
Hepatitis B virus	Cytomegalovirus
Hepatitis C virus	Enteroviruses other than
Hepatitis E virus	hepatitis A virus
Yellow fever virus	Leptospires
Epstein-Barr virus	(leptospirosis)
(infectious mononucleosis)	*Entamoeba histolytica*
Lassa, Marburg, and Ebola viruses	(amebic hepatitis)

of cases of viral hepatitis involve a limited number of hepatotropic viruses, named from A to G. Hepatitis F virus seems to be a variant of hepatitis B. Hepatitis G virus is 25% homologous with hepatitis C virus, but it does not lead to acute or chronic hepatitis.

The following discussion emphasizes the illnesses commonly termed *viral hepatitis*. The reader is referred to Chapter 9 for consideration of the other agents.

Hepatitis A Virus Is the Most Common Cause of Acute Hepatitis

Hepatitis A virus (HAV) is a small RNA-containing enterovirus of the picornavirus group (which includes the polio virus) (Fig. 14-18). The hepatocyte is the principal site of viral replication, although gastrointestinal epithelial cells may also be infected. Shedding of progeny virus into the bile accounts for its appearance in the feces. HAV is not directly cytopathic, and hepatic injury has been attributed to an immunological reaction to virally infected hepatocytes.

Epidemiology: The only reservoir for HAV is the acutely infected person, and transmission depends primarily on serial transmission from person to person by the fecal–oral route. Epidemics of hepatitis A occur under crowded and unsanitary conditions, such as exist in warfare, or by fecal contamination of water and food. Edible shellfish concentrate the virus in contaminated waters and may lead to infection if eaten after being inadequately cooked.

In the industrialized countries, which have low rates of infection, most cases of hepatitis A are seen in older children and adults. By contrast, in less-developed regions, where the disease is endemic, most of the population is infected before the age of 10 years.

In the United States, about 10% of the population younger than 20 years of age have serological evidence of previous HAV infection. **This circumstance indicates that most infections with HAV are anicteric.** Hepatitis A is common in day care centers, international travelers, and male homosexuals, the last reflecting oral–anal contact. However, in about half of all cases of hepatitis A, no source can be identified. An effective vaccine for hepatitis A confers long-term protection against the disease.

Clinical Features: Following an incubation period of 3 to 6 weeks, with a mean of about 4 weeks, persons infected with HAV develop nonspecific symptoms, including fever, malaise, and anorexia. Concomitantly, liver injury is evidenced by a rise in serum aminotransferase activity (Fig. 14-19). As the activities of aminotransferases begin to decline, usually 5 to 10 days later, jaundice may appear. It remains evident for an average of 10 days but may persist for more than a month. In most cases, the elevated levels of aminotransferases return to normal by the time jaundice has disappeared. **Hepatitis A never pursues a chronic course. There is no carrier state, and infection provides lifelong immunity.** Moreover, virtually all patients recover without hepatic encephalopathy, and fatal fulminant hepatitis occurs only rarely.

HAV can be detected in the liver about 2 weeks after infection. It reaches a maximum in another 2 weeks, and it disappears shortly thereafter (see Fig. 14-19). Fecal shedding of HAV follows its appearance in the liver by about a week and lasts for only a brief time. The period of viremia is also short, occurring early in the course of the disease.

The first detectable antibody response to HAV infection is the appearance of IgM anti-HAV in the blood during the acute illness (see Fig. 14-19). The antibody titer begins to fall within a few weeks and generally disappears by 3 to 5 months. IgG anti-HAV is detected as the patient recovers; it maintains peak levels after the IgM antibody has disappeared and persists for life. Finding IgM anti-HAV in the serum of a patient with acute hepatitis confirms HAV as the cause.

Hepatitis B Virus Is a Major Cause of Acute and Chronic Liver Disease

Hepatitis B virus (HBV) is a hepatotropic DNA virus that was the first of the so-called hepadnaviruses. The genomes of the hepadnaviruses are among the smallest of all known viruses. The DNA of HBV is predominantly double-stranded and consists of one long circular strand containing the entire genome, and a shorter complementary strand that varies from 50 to 85% of the length of the longer strand (Fig. 14-20). The HBV genome contains four genes:

- **Core (C) gene:** The core of the virus contains the **core antigen (HBcAg)** and the **e antigen (HBeAg),** both products of the C gene. The C gene includes two consecutive open reading frames, the precore and core regions. Transcription of the core frame alone yields HBcAg, whereas HBeAg is derived from the proteolysis of the translation product of the entire C gene.
- **Surface gene:** The core of HBV is enclosed in a coat that expresses an antigen termed **hepatitis B surface antigen (HBsAg).** The surface coat is synthesized by the infected hepatocyte independently from the viral core and is secreted into the blood in vast amounts. This material is visualized by electron microscopy in cen-

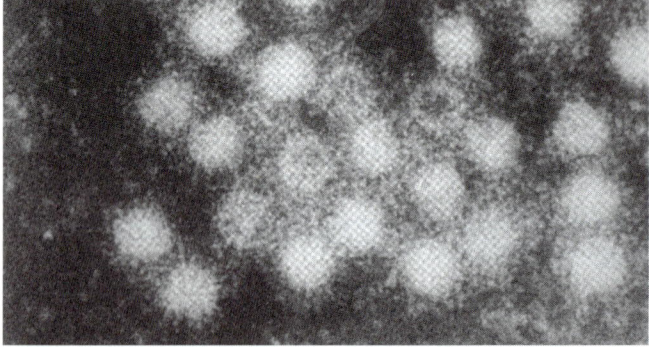

FIGURE 14-18
Electron micrograph of hepatitis A virus (HAV). A fecal extract was treated with convalescent serum containing anti-HAV.

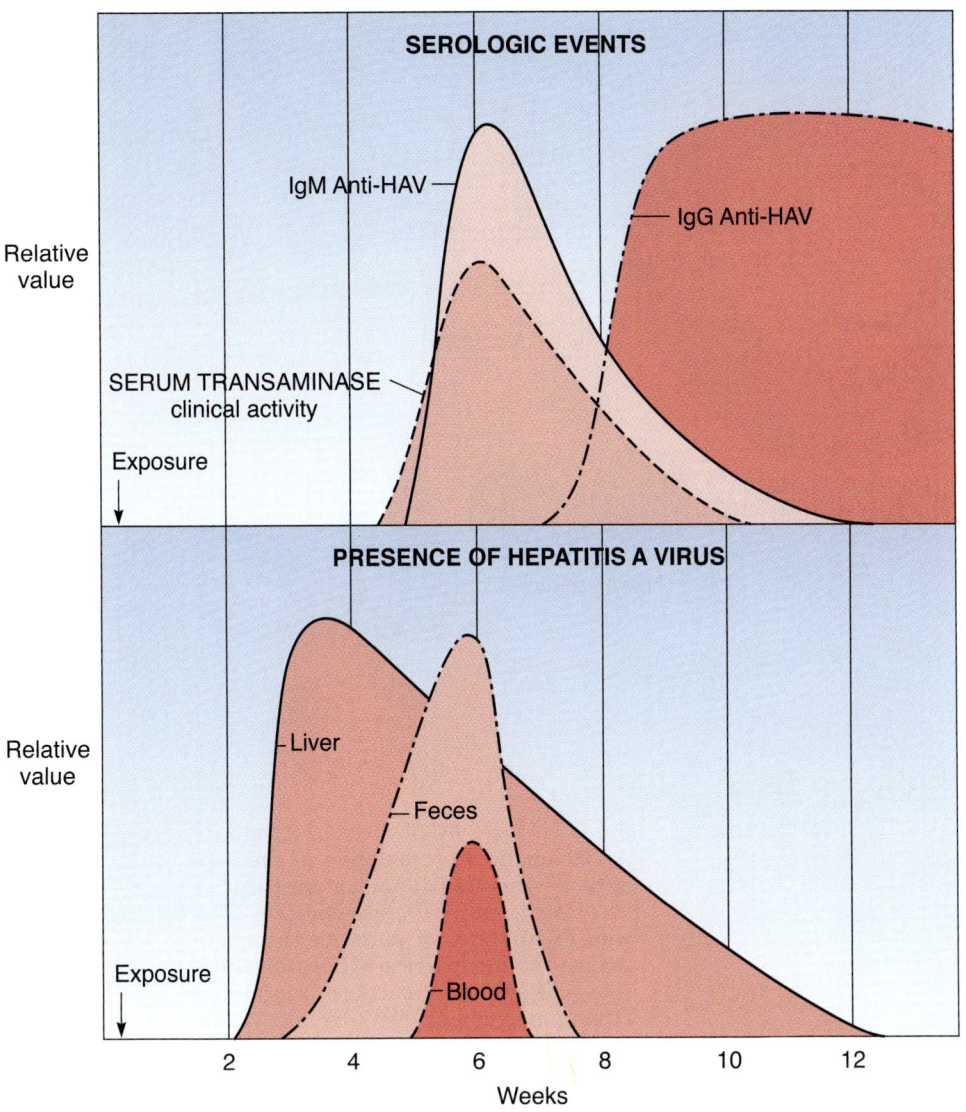

FIGURE 14-19
Typical serological events associated with hepatitis A.

trifuged serum as two distinct particles (see Fig. 14-20), one a 22-nm sphere and the other a tubular structure 22 nm in diameter and 40 to 400 nm in length. **HBsAg particles are immunogenic but not infectious. The intact and infectious virus** is also found in the same preparations as a 42-nm sphere *(Dane particle)* that contains viral DNA.
- **Polymerase gene:** The *P* gene encodes the DNA polymerase.
- **X gene:** The small X protein activates viral transcription and probably plays a role in the pathogenesis of hepatocellular carcinoma associated with chronic HBV infection.

Epidemiology: It is estimated that there are about 200 million chronic carriers of HBV in the world, constituting an enormous reservoir of infection. Depending on the incidence of primary infection with HBV, the carrier rates vary from as low as 0.3% (United States and western Europe) to 20% (Southeast Asia, sub-Saharan Africa, and Oceania). In the latter populations, an important avenue by which the high carrier rate is sustained is vertical transmission of the virus from a carrier mother to her newborn.

In the United States, it is estimated that there are between 500,000 and 1.5 million chronic HBV carriers, and 200,000 to 300,000 persons are newly infected with HBV annually. Of these new cases, only one fourth are clinically recognized because of jaundice. Fulminant hepatitis B results in 250 to 300 deaths a year. Before the advent of routine screening of blood for HBsAg, chronic HBV carriers posed a public health hazard as a source of posttransfusion hepatitis. This threat has been largely eliminated by routine screening for HBsAg.

Whereas no more than 10% of adults infected with HBV become carriers, neonatal hepatitis B is, as a rule, followed by persistent infection. Males exhibit an increased tendency to become carriers. In the United States, chronic HBV carriers are particularly common among male homosexuals and drug addicts.

Humans are the only significant reservoir of HBV. Unlike hepatitis A, hepatitis B is not transmitted by the fecal–oral route, nor does it contaminate food and water supplies. Al-

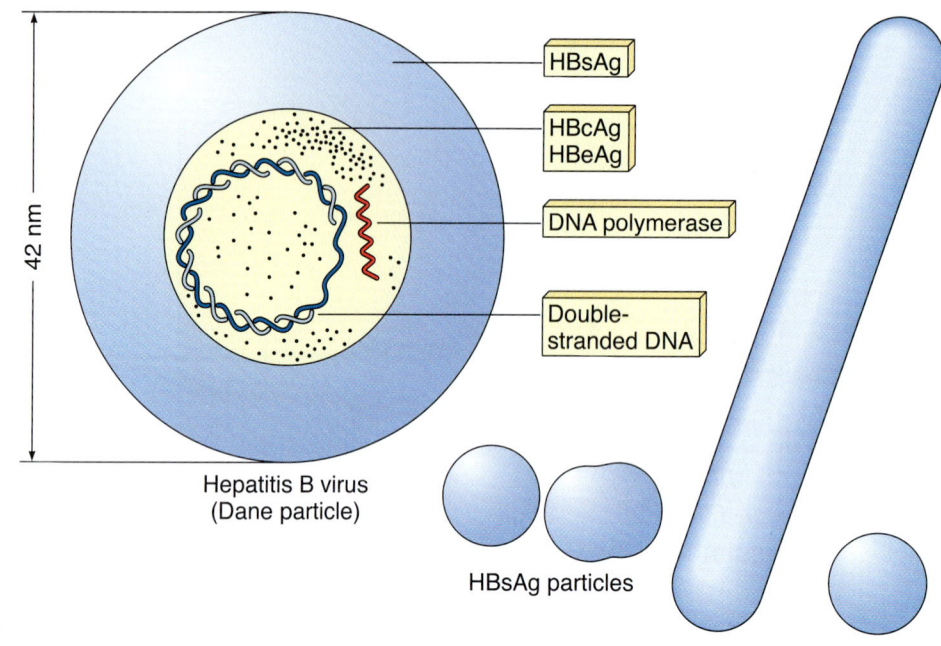

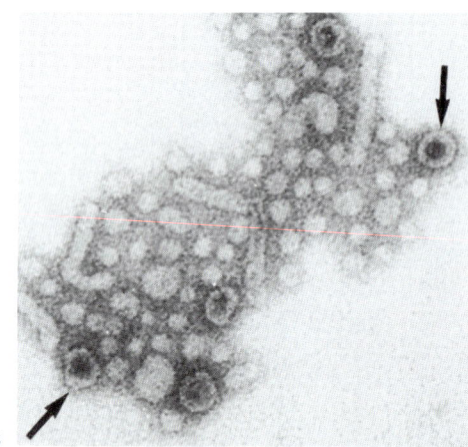

FIGURE 14-20
A. Schematic representation of the hepatitis B virus (HBV) and serum particles associated with HBV infection. B. Electron micrograph of particles from centrifuged serum in a case of hepatitis. Rod-like and spherical particles containing HBsAg are evident. The complete virion, composed of the viral core and its surrounding envelope, is represented by Dane particles *(arrows)*.

though HBsAg is found in most secretions, infectious virus has been demonstrated only in blood, saliva, and semen. Historically, transmission of hepatitis B was believed to be limited to direct transfer of blood products, either by transfusion or by the use of contaminated needles. However, it is now clear that most cases of hepatitis B result from transmission associated with intimate contact. The routes by which contact-transmission occurs are not entirely defined, but it seems probable that direct transfer of the virus through breaks in the skin or mucous membranes is most common. In this respect, sexual contact—occasionally heterosexual but particularly homosexual—is an important mode of transmission.

Synthetic vaccines for hepatitis B, composed of recombinant HbsAg or its immunogenic epitopes, are highly effective and confer lifelong immunity. In some regions where hepatitis B is endemic, its use has significantly reduced the prevalence of the disease. It is now routine in the United States to administer the vaccine to infants.

tious virus in the liver for years without functional or biochemical evidence of liver cell injury.

Cytotoxic ($CD8^+$) T lymphocytes (CTLs) directed against multiple HBV epitopes are the major mediators of the destruction of hepatocytes and consequent clinical liver disease. In conjunction with human leukocyte antigen (HLA) class I molecules, the target viral antigens are expressed on the surface of infected hepatocytes. In that location, they are recognized by $CD8^+$ CTLs that in turn kill the infected hepatocytes.

The infectivity of blood from patients with chronic hepatitis B tends to decline with the duration of the disease. This is due in large measure to a decline in episomal (extrachromosomal) replication of infectious virions. Although the intact viral genome is not integrated into the host DNA, genomic fragments are progressively integrated, after which they produce a variety of viral antigens. Thus, despite declining infectivity of the blood, chronic hepatitis tends to persist.

 Pathogenesis: HBV is not directly cytopathic, as reflected in the fact that asymptomatic chronic carriers of the virus maintain a large burden of infec-

 Clinical Features: There are three well-recognized clinical courses associated with HBV infection (Fig. 14-21):

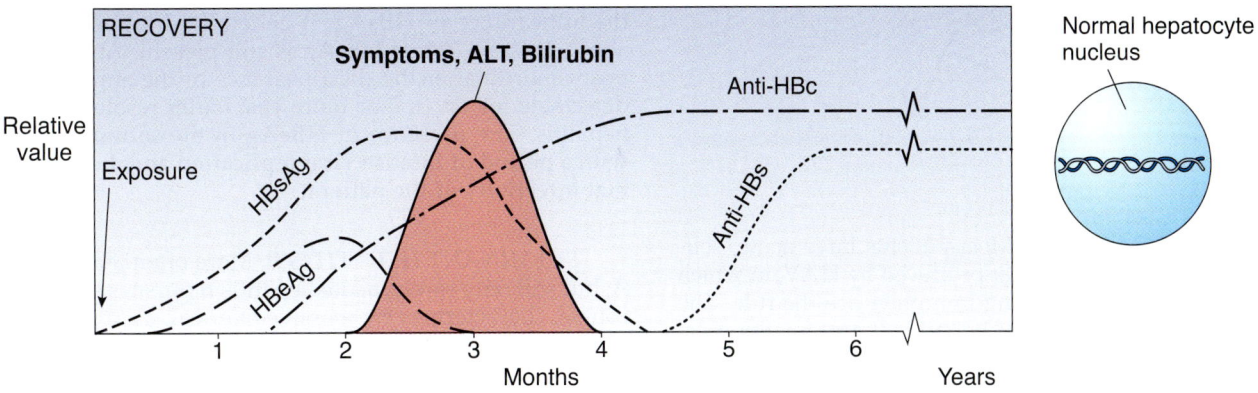
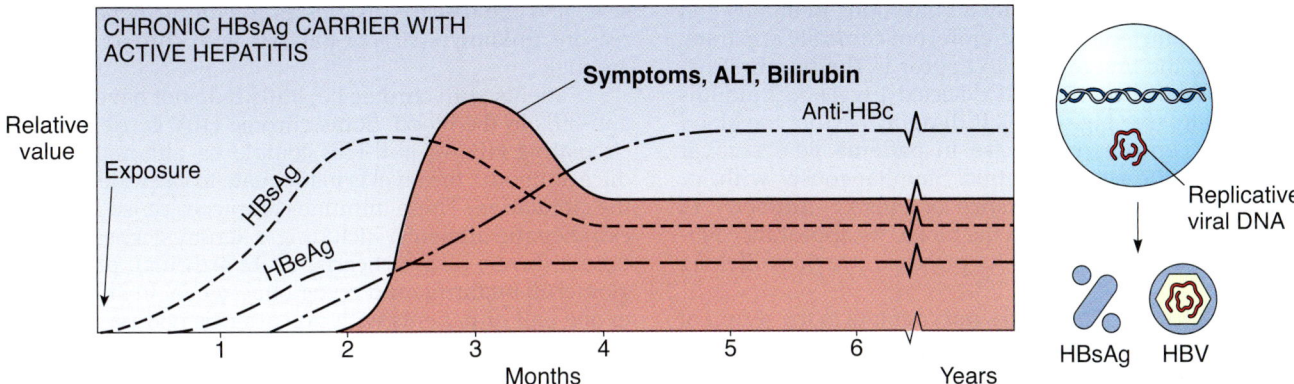
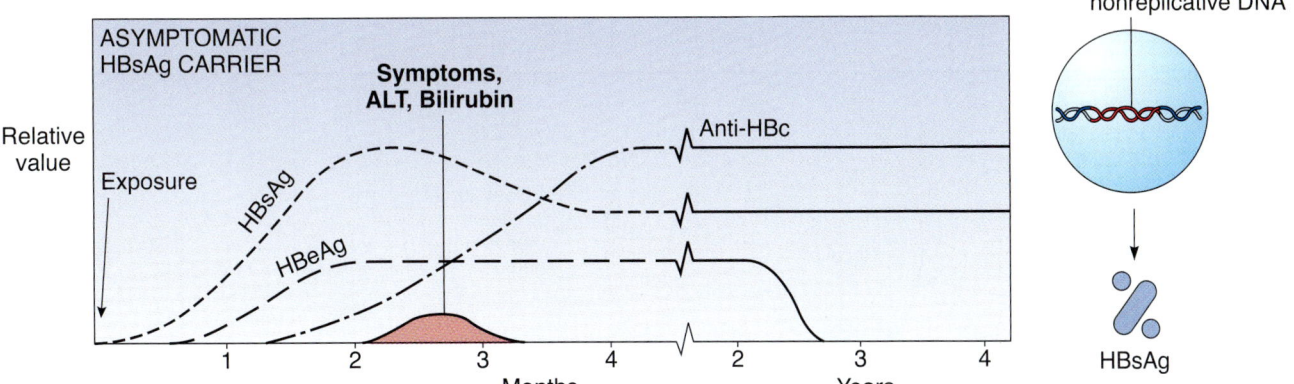

FIGURE 14-21
Typical serological events in three distinct outcomes of hepatitis B. *(Top panel)* In most cases, the appearance of anti-HBs ensures complete recovery. Viral DNA disappears from the nucleus of the hepatocyte. *(Middle panel)* In about 10% of cases of hepatitis B, HBs antigenemia is sustained for longer than 6 months, owing to the absence of anti-HBs. Patients in whom viral replication remains active, as evidenced by sustained high levels of HBeAg in the blood, develop active hepatitis. In such cases, the viral genome persists in the nucleus but is not integrated into host DNA. *(Lower panel)* Patients in whom active viral replication ceases or is attenuated, as reflected in the disappearance of HBeAg from the blood, become asymptomatic carriers. In these individuals, fragments of the HBV genome are integrated into the host DNA, but episomal DNA is absent.

- Acute hepatitis
- Fulminant hepatitis
- Chronic hepatitis

ACUTE HEPATITIS B: Most patients have acute, self-limited hepatitis similar to that produced by HAV, in which complete recovery and lifelong immunity are the rule. The acute onset and symptoms of hepatitis B are, for the most part, also similar to those of hepatitis A, although acute hepatitis B tends to be somewhat more severe. In addition, the incubation period is considerably longer. Typically, symptoms do not appear until 2 to 3 months after exposure, but incubation periods of less than 6 weeks and as long as 6 months are occasionally encountered. As in hepatitis A, many cases, including virtually all infections in infants and children, are anicteric and, therefore, not clinically apparent.

HBsAg, the first marker to appear in the serum of patients with acute hepatitis B, is detected 1 week to 2 months after exposure (see Fig. 14-21). It disappears from the blood during the convalescent phase in patients who recover rapidly from the acute hepatitis. Simultaneously with, or shortly after, the disappearance of HBsAg, antibody to HBsAg (anti-HBs) is found in the blood. Its appearance heralds complete recovery, and its presence provides lifelong immunity.

HBcAg (core antigen) does not circulate in the serum of persons with acute hepatitis B, but antibody to HBcAg (anti-HBc) appears shortly after HBsAg. This antibody does not clear the virus or protect against reinfection, although it is a marker of a previous HBV infection.

HBeAg, the second circulating antigen to appear in hepatitis B, is seen before the onset of clinical disease and after the appearance of HBsAg. It generally disappears within about 2 weeks, while HBsAg is still present. Anti-HBe appears shortly after the disappearance of the antigen and is detectable for up to 2 or more years after resolution of the hepatitis. **The presence of HBeAg in the serum correlates with a period of intense viral replication and, hence, maximal infectivity of the patient.**

FULMINANT HEPATITIS B: More often than hepatitis A, but still only rarely, acute hepatitis B pursues a fulminant course, characterized by massive liver cell necrosis, hepatic failure, and a high mortality.

CHRONIC HEPATITIS B: Chronic hepatitis refers to the presence of necrosis and inflammation in the liver for more than 6 months. In 5 to 10% of patients with hepatitis B, HBs antigenemia does not resolve. Accordingly, the infection persists, and the disease progresses to chronic hepatitis B. For reasons unknown, 90% of patients with chronic hepatitis B are male.

Patients with chronic hepatitis B do not have detectable anti-HBs in the blood. Some chronic HBV carriers manifest circulating HBsAg–anti-HBs complexes; although they produce antibody, the level is inadequate to clear the virus from the circulation. These immune complexes cause a variety of extrahepatic ailments, including a serum sickness-like syndrome (fever, rash, urticaria, acute arthritis), polyarteritis, glomerulonephritis, and cryoglobulinemia. In fact, one third to one half of patients with polyarteritis nodosa are carriers of HBV. Some chronic carriers who were initially negative for anti-HBs eventually develop measurable antibody (often after many years), clear the virus, and are restored to full health. Others (no more than 3% of all patients with hepatitis B) never develop anti-HBs and suffer from relentless and progressive chronic hepatitis that leads to cirrhosis. Hepati-

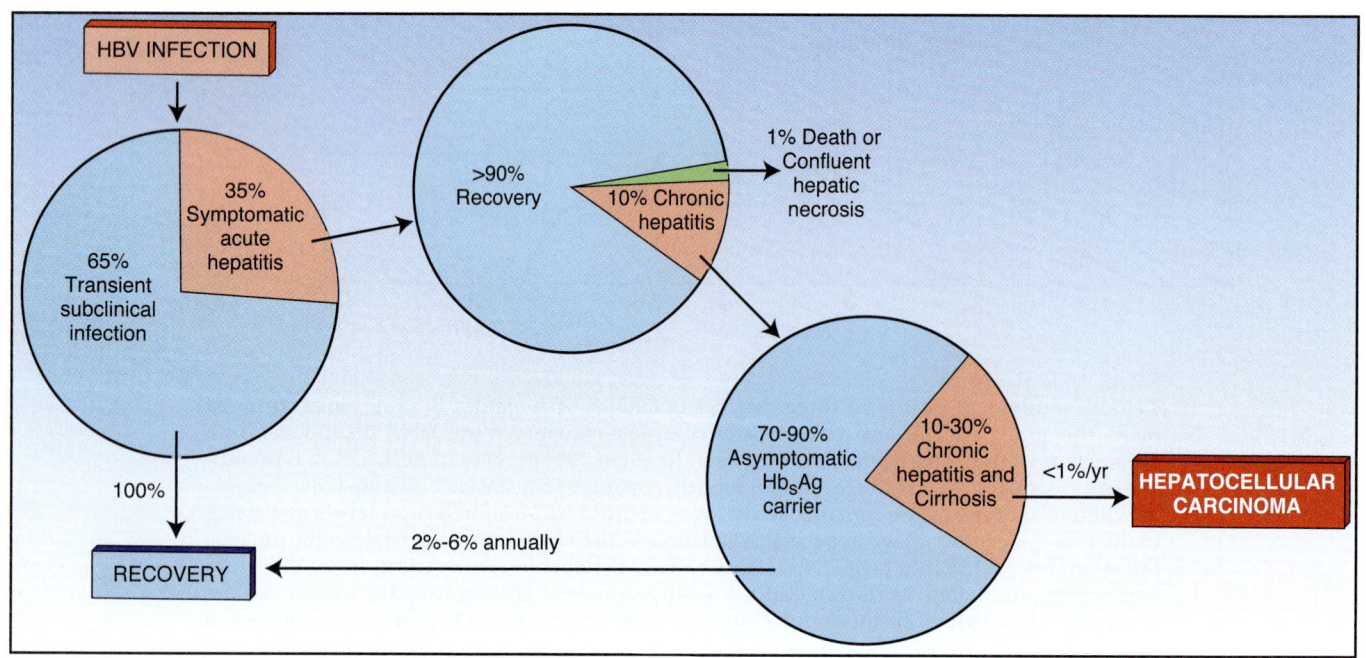

FIGURE 14-22
Possible outcomes of infection with the hepatitis B virus.

tis associated with persistent HBsAg antigenemia is often accompanied by the continued presence of HBeAg.

As is discussed in detail under the heading of hepatocellular carcinoma, chronic hepatitis B is associated with a significant risk of liver cancer. The possible outcomes of infection with HBV are summarized in Figure 14-22.

Hepatitis D Virus Is a Defective RNA Virus

Assembly of hepatitis D virus (HDV) in the liver requires the synthesis of HBsAg, and, therefore, infection with this agent is limited to persons infected with HBV. Infection with HDV may occur either simultaneously with HBV infection (coinfection) or following HBV infection (superinfection). HDV and HBsAg are cleared together, and the clinical course is generally no different from that of the usual acute hepatitis B. However, in some patients, coinfection with HDV leads to severe, fulminant, and often fatal hepatitis, particularly in intravenous drug abusers. **Superinfection of an HBV carrier with HDV typically increases the severity of an existing chronic hepatitis.** In fact, 70 to 80% of HBsAg carriers superinfected with HDV develop chronic hepatitis.

Hepatitis C Virus Is a Common Cause of Chronic Hepatitis and Cirrhosis

Hepatitis C virus (HCV) is classified as a flavivirus and contains a single strand of RNA. The genome consists of a single open reading frame that encodes a polyprotein of about 3000 amino acids. The transcript is cleaved into single proteins, including three structural proteins (one core and two envelope proteins) and four nonstructural proteins. Six different but related HCV genotypes are recognized, types 1, 2, and 3 being the most common (72% in the United States and Western Europe). Genotypes 2 and 3 are more responsive to antiviral therapy than is type 1.

Epidemiology: The prevalence of HCV is variable, ranging from less than 1% in Canada and 1.8% in the United States, to 22% in Egypt. It is estimated that 200 million people are infected worldwide. HCV infection is transmitted by contact with infected blood and is particularly associated with intravenous drug abuse, high-risk sexual behavior (particularly male homosexuals), and alcoholism. The risk from blood transfusions has been almost completely eliminated owing to screening of the blood supply for anti-HCV antibodies. Vertical transmission of HCV from an infected mother to her newborn baby is infrequent (about 5%), although it is more common in the case of HIV-infected women. A minority of cases occur in the absence of known risk factors.

Pathogenesis: HCV is not directly cytopathic, as evidenced by the fact that many chronic carriers of the virus often have no evidence of liver cell injury. Despite active humoral and cellular immune responses directed against all viral proteins, most patients display persistent viremia. Liver cell injury has been attributed to cytotoxic T-cell responses to virally infected hepatocytes.

Clinical Features: The incubation period of hepatitis C is similar to that of hepatitis B. Elevated serum aminotransferase activities (Fig. 14-23) are usually detected within 1 to 3 months of exposure to the virus (range, 2–26 weeks), and in most patients, anti-HCV becomes measurable a few weeks later. The presence of HCV RNA in the serum can be detected by polymerase chain reaction (PCR) within 2 weeks of infection. The clinical course of acute hepatitis C is surprisingly mild and is only very rarely complicated by fulminant hepatitis. In fact, only 10% of patients become jaundiced in the acute phase.

The major consequences of infection with HCV relate to chronic disease (Fig. 14-24). Despite complete recovery from clinical and biochemical acute liver disease, the probability of persistent HCV infection and chronic hepatitis is at least 80% and may be higher. Moreover, chronic hepatitis ensues in 50 to 70% of infected persons. Clinical morbidity in most patients remains mild for at least 10 years, and in many cases for 20 or more years. Importantly, some 20% of patients with chronic hepatitis C eventually develop cirrhosis. **In patients with well-established cirrhosis, up to 5% a year develop primary hepatocellular carcinoma.**

Liver disease in patients with chronic HCV infection tends to be more severe in the face of concurrent hepatitis B, alcoholic liver disease, hemochromatosis, and α_1-antitrypsin deficiency. Interestingly, a quarter of patients with advanced alcoholic liver disease have antibodies to HCV, although the rates vary in different geographical areas. Alcohol consumption has also been shown to worsen the course of chronic hepatitis C. The relationship is unexplained, and the possibility that HCV actually accounts for a proportion of cases otherwise classified as alcoholic cirrhosis is intriguing. Chronic HCV infection is also an important risk factor for the development of hepatocellular carcinoma, a topic discussed below.

Extrahepatic manifestations of hepatitis C are well recognized. Chronic HCV infection has been associated with essential mixed cryoglobulinemia, membranoproliferative glomerulonephritis, porphyria cutanea tarda, and sicca syndrome. A higher incidence of lymphoma has also been described in patients with chronic hepatitis C.

Treatment with α-interferon and antiviral agents has been beneficial in many patients with chronic hepatitis C.

Hepatitis E Virus Is a Major Cause of Epidemics of Hepatitis in Underdeveloped Countries

Hepatitis E virus (HEV) is an enteric RNA virus transmitted by the fecal–oral route. It accounts for more than half of cases of acute viral hepatitis in young to middle-aged persons in poor regions of the world. Large outbreaks have been reported in India, Nepal, Burma, Pakistan, the former Soviet Union, Africa, and Mexico. Most of these epidemics have followed heavy rains in areas with inadequate sewage disposal. Similar to hepatitis A, clinical illness from hepatitis E is far more common in adults than in children, suggesting that in-

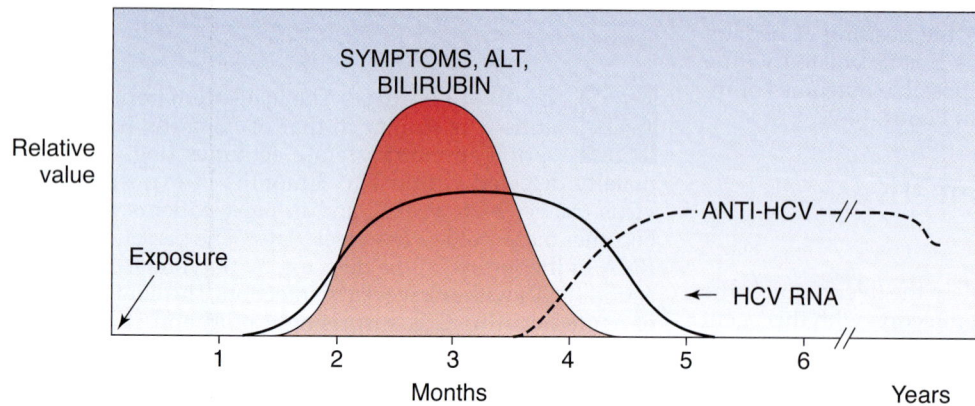

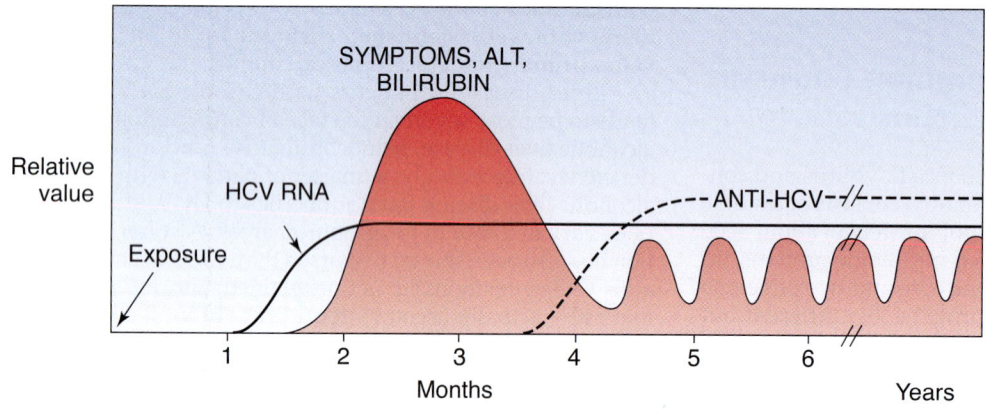

FIGURE 14-23
Clinical course of hepatitis C. Typical serological events in two distinct outcomes. *(Top panel)* About 20% of the patients with acute hepatitis C have a self-limited infection that resolves in a few months. Anti-HCV appears at the end of the clinical course and persists. *(Bottom panel)* The remaining patients with hepatitis C develop chronic illness, with exacerbations and remissions of clinical symptoms. The development of anti-HCV does not affect the clinical outcome. Chronic hepatitis often eventuates in cirrhosis.

fection in the latter is often subclinical. The disease is especially dangerous in pregnant women, with mortality rates as high as 20 to 40% reported. No chronic disease or carrier state has been identified. The close similarity of HEV to a virus in swine suggests that the latter may represent a reservoir of infection.

Hepatitis E is a self-limited, acute, icteric disease similar to hepatitis A. The average incubation period is 35 to 40 days. Jaundice, hepatomegaly, fever, and arthralgias are common and usually resolve within 6 weeks. Mortality rates range from 1 to 12%.

 PATHOLOGY OF VIRAL HEPATITIS

Acute Hepatitis Is Morphologically Similar in All Forms of Viral Hepatitis

The hallmark of acute viral hepatitis is liver cell death (Fig. 14-25). Within the hepatic lobule, scattered necrosis of single cells or of small clusters of hepatocytes is seen. A few apoptotic liver cells appear as small, deeply eosinophilic bodies *(Councilman or acidophilic bodies)*, sometimes containing pyknotic nuclear material, which have been extruded from the liver cell plate into the sinusoid. Although acidophilic bodies are characteristic of viral hepatitis, they are also encountered in other liver diseases. In acute viral hepatitis, many liver cells appear normal, but others show varying degrees of hydropic swelling and differences in size, shape, and staining qualities. Concomitantly, regenerative liver cells that display a larger nucleus and expanded basophilic cytoplasm are also seen. The resulting irregularity of the liver cell plates is termed *lobular disarray*.

Chronic inflammatory cells, principally lymphoid, infiltrate the lobule diffusely, surround individual necrotic liver cells, and accumulate in areas of focal necrosis. In addition to the lymphoid cells, macrophages may be prominent, and eosinophils and polymorphonuclear leukocytes are not uncommon. Characteristically, lymphoid cells infiltrate between the wall of the central vein and the liver cell plates, an appearance termed *central phlebitis*. Swelling and proliferation of the endothelial cells of the central vein *(endophlebitis)* often develop. The Kupffer cells are enlarged, project into the lumen of the sinusoid, and contain lipofuscin pigment and

Confluent Hepatic Necrosis

The term confluent hepatic necrosis *refers to particularly severe variants of acute viral hepatitis, which are characterized by the death of numerous hepatocytes in a geographical distribution and, in extreme cases, by the death of almost all the liver cells (massive hepatic necrosis).* The most common cause is acute hepatitis B, and only rarely does confluent hepatic necrosis result from infection with other hepatotropic viruses. Importantly, the lesions are not confined to viral hepatitis but may also be encountered after exposure to a variety of hepatotoxic agents and in autoimmune hepatitis (see below). In up to half of cases of severe confluent hepatic necrosis, the cause is undetermined. In contrast to the most common forms of acute viral hepatitis, in which the necrosis of hepatocytes appears to be random and patchy, **confluent hepatic necrosis typically affects whole regions of the lobule** (Fig. 14-26). The lesions of confluent hepatic necrosis, in order of increasing severity, are bridging necrosis, submassive necrosis, and massive necrosis.

BRIDGING NECROSIS: At the milder end of the spectrum of lesions that constitute confluent hepatic necrosis are bands of necrosis (bridging necrosis) that stretch between adjacent portal tracts, between adjacent central veins, and between portal tracts and central veins. The death of adjacent plates of hepatocytes results in the collapse of the collagenous stroma to form bands of connective tissue, best visualized with a reticulin stain. When such bands encircle an area of liver cells, a nodular pattern, similar to that seen in cirrhosis, may be apparent.

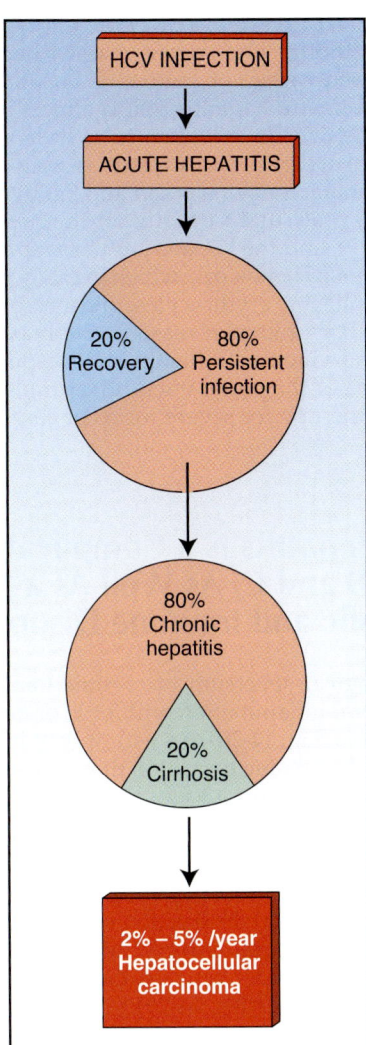

FIGURE 14-24
Possible outcomes of infection with the hepatitis C virus.

phagocytosed debris. Cholestasis is common and when severe is termed *cholestatic hepatitis*. In this situation, many liver cells are arranged around a lumen, thereby presenting an acinar or glandular appearance. The lumen of such an "acinus" may contain a large bile plug.

Chronic inflammatory cells accumulate within the portal tracts and mirror the distribution of those in the lobule. Occasionally, aggregates of lymphoid cells within the portal tracts assume a follicular form, particularly in hepatitis C. The limiting plate of hepatocytes around the portal tracts is usually intact. The portal tracts commonly exhibit only a few proliferated bile ductules, although occasionally this phenomenon may be more conspicuous. All of the pathological changes are gradually reversed during recovery, and the normal hepatic architecture is completely restored.

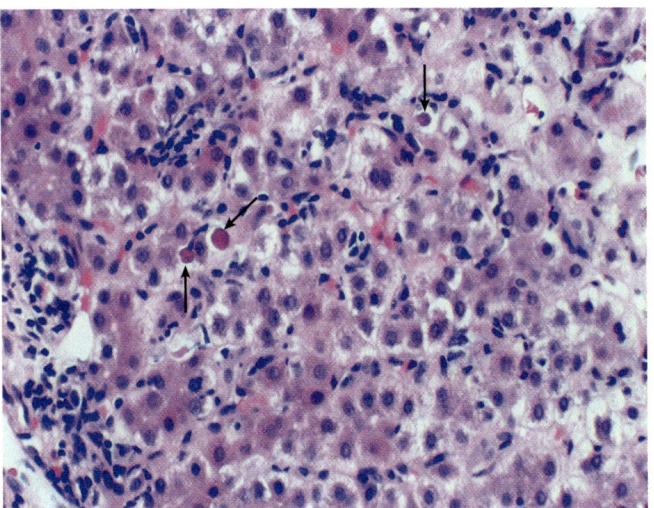

FIGURE 14-25
Acute viral hepatitis. A photomicrograph shows disarray of liver cell plates, swollen (ballooned) hepatocytes, and an infiltrate of lymphocytes and scattered mononuclear inflammatory cells. The remnants of necrotic hepatocytes have been extruded into the sinusoids, where they appear as acidophilic, or Councilman, bodies *(arrows)*.

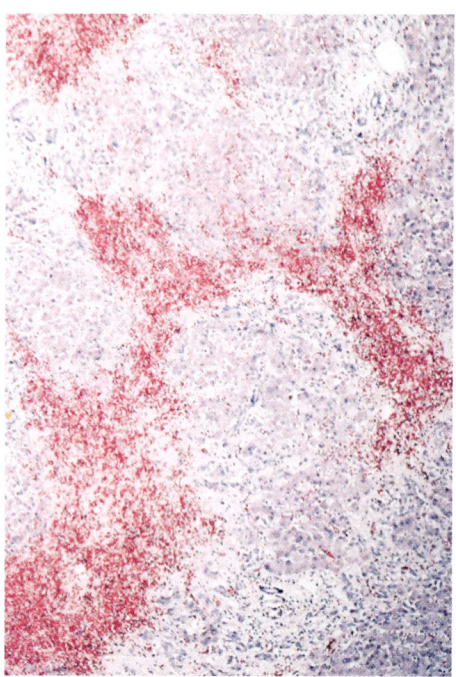

FIGURE 14-26
Confluent hepatic necrosis. Hemorrhagic zones of necrosis bridge adjacent portal tracts (bridging necrosis).

SUBMASSIVE CONFLUENT NECROSIS: This form of acute hepatitis defines an even more severe injury involving necrosis of entire lobules or groups of adjacent lobules. Clinically, these patients manifest severe hepatitis, which may rapidly proceed to hepatic failure, in which case the disease is classed clinically as *fulminant hepatitis.*

MASSIVE HEPATIC NECROSIS (ACUTE YELLOW ATROPHY): Although uncommon, massive hepatic necrosis is the most feared variant of acute viral hepatitis, because it is a form of fulminant hepatitis that is almost invariably fatal. Grossly, the liver is shrunken to as little as 500 g (one third of normal weight). The capsule is wrinkled, and the mottled, red-tan parenchyma is soft and flabby. Microscopic examination reveals that virtually all the hepatocytes are dead (Fig. 14-27), and the hepatic lobule is represented only by the collagenous framework, which in many areas has collapsed. Macrophages, erythrocytes, and necrotic debris fill the sinusoids. For unknown reasons, the massive necrosis does not elicit a vigorous inflammatory response in either the parenchyma or the portal tracts. Liver transplantation is a mainstay of therapy for severe forms of confluent hepatic necrosis.

Chronic Hepatitis Is a Complication of Hepatitis B and C, As Well As a Number of Metabolic and Immune Disorders

The morphological spectrum of chronic hepatitis ranges from mild, portal inflammation with little or no evidence of liver cell necrosis (Fig. 14-28) to a widespread inflammatory, necrotizing, and fibrosing condition that often eventuates in cirrhosis (Figs. 14-29 and 14-30).

PIECEMEAL NECROSIS: This lesion is essentially periportal and refers to focal destruction of the limiting plate of hepatocytes. A periportal chronic inflammatory infiltrate creates an irregular border between the portal tracts and the lobular parenchyma (see Fig. 14-29).

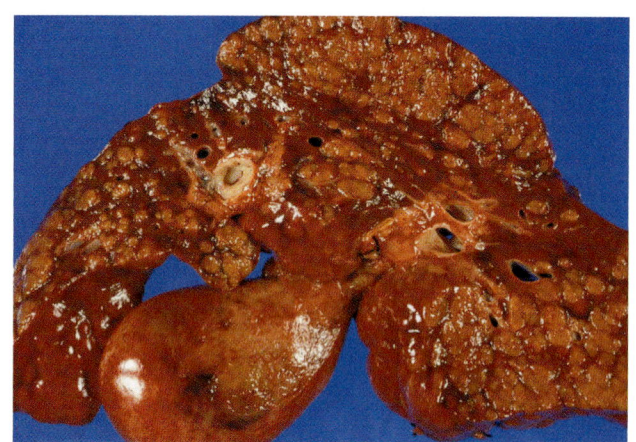
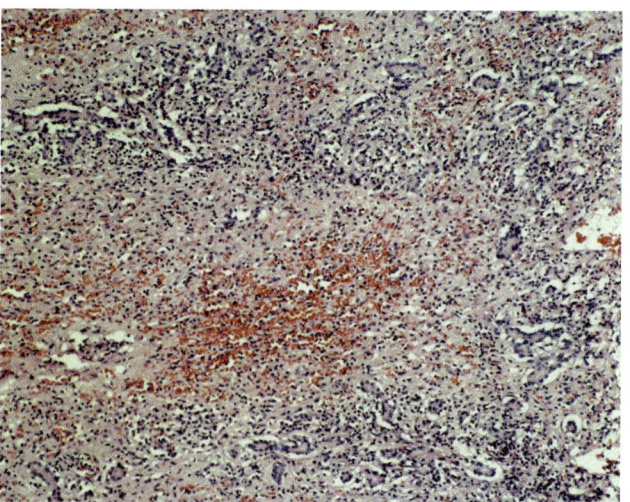

FIGURE 14-27
Massive hepatic necrosis. A. The liver is soft and reduced in size (note size of gallbladder) and shows a mottled, irregularly hemorrhagic cut surface. The surviving parenchyma appears as tan nodules. B. A photomicrograph shows the loss of most of the hepatocytes. Necrotic lobules are hemorrhagic, and the reticulin framework has collapsed. A sparse chronic inflammatory infiltrate is present within the lobules and portal tracts. The portal tracts are expanded and contain proliferated bile ducts.

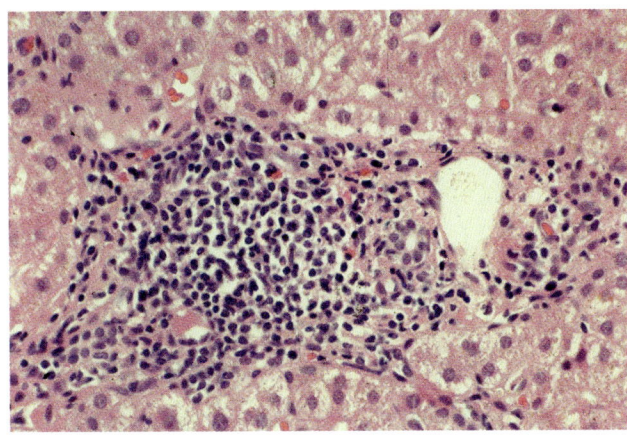

FIGURE 14-28
Mild chronic hepatitis. A photomicrograph shows a portal tract infiltrated by mononuclear inflammatory cells. The lobular parenchyma is intact.

PORTAL TRACT LESIONS: Chronic hepatitis is characterized by variable infiltration of the portal tracts by lymphocytes, plasma cells, and macrophages. The expanded portal tracts often display mild-to-severe proliferation of bile ductules, which represents a nonspecific response to chronic liver injury. In the case of chronic hepatitis C, lymphoid aggregates or follicles with reactive centers are often present (Fig. 14-31).

INTRALOBULAR LESIONS: Focal necrosis and inflammation within the parenchyma are typical of chronic hepatitis. Scattered acidophilic bodies are common, and enlarged Kupffer cells are seen within the sinusoids. The liver in chronic hepatitis B often exhibits scattered hepatocytes with a large granular cytoplasm containing abundant HBsAg *(ground-glass hepatocytes)* (Fig. 14-32).

PERIPORTAL FIBROSIS: The progressive erosion of the periportal hepatocytes by piecemeal necrosis leads to the deposition of collagen, which gives the portal tract a stellate (star-shaped) appearance. With time, the fibrosis may extend to adjacent portal tracts or into the lobule itself toward the central vein, ultimately developing into cirrhosis.

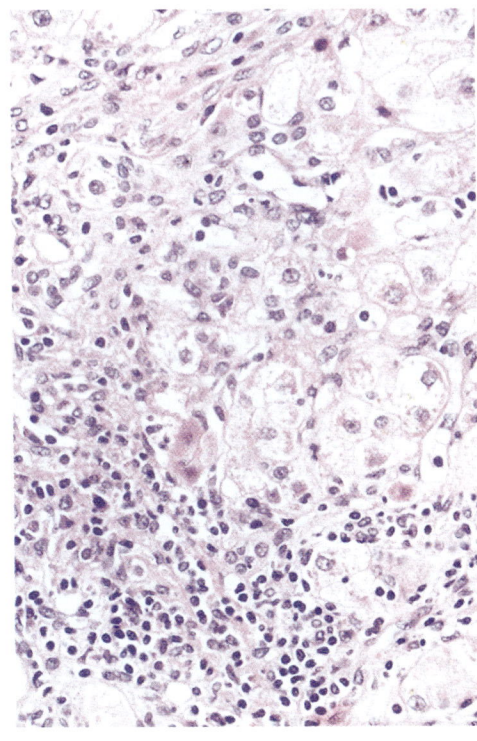

FIGURE 14-29
Severe chronic hepatitis. A photomicrograph discloses a mononuclear inflammatory infiltrate in an expanded portal tract. The inflammation penetrates the limiting plate and surrounds groups of hepatocytes at the border of the portal tract.

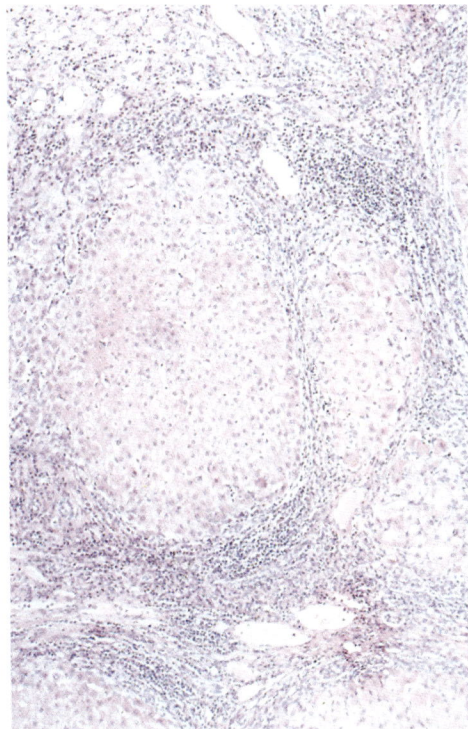

FIGURE 14-30
Chronic hepatitis with cirrhosis. A photomicrograph of the liver from a patient with long-standing chronic hepatitis B shows hepatocellular nodules and chronically inflamed fibrous septa.

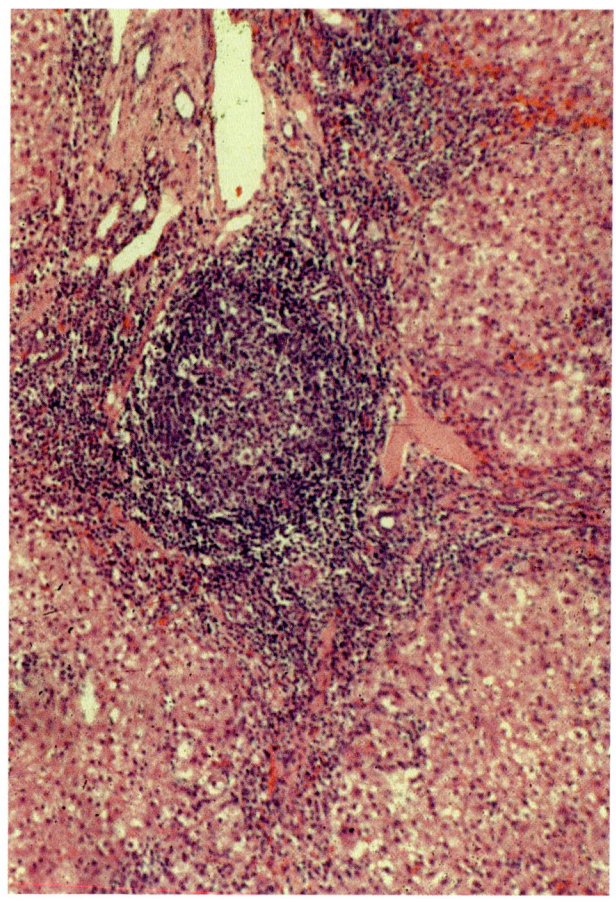

FIGURE 14-31
Chronic hepatitis C. A photomicrograph of the liver from a patient with long-standing hepatitis C exhibits an expanded portal tract containing a nodular aggregate of lymphoid cells.

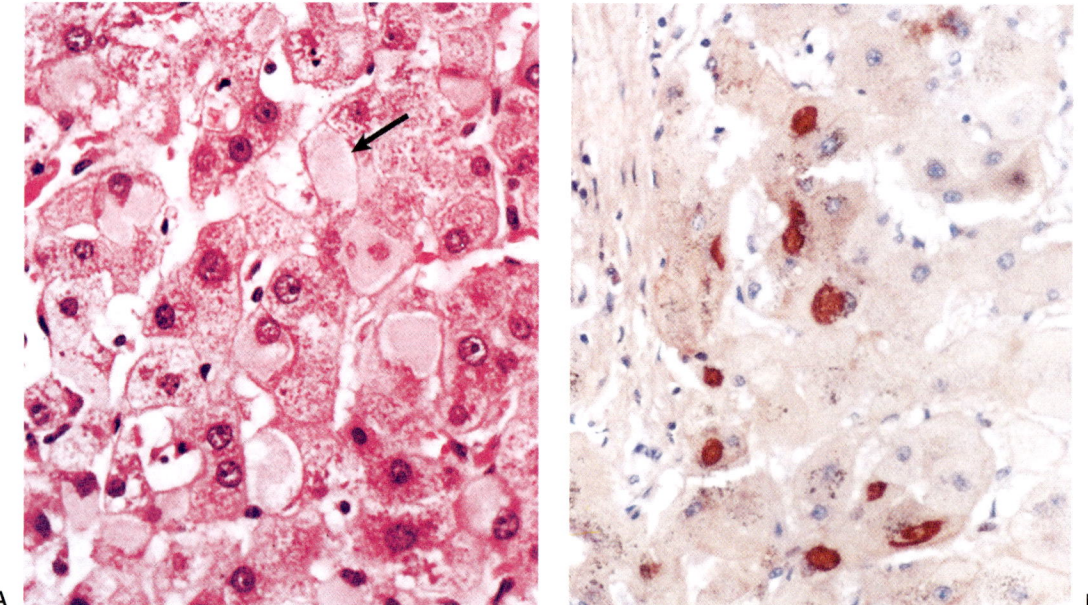

FIGURE 14-32
"Ground-glass" hepatocytes. A. A photomicrograph of liver from a patient with chronic hepatitis B shows scattered hepatocytes (arrow) with an abundant granular cytoplasm containing HBsAg. B. The same specimen has been stained for HBsAg by the immunoperoxidase method. The abundant cytoplasmic HBsAg appears brown.

TABLE 14-3 Comparative Features of the Common Forms of Viral Hepatitis

	Hepatitis A	Hepatitis B	Hepatitis C
Genome	RNA	DNA	RNA
Incubation period	3–6 weeks	6 weeks–6 months	7–8 weeks
Transmission	Oral	Parenteral	Parenteral
Blood	No	Yes	Yes
Feces	Yes	No	No
Vertical	No	Yes	5%
Fulminant hepatic necrosis	Very rare	Yes	Rare
Chronic hepatitis	No	10%	80%
Carrier state	No	Yes	Yes
Liver cancer	No	Yes	Yes

Table 14-3 compares the major features of the common forms of viral hepatitis.

AUTOIMMUNE HEPATITIS

Autoimmune hepatitis is a severe type of chronic hepatitis of unknown cause that is associated with circulating autoantibodies and high levels of serum immunoglobulins. The disorder occurs predominantly among young women, but up to one third of patients are men, and the disease may appear at any age. In the United States, autoimmune hepatitis affects some 200,000 persons and accounts for 6% of liver transplants.

Pathogenesis: Two distinct types of autoimmune hepatitis have been identified.

Type I autoimmune hepatitis is the most common form of the disease and features antinuclear and antismooth muscle antibodies. Some 70% of cases are women younger than 40 years of age, among whom a third have other autoimmune diseases, including thyroiditis and ulcerative colitis. Importantly, a quarter of patients with type I autoimmune hepatitis present with cirrhosis, indicating that the disease usually has a prolonged asymptomatic course. Antibodies against numerous cytosolic enzymes have been described, but the asialoglycoprotein receptor on the hepatocyte surface is the most likely target for antibody-dependent cell-mediated cytotoxicity. Susceptibility to type I autoimmune hepatitis resides within the *DRB1* gene.

Type II autoimmune hepatitis occurs principally in children aged 2 to 14 years and is recognized by the presence of antibody to liver and kidney microsomes (anti-LKM). However, the target autoantigen is a P450-type drug-metabolizing enzyme (CYP 2D6). These patients often suffer from other autoimmune diseases, especially type I diabetes and thyroiditis. The genetic background for this type of autoimmune hepatitis remains obscure.

Pathology: In general, the histological appearance of autoimmune hepatitis resembles that of chronic viral hepatitis.

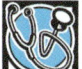

Clinical Features: In most patients, the disease begins insidiously. Eventually, serum aminotransferase levels become conspicuously elevated, and liver failure may ensue. In many patients, autoimmune hepatitis progresses to cirrhosis. Pronounced hyperglobulinemia is characteristic of the disease.

In contrast to viral hepatitis, autoimmune hepatitis often responds to therapy with corticosteroids, particularly when combined with immunosuppressive drugs. Liver transplantation is an option for patients whose disease progresses to end-stage cirrhosis.

ALCOHOLIC LIVER DISEASE

The deleterious effects of excess alcohol (ethanol, ethyl alcohol) consumption have been recognized since the early days of recorded history. The prophet Isaiah warned, "Woe to him that is mighty to drink wine." Although early investigators confused alcoholic liver injury with the effects of malnutrition, ethanol per se is today recognized as a hepatotoxin that acts both directly and indirectly.

Epidemiology: The prevalence of cirrhosis is highest in those countries with the highest per capita consumption of alcohol. This relationship is valid regardless of the specific nature of the preferred beverage (e.g., wine in France, beer in Australia, and spirits in Scandinavia). Although only a minority of chronic alcoholics develop cirrhosis, a dose–response relationship between the lifetime dose of alcohol (duration of exposure and the daily amount of alcohol consumed) and the appearance of cirrhosis has been established (Fig. 14-33).

It is estimated that some 10% of the adult male population in the United States abuse alcohol, and this figure is considerably higher in many other countries. **About 15% of alcoholics can be expected to develop cirrhosis, and many of these persons die in hepatic failure or from the extrahepatic complications of cirrhosis.** In fact, in many urban areas of the United States with high alcoholism rates, cirrhosis of the liver is the third or fourth leading cause of death in men younger than 45 years of age.

The amount of alcohol required to produce chronic liver disease varies widely, depending on body size, age, sex, and race, but the lower range seems to be about 80 g/day (8 ounces [240 mL] of 86 proof [43%] whiskey, two bottles of wine, or six 12-ounce bottles of beer). In general, more than 10 years of alcoholism are required to produce cirrhosis, although a few cirrhotic patients give shorter histories of heavy alcohol use.

The epidemiology of alcoholic liver disease has recently been complicated by the discovery of its association with hepatotropic viruses. The prevalence of serum HBV markers is two- to fourfold higher in alcoholics than in corresponding

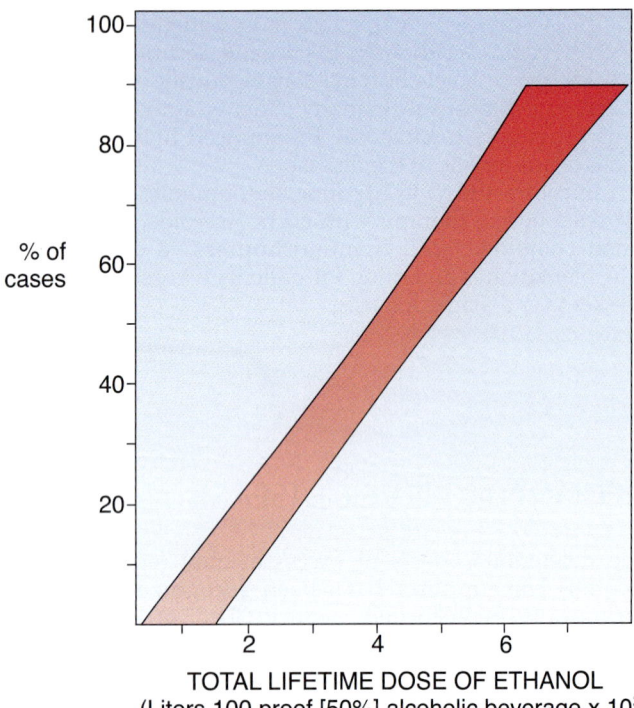

FIGURE 14-33
Dose–response relationship between the amount of alcohol consumed in a lifetime and the incidence of cirrhosis. Only a minority of all alcoholics develop cirrhosis, but those who drink very large amounts are at high risk of developing the disease.

A Spectrum of Liver Diseases Is Produced by Alcohol Consumption

Alcoholic liver disease spans three major morphological and clinical entities: **fatty liver, acute alcoholic hepatitis,** and **cirrhosis**. Although these lesions usually occur sequentially, they may coexist in any combination and may actually be independent entities.

Fatty Liver and Associated Lesions

 Pathogenesis: Virtually all chronic alcoholics accumulate fat in hepatocytes (steatosis). The pathogenesis of fatty liver is not precisely understood, and the relative contributions of different pathways may vary, depending on the amount of alcohol consumed, dietary lipid content, body stores of fat, hormonal status, and other variables. Nevertheless, the accumulation of fat clearly depends on the intake of ethanol, since it is fully and rapidly reversible on discontinuation of alcohol ingestion.

Dietary fat, in the form of chylomicrons and free fatty acids, is transported to the liver, where it is taken up by the hepatocytes. Triglycerides are then hydrolyzed to free fatty acids. These, in turn, undergo β-oxidation in the mitochondria or are converted to triglycerides in the endoplasmic reticulum. The newly synthesized triglycerides are secreted in the form of lipoproteins or are retained for storage.

Most of the fat deposited in the liver after chronic alcohol consumption is derived from the diet. Ethanol increases lipolysis and thus the delivery of free fatty acids to the liver. Within the hepatocyte, ethanol (1) increases fatty acid synthesis, (2) decreases mitochondrial oxidation of fatty acids, (3) increases the production of triglycerides, and (4) impairs the release of lipoproteins (Fig. 14-35). Collectively, these metabolic consequences produce a fatty liver.

control populations. The prevalence of anti-HCV antibodies is up to 10% among alcoholics and is considerably higher among alcoholics with chronic liver disease. The significance of these data with respect to the epidemiology of alcoholic cirrhosis deserves further study.

The Metabolism of Ethanol Occurs Primarily in the Liver

Ethanol is rapidly absorbed from the stomach and is eventually distributed in body water space. Almost all of the ethanol consumed is metabolized by the liver to acetaldehyde and acetate. Between 5 and 10% is excreted unchanged, principally in the urine and expired breath. The principal route of ethanol oxidation in the liver is through cytosolic alcohol dehydrogenase (ADH) (Fig. 14-34). A minor metabolic pathway is a microsomal ethanol-oxidizing system in the smooth endoplasmic reticulum, which is a mixed-function oxidase. In contrast to most drugs, the clearance of alcohol from the body is linear—that is, a fixed quantity is metabolized per unit time. A rough guide for the average man is 7 to 10 g of alcohol eliminated per hour. However, chronic alcoholics metabolize ethanol at a substantially higher rate, provided that they do not suffer from active liver disease.

 Pathology: In the alcoholic, the liver becomes yellow and enlarged, sometimes massively, to as much as three times the normal weight. The increased weight does not reflect fat accumulation alone, since protein and water content also increase. Microscopically, the extent of visible fat accumulation varies from minute droplets scattered in the cytoplasm of a few hepatocytes to distention of the entire cytoplasm of most cells by coalesced droplets (Fig. 14-36). In the latter situation, the liver cell is scarcely recognizable as such and bears a resemblance to an adipocyte, the cytoplasm being represented by a distended clear area, and the nucleus flattened and displaced to the periphery of the cell.

The ultrastructural appearance of the hepatocyte in alcohol-induced fatty liver reflects the cytotoxicity of ethanol rather than an effect of the fat per se. The mitochondria are enlarged, with occasional bizarre giant forms. The smooth endoplasmic reticulum exhibits hyperplasia resembling that produced by other inducers of microsomal drug-metabolizing enzymes. Initially, the fat accumulates as globules, which eventually merge to form large cytoplasmic bodies of variable electron density.

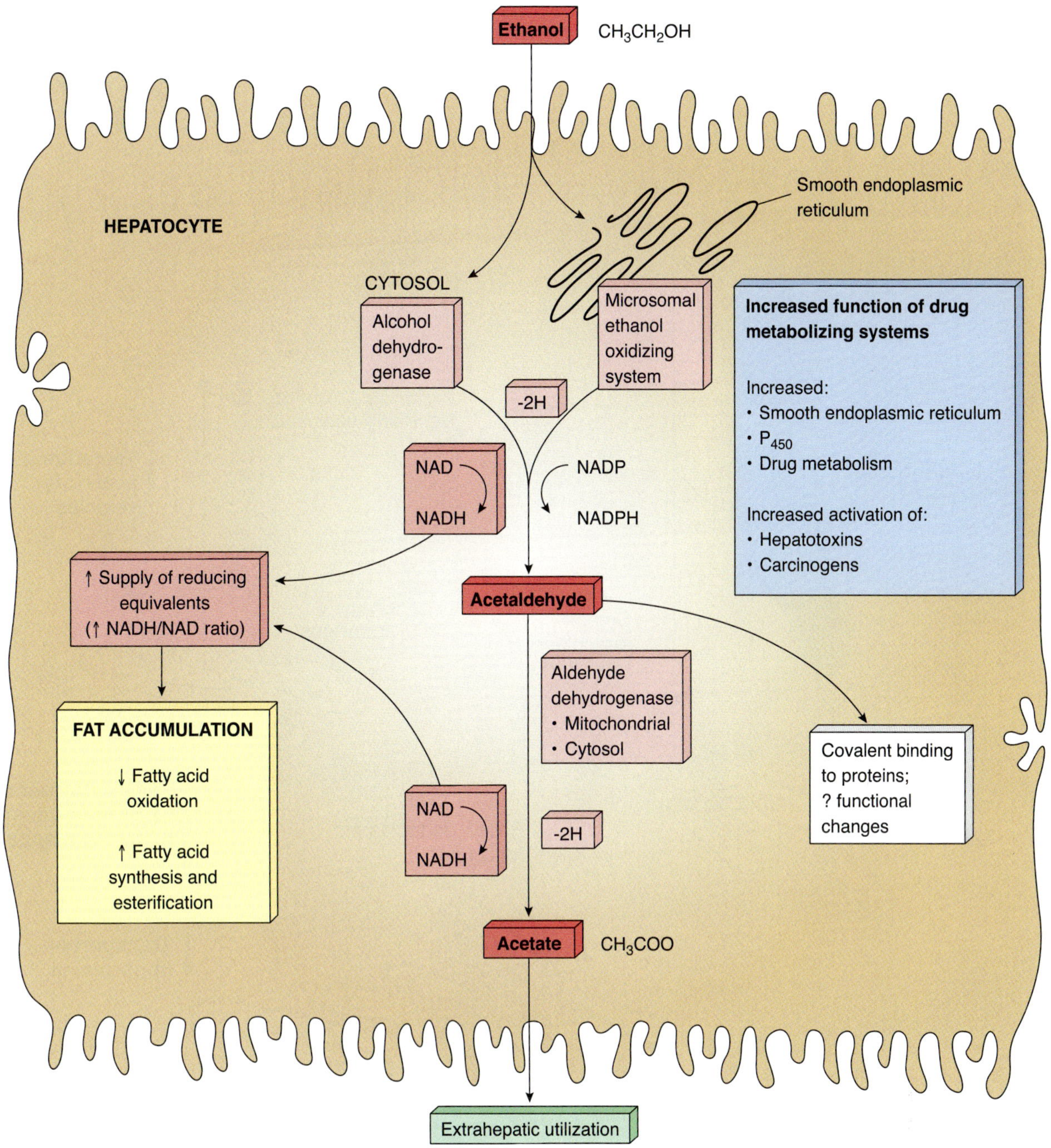

Alcoholic Liver Disease

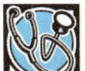

FIGURE 14-34
The metabolism of ethanol and its hepatocellular effects.

The ultrastructural changes in mitochondria and endoplasmic reticulum produced by chronic ethanol ingestion are paralleled by functional alterations. Hepatic mitochondria show decreased rates of substrate oxidation (e.g., of fatty acids) and impaired formation of ATP. Hyperplasia of the smooth endoplasmic reticulum is accompanied by an increase in the activity of the cytochrome P450-dependent mixed-function oxidases. Not only is the microsomal ethanol-oxidizing system induced, but the metabolism of a wide variety of drugs is also enhanced. The increased microsomal function also augments the metabolism of hepatic toxins, thereby exaggerating the danger produced by agents such as carbon tetrachloride and acetaminophen. In contrast to chronic alcohol consumption, which promotes microsomal functions, the presence of ethanol after acute alcohol ingestion inhibits the activity of mixed-function oxidases and acutely reduces the rate of clearance of drugs from the body.

Clinical Features: Patients with uncomplicated alcoholic fatty liver have surprisingly few symptoms of liver disease. Despite the striking morphological change in the liver, alcoholic fatty liver is a fully reversible lesion and does not by itself progress to more severe disease, notably cirrhosis. A fatty liver, although characteristic of alcoholism, is not restricted to that condition but

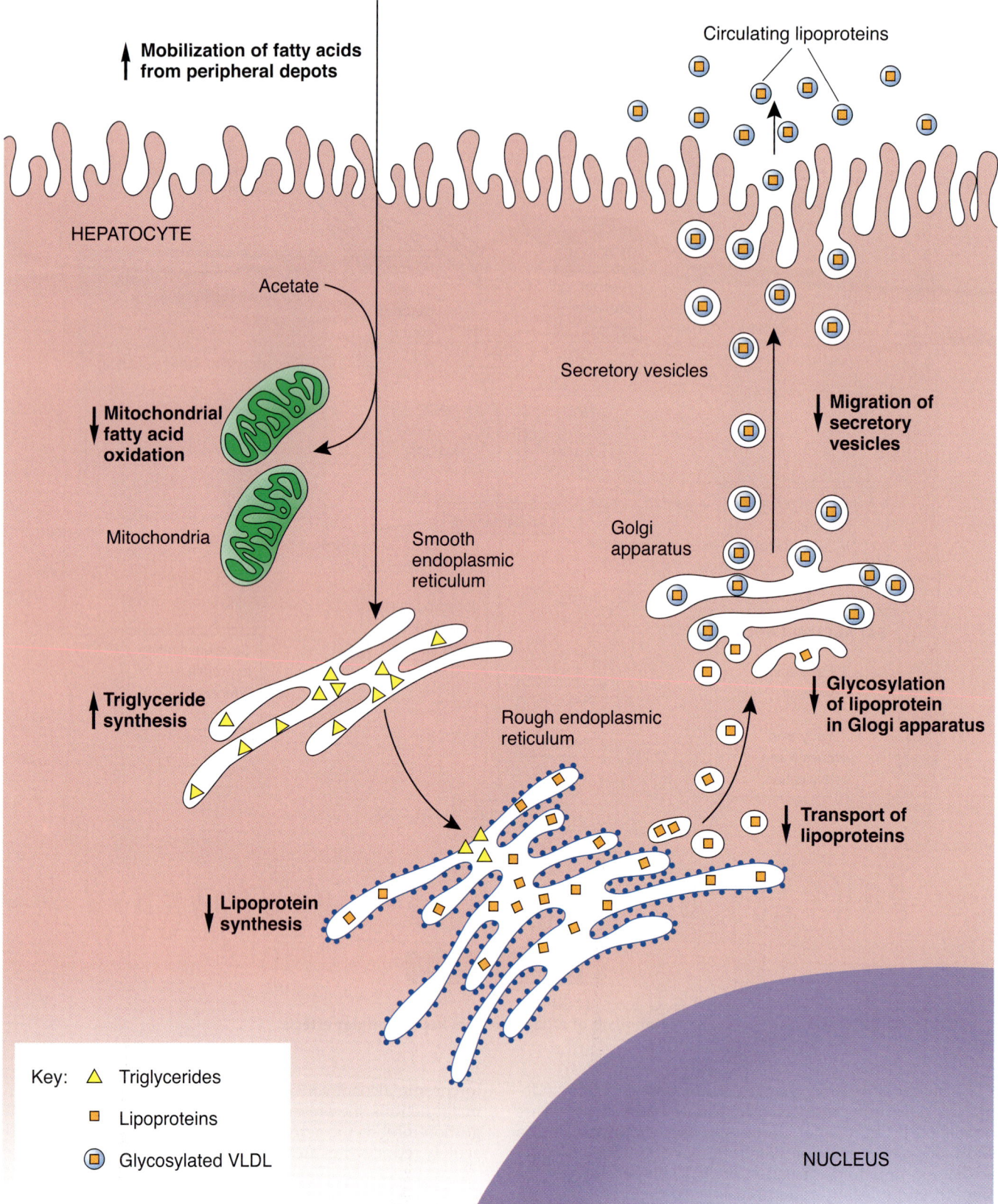

FIGURE 14-35
Pathogenesis of alcoholic fatty liver.

Alcoholic Liver Disease

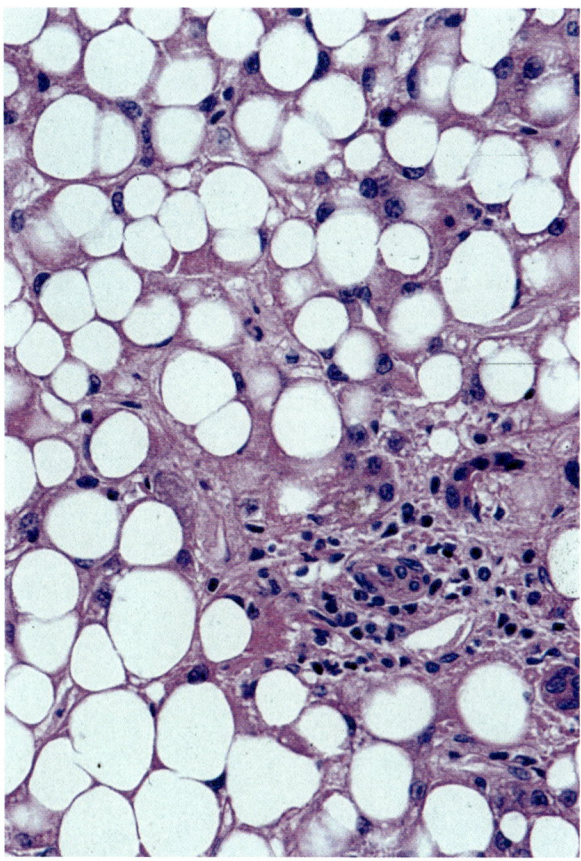

FIGURE 14-36
Alcoholic fatty liver. A photomicrograph shows the cytoplasm of almost all the hepatocytes distended by fat that displaces the nucleus to the periphery.

is also noted in nonalcoholic fatty liver disease (see below), in kwashiorkor, and following prolonged administration of corticosteroids.

Alcoholic Hepatitis

Alcoholic hepatitis is an acute necrotizing lesion characterized by (1) necrosis of hepatocytes, predominantly in the central zone; (2) cytoplasmic hyaline inclusions within hepatocytes; (3) a neutrophilic inflammatory response, and (4) perivenular fibrosis (Fig. 14-37). The pathogenesis of alcoholic hepatitis is mysterious. Alcoholics may have mild fatty liver for many years and, without any change in drinking habits, suddenly develop acute alcoholic hepatitis.

 Pathology: In the typical case of acute alcoholic hepatitis, the hepatic architecture is basically intact, with a normal relation of portal tracts to central venules. The hepatocytes show variable hydropic swelling, which gives them a heterogeneous appearance. Isolated necrotic liver cells or clusters of them exhibit pyknotic nuclei and karyorrhexis. Scattered hepatocytes contain Mallory bodies (alcoholic hyalin) (see Fig. 14-37). These cytoplasmic inclusions, which are more common in visibly damaged, swollen hepatocytes, are visualized as irregular skeins of eosinophilic material or as solid eosinophilic masses, often in a perinuclear location. Ultrastructurally, they are composed of aggregates of intermediate (cytokeratin) filaments (Fig. 14-38). The damaged, ballooned hepatocytes, particularly those containing Mallory bodies, are surrounded by neutrophils, although a more diffuse, intralobular inflammatory infiltrate is also present. Cholestasis, varying from mild to severe, is present in as many as one third of cases. Alcoholic hepatitis is usually superimposed on an existing fatty liver, although there is no evidence that fat accumulation predisposes or contributes to the development of alcoholic hepatitis.

Collagen deposition is a constant feature of alcoholic hepatitis, especially around the central vein (terminal hepatic venule). In severe cases, the venule and perivenular sinusoids are obliterated and surrounded by dense fibrous tissue, in which case the lesion has been termed *central hyaline sclerosis* (Fig. 14-39).

The appearance of the portal tracts in alcoholic hepatitis is highly variable. In some instances, they are virtually normal, whereas in others they are enlarged and contain a mononuclear infiltrate and proliferated bile ductules. The altered portal tracts often display spurs of fibrous tissue that penetrate the lobules.

 Clinical Features: Alcoholic hepatitis features malaise and anorexia, fever, right upper quadrant abdominal pain, and jaundice. A mild leukocytosis is common. The serum aminotransferase activities, particularly that of aspartate aminotransferase, are moderately elevated, but not to the levels often noted in viral hepatitis. Serum alkaline phosphatase activity is usually increased. In severe cases, the prothrombin time may be prolonged, a situation associated with an ominous prognosis.

The prognosis in patients with alcoholic hepatitis correlates with the severity of the liver cell injury. In some patients, the disease rapidly progresses to hepatic failure and death. The mortality in the acute stage of alcoholic hepatitis is about 10%. Among those who abstain from alcohol after recovery from acute alcoholic hepatitis, most recover. However, of those who continue to drink, up to 70% may ultimately develop cirrhosis. No specific treatment for acute alcoholic hepatitis is available, although corticosteroids and dietary supplementation may improve short-term survival.

Alcoholic Cirrhosis

In about 15% of alcoholics, hepatocellular necrosis, fibrosis, and regeneration eventually lead to the formation of fibrous septa surrounding hepatocellular nodules, the two features that define cirrhosis (Fig. 14-40). The other lesions of alcoholic liver disease—namely, fatty liver and acute or persistent alcoholic hepatitis—are often seen in conjunction with cirrhosis. The prognosis in cases of established alcoholic cir-

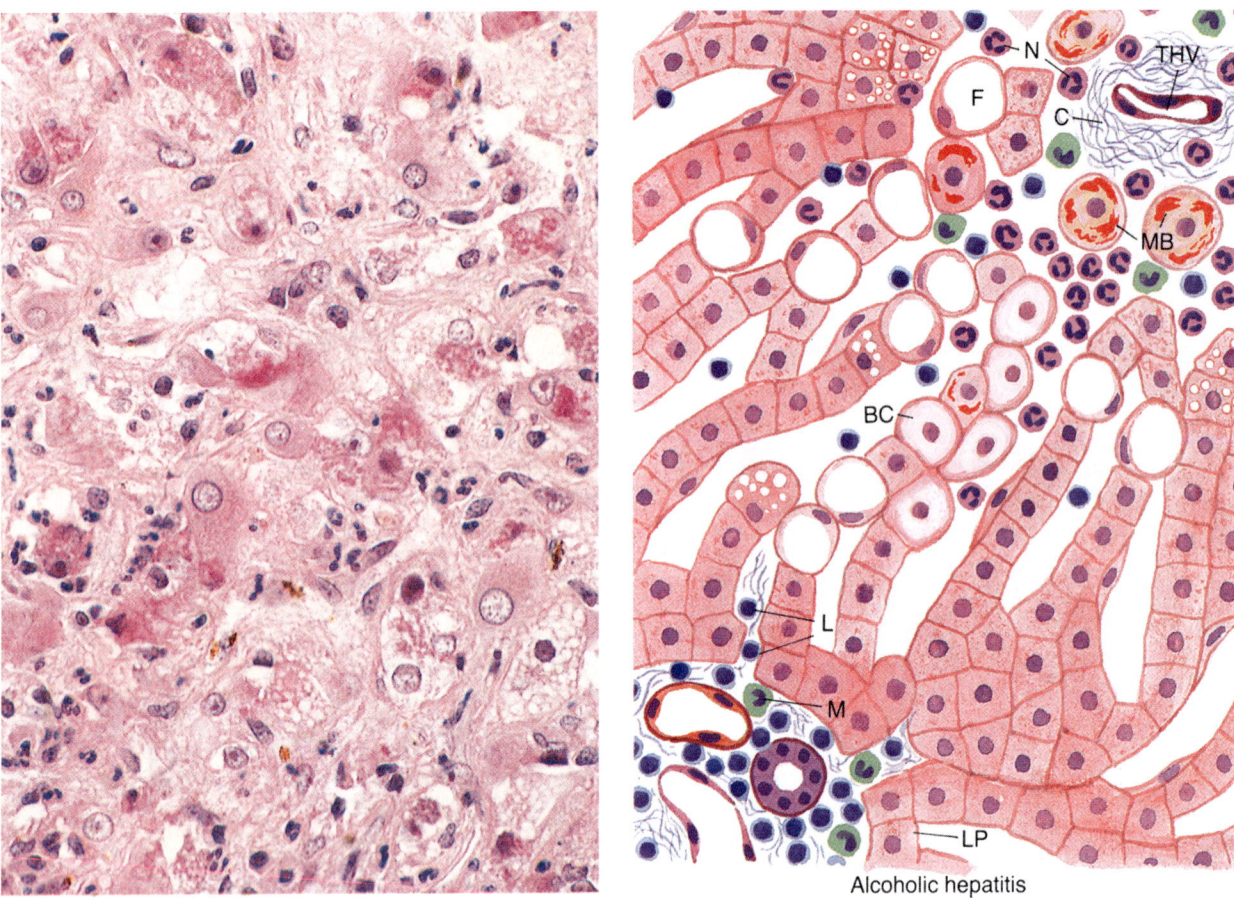

FIGURE 14-37

Alcoholic hepatitis. A. A photomicrograph shows necrosis and degeneration of hepatocytes; Mallory bodies (eosinophilic inclusions) in the cytoplasm of injured hepatocytes; and infiltration by neutrophils. **B.** Schematic representation of the major pathological features of alcoholic hepatitis. The lesions are predominantly centrilobular and include necrosis and loss of hepatocytes, ballooned cells *(BC)*, and Mallory bodies *(MB)* in the cytoplasm of damaged hepatocytes. The inflammatory infiltrate consists predominantly of neutrophils *(N)*, although a few lymphocytes *(L)* and macrophages *(M)* are also present. The central vein, or terminal hepatic venule *(THV)*, is encased in connective tissue *(C)* (central sclerosis). Fat-laden hepatocytes *(F)* are evident in the lobule. The portal tract displays moderate chronic inflammation, and the limiting plate *(LP)* is focally breached.

rhosis is considerably better in those who abstain from alcohol abuse. Nevertheless, many patients progress to end-stage liver disease, and alcoholic liver disease is a common indication for liver transplantation.

NONALCOHOLIC FATTY LIVER DISEASE

Nonalcoholic fatty liver disease (NAFLD) is so named because of its close resemblance to alcoholic liver disease. It represents a spectrum of liver injuries that initially display simple steatosis, with or without associated hepatitis (nonalcoholic steatohepatitis [NASH]), and progress to bridging fibrosis and cirrhosis. Risk factors for NAFLD include obesity, type 2 diabetes mellitus, and hyperlipidemia. Given the high prevalence of these conditions, NAFLD may affect as many as 25% of the general population worldwide, and 75% of conspicuously obese persons. Importantly, half of persons with both severe obesity and diabetes have NASH, and as many as a fifth of this population seems to develop cirrhosis.

Histologic features of NAFLD include steatosis, lobular and portal inflammation, hepatocyte necrosis, Mallory's hyaline, and fibrosis. As in alcoholic liver disease, centrilobular fibrosis is commonly observed. With the development of cirrhosis, steatosis often disappears. Thus, NAFLD is the likely cause of many cases of so-called cryptogenic cirrhosis. The pathogenesis of NAFLD is obscure, although insulin resistance, increased hepatic mitochondrial oxidation of free fatty acids, increased oxidative stress, and lipid peroxidation have been proposed as etiologic factors.

Progression to cirrhosis in NAFLD is often insidious, and many patients remain asymptomatic, with only moderate increases in serum liver enzymes. Weight loss tends to improve NAFLD, but no drug therapy is effective.

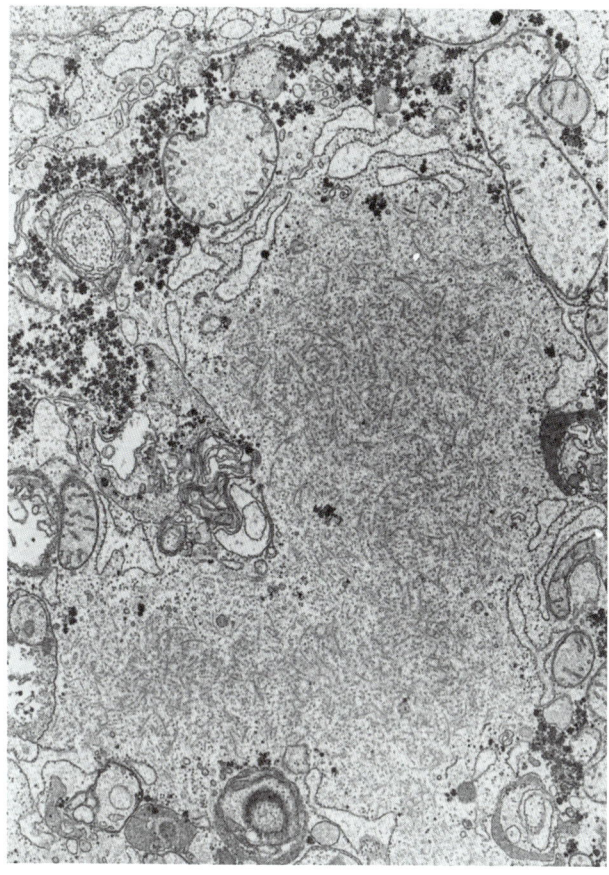

FIGURE 14-38
Mallory body. An electron micrograph shows an aggregate of filamentous material in the cytoplasm of a hepatocyte. The mass displaces the cytoplasmic organelles peripherally.

FIGURE 14-39
Central hyaline sclerosis. This photomicrograph (trichrome stain) from the liver of a patient with alcoholic liver disease shows the central terminal venule to be obliterated by fibrous tissue (blue).

PRIMARY BILIARY CIRRHOSIS

Primary biliary cirrhosis (PBC) is a chronic progressive cholestatic liver disease characterized by destruction of the intrahepatic bile ducts (nonsuppurative destructive cholangitis). PBC occurs principally in middle-aged women (10:1 female predominance). The use of the term *cirrhosis* in this context is somewhat misleading, in that cirrhosis is actually a late complication of the disease.

PBC accounts for up to 2% of deaths from cirrhosis. Cases are sporadic, although several familial clusters of the disease have been reported. The prevalence in families of patients with PBC is considerably higher than that in the general population, suggesting a hereditary predisposition.

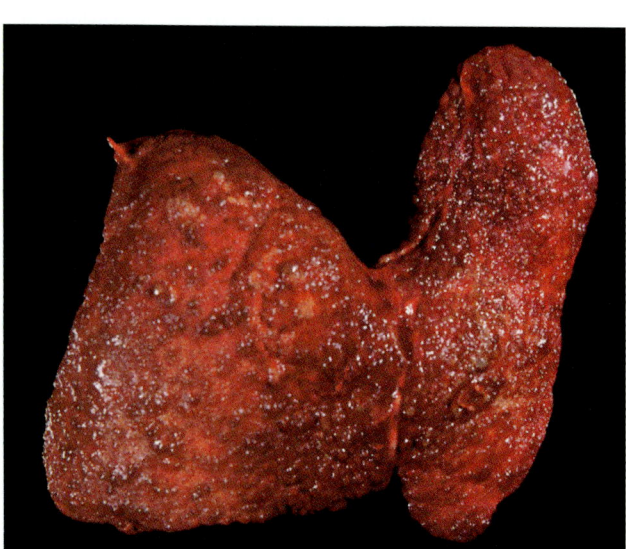
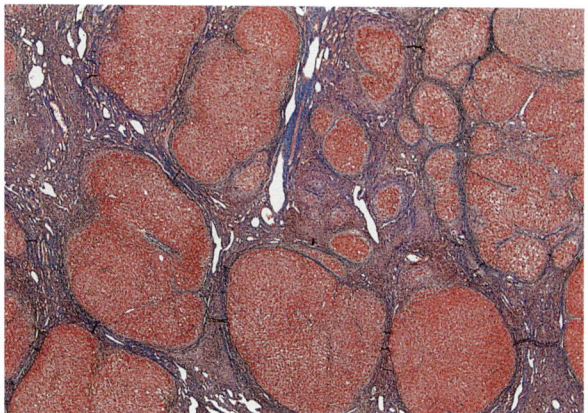

FIGURE 14-40
Alcoholic cirrhosis. A. The surface of the liver displays innumerable small, regular nodules.
B. A photomicrograph shows small regular nodules surrounded by uniform fibrous septa.

Pathogenesis: **PBC is associated with many immunological abnormalities and is, therefore, widely held to be an autoimmune disease.** Most (85%) patients with primary biliary cirrhosis have at least one other disease usually classed as autoimmune, and almost half (40%) have two or more such ailments. Among these disorders are chronic thyroiditis, rheumatoid arthritis, scleroderma, Sjögren syndrome, and systemic lupus erythematosus.

Both humoral and cellular immunity appear to be altered. Serum immunoglobulin levels are increased, especially the level of IgM. **More than 95% of patients have circulating antimitochondrial antibodies, a finding commonly used in the diagnosis of PBC.** These autoantibodies recognize epitopes associated with the mitochondrial pyruvate dehydrogenase complex. Despite the specificity of the antimitochondrial antibodies, they have no inhibitory effect on mitochondrial function and play no known role in the pathogenesis or progression of the disease. Other circulating autoantibodies are antinuclear, antithyroid, antiplatelet, anti-acetylcholine receptor, and antiribonucleoprotein antibodies. The complement system is also chronically activated.

The cells surrounding and infiltrating the sites of bile duct damage are predominantly suppressor/cytotoxic (CD8$^+$) lymphocytes, suggesting that they mediate the destruction of the ductal epithelium.

 Pathology: The pathological stages in the evolution of PBC are characterized by ductal lesions, scarring, and cirrhosis.

STAGE I: THE DUCT LESION. Early PBC features a unique lesion, namely a *chronic destructive cholangitis* affecting the intrahepatic small and medium-sized bile ducts (Fig. 14-41). The injury to the bile ducts is segmental and therefore appears focal in histological sections. The bile ducts are surrounded principally by lymphocytes, but plasma cells and macrophages are also seen. Characteristically, the bile duct epithelium is irregular and hyperplastic, with stratification of epithelial cells and occasional papillary ingrowths. **In some portal tracts, lymphoid follicles, occasionally containing germinal centers, are conspicuous.** Discrete epithelioid granulomas often occur in the portal tracts and may impinge on the bile ducts. In stage I PBC, the lobular parenchyma tends to be normal.

STAGE II: SCARRING. As a result of the destructive inflammatory process characteristic of stage I PBC, **the small bile ducts virtually disappear, and scarring of medium-sized bile ducts is common. Proliferation of bile ductules within the portal tracts is usual and may be florid.** Collagenous septa extend from the portal tracts into the lobular parenchyma and begin to encircle some lobules. Cholestasis, when present, may be severe and is located at the periphery of the portal tracts.

STAGE III: CIRRHOSIS. The end-stage of PBC is cirrhosis, characterized by a dark green bile-stained liver that exhibits fine nodularity. Microscopically, small bile ducts are

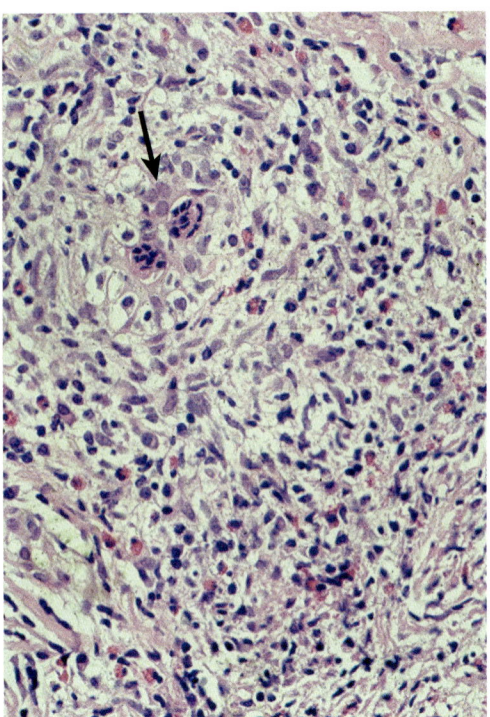

FIGURE 14-41
Primary biliary cirrhosis (PBC), stage 1. A photomicrograph shows a portal tract expanded by an inflammatory infiltrate consisting of lymphocytes, plasma cells, and macrophages. A bile duct *(arrow)* **is damaged by the inflammation.**

scarce and medium-sized ducts are conspicuously fewer in number. There is little inflammation within either the fibrous septa or the parenchymal nodules.

 Clinical Features: **Women, usually between 30 and 65 years of age, constitute some 90 to 95% of those afflicted with PBC.** A substantial proportion of patients with PBC have no symptoms during the early stages of the disease. Some remain asymptomatic and appear to have an excellent prognosis; others ultimately develop advanced cirrhosis and its complications.

In a typical case of PBC, high serum alkaline phosphatase activity is accompanied by a normal or only slightly elevated serum bilirubin level. The patient often suffers from severe pruritus, a symptom caused by the deposition of bile acids in the skin. As the disease advances, most patients have a progressive increase in serum bilirubin level. Serum aminotransferase activities are only moderately elevated. The serum cholesterol level increases strikingly, and an abnormal lipoprotein (lipoprotein-X) appears that is found in many forms of chronic cholestasis. Cholesterol-laden macrophages accumulate in the subcutaneous tissues, where they appear as localized lesions termed *xanthomas*. The impairment in the excretion of bile into the intestine often leads to severe **steatorrhea**, owing to fat malabsorption. Because of associated malabsorption of vitamin D and calcium, **osteomalacia** and **osteoporosis** are important complications of PBC. About one third of patients develop gallstones. Patients who eventually develop cirrhosis die in hepatic failure or of the complications of **portal hypertension**.

Primary biliary cirrhosis generally pursues an indolent course, which may be as long as 20 to 30 years. Liver transplantation is highly effective in end-stage PBC.

PRIMARY SCLEROSING CHOLANGITIS

Primary sclerosing cholangitis (PSC) is a chronic cholestatic liver disease of unknown cause, in which an inflammatory and fibrosing process narrows and eventually obstructs the intrahepatic and extrahepatic bile ducts. Most patients are men under the age of 40 years. **Progressive biliary obstruction typically leads to persistent obstructive jaundice and eventually to secondary biliary cirrhosis.**

Although the cause of PSC is unknown, about two thirds of patients also have ulcerative colitis. A few cases have been described in patients with Crohn disease of the colon. PSC has also been reported in association with retroperitoneal fibrosis, lymphoma, and the fibrosing variant of chronic thyroiditis (Riedel struma). In one fourth of cases, no associated disease is discerned.

Genetic and immunological factors contribute to the pathogenesis of PSC. The disease occasionally occurs in families and shows an association with certain HLA haplotypes, including HLA B8 and DR3. Hypergammaglobulinemia is common, as are circulating antineutrophil cytoplasmic antibodies (pANCAs), immune complexes in the serum, and activation of the complement system by the classic pathway. The portal tracts exhibit an increased number of T cells.

 Pathology: The liver disease associated with PSC can be divided into three histological stages.

- **Stage I:** The initial lesion is periductal inflammation and fibrosis in the portal tracts (Fig. 14-42).
- **Stage II:** Many bile ducts become obliterated, and fibrous septa extend into the parenchyma.
- **Stage III:** Secondary biliary cirrhosis eventually develops.

Similar inflammatory and fibrotic changes may be seen in the large intrahepatic and extrahepatic bile ducts, where they lead to obstruction of the lumen and true extrahepatic biliary obstruction. Since the disease tends to be segmental, a characteristic beaded appearance of the intrahepatic biliary tree is noted by contrast radiography. The same inflammatory process affects the wall of the gallbladder.

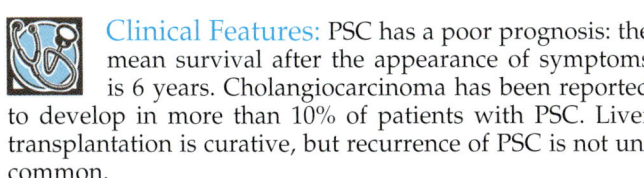 Clinical Features: PSC has a poor prognosis: the mean survival after the appearance of symptoms is 6 years. Cholangiocarcinoma has been reported to develop in more than 10% of patients with PSC. Liver transplantation is curative, but recurrence of PSC is not uncommon.

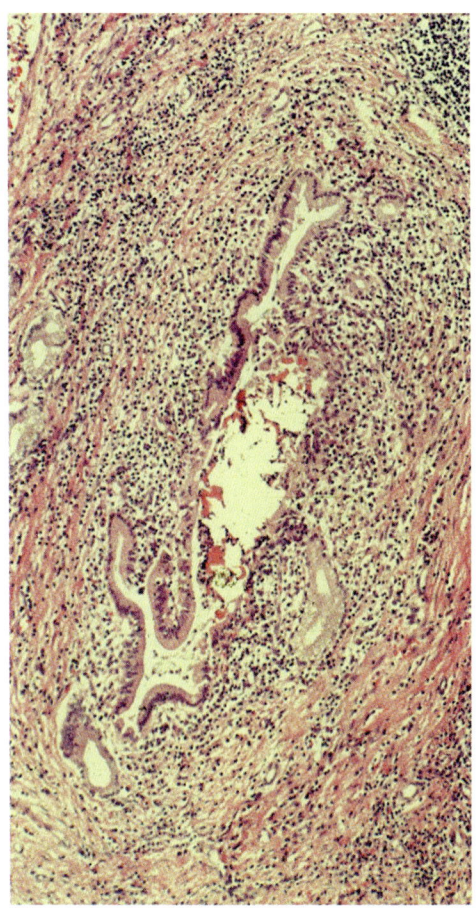

FIGURE 14-42
Primary sclerosing cholangitis. A photomicrograph of a liver removed for hepatic transplantation shows an edematous, fibrotic, and inflamed portal tract. Inflammatory debris is present within the lumen of the bile duct.

EXTRAHEPATIC BILIARY OBSTRUCTION

The extrahepatic biliary system may be obstructed by a number of lesions. These include gallstones passing through the cystic duct to lodge in the common bile duct, cancer of the bile duct or surrounding tissues (pancreas or ampulla of Vater), external compression by enlarged neoplastic lymph nodes in the porta hepatis (as in Hodgkin disease), benign strictures (postoperative scarring or primary sclerosing cholangitis), and congenital biliary atresia (Fig. 14-43).

 Pathology: Early in the precirrhotic stage of extrahepatic biliary obstruction, the liver is swollen and bile stained. In prolonged obstruction, the bile becomes almost colorless ("white bile") because of the suppression of bilirubin secretion, although the liver remains green. Initially, centrilobular cholestasis is accompanied by edema of the portal tracts. As obstruction proceeds, mononuclear inflammatory cells infiltrate the portal tracts. Tortuous and distended bile ductules, characterized by a high cuboidal ep-

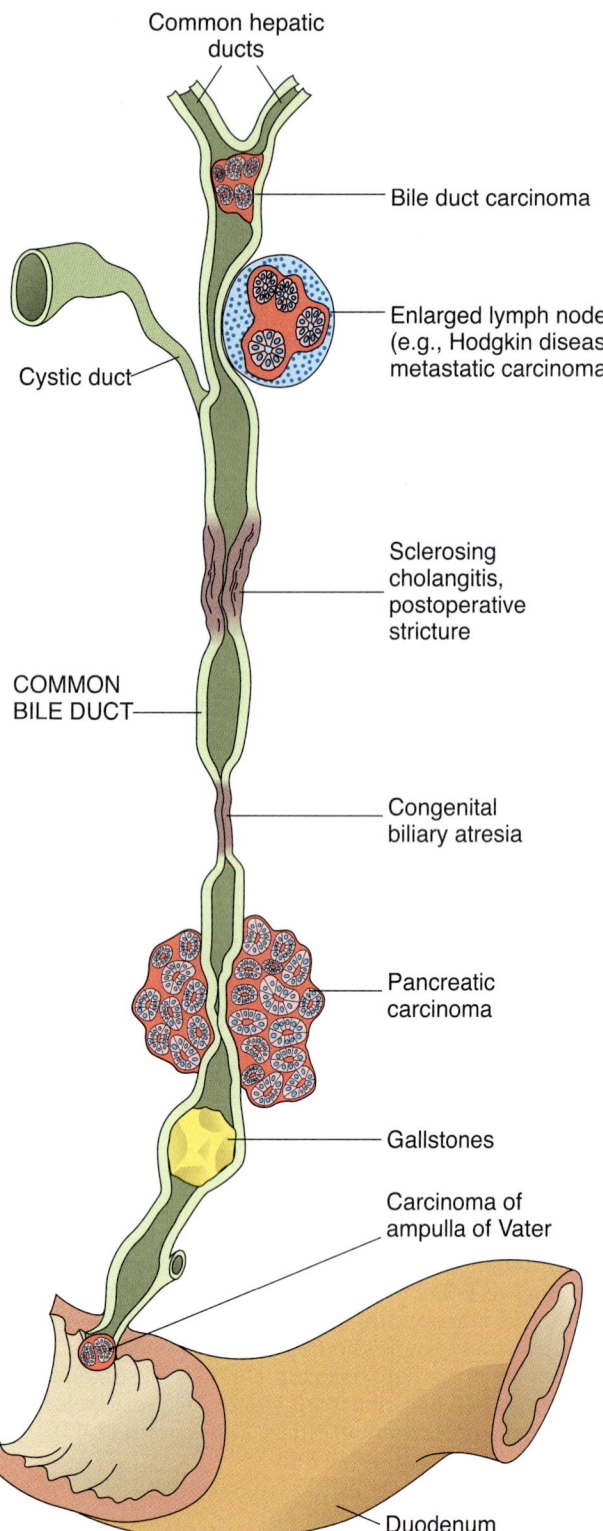

FIGURE 14-43
Major causes of extrahepatic biliary obstruction.

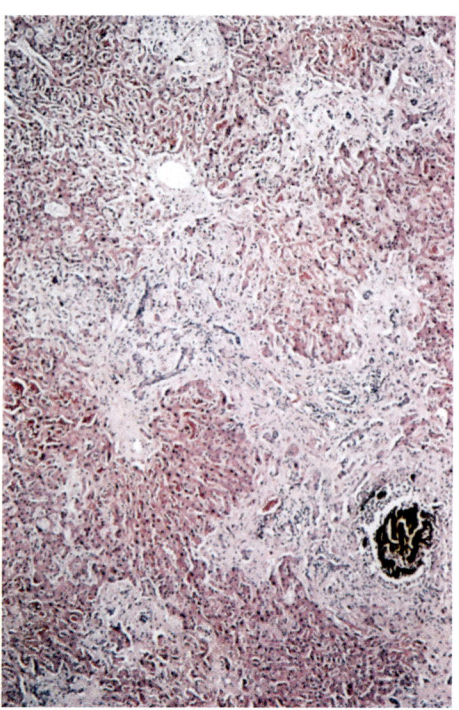

FIGURE 14-44
Secondary biliary cirrhosis. A photomicrograph of the liver from a patient with a carcinoma of the pancreas that obstructed the common bile duct. Irregular fibrous septa extend from an enlarged portal tract *(lower right)* containing a dilated interlobular bile duct that encloses a dense biliary concretion. Numerous proliferated bile ductules are seen within the septa.

ithelium, proliferate (Fig. 14-44). The cholestasis eventually extends to the periphery of the lobule. Dilated bile ducts may rupture, leading to the formation of *bile lakes* (see Fig. 14-10), which appear as focal, golden-yellow deposits that are surrounded by degenerating hepatocytes. Leakage of bile into the portal tracts also causes the appearance of foamy, lipid-laden macrophages, often aggregated as *granulomas*. Damaged hepatocytes containing large amounts of bile show a characteristic reticulated cytoplasm, termed *feathery degeneration*. Infection of the obstructed biliary passages often leads to a superimposed suppurative cholangitis, intraluminal pus, and even intrahepatic abscesses. Within bile ducts and proliferated ductules, biliary concretions may be conspicuous.

With time, the portal tracts become enlarged and fibrotic. Typically, the *periductal fibrosis* is concentric, giving rise to the term *onion-skin fibrosis*. In untreated extrahepatic biliary obstruction, septa eventually extend between the portal tracts of contiguous lobules to form **micronodular cirrhosis**.

IRON-OVERLOAD SYNDROMES

A number of conditions are characterized by the excessive accumulation of iron in the body (siderosis). Iron overload is divided into two major categories based on the etiology of the increased body iron. **Hereditary hemochromatosis** is caused by a common genetic alteration in the control of the intestinal absorption of iron. **Secondary iron overload** is a condition that (1) complicates certain hematological disorders; (2) is associated with parenteral iron overload, in which the iron is obtained from multiple blood transfusions or the parenteral administration of iron itself; or (3) is caused by an enormous dietary intake of iron.

Iron Metabolism

The body of a normal man contains 3 to 4 g of iron, two thirds of which is present in hemoglobin, myoglobin, and iron-containing enzymes. The remainder is represented by storage iron, which exists in two forms, soluble ferritin and insoluble hemosiderin. **Ferritin,** the primary iron storage protein, is present in the cytoplasm of all cells and, in small amounts, in the circulation. **Hemosiderin** is a product of the degradation of ferritin but, unlike the latter, is visualized by light microscopy as golden-yellow granules that stain with the Prussian blue reaction. The liver is an important organ for the storage of iron, although a comparable amount of storage iron exists in the bone marrow.

The absorption of iron from the gastrointestinal tract is controlled by the need to maintain appropriate iron stores. Thus, in the face of iron deficiency, small-intestinal absorption of iron increases. When body stores of iron are adequate, iron absorption is relatively constant. The obligatory daily iron loss through the urine and desquamated cells of the gut and skin is about 1 mg in men. Women suffer extra losses during menstruation and pregnancy. The possible range of daily iron absorption is from less than 0.5 mg in persons with a normal iron balance to an upper limit of 4 mg in those with iron deficiency. Dietary ascorbate is important in iron absorption because ferric iron in the diet is reduced by ascorbic acid to ferrous iron, the form in which it can be absorbed by the small intestine. The absence of dietary vitamin C significantly decreases the amount of iron that can be absorbed.

Hereditary Hemochromatosis (HH) Is a Common Disorder of Iron Metabolism

HH is characterized by excessive iron absorption and the toxic accumulation of iron in parenchymal cells, particularly of the liver, heart, and pancreas. In this disease, 20 to 40 g of iron (i.e., up to 10 times the normal content) accumulates in the body. The excess iron in HH is located exclusively within the storage compartment, and thus iron stores are increased up to 50 times normal. **The clinical hallmarks of advanced HH are cirrhosis, diabetes, skin pigmentation, and cardiac failure** (Fig. 14-45). The disease is most often manifested clinically in patients between 40 and 60 years of age, and men are afflicted 10 times as often as women. This striking male predilection may be attributed to the increased loss of iron in women during the reproductive years. However, given sufficient time to absorb additional iron, postmenopausal women also seem to be at risk for the development of hemochromatosis. Since maximum daily iron absorption is about 4 mg, hemochromatosis clearly takes years to develop.

Pathogenesis: HH is inherited as an **autosomal recessive** disorder, in which increased intestinal absorption of iron leads to its deposition in many organs. Lesser degrees of iron overload are often found in relatives of those with the disease.

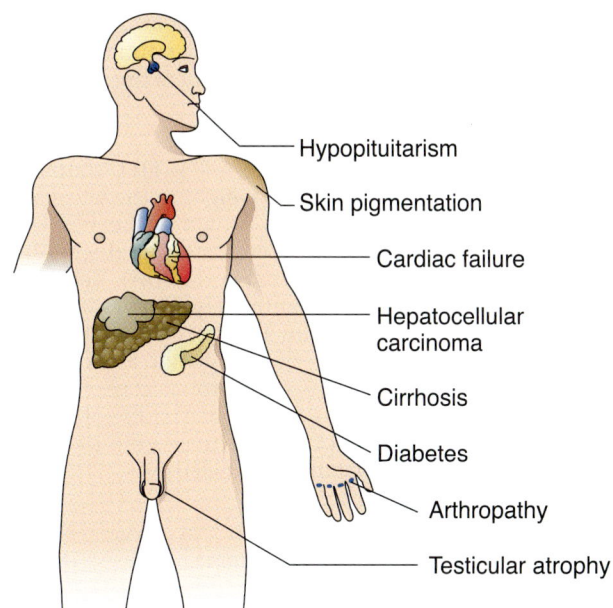

FIGURE 14-45
Complications of hemochromatosis.

The gene involved in HH, known as *HFe*, is located on the short arm of chromosome 6 and encodes a transmembrane protein that is similar to MHC class-1 molecules. The most common form of HH reflects a homozygous mutation (C282Y) in the *HFe* gene, although 10 to 15% of cases seem not to be caused by mutations in this gene. In populations of European descent, the heterozygous frequency is about 10%, and 1 of 200 to 400 persons is homozygous. Interestingly, some persons who are homozygous for the mutation do not have the HH phenotype and do not exhibit iron overload. Thus, only 1 in 400 persons develops clinically apparent hemochromatosis.

The iron content of the body is regulated by intestinal iron absorption. A divalent metal transporter (DMT-1) on the luminal surface of mucosal cells in the duodenum binds dietary ferrous iron and transfers it to the intracellular compartment, from which it is absorbed into the circulation. In the blood, most of the iron is bound to transferrin, but a lesser amount circulates bound to another protein(s). Iron is then transferred to all cells of the body through the transferrin receptor and, to a lesser extent, by the uptake of non-transferrin-bound iron. The HFe protein associates with the transferrin receptor and influences intracellular iron delivery to the cytoplasm, although the precise effect remains controversial. The mutant HFe protein, including that of the duodenal enterocytes, cannot promote iron uptake. As a result, duodenal crypt cells sense an iron deficiency and up-regulate DMT-1 expression, which then **increases absorption of dietary iron**. The transfer of iron across the mucosal cell is accelerated, leading to an increased concentration of non-transferrin-bound iron in the blood and its subsequent accumulation in parenchymal organs.

As noted in Chapter 1, iron is an essential factor in cellular injury mediated by activated oxygen species. The presence of excess iron in cells probably renders them more susceptible to oxidative injury.

Pathology: HH is characterized pathologically by the accumulation of very large amounts of iron in the parenchymal cells of a variety of organs and tissues.

LIVER: The liver is always affected in HH, containing more than 0.5 g iron per 100 g wet weight in the late stages. The liver is enlarged and reddish brown and exhibits micronodular cirrhosis. The hepatocytes and bile duct epithelium are filled with iron granules (Fig. 14-46A). The excess cellular iron is stored predominantly in lysosomes in the ferric form. Late in the disease, many Kupffer cells contain large deposits of iron derived from the phagocytosis of necrotic hepatocytes. Within the fibrous septa, iron is conspicuous in proliferated bile ductules and macrophages. Eventually, as in micronodular cirrhosis of other causes, the pattern is transformed to that of a macronodular cirrhosis.

SKIN: The skin in patients with HH is typically pigmented, but only half of patients exhibit increased iron deposition in the skin. Most patients display increased melanin in the basal melanocytes.

PANCREAS: Diabetes is a common complication of HH, and results from the deposition of iron in the pancreas (see Fig. 14-46B). Grossly, the organ appears rust colored and fibrotic. Both exocrine and endocrine cells contain excess iron, and there is degeneration of acinar cells and a reduction in the number of islets of Langerhans. The combination of pigmented skin and glucose intolerance in patients with HH is referred to as *bronze diabetes*.

HEART: Congestive heart failure is a common cause of death in patients with HH. The myocardial fibers contain iron pigment (see Fig. 14-46C), which is more extensive in the ventricles than in the atria. Necrosis of cardiac myocytes and accompanying interstitial fibrosis are common.

ENDOCRINE SYSTEM: Numerous endocrine glands are involved in HH, including the pituitary, adrenal, thyroid,

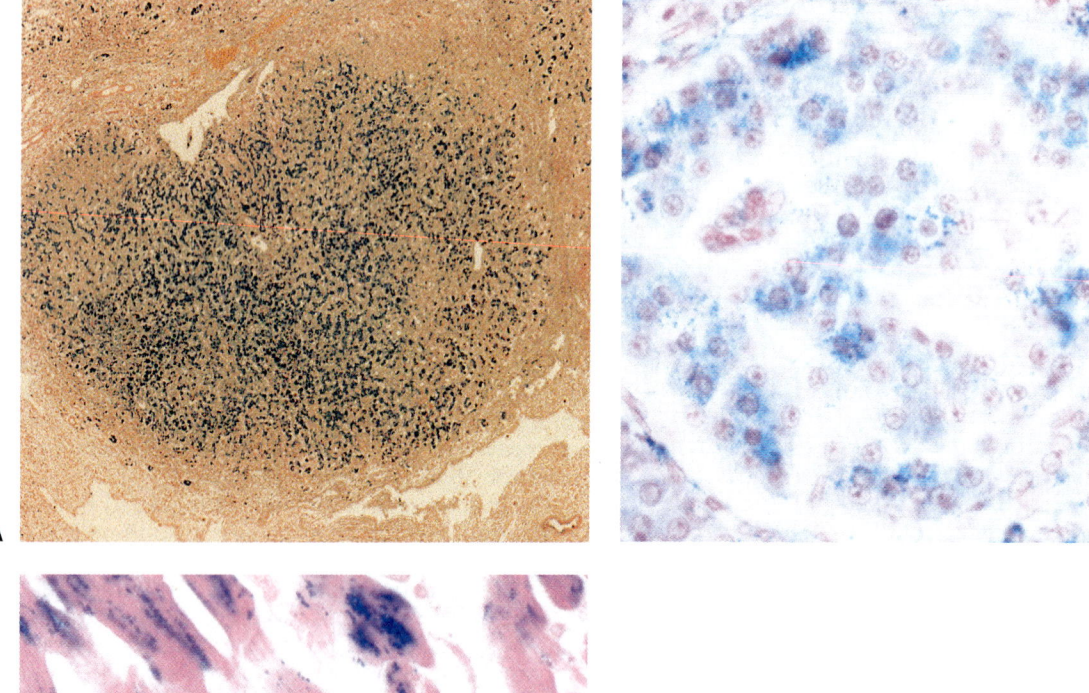

FIGURE 14-46

Hemochromatosis. A. Prussian blue stain demonstrates considerable iron in a nodule of a cirrhotic liver. B. Iron accumulation in a pancreatic islet of Langerhans and (C) in the myocardium.

and parathyroid glands. However, tissue damage is not a usual feature in these organs, except for the pituitary, in which the release of gonadotropins is impaired. As a result, testicular atrophy is seen in a fourth of male patients, even without iron deposition in the testes. The disturbance in the pituitary–gonadal axis is characterized by loss of libido and amenorrhea in women and impotence and sparse body hair in men.

JOINTS: Arthropathy, most severe in the fingers and hands, occurs in about half of patients with HH. When arthritis affects the larger joints, such as the knee, it may be severe enough to be disabling.

 Clinical Features: The liver disease in HH generally pursues an indolent and prolonged course, but among untreated patients, a fourth eventually die in hepatic coma or from gastrointestinal hemorrhage. **Hepatocellular carcinoma is a significant late complication of HH-induced cirrhosis.** In fact, among patients with cirrhosis, the 10-year cumulative probability of developing liver cancer is as high as 30%. By contrast, noncirrhotic patients with HH treated by phlebotomy are not at increased risk of hepatocellular carcinoma.

Laboratory Diagnosis

The normal value for plasma iron is 80 to 100 g/dL, and transferrin is normally about one third saturated. In patients with HH, the serum iron concentration is more than doubled, and transferrin is entirely saturated. The concentration of ferritin in the blood, which parallels the amount of storage iron, is greatly increased in HH.

Treatment

The treatment of HH is based on the removal of iron from the body, most effectively by repeated phlebotomy. Weekly phlebotomies for 2 to 3 years can remove 20 to 40 g of iron, after which phlebotomies every 2 to 3 months maintain iron balance. The beneficial effect of repeated phlebotomies is impressive. In homozygotes who have neither cirrhosis nor diabetes, iron depletion results in a life expectancy identical to that of the general population. By contrast, the 10-year survival of untreated patients with HH is a mere 6%.

Secondary Iron Overload Syndromes Occur in Persons Who Do Not Carry the Gene for HH

 Pathogenesis: Within certain limits, the amount of iron absorbed bears a relation to the amount of iron ingested. For example, a low iron content in the diet renders the development of hemochromatosis unlikely. Many patients with secondary iron overload (up to 40%) have a long history of **alcohol abuse,** and it is thought that alcohol may enhance both the accumulation of iron and its associated cell injury.

An interesting example of secondary hemochromatosis is presented by the well-recognized iron accumulation in blacks of sub-Saharan Africa, commonly misnamed *Bantu siderosis*. These populations show a high incidence of iron overload, presumably because of the consumption of large amounts of iron-containing alcoholic beverages. With the replacement of "home-brewed" beverages (low alcohol, high iron) by Western spirits (high alcohol, low iron), the incidence of siderosis has fallen while that of alcoholic cirrhosis has increased.

Massive iron overload occurs in patients with certain hemolytic anemias, such as sickle cell anemia, thalassemia major, and other anemias associated with ineffective erythropoiesis. The source of the excess iron is the patient's diet or transfused blood. Increased iron absorption occurs despite the saturation of transferrin; the release of iron by intravascular hemolysis adds a further burden of iron. Patients with thalassemia often develop secondary iron overload whether or not they have received blood transfusions. On the other hand, multiple blood transfusions alone are generally insufficient to produce secondary iron overload, even in patients with hypoplastic anemia given many transfusions (250 mg iron/500 mL unit of blood). In these patients, iron is concentrated principally in mononuclear phagocytes, and cirrhosis is rare.

The causes of iron overload are summarized in Table 14-4.

 Pathology: Cirrhosis with secondary iron overload shows varying degrees of iron accumulation, but iron deposition in the liver is generally less extensive than that in HH and is often restricted to the periphery of the nodules. Transfusional and other types of siderosis are characterized by the uniform, initial deposition of iron in Kupffer cells, with eventual spillover into the hepatocytes.

TABLE *14-4*   **Causes of Iron Overload**

Increased iron absorption	Parenteral iron overload
Hereditary hemochromatosis	Multiple blood
Chronic liver disease	transfusions
Iron-loading anemias	Injectable medicinal iron
Porphyria cutanea tarda	Focal iron overload
Congenital diseases	Idiopathic pulmonary
(e.g., atransferrinemia)	hemosiderosis
Dietary iron overload	Renal hemosiderosis
(Bantu siderosis)	
Excess medicinal iron	

HERITABLE DISORDERS ASSOCIATED WITH CIRRHOSIS

Wilson Disease (Hepatolenticular Degeneration) Is a Rare Disorder of Copper Metabolism

Wilson disease (WD) is an autosomal recessive malady in which excess copper is deposited in the liver and brain. The carrier rate is about 1 in 100, and the incidence of clinical disease is about 1 in 50,000 live births. The mutated gene has a worldwide distribution.

Pathogenesis: The intake of copper in the diet usually exceeds requirements, and the liver clears excess copper via excretion into the bile. In addition to biliary secretion, copper is normally bound to ceruloplasmin in the hepatocyte, and the complex is secreted into the blood. The gene for WD, *ATP7B*, codes for an ATP-dependent transmembrane cation channel that transports copper within the hepatocytes before it is excreted. **Mutations in the WD gene renders copper transport ineffective,** and both biliary excretion of copper and its incorporation into ceruloplasmin are deficient. Some 200 different mutations in the WD gene on chromosome 13 have been described. In European and North American populations, a single mutation, His1069Gln, accounts for up to 70% of WD, whereas this mutation is rare in India and Asia. Most patients are compound heterozygotes, possessing alleles with two different mutations.

Wilson disease is characterized by a striking reduction in the serum levels of ceruloplasmin. However, this deficiency is thought to be secondary to hepatic copper overload. After excess copper leads to the death of hepatocytes, copper is released into the blood and subsequently deposits in extrahepatic tissues. The primacy of the liver as the seat of WD is attested to by its cure with liver transplantation.

The mechanism by which excess copper injures cells remains elusive. Like iron, copper can catalyze the formation of potent oxidizing species from superoxide anions and hydrogen peroxide produced by normal oxygen metabolism. In this regard, copper can replace iron in the Fenton reaction, in which ferrous iron and hydrogen peroxide generate hydroxyl radicals (see Chapter 1).

Pathology: Liver disease in WD progresses from mild to severe **chronic hepatitis. Cirrhosis may develop rapidly, even in childhood.** The periportal hepatocytes often contain Mallory's hyaline, and cholestasis is not infrequent. An initial micronodular cirrhosis eventually assumes a macronodular pattern. Chemical measurement of liver copper in unfixed tissue from livers of patients with WD reveals more than 250 μg of copper per gram of dry weight.

In the brain, the corpus striatum and occasionally the subthalamic nuclei display a reddish brown discoloration. The central white matter of the cerebral or cerebellar hemispheres may manifest spongy softening or cavitation, in which case the overlying cortex is atrophic. The astrocytes proliferate in the putamen, and the number of neurons is decreased.

Clinical Features: Half of patients with WD display some symptoms by adolescence, and the remainder usually become ill in their early adult years. The presenting symptoms are referable to chronic liver disease in about half of patients, one third initially present with neurological complaints, and about one tenth are seen because of psychiatric manifestations.

LIVER: The liver disease begins insidiously with nonspecific symptoms and progresses to chronic liver disease indistinguishable from that of other forms of chronic hepatitis. Eventually, chronic hepatitis and cirrhosis result in jaundice, portal hypertension, and hepatic failure. Unlike hemochromatosis, WD is not associated with an increased risk of primary hepatocellular carcinoma.

BRAIN: The neurological disease begins with mild incoordination and tremors. In untreated patients, dysarthria and dysphagia appear, and in late stages, disabling dystonia and spasticity occur.

EYE: Ophthalmic manifestations invariably accompany the neurological disease. *Kayser-Fleischer ring* is a golden-brown, bilateral discoloration of the cornea that encircles the periphery of the iris and obscures its muscular pattern (Fig. 14-47). It represents a deposition of copper in Descemet membrane. In some patients, Kayser-Fleischer rings are accompanied by *sunflower cataracts,* which are green disks of copper deposition in the anterior capsule of the lens.

BONES: Skeletal lesions are commonly found on radiographic examination. They include osteomalacia, osteoporosis, spontaneous fractures, and various arthropathies.

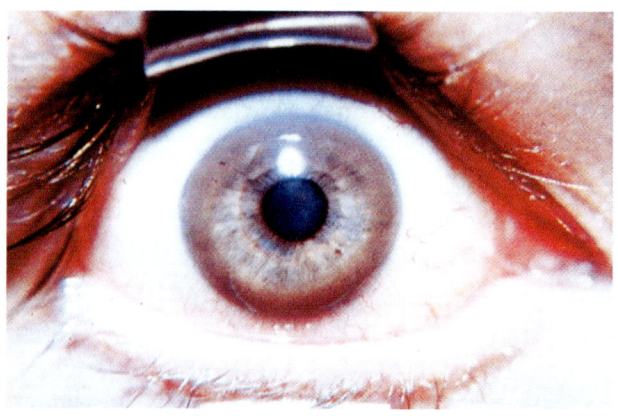

FIGURE 14-47

Kayser-Fleischer ring. The deposition of copper in Descemet membrane is reflected in a peripheral brown color, which obstructs the view of the underlying iris.

KIDNEY: Renal glomerular and tubular dysfunction, manifested by proteinuria, lowered glomerular filtration, aminoaciduria, and phosphaturia, is common in WD. These abnormalities are secondary to copper deposition in the renal tubules.

BLOOD: Transient acute hemolytic episodes, presumably related to a sudden release of free copper from the liver, occur in as many as 15% of patients with WD.

Treatment of WD not only prevents the accumulation of tissue copper but also extracts copper that has already been deposited. D-Penicillamine, a copper-chelating agent, augments the excretion of copper in the urine. Both central nervous system dysfunction and the symptoms of liver disease are often reversed by treatment. Liver transplantation is curative for WD.

Cystic Fibrosis May Cause Biliary Obstruction

Biliary obstruction results from the accumulation of tenacious mucous plugs in the intrahepatic biliary tree and may present in the first few weeks of life. Recovery typically occurs in 1 to 6 months, although some infants die in hepatic failure. **In children who survive to adolescence, clinically symptomatic liver disease develops in as many as 15%, and secondary biliary cirrhosis is found in 10% of patients who survive beyond the age of 25 years.**

α_1-Antitrypsin (α_1-AT) Deficiency Leads to Cirrhosis

α_1-AT deficiency is inherited as an autosomal recessive trait and was initially described as a cause of emphysema (see Chapter 12). Thereafter, cases of liver disease without pulmonary involvement were described, and disease of both organs has also been recognized. In infants and children, α_1-AT deficiency is the most common genetic cause of liver disease and the most frequent genetic disease for which liver transplantation is indicated. Although the disorder is found in 1 of 2000 live births, only 10 to 15% of those affected develop liver injury.

Pathogenesis: α_1-AT is synthesized in the liver, and both the pulmonary and hepatic disorders result from a defect in the secretion of a mutant variant by the liver. The α_1-AT gene locus is termed *Pi*, and over 75 isoforms have been identified. The two most frequent types are designated PiS and PiZ. The substitution of a lysine for a glutamate in the PiZ variant (95% of all cases) causes the mutant protein to fold abnormally and accumulate as an insoluble aggregate within the lumen of the endoplasmic reticulum of the hepatocyte, thereby damaging that cell.

Pathology: **The characteristic feature in the liver of patients with α_1-AT deficiency is the presence of faintly eosinophilic, PAS-positive cytoplasmic**

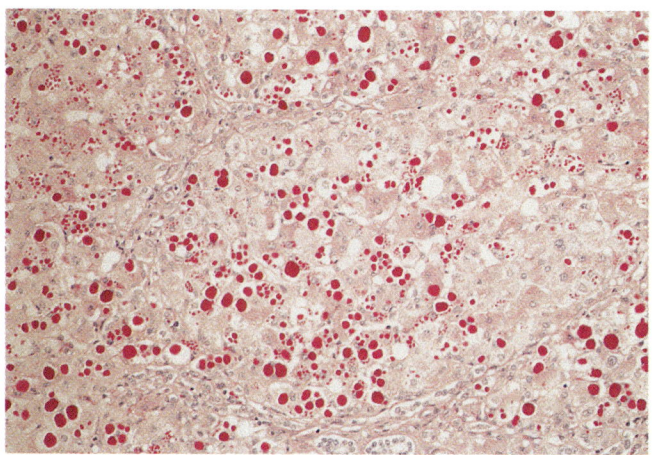

FIGURE 14-48
α_1-Antitrypsin deficiency. A photomicrograph of a section of liver stained by the periodic acid–Schiff (PAS) reaction with diastase digestion to remove glycogen reveals numerous cytoplasmic globules in the hepatocytes.

droplets (Fig. 14-48). Electron microscopy visualizes these inclusions as amorphous material within dilated cisternae of the endoplasmic reticulum. The disease often terminates in cirrhosis.

α_1-AT deficiency is a cause of hepatitis in the newborn (see below). **Micronodular cirrhosis develops by the age of 2 to 3 years in these children and may ultimately become macronodular.**

Clinical Features: The clinical expression of liver disease in α_1-AT deficiency is highly variable, ranging from a rapidly fatal neonatal hepatitis to an absence of any hepatic dysfunction. **Of those infants with the ZZ genotype—that is, those who are susceptible to the development of clinical disease—about 10% develop neonatal cholestatic jaundice (conjugated hyperbilirubinemia).** In fact, α_1-AT accounts for up to 30% of all cases of neonatal conjugated hyperbilirubinemia. Most infants recover within 6 months, but 10 to 20% develop permanent liver disease. Children with cirrhosis usually die before the age of 10 years from hepatic failure or other complications of α_1-AT deficiency. However, liver transplantation is curative.

Some patients are asymptomatic until early adulthood, when they may present with symptoms of cirrhosis as the initial complaint. **The cirrhosis of α_1-AT deficiency is complicated by a high incidence of hepatocellular carcinoma.**

Inborn Errors of Carbohydrate Metabolism Affect the Liver

Glycogen Storage Diseases

The biochemical basis of the glycogen storage diseases is discussed in Chapter 6. **Only glycogenosis type IV (brancher**

deficiency, Andersen disease) is usually complicated by cirrhosis. A slowly developing cirrhosis may occur in glycogenosis type III (debrancher deficiency, Cori disease) but is not inevitable. Glycogenosis type I (glucose-6-phosphatase deficiency, von Gierke disease) is associated with striking hepatomegaly, and type II (acid-glucosidase deficiency, Pompe disease) features mild hepatomegaly. Neither type I nor type II is complicated by cirrhosis.

GLYCOGENOSIS TYPE I: The hepatocytes are distended by large amounts of glycogen, which appears pale in sections stained with hematoxylin and eosin and red with PAS. Fat accumulation varies from mild to severe, but fibrosis is usually absent. Hepatic adenomas often develop in adolescence but regress with dietary therapy.

GLYCOGENOSIS TYPE III: Infants with this malady show severe hepatomegaly, and the liver morphologically resembles that seen in type I. Fat is less conspicuous, but fibrosis is present and may progress to cirrhosis.

GLYCOGENOSIS TYPE IV: Infants present with severe hepatomegaly and usually die of cirrhosis by the age of 4 years. Sharply circumscribed, PAS-positive inclusions are present in enlarged hepatocytes. By electron microscopy these inclusions consist of fibrillar material that represents abnormal glycogen. Deposits of mutant glycogen are also found in the heart, skeletal muscle, and brain. Liver transplantation is curative for glycogenosis type IV.

Galactosemia

Galactosemia, inherited as an autosomal recessive trait, is caused by a deficiency of galactose-1-phosphate uridyl transferase, the enzyme that catalyzes the second step in the conversion of galactose to glucose. As a result of this metabolic defect, galactose and its metabolites accumulate in the liver and other organs. Infants with this disorder who are fed milk rapidly develop **hepatosplenomegaly, jaundice,** and **hypoglycemia.** Cataracts and mental retardation are common.

Microscopically, within 2 weeks of birth the liver shows extensive and uniform fat accumulation and striking proliferation of bile ductules in and around the portal tracts. Cholestasis is often present in canaliculi and bile ductules. Bile plugs fill many of these pseudoacini. At about 6 weeks of age, fibrosis begins to extend from the portal tracts into the lobule and **within 6 months progresses to cirrhosis.** Institution of a galactose-free diet ameliorates the disease and reverses many of the morphological alterations.

Hereditary Fructose Intolerance

Hereditary fructose intolerance is an autosomal recessive disease caused by a deficiency of fructose-1-phosphate aldolase. When fructose is fed early in infancy, hepatomegaly, jaundice, and ascites develop. However, the feeding of fructose after the age of 6 months results in far less severe disease, and the only clinical impairment is spontaneous hypoglycemia. Infants who suffer from liver disease show many of the changes of neonatal hepatitis. Fat accumulation may be marked, in which case the appearance resembles that of galactosemia. Progressive fibrosis culminates in cirrhosis.

Tyrosinemia

Tyrosinemia is an autosomal recessive trait that interferes with the catabolism of tyrosine to fumarate and acetoacetate. The biochemical defect is a deficiency of fumarylacetoacetate hydrolase (FAH) in the liver caused by more than 30 mutations in the *FAH* gene. Damage to the liver and kidney is caused by the accumulation of succinyl acetone and succinyl acetoacetate, both of which are potent electrophiles that can react with the sulfhydryl groups of glutathione and proteins.

Acute tyrosinemia, which begins within a few weeks or months of birth, is characterized by hepatosplenomegaly and is associated with liver failure and death, usually before the age of 12 months. The appearance of the liver is remarkably similar to that in galactosemia, including progression to cirrhosis.

Chronic tyrosinemia begins in the first year of life and is characterized by growth retardation, renal disease, and hepatic failure. Death usually supervenes before the age of 10 years. **The incidence of hepatocellular carcinoma associated with chronic tyrosinemia is extraordinarily high.** Tyrosinemia is treated by liver transplantation.

Miscellaneous Inherited Causes of Cirrhosis

A wide variety of inborn errors of metabolism have been associated with cirrhosis, including storage diseases, such as Gaucher disease, Niemann-Pick disease, mucopolysaccharidoses, neonatal adrenoleukodystrophy, Wolman disease, and Zellweger syndrome.

INDIAN CHILDHOOD CIRRHOSIS

Indian childhood cirrhosis (ICC) is a fatal disorder largely restricted to preschool children on the Indian subcontinent. Similar cases have occasionally been described elsewhere. The disorder affects predominantly boys between the ages of 1 and 4 years from middle-class Hindu families. The liver displays micronodular cirrhosis and abundant Mallory bodies, similar to alcoholic liver disease.

The etiology and pathogenesis of ICC are not well understood. Familial cases have been reported, but no hereditary pattern has been established. Interestingly, children with this disease display a marked excess of copper and copper-binding protein in the liver, but the significance of these findings remains obscure.

TOXIC LIVER INJURY

Acute, chemically induced hepatic injury spans the entire spectrum of liver disease, from transient cholestasis to fulminant hepatitis. Chronic toxic injury to the liver is equally diverse; at one extreme is a mild chronic hepatitis and at the other, active cirrhosis. Although hepatic injury caused by drugs accounts for less than 5% of all cases of jaundice, it constitutes up to 25% of cases of fulminant hepatic failure.

Some hepatotoxic chemicals invariably produce liver cell necrosis—that is, their action is entirely predictable. Among such agents are substances as diverse as yellow phosphorus, the organic solvent carbon tetrachloride, the mushroom poison phalloidin, and the analgesic acetaminophen. The defining characteristics of the liver injury produced by "predictable" hepatotoxins are as follows:

- The agent, in sufficiently high doses, always produces liver cell necrosis.
- The extent of hepatic injury is dose dependent.
- These compounds produce the same lesions in different animal species.
- The liver necrosis is characteristically zonal—often, but not exclusively, centrilobular.
- The period between administration of the toxin and the development of liver cell necrosis is brief.

Chapter 1 includes a discussion of the possible mechanisms by which these toxins produce liver necrosis. Briefly, toxic liver necrosis is, in most cases, a consequence of the metabolism of the compound by the mixed-function oxidase system of the liver, by which activated oxygen species and reactive metabolites are produced. The rate of drug metabolism is influenced by many factors, including age, sex, nutritional status, interactions with other drugs, and prior induction of hepatic drug-metabolizing activity.

In contrast to the aforementioned classic poisons, **most reactions to therapeutic drugs are unpredictable** and seem to represent idiosyncratic events or manifestations of unusual sensitivity to a dose-related side effect. Sensitive persons may be predisposed to idiosyncratic reactions either because they possess metabolic pathways different from those of the general population or because they are particularly susceptible to a uniform pharmacological effect of the drug other than the desired therapeutic response.

Genetic variations in systems of biotransformation and in the production or detoxification of reactive metabolites may determine the toxicity of some drugs. An immunological reaction to drugs, their metabolites, or modified liver cells has not been ruled out. Drugs that are principally cholestatic do not necessarily depend on metabolism for their action.

With these considerations in mind, we shall discuss toxic liver injury in terms of the morphological patterns of the resulting reaction.

Zonal Hepatocellular Necrosis Is Caused by the Metabolites of Drugs and Chemicals

The centrilobular localization of necrosis presumably reflects the greater activity of drug-metabolizing enzymes in the central zones. Examples of agents that produce such injury agents are carbon tetrachloride, acetaminophen (Fig. 14-49), and the toxins of the mushroom *Amanita phalloides*.

In the affected zones, hepatocytes show coagulative necrosis, hydropic swelling, and variable amounts of fat. In-

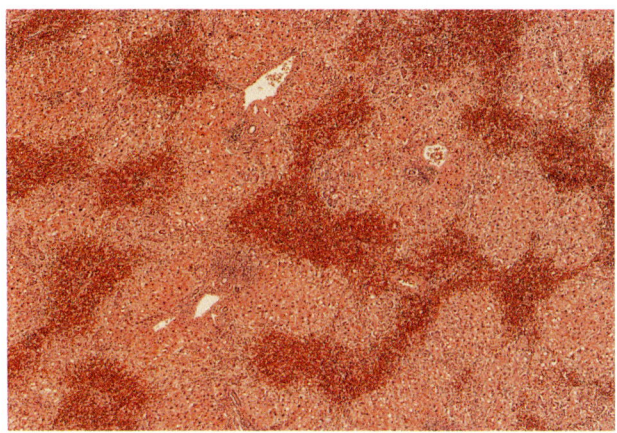

FIGURE 14-49
Toxic centrilobular necrosis. The autopsy specimen in a case of acetaminophen overdose discloses prominent hemorrhagic necrosis of the centrilobular zones of all liver lobules.

flammation tends to be sparse. If the dose of the hepatotoxin is sufficiently large, necrosis may extend to involve the entire lobule, leaving only a thin rim of viable hepatocytes surrounding the portal tracts. Patients either die in acute hepatic failure or recover without sequelae.

The chronic administration of hepatotoxins that cause zonal necrosis, exemplified by carbon tetrachloride, produces cirrhosis in experimental animals. However, this is generally not a problem in humans; once the acute toxic injury has been recognized, measures are usually taken to preclude reexposure to the offending agent.

Fatty Liver Is a Response to a Variety of Hepatotoxins

The accumulation of triglycerides within the hepatocytes (i.e., hepatic steatosis or fatty liver) generally occurs in a predictable fashion. Although substantial overlap may exist, two morphological patterns occur, namely macrovesicular and microvesicular steatosis.

Macrovesicular Steatosis

In macrovesicular steatosis, light microscopy shows the cytoplasm of the liver cell to be occupied by fat, seen as a large clear area that distends the cell and displaces the nucleus to the periphery. In addition to its association with chronic ethanol ingestion, macrovesicular fat results from the experimental administration of, or accidental exposure to, such direct hepatotoxins as carbon tetrachloride and the poisonous constituents of certain mushrooms. Moreover, corticosteroids and some antimetabolites, such as methotrexate, may cause macrovesicular steatosis. There is no reason to believe that the presence of fat per se is injurious to the hepatocyte. Rather, its accumulation reflects the underlying liver cell damage.

A puzzling variant of toxic macrovesicular steatosis that resembles alcoholic hepatitis, termed *steatohepatitis* (see above), occurs after the administration of certain drugs (e.g., amiodarone in the treatment of arrhythmias).

Microvesicular Steatosis

In contrast to macrovesicular steatosis, which by itself tends to be clinically inconsequential, microvesicular fatty liver is commonly associated with severe, and sometimes fatal, liver disease. Small fat vacuoles are dispersed throughout the cytoplasm of hepatocytes, and the nucleus retains its central position (Fig. 14-50). Again, it is not the presence of fat but the underlying metabolic defects that produce the liver dysfunction.

REYE SYNDROME: *This rare acute disease of children is characterized by microvesicular steatosis, hepatic failure, and encephalopathy.* Cerebral edema and fat accumulation are reported in the brain. The symptoms usually begin after a febrile illness, commonly influenza or varicella infection, and are claimed to correlate with the administration of **aspirin**. Clearly, Reye syndrome is more complex than simple aspirin toxicity, because the doses of aspirin consumed were far too small to produce liver injury. In any event, with the decline in the use of aspirin in children and possibly a reduced incidence of influenza, Reye syndrome is now distinctly uncommon.

FATTY LIVER OF PREGNANCY: Microsteatosis, not infrequently associated with hepatic failure, may occur during pregnancy and ordinarily improves on delivery. Women who have suffered fatty liver of pregnancy may complete subsequent pregnancies without untoward effects.

PHOSPHOLIPIDOSIS: Triglycerides are not the only lipids that can accumulate in the liver in response to toxic injury. Phospholipidosis, which resembles certain heritable disorders of lipid metabolism (e.g., Niemann-Pick and Tay-Sachs disease), occurs after the administration of drugs such as perhexiline maleate and amiodarone. By light microscopy, both hepatocytes and Kupffer cells are enlarged and show a foamy cytoplasm.

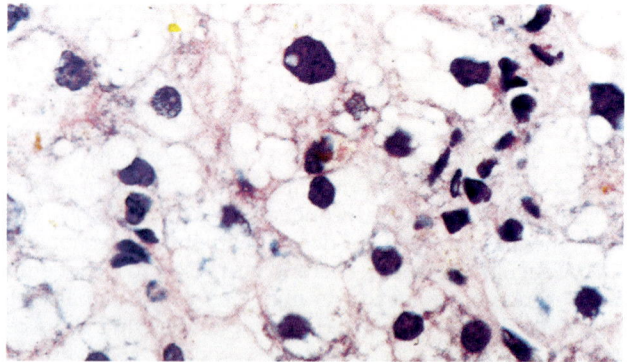

FIGURE 14-50
Microvesicular fatty liver. A liver biopsy specimen in a case of Reye syndrome shows small- droplet fat in hepatocytes and centrally located nuclei.

Acute Intrahepatic Cholestasis Is a Frequent Manifestation of Drug-Induced Liver Disease

Histologically, the lesions may range from bland centrilobular cholestasis with virtually no hepatocellular necrosis or inflammation to panlobular cholestasis with scattered foci of hepatocellular necrosis. Drugs incriminated in this type of liver injury include anabolic steroids and tranquilizing agents. Except for mild jaundice, pruritus, and an elevated serum alkaline phosphatase level, the patients feel well.

Lesions Resembling Viral Hepatitis Are Unpredictable

All the features of acute viral hepatitis occasionally occur after administration of a variety of drugs. The most widely appreciated examples are the inhalation anesthetic halothane, the antituberculosis agent isoniazid, and the antihypertensive drug methyldopa. Although the incidence of these viral hepatitis like reactions is low, they are far more dangerous than viral hepatitis itself, causing more severe disease and a much higher mortality rate. The entire range of acute liver injury, from mild anicteric hepatitis to rapidly fatal massive hepatic necrosis, is encountered.

Chronic Hepatitis Can Follow the Persistent Intake of Hepatotoxic Drugs

Like chronic hepatitis caused by persistent viral infection, drug-induced chronic hepatitis may progress to cirrhosis, albeit rarely. On discontinuation of drug administration, the lesion usually resolves, although this may require many months. In patients who have progressed to cirrhosis, the scarring remains, but the inflammatory and necrotizing activity is halted. Among the drugs incriminated in the production of chronic hepatitis are the antituberculosis drug isoniazid and certain sulfonamides.

Granulomatous Hepatitis Is a Reaction to Drugs

Noncaseating "sarcoid-like" granulomas may appear in the portal tracts and the lobular parenchyma after the intake of some drugs. The liver damage is transient and does not lead to chronic lesions. Among the many drugs that have been associated with granulomatous hepatitis are the antiinflammatory agent phenylbutazone, the antiarrhythmic drug quinidine, and allopurinol, used in the treatment of gout.

Vascular Lesions May Complicate Hormone Therapy

Occlusion of the hepatic veins (*Budd-Chiari syndrome*) has been reported to follow the use of oral contraceptive agents,

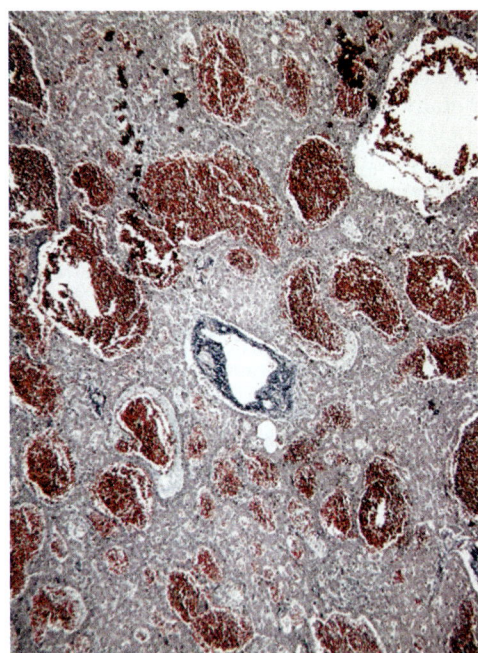

FIGURE 14-51
Peliosis hepatis. The liver contains numerous large, irregular, blood-filled spaces.

presumably reflecting the general hypercoagulable state associated with the use of these steroids.

Peliosis hepatis *is a peculiar hepatic lesion, characterized by cystic, blood-filled cavities that are not lined by endothelial cells* (Fig. 14-51). Anabolic sex steroids, contraceptive steroids, and the antiestrogen compound tamoxifen sometimes produce this lesion.

Neoplastic Lesions Are Rare Reactions to Drugs

Hepatic adenomas are uncommon benign tumors that arise after the use of oral contraceptives and (uncommonly) of anabolic steroids (see below).

Hemangiosarcomas of the liver appeared many years after the intravenous administration of thorium dioxide (Thorotrast), a radioactive compound used in the past to visualize the liver. This particulate isotope is engulfed by Kupffer cells, where it remains inert indefinitely, emits local radiant energy, and thereby produces neoplastic transformation. Chronic exposure to inorganic arsenic, usually in the form of insecticides, and the inhalation of vinyl chloride in an industrial setting have also been linked to the development of hemangiosarcoma of the liver.

THE PORPHYRIAS

The porphyrias comprise both acquired and inherited conditions; they are caused by deficiencies in the pathway of heme biosynthesis and are characterized by the accumulation of porphyrin intermediates (see Chapter 20). The porphyrias are divided into two types, hepatic and erythropoietic porphyrias, based on the location of defective heme metabolism and the accumulation of porphyrins and their precursors. The molecular genetics of the porphyrias is heterogeneous, with unique mutations usually occurring within individual families.

The hepatic porphyrias are inherited as autosomal dominant traits and are often precipitated by the administration of drugs, sex hormones, starvation, hepatitis C, HIV infection, and alcohol consumption. The liver in hepatic porphyrias variably displays steatosis, hemosiderosis, fibrosis, and cirrhosis. Needle-shaped cytoplasmic inclusions may be present.

ACUTE INTERMITTENT PORPHYRIA: This malady is the most common genetic porphyria and reflects a deficiency of porphobilinogen deaminase activity in the liver. However, only 10% of gene carriers suffer clinical symptoms, which generally affect young adults. Colicky abdominal pain and neuropsychiatric symptoms predominate.

PORPHYRIA CUTANEA TARDA: This chronic hepatic porphyria is the most frequent porphyria and is either acquired or inherited as an autosomal dominant trait. It reflects deficient uroporphyrinogen decarboxylase activity in the liver. The typical patient is middle-aged or elderly, displays cutaneous photosensitivity, and suffers from liver disease with hepatic iron overload.

Other inherited porphyrias, termed *erythropoietic porphyrias* **and** *congenital erythropoietic porphyria,* **are caused by enzyme deficiencies in cells of erythrocytic lineage. They are characterized by cutaneous photosensitivity and occasionally liver disease.**

VASCULAR DISORDERS

Congestive Heart Failure Is the Major Cause of Liver Congestion

Acute Passive Congestion

At autopsy, it is common for the liver to be acutely congested, presumably because of a failing heart in the agonal period. On cut section, the liver is diffusely speckled with small red foci. Microscopically, they represent centrilobular zones with dilated and congested sinusoids and terminal venules. These changes are not clinically significant.

Chronic Passive Congestion

In the face of persistent congestive heart failure, the pressure in the peripheral venous circulation increases, thereby impeding venous outflow from liver and producing chronic passive congestion of that organ. The chronically congested liver is often reduced in size. The cut surface exhibits an accentuated lobular pattern, with a mottled appearance of alternating light and dark areas (Fig. 14-52), termed *nutmeg liver*. In severe cases, the centrilobular terminal venules and adjacent sinusoids are markedly dilated and filled with erythrocytes, and the liver cell plates in this zone are thinned by pressure atrophy.

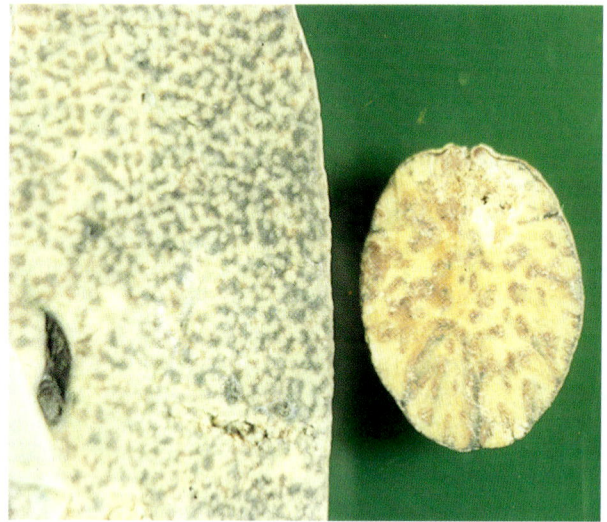

FIGURE 14-52
Chronic passive congestion of the liver. The surface of this fixed liver exhibits an accentuated lobular pattern, an appearance resembling that of a nutmeg *(right)*.

In cases of particularly severe and long-standing **right-sided heart failure** (e.g., tricuspid valvular disease or constrictive pericarditis), chronic passive congestion progresses to varying degrees of hepatic fibrosis. Delicate fibrous strands envelop terminal venules, and septa radiate from the centrilobular zones. Fibrous septa may link adjacent central veins, thereby producing a "reverse lobulation." Pressure atrophy of the centrilobular hepatocytes remains prominent. The older term *cardiac cirrhosis* is inappropriate, since the complete septa and regenerative nodules of true cirrhosis are rarely encountered.

Chronic passive congestion of the liver is of more pathological than clinical interest, since the condition has little effect on hepatic function. Features of portal hypertension, including splenomegaly and ascites, sometimes accompany chronic passive congestion of the liver.

Shock Results in Decreased Perfusion of the Liver

Shock from any cause often leads to ischemic necrosis of the centrilobular hepatocytes. The centrilobular zone, referred to as zone 3 in the functional concept of the hepatic acinus (see Fig. 14-2), is most distal to the blood supply from the portal tracts and is the area most vulnerable to ischemic insults. Microscopically, coagulative necrosis of centrilobular hepatocytes is accompanied by frank hemorrhage.

Infarction of the Liver Is Uncommon Because of Its Dual Blood Supply and the Anastomotic Structure of the Hepatic Sinusoids

Acute occlusion of the hepatic artery or its branches is unusual but can occur as a result of embolism, polyarteritis nodosa, or accidental ligation during surgery. Under such circumstances, irregular pale areas, often surrounded by a hyperemic zone, reflect the underlying ischemic necrosis.

Acute occlusion of intrahepatic branches of the portal vein, generally in the presence of elevated hepatic venous pressure, classically produces the *Zahn infarct*, a dark-red, triangular area with its base on the surface of the liver. Microscopically only dilation and congestion of the sinusoids are noted. Thus, the traditional term "infarct" is actually a misnomer.

BACTERIAL INFECTIONS

Bacterial infections are uncommon causes of liver disease in the industrialized countries and are for the most part complications of infections elsewhere. The characteristic reactions in the liver are granulomas, abscesses, and diffuse inflammation. Infections associated with granulomatous inflammation elsewhere (e.g., tuberculosis, tularemia, and brucellosis) also cause granulomatous hepatitis.

Pyogenic liver abscesses are produced by staphylococci, streptococci, and gram-negative enterobacteria. The morphological appearance of a pyogenic abscess in the liver is similar to that in other sites. Anaerobic inhabitants of the gastrointestinal tract, particularly *Bacteroides* species and microaerophilic streptococci, are common causes of liver abscesses. Organisms reach the liver in arterial or portal blood or through the biliary tract. In cases of septicemia, the liver is seeded with organisms from distant sites through the arterial blood.

Pylephlebitic abscesses (Fig. 14-53) result from intraabdominal suppuration, as in peritonitis or diverticulitis, with the organisms being transmitted to the liver in portal blood. At one time, pylephlebitis was the most common cause of hepatic abscesses, but the control of abdominal sepsis with antibiotics has rendered this route of infection uncommon.

Cholangitic abscesses in the liver are today the most common form of hepatic abscess in Western countries. Biliary obstruction from any cause is often complicated by bacterial infection of the biliary tree, termed *ascending cholangitis*. The retrograde biliary dissemination of organisms

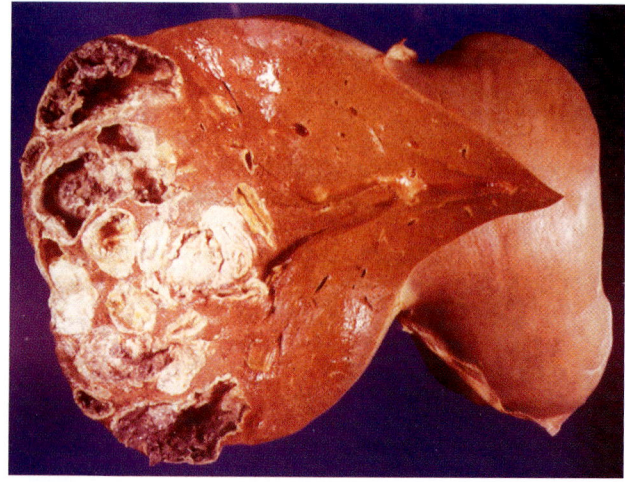

FIGURE 14-53
Pylephlebitic abscesses of the liver. The cut surface of the liver shows large, confluent, irregular abscess cavities.

(usually *Escherichia coli*) then leads to the formation of cholangitic abscesses.

Hepatic abscesses are more commonly located in the right lobe of the liver. Diffuse inflammation of the liver from bacterial infection is distinctly uncommon today but may be encountered in various septicemic states, particularly in immunocompromised patients. In about half of all cases of hepatic abscess, the source of infection cannot be demonstrated.

Clinical Features: A patient with a hepatic abscess typically presents with high fever, rapid weight loss, right upper quadrant abdominal pain, and hepatomegaly. Jaundice occurs in a fourth of cases, but the serum alkaline phosphatase level is almost always elevated. Solitary abscesses are treated with surgical drainage and antibiotics, but multiple abscesses present a difficult therapeutic problem. The complications of hepatic abscess relate principally to rupture and direct spread of the infection. Pleuropulmonary fistulas, from the rupture of an abscess through the diaphragm, and peritonitis, from leakage into the abdominal cavity, occur. The dissemination of organisms in the blood may lead to septicemia and metastatic abscesses in other parts of the body. The mortality from hepatic abscess, even in treated cases, remains high, ranging from 40 to 80%.

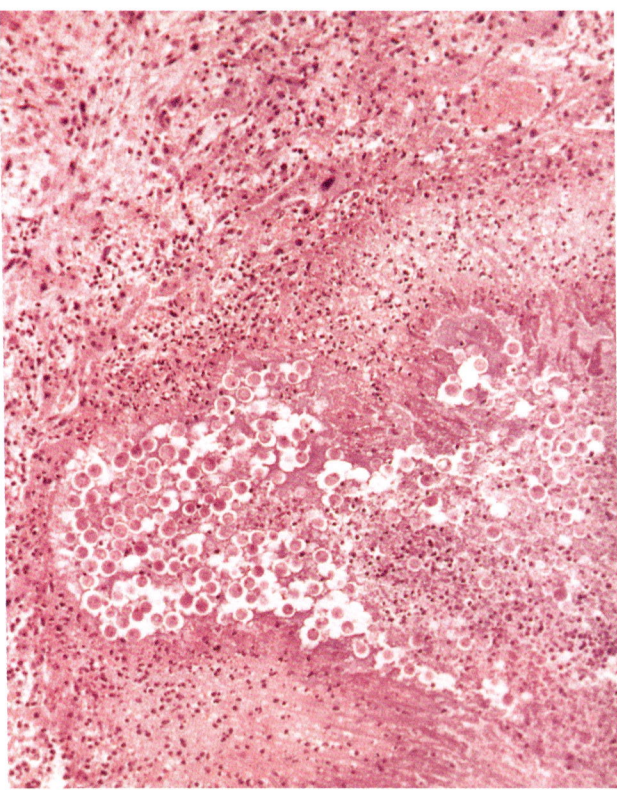

FIGURE 14-54
Amebic abscess of the liver. A photomicrograph of the margin of an amebic abscess shows fibroblastic proliferation surrounding the cavity and amebic trophozoites in the lumen.

PARASITIC INFESTATIONS

Parasitic infestations of the liver are a serious public health problem worldwide, although they are uncommon in industrialized countries. These diseases are discussed in Chapter 9. Here we summarize the major parasitic diseases that affect the liver.

Protozoal Diseases Frequently Involve the Liver

AMEBIASIS: In the United States, the carrier rate for *Entamoeba histolytica* is probably less than 5%, but a prevalence up to 35% has been reported in homosexual men. Amebiasis of the liver, the most common extraintestinal complication, leads to amebic abscesses, which are multiple in about half of cases (Fig. 14-54).

On gross examination, an amebic abscess typically ranges from 8 to 12 cm in diameter, appears well circumscribed, and contains thick, dark material that has been likened to anchovy paste or chocolate. Microscopically, the trophozoites can usually be visualized in the periphery of the necrotic debris.

The symptoms associated with amebic abscesses are similar to those that characterize pyogenic abscesses. With appropriate treatment (tissue amebicides), the abscess may heal and leave only residual scar tissue. Surgical drainage of large abscesses is important. If an amebic abscess continues to grow, it may rupture into the peritoneal cavity, where it produces peritonitis, a complication associated with a mortality rate as high as 40%. The amebae may also invade the blood, in which case abscesses of the brain and lung may ensue.

MALARIA: Hepatic involvement in malaria is a frequent cause of hepatomegaly in endemic areas. It reflects Kupffer cell hypertrophy and hyperplasia secondary to phagocytosis of the debris resulting from the rupture of parasitized erythrocytes. This hepatic involvement does not give rise to significant hepatic dysfunction.

VISCERAL LEISHMANIASIS (KALA AZAR): As in malaria, the hepatomegaly of chronic visceral leishmaniasis reflects hyperplasia of mononuclear phagocytes in the liver. In contrast to malaria, however, the Kupffer cells ingest the parasitic organisms themselves, which appear as *Donovan bodies*. Clinically, there is little evidence of hepatic dysfunction.

Helminthic Diseases Are Problems of Underdeveloped Areas

Diseases caused by helminths are described in Chapter 9, and *hepatic schistosomiasis* is discussed above in the context of portal hypertension.

ASCARIASIS: From the duodenum, the worms of *Ascaris lumbricoides* gain access to the biliary tree, where they may produce acute biliary colic. When the worms lodge in the intrahepatic biliary passages, their disintegration results in the liberation of innumerable eggs, which precipitate severe, suppurative cholangitis. The resulting cholangitic abscesses may rupture into the peritoneal cavity or into the pleural space. Spread of the infection into the hepatic or portal veins causes pylephlebitis, a highly dangerous complication.

At autopsy, the liver is enlarged and numerous irregular cavities contain foul-smelling material in which the remnants of degenerated parasites are found.

LIVER FLUKES: The major parasitic flukes that involve the human liver are *Clonorchis sinensis* and *Fasciola hepatica*. Humans are the definitive host for *C. sinensis*, whereas sheep and cattle are the principal reservoir of *F. hepatica*. Both parasites lodge in the intrahepatic biliary tree, where they provoke hyperplasia of the biliary epithelium, particularly severe in clonorchiasis (Fig. 14-55). In severe infestation with *C. sinensis*, the accumulation of material from degenerated worms, parasite eggs, and viscid mucus (secreted by metaplastic goblet cells in the biliary epithelium) obstructs intrahepatic bile flow and leads to intrahepatic pigment gallstones. Secondary infection of the bile with *E. coli* causes cholangitis and cholangitic abscesses, which are common causes of surgical emergencies in some Asian countries. **Biliary infestation with *C. sinensis* is an etiologic factor in the development of cholangiocarcinoma.**

ECHINOCOCCOSIS (CYSTIC HYDATID DISEASE): Infection with the tapeworms of the genus *Echinococcus*, principally *E. granulosus*, is an important zoonosis that involves the human liver. Echinococcal cysts expand slowly and produce symptoms only after many years. Within the liver, the cyst behaves as a space-occupying lesion; systemic manifestations reflect toxic or allergic reactions to the absorption of constituents of the organisms.

Leptospirosis (Weil Disease) Is an Accidental Infection from a Zoonosis

Leptospira spirochetes infect many animal species. Despite the animal reservoir of leptospira, fewer than one fifth of patients who contract leptospirosis give a history of direct contact with animals. **Weil syndrome** refers to leptospirosis complicated by prolonged fever and jaundice and in severe cases by azotemia, hemorrhages, and altered consciousness. Weil syndrome occurs in only 1 to 6% of all cases of leptospirosis. The morphological alterations of the liver in fatal cases are nonspecific and include focal necrosis, enlarged Kupffer cells, and centrilobular cholestasis. The organisms are generally not demonstrable in the liver.

Hepatic Lesions of Syphilis Were Common but Are Now Rare

Congenital syphilis causes neonatal hepatitis, which results in diffuse fibrosis in the portal tracts and around individual liver cells or groups of hepatocytes.

Tertiary syphilis is characterized by hepatic gummas (i.e., focal lesions resembling granulomas), which heal with dense scars. Retraction produces deep clefts and a gross pseudolobation of the liver, termed *hepar lobatum*, a condition that should not be confused with cirrhosis.

CHOLESTATIC SYNDROMES OF INFANCY

Diseases characterized by prolonged cholestasis and jaundice in infants represent either diseases primarily affecting the hepatocytes or obstruction of the biliary system.

Neonatal Hepatitis Is an Entity of Multiple Causes

Neonatal hepatitis features prolonged cholestasis, morphological evidence of liver cell injury, and inflammation.

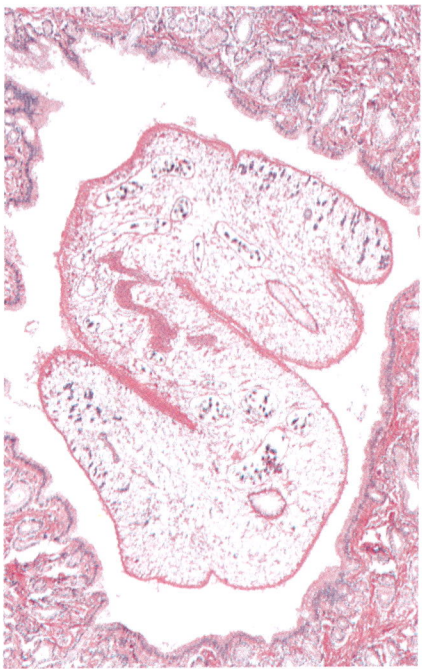

FIGURE 14-55
Infection of the liver by *Clonorchis sinensis*. The lumen of a bile duct contains an adult liver fluke, and the mucosa is hyperplastic.

 Pathogenesis: In about half of all cases of neonatal hepatitis, the cause is discernible (Table 14-5), and about 30% of cases are assigned to α_1-antitrypsin deficiency alone. Most of the other cases with known causes can be attributed to viral hepatitis B and infectious agents such as those of the TORCH group (*t*oxoplasmosis, "*o*ther", *r*ubella, *c*ytomegalovirus, and *h*erpes simplex). A few cases represent hepatic injury associated with metabolic defects, for instance, galactosemia or fructose intolerance.

TABLE 14-5 Causes of Neonatal Hepatitis

Idiopathic
   Idiopathic neonatal hepatitis
   Prolonged intrahepatic cholestasis
     Arteriohepatic dysplasia (Alagille syndrome)
     Paucity of intrahepatic bile ducts not associated with specific syndromes
     Zellweger syndrome (cerebrohepatorenal syndrome)
     Byler disease
Mechanical obstruction of the intrahepatic bile ducts
   Congenital hepatic fibrosis
   Caroli disease (cystic dilation of intrahepatic ducts)
Metabolic disorders
   Defects of carbohydrate metabolism
     Galactosemia
     Hereditary fructose intolerance
     Glycogenosis type IV
   Defects of lipid metabolism
     Gaucher disease
     Niemann-Pick disease
     Wolman disease
   Tyrosinemia (defect of amino acid metabolism)
   α_1-Antitrypsin deficiency
   Cystic fibrosis
   Parenteral nutrition
Hepatitis
   Hepatitis B
   TORCH agents
   Varicella
   Syphilis
   ECHO viruses
   Neonatal sepsis
Chromosomal abnormalities
   Down syndrome
   Trisomy 18
Extrahepatic biliary atresia

Occasional cases of neonatal hepatitis are seen in association with Down syndrome and other chromosomal disorders. The remaining half of all cases of neonatal hepatitis are of unexplained etiology.

 Pathology: The characteristic hepatic lesion of neonatal hepatitis is giant cell transformation of hepatocytes, hence the former term *giant cell hepatitis* (Fig. 14-56). The giant cells contain as many as 40 nuclei and may appear detached from other cells in the liver plate. The pale, distended cytoplasm contains large amounts of glycogen and iron. The number of giant cells decreases with time, and they are rare in children older than 1 year of age. Bile pigment is often prominent within canaliculi and hepatocytes. Ballooned hepatocytes, acinar transformation of hepatocytes, and acidophilic bodies are also typical of neonatal hepatitis. Extramedullary hematopoiesis is often conspicuous. Chronic inflammatory infiltrates are seen in the portal tracts as well as in the lobular parenchyma. Pericellular fibrosis around degenerating hepatocytes, singly or in groups, is common, and fibrous tissue septa extend from the portal tracts.

Biliary Atresia Refers to the Lack of a Lumen in the Biliary Tree

Both extrahepatic and intrahepatic biliary atresias are often associated with the morphological features of neonatal hepatitis.

Extrahepatic Biliary Atresia

Extrahepatic biliary atresia is a cholestatic disease characterized by obliteration of the lumen of all or part of the biliary tree external to the liver. It accounts for almost half of all cases of persistent cholestasis in the neonatal period. Of these, about 20% exhibit associated congenital anomalies, including abnormalities of the heart, intestine, and spleen. Other instances of extrahepatic biliary obstruction are associated with known causes of neonatal hepatitis, such as chromosomal abnormalities (trisomies) and a number of viral infections.

 Pathology: Extrahepatic biliary atresia may involve all the extrahepatic bile ducts or may be restricted to segments of the proximal or distal biliary tree. At one extreme, acute and chronic periluminal inflammation is prominent. Epithelial necrosis is evident, and cellular debris is found in the obstructed or narrow lumen. At the other extreme, the original lumen is completely replaced by mature connective tissue, and little or no inflammation is present. Histologically, cholestasis and periportal bile ductular proliferation in the liver are evident. A minority of cases

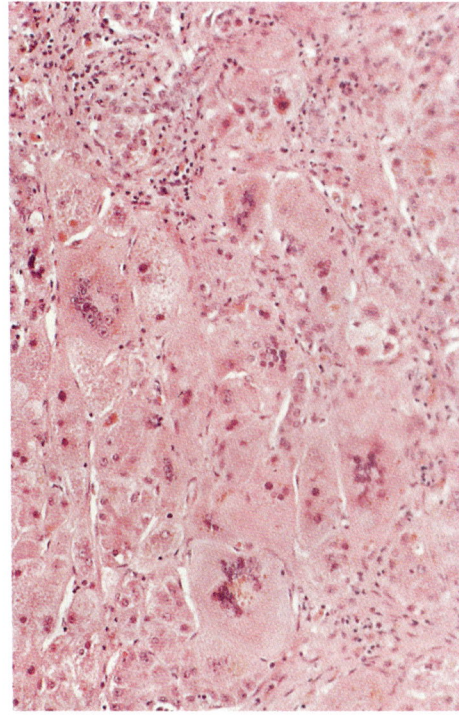

FIGURE 14-56
Neonatal hepatitis. A photomicrograph shows multinucleated giant hepatocytes, liver cell injury, and a mild chronic inflammatory infiltrate.

display multinucleated giant hepatocytes, identical to those seen in neonatal hepatitis. Although the intrahepatic bile ducts may initially appear normal, they are gradually obliterated with the persistence of cholestasis. Eventually, secondary biliary cirrhosis supervenes.

Intrahepatic Biliary Atresia

Intrahepatic biliary atresia refers to a paucity of bile ducts within the liver. The disorder occurs under three different circumstances:

- In association with known causes of neonatal hepatitis (e.g., α_1-AT deficiency, various chromosomal anomalies, and metabolic derangements)
- **Alagille syndrome** (syndromic bile duct paucity), an autosomal dominant disease, also characterized by congenital abnormalities of the heart, eye, skeleton, kidneys, and central nervous system, which involves mutation in the Notch signaling pathway
- Unassociated with other conditions (idiopathic)

Pathology: The major histological feature of intrahepatic biliary atresia is a scarcity of bile ducts in the liver. Cholestasis, giant cell transformation, and bile ductular proliferation are usual. However, cirrhosis is uncommon.

Many observations support the concept that neonatal hepatitis, intrahepatic biliary atresia, extrahepatic biliary atresia, and possibly choledochal cyst all result from a common inflammatory process (*infantile obstructive cholangiopathy*).

Clinical Features: Most patients who have uncomplicated neonatal hepatitis recover without sequelae. Intrahepatic biliary atresia associated with neonatal hepatitis carries a grave prognosis, since many of these children progress to biliary cirrhosis. By contrast, the outlook in Alagille syndrome is good. Uncorrected extrahepatic biliary atresia invariably results in progressive secondary biliary cirrhosis and is incompatible with survival. Although surgical correction has been successful in some anatomically favorable cases, most cases of both extrahepatic and intrahepatic biliary atresia are cured only by liver transplantation.

BENIGN TUMORS AND TUMORLIKE LESIONS

Hepatic Adenomas Are Benign Tumors of Hepatocytes That Occur Principally in Women

Hepatic adenomas were exceedingly rare before the availability of oral contraceptives, but since their introduction, many such neoplasms have been reported. The incidence has been reduced by the use of newer combinations of estrogen and progesterone.

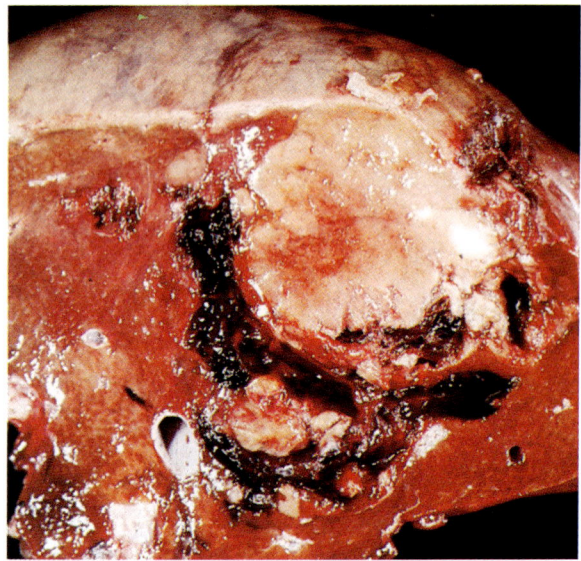
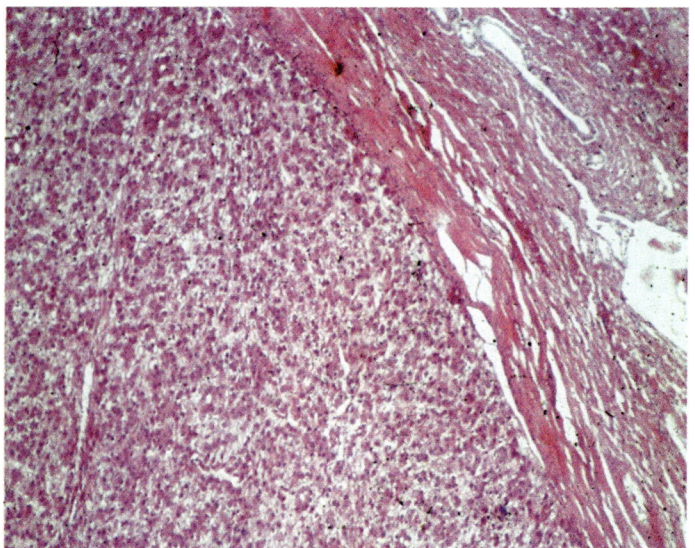

FIGURE 14-57
Hepatic adenoma. **A.** A surgically resected portion of liver shows a tan, lobulated mass beneath the liver capsule. Hemorrhage into the tumor has broken through the capsule and also into the surrounding liver parenchyma. The patient was a woman who had taken birth control pills for a number of years and presented with sudden intraperitoneal hemorrhage. **B.** A fibrous capsule separates normal liver and the adenoma *(left)*. The adenomatous hepatocytes are arranged without discernible lobular architecture and show a clear cytoplasm filled with glycogen.

Pathology: Hepatic adenomas usually occur as solitary, sharply demarcated masses, up to 40 cm in diameter and 3 kg in weight (Fig. 14-57). In a fourth of cases, multiple smaller adenomas are present. On gross examination, the tumor is encapsulated and paler than the surrounding parenchyma.

Microscopically, the neoplastic hepatocytes resemble their normal counterparts, except that they are not arranged in a lobular architecture (see Fig. 14-57). Portal tracts and central venules are absent. The cells making up the adenoma may be very large and eosinophilic or filled with glycogen, which makes the cytoplasm appear clear. The tumor is circumscribed by a fibrous capsule of variable thickness, and the adjacent hepatocytes appear compressed. Large, thick-walled arteries are often seen in the vicinity of the capsule, and arteries and veins traverse the tumor.

Clinical Features: In about one third of patients with hepatic adenomas (particularly in pregnant women who have used oral contraceptives), **the tumors bleed into the peritoneal cavity and require treatment as a surgical emergency.** Even large adenomas have been reported to disappear after discontinuation of oral contraceptive use. A few adenomas are encountered in men, and they have occasionally been reported in association with the use of anabolic steroids.

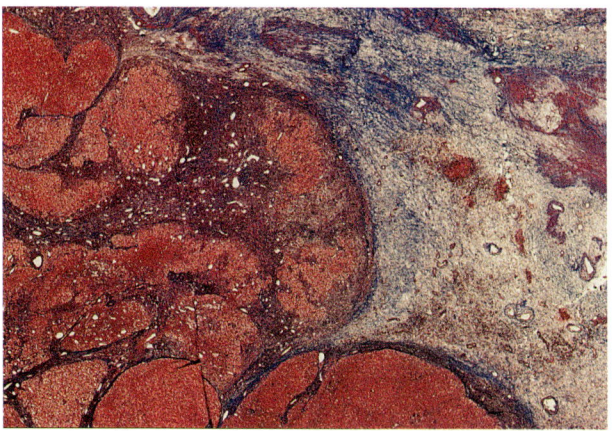

FIGURE 14-58
Focal nodular hyperplasia. A photomicrograph of a surgically resected mass from the liver shows a vascular central scar and irregular fibrous septa dissecting hepatic parenchyma, accounting for the resemblance to cirrhosis.

Focal Nodular Hyperplasia Is a Nodular Lesion That Resembles Cirrhosis

The lesion of focal nodular hyperplasia varies from 5 to 15 cm in diameter and weighs as much as 700 g. On occasion, it protrudes from the surface of the liver, and it may even be pedunculated. The cut surface exhibits a characteristic central scar from which fibrous septa radiate. The division of the mass by multiple fibrous septa accounts for the older term *focal cirrhosis.* Microscopically, hepatocytic nodules are circumscribed by fibrous septa (Fig. 14-58), which contain numerous tortuous bile ducts and mononuclear inflammatory cells. Within the nodules, lobular architecture is absent. The lesion exhibits large arteries and veins in the septa, but hemorrhage is uncommon.

Focal nodular hyperplasia occurs in both sexes and at all ages but most often in young women. It is not a neoplasm and is not associated with the use of oral contraceptives.

Nodular Regenerative Hyperplasia (Nodular Transformation of the Liver, Partial Nodular Transformation) Causes Portal Hypertension

Nodular regenerative hyperplasia is characterized by small, hyperplastic nodules without fibrosis in an otherwise normal liver. The lesion may be partial and located predominantly in the perihilar region or may be diffuse throughout the liver. The nodules are composed of liver cells arranged in plates that are two and three cells thick, which compress the surrounding parenchyma.

The clinical importance of nodular regenerative hyperplasia relates to its association with portal hypertension, which accounts for the older term *noncirrhotic portal hypertension.* The etiology is unknown, but it has been reported in association with the use of oral contraceptives or anabolic steroids, extrahepatic infections, neoplasms, chronic inflammatory disorders, and autoimmune diseases. Nodular regenerative hyperplasia is not preneoplastic.

Hepatic Hemangiomas Are the Most Common Tumors of the Liver

Benign hemangiomas in the liver occur at all ages and in both sexes and are found in up to 7% of autopsy specimens. They are ordinarily small and asymptomatic, although larger tumors have been reported to cause abdominal symptoms and even hemorrhage into the peritoneal cavity. Grossly, the tumor is usually solitary and less than 5 cm in diameter, but multiple hemangiomas and giant forms have been described. Microscopically, the tumor is similar to cavernous hemangiomas found elsewhere.

Infantile hemangioendothelioma, a rare cellular tumor that appears during the first 2 years of life (and sometimes at birth), contains arteriovenous shunts that may be large enough to cause congestive heart failure. Malignant transformation has been reported in a few cases.

Cystic Disease of the Liver Represents a Spectrum of Lesions

BILE DUCT MICROHAMARTOMAS (VON MEYENBURG COMPLEXES): These clinically inapparent lesions consist of anomalous, small cystic bile ducts embedded in a fibrous stroma. They are usually multiple and vary from barely visible grayish white foci to nodules 1 cm in diameter.

Microscopically, the cysts are lined by bile duct epithelium and sometimes contain inspissated bile.

SOLITARY AND MULTIPLE SIMPLE CYSTS: Simple cysts of the liver are lined by cuboidal to columnar epithelium and are occasionally associated with adult polycystic disease of the kidney (see Chapter 16). They are not infrequently seen in livers that contain von Meyenburg complexes.

CONGENITAL HEPATIC FIBROSIS: This recessively inherited disorder is marked by enlarged portal tracts that exhibit extensive fibrosis and numerous bile ductules. It is seen predominantly in children and adolescents. The bile ductules may be so dilated that they resemble microcysts, but even in these cases, they retain their communication with the biliary system. Regenerative nodules are absent, an appearance that distinguishes this condition from cirrhosis. The origin of the lesion is unknown, but it has been postulated that it may result from abnormal differentiation of primitive duct structures. **The principal complication of congenital hepatic fibrosis is severe portal hypertension with recurrent bleeding from esophageal varices.** *Infantile polycystic disease* of the liver resembles congenital hepatic fibrosis and is also inherited as an autosomal recessive trait.

MALIGNANT TUMORS OF THE LIVER

Hepatocellular Carcinoma (HCC) Is a Malignant Tumor That Derives from Hepatocytes or Their Precursors

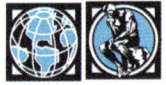

Epidemiology and Pathogenesis: HCC is probably the most common malignant tumor of humans. It occurs in all parts of the world, but its incidence shows a striking geographical variability. In Western industrialized countries, the tumor is uncommon, although the incidence of HCC has nearly doubled in the last 20 years; in sub-Saharan Africa, Southeast Asia, and Japan, the rates are up to 50 times greater. For example, in Mozambique, which seems to have the highest incidence in the world, two thirds of all cancers in men and one third in women are HCC. The incidence of HCC in the United States is expected to rise owing to the increased prevalence of HCV infection.

HEPATITIS B: **An association between HCC and infection with HBV is clearly established.** More than 85% of cases of HCC occur in countries with a high prevalence of chronic HBV infection. Most patients have chronic HBV infection for many years, the disease often being transmitted from an infected mother to her newborn child perinatally. Persistent HBV infection is indeed dangerous, since such persons are estimated to have as much as a 200-fold increased risk of developing HCC. One fourth of those with chronic hepatitis B acquired at or near birth ultimately develop HCC. The risk of HCC in men who are positive for HBsAg and HBeAg is about four times as great as in those who are positive only for HBsAg. Most (>80%) cases of HCC associated with HBV infection occur in patients with cirrhosis, although numerous instances are reported in noncirrhotic chronic hepatitis B.

The genome of HBV is integrated into the host DNA of both the nonneoplastic liver cells and the tumor cells. The X gene of HBV encodes a viral protein (HBxAg) that inactivates tumor suppressor proteins and transactivates certain oncogenes. The worldwide use of a vaccine for HBV should significantly decrease the prevalence of HCC in the future. The role of HBV itself in the pathogenesis of liver cancer is discussed in Chapter 5.

HEPATITIS C: Although hepatitis C has a lower global prevalence than hepatitis B, the former is associated with most cases of HCC in Europe and North America and has overtaken hepatitis B as a cause of HCC in Japan. As in hepatitis B, most patients with HCV who develop HCC have underlying cirrhosis. The cumulative rate for HCC in persons with HCV-induced cirrhosis is as high as 70% after 15 years.

The risk of liver cancer in persons who are infected with both HCV and HBV is three times higher than with either alone. The mechanism by which HCV leads to HCC is not understood, but experimental evidence suggests an important role for the interaction of HCV core protein with a variety of cellular proteins.

OTHER CAUSES OF HCC: **Alcoholic cirrhosis** has been considered by some to predispose to HCC. However, the high prevalence of infection with HBV and HCV in patients with alcoholic cirrhosis has called this association into question.

Liver diseases occurring in conjunction with **hemochromatosis** and **α_1-AT deficiency** carry a substantial risk of HCC; about 10% of patients with hemochromatosis may be expected to develop the tumor. On the other hand, HCC is rare in patients with "autoimmune" chronic hepatitis and cirrhosis, Wilson disease, and primary biliary cirrhosis.

Aflatoxin B_1, a fungal contaminant of many foods, particularly in less-developed countries, produces HCC in a number of mammalian species. The incidence of liver cancer in humans has also been roughly correlated with the content of aflatoxin in the diet. Studies in China have reported that the presence of urinary metabolites of aflatoxin B_1 is associated with a threefold increased risk of HCC, and the combination of these metabolites with HBV is synergistic, increasing the risk of HCC 60-fold.

Analyses of DNA from HCC in Africa and China, two areas with a high incidence of this cancer, revealed that as many as half of the samples had mutations in the *p53* gene. Interestingly, most of these mutations were G-to-T substitutions in one particular codon (249), a change known to be produced experimentally by aflatoxin B_1.

 Pathology: HCCs appear grossly as soft, hemorrhagic tan masses in the liver (Fig. 14-59). Occasionally, a green color is present, indicating bile staining. In some cases, a large solitary tumor occupies a portion of the liver; in other cases, many smaller tumors are found. Multiple lesions may indicate a multicentric origin of the tumor, although intrahepatic metastases from a single

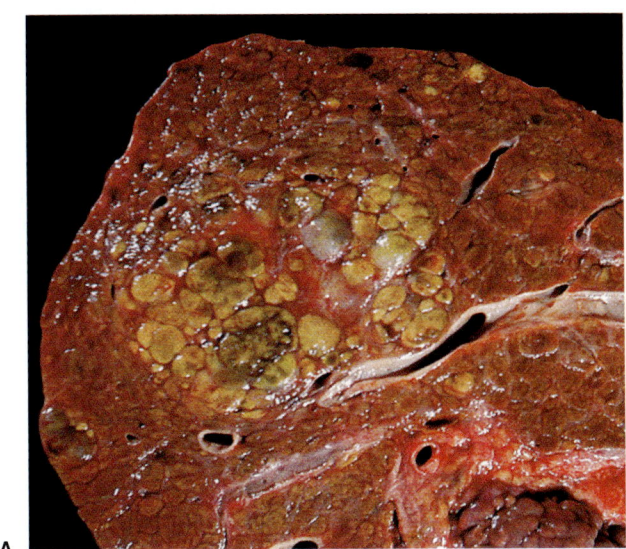
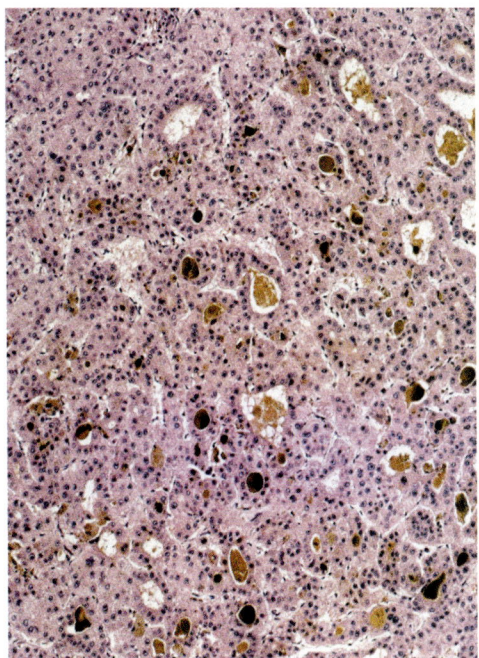

FIGURE 14-59
Hepatocellular carcinoma. A. Cross-section of a cirrhotic liver shows a poorly circumscribed, nodular area of yellow, partially hemorrhagic hepatocellular carcinoma. B. A photomicrograph of the tumor shows a trabecular pattern of malignant hepatocytes. Many cells are arranged in an acinar pattern and surround concretions of inspissated bile.

HCC cannot be excluded. The tumor has a tendency to grow into portal veins and may extend into the vena cava and even the right atrium through the hepatic veins. Metastases occur widely, but the most common sites are the lungs and portal lymph nodes.

The histological spectrum of HCC is variable, ranging from well-differentiated tumor difficult to distinguish from normal liver to an anaplastic or undifferentiated appearance. A number of histological patterns are recognized, but no prognostic significance can be attributed to any of them. Most HCCs exhibit a *trabecular pattern*, that is, the tumor cells are arranged in trabeculae or plates that resemble the normal liver (see Fig. 14-59). The plates are separated by endothelium-lined sinusoids. A second histological variant is termed the *pseudoglandular (adenoid, acinar) pattern*. In this variety, malignant hepatocytes are arranged around a lumen and thus resemble glands. The lumina may contain bile. The acini formed by the tumor cells are not true glands, and the lesion should not be confused with adenocarcinoma.

Fibrolamellar HCC is an uncommon variant that has a distinctive histological appearance and arises in an apparently normal liver, principally in adolescents and young adults. The tumor is composed of large, eosinophilic, neoplastic hepatocytes arranged in clusters and surrounded by delicate collagen fibers (Fig. 14-60). The prognosis is more favorable than in most cases of HCC.

Clinical Features: HCC usually presents as a painful and enlarging mass in the liver. The prognosis is dismal, and patients die of malignant cachexia, rupture of the tumor with catastrophic bleeding into the peritoneal cavity, or complications of cirrhosis.

HCC may be associated with a variety of paraneoplastic manifestations (e.g., polycythemia, hypoglycemia, hypercalcemia) as a result of hormone production by the tumor. α-Fetoprotein levels are often elevated in HCC (and may also be encountered in other neoplastic and nonneoplastic liver diseases and in some extrahepatic disorders).

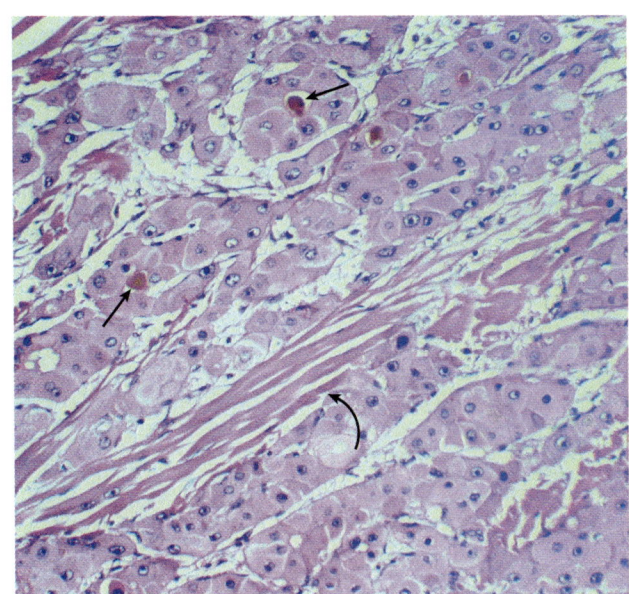

FIGURE 14-60
Fibrolamellar hepatocellular carcinoma. Eosinophilic tumor cells show a lamellar pattern. A fibrous band (curved arrow) traverses the tumor. Bile casts (straight arrows) are seen within neoplastic acinia.

In the cases of small tumors confined to one hepatic lobe, segmental resections of the liver have been successful in curing HCC in as many as half of patients. Hepatic transplantation has been used for larger tumors with disappointing results.

Cholangiocarcinoma (Bile Duct Carcinoma) Arises from Biliary Epithelium

Cholangiocarcinoma originates anywhere in the biliary tree, from the large intrahepatic bile ducts at the porta hepatis to the smallest bile ductules at the periphery of the hepatic lobule. The tumor occurs predominantly in older persons of both sexes, with an average age at presentation of 60 years. This cancer is particularly frequent in the parts of Asia in which the liver fluke *(C. sinensis)* is endemic, although cholangiocarcinoma is encountered in all parts of the world.

Pathology: Peripheral cholangiocarcinomas are composed of small cuboidal cells arranged in a ductular or glandular configuration (Fig. 14-61). Characteristically, they show substantial fibrosis, and on liver biopsy, they may be confused with metastatic scirrhous carcinoma of the breast or pancreas. A combined form of hepatocellular carcinoma and peripheral cholangiocarcinoma has been labeled *cholangiohepatocellular carcinoma*.

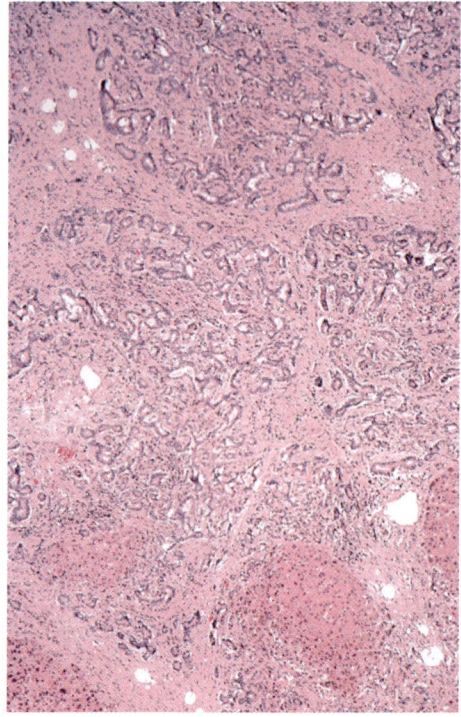

FIGURE 14-61
Cholangiocarcinoma. Well-differentiated neoplastic glands are embedded in a dense fibrous stroma.

Hilar cholangiocarcinomas are extrahepatic lesions that arise at the convergence of the right and left hepatic ducts. They present three histological patterns: (1) a small sclerosing tumor that obliterates the duct, (2) a tumor that spreads within the wall of the duct, and (3) a rare intraductal papillary variant. They produce symptoms of extrahepatic biliary obstruction.

Cholangiocarcinomas show less tendency to invade the portal and hepatic veins than do hepatocellular carcinomas. They metastasize to a wide variety of extrahepatic sites and show a greater predilection for the portal lymph nodes than do hepatocellular carcinomas. Liver transplantation has been attempted in patients with cholangiocarcinoma but is rarely successful in eradicating the tumor.

Hepatoblastoma Is a Rare Malignant Tumor of Children

Hepatoblastoma is usually discovered at birth or before the age of 3 years.

Pathology: Hepatoblastoma presents as a partially necrotic and hemorrhagic circumscribed mass up to 25 cm in diameter. Microscopically, cells of epithelial and mesenchymal appearance are seen, but occasionally the latter are missing. The epithelial component of hepatoblastoma includes cells resembling embryonal and fetal cells. The "embryonal" cells are small and fusiform and are arranged in ribbons or rosettes. The "fetal" cells more closely resemble hepatocytes, contain glycogen and fat, and are arranged in trabeculae with intervening sinusoids. Foci of squamous epithelium are occasionally encountered. The mesenchymal elements include those often present in teratomas, including connective tissue, cartilage, and osteoid.

Clinical Features: Attention is called to the presence of a hepatoblastoma by enlargement of the abdomen, vomiting, and failure to thrive. The serum α-fetoprotein level is almost invariably elevated, and occasionally secretion of ectopic gonadotropin leads to sexual precocity. Some of these children also exhibit congenital anomalies, including cardiac and renal malformations, hemihypertrophy, and macroglossia. Untreated hepatoblastomas are fatal, but liver transplantation or surgical resection by partial hepatectomy has been curative in many instances.

Hemangiosarcoma May Result from Exposure to Chemicals

Hemangiosarcoma is the only important sarcoma of the liver. As noted above, this malignant vascular tumor may result from exposure to thorium dioxide, vinyl chloride, or inorganic arsenic. Hemangiosarcoma of the liver is now distinctly uncommon.

 Pathology: On gross examination, hemangiosarcoma is characteristically multicentric, presenting as multiple hemorrhagic nodules that may coalesce. Microscopic examination reveals spindle-shaped, neoplastic, endothelial cells that line the sinusoids and compress the liver cell plates. The neoplasm may form cavernous blood spaces and solid masses of neoplastic cells. Widespread metastases are usual.

Clinical Features: Patients with hemangiosarcoma of the liver present with hepatomegaly, jaundice, and ascites. Hematological abnormalities, including pancytopenia and hemolytic anemia, are often prominent and in many cases reflect splenomegaly from noncirrhotic portal hypertension. The tumor may rupture and bleed vigorously into the abdominal cavity. The prognosis is poor.

Metastatic Cancer Is the Most Common Malignant Tumor of the Liver

The liver is involved in a third of all metastatic cancers, including half of those of the gastrointestinal tract, breast, and lung. Other tumors that characteristically metastasize to the liver are pancreatic carcinoma and malignant melanoma, although virtually any cancer may find its way to the liver.

 Pathology: The liver may show only a single nodule of tumor or may be virtually replaced by metastases (Fig. 14-62), and liver weights of 5 kg or more are not uncommon. **In fact, liver metastases are the most common cause of massive hepatomegaly.** Metastatic carcinomas are often seen on the surface of the liver as umbilicated masses, a reflection of central necrosis and hemorrhage. The metastatic deposits tend to be histologically similar to the primary tumor, but on occasion are so undifferentiated that the primary site cannot be determined.

 Clinical Features: Weight loss is a common early finding in cases of metastatic cancer in the liver. Portal hypertension with splenomegaly, ascites, and gastrointestinal bleeding may occur. Obstruction of the major bile ducts or replacement of most of the liver parenchyma leads to jaundice. If the patient lives long enough, hepatic failure may ensue. Often the first indication of a metastatic tumor is an unexplained increase in the serum alkaline phosphatase level. Most patients die within a year of the diagnosis of liver metastases. However, surgical resection of a solitary metastasis to the liver has often resulted in cures.

LIVER TRANSPLANTATION

The increasing availability of hepatic transplantation and the accompanying problems related to allograft rejection have focused attention on the morphological criteria by which the outcome can be assessed and therapy recommended. Despite immunosuppressive therapy, some patients subjected to hepatic transplantation develop graft rejection.

 Pathology: Acute rejection features distortion of the bile ducts by a portal inflammatory infiltrate, atypism of bile duct epithelial cells, and often inflammation of the ductal epithelium itself (Fig. 14-63). Lymphocytes often adhere to the endothelium of terminal venules and small branches of the portal veins, with or without subendothelial inflammation. This appearance has been termed *endothelialitis*.

Allograft rejection persisting for more than 2 months generally exhibits **damage to interlobular bile ducts.** As the lesion progresses, these small bile ducts are destroyed, and persistent cholestasis ensues. The end stage of this process is referred to as *vanishing bile duct syndrome*. Subintimal foam cells, intimal sclerosis, and myointimal hyperplasia may narrow or occlude these arteries (Fig. 14-64).

The Gallbladder and Extrahepatic Bile Ducts

ANATOMY

The gallbladder originates from the same foregut diverticulum that gives rise to the liver. It is a thin elongated sac

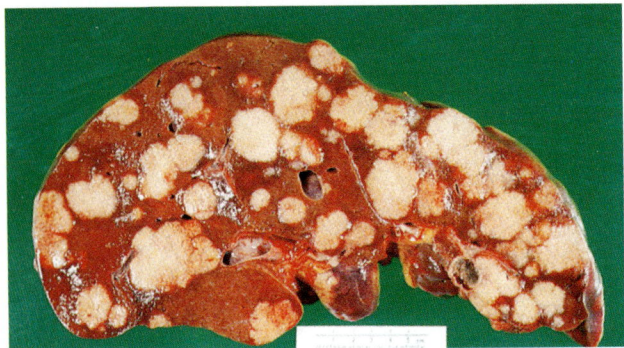

FIGURE 14-62
Metastatic carcinoma in the liver. The cut surface of the liver shows many firm, pale masses of metastatic colon cancer.

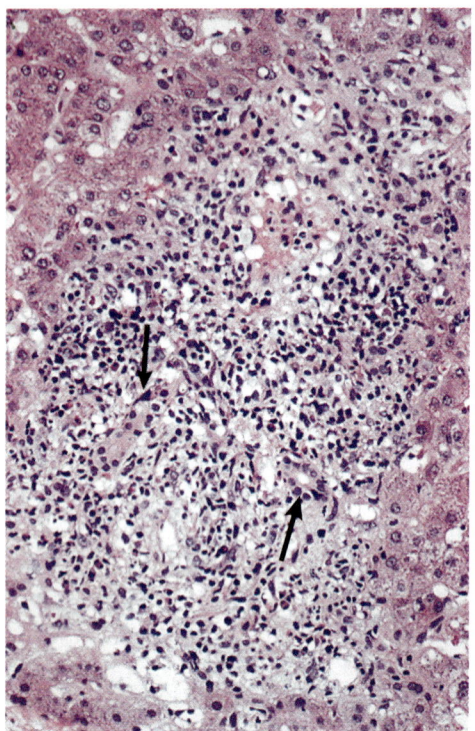

FIGURE 14-63
Acute rejection of a liver transplant. A portal tract is expanded by a polymorphous inflammatory infiltrate consisting of large and small lymphocytes, plasma cells, macrophages, and neutrophils. The bile ducts (arrows) are damaged.

about 8 cm long and about 50 mL in volume that occupies a fossa on the inferior surface of the liver between the right and the quadrate lobes. The primary function of the gallbladder is the storage, concentration, and release of bile. The cystic duct, which drains the gallbladder into the hepatic duct, is about 3 cm long. Dilute bile from the hepatic duct passes into the gallbladder through the cystic duct, where it is concentrated and subsequently discharged into the common bile duct.

The wall of the gallbladder is composed of a mucous membrane, a muscularis, and an adventitia and is covered by a reflection of the visceral peritoneum. The mucosa is thrown into folds and consists of a columnar epithelium and a lamina propria of loose connective tissue. Dipping into the wall of the gallbladder are mucosal diverticula, termed *Rokitansky-Aschoff sinuses*.

CONGENITAL ANOMALIES

Developmental anomalies of the gallbladder are rare and of little clinical significance except for the surgeon. Anomalies of the bile duct include **duplication** and **accessory bile ducts**. Congenital dilations of the bile duct are termed *choledochal cyst* (85% of all cases), *choledochal diverticulum*, and *choledochocele* (Fig. 14-65). Multiple cysts may occur as segmental dilations in the entire extrahepatic biliary tree. Similar multiple dilations in the intrahepatic portion of the biliary tree, termed *Caroli disease*, predispose to bacterial cholangitis. It has been suggested that choledochal cysts form part of the same complex as neonatal hepatitis and biliary atresia.

CHOLELITHIASIS

Cholelithiasis is defined as the presence of stones within the lumen of the gallbladder or in the extrahepatic biliary tree. Three fourths of gallstones in the industrialized countries consist primarily of cholesterol, and the remainder are composed of calcium bilirubinate and other calcium salts (pigment gallstones). However, pigment stones predominate in the tropics and the Orient. Most gallstones are not radiopaque, but they are readily visualized by ultrasound examination. Although gallstones are frequently asymptomatic, they often cause mild-to-severe pain *(biliary colic)* as a result of impaction in the cystic duct or (less frequently) in the common bile duct.

Cholesterol Stones Are the Most Common Gallstones

Cholesterol stones are round or faceted, yellow to tan, and single or multiple. They vary from 1 to 4 cm in greatest dimension (Fig. 14-66). Well over 50% of the stone is composed of cholesterol; the rest consists of calcium salts and mucin.

Epidemiology: Some 20% of American men and 35% of women older than the age of 75 years have gallstones at autopsy. **However, during their reproductive period, women are three times more likely to develop cholesterol gallstones than are men,** the incidence being higher in users of oral contraceptives and in women with several pregnancies. Interestingly, cholesterol gallstones are exceedingly common in Pima Indian women of the American Southwest, among whom 75% are affected by age 25 and 90% by the age of 60 years. This occurrence may reflect genetic factors.

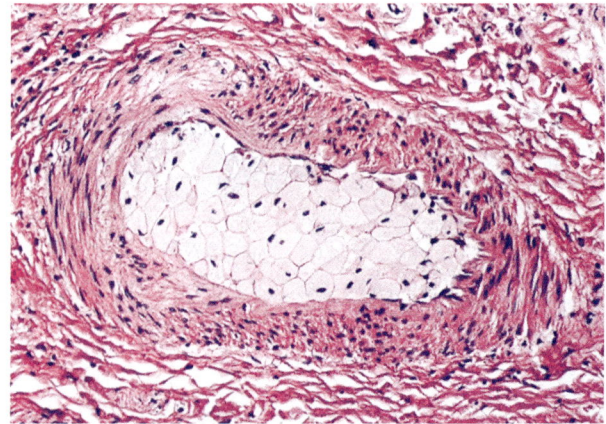

FIGURE 14-64
Arterial lesions in chronic rejection of a liver transplant. Subintimal foam cells, intimal sclerosis, and myointimal hyperplasia virtually obliterate the lumen of a hepatic artery.

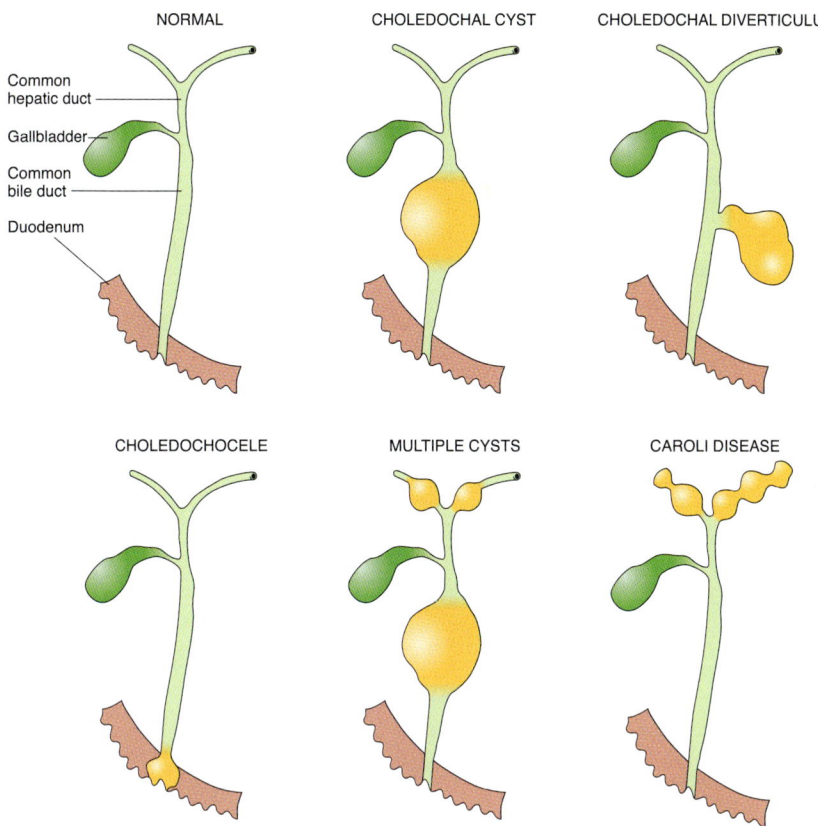

FIGURE 14-65
Congenital dilations of the bile ducts.

Pathogenesis: The pathogenesis of cholesterol gallstones is a multifactorial process that involves physicochemical qualities of bile and local factors within the gall bladder itself (Fig. 14-67):

Bile formation in the liver. Cholesterol is highly insoluble in water and is secreted by the hepatocytes into the bile. It is held in solution by the combined action of bile acids and lecithin and carried in the form of mixed lipid micelles. If the bile contains excess cholesterol or is deficient in bile acids, the bile becomes supersaturated with cholesterol. The bile of persons afflicted with cholesterol gallstones has more cholesterol and less bile salts as it leaves the liver than that of normal persons, and the supersaturated cholesterol precipitates as solid crystals and forms stones (lithogenic bile). In obese persons, cholesterol secretion by the liver is augmented, further adding to the supersaturation of the bile with cholesterol.

Local factors in the gallbladder. Bile in the gallbladder from patients with gallstones crystallizes more easily than normal. Pronucleating biliary proteins and hypersecretion of gallbladder mucus accelerate the rate of cholesterol precipitation from gallbladder bile.

Gallbladder motility. Impaired gallbladder motor function leads to bile stasis and permits the formation of biliary sludge, which then progresses to macroscopic stones.

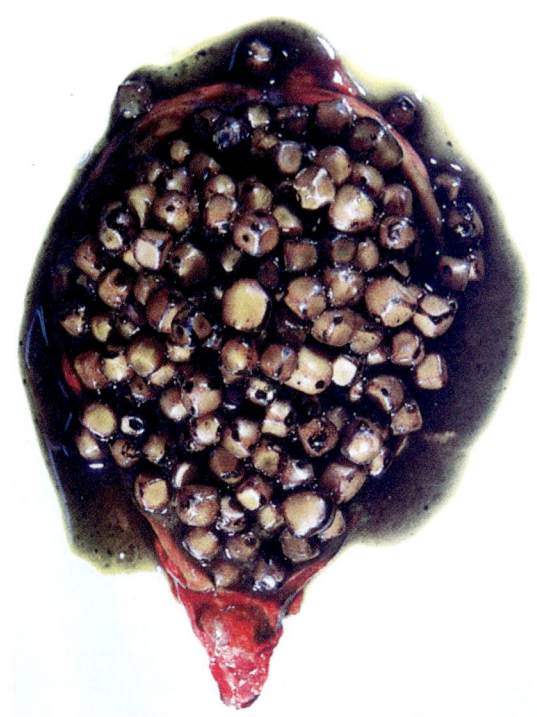

FIGURE 14-66
Cholesterol gallstones. The gallbladder has been opened to reveal numerous yellow cholesterol gallstones.

Risk Factors

The higher prevalence of gallstones in premenopausal women has been attributed to the fact that estrogens stimu-

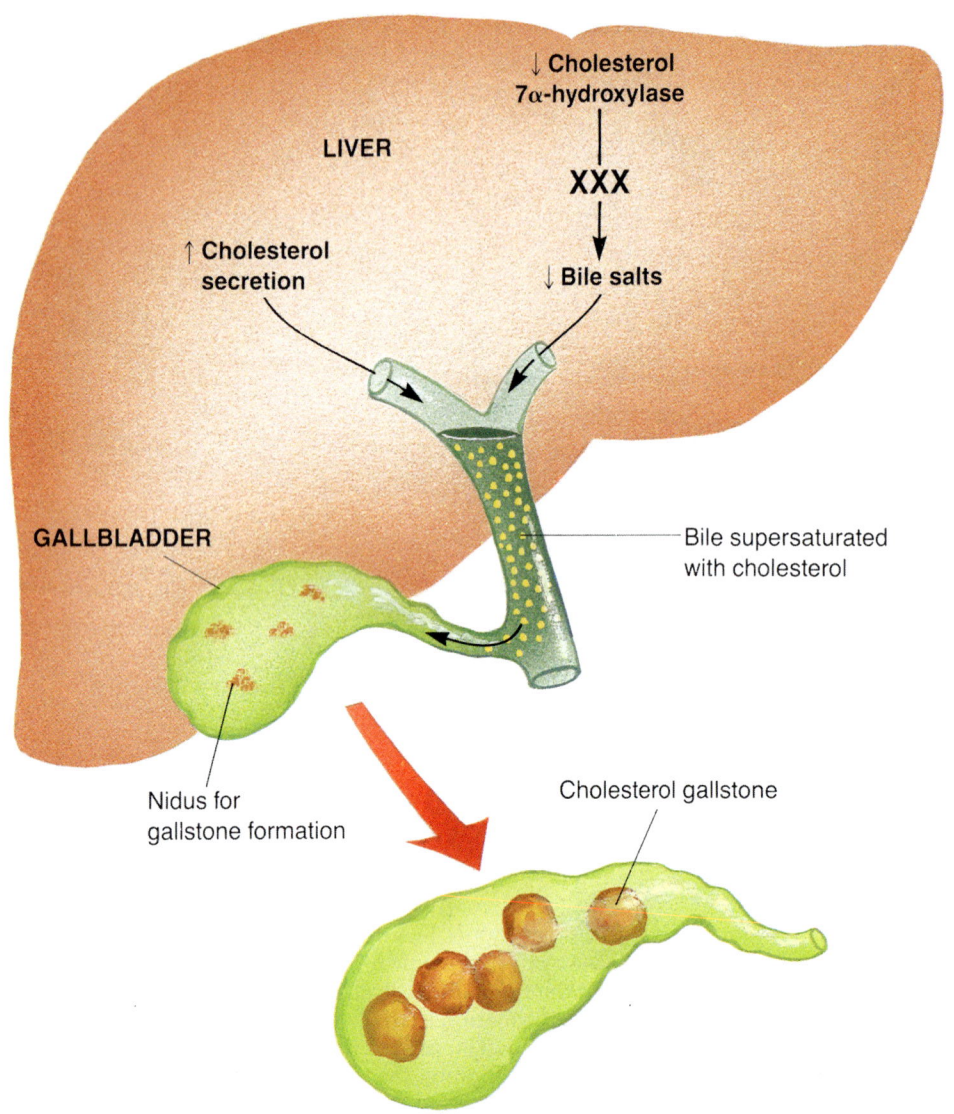

FIGURE 14-67
Pathogenesis of cholesterol gallstones.

late the formation of lithogenic bile by the liver. Estrogens increase the hepatic secretion of cholesterol and decrease the secretion of bile acids. These effects are augmented during pregnancy because the gallbladder empties more slowly in the last trimester, thereby causing stasis and increasing the opportunity for precipitation of cholesterol crystals. Indeed, progesterone, the predominant hormone of pregnancy, inhibits the discharge of bile from the gallbladder. These mechanisms are also invoked to explain the increased incidence of gallstones in users of oral contraceptives.

Other major risk factors for the development of cholesterol gallstones can be divided into those that relate to increased biliary cholesterol secretion, those that contribute to decreased secretion of bile salts and lecithin, and those that reflect a combination of the two.

Risk factors associated with **increased biliary cholesterol secretion** include the following:

- Increasing age
- Obesity
- Membership in certain ethnic groups (e.g., Chilean women, some northern European groups)
- Familial predisposition
- Diet high in calories and cholesterol
- Certain metabolic abnormalities associated with high blood cholesterol levels (e.g., diabetes, some genetic hyperlipoproteinemias, and primary biliary cirrhosis)

There is a linear correlation between the magnitude of obesity and the risk of symptomatic gallstones, reaching a value as high as five times the risk in nonobese persons. Hepatic cholesterol synthesis is stimulated by insulin, and the increased biliary excretion of cholesterol associated with obesity may relate to the hyperinsulinism that accompanies increased body fat.

Decreased secretion of bile salts and lecithin occurs in nonobese whites who develop gallstones. Gastrointestinal absorptive disorders that interfere with the enterohepatic circulation of bile acids (e.g., pancreatic insufficiency secondary to cystic fibrosis and Crohn disease) also decrease secretion of bile acids and favor gallstone formation.

In American Pima Indians and in those who take certain drugs (e.g., clofibrate), cholesterol synthesis increases, whereas that of bile salts and lecithin is reduced. The risk of gallstones is decreased by moderate alcohol consumption, probably because of reduced biliary cholesterol concentration.

Pigment Stones Are Classed As Black or Brown Stones

Black Pigment Stones

Black pigment stones are irregular and measure less than 1 cm across. On cross-section, the surface appears glassy (Fig. 14-68). Black stones contain calcium bilirubinate, bilirubin polymers, calcium salts, and mucin.

 Pathogenesis: The incidence of black stones is increased in old and undernourished persons, but no correlations with gender, ethnicity, or obesity have been made. Chronic hemolysis, such as occurs with sickle cell anemia and thalassemia, predisposes to the development of black pigment stones. Cirrhosis, either because it leads to increased hemolysis or because of damage to liver cells, is also associated with a high incidence of black stones. However, in most instances, no predisposing cause for the formation of black pigment stones is evident.

Unconjugated bilirubin is insoluble in bile and is usually present in only trace amounts. When increased amounts are secreted by the hepatocyte, the unconjugated bilirubin precipitates as calcium bilirubinate, probably around a nidus of mucinous glycoproteins. For unexplained reasons, patients without known predisposing factors who develop black pigment stones have increased concentrations of unconjugated bilirubin in the bile.

Brown Pigment Stones

Brown pigment stones are spongy and laminated and contain principally calcium bilirubinate mixed with cholesterol and calcium soaps of fatty acids. In contrast to the other types of gallstones, brown pigment stones are found more frequently in the intrahepatic and extrahepatic bile ducts than in the gallbladder.

 Pathogenesis: Brown stones are almost always associated with bacterial cholangitis, in which *E. coli* is the predominant organism. Rare or uncommon in Western countries, brown stones are not infrequent in Asia, where they are almost entirely restricted to persons infested with *A. lumbricoides* or *C. sinensis*, helminths that may invade the biliary tract. In the rare cases in Western countries, brown stones are found in patients with chronic mechanical obstruction to the flow of bile, as in sclerosing cholangitis or the presence of a catheter in the common bile duct after common bile duct surgery.

The pathogenesis of brown pigment stones also relates to an increased concentration of unconjugated bilirubin in the bile. Conjugated bilirubin is hydrolyzed to unconjugated bilirubin by the action of bacterial β-glucuronidase or other hydrolytic enzymes.

Clinical Features of Gallstones

Gallstones may remain "silent" in the gallbladder for many years, and few patients ever die of cholelithiasis itself. The 15-year cumulative probability that asymptomatic stones will lead to biliary pain or other complications is less than 20%. Medical treatment of gallstones, including the oral administration of bile acids, and extracorporeal lithotripsy (ultrasonic disruption of gallstones) have largely been replaced by laparoscopic cholecystectomy.

Most of the complications of cholelithiasis relate to the obstruction of the cystic duct or common bile duct by gallstones. Passage of a stone into the cystic duct often, but not invariably, causes severe biliary colic and may lead to acute cholecystitis. Repeated episodes of acute cholecystitis then produce chronic cholecystitis. The latter condition can also result from the presence of stones alone. Gallstones may pass into the common duct *(choledocholithiasis)*, where they may lead to obstructive jaundice, cholangitis, and pancreatitis. In fact, in populations in whom alcoholism is not a factor, gallstones are the most common cause of acute pancreatitis. Passage of a large gallstone into the small intestine has been known to cause intestinal obstruction, a condition called *gallstone ileus*. In obstruction of the cystic

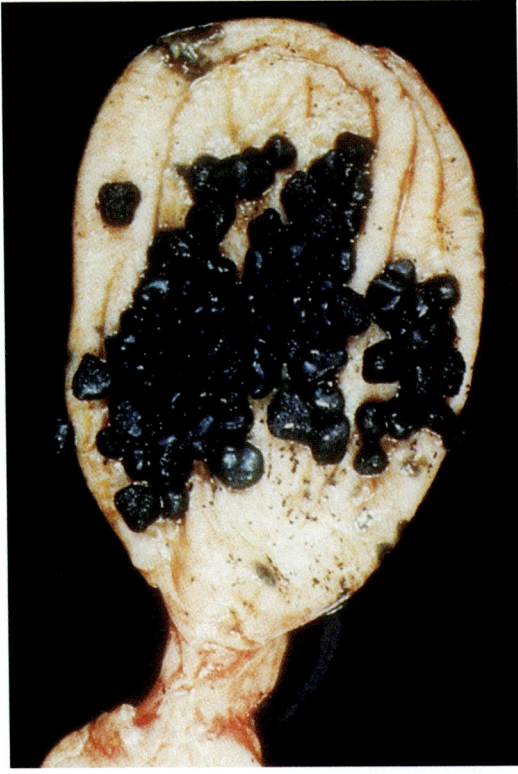

FIGURE 14-68
Pigment gallstones. The gallbladder has been opened to reveal numerous small, dark stones composed of calcium bilirubinate.

806 The Liver and Biliary System

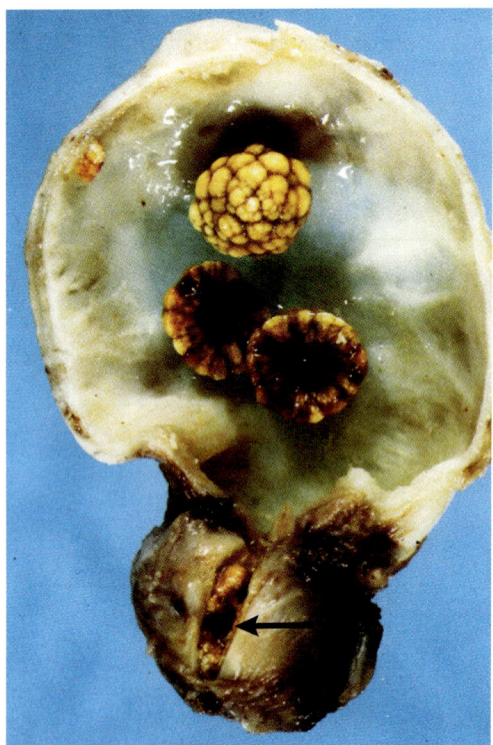

FIGURE 14-69
Hydrops of the gallbladder. The lumen of the dilated gallbladder is filled with clear mucus and contains cholesterol stones. Note the stone *(arrow)* obstructing the cystic duct.

duct, with or without acute cholecystitis, the bile in the gallbladder is reabsorbed, to be replaced by a clear mucinous fluid secreted by the gallbladder epithelium. The term *hydrops of the gallbladder (mucocele)* (Fig. 14-69) is applied to the distended and palpable gallbladder, which may become secondarily infected.

ACUTE CHOLECYSTITIS

Acute cholecystitis is a diffuse inflammation of the gallbladder, usually secondary to obstruction of the gallbladder outlet.

 Pathogenesis: **Some 90% of cases of acute cholecystitis are associated with the presence of gallstones.** The remaining cases *(acalculous cholecystitis)* occur in conjunction with sepsis, severe trauma, infection of the gallbladder with *Salmonella typhosa*, and polyarteritis nodosa. Bacterial infection is usually secondary to biliary obstruction, rather than a primary event.

It has been theorized that obstruction of the cystic duct by a gallstone leads to the release of phospholipase from the epithelium of the gallbladder. In turn, this enzyme may hydrolyze lecithin and release lysolecithin, a membrane-active toxin. At the same time, disruption of the mucous coat of the epithelium renders the mucosal cells vulnerable to damage by the detergent action of concentrated bile salts. Bile supersaturated with cholesterol may be toxic to the epithelium.

 Pathology: The external surface of the gallbladder in acute cholecystitis is congested and layered with a fibrinous exudate. The wall is remarkably thickened by edema, and opening the viscus reveals a fiery red or purple mucosa. Gallstones are usually found within the lumen, and a stone is often seen obstructing the cystic duct. On rare occasions, when obstruction of the cystic duct is complete and bacteria have invaded the gallbladder, the cavity may be distended by cloudy, purulent fluid, a condition termed *empyema of the gallbladder*.

Microscopically, edema and hemorrhage in the wall are striking, with accompanying acute and chronic inflammation (Fig. 14-70). Secondary bacterial infection may lead to suppuration in the gallbladder wall. The mucosa shows focal ulcerations or, in severe cases, widespread necrosis, in which case the term *gangrenous cholecystitis* is applied.

Perforation is a feared complication in severe cases and may occur after secondary bacterial infection, most commonly of the fundus. Discharge of bile into the abdominal cavity results in *bile peritonitis*. More commonly, the contents of the perforated gallbladder are localized by inflammatory adhesions, a lesion known as a *pericholecystic abscess*. The gallbladder contents may also erode into the small or large intestine, creating a *cholecystenteric fistula*.

 Clinical Features: The initial symptom of acute cholecystitis is abdominal pain in the right upper quadrant, and most patients have already experienced episodes of biliary colic. Mild jaundice, caused by stones in, or edema of, the common bile duct, is evident in 20% of patients. In most cases, the acute illness subsides within a week, but persistent pain, fever, leukocytosis, and shaking chills indicate progression of the acute cholecystitis

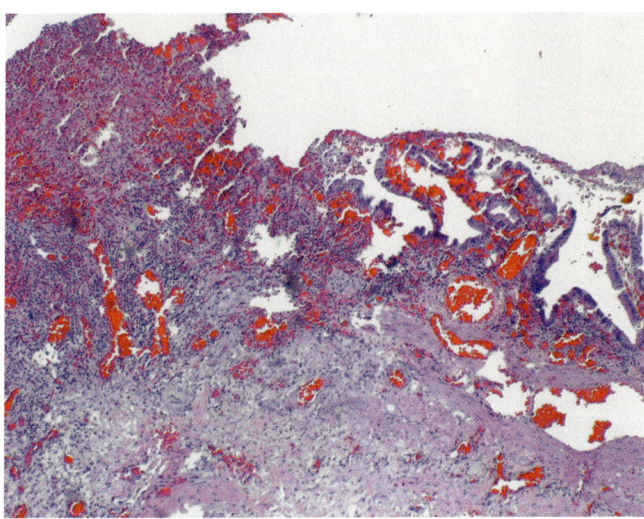

FIGURE 14-70
Acute cholecystitis. A photomicrograph of a gallbladder removed from a patient with acute cholecystitis demonstrates ulceration of the mucosa, edema, and acute and chronic inflammation.

and the need for cholecystectomy. As the inflammatory process resolves, the gallbladder wall becomes fibrotic and the mucosa heals. However, the function of the gallbladder usually remains impaired.

CHRONIC CHOLECYSTITIS

Chronic cholecystitis, the most common disease of the gallbladder, is a persistent inflammation of the gallbladder wall that is almost invariably associated with gallstones. Chronic cholecystitis may also result from repeated attacks of acute cholecystitis. In the latter case, the pathogenesis probably relates to chronic irritation and chemical injury to the gallbladder epithelium.

 Pathology: Grossly, the wall of the chronically inflamed gallbladder is thickened and firm (Fig. 14-71A), and the serosal surface may show fibrous adhesions to surrounding structures as a result of previous episodes of acute cholecystitis. Gallstones are usually found within the lumen, and the bile often contains *gravel or sludge* (i.e., fine precipitates of calculus material). The bile is infected with coliform organisms in about half of cases. The mucosa may be focally ulcerated and atrophic or may appear intact. Microscopically, the wall is fibrotic and often penetrated by sinuses of Rokitansky-Aschoff (see Fig. 14-71B). Chronic inflammation of variable degree may be seen in all layers. In long-standing chronic cholecystitis, the wall of the gallbladder may become calcified *(porcelain gallbladder)*.

Clinical Features: Many patients with chronic cholecystitis complain of nonspecific abdominal symptoms, although it is not at all clear that these are necessarily related to the gallbladder disease. On the other hand, pain in the right hypochondrium is typical and often episodic. The diagnosis is best made by ultrasound examination, which demonstrates gallstones in a thick, contracted gallbladder. Cholecystectomy is the definitive treatment.

CHOLESTEROLOSIS

Cholesterolosis of the gallbladder is defined as the accumulation of cholesterol-laden macrophages within the submucosa. It is a common incidental finding at autopsy but is not ordinarily associated with symptoms. Cholesterolosis is often associated with the presence of bile supersaturated with cholesterol. Grossly, the appearance of scattered, yellow mucosal flecks accounts for the term *strawberry gallbladder*. Micro-

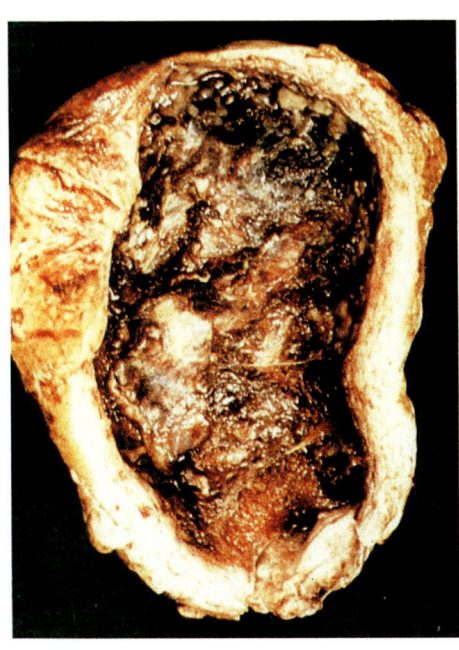
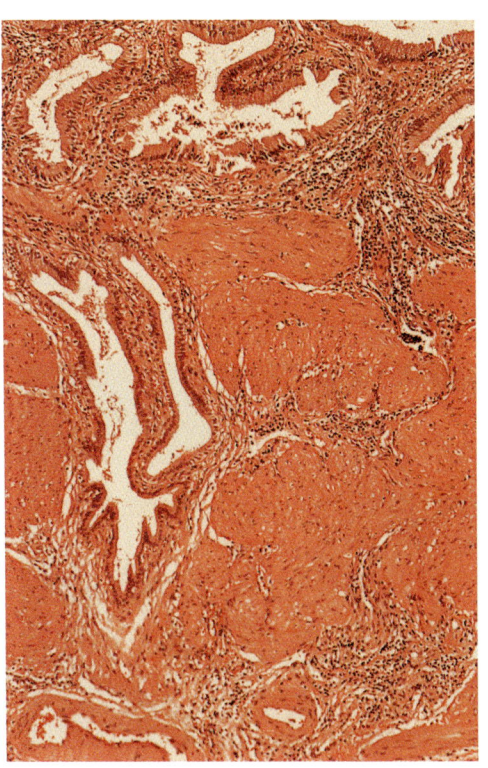

FIGURE 14-71
Chronic cholecystitis. A. The gallbladder is thickened and fibrotic, and the lumen contains several gallstones. B. A photomicrograph of (A) shows chronic inflammation of the gallbladder and a sinus of Rokitansky-Aschoff extending into the muscularis.

TUMORS

Benign Tumors of the Gallbladder and Extrahepatic Biliary Ducts Are Rare

Papillomas are the most common benign tumors of the gallbladder and may be single or multiple. In three fourths of cases, they are associated with gallstones. The combination of smooth muscle proliferation and an adenoma has been termed *adenomyoma*. Fibromas, lipomas, leiomyomas, and myxomas have also been recorded. The bile ducts are affected by the same benign tumors that occur in the gallbladder. Such tumors are clinically more important, since they may obstruct biliary flow and cause jaundice.

Adenocarcinoma Is the Most Common Tumor of the Gallbladder

Adenocarcinoma of the gallbladder is not rare, being incidentally found in 2% of patients who undergo gallbladder surgery. **Because this cancer is usually associated with cholelithiasis and chronic cholecystitis, it is considerably more common in women than in men.** In addition, populations that have a high incidence of cholelithiasis, such as Native Americans, have a higher risk of carcinoma of the gallbladder. The calcified gallbladder (porcelain gallbladder), which represents an extreme variant of chronic cholecystitis, is particularly prone to the development of gallbladder cancer.

Pathology: Gallbladder carcinoma may occur anywhere in the gallbladder but most frequently appears in the fundus. **The tumor is characteristically an infiltrative, well-differentiated adenocarcinoma** (Fig. 14-72). It is usually desmoplastic, and thus the wall of the gallbladder becomes thickened and leathery. Anaplastic, giant cell, and spindle cell forms of gallbladder carcinoma are reported. The rich lymphatic plexus of the gallbladder provides the most common route of metastasis, although vascular dissemination and direct spread into the liver and contiguous structures occur.

Clinical Features: The symptoms produced by carcinoma of the gallbladder are similar to those encountered with gallstone disease. However, by the time the tumor becomes symptomatic, it is almost invariably incurable, the 5-year survival rate being less than 3%. For practical purposes, surgical cure is obtained only in patients who undergo cholecystectomy for gallbladder disease in whom the cancer is an incidental finding.

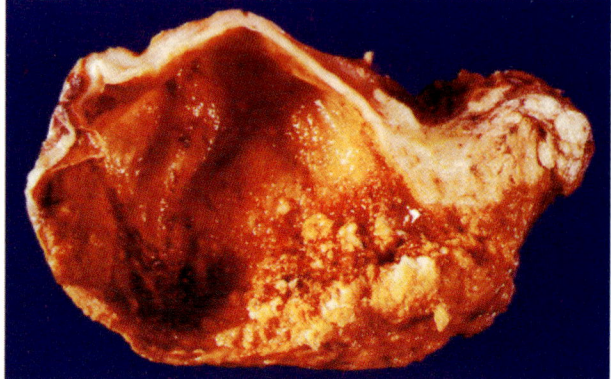
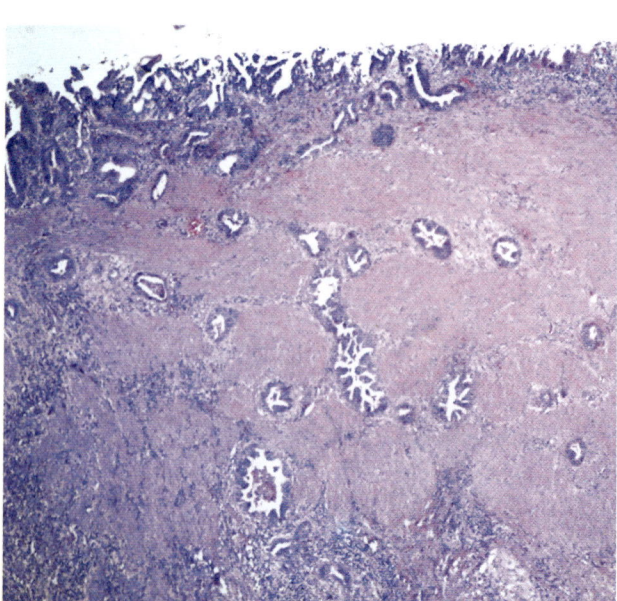

FIGURE 14-72
Carcinoma of the gallbladder. A. A surgically resected gallbladder has been opened to reveal a thickened wall infiltrated by adenocarcinoma, which also demonstrates exophytic growth into the lumen. B. The gallbladder wall is infiltrated by a moderately-differentiated adenocarcinoma, which has stimulated a desmoplastic response.

Carcinoma of the Bile Duct and the Ampulla of Vater Present As Obstructive Jaundice

Cancer of the extrahepatic bile ducts is almost always adenocarcinoma. It may occur anywhere along the length of the bile duct, including the location where the right and left hepatic ducts join to form the common hepatic duct.

The tumor is less common than gallbladder cancer, and the female predominance of gallbladder cancer is not evident. Gallstones are frequently found in those affected, and there is an association with inflammatory disease of the colon. The tumor has also been reported to arise in choledochal cysts and in Caroli disease. In the Orient, bile duct carcinoma is associated with biliary infestation by the fluke *C. sinensis*. As in carcinoma of the gallbladder, growth may be endophytic (into the lumen) or diffusely infiltrative. The prognosis is poor, but because symptoms arise early in the course of the disease, the outcome is somewhat better than that of gallbladder carcinoma.

Adenocarcinoma of the ampulla of Vater may also obstruct the bile duct. The initial symptom is again obstructive jaundice, although a few patients present with pancreatitis. In contrast to bile duct carcinoma, surgical treatment of cancer of the ampulla of Vater leads to a 35% 5-year survival rate.

SUGGESTED READING

Books

Bircher J, Benhamou J-P, McIntyre N, et al. (eds): *Oxford Textbook of Clinical Hepatology,* 2nd ed. Oxford: Oxford University Press, 1999.

Farrel GC: *Drug-induced liver disease.* Edinburgh: Churchill Livingstone, 1994.

Ishak KG, Goodman ZD, Stocker J. Tumors of the liver and intrahepatic bile ducts. In: *Atlas of tumor pathology,* series 3, fascicle 31. Washington, DC: Armed Forces Institute of Pathology, 2001.

MacSween RNM, Burt AD, Portmann BC, et al. (eds): *Pathology of the liver,* 4th ed. Edinburgh: Churchill Livingstone, 2002.

Schiff L, Schiff ER (eds): *Diseases of the liver,* 7th ed. Philadelphia: JB Lippincott, 1999.

Sherlock S, Dooley J: *Diseases of the liver and biliary system,* 11th ed. Oxford: Blackwell Scientific, 2002.

Zakim D, Boyer TD (eds): *Hepatology: A textbook of liver disease,* 3rd ed. Philadelphia: WB Saunders, 1996.

Zimmerman, HJ: Hepatotoxicity: the adverse effects of drugs and other chemicals on the liver. 2nd ed. Philadelphia: Lippincott Williams & Wilkins, 1999.

Review Articles

Al-Khalidi JA, Czaja A: Current concepts in the diagnosis, pathogenesis, and treatment of autoimmune hepatitis. *Mayo Clin Proc* 76:1237–1252, 2001.

Bacon BR: Hemochromatosis: Diagnosis and management. *Gastroenterology* 120:718–725, 2001.

Cuthbert JA: Hepatitis A: Old and new. *Clin Microbiol Rev* 14:38–58, 2001.

Dowling RH: Pathogenesis of gallstones. *Aliment Pharmacol Ther* 14:39–47, 2000.

Feitelson MA: Hepatocellular injury in hepatitis B and C virus infections. *Clin Lab Med* 16:307–324, 1996.

French SW: Mechanisms of alcoholic liver injury. *Can J Gastroenterol* 14:327–332, 2000.

Gish RG, Mason A: Autoimmune liver disease. Current standards, future directions. *Clin Liver Dis* 5:287–314, 2001.

Gochee PA, Powell LW: What's new in hemochromatosis. *Curr Opin Hematol* 8:98–104, 2001.

Hazell AS, Butterworth RF: Hepatic encephalopathy: An update of pathophysiologic mechanisms. *Proc Soc Exp Biol Med* 222:99–112, 1999.

Ko CW, Lee SP: Gallstone formation. *Gastroenterol Clin North Am* 28:99–115, 1999.

Lauer GM, Walker BD: Hepatitis C infection. *N Engl J Med* 345:41–51, 2001.

Lee WM: Drug-induced hepatotoxicity. *N Engl J Med.* 333:1118–1127, 1995.

Loudianos G, Gitlin J: Wilson's disease. *Semin Liver Dis* 20:353–364, 2000.

Lyon E, Frank E: Hereditary hemochromatosis since discovery of the HFE gene. *Clin Chem* 47:1147–1156, 2001.

Macdonald GA. Pathogenesis of hepatocellular carcinoma. *Clin Liver Dis* 5:69–85, 2001.

Portmann B, Koukoulis G: Pathology of the liver allograft. *Curr Top Pathol* 92:61–105, 1999.

Riordan SM, Williams R: The Wilson's disease gene and phenotypic diversity. *J Hepatol* 34:165–171, 2001.

Sherlock S: Primary biliary cirrhosis, primary sclerosing cholangitis, and autoimmune cholangitis. *Clin Liver Dis* 4:97–113, 2000.

Tanaka A, Borchers AT, Ishibashi H, et al.: Genetic and familial considerations of primary biliary cirrhosis. *Am J Gastroenterol* 96:8–15, 2001.

Thompson R, Jansen PLM: Genetic defects in hepatocanalicular transport. *Semin Liver Dis* 20:365–372, 2000.

Torok N. Gores GJ. Cholangiocarcinoma: *Semin Gastrointest Dis.* 12:125–132, 2001.

Trauner M, Fickert P, Zollner G: Genetic disorders and molecular mechanisms in cholestatic liver disease—A clinical approach. *Semin Gastrointest Dis* 12:66–88, 2001.

Tsukamoto H. Lu SC: Current concepts in the pathogenesis of alcoholic liver injury. *FASEB J* 15:1335–1349, 2001.

Wright TL, Monto A: The epidemiology and prevention of hepatocellular carcinoma. *Semin Oncol* 28:441–449, 2001.

Zein CO, Lindor KD: Primary sclerosing cholangitis. *Semin Gastrointest Dis* 12(2):103–112, 2001.

CHAPTER 15

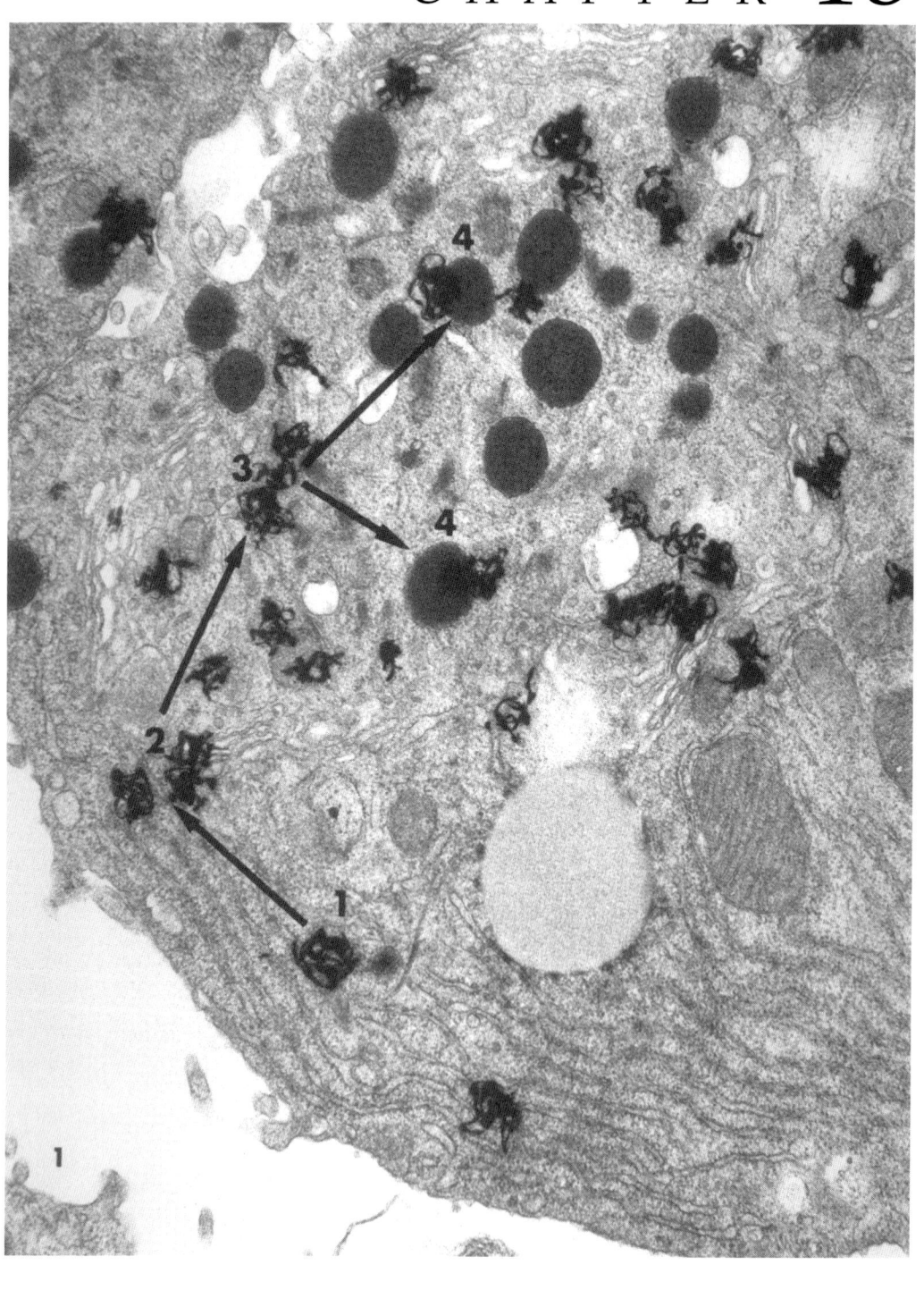

The Pancreas

Emanuel Rubin
Raphael Rubin

Anatomy and Physiology

Congenital Anomalies

Acute Pancreatitis

Chronic Pancreatitis

Pancreatic Cystadenoma

Pancreatic Cancer
Acinar Cell Carcinoma

Neoplasms of the Endocrine Pancreas
Normal Pancreatic Islets
Beta Cell Tumors (Insulinomas)
Pancreatic Gastrinomas (Zollinger-Ellison Syndrome)
Alpha Cell Tumors (Glucagonomas)
Delta Cell Tumors (Somatostatinomas)
D_1 Tumors (VIPomas, Verner-Morrison Syndrome)
Pancreatic Polypeptide-Secreting Tumors
Enterochromaffin Cell (Carcinoid) Tumors
Multiple Endocrine Neoplasia Syndrome Type I
Ectopic Hormone Syndromes

FIGURE 15-1 *(see opposite page)*
Protein synthesis in the pancreatic acinar cell. An electron microscopic autoradiograph of a rat pancreatic acinar cell 30 minutes after a pulse label of [^{3}H]leucine shows serpentine silver grains that delineate the localization of *(1)* synthesis, *(2)* intracellular transport, *(3)* concentration, and *(4)* storage of digestive proenzymes. The *arrows* show the vectorial movement of the secretory product. The electron dense bodies are zymogen granules.

ANATOMY AND PHYSIOLOGY

The pancreas begins as two endodermal outpouchings that arise on the dorsal and ventral sides of the embryonic duodenal tube. The duct systems of the two embryonic pancreases fuse, giving rise to a single duct *(the duct of Wirsung)*. The ducts branch into elongate ductules, which arborize to form a complex ductal system. Acinar cells arise from the ductules and acquire their complement of distinctive zymogen granules. Islet cells are also derived from larger ducts and acquire small, dense, secretory granules characteristic of the endocrine pancreas.

The pancreas is a mixed exocrine–endocrine gland that extends transversely in the upper abdomen and is cradled between the loop of the duodenum and the hilum of the spleen. It is retroperitoneal, lying behind the lesser omental sac and the stomach, a location that renders it largely inaccessible to physical examination. The adult pancreas is 10 to 15 cm long and weighs 60 to 150 g. It is divided into three anatomical subdivisions: (1) *the head* lies in the concavity of the duodenum and extends to the superior mesenteric vessels immediately behind the organ; (2) *the body* includes most of the gland; and (3) *a tapered tail* ends at the hilum of the spleen.

The secretions of the exocrine pancreas drain into the duct of Wirsung, which usually empties into the common bile duct immediately proximal to the ampulla of Vater. The common channel that carries bile and pancreatic secretions into the duodenum is invested with a circular complex of smooth muscle fibers that condense into the sphincter of Oddi as they pass through the duodenal wall.

Exocrine tissue makes up 80 to 85% of the pancreas and consists of secretory cells organized as acini that connect with ductules. Pancreatic acini are composed of a single layer of pyramidal cells, whose basophilic cytoplasm is filled with acidophilic zymogen granules. By electron microscopy, the acinar cells exhibit conspicuous rough endoplasmic reticulum and numerous electron-dense zymogen granules in the apical portion of the cell (Fig. 15-1). **Acinar cells synthesize some 20 different digestive enzymes, many in the form of inactive proenzymes (see below), which are secreted into the intestine following both neural and hormonal stimulation.** These include trypsin, chymotrypsin, amylase, carboxypeptidase, lipase, phospholipase, and elastase. The daily secretion of 1.5 to 3 liters of pancreatic juice attests to the remarkable synthetic and secretory capacity of the exocrine pancreas.

The endocrine pancreas consists of cells organized into islets that are distributed throughout the organ but make up only 2% of the total mass of the pancreas. Islets contain several cell types, each of which synthesizes one or more hormones, including, among others, insulin and glucagon. Following an appropriate stimulus, the hormones are secreted directly into the blood. The major endocrine disorder of the pancreas is diabetes mellitus, a disease that is accorded a separate chapter (see Chapter 22).

CONGENITAL ANOMALIES

Developmental defects of the pancreas occur but are rarely of clinical significance.

ABERRANT (ECTOPIC) PANCREAS: This anomaly, in which pancreatic tissue is present outside its normal location, is an incidental finding in 2% of autopsies and is most commonly localized in the wall of the duodenum, stomach, and jejunum. The tissue contains all the components of normal pancreas, namely, acini, ducts, and islets.

ANNULAR PANCREAS: This is an uncommon condition in which the head of the gland surrounds the second portion of the duodenum; encirclement may be complete or incomplete. Annular pancreas may be associated with duodenal atresia, an anomaly that requires surgery immediately after birth. Such infants frequently have other congenital anomalies, including trisomy 21 (Down syndrome). Many patients with annular pancreas do not require surgery in early life but develop symptoms at 60 or 70 years of age.

PANCREAS DIVISUM: Failure of the pancreatic rudiments to fuse results in two separate glands, each with its separate duct draining into the duodenum.

CYSTS: True cysts of the pancreas are believed to arise from faulty development of pancreatic ducts.

ACUTE PANCREATITIS

Pancreatitis is defined as an inflammatory condition of the exocrine pancreas that results from injury to acinar cells. In 1925, the devastation of acute pancreatitis was justly described as the "most terrible of all calamities that occur in connection with the abdominal viscera. The suddenness of its onset, the illimitable agony which accompanies it, and the mortality attendant upon it render it the most formidable of catastrophes." Sadly, for reasons unknown, the incidence of the disease has increased by an order of magnitude in the past few decades.

Depending on its severity and duration, pancreatitis presents in a variety of clinical forms. At one end of the spectrum is a mild, self-limited disease, consisting of acute inflammation and edema of the stroma, with little or no acinar cell necrosis. At the other extreme is a severe and sometimes fatal acute hemorrhagic pancreatitis with massive necrosis. In some cases, repeated episodes of acute pancreatitis lead to chronic pancreatitis, which is characterized by recurrent attacks of severe abdominal pain and progressive fibrosis, ultimately leading to pancreatic insufficiency. However, in about half the cases of chronic pancreatitis, no acute episodes are recognized clinically.

Interstitial or edematous pancreatitis is the mild and presumably reversible form of acute pancreatitis. An infiltrate of polymorphonuclear leukocytes and edema of the connective tissue between lobules of acinar cells constitute the initial lesion. There is no necrosis or hemorrhage.

Acute hemorrhagic pancreatitis is a condition of middle age, with a peak incidence at 60 years. It is often associated with alcoholism (more commonly in men) or chronic biliary disease (more often in women). Acute pancreatitis erupts abruptly, usually following a heavy meal or excessive alcohol intake.

Pathogenesis: Acinar cell injury and duct obstruction are the major factors involved in the initiation of acute pancreatitis. These processes allow the inappropriate extracellular leakage of activated digestive enzymes and the consequent autodigestion of pancreatic and extrapancreatic tissues. A number of factors have been implicated in acute pancreatitis.

ACTIVATED PANCREATIC ENZYMES: Acinar cells are shielded from the potentially destructive action of their digestive enzymes (proteases, nucleases, amylase, lipase, and phospholipase A) by 3 mechanisms.

1. An intricate, intracellular, cavitary system of endoplasmic reticulum, Golgi complex, and zymogen granule membranes physically isolates the various enzymes from other cytoplasmic components.
2. Many of the digestive enzymes are synthesized as inactive forms (e.g., chymotrypsinogen, proelastase, prophospholipase, and trypsinogen).
3. Specific enzyme inhibitors, such as that for trypsin, tend to protect the pancreas.

The activation of trypsin is central to the pathogenesis of acute pancreatitis. Although trypsin by itself does not produce cell necrosis, it does activate other pancreatic proenzymes, including prophospholipase A_2 and proelastase. Under the appropriate circumstances, phospholipase A_2 attacks membrane phospholipids to cause necrosis, and elastase digests the walls of blood vessels, thereby leading to hemorrhage. Moreover, the liberation of pancreatic lipase into the interstitium contributes to fat necrosis. **The inappropriate activation of pancreatic proenzymes is the common feature in the pathogenesis of all variants of pancreatitis.**

SECRETION AGAINST OBSTRUCTION: Most of the enzyme fluid secreted by acinar cells is discharged into the duct system and enters the duodenum. A small amount diffuses back into the periductular extracellular fluid and eventually into the plasma. Any condition that narrows the lumina of the pancreatic ducts or that impairs the easy outflow of exocrine secretions can raise the intraductal pressure and exacerbate back-diffusion across the ducts. This effect has been postulated to result in inappropriate activation of digestive proenzymes. A heavy meal leads to the release of pancreatic secretagogues, an effect that augments the production of pancreatic enzymes.

Gallstones can cause pancreatic duct obstruction. Some 45% of all patients with acute pancreatitis also have cholelithiasis, and **the risk of developing acute pancreatitis in patients with gallstones is 25 times higher than that in the general population.** Furthermore, unless the gallstones are eliminated after the first attack, recurrent pancreatitis can be expected in 50% of cases. However, fewer than 5% of patients with acute pancreatitis have an impacted stone at the ampulla of Vater, and the reason for the association between pancreatitis and cholelithiasis remains obscure. Neither ligation of the pancreatic duct nor its occlusion by tumor results in acute pancreatitis. It has been suggested that the reflux of bile or duodenal contents into the pancreatic duct may lead to pancreatitis, but there is little clinical evidence to support this theory.

PROTEASE INHIBITORS: The various inhibitors of proteolytic enzymes present in many body fluids and tissues constitute a defense against the inappropriate activation of the digestive proenzymes of the pancreas. Four potent protease inhibitors have been identified in human plasma: α_1-antitrypsin, α_2-macroglobulin, C_1 esterase inhibitor, and pancreatic secretory trypsin inhibitor. Despite the variety of trypsin inhibitors in different body compartments, clearly the protection they render is less than complete. Since trypsin activates other pancreatic proenzymes, its incomplete inhibition in pancreatic juice poses a hazard.

ETHANOL: **Chronic alcohol abuse accounts for one third of cases of acute pancreatitis,** although only 5% of chronic alcoholics develop this complication. Ethanol is well recognized as a chemical toxin, but a significant injurious effect on pancreatic acinar or duct cells has yet to be demonstrated. Ethanol consumption may adversely affect the pancreas by causing spasm or acute edema of the sphincter of Oddi, especially following an alcoholic binge. It also stimulates secretion from the small intestine, which in turn triggers the exocrine pancreas to release pancreatic juice. When these effects occur together (enhanced secretion into an obstructed duct), the results may be disastrous.

OTHER CAUSES OF PANCREATITIS: Other factors can cause acute pancreatitis, albeit uncommonly:

- **Viruses** such as mumps, coxsackievirus, and cytomegalovirus can cause pancreatitis. The incidence of acute pancreatitis is particularly high in patients with acquired immunodeficiency syndrome (AIDS), in whom the most common cause is cytomegalovirus infection.
- **Therapeutic drugs,** of which more than 85 have been reported to cause acute pancreatitis. These include immunosuppressive drugs (e.g., azathioprine), antineoplastic agents, sulfonamides, and diuretics. The pathogenetic mechanisms by which the pancreas is injured by these compounds are, in most instances, unclear.
- **Blunt trauma** to the upper abdomen can cause contusive injury to the pancreas, with leakage of digestive enzymes into the pancreas and peripancreatic tissues. Patients undergoing endoscopic retrograde cholangiopancreatography (ERCP) occasionally develop acute pancreatitis.
- **Acute ischemia** caused by shock, vasculitis, and thrombosis may injure the pancreas.
- **Hyperlipidemia** on occasion can precipitate the onset of acute pancreatitis. The mechanism is thought to involve

the hydrolysis of triglycerides in the extracellular space by lipase inappropriately leaked by pancreatic cells. The released free fatty acids are cytotoxic.
- **Hypercalcemia,** regardless of cause, may be associated with acute pancreatitis. In this context, Ca^{2+} is necessary for the activation of trypsinogen by trypsin.
- **Obesity** is a risk factor for pancreatitis, especially for severe disease. Obese persons have increased deposition of peripancreatic fat, which may predispose them to more extensive fat necrosis after the local release of pancreatic lipase.
- **Idiopathic pancreatitis** is still the third most common form of the disease, accounting for 10 to 30% of all cases.

Factors involved in the pathogenesis of acute hemorrhagic pancreatitis are shown in Figure 15-2.

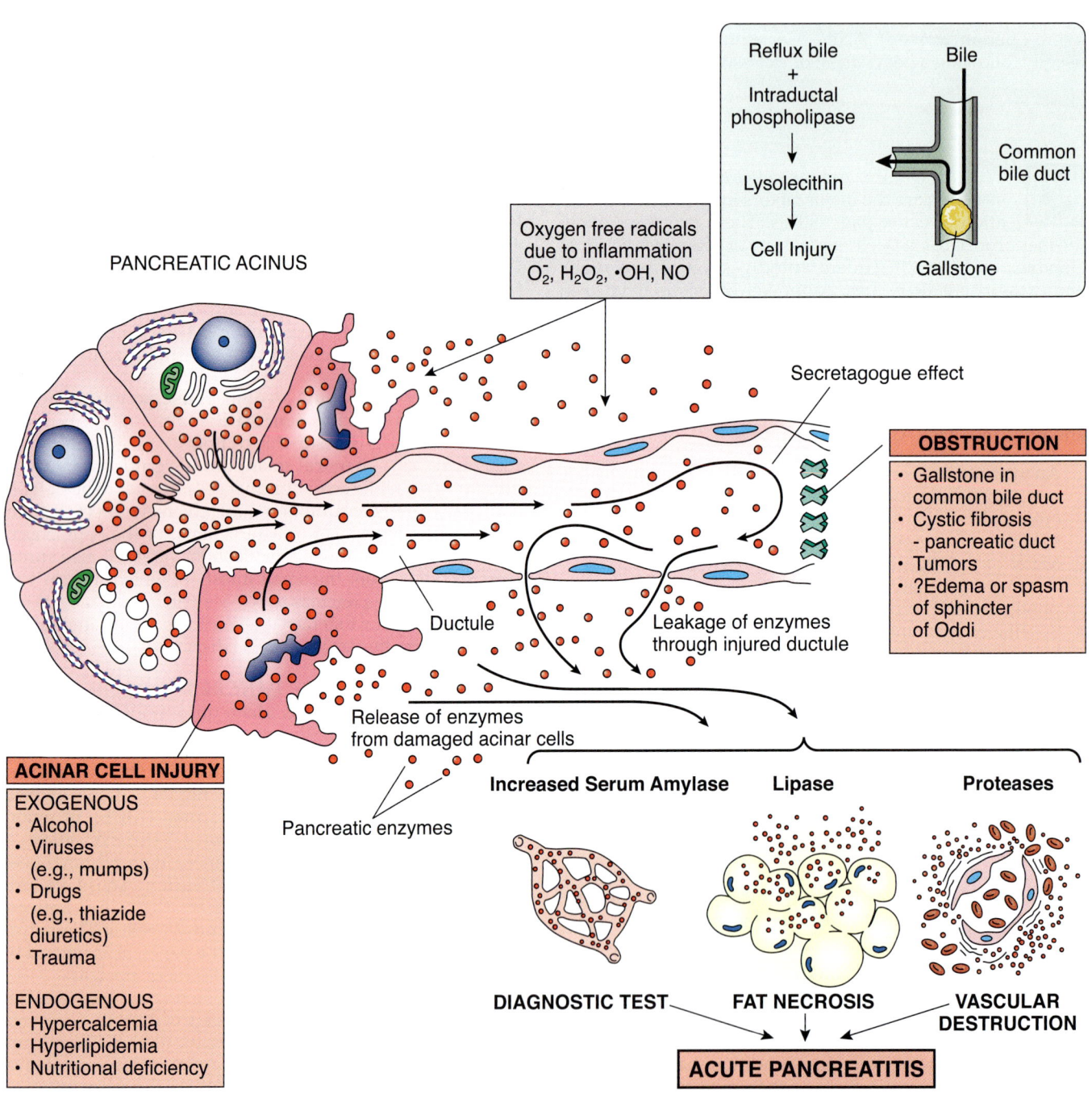

FIGURE 15-2
The pathogenesis of acute pancreatitis. Injury to the ductules or the acinar cells leads to the release of pancreatic enzymes. Lipase and proteases destroy tissue, thereby causing acute pancreatitis. The release of amylase is the basis of a test for acute pancreatitis.

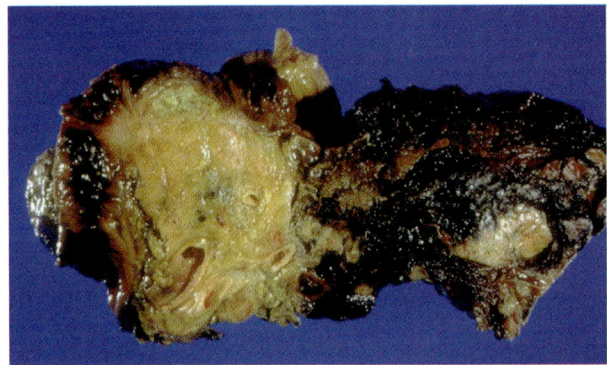
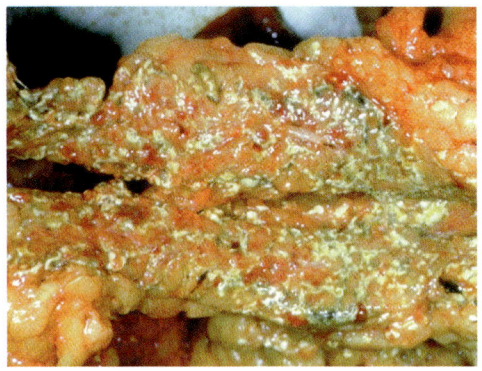

FIGURE 15-3
Acute hemorrhagic pancreatitis. A. Large areas of the pancreas are intensely hemorrhagic. B. The cut surface of the pancreas in a less severe case of acute pancreatitis, and at a somewhat later stage than in (A), shows numerous yellow-white foci of fat necrosis.

 Pathology: In acute hemorrhagic pancreatitis, the pancreas is initially edematous and hyperemic. Within a day, pale, gray foci appear, rapidly becoming friable and hemorrhagic (Fig. 15-3A). **In severe cases, these foci enlarge and become so numerous that most of the pancreas is converted into a large retroperitoneal hematoma, in which pancreatic tissue is barely recognizable.** Yellow-white areas of fat necrosis appear around the pancreas, including the adjacent mesentery (see Fig. 15-3B). These nodules of necrotic fat have a pasty consistency that becomes firmer and chalklike as more calcium and magnesium soaps are produced. Saponification reflects the interaction of cations with free fatty acids released by the action of activated lipase on triglycerides in fat cells. As a result, the level of blood calcium may be depressed, sometimes to the point of causing neuromuscular irritability.

The most prominent microscopic findings in acute pancreatitis are acinar cell necrosis, an intense acute inflammatory reaction, and foci of necrotic fat cells (Fig. 15-4). Irregular fibrosis of the pancreas and occasionally calcification are the residuals of healed acute pancreatitis.

PANCREATIC PSEUDOCYST: As many as half of patients who survive acute pancreatitis are at risk for the development of pancreatic pseudocysts (Fig. 15-5). These lesions exhibit large spaces limited by connective tissue, which contain degraded blood, debris of necrotic pancreatic tissue, and fluid rich in pancreatic enzymes. Pseudocysts may enlarge to compress and even obstruct the duodenum. They may become secondarily infected and form an abscess. Rupture of a pseudocyst is a rare complication that leads to a chemical or septic peritonitis or both.

Clinical Features: The patient with acute pancreatitis presents with severe epigastric pain that is referred to the upper back and is accompanied by nausea and vomiting. Within a matter of hours, catastrophic

FIGURE 15-4
Acute hemorrhagic pancreatitis. A photomicrograph of the pancreas shows areas of acinar cell necrosis, hemorrhage, and fat necrosis (lower right). An intact lobule is seen on the left.

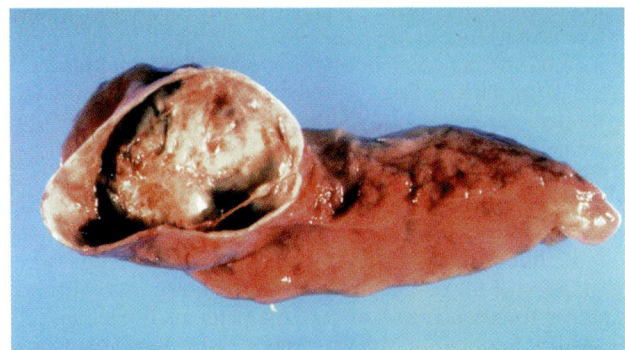

FIGURE 15-5
Pancreatic pseudocyst. A cystic cavity arises from the head of the pancreas.

peripheral vascular collapse and shock may ensue. When shock is sustained and profound, pancreatitis may be complicated within the first week of onset by the adult respiratory distress syndrome and acute renal failure. Early in the disease, pancreatic digestive enzymes are released from injured acinar cells into the blood and the abdominal cavity. **Elevation of serum amylase and lipase levels as early as 24 to 72 hours after onset is diagnostic for acute pancreatitis.** The necrotic pancreas becomes infected with gram-negative bacteria from the intestinal tract in half of cases of acute pancreatitis. This complication increases the mortality associated with abdominal surgery.

CHRONIC PANCREATITIS

Chronic pancreatitis is characterized by the progressive destruction of the pancreas with accompanying irregular fibrosis and chronic inflammation. Since the original description of the disease and its associated stones some two centuries ago, chronic pancreatitis "remains an enigmatic process of uncertain pathogenesis, unpredictable clinical course, and unclear treatment." Clinically, the disorder manifests as recurrent or persisting abdominal pain or simply as evidence of pancreatic exocrine or endocrine insufficiency.

Pathogenesis: Most of the factors that cause acute pancreatitis also cause chronic pancreatitis. The fact that chronic pancreatitis is often characterized by intermittent "acute" attacks followed by periods of quiescence suggests that in many patients the pathogenesis involves repeated bouts of acute pancreatitis, followed by scarring. However, about half of patients present without a history of acute episodes, and the pathogenesis of these cases of chronic pancreatitis may relate to persistent necrosis and insidious scarring, similar to the progression of cirrhosis of the liver.

- **Alcoholism** of long standing is the major cause of chronic pancreatitis, being responsible for two thirds of adult cases. In almost half of alcoholics who had no symptoms of chronic pancreatitis during life, autopsy reveals evidence of this disease. A comparable proportion of asymptomatic alcoholics manifest abnormal results of tests for pancreatic exocrine function. Although the etiological role of alcohol is undisputed, the mechanism by which it causes chronic pancreatitis is still debated.

  The earliest morphological abnormality in alcoholic chronic pancreatitis is the precipitation of protein plugs in the ducts, which serve as the nidus for subsequent calculi that obstruct the ductal system. Since alcohol is a secretagogue for the pancreas, early chronic pancreatitis features hypersecretion of enzyme proteins by acinar cells, without concomitantly increased fluid. As a result, protein plugs are precipitated in the small branches of the pancreatic ducts. These deposits, which are initially composed of degenerating cells within a reticular framework, enlarge to form laminar aggregates through the accretion of amorphous material. Intraductal stones then form when calcium carbonate is precipitated in the plugs.

- **Obstruction** by gallstones does not seem to be an etiologic factor in chronic pancreatitis, and cholecystectomy does not alter the course of the disease. Functional obstruction of the pancreatic duct caused by pancreas divisum or mechanical obstruction by cancer or by the inspissated mucus of cystic fibrosis leads to chronic pancreatitis.

- **Chronic injury to the acinar cells** (e.g., in hemochromatosis) is associated with fibrosis and atrophy of the pancreas.

- **Chronic renal failure** is linked to an increased incidence of acute and chronic pancreatitis.

- **Autoimmune chronic pancreatitis** occurs rarely and is occasionally associated with other autoimmune diseases, including Sjögren syndrome and inflammatory bowel disease.

- **Cystic fibrosis** (see Chapter 16) is briefly reviewed here because it manifests as a form of chronic pancreatitis. In the pancreas of a patient with cystic fibrosis, the intraductal secretions are abnormally viscid, accounting for the older name, *mucoviscidosis*. Plugs of inspissated mucus obstruct the pancreatic ducts, thereby leading to chronic pancreatitis and insufficiency of the exocrine pancreas. As a result, malabsorption is an important feature of cystic fibrosis in children, who may display bulky and fatty stools (steatorrhea). Death, however, usually results from the pulmonary complications of the disease.

- **Familial hereditary pancreatitis** is a rare autosomal dominant disease characterized by recurring episodes of severe abdominal pain. The condition often manifests in childhood. In some instances, hereditary pancreatitis is accompanied by aminoaciduria, although the two conditions are not necessarily linked etiologically. Some patients exhibit hypercalcemia, secondary to hyperplasia or adenomas of the parathyroid glands. About 15% of patients with hereditary pancreatitis subsequently develop ductal adenocarcinoma of the pancreas. The clinical and pathological features of hereditary pancreatitis are indistinguishable from those of other forms of chronic pancreatitis, including ductal stones and the late complications.

  Hereditary pancreatitis is associated with an arginine-to-histidine substitution at residue 117 of the trypsinogen molecule. Interestingly, the normal arginine 117 residue is a trypsin-sensitive site. Cleavage at this location is probably part of a fail-safe mechanism by which trypsin may be inactivated. Failure to inactivate trypsin allows its activation within the pancreas, resulting in autodigestion and pancreatitis.

- **Idiopathic chronic pancreatitis** exhibits a bimodal distribution. A juvenile form of the disease occurs, with a mean age of 25 years. In the older group of patients with chronic pancreatitis, the disease peaks at age 60 years. Mutations in the cystic fibrosis transmembrane conductance regulator *(CFTR)* gene have been identified in 10 to 30% of patients with idiopathic chronic pancreatitis. Mutations in the gene for pancreatic secretory trypsin inhibitor *(SPINK1)* have also been associated with chronic pancreatitis.

Pathology: By the time chronic pancreatitis becomes clinically evident, it is usually well advanced. Chronic calcifying pancreatitis is the most common type of the disease and is associated with chronic alcoholism in more than 90% of cases. On gross examination, the pancreas is firm, and the cut surface lacks the usual lobular appearance (Fig. 15-6A). Often the pancreatic duct and its tributaries are dilated, owing to obstruction by thick proteinaceous plugs, intraductal stones, or strictures. True cysts and poorly defined pseudocysts are common.

Microscopically, large regions of the pancreas display irregular areas of fibrosis, and the exocrine and endocrine elements are reduced in number and size (see Fig. 15-6B). Fibrotic areas exhibit activated fibroblasts, adjacent to which are infiltrates of lymphocytes, plasma cells, and macrophages, particularly around surviving pancreatic lobules. Pancreatic ducts of all sizes contain variably calcified proteinaceous material.

Clinical Features: Half of patients with chronic pancreatitis suffer from repeated episodes of acute pancreatitis. One third of cases are characterized by the gradual onset of continuous or intermittent pain, without any acute attacks (Fig. 15-7). In a few patients, chronic pancreatitis is initially painless but is heralded by the appearance of diabetes or malabsorption. By the time pancreatic calcifications are visible radiologically, most patients have developed diabetes, malabsorption, or both. Conspicuous weight loss is common, and unrelenting epigastric pain, radiating to the back, may cripple the patient. The mortality rate in chronic pancreatitis is 3 to 4% per year, and it approaches 50% within 20 to 25 years. One fifth of patients die of complications associated with attacks of acute pancreatitis. The remainder of the deaths are secondary to other causes, particularly alcohol-related disorders.

PANCREATIC CYSTADENOMA

Cystadenomas of the pancreas are large, multiloculated, cystic tumors, usually localized in the body or tail. They occur most frequently in women between the ages of 50 and 70 years. These neoplasms are of two types, depending on whether they are lined by serous or mucinous epithelium.

Serous cystadenomas, the rarer of the two types, are composed of numerous variably sized cysts lined by cuboidal epithelial cells with clear, glycogen-rich cytoplasm. The microcystic variant displays uniformly small cysts.

Mucinous cystadenomas account for 1% of all pancreatic exocrine tumors and feature multiloculated cysts lined by a high mucin-producing, columnar epithelium.

Both variants of pancreatic cystadenoma are believed to originate from the pancreatic duct system, the serous type from ductular cells and the mucinous form from cells lining the larger ducts. **Mucinous cystadenomas must be strictly separated from the serous variety because of the malignant potential of the former.** Pancreatic cystadenocarcinomas have recurred several years after the surgical removal of apparently benign mucinous cystadenomas.

PANCREATIC CANCER

In the United States, carcinoma of the pancreas is the fourth most common cause of cancer death in men and the fifth in women. Unfortunately, it remains virtually incurable. The incidence of pancreatic cancer seems to be increasing in all countries studied, and in the United States it has tripled in the past 50 years. Ductal adenocarcinoma accounts for 90% of all pancreatic cancers.

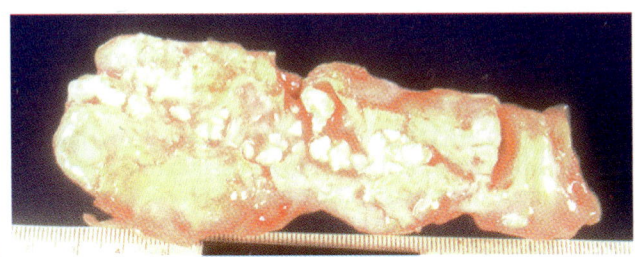

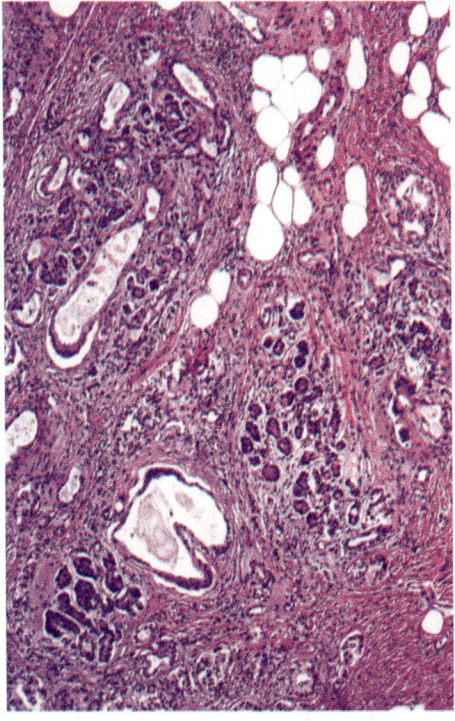

FIGURE 15-6
Chronic calcifying pancreatitis. A. The pancreas is shrunken and fibrotic, and the dilated duct contains numerous stones. B. Atrophic lobules of acinar cells are surrounded by dense fibrous tissue infiltrated by lymphocytes. The pancreatic ducts are dilated and contain inspissated proteinaceous material.

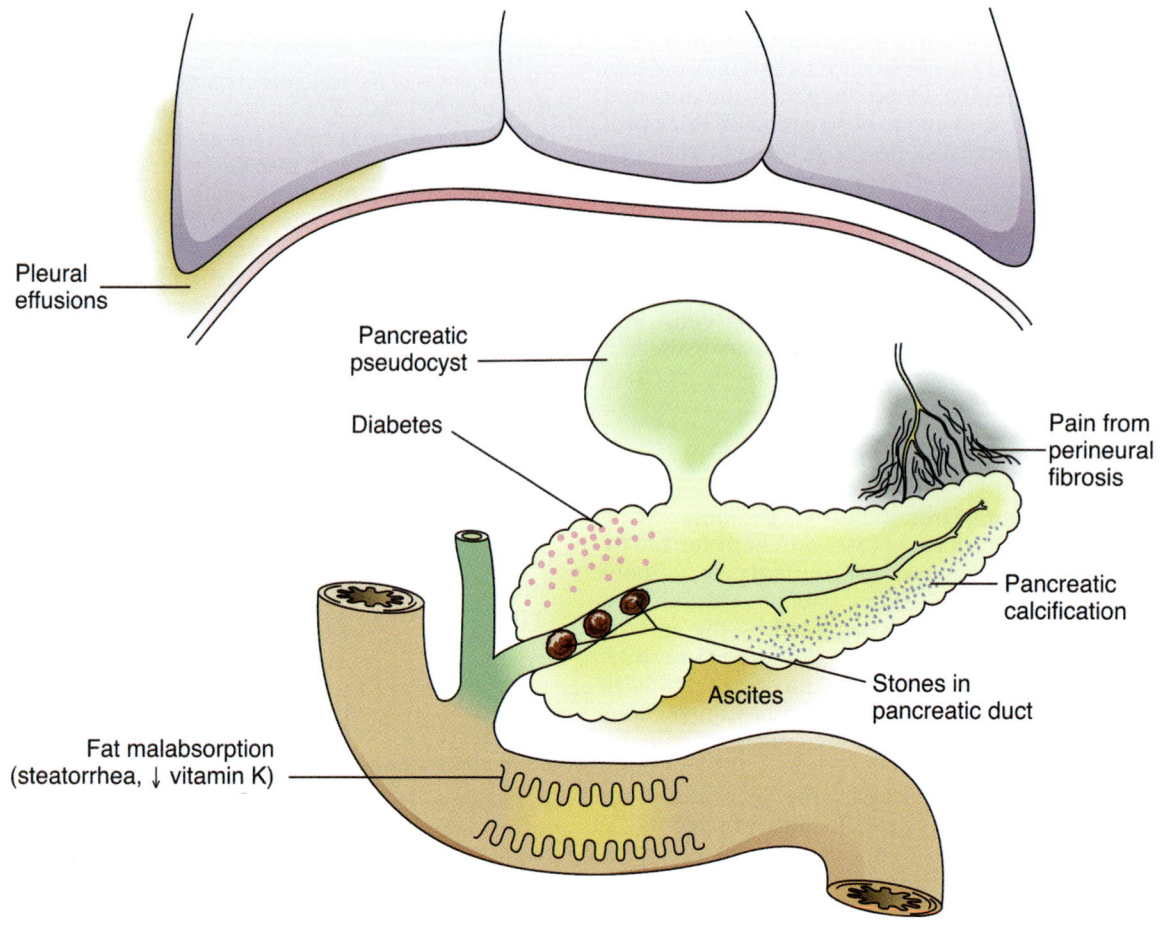

FIGURE 15-7
Complications of chronic pancreatitis.

Epidemiology: The distribution of pancreatic adenocarcinoma is worldwide, with the highest incidence (twice that in the United States) among male Maoris, Polynesian aborigines of New Zealand, and female natives of Hawaii. Cancer of the pancreas shows a significant male predominance (up to 3:1) in younger age groups but an almost equal distribution in old age. In the United States, the disease is more common in native Americans and blacks than in whites. Pancreatic carcinoma is a disease of late life, with the greatest incidence in persons older than 60 years of age, although its appearance as early as the third decade is not rare.

Pathogenesis: The factors involved in the causation of pancreatic cancer are obscure. Epidemiological studies have implicated both host and environmental factors as being of possible etiologic significance in cancer of the pancreas.

SMOKING: There is a two- to threefold increase in the risk of pancreatic cancer in cigarette smokers. A causal relationship is further implied by an apparent dose–response relationship associated with the number of cigarettes smoked per day and the demonstration of hyperplastic pancreatic ducts in autopsy studies of smokers.

CHEMICAL CARCINOGENS: Experimental studies in animals lend support to a possible role for chemical carcinogenesis in pancreatic cancer. Polycyclic hydrocarbons and a number of nitrosamines are pancreatic carcinogens in rodents.

DIETARY FACTORS: A high intake of meat and fat, especially the latter, may be a risk factor for pancreatic cancer.

DIABETES MELLITUS: Diabetics are at increased risk for the development of carcinoma of the pancreas. Up to 80% of patients with pancreatic cancer have evidence of diabetes mellitus at the time of cancer diagnosis. Patients with diabetes mellitus for five or more years are reported to exhibit a doubling of the risk for pancreatic cancer. In some patients, diabetes may be caused by pancreatic cancer, rather than the reverse. However, prospective studies of persons with abnormal glucose tolerance have documented a subsequent increase in the incidence of pancreatic cancer.

CHRONIC PANCREATITIS: Chronic pancreatitis is a risk factor for the development of pancreatic adenocarcinoma, although it accounts for only few cases. Since some cases of chronic pancreatitis are mild and clinically silent, its role in the development of pancreatic carcinoma may be underestimated.

MOLECULAR GENETICS: Pancreatic duct cancers exhibit a number of genetic alterations with considerable frequency. Mutational activation of K-*ras* (G to A transition in the second position of codon 12) is observed in most pancreatic carcinomas (up to 95%). In addition, mutational inactivation or deletion of tumor suppressor genes is common, including *p53* (50%), *p16 (MST1)* (85%), and *DPC-4* (deleted in pancreatic cancer, locus 4) (55%). Interestingly, deletions in chromosome 18 are present in 90% of pancreatic cancers. Although *DPC-4* is located on chromosome 18, only half of all pancreatic cancers show loss or inactivation of this gene, suggesting that another nearby tumor suppressor gene contributes to the development of the remaining 40%. Overactivity or inappropriate expression of several growth factors and their receptors is described, including epidermal growth factor (EGF) and its receptor, transforming growth factor-β (TGF-β), and fibroblast growth factor (FGF) and its receptor. Up to 10% of pancreatic carcinomas have inactivating mutations of *BRCA2*.

Pathology: Adenocarcinoma arises anywhere in the pancreas, the most frequent focus being in the head (60%), followed by the body (10%) and the tail (5%). In the remaining 25%, the pancreas is diffusely involved. Carcinomas of the head of the pancreas tend to be smaller than those of the body and tail and show more-limited spread to regional lymph nodes and more distant sites. In large part, these differences reflect earlier diagnosis of cancer of the head of the pancreas, which causes biliary obstruction and jaundice by compressing the ampulla of Vater and the common bile duct.

On gross examination, pancreatic carcinoma is a firm, gray, poorly demarcated multinodular mass (Fig. 15-8), often embedded in a dense connective tissue stroma. Tumors of the head of the pancreas may invade the common duct and the duodenal wall. They may also obstruct the duct of Wirsung and cause atrophy of the body and tail.

Microscopically, more than 75% of ductal adenocarcinomas of the pancreas are well differentiated, secrete mucin, and stimulate a florid deposition of collagen. The remaining 25% of cancers that originate from pancreatic ducts and ductules are giant cell carcinoma, adenosquamous carcinoma, and small cell carcinoma.

Pancreatic cancer metastasizes most commonly to the regional lymph nodes and the liver. Other frequent metastatic locations include the peritoneum, lungs, adrenals, and bones. Direct extension into neighboring organs (e.g., the stomach and duodenum) occasionally occurs. Perineural infiltration by tumor is characteristic of pancreatic cancer and accounts for the early and persistent pain of this disease.

Clinical Features: Early diagnosis of cancer of the pancreas is unusual, because the tumor is not ordinarily symptomatic until it is well advanced. Most pancreatic cancers have already metastasized by the time they have been diagnosed, and curative surgery is an option for only a trivial number of patients. Half of patients die within 6 months of diagnosis, and the overall 5-year survival rate is less than 1%. Serum levels of CA19-9, a Lewis blood group antigen, are increased in most cases.

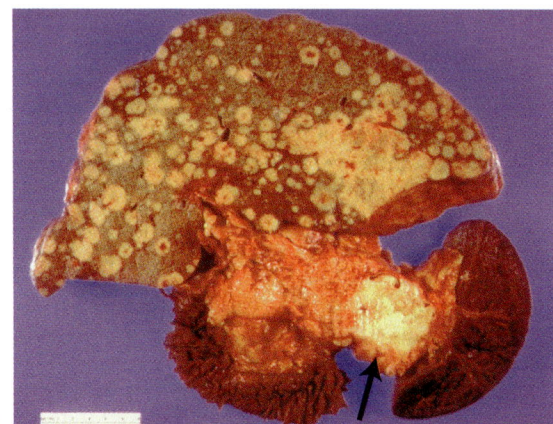
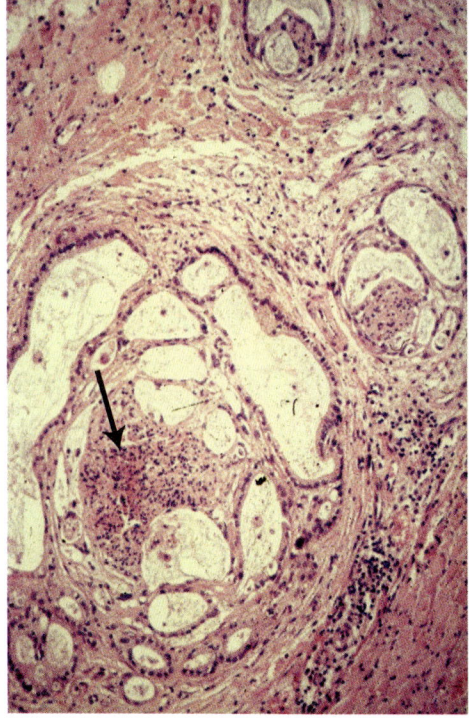

FIGURE 15-8
Carcinoma of the pancreas. A. An autopsy specimen shows a large tumor in the tail of the pancreas *(arrow)* and extensive metastases in the liver. B. A section of the tumor reveals malignant glands embedded in a dense fibrous stroma. A nerve (arrow) shows perineural invasion.

Patients with carcinoma of the pancreas present with anorexia, conspicuous weight loss, and a gnawing pain in the epigastrium, which often radiates to the back. Jaundice is present in about half of all patients with cancer localized to the head of the pancreas and in less than 10% of those in whom the body or tail is the site of the tumor. Progressive deterioration almost invariably ensues, with intractable pain, cachexia, and death.

Courvoisier sign refers to an acute painless dilation of the gallbladder accompanied by jaundice, owing to obstruction of the common bile duct by tumor. It may be the first indication of pancreatic cancer in about one third of patients but, unfortunately, does not identify potentially curable tumors.

Migratory thrombophlebitis (deep venous thrombosis) develops in 10% of patients with pancreatic cancer, especially when the tumor involves the body and tail of the pancreas. It is not uncommon for migratory thrombophlebitis, also known as *Trousseau syndrome*, to be the first evidence of an underlying pancreatic malignancy, although it may be seen with other cancers as well. In fact, unexplained thrombophlebitis in an otherwise healthy person mandates a careful search for an occult malignancy. Thrombi develop in multiple veins, including the deep veins of the legs, the subclavian vein, the inferior and superior mesenteric veins, and even the vena cava. Portal vein thrombosis may also occur, occasionally as the presenting event. Although the mechanisms responsible for the hypercoagulable state that leads to migratory thrombophlebitis are not completely understood, the following facts are known: (1) a serine protease synthesized and released by malignant tumor cells directly activates plasma factor X; (2) tumor cells spontaneously shed plasma membrane vesicles, which exhibit procoagulant activity; and (3) intracellular tissue thromboplastin is released from necrotic tumor.

The complications of pancreatic ductal carcinoma are summarized in Figure 15-9.

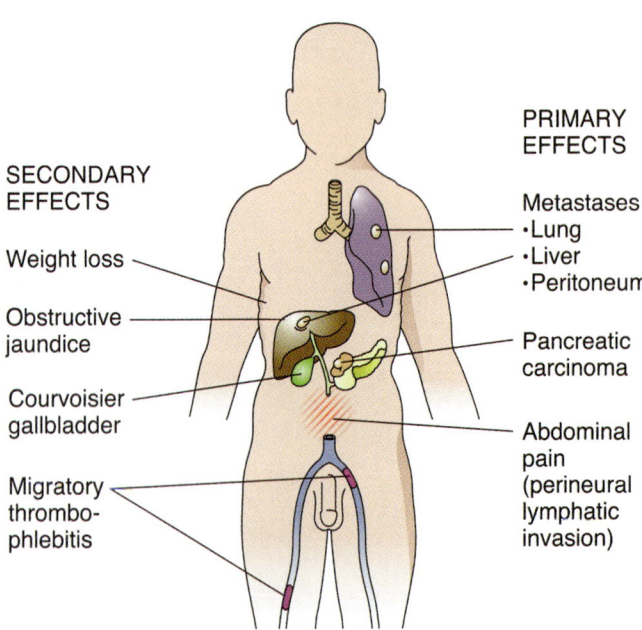

FIGURE 15-9
Complications of pancreatic carcinoma.

Acinar Cell Carcinoma Is an Uncommon Tumor of Mature Adults

Acinar cell cancers are usually large and tend to metastasize to regional lymph nodes and liver and more distantly to the lungs and other body sites. Some patients with this tumor develop a curious syndrome consisting of fat necrosis in subcutaneous tissues and bone marrow and polyarthralgia. The resemblance of this complication to the extrapancreatic lesions encountered in acute pancreatitis suggests that it is attributable to the unregulated release of pancreatic enzymes into the serum.

NEOPLASMS OF THE ENDOCRINE PANCREAS

Islet cell tumors are rare, comprising less than 10% of all pancreatic neoplasms. Of these, many are nonfunctional and are only discovered as incidental findings at autopsy. Functional islet cell tumors may occur alone or as part of the multiple endocrine neoplasia syndrome type I (MEN I). The secretion of hormones by endocrine tumors of the pancreas results in distinctive clinical syndromes. Before considering islet cell tumors, a brief discussion of normal islets is appropriate.

Pancreatic Islets Form the Endocrine Pancreas

The islets of Langerhans are scattered throughout the organ and consist of richly vascularized globular masses of cells. Six distinct cell types are correlated with specific hormones (Table 15-1).

- **Alpha cells** synthesize glucagon and are located in the outer rim of the islets. They constitute 15 to 20% of the total islet cell population (Fig. 15-10A). Glucagon induces glycogenolysis and gluconeogenesis in the liver, thereby raising the blood glucose level. Its secretion is stimulated by hypoglycemia and by the ingestion of a low-carbohydrate, high-protein meal. By virtue of these responses, glucagon, together with insulin, serves to maintain fuel homeostasis.
- **Beta cells** produce insulin and constitute 60 to 70% of all islet cells (see Fig. 15-10B). By electron microscopy, cellular insulin is resolved into characteristic polygonal and rhomboidal crystals enclosed in secretory vesicles. The major obligatory stimulus for insulin secretion is the binding of glucose to receptors on the surface of the beta cell.
- **Delta cells** are subdivided into D and D_1 types, secreting somatostatin and vasoactive intestinal polypeptide (VIP), respectively. They are fewer in number and slightly larger than alpha cells and, like them, tend to be localized at the periphery of the islets (see Fig. 15-10C). Delta cells are situated between the alpha and beta cells, so that the three cell types are often contiguous. Pancreatic somatostatin, a peptide identical to the one in the hypothalamus, inhibits the pituitary release of growth hormone. Somatostatin also inhibits secretion by alpha,

TABLE 15-1 Secretory Products of Islet Cells and Their Phsysiological Actions

Cell	Secretory Product	Mol. Wt.	Physiological Actions
Alpha	Glucagon	3500	Catabolic, stimulates glycogenolysis and gluconeogenesis, raises blood glucose
Beta	Insulin	6000	Anabolic, stimulates glycogenesis, lipogenesis, and protein synthesis, lowers blood glucose
Delta			Inhibits secretion of alpha, beta, D_1, and acinar cells
D	Somatostatin	1600	
D_1	Vasoactive intestinal polypeptide (VIP)	3800	Same as glucagon; also regulates tone and motility of GI tract and activates cAMP of intestinal epithelium
PP	Human pancreatic polypeptide (hpp)	4300	Stimulates gastric enzyme secretion, inhibits intestinal motility and bile secretion
EC	Serotonin, substance P (motilin)	176	Induces vasodilation, increases vascular permeability, stimulates motility of gastric muscle and tone of lower esophageal sphincter

beta, and D_1 cells, acinar cells of the exocrine pancreas, and certain hormone-secreting cells in the gastrointestinal tract. Coupled with the topographical cell–cell relations noted above, these hormonal interactions suggest that somatostatin plays a regulatory role in glucose homeostasis.

- **D_1 cells** are smaller than the other islet cell types and are rare in the islets of the normal human pancreas. Its hormone, VIP, has also been localized in ganglion cells and nerve fibers of the pancreas, gut, and brain. In a manner similar to that of glucagon, VIP induces glycogenolysis and hyperglycemia and regulates ion and water secretion by epithelial cells of the gastrointestinal tract.
- **Pancreatic polypeptide-secreting cells** are located primarily in the islets of the head of the pancreas and synthesize a polypeptide that appears to have variable and opposed functions. These include stimulation of the secretion of enzymes from the gastric mucosa and inhibition of a number of functions, such as smooth muscle contraction in the intestine and gallbladder, production of gastric acid, and secretion by the exocrine pancreas and biliary system.
- **Enterochromaffin cells** are rare components of the islet cell population in the head of the pancreas. They synthesize serotonin and the peptide *motilin*, a hormone that stimulates motility of gastric smooth muscle and increases the tone of the sphincter at the gastroesophageal junction.

Beta Cell Tumors (Insulinomas) Are the Most Common Islet Cell Neoplasms

Beta cell tumors (75% of islet cell neoplasms) may release enough insulin to induce severe hypoglycemia. Neoplastic beta cells, unlike their normal counterparts, are not regulated by the blood glucose level and continue to secrete insulin autonomously, even when the blood level of glucose is very low. Beta cell tumors and other islet cell neoplasms occur both sporadically and in the context of the MEN I syndrome (see Chapter 21).

 Pathology: *Most beta cell tumors are benign lesions in the body or tail of the pancreas* (Fig. 15-11). They are generally less than 3 cm in diameter and occasionally as small as 1 mm. Most (90%) are solitary and can be surgically excised. Only a minority (5–15%) demonstrate malignant behavior. Histologically, insulinoma cells resemble normal beta cells but are dispersed in trabecular or solid patterns (Fig. 15-12). The tumor often elicits a desmoplastic reaction, and amyloid (derived from a peptide hormone secreted with insulin and termed *amylin*) may be found in the stroma. Electron microscopy shows pleomorphic, paracrystalline granules surrounded by a clear halo, an appearance typical of insulin stored in normal beta cells. A

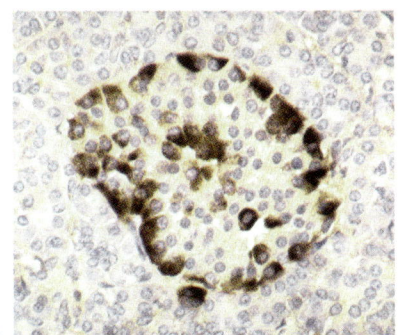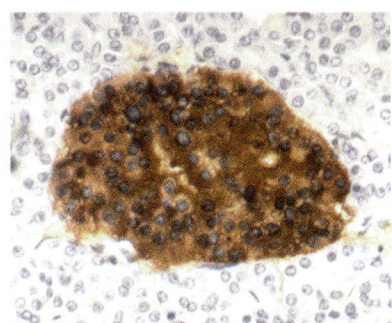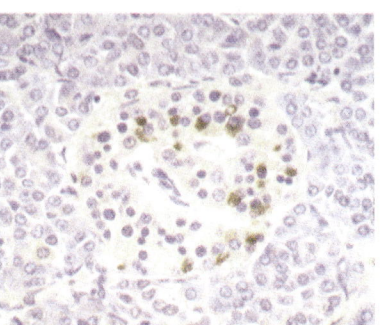

FIGURE 15-10
Localization of hormones of the pancreatic islet by specific antibodies. The immunoperoxidase technique reveals (A) glucagon in alpha cells at the periphery of the islet, (B) insulin in beta cells distributed throughout the islet, and (C) somatostatin in sparsely distributed delta cells.

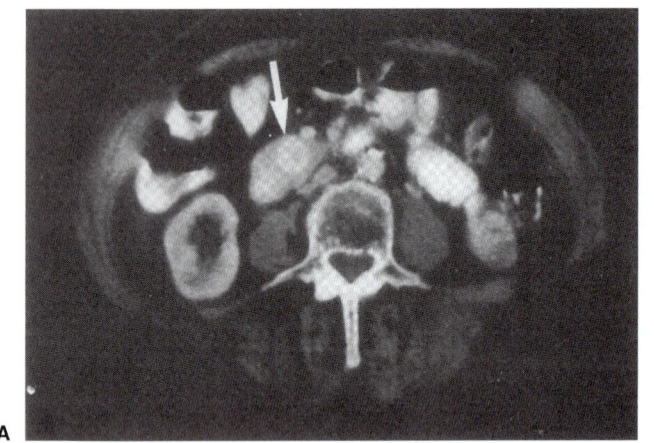
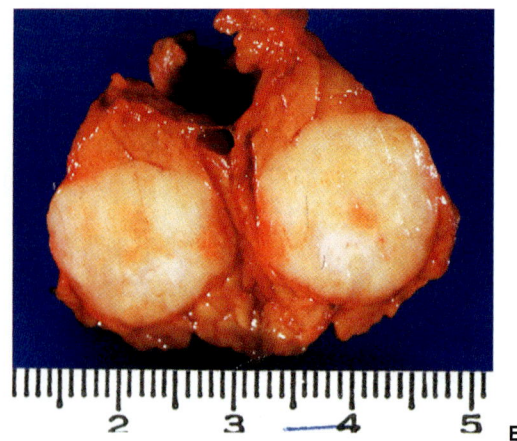

FIGURE 15-11
Insulinoma. A. A computed tomography (CT) scan of the abdomen shows a solitary insulinoma (arrow). B. An insulinoma is embedded in tan, lobular pancreatic tissue.

reliable distinction between benign and malignant insulinomas is usually not possible on histological grounds and in most cases awaits the appearance or absence of metastases.

Clinical Features: Low blood sugar produces a syndrome of sweating, nervousness, and hunger, which may progress to confusion, lethargy, and coma. Since these symptoms are relieved by eating, it is common for patients with insulinomas to be overweight. Frequently, the diagnosis is delayed by abnormal behavior that causes some patients to seek psychiatric care. Most cases are characterized by only a mild hypoglycemia, and in some, the tumor is not functional at all. The diagnosis is established by the demonstration of high levels of insulin in the blood and the tumor cells (see Fig. 15-12B).

Pancreatic Gastrinomas (Zollinger-Ellison Syndrome) Induce Gastric Acid Secretion

Pancreatic gastrinoma is an islet cell tumor consisting of so-called G cells, which produce gastrin, a potent hormonal stimulus for the secretion of acid by the stomach. The location of this tumor in the pancreas is curious, because gastrin-containing cells have not been demonstrated in normal islets. By electron microscopy, the tumor cells bear a strong resemblance to the gastrin-secreting cells that normally reside in the duodenal mucosa. The pancreatic tumor is believed to arise from multipotent primitive endocrine cells that have undergone inappropriate differentiation to form G cells in the islets. Pancreatic gastrinoma is the cause of *Zollinger-Ellison syndrome,* a disorder characterized by (1) intractable gastric hypersecretion, (2) severe peptic ulcera-

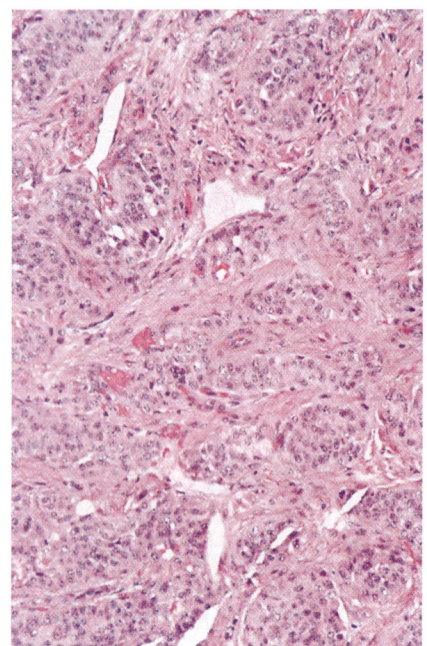
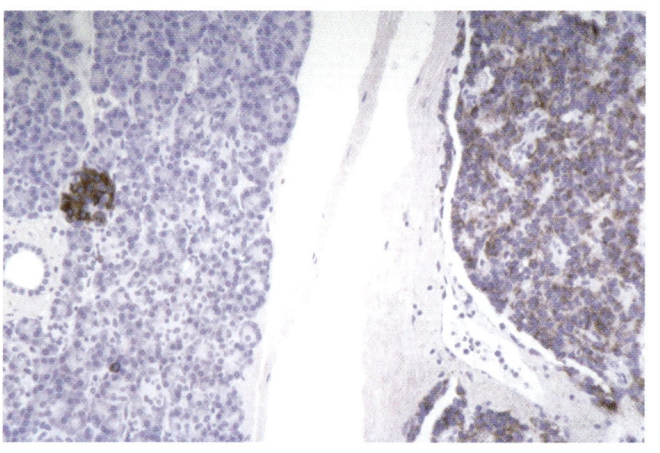

FIGURE 15-12
A functional insulinoma. A. Nests of tumor cells are surrounded by numerous capillaries. B. Immunochemical localization (brown staining) of insulin in an insulinoma (right) and in an islet in the adjacent normal pancreas.

tion of the duodenum and jejunum, and (3) high levels of gastrin in the blood.

Among islet cell tumors, pancreatic gastrinomas are second in frequency only to insulinomas, accounting for one fourth of islet cell tumors. They are most common between the ages of 30 and 50 years, with a slight male predominance. Fifteen percent of cases of the Zollinger-Ellison syndrome are due to gastrinomas outside the pancreas, particularly in the duodenum. Most gastrinomas are malignant (70–90%). The tumor may be solitary or multiple, the latter usually in the context of MEN I. Histologically, gastrinomas are remarkably similar to intestinal carcinoid tumors. Metastases to regional lymph nodes and the liver are often functional.

Alpha Cell Tumors Secrete Glucagon

Alpha cell tumors (glucagonomas) are associated with a syndrome consisting of (1) mild diabetes; (2) a necrotizing, migratory, erythematous rash; (3) anemia; (4) venous thromboses; and (5) severe infections. They are rare (1% of functional islet cell tumors) and occur between the ages of 40 and 70 years, with a slight female predominance. Two thirds of symptomatic glucagonomas are malignant.

Functional glucagonomas are usually large tumors that invade surrounding structures. Microscopically, they resemble the trabecular and solid patterns of insulinomas. The presence of glucagon within the tumor is demonstrated immunocytochemically and by the demonstration of characteristic alpha cell granules by electron microscopy (Fig. 15-13). In patients with alpha cell tumors, plasma glucagon levels are elevated up to 30 times above normal. In addition to the characteristic hyperglycemia, fasting plasma amino acid levels are decreased to as low as 20% of normal.

Delta Cell Tumors Produce Somatostatin

Delta cell tumors (somatostatinomas) are rare and produce a syndrome consisting of mild diabetes, gallstones, steatorrhea, and hypochlorhydria. These effects result from the inhibitory actions of somatostatin on other cells of the pancreatic islets and on neuroendocrine cells of the gastrointestinal tract. Thus, the levels of insulin and glucagon in blood are decreased. In addition to producing somatostatin, some delta cell tumors also secrete calcitonin or adrenocorticotropic hormone (ACTH). The tumor is usually solitary, and most are malignant, with metastases already present at the time of diagnosis.

D₁ Tumors Release Vasoactive Intestinal Peptide (VIP)

Verner-Morrison syndrome is caused by elevated levels of VIP and is characterized by explosive and profuse watery diarrhea, accompanied by hypokalemia and hypochlorhydria. The disorder has also been referred to as *pancreatic cholera*. VIPomas are rare tumors (less than 5% of all islet tumors), are usually large and solitary, and in most cases are malignant.

High levels of circulating VIP and severe diarrhea have also been encountered in patients with a variety of nonpancreatic neoplasms containing different types of neuroendocrine cells (e.g., ganglioneuroma, pheochromocytoma of the adrenal medulla, medullary thyroid carcinoma, and bronchogenic carcinoma). In some patients, the Verner-Morrison syndrome is caused by MEN I.

Pancreatic Polypeptide-Secreting Tumors Are Asymptomatic

No clinical syndrome occurs despite the fact that pancreatic polypeptide-secreting tumors secrete high levels of pancreatic polypeptide in the blood. The tumors are usually single and benign, although a few have metastasized to the liver. In addition to their own specific hormones, other islet cell tumors may secrete pancreatic polypeptide.

Enterochromaffin Cell (Carcinoid) Tumors Produce Serotonin

Carcinoid tumors of the pancreas are rare malignant neoplasms that resemble intestinal carcinoids and contain enterochromaffin cells. When confined to the pancreas, they may induce the so-called atypical carcinoid syndrome, consisting of a severe facial flush, hypotension, periorbital edema, and lacrimation. Carcinoid tumors that have metastasized to the liver cause the classic carcinoid syndrome (see Chapter 13).

The syndromes and complications of the major types of islet cell tumors are summarized in Figure 15-14.

Multiple Endocrine Neoplasia Syndrome Type I (MEN I) Is an Infrequent Familial Disorder

MEN I is characterized by multiple adenomas of the pituitary, parathyroids, and endocrine pancreas. It is frequently associated with the Zollinger-Ellison syndrome, in which

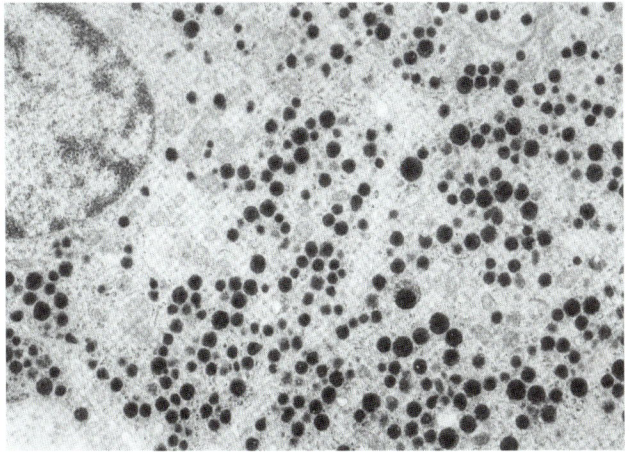

FIGURE 15-13
Alpha cells in a functional glucagonoma. The granules are indistinguishable from those of normal alpha cells.

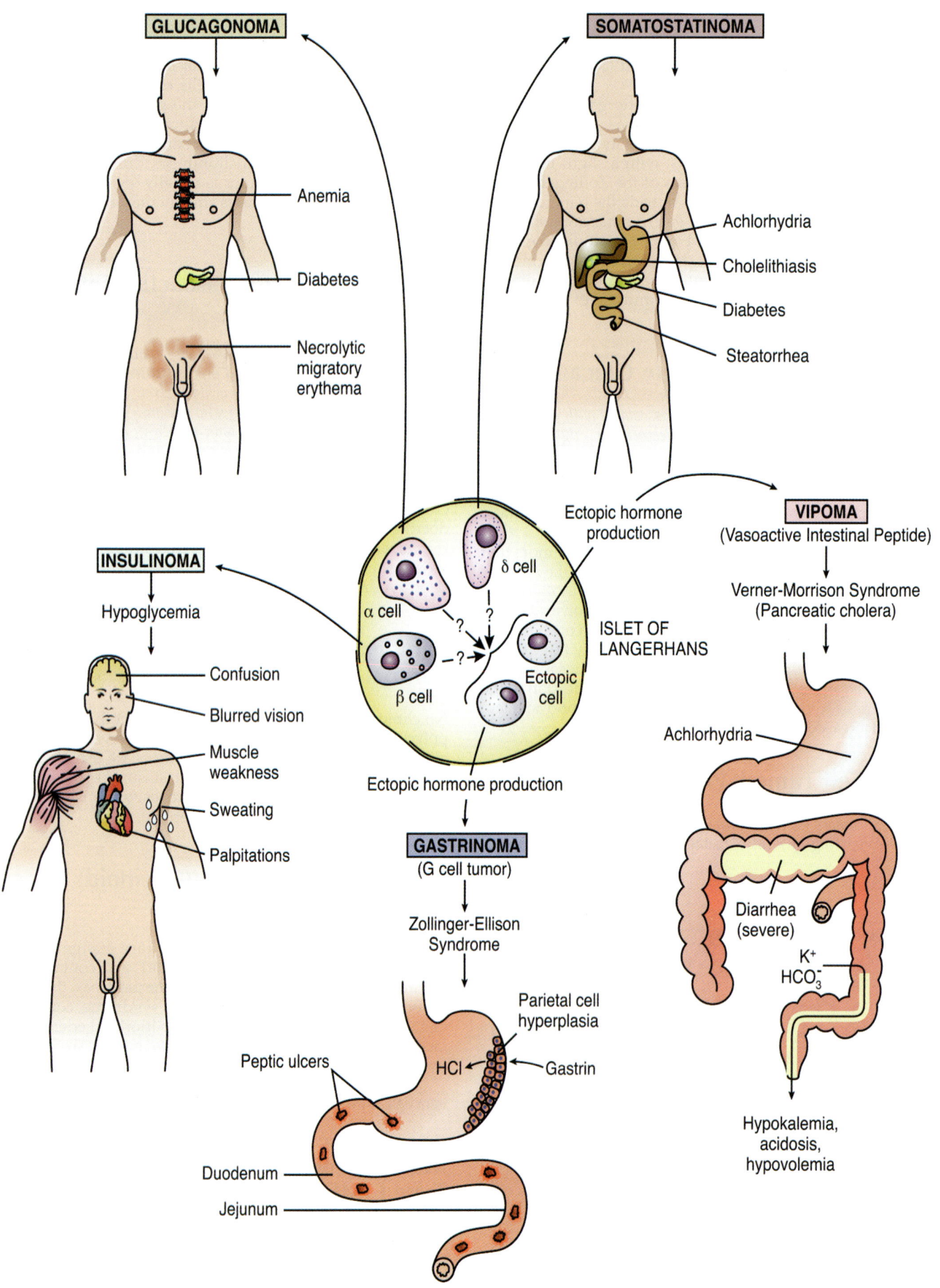

FIGURE 15-14
Syndromes associated with islet cell tumors of the pancreas.

case gastrin-secreting islet cell tumors are present. The MEN syndromes are described in detail in Chapter 21.

Ectopic Hormone Syndromes May Be Caused by Islet Cell Tumors

Islet cell tumors may secrete a variety of normal hormones that are not ordinarily produced in the pancreas (ectopic hormones), including ACTH, parathyroid hormone, calcitonin, and vasopressin. The ectopic hormone may be produced either alone or in combination with normally occurring pancreatic hormones. Endocrine tumors of the pancreas account for 10% of paraneoplastic Cushing syndrome, in this respect being second only to small cell carcinoma of the lung.

SUGGESTED READING

Books

Cruickshank, AH, Benbow EW: *Pathology of the pancreas.* New York: Springer, 1995.
Owen DA, Kelly JK: *Pathology of the gallbladder, biliary tract, and pancreas.* Philadelphia: WB Saunders, 2001.
Solcia E, Capella C, Kloppel G: Tumors of the pancreas. In: *Atlas of tumor pathology,* series 3, fascicle 20. Washington, DC: Armed Forces Institute of Pathology, 1997.

Review Articles

Baron R, Morgan DE: Acute necrotizing pancreatitis. *N Engl J Med* 340:1412–1417,1999.
Chen J-M, Ferec C. Molecular basis of hereditary pancreatitis. *Eur J Hum Genet* 8:473–479, 2000.
Choudari CP, Lehman GA, Sherman S: Pancreatitis and cystic fibrosis gene mutations. *Gastroenterol Clin North Am* 28:543–549,1999.
Cooperman AM: An overview of pancreatic pseudocysts *Surg Clin North Am* 81:391–397, 2001.
Efthimiou E, Crnogorac-Jurcevic T, Lemoine NR: Pancreatic cancer genetics. *Pancreatology* 1:571–575, 2001.
Etemad B, Whitcomb DC: Chronic pancreatitis: Diagnosis, classification, and new genetic developments. *Gastroenterology* 120:682–707, 2001.
Fernandez-del Castillo C, Warshaw AL: Cystic neoplasms of the pancreas. *Pancreatology* 1:641–647, 2001.
Gasslander T, Arnelo U, Albiin N, Permert J: Cystic tumors of the pancreas. *Dig Dis* 19(1):57–62, 2001.
Inoue S, Tezel E, Nakao A: Molecular diagnosis of pancreatic cancer. *Hepatogastroenterology* 48:933–938, 2001.
Levy MJ, Geenen JE: Idiopathic acute recurrent pancreatitis. *Am J Gastroenterol* 96:2540–2555, 2001.
Wick MR, Graeme-Cook FM: Pancreatic neuroendocrine neoplasms: A current summary of diagnostic, prognostic, and differential diagnostic information. *Am J Clin Pathol* 115(suppl):S28–45, 2001.

CHAPTER 16

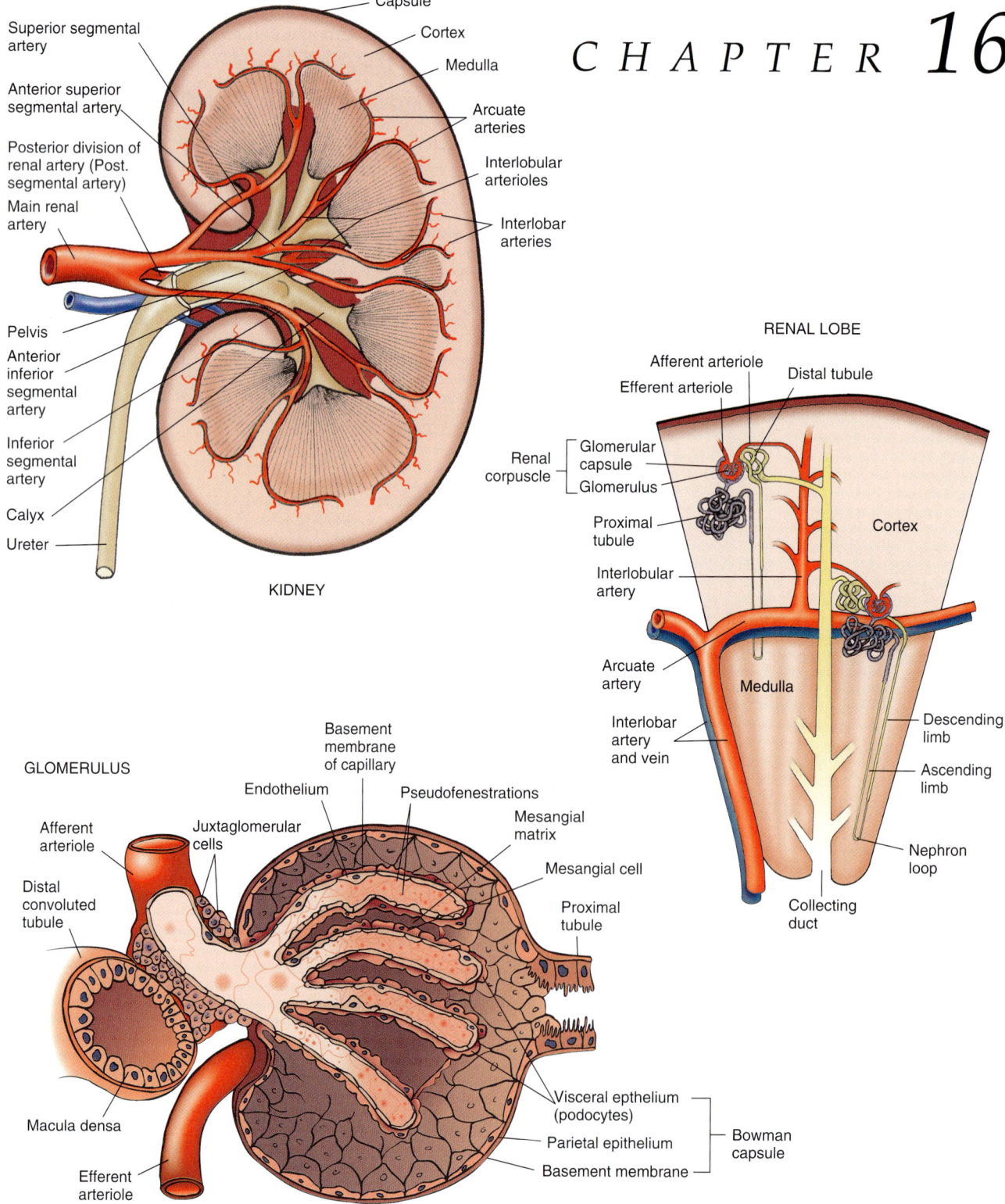

The Kidney

J. Charles Jennette

Anatomy
Blood Vessels
Glomerulus
Tubules
Juxtaglomerular Apparatus
Interstitium

Congenital Anomalies
Potter Sequence
Renal Agenesis
Renal Hypoplasia
Ectopic Kidney
Horseshoe Kidney
Renal Dysplasia
Autosomal Dominant Polycystic Kidney Disease
Autosomal Recessive Polycystic Kidney Disease
Glomerulocystic Disease
Nephronophthisis–Medullary Cystic Disease Complex
Medullary Sponge Kidney

Acquired Cystic Kidney Disease
Simple Renal Cysts
Acquired Cystic Disease

Glomerular Diseases
Nephrotic Syndrome
Nephritic (Glomerulonephritic) Syndrome
Pathogenesis of Glomerulonephritis
Pathology of Glomerular Diseases
Minimal-Change Glomerulopathy
Focal Segmental Glomerulosclerosis
Membranous Glomerulopathy
Diabetic Glomerulosclerosis
Amyloidosis
Light Chain and Heavy Chain Deposition Disease
Hereditary Nephritis (Alport Syndrome)
Thin Glomerular Basement Membrane Nephropathy
Acute Postinfectious Glomerulonephritis
Type I Membranoproliferative Glomerulonephritis
Type II Membranoproliferative Glomerulonephritis (Dense Deposit Disease)
Lupus Glomerulonephritis
IgA Nephropathy (Berger Disease)
Anti-Glomerular Basement Membrane (Anti-GBM)
ANCA Glomerulonephritis

(continued)

FIGURE 16-1 *(see opposite page)*
The gross and microscopic anatomy of the kidney.

Vascular Diseases

Renal Vasculitis

Hypertensive Nephrosclerosis (Benign Nephrosclerosis)

Malignant Hypertensive Nephropathy

Renovascular Hypertension

Renal Atheroembolism

Thrombotic Microangiopathy

Preeclampsia

Sickle Cell Nephropathy

Renal Infarcts

Cortical Necrosis

Diseases of Tubules and Interstitium

Acute Tubular Necrosis

Pyelonephritis

Analgesic Nephropathy

Drug-Induced (Hypersensitivity) Acute Tubulointerstitial Nephritis

Light-Chain Cast Nephropathy

Urate Nephropathy

Nephrocalcinosis

Renal Stones (Nephrolithiasis and Urolithiasis)

Obstructive Uropathy and Hydronephrosis

Renal Transplantation

Benign Tumors of the Kidney

Malignant Tumors of the Kidney

Wilms Tumor (Nephroblastoma)

Renal Cell Carcinoma

Transitional Cell Carcinoma

ANATOMY

The kidneys are paired, bean-shaped organs located on both sides of the vertebral column in the retroperitoneal space. The adult kidney weighs an average of 150 g and is approximately 11 cm long, 6 cm wide, and 3 cm thick. Each kidney consists of an outer cortex and an inner medulla (Fig. 16-1). When the kidney is bisected, the medulla is found to have approximately 12 pyramids, with their bases at the corticomedullary junction. Each medullary pyramid and the overlying cortex constitute a renal lobe. A pyramid has an inner and an outer zone. The inner zone, called the *papilla*, empties into a calyx, which is a funnel-shaped structure that conducts urine into the renal pelvis. The pelvis in turn empties into the ureter.

Blood Vessels

The kidney is one of the most vascularized organs in the body and receives about one fifth to one fourth of the cardiac output. The blood supply is derived from a single main renal artery that arises from the aorta, although a quarter of kidneys have one or more accessory renal arteries. Before entering the renal parenchyma, the main renal artery divides into anterior and posterior branches, which in turn give rise to the interlobar arteries (Fig. 16-1). The latter branch into the arcuate arteries, which course parallel to the renal surface between the medulla and the cortex. The interlobular arteries arise from the arcuate arteries and extend toward the renal surface. The interlobular arteries give off the afferent arterioles, each of which supplies a single glomerulus. After emerging from the glomerulus, the efferent arteriole branches into capillaries. The efferent arterioles of glomeruli in the outer cortex give rise to capillaries that supply blood to the parenchyma of the cortex. The efferent arterioles of glomeruli in the deep cortex, adjacent to the medulla, provide vessels that extend into the medulla to become the medullary peritubular vessels, namely, the *vasa recta*.

The Glomerulus is the Renal Filter

The nephron is the architectural unit of the kidney and includes the glomerulus and its tubule, the latter terminating at the common collecting system (see Fig. 16-1). The glomerulus is a specialized network of capillaries covered by epithelial cells and supported by modified smooth muscle cells called *mesangial cells* (Figs. 16-1 through 16-4). As it enters the glomerulus the afferent arteriole branches into capillaries, which form the convoluted glomerular tuft and eventually coalesce into the efferent arteriole that exits the glomerulus. The glomerular capillaries are lined by fenestrated endothelial cells lying on a basement membrane. The outer surface of this basement membrane is covered by specialized epithelial cells called *podocytes* or *visceral epithelial cells*. These visceral epithelial cells line the glomerular side of Bowman's space, whereas the parietal epithelial cells line Bowman's capsule on the opposite side.

Anatomy

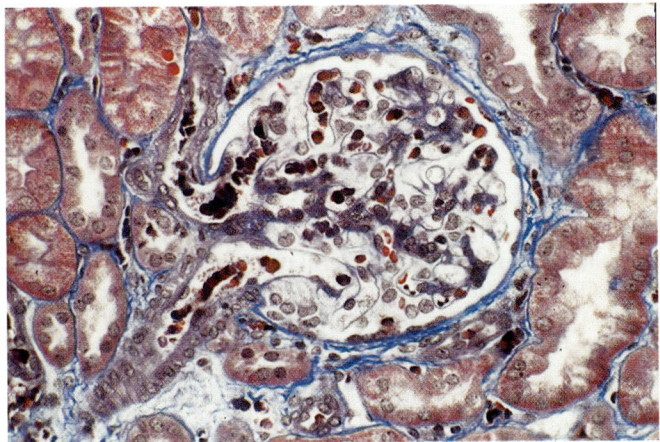

FIGURE 16-2
Normal glomerulus, light microscopy. The Masson trichrome stain shows a glomerular tuft with delicate blue capillary wall basement membranes, small amounts of blue matrix surrounding mesangial cells, and the hilum on the left. The afferent arteriole enters below and the efferent arteriole exits above.

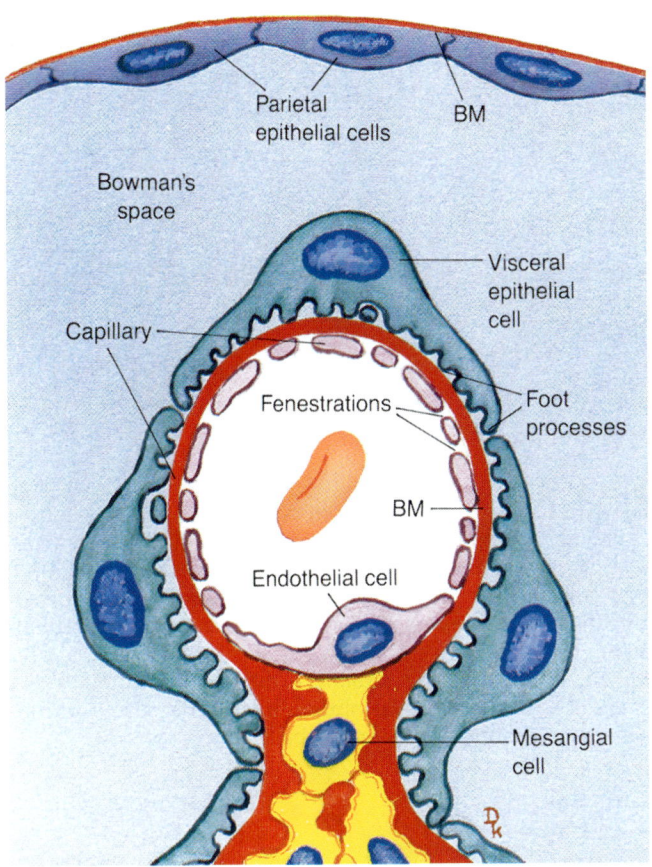

FIGURE 16-4
Normal glomerulus. The relationship of the different glomerular cell types to the basement membrane and mesangial matrix is illustrated using a single glomerular loop. The entire outer aspect of the glomerular basement membrane (BM) (peripheral loop and stalk) is covered by the visceral epithelial cell (podocyte) foot processes. The outer portions of the fenestrated endothelial cell are in contact with the inner surface of the basement membrane, whereas the central part is in contact with the mesangial cell and adjacent mesangial matrix. Compare this figure with Figure 16-3.

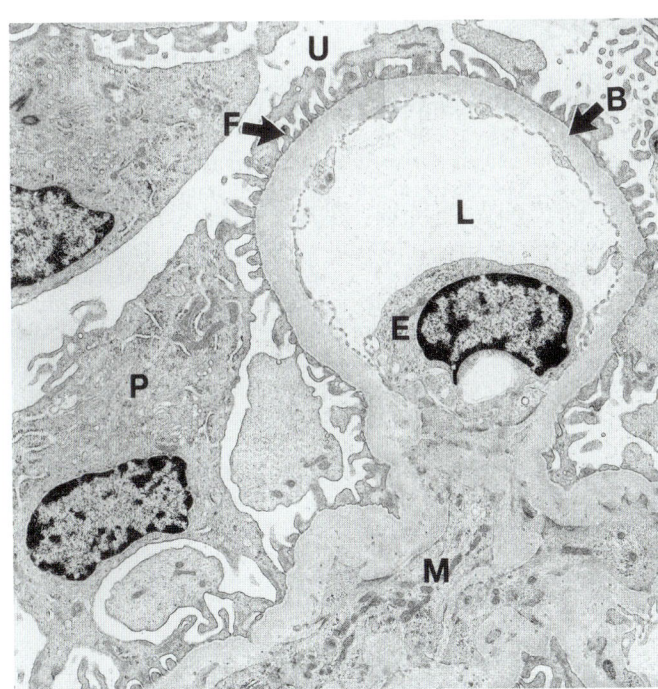

FIGURE 16-3
Normal glomerulus. In this electron micrograph of a single capillary loop and adjacent mesangium, the capillary wall portion of the lumen (L) is lined by a thin layer of fenestrated endothelial cytoplasm that extends out from the endothelial cell body (E). The endothelial cell body is in direct contact with the mesangium, which includes the mesangial cell (M) and adjacent matrix. The outer aspect of the basement membrane (B) is covered by foot processes (F) from the podocyte (P) that line the urinary space (U). Compare this figure with Figure 16-4.

Glomerular Basement Membrane

The glomerular basement membrane (GBM) (Figs. 16-3 through 16-5) lies between the endothelial cells and the podocytes in the peripheral capillary walls and between the mesangium and the podocytes. Thus, the GBM does not completely surround each capillary lumen but rather splays out over the mesangium as the paramesangial GBM. Thus a potential pathway exists for substances in the blood to enter the mesangium without crossing the GBM.

Although morphologically similar to many other basement membranes, the GBM is functionally and chemically distinct. Ultrastructurally, it is approximately 300 nm thick and has three definable layers (Fig. 16-5):

- **Lamina densa:** a central electron-dense zone
- **Lamina rara interna:** a thin inner electron-lucent zone
- **Lamina rara externa:** a thin outer electron-lucent zone

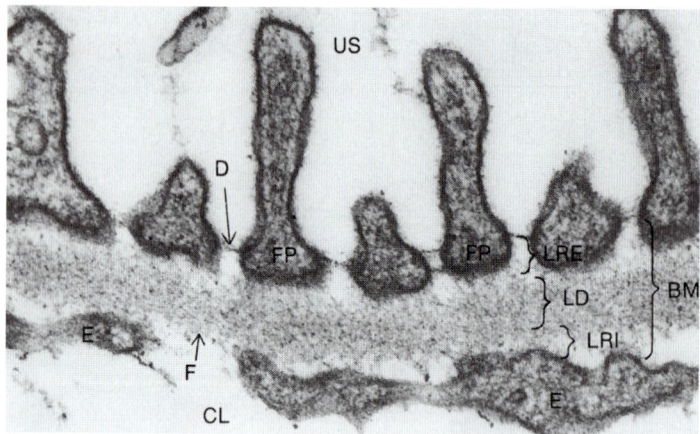

FIGURE 16-5
The glomerular filter. An electron micrograph illustrates the structures of the glomerular filter. Molecules that pass from the capillary lumen (CL) to the urinary space (US) traverse the fenestrations (F) of the endothelial cell (E), the trilaminar basement membrane (BM) (lamina rara interna [LRI], lamina densa [LD], and lamina rara externa [LRE]), and the slit pore diaphragm (D) that connects podocyte foot processes (FP).

The GBM is composed predominantly of type IV collagen. Other constituents include laminin, entactin, fibronectin, and glycosaminoglycans. The GBM has a strong negative charge because of the presence of polyanionic glycosaminoglycans, which are rich in heparan sulfate. This property allows charge-selective filtration of electrically neutral and cationic molecules and relative exclusion of negatively charged molecules such as albumin. The GBM also discriminates between molecules on the basis of size.

Endothelial Cells

Glomerular capillaries have a fenestrated endothelial layer, approximately 50 nm thick, with numerous 60- to 100-nm openings (Fig. 16-5). These pores are not a major filtration barrier to constituents of the plasma. Endothelial surface membrane proteins, such as adhesion molecules, and endothelial secretory products, such as prostaglandins and nitric oxide, play important roles in the pathogenesis of inflammatory and thrombotic glomerular diseases.

Podocytes

The podocytes rest on the outer aspect of the GBM and send cytoplasmic projections, termed *foot processes,* onto the lamina rara externa of the GBM (see Fig. 16-5). Between adjacent foot processes is a thin membrane called the *filtration slit diaphragm,* which is a modified adherens junction. The podocytes are the major size-selective glomerular filtration barrier, whereas the GBM is the major charge-selective barrier. Genetic abnormalities in the proteins that compose the slit diaphragm, such as *nephrin* and *podocin,* can result in abnormal protein loss into the urine (proteinuria).

Mesangium

The glomerulus is supported by a cellular and matrix network collectively termed the *mesangium.* Mesangial cells are modified smooth muscle cells situated in the center of the glomerular tuft between capillary loops. Important functions of the mesangium include:

- Mechanical support for the glomerulus
- Endocytosis and processing of plasma proteins, including immune complexes
- Maintenance of basement membrane and matrix elements
- Modulation of glomerular filtration by the contractility of mesangial cells
- Generation of molecular mediators (e.g., prostaglandins and cytokines)

The Tubules Comprise a Collecting System

The major segments of the tubule that arises from each glomerulus are the proximal tubule, loop of Henle, and distal tubule, which empties into the collecting duct. At the origin of the proximal tubule from the glomerulus, the flat parietal epithelium abruptly transforms into the tall columnar cells of the proximal tubule, which have numerous tall microvilli that form a brush border. The initial segment is the proximal tubule is very tortuous and thus is called the *proximal convoluted tubule.* As it descends into the medulla, the proximal tubule straightens into the thick descending limb of the loop of Henle. Further into the medulla, the thick descending limb flattens into the thin limb of the loop of Henle, which eventually loops back toward the cortex. As it approaches the cortex, the thin limb becomes the thick ascending limb. The thick ascending limb returns to the glomerulus from which the tubule arose, and contributes to the juxtaglomerular apparatus of that glomerulus. It then becomes the distal convoluted tubule. Several distal tubules unite to form a collecting duct, which ultimately empties into the ducts of Bellini, the structures that discharge urine through the papillae into the calyces.

The Juxtaglomerular Apparatus Secretes Hormones

The juxtaglomerular apparatus, located at the hilus of the glomerulus, is a complex that consists of the following:

- **Macula densa,** a region of the thick ascending limb of the loop of Henle that has closely packed nuclei
- **Extraglomerular mesangial cells,** located between the macula densa and the hilar arterioles
- **Terminal afferent arteriole and proximal efferent arteriole**

The wall of the afferent arteriole contains characteristic granular cells involved in the synthesis and secretion of renin and angiotensin.

Interstitium

The renal interstitium is composed of interstitial cells that resemble fibroblasts and surrounding collagenous matrix. The interstitium occupies only 10% of the cortical volume but constitutes 20 to 30% of medullary volume. The interstitium offers structural support. In addition, interstitial cells have homeostatic secretory functions. For example, some cortical interstitial cells secrete erythropoietin and some medullary cells elaborate prostaglandins.

CONGENITAL ANOMALIES

Potter Sequence Results from Insufficient Amniotic Fluid

Potter sequence (oligohydramnios sequence) is the syndrome of pathological abnormalities that are caused by markedly reduced intrauterine urine production (also see Chapter 6). Reduced urine production results in less amniotic fluid (oligohydramnios). The amniotic fluid normally cushions the fetus. With less fluid, the fetus is compressed by the uterus, which causes low-set ears, small receding chin, beaklike nose, and abnormally bent lower extremities. The most life-threatening component of Potter sequence is pulmonary hypoplasia, which is caused by inadequate maturational stimuli from amniotic fluid and by compression of the chest wall by the uterus. Because even neonates can be dialyzed, severe respiratory insufficiency secondary to Potter sequence (rather than renal insufficiency) may be the cause of death in infants with severe congenital renal anomalies.

Renal Agenesis Is the Complete Absence of Renal Tissue

Most infants born with bilateral renal agenesis are stillborn and have Potter sequence. Bilateral agenesis is often associated with other congenital anomalies, especially elsewhere in the urinary tract or in the lower extremities. Unilateral renal agenesis is not a serious matter if there are no associated anomalies, because the contralateral kidney undergoes sufficient hypertrophy to maintain normal renal function. Later in life, however, there is an increased risk for developing progressive glomerular sclerosis (secondary focal segmental glomerulosclerosis) because of overwork of the nephron.

Renal Hypoplasia Refers to a Congenital Reduction in Renal Mass

The kidney shows no histological malformation and is formed by six or fewer renal lobes (medullary pyramids with overlying cortex). Renal hypoplasia must be differentiated from small kidneys secondary to atrophy or scarring. A frequent variant of hypoplasia features enlargement of the too few glomeruli and thus is termed *oligomeganephronia*.

Ectopic Kidney Is an Abnormal Location of the Organ

The misplaced kidney is usually in the pelvis. Most commonly, this condition results from failure of the fetal kidney to migrate from the pelvis to the flank. Renal ectopia may involve only one kidney or it may be bilateral. In *simple ectopia*, the ureters drain into the appropriate side of the bladder. In *crossed ectopia*, the ectopic kidney is on the same side as its normal mate, and the ectopic ureter crosses the midline and drains into the contralateral side of the bladder.

Horseshoe Kidney Is a Single, Large, Midline Organ

The infant is born with fusion of the two kidneys, usually at the lower poles. (Fig. 16-6). This anomaly usually has no clinical consequences but does increase the risk for obstruction and pyelonephritis because the ureters must cross over the junction between the two kidneys when the organ is fused at the lower pole.

Renal Dysplasia Is a Developmental Disorder

Renal dysplasia is characterized by undifferentiated tubular structures surrounded by primitive mesenchyme, sometimes with heterotopic tissue such as cartilage. Cysts often form from the abnormal tubules.

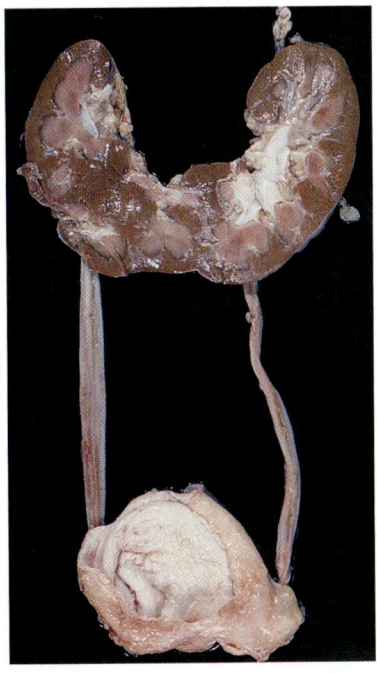

FIGURE 16-6
Horseshoe kidney. The kidneys are fused at the lower pole.

Pathogenesis: Renal dysplasia results from an abnormality in metanephric differentiation. There are multiple genetic and somatic causes. Some familial forms of dysplasia probably result from abnormal differential signals that affect the inductive interactions between the ureteric bud and the metanephric blastema. Many forms of dysplasia are accompanied by other urinary tract abnormalities, especially ones that cause obstruction of urine flow. This association suggests that an obstruction to the flow of urine in utero can cause dysplasia. Frequent associated anomalies include the following:

- Ureteral agenesis
- Ureteral atresia
- Ureteropelvic junction obstruction
- Ureterovesical stenosis or posterior urethral valves

 Pathology: Histologically, the hallmark of renal dysplasia is undifferentiated tubules and ducts lined by cuboidal or columnar epithelium. These structures are surrounded by mantles of undifferentiated mesenchyme that sometimes contain smooth muscle and islands of cartilage (Fig. 16-7). Rudimentary glomeruli may be present, and the tubules and ducts may be cystically dilated. Renal dysplasia can be unilateral or bilateral, and the involved kidney can be abnormally large or very small.

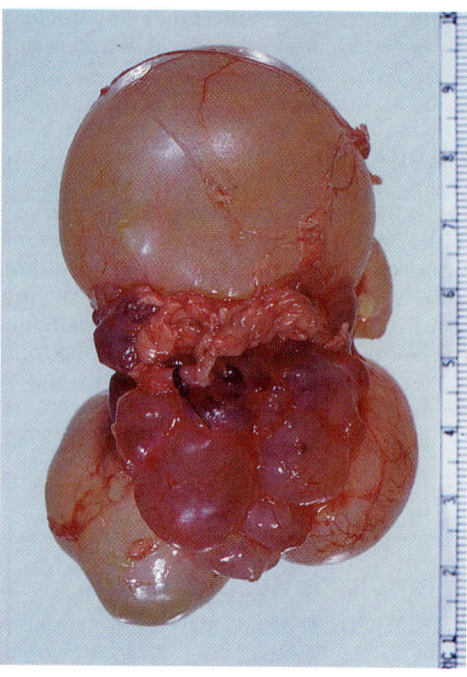

FIGURE 16-8
Multicystic renal dysplasia. An irregular mass of variably sized cysts does not have a reniform shape.

- **Aplastic renal dysplasia** results in very small misshapen dysplastic kidneys, which may be difficult to identify by gross examination.
- **Multicystic renal dysplasia** is usually unilateral and is characterized by renal enlargement by multiple cysts, ranging from microscopic to several centimeters in diameter. The kidney does not have the usual kidney shape, but is rather an irregular mass of cysts (Fig. 16-8).
- **Diffuse cystic renal dysplasia** features more-uniformly sized cysts and preservation of a kidney shape.
- **Obstructive renal dysplasia** is focal or diffuse, unilateral or bilateral dysplasia. It is caused by an overt intrauterine obstruction to urine flow, such as posterior urethral valves or ureteropelvic junction stenosis.

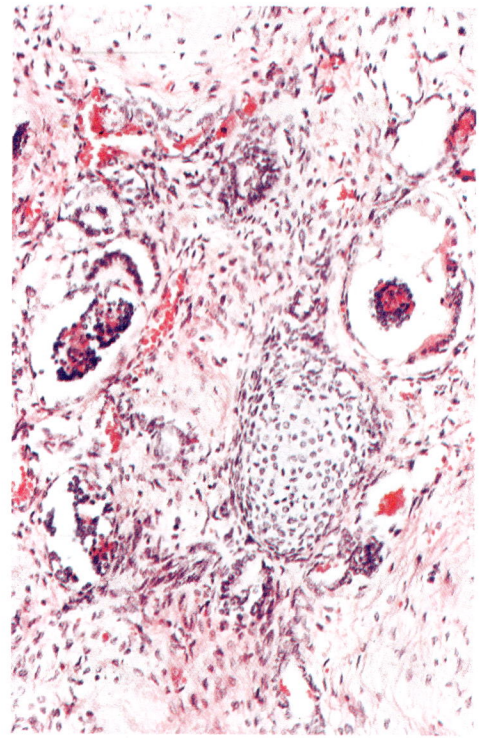

FIGURE 16-7
Renal dysplasia. Immature glomeruli, tubules, and cartilage are surrounded by loose, undifferentiated mesenchymal tissue.

 Clinical Features: In most patients with multicystic renal dysplasia, a palpable flank mass is discovered shortly after birth, although small multicystic kidneys may not become apparent until many years later. **Unilateral multicystic renal dysplasia is the most common cause of an abdominal mass in newborns.** Unilateral dysplasia is adequately treated by removal of the affected kidney. Bilateral aplastic dysplasia and diffuse cystic dysplasia cause oligohydramnios and the resultant Potter sequence and life-threatening pulmonary hypoplasia. Aplastic renal dysplasia and diffuse cystic dysplasia are more often hereditary than multicystic dysplasia, especially if they are associated with multiple anomalies in other organs, as in Meckel-Gruber syndrome.

Autosomal Dominant Polycystic Kidney Disease (ADPKD) Features Enlarged, Multicystic Kidneys

ADPKD is the most common of a group of congenital diseases that are characterized by numerous cysts within the renal parenchyma (Fig. 16-9). It affects 1:200 to 1:1000 persons in the United States. Half of all patients with this disease eventually develop end-stage renal failure. ADPKD is responsible for 10% of all cases of renal disease that require dialysis or transplantation. Only diabetes and hypertension cause more end-stage renal disease than does ADPKD.

Pathogenesis: Some 85% of ADPKD is caused by mutations in the polycystic kidney disease 1 gene (*PKD1*), 15% by mutations in *PKD2*, and less than 1% by mutations in *PKD3*. *PKD1* is a very large gene, which creates a substantial target for a variety of mutations. The function of the gene products, termed *polycystins*, has not been elucidated. However, evidence suggests that they are integral membrane proteins involved in cell–cell and cell–matrix interactions and the functions of the ion channels.

Although the precise pathogenesis of ADPKD remains unclear, it is held that cysts arise in segments of renal tubules from a few cells that proliferate abnormally. The wall of the tubule becomes covered by an undifferentiated epithelium composed of cells with a high nucleus-to-cytoplasm ratio and only few microvilli. Concomitantly, a defective basement membrane immediately underlying the abnormal epithelium allows dilation of the affected portion of the tubule. Initially, the fluid in the cysts is derived from the glomerular filtrate, but eventually most of the cysts become disconnected from the tubules, in which case the fluid accumulates by transepithelial secretion. Historically, end-stage renal disease in ADPKD has been attributed to the pressure exerted by the dilating cysts on the surrounding normal parenchyma. However, it is now appreciated that cysts originate in less than 2% of nephrons, and that factors other than crowding of normal tissue by the expanding cysts likely contribute to the loss of functioning renal tissue. Apoptotic loss of renal tubules and the accumulation of inflammatory mediators have been incriminated in the destruction of normal renal mass.

Pathology: The kidneys in ADPKD are markedly enlarged bilaterally, each weighing as much as 4500 g (Fig. 16-10). The external contours of the kidneys are distorted by numerous cysts, as large as 5 cm in diameter, which are filled with a straw-colored fluid. Microscopically, the cysts are lined by a cuboidal and columnar epithelium. They arise from virtually any point along the nephron, including glomeruli, proximal tubules, distal tubules, and collecting ducts. Areas of normal renal parenchyma are found between the cysts.

One third of patients with ADPKD also have **hepatic cysts,** whose lining resembles bile duct epithelium. Cysts oc-

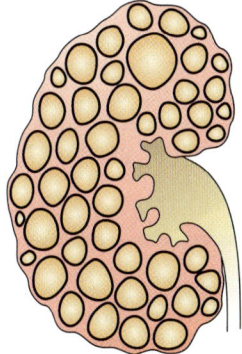
Autosomal dominant polycystic disease

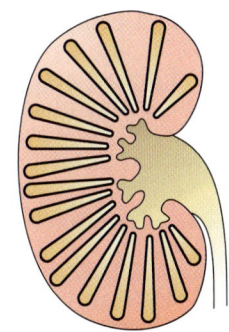
Autosomal recessive polycystic disease

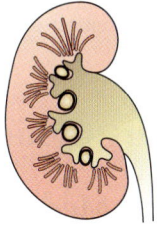
Medullary sponge kidney

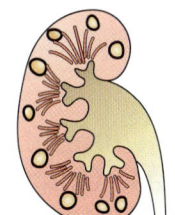
Medullary cystic disease complex

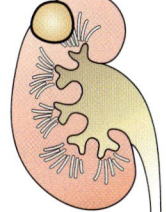
Simple cyst

FIGURE 16-9
Cystic diseases of the kidney.

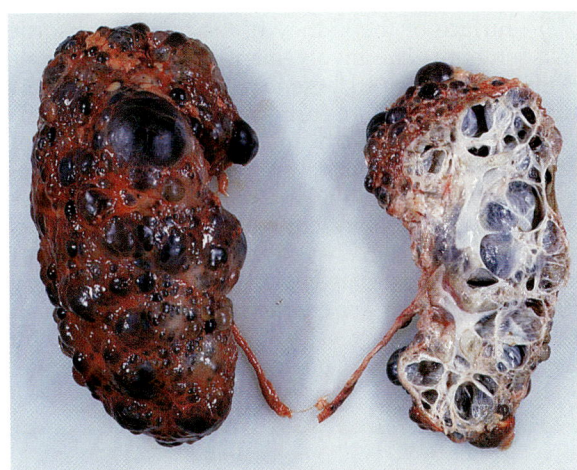

FIGURE 16-10
Adult polycystic disease. The kidney is enlarged, and the parenchyma is almost entirely replaced by cysts of varying size.

cur in the spleen in 10% of patients and in the pancreas in 5%. One fifth of patients have an associated cerebral aneurysm, and intracranial hemorrhage is the cause of death in 15% of patients with ADPKD. Interestingly, many patients with ADPKD also develop colonic diverticula.

 Clinical Features: Most patients with ADPKD do not develop clinical manifestations until the fourth decade of life, which is why this condition was once called *adult* polycystic kidney disease. A small minority of patients develop symptoms during childhood, and rare ones are symptomatic at birth. Symptoms include a sense of heaviness in the loins, bilateral flank and abdominal masses, and passage of blood clots in the urine. Azotemia (elevated blood urea nitrogen) is common, and in half of patients progresses to uremia (clinical renal failure) over a period of several years.

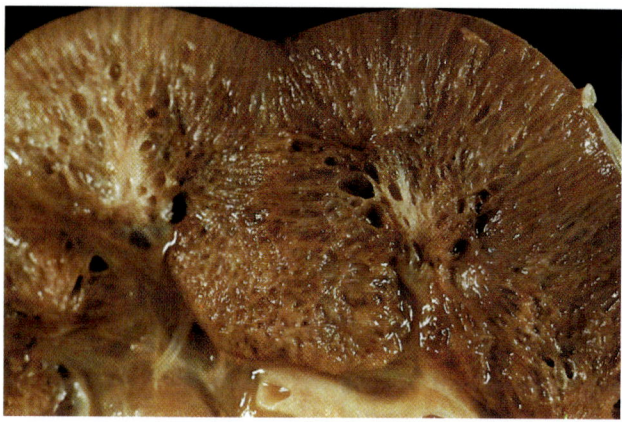

FIGURE 16-11
Infantile polycystic disease. The dilated cortical and medullary collecting ducts are arranged radially, and the external surface is smooth.

Autosomal Recessive Polycystic Kidney Disease (ARPKD) Occurs in Infants

ARPKD is characterized by cystic transformation of collecting ducts. It is rare compared with ADPKD, occurring in about 1 in 10,000 to 50,000 live births. Of these infants, 75% die in the perinatal period, often because of pulmonary hypoplasia caused by oligohydramnios (Potter sequence) and by the large size of the kidneys, which compromises expansion of the lungs. Exceptional cases of ARPKD manifest in older children and adults. ARPKD is caused by mutations in the *PKHD1* gene. The gene product, *fibrocystin,* is found in kidney, liver, and pancreas and appears to be involved in regulation of cell proliferation and adhesion. Mutations of *PKHD1* also result in ARPKD, pancreatic cysts, and hepatic biliary dysgenesis and fibrosis.

 Pathology: In contrast to ADPKD, the external surface of the kidney in the infantile disorder is smooth. The involvement is invariably bilateral. The kidneys are often so large that the delivery of the infant is impeded. The cysts are fusiform dilations of cortical and medullary collecting ducts and have a striking radial arrangement perpendicular to the renal capsule (Fig. 16-11). Interstitial fibrosis and tubular atrophy are common, particularly in children who present with the disorder at an older age. As in ADPKD, the calyceal system in ARPKD is normal. There are usually associated liver changes, termed *congenital hepatic fibrosis,* which are characterized by enlargement of portal areas, with an increase in connective tissue and proliferation of bile ducts (see Chapter 14).

Glomerulocystic Disease

Glomerulocystic disease exhibits dilation of Bowman's capsule in many glomeruli. The disorder occurs either as an isolated process or as a component of other cystic disease, such as ADPKD, nephronophthisis–medullary cystic disease complex, and diffuse cystic dysplasia. Thus, there are multiple causes for glomerulocystic disease. One form is autosomal dominant and is caused by mutations in the gene for hepatocyte nuclear factor-1 beta (HNF-1β).

 Pathology: Kidneys with primary glomerulocystic disease may be large or small. The cut surface reveals numerous small round cysts rarely more than 1 cm in diameter. Light microscopy shows dilation of Bowman's capsule in many glomeruli. The residual glomerular tuft is often distorted or appears immature.

Nephronophthisis–Medullary Cystic Disease Complex Displays Tubulointerstitial Injury and Medullary Cysts

Nephronophthisis–medullary cystic disease complex comprises a group of autosomal recessive and autosomal dominant diseases. The pathogenesis may involve a developmental defect in tubular basement membranes.

 Pathology: The kidneys are small and when sectioned display multiple, variably sized cysts (up to 1 cm) at the corticomedullary junction (see Fig. 16-9). The cysts arise from the distal portions of the nephron. Atrophic tubules with markedly thickened basement membranes and loss of tubules out of proportion to the glomerular loss are early histological features of the disease. Eventually, corticomedullary cysts develop, and the remainder of the parenchyma becomes increasingly atrophic. Secondary glomerular sclerosis, interstitial fibrosis, and a nonspecific inflammatory infiltrate dominate the late histological picture.

Clinical Features: Medullary cystic disease complex accounts for 10 to 25% of cases of renal failure in childhood. Patients present initially with deteriorating tubular function, such as impaired concentrating ability and sodium wasting, manifested as polyuria, polydipsia, and enuresis (bed wetting). Progressive azotemia and renal failure follow, usually within 5 years of the onset of symptoms. Nephronophthisis is an autosomal recessive disease with early onset that almost always progresses to end-stage renal disease by 25 years of age. Medullary cystic disease is autosomal dominant and usually does not terminate in renal failure until the third decade of life.

Medullary Sponge Kidney Is Distinguished by Cysts in the Papillae

Medullary sponge kidney is a disorder characterized by multiple small (<5 mm in diameter) cysts in one or more of the renal papillae (see Fig. 16-9). The cysts are lined by cuboidal or columnar epithelium and arise from the collecting ducts in the renal papillae. In 75% of patients, the disease is bilateral. A few familial cases have been described.

Medullary sponge kidney is asymptomatic in young adults. Symptomatic cases are usually discovered between the ages of 30 and 60, when the affected person complains of flank pain, dysuria, hematuria, or "gravel" in the urine caused by stone formation in the cysts. Although the disease itself does not pose a threat to health, the cysts may predispose to secondary pyelonephritis.

ACQUIRED CYSTIC KIDNEY DISEASE

Simple Renal Cysts Are Common Acquired Lesions

Simple renal cysts are found in about half of persons over 50 years of age. They are usually incidental findings at autopsy and rarely produce clinical symptoms unless they are very large. These fluid-filled cysts may be solitary or multiple and are usually located in the outer cortex, where they bulge the capsule. Less commonly, simple cysts occur in the medulla. Microscopically, they are lined by a flat epithelium.

Acquired Cystic Disease Follows Long-Term Dialysis

Acquired cystic disease is characterized by multiple cortical and medullary cysts that form in the kidneys of patients with end-stage renal disease who are maintained on dialysis. **After 5 years of dialysis, over 75% of patients acquire bilateral cystic kidneys.** The cysts are initially lined by flat-to-cuboidal epithelium, but hyperplastic and neoplastic epithelial proliferation may develop.

GLOMERULAR DISEASES

The functional complexity of the glomerulus and the varied pathogenetic mechanisms that can injure it cause a wide variety of renal disorders. A glomerular disease may be the only major site of disease (primary glomerular disease; e.g., IgA nephropathy) or may be a component of a disease that affects multiple organs (secondary glomerular disease; e.g., lupus glomerulonephritis). The signs and symptoms of glomerular disease fall into one of the following categories:

- Asymptomatic proteinuria
- Nephrotic syndrome
- Asymptomatic hematuria
- Acute nephritic syndrome
- Rapidly progressive nephritic syndrome
- Chronic nephritic syndrome

Nephrotic Syndrome Features Severe Proteinuria

Nephrotic syndrome is characterized by heavy proteinuria (>3.5 g of protein/24 hours), hypoalbuminemia, edema, hyperlipidemia, and lipiduria. The major pathogenetic abnormality is a permeability defect in the glomerular capillaries that allows protein to be lost from the plasma into the urine (proteinuria). Many different glomerular diseases cause proteinuria by a variety of mechanisms, most associated with reduced polyanionic charge of the glomerular basement membrane.

Severe proteinuria causes the nephrotic syndrome (Fig. 16-12), but lower levels of proteinuria may be asymptomatic. Table 16-1 lists the major causes of the nephrotic syndrome in adults and children and their approximate frequency. Important differences exist in the rates of specific glomerular diseases that produce the nephrotic syndrome in adults versus those in children. For example, minimal-change glomerulopathy is responsible for most (70%) cases of nephrotic syndrome in children but only 15% of cases in adults. The primary glomerular diseases that are the most frequent causes of

TABLE 16-1 **Frequency of Causes for the Nephrotic Syndrome Induced by Primary Glomerular Diseases in Children and Adults**

Cause	Children (%)	Adults (%)
Minimal-change glomerulopathy	75	15
Membranous glomerulopathy	5	30
Focal segmental glomerulosclerosis	10	30
Type I membranoproliferative glomerulonephritis	5	5
Other glomerular diseases[a]	5	20

[a] Includes many forms of mesangioproliferative and proliferative glomerulonephritis, such as IgA nephropathy, which often also cause nephritic features.

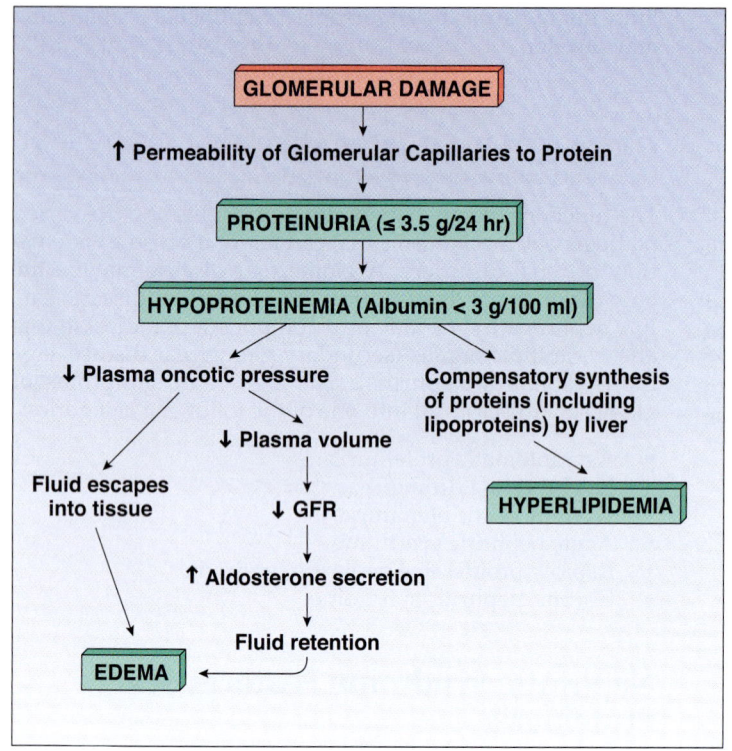

FIGURE 16-12
Pathophysiology of the nephrotic syndrome. (GFR, glomerular filtration rate).

nephrotic syndrome in adults are membranous glomerulopathy and focal segmental glomerulosclerosis. Membranous glomerulopathy is the most frequent cause in Caucasians and Asians, whereas focal segmental glomerulosclerosis is the most common etiology in American blacks. The incidence of focal segmental glomerulosclerosis has been increasing over the past decade. Systemic diseases that involve the kidney, such as diabetes, amyloidosis, and systemic lupus erythematosus, are responsible for many cases of nephrotic syndrome in adults. Membranoproliferative glomerulonephritis is a much more frequent reason for nephrotic syndrome in underdeveloped countries that have a high prevalence of chronic infectious diseases.

tis), or (3) persist continuously or intermittently for years and proceed slowly to renal failure (chronic glomerulonephritis).

As shown in Table 16-2, some glomerular diseases tend to cause the nephrotic syndrome, whereas others lead to the nephritic syndrome. However, with the possible exception of minimal-change glomerulopathy (which almost always causes the nephrotic syndrome), on occasion all glomerular diseases produce mixed nephritic and nephrotic manifestations that confound clinical diagnosis. Renal biopsy evaluation is the only means of definitive diagnosis for glomerular diseases, although clinical and laboratory data may provide presumptive evidence for a specific disease.

Nephritic (Glomerulonephritic) Syndrome Is an Inflammatory Disease

Nephritic syndrome is characterized by hematuria (either microscopic or visible grossly), variable degrees of proteinuria, and decreased glomerular filtration rate. It results in elevations in the levels of blood urea nitrogen and serum creatinine, oliguria, salt and water retention, edema, and hypertension. Glomerular diseases associated with the nephritic syndrome are caused by inflammatory changes in glomeruli, such as infiltration by leukocytes, hyperplasia of glomerular cells, and, in severe lesions, necrosis. Sufficient injury to the glomerular capillaries results in spillage of protein and blood cells into the urine (proteinuria and hematuria). The inflammatory damage may also impair glomerular flow and filtration, resulting in renal insufficiency, fluid retention, and hypertension. Nephritic manifestations may (1) develop rapidly and result in reversible renal insufficiency (acute glomerulonephritis), (2) progress rapidly, with renal failure that resolves only with aggressive treatment (rapidly progressive glomerulonephri-

TABLE 16-2 Tendencies of Glomerular Diseases to Manifest Nephrotic and Nephritic Features

Disease	Nephrotic	Nephritic
Minimal-change glomerulopathy	++++	−
Membranous glomerulopathy	++++	+
Focal segmental glomerulosclerosis	+++	++
Mesangioproliferative glomerulonephritis[a]	++	++
Membranoproliferative glomerulonephritis	++	++
Proliferative glomerulonephritis[a]	+	+++
Crescentic glomerulonephritis[a]	+	++++

[a] These histological phenotypes can be caused by many categories of glomerular disease, including IgA nephropathy, postinfectious glomerulonephritis, lupus glomerulonephritis, antineutrophil cytoplasmic autoantibody glomerulonephritis, and anti-glomerular basement membrane glomerulonephritis.

Pathogenesis: Glomerulonephritis is frequently caused by immunological mechanisms. Both antibody-mediated and cell-mediated types of immunity play roles in the production of glomerular inflammation. However, three mechanisms of antibody-induced inflammation have been incriminated as the major pathogenetic processes in most forms of glomerulonephritis (Fig. 16-13):

- In situ immune complex formation
- Deposition of circulating immune complexes
- Antineutrophil cytoplasmic autoantibodies

Immune complex formation in situ involves binding of circulating antibodies to intrinsic antigens or foreign antigens deposited within the glomeruli. For example, anti-GBM autoantibodies bind to type IV collagen in GBMs. The resultant immune complexes in the glomerular capillary walls attract leukocytes and activate complement and other humoral inflammatory mediator systems, resulting in inflammatory injury.

Immune complexes in the circulation can deposit in glomeruli and incite inflammation similar to that produced by immune complex formation in situ. For example, antigens released into the circulation by bacterial or viral infection can bind to circulating antibodies to produce immune complexes. If these complexes escape phagocytosis, they can deposit in the glomeruli and incite inflammation.

Immunofluorescence microscopy using antihuman antibodies detects the glomerular localization of immune complexes. Anti-GBM antibodies produce linear staining of GBMs, whereas other immune complexes produce granular staining in capillary walls, mesangium, or both.

Antineutrophil cytoplasmic autoantibodies (ANCAs) cause a severe glomerulonephritis that exhibits little or no glomerular immunofluorescent staining for immunoglobulins. These patients have a high frequency of circulating autoantibodies specific for antigens in the cytoplasm of neutrophils, which can mediate glomerular inflammation by activating neutrophils. Most ANCAs are directed against myeloperoxidase (MPO-ANCA) or proteinase-3 (PR3-ANCA). Even minor stimulation of neutrophils and monocytes, such as increased circulating levels of cytokines during viral infection, causes them to express MPO and PR3 on their surfaces, where these autoantigens can interact with ANCAs. This interaction leads to neutrophil and monocyte activation and results in leukocyte adhesion to endothelial cells in the microvasculature, especially glomerular capillaries. In that location they release injurious products that promote vascular inflammation, including glomerulonephritis, arteritis, and venulitis.

The formation of glomerular immune complexes in situ, the deposition of immune complexes, and the interaction of ANCA with leukocytes all initiate a final common pathway of glomerular inflammatory injury, which involves attraction and activation of leukocytes, especially neutrophils and monocytes (fig. 16-13).

Pathology: Many specific glomerular diseases have distinctive pathological features, as well as different natural histories and appropriate treatments.

Accurate pathological diagnosis of glomerular diseases requires evaluation of renal tissue by light, immunofluorescence, and electron microscopy, together with integration of the findings with clinical information. Table 16-3 lists pathological features that are useful for diagnosing glomerular diseases.

In general, the pathological features that indicate acute inflammation, such as endocapillary and extracapillary hypercellularity, leukocyte infiltration and necrosis, are more common in disorders that have predominantly nephritic features than in those with nephrotic attributes. **Glomerular crescent formation** (extracapillary proliferation) correlates with a more rapidly progressive course. Crescent formation is not specific for a particular cause of glomerular inflammation. It is rather a marker for severe injury that has resulted in extensive rupture of capillary walls, which allows inflammatory mediators to enter Bowman's space, where they stimulate macrophage infiltration and epithelial proliferation.

Minimal-Change Glomerulopathy Leads to Nephrotic Syndrome

Minimal-change glomerulopathy (minimal-change disease) is characterized clinically by the nephrotic syndrome and pathologically by the effacement of podocyte foot processes.

Pathogenesis: The pathogenesis of minimal-change glomerulopathy is unknown. Involvement of the immune system has been postulated because the disease frequently enters remission when treated with corticosteroids and because it may occur in association with an allergic disease or a lymphoid neoplasm. The occasional association with Hodgkin disease (a condition associated with T-cell dysfunction) and with T-cell lymphomas has led to the speculation that minimal-change glomerulopathy may be caused by a disorder of T lymphocytes, possibly production by T cells of a cytokine that increases glomerular permeability. The heavy proteinuria of minimal-change glomerulopathy is accompanied (and may be caused) by a loss of polyanionic sites on the GBM, which allows anionic proteins, particularly albumin, to pass more easily through the GBM.

Pathology: By definition, the light microscopic appearance of glomeruli in minimal-change glomerulopathy is essentially normal (Fig. 16-14). The presence of "normal" or "minimally changed" glomeruli in children with the nephrotic syndrome puzzled early investigators. Not until electron microscopic studies showed diffuse obliteration of the epithelial cell foot processes did speculation about a nonglomerular origin of proteinuria end. The loss of protein in the urine leads to hypoalbuminemia, and a compensatory increase in lipoprotein secretion by the liver results in hyperlipidemia. The loss of lipoproteins through the glomeruli causes accumulation of

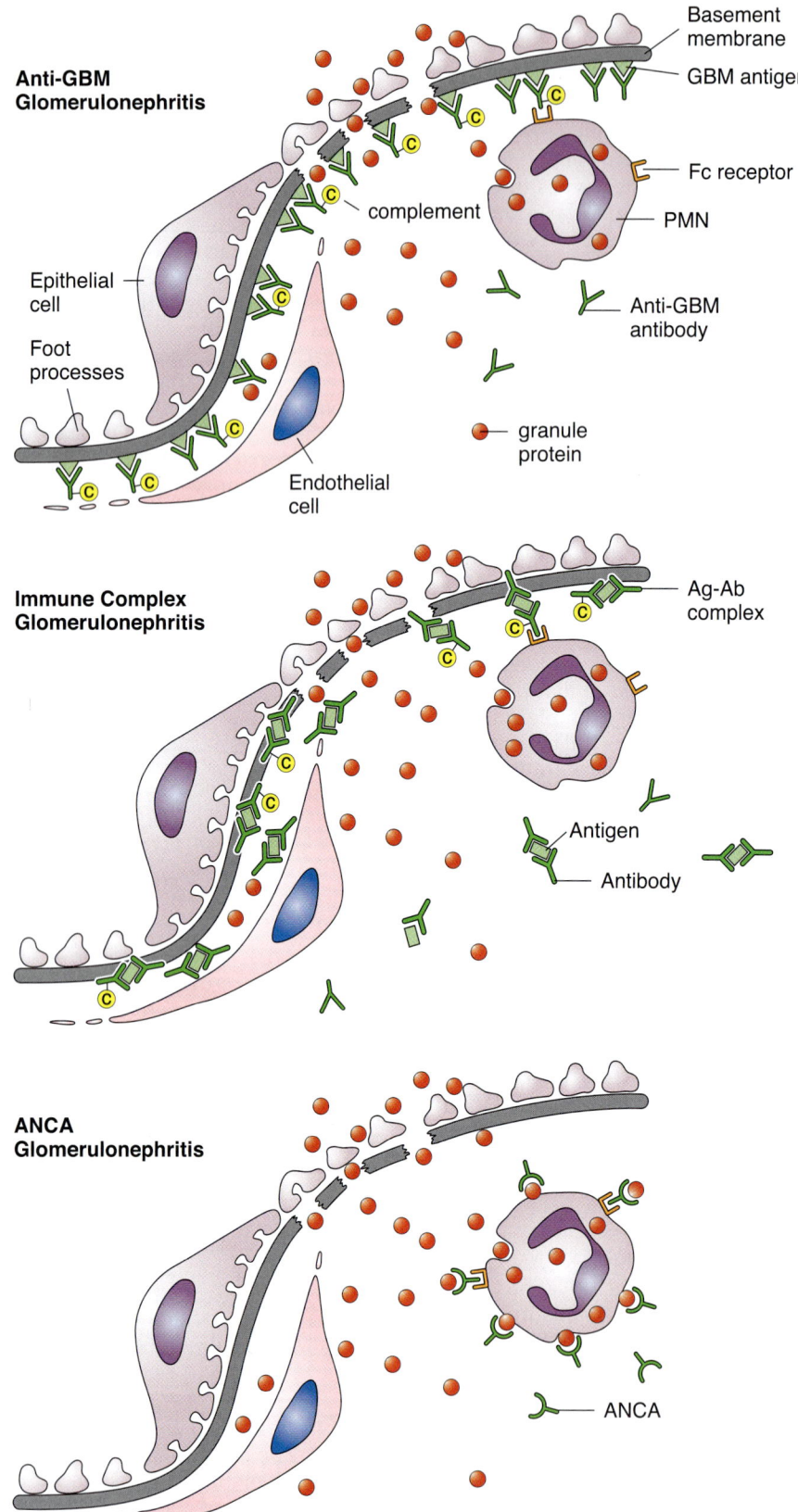

FIGURE 16-13

Antibody-mediated glomerulonephritis. *Top panel:* Anti-glomerular basement membrane (GBM) antibodies cause glomerulonephritis by binding in situ to basement membrane antigens. This activates complement and recruits inflammatory cells. *Middle panel:* Immune complexes that deposit from the circulation also activate complement and recruit inflammatory cells. *Bottom panel:* Antineutrophil cytoplasmic antibodies (ANCA) cause inflammation by activating leukocytes by direct binding of the antibodies to the leukocytes and by Fc receptor engagement of ANCA bound to antigen.

Glomerular Diseases

TABLE 16-3 Diagnostic Features of Glomerular Diseases

I. **Light microscopic features**
  A. Increased cellularity
   Infiltration by leukocytes (e.g., neutrophils, monocytes, macrophages)
   Proliferation of "endocapillary" cells (i.e., endothelial and mesangial cells)
   Proliferation of "extracapillary" cells (i.e., epithelial cells) (crescent formation)
  B. Increased extracellular material
   Localization of immune complexes
   Thickening or replication of glomerular basement membrane (GBM)
   Increases in collagenous matrix (sclerosis)
   Insudation of plasma proteins (hyalinosis)
   Fibrinoid necrosis
   Deposition of amyloid
II. **Immunofluorescence features**
  A. Linear staining of GBM
   Anti-GBM antibodies
   Multiple plasma proteins (e.g., in diabetic glomerulosclerosis)
   Monoclonal light chains
  B. Granular immune complex staining
   Mesangium (e.g., IgA nephropathy)
   Capillary wall (e.g., membranous glomerulopathy)
   Mesangium and capillary wall (e.g., lupus glomerulonephritis)
  C. Irregular (fluffy) staining
   Monoclonal light chains (AL amyloidosis)
   AA protein (AA amyloidosis)
III. **Electron microscopic features**
  A. Electron-dense immune complex deposits
   Mesangial (e.g., IgA nephropathy)
   Subendothelial (e.g., lupus glomerulonephritis)
   Subepithelial (e.g., membranous glomerulopathy)
  B. GBM thickening (e.g., diabetic glomerulosclerosis)
  C. GBM replication (e.g., membranoproliferative glomerulonephritis)
  D. Collagenous matrix expansion (e.g., focal segmental glomerulosclerosis)
  E. Fibrillary deposits (e.g., amyloidosis)

lipid in the proximal tubular cells, which is reflected histologically as glassy (hyaline) droplets in tubular epithelial cytoplasm. This appearance, together with lipid droplets in the urine, is responsible for the older term *lipoid nephrosis*. Droplets in the tubular epithelial cells are not specific for minimal-change glomerulopathy but are produced by any glomerular disease that causes the nephrotic syndrome.

Electron microscopic examination of the glomeruli reveals total **effacement of visceral epithelial cell foot processes,** an effect caused by their retraction into the parent epithelial cell bodies (Figs. 16-15 and 16-16). This retraction presumably results from extensive cell swelling and occurs in virtually all cases of proteinuria in the nephrotic range; it is not specific for minimal-change glomerulopathy. Numerous microvilli protrude from the surface of the epithelial cells. Immunofluorescence microscopy for immunoglobulins and complement are most often negative, but there is occasional weak mesangial staining for IgM and the complement component C3.

Clinical Features: Minimal-change glomerulopathy causes 90% of the nephrotic syndrome in young children, 50% in older children, and 15% in adults. Proteinuria is generally more selective (albumin > globulins) than in the nephrotic syndrome caused by other diseases, but

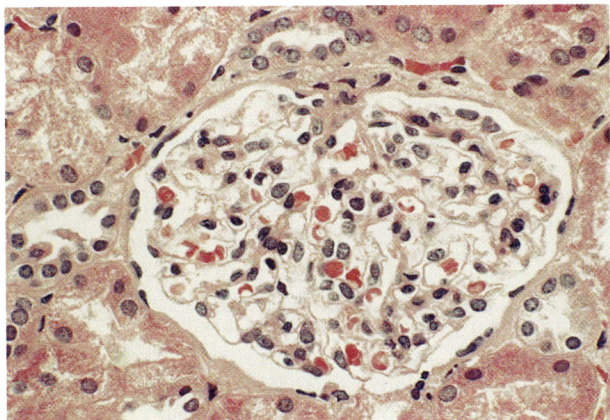

FIGURE 16-14
Minimal-change glomerulopathy. A light micrograph shows no abnormality.

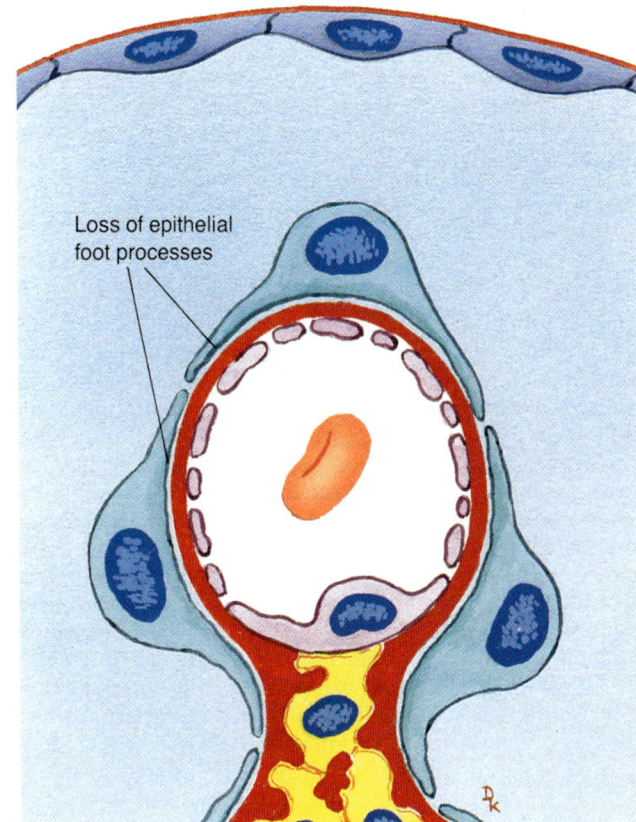

FIGURE 16-15
Minimal-change glomerulopathy. This condition is characterized predominantly by epithelial cell changes, particularly the effacement of the foot processes. All other glomerular structures appear intact.

The Kidney

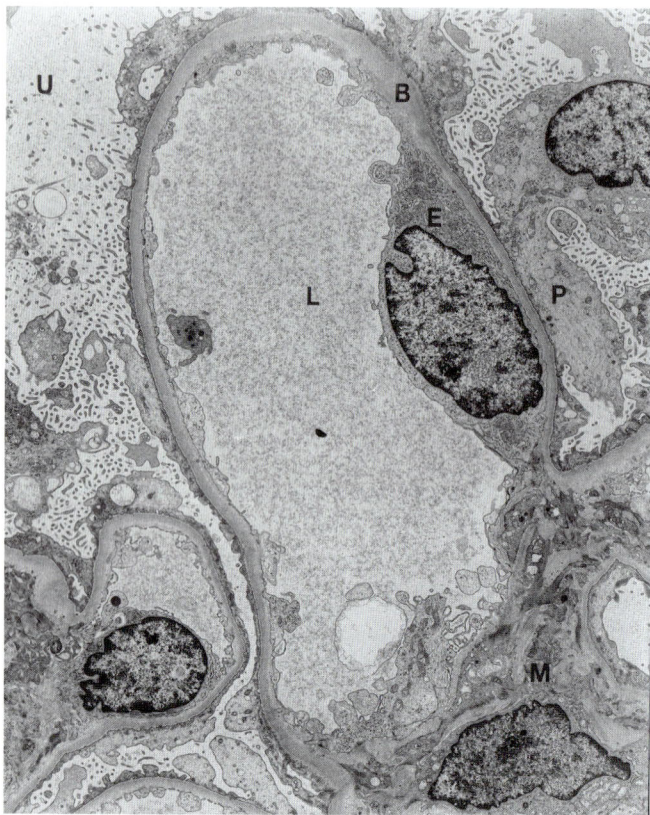

FIGURE 16-16
Minimal-change glomerulopathy. In this electron micrograph, the podocyte (P) displays extensive effacement of foot processes and numerous microvilli projecting into the urinary space (U). (B, basement membrane; E, endothelial cell; L, lumen; M, mesangial cell).

there is too much overlap for this selectivity to be used as a diagnostic criterion. Over 90% of children and fewer adults with minimal-change glomerulopathy have complete remission of proteinuria within 8 weeks of the initiation of corticosteroid therapy. Adults often require longer treatment with corticosteroids to induce remission. However, after withdrawal of corticosteroids, most patients suffer intermittent relapses for up to 10 years. A small subgroup of patients has only partial remission with corticosteroid therapy and continues to lose protein in the urine. In an even smaller group that is totally resistant to corticosteroid therapy, the diagnosis of minimal-change glomerulopathy may not be accurate, and focal segmental glomerulosclerosis that was not sampled in the initial biopsy specimen may be present.

Death from infection was frequent before antibiotics and corticosteroids became readily available, but a fatal outcome is now exceptional. The development of azotemia in a patient diagnosed as having minimal-change glomerulopathy should suggest an incorrect diagnosis, usually focal segmental glomerulosclerosis or perhaps a complication such as interstitial nephritis. In the absence of complications, the long-term outlook for patients with minimal-change glomerulopathy is no different from that of the general population.

Focal Segmental Glomerulosclerosis Reflects Glomerular Scarring

Focal segmental glomerulosclerosis is characterized by glomerular scarring (sclerosis) that affects some (focal), but not all, glomeruli and initially involves only part of an affected glomerular tuft (segmental). There are several primary and secondary forms of focal segmental glomerulosclerosis.

 Pathogenesis: The term *focal segmental glomerulosclerosis* (FSGS) is applied to a heterogeneous group of glomerular diseases that have different causes, different pathological features, different responses to treatment, and different outcomes. FSGS occurs as an idiopathic (primary) process or secondary to a number of conditions (Table 16-4). It is likely that multiple factors can lead to a final common pathway of injury. Pathological features and genetic evidence suggest that injury to podocytes may be common to all types of FSGS.

Several hereditary forms of FSGS have been traced to genetic abnormalities in podocyte proteins, for example, nephrin, podocin, and α-actinin-4. This supports the hypothesis that injury to, or dysfunction of, podocytes causes FSGS.

Congenital (e.g., unilateral agenesis) and acquired (e.g. reflux nephropathy) reductions in renal mass place adaptive stress on the reduced number of nephrons. In turn this strain appears to cause FSGS as a consequence of overwork, with increased glomerular capillary pressure and filtration and enlargement of glomeruli. A normal amount of renal tissue can also be stressed by excessive body mass (obesity), resulting in FSGS. Reduced oxygen in the blood (e.g., as caused by sickle cell disease or cyanotic congenital heart disease) also causes a similar pattern of glomerular injury. In all of these settings, glomerular enlargement reflects functional overwork, which places substantial stress on podocytes because of their limited proliferative capacity.

Viruses, drugs and serum factors have been implicated as causes of FSGS. Infection with human immunodeficiency virus (HIV), especially in blacks, is associated with a variant of FSGS that is characterized by a collapsing pattern of sclerosis. Such an appearance may also occur in idiopathic FSGS. There is speculation that collapsing FSGS is caused by viral

TABLE 16-4 Categories of Focal Segmental Glomerulosclerosis

Idiopathic (primary) focal segmental glomerulosclerosis
    Perihilar variant
    Collapsing variant
    Tip lesion variant
    Cellular variant
Secondary focal segmental glomerulosclerosis
    Obesity (perihilar variant)
    Reduced renal mass (perihilar variant)
    Cyanotic congenital heart disease (usually perihilar variant)
    Sickle cell nephropathy (usually perihilar variant)
    Human immunodeficiency virus (collapsing variant)
    Pamidronate (collapsing variant)
    Intravenous drug abuse (usually collapsing variant)

infection of podocytes. Pamidronate, a drug used to treat osteolytic bone disease in patients with cancer, causes collapsing FSGS in some patients. This drug has toxic effects on epithelial cells in vitro and probably causes FSGS by injuring podocytes. A serum permeability factor has been detected in some patients with FSGS, which suggests a systemic cause for the glomerular injury. This is further supported by the recurrence of FSGS in renal transplants, especially in patients who have the permeability factor.

Pathology: By light microscopy, varying numbers of glomeruli show segmental obliteration of capillary loops by increased collagen and the accumulation of lipid and proteinaceous material. The last is probably derived from insudation of plasma proteins and has a glassy appearance; the condition is, therefore, called *hyalinosis*. Adhesions to Bowman's capsule occur adjacent to the sclerotic lesions. Uninvolved glomeruli may appear entirely normal, although mild mesangial hypercellularity is occasionally present. Because uninvolved glomeruli usually appear normal, FSGS can be mistaken for minimal-change glomerulopathy in small biopsy specimens that contain only nonsclerotic glomeruli. A differential diagnostic consideration is focal glomerular scarring secondary to a prior inflammatory glomerular disease.

Several histological variants of segmental glomerulosclerosis have been recognized. In some patients, especially those with reduced renal mass or obesity, the sclerosis has a predilection for *perihilar* segments within glomeruli and for glomeruli in the deep cortex (juxtamedullary glomeruli) (Fig. 16-17). A *collapsing* pattern of sclerosis with hypertrophied podocytes adjacent to sclerotic segments is typical of HIV-associated nephropathy, and also occurs with intravenous drug abuse and pamidronate-induced disease and as an idiopathic process. This collapsing variant has a poor prognosis, and half of patients reach end-stage disease within 2 years. Sclerosis confined to the glomerular segment adjacent to the origin of the proximal tubule has been designated *tip lesion* and is most frequent in older patients with marked proteinuria. A *cellular variant* of FSGS has prominent lipid-laden cells within the sites of glomerular consolidation.

By electron microscopy, FSGS exhibits diffuse effacement of epithelial cell foot processes, with occasional focal detachment or loss of podocytes from the GBM. Increased matrix material, folding and thickening of the basement membranes, and capillary collapse are present in the sclerotic segments. Accumulation of electron-dense material within the sclerotic segments represents insudative trapping of plasma proteins, which corresponds to the hyalinosis seen by light microscopy. Immune complexes are not visualized.

Immunofluorescence microscopy demonstrates trapping of IgM and C3 in the segmental areas of sclerosis and hyalinosis. IgG, C4, and C1q are less frequently found in sclerotic segments. Nonsclerotic segments have no staining or only trace mesangial staining, usually for IgM and C3.

Clinical Features: FSGS is the cause of the nephrotic syndrome in 30% of adults and 10% of children. The disease is more common in blacks than in whites and is the leading cause of nephrotic syndrome in American blacks. For unknown reasons the frequency has been increasing over the past few decades. The clinical presentations and outcomes vary among the different patterns of injury. The most common clinical presentation is an insidious onset of asymptomatic proteinuria, which frequently progresses to the nephrotic syndrome. Many patients are hypertensive, and microscopic hematuria is frequent.

Most persons with FSGS manifest a persistent proteinuria and a progressive decline in renal function. Some, but not all, patients appear to improve with corticosteroid therapy. Many patients progress to end-stage renal disease after 5 to 20 years. Although renal transplantation is the preferred treatment for end-stage renal disease, FSGS recurs in half of transplanted kidneys.

Patients with FSGS secondary to obesity or reduced renal mass usually have a more indolent course that benefits from treatment with angiotensin-converting enzyme (ACE) inhibitors. Patients with the tip lesion variant often present with severe nephrotic syndrome but respond better to corticosteroids than those with other forms of FSGS. HIV-associated and idiopathic collapsing FSGS have the worst prognoses and typically manifest with severe nephrotic syndrome and renal failure, often progressing to end-stage renal disease within a year.

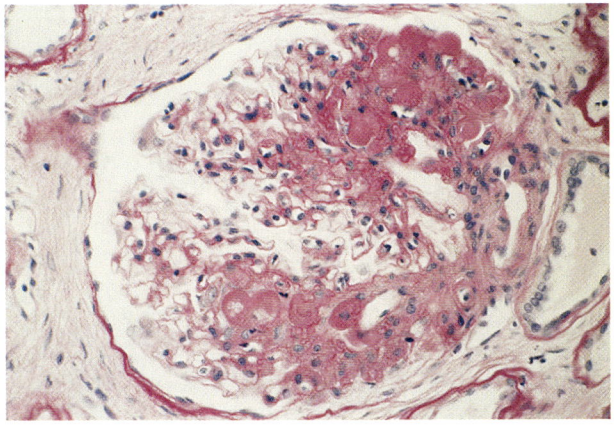

FIGURE 16-17
Focal segmental glomerulosclerosis. PAS staining shows perihilar areas of segmental sclerosis and adjacent adhesions to Bowman's capsule.

HIV-Associated Nephropathy

Nephropathy associated with HIV infection is a severe and rapidly progressive collapsing form of focal glomerular sclerosis.

Pathogenesis: The occurrence of nephropathy in patients with HIV infection has raised the possibility that it is caused by the virus within the renal parenchyma. A different hypothesis proposes that the nephropathy is caused by another virus that has infected the kidney of an immunocompromised person.

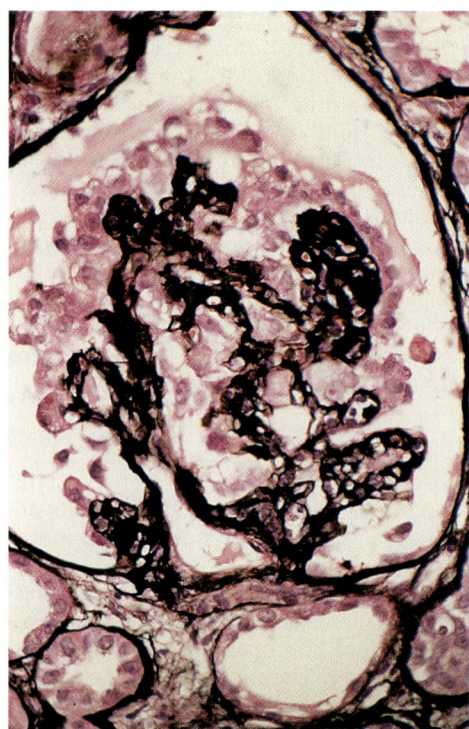

FIGURE 16-18
HIV-associated nephropathy. Silver staining shows a collapsing pattern of FSGS, with collapse of glomerular capillaries, increased matrix material (sclerosis), and hypertrophy of podocytes.

  Pathology: By light microscopy, HIV-associated nephropathy has a distinctive collapsing pattern of focal sclerosis that may be segmental or global (Fig. 16-18). Sclerotic segments display collapse of capillaries, frequently with adjacent swollen podocytes that contain numerous protein droplets. In addition to the glomerular injury, interstitial fibrosis and infiltration by mononuclear leukocytes are frequent. Tubular epithelial atrophy and degeneration are conspicuous, and cystically dilated tubules contain proteinaceous casts. By electron microscopy, numerous tubuloreticular inclusions are seen in endothelial cells, similar to those in lupus nephritis.

Clinical Features: Some 10% of HIV patients develop nephropathy, of whom over 90% are black. Idiopathic collapsing FSGS also occurs predominantly in blacks. The disease presents with severe proteinuria (>10 g/day) and renal insufficiency. Patients typically progress to end-stage renal disease in less than a year.

Membranous Glomerulopathy Is an Immune Complex Disease

Membranous glomerulopathy is a frequent cause of the nephrotic syndrome in adults and is caused by the accumulation of immune complexes in the subepithelial zone of glomerular capillaries.

  Pathogenesis: Membranous glomerulopathy exhibits localization of immune complexes in the **subepithelial zone** (between the visceral epithelial cell and the GBM) as a result of immune complex formation in situ or the deposition of circulating immune complexes. Formation in situ is the favored hypothesis because of the resemblance between membranous glomerulopathy and the experimental animal disease called *Heymann nephritis*. In the latter, mice are immunized with a renal epithelial antigen and develop autoantibodies. The antibodies cross GBMs and bind to antigens on podocytes. The resultant immune complexes are shed into the adjacent subepithelial zone and produce membranous glomerulopathy. An analogous pathogenesis has been postulated for human idiopathic membranous glomerulopathy, even though no comparable autoantibody has been identified.

Membranous glomerulopathy is also induced in animals by chronic injection of foreign proteins. This procedure results in the formation of circulating immune complexes and, in some circumstances, free antigens and antibodies that can form immune complexes in situ. The result is a chronic serum sickness model, which may be analogous to certain forms of secondary membranous glomerulopathy. The following are general causes of membranous glomerulopathy:

- Idiopathic (primary) membranous glomerulopathy
- Secondary membranous glomerulopathy
  —Autoimmune disease (systemic lupus erythematosus)
  —Infectious disease (hepatitis B)
  —Therapeutic agents (penicillamine)
  —Neoplasms (lung cancer)

  Pathology: By light microscopy, the glomeruli are slightly enlarged, yet normocellular. Depending on the duration of the disease, the capillary walls are normal or thickened (Fig. 16-19). In the early stages of the

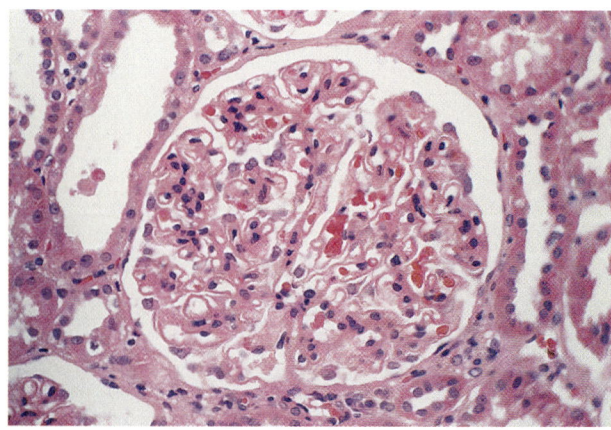

FIGURE 16-19
Membranous glomerulopathy. The glomerulus is slightly enlarged and shows diffuse thickening of the capillary walls. There is no hypercellularity.

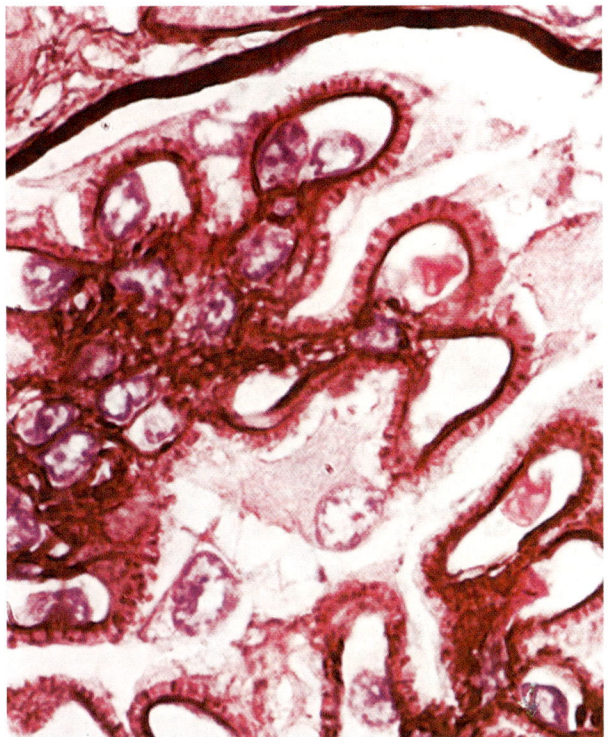

FIGURE 16-20
Membranous glomerulopathy. Silver staining reveals multiple "spikes" diffusely distributed in the glomerular capillary basement membranes. This pattern corresponds to the stage II lesion illustrated in Figure 16-22. The appearance is produced by the deposition of silver-positive basement membrane material around silver-negative immune complex deposits.

disease, silver stains (which demonstrate basement membrane material) reveal multiple projections or "spikes" of argyrophilic material on the epithelial surface of the basement membrane (Fig. 16-20). Such spikes are projections of basement membrane material that is deposited around the subepithelial immune complexes, which do not stain with silver. As the disease progresses, the capillary lumina are narrowed, and glomerular obsolescence eventually ensues. In advanced states of glomerular sclerosis, the lesions of membranous glomerulopathy cannot be distinguished from those in other forms of chronic glomerular disease. Atrophy of tubules and interstitial fibrosis parallel the degree of glomerular sclerosis.

By electron microscopy, immune complexes in the capillary walls appear as electron-dense deposits (Figs. 16-21 and 16-22). The progressive ultrastructural alterations that are induced by the subepithelial immune complexes are divided into stages:

- **Stage I:** Subepithelial dense deposits without adjacent projections of GBM material
- **Stage II:** Projections of GBM material around the subepithelial dense deposits (see Fig. 16-22)
- **Stage III:** Enclosure of the dense deposits within GBM material
- **Stage IV:** Rarefaction of the deposits within a thickened GBM

Mesangial electron-dense deposits are rare in idiopathic membranous glomerulopathy but are frequent in secondary membranous glomerulopathy (e.g., as seen in lupus erythematosus). This difference may reflect the fact that idiopathic disease is caused by antigens present only in the subepithelial zone (as in Heymann nephritis), whereas the secondary type is produced by circulating antigens.

Immunofluorescence microscopy reveals diffuse granular staining of capillary walls for IgG and C3 (Fig. 16-23). There is intense staining for terminal complement components, including the membrane attack complex, which participate in the induction of glomerular injury.

 Clinical Features: Membranous glomerulopathy is the most frequent cause of the nephrotic syndrome in white and Asian adults in the United States. The course of membranous glomerulopathy is highly variable, with a range of possible outcomes. When followed for 20 years, approximately 25% of patients have spontaneous remission, 50% have persistent proteinuria and stable or only partial loss of renal function, and 25% develop renal failure. The treatment of idiopathic membranous glomerulopathy is controversial. Patients who suffer progressive renal failure are treated with corticosteroids or cytotoxic drugs (e.g., cyclophosphamide) or both. The prognosis is better in children because of a higher rate of permanent spontaneous remission.

Diabetic Glomerulosclerosis Results in Proteinuria and Progressive Renal Failure

Pathogenesis: Diabetic glomerulosclerosis is a component of the vascular sclerosis that involves many small vessels throughout the body in patients with diabetes mellitus (see Chapter 22). Diabetes is complicated by a generalized increase in the synthesis of basement membrane material by the microvasculature, which in some way results from the abnormal metabolic state. One hypothesis proposes that abnormal **nonenzymatic glycosylation** of serum and matrix proteins, including those of the GBM and mesangial matrix, induces binding of plasma proteins, such as immunoglobulins, and thereby stimulates excessive matrix production. Less than half of patients with diabetes develop glomerulosclerosis, suggesting that, in addition to the diabetic state, synergistic factors are present in some, but not all, patients.

 Pathology: The earliest lesions of diabetic glomerulosclerosis are glomerular enlargement, GBM thickening, and expansion of the mesangial matrix (Fig. 16-24). Mild mesangial hypercellularity may

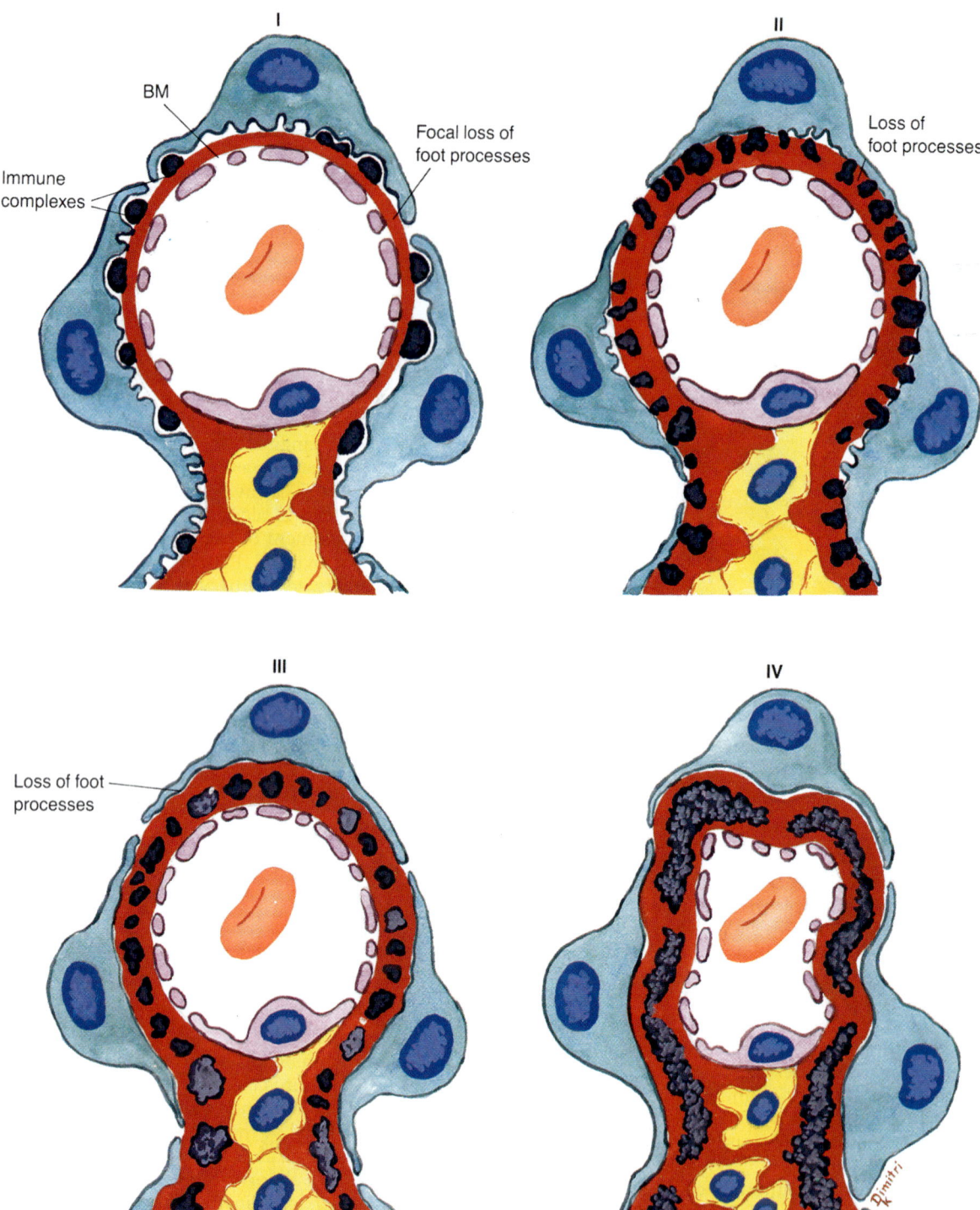

FIGURE 16-21

Membranous glomerulopathy. This disease is caused by the subepithelial accumulation of immune complexes and the accompanying changes in the basement membrane. Stage I exhibits scattered subepithelial deposits. The outer contour of the basement membrane remains smooth. Stage II disease has projections (spikes) of basement membrane material adjacent to the deposits. In stage III disease, newly formed basement membrane has surrounded the deposits. With stage IV disease, the immune-complex deposits lose their electron density, resulting in an irregularly thickened basement membrane with irregular electron-lucent areas.

Glomerular Diseases

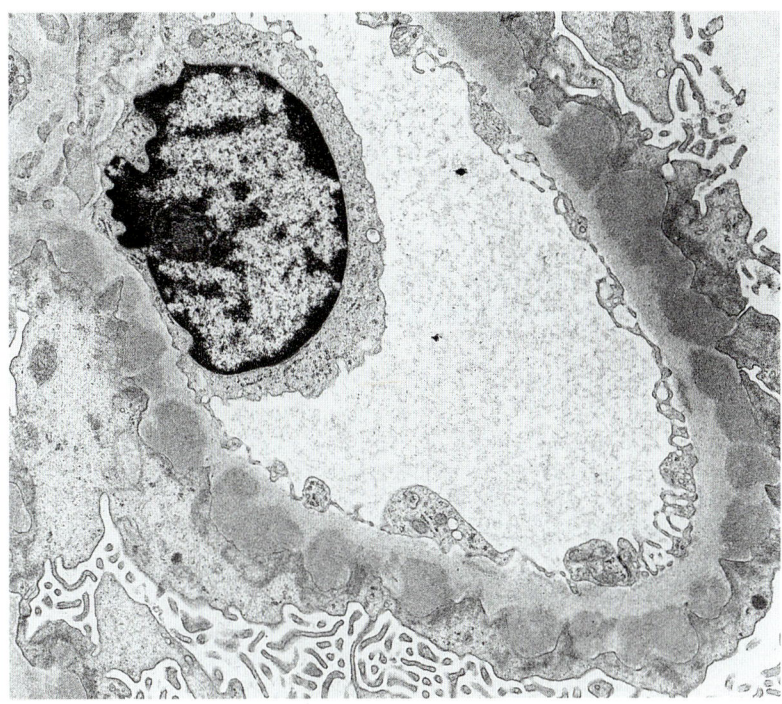

FIGURE 16-22
Stage II membranous glomerulopathy. An electron micrograph shows deposits of electron-dense material, with intervening delicate projections of basement membrane material.

also be present. In patients who develop symptomatic disease, GBM thickening and especially the expansion of the mesangial matrix result in changes that can be seen by light microscopy. Overt diabetic glomerulosclerosis is characterized by diffuse global thickening of GBMs and diffuse mesangial matrix expansion, accompanied by nodular sclerotic lesions termed *Kimmelstiel-Wilson nodules* (Fig. 16-25). These nodules have an acellular core, with mesangial cells and capillaries pushed to the periphery. Insudation of proteins forms rounded nodules between Bowman's capsule and the parietal epithelium ("capsular drops") or subendothelial accumulations along the capillary loops ("fibrin caps"). Tubular basement membranes are thickened. Scle-

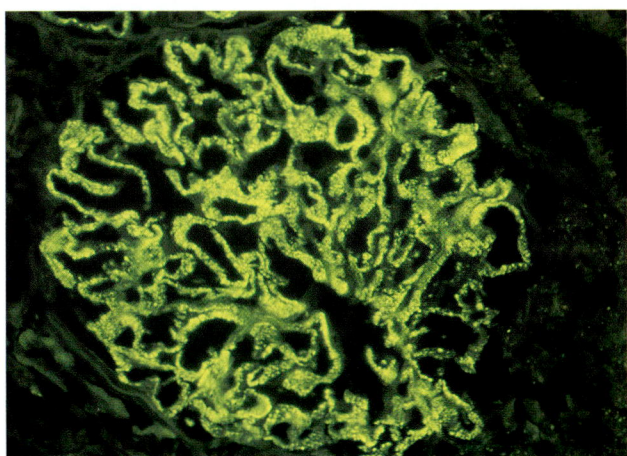

FIGURE 16-23
Membranous glomerulopathy. Immunofluorescence microscopy shows granular deposits of IgG outlining the glomerular capillary loops.

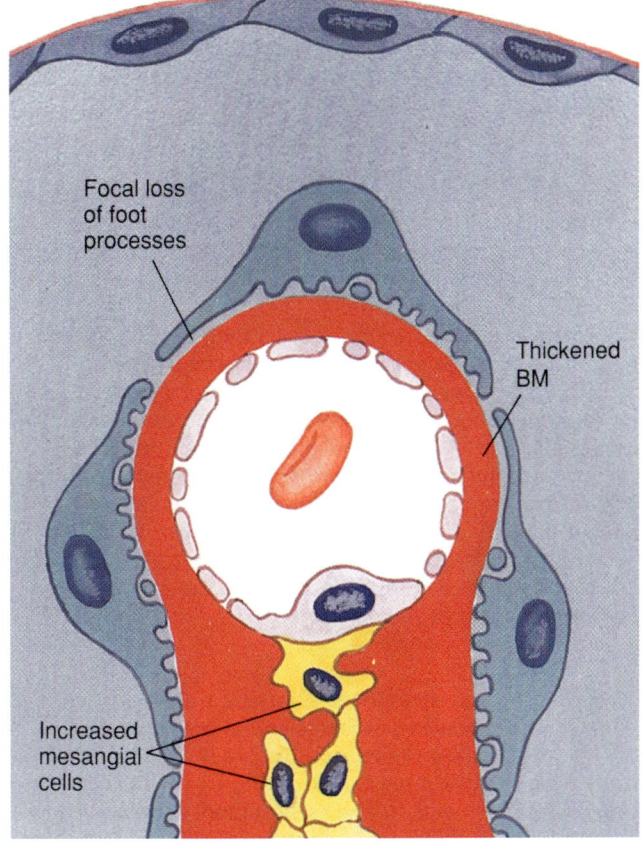

FIGURE 16-24
Diabetic glomerulosclerosis. The lamina densa of the glomerular basement membrane is thickened, and there is an increase in mesangial matrix material.

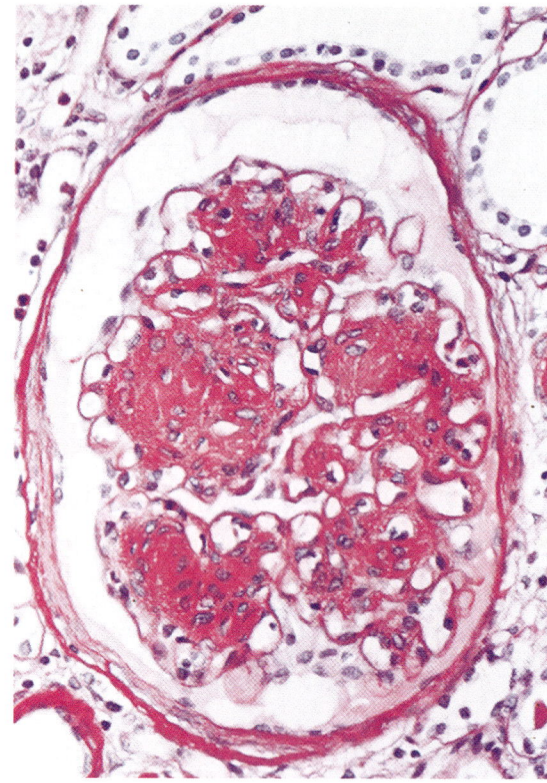

FIGURE 16-25
Diabetic glomerulosclerosis. PAS staining reveals a prominent increase in the mesangial matrix, forming several nodular lesions. Dilation of glomerular capillaries is evident, and some capillary basement membranes are thickened.

of blood glucose reduces the likelihood of developing diabetic glomerulosclerosis and retards progression once it develops. Control of hypertension and dietary protein restriction also slow progression of the disease.

Amyloidosis Leads to Nephrotic Syndrome and Renal Failure

Renal disease is a frequent complication of AA and AL amyloidosis (see Chapter 23).

 Pathogenesis: Amyloid may be formed from a number of different polypeptides. In each case, however, the amyloid has the same characteristic histological and ultrastructural appearance, and immunohistochemical tests are required to differentiate between the different forms. **AA amyloid** is derived from serum amyloid

rosing and insudative changes also occur in both the afferent and efferent arterioles, resulting in hyaline arteriolosclerosis. Generalized arteriosclerosis is usually present in the kidney. Reduced blood flow to the medulla predisposes to papillary necrosis and pyelonephritis.

Electron microscopy reveals widening of the basement membrane lamina densa, which may be thickened 5- to 10-fold. There is an increase in mesangial matrix, particularly in the nodular lesions (Fig. 16-26). The insudative lesions appear as electron-dense masses that contain lipid debris.

Immunofluorescence microscopy demonstrates diffuse linear trapping of IgG, albumin, fibrinogen, and other plasma proteins in the GBM. This finding reflects nonimmunological adsorption of these proteins to the thickened GBM, possibly as a result of nonenzymatic glycosylation of GBM and plasma proteins.

Clinical Features: Diabetic glomerulosclerosis is the leading cause of end-stage renal disease in the United States, accounting for a third of all patients with chronic renal failure. It occurs in both type I and type II diabetes mellitus. The earliest manifestation is microalbuminuria (slightly increased proteinuria below the usual detection range). Overt proteinuria occurs between 10 and 15 years after the onset of diabetes and often becomes severe enough to cause the nephrotic syndrome. In time, diabetic glomerulosclerosis progresses to renal failure. Strict control

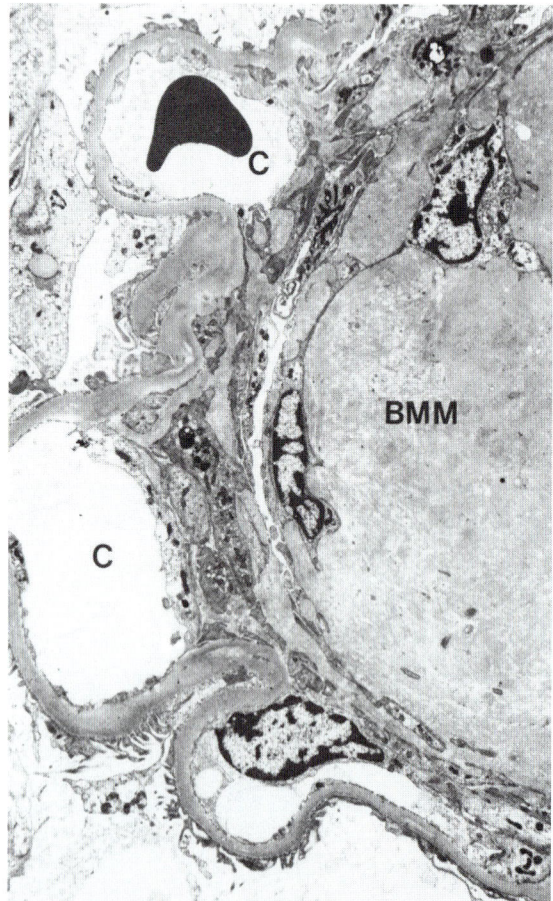

FIGURE 16-26
Advanced diabetic glomerulosclerosis. An electron micrograph shows a nodular aggregate of basement membrane material *(BMM)*. The peripheral capillary *(C)* demonstrates diffuse basement membrane widening but a normal texture.

A protein (SAA), which increases markedly during inflammatory processes. Thus, the deposition of AA amyloid is often associated with chronic inflammatory disorders (e.g., rheumatoid arthritis, chronic tuberculosis, and familial Mediterranean fever). AL amyloid is derived from λ or, less often, κ immunoglobulin light chains produced by a neoplastic clone of B cells or plasma cells. Thus, it frequently is associated with, or is a harbinger of, multiple myeloma.

 Pathology: Histologically, amyloid is an eosinophilic, amorphous material (Fig. 16-27) that has a characteristic apple-green color in sections stained with Congo red and examined by polarized light microscopy (Fig. 16-28). The acidophilic deposits initially are most apparent in the mesangium but later extend into capillary walls and may obliterate capillary lumens (Figs. 16-27, 16-29). In advanced amyloidosis, the glomerular structure is completely obliterated, and the glomeruli appear as large eosinophilic spheres.

By electron microscopy, amyloid is composed of nonbranching fibrils, approximately 10 nm in diameter. Amyloid fibrils are most prominent in the mesangium, but they often extend into capillary walls, especially in advanced cases (Figs. 16-29 and 16-30). The epithelial foot processes overlying the GBM are obliterated, and the epithelial cells may be tented by the amyloid fibrils, which are often oriented perpendicularly to the basement membrane.

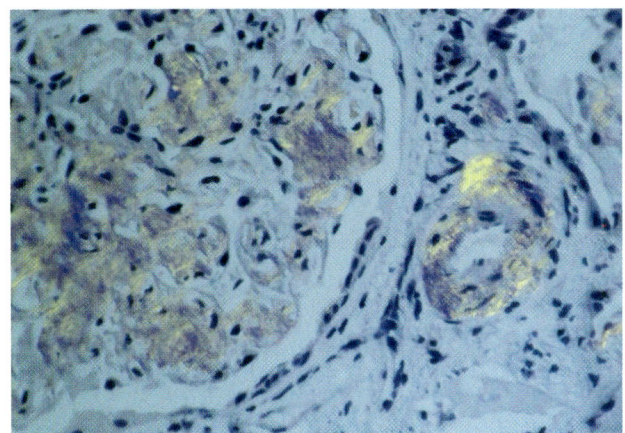

FIGURE 16-28
Amyloid nephropathy. In a section stained with Congo red and examined under polarized light, the amyloid deposits in the glomerulus and the adjacent arteriole show a characteristic apple-green birefringence.

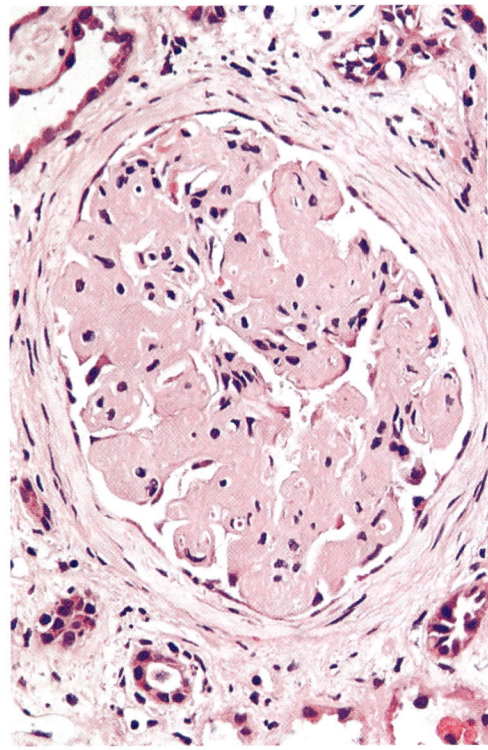

FIGURE 16-27
Amyloid nephropathy. Amorphous acellular material expands the mesangial areas and obstructs the glomerular capillaries. The deposits of amyloid may take on a nodular appearance, somewhat resembling those of diabetic glomerulosclerosis (see Fig. 16-25). However, amyloid deposits are not PAS positive and are identifiable by Congo red staining.

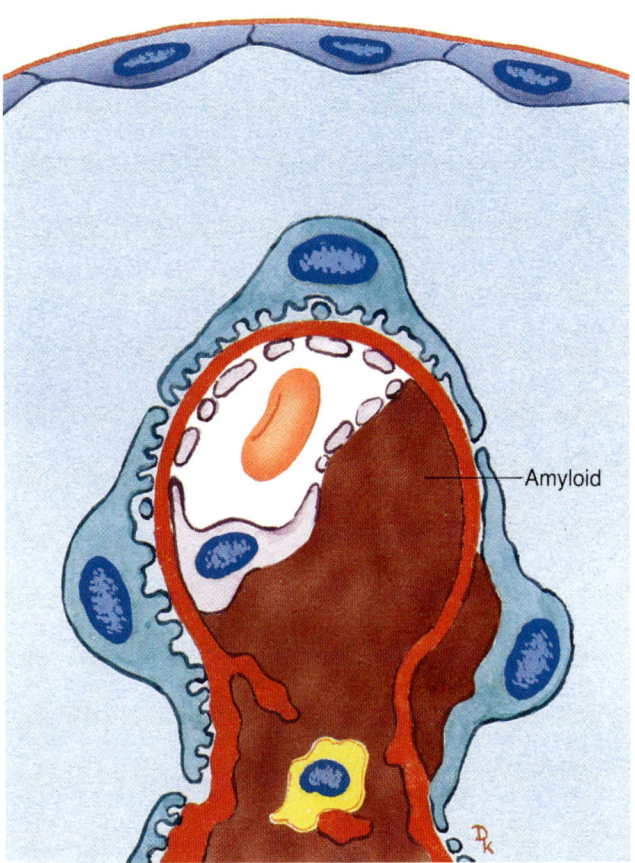

FIGURE 16-29
Amyloid nephropathy. This disorder is initially associated with the accumulation of characteristic fibrillar deposits in the mesangium. These inert masses, which are fibrillar by electron microscopy, extend along the inner surface of the basement membrane, frequently obstructing the capillary lumen. Focal extension of amyloid through the basement membrane may elevate the epithelial cell, in which case irregular spikes are seen along the outer surface of the basement membrane.

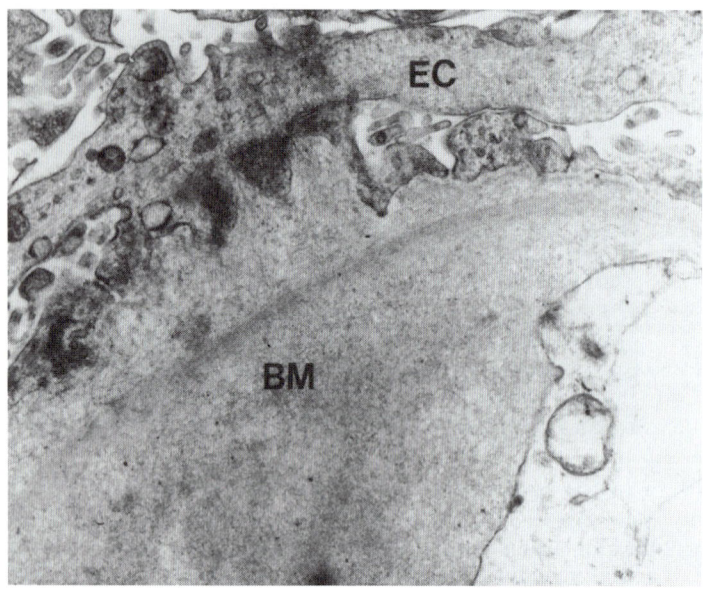

FIGURE 16-30
Amyloid nephropathy. Deposits of fibrils (10 nm diameter) accumulate in the mesangium and capillary walls of glomeruli. (*BM*, basement membrane; *EC*, epithelial cells).

 Clinical Features: Renal involvement is a prominent feature in most cases of systemic AL and AA amyloidosis. Proteinuria is commonly the initial manifestation. The proteinuria is nonselective (i.e., both albumin and globulins appear in the urine) and produces nephrotic syndrome in 60% of patients. Eventually, severe infiltration of the glomeruli and blood vessels by amyloid results in renal failure. AL amyloidosis is treated with chemotherapy analogous to that used for multiple myeloma. AA amyloidosis, especially when caused by familial Mediterranean fever, is ameliorated by colchicine therapy.

Light Chain and Heavy Chain Deposition Disease Occur in B-Cell Neoplasia

Both light chain and heavy chain deposition diseases reflect the deposition of monoclonal immunoglobulin light chains in GBMs, glomerular mesangial matrix, and tubular basement membranes. The underlying B-cell neoplasm may be occult or there may be overt multiple myeloma or lymphoma. The most common offender in light chain disease is κ light chains. The immunoglobulin heavy chains that cause this pattern of injury have deleted domains, so that they resemble light chains. The deposition of monoclonal immunoglobulin stimulates increased matrix production in basement membranes, causing thickening of glomerular and tubular basement membranes. Nodular expansion of mesangial regions resembles diabetic glomerulosclerosis. Importantly, the increased extracellular material does not stain with Congo red. Electron microscopy reveals a uniform, finely granular, electron-dense material along the glomerular and tubular basement membranes and within the mesangial matrix. Amyloid fibrils are not present. Immunofluorescence microscopy demonstrates linear staining for monoclonal immunoglobulin chains along the involved basement membranes. Light chain and heavy chain deposition disease usually manifest clinically as nephrotic syndrome and renal failure.

Hereditary Nephritis (Alport Syndrome) Reflects Abnormal Type IV Collagen in GBMs

Alport syndrome is a proliferative and sclerosing glomerular disease, often accompanied by defects of the ears or the eyes, that is caused by a genetic abnormality in type IV collagen.

 Pathogenesis: A variety of genetic mutations cause molecular defects in the GBM that produce the renal lesions of Alport syndrome. The most common defect is X-linked and is caused by a mutation in the gene for the α5 chain of type IV collagen (*COL4A5* gene). A deletion at the 5′ end of *COL4A5* that extends into the *COL4A6* gene, which codes for the α6 chain of type IV collagen, causes Alport syndrome and multiple leiomyomas in the gastrointestinal and genital tracts. An autosomal recessive form of Alport syndrome is caused by mutations in *COL4A3* and *COL4A4*.

Because of disturbed basement membrane structure in Alport syndrome, serum from patients with anti-GBM disease (e.g., Goodpasture syndrome) fails to react with GBMs from patients with Alport syndrome. Conversely, patients with Alport syndrome who are subjected to renal transplantation are at risk for developing antibodies to allograft GBMs, although this rarely causes significant disease.

Pathology: Early glomerular lesions of Alport syndrome show mild mesangial hypercellularity and matrix expansion. Progression of renal disease is associated with increasing focal and eventually diffuse glomerular sclerosis. Advanced glomerular lesions are accompanied by tubular atrophy, interstitial fibrosis, and the presence of foam cells in the tubules and interstitium. The most diagnostic morphological lesion is seen only by electron microscopy as an irregularly thickened GBM with splitting of the lamina densa into interlacing lamellae that surround electron-lucent areas (Fig. 16-31).

Clinical Features: Hematuria is present early in life in males with X-linked disease and in both sexes with autosomal recessive disease. Proteinuria, progressive renal failure, and hypertension develop later in the course of the disease. Virtually all men with the X-linked syndrome and both sexes with autosomal recessive disease develop end-stage renal disease by ages 40 to 50. Essentially all autosomal recessive and 80% of X-linked disease patients exhibit a progressive hearing impairment, initially manifested as high-frequency deafness. A quarter to a third of patients suffer ocular defects, most often involving the lens. Females with X-linked disease often display hematuria and occasionally have proteinuria, but rarely develop progressive renal failure.

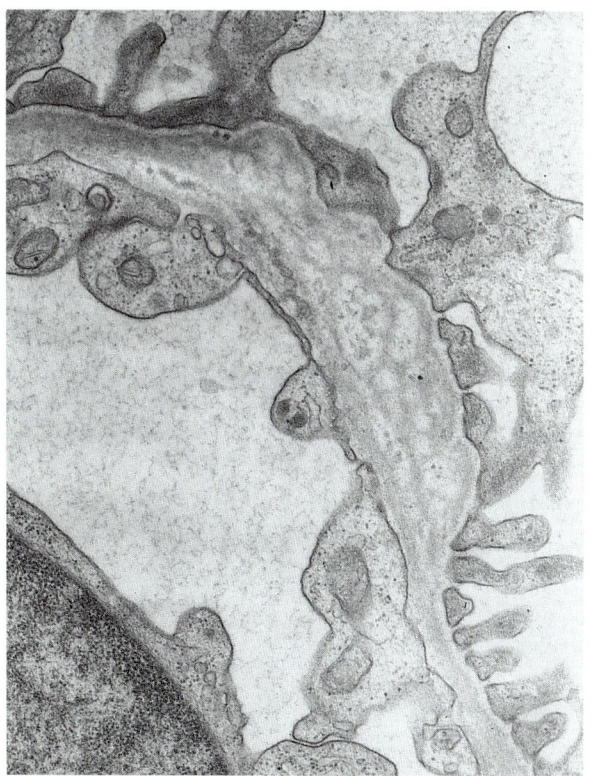

FIGURE 16-31
Hereditary nephritis (Alport syndrome). The lamina densa of the GBM is laminated rather than forming a single dense band (compare this electron micrograph with Fig. 16-5).

Thin Glomerular Basement Membrane Nephropathy Is a Benign Cause of Hematuria

Thin basement membrane nephropathy, also termed benign familial hematuria, *is a common hereditary disorder of GBMs that typically manifests as asymptomatic microscopic hematuria and occasionally with intermittent gross hematuria.* In fact, this disease and IgA nephropathy are the two major diagnostic considerations in patients with asymptomatic glomerular hematuria. Patients with thin basement membrane nephropathy usually do not develop renal failure or substantial proteinuria. By light microscopy, the glomeruli are unremarkable. Electron microscopy reveals a reduced thickness of the GBM (150 to 300 nm, compared with the normal 350 to 450 nm). The most common mode of inheritance is autosomal dominant. Heterozygous mutations in the COL4A3 and COL4A4 genes lead to thin basement membrane disease, and homozygous ones to Alport syndrome.

Acute Postinfectious Glomerulonephritis Is an Immune Complex Disease of Childhood

Acute postinfectious glomerulonephritis usually occurs after an infection with group A (β-hemolytic) streptococci and is caused by the deposition of immune complexes in glomeruli.

Pathogenesis: Acute postinfectious glomerulonephritis is most often caused by certain ***nephritogenic* strains of group A (β-hemolytic) streptococci.** Occasional examples are caused by staphylococcal infection (e.g., acute staphylococcal endocarditis, staphylococcal abscess), and rare cases result from viral (e.g., hepatitis B) or parasitic (e.g., malaria) infections. The exact mechanism by which infection causes the characteristic inflammatory changes in the glomeruli is not completely understood. Similarities to experimental acute serum sickness suggest that postinfectious glomerulonephritis is caused by glomerular localization of immune complexes generated by an antibody response to circulating antigens. Both poststreptococcal glomerulonephritis in patients and acute serum sickness caused by injecting foreign proteins into animals have a latent period of 9 to 14 days between the time of exposure to a new antigen and the occurrence of glomerulonephritis. The granular immunofluorescence pattern of immune-complex staining and the ultrastructural appearance of dense deposits are similar in the human and experimental diseases. Immune complexes could localize in glomeruli by deposition from the circulation or formation in situ as bacterial antigens trapped in the glomeruli bind circulating antibodies. The specific nephritogenic streptococcal antigens have not been conclusively identified. Candidates include streptokinase, endostreptosin, and streptococcal erythrogenic toxin B, which can activate complement even in the absence of antibodies.

Immune complexes within glomeruli initiate inflammation by activating complement, as well as other humoral and

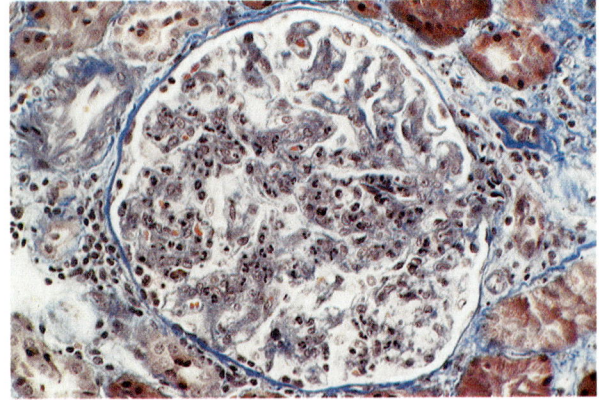

FIGURE 16-32
Acute poststreptococcal glomerulonephritis. The glomerulus of a patient who developed glomerulonephritis after a streptococcal infection contains numerous neutrophils (Masson trichrome stain)

cellular inflammatory mediator systems. Complement activation is so extensive that over 90% of patients develop hypocomplementemia. The inflammatory mediators attract and activate neutrophils and monocytes, and they stimulate the proliferation of mesangial and endothelial cells. These effects result in marked glomerular hypercellularity, which defines acute diffuse proliferative glomerulonephritis.

Pathology: The acute phase of postinfectious glomerulonephritis is characterized by diffuse enlargement and hypercellularity of the glomeruli (Fig. 16-32). Hypercellularity reflects the proliferation of both endothelial and mesangial cells (Fig. 16-33) and the infiltration of neutrophils and monocytes. Crescents are uncommon. Interstitial edema and mild infiltration of mononuclear leukocytes occur in parallel with the glomerular changes.

The acute phase begins 1 or 2 weeks after the onset of the nephritogenic infection and resolves in over 90% of patients after several weeks. Neutrophils and endothelial hypercellularity disappear first, leaving only mesangial hypercellularity and matrix expansion. After several months, most patients experience resolution of all histological abnormalities.

The most distinctive ultrastructural features of acute postinfectious glomerulonephritis are **subepithelial dense deposits that are shaped like "humps"** (Figs. 16-33 and 16-34). These deposits are invariably accompanied by mesan-

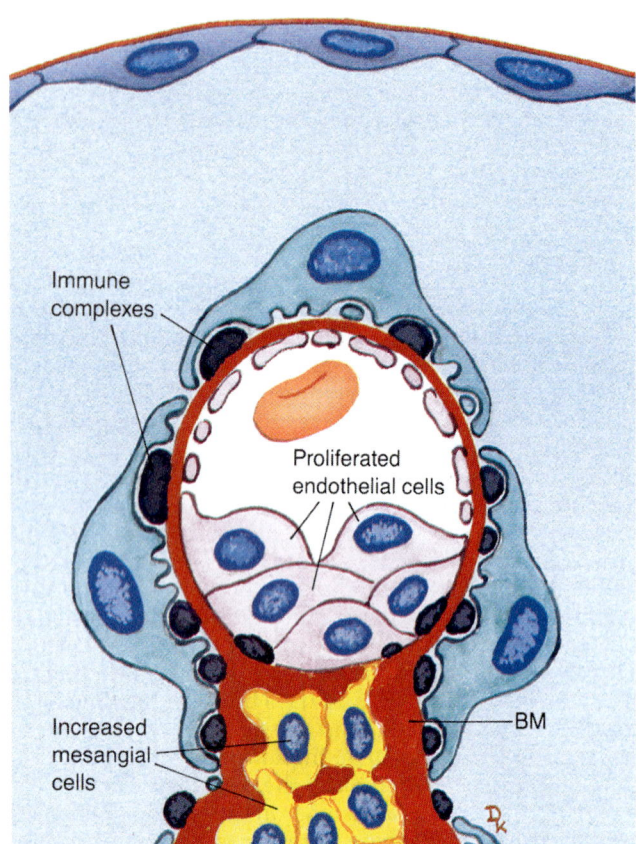

FIGURE 16-33
Postinfectious glomerulonephritis. Accumulation of numerous subepithelial immune complexes as humplike structures is a characteristic feature. Less prominent subendothelial immune complexes are associated with endothelial cell proliferation and are related to increased capillary permeability and narrowing of the lumen. Frequently, proliferation of mesangial cells and a thickened mesangial matrix (BM) result in widening of the stalk and conspicuous trapping of immune complexes.

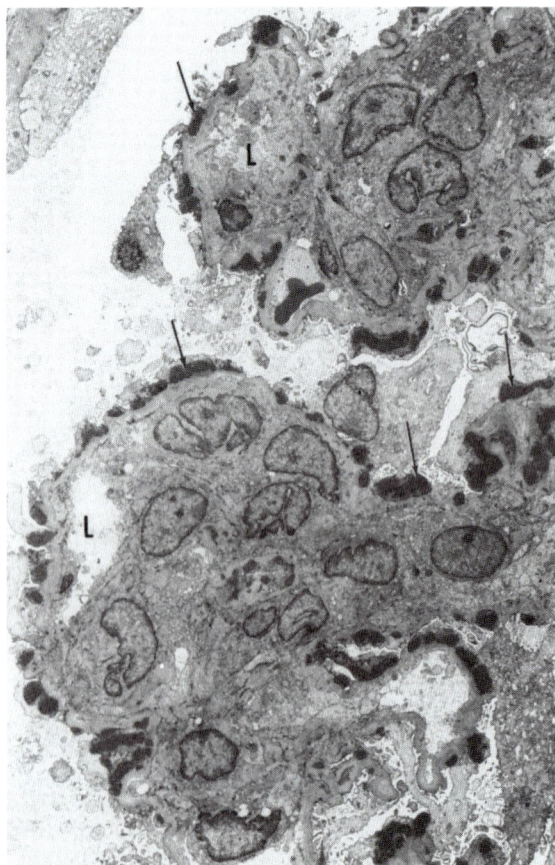

FIGURE 16-34
Acute postinfectious glomerulonephritis. An electron micrograph demonstrates numerous subepithelial humps (arrows). The capillary lumina (L) are markedly narrowed.

Glomerular Diseases

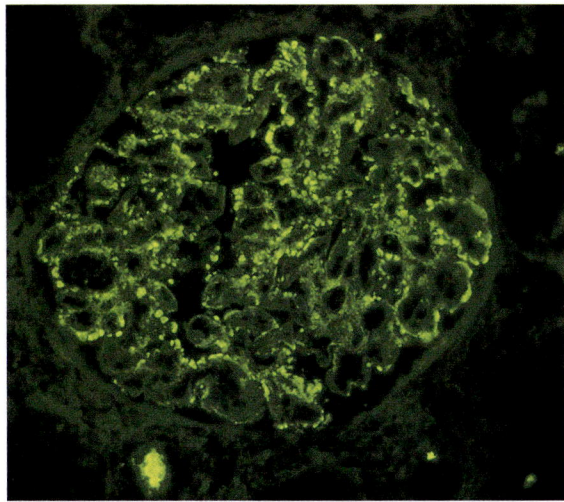

FIGURE 16-35
Acute postinfectious glomerulonephritis. An immunofluorescence micrograph demonstrates granular staining for C3 in capillary walls and the mesangium.

gial and subendothelial deposits, which may be more difficult to find but are probably more important in pathogenesis because of their proximity to the inflammatory mediator systems in the blood. The variably sized, dome-shaped humps are situated on the epithelial side of the basement membrane. They are not as diffusely distributed as the deposits of membranous glomerulopathy (compare Figs. 16-21 and 16-33).

In the first few weeks of disease, immunofluorescence microscopy typically reveals granular deposits corresponding to IgG and C3 along the basement membrane, in locations corresponding to the humps. Later in the disease, C3 is present without IgG, possibly because immune complexes containing IgG no longer accumulate in the glomeruli after the infection clears (Fig. 16-35).

Clinical Features: Acute poststreptococcal glomerulonephritis is not seen as frequently as in the past, but it remains one of the most common renal diseases in childhood. The primary infection involves the pharynx or, in hot and humid environments, the skin. In recent years, the proportion of cases of acute postinfectious glomerulonephritis caused by staphylococcal infection has been increasing. Because the organisms may not be recoverable at the time of the nephritis, the diagnosis depends on serological evidence of a rise in antibody titers to streptococcal products. The nephritic syndrome typically begins abruptly with oliguria, hematuria, facial edema, and hypertension. Typically, the level of serum C3 is depressed during the acute syndrome, but returns to normal within 1 to 2 weeks. Overt nephritis resolves after several weeks, although hematuria and especially proteinuria may persist for several months. A few patients have abnormal urinary sediment for years after the acute episode, and rare patients (particularly adults) develop progressive renal failure.

Type I Membranoproliferative Glomerulonephritis Is a Chronic Immune-Complex Disease That Is Idiopathic or Follows Infections

Type I membranoproliferative glomerulonephritis is characterized by hypercellularity and capillary wall thickening; deposition of mesangial and subendothelial immune complexes causes mesangial proliferation and extension into the subendothelial zone.

Pathogenesis: Type I membranoproliferative glomerulonephritis, also called *mesangiocapillary glomerulonephritis,* is caused by the localization of immune complexes to the mesangium and subendothelial zone of capillary walls. In most patients, the origin of the nephritogenic antigen is unknown, but some have associated conditions that are the apparent source of the antigen (Table 16-5).

Elimination of the associated condition, such as bacterial endocarditis or osteomyelitis, leads to resolution of the glomerulonephritis, which supports a causal relationship between the two. Unlike the agents that cause acute postinfectious glomerulonephritis, those that are responsible for type I membranoproliferative glomerulonephritis cause persistent, indolent infections that are associated with chronic antigenemia. This condition leads to chronic localization of immune complexes in glomeruli and resultant hypercellularity and matrix remodeling.

Pathology: The glomeruli in type I membranoproliferative glomerulonephritis are diffusely enlarged and exhibit conspicuous mesangial cell proliferation. The resulting lobular distortion ("hypersegmentation") of the glomeruli (Fig. 16-36) has in the past been termed *lobular glomerulonephritis.* Among these patients, 20% will have crescents, usually involving only a minority of glomeruli. Capillary walls are thickened, and silver stains show a doubling or complex replication of GBMs.

Electron microscopy demonstrates that the capillary wall thickening and replication of GBMs are a consequence of the marked expansion of the mesangial area, with extension of mesangial cytoplasm into the subendothelial zone and deposition of new basement membrane material between the mesangial cytoplasm and the endothelial cell

TABLE 16-5 **Classification of Type I Membranoproliferative Glomerulonephritis**

Primary (idiopathic)
Secondary
    Subacute bacterial endocarditis
    Infected ventriculoatrial shunt
    Osteomyelitis
    Hepatitis C virus infection
    Mixed cryoglobulinemia
    Neoplasia

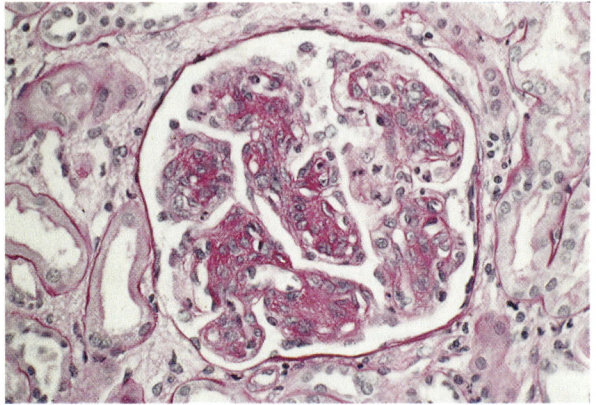

FIGURE 16-36
Type I membranoproliferative glomerulonephritis. The glomerular lobulation is accentuated. Increased cells and matrix in the mesangium and thickening of capillary walls are noted.

 Pathogenesis: Although the cause of the extensive localization of complement in the GBMs and mesangial matrix in this disease suggests that complement activation is a major mediator of the structural and functional abnormalities, the basis for complement deposition is unknown. The virtual absence of immunoglobulin in the glomeruli probably excludes mediation by immune complexes. Most patients have a circulating IgG autoantibody, termed *C3 nephritic factor,* that stabilizes the activated C3 convertase enzyme (C3bBb) of the alternative complement

(Figs. 16-37 and 16-38). Subendothelial and mesangial electron-dense deposits, corresponding to immune complexes, are the likely stimuli for the mesangial response. Variable numbers of subepithelial dense deposits may also be seen. Immunofluorescence microscopy demonstrates granular deposition of immunoglobulins and complement in glomerular capillary loops and mesangium (Fig. 16-39).

Clinical Features: Although it can occur at any age, type I membranoproliferative glomerulonephritis is most frequent in older children and young adults. It may manifest as either nephrotic or nephritic syndrome or a combination of both. Type I disease accounts for 5% of the nephrotic syndrome in children and adults in United States. It is much more frequent in underdeveloped countries that have a high prevalence of chronic infections. Patients often have low levels of C3. Acute postinfectious glomerulonephritis and lupus glomerulonephritis, both of which can cause nephritis with hypocomplementemia, are in the differential diagnosis. Type I membranoproliferative glomerulonephritis is usually a persistent but slowly progressive disease. Half of patients reach end-stage renal disease after 10 years.

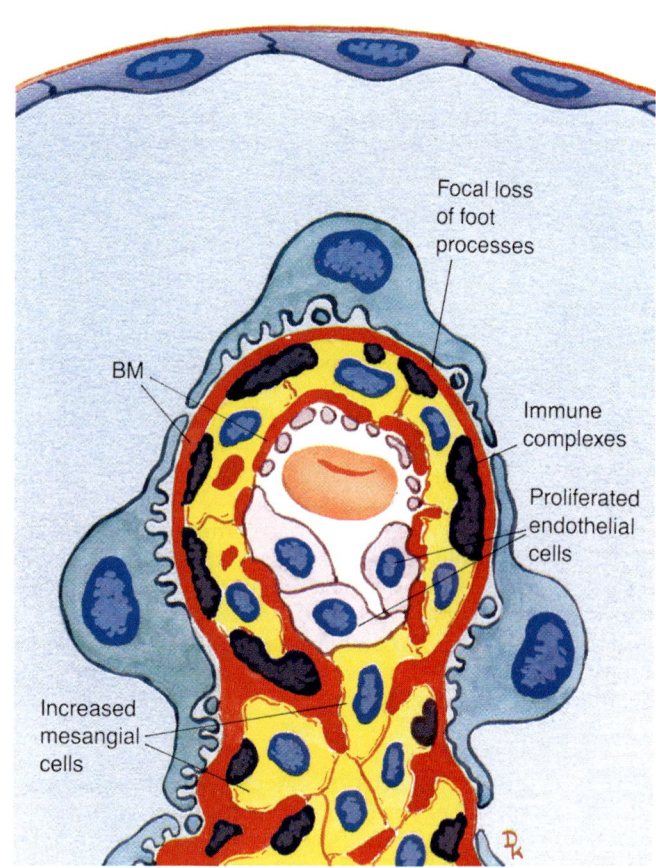

FIGURE 16-37
Membranoproliferative glomerulonephritis, type I. In this disease, the glomeruli are enlarged. Hypercellular tufts and narrowing or obstruction of the capillary lumen are seen. Large subendothelial deposits of immune complexes extend along the inner border of the basement membrane. The mesangial cells proliferate and migrate peripherally into the capillary. Basement membrane *(BM)* material accumulates in a linear fashion parallel to the basement membrane in a subendothelial position. The interposition of mesangial cells and basement membrane between the endothelial cells and the original basement membrane creates a double-contour effect. The accumulation of mesangial cells and stroma in the tufts narrows the capillary lumen. The proliferation of mesangial cells and the accumulation of basement membrane material also widen the mesangium. The entire process leads progressively to lobulation of the glomerulus. Note the proliferation of endothelial cells and focal effacement of foot processes.

Type II Membranoproliferative Glomerulonephritis (Dense Deposit Disease) Features Complement Deposition

Type II membranoproliferative glomerulonephritis is characterized by a pathognomonic electron-dense transformation of GBMs and extensive complement deposition.

Glomerular Diseases

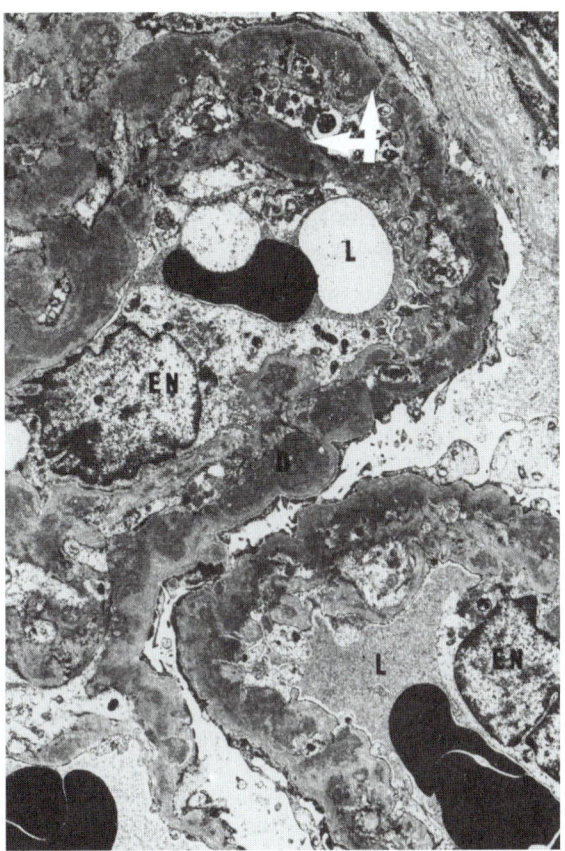

FIGURE 16-38
Type I membranoproliferative glomerulonephritis. An electron micrograph demonstrates a double-contour basement membrane (arrow), with mesangial interposition and prominent subendothelial deposits. EN, endothelial cell; L, capillary lumen.

activation pathway. The result is a prolongation of C3 cleaving activity. A similar C3 nephritic factor is also present in a minority of patients with type I membranoproliferative glomerulonephritis and lupus nephritis. The role of this factor, if any, in the pathogenesis of type II membranoproliferative glomerulonephritis remains obscure. However, the common recurrence of type II membranoproliferative glomerulonephritis in renal transplants suggests that glomerular injury is mediated through some unknown humoral factor.

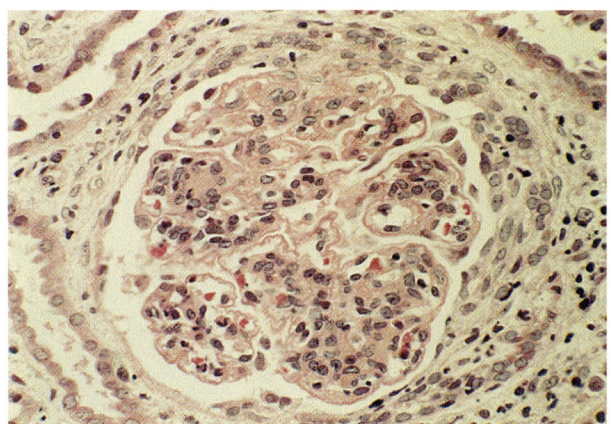

FIGURE 16-40
Type II membranoproliferative glomerulonephritis (dense deposit disease). Capillary wall thickening, hypercellularity, and a small crescent are evident.

 Pathology: The histological appearance of type II membranoproliferative glomerulonephritis may be similar to that of type I, with capillary wall thickening and hypercellularity (Fig. 16-40). However, many patients have less-pronounced or absent hypercellularity, which makes the term "proliferative" problematic. The distinctive ribbonlike zone of increased density in the center of a thickened GBM and in the mesangial matrix (Fig. 16-41), justifies the alternative name *dense deposit disease*. Areas of density may also be found in the membranes of peritubular capillaries and in the elastic laminae of arterioles. Immunofluorescence microscopy shows linear staining of capillary walls for C3, with little or no staining for immunoglobulins (Fig. 16-42).

 Clinical Features: Type II membranoproliferative glomerulonephritis is rare. The clinical presentation and course are similar to type I disease. The frequency of hypocomplementemia is, however, higher, and the prognosis is slightly worse. No effective treatment has been identified.

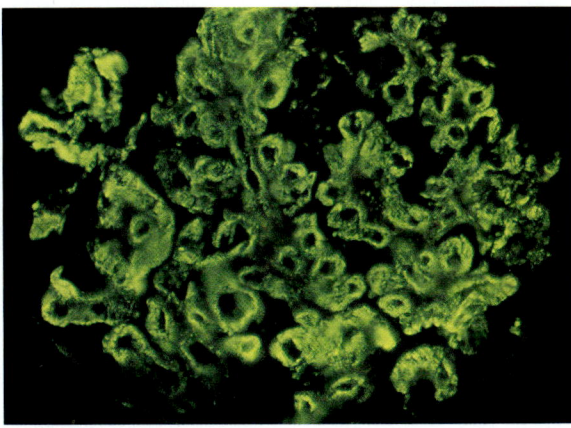

FIGURE 16-39
Type I membranoproliferative glomerulonephritis. An immunofluorescence micrograph demonstrates granular to bandlike staining for C3 in the capillary walls and mesangium.

Lupus Glomerulonephritis Is Associated with Many Autoantibodies

Systemic lupus erythematosus (SLE) is an autoimmune disease characterized by a generalized dysregulation and hyperactivity of B cells, with production of autoantibodies to a variety of nuclear and nonnuclear antigens, including DNA, RNA, nucleoproteins, and phospholipids. Nephritis is one of the most common com-

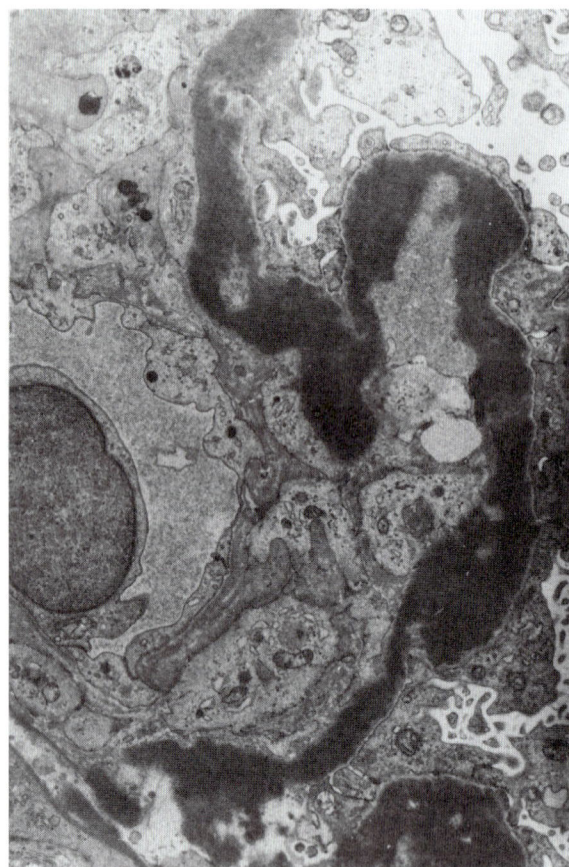

FIGURE 16-41
Type II membranoproliferative glomerulonephritis (dense deposit disease). An electron micrograph demonstrates thickening of the basement membrane and intramembranous dense deposits.

plications of SLE. There is a wide range of patterns of immune complex deposition in the glomeruli of lupus nephritis. Immune complexes confined to the mesangium cause less inflammation than do subendothelial immune complexes. The latter are more exposed to the cellular and humoral inflammatory mediator systems in the blood and are, therefore, more likely to initiate inflammation. Subepithelial localization of immune complexes causes proteinuria but does not stimulate overt glomerular inflammation.

 Pathogenesis: Immune complexes may localize in glomeruli by deposition from the circulation, formation in situ, or both. Circulating immune complexes formed by high-avidity antibodies deposit in the subendothelial and mesangial zones; low-affinity antibodies form immune complexes in situ in the subepithelial zone. Formation of immune complexes in situ may involve antigens such as DNA, which have been planted on GBMs or mesangial matrix by charge interactions. Glomerular immune complexes activate complement and initiate inflammatory injury. Complement activation in the kidneys and elsewhere often results in hypocomplementemia. Immune complexes also localize in the renal interstitium, in the walls of interstitial vessels, and along tubular basement membranes. These complexes may be involved in the production of tubulointerstitial inflammation in patients with lupus nephritis.

 Pathology: The pathological and clinical manifestations of lupus nephritis are highly variable because of variable patterns of immune complex accumulation in different patients (Table 16-6) and in the same patient over time.

- **Class I:** Immune complexes are confined to the mesangium and cause no changes by light microscopy or varying degrees of mesangial hypercellularity and matrix expansion.
- **Class II:** Varying degrees of mesangial hypercellularity and matrix expansion are seen. Immune complex accumulation in the subendothelial zone, which is always accompanied by mesangial immune complexes, stimulates inflammation with proliferation of mesangial and endothelial cells and the influx of neutrophils and monocytes. Necrosis and crescents develop. This overt glomerular inflammation is called *focal proliferative lupus glomerulonephritis* (Fig. 16-43).
- **Class III:** This class refers to more-severe disease. Overt glomerular inflammation, i.e., focal proliferative glomerulonephritis, involves less than 50% of glomeruli.
- **Class IV:** Also called *diffuse proliferative glomerulonephritis*, this type is similar to class III but shows involvement of more than 50% of glomeruli.
- **Class V:** Immune complexes are predominantly in the subepithelial zone, and the pathological phenotype is membranous glomerulopathy. Some patients have a background of class V injury and a concurrent class II, III, or IV injury because of the presence of numerous subepithelial immune complexes, as well as mesangial and subendothelial immune complexes. Even pure class V lupus nephritis has mesangial immune complexes that can be detected by electron microscopy. Lupus nephritis may progress to advanced chronic sclerosing disease.
- **Class VI:** Advanced chronic sclerosing disease

Electron microscopy demonstrates the varied locations of immune-complex dense deposits in mesangial, subendothe-

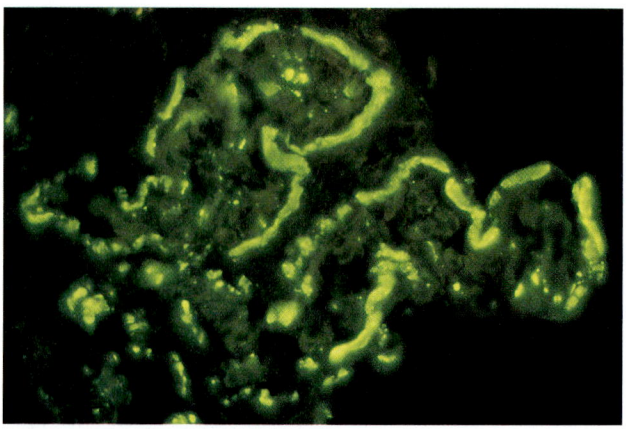

FIGURE 16-42
Type II membranoproliferative glomerulonephritis (dense deposit disease). An immunofluorescence micrograph demonstrates bands of capillary wall staining and coarsely granular mesangial staining for C3.

TABLE 16-6 Pathological and Clinical Features of Lupus Nephritis

Class	Location of Immune Complexes	Clinical Manifestations
I: No lesion by light microscopy	Mesangial	Mild hematuria and proteinuria
II: Mesangial proliferative	Mesangial	Mild hematuria and proteinuria
III: Focal proliferative	Mesangial and subendothelial	Moderate nephritis
IV: Diffuse proliferative	Mesangial and subendothelial	Severe nephritis
IV: Membranous	Subepithelial	Nephrotic syndrome
VI: Chronic	Variable	Chronic renal failure

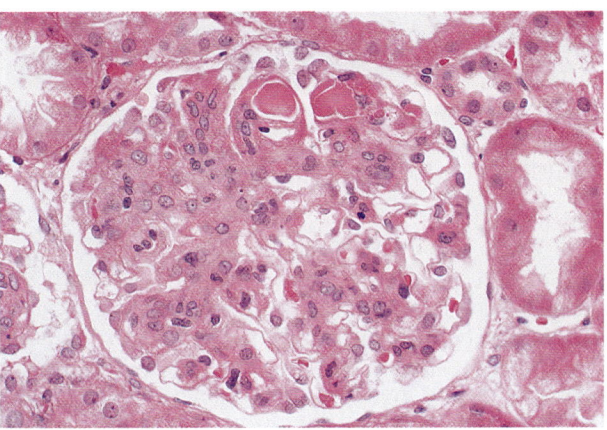

FIGURE 16-43
Proliferative lupus glomerulonephritis. Segmental endocapillary hypercellularity and thickening of capillary walls are present.

lial, and subepithelial locations. Class I and II lesions have only mesangial deposits. Classes III and IV have mesangial and subendothelial deposits, and usually scattered subepithelial deposits (Fig. 16-44). Class V lesions have numerous subepithelial dense deposits. The dense deposits of lupus glomerulonephritis occasionally have a patterned appearance that resembles a fingerprint. Some 80% of specimens have *tubuloreticular inclusions* in endothelial cells. Lupus nephritis and HIV-associated nephropathy are the only renal diseases with a high frequency of these structures.

Immunofluorescence microscopy also demonstrates the varied locations of immune complexes. The subepithelial complexes are granular, and the subendothelial deposits appear granular or bandlike (Fig. 16-45). The immune complexes often stain most intensely for IgG, but IgA and IgM are also almost always present. In addition, there is intense staining for C3, C1q, and other complement components. Granular staining along tubular basement membranes and interstitial vessels is present in over 50% of patients.

Clinical Features: Of all patients with SLE, 70% develop renal disease, which is the major cause for morbidity and mortality in many patients. The disease is most common in black women. As noted in Table 16-6, the clinical manifestations and prognosis of renal dysfunction are varied and depend on the pathological nature of the underlying renal disease. **Renal biopsy specimens from**

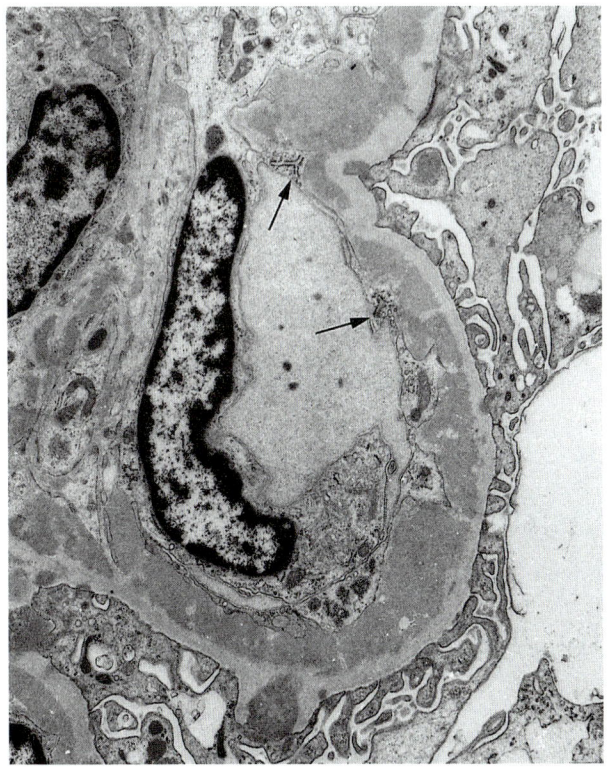

FIGURE 16-44
Diffuse proliferative lupus glomerulonephritis. An electron micrograph reveals large subendothelial and mesangial dense deposits and a few subepithelial deposits. Endothelial tubuloreticular inclusions *(arrows)* are present.

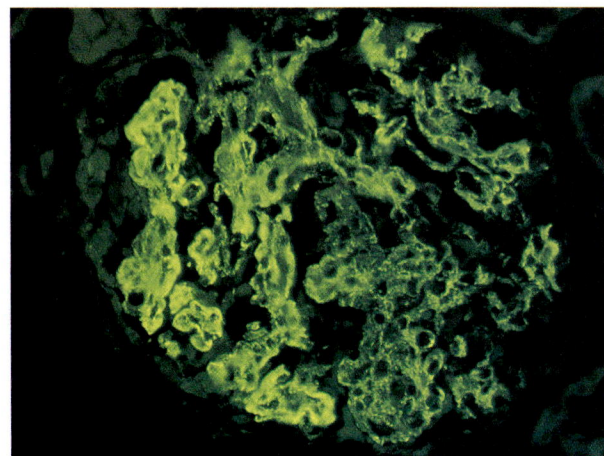

FIGURE 16-45
Diffuse proliferative lupus glomerulonephritis. An immunofluorescence micrograph demonstrates segmental staining for IgG in the capillary walls and mesangium.

lupus patients are usually evaluated to assess disease category, activity, and chronicity, rather than merely to make a diagnosis of lupus glomerulonephritis. Class III and class IV lupus nephritis have the poorest prognosis and are the categories that are treated most aggressively, usually with high doses of corticosteroids and other immunosuppressive drugs. Over time, sometimes prompted by treatment, there can be transitions from one type of lupus nephritis to another, with the expected changes in clinical manifestations. Prior to the use of current immunosuppressive regimens, more than 75% of patients with class IV disease reached end-stage renal failure within 5 years, compared to less than 25% with current treatment.

IgA Nephropathy (Berger Disease) Is Caused by Immune Complexes of IgA

Pathogenesis: Although the deposition of IgA-dominant immune complexes is the cause of IgA nephropathy, the constituent antigens and the mechanism of accumulation (deposition versus formation in situ) have not been determined. Patients with IgA nephropathy often have elevated blood levels of IgA, and circulating IgA-containing immune complexes have been detected. **Exacerbations of IgA nephropathy are often initiated by infections of the respiratory or gastrointestinal tracts.** A leading hypothesis proposes that mucosal exposure to viral, bacterial, or dietary antigens stimulates a nephritogenic, IgA-dominant, immune response that results in the glomerular accumulation of immune complexes. Possible involvement of dietary antigens is supported by the association between a small proportion of cases of IgA nephropathy and gluten-sensitive enteropathy and by the improvement in both diseases produced by eliminating dietary gluten. There is evidence for major histocompatibility complex (MHC)–linked susceptibility to IgA nephropathy, possibly mediated through dysregulation of IgA immune responses. Abnormal glycosylation of the hinge region of IgA appears to be an important predisposing factor in many patients with IgA nephropathy.

IgA-containing immune complexes within the mesangium most likely activate complement through the alternative pathway. This concept is supported by the demonstration of C3 and properdin in the IgA deposits, in the absence of C1q and C4.

Pathology: Immunofluorescence microscopy is essential for the diagnosis of IgA nephropathy. The diagnostic finding is mesangial staining that is more intense for IgA than for IgG or IgM (Fig. 16-46). This is almost always accompanied by staining for C3. IgA deposition in the glomerular capillary wall (in addition to the mesangium) may be present in more severe cases and suggests a less favorable prognosis.

Depending on the severity and duration of glomerular inflammation, IgA nephropathy manifests a continuum of histological appearances, ranging from (1) no discernible light microscopic changes, to (2) focal or diffuse mesangial hypercellularity, to (3) focal or diffuse proliferative glomerulonephritis (Fig. 16-47), to (4) chronic sclerosing glomerulonephritis. At the time of initial diagnosis, focal proliferative glomerulonephritis is the most frequent manifestation. Crescent formation is uncommon, except in unusually severe cases. This spectrum of pathological changes is analogous to that seen with lupus nephritis but tends to be less severe.

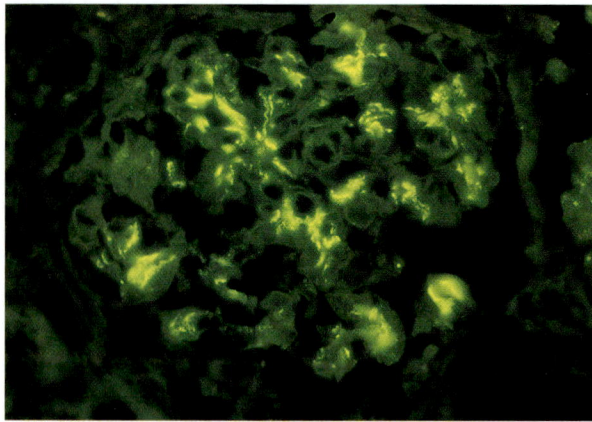

FIGURE 16-46
IgA nephropathy. An immunofluorescence micrograph shows deposits of IgA in the mesangial areas.

Ultrastructural examination reveals mesangial electron-dense deposits (Figs. 16-48 and 16-49). A minority of patients, usually those with severe disease, have dense deposits in the capillary walls.

Clinical Features: IgA nephropathy (Berger disease) is the most common form of glomerulonephritis in the world. It accounts for 10% of cases in the United States, 20% in Europe, and 40% in Asia.

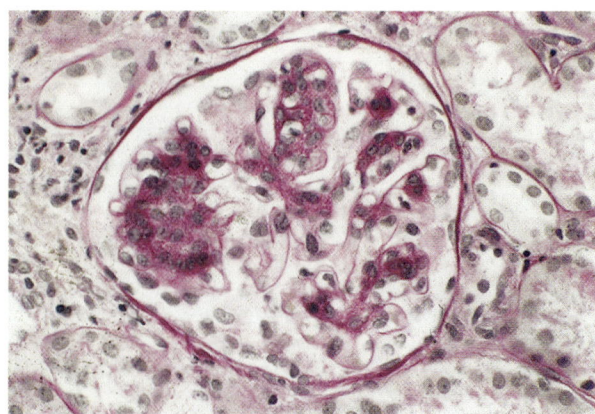

FIGURE 16-47
IgA nephropathy. Segmental mesangial hypercellularity and matrix expansion caused by the mesangial immune deposits. (PAS stain)

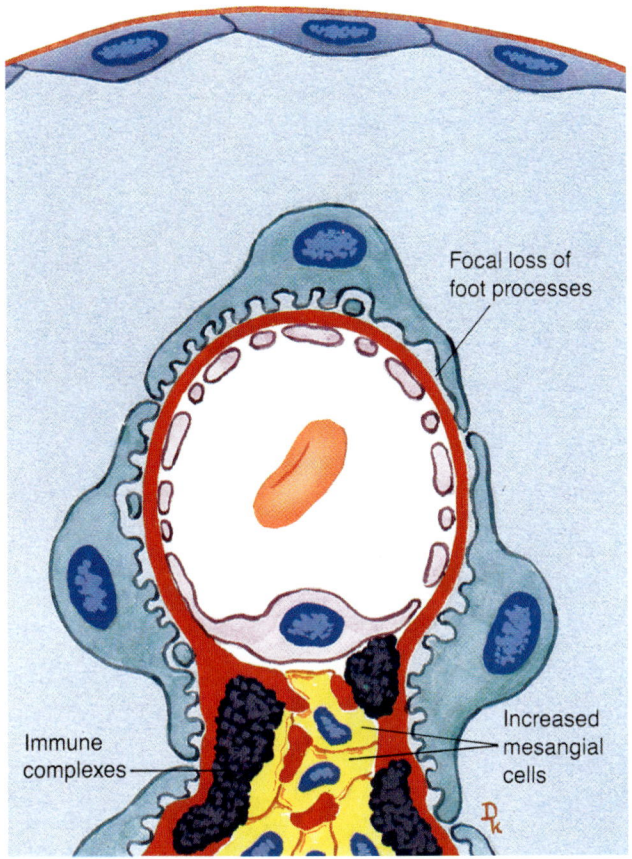

FIGURE *16-48*
IgA nephropathy. Significant accumulation of IgA is seen in the mesangium, most commonly, between the mesangial cells and the basement membrane.

IgA nephropathy has a high frequency in Native Americans and is rare in blacks. It is most common in young men, with a peak age of 15 to 30 years at diagnosis. The clinical presentations are varied, which reflects the varied pathological severity: 40% of patients have asymptomatic microscopic hematuria, 40% have intermittent gross hematuria, 10% have nephrotic syndrome, and 10% have renal failure. The disease rarely resolves completely but may follow an episodic course, with exacerbations often occurring at the time of an upper respiratory tract infection. IgA nephropathy has a slowly progressive course, with 20% of patients reaching end-stage renal failure after 10 years. When these patients are treated by renal transplantation, IgA deposits frequently recur in the allograft, although graft function is usually not impaired.

Anti-Glomerular Basement Membrane (Anti-GBM) Glomerulonephritis Is Often Associated with Pulmonary Hemorrhage

Anti-GBM antibody glomerulonephritis is an uncommon but aggressive form of glomerulonephritis that occurs as a renal-limited disease or combined with pulmonary hemorrhage (Goodpasture syndrome).

 **Pathogenesis:** Anti-GBM glomerulonephritis is mediated by an autoimmune response against a component of the GBM that is located within the **globular noncollagenous domain of type IV collagen.** Because of cross reactivity of the autoimmune response with pulmonary alveolar capillary basement membranes, half of patients also have pulmonary hemorrhages and hemoptysis, sometimes severe enough to be life threatening. When both the lungs and kidneys are involved, the eponym *Goodpasture syndrome* is used. Anti-GBM antibodies, anti-GBM T cells, or both may mediate the injury. The autoantibodies bind to the autoantigens in situ, and the resultant immune complexes could initiate acute inflammation by activating mediator systems, such as complement. Experimental observations suggest that T cells with specificity for GBM antigens may be involved in mediating the vascular injury. Genetic susceptibility to anti-GBM disease is associated with *HLA-DR2* genes. The onset of disease often follows viral upper respiratory tract infections, and the development of the pulmonary component of Goodpasture syndrome appears to require synergistic injurious agents, such as cigarette smoke.

 Pathology: The pathological sine qua non of anti-GBM glomerulonephritis is the presence of diffuse linear staining of GBMs for IgG, which indicates autoantibodies bound to the basement membrane (Fig. 16-50). Linear staining for IgG, however, is not entirely specific. For example, nonimmunological binding of IgG to basement membranes occurs in diabetic glomerulosclerosis. The diagnosis should, therefore, be confirmed by serological detection of anti-GBM antibodies. By light microscopy, over 90% of patients with anti-GBM glomerulonephritis have

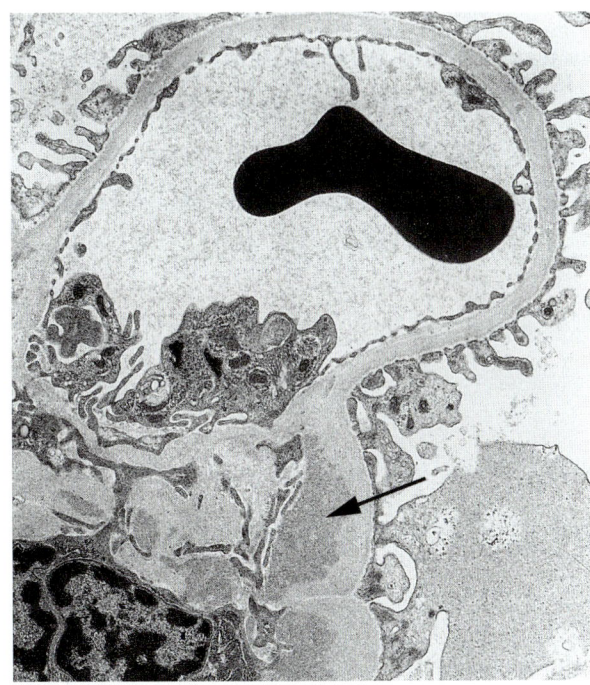

FIGURE *16-49*
IgA nephropathy. An electron micrograph demonstrates prominent dense deposits in the mesangial matrix.

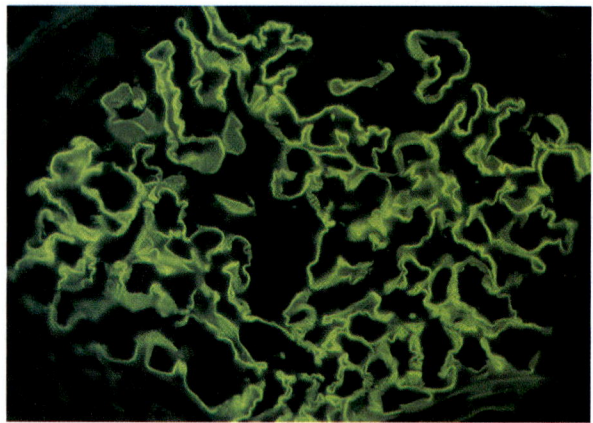

FIGURE 16-50
Anti-GBM glomerulonephritis. Linear immunofluorescence for IgG is seen along the glomerular basement membrane. Contrast this linear pattern of staining with the granular pattern of immunofluorescence typical for most types of immune complex deposition within capillary walls (see Fig. 16-35).

glomerular crescents *(crescentic glomerulonephritis)* (Figs. 16-51 and 16-52), usually involving over 50% of glomeruli. Focal glomerular fibrinoid necrosis is common. Involved lungs exhibit marked intraalveolar hemorrhage. Electron microscopy demonstrates focal breaks in GBMs, but no immune-complex-type electron-dense deposits.

Clinical Features: Anti-GBM glomerulonephritis typically presents with rapidly progressive renal failure and nephritic signs and symptoms. It accounts for 10 to 20% of rapidly progressive (crescentic) glomerulonephritis (see Table 16-7). Treatment consists of high-dose immunosuppressive therapy and plasma exchange, which are most effective when the disease is in an early stage before severe renal failure has occurred. If end-stage renal failure develops, renal transplantation is frequently successful, with little risk of loss of the allograft to recurrent glomerulonephritis.

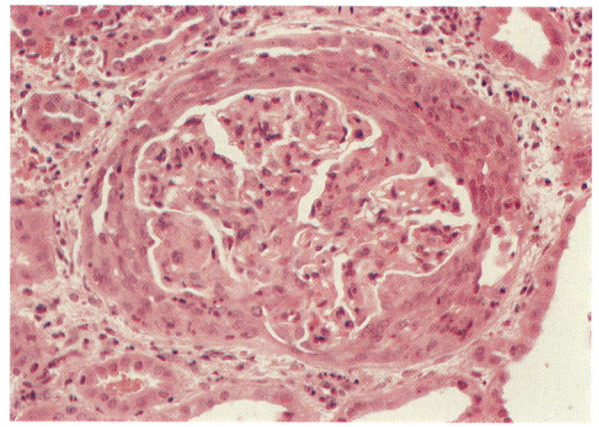

FIGURE 16-51
Crescentic anti-GBM glomerulonephritis. A crescent that surrounds the periphery of the glomerulus is composed of cells contiguous with the lining of the Bowman capsule.

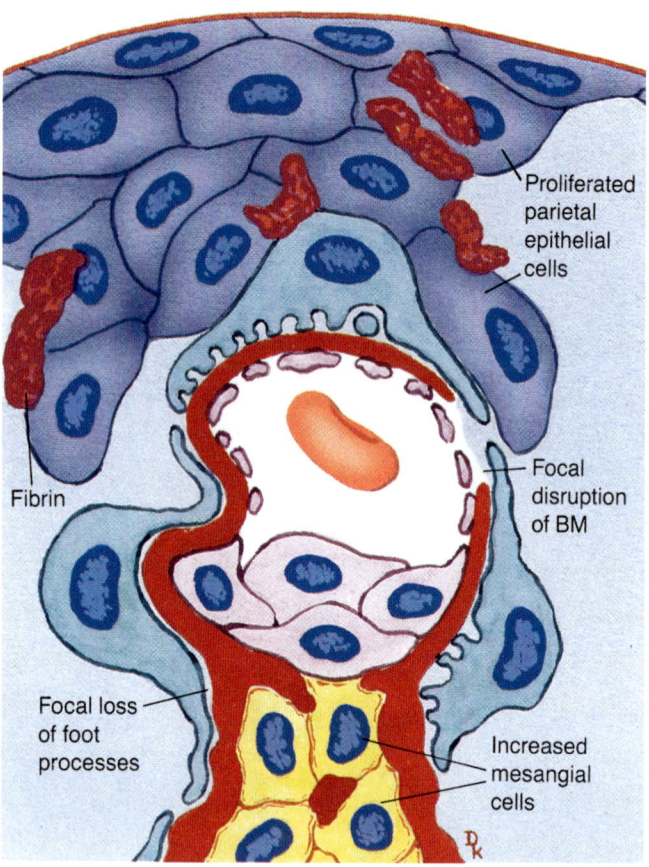

FIGURE 16-52
Crescentic (rapidly progressive) glomerulonephritis. A variety of different pathogenic mechanisms cause crescent formation by disrupting glomerular capillary walls. This allows plasma constituents into Bowman's space, including coagulation factors and inflammatory mediators. Fibrin forms, and there is proliferation of parietal epithelial cells and influx of macrophages resulting in crescent formation.

ANCA Glomerulonephritis Features Neutrophil-induced Injury

ANCA Glomerulonephritis is an aggressive, neutrophil-mediated disease that is characterized by glomerular necrosis and crescents.

Pathogenesis: Antineutrophil cytoplasmic autoantibody (ANCA) glomerulonephritis was once called *idiopathic crescentic glomerulonephritis* because immunofluorescence microscopy did not demonstrate evidence of glomerular deposition of anti-GBM antibodies or immune complexes. The discovery that 90% of patients with this pattern of glomerular injury have circulating ANCAs led to the demonstration that these autoantibodies cause the disease. **ANCAs are specific for proteins in the cytoplasm of neutrophils and monocytes, usually myeloperoxidase (MPO-ANCA) or proteinase 3 (PR3-ANCA).** These autoantibodies activate neutrophils and cause them to adhere to endothelial cells, release toxic oxygen metabolites, degranulate, and kill the endothelial cells.

TABLE 16-7 Frequency (%) of Immunopathological Categories of Crescentic Glomerulonephritis[a] in Different Age Groups

Category	Age (years)		
	<20	20–64	>65
Antiglomerular basement membrane	10	10	10
Immune complex	55	40	10
Antineutrophil cytoplasmic autoantibody (ANCA)	30	45	75
No evidence for the three categories above	5	5	5

[a] Glomerulonephritis with crescents in >50% of glomeruli.

Pathology: Over 90% of patients with ANCA glomerulonephritis have focal glomerular necrosis (Fig. 16-53) and crescent formation (Fig. 16-54). In many patients, over 50% of glomeruli exhibit crescents. Nonnecrotic segments may appear normal or have slight neutrophil infiltration or mild endocapillary hypercellularity. Immunofluorescence microscopy demonstrates an absence or paucity of staining for immunoglobulins and complement, a finding that distinguishes ANCA glomerulonephritis from anti-GBM glomerulonephritis and immune-complex glomerulonephritis. A minority of patients with crescentic glomerulonephritis have serological and pathological evidence for overlapping expression of ANCA glomerulonephritis with anti-GBM glomerulonephritis or immune-complex glomerulonephritis. Electron microscopy demonstrates no immune-complex-type dense deposits in ANCA glomerulonephritis.

Clinical Features: The most common clinical presentation for ANCA glomerulonephritis is rapidly progressive renal failure, with nephritic signs and symptoms. The disease accounts for 75% of rapidly progressive (crescentic) glomerulonephritis in patients over 60 years old, 45% in middle-aged adults, and 30% in young adults and children (see Table 16-7). **Three quarters of patients**

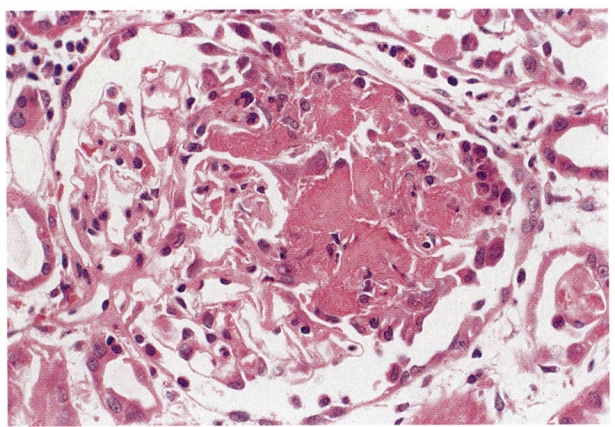

FIGURE 16-53
ANCA glomerulonephritis. Segmental fibrinoid necrosis is illustrated. In time, this lesion stimulates crescent formation.

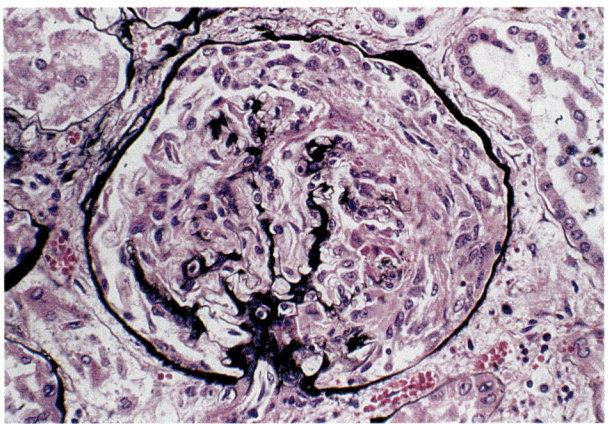

FIGURE 16-54
ANCA glomerulonephritis. Silver staining shows focal disruption of glomerular basement membranes and crescent formation within Bowman's space.

with ANCA glomerulonephritis have systemic small vessel vasculitis (see below), which has many manifestations, including pulmonary hemorrhage. ANCA glomerulonephritis with pulmonary vasculitis is actually a much more frequent cause of *pulmonary–renal vasculitic syndrome* than is Goodpasture syndrome. Without treatment, over 80% of patients with ANCA glomerulonephritis develop end-stage renal disease within 5 years. Immunosuppressive therapy decreases the development of end-stage disease at 5 years to less than 25%. Once remission of disease is induced with high-dose immunosuppressive treatment, patients are at risk for recurrent disease. ANCA glomerulonephritis recurs in 15% of patients who receive renal transplants.

VASCULAR DISEASES

Renal Vasculitis May Affect Vessels of All Sizes

The kidney is involved in many types of systemic vasculitis (Table 16-8). **In a sense, glomerulonephritis is a local form of vasculitis that affects glomerular capillaries.** The glomeruli may be the only site of vascular inflammation or the renal disease may be a component of a systemic vasculitis.

Small Vessel Vasculitis

Small vessel vasculitis affects small arteries, arterioles, capillaries, and venules. Glomerulonephritis is a frequent component of small vessel vasculitides. Other common manifestations include purpura, arthralgias, myalgias, peripheral neuropathy, and pulmonary hemorrhage. Immune complexes, anti-basement membrane antibodies, or ANCA (see Table 16-8) can cause small vessel vasculitides.

Henoch-Schönlein purpura is the most common type of childhood vasculitis and is caused by vascular localization

TABLE 16-8 Types of Vasculitis That Involve the Kidneys

Type of Vasculitis	Major Target Vessels in Kidney	Major Renal Manifestations
Small-vessel vasculitis		
Immune-complex vasculitis		
Henoch-Schönlein purpura	Glomeruli	Nephritis
Cryoglobulinemic vasculitis	Glomeruli	Nephritis
Anti-GBM vasculitis		
Goodpasture syndrome	Glomeruli	Nephritis
ANCA-vasculitis		
Wegener granulomatosis	Glomeruli, arterioles, interlobular arteries	Nephritis
Microscopic polyangiitis	Glomeruli, arterioles, interlobular arteries	Nephritis
Churg-Strauss syndrome	Glomeruli, arterioles, interlobular arteries	Nephritis
Medium-sized-vessel vasculitis		
Polyarteritis nodosa	Interlobar and arcuate arteries	Infarcts and hemorrhage
Kawasaki disease	Interlobar and arcuate arteries	Infarcts and hemorrhage
Large-vessel vasculitis		
Giant cell arteritis	Main renal artery	Renovascular hypertension
Takayasu arteritis	Main renal artery	Renovascular hypertension

ANCA, antineutrophil cytoplasmic autoantibody; GBM, glomerular basement membrane.

of immune complexes containing predominantly IgA. The glomerular lesion is identical with that of IgA nephropathy.

Cryoglobulinemic vasculitis causes proliferative glomerulonephritis, usually type I membranoproliferative glomerulonephritis. By light microscopy, aggregates of cryoglobulins ("hyaline thrombi") are often seen within capillary lumina (Fig. 16-55).

ANCA vasculitis involves vessels outside the kidneys in 75% of patients with ANCA glomerulonephritis. Based on clinical and pathological features, patients with systemic ANCA vasculitis are classified as follows:

- **Wegener granulomatosis,** if there is necrotizing granulomatous inflammation, usually in the respiratory tract
- **Churg-Strauss syndrome,** if there is eosinophilia and asthma
- **Microscopic polyangiitis,** if there is no asthma or granulomatous inflammation

In addition to causing necrotizing and crescentic glomerulonephritis, the ANCA vasculitides often display necrotizing inflammation in other renal vessels, such as arteries (Fig. 16-56), arterioles, and medullary peritubular capillaries.

Medium-Sized Vessel Vasculitis

Medium-sized vessel vasculitides affect arteries, but not arterioles, capillaries, or venules. **Polyarteritis nodosa,** which occurs mainly in adults, and **Kawasaki disease,** which principally afflicts young children, are rare causes of renal dysfunction. These diseases are characterized by necrotizing arteritis, which can involve renal arteries and result in pseudoaneurysm formation and renal thrombosis, infarction, and hemorrhage.

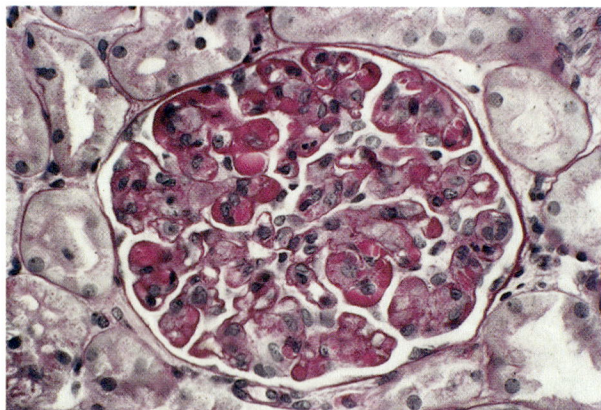

FIGURE 16-55
Cryoglobulinemic glomerulonephritis. The pattern of glomerular inflammation is similar to that of type I membranoproliferative glomerulonephritis. However, as in this specimen, there typically are conspicuous glassy aggregates ("hyaline thrombi") in the capillary lumina and subendothelial spaces. These are not true thrombi but rather are large aggregates of cryoglobulins. (PAS stain)

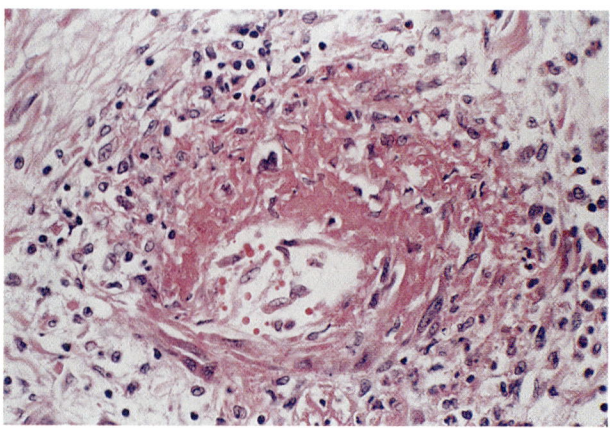

FIGURE 16-56
ANCA necrotizing arteritis. Fibrinoid necrosis and inflammation involve an interlobular artery in the renal cortex.

Large Vessel Vasculitis

Large vessel vasculitides, such as **giant cell arteritis** and **Takayasu arteritis,** affect the aorta and its major branches. These disorders may cause renovascular hypertension by involving the main renal arteries or the aorta at the origin of the renal arteries. Narrowing or obstruction of these vessels results in renal ischemia, which stimulates increased renin production and consequent hypertension (Table 16-8).

Hypertensive Nephrosclerosis (Benign Nephrosclerosis) Leads to Obliteration of Glomeruli

Pathogenesis: Although no precise definition is completely accepted for hypertension, a sustained systolic pressure of more than 140 mm Hg and a diastolic one of more than 90 mm are generally considered abnormal. The pathogenesis of hypertension is discussed in Chapter 10. Mild-to-moderate hypertension causes typical hypertensive nephrosclerosis and thus is not truly benign. In fact hypertensive nephrosclerosis is identified in approximately 15% of patients with "benign hypertension." Changes similar to those in hypertensive nephrosclerosis occasionally occur in older individuals who have never had hypertension, and are attributed to aging itself.

Pathology: The kidneys are smaller than normal (atrophic) and are usually affected bilaterally. The cortical surfaces have a fine granularity (Fig. 16-57), but coarser scars are occasionally present. On cut section, the cortex is thinned. Microscopically, many glomeruli appear normal; others show varying degrees of ischemic change. Initially, the glomerular capillaries are thickened because of thickening, wrinkling, and collapse of GBMs. Cells of the glomerular tuft are progressively lost, and collagen and matrix material are deposited within Bowman space. Eventually, the glomerular tuft is obliterated by a dense, eosinophilic globular mass enclosed in a scar, all within Bowman's capsule. Tubular atrophy, a consequence of the obsolescence of the glomerulus, is associated with interstitial fibrosis and infiltration by chronic inflammatory cells. Globally sclerotic glomeruli and surrounding atrophic tubules are often clustered in focal subcapsular zones, with adjacent areas of preserved glomeruli and tubules (Fig. 16-58), an effect that is the basis for the granular surfaces of nephrosclerotic kidneys.

The pattern of change in the blood vessels of the kidney depends on the size of the vessel involved. Large arteries down to the size of the arcuate arteries have fibrotic thickening of the intima, with replication of the elasticalike lamina and partial replacement of the muscularis with fibrous tissue. Interlobular arteries and arterioles may develop medial hyperplasia. Arterioles exhibit concentric hyaline thickening of the wall, often with the loss of smooth muscle cells or their displacement to the periphery. This arteriolar change is termed *hyaline arteriolosclerosis.*

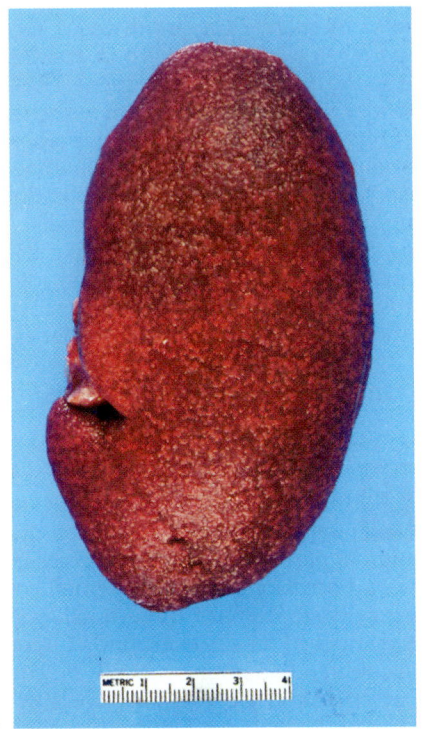
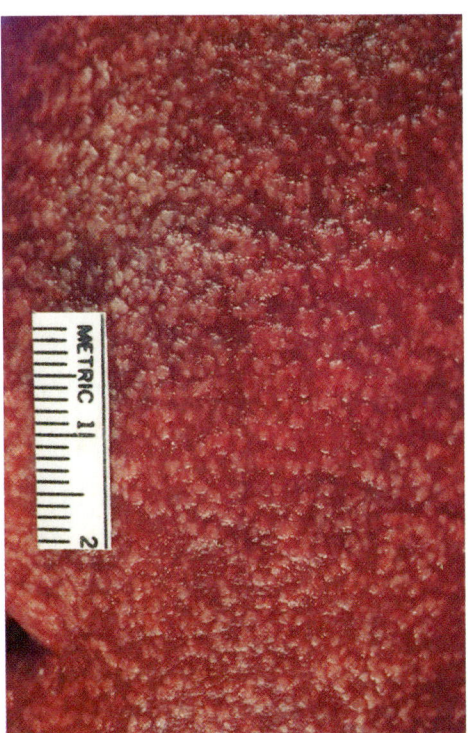

FIGURE 16-57

Hypertensive nephrosclerosis. A. The kidney is reduced in size, and the cortical surface exhibits fine granularity. B. High magnification of the renal surface.

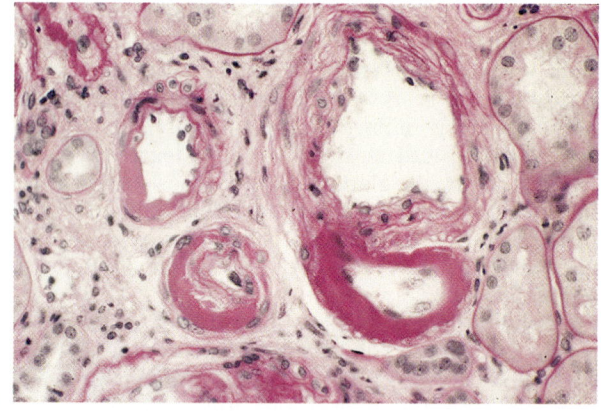
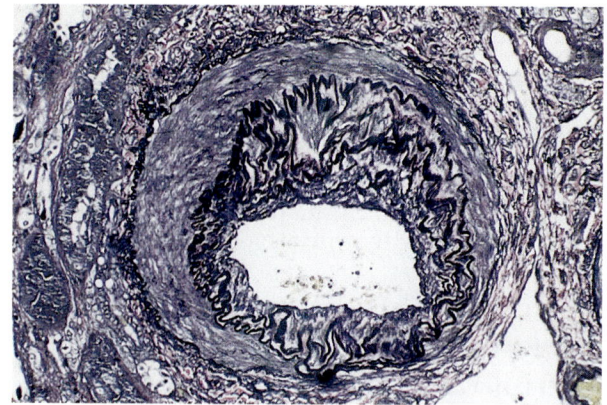
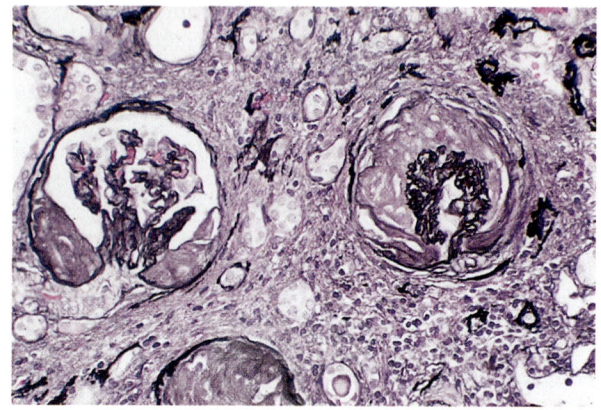

FIGURE 16-58
Hypertensive nephrosclerosis. A. Three arterioles with hyaline sclerosis. (PAS stain) B. Arcuate artery with fibrotic intimal thickening causing narrowing of the lumen. (silver stain) C. One glomerulus with global sclerosis and one with segmental sclerosis. Note also the tubular atrophy, interstitial fibrosis, and chronic inflammation. (silver stain)

Clinical Features: Although hypertensive nephrosclerosis is ordinarily not associated with significant abnormalities of renal function, a few of the many persons with "benign" hypertension develop progressive renal failure, which may terminate in end-stage renal disease. Because "benign" hypertension is so prevalent, even the small proportion of these patients who develop renal insufficiency amounts to one third of all patients with end-stage renal disease. Benign nephrosclerosis is most prevalent and aggressive among blacks. **In fact, among blacks in the United States, hypertension without any evidence of a malignant phase is the leading cause of end-stage renal disease.**

Malignant Hypertensive Nephropathy Is a Potentially Fatal Renal Disease

Pathogenesis: There is no specific blood pressure that defines malignant hypertension, but a diastolic pressure greater than 130 mm Hg, retinal vascular changes, papilledema, and renal functional impairment are usual criteria. About half of patients with malignant hypertension have an antecedent history of benign hypertension, and many others have a background of chronic renal injury caused by many different diseases. Occasionally, malignant hypertension arises de novo in apparently healthy persons, particularly young black men. The pathogenesis of the vascular injury in patients with malignant hypertension is not completely elucidated. One hypothesis proposes that extremely high blood pressures, combined with microvascular vasoconstriction, cause injury to endothelium as the blood slams into the narrowed small vessels. At sites of vascular injury, plasma constituents leak into the injured walls of arterioles (resulting in fibrinoid necrosis), into the intima of arteries (causing edematous intimal thickening), and into the subendothelial zone of glomerular capillaries (leading to glomerular consolidation). At these sites of vascular injury, thrombosis can result in focal cortical necrosis (infarcts) of the kidneys.

Pathology: The size of the kidneys in malignant hypertensive nephropathy varies from small to enlarged, depending on the duration of preexisting benign hypertension. The cut surface is mottled red and yellow and occasionally exhibits small cortical infarcts. Microscopically, malignant hypertensive nephropathy is often superimposed on a background of hypertensive nephrosclerosis, with edematous (myxoid, mucoid) intimal expansion in arteries and fibrinoid necrosis of arterioles. Variable glomerular changes range from capillary congestion to consolidation to necrosis (Fig. 16-59). Severe cases show thrombosis and focal ischemic cortical necrosis (infarction). Electron microscopy demonstrates electron-lucent expansion of

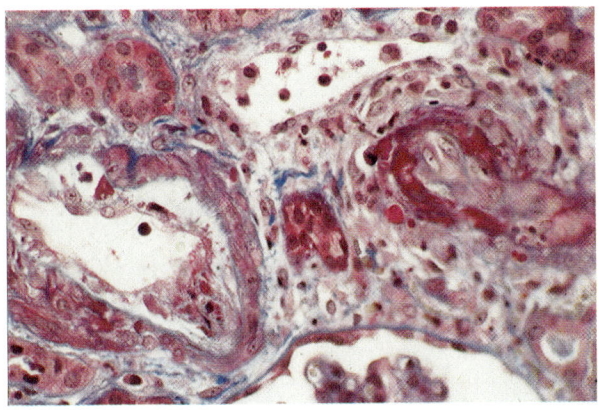

FIGURE 16-59
Malignant hypertensive nephropathy. Red fibrinoid necrosis in the wall of the arteriole on the right and clear edematous expansion in the intima of the interlobular artery on the left from a patient with malignant hypertension. (Masson trichrome stain)

the subendothelial zone in glomeruli. Immunofluorescence microscopy documents focal insudation of plasma proteins into injured vessel walls. These pathological changes are identical to those observed in other forms of thrombotic microangiopathy (see below).

 Clinical Features: Malignant hypertension occurs more frequently in men than in women, typically around the age of 40 years. Patients suffer headache, dizziness, and visual disturbances and may develop overt encephalopathy. Hematuria and proteinuria are frequent. Progressive deterioration of renal function develops if the malignant hypertension persists. The outlook for patients with malignant hypertension was previously dismal, but aggressive antihypertensive therapy now often controls the disease.

Renovascular Hypertension Follows Narrowing of a Renal Artery

 Pathogenesis: Stenosis or total occlusion of a main renal artery produces hypertension that is potentially curable by reconstitution of the arterial lumen. Goldblatt carried out the initial experiments that led to the understanding of this syndrome in rats more than a half century ago, and since that time, the kidney deprived of vascular supply has been known as the *Goldblatt kidney*. In patients with renal artery stenosis, hypertension reflects increased production of renin, angiotensin II, and aldosterone. Renal vein renin from the ischemic kidney is elevated, whereas it is normal in the contralateral kidney. Most (95%) cases are caused by atherosclerosis, which explains why this disorder is twice as common in men as in women and is seen primarily in older age groups (average age, 55 years). Fibromuscular dysplasia and vasculitis are less common causes overall but are the most frequent causes in children.

 Pathology: No matter what the cause of renal artery stenosis, the kidney parenchymal changes are the same. The size of the involved kidney is reduced. The glomeruli appear normal, but because the intervening tubules show marked ischemic atrophy without extensive interstitial fibrosis, the glomeruli are closer to each other than normal. Many glomeruli lose their attachment to the proximal tubule. The juxtaglomerular apparatus is prominent and reveals hyperplasia and increased granularity.

When vascular stenosis is caused by atherosclerosis, atherosclerotic plaques impinge on the aortic ostium or narrow the renal artery lumen, more frequently on the left than on the right. Occasionally, an atherosclerotic aneurysm of the abdominal aorta compromises the origin of the renal arteries. Takayasu arteritis and giant cell arteritis cause renal artery stenosis by producing inflammatory and sclerotic thickening of the artery wall with resultant narrowing of the lumen.

Fibromuscular dysplasia is characterized by fibrous and muscular stenosis of the renal artery. There are several patterns of renal artery involvement. The major categories are intimal fibroplasia, medial fibroplasia, perimedial fibroplasia, and periarterial fibroplasia. As the names imply, these disorders affect different layers of the artery, ranging from the intima to the adventitia. Medial fibroplasia is the most common and accounts for two thirds of all fibromuscular dysplasia. This process creates areas of medial thickening alternating with areas of atrophy and thus produces a "string of beads" pattern in angiograms.

 Clinical Features: Renovascular hypertension is characterized by mild-to-moderate elevations in blood pressure. A bruit may be heard over the renal artery. The diagnosis requires some type of imaging, such as angiography. In over half of patients, surgical revascularization, angioplasty, or nephrectomy cures hypertension. When there is long-standing renovascular hypertension, the uninvolved kidney may become damaged by hypertensive nephrosclerosis.

Renal Atheroembolism May Complicate Aortic Atherosclerosis

In patients with severe aortic atherosclerosis, embolization of atheromatous debris into the renal arteries and vascular tree as far as the glomerular capillaries may cause acute renal failure. Atheroembolization may be spontaneous or initiated by trauma, such as angiographic procedures. **Cholesterol clefts** are observed within vessel lumina (Fig. 16-60). Early lesions are surrounded by atheromatous material or thrombus. Later, they may elicit a foreign body reaction and may stimulate fibrosis in the adjacent vessel wall.

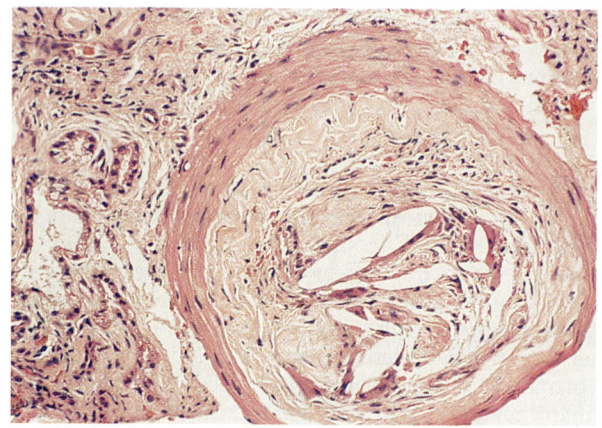

FIGURE 16-60
Atheroembolus. An atheroembolus obstructs an arcuate artery. Note the cholesterol clefts.

Thrombotic Microangiopathy Refers to Systemic Diseases with Similar Renal Lesions

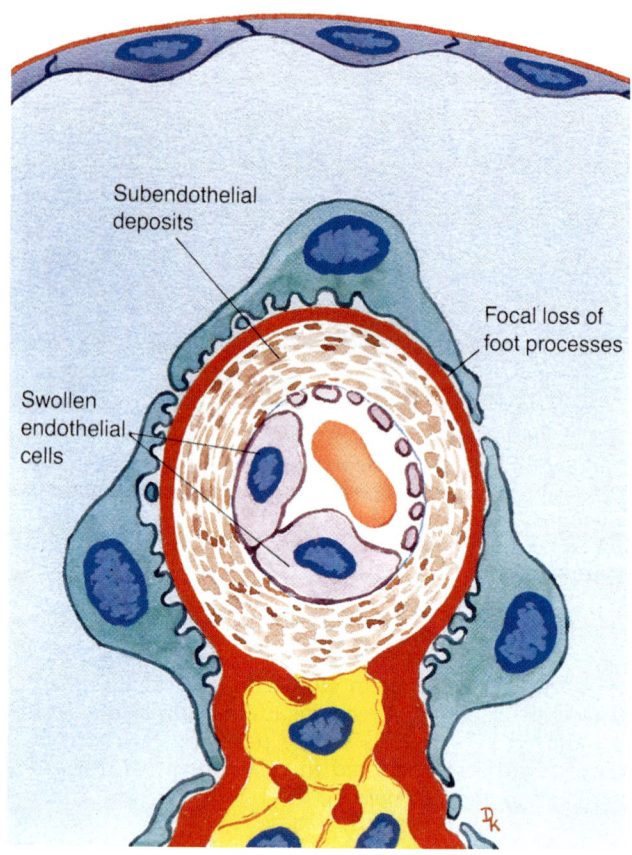

FIGURE 16-61
Hemolytic–uremic syndrome. A wide band of subendothelial electron-lucent material causes narrowing of the capillary lumen. Endothelial cell swelling also contributes to narrowing of the lumen.

Pathogenesis: Thrombotic microangiopathy has a variety of causes, all of which cause endothelial damage that initiates a final common pathway of vascular changes. A leading theory holds that endothelial damage allows plasma constituents to enter the intima of arteries, the walls of arterioles, and the subendothelial zone of glomerular capillaries, resulting in narrowing of vessel lumina and ischemia. The injured endothelial surfaces promote thrombosis, which worsens ischemia and may cause focal ischemic necrosis. The passage of blood through the injured vessels leads to a nonimmune (Coombs negative) hemolytic anemia, characterized by misshapen and disrupted erythrocytes (schistocytes) and thrombocytopenia. This condition is termed *microangiopathic hemolytic anemia*. The kidneys are ubiquitous targets of thrombotic microangiopathies, but other organs may also be injured.

Pathology: The pathological changes in the kidney are comparable to those in malignant hypertensive nephropathy, which is a form of thrombotic microangiopathy. The basic renal lesions are the following:

- Arteriolar fibrinoid necrosis
- Arterial edematous intimal expansion
- Glomerular consolidation, necrosis, or congestion
- Vascular thrombosis

Electron microscopy of glomeruli demonstrates electron-lucent expansion of the subendothelial zone (Figs. 16-61 and 16-62), which results from the insudation of plasma proteins under injured endothelial cells. Immunofluorescence microscopy reveals the accumulation of fibrin and insudation of plasma proteins in injured vessel walls.

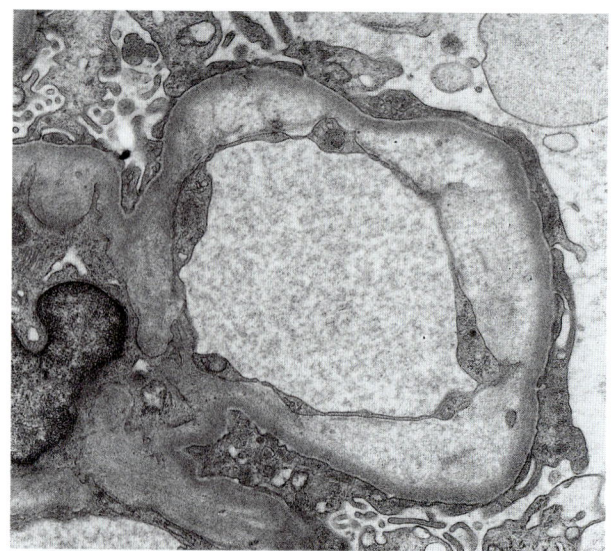

FIGURE 16-62
Thrombotic microangiopathy. An electron micrograph shows a wide band of lucent material in the subendothelial zone, which causes marked narrowing of the lumen.

Clinical Features: Various clinical presentations and causes allow the recognition of different categories of thrombotic microangiopathy. The various clinical disorders share microangiopathic hemolytic anemia, thrombocytopenia, hypertension, and renal failure, although these features are expressed to different degrees.

Hemolytic–Uremic Syndrome

Hemolytic–uremic syndrome (HUS) features microangiopathic hemolytic anemia and acute renal failure, with little or no evidence for significant vascular disease outside the kidneys. **HUS is the most common cause of acute renal failure in children.** Major causes for HUS are Shiga toxin-producing strains of *Escherichia coli*, which are ingested in contaminated food such as poorly cooked hamburger. The toxin injures endothelial cells, thereby setting in motion the sequence of events that produces thrombotic microangiopathy. These patients present with hemorrhagic diarrhea and rapidly progressive renal failure. Some of the causes of thrombotic microangiopathy that typically have the clinical and pathological features of HUS are listed in Table 16-9.

Thrombotic Thrombocytopenic Purpura

Thrombotic thrombocytopenic purpura (TTP) displays systemic microvascular thrombosis and is characterized clinically by thrombocytopenia, purpura, fever, and changes in mental status. Unlike HUS, renal involvement is often absent or less important than disease of other organs. The bleeding tendency caused by the consumptive thrombocytopenia is also more severe in TTP than it is in HUS. At least in some patients, the pathogenesis of TTP involves a genetic or acquired deficiency in the activity of a protease that cleaves

TABLE 16-9 Causes of Thrombotic Microangiopathy

Infections
  Escherichia coli
  Shigella spp.
  Pseudomonas spp.

Drugs
  Mitomycin
  Cisplatin
  Cyclosporin
  Tacrolimus

Autoimmune diseases
  Systemic sclerosis (scleroderma)
  Systemic lupus erythematosus
  Antiphospholipid antibody syndrome

Malignant hypertension

Pregnancy and postpartum factors

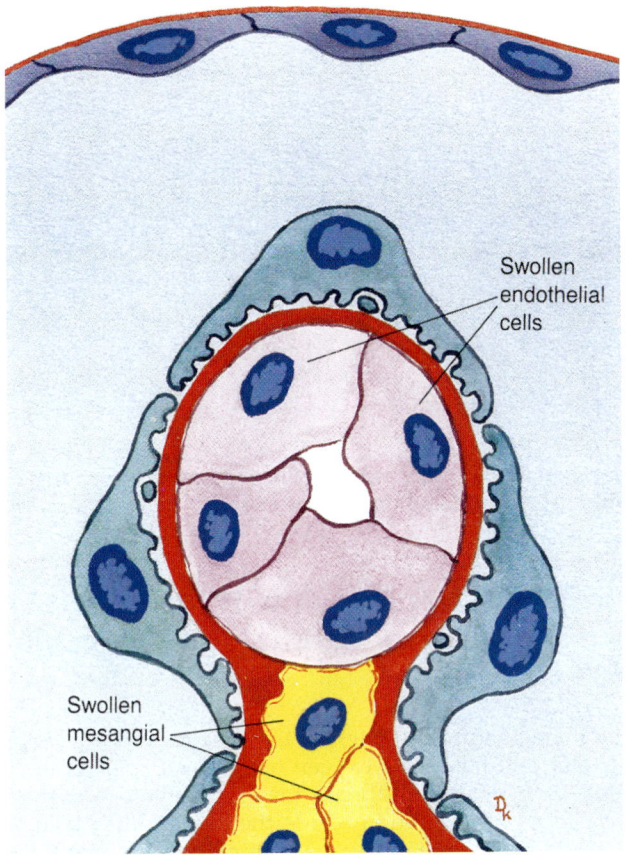

FIGURE 16-63
Preeclamptic nephropathy. Preeclamptic nephropathy, or pregnancy-induced nephropathy, exhibits marked swelling of endothelial cells with narrowing of the lumina. Both endothelial and mesangial cells are enlarged and have multiple vacuoles and vesicular structures.

multimers of von Willebrand factor. The large uncleaved multimers promote platelet aggregation and microvascular thrombosis.

Preeclampsia Complicates the Third Trimester of Pregnancy

Preeclampsia is characterized by the triad of hypertension, proteinuria, and edema. When these features are complicated by convulsions, the term **eclampsia** *is applied* (see Chapter 18). The kidney is by definition involved in preeclampsia. The glomeruli are uniformly enlarged, and the endothelial cells are swollen, an appearance that results in an apparently bloodless glomerular tuft (Fig. 16-63 and 16-64). Increased number and size of mesangial cells are usual. By electron microscopy, the swollen endothelial and mesangial cells contain large, irregular vacuoles. Vacuoles are also present in the foot processes and the trabeculae of the podocytes. Mild and moderate disease can be controlled with bed rest and antihypertensive agents. Severe cases may require induction of delivery. Hypertension and proteinuria typically disappear 1 to 2 weeks after delivery.

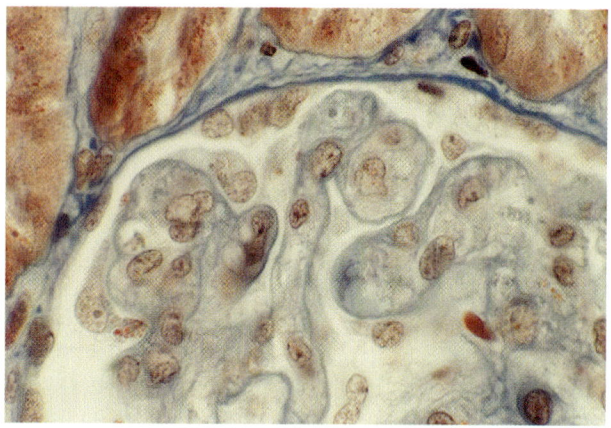

FIGURE 16-64
Preeclampsia. Capillary lumens are obliterated by swollen endothelial cells (Masson trichrome stain)

Sickle Cell Nephropathy Is the Most Common Organ Manifestation of Sickle Cell Disease

The interstitial tissue in which the vasa recta course is hypertonic and has a low oxygen tension. As a result, in patients with sickle cell disease the erythrocytes in the vasa recta tend to sickle and occlude the lumen. Infarcts in the medulla and papilla ensue, sometimes severe enough to cause papillary necrosis. Ischemic scarring of the medulla leads to focal tubular loss and atrophy. The glomeruli are conspicuously congested with sickle cells. Focal segmental glomerulosclerosis or, less commonly, membranoproliferative glomerulonephritis occurs in a minority of patients and may cause the nephrotic syndrome.

Renal Infarcts Usually Result from Embolization

Renal infarcts are, for the most part, caused by arterial obstruction, and most represent embolization to the interlobar or larger branches of the renal artery.

  Pathogenesis: The size of the infarct varies with the size of the occluded vessel. Common sources of emboli include the following:

- **Mural thrombi** overlying myocardial infarcts or caused by atrial fibrillation
- **Infected valves** in bacterial endocarditis
- **Complicated atherosclerotic plaques** in the aorta

Occasionally, a branch of the renal artery is occluded by thrombosis superimposed on underlying atherosclerosis or arteritis. The lumina of the small branches of the renal artery may be so severely compromised in malignant hypertension, scleroderma, or HUS that the blood supply is insufficient to maintain the viability of the tissue. Occlusion of small vessels by sickled erythrocytes in sickle cell anemia may cause renal infarcts, especially in the papillae. Hemorrhagic renal infarction caused by renal vein thrombosis may complicate severe dehydration, particularly in small infants, but it is also seen in adults with septic thrombophlebitis and conditions associated with hypercoagulability. Typically, an acute infarct causes sharp flank or abdominal pain and hematuria.

Infarction of an entire kidney by occlusion of the main renal artery is rare. When the main renal artery is occluded, it is more common for the kidney to remain viable because of collateral circulation. Clearly, in such a circumstance renal function ceases in that kidney.

  Pathology: Variably sized, wedge-shaped areas of pale ischemic necrosis, with the base on the capsular surface, are typical (Fig. 16-65). All structures within the affected zone show coagulative necrosis. A hemorrhagic zone borders acute infarcts. As in other tissues, the histological response to the infarct progresses through phases of acute inflammation, granulation tissue, and fibrosis. Healed infarcts appear as sharply circumscribed and depressed cortical scars containing ghosts of obliterated glomeruli, atrophic tubules, interstitial fibrosis, and a mild chronic inflammatory infiltrate. Dystrophic calcification is occasionally encountered in old infarcts. At the margins of a healed infarct, the viable tissue resembles that seen in chronic ischemia, with tubular atrophy, interstitial fibrosis, and infiltration by chronic inflammatory cells.

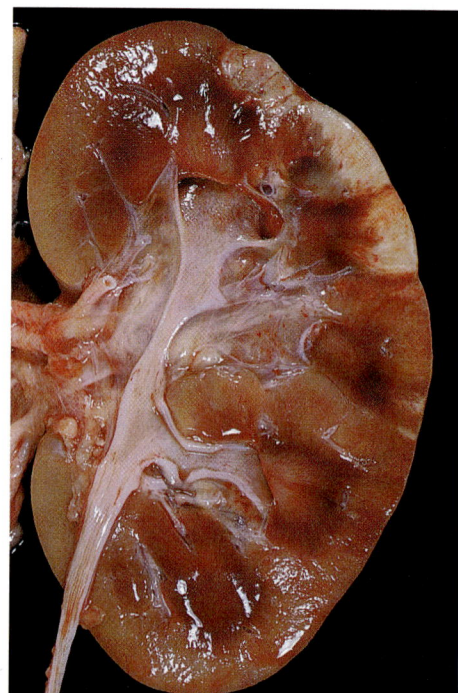

FIGURE 16-65
Renal infarct. A cross-section of the kidney shows multiple areas of infarction characterized by marked pallor, which extends to the subcapsular surface.

Cortical Necrosis Is Secondary to Shock

Cortical necrosis is ischemic necrosis of part or all of the renal cortex, with sparing of the medulla. The term *infarct* is used when there is one area (or a few areas) of necrosis caused by occlusion of arteries, whereas *cortical necrosis* implies more-widespread ischemic necrosis.

 Pathogenesis: Historically, the most common cause for renal cortical necrosis was premature separation of the placenta (abruptio placentae), a complication of the third trimester of pregnancy. Renal cortical necrosis can also complicate any clinical condition associated with hypovolemic or endotoxic shock. Since all forms of shock are associated with acute tubular necrosis, it is not surprising that there is an overlap between that condition and cortical necrosis, both clinically and pathologically.

The vasa recta that supply arterial blood to the medulla arise from the juxtamedullary efferent arterioles, proximal to the vessels supplying the outer cortex. Thus, occlusion of the outer cortical vessels, for example by vasospasm, thrombi, or thrombotic microangiopathy, leads to cortical necrosis and sparing of the medulla. Experimentally, vasoconstrictors such as vasopressin and serotonin produce cortical necrosis. The experimental Schwartzman phenomenon, which is characterized by disseminated intravascular coagulation with widespread fibrin thrombi, also results in cortical necrosis.

 Pathology: The extent of cortical necrosis varies from patchy to confluent (Fig. 16-66). In the most severely involved areas, all parenchymal elements exhibit coagulative necrosis. The proximal convoluted tubules are invariably necrotic, as are most of the distal tubules. In the adjacent viable portions of the cortex, the glomeruli and distal convoluted tubules are usually unaffected, but many of the proximal convoluted tubules have features of ischemic injury, such as epithelial flattening or necrosis.

With extensive necrosis, the cortex has a marked pallor. The cortex is diffusely necrotic, except for thin rims of viable tissue immediately beneath the capsule and at the corticomedullary junction, which are supplied by capsular and medullary collateral blood vessels, respectively. Patients who survive cortical necrosis may develop striking dystrophic calcification of the necrotic areas.

 Clinical Features: Severe cortical necrosis manifests as acute renal failure, which initially may be indistinguishable from that produced by acute tubular necrosis. However, the former is more often irreversible. A renal arteriogram or biopsy may be required for diagnosis. Recovery is determined by the extent of the disease, but there is a significant incidence of hypertension among survivors.

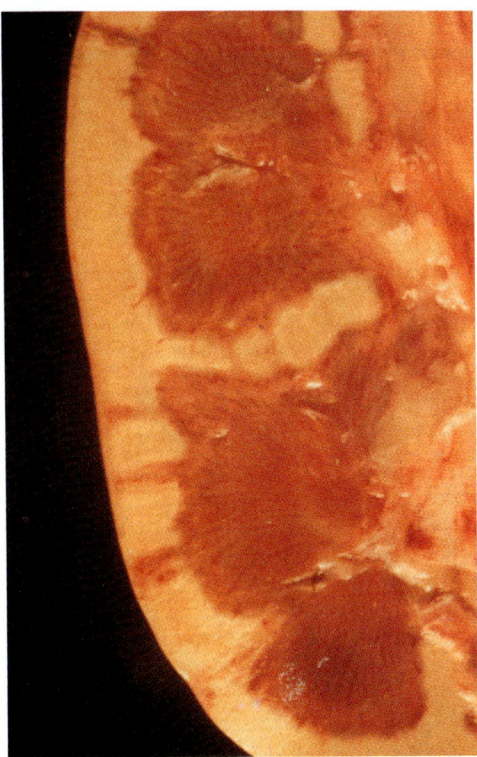

FIGURE 16-66
Renal cortical necrosis. The cortex of the kidney is pale yellow and soft owing to diffuse cortical necrosis.

DISEASES OF TUBULES AND INTERSTITIUM

Acute Tubular Necrosis Most Commonly Follows Shock

Acute tubular necrosis (ATN) is a severe, but potentially reversible, impairment of tubular epithelial function caused by ischemia or toxic injury, which results in acute renal failure.

 Pathogenesis: Some of the causes of ATN are listed in Table 16-10.

Ischemic ATN results from reduced renal perfusion, usually associated with hypotension. Tubular epithelial cells, with their high rate of energy-consuming metabolic activity and numerous organelles, are particularly sensitive to hypoxia and anoxia, which cause rapid depletion of intracellular ATP in the tubular epithelium. Tubular epithelial cells may be simplified (flattened) but not necrotic in some patients with typical clinical features of ATN.

Nephrotoxic ATN is caused by chemically induced injury to epithelial cells. Tubular epithelial cells are preferred targets for certain toxins because they absorb and concentrate the toxins. The high rate of energy consumption by epithelial cells also makes them susceptible to injury by toxins that perturb oxidative or other metabolic pathways. Hemoglobin and myoglobin can be considered endogenous

TABLE 16-10 Causes of Acute Tubular Necrosis

Ischemia
  Massive hemorrhage
  Septic shock
  Severe burns
  Dehydration
  Prolonged diarrhea
  Congestive heart failure
  Volume redistribution (e.g., pancreatitis, peritonitis)

Nephrotoxins
  Antibodies (e.g., aminoglycosides, amphotericin B)
  Radiographic contrast agents
  Heavy metals (e.g., mercury, lead, cisplatin)
  Organic solvents (e.g., ethylene glycol, carbon tetrachloride)
  Poisons (e.g., paraquat)

Heme proteins
  Myoglobin (from rhabdomyolysis, e.g., with crush injury)
  Hemoglobin (from hemolysis, e.g., with transfusion reaction)

toxins that can induce ATN *(pigment nephropathy)* when they are present in the urine in high concentrations.

The pathophysiology of ATN appears to involve some or all of the following perturbations (Fig. 16-67), various combinations of which result in a reduced glomerular filtration rate and tubular epithelial dysfunction:

- Intrarenal vasoconstriction
- Alteration of arteriolar tone by tubuloglomerular feedback
- Decreased glomerular hydrostatic pressure
- Decreased glomerular capillary permeability (K_f)
- Tubular obstruction by cellular debris, with increased hydrostatic pressure
- Backleakage of glomerular filtrate into the interstitium through damaged tubular epithelium

Pathology: Ischemic ATN is characterized by swollen kidneys that have a pale cortex and a congested medulla. No pathological changes are seen in the glomeruli or blood vessels. Tubular injury is focal and is most pronounced in the proximal tubules and in the thick limbs of the loop of Henle in the outer medulla. The proximal tubules display focal flattening of the epithelium, with dilation of the lumina and loss of the brush border (epithelial simplification). This effect results in part from sloughing of the apical cytoplasm, which appears in the distal tubular lumina and urine as brown granular casts. The color reflects renal cytochrome pigments. Electron microscopy confirms the loss of the proximal tubular brush border and also demonstrates decreased infoldings at the basolateral membrane of proximal tubular epithelial cells. A characteristic feature of ischemic ATN is the absence of widespread necrosis of tubular epithelial cells, although simplification may be prominent. Instead,

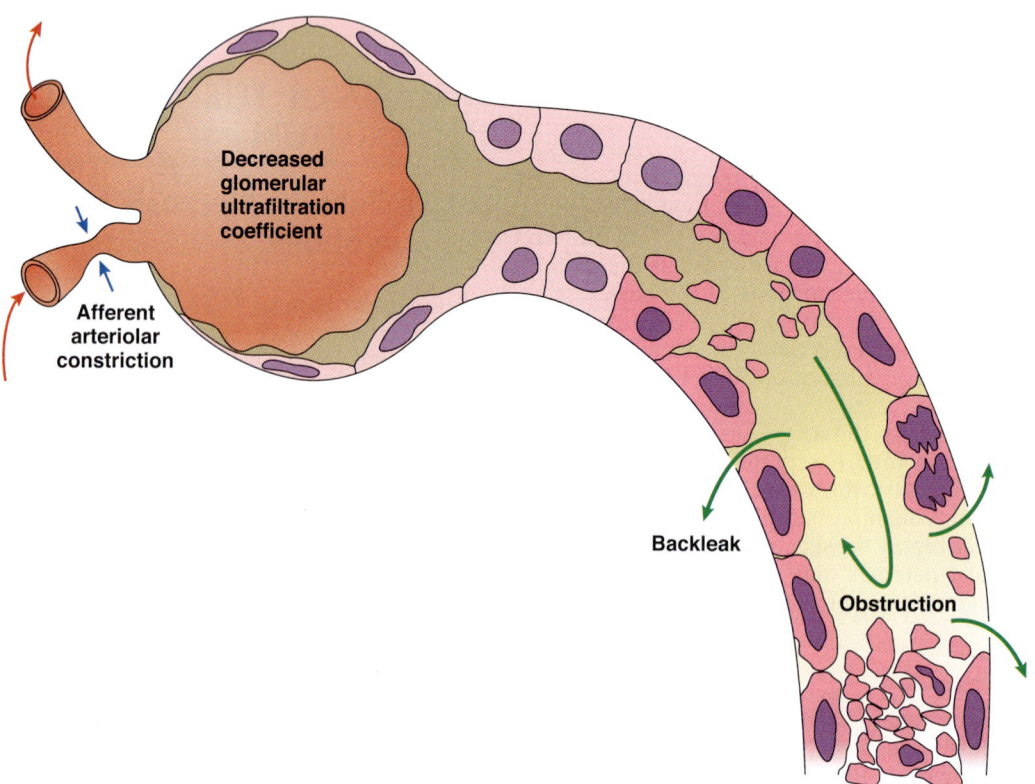

FIGURE 16-67
Pathogenesis of acute tubular necrosis. Sloughing and necrosis of epithelial cells result in cast formation. The presence of casts leads to obstruction and increased intraluminal pressure, which reduces glomerular filtration. Afferent arteriolar vasoconstriction, caused in part by tubuloglomerular feedback, results in decreased glomerular capillary filtration pressure. Tubular injury and increased intraluminal pressure cause fluid backleakage from the lumen into the interstitium.

Diseases of Tubules and Interstitium   869

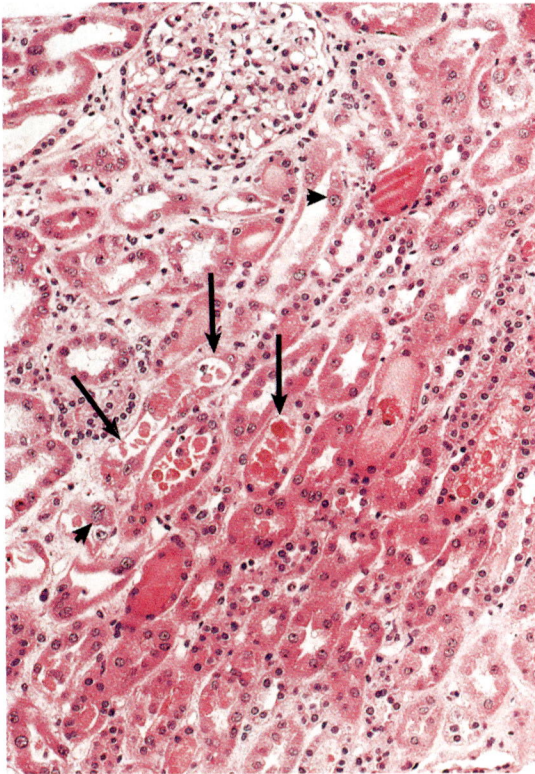

FIGURE 16-68
Ischemic acute tubular necrosis. Necrosis of individual tubular epithelial cells is evident both from focal denudation of the tubular basement membrane (arrows) and from the individual necrotic epithelial cells present in some tubular lumina. Some enlarged, regenerative-appearing epithelial cells are also present (arrowheads). Note the lack of significant interstitial inflammation.

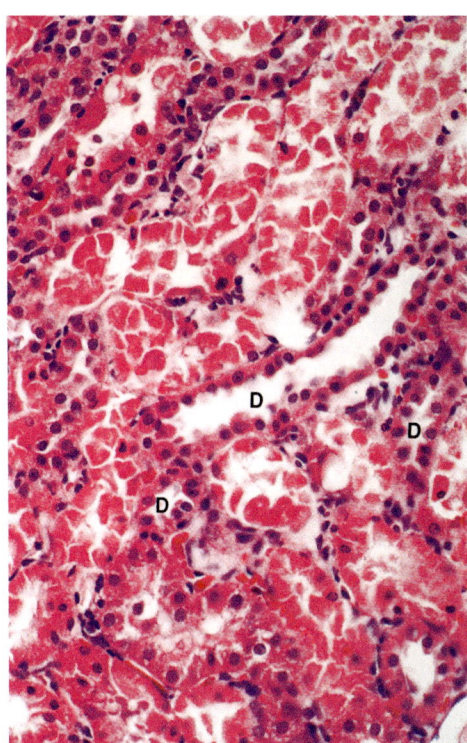

FIGURE 16-69
Toxic acute tubular necrosis due to mercury poisoning. There is widespread necrosis of proximal tubular epithelial cells, with sparing of distal and collecting tubules (D). Interstitial inflammation is minimal.

"necrosis" is more subtle and is reflected in individual necrotic cells within some proximal or distal tubules. These single necrotic cells as well as a few viable cells are shed into the tubular lumen, with resulting focal denudation of the tubular basement membrane (Fig 16-68). Interstitial edema is common. The vasa recta of the outer medulla are congested and frequently contain nucleated cells, which are predominantly mononuclear leukocytes.

Toxic ATN shows more-extensive necrosis of the tubular epithelium than is usually caused by ischemic ATN (compare Figs. 16-68 and 16-69). In most cases, however, the necrosis is limited to certain tubular segments that are most sensitive to the particular toxin. The most common site of injury is the proximal tubule. ATN caused by hemoglobin or myoglobin has the added feature of numerous red-brown tubular casts that are colored by heme pigments.

During the recovery phase of ATN, the tubular epithelium regenerates, leading to the appearance of mitoses, increased size of cells and nuclei, and cell crowding. Survivors eventually display complete restoration of normal renal architecture.

 Clinical Features: **ATN is the leading cause of acute renal failure**. It manifests as a rapidly rising serum creatinine level, which is usually associated with decreased urine output (oliguria). Less commonly, ATN induces nonoliguric acute renal failure. Urinalysis demonstrates degenerating epithelial cells and **"dirty brown" granular casts** (acute renal failure casts) that contain cellular debris that is rich in cytochrome pigments. Urinalysis is useful in differentiating among the three major intrinsic renal diseases that cause acute renal failure (Table 16-11).

The duration of renal failure in patients with ATN depends on many factors, especially the nature and reversibility of the cause. Many patients, at least transiently, develop uremia (azotemia, fluid retention, metabolic acidosis, hyperkalemia) and may require dialysis. If the cause is immediately removed after the initiation of the injury, recovery of renal function often occurs within 1 to 2 weeks, although it may be delayed for months. Increased urine output and a fall in serum creatinine herald the recovery phase.

TABLE 16-11 Urinalysis in Acute Renal Failure

Causes of Acute Renal Failure	Urinalysis Findings
Acute tubular necrosis	Dirty brown casts and epithelial cells
Acute glomerulonephritis	Red blood cell casts and proteinuria
Acute tubulointerstitial nephritis	White blood cell casts and pyuria

Pyelonephritis Refers to Bacterial Infection of the Kidney

Acute Pyelonephritis

Pathogenesis: Gram-negative bacteria from the feces, most commonly E. coli, cause 80% of acute pyelonephritis. The infection reaches the kidney by ascending through the urinary tract, a process that depends on several factors:

- Bacterial infection of the urine
- Reflux of the infected urine up the ureters into the renal pelvis and calyces
- Entry of the bacteria through the papillae into the renal parenchyma

Infection of the bladder precedes acute pyelonephritis. Bladder infection is more common in females because of a short urethra, lack of antibacterial prostatic secretions, and facilitation of bacterial migration by sexual intercourse. The normal commensal flora of the urethra is replaced by fecal organisms in some women who are unusually vulnerable to recurrent attacks of urinary tract infection. This change in bacterial flora may reflect poor hygiene, hormonal effects, and genetic predisposition (e.g., increased numbers of receptors for *E. coli* on urothelial cells).

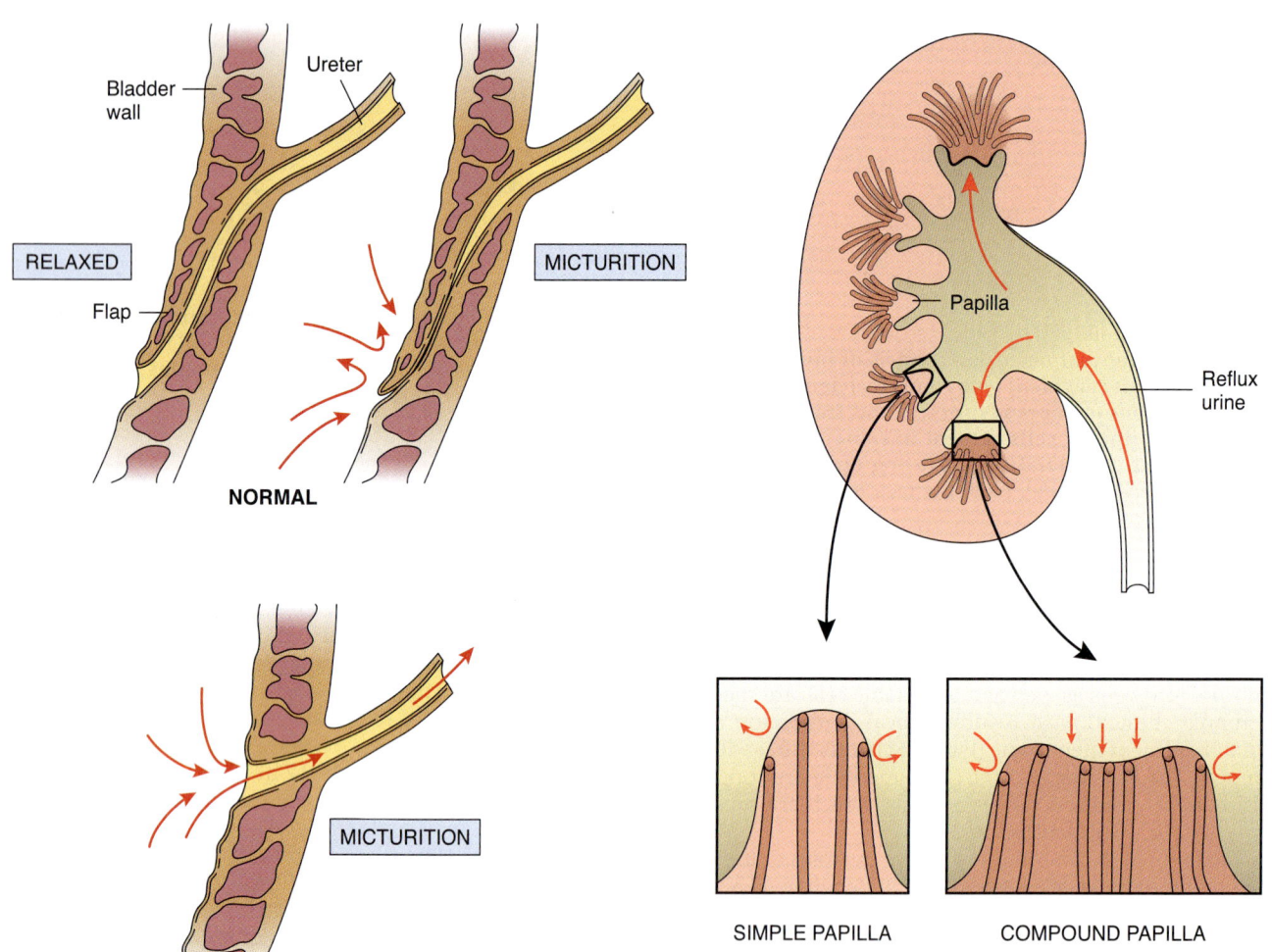

FIGURE 16-70

Anatomical features of the bladder and kidney in pyelonephritis caused by ureterovesical reflux. In the normal bladder, the distal portion of the intravesical ureter courses between the mucosa and the muscularis, forming a mucosal flap. On micturition, the elevated intravesicular pressure compresses the flap against the bladder wall, thereby occluding the lumen. Persons with a congenitally short intravesical ureter have no mucosal flap, because the angle of entry of the ureter into the bladder approaches a right angle. Thus, micturition forces urine into the ureter. In the renal pelvis, simple papillae of the central calyces are convex and do not readily allow reflux of urine. By contrast, the peripheral compound papillae are concave and permit entry of refluxed urine.

Asymptomatic bacteriuria occurs in 10% of pregnant women, one fourth of whom develop acute pyelonephritis. This increased incidence of acute pyelonephritis in pregnancy can also be attributed to an increased residual urine volume. Under the influence of high levels of progesterone, the bladder musculature becomes flaccid and does not expel the urine with its customary efficiency.

During micturition, the bladder normally empties all but 2 to 3 mL of residual urine. The subsequent addition of sterile urine from the kidneys dilutes any bacteria that may have found their way into the bladder. Under some circumstances, the residual urine volume is increased, for example, in prostatic obstruction or in an atonic bladder caused by neurogenic disorders such as paraplegia or diabetic neuropathy. As a result, the bladder contents are not sufficiently diluted with sterile urine from the kidneys to prevent the accumulation of bacteria. The glycosuria of diabetes also predisposes to infection by providing a rich medium for bacterial growth.

Bacteria in the bladder urine usually do not gain access to the kidneys. The ureter commonly inserts into the bladder wall at a steep angle (Fig. 16-70) and in its most distal portion courses parallel to the bladder wall between the mucosa and muscularis. The intravesicular pressure produced by micturition occludes the distal lumen of the ureter, thereby preventing reflux of urine. In many persons who are particularly susceptible to pyelonephritis, an abnormally short passage of the ureter within the bladder wall is associated with an angle of insertion that is more perpendicular to the mucosal surface of the bladder. Thus, on micturition, rather than occluding the lumen, intravesicular pressure forces urine into the patent ureter. This reflux is powerful enough to force the urine into the renal pelvis and calyces.

Even when present in the calyces, bacteria are not necessarily carried into the renal parenchyma by the reflux pressure. The simple papillae of the central calyces are convex and do not readily admit reflux urine (see Fig. 16-70). By contrast, the concave shape of the peripheral compound papillae allows easier access to the collecting system. However, if the pressure is prolonged, as in obstructive uropathy, even the simple papillae are eventually rendered vulnerable to the retrograde entry of urine. From the collecting tubules, the bacteria gain access to the interstitial tissue and other tubules of the kidney.

In addition to ascending through the urine, bacteria and other pathogens can gain access to the renal parenchyma through the blood. For example, gram-positive organisms, such as staphylococci, can disseminate from an infected valve in bacterial endocarditis and establish a focus of infection in the kidney. The kidney is commonly involved in miliary tuberculosis. Fungi, such as *Aspergillus,* can seed the kidney in an immunocompromised host. Hematogenous infections of the kidney preferentially affect the cortex.

Pathology: On gross examination, the kidneys of acute pyelonephritis have small white abscesses on the subcapsular surface and on cut surfaces. The urothelium of the pelvis and calyces may be hyperemic and covered by a purulent exudate. **Acute pyelonephritis is often a focal disease, and much of the kidney may appear normal.** Most infections involve only a few papillary systems. Microscopically, the parenchyma, particularly the cor-

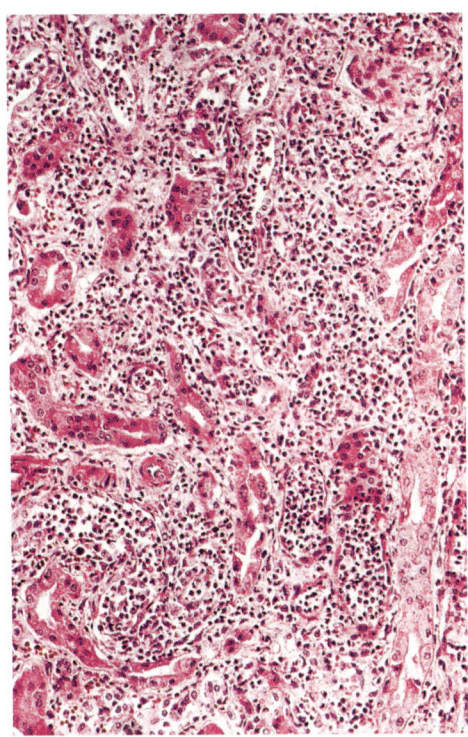

FIGURE 16-71
Acute pyelonephritis. An extensive infiltrate of neutrophils is present in the collecting tubules and interstitial tissue.

tex, typically shows extensive focal destruction by the acute inflammatory process, although vessels and glomeruli often are preferentially preserved. The inflammatory infiltrates contain predominantly neutrophils. Tubules, especially collecting ducts, are often filled with neutrophils (Fig. 16-71). In severe cases of acute pyelonephritis, necrosis of the papillary tips may occur (Fig. 16-72) or the infection may extend beyond the renal capsule, resulting in perinephric abscess formation.

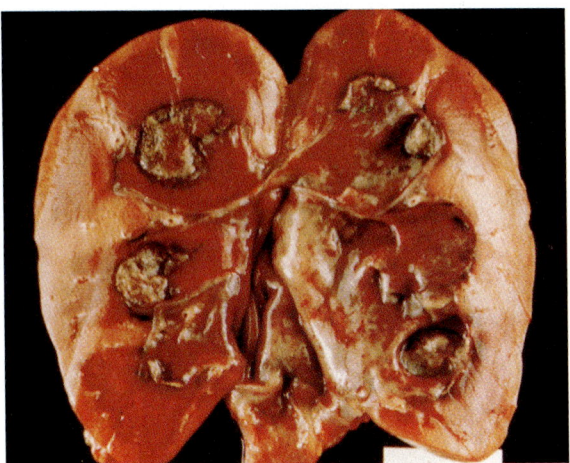

FIGURE 16-72
Papillary necrosis. The bisected kidney shows a dilated renal pelvis and dilated calyces secondary to urinary tract obstruction. The papillae are all necrotic and appear as sharply demarcated, ragged, yellowish areas.

Clinical Features: Symptoms of acute pyelonephritis include fever, chills, sweats, malaise, flank pain, and costovertebral angle tenderness. Leukocytosis with neutrophilia is common. The differentiation of upper from lower urinary tract infection is often clinically difficult, but the finding of **leukocyte casts** in the urine supports a diagnosis of pyelonephritis.

Chronic Pyelonephritis

Pathogenesis: Chronic pyelonephritis is caused by recurrent and persistent bacterial infection secondary to urinary tract obstruction, urine reflux, or both (Fig. 16-73). Whether urine reflux in the absence of infection can produce pathological changes identical to chronic pyelonephritis is controversial.

In chronic pyelonephritis caused by reflux or obstruction, the medullary tissue and overlying cortex are preferentially injured by recurrent acute and chronic inflammation. Progressive atrophy and scarring ensue, with resultant contraction of the involved papillary tip (or sloughing if there is papillary necrosis) and thinning of the overlying cortex. **This process results in the distinctive gross appearance of a broad depressed area of cortical fibrosis and atrophy overlying a dilated calyx** (*caliectasis*) (Fig. 16-74).

Pathology: The microscopic appearance of chronic pyelonephritis is nonspecific. Many diseases that cause chronic injury to the tubulointerstitial compartment induce chronic interstitial inflammation, interstitial fibrosis, and tubular atrophy. Thus, chronic pyelonephritis is only one of many causes of the pattern of injury termed *chronic tubulointerstitial nephritis*. The gross appearance of chronic pyelonephritis is more distinctive. Only chronic pyelonephritis and analgesic nephropathy produce a combination of calyceal deformity and dilation (*caliectasis*) with overlying corticomedullary scarring. In obstructive uropathy, all of the calyces and the renal pelvis are dilated, and the parenchyma is uniformly thinned (see Fig. 16-74). In cases associated with vesicoureteral reflux, the calyces at the poles of the kidney are preferentially expanded and are associated with overlying discrete, coarse scars that cause indentation of the renal surface. Microscopically, the scars have atrophic dilated tubules surrounded by interstitial fibrosis and infiltrates of chronic inflammatory cells (Fig. 16-75). The most characteristic (but not specific) tubular change is severe atrophy of the epithelium, with diffuse, eosinophilic, hyaline casts. Such tubules, which are "pinched-off" spherical segments, resemble colloid-containing thyroid follicles, a pattern called "thyroidization." This appearance results from the breakup of tubules, with residual segments forming spherules. The glomeruli may be completely uninvolved, may have periglomerular fibrosis, or may be sclerotic. The loss of most functioning nephrons may induce secondary focal segmental glomerulosclerosis. Fibrosis of the walls of arteries and arterioles is common. There is marked scarring and chronic inflammation of the calyceal mucosa.

Xanthogranulomatous Pyelonephritis

Xanthogranulomatous pyelonephritis is an uncommon form of chronic pyelonephritis that is often caused by *Proteus* infection. The name derives from the yellow gross appearance of the nodular renal lesions, which results from the presence of numerous lipid-laden foamy macrophages (*xanthoma cells*). The disease is usually unilateral. The clini-

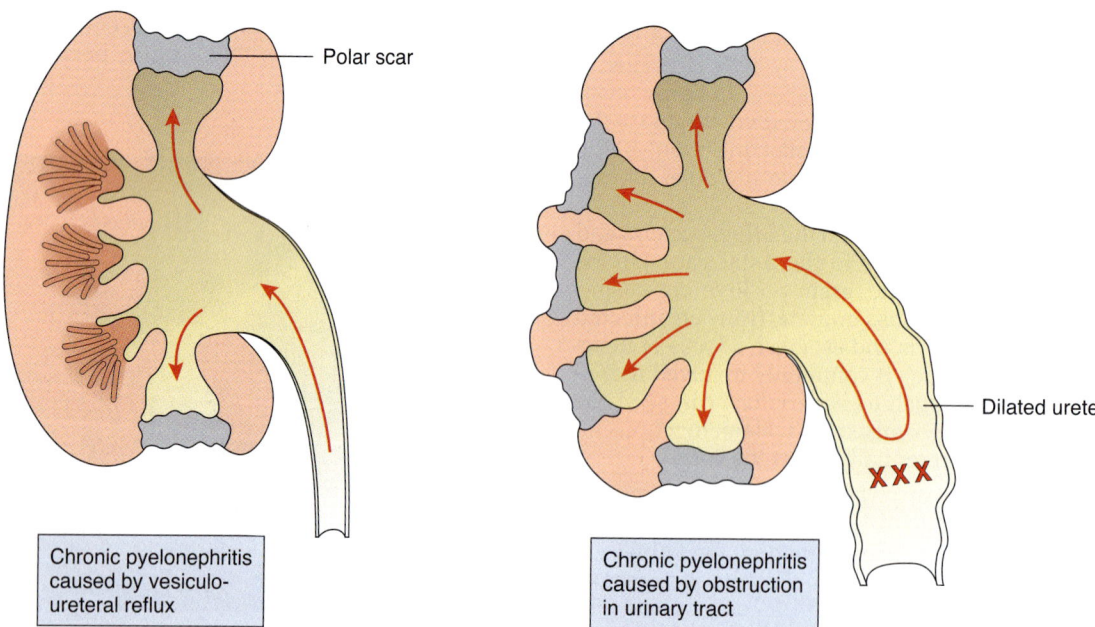

FIGURE 16-73

The two major types of chronic pyelonephritis. *(Left)* Vesicoureteral reflux causes infection of the peripheral compound papillae and, therefore, scars in the poles of the kidney. *(Right)* Obstruction of the urinary tract leads to high-pressure backflow of urine, which causes infection of all papillae, diffuse scarring of the kidney, and thinning of the cortex.

Diseases of Tubules and Interstitium   873

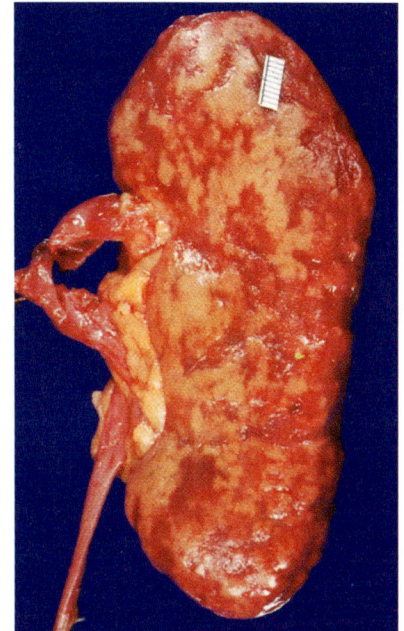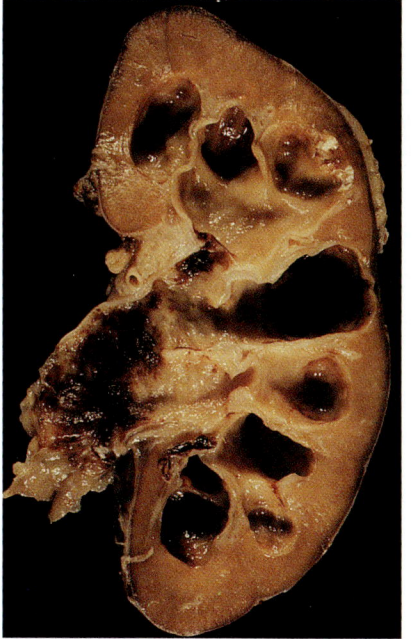

FIGURE 16-74
Chronic pyelonephritis. A. The cortical surface contains many irregular, depressed scars (reddish areas). B. There is marked dilation of calyces (caliectasis) caused by inflammatory destruction of papillae, with atrophy and scarring of the overlying cortex.

cal and pathological features can be confused with renal cell carcinoma.

Clinical Features: Most patients with chronic pyelonephritis suffer episodic manifestations of urinary tract infection or acute pyelonephritis, such as recurrent fever and flank pain. Occasional patients have a silent course until end-stage renal disease develops. Urinalysis demonstrates leukocytes, and imaging studies reveal caliectasis and cortical scarring.

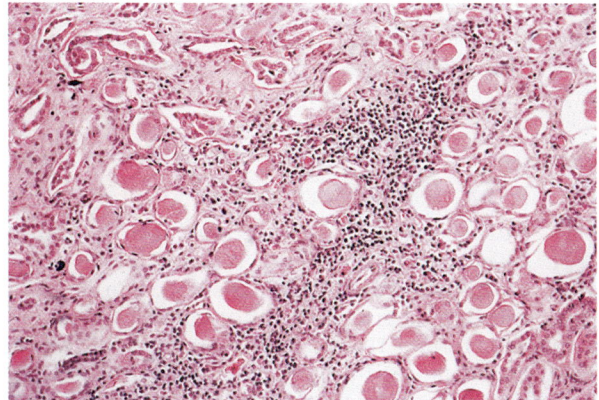

FIGURE 16-75
A light micrograph shows tubular dilation and atrophy, with many tubules containing eosinophilic hyaline casts resembling the colloid of thyroid follicles (so-called thyroidization). The interstitium is scarred and contains a chronic inflammatory cell infiltrate.

Analgesic Nephropathy Results from Chronic Overdosage of Drugs

Patients with analgesic nephropathy typically have consumed more than 2 kg of analgesic compounds. Incriminated analgesics often occur in combinations, such as aspirin and phenacetin, or aspirin and acetaminophen. Phenacetin has been recognized as the drug that carries the greatest risk for developing nephropathy and has been banned in many countries, including the United States. Acetaminophen poses a higher risk for inducing nephropathy than aspirin or nonsteroidal antiinflammatory drugs. The pathophysiological basis for analgesic nephropathy is not clear. Possibilities include direct nephrotoxicity or ischemic damage as a result of drug-induced vascular changes, or both.

Pathology: Medullary injury with papillary necrosis appears to be the earliest event in analgesic nephropathy, followed by atrophy, chronic inflammation, and scarring of the overlying cortex. The earliest histological abnormality is a distinctive **homogeneous thickening of the walls of the capillaries immediately beneath the transitional epithelium of the urinary tract**. Early parenchymal changes are confined to the papillae and the inner medulla and consist of focal thickening of tubular and capillary basement membranes, interstitial fibrosis, and focal coagulative necrosis. These necrotic areas eventually become confluent and extend to the corticomedullary junction, after which the collecting ducts become involved. Few inflammatory cells are found around the necrotic foci. Eventually, the entire papilla becomes necrotic *(papillary necrosis)*, often remaining in place as a structureless mass. In such circumstances, dystrophic calcification of the necrotic papilla is common. Papillae may have incomplete detachment at the demarcation zone or they may be completely sloughed. There is secondary tubular atrophy, interstitial fibrosis, and chronic inflammation in the overlying cortex.

 Clinical Features: Signs and symptoms occur only in the late stages of analgesic nephropathy and include an inability to concentrate the urine, distal tubular acidosis, hematuria, hypertension, and anemia. Sloughing of necrotic papillary tips into the renal pelvis may result in colic as they pass through the ureters. Progressive renal failure often develops and may lead to end-stage renal disease.

Drug-Induced (Hypersensitivity) Acute Tubulointerstitial Nephritis Is a Cell-Mediated Immune Response

 Pathogenesis: Acute drug-induced tubulointerstitial nephritis is characterized histologically by infiltrates of activated T lymphocytes and admixed eosinophils, a pattern that indicates a type IV cell-mediated immune reaction. The immunogen could be the drug itself, the drug bound to certain tissue components, a drug metabolite, or a tissue component altered in response to the drug. Drugs that are most commonly implicated include nonsteroidal antiinflammatory drugs, diuretics, and certain antibiotics, especially β-lactam antibiotics, such as synthetic penicillins and cephalosporins.

 Pathology: Microscopically, there is patchy infiltration of the cortex and (to a much lesser extent) the medulla by lymphocytes and a small number of eosinophils (5–10% of the total leukocytes in the tissue) (Fig. 16-76). The eosinophils tend to be concentrated in small foci and may be seen within tubular lumina and in the urine. Neutrophils are rare, and their presence should raise suspicion of the possibility of pyelonephritis or hematogenous bacterial infection. Foci of granulomatous inflammation may be present, especially in the later phase of the disease. Proximal and distal tubules are focally invaded by white blood cells ("tubulitis"). Glomeruli and vessels are not inflamed, although some instances of drug-induced tubulointerstitial nephritis, usually caused by nonsteroidal antiinflammatory drugs, are accompanied by minimal-change glomerulopathy.

 Clinical Features: Acute tubulointerstitial nephritis usually manifests as acute renal failure, typically about 2 weeks after drug administration is started. The urine contains erythrocytes, leukocytes (including eosinophils), and sometimes leukocyte casts. Tubular defects

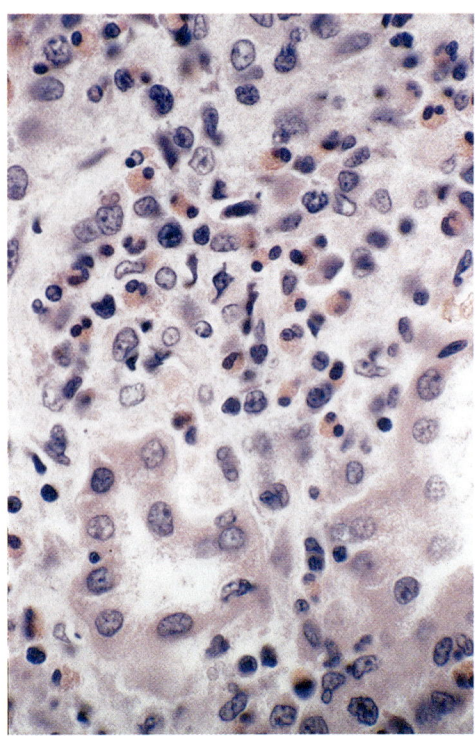

FIGURE 16-76
Hypersensitivity tubulointerstitial nephritis. There is interstitial edema and infiltration by mononuclear leukocytes, with admixed eosinophils.

are common, including sodium wasting, glucosuria, aminoaciduria, and renal tubular acidosis. Systemic allergic symptoms such as fever and rash may also be present. Most patients recover fully within several weeks or months if the drug is discontinued.

Light-Chain Cast Nephropathy May Complicate Multiple Myeloma

Light-chain cast nephropathy is renal injury caused by monoclonal immunoglobulin light chains in the urine, which produce tubular epithelial injury and numerous tubular casts.

 Pathogenesis: As discussed above, multiple myeloma may produce AL amyloidosis, light-chain deposition disease, heavy-chain deposition disease, and light-chain cast nephropathy. The last is the most common form of renal disease associated with multiple myeloma and is caused by glomerular filtering of circulating light chains. At the acidic pH typical of urine, the light chains bind to Tamm-Horsfall glycoproteins, which are secreted by distal tubular epithelial cells, and form casts. Renal dysfunction results from the toxic effects of free light chains on tubular epithelial cells and obstruction from the casts. The molecular structure of light chains determines whether they will

Urate Nephropathy Displays Urate Crystals in the Tubules and Interstitium

Any condition associated with elevated levels of uric acid in the blood may cause urate nephropathy. The classic chronic disease in this category is primary gout (see Chapter 26).

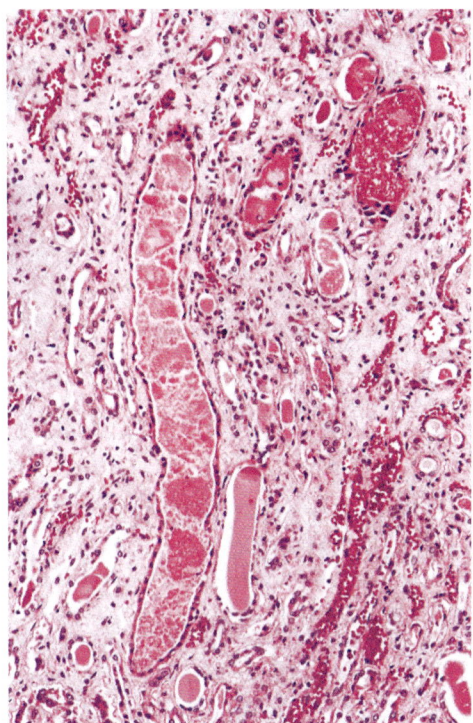

FIGURE 16-77
Light-chain cast nephropathy. A light micrograph shows numerous casts within tubular lumina.

induce disease by causing light-chain cast nephropathy, AL amyloidosis, or light-chain deposition disease. Occasional patients have more than one of these renal diseases.

Pathology: The characteristic tubular lesion exhibits numerous dense, hyaline casts in the distal tubules and collecting ducts (Fig. 16-77). These casts are brightly eosinophilic and glassy (hyaline) and often have fractures and angular borders. Occasionally, they have a crystalline appearance. The casts may induce a foreign body reaction, characterized by macrophages and multinucleated giant cells. Interstitial infiltrates of chronic inflammatory cells, as well as interstitial edema, typically accompany the tubular lesions. More chronic lesions show interstitial fibrosis and tubular atrophy. Focal calcium deposits (nephrocalcinosis) are also frequently noted in the fibrotic interstitium of the tubules. Immunohistochemical staining shows that the casts contain light chains and Tamm-Horsfall proteins.

Clinical Features: Light-chain cast nephropathy may manifest as either acute or chronic renal failure. Proteinuria is usually present, although not necessarily in the nephrotic range, and most often consists predominantly of immunoglobulin light chains. If nephrotic-range proteinuria is present in a patient with multiple myeloma, either AL amyloidosis or light-chain deposition disease is more likely than light-chain cast nephropathy.

Pathogenesis: Chronic urate nephropathy caused by gout is characterized by tubular and interstitial deposition of crystalline monosodium urate. **Acute urate nephropathy** can be caused by increased cell turnover (e.g., leukemia or polycythemia). For example, chemotherapy for malignant neoplasms results in a sudden increase in blood uric acid because of the massive necrosis of cancer cells *(tumor lysis syndrome)*. Hepatic catabolism of large amounts of purines released from the DNA of necrotic cells leads to hyperuricemia. Acute renal failure reflects the obstruction of the collecting ducts by precipitated crystals of uric acid, a result of increased concentrations of uric acid in the acidic pH of the urine. Conditions that interfere with the excretion of uric acid can also result in hyperuricemia, for example, the chronic intake of certain diuretics. Chronic lead intoxication interferes with the secretion of uric acid by proximal tubules and leads to *saturnine gout*.

Pathology: In acute urate nephropathy, the precipitated uric acid in the collecting ducts is seen grossly as yellow streaks in the papillae. Histologically, the tubular deposits appear amorphous, but in frozen sections, birefringent crystals are apparent (Fig. 16-78). The tubules proximal to the obstruction are dilated. Penetration of collecting ducts by uric acid crystals may provoke a foreign-body giant cell reaction.

The basic disease process of chronic urate nephropathy is similar to that of the acute form, but the prolonged course results in more substantial deposition of urate crystals in the interstitium, interstitial fibrosis, and cortical atrophy. The most diagnostic feature is the *gouty tophus*. Tophi are focal accumulations of urate crystals surrounded by inflamma-

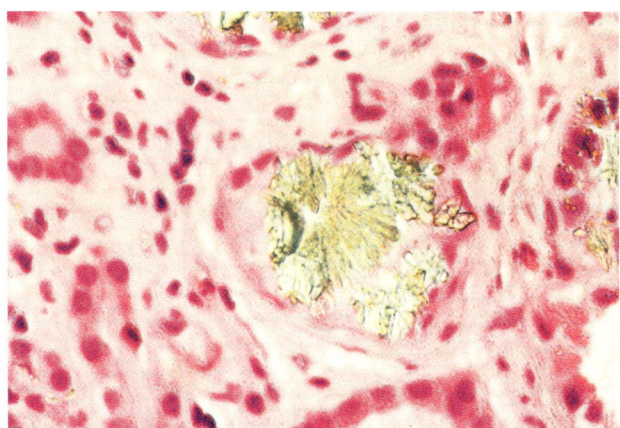

FIGURE 16-78
Urate nephropathy. A frozen section demonstrates tubular deposits of uric acid crystals.

tory cells, which may appear granulomatous and include multinucleated giant cells. Uric acid stones, which account for one tenth of all cases of urolithiasis, occur in 20% of patients with chronic gout and in 40% of those with acute hyperuricemia.

 Clinical Features: Acute urate nephropathy manifests as acute renal failure, whereas chronic urate nephropathy causes chronic renal tubular defects. Although histological renal lesions are found in most persons with chronic gout, significant compromise of renal function is seen in fewer than half.

Nephrocalcinosis Is the Deposition of Calcium in the Renal Parenchyma

 Pathogenesis: Hypercalciuria may result in nephrocalcinosis (Table 16-12) or the formation of calcium-containing stones (nephrolithiasis) or both. Nephrocalcinosis may cause abnormal renal function, especially tubular defects such as impaired concentrating ability, salt wasting, and renal tubular acidosis. When nephrocalcinosis is caused by hypercalcemia, it is categorized as *metastatic calcification*, in contrast to calcification at sites of renal parenchymal injury (e.g., infarcts or cortical necrosis), which is representative of *dystrophic calcification*.

 Pathology: One fifth of kidneys at autopsy have small calcium deposits that have no functional significance or recognized association with hypercalcemia. In patients with nephrocalcinosis caused by hypercalcemia, the extent of calcification varies from microscopic deposits to marked calcium accumulation visible grossly and radiologically. In the presence of severe hypercalcemia (e.g., caused by primary hyperparathyroidism), gross examination characteristically reveals wedge-shaped scars interspersed with relatively normal renal tissue. These scars reflect parenchymal atrophy and interstitial fibrosis caused by

TABLE **16-12 Causes of Hypercalcemia That Lead to Nephrocalcinosis**

Increased resorption of calcium from bone
Renal osteodystrophy
Primary hyperparathyroidism
Neoplasms producing parathormone or parathormone-like protein
Osteolytic neoplasms and metastases
Increased intestinal absorption of calcium
Idiopathic hypercalcenia
Vitamin D excess
Milk-alkali syndrome
Sarcoidosis

the calcification. Histologically, there is striking calcification of the basement membranes of the renal tubules, particularly those of the proximal convoluted tubules. The interstitial tissue also contains calcium deposits. Such deposits also accumulate in the cytoplasm of tubular epithelial cells, which eventually degenerate and are sloughed into the lumina to aggregate as calcified casts. Scattered glomeruli show calcification of Bowman's capsule. The walls of intrarenal arteries may also be calcified. With hematoxylin, renal calcium deposits are deeply basophilic; with the more specific von Kossa stain, they are black. By electron microscopy, the mitochondria of renal tubular epithelial cells contain abundant calcium deposits.

RENAL STONES (NEPHROLITHIASIS AND UROLITHIASIS)

Nephrolithiasis and urolithiasis are stones within the collecting system of the kidney (nephrolithiasis) or elsewhere in the collecting system of the urinary tract (urolithiasis). The pelvis and calyces of the kidney are common sites for the formation and accumulation of calculi. Stones vary in composition, depending on individual factors, geography, metabolic alterations, and the presence of infection. For unknown reasons, renal stones are more common in men than in women. They vary in size from gravel (<1 mm in diameter) to large stones that dilate the entire renal pelvis. Kidney stones may be well tolerated, but in some cases, they lead to severe hydronephrosis and pyelonephritis. Moreover, they can erode the mucosa and cause hematuria. The passage of a stone into the ureter causes excruciating flank pain, termed *renal colic*. Until recently, most kidney stones required surgical methods for their removal, but ultrasonic disintegration (lithotripsy) and endoscopic removal are now effective alternatives.

In most cases, the presence of a urinary stone is associated with an increased blood level and urinary excretion of its principal component. This is clearly the case with uric acid and cystine stones. However, in many patients with calcium stones, hypercalciuria occurs in the absence of hypercalcemia. Mixed uric acid and calcium stones are common in the presence of increased uric acid excretion, because urate crystals act as a nidus around which calcium salts precipitate.

Calcium stones: Most (75%) kidney stones contain calcium complexed with oxalate or phosphate or a mixture of these anions. In the United States, calcium oxalate is more common, whereas in England, calcium phosphate predominates. A calcium oxalate stone is hard and occasionally dark, because it is covered by hemorrhage from the mucosa of the renal pelvis injured by the sharp calcium oxalate crystals. Calcium phosphate stones tend to be softer and paler.

Infection stones: Some 15% of stones are caused by infection. In the presence of urea-splitting bacteria, usually *Proteus* or *Providencia* species, the resulting alkaline urine favors the precipitation of magnesium ammonium phosphate *(struvite)* and calcium phosphate *(apatite)*. These stones vary in consistency from hard to soft and friable. Infection stones occasionally fill the pelvis and calyces to form a cast of these spaces, referred to as a *staghorn calculus* (Fig. 16-79). Infection stones are the most troublesome category of stones because

Renal Transplantation

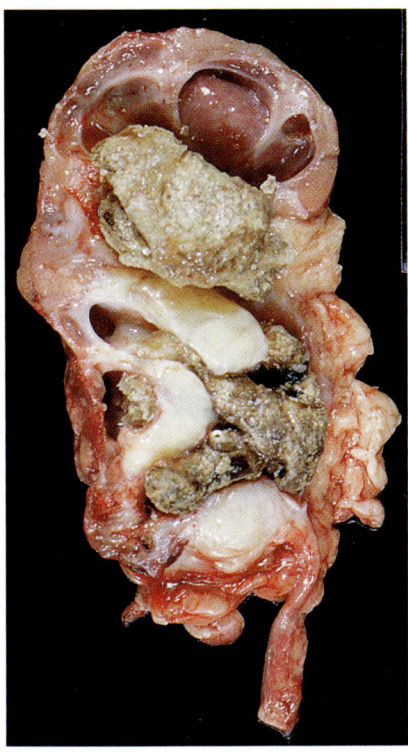

FIGURE 16-79
Staghorn calculi. The kidney shows hydronephrosis and stones that are casts of the dilated calyces.

they cause frequent complications, such as intractable urinary tract infection, pain, bleeding, perinephric abscess, and urosepsis.

Uric acid stones: These stones occur in 25% of patients with hyperuricemia and gout, but most patients with uric acid stones do not have either condition *(idiopathic urate lithiasis)*. The stones are smooth, hard, and yellow and are usually less than 2 cm in diameter. Importantly, in contrast to calcium-containing stones, pure uric acid stones are radiolucent.

Cystine stones: These stones account for only 1% of stones overall but represent a significant proportion of childhood calculi and occur exclusively with hereditary cystinuria. Although the stones are composed entirely of cystine, they may be enveloped by a layer of calcium phosphate.

OBSTRUCTIVE UROPATHY AND HYDRONEPHROSIS

Obstructive uropathy is caused by structural or functional abnormalities in the urinary tract that impede urine flow, which may cause renal dysfunction (obstructive nephropathy) and dilation of the collecting system (hydronephrosis). The causes of urinary tract obstruction are discussed in detail in Chapter 17.

 Pathology: In early hydronephrosis, the most prominent microscopic finding is dilation of the collecting ducts, followed by dilation of the proximal and distal convoluted tubules. Eventually, the proximal tubules become widely dilated, and loss of tubules is common. The glomeruli are usually spared. Grossly, progressive dilation of the renal pelvis and calyces occurs, and atrophy of the renal parenchyma ensues (Fig. 16-80). In the presence of hydronephrosis, the kidney is more susceptible to pyelonephritis, which causes additional injury.

 Clinical Features: Bilateral acute urinary tract obstruction causes acute renal failure *(postrenal acute renal failure)*. Unilateral obstruction is frequently asymptomatic. Because many causes of acute obstruction are reversible, prompt recognition is important. Left untreated, an obstructed kidney undergoes atrophy, and in the case of bilateral obstruction, chronic renal failure ensues.

RENAL TRANSPLANTATION

Renal transplantation is the treatment of choice for most patients with end-stage renal disease. The major obstacle is immunological rejection, but recurrence of the disease that destroyed the native kidneys and nephrotoxicity from immunosuppressive drugs also injure the renal allograft. Table 16-13 lists distinct, but often coexisting, patterns of humoral and cellular renal allograft rejection.

ABO blood group antigens and **human leukocyte antigens (HLAs)** are the two major groups of tissue antigens that are the principal targets of immune attack directed against the transplanted kidney. Incompatible ABO blood group antigens, expressed on endothelial cells and erythrocytes, are absolute barriers to a successful transplant. ABO-incompatible grafts encounter preformed, circulating antibodies that bind to endothelial cells and cause immediate (hyperacute) rejection. The more commonly encountered (and more gradual) patterns of acute rejection and chronic rejection are caused primarily by donor–recipient differences in

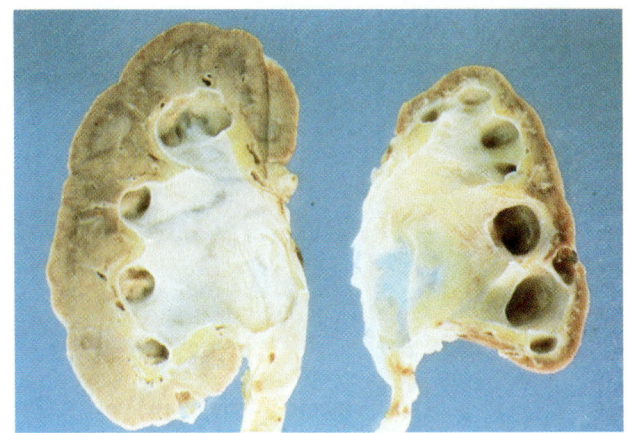

FIGURE 16-80
Hydronephrosis. Bilateral urinary tract obstruction has led to conspicuous dilation of the ureters, pelves, and calyces. The kidney on the right shows severe parenchymal atrophy.

TABLE 16-13 Categories of Renal Allograft Rejection

Category	Most Characteristic Lesion
Hyperacute humoral rejection	Neutrophils, hemorrhage and necrosis
Acute cellular rejection	
Acute tubulointerstitial rejection	Tubulitis (mononuclear leukocytes in tubules)
Acute cellular vascular rejection	Endarteritis (mononuclear leukocytes in intima)
Acute humoral rejection	
Acute humoral capillary rejection	Neutrophils and C4d in capillaries
Acute necrotizing vascular rejection	Arterial fibrinoid necrosis
Chronic rejection	Arterial intimal fibrosis, cortical atrophy

HLAs (major histocompatibility complex antigens, MHCs), which are expressed on most cell membranes and are controlled by several closely related loci on chromosome 6. Sensitization of kidney allograft recipients to HLAs produces both cell-mediated and antibody-mediated reactions (Chapter 4). Renal allograft rejection can be classified on the basis of the clinical course, pathological features, and presumed pathogenesis, as shown in Table 16-13. However, more than one type of rejection can involve the allograft at the same time.

HYPERACUTE HUMORAL REJECTION: This form of rejection is rare because of current compatibility testing; it occurs in less than 0.5% of allografts. When recipient blood containing antibodies to major alloantigens (usually ABO or class I HLAs) begins flowing through allograft vessels, immediate binding of the antibodies to endothelial cells causes prompt and irreversible injury in minutes, which may become apparent intraoperatively by mottling, cyanosis, and poor tissue turgor of the graft. The complexing of antibodies with endothelial alloantigens induces complement activation, which attracts neutrophils. The cytotoxic effects of complement and neutrophil activation cause endothelial cell swelling, vacuolization, and lysis. The accumulation of neutrophils in glomerular capillaries is regarded as a sign of impending rejection. Endothelial cell changes are followed by platelet thrombi and later by fibrin thrombi. Interstitial edema, hemorrhage, and cortical necrosis develop over the following 12 to 24 hours.

ACUTE HUMORAL REJECTION: The most common type of acute humoral rejection is directed primarily at capillaries and may cause only subtle or no pathological changes by light microscopy. The most common feature is increased neutrophils in peritubular and glomerular capillaries and in tubules. The most consistent finding is localization of complement activation products, especially C4d, in the walls of peritubular and glomerular capillaries (Fig. 16-81A). The most severe, but least common, pattern of acute humoral rejection is characterized by **necrotizing arteritis** with fibrinoid necrosis involving the media (Fig. 16-81B). It occurs in less than 1% of allografts in patients whose immunosuppression includes a calcineurin inhibitor, although it occurred in 5% of renal allografts prior to the introduction of this therapy. Once necrotizing arteritis develops, the chances of graft survival for 1 year are less than 25%, even with aggressive immunosuppressive treatment.

ACUTE CELLULAR REJECTION: This reaction is the most common form of acute rejection and is characterized by infiltration of the interstitium, tubules, arteries, arterioles, or glomeruli by T lymphocytes and macrophages. The nuclei of

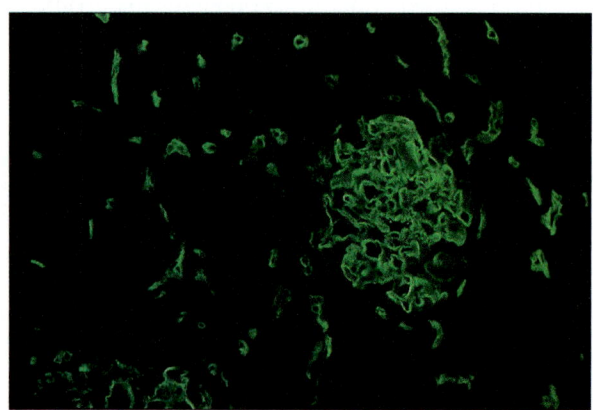
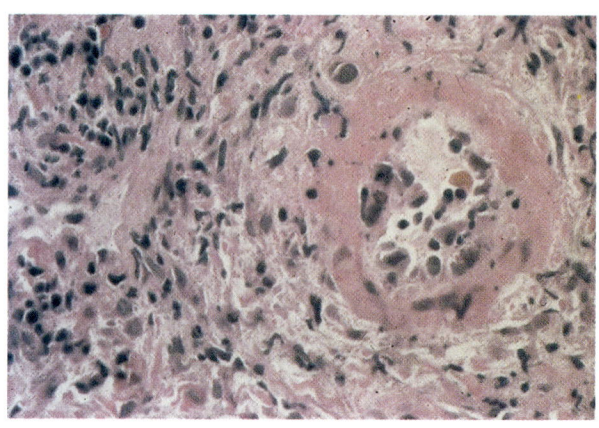

FIGURE 16-81
Acute humoral allograft rejection. A. Staining of peritubular and glomerular capillaries with a fluoresceinated anti-C4d antibody showing evidence of complement activation by antibodies directed against donor antigens on endothelial cells. B. Acute humoral necrotizing acute vasculitis in an interlobular artery with extensive fibrinoid necrosis of the muscularis. The vascular and interstitial infiltrates of mononuclear leukocytes indicate concurrent acute cellular rejection.

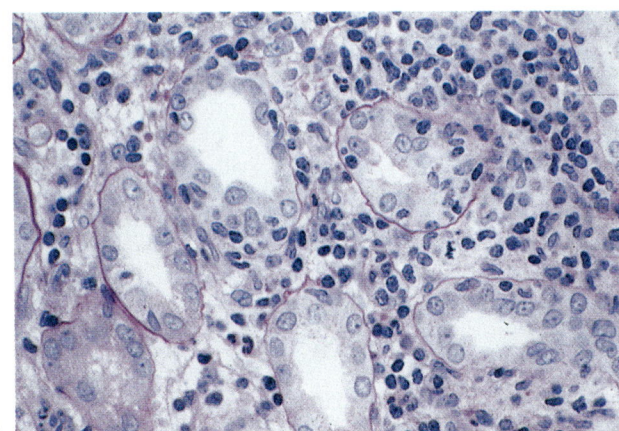
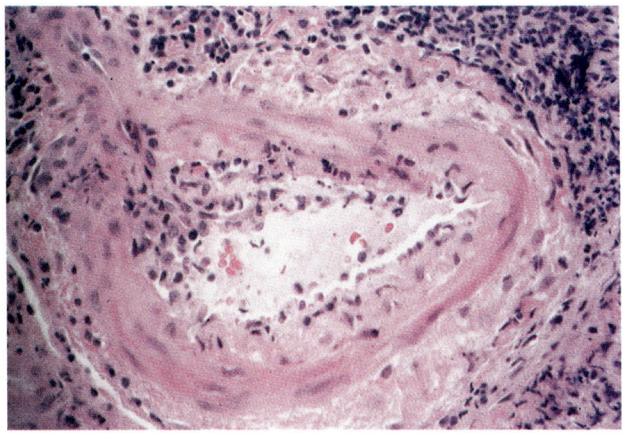

FIGURE 16-82
Acute cellular allograft rejection. A. Acute tubulointerstitial cellular rejection with tubulitis indicated by the lymphocytes on the epithelial side of the basement membrane (PAS stain). B. Acute cellular vascular rejection with endarteritis indicated by the mononuclear leukocytes infiltrating into the intima of an arcuate artery.

the infiltrating lymphocytes are of variable sizes and shapes because the cells are at various stages of activation. Occasional cells are completely transformed into immunoblasts. Interstitial infiltrates are typically patchy rather than diffuse. Involvement of tubules *(tubulitis)* is manifested by lymphocytes crossing tubular basement membranes and lying between tubular epithelial cells (see Fig. 16-82A). Arterial involvement by cellular rejection leads to the penetration of T lymphocytes and monocytes across the endothelium, resulting in an expanded intima filled with mononuclear leukocytes *(intimal arteritis, or endarteritis)* (Fig. 16-82B). Arterioles are occasionally involved by similar infiltration. Glomerular infiltration by mononuclear leukocytes with obliteration of capillary lumens *(acute transplant glomerulopathy)* is an uncommon manifestation of acute cellular rejection. Renal transplants found to have tubulitis without endarteritis have an 80% chance for 1-year graft survival, compared with 60% for allografts with endarteritis.

CHRONIC REJECTION: The pathological changes attributed to chronic rejection are listed in Table 16-14.

The arterial changes of chronic rejection affect a wide spectrum of vessels, ranging from small arteries to the main renal artery. There is prominent initial widening, caused by stromal cell proliferation and matrix deposition (Fig. 16-83). Mononuclear leukocytes within the vessel wall are much less prominent than with active intimal arteritis. Foam cells may be conspicuous, and there may be interruption of the internal elastic lamina. Peritubular capillaries demonstrate thickening and replication of basement membranes. Tubular atrophy and interstitial fibrosis may be caused at least in part by ischemia secondary to the narrowing of arteries and peritubular capillaries. Tubulointerstitial injury may also result from indolent tubulitis. Glomerular involvement *(chronic transplant glomerulopathy)* manifests as thickening of capillary walls and mesangial widening. Electron microscopy demonstrates electron-lucent expansion of the subendothelial zone and occasional mesangial interposition and replica-

TABLE 16-14 Histological Features of Chronic Renal Allograft Rejection

Fibrotic intimal thickening of arteries
Tubular atrophy
Interstitial fibrosis
Interstitial mononuclear leukocytes
Glomerular capillary wall thickening and mesangial expansion
Glomerular sclerosis

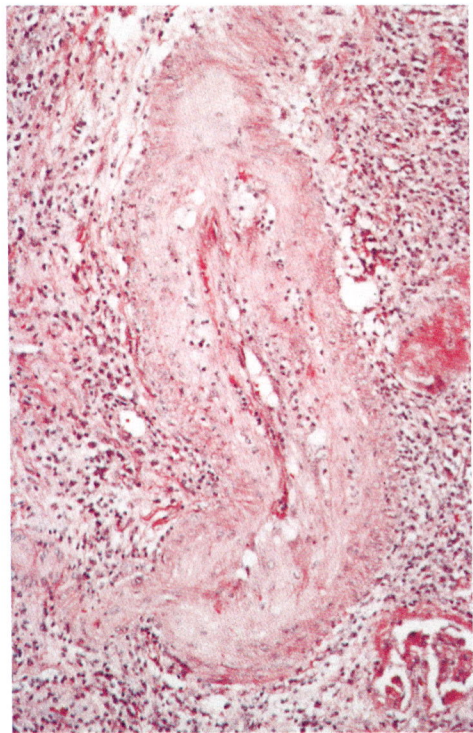

FIGURE 16-83
Chronic allograft rejection. The lumen of this medium-sized artery is occluded by a thickened and fibrotic intima, which contains a few inflammatory cells.

TABLE 16-15 Recurrence of Disease in Renal Allografts

Disease	Recurrence Rate (%)	Rate of Graft Loss (%)
Type II membranoproliferative glomerulonephritis	>90	15
Diabetic glomerulosclerosis	>90	<5
IgA nephropathy	40	<10
Focal segmental glomerulosclerosis	35	30
Type I membranoproliferative glomerulonephritis	30	<10
Membranous glomerulopathy	20	<5
ANCA glomerulonephritis	15	<5
Anti-GBM glomerulonephritis	5	<5
Lupus glomerulonephritis	5	<5

ANCA, antineutrophil cytoplasmic autoantibody; GBM, glomerular basement membrane.

tion of basement membranes. The arterial, peritubular capillary, and glomerular injury all may result from persistent, low-level, immune injury to the vascular endothelium.

RECURRENCE OF KIDNEY DISEASE: The same disease that caused end-stage disease in the native kidneys can recur in a renal transplant. The frequency and significance of recurrence varies among different types of glomerular disease (Table 16-15).

NEPHROTOXICITY OF CYCLOSPORINE AND TACROLIMUS (FK506): Cyclosporine and tacrolimus, which are calcineurin inhibitors, are effective immunosuppressive drugs that have dramatically improved the survival of not only kidney allografts, but also other allografts (e.g., liver, heart, and lungs). Unfortunately, both drugs injure kidney allografts, as well as the native kidneys of patients who are receiving immunosuppressive treatment for other reasons. The toxicity can cause acute or chronic renal failure.

The most characteristic renal lesion is an *arteriolopathy* that begins with smooth muscle cell degeneration and necrosis. The destroyed arteriolar muscle cells are replaced by acidophilic hyaline material (Fig. 16-84). In fulminant cases, the vascular lesions take on the appearance of a full-blown thrombotic microangiopathy, with circumferential fibrinoid necrosis of arterioles. Chronic toxicity has zones of interstitial fibrosis and tubular atrophy ("striped fibrosis").

BENIGN TUMORS OF THE KIDNEY

RENAL ADENOMA: Whether any renal epithelial cell neoplasm should be designated an *adenoma*, a term that signifies no malignant potential, is controversial. Tumor size has been used as a criterion to separate adenomas from carcinomas, but this is problematic because all carcinomas begin as small lesions. Renal epithelial neoplasms less than 3 cm in diameter rarely metastasize, but "rarely" is not "never." Such small tumors are termed *adenomas* when they have well-demarcated margins and are composed of small cuboidal cells with round, regular nuclei. The cells may be arranged in closely packed tubules or papillary configurations (papillary adenoma). Neoplasms with clear cells that resemble renal cell carcinomas (clear cells) or oncocytomas (oncocytes) should not be designated adenomas even if they are small. When these criteria are used, most renal adenomas are in the outer cortex and are less than 1 cm in diameter. Renal adenomas increase in frequency with age and are found at autopsy in 40% of patients over 70 year of age.

RENAL ONCOCYTOMA: This tumor is composed of plump cells with abundant, finely granular, acidophilic cytoplasm and round nuclei without atypia. Electron microscopy demonstrates numerous mitochondria as the basis for the distinctive appearance of the cytoplasm. Grossly, oncocytomas have a characteristic mahogany-brown color, caused by the lipochrome pigments in the mitochondria. These tumors rarely metastasize.

MEDULLARY FIBROMA: Medullary fibromas (renomedullary interstitial cell tumors) are typically small (<0.5 cm in diameter), pale gray, well-circumscribed tumors that are usually located in the midportion of the medullary pyramid. Histologically, the neoplasms are composed of small stellate to polygonal cells lying in a loose stroma. Renal medullary fibromas can be identified in half of all adult autopsies.

ANGIOMYOLIPOMA: These lesions exhibit an admixture of well-differentiated adipose tissue, smooth muscle, and thick-walled vessels. Grossly, the tumors are yellow and bosselated and may resemble renal cell carcinoma. However, they are always well encapsulated and lack areas of necrosis. **Angiomyolipomas have a strong association with tuberous sclerosis.** Fully 80% of patients with tuberous sclerosis have angiomyolipomas, although less than 50% of patients with angiomyolipomas have tuberous sclerosis.

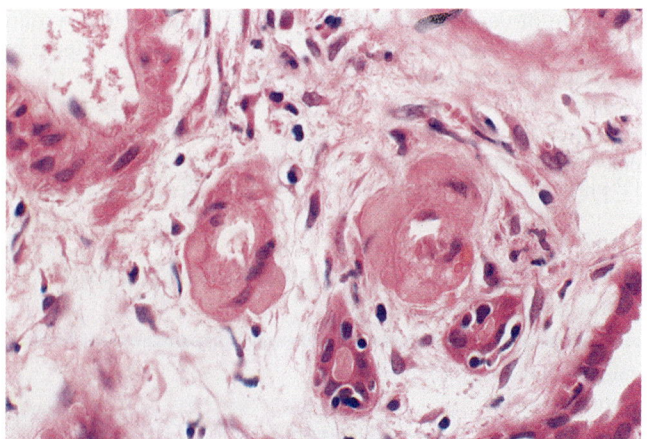

FIGURE 16-84
Cyclosporine nephrotoxicity and arteriolopathy. Marked destructive hyalinosis of arterioles is present.

MESOBLASTIC NEPHROMA: Mesoblastic nephromas are congenital benign neoplasms or hamartomas that are usually recognized during the first 3 months of life and must be differentiated from Wilms tumor. The lesions range from less than 1 cm in diameter to over 15 cm. Histologically, they are composed of spindle cells of fibroblastic or myofibroblastic lineage. Characteristically, the tumor margins are irregular, with bands of cells interdigitating with adjacent parenchyma. If some of these tongues of tumor tissue are left behind after surgical resection, local recurrence is possible.

MALIGNANT TUMORS OF THE KIDNEY

Wilms Tumor (Nephroblastoma) Is Composed of Embryonal Elements

Wilms tumor is a malignant neoplasm of embryonal nephrogenic elements composed of mixtures of blastemal, stromal, and epithelial tissue. It is the most frequent abdominal solid tumor in children, with a prevalence of 1 in 10,000.

Pathogenesis: In most (90%) cases of Wilms tumor, the neoplasm is sporadic and unilateral. In 5% of cases, however, Wilms tumor arises in the context of three different congenital syndromes, all of which include an increased risk for the development of this cancer at an early age and often bilaterally:

- **WAGR syndrome**—for **W**ilms tumor, **a**niridia, **g**enitourinary anomalies, mental **r**etardation
- **Denys-Drash syndrome (DDS)**—Wilms tumor, intersexual disorders, glomerulopathy
- **Beckwith-Wiedemann syndrome (BWS)**—Wilms tumor, overgrowth ranging from gigantism to hemihypertrophy, visceromegaly, and macroglossia

Some 6% of cases of Wilms tumor are familial, have an early onset, and are bilateral but are not associated with any other syndrome.

Two decades ago, karyotypic analysis of children with WAGR syndrome revealed a deletion in the short arm of one copy of chromosome 11 (11p13). We now understand that the WAGR deletion affects contiguous genes, including *PAX6*, the aniridia gene, and ***WT1*, the Wilms tumor gene**. The loss or mutation of one *WT1* allele leads to genitourinary anomalies, whereas a defect in the *PAX6* gene is responsible for aniridia. One third of children with WAGR syndrome eventually develop Wilms tumor. The presence of a germline mutation in one *WT1* allele and loss of heterozygosity at this locus in the tumors of WAGR syndrome imply that a second mutation in the normal *WT1* allele is responsible for the appearance of Wilms tumor (similar to the pathogenesis of hereditary retinoblastoma; see Chapter 5). In contrast to the deletions in WAGR syndrome, specific mutations of the *WT1* gene characterize DDS. The fact that the phenotypic expression of the abnormalities in DDS is far more severe than that in WAGR syndrome suggests that mutated *WT1* is actually a dysfunctional gene (dominant negative mutation).

WT1 is a tumor suppressor gene that functions as a regulator of the transcription of a number of other genes, including IGF-2 and PDGF. The *WT1* gene protein also forms a complex with the p53 protein. **Whereas Wilms tumors arising in the context of WAGR syndrome all display defects of *WT1*, less than 10% of sporadic tumors exhibit such abnormalities.** Thus, it is believed that other genes play a more critical role than does *WT1* in the genesis of sporadic Wilms tumors.

A second gene for susceptibility to Wilms tumor (**WT2**) was discovered in sporadic tumors that showed loss of heterozygosity (LOH) on chromosome 11 (11p15), a site distinct from, but close to, the *WT1* gene. *WT2* is also linked to BWS. Interestingly, in loss of heterozygosity at the *WT2* locus in sporadic Wilms tumors, the allele lost is invariably the maternal one. Importantly, some patients with BWS show a germline duplication of the paternal *WT2* allele, and others have inherited both apparently normal copies of this gene from the father and none from the mother (*paternal uniparental isodisomy*). One possibility is that *WT2* is normally expressed only by the paternal allele (*genomic imprinting*), and, therefore, overexpression of *WT2* may be responsible for the overgrowth characteristic of BWS. Since the *IGF-2* gene has also been mapped to chromosome 11p15 and is also paternally imprinted, it is possible that increased dosage of *IGF-2* might contribute both to BWS and to tumorigenesis. Another possibility is that *WT2* is expressed only by the maternal allele acting as a tumor suppressor. Thus, loss of the maternal allele would contribute to tumorigenesis.

Nephrogenic rests (small foci of persistent primitive blastemal cells) are found in the kidneys of all children with syndromic Wilms tumors and in one third of sporadic cases. Since such rests in the nontumorous kidney contain the same somatic mutations in *WT1* as are present in the tumors, it is thought that these rests represent clonal precursor lesions that are at least one step along the pathway to tumor formation.

Pathology: Wilms tumor tends to be large when detected, with a bulging, pale tan, cut surface enclosed within a thin rim of renal cortex and capsule (Fig. 16-85). Histologically, the tumor is composed of elements that resemble normal fetal tissue (Fig. 16-86), including (1) metanephric blastema, (2) immature stroma (mesenchymal tissue), and (3) immature epithelial elements.

Although most Wilms tumors contain all three elements in varying proportions, occasional ones contain only two elements or even only one. The component corresponding to blastema is composed of small ovoid cells with scanty cytoplasm, growing in nests and trabeculae. The epithelial component appears as small tubular structures. In some cases, structures resembling immature glomeruli are found. The stroma between the other elements is composed of spindle cells, which are mostly undifferentiated but occasionally display smooth muscle or fibroblast differentiation. Skeletal muscle is the most common heterotopic stromal element, although bone, cartilage, fat, or neural tissue may rarely be encountered.

Clinical Features: Wilms tumor usually presents between 1 and 3 years of age, and 98% occur before 10 years of age. The few familial cases usually exhibit autosomal dominant inheritance. Only 5% of sporadic

882   The Kidney

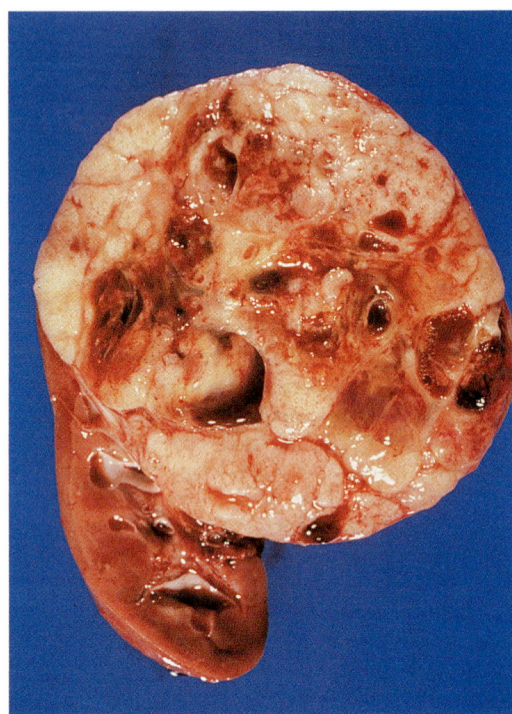

FIGURE 16-85
Wilms tumor. A cross-section of a pale tan neoplasm attached to a residual portion of the kidney.

cases are bilateral, contrasted with 20% of familial cases. Most often, the diagnosis is made after the recognition of an abdominal mass. Additional manifestations include abdominal pain, intestinal obstruction, hypertension, hematuria, and symptoms of traumatic rupture of the tumor.

A number of histological and clinical parameters have been used with varying success to predict the behavior of Wilms tumor. Patients younger than 2 years of age tend to have a better prognosis. Invasion of the tumor beyond the renal capsule, noted at the time of surgery, is a negative prognostic indicator. Anaplasia (nuclear enlargement, hyperchromasia, and atypical mitotic figures) also indicates a poorer prognosis. Anaplasia is more common in older patients, a feature that contributes to the overall worse prognosis in these cases. Chemotherapy and radiation therapy, combined with surgical resection, have dramatically improved the outlook of patients with this tumor, and many centers now report an overall long-term survival rate of 90%.

Renal Cell Carcinoma Is the Most Common Cancer of the Kidney

Renal cell carcinoma (RCC) is a malignant neoplasm of renal tubular or ductal epithelial cells. It accounts for 90% of all renal cancers and more than 11,000 cases a year in the United States. The incidence of this tumor worldwide has recently been increasing 2% annually.

 Pathogenesis: Most cases of RCC are sporadic, but about 5% are inherited. Hereditary RCC occurs in the context of three distinct syndromes:

- **Autosomal dominant RCC,** in which a clear cell tumor is the primary manifestation and occurs in half of the persons at risk
- **von Hippel-Lindau (VHL) disease,** an autosomal dominant cancer syndrome, characterized by the development of hemangioblastomas in the brain, retinal angiomas, clear cell RCC (40% of all cases of VHL disease), pheochromocytoma, and cysts in various organs
- **Hereditary papillary RCC**

All forms of hereditary RCC tend to be multifocal and bilateral, and they appear at a younger age than sporadic RCC. It is estimated that some 5% of cases of RCC are hereditary, and a family history of RCC places a person at a four-to five-fold increased risk for this malignancy.

In genetic studies of autosomal dominant RCC, a variety of translocations involving a breakpoint on chromosome 3 were recognized. Subsequently, studies of patients with sporadic RCC demonstrated consistent deletions and LOH in the short arm of chromosome 3 (3p) in the tumor tissue. Finally, the position of the *VHL* gene was similarly localized to 3p. *VHL* is a tumor suppressor gene. **Loss of one allele of the *VHL* gene occurs in virtually all (98%) sporadic clear cell RCC, and mutations in the gene are found in more than half of these tumors.** Thus, the evi-

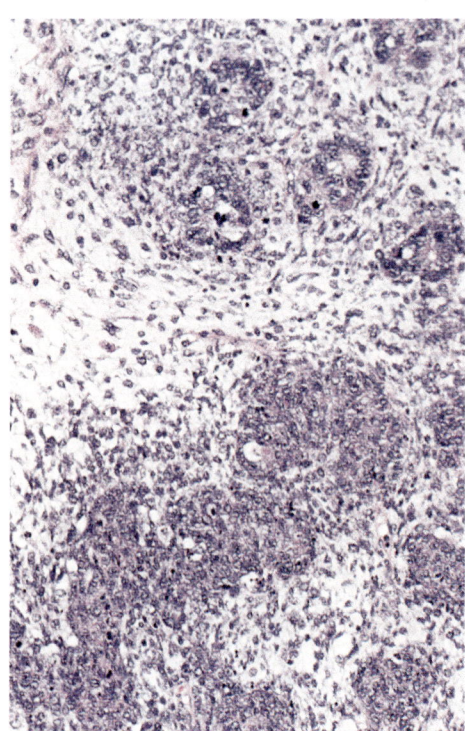

FIGURE 16-86
Wilms tumor (nephroblastoma). This photomicrograph of the tumor shows highly cellular areas composed of undifferentiated blastema, loose stroma containing undifferentiated mesenchymal cells, and immature tubules.

TABLE 16-16 **Categories of Renal Cell Carcinoma**

Category	Frequency (%)
Clear cell type	70–80
Papillary type	10–15
Chromophobe type	5
Collecting duct type	1

dence strongly suggests that loss of the tumor suppressive function of *VHL* is an important event in the genesis of clear cell RCC.

Unlike clear cell RCC, hereditary papillary RCC shows no association with the *VHL* gene. Trisomies of chromosomes 7, 16, and 17 and loss of the Y chromosome have been demonstrated in many cases. Mutations in the c-*met* protooncogene *(MET)* are implicated in the development of hereditary papillary RCC.

Tobacco, whether smoked or chewed, is associated with an increased risk of RCC, and one third of these tumors are linked to tobacco use. Both inherited and acquired cystic diseases of the kidney may be complicated by the development of renal cell carcinoma, especially papillary RCC. The cancer has also been tied to analgesic nephropathy.

Pathology: There are pathological variants of RCC that reflect differences in histogenesis and predict different outcomes. The various histological categories are shown in Table 16-16.

Clear cell RCC is the most common type and arises from proximal tubular epithelial cells. It is typically yellow-orange and often shows conspicuous focal hemorrhage and necrosis (Fig. 16-87). The tumors are solid or focally cystic.

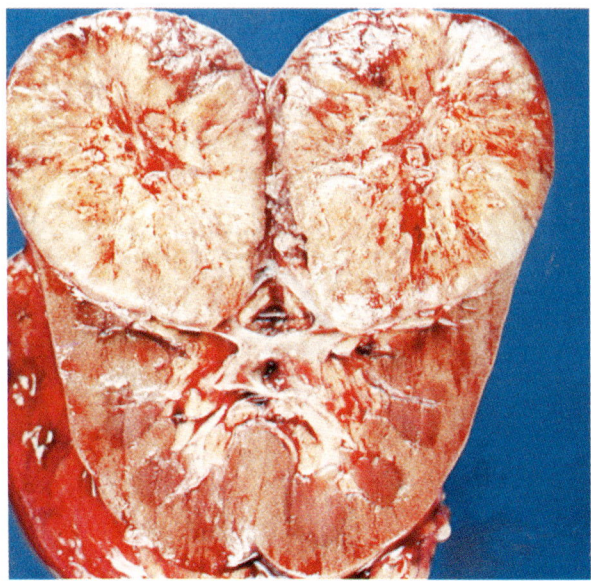

FIGURE 16-87
Clear cell renal cell carcinoma. The kidney contains a large irregular neoplasm with a variegated cut surface. Yellow areas correspond to lipid-containing cells.

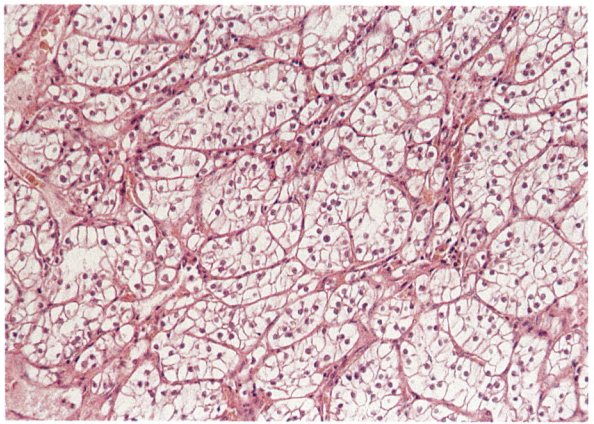

FIGURE 16-88
Clear cell renal cell carcinoma. Photomicrograph showing islands of neoplastic cells with abundant clear cytoplasm.

The clear cytoplasm of the neoplastic cells (Fig. 16-88) reflects the removal of abundant cytoplasmic lipids and glycogen by the water and solvents used in the preparation of the tissue. The cells are often arranged in round or elongated collections demarcated by a network of delicate vessels, and little cellular or nuclear pleomorphism is present. By electron microscopy, the neoplastic cells often resemble proximal tubular epithelial cells, with microvilli, membrane-associated vesicles involved in pinocytosis, and infolding of the plasma membrane.

Papillary RCC is characterized by neoplastic cells arranged on fibrovascular stalks. The tumor cells are typically cuboidal, with small round nuclei. The cytoplasm may be eosinophilic or basophilic. These tumors arise from proximal tubular epithelial cells.

Chromophobe RCC shows a mixture of acidophilic granular cells and pale transparent cells with prominent cell borders, which impart a plant cell-like appearance. The cytoplasm contains numerous vesicles filled with a distinctive type of mucopolysaccharide that can be stained with the Hale colloidal iron technique. In the pale cells, these vesicles displace other organelles to the periphery, causing a central cytoplasmic pallor. Chromophobe RCC appears to arise from the intercalated cells of renal collecting ducts.

Collecting duct RCC is a rare variety that arises from medullary collecting ducts but may extend into the cortex. Histologically, it is composed of tubular and papillary structures lined by a single layer of cuboidal cells that may have a hobnail appearance. Renal medullary carcinomas are a variant of collecting duct carcinomas that develop almost exclusively in African Americans with sickle cell trait or disease.

"Sarcomatoid" changes may occur in any variant of RCC and portends a worse clinical outcome. The recommended histological grading system for RCC is the Fuhrman system:

- **Grade I:** Nuclei round, uniform, 10 μm; nucleoli inconspicuous or absent
- **Grade II:** Nuclei irregular, 15 μm; nucleoli evident
- **Grade III:** Nuclei very irregular, 20 μm; nucleoli large and prominent
- **Grade IV:** Nuclei bizarre and multilobated, 20 μm or more; nucleoli prominent

Clinical Features: The incidence of RCC peaks in the sixth decade and is twice as frequent in men as in women. **The classic clinical triad of hematuria, flank pain, and a palpable abdominal mass** occurs in less than 10% of patients. Hematuria is the single most common presenting sign. Known in clinical medicine as one of the great mimics, RCC is a potential source of ectopic hormone production and is frequently associated with paraneoplastic syndromes. For example, secretion of a parathormone-like substance leads to hyperparathyroidism; production of erythropoietin causes erythrocytosis; the release of renin results in hypertension. Often a patient with RCC initially presents with symptoms due to a metastasis. For instance, a sudden convulsion or development of a cough in a previously healthy person leads to the discovery of an unsuspected tumor in the brain or lung, which proves on further examination to be RCC.

The prognosis for RCC is influenced by many factors, including tumor size, extent of invasion and metastasis, histological type, and nuclear grade. Few patients with prominent sarcomatoid features survive for more than 1 year. By contrast, 1-year overall survival after nephrectomy for clear cell RCC is 50%. The papillary and chromophobe types have a better prognosis than the clear cell type. Tumor stage (a measure of invasion and metastasis) is the most important prognostic factor. The 5-year survival is 90% if the RCC has not extended beyond the renal capsule; survival drops to 30% if there are distant metastases. The tumor spreads most frequently to the lung and the bones.

Transitional Cell Carcinoma

Between 5 and 10% of primary neoplasms of the kidney are transitional cell carcinomas of the renal pelvis or calyces (see Chapter 17). These are morphologically identical to the more common transitional cell carcinomas of the urinary bladder and are associated with them in half of cases. Less than 5% of transitional cell carcinomas occur in the collecting system proximal to the bladder.

SUGGESTED READING

Books

Jennette JC, Olson JL, Schwartz MM, Silva FG: *Heptinstall's pathology of the kidney*, 5th ed. Boston: Little, Brown, 1998.

Murphy WM: *Urological pathology*, 2nd ed. Philadelphia: WB Saunders, 1997.

Murphy WM, Beckwith JB, Farrow GM: *Tumors of the kidney, bladder and related urinary structures.* Washington, DC: Armed Forces Institute of Pathology, 1994.

Silva FG, D Agati VD, Nadasdy T: *Renal biopsy interpretation.* New York: Churchill Livingstone, 1996.

Review Articles

Colvin RB: The renal allograft biopsy. *Kidney Int* 50:1069–1082, 1996.

Couser WG: Pathogenesis of glomerulonephritis. *Kidney Int* 44(suppl 42):S19–S26, 1993.

D'Agati VD: Morphologic features of cyclosporin nephrotoxicity. *Contrib Nephrol* 114:84–110, 1995.

Freedman BI, Iskandar SS, Appel RG: The link between hypertension and nephrosclerosis. *Am J Kidney Dis* 25:207–221, 1995.

Glassock RJ, Cohen AH: The primary glomerulopathies. *Disease-A-Month* 42:329–383, 1996.

Harris PC, Ward CJ, Peral B, Hughes J: Polycystic kidney disease 1: Identification and analysis of the primary defect. *J Am Soc Nephrol* 6:1125–1133, 1995.

Jennette JC, Falk RJ: Small Vessel Vasculitis. *N Engl J Med* 337:1512–1523, 1997.

Jennette JC, Falk RJ: Diagnosis and management of glomerular diseases. *Med Clin N Am* 81:653–677, 1997.

Linehan WM, Lerman MI, Zbar B: Identification of the von Hipple-Lindau (VHL) gene. Its role in renal cancer. *JAMA* 273:564–570, 1995.

Mauiyyedi S, Crespo M, Collins AB, et al.: Acute humoral rejection in kidney transplantation: II. Morphology, immunopathology, and pathological classification. *J Am Soc Nephrol* 13:779–787, 2002.

Pantuck AJ, Zisman A, Belldegrun A: Biology of renal cell carcinoma: Changing concepts in classification and staging. *Semin Urol Oncol* 19:72–79, 2001.

Reddy JC, Licht JD: The WT1 Wilms tumor suppressor gene. How much do we really know? *Biochim Biophys Acta* 1287:1–28, 1996.

Ruggenenti P, Remuzzi G: Malignant vascular disease of the kidney: Nature of the lesion, mediators of disease progression, and the case for bilateral nephrectomy. *Am J Kidney Dis* 27:459–475, 1996.

Silva FG, Hogg RJ: Glomerular lesions associated with the acute nephritic syndrome and hematuria. *Semin Diagn Pathol* 5:4–38, 1988.

Weber M: Rapidly progressive glomerulonephritis: Recent advances in pathogenesis, diagnosis and therapy. *Clin Invest* 71:825–829, 1993.

CHAPTER 17

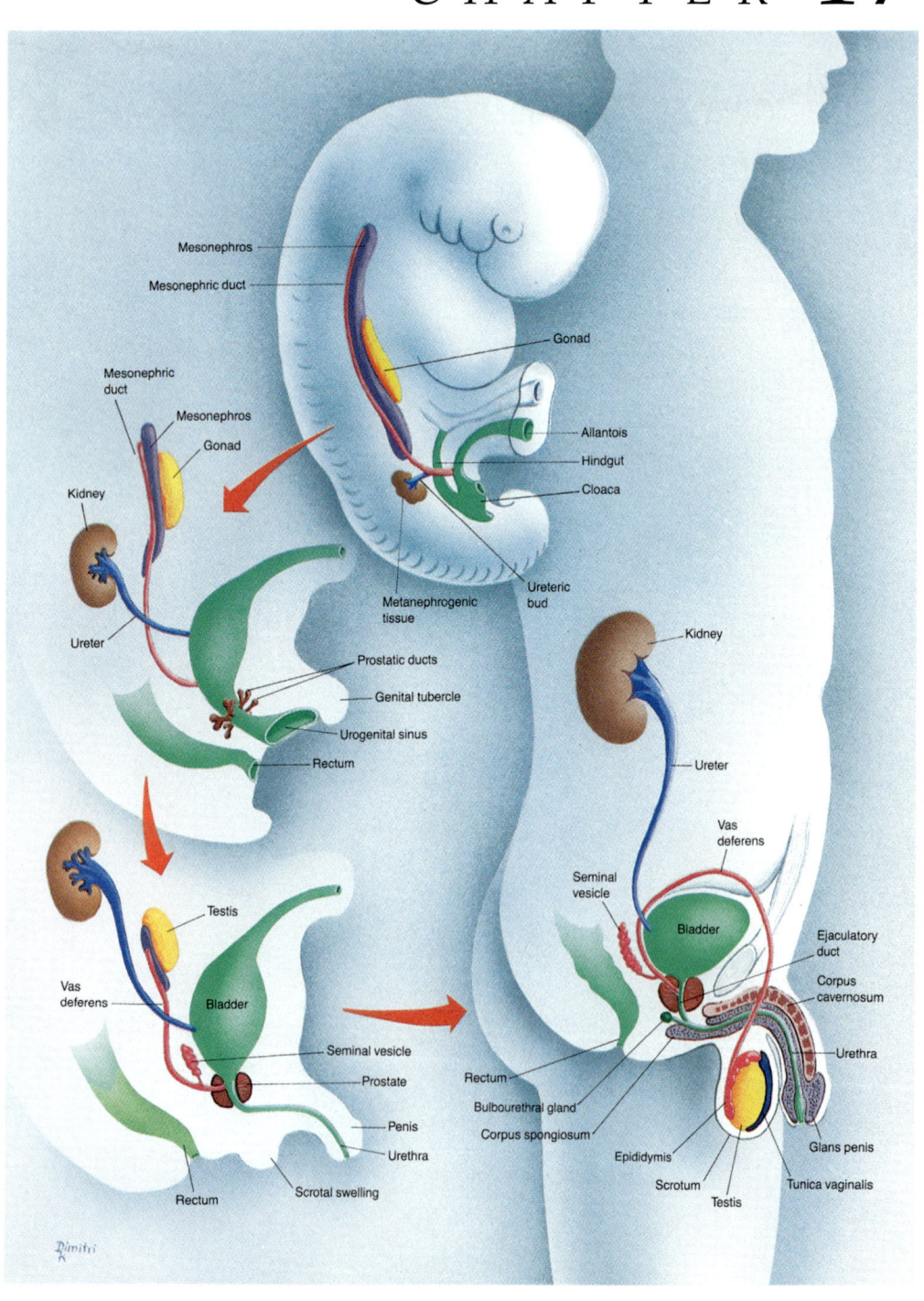

The Lower Urinary Tract and Male Reproductive System

Ivan Damjanov

Anatomy and Embryology

Lower Urinary Tract
Urinary Bladder
Ureters
Urethra
Histological Features
Embryology

Male Reproductive System
Embryology

Renal Pelvis and Ureter

Congenital Disorders

Ureteritis and Ureteral Obstruction

Tumors

Urinary Bladder

Congenital Disorders

Cystitis
Special Forms of Chronic Cystitis

Benign Proliferative and Metaplastic Urothelial Lesions

Tumors
Transitional (Urothelial) Cell Papilloma
Transitional Cell Carcinoma in Situ
Transitional Cell Carcinoma
Rare Forms of Bladder Cancer

Penis, Urethra, and Scrotum

Congenital Disorders of the Penis

Scrotal Masses

Circulatory Disturbances

Inflammatory Disorders
Balanitis

Urethritis and Related Conditions

(continued)

FIGURE 17-1 *(see opposite page)*
Embryological development of the urinary tract and male reproductive system.

Tumors

Cancer of the Urethra

Cancer of the Scrotum

Testis, Epididymis, and Vas Deferens

Cryptorchidism

Abnormalities of Sexual Differentiation

Epididymitis

Orchitis

Tumors of the Testis

Intratubular Germ Cell Neoplasia

Seminoma

Prostate

Prostatitis

Nodular Hyperplasia of the Prostate

Adenocarcinoma of the Prostate

Anatomy and Embryology

LOWER URINARY TRACT

The ureters, urinary bladder and the urethra, also known as the lower urinary tract, form the outflow part of the urinary system (Fig. 17-1). In males, the lower urinary tract is closely related to the reproductive system.

Urinary Bladder

The urinary bladder is located in the retroperitoneal space of the lower abdominal cavity In males, the bladder is anterior to the rectum and superior to the prostate. In females, it is anterior to the lower uterine corpus and anterior vaginal fornix.

The urinary bladder can be subdivided anatomically into several parts: the apex (dome), the midportion, and the base, the last comprising the trigone and the bladder neck. The apex is located behind the margin of the symphysis pubis and is linked in the midline to the umbilicus by the umbilical ligament, a fibrous strand representing the involuted fetal *urachus*. In males, the neck of the bladder rests on the upper surface of the prostate, where the smooth muscle fibers of the two organs intertwine. Inside the bladder, the posterior aspect of the base of the bladder has a triangular shape and is called the *trigone*, a region that is devoid of mucosal folds and appears flattened. Superiorly, the trigone is bound by a muscular ridge joining the laterally placed orifices of the ureters. The inferior tip of the trigone is formed by the funnel-shaped internal orifice of the urethra.

Ureters

The ureters are paired organs linking each renal pelvis with the bladder. Like the kidneys, they are located in the posterior retroperitoneal space lateral to the vertebral column. The lowermost part of the ureters is embedded in the wall of the urinary bladder, which forms the *ureterovesical valves*. These valves allow the passage of urine downward from the ureters into the urinary bladder but not passage in the opposite direction.

Urethra

The urethra is the terminal part of the urinary outflow tract. The male urethra, on average 20 cm long, is divided into (1) the prostatic urethra, extending through the prostate; (2) the membranous urethra, penetrating through the pelvic floor; and (3) the spongy or penile urethra, occupying the central portion of the penis. The prostatic urethra contains the ostia of the ejaculatory and prostatic ducts. The posterior part of the penile urethra, also labeled *bulbous urethra,* receives the secretions from the mucous bulbourethral (Cowper) glands. The penile urethra terminates in the fossa navicularis, immediately proximal to the external orifice, or meatus, located on the tip of the penis.

The female urethra is shorter than the male urethra, measuring only 3 to 4 cm in length. It extends from its internal orifice at the urinary bladder to its external orifice in the vulva, immediately below the clitoris. The wall of the female urethra also contains mucous glands.

Histological Features

The ureters, the urinary bladder, and the posterior urethra are lined by transitional epithelium, also known as *urothelium*. The terminal parts of the urethra are lined by squamous epithelium. The urothelium consists of three epithelial zones. The basal layer lies on a basement membrane and contains cells that can divide and replace damaged superficial cells. Above the basal layer are 3 to 4 layers of polygonal cells that form the intermediate zone. Both the basal and the polygonal cells can flatten when the bladder dilates. The superficial layer of the urothelium consists of "umbrella cells," which are resistant to the urine that constantly bathes them.

Underneath the epithelium lies the lamina propria, composed principally of loose connective tissue and blood vessels. The muscularis mucosae is incomplete and poorly developed. The lamina propria is externally surrounded by a thick muscle layer that is covered by adventitia. Since the urinary bladder, ureters, and urethra are retroperitoneal, they do not have an external serosa. The only part of the lower urinary tract that has serosa is the dome of the bladder.

Embryology

The lower urinary tract develops to a large extent from the cloaca, a fetal structure that is partitioned early during ontogenesis into an anterior part, the urogenital sinus, and the posterior part, which is the primordium of the rectum. The urogenital sinus is the anlage of the urinary bladder, the proximal urethra, and the urachus, a temporary fetal structure connecting the urinary tract with the umbilicus. The caudal urogenital sinus makes contact with an invagination of the urogenital membrane, thereby forming the urethra. The urachus gradually involutes into the umbilical ligament. The fetal urinary bladder forms symmetrical lateral outpouchings that grow cranially as ureteric buds. When these epithelial buds reach the nephrogenic zone, they induce the formation of the metanephros, the primordium of the kidneys.

MALE REPRODUCTIVE SYSTEM

The male reproductive system comprises the testis, epididymis, ductus (vas) deferens, seminal vesicles, prostate and penis (Fig. 17-1). The adult testis is located in the scrotum and measures 4 by 3 by 3 cm. Along the lateral–posterior aspect of the testis lies the epididymis, which extends into the ductus deferens. The testis is invested with the *tunica vaginalis,* a layer of mesothelial cells that covers the outer fibrous capsule of the testis, the *tunica albuginea.* This capsule has internal septal ramifications that divide the testis into about 250 lobules. Each lobule consists of coiled seminiferous tubules and loose interstitial tissue containing blood vessels and interstitial cells of Leydig.

The *arterial supply* to the testis is through the testicular arteries, which originate from the abdominal aorta. The *venous drainage* is a dual system: the right internal spermatic vein empties into the vena cava, and the left drains into the ipsilateral renal vein. This anatomical difference has several clinical implications discussed below.

Seminiferous tubules, the principal functional unit of the testis, contain the seminiferous epithelium and Sertoli cells, which provide support to *spermatogenesis.* **Sertoli cells** also secrete *inhibin,* which provides feedback information to the pituitary, thereby regulating the secretion of *gonadotropins,* namely, follicle-stimulating hormone (FSH) and luteinizing hormone (LH). The interstitial spaces of the testis contain **Leydig cells,** the primary source of *testosterone.*

In prepubertal testes the seminiferous tubules contain two cell types: **germ cells** at the stage of spermatogonia and **Sertoli cells.** At puberty, LH stimulates Leydig cells to produce testosterone and initiate spermatogenesis, and FSH acts on both germ cells and Sertoli cells to support spermatogenesis.

Hormonal stimuli lead to an increased number of germ cells, primarily *spermatogonia,* which also begin differentiating into primary *spermatocytes.* The meiotic division of primary spermatocytes leads to the formation of *secondary spermatocytes,* which contain a haploid number (23) of chromosomes. Secondary spermatocytes mature to *spermatids,* and the latter to *spermatozoa,* which are discharged through the channels of rete testis into the epididymal ducts. In the **epididymis,** spermatozoa are admixed with the fluid secreted by the epididymal lining cells and are carried through the **vas deferens,** which empties its contents into the urethra. The final semen to be *ejaculated* through the penile urethra is formed by the mixing of the spermatozoa in the epididymal secretions with the fluids produced by the **accessory glands,** namely, the seminal vesicles, prostate, Cowper bulbourethral glands, and urethral glands.

The prostate is the largest and the most important accessory gland. It is located in the pelvis in contact with the posterior and inferior external layers of the urinary bladder, close to the rectum. Anatomically, the prostate can be divided into five parts: anterior, middle, posterior, and two lateral lobes. Microscopically it is a tubuloalveolar gland with a rich fibromuscular stroma. The prostate develops under the influence of testosterone, which is essential for maintaining its production of seminal fluid.

Embryology

The embryology of the male reproductive system is complex because it develops from several embryological anlagen. The testes develop from the *genital ridges,* which form on the posterior surface of the celomic cavity. These ridges are populated by migratory *primordial germ cells* (formed initially in the yolk sac) that enter the fetal body through the midline and then migrate laterally into the right and left genital ridges. Complex interactions of germ cells and stromal cells in the genital ridges lead to formation of the fetal testes, which are located on the posterior wall of the midabdomen. At the same time, the testes connect with the future epididymis and the vas deferens, which develop from the *wolffian ducts.* At that point the testes begin their gradual descent into the inguinal canal, through which they finally reach the scrotum.

The scrotum and the penis develop simultaneously with the testes but from another anlage that corresponds predominantly to the *genital tubercle* and partly to the anterior *urogenital sinus.* These primordia of the external genital organs are initially identical in both sexes. In the male fetus they develop under the influence of testosterone into the penis, penile urethra, and scrotum, whereas in the female they give rise to the clitoris, labia minora, and labia majora.

Renal Pelvis and Ureter

CONGENITAL DISORDERS

Developmental anomalies of the renal pelvis and ureters are found in 2 to 3% of all persons. In most instances they cause no clinical problems, but on occasion they predispose to obstruction and infections of the urinary tract. The most important developmental anomalies of the renal pelves and ureters include agenesis, ectopia, duplications, obstructions, and dilations (Fig. 17-2).

AGENESIS OF THE RENAL PELVIS AND URETERS: This rare anomaly is always associated with agenesis of the corresponding kidney. Unilateral agenesis is usually asymp-

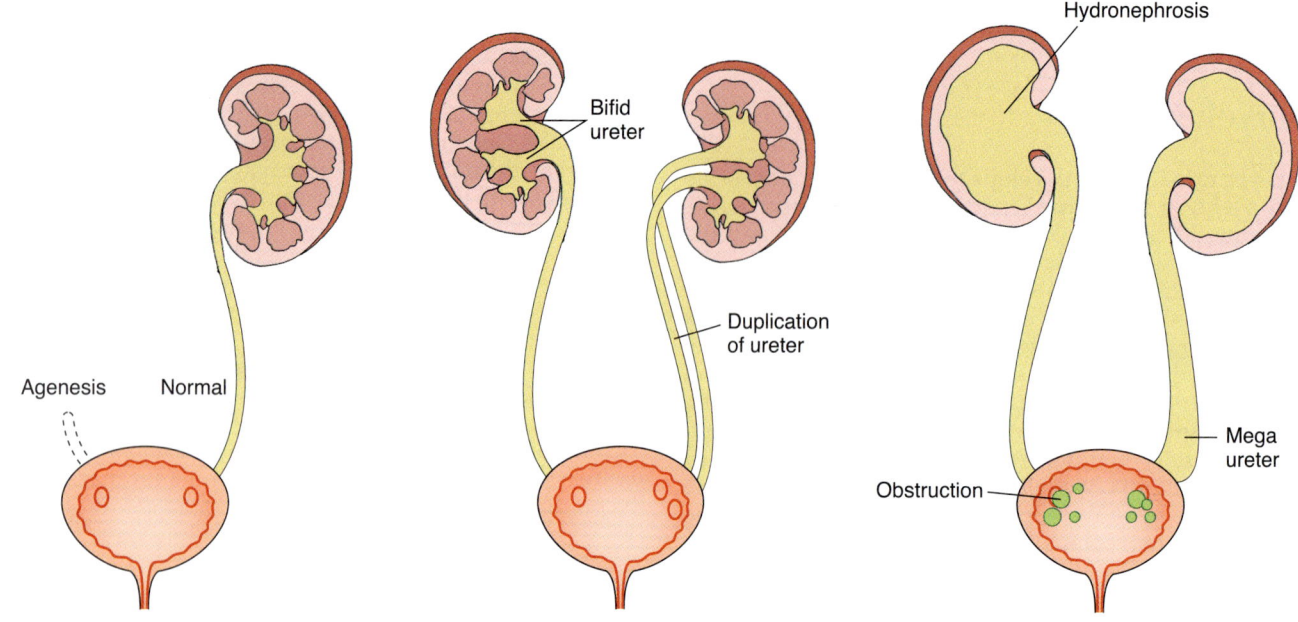

FIGURE 17-2
Anomalies of the renal pelves and ureters.

tomatic. Bilateral agenesis of the ureters and kidneys, a feature of *Potter syndrome*, is incompatible with life.

ECTOPIC URETERS: Ureteric buds may develop at the wrong anatomical site during embryogenesis. The lower orifices of ectopic ureters can be found in many anomalous places, such as midportion of the urinary bladder, the seminal vesicles, urethra, or vas deferens.

DUPLICATIONS: Single or multiple ureteric buds may be duplicated on the side of the fetal urinary bladder. The duplications may be unilateral or bilateral, complete or partial. Usually there are two parallel ureters, each with its own renal pelvis and separate vesical orifice. *Bifid ureters* (subdivided by a septum), *bifurcate ureters*, and many other variations of this anomaly can be encountered, but most are of no clinical significance.

OBSTRUCTIONS OF THE URETERS: Obstructions can be traced to congenital *atresia* or abnormal *ureteral valves*. However, congenital *obstruction of the ureteropelvic junction*, the most common form of hydronephrosis in infants and children, cannot be explained in those terms. It is thought to be related to abnormal layering of smooth muscle cells and/or fibrosis replacing the smooth muscle cells at the site of the ureteropelvic junction. Urinary obstruction in these children is usually unilateral, but in 20% of cases it is bilateral. This form of hydronephrosis is often associated with other urinary tract anomalies and, in some cases, with agenesis of the contralateral kidney.

DILATIONS OF THE RENAL PELVIS OR THE URETERS: can be localized in the form of *diverticula* or generalized. The dilation involving the entire ureter, known as *congenital megaureter*, may be unilateral or bilateral. The possible causes or the pathogenesis of congenital megaureters are mostly unknown. The ureters are tortuous and lack peristalsis. The resulting stagnation of urine *(hydroureter)* is typically associated with progressive hydronephrosis that ultimately leads to renal failure.

URETERITIS AND URETERAL OBSTRUCTION

Ureteritis is an inflammation of the ureters, which occurs as a complication of descending infections of the kidneys or may be due to ascending infections in vesicoureteric reflux. Ureteritis is often associated with ureteral obstruction, which may be either intrinsic or extrinsic (Fig. 17-3).
   Intrinsic causes of ureteral obstruction include calculi, intraluminal blood clots, fibroepithelial polyps, inflammatory strictures, amyloidosis, and tumors of the ureter.
   Extrinsic causes of ureteral obstruction include aberrant renal vessels to the lower pole of the kidney that cross the ureter, endometriosis, and tumors in adjacent lymph nodes. In addition, the pregnant uterus can compress the ureters.
   Ureteral obstruction may also result from diseases that involve the urinary bladder, prostate, and urethra. Such disorders include cancer of the bladder in the vicinity of the ureteral orifice or bladder neck, neurogenic bladder, and prostatic hyperplasia. Proximal causes of ureteral obstruction tend to be unilateral, whereas more distal ones, such as prostatic hyperplasia, lead to bilateral hydronephrosis, with the possibility of renal failure in untreated cases.
   Idiopathic retroperitoneal fibrosis is *a distinctly uncommon cause of ureteral obstruction, which is characterized by dense fibrosis of the retroperitoneal soft tissues and a modest, nonspecific, chronic inflammatory reaction.* As the name implies, the etiology is unknown, although the use of certain drugs (methysergide, β-adrenergic blockers) and autoimmunity have been proposed as causes. On occasion, idiopathic retroperitoneal fibrosis is accompanied by inflammatory fibrosis in

Congenital Disorders

"target organ." The renal pelvis and ureters are the site of origin of 5% of all urothelial tumors.

Patients most frequently present in their sixth and seventh decades with hematuria (80%) and flank pain (25%). Transitional cell carcinoma of the ureter or renal pelvis requires radical nephroureterectomy. Excision of the entire ureter is necessary because of the high frequency of concurrent and subsequent transitional cell carcinomas. The prognosis is related to the tumor stage at the time of diagnosis.

Urinary Bladder

CONGENITAL DISORDERS

Congenital malformations of the urinary bladder include (1) exstrophy of the bladder, (2) diverticula, (3) urachal remnants, and (4) congenital incompetence of the vesicoureteral valve.

EXSTROPHY OF THE BLADDER: *This developmental abnormality is characterized by the absence of the anterior wall bladder and a portion of the anterior abdominal wall.* The estimated frequency of this anomaly is 1 per 50,000 births. In some male infants it is associated with *epispadias* (i.e., incomplete formation of the penile urethra).

Exstrophy of the bladder develops from incomplete resorption of the anterior cloacal membrane. In normal embryogenesis this membrane is replaced by smooth muscle, but if it persists, it forms the anterior vesical wall. Since the membrane is thin, it ultimately ruptures, leaving a large defect that is accompanied by defective closure of the anterior muscular wall of the abdominal cavity. These two defects expose the posterior wall of the bladder to the exterior and transform the bladder into a cuplike organ that cannot hold urine (Fig. 17-4). The posterior wall of the bladder exposed to mechanical injury undergoes squamous or glandular metaplasia and is prone to frequent infections. Although exstrophy can be surgically repaired, the metaplastic bladder mucosa remains at increased risk for malignant transformation. In fact, a greater than expected incidence of bladder

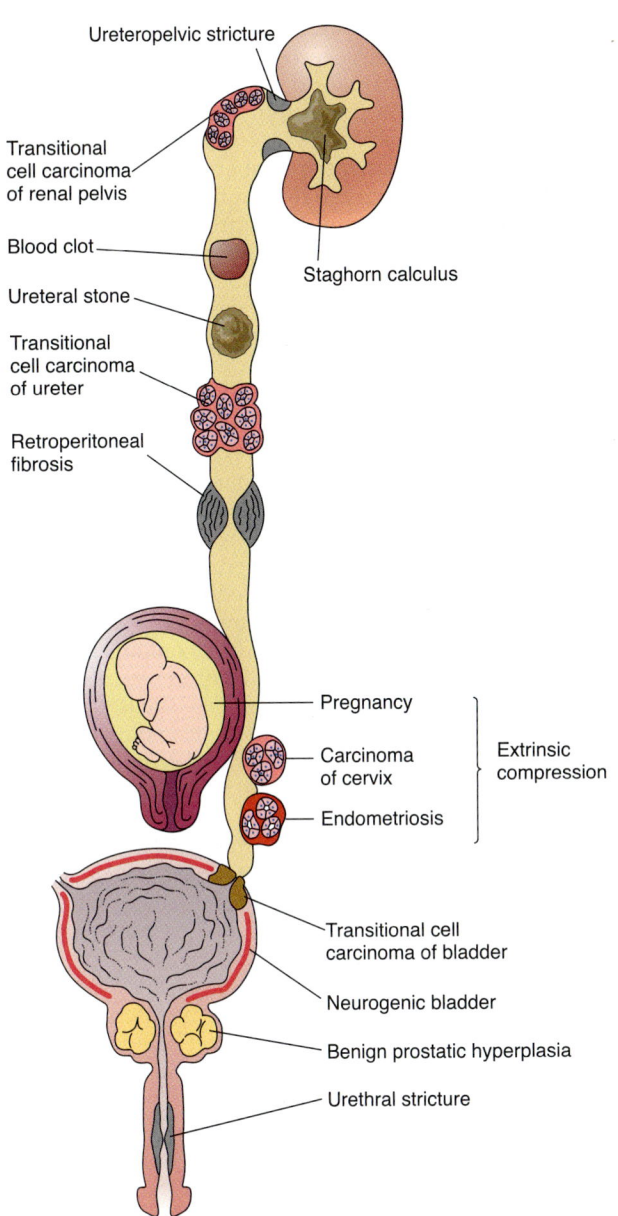

FIGURE 17-3
Most common causes of ureteral obstruction.

other areas, including Riedel struma (thyroid), sclerosing cholangitis (liver), and mediastinal fibrosis. The disease may respond to treatment with corticosteroids and immunosuppressive agents.

TUMORS

Tumors of the renal pelvis and ureter resemble those of the urinary bladder except for the fact that they are much less common. Histologically, most (>90%) are **transitional cell carcinomas.** The etiologic factors associated with epithelial tumors of the renal pelvis and ureter are similar to those observed in bladder cancer, suggesting a "field effect" in which the entire urothelial mucosa represents a continuous

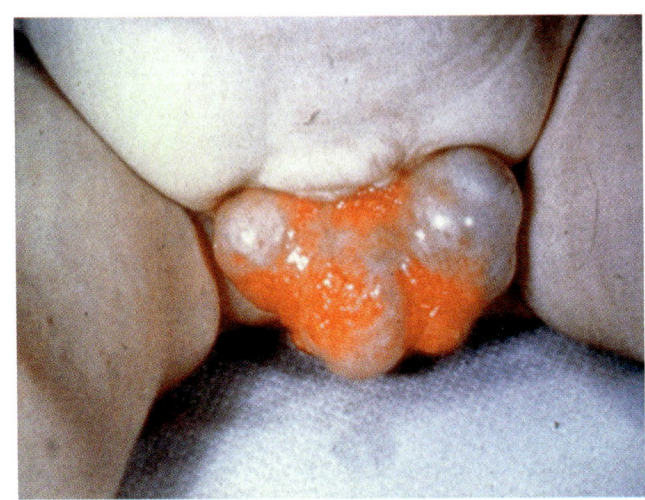

FIGURE 17-4
Exstrophy of the urinary bladder.

cancer has been reported in persons who have lived for 50 to 60 years after surgical repair of exstrophy.

DIVERTICULA: *These saclike outpouchings of the bladder wall are related to incomplete formation of the muscular layers.* They can be solitary or multiple. Urine retained inside such diverticula is commonly infected, a complication that may lead to the formation of urinary stones. Congenital diverticula must be distinguished from *acquired vesical diverticula* that typically occur in long-standing urinary tract obstruction caused by prostatic hyperplasia.

URACHAL REMNANTS: *The urachus (i.e., the fetal allantoic stalk connecting the urinary bladder and the umbilicus) may undergo incomplete involution..* If the urachus remains patent throughout, it forms a *vesical–umbilical fistula.* Incomplete regression of the urinary end, midportion, or umbilical end of the urachus results in an *urachal diverticulum, umbilical–urachal sinus,* or *urachal cyst,* respectively. The columnar epithelium of the urachal remnants may give rise to *adenocarcinoma.* Although these tumors account for only 0.2% of the bladder cancers, they represent one third of bladder adenocarcinomas.

CONGENITAL INCOMPETENCE OF THE VESICOURETERAL VALVE: *This anomaly results from an abnormal junction between the ureters and the urinary bladder.* The ureters normally enter the wall of the bladder obliquely and have a long intravesical portion. The muscle layer of the urinary bladder serves as a sphincter that prevents the backflow of urine into the normal ureters during micturition. By contrast, ureters that enter the bladder perpendicularly have a short intravesical segment, which does not adequately protect against backflow of urine during micturition. **Vesicoureteric reflux** (VUR) is more common in young girls than boys and is often familial. In 75% of cases, VUR is asymptomatic, but in the remaining cases, it is an important cause of reflux pyelonephritis. Congenital VUR is distinguished from the acquired form that occurs during pregnancy or in conditions associated with bladder hypertrophy.

CYSTITIS

Cystitis is an inflammation of the urinary bladder that may be acute or chronic. It is the most frequent urinary tract infection and is a common nosocomial infection in hospitalized patients.

Pathogenesis: In most cases cystitis is secondary to infection of the lower urinary tract. Factors related to bladder infection include the age and sex of the patient, presence of bladder calculi, bladder outlet obstruction, diabetes mellitus, immunodeficiency, prior instrumentation or catheterization, radiation therapy, and chemotherapy. The risk of cystitis in females is increased because of a short urethra, especially during pregnancy. Bladder outlet obstruction secondary to prostatic hyperplasia predisposes men to cystitis. Introduction of pathogens into the bladder may also occur during instrumentation (cystoscopy) and is particularly common in patients in whom indwelling catheters remain for prolonged periods.

In most cases, coliform bacteria are the cause of cystitis, most frequently *Escherichia coli, Proteus vulgaris, Pseudomonas aeruginosa,* and *Enterobacter* spp. Tuberculosis of the bladder is almost always secondary to renal tuberculosis. Fungal cystitis may be seen in immunosuppressed patients. Gas-forming bacilli, usually in persons with diabetes, may produce characteristic interstitial bubbles in the lamina propria of the urinary bladder *(emphysematous cystitis).* Virtually unknown in the Western world, schistosomiasis as a cause of cystitis is common in areas where *Schistosoma haematobium* is endemic, namely, North Africa and the Middle East.

Pathology: Stromal edema, hemorrhage, and a neutrophilic infiltrate of variable intensity are typical of acute cystitis (Fig. 17-5). Lack of resolution of the inflammatory reaction is associated with the hallmarks of chronic inflammation, including a predominance of lymphocytes (Fig. 17-6) and fibrosis of the lamina propria. Occasionally, the mucosa of the inflamed bladder contains numerous lymphocytic follicles *(follicular cystitis)* or dense infiltrates of eosinophils *(eosinophilic cystitis).* Granulomatous *cystitis* is a feature of tuberculosis. Ova of *S. hematobium* can cause simultaneous granulomatous reactions and eosinophilic infiltrates. The specific pathological forms of chronic cystitis include the following:

Hemorrhagic cystitis: Focal petechial hemorrhages in the mucosa are often seen in acute bacterial cystitis. Bleeding diatheses (e.g., leukemia or treatment with cytotoxic drugs) and disseminated intravascular coagulation often cause extensive hemorrhagic cystitis.

Ulcerative cystitis: Chronic irritation, caused for example by indwelling catheters or traumatic cystoscopy, may be followed by ulceration and focal mucosal hemorrhage. *Solitary mucosal ulcer* is also found in interstitial cystitis (see below).

Suppurative cystitis: Pus may cover the bladder mucosa, fill the lumen or permeate the wall. Suppurative cystitis may develop in the course of local infection, but more often it is a complication of sepsis, pyelonephritis, or purulent infections secondary to bladder surgery.

Pseudomembranous cystitis: Pseudomembranes (i.e., shaggy layers of necrotic, gray, or yellow material) sometimes cover the mucosa of the urinary bladder. They can be removed to expose the underlying hemorrhagic ulcerated mucosa. Typically, pseudomembranous cystitis is a complication of infection that follows treatment with cytotoxic drugs, most often cyclophosphamide. Pseudomembranes consist of cell detritus, fibrin, inflammatory cells, and blood.

Calcific cystitis: This form of chronic inflammation is typically found in schistosomiasis. Calcification of ova produces encrustations of the bladder wall similar to grains of sand. These grains gradually coalesce and transform the entire urinary bladder into a calcified rigid vessel.

Clinical Features: Virtually all patients with acute or chronic cystitis complain of excessive frequency of urination, pain on urination *(dysuria),* and lower abdominal or pelvic discomfort. Examination of the urine usually reveals inflammatory cells, and the causative

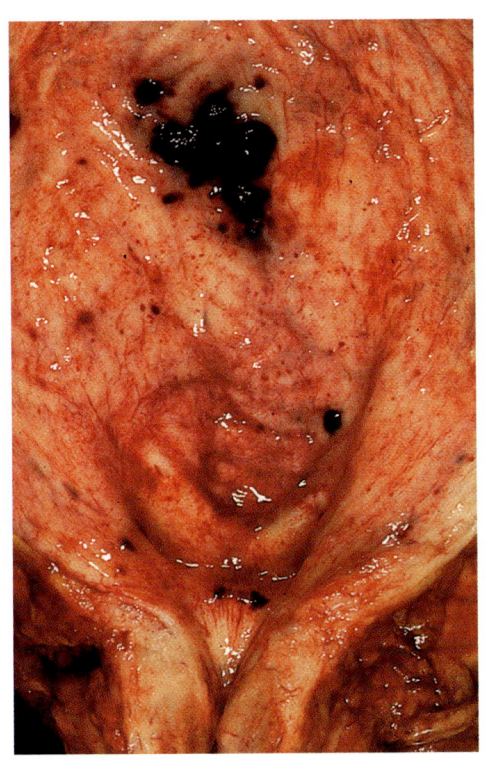
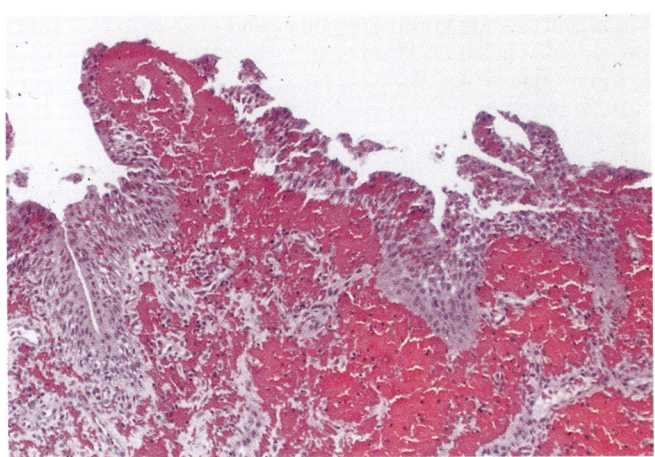

FIGURE 17-5
Acute hemorrhagic cystitis. The patient died 2 days after surgery, and the cystitis was obviously caused by an indwelling catheter. A. Several foci of hemorrhage are seen on the hyperemic bladder mucosa. B. Microscopic foci of mucosal hemorrhage.

agent can be identified by urine culture. Most cases of cystitis respond well to treatment with antimicrobial agents.

Special Forms of Chronic Cystitis

CHRONIC INTERSTITIAL CYSTITIS: This disorder of unknown cause, typically affects middle-aged women, and features transmural inflammation of the bladder wall, which is occasionally associated with mucosal ulceration **(Hunner ulcer)** *(Fig. 17-7).* Chronic inflammation, including an increased number of

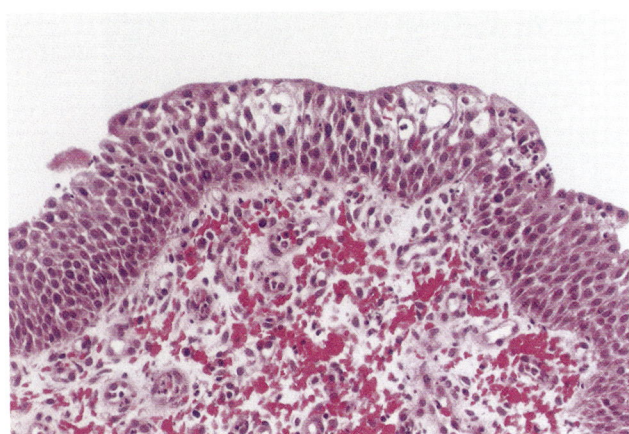

FIGURE 17-6
Chronic cystitis. A nonspecific inflammatory infiltrate composed of lymphocytes and plasma cells is present in the edematous lamina propria.

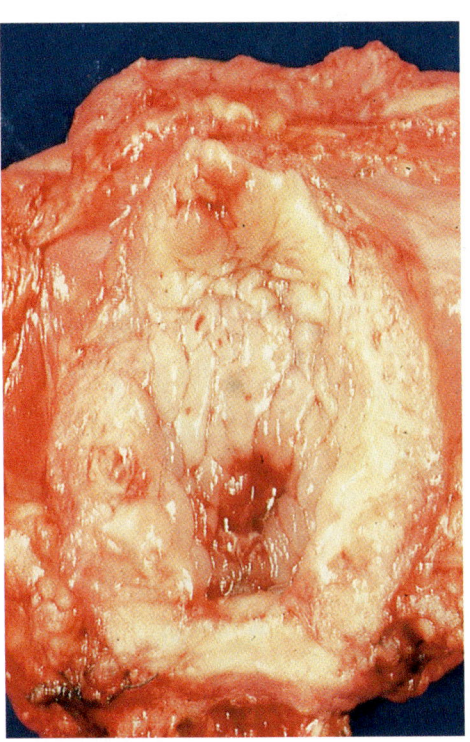

FIGURE 17-7
Interstitial cystitis. The hemorrhagic defect in the edematous mucosa of the posterior wall of the bladder is clinically known as Hunner ulcer.

mast cells, and fibrosis are commonly observed within the mucosa and the muscularis. A Hunner ulcer displays an intense acute inflammatory reaction.

The most common symptoms of chronic interstitial cystitis are long-standing suprapubic pain, frequency, and urgency, with or without hematuria. At cystoscopy, mucosal edema, focal petechiae, and irregular hemorrhagic areas, most often in the dome and posterior wall, are characteristic. Urine cultures are usually negative. The disease is typically persistent and refractory to all forms of therapy

MALAKOPLAKIA (Gk. malakos, soft; plax, plaque): *An uncommon inflammatory disorder of unknown etiology, malakoplakia is identified by the accumulation of characteristic macrophages.* The disorder was originally described in the bladder, but it has since been observed in numerous other sites, both within and outside the urinary tract. Malakoplakia is found in all age groups, the peak frequency occurring in the fifth to seventh decades. There is a marked preponderance of cases in women, regardless of the site.

Malakoplakia is often associated with an infection of the urinary tract by *E. coli*, although a direct causal relationship is dubious. A clinical background of immunosuppression, chronic infections, or cancer is common.

Pathology: Malakoplakia is characterized by soft, yellow plaques on the mucosal surface of the bladder (Fig. 17-8). Histologically, the most striking feature is a chronic inflammatory cell infiltrate composed predominantly of large macrophages with abundant, eosinophilic cytoplasm containing periodic acid–Schiff (PAS)-positive granules *(von Hansemann cells)*. Some of these macrophages exhibit laminated, basophilic calcospherites, termed *Michaelis-Gutmann bodies*. Ultrastructurally, the granules of the von Hansemann cells are engorged lysosomes that contain fragments of bacteria, suggesting that malakoplakia may reflect an acquired defect in lysosomal degradation. The Michaelis-Gutmann bodies result from the deposition of calcium salts in these enlarged lysosomes.

The urinary bladder is the most common site of malakoplakia, with half of cases occurring in this organ. This enigmatic disorder has also been reported in other regions of the genitourinary system, including the kidney, renal pelvis, ureter, testis, epididymis, and prostate. The colon, bones, and lungs have also been sites of malakoplakia. The clinical symptomatology of malakoplakia is indistinguishable from that of other forms of chronic cystitis, and treatment is ineffective.

BENIGN PROLIFERATIVE AND METAPLASTIC UROTHELIAL LESIONS

Benign proliferative and metaplastic lesions of the urothelium occur most often in the urinary bladder but may be found in the entire urinary tract, from the renal pelvis to the urethra. These nonneoplastic lesions are characterized either by hyperplasia or by combined hyperplasia and metaplasia (Fig. 17-9). They are mostly found in association with chronic inflammation caused by urinary tract infections, calculi, neurogenic bladder, and (rarely) bladder exstrophy. They are also occasionally observed in the absence of any preexisting inflammatory condition.

Brunn buds are bulbous invaginations of the surface urothelium into the lamina propria. They are found in over 85% of bladders and are considered normal variants of the epithelium.

Brunn nests are similar to Brunn buds, but the urothelial cells have detached from the surface and are seen within the lamina propria.

Cystic lesions of the urinary bladder (cystitis cystica) appear as fluid-filled grouped cysts. Similar cysts can be

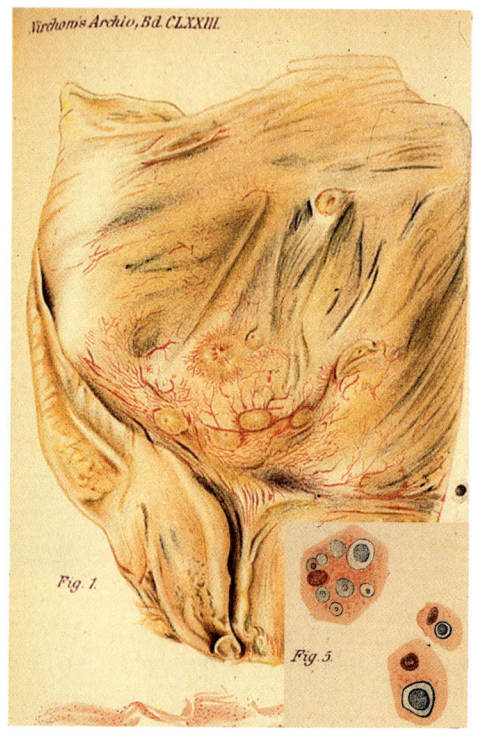

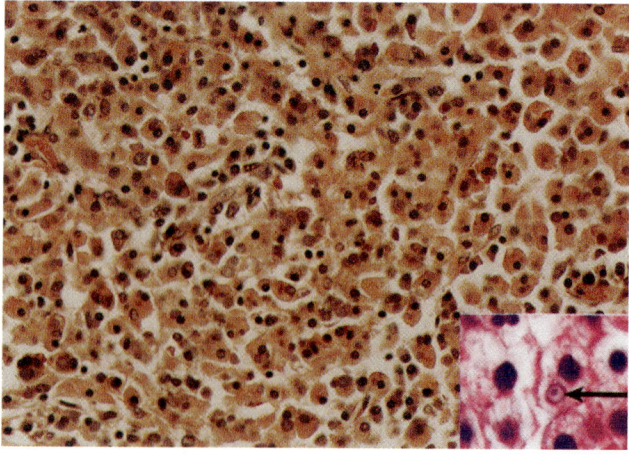

FIGURE 17-8
A. Malakoplakia. This color drawing of the original case reported by von Hansemann in 1903 illustrates the plaquelike indurations of the bladder mucosa and the bluish Michaelis-Gutmann bodies in the cytoplasm of the inflammatory cells *(inset)*. B. A photomicrograph shows numerous Michaelis-Gutmann bodies are seen as well-defined spherical structures in the cytoplasm. The background inflammatory cells are composed principally of macrophages, with fewer lymphocytes. *(inset)* A Michaelis-Gutmann body *(arrow)* is seen at high magnification.

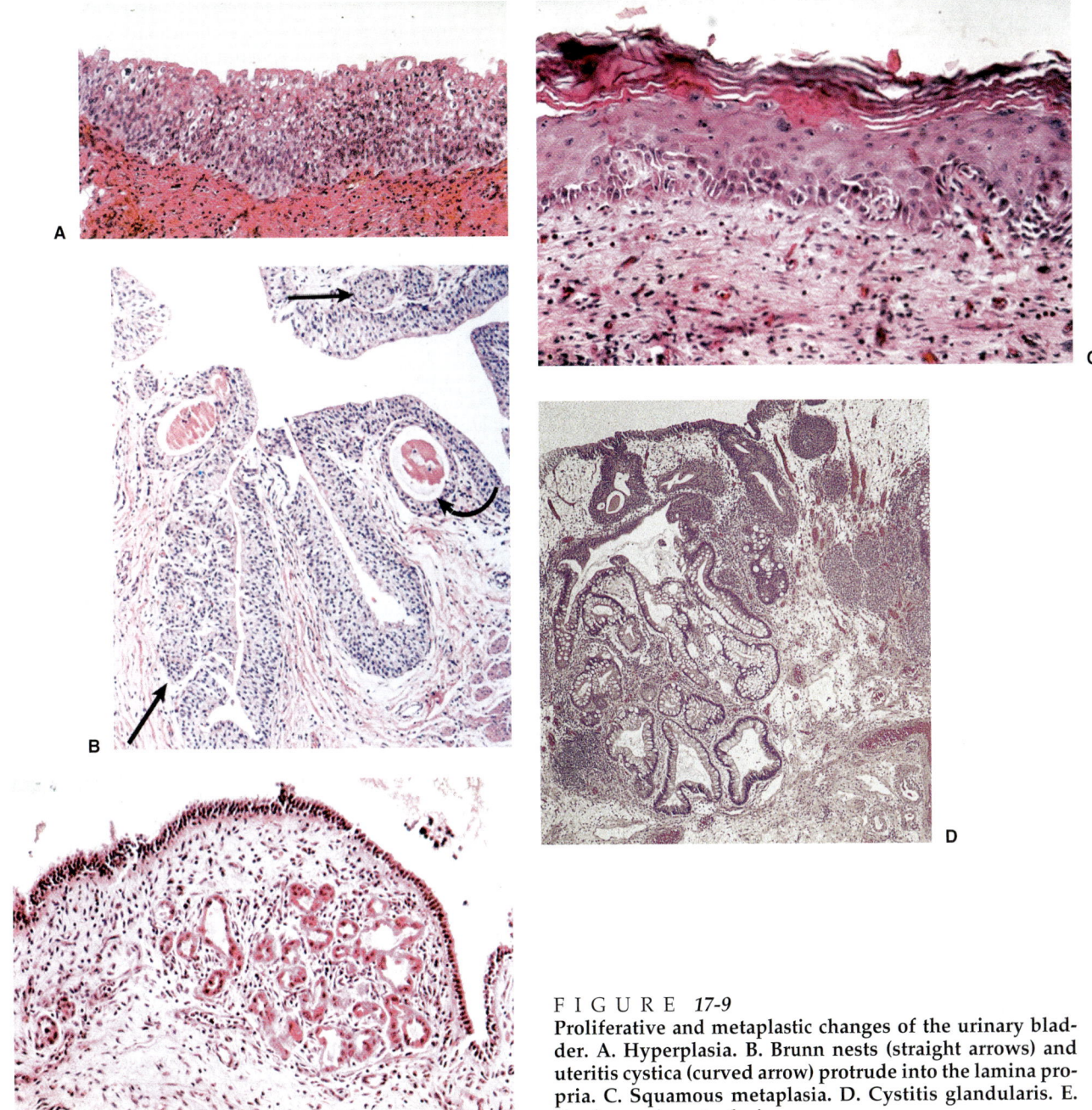

FIGURE 17-9
Proliferative and metaplastic changes of the urinary bladder. A. Hyperplasia. B. Brunn nests (straight arrows) and uteritis cystica (curved arrow) protrude into the lamina propria. C. Squamous metaplasia. D. Cystitis glandularis. E. Nephrogenic metaplasia.

seen in the urethra or the ureter (**urethritis cystica, ureteritis cystica**) (Fig. 17-10). Cystitis cystica is actually common, being found histologically in 60% of otherwise normal bladders. These cysts may become large enough to be apparent on cystoscopy. Histologically, all these lesions correspond to cystic Brunn nests and are lined by normal transitional epithelium. Eosinophilic, proteinaceous material may be present within the lumina of the cysts.

Cystitis glandularis is a mucosal lesion characterized by glandular structures lined by mucin-secreting, columnar epithelial cells, frequently in proximity to Brunn nests and cystitis cystica. Cystitis glandularis differs from cystitis cystica only in the nature of the lining cells. In fact, structures with both columnar cells of cystitis glandularis and transitional cells of cystitis cystica are not uncommon.

Squamous metaplasia is a reaction to chronic injury and inflammation, particularly when it is associated with calculi. It is now apparent that squamous metaplasia of the urinary tract, presumably associated with infections, is considerably more common than previously appreciated and is present in as many as 50% of normal adult women and 10% of men.

Nephrogenic metaplasia is a lesion caused by transformation of transitional epithelium into epithelium resembling renal tubules. It occurs most frequently in the urinary bladder but has been reported uncommonly in the urethra and in the ureter. Numerous small tubules clustered in the lamina propria produce a papillary exophytic nodule. The histogenesis of nephrogenic metaplasia is unsettled, but it seems that in some cases, the lesions result from implants of detached renal tubular cells carried downstream by

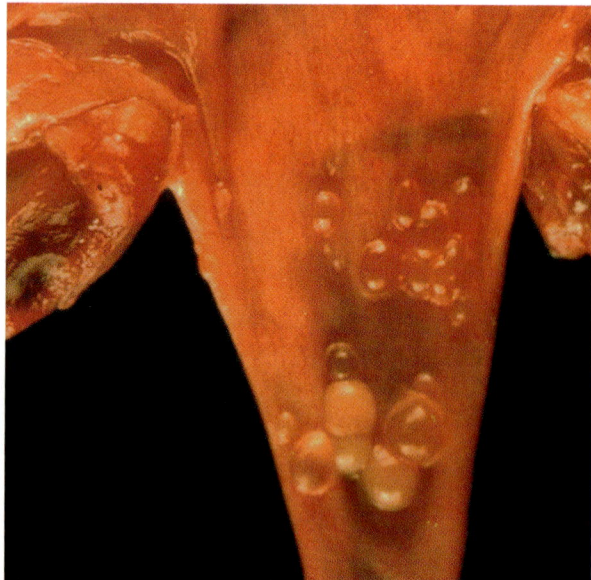

FIGURE 17-10
Ureteritis cystica. The mucosa of the proximal ureter exhibits small cystic structures.

urine. The lesion may produce tumorlike protrusions in the urinary bladder. These may obstruct the ureters, in which case they require surgical treatment.

 Clinical Features: The proliferative and metaplastic lesions of the urothelium are of limited clinical significance. Most importantly, such lesions should not be confused with cancer. However, patients with these changes have a significantly increased risk for the development of transitional cell carcinoma of the bladder and, in the case of cystitis glandularis, of adenocarcinoma as well. Yet, there is no evidence to suggest that these lesions themselves are preneoplastic. Rather, the persistence of the injury related to the development of proliferative and metaplastic urothelial lesions is more likely the important factor in the pathogenesis of bladder cancer.

TUMORS

The most important facts about bladder cancer are as follows:

- The urinary bladder is the most common site of urinary tract tumors.
- Most bladder tumors occur in older patients (median age 65 years) and are rare under the age of 50 years.
- Cancers are more common in men than in women.
- Most tumors are microscopically classified as transitional cell (urothelial) neoplasms.
- Most tumors are cancerous, but the degree of malignancy varies, depending on the clinical stage and microscopic grade of each tumor.
- Tumors are often multifocal and can occur in any part of the urinary tract lined by transitional epithelium, from the renal pelvis to the posterior urethra.
- Surgical treatment is often followed by tumor recurrence.

 Epidemiology: Some 50,000 new cases of bladder cancer are diagnosed every year in the United States, accounting for 3 to 5% of all cancer-related deaths. The incidence of bladder cancer shows significant geographical and sex differences throughout the world. The highest frequencies are recorded among urban whites in the United States and western Europe, whereas a low prevalence obtains in Japan and among American blacks.

A high incidence of bladder cancer in Egypt, Sudan, and other African countries is attributed to endemic schistosomiasis. In 70% of cases, tumors complicating schistosomiasis are squamous cell carcinomas.

Bladder cancer may be encountered at any age, but most patients (80%) are 50 to 80 years old. Men are affected three times as often as women. The most important risk factors are

- Cigarette smoking (fourfold increased risk)
- Industrial exposure to azo dyes
- Infection with *S. haematobium*
- Drugs, such as cyclophosphamide and analgesics
- Radiation therapy (cervical, prostate, or rectal cancer)

 Pathogenesis: The association of bladder cancer with occupational exposure to certain organic chemicals among workers in the German aniline dye industry was described in 1895 and was subsequently confirmed in similar workers in the United States. Later, an increased risk of bladder cancer was identified in the leather, rubber, paint, and organic chemical industries. Improved industrial hygiene has reduced this risk.

A role for chemicals in the origin of bladder cancer has been strengthened by the demonstration that the administration of β-naphthylamine, a compound to which the dye industry workers were exposed, produces bladder cancer in dogs. The metabolic pathway of naphthylamines explains their organ specificity. Arylamines are conjugated with glucuronic acid in the liver, after which the conjugates are excreted in the urine. In the bladder, β-glucuronidase hydrolyzes the glucuronic acid conjugate at the acidic pH of urine, thereby producing reactive arylnitrenium ions. These species are presumably carcinogenic to the mucosal cells by virtue of their ability to bind to the guanine moiety of DNA.

Specific cytogenetic abnormalities have been observed in 50% of bladder cancers. These include most often deletion of chromosome 9 or its short or long arm (9p-, or 9q-) and deletions of 11p, 13p, 14q, or 17p. Chromosomal deletions in 9p, which contains the **tumor-suppressor gene *p16***, are the only consistent finding in low grade papillary tumors and flat carcinomas in situ. Deletions in 17p, the site of the *p53* **gene**, are often found in invasive bladder cancers.

There is evidence that multiple bladder tumors, whether they arise simultaneously or at different times, are all derived from the same **clone of neoplastic cells** and thus represent seeding of additional sites within the vesical mucosa from a single original tumor. The presence of multiple tumors was

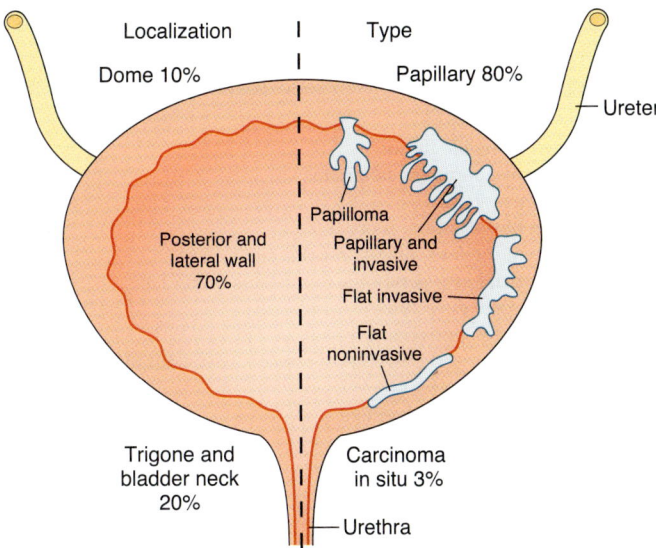

FIGURE 17-11
Urothelial neoplasms. Most tumors occur in the urinary bladder and are classified histologically as transitional cell carcinomas (TCCs). Ureters and the posterior urethra are also lined by transitional epithelium and can give rise to TCC. TCCs can be flat, papillary, papillary and invasive, or simply invasive. Benign transitional cell papillomas are rare.

previously regarded as a "**field effect**" on a urothelial mucosa "not at rest." The "field effect theory" is supported by the fact that identical tumors may originate simultaneously in the renal pelvis, ureters, and the posterior part of the urethra, all of which are lined by transitional epithelium. Thus the "field effect theory" cannot be dismissed entirely.

 Pathology: Epithelial tumors, most of which are transitional cell carcinomas, constitute more than 98% of all primary tumors of the bladder. Neoplastic transitional cell epithelial lesions arising from the bladder mucosa comprise a spectrum that at one end includes benign papillomas and low-grade exophytic papillary carcinomas and at the other, invasive transitional cell carcinomas and highly malignant tumors (Fig. 17-11). Other tumors listed in Table 17-1 are less common.

Transitional (Urothelial) Cell Papilloma Is a Benign Lesion

Transitional cell papilloma of the urinary bladder is uncommon and is often encountered incidentally or after painless hematuria. Papillomas make up 2 to 3% of bladder epithelial tumors and occur most frequently in men above the age of 50 years. Two forms are classical exophytic papilloma and inverted papilloma.

Exophytic papilloma features papillary fronds that are lined by transitional epithelium that is virtually indistinguishable from normal urothelium. Papillary tumors that meet this criterion are uncommon, and they have been only recently accepted as papillomas rather than low-grade transitional cell carcinomas. On cystoscopy, most patients show single lesions, 2 to 5 cm in diameter, although multiple papillomas are not unusual. Recurrent exophytic papillomas are common (70%), and invasive carcinoma develops in 7% of patients.

TABLE 17-1 Tumors of the Urinary Bladder

Transitional cell papilloma
   Exophytic papilloma
   Inverted papilloma
Transitional cell carcinoma in situ
Papillary transitional cell carcinoma, grades I–III
Squamous cell carcinoma
Adenocarcinoma
Neuroendocrine (small cell) carcinoma
Carcinosarcoma
Sarcoma

Although transitional cell papillomas are not malignant, they arise in a urothelial mucosa that is not at rest, and evolving tumors may be detected by repeated examinations for many years. In most instances, "recurrences" represent new tumors that develop elsewhere in the urinary bladder.

Inverted papillomas are rare and typically present as nodular mucosal lesions in the urinary bladder, usually in the trigone region. They have also been observed in the renal pelvis, ureter, and urethra. Inverted papillomas are covered by normal urothelium, from which cords of transitional epithelium descend into the lamina propria. These lesions are more frequent in men, with a peak incidence in the sixth and seventh decades. Hematuria of recent onset is the usual clinical presentation.

Transitional Cell Carcinoma in Situ Is Confined to Flat Urothelium

The term carcinoma in situ *is reserved for full-thickness, malignant changes confined to flat urothelium in nonpapillary bladder mucosa.* The lesion is characterized by a urothelium of variable thickness that exhibits cellular atypia of the entire mucosa, from the basal layer to the surface (Fig. 17-12). Atypia

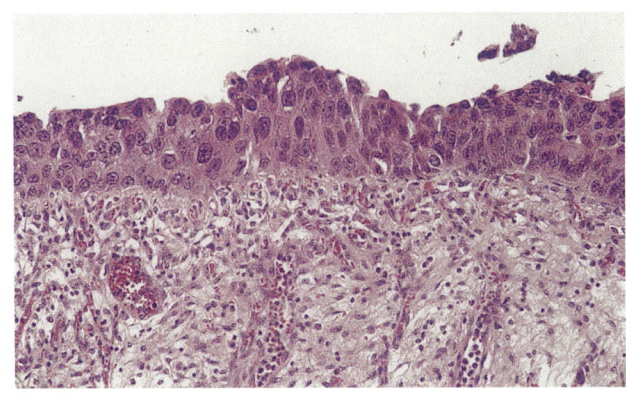

FIGURE 17-12
Transitional cell carcinoma in situ. The urothelial mucosa shows nuclear pleomorphism and lack of polarity from the basal layer to the surface, without evidence of maturation.

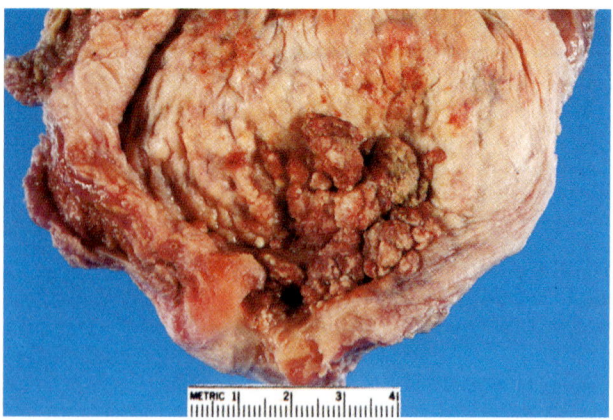

FIGURE 17-13
Transitional cell carcinoma of the urinary bladder. A large exophytic tumor is situated above the bladder neck.

TABLE 17-2 TNM Staging of Transitional Carcinoma of the Urinary Bladder

T—Primary tumor
  T0 No grossly visible tumor
  Ta Noninvasive papillary carcinoma
  Tis Carcinoma in situ
  T1 Invasion of the lamina propria
  T2 Invasion of the muscularis propria
    T2a Superficial invasion of the muscularis (inner half)
    T2b Invasion of deep muscle (outer half)
  T3 Invasion of the perivesical tissue
  T4 Extravesical spread into adjacent organs or distant metastases
N—Regional lymph nodes
  N0 No lymph node involvement
  N1 Single lymph node metastasis
  N2, N3 More lymph nodes involved
M—Distant metastases
  M0 No metastases
  M1 Distant metastases

features nuclear changes, including enlargement, hyperchromatism, irregular shape, prominent nucleoli, and coarse chromatin. Occasional multinucleated cells are present. A disorganized appearance reflecting variation in nuclear polarity is a constant feature.

In one third of cases carcinoma in situ of the bladder is associated with subsequent invasive carcinoma. In turn, most invasive transitional cell carcinomas arise from carcinoma in situ rather than from papillary transitional cell cancers. Confined to the mucosal surface, the in situ lesion is most frequently observed endoscopically as multiple, red, velvety, flat patches topographically close to exophytic papillary transitional cell carcinoma (see below). Concurrent involvement with in situ cancer elsewhere in the bladder or in the ureters, urethra, and prostatic ducts is common. Carcinoma in situ is often multifocal when it is discovered or similar lesions may develop shortly thereafter. When confined to the urinary bladder, transitional cell carcinoma in situ is currently treated with intravesical chemotherapy agents or BCG. Patients are followed closely, and radical surgery is performed only when repeat biopsy indicates progression (bladder wall invasion or prostate involvement). However, the growing respect for the aggressive nature of carcinoma in situ of the bladder has prompted some to advocate radical cystectomy for such lesions.

Transitional Cell Carcinoma Ranges from Superficial Papillary to Deeply Invasive

By cystoscopy, bladder cancers vary from exophytic and with no invasion to flat and deeply penetrating.

 Pathology: Papillary cancer arises most frequently from the lateral walls of the bladder and less often from the posterior wall. At cystoscopy, the tumors may be small, delicate, low-grade papillary lesions that are limited to the mucosal surface or larger, higher-grade, solid invasive masses that are often ulcerated (Fig. 17-13). The papillary and exophytic cancers tend to be more differentiated; the infiltrating tumors are usually more anaplastic.

Bladder cancers are staged according to the TNM classification system (Table 17-2; Fig. 17-14). In order of decreasing frequency, metastases of bladder cancer occur in regional and periaortic lymph nodes, liver, lung, and bone.

Histologically, transitional cell carcinomas of the bladder are classified according to the following grading system (Fig. 17-15A–D):

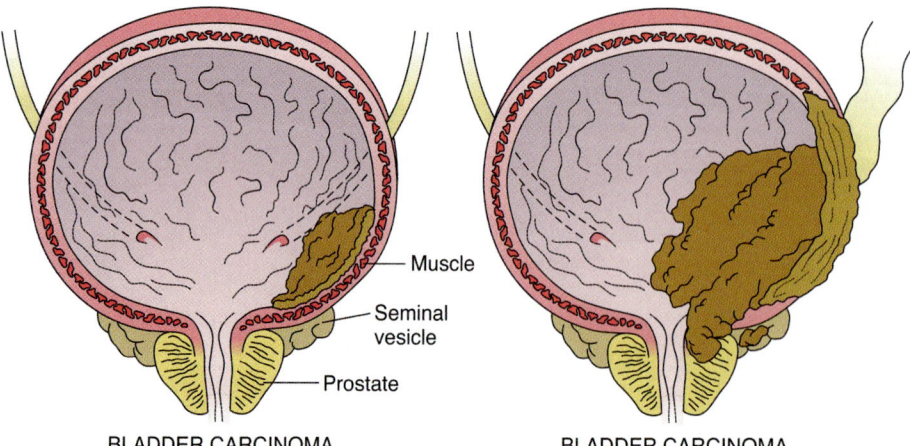

FIGURE 17-14
Staging of urothelial carcinoma of the urinary bladder. Stage T0 tumors (carcinoma in situ) are limited to the epithelium of the mucosa. T1 tumors show invasion of the lamina propria. T2 tumors invade the muscle layer superficially. T3 tumors invade the perivesical tissue. T4 tumors invade into the adjacent organs or show local and distant metastases.

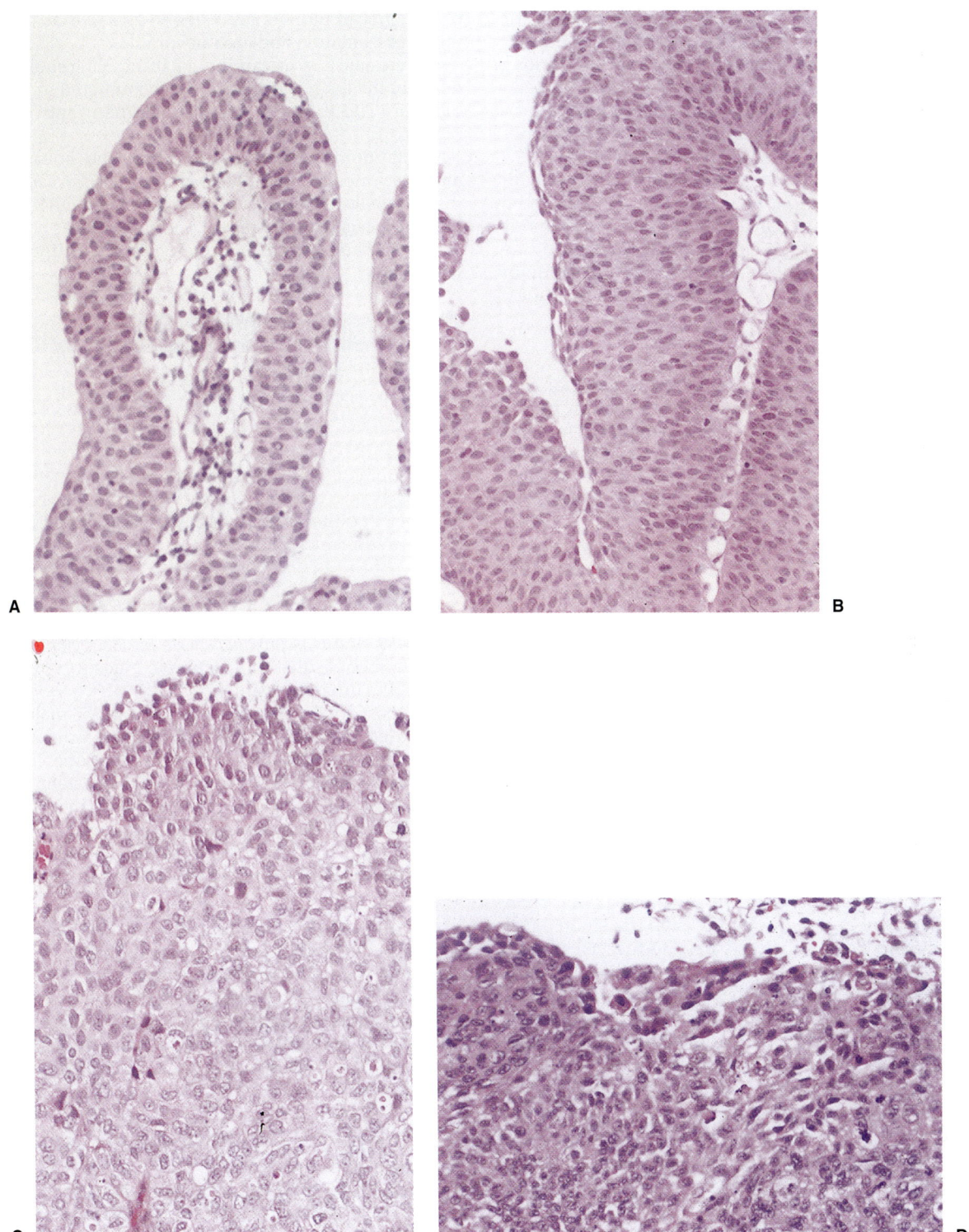

FIGURE 17-15
Urothelial tumors of the urinary bladder. A. Papilloma. The papilla contains a vascular core lined by benign epithelium that is only several cells thick. B. Transitional cell carcinoma grade 1. The papilla is lined by a thickened transitional epithelium composed of relatively uniform cells. C. Transitional cell carcinoma grade 2. The epithelium lining the papilla shows moderate atypia, and cells vary in size and shape. D. Transitional cell carcinoma grade 3. The disorganized epithelium is composed of hyperchromatic cells that show considerable atypia and vary in size and shape.

- **Grade 1:** Papillary projections are lined by neoplastic transitional epithelial cells that show minimal nuclear pleomorphism and mitotic activity. The papillae are long and delicate, and fusion of papillae is focal and limited.
- **Grade 2:** The histological and cytological features are intermediate between those of grade 1 (the best differentiated) and grade 3 (the most poorly differentiated).
- **Grade 3:** Significant nuclear pleomorphism, frequent mitoses, and fusion of papillae are typical. Occasional bizarre cells may be present, and focal sites of squamous differentiation are often seen. Although invasion of the underlying bladder wall may occur with any grade of transitional cell carcinoma, it is most frequent in grade 3 tumors.

 Clinical Features: Transitional cell carcinoma of the bladder typically manifests as sudden **hematuria** and less frequently as **dysuria**. Cystoscopy reveals single or multiple tumors. At the time of initial presentation, 85% of patients have tumor confined to the urinary bladder and 15% have regional or distant metastases. Papillary lesions limited to the mucosa (stage T0) or lamina propria (stage T1) are commonly treated conservatively by transurethral resection. Radical cystectomy is performed on patients who demonstrate muscle invasion and occasionally on those with advanced-stage tumors.

The probability of tumor extension and subsequent recurrence correlates with a number of factors:

- Large size
- High stage
- High grade
- Presence of multiple tumors
- Vascular or lymphatic invasion
- Urothelial dysplasia (including carcinoma in situ) at other sites in the bladder

The estimated 5-year survival of patients with T0 and T1 tumors is 80%, T2 60%, T3 30 to 50%, and T4 less than 20%. Noninvasive or superficially invasive transitional cell tumors are treated conservatively, despite the fact that as many as 30% of such patients eventually exhibit extension of the tumor. The invasion of the tumor into the muscle layer and beyond worsens the prognosis. However, recent advances in chemotherapy have significantly improved the outcome of treatment. The most common causes of death are uremia (from obstruction of the urinary outflow tract) and carcinomatosis.

Rare Forms of Bladder Cancer

Squamous cell carcinoma of the bladder as a consequence of schistosomiasis develops in foci of squamous metaplasia. Virtually all patients with this tumor demonstrate invasion of the bladder wall at the time of initial presentation and thus have a poor prognosis.

Adenocarcinoma of the bladder accounts for only 1% of all malignant tumors of the bladder. It originates from foci of cystitis glandularis or intestinal metaplasia or from remnants of urachal epithelium in the bladder dome. Most bladder adenocarcinomas are deeply invasive at the time of initial presentation and are not curable.

Neuroendocrine carcinoma, resembling small cell carcinoma of the lung, is occasionally encountered in the urinary bladder. The tumor is highly malignant and has a poor prognosis.

Rhabdomyosarcoma, typically of the embryonal type, manifests most commonly in children as *sarcoma botryoides* (i.e., edematous, mucosal, polypoid masses that have been likened to a cluster of grapes). Combined treatment with radiation therapy and chemotherapy has greatly increased survival rates.

Penis, Urethra, and Scrotum

CONGENITAL DISORDERS OF THE PENIS

Developmental anomalies of the penis include rare conditions such as agenesis, occasional abnormalities such as hypoplasia, and the more frequent anomalies that involve the penile urethra and prepuce.

HYPOSPADIAS: This term refers to a congenital anomaly in which the urethra opens on the underside (ventral) of the penis, so that the meatus is proximal to its normal glandular location. The condition results from incomplete closure of the urethral folds of the urogenital sinus.

Hypospadias has a frequency of 1 in 350 male neonates. Most cases are sporadic but a familial occurrence has been noted. Hypospadias also shows an association with other urogenital anomalies and complex, multisystemic, developmental syndromes. In 90% of cases, the meatus is located on the underside of the glans or the corona. Less often it is found along the midshaft of the penis, in the scrotum, and even in the perineum. Surgical repair is usually uncomplicated.

EPISPADIAS: In this rare congenital anomaly the urethra opens on the upper side (dorsal) of the penis. In the most common form of epispadias, the entire penile urethra is open along the entire shaft. Severe epispadias may be associated with exstrophy of the bladder (see Fig. 17-4). In the mildest form, the defect is limited to the glandular urethra. The surgical treatment of epispadias is more complicated than that of hypospadias.

PHIMOSIS: The orifice of the prepuce may be too narrow to allow retraction over the glans penis. Phimosis predisposes the penis to infections. If the narrow prepuce is forcefully retracted, it may strangulate the glans and impede the outflow of venous blood, a condition termed *paraphimosis*. Congenital phimosis must be distinguished from acquired phimosis, which is usually a consequence of recurrent infections or trauma of the prepuce in uncircumcised men. Circumcision cures both phimosis and paraphimosis.

SCROTAL MASSES

Scrotal masses and conditions that lead to swelling or enlargement of the scrotum often reflect abnormalities of testicular, epididymal, and scrotal development. Clinical problems related to these pathological conditions are most often encountered in children but may be found in adults (Figure 17-16A–D).

HYDROCELE: This term refers to a collection of serous fluid in the scrotal sac between the two layers of the tunica vaginalis. The cavity is lined by mesothelium. Hydrocele may be congenital or acquired.

Congenital hydrocele reflects a patent processus vaginalis testis or its incomplete obliteration. It is the most common cause of scrotal swelling in infants and is often associated with inguinal hernia.

Acquired hydrocele in adults is secondary to some other disease affecting the scrotum, such as infection, tumor, or trauma. The cause cannot be found. The diagnosis is made by ultrasound or by transluminating the fluid in the cavity. Hydrocele is a benign condition that disappears once the causal disease has been eliminated. However, long-standing hydrocele may cause testicular atrophy or compression of the epididymis, or the fluid may become infected and lead to **periorchitis.**

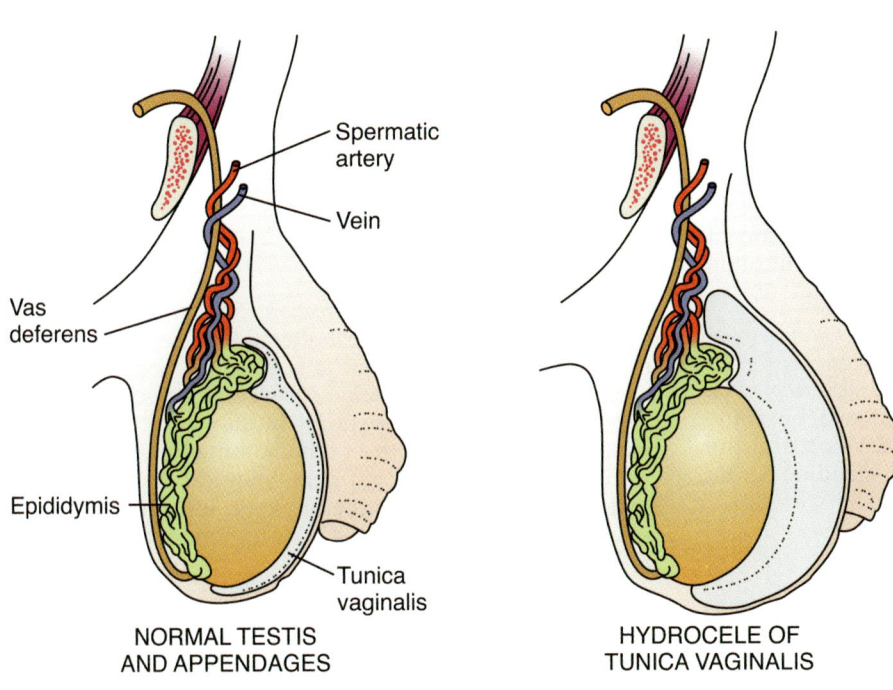
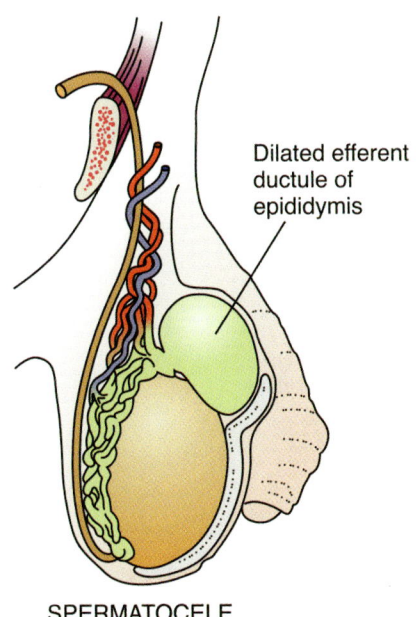
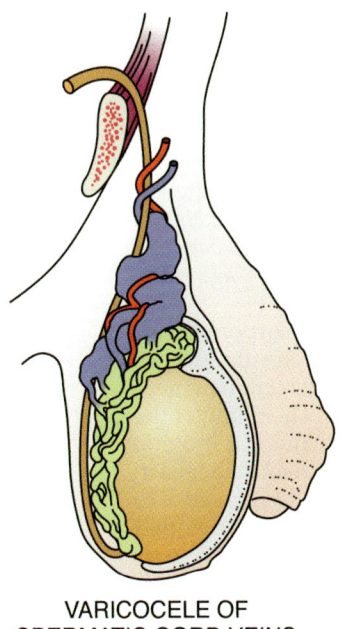

FIGURE 17-16
Scrotal masses. A. Normal testis. B. Hydrocele. C. Spermatocele. D. Varicocele.

HEMATOCELE: *An accumulation of blood between the layers of tunica vaginalis* may develop after trauma or hemorrhage into a hydrocele. Testicular tumors and infections may also lead to a hematocele.

SPERMATOCELE: *This mass is a cyst formed from the protrusions of widened efferent ducts of the rete testis or epididymis.* It manifests as a hilar paratesticular nodule or as a fluctuating mass filled with milky fluid. Microscopic examination reveals a cyst lined by cuboidal epithelium that contains spermatozoa in various stages of degeneration.

VARICOCELE: *A dilation of testicular veins appears as a nodularity on the lateral side of the scrotum.* Most varicoceles are asymptomatic and are discovered during physical examination of infertile men. Massive varicocele is mentioned in clinical texts as resembling a "bag of worms." Varicocele is considered a common cause of infertility and oligospermia, although it is not clear why dilation of veins should have such consequences. Testicular atrophy is found only rarely and only in long-standing disease. Surgical resection of varicocele by ligation of the internal spermatic vein often improves reproductive function.

SCROTAL INGUINAL HERNIA: *A protrusion of the intestines into the scrotum through the inguinal canal is recognized as a mass.* The intestinal loops can be repositioned, but if the condition remains untreated, adhesions develop and the hernia can only be repaired surgically. Long-standing hernia may cause testicular atrophy.

CIRCULATORY DISTURBANCES

SCROTAL EDEMA: *Lymph or serous fluid may accumulate in the scrotum owing to obstruction of lymphatic or venous drainage.* **Lymphedema** due to obstruction of the lymphatics can be caused by pelvic or abdominal tumors, surgical scars, or infections such as filariasis. **Transudation** of plasma is common in patients who have heart failure, anasarca secondary to cirrhosis, or nephrotic syndrome. Fluid accumulates both in the loose connective tissue and the cavity lined by the tunica vaginalis testis.

ERECTILE DYSFUNCTION: Also known as impotence, this condition is defined as *"the inability to achieve or maintain an erection sufficient for satisfactory sexual performance."* Its prevalence increases with age, from 20% at the age of 40 years to 50% by the age of 70 years.

Erection requires adequate filling of the corpora cavernosa and spongiosa of the penis with blood. The tumescence of the penis is the end result of a complex interaction of mental, neural, hormonal, and vascular factors. The filling of the vascular spaces of the penis depends on the nitric oxide (NO)-mediated relaxation of vascular smooth muscle cells in the erectile cylinders. Since the release of NO is related to cyclic guanosine 3′,5′-monophosphate (cGMP), drugs that inhibit the phosphodiesterase that degrades cGMP (e.g., sildenafil [Viagra]) are used for the treatment of erectile dysfunction. Disorders associated with erectile dysfunction are listed in Table 17-3.

TABLE 17-3 Erectile Dysfunctions

Neuropsychiatric
   Psychiatric disorders (e.g., depression)
   Spinal cord injury
   Nerve injury during surgery (e.g. pelvic or perineal surgery)
Endocrine
   Hypogonadism
   Pituitary diseases (e.g., hyperprolactinemia)
   Hypothyroidism, Cushing syndrome, Addison disease
Vascular
   Diabetic microangiopathy
   Hypertension
   Atherosclerosis
Drugs
   Antihypertensives
   Psychotropic drugs
   Estrogens, anticancer drugs, etc.
Idiopathic
   "Performance anxiety"
   Age-related "impotence"

PRIAPISM: *Continuous erection of the penis unrelated to sexual excitation is painful.* Most often the cause of priapism is unknown, and its treatment is ineffective. Secondary priapism occurs as a complication of several diseases, including (1) pelvic diseases that impede the outflow of blood from the penis (e.g., pelvic tumors or hematomas, thrombosis of pelvic veins, infections), (2) hematological disorders (e.g., sickle cell anemia, polycythemia vera, leukemia), and (3) brain and spinal cord diseases (e.g., tumors, syphilis).

INFLAMMATORY DISORDERS

The most important inflammatory conditions affecting the penis are (1) sexually transmitted diseases, (2) nonspecific infections, (3) diseases of unknown etiology, such as balanitis xerotica obliterans, (4) dermatoses, and 5) dermatitis involving the shaft of the penis and scrotum (Table 17-4).

TABLE 17-4 Inflammatory Lesions of the Penis

Sexually transmitted diseases
   Herpes genitalis
   Syphilis
   Chancroid
   Granuloma inguinale
   Lymphogranuloma venereum
   Human papillomavirus infections
Nonspecific infectious balanoposthitis
   Bacterial, fungal, viral
Diseases of unknown etiology
   Balanitis xerotica obliterans
   Circinate balanitis
   Plasma cell balanitis (Zoon balanitis)
   Peyronie disease
Dermatitis involving the shaft of the penis and scrotum
   Infectious (bacterial, viral, fungal)
   Noninfectious (e.g., lichen planus, bullous skin diseases)

Sexually Transmitted Diseases Cause Discrete Penile Lesions

Sexually transmitted diseases (STDs) are discussed in greater detail in Chapter 9 and are reviewed here briefly in the context of other infections of the lower urinary tracts (Fig. 17-17).

Genital herpes (HSV-2) is the most common STD affecting the glans. It manifests typically as grouped vesicles that ulcerate and transform into crusts.

Syphilis (*Treponema pallidum*) manifests as a solitary, soft ulcer (*chancre*).

Chancroid (*Haemophilus ducreyi*) manifests as a papule that transforms into a pustule and finally ulcerates. Shallow ulcers on the glans or the skin of the shaft are often associated with painful suppurative inguinal lymphadenitis.

Granuloma inguinale, a tropical disease caused by *Calymmatobacterium granulomatis*, manifests as a raised ulceration filled with a copious chronic inflammatory exudate and granulation tissue. Such ulcerations tend to enlarge and heal very slowly.

Lymphogranuloma venereum (*Chlamydia trachomatis*) appears as a small, often innocuous, vesicle that ulcerates. It is typically accompanied by tender enlargement of the inguinal lymph nodes, which adhere to the skin and form sinuses draining pus and serosanguinous fluid.

Condylomata acuminata (human papillomavirus) feature flat topped warts on the shaft (Fig. 17-18) small polyps on the glans and the urethral meatus, or larger cauliflower-like tumors that may be confused with verrucous carcinoma.

Balanitis Is an Inflammation of the Glans

In uncircumcised men, balanitis usually extends from the glans of the penis to the foreskin and is called *balanoposthitis*. Most often it is caused by bacteria, but in immunosuppressed persons and in diabetics it can also be caused by fungi. Typically, balanitis is a consequence of poor hygiene. Significant complications of chronic balanoposthitis are stricture of the meatus, phimosis, and paraphimosis.

BALANITIS XEROTICA OBLITERANS: *This chronic inflammatory condition of unknown origin is characterized by fibrosis and sclerosis of subepithelial connective tissue.* The affected portion of the glans appears white and indurated. Fibrosis may constrict the urethral meatus or cause phimosis. This condition is equivalent to lichen sclerosus et atrophicus of the vulva (See Chapter 18).

CIRCINATE BALANITIS: *In the course of* **Reiter syndrome** *(see below), the glans may show circular, linear, or confluent, plaquelike discolorations, occasionally associated with superficial ulcerations.*

PLASMA CELL BALANITIS: Also known as ***zoon balanitis****, this disease of unknown origin causes macular discol-*

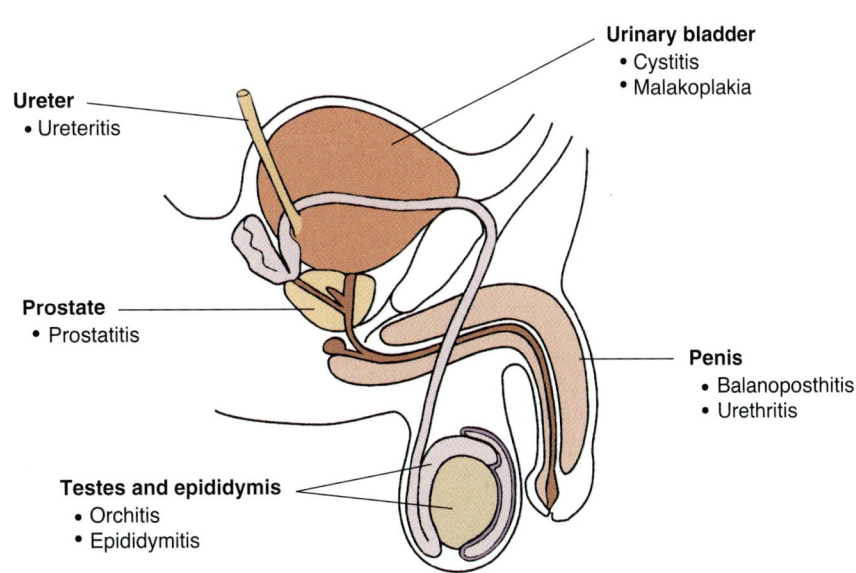

FIGURE 17-17
Infections of the lower urinary tract and male reproductive system.

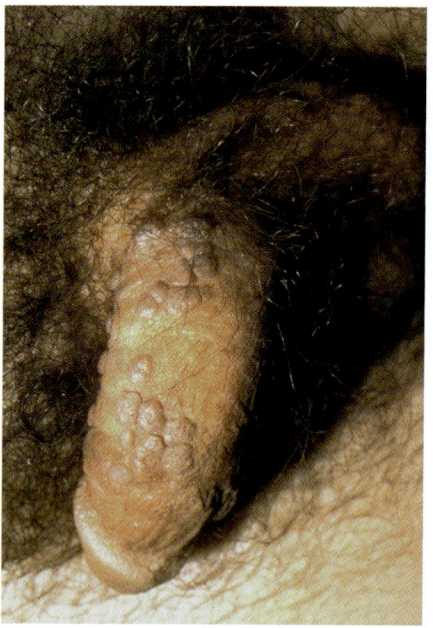
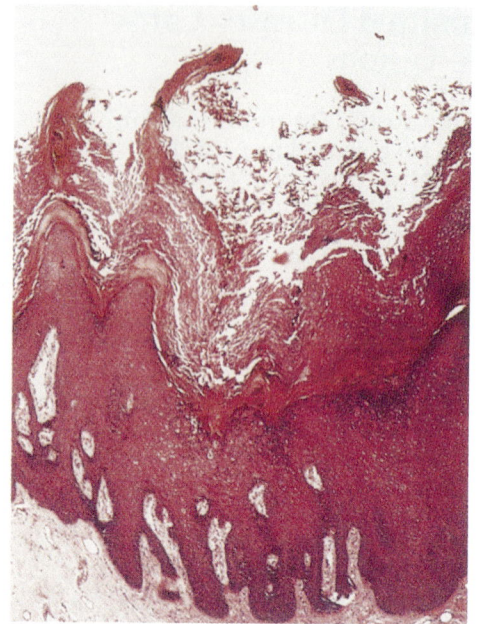

FIGURE 17-18
Condylomata acuminata of the penis. A. Raised, circumscribed lesions are seen on the shaft of the penis. B. Section of a lesion shows epidermal hyperkeratosis, parakeratosis, acanthosis, and papillomatosis.

oration or painless papules on the glans. Histologically, the connective tissue shows infiltrates of plasma cells and lymphocytes, and the overlying epithelium is thickened. The disease is chronic but innocuous.

DERMATOSES: Many inflammatory skin diseases may involve the penis. Such conditions are discussed in Chapter 24.

Peyronie Disease Is an Induration of the Penis

Peyronie disease is a malady of unknown etiology characterized by focal, asymmetric fibrosis of the shaft of the penis. The resulting penile curvature (penile strabismus) is accompanied by pain during erection. The typical case is an ill-defined induration of the penile shaft in a young or middle-aged man, without any change in the overlying skin. On microscopic examination, dense fibrosis is associated with a sparse, nonspecific, chronic inflammatory cell infiltrate. Collagen focally replaces muscle in the septum of the corpus cavernosum.

Peyronie disease affects 1% of men over the age of 40 years, but in most instances, it occurs in a mild form that does not interfere with sexual function. Severe penile curvature may be incapacitating and require surgical treatment, although the outcome is not always satisfactory.

URETHRITIS AND RELATED CONDITIONS

Urethritis is an inflammation of the urethra that can occur in an acute or chronic form.

SEXUALLY TRANSMITTED URETHRITIS: *Urethritis is the most common manifestation of sexually transmitted diseases (STD) in men, in whom it typically presents with urethral discharge.* Women rarely notice distinct urethral discharge and usually complain of vaginal discharge.

Both **gonococcal and nongonococcal** urethritis have an acute onset and are related to recent sexual intercourse. The infection manifests with urethral discharge, typically purulent and greenish yellow. Symptoms include pain or tingling at the meatus of the urethra and pain on micturition *(dysuria).* Redness and swelling of the urethral meatus are usually seen in both sexes. Acute gonococcal and nongonococcal urethritis can both become chronic.

The final diagnosis is made by identifying the causative pathogen. In gonococcal urethritis the urethral discharge contains *Neisseria gonorrhoeae,* which can be identified microscopically in smears of the urethral exudates. Nongonococcal urethritis is most often caused by *C. trachomatis* or *Ureaplasma urealyticum* but may be related to a variety of other pathogens.

NONSPECIFIC INFECTIOUS URETHRITIS: *Uropathogens such as* E. coli *and* Pseudomonas *can cause urethritis.* Typically the infection is associated with cystitis but it may be related to other diseases (e.g., prostatic hyperplasia or urinary stones). In men, infectious urethritis may be the only sign of prostatitis; in women, it may be a complication of vaginitis and vulvitis. In hospitalized patients it is a common consequence of cystoscopy and other urological procedures and is almost inevitable in patients who have indwelling urethral catheters.

Clinically, nonspecific infectious urethritis manifests with urgency and a burning sensation during urination. Usually there is no discharge, although men can express some milky fluid by "stripping" or "milking" the urethra.

URETHRAL CARUNCLES: *Polypoid inflammatory lesions near the female urethral meatus produce pain and bleeding.* They occur exclusively in women, most frequently after menopause. The etiology and pathogenesis are unclear; prolapse of the urethral mucosa and associated chronic inflammation have been suggested as the cause.

Urethral caruncle presents as an exophytic, often ulcerated, polypoid mass, 1 to 2 cm in diameter, at or near the urethral meatus. Microscopically, the lesion exhibits acutely and chronically inflamed granulation tissue and ulceration and hyperplasia of transitional cell or squamous epithelium. Although complex patterns of papillomatosis and occasional dysplastic epithelium may give this inflammatory lesion a superficial resemblance to carcinoma, it does not lead to cancer. Treatment is surgical excision.

REITER SYNDROME: *This condition features a triad of* **urethritis, conjunctivitis, and arthritis** *of weight-bearing joints* (e.g., knee, sacroiliac, and vertebral joints). Other clinical findings encountered in variable proportions are circinate balanitis, cervicitis, and skin eruptions. Reiter syndrome tends to affect young adults who have an HLA-B27 haplotype. Symptoms usually appear a few weeks after a chlamydial urethritis or an enteric infection caused by a variety of pathogens such as *Shigella, Salmonella,* or *Campylobacter.* Hence, the syndrome is thought to represent an inappropriate immune reaction to some microbial antigen(s). In most patients, symptoms usually disappear spontaneously over a period of 3 to 6 months. However, arthritis recurs in half of patients.

TUMORS

Cancer of the Urethra Arises from Squamous or Transitional Epithelium

Urethral carcinoma has a female predominance of 2:1. The tumor may be associated with strictures caused by prior instrumentation or venereal disease and, most importantly, prior or concomitant bladder cancer.

Pathology: Most urethral cancers are squamous cell carcinomas originating in the distal urethra. Transitional cell carcinoma similar to that in the bladder arises in the proximal urethra.

Clinical Features: Urethral cancer is most frequently observed in the sixth and seventh decades. Most patients present with urethral bleeding and dysuria. In spite of the accessible location and associated symptoms, most have spread to adjacent tissues or regional lymph nodes at the time of presentation. The primary therapy is radical surgery.

Cancer of the Penis Occurs in Uncircumcised Men

Cancer of the penis originates from the squamous mucosa of the glans and contiguous urethral meatus or the prepuce and the skin covering the shaft of the penis.

Epidemiology: In the United States, invasive squamous cell carcinoma of the penis is an uncommon tumor, accounting for less than 0.5% of all cancers in men. The average age of patients with this tumor is 60 years. Penile cancer is much more common in less-developed countries, and in some parts of Africa and Asia it constitutes 10% of male cancers. Since this malignancy is virtually unknown in men circumcised at birth, these geographical variations have been attributed to differences in the frequency of circumcision.

No single agent has been identified as the cause of cancer of the penis. Current interest centers on the possible influence of accumulated keratin debris and the inflammatory exudate *(smegma)* that accumulates beneath the prepuce. More than half of patients with cancer of the penis have had phimosis since an early age, suggesting that prolonged contact between smegma and the penile epithelium may play a role. Human papillomavirus (HPV) types 16 and 18 have also been suggested as factors in the pathogenesis of penile cancer.

Pathology: Penile carcinoma occurs in a preinvasive form (carcinoma in situ) and an invasive variety.

SQUAMOUS CELL CARCINOMA IN SITU: Historically, carcinoma in situ of the penis was described in two forms: Bowen disease and erythroplasia of Queyrat.

Bowen disease appears as a sharply demarcated, erythematous or grayish white plaque on the shaft.

Erythroplasia of Queyrat manifests as solitary or multiple, shiny, soft, erythematous plaques on the glans and foreskin.

Both of these conditions appear microscopically as squamous cell carcinoma in situ similar to that in other sites. The lesions show cytological atypia of the keratinocytes of all layers of the epidermis, with parakeratosis or hyperkeratosis, papillomatosis with broad epidermal papillae, and thinning of the granular layer. By definition, the atypical keratinocytes do not invade the underlying dermis. A chronic inflammatory cell infiltrate within the subjacent dermis may be present. The frequency with which Bowen disease and erythroplasia of Queyrat progress to invasive squamous cell carcinoma remains unsettled but is estimated to be less than 10% of cases.

Bowenoid papulosis of the penis is caused by HPV and affects young, sexually active men. In contrast to the solitary lesion of Bowen disease, bowenoid papulosis manifests with multiple brownish or violaceous papules. Microscopically, the disorder resembles other variants of carcinoma in situ, but occasionally there are some differences. In contrast to true carcinoma in situ, which at the margins slowly merges with normal epithelium, the lesions of bowenoid papulosis are sharply demarcated from normal epidermis and thus resemble HPV-induced warts. The altered epidermis shows some superficial stratification and maturation and may contain giant keratinocytes with multinucleated atypical nuclei. HPV type 16 can be demonstrated in 80% of patients. Virtually all lesions of bowenoid papulosis regress spontaneously and do not progress to invasive carcinoma.

INVASIVE SQUAMOUS CELL CARCINOMA: The tumor presents as (1) an ulcer, (2) an indurated crater, (3) a friable hemorrhagic mass, or (4) an exophytic, fungating, papillary tumor. Squamous cell carcinoma usually involves the glans or the prepuce and less commonly the shaft of the penis. Extensive destruction of penile tissue, including the urethral meatus, is observed in neglected cases. Microscopically, the typical example is a well-differentiated, focally keratinizing, squamous cell carcinoma. Invasive tumors are associated with a dense, chronic inflammatory cell infiltrate in the dermis. The adjacent epidermis often shows dysplastic changes. The tumor may invade deeply along the penile shaft and may spread to inguinal lymph nodes, then to the iliac nodes, and ultimately to distant organs.

VERRUCOUS CARCINOMA: This tumor deserves to be separated from other penile cancers because it is a cytologically benign but clinically malignant exophytic squamous cell carcinoma (Fig. 17-19). It is also known as **Buschke and Löwenstein tumor,** so named in honor of the two physicians who first described it, in 1925. This penile lesion is grossly and cytologically similar to condyloma acuminatum, but unlike the latter, it shows local invasion. This low-grade squamous cell carcinoma usually does not metastasize, and surgical removal is curative.

Clinical Features: Most squamous cell cancers are confined to the penis at the time of initial presentation, but occult metastases to inguinal lymph nodes are not uncommon. Conversely, half of patients with clinically enlarged regional lymph nodes have no nodal metastases but only reactive changes secondary to the inflammation associated with the cancer.

The survival of patients with penile cancer is related to the clinical stage and, to a lesser degree, to the histological grade of the tumor. Amputation of the penis is usually necessary. Patients with superficially invasive cancer have a 90% 5-year survival; those with inguinal lymph node metastases experience a 20 to 50% 5-year survival, depending on the extent of spread.

Cancer of the Scrotum Is of Historical Interest

The identification in 1775 of scrotal cancer as an occupational disease of chimney sweeps by Sir Percival Pott introduced the concept of chemical carcinogenesis (see Chapter 5). Pott implicated constant exposure to soot as the causative agent, but later investigators incriminated a large variety of industrial chemicals in the pathogenesis of this tumor. Owing to refinements in industrial hygiene, scrotal cancer is today distinctly uncommon.

Squamous cell carcinoma of the scrotum typically affects older men and is most frequent in the sixth and seventh decades. At initial presentation, many patients demonstrate invasion of the scrotal contents and metastases to regional nodes. Therapy is surgical excision.

Testis, Epididymis, and Vas Deferens

CRYPTORCHIDISM

Cryptorchidism, clinically known as undescended testis, is a congenital abnormality in which one or both testes are not found in their normal position in the scrotum. It is the most common urologic condition requiring surgical treatment in infants. In 5% of male infants born at term and 30% of those born prematurely, the testes are not located in the scrotum or are easily retracted. In the large majority of these infants, the testis will descend into the scrotum during the first year of life. Accordingly, the prevalence of cryptorchidism from the end of the first year of life into adulthood is in range of 1%. Cryptorchidism is usually unilateral but is bilateral in 30% of affected men.

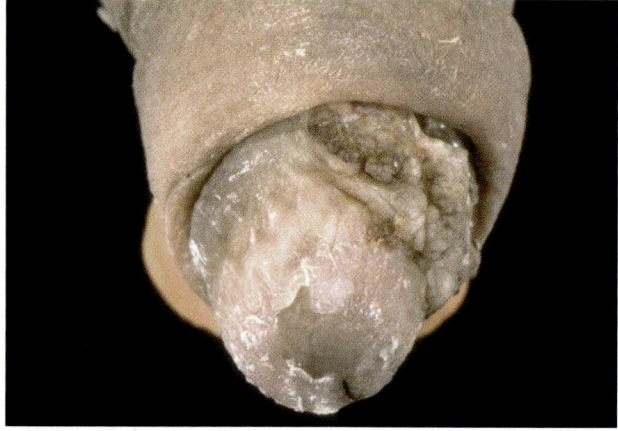

FIGURE 17-19
Carcinoma of the penis. This verrucous carcinoma arises on the glans and appears as an exophytic mass.

Pathogenesis: The causes of testicular maldescent are usually unknown, but theoretically the condition could be related to (1) developmental disorders of the gonad, (2) endocrine factors, or (3) mechanical factors that prevent the passage of the fetal testis through the inguinal canal. It is usually an isolated developmental disorder, but in rare instances, it is associated with other congenital anomalies.

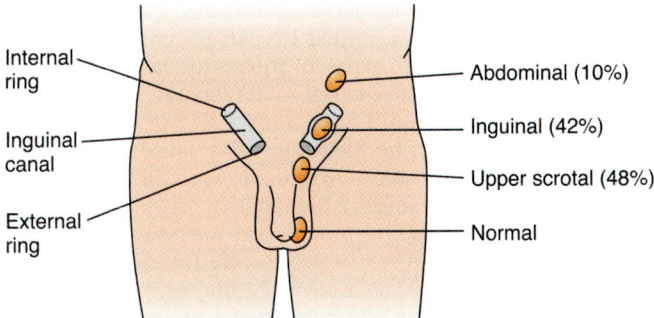

FIGURE 17-20
Cryptorchidism. In most instances, the testis has an upper scrotal location or is retained in the inguinal canal.

 Pathology: The descent of the testis may be arrested at any point from the abdominal cavity to the upper scrotum (Fig. 17-20). According to their location, the cryptorchid testes can be classified as **abdominal, inguinal, or upper scrotal**. In rare cases of ectopic testes, the testes are located in unusual locations, such as the perineum or the calf.

Cryptorchid testes are smaller than normal even at an early age, and the difference between the affected and the normal testis becomes more prominent with age. Such testes appear firm, owing to fibrosis of the parenchyma.

The microscopic changes in the cryptorchid testis are also age-related. In infancy and early childhood, the seminiferous tubules in the affected testes are smaller than normal and contain fewer germ cells. Postpubertal testes contain fewer germ cells than normal, and spermatogenesis is limited to a minority of tubules. Hyaline thickening of the tubular basement membranes and prominent stromal fibrosis are observed (Fig. 17-21). Eventually, the tubules become devoid of spermatogenic cells and become entirely hyalinized. *Orchiopexy* (surgical placement of the testis into the scrotum) performed either in childhood or after puberty does not prevent the loss of seminiferous epithelium and tubules; both the untreated and the repositioned testes show no signs of spermatogenesis in half of the cases. A few adult cryptorchid testes (2%) contain atypical germ cells corresponding to carcinoma in situ.

 Clinical Features: The clinical significance of undescended testes is not related to the abnormal position of the gonad per se (patients are asymptomatic) but to an increased incidence of **infertility** and **germ cell neoplasia**. All men with bilateral cryptorchid testes have *azoospermia* and are infertile. Unilateral cryptorchidism is associated in 40% of cases with *oligospermia*, defined as a sperm count below 20 million/mL. Even though oligospermia is a cause of reduced fertility, most men who have one normal testis have a reasonable chance of fathering a child. Orchiopexy performed in childhood or after puberty has no effect on the sperm count. Most urologists recommend early orchiopexy between the age of 6 months and 1 year, but there are no reliable data to indicate whether this treatment improves the sperm count.

Cryptorchidism is associated with a 20- to 40-fold greater than normal risk for testicular cancer. Conversely, 10% of patients with germ cell neoplasia have cryptorchid testes. Intraabdominal testes are at higher risk than those retained in the inguinal canal; in turn, inguinal testes are at higher risk than those located high in the scrotum. The contralateral, normally descended testis is also at risk, but the incidence of cancer in these testes is only four times higher than in normal men. Unfortunately, orchiopexy does not reduce the cancer risk, and patients are instructed to perform regular self-examinations.

ABNORMALITIES OF SEXUAL DIFFERENTIATION

Disorders of gonadogenesis and the formation of the external genital organs, as well as the development of secondary sex characteristics, can be explained as pertaining to:

- Genetic sex; the presence or absence of X and Y chromosomes
- Gonadal sex; the presence or absence of testes or ovaries
- Genital sex; the appearance of external genital organs
- Psychosocial sexual orientation

Various conditions are listed in Table 17-5. Some of these, such as Klinefelter and Turner syndromes, are discussed in Chapter 6.

HERMAPHRODITISM: This rare developmental disorder is characterized by ambiguous genitalia in a person who has both male and female gonads. The gonads may develop into ovotestes (combination of ovary and testis) or one gonad may be testis and the other ovary. Half of these persons have

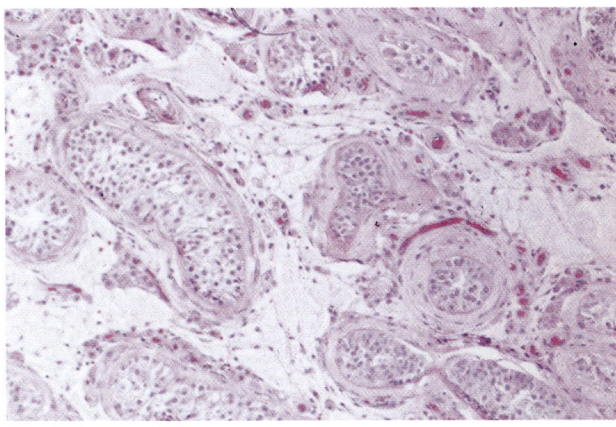

FIGURE 17-21
Cryptorchidism. This testis removed from a postpubertal man shows focal hyalinization of tubules and interstitial fibrosis separating the seminiferous tubules one from another. The tubules contain no spermatozoa.

TABLE 17-5 Disorders of Sexual Differentiation

Sex chromosomal abnormalities
    Klinefelter syndrome and its variants
    Turner syndrome
    46,XX males
Single gene defects
    Adrenogenital syndromes
    Androgen insensitivity syndromes
    Müllerian inhibitory substance deficiency
Prenatal hormonal effects
    Exogenous hormones during pregnancy
    Maternal hormone-producing tumors
Idiopathic conditions
    Hermaphroditism
    Gonadal dysgenesis

a female karyotype (46,XX), and the remaining persons are genetic males (46,XY) or mosaics, or have a missing sex chromosome (45,X).

FEMALE PSEUDOHERMAPHRODITISM: *Virilization of the external genital organs may occur in genetic females (46,XX) who have normal ovaries and internal female genital organs.* Virilization of the vulva, which may show fusion into scrotal folds and is associated with clitoromegaly, is most often found in the adrenogenital syndrome caused by 21-hydroxylase deficiency. Lack of this enzyme leads to overproduction of androgens in the adrenal gland during fetal life, and the ambiguous genitalia are seen at birth. Excess androgens in a pregnant woman can have the same effects on the external genitalia of the baby.

The karyotype 46,XX is found in 1 of 25 patients with classical signs of Klinefelter syndrome. These *46,XX males* have been show to carry the locus for the sex-determining region of chromosome Y (SRY) on one of the X chromosomes. It is not known how this translocation occurs, but it is probably related to the cross-over that occurs during male meiosis.

MALE PSEUDOHERMAPHRODITISM: *A spectrum of congenital disorders affects genetically male persons who have a normal 46,XY karyotype. The gonads are cryptorchid testes, but the external genital organs appear feminine or ambiguously female with signs of virilization.* Male pseudohermaphroditism is most often encountered in *androgen insensitivity syndromes* due to a congenital deficiency of the androgen receptor, also known as *testicular feminization syndrome.*

MALE INFERTILITY

Infertility is empirically defined as the inability to conceive after 1 year of coital activity with the same sexual partner without contraception. Some 15% of couples are childless in the United States, but the true prevalence of infertility is difficult to assess because it is confounded by various cultural and social, determinants. The causes of infertility can be found in the male partner in 20% of cases, in the female in 40%, and in both partners in 20%. In the remaining 20% of infertile couples, the cause cannot be identified. The causes of male infertility are listed in Table 17-6 and shown in Figure 17-22.

Supratesticular causes of infertility are factors that influence or regulate the hormonal and metabolic aspects of spermatogenesis. The best examples are injuries of the hypothalamic–pituitary area. Infertility can result from transection of the pituitary stalk, destruction of the hypothalamus by a brain tumor, or pressure on the pituitary by a craniopharyngioma. A pituitary tumor secreting prolactin (prolactinoma) may act as a mass lesion that destroys the gonadotropin-secreting pituitary cells or compresses the pituitary stalk. It also secretes prolactin, which suppresses spermatogenesis.

Testicular infertility, the most common variety of male infertility, is related to pathological changes in the testis. A male infertility (andrologic) work-up includes urological examination, sonography, semen analysis, hormonal studies, and in some cases testicular biopsy.

Post-testicular infertility refers to blockage of the excretory ducts through which the sperm reaches the urethra. Chronic infections of the epididymis or the vas deferens are often responsible. Less frequently, excretory duct obstruction is due to previous trauma or congenital atresia. Voluntary vasectomy, performed yearly on millions of Americans, is the most common cause of post-testicular infertility.

 Pathology: Morphological alterations in the testicular biopsy that may identify the cause of infertility include the following:

TABLE 17-6 Causes of Male Infertility

Supratesticular causes
    Disorders of the hypothalamic–pituitary–gonadal axis
    Endocrine disease of the adrenal, thyroid; diabetes
    Metabolic disorders
    Major organ diseases (e.g., renal, hepatic, cardiopulmonary diseases)
    Chronic infectious and debilitating diseases (e.g., tuberculosis, AIDS)
    Drugs and substance abuse
Testicular causes
    Idiopathic hypospermatogenesis or azoospermia
    Developmental (cryptorchidism, gonadal dysgenesis)
    Genetic diseases affecting gonads (Klinefelter syndrome)
    Orchitis (immune and infectious)
    Iatrogenic testicular injury (radiation, cytotoxic drugs)
    Trauma of the testis and surgical injury
    Environmental (phytoestrogens)
Post-testicular causes
    Congenital anomalies of the excretory ducts
    Inflammation and scarring of excretory ducts
    Iatrogenic or posttraumatic lesions of excretory ducts

Male Infertility

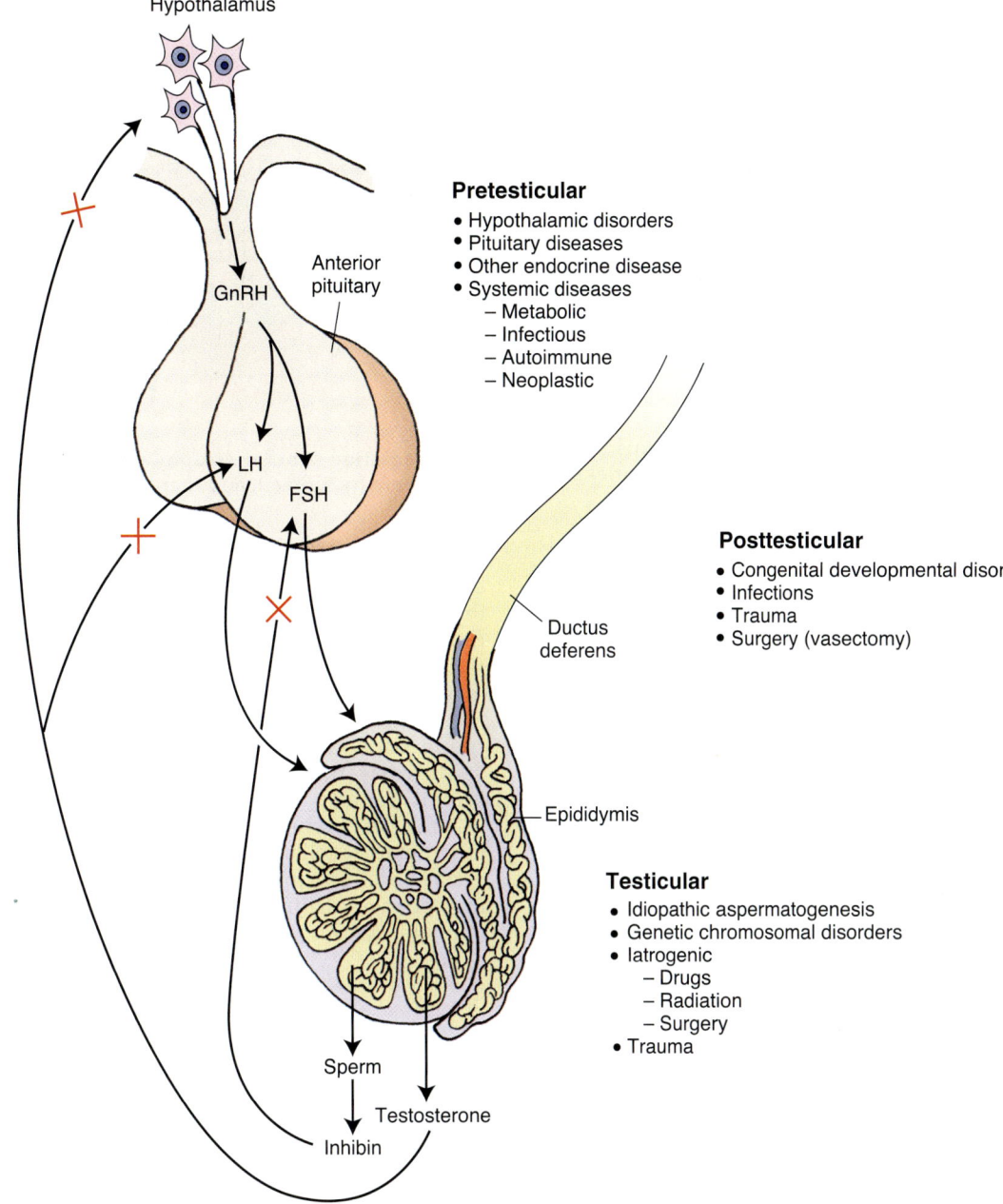

FIGURE 17-22
Causes of male infertility. A. Pretesticular infertility. B. Testicular infertility. C. Post-testicular (obstructive) infertility.

- **Immaturity of the seminiferous tubules** is typically found in hypogonadotropic hypogonadism caused by pituitary or hypothalamic diseases (Fig. 17-23). The seminiferous tubules show no signs of spermatogenic differentiation and resemble those of prepubertal testes.
- **Decreased spermatogenesis (hypospermatogenesis)** occurs in a variety of systemic and endocrine diseases, including malnutrition and AIDS. Hypospermatogenesis is also found in cryptorchid testes and following vasectomy.
- **Germ cell maturation arrest** is usually idiopathic. It can occur at the level of spermatogonia, spermatocytes, or spermatids.
- **Germ cell aplasia** (Sertoli cells only) is mostly idiopathic but can be seen in drug-induced and toxic injury (Fig. 17-24).
- **Orchitis** is caused by viruses (e.g., mumps) or autoimmune diseases.
- **Peritubular and tubular fibrosis** may be related to congenital disorders such as cryptorchidism or to previous infection, ischemia, or radiation (Fig. 17-25).

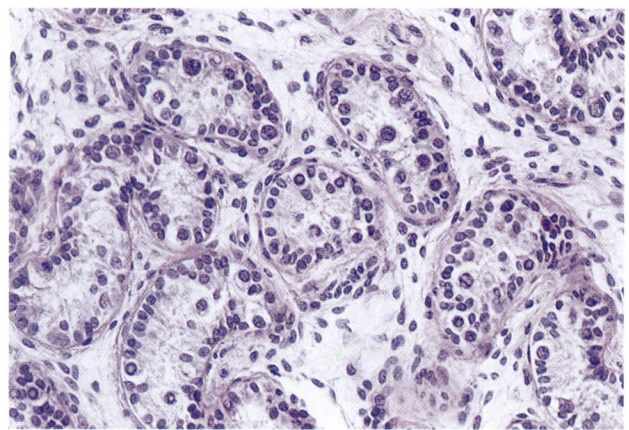

FIGURE 17-23
Hypogonadotropic hypogonadism. The testis of this 25-year-old man is composed of immature seminiferous tubules similar to those seen in prepubertal boys.

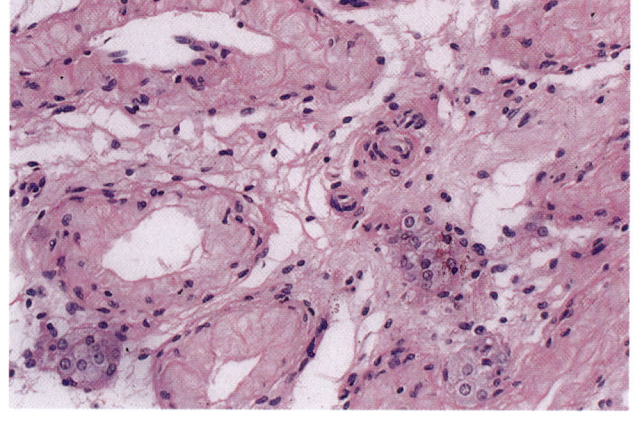

FIGURE 17-25
Postirradiation tubular atrophy of the testis. Seminiferous tubules are hyalinized, and there is no evidence of spermatogenesis.

EPIDIDYMITIS

Epididymitis is an inflammation of the epididymis, usually caused by bacteria, which may be acute or chronic.

Bacterial epididymitis in young men most often occurs in an acute form as a complication of gonorrhea or as a sexually acquired infection with *Chlamydia*. It is characterized by suppurative inflammation (Fig. 17-26). In older men, *E. coli* from associated urinary tract infections is the most common causative agent. Patients present with intrascrotal pain and tenderness, with or without associated fever. Epididymitis of recent origin shows the usual hallmarks of acute inflammation. Persistent chronic epididymitis is associated with the accumulation of plasma cells, macrophages, and lymphocytes and, ultimately, with fibrotic obstruction of the infected ducts. In fact, epididymal inflammation caused by gonorrhea is a common cause of male infertility.

Tuberculous epididymitis is now infrequent and is usually associated with previously established pulmonary and renal tuberculosis. The infection is manifested clinically by a palpable enlargement of the epididymis and beading of the vas deferens. Microscopically, the nodules consist of confluent caseating granulomas.

Spermatic granulomas result from an intense inflammatory response to sperm that have gained entrance to the interstitium of the epididymis. The underlying cause of sperm extravasation is obscure, but traumatic rupture of the epididymal ducts may play a role. Patients present with scrotal pain and swelling, frequently lasting weeks or months. Microscopically, the epididymis displays a mixed inflammatory cell infiltrate that is associated with numerous extravasated sperm fragments and phagocytosis of sperm by macrophages. Ultimately, the inflammatory process results in interstitial fibrosis, ductal obstruction, and infertility.

ORCHITIS

Orchitis is an acute or chronic inflammation of the testis. It may be part of epididymo-orchitis, usually caused by ascending

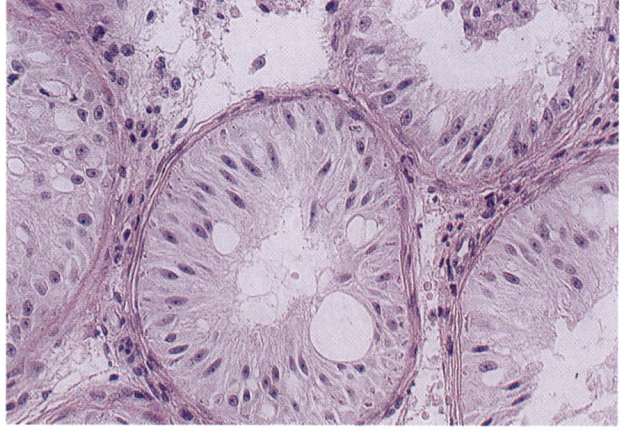

FIGURE 17-24
Germ cell aplasia–Sertoli cell only syndrome. The seminiferous tubules are lined by Sertoli cells and do not contain germ cells.

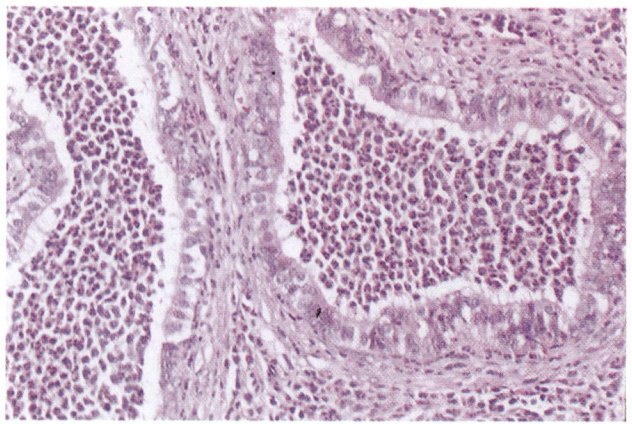

FIGURE 17-26
Bacterial epididymitis. The epididymal ducts contain numerous polymorphonuclear leukocytes.

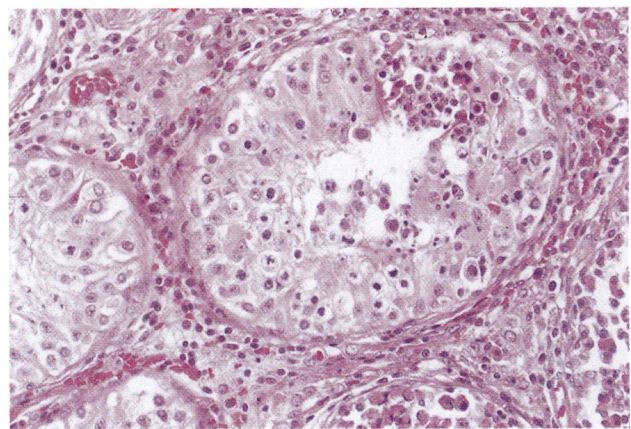

FIGURE 17-27
Viral orchitis. The interstitial spaces are infiltrated with mononuclear cells that spill focally into the lumen of seminiferous tubules. Note that the inflammation has interrupted normal spermatogenesis and that the seminiferous tubules do not contain sperm.

infection, or it may occur as an isolated testicular inflammation. Orchitis is usually secondary to hematogenous spread of pathogens or is an immune-mediated disease.

Gram-negative bacterial orchitis is the most common form of the disease and is often secondary to urinary tract infections. It is typically associated with epididymitis. Infection may also manifest as intratesticular abscess or peritesticular suppuration and fibrosis.

Syphilitic orchitis manifests microscopically in two forms: (1) interstitial perivascular inflammation, characterized by infiltrates of lymphocytes, macrophages and plasma cells, or (2) a granulomatous inflammation of the testis in the form of gummas.

Mumps orchitis occurs in 20% of adult males with mumps, but widespread immunization against mumps has reduced the incidence of the disorder. Viral infection is characterized by testicular pain and gonadal swelling, most commonly unilateral. Microscopically, it appears as an interstitial inflammation that also leads to destruction and loss of seminiferous epithelium (Fig. 17-27).

Granulomatous orchitis of unknown cause is an infrequent disorder of middle-aged men that presents acutely as painful enlargement of the testis or insidiously as testicular induration. The disease is characterized microscopically by noncaseating granulomas that fail to reveal any organisms or the presence of sperm remnants that might act as inciting agents. Variable numbers of seminiferous tubules are destroyed by the granulomatous inflammatory process, which is considered to be a type IV (cell-mediated) hypersensitivity reaction.

Malakoplakia of the testis has the same microscopic features and presumably the same histogenesis as malakoplakia elsewhere.

TUMORS OF THE TESTIS

Tumors of the testis account for less than 1% of all malignancies in adult males. More than 90% of these tumors show the following features:

- Diagnosis between 25 and 45 years of age.
- Germ cell origin.
- Malignancy
- Curable by a combined surgical–chemotherapy approach
- Cytogenetic marker, namely i(p12).
- Metastasize first to periaortic abdominal lymph nodes
- Most (65%) of testicular tumors release markers detectable in the blood.

 Pathogenesis: The etiology of testicular tumors remains unknown and the search for possible environmental or genetic causes has yielded no significant leads for further studies. However, there is a geographical variation in the incidence of testicular cancer. The incidence is highest in Denmark, Sweden, and Norway, but is low in Finland and southern European countries. The tumors are five times more common among Americans of European descent than those of African heritage. Familial occurrence of testicular cancer in brothers or sons and fathers are on record but are rare and provide no support for a genetic theory of tumorigenesis. The only consistent cytogenetic abnormality is an additional fragment of the chromosome 12 (isochromosome p12). As discussed previously, the only documented risk factors for testicular tumors are **cryptorchidism and gonadal dysgenesis**.

 Pathology: Testicular tumors are classified histogenetically on the basis of their cell of origin into several groups (Table 17-7).

 Pathogenesis: It has been proposed that malignant transformation of germ cells could occur during fetal development and involve (1) migrating primordial germ cells, (2) fetal germ cells interacting with

TABLE 17-7 Testicular Tumors

Germ cell tumors—**90%**
   Seminoma (40%)
   Nonseminomatous germ cell tumors
     Embryonal carcinoma (5%)
     Teratocarcinoma (35%)
     Choriocarcinoma (<1%)
   Mixed germ cell tumors (15%)
   Teratoma (1%)
   Spermatocytic seminoma (1%)
   Yolk sac tumor of infancy (2%)
Sex cord cell tumors—**5%**
   Leydig cell tumors (60%)
   Sertoli cell tumors
Metastases—**5%**

Note: The percentages in bold letters refer to the three major groups of tumors. Percentages given in parentheses refer to the frequency of tumor types in each group.

stromal cells in the genital ridge, or (3) early fetal spermatogonia. Since germ cell tumors rarely occur before puberty, some investigators believe that the malignant transformation occurs in the peripubertal period and involves spermatogonia that are stimulated hormonally to proliferate and differentiate into spermatocytes. Despite controversies about the initial events that lead to the onset of neoplasia, a consensus holds that the histogenesis of germ cell tumors progresses through two pathways (Fig. 17-28). The most common pathway involves a carcinoma in situ stage, also known as **intratubular testicular germ cell neoplasia** (ITGCN), which subsequently progresses to invasive carcinoma (see below). This pathway accounts for the development of most adult germ cell tumors, although ITGCN is not found in spermatocytic seminomas, teratomas of prepubertal testes, and yolk sac tumors of infancy, which develop directly from germ cells without an in situ lesion. It is possible that some migratory primordial germ cells have not found their way into the seminiferous tubules during fetal testicular organogenesis and that such "misplaced" cells become the progenitors of yolk sac tumors and teratomas. Such germ cells can also give rise to extragonadal germ cell tumors in the retroperitoneum, sacral region, anterior mediastinum, and the area of the pineal.

Tumor cells of ITGCN resemble spermatogonia or fetal germ cells but have much larger polyploid nuclei (Fig.17-29).

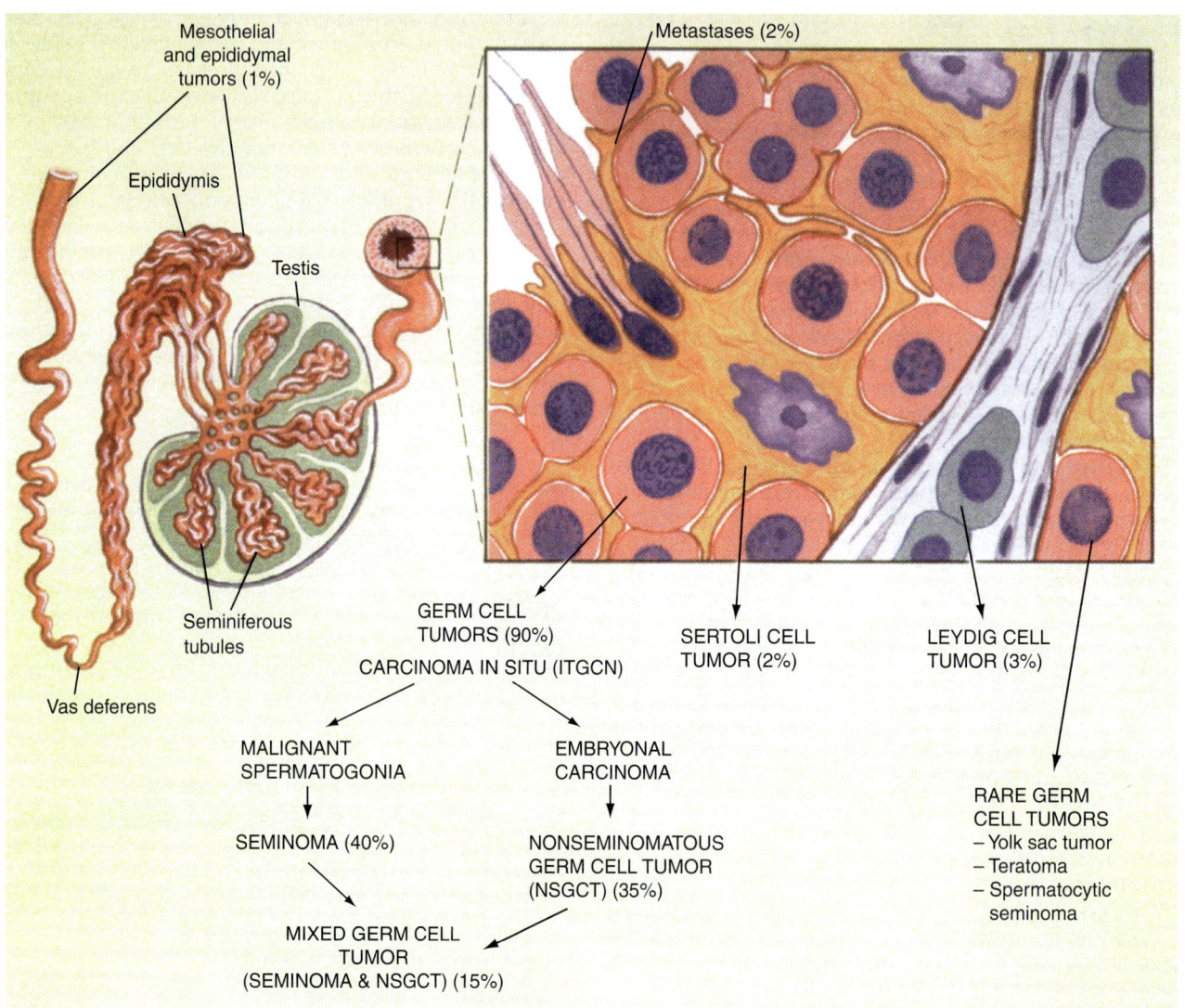

FIGURE 17-28
Tumors of the testis, epididymis, and related structures. Most testicular tumors originate from germ cells and are preceded by a carcinoma in situ stage known as intratubular germ cell neoplasia (ITGCN). Germ cell tumors of adult testis can be classified as seminomas (40%) or nonseminomatous germ cell tumors (NSGCTs) (35%). In 15% of cases seminomatous elements are intermixed with NSGCT, forming mixed germ cell tumors. Some germ cell tumors (yolk sac tumor of childhood, childhood teratomas, and spermatocytic seminomas) develop without passing through a preinvasive ITGCN stage. Tumors originating from sex cord stromal cells (Leydig and Sertoli cell tumors), epididymal tumors, tumors of the mesothelial lining of the tunica vaginalis (adenomatoid tumors), and metastases are rare.

Tumors of the Testis 913

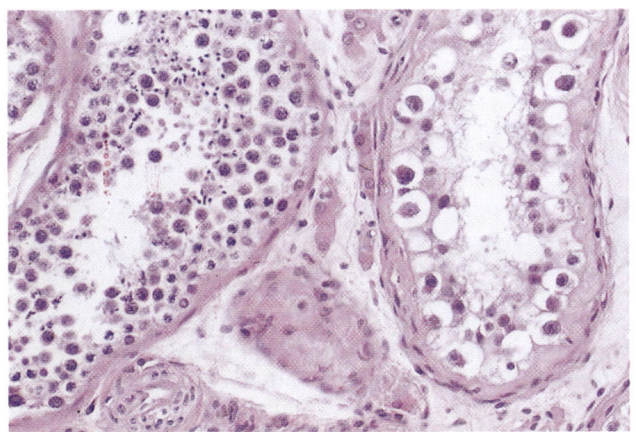

FIGURE 17-29
Intratubular germ cell neoplasia (ITGCN). The seminiferous tubule to the right contains large atypical cells corresponding to intratubular carcinoma in situ. Compare these cells with the normal spermatogonia in the adjacent tubule *(to the left)*, which show normal spermatogenesis.

Like fetal germ cells, these cells express on their surface placental-like alkaline phosphatase. In infertile men with a history of cryptorchid testes, ITGCN can persist unchanged for 5 to 10 years, after which the neoplastic cells acquire invasive properties, penetrate through the tubular basement membrane, and give rise to infiltrating malignant tumors.

The malignant cells that retain the phenotypic features of spermatogonia give rise to **seminomas**. Alternatively, the neoplastic germ cells can differentiate into malignant embryonic cells **(embryonal carcinoma)** by a process that resembles *parthenogenetic activation* of oocytes in the female gonads of amphibians and reptiles.

In some cases, embryonal carcinoma cells proliferate in an undifferentiated form. In others, they differentiate into the three embryonic germ layers (ectoderm, mesoderm, endoderm) or extraembryonic tissues that form the fetal membranes and the placenta. Further differentiation of germ layer cells leads to the formation of various somatic tissues. Ectoderm differentiates into skin, central nervous system, retinal pigment, and other related tissues; mesoderm gives rise to smooth and striated muscle, cartilage, bone, etc.; endoderm forms intestinal tissue, bronchial epithelium, salivary glands, etc. The extraembryonic derivatives of embryonal carcinoma cells give rise to chorionic epithelium (cytotrophoblast and syncytiotrophoblast) and yolk sac-like epithelium. These complex tumors composed of malignant undifferentiated embryonal carcinoma cells and their somatic and extraembryonic derivatives are called **teratocarcinomas** or **malignant teratomas**. When embryonal carcinoma cells proliferate without further differentiating and exhibit a single histological pattern, the tumor is labeled *embryonal carcinoma*. In rare instances, the extraembryonic components of teratocarcinomas overgrow and destroy all other components. Such tumors are composed of a single tumor type and are classified as **yolk sac carcinoma** or **choriocarcinoma**.

For clinical purposes, all germ cell tumors containing embryonal carcinoma as their malignant stem cells are grouped as **nonseminomatous germ cell tumors,** to distinguish them from seminomas. Pure yolk sac carcinomas of the adult testis and choriocarcinomas are also included in this group because

it is assumed that these tumors must contain a few embryonal carcinoma cells that are not readily recognizable.

In 15% of cases, germ cell tumors contain both seminoma and nonseminomatous elements. Such **mixed germ cell tumors** are treated clinically as nonseminomatous neoplasms.

Intratubular Germ Cell Neoplasia Refers to Testicular Carcinoma in Situ

ITGCN represents a preinvasive form of germ cell tumors.

 Epidemiology: ITGCN can be encountered as (1) an isolated focal histological change in 2% of cryptorchid testes or testicular biopsies performed for infertility, (2) widespread carcinoma in situ adjacent to almost all invasive germ, and (3) lesions in 5% of contralateral testes in patients who had an orchiectomy for a testicular germ cell neoplasm.

 Pathology: ITGCN involves testes in a patchy manner, usually affecting not more than 10 to 30% of the tubules. The seminiferous tubules harboring ITGCN have thick basement membranes and do not contain sperm. The normal germ cells are replaced by neoplastic germ cells that are broadly attached to the basal lamina (see Fig. 17-32). The neoplastic cells appear larger than normal spermatogonia. Their nuclei are large, have finely dispersed chromatin, and display prominent nucleoli. The nuclei are centrally located and surrounded by abundant, clear cytoplasm that contains large amounts of glycogen. The nuclear DNA content is increased, suggesting that the cells are triploid. The plasma membrane is distinct and stains with antibodies to placental alkaline phosphatase (PLAP).

 Clinical features: ITGCN diagnosed in testicular biopsy specimens is a precursor of invasive carcinoma, which develops at an unpredictable pace. Half of men diagnosed with ITGCN will develop invasive cancer within 5 years, and 70% in 7 years. Microscopic diagnosis of ITGCN in a testicular biopsy specimen is an indication for prophylactic orchiectomy.

Seminoma Contains Monomorphous Cells That Resemble Spermatogonia

 Epidemiology: Seminoma is the most common testicular cancer, accounting for 40% of all germ cells tumors in that organ. The peak incidence occurs in men between 30 and 40 years of age. Seminomas are never found in prepubertal children, except in those who have dysgenetic gonads.

 Pathology: On gross examination, seminomas appear as solid, rubbery-firm, bosselated masses. Tumor tissue is usually sharply demarcated from the normal testicular tissue, which may be compressed, atrophic, and fibrotic. On cross section the tumors appear lobulated, and homogeneously tan or grayish yellow (Fig. 17-30). Areas of necrosis or hemorrhage are usually inconspicuous but may be seen in larger tumors.

Microscopically, seminoma is equivalent to ovarian dysgerminoma. The tumor features a single population of uniform polygonal cells that have centrally located vesicular nuclei. The ample cytoplasm appears clear in standard histological sections because it contains large amounts of glycogen and some lipid. Tumor cells are arranged as nests or sheets that are separated by fibrous septa infiltrated with lymphocytes, plasma cells, and macrophages. Occasionally, the septa contain granulomas with giant cells. Tumor cells invade the parenchyma of the testis but also spread through the seminiferous tubules and into the rete testis. Invasion of the epididymis is seen later in the course of the disease, usually preceding the spread to the abdominal lymph nodes.

Seminoma cells resemble immature spermatogonia. Like fetal spermatogonia and primordial germ cells in the fetus, they express PLAP on the plasma membrane. PLAP is shed into the blood in small amounts but cannot be used for diagnostic purposes.

Pathologists recognize two additional subtypes of seminoma: (1) seminoma with syncytiotrophoblastic giant cells and (2) anaplastic seminoma. The first subgroup includes 20% of tumors that contain syncytiotrophoblastic cells. These multinucleated giant cells are best demonstrated with antibodies to human chorionic gonadotropin (hCG). Although syncytiotrophoblastic cell secrete hCG, this potential serological tumor marker rarely becomes detectable in the systemic circulation. Some 5% of seminomas show brisk mitotic activity and nuclear pleomorphism and are classified as *anaplastic seminoma.*

 Clinical Features: Seminoma manifests as a progressively growing scrotal mass and is usually diagnosed while it can still be cured by orchiectomy, with or without abdominal lymph node dissection. Seminomas are extremely radiosensitive, and radiotherapy plays an important role in the treatment of tumors that cannot be cured by surgery alone. Seminomas in advanced stages of dissemination are treated with additional chemotherapy. **The cure rate is over 90% in all histological types of seminoma.**

Spermatocytic seminoma is a rare tumor related to classical seminoma only in name. Spermatocytic seminomas are benign tumors of men older than 40 years of age. These tumors are not associated with ITGCN and do not elicit a lymphocytic reaction. Spermatocytic seminomas contain three cell types, namely, large, small, and intermediate cells. Orchiectomy is curative.

Nonseminomatous Germ Cell Tumors Are Derived from Embryonal Cells

Nonseminomatous germ cell tumors (NSGCTs) of the testis include several pathological entities, two of which account for most of the cases: (1) pure embryonal carcinomas and (2) teratocarcinomas, also known as *malignant teratomas* or *mixed germ cell tumors*. Pure choriocarcinoma, pure yolk sac carci-

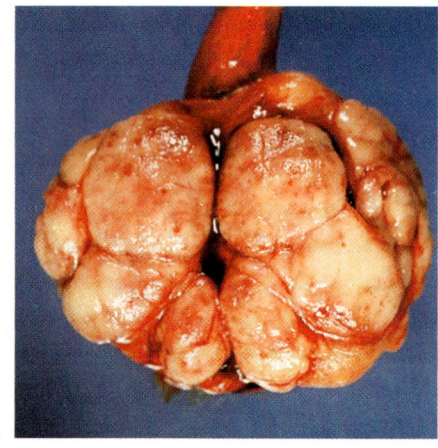

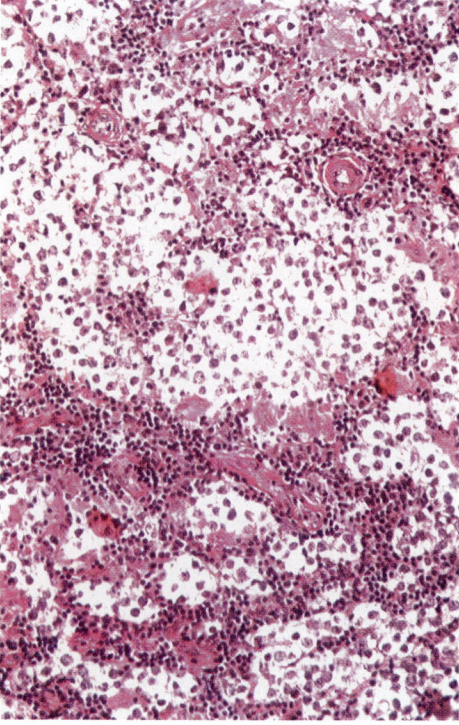

FIGURE 17-30
Seminoma. A. The cut surface of this nodular tumor is tan and bulging, suggesting that the tumor is firm and rubbery. **B.** Groups of cells are surrounded by fibrous septa infiltrated with lymphocytes.

noma of the adult testis, and the so-called growing benign teratoma are rare NSGCTs. Mixed germ cell tumors are NSGCTs combined with seminomas.

 Epidemiology: NSGCTs constitute 55% of all testicular germ cell tumors. Teratocarcinomas account for two thirds of all NSGCTs, followed by mixed germ cell tumors and pure embryonal carcinomas. All other tumors of this group are extremely rare. Like seminomas, NSGCTs have a peak incidence in the 25- to 40-year-old age group, but at the time of diagnosis, patients with NSGCTs are somewhat younger than those with seminomas.

Pathology: On gross examination, nonseminomatous tumors vary in size and shape. On cross section they are solid or partially cystic. The solid areas vary in color from white to yellow to red, indicating that they are composed of viable tumor cells, foci of necrosis, and hemorrhage, respectively (Fig. 17-31).

Microscopic features of NSGCTs are highly variable. In pure embryonal carcinoma, the tumor is composed exclusively of undifferentiated embryonal carcinoma cells that are similar to cells from preimplantation-stage embryos (Fig. 17-32). Since the tumor cells have little cytoplasm, their hyperchromatic, disproportionately large nuclei seem to overlap. Embryonal carcinoma cells may be arranged as broad solid sheets, cords, glandlike tubules, and acini and sometimes even line papillary structures. Numerous mitoses and apoptotic cells are characteristic. Antibodies to keratins are used to distinguish keratin-rich embryonal carcinoma from seminoma, lymphoma, sarcoma, and melanoma, which are de-

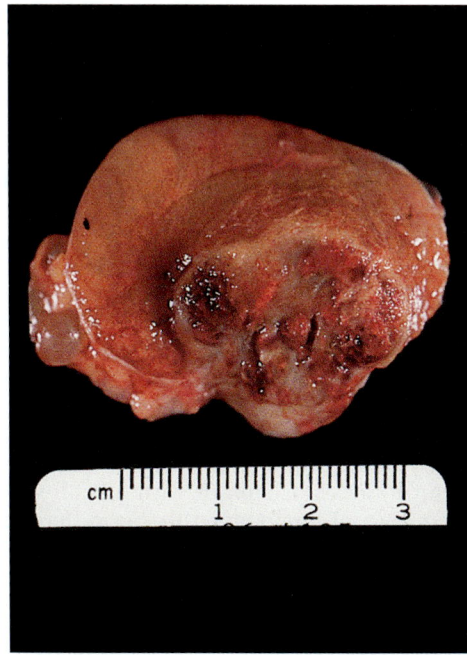

FIGURE 17-31
Nonseminomatous germ cell tumor of the testis. The cut surface of this small testicular tumor shows considerable heterogeneity, varying in color from white to dark red.

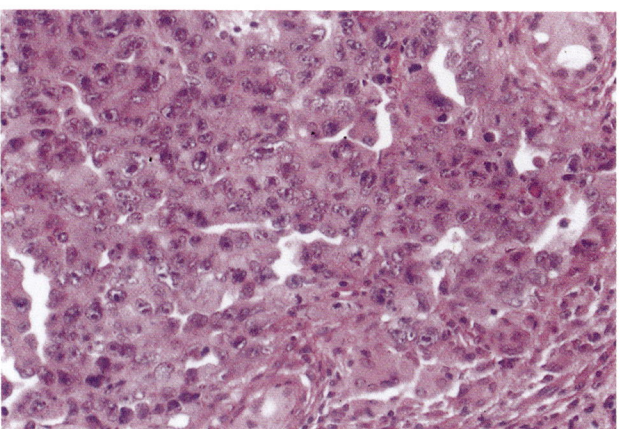

FIGURE 17-32
Embryonal carcinoma component of a NSGCT. Because these undifferentiated cells have scant cytoplasm, their hyperchromatic nuclei appear crowded and seem to overlap each other. The cells form solid sheets, focally interrupted by clefts.

void of keratin. Embryonal carcinoma invades the testis, epididymis, and blood vessels and metastasizes to abdominal lymph nodes, lungs, and other organs.

Embryonal carcinoma cells are the stem cells of **teratocarcinomas** (malignant teratomas), which feature differentiated somatic elements (i.e., tissues that are normally found in various organs, and extraembryonic elements, including yolk sac cells and trophoblastic cells). Microscopic examination of such nonseminomatous tumors thus reveals foci of embryonal carcinoma and a variety of other tissues (Fig. 17-33). For example, in the shorthand form used by some pathologists, a tumor might be labeled NSGCT (EC+YS+Ch), indicating that it is composed of embryonal carcinoma yolk sac components and trophoblastic components corresponding to choriocarcinoma. A similar tumor that also contains seminoma cells would, however, be called **mixed germ cell tumor,** and the abbreviation would be NSGCT (EC+YS+Ch+Se). In most tumors, malignancy resides in embryonal carcinoma cells. Interestingly, when these cells metastasize, they can differentiate into somatic or extraembryonic tissues, in which case the metastatic tumor can resemble the original one.

NSGCTs can give rise to clones of highly malignant cytotrophoblastic and syncytiotrophoblastic cells that overgrow the other elements. Tumors composed exclusively of malignant chorionic epithelium are termed *choriocarcinomas*. Likewise, clones of malignant yolk sac epithelium produce **yolk sac carcinoma.**

Some histologically benign teratomas of postpubertal young men may have a malignant clinical course, even though they appear to be composed of mature, nonproliferating somatic tissues, without embryonal elements (Fig.17-34). In some instances it is assumed that the tumor was actually a teratocarcinoma in which almost all embryonal cells have differentiated into mature somatic tissues but that a few remaining malignant cells were undetected by the pathologist or had metastasized before the tumor was resected. These tumors are clinically known as the **growing teratoma syndrome.** In other cases, the teratoma tissues remain undifferentiated and resemble embryonic organs or embryonic tumors such as neuroblastoma. These **immature teratomas** are also potentially malignant tumors.

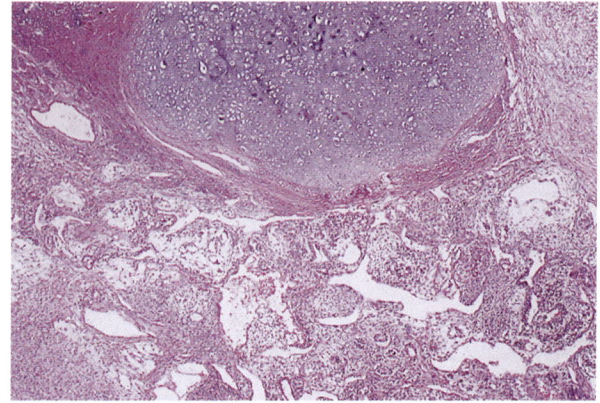
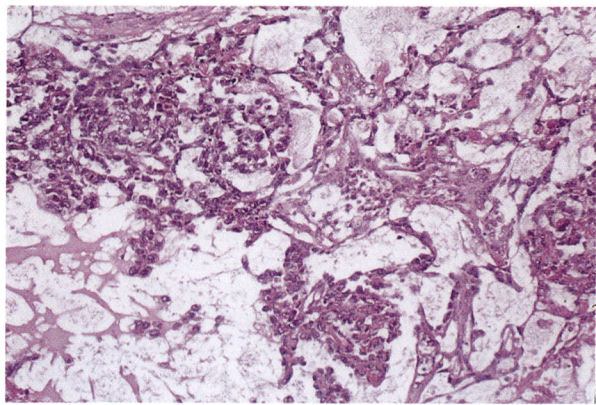
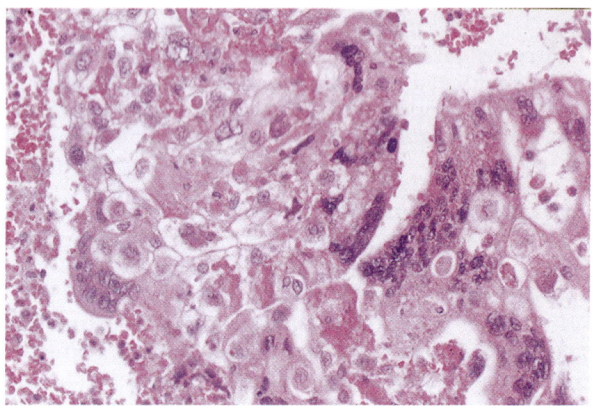

FIGURE 17-33
Nonseminomatous germ cell tumor. A. Somatic tissue of this tumor includes well-differentiated cartilage *(top)* and nondescript connective tissue *(bottom)*. **B.** Yolk sac component consists of interlacing cord of epithelial cells surrounded by loose stroma resembling the early yolk sac. **C.** Choriocarcinoma component of the NSGCT consists of multinucleated syncytiotrophoblastic giant cells and mononuclear cytotrophoblastic cells. Invasive growth of trophoblasts is usually associated with hemorrhage.

 Clinical Features: Most NSGCTs manifest as a testicular mass. They tend to grow faster than seminomas and metastasize more readily and more widely. Hence, in some NSGCTs metastases may be the first sign of the neoplastic disease.

In contrast to seminomas, NSGCTs often contain yolk sac components and syncytiotrophoblastic cells. Yolk sac cells secrete a-fetoprotein (AFP), a fetal plasma protein that is not normally found in the blood. Syncytiotrophoblastic cells release hCG, a hormone of pregnancy, that is also not found in males. **Elevated levels of serum AFP or hCG are found in 70% of patients harboring NSGCTs and are thus reliable tumor markers.** These antigens are most useful in the postoperative follow-up of patients who have been treated for NSGCT. Persistently elevated levels of AFP or hCG or both indicate that the patient is not tumor free. Patients whose initially high levels of AFP and hCG normalize after treatment but subsequently rise again have metastases.

The treatment of NSGCT includes orchiectomy to remove the primary tumor, followed by platinum-based chemotherapy and, if indicated, surgical dissection of abdominal lymph nodes. Chemotherapy usually eliminates metastatic embryonal carcinoma cells, but differentiated tissues originating from them are resistant. However, such tissues do not grow and are not likely to endanger the patient. Nevertheless, it is better to remove any residual neoplasia than to take a chance that a few malignant tumor cells might be hiding in the residuals tumors. Only 3 decades ago, patients with NSGCTs had only a 35% chance for 5-year survival. **By contrast, complete cures are now recorded in over 90% of cases.**

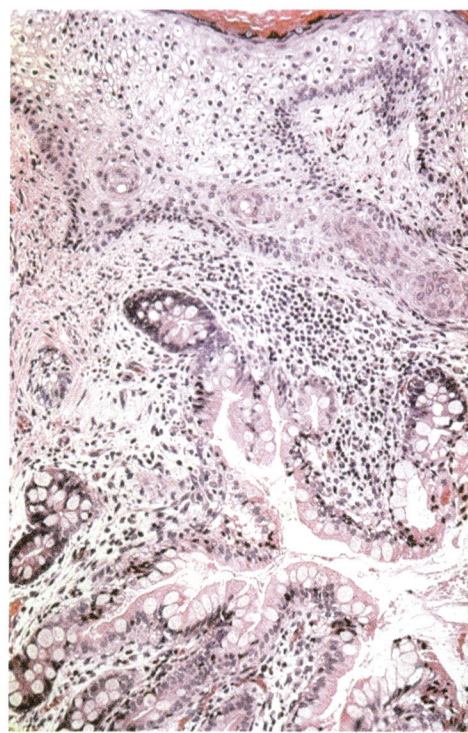

FIGURE 17-34
Teratoma. The main cavity of this cystic tumor is lined by squamous epithelium *(top)*. Adjacent to the squamous epithelium, the wall of the cyst contains mucus-secreting epithelium resembling colonic mucosa.

Testicular Tumors of Infancy and Childhood

Testicular tumors are rare in prepubertal boys. In the first 4 years of life, most testicular neoplasms are classified histologically as yolk sac tumors. Benign teratomas are the most common testicular tumor in the age group between 4 and 12 years.

YOLK SAC TUMORS: These neoplasms are composed of cells arranged into structures reminiscent of parts of the fetal yolk sac. The diagnosis is based on recognizing multiple microscopic tumor patterns and the so-called glomeruloid *Schiller-Duval bodies* (Fig. 17-35). The histological features of neonatal tumors are similar to those of the yolk sac elements in NSGCTs. Yolk sac tumors of infancy and childhood are considered malignant, but a timely orchiectomy and removal of the tumor is associated with a greater than 95% complete cure rate.

TERATOMAS: These tumors of prepubertal testes are benign and are composed of mature somatic tissues. Simple orchiectomy and even testis-sparing surgery are curative.

Gonadal Stromal/Sex Cord Tumor

Gonadal stroma/sex cord tumors are composed of cells that resemble Sertoli or Leydig cells. These neoplasms constitute 5% of all testicular tumors.

LEYDIG CELL TUMORS: *Rare neoplasms are composed of cells resembling interstitial (Leydig) cells of the testis.* They can be hormonally active and secrete androgens, estrogens, or both.

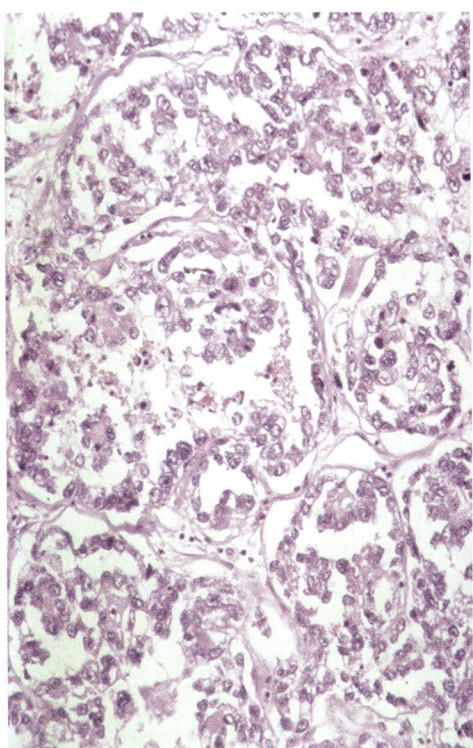

FIGURE 17-35
Yolk sac tumor. This childhood tumor is composed of interlacing strands of epithelial cells surrounded by loose connective stroma. The lobular arrangement of cells surrounded by empty spaces leads to the formation of glomeruloid structures (Schiller-Duval bodies).

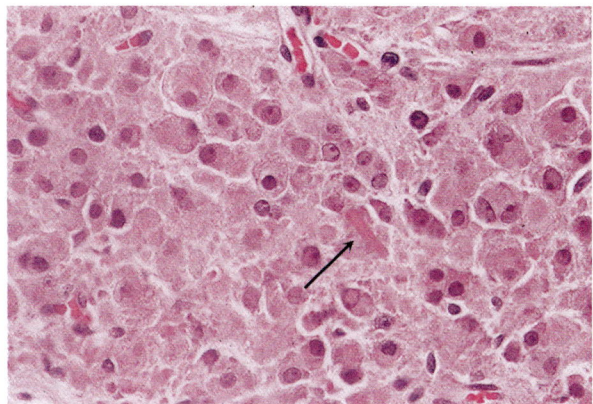

FIGURE 17-36
Leydig cell tumor. The tumor cells have uniform round nuclei and well-developed eosinophilic cytoplasm. A cytoplasmic Reinke crystal is seen in the center of the field *(arrow)*.

Leydig cell tumors can occur at any age, with two distinct peaks, one in childhood and one in adults from the third to the sixth decade.

 Pathology: Leydig cell tumors are well circumscribed, and some appear encapsulated. They vary in size from 1 to 10 cm in diameter. The cut surface is yellow to brown, and the larger tumors have fibrous trabeculae, which impart a lobular appearance. Microscopically, Leydig cell tumor is composed of uniform cells that have round nuclei and well-developed eosinophilic or vacuolated cytoplasm (Fig. 17-36). *Reinke crystals,* rectangular, eosinophilic, cytoplasmic inclusions, are typically found in normal Leydig cells and are present in 30% of tumors. Although most (90%) of Leydig cell tumors are benign (only 10% are malignant), it is difficult to predict the biological behavior on histological grounds.

 Clinical Features: The androgenic effects of testicular Leydig cell tumors in prepubertal boys lead to precocious physical and sexual development. By contrast, feminization and gynecomastia are observed in some adults with this tumor. Either estrogen or testosterone levels may be elevated, but there is no characteristic pattern. All Leydig cell tumors in children and almost all tumors in adults are cured by orchiectomy.

SERTOLI CELL TUMORS: *Some testicular sex cord stromal cell tumors are composed of neoplastic Sertoli cells.* Most (90%) tumors are benign and produce few if any hormonal symptoms.

 Pathology: Sertoli cell tumors tend to be small (1–3 cm), solid, well-circumscribed yellow–gray nodules. Microscopically, they are composed of columnar tumor cells arranged into tubules or cords in a fibrous trabecular framework (Fig. 17-37). The rare malignant variant exhibits greater cellular pleomorphism, areas of necrosis, and little tendency to form cords and tubules.

 Clinical Features: Most patients with Sertoli cell tumors are younger than 40 years of age and come to medical attention because of a mass in the scro-

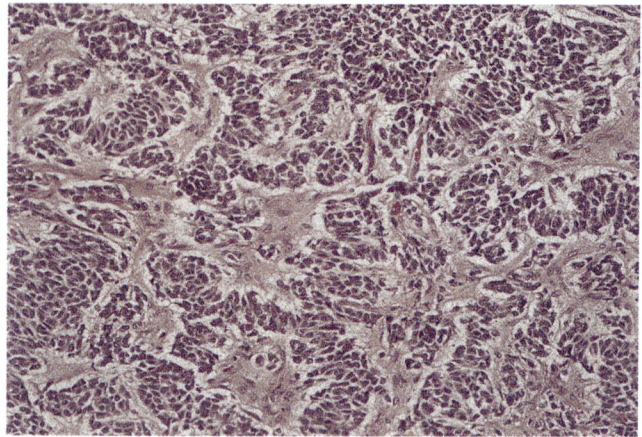

FIGURE 17-37
Sertoli cell tumor. The neoplastic cells are arranged in cords of variable size in a fibrous stroma.

tum. Endocrine effects are uncommon and, if present, are vague. Orchiectomy is curative.

Other Testicular Tumors

METASTASES: Involvement of the testis with metastases is rare and accounts for only 5% of all testicular tumors. Most often these tumors are secondary to primary cancers of the prostate, large intestine, or bladder.

MALIGNANT LYMPHOMA: This cancer is the most frequently encountered neoplasm in the testes of men older than 60 years. It usually occurs in the context of systemic disease, but a few cases of primary lymphoma of the testis have been reported. Most but not all patients with lymphomatous involvement of the testis have a poor prognosis.

Adenomatoid tumor (*benign mesothelioma*) *is a benign tumor that originates from the mesothelial layer of the testicular tunica vaginalis.* These neoplasms are usually located in the upper pole of the epididymis, with fewer cases involving the tunica vaginalis of the testis or the spermatic cord. The lesions are well-demarcated tan nodules that vary in size from a few millimeters to 2 cm, although rare examples have been reported up to 6 cm. Three microscopic patterns have been recognized: plexiform, tubular, and mixed.

Prostate

PROSTATITIS

Prostatitis is an inflammation of the prostate that can occur in acute and chronic forms. It is usually caused by coliform uropathogens, but in many instances, the cause cannot be determined.

ACUTE PROSTATITIS: *Typically a complication of other urinary tract infections, acute prostatitis results from the reflux of infected urine into the prostate.* Microscopically, an acute inflammatory infiltrate is seen in the prostatic acini and stroma. The disorder causes intense discomfort on urination and is often associated with fever, chills, and perineal pain. Most patients respond well to standard antibiotic treatment.

CHRONIC BACTERIAL PROSTATITIS: *This infection of longer duration that may or may not be preceded by an episode of acute prostatitis.* Most patients with chronic prostatitis complain of dysuria and burning at the urethral meatus. Suprapubic, perineal, and low back pain or discomfort and nocturia may be also present. The urine usually contains bacteria. In addition to reflux of urine, additional factors such as prostatic calculi and local prostatic duct obstruction may contribute to the development of chronic bacterial prostatitis. Microscopically, infiltrates of lymphocytes, plasma cells, and macrophages are the rule. Prolonged antibiotic therapy is often, but not necessarily, curative.

NONBACTERIAL PROSTATITIS: *There exists a form of chronic prostatitis in which no causative organism is identified.* It is the most common form of inflammation in prostatic biopsy or prostatectomy specimens or at autopsy. Nonbacterial prostatitis typically affects men older than 50 years of age, but it has been reported in virtually all age groups. It has been hypothesized that some cases may be due to *C. trachomatis, Mycoplasma, U. urealyticum* and *Trichomonas vaginalis*. However, in clinical practice it is a diagnosis of exclusion.

The most common histological pattern consists of dilated glands filled with neutrophils and foamy macrophages and surrounded by chronic inflammatory cells. The condition may be asymptomatic or cause symptoms similar to those in chronic bacterial prostatitis. The diagnosis requires fractionated collection of urine combined with transrectal prostatic massage. In most cases no specific therapy is available.

GRANULOMATOUS PROSTATITIS: *This chronic inflammation is characterized by the presence of granulomas.* In most cases, the cause cannot be established. On rare occasions, granulomatous prostatitis can be traced to specific causative agents, including *M. tuberculosis* and a wide variety of fungal pathogens such as *Histoplasma capsulatum*. A granulomatous lesion resembling rheumatoid nodules has been recognized and related to previous transurethral resection of a portion of the prostate gland. The symptoms of chronic granulomatous prostatitis are vague, and the diagnosis is made histologically. Caseating or noncaseating granulomas are associated with localized destruction of prostatic ducts and acini and, in later stages, with fibrosis.

 Clinical Features: As indicated above, the symptoms of chronic prostatitis are highly variable and the treatment may be quite frustrating. Most importantly, chronic prostatitis may cause an elevation of serum prostate-specific antigen (PSA), raising the possibility of prostatic malignancy. Accordingly, the diagnosis is often made by biopsy performed to exclude carcinoma.

NODULAR HYPERPLASIA OF THE PROSTATE

Nodular hyperplasia of the prostate, also termed benign prostatic hyperplasia *(BPH), is a common disorder characterized clinically by enlargement of the gland and obstruction to the flow of urine through the bladder outlet and pathologically by the proliferation of glands and stroma.*

Epidemiology: BPH is most frequent in western Europe and the United States and least common in the Orient. The prevalence of the disorder in the United States is higher among blacks than among whites. Clinical prostatism (i.e., BPH severe enough to interfere with urination) peaks in the seventh decade. However, the prevalence of BPH is far greater at autopsy than is suggested by clinically apparent prostatism. In fact, 75% of men 80 years of age or older have some degree of prostatic hyperplasia. The disorder is rarely observed in men younger than 40 years of age (Fig. 17-38).

Pathogenesis: The earliest histogenetic events in the evolution of BPH are still not understood. Although noted previously, prepubertal castration prevents the subsequent development of BPH, exogenous testosterone has no effect on either the histological appearance of the hyperplastic nodules or the areas of the prostate that show evidence of senile atrophy. Advancing age is associated with a comparable reduction in circulating testosterone in men with and without BPH. Moreover, no change in the serum level of dihydrotestosterone (DHT) is observed in men with BPH, although the ratio of circulating testosterone to DHT may be abnormally low. Interestingly, changes resembling BPH have been produced in dogs by the administration of DHT, and the intake of a drug that blocks 5α-reductase (finasteride) has reduced the size of the prostate in men with BPH.

Pathology: Early nodular hyperplasia of the prostate begins in the submucosa of the proximal urethra **(the transitional zone).** The developing prostatic nodules compress the centrally located urethral lumen and the more peripherally located normal prostate (Fig. 17-39). In well-developed BPH, the normal gland is actually limited to an attenuated rim of tissue beneath the capsule. On cut section, an individual nodule is clearly demarcated by an enveloping fibrous pseudocapsule (Fig. 17-40). Focal hemorrhage and infarction may be present, especially in the larger nodules. On occasion, small stones are present within the dilated hyperplastic acini. The secondary changes reflect bladder outlet obstruction (Fig. 17-41).

Histologically, BPH features the proliferation of epithelial cells of the acini and ductules, smooth muscle cells, and stromal fibroblasts, all in variable proportions. Accordingly, five types of nodules have been described: (1) stromal (fibrous), (2) fibromuscular, (3) muscular, (4) fibroadenomatous, and (5) fibromyoadenomatous, the most common type.

In the typical fibromyoadenomatous nodule, variably sized hyperplastic prostatic acini are randomly scattered throughout the stroma of the nodule. The epithelial (adenomatous) component is composed of a double layer of cells, with tall columnar cells overlying the basal layer (see Fig. 17-40B). Papillary hyperplasia of the glandular epithelium is characteristic. Hyperplastic nodules often contain chronic inflammatory cells, and *corpora amylacea* (eosinophilic laminated concretions) are frequently seen within the acini. The glands of the uninvolved peripheral region of the prostate are frequently atrophic and compressed by the expanding nodules. The stroma of each type of nodule differs in composition, but elastic fibers are always absent. Immunoperoxidase staining of the hyperplastic epithelium is consistently positive for PSA and prostatic acid phosphatase.

Nonspecific prostatitis is frequently encountered in specimens that exhibit nodular hyperplasia. There is a dense intraglandular and periglandular infiltrate of lymphocytes, plasma cells, and macrophages, frequently accompanied by acute inflammatory cells and focal gland destruction. Focal infarcts of varying age are observed in 20% of cases. Squamous metaplasia of the epithelium of ducts at the periphery of infarcts is typical. Incidental foci of prostatic adenocarci-

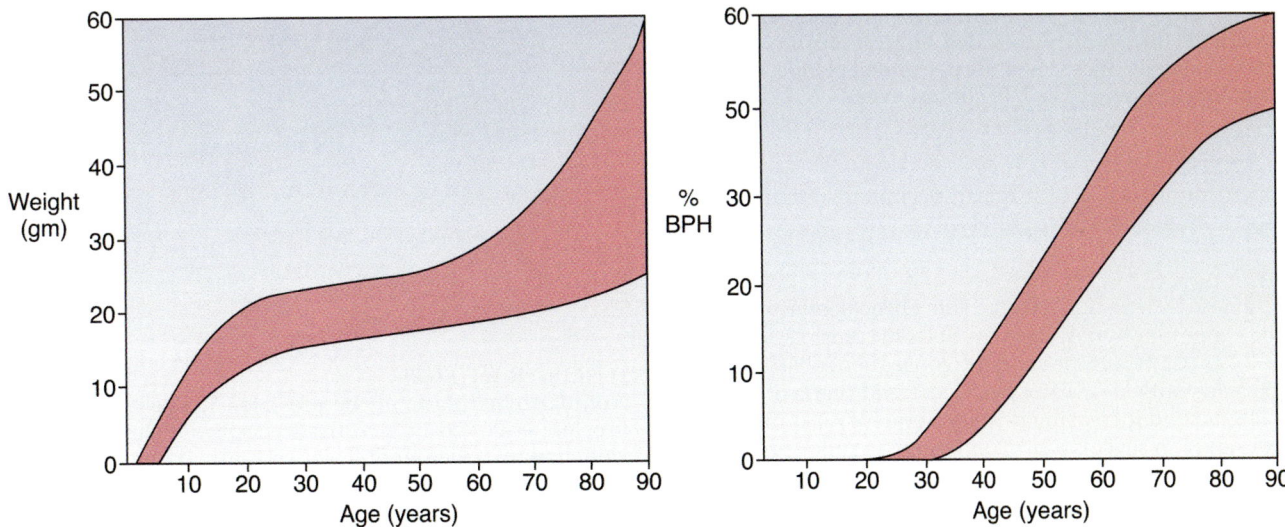

FIGURE 17-38
Growth of the prostate *(left)* **and frequency of nodular hyperplasia** *(right).* **By 80 years of age, most men have benign prostatic hyperplasia (BPH).**

920 The Lower Urinary Tract and Male Reproductive System

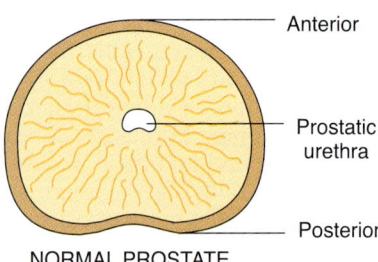

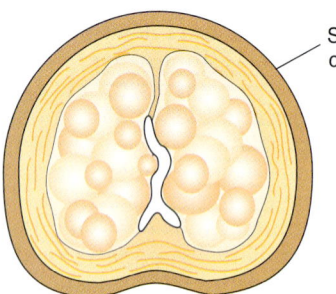

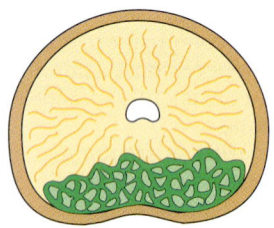

FIGURE 17-39
Normal prostate, nodular hyperplasia, and adenocarcinoma. In prostatic hyperplasia, which involves predominantly the periurethral part of the gland, the nodules compress and distort the urethra. The expansion of the central prostatic glands leads to compression of the peripheral parts and fibrosis, resulting in the formation of so-called surgical capsule. Prostatic carcinoma usually arises from the peripheral glands, and compression of the urethra is a late clinical event.

noma are found in 10% of surgical specimens submitted with a preoperative diagnosis of BPH.

Clinical Features: The clinical symptoms of nodular hyperplasia result from compression of the prostatic urethra and the consequent obstruction to the bladder outlet. A history of decreased vigor of the urinary stream and increasing urinary frequency is typical. Rectal examination reveals a firm, enlarged, nodular prostate. If the duration of severe obstruction is prolonged, backpressure results in hydroureter, hydronephrosis, and ultimately renal failure and death.

The classic treatment of BPH was surgical. Transurethral resection of the prostate or, less commonly, suprapubic enucleation of the hyperplastic tissue alleviated the symptoms of prostatism. Both procedures result in the surgical excision of the central hyperplastic nodules, leaving behind the more peripheral (subcapsular) prostatic glandular tissue. Currently, the surgical treatment of nodular hyperplasia has largely been replaced by administration of drugs that inhibit 5α-reductase, with resultant diminution of prostate size. α-Adrenergic blockers decrease muscular tone in the prostate and ameliorate the symptoms of urinary obstruction.

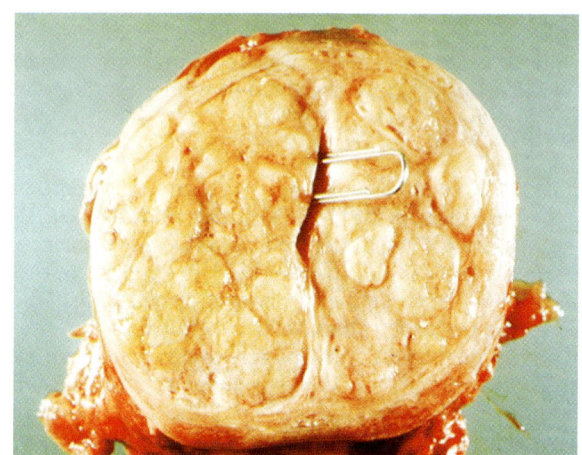

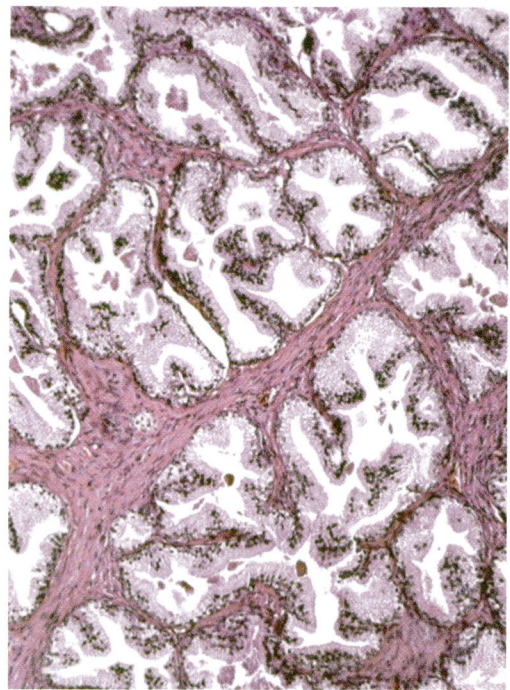

FIGURE 17-40
Nodular hyperplasia of the prostate. A. The cut surface of a prostate enlarged by nodular hyperplasia shows numerous well-circumscribed nodules of prostatic tissue. The prostatic urethra *(paper clip)* has been compressed to a narrow slit. B. The columnar epithelium lining the acini is composed of two cell layers: polarized clear cuboidal cells lining the acinar lumen and flattened basal cells interposed between the cuboidal acinar cells and the stroma. Hyperplastic cells line papillary projections protruding into the lumina of the acini.

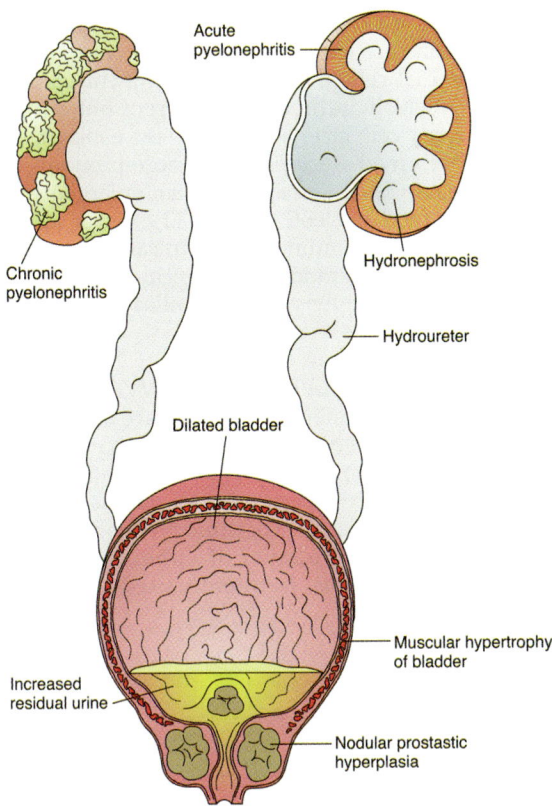

FIGURE 17-41
Complications of nodular prostatic hyperplasia.

ADENOCARCINOMA OF THE PROSTATE

 Epidemiology: In 1990, prostatic adenocarcinoma became the cancer most frequently diagnosed in American men, surpassing the incidence of lung cancer for the first time. An estimated 30,000 American men die annually of this malignancy, a figure that is still far lower than the mortality from lung cancer. Prostate cancer is a disease of elderly men, and of all patients with this diagnosis, 75% are 60 to 80 years of age. Patients younger than 50 years of age constitute less than 1% of cases in the United States. At the age of 50 years, the estimated lifetime probability of developing clinically apparent prostatic carcinoma is 10% for American men.

Autopsy studies have shown that the true frequency of prostatic carcinoma is actually considerably higher than is indicated by its clinical incidence. Most cases (70–90%) are incidental microscopic findings at autopsy or are discovered in a specimen resected for prostatic hyperplasia. **The prevalence of prostatic carcinoma at autopsy increases progressively with age, rising from less than 10% among men 40 to 50 years of age to between one third and one half of those older than 80 years of age.**

Considerable geographical variation in the age-related death rates exists for adenocarcinoma of the prostate throughout the world. The highest frequencies are reported in the United States and the Scandinavian countries; the lowest are described in Mexico, Greece, and Japan. Most western European countries have intermediate rates. The highest incidence in the world is recorded in American blacks, who exhibit a rate twice as high as that of white Americans. Migrant studies have shown that in the United States, the descendants of Polish and Japanese immigrants demonstrate a higher incidence of prostatic carcinoma than do men in their original countries. Similarly, the mortality rate from prostatic carcinoma among black American men exceeds that among blacks in Africa.

In addition to geographical, racial, and age differences, heredity and possibly diet influence the risk of prostate cancer. One tenth of cases are familial, with a significantly increased risk in persons whose first-degree relatives are afflicted with prostate cancer. There is some evidence that dietary fat content may increase the risk of developing prostate cancer, but further studies are required to confirm this relationship.

 Pathogenesis: The cause of prostatic adenocarcinoma is unknown, but the principal focus of research interest is directed toward endocrine influences. The androgenic control of normal prostatic growth and the responsiveness of prostate cancer to castration and exogenous estrogens support a role for male hormones. However, higher levels of serum androgens have not been demonstrated consistently in patients with prostate cancer. Elevated urinary estrone-to-testosterone ratios have been reported. Prostatic adenocarcinoma has been produced experimentally by a chemical carcinogen (3,2'-dimethyl-4-aminobiphenyl [DMAB]). In addition, rats have developed the tumor following prolonged administration of testosterone.

There is no evidence that prostatic adenocarcinoma originates from hyperplastic nodules. Current attention addresses intraductal dysplastic foci termed *prostatic intraepithelial neoplasia (PIN)*. *PIN refers to resident prostatic ducts lined by cytologically atypical luminal cells and a concomitant diminution in the number of the basal cells.* **Substantial evidence now supports the contention that PIN lesions are premalignant changes that progress to prostatic adenocarcinoma.** Such lesions precede the appearance of invasive cancer by two decades, and their severity increases with increasing age.

Morphological evidence linking PIN to invasive prostate cancer includes (1) the preponderance of the peripheral location of both lesions, (2) the cytological similarity of high-grade PIN to invasive cancer, and (3) the close topographical proximity of high-grade PIN to invasive cancer. Finally, PIN lesions are observed more frequently in prostates harboring cancer than in those without tumors. Certain markers are similar in high-grade PIN and invasive cancer (e.g., aneuploidy, TGF-α, type IV collagenase, and the expression of the *bcl*-2 and c-*erb*-2 oncogenes).

High-grade PIN functions as an important marker for carcinoma when identified in needle biopsies of the prostate. Many patients who show only high-grade PIN on initial biopsy are demonstrated to harbor invasive carcinoma in subsequent follow-up biopsies performed within weeks to months.

 Pathology: Prostatic adenocarcinomas, which account for 98% of all primary prostatic tumors, are commonly multicentric and located in the peripheral zones. The cut surface of the prostate shows irregular, yellow–white, indurated subcapsular nodules.

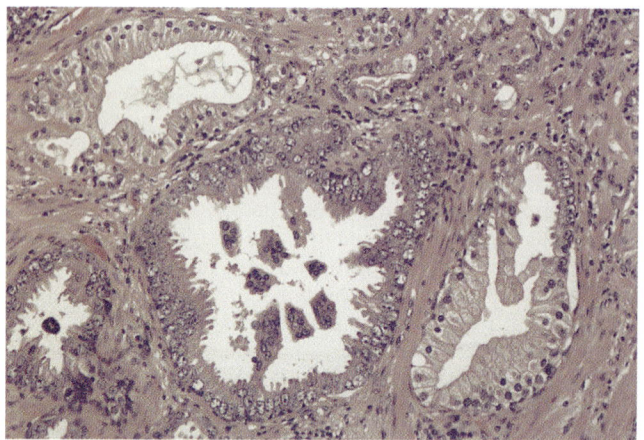

FIGURE 17-42
High-grade prostatic intraepithelial neoplasia (PIN). The large duct in the center is lined by atypical cells with enlarged nuclei and prominent nucleoli. Two normal ducts are located adjacent to the neoplastic one.

PROSTATIC INTRAEPITHELIAL NEOPLASIA: **Low-grade PIN** lesions are characterized by crowding and overlapping of luminal cells that exhibit prominent variation in nuclear size. Nucleoli are frequently present but are not enlarged. The basal cell layer is present. By contrast, foci of **high-grade PIN** are characterized by more-pronounced cell crowding, greater prevalence of nuclear enlargement, and prominent, enlarged nucleoli (Fig. 17-42). Fewer basal cells are demonstrated by immunohistochemical stains for high-molecular-weight cytokeratin. The atypical cells within PIN-affected ducts may show a flat, papillary, or cribriform pattern.

HISTOLOGICAL FEATURES OF INVASIVE CARCINOMA: Most prostatic adenocarcinomas are of acinar origin and feature small to medium-sized glands that lack organization and infiltrate the stroma. Well-differentiated tumors show uniform medium-sized or small glands (Fig. 17-43) that are lined by a single layer of uniform neoplastic epithelial cells. **In fact, a single layer of cuboidal cells lining neoplastic acini is the most frequently used criterion to es-**

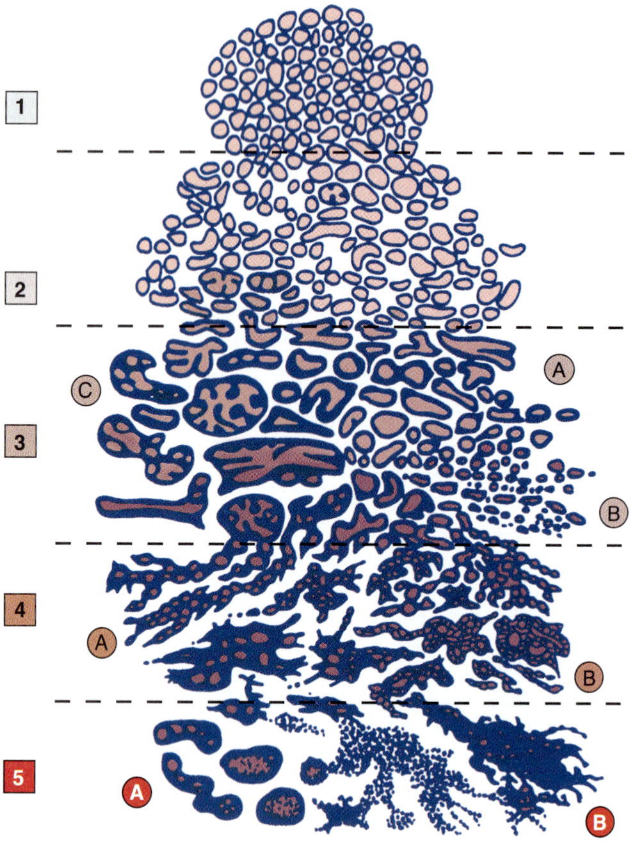

GLANDS

	Differentiation	Distribution
1	'Round,' lined by single layer of cuboidal cells	Close packed in rounded masses; definite edge
2	More variable in size and shape	Separated up to one gland diameter; 'loose' edge
3a	Irregular shape; medium to large size	Irregularly spaced apart; poorly defined 'edge'; surround normal strucutres
3b	Small to minute glands, not fused or 'chained'	
3c	Masses of cribriform or papillary epithelium with smooth outer surfaces	Very irregular spacing and distribution; no 'edge'; surround normal structures
4a	Ragged masses of fused glandular epithelium; bare tumor cells in stroma	Ragged infiltrating masses that overrun normal structures; No smooth surfaces against stroma
4b	Same as 4a; large clear cells	
5a	Smooth, cribriform to solid masses; often central necrosis 'comedocarcinoma'	Ragged infiltrating masses that infiltrate stromal fibers
5b	Anaplastic carcinoma with vacuoles and glands that suggest adenocarcinoma	

FIGURE 17-43
Prostate carcinoma. Gleason grading system.

tablish the diagnosis of prostatic adenocarcinoma. Progressive loss of differentiation of prostatic adenocarcinomas is characterized by the following microscopic changes:

- Increasing variability of gland size and configuration
- Papillary and cribriform patterns
- Rudimentary (or no) gland formation, with only solid cords of infiltrating tumor cells. Uncommonly, a prostate cancer is composed of small undifferentiated cells growing individually or in sheets, without evidence of any structural organization.

CYTOLOGICAL FEATURES: The prominence of pleomorphic and hyperchromatic nuclei is highly variable. One or two conspicuous nucleoli in a background of chromatin clumped near the nuclear membrane is the most frequent nuclear feature. The cytoplasm stains slightly eosinophilic or may be so vacuolated that it simulates the clear cells of renal cell carcinoma. Cell borders are distinct in the better-differentiated tumors but are not well demarcated in the more poorly differentiated ones.

GRADING: Prostatic adenocarcinoma is most commonly classified according to the **Gleason grading system** (Fig. 17-44), which is based on five histological patterns of tumor gland formation and infiltration. Recognizing the high frequency of mixed tumor patterns, the Gleason score is the sum of the grades (1–5) attributed to the most prominent pattern and that of the minority pattern. The best-differentiated tumors have a Gleason score of 2 (1 + 1), whereas the most poorly differentiated cancers yield a Gleason score of 10 (5 + 5). Most prostate cancers have Gleason scores of 4 to 7 (2 + 2, to 3 + 4 or 4 + 3). When combined with the tumor stage, the Gleason grading system has prognostic value: the lower the score, the better the outlook.

INVASION AND METASTASIS: The high frequency of invasion of the prostatic capsule by adenocarcinoma relates to the subcapsular location of the tumor. Perineural tumor invasion within the prostate and adjacent tissues is usual. Since peripheral nerves are devoid of perineural lymphatic channels, this mode of invasion represents contiguous spread of the tumor along a tissue space that offers the plane of least resistance.

The seminal vesicles are almost always involved by direct extension of prostate cancer. Invasion of the urinary bladder is less frequent until late in the clinical course. The earliest metastases occur in the obturator lymph node, with subsequent dissemination to the iliac and periaortic lymph nodes. Metastases to the lung reflect further lymphatic spread through the thoracic duct and through dissemination from the prostatic

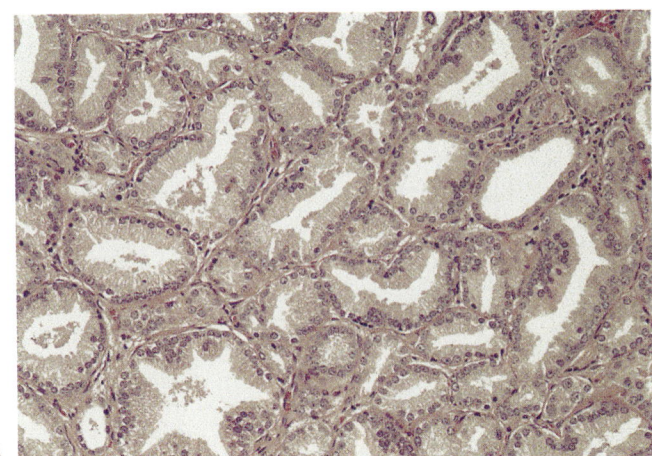
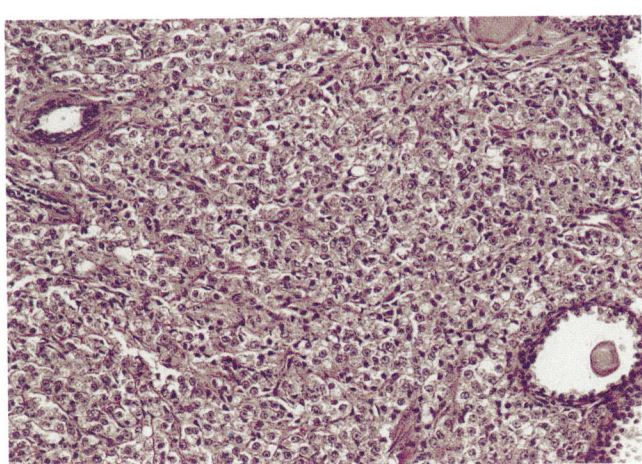
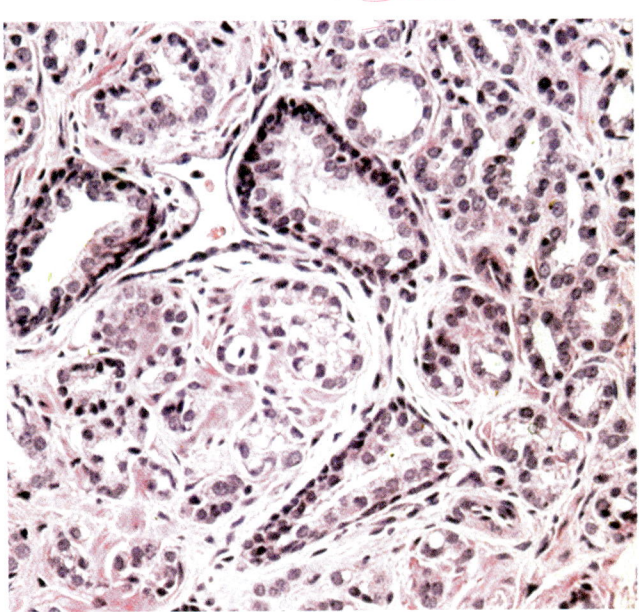

FIGURE *17-44*
Gleason grading system. A. Gleason grade 1. B. Gleason grade 3. C. Gleason grade 5.

924 The Lower Urinary Tract and Male Reproductive System

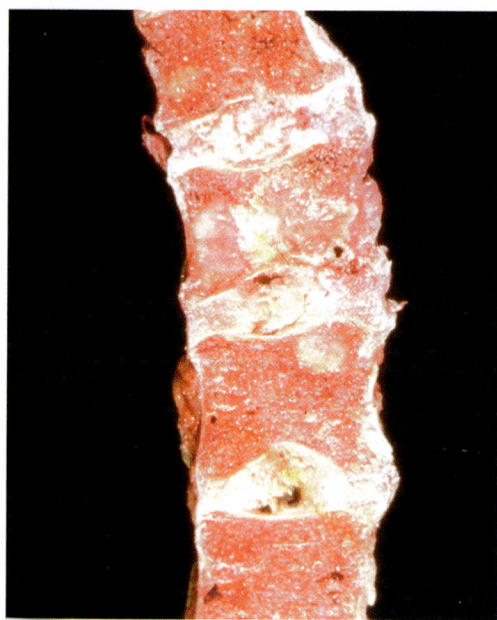

FIGURE 17-45
Prostatic carcinoma metastatic to the spine. The vertebral bodies contain several nodular osteoblastic metastases.

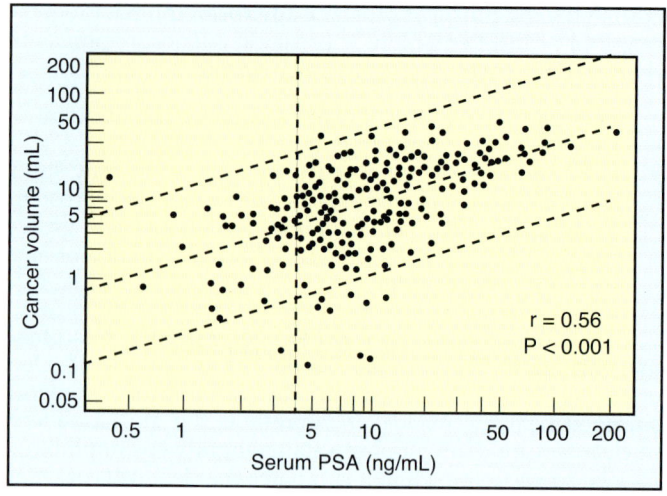

FIGURE 17-46
Preoperative prostate-specific antigen (PSA) correlates positively with cancer volume.

venous plexus to the inferior vena cava. Bony metastases, particularly to the vertebral column (Fig. 17-45), ribs, and pelvic bones, are painful and present a thorny clinical problem.

 Clinical Features: One tenth of all cases of prostate cancer are initially discovered in the fragments of tissue obtained at the time of transurethral resection for prostatic hyperplasia. The current widespread screening programs for prostate cancer that use digital rectal examination in combination with serum PSA serve to detect this malignancy in most cases. Patients who demonstrate elevated serum PSA are further evaluated by needle biopsies of the prostate. Preoperative PSA levels are correlated with cancer volume (Fig. 17-46). Uncommonly, patients with prostate cancer present with bladder outlet obstruction or symptoms referable to metastatic tumor.

The principles of clinical staging of prostate cancer are shown in Figure 17-47 and Table 17-8. At the time of initial presentation, 10% of prostate cancers are stage T1. In patients with tumors clinically judged to be localized to the prostate (stage T2), 60% show microscopic evidence of capsular penetration or seminal vesicle invasion (stage T3). Metastases of prostate cancer, in order of decreasing frequency, are observed in lymph nodes, bones, lung, and liver. Widespread

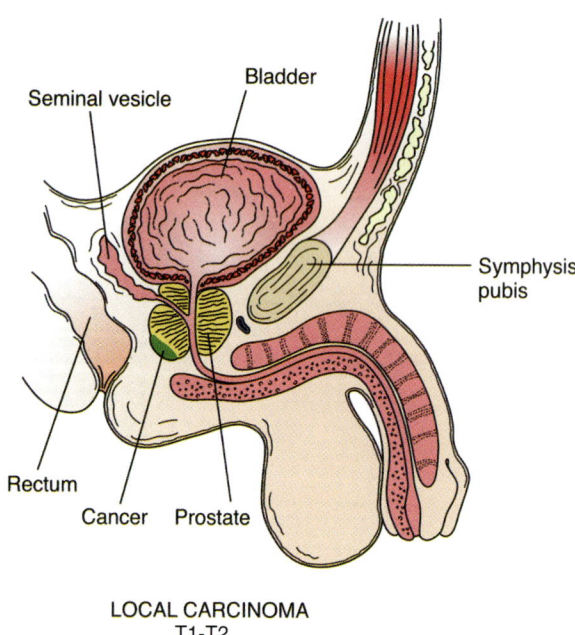
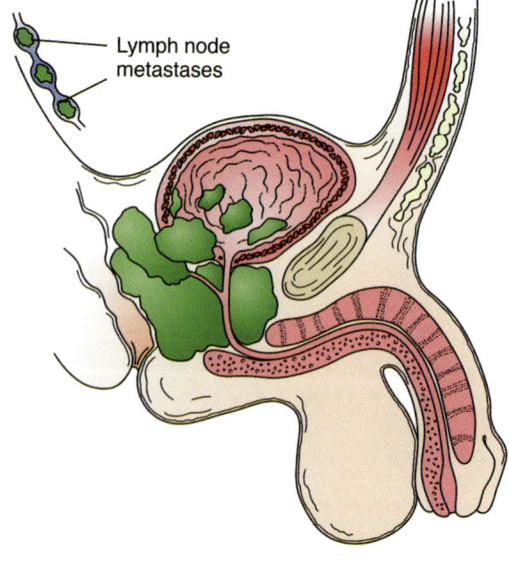

FIGURE 17-47
TNM staging of prostatic carcinoma.

TABLE 17-8 **TNM Staging of Prostatic Carcinoma**

T—Primary tumor
  T1 No clinically detectable tumor
    T1a Histological tumor found in 5% or less of tissue examined
    T1b Histological tumor found in more than 5% of tissue examined
  T2 Tumor confined to the prostate
    T2a Tumor in one lobe only
    T2b Tumor in both lobes
  T3 Tumor extends through the capsule
    T3a Extracapsular extension only
    T3b Tumor extends into seminal vesicles
  T4 Tumor invades adjacent structures other than seminal vesicles
N—Regional lymph nodes
  N0 No regional lymph node involvement
  N1 Regional lymph node metastases present
M—Distant metastases
  M0 No distant metastases
  M1 Distant metastases present

dissemination of the tumor (carcinomatosis), frequently with terminal pneumonia or sepsis, is the most common cause of death.

The demonstration of PSA and prostatic acid phosphatase by immunoperoxidase staining of biopsy specimens of metastatic sites has proved valuable in identifying the prostate as the primary site of the tumor. These tumor markers are also detectable in the serum of patients with prostate cancer. Serum PSA serves as a useful screening test for the presence of the disease and as an indicator of response to treatment. Serum prostatic acid phosphatase levels are elevated only in cases of metastatic prostate cancer, especially in patients with osteoblastic bony metastases.

Therapy for prostate cancer is stage-dependent. Patients with stage T1 and T2 cancers are treated by radical prostatectomy or radiation therapy. In stage T3 tumors, radiation therapy is the treatment of choice, acknowledging that half of these patients have occult pelvic lymph node metastases (and possibly further systemic dissemination), which cannot be cured by surgical means.

For patients whose tumors progress clinically and for all patients judged to have regional or distant metastases at initial presentation, the principal form of therapy is hormonal. This treatment involves orchiectomy or the administration of antagonists of pituitary luteinizing hormone (LH) or releasing hormone (LHRH). In either case, the goal is androgen deprivation.

The 5-year survival rates depend on the stage and Gleason grade. Using only the staging data, the survival is as follows: stages T1 and T2, 90%; stage T3, 40%; and stage T4, 10%.

SUGGESTED READING

Books

Bostwick DG, Eble JN (eds): Urologic surgical pathology. St.Louis: Mosby, 1997.
Epstein JI, Yang XJ: Prostate biopsy interpretation, 3rd ed. Philadelphia: Lippincott Williams & Wilkins, 2002.
Petersen RO: Urologic pathology, 2nd ed. Philadelphia: JB Lippincott, 1992.
Teichman JMH (ed): 20 Common problems in urology. New York: McGraw-Hill, 2001.
Ulbright TM, Amin MB, Young RH: Atlas of tumor pathology: Tumors of the testis, adnexa, spermatic cord and scrotum. Washington, DC: Armed Forces Institute of Pathology, 1999.

Review Articles

Bostwick DG, Mikuz G: Urothelial papillary (exophytic) neoplasms. *Virchows Arch* 441:109., 2002.
Bostwick DG, Ramnani D, Cheng L: Diagnosis and grading of the bladder cancer and associated lesions. *Urol Clin North Am* 26:493, 1999.
Buechner SA: Common skin disorders of the penis. *Brit. J. Urol. Internat* 90:498, 2002.
Emberton M, Andriole GL, de la Rosette J, et al.: Benign prostatic hyperplasia: A progressive disease of aging men. *Urology* 61:267–273, 2003.
Epstein JI: Pathological assessment of the surgical specimen. *Urol Clin North Am* 28:567, 2001.
Frankel S, Smith GD, Donovan J, Neal D. Screening for prostate cancer. *Lancet* 361:1122–1128, 2003.
Hughes IA: Intersex. *Brit. J. Urol. Internat* 90:769, 2002.
Jones RH, Vasey PA: New directions in testicular cancer: Molecular determinants of oncogenesis and treatment success. *Eur J Cancer* 39:147–156, 2003.
Krieger JN: Urinary tract infections: What's new? *J Urol* 168:2351, 2002.
Leissner J, Koeppen C, Wolf HK: Prognostic significance of vascular and perineural invasion in urothelial bladder cancer treated with radical cystectomy. *J Urol* 169:955–960, 2003.
Looijenga LH, Oosterhuis JW: Pathogenesis of testicular germ cell tumors. *Rev Reprod* 4:90, 1999.
Marker PC, Donjacour AA, Dahiya R, Cunha GR: Hormonal, cellular, and molecular control of prostatic development. *Dev Biol* 253:165–174, 2003.
Oberpenning F, van Ophoven A, Hertle L: Interstitial cystitis: An update. *Curr Opin Urol* 12:321–332, 2002.
Oottamasathien S, Crawford ED: Should routine screening for prostate-specific antigen be recommended? *Arch Intern Med* 163:661–662, 2003.
Pollack A, Cowen D, Troncoso P, et al.: Molecular markers of outcome after radiotherapy in patients with prostate carcinoma: Ki-67, bcl-2, bax, and bcl-x. *Cancer* 97:1630–1638, 2003.
Ronald A. The etiology of urinary tract infection: traditional and emerging pathogens. *Am J Med* 113(suppl 1A):14S–19S, 2002.
Sirovich BE, Schwartz LM, Woloshin S: Screening men for prostate and colorectal cancer in the United States: Does practice reflect the evidence? *JAMA* 289:1414–1420, 2003.
Smith ND, Rubenstein JN, Eggener SE, Kozlowski JM: The p53 tumor suppressor gene and nuclear protein: Basic science review and relevance in the management of bladder cancer. *J Urol* 169:1219–1228, 2003.
Theodorescu D. Molecular pathogenesis of urothelial bladder cancer. *Histol Histopathol* 18:259–274, 2003.
Thorpe A, Neal D: Benign prostatic hyperplasia. *Lancet* 361:1359–1367, 2003.
Toner GC, Frydenberg M: Poor prognosis germ-cell tumors: An unresolved challenge. *Semin Urol Oncol* 20:251–261, 2002.

CHAPTER 18

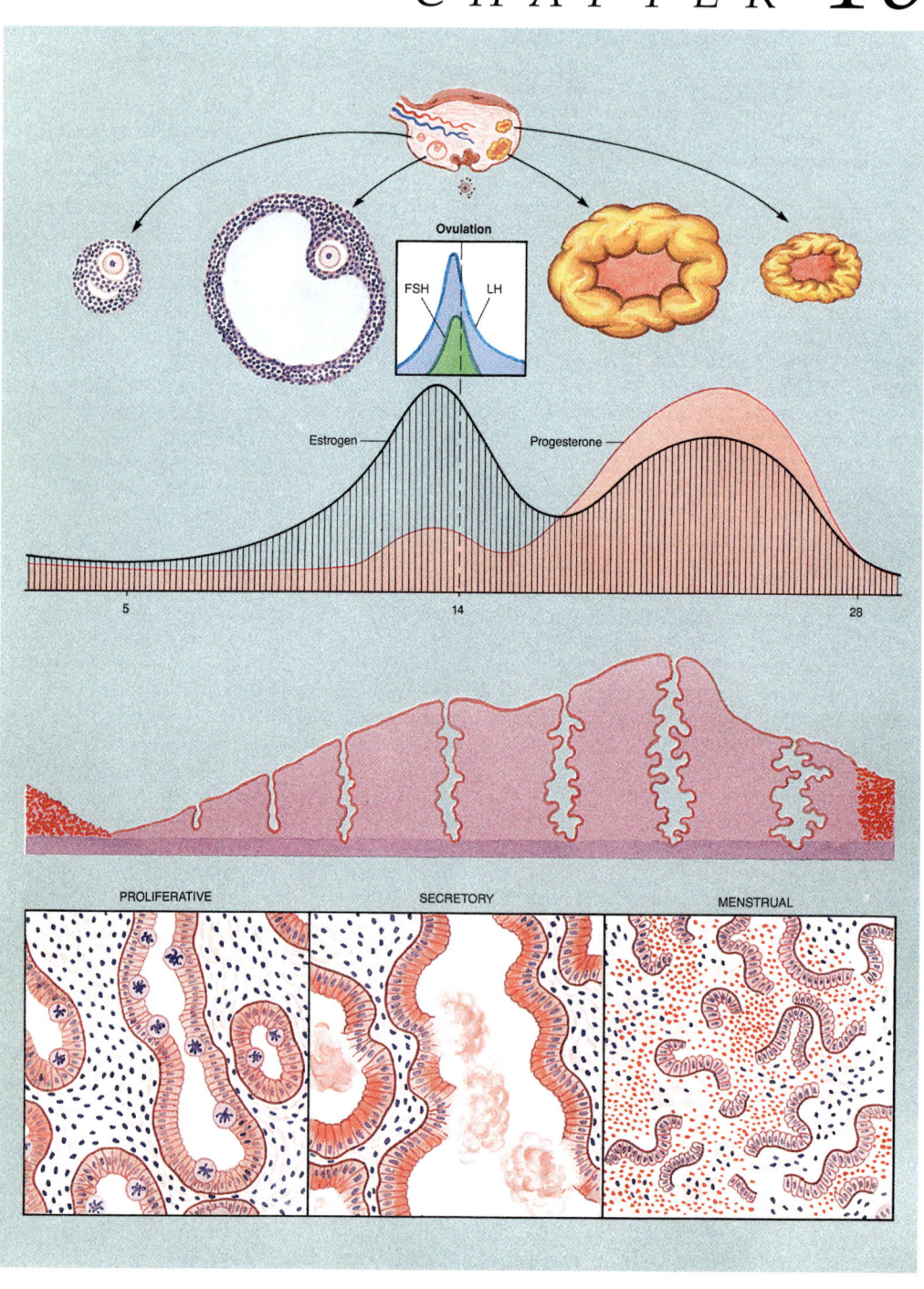

The Female Reproductive System

Stanley J. Robboy
Robert J. Kurman
Maria J. Merino

Embryology

Genital Infections
Sexually Transmitted Genital Infections
Genital Infections Not Transmitted Sexually
Toxic Shock Syndrome

Vulva

Anatomy

Developmental Anomalies and Cysts

Dermatoses
Acute Dermatitis
Chronic Dermatitis

Benign Tumors

Malignant Tumors and Premalignant Conditions
Vulvar Intraepithelial Neoplasia
Squamous Cell Carcinoma
Malignant Melanoma
Extramammary Paget Disease

Vagina

Anatomy

Nonneoplastic Conditions and Benign Tumors
Congenital Anomalies
Atrophic Vaginitis
Vaginal Adenosis
Fibroepithelial Polyp
Benign Mesenchymal Tumors

Malignant Tumors
Squamous Cell Carcinoma
Clear Cell Adenocarcinoma
Embryonal Rhabdomyosarcoma (Sarcoma Botryoides)

Cervix

Anatomy
The Transformation Zone

Cervicitis

Benign Tumors and Tumorlike Conditions
Endocervical Polyp
Microglandular Hyperplasia
Leiomyoma

Squamous Cell Neoplasia
Cervical Intraepithelial Neoplasia (CIN)
Microinvasive Squamous Cell Carcinoma

(continued)

FIGURE 18-1 *(see opposite page)*
Menstrual cycle with correlation of hormonal, ovarian, and endometrial changes.

Invasive Squamous Cell Carcinoma

Adenocarcinoma

Uterus

Anatomy

The Menstrual Cycle

Endometrium of Pregnancy

Congenital Anomalies

Endometritis

Traumatic Lesions

Adenomyosis
Contraceptive Steroids
Dysfunctional Uterine Bleeding
Anovulatory Bleeding
Luteal Phase Defect

Tumors
Endometrial Polyp
Endometrial Hyperplasia and Adenocarcinoma
Endometrial Stromal Tumors
Leiomyoma
Intravenous Leiomyomatosis
Leiomyosarcoma

Fallopian Tube

Anatomy

Salpingitis

Ectopic Pregnancy

Tumors

Ovary

Anatomy and Embryology

Cystic Lesions

Follicle Cyst
Corpus Luteum Cyst
Theca Lutein Cysts

Polycystic Ovary Syndrome

Stromal Hyperthecosis

Tumors
Epithelial Tumors
Germ Cell Tumors
Sex Cord/Stromal Tumors
Tumors Metastatic to the Ovary

Peritoneum

Endometriosis

Mesothelial Tumors
Adenomatoid Tumor
Well-Differentiated Papillary Mesothelioma
Diffuse Malignant Mesothelioma

Serous Tumors (Primary and Metastatic)
Serous Adenocarcinoma

Pseudomyxoma Peritonei

Placenta and Gestational Disease

Development

Anatomy

Infections
Chorioamnionitis
Villitis

Preeclampsia and Eclampsia

Retroplacental Hematoma

Placenta Accreta

Multiple Gestations

Spontaneous Abortion

Gestational Trophoblastic Disease

Complete Hydatidiform Mole

Partial Hydatidiform Mole

Invasive Hydatidiform Mole

Choriocarcinoma

Placental Site Trophoblastic Tumor

EMBRYOLOGY

The anlage of the human gonad, which forms as a swelling of the embryonic urogenital ridge, is initially in an indifferent state. Both sex chromosomes and autosomal chromosomes in the stromal cells of the gonad determine whether it will differentiate into a testis or an ovary. If the gonadal stroma is male, a gene on the Y chromosome (testis-determining gene) interacts with somatic components in the primitive gonad and initiates the development of seminiferous tubules. If the gonadal stroma is female and there is no stimulation to form a testis, an ovary develops. The ovary is derived from mesoderm, except for the germ cells, which are endodermal. By about the 40th day, the ovaries and testes are histologically distinct.

The wolffian (mesonephric) ducts begin their development at about day 25, regardless of the embryo's sex. If stimulated by testosterone (secreted by Leydig cells starting at about day 70), the ducts differentiate into vas deferens, epididymis, and seminal vesicle. If not stimulated by day 84, the ducts regress and remain as vestigial rests in the female. They may form cysts in the cervix or vagina (mesonephric cyst).

The müllerian (paramesonephric) ducts comprise the anlage of the fallopian tubes, uterus, and vaginal wall. They appear at about day 37 as funnel-shaped openings of celomic epithelium. These develop into paired, undifferentiated tubes, using the wolffian ducts as "guide wires" to reach the region of the future hymen. If the wolffian duct is absent, as in renal agenesis, the vagina and cervix are almost always abnormal or absent. At day 54, the müllerian ducts fuse to become a straight uterovaginal canal.

A central tenet of genital tract development in both sexes is that the müllerian tubes will develop along female lines unless specifically impeded by embryonic testicular factors. In males, Sertoli cells in the developing testis produce *müllerian-inhibiting substance,* a protein that causes the müllerian ducts to regress.

The development of the external genitalia into a masculine form depends on the local conversion of testosterone to dihydrotestosterone. A lack of dihydrotestosterone (i.e., a state of relative estrogen excess) results in the persistence of female external genitalia. The genital tubercle develops into the clitoris, the genital folds into the labia minora, and the genital swellings into the labia majora. The basic architecture of the female genital tract is completed by day 120.

GENITAL INFECTIONS

Genital Infections Are Commonly Sexually Transmitted

Infectious diseases of the female genital tract are common and are caused by a wide variety of pathogenic organisms (Table 18-1), which are also discussed in Chapter 9. Most of the important infectious diseases affecting the female genital tract are sexually transmitted.

Bacterial Infections

Gonorrhea

Gonorrhea is caused by *Neisseria gonorrhoeae,* a fastidious, gram-negative diplococcus. A million cases of gonorrhea occur yearly in the United States. The infection is a frequent cause of acute salpingitis and pelvic inflammatory disease (PID) (Fig. 18-2).

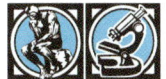

Pathogenesis and Pathology: The organisms ascend through the cervix and the endometrial cavity, where they cause an acute endometritis. The bacteria then attach to mucosal cells in the fallopian tube and elicit an acute inflammatory reaction, which is confined to the mucosal surface (*acute salpingitis*). From the tubal lumen, the infection spreads to involve the ovary, sometimes resulting in a *tuboovarian abscess.* It may also involve the pelvic and abdominal cavities, with the formation of subdiaphragmatic and pelvic abscesses.

Systemic complications of gonorrhea include septicemia and septic arthritis. The organisms induce a purulent inflammatory reaction at all sites of infection. Resolution is rarely complete, and dense fibrous adhesions remain. The healing process distorts and destroys the plicae of the fallopian tube, often leading to sterility.

Syphilis

Syphilis is a venereal disease caused by *Treponema pallidum,* a thin, motile, spiral-shaped bacterium, commonly known as a spirochete. The disease is acquired through sexual contact with an infected person or as a result of transplacental spread (congenital syphilis). *T. pallidum* penetrates small abrasions in the skin or normal mucosal membranes. Because of a complex immunological reaction to the bacterium, which results in a chronic host–parasite relationship, untreated syphilis may wax and wane, progressing through primary, secondary, and tertiary stages.

- **The primary stage** features the *chancre,* which usually appears after an incubation period of about 3 weeks, be it on the penis, vulva, tongue, or other portals of bacterial entry. The chancre manifests as a painless, indurated papule, 1 cm to several centimeters in diameter. It is

TABLE 18-1 Infectious Diseases of the Female Genital Tract

Organism	Disease	Diagnostic Feature
Sexually Transmitted Diseases		
Gram-negative rods and cocci		
Calymmatobacterium granulomatis	Granuloma inguinale	Donovan body
Gardnerella vaginalis	*Gardnerella* infection	Clue cell
Haemophilus ducreyi	Chancroid (soft chancre)	
Neisseria gonorrhoeae	Gonorrhea	Gram-negative diplococcus
Spirochetes		
Treponema pallidum	Syphilis	Spirochete
Mycoplasmas		
Mycoplasma hominis	Nonspecific vaginitis	
Ureaplasma urealyticum	Nonspecific vaginitis	
Rickettsiae		
Chlamydia trachomatis type D–K	Various forms of PID*	
Chlamydia trachomatis type L_{1-3}	Lymphogranuloma venereum	
Viruses		
Human papillomavirus (HPV)	Condyloma acuminatum/planum	Koilocyte
	Neoplastic potential	
Types 6, 11, 40, 42, 43, 44, 57	Low risk	
Types 16, 18, 31, 33, 35, 39, 45, 51, 52, 56, 58, 66	High risk	
Herpes simplex, type 2	Herpes genitalis	Multinucleated giant cell with intranuclear homogenization and inclusion bodies
Cytomegalovirus (CMV)	Cytomegalic inclusion disease	Bulbous intranuclear inclusion body
Molluscum contagiosum	Molluscum infection	Molluscum body
Protozoa		
Trichomonas vaginalis	Trichomoniasis	Trichomonad
Selected Nonsexually Transmitted Diseases		
Actinomyces and related organisms		
Actinomyces israelii	PID (one of many organisms)	Sulfur granules
Mycobacterium tuberculosis	Tuberculosis	Necrotizing granulomas
Fungi		
Candida albicans	Candidiasis	*Candida* species

*PID, pelvic inflammatory disease.

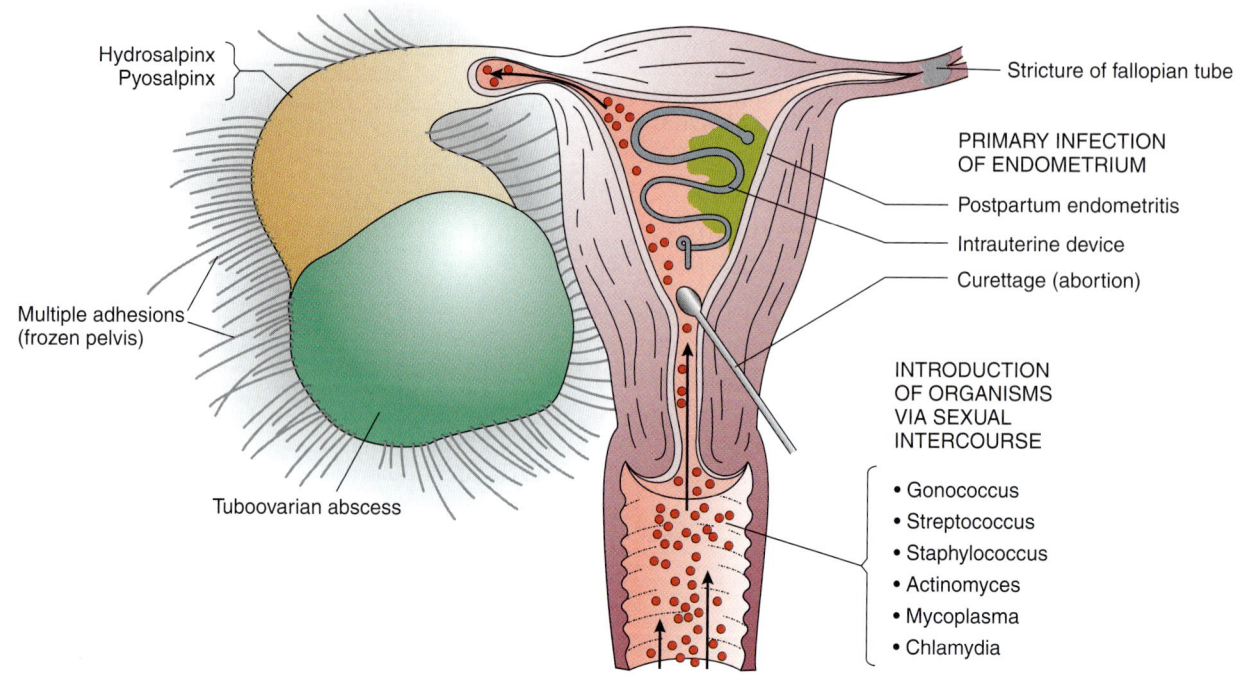

FIGURE 18-2
Pelvic inflammatory disease.

surrounded by an inflammatory cuff that breaks down to form an ulcer. The chancre may persist for 2 to 6 weeks and then heals spontaneously.
- **The secondary stage** appears after a latent period of several weeks to months. Common features include low-grade fever, headache, malaise, lymphadenopathy, and the appearance of highly contagious syphilitic lesions called *condylomata lata* (syphilitic warts). The secondary infectious lesions heal after 2 to 6 weeks, and the symptoms disappear spontaneously.
- **The tertiary stage** develops any time thereafter and may be complicated by severe damage to the cardiovascular and nervous systems.

Pathology: The hallmark of syphilis in biopsy specimens is the dense infiltrate with lymphocytes and plasma cells, particularly adjacent to blood vessels, and prominent endothelial swelling. Silver impregnation techniques (Warthin-Starry stain or its modifications) help demonstrate the spirochetes. The more advanced stages of disease show greater obliterative endarteritis and subsequent tissue destruction.

Granuloma Inguinale

Granuloma inguinale is caused by *Calymmatobacterium granulomatis*, a sexually transmitted, gram-negative, encapsulated rod. The disease occurs with equal frequency in men and women.

Pathology: The primary lesion begins as a painless, ulcerated nodule involving the genital, inguinal, or perianal skin. The organisms invade through skin abrasions and spread locally by direct extension, destroying the skin and its underlying tissues. Extensive local spread and lymphatic permeation occur later. Vacuolated macrophages teem with characteristic intracellular bacteria *(Donovan bodies)*. The organism, best seen with the Wright stain, resembles a closed safety pin. The squamous epithelium overlying the involved area may demonstrate conspicuous hyperplasia, sometimes exuberant enough to be misinterpreted as a squamous cell carcinoma. Relapses are common following antibiotic therapy.

Chancroid

Chancroid, also called *soft chancre*, is caused by *Haemophilus ducreyi*, a gram-negative bacillus. This disease is rare in the United States but is common in underdeveloped countries.

Pathology: Usually 3 to 5 days after sexual congress with an infected partner, single or sometimes multiple small, vesiculopustular lesions appear on the cervix, vagina, vulva, or perianal region. Histological examination reveals a granulomatous inflammatory reaction. The lesion often ruptures to form a purulent ulcer that is painful and bleeds easily. There may be associated inguinal lymphadenopathy, fever, chills, and malaise. A major complication is scar formation during the healing phase, an outcome that sometimes causes urethral stenosis.

Gardnerella

Sexual transmission of *Gardnerella vaginalis*, a gram-negative coccobacillus, causes a substantial proportion of cases classified as nonspecific vaginitis. A biopsy specimen is usually normal, because the organism neither penetrates the mucosa nor elicits an inflammatory reaction. The diagnosis of *Gardnerella* infection is best established by identifying the organisms either in a wet mount specimen of a vaginal discharge or in a Papanicolaou-stained smear. The *clue cell* is pathognomonic and shows squamous cells covered by coccobacilli. Other aids to the diagnosis are a thin, homogeneous, milk-like vaginal discharge, a vaginal pH above 4.5, and the presence of a fishy odor from the discharge once alkalinized with 10% potassium hydroxide.

Mycoplasma

Mycoplasmas are minute pleomorphic organisms that resemble the so-called L bacterial forms but differ by having no cell wall. They are the smallest known free-living organisms. Mycoplasmas are common commensals of the oropharyngeal and urogenital tracts. Colonization of the lower genital tract by mycoplasmas occurs through sexual contact. *Ureaplasma urealyticum* can be isolated from the lower genital tract in 40% of healthy women and may cause infertility, adverse effects on pregnancy, and perinatal infections. *Mycoplasma hominis*, found in the lower genital tract of 5% of healthy women, is responsible for a small proportion of cases of symptomatic cervicitis and vaginitis. *M. hominis* is frequently cultivated in association with *G. vaginalis* or *Trichomonas vaginalis* infection. Although the role of mycoplasma in genital tract infection is not completely understood, the organisms are encountered in PID, acute salpingitis, spontaneous abortion, and puerperal fever. The histological appearance of the affected tissue is usually unremarkable.

Chlamydia Infections

Chlamydia trachomatis is a common, venereally transmitted organism, which is a gram-negative obligate, intracellular rickettsia. Fifteen serotypes are known. Infection with *C. trachomatis* results in a wide variety of disorders in women, men, and infants. This organism has been found in the genital tract of about 8% of asymptomatic women and in 20% of women presenting with symptoms of a lower genital tract infection.

Pathology: In the more common genital infections, which involve serotypes D through K, the cervical mucosa is severely inflamed and the endocervical and metaplastic squamous cells reveal small inclusion bodies. By cytological examination, chlamydia infection manifests as perinuclear intracytoplasmic inclusions with distinct borders and intracytoplasmic *coccoid bodies*. Complications include ascending infection of the endometrium, fallopian tube, and ovary, which may result in tubal occlusion and infertility. Chlamydia also gives rise to infected Bartholin glands and acute urethritis. Infants delivered vaginally from infected mothers may develop conjunctivitis, otitis media, and pneumonia.

Lymphogranuloma Venereum

Lymphogranuloma venereum is a sexually transmitted infection in both men and women that is endemic in tropical countries. The disease is caused by the L form of *C. trachomatis*, serotypes L1 through L3.

Pathology: After a few days to a month, a small painless vesicle forms at the site of inoculation. It heals rapidly, and in many instances the vesicle is not even noticed. The second stage presents with bilaterally enlarged inguinal lymph nodes that may rupture and form suppurative fistulas. The inguinal nodes in men and perirectal nodes in women become matted and painful. In some untreated patients, a third stage appears after a latency of several years. This chronic phase shows scarring, which causes lymphatic obstruction and resulting genital elephantiasis and rectal strictures. In the second and third stages, infected tissues contain necrotizing granulomas, neutrophilic infiltrates, and, occasionally, inclusion bodies within macrophages.

Viral Infections

Human Papillomavirus

Human papillomavirus (HPV) is a DNA virus that infects a wide variety of skin and mucosal surfaces to produce wartlike lesions, referred to as *verrucae* and *condylomata*. Over 100 types of this virus are known, one third of which cause genital tract lesions. The median time from infection to first detection of HPV is 3 months. In the United States, as many as two thirds of graduating college women have genital HPV infections, which result from sexual contact with an infected person. Even in women who have had only one sexual partner, by 3 years after first intercourse, the risk of acquiring cervical HPV was 50% in one study. HPV types 6 and 11 are detected in over 80% of the macroscopically visible condylomata.

Several strains of HPV are now considered the major etiological factor in the development of squamous cell cancer in the female lower genital tract. Types 16, 18, 31, and 45 are the most representative high-risk types linked to intraepithelial neoplasia and to invasive cancer (see section on cervix for further discussion).

Condyloma Acuminatum

Condyloma acuminatum is caused by HPV infection. It is a benign, exophytic, papillomatous lesion on the skin or mucous membranes of the lower female genital tract, which is often visible to the naked eye, but sometimes requires the colposcope to be seen.

Pathology: Condylomata acuminata occur on the vulva, perianal region, perineum, vagina, and cervix. They may also involve the urethra, bladder, and rectum. Condylomata grow as papules, plaques, or nodules and eventually as spiked or cauliflower-like excrescences (Fig. 18-3A). Microscopic examination reveals a striking papillomatous proliferation of squamous epithelium. A characteristic finding is the *koilocyte* (Greek *koilos*, hollow), an epithelial cell with a perinuclear halo and a wrinkled nucleus that contains HPV particles (Fig. 18-3B). The organisms typically remain in an episomal state and replicate within the cell. The large numbers of particles cause extensive cytoplasmic destruction, creating the koilocyte (Fig. 18-3C).

Herpesvirus

Herpes simplex type 2 is a double-stranded DNA virus that is a common cause of sexually transmitted genital infections. After an incubation period of 1 to 3 weeks, small vesicles develop on the vulva and erode into painful ulcers. Similar lesions occur in the vagina and cervix. Epithelial cells adjacent to intraepithelial vesicles show ballooning degeneration, and many contain large nuclei with eosinophilic inclusions.

Genital herpes tends to become latent, and the virus remains in the sacral ganglia. Reactivation of the virus during pregnancy can result in its transmission to the newborn during passage through the birth canal, a complication that can be fatal.

Cytomegalovirus

Cytomegalovirus is a double-stranded DNA virus of the herpesvirus family. The virus is ubiquitous, and more than 80% of persons over the age of 35 years have antibodies to it. Several lines of evidence suggest that many cases are sexually transmitted: (1) the seroprevalence of cytomegalovirus has risen in young adults, (2) the virus is recovered more frequently from cervical secretions and semen than from any other body sites, and (3) viral titers in semen are 100,000 times higher than those in urine. Nevertheless, cytomegalovirus only rarely causes genital infections in women. Infection in the endometrium may result in spontaneous abortion or infection of the newborn. Infected cells exhibit characteristic large, eosinophilic, intranuclear inclusions and, occasionally, cytoplasmic inclusions.

Molluscum Contagiosum

Molluscum contagiosum is a double-stranded DNA virus of the highly contagious poxvirus group. Infection with this virus leads to the appearance of multiple smooth, gray-white nodules that are centrally umbilicated and exude a cheesy material. The lesions occur predominantly in the genital region but may be found elsewhere on the body. Characteristic large, cytoplasmic viral inclusions (*molluscum bodies*) are found in the infected epithelial cells. Most lesions regress spontaneously, but untreated ones may persist for years.

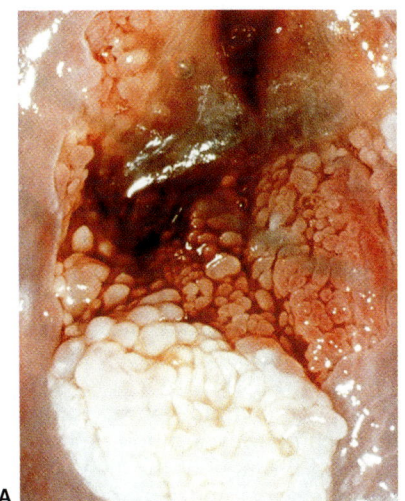
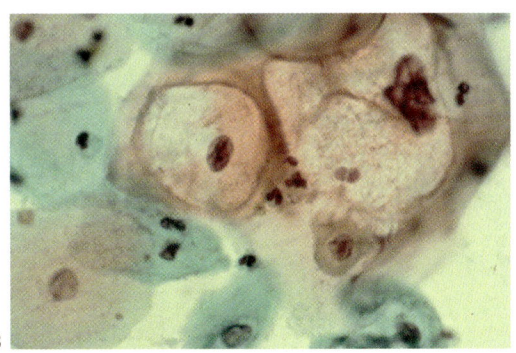
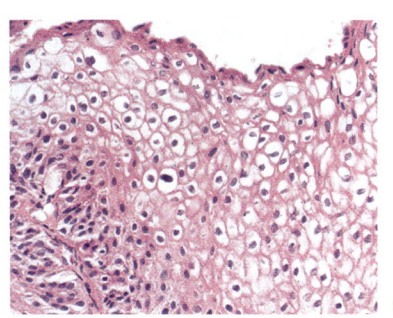

FIGURE 18-3
Human papillomavirus-induced condylomatous infections. **A.** Condyloma acuminatum on the cervix, visible with the naked eye as cauliflower-like excrescences. **B.** A cervical smear contains characteristic koilocytes, with a perinuclear halo and a wrinkled nucleus that contains viral particles. **C.** Biopsy of the condyloma shows koilocytes with perinuclear halos but lacking nuclear atypia.

Trichomoniasis

T. vaginalis is a large, pear-shaped, flagellated protozoan that commonly causes vaginitis. The disease is sexually transmitted, and 25% of infected women are asymptomatic carriers. The infection manifests as a heavy, yellow-gray, thick, foamy discharge that is accompanied by severe itching, dyspareunia (painful intercourse), and dysuria (painful urination). The diagnosis is confirmed by a wet mount preparation in which the motile trichomonads are seen. The organisms are also demonstrated in Papanicolaou-stained cervical smears.

Pelvic Inflammatory Disease

PID describes an infection of the pelvic organs that follows the extension of any of a variety of microorganisms beyond the uterine corpus (see Fig. 18-2). Ascent of the infection results in bilateral acute salpingitis, pyosalpinx, and tuboovarian abscesses. *N. gonorrhoeae* and chlamydia are the principal organisms causing PID, but most infections are polymicrobial. The incidence of PID is far greater in sexually promiscuous women than in those who are monogamous. Occasionally, PID is a sequel to postpartum endometritis or an infection after endometrial curettage.

Patients with PID typically present with lower abdominal pain. Physical examination reveals bilateral adnexal tenderness and marked discomfort when the cervix is manipulated (*chandelier sign*). Complications of PID include (1) rupture of a tuboovarian abscess, which may result in life-threatening peritonitis; (2) infertility from scarring of the healed tubal plicae; (3) increased rates of ectopic pregnancy; and (4) intestinal obstruction from fibrous bands and adhesions.

Some Genital Infections Are Not Transmitted Sexually

Tuberculosis

Mycobacterium tuberculosis may infect any segment of the female genital tract. Genital tuberculosis is found in 1% of infertile women in the United States and in more than 10% of such women in less-developed countries.

 Pathology: TUBERCULOUS SALPINGITIS: Inflammation of the fallopian tube is the initial lesion in most cases of tuberculous genital infection. The mycobacteria usually reach the tube by hematogenous dissemination from the lung. Tuberculous salpingitis results in fibrinous adhesions and scarring of the fallopian tube. In turn, these complications lead to multiple functional abnormalities (e.g., infertility, ectopic gestation, pelvic pain). The tubes may become nodular and mimic salpingitis isthmica nodosa. *Pyosalpinx* (fallopian tube distended with pus) and *hydrosalpinx* (fluid-filled tube) are late sequelae, and the adjacent ovary may become infected.

TUBERCULOUS ENDOMETRITIS: This condition complicates half of cases of tubal tubercular infection. Noncaseating, poorly formed granulomas with rare giant cells are typical. In other areas of the body afflicted with this infection, granulomas have time to develop caseous necrosis and characteristic Langhans giant cells. By contrast, tuberculous granulomas that develop in the endometrium are no more than one cycle old, owing to menstrual shedding, and thus are at an earlier stage of development.

Candidiasis

Ten percent of women are asymptomatic carriers of fungi in the vulva and vagina, with *Candida albicans* being the most common offender. However, only 2% of women present with clinically apparent candidal vulvovaginitis. Pregnant women are considerably more susceptible, and 10% of such women are symptomatic. Diabetes mellitus and use of oral contraceptives also promote vaginal candidiasis. The infection manifests as vulvar itching and a white discharge. Clinical examination reveals firmly adherent, small white plaques on the mucous membranes ("thrush"). Biopsy discloses submucosal edema and a chronic inflammatory infiltrate. The fungi do not penetrate the epithelium, and the white patches correspond to foci of desquamated, necrotic epithelial cells, cellular debris, bacterial flora, and the candidal spores and pseudohyphae. If untreated, the infection waxes, wanes, and frequently disappears following delivery. The diagnosis is made by finding characteristic spores and pseudohyphae in a wet mount preparation or with a Papanicolaou stain.

Actinomycosis

Genital tract actinomycosis is uncommon but has been increasingly reported in association with the use of intrauterine devices (IUDs). *Actinomyces israelii*, the causative organism, is a gram-positive rod found in 4% of normal genital tracts. The bacterium is believed to enter the uterine cavity by way of the tail of the IUD. It ascends to infect the fallopian tube, ovary, and broad ligaments and forms a tuboovarian abscess. Suppurating lesions display drainage tracts that contain dense microcolonies of organisms ("sulfur granules"). Actinomycosis results in extensive fibrosis and scarring of the female genital tract.

Toxic Shock Syndrome Is Associated with Vaginal Staphylococcal Infection

Toxic shock syndrome is an acute, sometimes fatal disorder characterized by fever, shock, and a desquamative erythematous rash. In addition, vomiting, diarrhea, myalgias, neurological signs, and thrombocytopenia are common. Certain strains of *Staphylococcus aureus* release an exotoxin called toxic shock syndrome toxin-1. This toxin exerts its own effects and also alters the function of mononuclear phagocytes, thereby impairing the clearance of other potentially toxic substances, such as endotoxin. In addition to the pathological alterations characteristic of shock, the lesions of disseminated intravascular coagulation are usually prominent. The disease was first recognized when long-acting tampons were first introduced, providing sufficient time for the staphylococcal organisms to proliferate. The contraceptive "sponge" was also associated. The occurrence of toxic shock syndrome has decreased markedly since the recognition of the role of tampons in promoting colonization of the vagina by *S. aureus*.

Vulva

ANATOMY

The vulva comprises the mons pubis, labia majora and minora, clitoris, and vestibule. With the onset of puberty, the mons pubis and the lateral borders of the labia majora acquire increased subcutaneous fat and grow coarse hair. The sebaceous and apocrine glands in these regions develop concomitantly. The paired external openings of the paraurethral glands *(Skene glands)* lie on either side of the urethral meatus. *Bartholin glands,* located immediately posterolateral to the introitus, are branching, mucus-secreting, tubuloalveolar glands drained by a short duct lined by transitional epithelium. In addition, microscopic mucous glands are scattered throughout the area bounded by the labia minora. The inguinal and femoral lymph nodes provide the primary lymph drainage routes, except for the clitoris (the homologue of the penis), which shares the lymphatic drainage of the urethra.

DEVELOPMENTAL ANOMALIES AND CYSTS

ECTOPIC BREAST TISSUE: Small, isolated nodules of ectopic breast tissue may extend in the "milk line" to the vulva and enlarge during pregnancy.

BARTHOLIN GLAND CYST: The paired Bartholin glands produce a clear mucoid secretion that continuously lubricates the vestibular surface. The ducts are prone to obstruction and consequent cyst formation (Fig. 18-4). In turn, infection of the cyst leads to abscess formation. Bartholin gland abscess was formerly associated with gonorrhea, but staphylococci, chlamydia, and anaerobes are now more frequently the cause. Treatment consists of incision, drainage, marsupialization, and appropriate antibiotics.

FOLLICULAR CYSTS: The follicular cyst recapitulates the most distal portion of the hair follicle. Also termed *epithelial inclusion cysts* or *keratinous cysts,* follicular cysts frequently appear on the vulva, especially the labia majora. They contain a white cheesy material and typically are lined by stratified squamous epithelium.

MUCINOUS CYSTS: Mucinous glands of the vulva, a normal but generally unrecognized finding, occasionally become obstructed and subsequently cystic. Mucinous columnar cells line the cyst and may become infected.

DERMATOSES

Acute Dermatitis

Acute dermatitis of the vulva appears as reddened vesiculated skin (Fig. 18-5).

Dermatoses 935

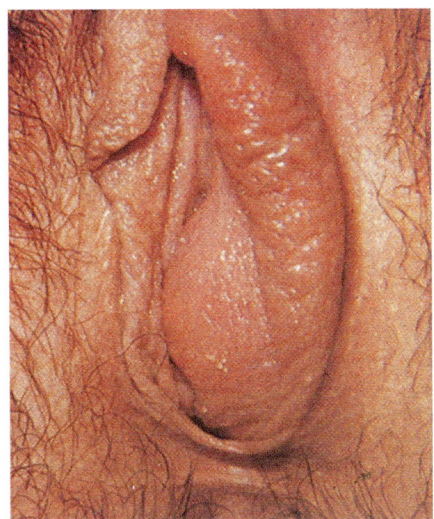

FIGURE 18-4
Bartholin gland cyst. The 4-cm lesion is located to the right of and posterior to the vaginal introitus.

manifested by separation of collagen fibers. Telangiectatic lymphatics and dilated capillaries are typical.

The most common endogenous types of acute dermatitis are atopic (hypersensitivity) dermatitis and seborrheic dermatitis, seen as a scaly macular eruption. Dermatitis with an exogenous cause that manifests as acute or chronic dermatitis includes irritant dermatitis (urine on the vulvar skin) and contact allergic dermatitis (a type 4 delayed hypersensitivity reaction).

Chronic Dermatitis

Lichen simplex chronicus (Fig. 18-6), or chronic dermatitis, is an "end-stage" of many inflammatory vulvar diseases that in their active phase are clinically pruritic and therefore subject to repeated scratching. It may also occur in other disorders such as lichen planus, psoriasis, and lichen sclerosus. The skin is thickened with exaggerated skin markings ("lichenification") and white, owing to marked hyperkeratosis. Scaling is generally present, and excoriations due to recent scratching can often be seen.

LICHEN SCLEROSUS: Lichen sclerosus is an inflammatory disease of the vulva associated with autoimmune disorders such as vitiligo, pernicious anemia, and thyroiditis.

Pathology: As vesicles rupture onto the surface, the fluid forms a crust on the skin surface. Histologically, the epidermis shows a range of inflammatory cells, and spongiotic areas form spongiotic vesicles that rupture to produce the exudative lesions. The dermis shows a perivascular lymphocytic infiltrate and edema,

Pathology: The condition is represented by white plaques, atrophic skin, a parchmentlike or crinkled appearance, and, occasionally, marked contracture of the vulvar tissues (Fig. 18-7A). Histologically, there is hyperkeratosis, loss of rete ridges, and a homogeneous, acellu-

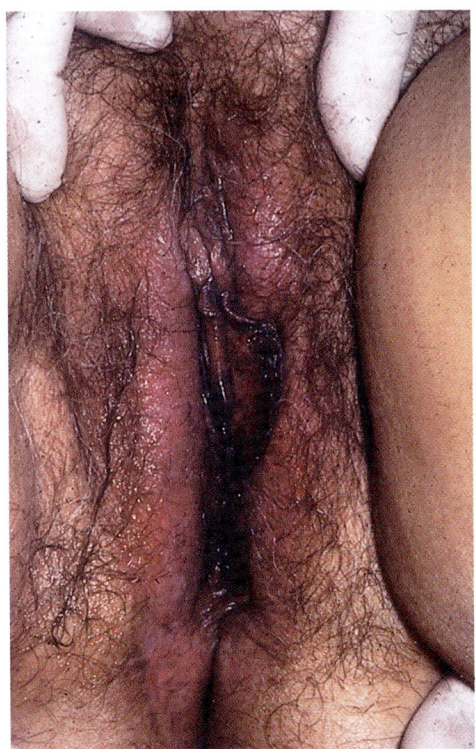

FIGURE 18-5
Vulvar acute dermatitis (eczema). Erythema and edema are present, with linear excoriations due to scratching.

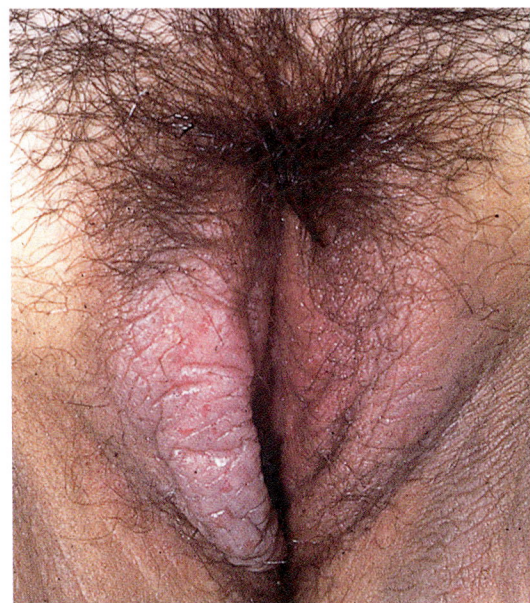

FIGURE 18-6
Lichen simplex chronicus of the right labium majus. There is thickening and accentuation of skin markings, with surface excoriation due to recent scratching.

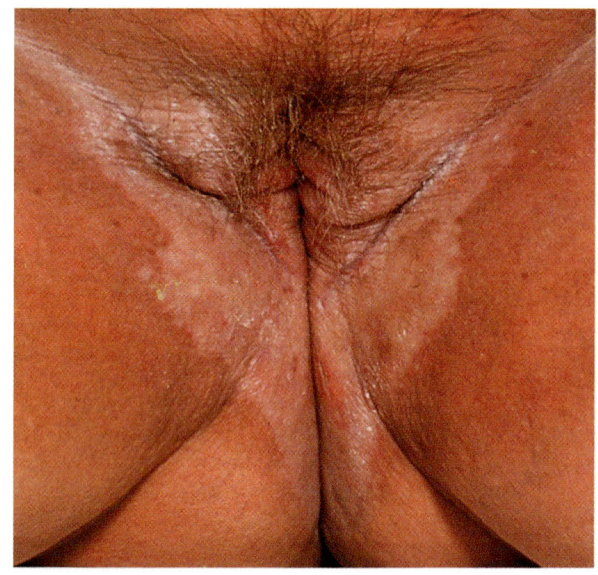
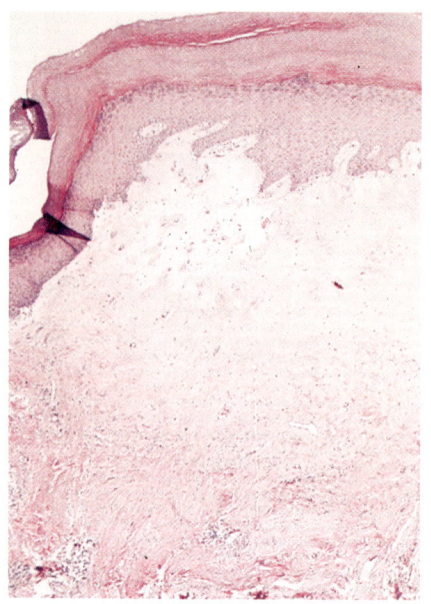

FIGURE 18-7
Lichen sclerosus of vulva. A. The sharply demarcated white lesion affects the vulva and perineum. B. The epidermis is thin and exhibits hyperkeratosis and a lack of the normal rete pattern. The dermis displays an acellular, homogeneous zone overlying a mild chronic inflammatory infiltrate.

lar zone in the upper dermis (Fig. 18-7). A band of chronic inflammatory cells typically lies beneath this layer. Itching is the most common symptom, and dyspareunia is frequent. The disease develops insidiously and is progressive. Women with symptomatic lichen sclerosus have a 15% chance of developing squamous cell carcinoma.

BENIGN TUMORS

HIDRADENOMA: This benign tumor of apocrine sweat gland origin appears chiefly in the labia majora as a sharply circumscribed nodule, rarely larger than 1 cm. Microscopically, the lesion is composed of papillary tubules and acini lined by two layers of cells: an inner layer of apocrine columnar cells and an outer one of myoepithelial cells.

SYRINGOMA: An adenoma of eccrine glands, syringoma manifests as a flesh-colored papule within the dermis of the labia majora. This asymptomatic tumor is composed of two layers of cells: an inner layer of serous cells and an outer one of myoepithelial cells.

CONNECTIVE TISSUE TUMORS: Senile hemangiomas (cherry hemangiomas) are small, purple skin papules, which on surface trauma may bleed. *Pyogenic granuloma,* previously thought to be a reaction to superficial wound infection, is a variant of hemangioma. Secondary infection occurs, as the surface of the lesion is fragile and easily traumatized. Soft tissue tumors found elsewhere in the body also occur in the vulva, including granular cell tumor, leiomyoma, fibroma, lipoma, and histiocytoma.

MALIGNANT TUMORS AND PREMALIGNANT CONDITIONS

Vulvar Intraepithelial Neoplasia (VIN) Is a Precursor of Invasive Cancer

VIN reflects a spectrum of neoplastic changes that range from minimal cellular atypia to the most marked cellular changes short of invasive cancer. Since 1980, there has been a 5- to 10-fold increase in the frequency of VIN and a 10-fold increase in the number of women with the disease who are younger than 40 years of age. In addition, younger women have increasingly developed an undifferentiated form of VIN, sometimes called *warty* or *basaloid dysplasia,* which typically displays HPV 16. A second form of VIN, which is found more frequently in older women, is more differentiated. If left untreated, some of these women develop invasive squamous cell carcinoma after 6 to 7 years. Thus, like comparable lesions in the cervix (CIN), **VIN is a precursor of squamous cell carcinoma, of which at least 30 to 40% are caused by HPV.**

 Pathology: The lesions of VIN may be single or multiple, and macular, papular, or plaquelike. Microscopically, the grades are labeled VIN I, II, and III, corresponding to mild, moderate, and severe dysplasia. Grade III also includes squamous cell carcinoma in situ. The criteria used in establishing the grade of VIN include (1) nuclear size and atypia, (2) number and degree of atypical mitoses, and (3) loss of cytoplasmic differentiation toward the epithelial surface. In the undifferentiated form seen in younger women, the entire epithelium consists of cells with highly atypical nuclei and negligible cytoplasm. Mitoses, including many atypical forms, are frequent. The more differentiated form in older women shows atypia confined to the basal or parabasal walls, with keratin pearls in the rete pegs. This type is more frequently associated with invasive carcinoma but less commonly with HPV infection. *Bowen disease,* a term still common in the dermatological literature, is a synonym for VIN III.

VIN, even if locally excised, often recurs (25%), in which case it may progress to invasive squamous cell carcinoma (6%). Women with VIN may have squamous neoplasms similar to VIN elsewhere in the lower genital tract.

Squamous Cell Carcinoma follows VIN

Squamous cell carcinoma of the vulva (Fig. 18-8) is the end result of a multistep process that has its origin in VIN. This tumor accounts for 3% of all genital cancers in women and is the most common cancer of the vulva (86%). In the past, it mainly affected older women, but like VIN it now occurs with increasing frequency in younger women. Two thirds of larger tumors are exophytic; the others are ulcerative and endophytic. Pruritus of long duration is commonly the first symptom. Ulceration, bleeding, and secondary infection may develop. The tumors grow slowly and then extend to the contiguous skin, vagina, and rectum. They metastasize to the superficial inguinal and then the deep inguinal, femoral, and pelvic lymph nodes.

A staging system for vulvar cancer uses 2 cm in greatest dimension as the critical size that differentiates stage I and stage II lesions (Table 18-2). In one series, each centimeter of tumor size increased the risk of death by 50%. In addition to increased size, factors affecting patient survival include tumor grade and the presence and location of lymph node metastases. More-differentiated tumors have a higher mean survival, approaching 90% when nodes are uninvolved. Two thirds of women with inguinal node metastases survive for at least 5 years, whereas only a fourth of those with pelvic node metastases live that long.

Verrucous Carcinoma

Verrucous carcinoma of the vulva is a distinct variety of squamous cell carcinoma that manifests as a large fungating mass resembling a giant condyloma acuminatum. HPV, usu-

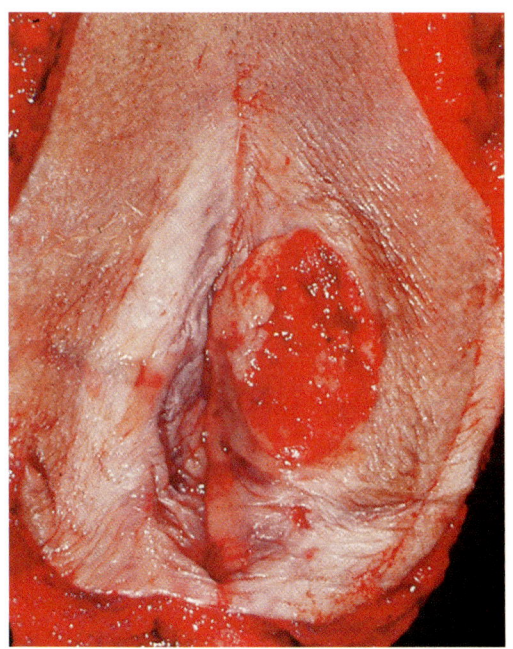
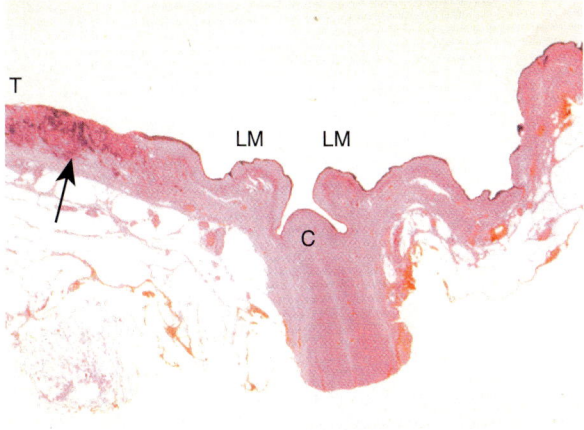
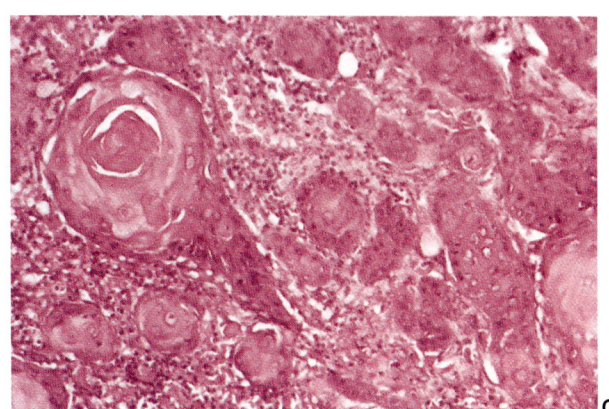

FIGURE 18-8

Squamous cell carcinoma of vulva. **A.** The tumor is situated in an extensive area of lichen sclerosus *(white)*. **B.** A cross-section of the vulva with a small squamous cell carcinoma *(arrow)* shows both halves of the perineum, including labia minora *(LM)* and clitoris *(C)*. A 1-cm tumor *(T)* is confined to the dermis. **C.** Small nests of neoplastic squamous cells, some with keratin pearls, are evident in this well-differentiated tumor.

TABLE 18-2 Clinical Staging of Carcinoma of Vulva

Stage	Description
0	Carcinoma in situ
I	Tumor ≤2 cm, confined to vulva
Ia	Stromal invasion ≤1 mm
Ib	Stromal invasion >1 mm
II	Tumor >2 cm confined to vulva
III	Tumor of any size extending to the lower urethra, vagina, or anus; or ulilateral regional lymph node metastasis
IV	Tumor extension
IVa	Mucosa of bladder or rectum; bone or upper urethra; or bilateral regional lymph nodes
IVb	Distant metastases, including pelvic lymph nodes

ally type 6 or 11, is commonly identified. The tumor is very well differentiated, being composed of large nests of squamous cells with abundant cytoplasm and small, bland nuclei. Squamous pearls are common, and mitoses are rare. The tumor "invades" with broad tongues, and the stromal interface frequently exhibits a heavy infiltrate of lymphocytes and plasma cells. Verrucous carcinoma rarely metastasizes. Wide local surgical excision is the treatment of choice, but other forms of therapy (cryosurgery and retinoids) have been used successfully.

Malignant Melanoma

Although uncommon, malignant melanoma is the second most frequent cancer of the vulva (5%). It occurs in the sixth and seventh decades but occasionally is found in younger women. The tumor has biological and microscopic characteristics of melanoma occurring elsewhere in the body. It is highly aggressive, and the prognosis is poor.

Extramammary Paget Disease Exhibits Intraepithelial Cells with Copious Pale Cytoplasm

Paget disease of the vulva is named after similar-appearing tumors in the nipple and extramammary sites, such as the axilla and perianal region. The disorder usually occurs on the labia majora in older women. Women with Paget disease of the vulva complain of pruritus or a burning sensation for many years.

Pathology: The lesion of Paget disease is large, red, moist, and sharply demarcated. The exact origin of the diagnostic cells (Paget cells) remains controversial; they are thought to arise in the epidermis or in epidermally derived adnexal structures. Paget cells are usually confined to the epidermis and appear as large single cells or, less commonly, clusters of cells that lack intercellular bridges. The typical Paget cell has a pale, vacuolated cytoplasm (Fig. 18-9) that contains glycosaminoglycans; it stains with periodic acid–Schiff (PAS) and mucicarmine and expresses carcinoembryonic antigen (CEA).

Intraepidermal Paget disease may have been present for many years and is often far more extensive throughout the epidermis than preoperative biopsies indicate. In contrast to Paget disease of the breast, which is almost always associated with an underlying duct carcinoma, extramammary Paget disease is only rarely associated with an adenocarcinoma of the skin adnexa. Since metastases rarely occur,

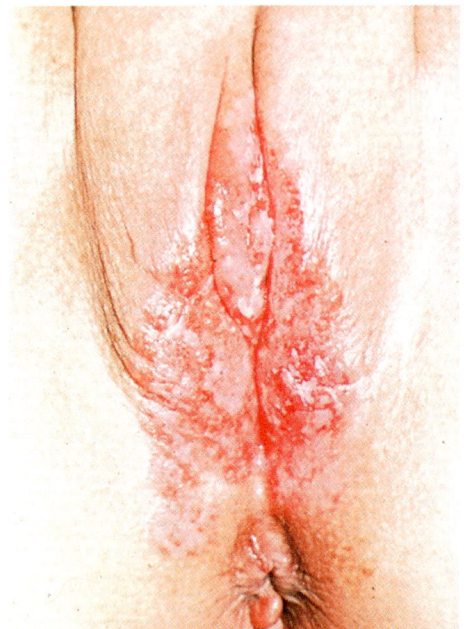
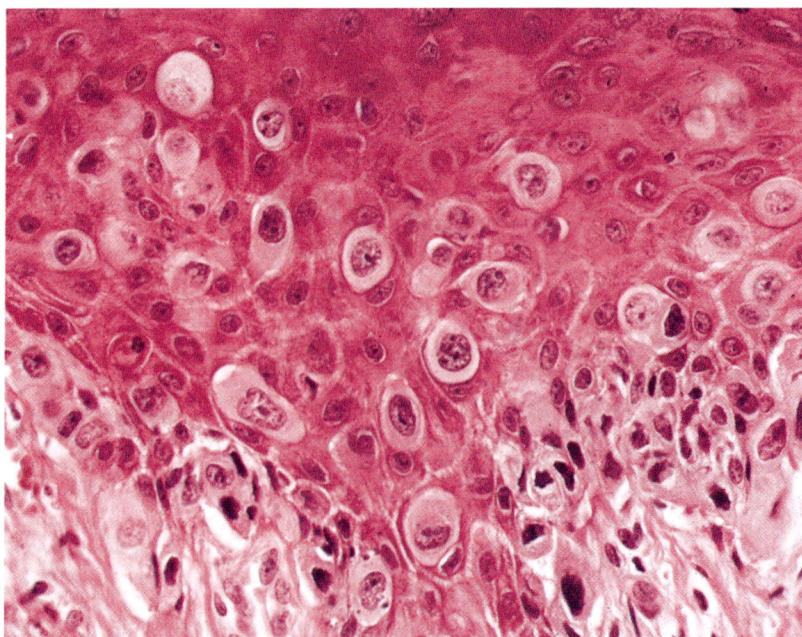

FIGURE 18-9
Paget disease of the vulva. A. The lesion is red, moist, and sharply demarcated. B. Individual Paget cells, characterized by an abundant pale cytoplasm, infiltrate the epithelium and are interspersed among normal keratinocytes.

treatment requires only wide local excision or simple vulvectomy.

Vagina

ANATOMY

The vagina extends from the uterus to the vestibule of the vulva and is lined by a hormone-responsive squamous epithelium. Estrogens stimulate the proliferation and maturation of vaginal epithelial cells. Maturation is marked by the accumulation of glycogen, which imparts a clear appearance to the cytoplasm of the epithelial cells. By contrast, the maturation of vaginal epithelium is inhibited by progesterone. As a result, during the secretory phase of the menstrual cycle or during pregnancy, when progesterone levels are high, the intermediate cells, rather than the superficial ones, predominate in vaginal smears.

Lymph drains through the lateral perivaginal plexus. The lymphatics from the vaginal vault and upper vagina communicate with branches from the cervix to drain into the pelvic and then the paraaortic nodes. The lower vagina also drains to the inguinal and femoral nodes.

NONNEOPLASTIC CONDITIONS AND BENIGN TUMORS

Congenital Anomalies of the Vagina Are Rare

Congenital absence of the vagina is generally associated with anomalies of the uterus and urinary tract. In the presence of a functional uterus, the absence of a vagina may lead to the accumulation of menstrual blood in the uterus.

Septate vagina results from the failure of the embryonic müllerian ducts to fuse properly, and the resulting median wall does not resorb.

Vaginal atresia and imperforate hymen prevent the transformation of the embryonic lining of the vagina from a müllerian to a squamous epithelium, an effect that is a cause of vaginal adenosis.

Atrophic Vaginitis Results from Diminished Estrogenic Stimulation

Atrophic vaginitis is thinning and atrophy of the vaginal epithelium. The thinned epithelium in an estrogen-deficient woman is a poor barrier to infections or abrasions. Atrophic vaginitis occurs most commonly in postmenopausal women in whom estrogen levels are low. Dyspareunia and vaginal spotting are common symptoms.

Vaginal Adenosis Occurs in Daughters Exposed in Utero to Diethylstilbestrol (DES)

Vaginal adenosis refers to failure of the normal glandular epithelium that lines the embryonic vagina to be replaced during fetal life by squamous epithelium. Prior to the use of DES for the treatment of high-risk pregnancies, which began in the 1940s, vaginal adenosis was a curiosity. However, in the 1970s, there was a substantial increase in the incidence of this disorder in young daughters of women who had received DES during pregnancy. Many of these lesions have disappeared as the young women have grown older. Rare cases of clear cell adenocarcinoma of the vagina have also occurred in the daughters of women treated with DES.

 Pathogenesis: At the 10th week of gestation, the upgrowth of a squamous epithelium derived from the urogenital sinus replaces the glandular (müllerian) epithelium lining the vagina and exocervix. DES exposure at any time during this critical window, which lasts until about the 18th week, arrests the transformation process. Hence, some glandular tissue (i.e., adenosis) remains.

 Pathology: Adenosis manifests as red, granular patches on the vaginal mucosa. Microscopically, it comprises two types of cells: mucinous columnar cells, resembling those lining the endocervix, and ciliated cells with eosinophilic cytoplasm, similar to those lining the endometrium and fallopian tubes (Fig. 18-10). The glandular cells ultimately undergo squamous metaplasia.

Fibroepithelial Polyp

Vaginal polyps are uncommon benign growths composed of a connective tissue core and an outer lining of vaginal squamous epithelium. They are usually single, gray-white, and less than 1 cm in diameter. Simple excision is usually curative.

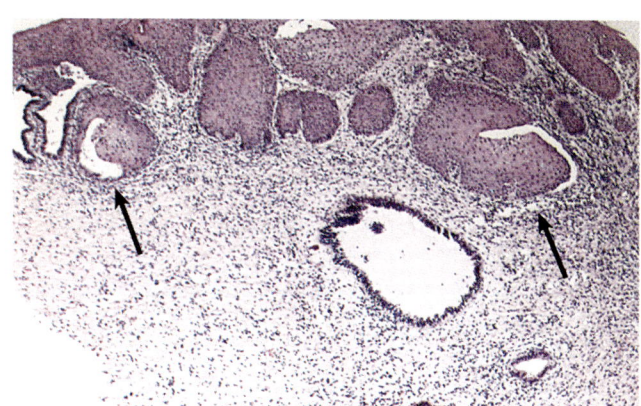

FIGURE 18-10
Vaginal adenosis. A section of the vagina shows glands in the chronically inflamed lamina propria, lined by ciliated, darkly staining cells similar to tubal or endometrial epithelium. Some glands merge with metaplastic squamous pegs (*arrows*). **The surface epithelium consists of metaplastic glycogen-free squamous cells, accounting for the abnormal iodine staining.**

Benign Mesenchymal Tumors

Most benign tumors in the vagina resemble those in other parts of the female genital tract and include leiomyomas, rhabdomyomas, and neurofibromas. These are solid submucosal tumors usually less than 2 cm in diameter. *Granular cell tumor* is an unusual tumor of Schwann cell origin that impinges on the overlying squamous epithelium.

MALIGNANT TUMORS

Primary malignant tumors of the vagina are uncommon, constituting about 2% of all genital tract tumors. Most (80%) vaginal malignancies represent secondary spread. The most common symptoms are a vaginal discharge, and bleeding during coitus, but advanced tumors may cause pelvic or abdominal pain and edema of the legs. Tumors that are confined to the vagina are usually treated by radical hysterectomy and vaginectomy.

Squamous Cell Carcinoma Is the Major Vaginal Cancer

Squamous cell carcinoma of the vagina accounts for over 90% of all primary malignant tumors of the vagina. It is generally a disease of older women, with a peak incidence between the ages of 60 and 70 years. Squamous cell carcinoma appears most commonly in the anterior wall of the upper third of the vagina, where it usually manifests as an exophytic mass. *Vaginal intraepithelial neoplasia* (VAIN), a term replacing both *vaginal dysplasia* and *carcinoma in situ*, frequently precedes the development of invasive carcinoma. Not infrequently, squamous cell carcinoma of the vagina develops some years after cervical or vulvar carcinoma, a sequence that supports the concept of a carcinogenic field effect in the lower genital tract related to HPV infection.

Since most preinvasive and early invasive cancers are clinically silent, the routine use of vaginal cytology remains the most effective method to detect squamous cell carcinoma of the vagina. The prognosis is related to the spread of the tumor at the time of its discovery (Table 18-3). The 5-year survival rate for tumors confined to the vagina (stage I) is 80%, whereas it is only 20% for those with extensive spread (stages III/IV).

TABLE 18-3 **Clinical Staging of Carcinoma of Vagina**

Stage	Description
0	Carcinoma in situ
I	Limited to vaginal wall
II	Involves subvaginal tissue, but does not extend to pelvic wall
III	Extends to pelvic wall
IV	Extends beyond true pelvis or involves mucosa of bladder or rectum
IVa	Spread to adjacent organs
IVb	Spread to distant organs

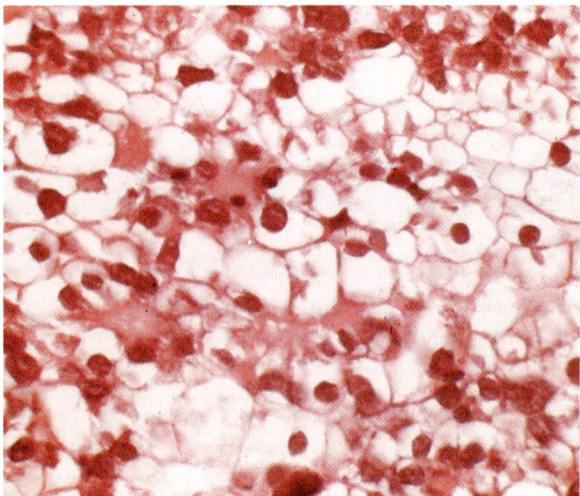

FIGURE 18-11
Clear cell adenocarcinoma of the vagina in the daughter of a woman treated with diethylstilbestrol.

Clear Cell Adenocarcinoma Follows in Utero DES Exposure

Clear cell adenocarcinoma is most frequent on the anterior wall of the upper third of the vagina. The tumor is unusual before age 13 and is most common between ages 17 and 22. Almost all clear cell adenocarcinomas are associated with vaginal adenosis, but very few women with adenosis develop this cancer. The abundant clear cytoplasm, reflecting the presence of glycogen, accounts for the name *clear cell adenocarcinoma* (Fig. 18-11). Its other pattern shows cells with bulbous nuclei that line the glandular lumina *(hobnail cells)*. Clear cell adenocarcinomas are almost invariably curable when they are small and asymptomatic, but in more advanced stages, they may spread by hematogenous or lymphatic routes.

Embryonal Rhabdomyosarcoma (Sarcoma Botryoides) Is a Malignant Childhood Tumor

Embryonal rhabdomyosarcoma is a rare vaginal tumor that appears as confluent polypoid masses resembling a bunch of grapes, hence the name sarcoma botryoides *(Greek* botrys, *grapes)* (Fig. 18-12). It occurs almost exclusively in girls younger than 4 years of age.

 Pathology: The tumor arises in the lamina propria of the vagina and consists of primitive spindle rhabdomyoblasts, some of which display cross striations. Myofibrils composed of myosin and actin are often demonstrable. A dense zone of round rhabdomyoblasts (the cambium layer) is present beneath the vaginal epithelium. Deep to this layer the stroma is myxomatous and shows fewer neoplastic rhabdomyoblasts.

 Clinical Features: The tumor is usually detected because of spotting on the child's diaper. Tumors less than 3 cm in greatest dimension tend to be local-

Anatomy

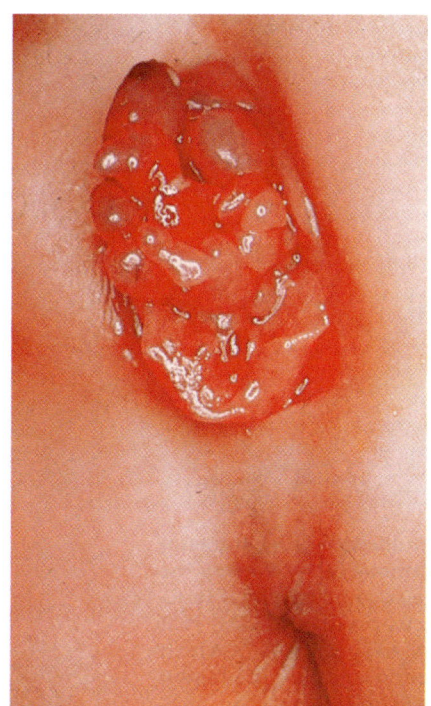
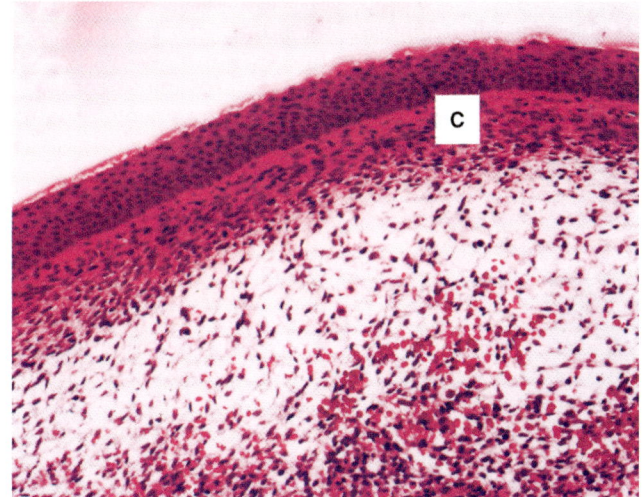
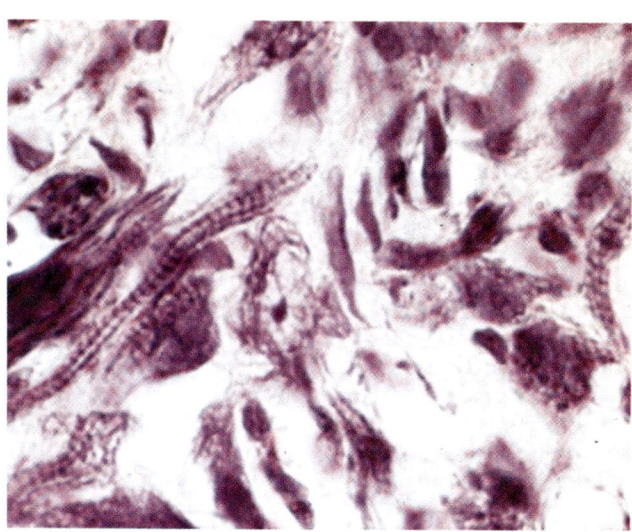

FIGURE 18-12
Embryonal rhabdomyosarcoma (sarcoma botryoides) of vagina. **A.** The grapelike tumor protrudes through the introitus. **B.** A section of the tumor shows a dense layer of neoplastic stroma termed the *cambium layer (c)* beneath the surface epithelium of the vagina. A loose neoplastic stroma is present beneath the cambium layer. **C.** The tumor contains rhabdomyoblasts characterized by cross striations (PTAH stain).

ized and may be cured by wide excision and chemotherapy. Larger tumors are likely to have invaded adjacent structures, metastasized to regional lymph nodes, and spread hematogenously to distant sites. Even in advanced cases, half of patients survive following radical surgery and chemotherapy.

Cervix

ANATOMY

The cervix (Latin *collare,* neck) is the inferior portion of the uterus that connects the corpus to the vagina (Fig. 18-13). Its exposed portion (also termed the *exocervix, ectocervix,* or *portio vaginalis*) protrudes into the upper vagina and is covered by glycogen-rich squamous epithelium. The endocervix is the canal that leads to the endometrial cavity. It is lined by longitudinal mucosal ridges that are composed of fibrovascular cores lined by a single layer of mucinous columnar cells. Occasionally, the outlet of the endocervical glands becomes blocked. As a result, mucin is retained and produces macroscopically visible cystic dilations of these glands, termed *nabothian cysts.* The external os is the *macroscopically* visible junction between the exocervix and endocervix. The squamocolumnar junction is the *microscopic* anatomical junction of the squamous and mucinous columnar epithelia. The area between the endocervix and endometrial cavity is called the *isthmus* or *lower uterine segment.*

The Transformation Zone Is the Site of Squamous Carcinoma

The exocervix remodels continuously during life. During embryonic development, the upward migration of squamous cells meets the columnar epithelium of the endocervix to form

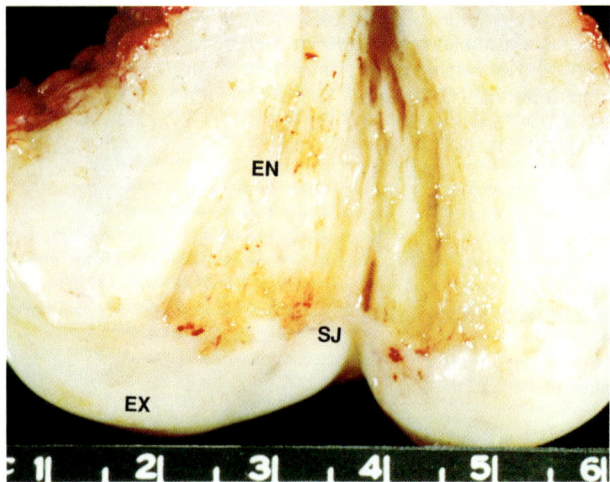
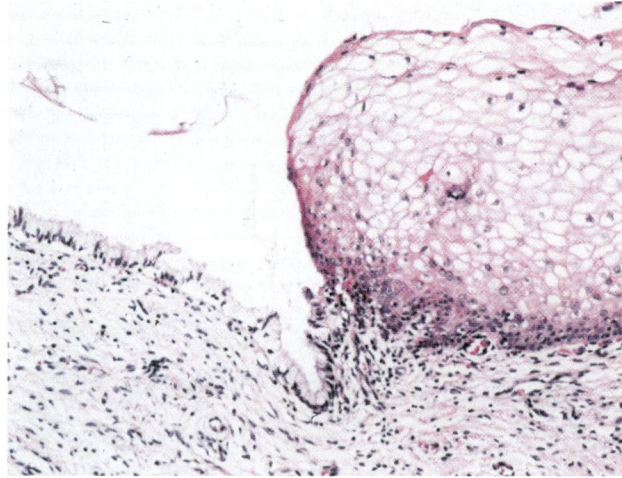

FIGURE 18-13
Anatomy of the cervix. A. The cervix has been opened to show the endocervix *(EN)*, squamocolumnar junction *(SJ)*, and exocervix *(EX)*. The thick layer of squamous cells covering the exocervix accounts for its white color. B. A microscopic view of the squamocolumnar junction. The endocervix is lined by a single layer of columnar mucus-producing cells that abruptly meets the exocervix lined by mature squamous cells. *Note:* In specimens in which the squamocolumnar junction is on the ectocervix or in the endocervical canal, the region between it and the external os is called the *transformation zone* (see Fig. 18-14).

the initial squamocolumnar junction (Fig. 18-14). In some young women, this "original" squamocolumnar junction is located at the internal os. In most young women, however, the columnar epithelium extends onto the exocervix, in which case the squamocolumnar junction is also located on the exocervix. In the latter situation, the areas of the exocervix lined by columnar epithelium are referred to as *endocervical ectropion* and appear by colposcopic examination as reddish discolorations. With age, the columnar epithelium of the ectropion undergoes squamous metaplasia, and the new squamocolumnar junction is located at the internal os. **The area between the most distal squamocolumnar junction and the external os is termed the *transformation zone*.**

The immature squamous epithelium of the transformation zone displays progressive nuclear maturation and increasing amounts of glycogen-free cytoplasm toward the surface. Colposcopy reveals the development of a thin white membrane, which eventually becomes thicker and whiter as the squamous epithelium matures (Fig. 18-15). Subsequently, the cells accumulate glycogen and are indistinguishable from the normal squamous epithelium lining the exocervix.

Examination of the transformation zone by iodine staining forms the basis of the *Schiller iodine test*. If the squamous cells lining the exocervix are mature (glycogen rich), which is normal, they stain with iodine, and the exocervix appears mahogany brown. If the cells lining the exocervix are immature (glycogen poor), no iodine staining occurs, and the exocervix is pale.

CERVICITIS

Inflammation of the cervix is common and is related to constant exposure to bacterial flora in the vagina. Acute and chronic cervicitis result from infection with many microorganisms, particularly the endogenous vaginal aerobes and anaerobes, *Streptococcus, Staphylococcus,* and *Enterococcus.*

Other specific organisms include *C. trachomatis, N. gonorrhoeae,* and occasionally herpes simplex, type 2. Some agents are sexually transmitted; others may be introduced by foreign bodies, such as residual fragments of tampons and pessaries.

 Pathology: In **acute cervicitis,** the cervix is grossly red, swollen, and edematous, with copious pus "dripping" from the external os. Microscopically, the tissues exhibit an extensive infiltrate of polymorphonuclear leukocytes and stromal edema.

In **chronic cervicitis,** which is more common, the cervical mucosa is hyperemic (Fig. 18-16), and there may be true epithelial erosions. Microscopically, the stroma is infiltrated by mononuclear cells, principally lymphocytes and plasma cells. The metaplastic squamous epithelium of the transformation zone may extend into the endocervical glands, forming clusters of squamous epithelium with slightly enlarged nuclei, which must be differentiated from carcinoma.

BENIGN TUMORS AND TUMORLIKE CONDITIONS

Endocervical Polyp

Endocervical polyp, the most common cervical growth (Fig. 18-17), appears as a single smooth or lobulated mass, typically less than 3 cm in greatest dimension. It typically manifests as vaginal bleeding or discharge. The lining epithelium is mucinous, with varying degrees of squamous metaplasia,

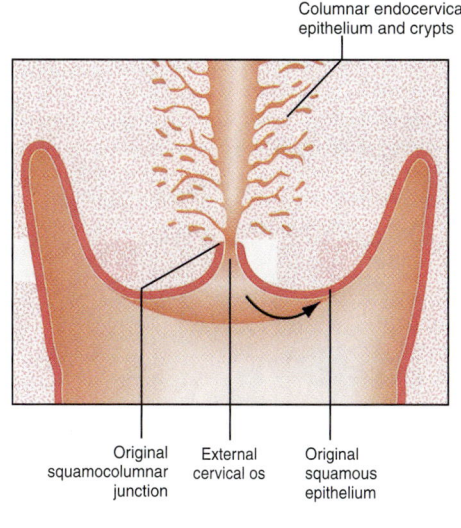
A. Prepubertal

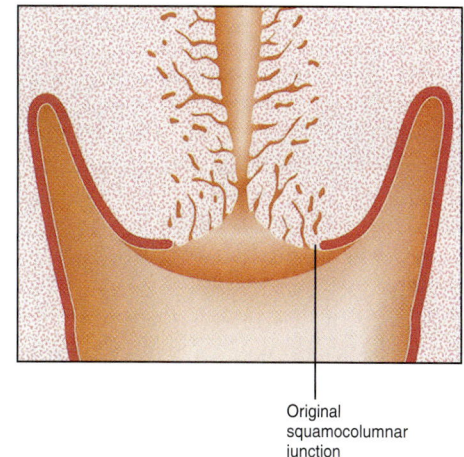
B. Eversion

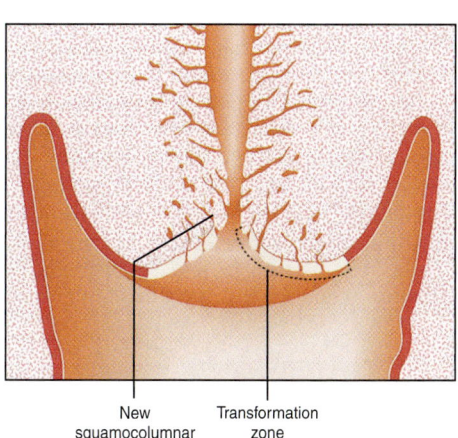
C. Postadolescent

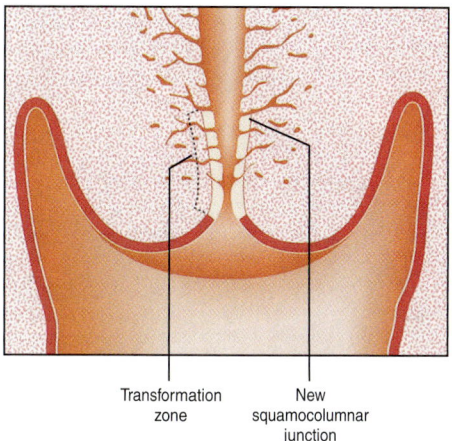
D. Postmenopausal

FIGURE 18-14
The transformation zone of the cervix. A. Prepubertal cervix. The squamocolumnar junction is situated at the external cervical os. The leaders show the direction of the movement that takes place as a result of the increase in bulk of the cervix during adolescence. B. The process of eversion. On completion, endocervical columnar tissue lies on the vaginal surface of the cervix and is exposed to the vaginal environment. C. Postadolescent cervix. The acidity of the vaginal environmental is one of the factors that encourage squamous metaplastic change, replacing the exposed columnar epithelium with squamous epithelium. D. Postmenopausal cervix. At this time, cervical inversion occurs. This phenomenon is the reverse of eversion, which was so important in adolescence. The transformation zone is now drawn into the cervical canal, often making it inaccessible to colposcopic examination.

but may feature erosions and granulation tissue in women with symptoms. Simple excision or curettage is curative. Cancer rarely arises in an endocervical polyp (0.2% of cases).

Microglandular Hyperplasia Reflects Progestational Stimulation

Microglandular hyperplasia of the cervix is a benign condition showing closely packed glands that lack an intervening stroma and display a neutrophilic infiltrate. It should not be confused with well-differentiated adenocarcinoma. Microglandular hyperplasia is usually asymptomatic and is typically associated with progestin stimulation. It usually occurs during pregnancy and the postpartum period, and in women taking oral contraceptives.

Leiomyoma

Leiomyomas of the cervix can bleed or prolapse into the endocervical canal, an event that leads to uterine contractions

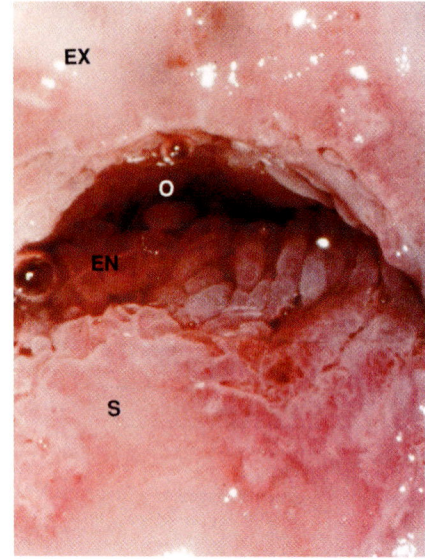
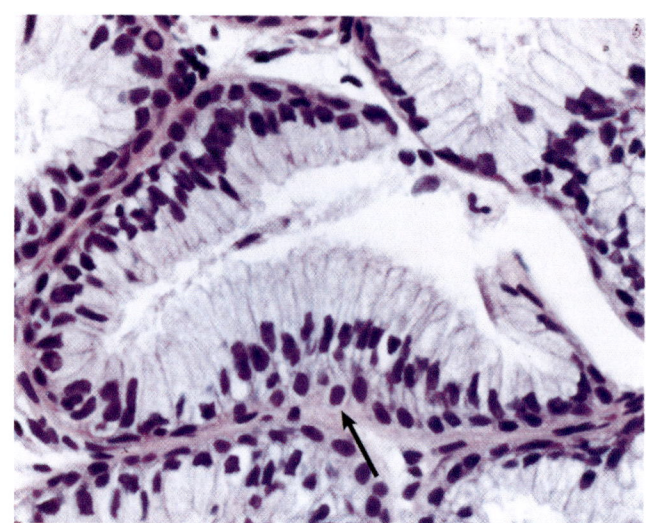
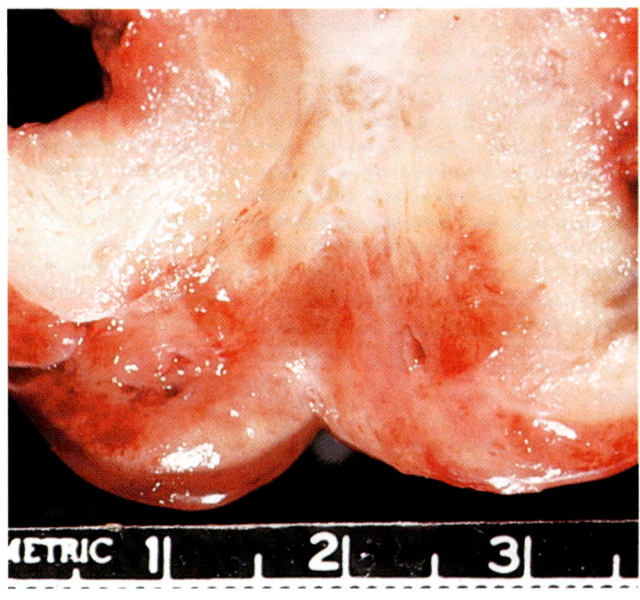

FIGURE 18-15
Squamous metaplasia in the transformation zone. A. In this colposcopic view of the cervix, a white area of metaplastic squamous epithelium (S) is situated between the exocervix (EX) and the mucinous endocervix (EN), which terminates at the internal os (O). B. In the early stages of squamous metaplasia of the transformation zone, the reserve cells, which normally constitute a single layer, begin to proliferate (arrow). C. At a later stage, the proliferating reserve cells displace the glandular epithelium. As a final step, the metaplastic cells mature into glycogen-rich squamous cells, resembling those in Figure 18-13B.

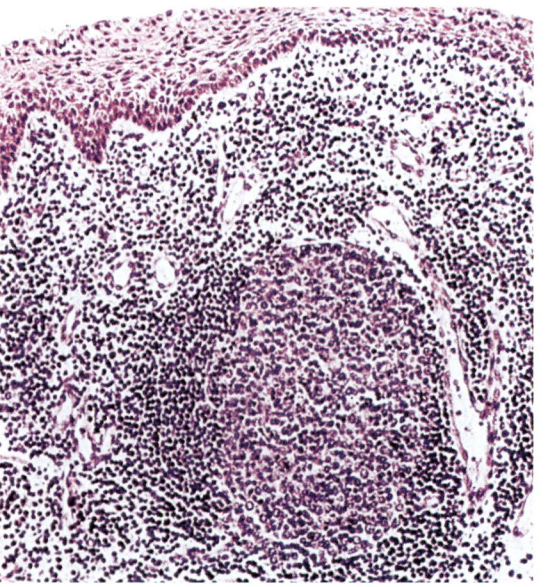

FIGURE 18-16
Chronic cervicitis. A. The cervix has been opened to reveal the reddened exocervix. B. Microscopic examination discloses chronic inflammation and the formation of a lymphoid follicle.

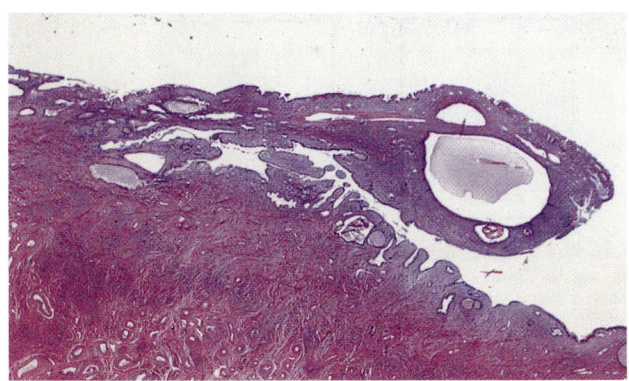

FIGURE 18-17
Endocervical polyp. A low-power photomicrograph shows cystic endocervical glands in a chronically inflamed stroma.

and pain resembling the early phases of labor. The appearance is similar to that of uterine leiomyomas (see below).

SQUAMOUS CELL NEOPLASIA

Fifty years ago, cervical cancer was the leading cause of cancer death in American women. With the introduction and widespread application of cytological screening, the incidence of cervical cancer has decreased by 50 to 85% in Western countries. It is the sixth most common female cancer in the United States, where the mortality rate has fallen by 70%. Nevertheless, worldwide, cervical cancer remains the second most common cancer in women.

Cervical Intraepithelial Neoplasia (CIN) Is the Precursor of Invasive Cancer

CIN is defined as a spectrum of intraepithelial changes that begins with minimal atypia and progresses through stages of more-marked intraepithelial abnormalities to invasive squamous cell carcinoma (Fig. 18-18). CIN, dysplasia, carcinoma in situ, and *squamous intraepithelial lesion* (SIL) are commonly used interchangeably (see Chapter 30).

Dysplasia in the cervical epithelium carries a risk for malignant transformation (Fig. 18-19). The concept of CIN emphasizes that dysplasia and carcinoma in situ are points on a disease spectrum rather than separate entities.

The grades of CIN are as follows:

- CIN-1: mild dysplasia
- CIN-2: moderate dysplasia
- CIN-3: severe dysplasia and carcinoma in situ

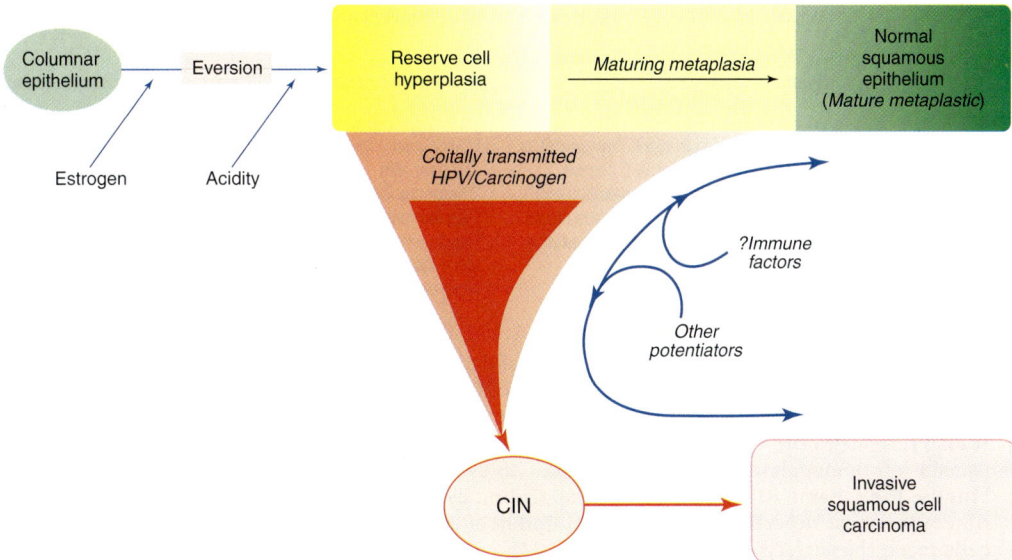

FIGURE 18-18
Pathophysiology of squamous cell carcinoma of the cervix. Hormonally induced eversion of the cervix and an acidic vaginal environment encourage the development of the transformation zone. In physiological conditions, benign squamous metaplasia is the eventual outcome. In the presence of a sexually transmitted agent (HPV), the benign metaplastic process is diverted into a malignant transformation, resulting first in increasingly severe cervical intraepithelial neoplasia (CIN) and then, in an unknown proportion of women, progressing to invasive squamous cell carcinoma. *Note:* The broad base of this arrow reflects uncertainty concerning how far along the process the metaplastic squamous cells remain susceptible to change by the carcinogen. Cells at the early reserve cell hyperplasia stage are usually considered to be at greatest risk and mature metaplastic squamous epithelium at no risk. The potential for transformation of the cells between these two extremes is unknown. Whether all agents act in unison or sequentially as initiators and promoters is unclear. It is also not known whether continued exposure to the carcinogen (or other potentiators) is necessary for the progression from mild to severe CIN or for the establishment of an invasive carcinoma. Local and systemic immune defenses are probably important in counteracting the changes generated by the carcinogenic agents.

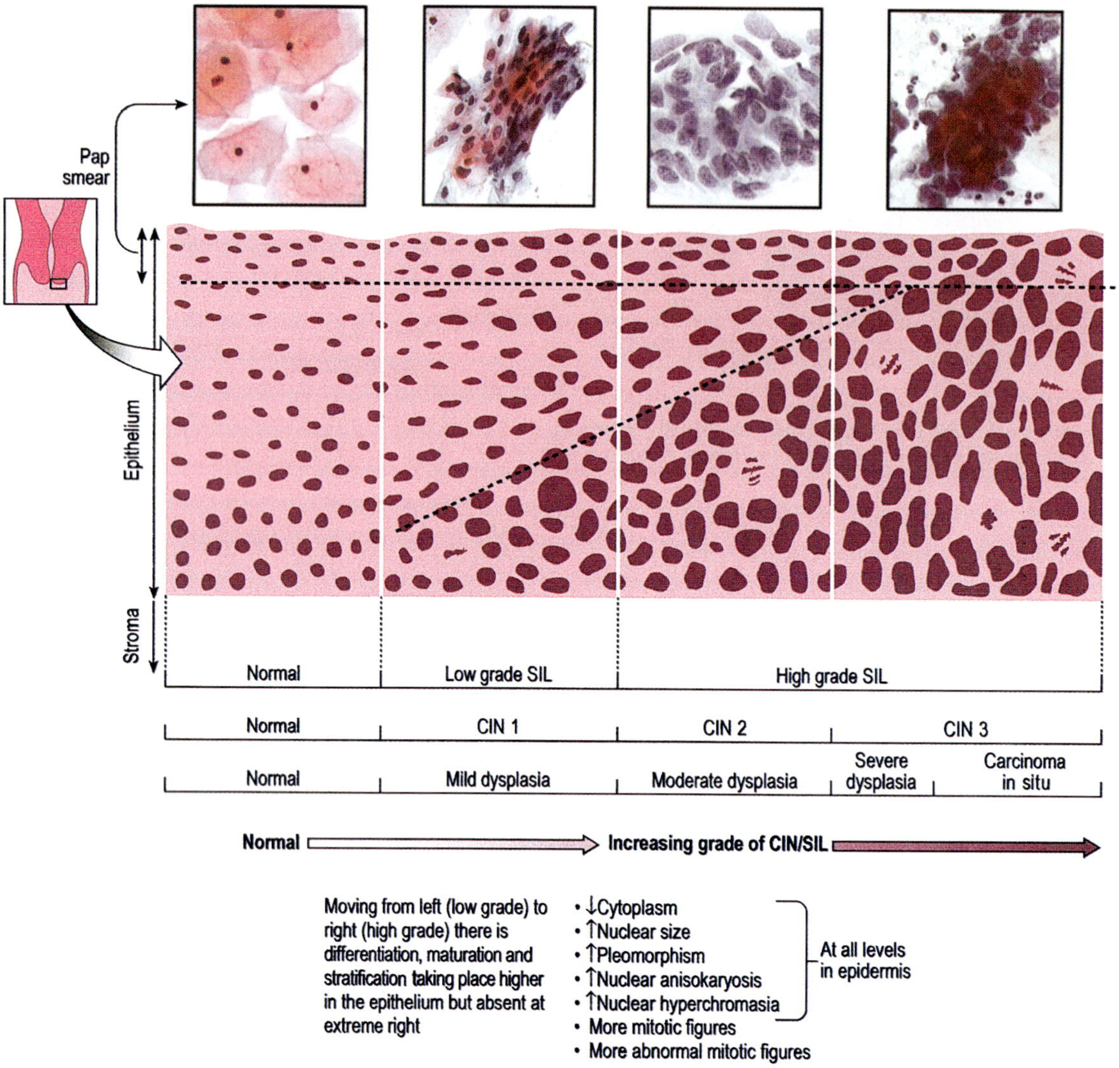

FIGURE 18-19
Interrelations of naming systems in preneoplastic cervical disease. This complex chart integrates multiple aspects of the disease complex. It lists the qualitative and quantitative features that become increasingly abnormal as the preneoplastic disease advances in severity. It also illustrates the changes in progressively more abnormal disease states and provides translation nomenclature for the dysplasia/CIS system, CIN system, and Bethesda system. Finally, the scheme illustrates the corresponding cytological smear resulting from exfoliation of the most superficial cells, indicating that even in the mildest disease state, abnormal cells reach the surface and are shed.

The recently promulgated "Bethesda System for Reporting Cervical/Vaginal Cytologic Diagnoses" groups these lesions slightly differently, calling them low- and high-grade squamous intraepithelial lesions. Low-grade SIL (LSIL) reflects conditions that should rarely progress in severity and commonly disappear (CIN-1, mild dysplasia). High-grade SIL (HSIL) corresponds to more severe histological lesions (CIN-2 and CIN-3), which tend to progress and require treatment. There is accumulating evidence that changes produced by oncogenic types of HPV may often appear initially as CIN-2, whereas lesions associated with nononcogenic types often progress no further than CIN-1 and then disappear.

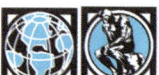

Epidemiology and Pathogenesis: The epidemiological features of CIN and invasive cancer are similar. Cervical cancer usually manifests between the ages of 40 and 60 years (mean 54), but CIN generally occurs under the age of 40. **The critical factor is HPV infection, which reflects multiple sexual partners and early age at first coitus.** Thus CIN is a **sexually transmitted disease.** Smoking seems to increase the incidence of cancer of the cervix, but the mechanism is obscure.

HUMAN PAPILLOMAVIRUS INFECTION: An HPV infection is etiological in the pathogenesis of CIN and cervical cancer (Fig. 18-20). Low-grade CIN is an example of a permissive infection, in which HPV is episomal and freely replicates, thereby causing cell death. Massive numbers of viral copies must accumulate in the cytoplasm of the cell before it can be seen microscopically as a *koilocyte.*

In most cases of higher-grade CIN, viral integration into the cell genome occurs. Proteins encoded by the *E6* and *E7* genes of HPV 16 bind p53 and Rb proteins, respectively, thereby inactivating important tumor suppressor functions (see Chapter 5).

After HPV integrates into the host DNA, the capsid of the virus becomes superfluous. As a result, copies of the whole virus do not accumulate, and koilocytes are absent in many cases of high-grade dysplasia and all invasive cancers.

Some 85% of low-grade CIN lesions harbor high-risk HPV. Many genital warts (condylomata acuminata) on the cervix contain HPV 6 or 11, which are regarded as low-risk HPV types. By contrast, cells in high-grade CIN usually contain HPV types 16, 18, 31, 33, 35, 39, 45, 51, 52, 56, 58, 59, and 68. **HPV types 16 and 18 are found in 70% of invasive cancers, and the other high-risk types account for another 25%.**

 Pathology: **CIN is nearly always a disease of the metaplastic squamous epithelium in the transformation zone or the endocervix. Practically, the extent of the transformation zone determines the distribution of CIN, and hence cervical cancer, on the exposed portion of the cervix.**

The normal process by which the cervical squamous epithelium matures is disturbed in CIN, as evidenced morphologically by changes in cellularity, differentiation, polarity, nuclear features, and mitotic activity. In CIN-1 (mild dysplasia), the most pronounced changes are seen in the basal third of the epithelium. However, abnormal cells are present throughout the entire thickness of the epithelium. Substantial cytoplasmic differentiation proceeds as the abnormal cells migrate through the upper two thirds of the epithelium, but the nuclei in the upper levels are still morphologically abnormal. Thus, the sloughed cells can be detected as abnormal in Papanicolaou smears. In CIN-2 (moderate dysplasia), most of the cellular abnormalities are in the lower and middle thirds of the epithelium. Cytodifferentiation occurs in cells in the upper third, but it is less than in CIN-1.

CIN-3 is synonymous with severe dysplasia and carcinoma in situ (CIS). In severe dysplasia, the cells in the superficial (upper) epithelium disclose some, albeit minimal, differentiation, whereas CIS shows none at all. The sequence of histological changes from CIN-1 to CIN-3 is illustrated in Figure 18-21.

Dysplasia and carcinoma in situ can often be detected on colposcopic examination by signs associated with their altered vasculature and epithelial changes. Mosaicism (irregu-

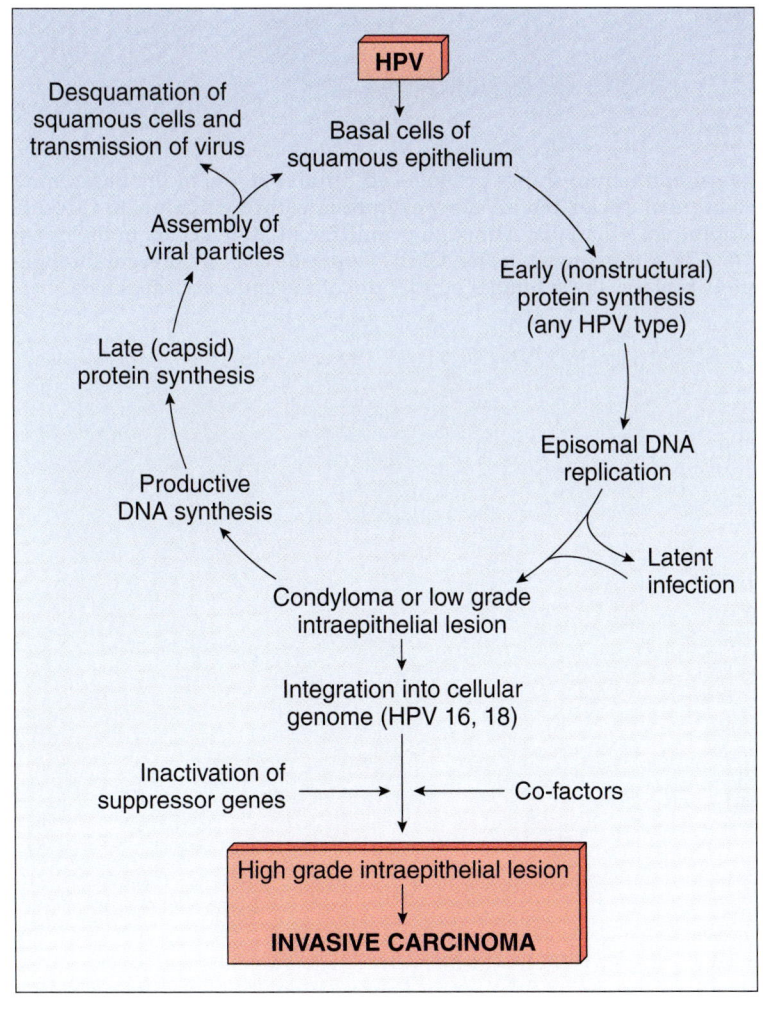

FIGURE *18-20*
Role of human papillomavirus (HPV) in the pathogenesis of cervical neoplasia.

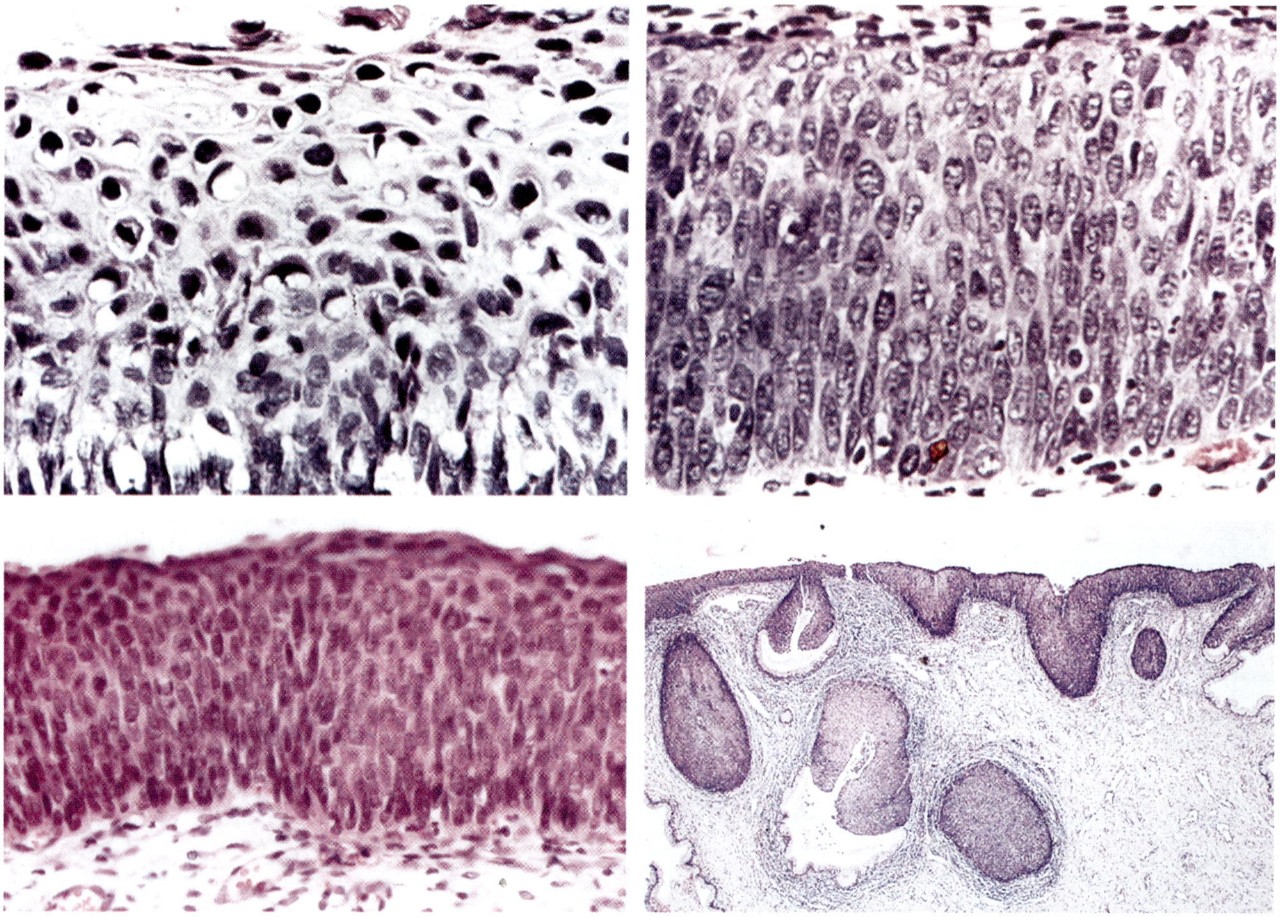

FIGURE 18-21

Cervical intraepithelial neoplasia (CIN). **A. CIN-1:** The cervical epithelium shows pronounced cellular atypia in the basal third. Some cells in the upper two thirds of the epithelium have abnormal nuclei, but all show cytoplasmic differentiation. **B. CIN-2 to CIN-3:** The lower two thirds of the epithelium displays pronounced cell atypia. Although cytodifferentiation occurs in the upper third of the epithelium, it is less pronounced than in CIN-1. **C. CIN-3 (carcinoma in situ, CIS):** Neoplastic cells are present throughout the entire epithelium. **D. CIN-3:** CIS partially or completely replaces the columnar epithelium of the endocervical glands.

lar surface resembling inlaid woodwork) (Fig. 18-22) (dots differentiated from the surrounding tissue surface by color and texture) are the two patterns most often found in high-grade CIN. The neoplastic process occurs more commonly on the anterior than on the posterior cervical lip of the cervix and often extends to involve the endocervical glands.

The mean age at which women develop CIN is 24 to 27 years for CIN-1 and CIN-2 and 35 to 42 for CIN-3. Based on morphological criteria, half of cases of CIN-1 regress, 10% progress to CIN-3, and less than 2% eventuate in invasive cancer. The frequency is much greater and the time required much shorter for progression to CIS for initially higher grades of CIN. The average time for all grades of dysplasia to progress to carcinoma in situ is about 10 years. **At least 20% of cases of CIN-3 progress to invasive carcinoma within that time.**

Clinical Features: When CIN is discovered, colposcopic examination in combination with a Schiller test is important to delineate the extent of the lesion and to indicate the areas to be biopsied. Diagnos-

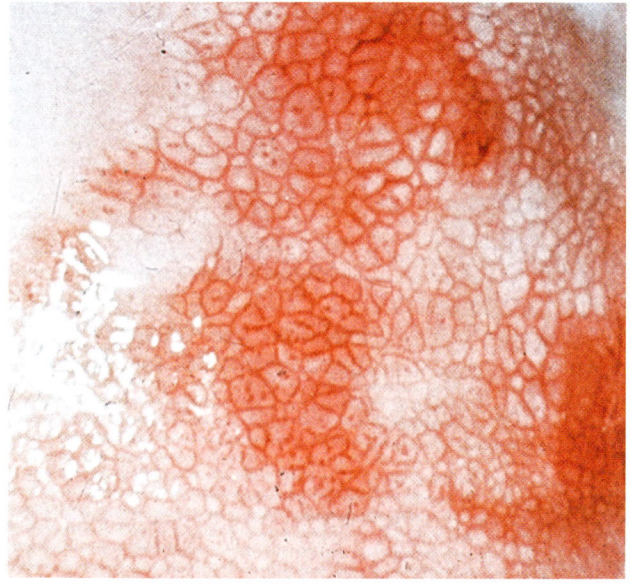

FIGURE 18-22
Dysplasia of the cervix. Examination with the colposcope discloses a mosaic pattern resembling inlaid woodwork.

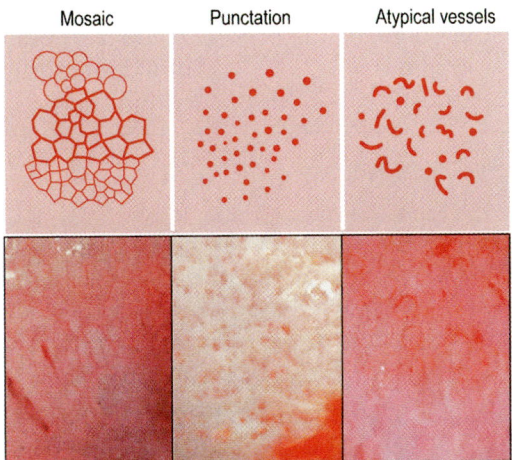

FIGURE 18-23
Abnormal vessels in colposcopy.

tic endocervical curettage is also useful for determining the extent of endocervical involvement. Women with CIN-1 are often followed conservatively (i.e., repeated Papanicolaou smears plus close follow-up), although some gynecologists now advocate local ablative treatment. High-grade lesions are treated according to the extent of disease. LEEP (loop electrosurgical excision procedure), which can be performed on an outpatient basis, is commonly used. In certain situations, cervical conization (removal of a cone of tissue around the external os), cryosurgery, and (rarely) hysterectomy are performed. Follow-up smears and clinical examinations should continue for life, since vaginal or vulvar squamous cancer may develop later.

Microinvasive Squamous Cell Carcinoma Is the Earliest Stage (Ia) of Invasive Cervical Cancer

Microinvasive cancer features neoplastic cells that minimally invade the stroma (Fig. 18-24). About 7% of specimens removed for carcinoma in situ demonstrate foci of microinvasive cancer. Small clusters of cells or solid lesions in the stroma have the following characteristics (see Table 18-5 and Fig. 18-25):

- Invasion to a depth of less than 3 mm (stage 1a1) or 5 mm (stage 1a2) below the basement membrane
- 7 mm maximum lateral extension

Most American gynecological oncologists further limit the definition to

- Lack of vascular invasion
- No lymph node metastases

Conization or simple hysterectomy generally suffices for the cure of microinvasive cancers less than 3 mm deep.

Invasive Squamous Cell Carcinoma Is Still Common Worldwide

 Epidemiology: Squamous cell carcinoma is by far the most common type of cervical cancer. Despite its declining frequency in the United States (Table 18-4), owing to the widespread use of cytological smears, it still accounts for some 13,000 new cases annually, which is less than the incidence of either endometrial or ovarian cancer. However, in underdeveloped areas, where cytological screening is not readily available, squamous cell cancer of the cervix remains a major cause of cancer death.

 Pathology: Cervical cancer in its early stages often manifests as a poorly defined, granular, eroded lesion or as a nodular and exophytic mass (Fig. 18-26A). If it is predominantly within the endocervical canal, it may appear as an endophytic mass, infiltrating the stroma and causing diffuse enlargement and hardening of the cervix (barrel-shaped cervix). On microscopic examination, most tumors display a nonkeratinizing pattern that is characterized by solid nests of large malignant squamous cells, with no more than individual cell keratinization. Most of the remaining cancers exhibit nests of keratinized cells organized in concentric whorls, so-called keratin pearls (Fig. 18-26B).

The least common pattern of squamous cell cancer is small cell carcinoma, the most aggressive cancer of the cervix and the one associated with the poorest prognosis. It consists of infiltrating masses of small, cohesive, nonkeratinized, malignant cells.

Cervical cancer spreads by direct extension and through lymphatic vessels (Fig. 18-27) and only rarely by the hematogenous route. Local extension into surrounding tissues (parametrium) results in ureteral compression

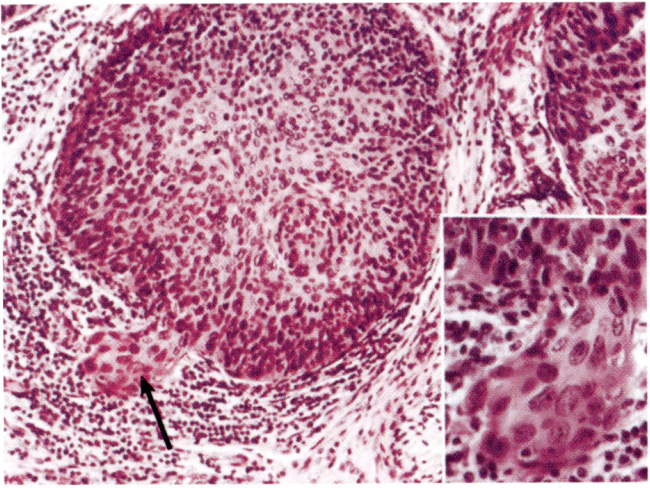

FIGURE 18-24
Microinvasive squamous cell carcinoma. Section of the cervix shows that carcinoma in situ in an endocervical gland has broken through the basement membrane *(arrow)* to invade the stroma. *(Inset)* A higher-power view of the microinvasive focus.

FIGURE 18-25
Comparison of microinvasive carcinomas of cervix.

(stage IIIb, Table 18-5); the corresponding clinical complications are hydroureter, hydronephrosis, and renal failure, the last being the most common cause of death (50% of patients). Bladder and rectal involvement (stage IVa) may lead to fistula formation. Metastases to regional lymph nodes involve the paracervical, hypogastric, and external iliac nodes. Overall, the cancer's growth and spread are relatively slow, since the average age for patients with stage 0 tumor (CIN-III) is 35 to 40 years; for stage 1A, 43 years; and for stage IV, 57 years.

Clinical Features: In the earliest stages of cervical cancer, patients complain most frequently of vaginal bleeding after intercourse or douching. With more-advanced tumors, the symptoms are referable to the route and degree of spread. Although the Papanicolaou smear remains the most reliable screening test for the detection of cervical cancer, a newer assay for squamous cell carcinoma antigen (SCC-Ag) on Papanicolaou smear is positive in one third of cases of stage I tumor and in over half of higher-stage cases.

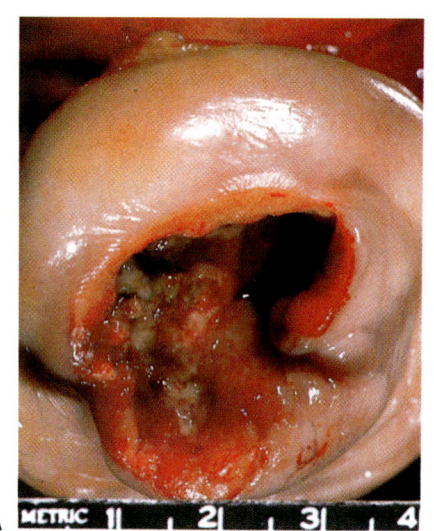
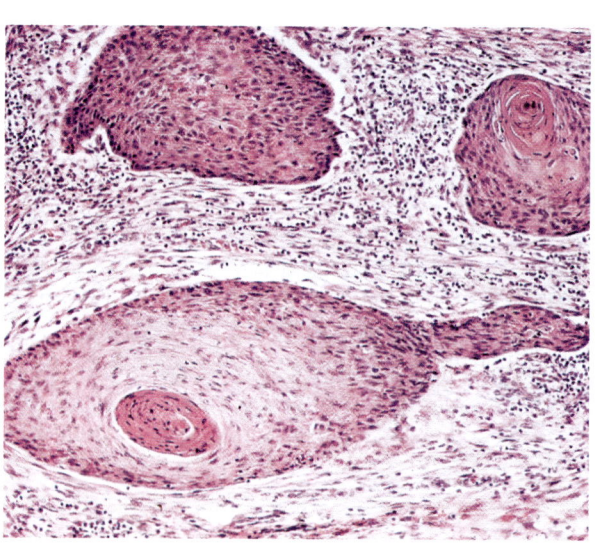

FIGURE 18-26
Squamous cell cancer. A. The cervix is distorted by the presence of an exophytic, ulcerated squamous cell carcinoma. B. The keratinizing pattern of the tumor is manifested as whorls of keratinized cells ("keratin pearls").

TABLE 18-4 Incidence of Gynecological Cancer in the United States

	New Cases		Death	
	Cases	%	Cases	%
Endometrium	34,000	6	6000	2
Ovary	27,000	4	15,000	6
Cervix, invasive	16,000	3	5000	2
Vulva, invasive	3000	<1		
Vagina, invasive	1000	<1		
Other	2000	<1		

Carcinoma in situ of cervix >50,000 new case/year.
%, percentage of all cases of cancer in females.

The clinical stage of cervical cancer is the best prognostic index of survival (see Table 18-5). The overall 5-year survival rate is 60%, and for each stage it is as follows: I, 90%; II, 75%; III, 35%; and IV, 10%. About 15% of patients develop recurrences on the vaginal wall, bladder, pelvis, or rectum within 2 years of therapy. Radical hysterectomy is favored for localized tumor, especially in younger women; radiation therapy or combinations of the two are used for more advanced tumors.

Adenocarcinoma of the Endocervix Accounts for 20% of Malignant Cervical Tumors

An increased incidence of cervical adenocarcinoma has been reported recently, with a mean age at presentation of 56 years.

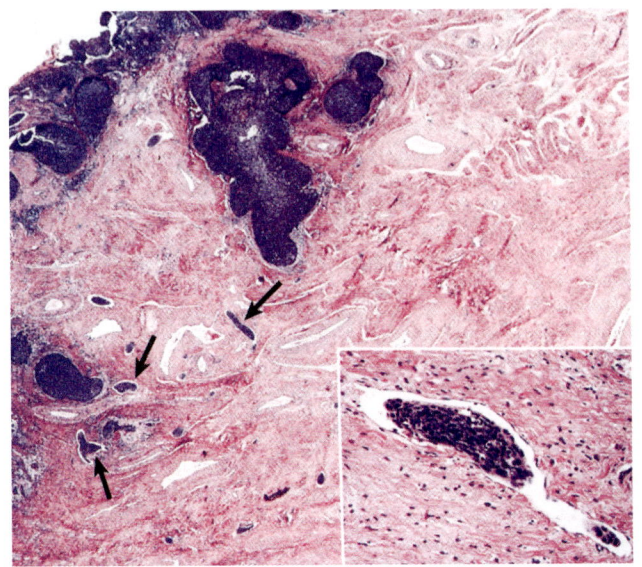

FIGURE 18-27
Squamous cell cancer of the cervix with lymphatic invasion. Low magnification shows a squamous cell carcinoma that has invaded the stroma and permeated the lymphatics *(arrows).* **(Inset)** A high-power view of lymphatic invasion.

TABLE 18-5 Clinical Staging of Cervical Cancer (FIGO)

Stage	Description
0	Carcinoma in situ (cervical intraepithelial neoplasia III)
I	Carcinoma confined to cervix (extension to corpus disregarded)
Ia	Invasive cancer identified *only* microscopically. Maximum depth, 5.0 mm; maximum width, 7.0 mm.
1a1	Depth ≤3.0 mm
1a2	Depth >3.0 mm
Ib	Any cancer *grossly* visible
1b1	Clinical size ≤4.0 cm
1b2	Clinical size >4.0 cm
II	Carcinoma extending beyond cervix, but not to lateral pelvic wall; involvement of vagina limited to upper two thirds
IIa	Paracervical extension not suspected
IIb	Paracervical extension suspected
III	Invasive carcinoma extending to lateral pelvic wall or lower one third of vagina
IIIa	No extension to pelvic wall
IIIb	Extension to pelvic wall, hydronephrosis, or nonfunctioning kidney
IV	Extended spread involving
IVa	Mucosa of urinary bladder or rectum
IVb	Tissues beyond true pelvis

Most of the tumors are of the endocervical cell (mucinous) type, but the various subtypes have little importance for overall survival. Adenocarcinoma shares epidemiological factors with squamous cell carcinoma of the cervix and spreads similarly. The tumors are often associated with adenocarcinoma in situ and are frequently infected with HPV types 16 and 18.

 Pathology

ADENOCARCINOMA IN SITU: This lesion, also called *cervical glandular intraepithelial neoplasia* (CGIN), generally arises in the region of the squamocolumnar junction and extends into the endocervical canal. It displays tall columnar cells with eosinophilic or mucinous cytoplasm, sometimes resembling goblet cells. The pattern of spread and involvement of endocervical glands resemble those of CIN. Adenocarcinoma in situ typically is an intraepithelial proliferation, and the normal architecture of the endocervical glands is maintained. The cells show slight enlargement, atypical hyperchromatic nuclei, an increased nuclear-to-cytoplasmic ratio, and variable numbers of mitoses. Abrupt transitions help distinguish neoplastic from neighboring normal endocervical cells. Associated high-grade squamous cell CIN occurs in 40% of cases of adenocarcinoma in situ.

INVASIVE ADENOCARCINOMA: This tumor typically manifests as a fungating polypoid or papillary mass. Microscopically, exophytic tumors often have a papillary pattern, whereas endophytic ones display tubular or glandular patterns. Poorly differentiated tumors are predominantly composed of solid sheets of cells.

Invasive adenocarcinoma of the endocervix spreads by local invasion and lymphatic metastases, but the overall survival is somewhat less than that for squamous carcinoma. The tumor is treated in a manner similar to that of squamous carcinoma.

Uterus

ANATOMY

The uterine corpus (body) is smaller than the cervix at birth and during childhood, but increases rapidly in size after puberty. The endometrium, composed of glands and stroma, is thin at birth, when it consists of a continuous surface of cuboidal epithelium that dips to line a few sparse tubular glands. After puberty, the endometrium thickens. The superficial two thirds, the *zona functionalis*, respond to hormones and is shed with each menstrual phase. The deepest third, the basal layer, is the germinative portion and with each cycle regenerates a new functional zone.

The endometrium is supplied by arcuate arteries that traverse the outer myometrium and give off two sets of vessels, one to the myometrium and the other, the radial arteries, to the endometrium. In turn, the radial arteries branch into two types of vessels. The basal arteries supply the basal endometrium, and the spiral arteries nourish the superficial two thirds.

THE MENSTRUAL CYCLE

The normal endometrium undergoes a series of sequential changes that support the growth of the implanted fertilized ovum (*zygote*) (Fig. 18-28). In the absence of conception, the endometrium is shed and then regenerated to support a fertilized ovum during the next cycle.

PROLIFERATIVE PHASE: During the first 14 days of the menstrual cycle, the endometrium is under estrogenic stimulation. The functional zone exhibits tubular to coiled glands, which are evenly distributed and supported by a cellular, monomorphic stroma (Fig. 18-28). Early during the proliferative phase, the glands are of narrow diameter, but as

Day of Cycle		Before 14	15–16	17	18	19–22	23	24–25	26–27	28+
Post-ovulatory day			1–2	3	4	5–8	9	10–11	12–13	14+
Cycle phases		Proliferative	Interval	Early secretory		Mid-secretory			Late secretory	Menstrual
Key feature		Mitoses	Mitoses and subnuclear vacuoles	Maximum subnuclear vacuoles	Subnuclear vacuoles present	Stromal edema	Focal decidua around spiral arteries	Patchy decidua	Extensive decidua	Stromal crumbling
Microscopic features of functional zone	Stroma	Loose stroma. Mitoses	Same as proliferative	Loose stroma. Scanty mitoses	Loose stroma	Stromal edema	Focal decidua around spiral arteries. Edema prominent	Decidua throughout stroma. Some edema	Extensive decidua. Prominent granulated lymphocytes	Stromal crumbling. Hemorrhage
	Glands	Straight to tightly coiled tubules. Mitoses	Some subnuclear vacuoles, otherwise as proliferative	Extensive subnuclear vacuoles	Dilated glands. Some subnuclear vacuoles	Dilated glands with irregular outline. Luminal secretion		'Saw tooth' glands	Prominent 'saw tooth' glands	Disrupted glands. Secretory exhaustion. Regenerating epithelium
Appearances		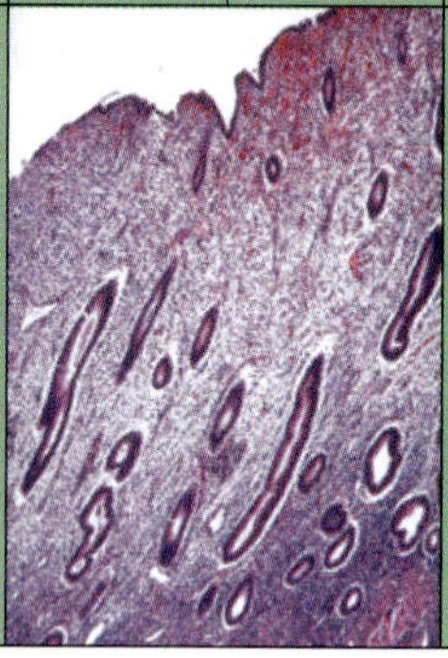		A		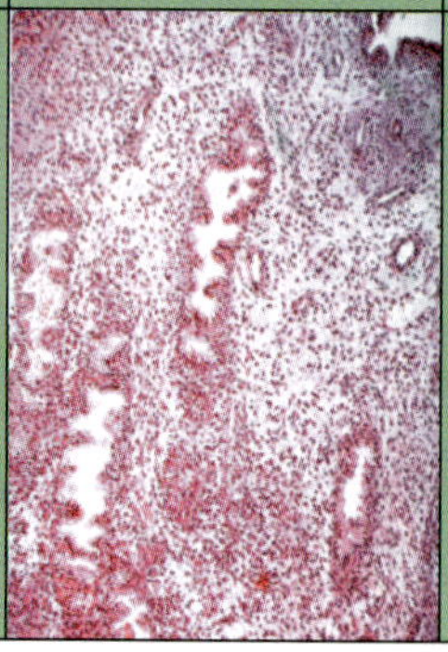	B		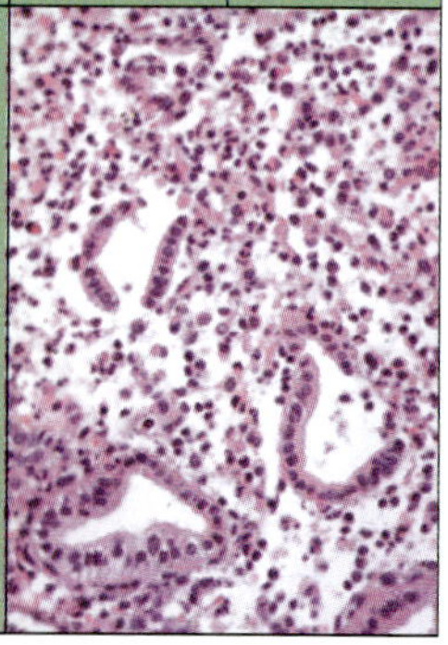	C

FIGURE 18-28

Main histological features of the endometrial phases of the normal menstrual cycle. A. Proliferative phase. Straight tubular glands are embedded in a cellular monomorphic stroma. B. Secretory phase, day 24. Dilated tortuous glands with serrated borders are situated in a predecidual stroma. C. Menstrual endometrium. Fragmented glands, dissolution of the stroma, and numerous neutrophils are evident.

proliferation progresses, the glands coil more and increase slightly in caliber. The columnar cells lining the tubules increase from one layer in thickness to a pseudostratified epithelium that is mitotically active. The glands produce a watery alkaline secretion that facilitates passage of the sperm through the endometrial cavity into the fallopian tubes. The stroma is also mitotically active. The spiral arteries are narrow and usually inconspicuous.

SECRETORY PHASE: After ovulation, which occurs about 14 days after the last menstrual period, the graafian follicle that has discharged its ovum becomes a corpus luteum. The granulosa cells of the corpus luteum luteinize and begin to secrete progesterone, the hormone that transforms the endometrium from a proliferative into a secretory state.

- **Days 17 to 19 (postovulatory days 3–5):** The endometrial glands enlarge, dilate, and become more coiled. The lining cells develop abundant and prominent, glycogen-rich, subnuclear vacuoles (day 17). Over the next several days, the glandular cells produce copious secretions that can support a zygote while it develops early chorionic villi capable of invading the endometrium.
- **Days 20 to 22 (postovulatory days 6–8):** The endometrium displays prominent glandular secretions and stromal edema. The glands dilate and are more tortuous.
- **Day 23 (postovulatory day 9):** The stromal cells enlarge and exhibit large, round, vesicular nuclei and abundant eosinophilic cytoplasm. These cells, which normally appear first about the spiral arterioles, are the precursors of the decidual cells of pregnancy and are referred to as *"predecidual"* or *"pseudodecidual."*
- **Day 27 (postovulatory day 13):** The full thickness of the stroma is now predecidualized and prepared for menstruation. The tubular glands continue to dilate and develop serrated (saw-toothed) borders.

MENSTRUAL PHASE: In the absence of pregnancy, a series of regressive events occurs. Without a blastocyst to elaborate human chorionic gonadotropin (hCG), the granulosa and thecal cells of the corpus luteum degenerate. As the corpus luteum degenerates, progesterone levels fall, the endometrium becomes desiccated, the spiral arteries collapse, and the stroma disintegrates. Menses commence on day 28, last 3 to 7 days, and result in a flow of about 35 mL of blood. The denuded surface is reepithelialized by extension of the residual glandular epithelium.

ATROPHIC ENDOMETRIUM: After the menopause, the number of glands and the quantity of stroma progressively decrease. The remaining glands often are oriented parallel to the surface, and the stroma contains abundant collagen. The glands of the atrophic endometrium are often conspicuously dilated, an appearance termed *senile cystic atrophy of the endometrium.*

ENDOMETRIUM OF PREGNANCY

The maintenance of the corpus luteum of pregnancy depends on continuous stimulation by hCG secreted by the placental trophoblast of the developing embryo. The tro-

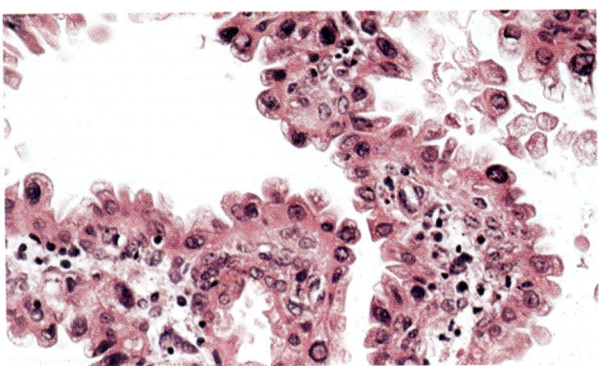

FIGURE 18-29

Arias-Stella reaction of pregnancy associated with human chorionic gonadotropin (hCG) stimulation. A section of endometrium shows enlarged, bulbous nuclei that protrude into the gland lumen.

phoblast begins to develop about day 23. Under the influence of hCG, the corpus luteum then increases its output of progesterone, thereby stimulating secretion of fluid by the endometrial glands. The hypersecretory endometrium of pregnancy shows widely dilated glands lined by cells with abundant glycogen. These features can persist for up to 8 weeks after delivery.

The hypersecretory response may become exaggerated with intrauterine pregnancy, ectopic pregnancy, or trophoblastic disease. In this circumstance, the nuclei of the glandular cells become enlarged, bulbous, and polyploid, because the DNA has replicated, but the cells have not divided. The nuclei protrude beyond the apparent cytoplasmic limits of the cell into the gland lumen, an appearance referred to as the *Arias-Stella reaction* (Fig. 18-29). The cells are not aneuploid, and this change should not be confused with adenocarcinoma or its preneoplastic precursors.

CONGENITAL ANOMALIES

Congenital anomalies of the uterus are rare. **Congenital absence of the uterus (agenesis)** reflects failure of the müllerian ducts to develop. Since elongation of the müllerian ducts during embryonic life depends on the presence of the wolffian ducts as guide wires, uterine agenesis is almost always accompanied by other anomalies of the urogenital tract as well as an absent vagina and fallopian tubes.

Uterus didelphys refers to a double uterus, which reflects the failure of the two müllerian ducts to fuse during early embryonic life. A double vagina commonly accompanies this anomaly.

Uterus duplex bicornis is a uterus with a common fused wall between two distinct endometrial cavities. In this condition, the common wall between the apposed müllerian ducts fails to degenerate and form a single uterine cavity.

Uterus septus is a single uterus with a partial remaining septum, owing to a failure of the wall of the fused müllerian ducts to resorb completely. Patients with a uterine septum are at increased risk for habitual abortion.

Bicornuate uterus refers to a uterus with two cornua (horns) and a common cervix. Didelphic and bicornuate uterine fusion defects lead to a small increase in the incidence of premature birth.

ENDOMETRITIS

Endometritis, or an inflamed endometrium, is a histological diagnosis based on the finding of an abnormal inflammatory cell infiltrate in the endometrium. It must be distinguished from the normal presence of polymorphonuclear leukocytes during menstruation and a mild lymphocytic infiltrate at other times. The findings in most cases of endometritis are nonspecific, and rarely point to a specific cause.

ACUTE ENDOMETRITIS: This condition is defined as the abnormal presence of polymorphonuclear leukocytes in the endometrium. Most cases result from an ascending infection from the cervix, such as occurs after the usually impervious cervical barrier is compromised by abortion, delivery, or medical instrumentation. Curettage is diagnostic and often curative, because it removes the necrotic tissue that has served as the nidus of the ongoing infection. Nowadays, the condition is of little significance, contrasted with the dangers that it presented before the antibiotic era.

CHRONIC ENDOMETRITIS: Plasma cells in the endometrium typify chronic endometritis (Fig. 18-30). Although lymphocytes and lymphoid follicles are occasionally found scattered in the normal endometrium, their presence alone is not considered diagnostic of chronic endometritis. The disorder is associated with intrauterine devices (IUDs), PID, and retained products of conception after an abortion or delivery. In the absence of culture, the pathological findings alone are insufficient to distinguish between infective and noninfective causes. Patients usually complain of bleeding, pelvic pain, or both. The condition is generally self-limited.

PYOMETRA: Defined as pus in the endometrial cavity, pyometra is associated with any lesion that causes cervical stenosis, such as a tumor or scarring from surgical treatment (conization) of the cervix. Long-standing pyometra may be associated with the rare development of endometrial squamous cell cancer.

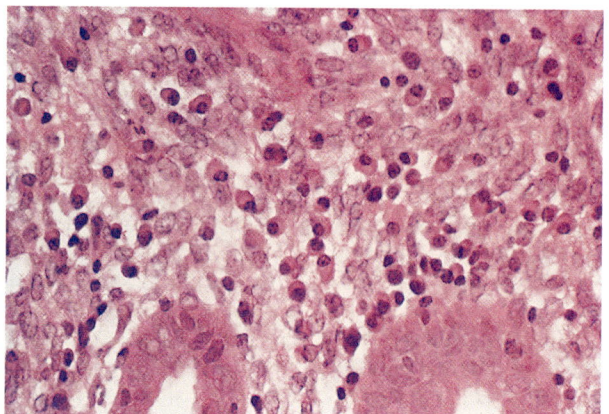

FIGURE 18-30
Chronic endometritis. The inflammatory infiltrate is composed largely of lymphocytes and plasma cells.

TRAUMATIC LESIONS

INTRAUTERINE DEVICE: IUDs predispose bearers to increased menstrual flow, (2) uterine perforation, and (3) spontaneous abortion when conception occurs with the IUD in place. Much of the adverse publicity about IUDs relates to early devices, and only 1% of women who desire contraception now use an IUD.

INTRAUTERINE ADHESIONS (ASHERMAN SYNDROME): Intrauterine fibrous adhesions sometimes develop after the uterus has been curetted, particularly for postpartum complications or therapeutic abortion. These bands traverse, but do not necessarily obliterate, the endometrial cavity. Additional complications include amenorrhea or, in the event of a subsequent pregnancy, increased abortion rates, preterm labor, and placenta accreta.

ADENOMYOSIS

Adenomyosis refers to the presence of endometrial glands and stroma within the myometrium (Fig. 18-31). While commonly but erroneously defined as glands more than 3 mm beneath the endometrial–myometrial junction, more than two thirds of women symptomatic with pain, dysmenorrhea, or menorrhagia show glands located as little as 1 mm deep to the basalis, indicating that the definition is in error. The most clinically significant correlation occurs if the glands are located 2 mm or more into the myometrium. One fifth of all uteri removed at surgery show some adenomyosis.

Pathology: On gross examination, the myometrium discloses small, soft, red areas, some of which are cystic. Microscopic examination of these lesions reveals glands lined by mildly proliferative to inactive endometrium and surrounded by endometrial stroma with varying degrees of fibrosis. Secretory changes are rare, except during pregnancy and in patients treated with progestins. Sometimes the uterus is enlarged by smooth muscle that has hypertrophied about the adenomyotic foci. Over time, the uterus may also become enlarged from cyclic bleeding into these foci. Varying degrees of glandular hyperplasia may be seen, and occasionally hyperplastic surface endometrium extends into the foci of adenomyosis.

Clinical Features: Although many patients with adenomyosis are asymptomatic, it is not uncommon for patients to exhibit varying degrees of pelvic pain, dysfunctional uterine bleeding, dysmenorrhea, and dyspareunia. These symptoms appear in parous women of reproductive age and regress after the menopause.

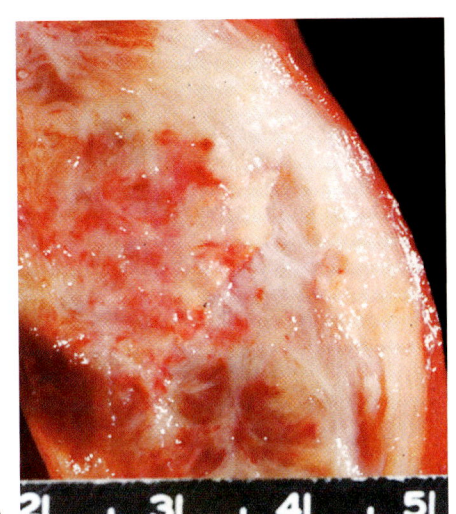
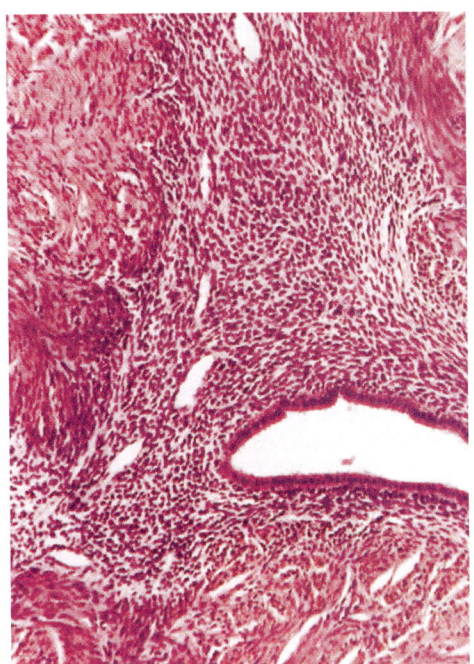

FIGURE 18-31
Adenomyosis. A. The cut surface of the uterus reveals small, red areas corresponding to endometrial glands in the myometrium. B. A microscopic view shows an endometrial gland and stroma in the myometrium.

HORMONAL EFFECTS

Contraceptive Steroids Prevent Pregnancy and Many Gynecological Cancers

Oral contraceptive agents induce a wide variety of endometrial changes that reflect the types, potencies, and dosages of estrogens and progestins used in these formulations. Combined preparations generally contain potent progestins and weak estrogens. The decidual change, therefore, appears early and overshadows the weak glandular growth. Over time (i.e., after a number of cycles), the endometrial glands atrophy. More recently developed contraceptive combinations contain lower doses of hormones and correspondingly elicit less change. **Women who use contraceptive steroids have significantly reduced rates of both endometrial and ovarian cancer, effects that reflect the growth-inhibiting properties of progesterone, and in the ovary, a reduction in the number of ovulations.**

Dysfunctional Uterine Bleeding Occurs during or between Menstrual Periods

In dysfunctional bleeding, the cause lies outside the uterus. It is one of the most common gynecological disorders of women of reproductive age but is still poorly understood. Most cases are related to an endocrine disturbance that involves an aspect of the hypothalamic–pituitary–ovarian axis (Table 18-6). Ovarian dysfunction is usual, especially in the presence of anovulation.

Some causes of menstrual irregularity are intrinsic to the uterus and are not considered dysfunctional. These include (1) growths (e.g., carcinoma, hyperplasia, and polyps), (2) inflammation (e.g., endometritis), (3) pregnancy (e.g., complications of intrauterine or ectopic pregnancy), and (4) the effects of IUDs (see Table 18-6).

Anovulatory Bleeding Is the Most Common Dysfunctional Bleeding

Anovulatory bleeding is a complex syndrome of many causes that manifests as the absence of ovulation during the reproductive years. It is most often noted at either end of reproductive life (i.e., menarche and menopause).

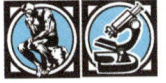 Pathogenesis and Pathology: In an anovulatory cycle, the failure of ovulation leads to excessive and prolonged estrogen stimulation, without the postovulatory rise in progesterone levels. The end result is an endometrium that remains in a proliferative state but exhibits a disordered and fragmented appearance. In the absence of adequate progesterone, the spiral arteries of the endometrium do not develop normally. When the estrogen level falls, "breakthrough bleeding" occurs. Since estrogen maintains the stromal fluid turgescence that supports the endometrial blood vessels, a fall in the estrogen level results in stromal fluid loss and hence a loss of vascular support. The subsequent compression of the poorly developed spiral arteries leads in turn to stasis, thrombosis, infarction, and hemorrhage. Bleeding can also occur if the

TABLE 18-6 Causes of Abnormal Uterine Bleeding (Including Uterine and Extrauterine Causes)

Newborn	Maternal estrogen
Childhood	Iatrogenic (trauma, foreign body, infection of vagina)
	Vaginal neoplasms (sarcoma botryoides)
	Ovarian tumors (functional)
Adolescence	Hypothalamic immaturity
	Psychogenic and nutritional problems
	Inadequate luteal function
Reproductive age	Anovulatory
	Central: psychogenic, stress
	Systemic: nutritional and endocrine disease
	Gonadal: functional tumors
	End-organ: endometrial hyperplasia
	Pregnancy: ectopic, retained placenta, abortion, mole
	Ovulatory
	Organic: neoplasia, infections (PID), leiomyomas
	Polymenorrhea: short follicular or luteal phases
	Iatrogenic: anticoagulants, IUD
	Irregular shedding
Menopause	Organic: carcinoma, hyperplasias, polyps
Postmenopause	Organic: carcinoma, hyperplasias, polyps
	Endometrial atrophy

IUD, intrauterine device; PID, pelvic inflammatory disease.

endometrium continues to proliferate in the presence of an unchanged estrogen level. In this case, the proliferative endometrium is inadequately nourished, and withdrawal bleeding ensues.

On microscopic examination, the glands in anovulatory bleeding are frequently disordered and appear crowded because of severe stromal necrosis and collapse of the proliferative endometrium. Fragments of menstrual-type endometrium are also present.

Luteal Phase Defect Relates to Inadequate Progesterone

Luteal phase defect results in an abnormally short menstrual cycle in which menses occur 6 to 9 days after the surge of luteinizing hormone associated with ovulation. A luteal phase defect occurs when the corpus luteum develops improperly or regresses prematurely. The disorder is primarily of interest in infertility investigations and occasionally in the analysis of abnormal uterine bleeding. In fact, luteal phase defects are responsible for 3% of cases of infertility. The diagnosis of a luteal phase defect is confirmed by endometrial biopsy in which the microscopic findings are more than 2 days out of synchrony with the chronological day of the menstrual cycle.

TUMORS

Endometrial Polyp Is a Benign Overgrowth in the Endometrial Cavity

Endometrial polyps occur most commonly in the perimenopausal period and are virtually unknown before menarche. They are thought to arise from endometrial foci that are hypersensitive to estrogenic stimulation or unresponsive to progesterone. In either case, such foci do not slough during menstruation and continue to grow.

Pathology: Most endometrial polyps arise in the fundus (Fig. 18-32), although they may originate in any location within the endometrial cavity. They vary from several millimeters in length to a growth filling the entire endometrial cavity. Most are solitary, but 20% are multiple.

Microscopically, the core of a polyp is composed of (1) endometrial glands, which often are cystically dilated and hyperplastic; (2) a fibrous endometrial stroma; and (3) thick-walled, coiled, dilated blood vessels, derived from a straight

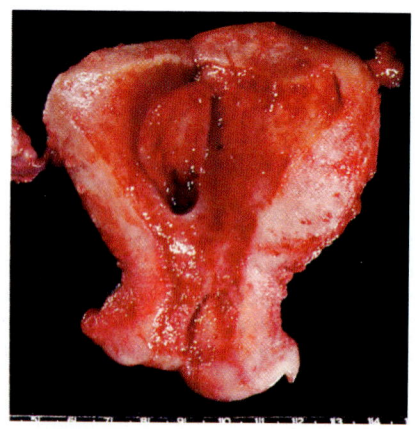
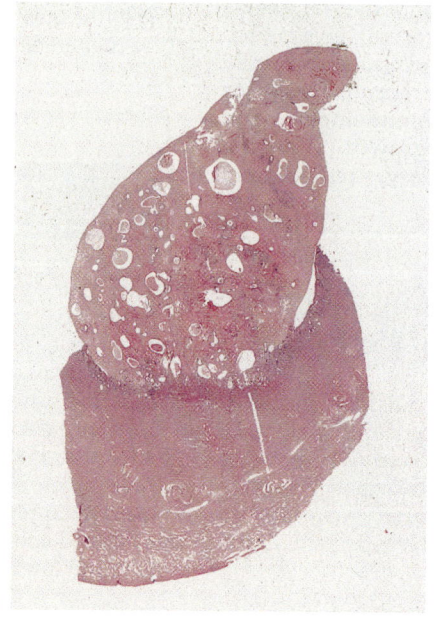

FIGURE 18-32
Endometrial polyp. A. A single polyp extends into the endometrial cavity. The necrotic tip is responsible for clinical bleeding. B. On microscopic section, a polyp (from a different patient) exhibits slightly dilated endometrial glands embedded in a markedly fibrous stroma.

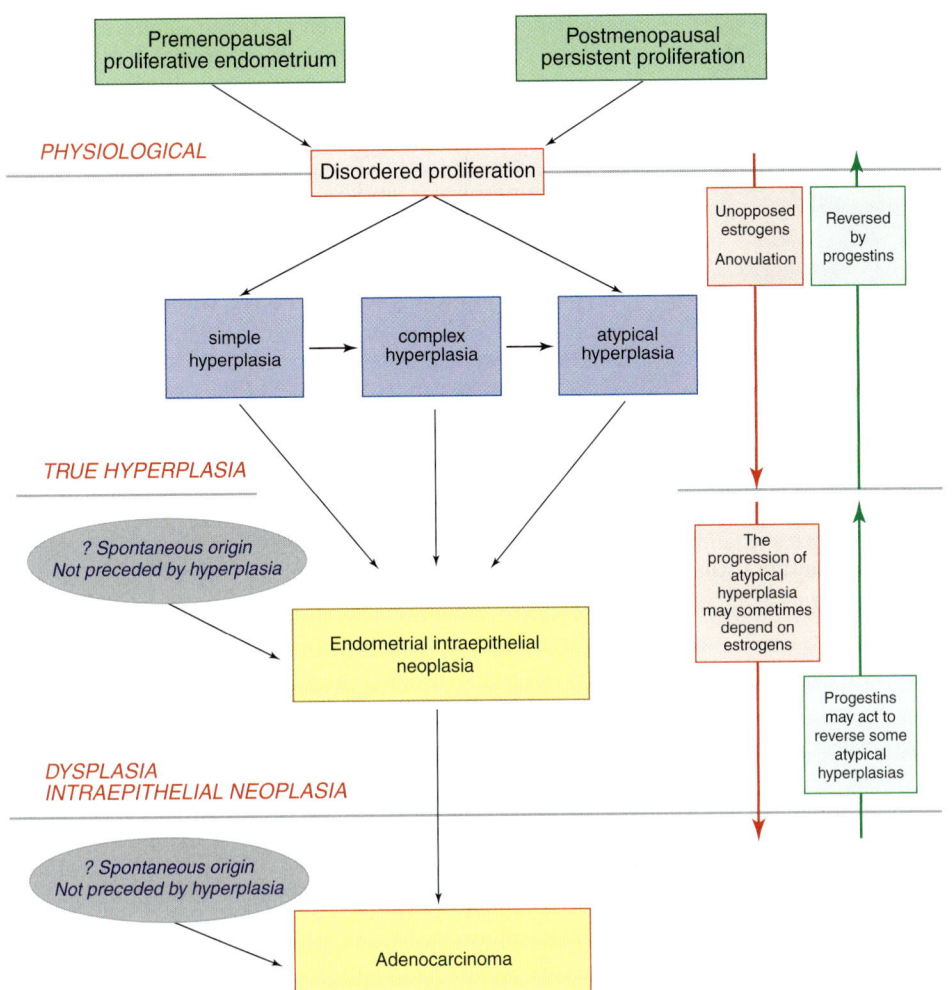

FIGURE 18-33
Relations among proliferation, hyperplasia, atypical hyperplasia, and carcinoma of the endometrium.

artery that normally would have supplied the basal zone of the endometrium. A mantle of endometrial epithelium covers the polyp. The glandular epithelium uncommonly is at the same stage of the cycle as that of the adjacent, normal endometrium.

 Clinical Features: Endometrial polyps typically manifest with intermenstrual bleeding, owing to surface ulceration or hemorrhagic infarction. Since bleeding in an older woman is not uncommonly due to cancer, the presence of this sign must be thoroughly evaluated. Endometrial polyps are not ordinarily preneoplastic, but up to 0.5% harbor adenocarcinoma.

Endometrial Hyperplasia and Adenocarcinoma Are Points on a Continuum

Endometrial hyperplasia and adenocarcinoma represent a broad spectrum of proliferative disease that constitutes a morphological and biological continuum, similar to multistep carcinogenesis in other tissues (Fig. 18-33). Thus, the lesions progress from the mildest hyperplasia of endometrial glands to invasive cancer. Proliferative lesions often result from endogenous estrogens produced by hormonally functioning tumors, such as granulosa cell tumor of the ovary, or in polycystic ovary syndrome. Hyperestrinism also results from exogenous estrogens administered to control menopausal symptoms.

Endometrial Hyperplasia

Endometrial hyperplasia refers to a spectrum that ranges from simple glandular crowding to conspicuous proliferation of atypical glands, which are difficult to distinguish from early carcinoma. It is generally agreed that the risk of developing endometrial cancer increases with progressively higher degrees of endometrial hyperplasia. The progression from hyperplasia free of atypia to invasive cancer requires some 10 years, but the corresponding time for hyperplasia with atypia is only 4 years. The cancers that develop in women with hyperplasia are usually endometrioid adenocarcinoma. Commonly, there is a relationship to estrogen exposure.

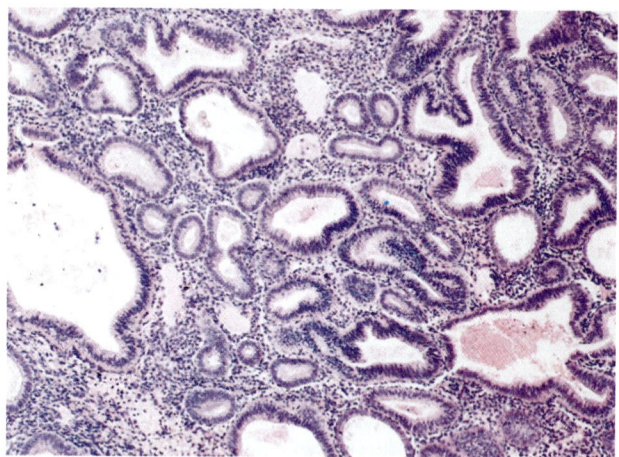

FIGURE 18-34
Complex endometrial hyperplasia. The endometrial glands, which are in the proliferative phase, are closely packed and display moderate architectural disarray (budding and branching). No cytological atypia is present.

 Pathology: There are now two classifications of endometrial hyperplasia. The older classification centered on the presence of cytological atypia and abnormal glandular architecture. **Cytological atypia is the most important prognostic feature.**

- **Simple hyperplasia:** This proliferative lesion shows minimal glandular complexity and crowding and no cytological atypia. The epithelial lining is usually one cell layer thick, and the stroma between the glands is abundant. One percent of cases of simple endometrial hyperplasia progress to adenocarcinoma.
- **Complex hyperplasia:** This variant exhibits marked glandular complexity and crowding but no cytological atypia (Figure 18-34). The glands are increased in number and may vary in size. The stroma between the glands is scanty. Three percent develop adenocarcinoma.
- **Atypical hyperplasia:** This lesion displays cytological atypia and marked glandular crowding, frequently as back-to-back glands. The glands may have a complex architecture, with an intraluminal papillary arrangement or the appearance of budding glands in the stroma. The epithelial cells are enlarged and hyperchromatic and have prominent nucleoli and an increased nuclear-to-cytoplasmic ratio. One fourth of these cases progress to adenocarcinoma, which is almost always of the endometrioid type. Commonly these women have had prior estrogen exposure, whether endogenous or exogenous (see below).

Endometrial intraepithelial neoplasia (EIN) is a newer classification that **is based on the concept that the most common precursors to endometrial cancer are monoclonal benign neoplasms that are prone to malignant transformation and show a continuity of acquired genetic markers during transformation into a malignant phase.** The most important architectural feature of EIN is the area occupied by glands, which exceeds that of the stroma. The abnormal focus must exceed 1 mm and should differ cytologically from the background endometrium. In keeping with a proliferative monoclonal origin, EIN lesions originate focally and expand in size over time, being diagnosed as cancer when mazelike glands, solid areas, or a significant cribriform arrangement appear. Unlike the benign and diffuse architectural changes usually associated with unopposed estrogen, EIN originates focally, only later progressing to a diffuse state. When correlated with the older system (described above), 5% of simple hyperplasias, 44% of complex hyperplasias, and 79% of atypical hyperplasias can be rediagnosed as EIN. Morphometric diagnosis of EIN predicts a patient's future likelihood of developing endometrial cancer with 100% sensitivity and 78% specificity.

The *PTEN* tumor suppressor gene, which is hormonally regulated in normal endometrium, is an informative biomarker for endometrial carcinogenesis. Loss of gene function occurs clonally in two thirds of EIN lesions, and a comparable fraction of subsequent endometrial carcinomas. Additional evidence that the *PTEN* gene has a functional role comes from heterozygous *PTEN* knockout mice, which uniformly develop an "endometrial hyperplasia" that evolves to carcinoma in one fifth of the animals.

 Clinical Features: Endometrial hyperplasia may result from anovulatory cycles, polycystic ovary syndrome, an estrogen-producing tumor, or obesity. In such cases, therapy aimed at the primary disease may alleviate the estrogenic stimulation. Treatment with large doses of progestins can produce objective remissions, although more than 60% of cases recur when the initial hyperplasia is severe. Hysterectomy is usually considered the therapy of choice in a woman who has completed child bearing and in whom curettage reveals significant hyperplasia. About one sixth of uteri harbor small foci of adenocarcinoma when endometrial curettage discloses only advanced hyperplasia.

Endometrial Adenocarcinoma

 Epidemiology: Endometrial carcinoma is the fourth most frequent cancer in American women and the single most common gynecological cancer. An estimated 6000 deaths occurred in the United States in 2002 (7% of all cancers in women). The incidence of this cancer was stable between 1950 and 1970 but then increased by 40% by 1975. The rise was attributed to the common practice of prescribing estrogens for menopause. By 1985, the rates had returned nearly to 1950 levels, a trend that reflected the administration of lower doses of estrogen, the incorporation of progestins (estrogen antagonists) into estrogen replacement regimens, and increased surveillance of women treated with estrogens.

The occurrence of endometrial cancer varies with age. Whereas the incidence is 12 cases per 100,000 women at 40 years of age, it is sevenfold higher at age 60. Three quarters of women with endometrial cancer are postmenopausal, and the median age at diagnosis is 63 years.

 Pathogenesis: The major form of endometrial cancer, endometrioid adenocarcinoma, is linked to prolonged estrogenic stimulation of the en-

dometrium. In addition to treatment with exogenous estrogens, the most common risk factors are obesity, diabetes, nulliparity, early menarche, and late menopause. Each risk factor points to relative hyperestrinism. Women with ovarian agenesis do not develop endometrial cancer unless treated with exogenous estrogens. A high frequency of endometrial cancer is also found in women with estrogen-secreting granulosa cell tumors. In the case of obesity, the incidence correlates with body weight, the risk being increased 10-fold for women who are more than 23 kg (50 lb) overweight. This effect of obesity is related to the enhanced aromatization of androstenedione to estrone in adipocytes. Cigarette smoking, which interferes with the hepatic conversion of estrone to its active metabolite estriol (see Chapter 8), is associated with a reduced risk of endometrial cancer. Treatment of breast cancer with tamoxifen, a synthetic antiestrogen that also has agonist activity, may slightly increase the risk of endometrial cancer.

Nonendometrioid cancers, especially serous and clear cell adenocarcinoma, are unrelated to estrogen exposure and usually occur in women in their 60s and 70s. The adjacent endometrium is usually atrophic, a sign of estrogen deficiency. Occasionally, the tumor may show a precursor form, termed *endometrial intraepithelial carcinoma* (see below).

Endometrial cancer also occurs in association with a higher incidence of both breast and ovarian cancer in closely related women, suggesting a genetic predisposition. Moreover, it is the most common extracolonic cancer in women with the hereditary nonpolyposis syndrome *(Lynch syndrome II)*, which is also associated with breast and ovarian cancers.

Pathology: Endometrial cancer grows in a diffuse or polypoid pattern (Fig. 18-35). Regardless of its site of origin, the tumor often tends to involve multiple areas, since the anterior and posterior walls of the endometrium are in contact. Large tumors are usually hemorrhagic and necrotic.

ENDOMETRIOID ADENOCARCINOMA OF THE ENDOMETRIUM: This type of endometrial cancer is composed entirely of glandular cells and is the most common histological variant (60%). The FIGO system divides this tumor into three grades on the basis of the ratio of glandular to solid elements, the latter being a sign of decreasing differentiation (Table 18-7; (Fig. 18-36).

- **Grade 1:** Highly differentiated; composed almost exclusively of neoplastic glands, with only minimal (<5%) solid areas
- **Grade 2:** Moderately differentiated; formed partly of glandular elements and partly (<50%) of solid tumor
- **Grade 3:** Poorly differentiated; shows large (>50%) areas of solid tumor

The nuclei of endometrial adenocarcinoma are vesicular and may be markedly pleomorphic and show prominent nucleoli. Mitotic figures are abundant and frequently abnormal. Tumor cells that grow in solid sheets generally are poorly differentiated.

ENDOMETRIOID ADENOCARCINOMA WITH SQUAMOUS DIFFERENTIATION: One third of all endometrial carcinomas contain squamous cells in addition to the glandular element. If the squamous element is well differentiated and exhibits no more than minimal atypia, the tumor is called *well-differentiated adenocarcinoma with squamous differentiation* (previously termed *adenoacanthoma*) (Fig. 18-37). If the squamous element appears malignant, the tumor is labeled *poorly differentiated adenocarcinoma with squamous differentiation* (also known as *adenosquamous carcinoma*). These two variants represent 22% and 7% of all endometrial cancers, respectively. They frequently coexist with synchronous ovarian cancer of the same histology and are thought to reflect synchronous primary tumors (i.e., field effects).

TABLE 18-7 Surgical Staging and Histopathological Grading of Endometrial Cancer

Stage	Description
O	Atypical hyperplasia or carcinoma in situ
I	Confined to corpus
Ia	Confined to endometrium
Ib	Invades $<\frac{1}{2}$ myometrium
Ic	Invades $>\frac{1}{2}$ myometrium
II	Involves cervix
IIa	Endocervical glandular involvement only (i.e., in situ in glands)
IIb	Cervical stromal invasion
III	Extends beyond uterus but not outside true pelvis
IIIa	Involves serosa or adnexa, or has positive peritoneal cytology
IV	Extends beyond true pelvis or involves the mucosa of bladder or rectum
IVa	Spread to adjacent organs
IVb	Spread to distant organs

Grading (FIGO) of glandular tissue: G1, <5% solid (highly differentiated); G2, 5%–50% solid (differentiated with partly solid areas); G3, >50% solid (predominantly solid or entirely undifferentiated).

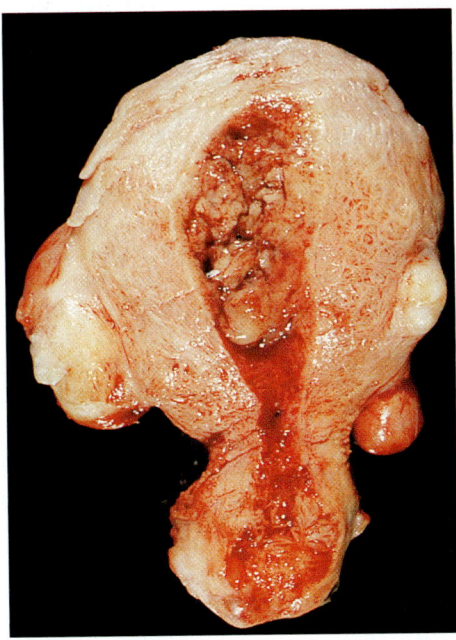

FIGURE 18-35
Adenocarcinoma of the endometrium. The uterus has been opened to reveal a partially necrotic, polypoid endometrial cancer.

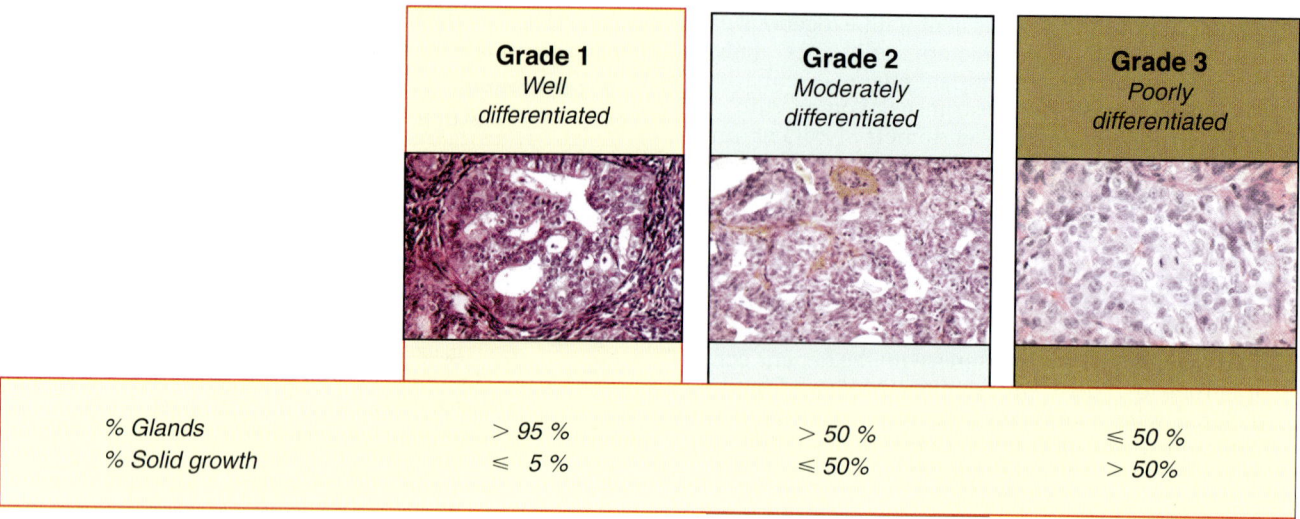

FIGURE 18-36
Grading of endometrial adenocarcinoma. The grade depends primarily on the architectural pattern, but significant nuclear atypia changes a grade 1 tumor to grade 2, and a grade 2 tumor to grade 3.

OTHER TYPES OF ENDOMETRIAL CARCINOMA: Other types of endometrial carcinoma are less common and include the following:

- **Serous adenocarcinoma** histologically resembles serous adenocarcinoma of the ovary (Fig. 18-38A). It also behaves more like an ovarian carcinoma than an endometrial tumor, often showing transcelomic spread. An in situ form has been termed "endometrial intraepithelial carcinoma" (EIC), which is not to be confused with EIN, described above.
- **Clear cell adenocarcinoma** is a tumor of elderly women. It is composed of large cells with copious cytoplasmic glycogen *(clear cells)* or of cells with bulbous nuclei that line glandular lumina *(hobnail cells)* (Fig. 18-38B). Serous and clear cell carcinomas and poorly differentiated adenocarcinoma with squamous differentiation are associated with adverse outcomes.
- **Secretory carcinoma** describes cells with subnuclear vacuolization, usually in premenopausal women. The tumor is an extremely well differentiated but otherwise typical endometrial adenocarcinoma. The cancer cells respond to progesterone by forming large subnuclear vacuoles of glycogen. Secretory carcinoma has the most favorable outcome of any adenocarcinoma, presumably because the cells are well differentiated.

Although most endometrial carcinomas arise in the uterine corpus, a small proportion originate in the lower uterine segment (isthmus). These tumors often occur in women under the age of 50 years and are often high grade and deeply invasive.

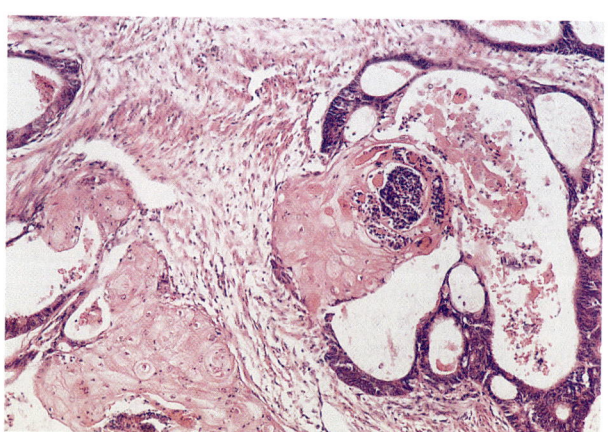

FIGURE 18-37
Squamous differentiation in endometroid adenocarcinoma of the endometrium. The well-differentiated squamous cells show minimal atypia, a pattern that has also been called adenoacanthoma.

 Clinical Features: Endometrial carcinoma typically occurs in perimenopausal or postmenopausal women. The chief complaint is usually abnormal uterine bleeding, especially when the tumor is in its early

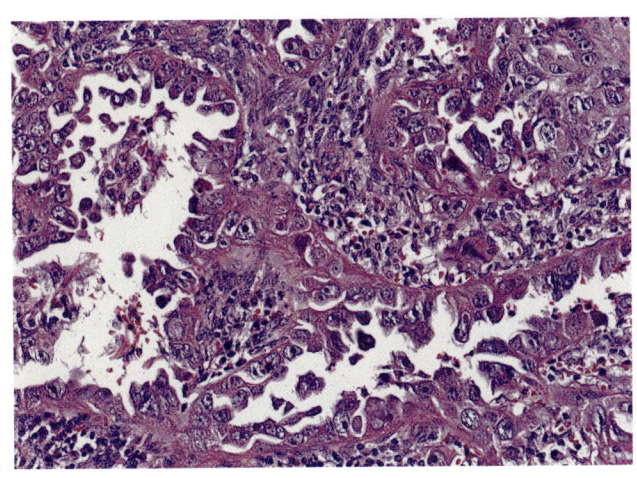 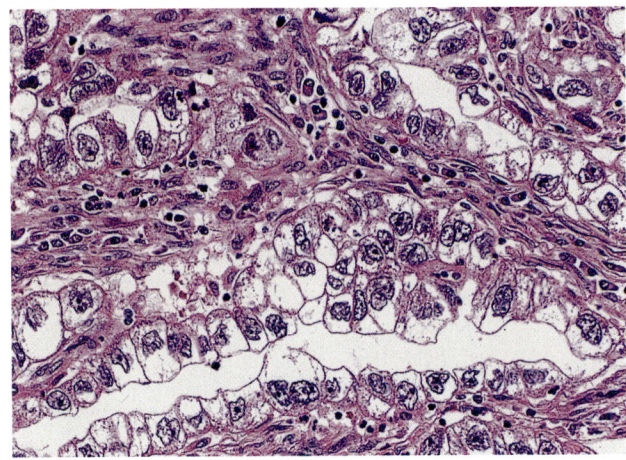

FIGURE 18-38
Variants of endometrial adenocarcinoma. A. Serous adenocarcinoma. Large cells with bulbous, pleomorphic nuclei grow in a papillary configuration. B. Clear cell adenocarcinoma. The clear appearance of the cytoplasm is due to the dissolution of glycogen when the specimen was processed for microscopic examination. Hobnail cells with bulbous nuclei line glandular lumina.

stages of growth (i.e., confined to the endometrium). Unfortunately, cervicovaginal cytological screening is unsuitable for the early detection of endometrial carcinoma. Fractional curettage is necessary to assess spread to the cervix, whereas peritoneal washing detects tubal reflux and abdominal contamination. Transvaginal ultrasonography is a valuable diagnostic modality; endometrium more than 5 mm thick is considered highly suspicious. Unlike cervical cancer, endometrial cancer may spread directly to paraaortic lymph nodes, thereby skipping the pelvic nodes. Patients with advanced cancers may also develop pulmonary metastases (40% of cases with metastases).

Women with well-differentiated cancers confined to the endometrium are usually treated by simple hysterectomy. Postoperative radiation is administered if (1) the tumor is poorly differentiated, (2) the myometrium is more than superficially invaded, (3) the cervix is involved, or (4) the lymph nodes contain metastases.

Survival in endometrial carcinoma is related to multiple factors, including (1) the stage and grade, (2) age, and (3) other measurable risk factors, such as progesterone receptor activity, depth of myometrial invasion, extent of lymphovascular invasion, and results of peritoneal washings. High levels of estrogen and progesterone receptors in the tumor and low levels of proliferative activity correlate with a better prognosis. The actuarial survival rate of all patients with endometrial cancer following treatment is 80% after the second year, decreasing to 65% after 10 years. Tumors that penetrate into the myometrium or invade lymphatics are more likely candidates for extrauterine dissemination. Endometrial cancers involving the cervix have a poorer prognosis, and those that extend outside the uterus have the worst outlook (Table 18-8).

Endometrial Stromal Tumors Account for Fewer Than 2% of All Uterine Cancers

Some endometrial stromal tumors are pure sarcomas; others exhibit intimate admixtures of sarcomatous (stromal) and carcinomatous (epithelial) elements. In the latter case, the prognosis depends on the relative maturity or malignancy of each component. The nomenclature of these tumor types, the spectrum of their histological components, and the correlation of each tumor type with its potential for malignant behavior are presented in Table 18-9.

Endometrial Stromal Sarcoma

Pure stromal tumors are divided into two major categories, based on whether the tumor margin is expansile or infiltrating. Expansile lesions that do not invade are *benign stromal nodules,* which have little clinical significance. Tumors with infiltrating margins are termed *stromal sarcomas.*

TABLE 18-8 Stage, Grade, and Survival for Endometrial Cancer

Stage	5-Year Survival (%)		
	G-1*	G-2	G-3
I	90	69	52
II	80	42	12
III, IV	25	33	17

*G, FIGO grade.

 Pathology: Endometrial stromal sarcoma may be polypoid and fill the endometrial cavity or may diffusely invade the myometrium. Large masses of spindle cells with scant cytoplasm dissect the myometrium and invade vascular channels. The neoplastic cells resemble endometrial stromal cells in the proliferative phase. A characteristic feature of all endometrial stromal tumors is a rich

TABLE 18-9 Nomenclature of Uterine Tumors

Tumor	Epithelium	Stroma	Clinical Behavior
Epithelium and Stroma			
Endometrial hyperplasia	Hyperplastic	—	Benign
Endometrial adenocarcinoma	Malignant	—	Malignant
Endometrial stromal nodule	—	Benign	Benign
Endometrial stromal sarcoma			
Low grade	—	Malignant	Low-grade malignant
High grade	—	Malignant	Malignant
Adenosarcoma	Benign	Malignant	Low-grade malignant
Carcinosarcoma			
Homologous type	Malignant	Malignant	Malignant
Heterologous type[a]	Malignant	Malignant	Malignant
Smooth Muscle			
Leiomyoma	—	Benign	Benign
Cellular leiomyoma	—	Benign	Benign
Intravenous leiomyomatosis	—	Benign	Benign
Leiomyosarcoma	—	Malignant	Malignant

[a] Formerly called rhabdomyosarcoma if composed predominantly of embryonal rhabdomyoblasts, or malignant mixed mesodermal tumor if other heterologous components (e.g., cartilage, bone) were present.

vascular supporting framework, with the neoplastic cells concentrically arranged around blood vessels (Fig. 18-39). Nuclear atypism may be minimal to severe, and mitotic activity may be restrained (low-grade stromal sarcoma) or exuberant (high-grade stromal sarcoma). As the tumor becomes progressively less differentiated, it tends to lose its resemblance to endometrial stroma and appears as an undifferentiated sarcoma. Expression of undifferentiated CD-10 helps confirm the diagnosis.

Clinical Features: Endometrial stromal sarcoma may recur even if confined to the uterus at initial surgery. Recurrences usually involve the pelvis initially and are followed later by pulmonary metastases. In small tumors or low-grade sarcomas (also called *endolymphatic stromal myosis*), many years may elapse before recurrent disease becomes clinically evident. In these cases, prolonged survival and even cure are feasible, despite metastases. By contrast, high-grade sarcomas recur early, generally with widespread metastases, even if there has been little myometrial invasion.

UTERINE ADENOSARCOMA: Uterine (müllerian) adenosarcoma is a distinctive low-grade tumor characterized by a combination of benign (but neoplastic) glandular epithelium and malignant stroma. It should be distinguished from carcinosarcoma, which has both malignant epithelial and stromal elements and is highly aggressive.

Adenosarcoma typically presents as a polypoid mass within the endometrial cavity. The glandular epithelium resembles endometrial glands in the proliferative phase, but occasionally squamous epithelium and mucinous-type epithelium may be encountered. The stroma is cellular, may exhibit mitotic activity, and is often densest about the glandular epithelium (periglandular cuffing). The stromal cells are malignant and resemble endometrial stromal cells in the proliferative phase of the cycle. One fourth of patients with adenosarcoma eventually succumb to local recurrence or metastatic spread.

CARCINOSARCOMA (MALIGNANT MIXED MESODERMAL TUMOR): In this mixed tumor, the epithelial and stromal components are both highly malignant. These neoplasms are derived from multipotential stromal cells. In the past they were subdivided as *heterologous* if they contained mesenchymal components foreign to the uterus, such as striated muscle, bone, osteoid, cartilage, and fat. They were labeled *homologous* if the stromal component lacked such an admixture. This distinction is no longer considered useful, since no component has any prognostic significance or unique clinical correlate. The overall 5-year survival is 25%.

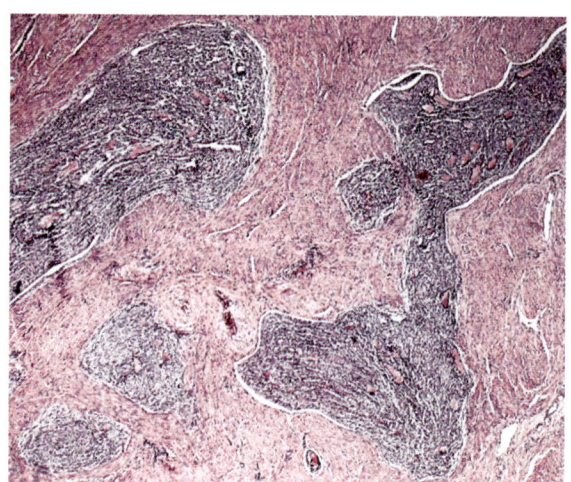

FIGURE 18-39
Endometrial stromal sarcoma. The myometrium is irregularly invaded by the tumor, which displays a rich vascular network.

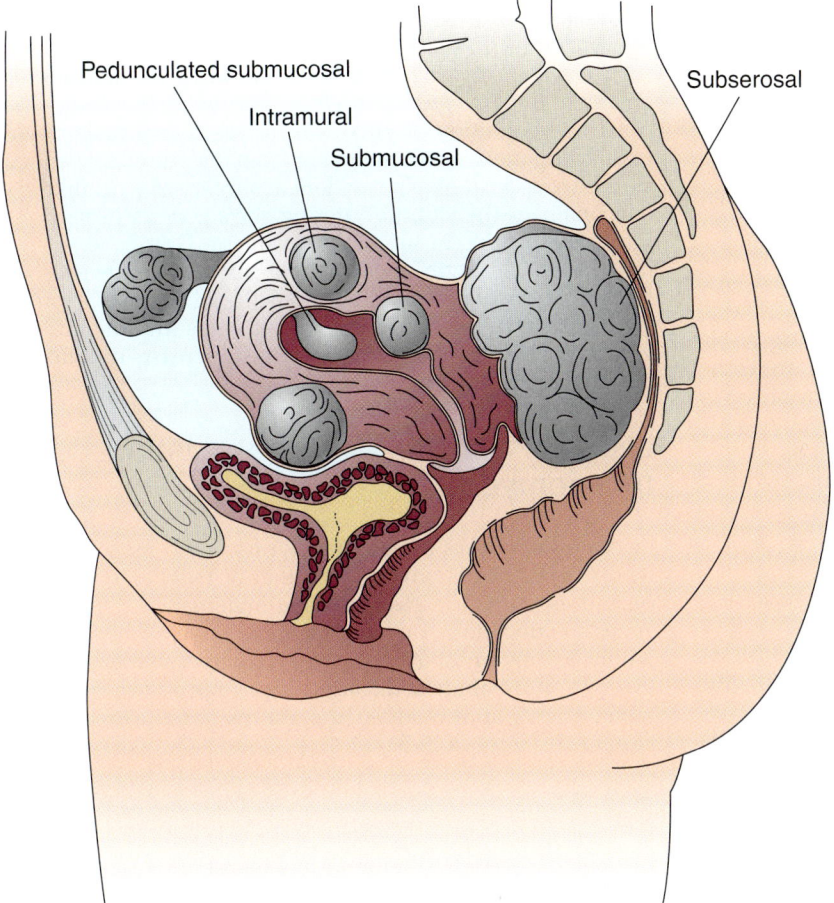

FIGURE 18-40
Leiomyomas of the uterus. The leiomyomas are intramural; submucosal (a pedunculated one appearing in the form of an endometrial polyp) and subserosal (one compressing the bladder and the other the rectum).

Leiomyoma Is the Most Common Tumor of the Female Genital Tract

Leiomyoma, defined as a benign tumor of smooth muscle origin, is colloquially known as a "myoma" or "fibroid." If minute tumors are included, leiomyomas occur in 75% of women older than 30 years of age. They are rare before age 20, and most regress after the menopause. Although often multiple, each leiomyoma is monoclonal (see Chapter 5). Estrogen promotes the growth of leiomyomas, although it does not initiate them.

 Pathology: Grossly, leiomyomas are firm, pale gray, whorled, and without encapsulation (Figs. 18-40 and 18-41). They range in size from 1 mm to more

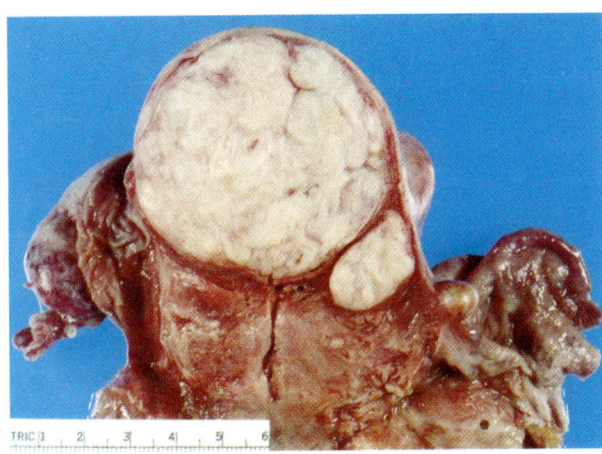
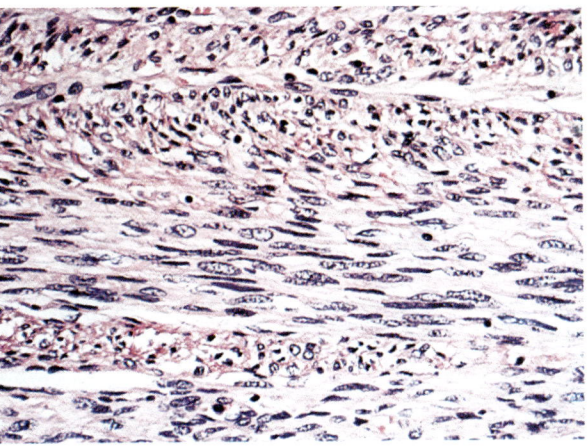

FIGURE 18-41
Leiomyoma of the uterus. A. A bisected uterus displays a prominent, sharply circumscribed, fleshy tumor. B. Microscopically, smooth muscle cells intertwine in bundles, some of which are cut longitudinally (elongated nuclei) and others transversely.

than 30 cm in diameter. The cut surface bulges, and the borders are smooth and distinct from the neighboring myometrium. Most leiomyomas are intramural, but some are submucosal, subserosal, or pedunculated. Many leiomyomas, especially those that are larger, show areas of degenerative hyalinization that are sharply demarcated from the adjacent normal myometrium. By contrast, geographical ("coagulative") necrosis is common in leiomyosarcoma, in which small islands of viable tumor persist around small blood vessels. Leiomyomas that display low mitotic activity (≤4 mitoses per 10 high-power fields [HPFs]) and lack nuclear atypia and geographical necrosis have little or no malignant potential.

Microscopically leiomyomas exhibit interlacing fascicles of uniform spindle cells, in which the nuclei are elongated and have blunt ends (see Fig. 18-41). The cytoplasm is abundant, eosinophilic, and fibrillar. The myocytes of leiomyomas and adjacent myometrium are cytologically identical, but leiomyomas are easily distinguished by their circumscription, nodularity, and denser cellularity.

 Clinical Features: Submucosal leiomyomas may cause bleeding, an effect due to ulceration of the thinned, overlying endometrium. Some submucosal leiomyomas become pedunculated and protrude through the cervical os, thereby eliciting cramping pains. Many intramural leiomyomas are symptomatic because of sheer bulk, and large ones may interfere with bowel or bladder function or cause dystocia in labor. Pedunculated leiomyomas on the uterine serosa may interfere with the function of neighboring viscera. Leiomyomas may also infarct and become painful if they undergo torsion.

Leiomyomas usually grow slowly, but occasionally they enlarge rapidly during pregnancy. Large symptomatic leiomyomas are removed by myomectomy or hysterectomy. Ablation by arterial thrombosis has also been used recently.

Intravenous Leiomyomatosis

Intravenous leiomyomatosis is a rare condition that features the growth of benign smooth muscle within the uterine and pelvic veins. The condition originates from vascular invasion by a preexisting uterine leiomyoma or from the growth of venous smooth muscle. It may be evident at surgery as wormlike extensions near the external uterine surface or as projections into uterine veins in the broad ligament. Despite extensive intravascular growth, these neoplasms do not metastasize. Rare fatalities have resulted from the direct extension of leiomyomatous tissues within pelvic veins into the inferior vena cava and right atrium. Treatment consists of total abdominal hysterectomy.

Leiomyosarcoma Is Rare in Comparison to Leiomyoma

Leiomyosarcoma is a malignancy of smooth muscle origin whose incidence is only 1/1000 that of its benign counterpart. It accounts for 2% of uterine malignancies. Its pathogenesis is uncertain, but at least some appear to arise from within leiomyomas. Women with leiomyosarcomas are on average more than a decade older (age above 50) than women with leiomyomas, and the malignant tumors are larger (10–15 cm vs. 3–5 cm).

 Pathology: Leiomyosarcoma should be suspected if an apparent leiomyoma is soft, shows areas of necrosis on gross examination, has irregular borders (invasion into neighboring myometrium), or does not bulge above the surface when cut (Fig. 18-42). Mitotic activity, cellular atypia, and geographical necrosis are the best diagnostic criteria (Fig. 18-43). There is usually a sharp transi-

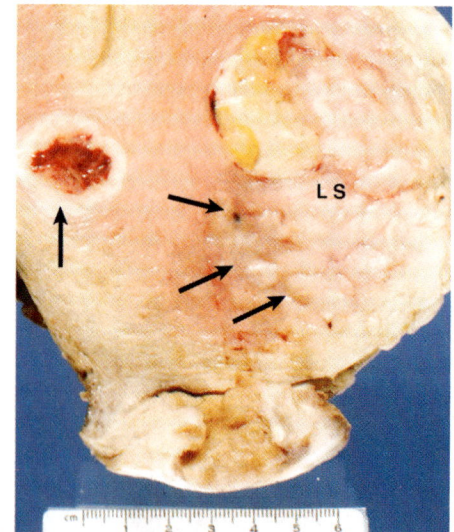
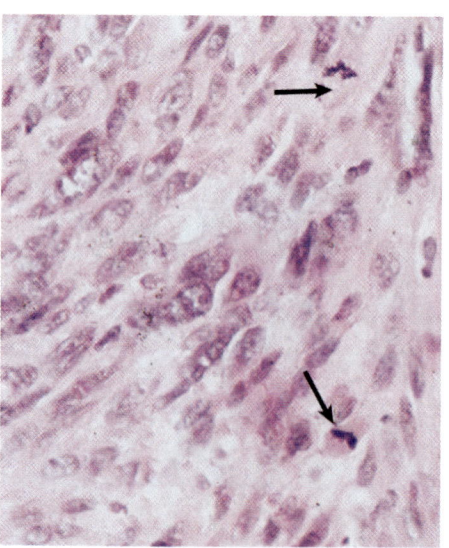

FIGURE 18-42
Leiomyosarcoma of the uterus. A. The uterus has been opened to reveal a large, soft leiomyosarcoma *(LS)* that has irregular borders *(horizontal arrows)* and invades the surrounding myometrium. By comparison, a small, firm leiomyoma *(vertical arrow)* with a hemorrhagic center is sharply demarcated. B. The malignant cells are moderately disorganized in arrangement, they are irregular in shape, and display numerous mitoses *(arrows)*.

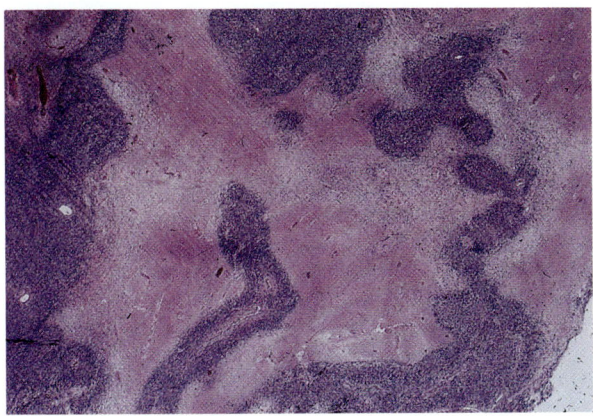

FIGURE 18-43
Leiomyosarcoma with coagulative necrosis. At low magnification, areas of necrosis are sharply demarcated from the viable tumor.

tion from viable tumor to large zones of necrosis, with an intervening rim of partially viable tumor cells. Blood vessels, if present, may be surrounded by a thin rim of viable tumor cells. The following features are considered evidence for the diagnosis of leiomyosarcoma: (1) 10 or more mitoses per 10 HPFs; (2) 5 or more mitoses per 10 HPFs, with nuclear atypia and geographical necrosis; and (3) myxoid and epithelioid smooth muscle tumors with 5 or more mitoses per 10 HPFs. Size is an important prognostic feature, since tumors less than 5 cm in diameter almost never recur.

Most leiomyosarcomas are large and at an advanced stage when detected and thus are usually fatal despite combinations of surgery, radiation therapy, and chemotherapy. Nearly half recur initially in the lung, and the 5-year survival rate is about 20%.

Fallopian Tube

ANATOMY

The fallopian tubes extend from the uterine fundus to the ovaries. An interstitial portion, termed *the isthmus*, lies within the cornua of the uterus and connects the uterine cavity with the straight portion of the tube. As the tube extends to the ovary, it increases in diameter to form the ampulla, which merges with the infundibulum. The fimbriated end opens like the bell of a trumpet and has numerous fingerlike extensions that envelop the ovary and facilitate passage of the ovum from the ruptured graafian follicle. Cells lining the fallopian tube are ciliated and play an important role in transport of the ovum.

SALPINGITIS

Salpingitis refers to inflammation of the fallopian tubes, typically the result of ascending infections of the lower genital tract. The most common causative organisms are *N. gonorrhoeae, Escherichia coli, Chlamydia,* and *Mycoplasma.* The infection is typically polymicrobial. Acute episodes of salpingitis (particularly those associated with chlamydial infection) may be asymptomatic. A fallopian tube damaged by prior infection is particularly susceptible to reinfection. In most cases, chronic salpingitis develops only after repeated episodes of acute salpingitis.

 Pathology and Clinical Features: In acute salpingitis, microscopic examination reveals a marked inflammatory infiltrate of polymorphonuclear leukocytes, in association with pronounced edema and congestion of the mucosal folds (plicae). The inflammatory infiltrate in chronic salpingitis consists of lymphocytes and plasma cells, and edema and congestion tend to be minimal. In late stages, the fallopian tube may seal and become distended with pus (*pyosalpinx*) or a transudate (*hydrosalpinx*).

The fallopian tube allows ascending microorganisms from the lower genital tract to reach the peritoneal cavity, a journey that leads to peritonitis and PID. Fibrinous adhesions between the serosa of the fallopian tube and surrounding peritoneal surfaces organize into thin fibrous adhesions (*"violin string" adhesions*). The adjacent ovary may also be involved in the process, sometimes giving rise to a *tuboovarian abscess*.

Complications also ensue from damage to the fallopian tube itself. Destruction of the epithelium or deposition of fibrin on the mucosa results in the formation of fibrin bridges, which cause adherence of the plicae to one another. In severe cases of chronic salpingitis, the adhesions are dense and form a blunted, clubbed end of the tube. The consequence of the blocked lumen may be hydrosalpinx or pyosalpinx. **The damage wrought by chronic salpingitis often impairs general tubal motility and possibly the passage of sperm, in which case infertility results. Chronic salpingitis is a common cause of ectopic pregnancy,** since adherent mucosal plicae create pockets in which ova are entrapped.

ECTOPIC PREGNANCY

Ectopic pregnancy refers to implantation outside the endometrium. The frequency of ectopic pregnancy in the United States has increased threefold to 1.5% of live births during the past two decades, although mortality has sharply declined. **Over 95% of ectopic pregnancies occur in the fallopian tube, mostly in the distal and middle thirds** (Fig. 18-44).

 Pathology: Ectopic pregnancy results when the passage of the conceptus along the fallopian tube is impeded, for example, by mucosal adhesions or abnormal tubal motility secondary to inflammatory disease or endometriosis. The trophoblast readily penetrates the mucosa and tubal wall. Thus, ectopic pregnancy resembles placenta increta or placenta percreta of the uterus (see below). Blood from the implantation site in the tube enters the peritoneal cavity, causing abdominal pain. In addition, ectopic

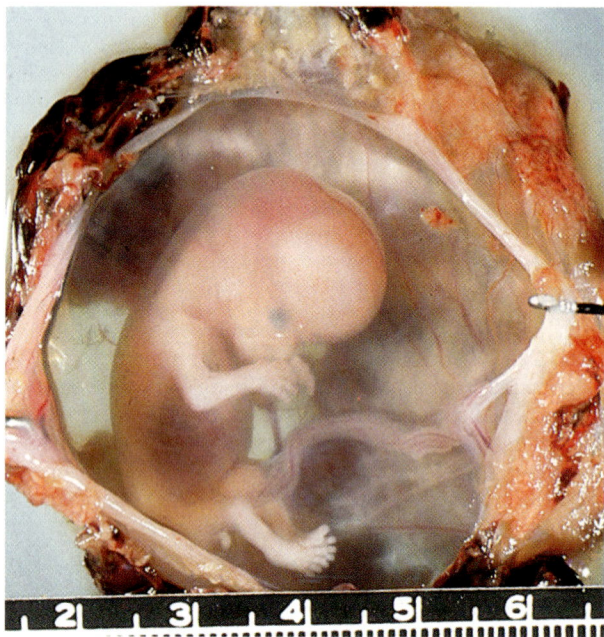

FIGURE 18-44
Ectopic pregnancy. An enlarged fallopian tube has been opened to disclose a minute fetus.

pregnancy is often associated with anomalous uterine bleeding following a period of amenorrhea and the presence of Arias-Stella cells in the endometrium. The thin tubal wall usually ruptures by the 12th week of gestation. **Tubal rupture is life-threatening because it can result in rapid exsanguination.**

Rupture of the tube's interstitial portion produces greater intraabdominal hemorrhage than rupture in other locations because the vasculature there is richer and the rupture occurs later in gestation. In the isthmus, the tube ruptures early (within the first 6 weeks), because its thick muscular wall does not allow much distension. Tubal pregnancies in the ampulla tend to be of longer duration, since the distensible tubal wall can accommodate a growing pregnancy for a longer time.

Ectopic pregnancy must be treated promptly with surgical or chemotherapeutic intervention. The administration of methotrexate terminates ectopic pregnancy and is used when the conceptus is smaller than 4 cm.

TUMORS

Tumors of the fallopian tube are rare. The most common is the small, circumscribed *adenomatoid tumor*, which is of mesothelial origin. It arises in the mesosalpinx and shows benign mesothelial cells that line slitlike spaces.

Tubal involvement by metastases or implants from adjacent ovarian and uterine neoplasms far exceeds the frequency of the rare primary cancer of the fallopian tube. Most primary malignancies are adenocarcinomas, and the peak incidence is in the 50- to 60-year-old age group. The tumor is bilateral in 25% of cases. The prognosis is poor, as the disease is almost always detected at a late stage.

Ovary

ANATOMY AND EMBRYOLOGY

The ovaries are paired organs that lie on both sides of the uterus. They are attached to the posterior surface of the broad ligament in a shallow peritoneal fossa between the external iliac vessels and the ureter. Each ovary consists of (1) an epithelial surface, (2) a mesenchymal stroma containing steroid-producing cells, and (3) germ cells. It has an outer cortex and inner medulla.

The ovaries appear early in fetal life as swellings of the genital ridges. At the 19th day of gestation, germ cells migrate from the primitive yolk sac to the gonads and multiply by mitotic division. By the 40th day, the ovaries and testes are histologically distinct. Toward the third trimester of fetal life, the germ cells stop multiplying and instead continue to develop by meiosis. Of the 1 million primordial follicles present at birth, only 70% remain by puberty, and fewer than 15% persist to age 25 years. Only some 450 ova are actually shed during a reproductive lifetime of 35 years.

The mesenchyme of the ovarian cortex consists of spindle-shaped, fibroblast-like cells. These give rise to the granulosa and theca cells, which form the functional unit about each ovum (theca interna and theca externa). The complex of the germ cell and supporting granulosa cells is known first as a *primordial follicle*. During the reproductive period, a dominant follicle develops every month into a *graafian follicle*, which then ruptures during ovulation. Ovulation itself is often associated with mild cramping pain and, if severe, is called *mittelschmerz* (i.e., midcycle pain). It is frequently confused with appendicitis. Following ovulation the granulosa cells of the follicle luteinize, a change characterized by hypertrophy and lipid accumulation At that time they secrete progesterone in addition to estrogens. The collapsed follicle turns bright yellow and becomes the *corpus luteum* (yellow body).

The cells of ovarian stromal origin include hilus cells and those resembling luteinized cells of the theca interna, both of which respond to pituitary hormones. These specialized cells synthesize and secrete both androgenic and estrogenic hormones, which stimulate proliferation in end organs, (e.g., uterus). They inhibit hypothalamic function by negative feedback loops.

CYSTIC LESIONS

Cysts are the most common cause of enlarged ovaries. Excluding cysts that arise from the invaginated surface epithelium (serous cysts), which are quite common, almost all of the rest arise from ovarian follicles.

Follicle Cysts Tend to be Asymptomatic

Follicle cysts are thin-walled, fluid-filled structures that are lined internally by granulosa cells and externally by a layer of theca interna cells. They occur at any age up to the menopause. Follicular cysts are unilocular and may be single or multiple, unilateral or bilateral. They arise from ovarian follicles and are probably related to abnormalities in the release of pituitary gonadotropins.

Pathology: Follicle cysts rarely exceed 5 cm greatest dimension. In an unstimulated state, the granulosa cells of the cyst have uniform, round nuclei and little cytoplasm. The thecal cells are small and spindle shaped. Occasionally, the layers may be luteinized, in which case the lumen contains fluid with a high estrogen or progesterone content. If the cyst persists, the hormonal output can cause precocious puberty in a child and menstrual irregularities in the adult. The only significant complication is mild intraperitoneal bleeding (fig. 18-45).

Corpus Luteum Cyst Can Bleed

A corpus luteum cyst results from the delayed resolution of a corpus luteum's central cavity. Continued progesterone synthesis by the luteal cyst leads to menstrual irregularities. Rupture of a cyst can cause mild hemorrhage into the abdominal cavity. A corpus luteum cyst is typically unilocular, 3 to 5 cm in size, and possessed of a yellow wall. The contents of the cyst vary from serosanguineous fluid to clotted blood. Microscopic examination shows numerous large, luteinized granulosa cells. The condition is self-limited.

Theca Lutein Cysts Relate to High Gonadotropin Levels

Theca lutein cysts are also known as hyperreactio luteinalis and are commonly multiple and bilateral. They are associated with high levels of circulating gonadotropin (e.g., in pregnancy, hydatidiform mole, choriocarcinoma, and exogenous gonadotropin therapy). The excessive gonadotropin levels lead to exaggerated stimulation of the theca interna and extensive cyst formation.

 Pathology: Multiple thin-walled cysts filled with clear fluid replace both ovaries. Microscopically, the cysts show a markedly luteinized layer of theca interna. The ovarian parenchyma shows edema and foci of luteinized stromal cells. Intraabdominal hemorrhage secondary to torsion or rupture of the cyst may require surgical intervention.

POLYCYSTIC OVARY SYNDROME

Polycystic ovary syndrome, known as **Stein-Leventhal syndrome,** *describes (1) clinical manifestations related to the secretion of excess androgenic hormones, (2) persistent anovulation, and (3) ovaries containing many small subcapsular cysts.* It was described initially as a syndrome of *secondary amenorrhea, hirsutism, and obesity.* However, the clinical presentation is now recognized to be far more variable and includes amenorrheic women who appear otherwise normal and, even rarely, have ovaries lacking polycystic features. Up to 7% of women experience the polycystic ovary syndrome, making this condition a common cause of infertility.

Pathogenesis: Polycystic ovary syndrome represents a state of functional ovarian hyperandrogenism associated with increased levels of luteinizing hormone (LH), although the increase in LH is probably a result rather than a cause of the ovarian dysfunction (Fig. 18-46).

1. The central abnormality is thought to be increased ovarian production of androgens, although adrenal hypersecretion of androgens may contribute to the clinical manifestations. There is ample evidence for abnormal regulation of the rate-limiting enzyme in the biosynthesis of androgens, namely, cytochrome $P450_{c17\alpha}$ (17α-hydroxylase), an enzyme expressed in both the ovary and the adrenal gland.
2. Excess ovarian androgens act locally to cause (a) premature follicular atresia, (b) multiple follicular cysts, and (c) a persistent anovulatory state. The impaired follicular maturation results in lower secretion of progesterone. Peripherally, hyperandrogenism leads to hirsutism, acne, and male-pattern (androgen-dependent) alopecia.
3. Excess androgens are converted to estrogens in peripheral adipose tissue, an effect exaggerated by obesity. Acyclical estrogen production and progesterone deficiency increase the pituitary secretion of LH.
4. Women with polycystic ovary syndrome exhibit marked peripheral insulin resistance, which is out of proportion to the degree of obesity. The mechanism appears to involve a post–insulin receptor defect, possibly related to decreased expression of a glucose transporter. In any event, the resulting hyperinsulinemia seems to contribute to

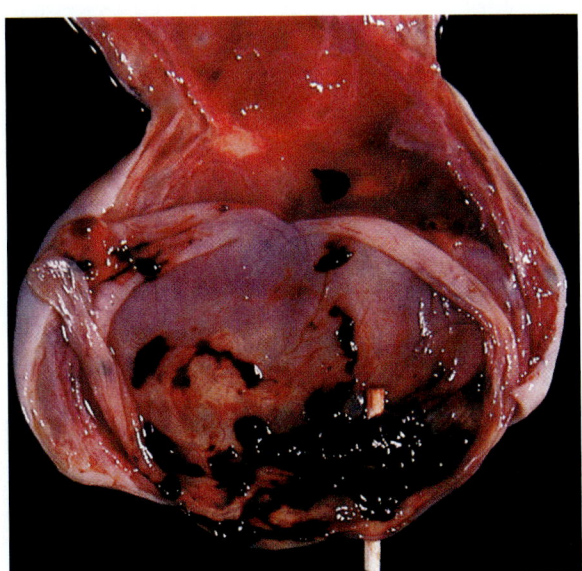

FIGURE 18-45
Follicle cyst of the ovary. The rupture of this thin-walled follicular cyst (dowel stick) led to intraabdominal hemorrhage.

968 The Female Reproductive System

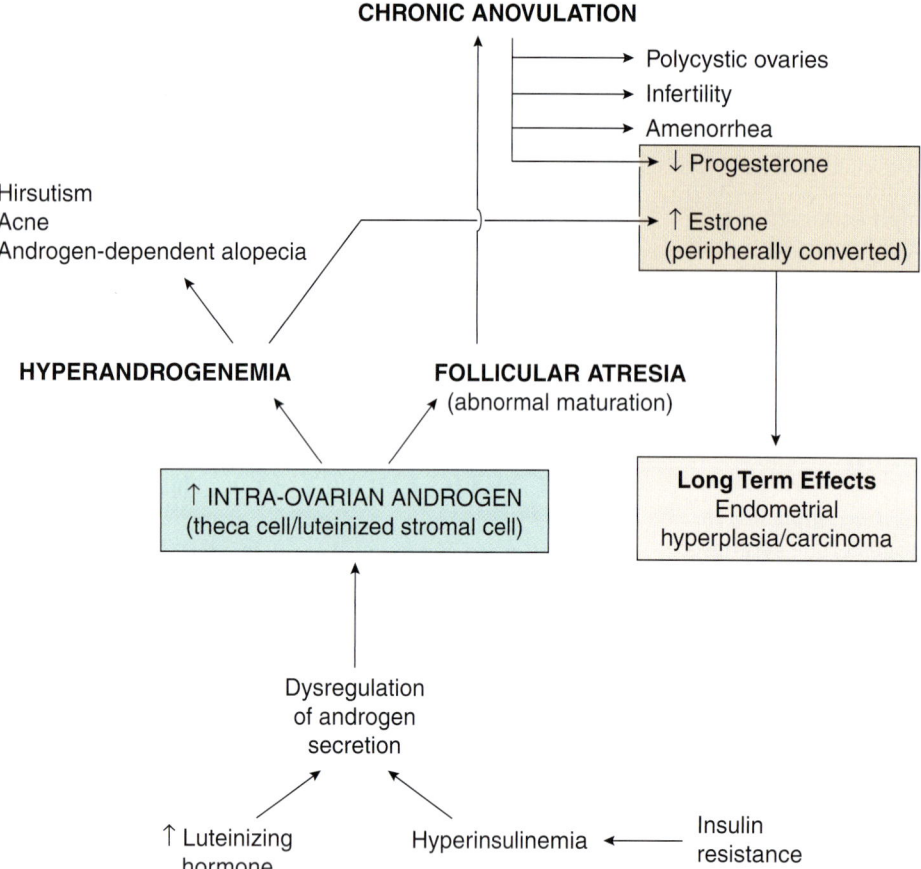

FIGURE 18-46
Pathogenesis of the polycystic ovary syndrome.

both increased ovarian hypersecretion of androgens and a direct stimulation of pituitary LH production.

  Pathology: On gross examination, both ovaries are enlarged. The surface is smooth, reflecting the absence of ovulation. On cut section, the cortex is thickened and discloses numerous cysts, typically 2 to 8 mm in diameter, arranged peripherally around a dense core of stroma or scattered throughout an increased amount of stroma (Fig. 18-47). Microscopically, the following features are present: (1) numerous follicles in early stages of development; (2) follicular atresia; (3) increased stroma, occasionally with luteinized cells (hyperthecosis); and (4) morphological signs of an absence of ovulation (thick, smooth capsule and absence of corpora lutea and corpora albicantiae). Many subcapsular cysts show thick zones of theca interna, in which some cells may be luteinized.

  Clinical Features: Infertility afflicts 15% of married couples in the United States. Of those with anovulatory infertility, nearly three quarters have polycystic ovary syndrome. Patients are typically in their twenties and tell of early obesity, menstrual problems, and hirsutism. Half of women with polycystic ovary syndrome are amenorrheic, and most of the others have irregular menstrual periods. Only 75% of affected women are actually infertile, indicating that some do occasionally ovulate. Unopposed acyclic estrogen secretion results in an increased incidence of endometrial hyperplasia and adenocarcinoma.

The treatment of the polycystic ovary syndrome encompasses two common problems in reproductive endocrinology—hirsutism and anovulation. Therapy is mostly hormonal and is directed toward interruption of the steady state of excess androgen production. Wedge resection of the ovary

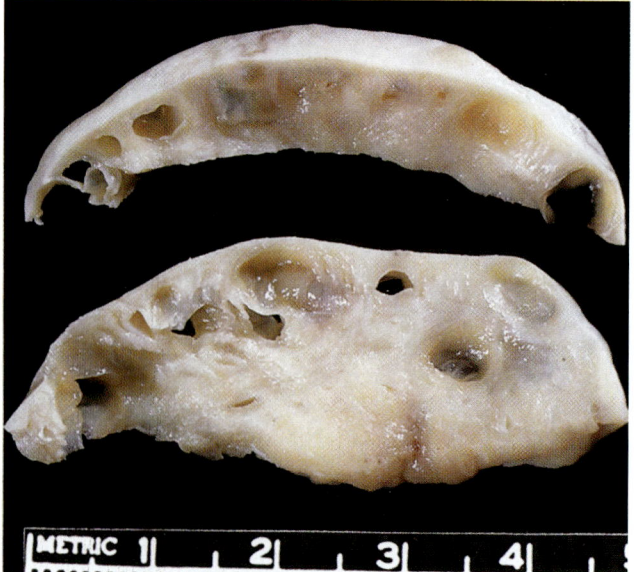

FIGURE 18-47
Polycystic disease of the ovary. Cut sections of an ovary show numerous cysts embedded in a sclerotic stroma.

has provided temporary remission of the syndrome, but is rarely used today.

STROMAL HYPERTHECOSIS

Stromal hyperthecosis refers to focal luteinization of ovarian stromal cells. The luteinized stromal cells are often functional and cause **virilization.** The condition occurs most commonly in postmenopausal women and, in a microscopic form, is found in one third of postmenopausal ovaries.

 Pathology: In women in whom stromal hyperthecosis is detected clinically, usually on the basis of masculinizing signs, both ovaries. may be enlarged, sometimes up to 8 cm in greatest dimension. The ovarian serosa is smooth, and the cut surface is homogeneous, firm, and brown to yellow. Microscopically, single nests or nodules of luteinized stromal cells are present in the cortex or medulla (Fig. 18-48). The cytoplasm of these cells is deeply eosinophilic and often vacuolated. The luteinized cells have a central large nucleus with a prominent nucleolus, a feature shared with all hormonally active stromal cells in the ovary.

TUMORS

Cancer of the ovary is the second most frequent gynecological malignancy after endometrial cancer, but in the United States it carries a higher mortality rate than all other female genital cancers combined (see Table 18-4). Unfortunately, it is difficult to detect this cancer early in its evolution when it is still curable. More than three fourths of patients already have extragonadal spread of tumor to the pelvis or abdomen at the time of diagnosis.

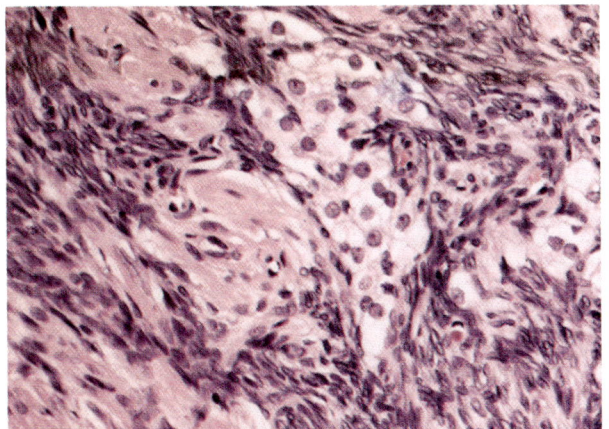

FIGURE *18-48*
Hyperthecosis of the ovary. Nests of luteinized (lipid-rich) stromal cells are present.

There are more than 25 major types of ovarian neoplasms. With variants and rare entities, they number over 100. The most common malignant tumor, serous adenocarcinoma (also termed *serous cystadenocarcinoma*), occurs in 1 to 2% of women.

The broad range of histological features in these tumors reflects the diverse anatomical structure of the ovary itself. The classification of ovarian tumors identifies them by the tissue of origin (Fig. 18-49). The most frequently encountered tumors arise from the surface epithelium and are termed *common epithelial tumors.* Other important groups include germ cell tumors, sex cord/stromal tumors, steroid cell tumors, and tumors metastatic to the ovary. About one sixth of ovarian tumors are of a mixed type.

Epithelial Tumors Account for over 90% of Ovarian Cancers

Tumors of common epithelial origin can be broadly classified as (1) benign, (2) of borderline malignancy (also called *atypical proliferating* or *low malignant potential*), and (3) malignant.

 Epidemiology: Epidemiological studies suggest that common epithelial neoplasms are related to repeated disruption and repair of the epithelial surface, which is part of cyclic ovulation. Thus, the tumors most commonly afflict women who are nulliparous and, conversely, occur least often in women in whom ovulation has been suppressed (e.g., by pregnancy or oral contraceptives). Irritants, such as powder used for feminine hygiene, have also been implicated, since they may be transported up the reproductive tract and reach the ovaries.

A family history of ovarian carcinoma is occasionally elicited. Women with a first-degree relative with ovarian cancer have a 3.5-fold increased risk of developing the same disease. Women who have a history of ovarian carcinoma are also at greater risk for breast cancer, and vice versa. The same gene implicated in hereditary breast cancers, namely *BRCA-1* (17q12-q23), has been incriminated in the pathogenesis of familial ovarian cancers. As for endometrial carcinoma, women who suffer from hereditary nonpolyposis colon cancer (HNCC) are also at greater risk for ovarian cancer. Women who bear *BRCA-1* tend to develop ovarian cancer considerably earlier than women who have sporadic ovarian cancer, but their prognosis is considerably better. Ovaries that are clinically normal in a woman who is a *BRCA-1* heterozygote rarely show any evidence of premalignant alterations, suggesting that prophylactic oophorectomy may not be warranted in such women.

 Pathogenesis: Most common epithelial tumors, especially serous carcinomas, arise from the surface epithelium, or serosa, of the ovary. A few, especially Brenner tumor, arise elsewhere in the ovary. During embryonic life, the celomic cavity is lined by a mesothelium, parts of which become specialized to form the serosal epithelium covering the gonadal ridge. The same mesothelial lining gives rise to the müllerian ducts, from which arise the fallopian tubes, uterus, and vagina (Fig. 18-50).

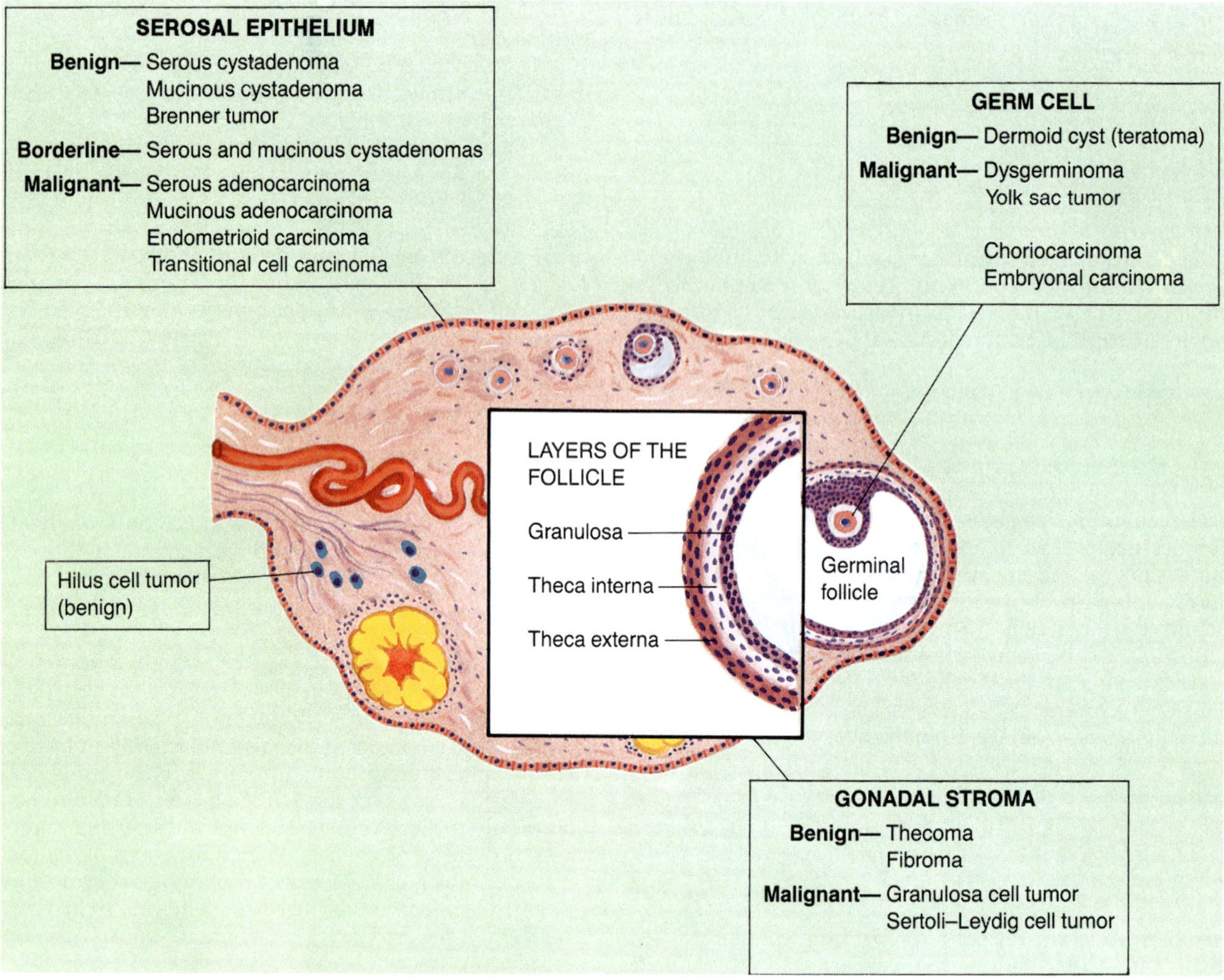

FIGURE 18-49
Classification of ovarian neoplasms based on cell of origin.

As the ovary develops, the surface epithelium may extend into the ovarian stroma to form glands and cysts. In some cases, these inclusions become neoplastic and exhibit a variety of müllerian-type differentiations (Fig. 18-51).

 Pathology: In order of decreasing frequency, the **common epithelial tumors** are as follows:

- **Serous tumors** that resemble the epithelium of the fallopian tube
- **Mucinous tumors** that mimic the mucosa of the endocervix
- **Endometrioid tumors** that are similar to the glands of the endometrium
- **Clear cell tumors** that display glycogen-rich cells that resemble endometrial glands in pregnancy
- **Transitional cell tumors** that resemble the mucosa of the bladder
- **Mixed**

Cystadenomas

Benign common epithelial tumors are almost always serous or mucinous adenomas and generally arise in women between the ages of 20 and 60 years. The neoplasms are frequently large, often 15 to 30 cm in diameter. Some of these tumors, particularly the mucinous variety, reach truly massive proportion, exceeding 50 cm in diameter, in which case they may mimic the appearance of a term pregnancy. Benign epithelial tumors are typically cystic, hence the term *cystadenoma*. Serous cystadenomas are more commonly bilateral (15%) than mucinous cystadenomas and tend to be unilocular (Fig. 18-52). By contrast, *mucinous tumors* characteristically show hundreds of small cysts (locules) (Fig. 18-53). As opposed to their malignant counterparts, benign epithelial tumors of the ovary tend to have thin walls and lack solid areas. Microscopically, a single layer of tall columnar epithelium lines the cysts. Papillae, when present, consist of a fibrovascular core covered by a single layer of tall columnar epithelium identical to that of the cyst lining.

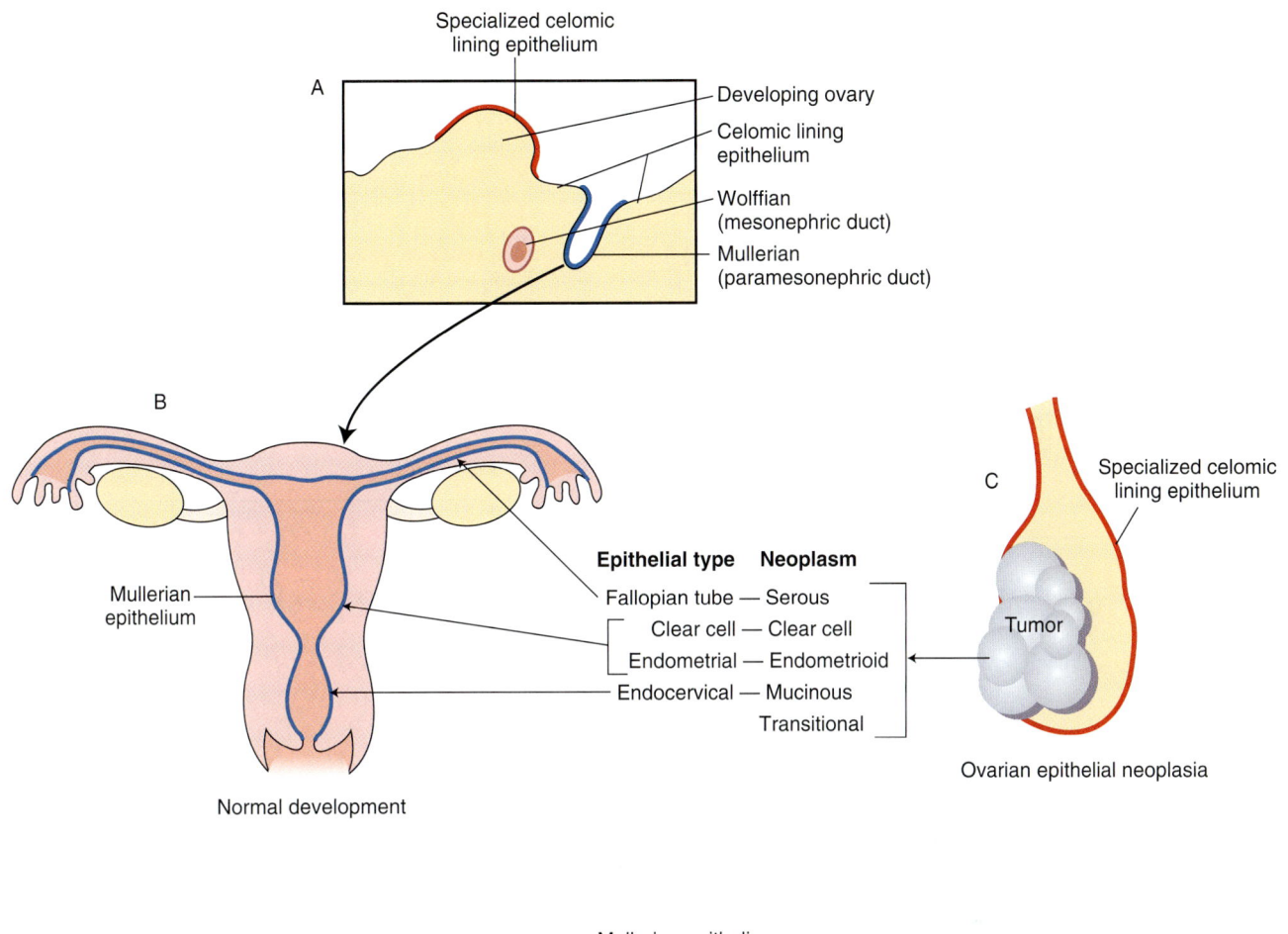

FIGURE 18-50
The müllerian relations of epithelial/stromal tumors of the ovaries.

Transitional Cell Tumor (Brenner Tumor)

The typical Brenner tumor is benign and occurs at all ages, with half of cases presenting in women over 50 years of age. The size varies from a microscopic focus to masses as large as 8 cm or more in diameter. Unlike other common epithelial tumors, Brenner tumor has two components. Histologically, it shows solid nests of transitional-like (urothelium-like) cells encased in a dense, fibrous stroma (Fig. 18-54). The most superficial epithelial cells may exhibit mucinous differentiation.

Borderline Tumors (Tumors of Low Malignant Potential) or Atypical Proliferative Tumors

The designation "borderline tumor" refers to a well-defined group of ovarian tumors that share an excellent prognosis, despite histological features suggesting cancer. Borderline tumors generally occur in women between the ages of 20 and 40 years but may also be encountered in older women. In terms of biological behavior, the tumor is "of low malignant potential," but from the morphological point of view it is atypical and proliferating. Chromosomal abnormalities have been found in borderline tumors that are different from those in the common forms of cancer. A surgical cure is almost always possible if the tumor is confined to the ovaries. Even when it has spread to the pelvis or abdomen, 80% of patients are alive after 5 years, although there is a significant rate of late recurrence.

Serous tumors of borderline malignancy are more commonly bilateral (34%) than mucinous ones (6%) or other types. The tumors vary in size, although mucinous ones sometimes achieve gigantic size (100+ kg). In serous tumors of borderline malignancy, it is common to find papillary projections, ranging from fine and exuberant to grapelike clusters arising from the cyst wall (Fig. 18-55). Microscopically, these structures resemble the papillary fronds in benign cystadenomas, but they are distinguished from them by (1) epithelial stratification, (2) nuclear atypism, and (3) mitotic activity. The same criteria apply to borderline mucinous tumors, although papillary projections are less conspicuous. **By definition, the presence of more than focal microinvasion (i.e., discrete nests of epithelial cells that invade less than 3 mm into the ovarian stoma) removes it from the category of borderline malignancy and identifies it as frankly**

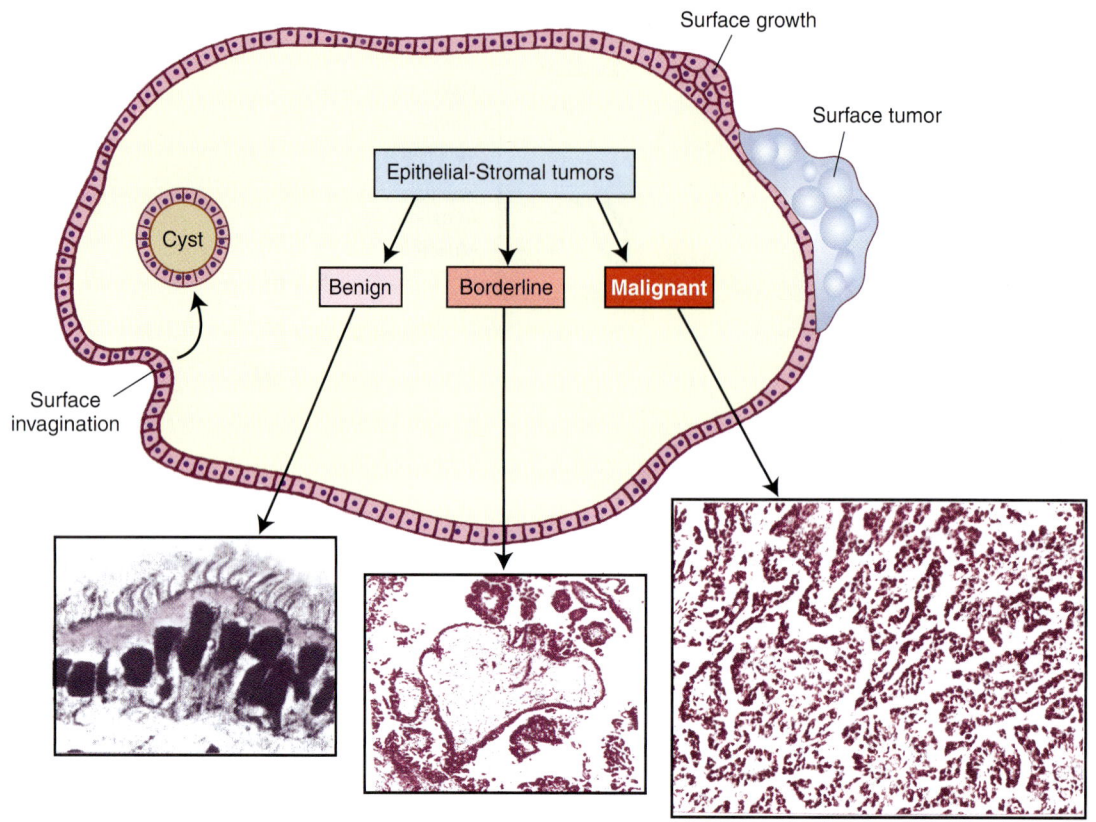

FIGURE 18-51
Histogenesis of ovarian epithelial-stromal tumors.

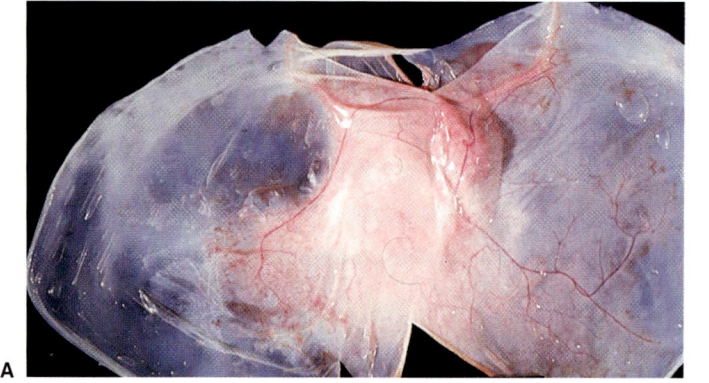
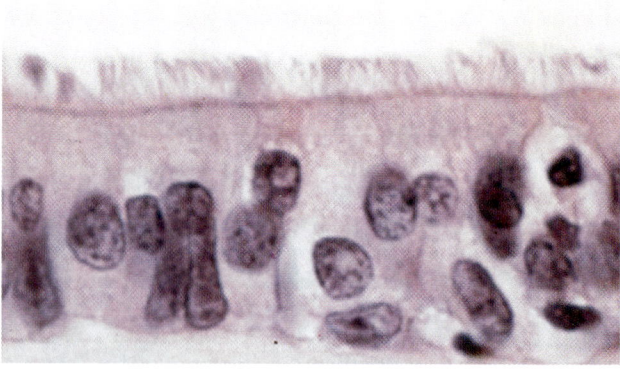

FIGURE 18-52
Serous cystadenoma of the ovary. A. The fluid has been removed from this huge unilocular serous cystadenoma. The wall is thin and translucent. B. On microscopic examination, the cyst is lined by a single layer of ciliated tubal-type epithelium.

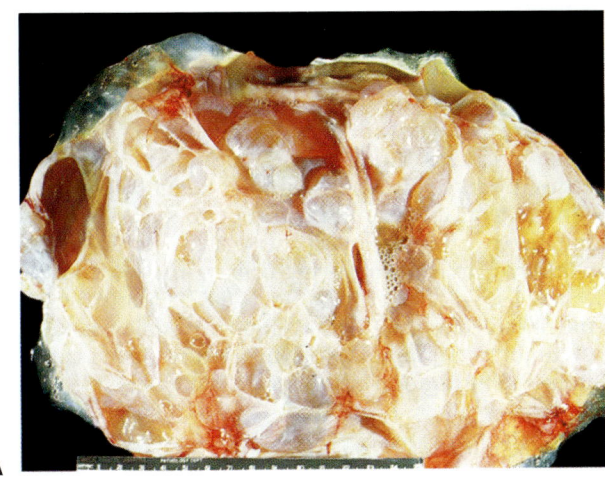
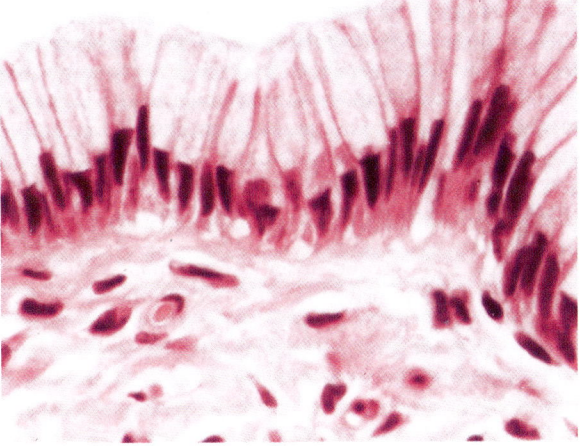

FIGURE 18-53
Mucinous cystadenoma of the ovary. A. The tumor is characterized by numerous cysts filled with thick, viscous fluid. B. A single layer of mucinous epithelial cells lines the cyst.

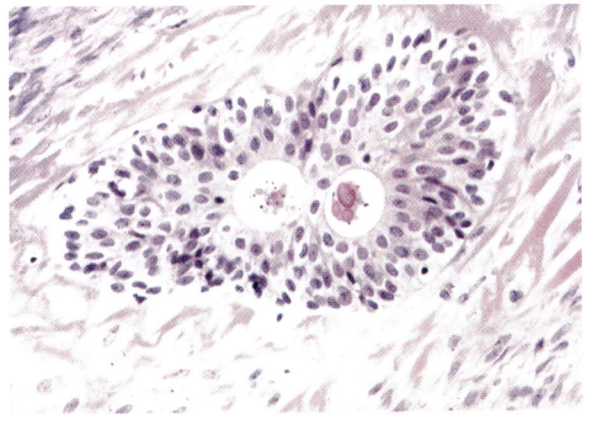

FIGURE 18-54
Brenner tumor. A nest of transitional-like cells is embedded in a dense, fibrous stroma.

malignant. As described below in the section on the peritoneum, borderline tumors with lymph node metastases or implants in the peritoneum, whether noninvasive or invasive, are still classified as "borderline," reflecting that this category is well defined and carries a prognosis far better than the usual adenocarcinoma.

Malignant Epithelial Tumors

Malignant epithelial tumors of the ovary are most common between the ages of 40 and 60 years and are rare under the age of 35. By the time an ovarian cancer has attained a size of 10 to 15 cm, it has often spread beyond the ovary and seeded the peritoneum.

SEROUS ADENOCARCINOMA: This tumor (commonly called "cystadenocarcinoma") is the most common

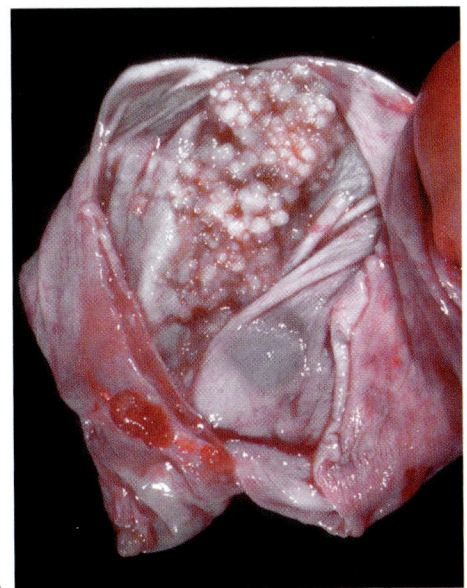
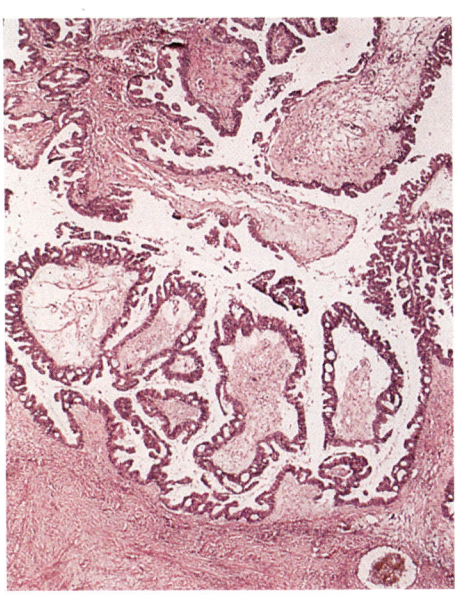

FIGURE 18-55
Serous ovarian tumor of borderline malignancy. A. Papillary excrescences project from the cyst wall. B. A microscopic view demonstrates the papillary structure of the tumor.

malignancy of the ovary, accounting for a third of all ovarian cancers. Since tumors of advanced stage are bilateral more than twice as often as those of low stage, it seems that the cancer commonly spreads to the contralateral ovary by implantation. In fact two thirds of serous cancers with extragonadal spread are bilateral. On gross examination, serous adenocarcinomas are usually uniloculated or pauciloculated tumors, with soft, delicate papillae lining the entire surface. Solid areas, often with necrosis and hemorrhage, are common (Fig. 18-56).

Microscopically, serous adenocarcinomas vary from well differentiated to poorly differentiated. In the latter, the papillary pattern may be inconspicuous, with most areas being composed of solid sheets of malignant cells. Stromal and capsular invasion by the tumor cells is evident. Laminated calcified concretions, referred to as *psammoma bodies,* are present in a third of cases (see Fig. 18-56c).

MUCINOUS ADENOCARCINOMA: Mucinous cystadenocarcinoma constitutes about 10% of all ovarian cancers. When confined to the ovary, one sixth of cases are bilateral. Mucinous cancers are typically multilocular, with small cysts often ranging into the hundreds to thousands. Unlike serous tumors that are grossly uniform throughout, mucinous tumors often contain some solid areas or others with papillary projections. The cystic areas typically appear as benign or borderline tumors, and clearly malignant features are found only in the solid regions. Microscopically, the same mucinous tumor may display a full range of appearances, from well to poorly differentiated By contrast, serous tumors tend to be uniform throughout. Well-differentiated mucinous tumors contain neoplastic glands lined by tall columnar, mucin-producing cells, usually with some areas that are solid or cribriform (Fig. 18-57). Poorly differentiated mucinous adenocarcinomas exhibit irregular nests and cords of tumor cells and numerous mitoses. Stromal invasion is the rule, and infiltration of the serosa is common.

ENDOMETRIOID ADENOCARCINOMA: Endometrioid adenocarcinoma histologically resembles its endometrial counterpart and is second only to serous adenocarcinoma in frequency, accounting for 20% of all ovarian cancers. The tumor occurs most commonly after the menopause. In contrast to serous and mucinous neoplasms, most endometrioid tumors are malignant. Up to one half of these cancers are bilateral.

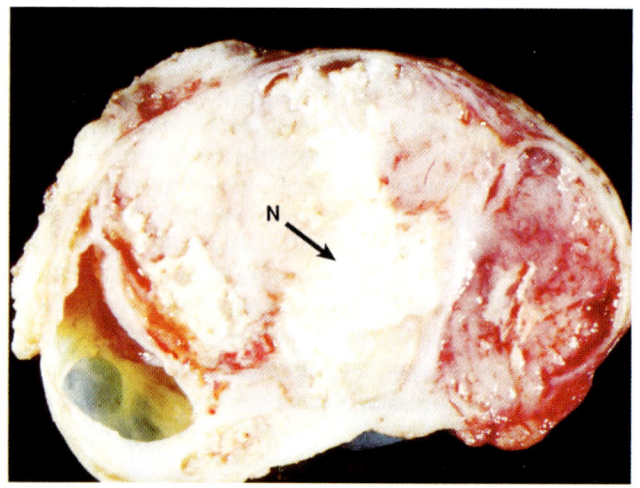

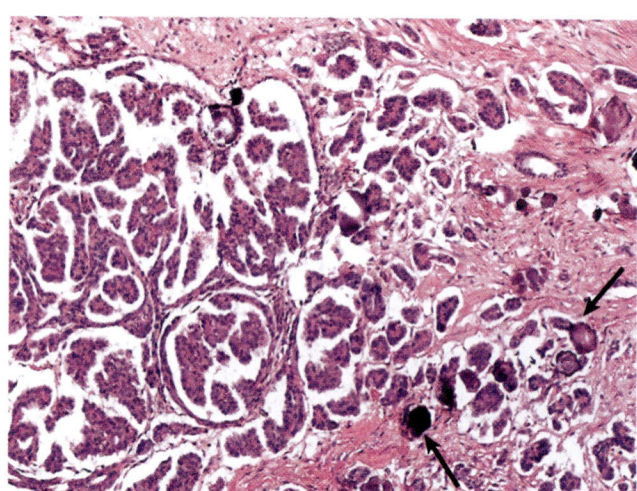

FIGURE 18-56
Serous cystadenocarcinoma. A. The ovary is enlarged by a solid tumor that exhibits extensive necrosis (*N*). **B.** Microscopic examination shows a papillary cancer invading the ovarian stroma. Several psammoma bodies are present (*arrows*). **C.** A higher-power view shows the laminated structure of a psammoma body.

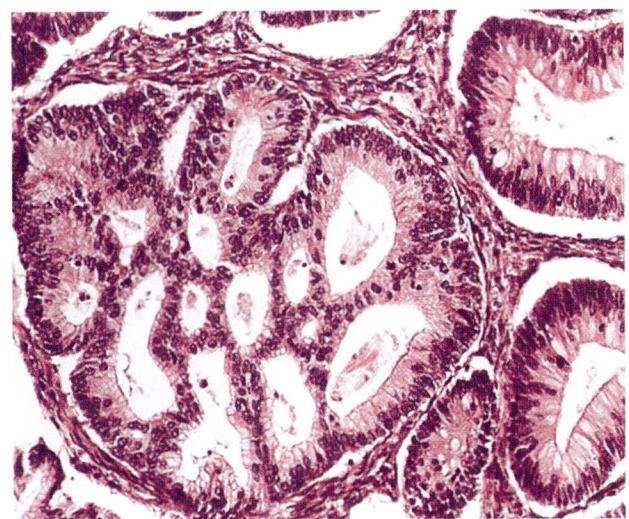

FIGURE 18-57
Mucinous cystadenocarcinoma. The malignant glands are arranged in a cribriform pattern and are composed of mucin-producing columnar cells.

On gross examination, endometrioid carcinomas vary in size from 2 cm to more than 30 cm in greatest dimension. Most are largely solid and exhibit necrotic areas, although they may be cystic. Microscopically, the tumors are graded according to the same scheme used for endometrial adenocarcinoma. Many patients with endometrioid carcinoma of the ovary also harbor an endometrial cancer, the rates in various series ranging from 15 to 50%. Strong evidence suggests that both the ovarian and endometrial cancers arise independently, rather than as metastases from one or the other. Accordingly, the 5-year survival exceeds 85% in such synchronous tumors. As with all malignant epithelial tumors of the ovary, the prognosis depends on the stage at which it presents.

CLEAR CELL ADENOCARCINOMA: This ovarian cancer, which is closely related to endometrioid adenocarcinoma, often occurs in association with endometriosis. It constitutes 5 to 10% of all ovarian cancers usually occurring after the menopause. The size ranges from 2 to 30 cm in diameter, and 40% are bilateral. Most of these tumors are partially cystic and exhibit necrosis and hemorrhage in the solid areas.

Microscopically, clear cell adenocarcinoma of the ovary displays sheets or tubules of malignant cells with clear cytoplasm. In the tubular form, the malignant cells often display bulbous nuclei that protrude into the lumen of the tubule *(hobnail cell),* an appearance similar to the Arias-Stella reaction in the gestational endometrium. The microscopic appearance of clear cell adenocarcinoma resembles that of its counterpart in the vagina. The clinical course parallels that of endometrioid carcinoma.

Clinical Features: The vast majority of ovarian tumors are nonfunctional, that is, they do not secrete hormones. However, an antibody to a cancer antigen (CA-125) in the serum detects about half of the epithelial tumors that are confined to the ovary and about 90% that have already spread. The specificity of this test is 90%; the sensitivity is 75%.

Ovarian masses rarely cause symptoms until they are large. When they distend the abdomen, they cause pain, pelvic pressure, or compression of regional organs. By the time ovarian cancers are diagnosed, many have metastasized (implanted) to the surfaces of the pelvis, abdominal organs, or bladder. Evaluation of a patient with an ovarian cancer of epithelial origin requires an intimate knowledge of staging, grading, and routes of tumor spread. For example, ovarian tumors have a tendency to implant in the peritoneal cavity on the diaphragm, paracolic gutters, and omentum. Lymphatic dissemination carries malignant cells preferentially to the paraaortic lymph nodes near the origin of the renal arteries and to a lesser extent to the external iliac (pelvic) or inguinal lymph nodes. In addition to specific symptoms, metastatic cancers are associated with ascites, weakness, weight loss, and cachexia.

In general, survival for patients with malignant ovarian tumors is poor. The single most important prognostic index is the surgical stage of the tumor at the time it is first detected (Table 18-10). Overall, the 5-year survival is only 35%, because more than half the tumors have spread to the abdominal cavity (stage 3) or elsewhere by the time they are discovered. Prognostic indices for epithelial tumors also include grade, histological type, and the size of the residual neoplasm.

The cornerstone to managing ovarian cancer is surgery, because it not only removes the primary tumor but also establishes the diagnosis and assesses the extent of spread. At laparotomy, the surgeon must examine the peritoneal surfaces, omentum, liver, subdiaphragmatic recesses, and all abdominal regions, so as to remove as much of the metastatic tumor as possible. Adjuvant chemotherapy is used to treat distant occult sites of tumor spread.

At some time after the initial operation, another exploratory laparotomy (second-look laparotomy) has been used

TABLE 18-10 Clinical Staging of Ovarian Cancer

Stage	Description
I	Limited to ovaries; capsule intact; no tumor on the external surface
Ia	Limited to one ovary; ascitic fluid, if present, lacks malignant cells
Ib	Limited to both ovaries; capsule intact; no tumor on the external surface; ascitic fluid, if present, lacks malignant cells
Ic	Any of above, but with ascites or positive peritoneal washings
II	With pelvic extension
IIa	Extension or metastases to uterus or tubes
IIb	Extension to other pelvic tissues
IIc	Any of above, but with ascites or positive peritoneal washings
III	With intraperitoneal metastases outside the pelvis, or positive retroperitoneal nodes, or both. Tumor limited to true pelvis with histologically proven malignant extension to small bowel or omentum.
IIIa	Microscopic seeding on abdominal-peritoneal surface
IIIb	Implants ≤2 cm on abdominal peritoneal surface
IIIc	Implants >2 cm on abdominal peritoneal surface
IV	With distant metastases. If pleural effusion present, positive cytology required. Liver metastases must be parenchymal.

Germ Cell Tumors Tend to Be Benign in Adults and Malignant in Children

Tumors derived from germ cells constitute a fourth of all ovarian tumors. In adult women, germ cell tumors are virtually all benign (mature cystic teratoma, dermoid cyst), whereas in children and young adults, they are largely cancerous. In children, germ cell tumors are the most common form of ovarian cancer (60%); they are rare after the menopause.

The neoplastic germ cell may follow one of several lines of differentiation, giving rise to tumors analogous to those found in the male testis (Fig. 18-58).

Dysgerminoma is composed of neoplastic germ cells, resembling the oogonia of the fetal ovary.
Teratoma differentiates toward somatic (embryonic) tissues.
Yolk sac tumor differentiates toward extraembryonic tissue and resembles the placental mesenchyme or its precursors.
Choriocarcinoma features cells that are similar to those covering the placental villi.

Germ cell tumors in infants tend to be solid and immature (e.g., yolk sac tumor and immature teratoma). Tumors in young adults show greater differentiation, as in mature cystic teratoma. Malignant germ cell tumors in women older than 40 years of age usually result from the transformation of one of the components of a benign cystic teratoma.

Malignant germ cell tumors tend to be highly aggressive. At one time, solid germ cell tumors of the ovary were uniformly fatal, but with the advent of chemotherapy, survival rates for many exceed 80%.

Dysgerminoma

Dysgerminoma is the ovarian counterpart of testicular seminoma and is composed of primordial germ cells. Although it accounts for less than 2% of all ovarian cancers, dysgerminoma constitutes 10% of these malignancies in women younger than 20 years of age. Most patients are between 10 and 30 years of age. The tumors are bilateral in about 15% of cases.

Pathology: On gross examination, dysgerminomas are often large and firm and have a bosselated external surface. The cut surface is soft and fleshy. Microscopic examination reveals large nests of monotonously uniform tumor cells, which have a clear glycogen-filled cytoplasm and irregularly flattened central nuclei (Fig. 18-59). Fibrous septa containing lymphocytes traverse the tumor.

Dysgerminoma is treated surgically, and the 5-year survival rate for patients with stage I tumor approaches 100%. Because the tumor is highly radiosensitive, 5-year survival rates for higher-stage tumors still exceed 80%.

Teratoma

Teratoma is a tumor of germ cell origin that differentiates toward somatic structures. Most teratomas contain tissues representing at least two, and usually all three, embryonic layers.

MATURE TERATOMA (MATURE CYSTIC TERATOMA, DERMOID CYST): This benign neoplasm accounts for one fourth of all ovarian tumors with a peak incidence in the third decade. Mature teratomas develop by parthenogenesis. Haploid (postmeiotic) germ cells autofertilize to give rise to diploid tumor cells that are genetically female (46,XX).

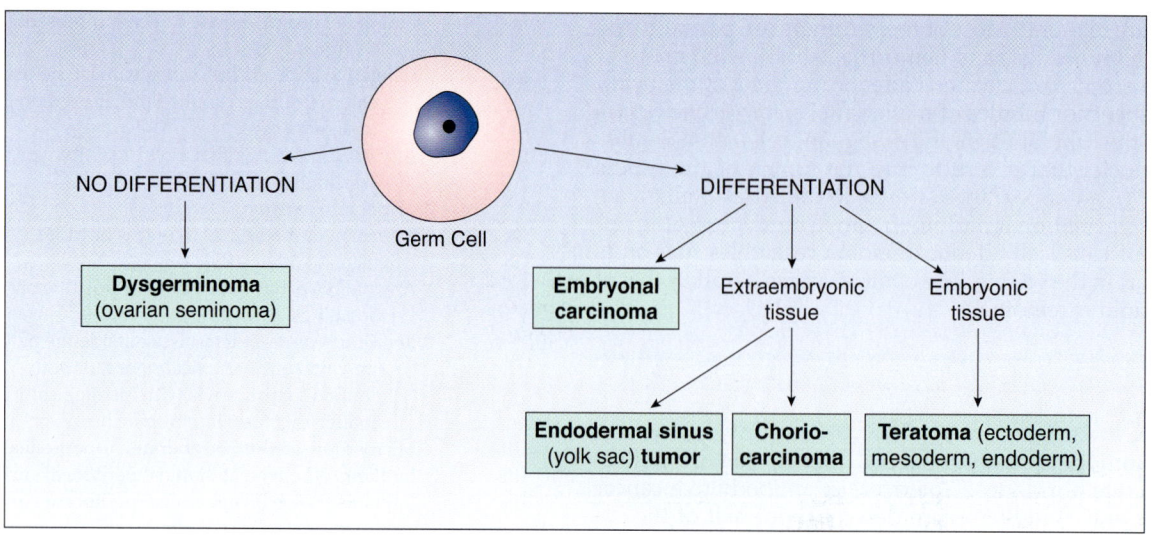

FIGURE 18-58
Classification of germ cell tumors of the ovary.

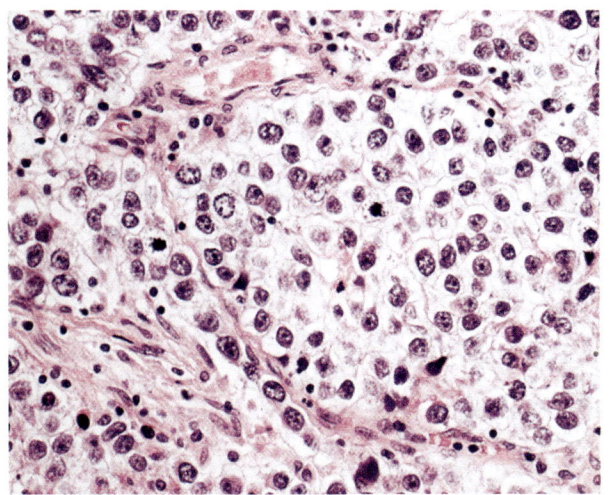

FIGURE 18-59
Dysgerminoma. The neoplastic germ cells have clear, glycogen-filled cytoplasm and central nuclei. Fibrous septa containing lymphocytes traverse the tumor.

Pathology: Mature teratoma is cystic, and more than 90% contain skin, sebaceous glands, and hair follicles (Fig. 18-60). Half of the tumors exhibit smooth muscle, sweat glands, cartilage, bone, teeth, and respiratory tract epithelium. Tissues such as gut, thyroid, and brain are encountered less frequently. When present, nodular foci in the cyst wall ("mammary tubercles" or "Rokitansky nodules") contain tissue elements of all three germ cell layers, namely (1) ectoderm (e.g., skin and glia), (2) mesoderm (e.g., smooth muscle or cartilage), and (3) endoderm (e.g., respiratory epithelium).

Struma ovarii refers to a cystic lesion composed predominantly of thyroid tissue (5–20% of mature cystic teratomas). Rare cases of hyperthyroidism have been associated with struma ovarii.

A small minority (1%) of dermoid cysts undergo malignant transformation. These cancers usually occur in older women and correspond to the tumors that arise in other differentiated tissues of the body. Three fourths of all cancers that arise in dermoid cysts are squamous cell carcinomas. The remainder include carcinoid tumor, basal cell carcinoma, thyroid cancer, adenocarcinoma, and others. In rare cases, derivatives of gut may be functional and produce carcinoid syndrome. The prognosis of patients with malignant transformation of mature cystic teratoma is related largely to the stage of the cancer.

IMMATURE TERATOMA: Immature teratoma of the ovary is composed of elements derived from the three germ layers. However, unlike mature cystic teratoma, the immature variety contains embryonal tissues. Immature teratoma accounts for 20% of malignant tumors at all sites in women under the age of 20 and becomes progressively less common in older women.

Pathology: Immature teratoma is predominantly solid and lobulated and contains numerous small cysts. The solid areas may contain grossly recog-

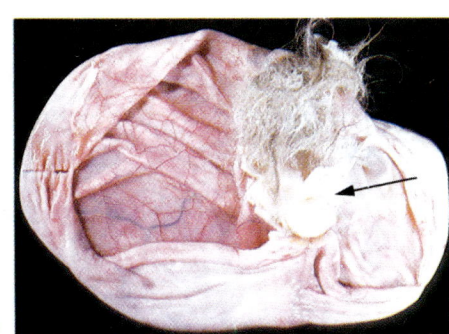
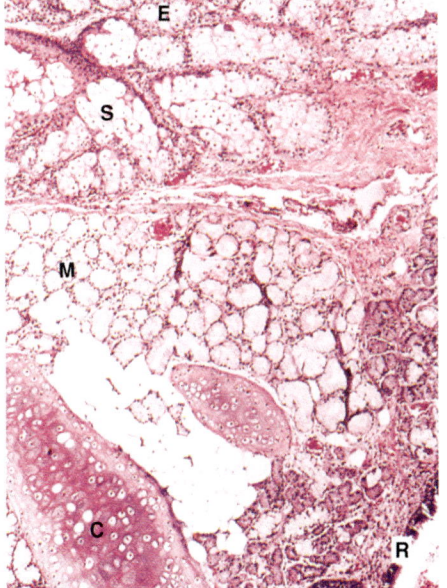

FIGURE 18-60
Mature cystic teratoma of the ovary. A. A mature cystic teratoma has been opened to reveal a solid knob *(arrow)* from which hair projects. B. A photomicrograph of the solid knob shows epidermal and respiratory components. Tissue resembling the skin exhibits an epidermis *(E)* with underlying sebaceous glands *(S)*. The respiratory tissue consists of mucous glands *(M)*, cartilage *(C)*, and respiratory epithelium *(R)*.

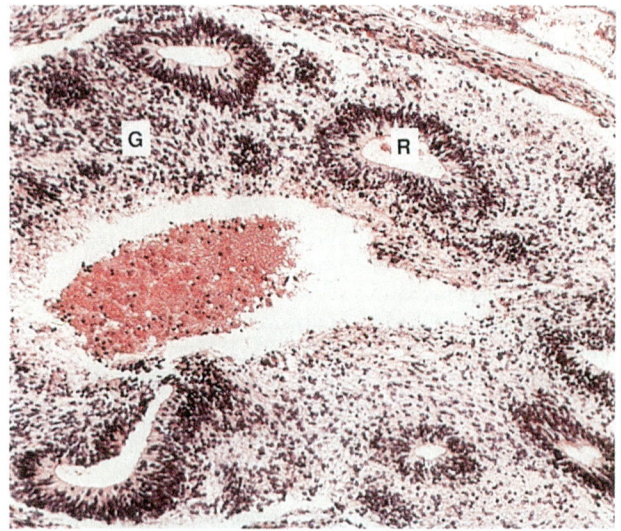

FIGURE 18-61
Immature teratoma of the ovary. Immature neural tissue exhibits rosettes *(R)* with multilayered nuclei. Embryonal glia *(G)* display densely packed, atypical nuclei.

nizable immature bone and cartilage. Microscopically, multiple tumor components are usually found, including those differentiating toward nerve (neuroepithelial rosettes and immature glia) (Fig. 18-61), glands, and other structures found in mature cystic teratomas. The metastases of immature teratoma are composed of embryonal, usually stromal, tissues. By contrast, the rare metastases of mature cystic teratomas, resemble epithelial adult-type malignancies.

Survival correlates with the grade of the tumor. Well-differentiated immature teratomas generally have a favorable outcome, whereas high-grade tumors (predominantly embryonal tissue) have a poor prognosis.

Yolk Sac Tumor

Yolk sac tumor is a highly malignant tumor of women under the age of 30 that histologically resembles the mesenchyme of the primitive yolk sac.

 Pathology: Typically, the neoplasm is large and displays extensive necrosis and hemorrhage. Microscopic examination reveals multiple patterns. The most common appearance is a reticular, honeycombed structure of communicating spaces lined by primitive cells. *Schiller-Duval bodies* (Fig. 18-62), which resemble the endodermal sinus of the rodent placenta, are found sparingly in a few tumors, but are characteristic. These structures consist of papillae that protrude into a space lined by tumor cells, resembling the glomerular Bowman space. The papillae are covered by a mantle of embryonal cells and contain a fibrovascular core and a central blood vessel.

Yolk sac tumor should not be confused with embryonal cell carcinoma, which is common in the testis. The former secretes α-fetoprotein, which can be demonstrated histochemically within eosinophilic droplets. Detection of α-fetoprotein in the blood is useful both for diagnosis and for monitoring the effectiveness of therapy. Prior to the era of chemotherapy, yolk sac tumor was nearly always fatal. Now 5-year survival rates for stage I tumors exceed 80%.

Choriocarcinoma

Choriocarcinoma of the ovary is a rare tumor that mimics the epithelial covering of placental villi, namely, cytotrophoblast and syncytiotrophoblast. A derivation from ovarian germ cells is assumed if the tumor arises before puberty or in combination with another germ cell tumor. In women of reproductive age, however, ovarian choriocarcinoma may also represent metastasis from an intrauterine gestational tumor. Choriocarcinoma of germ cell origin manifests in young girls as precocious sexual development, menstrual irregularities, or rapid breast enlargement.

 Pathology: Choriocarcinoma is unilateral, solid, and extensively hemorrhagic. Microscopically, it displays an admixture of malignant cytotrophoblast and syncytiotrophoblast (see placenta, choriocarcinoma, below). The syncytial cells secrete human chorionic gonadotropin (hCG), which accounts for the frequent finding of a positive pregnancy test result. Bilateral theca lutein cysts, a result of hCG stimulation, may also be found.

Serial determinations of serum hCG levels are useful for both diagnosis and follow-up. The tumor is highly aggressive but responds to chemotherapy.

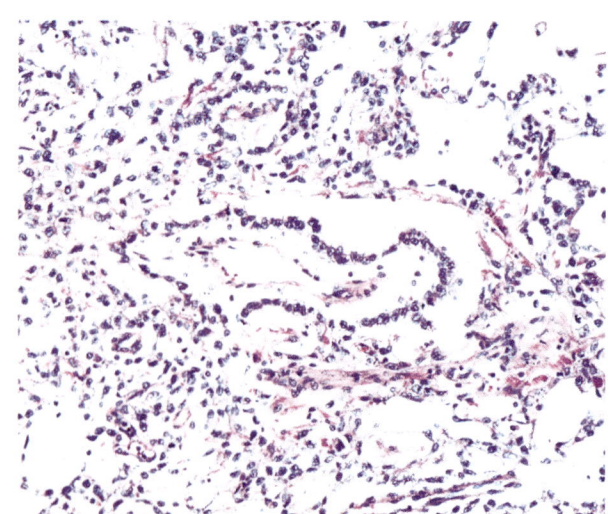

FIGURE 18-62
Yolk sac carcinoma of ovary. The tumor cells are arrayed in a reticular pattern. A Schiller-Duval body *(center)* resembles the endodermal sinuses of the rodent placenta and consists of a papilla protruding into a space lined by tumor cells.

Gonadoblastoma

Gonadoblastoma is a rare ovarian tumor that is distinctive because of its association with various types of gonadal dysgenesis, especially in women who bear a Y chromosome. It occurs in phenotypic women under 30 years of age, although 20% are found in phenotypic men with cryptorchidism, hypospadias, and female internal sex organs. Most affected women are virilized and suffer from primary amenorrhea and developmental abnormalities of the genitalia.

 Pathology: The tumor is solid and often extensively calcified. Microscopically, cellular nests show a mixture of germ cells and sex cord derivatives that resemble immature Sertoli and granulosa cells, which is why some consider the tumor to be an in situ form of germinoma. In half of cases, gonadoblastoma is overgrown by dysgerminoma. The gonadoblastoma itself does not metastasize, but its overgrowths do.

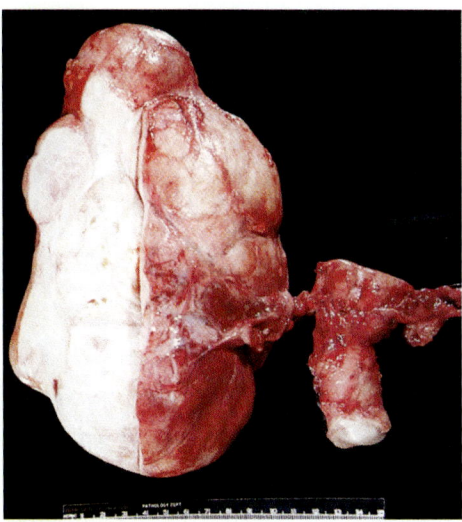

FIGURE 18-63
Fibroma of ovary. The ovary is conspicuously enlarged by a firm, white, bosselated tumor.

Sex Cord/Stromal Tumors Are Clinically Functional

Tumors of the sex cord and stroma originate from either primitive sex cords or from mesenchymal stroma of the developing gonad. They account for 10% of all ovarian tumors. The tumors range from benign to low-grade malignant and may differentiate toward female (granulosa and theca cells) or male (Sertoli and Leydig cells) structures.

Fibroma

Fibromas are the most common ovarian stromal tumors, accounting for 75% of all stromal tumors and 7% of all ovarian tumors. They occur at all ages, with a peak in the perimenopausal period, and are virtually always benign.

 Pathology: The tumors are solid, firm, and white (Fig. 18-63). Microscopically, the cells resemble the stroma of the normal ovarian cortex, being composed of well-differentiated fibroblasts and variable amounts of collagen. Half of the larger tumors are associated with ascites and, rarely, with ascites and pleural effusions *(Meigs syndrome)*.

Thecoma

Thecomas are functional ovarian tumors that arise in postmenopausal women. In most cases, they produce signs of estrogen production.

 Pathology: Thecomas are solid tumors, mostly 5 to 10 cm in diameter. The cut section is yellow, owing to the presence of many lipid-laden theca cells. Microscopically, the cells are large and oblong to round, with a vacuolated cytoplasm that contains lipid. Bands of hyalinized collagen separate nests of theca cells. Thecomas are almost always benign.

Because of estrogen output by the tumor, thecomas in premenopausal women commonly cause irregularity in menstrual cycles and breast enlargement. Endometrial hyperplasia and cancer are well-recognized complications.

Granulosa Cell Tumor

Granulosa cell tumor is the prototypical functional neoplasm of the ovary associated with estrogen secretion. This tumor should be considered malignant because of its potential for local spread and the rare occurrence of distant metastases.

 Pathogenesis: Most granulosa cell tumors occur after the menopause (adult form), and they are unusual before puberty. The juvenile form occurs in children and young women and has distinct clinical and pathological features (hyperestrogenism and precocious puberty. In contrast to common epithelial tumors, in which repeated ovulation is a contributing factor, experimental evidence suggests that the development of granulosa cell tumors is linked to the loss of oocytes. Oocytes appear to regulate granulosa cells, and tumorigenesis occurs when the follicles are disorganized or atretic.

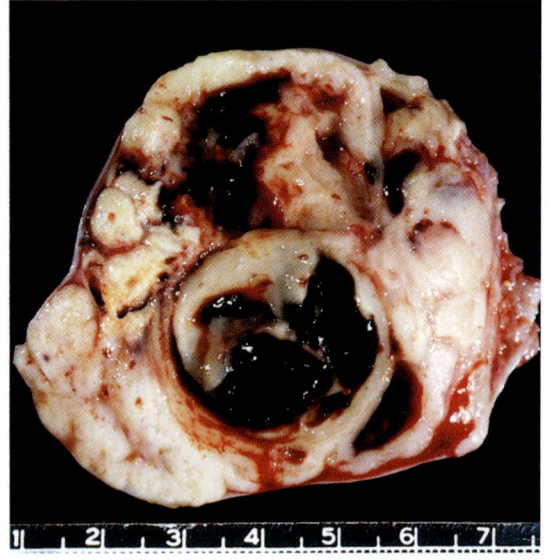
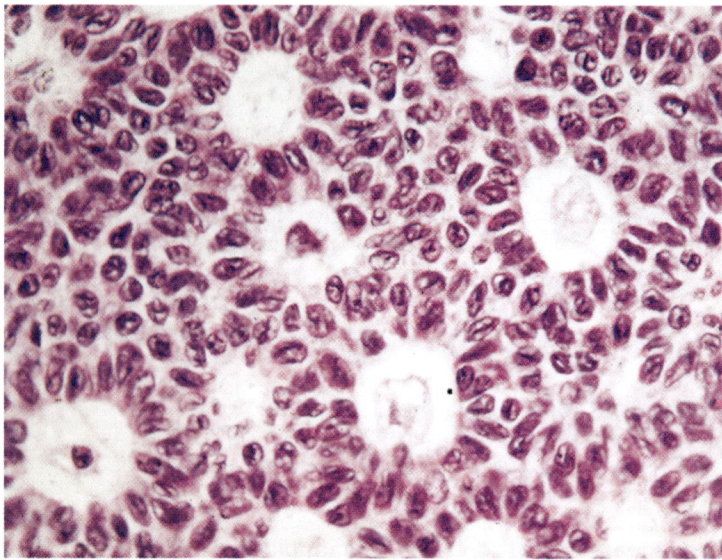

FIGURE 18-64
Granulosa cell tumor of the ovary. A. Cross-section of the enlarged ovary shows a variegated solid tumor with focal hemorrhages. The yellow areas represent collections of lipid-laden luteinized granulosa cells. B. The orientation of tumor cells about central spaces results in the characteristic follicular pattern (Call-Exner bodies).

Pathology: Adult-type granulosa cell tumors, like most ovarian tumors, are large and focally cystic to solid. The cut surface shows yellow areas, representing lipid-laden luteinized granulosa cells, and white zones of stroma and focal hemorrhages (Fig. 18-64). Microscopically, granulosa cell tumors display an array of growth patterns: (1) diffuse (sarcomatoid), (2) insular (islands of cells), or (3) trabecular (anastomotic bands of granulosa cells). Haphazard orientation of the nuclei about a central degenerative space *(Call-Exner bodies)* results in a characteristic follicular pattern (Fig. 18-64). The tumor cells are typically spindle-shaped and commonly have a cleaved, elongated nucleus (coffee bean appearance). They secrete inhibin, a protein that suppresses pituitary release of follicle-stimulating hormone (FSH).

Clinical Features: Three fourths of granulosa cell tumors are functional, that is, they secrete estrogens. Consequently, endometrial hyperplasia is a common presenting sign. It may progress to endometrial adenocarcinoma if the functioning granulosa cell tumor remains undetected. When detected clinically, 90% of granulosa cell tumors are confined to the ovary (stage I). These patients have a greater than 90% 10-year survival. Tumors that have extended into the pelvis and lower abdomen have a poorer prognosis. Late recurrence after surgical removal is not uncommon after 5 to 10 years and is usually fatal.

Sertoli-Leydig Cell Tumors

Sertoli-Leydig cell tumor (arrhenoblastoma or androblastoma) is a rare mesenchymal neoplasm of the ovary of low malignant potential that resembles the embryonic testis. It is the prototypical functional tumor associated with androgen secretion. The neoplastic cells typically secrete weak androgens (dehydroepiandrosterone), which accounts for the large tumor size required to achieve masculinizing signs. Sertoli-Leydig cell tumor occurs at all ages but is most common in young women of childbearing age.

Pathology: Sertoli-Leydig cell tumors are unilateral, most measuring between 5 and 15 cm in diameter. They tend to be lobulated, solid, and brown to yellow. Microscopically, the tumors vary from well differentiated to poorly differentiated, and some exhibit heterologous elements (e.g., mucinous glands and, rarely, even cartilage). The most characteristic features are large Leydig cells, which have abundant eosinophilic cytoplasm and a central round to oval nucleus with a prominent nucleolus. The tumor cells are embedded in a sarcomatoid stroma (Fig. 18-65).

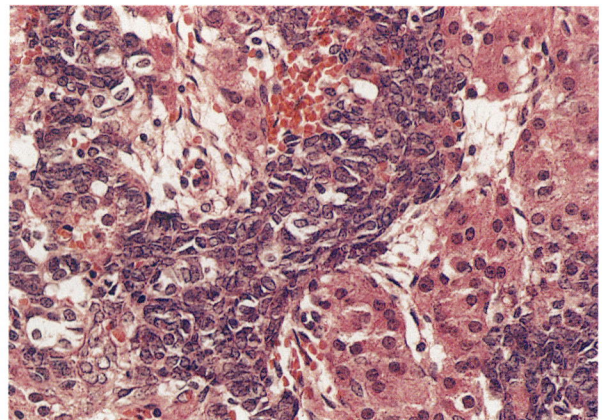

FIGURE 18-65
Sertoli-Leydig cell tumor. Immature solid tubules of embryonic Sertoli cells are adjacent to clusters of Leydig cells that exhibit abundant eosinophilic cytoplasm.

The stroma in some areas often differentiates into immature solid tubules of embryonic Sertoli cells.

 Clinical Features: Nearly half of all patients with Sertoli-Leydig cell tumors exhibit androgenic effects (i.e., signs of virilization, evidenced by hirsutism, male escutcheon, enlarged clitoris, and deepened voice). The initial signs are often defeminization, manifested as breast atrophy, amenorrhea, and loss of hip fat. Once the tumor is removed, the signs disappear or are at least ameliorated. Well-differentiated tumors are virtually always cured by surgical resection, but poorly differentiated ones may metastasize.

Steroid Cell Tumor

Steroid cell tumors of the ovary, also known as *lipid cell* and *lipoid cell tumors,* are composed of cells that resemble lutein cells, Leydig cells, and adrenal cortical cells. Most steroid cell tumors are hormonally active, usually with androgenic manifestations. Some secrete testosterone; others synthesize weaker androgens.

Hilus Cell Tumor

Hilus cell tumor is a specialized form of steroid cell tumor that is typically a benign neoplasm composed of Leydig cells. It arises in the hilus of the ovary, usually after the menopause, and secretes testosterone, which is the most potent of the common androgens. As a result, masculinizing signs are frequent (75%), despite the typically small size of the tumor. Most hilus cell tumors contain *crystalloids of Reinke* (rodlike cytoplasmic structures).

Tumors Metastatic to the Ovary May Mimic a Primary Tumor

About 3% of ovarian cancers arise outside the ovary, the most common primary sites being breast, large intestine, endometrium, and stomach, in descending order. The tumors vary in size from microscopic lesions to large masses. Metastases from the breast are in most cases microscopic and are found in 10% of ovaries removed prophylactically in cases of advanced breast cancer. Of those metastatic tumors large enough to manifest clinically, the colon is the most frequent site of origin. Commonly, the tumor cells stimulate the ovarian stroma to differentiate into hormonally active cells (luteinized stromal cells), thereby inducing androgenic and sometimes estrogenic symptoms.

Krukenberg tumors are ovarian metastases in which the tumor appears as nests of mucin-filled "signet-ring" cells within a cellular stroma derived from the ovary (Fig. 18-66). The stomach is the primary site in 75% of cases, and most of the other Krukenberg tumors are from the colon.

Bilateral ovarian involvement and multinodularity are important clues to the diagnosis of metastatic carcinoma. Both ovaries are grossly involved in 75% of cases. In metastatic disease that is clinically unilateral, the seemingly normal ovary may also contain implants on the surface or

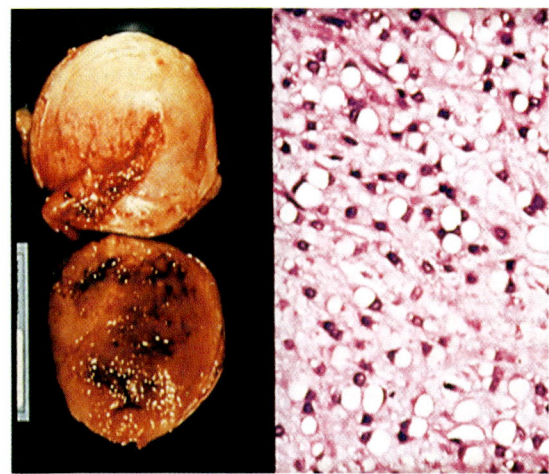

FIGURE 18-66
Krukenberg tumor. A. The ovary is enlarged and partially hemorrhagic. B. A microscopic section of *A* reveals mucinous (signet-ring) cells infiltrating the ovary.

minute foci of tumor within the parenchyma. Thus, when metastasis to one ovary is documented, the surgeon must remove the contralateral ovary as well.

Peritoneum

The peritoneum is a nearly continuous membrane that lines the peritoneal cavity and separates the viscera from the abdominal wall. In men, the peritoneal cavity forms a closed system. In women, the peritoneum is an "open system" that is interrupted in the pelvis by the fallopian tubes. The fallopian tubes provide a final conduit for the transmission of pathogens and chemicals from the genital tract to the peritoneal cavity.

The cells that line the peritoneal cavity and those that form the serosa of the ovary are both of celomic epithelial origin. Thus, whether tumors and tumorlike lesions of the peritoneum and ovary (i.e., müllerian epithelial lesions) are the same entity in both locations remains an open question.

The peritoneum is the site of a wide range of inflammatory lesions, including granulomatous peritonitis as a response to suture materials, surgical glove powder, contrast media, intestinal contents following perforation (e.g., in Crohn disease or diverticulitis), rupture of a mature cystic teratoma (dermoid cyst) of the ovary, and of course, tuberculosis. It is also the site of reactive mesothelial proliferation, which occurs with the slightest irritation. Peritonitis is discussed in Chapter 13.

ENDOMETRIOSIS

Endometriosis refers to the presence of benign endometrial glands and stroma outside the uterus. It afflicts 5 to 10% of women of reproductive age and regresses following natural or artificial menopause. The mean age at diagnosis is between the late 20s and early 30s, although it may appear at any time after menarche. The sites most frequently involved are the ovaries (>60%), other uterine adnexae (uterine ligaments, rectovaginal septum, pouch of Douglas), and the pelvic peritoneum covering the uterus, fallopian tubes, rectosigmoid colon, and

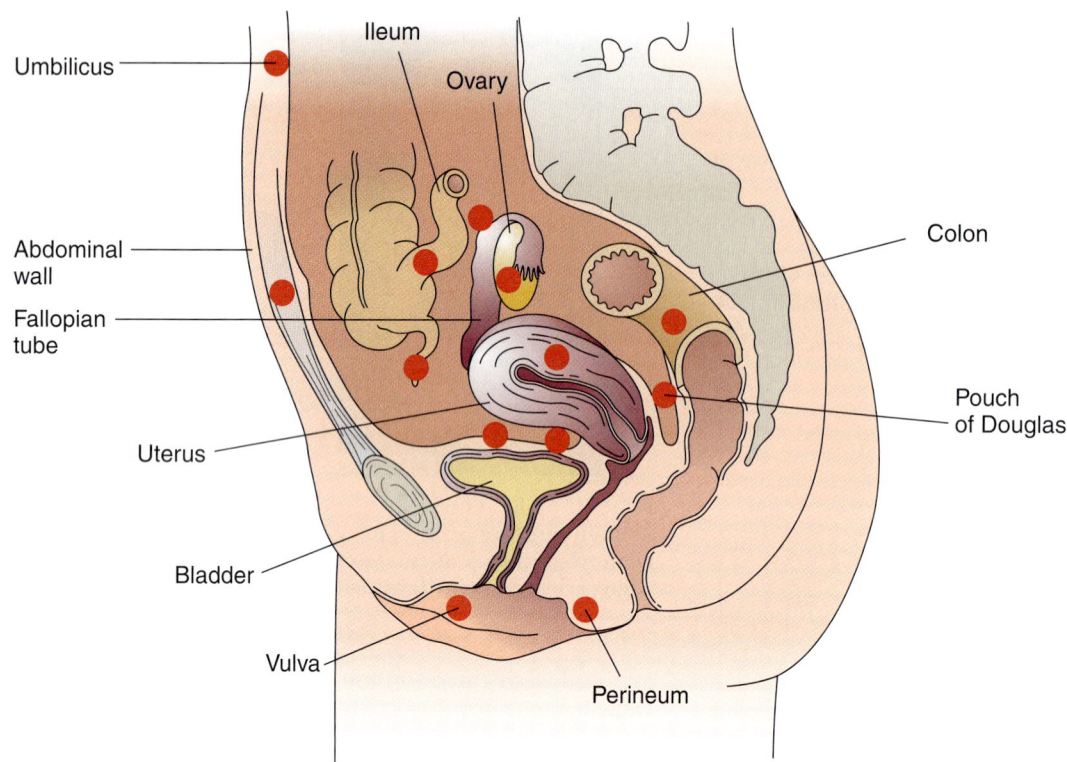

FIGURE 18-67
Sites of endometriosis.

bladder (Fig. 18-67). Endometriosis can be even more widespread and occasionally affects the cervix, vagina, perineum, bladder, and umbilicus. Even the pelvic lymph nodes may contain foci of endometriosis. On rare occasions, distant areas such as lungs, pleura, small bowel, kidneys, and bones contain lesions.

 Pathogenesis: Theories to explain the histogenesis of endometriosis include the following:

Transplantation of endometrial fragments to ectopic sites
Metaplasia of the multipotential celomic peritoneum
Induction of undifferentiated mesenchyme in ectopic sites to form lesions after exposure to substances released from shed endometrium.

TRANSPLANTATION: The most widely accepted theory holds that foci of menstrual endometrium reflux through the fallopian tubes and implant at ectopic sites. In this context, retrograde menstruation through the fallopian tubes occurs in 90% of women. An extension of the transplantation theory is lymphatic and hematogenous dissemination, which would explain the occurrence of endometriosis at distant sites such as the lungs and kidneys. The observation that pulmonary endometriosis occurs almost exclusively in women who have been subjected to uterine surgery supports this contention. The presence of endometriosis in lymph nodes is consistent with similar lymphatic dissemination.

CELOMIC METAPLASIA: The metaplastic theory proposes that endometriosis arises in the pelvis and elsewhere by endometrial metaplasia of the peritoneal serosa or serosa-like structures. According to this concept, the pelvic peritoneum can potentially differentiate, if appropriately stimulated, into any type of müllerian epithelium.

INDUCTION THEORY: This concept offers an alternative to the transplantation postulate and suggests that some substance secreted by the endometrium induces the development of endometrial epithelium and stroma in ectopic sites.

 Pathology: On gross examination, the lesions of endometriosis vary in color. Yellow-red stains, when confined to the serosa, reflect breakdown of blood products and often are the earliest detectable lesions. Red lesions also reflect an early form of the disease, in which foci of endometriosis are actively growing. Pathologists usually see black lesions in operative specimens, which show some degree of resolution. Such foci on the ovary and peritoneal surfaces, termed "mulberry" nodules, are 1 to 5 mm in diameter. With repeated cycles, hemorrhage, and the onset of fibrosis, the affected surface may show scarring and take on a grossly brown discoloration ("powder burns"). Over time, fibrous adhesions may become more pronounced. Sometimes, the scarring leads to complications, such as intestinal obstruction. In the ovaries, repeated hemorrhage may cause the endometriotic foci to form cysts up to 15 cm in diameter, which contain inspissated, chocolate-colored material *(chocolate cysts)*.

Microscopically, endometriosis shows ectopic endometrial glands and stroma (Fig. 18-68). Occasionally, healed foci of endometriosis may consist only of fibrous tissue and hemosiderin-laden macrophages, features that by them-

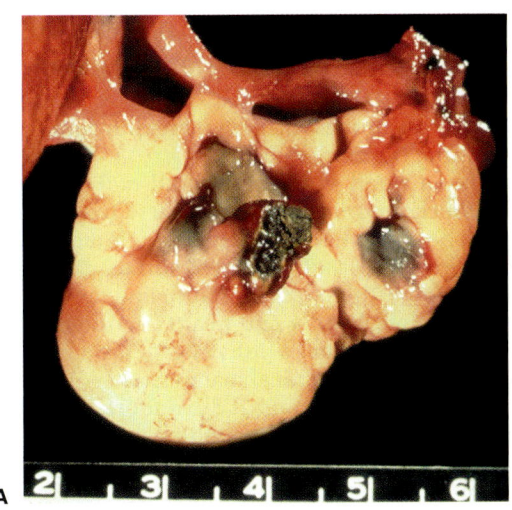
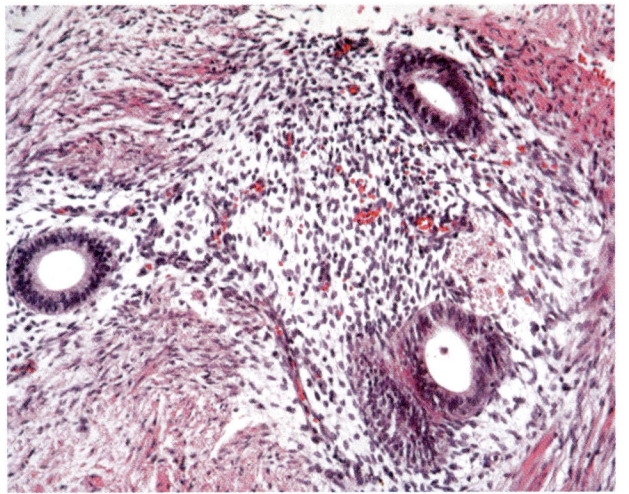

FIGURE 18-68
Endometriosis. A. Implants of endometriosis on the ovary appear as red-blue nodules. B. A microscopic section shows endometrial glands and stroma in the ovary.

selves are not diagnostic. Demonstration of CD-10 expression can be diagnostic.

 Clinical Features: The signs and symptoms of endometriosis depend on the location of the implants. The most common complaint is dysmenorrhea, related to implants on the uterosacral ligaments. These lesions swell immediately before or during menstruation, producing pelvic pain. In fact, half of all women with dysmenorrhea have endometriosis. Dyspareunia and cyclical abdominal pain may be troublesome.

Infertility is the primary complaint in a third of women with endometriosis (Fig. 18-69). The hormonal mi-

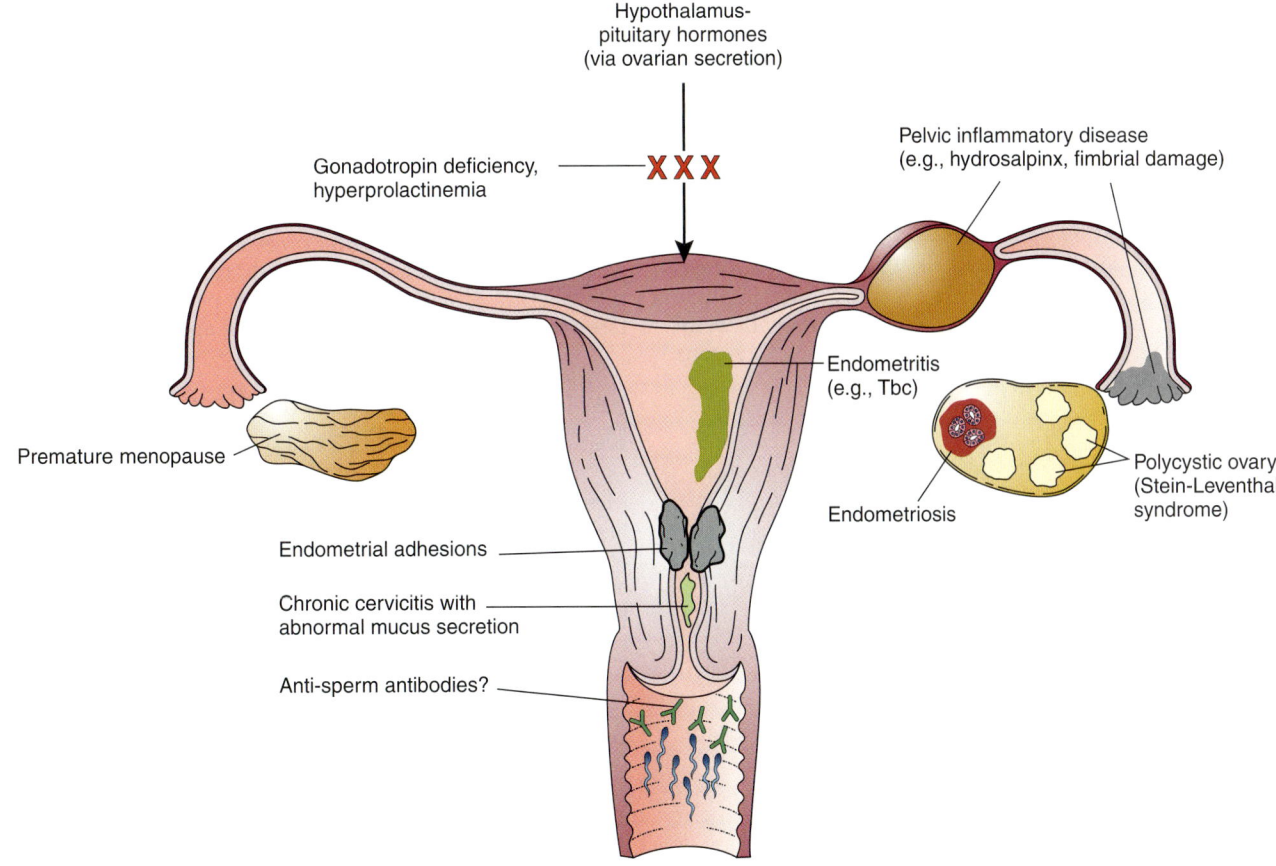

FIGURE 18-69
Causes of acquired infertility.

lieu in a woman who does not achieve pregnancy encourages the development of endometriosis. In turn, once endometriosis develops, its presence contributes to the infertile state, and a vicious circle is established. Conversely, pregnancy often has a beneficial effect on the disease. With conservative surgery to restore the pelvic anatomy, many of women who suffer from endometriosis eventually become pregnant.

Malignant transformation occurs in about 1 to 2% of cases of endometriosis. Clear cell and endometrioid tumors are the most frequent forms. Adenosarcoma, although rare, is the most common sarcoma.

MESOTHELIAL TUMORS

Tumors of mesothelial origin range from neoplastic but benign to multicentric and aggressive malignancies.

Adenomatoid Tumor Is a Benign Mesothelial Neoplasm

Adenomatoid tumor is encountered in the fallopian tube and in the subserosal tissue of the uterine corpus near the fallopian tube. It is seldom encountered elsewhere in the peritoneal cavity.

Well-Differentiated Papillary Mesothelioma Is Benign

A rare form of peritoneal mesothelioma, well-differentiated papillary mesothelioma is a rare neoplasm of women in the reproductive age. The lesions are typically asymptomatic and usually found incidentally at operation. The tumors are typically solitary, small, broad-based, wartlike excrescences that are polypoid or nodular. Microscopically, thick papillae are covered by a single layer of small cuboidal cells with bland nuclei (Fig. 18-70). These lesions often resemble serous epithelial tumors, but the two are treated differently.

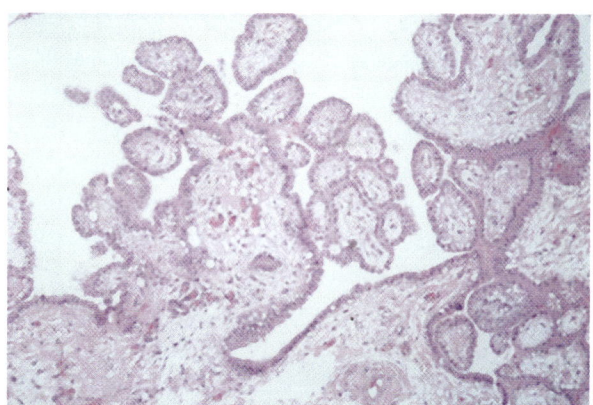

FIGURE 18-70
Well-differentiated peritoneal mesothelioma.

Diffuse Malignant Mesothelioma Is an Invariably Fatal Peritoneal Tumor

Diffuse malignant mesothelioma, arises from the mesothelium covering the peritoneum. It is rare in women and comprises only a small proportion of all malignant mesotheliomas, which are mostly pleural. These tumors need to be distinguished from serous adenocarcinomas, including those arising from the peritoneal surface itself and those metastatic from the ovary, because the survival rates of mesothelioma are so poor and treatment differs from that of serous adenocarcinoma. Most patients are middle-aged or postmenopausal. The clinical manifestations are nonspecific and include ascites, abdominal discomfort, digestive disturbances, and weight loss. Although asbestos exposure is uncommon in women with peritoneal mesothelioma compared to pleural tumors, as many as 2 million fibers per gram of wet weight have been reported in some tumors.

 Pathology: Diffuse malignant mesothelioma extensively involves and thickens the peritoneum and the serosa of the various abdominal and pelvic organs. On microscopic examination, it has a tubulopapillary to solid pattern. Unlike pleural mesothelioma, the sarcomatoid type is rare. The epithelial variant displays polygonal or cuboidal neoplastic cells with abundant cytoplasm. No effective treatment is available.

SEROUS TUMORS (PRIMARY AND METASTATIC)

Unlike the ovary, which features a wide range of tumors, serous tumors are virtually the only type encountered in the peritoneum. Mucinous tumors in the peritoneum are metastases from a primary neoplasm in the appendix or ovary.

Serous Tumor of Borderline Malignancy Resembles the Ovarian Neoplasm

Most serous borderline tumors in the peritoneum are metastases from the ovary, but some may be primary in the peritoneum. In the latter case, serous peritoneal tumors without evidence of invasion usually follow a benign course; those that are invasive carry a worse prognosis.

 Pathology: Whether it is in the ovary or the peritoneum, a serous tumor of borderline malignancy is characterized by papillary processes, small clusters of cells, cell stratification, detached cellular clusters, nuclear atypia, and mitotic activity in the absence of invasion. Grossly, the implants appear as fine granularities or small nodules on the peritoneum. Microscopic examination dis-

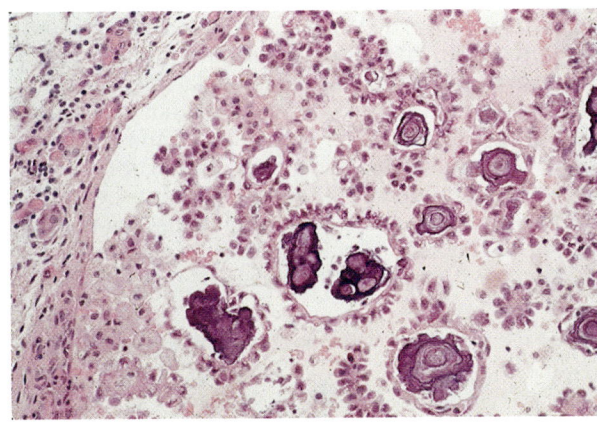

FIGURE 18-71
Noninvasive implants of borderline serous tumor on the peritoneum exhibit epithelial tufts and psammoma bodies.

closes clusters of blunt papillae or glandular structures, often with complex cellular tufts (Fig. 18-71). Psammoma bodies are common and may fill the core of the papillae. Mild-to-severe cytological atypia with some stratification is common but is substantially less than that seen in adenocarcinoma.

Serous Adenocarcinoma Occurs in Women With Normal Ovaries

The frequency of serous adenocarcinoma arising de novo in the peritoneum is estimated as 10% of its counterpart in the ovary. The mean age of women with this tumor is 50 to 65 years. The diagnosis of a primary peritoneal tumor requires the demonstration of normal ovaries. Abdominal pain and ascites are frequent presentations. Like ovarian cancer, serous adenocarcinoma primary in the peritoneum may have a familial basis and can metastasize to distant locations.

PSEUDOMYXOMA PERITONEI

Pseudomyxoma peritonei *refers to the accumulation of jellylike mucus in the pelvic or peritoneal cavity.* Although historically interpreted as stage 3 spread from mucinous ovarian tumors, it is now recognized that many if not most of the tumors are actually mucus-producing adenocarcinomas of the appendix.

 Pathology: The condition may be extensive and appear as semisolid gelatin covering all of the abdominal structures or there may be little more than a slightly thickened gelatinous coat over a focal area of bowel or omentum. During surgery, the appendix will commonly be found to be enlarged or adherent to omentum that is covered with the gelatinous material. Microscopically, the gelatin discloses strips of extremely well differentiated, intestinal-type, mucinous epithelium (Fig. 18-72). If only isolated foci are present, the epithelium may be so well differ-

entiated that it resembles a simple mucinous adenoma. Occasionally, cribriform patterns or other histological features of malignancy, such as signet-ring cells, warrant a diagnosis of adenocarcinoma.

Low-grade tumors are usually treated for cure, which consists of aggressive surgical debulking and intraperitoneal chemotherapy. The 5-year survival rate is less than 50%.

Placenta and Gestational Disease

DEVELOPMENT

The fertilized ovum implants in the endometrium about 5 days after ovulation. The blastocyst gives rise to three layers of trophoblast:

- **The cytotrophoblast** constitutes the germinative layer of the placenta and is devoid of hormones. The cells are small and mononuclear.
- **The syncytiotrophoblast,** the most differentiated form of trophoblast, is composed of large multinucleated cells. These cells contain numerous hormones, among them hCG and human placental lactogen (hPL).
- **The intermediate trophoblastic cells** are a transitional form between cytotrophoblasts and syncytiotrophoblasts. These are mononuclear cells but have an eosinophilic cytoplasm closely resembling syncytiotrophoblast. Intermediate cells contain mainly hPL and small quantities of hCG.

Trophoblast functions to (1) foster implantation of the blastocyst, (2) develop the uteroplacental circulation, and (3) synthesize hormones.

Chorionic villi develop on day 21 from the primary villous stems that extend into the intervillous space. By the fourth month of gestation, the definitive placenta is developed, and no further anatomical alterations occur, although growth continues until parturition.

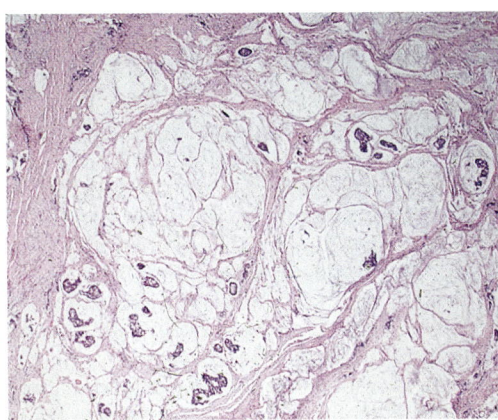

FIGURE 18-72
Pseudomyxoma peritonei. Multiple clusters of tumor cells are present in the mucinous material.

ANATOMY

The placenta contains some 200 subunits called *lobules*. The primary stem villi originate from the chorionic plate and branch into secondary and then tertiary stem villi. The lobules form from the tertiary stem villi, which course through the intervillous space toward the basal plate. There they insert and reenter the intervillous space, dividing into a complex terminal villous network. Fetal blood enters the placenta through two umbilical arteries that spiral around the umbilical vein. Each artery supplies one half of the placenta.

The terminal villus is the placenta's functional unit and is composed of an inner layer of cytotrophoblast *(Langhans cells)*, a middle layer of intermediate trophoblast, and an outer layer of syncytiotrophoblast. The villous stroma consists of loose mesenchyme that contains macrophages *(Hofbauer cells)*. During the second trimester, the villi become smaller and more numerous, the cytotrophoblastic cells and intermediate trophoblast become less prominent, and the syncytiotrophoblast attenuates. The villous capillaries grow larger and more numerous and remain mainly within the center of the villi. This process continues until term.

In the third trimester, syncytiotrophoblastic nuclei aggregate to form multinuclear protrusions referred to as *syncytial knots*. In other areas along the villous surface, the syncytium between the knots thins markedly and attenuates. At these points, the trophoblastic cytoplasm comes into direct contact with the endothelium of the fetal capillaries to form the *vasculosyncytial membrane*. These specialized zones facilitate gas and nutrient transfer across the placenta. Nonmembranous areas play a role in hormone synthesis.

INFECTIONS

Chorioamnionitis Results from Ascending Infection

Chorioamnionitis refers to inflammation of the placental amnion and chorion and the extraplacental membranes. Infectious organisms ascend from the maternal birth canal, commonly owing to premature rupture of the membranes. The inflammatory process affects primarily the membranes (chorioamnionitis) rather than the chorionic villi.

 Pathology: The amniotic fluid is usually cloudy. The membrane walls are slightly opaque, malodorous, and edematous. Microscopically, they disclose a neutrophilic infiltrate, often with fibrin deposition. With more-extensive spread, the umbilical cord may become infected *(funisitis)* and may exhibit vasculitis of one or more umbilical vessels or inflammation of the cord mesenchyme *(Wharton jelly)*. Generally, the chorionic villi remain free of the inflammatory infiltrate. Microorganisms isolated from placentas with chorioamnionitis, in descending frequency, are the genital mycoplasmas (*U. urealyticum, M. hominis*) anaerobic organisms of the *Bacteroides* group, and aerobes (group B streptococci, *E. coli,* and *G. vaginalis*).

 Clinical Features: Acute chorioamnionitis is found in 10% of placentas and is associated with preterm labor, fetal and neonatal infections, and intrauterine hypoxia. The risks of chorioamnionitis to the fetus include (1) pneumonia after inhalation of infected amniotic fluid, (2) skin or eye infections from direct contact with organisms in the fluid, and (3) neonatal gastritis, enteritis, or peritonitis from ingestion of infected fluid. Major risks to the mother are intrapartum fever, postpartum endometritis, and pelvic sepsis with venous thrombosis.

Villitis May Reflect Hematogenous Infection

Infection of chorionic villi results from endometritis or transplacental passage of organisms delivered by way of the maternal circulation. The process is frequently focal. Although the infection cannot be demonstrated in most cases, the microorganisms include (1) bacteria (*T. pallidum, M. tuberculosis, Mycoplasma* spp., *Chlamydia* spp.), (2) viruses (rubella, cytomegalovirus, herpes), (3) parasites and protozoa (*Toxoplasma* spp.), and (4) fungi (*Candida* spp.). The most important consequence of hematogenous placental infection is the establishment of an inflammatory focus that can then secondarily infect the fetus. Approximately 30% of the villi must be destroyed before perinatal mortality significantly increases.

PREECLAMPSIA AND ECLAMPSIA

The hypertensive disorders of pregnancy, known as preeclampsia and eclampsia, define a syndrome of hypertension, proteinuria, and edema, and in its most advanced stage, convulsions. Preeclampsia occurs in 6% of pregnant women during the last trimester, especially with the first child. The disorder is termed *eclampsia* if convulsive seizures appear.

 Pathogenesis: In the past eclampsia was called toxemia of pregnancy, but that term is a misnomer, since no toxin has been identified. The pathogenesis of preeclampsia and eclampsia is still not resolved. Immunological and genetic factors have been invoked as well as altered vascular reactivity, endothelial injury, and coagulation abnormalities. (Fig. 18-73). Regardless of the precise cause, certain features are characteristic:

- Preeclampsia occurs with hydatidiform mole (see below), which suggests that the trophoblast is the most likely responsible tissue and that preeclampsia is a trophoblastic disease. Even though the hemodynamic, renal, and endothelial systems are essential for this disorder to develop, preeclampsia is not a primary disease in any of these systems.

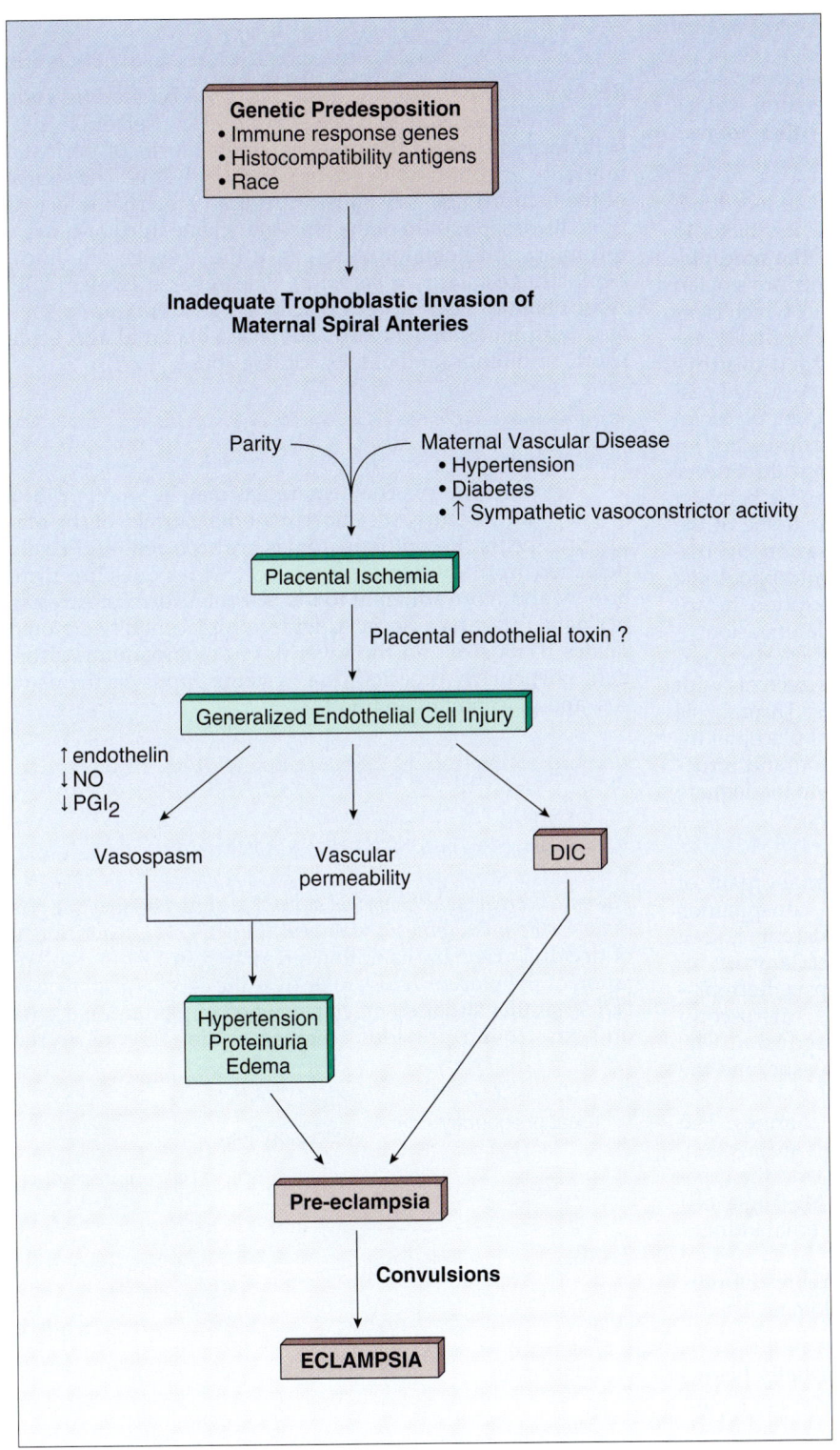

FIGURE 18-73
Pathogenesis of preeclampsia and eclampsia.

- Maternal blood flow to the placenta is markedly reduced because the normal changes in the maternal spiral arteries of the placental bed do not take place.
- Renal involvement in preeclampsia contributes to hypertension and proteinuria.
- Disseminated intravascular coagulation is a prominent feature of preeclampsia, manifested as fibrin thrombi in the liver, brain, and kidneys. Treatment with antiplatelet agents, particularly aspirin in low doses, ameliorates or prevents preeclampsia.
- The first pregnancy presents a risk for the syndrome that is many-fold higher than that associated with subsequent pregnancies. The incidence is also increased in women whose current pregnancy was conceived with a different partner than the first pregnancy, and in women with a history of using barrier contraception. These findings sug-

gest that previous antigen exposure may protect against the disease.

- Eclampsia is a cerebrovascular malady characterized by seizures, worsening hypertension, and cerebral edema. It is often the first sign of preeclampsia but does not necessarily evolve from that condition.

The pathological changes in the placenta reflect reduced maternal blood flow to the uteroplacental unit. **The key factor in preeclampsia resides in the spiral arteries of the uteroplacental bed, which never fully dilate.** The arteries are smaller than normal and retain their musculoelastic wall, which is ordinarily attenuated by infiltrative trophoblasts. Normally, extravillous trophoblast invades these arteries and destroys their vascular tone. As a result, the vessels become dilated passive conduits of blood from the mother to the fetoplacental unit. In preeclampsia, up to half of the spiral arteries escape invasion by endovascular trophoblastic tissue and thus never dilate. There is an inappropriate immune response between the trophoblastic tissue and the musculoelastic tissue of the spiral artery that prevents appropriate invasion by trophoblast. There are also data to suggest that cytotrophoblastic cells do not differentiate properly and do not express the appropriate adhesion molecules that allow vascular invasion.

In women with preeclampsia, the spiral arteries commonly exhibit *acute atherosis*, namely fibrinoid necrosis with the accumulation of lipid-laden macrophages. Thrombosis of these vessels is frequent and results in focal placental infarctions. The combination of vasoconstriction and structural changes in the spiral arteries contributes to inadequate blood flow and placental ischemia.

 Pathology: The placenta and maternal organs of women with preeclampsia show conspicuous changes. Extensive infarction of the placenta is seen in nearly one third of women with severe preeclampsia, although it is often negligible in mild preeclampsia. Retroplacental hemorrhage occurs in 15% of patients. Microscopically, the chorionic villi show signs of underperfusion. The cytotrophoblastic cells lining them are hyperplastic, and the basement membrane is thickened.

The kidneys always show glomerular changes. The glomeruli are enlarged, and the endothelial cells are swollen. Fibrin is present between the endothelial cells and the basement membrane of the glomerular capillaries. Mesangial cell hyperplasia is the rule. The changes in the maternal kidneys are reversible with therapy or after delivery.

Fatal cases of eclampsia often show cerebral hemorrhages, ranging from petechiae to large hematomas.

 Clinical Features: Preeclampsia usually begins insidiously after the 20th week of pregnancy with (1) excessive weight gain occasioned by fluid retention, (2) increased maternal blood pressure, and (3) the appearance of proteinuria. As the disease progresses from mild to severe preeclampsia, the diastolic pressure persistently exceeds 110 mm Hg. Proteinuria is greater than 3 g/day, and renal function declines. Disseminated intravascular coagulation often supervenes. Preeclampsia is treated with antihypertensive agents and antiplatelet drugs, but the definitive therapy is the removal of the placenta, hopefully by normal delivery. Eclampsia is treated with magnesium sulfate, which reduces cerebrovascular tone.

RETROPLACENTAL HEMATOMA

Retroplacental hematoma is defined as blood between the basal plate of the placenta and the uterine wall. Retroplacental hematoma is one of the most common causes of perinatal mortality, accounting for 8% of perinatal deaths. The source of the hemorrhage is usually a ruptured maternal artery or premature separation of the placenta. In one third of cases, a retroplacental hematoma occurs in the absence of clinical hemorrhage *(abruptio placenta)*. The reverse is also true. About half of cases of retroplacental hematoma are associated with maternal smoking, advanced maternal age, acute chorioamnionitis, and of late, cocaine abuse.

 Pathology: The hematomas may be small or they may occupy the entire maternal surface of the placenta. Recent hematomas are soft, red, and easily detached from the maternal surface. Older ones are firm, brown, and more adherent to the placental surface. Adverse perinatal outcome associated with retroplacental hematoma relates to its size and the severity of accompanying disorders, particularly preeclampsia, systemic lupus erythematosus, and placental infarction.

PLACENTA ACCRETA

Placenta accreta is the abnormal adherence of part or all of the placenta to the underlying uterine wall (Fig. 18-74). A deficiency of decidua at the implantation site may result from implantation of the placenta close to or over the cervix *(placenta previa)*. A similar situation may arise when implantation occurs on scars from a previous cesarean section. Owing to the

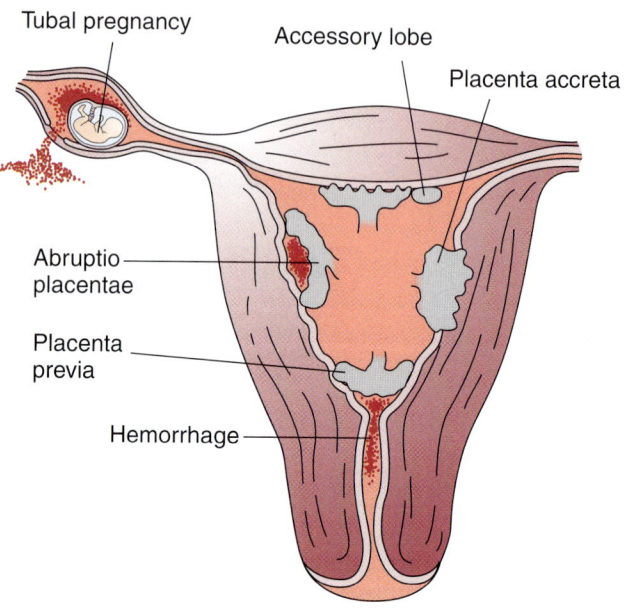

FIGURE 18-74
Uteroplacental abnormalities.

absence of decidua, the placenta does not separate normally from the underlying uterine wall following parturition, an event that can result in life-threatening bleeding.

 Pathology: Placenta accreta is subclassified according to the depth of villous invasion into the myometrium:

- **Placenta accreta** refers to the attachment of villi to the myometrium without further invasion.
- **Placenta increta** defines villi invading the underlying myometrium.
- **Placenta percreta** describes villi penetrating the full thickness of the uterine wall.

The placental villi in these placental disorders are normal and show no evidence of hyperplastic trophoblastic proliferation.

 Clinical Features: Most patients with placenta accreta have a normal pregnancy and delivery. However, complications may occur during pregnancy, delivery, or especially in the immediate postpartum state. Bleeding in the third trimester is the most common presenting sign before delivery. Uterine rupture before, during, or after labor occurs in 15% of patients. Substantial fragments of placenta may remain adherent following delivery and are a source of postpartum hemorrhage. The bleeding can be difficult to control and not uncommonly requires emergency hysterectomy. An attempt to remove the attached placental fragments can itself cause hemorrhage and even uterine inversion. Placenta accreta is a serious complication of pregnancy and is associated with a maternal death rate of 2%.

MULTIPLE GESTATIONS

Twinning occurs in slightly under 1% of pregnancies and may be dizygotic or monozygotic (Fig. 18-75).

DIZYGOTIC TWINS: The fertilization of two separate ova results in twins that are genetically different; they may be of the same or opposite sex. Dizygotic twinning has a strong hereditary component, which is confined to the maternal side. The frequency of dizygotic twinning and multiple gestations is increased in women who have used hormones to artificially induce ovulation or who have been impregnated after in vitro fertilization.

Separate placentas develop when two fertilized ova implant apart from one another. If the ova implant near each other, the two placentas show varying degrees of fusion and may appear as one. When the ova implant apart, there are discrete conceptuses, each placenta having its own amniotic sac. In the case of placental fusion, microscopic examination of the intervening membranes between the two fetuses discloses two amnions and two chorions (diamnionic, dichorionic gestation).

MONOZYGOTIC TWINS: Early division of a single fertilized ovum results in twins that are genetically identical and therefore of the same sex. If a single fertilized ovum divides within 2 days of fertilization, before the trophoblast has differentiated, two separate embryos develop, each with its own placenta and amniotic sac (dichorionic, diamniotic twinning). Hence, scrutiny of the placenta cannot always distinguish between monozygotic and dizygotic twinning. If division occurs between the 3rd and 8th days after conception, the trophoblast (but not the amniotic cavity) has already differentiated. A single placenta with two amniotic sacs develops (monochorionic, diamniotic twinning). A monochorionic, monoamniotic placenta is formed if division occurs between the 8th and 13th day after conception, because the amniotic cavity has already developed. Division at later periods results in conjoint (Siamese) twins.

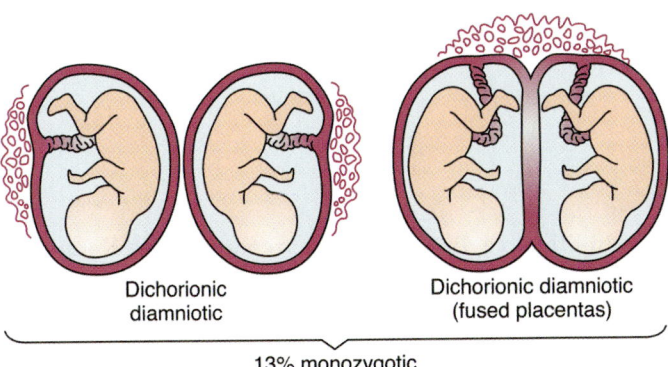
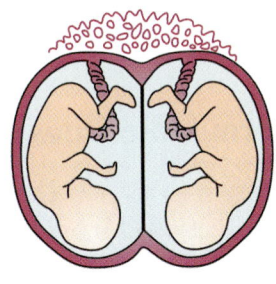
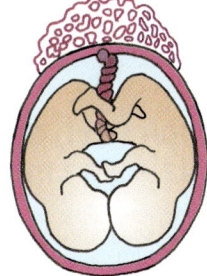

FIGURE 18-75

Placental structure in twin pregnancies. The percentages in the figure refer to the proportion of total twin pregnancies (100%) accounted for by each variant.

SPONTANEOUS ABORTION

The term spontaneous abortion *applies to a pregnancy that terminates before the fetus is capable of extrauterine life, which currently is about the 22nd week of gestation.* Some 15% of recognized pregnancies abort spontaneously, and an additional 30% of women abort without being aware that pregnancy has occurred. **Thus, the overall spontaneous abortion rate is estimated to be 45%.**

Pathogenesis: The principal factors responsible for abortion are maternal and fetal and include the following:

- Infection early in pregnancy
- Mechanical factors (e.g., submucous uterine leiomyoma or cervical incompetence)
- Endocrine factors (e.g., inadequate progesterone production)
- Immunological factors
- Fetal congenital abnormalities (e.g., neural tube defects)
- Chromosomal abnormalities

Pathology: Pathological examination of the abortus and placenta is often difficult because the aborted tissue is often fragmented and/or macerated by the time the pathologist receives it. Fetal products, if identified, should be examined for changes suggesting chromosomal anomalies. An empty gestational sac with hydropic swelling of the chorionic villi (blighted ovum) suggests early demise of the fetus. Microscopically, the chorionic villi in spontaneous abortion may appear normal for gestational age or show intravillous fibrosis or hydropic change.

GESTATIONAL TROPHOBLASTIC DISEASE

The term *gestational trophoblastic disease* embraces the spectrum of trophoblastic disorders that exhibit abnormal proliferation and maturation of trophoblast, as well as neoplasms derived from the trophoblast (Fig. 18-76).

Complete Hydatidiform Mole Does Not Contain an Embryo

Complete hydatidiform mole is a placenta that has grossly swollen chorionic villi, resembling bunches of grapes, in which there are varying degrees of trophoblastic proliferation. The villi are enlarged, often exceeding 5 mm in diameter (Fig. 18-77).

Pathogenesis: Complete mole results from the fertilization of an empty ovum that lacks functional DNA. The haploid (23,X) set of paternal chromo-

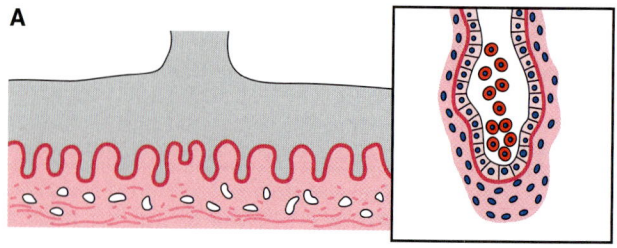
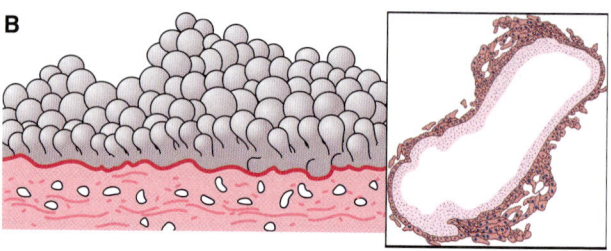
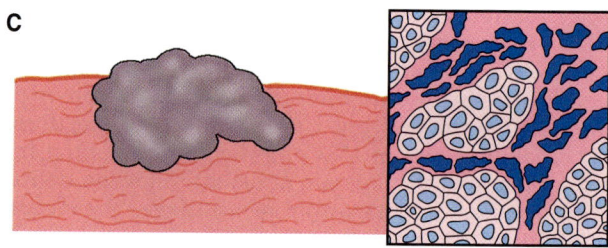
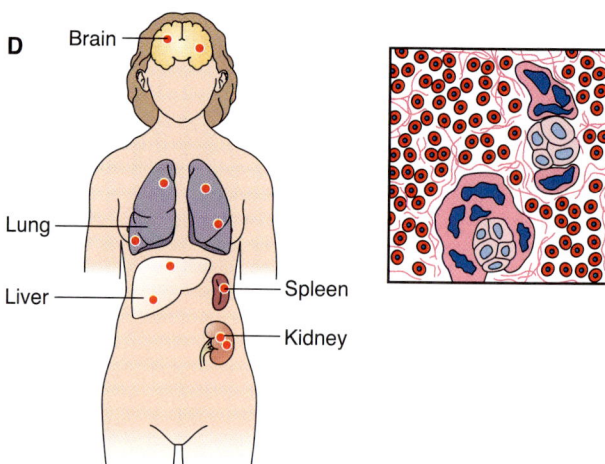

FIGURE 18-76
Proliferative disorders of the trophoblast. **A.** Normal chorionic villus of 8-week fetus, with blood vessel containing nucleated red blood cells. **B.** Complete hydatidiform mole with hydropic villi. The villi are enlarged by an edematous stroma devoid of blood vessels. The trophoblastic epithelium is hyperplastic and exhibits variable atypia. **C.** Choriocarcinoma that has arisen in a molar pregnancy invades the myometrium and consists of admixed syncytiotrophoblastic and cytotrophoblastic elements. **D.** Common sites of metastasis from choriocarcinoma.

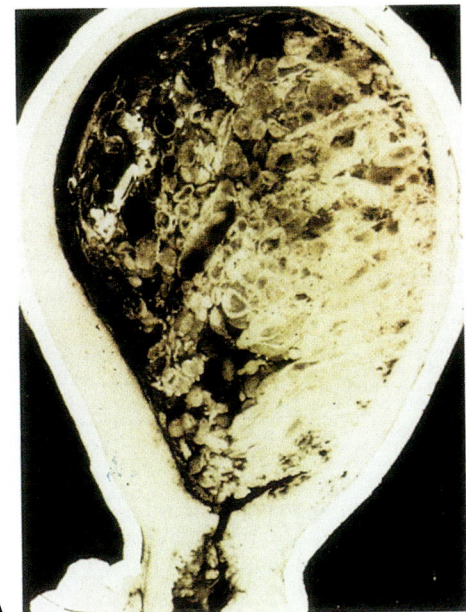
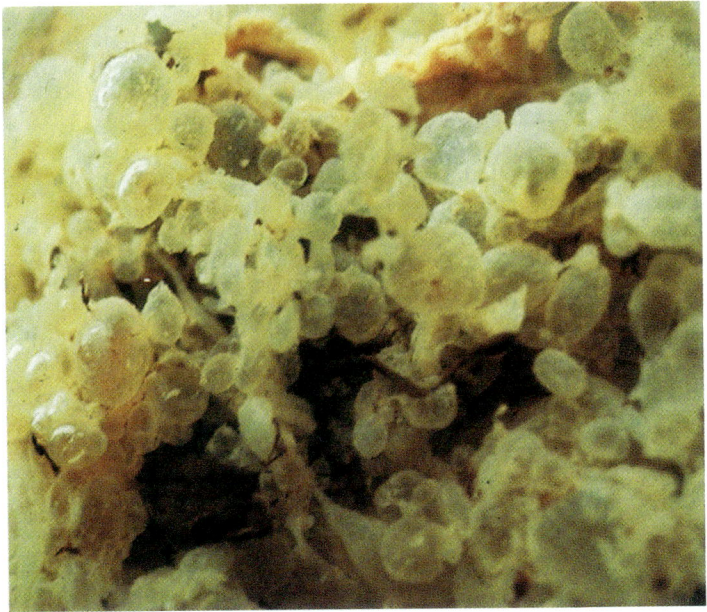
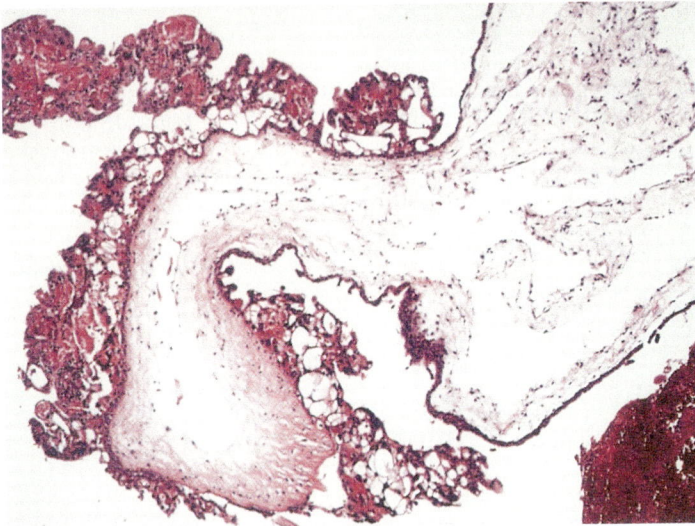

FIGURE 18-77
Complete hydatidiform mole. A. Complete mole in which the entire uterine cavity is filled with swollen villi. **B.** The villi are each 1 to 3 mm in diameter and appear grapelike. **C.** Individual molar villi, many of which have cavitated central cisterns, exhibit considerable trophoblastic hyperplasia and atypia. The blood vessels of the villi have atrophied and disappeared.

somes duplicates to 46,XX. Hence, most complete moles are homozygous 46,XX, but all the chromosomes are of paternal origin. Since the embryo dies at a very early stage, before placental circulation has developed, few chorionic villi develop blood vessels, and fetal parts are absent.

RISK FACTORS: The risk for developing hydatidiform mole relates to maternal age and has two peaks. Girls younger than 15 years of age have a 20-fold higher risk than women of ages 20 to 35 years. The risk increases progressively for women older than 40 years of age. In fact, women older than 50 years of age have a risk 200 times greater than those between 20 and 40 years of age. Ethnic background and obstetric history also influence the risk of developing hydatidiform mole. The incidence is many-fold higher in Asian women than among white women, reaching a frequency in Taiwan 25 times that in the United States. Women who have had a previous hydatidiform mole have a 20-fold greater risk than the general population to develop a subsequent molar pregnancy.

 Pathology: Molar tissue is voluminous and consists of macroscopically visible villi that are obviously swollen. Microscopically, many individual villi have cisternae, which are central, acellular, fluid-filled spaces devoid of mesenchymal cells. The trophoblast is hyperplastic and composed of syncytiotrophoblast, cytotrophoblast and intermediate trophoblast. Considerable cellular atypia is present.

 Clinical Features: Patients with complete moles commonly present between the 11th and 25th weeks of pregnancy and complain of excessive uterine enlargement and often abnormal uterine bleeding. Passage of tissue fragments, which appear as small grapelike masses, is common. The serum hCG concentration is markedly elevated, and serial determinations disclose rapidly increasing levels.

Complications of complete mole include uterine hemorrhage, disseminated intravascular coagulation, uterine perforation, trophoblastic embolism, and infection. **The most**

important complication is the development of choriocarcinoma, which occurs in about 2% of patients after the mole has been evacuated.

Treatment of hydatidiform mole consists of suction curettage of the uterus and subsequent monitoring of serum hCG levels. As many as 20% of patients require adjuvant chemotherapy for persistent disease, as judged by stable or rising hCG levels. The presence of aneuploidy in the molar tissue may help to identify patients who will require adjuvant treatment. With such management, the survival rate approaches 100%.

Partial Hydatidiform Mole Features Triploid Cells

Partial hydatidiform mole is a distinct form of mole that almost never evolves into choriocarcinoma (see Table 18-11). Partial hydatidiform moles have 69 chromosomes (triploidy). This abnormal chromosomal complement results from the fertilization of a normal ovum (23,X) by two normal spermatozoa, each carrying 23 chromosomes, or a single spermatozoon that has not undergone meiotic reduction and bears 46 chromosomes. The fetus associated with a partial mole usually dies after 10 weeks gestation, and the mole is aborted shortly thereafter. In contrast to a complete mole, fetal parts are commonly present.

 Pathology: Partial moles have two populations of chorionic villi. Some villi are normal; others are enlarged by hydropic swelling and show central cav-

TABLE 18-11 Comparative Features of Complete and Partial Hydatidiform Mole

Features	Complete Mole	Partial Mole
Karyotype	46,XX	47,XXY or 47,XXX
Preoperative diagnosis	Mole	Missed abortion
Marked vaginal bleeding	3+	1+
Uterus	Large	Small
Serum hCG	High	Less elevated
Hydropic villi	All	Some
Trophoblastic proliferation	Diffuse	Focal
Atypia	Diffuse	Minimal
hCG in tissue	3+	1+
Embryo present	No	Some
Blood vessels	No	Common
Nucleated erythrocytes	No	Sometimes
Persists after initial therapy	20%	7%
Choriocarcinoma	2% after mole	No choriocarcinoma

hCG, human chorionic gonadotropin.

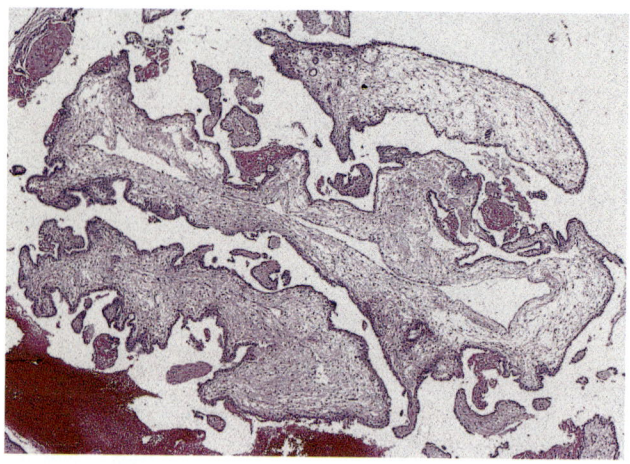

FIGURE 18-78
Partial hydatidiform mole. Two populations of chorionic villi are evident. Some are normal; others are conspicuously swollen. Trophoblastic proliferation is focal and less conspicuous than in a complete mole.

itation, resulting from tangential histological sections of invaginated surface epithelium ("fjord-like") (Fig. 18-78). Trophoblastic proliferation is focal and much less pronounced than in the complete mole. Blood vessels are typically found within the chorionic villi and contain fetal (nucleated) erythrocytes.

Invasive Hydatidiform Mole Penetrates the Underlying Myometrium

 Pathology: Villi of a hydatidiform mole may extend only superficially into the myometrium or may invade the uterus and even involve the broad ligament. The mole tends to enter dilated venous channels in the myometrium, and a third of them spread to distant sites, most frequently the lungs. Unlike choriocarcinoma (see below), distant deposits of an invasive mole do not penetrate beyond the confines of the blood vessels in which they are lodged, and death from such spread is unusual. The clinical distinction between invasive mole and choriocarcinoma is often difficult.

Histologically, invasive moles show less hydropic change than complete moles. Trophoblastic proliferation is usually prominent. Uterine perforation is a major complication, but occurs in only a minority of cases. Theca lutein cysts, which may occur with any form of trophoblastic disease as a result of hCG stimulation, are prominent with invasive moles.

Choriocarcinoma Is a Tumor Allograft in the Host Mother

Gestational choriocarcinoma is a malignant tumor derived from trophoblast.

 Epidemiology: Choriocarcinoma occurs in 1 in 30,000 pregnancies in the United States; in the Orient, the frequency is far greater. The incidence of choriocarcinoma seems related to abnormalities of pregnancy. Thus, the incidence is 1 in 160,000 normal gestations, 1 in 15,000 spontaneous abortions, 1 in 5000 ectopic pregnancies, and 1 in 40 molar pregnancies. In Caucasians, 25% of choriocarcinomas arise from term deliveries, 25% from spontaneous abortions, and 50% from hydatidiform moles. Although the risk that a hydatidiform mole will transform into a choriocarcinoma is only 2%, it is still several orders of magnitude higher than if the pregnancy were normal.

 Pathology: The uterine lesions of choriocarcinoma range from microscopic foci to huge necrotic and hemorrhagic tumors. Viable tumor is usually confined to the rim of the neoplasm because, unlike most other cancers, choriocarcinoma lacks an intrinsic tumor vasculature. Histologically, choriocarcinoma consists of a dimorphic population of cytotrophoblast and syncytiotrophoblast, with varying degrees of intermediate trophoblast (Fig. 18-79). The tumor resembles the trophoblast in the early implanting blastocyst. Rims of syncytiotrophoblast surround central cores of cytotrophoblast, in addition to being arranged around maternal blood spaces, which resemble the intervillous space of normal placentation. hCG is localized to the syncytiotrophoblastic element. By definition, tumors containing any villous structures, even if metastatic, are considered hydatidiform mole and not choriocarcinoma.

Choriocarcinoma invades primarily through venous sinuses in the myometrium. It metastasizes widely by the hematogenous route, especially to lung (over 90%), brain, gastrointestinal tract, liver, and vagina (Table 18-12).

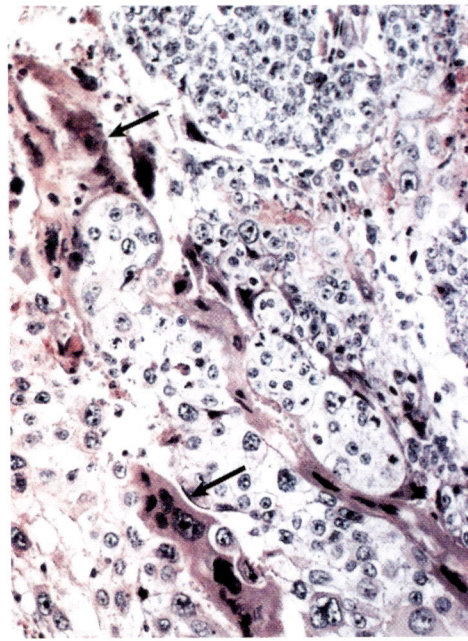

FIGURE 18-79
Choriocarcinoma. Malignant cytotrophoblast and syncytiotrophoblast (*arrows*) **are present.**

TABLE 18-12 Clinical Staging of Gestational Trophoblastic Tumors

I		Confined to the uterus
	Ia	0 risk factors
	Ib	1 risk factor
	Ic	2 risk factors
II		Extends outside of the uterus but limited to genital structures
III		Extends to lungs
IV		All other metastatic sites

Risk factors affecting stage include (1) hCG > 100,000 mIU/mL, and (2) duration of disease >6 months from termination of antecedent pregnancy.

 Clinical Features: Abnormal uterine bleeding is the most frequent initial indication that heralds choriocarcinoma. Occasionally, the first sign relates to metastases to the lungs or brain. In some cases, choriocarcinoma only becomes evident 10 or more years after the last pregnancy.

Prior to the era of chemotherapy, the cure rate for choriocarcinoma limited to the uterus was only 20%, and metastatic choriocarcinoma was virtually always fatal. Today, with recognition of risk factors (high hCG levels and prolonged interval since antecedent pregnancy) and early treatment, most patients are cured. Survival rates above 70% are now achieved with chemotherapy for tumors that have metastasized, and virtually 100% remission rates are expected if the tumor is localized. Serial serum hCG levels monitor the effectiveness of treatment.

Placental Site Trophoblastic Tumor Is Usually Benign

Placental site trophoblastic tumor, the least common of the various forms of trophoblastic disease, is composed predominantly of intermediate trophoblastic cells.

 Pathology: The gross appearance of placental site trophoblastic tumor is more variable than that of choriocarcinoma. Often, the myometrium shows an ill-defined, yellowish tumor mass that does not display conspicuous hemorrhage. The degree of myometrial invasion varies. Microscopically, the pattern of infiltration resembles that of normal trophoblast in the placental bed. Since intermediate trophoblast in the normal developing pregnancy functions to anchor the pregnancy into the superficial myometrium, the microscopic appearance of the tumor is typically that of an exaggerated placental site. Mononuclear and multinuclear trophoblast may be present as single cells or as cords, islands, and sheets of cells interspersed among myometrial cells. Neither necrosis nor chorionic villi is present. Placental site trophoblastic tumor is also distinguished from choriocarcinoma by its monomorphic (intermediate) trophoblastic proliferation, contrasted with the dimorphic pattern of trophoblast in choriocarcinoma. Most trophoblastic cells are positive for hPL, but a few express hCG.

Clinical Features: The age and parity of patients with placental site trophoblastic tumor resemble those of patients with choriocarcinoma. Half of patients with placental site trophoblastic tumor report amenorrhea, whereas vaginal bleeding usually occurs with choriocarcinoma. Compared with patients with choriocarcinoma, many fewer women with placental site trophoblastic tumor have had a preceding molar pregnancy (5% vs. 50%).

Placental site trophoblastic tumor generally behaves in a benign fashion, but it sometimes metastasizes and may prove fatal. Adverse features are large tumors and a mitotic index of more than 5 mitoses/10 HPFs. Because of the short half-life of hPL, serum levels of hCG are more useful in monitoring the response to treatment. Generally, conservative management suffices. If hCG persists, even at low levels, or the mitotic count is elevated, aggressive treatment with hysterectomy or chemotherapy is indicated.

SUGGESTED READING

Books

Dabbs DJ: *Diagnostic immunohistochemistry*. London: Churchill Livingstone, 2001.

Fox H, Wells M: *Haines and Taylor's Gynecopathologic and obstetrical pathology*, 4th ed. London: Churchill Livingstone, 2002.

Kurman RJ: *Blaustein's pathology of the female genital tract*, 5th ed. New York: Springer-Verlag, 2002.

Robboy SJ, Anderson MC, Russell P: *Pathology of the female reproductive tract*. London: Churchill Livingstone, 2002.

Tavassoli FA, Stratton MR: *Tumors of the breast and female genital organs*. Lyon: IARC Press, 2002.

Review Articles

Nielsen GP, Young RH: Mesenchymal tumors and tumor-like lesions of the female genital tract: A selective review with emphasis on recently described entities. *Int J Gynecol Pathol* 20:105–127, 2001.

Scully R, Young RH: A half century in gynecological pathology: Reminiscences of Robert E. Scully on his career—An interview with Robert H. Young. *Int J Gynecol Pathol* 20: 2–15, 2001.

Embryology

Ali S, Hasnain SE: Molecular dissection of the human Y-chromosome. *Gene* 283:1–10, 2002.

Vulva

Hart WR: Vulvar intraepithelial neoplasia: Historical aspects and current status. *Int J Gynecol Pathol* 20:16–30, 2001.

McCluggage WG: Recent advances in immunohistochemistry in gynaecological pathology. *Histopathology* 40:309–326, 2002.

Rogstad KE: Vulvar vestibulitis: Aetiology, diagnosis and treatment. *Int J STD AIDS* 11:557–562, 2000.

Vagina

Hatch EE, Herbst AL, Hoover RN, et al.: Incidence of squamous neoplasia of the cervix and vagina in women exposed prenatally to diethylstilbestrol (United States). *Cancer Causes Control* 12:837–845, 2001.

Titus-Ernstoff L, Hatch EE, Hoover RN, et al.: Long-term cancer risk in women given diethylstilbestrol (DES) during pregnancy. *Br J Cancer* 84:126–133, 2001.

Cervix

Alfsen GC, Kristensen GB, Skovlund E, et al.: Histologic subtype has minor importance for overall survival in patients with adenocarcinoma of the uterine cervix—A population-based study of prognostic factors in 505 patients with nonsquamous cell carcinomas of the cervix. *Cancer* 92:2471–2483, 2001.

Pinto AP, Crum CP: Natural history of cervical neoplasia: defining progression and its consequence. *Clin Obstet Gynecol* 43:352–362, 2000.

Stoler MH: Human papillomaviruses and cervical neoplasia: A model for carcinogenesis. *Int J Gynecol Pathol* 19:16–28, 2000.

Uterine Body

Clement PB: The pathology of uterine smooth muscle tumors and mixed endometrial stromal-smooth muscle tumors: A selective review with emphasis on recent advances. *Int J Gynecol Pathol* 19:39–55, 2000.

Clement PB, Young TH: Endometrioid carcinoma of the uterine corpus: A review of its pathology with emphasis on recent advances and problematic aspects. *Adv Anat Pathol* 9:145–184, 2002.

Mutter GL: Diagnosis of premalignant endometrial disease. *J Clin Pathol* 55:326–331, 2002.

Robboy SJ, Bentley RC, Butnor K, Anderson MC: Pathology and pathophysiology of uterine smooth-muscle tumors. *Environ Health Perspect* 108:779–784, 2000.

Fallopian Tube

Agoff SN, Mendelin JE, Grieco VS, Garcia RL: Unexpected gynecologic neoplasms in patients with proven or suspected BRCA-1 or-2 mutations—Implications for gross examination, cytology, and clinical follow-up. *Am J Surg Pathol* 26:171–178, 2002.

Demopoulos RI, Aronov R, Mesia A: Clues to the pathogenesis of fallopian tube carcinoma: A morphological and immunohistochemical case control study. *Int J Gynecol Pathol* 20:128–132, 2001.

Ovary

Bell KA, Kurman RJ: A clinicopathologic analysis of atypical proliferative (borderline) tumors and well-differentiated endometrioid adenocarcinomas of the ovary. *Am J Surg Pathol* 24:1465–1479, 2000.

Dietel M, Hauptmann S: Serous tumors of low malignant potential of the ovary. 1. Diagnostic pathology. *Virchows Archiv* 2000;436:403–412.

McGuire V, Jesser CA, Whittemore AS: Survival among US women with invasive epithelial ovarian cancer. *Gynecol Oncol* 84:399–403, 2002.

Seidman JD, Kurman RJ: Ovarian serous borderline tumors: A critical review of the literature with emphasis on prognostic indicators. *Hum Pathol* 31:539–557, 2000.

Silverberg SG: Histopathologic grading of ovarian carcinoma: A review and proposal. *Int J Gynecol Pathol* 19:7–15, 2000.

Placenta and Gestational Disease

Benirschke K, Masliah E: The placenta in multiple pregnancy: Outstanding issues. *Reprod Fertil Dev* 13:615–622, 2001.

Katz VL, Farmer R, Kuller JA: Preeclampsia into eclampsia: toward a new paradigm. *Am J Obstet Gynecol* 182:1389–1396, 2000.

Shih IM, Kurman RJ: The pathology of intermediate trophoblastic tumors and tumor-like lesions. *Int J Gynecol Pathol* 20:31–47, 2001.

Shih IM, Kurman RJ: Placental site trophoblastic tumor—Past as prologue. *Gynecol Oncol* 82:413–414, 2001.

Peritoneum

Kerrigan SAJ, Turnnir RT, Clement PB, et al.: Diffuse malignant epithelial mesotheliomas of the peritoneum in women—A clinicopathologic study of 25 patients. *Cancer* 94:378–385, 2002.

Stern RC, Dash R, Bentley RC, et al.: Malignancy in endometriosis: Frequency and comparison of ovarian and extraovarian types. *Int J Gynecol Pathol* 20:133–139, 2001.

Witz CA: Pathogenesis of endometriosis. *Gynecol Obstet Invest* 53:52–60, 2002.

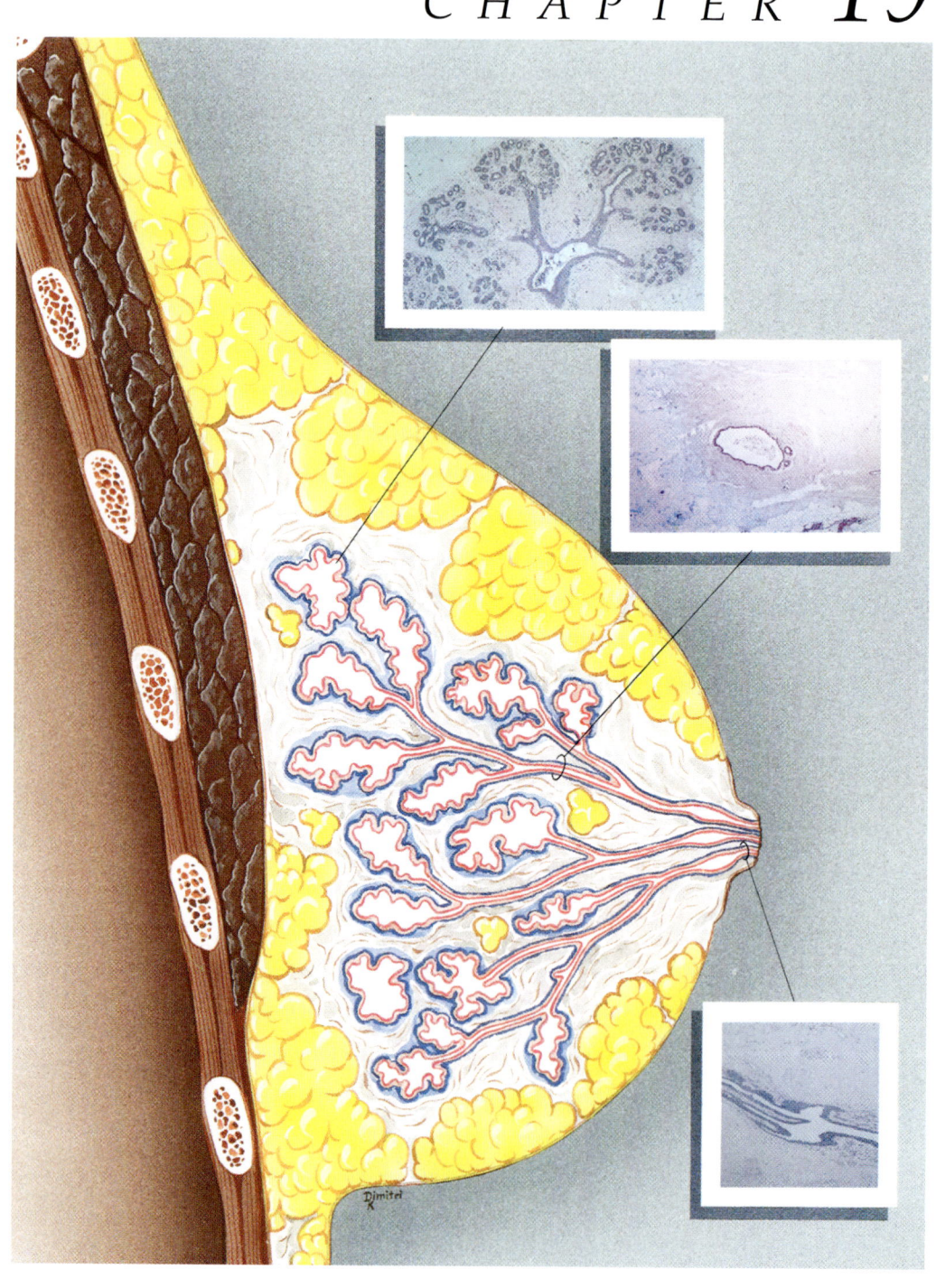

CHAPTER 19

The Breast

Ann D. Thor
Jianzhou Wang
Sue A. Bartow

Anatomy and Development

Hormonal Control of Development and Function

Congenital Anomalies

Juvenile Hypertrophy

Gynecomastia

Acute Mastitis

Duct Ectasia

Fat Necrosis

Granulomatous Mastitis

Fibrocystic Change
Nonproliferative Fibrocystic Change
Proliferative Fibrocystic Change

Benign Tumors
Fibroadenoma
Intraductal Papilloma

Carcinoma of the Breast
Carcinoma in Situ
Invasive Carcinoma
Metastatic Patterns
Prognostic Factors
Treatment
Cancer of the Male Breast

Phyllodes Tumor

FIGURE 19-1 *(see opposite page)*
Anatomy of the breast. The terminal duct lobular units *(top)* are the functional units of the breast. The conduits for the secretory products are the intermediate ducts *(center)* and the lactiferous sinuses *(bottom)*. The lobular, ductal, and fibrous stromal components of the parenchyma are dispersed within the fatty tissue of the organ.

The breast has become biologically superfluous in advanced societies, and it is now a matter of choice whether to make use of its sole function of nursing the young. Nevertheless, cancer of the breast is common and remains one of the leading causes of death in women. It is, therefore, important to understand the biology of malignant tumors and of benign changes that are associated with an increased risk of cancer.

ANATOMY AND DEVELOPMENT

The human breast is first recognizable at about 6 weeks of embryonic development as an ectodermal, ridgelike thickening extending from the anterior limb bud to the posterior limb bud along either side of the ventral surface of the fetus. Most of this ridge undergoes regression. By the ninth week of gestation, solid epithelial cords begin to extend from the epidermis into the underlying mesenchyme and gradually form branching primary mammary ducts.

Breast development is still rudimentary at birth, and the ducts continue to elongate and branch throughout childhood. In the female breast, this development accelerates at puberty. Under the influence of increasing estrogen production, the large and intermediate-sized ducts and connective tissue stroma proliferate in the perimenarchal breast. The branching duct system consists of approximately 20 lobes that are radially distributed around the nipple. These lobes are further divided into *terminal duct lobular units* (TDLUs) that do not fully develop until after menarche. The TDLUs consist of (1) the terminal ductules, whose epithelium differentiates into the secretory "acini" of the pregnant or lactating breast; (2) the intralobular collecting duct; and (3) the specialized intralobular stroma. Each of the lobes drains into its own lactiferous duct, which opens onto the surface of the nipple (Fig. 19-1).

The parenchyma of the female breast consists of the ducts and lobules (Fig. 19-1) together with their surrounding interlobular fibrous tissue. The parenchyma is diffusely distributed within the adipose tissue of the breast. The amount of adipose tissue varies considerably, depending on the age and general habitus of the woman. Whereas adolescent women typically have dense, fibrous breasts, postmenopausal women generally have predominantly fatty breasts. Women of reproductive age, between the ages of 20 and 50, have much more variable patterns. In half of these women, fibrous parenchyma constitutes more than 25% of the breast. Breasts containing abundant fibrous tissue are more difficult to evaluate radiologically than fatty breasts, because tumors of the breast also contain fibrous tissue and may be difficult to distinguish from normal fibrous parenchyma in a mammogram.

The lymphatic channels of the breast communicate with the lower pectoralis group of axillary nodes, which receive 75% of the drainage. The remaining 25% of the lymphatic flow leads into the parasternal nodes (internal mammary nodes).

The nipple consists predominantly of dense fibrous tissue mixed with fascicles of smooth muscle. The latter component gives the nipple its "erectile" capability and contributes to the expression of the milk. The skin immediately surrounding the nipple is the areola, which becomes pigmented during pregnancy. In this area the skin has pilosebaceous units, and it is one of the few areas of the body that contains apocrine as well as eccrine sweat glands (Fig. 19-2).

HORMONAL CONTROL OF DEVELOPMENT AND FUNCTION

With the onset of menarche and the attendant increase in estrogen and progesterone, the terminal duct lobular units (TDLUs) develop more fully (Fig. 19-2A). Once formed, the large and intermediate duct systems of the breast are unaffected by the fluctuating hormone levels of the menstrual cycle, pregnancy, or lactation. By contrast, the TDLUs are dynamic structures that undergo marked alterations, not only at the time of pregnancy but, to a lesser degree, also during the regular menstrual cycles. These cyclical changes involve not only the epithelial cells of the lobule but also the intralobular stromal components. Thus, the TDLUs are the functional components of the adult female breast (Fig. 19-2B,C).

The female breast and endometrium are governed by many of the same hormones. The endometrium shows mitotic activity during the first half of the menstrual cycle, but the breast epithelium undergoes its greatest proliferation during the second half of the menstrual cycle.

- **Follicular phase:** During the first half, or follicular phase, of the cycle, the terminal ducts are few and lined by a simple, two-cell layer of epithelium surrounded by a layer of myoepithelial cells.
- **Luteal phase:** After ovulation, enhanced mitotic activity in the terminal duct epithelium results in a conspicuous increase in the number of terminal ducts within a lobule. Simultaneously, the basal layer of epithelial cells becomes vacuolated. The intralobular stroma becomes edematous and distinct from the dense fibrous tissue that surrounds each lobule. Clinically, women perceive progressive fullness and tenderness of the breast during the luteal phase of the menstrual cycle.
- **Menses:** With the onset of menstruation, as the levels of estrogen and progesterone fall, apoptotic cell death in-

Hormonal Control of Development and Function

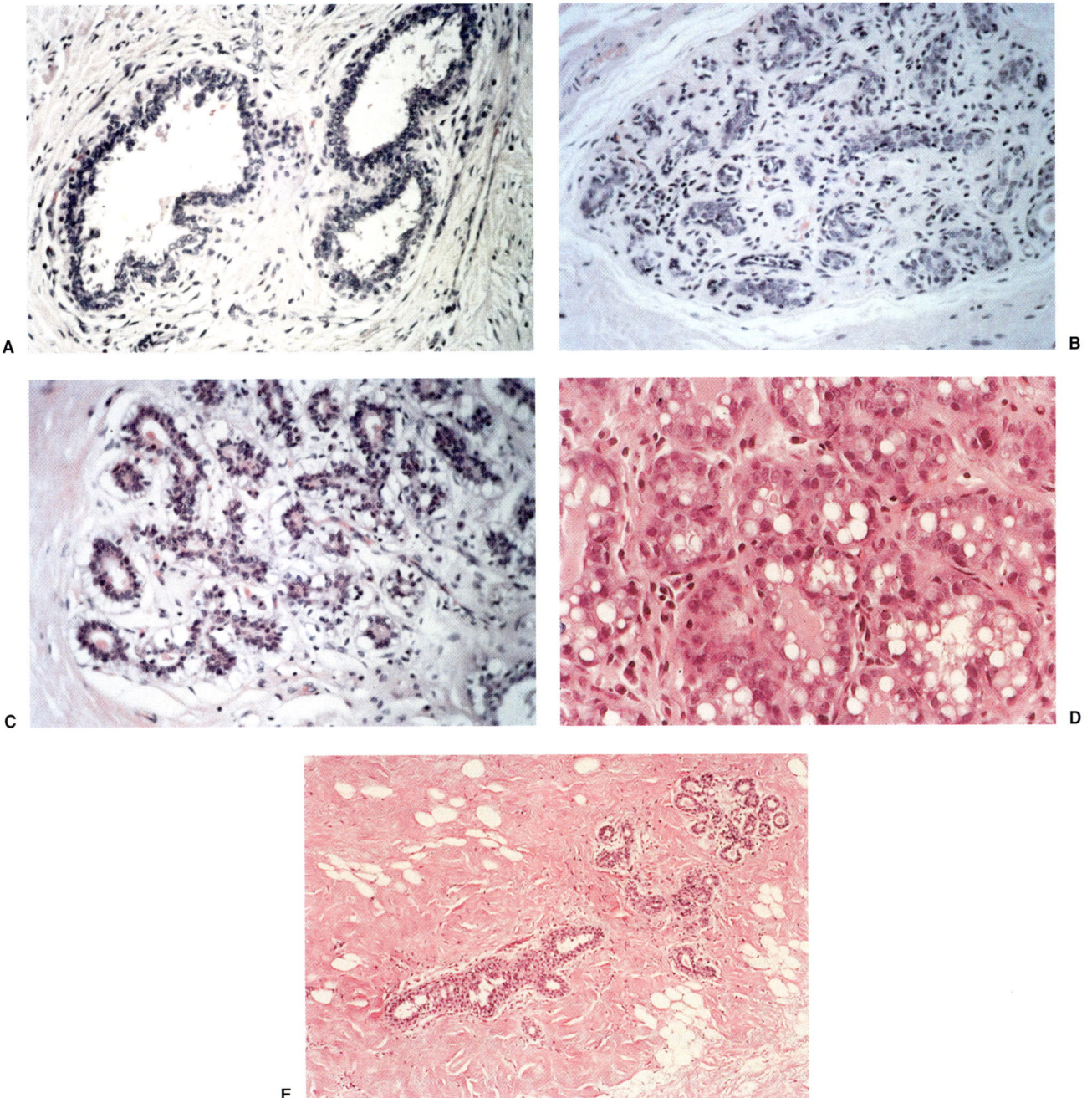

FIGURE 19-2
Normal breast architecture at various ages. A. Adolescent breast. Large and intermediate-size ducts are seen within a dense fibrous stroma. No lobular units are present. B. Postpubertal breast, first half of the menstrual cycle. The terminal duct lobular unit consists of small ductules arrayed around an intralobular duct. The two cell-layered epithelium shows no secretory or mitotic activity. The intralobular stroma is dense and confluent with the interlobular stroma. C. Postpubertal breast, second half of the menstrual cycle. The terminal duct lobular units are enlarged, with increased numbers of terminal ducts. The basal epithelial cells are vacuolated, and mitoses are present. The intralobular stroma is edematous and distinct from the interlobular stroma. D. Lactating breast. The terminal duct lobular units are conspicuously enlarged, with inapparent interlobular and intralobular stroma. The individual terminal ducts (now termed *acini*) show prominent epithelial secretory activity (cytoplasmic vacuolization). The acinar lumina contain secretory material. E. Postmenopausal breast. The terminal duct lobular units are absent. The remaining intermediate ducts and larger ducts are commonly dilated. There is little interlobular fibrous connective tissue, and much of the breast is composed of fat.

creases in the terminal duct epithelium. Progressive lymphocytic infiltration occurs in the intralobular stroma. The TDLUs ultimately regress to the state of the follicular phase of the menstrual cycle.
- **Pregnancy:** In pregnancy, there is a pronounced hormonally induced increase in the number of terminal ducts. The lobular epithelium is increased to such a point that it is the major component of the breast tissue.
- **Lactation:** During lactation, the breast epithelial cells become vacuolated, and the ductal lumina are distended with secretions. When lactation ceases, the lobular units involute and revert to their former state (Fig. 19-2D).
- **Postmenopause:** After menopause, the TDLUs atrophy, but large and intermediate duct systems remain, and minor cystic dilation of residual ducts is common, accompanied by a concomitant loss of the dense, interlobular, fibrous connective tissue. Thus, the amount of adipose tissue is relatively increased. By 80 years of age, 80% of women have predominantly fatty breasts. In some older women, cuffs of dense fibrous tissue persist around the remaining ducts (Fig. 19-2E).
- **The male breast:** Until puberty the male breast develops in a manner similar to that of the female breast, at which time further development is arrested. Thus, the adult male breast consists of large to intermediate-sized ducts that are similar to those of the immature female breast.

CONGENITAL ANOMALIES

It is common for a tail of breast tissue to extend to the lower edge of the axilla. Uncommonly, breast or nipple tissue may be present elsewhere along the original embryonic breast ridge *(milk line).* Thus, accessory breast tissue may be found along the anterior trunk, superior or inferior to the main breast, all the way to the inguinal area, and even occasionally into the vulva. The most frequent variant of the normal breast is *inversion of the nipple.* It is of clinical significance because of the difficulty it may cause in nursing and because secondary nipple inversion may be caused by traction from an underlying carcinoma.

JUVENILE HYPERTROPHY

NEONATAL HYPERTROPHY: Hypertrophy of the breast in the neonatal period is induced by maternal hormones and resolves as levels of these hormones fall after birth.

JUVENILE (PUBERTAL) HYPERTROPHY: Hypertrophy of the breast at the time of puberty may occur in both girls and boys and may be bilateral or unilateral.

 Pathology: Morphologically, the fibrous stroma expands and the ducts increase in number. The duct epithelium becomes hyperplastic, and the branching structures become more exaggerated. Since lobules are not yet formed, they do not participate in the hyperplastic process. Juvenile hypertrophy usually presents no major problem, except to the psyche of the adolescent girl or boy, and most often regresses spontaneously.

SECONDARY HYPERTROPHY: Hypertrophy of the breast may be secondary to abnormally high hormone levels, such as those induced by functioning ovarian, adrenocortical, or pituitary tumors.

GYNECOMASTIA

Gynecomastia refers to an enlargement of the adult male breast and is morphologically similar to juvenile hypertrophy of the female breast (Fig. 19-3).

 Pathogenesis: In the adult man, gynecomastia is caused by an absolute increase in circulating estrogens or by a relative increase in the estrogen/androgen ratio. Gynecomastia associated with excess estrogens occurs with (1) the intake of exogenous estrogens or estrogen-like agents (e.g., digitalis, opiates); (2) the presence of hormone-secreting adrenal or testicular tumors; (3) the paraneoplastic production of gonadotropins by cancers of the liver, lung, and other organs; and (4) metabolic disorders such as liver disease and hyperthyroidism that are characterized by increased conversion of androstenedione into estrogens. Low levels of androgens may be due to inadequate testicular secretion of testosterone (Klinefelter syndrome, castration, orchitis) or to androgen insensitivity (testicular feminization). Gynecomastia is often idiopathic, in which case it is commonly unilateral. There is no evidence that gynecomastia is associated with an increased risk of cancer.

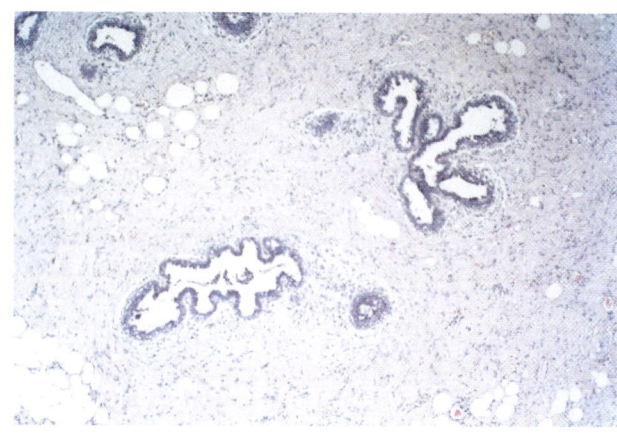

FIGURE 19-3

Gynecomastia. There is proliferation of branching, intermediate-sized ducts. The ductal epithelium is hyperplastic, and mitoses are present. A concomitant increase in the surrounding fibrous tissue causes a palpable mass. Note the resemblance to the normal adolescent breast.

ACUTE MASTITIS

Acute mastitis is a bacterial infection of the breast. It may be seen at any age, but by far the most frequent setting is in the postpartum lactating or involuting breast. This disorder is usually secondary to obstruction of the duct system by inspissated secretion, with stasis of secretions. The most common organisms isolated are *Staphylococcus* and *Streptococcus.* Untreated, the infection may progress to abscess formation, a complication that necessitates surgical intervention. A firm, walled-off, nontender abscess may be mistaken for cancer. Acute bacterial mastitis may be treated successfully by aggressive mechanical suction, with frequent emptying of the breasts, and by the administration of antibiotics.

DUCT ECTASIA

Duct ectasia refers to the presence of dilated large and intermediate ducts of the breast containing pasty, inspissated material, with accompanying periductal inflammation and fibrosis. It is a common lesion in elderly women, in whom it affects the large collecting ducts immediately under the areola. Morphologically, the involved ducts are dilated and contain acellular debris and foamy macrophages. These dilated ducts may rupture, and the escape of grumous material incites chronic inflammation, often with foreign body granulomas, in the surrounding stroma. Duct ectasia may be subjected to biopsy because it is clinically difficult to distinguish from cancer.

FAT NECROSIS

A history of trauma can usually be elicited in cases of fat necrosis occurring in the breast.

Pathology: Initially, the lesion consists of necrosis of adipocytes and hemorrhage, after which, inflammatory cells phagocytize the lipid debris. Fibroblastic proliferation during healing leads to fingers of fibrous scar tissue that extend into the adjacent breast. **As a result, an irregular, fixed, hard mass may ensue and clinically resemble breast cancer.** Dystrophic calcification, a common feature of breast cancer, may also be detected radiographically in areas of fat necrosis. Thus, the lesions of fat necrosis often require biopsy to establish their benign character.

GRANULOMATOUS MASTITIS

Granulomatous inflammation is uncommon in the breast but is found in two settings. The first is in association with foreign material. Breast implants made of silicone, even when there is no evidence of rupture, slowly leak into the surrounding breast tissue, resulting in the formation of a fibrous capsule with associated macrophages and foreign body giant cells. The second diagnosis to be considered in granulomatous breast inflammation is infection, usually of the mycobacterial type. Fungal infection is much less common.

FIBROCYSTIC CHANGE

Fibrocystic change of the breast refers to a constellation of morphological features characterized by (1) cystic dilation of terminal ducts, (2) relative increase in fibrous stroma, and (3) variable proliferation of terminal duct epithelial elements. It is most often diagnosed in women from their late 20s to the time of menopause, and some fibrocystic change occurs in 75% of adult women in the United States. Symptomatic fibrocystic change, in which large, clinically detectable cysts are formed, is much less common, occurring in 10% of adult women between the ages of 35 and 55 years. The frequency of fibrocystic change decreases progressively after menopause.

Fibrocystic change with giant cysts and proliferative epithelial lesions is more common in populations that have an increased risk of breast cancer, but progression to carcinoma has not been documented. However, some of the florid manifestations appear to be indicators for women at increased risk for breast cancer. Such lesions are designated *proliferative* fibrocystic change. The forms of fibrocystic change that do not carry an increased risk for the development of cancer, termed *nonproliferative* fibrocystic change, are far more prevalent. (See Fig. 19-4 A–C)

Pathology: Fibrocystic change of both the nonproliferative and proliferative types involves the terminal duct lobular units.

Nonproliferative Fibrocystic Change Is Not Preneoplastic

The morphological hallmarks of nonproliferative fibrocystic change are an increase in dense, fibrous stroma and some cystic dilation of the terminal ducts (Fig. 19-5). Although the degree may vary from one area to another, fibrocystic change always occurs in multiple areas of both breasts. Most often, cystic changes are minor and are not the cause of discrete masses. However, a dominant cyst or aggregate of fibrous connective tissue containing smaller cysts may manifest as a discrete "mass," prompting biopsy to exclude the possibility of cancer.

The large cysts, up to 5 cm in diameter, often contain dark, thin fluid that imparts a blue color to the unopened cysts—the so-called *blue-domed cysts of Bloodgood.* Aspiration of a large cyst will usually cause it to collapse and the mass to disappear.

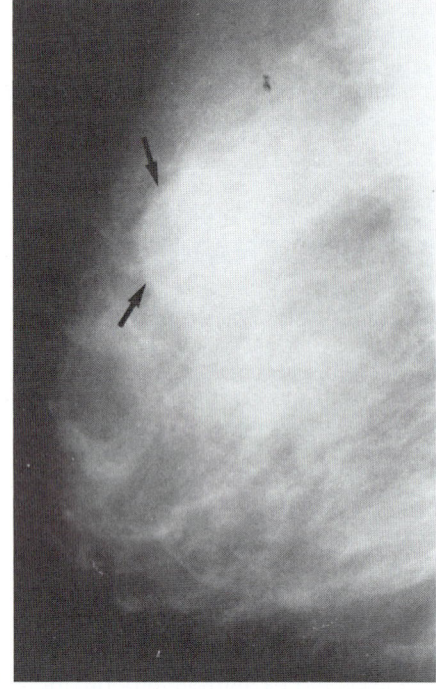
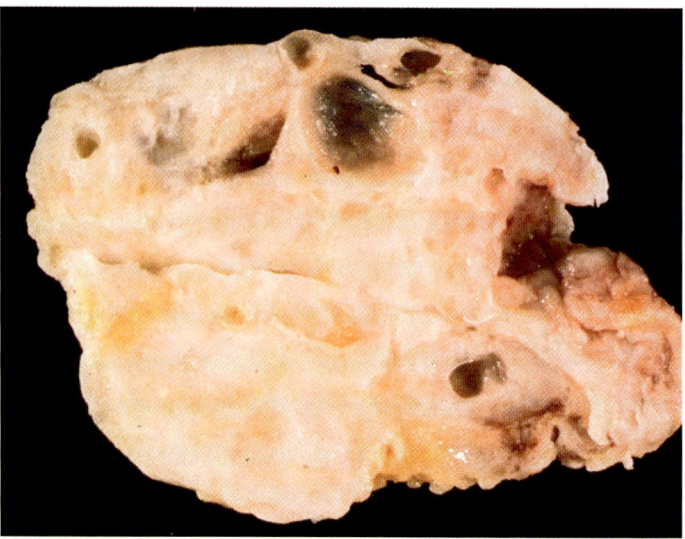
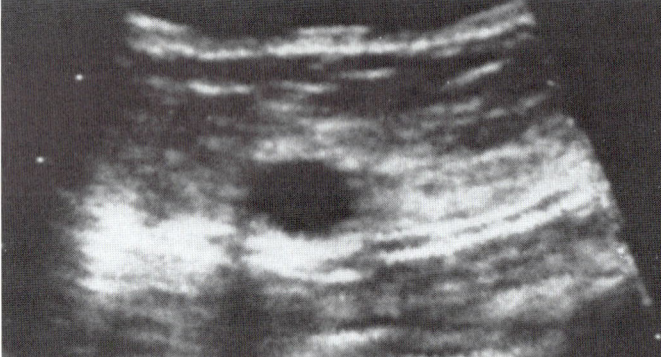

FIGURE 19-4
Fibrocystic change. A. Mammogram: Irregular densities are present, including one dominant mass *(arrows)*. B. Ultrasonogram: White areas are solid tissue. The central round dark area is a sonolucent cyst, corresponding to the dominant mass in the mammogram *(A)*. C. Surgical specimen: Cysts of various sizes are dispersed in dense, fibrous connective tissue.

On microscopic examination, the epithelium lining the cysts varies from columnar to flattened or may be entirely absent. A frequent concomitant of nonproliferative fibrocystic change is an alteration of the epithelial lining, termed *apocrine metaplasia* (Fig. 19-5B). The metaplastic cells are larger and more eosinophilic than the cells that usually line the ducts and resemble apocrine sweat gland epithelium.

Proliferative Fibrocystic Change Increases the Risk of Cancer

Proliferative fibrocystic change refers to several forms of epithelial proliferation that occur in the context of nonproliferative fibrocystic change. The most common proliferative change is an increase in the number of cells lining the dilated terminal ducts, described as *ductal epithelial hyperplasia*. The proliferation can at times become exuberant and form papillary structures within the lumen of the distended ductule *(papillomatosis)*.

The morphological spectrum of ductal hyperplasia includes (1) minor degrees of hyperplasia; (2) florid, but cytologically benign, hyperplasia; (3) hyperplasia with cytological atypia not sufficient to warrant a diagnosis of malignancy *(atypical hyperplasia)*; and (4) ductal carcinoma in situ.

SCLEROSING ADENOSIS: *This condition is a less common variant of proliferative fibrocystic change, which is characterized by a proliferation of small ducts and myoepithelial cells in the region of the TDLU (adenosis)* (Fig. 19-6). It is almost always associated with other forms of proliferative fibrocystic change. Because the lesion is commonly associated with fibrosis, the term *sclerosing* is added. Microscopically, the lobular units are deformed and enlarged by the proliferated epithelial cells, which appear as whorls and cords of tubules surrounded by fibrous stroma (Fig. 19-6).

Sclerosing adenosis is of significance primarily to the surgical pathologist, who must distinguish it histologically from invasive carcinoma. **The condition is occasionally so florid that it gives rise to a distinct mass that can be mistaken clinically for cancer.**

Fibrocystic Change

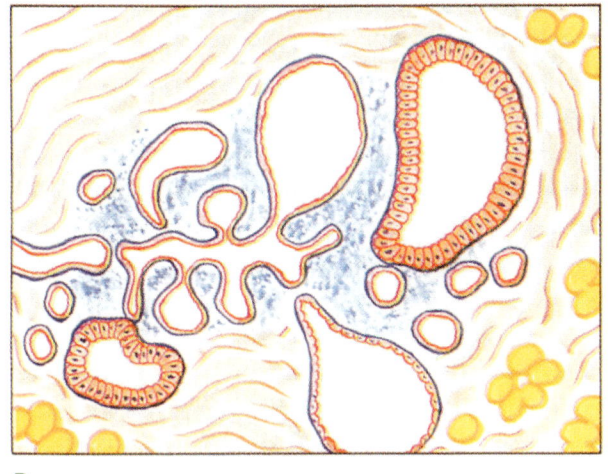
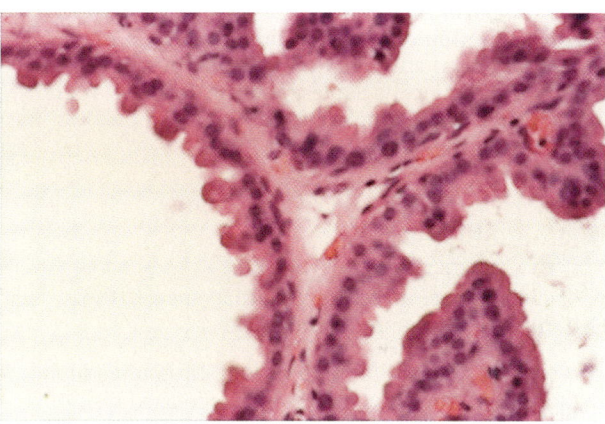
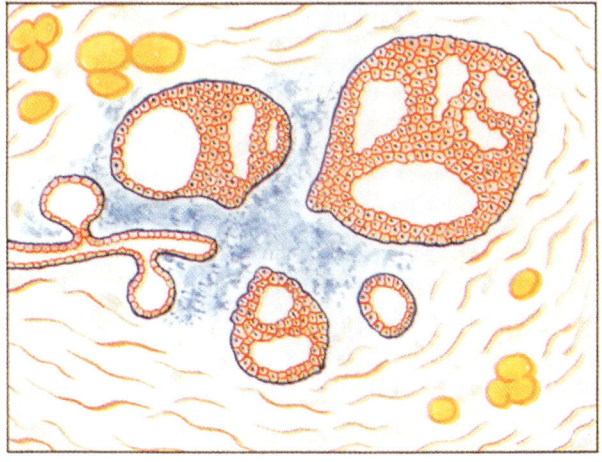
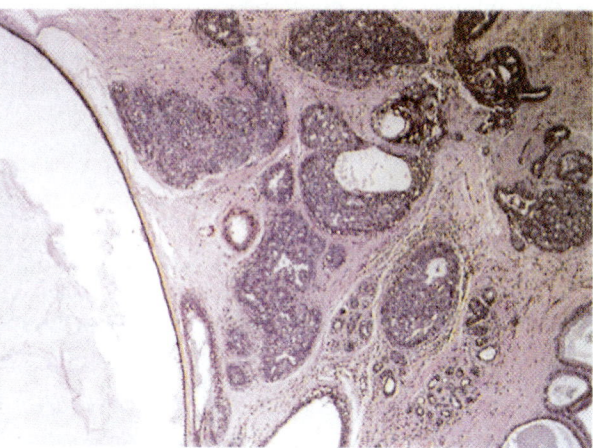

FIGURE 19-5
Histology of fibrocystic change. **A.** The normal terminal lobular unit. **B.** Nonproliferative fibrocystic change: This lesion combines cystic dilation of the terminal ducts with varying degrees of apocrine metaplasia of the epithelium and increased fibrous stroma. **C.** Proliferative fibrocystic change: Terminal duct dilation and intraductal epithelial hyperplasia are present.

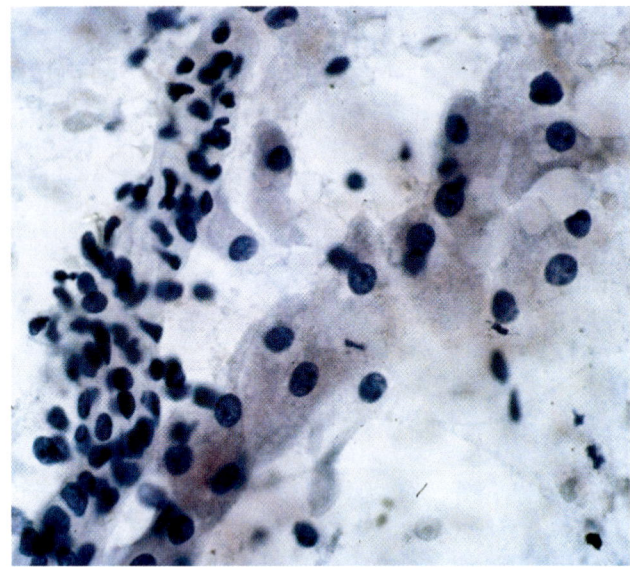

FIGURE 19-5 (continued)
D. Fine-needle aspiration cytology: In this cytological preparation, the normal ductal epithelial cells display small, bland nuclei. Some epithelial cells have apocrine features with eosinophilic cytoplasm and single nucleoli.

Prognostic Significance

A number of conclusions can be drawn with respect to the relationship of fibrocystic change to breast cancer.

- The presence of nonproliferative fibrocystic change in a biopsy specimen does not indicate an increased risk of developing invasive breast cancer.
- The demonstration of proliferative fibrocystic change in a biopsy places a woman at a 1.5- to 2-fold increased risk for the development of invasive cancer.
- **"Atypical hyperplasia" increases the risk for the subsequent development of invasive carcinoma of the breast to four to five times that of the general population.**
- Proliferative lesions increase the risk of subsequent cancer equally in both breasts.

BENIGN TUMORS

Fibroadenoma Is Hormonally Responsive

Fibroadenoma is the most common benign neoplasm of the breast and is composed of epithelial and stromal elements that originate from the terminal duct lobular unit. The tumors are usually found in women between the ages of 20 and 35, although they also occur in adolescent girls. Some juvenile fibroadenomas attain great size, in which case they are termed *giant fibroadenomas*. They do not regress spontaneously and may not be detected until the woman is in her 40s or 50s.

Fibroadenomas commonly enlarge more rapidly during pregnancy and cease to grow after the menopause. Although they are hormonally responsive, a causal relationship between hormones and the development of fibroadenomas has not been established. Fibroadenomas are ordinarily solitary, but they are occasionally multiple. Interestingly, the risk of subsequent invasive cancer in a breast from which a fibroadenoma has been removed has been reported to be doubled.

 Pathology: Fibroadenoma is a round, rubbery tumor that is sharply demarcated from the surrounding breast and is thus freely movable. The cut surface appears glistening gray-white. Although it may vary in size from a microscopic lesion to a large tumor, it is usually 2 to 4 cm in diameter when first detected. (Fig 19-7A and B)

On microscopic examination, fibroadenomas are composed of a mixture of fibrous connective tissue and ducts (Fig. 19-7C). The ducts may be either simple and round or elongate and branching and are dispersed within a characteristic fibrous stroma that varies from loose and myxomatous to hyalinized collagen. This connective tissue, which forms most of the tumor, often compresses the proliferated ducts, reducing them to curvilinear slits. In other areas, the ducts remain patent because the stroma proliferates circumferentially around them. The appearance of the epithelium ranges from the double layer of epithelium of normal lobules to varying degrees of hyperplasia.

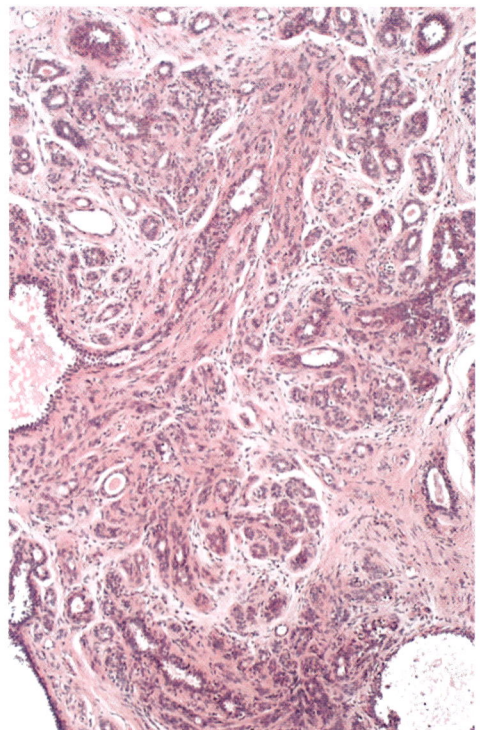

FIGURE 19-6
Sclerosing adenosis. A proliferation of small, abortive, duct-like structures and myoepithelial cells expands and distorts the lobule in which it arises.

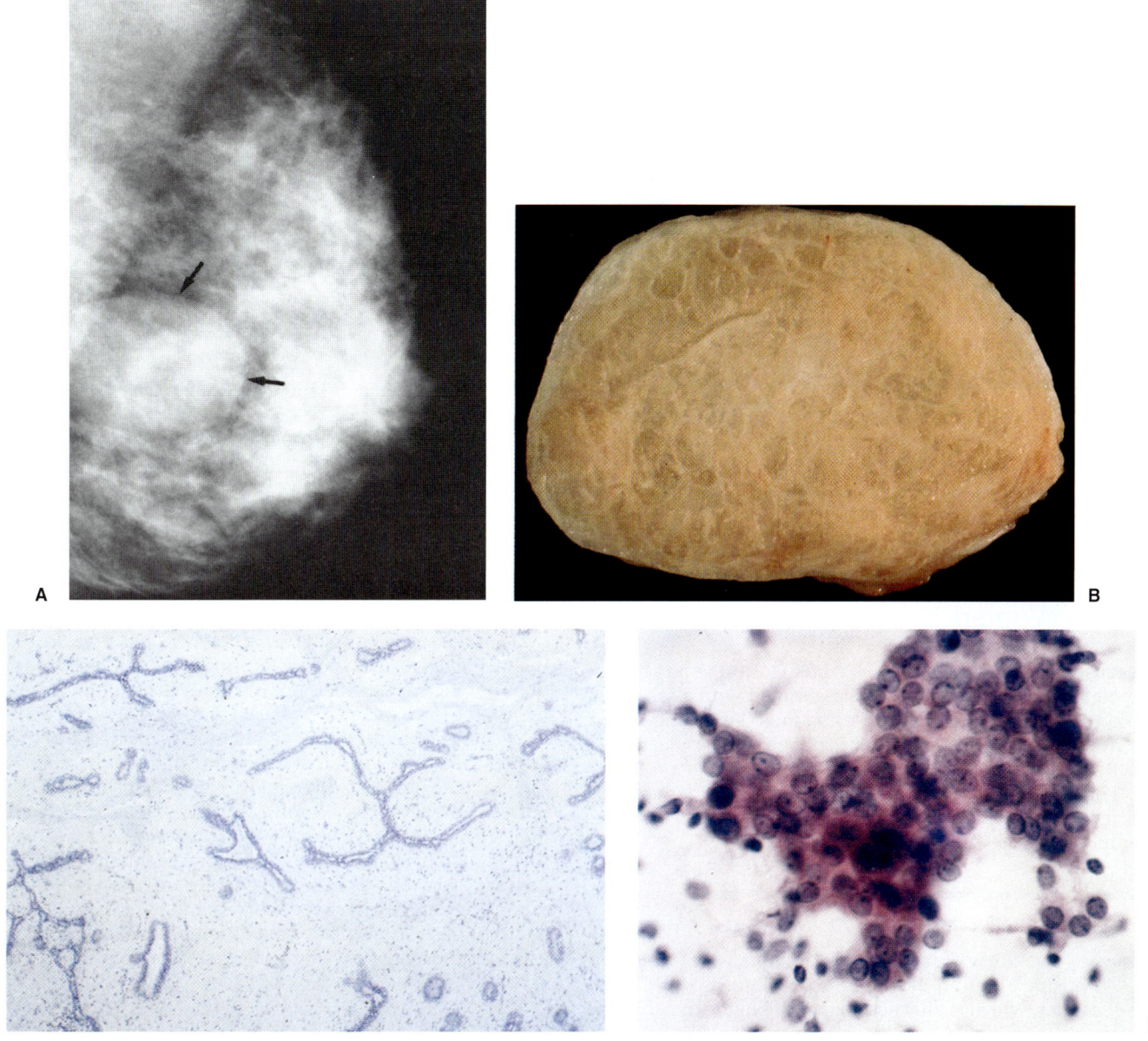

FIGURE 19-7
Fibroadenoma. A. Mammogram. A dominant mass *(arrows)* with smooth borders is the same density as that of normal breast tissue in a young woman. B. Surgical specimen. This well-circumscribed tumor was easily enucleated from the surrounding tissue. The cut surface is characteristically glistening tannish-white and has a septate appearance. C. Microscopic section. Elongated epithelial duct structures are situated within a loose, myxoid stroma. D. Fine-needle aspiration. This cytological preparation shows bland ductal cells arranged in cohesive clusters that have an irregular "staghorn" shape.

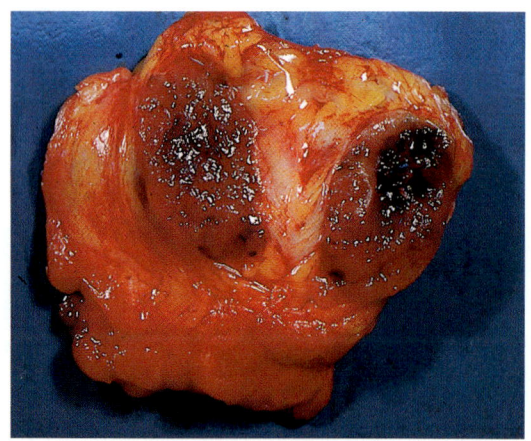
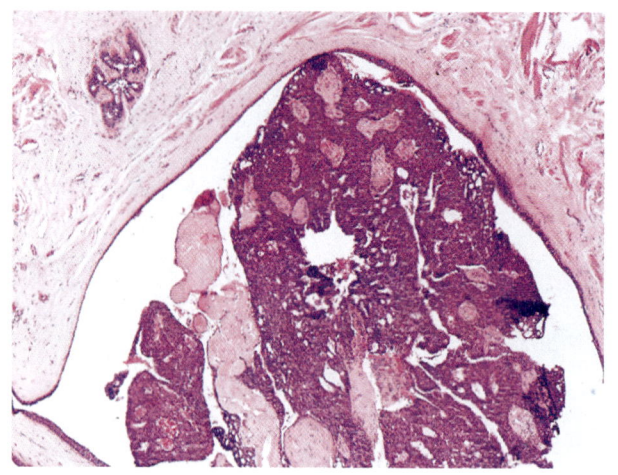

FIGURE 19-8
Intraductal papilloma. A. A large papillary mass is seen within dilated ducts. B. A photomicrograph shows a benign papillary growth in a subareolar duct.

Intraductal Papilloma Occurs in the Lactiferous Ducts of Middle-Aged and Older Women

Because intraductal papilloma is situated in the large, subareolar ducts, the lesion may be associated with a serous or bloody nipple discharge. This lesion must be distinguished from papillomatosis, the form of epithelial hyperplasia that occurs in the peripheral ducts as a component of proliferative fibrocystic change. Solitary intraductal papilloma is not a premalignant lesion or a marker for increased risk of cancer in the breast.

 Pathology: Intraductal papilloma (Fig. 19-8) is a single tumor, usually a few millimeters in diameter, which is attached to the wall of the duct by a fibrovascular stalk. The papillomatous portion consists of a double layer of epithelial cells, an outer one of cuboidal or columnar cells and an inner layer of more-rounded myoepithelial cells.

CARCINOMA OF THE BREAST

Breast cancer is the most common malignancy of women in the United States, and the mortality from this disease among women is second only to that of lung cancer.

 Epidemiology: The incidence of cancer of the breast has slowly increased over the past 50 years. Currently, one in nine American women may be expected to develop breast cancer, of whom one third will die of the disease. In Western industrialized countries with high rates of breast cancer, the incidence of this tumor continues to increase throughout life, albeit at a slower rate in elderly women. In populations at low risk for breast cancer, the incidence reaches a plateau prior to menopause and then does not increase further. Breast cancer is uncommon before the age of 35 years.

There is a fourfold to fivefold greater incidence of breast cancer in Western industrialized countries than in less-developed countries and in Native Americans in the United States. Furthermore, women who migrate to the United States from countries where the incidence of breast cancer is low (e.g., Japan), within one or two generations manifest a cancer risk as high as that of the white American population. It has been suggested that dietary factors, particularly the fat content, are responsible for the differences in the geographical distribution of breast cancer, but the concept remains controversial.

 Pathogenesis: The pathogenesis of breast cancer is poorly understood, but epidemiological and molecular and clinical genetic studies have implicated factors that are associated with an increased risk of breast cancer.

HEREDITARY FACTORS: **The strongest association with an increased risk for breast cancer is a family history, specifically breast cancer in first-degree relatives (mother, sister, daughter).** The risk is greater when the relative is afflicted at a young age or with bilateral breast cancer. A woman who has two sisters with breast cancer, one of whom had bilateral tumors, or a mother and sister who show the same pattern, has a greater than 25% chance of developing breast cancer by age 70.

The *BRCA1* **gene** (breast cancer 1), a tumor suppressor gene located on chromosome 17 (17q21), has been implicated in the pathogenesis of hereditary breast and ovarian cancers. Mutations in this tumor-suppressor gene are thought to be carried by 1 in 200 to 400 people in the United States.

Germline point mutations and deletions in *BRCA1* place a woman at a remarkable 60 to 85% lifetime risk for breast cancer. Moreover, breast cancer develops in more than half these women before the age of 50 years. Thus, although inherited *BRCA1* mutations seem to be responsible for less than 2% of cases of breast cancer discovered after 70 years of age, some 30% of women in whom the tumor is detected before the age of 45 are carriers of these mutations. It is currently suspected that mutated *BRCA1* is responsible for 20% of all cases of *inherited* breast cancer (about 3% of all breast cancers). Somatic mutations in *BRCA1* are uncommon in *sporadic* (nonfamilial) breast cancers.

Women with *BRCA1* mutations are also at greater lifetime risk of ovarian cancer, which has been estimated to range from 15 to 40%. There is some evidence that persons with mutations in this gene may also be at increased risk of prostate and colon cancers.

The **BRCA2 gene**, located on chromosome 13q12, is incriminated in some 20% of cases of inherited breast cancer that are not secondary to mutations in *BRCA1*. Women with one copy of a mutated *BRCA2* gene have a 30 to 40% lifetime chance of developing breast cancer. Like the situation with *BRCA1*, these women also exhibit an increased risk of ovarian cancer. Moreover, *BRCA2* mutations place men at increased risk of breast cancer. Mutations in *BRCA2* are particularly common among Ashkenazi Jewish women.

The **p53 gene** is mutated in the Li-Fraumeni syndrome. This rare familial cancer syndrome features tumors of the brain and adrenals in children and breast cancer in young women. It is estimated that germline (inherited) mutations in *p53* account for 1% of breast cancers among women in whom the tumor is detected before the age of 40 years. However, almost all (90%) women with Li-Fraumeni syndrome who survive childhood cancers linked to this disorder can expect to develop breast cancer. Somatic *p53* mutations are commonly found in the breast cancers that arise in women who do not evidence a family history of this disease.

The **CHEK2 (cell-cycle–checkpoint kinase) gene** is mutated in 5% of women with breast cancer who have two or more family members who developed breast cancer before the age of 60 years. The individual risk for women who carry the mutation is less than 20%. This mutation doubles the risk of breast cancer among women and increases the risk among men by a factor of 10. *CHEK2* is phosphorylated by *ATM*, another checkpoint gene, and in turn activates *BRCA1*.

HORMONAL STATUS: A link between breast cancer and the hormonal status of women is strongly suggested by the conspicuous association between the incidence of this tumor and the age of menarche, menopause, and first pregnancy. **Early menarche, late menopause, and older age at first-term pregnancy all increase the risk of breast cancer.** Oophorectomy before age 35, but not after, dramatically lowers the risk of breast cancer. Nulliparous women, or those who become pregnant for the first time after age 35, have a twofold to threefold higher risk of breast cancer than women whose first pregnancy occurred before age 25. The use of oral contraceptive agents has not been associated with an increased risk of breast cancer, although postmenopausal hormone supplementation slightly augments the risk.

RADIATION: The female breast is susceptible to radiation-induced neoplasia. The risk of breast cancer was increased in survivors of atomic bomb explosions, women irradiated for postpartum mastitis, and women subjected to multiple fluoroscopic examinations during treatment of tuberculosis. The increased risk of breast cancer is highest when exposure occurs in young children and pre- and perimenarchal women; there is little hazard when women are exposed to radiation after the age of 40. Modern mammographic techniques use extremely low doses of radiation that do not pose a hazard.

FIBROCYSTIC CHANGE: Women with fibrocystic change have an increased risk of breast cancer only when specific proliferative lesions are identified in biopsy tissue. As discussed above, the strongest association with increased risk appears to be in women with "atypical" hyperplasia. Women with both a first-degree family history of breast cancer and "atypical" hyperplasia have a 10-fold increased risk of developing cancer.

PREVIOUS CANCER: Women who have previously had breast cancer have a 10-fold increased risk of developing a second primary breast cancer.

 Pathology: Cancers of the breast (Fig. 19-9) are almost all adenocarcinomas that are derived from the glandular epithelium of the terminal duct lobular unit. The various subtypes derive their names from a combination of their histological patterns and cytological characteristics, not their site of origin (Table 19-1).

Carcinoma in Situ Is Often a Preinvasive Lesion

The term carcinoma in situ *refers to the presence of apparently malignant epithelial cells that have not penetrated the basement membrane.* The name carcinoma in situ implies that these lesions are obligate precursors of invasive carcinoma, and histologically, the various subtypes of carcinoma in situ do have invasive counterparts. However, only 20 to 30% of women who have demonstrated these lesions in a breast biopsy but have received no further therapy subsequently developed invasive cancer. The likelihood of an invasive cancer arising after the diagnosis of "in situ carcinoma" varies with the histological subtype of this lesion.

Intraductal Carcinoma in Situ

Intraductal carcinoma in situ arises in the TDLU, greatly distending and distorting the ducts by its growth. The terminal ducts may become markedly enlarged, thereby resembling large ducts. Intraductal carcinoma in situ has two main histological types, namely, comedocarcinoma and noncomedo carcinoma.

DUCTAL CARCINOMA IN SITU—COMEDO TYPE: This subtype is composed of very large, pleomorphic cells that have abundant eosinophilic cytoplasm and irregular

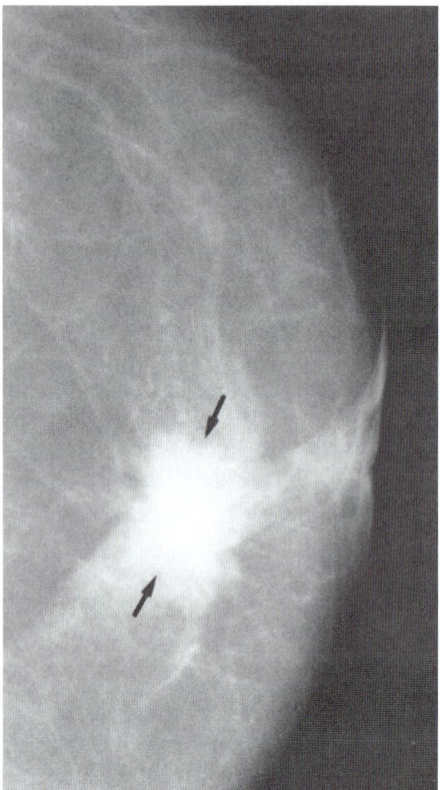
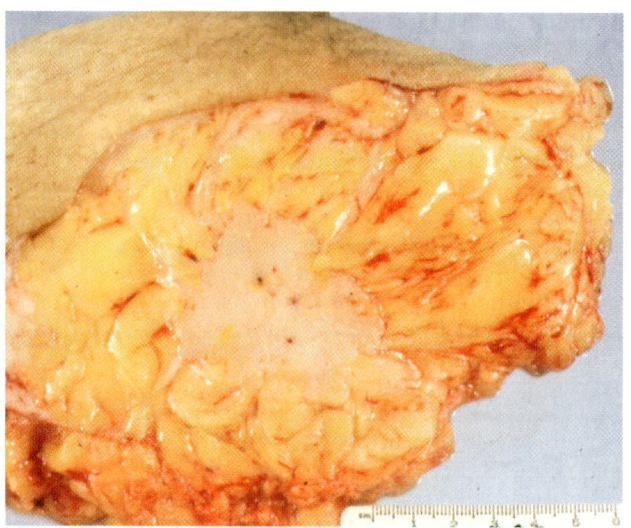

FIGURE 19-9
Carcinoma of the breast. A. Mammogram. An irregularly shaped, dense mass (arrows) is seen in this otherwise fatty breast. B. Mastectomy specimen. The irregular white, firm mass in the center is surrounded by fatty tissue.

nuclei, commonly with prominent nucleoli, and typically grows in a solid pattern. Central necrosis is a prominent factor (Fig. 19-10A). The necrotic debris may undergo dystrophic calcification. On gross examination, the cut surface shows distended ducts containing pasty necrotic debris resembling comedos, hence the term *comedocarcinoma*. Even though the malignant cells do not invade through the basement membrane of the ducts, this form of carcinoma in situ commonly incites a chronic inflammatory and fibroblastic response in the surrounding stroma.

The stromal inflammation and fibrosis in comedocarcinoma sometimes suffice to cause a clinically palpable or radiographically detectable mass. In addition, the microcalcifications that occur in the necrotic debris within the ducts have a distinctive, branching appearance by mammography. The cancer may extend within the duct system beyond the clinically detectable tumor growth. The consequent difficulties in obtaining complete excision of the primary tumor frequently necessitates mastectomy rather than "lumpectomy."

DUCTAL CARCINOMA IN SITU—NONCOMEDO TYPE: This tumor has multiple architectural patterns, which are often intermixed and exhibit a spectrum of cytological atypia. The patterns are classified as micropapillary, cribriform, and solid. The tumor cells and nuclei are smaller and more regular than those of the comedo type. Noncomedo intraductal carcinoma in situ is less likely than the comedo type to incite a desmoplastic response in the surrounding tissue. Necrosis is minimal or absent (Fig. 19-10B).

Ductal carcinoma in situ, treated only by biopsy, carries a 30% risk of developing invasive carcinoma in the same breast over the ensuing 20 years. The risk of cancer in the contralateral breast is also increased, but not to the same degree. The chances of local recurrence as either in situ or invasive cancer is substantially greater in the case of the comedo than in noncomedo subtypes.

Lobular Carcinoma in Situ

Lobular carcinoma in situ also arises in the TDLU. In this tumor the cells tend to be smaller and more monotonous than those of the ductal type, with round, regular nuclei and minute nucleoli (see Fig. 19-12A). The malignant cells appear as solid clusters that pack and distend the terminal ducts, but not to the extent of ductal carcinoma in situ. Lobular carcinoma in situ may also have microcalcifications in

TABLE 19-1 Frequency of Histological Subtypes of Invasive Breast Cancer

Subtype	Frequency (%)
Invasive ductal carcinoma	
Pure	55
Mixed with other types (including lobular)	25
Invasive lobular carcinoma (pure)	10
Medullary carcinoma (pure)	<5
Mucinous carcinoma (pure)	2
Other pure types	2
Other mixed types	1

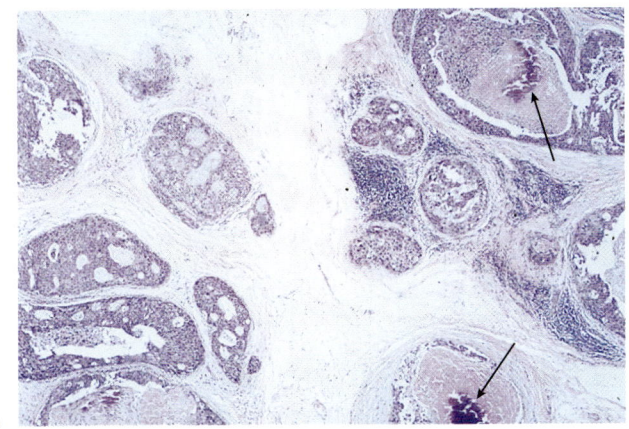
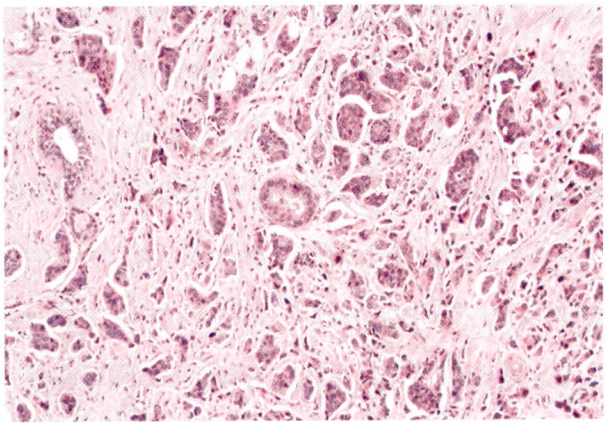
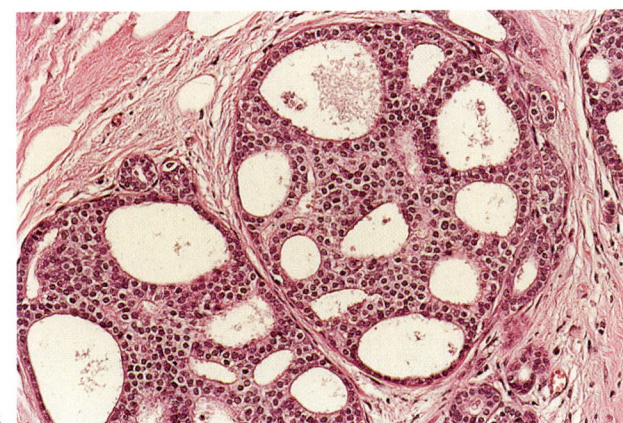

FIGURE 19-10
Ductal carcinoma. **A.** Ductal carcinoma in situ-comedo type. The terminal ducts are distended by carcinoma in situ (intraductal carcinoma). The centers of the tumor masses are necrotic and display dystrophic calcification (arrows). **B.** Ductal carcinoma in situ-noncomedo type. A cribriform arrangement of tumor cells is evident. **C.** Invasive Ductal Carcinoma. Irregular cords and nest of tumor cells, derived from the same cells that compose the intraductal component (A), invade the stroma. Many of the cells form ductlike structures. **D.** Fine-needle aspiration. This cytological preparation shows tumor cells that exhibit nuclear pleomorphism and prominent nucleoli.

the ducts that can be detected radiographically. The lesion does not usually incite the dense fibrosis and chronic inflammation so characteristic of intraductal carcinoma in situ and is, therefore, less likely to cause a detectable mass. It is not uncommon for lobular carcinoma in situ to be an "incidental" finding in a biopsy that was prompted by benign changes.

As with intraductal carcinoma in situ, 20 to 30% of women with lobular carcinoma in situ receiving no further treatment after biopsy will develop invasive cancer within 20 years of diagnosis. However, about half of these invasive cancers will arise in the contralateral breast and may be either lobular or ductal cancers. Thus, lobular carcinoma in situ, more than ductal carcinoma in situ, serves as a marker for an enhanced risk of subsequent invasive cancer in both breasts.

Papillary Carcinoma in Situ

Papillary carcinoma in situ is far less common than either intraductal carcinoma or lobular carcinoma in situ. This neoplasm is unusual in that it originates in the larger branches of the duct system. The tumor is very well differentiated and exhibits a papillary configuration. The cells are typically small and regular, making it in some instances difficult to distinguish this form of carcinoma from a benign intraductal papilloma. Papillary carcinoma in situ does not carry an increased risk of subsequent invasive cancer after its complete local excision.

Invasive Carcinoma Carries a Stage-Dependent Prognosis

Ductal Carcinoma

Invasive, or infiltrating, ductal carcinoma is the most common form of breast cancer. In this cancer, stromal invasion by malignant cells usually incites a pronounced fibroblastic proliferation. This "desmoplasia" creates a palpable mass, which is the most common initial sign of ductal carcinoma. Invasive ductal carcinoma usually manifests as a hard, fixed mass, which is often referred to as *scirrhous carcinoma* (see Fig. 19-9). On gross examination, the tumor is typically firm and shows irregular margins. The cut surface is pale gray and gritty and flecked with yellow, chalky streaks.

Microscopically, invasive ductal carcinoma grows as irregular nests and cords of epithelial cells, usually within a dense fibrous stroma (Fig. 19-10C). The well-differentiated cancers may form abortive glands, whereas the less-differentiated forms consist of solid sheets of neoplastic cells. The cells show a variable degree of differentiation and mitotic activity and are cytologically indistinguishable from those of ductal carcinoma in situ (Fig.19-10A and D). Poorly differentiated, rapidly growing cancers may display extensive necrosis.

PAGET DISEASE OF THE NIPPLE: Paget disease of the nipple refers to an uncommon variant of ductal carcinoma, either

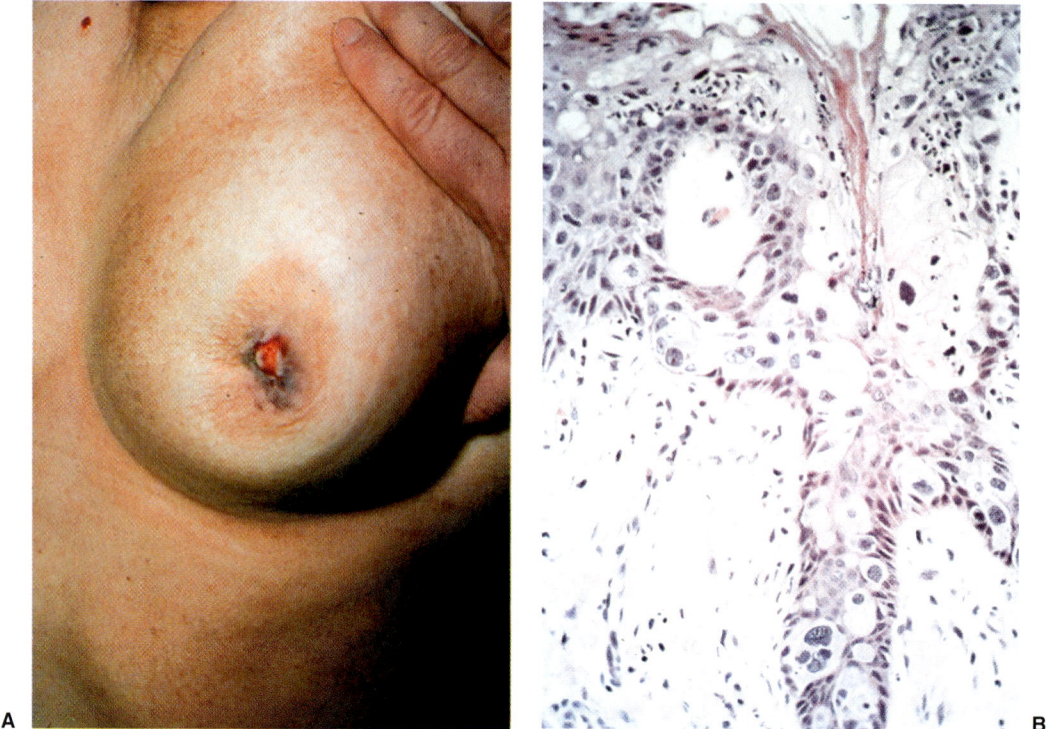

FIGURE 19-11
Paget disease of the nipple. A. An erythematous, scaly, and weeping "eczema" involves the nipple. B. The epidermis contains clusters of ductal type carcinoma cells that are larger and have more abundant pale cytoplasm than the surrounding keratinocytes.

in situ or invasive, that extends to involve the epidermis of the nipple and areola (Fig. 19-11A). This condition usually comes to medical attention because of an eczematous change in the skin of the nipple and areola. Microscopically, large cells with clear cytoplasm *(Paget cells)* are found singly or in groups within the epidermis (Fig. 19-11B). The prognosis of Paget disease is related to that of the underlying ductal cancer.

Lobular Carcinoma

Invasive lobular carcinoma is the second most common form of invasive breast cancer (Fig. 19-12). Because the amount of fibrosis is variable, the clinical presentation of invasive lobular carcinoma varies from a discrete firm mass, similar to ductal carcinoma, to a more subtle, diffuse, indurated area. Microscopically, the classic invasive lobular carcinoma consists of single strands of malignant cells infiltrating between stromal fibers, a feature termed *Indian filing* (Fig. 19-12B). Occasionally, a more solid or trabecular growth pattern is observed. The small, bland cells are cytologically identical to those of the in situ form, and mitotic activity is rare. In spite of the innocuous cytological characteristics of this form of invasive carcinoma, it is biologically as aggressive as the invasive ductal type.

Variants of classical lobular carcinoma display an overall growth pattern that is identical to that of the ordinary invasive lobular carcinoma. However, the nuclear characteristics are different. In one form, the small, regular tumor cells possess intracellular mucin. The mucin commonly compresses the nucleus to one side, giving the cell a "signet ring" appearance, hence the term *signet ring carcinoma* (Fig. 19-12C). Another variant maintains the usual lobular growth pattern, but has more marked nuclear pleomorphism, and is referred to as *pleomorphic lobular carcinoma.* Twenty-five percent of invasive carcinomas have features of both ductal and lobular carcinoma (see Table 19-1).

Uncommon Types of Invasive Breast Cancer

COLLOID (MUCINOUS) CARCINOMA: This invasive variant tends to occur in older women. On cut section, colloid carcinoma has a glistening surface and mucoid consistency. Histologically, it is composed of small clusters of epithelial cells, occasionally forming glands, floating in pools of extracellular mucin (Fig. 19-13). In its pure form, colloid carcinoma has a considerably better prognosis than infiltrating ductal or lobular carcinoma. However, it is often admixed with infiltrating ductal carcinoma, in which circumstance the prognosis is determined by the ductal component.

TUBULAR CARCINOMA: Also known as well-differentiated carcinoma, invasive tubular carcinoma is composed of randomly arranged, infiltrating, well-formed small ducts that consist of only one or two layers of small, regular cells. The prognosis of this cancer, when it is not admixed with other types, is excellent, and it is virtually always cured by mastectomy or wide excision.

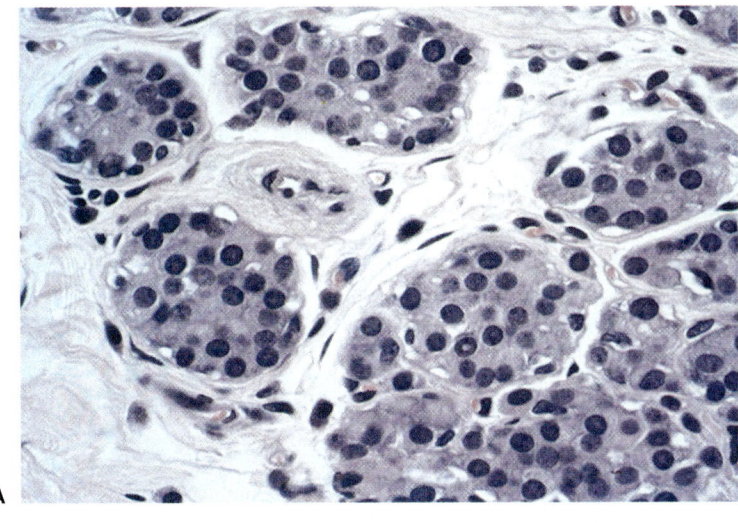
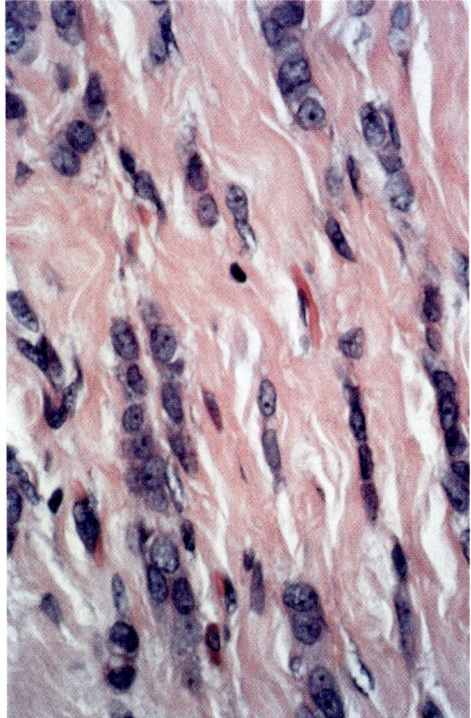
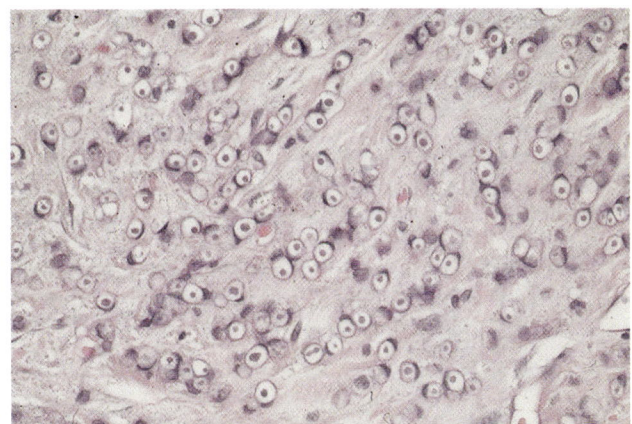

FIGURE 19-12
Lobular carcinoma. **A.** Lobular carcinoma in situ. The lumina of the terminal duct lobular units are distended by tumor cells, which exhibit round nuclei and small nucleoli. The cancer cells in the lobular form of carcinoma in situ are smaller and have less cytoplasm than those in the ductal type. **B.** Invasive lobular carcinoma. In contrast to invasive ductal carcinoma, the cells of lobular carcinoma tend to form single strands that invade between collagen fibers in a single pattern. The tumor cells are similar to those seen in lobular carcinoma in situ. **C.** Signet ring carcinoma. The tumor cells contain large amounts of clear mucin.

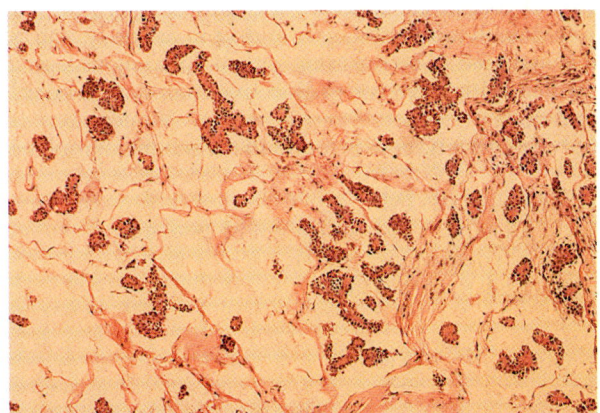

FIGURE 19-13
Colloid (mucinous) carcinoma. Clusters of malignant cells float in large pools of extracellular mucin.

MEDULLARY CARCINOMA: Clinically and by mammography, this invasive tumor presents as a circumscribed mass that lacks calcifications. Medullary carcinoma has a distinctive gross appearance, being a well-circumscribed, fleshy, pale gray mass. Microscopically, it is composed of sheets of cells that are highly pleomorphic and have a high mitotic index (Fig. 19-14). The pathological definition of medullary carcinoma includes a lymphoid infiltrate encompassing the periphery of the tumor. In spite of the highly malignant histological appearance of this neoplasm, it has a distinctly better prognosis than infiltrating ductal or lobular carcinoma.

METAPLASTIC CARCINOMA: This is a rare invasive variant in which the malignant epithelium has partially differentiated into either another type of epithelium or mesenchymal tissue. Such tumors may show areas of malignant squamous, fibrous, cartilaginous, or bony tissue, admixed with the malignant glandular component.

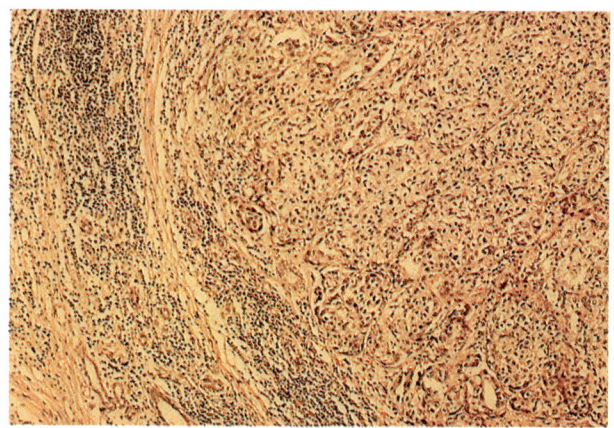

FIGURE 19-14
Medullary carcinoma. The malignant cells are pleomorphic and grow in solid sheets, forming a blunt margin. There is no gland formation. Numerous mitoses are present. The tumor is surrounded by a dense lymphocytic infiltrate.

Metastatic Patterns of Breast Cancer

Invasive breast cancer spreads primarily through the lymphatics to regional lymph nodes, including the axillary, internal mammary, and supraclavicular nodes. In about half of all patients with breast cancer, the tumor has already metastasized to the axillary nodes at the time of diagnosis. The probability of spread to the axillary nodes is directly related to the size of the primary tumor. Involvement of the internal mammary and the supraclavicular lymph nodes is uncommon in the absence of metastases to the axillary nodes. Breast cancer also spreads to distant sites, most commonly the lung and pleura, liver, bone, adrenals, skin, and brain.

Prognostic Factors

Stage at Diagnosis

The most important prognostic factor in breast cancer is the stage (i.e., the extent of tumor spread) at the time of diagnosis. In general, small tumors localized to the breast have an excellent prognosis, whereas those that have spread to distant organs are incurable. Larger primary tumors and those that have metastasized to regional lymph nodes have an intermediate prognosis.

- **Stage I:** Tumors 2 cm or less in diameter without direct extension or nodal metastases
- **Stage II:** Tumors between 2 and 5 cm in diameter without nodal metastases or any tumor less than 5 cm with ipsilateral axillary metastases in which the lymph nodes remain movable
- **Stage III:** A tumor more than 5 cm in diameter with or without lymph node metastases; any tumor with metastases in axillary lymph nodes and nodes fixed to one another or other structures; any tumor with involvement of the underlying pectoral muscle or fascia (not including the chest wall)
- **Stage IV:** Any tumor with involvement of the chest wall (ribs and intercostal muscles) skin of the breast (including inflammatory carcinoma); any tumor with metastases to ipsilateral supraclavicular or infraclavicular nodes, or edema of the arm, or any distant metastases

Most breast cancers present as small tumors localized in the breast (stage I or II). There is a significant difference in survival between women who are seen with stage I disease and those with axillary node metastases (stage II). Within stage II disease, survival decreases as the number of involved axillary nodes increases. Women with advanced local or regional disease (stage III) can be palliated but usually not cured. The prognosis for women with distant metastases (stage IV) is poor in terms of survival, but palliative treatment may significantly prolong life.

With growing public awareness of breast cancer and the expanding use of screening mammography, more than half of the breast cancers currently diagnosed in the United States manifest as stage I disease. Some 70% of these women will be cured by surgery; the remaining 30%, if treated with surgery alone, will have recurrent disease. Clinical studies have shown that the benefit of routinely adding chemotherapy to surgery in the treatment of all stage I patients is marginal and not without morbidity. Thus, there is an impetus to identify specific subsets of women who might particularly benefit from chemotherapy in addition to surgery.

The stage of a neoplasm is also expressed in terms of the TMN classification, which describes the clinical or pathological extent of the neoplasm and the degree of cellular differentiation. A simplified scheme is noted below.

Primary tumor (T)

Tis	Carcinoma in situ
T1	Diameter equal to 2 cm or less in greatest dimension
T1cs	Diameter more than 1 cm, not more than 2 cm
T2	Diameter more than 2 cm but not more than 5 cm

Regional lymph nodes (N)

N0	No regional lymph node metastasis
N1	Metastasis to movable ipsilateral axillary lymph node(s)
N2	Metastases in ipsilateral axillary lymph nodes fixed or matted

A "sentinel node" assessment often is performed intraoperatively to assess the status of the ipsilateral lymph nodes. The sentinel lymph node is the most proximate lymph node and is assumed to be the initial site of nodal metastasis. It is identified with a dye or radioactive material. An axillary lymph node dissection is performed only if microscopic evidence of metastatic cells is found in the sentinel lymph node.

Distant metastasis (M)

MX	Distant metastasis cannot be assessed
M0	No distant metastasis
M1	Distant metastasis

Histological Grade

In addition to the histological subtype and stage of the cancer, the histological grade of the primary tumor is also a useful prognostic indicator. The histological grade includes (1) the degree of glandular differentiation, (2) the degree of nuclear atypia, and (3) the mitotic index. In the standard grading system, each of these parameters is given a score of 1 to 3. The sum of the scores of these three parameters results in an overall grade as follows: 3 to 5, well-differentiated; 6 to 7, moderately differentiated; 8 to 9, poorly differentiated. Less differentiated tumors tend to have a worse prognosis.

Estrogen and Progesterone Receptors

Over half of breast cancers exhibit nuclear estrogen-receptor protein. A slightly smaller proportion also have progesterone receptors. Women whose cancers possess hormone receptors have a longer disease-free survival and overall survival than those with early stage cancers who are negative for these receptors.

The beneficial effects of oophorectomy on survival in patients with breast cancer led to the use of estrogen antagonists in the treatment of breast cancer. In general, antiestrogen therapy seems to prolong disease-free survival, particularly in postmenopausal and node-positive women. It also lowers the risk of cancer in the contralateral breast. The latter discovery has led to the use of antiestrogens as chemoprevention in women at "high risk" for developing breast cancer.

Proliferative Capacity and Ploidy

The measurement of proliferative capacity of breast cancers has prognostic value. In general, increased proliferative capacity is associated with a poorer prognosis. There are several methods used to evaluate the proliferative capacity of breast cancers, including (1) mitotic index, as judged by histological evaluation; (2) estimation of the proportion of cells in the S phase of the cell cycle by flow cytometry; and (3) immunohistochemical staining for nuclear proteins expressed in cells that are actively proliferating (Ki67 or mib1 antigens). When proliferative capacity is evaluated by flow cytometry, cell cycle analysis can also detect the presence of aneuploid cell populations. The presence of aneuploidy, which is found in two thirds of breast cancers, has also been associated with a worse prognosis.

Lymphatic and Vascular Invasion

The presence of lymphatic and vascular invasion within the breast is associated with a poorer prognosis. *Inflammatory carcinoma of the breast* describes dermal lymphatic invasion, a condition that carries a particularly bad prognosis. Such invasion causes obstruction of lymphatic drainage and, therefore, commonly correlates with clinical erythema and induration of the skin of the breast, so-called *peau d'orange* (because of the resemblance to the skin of an orange).

Oncogene Expression

Overexpression of *HER2/neu* is identified in 10 to 35% of primary breast tumors and is mostly attributable to gene amplification. Amplification or overexpression of *HER2/neu* has also been described in cancers of the lung, ovary, and stomach. Overexpression can be determined by immunohistological detection of the c-erbB2 protein on the cell membrane (Fig. 19-15A) or by analysis of the *HER2/neu* gene using fluorescent in situ hybridization (FISH) (Fig. 19-15B). Patients whose tumors demonstrate *HER2* gene amplification benefit from therapy with a monoclonal antibody that selectively binds to the extracellular domain of the protein. Mutation and overexpression of the *p53* tumor suppressor gene correlates with recurrence of breast cancer and shortened survival.

Other Factors Related to Invasion and Metastasis

A number of enzymes, cell adhesion molecules, and angiogenic markers have been reported to bear some relationship to breast cancer metastasis and recurrence. These include stromelysin, urokinase-plasminogen activator, laminin receptor, and high vascular density. However, these markers have demonstrated only limited predictive power, and their significance remains to be established. Recent studies have reported that the "gene expression signature" of a tumor can be a significant predictor of survival in breast can-

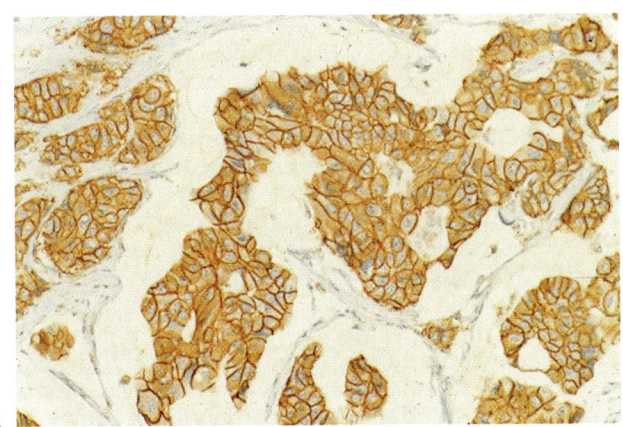
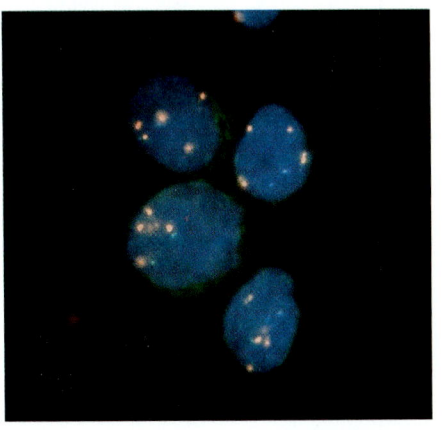

FIGURE 19-15
HER2/neu in breast cancer. A. Immunoperoxide staining of invasive ductal carcinoma shows over expression of HER2/neu protein. B. Flourescence in situ hybridization (FISH) demonstrates genetic amplification of HER2/neu.

cer. In one such study, microarray analysis of 70 candidate genes encoding tumor suppressor proteins, growth factors, and hormonal receptors, together with genes expressed primarily by B and T cells of infiltrating lymphocytes, permitted the separation of patients with stage I and stage II disease into either good or poor prognostic groups, regardless of the lymph node status of the patient. (Fig 19-16). Other studies of prostatic, lung, and colonic adenocarcinoma have demonstrated similar gene expression profiles that provide prognostic information.

Treatment

The cornerstone of effective treatment of breast cancer is early detection. Regular self-examination of the breasts, adherence to recommended guidelines for screening mammograms, and periodic examinations by a physician decrease mortality from breast cancer by 30%.

It is useful to evaluate a suspicious mass in as minimally invasive a way as possible, so that the greatest number of options for definitive therapy are maintained, not only for curing the cancer but also for preservation of the woman's breast. Fine-needle aspiration is now a widely accepted modality for evaluating a clinically palpable mass. This technique has a sensitivity of 80 to 90%, with virtually no false-positive results.

The treatment of breast cancer remains controversial. Historically, a significant advance in the treatment of this cancer was radical mastectomy (en bloc removal of the breast, all axillary lymph nodes, and underlying chest wall muscles). Although early detection has increased the proportion of tumors that are treated at more favorable stages, subsequent developments in the therapy for breast cancer have not greatly improved the prognosis of women with this disease. Today, the modified radical mastectomy, which differs from radical mastectomy in leaving the chest wall muscles intact and foregoing dissection of the superior axillary lymph nodes, is the treatment of choice for many breast cancers. In early-stage breast cancer, an acceptable alternative to mastectomy is the complete excision of the primary cancer ("lumpectomy" or segmental excision), leaving most of the breast intact. Separate surgical excision of the nearby axillary nodes is performed, followed by irradiation of the breast. In terms of the 10-year survival for appropriately selected cases, this approach is as successful as a modified radical mastectomy.

Cancer of the Male Breast Is Distinctly Uncommon

Cancer in the male breast accounts for less than 1% of all cases of breast cancer. As in women, by far the most common subtype is infiltrating ductal carcinoma. Because there is less fat in the breast, invasion of chest wall muscles is more frequent at the time of diagnosis in men. For tumors of the same stage, however, the prognosis for male breast cancer is similar to that of the female. Predisposing factors for the development of breast cancer in men are largely unknown, although mutations in the *BRCA2* gene (see above) increase the risk of this tumor.

PHYLLODES TUMOR

Phyllodes tumor of the breast is a proliferation of stromal elements accompanied by a benign growth of ductal structures (Fig. 19-17). These tumors usually occur in women between 30 and 70 years of age, with a peak in the fifth decade. The original term for this tumor, *cystosarcoma phyllodes,* implies malignant behavior, although only a minority of these tumors are capable of invasion and metastasis. Thus, current terminology refers to *phyllodes tumor,* with the additional designation of benign or malignant.

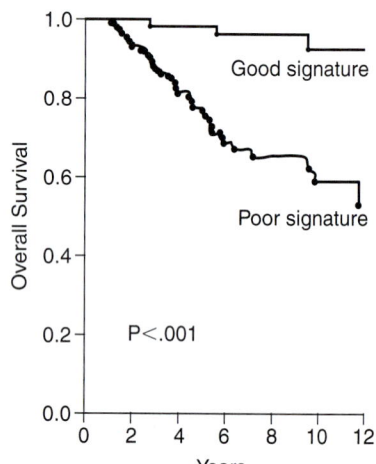

Pathology: Phyllodes tumors resemble fibroadenomas in their overall architecture and the presence of glandular and stromal elements. Like fibroadenoma, benign phyllodes tumor is sharply circumscribed, and the cut surface is firm, glistening, and grayish white. Benign and malignant phyllodes tumor is similar in gross appearance. Although in the past they were described as very large tumors, the average size today is 5 cm in diameter, and many smaller tumors are encountered.

Microscopically, the stroma of a benign phyllodes tumor is hypercellular and has mitotic activity. The distinction from fibroadenoma is made not on the size, but on the histological and cytological characteristics of the stromal component.

The diagnosis of a malignant phyllodes tumor is based on the appearance of the stromal component. Malignant phyllodes tumors have an obviously sarcomatous stroma with abundant mitotic activity, and the stromal component is increased out of proportion to the benign duct elements. They are usually poorly circumscribed, with invasion into the surrounding breast tissue. Malignant tumors may exhibit various sarcomatous tissue types, such as malignant fibrous histiocytoma, chondrosarcoma, and osteosarcoma.

FIGURE 19-16
Genomic expression and prognosis of breast cancer. Microarray analysis of gene expression in patients with lymph node metastases demonstrates prognostic differences.

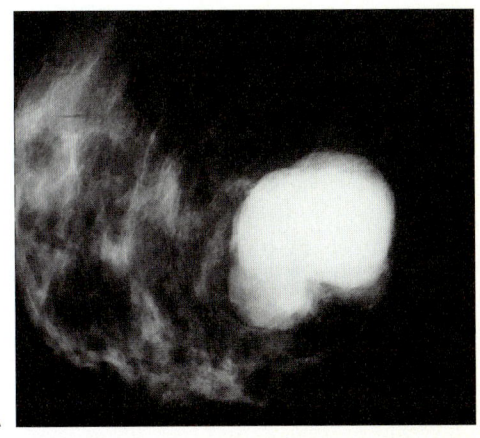
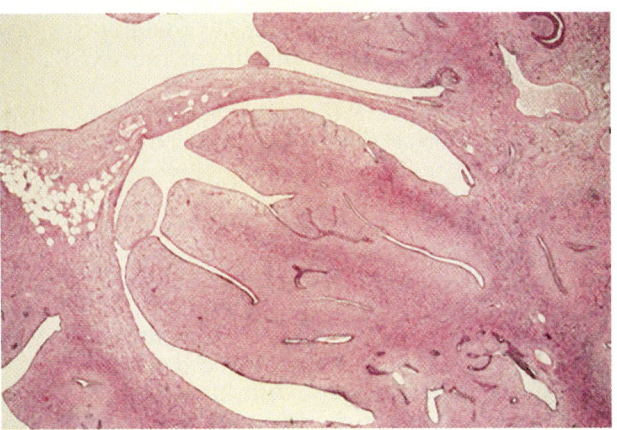
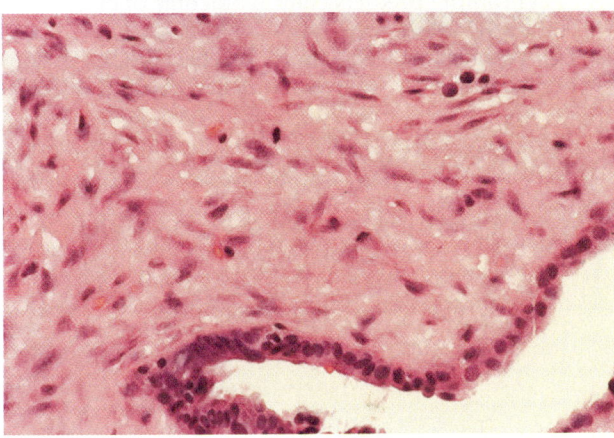

FIGURE 19-17
A. A mammogram demonstrates a large, circumscribed phyllodes tumor with an irregular contour. B. A polypoid tumor with a leaflike pattern expands a duct. C. The stromal component adjacent to ductal epithelium is similar to a fibroadenoma, but is more cellular. The residual ductal structure is benign.

Clinical Features: Benign phyllodes tumors are adequately treated by local excision. The initial treatment of a malignant phyllodes tumor is wide excision if the tumor is small or a simple mastectomy if the tumor is large. An axillary lymph node dissection is not indicated. Malignant phyllodes tumors tend to recur locally, and 15% eventually metastasize to both distant sites and axillary lymph nodes.

SUGGESTED READING

Books

Harris JR, Lippman ME, Morrow M, Hellman S: *Diseases of the breast.* Philadelphia: Lippincott–Raven, 1996.

Rosai J: Breast. In: *Ackerman's surgical pathology,* 9th ed. St. Louis: Mosby, 2002.

Rosen PP: *Rosen's breast pathology.* Philadelphia: Lippincott Williams & Wilkins, 2001.

Sharkey FE, Allred DC, Valente PT: Breast. In: Damjanov I, Linder J (eds): *Anderson's pathology,* 10th ed. St. Louis: Mosby, 1996.

Tavassoli FA: *Pathology of the breast,* 2nd ed. New York: Elsevier, 1999.

Review Articles

Armstrong K, Eisen A, Weber B: Assessing the risk of breast cancer. *N Engl J Med* 342(8):564–570, 2000.

Association of Directors of Anatomic and Surgical Pathology: Recommendations in the reporting of breast carcinoma. *Am J Clin Path* 104:614–619, 1995.

Balmain A, Gray J, Ponder B: The genetics and genomics of cancer. *Nat Genet* 33(suppl):238–244, 2003.

Braunstein GD: Gynecomastia. *N Engl J Med* 328:490–495, 1993.

Clemons M, Goss P: Estrogen and the risk of breast cancer. *N Engl J Med* 344(4):276–85, 2001.

Domchek SM, Weber BL: Recent advances in breast cancer biology. *Curr Opin Oncol* 14(6):589–593, 2002.

Fechner RE: One century of mammary carcinoma *in situ.* What have we learned. *Am J Clin Path* 100:654–661, 1993.

International conference series on nutrition and health promotion. Breast cancer research: Current issues—Future directions. *Cancer* 74(suppl):991–1192, 1994.

Jakub JW, Pendas S, Reintgen DS: Current status of sentinel lymph node mapping and biopsy: facts and controversies. *Oncologist* 8(1):59–68, 2003.

Keen JC, Davidson NE: The biology of breast carcinoma. *Cancer* 97(3 suppl):825–833, 2003.

Key TJ, Allen NE: Hormones and breast cancer. *IARC Sci Publ* 156:273–276, 2002.

Popescu NC, Zimonjic DB: Chromosome and gene alterations in breast cancer as markers for diagnosis and prognosis as well as pathogenetic targets for therapy. *Am J Med Genet* 115(3):142–149, 2002.

Sauer G, Deissler H: Angiogenesis: Prognostic and therapeutic implications in gynecologic and breast malignancies. *Curr Opin Obstet Gynecol* 15(1):45–49, 2003.

Skolnick AA: New data suggest needle biopsies could replace surgical biopsy for diagnosing breast cancer. *JAMA* 271:1724–1728, 1994.

Terribile D, Palumbo F, Nardone L: Prognostic role of sentinel lymph node biopsy in breast cancer. *Rays* 27(4):291–294, 2002.

Original Articles

Bellamy COC, McDonald C, Salter DM, et al.: Non-invasive ductal carcinoma of the breast. The relevance of histologic categorization. *Hum Pathol* 24:16–23, 1993.

Fisher B, Anderson S, Redmond CK, et al: Reanalysis and results after 12 years of follow-up in a randomized clinical trial comparing total mastectomy with lumpectomy with or without irradiation in the treatment of breast cancer. *N Engl J Med* 333:1456–1461, 1995.

Kallioniemi A: Molecular signature of breast cancer—Predicting the future (editorial) *N Engl J Med* 347:25, 2067–2068, (2002).

Page DL, Jensen RA: Ductal carcinoma *in situ* of the breast. Understanding the misunderstood stepchild (editorial). *JAMA* 275:948, 949, 1996.

Sandias EE, DeBree E, Tsiftsis DD: How many cases are enough for accreditation in sentinel lymph node biopsy in breast cancer: *Am J Surg* 185(3):202–210, 2003.

Shattuck-Eidens D, McClure M, Simard J, et al.: A collaborative survey of 80 mutations in the BRCA1 breast and ovarian cancer susceptibility gene. Implications for presymptomatic testing and screening. *JAMA* 273: 535–541, 1995.

Van de Vijver M, et al.: A gene expression signature as a predictor of survival in breast cancer. *N Engl J Med* 347: 1999–2009, 2002.

Van't Veer LJ, Dai H, van de Vijver MJ, et al.: Gene expression profiling predicts clinical outcome of breast cancer. *Nature* 415:2002.

Yang Q, Yoshimura G, Nakamura M, et al.: BRCA1 in non-inherited breast carcinomas. *Oncol Rep* 9(6):1329–1333, 2002.

CHAPTER 20

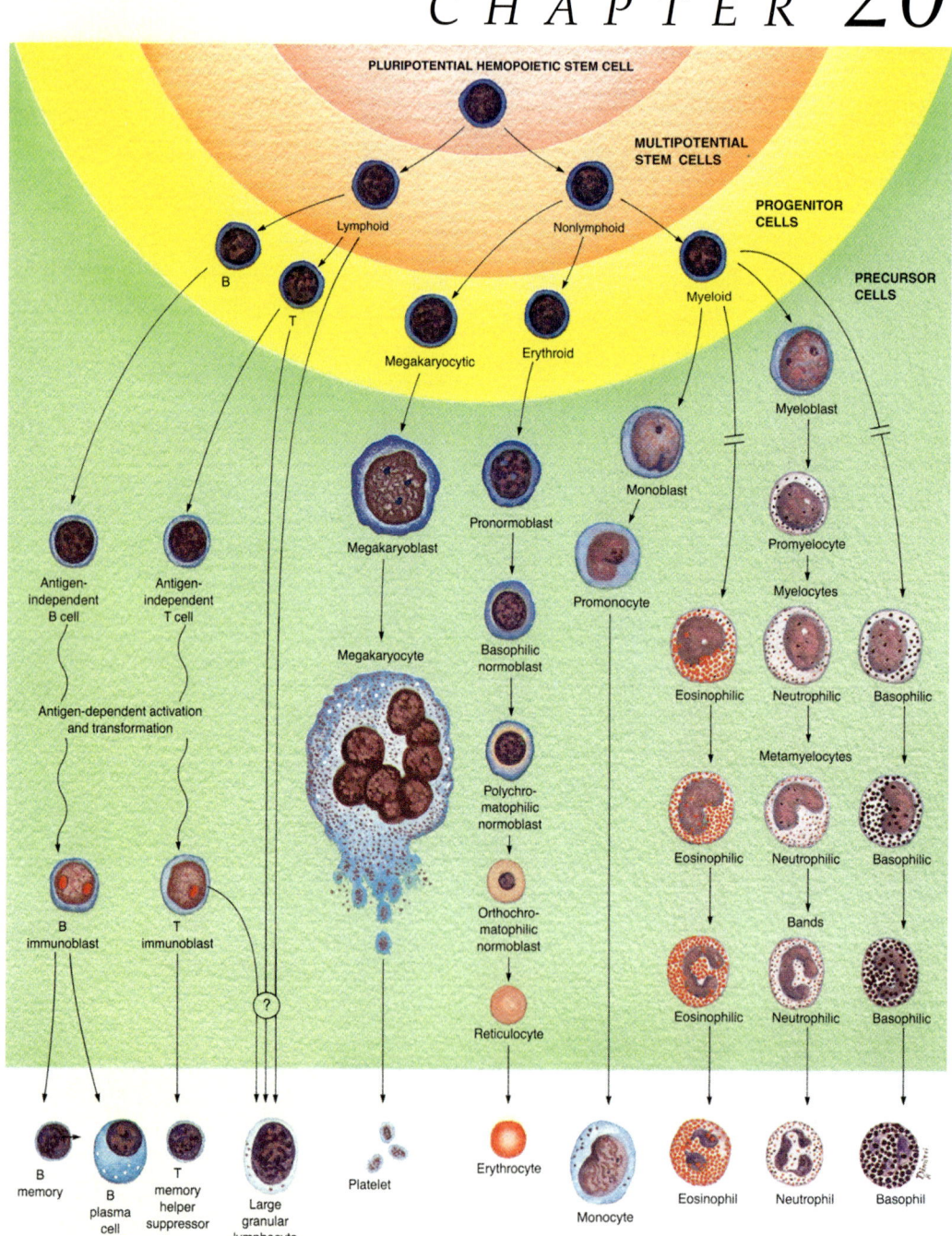

Hematopathology

Roland Schwarting
William D. Kocher
Steven McKenzie
Mohammad Alomari

Bone Marrow and Normal Myelopoietic Cells

Embryology

Bone Marrow

Bone Marrow Disorders

Functional Kinetics

Peripheral Myelopoietic Cells

Granulocytes

Basophils

Monocytes

Red Blood Cells

Normal Structure and Function

Red Blood Cell Disorders

Anemia

Decreased Red Blood Cell Production

Ineffective Red Cell Production

Hemolytic Anemias

Acute Blood Loss Anemia

Polycythemia

Platelets and Hemostasis

Normal Hemostasis

Platelets

Blood Vessels and Endothelial Cells

Activation of the Coagulation Cascade

Thrombolysis

Hemostatic Disorders

Hemostatic Disorders of Blood Vessels

Platelet Disorders

Coagulopathies

Hypercoagulability

White Blood Cells

Nonmalignant Disorders

Neutropenia

Neutrophilia

Qualitative Disorders of Neutrophils

Eosinophilia

Basophilia

Monocytosis

Langerhans Cell Histiocytosis

Proliferative Disorders of Mast Cells

(continued)

FIGURE 20-1 *(see opposite page)*
Cellular differentiation and maturation of the lymphoid *(left)* and myeloid *(right)* components of the hematopoietic system. Only the precursor cells (blasts and maturing cells) are identifiable by light microscopic evaluation of the bone marrow.

Ancillary Techniques in the Diagnosis of Hematological Malignancies

Leukemias and Myelodysplastic Syndromes

Chronic Myeloproliferative Diseases

Myelodysplastic Syndromes

Acute Myeloid Leukemia

Disorders of the Lymphopoietic System

Normal Lymphocytes

Lymph Nodes

Lymphoid Tissue of the Intestine and Bronchus

Benign Disorders of the Lymphopoietic System

Lymphocytosis

Plasmacytosis

Lymphocytopenia

Reactive Hyperplasia of Lymph Nodes

Sinus Histiocytosis

Sinus Histiocytosis with Massive Lymphadenopathy

Dermatopathic Lymphadenopathy

Infection-Induced Hemophagocytic Syndrome

Malignant Lymphomas

B Acute Lymphoblastic Leukemia/Lymphoma

Precursor T Cells in Lymphoblastic Lymphomas

Mature (Peripheral) B-Cell Lymphomas

Mature T-Cell and NK-Cell Malignancies

Hodgkin Lymphoma

Histological Classification of Hodgkin Lymphoma

Posttransplant Lymphoproliferative Disorder

Spleen

Anatomy and Function

Disorders of the Spleen

Splenomegaly

Thymus

Hyperplasia

Thymoma

Malignant Thymoma

Other Tumors of the Thymus

Bone and Normal Myelopoietic Cells

EMBRYOLOGY

Hematopoiesis, or blood cell formation, first occurs in the fetal yolk sac (Fig. 20-2). After the third week of embryogenesis, erythrocyte formation shifts to the liver and spleen, where the cells contain fetal hemoglobins rather than the embryonic hemoglobins produced during the yolk sac phase. At term, erythropoiesis in the liver and spleen has ceased, and marrow erythropoiesis has become fully established.

From birth until 4 years of age, all bone cavities are densely packed with hematopoietic tissue. After that time, the size of the bone cavities outgrows the volume required for hematopoiesis, and in adults, fat cells are intermixed in the available space. The cavities in the axial skeleton continue to be active and full of "red marrow" until old age, when resorption of cancellous bone further enlarges the marrow cavities and leads to replacement by fat.

Local expansion of red (cellular) marrow and reactivation of peripheral yellow marrow provide the hematopoietic system with a capacity to meet demands for increased blood cell formation. Reactivation of hepatic and splenic hematopoiesis rarely occurs during adult life. **The finding of extramedullary hematopoiesis in soft tissue sites usually suggests a clonal (malignant) disorder, rather than a reactive one.**

BONE MARROW

The bone marrow consists of a complex network of solid cords separated by sinusoids (Fig. 20-3). The cords are composed of stromal and hematopoietic cells, knitted together by extracellular matrix. The semipermeable barrier between the sinusoids and the cords consists of a layer of endothelial cells, a thin basement membrane, and an outer interrupted layer of reticular adventitial cells. These reticular cells branch extensively throughout the cords and provide a scaffold for stromal and hematopoietic cells. The other stromal cells include macrophages, endothelial cells, lymphocytes, and fibroblasts.

Within the cords are islands of erythroblasts, usually located in concentric rings around a macrophage (inappropri-

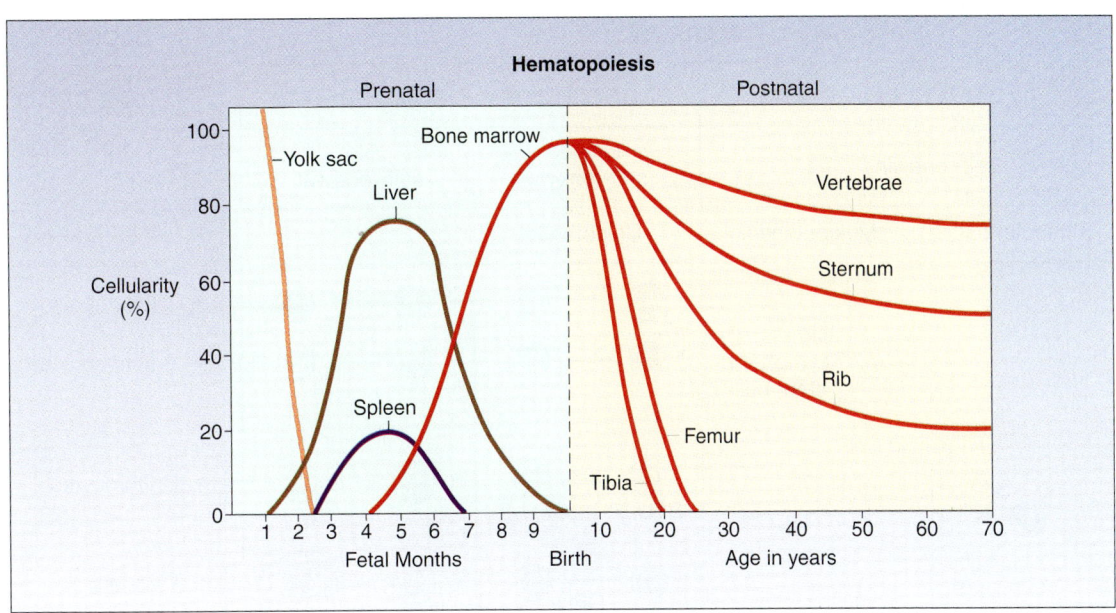

FIGURE 20-2
Hematopoiesis in various organs before and after birth.

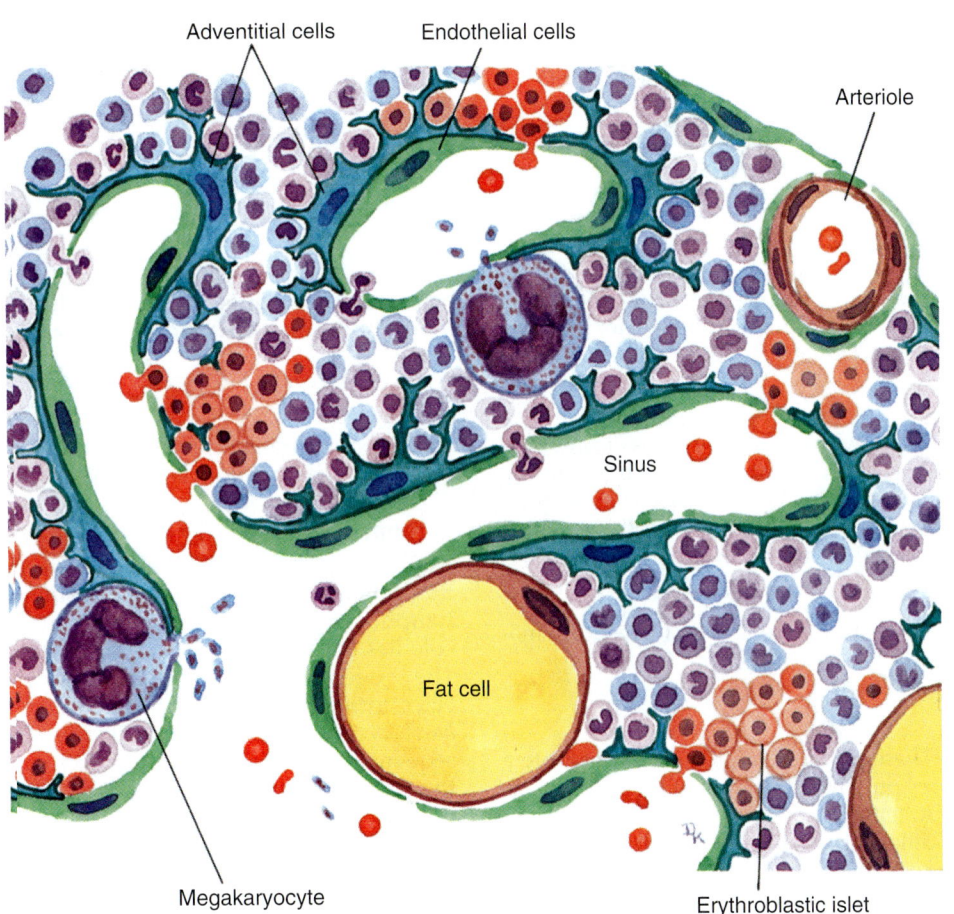

FIGURE 20-3
Structure of normal bone marrow.

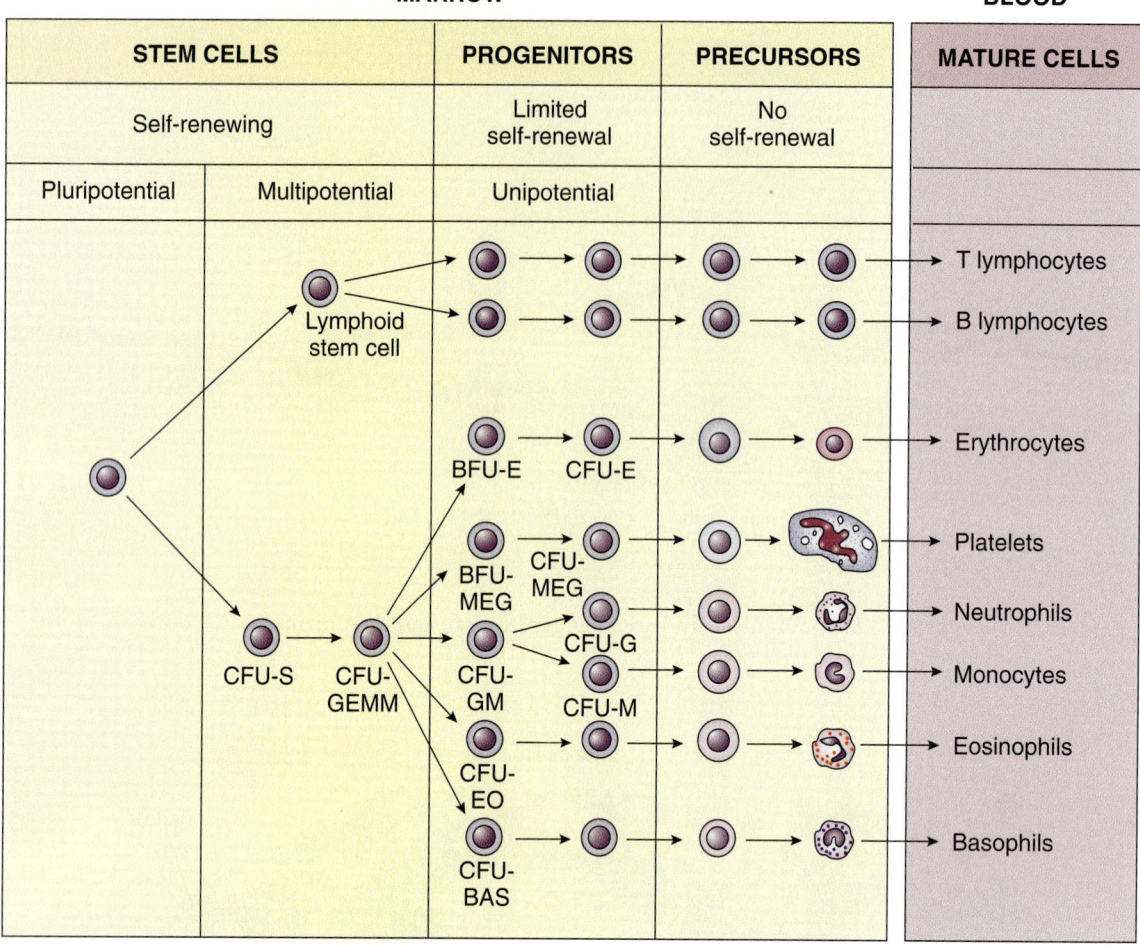

FIGURE 20-4
Differentiation of formed elements of the blood, with a simplified schema of some sites of action (→) of selected cytokines, interleukins, and colony-stimulating factors. Note that the stem cells and progenitors are not readily identifiable in the routine examination of a bone marrow aspirate.

ately termed a *nurse cell*), which removes excess iron or extruded nuclei. These islands lie in close proximity to the walls of the sinusoids, as do the megakaryocytes. The granulocyte precursors are located deeper in the cords.

There are three critical components of hematopoiesis:

- Stem cells (*seed*)
- Stroma, consisting of stromal cells and extracellular matrix (*soil*)
- Growth factors (*fertilizer*)

STEM CELLS: These undifferentiated cells constitute a self-perpetuating pool, in which differentiation and exit are carefully balanced by self-renewal (Fig. 20-4). Stem cells are small mononuclear cells that cannot be easily identified morphologically. However, they can be isolated by injecting marrow elements into radiated mice, in which the stem cells form visible colonies in the spleen (*colony-forming unit, spleen; CFU-S*). In bone marrow that is cultured in semisolid medium, stem cells also form colonies composed of multiple cell types, including *g*ranulocyte, *e*rythroid, *m*acrophage, and *m*egakaryocyte elements *(CFU-GEMM)*. Stem cells are semidormant (noncycling), but on demand undergo differentiation to progenitor cells of specific cell lines.

PROGENITOR CELLS: Similar to stem cells, the progenitor cells are small to medium-sized mononuclear cells that cannot be morphologically distinguished from mature lymphocytes. When cultured in vitro, they give rise to colonies consisting of thousands of differentiated progeny. The progenitor cell committed to the production of erythrocytes forms luxuriant burst-shaped colonies and is named *burst-forming unit, erythroid (BFU-E)* (Fig. 20-5). Each subsequent generation of BFU-E makes smaller colonies, until the final progenitor cell, the *colony-forming unit, erythroid (CFU-E)*, produces only a small clone of mature erythroblasts.

The granulocytic and monocytic cell lines originate from a single progenitor cell. When grown in vitro, this cell, named *colony-forming unit, granulocyte-monocyte (CFU-GM)*, forms a colony consisting of both granulocytic and monocytic cells. As the cell matures, its progeny become increasingly committed to one or the other cell line.

Eosinophils and basophils also have specific progenitor cells, although they appear to branch off during the matura-

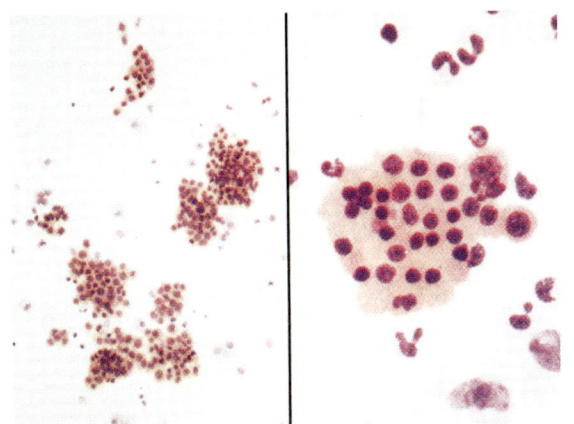

FIGURE 20-5
(Left) When grown in vitro, erythroid progenitor cells give rise to burst-shaped colonies consisting of differentiated progeny. *(Right)* A higher-power view. The progenitor cell committed to the production of erythrocytes forms luxuriant burst-shaped colonies and is named *burst-forming unit, erythroid* (BFU-E).

tion of precursor cells. The *megakaryocytic progenitor cells* (CFU-Meg) produce colonies in vitro consisting of four to eight megakaryocytes.

PRECURSOR CELLS: The next step in hematopoiesis is the transformation of progenitor cells to precursor cells termed *blasts* (Fig. 20-1). It is only at this stage and beyond that the cells become morphologically recognizable in terms of their lineage.

The erythroid precursor cell: The *proerythroblast* is a large cell with intense blue cytoplasm and a round homogeneous nucleus, containing a few nucleoli. The proerythroblast matures sequentially as follows:

1. *Basophilic erythroblasts* without nucleoli
2. *Polychromatic erythroblasts* with grayish cytoplasm (owing to hemoglobin synthesis) and a nucleus with coarsely clumped chromatin
3. *Orthochromatic erythroblasts* with red hemoglobin-containing cytoplasm and a dense pyknotic nucleus
4. *Reticulocytes,* nonnucleated cells that represent the last stage before mature erythrocytes. The nucleus is extruded from the orthochromatic erythroblast, leaving mitochondria and hemoglobin-producing polyribosomes in the reticulocyte. After release from the bone marrow, the reticulocyte loses its capacity for aerobic metabolism and hemoglobin synthesis, and after 1 or 2 days becomes a mature erythrocyte.

The granulocytic precursor cell: The *myeloblast* has a round to oval nucleus, with delicate chromatin and a few nucleoli, and a blue-gray cytoplasm. The next stage, the *promyelocyte,* has a similar nucleus, but the cytoplasm contains a number of primary (azurophilic) granules. Subsequent maturation from *myelocyte* to mature *neutrophil* involves (1) the progressive condensation of nuclear chromatin, (2) increasing lobulation of the nucleus, and (3) the appearance of secondary (specific) granules, which are neutrophilic, basophilic, or eosinophilic.

The monocytic precursor cell: The parallel formation of monocytes from monoblasts also involves a nuclear condensation, but less prominent formation of nuclear lobes. The cytoplasm becomes grayish, containing only a few pink or purple granules. Subsequently, after the monocyte leaves the bloodstream and becomes a member of the mononuclear phagocyte system. It then undergoes further morphological changes, depending on its tissue location and its function as either a phagocyte (fixed or wandering) or an immunoregulator (Fig. 20-6).

The megakaryocytic precursor: Megakaryocytes in the bone marrow mature into multilobed giant cells by a number of endomitotic divisions. After reaching a certain ploidy, the cytoplasm becomes stippled and azurophilic and is eventually released into the sinusoids in long platelet-containing ribbons. Some intact megakaryocytes are also released, and platelet production occurs after they have been trapped in the pulmonary microcirculation.

The Bone Marrow Is Examined by Biopsy and Aspirate Smear

The cellular elements of the bone marrow are commonly evaluated by both needle biopsy and aspiration of marrow from the posterior iliac crest. Marrow can also be obtained in infants from the anterior tibial bone and in adults from the sternum. The cellularity and histological architecture of the bone marrow is evaluated on examination of biopsy sections (Fig. 20-7A), whereas specific precursor cells are identified in a smear of the aspirate (Fig. 20-7B). In a normal adult, about half of the biopsy surface area consists of fat cells and half of active hematopoietic tissue. The proportion of hematopoietic cells is referred to as the *cellularity.* The cellularity is high in children and decreased in the elderly.

The normal proportions of granulocytic precursors (myeloid cells) and erythroblastic precursors (erythroid cells), or the *myeloid-to-erythroid ratio,* is between 2:1 and 7:1 (Table 20-1). Blast cells are few, and the most mature cells are plentiful. Changes in this distribution are designated as a "left shift" (toward immaturity) or a "right shift" (toward maturity). Two to five megakaryocytes per high-power field are present. The normal bone marrow contains fewer than 3% plasma cells, up to 20% lymphocytes, and only rare mast cells and macrophages. The reticulin silver stain reveals scattered fibers in the hematopoietic stroma. With the trichrome stain for collagen, delicate perivascular fibrosis is usually observed.

Evaluation of bone marrow iron stores uses the Prussian blue stain, which demonstrates blue hemosiderin granules in macrophages and in the interstitium. Minute hemosiderin granules are found in the cytoplasm of 10% of erythroid precursors *(sideroblasts).*

Functional Kinetics Is Regulated by Growth Factors

The hematopoietic cells in the bone marrow maintain the size of the circulating blood cell mass, adjusting to compensate for senescence of blood cells. Such regulation is mediated by a number of growth factors that affect the rate of cellular proliferation, primarily within the progenitor cell compartment.

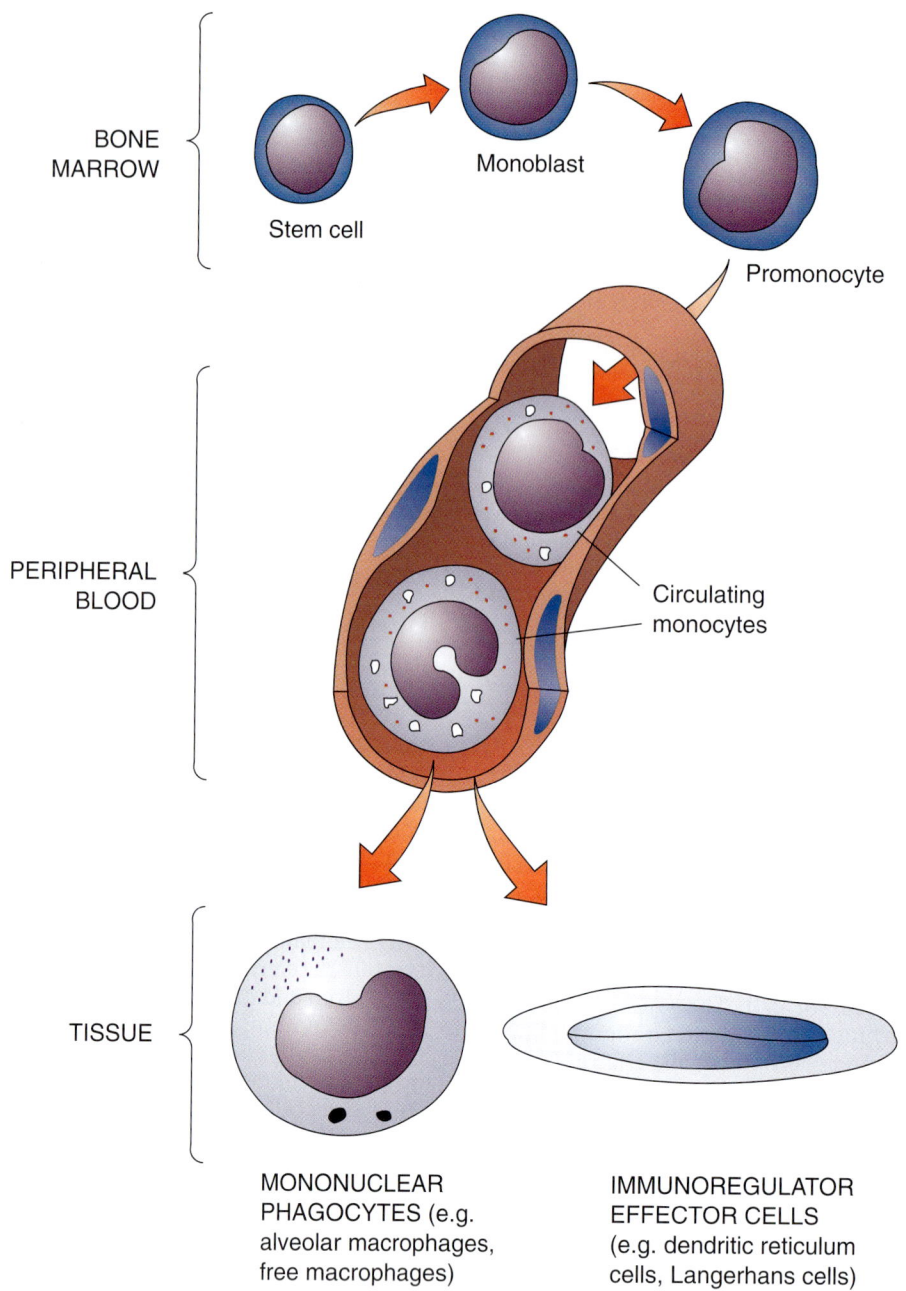

FIGURE 20-6
The mononuclear phagocyte and immune regulator effector (M-PIRE) system. The cells of this system originate in the bone marrow from hematopoietic stem cells that give rise to monoblasts and then promonocytes. The latter mature into monocytes, which circulate in the peripheral blood. These monocytes then exit the peripheral blood and enter the tissues, where they become the various specialized phagocytes or immunoregulator cells.

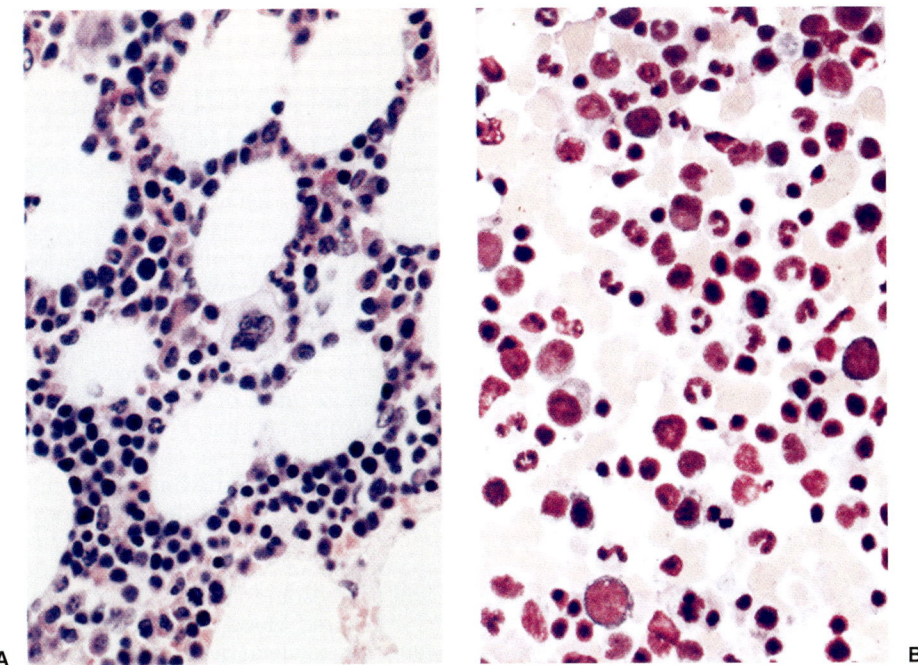

FIGURE 20-7
Normal bone marrow. A. A photomicrograph of a tissue section shows the normal relationship (1:1) of cellular elements to fat, a normal myeloid-to-erythroid ratio, and a megakaryocyte in the center. B. A smear of the bone marrow aspirate from the same patient demonstrates normal hematopoietic elements and varying stages of differentiation.

GROWTH FACTORS: Interleukin-1 (IL-1), IL-3, IL-6, IL-11, and stem cell factor (SCF) support the survival and proliferation of stem cells. The subsequent proliferation and maturation of the progenitor cells is affected by the specific colony-stimulating factors mentioned above.

Erythropoietin is released by the interstitial peritubular cells of the kidney in response to hypoxia and activates specific receptors on the cell membrane of erythroid progenitor cells. In conjunction with IL-3 and GM-CSF, this growth factor promotes the growth of early erythroid progenitor cells (BFU-E). However, erythropoietin alone determines the transformation of the late erythroid progenitor cells (CFU-E) to erythroblasts.

Whereas IL-3, IL-6, and IL-11, among others, affect the growth and differentiation of megakaryocytes, a more specific regulator of megakaryopoiesis, namely *thrombopoietin*, facilitates the production and maturation of megakaryocytes.

RELEASE FROM THE MARROW: Mature blood cells form a narrow migration channel through the endothelium, which participates in the extrusion of the nondeformable pyknotic nucleus of the orthochromatic erythroblast. By contrast, the nuclei of other precursor cells can change their shape to accommodate even an extremely narrow opening. The release mechanism can, in an emergency situation, provide the circulation with a boost of mature cells stored in the bone marrow, particularly short-lived granulocytes.

PERIPHERAL MYELOPOIETIC CELLS

Granulocytes Are the First Defense against Microorganisms

Because of their nuclear configuration, mature granulocytes are also termed *polymorphonuclear leukocytes*. Subtypes are defined by the staining characteristics of specific cytoplasmic granules and are labeled neutrophils, eosinophils, and basophils.

NEUTROPHILS: The neutrophilic granulocyte has a pink, finely granulated cytoplasm and a nucleus composed of two to four interconnected lobes. Immature neutrophils *(band cells)* have indented, nonlobulated nuclei. There is a

TABLE 20-1   Normal Adult Bone Marrow (Age 18–70 Years)

Fat:cell ratio, 50:50 ± 15%
Myeloid-to-erythroid ratio, 2:1 to 7:1
Cell distribution (% surface area)
    Fat cells, 35–65%
    Erythroid series, 10–20%
    Granulocytic (myeloid) series, 40–65%
Megakaryocytes, 2–5/high-power field
Plasma cells, <3% of nucleated cells
Lymphocytes, <20% of nucleated cells
No fibrosis

considerable storage pool of these cells in the bone marrow, as well as a pool of temporarily marginated neutrophils along the vascular walls. This reserve can be mobilized acutely and released to the circulating blood by endotoxin, epinephrine, or corticosteroids. Sporadic releases contribute to the day-to-day variations in the neutrophil counts. The local destruction of cells at sites of infection causes the release of chemotactic molecules that recruit neutrophils.

EOSINOPHILS: The eosinophilic granulocytes contain large granules that stain red with eosin because of their content of basic proteins. The nucleus is usually bilobed, with a thin connecting filament. Eosinophils are mostly tissue cells, with only a short intravascular stay. They are present primarily in the mucosa of the gastrointestinal, bronchial, and lower genitourinary tracts. Here their IgA receptors and toxic cationic proteins contribute to the defense against parasites and participate in allergic reactions.

Basophils Contain Inflammatory Mediators

Basophilic granulocytes feature prominent blue-black granules that often overlie and obscure the nucleus. The granules contain histamine and other substances, and their release is an important component of certain allergic disorders. Other inflammatory mediators, for example leukotrienes (SRS-A), are produced upon appropriate stimulation.

Monocytes Exert Immunoregulatory and Phagocytic Functions

Monocytes are medium-sized to large cells that exhibit a kidney-shaped or lobed nucleus and abundant gray cytoplasm with few granules. They are potentially phagocytic, but they do not become truly functional macrophages until they enter tissues and undergo a number of morphological changes. Fully differentiated monocytes perform either phagocytic or immunoregulatory functions, accounting for the term *M-PIRE system* (*m*ononuclear-*p*hagocyte and *i*mmuno*r*egulatory *e*ffector) (Fig. 20-6). The immunoregulatory arm includes Langerhans cells and other dendritic cells. The functions of these versatile M-PIRE cells include the following:

- Production of factors that control cellular proliferation and maturation. These cells are thus referred to as the *conductors of the immune system*.
- Phagocytosis and processing of foreign antigens. Class I and class II human leukocyte antigen (HLA) proteins on the surface of monocytes facilitate the presentation of processed antigenic fragments for the activation of lymphocytes.
- Removal of abnormal or senescent erythrocytes and salvage of iron for reuse by erythroid precursors.
- Clearance from the blood and tissues of neoplastic or foreign cells.

Red Blood Cells

NORMAL STRUCTURE AND FUNCTION

The function of red blood cells, or erythrocytes, is the transport of oxygen to tissues. Mature erythrocytes are nonnucleated and assume the shape of a 7- to 8-μm biconcave disk, which is equal in size to the nucleus of a small lymphocyte (Fig. 20-8). On Wright-stained blood smears, they appear round and have reddish, eosinophilic cytoplasm. The red color is imparted by hemoglobin, which is the main cytoplasmic component. Because of their biconcave disk shape, red blood cells display an area of central pallor that is approximately one third the diameter of the cell. Red blood cells are released from the bone marrow at the reticulocyte stage. Compared with mature erythrocytes, reticulocytes are larger and have more diffusely basophilic gray cytoplasm. This polychromatophilia of reticulocytes is secondary to their higher content of ribosomes, as these cells still synthesize hemoglobin.

The red blood cell membrane is attached to an underlying cytoskeletal network (Fig. 20-9). Inserted into the lipid bilayer are a variety of transmembrane proteins that serve as receptors, channels, and anchors for other membrane components and the underlying cytoskeleton. The addition of carbohydrate groups to some membrane proteins results

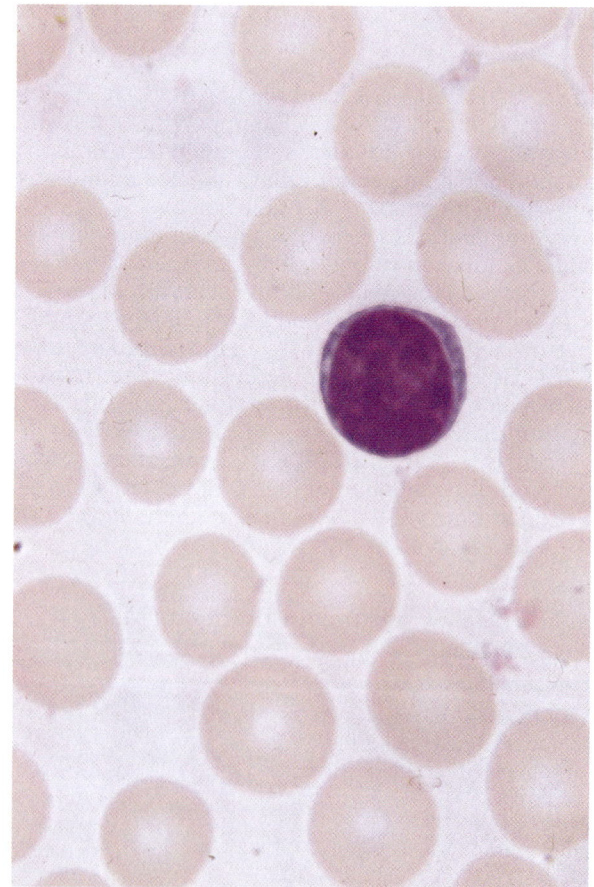

FIGURE *20-8*
Normal red blood cells are approximately the same size as the nucleus of a lymphocyte.

Normal Structure and Function

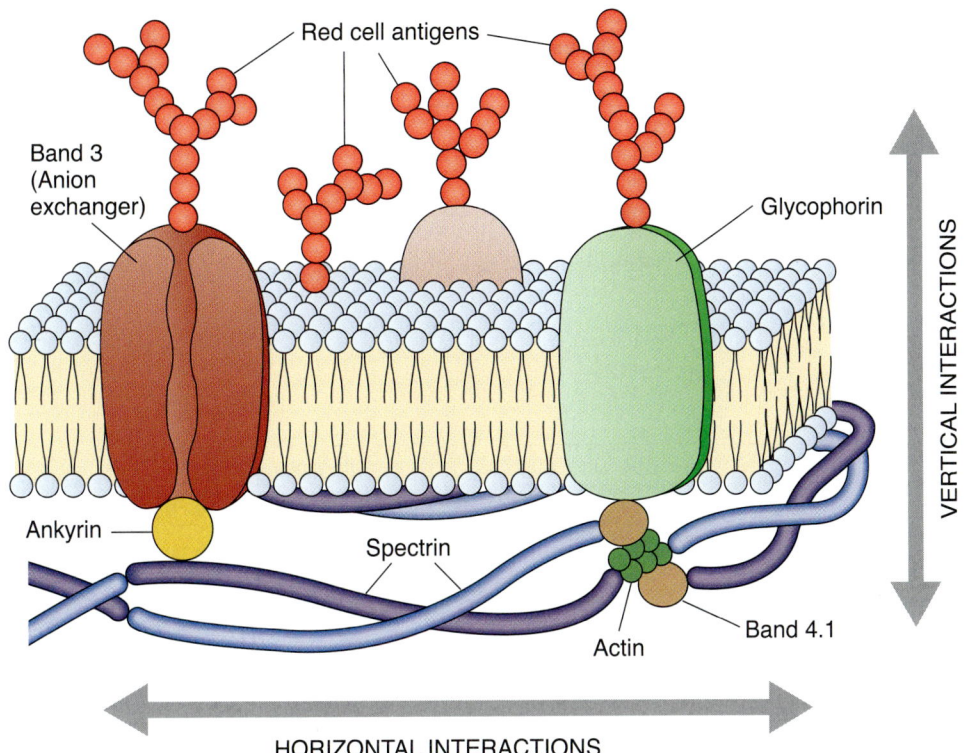

FIGURE 20-9
Structure of the erythrocyte plasma membrane. The membrane is stabilized by a number of interactions. The two vertical ones are spectrin-ankyrin–band 3 and spectrin-protein 4.1–glycophorin. The two horizontal interactions are spectrin heterodimer assembly and spectrin-actin–protein 4.1.

in the formation of different red cell antigen groups. The erythrocyte cytoskeleton is composed of interconnected spectrin dimers and other stabilizing proteins (ankyrin, actin, band 4.1). This complex arrangement allows for the inherent deformability characteristic of red blood cells. Alterations in this membrane-cytoskeletal unit lead to increased cell rigidity and premature destruction of circulating erythrocytes.

The cytoplasm of erythrocytes contains few organelles, and metabolism and energy generation are accomplished anaerobically through the glycolytic pathway. Some 10% of erythrocyte glucose is alternatively metabolized through the hexose monophosphate shunt, which uses the enzyme glucose-6-phosphate dehydrogenase (G6PD). This pathway is ultimately responsible for reducing glutathione, which protects red cells from oxidative stress. The Rapoport-Luebering shunt, another alternate pathway during glycolysis, generates 2,3-diphosphoglycerate (2,3-DPG) at the expense of ATP production. 2,3-DPG enhances oxygen delivery to tissues by regulating the slope of the oxygen dissociation curve (Fig. 20-10).

Hemoglobin accounts for the oxygen-carrying capacity of red blood cells. Each hemoglobin molecule is composed of four heme groups and four globin chains and, when fully saturated, transports four molecules of oxygen. The heme portion of the molecule consists of a porphyrin ring (protoporphyrin IX), into which a ferrous iron atom (Fe^{2+}) has been inserted. The globin portion of the molecule consists of pairs of two different protein chains. The most abundant normal hemoglobin, hemoglobin A, contains two alpha (α) and two beta (β) globin chains. Other hemoglobins are normally present in minor amounts and include hemoglobin F and hemoglobin A_2. These have two gamma (γ) and two delta (δ) globin chains, respectively, substituted for the β globin chains.

Each heme group interacts with a hydrophobic pocket of one of the globin chains, and the entire molecule attains a globular tertiary structure. Deoxygenated hemoglobin has low oxygen affinity and requires increased oxygen tension for heme–oxygen binding to occur. Following this initial interaction, the hemoglobin molecule undergoes a conformational change that facilitates subsequent oxygen binding to the remaining three heme groups. This progressive increase

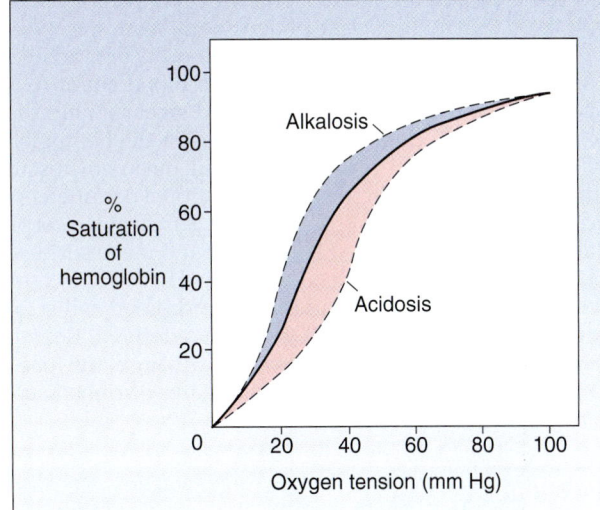

FIGURE 20-10
Oxygen dissociation curve of hemoglobin. With decreasing pH (acidosis) the oxygen affinity declines (shifts right); with increasing pH (alkalosis) the affinity increases (shifts left). Oxygen affinity is also increased by 2,3-DPG and lower temperatures.

TABLE 20-2 Complete Blood Count (CBC): Normal Adult Values

Erythrocytes	
Hemoglobin	Male, 14–18 g/dL
	Female, 12–16 g/dL
Hematocrit	Male, 40–54%
	Female, 35–47%
Red blood cell (RBC) count	Male, 4.5–6 × 10^6/μL
	Female, 4–5.5 × 10^6/μL
Reticulocytes	0.5–2.5%
Indices	
Mean corpuscular volume	82–100 μm^3
Mean corpuscular hemoglobin	27–34 pg
Mean corpuscular hemoglobin concentration	32–36%
Leukocytes	

	Absolute Count/μL	Differential Count (%)
White blood cells (WBC)	4000–11,000	
Neutrophil granulocytes	1800–7000	50–60
Neutrophil bands	0–700	2–4
Lymphocytes	1500–4000	30–40
Monocytes	0–800	1–9
Basophils	0–200	0–1
Eosinophils	0–450	0–3
Platelets		

Quantitative normal value: 150,000–400,000/μL
Qualitative estimation on smear: Number of platelets/oil immersion field × 10,000 = estimated platelet count
Normal ratio of RBC to platelets = 15:1 to 20:1

---

in oxygen affinity is reflected in the sigmoid shape of the oxygen dissociation curve (Fig. 20-10). The slope of the oxygen dissociation curve can be shifted to the right by acidosis or an increase in 2,3-DPG levels, thereby enhancing oxygen delivery to the tissues. The curve is shifted to the left by alkalosis and results in increased oxygen binding by hemoglobin.

Following release from the bone marrow, the average life span of the erythrocyte in circulation is 120 days. Changes in membrane proteins and phospholipids appear in aged red cells and are likely signals for removal of the erythrocyte by the mononuclear phagocyte system.

The erythroid component of the blood is best analyzed through the combination of a complete blood count (CBC) and microscopic examination of a blood smear (Table 20-2). The CBC includes direct determinations of the hemoglobin (HGB), red blood cell count (RBC), and mean corpuscular volume (MCV). From these values, additional parameters including the hematocrit (HCT = MCV × RBC), mean corpuscular hemoglobin (MCH = HGB/RBC), and mean corpuscular hemoglobin concentration (MCHC = HGB/HCT) can be calculated. The degree of variation in red blood cell size or red cell distribution width (RDW) is also derived. Reticulocytes can be quantitated accurately through the use of supravital dyes, which stain the aggregates of ribosomes in their cytoplasm.

Red Blood Cell Disorders

ANEMIA

Anemia refers to a reduction in the total circulating erythrocyte mass. A diagnosis of anemia is made by the demonstration of a reduction in hemoglobin, hematocrit, or red blood cell count. Anemia leads to decreased oxygen transport by the blood and ultimately tissue hypoxia.

Classification of Anemias

Anemias are classified according to morphological or pathophysiological criteria. The morphological classification of anemia is based on the appearance of the erythrocytes as determined by automated blood counters and microscopic evaluation of a blood smear. Red blood cell size, which is reflected in the CBC by the MCV, allows division of anemias into three groups: (1) microcytic (decreased MCV), (2) normocytic, and (3) macrocytic (increased MCV) (Table 20-3).

TABLE 20-3 Morphological Classification of Anemia

Macrocytic
  Megaloblastic
  Alcohol use
  Liver disease
  Hypothyroidism
  Reticulocytosis
  Primary bone marrow disease
Microcytic
  Iron deficiency
  Anemia of chronic disease/inflammation
  Thalassemias
  Sideroblastic anemias
Normocytic
  Anemia of chronic disease/inflammation
  Anemia of renal disease
  Acute blood loss

Examination of a blood smear is also useful in the morphological classification of anemia. Abnormally shaped red blood cells *(poikilocytes)* can be seen in a wide variety of anemias, and the particular type of poikilocyte observed can aid in the formulation of an etiologic diagnosis (Fig. 20-11).

On a pathophysiological basis, anemia can be classified into four major groups (Table 20-4): (1) decreased production of red blood cells by the bone marrow, (2) ineffective production of red blood cells in the bone marrow, (3) increased destruction of red blood cells after release from the bone marrow, and (4) acute blood loss. In general, anemias associated with either decreased or ineffective production of red cells can be distinguished from those due to increased destruction of red cells by the absence or presence, respectively, of increased numbers of circulating reticulocytes (reticulocytosis).

 Clinical Features: In the face of anemia, the body has several compensatory mechanisms, to enhance oxygen delivery to tissues.

- Increased cardiac output
- Increased respiratory rate

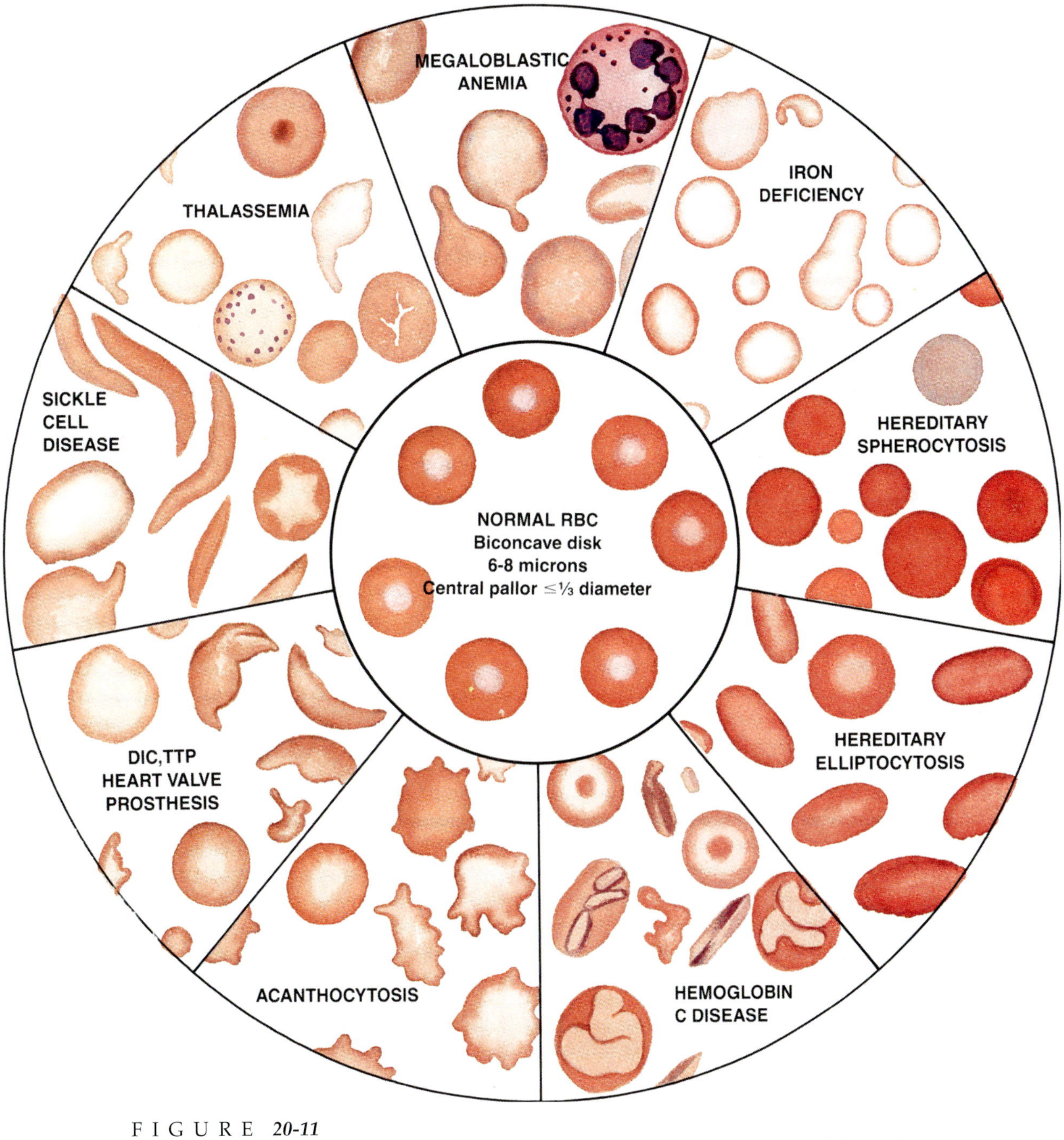

FIGURE *20-11*
The anemias. The pathophysiology of characteristic morphological features of the various anemias are shown. The morphology of normal erythrocytes is contrasted in the central circle.

DISORDER	PATHOPHYSIOLOGY	MORPHOLOGY
Megaloblastic anemia	Disturbance in DNA synthesis	Oval macrocytes, teardrop poikilocytosis, hypersegmented polys
Iron deficiency	Disturbance in hemoglobin synthesis (lack of iron)	Hypochromic, microcytic
Hereditary spherocytosis	Membrane defect	Spherocytes
Hereditary elliptocytosis	Membrane defect	Elliptocytes
Hemoglobin C disease	Abnormal globin chain	Target cells, rhomboid crystals (HbC)
Acanthocytosis	Membrane lipid defect (abetalipoproteinemia)	Irregular spiculation (similar to spur cells of liver disease)
DIC, TTP, heart valve prosthesis sequela	Mechanical damage to erythrocytes	Schistocytes
Sickle cell disease	Abnormal globin chain	Sickle cells
Thalassemia	Disturbance in hemoglobin synthesis (defect of globin chain)	Hypochromic, microcytic, poikilocytosis, basophilic stippling
Myelophthisic anemia	Marrow replacement or infiltration	Teardrop poikilocytosis, immature WBC and RBC, large platelets
Anemia of chronic disease	Block in utilization of storage iron	Normochromic, normocytic to mild hypochromic, microcytic
Sideroblastic anemia	Defect in porphyrin and heme synthesis	Bimorphic population (normal and microcytic), Pappenheimer bodies
Anemia of renal disease	Multifactorial	Burr cells (uniform marginal scalloping)
Autoimmune hemolytic anemia	RBC destruction mediated by antibodies	Spherocytes
Acute blood loss anemia	Hemorrhage	Polychromasia (increased reticulocytes)

FIGURE 20-11 (continued)

TABLE 20-4 Pathophysiologic Classification of Anemia

Decreased Production	Increased Destruction

Stem cell- and progenitor cell-based
  Aplastic anemia
  Pure red cell aplasia
  Paroxysmal nocturnal hemoglobinuria
  Leukemia
  Myelodysplastic syndromes
  Marrow infiltration
  Anemia of chronic disease/inflammation
  Anemia of renal disease
Nutritional deficiency
  Megaloblastic anemia (vitamin B$_{12}$ and folic acid)
  Iron deficiency
	Intracorpuscular
	  Membrane defect
	  Enzyme deficiency
	  Hemoglobinopathies
	Extracorpuscular
	  Immunological
	    Autoimmune
	    Alloimmune
	  Nonimmunological
	    Mechanical
	    Hypersplenism
	    Infectious
	    Chemical
	    Acute blood loss

- Shunting of blood flow to provide increased tissue perfusion of vital organs
- Decreased hemoglobin–oxygen affinity
- Increased erythrocyte production in the bone marrow secondary to erythropoietin stimulation

Clinical signs and symptoms (tachycardia, shortness of breath, and systolic murmurs) may develop secondary to these compensatory processes. If the anemia is sufficiently severe (generally hemoglobin levels below 7 g/dL), tissue hypoxia remains uncompensated, and additional clinical findings appear, including easy fatigability, faintness, angina, and dyspnea on exertion.

Decreased Red Blood Cell Production Characterizes Varied Types of Anemia

Aplastic Anemia

Aplastic anemia is a disorder of pluripotential stem cells that leads to bone marrow failure. The disorder features hypocellular bone marrow and pancytopenia (decreased circulating levels of all formed elements in the blood).

 Pathogenesis: Aplastic anemia results from injury to stem cells in the bone marrow. Most cases are idiopathic, and no specific initiating etiology can be identified (Table 20-5). Two main mechanisms can lead to stem cell injury. The first is a predictable, dose-dependent, toxic injury, typified by exposure to certain chemotherapeutic drugs, chemicals, and ionizing radiation. The other mechanism is an idiosyncratic, dose-independent, immunological injury, as seen in idiopathic cases or after certain drug exposures or viral infections. Rare cases of aplastic anemia (Fanconi anemia) have an inherited basis. Depending on the underlying cause, the stem cell injury may or may not be reversible.

The immunological nature of stem cell injury in some patients is supported by the clinical response to antithymocyte globulin or other immunosuppressive agents. An intrinsic abnormality of stem cells in other cases of aplastic

TABLE 20-5 **Etiology of Aplastic Anemia**

Idiopathic ($\frac{2}{3}$ of cases)
Ionizing radiation
Drugs
    Chemotherapeutic agents
    Chloramphenicol
    Anticonvulsants
    Nonsteroidal antiinflammatory agents
    Gold
Chemicals
    Benzene
Viruses
    Hepatitis (HCV)
    Epstein-Barr virus (EBV)
    HIV
    Parvovirus B19
Hereditary
    Fanconi anemia

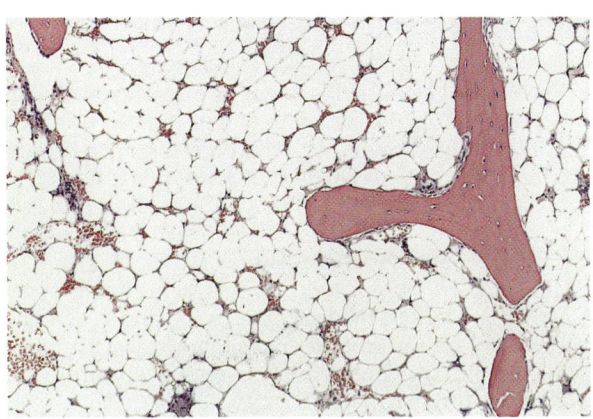

FIGURE 20-12
Aplastic anemia. The bone marrow consists largely of fat cells and lacks normal hematopoietic activity.

anemia is suggested by the subsequent evolution of clonal stem cell disorders (paroxysmal nocturnal hemoglobinuria, myelodysplasia, acute leukemia). In cases of **Fanconi anemia**, germline mutations in *FAC* (Fanconi anemia complementation) genes lead to chromosomal instability upon exposure to ionizing radiation or alkylating agents.

 Pathology: The bone marrow in aplastic anemia shows variably reduced cellularity, depending on the clinical stage of the disease (Fig. 20-12). There is a decrease in the number of cells of myeloid, erythroid, and megakaryocytic lineage, with a relative increase in lymphocytes and plasma cells. As the cellularity decreases, there is a corresponding increase in bone marrow fat.

Anemia, leukopenia (primarily granulocytopenia) and thrombocytopenia characterize aplastic anemia. Circulating red cells have a normal shape but are often mildly macrocytic. Despite elevated erythropoietin levels, reticulocytosis is not present. Increased fetal hemoglobin can be demonstrated in the red cells in some cases. As in the bone marrow, a relative lymphocytosis is observed in the blood.

 Clinical Features: Patients with aplastic anemia present with signs and symptoms attributable to pancytopenia, namely, weakness, fatigue, infection, and bleeding. Fanconi anemia often manifests in the first decade of life and has a variety of associated malformations, including hypoplastic thumbs, absent radii, and skin pigmentation and renal anomalies. Increased bone marrow fat is readily demonstrated by nuclear magnetic resonance imaging studies. For untreated aplastic anemia, the prognosis is grim, with a 3- to 6-month median survival and only 20% survival after 1 year. Immunosuppressive therapy often leads to transient remissions, and transplantation of bone marrow or stem cells may be curative.

Pure Red Cell Aplasia

Pure red cell aplasia (PRCA) is the selective suppression of committed erythroid precursors in the bone marrow. White blood cells and platelets are unaffected.

Pathogenesis: PRCA most often results from an immunological suppression of red cell production without known cause. On occasion, it is secondary to viral infections (parvovirus B19) or thymic lesions. The P antigen system on the red cell membrane serves as a receptor for parvovirus and explains the restricted infection of erythroid precursors by this agent.

Diamond-Blackfan syndrome is a heritable type of PRCA that appears in the first year of life and is associated with defective erythroid precursors that show a diminished response to erythropoietin and decreased erythroid burst and colony-forming capacities.

 Pathology: In PRCA, the overall marrow cellularity is normal, but there is a selective absence of erythroid precursors. Erythroid precursors are completely absent or are arrested at the erythroblast stage. In cases secondary to parvovirus B19, intranuclear viral inclusions can be observed. Myeloid and megakaryocytic precursors are present in adequate numbers and show normal maturation.

Patients with PRCA develop moderate to severe anemia that often has macrocytic indices. Despite increased erythropoietin levels, there is no accompanying reticulocytosis.

 Clinical Features: Acquired PRCA manifests as either an acute self-limited illness or a chronic relapsing process.

Acute self-limited PRCA often arises secondary to parvovirus B19 infection. This condition may not be clinically apparent unless the patient suffers from an underlying chronic hemolytic anemia (e.g. hereditary spherocytosis, sickle cell anemia). Such cases may be complicated by a so-called aplastic crisis, with sudden worsening of anemia. Immunocompromised patients cannot clear the parvovirus infection, and anemia may become prolonged.

Chronic relapsing PRCA is seen in idiopathic cases or may be associated with an underlying thymic lesion (thymoma, thymic hyperplasia). In these cases, thymectomy can lead to resolution of the condition and subsequent correction of the anemia.

Transfusion support is often necessary in all forms of PRCA.

Iron Deficiency Anemia

Iron deficiency interferes with normal heme (hemoglobin) synthesis and thereby leads to impaired erythropoiesis and anemia. Iron deficiency is the most common cause of anemia worldwide.

 Pathogenesis: The normal Western adult diet contains about 20 mg of iron, of which only 1 to 2 mg is absorbed by the duodenum and proximal jejunum (see Chapter 14). The rate of iron absorption is regulated by normal losses, but with anemia (especially in cases of ineffective erythropoiesis) intestinal absorption is increased and may ultimately lead to iron overload. Following absorption, about 85% of absorbed iron is transported in the blood by a carrier protein, transferrin, and is then incorporated into developing red cells through specific transferrin receptors on their surface. As senescent red cells are removed from circulation, hemoglobin is broken down into component parts, and the iron is recycled. Excess iron is stored in the body in two forms, hemosiderin and ferritin. Hemosiderin consists of large aggregates of iron with a disorganized structure, whereas ferritin is complexed with protein (apoferritin) and appears highly organized.

Many underlying conditions give rise to iron deficiency. In infants and children, dietary iron sources may be inadequate for growth and development. An increased demand for iron is also encountered with pregnancy and lactation. In adults, iron deficiency typically results from chronic blood loss or, less commonly, intravascular hemolysis. One milligram of iron is contained in 2 mL of whole blood lost from the body. In women of reproductive age, the blood loss most frequently has a gynecological source (menstruation, parturition, vaginal bleeding). In men and postmenopausal women, unexplained iron deficiency should prompt an investigation of the gastrointestinal tract for tumors or vascular lesions, since this is the most common site of chronic blood loss.

 Pathology: Iron deficiency anemia is characterized by a microcytic, hypochromic anemia (Fig. 20-13). Variation in the size and shape of the erythrocytes *(anisopoikilocytosis)* is reflected in an increased RDW. Ovalocytes may be encountered, some of which are very thin and are designated *pencil cells.* Because of the production defect in the marrow, there is no associated reticulocytosis. Frequently, iron deficiency anemia is accompanied by a mild thrombocytosis. The bone marrow displays erythroid hyperplasia, and many of the developing normoblasts have ragged cytoplasmic borders. Prussian blue staining demonstrates an absence of storage iron.

Serum iron and ferritin levels are decreased by iron deficiency, whereas the total iron-binding capacity (a reflection of

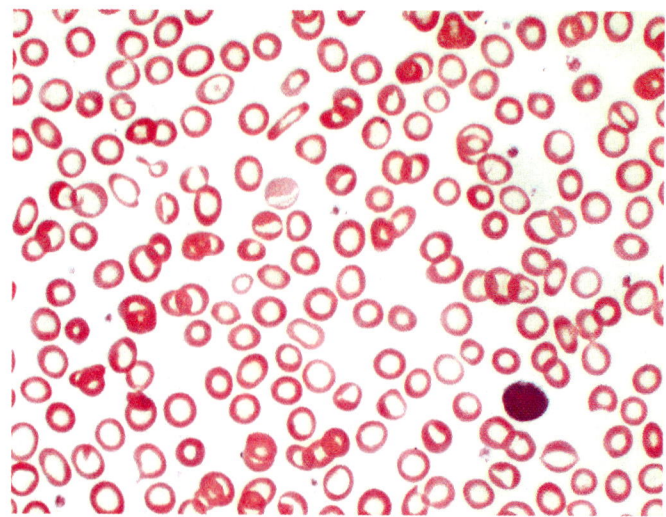

FIGURE 20-13

Microcytic hypochromic anemia caused by iron deficiency. Red blood cells are significantly smaller than the nucleus of a lymphocyte.

the serum transferrin level) is increased. As a result, the percent saturation of transferrin is conspicuously lowered (often less than 5%). Increased levels of free erythrocyte protoporphyrin and zinc protoporphyrin are characteristic because of the impaired incorporation of iron into protoporphyrin IX.

Clinical Features: The symptoms of iron deficiency are those of anemia in general. With advanced disease, atrophic glossitis and angular stomatitis may be encountered, as well as a spoon-shaped deformity of the fingernails *(koilonychia)*. Treatment of iron deficiency involves correcting the source of chronic blood loss and oral iron supplementation. Parenteral iron is available for patients who are not compliant.

Anemia of Renal Disease

Anemia of chronic renal insufficiency reflects decreased production of erythropoietin by the damaged kidneys.

Pathogenesis: Renal disease of varying causes is associated with decreased production of erythropoietin and subsequent development of anemia. Additionally, the presence of a "uremic toxin," which suppresses erythroid precursors, as well as a minor hemolytic component have been suggested (but poorly proven) as contributing to the anemia of chronic renal disease.

Pathology: The anemia of chronic renal disease is normocytic and normochromic. In some cases, *echinocytes* (crenated cells, burr cells) with scalloped cell membranes can be seen. If the renal insufficiency is secondary to malignant hypertension, red cell fragmentation with formation of schistocytes may be seen.

Clinical Features: The severity of anemia is proportional to the underlying degree of renal insufficiency. Administration of recombinant erythropoietin is the treatment of choice.

Anemia of Chronic Disease

Anemia of chronic disease arises in association with chronic inflammatory and malignant conditions.

Pathogenesis: Chronic disease leads to ineffective use of iron from macrophage stores in the bone marrow, resulting in a functional iron deficiency, although storage iron is normal or even increased. Other factors that may contribute to anemia are decreased erythrocyte life span, blunted erythropoietin production by the kidney in response to tissue hypoxia, and impaired bone marrow response to erythropoietin. It is thought that inflammatory cytokines (lactoferrin, IL-1, tumor necrosis factor-α [TNF-α], and interferon) interfere with iron mobilization.

Pathology: The anemia of chronic disease is mild to moderate, and the red cells are often microcytic. Prussian blue staining demonstrates normal or often increased amounts of storage iron. Serum iron levels tend to be reduced. However, in contrast to iron deficiency anemia, total iron binding capacity also tends to be decreased (as is the serum albumin level). Successful treatment of the underlying chronic disease is associated with restoration of normal hemoglobin levels.

Anemia Associated with Marrow Infiltration (Myelophthisic Anemia)

Myelophthisic anemia refers to hypoproliferative anemia associated with infiltration of the bone marrow by a variety of processes.

Pathogenesis: Any infiltrative process, such as myelofibrosis, hematological malignancies, metastatic carcinoma, or granulomatous disease, can replace normal hematopoietic elements and cause anemia (and often leukopenia and thrombocytopenia). In an attempt to maintain blood cell production, foci of extramedullary hematopoiesis may appear, most prominently in the spleen and liver.

Pathology: Bone marrow infiltration results in moderate to severe normocytic anemia, with anisopoikilocytosis and teardrop cells. Circulating immature granulocytes and nucleated red blood cells *(leukoerythroblastosis)* are frequently identified.

Anemia of Lead Poisoning

Lead poisoning results in anemia through interference with several of the enzymes involved in heme synthesis.

Pathogenesis: Most of the enzymes in the heme synthetic pathway are susceptible to lead toxicity, but aminolevulinic acid (ALA) dehydratase and

Pathology: The degree of anemia in lead poisoning varies but is frequently more severe in affected children. Blood smear examination reveals microcytic, hypochromic red cells with prominent basophilic stippling. Within the bone marrow, ringed sideroblasts reflect impaired use of iron in erythroid precursors.

ferrochelatase are the most sensitive. The end result is decreased heme (and ultimately hemoglobin) synthesis. Lead also inhibits pyrimidine 5′-nucleotidase, thereby producing basophilic stippling in circulating erythrocytes. Lead poisoning most commonly develops from ingestion of lead-painted materials (children) or occupational exposure (adults) (see Chapter 8).

Ineffective Red Cell Production Is Reflected in Fewer Circulating Erythrocytes

Megaloblastic Anemias

Megaloblastic anemias are caused by impaired DNA synthesis, usually owing to a deficiency of either vitamin B_{12} or folic acid.

Pathogenesis: Impaired DNA synthesis results in abnormal nuclear development, which in turn leads to ineffective erythrocyte maturation and anemia. Megaloblastic anemia is also seen following administration of certain chemotherapeutic agents (methotrexate, hydroxyurea) or antiretroviral drugs (5-azacytidine). Less commonly, an inherited defect in purine or pyrimidine metabolism is characterized by megaloblastic anemia.

In the synthesis of DNA, uridylate molecules are converted to thymidylate (Fig. 20-14) through the action of thymidylate synthetase, which uses tetrahydrofolate as a cofactor. Tetrahydrofolate is converted from methyl tetrahydrofolate by methyl tetrahydrofolate reductase and vitamin B_{12}, which serves as a cofactor. Vitamin B_{12} is also required for the conversion of homocysteine to methionine.

In the face of defective DNA synthesis, nuclear development is impaired, whereas cytoplasmic maturation proceeds normally. This situation, termed *nuclear to cytoplasmic asynchrony*, results in the formation of megaloblasts. Since the megaloblastic precursors do not mature enough to be released into the blood, they undergo intramedullary destruction.

Vitamin B_{12} (cyanocobalamin) is found in a wide variety of animal food sources and is also synthesized by intestinal microorganisms. Proper absorption of vitamin B_{12} requires binding to intrinsic factor, which protects vitamin B_{12} from degradation by intestinal enzymes (Fig. 20-15). Intrinsic fac-

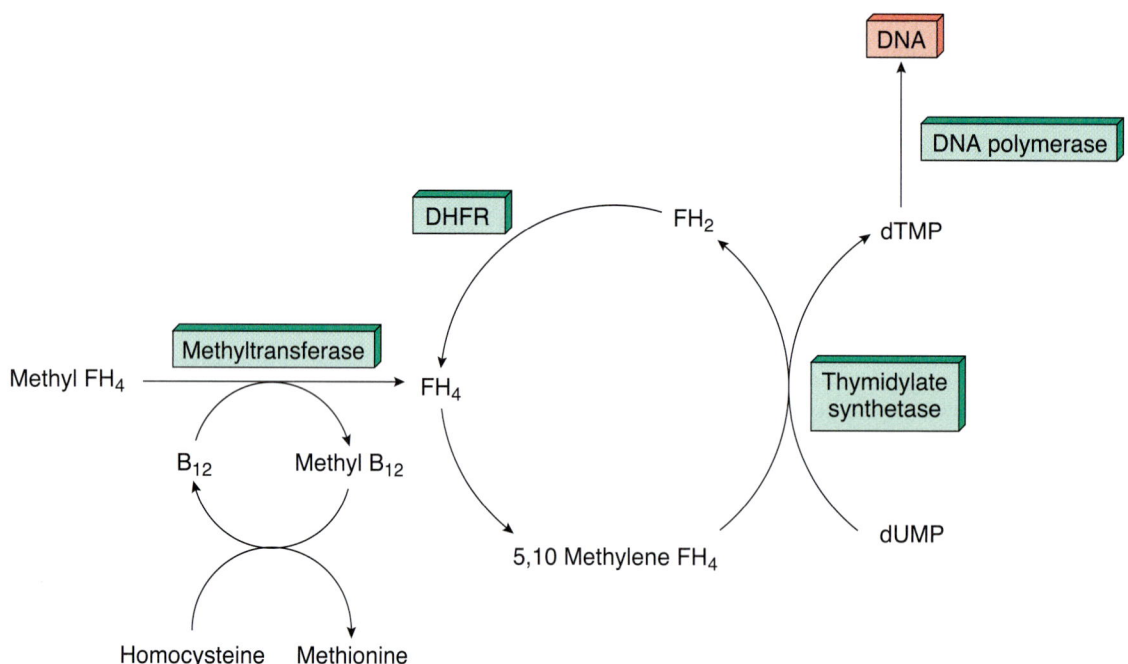

FIGURE 20-14
Relationship of folic acid to vitamin B_{12}. A 1-carbon transfer mediated by folic acid, methylates dUMP to dTMP, which is then used for the synthesis of DNA. To enter this cycle, folate (methyl FH_4) is demethylated to FH_4, vitamin B_{12} acting as the cofactor. Thus, both vitamin B_{12} and folic acid deficiencies lead to impaired DNA synthesis and megaloblastic anemia. FH_4, tetrahydrofolate; dUMP, deoxyuridine monophosphate; dTMP, deoxythymidine monophosphate; FH_2, dihydrofolate; DHFR, dihydrofolate reductase.

Anemia   1035

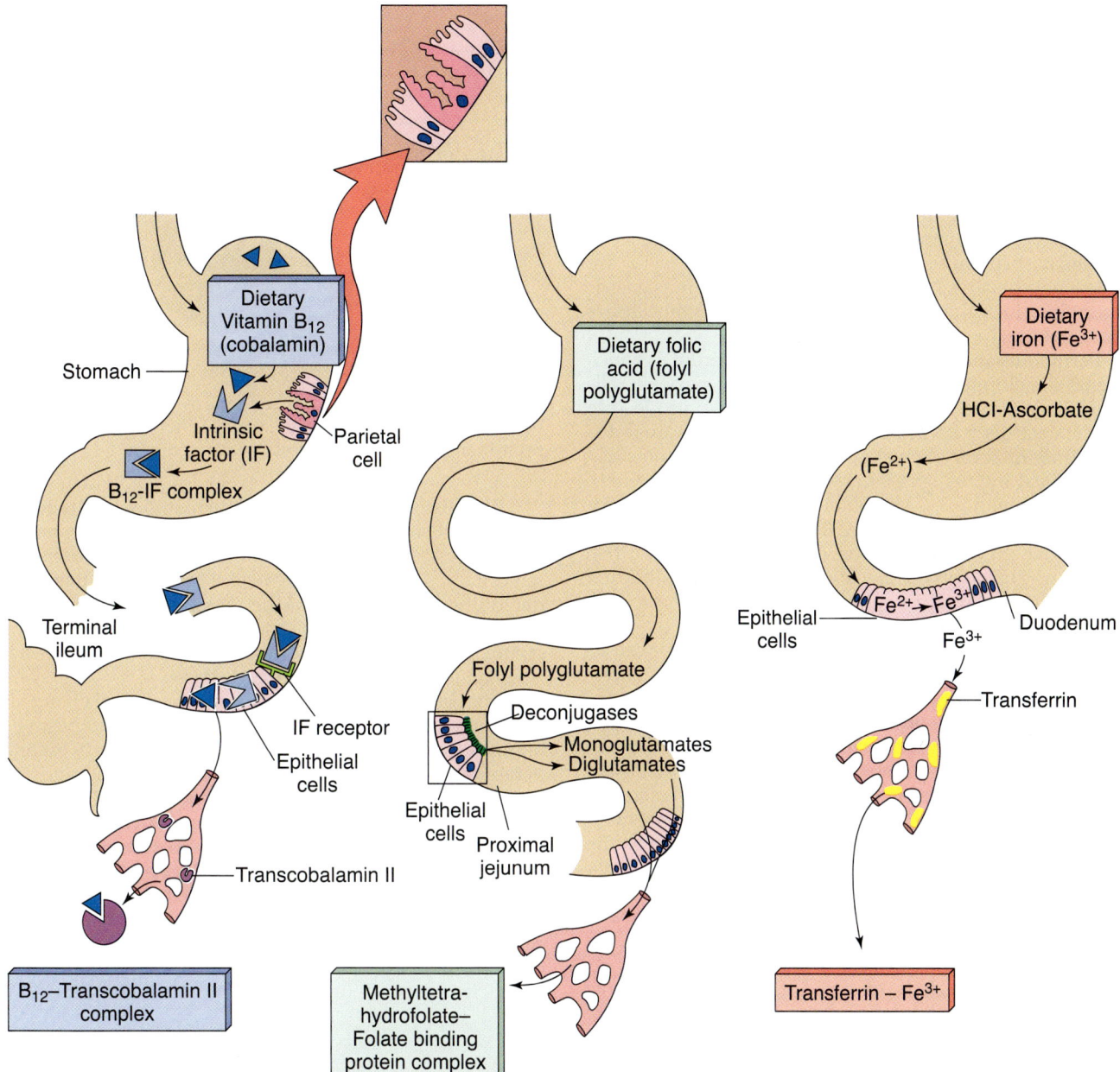

FIGURE 20-15
Absorption of vitamin B_{12}, folic acid, and iron. Absorption of vitamin B_{12} requires initial complexing with intrinsic factor (IF), which is produced by the parietal cells of the gastric mucosa. Absorption then occurs in the terminal ileum, where there are receptors for the IF–B_{12} complex. Dietary folic acid is conjugated by conjugase enzymes to polyglutamate. Absorption occurs in the jejunum following deconjugation in the intestinal lumen. Reduction and methylation result in the generation of methyl tetrahydrofolate, which is then transported by folate-binding protein. Dietary ferric iron is reduced to ferrous iron in the stomach and absorbed principally in the duodenum. Iron is transported by transferrin in the circulation.

tor is produced, along with hydrochloric acid, by the gastric parietal cells. Vitamin B_{12} is absorbed via specific receptors in the distal ileum. In the blood, vitamin B_{12} is transported by a group of proteins called *transcobalamins*, of which transcobalamin II is the most important. The daily requirement for vitamin B_{12} is 1 μg, and therefore, normal body stores of 1000 to 5000 μg provide several years of vitamin reserve. Vitamin B_{12} deficiency arises from diverse causes.

Inadequate dietary intake of vitamin B_{12} occurs rarely and is usually encountered only in strict vegetarians (vegans). The most common cause of vitamin B_{12} deficiency is impaired absorption secondary to lack of intrinsic factor. Intrinsic factor may be deficient as a result of previous gastric surgery in which the parietal cell mass of the stomach has been removed.

Pernicious anemia is an autoimmune disorder in which patients develop antibodies directed against parietal cells and intrinsic factor. The parietal cell antibodies also lead to atrophic gastritis with achlorhydria. Primary intestinal disorders (inflammatory bowel disease) or previous intestinal surgery (ileal bypass) can be associated with impaired absorption of vitamin B_{12}. Microbiological competition for vitamin B_{12} may lead to deficiency. This may arise from bacterial overgrowth of a blind loop or infestation by the fish tapeworm, *Diphyllobothrium latum*. Rarely, an inherited defect in the intestinal receptor for vitamin B_{12} (*Imerslund-Grasbeck syndrome*) is the cause of the deficiency.

Folic acid is contained in leafy vegetables, as well as meat and eggs. Dietary folic acid exists in a polyglutamate form but is deconjugated to monoglutamates in the intestines and primarily absorbed in the jejunum. Following absorption, the folate is reduced and methylated to form 5-methyl tetrahydrofolate, which is then transported in the blood by folate-binding protein. The daily requirement for folic acid is approximately 50 μg. Body stores of folate average 2000 to 5000 μg, providing a few months reserve before signs of deficiency develop.

The most common cause of folic acid deficiency is inadequate dietary intake. This scenario most often develops in patients with poorly balanced diets (alcoholics, recluses). An increased demand for folic acid is encountered with pregnancy, lactation, periods of rapid growth, and chronic hemolytic processes, and deficiency may result unless folate supplementation is provided. Primary intestinal diseases (inflammatory bowel disease, sprue) may interfere with absorption of folic acid. Various medications can also impair folic acid absorption (phenytoin) or metabolism (methotrexate).

 Pathology: The hematological manifestations, in both bone marrow and blood, are identical for either folic acid or vitamin B_{12} deficiency. Although the bone marrow tends to be hypercellular, the blood demonstrates pancytopenia because of ineffective hematopoiesis. Megaloblastic maturation, characterized by cellular enlargement with asynchronous maturation between the nucleus and cytoplasm (Fig. 20-16), is noted in bone marrow precursors from all lineages.

The degree of anemia varies but may be severe. Erythrocytes are macrocytic and many assume an oval shape (oval macrocytes). Anisopoikilocytosis is usually prominent, and teardrop cells may be seen. Circulating neutrophils often show hypersegmentation (more than five lobes) of their nuclei (Fig. 20-17). No increase in reticulocytes occurs.

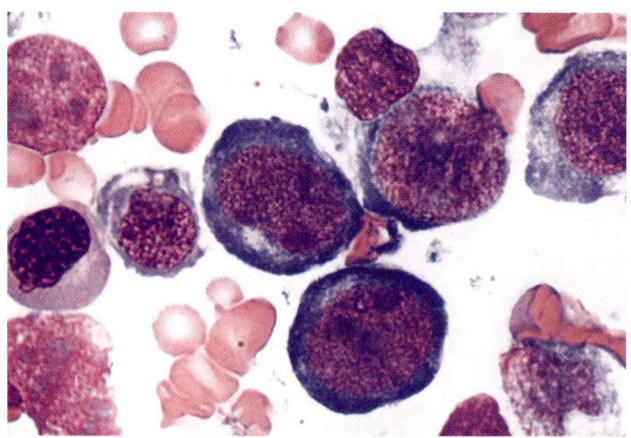

FIGURE 20-16
Megaloblastic anemia. A. A bone marrow aspirate from a patient with vitamin B_{12} deficiency (pernicious anemia) shows prominent megaloblastic erythroid precursors.

The distinction between folic acid and vitamin B_{12} deficiency can usually be established by measuring serum levels of these compounds. Occasionally, specific measurement of red cell folate provides more useful information than serum determinations. Because of the massive intramedullary destruction of red cell precursors in megaloblastic anemia, serum levels of lactate dehydrogenase (LDH), especially isoenzyme 1, are conspicuously elevated.

The Schilling test measures the absorption of vitamin B_{12}. In this test, the patient is orally administered radioactive vitamin B_{12} with or without intrinsic factor. Urinary excretion of radioactivity is measured over a 24-hour period, and based on the results, the cause of the vitamin B_{12} deficiency can be suggested. The Schilling test is no longer commonly used, owing to difficulties in working with radiolabeled compounds. Demonstration of elevated levels of homocysteine and methyl malonic acid may prove useful in cases of vitamin B_{12} deficiency. Circulating antibodies against gastric parietal cells or intrinsic factor can be detected in the setting of pernicious anemia. The former antibody is more frequently detected; the latter is more specific for pernicious anemia.

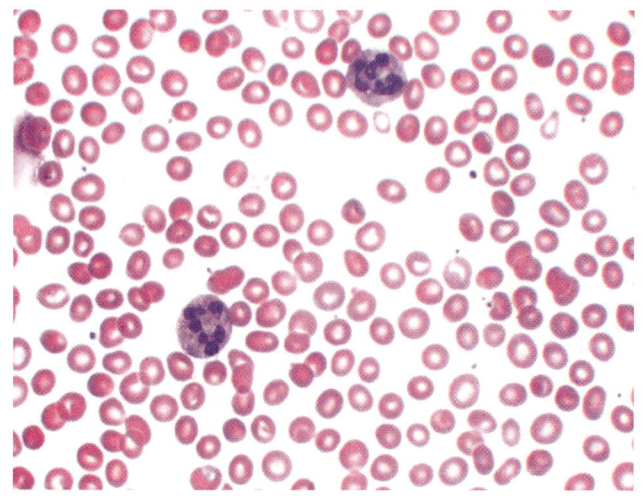

FIGURE 20-17
Hypersegmented granulocytes in a patient with vitamin B_{12} deficiency.

Clinical Features: Whether due to deficiency of vitamin B_{12} or folic acid, the clinical presentation of megaloblastic anemia is similar. In general, folate deficiency develops more rapidly (months) than does vitamin B_{12} deficiency (years). The most important difference clinically is the development of neurological symptoms in cases of vitamin B_{12} deficiency, secondary to degeneration of the posterior and lateral columns of the spinal cord (see Chapter 28). Unless appropriate and prompt therapy is instituted, the neurological symptoms may become irreversible. These neurological findings are not encountered with folate deficiency.

Thalassemia

Thalassemias are anemias that result from defective globin chains.

 Epidemiology: Thalassemia is derived from the Greek word *thalassa*, meaning sea, because of its high incidence around the Mediterranean Sea, especially in Italy and Greece. Thalassemia does, however, have a more worldwide distribution, particularly in areas where malaria has historically been endemic (Middle East, India, Southeast Asia, and China). A heterozygous state for thalassemia may provide a protective effect against malaria and increase the reproductive potential of heterozygotes, thereby explaining the persistence of thalassemic disorders. Many of the geographical areas that have a higher incidence of thalassemia also exhibit an increased prevalence of structural hemoglobin defects (e.g., hemoglobin S). This situation leads to the occurrence of double heterozygosity (e.g., sickle thalassemia), which demonstrates features of both disorders.

A normal hemoglobin molecule contains four globin chains, consisting of two α and two non-α chains. Three normal variants of hemoglobin are encountered, based on the nature of the non-α chains (Fig. 20-18). Hemoglobin A ($\alpha_2\beta_2$) accounts for 95 to 98% of the total hemoglobin in adults; only minor amounts of hemoglobin F ($\alpha_2\gamma_2$) and hemoglobin A_2 ($\alpha_2\delta_2$) are present.

A total of four α genes, paired on each chromosome 16, are normally present. The non-α genes are located on chromosome 11, and consist of two γ, one δ, and one β gene per chromosome. Also present are embryonic globin genes zeta (ζ) (α equivalent) and epsilon (ϵ) (non-α equivalent), which are located on chromosomes 16 and 11, respectively.

Thalassemias are generally classified according to the affected globin chain, and the two most clinically significant forms involve deficits of α and β chains. Thalassemias involving γ and δ globin chain synthesis have also been described but are not common.

β Thalassemia

 Pathogenesis: β Thalassemias are a heterogeneous group of disorders that most often arise secondary to point mutations affecting the β globin gene. The mutation may be located in the promoter region of the gene, a splice site, or other coding regions, or may lead to the creation of an inappropriate stop codon. In any event, transcription of the gene is either entirely (β^0) or partially (β^+) suppressed. Occasionally, a mutation may also affect the adjacent δ globin gene, leading to a β-δ thalassemia.

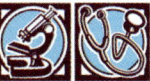 **Pathology and Clinical Features:** Homozygous β thalassemia *(Cooley anemia)* is characterized by moderate-to-severe, microcytic and hypochromic anemia (Fig. 20-19). There is a marked excess of α chains, which form unstable tetramers (α_4) that precipitate in the cytoplasm of the developing erythroid precursors. In the β^0 type, fetal hemoglobin accounts for most of the hemoglobin, although increased levels (5–8%) of hemoglobin A_2 are also present. In the case of β^+ type,

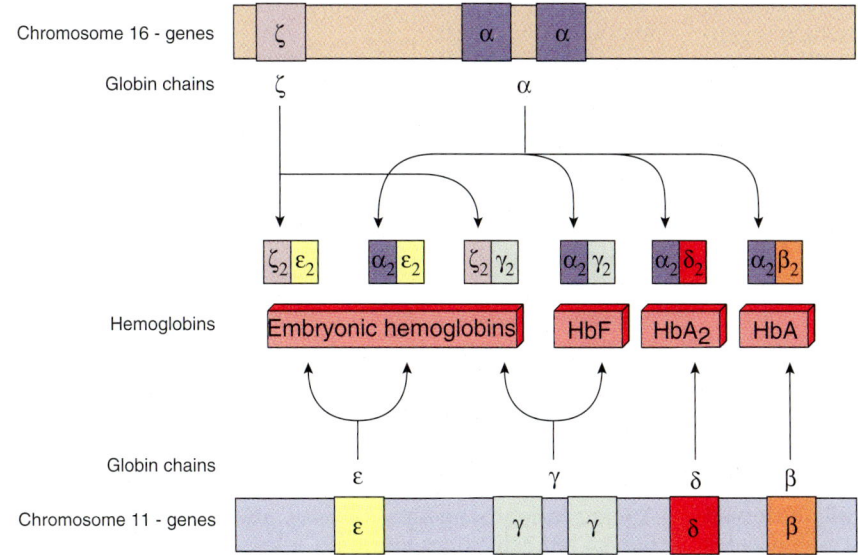

FIGURE 20-18
Assembly of subunit chains to form different hemoglobins.

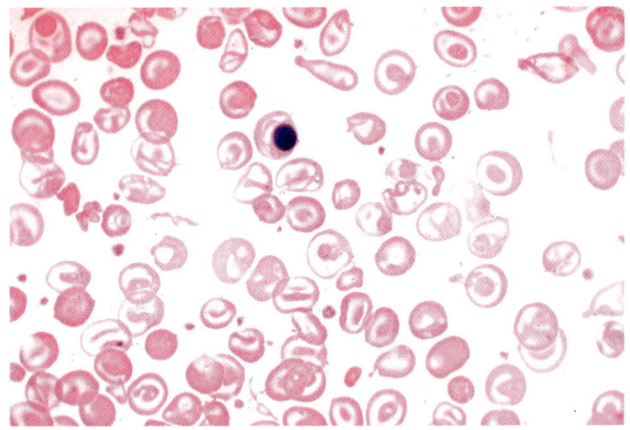

FIGURE 20-19
Thalassemia. The peripheral blood erythrocytes are hypochromic and microcytic and show anisocytosis, poikilocytosis, and target cells.

some hemoglobin A may be detected (depending on the nature of the underlying defect), and hemoglobin A_2 is mildly increased. A modest increase in hemoglobin A_2 is characteristic of all forms of β thalassemia, owing to upregulation of δ globin genes.

In addition to microcytosis and hypochromia, striking anisopoikilocytosis with target cells, basophilic stippling, and circulating normoblasts (especially following splenectomy) can be identified in the blood. A combination of the increased oxygen affinity of hemoglobin F and the underlying anemia leads to decreased oxygen delivery and increased production of erythropoietin, which causes marked erythroid hyperplasia in the bone marrow. The marrow space is thus expanded, with resultant facial and cranial bone deformities. Extramedullary hematopoiesis contributes to hepatosplenomegaly and the formation of soft tissue masses.

Excess erythropoiesis leads to increased iron absorption, which, together with repeated transfusions, creates iron overload. Excess iron deposition in tissues is a major cause of morbidity and mortality in thalassemic patients and often requires aggressive chelation therapy.

Heterozygous β thalassemia is associated with microcytosis and hypochromia, and the degree of microcytosis is disproportionate to the severity of the anemia, which is generally mild. There is often an accompanying erythrocytosis (increased red blood cell count) but minimal anisocytosis (normal RDW). Target cells, basophilic stippling, and a mild increase in hemoglobin A_2 are present. Most patients are entirely asymptomatic.

α Thalassemia

 Pathogenesis: Unlike β thalassemias, α thalassemias arise most frequently as a result of gene deletions. More syndromes are clinically observed because of the potential number (up to four) of α globin genes

that may be affected. α Thalassemia is associated with excess β or γ chains, which can then form the tetrameric hemoglobin H ($β_4$) and hemoglobin Bart ($γ_4$). Hemoglobin H and hemoglobin Bart are both unstable and precipitate in the cytoplasm, forming Heinz bodies, but to a lesser degree than $α_4$ tetramers. Hemoglobin H and Bart have high oxygen affinities and lead to decreased tissue oxygen delivery. The relative amount of these tetrameric hemoglobins depends on the number of α genes involved and the patient's age. Because of the underlying impairment in hemoglobin synthesis, circulating red cells usually exhibit microcytosis and hypochromia.

 Pathology and Clinical Features: **Silent carrier α thalassemia (one gene affected)** is difficult to diagnose, because patients have no hematological abnormalities, except for slight amounts of hemoglobin Bart, which are detectable only in infancy. Clinically, there is no anemia, and patients are asymptomatic.

α Thalassemia trait (two genes affected) is associated with a mild microcytic anemia. Like heterozygous β thalassemia, the degree of microcytosis is disproportionately low compared with the degree of anemia. Erythrocytosis is observed, and there is minimal anisopoikilocytosis. There is no elevation of hemoglobin A_2, allowing for distinction between α and β thalassemia traits. Up to 5% hemoglobin Bart can be seen during infancy. Two different genotypes are possible in heterozygous α thalassemia. There may be a single gene deleted from each chromosome 16, or alternatively, both genes may be deleted from the same chromosome 16. The former scenario is more common in persons of Mediterranean and African descent; the latter is more frequent in Southeast Asia. Clinically, both genotypes have similar presentations, but the potential for development of homozygous α thalassemia is possible only if both genes are deleted from the same chromosome.

Hemoglobin H disease (three genes affected) is associated with moderate microcytic anemia. Circulating erythrocytes display moderate anisopoikilocytosis and some target cells. Increased amounts of hemoglobin Bart (up to 25% in infancy) and variable levels of hemoglobin H can be detected. Both hemoglobin H and hemoglobin Bart can be recognized by hemoglobin electrophoresis, because of their fast migration relative to hemoglobin A. Precipitated hemoglobin H (Heinz bodies) can also be demonstrated by supravital staining of a blood smear.

Homozygous (four genes affected) α thalassemia, also termed α *hydrops fetalis,* is incompatible with life. Affected infants die either in utero or shortly after birth with severe anemia, marked anisopoikilocytosis, and large amounts of hemoglobin Bart. Severe impairment in tissue oxygen delivery is associated with heart failure and generalized edema. Massive hepatosplenomegaly is secondary to extramedullary hematopoiesis.

Hemolytic Anemias Feature Increased Red Cell Destruction

A wide variety of anemias develop due to increased destruction of red cells following their release from the bone marrow. Premature elimination of circulating erythrocytes is called *hemolysis,* and the resulting anemias are termed *hemolytic anemias.* These anemias are classified according to the site of red cell destruction. *Extravascular* hemolysis is accomplished by cells of the monocyte/macrophage system in the spleen and, to a lesser extent, the liver. In *intravascular* hemolysis, erythrocytes are destroyed in the circulation.

Hemolytic anemias are characterized by a compensatory increase in production and release of red cells by the bone marrow, manifested in the blood by polychromasia of red cells and an increased reticulocyte count. Other laboratory findings commonly associated with hemolysis include increased unconjugated (indirect) bilirubin, decreased haptoglobin, increased LDH (particularly isoenzyme 1), free (extracellular) hemoglobin in the blood and urine, increased urobilinogen, and urine hemosiderin.

Membrane Defects

The erythrocyte membrane normally has remarkable flexibility and can deform to allow red cells to circulate unimpaired through the microcirculation and the splenic vasculature. The red cell membrane consists of a lipid bilayer, which is attached to an underlying cytoskeleton (Fig. 20-9). The main component of the cytoskeleton is spectrin, which is a dimer composed of α and β subunits. The genes for the α and β subunits of spectrin are located on chromosomes 1 and 14, respectively. Ankyrin (band 2.1) anchors spectrin to transmembrane proteins (band 3, anion exchanger proteins), whereas spectrin is bound to actin and glycophorin by protein 4.1. Alterations in any portion of the red cell membrane can reduce the normal plasticity and render the erythrocytes susceptible to hemolysis.

Hereditary Spherocytosis

Hereditary spherocytosis (HS) represents a heterogeneous group of inherited disorders of the erythrocyte cytoskeleton, characterized by a deficiency of spectrin or another cytoskeletal component (ankyrin, protein 4.2, band 3).

 Pathogenesis: The deficiency of a cytoskeletal protein in HS leads to a *vertical* defect in the red cell membrane, with uncoupling of the lipid bilayer from the underlying cytoskeleton. The defect results in progressive loss of membrane surface area and formation of spherocytes. These abnormal red cells are more rigid and cannot easily traverse the spleen. While circulating through the spleen, spherocytes become "conditioned" and lose additional surface membrane before they ultimately succumb to extravascular hemolysis. Most forms of HS are inherited as autosomal dominant traits, and the rare recessive cases all involve the α subunit of spectrin.

 Pathology: Most patients with HS have a moderate normocytic anemia. Conspicuous spherocytes that appear hyperchromic (no central pallor) are typical, and along with polychromasia and reticulocytosis, are invariable (Fig. 20-20). The bone marrow demonstrates erythroid hyperplasia.

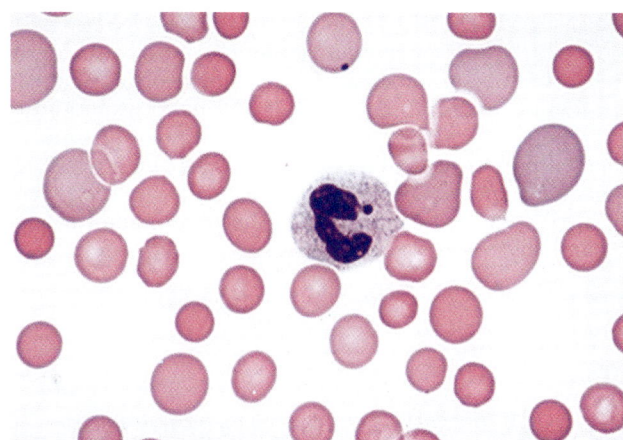

FIGURE 20-20
Hereditary spherocytosis. The peripheral blood smear shows many erythrocytes with decreased diameter, intense staining, and no central pallor (spherocytes).

MCHC is mildly increased, reflecting the loss of surface area that characterizes spherocytes. When placed in salt solutions of decreasing concentration, spherocytes demonstrate more osmotic fragility than normal erythrocytes. Laboratory findings typical of hemolysis (decreased haptoglobin, increased indirect bilirubin, increased LDH) are often present.

 Clinical Features: Most patients demonstrate splenomegaly secondary to chronic extravascular hemolysis. They may appear jaundiced, and up to 50% of these patients develop cholelithiasis, with pigmented (bilirubin) gallstones. Despite chronic hemolysis, transfusion is generally not required. An exception is a sudden decline in hemoglobin and reticulocytes, which heralds an aplastic crisis (usually due to infection by parvovirus B19). Anemia may also become more severe in so-called hemolytic crisis, during which there is a transient acceleration of the hemolysis. HS patients can be managed effectively by splenectomy, although spherocytes still persist in the circulation.

Hereditary Elliptocytosis

Hereditary elliptocytosis (HE) refers to a heterogeneous group of inherited disorders involving the erythrocyte cytoskeleton.

 Pathogenesis: HE features a *horizontal* abnormality within the cytoskeleton. More-commonly described variants of HE include defects in self-assembly of spectrin, spectrin–ankyrin binding, protein 4.1, and glycophorin C. Regardless of the underlying molecular abnormality, most circulating red cells assume an elliptical or oval shape. These elliptocytes still have an area of central pallor, because there is no loss of the lipid bilayer (as seen in HS). Most forms of HE are autosomal dominant. Interestingly, the red cells of camels and llamas are elliptical.

Pathology and Clinical Features: HE usually manifests with only mild normocytic anemia, and many patients are completely asymptomatic. Blood smear examination demonstrates numerous elliptocytes with only minimal reticulocytosis (Fig. 20-21). Generally, less hemolysis and subsequent anemia are seen than are seen with HS. Occasional patients with more severe hemolysis may require splenectomy.

Acanthocytosis

Acanthocytosis results from a defect within the lipid bilayer of the red cell membrane and features spiny projections of the surface, which may be associated with hemolysis.

 Pathogenesis: The most common cause of acanthocytosis is chronic liver disease, in which increased free cholesterol is deposited within the cell membrane. Acanthocytes are also a prominent feature in cases of abetalipoproteinemia, an autosomal recessive disorder associated with lipid membrane abnormalities (see Chapter 13).

 Pathology and Clinical Features: Abnormalities in the lipid membrane cause erythrocytes to become deformed and develop irregular spiny surface projections and centrally dense cytoplasm (no central pallor) (Fig. 20-22). These red cell are referred to as *acanthocytes* (spur cells). Acanthocytes need to be distinguished from burr cells (crenated cells, echinocytes), which have more-uniform scalloping of the red cell membrane and maintain an area of central pallor. Hemolysis and anemia associated with acanthocytosis are mild.

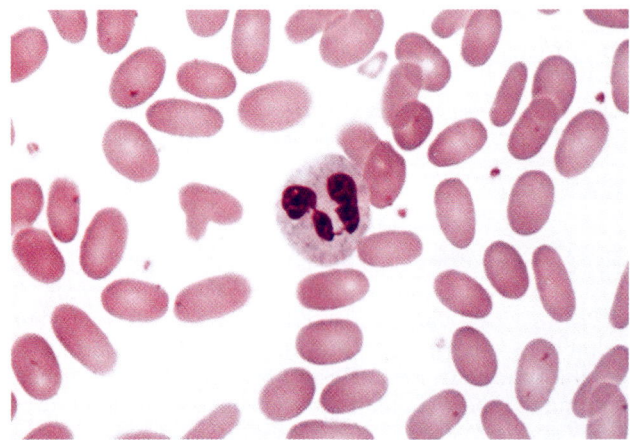

FIGURE 20-21
Hereditary elliptocytosis. A smear of peripheral blood reveals that virtually all of the erythrocytes are elliptical.

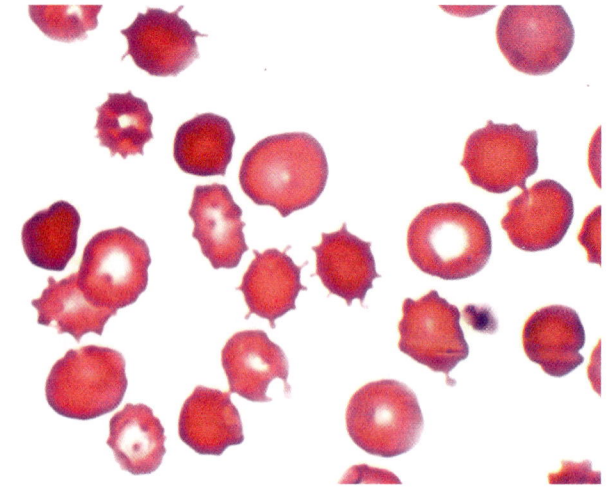

FIGURE 20-22
Acanthocytes. The red cells lack central pallor and display spikes on the surface.

Enzyme Defects

Energy generation within erythrocytes occurs primarily through the process of glycolysis. Inherited defects of enzymes involved in the glycolytic pathway can predispose the circulating red cells to hemolysis. The most common enzyme defect involves glucose-6-phosphate dehydrogenase (G6PD), which catalyzes the conversion of glucose-6-phosphate to 6-phosphogluconate (see below). Deficiencies of the remaining glycolytic enzymes are rare and autosomal recessive, and among these, pyruvate kinase deficiency is the most frequent. Clinically, these enzyme deficiencies manifest with a variable degree of anemia and are grouped together under the designation *hereditary nonspherocytic anemias*.

G6PD Deficiency

G6PD deficiency is an X-linked disorder that causes a hemolytic anemia characterized by abnormal sensitivity of red cells to oxidative stress. G6PD deficiency has a variable worldwide distribution and has its highest prevalence in areas in which malaria is historically endemic, notably Africa and the Mediterranean region. G6PD mutations appear to provide some protective effect against malaria.

 Pathogenesis: Because of the role of G6PD in recycling reduced glutathione, red cells deficient in this enzyme are susceptible to oxidative stress (e.g., infections, drugs, or fava bean ingestion [favism]). Oxidation of hemoglobin leads to the formation of methemoglobin, in which ferrous (Fe^{2+}) iron is converted to the ferric (Fe^{3+}) state. Methemoglobin, which cannot transport oxygen, is unstable and precipitates in the cytoplasm as Heinz bodies. The precipitated methemoglobin increases cell rigidity and leads to hemolysis.

Pathology: In quiescent periods, the erythrocytes of G6PD deficiency appear normal. However, during a hemolytic episode precipitated by oxidative stress, Heinz bodies can be demonstrated by supravital staining. As a result of previous passage through the spleen, circulating red cells may have a portion of the membrane removed, forming so-called *bite cells*. Testing for low enzyme activity should ideally be performed when the patient is not experiencing hemolysis, since young erythrocytes (reticulocytes) normally have higher enzyme levels, which may lead to a false-negative result.

 Clinical Features: Full expression of G6PD deficiency is seen only in males, with females being asymptomatic carriers. The A–variant of G6PD is seen in 10 to 15% of American blacks and is associated with reduced enzyme activity (10% of normal) because of instability of the molecule. In affected patients, exposure to oxidant drugs, such as the antimalarial agent primaquine, may result in hemolysis.

In the Mediterranean type of G6PD mutation, enzyme activity is absent and, therefore, with exposure to oxidant stress, hemolysis is more sustained and severe. Potentially lethal hemolysis may follow ingestion of fava beans *(favism)* in susceptible patients.

Hemoglobinopathies

Most clinically relevant hemoglobinopathies are caused by point mutations affecting the β globin chain gene.

Sickle Cell Disease

Sickle cell disease is characterized by the presence of an abnormal hemoglobin, hemoglobin S, which upon deoxygenation transforms the erythrocyte into a sickle shape.

 Epidemiology: The presence of hemoglobin S has its highest incidence in persons of African ancestry, although the gene is also encountered in Mediterranean, Middle Eastern, and Indian populations. In some regions of Africa, up to 40% of the population is heterozygous for hemoglobin S. Ten percent of American blacks are heterozygous, and 1 in 650 is homozygous. Heterozygosity for hemoglobin S is thought to provide some protection against falciparum malaria. Infected erythrocytes selectively sickle and are removed from the circulation by splenic and hepatic macrophages, effectively destroying the organism.

 Pathogenesis: Hemoglobin S results from a point mutation in the gene encoding the β globin chain gene, with substitution of a valine for the normal glutamic acid at the sixth amino acid position. This single change results in a structurally abnormal molecule that polymerizes within the cytoplasm under conditions of deoxygenation. Polymerization of hemoglobin S transforms the cytoplasm into a rigid filamentous gel and leads to the formation of less deformable sickled erythrocytes.

The increased rigidity of sickled erythrocytes results in obstruction of the microcirculation, with subsequent tissue hypoxia and ischemic injury in many organs. The inflexible nature of sickle cells also renders them susceptible to destruction (hemolysis) during circulation through the spleen. Thus, the two primary manifestations of sickle cell disease are recurrent ischemic events and chronic extravascular hemolytic anemia.

Erythrocyte sickling is initially reversible with reoxygenation, but after several cycles of sickling and unsickling, the process becomes irreversible. Sickled erythrocytes also demonstrate changes in the phospholipid component of the membrane, leading to increased adherence to endothelial cells and further complicating capillary blood flow.

Persons who are homozygous for the hemoglobin S mutation show the full clinical presentation of sickle cell disease. A sickling disorder is also observed in patients who are doubly heterozygous for two β chain mutations (e.g. hemoglobin SC disease, sickle/β-thalassemia). Heterozygotes for hemoglobin S (sickle cell trait), however, do not develop red cell sickling, because the presence of hemoglobin A effectively blocks the ability of hemoglobin S to polymerize. Hemoglobin F also interferes with hemoglobin S polymerization, and homozygous patients with increased levels of hemoglobin F suffer a milder form of disease.

 Pathology: Homozygous patients (hemoglobin SS) have severe normocytic or macrocytic anemia. The macrocytosis can be attributed to an increased number of reticulocytes, secondary to chronic hemolysis. Blood smear examination reveals marked anisopoikilocytosis and polychromasia. Classic sickle cells and target cells, as well as a variety of other abnormally shaped erythrocytes, are observed (Fig. 20-23). Howell-Jolly bodies, representing nuclear remnants, are seen in most patients beyond childhood and reflect hyposplenism caused by ischemic loss of splenic tissue.

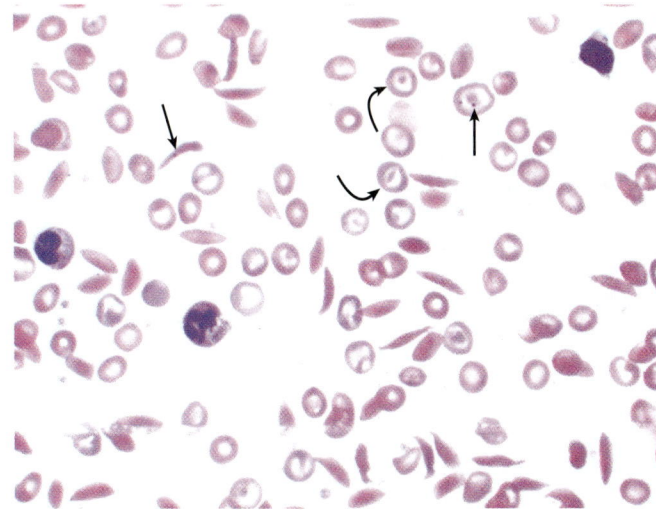

FIGURE 20-23

Sickle cell anemia. Howell-Jolly bodies (straight arrows) and target cells (curved arrows) are evident.

Hemoglobin electrophoresis demonstrates the absence of hemoglobin A, and hemoglobin S accounts for 80 to 95% of the total hemoglobin. The remaining hemoglobin consists of a combination of hemoglobins F and A_2.

Clinical Features: Affected infants with SS hemoglobin are asymptomatic for the first 8 to 10 weeks of life, owing to high levels of hemoglobin F. Clinical symptoms first manifest in childhood when the synthesis of γ globin chains is downregulated, an event that is somewhat delayed in homozygous S patients. Although patients suffer from lifelong hemolysis, adaptation occurs over time, and most may not require regular transfusions. Instead, the clinical picture is dominated by sequelae of repeated vasoocclusive disease. In an attempt to minimize these complications by decreasing the amount of hemoglobin S in circulation, a chronic exchange transfusion program may become necessary. Sickle cell anemia is a systemic disorder and is eventually responsible for impaired function in most organ systems and tissues throughout the body (Fig. 20-24).

Patients with sickle cell disease develop episodic painful crises, the number of which varies. Capillary occlusion leads to ischemia and hypoxic cell injury, which are associated with severe pain, especially in the chest, abdomen, and bones. Painful crises can be triggered by a variety of stimuli (e.g. underlying infection, acidosis, or dehydration).

APLASTIC CRISIS: This condition arises when there is a cessation of compensatory events in the bone marrow. Such crises are characterized by a rapid drop in the hemoglobin level and the absence of an appropriate reticulo-

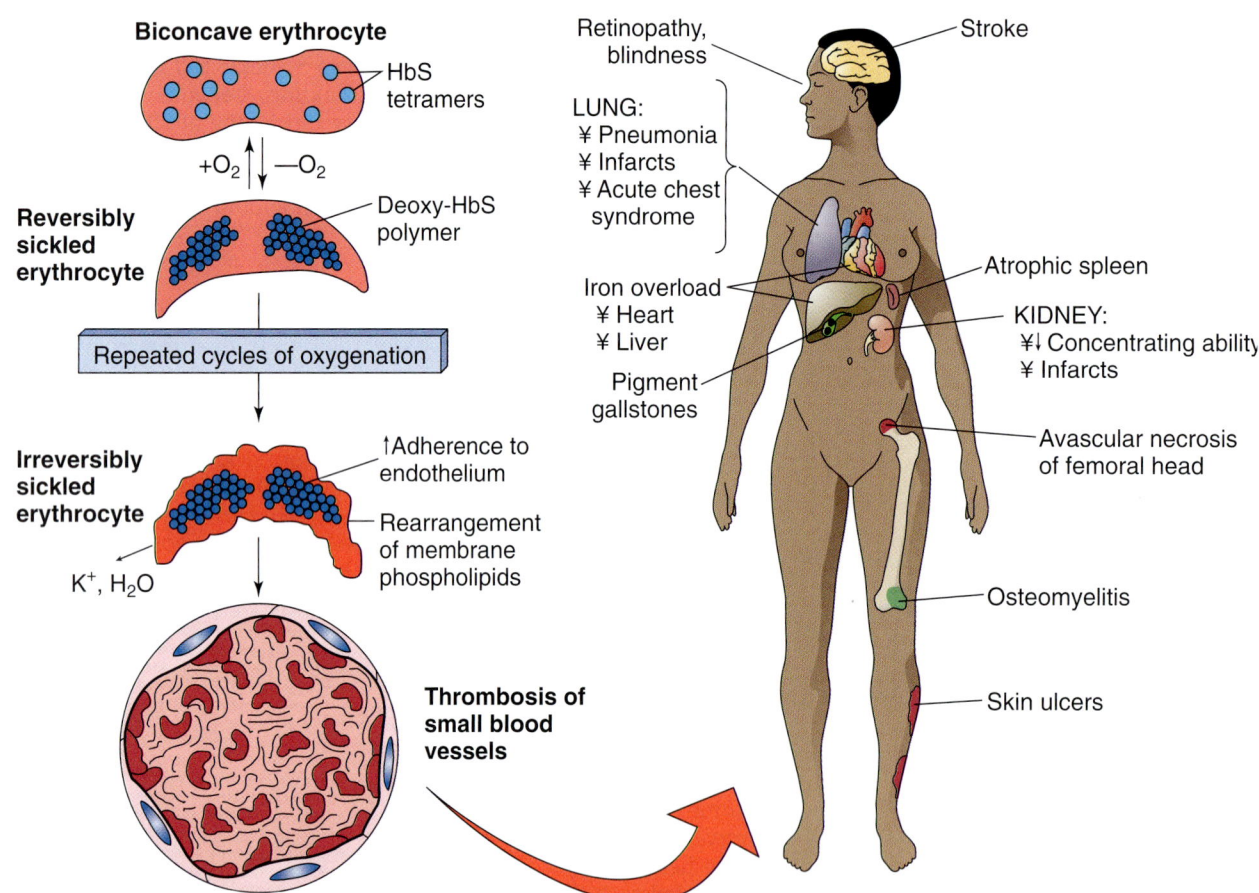

FIGURE 20-24
Pathogenesis of the vascular complications of sickle cell anemia. Substitution of valine for glutamic acid leads to an alteration in the surface charge of the hemoglobin molecule. Upon deoxygenation, sickle hemoglobin tetramers aggregate to form poorly soluble polymers. The erythrocyte change shape from a biconcave disk to a sickle form with the polymerization of sickle hemoglobin (HbS). This process is initially reversible upon reoxygenation, but with repeated cycles of deoxygenation and reoxygenation, the erythrocytes become irreversibly sickled. Irreversibly sickled cells display a rearrangement of phospholipids between the outer and inner monolayers of the cell membrane, in particular an increase in aminophospholipids in the outer leaflet. Potassium and water are lost from the cells. The erythrocytes are no longer deformable and are more adherent to endothelial cells, properties that predispose to thrombosis of small blood vessels. The resulting vascular occlusions lead to widespread ischemic complications.

cyte response. Infection by parvovirus B19 is the most frequent cause of an aplastic crisis, although other viral and bacterial infections may also be associated with transient bone marrow suppression.

SEQUESTRATION CRISIS: This term applies to sudden pooling of erythrocytes, especially in the spleen. It results in a decreased circulating blood volume and low hemoglobin levels. The etiology of this process is not well understood, but it most frequently develops in younger children, who still have a functioning spleen. This complication is followed by hypovolemic shock and is the most frequent cause of death during the early years of life.

Heart: A chronic demand for increased cardiac output may lead to the development of cardiomegaly and congestive heart failure. In addition, obstruction of the coronary microcirculation may cause myocardial ischemia. Myocyte function may also be impaired by excess iron deposition, secondary to chronic hemolysis and repeated blood transfusions.

Lungs: Up to one third of patients with sickle cell anemia develop a rapid decrease in respiratory function, which is associated with pulmonary infiltrates on chest x-ray. The situation is referred to as *acute chest syndrome* and may be fatal. Pulmonary infarction may be caused by sickle cell disease, and there is an increased susceptibility to a variety of pulmonary infections.

Spleen: Although splenomegaly is often encountered in childhood, repeated infarction leads to a functional autosplenectomy, and in most adults, only a small fibrous remnant of the spleen remains. The asplenic state renders the patient susceptible to infections by encapsulated bacteria, especially *Streptococcus pneumoniae*.

Brain: Patients with sickle cell anemia develop a variety of neurological complications related to vascular obstruction, including transient ischemic attacks, overt strokes, and cerebral hemorrhages. Occlusion of the microvasculature of the retina may lead to retinal hemorrhage and detachment, proliferative retinopathy, and blindness.

Kidney: Sickling commonly occurs in the renal medulla because of the hypoxic, acidotic, and hypertonic environment that normally exists there. Complications include the inability to form concentrated urine, renal infarcts, and papillary necrosis. Male patients may develop priapism, which, if not treated promptly, may lead to permanent erectile dysfunction.

Liver: As in any form of chronic hemolytic anemia, patients with sickle cell anemia have increased levels of unconjugated (indirect) bilirubin, which predisposes to the development of pigmented bilirubin gallstones. Cholelithiasis may lead to cholecystitis, which then may require cholecystectomy. Hepatomegaly and increased hepatic iron deposition are also seen.

Extremities: Cutaneous ulcers over the lower extremities, especially in the region of the ankles, are common and reflect obstruction of dermal capillaries. *Hand–foot syndrome*, with self-limited swelling of the hands and feet, may develop in children because of underlying bone infarcts. Avascular necrosis of the femoral head necessitates corrective hip surgery. Sickle cell disease is also associated with an increased incidence of osteomyelitis, particularly with *Salmonella typhimurium*, possibly related to the underlying impairment in splenic function.

Sickle Cell Trait

Heterozygosity for the hemoglobin S mutation is referred to as sickle cell trait.

Pathogenesis: In persons with sickle cell trait, hemoglobin A in the red cells prevents polymerization of hemoglobin S and therefore, sickling. Sickling of erythrocytes may, however, occur under extreme conditions (flight at high altitude in unpressurized aircraft, deep sea diving). Heterozygotes are clinically asymptomatic, do not develop hemolytic anemia, and have a normal life span.

Pathology: On blood smear examination, erythrocyte morphology is normal, except for occasional target cells. Hemoglobin electrophoresis reveals approximately 60% hemoglobin A and 40% hemoglobin C. Although normal and abnormal β globin chains are synthesized at equal rates, preferential pairing between α chains and normal β chains leads to higher amounts of hemoglobin A.

Double Heterozygosity for Hemoglobin S and Other Hemoglobinopathies

Some patients who present with a sickling disorder actually represent compound heterozygotes for hemoglobin S and other structurally abnormal hemoglobin molecules (e.g., hemoglobin C, hemoglobin D) or thalassemia.

Pathogenesis: The presence of an additional abnormal hemoglobin or thalassemic gene does not prevent the polymerization of hemoglobin S, and the clinical expression and severity of disease may be affected. Doubly heterozygous individuals may have less frequent crises, higher baseline hemoglobin values, microcytic red cell indices, or persistent splenomegaly into adult life.

Hemoglobin C Disease

Hemoglobin C disease results from homozygous inheritance of a structurally abnormal hemoglobin, which leads to increased erythrocyte rigidity and mild chronic hemolysis.

Pathogenesis: The mutation that results in hemoglobin C involves the substitution of a lysine for the normal glutamic acid molecule at the sixth amino acid position of the β globin chain. Hemoglobin C precipitates in the erythrocyte cytoplasm and leads to cellular dehydration and decreased deformability. Upon passage through the spleen, the abnormal red cells are removed from the circulation, and mild anemia and splenomegaly ensue. Hemoglobin C has reduced oxygen affinity, which leads to increased tissue oxygen delivery and lessens the overall severity of disease. Hemoglobin C is most commonly found in the same populations as hemoglobin S, although the overall incidence is less.

Pathology: Homozygous hemoglobin C disease (CC) is associated with a mild normocytic anemia. Blood smear examination reveals numerous target cells and mild polychromasia. Hemoglobin may be unevenly distributed within the red cells, and dense, rhomboidal crystals (representing precipitated hemoglobin C) are present in some erythrocytes. Hemoglobin electrophoresis reveals no hemoglobin A and more than 90% hemoglobin C.

Two to 3% of American blacks are heterozygous for hemoglobin C and remain asymptomatic (hemoglobin C trait). About 40% of the total hemoglobin consists of hemoglobin C. Red cell morphology is normal, except for some target cells.

Hemoglobin E Disease

Hemoglobin E disease results from homozygous inheritance of structurally abnormal hemoglobin, which creates a thalassemia-like defect and is associated with mild chronic hemolysis.

Pathogenesis: The mutation in hemoglobin E involves the substitution of a lysine for the normal glutamic acid at the twenty-sixth amino acid position of the β globin chain. This position is at a splice site in the gene, and the mutation results not only in a structurally abnormal molecule, but also in decreased transcription of the gene and unstable messenger RNA. The latter defects diminish synthesis of hemoglobin E, creating a situation akin to that seen with thalassemia. Hemoglobin E is relatively unstable and may precipitate within the cell, contributing to the hemolysis. Hemoglobin E is most prevalent in regions of Southeast Asia and globally is second only to hemoglobin S in terms of overall incidence. The presence of hemoglobin E in erythrocytes is believed to exert a protective effect against malaria.

Pathology: Homozygous hemoglobin E disease (EE) is associated with mild microcytic anemia. The MCV is decreased, and there is often erythrocytosis because of the thalassemia-like component. Blood smear examination reveals microcytic, hypochromic red cells and target cells. Hemoglobin electrophoresis demonstrates more than 90% hemoglobin E.

Heterozygosity for hemoglobin E (hemoglobin E trait) is generally asymptomatic, although erythrocytes from affected patients are microcytic. Only about 30% of the total hemoglobin is hemoglobin E.

Other Hemoglobinopathies

Several hundred additional hemoglobin variants have been described that result from mutations in either the α or β globin genes. These mutations may lead to structural abnormalities or to a functional derangement of the hemoglobin molecule.

Pathogenesis: Some mutations result in alteration of the tertiary structure of hemoglobin, leading to destabilization of the molecule and cytoplasmic precipitation. As a group, these hemoglobins are referred to as *unstable hemoglobins* and are often named after the geographical location in which they were first discovered (e.g., hemoglobin Köln). Unstable hemoglobins precipitate and form Heinz bodies within the erythrocytes that can be demonstrated with supravital staining. The Heinz bodies bind to the cell membrane, increasing their rigidity and leading to mild chronic hemolysis. Patients may suffer jaundice and splenomegaly.

Other hemoglobin mutations are associated with *abnormal hemoglobin oxygen affinity*. Increased oxygen affinity is clinically associated with decreased oxygen delivery at the tissue level, resulting in hypoxia. Hypoxia leads to increased erythropoietin production and erythroid hyperplasia in the bone marrow, which in turn causes erythrocytosis. Although patients are mostly asymptomatic, in some cases they may have symptoms related to hyperviscosity.

Abnormal hemoglobins with decreased oxygen affinity readily release oxygen at the tissue level. Erythropoietin levels are low, and most patients have mild anemia. Because of increased concentrations of deoxyhemoglobin, patients appear cyanotic.

Immune Hemolytic Anemias

Immune hemolytic anemias are characterized by increased red cell destruction (hemolysis) secondary to antibodies directed against antigens on the erythrocyte surface. In these disorders, the red cell itself is intrinsically normal but becomes the target of an immune-mediated attack. Immune hemolytic anemia can develop secondary to either auto- or alloantibodies, and the site of hemolysis may be either extra- or intravascular.

Autoimmune Hemolytic Anemia

Autoimmune hemolytic anemia (AIHA) features autoantibodies against red cells.. Autoantibodies can be classified as either warm or cold antibodies.

Warm Antibody AIHA

Pathogenesis: Warm autoantibodies have optimal reactivity at 37°C and account for 80% of all cases of AIHA. They are usually IgG and have a general specificity directed against Rh determinants on the erythrocyte. Warm antibodies do not bind complement and, therefore, extravascular hemolysis occurs primarily in the spleen. Splenic macrophages have Fc receptors that recognize erythrocyte-bound warm antibodies and remove segments of the membrane with attached antibody. Progressive loss of membrane leads to the formation of spherocytes, which ultimately undergo hemolysis.

Warm antibody AIHA affects women more frequently than men, and half of cases are idiopathic. In remaining cases, warm antibody develops secondary to an underlying condition, such as infection, collagen vascular disease, lymphoproliferative disorders, and drug reactions.

Drug-induced warm antibodies may arise by several different mechanisms. In the "hapten" mechanism, a drug such as penicillin binds to the erythrocyte surface, which then becomes modified and evokes an autoantibody response. In the "immune complex" mechanism, a drug such as quinidine reacts with specific circulating antibody to form immune complexes, which then become bound to the red cell membrane. In the "autoantibody" mechanism, a drug (e.g., α-methyldopa) leads to the formation of antibodies that cross-react with components of the red cell membrane. In the hapten and immune-complex models, the presence of the offending drug is required for the development of hemolysis, whereas in the autoantibody model, hemolysis occurs in the absence of the initiating drug.

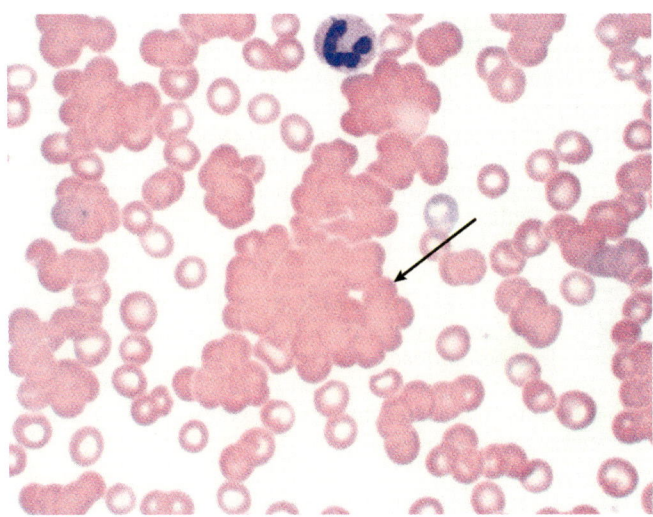

FIGURE 20-25
Clumped red cells (*arrow*) caused by cold agglutinins.

 Pathology: Warm antibody AIHA is associated with normocytic or occasionally macrocytic anemia, with spherocytes and polychromasia. The direct antiglobulin (Coombs) test is usually positive and is useful in distinguishing cases of immune spherocytosis from those that are nonimmune. In the direct Coombs test, the patient's red cells are incubated with anti-human globulin serum. Agglutination indicates antibody molecules on the cell surface.

 Clinical Features: Warm antibody AIHA is treated with corticosteroids or other immunosuppressive agents. Refractory cases may require splenectomy or transfusion support.

Cold Antibody AIHA

Cold antibodies have maximal reactivity at 4°C. Some 20% of cases of AIHA are caused by cold IgM or IgG antibodies, which occur as cold agglutinins or hemolysins.

Cold Agglutinin Disease

 Pathogenesis: Cold agglutinins are mostly IgM and are directed against the I/i antigen system on red cells. At cooler temperatures in the peripheral circulation, these antibodies bind to and agglutinate red cells (Fig. 20-25). Cold agglutinins also fix complement. Upon rewarming in the central circulation, the antibody dissociates from the erythrocyte surface, leaving unactivated complement attached. These complement-coated red cells may undergo extravascular hemolysis in the liver, because Kupffer cells have more complement receptors than do splenic macrophages. Occasionally, the thermal amplitude of a cold agglutinin is high enough for the antibody to remain attached; complement becomes activated, and intravascular hemolysis occurs.

Cold agglutinins may be idiopathic or develop secondary to an underlying condition, most frequently infections (Epstein-Barr virus [EBV], mycoplasma) or lymphoproliferative disorders. Significant hemolysis is uncommon with cold agglutinins, and patients are more likely to develop peripheral vascular symptoms (Raynaud phenomenon) upon cold exposure, because of red cell agglutination.

 Pathology: Cold agglutinins often become activated upon cooling of blood to room temperature, and erythrocyte agglutination in vitro can be noted on blood smears (Fig. 20-25). Agglutination leads to falsely low RBCs and HCT and falsely elevated MCV and MCHC. Warming the blood sample to 37°C prior to analysis corrects the spurious results. The direct Coombs test is positive but usually only for the presence of complement on red cells.

Cold Hemolysin Disease (Paroxysmal Cold Hemoglobinuria)

 Pathogenesis: Cold hemolysins (Donath-Landsteiner antibodies) are usually IgG and have specificity directed against the P antigen system on red cells. Cold hemolysins have biphasic activity and rarely cause AIHA. The antibody binds to erythrocytes at low temperatures and fixes complement. Because the antibody is IgG, red cell agglutination does not occur. Upon warming, the cold hemolysin remains attached, complement is activated, and intravascular hemolysis occurs.

The clinical syndrome related to cold hemolysins is designated *paroxysmal cold hemoglobinuria* (PCH). Historically, PCH was commonly associated with syphilis, but today it most often follows a viral illness. Immunosuppressive therapy and splenectomy are usually ineffective, and supportive therapy is required.

 Pathology: Patients with PCH may develop severe anemia, decreased haptoglobin levels, and hemoglobinuria secondary to intravascular hemolysis. The direct Coombs test is positive for complement but may be negative for IgG, since cold hemolysins may readily dissociate from red cells in vitro.

Alloimmune Hemolytic Anemia

Alloimmune hemolytic anemia refers to the destruction of circulating foreign red cells by alloantibodies.

 Pathogenesis: Alloimmune hemolytic anemia develops under two circumstances, transfusion of incompatible blood products (hemolytic transfusion reaction) and hemolytic disease of the newborn. Alloantibodies in the ABO system are naturally occurring, whereas those directed against other erythrocyte antigens (including the Rh system) require prior exposure through transfusion or pregnancy.

Hemolytic Transfusion Reactions

An immediate hemolytic transfusion reaction occurs when grossly incompatible blood is administered to a patient with preformed alloantibodies, usually because of a clerical error. Massive hemolysis of the transfused blood may be associated with severe complications, including hypotension, renal failure, and even death.

Delayed hemolytic transfusion reactions usually involve antibodies to minor red cell antigens. Over time, alloantibody levels may decline to the point where they become undetectable in routine pretransfusion screening tests. With subsequent reexposure to the offending antigen, an anamnestic antibody response follows, with hemolysis occurring several days later. Delayed hemolytic transfusion reactions are usually less severe than immediate reactions and may be clinically undetectable. In both types of hemolytic transfusion reactions, the direct antiglobulin test is positive.

Hemolytic Disease of the Newborn

Hemolytic disease of the newborn (HDN) reflects an incompatibility of blood types between the mother and developing fetus; the mother lacks an antigen that is expressed by the fetus. Maternal IgG alloantibodies can then cross the placenta and cause hemolysis of fetal erythrocytes and erythroblastosis detectable in peripheral blood smears (Fig. 20-26). Most commonly, HDN is usually ABO or Rh in type.

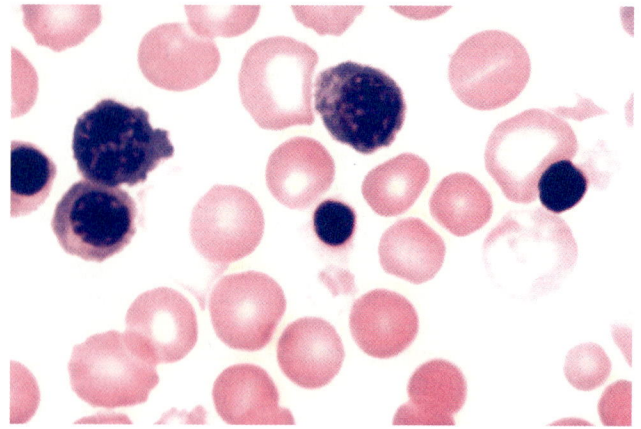

FIGURE 20-26
Hemolytic disease of the newborn. The peripheral blood contains numerous erythroid precursors (erythroblasts), which are normally confined to the bone marrow.

With ABO-type HDN, the mother is type O and the fetus is usually type A. Naturally occurring maternal anti-A antibodies cause hemolysis in the fetus. No prior exposure through pregnancy or transfusion is required for hemolysis to develop. The anemia associated with ABO incompatibility is usually mild, and affected babies develop hyperbilirubinemia, spherocytosis, and a positive direct antiglobulin test.

With Rh-type HDN, the mother is Rh-negative and the fetus is Rh-positive. The D antigen is most frequently involved, although minor Rh antigens can also cause disease. Because Rh antigens are not naturally occurring, prior maternal exposure through pregnancy or transfusion is necessary. The severity of the disease varies, but the hemolysis in Rh incompatibility is generally more significant than that seen with ABO- type HDN. Severely affected fetuses may develop *hydrops fetalis*, characterized by heart failure, generalized edema, and intrauterine death. Fortunately, today most cases of D-related HDN are preventable by passive immunization of Rh-negative mothers during pregnancy with injections of Rh immune globulin. Laboratory findings are similar to those described above for ABO HDN.

Mechanical Red Cell Fragmentation Syndromes

Red cell fragmentation syndromes are disorders in which intrinsically normal erythrocytes are subjected to mechanical disruption as they circulate in the blood (intravascular hemolysis).

 Pathogenesis. These disorders are classified as either macroangiopathic (large vessels) or microangiopathic (capillaries), according to the site of hemolysis. Mechanical fragmentation of red cells is due to either alteration of the endothelial surface of blood vessels or disturbances in blood flow patterns that lead to turbulence and increased shear stress.

Macroangiopathic hemolytic anemia most commonly results from direct red cell trauma, owing to an abnormal vascular surface (e.g., prosthetic heart valve, synthetic vascular graft).

Microangiopathic hemolytic anemia more frequently results from abnormalities in the microcirculation that cause turbulent blood flow patterns. The classic examples of microangiopathic hemolysis are disseminated intravascular coagulation (DIC) and thrombotic thrombocytopenic purpura (TTP), both of which feature generalized thrombosis of capillary vessels (see below). Long distance running or walking *(march hemoglobinuria)* or prolonged vigorous exercise can cause repetitive trauma to red cells in the microcirculation and lead to hemolysis. Alterations in blood flow, as are encountered in malignant hypertension or vasculitis syndromes, may also lead to mechanical fragmentation of erythrocytes.

Pathology: The laboratory findings are similar for patients with either macro- or microangiopathic hemolytic anemias. Anemia is mild to moderate and is accompanied by an appropriate reticulocyte response. Blood smear examination reveals fragmented red blood cells (schistocytes) and polychromasia (Fig. 20-27). Abnormalities in coagulation and thrombocytopenia characterize DIC, whereas thrombocytopenia alone is seen in cases of TTP (see below).

Paroxysmal Nocturnal Hemoglobinuria

Paroxysmal nocturnal hemoglobinuria (PNH) is an acquired clonal stem cell disorder characterized by episodic intravascular hemolytic anemia that is secondary to increased sensitivity of erythrocytes to complement-mediated lysis.

Pathogenesis: The underlying defect in cases of PNH involves somatic mutation of the phosphatidylinositol glycan-class A *(PIG-A)* gene, which is located on the short arm of the X chromosome (Xp22.1) in multipotential hematopoietic stem cells. Mutation of the *PIG-A* gene leads to disrupted synthesis of glycosyl phosphatidylinositol (GPI), which normally anchors a variety of proteins to the red cell membrane (e.g., CD14, CD16, CD55, CD59). Subsequent loss of *decay acceleration factor* (CD55) and more importantly *membrane inhibitor of reactive lysis* (CD59) from the erythrocyte surface renders the cell susceptible to complement-mediated hemolysis. Leukocytes and platelets derived from the abnormal stem cells also demonstrate loss of GPI-linked membrane proteins.

PNH may develop as a primary disorder or evolve from preexisting cases of aplastic anemia. Because of the clonal nature of the defect, progression to myelodysplasia or overt acute leukemia can occur. Some patients exhibit several abnormal clonal erythrocyte populations, with varying susceptibility to complement.

Pathology: During hemolytic episodes, patients develop normocytic or macrocytic anemia of varying severity, accompanied by an appropriate reticulocyte response. Because of the intravascular nature of the hemolysis, hemoglobinuria is present, and over time iron deficiency may develop secondary to recurrent iron loss in the urine. Traditionally, a diagnosis of PNH was suggested by observing increased lysis of patient red cells when incubated with sugar (sucrose hemolysis test) or acidified serum (Ham test), both of which enhance complement binding to red cells. Today, PNH is more easily diagnosed by demonstrating loss of GPI-anchored proteins on blood cells by flow cytometry. Leukopenia and thrombocytopenia are frequently detected, and sensitivity to complement may lead to inappropriate platelet activation.

Clinical Features: Patients with PNH develop intermittent intravascular hemolysis, although it is nocturnal in only a minority of cases. There is an increased incidence of venous and arterial thrombosis, notably Budd-Chiari syndrome (hepatic vein thrombosis), in cases of PNH due to complement-mediated platelet activation. Bleeding may arise secondary to thrombocytopenia. Treatment is supportive, and bone marrow transplantation is curative.

Hypersplenism

A mild hemolytic anemia may develop in patients with hypersplenism and congestive splenomegaly.

Pathogenesis: Splenic enlargement causes pooling of blood and delayed transit of blood cells through the splenic circulation. Prolonged exposure of red cells to splenic macrophages is associated with their premature destruction.

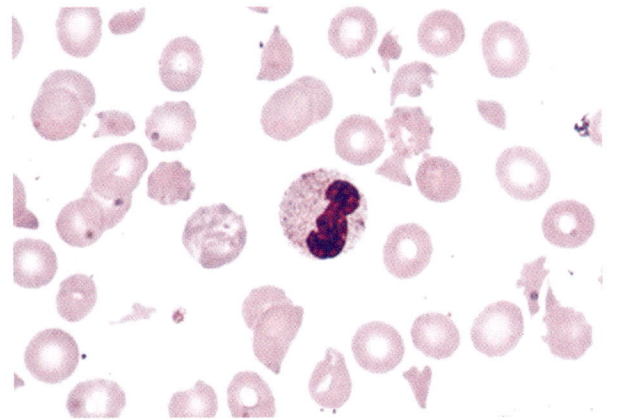

FIGURE 20-27
Microangiopathic hemolytic anemia. Irregular, fragmented erythrocytes (schistocytes) are seen in the blood smear of a patient with disseminated intravascular coagulation.

Pathology and Clinical Features: The anemia associated with hypersplenism shows no specific morphological features. Some leukopenia and thrombocytopenia is often encountered, but this is due to sequestration, rather than destruction, of these elements within the enlarged spleen. Bone marrow examination demonstrates compensatory hyperplasia of all cell lines. If the patient is sufficiently symptomatic, splenectomy can be performed.

Other Hemolytic Anemias

Severe thermal burns lead to intravascular hemolysis of erythrocytes. Normal red cells undergo membrane disruption and fragmentation when exposed to temperatures in excess of 49°C. Blood smear examination in burn patients reveals numerous schistocytes and microspherocytes, as well as polychromasia. The direct Coombs test is negative.

Several infectious microorganisms specifically parasitize erythrocytes and can be associated with significant hemolysis. All species of *Plasmodium* have an intraerythrocytic life cycle, which upon completion results in lysis of the red cell (see Chapter 9). Infected red cells are also removed from circulation by splenic macrophages. *Babesiosis*, found in more temperate climates (northeastern United States), is also associated with hemolysis following completion of an intraerythrocytic life cycle. In both cases, blood smear examination reveals the presence of parasites within red cells.

Acute Blood Loss Leads to Normocytic Normochromic Anemia

Acute anemia reflects the loss of blood from the intravascular compartment.

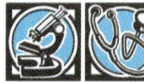**Pathology and Clinical Features:** The initial manifestations of acute blood loss are related to volume depletion and decreased tissue perfusion. Since whole blood is lost, the severity of the anemia may not be appreciated initially. Within the first 24 to 48 hours following significant hemorrhage, however, fluid is mobilized from extravascular locations into the intravascular space to restore the overall blood volume. Because red cell replacement does not occur as promptly, the true degree of anemia becomes apparent at this time. If the underlying bleeding is stopped, erythropoietin-driven erythroid hyperplasia in the bone marrow will gradually correct the anemia. Examination of the blood smear reveals no specific red cell abnormalities, but polychromasia is present during the recovery phase.

POLYCYTHEMIA

Polycythemia (erythrocytosis) refers to an increase in the red blood cell mass.

Pathogenesis: Polycythemia can be arbitrarily defined as a HCT value greater than 54% in men and 47% in women. As HCT levels rise above 50%, blood viscosity increases exponentially, and cardiac function and peripheral blood flow may become impaired. With a HCT above 60%, blood flow may become so severely compromised as to lead to tissue hypoxia.

Polycythemia can be further divided on the basis of overall red cell mass into relative and absolute categories. *Relative polycythemia*, characteristic of dehydration, is characterized by decreased plasma volume with a normal red cell mass. *Gaisbock syndrome* (spurious polycythemia) is seen in middle-aged, overweight, hypertensive smokers and is due to a combination of plasma volume depletion and increased red cell production. Nicotine in cigarettes acts as a diuretic and leads to the reduction in plasma volume, while increased carbon monoxide levels cause hypoxia and a compensatory increase in erythropoiesis.

Absolute polycythemia is associated with a true increase in red cell mass and can be further subdivided into primary and secondary categories. *Primary polycythemia*, or **polycythemia vera,** is an autonomous, erythropoietin-independent, proliferation of erythroid cells that results from an acquired, clonal, hematopoietic stem cell disorder. Polycythemia vera is considered one of the chronic myeloproliferative disorders and is discussed below.

Secondary polycythemias arise from erythropoietin-dependent stimulation of erythropoiesis in the bone marrow, usually as a compensatory response to generalized tissue hypoxia. Causes of tissue hypoxia, include chronic lung disease, cigarette smoking, residence at high altitudes, a right-to-left shunt in the heart, and the presence of an abnormal hemoglobin with high oxygen affinity.

Secondary polycythemia can also develop under certain circumstances that are unrelated to generalized tissue hypoxia. A variety of neoplasms can inappropriately produce erythropoietin as a paraneoplastic syndrome. Tumors most commonly implicated in causing secondary polycythemia include renal cell carcinoma, hepatocellular carcinoma, cerebellar hemangioblastoma, and uterine leiomyoma. Nonneoplastic conditions involving the kidney may cause secondary polycythemia. Renal cysts or hydronephrosis may exert direct pressure on the kidney, thereby leading to localized hypoxia and increased erythropoietin production.

Platelets and Hemostasis

NORMAL HEMOSTASIS

Platelets, endothelium, and coagulation factors participate in hemostasis. Hemostasis is normally achieved by clot formation. Initially, platelets *adhere* to the vascular endothelium, and subsequently they form platelet *aggregates* that are stabilized by fibrin after activation of the coagulation cascade. Blood clots can be dissolved by the *fibrinolytic system*.

Platelets Form the First Line of Defense in Hemostasis

Hematopoietic stem cells proliferate and differentiate in the bone marrow to form megakaryocytes, under the influence of *thrombopoietin* (TPO), which is produced by the liver. Each megakaryocyte releases 1000 to 4000 anucleate platelets.

Morphology and Function

At rest, platelets are small discoid cells, 2 to 3 μm in diameter. Platelets circulate freely for about 10 days at a concentration of 150,000 to 400,000/μL. On a Wright-stained smear they appear pale blue and contain faint pink granules. By electron microscopy, they exhibit mitochondria, glycogen particles, dense granules, and alpha granules. Dense granules contain various nucleotides, including the potent aggregating molecule ADP. α Granules contain many polypeptides, including adhesive proteins, such as fibrinogen, von Willebrand factor, fibronectin, and thrombospondin, as well as the chemokines platelet factor 4 and neutrophil-activating peptide 2. When the vascular endothelium has been disrupted, platelets respond by creating a platelet plug to minimize bleeding. Platelets are particularly important in sealing damaged blood vessels that are subjected to high shear rate, such as arteries and arterioles. In pathological circumstances, platelets also respond to activated leukocytes and endothelial cells (see Chapter 2) (Fig. 20-28).

Platelet Activation

There are multiple sequential steps in the activation of platelets following blood vessel injury and loss of an intact endothelial cell layer (Fig. 20-29).

1. **Adhesion of the platelets** to the subendothelial matrix proteins, such as collagen and von Willebrand factor (vWF), by specific glycoprotein receptors on the platelet surface. GP Ib/IX binds vWF, and GP Ia/IIa and GPVI bind collagen.
2. **Shape change,** from discoid to spherical to stellate
3. **Secretion of platelet granule contents,** including ADP, epinephrine, calcium, vWF, and platelet-derived growth factor (PDGF)
4. **Generation of thromboxane A$_2$** by cyclooxygenase 1

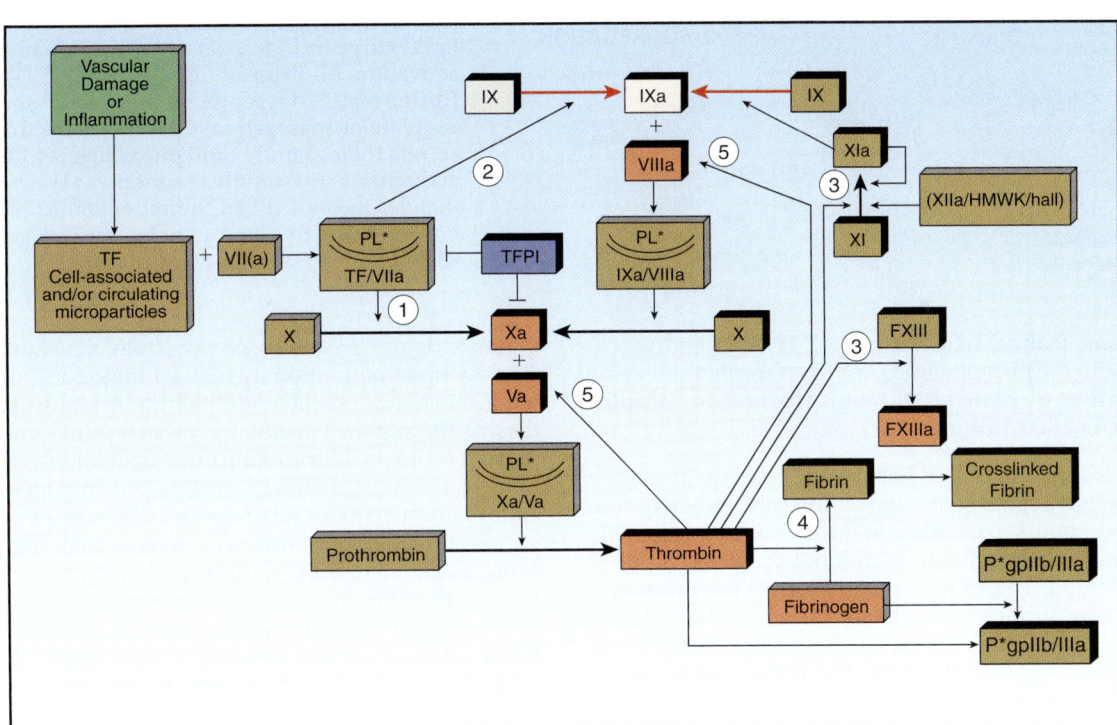

FIGURE 20-28

Hemostasis and thrombosis. Following injury to a vessel, rupture of an atherosclerotic plaque, or the presence of major inflammation, coagulation is initiated when tissue factor (TF) binds to circulating factor VII, a small proportion of which is activated (VIIa). TF is located on cells (subendothelial or activated endothelial cells or leukocytes) or circulating microparticles. The TF/VIIa complex is activated by localizing to an activated phospholipid surface (PL*) such as that provided by activated platelets. TF/VIIa activates factor X to form Xa *(1)* and IX to form IXa *(2)*. However, TF pathway inhibitor (TFPI) inhibits both *(1)* and *(2)*. Sustained amplification is achieved through the actions of factors XI, IX, and VIII. Factor XI is activated through the small amount of initial thrombin formed and, to a limited extent, by autoactivation or factor XIIa. Cofactors II and VIII, when activated by thrombin, form complexes with X (Xa/Va) and IX (IXa/VIIIa), respectively, on activated PL surfaces. Note the central and multiple roles for thrombin *(4)*, which converts fibrinogen to fibrin, *(5)* activates cofactors V and VIII, *(3)* activates factors XI and XIII, and activates platelets. Fibrinogen binds to the gpIIb/IIIa integrin receptor on activated platelets (P*). Note the extensive control in time and space of these concerted surface reactions. The combined result is the platelet–fibrin thrombus.

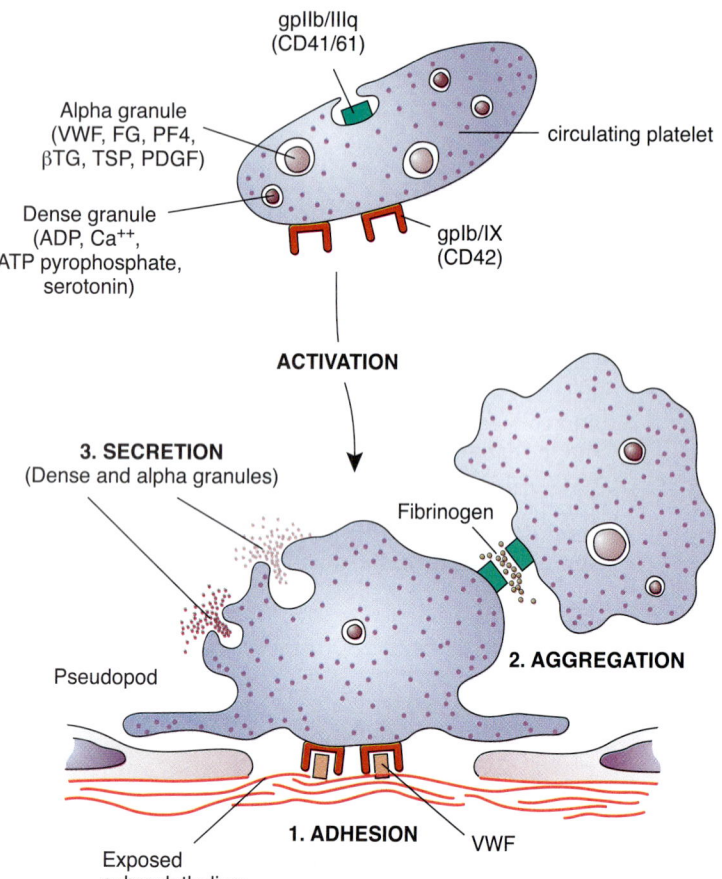

FIGURE 20-29
Platelet activation involves three overlapping mechanisms. (1) Adhesion to the exposed subendothelium is mediated by the binding of von Willebrand factor (VWF) to gpIb/IX (CD42) and is the initiation signal for activation. (2) Exposure of gpIIb/IIIa (CD41/61) to the fibrinogen (FG) receptor on the platelet surface allows for platelet aggregation. (3) At the same time, platelets secrete their granule contents, which facilitates further activation. α-Granules contain vWF, fibrinogen, platelet factor 4 (PF4), thromboglobulin (TG), thrombospondin (TSP), and platelet-derived growth factor (PDGF).

5. **Membrane change,** which exposes P-selectin and procoagulant anionic phospholipids such as phosphatidylserine
6. **Aggregation of platelets through fibrinogen receptor GP IIb/IIIa cross-linking**

Each of these functional steps has specific consequences. The initial adhesive events send signals for further activation. The secreted granule contents and thromboxane A_2 provide positive feedback to activate additional platelets via their surface receptors. The stellate shape projects the procoagulant membrane surface and activated GP IIb/IIIa/ fibrinogen to the site of interaction with coagulation factors and other platelets, respectively. Thus the surface of activated platelets is an optimal environment for propagating the assembly of the coagulation-factor complex, including the prothrombinase complex. The resulting thrombin has pleiotropic effects, particularly additional platelet activation. Finally, P-selectin participates in binding leukocytes and localizing them to participate in healing, together with substances secreted by platelets such as PDGF. As a result of these concerted steps, activated platelets form a strong primary *plug* and then an *aggregate* within a platelet–fibrin meshwork, which stops bleeding and initiates healing.

Blood Vessels and Endothelial Cells Interact with Platelets

Blood vessels are covered internally by a smooth, nonthrombogenic monolayer of endothelial cells. Unstimulated platelets do not adhere to, or penetrate, the endothelial barrier, owing to regulation by platelet inhibitors and anticoagulant molecules on the endothelium. Endothelial cells synthesize the potent vasodilator prostacyclin, which inhibits platelet function. Nitric oxide exerts similar effects. These actions maintain the blood in a fluid state until an injury to the endothelium exposes subendothelial tissue.

Endothelial cells rest on a matrix that contains collagens, elastin, laminin, fibronectin, vWF, and other structural and adhesive proteins. The subendothelial cells are also a potent source of tissue factor (TF). When exposed, the matrix of the intima is intensely thrombogenic. Its adhesive proteins bind the corresponding glycoprotein receptors on platelet membranes and cause their adherence to the exposed matrix. TF serves to bind circulating activated factor VIIa to initiate the generation of activated factor X and activated factor IX.

Activation of the Coagulation Cascade Completes Blood Clot Formation

Platelets and leukocytes circulate in an inactive state. Similarly, the coagulation proteins are present as inactive zymogen forms. The activation of platelets and the generation of activated coagulation factors are concerted and highly constrained in space and time to limit the dissemination of clots through the circulation. The localization of coagulation-factor complexes to activated surfaces of blood cells, especially platelets, accelerates the activation of coagulation factors, thereby avoiding the many anticoagulant factors in plasma. Four main complexes are essential, three *procoagulant* and one *anticoagulant* (Fig. 20-28). As a general rule, each active enzyme in the cascade is assisted by a cofactor and localized to a phospholipid surface (PL). There are two complexes that activate factor X, the so-called Xase complexes.

The complex of TF and factor VIIa is the initiator of coagulation. Its activation is controlled by exposure to subendothelial cells or activated monocytes and endothelial cells. Microparticles derived from activated leukocytes and endothelial cells contribute to a pool of circulating TF that participates in hemostasis and thrombosis. The TF/VIIa/PL complex also cleaves and thus activates a small amount of factor IX. Factor Xa, together with its cofactor Va, cleaves factor II (prothrombin) into IIa (thrombin). Thrombin has the interesting property of feeding back to activate factors XI, VIII, and V.

The second complex for activating factor X is the IXa/VIIIa/PL complex. TF/VIIa/PL initiates factor X activation but is then rapidly shut off by TF pathway inhibitor (TFPI). The larger-scale propagation of factor X activation is then carried out by the IXa/VIIIa/PL complex, with the ongoing activation of factor IX by XIa.

In summary, the three procoagulant complexes are two Xase complexes, namely TF/VIIa/PL and IXa/VIIIa/PL, and the prothrombinase complex, Xa/Va/PL. The anticoagulant complex functions to activate protein C. The protein C_{ase} complex is composed of thrombin and thrombomodulin in the endothelial cell plasma membrane. Activated Protein C, together with its cofactor Protein S, then inactivates the key cofactors VIIIa and Va, thereby limiting further generation of Xa and IIa.

Antithrombin (formerly known as antithrombin III) inhibits thrombin activity. In addition to its inhibition of thrombin, antithrombin cleaves a number of activated factors, namely IXa, Xa, XIa, and XIIa. In vivo this effect is accentuated by heparan sulfate proteoglycans and, most dramatically, by the therapeutic administration of heparin.

Thrombolysis Is Mediated by Plasminogen Activation

After the thrombus has become firmly established, further growth is curtailed by the removal of platelet-activating factors and coagulation proteins. The endothelial cells in the vicinity of the thrombus produce plasminogen activators, which in turn activate circulating plasminogen to plasmin and initiate thrombolysis (also known as *fibrinolysis*). There are two major plasminogen activators, tissue plasminogen activator (t-PA), and urokinase-type plasminogen activator (u-PA). Plasminogen cleavage to plasmin and plasmin action are tightly regulated by several naturally occurring inhibitors. These include plasminogen activator inhibitor-I (PAI-I), antiplasmin, and thrombin-activatable fibrinolysis inhibitor (TAFI). The dissolution of the thrombus is accomplished by the protease plasmin and the activity of macrophages. Plasmin targets specific sites in the fibrin meshwork for degradation, helping to localize its activity to sites where it is needed. Thrombolysis is also coincident with the beginning of the wound repair process. The latter involves migration and proliferation of fibroblasts and endothelial cells, secretion of new extracellular matrix, and restoration of the patency of the blood vessel if it has been occluded. Angiogenesis (i.e., the budding of new blood vessels from existing ones) occurs in the setting of tissue ischemia or damage. Many of the products of the coagulation and fibrinolysis pathways are potently angiogenic.

HEMOSTATIC DISORDERS

Defects of the system for maintaining fluid blood passage through intact vessels fall into two categories: *hemostatic* disorders and *thrombotic* disorders. Failure of the hemostatic system to restore the integrity of an injured vessel causes *bleeding*. Inability to maintain the fluidity of blood results in *thrombosis*.

The clinical manifestations of hemorrhage associated with disorders of each component of the hemostatic system tend to be distinctive (Table 20-6). Platelet abnormalities result in both petechiae and purpuric hemorrhages in the skin and mucous membranes. Deficiencies of coagulation factors lead to hemorrhage into muscles, viscera, and joint spaces. Disorders of the blood vessels usually cause purpura.

Hemostatic Disorders of Blood Vessels Reflect Dysfunction of Vascular or Extravascular Tissues

Dysfunction of the extravascular or vascular tissues may cause hemorrhages ranging from cosmetic blemishes to life-threatening blood loss.

T A B L E 20-6   **Principal Causes of Bleeding**

Vascular disorders
  Senile purpura
  Purpura simplex
  Glucocorticoid excess
  Dysproteinemias
  Allergic (Henoch-Schönlein) purpura
  Hereditary hemorrhagic telangiectasia
Platelet abnormalities
  Thrombocytopenia (see Table 20-7)
  Qualitative disorders
    Inherited
      Glycoprotein IIb/IIIa deficiency (Glanzmann thrombasthenia)
      Glycoprotein Ib/IX/V deficiency (Bernard-Soulier syndrome)
      Storage pool diseases (α and δ)
      Abnormal arachidonic acid metabolism
    Acquired
      Uremia
      Drugs
      Cardiopulmonary bypass
      Myeloproliferative disorders
      Liver disease
Coagulation factor deficiencies
  Inherited
    Von Willebrand disease
    Hemophilia A
    Hemophilia B
  Acquired
    Vitamin K deficiency/antagonism
    Liver disease
    Disseminated intravascular coagulation

Extravascular Dysfunction

SENILE PURPURA: The most common disorder in extravascular dysfunction is age-related atrophy of the supporting connective tissues. Termed *senile purpura*, it is associated with superficial, sharply demarcated, persistent purpuric spots on the forearms and other sun-exposed areas.

PURPURA SIMPLEX: A similar type of purpura occurs principally in women at the time of the menses. Purpura simplex is present in the deeper layers of the dermis and resolves quickly.

SCURVY: Collagen synthesis is disturbed in vitamin C deficiency, and purpura is a common manifestation. Perifollicular hemorrhages are particularly characteristic of scurvy.

Vascular Dysfunction

The deposition of immunoglobulin fragments in vessel walls may occur in **amyloidosis, cryoglobulinemia, and other paraproteinemias** and can cause vessel wall weakness and purpura. Certain types of arteritis also injure the vessel wall and may lead to hemorrhage.

Hereditary Hemorrhagic Telangiectasia (Rendu-Osler-Weber Syndrome)

Hereditary hemorrhagic telangiectasia is an autosomal dominant disorder of blood vessel walls (venules and capillaries) that results in tortuous, dilated vessels (telangiectasias). The underlying defect is a thinning of the vessel walls, in which inadequate elastic tissue and smooth muscle permit dilation of the vessels. Telangiectasias appear initially as punctate reddish spots on the lips and nose, measuring up to 0.5 cm in diameter. They can remain as telangiectasias or progress to arteriovenous malformations or aneurysmal dilations throughout the body.

Clinical Features: Patients with hereditary hemorrhagic telangiectasia experience recurrent hemorrhage, which may be spontaneous or secondary to trivial trauma, and anemia. Although bleeding may occur at the site of any lesion, recurrent epistaxis ensues in over 80% of patients, beginning at an early age. Later in life, gastrointestinal hemorrhage may be the dominant symptom. Arteriovenous fistulas in the lung, brain, and retina may be troublesome and associated with hemorrhage or clinically significant shunting of blood. The patient's activities may be restricted by recurrent bleeding, but death from exsanguination is rare.

Allergic Purpura (Henoch-Schönlein Purpura)

Allergic purpura is a vascular disease that results from immunological damage to the blood vessel wall (see Chapter 16). In children, the disorder is self-limited and often follows a viral infection. In adults, it is associated with exposure to a variety of drugs and may be chronic.

Pathology: Histologically, Henoch-Schönlein purpura is characterized by *leukocytoclastic vasculitis*, with a perivascular infiltration of neutrophils and eosinophils. Fibrinoid necrosis of the vessel wall and plugging of the vascular lumen by platelets are observed. IgA and complement are often deposited in the vessel wall, and IgA complexes have been found in the circulating blood. The purpuric spots are often accompanied by raised urticarial lesions. Gastrointestinal involvement is indicated by intestinal cramps and bleeding, and renal involvement may lead to renal failure.

Platelet Disorders Impair Hemostasis

The most common platelet disorders are associated with bleeding. Patients may have a history of easy bruisability or life-threatening bleeding. Although bleeding can occur in any damaged vascular bed, a particular pattern of mucocutaneous bleeding is often seen, including gingival bleeding, epistaxis, and menorrhagia. More-severe manifestations are bleeding into the gastrointestinal tract, genitourinary tract, and brain. Petechiae, which are characteristic of platelet disorders, are nonblanching red lesions that are less then 2 mm in size. They usually occur in lower extremities, in dependent regions of the body, on the buccal mucosal and soft palate, and at pressure points (waistband, wristwatch band). Petechiae may also occur in vascular disorders. Platelet disorders reflect (1) decreased production, (2) increased destruction, or (3) impaired function of platelets.

Thrombocytopenia

Thrombocytopenia is defined as platelet counts less than 150,000/μL. The lower the platelet count, the greater the risk of traumatic and perioperative bleeding. Patients with fewer than 10,000 platelets/μL are at increased risk of spontaneous hemorrhage (Table 20-7).

Decreased platelet production is caused by infiltration of the bone marrow with leukemic cells or metastatic cancer, which impair megakaryopoiesis. Ineffective megakaryopoiesis in myelodysplasia also results in thrombocytopenia. Bone marrow failure in patients with aplastic anemia or in those who have received radiotherapy or chemotherapy produces pancytopenia, including thrombocytopenia. Certain viral infections such as cytomegalovirus or any megaloblastic anemia can be associated with severe thrombocytopenia.

May-Hegglin anomaly is a hereditary defect in megakaryocyte maturation in which thrombocytopenia is associated with circulating giant platelets and Döhle-like bodies in neutrophils (Fig. 20-35).

Increased platelet destruction reflects immune-mediated damage and removal of circulating platelets, as in idiopathic thrombocytopenic purpura and drug-induced

TABLE 20-7 Principal Causes of Thrombocytopenia

Decreased production
    Aplastic anemia
    Bone marrow infiltration (neoplastic, fibrosis)
    Bone marrow suppression by drugs or radiation
Ineffective production
    Megaloblastic anemia
    Myelodysplasias
Increased destruction
    Immunological (idiopathic, HIV, drugs, alloimmune, posttransfusion purpura, neonatal)
    Nonimmunological (DIC, TTP, HUS, vascular malformations, drugs)
Increased sequestration
    Splenomegaly
Dilutional
    Blood and plasma transfusions

thrombocytopenia. Alternatively, intravascular platelet aggregation may produce thrombocytopenia (e.g., in TTP).

Idiopathic (Immune) Thrombocytopenic Purpura

Idiopathic thrombocytopenic purpura (ITP) is a quantitative disorder of platelets caused by antibodies directed against platelet or megakaryocytic antigens. It is, therefore, more appropriate to speak of *immune* thrombocytopenic purpura. ITP occurs in two forms, an acute, self-limited, hemorrhagic syndrome in children and a chronic bleeding disorder in adults.

Pathogenesis: Similar to autoimmune hemolytic anemia, the etiology of ITP is related to antibody-mediated immune destruction of platelets or their precursors. In most patients, the autoantibodies are of the IgG class, but IgM antiplatelet antibodies have also been reported in a few patients, although their clinical significance remains to be clarified.

Acute ITP typically appears in children of either sex after a viral illness and is likely caused by virus-induced changes in platelet antigens that elicit autoantibodies. Complement is then bound at the surface, after which the platelets are lysed in the blood or phagocytosed and destroyed by splenic and hepatic macrophages.

Chronic ITP occurs predominantly in adults (male to female ratio of 1:2.6) and may be associated with a collagen vascular disease (e.g., systemic lupus erythematosus) or a malignant lymphoproliferative disease, especially chronic lymphocytic leukemia. It is also common in persons infected with HIV. The extent of thrombocytopenia in ITP is determined by the balance between three mechanisms: (1) the level of antiplatelet antibodies; (2) the degree of inhibition of platelet production in the bone marrow, since some antibodies may be directed against megakaryocytes; and (3) the expression of Fc and complement receptors on the surface of macrophages. This expression is up-regulated in infection and pregnancy but is ameliorated by certain drugs, for example, corticosteroids, danazol, and intravenous gamma globulin, all of which are used to treat ITP.

Pathology: In acute ITP, the platelet count is typically less than 20,000/μL. In chronic adult ITP, the platelet count varies from a few thousand to 100,000/μL. The peripheral blood smear in ITP exhibits numerous large platelets, which reflect an increased number of young platelets released by bone marrow actively engaged in platelet production. Accordingly, examination of the bone marrow reveals a compensatory increase in megakaryocytes (Fig. 20-30). IgG is present on the platelets in more than 80% of patients with chronic ITP, and in half of them, increased levels of platelet-associated C3 can be demonstrated.

Clinical Features: Children with acute ITP experience the sudden onset of petechiae and purpura but are otherwise asymptomatic. Spontaneous recovery can be expected in more than 80% of cases within 6 months. The major threat (1% of cases) is intracranial hemorrhage. In most cases, no treatment is necessary, but with serious disease, corticosteroids and intravenous immunoglobulin may be needed. Glucocorticoids decrease the production of the antiplatelet antibodies and down-regulate Fc receptors on macrophages. γ-Globulin interferes with the clearance of IgG-coated platelets from the circulation.

Chronic ITP in adults manifests as bleeding episodes, such as epistaxis, menorrhagia, or ecchymoses. Although life-threatening hemorrhages may occur, they are uncommon. Occasionally, asymptomatic persons are discovered to have thrombocytopenia on a routine blood cell count. Most adults with chronic ITP are improved by corticosteroid treatment and intravenous administration of γ-globulin. Danazol (a synthetic anabolic steroid) acts in a manner similar to that of glucocorticoids. In patients who fail to respond adequately to drug therapy within 2 to 3 months, splenectomy produces a complete or partial remission in 70% of cases.

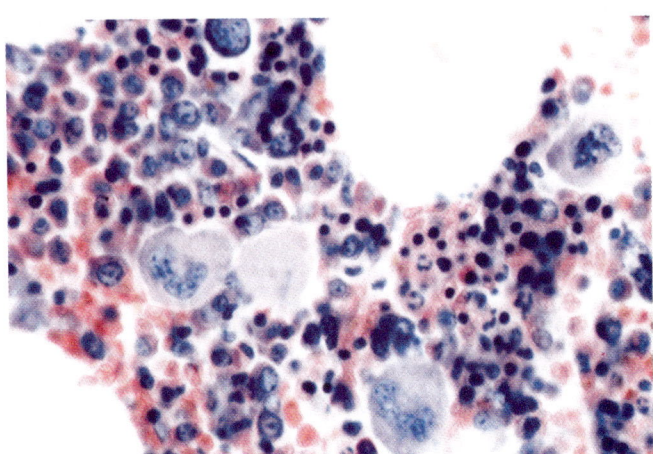

FIGURE 20-30
Idiopathic thrombocytopenic purpura. A section of the bone marrow reveals increased megakaryocytes.

Drug-Induced Thrombocytopenia

Drugs can cause immune-mediated platelet destruction. Examples include quinine, quinidine, heparin, sulfonamides, gold salts, antibiotics, sedatives, tranquilizers, and anticonvulsants. In many cases, the drug forms a complex with a platelet-related protein to form a neoepitope that elicits antibody production. By contrast, chemotherapeutic agents, ethanol, and thiazides cause thrombocytopenia by suppression of platelet production.

In *heparin-induced thrombocytopenia,* a mild, transient thrombocytopenia occurs within the first 2 to 5 days in 25% of patients treated with this drug. However, 1 to 3% develop a profound thrombocytopenia after 1 to 2 weeks of heparin therapy. These patients are predisposed to arterial and venous thromboembolic events that may be lethal. The diagnosis of heparin-induced thrombocytopenia is supported by the demonstration of antibodies to the complex of heparin and platelet factor 4.

Pregnancy-Associated Thrombocytopenia

Minimal thrombocytopenia occurs frequently during the 3rd trimester of pregnancy. It is due to dilution of platelets, and since the platelet count is usually above 100,000/µL, it does not require any special management. The preeclampsia/eclampsia syndromes can result in maternal thrombocytopenia. A related condition is called *HELLP,* which stands for *h*emolysis, *e*levated *l*iver enzyme tests, and *l*ow *p*latelets.

Neonatal thrombocytopenia

Neonatal thrombocytopenias can be classified as *inherited* or *acquired.*

Inherited causes associated with increased platelet destruction include **Wiskott-Aldrich syndrome** (WAS), which is caused by a defect in the *WASP* gene on the X-chromosome. Affected boys have small platelets, eczema, and immunodeficiency. A variant of WAS is *X-linked thrombocytopenia,* which displays defects in the same gene but features only thrombocytopenia.. Inherited causes associated with poor production include **amegakaryocytic thrombocytopenia, thrombocytopenia-absent radius syndrome, Fanconi anemia,** and other genetic defects in platelet development. Thrombocytopenia can also be seen in infants with trisomy 13, 18, or 21.

Fanconi anemia is a genetic bone marrow failure disorder manifesting often with thrombocytopenia and red blood cell macrocytosis. There is a high incidence of associated congenital anomalies, such as skin hypopigmentation and hyperpigmentation, short stature, microcephaly, microphthalmia and radial/thumb abnormalities. Defects in a family of genes responsible for Fanconi anemia have been identified.

Neonatal alloimmune thrombocytopenia (NAIT) is due to increased destruction of platelets. It is caused by alloimmunization to HPA-1a and other platelet-specific antigens that occur during pregnancy. The mechanism for alloimmunization in this condition is similar to Rh alloimmunization in that the fetus is HPA-1a positive, whereas the mother is negative. In NAIT, the fetus or neonate but not the mother is thrombocytopenic. NAIT predisposes to fetal and neonatal intracranial hemorrhage. In persons at high risk for NAIT, such as a history suggesting alloimmunization or differences in maternal and paternal platelet typing (e.g., HPA 1a/1b), percutaneous umbilical cord blood sampling (PUBS) and possibly treatment of the mother with intravenous immunoglobulin or corticosteroids are indicated. After delivery, an additional therapeutic option is transfusion with platelets that are negative for the antigen to which the maternal antibody is directed.

Nonimmune causes of thrombocytopenia in the neonate are similar to those in adults, with additional considerations such as birth asphyxia, hypoxic injury, sepsis, and DIC, necrotizing enterocolitis, hemangiomas, and thrombosis.

Posttransfusion Purpura

As a consequence of a prior transfusion, HPA-1–negative persons may develop alloantibodies to HPA-1–positive platelets. Newly infused HPA-1–positive platelets are destroyed by these antibodies. Curiously, the patient's own HPA-1–negative platelets are also destroyed, perhaps related to the passive acquisition of the antigen by these platelets or the development of immune complexes. In any event, a self-limited thrombocytopenia occurs about a week after the transfusion.

Thrombotic Thrombocytopenic Purpura

TTP is a rare syndrome featuring the pentad of thrombocytopenia, microangiopathic hemolytic anemia, neurological symptoms, fever, and renal impairment. Platelet aggregation leads to widespread deposition of platelets in the microvasculature as characteristic hyaline thrombi.

Pathogenesis: The pathogenesis of TTP is obscure, but the most tenable hypothesis holds that it results from the introduction of one or more platelet-aggregating substances into the circulation. The theory that has received the most attention is the cross-linking of platelets by inappropriate vWF multimers from injured endothelial cells. vWF monomers are normally assembled into multimeric molecules of varying size (up to millions of daltons) within endothelial cells and released locally in response to endothelial stimulation. For unknown reasons, in TTP, unusually large multimers of vWF are present in the plasma, where they presumably mediate intravascular platelet aggregation. A protease that cleaves vWF is genetically absent or defective in familial TTP and is inactivated by autoantibodies against it in sporadic TTP. Thus plasma infusion is best in familial forms of TTP, and plasma exchange is preferred in acquired types.

Although most cases of TTP arise in otherwise normal persons, the disease may also complicate autoimmune collagen vascular disorders (systemic lupus erythematosus, rheumatoid arthritis, Sjögren syndrome) and drug-induced hypersensitivity reactions. TTP has also been triggered by infections, cancer chemotherapy, bone marrow transplantation, and pregnancy. Occurrence of the disease in siblings suggests a hereditary predisposition.

Pathology: The morphological hallmark of TTP is the deposition throughout the body of PAS-positive hyaline microthrombi in arterioles and capillaries, principally in the heart, brain, and kidneys. The microthrombi contain platelet aggregates, fibrin, and a few erythrocytes and leukocytes. TTP is clearly distinguished from immune-mediated vasculitis by a lack of inflammation. On the peripheral blood smear, fragmented erythrocytes (schistocytes) are always evident (Fig. 20-31), and numerous reticulocytes are present.

Clinical Features: TTP occurs at virtually any age, but is most common in women in the fourth and fifth decades of life. The disease may be chronic and recurrent over a period of years or more frequently occurs as an acute, fulminant disease that is often fatal. Most patients present with neurological symptoms, including seizures, focal weakness, aphasia, and alterations in the state of consciousness. Widespread purpura is often present, and vaginal bleeding may occur in women. Anemia is a constant feature, often with a hemoglobin level below 6 g/dL. Jaundice secondary to hemolysis may be pronounced. Renal dysfunction is often prominent, half of patients being azotemic.

More than half of patients with TTP have platelet counts below 20,000/μL. Despite the presence of aggregated platelets, activation of the coagulation cascade does not occur. Consequently, the prothrombin time, partial thromboplastin time (PTT), and fibrinogen concentration remain normal, distinguishing this syndrome from DIC (see below). Prior to modern therapy, acute TTP was ordinarily fatal. However, with the use of plasma infusion and plasmapheresis, the cure rate has increased to 80%.

Hemolytic–Uremic Syndrome

Hemolytic–uremic syndrome (HUS) is similar to TTP and in its adult form is a variant of the latter. Classic HUS occurs in children, usually after an acute enteric infection. It seems to be the consequence of glomerular endothelial cell injury produced by verotoxins elaborated by the offending microorganism (usually *Escherichia coli* or *Shigella dysenteriae*) (see Chapter 16). In HUS, aggregated platelet thrombi are found primarily in the renal microvasculature, and renal failure, rather than neurological abnormalities, is the characteristic clinical feature. Adult HUS has not been linked to enteric infections, and the pathogenesis of the underlying endothelial injury has not been elucidated.

Splenic Sequestration of Platelets

Many patients with splenomegaly, irrespective of the cause, manifest *hypersplenism,* a syndrome that includes sequestration of platelets in the spleen. Whereas one third of platelets produced are normally stored temporarily in the spleen, in massive splenomegaly, up to 90% of the total platelet pool may be captured in that organ. Interestingly, the platelet life span is normal or only slightly reduced. Thrombocytopenia associated with hypersplenism is rarely severe and by itself does not produce a hemorrhagic diathesis.

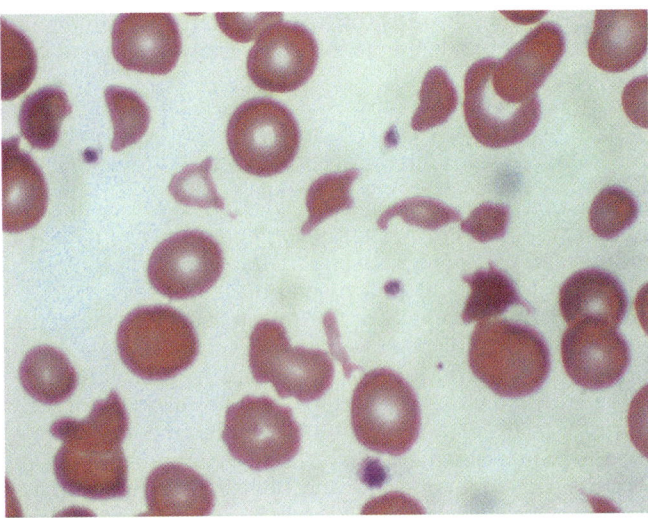

FIGURE 20-31
Microangiopathic hemolytic anemia. Numerous schistocytes are present in a patient with thrombotic thrombocytopenic purpura.

Other Causes of Thrombocytopenia

Vascular malformations can result in thrombocytopenia, including hemangiomas and arteriovenous malformations. In hemangiomas, consumption of platelets has been called the *Kasabach-Merritt syndrome.* Platelet loss occurs in patients who have massive hemorrhage, as occurs in bleeding from a peptic ulcer or during surgery with heavy blood loss. Blood given as a transfusion does not contain viable platelets since it is stored at 4°C in the blood bank. Thus, thrombocytopenia occurs in transfused patients due to platelet loss and dilution. Platelet transfusion may be indicated to prevent development of thrombocytopenia.

Hereditary Disorders of Platelets

Bernard-Soulier Syndrome (Giant Platelet Syndrome)

Bernard-Soulier Syndrome is an autosomal recessive trait in which platelets have a quantitative or qualitative defect in the membrane glycoprotein complex (GPIb/IX [CD42] and sometimes [GPV]) that serves as a receptor for vWF. The complex plays a prominent role in the adhesion of normal platelets to vWF in injured subendothelial tissues. The platelets in Bernard-Soulier syndrome vary widely in size and shape, and the diagnosis is suggested by the presence of thrombocytopenia and giant platelets on the blood smear.

Clinical Features: Bernard-Soulier syndrome manifests in infancy or childhood with a bleeding pattern characteristic of abnormal platelet function, namely, ecchymoses, epistaxis, and gingival bleeding. At a later age, traumatic hemorrhage, gastrointestinal bleeding, and menorrhagia occur. Although many patients have only a mild bleeding disorder, others suffer more severe hemorrhage that demands frequent platelet transfusions and may even be fatal.

Glanzmann Thrombasthenia

Glanzmann thrombasthenia is an autosomal recessive defect in platelet aggregation caused by a quantitative or qualitative abnormality in the glycoprotein complex IIb/IIIa (CD41/61). In normal platelets, this complex is activated during platelet adhesion and serves as a receptor for fibrinogen and vWF, mediating platelet aggregation and the generation of a solid plug. In addition, the IIb/IIIa complex is linked to the platelet cytoskeleton and transmits the force of contraction to adherent fibrin, a mechanism that promotes clot retraction. In Glanzmann thrombasthenia the lack of aggregation and clot retraction impairs hemostasis and causes bleeding, despite a normal platelet count.

Clinical Features: The disease becomes clinically apparent shortly after birth when the infant manifests mucocutaneous or gingival hemorrhage, epistaxis, or bleeding after circumcision. Later, patients may suffer unexpected hemorrhage after trauma or surgery. The severity of the disease varies, and only a few patients experience life-threatening hemorrhage. Platelet transfusions temporarily correct the condition.

Alpha Storage Pool Disease (Grey Platelet Syndrome)

A rare inherited malady, alpha storage pool disease is characterized by the absence of morphologically recognizable α granules in the platelets. The defect resides in abnormal granule membranes. Thrombocytopenia is common, and the platelets are large and pale. The bleeding diathesis tends to be mild.

Delta Storage Pool Disease

This heterogeneous malady affects the dense granules of platelets. The disease is sometimes associated with other multisystem hereditary disorders, including Chediak-Higashi syndrome or Hermansky-Pudlak syndrome (a type of oculocutaneous albinism; see Chapter 6). Bleeding manifestations are mild to moderate.

Acquired Qualitative Disorders of Platelets

A variety of acquired disorders may adversely affect platelet function (see Table 20-7).
  Drugs: A number of drugs can impair platelet function. Aspirin irreversibly acetylates cyclooxygenase, primarily COX-1, and thus blocks the production of platelet thromboxane A_2, which is an important platelet aggregator. Platelets cannot synthesize cyclooxygenase, and therefore the aspirin effect lasts for the life span of platelets (7–10 days). Nonsteroidal analgesics, such as indomethacin or ibuprofen, can impair platelet function, but their inhibition of cyclooxygenase is reversible, and the duration of their effect on platelets is short. Antibiotics, particularly those that share a β-lactam ring (penicillin and cephalosporins), can cause platelet dysfunction. Ticlopidine, an agent used to suppress platelet function in patients with thromboembolic disease, causes marked impairment of platelet function and even TTP.
  Renal failure: End-stage kidney disease is often accompanied by a qualitative platelet defect that results in a prolonged bleeding time and a hemorrhagic tendency. The platelet abnormality is heterogeneous and is aggravated by uremic anemia. Restoration of a normal hematocrit by erythropoietin administration may return the bleeding time to normal without affecting the degree of azotemia.
  Cardiopulmonary bypass surgery: Platelet dysfunction due to platelet activation and fragmentation occurs within the extracorporeal circuit during bypass surgery.
  Hematological malignancies: In chronic myeloproliferative disorders and myelodysplastic syndromes, platelet dysfunction is due to intrinsic platelet defects. In dysproteinemias, platelets are impaired because they are coated with plasma paraprotein.

Thrombocytosis

Reactive Thrombocytosis

An increase in platelets occurs frequently in association with the following conditions: (1) iron deficiency anemia, especially in children; (2) splenectomy; (3) cancer; and (4) chronic inflammatory disorders. Reactive thrombocytosis is rarely symptomatic, although it has been associated with thrombotic episodes, especially in bedridden patients after splenectomy.

Clonal Thrombocytosis

Patients with chronic myeloproliferative syndromes, such as polycythemia vera and essential thrombocythemia, suffer a malignant proliferation of megakaryocytes. The resulting increase in circulating platelets may be associated with episodes of thrombosis or bleeding (see below).

Coagulopathies Are Caused by Deficient or Abnormal Coagulation Factors

Quantitative and qualitative disorders of all of the coagulation factors have been identified. These conditions may be hereditary or acquired. Of the hereditary deficiencies, only those of factor VIII (hemophilia A), factor IX (hemophilia B), and vWF are common. Most of these disorders are the result of deficiency of the protein factor, leading to inadequate hemostasis and concomitant bleeding. Occasionally the protein factor is present but dysfunctional.
  Hemophilia A is discussed in Chapter 6.

Hemophilia B

Pathogenesis: *Hemophilia B is an X-linked heritable disorder of factor IX deficiency.* At 1 in 20,000 male births, hemophilia B is four times less common than hemophilia A and accounts for 15% of all cases of hemophilia. Factor IX is a liver-synthesized, Vitamin K-dependent protein that circulates as a zymogen and is initially activated by TF/VIIa. After TFPI inactivates TF/VIIa, factor IX is activated by XIa, which itself was activated by an initial burst of thrombin. Factor IX works with factor VIIIa, PL, and Ca^{2+} on activated platelet surfaces to activate factor X into Xa.

The factor IX gene is located at Xq27.1, telomeric to the factor VIII gene. The N-terminal Gla domain of the protein is the site for vitamin K-dependent carboxylation of glutamic acid residues, yielding the domain that is optimized for interactions with phospholipids and Ca^{2+} at membrane surfaces. Many different mutations, ranging from single nucleotide substitutions to gross deletions, have been noted.

Clinical Features: The bleeding manifestations in hemophilia B, mirror those of hemophilia A. Treatment of factor IX deficiency relies on the infusion of purified or recombinant protein. Recent reports indicate that hemophilia B can be treated successfully with somatic gene therapy in vivo, using specially modified viral vectors.

von Willebrand Disease

von Willebrand disease (vWD) denotes a heterogeneous complex of hereditary bleeding disorders related to a deficiency or abnormality of vWF. Over 20 distinct subtypes have been described. A simplified classification (see below) recognizes three major categories. Variable expression of vWF (especially type I) confounds estimates of prevalence, although some hold that vWD is the most common inherited coagulopathy (1–2% of the population).

vWF, an adhesive molecule, is synthesized by endothelial cells and megakaryocytes as a 250-kd monomer that undergoes polymerization to multimers with molecular weights in the millions. It is stored in the cytoplasmic Weibel-Palade bodies of endothelial cells and is released into the subendothelial tissues and the plasma. After endothelial injury, subendothelial vWF binds to platelet glycoprotein receptors (Ib/IX or D42), thereby promoting the adherence of platelets and sealing off the endothelial injury. It can also bind to GPIIb/IIIa (CD41/61) to promote platelet aggregation. **In plasma, vWF binds to and protects factor VIII; its absence is always associated with a deficiency in the activity of factor VIII.**

Pathogenesis: As an autosomal disorder, vWD affects men and women. The *vWF* gene on chromosome 12 is large and complex (180 kb with 52 exons). Three types of the disease are recognized, each of which represents a heterogeneous group of defects.

TYPE I vWD: These variants constitute 75% of all cases of vWD and are inherited as autosomal dominant traits with variable penetrance. Type I vWD is a *quantitative* deficiency in vWF, in which the levels of *all* the multimers are reduced, although their relative concentrations remain unchanged.

TYPE II vWD: Qualitative defects in vWF characterize the type II variants, which account for 20% of all cases of vWD. In type II disease, the interactions of vWF and the blood vessel wall are defective. The plasma activities of both vWF and factor VIII are reduced. In type IIa, the higher-molecular-weight multimers are *absent* from the platelets and the plasma. Type IIb is caused by the synthesis of an *abnormal* vWF with an increased affinity for platelets and may be associated with thrombocytopenia.

TYPE III vWD: This severe form of vWD is the least common variety and is inherited as an autosomal recessive trait. Some patients exhibit compound heterozygosity (different mutations in the two vWF alleles). vWF activity is absent, and the plasma levels of factor VIII are less than 10% of normal.

Clinical Features: Most cases of vWD are associated with only a mild bleeding diathesis, with the exception of type III. Easy bruising, epistaxis, gastrointestinal bleeding, and (in women) menorrhagia are frequent. The presenting symptom is often excessive hemorrhage after trauma or surgery. Patients with type III vWD may experience life-threatening hemorrhage from the gastrointestinal tract, and hemarthroses comparable to those in hemophilia are not infrequent.

The bleeding tendency in all forms of vWD is treated successfully with factor VIII, vWF concentrates, or cryoprecipitate. The vasopressin analogue DDAVP is the treatment of choice in types I and IIa vWD because it increases the release of preformed VWF from its endothelial storage pools. Intranasal sprays of DDAVP are now available.

Other Coagulation Factor Deficiencies

Deficiencies of all of the coagulation factor proteins have been noted in humans, including those of factors VII, X, V, XI, II (prothrombin), and fibrinogen. As expected, the severity of bleeding usually correlates with the level of functional protein activity detected in laboratory tests in vitro. Prolongation of the prothrombin time (PT) or partial thromboplastin time (PTT) in patients with bleeding manifestations helps to identify a problem with coagulation factors. Factor-specific assays confirm the diagnosis. There are rare deficiencies of more than one coagulation factor. For example, defects in γ-carboxylase result in low levels of several vitamin-K-dependent factors, including II, VII, IX, and X. The thrombin time helps to screen for deficiency or dysfunction of fibrinogen. Deficiency of fibrinogen causes bleeding. By contrast, dysfibrinogenemia may cause bleeding but more often leads to thrombosis.

Liver Disease

Many of the coagulation factors are produced in the liver. Impaired secretion of these proteins occurs in severe liver disease as a manifestation of the general protein synthetic defect. In this case, the levels of all of the liver-synthesized coagulation factors are low, and both the PT and PTT are prolonged.

Vitamin K Deficiency

Coagulation factors II, VII, IX, and X are synthesized in the liver and depend on vitamin K as an essential cofactor in γ-carboxylation of glutamic acid residues to Gla residues. Only when Gla residues are present are the secreted proteins functional. By contrast, factor V is synthesized in the liver but does not require vitamin K. Thus, vitamin K deficiency is associated with low activity of factors II, VII, IX, and X but normal factor V activity. **However, in severe liver disease, all of these factors have low activity.**

Clinical Features: The level of vitamin K is physiologically low in the neonate, and it is standard practice to administer vitamin K to newborn infants to prevent hemorrhagic disease. In adults, vitamin K deficiency may reflect inadequate dietary intake. Since bacteria in the colon produce the form of vitamin K that is best absorbed, prolonged intake of antibiotics or large colonic resections may lead to vitamin K deficiency.

Inhibitors of Coagulation Factors

Acquired inhibitors of coagulation factors, also termed *circulating anticoagulants*, are usually IgG autoantibodies. Most are directed against factor VIII and vWF, although rare cases of antibodies against most of the other coagulation factors are reported. In hereditary coagulation disorders, especially hemophilia, circulating anticoagulants arise in response to the administration of plasma concentrates containing the deficient factor. Anticoagulants also develop in some patients with autoimmune disorders (e.g., systemic lupus erythematosus, rheumatoid arthritis), presumably as a result of abnormal immune regulation. Finally, many cases of acquired anticoagulants appear in apparently normal persons.

Clinical Features: The consequences of acquired anticoagulants vary from an asymptomatic laboratory finding to life-threatening hemorrhage. These autoantibodies are difficult to eliminate, but one third of patients experience spontaneous remission. The condition is treated by the administration of plasma concentrates, corticosteroids, or immunosuppressive agents.

Lupus anticoagulants are antiphospholipid antibodies in patients with systemic lupus erythematosus and other autoimmune conditions or in otherwise asymptomatic persons. Bleeding is distinctly uncommon, but these patients have a hypercoagulable (thrombotic) tendency (see below).

Disseminated Intravascular Coagulation (DIC)

DIC refers to widespread ischemic changes secondary to microvascular fibrin thrombi, which are accompanied by the consumption of platelets and coagulation factors and a hemorrhagic diathesis. DIC is a serious and often fatal disorder and typically occurs as a complication of massive trauma, septicemia from numerous organisms, and obstetric emergencies. It is also associated with metastatic cancer, hematopoietic malignancies, cardiovascular and liver disease, and numerous other conditions.

Pathogenesis: The central event in the initiation of DIC is the activation of the clotting cascades within the vascular compartment by tissue injury or damage to the endothelium or both. **The subsequent generation of substantial amounts of thrombin** (Fig. 20-28), **combined with the initial failure of the natural inhibitory mechanisms that neutralize thrombin, is responsible for triggering DIC. With the consequent uncontrolled intravascular coagulation, the delicate balance between coagulation and fibrinolysis is disrupted. This event leads to the consumption of clotting factors, platelets, and fibrinogen and a consequent hemorrhagic diathesis** (Fig. 20-32).

Procoagulant tissue factor (TF) is released into the circulation following injury in a variety of circumstances, including direct trauma, brain injury, and obstetric accidents (e.g., premature separation of the placenta) (see Chapter 18). **Bacterial endotoxin** also stimulates macrophages to release TF. **Certain neoplasms** are associated with DIC, owing to the release of TF by the cancer cells. As a consequence of the activation of the clotting cascade, intravascular fibrin is deposited as microthrombi in the smallest blood vessels. The stimulation of the fibrinolytic system by fibrin generates fibrin split products, which possess anticoagulant properties and contribute to the bleeding diathesis.

Endothelial injury plays an important role in the pathogenesis of many cases of DIC. The normal endothelium has anticoagulant properties (Fig. 20-33) and shields platelets from activation by contact with the subendothelial connective tissue (see Chapters 2 and 10). The anticoagulant properties of the endothelium are impaired by widely varying injuries, including (1) TNF in gram-negative sepsis; (2) other inflammatory mediators, such as activated complement, IL-1 or neutrophil proteases; (3) viral or rickettsial infections; and (4) trauma (e.g., burns). As a result, platelet aggregates form in the microvasculature.

Pathology: Arterioles, capillaries, and venules in many parts of the body are occluded by **microthrombi** composed of fibrin and platelets (Fig. 20-34). However, owing to the enhancement of fibrinolysis, these thrombi may no longer be visualized at the time of autopsy. Microvascular obstruction is associated with **widespread ischemic changes,** particularly in the brain, kidneys, skin, lungs, and gastrointestinal tract. These organs are also the sites of bleeding, which in the case of the brain and gastrointestinal tract may be fatal.

Erythrocytes become fragmented *(schistocytes)* by passage through webs of intravascular fibrin strands, resulting in **microangiopathic hemolytic anemia.** The consumption of activated platelets leads to **thrombocytopenia,** whereas the **depletion of clotting factors** is reflected in prolonged PT and PTT and a decreased plasma fibrinogen level. Plasma fibrin split products prolong the thrombin time. Laboratory tests that are useful in the diagnosis of DIC include the measurement of fibrinopeptide A and D-dimers, the levels of which are elevated (as markers of coagulation and fibrinolytic activation, respectively).

Clinical Features: The symptoms of DIC reflect both microvascular thrombosis and a bleeding tendency. Ischemic changes in the brain lead to seizures and coma. Depending on the severity of DIC, renal symptoms range from mild azotemia to fulminant acute renal failure. The acute respiratory distress syndrome may supervene, and acute ulcers of the gastrointestinal tract may bleed. The bleeding diathesis is evidenced by cerebral hemorrhage, ecchymoses, and hematuria. Patients with DIC are treated with (1) heparin anticoagulation to interrupt the cycle of intravascular coagulation and (2) replacement of platelets and clotting factors to control the bleeding.

Fibrinolysis and Bleeding

Fibrinolysis is the process by which fibrin clots are dissolved. Inactive plasminogen is converted to proteolytically active plasmin by the plasminogen activators t-PA and u-PA. Plasminogen activator inhibitor I (PAI-I) is the primary inhibitor of plasminogen activation, and α_2-antiplasmin inhibits plasmin itself. Rare inherited deficiencies of either α_2-antiplasmin or PAI-I result in hemorrhage, which is presumed to result from rapid breakdown of clots secondary to the uninhibited generation or activity of plasmin.

Hypercoagulability Causes Widespread Thrombosis

Hypercoagulability is defined as an increased risk of thrombosis in circumstances that would not cause thrombosis in a normal person. Laboratory evaluation of an underlying hypercoagulable

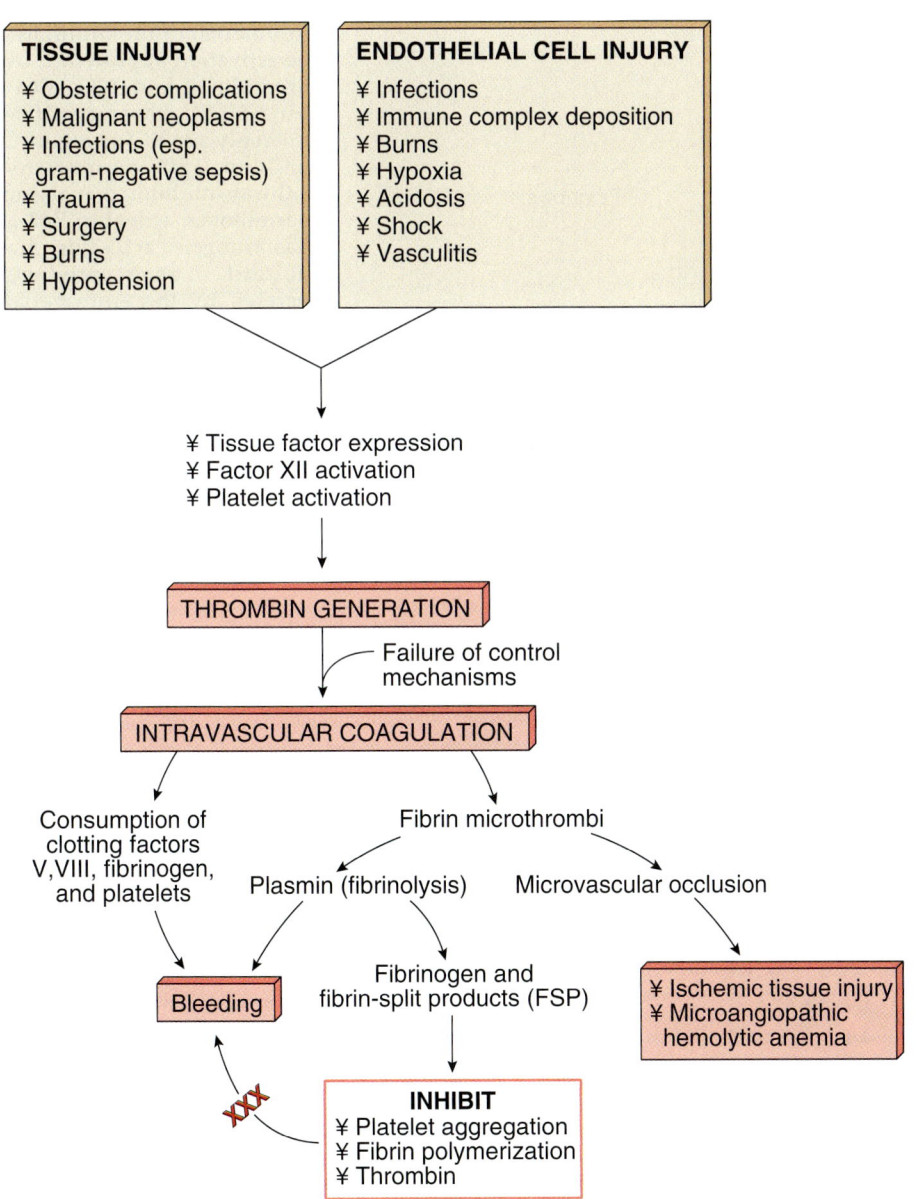

FIGURE 20-32

The pathophysiology of disseminated intravascular coagulation (DIC). The DIC syndrome is precipitated by tissue injury, endothelial cell injury, or a combination of the two. These injuries trigger increased expression of tissue factor on cell surfaces, and activation of clotting factors (including XII and V) and platelets. With the failure of normal control mechanisms, generation of thrombin leads to intravascular coagulation.

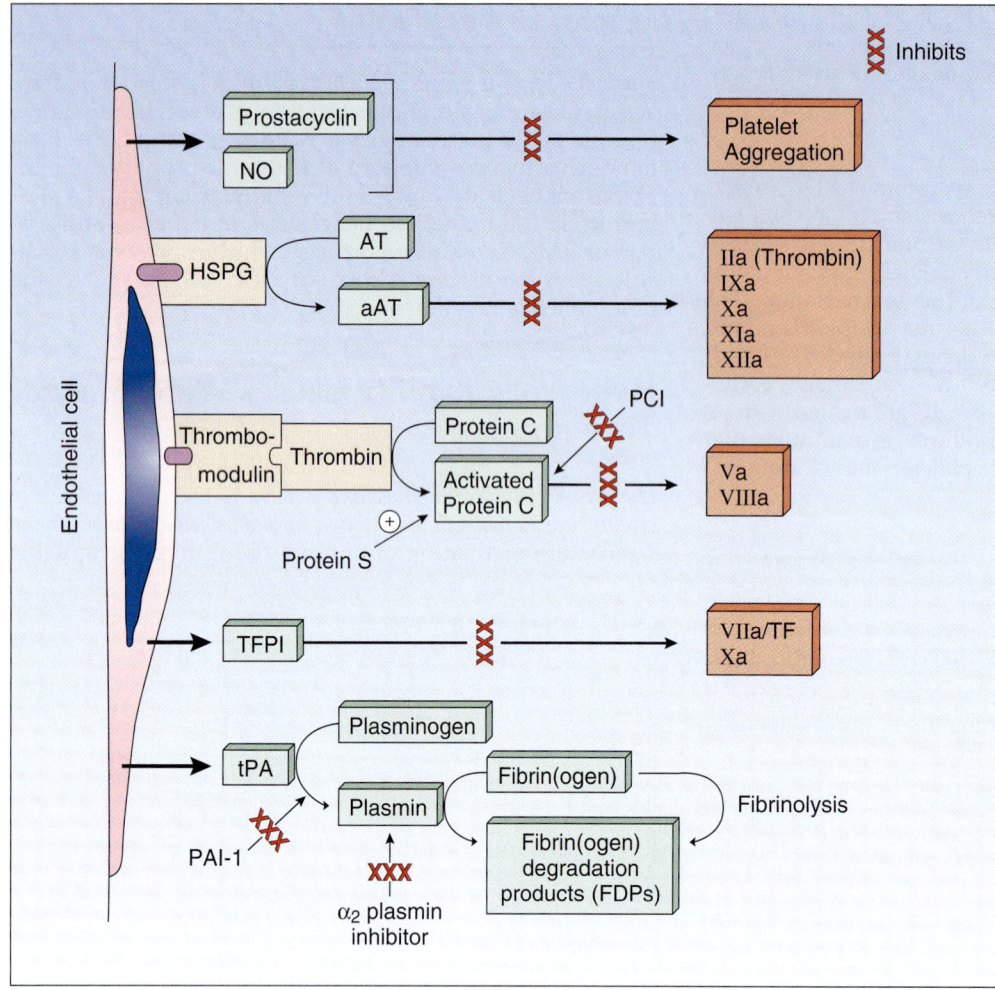

FIGURE 20-33
The role of endothelium in anticoagulation, platelet inhibition, and thrombolysis. The endothelial cell plays a central role in the inhibition of various components of the clotting mechanism. Heparan sulfate proteoglycan potentiates the activation of antithrombin (AT) 15-fold. Thrombomodulin stimulates the activation of protein C by thrombin 30-fold. NO, nitric oxide; HSPG, heparan sulfate proteoglycan; PCI, protein C inhibitor; TFPI, tissue factor pathway inhibitor; tPA, tissue plasminogen activator; PAI-I, plasminogen activator inhibitor-I. *Arrows*, products secreted by the endothelial cell; *bars*, molecules bound to the cell surface; +, potentiation; XXX, inhibition.

state is warranted in persons who have unexplained thrombotic episodes that show one or more of the following:

- Recurrence
- Development at a young age
- Family history of thrombotic episodes
- Thrombosis in unusual anatomical locations
- Difficulty in controlling with anticoagulants

Hypercoagulable states are divided into inherited and acquired forms (Table 20-8).

Inherited Hypercoagulability

Inherited hypercoagulable states are due to genetic mutations that affect one of the natural anticoagulant mechanisms. The hereditary tendency to develop thrombosis, irrespective of its origin, is referred to as *thrombophilia*.

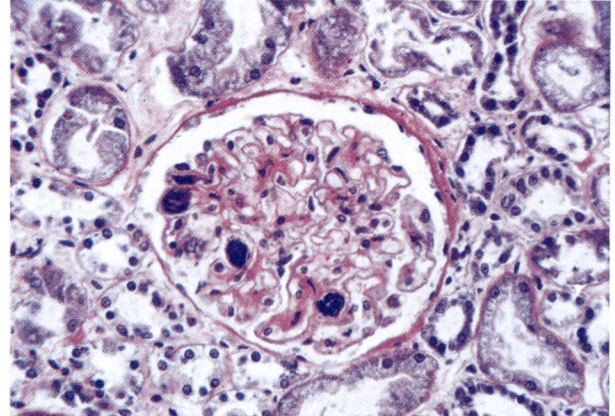

FIGURE 20-34
Disseminated intravascular coagulation. A section of a glomerulus stained with phosphotungstic acid hematoxylin (PTAH), which colors fibrin deep purple, demonstrates several microthrombi.

TABLE 20-8 **Principal Causes of Hypercoagulability**

Inherited
    Activated protein C resistance (factor V Leiden)
    Antithrombin deficiency
    Protein C deficiency
    Protein S deficiency
    Dysfibrinogenemias
Acquired
    Lupus inhibitor
    Malignancy
    Nephrotic syndrome
    Therapy
        Factor concentrates
        Heparin
        Oral contraceptives
    Hyperlipidemia
    Thrombotic thrombocytopenic purpura

Activated protein C (APC) resistance—factor V Leiden: A point mutation in the gene encoding factor V (factor V Leiden) renders it resistant to the inhibitory effect of APC. *Resistance to the action of APC is the most common genetic disorder associated with hypercoagulability, and its prevalence in patients with venous thrombosis has been reported to be as high as 65%.* The factor V Leiden mutation is found worldwide, but more so in Caucasians (up to 5% of the general population) and much less so in Africans (near 0%). Compared with normal persons, the risk for deep venous thrombosis is increased 7-fold in heterozygotes and 80-fold in homozygotes.

Antithrombin deficiency: This autosomal dominant disorder, which has incomplete penetrance, occurs in 0.2 to 0.4% of the general population and can result in either a quantitative or a qualitative effect on antithrombin. The risk of a thrombotic event (usually venous) ranges between 20 and 80% in different families.

Protein C and protein S deficiencies: Homozygous protein C deficiency causes life-threatening neonatal thrombosis with *purpura fulminans.* Up to 0.5% of the general population has heterozygous protein C deficiency, but many of these persons are symptom free. The clinical presentations for deficiencies of protein C and protein S are similar to that for ATIII deficiency.

Other causes of hypercoagulability: Prothrombin also has a known genetic variant (G20210A) in the 3′ untranslated region of the mRNA that is associated with thrombosis. The mechanism is not defined but may involve excessively high prothrombin levels in persons with the variant. Unusually high levels of fibrinogen, factor VII, and factor VIII are associated with thrombosis, although the molecular basis for the elevated levels remains to be elucidated. Some dysfibrinogenemias are also associated with thrombosis.

Acquired Hypercoagulability

Venous stasis contributes to the hypercoagulability associated with prolonged immobilization and congestive cardiac failure. Increased platelet activation probably accounts for the clotting tendency in patients with myeloproliferative disorders, heparin-associated thrombocytopenia, and TTP.

Antiphospholipid Antibody Syndrome

Antibodies directed against several negatively charged phospholipids are associated with the development of antiphospholipid antibody syndrome. This disorder features (1) thromboembolic events, (2) spontaneous abortions, and (3) thrombocytopenia. Combinations of laboratory tests help to confirm the diagnosis of antiphospholipid syndrome. Antibodies (IgG primarily but not exclusively) react with proteins that bind anionic phospholipids such as phosphatidylserine (PS) or cardiolipin. These membrane lipids are only exposed when cells such as platelets are activated. Many plasma proteins, and Gla-domain-containing procoagulant proteins (e.g., prothrombin) bind to PS and related anionic phospholipids. The laboratory tests are (1) detection of lupus-type anticoagulant activity, (2) anticardiolipin antibodies, and (3) antibodies to plasma protein β2-GPI. Anticardiolipin antibodies bind to β2-GPI in the presence of cardiolipin.

The antiphospholipid antibody syndrome is the leading acquired hematological cause of thrombosis. The thrombosis in this syndrome has several proposed mechanisms, including platelet activation, endothelial cell activation, and alterations in the coagulation factor assembly on membranes. Interference with placental vascular function is the likely mechanism in recurrent fetal loss.

The lupus anticoagulant (which is not restricted to patients with systemic lupus erythematosus) is an antiphospholipid antibody that results in paradoxical prolongation of PTT in vitro (due to phospholipid inhibition) but hypercoagulability in vivo (probably through platelet activation). The latter accounts for the frequent occurrence of arterial thrombosis and is the most common of the acquired blood protein defects that cause thrombosis.

Impaired Platelet Function

Abnormal platelet activity has been implicated in recurrent arterial thrombosis and postcoronary angioplasty stenosis. *Primary thrombocytosis,* as occurs in the myeloproliferative syndromes, has been implicated in thrombosis. *Secondary thrombocytosis* is associated with solid tumors, the postsplenectomy state, iron deficiency, and sepsis. Platelet counts are generally higher in primary than in secondary thrombosis, and the incidence of thrombosis is greater in the former. Myeloproliferative disorders, such as essential thrombocythemia and polycythemia vera, may result in platelet counts well in excess of 1,000,000/μL.

The recognition that platelets play a major role in acute coronary syndromes and in cerebrovascular disease has let to the development of important drugs that are used to prevent complications of atherosclerosis. Ruptured atherosclerotic plaques activate platelets, and the platelet plug and platelet–fibrin meshwork that ensue cause vascular obstruction and ischemia. There are several options in antiplatelet therapy. Aspirin, an irreversible inhibitor of platelet cyclooxygenase, is the gold standard for antiplatelet therapy. Ticlopidine and Clopidogrel (thienopyridine derivatives) inhibit ADP-mediated platelet aggregation, but their full effect occurs only after 3 to 5 days. ABCIXIMAB (ReoPro), is a GPIIa/IIIb inhibitor. This chimeric antibody blocks the fibrinogen receptor, thereby preventing platelet aggregation.

Vascular injury

On the arterial side, atherosclerosis is by far the leading cause of thrombosis. Diabetes, hypercholesterolemia, hypertension, and tobacco use are the major risk factors. Other causes include arteritis, aneurysm, and arteriovenous malformations. Elevated homocysteine levels contribute to altered endothelial cell function and resultant thrombosis (see Chapter 10).

On the venous side, vasculitis, tortuous vessels, mechanical injury, and stasis contribute to thrombosis. These disorders are often exacerbated by inherited abnormalities of the coagulation proteins.

White Blood Cells

NONMALIGNANT DISORDERS

Neutropenia Refers to an Absolute Neutrophil Count below 1800/μL

In most patients with neutropenia (granulocytopenia), the number of neutrophils is adequate to defend against microorganisms. When the number declines to 1000/μL, the patient becomes vulnerable to microbial infections, but a serious risk is experienced with absolute counts below 500/μL. The term *agranulocytosis* is reserved for a virtual absence of neutrophils caused by depletion of both the marginated pool and the bone marrow reserve.

Neutropenia reflects decreased production or increased destruction of neutrophils (Table 20-9). Most cases of neutropenia are asymptomatic and unexplained, and the term *chronic benign neutropenia* is used. In some cases, the total granulocyte pool is normal, but excessive neutrophils are stored in the marrow or marginated in blood vessels.

DECREASED PRODUCTION OF NEUTROPHILS: Radiation or chemotherapeutic drugs interfere with the generation of neutrophils in a general suppression of cellular proliferation in the marrow. Certain drugs, such as phenothiazines, phenylbutazone, antithyroid drugs, and indomethacin, can cause an *idiosyncratic* suppression of the bone marrow. Viral infection and alcohol intake have also been associated with suppression of myelopoiesis. Decreased production of granulocytes is a feature of a number of hereditary disorders, including *Kostmann syndrome* and infantile genetic agranulocytosis. Ineffective myelopoiesis is involved in the neutropenia of megaloblastic anemias and myelodysplastic syndromes. In *cyclic neutropenia,* episodes recur regularly about every 21 days.

INCREASED PERIPHERAL DESTRUCTION OF GRANULOCYTES: Accelerated elimination of granulocytes is caused by the following:

- Increased consumption of neutrophils in overwhelming infections
- Increased sequestration in hypersplenism
- Increased destruction by antibodies

Neutropenia is a common feature in AIDS and is multifactorial. Virus-induced depression of neutrophil production is aggravated by infectious consumption of neutrophils and often by drug-related mechanisms (e.g., zidovudine).

Another type of drug-induced neutropenia is immunologically mediated. Many drugs lead to this form of neutrophil destruction, especially sulfonamides, phenylbutazone, and indomethacin. The toxic effect results from the attachment of circulating antigen–antibody complexes to the granulocyte surface, with subsequent complement-mediated injury.

Neutrophilia Is an Absolute Neutrophil Count above 7000/μL

Neutrophilia has many causes (Table 20-10) and reflects (1) increased mobilization of neutrophils from the bone marrow

TABLE **20-9** Principal Causes of Neutropenia

Decreased production
  Irradiation
  Drug induced (long and short term)
  Viral infections
  Congenital
  Cyclic
Ineffective production
  Megaloblastic anemia
  Myelodysplastic syndromes
Increased destruction
  Isoimmune neonatal
  Autoimmune
    Idiopathic
    Drug induced
    Felty syndrome
    Systemic lupus erythematosus
    Dialysis (complement activation induced)
  Splenic sequestration
  Increased margination

TABLE **20-10** Principal Causes of Neutrophilia

Infections
  Primarily bacterial
Immunological inflammatory
  Rheumatoid arthritis
  Rheumatic fever
  Vasculitis
Neoplasia
Hemorrhage
Drugs
  Glucocorticoids
  Colony-stimulating factors (CSFs)
  Lithium
Hereditary
  CD18 deficiency
Metabolic
  Acidosis
  Uremia
  Gout
  Thyroid storm
Tissue necrosis
  Infarction
  Trauma
  Burns

storage pool, (2) enhanced release from the peripheral blood marginal pool, or (3) stimulation of granulopoiesis in the bone marrow. Increased mobilization of neutrophils from the bone marrow pool or from the peripheral marginal pool occurs in acute traumatic or infectious disorders. A mild neutrophilia occurs in 20% of women during the third trimester of pregnancy, but the mechanism is poorly defined.

LEUKEMOID REACTION: In acute infections, neutrophilia may be so pronounced that it may be mistaken for leukemia, especially chronic myeloid leukemia (CML), in which case it is termed a *leukemoid reaction.* Clues to the benign (or reactive) nature of a leukemoid reaction include the following: (1) the cells in the peripheral blood are usually more mature than myelocytes; (2) leukocyte alkaline phosphatase activity is high in a leukemoid reaction, but low in CML; and (3) benign neutrophils often contain large blue cytoplasmic inclusions *(Döhle bodies)* or toxic granulation (see Fig. 20-35).

Qualitative Disorders of Neutrophils Are Associated with Impaired Function

If the functional competence of granulocytes is impaired, resistance to infection may decrease despite a normal granulocyte count. A number of rare hereditary disorders of granulocytes have been described.

CHRONIC GRANULOMATOUS DISEASE (CGD): *CGD refers to a group of rare, inherited, X-linked or autosomal recessive disorders characterized by a defect in bactericidal function of neutrophils and macrophages.*

 Pathogenesis: All forms of CGD reflect the inability of these cells to undergo a respiratory burst and generate hydrogen peroxide on phagocytosis of mi-

NEUTROPHILS

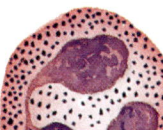 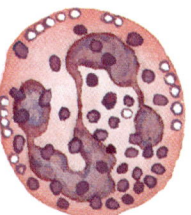 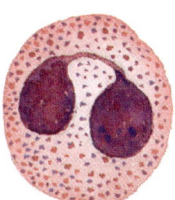

| Normal | With Döhle body | With toxic granulation | In mucopolysaccharidosis | With Pelger-Huët anomaly |

LYMPHOCYTES

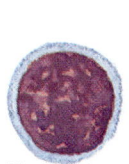
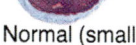
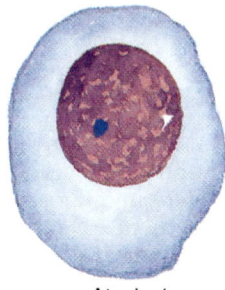 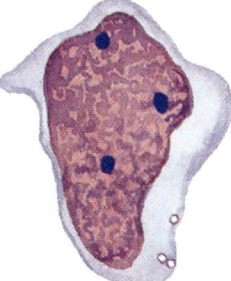 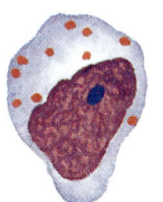 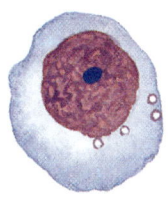

| Normal (small) | Atypical | Atypical | Granular (large) | Plasmacytoid |

FIGURE 20-35

Abnormal leukocyte morphology. Abnormal neutrophils and lymphocytes are contrasted with normal cells. *Döhle bodies* are blue cytoplasmic inclusions that represent ribosome-associated endoplasmic reticulum. In *toxic granulation,* there is prominent blue-black granulation in the cytoplasm. This represents persistence of primary or azurophilic granules. Both Döhle bodies and toxic granulation are characteristic of benign or reactive processes. In the storage diseases such as mucopolysaccharidoses, large, blocklike cytoplasmic inclusions are seen. The *Pelger-Huet anomaly* consists of nuclear hyposegmentation, frequently with bilobed nuclei, and dense chromatin. *Atypical lymphocytes* are large and exhibit deep blue to pale gray cytoplasm; they are seen in benign reactive processes. *Large granular lymphocytes* are medium-to-large lymphoid cells with some pink cytoplasmic granules. They are suppressor T lymphocytes, some with natural killer function, and may be increased in benign or malignant disorders. *Plasmacytoid lymphocytes* have abundant blue cytoplasm and are seen in some reactive disorders.

croorganisms. The basic defect in the X-linked variant is a deficiency of the membrane-bound cytochrome b moiety of NADPH oxidase. In autosomal recessive CGD, a cytosolic factor necessary for the activation of NADPH oxidase is lacking.

In CGD, neutrophils and macrophages can phagocytose microorganisms. However, they cannot kill catalase-positive microorganisms (e.g., *Staphylococcus aureus*, *Serratia marcescens*, *Salmonella* spp.), which are protected from their own endogenous hydrogen peroxide by catalase. As a result of the inability to generate hydrogen peroxide, hypochlorous acid is not formed, and the microorganisms are not killed. However, catalase-negative microorganisms, such as *Lactobacillus*, are eliminated in a normal fashion.

Clinical Features: CGD becomes symptomatic at any age from infancy to adulthood, and recurrent infections lead to widespread microabscesses and granulomas. The neutrophils are morphologically normal in CGD. The diagnosis is made by measuring respiratory burst activity in the nitroblue tetrazolium (NBT) test.

MYELOPEROXIDASE DEFICIENCY: This inherited autosomal recessive disorder is characterized by a lack of neutrophilic lysosomal myeloperoxidase. Bacterial infections are rarely observed, however, because there is a compensatory increase in intracellular hydrogen peroxide. Candidal infections are a significant problem in diabetic patients with this deficiency.

CHÉDIAK-HIGASHI SYNDROME: This rare, autosomal recessive condition is characterized by giant lysosomes in leukocytes and many cells in other tissues. In neutrophils, monocytes, and lymphocytes, the defect is manifested morphologically by the presence of huge cytoplasmic granules. Functionally, neutropenia, decreased chemotaxis, impaired degranulation, and ineffective bactericidal activity are seen. The disorder is attributed to a generalized increase in the fusion of cytoplasmic granules (lysosomes).

Clinical Features: Clinically, patients with Chédiak-Higashi syndrome suffer recurrent **bacterial and fungal infections** involving principally the skin, mucous membranes, and respiratory tract. Defective platelet aggregation is reflected in **prolonged bleeding times**. **Oculocutaneous albinism** (see Chapter 6) is related to the segregation of melanin in giant melanosomes. The disease may progress to a fatal *accelerated phase,* in which a lymphoproliferative syndrome (likely a consequence of EBV infection) leads to pancytopenia. In a few patients, bone marrow transplantation has cured Chédiak-Higashi syndrome.

Eosinophilia Occurs with Allergic Reactions and Malignancies

Eosinophils differentiate in the bone marrow under the influence of one or several eosinophil growth factors (e.g., IL-5). They circulate briefly in the peripheral blood and then migrate preferentially to the gastrointestinal and respiratory tracts and the skin. Eosinophils respond to chemotactic substances produced by mast cells or are induced by the presence of persistent antigen–antibody complexes, such as occur in chronic parasitic, dermatological, and allergic conditions. The principal causes of eosinophilia are listed in (Table 20-11).

IDIOPATHIC HYPEREOSINOPHILIC SYNDROME: This term refers to an increase in circulating eosinophils above 1500/µL for more than 6 months without evident underlying disease. The accumulation of eosinophils in tissue often leads to necrosis, particularly in the myocardium, where it produces endomyocardial disease (see Chapter 11). Neurological dysfunction may also develop. The eosinophil-mediated cell injury is related to constituents of the eosinophil granules, particularly major basic protein and cationic protein (see Chapter 2). The prognosis of untreated idiopathic hypereosinophilic syndrome is serious, and only 10% of untreated patients survive for 3 years. Aggressive therapy with corticosteroids has markedly improved this situation, and even in patients with cardiac involvement, 70% survive for more than 5 years.

Basophilia Is Associated with Allergic Reactions and Myeloproliferative Diseases

The basophil, the least numerous of all leukocytes, differentiates in the bone marrow, circulates briefly in the peripheral blood, and then passes to the tissues. Its relationship to mast cells is controversial. Basophil granules contain a number of preformed mediators of the inflammatory response, including histamine and chondroitin sulfate. Upon stimulation, these cells also synthesize leukotriene and other mediators. The principal causes of basophilia are listed in (Table 20-12). Basophilia is most commonly observed in immediate-type hypersensitivity reactions and in the chronic myeloproliferative syndromes.

Monocytosis Is Seen in Malignant and Inflammatory Conditions

Monocytosis is defined as a peripheral blood monocyte count above 800/µL. The principal causes of monocytosis include hematological disorders, immunological and inflammatory conditions, infectious diseases, and solid cancers. Hematological diseases account for at least half of the peripheral blood

TABLE 20-11 **Principal Causes of Eosinophilia**

Allergic disorders
Skin diseases
Parasitic (helminth) infestations
Malignant neoplasms
   Hematopoietic
   Solid tumors
Collagen vascular disorders
Miscellaneous
   Hypereosinophilic syndromes
   Eosinophilia–myalgia syndrome
   IL-2 therapy

TABLE 20-12 Principal Causes of Basophilia

Allergic (drug, food)
Inflammation
   Juvenile rheumatoid arthritis
   Ulcerative colitis
Infection
   Viral (chickenpox, influenza)
   Tuberculosis
Neoplasia
   Myeloproliferative syndromes
   Basophilic leukemia
   Carcinoma
Endocrine
   Diabetes mellitus
   Myxedema
   Estrogen administration

monocytoses. For example, monocytes may constitute a component of acute or chronic myelogenous leukemia. In such cases, they may be either morphologically normal or they may exhibit immature and dyspoietic cytological features. Monocytosis often occurs in neutropenic states, probably as a compensatory mechanism. Peripheral blood monocytosis may also accompany malignant lymphomas and Hodgkin lymphoma.

Langerhans Cell Histiocytosis Is Usually a Juvenile Neoplastic Proliferation

Langerhans cell histiocytosis (LCH) refers to a spectrum of uncommon proliferative disorders of Langerhans cells. The diseases range from an asymptomatic involvement of a single site, such as bone or lymph nodes, to an aggressive systemic disorder that involves multiple organs.

Langerhans cells are components of the mononuclear phagocyte system derived from precursor cells in the bone marrow. They are found in the epidermis and in other sites such as the lymph nodes, spleen, thymus, and mucosal tissues. Langerhans cells ingest, process, and present antigens to T lymphocytes.

The etiology and pathogenesis of LCH are unknown. It has been thought that the disease may represent an atypical immunological reaction or an unusual manifestation of an autoimmune disorder, but the recent demonstration of clonal proliferation of Langerhans cells in all forms of LCH suggests the possibility of a neoplastic disorder. In turn, the production of cytokines by neoplastic Langerhans cells may account for the polymorphous appearance of the lesions of LCH. Infants, children, and young adults are most commonly affected. The extent of the disease and the rate of progression correlate inversely with the age at presentation. Certain eponyms were traditionally attached to the various presentations of LCH.

- **Eosinophilic granuloma** is the localized, usually self-limited, disorder of older children (5–10 years old) and young adults (below the age of 30 years). It accounts for almost 75% of all cases of LCH and afflicts males four times as frequently as females. The bones (Fig. 20-36) and the lungs are the principal organs affected.
- **Hand-Schüller-Christian disease** is a multifocal and typically indolent disorder, usually in children between 2 and 5 years of age, which represents about one fourth of all cases of LCH. Boys and girls are affected equally. Bony lesions tend to predominate, although involvement of endocrine glands may be prominent.
- **Letterer-Siwe disease** is a rare (less than 10% of cases), acute, disseminated variant of LCH in infants and children younger than 2 years of age. There is no sex predominance. Skin lesions and involvement of visceral organs and the hematopoietic system are characteristic (Fig. 20-37).

Pathology: Despite the clinical heterogeneity of the LCHs, there are common histopathological findings. The cells that accumulate in this disorder are large (15–25 μm in diameter), with round to indented nuclei, delicate vesicular chromatin, and small nucleoli. Marked nuclear folds and prominent grooves or creases are cytological features lacking in other disorders of mononu-

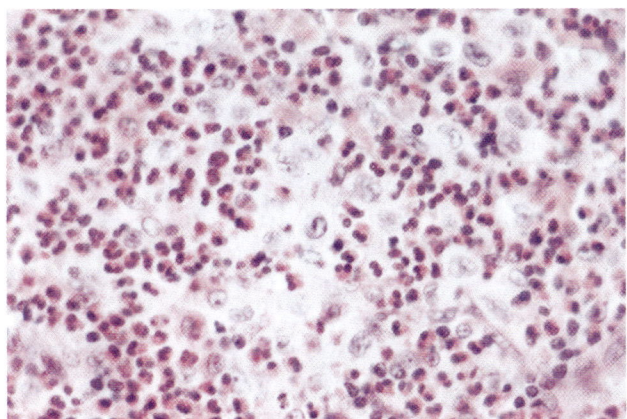

FIGURE 20-36
Eosinophilic granuloma. A section of an affected rib shows proliferated Langerhans cells and numerous eosinophils.

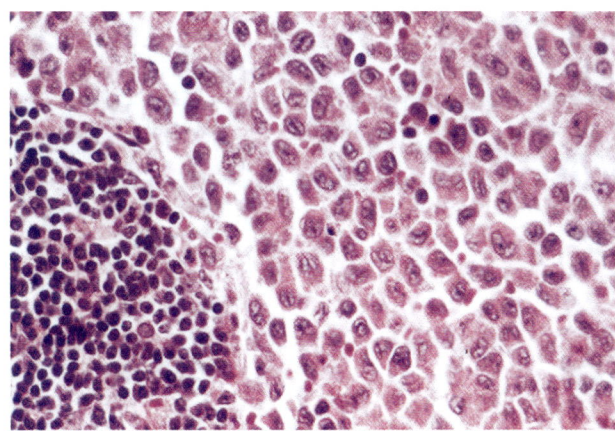

FIGURE 20-37
Letterer-Siwe disease. A section of the spleen illustrates sheets of proliferated Langerhans cells.

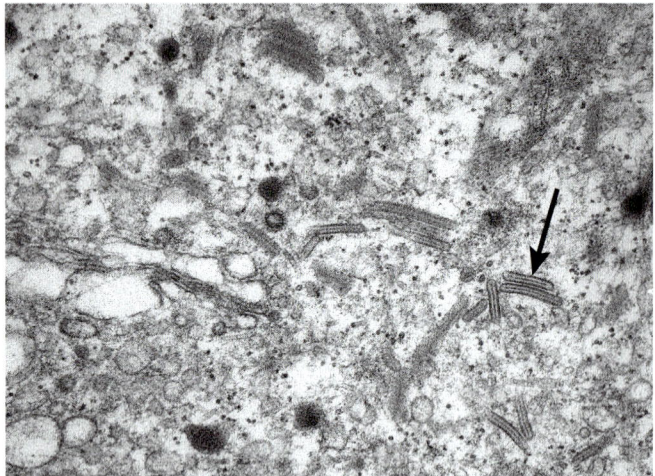

FIGURE 20-38
Electron micrograph showing a Birbeck granule in Langerhans histiocytosis.

phadenopathy and hepatosplenomegaly are frequent. Lytic lesions of bone cause pain or tenderness to palpation. Proptosis (protrusion of the eyeball) may be a complication of infiltration of the orbit. Diabetes insipidus occurs when the hypothalamic–pituitary axis is affected. **The classic triad of diabetes insipidus, proptosis, and defects in membranous bones occurs in only 15% of cases of Hand-Schüller-Christian disease.**

The prognosis in LCH depends principally on the age at presentation, the extent of disease, and the rate of progression. In general, the disorder is self-limited and benign in older persons (eosinophilic granuloma), whereas children younger than the age of 2 years (Letterer-Siwe disease) tend to do poorly. Rarely, the clinical course is aggressive and indistinguishable from that of a malignant neoplasm.

clear phagocytes. The abundant cytoplasm is pink to red and in chronic disease may contain lipid vacuoles. Binucleated or multinucleated Langerhans cells may be identified.

By electron microscopy, a distinctive cytoplasmic inclusion, the *Birbeck granule* (Fig. 20-38), is commonly observed in the Langerhans cells. This inclusion is rod-shaped or tubular, with a dense core and a double outer sheath. Frequently, one end is bulbous, in which case the granule resembles a tennis racket. Characteristic immunological cell markers identical to those of epidermal Langerhans cells include S-100 protein and CD1 (Fig. 20-39).

The infiltrating Langerhans cells are accompanied by variable numbers of inflammatory cells, principally eosinophils, and less commonly plasma cells and neutrophils. Foci of necrosis with surrounding eosinophils are called *eosinophilic microabscesses*. There are characteristic histopathological patterns of histiocytic infiltration in different organs.

- The **skin** initially shows involvement of the superficial papillary dermis. Invasion of the epidermis by Langerhans cells leads to secondary ulceration.
- The **lymph nodes** first exhibit involvement of the sinuses, although subsequent infiltration of the stroma is common.
- The **spleen** is infiltrated by Langerhans cells, predominantly in the red pulp.
- The **liver** displays Langerhans cells in the sinusoids.
- The **lungs** initially show infiltration in the alveolar septa and in peribronchial and perivascular areas.
- The **bone marrow** is infiltrated in the hematopoietic stroma.

Clinical Features: The clinical manifestations of LCH reflect the sites of tissue involvement. Skin involvement, principally in the Letterer-Siwe variant, takes the form of seborrheic or eczematoid dermatitis, most prominently on the scalp, face, and trunk. Otitis media is a common finding. Painless localized or generalized lym-

Proliferative Disorders of Mast Cells Release Inflammatory Mediators

Mast cells derive from precursor cells in the bone marrow and are found in the connective tissues, usually in close proximity to blood vessels. In sections stained with hematoxylin and eosin, mast cells are indistinguishable from fibroblasts or tissue macrophages. They are elongate or spindle-shaped but may be polygonal or stellate. The nucleus is centrally situated, round to elongate, and frequently indented. The cytoplasm is pale pink and finely granular. With Giemsa or metachromatic stains, such as toluidine blue, mast cell granules are basophilic (blue-purple). The chloroacetate esterase (CAE) reaction stains the granules red.

Mast cell granules contain inflammatory mediators, such as histamine, heparin, eosinophil and neutrophil chemotactic factors, and certain proteases. The symptoms of mast cell proliferative diseases are due to the release of these substances and

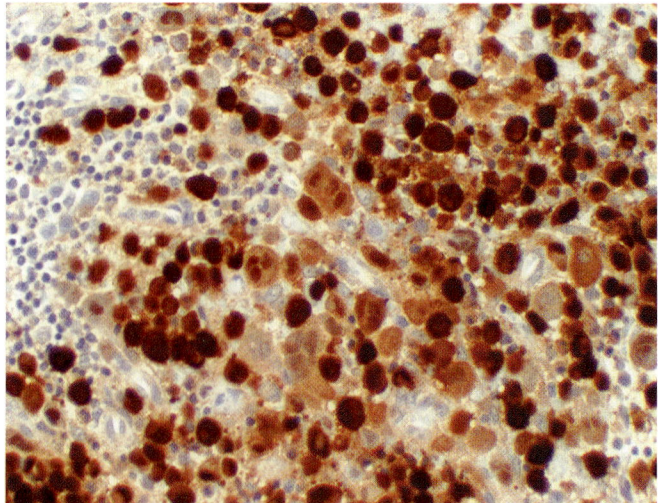

FIGURE 20-39
Eosinophilic granuloma. Langerhans cells are positive for CD1 by immunoperoxidase staining.

include flushing, pruritus, and hives. The secretion of heparin also causes bleeding from the nasopharynx or gastrointestinal tract. The spectrum of mast cell proliferative disorders comprises a variety of benign and malignant conditions.

MAST CELL HYPERPLASIA (REACTIVE MASTOCYTOSIS): This process occurs in immediate- and delayed-type hypersensitivity reactions and in lymph nodes that drain the sites of malignant tumors. It is also observed in Waldenström macroglobulinemia, in the bone marrow of women with postmenopausal osteoporosis, in myelodysplastic syndromes, and after chemotherapy for leukemia.

LOCALIZED MASTOCYTOSIS (MASTOCYTOMA): This lesion presents either as a single, tan-brown, cutaneous nodule in newborns or as several groups of skin nodules in young children. Microscopically, a diffuse dermal infiltrate of mast cells is noted. The disorder resolves spontaneously, and secondary extracutaneous involvement is rare.

URTICARIA PIGMENTOSA: This entity presents as multiple, symmetrically distributed, tan-brown, cutaneous macules or papules, most commonly in infants and young children. The skin of the trunk is predominantly affected, but any cutaneous site may be involved. Microscopically, a diffuse dermal infiltrate of mast cells is observed. Spontaneous resolution usually occurs at puberty, and systemic involvement is unusual.

SYSTEMIC MASTOCYTOSIS: This rare disorder is characterized by infiltration of many organs with mast cells, including the skin, lymph nodes, spleen, liver, bones and bone marrow, and gastrointestinal tract. Systemic mastocytosis occurs at any age, but adults in the sixth and seventh decades of life are most commonly affected. Systemic mastocytosis may accompany urticaria pigmentosa. It is not clear whether the disorder is a reactive process or represents a neoplastic proliferation of mast cells.

Pathology: In systemic mastocytosis, the lymph nodes initially show perifollicular and perivascular infiltration by mast cells. The spleen exhibits nodular aggregates of mast cells with accompanying dense fibrosis in the red pulp, particularly in relation to the fibrous trabeculae and the capsule. In the liver, the portal triads are first involved. Involvement of the bone marrow may be peritrabecular, perivascular, or diffuse (Fig. 20-40), and there is often accompanying fibrosis.

On roentgenological examination, both osteolytic and osteoblastic lesions may be identified in systemic mastocytosis. The central axial skeleton, which includes the ribs, vertebrae, pelvis, skull, and proximal long bones, is most commonly affected.

Clinical Features: Patients with systemic mastocytosis suffer symptoms related to the overproduction of a number of mediators normally produced by mast cells and basophils, including histamine, prostaglandin D_2 and thromboxane B_2. Most experience gastrointestinal pain and diarrhea. Anaphylactic episodes, with pruritus, flushing, and asthmatic symptoms, are common. Extensive mast cell infiltration of the bone marrow leads to secondary anemia, leukopenia, and thrombocytopenia.

Systemic mastocytosis follows a chronic, indolent course, with about half of patients surviving for 5 years. Symptomatic relief is obtained, at least partially, with H_1- and H_2-receptor antagonists. There is no effective therapy for the underlying disease process.

MAST CELL LEUKEMIA: This complication develops in 15% of cases of systemic mastocytosis. The circulating cells exhibit the typical cytological features of mast cells or of less-differentiated variants. The leukocyte count may be markedly increased.

MAST CELL SARCOMA: This cancer is a rare malignant disorder of mast cells that is characterized by extensive infiltration of cutaneous and extracutaneous sites by anaplastic mast cell variants. The disease is rapidly progressive, and the prognosis is poor.

Ancillary Techniques Assist in the Diagnosis of Hematological Malignancies

For many years, conventional morphology, in conjunction with a limited number of cytochemical tests, has been the sole basis for diagnosing hematological malignancies (leukemias and lymphomas). A number of techniques are now available for the characterization of these cancers at a molecular level.

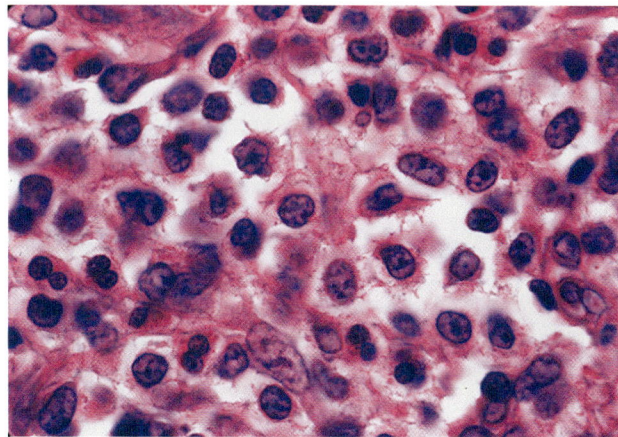

FIGURE 20-40
Mastocytosis. A section of lymph node shows effacement of the normal architecture by sheets of mast cells. The centrally situated nuclei are round to elongated, and occasionally indented. The cytoplasm is pale pink and finely granular.

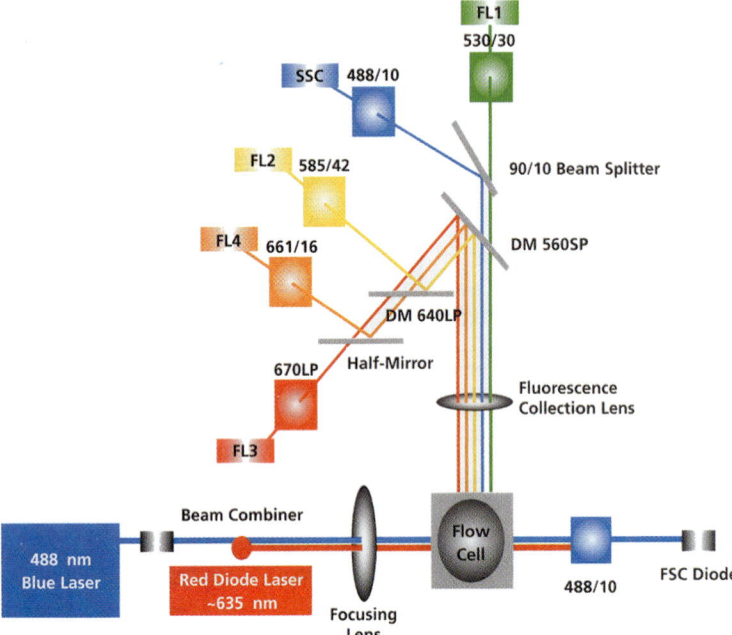

FIGURE 20-41
Diagram of a six-parameter flow cytometer. Cells labeled with various fluoresceinated antibodies running through the flow cell are analyzed for cell size (forward scatter, *FSC*), internal granularity (side scatter, *SSC*) and labeling with four additional antibodies. Different fluorescent dyes attached to four antibodies are excited with 488-nm and 635-nm monochromatic light, and their emission spectrum is detected by four individual light detectors. The system detects cells with abnormal immunophenotypes.

Flow Cytometry

Tumor cell suspensions stained with fluoresceinated antibodies are analyzed for marker expression by flow cytometry (Fig. 20-41). Most instruments assess six parameters simultaneously—cell size, internal granularity, and four different markers—with the goal of identifying and defining abnormal cell populations. Figure 20-42 depicts the histograms of a patient with chronic lymphocytic leukemia. The tumor cells express the B-cell markers CD19/20/23, show aberrant coexpression for the T cell marker CD5, and are positive for λ light chain. In a normal person, B cells do not coexpress CD5, and a mixture of B cells positive for κ and λ light chains would be expected (normal κ/λ ratio is 2:1).

Immunohistochemistry

Antibodies directed against the same target have the same cluster designation (CD). For most hematological malignancies, a panel of several antibodies is used to assess an abnormal pattern of expression, which often has diagnostic and prognostic significance.

Cytogenetics

There is an increasing number of hematological malignancies whose diagnosis is defined and whose prognosis is determined by genetic abnormalities. Conventional banding techniques reveal numerical chromosomal aberrations and translocations. Chromosomal translocations can also be identified by fluorescence in situ hybridization (FISH) (Fig. 20-43).

Molecular Diagnostics

T and B cell clonality in lymphoid malignancies is assessed by polymerase chain reaction (PCR)-based techniques. Amplifying parts of the immunoglobulin heavy chain gene results in a polyclonal ladder in benign conditions; a dominant band suggests an expanded B-cell clone frequently seen in lymphomas (Fig. 20-44).

FIGURE 20-42
Flow cytometric analysis of peripheral blood obtained from a patient with chronic lymphocytic leukemia of B cell type (CD19+ CD20+ CD5+ CD23+ κ−λ+).
   A) Lymphocytes are gated for analysis (R1 gate)
   B) The tumor cells coexpress B-cell markers CD23 and CD20 (right upper quadrant)
   C) The tumor cells aberrantly coexpress T-cell marker CD5 and B-cell marker CD20 (right upper quadrant)
   D) The tumor cells coexpress T-cell marker CD5 and B-cell marker CD23 (right upper quadrant)
   E) The tumor cells express surface λ light chain (left upper quadrant) but no κ light chain (right lower quadrant).
   F) and G) show reactivity of κ and λ light chains versus B-cell marker CD19.

Nonmalignant Disorders

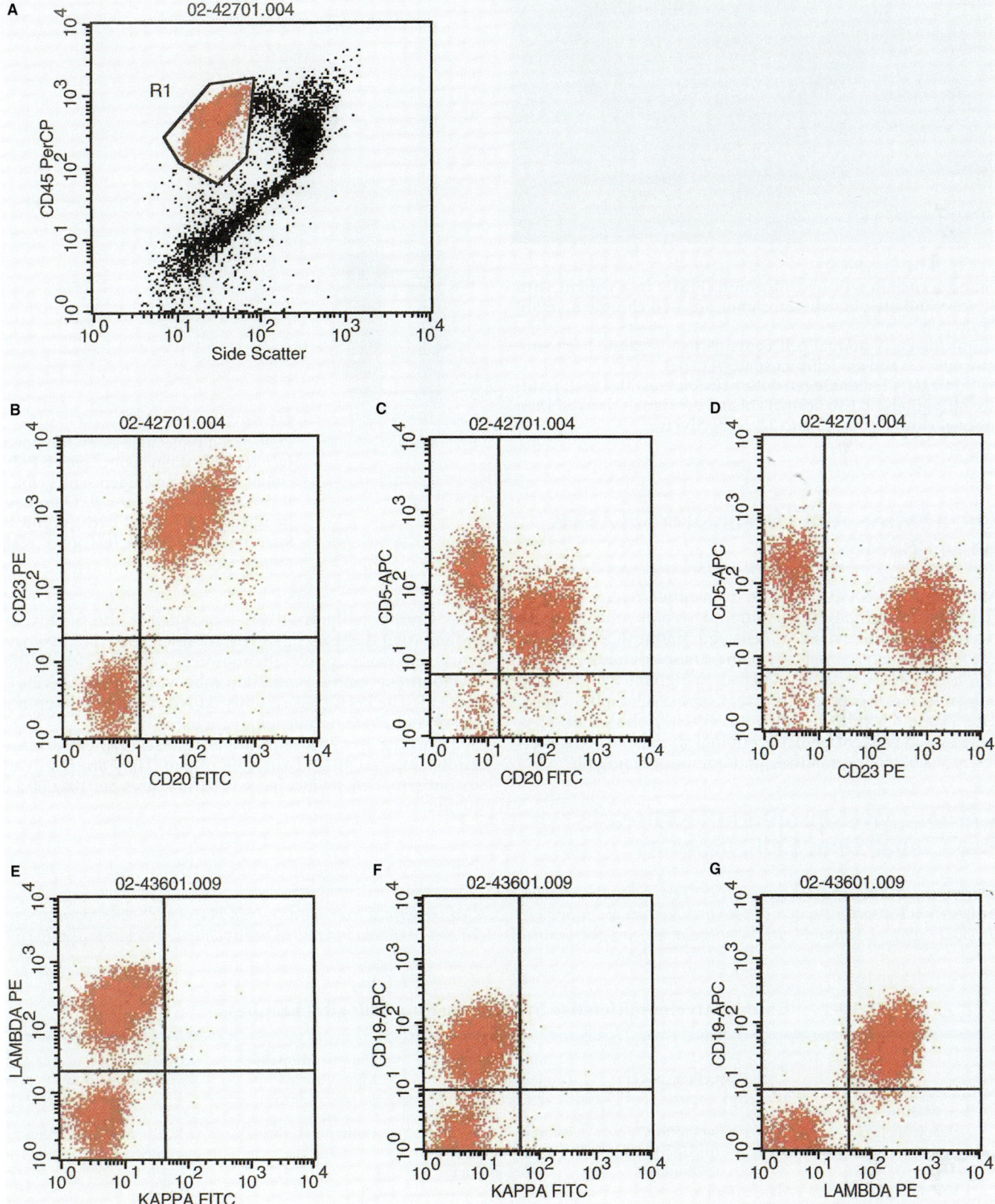

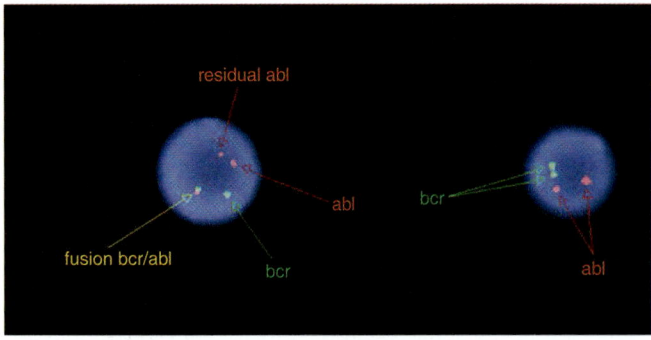

FIGURE 20-43
Fluorescence in situ hybridization (FISH) in a patient with t(9;22) (Philadelphia chromosome) positive chronic myeloid leukemia.
Right image: A normal cell contains two separate bcr (chromosome 22) and abl (chromosome 9) genes
Left image: A leukemic cell with a fusion bcr/abl signal, residual abl signal and two normal abl and bcr signals derived from normal chromosomes 9 and 22, respectively

LEUKEMIAS AND MYELODYSPLASTIC SYNDROMES

Malignant leukocytes originate from either myeloid cells or lymphoid cells. Malignant proliferations of myeloid cells are derived from bone marrow cells and manifest as *myelodysplastic syndromes, chronic myeloproliferative diseases,* or *acute myelogenous leukemias.* By contrast, malignant lymphocytes can arise in any compartment that contains lymphoid cells. The World Health Organization (WHO) classification is based upon conventional morphological criteria, cytogenetics, molecular abnormalities, and immunophenotype.

Chronic Myeloproliferative Diseases Are Clonal Stem Cell Disorders

Chronic myeloproliferative diseases are defined as clonal hematogenous stem cell disorders with increased proliferation of one or more myeloid lineages (granulocytic, erythroid, or megakaryocytic

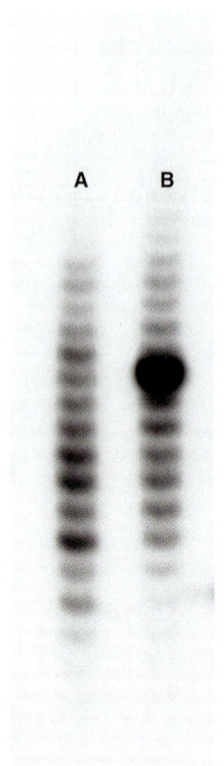

FIGURE 20-44
PCR-based molecular assay for clonal *IgH* gene rearrangement. *Lane A:* Polyclonal ladder—no evidence of a clonal B cell population. *Lane B:* Dominant band in a polyclonal background in keeping with clonal *IgH* gene rearrangement.

cells). Traditionally, four different types of chronic myeloproliferative diseases have been defined: chronic myelogenous leukemia, polycythemia vera, chronic idiopathic myelofibrosis, and essential thrombocythemia (Tables 20-13 to 20-15) The WHO has recently added chronic neutrophilic and chronic eosinophilic leukemia to the list.

Chronic myeloproliferative diseases typically affect adults between 40 and 80 years of age. They are relatively uncommon, with an incidence of 5 to 10 cases per 100,000 annually.

Chronic Myelogenous Leukemia (CML)

CML is derived from an abnormal pluripotent bone marrow stem cell and results in prominent neutrophilic leukocytosis over the full

TABLE 20-13   Chronic Myeloproliferative Syndromes: Morphological Features

	Polycythemia Vera	Chronic Myelogenous Leukemia	Chronic Idiopathic Myelofibrosis	Essential Thrombocythemia
Bone Marrow				
Histopathology	Panhyperplasia (predominantly erythroid)	Panhyperplasia (predominantly granulocytic)	Panhyperplasia with fibrosis	Atypical megakaryocytes predominate
M:E ratio	<=2:1	10:1 to 50:1	2:1 to 5:1	2:1 to 5:1
Marrow iron	↓ or absent	Normal or ↑	Normal or ↑	Normal to absent
Marrow fibrosis	15–20%	<10%	90–100%	<5%
Liver, Spleen				
Extramedullary hematopoiesis (myeloid metaplasia)	Moderate (predominantly erythroid)	Moderate to marked (predominantly granulocytic)	Moderate to marked	Slight (predominantly megakaryocytic)

Leukemias and Myelodysplastic Syndromes

TABLE 20-14   Chronic Myeloproliferative Syndromes: Laboratory Features

	Polycythemia Vera	Chronic Myelogenous Leukemia	Chronic Idiopathic Myelofibrosis	Essential Thrombocythemia
Hemoglobin	>20 g/dL	Mild anemia	Mild anemia	Mild anemia
RBC morphology	Slight aniso- and poikilocytosis	Slight aniso- and poikilocytosis	Immature erythrocytes and marked aniso- and poikilocytosis	Hypochromic microcytes
Granulocytes	Normal to mildly increased; may show a few immature forms	Moderate to markedly increased with spectrum of maturation	Normal to moderately increased; some immature WBC	Normal to slightly increased
Platelets	Normal to moderately increased	Normal to moderately increased	Increased to decreased	Markedly increased with abnormal forms
Leukocyte alkaline phosphatase (LAP)	Normal to increased	Decreased to absent	Variable	Variable
Cytogenetics	Nonspecific	Philadelphia chromosome (Ph¹); BCR/ABL gene rearrangement	Nonspecific	Nonspecific

RBC, red blood cells; WBC, white blood cells.

range of myeloid maturation. By definition, the presence of the Philadelphia chromosome or molecular demonstration of the *BCR/ABL* fusion gene is required to establish the diagnosis.

Epidemiology: CML is the most common myeloproliferative disease and accounts for 15 to 20% of all cases of leukemia. The peak incidence occurs in the fifth and sixth decades of life, with a slight male predominance.

Pathogenesis: The cause in most cases of CML is unknown. Radiation exposure and myelotoxic agents such as benzene have been implicated in a small number of cases. The leukemic cells represent transformed pluripotent stem cells with predominantly granulocytic differentiation. In 95% of all CML cases, the Philadelphia chromosome, which results from t(9:22)(q34:q11) translocation, can be demonstrated by conventional cytogenetics (Fig. 20-45). The Philadelphia chromosome itself is a derived

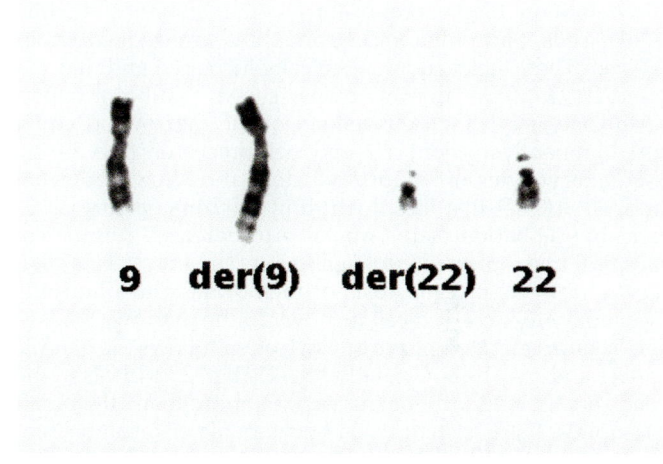

FIGURE 20-45
Chronic myelogenous leukemia. The Philadelphia chromosome der(22) is shown.

TABLE 20-15   Chronic Myeloproliferative Syndromes: Clinical Features

	Polycythemia Vera	Chronic Myelogenous Leukemia	Chronic Idiopathic Myelofibrosis	Essential Thrombocythemia
Male-to-female ratio	1.2:1	3:2	1:1	1.2:1
Peak age range (years)	40–60	25–60	50–70	50–70
Clinical symptoms	Headache, dizziness, pruritus	Asymptomatic or LUQ discomfort, fatigability	Asymptomatic or LUQ discomfort, fatigability	Asymptomatic or LUQ discomfort
Splenomegaly	75%	90%	100%	30% (slight)
Hepatomegaly	40%	50%	80%	40% (slight)
Acute leukemic conversion	5–10%	80%	5–10%	2–5%
Median survival (years)	13	3–4	5	>10

LUQ, left upper quadrant.

(shortened) chromosome 22 [DER(22q)]. The *BCR* (break point cluster region) gene on chromosome 22 is fused to the *ABL* gene on chromosome 9. A small number of cases involve additional chromosomal abnormalities or cryptic translocation of 9q34 and 22q11 that cannot be identified by conventional cytogenetics. In these cases, the *BCR/ABL* fusion gene is detected by FISH (Fig. 20-43), PCR, or Southern blot techniques, which demonstrate a fused *BCR/ABL* gene or fusion transcripts on chromosome 22. The *BCR/ABL* gene encodes a fusion protein, p210, which acts as a constitutively activated tyrosine kinase. Much less commonly, *BCR/ABL* fusion genes result from breakage in the minor break point cluster region and produce a fusion protein termed p190. P190 is most commonly seen in Philadelphia chromosome-positive *acute lymphoblastic leukemia*. Acquisition of additional chromosomal abnormalities (e.g., second Philadelphia chromosome or trisomy 8) is associated with a more aggressive clinical course.

Pathology: CML may present in *chronic, accelerated, or blast phases.*

The **chronic phase of CML** features conspicuous leukocytosis, consisting mainly of maturing neutrophils. By definition, blasts account for less than 10% of the white blood cells. Basophilia and eosinophilia are frequently observed. The platelet count is typically increased and may exceed $10^6/\mu L$. Bone marrow biopsy shows significant hypercellularity, with total effacement of the marrow space by predominantly myeloid cells and their precursors (Fig. 20-46). Megakaryocytes often form clusters and show abnormal morphological features, including micromegakaryocytes and hypolobation of the nuclei. An increased number of atypical macrophages *(pseudo-Gaucher cells and sea-blue histiocytes)* reflects phagocytosis of membrane phospholipids secondary to increased cell turnover in the marrow.

The **accelerated phase of CML** often follows the chronic phase and may be associated with (1) 10 to 20% blasts in the peripheral blood or bone marrow, (2) more than 20% blood basophils, (3) persistent thrombocytopenia or thrombocytosis unresponsive to therapy, (4) splenomegaly, (5) increasing white blood cell count unresponsive to therapy, and (6) additional chromosomal abnormalities.

The **blast phase of CML** is the ultimate outcome and features (1) at least 20% blasts in the bone marrow, (2) extramedullary proliferation of blasts (skin, lymph nodes, spleen, bone, central nervous system [CNS]), and (3) clusters of blasts in the bone marrow biopsy. In most cases (70%), the leukemic cells in blast phase exhibit morphological and immunophenotypic features of myeloid lineage; in 30%, they have the appearance of lymphoblasts. In most cases of lymphoblastic blast phase, the malignant lymphoblasts demonstrate a B-cell precursor immunophenotype, with the expression of CD10, CD19, CD34, and terminal deoxynucleotidyl transferase TdT. On occasion, the lymphoblasts show a precursor T-cell immunophenotype that stains for CD3, CD7, and TdT. The blast phase heralds a poor prognosis.

Clinical Features: In the long term, CML is uniformly fatal. However, with improved treatment modalities, median survival times of 5 to 7 years are commonly reported.

CML is a paradigm for a malignancy with a well-defined cytogenetic abnormality that can be targeted by specific drug therapy. A newly developed drug, Gleevec, blocks the ATP-binding site on the *BCR/ABL* tyrosine kinase, thereby inactivating it. Significant remissions of CML are observed after treatment with the drug. However, allogenic bone marrow transplantation is currently the only hope for cure.

Polycythemia Vera

Polycythemia vera (PV) is a myeloproliferative disease that arises from a clonal hematopoietic stem cell and results in uncontrolled production of red blood cells. The increase in erythrocytes in PV is autonomous and is not regulated by erythropoietin. The WHO has established major and minor diagnostic criteria for polycythemia.

Major criteria

- Increased red blood cell mass (hemoglobin >18.5 g/dL in men and >16.5 g/dL in women)

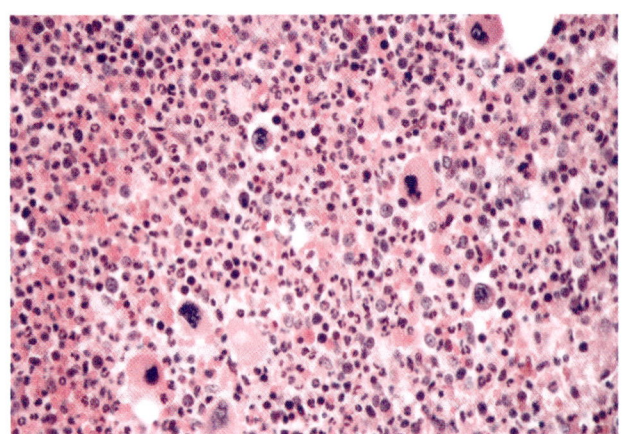
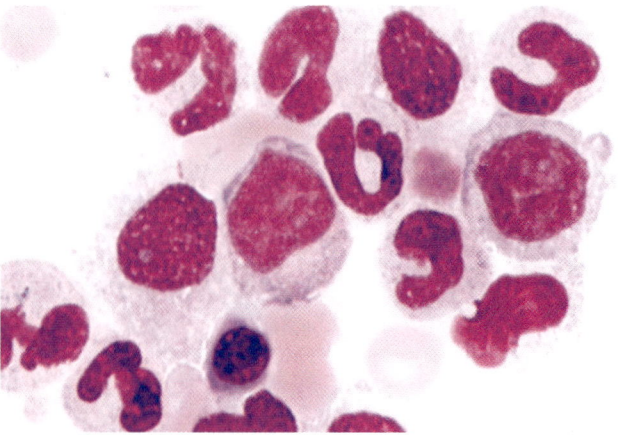

FIGURE 20-46

Chronic myelogenous leukemia. A. The bone marrow is conspicuously hypercellular, owing to an increase in granulocyte precursors, mature granulocytes, and megakaryocytes. B. A smear of the bone marrow aspirate from the same patient reveals numerous granulocytes at various stages of development.

- No elevation of erythropoietin level
- No cause of secondary erythrocytosis
- Splenomegaly
- Demonstration of a clonal genetic abnormality other than the Philadelphia chromosome
- Erythroid colony formation in vitro in the absence of growth factor stimulation

Minor criteria

- Thrombocytosis >400 × 10^9/L
- Leukocytosis >12 × 10^9/L
- Prominent erythropoiesis and megakaryopoiesis in the bone marrow
- Low serum erythropoietin levels.

Epidemiology: In North America, 8 to 10 cases of PV per million are seen annually. The mean age at diagnosis is 60 years.

Pathogenesis: Polycythemia vera derives from the malignant transformation of a single hematopoietic stem cell with primary commitment to the erythroid lineage. Proliferation of the neoplastic clone occurs predominantly in the bone marrow but may involve such extramedullary sites as the spleen, lymph nodes, and liver (myeloid metaplasia).

The neoplastic erythroid progenitor cells of polycythemia vera are sensitive to erythropoietin like their normal counterparts. In semisolid culture media, they form luxuriant clusters of erythroid cells (BFU-E) when exposed to erythropoietin. However, at the more mature colony-forming stage (CFU-E), the neoplastic cells form erythroid colonies in semisolid culture media even in the absence of exogenous erythropoietin stimulation. These autonomous erythroid colonies are called *endogenous* CFU-E and are characteristic of polycythemia vera during the entire course of the disease. By contrast, CFU-E formation in normal erythroid progenitor cells is erythropoietin dependent (*exogenous* CFU-E). The autonomous proliferation of the more mature cells confers a proliferative advantage to the neoplastic clones, since the increased erythrocyte mass suppresses normal erythropoietin secretion and the function of the remaining normal progenitors. As a result, serum erythropoietin levels are either normal or low in PV, unlike secondary (functional) erythrocytosis, in which erythropoietin levels are increased. No specific recurrent genetic defect has been identified in PV, although some cytogenetic abnormalities have been described.

Pathology: The bone marrow in PV is homogeneously red-purple. The spleen is moderately enlarged, and its cut surface is uniformly dark red, with expansion of the red pulp and obliteration of the white pulp. The liver tends to be enlarged. The lymph nodes may be slightly enlarged, owing to myeloid metaplasia. The principal morphological features in PV are outlined in Table 20-13.

The bone marrow is hypercellular, with hyperplasia of all elements. However, erythroid precursor cells predominate, and the myeloid-to-erythroid ratio is less than 2:1. Erythroid maturation is normal (normoblastic). There is normal maturation of the granulocytic cell lineage. Megakaryocytes are typically increased in number and size and tend to be clustered. In 90% of cases, marrow stainable iron is decreased or absent. A mild-to-moderate increase in reticulin fibrosis is common, and 10% of cases progress to severe collagenous fibrosis.

The spleen exhibits a prominent accumulation of erythrocytes in the red pulp cords and sinuses. There may be myeloid metaplasia, characterized by erythroid precursor cells, immature granulocytes, and megakaryocytes. The lymphoid white pulp is atrophic or obliterated. Myeloid metaplasia is also common in the sinusoids of the liver and in the sinuses and paracortex of the lymph nodes.

The peripheral blood smear reveals normal erythrocytes, although hypochromia and microcytosis are observed if iron deficiency is present. Iron deficiency anemia is a characteristic feature of polycythemia vera because of (1) diversion of storage iron to the increased red cell mass, (2) loss of iron in the gastrointestinal tract as a complication of gastric and duodenal ulcers, and (3) therapeutic phlebotomy. If splenomegaly causes hypersplenism, the erythrocytes exhibit marked anisocytosis and poikilocytosis, with characteristic teardrop forms.

The common initial laboratory findings in PV are outlined in Table 20-15. The hemoglobin concentration may exceed 20 g/dL, and the hematocrit surpass 60%. The erythrocyte count is 6 to 10 ×10^6/L. Serum iron is usually decreased, and the total iron-binding capacity is increased. In the blood smear, formed elements are usually increased in PV. A mild-to-moderate leukocytosis of 10,000 to 25,000/μL occurs initially in two thirds of cases, but on rare occasions, neutrophil counts of more than 100,000/μL are observed. A mild increase in circulating immature granulocytes (left shift) is common. Circulating basophils and eosinophils also tend to be increased. A mild-to-moderate thrombocytosis (400,000–800,000 platelets/μL) occurs initially in half of cases. The platelets often exhibit abnormal morphological features, including giant and hypogranulated forms. Abnormal aggregation of platelets on exposure to ADP, epinephrine, and collagen is observed in many cases. The leukocyte alkaline phosphatase (LAP) score is normal in 30% of cases and increased in 70%. The LAP score is sometimes useful in distinguishing the subtypes of the chronic myeloproliferative syndromes (Table 20-14). Hyperuricemia and secondary gout may be present and are related to rapid cell turnover.

Clinical Features: The onset of polycythemia vera tends to be insidious, and the symptoms are generally nonspecific, typically relating to the increased erythrocyte mass. Plethora and splenomegaly are early findings. Headache, dizziness, and visual problems result from vascular disturbances in the brain and retina. Angina pectoris, secondary to slowing of coronary artery blood flow, and intermittent claudication caused by sluggish peripheral blood flow in the lower extremities may be observed. Gastric or duodenal ulcers may result from circulatory problems in the gastrointestinal tract and possibly (in part) from histamine release by basophils. Major thrombotic complications occur in a third of cases, including stroke and myocardial infarction. The clinical features of polycythemia vera are outlined in Table 20-15.

The clinical course of polycythemia vera proceeds as a series of phases.

- **Proliferative phase:** Most patients experience a prolonged proliferative phase that is dominated by erythroid proliferation and an increased erythrocyte mass. This phase often persists unchanged until the patient succumbs to complications or dies of extraneous causes. In one third of patients, the disease progresses to other stages.
- **Spent phase:** In 10% of cases, the excessive proliferation of erythroid cells ceases, resulting in a stable or decreased erythrocyte mass.
- **Postpolycythemic myelofibrosis with myeloid metaplasia:** Some 10% of cases show progression to myelofibrosis, which is similar to that observed in other chronic myeloproliferative syndromes. Such patients display (1) progressively severe anemia, (2) increasing splenomegaly owing to myeloid metaplasia, (3) a peripheral blood leukoerythroblastic reaction with circulating immature erythroid and granulocytic cells, and poikilocytosis and anisocytosis of erythrocytes, and (4) severe myelofibrosis with depletion of hematopoietic cells. At this stage, the prognosis is poor, with a mean survival of only 2 years.
- **Acute myelogenous leukemia:** AML develops in 5 to 10% of cases of PV. The risk of progression to AML appears to be increased if there has been prior treatment with ^{32}P or alkylating agents. However, it may also reflect the natural history of the disease, with treated patients surviving longer.

The median survival in PV is 13 years, and the most common causes of death are those associated with old age. Specific causes of death related to the disease itself include thrombosis, hemorrhage, AML, and the spent phase. Therapeutic reduction of the erythrocyte mass, by either repeated phlebotomy or chemotherapy, constitutes effective management in most cases.

Chronic Idiopathic Myelofibrosis

Chronic idiopathic myelofibrosis is a clonal myeloproliferative disease in which marrow fibrosis is accompanied by prominent megakaryopoiesis and granulopoiesis.

Epidemiology: The annual incidence of idiopathic myelofibrosis is estimated to be between 0.5 and 1.5 per 100,000. It is a disease of the elderly, with a peak incidence in the 7th decade of life.

Pathogenesis: As in other types of myeloproliferative disease, some exposure to benzene or radiation has occasionally been implicated in chronic idiopathic myelofibrosis. The malignant megakaryocytes produce PDGF and TGF-β, both of which are powerful fibroblast mitogens. Ultimately, the entire marrow space is displaced by connective tissue, although the fibroblasts are not part of the clonal stem cell disorder. In the *fibrotic phase,* malignant stem cells enter the circulation and give rise to extramedullary hematopoiesis at multiple anatomical sites. No genetic defect has been identified.

Pathology: Most patients are diagnosed at the fibrotic stage, but 25% are first detected in the cellular phase. The **prefibrotic stage** features a hypercellular bone marrow, with predominant neutrophilic and megakaryocytic proliferation. The megakaryocytes are clustered and atypically lobated. In the **fibrotic stage,** the peripheral blood shows either leukopenia or marked leukocytosis, and myeloid precursors and nucleated red blood cells (leukoerythroblastosis) are usually present. The red cells exhibit poikilocytosis and teardrop forms. Conspicuous reticulin or collagen fibrosis in the marrow defines this stage (Fig. 20-47). As in the cellular phase, many atypical megakaryocytes are present. Extramedullary hematopoiesis results in splenomegaly, hepatomegaly, and lymphadenopathy and may be present in other organs.

Clinical Features: A quarter of patients with idiopathic myelofibrosis are asymptomatic at diagnosis. In these cases, the disease is detected by splenomegaly on physical examination or by demonstration of teardrop red cells or thrombocytosis. The early clinical symptoms are nonspecific and include fatigue, low-grade fever, night sweats, and weight loss. Platelet function may be impaired and associated with either increased platelet aggregation and thrombosis or decreased platelet aggregation with a bleeding diathesis. Transformation to AML occurs in 15% of cases.

Essential Thrombocythemia

Essential thrombocythemia is an uncommon neoplastic disorder of hematopoietic stem cells that is characterized by uncontrolled proliferation of megakaryocytes. A marked increase in circulating platelets is accompanied by recurrent episodes of thrombosis

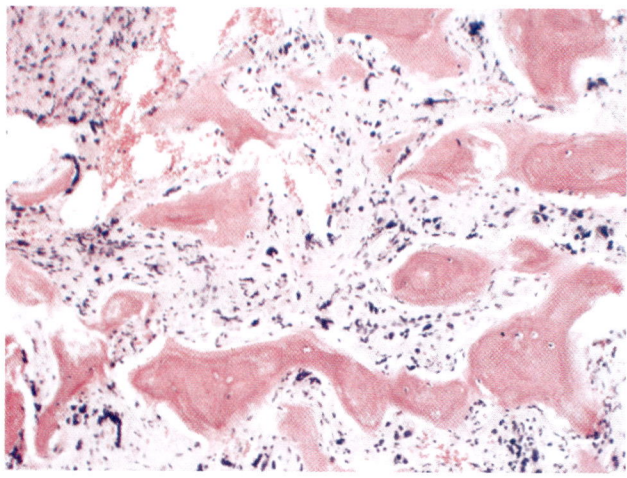

FIGURE 20-47
Chronic idiopathic myelofibrosis. A section of bone marrow shows collagenous fibrosis, osteosclerosis, and numerous abnormal megakaryocytes.

and hemorrhage. The disease affects middle-aged persons, with a slight male predominance. The WHO criteria require a sustained platelet count above 600,000/μL and prominent megakaryocytic proliferation in the bone marrow. Criteria of exclusion include no evidence for the following:

Polycythemia (normal red cell mass)
Chronic myelogenous leukemia
Idiopathic myelofibrosis
Chromosomal abnormalities
Dysplastic morphological features
Reactive thrombocytosis

Pathogenesis: Essential thrombocythemia is a clonal disorder that is believed to derive from the malignant transformation of a single hematopoietic stem cell with principal, but not exclusive, commitment to the megakaryocytic lineage. The disease features marked proliferation of megakaryocytes, with up to a 15-fold or greater increase in platelet production. Megakaryocyte colony-forming units (CFU-Mega) increase in number and can proliferate autonomously without the addition of specific growth factors. In some cases, the number of BFU-E also increase, a finding that may explain some features that overlap with PV. Unlike PV, the erythrocyte mass in thrombocythemia is not increased.

Pathology: Abnormalities of platelet function are common in primary thrombocythemia. Recurrent episodes of thrombosis are attributed to severe thrombocytosis, and hemorrhage reflects defects in platelet function. Iron deficiency anemia follows hemorrhage from the gastrointestinal and urogenital tracts.

Thrombosis may occur in any organ or tissue and may involve arteries or veins. Thromboses in the spleen, with subsequent infarctions, may result in splenic atrophy. In turn, this effect reduces the size of the principal sequestration site for the increased blood platelet pool, and the consequent enhancement of thrombocytosis worsens the prognosis. Similarly, splenectomy is generally contraindicated because it produces a conspicuous increase in the platelet count.

The bone marrow is markedly hypercellular, with a decreased number of fat cells and increased number of megakaryocytes (Fig. 20-48). Less commonly, hyperplasia of all three hematopoietic cell lineages occurs, but the megakaryocytic lineage predominates. Megakaryocytes are distributed in cohesive clusters or sheets and exhibit atypical morphological features. These include forms with large, bizarre, hyperchromatic and hyperlobulated nuclei and abundant cytoplasm, as well as smaller micromegakaryocytic forms. Large clusters of free platelets are a characteristic finding. Reticulin fibers in the marrow are increased in one third of cases, but overt fibrosis is rare. Iron stores are normal or decreased.

The spleen is mildly enlarged in half the cases of primary thrombocythemia. The cut surface of the spleen is homogeneously red-purple, with expansion of the red pulp and atrophy of the white pulp. Microscopically, myeloid metaplasia is common. Myeloid metaplasia of the hepatic sinusoids and of the lymph nodes is occasionally observed. The principal morphological findings in primary thrombocythemia are summarized in Table 20-13.

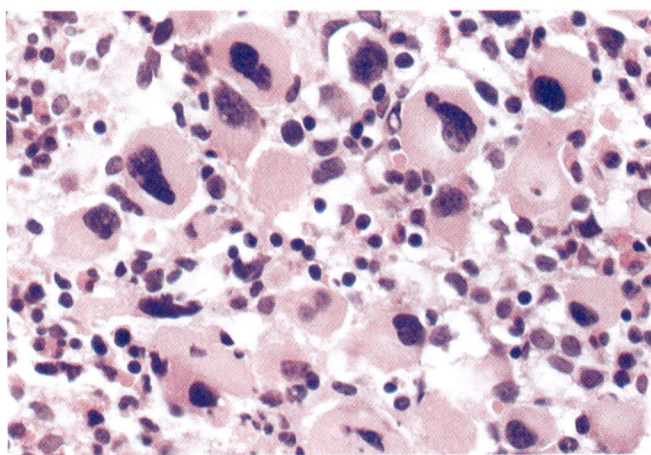

FIGURE 20-48
Essential thrombocythemia. A section of bone marrow exhibits a conspicuous increase in the number of megakaryocytes, which display atypical features and hypolobated forms.

Clinical Features: The clinical course of primary thrombocythemia is protracted, with a median survival of over 10 years. In untreated cases, thrombosis of large arteries and veins is a common complication, especially in the lower extremities, heart, intestine, and kidneys. Hemorrhage is usually mild and not life-threatening. AML supervenes in up to 5% of cases, the neoplastic blast cells being of either granulocytic or megakaryocytic lineage. In a small minority of patients, primary thrombocythemia becomes transformed into another chronic myeloproliferative syndrome. The disease is treated with plateletpheresis and myelosuppressive chemotherapy. The clinical features of primary thrombocythemia are listed in Table 20-15.

Neutrophilic Leukemia

Chronic neutrophilic leukemia is a rare myeloproliferative disease that has been recently acknowledged by the WHO as a separate disease entity. *It is characterized by sustained peripheral blood neutrophilia and bone marrow hypercellularity and features neutrophilic granulocyte proliferation and hepatosplenomegaly.* By definition, there is no Philadelphia chromosome or *BCR/ABL* fusion gene. The most difficult differential diagnosis is reactive neutrophilia. To establish a diagnosis of chronic neutrophilic leukemia, all identifiable causes for physiological neutrophilia, such as infection or any other type of inflammatory process, need to be excluded. More than 80% of the white blood cells in the peripheral blood must be segmented neutrophils, in contrast to CML, in which the full spectrum of myeloid maturation is noted.

Chronic Eosinophilic Leukemia and Hypereosinophilic Syndrome

Chronic eosinophilic leukemia is a myeloproliferative disease with clonal proliferation of eosinophilic precursors. The disorder shows persistently increased eosinophils in the blood

(>1500/μL), bone marrow, and peripheral tissues. Cardiac and pulmonary organ damage results from eosinophilic infiltration, which releases cytokines and cytotoxic proteins. Causes of secondary hypereosinophilia (allergies, parasites, etc.) need to be excluded. Cases of idiopathic eosinophilia with no molecular demonstration of clonality and no abnormal karyotype are best designated *hypereosinophilic syndrome*.

Myelodysplastic Syndromes Are Clonal Disorders That Cause Ineffective Hematopoiesis

Myelodysplastic syndromes (MDS) are clonal hematopoietic stem cell disorders in which dysplastic morphological features in one or more hematopoietic lineages are accompanied by ineffective hematopoiesis (Table 20-16). The disease is most common in the elderly. There is a discrepancy between the paucity of peripheral blood elements and the marked hyperplasia seen in the bone marrow. All types of MDS manifest refractory anemia or other types of cytopenia. Some cases are associated with an increase in myeloblasts. In contrast to myeloproliferative diseases, MDS displays neither leukocytosis nor thrombocytosis. MDS also must be distinguished from AML, which exhibits at least 20% blasts in the bone marrow. Because MDS frequently converts to AML, it is also referred to as *preleukemic syndrome*.

Pathogenesis: MDS may be either primary (de novo) or secondary (therapy related). Patients with secondary myelodysplasia usually have a history of chemotherapy, especially alkylating agents or radiation therapy for the treatment of cancer. Other risk factors for MDS include viruses, benzene exposure, cigarette smoking, and Fanconi anemia.

TABLE 20-16 WHO Classification of Peripheral Blood and Bone Marrow Findings in Myelodysplastic Syndromes.

Disease	Blood Findings	Bone Marrow Findings
Refractory anemia (RA)	Anemia No or rare blasts	Erythroid dysplasia only <5% blasts <15% ringed sideroblasts
Refractory anemia with ringed sideroblasts (RARS)	Anemia No blasts	≥15% ringed sideroblasts Erythroid dysplasia only <5% blasts
Refractory cytopenia with multilineage dysplasia (RCMD)	Cytopenia (bicytopenia or pancytopenia) No or rare blasts No Auer rods <1 × 10⁹/L monocytes	Dysplasia in ≥10% of the cells of two or more myeloid cell lines <5% blasts in marrow No Auer rods <15% ringed sideroblasts
Refractory cytopenia with multilineage dysplasia and ringed sideroblasts (RCMD-RS)	Cytopenias (bicytopenia or pancytopenia) No or rare blasts No Auer rods <1 × 10⁹/L monocytes	Dysplasia in ≥10% of the cells in two or more myeloid cell lines ≥15% ringed sideroblasts <5% blasts No Auer rods
Refractory anemia with excess blasts-1 (RAEB-1)	Cytopenias <5% blasts No Auer rods <1 × 10⁹/L monocytes	Unilineage or multilineage dyslasia 5–9% blasts No Auer rods
Refractory anemia with excess blasts-2 (RAEB-2)	Cytopenias 5–19% blasts Auer rods ± <1×10⁹/L monocytes	Unilineage or multilineage dysplasia 10–19% blasts Auer rods ±
Myelodysplastic syndrome-unclassified (MDS-U)	Cytopenias No or rare blasts No Auer rods	Unilineage dysplasia: one myeloid cell line <5% blasts No Auer Rods
MDS associated with isolated del(5q)	Anemia Usually normal or increased platelet count <5% blasts	Normal to increased megakaryocytes with hypolobated nuclei <5% blasts Isolated del(5q) cytogenetic abnormality No Auer rods

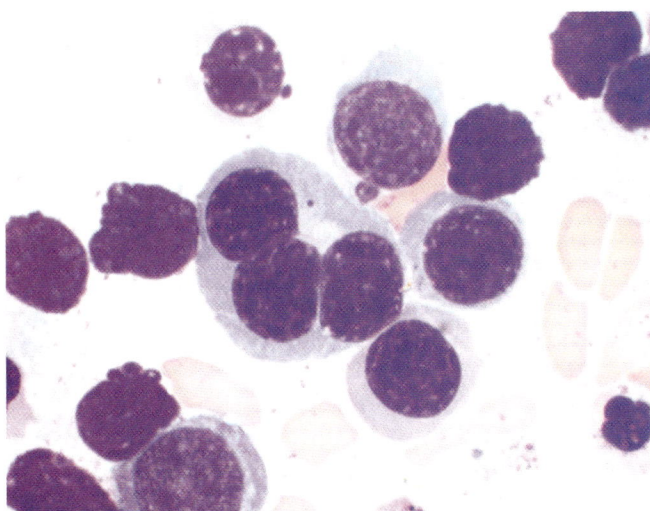

FIGURE 20-49
Myelodysplastic syndrome. Dysplastic, multinucleated, megaloblastoid red cells are shown.

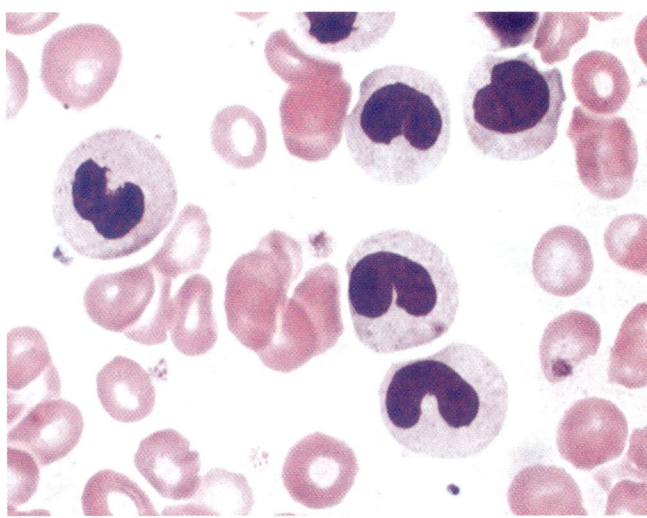

FIGURE 20-51
Myelodysplastic syndrome. Hypogranular granulocytes.

Pathology: The morphological classification of MDS is based upon the presence of abnormally shaped hematopoietic cells and the proportion of myeloblasts (Table 20-16). Dysplastic features may be present in one or more hematopoietic lineages. They are most frequent in erythroid precursors, which show megaloblastoid changes, multinucleation, nuclear budding, bridging between nuclei, and karyorrhexis (Fig. 20-49). Ringed sideroblasts are common (Fig. 20-50). Dysgranulopoietic features include nuclear hypersegmentation or hyposegmentation (*pseudo Pelger-Huët cells*) and cytoplasmic hypogranulation (Fig. 20-51). Dysplastic megakaryocytes include mononuclear or hypolobated forms and cells with nuclear separation (Fig. 20-52).

MDS with more than 15% ringed sideroblasts (RS) are designated MDS-RS. Cases with more than 5% blasts are termed *refractory anemia with excess blasts (RAEB)*. Increased blasts in the marrow that are accompanied by clusters of immature cells in the interstitium are called *atypical localization of immature precursors* (ALIP).

Cytogenetic and molecular studies are essential for the diagnosis and prognosis of myelodysplastic syndromes. Isolated deletion of chromosome 5 (5q-) occurs primarily in women and indicates a more favorable prognosis. Unlike other types of MDS, 5q- syndrome features normal or increased platelet counts. Other favorable chromosomal abnormalities are -y, and 20q-. By contrast, deletion of chromosome 7 (7q-) carries an unfavorable prognosis. The more

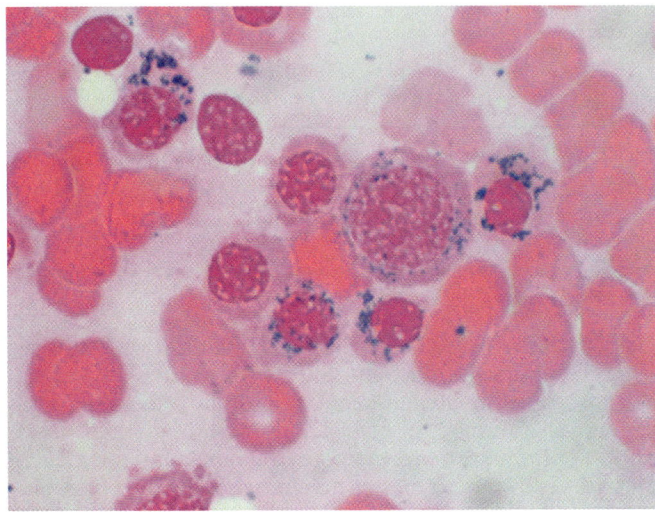

FIGURE 20-50
Ringed sideroblast. Smear of a bone marrow aspirate stained with Prussian blue shows an erythroid precursor cell containing iron-laden mitochondria that encircle the nuclei.

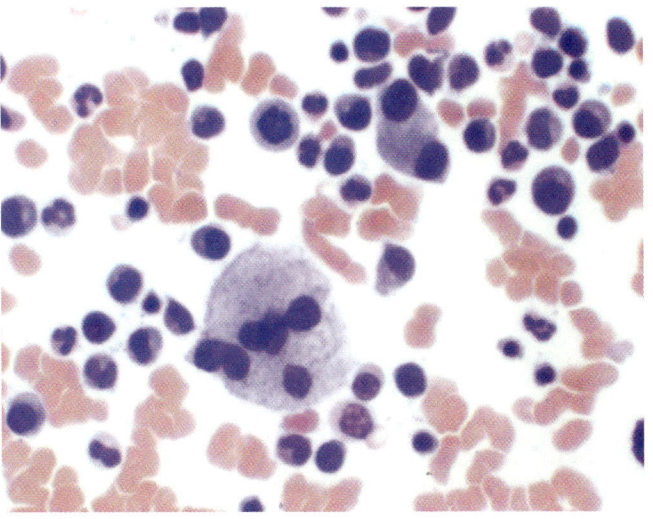

FIGURE 20-52
Myelodysplastic syndrome. Dysplastic megakaryocyte with nuclear separation.

chromosomal abnormalities present, the less favorable is the outcome of disease.

Clinical Features: MDS presents with anemia, neutropenia, and thrombocytopenia. Patients with the disease are at increased risk for acute leukemia, and the higher the proportion of blasts in the bone marrow, the greater is the risk.

Refractory Anemia

Refractory anemia (RA) is a type of MDS defined as ineffective erythropoiesis with dysplastic features. It is a disease of the elderly, accounting for 5 to 10% of all cases of MDS. There is no increase in blasts or ringed sideroblasts. RA is a diagnosis of exclusion, and other conditions that produce abnormal erythroid precursors (e.g., alcohol, drugs and toxins, viruses, and vitamin deficiencies) must be ruled out.

Pathology: Bone marrow biopsy shows higher than expected cellularity, with marked erythropoietic proliferation. This discrepancy with the anemia reflects ineffective erythropoiesis. Iron stains demonstrate increased iron in macrophages, but less than 15% ringed sideroblasts.

There are no specific immunophenotypical abnormalities in RA, but an abnormal karyotype is determined in 25% of cases, including 5q-, 7q-, 20q-, and trisomy 8.

Clinical Features: The median survival in RA is 5 years. Progression to acute leukemia occurs in 5 to 10% of cases.

Refractory Anemia with Ringed Sideroblasts (RARS)

A diagnosis of RARS requires that 15% or more nucleated red blood cells be ringed sideroblasts (Fig. 20-50). In iron stains, the nucleus of ringed sideroblasts is encircled by at least 10 siderotic granules, representing accumulation of iron in mitochondria. RARS accounts for 10% of all cases of MDS and is typically seen in the elderly. The etiology of the disorder is unknown.

Pathology: Morphological findings in the bone marrow in patients with RARS are similar to those noted in patients with RA who present with marked erythroid hyperplasia. Red cells in the blood smear may exhibit a dimorphic pattern, namely a mixture of normochromic and hypochromic cells. Signs of iron overload are common, with abundant siderophages in the bone marrow and increased iron deposits in the liver and spleen.

Clinical Features: The symptoms of RARS are mainly related to moderate anemia and progressive iron overload. Of all the different types of MDS, RARS has the lowest risk for AML (1–2%). The median survival is 6 years.

Refractory Cytopenia with Multilineage Dysplasia (RCMD)

RCMD is a MDS characterized by dysplastic erythroblasts and dysplastic features in at least 10% of the cells of one additional hematopoietic lineage.

Pathology: Dysplastic changes are present in 10% or more of cells of at least two hematopoietic lineages. In addition to the changes in erythroid precursors, neutrophilic precursors may demonstrate hypogranulation and nuclear hyposegmentation or hypersegmentation. Abnormalities of megakaryocytes may also be present. Chromosomal abnormalities are seen in half of patients with RCMD or RCMD-RS.

Clinical Features: Most patients with RCMD show evidence of bone marrow failure. A discrepancy between a hypercellular bone marrow and a striking peripheral cytopenia indicates ineffective hematopoiesis. Ten percent of patients proceed to acute leukemia, and the median survival is less than 3 years.

Refractory Anemia with Excess Blasts (RAEB)

RAEB shows up to 20% myeloblasts in the bone marrow and accounts for more than one third of all cases of MDS. Persons above the age of 50 years are affected.

Pathology: The dysplastic features of RAEB are similar to those in other types of myelodysplasia. Since the myelopoietic cells show a left shift, with an increased number of blasts, abnormal (interstitial) localization of immature precursors in the bone marrow may be present. As in other types of myelodysplasia, the bone marrow is usually hypercellular, although hypocellular variants are seen in 10% of patients. Cytogenetic abnormalities are the same as described in other types of myelodysplasia. The immunophenotype of the blasts detected by flow cytometry are the same as those in many types of AML.

Clinical Features: Patients with RAEB present with symptoms of peripheral pancytopenia and bone marrow failure. The prognosis deteriorates with an increasing number of blasts, and the median survival is 1 to 2 years.

5q-Syndrome

The 5q- MDS is associated with isolated del(5q) and shows less than 5% blasts in the bone marrow. Patients present with symptoms of refractory anemia. This disorder is typically seen in middle-aged women, as opposed to older persons in other types of MDS. The 5q- syndrome has a relatively favorable prognosis.

Acute Myeloid Leukemia (AML) Features Myeloblasts with Maturation Arrest

AML is characterized by clonal expansion of myeloblasts in the bone marrow and their subsequent appearance in blood and tissues. According to the WHO classification, **more than 20% blasts should be present in the bone marrow to establish a diagnosis of AML.** If less than 20% blasts are present, the process should be designated RAEB. The blasts should have cytochemical and immunophenotypic characteristics of myeloid cells. Four types of AML are recognized (Table 20-17):

AML with recurrent genetic abnormalities
AML evolving from multilineage dysplasia
AML—therapy related
AML not otherwise categorized. (Overlaps with the M-types of the old FAB classification, see Fig. 20-53, see Table 20-17)

 Epidemiology: Of all acute leukemias, 70% are myeloid leukemias, and the remaining 30% are lymphoblastic leukemias. Most cases of AML are seen in adults, with a median age of 60 years at onset.

 Pathogenesis: Most cases of AML are of unknown etiology, but in a few instances a causal relationship between radiation, cytotoxic chemotherapy, or benzene exposure has been documented. An increase in AML was noted following the detonation of atomic bombs in Hiroshima and Nagasaki (see Chapter 8). Cigarette smoking doubles the risk for AML. **The major problems associated with AML relate principally to progressive accumulation in the marrow of immature myeloid cells that lack the potential for further differentiation and maturation.** Whereas leukemic myeloblasts replicate at a slower rate than do normal hematopoietic precursor cells, the frequency of spontaneous cell death is less than normal. The expanded pool of abnormal leukemic blasts encroaches on the marrow and suppresses normal hematopoiesis. As a consequence, the major clinical problems in AML are **granulocytopenia, thrombocytopenia, and anemia.**

 Pathology: Malignant myeloblasts of AML are detectable in the bone marrow and in most instances in peripheral blood. Typically, the malignant cells pack the bone marrow and displace normal hematopoietic cells (Fig. 20-54). Myeloblasts are medium-sized to large cells with round or slightly irregular nuclei. Depending on the subtype, Auer rods may be present in the cytoplasm (Fig. 20-55). These inclusions are specific for the myeloid lineage and preclude a diagnosis of lymphoblastic leukemia.

Immunophenotyping by flow cytometry and cytogenetic studies are essential for the correct classification of AML. Myeloid markers that are frequently expressed include CD13, CD15, CD33, CD34, and CD117. AML with megakaryoblastic differentiation may exhibit the platelet/megakaryocyte markers CD41 and CD61 (platelet GPIIb/IIIa complex).

Important cytochemical markers include myeloperoxidase, Sudan black, and nonspecific esterase (NSE). Myeloperoxidase and Sudan black decorate myeloid cells and their precursors with increased staining intensity in the more mature forms. Nonspecific esterase labels monoblasts and promonocytes and is a marker for AML with monocytoid differentiation (Fig. 20-56).

Acute Myeloid Leukemia with Recurrent Genetic Abnormalities

The WHO classification of AML defines four different types with recurrent genetic abnormalities:

AML with t(8;21) (AML1/ETO)
AML with inv(16) or t(16;16)(CBFβ/MYH11)
Acute promyelocytic leukemia (AML with t(15;17)(PML/RARα)
AML with 11q23 (MLL) abnormalities

Acute Promyelocytic Leukemia

Acute promyelocytic leukemia (APL) is defined by a chromosomal translocation involving the PML1 *gene and the retinoic acid receptor (RAR) gene.* The disease affects mainly middle-aged patients and accounts for 5 to 10% of all cases of AML.

 Pathogenesis: The underlying genetic defect in APL is a translocation involving the *PML* gene on chromosome 15 and the *RARα* gene on chromosome 17. The resulting *PML/RARα* fusion gene encodes a functional retinoic acid receptor. The receptor can be targeted by all-*trans*-retinoic acid (ATRA), which mediates maturation of the tumor cells (see below).

 Pathology: The bone marrow is packed with tumor cells that have promyelocytic morphological features. Auer rods are abundantly present (Fig. 20-55). The leukemic cells show strong reactivity for myeloperoxidase or Sudan black. Myeloid markers CD13 and CD33

MORPHOLOGY	CLASSIFICATION	NUCLEUS	NUCLEOLUS	CHROMATIN	CYTOPLASM
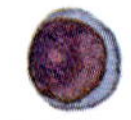	L1 ACUTE LYMPHOBLASTIC (principally pediatric)	Uniformly round, small	Single, indistinct	Slightly reticulated with perinucleolar clumping	Scant, blue
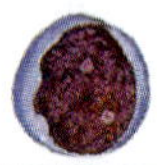	L2 LYMPHOBLASTIC (principally adult)	Irregular	Single to several, indistinct	Fine	Moderate, pale
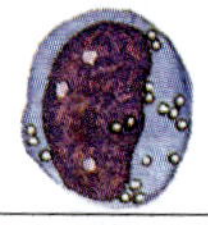	L3 BURKITT-TYPE	Round to oval	Two to five	Coarse with clear parachromatin	Moderate blue, prominently vacuolated
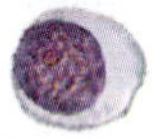	M0 MYELOBLASTIC (minimally differentiated)	Round to oval	Single to multiple, distinct	Fine to coarse	Scant, non-granulated
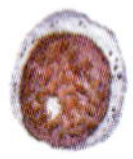	M1 MYELOBLASTIC (without maturation)	Round to oval	Single to multiple, distinct	Fine	Scant, variably granulated
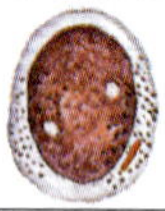	M2 MYELOBLASTIC (with maturation)	Round to oval	Single to multiple, distinct	Fine	Moderate azurophilic granules with or without Auer rods
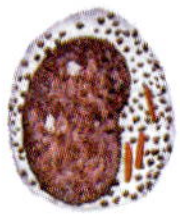	M3 MYELOCYTIC	Round to indented to lobed, cottage-loaf	Single to multiple, (granules may obscure)	Fine	Prominent azurophilic granules and/or multiple Auer rods
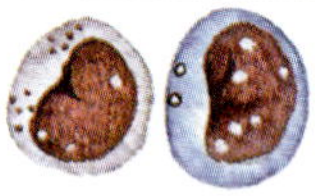	M4 MYELOMONOBLASTIC (biphasic M1 and M5)	Round to indented, folded	Single to multiple, distinct	Fine	Moderate, blue to gray, may be granulated
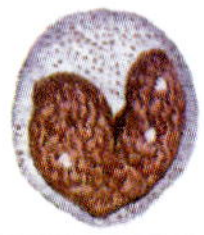	M5 MONOBLASTIC	Round to indented, folded	Single to multiple, distinct	Variable, lacy or ropy	Scant to moderate, gray-blue, dustlike lavender granules
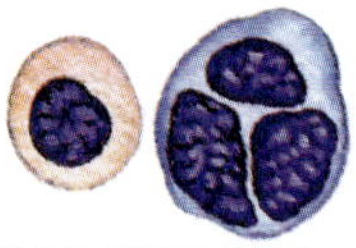	M6 ERYTHROBLASTIC	Single to bizarre multinucleated, multilobed	Single to multiple, distinct	Open megaloblastoid	Abundant, red to blue
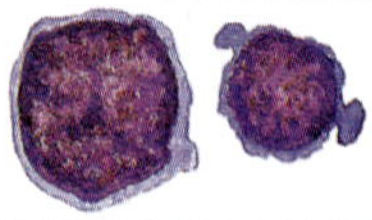	M7 MEGAKARYOBLASTIC	Round to oval	Single to multiple, distinct	Slightly to moderately reticulated	Scant to moderate, gray-blue, with blebbing

FIGURE 20-53
Morphology of acute leukemia in the traditional French-American-British (FAB) classification scheme. The acute myeloid leukemias in the FAB classification (M0–M7) largely overlap with "AML-not otherwise categorized" in the new WHO classification.

may be positive. Unlike in mature forms of AML, HLA-DR and CD34 are negative.

Clinical Features: Patients with APL frequently present with DIC. Senescent leukemic cells degranulate and activate the coagulation cascade. Treatment with ATRA induces maturation of the tumor cells and prevents both degranulation and DIC. APL is a paradigm for a molecularly defined disease in which the underlying genetic defect determines the type of treatment.

Therapy-Induced Acute Myeloid Leukemias and Myelodysplastic Syndromes

Treatment of solid tumors with chemotherapy or radiation therapy can induce later hematopoietic cancers. The most common therapy-induced secondary malignancies are MDS and AML. Alkylating agents and topoisomerase II inhibitors (epipodophylotoxins) most often give rise to AML. AML or MDS following treatment with alkylating agents or radiation occur with a median latency period of approximately 6 years, whereas AML after treatment with topoisomerase II inhibitor occurs on average 3 years after treatment.

TABLE 20-17 WHO Classification of Acute Myeloid Leukemia (AML)

Acute myeloid leukemia with recurrent genetic abnormalities
    Acute myeloid leukemia with t(8;21)(q22;q22);(AML1/ETO)
    Acute myeloid leukemia with abnormal bone marrow eosinophils inv(16)(p13q22) or t(16;16)(p13;q22);(CBFβ/MYH11)
    Acute promyelocytic leukemia (AML with t(15;17)(q22;q12)(PML/RARα) and variants (FAB-M3)
    Acute myeloid leukemia with 11q23 (MLL) abnormalities
Acute myeloid leukemia with multilineage dysplasia
    Following a myelodysplastic syndrome or myelodysplastic syndrome/myeloproliferative disorder
    Without antecedent myelodysplastic syndrome
Acute myeloid leukemia and myelodysplastic syndromes, therapy related
    Alkylating agent related
    Topoisomerase type II inhibitor related (some may be lymphoid)
    Other types
Acute myeloid leukemia not otherwise categorized
    Acute myeloid leukemia minimally differentiated (FAB M0)
    Acute myeloid leukemia without maturation (FAB M1)
    Acute myeloid leukemia with maturation (FAB-M2)
    Acute myelomonocytic leukemia (FAB-M4)
    Acute monoblastic and monocytic leukemia (FAB-M5)
    Acute erythroid leukemia (FAB-M6)
    Acute megakaryoblastic leukemia (FAB-M7)
    Acute basophilic leukemia
    Acute panmyelosis with myelofibrosis
    Myeloid sarcoma

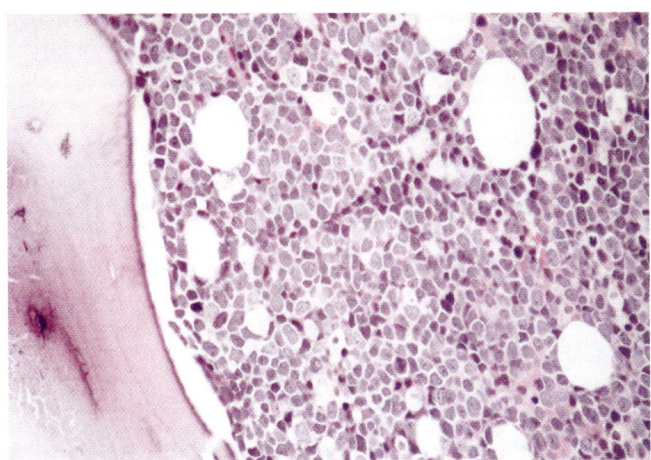

FIGURE 20-54
Acute myelogenous leukemia. A bone marrow section is hypercellular, owing to effacement of the normal architecture by myeloblasts.

 Pathology: Secondary AML is often associated with monocytoid morphology and immunophenotype. The most common translocations in this type of AML involve the *MLL* (mixed lineage leukemia) gene (11q23).

positive for t(8;21) is classified as AML with recurrent cytogenetic abnormalities.

M3—APL: Many of the leukemic cells in acute promyelocytic leukemia resemble normal promyelocytes. Auer rods are common. APL associated with chromosome translocations involving the retinoic acid receptor gene on chromosome 17 now belongs in the group of leukemias with recurrent cytogenetic abnormalities (see above).

M4—Acute myelomonocytic leukemia (AMML): Some 20 to 80% of tumor cells show monocytoid features. AMML accounts for 20% of all AMLs, with a median age at onset of 50 years. Extramedullary infiltration of leukemic cells is common.

M5—Acute monoblastic/monocytic leukemia (AMoL): At least 80% of the myeloid cells have monocytoid differentiation (Fig. 20-57). AmoL constitutes 5 to 8% of all cases of AML and is seen in younger patients. It is also a common leukemia in infancy, in which case it is associated with 11q23 translocations and is classified as AML with recurrent cytogenetic abnormality. Extramedullary masses are

Acute Myeloid Leukemia, Not Otherwise Categorized

The varieties of AML not otherwise categorized do not demonstrate recurrent cytogenetic abnormalities and are not therapy related. Subtypes in this type of AML essentially follow the old French–American–British (FAB) morphological classification for AMLs.

M0—AML, minimally differentiated: The leukemic cells are immature myeloblasts with no defining morphological criteria of the myeloid lineage. Immunophenotyping by flow cytometry establishes the myeloid nature of the tumor cells. The prognosis is unfavorable.

M1—AML without maturation: Less than 10% of the myeloid cells are promyelocytes or more mature myeloid cells. The disease occurs most often in middle-aged persons. Occasional Auer rods may be seen.

M2—AML with maturation: More than 10% maturing myeloid cells (promyelocytes and later) are present. The disease occurs in all age groups. AML with maturation

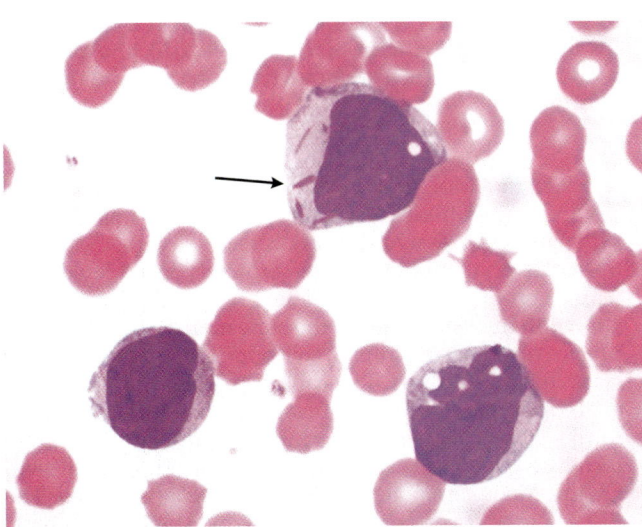

FIGURE 20-55
Acute promyelocytic leukemia. Auer rods are prominent.

Reaction	LYMPHOID	MYELOID	MONOCYTOID
PAS			
CAE			
SBB			
APh			
ANAE			
ANAE/NaF			

FIGURE 20-56
Acute lymphoblastic, myeloblastic, and monocytic leukemias: cytochemical stains. *PAS*, periodic acid–Schiff; *CAE*, chloracetate esterase; *SBB*, Sudan black B; *APh*, acid phosphatase; *ANAE*, α-naphthol acetate esterase (with and without fluoride inhibition).

common in AMoL and may involve the skin, gingiva, and CNS. Some patients exhibit bleeding disorders. AMoL pursues an aggressive clinical course.

M6—Acute erythroid leukemia: Acute erythroid leukemias feature prominent erythropoietic proliferation; more than 50% of all nucleated cells in the bone marrow are erythroid precursors. The remaining cell population consists of at least 20% myeloblasts. Typically, the disease progresses to a predominance of myeloblasts. A rare, more chronic, form of this disease displays pure erythroblasts and is referred to as *erythremic myelosis* or *di Guglielmo syndrome*. Erythroid leukemia may present with severe anemia. The disease may evolve de novo or follow MDS. The clinical course is aggressive.

M7—Acute megakaryoblastic leukemia (AMegL): At least 50% of the blasts demonstrate a megakaryocytic immunophenotype.

Epidemiology: AMegL is an uncommon leukemia that makes up less than 5% of all types of AML. It is a distinct childhood leukemia associated with t(1;22) and hepatosplenomegaly. It occurs as a late complication in young adult men suffering from mediastinal germ cell tumors.

Pathology: In peripheral blood, micromegakaryocytes, megakaryocytic fragments, atypical platelets, or blasts can be seen. The bone marrow often shows marked fibrosis resulting from the release of PDGF, which stimulates fibroblasts to deposit collagen.

Cytogenetic abnormalities include t(1;22) and chromosome 3 abnormalities. The tumor blasts may express the platelet-associated markers CD41 and CD61 (platelet GPIIb/GPIIIa complex), CD42(platelet GPIb) or factor VIII-related antigen (vWF). Myeloid markers CD13 and CD33 are present.

The prognosis is uniformly dismal, particularly in children with t(1;22). A variant of AMegL is seen in children with Down syndrome.

Myeloid sarcoma

Myeloid sarcoma is an extramedullary solid tumor consisting of myeloblasts or monoblasts (Fig. 20-58). Another term for this entity is *chloroma* because of its greenish color. The term *granulocytic sarcoma* applies to lesions that are composed predominantly of myeloblasts. *Monoblastic sarcoma* is less common

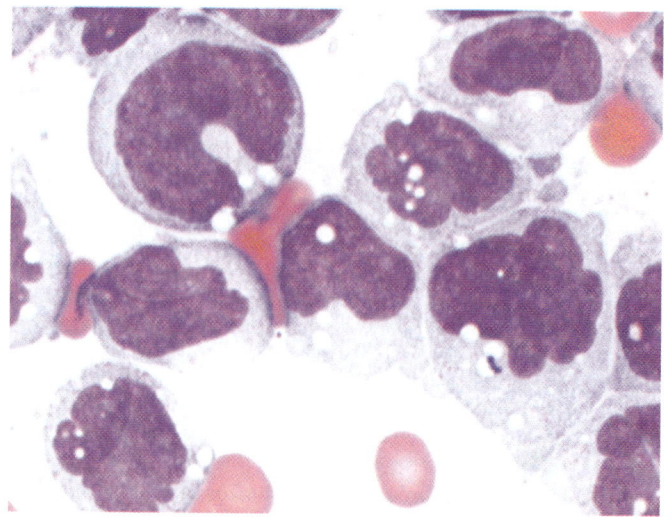

FIGURE 20-57
Acute monoblastic leukemia.

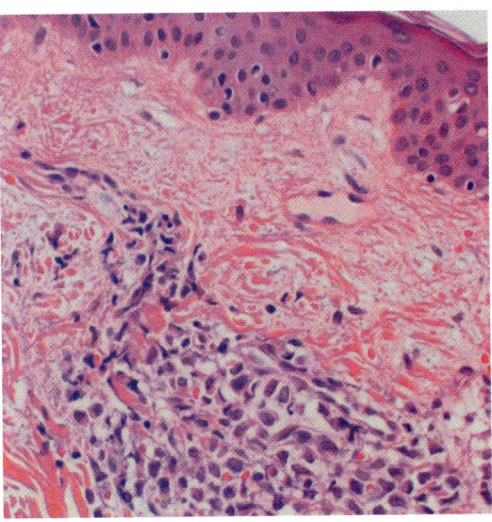

FIGURE 20-58
Myeloid sarcoma. The skin from a patient with acute monoblastic leukemia (leukemia cutis) shows neoplastic myeloid cells.

than granulocytic sarcoma and is most commonly associated with translocations involving the MLL gene (11q23).

Myeloid sarcoma may evolve de novo or in association with AML, or it may represent the blast phase in myeloproliferative disorders. The prognosis is determined by the underlying leukemic process.

Disorders of the Lymphopoietic System

NORMAL LYMPHOCYTES

The lymphopoietic system consists of circulating B and T lymphocytes and lymphoid organs, including lymph nodes, spleen, thymus, and mucosa-associated lymphoid tissue (MALT). MALT comprises the oropharyngeal lymphoid tissue (Waldeyer's ring), the gut-associated lymphoid tissue (GALT), and the bronchus-associated lymphoid tissue (BALT).

Lymphocytes are all derived from bone marrow stem cells. Cells that undergo differentiation and maturation in the thymus are termed *T cells;* those that develop in the bone marrow are called *B cells*. The differentiation and maturation of lymphocytes are associated with a sequential gain and loss of a number of cytoplasmic and surface antigens. The pattern of expression of these antigens identifies the character of the cells or the maturation stage of a neoplastic clone.

T lymphocytes: the lymphocytic stem cells that migrate to the thymus are exposed to a number of thymic hormones that first induce the expression of CD2 surface receptors that bind sheep erythrocytes. At this point, recombination of the T-cell receptor genes leads to the production of many different receptors, each of which recognizes a single antigen. The T-cell receptor is present on the membrane in association with a CD3 molecule; the CD2 and CD3 markers define the cells as T cells. Other markers appear, such as CD5 and particularly CD4 (helper) or CD8 (suppressor). The cells then migrate from the thymus to lymph nodes, spleen, and peripheral blood.

When exposed to antigens specific for their receptors, $CD4^+$ cells become activated. These antigens are peptide fragments derived from the partial digestion of proteins by macrophages or antigen-presenting cells. When such antigens are presented in association with a class 2 HLA molecule, $CD4^+$ cells become activated, release mitogenic growth factors (IL-1 and IL-2), and undergo transformation to a helper/inducer cell. In turn these T cells interact with B lymphocytes that express the same antigenic specificity, thereby promoting proliferation of the latter and inducing their differentiation to immunoglobulin-producing plasma cells.

$CD8^+$ cells are activated when their receptors recognize peptides presented in association with a class I HLA antigen, after which they become suppressor/cytotoxic cells. $CD8^+$ cells limit the expansion of activated B cells and terminate their immune response.

A subpopulation of T lymphocytes activated by antigenic peptides becomes cytotoxic lymphocytes (killer cells), which eliminate foreign cells or viruses bearing the recognized antigen.

B lymphocytes: the precursor cells of B lymphocytes acquire their repertoire of cytoplasmic and cell surface antigens in the bone marrow. The earliest B-cell marker to appear on the cell surface is CD19, followed by CD20, CD22, and CD79a. Like the surface membrane of all cells, the surface membrane of B cells expresses HLA class I antigen. However, it also displays an HLA class II antigen, a feature shared only by antigen-processing and presenting cells. Early in B-cell maturation, the antigen CALLA (common acute leukemia/lymphoma antigen, CD10) is present for a short time, as is the nuclear antigen TdT.

As the B lymphocytes mature, the genes for the immunoglobulin heavy chains are rearranged in preparation for the synthesis of IgM molecules. In pre-B cells, IgM is expressed in the cytoplasm.

Mature B cells express surface pan B-cell markers CD19, CD20, CD22, as well as heavy and light Ig chains. When activated by an antigen and stimulated by an appropriate T-helper cell, B cells transform into plasma cells that synthesize and export immunoglobulins. At this stage, they no longer display heavy or light Ig chains on the surface membrane.

Null cells: a small proportion of lymphocytes do not express either B- or T-lymphocyte differentiation antigens and are, therefore, termed *null cells*. They may function as cytotoxic or natural killer cells (*NK cells*), which do not require antigenic recognition for their function. Morphologically, NK cells are recognized by their granular cytoplasm (*large granular lymphocytes*).

Lymphocytes exhibit a heterogeneous morphological appearance. Small to medium-sized lymphocytes may be primitive, antigen-independent B and T cells or antigen-dependent, committed cells that have not been reexposed to the specific sensitizing antigen. When activated by an antigen, both B and T lymphocytes undergo transformation to large, protein-synthesizing cells, called *atypical lymphocytes* in peripheral blood smears and *immunoblasts* in tissue sections. Atypical lymphocytes in smears visualized with the Wright-Giemsa stain tend to have abundant blue-gray cytoplasm and multiple nucleoli. The same cells in tissue sections stained with hematoxylin and eosin have a round to oval nucleus with clear or vesicular chromatin, one to several eosinophilic nucleoli apposed to the nuclear membrane, and abundant clear to purple cytoplasm. In tissues affected by infections and immune reactions, the size and appearance of lymphocytes varies widely, owing to lymphocyte transformation and modulation. Small lymphocytes, partially activated (transformed) lymphocytes, and large activated lymphocytes (immunoblasts) are all observed.

Normal germinal centers of lymph follicles exhibit a spectrum of B cells. The cell population varies from small lymphocytes with irregularly indented or "cleaved" nuclei *(centrocytes)* to large lymphocytes with vesicular, irregular to round nuclei *(centroblasts)*. In lymphoid tissue other than germinal centers, B lymphocytes are more regular and have round-to-oval hyperchromatic nuclei and blue-purple cytoplasm. Immunoblast-like cells with prominent blue-purple cytoplasm are termed *plasmacytoid immunoblasts*.

Terminally differentiated, effector B lymphocytes are recognized as *plasma cells* in both smears and tissue sections. These cells have an eccentric nucleus with clumped chromatin marginated on the nuclear membrane, traditionally described as "clockface chromatin." The abundant blue-purple cytoplasm of plasma cells often displays a clear paranuclear clear zone representing the Golgi complex.

T lymphocytes are usually indistinguishable from B cells in tissue sections. Infrequently, they show an irregularly contoured nuclear membrane and pale, clear cytoplasm. In peripheral blood, 60 to 80% of circulating lymphocytes are of T-cell lineage and 10 to 15% are of B-cell origin. The remainder are null cells lacking both B- and T-cell lineage differentiation markers.

LYMPH NODES

Lymph nodes consist of organized collections of lymphoid tissue located along the lymphatic vessels. Typically grayish white and ovoid or bean-shaped, they vary from 2 mm to 2 cm in diameter. A fibrous capsule and radiating trabeculae provide a supporting structure, and a delicate reticular network contributes internal support. Architecturally, lymph nodes exhibit an outer cortex and an inner medulla. The cortex contains defined B-cell and T-cell domains (Fig. 20-59).

The B cell-dependent cortex consists of two types of follicles. Immunologically inactive follicles are termed *primary follicles;* active ones that contain germinal centers are referred to as *secondary follicles*. Primary follicles consist of cohesive aggregates of small, normal-appearing lymphocytes. Germinal centers contain large lymphocytes (centroblasts) and small lymphocytes with cleaved nuclei (centro-

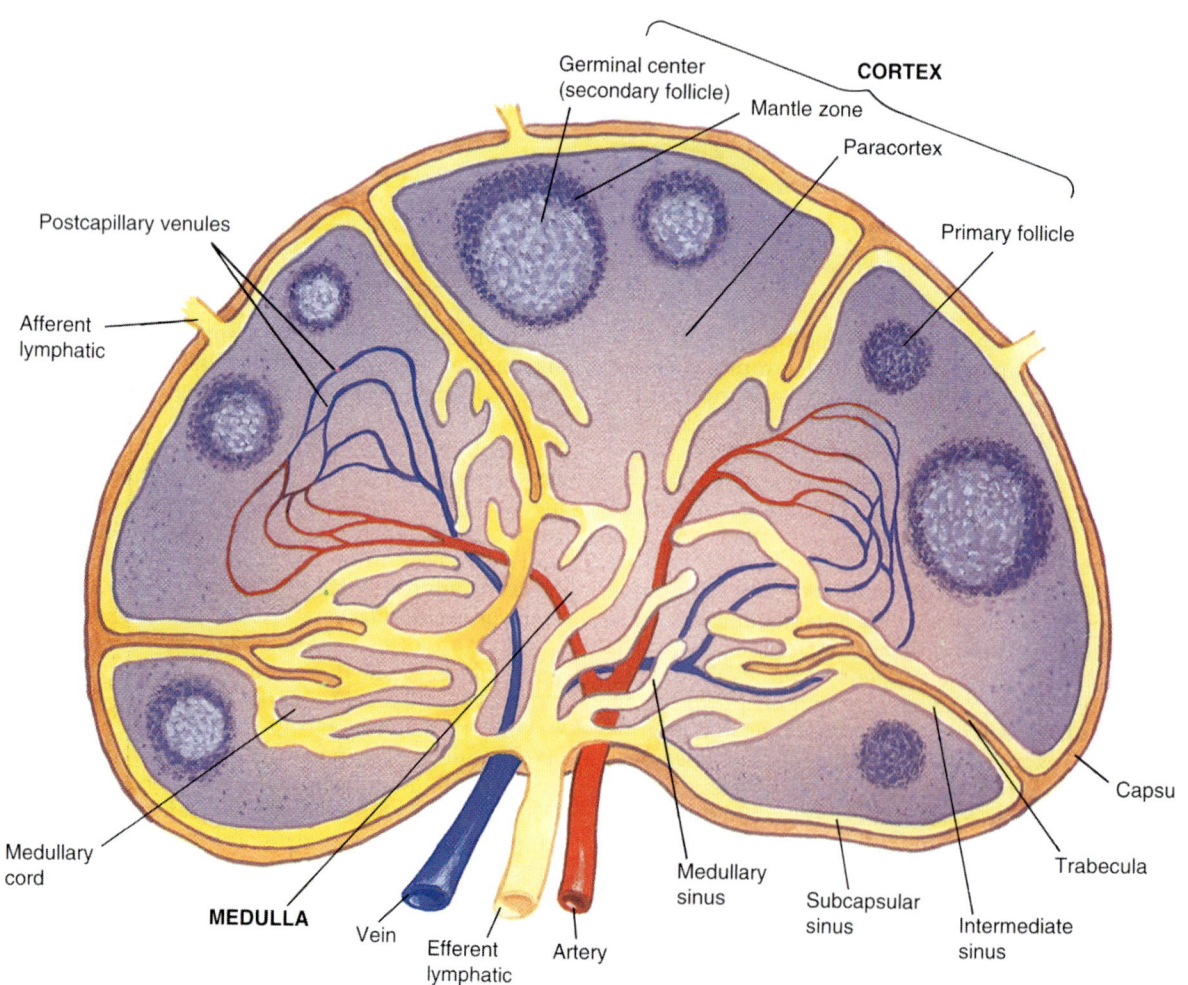

FIGURE 20-59
Structure of a normal lymph node.

cytes). There are also scattered macrophages that contain phagocytized nuclear and cytoplasmic debris ("tingible body" macrophages). The follicular dendritic cells (FDCs) are stellate cells with long cytoplasmic processes, which form a meshwork of cells that present antigens to follicular B cells. Macrophages and, to a lesser extent, dendritic cells provide growth factors for activated B cells. Following activation and clonal expansion in the germinal centers, B lymphocytes migrate to the B cell-dependent medullary cords of the lymph nodes and either become immunoglobulin-secreting plasma cells or exit the lymph nodes as memory B lymphocytes.

The T cell-dependent paracortex, also known as the deep cortex, is situated between the B-cell follicles and deep to them. In addition to T lymphocytes, scattered macrophages and interdigitating reticulum cells (IDCs) are found in the paracortex. IDCs process and present antigens to T lymphocytes, which in turn proliferate and induce the transformation of both T cells and B cells.

Circulating B lymphocytes and T lymphocytes enter the lymph nodes by migrating through the tall endothelial cells of the postcapillary venules in the paracortex. T lymphocytes tend to remain in the paracortex; B lymphocytes home to the germinal centers.

Lymph or interstitial fluid enters the lymph nodes through afferent lymphatics in the convexity of the cortex. Percolating first through the subcapsular sinuses and then the radial sinuses, lymph exits through efferent lymphatics. The sinuses are lined by cells that belong to the mononuclear phagocyte system. The arrangement of the sinuses maximizes the exposure of foreign antigens in lymph to macrophages and to immunoreactive B cells and T cells.

LYMPHOID TISSUE OF THE INTESTINE AND BRONCHUS

Aggregates of lymphoid tissue are present along the course of the gastrointestinal tract, with prominent accentuation in the oropharynx and nasopharynx *(Waldeyer ring)* and in Peyer patches of the terminal ileum. Less prominent aggregates of lymphocytes are also distributed in the lamina propria of the bronchial tree *(BALT)*. In sites such as the tonsils and Peyer patches, lymphocytes arrive by migration through tall endothelial cells of vessels that are comparable to the postcapillary venules of the lymph nodes. *(MALT)* plays an important role in immunological protection of the host in areas vulnerable to potential invaders. IgA secretion is a prominent component of this protective function.

BENIGN DISORDERS OF THE LYMPHOPOIETIC SYSTEM

Lymphocytosis Reflects Infections or Lymphoproliferative Conditions

Peripheral blood lymphocytosis is defined as an increase in the absolute peripheral blood lymphocyte count above the normal range (>4000/μL in adults, 7000/μL in children, and 9000/μL in infants). The principal causes of absolute peripheral blood lymphocytosis are (1) acute infections (infectious mononucleosis, whooping cough, acute infectious lymphocytosis), (2) chronic bacterial infections (tuberculosis, brucellosis), and (3) lymphoproliferative diseases.

In addition to lymphocytosis, **atypical lymphocytes** are a hallmark of viral infections, particularly infectious mononucleosis, and some immunological disorders, such as drug reactions and serum sickness. Atypical lymphocytes are large cells (Fig. 20-60) with round to irregular nuclei, coarsely clumped chromatin, one to several distinct nucleoli, and abundant blue cytoplasm. Occasionally, the cytoplasm is vacuolated. Frequently, the cytoplasmic membrane is indented by surrounding erythrocytes (ballerina-skirt phenomenon). Most atypical lymphocytes are of the T-cell lineage (CD8$^+$ cytotoxic/suppressor cells).

Acute infectious lymphocytosis is a rare, self-limited, childhood disorder in which there is a marked peripheral blood lymphocytosis, principally T cells. Although lymphocytosis may persist for several weeks, affected children are usually asymptomatic. In a few cases of acute infectious lymphocytosis, mild fever, abdominal pain, and diarrhea occur. The etiology is unknown.

In **reactive lymphoid hyperplasia of the bone marrow,** an increased number of lymphocytes in the marrow may accompany peripheral blood lymphocytosis, although either may occur alone. In normal bone marrow, lymphocytes are distributed interstitially in the hematopoietic stroma or in cohesive aggregates called *lymphoid nodules*. In biopsy sections of the marrow, lymphoid hyperplasia has been defined as four or more lymphoid aggregates in any low-power (4×) microscopic field or as the presence of a single aggregate that measures at least 0.6 cm in diameter. An adult with more than 20% lymphocytes in either bone marrow aspirates or biopsy sections is considered to have lymphocytosis.

Plasmacytosis Is Most Common in End-Stage Multiple Myeloma

Peripheral blood plasmacytosis: An increase in plasma cells in the blood is uncommon. The most frequent cause is plasma cell neoplasia (multiple myeloma), usually in the terminal stages of the disease. Peripheral plasmacytosis is occa-

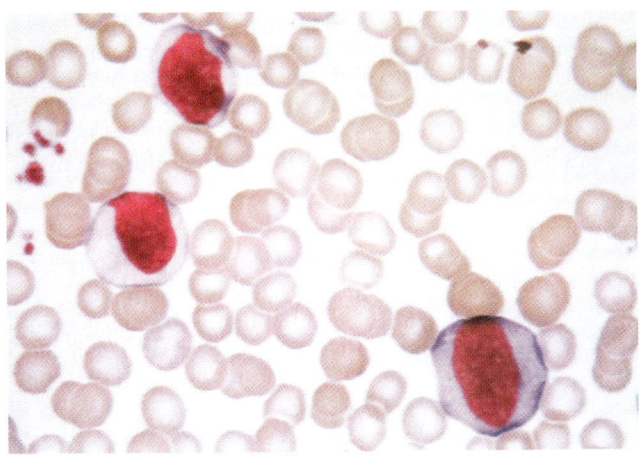

FIGURE **20-60**
Infectious mononucleosis. Atypical lymphocytes are characteristic.

sionally identified in some systemic immunological reactions and viral infections. Atypical lymphocytes sometimes resemble plasma cells, in which case they are called *Türk cells*.

Reactive bone marrow plasmacytosis: An increase in plasma cells in the marrow occurs in a variety of infectious, inflammatory, and neoplastic disorders. For example, it accompanies infections as diverse as bronchopneumonia and viral hepatitis. It also occurs in association with collagen vascular diseases and with epithelial cancers, such as carcinoma of the lung. Reactive bone marrow plasmacytosis is present when plasma cells constitute more than 3% of the total nucleated cell population in the bone marrow. In both reactive and neoplastic proliferation of plasma cells, immunoglobulin may accumulate in the cytoplasm to form a prominent eosinophilic globule called the *Russell body*. The invagination of immunoglobulin-containing cytoplasm into the nucleus, usually in plasma cell neoplasia, appears in cross section as an intranuclear eosinophilic globule called a *Dutcher body*.

Lymphocytopenia Usually Reflects a Decrease in T-Helper Lymphocytes

Peripheral blood lymphocytopenia is defined as a decrease in the peripheral blood lymphocyte count to less than 1500/μL in adults or less than 3000/μL in children. Since the predominant lymphocyte in the peripheral blood is the T helper-inducer (CD4$^+$) lymphocyte, lymphocytopenia generally indicates a decrease in these cells. There are several mechanisms by which lymphocytopenia occurs:

- **Decreased production of lymphocytes:** A variety of congenital and acquired immunodeficiency syndromes are characterized by reduced production of lymphocytes. Decreased production of T lymphocytes occurs in Hodgkin lymphoma, particularly in advanced stages.
- **Increased destruction of lymphocytes:** Lymphocytes are destroyed by a number of medical treatments, including x-irradiation, chemotherapy for malignant tumors, and the administration of antilymphocyte globulin, ACTH, or corticosteroids. Some viral infections, particularly AIDS, are characterized by the destruction of T cells.
- **Loss of lymphocytes:** Intestinal disorders that are associated with damage to lymphatics result in the loss of lymph and its lymphocytes into the intestinal lumen. Such maladies include the protein-losing enteropathies, Whipple disease, and disorders associated with increased central venous pressure (e.g., right-sided heart failure and chronic constrictive pericarditis). Immunological damage to lymphocytes may occur in the collagen vascular diseases, such as systemic lupus erythematosus.

Reactive Hyperplasia of Lymph Nodes Is a Response to Infections, Inflammation or Tumors

The lymph nodes may exhibit hyperplasia of all cellular components or any combination of B lymphocytes, T lymphocytes, and mononuclear phagocytic cells in response to a variety of infectious, inflammatory, and neoplastic disorders (Fig. 20-61).

- **Hyperplasia of the secondary follicles** (germinal centers) and plasmacytosis of the medullary cords indicate B-lymphocyte immunoreactivity.
- **Hyperplasia of the deep cortex or paracortex** (interfollicular or diffuse hyperplasia) is characteristic of T-lymphocyte immunoreactivity.

The histopathological features and degree of lymph node enlargement in immunoreactive hyperplasias reflect (1) the age of the patient (children tend to exhibit more pronounced immunoreactivity than adults), (2) the immunological competence of the host, and (3) the type of infectious agent or inflammatory disorder.

Acute suppurative lymphadenitis occurs in the lymph nodes that drain a site of acute bacterial infection. Suppurative lymph nodes enlarge rapidly because of edema and hyperemia and are tender, owing to distention of the capsule. Microscopically, infiltration of the lymph node sinuses and stroma by polymorphonuclear leukocytes and prominent follicular hyperplasia are noted.

The anatomical site of lymphadenopathy often provides a clue to its cause. For example, the posterior auricular lymph nodes are commonly enlarged in rubella infection; the occipital lymph nodes in scalp infections; the posterior cervical lymph nodes in toxoplasmosis; the axillary lymph nodes in infections of the upper extremities or chest wall; and the inguinal lymph nodes in venereal infections and infections of the lower extremities. Generalized lymphadenopathy may occur in systemic infections, hyperthyroidism, drug reactions, and collagen vascular diseases.

Follicular Hyperplasia

In **nonspecific reactive follicular hyperplasia,** a benign condition, prominent hyperplastic follicles occur principally in

FIGURE 20-61

Lymph nodes. Patterns of benign reactive hyperplasia are contrasted with the structure of a normal lymph node. *Follicular hyperplasia* with prominent enlarged and irregular benign follicles, is characteristic of B-cell immunoreactivity. *Interfollicular hyperplasia* is typical of T-cell immunoreactivity. The *sinusoidal pattern* with expansion of sinuses by benign macrophages is seen in reactive proliferations of the mononuclear–phagocyte system. Mixed patterns of follicular, interfollicular, and sinusoidal hyperplasia are common in a variety of complex immune reactions. In *necrotizing lymphadenitis,* variable necrosis of the lymph node architecture with residual cell debris is present. In *granulomatous inflammation,* cohesive clusters of macrophages and occasional multinucleated giant cells are characteristic.

Benign Disorders of the Lymphopoietic System

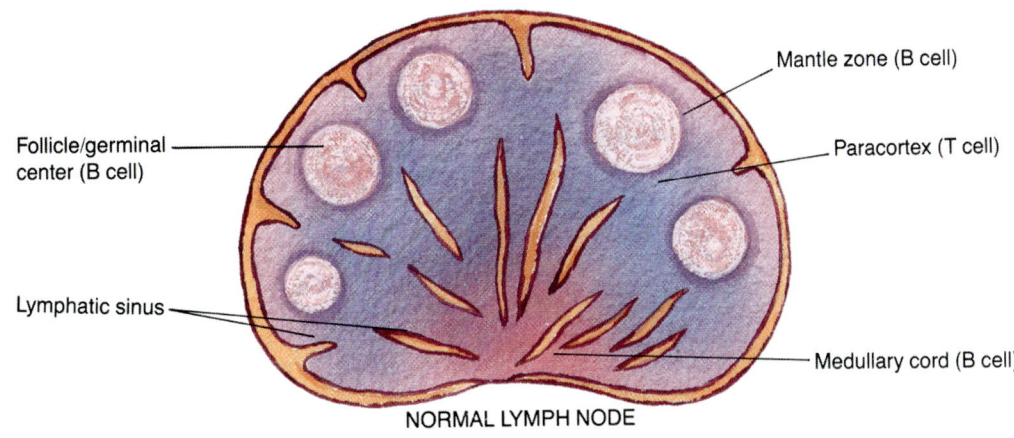

NORMAL LYMPH NODE

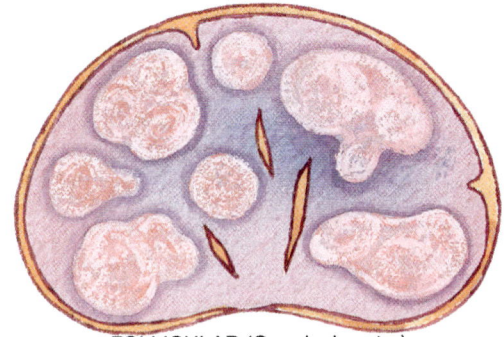

FOLLICULAR (Germinal center)

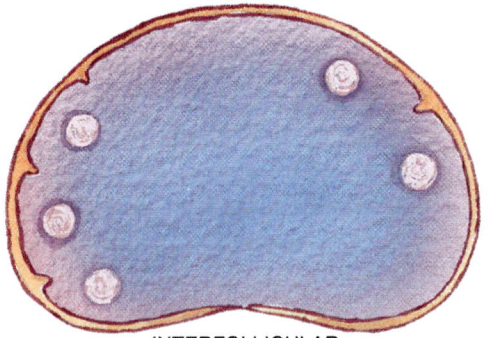

INTERFOLLICULAR

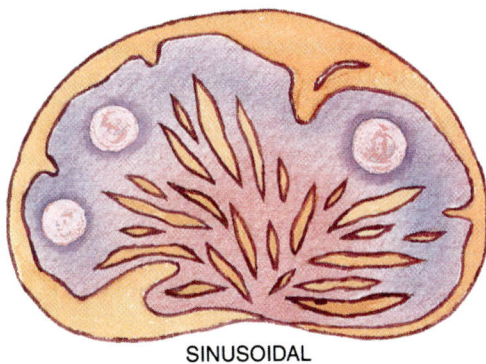

SINUSOIDAL

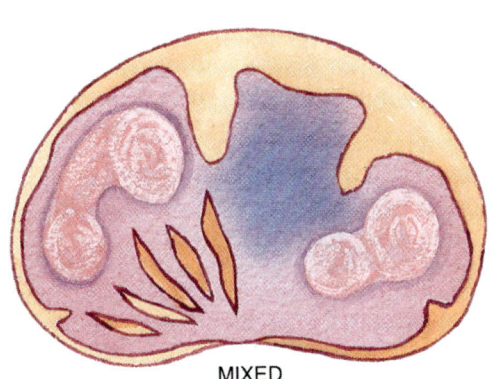

MIXED

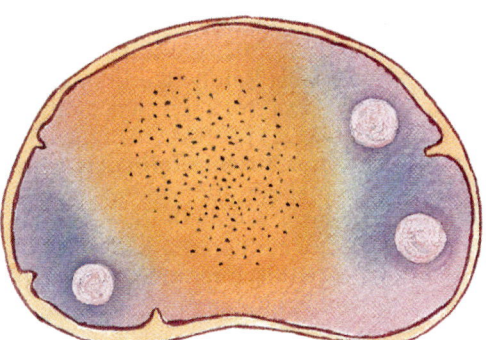

NECROTIZING

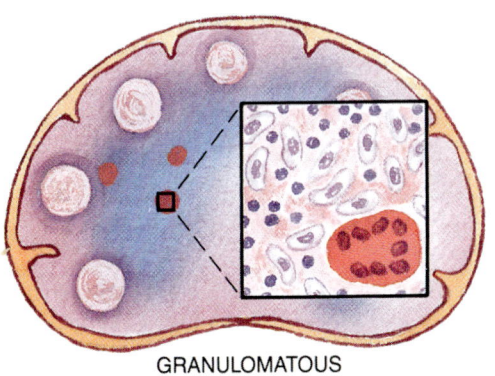

GRANULOMATOUS

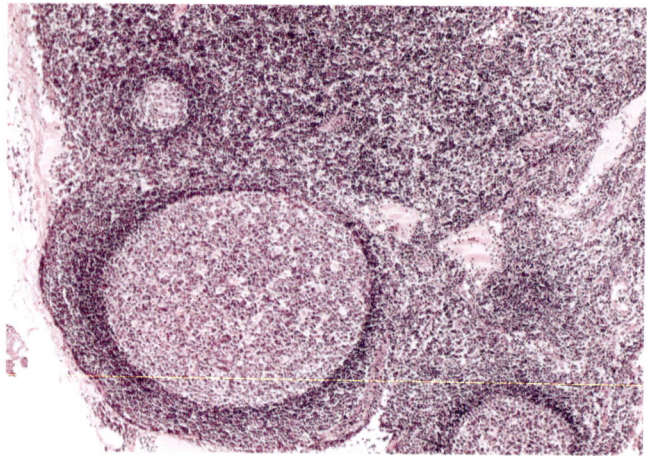

FIGURE 20-62
Lymph node with reactive follicular hyperplasia. A section of a hyperplastic lymph node shows prominent follicles (germinal centers) containing numerous macrophages with pale cytoplasm.

the cortex of the lymph node (Fig. 20-62). The follicles are round or irregular and may be confluent. The activated B lymphocytes in the follicles range from small cells with irregular, cleaved nuclei to large immunoblasts. Benign lymphoid follicles are characterized by "polarization" (i.e., a predominance of transformed lymphocytes or immunoblasts at one pole). Numerous mitotic figures reflect the rapid proliferation of activated B lymphocytes. Scattered benign macrophages, with abundant pale cytoplasm containing pyknotic nuclear and cytoplasmic debris, impart the characteristic "starry sky" pattern of benign follicles. Isolated dendritic reticulum cells, with round vesicular nuclei and abundant pink cytoplasm, may be identified near the margin of the follicle. A well-defined mantle of normal small B lymphocytes surrounds the follicles, sharply demarcating them from the interfollicular regions. A few partially transformed lymphocytes and immunoblasts and nonspecific inflammatory cells inhabit the interfollicular zone, and plasma cells may be increased in the medullary cords.

The cause of nonspecific reactive follicular hyperplasia is frequently not known, although a viral or inflammatory etiology is often suspected. The clinical course features rapid and complete resolution of the lymphadenopathy.

Lymphadenopathy, either localized or generalized, is a common finding in rheumatoid arthritis. Conspicuous follicular hyperplasia primarily involves the cortex, but occasionally may extend to the medulla. Prominent interfollicular plasmacytosis is also characteristic. Lymphadenopathy with histological features indistinguishable from those of rheumatoid arthritis may also occur in related disorders, such as Sjögren syndrome and Felty syndrome, and in unrelated diseases such as syphilis.

Angiofollicular lymph node hyperplasia (Castleman disease)

This distinctive disorder of unknown etiology involves both lymph nodes and extranodal tissues. Two histopathological subtypes are recognized:

Hyaline-vascular angiofollicular lymph node hyperplasia makes up 90% of cases of Castleman disease. It manifests as an asymptomatic mass, most commonly in the mediastinum, but also in other soft tissues. Young adult men are most commonly affected. Characteristic histopathological features include (1) numerous, small, follicle-like structures, frequently with radially penetrating, thick-walled, hyalinized vessels; (2) concentrically arranged small lymphocytes around the follicular structures, called "onion skinning"; and (3) extensive proliferation of capillaries in the interfollicular areas.

Plasma cell angiofollicular lymph node hyperplasia accounts for 10% of cases of Castleman disease and appears as either a localized mass or a multicentric systemic disorder.

The **localized variety** of the plasma cell type, which may actually consist of multiple matted lymph nodes, displays (1) large hyperplastic follicles with less prominent penetrating vessels than in the hyaline-vascular type, (2) pronounced interfollicular plasmacytosis, and (3) prominent vascularity.

The **multicentric form** of the plasma cell variant of Castleman disease is more aggressive and occasionally exhibits a chronic course. Affected patients are at some risk for the development of Kaposi sarcoma or immunoblastic lymphoma. Herpesvirus 8 has been detected in all HIV-positive patients with multicentric Castleman disease. Clinical features of plasma cell angiofollicular hyperplasia include fever, polyclonal hypergammaglobulinemia, elevated sedimentation rate, and anemia.

AIDS lymphadenopathy

This disorder is characterized by (1) marked follicular hyperplasia, with a distinctive loss of mantle zones; (2) infiltration of follicles by clusters of small lymphocytes; (3) foci of intrafollicular hemorrhage ("follicle lysis"); and (4) focal perisinusoidal, monocytoid, B-cell hyperplasia. Variable degrees of vascular proliferation, with subsequent depletion of lymphocytes in both follicles and interfollicular areas, may occur. Additionally, the lymph nodes in AIDS show a high incidence of superimposed malignant neoplasms, including diffuse B-cell lymphomas, Burkitt lymphoma, Hodgkin lymphoma, and Kaposi sarcoma.

Interfollicular Hyperplasia

In **nonspecific interfollicular hyperplasia,** the lymph nodal paracortex is expanded by a heterogeneous, reactive cell population. On low-power microscopy, the infiltrate imparts a typical mottled ("salt and pepper") appearance, reflecting an admixture of small lymphocytes, variably activated lymphocytes, immunoblasts, and scattered macrophages. Isolated interdigitating reticulum cells with grooved nuclei can be identified. Prominent postcapillary venules exhibit conspicuous endothelial lining cells. Rarely, the immunoblastic component is so florid that reactive interfollicular hyperplasia must be distinguished from an evolving malignant lymphoma.

Reactive nonspecific interfollicular hyperplasia (Fig. 20-63) is most commonly due to viral infections or to immunological reactions. Although the precise cause is often not determined, the condition resolves promptly.

Viral lymphadenitis: Interfollicular lymph node hyperplasia is a common finding in viral diseases, a few of which are characterized by specific histological features:

Infectious mononucleosis shows immunoblastic cells in lymph node sinuses. Rarely, extensive or even complete

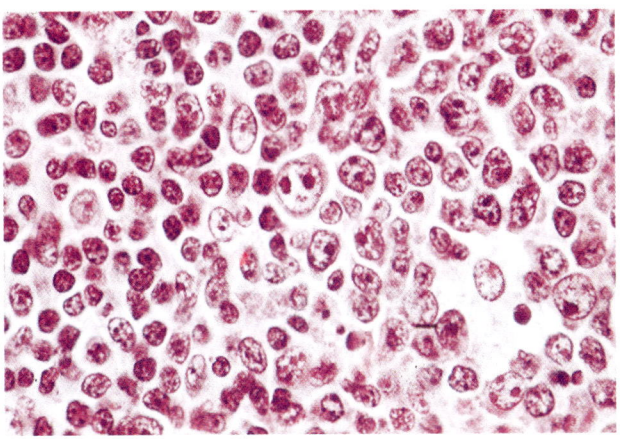

FIGURE 20-63
Lymph node with reactive interfollicular hyperplasia. High-power view of the T-dependent paracortex shows an admixture of small lymphocytes, variably activated lymphocytes, immunoblasts, and scattered macrophages.

obliteration of the normal nodal architecture by proliferating immunoblasts occurs. Bizarre binucleated or multinucleated immunoblasts that may be mistaken for the Reed-Sternberg cells of Hodgkin lymphoma, may be noted.
- **Varicella-herpes zoster infection** features eosinophilic intranuclear inclusions surrounded by a clear zone or halo (Cowdry type A inclusions) in endothelial cells.
- **Measles** in the prodromal phase is characterized by scattered multilobed or multinucleated lymphoid cells. These cells *(Warthin-Finkeldey cells)* display delicate chromatin, small punctate nucleoli, and scant pale cytoplasm.
- **Cytomegalovirus lymphadenitis** is distinguished by the presence in endothelial cells of large, round, eosinophilic, intranuclear inclusions with a surrounding clear halo.

Histiocytic necrotizing lymphadenitis (Kikuchi disease) is an unusual lymphadenitis of young women that most commonly involves the cervical lymph nodes. Focal infiltrates of immunoblasts and macrophages, both with distinctive angulated and twisted nuclei, are noted in the cortex and paracortex. Prominent karyorrhexis and cytoplasmic debris are characteristic, but granulocytes are absent. The lymphadenitis is usually self-limited and resolves in 3 to 4 months. A viral etiology is suspected.

Phenytoin (Dilantin) is a drug commonly used in the treatment of epilepsy. Some patients chronically treated with this drug develop **phenytoin-induced lymphadenopathy** characterized by interfollicular hyperplasia with variable effacement of the lymph nodal architecture. A polymorphous cell population, consisting of small lymphocytes, immunoblasts, eosinophils, and plasma cells, is characteristic. Atypical binucleated immunoblasts, which are similar to the Reed-Sternberg cells of Hodgkin lymphoma, may be observed. Focal areas of necrosis are common. Systemic abnormalities include fever, rash, polyclonal hypergammaglobulinemia, and peripheral blood eosinophilia. Resolution usually occurs after withdrawal of the drug. Whether there is an increased incidence of Hodgkin lymphoma or malignant lymphoma associated with phenytoin-induced lymphadenopathy is controversial.

Systemic lupus erythematosus is often associated with lymphadenopathy characterized by interfollicular hyperplasia with prominent immunoblasts and plasma cells and focal-to-massive necrosis. Arteriolitis, with fibrinoid necrosis of vessel walls, is frequently observed. Hematoxylin bodies (see Chapter 4) are found in relation to foci of necrosis or in nodal sinuses.

Mixed Patterns of Reactive Hyperplasia of Lymph Nodes

Some infectious diseases are associated with mixed patterns of lymph node hyperplasia, in which several different features are prominent.

TOXOPLASMOSIS: This form of lymphadenitis is characterized by (1) prominent follicular hyperplasia; (2) small collections of epithelioid macrophages in the interfollicular regions of the lymph node (Fig. 20-64) that encroach on the follicles *(Piringer-Kuchinka lesion)*; and (3) perisinusoidal monocytoid B-cell hyperplasia. Monocytoid B lymphocytes are medium-sized lymphoid cells with round-to-indented nuclei, bland chromatin, and moderately pale cytoplasm.

CAT-SCRATCH DISEASE: This malady typically presents with lymphadenitis of the axillary and cervical lymph nodes, characterized by follicular hyperplasia and suppurative granulomatous foci. The latter areas consist of elongated or stellate abscesses with central necrosis, containing polymorphonuclear leukocytes and cell debris and surrounded by palisaded macrophages and fibroblasts. Monocytoid B-cell hyperplasia and scattered immunoblasts may be observed in the interfollicular regions. The histological features of lymphadenitis caused by **lymphogranuloma venereum** and **tularemia** (see Chapter 9) are indistinguishable from those of cat-scratch disease.

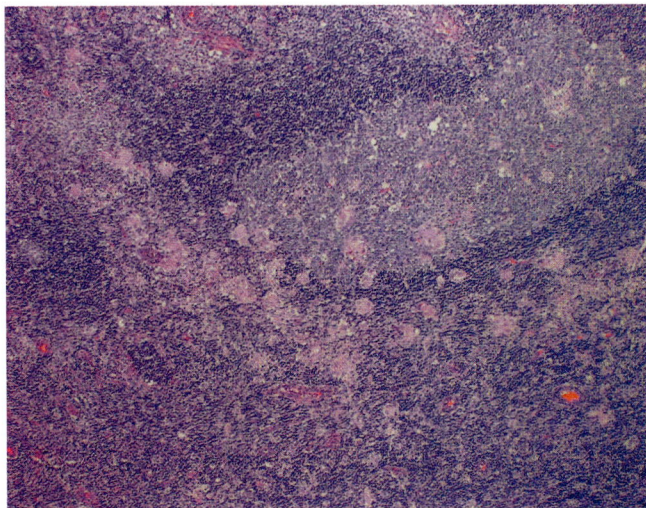

FIGURE 20-64
Toxoplasmosis. A section of a lymph node displays clusters of pink epithelioid macrophages and follicular hyperplasia.

Sinus Histiocytosis Represents an Increase in Macrophages

Sinus histiocytosis refers to an increase in tissue macrophages (histiocytes) of the subcapsular and trabecular sinuses of the lymph nodes (Fig. 20-65). The sinus histiocytes are derived from the sinus lining cells, which in turn originate from blood monocytes. Sinus histiocytes have eccentric, round-to-oval, indented nuclei, with delicate chromatin, punctate nucleoli, and abundant pink cytoplasm. Free macrophages and multinucleated giant cells may be observed in the expanded sinuses.

Sinus histiocytosis is a common finding in lymph nodes draining sites of cancer and, less commonly, inflammatory and infectious foci. The character of the phagocytic debris in the cytoplasm of the macrophages helps identify the origin of the sinus histiocytosis. For example, anthracotic pigment is frequently seen in the macrophages of mediastinal lymph nodes that exhibit sinus histiocytosis. Macrophages containing erythrocytes and hemosiderin pigment occur with autoimmune hemolytic anemia. Radiopaque contrast material is observed in the macrophages of enlarged pelvic and abdominal lymph nodes after lymphangiographic staging of malignant lymphoma.

Sinus Histiocytosis with Massive Lymphadenopathy Is Benign

Sinus histiocytosis with massive lymphadenopathy (SHML), also known as **Rosai-Dorfman disease,** *is a rare, self-limited disorder of unknown etiology characterized by striking, bilateral, painless, cervical lymphadenopathy.* Other peripheral and central lymph node groups may also be involved, and in over a fourth of cases, extranodal soft tissue sites are affected. SHML occurs most commonly in blacks in the first two decades of life, although it may be encountered at any age.

 Pathology: On gross examination, the involved lymph nodes are enlarged and orange-brown. Characteristic histopathological features include (1) capsular and pericapsular fibrosis and chronic inflammation; (2) marked sinus histiocytosis, with dilation of the subcapsular and trabecular sinuses and variable distortion of the lymph node architecture; and (3) prominent plasmacytosis of the intersinusoidal stroma. The sinus histiocytes have large, oval-or-indented, vesicular nuclei, with one to

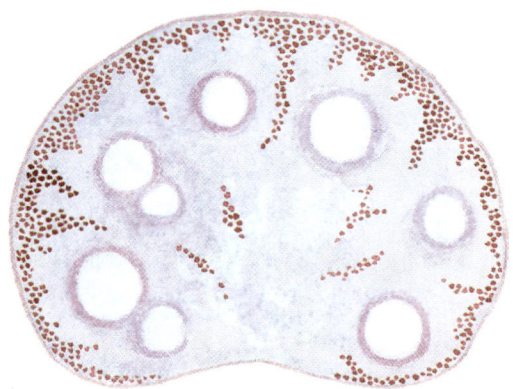

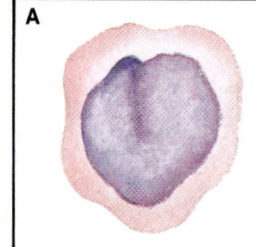 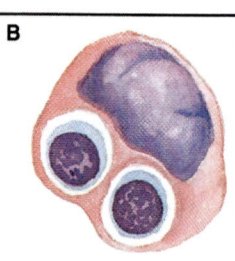 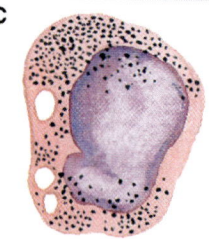 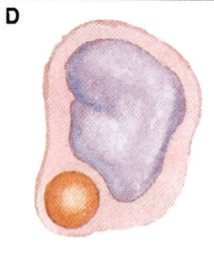 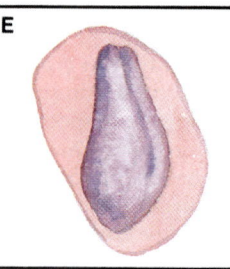

FIGURE 20-65
Benign disorders of the mononuclear phagocyte system. In the lymph nodes, benign proliferations of mononuclear phagocytes first involve the nodal sinuses *(blue dots in lymph node cross-section)* but may subsequently extend to involve the nodal stroma. A. In *benign sinus histiocytosis*, the nodal sinuses are expanded by bland histiocytes or phagocytic macrophages. B. In *sinus histiocytosis with massive lymphadenopathy*, the macrophages contain lymphocytes in cytoplasmic vacuoles. C. In *dermatopathic lymphadenopathy* the macrophages contain cytoplasmic lipid and melanin pigment. D. In *infection-induced hemophagocytic reticulosis*, the macrophages contain phagocytosed red cells. E. In the *differentiated histiocytoses* the cells are bland, and a deep nuclear crease or fold is characteristic.

several small nucleoli. The abundant cytoplasm is pink and occasionally vacuolated. Numerous lymphocytes and, less commonly, erythrocytes and plasma cells are typically seen in the cytoplasm of the sinus histiocytes (see Fig. 20-64). This phenomenon may reflect phagocytosis but may also represent active penetration of the cytoplasm of sinus histiocytes by these cells *(emperipolesis)*. The sinus histiocytes of SHML exhibit the usual immunological and cytochemical cell markers of mononuclear phagocytes. Additionally, they demonstrate strong immunohistochemical reactivity for S-100 protein.

Common accompanying clinical signs of inflammation include fever, an elevated erythrocyte sedimentation rate, neutrophilic leukocytosis, and polyclonal hypergammaglobulinemia. The clinical course is benign, with spontaneous resolution in months to years. There is no effective therapy.

Dermatopathic Lymphadenopathy Features Paracortical T-cell Proliferation

Dermatopathic lymphadenopathy refers to specific reactive changes in lymph nodes that are secondary to a variety of chronic dermatoses. This reaction is due to the drainage of lipid, melanin, and hemosiderin from the affected skin to the regional lymph nodes. The lymph nodes demonstrate an immunological reaction to antigenic material draining from the skin, which accumulates principally in paracortical macrophages. The paracortex is expanded by a heterogeneous cell population that consists principally of macrophages whose cytoplasm contains lipid or granular, brown, melanin pigment (Fig. 20-64). There are increased Langerhans cells and interdigitating reticulum cells, whose nuclei are folded and contain delicate chromatin. The paracortex also contains lymphocytes and some eosinophils, plasma cells, and immunoblasts. On low-power microscopy of the lymph node, the heterogeneous cell population imparts a characteristic mottled appearance to the paracortex.

Infection-Induced Hemophagocytic Syndrome Is Caused by Activated Macrophages

Infection-induced hemophagocytic syndrome is a rare disorder in immunodeficient persons, which is characterized by generalized activation of tissue macrophages. It occurs in a variety of viral, bacterial, fungal, and parasitic infections and (rarely) in some T-cell lymphomas. The common pathophysiological mechanism may be lymphokine-induced activation of tissue macrophages.

The principal histopathological feature of infection-induced hemophagocytic syndrome is a generalized hyperplasia of tissue macrophages in the splenic red pulp, hepatic sinusoids, lymph node sinuses, and bone marrow. The macrophages exhibit active phagocytosis, principally of erythrocytes (Fig. 20-65), but also of neutrophils and platelets.

Infection-induced hemophagocytic reticulosis is characterized by the acute onset of fever, hepatosplenomegaly, lymphadenopathy, rash, pulmonary infiltration, and pancytopenia. The disorder is generally self-limited but (rarely) may be fatal.

MALIGNANT LYMPHOMAS

Lymphomas are malignant proliferations of lymphocytes or lymphoblasts. The WHO classification distinguishes between Hodgkin lymphoma and *B-cell and T-cell lymphomas* (commonly referred to as non-Hodgkin lymphomas) (Tables 20-18 and 20-19). *B-cell and T-cell lymphomas* are further categorized as derived from *immature* (precursor) cells or from *mature* (peripheral) effector cells.

Malignant lymphomas comprise the most heterogeneous group of tumors in man. The WHO classification of lymphomas is based upon their normal cellular counterparts, which may represent (1) *immature* or *mature* lymphocytes, (2) *B cells* or *T cells*, and (3) lymphocytes *homing to different anatomical sites*. Malignant lymphomas also exhibit characteristic immunophenotypic, cytogenetic, and molecular abnormalities. In many instances, the new WHO classification does not distinguish between *lymphoma* and *leukemia*. For example, no distinction in principle is made between chronic lymphocytic *leukemia* (CLL) and small lymphocytic *lymphoma* (SLL).

B Acute Lymphoblastic Leukemia/Lymphoma (B-ALL/LBL) Is the Most Common Childhood Leukemia

Immature (precursor) B lymphoblasts are the malignant cells in B-ALL/LBL. Most precursor B-cell malignancies involve primarily bone marrow and peripheral blood, and are termed *B lymphoblastic leukemia*. However, nodal involvement can occur, in which case the disease is referred to as *B lymphoblastic lymphoma*.

TABLE 20-18 WHO Histological Classification of B-Cell Neoplasms

Precursor B-cell neoplasm
  Precursor B lymphoblastic leukemia/lymphoma
Mature B-cell neoplasms
  Chronic lymphocytic leukemia/small lymphocytic lymphoma
  B-cell prolymphocytic leukemia
  Lymphoplasmacytic lymphoma
  Splenic marginal zone lymphoma
  Hairy cell leukemia
  Plasma cell myeloma
  Monoclonal gammopathy of undetermined significance (MGUS)
  Solitary plasmacytoma of bone
  Extraosseous plasmacytoma
  Primary amyloidosis
  Heavy-chain diseases
  Extranodal marginal zone B-cell lymphoma of mucosa-associated lymphoid tissue (MALT lymphoma)
  Nodal marginal zone B-cell lymphoma
  Mediastinal (thymic) large B-cell lymphoma
  Intravascular large B-cell lymphoma
  Primary effusion lymphoma
  Burkitt lymphoma/leukemia

TABLE 20-19 WHO Histological Classification of T-Cell and NK-Cell Neoplasms

Precursor T-cell neoplasm
  Precursor T-lymphoblastic leukemia/lymphoma
Mature T-cell neoplasms
  Leukemic/disseminated
    T-cell prolymphocytic leukemia
    T-cell large granular lymphocytic leukemia
    Aggressive NK-cell leukemia
    Adult T-cell leukemia/lymphoma
  Cutaneous
    Mycosis fungoides
    Sézary syndrome
    Primary cutaneous anaplastic lymphoma
    Large cell lymphoma
    Lymphomatoid papulosis
  Other extranodal
    Extranodal NK/T-cell lymphoma, nasal type
    Enteropathy-type T-cell lymphoma
    Hepatosplenic T-cell lymphoma
    Subcutaneous panniculitis-like T-cell lymphoma
  Nodal
    Angioimmunoblastic T-cell lymphoma
    Peripheral T-cell lymphoma, unspecified
    Anaplastic large cell lymphoma
Neoplasm of uncertain lineage and stage of differentiation
  Blastic NK cell lymphoma

Epidemiology: Most childhood leukemias are acute lymphoblastic leukemias of B-cell type (B-ALL). Some 75% of cases occur in children under the age of 6. Almost all the precursor B-cell malignancies are predominantly *leukemic*, and lymphoblastic *lymphoma* is an uncommon type.

Pathology: The malignant lymphoblasts (at least 20% in bone marrow) are small to medium-sized cells with an increased nuclear-to-cytoplasmic ratio and inconspicuous nucleoli (morphologically mostly L1 type according to the old FAB classification (Fig. 20-53)).

The **immunophenotypes** of B-ALL reflect different stages of B-cell maturation (Fig. 20-66). The earliest markers that indicate B-cell differentiation are CD19 and cytoplasmic CD79A, usually accompanied by cytoplasmic expression of CD22, which is B-cell lineage specific. B-ALL that expresses these markers but shows no cytoplasmic μ chains is called *progenitor, pre-pre-B, or early precursor B-cell leukemia*.

The advent of cytoplasmic μ chain expression is characteristic of *pre-B-cell leukemias*. Both, progenitor B-cell leukemia and pre-B-cell leukemia are positive for nuclear expression of TdT (Fig. 20-67). CD10 (CALLA) may be expressed in either type. **B-cell malignancies that express immunoglobulin on the cell surface are not regarded as precursor leukemias.**

Cytogenetic abnormalities are involved. B-ALL features *numerical aberrations* and *chromosomal translocations* including the Philadelphia chromosome. In childhood ALL, a

FIGURE 20-66
B-cell maturation: Immunophenotypes and neoplastic counterparts. *H*, immunoglobulin heavy-chain gene; *L*, immunoglobulin light-chain gene; Cμ, cytoplasmic μ chain; sIg, surface immunoglobulin; cIg, cytoplasmic immunoglobulin

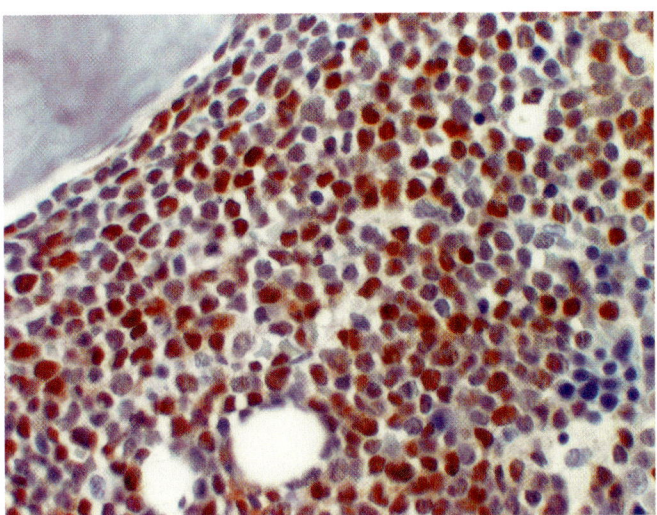

FIGURE 20-67
Acute lymphoblastic leukemia. The bone marrow contains TdT-positive cells (immunoperoxidase).

BCR/ABL fusion protein, P190, is produced, in contrast to the *CML* fusion protein (P210) that is seen in half of adult cases of ALL or CML. Progenitor B-ALL may present with t(4;11) involving the *MLL* gene at 11q23. About 25% of childhood pre-B-ALL patients are positive for t(1;19), which involves *PBX/E2A*.

 Clinical Features: The leukemic cells of B-ALL displace normal hematopoietic elements in the bone marrow, resulting in anemia, thrombocytopenia, and neutropenia. Organomegaly and involvement of the CNS are common. The rapidly growing tumor cells in the marrow cause bone pain and arthralgias. In general, childhood B-ALL treated with chemotherapy has an excellent prognosis, with complete remission rates of better than 90%. However, very young age (less than 1 year), t(9;22), t(1;19), and t(4;11) are bad prognostic indicators. All translocations involving the *MLL* gene at 11q23 are associated with a poor prognosis irrespective of age. *Hyperdiploidy* (>50 chromosomes) carries a good prognosis, whereas *hypodiploid* karyotypes portend an unfavorable outcome.

Precursor T Cells Compose Most Lymphoblastic Lymphomas

Precursor T-acute lymphoblastic leukemia (T-ALL) and T-lymphoblastic lymphoma (T-LBL) are immature T-cell neoplasms. Whether the terms *leukemia* or *lymphoma* apply is arbitrary in many instances, and the considerations are similar to those described for B-ALL.

 Epidemiology: Most childhood ALL is derived from B cells, and only 15% originates from T cells. In adults, the percentage of T-lymphoblastic leukemia is higher. Lymphoblastic lymphoma, a tumor mass consisting of precursor lymphocytes, is 90% of T-cell origin.

 Pathology: The morphological appearance of T lymphoblasts is similar to that of B lymphoblasts. In T-LBL, a "starry sky" pattern of macrophages may be present, resembling Burkitt lymphoma. Most T-ALLs have L2 morphology in the old FAB classification (Fig. 20-53) (larger blasts with more prominent nucleoli and variation in cell size) (Fig. 20-68).

Immunophenotypes: The expression of markers in T-ALL reflects normal T-cell differentiation and maturation in the bone marrow and thymus (Fig. 20-69). The earliest T-cell marker is CD7, followed by CD2 and CD5. During thymic differentiation, T cells become positive for CD1a and cytoplasmic CD3 (cCD3), CD4, and CD8. The immunophenotypes in T-ALL reflect that sequence of marker expression. Frequently, thymic-derived T-ALL coexpresses CD4 and CD8. As with B-ALL, T-ALL is positive for TdT.

Cytogenetic abnormalities: The genes encoding the four T-cell receptor chains ($\alpha, \beta, \gamma, \delta$ chains) often participate in chromosomal translocations with transcription factor genes such as *MYC, TAL1, RBTN1, RBTN2,* and *HOX11*. Juxtaposition of the T-cell receptor loci to one of the transcription partner genes often results in disturbed regulation of transcription. Another common chromosomal abnormality is del(9p), with the loss of *CDKN2A*, which functions as a *CDK* inhibitor.

 Clinical Features: Blood and bone marrow are most commonly involved in T-ALL. The leukemia frequently infiltrates peripheral lymph nodes, brain, gonads, spleen, and liver. Precursor T-cell malignancies that originate from thymic T cells most often manifest as a mediastinal mass.

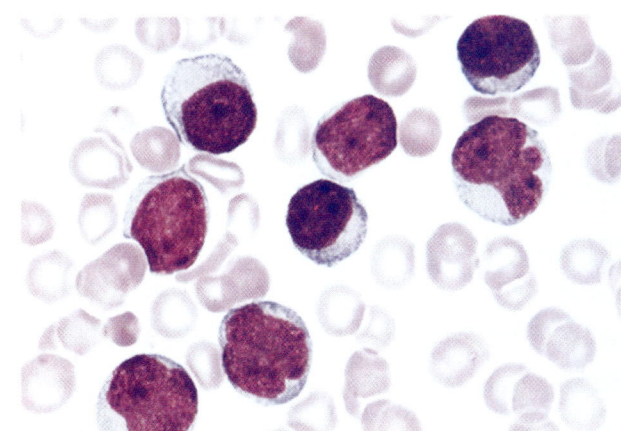

FIGURE 20-68
Acute lymphoblastic leukemia (L2 ALL). The lymphoblasts in peripheral blood contain irregular and indented nuclei with prominent nucleoli and a moderate amount of cytoplasm.

FIGURE 20-69
T-cell maturation: Immunophenotypes and their neoplastic counterparts. TrR, T cell receptor rearrangement

Mature (Peripheral) B-cell Lymphomas Are the Most Common Type in the Western World

Mature B-cell malignancies are derived from the clonal proliferation of peripheral B cells.. As B cells go through multiple steps of differentiation and maturation from naïve B cells to mature plasma cells, lymphomas may arise at every step of the way.

 Epidemiology: The incidence of malignant lymphomas in the United States is 15 per 100,000 annually. B-cell neoplasms by far outnumber T-cell malignancies, particularly in the Western world. The most common B-cell lymphomas are follicular lymphoma and diffuse large cell lymphoma (Table 20-20), which alone account for 50% of all malignant lymphomas in the Western world. With the exception of mediastinal B-cell and Burkitt lymphoma, most mature B-cell lymphomas occur in the 6th and 7th decades. Peripheral B-cell lymphomas are distinctly uncommon in children with the exception of Burkitt lymphoma and large cell B-cell lymphoma.

 Pathogenesis: Most peripheral B-cell lymphomas occur without apparent cause. However, impairment of the immune system and certain infectious agents may give rise to malignant lymphomas (Table 20-21). Immunodeficiency caused by HIV infection and therapeutic immunosuppression in allograft recipients promote the development of large B-cell lymphoma or Burkitt lymphoma. In patients with certain types of autoimmune disease, low-grade malignant B-cell lymphomas can develop.

For example, patients with *Sjögren disease* or *Hashimoto thyroiditis* (see Chapter 21) may develop extranodal marginal zone lymphoma (MALT lymphoma). *EBV* is linked to endemic Burkitt lymphoma and HIV-associated lymphomas. Other viruses that predispose to B-cell malignancies include *human herpesvirus 8* (HHV-8) in primary effusion lymphoma and *hepatitis C virus* in lymphoplasmacytic lymphoma associated with type 2 cryoglobulinemia. MALT lymphoma is frequently associated with *Helicobacter pylori* infection of the stomach (see Chapter 13) and often regresses upon antibiotic treatment.

Pathology: Immunophenotypes: Following the precursor stage, B cells undergo immunoglobulin *VDJ* gene arrangements and mature to surface

TABLE 20-20 Frequency of B- and T/NK-Cell Lymphomas

Diagnosis	% of Total Cases
Diffuse large B-cell lymphoma	30.6%
Follicular lymphoma	22.1%
MALT lymphoma	7.6%
Mature T-cell lymphomas (except ALCL)	7.6%
Chronic lymphocytic leukemia/ small lymphocytic lymphoma	6.7%
Mantle cell lymphoma	6.0%
Mediastinal large B-cell lymphoma	2.4%
Anaplastic large cell lymphoma	2.4%
Burkitt lymphoma	2.50%
Nodal marginal zone lymphoma	1.8%
Precursor T-lymphoblastic lymphoma	1.7%
Lymphoplasmacytic lymphoma	1.2%
Other types	7.4%

TABLE 20-21 **Disorders with Increased Risk of Secondary Malignant Lymphoma**

Sjögren syndrome
Hashimoto thyroiditis
Renal and cardiac transplant recipients
Acquired immunodeficiency syndrome (AIDS)
EBV infection
HHV-8 infection
Helicobacter pylori-positive gastritis
Hepatitis C
Congenital immune deficiency syndromes
    Chediak-Higashi
    Wiskott-Aldrich
    Ataxia telangiectasia
    IgA deficiency
    Severe combined immune deficiency
α Heavy-chain disease
Celiac disease
Hodgkin lymphoma (post-treatment)

IgM- and IgD-positive naïve B cells that often express CD5 (Fig. 20-70). Two B-cell malignancies are derived from naïve B cells, namely, B-CLL and mantle cell lymphoma.

Naïve B cells become activated upon antigenic stimulation and populate the germinal centers of lymph follicles, where they ultimately mature into IgG- or IgA-secreting plasma cells and memory cells. The large activated B cells that home to germinal centers are called *centroblasts*. In the germinal center, centroblasts mature into smaller cells with cleaved nuclei, termed *centrocytes*. Centroblasts and centrocytes lack the apoptosis inhibitor BCL-2 (Fig. 20-71); they express *BCL6* and *CD10*. Somatic mutations in the Ig variable region take place in the germinal center, resulting in remarkable diversity of antibody specificity. Follicular lymphomas are derived from germinal center B cells and consist of a mixture of centroblasts and centrocytes. Burkitt lymphoma and some large B-cell lymphomas are also derived from germinal center lymphocytes.

Late-stage memory B cells reside in *the marginal zone*, the outermost compartment of the lymph follicle. Variants of marginal zone lymphomas include splenic marginal zone lymphoma and MALT lymphomas of the stomach and other mucosal surfaces.

Ultimately, some B cells differentiate into plasma cells. These cells are the only B cells that secrete immunoglobulins, although they lack Ig expression on the cell surface. Plasma cells home to bone marrow, where they may give rise to multiple myeloma.

Classification of mature B cell lymphomas: The WHO lymphoma classification distinguishes three groups of B-cell lymphomas:

Lymphomas with predominant involvement of bone marrow
Lymphomas with predominant extranodal involvement
Lymphomas with predominant lymphadenopathy

Clinical Features: *Indolent* lymphomas are distinguished from *aggressive* B-cell lymphomas. Typical indolent lymphomas are B-CLL and follicular lymphoma; aggressive B-cell lymphomas tend to be large B-cell lymphoma and Burkitt lymphoma. Although indolent lymphomas follow a prolonged clinical course, they are usually incurable. By contrast, aggressive lymphomas progress rapidly, but many of them are curable. Not all malignant lymphomas fall unequivocally into either category. MALT lymphomas, for example, are indolent lymphomas that can sometimes be cured by local irradiation.

Chronic Lymphocytic Leukemia/Small Lymphocytic Lymphoma (CLL/SLL)

CLL/SLL is a malignant B-cell proliferation of small, mature-appearing, lymphocytes and a variable number of larger cells (prolymphocytes and paraimmunoblasts). A diagnosis of CLL is made if bone marrow and peripheral blood are primarily involved. If the tumor cells predominantly give rise to lymphadenopathy or solid tumor masses, the term small lymphocytic lymphoma is more appropriate.

Epidemiology: CLL/SLL is a typical indolent malignant lymphoma of the elderly (median age 65) and accounts for 7% of malignant lymphomas.

Pathology: Lymph nodes infiltrated by CLL show complete effacement of the architecture (Fig. 20-72). At low magnification, ill-defined lighter areas, termed *pseudofollicles* or *proliferation centers,* represent an admixture of larger, more immature-appearing lymphocytes (paraimmunoblasts or prolymphocytes).

In the spleen, the white pulp is expanded (Fig. 20-73), although tumor cells may also extend into the red pulp. Bone marrow involvement ranges from complete effacement of the marrow space to more patchy distribution. In peripheral blood smears (Fig. 20-74), some leukemic lymphocytes are destroyed and show ill-defined nuclear remnants (*"smudge" cells*). A variable number of larger cells with prominent nucleoli (*prolymphocytes*) can be seen. An increasing number of prolymphocytes may indicate a more aggressive course. If more than 55% prolymphocytes are present, the criteria of *prolymphocytic transformation* are met. Transformation of CLL/SLL into diffuse large cell lymphoma is labeled *Richter syndrome*, which is characterized by sheets of large lymphocytes (centroblasts or immunoblasts).

Immunophenotypes: SLL/CLL features a mature B-cell population that expresses CD19, CD20, CD22, and CD79. Coexpression of CD23 and the T-cell marker CD5 sets CLL apart from other types of B-cell lymphomas. There is only dim expression for surface IgM or IgG. Expression of the plasma cell marker CD38 or ZAP-70 carries an unfavorable prognosis.

Genotypes: Half of cases of B-CLL have not undergone somatic mutations in the variable-region genes and therefore resemble the genotype of naïve B cells. The other half are derived from B cells that have undergone *VH* gene mutations and resemble post-germinal center B cells. Common karyotypic abnormalities include trisomy 12 and deletions of 13q14 and of 11q23.

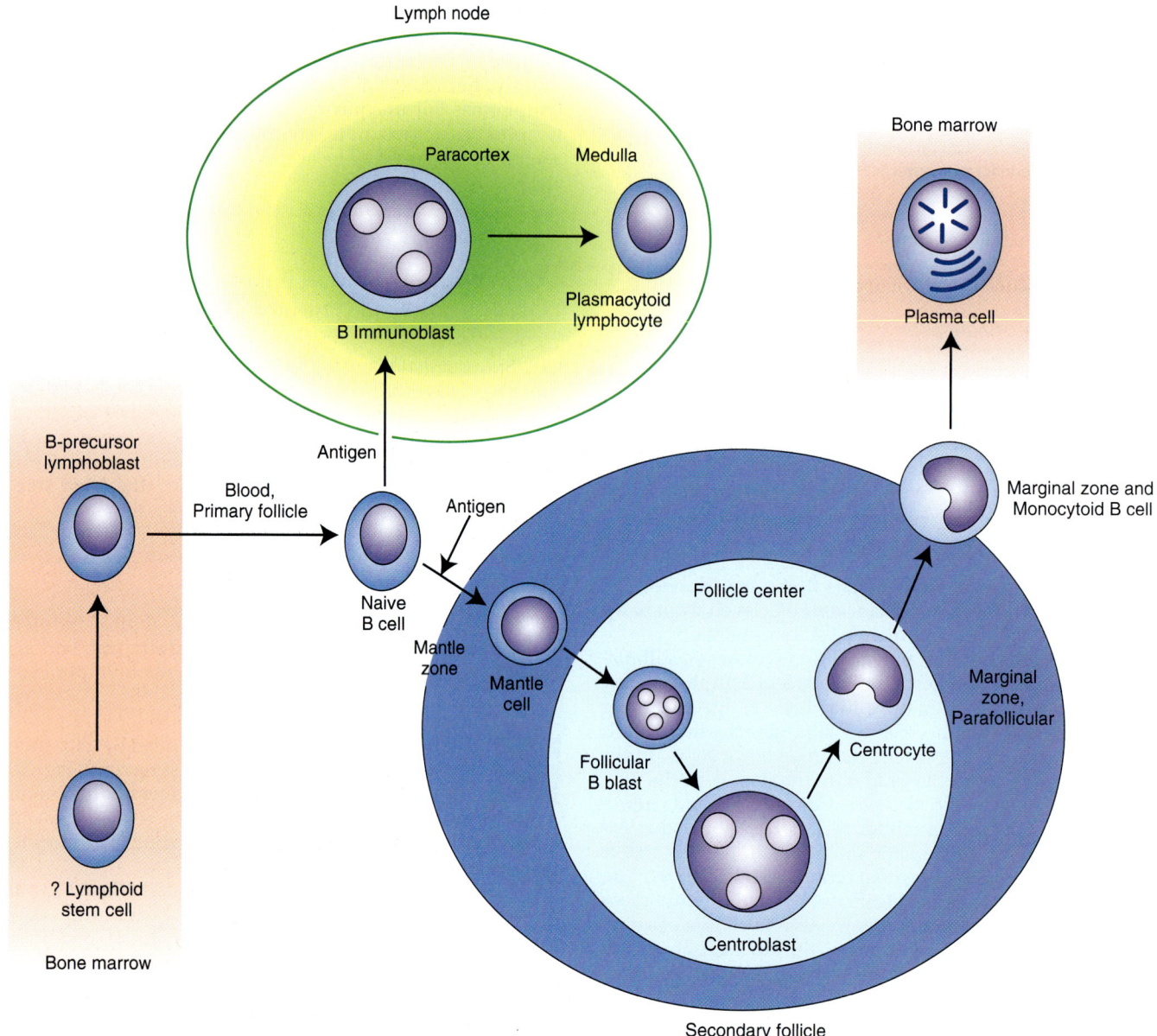

FIGURE 20-70
Schematic pathway of B cell differentiation. Following the precursor status, B cells mature into naive B lymphocytes. The germinal-center response represents an important turntable for immunoglobulin variable region gene mutations, Ig heavy-chain switch, and differentiation into plasma cells and memory cells.

Clinical Features: The diagnosis of B-CLL is established by the demonstration of a sustained peripheral blood lymphocytosis, generally more than 15,000/μL, and a bone marrow lymphocytosis exceeding 40% of the nucleated cell elements. If the blood lymphocyte count is between 5,000 and 15,000/μL, the demonstration of monoclonality (light-chain restriction or clonal rearrangement of a light-chain gene) confirms the diagnosis of B-CLL.

The erythrocyte and platelet counts are initially normal, but with advanced disease, severe anemia, thrombocytopenia, and neutropenia develop. A positive Coombs test is observed at some time in up to 20% of cases.

Immunological deficiencies, principally of B cells but also of T cells, are common. Although the precise cause of B-cell dysfunction is not known, hypogammaglobulinemia occurs in 50 to 75% of cases at some time during the course of the disease. The degree of hypogammaglobulinemia generally correlates with the disease stage and is responsible for infectious complications.

Patients with B-CLL also exhibit an increase in peripheral blood T cells (>3,000/μL). There is an increase in $CD8^+$ T cells and a corresponding decrease in $CD4^+$ cells, with a resulting decrease in the $CD4^+$/$CD8^+$ cell ratio. The T cells often show impaired delayed-type hypersensitivity in vitro, which also contributes to the increased risk of infection. A small amount of monoclonal immunoglobulin, most commonly IgM κ, is found in the serum in a minority of patients with B-CLL.

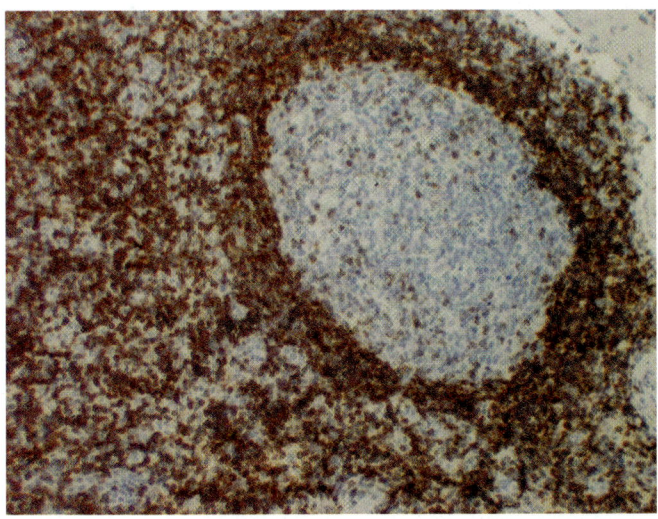

FIGURE 20-71
Lymph follicle stained with an antibody against BCL-2. The absence of staining in the germinal center favors a benign follicle.

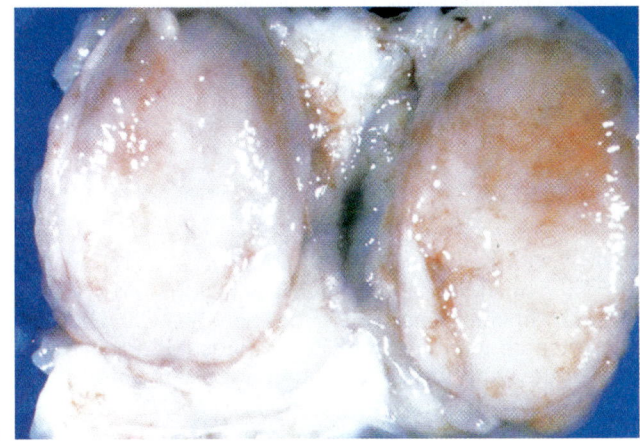

FIGURE 20-72
Small lymphocytic lymphoma/leukemia. A. A bisected, enlarged lymph node shows the characteristic uniform, glistening, gray color that imparts a fish-flesh appearance. B. On microscopic examination, the lymph nodal architecture is replaced by a diffuse infiltration of normal-appearing small lymphocytes.

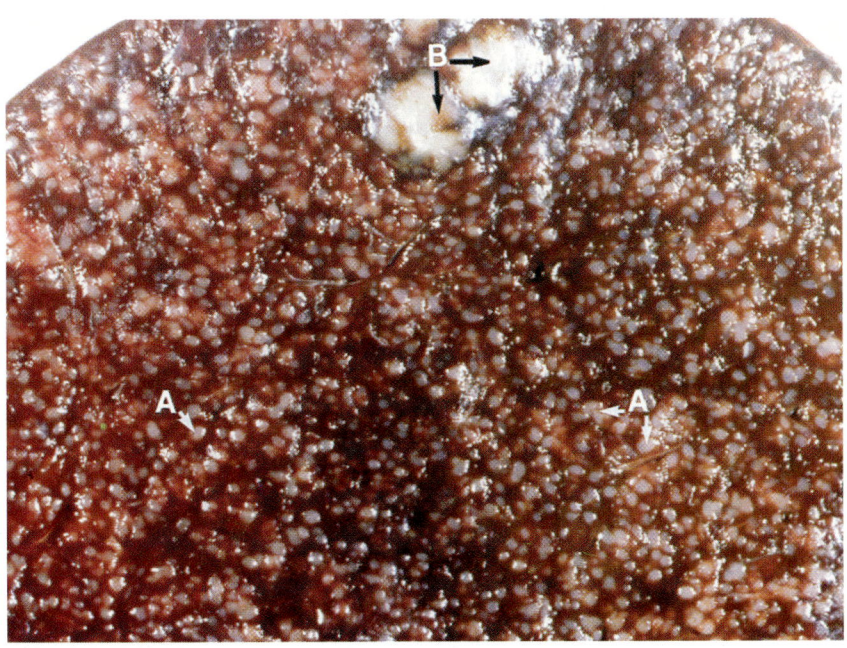

FIGURE 20-73
The spleen in chronic lymphocytic leukemia. There is diffuse enlargement of the white pulp (A) with focally prominent tumor nodules (B).

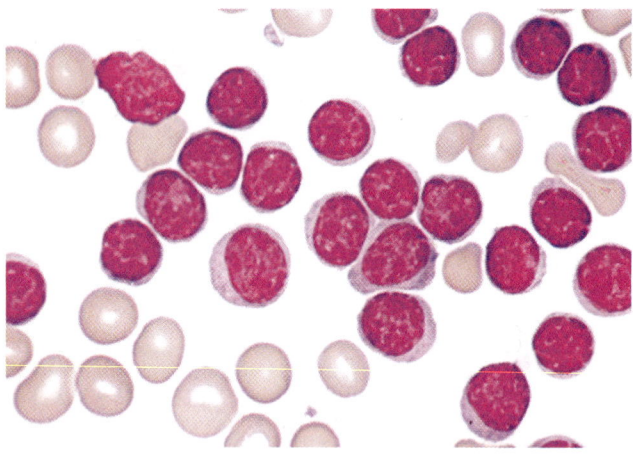

FIGURE 20-74
Chronic lymphocytic leukemia. A smear of peripheral blood exhibits numerous small-to-medium sized lymphocytes. A smudge cell is seen upper left.

Initially, most patients with B-CLL are asymptomatic, and the diagnosis is suggested by finding lymphadenopathy and splenomegaly in a routine physical examination or lymphocytosis on a blood cell count. The subsequent clinical course is highly variable. In some cases, the disease progresses rapidly, and the patients die within 2 to 3 years. Other patients remain asymptomatic for 10 to 20 years. The most common complications are bacterial infections and, less frequently, fungal and viral ones. Coombs-positive, autoimmune hemolytic anemia and hemorrhagic episodes secondary to thrombocytopenia are often observed.

The overall mean survival in B-CLL is 6 years. The prognosis is related principally to (1) the extent of tumor burden at the time of initial diagnosis, (2) the pattern of bone marrow infiltration, and (3) the presence of cytogenetic abnormalities. Adverse prognostic findings include (1) advanced disease; (2) diffuse rather than interstitial or nodular patterns of marrow involvement; and (3) the presence of chromosomal abnormalities, particularly multiple ones.

Patients with trisomy 12 have a worse than average prognosis, whereas those with 13q14 deletion have a longer mean survival. Patients with CLL that originates from naïve B cells have a poor prognosis and are more likely to have tumor cells that express CD38.

Conversion to prolymphocytic leukemia occurs in 10% of cases of B-CLL and is characterized by a marked elevation in the blood lymphocyte count, 15 to 50% prolymphocytes, and increasing splenomegaly. Prolymphocytic conversion predicts a more aggressive clinical course, with a mean survival of less than 2 years. Rare instances of conversion to acute lymphoblastic leukemia have been described, with a rapidly fatal course. There is more than a twofold increase in the expected incidence of second cancers in B-CLL, including lung tumors, malignant melanoma, soft tissue sarcomas, and plasma cell neoplasms.

Richter syndrome, a large cell lymphoma (see below), is superimposed in 5% of cases of B-CLL. Patients with this complication present with a rapid onset of fever, abdominal pain, and progressive lymphadenopathy and hepatosplenomegaly. Prominent enlargement of the retroperitoneal lymph nodes and neoplastic involvement of the gastrointestinal tract are common findings. Richter syndrome is aggressive and refractory to therapy, with a mean survival of 2 months.

Asymptomatic patients with B-CLL who have stable lymphocyte counts are ordinarily not treated. More-advanced disease is treated with chemotherapeutic agents and antilymphocyte antibody. Corticosteroids are used to control autoimmune hemolytic anemia and thrombocytopenia. Splenectomy or splenic irradiation may be needed to manage refractory hypersplenism.

Lymphoplasmacytic Lymphoma/Waldenström Macroglobulinemia

Lymphoplasmacytic lymphoma (LPL) / Waldenström disease is a neoplastic proliferation of small lymphocytes and a variable number of IgM-secreting plasma cells of the same malignant clone. Waldenström disease is not a variant of multiple myeloma, but rather an indolent malignant lymphoma that mainly affects the elderly.

 Pathogenesis: The etiology of LPL is obscure. In a small subset of patients with LPL and cryoglobulinemia who suffer from hepatitis C, HCV protein can often be demonstrated in lymphocytes. Partial regression of the lymphoma occurs after antiviral treatment of the hepatitis with interferon α.

 Pathology: Waldenström disease, or LPL, primarily involves the bone marrow, but the disease can also be seen in lymph nodes, spleen, and peripheral blood. In lymph nodes, LPL shows an interfollicular lymphocytic infiltrate with plasma cells. The leukemic bone marrow infiltrates are similar to those in CLL, although there may be more plasma cells. Transformation from LPL into a large cell lymphoma may occur.

LPL expresses common B-cell markers, and CD5 and CD23 are negative. The most common translocation is t(9;14). As in other lymphomas with plasma cell differentiation, rearrangement of the *PAX-5* gene, which encodes B-cell-specific activator protein (BSAP), is common.

Clinical Features: Eighty percent of patients with Waldenström macroglobulinemia present with a monoclonal IgM spike on serum electrophoresis (>3 g/dL). Many of the clinical symptoms result from hyperviscosity. Sludging and rouleaux formation of red blood cells in the microvascular system may lead to visual disturbances and stroke. Complications associated with hyperviscosity are treated with plasmapheresis. Excess IgM in the serum may cause a coagulopathy by binding to clotting factors, platelets, and fibrin. The clinical outcome of the disease is comparable to that of other indolent lymphomas such as B-CLL.

Hairy Cell Leukemia

Hairy cell leukemia is a clonal B-cell proliferation of small to medium-sized lymphocytes that display abundant cytoplasm and hairlike protrusions of the cell membrane. The disease involves primarily the monocyte/macrophage system of the bone marrow, spleen, and liver.

Hairy cell leukemia is rare and affects mainly middle-aged to elderly persons, with a markedly increased male-to-female ratio of 5:1.

 Pathology: Hairy cell leukemia exhibits subtle interstitial infiltrates that do not disturb the normal bone marrow architecture. Hairy cells have more-abundant cytoplasm than normal small lymphocytes, which lends them a "fried egg" appearance (Fig. 20-75). Silver stain of the bone marrow demonstrates an increase in reticulin fibers, and bone marrow aspirations are often unsuccessful because of a "dry tap." Unlike B-CLL, hairy cells in the spleen infiltrate the red pulp, and the white pulp is atrophic. The liver shows densely packed sinusoidal infiltrates.

Immunophenotypes: The normal cellular counterpart of hairy cell leukemia is not known. The cells are positive for all established B-cell markers and are negative for CD5, CD10, and CD23. The malignant cells also strongly express CD11c, CD25, FMC7, and CD103. The cytochemical or immunohistochemical demonstration of tartrate-resistant acid phosphatase (TRAP) is an additional marker (Fig. 20-76).

 Clinical Features: Most patients with hairy cell leukemia present with splenomegaly and peripheral monocytopenia or pancytopenia. The disorder is an indolent lymphoma with a prolonged clinical course. Chemotherapeutic drugs that specifically target low-grade malignant lymphomas, such as deoxycoformycin or 2-chlorodeoxyadenosine (2-CDA), can achieve long term remissions.

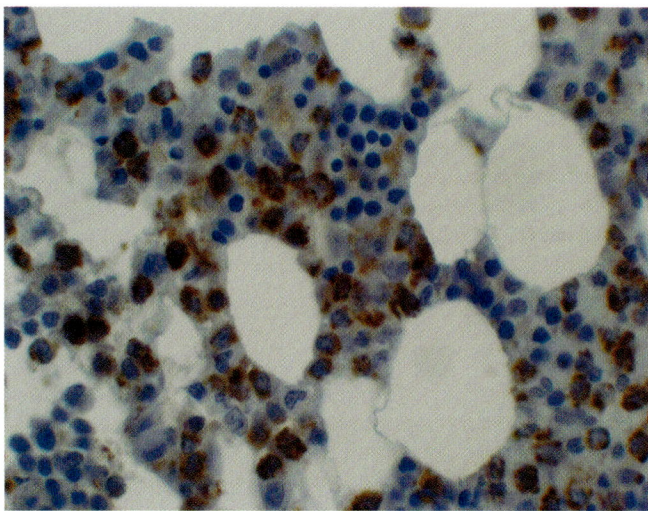

FIGURE 20-76
Hairy cells positive for antibody against tartrate-resistant acid phosphatase (TRAP) in bone marrow.

Plasma Cell Neoplasia

Plasma cell neoplasia comprises a group of related malignant disorders of terminally differentiated B lymphocytes (plasma cells).

Plasma cell myeloma or multiple myeloma (90% of cases) is characterized by a multifocal infiltration of malignant plasma cells in the bone marrow. In this condition, there are typically multiple destructive (lytic) lesions or diffuse demineralization of bone. The WHO diagnostic criteria for plasma cell myeloma are summarized in Table 20-22.

Solitary osseous myeloma (5% of cases) is a single destructive lesion of bone.

Extramedullary plasmacytoma (5% of cases) presents as a soft tissue mass, most frequently in the upper respiratory tract.

In most cases of plasma cell neoplasia, the neoplastic cells secrete a homogeneous, complete or partial, immunoglobulin molecule, termed an *M-component* or *parapro-*

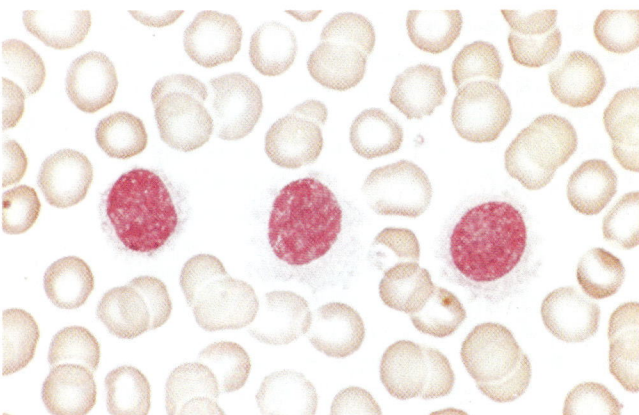

FIGURE 20-75
Hairy cell leukemia. Hairy cells with fine, irregular cytoplasmic projections are seen in the peripheral blood.

TABLE 20-22 WHO Diagnostic Criteria for Plasma Cell Myeloma

The diagnosis of myeloma requires a minimum of one major and one minor criterion or three minor criteria which must include at least the first two.
A. Major criteria:
  1. Marrow plasmacytosis (>30%)
  2. Plasmacytoma on biopsy
  3. M-component:
    Serum: IgG > 3.5g/dL, IgA >2 g/dL
    Urine >1g/24 hr of Bence-Jones (BJ) protein
B. Minor criteria:
  1. Marrow plasmacytosis (10–30%)
  2. M-component present but less than above
  3. Lytic bone lesions
  4. Reduced normal immunoglobulins (<50% normal):
    IgG <600 mg/dL, IgA <100 mg/dL, IgM <50 mg/dL

tein. Based on the type of M-component, multiple myeloma can be divided into the following types:

- **IgG, IgA, IgD, IgE, and IgM types**
- **Light-chain disease**, in which only κ or λ light chains are synthesized
- **Biclonal multiple myeloma**, in which two distinct M-components are secreted (rare)
- **Nonsecretory myeloma**, in which no M-component is secreted (1%)

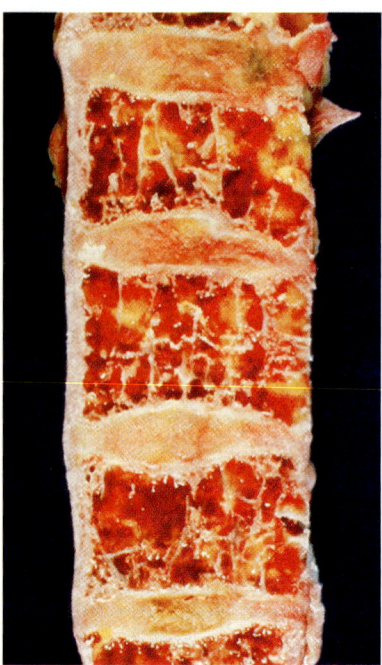

FIGURE 20-77
Multiple myeloma. Multiple lytic bone lesions are present in the vertebra.

 Epidemiology: Plasma cell neoplasia constitutes 10% of all hematological malignancies. About 7500 cases are reported annually in the United States, yielding an overall incidence of 3 per 100,000 population. The disorder is more than twice as common in blacks (8 per 100,000 population) than in whites. The frequency of plasma cell neoplasia increases with age, the mean age at diagnosis of multiple myeloma being 65 years and that of solitary osseous myeloma and extramedullary plasmacytoma a decade earlier. Plasma cell neoplasia is distinctly uncommon before the age of 40 years. There is a slight male predominance in multiple myeloma, with an overall male-to-female ratio of 1.5:1. This male predominance is even more pronounced for solitary osseous myeloma and extramedullary plasmacytoma, each with a male-to-female ratio of 3:1.

 Pathogenesis: A number of risk factors for plasma cell neoplasia have been identified.

- A **genetic predisposition** is suggested by an increased incidence of multiple myeloma in first-degree relatives of patients with plasma cell neoplasia and the higher frequency of multiple myeloma in blacks.
- **Ionizing radiation** has been incriminated in the etiology of plasma cell neoplasia. Long-term survivors of the bombing of Hiroshima and Nagasaki suffered a fivefold increased incidence of multiple myeloma.
- **Chronic antigenic stimulation** may constitute a risk factor. For example, in Balb-C mice, intraperitoneal instillation of mineral oil or solid plastic material commonly induces the formation of a plasmacytoma. In humans, some cases of multiple myeloma have been associated with chronic infections, such as HIV and chronic osteomyelitis, and with chronic inflammatory disorders (e.g., rheumatoid arthritis). A two-hit hypothesis is proposed by which (1) antigenic stimulation leads to reactive, polyclonal proliferation of B lymphocytes and (2) a subsequent mutagenic event establishes a single malignant clone.

 Pathology: On gross examination, the osseous and extraosseous tumors of plasma cell neoplasia are variably red, tan, or gray and have a consistency that ranges from fleshy to gelatinous. The bony lesions are well demarcated from the surrounding normal tissue (Fig. 20-77). The cortical bone may be destroyed, with direct tumor extension into the surrounding soft tissues. In multiple myeloma, moderate enlargement of the lymph nodes, spleen, and liver is occasionally observed, although the gross appearance of these organs is not distinctive. The kidneys are often contracted in size.

Bone marrow: Microscopically, the morphological hallmark of multiple myeloma in the bone marrow is the presence of diffuse sheets or nodular aggregates of plasma cells. A characteristic early feature is the encircling of fat cells by plasma cells. Ultimately, both normal hematopoietic tissues and fat cells are replaced by neoplastic plasma cells.

In smears of marrow aspirates, neoplastic plasma cells usually exceed 30% of the nucleated cell elements (Table 20-22). The malignant cells may be morphologically normal, but more commonly they demonstrate cytological atypia (Fig. 20-78). The atypical cytological features include (1) prominent nucleoli, (2) irregular chromatin distri-

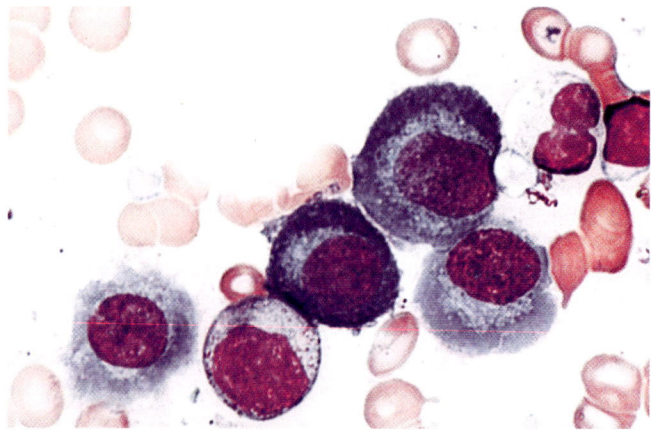

FIGURE 20-78
Multiple myeloma. A smear of a bone marrow aspirate shows a cluster of three neoplastic plasma cells.

bution, (3) binucleation and bizarre multinucleation, and (4) nuclear–cytoplasmic asynchrony, with immature nuclei and mature cytoplasm. Plasmablasts, characterized by large central nuclei, finely dispersed chromatin, prominent nucleoli, and scant blue cytoplasm, may be observed and in some cases constitute the predominant cell type. A distinctive reddish tint of the peripheral cytoplasm of the neoplastic plasma cells *(flame cells)* is commonly seen in IgA myeloma.

Cytoplasmic and nuclear inclusions, representing immunoglobulin accumulation, may be observed in neoplastic plasma cells. *Russell bodies* are globular, eosinophilic, refractile, cytoplasmic inclusions, and *Dutcher bodies* are similar nuclear invaginations. *Moth cells* contain grapelike eosinophilic accumulations of immunoglobulin. Precipitates of crystalline immunoglobulin may also be observed in the cytoplasm of the neoplastic plasma cells.

Bones: Increased osteoclasts are commonly present in resorption lacunae along the scalloped margins of bony trabeculae. Mild myelofibrosis or thickening of the bony trabeculae (osteosclerosis) is occasionally encountered.

Kidneys: A constellation of renal abnormalities is seen in over half of cases of plasma cell neoplasia (see Chapter 16).

Light-chain cast nephropathy is the most characteristic finding and is characterized by the precipitation of finely granular or lamellar protein casts containing light chains and other proteins, in the distal convoluted and collecting tubules. Secondary injury to the tubules by the protein casts leads to tubular epithelial cell atrophy or hyperplasia, with the formation of epithelial cell syncytia. Destruction of tubular basement membranes induces renal tubulointerstitial inflammation and secondary interstitial fibrosis.

Glomerulopathy is the other important renal abnormality in plasma cell neoplasia. A diffuse deposition of M-component occurs in the renal glomeruli, tubular basement membranes, and the vasculature. The glomerulopathy is characterized by proliferation of mesangial cells and increased mesangial matrix. Additionally, there may be damage to both renal tubules and blood vessels.

Additional renal findings in multiple myeloma include the deposition of (1) amyloid in the glomeruli and blood vessels, (2) calcium (nephrocalcinosis), and (3) uric acid crystals (urate nephropathy). Acute and chronic pyelonephritis may be seen. Focal or (rarely) massive neoplastic plasma cell infiltration may occur in the interstitium.

Lymph nodes: The lymph nodes may be infiltrated by neoplastic plasma cells, initially in the B cell-dependent medullary cords. This process may progress to a total obliteration of the normal nodal architecture.

Spleen and liver: The spleen shows variable infiltration of the red pulp cords and sinuses. In the liver, the portal triads may contain plasma cells, and in the case of a leukemic distribution, they are identified in the hepatic sinusoids.

Immunophenotypes: Most cases of multiple myeloma present with secretion of monoclonal IgG or IgA. Rarely, secretion of IgD or IgE is noted. In 85% of cases, complete immunoglobulin is secreted, but in 15%, only light chains are produced *(light chain disease)*. Surface Ig is absent from the tumor cells. Many of the B-cell markers that are expressed on the cell surface of mature B cells are absent in plasma cells, with the exception of CD79A.

Genotypes: Clonal rearrangement for IgH can be demonstrated by molecular studies. Multiple chromosomal abnormalities have been described in multiple myeloma, including monosomy or partial deletion of chromosome 13 in 25% of cases. As in mantle cell lymphoma, t(11;14) gene rearrangement of the *BCL-1* gene locus may occur. Similar to other clonal plasma cell proliferations, *PAX-5* abnormalities on chromosome 9 have been described. Genetic abnormalities associated with an unfavorable prognosis are deletions of 30q14 and 17p13 (loss of *p53*).

Clinical Features: Criteria for the diagnosis of multiple myeloma are summarized in Table 20-22. Lytic bone lesions of the skull and other flat bones, including the spine and ribs, are a characteristic (but not diagnostic) radiological finding in multiple myeloma (Fig. 20-79).

The most important disorder to consider in the differential diagnosis of multiple myeloma is the more common *monoclonal gammopathy of unknown significance (MGUS)* (Fig. 20-80). Also known as *benign essential gammopathy*, the term *monoclonal gammopathy of unknown significance* is preferred because the disorder is not necessarily benign. About 2% of patients with MGUS per year progress to a B-cell neoplasm (lymphoplasmacytic disorder or multiple myeloma). The strong link between MGUS and multiple myeloma supports the two-hit hypothesis in which a first oncogenic event causes MGUS and a second event results in multiple myeloma.

Common initial laboratory findings in multiple myeloma include normocytic, normochromic anemia, hypercalcemia, and hyperuricemia. A sharp peak or spike representing the M-component is observed with serum or urine protein electrophoresis (Fig. 20-80). Immunofixation with antibodies directed against heavy and light chain immunoglobulins allows better characterization of the abnormal protein (Fig. 20-81). The erythrocyte sedimentation rate is elevated, owing to the M-component. On the peripheral blood smear, the erythrocytes may appear stacked and clumped (rouleaux formation) (Fig. 20-82), which also reflects the M-component.

The type of M-component is clinically relevant because of some commonly observed clinicopathological associations.

- **IgG myeloma** is "typical" myeloma, with a mean survival of 3 to 4 years. Infections are a common complication.
- **IgA myeloma** shows symptoms and signs due to serum hyperviscosity because of the tendency of the IgA molecule to form dimers.
- **IgD myeloma** is an aggressive clinical disorder that tends to occur in middle-aged men. The mean survival is 1 year. Extramedullary involvement with soft tissue masses is common. Renal disease is also frequent, possibly because IgD heavy chains are almost invariably associated with an unbalanced synthesis of nephrotoxic λ light chains.
- **IgE myeloma** is an uncommon and aggressive clinical disorder that also tends to occur in young adult men. A leukemic phase, with peripheral blood plasma cell counts exceeding 2000/μL, occurs in a fourth of cases. Other than in IgE myeloma, plasma cell leukemia is an uncommon and usually preterminal manifestation of plasma cell neoplasia.

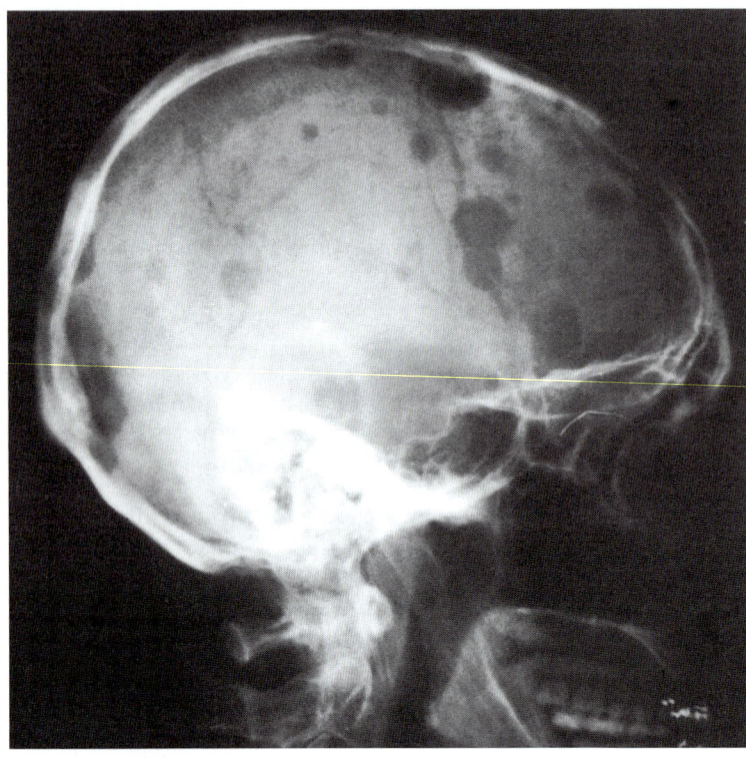

FIGURE 20-79
Multiple myeloma. A radiograph of the skull shows numerous punched-out radiolucent areas.

- **Light-chain disease** is an aggressive variant of multiple myeloma in which only κ or λ light chains are synthesized. The κ chain disease is twice as common as the λ chain disease. The serum protein pattern is normal until secondary renal disease prevents glomerular filtration of light chains.

Multiple myeloma typically presents with bone pain, most commonly involving the vertebrae and ribs. Symptoms due to anemia, hypercalcemia, and renal insufficiency are frequent. Amyloidosis of light-chain origin (principally λ) occurs in 15% of cases, and the hyperviscosity syndrome is observed in less than 5%. There is a "primary" distribution of

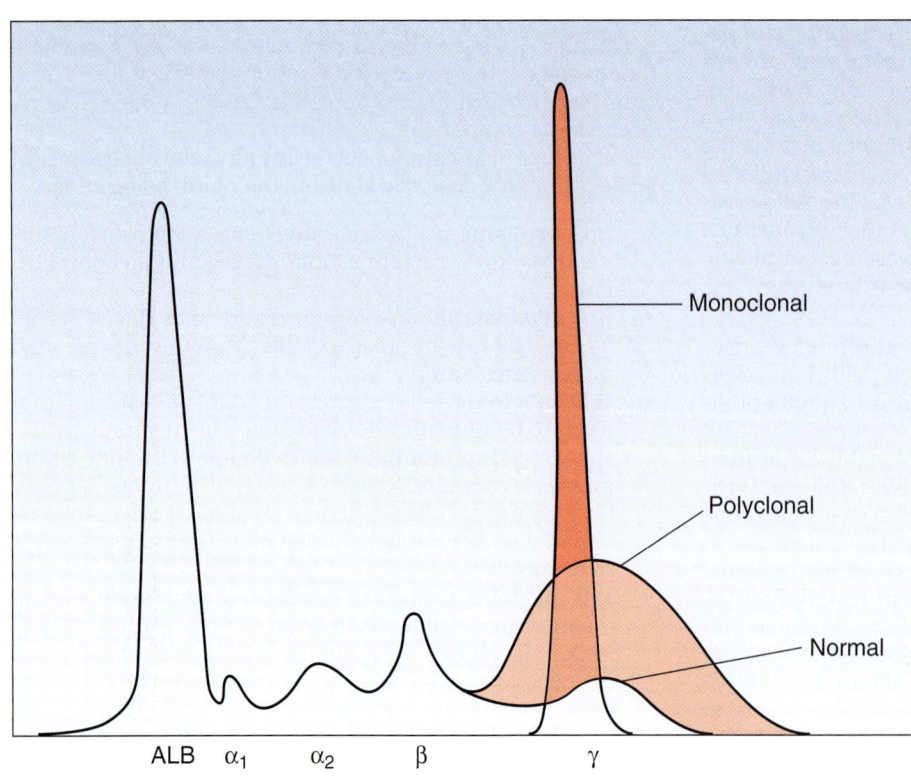

FIGURE 20-80
Abnormal serum protein electrophoretic patterns contrasted with a normal pattern. Polyclonal hypergammaglobulinemia, characteristic of benign reactive processes, shows a broad-based increase in immunoglobulins, owing to immunoglobulin secretion by a myriad of reactive plasma cells. Monoclonal gammopathy of unknown significance or plasma cell neoplasia shows a narrow peak, or spike, owing to the homogeneity of the immunoglobulin molecules secreted by a single clone of aberrant plasma cells.

Malignant Lymphomas

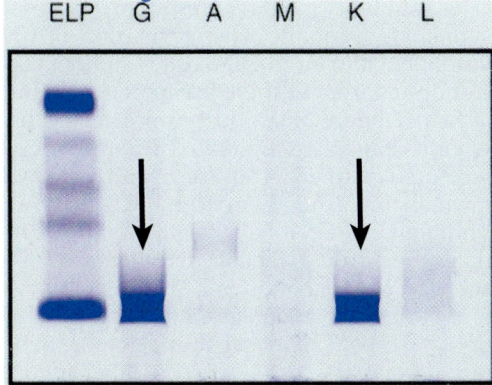

FIGURE 20-81
Serum protein electrophoresis and immunofixation in a patient with an IgGκ spike. Serum proteins are separated by standard serum protein electrophoresis (lane ELP). A distinct band is noted in the gamma fraction at the bottom of lane ELP. Subsequently, individual lanes are incubated with antibodies directed against IgG,A,M and κ and λ light chains. Reagents directed against IgG and κ light chain are positive. (arrows).

amyloid, with deposition in such sites as the tongue, the gastrointestinal tract, and the heart.

The clinical course in multiple myeloma tends to be biphasic. An initial chronic stable phase is followed by an aggressive or accelerated preterminal phase. The prognosis depends on (1) the total body tumor burden at the time of diagnosis and (2) the status of renal function. A high total body tumor burden is indicated by (1) a hemoglobin level below 8.5 g/dL; (2) serum calcium concentration above 12 mg/dL; (3) an M-component higher than 5 g/dL; (4) high levels of serum LDH or $β_2$-microglobulin, both reflecting turnover of nucleated cells; and (5) extensive lytic bone lesions.

Bone destruction in multiple myeloma is due to both progressive tumor growth and secretion by neoplastic plasma cells of osteoclast-activating factor. Osteoclasts may also be activated by the IL-6 system, whose activity is increased in patients with multiple myeloma. Common complications of bone destruction include vertebral collapse and pathological fractures of long bones. Additionally, calcium released from the injured bone may precipitate in the kidneys and cause renal damage (nephrocalcinosis).

The hyperviscosity syndrome (see macroglobulinemia) is particularly common in IgG and IgA myelomas, although it is far less frequent than in macroglobulinemia. An increase in serum viscosity to over 4 cp units (normal, 1.4 to 1.8) results in abnormalities of blood flow, with secondary complications in multiple organ systems. Neurological abnormalities and spontaneous bleeding episodes are observed.

Some M-components function as cryoglobulins, which are proteins that precipitate in the cold. As a consequence, blood flow to the distal extremities may be impaired, with resultant acrocyanosis and Raynaud phenomenon.

Coagulation abnormalities result from (1) complexes formed between the M-component and coagulation factors, (2) coprecipitation of M-component cryoglobulins with coagulation complexes, and (3) coating of platelets with the M-component.

Monoclonal light chains are present in the urine (Bence-Jones protein) in up to 75% of cases of multiple myeloma and in a minority of solitary osseous myelomas and extramedullary plasmacytomas. The neoplastic clone of plasma cells may secrete excess light chains, owing to unbalanced synthesis of heavy and light chains. The light chains are rapidly filtered through the glomeruli and appear in the urine as Bence-Jones protein.

Humoral immune deficiency, with decreased levels of normal serum immunoglobulins, is characteristic of multiple myeloma. This defect is due to (1) suppression of normal B lymphocytes by the neoplastic clone, and (2) increased catabolism of normal IgG. Because of the low levels of normal antibodies, patients with multiple myeloma are susceptible to a variety of infectious complications, particularly pneumonia and pyelonephritis.

Multiple myeloma is an incurable disease, with a mean survival of 6 months in untreated patients and 3 years with appropriate chemotherapy. Death is usually due to either infection or renal failure. The disease may be complicated by superimposed MDS or AML, usually attributed to the leukemogenic effect of treatment with alkylating agents. After treatment, the risk of AML occurring in 5 years is 14% and in 10 years, 20%.

Solitary osseous myeloma presents as a single lytic skeletal lesion, most commonly involving the ribs, vertebrae, or pelvic bones. The natural history of solitary osseous myeloma is progression to multiple myeloma (70%), local extension or recurrence (15%), or extension to a distant skeletal site (15%). The overall 10-year survival is 20%. Solitary osseous myeloma is treated with irradiation.

Extramedullary plasmacytomas occur in the upper respiratory tract in 80% of cases, including the nasal sinuses, nasopharynx, and the tonsils. The remaining 20% occur in other soft tissue sites, such as the lungs, breast, and lymph nodes. Extramedullary plasmacytoma is eradicated by surgery or local radiation therapy. In 20% of cases progression to multiple myeloma occurs.

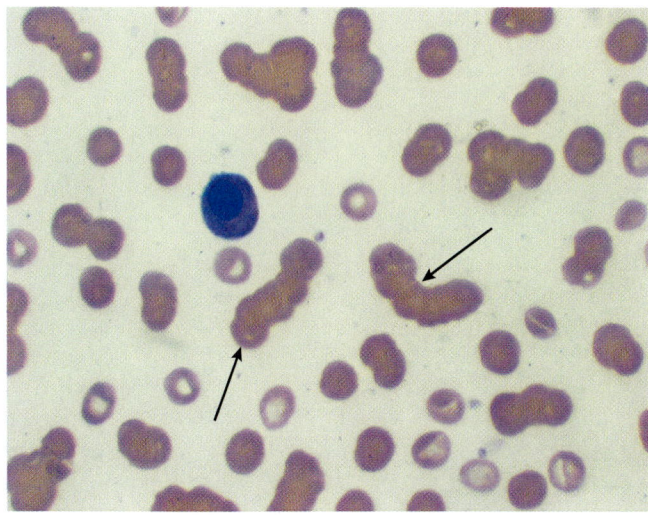

FIGURE 20-82
Multiple myeloma. Rouleaux formation (arrows) and a circulating plasma cell are seen.

Extranodal Marginal-Zone B-cell Lymphoma of Mucosa-Associated Lymphoid Tissue

MALT lymphomas are indolent, malignant lymphocyte proliferations that consist of small to medium-sized lymphocytes, with frequent monocytoid features and variable admixtures of plasma cells. The malignant lymphocytes appear to originate from marginal-zone B cells.

Epidemiology: MALT lymphomas constitute 5 to 10% of all B-cell lymphomas, with a mean incidence at age 60 years. Most primary gastric lymphomas are MALT lymphomas.

Pathogenesis: MALT lymphomas occur either in glandular organs or along mucosal surfaces. They commonly arise in the context of a chronic inflammatory process or autoimmune disease. The prototype of an infection-driven MALT lymphoma is gastric lymphoma secondary to *H. pylori*-associated gastritis.. Examples of MALT lymphomas in autoimmune diseases include salivary gland lymphoma in Sjögren syndrome and thyroid lymphoma associated with Hashimoto thyroiditis.

Pathology: Early-stage MALT lymphomas present microscopically with expanded marginal zone lymphocytes around reactive B-cell follicles. The spectrum of malignant lymphocytes ranges from small lymphocytes to medium-sized, monocytoid lymphocytes with more abundant cytoplasm and a variable admixture of clonal plasma cells. The tumor cells invade glandular epithelium or epithelia of mucosal surfaces, where they form *lymphoepithelial lesions* (Fig. 20-83). *Immunoproliferative small intestinal disease*, also termed *alpha chain disease* or *Mediterranean lymphoma*, is a subtype of MALT lymphoma that produces α heavy chains. Occasionally, transformation of (indolent) MALT lymphoma into large cell B cell lymphoma occurs.

Immunophenotypes: There is no specific immunophenotype of MALT lymphoma. Most tumor cells express IgM and show light chain restriction. MALT lymphomas express B cell-associated antigens and are negative for CD5 and CD23, which distinguishes them from B-CLL/SLL and mantle cell lymphoma. They are also negative for CD10, which differentiates them from follicular lymphoma.

Genotypes: MALT lymphoma typically shows somatic mutation of variable region genes and is believed to derive from memory B cells. The most common cytogenetic abnormalities are trisomy 3 and t(11;18), the latter involving the apoptosis inhibitor gene *API2* and a novel gene termed *MLT*. In cases with subtle lymphocytic infiltrates in the gastric mucosa, demonstration of clonal *IgH* gene rearrangement helps to establish the diagnosis.

Clinical Features: Most MALT lymphomas involve the stomach or other mucosal sites, including the respiratory tract. They may also be seen in the head and neck region, ocular adnexal sites, skin, thyroid, and breast. MALT lymphomas remain localized for prolonged periods and tend to follow an indolent clinical course. MALT lymphomas involving the parotid are sensitive to radiation therapy; gastric MALT lymphomas secondary to *H. pylori* infection respond to antibiotic therapy.

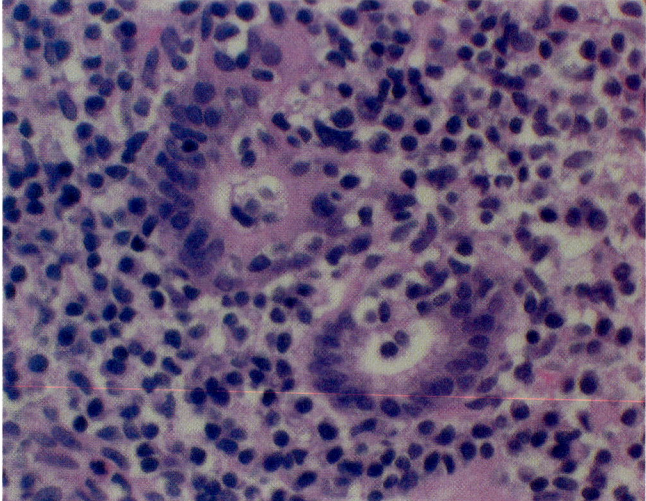

FIGURE 20-83
Mucosa-associated lymphoid tissue (MALT) lymphoma. Lymphoepithelial lesions of the stomach are present.

Follicular Lymphoma

Follicular lymphoma (FL) is the malignant counterpart of lymphocytes derived from follicle centers. Follicle (germinal) centers are composed of large round cells (centroblasts) and smaller cells with irregular or cleaved nuclei (centrocytes). Unlike any other type of lymphoma, follicular lymphoma mimics an entire functional unit of lymphocytes, including their ancillary cells. The opposite of *follicular* lymphoma is *diffuse* lymphoma. Depending on the percentage of centroblasts, follicular lymphoma is divided into three grades. The more centroblasts present, the higher the grade.

Epidemiology: FL is a particularly common neoplasm in the United States, where it constitutes 35% of all adult malignant lymphomas. The disease shows a peak incidence at 60 years of age and is somewhat more common in women than in men.

Pathology: FL (Fig. 20-84) predominantly involves lymph nodes and resembles benign follicular hyperplasia. FL is distinguished from the latter by (1) ill-defined mantle zones, (2) lack of polarization within the germinal center, (3) absence of "starry sky" macrophages, and (4) extracapsular invasion into perinodal fat. FL may transform into a more aggressive diffuse lymphoma consisting of a mixture of centroblasts and centrocytes.

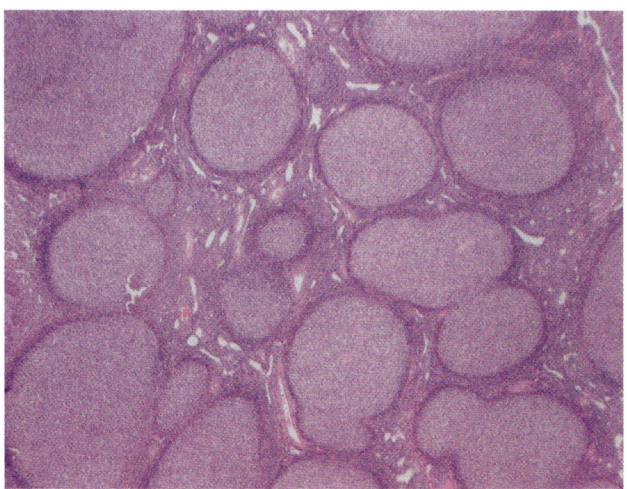

FIGURE 20-84
Follicular lymphoma.

Immunophenotypes: FL usually displays surface Ig and is light-chain restricted. The tumor cells are positive for most B-cell markers and CD10 but negative for CD5. In contrast to benign germinal center B lymphocytes (Fig. 20-71), FL expresses BCL-2 protein (Fig. 20-85).

Genotypes: The most common cytogenetic translocation in FL is t(14:18)(q32:q21), with *IgH* and *BCL-2* as partner genes. BCL-2 protein is localized in the mitochondrial membrane and functions as an apoptosis inhibitor. Clonal rearrangement of the *BCL-6* oncogene is common.

Clinical Features: FL predominantly affects lymph nodes. Other sites of involvement include the spleen, bone marrow, peripheral blood, head and neck region, gastrointestinal tract, soft tissue, and skin. Most patients have advanced disease at presentation. Low-grade FL is an indolent, but usually incurable, malignancy, whereas grade 3 FL is more aggressive but has the potential for cure. The prognosis deteriorates with the number of genetic abnormalities. One third of patients with FL progress to (diffuse) large B-cell lymphoma, which retains expression of CD10 (CALLA) even if the typical nodular architecture of FL is lost.

Mantle Cell Lymphoma

Mantle cell lymphoma is a B-cell neoplasm consisting of small to medium-sized lymphocytes with irregular nuclear features.

Epidemiology: Mantle cell lymphoma constitutes less than 10% of all malignant lymphomas. It does not occur in children, but affects older persons, with a median age of 60 years. Men are more likely to be affected than women.

Pathology: Small to medium-sized lymphocytes with irregular nuclear features diffusely infiltrate lymph nodes. In one variant, an expanded (malignant) follicular mantle is wrapped around (benign) germinal centers *(mantle zone lymphoma)*. In another, more aggressive variant, the tumor cells appear larger and more immature *(blastoid mantle cell lymphoma)*. The spleen, bone marrow, and gastrointestinal tract may be involved. In the gastrointestinal tract, mantle cell lymphoma produces nodular alterations of the mucosal surface, termed *lymphomatous polyposis*.

Immunophenotypes: Mantle cell lymphoma has a B-cell immunophenotype, and the tumor cells express CD5 but are negative for CD23 and CD10. The tumor cells are positive for nuclear BCL-1 protein (Fig. 20-86).

Genotypes: The variable-region genes are normally not mutated, indicating derivation from a pre-germinal center B

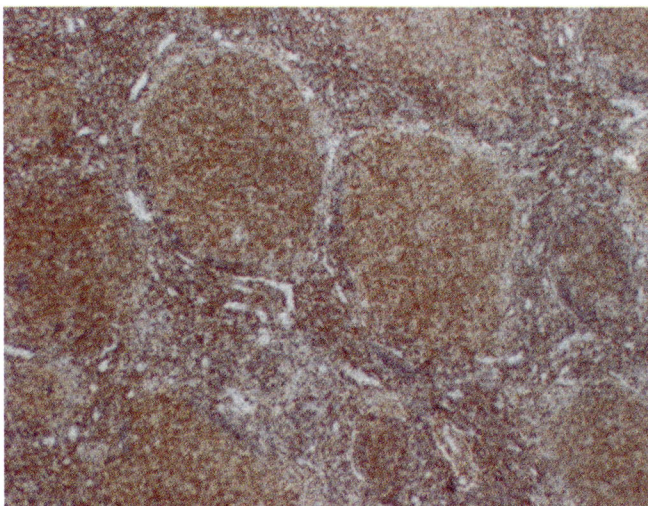

FIGURE 20-85
Follicular lymphoma. Malignant lymph follicles are marked with an antibody against BCL-2 (compare with negative stain in follicular hyperplasia in Fig. 20-70).

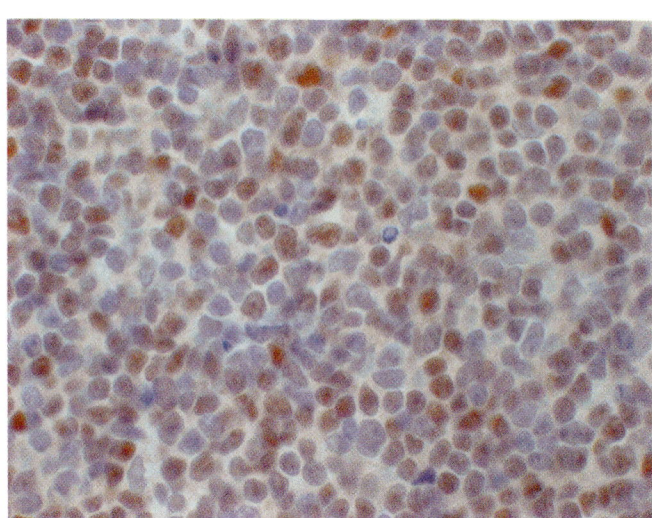

FIGURE 20-86
Mantle cell lymphoma. A nuclear stain for BCL-1 is positive.

cell. The most important cytogenetic abnormality is t(11:14)(q13:q32), which involves the cyclin D1 *(BCL-1, PRAD1)* gene on chromosome 11 and the *IgH* gene on chromosome 14. Cyclin D1 exerts cell cycle control at the transition from G1 to S by complexing with CDK 4/6. This event results in the phosphorylation of RB and subsequent activation of transcription factors (see Chapter 5). In many cases, abnormalities of the *ATM* (**a**taxia **t**elangiectasia **m**utated) gene have been described.

 Clinical Features: Mantle cell lymphoma progresses relentlessly, and half the patients do not survive 3 years.

Diffuse Large B-cell Lymphoma

Diffuse large B-cell lymphoma (DLBCL) encompasses a heterogeneous group of aggressive, potentially curable B-cell neoplasms. The disease occurs in all age groups but is most prevalent between the ages of 60 and 70 years. The cause of DLBCL is unknown, but it may be seen in association with EBV and HIV infections.

Pathology: DLBCL may involve lymph nodes or extranodal sites. The tumor cells resemble immunoblasts or centroblasts (Fig. 20-87) or appear as anaplastic bizarre cells with marked nuclear irregularities. Immunoblasts are large B cells (Fig. 20-88) whose nuclei exhibit prominent central nucleoli. Centroblasts are large germinal center-derived cells (Fig. 20-88). A variant of DLBCL is *T-cell rich B-cell lymphoma*, in which a few tumor cells are surrounded by normal small T cells.

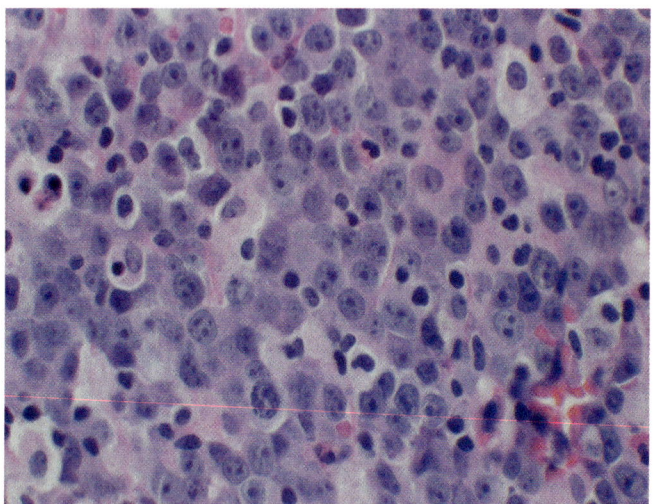

FIGURE 20-87
Diffuse large B-cell lymphoma. Tumor cells show prominent nucleoli.

The tumor cells of DLBCL express various B-cell markers, with occasional reactivity for CD5 or CD10. As in FL, clonal *BCL2* gene rearrangements are often seen, indicating a potential germinal center origin in some cases. DLBCL associated with immunodeficiency is usually positive for EBV.

 Clinical Features: Rapidly evolving, multifocal, nodal and extranodal tumor manifestations are typically seen at the time of presentation. DLBCL is potentially curable, but a high proliferation rate conveys an adverse prognosis.

Mediastinal (Thymic) Diffuse Large B-cell Lymphoma

Mediastinal diffuse large B-cell lymphoma (MED-DLBCL) features a locally invasive tumor of the anterior mediastinum, most commonly affecting young women. The tumor often displays marked fibrosis. The tumor cells derive from thymic medullary B cells and are positive for most B-cell markers. MED-DLBCL confined to the mediastinum can be treated successfully with combination radiation therapy and chemotherapy, but disseminated disease carries a less favorable prognosis.

Primary Effusion Lymphoma

Primary effusion lymphoma (PEL) is a newly recognized entity that mainly occurs in HIV-infected immunocompromised persons and is characterized by tumor cell suspensions in the pleural, pericardial or peritoneal cavities. HHV 8 is detectable in all instances, and EBV is a common coinfectant. Although most tumors feature B cells with clonal *IgH* gene rearrangements, B-cell surface markers are usually absent. The normal counterpart of PEL is a post-germinal-center B cell. Survival is usually less than 6 months after diagnosis.

Burkitt Lymphoma

Burkitt lymphoma (BL), one of the most rapidly growing malignancies, is defined by a chromosomal translocation involving 8q24, which harbors the *MYC* oncogene (see Chapter 5).

Epidemiology: **Endemic Burkitt lymphoma** is the most common childhood malignancy in Central Africa, with a peak incidence at ages 3 to 7. **Sporadic Burkitt lymphoma** affects mainly children and young adults in the Western world, where it accounts for 1 to 2% of all lymphomas. As in endemic Burkitt lymphoma, males are more often affected than females. **Immunodeficiency-associated Burkitt lymphoma** mainly occurs in HIV-infected persons.

 Pathogenesis: EBV is present in virtually all cases of endemic BL, but is detected in less than 30% of sporadic types. EBV-positive sporadic BL is as-

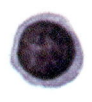 **SMALL LYMPHOCYTIC**
Nucleus: round
Chromatin: dense
Nucleolus: indistinct
Cytoplasm: scant, blue

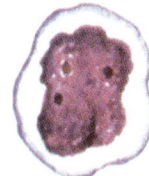 **T-CELL**
Nucleus: round to irregular
Chromatin: variable
Nucleoli: variable
Cytoplasm: clear

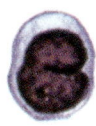 **MANTLE CELL or FOLLICULAR**
(Centrocytic)
Nucleus: indented
Chromatin: coarse
Nucleolus: small
Cytoplasm: scant

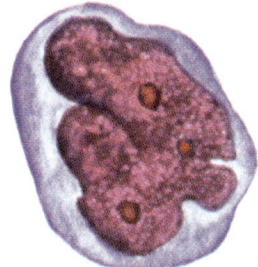 **ANAPLASTIC LARGE CELL**
Nucleus: pleomorphic
Chromatin: variable
Nucleoli: variable
Cytoplasm: moderate

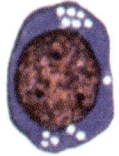 **BURKITT**
Nucleus: round to oval
Chromatin: coarsely reticulated
Nucleoli: small, 2-5
Cytoplasm: blue, vacuolated

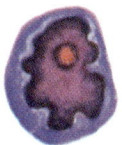 **LYMPHOBLASTIC, CONVOLUTED**
Nucleus: irregular
Chromatin: delicate
Nucleolus: variable
Cytoplasm: blue, scant

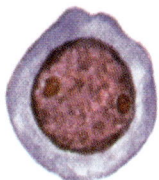 **LARGE CELL (Centroblastic)**
Nucleus: round to oval
Chromatin: vesicular
Nucleoli: contiguous to membrane
Cytoplasm: moderate

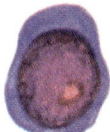 **LYMPHOBLASTIC, NONCONVOLUTED**
Nucleus: round to oval
Chromatin: delicate
Nucleolus: variable
Cytoplasm: scant, blue

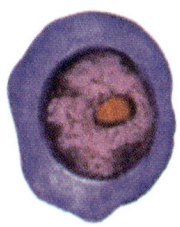 **LARGE CELL (Immunoblastic)**
Nucleus: round to oval
Chromatin: vesicular
Nucleolus: prominent
Cytoplasm: moderate, dense, blue

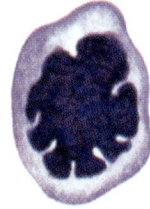 **MYCOSIS FUNGOIDES**
Nucleus: irregular, convoluted
Chromatin: dense
Nucleolus: indistinct
Cytoplasm: scant

FIGURE 20-88
Malignant lymphomas: Neoplastic cells.

sociated with low socioeconomic status. Many patients experience a prodromal stage of polyclonal B-cell activation caused by bacterial, viral, or parasitic infections (malaria) (see Chapter 5).

 Pathology: BL typically produces extranodal tumors rather than lymphadenopathy. All types of this lymphoma have a high risk for CNS involvement. The classic presentation for endemic BL is a destructive tumor in the jaws or other facial bones. Patients suffering from sporadic BL typically present with abdominal masses. All types may involve ovaries, kidneys, and breast. Patients with sizable bulky tumors sometimes present with Burkitt leukemia and extensive bone marrow involvement. Immunodeficiency-associated BL involves lymph nodes more often than other types of BL.

Microscopically, BL cells are medium-sized and lack significant cytological atypia. Tissue sections reveal a high number of mitotic figures, which attests to the extremely high proliferation rate in this tumor. The cellular debris of apoptotic tumor cells is cleared by macrophages, whose scattered appearance is termed "starry sky macrophage" (Fig. 20-89). Aspirate smears stained with Wright-Giemsa demonstrate numerous lipid vacuoles in the deeply basophilic cytoplasm of the tumor cells (L3 morphology in the old FAB classification) (Figs. 20-88 and 20-53).

Immunophenotypes: Burkitt cells express surface IgM and are positive for common B cell antigens (CD19, CD20, CD22). They mark for CD10 and BCL-6, and are thus thought to be of germinal center origin. Since Burkitt cells express surface Ig but are negative for TdT, they do not represent precursor B cells.

Genotypes: Clonal *IgH* gene arrangement can be demonstrated for heavy- and light-chain genes. Somatic mutations of the *IgH* genes point toward a more mature type of B cell. Immunoglobulin heavy-chain genes and *MYC* genes participate in t(8;14). In endemic cases, the breakpoint on chromosome 14 occurs in the heavy chain joining region, as seen in early B cells. In sporadic BL, the translocation occurs in the Ig switch region, which is more characteristic of mature B lymphocytes. In these cases, regulation of the *MYC* gene by the Ig heavy-chain promoter leads to uncontrolled growth of the tumor cells. Less commonly, the *MYC* gene is translocated to the λ light-chain gene on chromosome 22 or the κ light-chain gene on chromosome 2.

Clinical Features: Most patients present with bulky extranodal tumors that emerge in a short time and respond to aggressive chemotherapy. Both endemic and sporadic BL are curable in up to 90% of the patients.

Mature T-cell and NK-Cell Lymphomas Have a Poor Prognosis

Mature (peripheral) T-cell and NK-cell malignancies originate from postthymic T-cells.

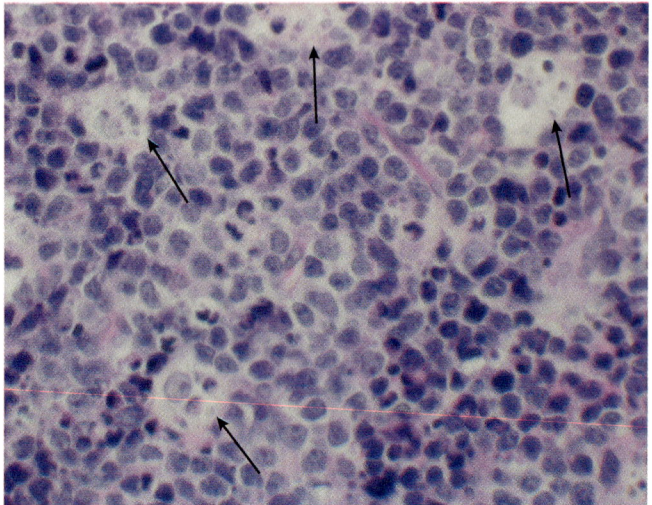

FIGURE 20-89
Burkitt lymphoma with several starry sky macrophages (arrows).

Epidemiology: Worldwide, T-cell malignancies account for 12% of all non-Hodgkin lymphomas. T-cell and NK-cell lymphomas are more common in Asia than in the Western world. In Japan, a major group of T-cell malignancies is attributed to infection with human T-cell leukemia virus (HTLV-1).

Pathology: The immunophenotype of mature T-cell malignancies is uniformly characterized by the expression of α,β or γ,δ pairs of T-cell receptors, both of which are linked to CD3 protein. By definition, NK cells lack complete T-cell receptor gene expression, but they are positive for the intracellular ε chain of CD3. γ,δ T cells constitute less than 5% of the T-cell repertoire and are mainly found in association with epithelial surfaces and within the splenic red pulp. These T cells do not express CD4, CD8, and CD5, whereas α,β T cells are (CD4$^+$) helper or CD8$^+$ (cytotoxic).

NK cells express CD2, CD7, and CD8 and are also positive for CD16, CD56, and CD57. Both NK and cytotoxic T-cell malignancies demonstrate the granule-associated proteins *perforin, granzyme B,* and *T-cell intracellular antigen (TIA-1).*

Clinical Features: T-cell and NK-cell malignancies are clinically grouped into leukemic or nodal, extranodal, and cutaneous malignancies. As a rule of thumb, these neoplasms and NK cell lymphomas are more aggressive than most B-cell malignancies and Hodgkin lymphoma. They are treated with standard chemotherapy for B-cell lymphomas. Many T-cell neoplasms respond poorly to treatment, with an overall 5-year survival in the range of 20 to 30%.

T-cell Prolymphocytic Leukemia

T-cell prolymphocytic leukemia (T-PLL) is a rare, aggressive, T-cell leukemia characterized by proliferation of medium-sized lymphocytes. Hepatosplenomegaly with peripheral leukocytosis is common. Chromosomal abnormalities involving the T-cell oncogenes *TCL1* at 14q32.1 are most common. The prognosis is favorable.

T-cell Large Granular Lymphocyte Leukemia (T-LGL)

T-LGL is a rare, chronic proliferation of large granular lymphocytes involving peripheral blood, bone marrow, liver, and spleen. It is the prototype of an indolent lymphoproliferative disorder. T-LGL is frequently associated with splenomegaly, rheumatoid arthritis, autoantibodies, and hypergammaglobulinemia. Leukopenia and severe anemia are other common associations.

Aggressive NK-Cell Leukemia

Aggressive NK-cell leukemia is a rare, systemic lymphoproliferative disorder, most commonly seen in young adult Asians. Most cases are associated with EBV infection. Patients present with fever, hepatosplenomegaly, and leukemia. Survival is short, usually not exceeding 2 years.

Adult T-cell Leukemia/Lymphoma

Adult T-cell leukemia/lymphoma (ATLL) is caused by HTLV-1.

 Epidemiology: Geographically, ATLL parallels the endemic prevalence of HTLV-1 infection in Japan, the Caribbean basin, and Central Africa. Only a few persons (2%) who harbor the virus develop ATLL.

 Pathology: ATLL is caused by gene activation mediated through HTLV-1 viral protein P40 tax. The leukemic cells in ATLL are markedly atypical and contain multilobulated nuclei *(flower cells)*. Peripheral blood, bone marrow, and skin are common sites of involvement.

Immunophenotypes: T-cell markers in ATLL are positive for CD2, CD3, and CD5. As in many other peripheral T-cell lymphomas, CD7 is often absent. Most patients have a T-cell helper immunophenotype (CD4$^+$). In some, the tumor cells are positive for the low-molecular-weight IL-2 receptor (CD25) and CD30.

Genotypes: The tumor cells show a clonal T-cell receptor gene rearrangement pattern and are positive for clonally integrated HTLV-1. The normal counterpart of ATLL is a mature, activated, CD4$^+$ T cell.

 Clinical Features: ATLL is a systemic disease with multiorgan manifestations and peripheral leukocytosis. Acute, smoldering, and chronic variants are recognized. Hypercalcemia, with or without lytic bone lesions, is typical. The skin represents the most important extranodal involvement. Acute ATLL has an unfavorable prognosis. Death frequently occurs from infectious complications, similar to those seen in HIV-infected patients. Chronic and smoldering forms have a somewhat better prognosis.

Extranodal NK/T-cell Lymphoma, Nasal Type

NK/T-cell lymphoma is a highly aggressive, predominantly extranodal malignancy characterized by an angiocentric, necrotizing, vascular infiltrate. The disease combines NK-cell (CD56$^+$) and T-cell features and is usually positive for EBV. The prototype of this malignancy is seen in and around the nasal cavity. Skin, soft tissue, gastrointestinal tract, and testis are other common sites of involvement.

Enteropathy-Associated T-cell Lymphoma

Enteropathy-associated type T-cell lymphoma is an uncommon, malignant disorder that arises from intraepithelial T lymphocytes in patients with celiac disease (see Chapter 13). The tumor is most commonly seen in the jejunum and ileum, and manifestations outside the gastrointestinal tract are rare. The tumor cells show variable expression for T-cell antigens. The most specific marker is CD103, which is expressed in normal CD8$^+$ intraepithelial lymphocytes along mucosal surfaces. Enteropathy-associated T-cell lymphoma and hairy cell leukemia, a B-cell malignancy, are the lymphoid neoplasms with consistent expression of CD103. The disease has a poor prognosis.

Hepatosplenic T-cell Lymphoma

Hepatosplenic T-cell lymphoma is a rare malignancy derived from cytotoxic T cells. The spleen, liver, and bone marrow are the main sites of involvement. In most cases, the disease occurs in young men and exhibits cells that express the γ,δ T-cell receptor. Most patients exhibit marked hepatosplenomegaly, with involvement of the monocyte/macrophage system in the liver and spleen, a situation also seen in hairy cell leukemia. Isochromosome 7q is a consistent genetic abnormality. The disease is clinically aggressive, with a median survival of less than 2 years.

Subcutaneous Panniculitis-Like T-cell Lymphoma

Subcutaneous panniculitis-like T-cell lymphoma originates from cytotoxic T cells and infiltrates subcutaneous tissue, with characteristic rimming of the tumor cells around fat vacuoles. The disease takes an aggressive clinical course, and hemophagocytic syndrome is a common complication. Most of these lymphomas express α,β cell receptors.

Mycosis Fungoides and Sézary Syndrome

Mycosis fungoides is a cutaneous T-cell lymphoma that features epidermal tropism.

 Epidemiology: The disease occurs mainly in adults and the elderly, and more men than women are affected.

 Pathology: Mycosis fungoides displays lymphocytic infiltrates at the dermal–epidermal junction and, in some cases, intraepidermal accumulations of tumor cells *(Pautrier microabscesses)* (see Chapter 24).

Immunophenotypes and Genotype: Most tumors show a mature T-helper cell immunophenotype (CD2$^+$, CD3$^+$, CD5$^+$, CD4$^+$, CD8$^-$ and TCRα,β^+). As with other peripheral T-cell lymphomas, CD7 is absent. Clonal T-cell receptor gene rearrangements are common, which helps to distinguish subtle cases of mycosis fungoides from inflammatory infiltrates.

 Clinical Features: Mycosis fungoides is an indolent lymphoma.

- **The premycotic or eczematous stage** lasts some years and is not distinguishable from a variety of benign chronic dermatoses. A skin biopsy specimen is not diag-

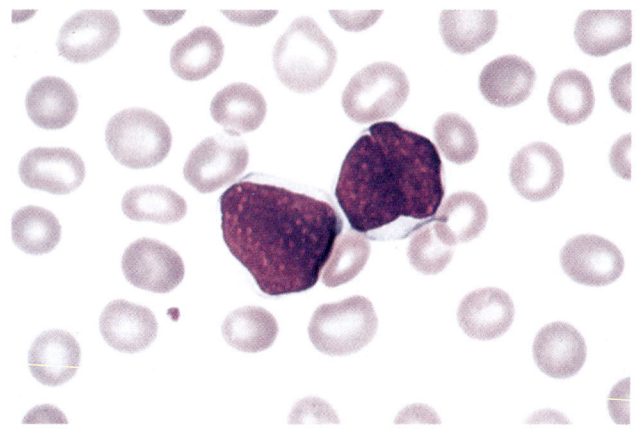

FIGURE 20-90
Sézary cells. Two circulating, neoplastic, T- helper cells with irregular nuclei and a thin rim of cytoplasm are seen.

nostic of lymphoma and shows a nonspecific perivascular and periadnexal lymphocytic infiltration with accompanying eosinophils and plasma cells.
- **The plaque stage,** which follows the premycotic stage, is characterized by well-demarcated, raised cutaneous plaques. A definitive diagnosis of CTCL can usually be made in this stage. There is a dense subepidermal band-like infiltrate of lymphoid cells, with irregular nuclear contours and a spectrum of cell sizes. Distinctive medium-to-large lymphoid cells with hyperchromatic nuclei and cerebriform nuclear contours, called *mycosis cells,* are typical. Often, Pautrier microabscesses in intraepidermal clear spaces are observed.
- **The tumor stage** features raised cutaneous tumors, most commonly on the face and in the body folds, which frequently ulcerate and become secondarily infected. The name *mycosis fungoides* derives from the raised, fungating, mushroomlike appearance of these cutaneous tumors. Extracutaneous involvement, particularly of the lymph nodes, spleen, liver, bone marrow, and lungs, occurs commonly.

Spread of mycosis fungoides to other organs, including lung, spleen, liver, and peripheral blood, is termed *Sézary syndrome.* Sézary syndrome arises after extensive cutaneous lesions have existed for a long time. Small *(Lutzner)* cells or large *(Sézary)* tumor cells are found in the peripheral blood (Fig. 20-90).

Angioimmunoblastic T-cell Lymphoma

Angioimmunoblastic T-cell lymphoma (AILT) presents with generalized lymphadenopathy and shows T zones expanded by a polymorphic T-cell infiltrate and proliferation of high endothelial venules. EBV can be demonstrated in atypical B cells, but for the most part not in the malignant T cells.

 Clinical Features: Most patients with AILT present with generalized lymphadenopathy, hepatosplenomegaly, bone marrow involvement, hypergammaglobulinemia, and often effusions from serosal surfaces. Other laboratory findings include cold hemagglutinins, hemolytic anemia, circulating immune complexes, and positive rheumatoid factor. In contrast to previous views, AILT is now regarded as an aggressive malignant lymphoma, with a median survival of less than 3 years.

Peripheral T-Cell Lymphoma, unspecified

T-cell lymphomas without specific defining features fall collectively into the category of "unspecified." They account for approximately half of all T-cell lymphomas in the Western world. They may be nodal or extranodal. They may be associated with eosinophilia, pruritus or hemophagocytic syndrome. There is variable expression of T-cell antigens, with most nodal cases exhibiting a T-helper immunophenotype (CD4+). Peripheral T-cell lymphomas as a group are aggressive malignancies with low 5 year survival (20–30%).

Anaplastic Large Cell Lymphoma

Anaplastic large cell lymphoma (ALCL) is characterized by large atypical tumor cells that universally express the activation marker CD30. Most cases are characterized by t(2;5) involving the *nucleophosmin (NPM)* and *anaplastic lymphoma kinase (ALK)* genes. NPM is a nuclear transfer protein and ALK is a transmembranous tyrosine kinase receptor of the insulin receptor superfamily. The fusion protein resulting from this translocation is silent in normal lymphocytes, but is up-regulated in ALCL.

 Epidemiology: ALCL follows a bimodal age distribution; the first peak occurs in young adulthood and the second in older persons. A sizable number of cases occur in childhood.

 Pathology: ALCL is characterized by highly irregular tumor cells (Fig. 20-91) that contain kidney- or horseshoe-shaped nuclei. Multinucleated tumor cells with prominent nucleoli, resembling Reed-Sternberg cells, are sometimes present. ALCL shows variable expression of T-cell markers, and most patients are positive for cytotoxic granule-associated proteins, granzyme B, TIA-1, and perforin.

 Clinical Features: Both nodal and extranodal sites are commonly involved. Many patients exhibit fever. Within the spectrum of T-cell malignancies, ALK-positive ALCL has a favorable prognosis, with a median 5-year survival of 80%; the outlook for ALK-negative patients is worse.

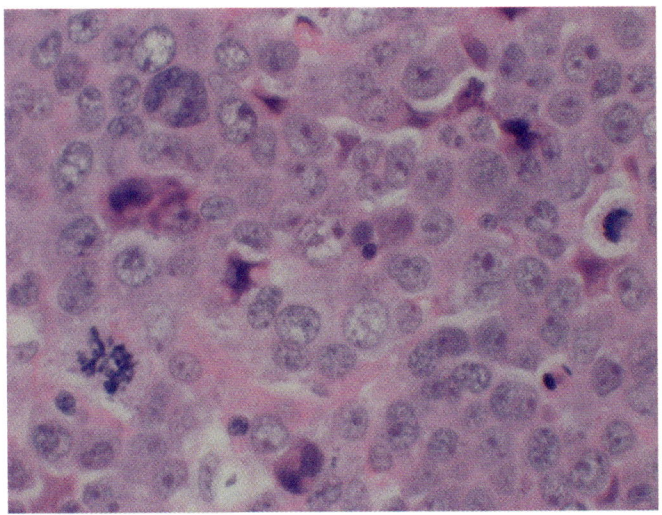

FIGURE 20-91
Anaplastic large cell lymphoma.

Hodgkin Lymphoma (HL) Features Hodgkin Cells and Reed-Sternberg Cells against an Inflammatory Background

Large atypical mononuclear or multinucleated tumor cells termed Hodgkin and Reed-Sternberg cells *are the diagnostic hallmark of Hodgkin lymphoma* (Figs. 20-92 and 20-93). Hodgkin disease was first recognized by Thomas Hodgkin of Guy's Hospital, London, in 1832. The first descriptions of the distinctive malignant cell were by Sternberg in 1898 and by Reed in 1902. HL has traditionally been included with the malignant lymphomas and the terms *Hodgkin lymphoma* and *non-Hodgkin lymphoma* are commonly encountered. Historically, there has been uncertainty as to the histogenesis of HL. There is now accumulating evidence that most cases of HL are neoplasms of B lymphocytes. However, its unique clinicopathological features warrant its recognition as a distinctive neoplastic disorder.

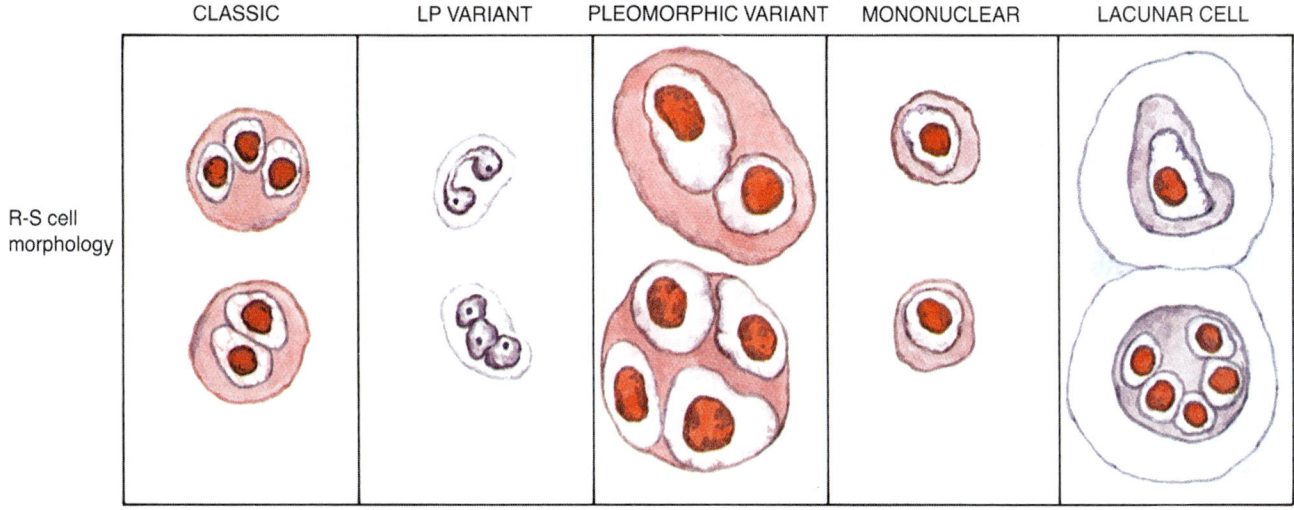

	CLASSIC	LP VARIANT	PLEOMORPHIC VARIANT	MONONUCLEAR	LACUNAR CELL
Nuclear Configuration	Binucleated to multinucleated to multilobulated	Single to multilobed	Single to multinucleated or multilobed	Single	Single to multilobed
Nucleoli	large (≥1/3 diameter of nucleus), eosinophilic	Small, punctate	Variable, prominent	large (≥1/3 diameter of nucleus), eosinophilic	Variable (generally <1/3 diameter of nucleus), eosinophilic
Chromatin	Clear parachromatin	Delicate	Variable, clear parachromatin to hyperchromatic	Abundant, clear parachromatin	delicate to clear parachromatin
Cytoplasm	Moderate to abundant, pale to pink	Scant, nodular	Moderate to abundant, eosinophilic	Moderate, pale to pink	Abundant, pale[†]
Associated histologic subtype	Diagnostic in mixed cellularity, may be seen (diagnostic) in lymphocyte depleted, nodular sclerosis	Lymphocyte predominance	Lymphocyte depleted[‡]	May be seen in any subtype	Nodular sclerosis[§]

Mononuclear R-S cell variants are not diagnostic of Hodgkin's disease. However, these cells, in the appropriate environment, indicate involvement either in the staging work-up or in relapse
[†] Formalin fixation artifact: the cytoplasm of these cells may retract and the cell appears to lie in a clear space (lacuna or lake).
[‡] Pleomorphic large cell lymphoma of T-cell type must be ruled out
[§] Similar cells may occasionally be seen in mixed cellularity

FIGURE 20-92
Reed-Sternberg cells in Hodgkin lymphoma. The table lists criteria for the identification of each cell type.

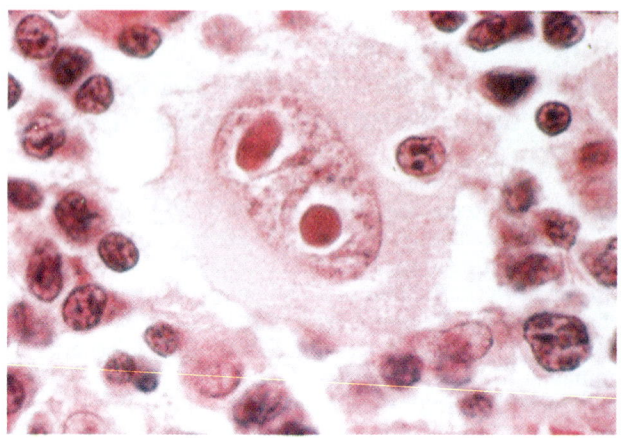

FIGURE 20-93
Classic Reed-Sternberg cell. Mirror-image nuclei contain large eosinophilic nucleoli.

 **Epidemiology and Pathogenesis:** HL is the most common malignant neoplasm of Americans between the ages of 10 and 30 years. Some 8000 cases are reported annually in the United States, for an incidence of 3 per 100,000 population. The disorder is somewhat more common in men than in women (4:2.5) and in whites than in blacks (3.5:2). There is a distinctive **bimodal age distribution in developed countries,** with a peak in the late 20s, a decrease in frequency during the fourth and fifth decades, and a gradually increasing incidence after the age of 50 years.

Epidemiological patterns in HL suggest that early and increased exposure to an unidentified agent of low oncogenic potential may be important in its development. In underdeveloped countries and less advanced regions of developed countries, the overall incidence is low, but there is an increased frequency in children. There is also a different distribution of subtypes of HL in different areas. Compared with affluent societies, less-developed regions show an increased frequency of the more aggressive "mixed cellularity" and "lymphocyte depletion" subtypes. In developed countries, less aggressive variants (nodular sclerosis and lymphocyte predominant) are more common in young adults from small families with few neighborhood playmates during childhood.

These epidemiological patterns suggest the possibility that early exposure to an unidentified etiologic agent may predispose children to aggressive HL. According to this theory, delayed exposure results in a predisposition to indolent HL in young adults. This scheme does not explain whether the increasing incidence of HL after the age of 50 years reflects exposure to the same hypothetical etiologic agent or has a different cause.

The **geographical variation** in the incidence of HL and some clinicopathological features that simulate an infectious process suggest a viral etiology, but proof is still lacking. The possibility of horizontal transmission (transmission by interpersonal contact) of an infectious agent has been suggested by several self-limited "mini-epidemics" of HL in children. However, such apparent case clustering is predictable on statistical grounds and has not been confirmed by broader epidemiological studies. A possible relationship between HL and infection with EBV has been suggested. Young adults who have experienced EBV infection (infectious mononucleosis) have a threefold increased risk of developing HL, and the EBV genome is frequently identified in the Reed-Sternberg cell (Fig. 20-94).

Genetic factors may play a role. The frequency of certain HLA subtypes, particularly HLA-B18, is higher in patients with HL. Moreover, there is a 7-fold increased risk of HL in siblings of patients with this disorder, and a 100-fold increased risk when the sibling is a monozygotic twin.

Immune status seems to be a factor in at least some cases of HL. There is an increased incidence of HL in patients with compromised immunity and in persons with autoimmune diseases, such as rheumatoid arthritis. In fact, in patients with ataxia telangiectasia, who have a 100-fold increased incidence of cancer, 7% of the malignancies are HL.

Historically, the pathogenesis of HL has been difficult to study, in part because of the inability to define the lineage and clonality of the Reed-Sternberg cell. In this context Reed-Sternberg cells frequently constitute less than 1% of the total cell population. In fact, a salient feature of HL is the predominance in tumor tissue of reactive benign tissue components. Recent studies have indicated that in most patients with HL, EBV is present in Reed-Sternberg cells. EBV antigens can be demonstrated in situ in the tumor cells by immunohistochemistry or in situ hybridization. Mixed-cellularity HL is associated with EBV in 70 to 80% of cases, but in less than 40% of those of the nodular sclerosing type.

The clonality of the Reed-Sternberg cell has been confirmed, suggesting that it is, indeed, the neoplastic cell of HL. Many of the normal cell components of lymph nodes have been proposed as candidates for the origin of the Reed-Sternberg cell. These include B and T lymphocytes and cells of the mononuclear phagocyte system, including macrophages, dendritic reticulum cells of the lymphoid follicles, and the interdigitating reticulum cells of the T cell-

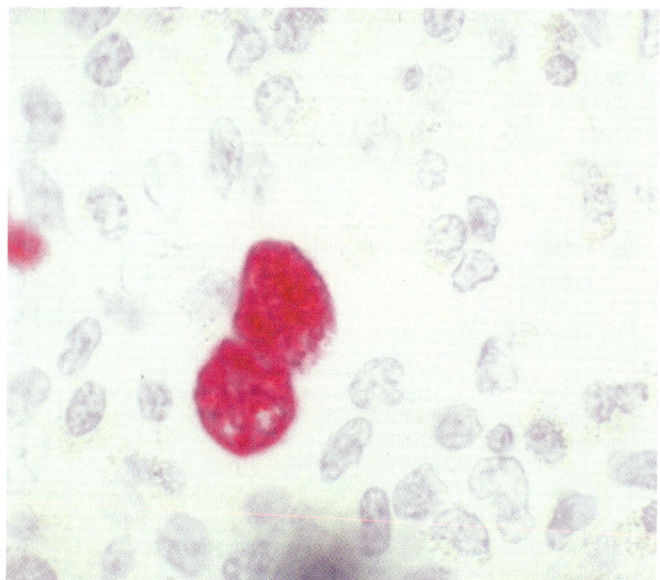

FIGURE 20-94
EBV genome in a Reed-Sternberg cell. EBV-RNA is visualized as red by in situ hybridization.

dependent paracortex. Cell markers characteristic of each of these cell lineages have been demonstrated in some, but not all, Reed-Sternberg cells.

Nodular lymphocyte-predominant HL is now recognized as a neoplasm of B-lymphocyte origin, and the Reed-Sternberg cells of this variant express specific B-lymphocyte lineage markers. They lack the immunological cell markers CD15 (Leu-M1) and CD30 (Ki-1), which are usually but not always identified on the Reed-Sternberg cells of all other subtypes of HL. Nevertheless, cases of classical HL are thought to be neoplasms of aberrant B lymphocytes. The expression of B-cell-specific activator protein (BSAP) in the vast majority of cases favors this interpretation. The *PAX5* gene encodes BSAP, a B-cell specific transcription factor. Clonal *IgH* gene rearrangement in the tumor cells is observed in almost all cases. The rearranged *IgG* genes are positive for mutations in the variable region of the IgG heavy chain, indicating that they are most likely of germinal center B-cell origin. In a few cases, the normal counterpart appears to be a postthymic T cell.

Pathology: Most patients with HL present with lymphadenopathy. After an initial diagnosis of HL, a comprehensive evaluation is commonly performed to establish the extent, or stage, of the disease. In selected cases, an abdominal exploratory operation (staging laparotomy) is performed, in which the spleen is removed and biopsies of lymph nodes, liver, and bone marrow are taken to search for abdominal involvement.

Lymph nodes: On clinical examination, lymph nodes involved by HL are described as firm or rubbery, but on gross examination in the laboratory, the consistency varies. When fibrosis is not a prominent feature, and when there are broad areas of cell necrosis, the lymph nodes may even be soft. The cut surface is homogeneously gray-white, producing a "fish flesh" appearance. If tumor tissue extends beyond the confines of individual lymph nodes, groups of nodes may be matted together.

Spleen: The spleen is involved in one third of cases of HL at the time of diagnosis and in most patients at autopsy. On cut section, the splenic white pulp is enlarged by HL, and the red pulp is affected only secondarily by direct extension from the white pulp. The incidence of splenic involvement correlates directly with the size of the organ. A spleen that weighs more than 400 g is almost invariably involved by HL. By contrast, a smaller spleen may show HL or may exhibit only benign reactive hyperplasia.

In the spleen, HL occurs first in the T cell-dependent, periarteriolar lymphoid sheath of the white pulp or in the marginal zone between the white pulp and the red pulp. As the disease progresses, single or multiple discrete tumor nodules or confluent multinodular tumor masses in the spleen are common (Fig. 20-95). The prognosis in HL is adversely affected by multiple discrete tumor nodules in the spleen.

Liver: At autopsy, the liver is involved with HL in two thirds of patients with residual disease, although it is unusual at the time of presentation. The portal areas are first involved, without significant macroscopic findings. With time, multiple gray-white tumor nodules, often resembling metastatic carcinoma, may appear in the liver.

Bone marrow: The bone marrow is only rarely involved initially. The early changes in the bone marrow are characterized macroscopically by discrete foci of fibrotic tumor, without destruction of bony trabeculae. As the disease progresses, destruction of bone may produce an osteolytic appearance on radiological examination. Rarely, thickening of bony trabeculae (osteosclerosis) occurs. When present, osteosclerosis may be particularly prominent in the vertebrae, producing a densely sclerotic radiological appearance described as "ivory vertebrae."

Other systems: Pulmonary involvement is discovered at autopsy in more than half the patients with residual disease, and epidural spread of HL from paravertebral nodes through intervertebral foramina is a frequent neurological complication.

Clinical Features: HL usually manifests as nontender peripheral adenopathy involving a single lymph node or groups of lymph nodes. The cervical and mediastinal nodes are involved in over half of cases, and the anterior mediastinum is frequently involved, especially in the nodular sclerosis type. Less commonly, the axillary, inguinal, and retroperitoneal lymph nodes are initially enlarged. Peripheral lymph node groups, such as the antecubital, popliteal, and mesenteric lymph nodes, tend to be spared.

Initially, HL spreads predictably between contiguous lymph node groups by way of the efferent lymphatics. As the disease progresses, spread is frequently unpredictable, owing to vascular invasion and hematogenous dissemination.

Constitutional ("B") symptoms are found in 40% of patients with HL. These include low-grade fever, which is occasionally cyclical (*Pel-Ebstein* fever), night sweats, and weight loss exceeding 10% of body weight. Pruritus may occur with disease progression. For unknown reasons, ingestion of alcohol induces pain in involved sites in 10% of patients with HL.

The laboratory findings in HL are nonspecific. They include mild normocytic, normochromic anemia and moderate neutrophilia and eosinophilia. Elevation of the erythrocyte sedimentation rate correlates with disease activity.

Deficient T-lymphocyte function is characteristic of HL. Subtle defects of delayed-type hypersensitivity, which can be detected in most patients even at the time of initial diagnosis, tend to become more pronounced as the disease progresses. Anergy to skin test antigens is often noted early

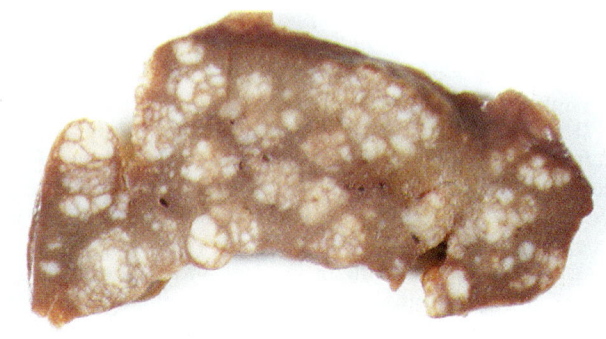

FIGURE *20-95*
Hodgkin lymphoma involving the spleen. Multinodular tumor masses replace the normal splenic parenchyma.

in the course of HL. Such immune dysfunction is exacerbated by the immunosuppressive effects of therapy. An absolute lymphocytopenia (<1500 per µL) is observed in half of cases, most commonly in advanced HL. Humoral immunity usually remains intact until late in the course of the disease.

Lymphocyte-predominant HL (LPHL) is the most indolent type. Adult men under 35 years of age are most commonly affected (male-to-female ratio, 4:1). At the time of initial diagnosis, the disease is usually localized (stage I), with the high cervical, axillary, or inguinal lymph nodes most commonly involved. B signs and symptoms are typically lacking, being present in only 20% of cases. Visceral involvement is uncommon. In contrast to classical types of HL, lymphocyte-predominant disease tends to skip anatomical lymph node regions. Mediastinal involvement is rare. The overall survival is excellent, with more than 80% 10-year survival at stage I and stage II. However, lymphocyte-predominant HL has a high recurrence rate.

Mixed-cellularity HL (MCHL) is most common in the fourth and fifth decades of life, although any age group may be affected. The left cervical lymph nodes are the most common site of initial involvement. However, after staging, most patients are found to have stage II or III disease, and a minority have visceral involvement (stage IV). B signs and symptoms are present in half of the cases of MCHL. The prognosis is intermediate, with a cure rate of 75%.

Lymphocyte-depleted HL (LDHL) is the most clinically aggressive type. Middle-aged to elderly men are most commonly affected. Advanced clinical stage (III–IV) and B signs and symptoms are present in two thirds of patients. Those with the diffuse fibrosis subtype of LDHL commonly present with fever of undetermined origin, pancytopenia, and wasting. There is usually no peripheral or mediastinal adenopathy. However, retroperitoneal adenopathy is frequently prominent, and involvement of the spleen, liver, and bone marrow is common. Profound immunodeficiency develops, and death commonly results from inanition or secondary infections. The reticular subtype of LDHL is characterized by bulky peripheral adenopathy, which is most frequent above the diaphragm. Patients usually succumb because of tumor progression. The overall cure rate in both types of LDHL is 40 to 50%.

Nodular sclerosis HL (NSHL) is the most common form of HL and is often found in adolescent and young adult women, ages 15 to 35 years. It tends to manifest as lower cervical, supraclavicular, and mediastinal adenopathy (stage II). B symptoms (Table 20-23) occur in up to 40% of patients. The prognosis is good, with a cure rate of 80 to 85%.

If untreated, HL is a lethal disorder, with a 10-year survival rate of only 1%. With modern radiation therapy and chemotherapy, an overall 70% cure rate can be achieved. **The prognosis in HL depends principally on the age of the patient and the anatomical extent of the disease or the stage.** A better prognosis is associated with (1) younger age, (2) lower clinical stage (localized disease), and (3) the absence of B signs and symptoms. In the assessment of stage, the comprehensive Ann Arbor staging system (Table 20-23), which is based on both clinical evaluation and the pathological findings from staging laparotomy, is used.

Complications of HL include compromise of vital organs by progressive tumor growth and secondary infections, owing to both the primary defect in delayed type hypersensitivity and the immunosuppressive effects of therapy. The development of second malignancies as a consequence of therapy is of special concern, since more than 15% of treated patients may eventually suffer this complication. AML develops in 5% of patients, and aggressive large cell lymphomas occur somewhat less frequently.

Histological Classification of Hodgkin Lymphoma

Two major types of HL are distinguished, *nodular lymphocyte-predominant HL* (NLPHL) and *classical* HL (CHL) (Fig. 20-96).

Nodular Lymphocyte-Predominant Hodgkin Lymphoma

NLPHL features Reed-Sternberg cell variants called "popcorn" or L&H (lymphohistocytic) cells. The tumor cells consistently express membranous B-cell antigens. NLPHL represents only a small proportion of all cases of HL.

Pathology: The tumor completely effaces the lymph node architecture in a vaguely nodular pattern. The usual inflammatory background of eosinophils and plasma cells is missing. In contrast to classical types of HL, the tumor cells are positive for B-cell surface antigens and surface Ig. They are negative for both CD15 and

TABLE 20-23 **Ann Arbor Staging System**

Stage I A or B[a]	I	Involvement of a single lymph node region
		or
	I$_E$	A single extralymphatic organ or site
Stage II A or B	II	Involvement or two or more lymph node regions on the same side of the diaphragm
		or
	II$_E$	with localized contiguous involvement of an extralymphatic organ site
Stage III A or B	III	Involvement of lymph node regions on both sides of the diaphragm
		or
	III$_E$	with localized contiguous involvement of an extralymphatic organ or site
		or
	III$_S$	with involvement of spleen
		or
	III$_{ES}$	both extralymphatic organ or site and spleen involvement
Stage IV A or B	IV	Diffuse or disseminated involvement of one or more extralymphatic organs with or without associated lymph node involvement

[a] A, asymptomatic; B, presence of constitutional symptoms (fever, night sweats, and weight loss exceeding 10% of baseline body weight in preceding 6 months).

CD30, which define classical types of HL. Genotypically, the tumor cells resemble germinal center B cells. The tumor cells in NLPHL are negative for EBV.

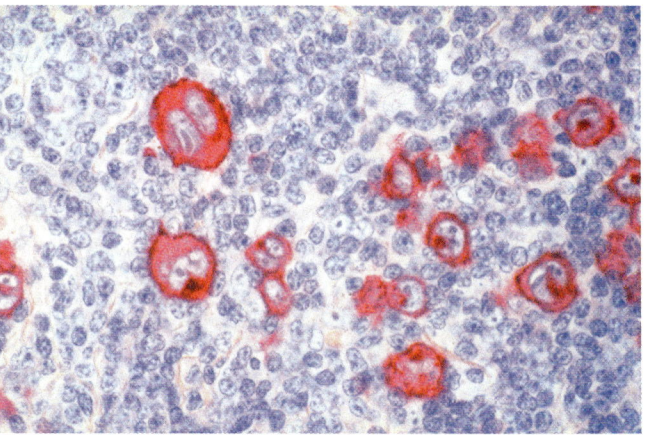

FIGURE 20-97
Reed-Sternberg and Hodgkin cells. The cells are positive for CD30.

Classical Hodgkin Lymphoma

CHL is characterized by clonal proliferation of typical mononuclear Hodgkin cells and multinucleated Reed-Sternberg cells (HRS), with invariable expression of CD30 (Fig. 20-97). A variable inflammatory background consisting of lymphocytes, eosinophils, macrophages, neutrophils, plasma cells, fibroblasts, and collagenous tissue determines the morphological appearance. Four different types of classical HL have been defined: lymphocyte-rich, nodular-sclerosis, mixed-cellularity, and lymphocyte-depleted variants.

 Pathology: Typical mononuclear or multinucleated Reed-Sternberg cells with large nucleoli are immersed in a rich inflammatory background. Occasionally, HRS cells undergo apoptosis, resulting in ghost cells with condensed cytoplasm and pyknotic nuclei (mummified cells). In nodular sclerosis, *lacunar cells* result from a retraction artifact in formaldehyde-fixed tissue. Expression for the lymphocytic activation marker CD30 unites the different types of classical HL. Most patients are also positive

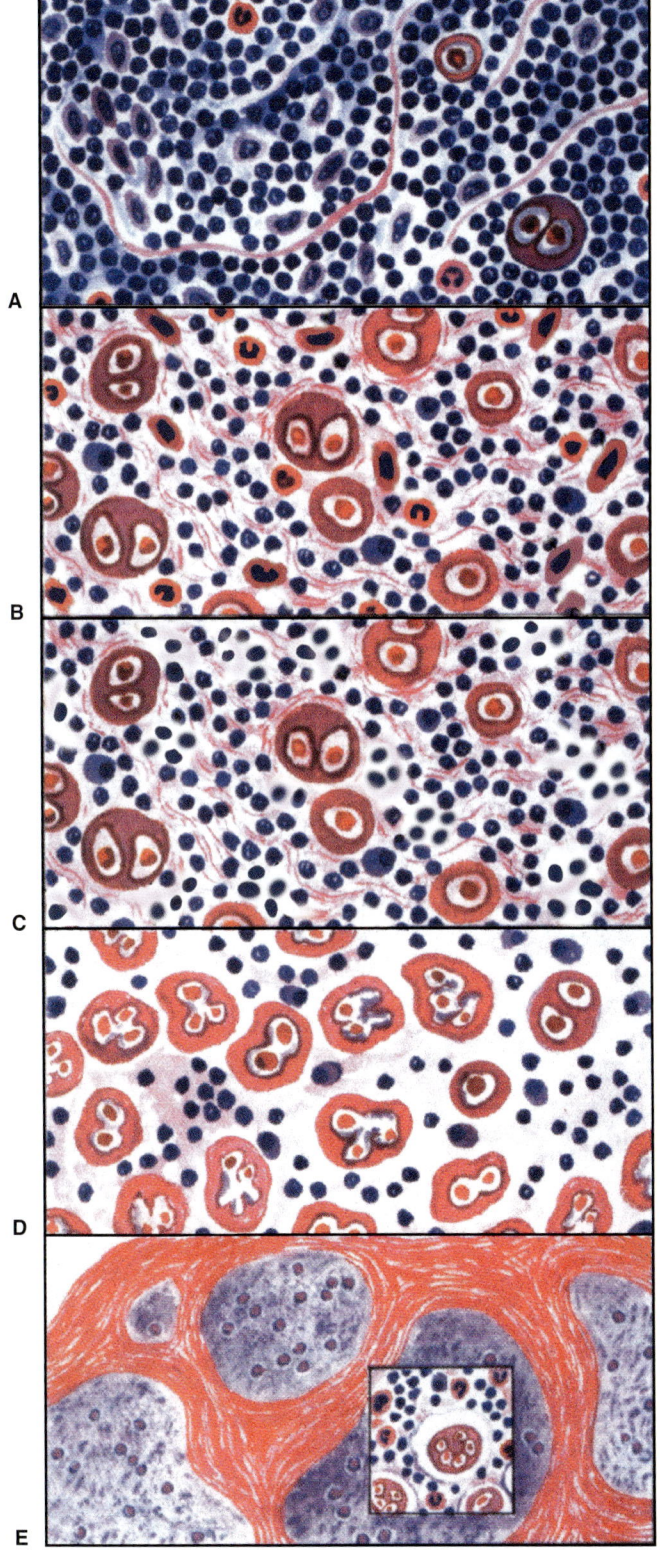

FIGURE 20-96
Histopathological subtypes of Hodgkin lymphoma. A. Lymphocyte predominant. B. Mixed cellularity. C. Lymphocyte rich. D. Lymphocyte depleted. E. Nodular sclerosis. The sequence from lymphocyte-predominant HL to the lymphocyte-depleted variant is characterized by progressively fewer normal lymphocytes and increasing numbers of Reed-Sternberg cells. The subtype of lymphocyte-depleted diffuse fibrosis features only few lymphocytes, and Reed-Sternberg cells and abundant loose fibrosis. Nodular sclerosis Hodgkin lymphoma is distinctive because of dense, bandlike, collagenous fibrosis that envelops cellular aggregates that contain lymphoid and inflammatory cells, and the specific lacunar cell variant of the Reed-Sternberg cell.

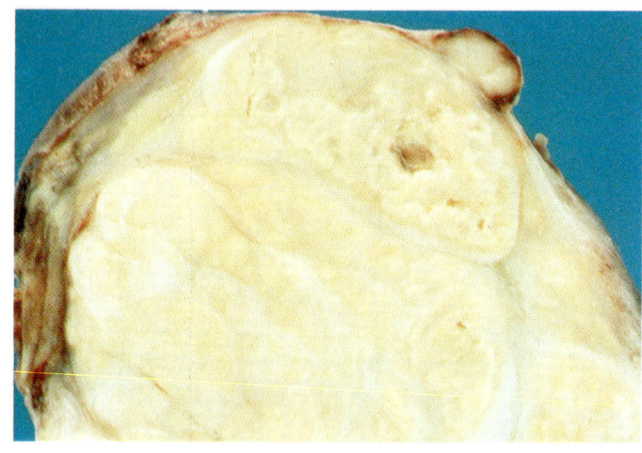
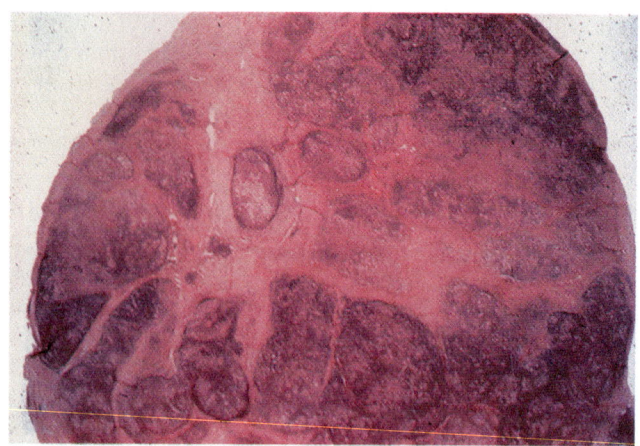

FIGURE 20-98
Hodgkin lymphoma; nodular sclerosis. **A.** A cut section of matted lymph nodes shows broad bands of fibrosis that divide the parenchyma into distinct nodules. Several foci of necrosis are evident. **B.** A low-power photomicrograph demonstrates broad bands of fibrosis.

for CD15, whereas leukocyte common antigen (CD45) is negative. Common T- and B-cell markers are missing, with the exception of CD20, which is occasionally detected.

HRS cells produce a number of cytokines that elicit characteristic tissue effects. Eosinophils are attracted by the combined effects of IL-5 and eotaxin, and IL-6 can attract plasma cells. TGFβ activates fibroblasts and may be accountable for nodular fibrosis. Other growth factors and cytokines produced by the tumor cells include interleukins 2, 7, 9, 10, and 13.

Nodular-Sclerosis Hodgkin Lymphoma

NSHL features nodular architecture in which lymphoid tissue is surrounded by fibrosis (Fig. 20-98). Classical HRS cells with lacunar variants are typical. NSHL accounts for 70% of classical HL, with most cases occurring between the ages of 20 and 30 years. Mediastinal involvement is most common in this type of HL.

Mixed-Cellularity Hodgkin Lymphoma

MCHL is characterized by HRS cells and a mixed inflammatory background consisting of eosinophils, neutrophils, macrophages, and plasma cells (Fig. 20-99). The histological appearance is like that of the nodular-sclerosis variety, but collagen bands are missing. MCHL is the most frequent histological subtype in HIV- infected patients with HL and demonstrates the highest association with EBV (Fig. 20-94). Mediastinal involvement is uncommon.

Lymphocyte-Rich Hodgkin Lymphoma (LRHL)

LRHL has recently been added to the list of Hodgkin lymphomas. It is characterized by classical HRS cells in an abundant background of small lymphocytes. Mixed inflammatory cells and collagen bands are missing.

Lymphocyte-Depleted Hodgkin Lymphoma

LDHL is the least common type of classical HL. The histological appearance demonstrates a predominance of tumor cells and a marked absence of background lymphocytes (Fig. 20-100). LDHL is frequently associated with HIV infection. Without treatment, this type of Hodgkin disease has the least favorable prognosis. Advanced stage and B symptoms are seen in more than 70% of patients and most are positive for EBV.

Posttransplant Lymphoproliferative Disorder Is Often Associated with EBV Infection

Posttransplant lymphoproliferative disorder (PTLD) results from immunosuppression. In most cases, PTLD is an EBV-driven, monoclonal, lymphocyte proliferation with variable morphology.

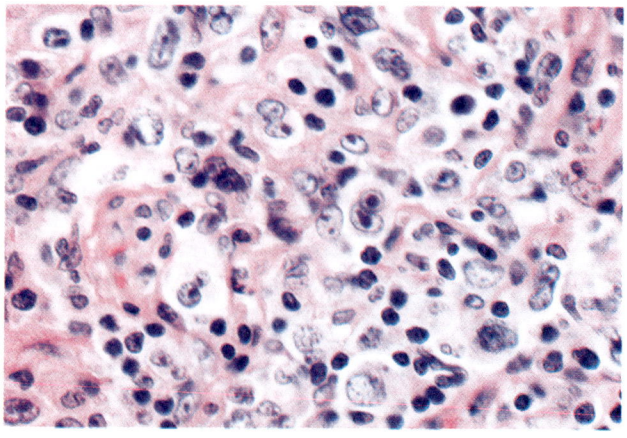

FIGURE 20-99
Hodgkin lymphoma; mixed cellularity. A photomicrograph of a lymph node shows classic, binucleated and mononuclear Reed-Sternberg cells, lymphocytes, and mild diffuse fibrosis.

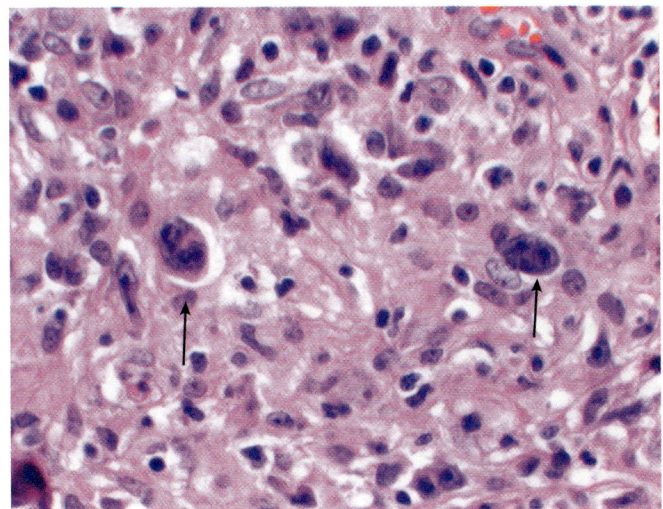

FIGURE 20-100
Hodkgin lymphoma; lymphocyte depleted type. Two tumor cells are seen (arrows). The number of reactive lymphocytes in the fibrotic background is markedly reduced.

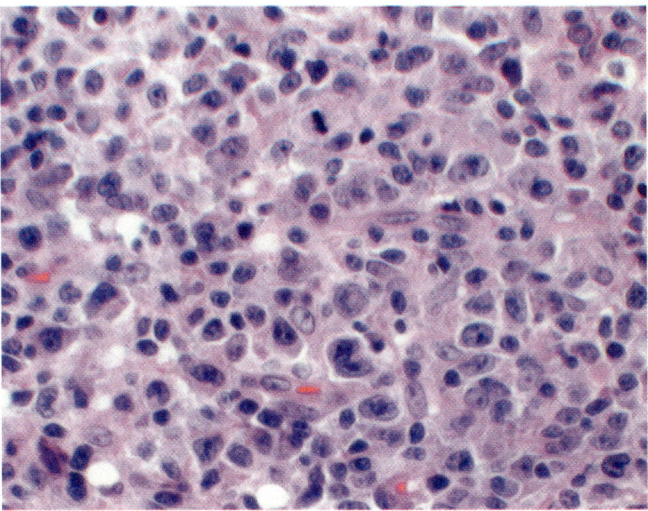

FIGURE 20-102
Posttransplant lymphoproliferative disorder (PTLD). Highly atypical lymphocytes are shown.

 Epidemiology: The incidence of PTLD parallels the extent of immunosuppression. Liver transplant recipients have a higher incidence of PTLD than do those who receive kidney transplants (5% vs. 1%). Recipients of matched bone marrow allografts show a low incidence of PTLD (1%), whereas unmatched recipients have a much higher incidence, owing to higher levels of immunosuppression.

 Pathogenesis: Most cases of PTLD are causally related to EBV (Fig. 20-101), with an average latency period of less than 1 year. However, EBV-negative cases may evolve more than 5 years after transplantation. Whereas in solid organ recipients, *host* lymphocytes become infected with EBV, in bone marrow allograft recipients, PTLD is caused by infected *donor* lymphocytes.

 Pathology: Early lymph node lesions of PTLD are characterized by increased plasma cells or an appearance similar to that of *infectious mononucleosis*. The proliferation of lymphocyte and plasma cells at this stage is not clonal.

Polymorphic PTLD is the next step in the evolution of the disease and features a mixture of immunoblasts, plasma cells, and medium-sized lymphocytes in lymph nodes or other organs (Fig. 20-102). B cells that demonstrate the full range of maturation and have numerous mitotic figures infiltrate the tissue. In spite of the polymorphic appearance of the lymphocytes, clonal *IgH* gene arrangements are almost always demonstrated by PCR. Some patients may spontaneously regress when the level of immunosuppressive therapy is reduced.

PTLD eventually acquires a *monomorphic* appearance indistinguishable from that of *malignant lymphoma*. Histological types include diffuse large B-cell lymphoma, Burkitt lymphoma, HL, plasma cell myeloma or, rarely, T-cell lymphoma.

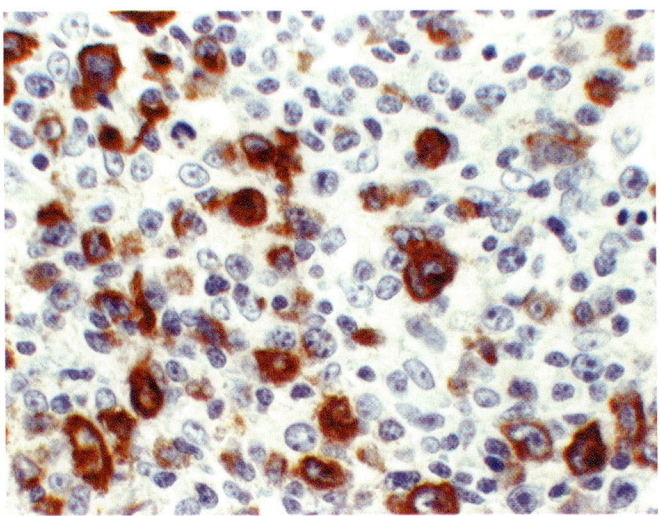

FIGURE 20-101
Posttransplant lymphoproliferative disorder (PTLD). Atypical lymphocytes are positive for latent membrane protein (LMP) of EBV.

 Clinical Features: In PTLD, neoplastic lymphocytes can be seen at any nodal or extranodal site. Solid organ recipients treated with azathioprine present with PTLD after an average latency period of 48 months, whereas those given cyclosporine develop the disease within 15 months. PTLD in bone marrow allograft recipients occurs within the first 6 months. EBV-positive cases occur much earlier than EBV-negative ones. Early PTLD has an excellent prognosis and may regress at a decreased level of immunosuppression. Late-stage PTLD, with full-blown malignant lymphoma, has a mortality rate of 70%. Treatment with an anti-CD20 antibody (Rituxan) has been successful in eliminating clonal B-cell proliferations.

Spleen

ANATOMY AND FUNCTION

The spleen is a lymphoid organ that also serves as a versatile filter for abnormal or senescent cells. The normal weight of the spleen is 100 to 170 g; it is normally not palpable on clinical examination. The supporting structure of the organ consists of a fibrous capsule, radiating fibrous trabeculae, and a delicate stromal framework of reticulum fibers. The splenic artery enters at the hilum and branches into the trabecular arteries, following the course of the fibrous trabeculae.

The white pulp: Leaving the trabeculae, the central arteries become ensheathed by lymphocytes, which constitute the white pulp. The white pulp is further subdivided into a T-cell domain, located in the periarteriolar lymphoid sheath, and a B-cell domain that comprises the follicles and perifollicular mantle zone (Fig. 20-103). Like the lymph nodes, the follicles are either inactive or activated, the latter being associated with germinal-center formation. Arising from the central artery, follicular arteries enter the B-cell follicles and terminate in the marginal sinus at the junction between the white and red pulp. Circulating lymphocytes exit the vascular system from the marginal sinus and travel to their respective B-cell and T-cell domains. Lymphocytes leave the white pulp and enter the red pulp by way of the same marginal sinuses.

The red pulp: this region comprises a network of stromal cords and vascular sinuses. Most of the blood from the penicilliary arteries empties directly into the sinuses (closed circulation), with subsequent drainage to the trabecular veins and ultimately to the splenic vein. A small fraction (5–10%) is diverted into the splenic cords (open circulation) and slowly percolates through a meshwork studded with phagocytic macrophages. The blood then reenters the sinusoids through narrow slits composed of longitudinally oriented, slender endothelial cells and radially oriented ring fibers.

In the splenic cords, erythrocytes are subjected to the sustained scrutiny of mononuclear phagocytes and must be deformable to traverse the narrow interstices between the lining endothelial cells. The erythrocytes must also be able to withstand the hypoxia, hypoglycemia, and acidosis that are characteristic of the stromal cord microenvironment. Most normal erythroid cells survive, as do granulocytes and platelets. They ultimately enter the trabecular veins and leave the hilum by way of the splenic vein.

As part of the peripheral lymphoid system, effector B and T lymphocytes of the white pulp perform an immunological function for the circulatory system comparable to the

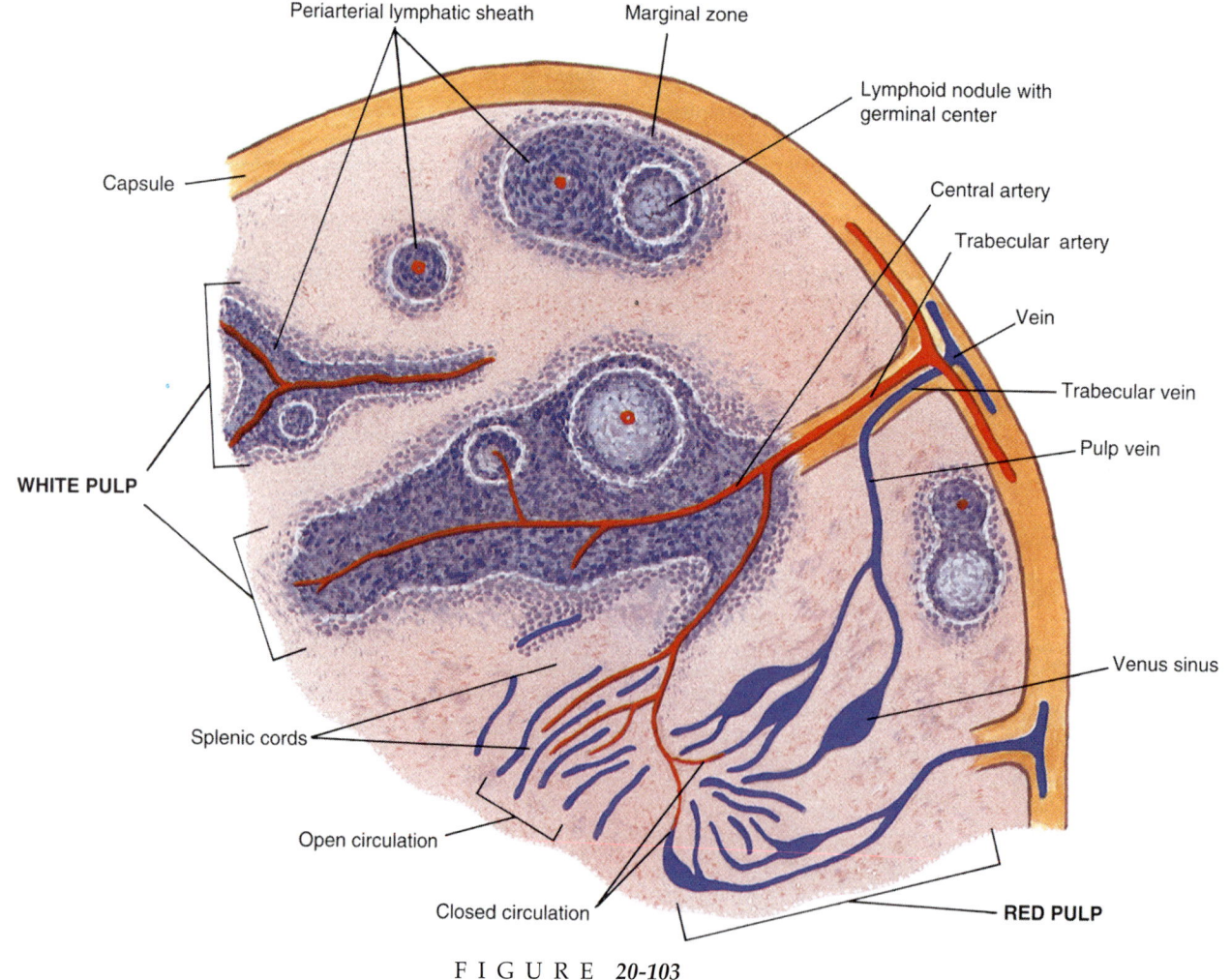

FIGURE 20-103
Structure of the normal spleen.

immunological function of the lymph nodes. The white pulp is (1) the source of protection from blood-borne infection, (2) a major locale for the synthesis of opsonizing IgM antibody, and (3) a site of production of lymphocytes and plasma cells.

The red pulp is primarily a filter designed to screen and eliminate defective or foreign cells. Senescent and damaged erythrocytes are recognized and phagocytosed by splenic macrophages. The spleen ordinarily accounts for the removal of about half of aged erythrocytes, the remainder being destroyed in the liver, bone marrow, and other components of the mononuclear phagocyte system. Following phagocytosis and breakdown of erythrocytes, the iron is first stored as hemosiderin in macrophages. It is then released, bound to transferrin, and transported to the bone marrow for reuse in erythrocyte production. Abnormal erythrocyte inclusions, such as Howell-Jolly bodies (remnants of nuclear DNA), Heinz bodies (denatured hemoglobin), and sideritic granules (iron), are recognized and removed (pitted) by macrophages, without destruction of the erythrocyte.

Some membrane lipids of the maturing erythrocyte are removed in the red pulp. In the absence of this function, such as after splenectomy, there may be excess erythrocyte membrane in relation to hemoglobin content, a situation that leads to central pooling of hemoglobin and a "target cell" appearance.

One third of the peripheral blood platelet pool and a small fraction of granulocytes are normally sequestered in the spleen without causing any damage to the cells. By contrast, there is no significant splenic sequestration of erythrocytes, and splenectomy is followed only by an increase in platelet and granulocyte counts.

DISORDERS OF THE SPLEEN

Hypersplenism is a functional disorder, which, as noted above (see hemolytic anemia), is characterized by anemia, leukopenia, thrombocytopenia, and compensatory bone marrow hyperplasia. Hyposplenism refers to a situation in which normal splenic functions are reduced by disease or are absent after splenectomy. Impaired filtering leads to increased risk of severe bacteremia and mild leukocytosis and thrombocytosis. Nuclear remnants and Howell-Jolly bodies are found in many of the circulating erythrocytes.

Congenital absence of the spleen (asplenia) is rare and is often associated with other congenital anomalies. **Acquired asplenia** is seen most commonly in young adults with sickle cell anemia. Multiple infarctions eventually result in atrophy and hyposplenism. The infarctions are often painful, owing to the complication of fibrinous perisplenitis. As the result of the absence of splenic sequestration of erythrocytes, with consequent lack of removal of excess membrane and intracellular debris, many erythrocytes become target cells and contain nuclear remnants, Howell-Jolly bodies, or even intact nuclei.

Accessory spleens are common, occurring in 10% of normal persons. They may measure up to several centimeters in diameter and are most frequently found in the tail of the pancreas or in the gastrosplenic ligament. Following splenectomy, accessory spleens may increase considerably in size, but they rarely become large enough to restore the functions of the lost spleen.

Splenomegaly Is Caused by Functional, Infectious, and Infiltrative Processes

The spleen is a prominent member of the lymphopoietic and mononuclear phagocyte systems, and splenomegaly is a common finding in a variety of unrelated pathological situations (Table 20-24).

Reactive Splenomegaly

Reactive hyperplasia of the spleen occurs in a number of acute and chronic inflammatory conditions. It is probably caused by phagocytosis of blood-borne bacteria, which leads to the release of growth factors and other products of the inflammatory response. The spleen is moderately enlarged (up to 400 g), and macrophages and neutrophils abound in the red pulp. Mild hyperplasia of the lymphoid white pulp is common.

In **acute and chronic parasitemias,** the red pulp may be engorged with parasites and their breakdown products. The spleen is often massively enlarged in chronic malarial infections (up to 10 kg). It shows fibrous thickening of the capsule and trabeculae, with a slate gray to black coloration of the pulp, owing to the presence of phagocytosed malarial pigment (hematin).

In **chronic immunological inflammatory disorders,** splenomegaly is caused by hyperplasia of the white pulp. Germinal centers are prominent, as in rheumatoid arthritis, and the red pulp displays an associated increase in mononuclear phagocytes, immunoblasts, plasma cells, and eosinophils.

TABLE 20-24 **Principal Causes of Splenomegaly**

Infections
   Acute
   Subacute
   Chronic
Immunological inflammatory disorders
   Felty syndrome
   Lupus erythematosus
   Sarcoidosis
   Amyloidosis
   Thyroiditis
Hemolytic anemias
Immune thrombocytopenia
Splenic vein hypertension
   Cirrhosis
   Splenic or portal vein thrombosis or stenosis
   Right-sided cardiac failure
Primary or metastatic neoplasm
   Leukemia
   Lymphoma
   Hodgkin disease
   Myeloproliferative syndromes
   Sarcoma
   Carcinoma
Storage diseases
   Gaucher
   Niemann-Pick
   Mucopolysaccharidoses

Systemic lupus erythematosus is characterized by fibrinoid necrosis of capsular and trabecular collagen and concentric, or "onion skin," thickening of the penicilliary arteries and central arterioles of the white pulp.

In **infectious mononucleosis**, transformed lymphocytes (immunoblasts) prominently infiltrate the red pulp, whereas the white pulp may no longer be evident. Infiltration of the capsular and trabecular systems and of blood vessels by lymphoid elements weakens the supporting structure of the spleen and accounts for **traumatic splenic rupture** in infectious mononucleosis.

Congestive Splenomegaly

Chronic passive congestion of the spleen causes splenomegaly and hypersplenism. This is most common in patients with portal hypertension due to cirrhosis, thrombosis of the portal or splenic veins, or right-sided heart failure.

 Pathology: The spleen is modestly enlarged (300–700 g) and has a thickened, fibrotic capsule. Focal accentuation of the capsular fibrosis leads to a "sugar-coated" appearance. The cut surface is firm, and the color varies from pink to deep red, depending on the extent of fibrosis. Microscopically, the red pulp initially shows dilated sinuses and an increased number of macrophages. Later, the parenchyma becomes fibrotic, and the red pulp is hypocellular. Foci of old hemorrhages persist as *Gamna-Gandy bodies*, which are fibrotic nodules containing iron and calcium salts encrusted on collagenous and elastic fibers. The white pulp tends to be atrophic.

Infiltrative Splenomegaly

The spleen may be enlarged by an increase in the number of cellular elements or by the deposition of extracellular material, as in amyloidosis. Splenic macrophages accumulate in chronic infections, hemolytic anemias, and a variety of storage diseases, Gaucher disease being the prototype (see Chapter 6). A variety of neoplastic and reactive bone marrow disorders are accompanied by extramedullary hematopoiesis and a corresponding increase in the size of the spleen. Splenomegaly is also caused by the infiltration of malignant cells in hematological proliferative disorders, such as leukemias and lymphomas.

Splenomegaly Due to Cysts and Tumors

Splenic cysts are rare, and the most common are actually pseudocysts. The latter are lined by a fibrous wall and are the residue of previous hemorrhage or infarction. *Hydatid cysts* are encountered in areas endemic for *Echinococcus granulosus* (see Chapter 9).

Primary splenic tumors are also distinctly uncommon. The most common primary benign tumors of the spleen are hemangiomas and lymphangiomas. Usually of the cavernous type, they contain large endothelial-lined spaces and vary from minute foci to lesions that occupy most of the spleen. The spaces in hemangiomas are occupied by erythrocytes, and in lymphangiomas by lymph.

Malignant tumors, such as malignant lymphomas or HL, are usually not primary in the spleen but rather part of a generalized disease. *Splenic hemangiosarcoma* is a rare, highly malignant neoplasm of vascular endothelial cells that tends to metastasize to the liver by way of the portal drainage.

Despite its large blood supply and filtering function, the spleen is only rarely involved by metastatic tumors. The microenvironment, with its abundance of macrophages and lymphocytes, is apparently not favorable for tumor growth. Metastatic tumors are usually observed only late in the course of a widely metastasizing neoplasm.

Thymus

HYPERPLASIA

Thymic hyperplasia refers to the presence of lymphoid follicles in the thymus irrespective of the size of the gland (Fig. 20-104). The total weight of the thymus is usually within the normal range, although it may be increased. The follicles contain germinal centers and are composed largely of B lymphocytes that contain IgM and IgD. The follicles tend to occupy and distort the medullary zones.

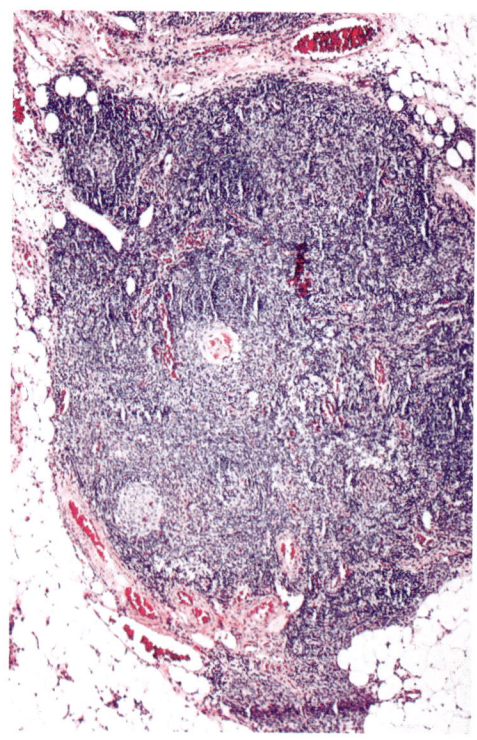

FIGURE 20-104
Thymic hyperplasia. This thymus removed from a patient with myasthenia gravis shows lymphoid follicles with germinal centers.

The best known association of thymic hyperplasia is with **myasthenia gravis** (see Chapter 27), in which two thirds of patients exhibit this thymic abnormality. Interestingly, thymic epithelial and myoid cells contain nicotinic acetylcholine receptor protein, suggesting a potential source for the development of antibodies directed against this receptor. Thymic follicular hyperplasia may also be found in other diseases in which autoimmunity is believed to play a role, including Graves disease, Addison disease, systemic lupus erythematosus, scleroderma, and rheumatoid arthritis.

THYMOMA

Thymoma is a neoplasm of thymic epithelial cells, without regard to the presence or number of lymphocytes. This tumor almost always occurs in adult life, and most (80%) are benign.

Pathology: Most thymomas are located in the anterosuperior mediastinum, although a few have been described in other locations where thymic tissue is found, including the neck, middle and posterior mediastinum, and pulmonary hilus. Benign thymomas are irregularly shaped masses that range from a few centimeters to 15 cm or more in greatest dimension. They are encapsulated, firm, and gray to yellow tumors that are divided into lobules by fibrous septa (Fig. 20-105). Large tumors show foci of hemorrhage, necrosis, and cystic degeneration. In some instances, the entire thymoma becomes cystic, and multiple sections are required to identify the true nature of the lesion.

On microscopic examination, thymomas consist of a mixture of neoplastic epithelial cells and nontumorous lymphocytes. The proportions of these elements vary in individual cases and even among different lobules. The epithelial cells are plump or spindle shaped and show vesicular nuclei. In cases in which epithelial cells predominate, they may exhibit an organoid differentiation, including perivascular spaces containing lymphocytes and macrophages, tumor cell rosettes, and whorls suggesting abortive Hassall corpuscle formation.

MYASTHENIA GRAVIS: Fifteen percent of patients with myasthenia gravis have thymoma. Conversely, one third to one half of patients with thymoma develop myasthenia gravis. The occurrence of thymoma in persons with myasthenia gravis is more common in men older than 50 years of age.

In cases of thymoma associated with myasthenic symptoms, the epithelial cells are of the plump, rather than the spindle cell, variety. Antigens related to the nicotinic acetylcholine receptor have also been detected in thymomas. Thymic hyperplasia is almost always present in the nontumorous thymic tissue, and lymphoid follicles may even be present in the thymoma itself.

OTHER ASSOCIATED DISEASES: Thymoma is also associated with many other immune disorders. More than 10% of patients with thymoma have hypogammaglobulinemia, and 5% have erythroid hypoplasia. In contrast to the situation with myasthenia gravis, the epithelial component of the thymoma is spindle shaped in these cases. Other associated diseases include myocarditis, dermatomyositis, rheumatoid arthritis, lupus erythematosus, scleroderma, and Sjögren syndrome. Certain malignant tumors have also been associated with thymoma, including T-cell leukemia-lymphoma and multiple myeloma.

Malignant Thymoma Invades Locally and May Metastasize

One fourth of thymomas are not encapsulated and exhibit malignant features.

Pathology: **Type I malignant thymoma** is the most common cancer of the thymus and is virtually indistinguishable histologically from encapsulated,

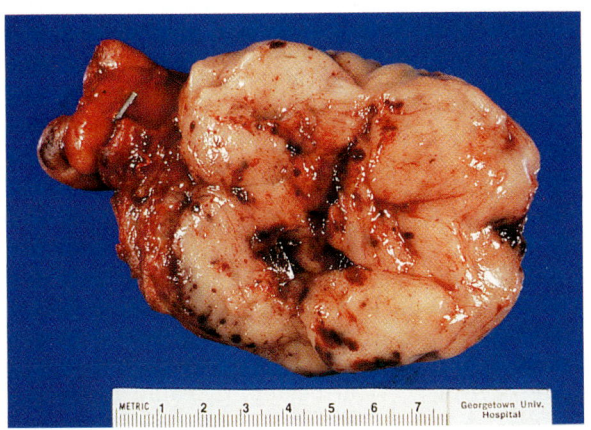
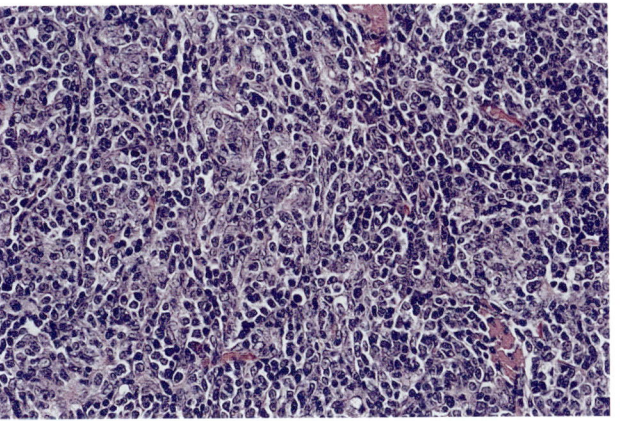

FIGURE 20-105

Thymoma. **A.** The tumor in cross section is whitish and has a bulging surface with areas of hemorrhage. Note the attached portion of normal thymus. **B.** Microscopically, the tumor consists of a mixture of neoplastic epithelial cells and nontumorous lymphocytes.

benign thymoma. However, it penetrates the capsule, implants on pleural or pericardial surfaces, and metastasizes to lymph nodes, lung, liver, and bone.

Type II malignant thymoma is a distinctly uncommon, invasive tumor, that is also termed *thymic carcinoma*. The morphological appearance of this tumor is highly variable and takes the form of squamous cell carcinoma, lymphoepithelioma-like carcinoma (identical to that found in the oropharynx; see Chapter 25), a sarcomatoid variant (carcinosarcoma), and a number of other rare patterns. These variants share a distinct epithelial appearance, and a mediastinal tumor that lacks this feature is probably not a thymic carcinoma.

Clinical Features: Malignant thymoma is treated by surgical excision and radiation therapy. Chemotherapy is added in cases with distant metastases. The prognosis for benign thymoma is excellent, and the presence or absence of myasthenic symptoms has little prognostic value. In the case of type I malignant thymomas, the prognosis correlates with the extent of the disease. Most patients with type II thymomas die within 5 years of the diagnosis.

Other Tumors of the Thymus Are Uncommon

CARCINOID TUMOR: The thymus gives rise to carcinoid tumor, which is similar in its morphological appearance and natural history to comparable tumors elsewhere. Thymic carcinoid tumors tend to invade locally and metastasize widely, although well-circumscribed tumors may be cured by local excision. Interestingly, one third of patients manifest Cushing syndrome, and carcinoid syndrome does not occur. A thymic carcinoid tumor may also arise in the context of MEN-1 and 2A.

SMALL CELL CARCINOMA: The thymus may also be the site of another neuroendocrine tumor, namely, small cell carcinoma, which is indistinguishable from its counterpart in the lung.

GERM CELL TUMORS: Germ cell tumors in the thymus account for 20% of all mediastinal tumors. It is thought that the migration of germ cells during embryogenesis leaves misplaced germ cells in this location that eventually give rise to germ cell neoplasms. The spectrum of germ cell tumors in the mediastinum parallels that in the gonads (see Chapters 17 and 18). Mature cystic teratoma is the most common of these thymic tumors. Seminoma, embryonal carcinoma, endodermal sinus tumor, teratocarcinoma, and choriocarcinoma all occur. With the exception of mature cystic teratoma, which afflicts both sexes equally, all the other tumors show a substantial male predilection, and thymic seminoma occurs only in men. In general, the prognosis is similar to that of comparable gonadal tumors.

SUGGESTED READING

Beutler E, Lichtman MA, Coller BS, et al.: *Williams hematology*, 6th ed. New York: McGraw Hill, 2001.

Brunning RD, McKenna RW: *Tumors of the bone marrow*. Washington, DC: Armed Forces Institute of Pathology, 1994.

Colman R, Hirsh J, Marder VJ, et al.: *Hemostasis and thrombosis*, 4th ed. Philadelphia: Lippincott Williams & Wilkins, 2001.

Ferry JA, Harris NL: *Atlas of lymphoid hyperplasia and lymphoma*. Philadelphia: WB Saunders, 1997.

Foucar K: *Bone marrow pathology*. Chicago: ASCP (American Society of Pathology) Press, 2001.

Harmening D: *Clinical hematology and fundamentals of hemostasis*, 4th ed. Philadelphia: FA Davis, 2001.

Hoffbrand AV, Pettit JE: *Color atlas of clinical hematology*, 3rd ed. London: Mosby-Wolfe, 2000.

Jaffe ES, Harris NL, Stein H, Vardiman JW: *World Health Organization classification of tumours. pathology and genetics. Tumours of haematopoietic and lymphoid tissues*. Lyon: IARC Press, 2001.

Jandl JH: *Textbook of hematology*, 2nd ed. Boston: Little, Brown & Co, 1996.

Keren DF, McCoy JP, Carey JL: *Flow cytometry in clinical diagnosis*, 3rd ed. Chicago: ASCP (American Society of Pathology) Press, 2001.

Knowles DM: *Neoplastic hematology*, 2nd ed. Philadelphia: Lippincott Williams & Wilkins, 2001.

McKenzie SB: *Textbook of hematology*, 2nd ed. Baltimore: Williams & Wilkins, 1996.

Warnke RA, Weis LM, Chan JKC, et al.: *Tumors of the lymph nodes and spleen*. Washington, DC: Armed Forces Institute of Pathology, 1995.

Review Articles

Alizadeh AA, Eisen MB, Davis RE, Ma C, Lossos IS, Rosenwald A, Boldrick JC, Sabet H, Tran T, Yu X, Powell JI, Yang L, Marti GE, Moore T, Hudson J, Jr., Lu L, Lewis DB, Tibshirani R, Sherlock G, Chan WC, Greiner TC, Weisenburger DD, Armitage JO, Warnke R, Levy R, Wilson W, Grever MR, Byrd JC, Botstein D, Brown PO, Staudt LM (2000). Distinct types of diffuse large B-cell lymphoma identified by gene expression profiling. Nature 403, 503–511.

Bennett JM (2000). World Health Organization classification of the acute leukemias and myelodysplastic syndrome. Int J Hematol 72, 131–133.

Bick RL (1995). Laboratory evaluation of platelet dysfunction. Clin Lab Med 15, 1–38.

Chan JK (2001). The new World Health Organization classification of lymphomas: the past, the present and the future.

Giardini C, Galimberti M, Lucarelli G (1995). Bone marrow transplantation in thalassemia. Annu Rev Med 46, 319–330.

Harris NL, Jaffe ES, Stein H, Banks PM, Chan JK, Cleary ML, Delsol G, Wolf-Peeters C, Falini B, Gatter KC (1994). A revised European-American classification of lymphoid neoplasms: a proposal from the International Lymphoma Study Group. Blood 84, 1361–1392.

..., Rauch J (2002). The antiphospholipid ... Engl J Med 346, 752–763.
...khani SR (2000). How diagnosis with microar-... help cancer patients. Nature 404, 921–•••
...NF (1999). The beta-thalassemias. N Engl J Med 341, ...9–109.
...odak BF, Leclair SJ (2002). The new WHO nomenclature: introduction and myeloid neoplasms. Clin Lab Sci 15, 44–54.

Rosenwald A, Staudt LM (2002). Clinical translation of gene expression profiling in lymphomas and leukemias. Semin Oncol 29, 258–263.

Tefferi A (2003). Anemia in adults: a contemporary approach to diagnosis. Mayo Clin Proc 78, 1274–1280.

Vardiman JW, Harris NL, Brunning RD (2002). The World Health Organization (WHO) classification of the myeloid neoplasms. Blood 100, 2292–2302.

CHAPTER 21

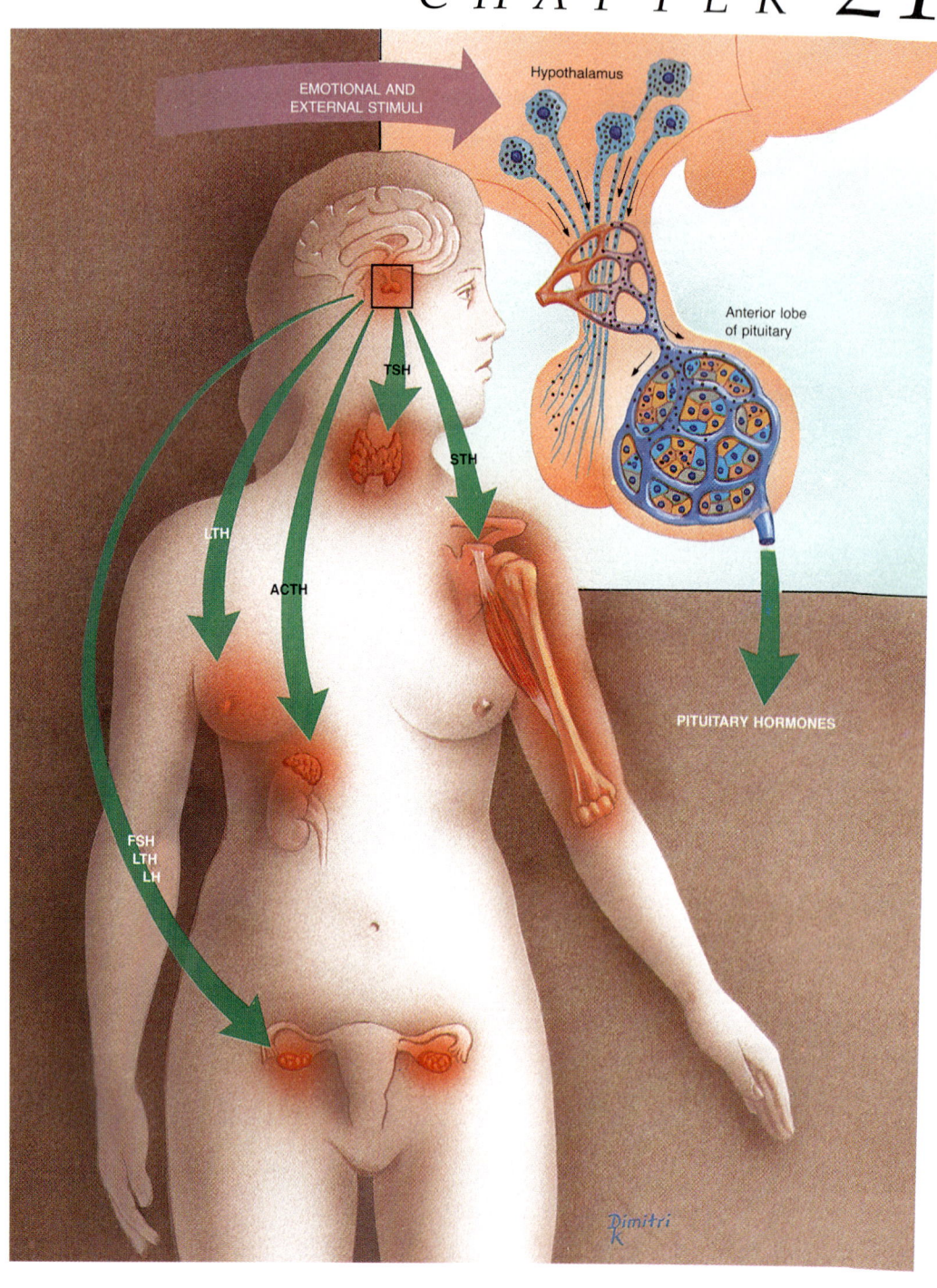

The Endocrine System

Raphael Rubin
Emanuel Rubin

Pituitary Gland

Anatomy

Hypopituitarism

Pituitary Adenomas
Lactotrope Adenoma (Prolactinomas)
Somatotrope Adenoma
Corticotrope Adenoma
Gonadotrope Adenoma
Thyrotrope Adenomas
Nonfunctional Pituitary Adenomas

Posterior Pituitary

Hypothalamic–Pituitary Axis

Thyroid Gland

Anatomy

Function

Congenital Anomalies

Nontoxic Goiter

Hypothyroidism
Primary (Idiopathic) Hypothyroidism
Goitrous Hypothyroidism
Congenital Hypothyroidism

Hyperthyroidism
Graves Disease
Toxic Multinodular Goiter
Toxic Adenoma

Thyroiditis
Chronic Autoimmune Thyroiditis (Hashimoto Thyroiditis)
Subacute Thyroiditis (de Quervain, Granulomatous, or Giant Cell Thyroiditis)
Silent Thyroiditis
Riedel Thyroiditis

Follicular Adenoma of the Thyroid

Thyroid Cancer
Papillary Thyroid Carcinoma
Follicular Thyroid Carcinoma
Medullary Thyroid Carcinoma
Anaplastic (Undifferentiated) Thyroid Carcinoma
Lymphoma of the Thyroid

(continued)

FIGURE 21-1 *(see opposite page)*
The pituitary releases a variety of hormones that stimulate hormone secretion by other endocrine glands or act directly. Pituitary activity is modulated by releasing factors from the hypothalamus, which in turn responds to emotional and external stimuli. *ACTH*, adrenocorticotropic hormone; *FSH*, follicle-stimulating hormone; *LH*, luteinizing hormone; *LTH*, luteotropic hormone (prolactin); *STH*, somatotropin (growth hormone); *TSH*, thyroid-stimulating hormone.

Parathyroid Glands

Anatomy and Physiology

Hypoparathyroidism

Decreased Secretion of Parathyroid Hormone

Pseudohypoparathyroidism

Primary Hyperparathyroidism

Primary Parathyroid Hyperplasia

Parathyroid Carcinoma

Clinical Features of Hyperparathyroidism

Secondary Hyperparathyroidism

Adrenal Cortex

Anatomy

Congenital Adrenal Hyperplasia

21-Hydroxylase Deficiency

11β-Hydroxylase Deficiency

Adrenal Cortical Insufficiency

Primary Chronic Adrenal Insufficiency (Addison Disease)

Acute Adrenal Insufficiency

Secondary Adrenal Insufficiency

Adrenal Hyperfunction

ACTH-Dependent Adrenal Hyperfunction

ACTH-Independent Adrenal Hyperfunction

Clinical Features of Cushing Syndrome

Primary Aldosteronism (Conn Syndrome)

Miscellaneous Adrenal Tumors

Adrenal Medulla and Paraganglia

Anatomy and Function

Pheochromocytoma

Paraganglioma

Neuroblastoma

Ganglioneuroma

Thymus

Anatomy and Function

Agenesis and Dysplasia

Pineal Gland

Anatomy and Physiology

Neoplasms

Multicellular organisms use two seemingly distinct systems for intercellular communication. It was recognized almost a century ago that one, the nervous system, is a structurally fixed network designed for rapid signaling. The other, the endocrine system, was described as acting more slowly and using mobile chemical messengers that are effective at a distance from their site of production (Fig. 21-1). With the discovery of neurotransmitters and the recognition that signaling molecules can act locally on adjacent cells or even on the producing cell itself, it is today understood that a rigid distinction between the nervous and endocrine systems is inappropriate and that in many ways they act in an integrated manner as a *neuroendocrine system*.

The term *hormone* (Greek, "set in motion") originally referred to a chemical secreted in one location that produces effects, often at a distance, on another part of the body. The notion of "ductless" (i.e., endocrine) glands implied that the chemical messenger enters the circulation, which carries it to the target organ. Many hormones, such as thyroid hormone, corticosteroids, and pituitary hormones, conform to this classic definition. By contrast, some traditionally recognized hormones, such as catecholamines, are produced in a variety of sites and act either locally or through the circulation. Other mediators function only in restricted compartments. For example, hypothalamic hormones act only on the pituitary and reach this gland through portal tributaries without entering the systemic circulation. Finally, many hormones exert their effects in the same tissues in which they are formed, such as müllerian-inhibiting substance. These diverse forms of chemically mediated cell-to-cell communication are summarized in Figure 21-2.

To qualify as a hormone, a chemical messenger must bind to a receptor, either on the surface of the cell or within it. Hormones act either on the final effector target or on other glands that in turn produce another hormone. For instance, thyroid hormone acts directly on many types of peripheral

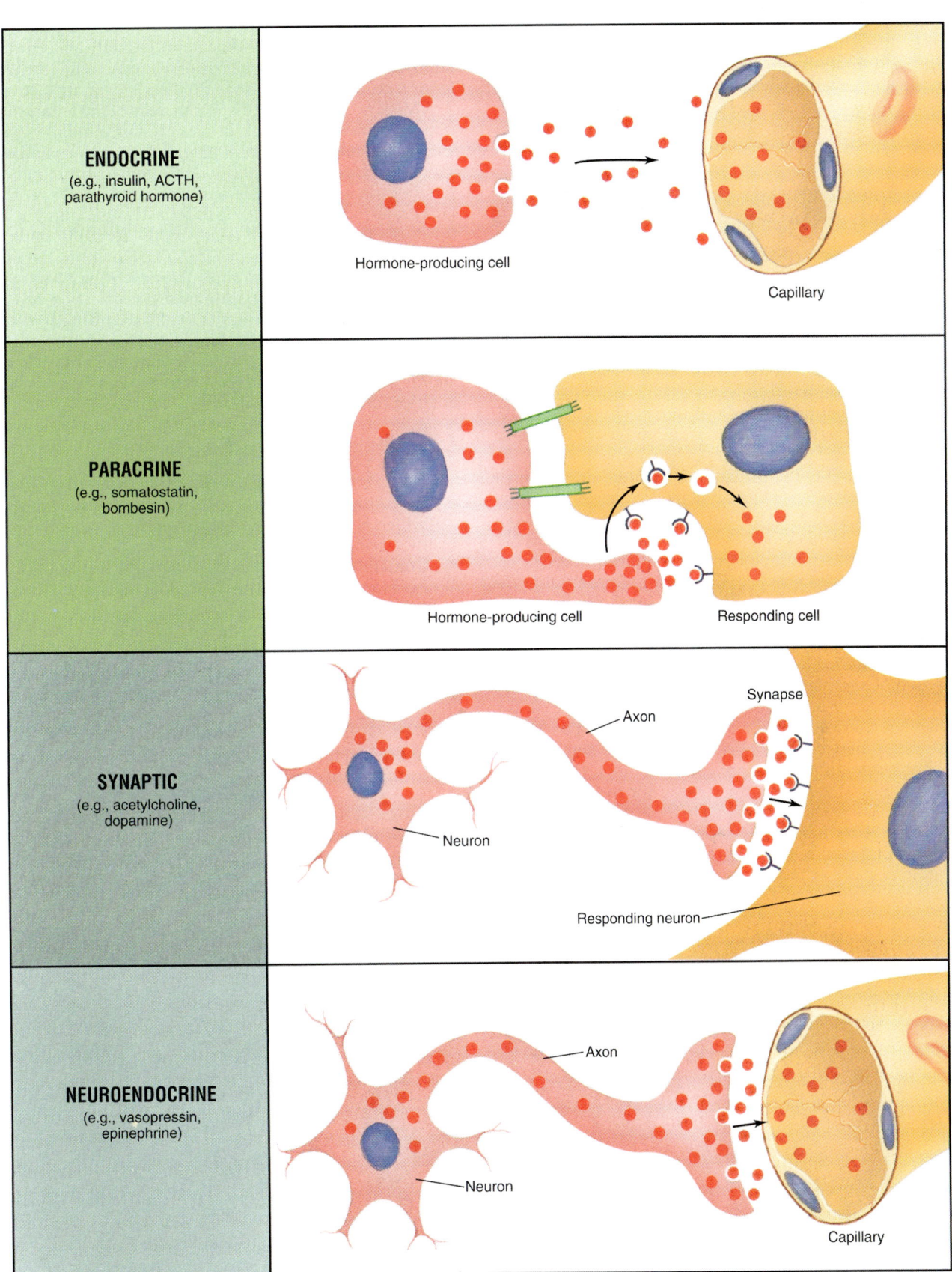

FIGURE 21-2
Mechanisms of chemically mediated cell-to-cell communication. Biological messages may be transmitted by mechanisms other than the classic endocrine pathway via the circulation. These include paracrine, synaptic, and neuroendocrine modes of communication.

cells, whereas thyroid-stimulating hormone (TSH) is released by the pituitary and thereafter promotes the secretion of thyroid hormone by the thyroid gland. Diseases of the endocrine system result in overproduction or underproduction of hormones. In addition, insensitivity of target tissues leads to effects similar to those associated with underproduction of hormones.

Pituitary Gland

ANATOMY

The pituitary gland, also termed the *hypophysis,* resides within the sella turcica, located at the base of the skull within the sphenoid bone. The anterior lobe, which makes up 80% of the gland, is known as the *adenohypophysis,* and the posterior lobe is termed the *neurohypophysis.* The pituitary is in proximity to the optic chiasm and cranial nerves III, IV, V, and VI; thus, tumors of the gland may produce blindness or a number of cranial nerve palsies.

The two lobes of the pituitary are anatomically distinct and derived from different embryological anlagen. The anterior lobe develops from ectoderm that grows upward from the oral cavity (Rathke duct). Along its tract, this craniopharyngeal duct leaves intrasphenoidal squamous epithelial rests that may later serve as the origin of craniopharyngioma. The neurohypophysis (posterior lobe) originates as a downward projection of the brain and remains connected to the hypothalamus by the hypophyseal stalk. Between the anterior and posterior lobes is the vestigial intermediate lobe, composed of a few colloid-filled follicles.

The pituitary has a dual circulation, composed on the one hand of arteries and veins and on the other of a portal venous system between the hypothalamus and the anterior lobe. The latter supplies 80 to 90% of the blood to the pituitary. This portal system is the conduit for the transport of hypothalamic releasing hormones to the anterior pituitary.

The posterior lobe is controlled by unmyelinated nerve fibers that originate in the hypothalamus and proceed along the pituitary stalk to the neurohypophysis. In addition to their conventional neural action, these nerves also secrete arginine vasopressin (antidiuretic hormone [ADH]) and oxytocin, which are synthesized in the hypothalamus, stored in the posterior lobe, and then released into the systemic circulation.

Microscopically, the glandular cells of the anterior pituitary are arranged in cords or nests within a highly vascular stroma. On the basis of staining with hematoxylin and eosin, these cells were classically divided into two groups of equal number, namely, stainable and unstainable cells, with the latter referred to as *chromophobe cells.* The cytoplasmic granules of the stainable cells were termed *acidophilic* (eosinophilic) (40%) or *basophilic* (10%). **However, the tinctorial properties of the granules proved to be unrelated to their function, and the histological classification has been replaced by one that defines the cells according to the hormone secreted.** The cellular localization of specific pituitary hormones is determined by means of immunohistochemical staining (Fig. 21-3). The hormone-producing cells in the anterior pituitary are as follows:

- **Corticotropes:** These basophilic cells secrete adrenocorticotropic hormone (ACTH, corticotropin), which controls the adrenal secretion of corticosteroids.
- **Lactotropes:** Certain acidophilic cells secrete prolactin, which is essential for lactation and has numerous other metabolic activities.
- **Somatotropes:** These acidophilic cells elaborate growth hormone and constitute half of all hormone-producing cells of the adenohypophysis.
- **Thyrotropes:** TSH is produced by pale basophilic or amphophilic cells, which constitute only 5% of the cells of the anterior lobe.
- **Gonadotropes:** Follicle-stimulating hormone (FSH) and luteinizing hormone (LH) are secreted by the same basophilic cell. FSH stimulates the formation of graafian follicles in the ovary, and LH induces ovulation and the formation of corpora lutea in the ovary.

Histologically, the posterior lobe of the pituitary is composed of pituicytes, a type of glial cell without secretory function, and unmyelinated nerve fibers containing ADH and oxytocin. Both of these hormones are formed in the

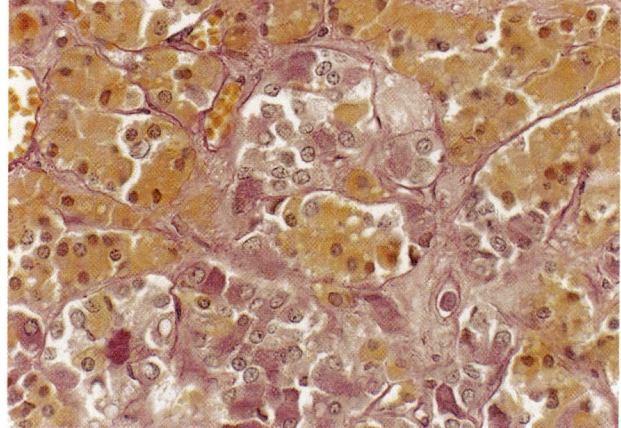 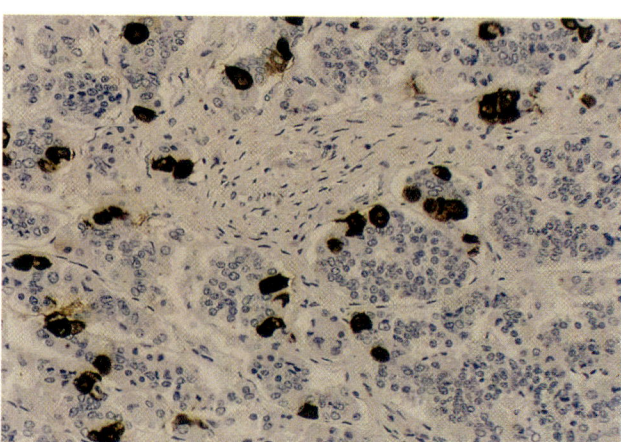

FIGURE 21-3
Normal anterior lobe of pituitary. A. In a PAS-orange G stain, the cytoplasm of somatotropic and prolactin-secreting cells take up the orange G stain. Most of the cells with a lavender cytoplasm produce ACTH (corticotropes). B. An immunohistochemical stain demonstrates cells that synthesize growth hormone (somatotropes).

bodies of the nerve cells in the hypothalamus and transported axonally to the neurohypophysis. ADH promotes water resorption from the distal renal tubules; oxytocin stimulates the pregnant uterus to contract at term.

HYPOPITUITARISM

Hypopituitarism refers to the deficient secretion of one or more of the hormones secreted by the pituitary. In the most common situation, only one or a few of the pituitary hormones are deficient. Occasionally, a total failure of pituitary function occurs, in which case the term *panhypopituitarism* is applied. The effects of hypopituitarism vary with (1) the extent of the loss, (2) the specific hormones involved, and (3) the age of the patient. In general, the symptoms relate to deficient function of the thyroid and adrenal glands and the reproductive system. In children, growth retardation and delayed puberty are additional problems.

PITUITARY TUMORS: More than half of all cases of hypopituitarism in adults are caused by pituitary tumors, usually an adenoma. Even though the tumor itself may be functional, symptoms of hypopituitarism often result from the compression of adjacent tissue by the mass.

SHEEHAN SYNDROME: In this situation, panhypopituitarism is caused by ischemic necrosis of the gland, commonly (but not exclusively) after hypotension induced by postpartum hemorrhage. The pituitary is particularly susceptible at this time, because its enlargement during pregnancy renders it vulnerable to a reduction in blood flow. Amenorrhea, hypothyroidism, and inadequate adrenal function are frequent consequences (Fig. 21-4). With modern obstetric care, Sheehan syndrome has become rare.

PITUITARY APOPLEXY: Hemorrhagic infarction of a pituitary adenoma is usually without endocrine effects because sufficient functioning tissue remains. However, on occasion, pituitary apoplexy leads to hypopituitarism.

IATROGENIC HYPOPITUITARISM: Radiation therapy to the pituitary itself or to lesions of the adjacent head and neck regions can result in hypopituitarism. Similarly, neurosurgical procedures may damage the pituitary.

TRAUMA: Basal skull fractures and other trauma to the sella turcica may injure the pituitary.

INFILTRATIVE DISEASES: Bacterial and viral infections that lead to inflammation of the pituitary area can damage the gland. Hand-Schüller-Christian disease is associated with diabetes insipidus but may also cause hypopituitarism. Hemochromatosis leads to iron deposition in the pituitary and may result in panhypopituitarism.

GENETIC ABNORMALITIES OF PITUITARY DEVELOPMENT: In some instances, children suffer from isolated growth hormone deficiency (IGHD), for which deletions and inactivating mutations of the growth hormone gene are

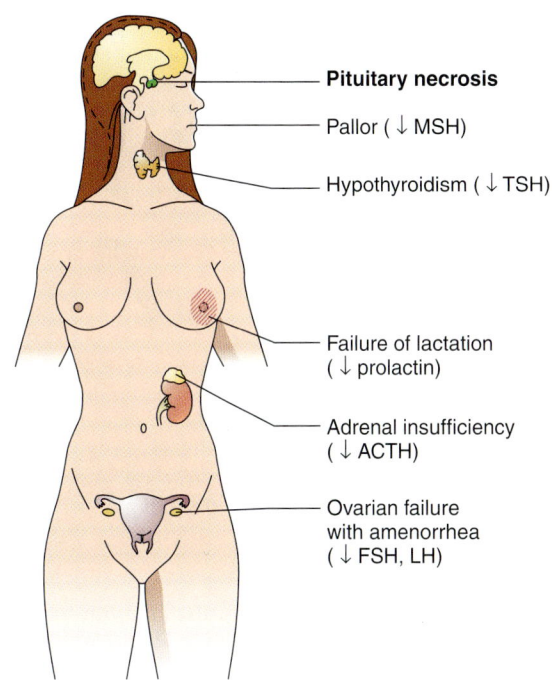

FIGURE 21-4
Major clinical manifestations of panhypopituitarism.

responsible. The availability of recombinant human growth hormone has permitted the safe and effective treatment of these children. In other situations, individuals suffer from multiple pituitary hormone deficiencies. A number of mutations in transcription factors that are involved in embryological development of the pituitary have been identified:

Pit-1: Mutations in this gene (3p11) lead to deficiencies of growth hormone (GH), prolactin (PRL), and TSH.

PROP1 (5q): Mutations in this transcription factor inactivate LH, FSH, GH, PRL, and TSH.

HSEX1 (3p21): This gene is important for the development of the optic nerve as well as the pituitary. Its expression begins before that of the other developmental genes. Mutations result in a small pituitary that releases insufficient GH and ADH.

GROWTH HORMONE INSENSITIVITY (LARON SYNDROME): *Laron dwarfism is a rare, autosomal recessive form of short stature due to extreme resistance to GH secondary to abnormalities in the growth hormone receptor* (GHR). Clinically, these dwarfs tend to be obese and display high levels of serum GH and low concentrations of insulin-like growth factor-I (IGF-I). The condition is seen predominantly in people of Mediterranean origin, especially Sephardic Jews. Interestingly, the same lesion is responsible for the dwarfism of African pygmies.

Laron syndrome is caused by more than 30 *GHR* mutations, all of which involve the extracellular domain of the receptor. The clinical presentation is heterogeneous, and most cases are unique to particular families or geographical areas. Since GH exerts its effects by promoting the secretion of IGF-I, the latter hormone provides effective replacement therapy for Laron syndrome, mimicking most effects ascribed to GH itself.

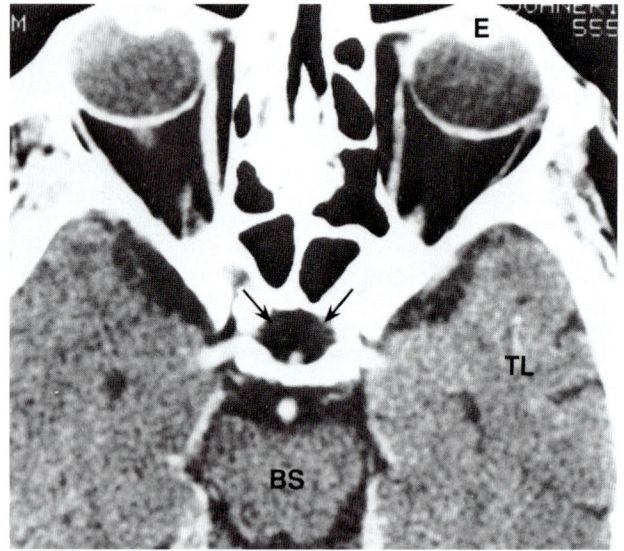

FIGURE 21-5
Empty sella syndrome. A CT scan of the cranium in an axial section demonstrates an empty sella turcica (arrows). E, eye; TL, temporal lobe; BS, brainstem.

ISOLATED GONADOTROPIN DEFICIENCY (KALL-MANN SYNDROME): *Kallmann syndrome is characterized by hypogonadism secondary to a deficiency of gonadotropin and anosmia (absent sense of smell).* Cleft palate and other anomalies may also be present. Kallmann syndrome is usually diagnosed at puberty because of a delay in the appearance of secondary sex characteristics. The prevalence of Kallmann syndrome is 1/10,000 in boys, and much lower in girls. Most cases are sporadic, although familial forms of the disease have been described. All cases reflect mutations in the *KAL* gene family, some of which are X-linked and others of which are autosomal dominant or autosomal recessive. The *KAL* gene codes for an extracellular matrix component with putative antiprotease activity and cell adhesion function. As a result of this mutation, neurons destined to secrete gonadotropin-releasing hormone (GnRH) fail to migrate from their origin in the olfactory anlage to their normal location in the hypothalamus.

EMPTY SELLA SYNDROME: This is a radiological term that describes an enlarged sella containing a thin, flattened pituitary at the base (Fig. 21-5). Empty sella syndrome is secondary to a congenitally defective or absent diaphragma sella, which permits the transmission of cerebrospinal fluid pressure into the sella. Hormonal abnormalities are usually minor, although some women develop mild hypopituitarism.

PITUITARY ADENOMAS

Pituitary adenomas are benign neoplasms of the anterior lobe of the pituitary and are often associated with excess secretion of pituitary hormones and evidence of corresponding endocrine hyperfunction (Table 21-1). They occur in both sexes at almost any age but are more common in men between the ages of 20 and 50 years. Small, apparently nonfunctioning pituitary adenomas are found incidentally in as many as 25% of adult autopsies.

 Pathogenesis: The etiology of pituitary adenomas is obscure. In rare instances, they occur in the context of multiple endocrine neoplasia (MEN) type 1, a hereditary disposition to the formation of adenomas of the pituitary, parathyroid hyperplasia or adenoma, and islet cell adenomas of the pancreas (see Chapter 15). Acquired activating point mutations in the stimulatory subunit of the G_s protein that activates adenylyl cyclase have been reported in 40% of pituitary adenomas that secrete growth hormone. The resultant elevation of intracellular cyclic adenosine monophosphate (cAMP) levels has been suggested to lead to hypersecretion of GH and cellular proliferation. Mutations or overexpression of a number of regulatory genes have been described in a number of pituitary adenomas, including cyclin D_1, *CREB, ras,* and the recently described pituitary tumor transforming gene *(PTTG).*

 Pathology: Pituitary adenomas have classically been subdivided histologically according to the tinctorial properties of their cells. Thus, they have been classified as acidophil, basophil, or chromophobe adenomas. In this scheme, acidophil adenomas were associated with overproduction of GH, basophil adenomas with excess secretion of ACTH, and chromophobe adenomas with no endocrine hyperfunction. In view of the lack of correlation between the staining properties of the tumor cells and the type of hormone secreted, pituitary adenomas are today classified according to the hormone(s) elaborated by the neoplastic cells.

Pituitary adenomas range from small lesions that do not enlarge the gland to expansive tumors that erode the sella turcica and impinge on adjacent cranial structures (Fig. 21-6). In general, adenomas less than 10 mm in diameter are referred to as *microadenomas,* and larger ones are termed *macroadenomas.* Microadenomas do not produce symptoms unless they secrete hormones. However macroadenomas tend to cause local symptoms, by virtue of their size, and systemic manifestations, as a result of the overproduction of hormones.

 Clinical Features: The mass effects of pituitary macroadenomas include impingement on the optic chiasm, often with bitemporal hemianopsia and

TABLE 21-1 Frequency of Adenomas of the Anterior Pituitary

Cell Type	Hormone	Frequency (%)
Lactotrope	Prolactin	26
Null cell	None	17
Corticotrope	ACTH (corticotropin)	15
Somatotrope	Growth hormone	14
Plurihormonal	Multiple	13
Gonadotrope	FSH, LH	8
Oncocytoma	None	6
Thyrotrope	TSH	1

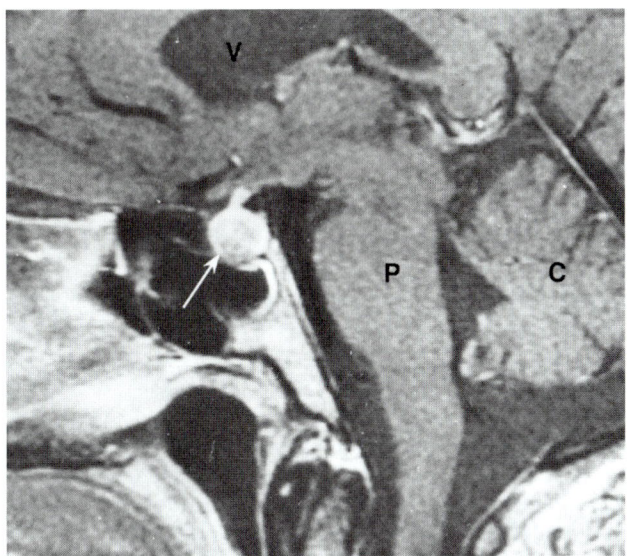

FIGURE 21-6
Pituitary adenoma. A magnetic resonance sagittal view of the brain shows a distinct pituitary tumor *(arrow)*. *V*, lateral ventricle; *P*, pons; *C*, cerebellum.

loss of central vision, oculomotor palsies when the tumor invades the cavernous sinuses, and severe headaches. Large adenomas may invade the hypothalamus and lead to loss of temperature regulation, hyperphagia, and hormonal syndromes caused by interference with the normal hypothalamic input to the pituitary.

Lactotrope Adenoma (Prolactinomas) Leads to the Most Common Pituitary Endocrinopathy

Hyperprolactinemia is the most common endocrinopathy associated with pituitary adenomas. Almost half of all pituitary microadenomas contain prolactin (PRL), but many fewer appear to secrete this hormone. PRL-producing microadenomas are most often symptomatic in young women, but more than half of all macroadenomas that elaborate PRL are found in men. This difference in sex distribution is related to the more frequent occurrence of endocrinological symptoms in women, and the true incidence in unselected autopsies is similar in both sexes. In general, the larger the adenoma the more PRL is secreted.

 Pathology: Lactotrope adenomas tend to be chromophobic and stain for PRL by immunohistochemistry. The deposition of endocrine amyloid (see Chapter 23) and the presence of psammoma bodies (calcospherites) are characteristic of lactotrope adenoma but are not pathognomonic.

 Clinical Features: In women, functional lactotrope adenomas lead to amenorrhea, galactorrhea, and infertility. The consistently elevated blood PRL levels inhibit the surge in the secretion of pituitary LH necessary for ovulation. Men tend to suffer from decreased libido and erectile dysfunction. Functional lactotrope microadenomas are successfully treated with dopamine agonists (bromocriptine) to inhibit PRL secretion, whereas macroadenomas may require surgery or radiation therapy. Excess secretion of PRL may be caused by factors other than pituitary adenomas, including pregnancy, lactation, administration of certain drugs, or pressure effects on the hypothalamus by other tumors.

Somatotrope Adenomas Secrete Growth Hormone

The excess secretion of growth hormone (GH) produces dramatic bodily changes. A somatotrope adenoma that arises in a child or adolescent before the epiphyses close results in *gigantism*. By contrast, after the epiphyses of the long bones have fused and adult height has been achieved, the same tumor produces *acromegaly*.

Pathology: Of patients with acromegaly, 75% have a somatotrope macroadenoma, and most of the remainder have microadenomas. By light microscopy, somatotrope adenomas are either acidophilic or chromophobic. By electron microscopy, acidophilic tumors tend to contain abundant secretory granules, whereas the chromophobic ones are sparsely granular. Acidophilic somatotrope adenomas usually grow slowly and remain within the sella.

Microscopically, sheets or trabeculae of regular eosinophilic cells are noted (Fig. 21-7). The chromophobic variant is typically faster growing and invasive and microscopically manifests cellular and nuclear pleomorphism.

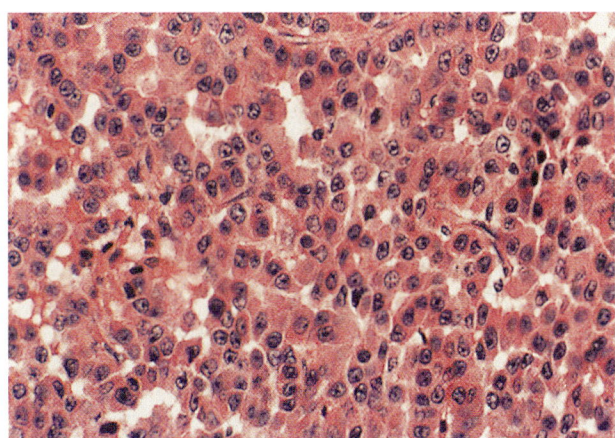

FIGURE 21-7
Pituitary somatotrope adenoma from a man with acromegaly. The tumor cells are arranged in thin cords and ribbons.

Clinical Features: Acromegaly is an uncommon disorder, with an annual incidence of only three cases per million. Over the course of many years, patients with acromegaly gradually develop coarse facial features (Fig. 21-8). They exhibit overgrowth of the mandible (prognathism) and maxilla, with spaces between the upper incisor teeth, and a thickened nose. The hands and feet enlarge, and the hat size increases.

Acromegaly has more implications for the health of the patient than simple cosmetic disfigurement. The incidence of cardiovascular, cerebrovascular, and respiratory deaths increases. Most acromegalics suffer from neurological and musculoskeletal symptoms, including headaches, paresthesias, arthralgias, and muscle weakness. One third have hypertension, and even half of normotensive persons with acromegaly have an increased left ventricular mass and may develop congestive heart failure in the absence of a defined cardiac condition. The viscera also hypertrophy. Diabetes occurs in as many as 20%, and hypercalciuria and renal stones are present in another fifth of patients. In half of patients with acromegaly, hyperprolactinemia is severe enough to be symptomatic (see above).

The treatment of choice for somatotrope adenomas is transsphenoidal removal of the pituitary, after which circulating GH levels may decline to normal levels within hours. Radiation therapy is an alternative when surgery is contraindicated. A long-acting analogue of somatostatin, an antagonist of GH, is a useful adjunct to treatment.

Corticotrope Adenoma Produces ACTH

Excess ACTH induces adrenal cortical hypersecretion to produce *Cushing disease* (see below). In most cases, the tumor is a microadenoma that is intensely basophilic and periodic acid–Schiff (PAS) positive. Immunohistochemical analysis reveals the presence of not only ACTH but also of related peptides, such as endorphins and lipotropin, in the cytoplasm. A few functional corticotrope adenomas are chromophobic and tend to be more aggressive than their basophilic counterparts.

By electron microscopy, basophilic adenomas contain numerous secretory granules and perinuclear bundles of fine, keratin-positive, intermediate filaments (type I filaments). These filaments may be abundant enough to be visible by light microscopy as *Crooke hyalinization,* a change related to the suppression of ACTH secretion by high levels of circulating cortisol.

Gonadotrope Adenoma Secretes LH and FSH

Most of these tumors are macroadenomas and manifest in middle-aged men as headache, visual disturbance, and acquired hypogonadism. Since LH normally stimulates testosterone production in the testis, the hypogonadism in men with gonadotrope adenomas is seemingly paradoxical. This effect has been attributed to inadequate bioactivity of the secreted LH or abnormalities in the normal pulsatile pattern of LH release.

Gonadotrope adenomas are chromophobic or somewhat acidophilic. The tumor cells exhibit strong immunoreactivity for FSH, LH, or both. Surgical resection is the treatment of choice.

Thyrotrope Adenomas Produce TSH

Thyrotrope adenoma, the rarest of all pituitary adenomas, comes to medical attention because of symptoms of hyperthyroidism, goiter, or a pituitary mass lesion. Typically, circulating levels of TSH and thyroid hormone both increase, a situation unique to this tumor. Thyrotrope adenomas are chromophobic, with polyhedral or columnar cells that form pseudorosettes around blood vessels. They stain for TSH, and by electron microscopy, the secretory granules are often

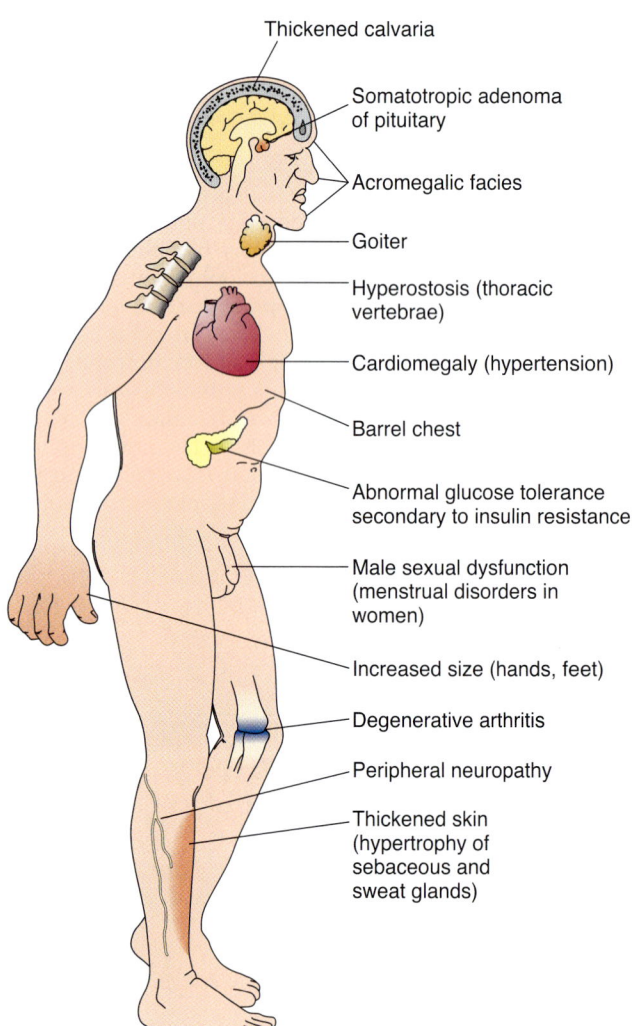

FIGURE 21-8
Clinical manifestations of acromegaly.

Posterior Pituitary

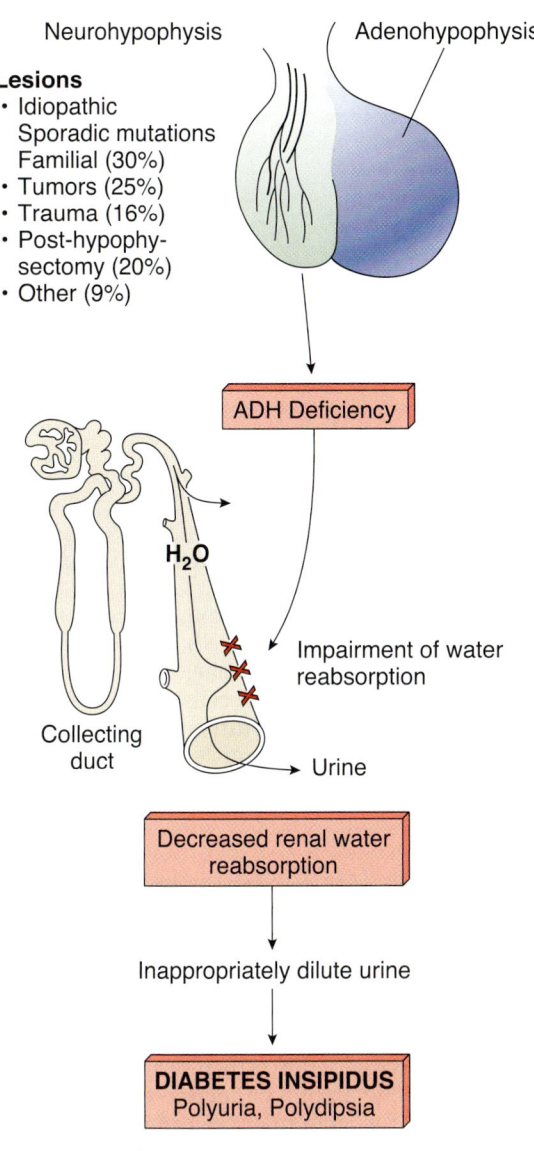

FIGURE 21-9
Mechanism of diabetes insipidus.

arranged in a single row immediately beneath the plasma membrane.

In patients with long-standing hypothyroidism, hyperplasia of pituitary thyrotropes (thyroid deficiency cells) is a well-described entity and is presumably secondary to inadequate feedback inhibition by thyroid hormones.

Nonfunctional Pituitary Adenomas Are Not Associated with Endocrinopathies

One fourth of all pituitary tumors removed surgically do not secrete excess hormones. The tumors are slowly growing macroadenomas that are diagnosed in older persons because of their mass effects.

Null cell adenomas are chromophobic and PAS-negative. By immunohistochemistry, the cells are either negative for all hormones of the anterior pituitary or display a few immunoreactive cells.

Oncocytoma is a variant of nonfunctional null cell adenoma characterized by enlarged, eosinophilic, and often granular tumor cells. By electron microscopy, they are packed with mitochondria but are otherwise similar to other null cell adenomas.

Silent adenomas are distinguished from other nonfunctional pituitary adenomas by their well-differentiated appearance under the electron microscope and in many cases by immunoreactivity for ACTH and other hormones. The reasons for the lack of hormone secretion are not understood.

POSTERIOR PITUITARY

Central diabetes insipidus (Fig. 21-9) is the only significant condition associated with disease of the posterior pituitary. This disorder is characterized by an inability to concentrate the urine and consequent chronic water diuresis (polyuria), thirst, and polydipsia. The biochemical basis of the disease is a deficiency of ADH (vasopressin), which is secreted by the posterior pituitary under the influence of the hypothalamus. One third of cases of central diabetes insipidus are still of unknown etiology or can be attributed to sporadic or familial mutations in the vasopressin–neurophysin II gene. Mutations in the vasopressin receptor and the vasopressin-sensitive water channel genes have also been described in the context of *nephrogenic diabetes insipidus*.

One fourth of cases of central diabetes insipidus are associated with brain tumors, particularly *craniopharyngioma* (Fig. 21-10). This tumor arises above the sella turcica from remnants of Rathke pouch and invades and compresses adjacent tissues (see Chapter 28). Trauma and hypophysectomy for anterior pituitary tumors account for most of the remaining cases of diabetes insipidus. Uncommonly, localized hemorrhage or infarction, Langerhans cell histiocytosis, or granulomatous infiltrates involve the posterior pituitary stalk or body. Polyuria may be controlled by powdered posterior pituitary or vasopressin administered as snuff. Ectopic secretion of ADH and a syndrome of inappropriate ADH secretion (SIADH) may be caused by paraneoplastic secretion of ADH by tumor cells.

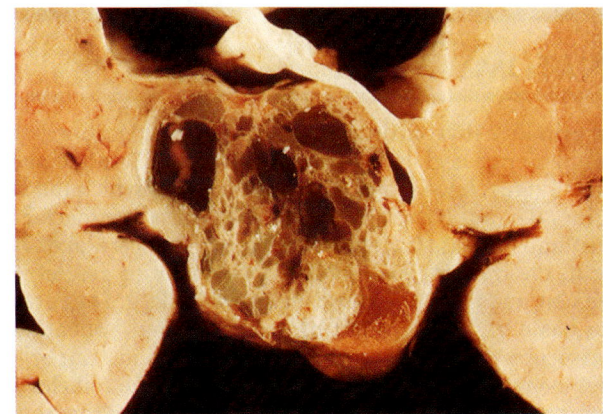

FIGURE 21-10
Craniopharyngioma. Coronal section of the brain shows a large, cystic tumor mass replacing the midline structures in the region of the hypothalamus.

TABLE 21-2 Hormones of the Hypothalamic–Pituitary–Target Gland Axis

Hypothalamus	Pituitary	Target Gland	Peripheral Inhibitory Hormone
CRH	ACTH	Adrenal	Corticosteroids
TRH	TSH	Thyroid	T_3, T_4
GHRH	Growth hormone	Varied	IGF-I
Somatostatin	Growth hormone	Varied	IGF-I
LHRH	LH	Gonads	Estradiol, testosterone
	FSH	Gonads	Inhibin, estradiol, testosterone
Dopamine	Prolactin	Breast	Unknown

CRH, corticotropin (ACTH)-releasing hormone; GHRH, growth hormone-releasing hormone; IGF-I insulin-like growth factor-I; LHRH, luteinizing hormone-releasing hormone; TRH, thyrotropin-releasing hormone.

HYPOTHALAMIC–PITUITARY AXIS

The hypothalamus, pituitary stalk, and pituitary gland constitute an integrated "neuroendocrine system," both anatomically and functionally. Neuron groups in the hypothalamus secrete a number of factors that stimulate the anterior pituitary lobe (Table 21-2). Secretion of these hypothalamic factors is, in turn, antagonized by the hormones secreted by the peripheral target organs, thereby completing a feedback loop. In addition, specific hypothalamic inhibitory hormones have been identified. For example, dopamine inhibits the pituitary secretion of prolactin.

The hypothalamus may be damaged by a variety of primary and metastatic tumors, viral infections and granulomatous inflammations and several types of degenerative and hereditary disorders. In many instances, hypothalamic dysfunction occurs in the absence of an identifiable anatomical abnormality. Diverse conditions result from disturbances of hypothalamic function and include, among others, hypogonadism, precocious puberty, amenorrhea, and eating disorders (obesity or anorexia). Some pituitary disorders characterized by increased or decreased hormone secretion have their origin in hypothalamic dysfunction. A detailed description of the hypothalamic syndromes is beyond the scope of this chapter, and the reader is referred to the textbooks of endocrinology listed under "Suggested Reading."

Thyroid Gland

ANATOMY

The primitive thyroid descends to its eventual location in the lower anterior neck by elongation of its tubular attachment to the tongue, known as the *thyroglossal duct*, which then atrophies. The adult thyroid comprises two lobes connected by an isthmus and is situated below the thyroid cartilage anterior to the trachea. Each lobe is about 4 cm in greatest dimension, and the entire gland weighs some 20 g. The cut surface has a glistening, light brown, lobulated appearance. Microscopically, the parenchyma is arranged in acini or follicles averaging about 200 μm in diameter. The follicles are lined by an epithelium whose appearance depends on the demand for thyroid hormone. The lining cells are columnar when the gland is actively secreting hormone and flatter when the thyroid is less active. The epithelial cells display glycoprotein globules composed of thyroglobulin. The lumen of the follicle contains a glassy, eosinophilic proteinaceous material termed *colloid*. This substance represents secreted thyroglobulin, from which active thyroid hormones are released.

In addition to the follicular epithelial cells, the thyroid also contains parafollicular or *C cells*, which produce calcitonin, a calcium-lowering hormone. These cells are interspersed with follicular epithelial cells or in the interstitium. With routine stains, C cells are difficult to identify, but they are readily visualized with immunostaining for calcitonin.

FUNCTION

The principal metabolic products of the thyroid gland are triiodothyronine (T_3) and tetraiodothyronine (thyroxine, T_4). T_4 is principally a prohormone; the major effector of thyroid function is T_3. These molecules are formed by the iodination of tyrosine residues of thyroglobulin within the follicular cells. Iodinated thyroglobulin is then secreted into the lumen of the follicle. Alone among endocrine glands, the thyroid can thus store a large amount of preformed hormone.

On demand, thyroglobulin is reabsorbed by the follicular cells, after which T_4 and T_3 are liberated by proteolytic cleavage and released to the blood. Most of the secreted hormone is T_4, which is deiodinated in peripheral tissues to the more active form, T_3. In the blood, thyroid hormones circulate both free and bound to thyronine-binding globulin (TBG). Peripheral cells take up only free hormone, which binds to nuclear receptors and initiates specific protein synthesis.

Thyroid hormone affects almost all organs in the body. It stimulates the basal metabolic rate and the metabolism of carbohydrates, lipids, and proteins. Thyroid hormone augments thermogenesis and hepatic glucose production through enhanced gluconeogenesis and glycogenolysis. It promotes the synthesis of numerous structural proteins, enzymes, and other hormones. Glucose use, fatty acid synthesis in the liver, and adipose tissue lipolysis are all increased. In general, the overall metabolic activities of the body, both anabolic and catabolic, are up-regulated by thyroid hormone.

Thyroid structure and function are governed principally by TSH secreted by the pituitary. In turn, thyroid hormone suppresses TSH secretion, to complete an autoregulatory feedback loop. The maintenance of a normal rate of thyroid hormone production depends on an adequate dietary supply of iodine.

CONGENITAL ANOMALIES

LINGUAL THYROID: If the thyroid fails to descend during embryogenesis, it remains at its origin as a nodule at the base of the tongue. Its removal results in total hypothyroidism.

HETEROTOPIC THYROID TISSUE: Nests of thyroid tissue may be found anywhere along the pathway of its descent into the lower neck. Thyroid tissue is also occasionally encountered in the pericardium or mediastinum.

LATERAL ABERRANT THYROID: Ectopic thyroid tissue occasionally occurs in the lymph nodes and soft tissue adjacent to the normal gland. The origin of lateral aberrant thyroid tissue is controversial. Some hold that all of these cases actually represent well-differentiated metastases from an occult thyroid cancer; others accept the concept of embryonal rests lateral to the thyroid. In any event, finding thyroid follicles in enlarged lymph nodes must be treated as suggestive evidence for a primary thyroid cancer.

THYROGLOSSAL DUCT CYST: Failure of the thyroglossal duct to involute completely can result in a cystic, fluid-filled remnant anywhere along the route of the duct. The cysts, which are most common in children, are 1 to 3 cm in diameter and are lined by squamous or respiratory-type epithelium. Surgical excision is curative.

NONTOXIC GOITER

Nontoxic goiter (Latin, guttur, "throat"), *also termed simple, colloid, or multinodular goiter, refers to an enlargement of the thyroid that is not associated with functional, inflammatory, or neoplastic alterations.* Thus, patients with nontoxic goiter are neither hyperthyroid nor hypothyroid and do not suffer from any form of thyroiditis (see below). The disease is far more common in women than in men (8:1). The diffuse form is frequent in adolescence and during pregnancy, whereas the multinodular type usually occurs in persons older than 50 years of age.

Pathogenesis: In nontoxic goiter, the capacity of the thyroid to produce thyroid hormone is impaired. The resulting increased secretion of TSH leads to enlargement of the gland, a situation that maintains the euthyroid state. The etiology of the decrease in thyroid hormone production is not established.

Simple nodular enlargement of the thyroid tends to be familial, suggesting a genetic contribution to the disorder. Indeed, mutations in the thyroglobulin gene have been detected in a number of families affected by simple goiter.

Pathology: The size of nontoxic goiters ranges from a doubling in the size of the gland (40 g) to a massive enlargement in which the thyroid weighs a few hundred grams (Fig. 21-11).

Diffuse nontoxic goiter characterizes the early stages of the disease. The gland is diffusely enlarged and microscopically exhibits hypertrophy and hyperplasia of the follicular epithelial cells. On occasion, the epithelium has a papillary appearance. At this stage, the amount of colloid in the follicles is decreased.

Multinodular nontoxic goiter evolves as the disease becomes more chronic. The enlarged thyroid assumes an increasingly nodular configuration, and the cut surface is typically studded with numerous irregular nodules. When they contain large amounts of colloid, nodules tend to be soft, glistening, and reddish. Those composed of smaller follicles containing little colloid are typically grayish white and fleshy. Hemorrhagic, necrotic, and cystic areas are common, and fibrous bands often traverse the gland. Calcific foci, which impart a gritty surface, are frequent.

Microscopically, the nodules vary considerably in size and shape. Some are distended with colloid; others are collapsed. Large colloid-containing follicles may fuse to form even larger "colloid cysts." The lining epithelial cells are flat to cuboidal and are occasionally arrayed as papillae that project into the follicular lumen. Hemosiderin deposition and cholesterol granulomas are evidence of old hemorrhage. The individual follicles or groups of follicles are separated by dense fibrosis, and dystrophic calcification of necrotic foci is often noted.

Clinical Features: Patients with nontoxic goiter are typically asymptomatic and come to medical attention because of a mass in the neck. Large goiters may cause dysphagia or inspiratory stridor by compressing the esophagus or the trachea. Pressure by the goiter on the neck veins leads to venous congestzion of the head and face. Hoarseness may result from compression of the recurrent laryngeal nerve. Occasionally, local pain is produced by hemorrhage into a nodule or cyst. Importantly, the blood concentrations of T_4, T_3, and (usually) TSH are normal.

Nontoxic goiter is most commonly treated by administration of thyroid hormone to reduce TSH levels and, thus, the stimulation to thyroid growth. In older patients with low TSH levels, further suppression by exogenous thyroid hormone may be ineffective, and radioactive iodine therapy is indicated. Although surgery is ordinarily contraindicated, it may become necessary if local obstructive symptoms become troublesome. Many patients with nontoxic goiter eventually develop hyperthyroidism, in which case the term *toxic multinodular goiter* is applied (see below).

HYPOTHYROIDISM

Hypothyroidism refers to the clinical manifestations of thyroid hormone deficiency. It can be the consequence of three general processes:

- **Defective synthesis of thyroid hormone,** with compensatory goitrogenesis (goitrous hypothyroidism)

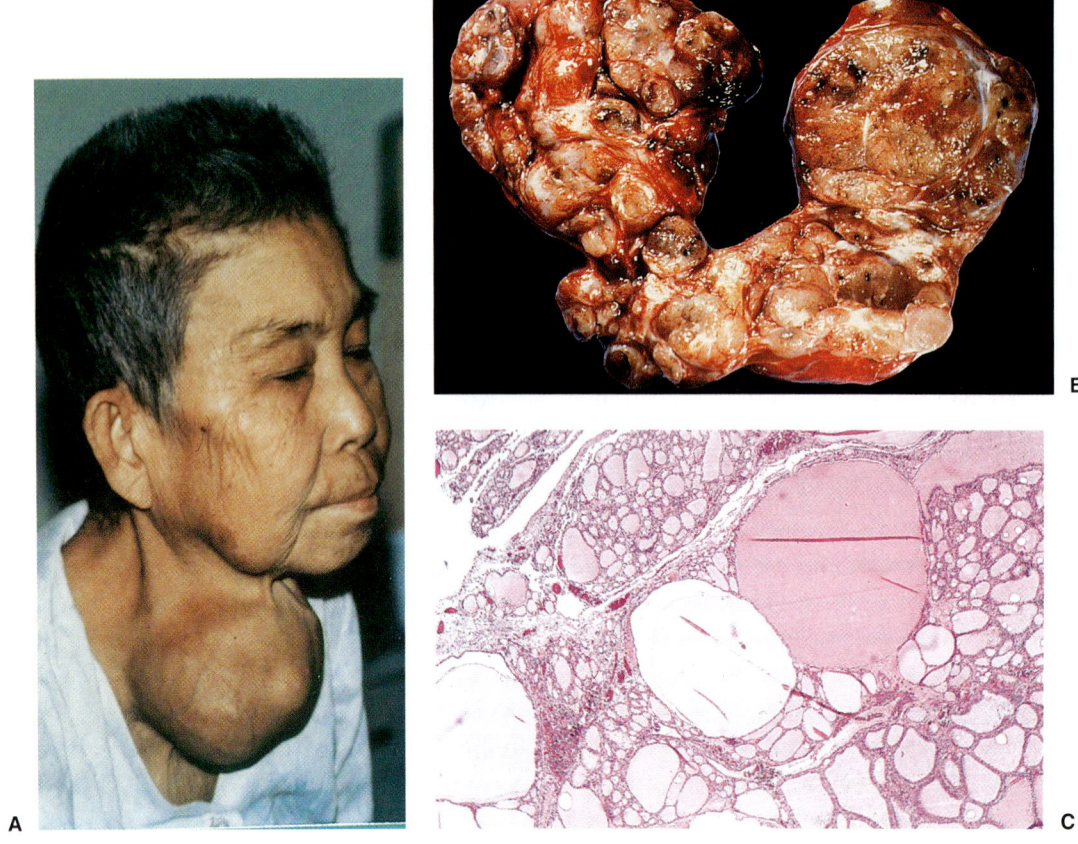

FIGURE 21-11
Nontoxic goiter. A. In a middle-aged woman with nontoxic goiter, the thyroid has enlarged to produce a conspicuous neck mass. B. Coronal section of the enlarged thyroid gland shows numerous irregular nodules, some with cystic degeneration and old hemorrhage. C. Microscopic view of one of the macroscopic nodules shows marked variation in the size of the follicles.

- **Inadequate function of thyroid parenchyma,** usually as a result of thyroiditis or surgical resection of the gland or the therapeutic administration of radioiodine
- **Inadequate secretion of TSH** by the pituitary or of thyroid-releasing hormone (TRH) by the hypothalamus

The clinical symptomatology of hypothyroidism reflects decreased levels of circulating thyroid hormone. Symptoms of hypothyroidism (Fig. 21-12) develop insidiously, and often the first manifestations are tiredness, lethargy, sensitivity to cold, and an inability to concentrate. Many organ systems in the body are affected, but all are hypofunctional. Hypothyroidism is treated effectively by the administration of thyroid hormone.

SKIN: Alterations in the skin are almost universal in patients with clinically apparent hypothyroidism. Proteoglycans accumulate in the extracellular matrix and bind water, resulting in a peculiar form of edema termed *myxedema*. Myxedematous patients have boggy facies, puffy eyelids, edema of the hands and feet, and an enlarged tongue. Thickening of the mucous membranes of the larynx causes patients to be hoarse. A pale, cool skin reflects cutaneous vasoconstriction. The skin is also dry and coarse, because the secretions of the sebaceous and sweat glands are inadequate. Ecchymoses are common because of increased capillary fragility, and skin wounds heal slowly.

NERVOUS SYSTEM: Hypothyroidism in pregnant women has grave neurological consequences for the fetus, expressed after birth as cretinism (see below). The hypothyroid adult is lethargic and somnolent and suffers from memory loss and a general slowing of mental processes. Paranoid ideation or depression is frequent, and severe agitation, termed *myxedema madness,* may develop. Sensory defects, including deafness and night blindness, occur. A cerebellar ataxia may appear, and tendon reflexes are dulled. Microscopic examination of the brain shows mucinous accumulations in nerve fibers and in the cerebellum.

HEART: In early hypothyroidism the heart rate and stroke volume are both reduced, resulting in decreased cardiac output. In untreated hypothyroidism, so-called *myxedema heart* develops, which is characterized by a dilated heart and a pericardial effusion. On pathological exam-

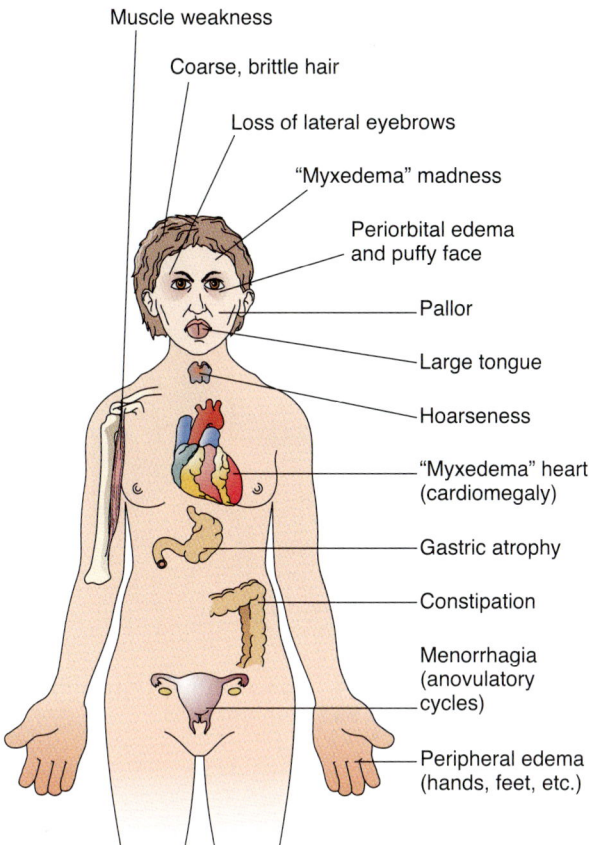

FIGURE 21-12
Dominant clinical manifestations of hypothyroidism.

ination, the heart is flabby and microscopically shows interstitial edema and swelling of the myocytes. Coronary atherosclerosis is a common finding.

GASTROINTESTINAL TRACT: Constipation, owing to decreased peristalsis, is a common complaint and may be severe enough to lead to fecal impaction (*myxedema megacolon*).

REPRODUCTIVE SYSTEM: Women with hypothyroidism suffer ovulatory failure, progesterone deficiency, and irregular and excessive menstrual bleeding. In men, erectile dysfunction and oligospermia are common.

Primary (Idiopathic) Hypothyroidism Is Often Autoimmune

Primary hypothyroidism is most common in the fifth and sixth decades and, like most thyroid disorders, is more common in women than in men. Three fourths of patients have circulating antibodies to thyroid antigens, suggesting that these cases represent the end stage of autoimmune thyroiditis (see below). Nongoitrous hypothyroidism may also result from antibodies that block TSH itself or the TSH receptor without activating the thyroid. Some cases of primary hypothyroidism are part of multiglandular autoimmune syndrome, including insulin-dependent diabetes, pernicious anemia, hypoparathyroidism, adrenal atrophy, and hypogonadism (see below).

Goitrous Hypothyroidism Reflects Inadequate Secretion of Thyroid Hormone

There are a number of conditions in which thyroid enlargement (goiter) is associated with hypothyroidism. The etiology of goitrous hypothyroidism includes iodine deficiency, antithyroid agents (drugs or dietary goitrogens), long-term iodide intake, and a number of hereditary defects in the synthesis of thyroid hormone. **The evolution of the pathological changes in goitrous hypothyroidism is similar to that described earlier for nontoxic goiter.**

Endemic Goiter

Endemic goiter refers to the goitrous hypothyroidism of dietary iodine deficiency in locales with a high prevalence of the disease. In areas far from salt water and seafood, which are rich sources of iodides, goiters are (or were) common. The Great Lakes region of the United States, alpine Europe, central Africa, parts of China, and the Himalayas are such places. Iodized salt is an effective preventive dietary measure, and its wide availability has essentially eliminated endemic goiter in many areas. Nevertheless, it has been estimated that more than 200 million persons worldwide are still afflicted with the disease.

The pathological evolution of endemic goiter is comparable to that of nontoxic goiter discussed above. However, in contrast to the latter, endemic goiter rarely eventuates in hyperthyroidism. Although the administration of iodine may reverse the early, diffuse stage of endemic goiter, such therapy has little effect on a fully developed multinodular goiter. Replacement therapy with thyroid hormone is indicated, and surgical resection may be necessary if local symptoms are severe.

Goiter Induced by Antithyroid Agents

A number of drugs and naturally occurring chemicals in foods are goitrogenic, owing to their suppression of thyroid hormone synthesis. Such goiters may or may not be associated with hypothyroidism. The most commonly used goitrogenic drug is **lithium,** which is used in the management of manic-depressive states. Other common goitrogenic drugs include phenylbutazone and *p*-aminosalicylic acid. Certain cruciferous vegetables (turnips, rutabaga, cassava) contain goitrogens, and their ingestion can potentiate an iodine-deficient diet to produce goitrous hypothyroidism.

Iodide-Induced Goiter

Goiter and hypothyroidism, or either alone, may occur in persons who consume large amounts of iodide, either as a medicinal component (potassium iodide-containing expectorants) or in foods particularly rich in this halide (e.g., seaweed in Japan). In most cases, iodide-induced goiter develops in the context of preexisting thyroid disease, such as thyroiditis. Women given large doses of iodine during pregnancy may deliver goitrous infants.

Congenital Hypothyroidism Is Also Termed *Cretinism*

Cretinism may be endemic, sporadic, or familial and is twice as frequent in girls as boys. In nonendemic regions, 90% of cases result from developmental defects of the thyroid *(thyroid dysgenesis)*. The remainder principally have a variety of inherited metabolic defects, including mutations in the genes for TRH and its receptor, TSH and its receptor, sodium-iodide symporter, thyroglobulin, and thyroid oxidase.

 Clinical Features: Symptoms of congenital hypothyroidism appear in the early weeks of life. The infants are apathetic and sluggish. The abdomen is large and often exhibits an umbilical hernia. The body temperature is often below 35°C (95°F), and the skin is pale and cold. Refractory anemia and a dilated heart are frequent. By the age of 6 months, the clinical syndrome of congenital hypothyroidism is well developed. Mental retardation, stunted growth (owing to defective osseous maturation), and characteristic facies are evident. The serum levels of T_4 and T_3 are low, and the serum TSH level is high (unless the problem relates to a lack of TSH secretion itself).

If thyroid hormone replacement therapy is not promptly provided, congenital hypothyroidism results in mentally retarded dwarfs. Although treatment may prevent dwarfism, the effects on mental development are more variable. Children in whom hypothyroidism is detected early in neonatal screening programs respond well to treatment with thyroid hormone and develop apparently normal mental capacity. By contrast, children treated at a later age may be left with irreversible brain damage.

Endemic Cretinism

Endemic cretinism refers to congenital hypothyroidism in areas of endemic goiter. Both parents are usually goitrous. The disease encompasses two overlapping clinical presentations, a neurological syndrome and a predominantly hypothyroid one.

Neurological cretinism features mental retardation, ataxia, spasticity, and deaf-mutism. In the pure form of neurological cretinism, the children may be of normal stature and virtually euthyroid. Thus, it is postulated that iodine deficiency in the first trimester of pregnancy may damage the developing nervous system independently of its effect on thyroid hormone production.

Hypothyroid cretinism is thought to arise from iodine deficiency in late fetal life and in the neonatal period. The clinical course in these children is similar to that of other forms of congenital hypothyroidism.

HYPERTHYROIDISM

Hyperthyroidism refers to the clinical consequences of an excessive amount of circulating thyroid hormone. In general, the signs and

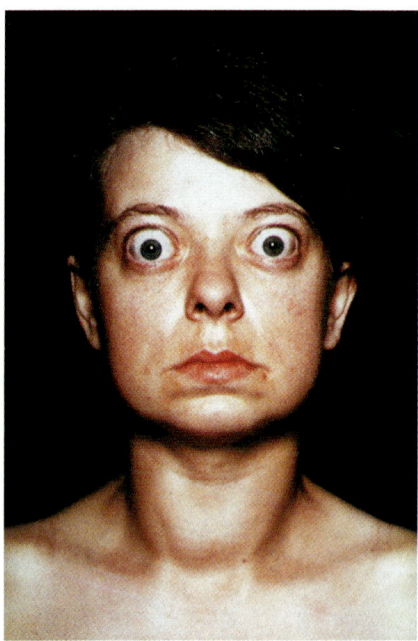

FIGURE 21-13
Graves disease. A young woman with hyperthyroidism displays a mass in the neck and exophthalmos.

symptoms of hyperthyroidism reflect a hypermetabolic state of the target tissues. Prolonged hypersecretion of thyroid hormone can result from (1) the presence of an abnormal thyroid stimulator (Graves disease), (2) intrinsic disease of the thyroid gland (toxic multinodular goiter or functional adenoma), and (3) excess production of TSH by pituitary adenoma (rare).

Graves Disease Is the Most Frequent Cause of Hyperthyroidism in Young Adults

Also known as *Basedow disease* in continental Europe, Graves disease is an autoimmune disorder characterized by diffuse goiter, hyperthyroidism, and exophthalmos (Fig. 21-13). The disorder is the most prevalent autoimmune disease in the United States, affecting 0.5 to 1% of the population under 40 years of age.

 Pathogenesis: The etiology of Graves disease is not fully understood and seems to involve an interplay between immune mechanisms, heredity, sex, and possibly emotional factors.

IMMUNE MECHANISMS: Patients with Graves disease are hyperthyroid owing to the presence of IgG antibodies that bind to the TSH receptor expressed on the plasma membrane of thyrocytes (Fig. 21-14). These antibodies function as agonists; that is, they stimulate the TSH receptor, thereby activating adenylyl cyclase and increasing

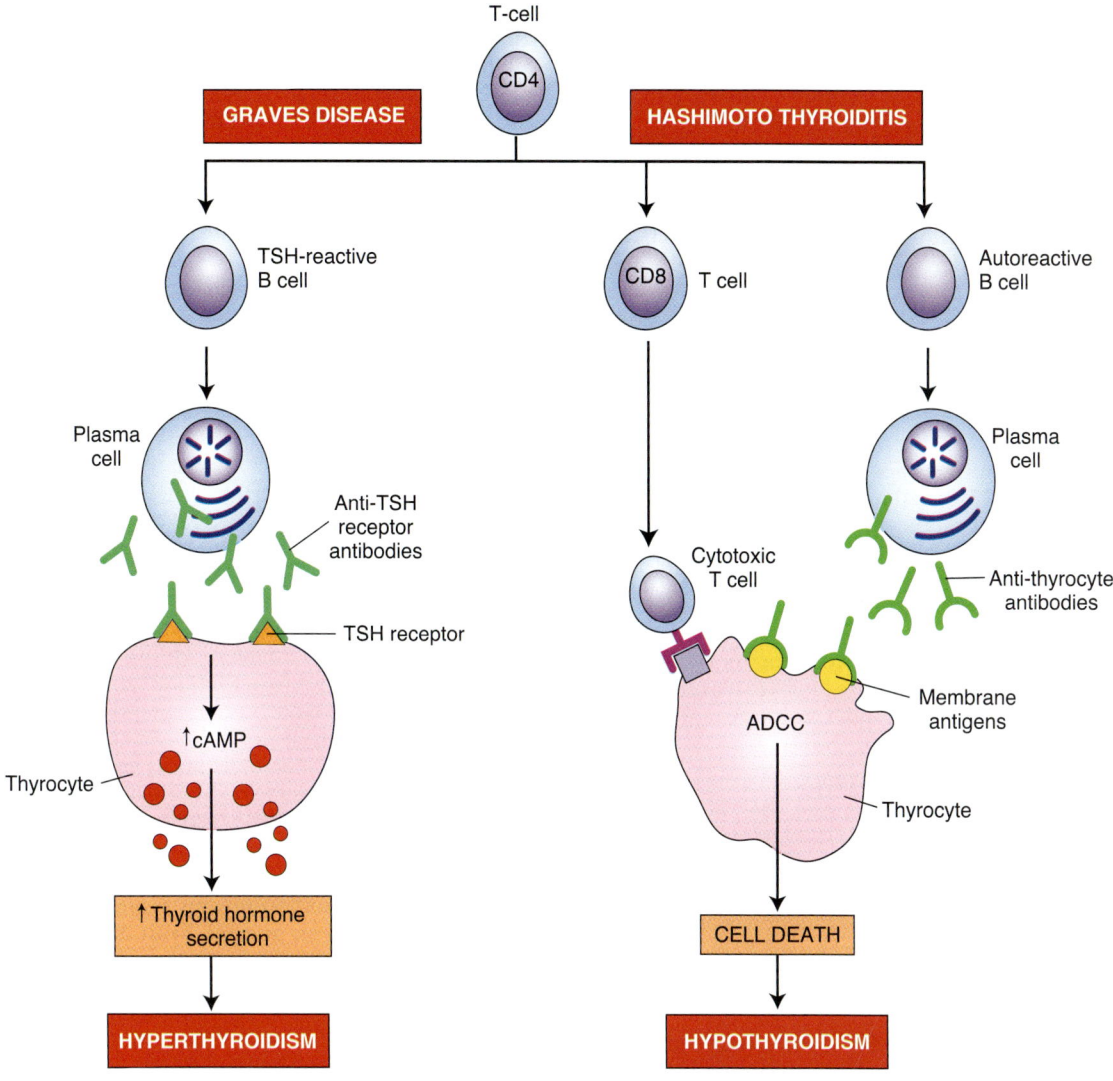

FIGURE 21-14
Immune mechanisms of Graves disease and Hashimoto thyroiditis. CD4+ T cells stimulate antibody production by autoreactive B cells. Anti-TSH receptor antibodies stimulate thyroid hormone synthesis in Graves disease. Antibodies induce thyrocyte cell death in Hashimoto thyroiditis by complement-dependent cytotoxicity and antibody-dependent cell-mediated cytotoxicity. Thyrocyte death also results from attack by CD8+ (cytotoxic) T cells.

thyroid hormone secretion. Under this continued stimulation, the thyroid becomes diffusely hyperplastic and excessively vascular.

The elaboration of thyroid-stimulating antibodies depends on the activation of thyroid-specific helper (CD4+) T cells that recognize multiple epitopes of the TSH receptor. These T cells stimulate autoreactive B cells, which then produce thyroid-stimulating immunoglobulins. Graves autoantibodies are actually heterogeneous, and those that stimulate thyroid hormone secretion represent only one component. Other antibodies seem to be cytotoxic and may account for the thyroid failure that often follows long-standing Graves disease. These include antibodies directed against thyroglobulin, thyroid peroxidase, and the sodium–iodide symporter, all of which have also been postulated to play a role in the pathogenesis of chronic lymphocytic thyroiditis (Hashimoto disease; see below)

GENETIC FACTORS: The strongest risk factor for the development of Graves disease is a positive family history. No single gene is responsible for Graves diseases or is necessary for its development. The concordance rate in monozygotic twins is far less than 100%, ranging from 30 to 50%. By contrast, dizygotic twins display a concordance rate of only 5%. Thus, both genetic and environmental factors are involved in the pathogenesis of Graves disease. With respect to the genetic contribution, HLA class II molecules exposed on thyrocytes (e.g., HLA-DR3, HLA-DQA1) have been established as susceptibility loci, with a number of loci carrying a relative risk of Graves disease of up to 4. Graves disease is also associated with polymorphism of cytotoxic T-lymphocyte antigen-4 (CTLA-4), which indicates the importance of autoreactive T cells. Patients with Graves disease and their relatives have a considerably higher incidence of other autoimmune diseases, including pernicious anemia and Hashimoto thyroiditis.

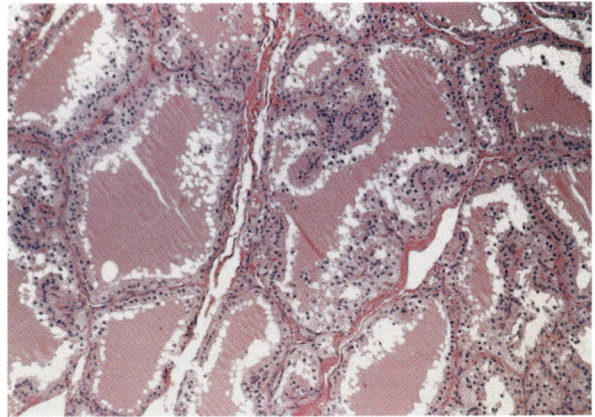

FIGURE 21-15
Graves disease. The follicles are lined by hyperplastic, tall columnar cells. Colloid is pink and scalloped at the periphery adjacent to the follicular cells.

Some asymptomatic, first-degree relatives of these patients also have an increased uptake of ^{131}I. White patients with Graves disease display an increased frequency of HLA-B8 and HLA-DR3, Chinese patients are more likely to manifest HLA-Bw46, and Japanese ones to exhibit HLA-Bw35.

SEX: Like other autoimmune diseases, Graves disease is far more common (7–10 times) in women than in men. Interestingly, the disorder tends to arise during periods of hormonal imbalance, including puberty, pregnancy, and menopause. Men with Graves disease are usually older, and although the degree of thyroid hyperfunction is often greater in men than in women, the symptoms tend to be less severe in men.

EMOTIONAL INFLUENCES: Quantitative data are lacking, but endocrinologists have long observed that the onset of Graves disease often follows a period of emotional stress, such as separation anxiety, death of a loved one, or near injury in an accident.

SMOKING: Smoking is associated with an increased risk of contracting Graves disease, and it increases the severity of the eye disease in patients who develop ophthalmopathy.

OPHTHALMOPATHY: Although exophthalmos (protrusion of the eyeballs) is a common complication of Graves disease, its occurrence and severity correlate poorly with the levels of thyroid hormone. It seems likely that a combination of humoral and cell-mediated immune mechanisms is involved. T lymphocytes that are sensitized to antigens shared by thyroid follicular cells and orbital fibroblasts (possibly the TSH receptor) accumulate around the eye, where they secrete cytokines that activate fibroblasts. There is also evidence for systemic or local production of antibodies that stimulate orbital fibroblasts to proliferate and produce collagen and glycosaminoglycans.

 Pathology: The thyroid in Graves disease is symmetrically enlarged, usually weighing 35 to 40 g. The cut surface is firm and dark red. The tan translucence of the normal cut surface of the thyroid, attributable to stored colloid, is notably absent. Microscopically, the thyroid is diffusely hyperplastic and highly vascular. The epithelial cells are tall and columnar and are often arranged as papillae that project into the lumen of the follicles. The colloid tends to be depleted and presents a scalloped or "moth-eaten" appearance where it abuts the epithelial cells (Fig. 21-15). Scattered lymphocytes and plasma cells infiltrate the interstitial tissue and may even aggregate to form germinal follicles.

Therapy with antithyroid medication (e.g., methimazole or propylthiouracil) commonly results in increased thyroid hyperplasia and a complete absence of colloid.

Exophthalmos is caused by enlargement of the extraocular muscles within the orbit. The muscles themselves are normal, but they are swollen by mucinous edema, the accumulation of fibroblasts, and infiltration by lymphocytes. The increased orbital contents cause forward displacement of the eye *(proptosis).*

 Clinical Features: Patients with Graves disease note the gradual onset of nonspecific symptoms, such as nervousness, emotional lability, tremor, weakness, and weight loss (Fig. 21-16). They are intolerant of heat, seek cooler environments, tend to sweat profusely, and may report palpitations. Excess thyroid hormone reduces systemic vascular resistance, enhances cardiac contractility, and increases the heart rate. In patients with preexisting heart disease, congestive heart failure may ensue. Women develop oligomenorrhea, which may progress to amenorrhea.

Physical examination reveals a symmetrically enlarged thyroid, often with an audible bruit and a palpable thrill.

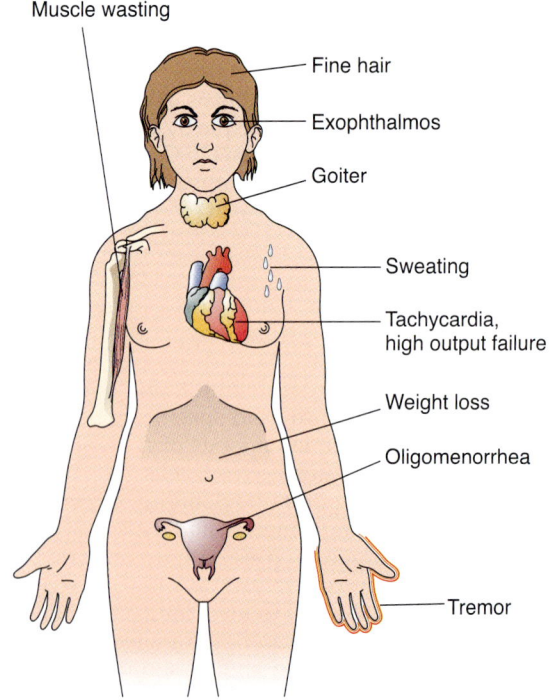

FIGURE 21-16
Major clinical manifestations of Graves disease.

Protrusion of the eyeball and retraction of the eyelids expose the sclera above the superior margin of the limbus. The skin is warm and moist, and some patients exhibit *Graves dermopathy*, a peculiar pretibial edema caused by the accumulation of fluid and glycosaminoglycans. The diagnosis of Graves disease is documented by increased uptake of radioactive iodine by the thyroid and elevated serum levels of T_4 and T_3.

The course of Graves disease is characterized by exacerbations and remissions. In untreated cases, hyperthyroidism may eventually be replaced by progressive thyroid failure and hypothyroidism, presumably as a result of chronic thyroiditis. Treatment of the disorder depends on many individual factors and includes the use of antithyroid medication, destruction of thyroid tissue with radioactive iodine, and adjunctive therapy with corticosteroids and adrenergic antagonists. Surgical ablation is not commonly performed today. Unfortunately, despite successful relief of hyperthyroidism, exophthalmos often persists and may even worsen.

Toxic Multinodular Goiter Results from Functional Autonomy of Thyroid Nodules

Many patients with nontoxic multinodular goiter, usually over the age of 50 years, eventually develop a toxic form of the disease. Like its precursor disease, toxic goiter is 10 times more frequent in women than in men.

 Pathogenesis and Pathology: The precise mechanisms by which nontoxic multinodular goiter assumes functional autonomy are not clear, but two patterns are noted. In some patients, the uptake of iodine is diffuse and not affected by the administration of thyroid hormone. Microscopic examination of the thyroid shows groups of small hyperplastic follicles mixed with other nodules of varying size that appear to be inactive. The second pattern is characterized by focal accumulation of radiolabeled iodine in one or more nodules. Hyperfunction of these nodules suppresses the function of the remainder of the thyroid. Exogenous thyroid hormone produces no further suppression of iodine uptake, although the previously inactive areas will respond to TSH by sequestering iodine. On microscopic examination, the functional nodules are clearly demarcated from the inactive areas and consist of large hyperplastic follicles, thus resembling adenomas. Although there is little evidence to suggest that the functional nodules have neoplastic characteristics, the clinical presentation is similar to that of a normal thyroid with a single hyperfunctioning adenoma.

 Clinical Features: Patients with toxic multinodular goiter usually have less severe symptoms of hyperthyroidism than those with Graves disease and never develop exophthalmos. Since patients with toxic goiter tend to be older, cardiac complications, including atrial fibrillation and congestive heart failure, may dominate the clinical presentation. Serum T_4 and T_3 levels are frequently only minimally elevated, and the uptake of radiolabeled iodine may be within the normal range or only slightly above it. Radiolabeled iodine administration after a course of antithyroid therapy is the most common therapy for toxic multinodular goiter.

Toxic Adenoma Is a Functional Neoplasm

Toxic adenoma is defined as a benign, solitary, hyperfunctioning, follicular tumor in an otherwise normal thyroid. It is an infrequent cause of hyperthyroidism. Such tumors (1) display autonomous function, (2) do not depend on TSH, and (3) are not suppressed by administration of thyroid hormone. Hyperfunction of the toxic adenoma eventually suppresses the remainder of the thyroid, which then atrophies. Under these circumstances, a ^{131}I scintiscan shows a solitary focus of iodine uptake ("hot nodule") in a background of minimal uptake. Many, but not all, toxic adenomas exhibit a variety of somatic activating mutations of the TSH-receptor gene, which result in constitutive up-regulation of the cAMP cascade and less commonly the inositol phosphate-diacylglycerol system.

 Clinical Features: Toxic adenoma of the thyroid is most common in the fourth and fifth decades of life. Most patients do not suffer symptoms of hyperthyroidism until the adenoma has grown to a diameter of about 3 cm. On occasion, spontaneous necrosis and hemorrhage within the adenoma relieves the hyperthyroidism, after which the remainder of the gland resumes its normal function. In such cases, the adenoma appears as a "cold" nodule in a scintigram and may simulate thyroid cancer.

Since the normal thyroid tissue is suppressed, toxic adenoma is treated effectively with radiolabeled iodine. Alternatively, large nodules may be excised surgically, especially in young patients who are at risk for the development of thyroid cancer many years after radiolabeled iodine administration.

THYROIDITIS

Thyroiditis is a term that encompasses a heterogeneous group of inflammatory disorders of the thyroid gland, including those that are caused by autoimmune mechanisms and infectious agents.

Chronic Autoimmune Thyroiditis (Hashimoto Thyroiditis) Is a Common Cause of Goitrous Hypothyroidism

Hashimoto thyroiditis is characterized by the presence of circulating antibodies to thyroid antigens and features of cell-mediated immunity to thyroid tissue. The disease arises most commonly in the fourth and fifth decades, and women are six times more likely to be afflicted than are men. Although autoimmune thyroiditis is rare in children, it accounts for half of the cases of adolescent goiter.

 Pathogenesis: The mechanism underlying the pathogenesis of Hashimoto thyroiditis involves both cellular and humoral immunity. The autoimmune process in Hashimoto thyroiditis arises from the activation of CD4 (helper) T lymphocytes that have been sensitized to thyroid antigens (see Fig. 21-14). In turn, the $CD4^+$ cells stimulate the proliferation of autoreactive cytotoxic ($CD8^+$) T cells, which attack thyrocytes. Thyrocytes are also induced to express MHC class II molecules (HLA-DR, DP, DQ) by activated lymphocytes that secrete interferon-γ, thereby expanding the autoreactive T cell population. These effects account for the striking accumulation of lymphocytes in the glands of patients with autoimmune thyroiditis.

Activated CD4 cells also recruit autoreactive B cells that produce antibodies against thyroid antigens. These include antibodies against thyroid microsomal peroxidase (95%), thyroglobulin (60%), and the TSH receptor. Cytotoxic antibodies capable of fixing complement have been described in some patients, and antibody-dependent cell-mediated cytotoxicity (ADCC) may contribute to thyroid injury. In contrast to the agonist function of the anti-TSH receptor antibodies in Graves disease, the comparable antibodies in Hashimoto thyroiditis block the action of TSH. Such blocking antibodies have been described in 10% of patients with goitrous autoimmune thyroiditis and in 20% of those with end-stage atrophy of the gland.

A **genetic predisposition** to autoimmune thyroiditis is suggested by the familial nature of the disease. Half of all first-degree relatives of patients with this condition display thyroid antibodies, apparently transmitted as a dominant trait. Moreover, both Graves disease and chronic autoimmune thyroiditis have been described in these family members. A familial tendency for Hashimoto thyroiditis is further suggested by the higher prevalence of other autoimmune disorders in patients and their relatives, including multiple endocrine neoplasia syndrome type 2 (MEN 2), insulin-dependent diabetes, pernicious anemia, Addison disease, and myasthenia gravis. The high incidence of autoimmunity and thyroiditis in persons with Down syndrome and familial Alzheimer disease has attracted attention to genes on chromosome 21, but none have yet been identified as causes of the disorders. Interestingly, half of all adult patients with Turner syndrome, especially those with an X isochromosome, exhibit antithyroid antibodies, and a third develop hypothyroidism. The only hereditary risk factors that have been found consistently are HLA and CTLA-4 genes, but the mechanisms by which they contribute to autoimmune thyroiditis remain obscure.

Iodine intake is linked to the prevalence of Hashimoto thyroiditis, which is highest in regions with the greatest intake of iodine, for example, Japan and the United States. In iodine-deficient areas, iodine supplementation significantly increases the prevalence of chronic inflammation of the thyroid and the presence of thyroid autoantibodies.

 Pathology: On gross examination, the gland in patients with Hashimoto thyroiditis is diffusely enlarged and firm, weighing 60 to 200 g. The cut surface is pale tan and fleshy and exhibits a vaguely nodular pattern (Fig. 21-17). Microscopically, the thyroid displays (1)

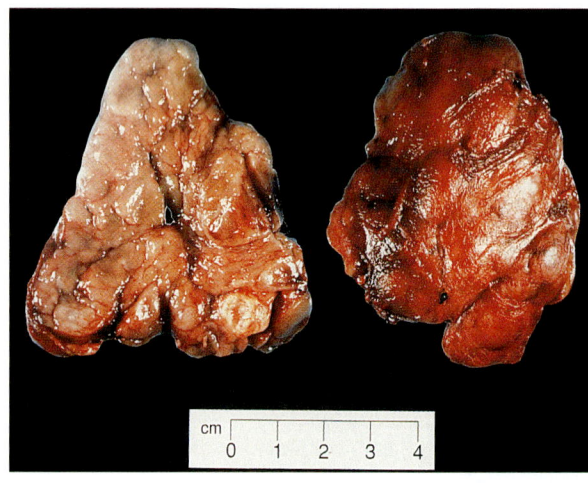
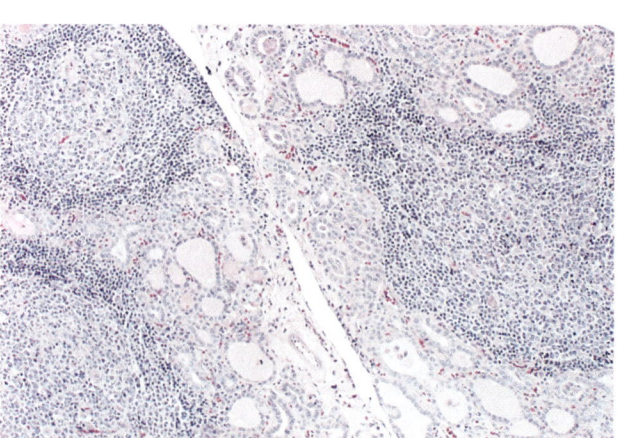

FIGURE 21-17
Chronic autoimmune (Hashimoto) thyroiditis. The thyroid gland is symmetrically enlarged and coarsely nodular. **A.** A coronal section of the right lobe shows irregular nodules and an intact capsule. **B.** A microscopic section of the thyroid reveals a conspicuous chronic inflammatory infiltrate and many atrophic thyroid follicles. The inflammatory cells form prominent lymphoid follicles with germinal centers.

a conspicuous infiltrate of lymphocytes and plasma cells, (2) destruction and atrophy of the follicles, and (3) oxyphilic metaplasia of the follicular epithelial cells (*Hürthle* or *Askanazy cells*). The inflammatory infiltrates are focally arranged in lymphoid follicles, often with germinal centers. The Askanazy cells are filled with mitochondria and frequently display nuclear atypia, which may be mistaken for cancer. Interstitial fibrosis is present to a varying extent and in 10% of cases is particularly conspicuous (fibrous variant). The thyroid eventually undergoes atrophy in some patients, and they are left with a small, fibrotic gland infiltrated by lymphocytes.

 Clinical Features: In most cases of Hashimoto thyroiditis, the patient notes the gradual onset of a goiter, although in a few cases the thyroid enlarges rapidly. Most of these patients are initially euthyroid, but a few are hypothyroid when they seek medical attention. Eventually, one third to a half of all patients progress to an overt hypothyroid state, the risk being considerably greater among men than among women. On rare occasions, hyperthyroidism may develop *(hashitoxicosis)*. The diagnosis of Hashimoto thyroiditis is now made by the detection of circulating antithyroid antibodies and an elevated TSH level.

Many patients require no treatment for Hashimoto thyroiditis. Thyroid hormone is administered to alleviate hypothyroidism and to decrease the size of the gland. Surgery is reserved for patients who do not respond to suppressive hormone therapy or in whom pressure symptoms are troublesome.

Subacute Thyroiditis (de Quervain, Granulomatous, or Giant Cell Thyroiditis) Is Caused by a Viral Infection

Subacute thyroiditis is an infrequent, self-limited disorder of the thyroid characterized by granulomatous inflammation. The disease typically occurs after upper respiratory tract infections, including those caused by influenza virus, adenovirus, echovirus, and coxsackievirus. Mumps virus has also been incriminated in some cases. de Quervain thyroiditis principally affects women between the ages of 30 and 50 years.

Pathology: The thyroid gland is enlarged to 40 to 60 g, and the cut surface is firm and pale. Initially, microscopic examination reveals an acute inflammatory reaction, often with microabscesses. This is followed by the appearance of a patchy infiltrate of lymphocytes, plasma cells, and macrophages throughout the thyroid. Destruction of follicles allows the release of colloid, which elicits a conspicuous granulomatous reaction (Fig. 21-18). Numerous multinucleated giant cells of the foreign body type, often containing colloid, are present. Fibrosis of the thyroid may follow resolution of the inflammatory reaction, but the normal thyroid architecture is usually restored.

 Clinical Features: Patients with subacute thyroiditis typically notice pain in the anterior neck, sometimes accompanied by fever. The disorder is often mistaken for a pharyngitis, because of a preceding respiratory tract infection and the presence of hoarseness and dysphagia. On physical examination, the thyroid is moderately enlarged and exquisitely tender. Subacute thyroiditis generally resolves within a few months without any clinical sequelae.

The release of preformed thyroid hormone by destruction of the follicles often elevates serum T_4 and T_3 levels, occasionally high enough to produce transient clinical hyperthyroidism. The consequent suppression of TSH leads to decreased uptake of radiolabeled iodine. This phase is followed by decreased serum T_4 and T_3 levels, but as subacute thyroiditis resolves, a euthyroid state is restored.

Silent Thyroiditis Causes Transient Hyperthyroidism

Silent thyroiditis, also termed *painless subacute thyroiditis* or *lymphocytic thyroiditis,* is characterized by painless enlargement of the thyroid, self-limited hyperthyroidism, and destruction of thyroid parenchyma with a lymphocytic infiltrate. Thus, it clinically resembles subacute thyroiditis but pathologically is more similar to Hashimoto thyroiditis. Importantly, silent thyroiditis is distinguished from the latter by the lack of antithyroid antibodies or other evidence of autoimmune thyroiditis. However, an association with HLA-DR3 has been reported. As in subacute thyroiditis, the hyperthyroid state reflects the release of preformed thyroid hormone from the injured gland.

Silent thyroiditis predominantly affects women, often in the postpartum period. Hyperthyroidism usually persists for 2 to 4 months. Treatment is symptomatic, and most patients become euthyroid.

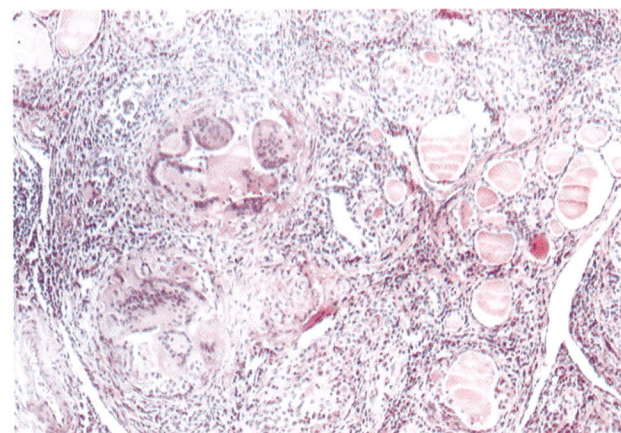

FIGURE 21-18
Subacute thyroiditis. The release of colloid into the interstitial tissue has elicited a prominent granulomatous reaction, with numerous foreign body giant cells.

Riedel Thyroiditis Causes Fibrosis of the Thyroid

The term *thyroiditis* in Riedel thyroiditis is something of a misnomer, since this rare disease also involves extrathyroidal soft tissues of the neck and is often associated with progressive fibrosis in other locations, including the retroperitoneum, mediastinum, and orbit. Riedel thyroiditis is primarily a disease of middle age, with a female-to-male ratio of 3:1. The etiology is unknown, but it does not appear to be related to other forms of thyroiditis.

Pathology: On gross examination, part or all of the thyroid is stony hard and is described as "woody." In most instances, the process is asymmetric and often affects only one lobe. Characteristically, fibrosis extends beyond the borders of the gland, and the surgeon may have extreme difficulty in identifying a tissue plane. Microscopic examination reveals dense, hyalinized fibrous tissue and a chronic inflammatory infiltrate replacing the parenchyma in the involved portions of the thyroid (Fig. 21-19). The follicles are normal in the unaffected portions of the gland. Fibrous tissue also surrounds and infiltrates other tissues, including skeletal muscle, nerves, fat, and blood vessels. In some cases, the parathyroids are also embedded in the fibrosis.

Clinical Features: Patients with Riedel thyroiditis notice the gradual onset of a painless goiter. Subsequently, they may suffer from the consequences of compression of the trachea (stridor), esophagus (dysphagia), and recurrent laryngeal nerve (hoarseness). In the unusual cases that involve the entire thyroid, hypothyroidism ensues. Treatment is primarily surgical to relieve the compression of the local organs.

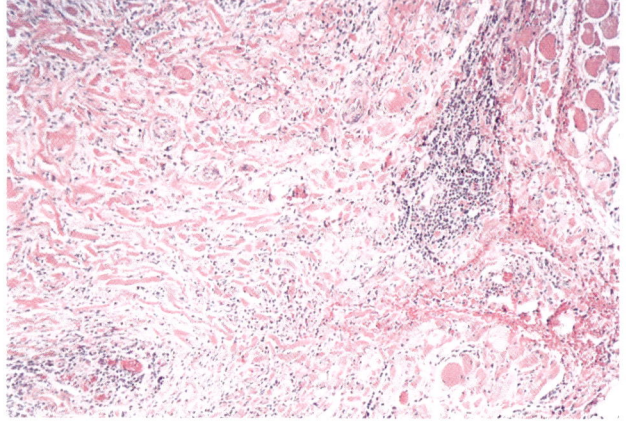

FIGURE 21-19
Riedel thyroiditis. The thyroid parenchyma is largely replaced by dense, hyalinized fibrous tissue and a chronic inflammatory infiltrate.

FOLLICULAR ADENOMA OF THE THYROID

Follicular adenoma refers to a benign neoplasm that exhibits follicular differentiation. It is the most common tumor of the thyroid and typically presents in euthyroid persons as a solitary "cold" nodule, that is, a tumor that does not take up radiolabeled iodine. Follicular adenoma is an encapsulated neoplasm in which the cells are either arranged in follicles resembling normal thyroid tissue or mimic stages in the embryonic development of the gland. Up to 90% of palpable, solitary follicular lesions are actually the dominant nodule in a multinodular goiter, and follicular adenomas are correspondingly infrequent. Follicular adenoma is most common in the fourth and fifth decades, with a female-to-male ratio of 7:1. The clonal origin of follicular adenomas has been established.

Pathology: On gross examination, follicular adenoma is a solitary, circumscribed nodule, 1 to 3 cm in diameter, which protrudes from the surface of the thyroid. The cut surface of the tumor is soft and paler than the surrounding parenchyma. Hemorrhage, fibrosis, and cystic change are common. Histologically, a number of distinctive patterns are observed (Fig. 21-20). Although these variants are of no particular clinical significance, their recognition may be important in separating them from thyroid cancers.

- **Embryonal adenoma** is distinguished by a trabecular pattern in which poorly formed follicles contain little or no colloid.
- **Fetal adenoma** displays cells that are similar to those of embryonal adenoma but tend to be arranged in microfollicles containing little colloid.
- **Simple adenoma** exhibits mature follicles with a normal amount of colloid.
- **Colloid adenoma** is similar to simple adenoma except that the follicles are larger and contain more abundant colloid.
- **Hürthle cell adenoma** is a solid tumor characterized by oxyphil cells, small follicles, and scanty colloid.
- **Atypical adenoma** is a follicular tumor that displays mitoses, excessive cellularity, nuclear atypism, or equivocal capsular invasion but for which a diagnosis of carcinoma cannot be established with certainty.

THYROID CANCER

The topic of thyroid neoplasia has aroused the interest of clinicians and pathologists out of proportion to its incidence. This attention can be attributed to the frequency of nontoxic thyroid nodules and the difficulty of distinguishing clinically between nonneoplastic lesions, benign tumors, and thyroid cancer. Whereas thyroid nodules are found in as many as 1 to 10% of the population, malignant tumors of the thyroid account for only about 1% of all cancers. Nevertheless, thyroid cancer is the most common malignant endocrine tumor.

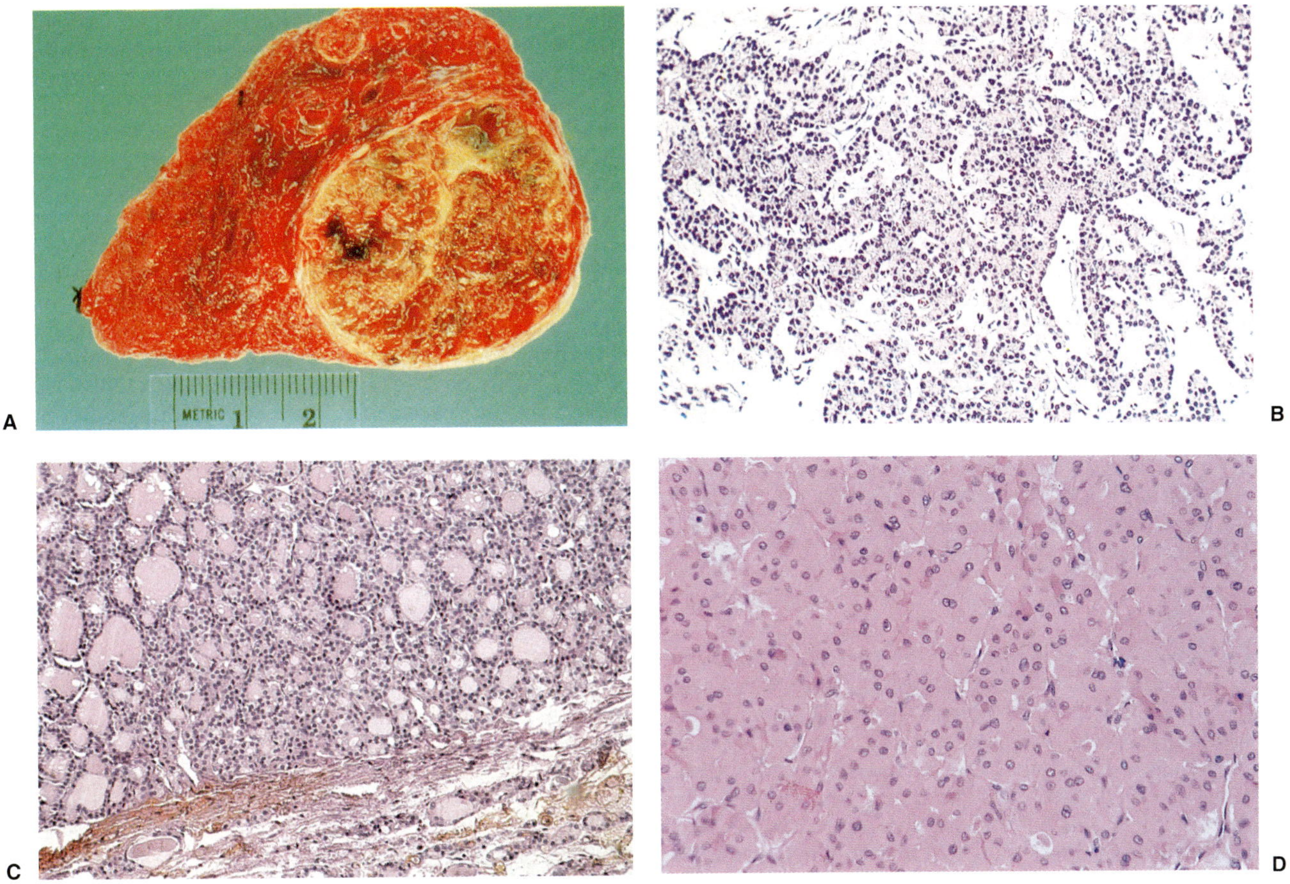

FIGURE 21-20
Follicular adenoma. **A.** Colloid adenoma. The cut surface of an encapsulated mass reveals hemorrhage, fibrosis, and cystic change. **B.** Embryonal adenoma. The tumor features a trabecular pattern with poorly formed follicles that contain little if any colloid. **C.** Fetal adenoma. A regular pattern of small follicles is noted. **D.** Hurthle cell adenoma. The tumor is composed of cells with small, regular nuclei and abundant eosinophilic cytoplasm.

Most cases of carcinoma of the thyroid occur between the third and seventh decades. Fine-needle biopsy of thyroid nodules provides a diagnosis in most cases. The prognosis is related to the morphological features of the tumor, ranging from a virtually benign clinical course to a rapidly fatal disease. The latter outcome is fortunately uncommon.

Papillary Thyroid Carcinoma (PTC) Is the Most Common Thyroid Cancer

PTC constitutes up to 90% of sporadic cases of thyroid cancer in the United States. The tumor is most frequent between the ages of 20 and 50 years, with a female-to-male ratio of 3:1. However, PTC may arise at any age, even in children. The reported incidence of this tumor has varied from 35 to 90% of all thyroid cancers. Some pathologists consider the most mature variant to be a papillary adenoma, and others classify papillary tumors with follicular elements as follicular carcinoma. **In this context, we consider all neoplasms with papillary elements to be papillary cancers.** Such a classification is of more than academic interest, since the biological behavior of papillary cancers differs from that of other malignant tumors of the thyroid.

 Pathogenesis: Although the etiology of PTC remains to be established, a number of associations have been identified.

- **Iodine excess:** PTC has been produced in animals by administering excess iodine. In endemic goiter regions, the addition of iodine to the diet has increased the proportion of papillary carcinoma compared with follicular cancer.
- **Radiation:** External radiation to the neck of children and adults increases the incidence of later PTC. Survivors of the atomic bomb explosions in Japan suffered more papillary cancers than would otherwise be expected. A substantially higher incidence of PTC has occurred in children living in contaminated areas surrounding Chernobyl, the site in Ukraine of a nuclear reactor catastrophe in 1986. On the other hand, treatment with radiolabeled iodine has not been shown to increase the risk of this tumor.
- **Genetic factors:** Epidemiological studies have reported a 4- to 10-fold higher risk for PTC in first-degree relatives of persons with that tumor. A concordance for PTC has been described in monozygotic twins. A familial

form of PTC accounts for some 5% of all cases, but the genes responsible have not been definitively identified.
- **Somatic mutations:** The risk for PTC is higher in patients with familial adenomatous polyposis. Somatic rearrangements of the *RET* protooncogene on chromosome 10 (10q11.2) are common in PTC, and 60% of such tumors in children exposed to radiation from the Chernobyl accident displayed this mutation. The same mutation occurs after external radiation to the thyroid. These rearrangements cause the fusion of the tyrosine kinase domain of *RET* to various other genes, creating the *RET/PTC* fusion oncogenes. Interestingly, the frequency of *RET/PTC* rearrangements in patients with PTC displays a pronounced geographical distribution, ranging from none in Korea to 2% in Saudi Arabia and 60% in the United States and Great Britain. Illegitimate recombination of the *NTRK1* gene on chromosome 1, which encodes the high-affinity nerve growth factor receptor (*NGFR*), with another gene on the same chromosome (*TPM3*) has also been described in some PTCs.

Pathology: PTCs vary from microscopic lesions to tumors larger than the normal gland. Serial sections of ostensibly normal thyroids obtained at autopsy have revealed a high proportion of papillary cancers that measure less than 1 mm across, but lymph node metastases in such cases are distinctly uncommon. On gross examination, most PTCs are pale and firm or hard and gritty lesions, and less than 10% are truly encapsulated (Fig. 21-21A).

Microscopic examination reveals branching papillae that are composed of a central fibrovascular core and a single or stratified lining of cuboidal to columnar cells (see Fig. 21-21B). In most instances, irregularly shaped or tubular neoplastic follicles are present within the tumor, but the proportions of the papillary and follicular elements are highly variable. Nuclear atypism is an important diagnostic feature and includes clear (*ground-glass* or *Orphan Annie*) nuclei, eosinophilic pseudoinclusions (which represent invaginations of the cytoplasm into the nucleus), and nuclear grooves. Many papillary cancers show dense fibrosis, and calcospherites (*psammoma bodies*) are present in half the cases. The latter feature is virtually diagnostic of papillary carcinoma, being rare in other conditions. The stroma may be infiltrated by lymphocytes and Langerhans cells. In over three fourths of cases of PTC, careful sectioning of the resected thyroid reveals multiple microscopic foci of tumor, but it is not clear whether this represents a multifocal origin of the tumor or lymphatic spread from a solitary primary. Vascular invasion is distinctly uncommon.

PTC typically invades lymphatics and spreads to the regional cervical lymph nodes. The lymph node metastases vary from microscopic foci in otherwise normal lymph nodes to large masses that dwarf the primary lesion. Direct extension of PTC into the soft tissues of the neck occurs in one fourth of cases. Although hematogenous metastases are less common than in other varieties of thyroid cancer, they occasionally occur, most commonly to the lungs.

Clinical Features: PTC presents as (1) a painless, palpable nodule in an otherwise normal gland; (2) a nodule with enlarged cervical lymph nodes; or (3) cervical lymphadenopathy in the absence of a palpable thy-

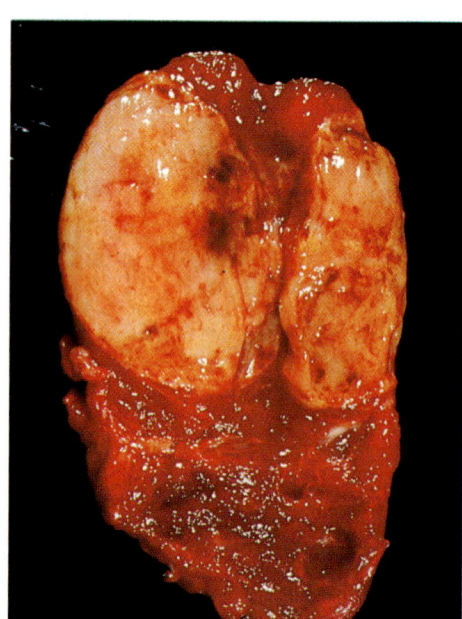
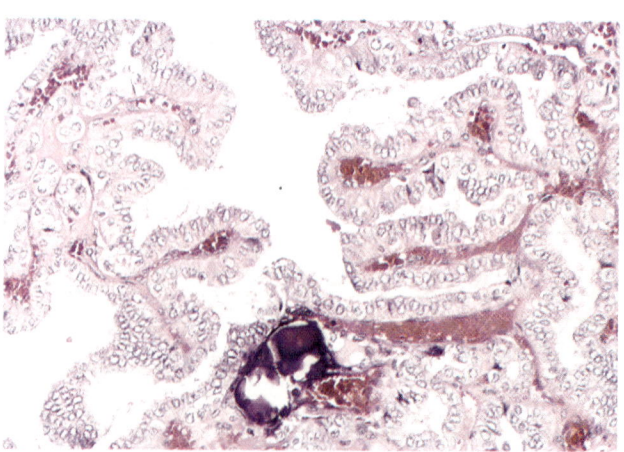

A   B

FIGURE *21-21*

Papillary carcinoma of the thyroid. A. The cut surface of a surgically resected thyroid displays a circumscribed pale tan mass with foci of cystic change. B. Branching papillae are lined by neoplastic columnar epithelium with clear nuclei. A calcospherite, or psammoma body, is evident.

roid nodule. Tumors larger than 0.5 cm can be detected as cold areas in a thyroid scintiscan.

In general, the prognosis of PTC is excellent, and life expectancy for these patients differs little from that of the general population. The prognosis is more serious in patients older than 50 years of age, whereas in children, the outlook is good even when lung metastases are detected. PTC tends to be more aggressive in men than in women.

As a rule, the larger the primary tumor, the more aggressive it is, and direct extension into the adjacent soft tissues points to a poorer prognosis. The proportion of papillary and follicular elements contributes little to the prognosis, but less-differentiated papillary carcinomas tend to be more aggressive. The presence of metastases to cervical nodes at the time or surgery does not change the prognosis, and less than 10% of these patients succumb to the tumor. In fatal cases of PTC, death is caused principally by metastases to the lungs or brain or by obstruction of the trachea or esophagus.

Follicular Thyroid Carcinoma (FTC) Is Rarely Fatal

FTC is defined as a malignant neoplasm that is purely follicular and does not contain any papillary or other elements. Most patients are above 40 years of age, and the female-to-male ratio is 3:1. The incidence of follicular carcinoma is increased in endemic goiter areas among persons who do not receive iodine supplements. However, in areas where iodine is added to salt, such as the United States, FTC has become uncommon, constituting as few as 2% of all thyroid cancers.

Pathology: FTCs are subdivided into minimally invasive and widely invasive variants.

Minimally invasive FTC is seen grossly as a well-defined, encapsulated tumor, which on cut section is soft and pale tan to pink and bulges from the confines of its capsule. Microscopically, most lesions resemble follicular adenoma, although they tend more to a microfollicular or trabecular pattern. Occasionally, hemorrhagic necrosis is present in the center of the tumor. Mitoses are commonly encountered, a feature that distinguishes follicular cancer from a benign adenoma. The principal distinction from adenoma is in the interface of the capsule and the normal parenchyma. Minimally invasive cancer is diagnosed when the tumor extends into, but not entirely through, the capsule (Fig. 21-22).

Invasive FTC usually presents few diagnostic problems, since it extends through the capsule or shows vascular invasion (see Fig. 21-22), often within or adjacent to the capsule. The tumor may also extend into the surrounding soft tissues.

FTC differs from PTC in that metastases in the former are blood borne rather than lymphatic and are directed principally to the bones of the shoulder and pelvic girdles, sternum, and skull.

Clinical Features: Most follicular cancers are detected clinically as a palpable nodule or as an enlarged thyroid, but in some cases, the presenting sign is a pathological fracture through a bony metastasis or a pulmonary lesion. Both the primary tumor and the metastases have an affinity for radiolabeled iodine, although the thyroid scintiscan may indicate a cold nodule because the normal thyroid accumulates iodine more efficiently. However, the affinity for ^{131}I may be used therapeutically. Minimally invasive follicular tumors have a cure rate of at least 95%, compared with a survival of about 50% for the widely invasive form.

Medullary Thyroid Carcinoma (MTC) Is Derived from C Cells of the Thyroid

MTC is distinguished by its secretion of the calcium-lowering hormone calcitonin. This tumor represents no more than 5% of all thyroid cancers, although the proportion in referral centers is higher. The disease occurs in sporadic and familial forms, the latter accounting for 20% of cases. Patients with the familial form of medullary carcinoma are often afflicted with MEN type 2, which includes pheochromocytoma of the adrenal medulla and parathyroid hyperplasia or adenoma.

Somatic mutations in the *RET* protooncogene have been detected in 25 to 70% of cases of sporadic MTC. Most of these occur at codon 918 (ATG to ACG) in the tyrosine kinase domain of the RET protein and indicate a poorer prognosis than that in tumors without a *RET* mutation. The *RET* gene is discussed more fully in the section on MEN syndromes (see below).

The mean age of patients with MTC is 50 years, but familial cases appear earlier (mean age, 20 years). There is a slight female predominance (1.5:1); in familial cases, the inheritance is autosomal dominant, and the sex distribution is equal.

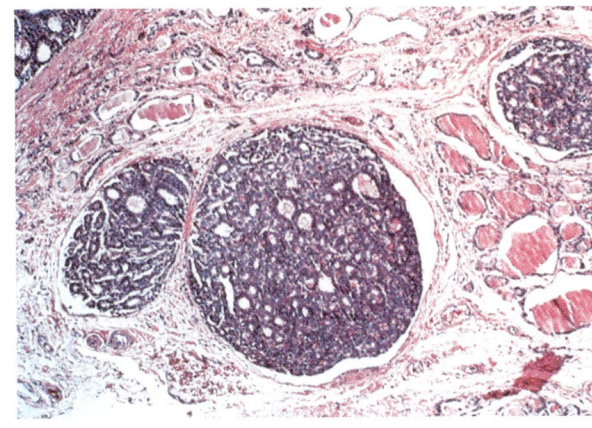

FIGURE 21-22
Follicular carcinoma of the thyroid. A microfollicular tumor has invaded veins in the thyroid parenchyma.

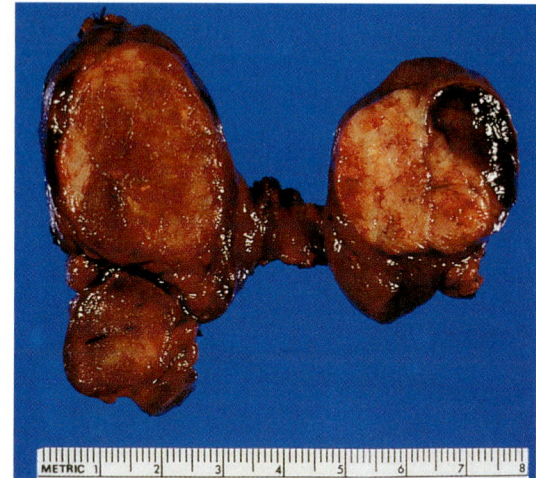
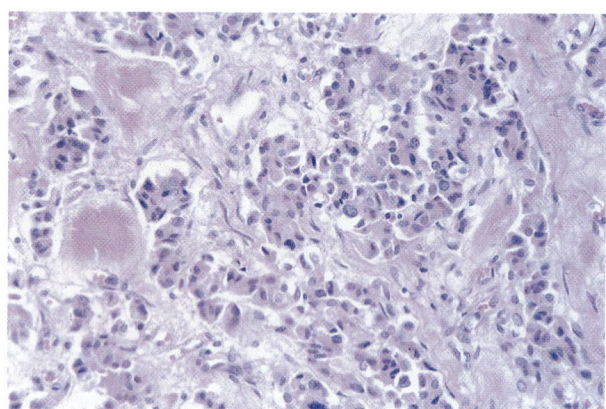
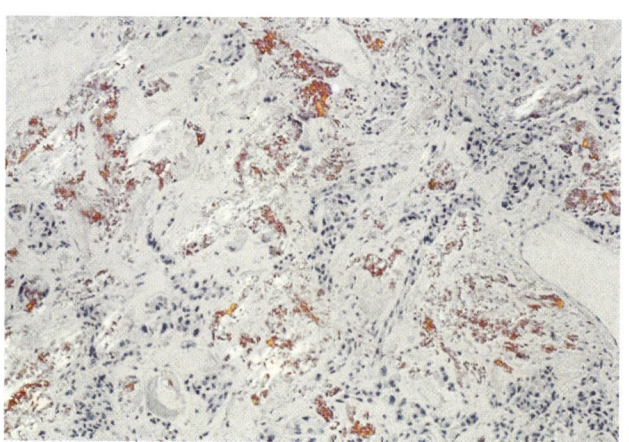

FIGURE 21-23
Medullary thyroid carcinoma. A. Coronal section of a total thyroid resection shows bilateral involvement by a firm, pale tumor. B. The tumor features nests of polygonal cells embedded in a collagenous framework. The connective tissue septa contain eosinophilic amyloid. C. A section stained with Congo red and viewed under polarized light demonstrates the pale green birefringence of amyloid.

Pathology: On gross examination, MTC tends to arise in the superior portion of the thyroid, the regions that are richest in C cells. In the setting of MEN type 2, the tumors are often multicentric and bilateral. Although MTCs are not encapsulated, they are usually circumscribed. The cut surface is firm and grayish white. The histological appearance is highly variable. Characteristically, the tumor is solid and composed of polygonal, granular cells that are separated by a distinctly vascular stroma (Fig. 21-23). However, the architectural patterns and appearances of the cells are highly variable. **A conspicuous feature is the presence of stromal amyloid, representing the deposition of procalcitonin.** The nests of tumor cells are embedded in a hyalinized collagenous framework. Focal calcification is often present and may be extensive enough to be detected radiologically.

By electron microscopy, the neoplastic C cells show dense-core secretory granules that stain immunohistochemically for a variety of endocrine markers, including calcitonin, synaptophysin, chromogranin, and neuron-specific enolase. Almost all of these tumors are positive for carcinoembryonic antigen (CEA). Many patients are also positive for ACTH, serotonin, substance P, glucagon, insulin, and human chorionic gonadotropin (hCG).

MTC extends by direct invasion into soft tissues and metastasizes to the regional lymph nodes and to lung, liver, and bone. In some instances, metastatic disease is responsible for the initial presentation. The metastatic deposits resemble the primary tumor and also tend to contain amyloid.

The precursor lesion of the familial variety of MTC is C cell hyperplasia. Thus, patients with MEN types 2A and 2B (see section on adrenal medulla) who are at risk for the development of MTC are monitored by periodic measurements of serum calcitonin, CEA, and sometimes chromogranin. When levels of these markers are elevated, the patient is subjected to a total thyroidectomy.

Clinical Features: Patients with MTC often suffer a number of symptoms related to endocrine secretion, including carcinoid syndrome (serotonin) and Cushing syndrome (ACTH). Watery diarrhea in one third of patients is caused by the secretion of vasoactive intestinal peptide, prostaglandins, and several kinins. In cases of familial MTC, patients may exhibit hyperparathyroidism, episodic hypertension, and other symptoms attributable to the secretion of catecholamines by pheochromocytoma.

The tumor usually manifests as a firm thyroid nodule or cervical lymphadenopathy. By scintiscan, a cold nodule is characteristic. The treatment is total thyroidectomy, but local recurrences follow in one third of patients. The 5-year survival rate is 75%.

Anaplastic (Undifferentiated) Thyroid Carcinoma Is Usually Fatal

Anaplastic thyroid cancer principally afflicts women (female-to-male ratio of 4:1) over the age of 60 years. The tumor constitutes 10% of thyroid cancers and is more common in endemic goiter areas. In fact, overall, at least half of patients suffer from long-standing goiter. In addition, many patients with anaplastic carcinoma have a history of a lower-grade thyroid cancer. Thus, it seems likely that the anaplastic variant often represents the transformation of a benign or low-grade thyroid neoplasm into a poorly differentiated and highly aggressive cancer. There is evidence that the risk of such an event is enhanced by external radiation. Mutations in the *p53* tumor suppressor gene are common in anaplastic cancers, but *RET* activation has not been observed.

 Pathology: Anaplastic carcinoma of the thyroid manifests as large masses in the gland that are poorly circumscribed and frequently extend into the soft tissues of the neck. The cut surface is hard and grayish white. The histological appearance is highly variable. The most common pattern is a sarcoma-like proliferation of bizarre spindle and giant cells, with polyploid nuclei, many mitoses, necrosis, and stromal fibrosis (Fig. 21-24). Other specimens reveal distinct epithelial differentiation. The tumor tends to invade veins and arteries, often occluding the vessels and producing foci of infarction within the tumor.

Clinical Features: These highly malignant tumors compress and destroy local structures. Dysphagia and dyspnea are caused by tracheal compression or invasion. The prognosis is dismal, and widespread metastases are frequent. Less than 10% of patients survive for 5 years.

Lymphomas of the Thyroid Are Largely B-Cell Tumors

Lymphoma originating in the thyroid is distinctly uncommon, accounting for 2% of all thyroid cancers. Most if not all cases arise in the setting of chronic thyroiditis, and in regions where this disorder is frequent, up to 10% of malignant tumors of the thyroid are lymphomas. Like chronic thyroiditis, thyroid lymphoma is more common in women than in men (4:1), but the mean age at presentation (seventh decade) is older.

Thyroid lymphomas manifest as large, soft, tannish masses in the thyroid, usually extending beyond the confines of the gland. Microscopically, they show the spectrum of lymphomas seen at other sites; the most common subtype is the diffuse large cell pattern.

The prognosis of thyroid lymphoma depends on the stage at the time of diagnosis. If restricted to the thyroid gland, the prognosis is excellent, and three fourths of patients now survive for 10 years. The outlook for patients with disseminated disease is similar to that for other lymphomas.

Parathyroid Glands

ANATOMY AND PHYSIOLOGY

The parathyroid glands are derivatives of branchial clefts III and IV. Most persons have 4 glands, but the number varies from 1 to 12. Normally, they are found on the posterior thy-

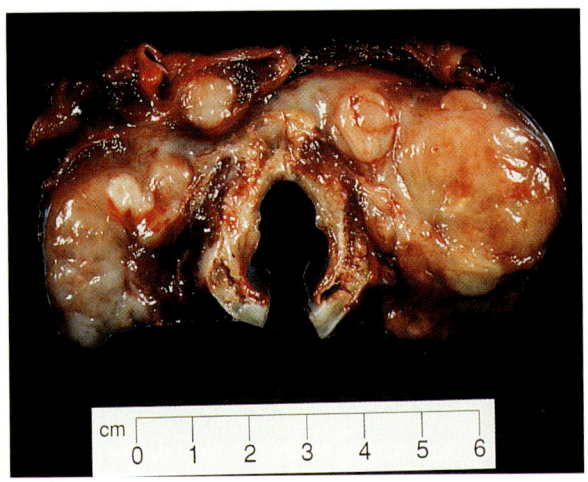 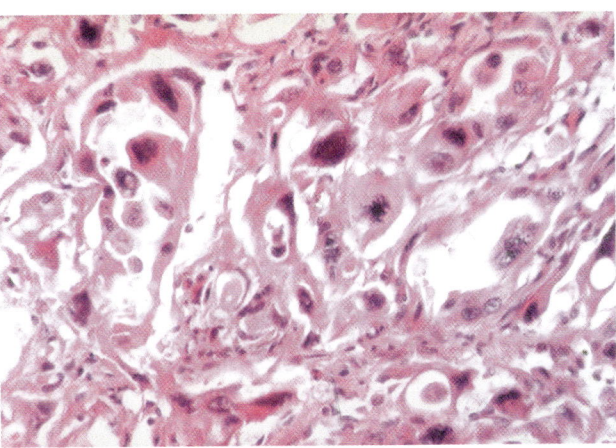

FIGURE 21-24
Anaplastic carcinoma of the thyroid. **A.** The tumor in transverse section partially surrounds the trachea and extends into the adjacent soft tissue. **B.** The tumor is composed of bizarre spindle and giant cells with polyploid nuclei and numerous mitoses.

roid surface, although they occasionally occur in ectopic locations.

The parathyroid glands are the size and color of a grain of saffron-cooked rice. The combined weight of all the glands is about 130 mg. The weight of an individual gland varies considerably, but anything in excess of 50 mg probably represents enlargement. Microscopically, about three fourths of the parathyroids are composed of chief cells and oxyphil cells, with the remainder being adipose tissue scattered throughout the parenchyma.

Chief cells are responsible for the secretion of parathyroid hormone (PTH). They are polyhedral cells that are characterized by a pale, eosinophilic-to-amphophilic cytoplasm that contains glycogen and fat droplets. Electron microscopy reveals membrane-bound secretory granules in the cytoplasm.

Clear cells are chief cells whose cytoplasm is packed with glycogen.

Oxyphil cells, which appear after puberty, are larger than chief cells and display a deeply eosinophilic cytoplasm, owing to the presence of numerous mitochondria. They do not contain secretory granules and do not secrete PTH.

The parathyroids respond to the level of ionized calcium and magnesium in the blood. In turn, PTH controls the level of plasma calcium. Magnesium, a cation closely related to calcium, acts as a brake on PTH secretion.

HYPOPARATHYROIDISM

Hypoparathyroidism results from decreased secretion of PTH or end-organ insensitivity to the hormone (pseudohypoparathyroidism).

Decreased Secretion of Parathyroid Hormone Is Most Commonly Iatrogenic

The most common cause of hypoparathyroidism is surgical resection of the parathyroids as a complication of -thyroidectomy. Of patients undergoing surgery for primary hyperparathyroidism, 1% develop irreversible hypoparathyroidism. The symptoms of hypoparathyroidism relate to hypocalcemia. Increased neuromuscular excitability is reflected in symptoms that range from mild tingling in the hands and feet to severe muscle cramps, laryngeal stridor, and convulsions. Neuropsychiatric manifestations include depression, paranoia, and psychoses. A high cerebrospinal fluid pressure and papilledema may mimic a brain tumor. Patients with all forms of hypoparathyroidism are successfully treated with vitamin D and calcium supplementation.

Familial hypoparathyroidism may be part of a polyglandular syndrome that also includes adrenal insufficiency and mucocutaneous candidiasis (see below). *Familial isolated hypoparathyroidism* is a rare disorder characterized by deficient secretion of PTH, which has variable inheritance patterns. *Idiopathic hypoparathyroidism* is a heterogeneous group of rare disorders, sporadic and familial, that share deficient secretion of PTH. *Agenesis of the parathyroid glands* occurs as part of DiGeorge syndrome (see Chapter 4).

Pseudohypoparathyroidism Reflects Target Organ Insensitivity to PTH

Pseudohypoparathyroidism designates a group of hereditary conditions characterized by hypocalcemia. The defect in these patients has been traced to mutations in the *GNAS1* gene on the long arm of chromosome 20 that result in decreased activity of G_s, the G protein that couples hormone receptors to the stimulation of adenylyl cyclase. Consequently, in the renal tubular epithelium the production of cAMP in response to PTH is impaired, and inadequate resorption of calcium from the glomerular filtrate ensues. Patients with pseudohypoparathyroidism are also often resistant to the other hormones that are coupled to cAMP, including TSH, glucagon, and the gonadotropins FSH and LH. These patients demonstrate a characteristic phenotype *(Albright hereditary osteodystrophy),* including short stature, obesity, mental retardation, subcutaneous calcification, and a number of congenital anomalies of bone, particularly abnormally short metacarpals and metatarsals (Fig. 21-25).

Some patients with pseudohypoparathyroidism display normal G_S activity and have a normal phenotype. The basis for the resistance to PTH in these patients probably resides in a mutation in or near *GNAS1*.

Pseudopseudohypoparathyroidism reads like a typographical error, but the term refers to rare cases in which the phenotype of Albright hereditary osteodystrophy is associated with a normal cAMP response to PTH. Paradoxically, these patients also have reduced G_S activity comparable to that reported in cases of pseudohypoparathyroidism. No *GNAS1* mutations have been found in this condition, although a candidate gene has been mapped to a nearby region on chromosome 20.

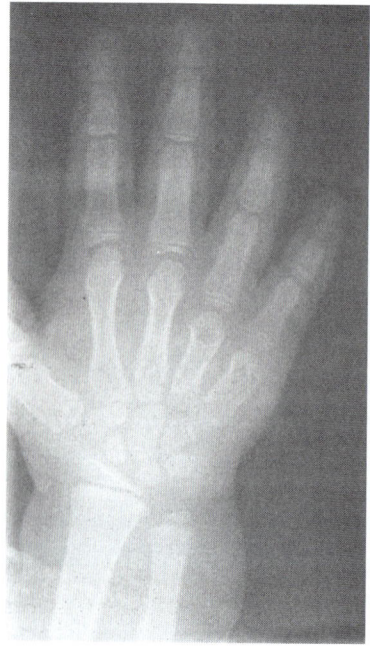

FIGURE 21-25
Pseudohypoparathyroidism. A radiograph of the hand reveals the characteristic shortness of the fourth and fifth metacarpal bones.

PRIMARY HYPERPARATHYROIDISM

Primary hyperparathyroidism refers to the syndrome caused by excessive secretion of PTH by a parathyroid adenoma, primary hyperplasia of all the parathyroids, or (in rare cases) parathyroid carcinoma.

Parathyroid Adenoma Accounts for Most Cases of Hyperparathyroidism

Parathyroid adenoma is the cause of 85% of all cases of primary hyperparathyroidism. The tumor arises sporadically or (in 20%) in the context of MEN-1 (see below). In a small minority of cases of sporadic adenoma, genetic analysis has identified rearrangement and overexpression of the cyclin D_1 *(PRAD1)* protooncogene on chromosome 11.

 Pathology: A parathyroid adenoma is a circumscribed, reddish brown, solitary mass, measuring 1 to 3 cm in diameter. Hemorrhagic areas are common, and cystic changes are occasionally noted. On microscopic examination, parathyroid adenoma is composed of sheets of neoplastic chief cells embedded in a rich capillary network. A rim of normal parathyroid tissue is usually evident outside the capsule and serves to distinguish an adenoma from parathyroid hyperplasia (Fig. 21-26). For the most part, the cells resemble normal chief cells. Positive immunohistochemical stains for PTH attest to the secretory activity of the tumor. In the presence of a functioning parathyroid adenoma, the other three glands tend to be atrophic. Surgical resection of the tumor relieves the symptoms of hyperparathyroidism.

Primary Parathyroid Hyperplasia Is a Minor Cause of Hyperparathyroidism

Chief cell hyperplasia is responsible for some 15% of cases of primary hyperparathyroidism. Of these, about 20% are associated with familial hyperparathyroidism or MEN syndromes (MEN types 1 and 2A). One third of the sporadic instances of primary parathyroid hyperplasia demonstrate monoclonality, suggesting a neoplastic basis for the proliferation of chief cells in these cases. In such instances, both chief cell hyperplasia and multiple small adenomas are present in the same gland. Factors associated with sporadic primary hyperparathyroidism include external radiation and the intake of lithium. About 75% of cases occur in women.

 Pathology: On gross examination, all four parathyroid glands are enlarged, the combined weights ranging from less than 1 g to as much as 10

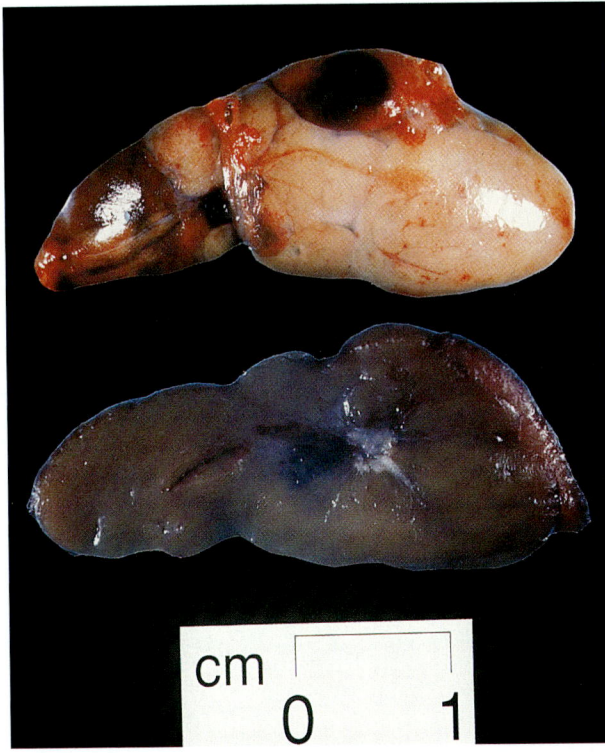
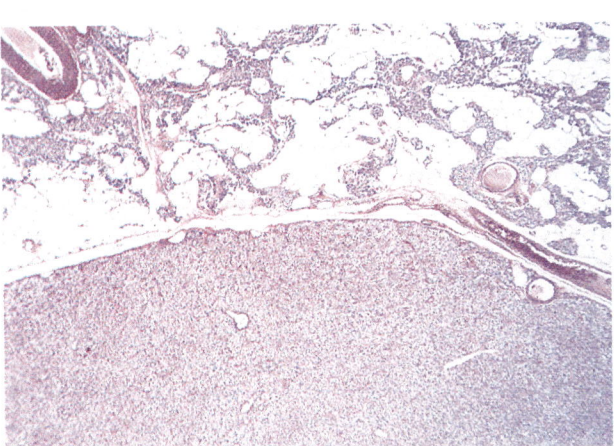

FIGURE 21-26
Parathyroid adenoma. A. External *(top)* and cross-section views *(bottom)* show a tan fleshy tumor. B. The tumor consists of sheets of neoplastic chief cells and is separated from normal parenchyma by a thin capsule.

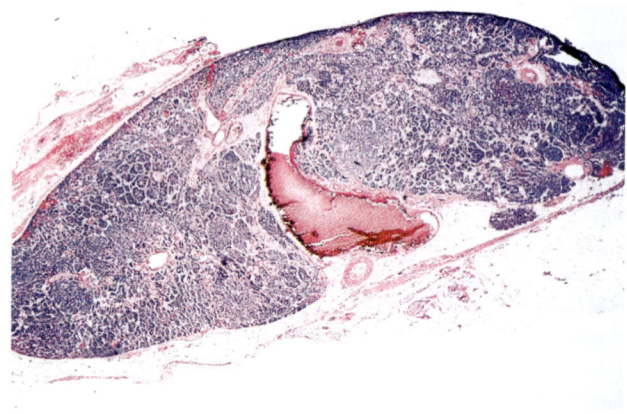

FIGURE 21-27
Primary parathyroid hyperplasia. The normal adipose tissue of the gland has been replaced by sheets and trabeculae of hyperplastic chief cells.

g. In half the patients, one gland is noticeably larger than the others, in which case the distinction from adenoma may be difficult. Microscopically, the normal adipose tissue of the gland is replaced by hyperplastic chief cells arranged as sheets or in trabecular or follicular patterns (Fig. 21-27). Scattered oxyphil cells are common, and small foci of adipose tissue may remain. An important feature that distinguishes hyperplasia from adenoma is the lack of cellular pleomorphism in the former.

Parathyroid Carcinoma Is a Rare Cause of Hyperparathyroidism

Parathyroid carcinoma accounts for 1% of all cases of primary hyperparathyroidism, occurring principally between the ages of 30 and 60 years in both sexes. It is usually a functioning tumor, and most patients present with symptoms of hyperparathyroidism. Similar to functioning parathyroid adenomas, overexpression of cyclin D_1 has also been described in some parathyroid carcinomas, suggesting that deregulation of this protooncogene is an important feature of parathyroid neoplasia in general. Most parathyroid carcinomas do not stain for retinoblastoma protein (another cell cycle regulator); adenomas usually display normal staining.

Pathology: Carcinomas tend to be somewhat larger than adenomas and appear as lobulated, firm, tannish, unencapsulated masses, often adherent to the surrounding soft tissues. Microscopically, most cases show a trabecular pattern, with significant mitotic activity and thick fibrous bands. Capsular or vascular invasion is occasionally noted. Importantly, the cell atypism often encountered in parathyroid adenoma is unusual in parathyroid carcinoma.

Despite surgical removal of the tumor, local recurrence is common, and about a third of patients develop metastases to regional lymph nodes, lungs, liver, and bone. In fatal cases, the cause of death is most often hyperparathyroidism rather than carcinomatosis.

Clinical Features of Hyperparathyroidism Are Highly Variable

The clinical manifestations of primary hyperparathyroidism range from asymptomatic hypercalcemia detected on routine blood analysis to florid systemic, renal, and skeletal disease (Fig. 21-28). Hypercalcemia and hypophosphatemia are the characteristic biochemical abnormalities. Excessive PTH leads to excessive loss of calcium from the bones and enhanced calcium resorption by the renal tubules. The production of the activated form of vitamin D (1,25[OH]$_2$D) by the renal tubules is also stimulated by PTH, an effect that increases intestinal absorption of calcium. The action of PTH on the kidney, together with hypercalcemia, leads to hypophosphatemia.

SKELETAL SYSTEM: The classic bone lesions of hyperparathyroidism, known as *osteitis fibrosa cystica* (see Chapter 26), are encountered in a minority of patients who follow an accelerated and serious form of the disease. Briefly, these patients present with bone pain, bone cysts, pathological fractures, and localized bone swellings (brown tumors and epulis of the jaw). Chondrocalcinosis may be a complication of hyperparathyroidism.

KIDNEY: Ten percent of patients with primary hyperparathyroidism present with renal colic as a result of kidney stones. Nephrocalcinosis, observed radiologically as diffuse renal calcification, may also occur (see Chapter 16). Polyuria is related to hypercalciuria, an effect that also leads to polydipsia.

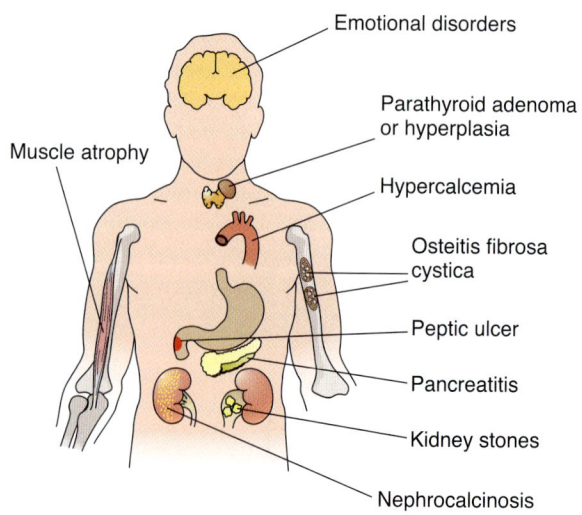

FIGURE 21-28
Major clinical features of hyperparathyroidism.

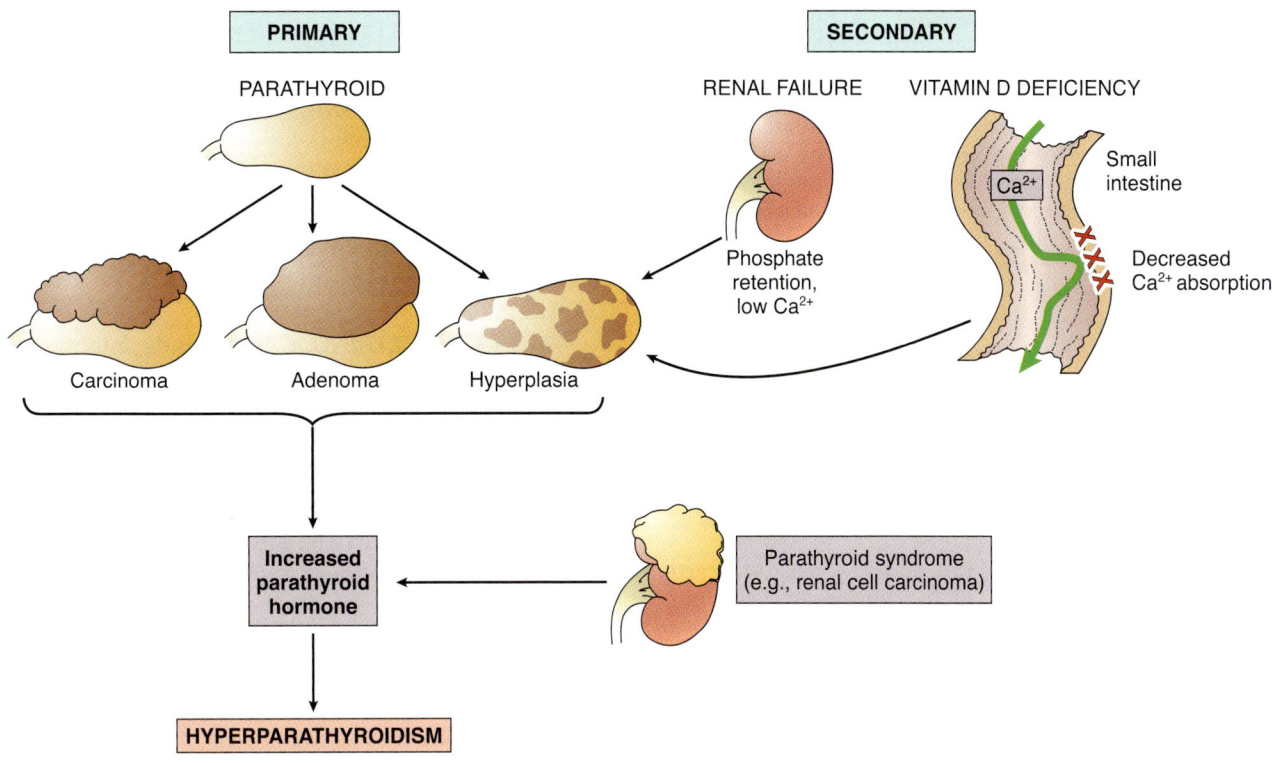

FIGURE 21-29
Major pathogenetic pathways leading to clinical primary and secondary hyperparathyroidism.

NERVOUS SYSTEM: Hyperparathyroidism is often accompanied by mental changes, including depression, emotional lability, poor mentation, and memory defects. Hyperactive reflexes are common. Peripheral neuropathy results in type 2 fiber atrophy of skeletal muscles and consequent weakness.

GASTROINTESTINAL TRACT: The incidence of peptic ulcer disease is increased in patients with hyperparathyroidism, possibly because hypercalcemia increases serum gastrin, thereby stimulating gastric acid secretion. Peptic ulcers in the context of MEN type 1, which includes parathyroid hyperplasia or adenoma, may be secondary to Zollinger-Ellison syndrome (see Chapter 15). Chronic pancreatitis is also a recognized complication of prolonged hypercalcemia, but the pathogenesis is not understood. Hypercalcemia is also a cause of constipation.

OTHER SYSTEMS: Hypertension occurs in up to half of patients with hyperparathyroidism, although the underlying mechanism is not clear. Anemia of unknown cause is also frequent.

SECONDARY HYPERPARATHYROIDISM

Secondary parathyroid hyperplasia is encountered principally in patients with chronic renal failure, although the disorder also occurs in association with vitamin D deficiency, intestinal malabsorption, Fanconi syndrome, and renal tubular acidosis (Fig. 21-29). Chronic hypocalcemia owing to renal retention of phosphate, inadequate production of 1,25(OH)$_2$D by the diseased kidneys, and some skeletal resistance to PTH all lead to compensatory hypersecretion of PTH. As a result, secondary hyperplasia of all four parathyroids occurs. In turn, the excess levels of PTH cause osseous manifestations of hyperparathyroidism, termed *renal osteodystrophy* (see Chapter 26). The morphological appearance of the parathyroids in secondary hyperplasia is similar to that in primary hyperplasia.

Tertiary hyperparathyroidism refers to the development of autonomous parathyroid hyperplasia after long-standing hyperplasia secondary to renal failure. In such instances parathyroid hyperplasia may not regress following renal transplantation, and surgical intervention to remove parathyroid tissue is required. In this context, monoclonality of hyperplastic parathyroid lesions has been described in two thirds of patients with long-standing uremia.

Adrenal Cortex

ANATOMY

Each adrenal gland consists of two independent endocrine organs, namely, the cortex and the medulla. Both components are distinct not only anatomically and functionally but also embryologically. The adrenal cortex arises from celomic mesenchymal cells near the urogenital ridge. The medulla is formed when the fetal adrenal is invaded by neuroectodermal cells.

The adult adrenal glands are pyramidal organs situated at the upper pole of each kidney. Each gland is 4 to 6 cm in greatest dimension and weighs about 4 g. Microscopically, the cortex exhibits three layers or zones.

- The **zona glomerulosa** is the outermost layer and is the site of aldosterone secretion. It is stimulated by angiotensin and potassium and inhibited by atrial natriuretic peptide and somatostatin. The zona glomerulosa makes up 15% of the cortex and is composed of indistinct spherical nests of cells with dark-staining nuclei and a moderate number of fat droplets in the cytoplasm.
- The **zona fasciculata** accounts for 75% of the cortex and is not distinctly separated from the zona glomerulosa. Radial cords of cells, each containing a small nucleus and a large, foamy, clear cytoplasm, representing stored lipid, are readily appreciated.
- The **zona reticularis** is the innermost layer adjacent to the medulla. Irregular anastomosing cords are composed of compact cells with a lipid-poor, slightly granular cytoplasm and bland nuclei.

The cells of the fasciculata and reticularis secrete glucocorticoids under the control of ACTH. In addition, ACTH stimulates adrenal growth. These zones also produce dehydroepiandrosterone, a weak adrenal androgen.

CONGENITAL ADRENAL HYPERPLASIA

Congenital adrenal hyperplasia (CAH) is a syndrome that results from a number of autosomal recessive, enzymatic defects in the biosynthesis of cortisol from cholesterol (Fig. 21-30). The extent of the defects is highly variable, ranging from mild to complete deficiencies. In general, a deficiency in the synthesis of corticosteroids results in the unopposed action of ACTH and, hence, adrenal hyperplasia. CAH is the most common cause of ambiguous genitalia in newborn girls (Fig. 21-31A).

 Pathology: The adrenal glands are enlarged, weighing as much as 30 g (see Fig. 21-31B). The cut surface is soft, tan to brown, and either diffusely enlarged or nodular. Microscopically, the cortex is widened between the medulla and the zona glomerulosa (see Fig. 21-31C). The hyperplastic zone is filled by compact, granular, eosinophilic cells. In most cases, the zona glomerulosa is also hyperplastic, although not to the extent of the other zones.

21-Hydroxylase Deficiency Is the Major Cause of CAH

More than 90% of cases of CAH represent an inborn deficiency of 21-hydroxylase, more specifically termed P450$_{C21}$. The gene for P450$_{C21}$ is linked to the *MHC* locus on the short arm of chromosome 6 and is closely associated with *HLA-B* and the *C4A* and *C4B* complement genes. The incidence of this disease varies from about 1 in 10,000 among whites to 1 in 500 in Alaskan Eskimos.

P450$_{C21}$ is a microsomal enzyme that converts 17-hydroxyprogesterone to 11-deoxycortisol. A deficiency in this enzymatic activity impairs cortisol biosynthesis, and the accumulated precursors are instead converted to androgens.

 Clinical Features: Classic CAH caused by 21-hydroxylase deficiency manifests as several genetically distinct syndromes. Two variants affect newborns. One is simple virilizing CAH; the other is the salt-wasting form, which is linked to HLA-Bw47. There is also a late-onset (nonclassic) variant, which is less severe. Mutations that result in complete inactivation of 21-hydroxylase lead to salt-wasting CAH, whereas those that reduce this activity to 2% correlate with simple virilizing CAH. Late-onset CAH features intermediate values.

SIMPLE VIRILIZING CAH: Female infants exhibit pseudohermaphroditism, whereas males exhibit no abnormalities of the sexual organs. The conversion of cortisol precursors into adrenal androgens is amplified by the ACTH-dependent increase in the size of the gland. Female newborns exposed to a large excess of adrenal androgens in utero are born with fused labia, an enlarged clitoris, and a urogenital sinus that may be mistaken for a penile urethra. The sexual ambiguity may be so severe that the infant is mislabeled male.

The female external genitalia are not necessarily abnormal at birth, but infant girls may develop a syndrome of androgen excess, characterized by enlargement of the clitoris and the presence of pubic hair. Infant boys exhibit sexual precocity. Eventually, the high levels of adrenal androgens lead to closure of the epiphyses and stunted growth. Adult women with CAH tend to be infertile because the elevated levels of androgens and progestogens interfere with the hypothalamic–pituitary–gonadal axis and thus inhibit ovulation and disturb the menstrual cycle. By contrast, men with CAH may be fertile, although some exhibit azoospermia.

SALT-WASTING CAH: Owing to 21-hydroxylase deficiency, aldosterone synthesis may be impaired. As a result, hypoaldosteronism develops within the first few weeks of life in two thirds of newborns with CAH, manifested as hyponatremia, hyperkalemia, dehydration, hypotension, and increased renin secretion. These effects may be rapidly fatal if the disease remains untreated.

Both infantile variants of CAH caused by 21-hydroxylase deficiency are treated by the administration of glucocorticoids and mineralocorticoids to suppress ACTH secretion and to provide replacement steroids. Reconstructive surgery is necessary for virilized females with ambiguous external genitalia.

LATE-ONSET CAH: Patients with nonclassic variants of 21-hydroxylase deficiency show no abnormalities at birth but exhibit virilizing symptoms at the time of puberty. In young women, late-onset CAH may be difficult to distinguish from polycystic ovary syndrome. By contrast, most young men with the disorder are asymptomatic. This form of CAH is probably more common than is classic CAH, particularly among Ashkenazi Jews, Italians, and persons from the former Yugoslavia.

11β-Hydroxylase Deficiency Is a Minor Cause of CAH

A deficiency in 11β-hydroxylase is responsible for 5% of cases of CAH. Although the disorder is distinctly uncommon in the general population, among Jews of Iranian or

Congenital Adrenal Hyperplasia

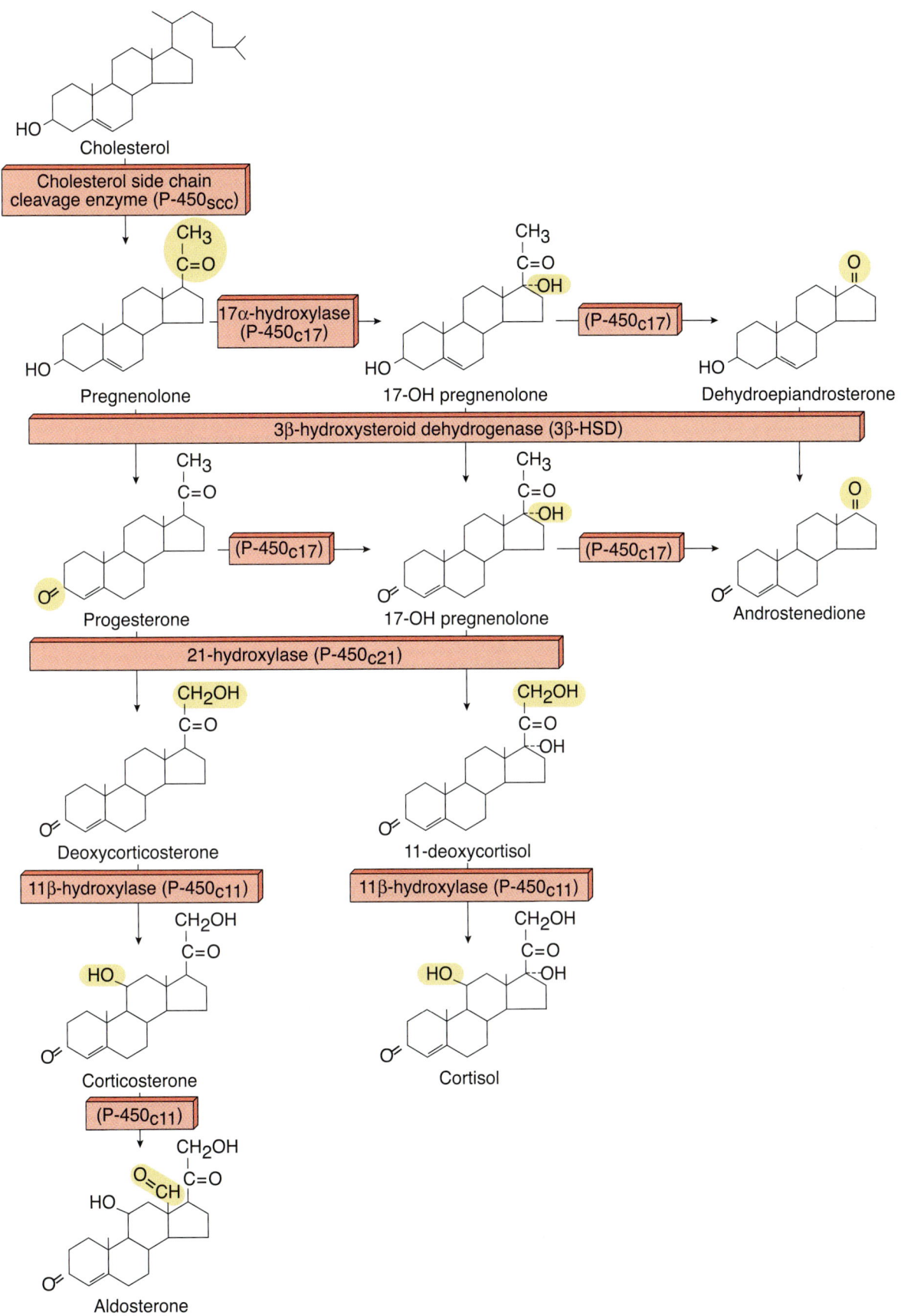

FIGURE 21-30
Biosynthetic pathways in the synthesis of adrenal corticosteroids.

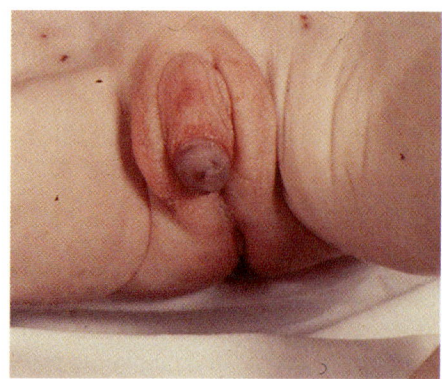
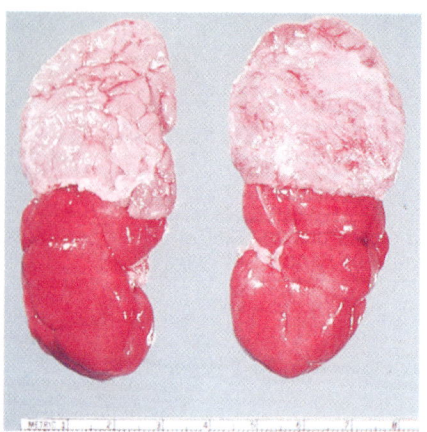
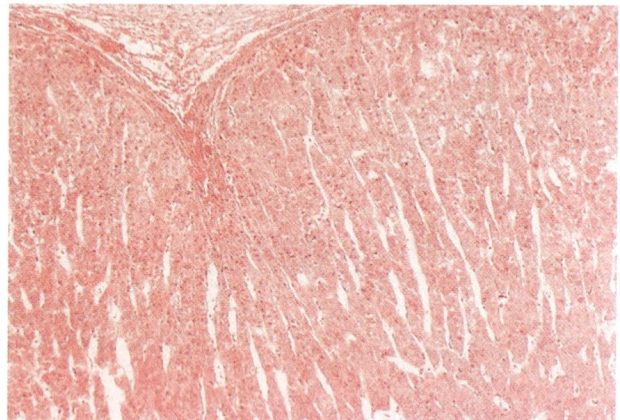

FIGURE 21-31
Congenital adrenal hyperplasia. **A.** A female infant is markedly virilized with hypertrophy of the clitoris and partial fusion of labioscrotal folds. **B.** A 7-week-old male died of severe salt-wasting congenital adrenal hyperplasia. At autopsy, both adrenal glands were markedly enlarged. **C.** A microscopic view shows a widened cortex containing compact eosinophilic cells.

Moroccan ancestry in Israel, 11β-hydroxylase deficiency is the most common cause of CAH. The gene for 11β-hydroxylase is located on chromosome 8, and thus, there is no linkage to the *HLA* locus. 11β-Hydroxylase is the enzyme responsible for the terminal hydroxylation in the biosynthesis of cortisol. In addition to the androgenic complications of CAH, the presence of high levels of 11-deoxycortisol, a weak mineralocorticoid, often causes sodium retention and accompanying hypertension.

Rare forms of CAH have been described, including deficiencies of a variety of enzymes involved in the biosynthesis of adrenocorticosteroids. These result in variable combinations of electrolyte abnormalities and anomalies of the sex organs.

ADRENAL CORTICAL INSUFFICIENCY

Deficient production of adrenal cortical hormones can result from (1) destruction of the adrenal gland, (2) pituitary or hypothalamic dysfunction, or (3) the intake of corticosteroids in the treatment of chronic inflammatory diseases.

Primary Chronic Adrenal Insufficiency (Addison Disease) Often Reflects an Autoimmune Destruction of the Adrenal

Addison disease is a fatal wasting disorder caused by the failure of the adrenal glands to produce glucocorticoids, mineralocorticoids, and androgens. If untreated, the disease is characterized by weakness, weight loss, gastrointestinal symptoms, hypotension, electrolyte disturbances, and hyperpigmentation.

 Pathogenesis: When Addison described primary adrenal insufficiency in 1855, the most common cause of the syndrome that carries his name was tuberculosis of the adrenal glands. Worldwide, tuberculosis probably remains the most common cause of chronic adrenal insufficiency, but in advanced societies, autoimmune adrenalitis is responsible for 75% of cases. Autoimmune adrenalitis occurs as an isolated disorder or as a part of two different polyglandular autoimmune syndromes. There is evidence that sporadic cases may in fact be a variant of type II polyglandular autoimmune syndrome (see below). Other causes of adrenal destruction include metastatic carcinoma, amyloidosis, adrenal hemorrhage, sarcoidosis, and fungal infections. In idiopathic Addison disease, the biochemical defect of adrenoleukodystrophy (see Chapter 28) is often detected. Rarely, adrenal insufficiency is the result of congenital adrenal hypoplasia or familial glucocorticoid deficiency (defective ACTH receptor).

The autoimmune pathogenesis of most cases of Addison disease is supported by the following:

- Lymphoid infiltrates in the adrenal gland
- The presence of circulating antibodies to adrenal antigens
- Abnormalities of cellular immunity
- Associations with other autoimmune endocrinopathies
- Genetic linkage with *HLA* loci

IMMUNE MECHANISMS: Antiadrenal antibodies that react with tissue from all three zones of the adrenal cortex have been reported in two thirds of patients with chronic adrenal insufficiency that could not be attributed to a specific cause. The major autoantigens are adrenal steroidogenic enzymes, particularly 21-hydroxylase, which is located in the class III segment of the major histocompatibility complex (MHC). Although autoantibodies are characteristic of Addison disease, they are not thought to result in tissue injury. Rather, cell-mediated immunity is probably responsible for the destruction of the adrenal gland. Increased numbers of Ia$^+$ T lymphocytes and decreased suppressor T-cell function have been detected in blood from patients with the disorder.

POLYGLANDULAR ENDOCRINOPATHIES: Half of patients with autoimmune adrenal insufficiency suffer from other autoimmune endocrine diseases. These disorders are grouped into two polyglandular endocrine syndromes.

Type I polyglandular autoimmune syndrome is a rare autosomal recessive condition that exhibits a slight female predominance and is seen in older children and adolescents. In addition to adrenal insufficiency, most (60%) patients are afflicted with hypoparathyroidism and chronic mucocutaneous candidiasis. Insulin-dependent diabetes (type I) is also frequent. Premature ovarian failure is common, and hypothyroidism, malabsorption syndromes, pernicious anemia, chronic hepatitis, alopecia totalis, and vitiligo are also encountered.

Type I polyglandular disease is prevalent among the Finnish population and Iranian Jews. The gene associated with type I disease has been identified as *AIRE* (autoimmune regulator), which is expressed in the thymus, lymph nodes, and fetal liver, all tissues that are involved in the maturation of the immune system and immune tolerance. Similar to the common form of autoimmune Addison disease, sera from patients with type I polyglandular disease recognize steroidogenic autoantigens and other targets.

Type II polyglandular autoimmune syndrome (*Schmidt syndrome*) is more common than type I and always includes adrenal insufficiency. Women are affected twice as often as men, and the disorder usually manifests between 20 and 40 years of age. Half of the cases are familial, but several modes of inheritance are known. Hashimoto thyroiditis and occasionally Graves disease occur in more than two thirds of cases. Insulin-dependent diabetes mellitus and premature ovarian failure are common. Only rarely are other autoimmune diseases present.

GENETIC FACTORS: Half of patients with autoimmune adrenal insufficiency as part of a polyglandular syndrome have a familial history of an autoimmune endocrinopathy. In instances in which Addison disease occurs in the absence of other endocrinopathies, a third have an affected relative. There is a strong linkage between autoimmune adrenalitis and *HLA-B8*, *HLA-DR3*, and *HLA-DR4*, with the exception of cases occurring as part of polyglandular syndrome type I, which is not linked to any *HLA* alleles.

 Pathology: More than 90% of the adrenal gland must be destroyed before the symptoms of chronic adrenal insufficiency surface. Cases attributed to

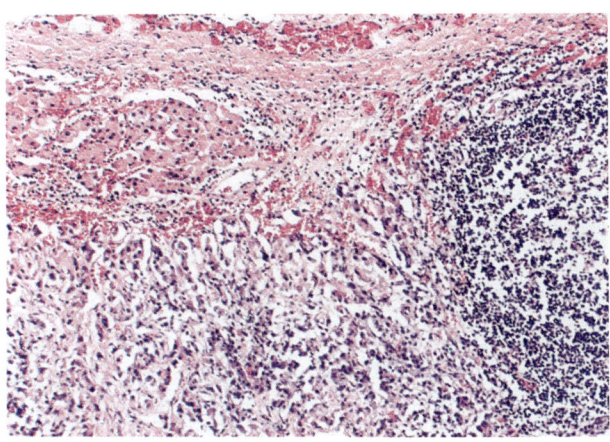

FIGURE 21-32
Autoimmune adrenalitis. A section of the adrenal gland from a patient with Addison disease shows chronic inflammation and fibrosis in the cortex, an island of residual atrophic cortical cells, and an intact medulla.

specific infectious, neoplastic, or metabolic disorders show corresponding evidence of the underlying disorder in the adrenals. Autoimmune adrenalitis leads to a pale, irregular, shrunken gland, weighing 2 to 3 g or less. Microscopically, an intact medulla is surrounded by fibrous tissue containing small islands of atrophic cortical cells (Fig. 21-32). Depending on the stage of the disease, lymphoid infiltrates of varying density are encountered.

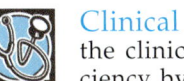 **Clinical Features:** The original description of the clinical features of chronic adrenal insufficiency by Addison remains valid for untreated cases today. The patients were reported as having "general languor and debility, remarkable feebleness of the heart's action, irritability of the stomach and a peculiar change of the colour of the skin." In the typical case, the first symptom is the insidious onset of weakness, which may become so profound that the patient becomes bedridden. Anorexia and weight loss are invariable features of the disease. A diffuse, tan pigmentation usually, but not invariably, develops on the skin, and dark patches may appear on the mucous membranes. The hyperpigmentation is related to the stimulation of skin melanocytes by pituitary proopiomelanocortin (POMC). Hypotension, with blood pressures in the range of 80/50 mm Hg, is the rule. A variety of gastrointestinal symptoms, including vomiting, diarrhea, and abdominal pain, affects most patients and may be the presenting complaint. Patients with Addison disease often exhibit marked personality changes and even organic brain syndromes.

The lack of mineralocorticoid secretion, together with other metabolic derangements, leads to low serum levels of sodium and high potassium levels. The absence of glucocorticoids is reflected in lymphocytosis and mild eosinophilia. The diagnosis of chronic adrenal insufficiency is established by measuring corticosteroid blood levels after stimulation by ACTH. Prior to the availability of corticosteroids, less than 20% of patients with a diagnosis of Addison disease survived for 2 years. Today, such patients live a normal life when treated with glucocorticoids and mineralocorticoids.

Acute Adrenal Insufficiency Is a Life-Threatening Emergency

Acute adrenal insufficiency, or adrenal crisis, reflects a sudden loss of adrenal cortical function. The symptoms are related more to mineralocorticoid deficiency than to inadequate glucocorticoids. Adrenal crisis occurs in three settings:

- Abrupt withdrawal of corticosteroid therapy in patients with adrenal atrophy secondary to long-term administration of these steroids is the most common cause of acute adrenal insufficiency.
- A sudden, devastating worsening of chronic adrenal insufficiency may be precipitated by the stress of infection or surgery.
- *Waterhouse-Friderichsen syndrome* is acute, bilateral, hemorrhagic infarction of the adrenal cortex, most commonly secondary to meningococcal or pseudomonal septicemia (see Fig. 7-24). Adrenal hemorrhage in these circumstances is thought to be a local manifestation of a generalized Shwartzman reaction with disseminated intravascular coagulation. Acute adrenal insufficiency secondary to adrenal hemorrhage is also seen in newborns who have been subjected to birth trauma.

Clinical Features: The initial manifestations of adrenal crisis are usually hypotension and shock. Nonspecific symptoms are also common, including weakness, vomiting, abdominal pain, and lethargy, which may progress to coma. In the typical case of Waterhouse-Friderichsen syndrome, a young person suddenly develops hypotension and shock, together with abdominal or back pain, fever, and purpura. Adrenal crisis is almost invariably fatal unless the patient is promptly and aggressively treated with corticosteroids and supportive measures.

Secondary Adrenal Insufficiency Reflects a Lack of ACTH

Destruction of the pituitary and consequent panhypopituitarism result in secondary adrenal insufficiency. Such lesions include pituitary tumors, craniopharyngioma, empty sella syndrome, and pituitary infarction. Trauma, surgery, and radiation therapy also may result in loss of pituitary function. Isolated ACTH deficiency is often associated with autoimmune endocrinopathies.

Any disorder that interferes with the secretion of corticotropin (ACTH)-releasing hormone (CRH) by the hypothalamus (e.g., tumors, sarcoidosis) can result in inadequate secretion of ACTH. Secretion of glucocorticoids in response to ACTH serves to distinguish secondary from primary adrenal insufficiency. Pigmentary and electrolyte abnormalities are typically absent in secondary adrenal insufficiency since these processes are not regulated by ACTH.

ADRENAL HYPERFUNCTION

Excess secretion of corticosteroids occurs in the context of adrenal hyperplasia or neoplasia (Fig. 21-33). Such hyperfunction may take one of two forms, namely, hypercortisolism (Cushing syndrome) or hyperaldosteronism (Conn syndrome), disorders reflecting the two major classes of adrenal steroid hormones.

In the early part of the 20th century, the neurosurgeon Harvey Cushing associated "painful obesity, hypertrichosis and amenorrhea" with the presence of a pituitary tumor. The combination of pituitary hyperfunction and the signs and symptoms produced by chronic glucocorticoid excess was termed *Cushing disease*. It is now recognized that the constellation of clinical features caused by high glucocorticoid levels can also result from an adrenal adenoma or carcinoma, ectopic production of ACTH or CRH by a tumor, or the exogenous administration of corticosteroids. *Thus, the clinical features of hypercortisolism from any cause are now referred to as* **Cushing syndrome,** *and the term* **Cushing disease** *is reserved for excessive secretion of ACTH by pituitary corticotrope tumors.*

The most common cause of Cushing syndrome in the United States is the chronic administration of corticosteroids in the treatment of immunological and inflammatory disorders. The second most common cause is a paraneoplastic effect associated with nonpituitary cancers that inappropriately produce ACTH. Cushing disease is five times more frequent than the type of Cushing syndrome associated with adrenal tumors.

ACTH-Dependent Adrenal Hyperfunction Is of Pituitary or Ectopic Origin

Pathogenesis: Women, usually between the ages of 25 and 45 years, are five times more likely than men to develop Cushing disease. Excessive secretion of ACTH leads to adrenal cortical hyperplasia. ACTH-dependent adrenal hyperfunction results from one of the following:

- Ectopic ACTH production by a nonpituitary tumor
- Primary hypersecretion of ACTH by the pituitary (Cushing disease)
- Inappropriate secretion of CRH by tumors arising outside the hypothalamus, with secondary pituitary hypersecretion of ACTH

ECTOPIC PRODUCTION OF ACTH: Inappropriate secretion of ACTH by a malignant tumor accounts for most cases of ACTH-dependent hyperadrenalism. Cancer of the

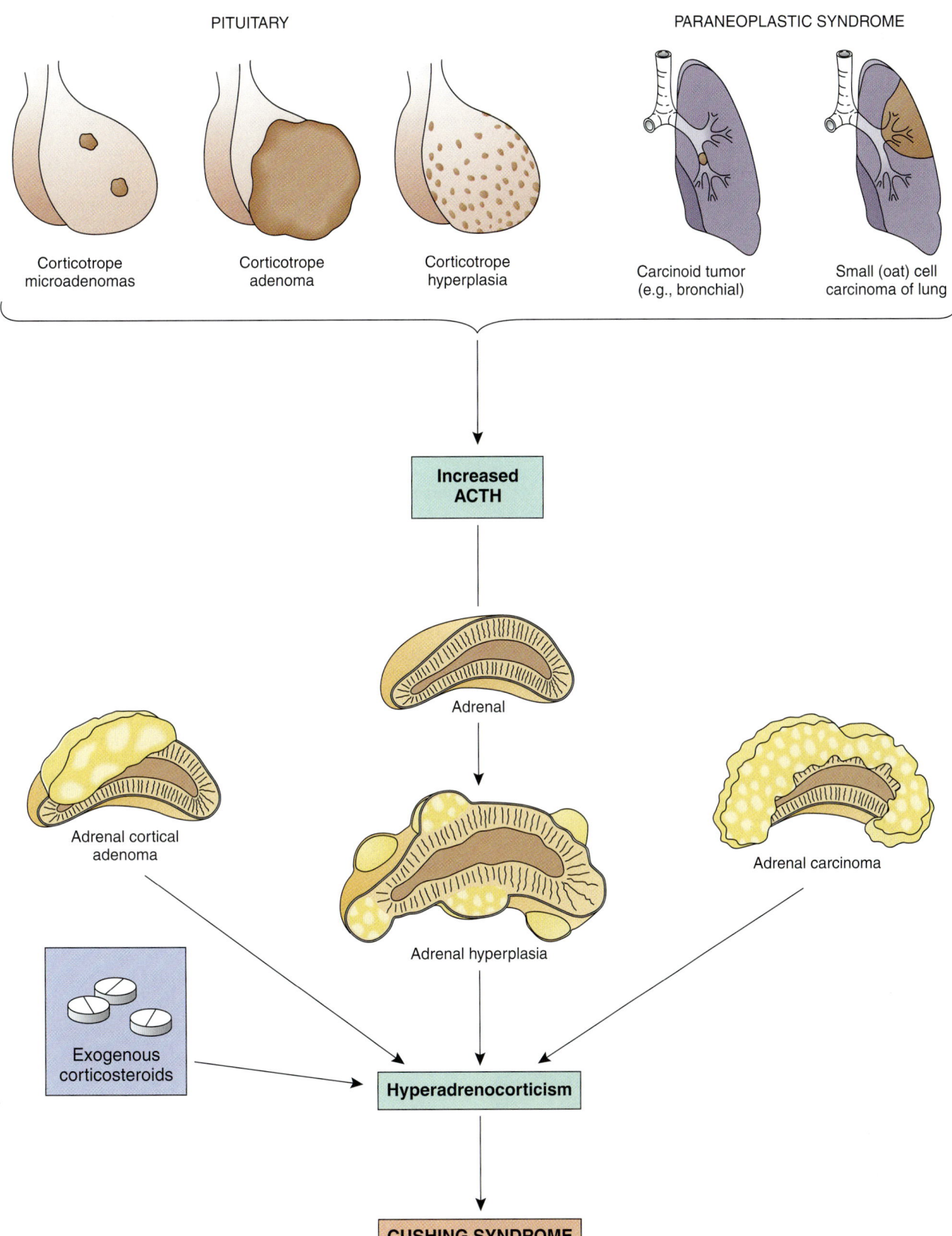

FIGURE 21-33
The pathogenetic pathways of Cushing syndrome. The ACTH-dependent pathway is referred to as Cushing disease.

lung, particularly small cell carcinoma, is responsible for more than half of the cases of ectopic ACTH syndrome. The remainder are attributable principally to carcinoids and neural crest tumors (pheochromocytoma, neuroblastoma, medullary carcinoma of the thyroid), thymoma, and islet cell adenoma of the pancreas.

PRIMARY HYPERSECRETION OF ACTH: Cushing disease usually results from corticotrope microadenomas of the pituitary, although it is occasionally secondary to a macroadenoma or, in a few patients, diffuse corticotrope hyperplasia. Whereas adenomas are clearly monoclonal, arising from a single progenitor cell, corticotrope hyperplasia is caused by chronic CRH hypersecretion.

ECTOPIC PRODUCTION OF CRH: The ectopic CRH syndrome is similar to the ectopic ACTH syndrome, except that a malignant tumor secretes CRH. In turn, CRH stimulates ACTH secretion by the pituitary, thereby leading to adrenal hyperplasia.

Pathology: Cushing disease is characterized by bilateral, diffuse (75%) or nodular (25%) hyperplasia of the adrenal glands. Each gland usually weighs 8 to 10 g but occasionally as much as 20 g.

Diffuse adrenal hyperplasia features a grossly visible, broadened cortex composed of an inner brown layer and a yellow, lipid-rich cap. Microscopically, the inner third of the cortex is composed of a compact cell layer, and the outer zone, corresponding to the zona fasciculata, displays large clear cells packed with lipid. The appearance of the zona glomerulosa varies, sometimes being prominent and at other times difficult to identify.

Nodular adrenal hyperplasia is a term reserved for grossly visible nodules up to 2.5 cm in diameter, since microscopic nodules are common in diffuse hyperplasia. Bilateral, multiple nodules compress the overlying cortex, and the intervening parenchyma exhibits diffuse hyperplasia. However, nodular hyperplasia may be asymmetric, and the two glands may differ significantly in weight. Microscopically, the nodules are composed of large, lipid-laden, clear cells.

ACTH-Independent Adrenal Hyperfunction is Caused by Adrenal Tumors

In adults, the incidence of adrenal carcinoma peaks at 40 years of age and that of adenoma a decade later. In children, adrenal carcinoma accounts for fully one half of cases of Cushing syndrome, whereas 15% are caused by adenoma. At all ages, the female-to-male ratio is 4:1.

Adrenal Adenoma

Pathology: Adenomas of the adrenal gland are uncommon, provided that minute nodules of the adrenal cortex are excluded. The typical adenoma is an encapsulated, firm, yellow, slightly lobulated mass, measuring about 4 cm in diameter (Fig. 21-34). These tumors usually weigh between 10 and 50 g, although weights up to 100 g have been recorded. On cut section, the surface is mottled yellow and brown and occasionally black, owing to the deposition of lipofuscin pigment. A thin rim of compressed normal adrenal cortex surrounds the tumor. Necrosis and calcification may be present, even in small tumors. Microscopically, adenomas exhibit clear, lipid-laden (fasciculata type) cells arranged in sheets or nests, often with interspersed clusters of compact, lipid-depleted, eosinophilic (reticularis type) cells. The nontumorous cortex of the involved and contralateral gland is generally atrophic.

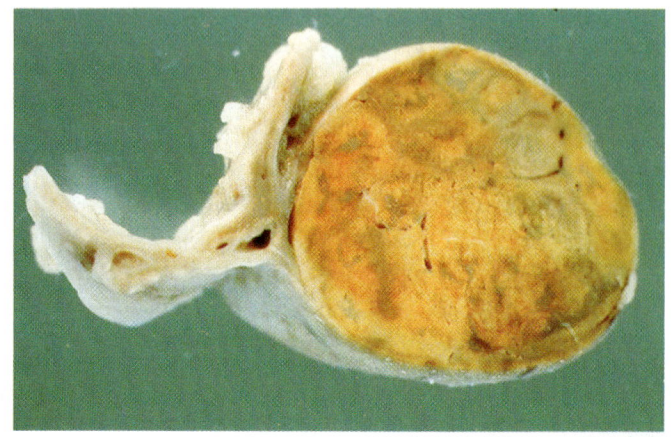
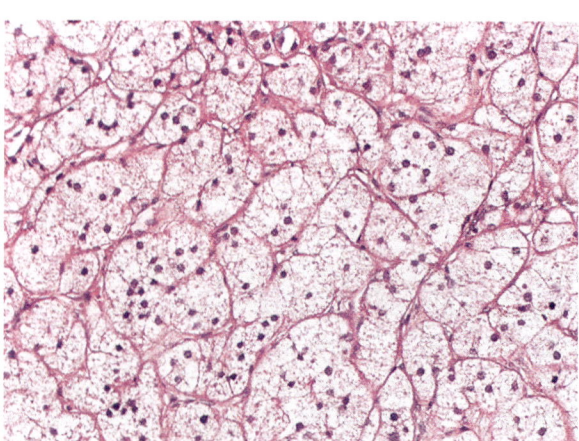

FIGURE 21-34

Adrenal adenoma. A. The cut surface of an adrenal tumor removed from a patient with Cushing syndrome is a mottled yellow with a rim of compressed normal adrenal tissue. B. A microscopic view reveals nests of clear, lipid-laden cells.

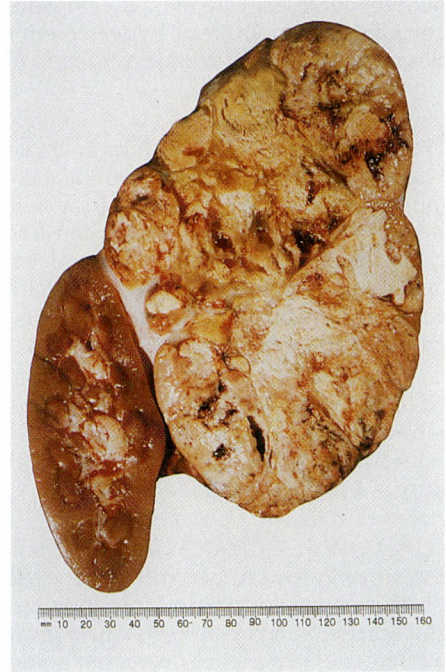
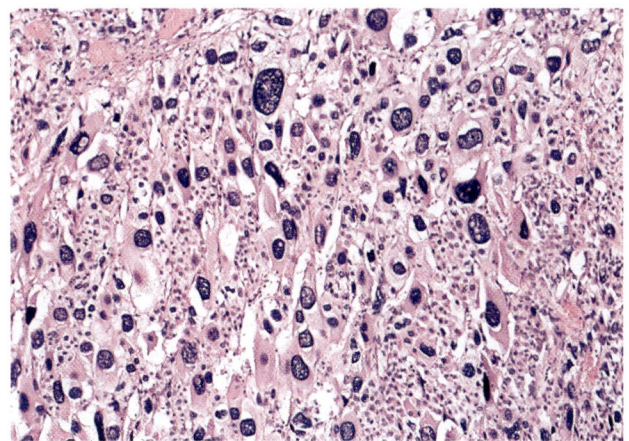

FIGURE 21-35
Adrenal cortical carcinoma. A. The bulky tumor on section is yellow to tan with areas of necrosis and cystic degeneration. B. A microscopic section demonstrates marked anisocytosis and nuclear pleomorphism.

Nonfunctional adrenal cortical adenoma is observed in as many as 5% of adult autopsies, but less than 10% of surgically removed benign tumors of the adrenal are hormonally silent. On morphological grounds alone, nonfunctional adenomas cannot be distinguished from their functional counterparts.

Adrenal Cortical Carcinoma

Adrenal cortical carcinoma is a rare and aggressive tumor that has an incidence of 1 case per million per year. Eighty percent of adrenal cortical carcinomas are functional.

 Pathology: The tumors weigh more than 100 g, and weights up to 5 kg have been recorded. Adrenal carcinomas are soft, encapsulated, lobulated, bulky tumors (Fig. 21-35). The cut surface has a variegated pink, brown, or yellow color, often with necrosis, hemorrhage, and cystic change. The tumor commonly invades locally, and remnants of normal adrenal tissue are difficult to identify. Microscopically, both clear and compact cells are present. Varying degrees of nuclear pleomorphism are seen. Mitotic figures and vascular invasion may or may not be apparent. In functional carcinomas, the contralateral adrenal cortex is atrophic.

Most adrenal cortical carcinomas cannot be resected completely, and even when the surgeon believes that the entire tumor has been removed, micrometastases in other organs are already present. Even with surgery, most patients survive for only 1 to 3 years.

Nonfunctional adrenal cortical carcinomas tend to be highly malignant tumors, with weights exceeding 1 kg. They are morphologically identical to functional cancers.

Adrenal carcinomas are monoclonal, whereas one third of adenomas are polyclonal. Several hereditary tumor syndromes are associated with benign and malignant tumors of the adrenal including Li-Fraumeni syndrome, Beckwith-Wiedemann syndrome, MEN type 1, and a few other rare conditions.

Other Causes of ACTH-Independent Cushing Syndrome

Chronic administration of corticosteroids in the treatment of a variety of immunological and inflammatory diseases is today by far the most common cause of Cushing syndrome. The synthetic hormones ordinarily used (e.g., dexamethasone, prednisone) have only glucocorticoid activity and few or no mineralocorticoid or androgen effects. As a result, hypertension and hirsutism, features commonly seen with Cushing syndrome secondary to adrenal hyperplasia or neoplasia, are usually absent in this iatrogenic disorder.

Bilateral micronodular hyperplasia of the adrenal cortex *(Carney complex or primary pigmented nodular adrenocortical disease)* is a rare cause of ACTH-independent Cushing syndrome. The patients are children or young adults. Half have an autosomal dominant disease characterized by pigmented skin lesions over much of the body, a variety of myxomas, testicular tumors, and somatotrope adenomas of the pituitary. The adrenal glands contain small, brown or black nodules, up to 0.5 cm in diameter, which consist of large eosinophilic cells laden with lipofuscin granules. Half of the patients with Carney complex demonstrate a mutation in a tumor suppressor gene (17q22-24) that codes for a regulatory subunit of protein kinase A. Another gene in 2p16 has also been mapped to the disease.

1162 The Endocrine System

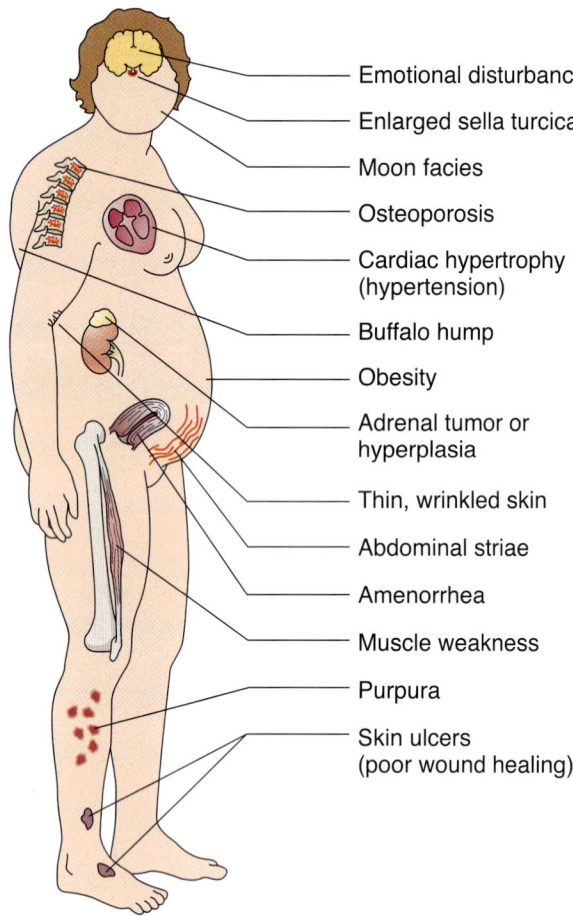

FIGURE 21-36
Major clinical manifestations of Cushing syndrome.

Clinical Features of Cushing Syndrome Are Manifested in Many Organ Systems

Clinical Features: The clinical manifestations of Cushing syndrome (Fig. 21-36) depend on the degree and duration of excessive corticosteroid levels, as well as on the levels of adrenal androgens and mineralocorticoids.

OBESITY: Typically, the patient notes the gradual onset of obesity of the face (moon face), neck (buffalo hump), trunk, and abdomen (Fig. 21-37). The extremities are characteristically unaffected or even wasted.

SKIN: The skin is atrophic, and there is a loss of subcutaneous fat. Enlargement of the abdomen and other areas of fat deposition stretches the thin skin and produces purplish striae, which represent venous channels that are visible through the attenuated dermis. Hyperpigmentation of the skin, similar to, but less severe than, that in Addison disease, may occur because of pituitary hypersecretion of POMC. Acanthosis nigricans is seen with increased frequency in patients with Cushing syndrome.

MUSCULOSKELETAL SYSTEM: Increased bone resorption causes osteoporosis. Back pain is a common complaint, and up to a fifth of patients with Cushing syndrome have radiological evidence of compression fractures of the vertebrae. Fractures of the ribs and occasionally the long bones may occur. Proximal muscle wasting (*steroid myopathy*) causes weakness, which may be so severe that the patient cannot rise from a sitting position or climb a flight of stairs.

CARDIOVASCULAR SYSTEM: Hypertension is a frequent feature of Cushing syndrome, often reflecting excessive mineralocorticoid activity. In older patients, congestive heart failure is a common sequel.

SECONDARY SEX CHARACTERISTICS: Women with Cushing syndrome tend to be virilized, showing increased facial hair, thinning of scalp hair, acne, and oligomenorrhea. Excess glucocorticoid levels in men cause erectile dysfunction, and both sexes experience decreased libido.

EYES: One fourth of patients have increased intraocular pressure, which may be a problem in the presence of preexisting glaucoma.

GLUCOSE INTOLERANCE: The stimulation of gluconeogenesis by glucocorticoids leads to glucose intolerance and hyperinsulinemia. Diabetes mellitus supervenes in 15% of patients, usually in those with a family history of diabetes.

PSYCHOLOGICAL CHANGES: Most patients with Cushing syndrome, both endogenous and iatrogenic, suffer distinct personality changes. These include irritability, emotional lability, depression, and paranoia. The disturbance in mentation may be so severe that the patient becomes suicidal.

LABORATORY FINDINGS: Half of patients exhibit an absolute lymphopenia, and one third have abnormally low

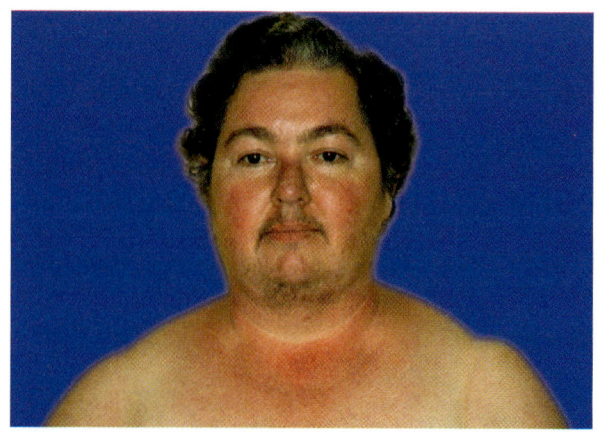

FIGURE 21-37
Cushing syndrome. A woman who had a pituitary adenoma that produced ACTH exhibits a moon face, buffalo hump, increased facial hair, and thinning of the scalp hair.

eosinophil counts. Hypercalciuria is common, although serum calcium levels remain unchanged. Serum cholesterol and triglyceride levels are frequently elevated.

All forms of Cushing syndrome are characterized by increased glucocorticoid levels. The dexamethasone suppression test is used to distinguish ACTH-dependent from ACTH-independent forms of Cushing syndrome. Dexamethasone suppresses pituitary ACTH secretion, and hence hypercortisolism, whereas it is without effect on adrenal tumors.

Cushing syndrome is treated by (1) extirpation (surgery or irradiation) of pituitary, adrenal, or ectopic ACTH-producing tumors; (2) discontinuation of corticosteroid therapy; or (3) administration of adrenal enzyme inhibitors (e.g., aminoglutethimide, ketoconazole, metapyrone). At one time, the 5-year mortality for Cushing syndrome was 50%, but the prognosis is considerably better today. With the exception of ectopic ACTH syndrome and adrenal carcinoma, in which patients die of the cancer rather than of hypercortisolism, Cushing syndrome is highly curable.

Primary Aldosteronism (Conn Syndrome) Leads to Hypertension and Hypokalemia

The inappropriate secretion of aldosterone is caused by an adrenal adenoma or hyperplastic adrenal glands. Aldosterone-secreting adenomas are more common in women than in men (3:1) and usually occur between the ages of 30 and 50 years.

Pathogenesis: About 75% of the causes of primary aldosteronism are caused by a solitary adrenal adenoma (aldosteronoma). In a quarter of cases, the condition is associated with adrenal hyperplasia. The remainder reflect bilateral hyperplasia of the adrenal zona glomerulosa. Only a few cases of primary aldosteronism are caused by adrenal carcinoma.

Two types of familial hyperaldosteronism have been defined. Type I (glucocorticoid-suppressible) is an autosomal dominant disease in which the fusion of the ACTH-responsive regulatory elements of the 11β-hydroxylase gene to the aldosterone synthase gene results in a hybrid gene. This gene is ectopically and constitutively activated in the zona fasciculata, with resulting bilateral hyperplasia of this zone. By suppressing the release of ACTH, glucocorticoids ameliorate type I disease. In contrast to type I disease, type II familial hyperaldosteronism is associated with adrenal cortical adenomas and is, therefore, not suppressible by glucocorticoids.

The hypersecretion of aldosterone enhances sodium reabsorption by the renal tubules, thereby increasing body sodium. Hypertension is caused not only by the retention of sodium and consequent volume expansion but also by increased peripheral vascular resistance. Hypokalemia reflects aldosterone-induced loss of potassium in the distal renal tubule.

Pathology: Most aldosterone-secreting adenomas measure less than 3 cm in diameter, weigh less than 6 g, and are yellow. However, the size varies, and tumors up to 50 g are reported. On microscopic examination, the dominant cells are clear, lipid-rich, and arranged in cords or alveoli. Little nuclear pleomorphism is noted. In contrast to cortisol-producing adenomas, the nontumorous cortex in cases of hyperaldosteronism is not atrophic, because aldosterone does not inhibit ACTH secretion by the pituitary.

Bilateral nodular adrenal hyperplasia in Conn syndrome is characterized by yellow cortical nodules less than 2 cm in diameter. Microscopically, they are formed by clear cells that show no nuclear pleomorphism.

Clinical Features: Most patients with primary aldosteronism are diagnosed after the detection of asymptomatic diastolic hypertension. Muscle weakness and fatigue are produced by the effects of potassium depletion on skeletal muscle. Polyuria and polydipsia result from a disturbance in the concentrating ability of the kidney, probably secondary to hypokalemia. Metabolic alkalosis and an alkaline urine are common.

Primary aldosteronism caused by an adenoma is cured by surgical removal of the tumor. Dietary sodium restriction and treatment with the aldosterone antagonist spironolactone are also frequently effective. Bilateral adrenal hyperplasia in Conn syndrome is treated medically with aldosterone antagonists and sometimes with dexamethasone in the case of glucocorticoid-suppressible hyperaldosteronism.

MISCELLANEOUS ADRENAL TUMORS

Adrenal myelolipoma is a mixture of mature adipose tissue and hematopoietic marrow and is notable for its occasional large size.

Adrenal cysts are rare, and most are actually pseudocysts that have developed secondary to degenerative changes in benign adrenal tumors or the resolution of hemorrhage. In some cases, they represent the remnants of an underlying vascular lesion.

Metastatic cancer to the adrenal glands commonly originates from carcinomas of the lung or breast or from malignant melanoma. The glands may be unilaterally or bilaterally massively enlarged, up to 20 to 45 g each. They are largely replaced by carcinoma and often display necrosis and hemorrhage. Usually, enough adrenal cortical parenchyma remains to ensure that Addison disease does not develop, particularly in view of the limited survival of these patients.

Adrenal Medulla and Paraganglia

ANATOMY AND FUNCTION

The adrenal medulla is entirely contained within the adrenal cortex and accounts for 10% of the weight of the gland. It consists of neuroendocrine cells, termed *chromaffin cells,* which are derived from primitive pheochromoblasts of the developing sympathetic nervous system (Fig. 21-38). Chromaffin cells are so named because the catecholamines contained in their cytoplasmic granules have an affinity for chromium salts and darken on oxidation by potassium dichromate.

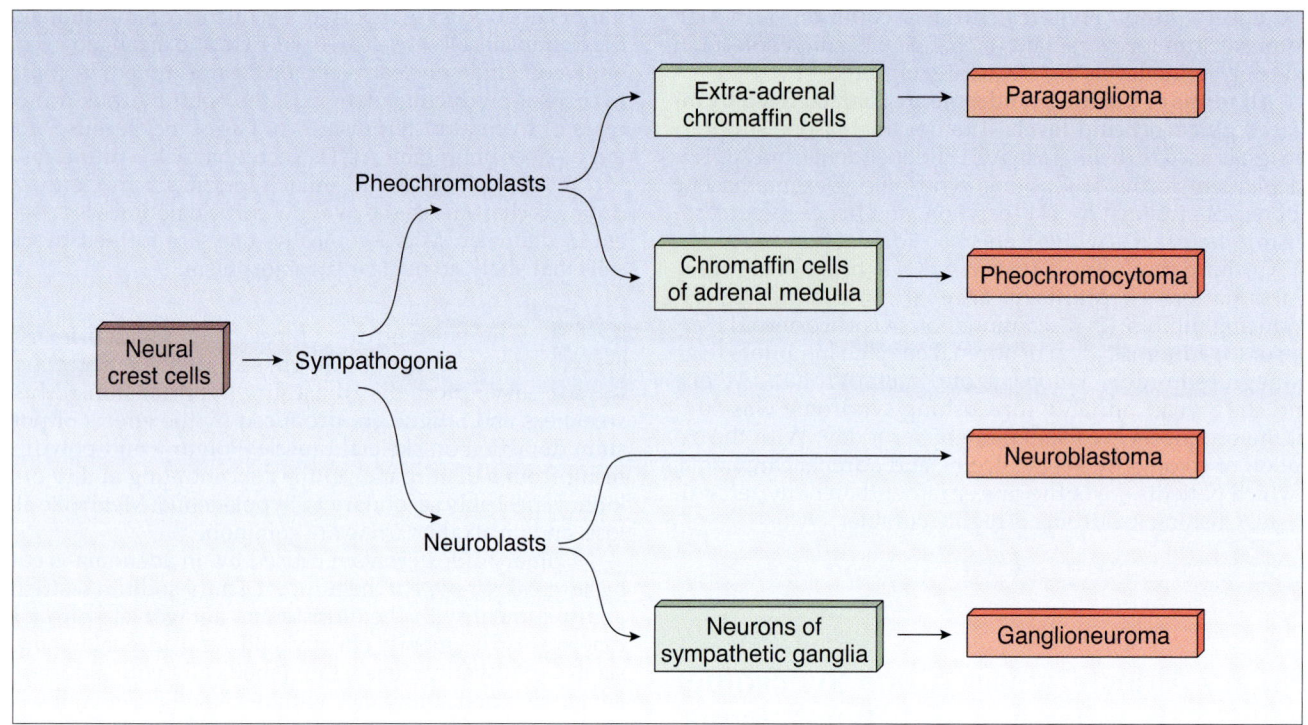

FIGURE 21-38
Histogenesis of tumors of the adrenal medulla and extraadrenal sympathetic nervous system.

These cells are also present at extraadrenal sites of the sympathetic nervous system, such as the preaortic sympathetic plexuses and the paravertebral sympathetic chain.

Chromaffin cells appear as nests of small polyhedral cells that display pale amphophilic cytoplasm and vesicular nuclei. The cells of the adrenal medulla contain numerous, electron-dense chromaffin (catecholamine-containing) granules that are 100 to 300 nm in diameter and resemble those of the sympathetic nerve endings. Epinephrine constitutes 85% of the contents of the granules, with norepinephrine and a number of noncatecholamine hormones representing the remainder. Interspersed among the chromaffin cells are postganglionic neurons and small autonomic nerve fibers. Stored catecholamines are secreted on sympathetic stimulation as an arousal response to stress (exercise, cold, fasting, trauma) and to emotional excitation accompanying fear and anger.

The adrenal medulla is supplied by both arterial and portal venous circulations that originate in the zona reticularis of the cortex. Most of the blood to the hormonally active cells of the medulla is derived from the portal blood. The medulla is innervated from the splanchnic nerves by cholinergic preganglionic sympathetic neurons.

PHEOCHROMOCYTOMA

Pheochromocytoma is a rare tumor of chromaffin cells of the adrenal medulla that secretes catecholamines. Such tumors also originate in extraadrenal sites, in which case they are termed *paraganglioma*. Other catecholamine-producing tumors (e.g., chemodectoma and ganglioneuroma) may also cause a syndrome similar to that associated with pheochromocytoma.

Pheochromocytomas are somewhat more frequent in women than in men and are observed at any age, including infancy, although they are uncommon after 60 years of age. **The presenting symptoms are related to sustained or episodic hypertension.** Despite the fact that pheochromocytoma accounts for less than 0.1% of cases of hypertension, it is important to consider this tumor in the evaluation of any hypertensive patient. When detected early, pheochromocytoma is amenable to surgical resection, but when left untreated, patients can die of the complications of prolonged hypertension. This problem is emphasized by the observation that most pheochromocytomas are found unexpectedly at autopsy, indicating that some curable cases of hypertension escaped clinical detection.

 Pathogenesis: Most pheochromocytomas are sporadic; a minority of cases are familial and arise alone or as part of several hereditary syndromes, including MEN types 2A and 2B, von Hippel-Lindau disease, neurofibromatosis type 1, and McCune-Albright syndrome.

The features of the autosomal dominant MEN syndromes are as follows:

- **MEN type 1 (Wermer syndrome)** includes (1) adenoma of the pituitary, (2) parathyroid hyperplasia or adenoma, and (3) islet cell tumors of the pancreas (insulinoma, gastrinoma). The pancreatic neoplasms tend to be multicentric and more malignant than sporadic cases. Two thirds of patients have adenomas of two or more endocrine systems, and one fifth develop tumors of three or more systems. Carcinoid, adrenocortical, and lipoid tumors may also occur in MEN-1. Almost all persons with MEN type 1 (>95%) suffer from primary hyperparathyroidism. The disease is caused by a mutation in the MEN1 tumor sup-

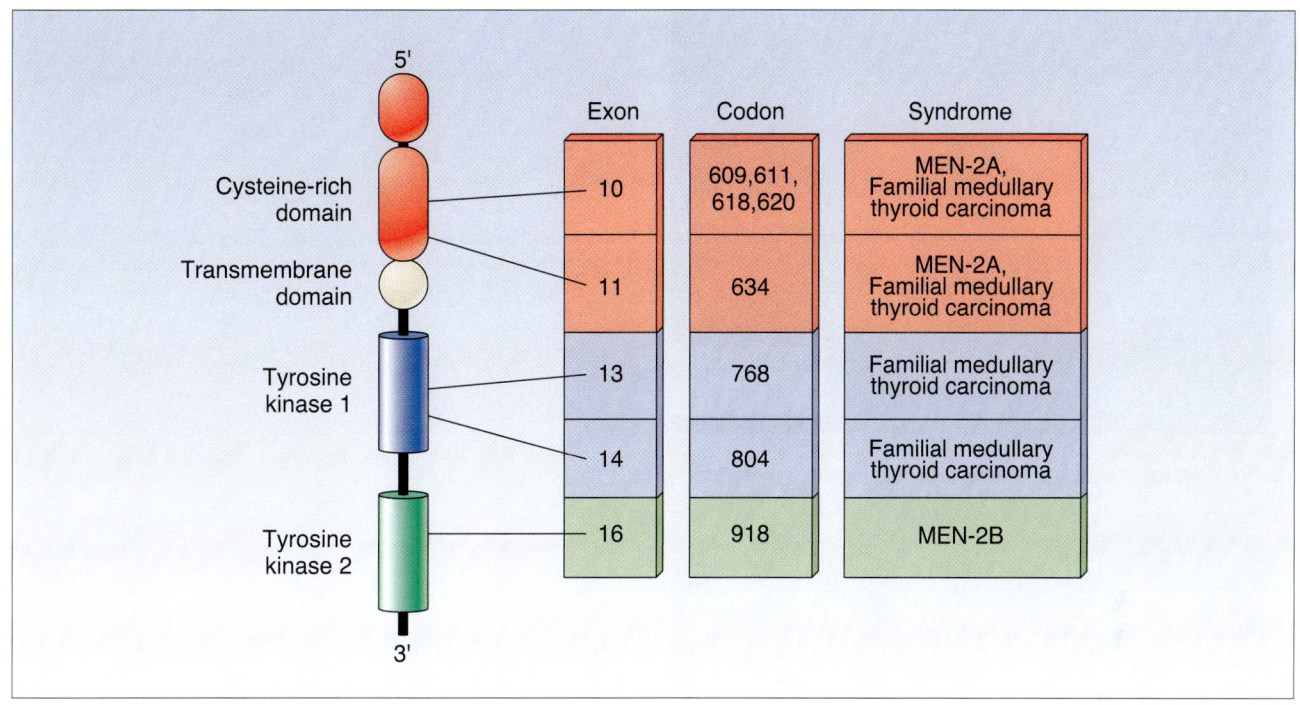

FIGURE 21-39
Representative *RET* protooncogene mutations in multiple endocrine neoplasia, type 2 (MEN-2).

pressor gene (chromosome 11), which encodes a protein termed *menin*. This nuclear protein is thought to interact with the transcription factor *junD*.
- **MEN type 2 syndromes** feature medullary thyroid carcinoma in virtually all patients and pheochromocytoma in about half.

MEN-2A (SIPPLE SYNDROME): Most (95%) MEN-2 patients are classified as 2A. In addition to medullary thyroid carcinoma and pheochromocytoma, a third of these patients exhibit hyperparathyroidism as a result of parathyroid hyperplasia or adenoma. A variety of neural crest tumors are occasionally seen in patients with MEN type 2A, including gliomas, glioblastomas, and meningiomas. Hirschsprung disease is also associated with MEN type 2A.

MEN-2B: This disorder is similar to MEN-2A, but it develops some 10 years earlier and parathyroid disease is uncommon. The *mucosal neuroma syndrome* (ganglioneuromas of the conjunctiva, oral cavity, larynx, and gastrointestinal tract) is a feature of MEN-2B. Mucosal neuromas are always encountered, but only half of patients express the full phenotype. Many patients have a habitus similar to that in Marfan syndrome.

FAMILIAL MEDULLARY THYROID CARCINOMA: There are families who have at least four members with this tumor and no evidence of other features of MEN-2.

Adrenal medullary hyperplasia has been reported in some patients with both MEN-2A and 2B. Like C-cell hyperplasia as a precursor of medullary carcinoma of the thyroid, adrenal medullary hyperplasia is thought to antedate pheochromocytoma in these cases. Cut section of the enlarged adrenal shows an expanded medulla. Microscopically, the chromaffin cells are not unusual but are larger than normal and are arranged in distinct nests or cords.

The **RET protooncogene** on chromosome 10q11.2 is responsible for MEN-2 syndromes. This gene codes for a transmembrane receptor of the tyrosine kinase family. Glia-derived growth factor and neurturin are ligands for the RET receptor. A variety of germline, missense, and activating mutations in the cysteine-rich extracellular domain of RET have been identified in 95% of families with MEN-2A and in 85% of those with familial thyroid carcinoma (Fig. 21-39). The most common mutation (codon 634) constitutively activates the receptor by promoting the dimerization of its monomer, thereby reproducing the effect caused by the ligand binding.

A point mutation at codon 918 of the tyrosine kinase domain of *RET* has been found in 95% of patients with MEN-2B. This mutation not only constitutively activates the tyrosine kinase function of the receptor, but also causes it to phosphorylate substrates ordinarily preferred by other kinases (e.g., c-*src* and c-*abl*).

Identification of *RET* mutations is now used to confirm the diagnosis of MEN-2 and to identify asymptomatic family members. Persons who carry *RET* mutations are screened for thyroid cancer, pheochromocytoma, and hyperparathyroidism from the age of 6 years to the age of 35 and are offered prophylactic thyroidectomy.

Somatic mutations in *RET* have been found in a minority (10–20%) of patients with sporadic pheochromocytomas. In addition, some sporadic pheochromocytomas exhibit mutations in the von Hippel-Lindau *(VHL)* and neurofibromatosis, type 1 *(NF1)* genes.

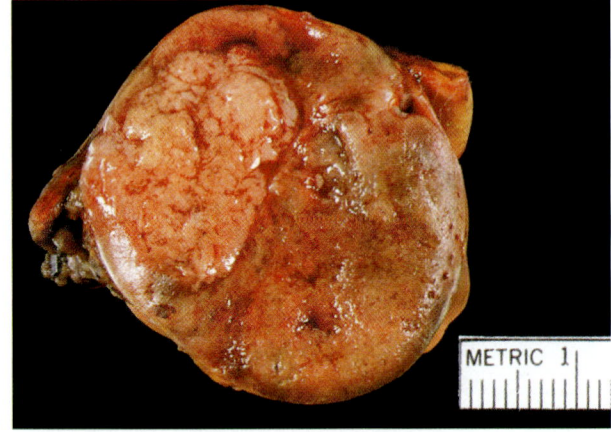
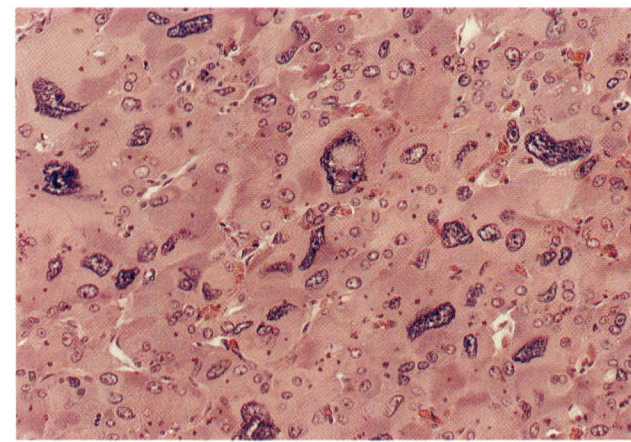
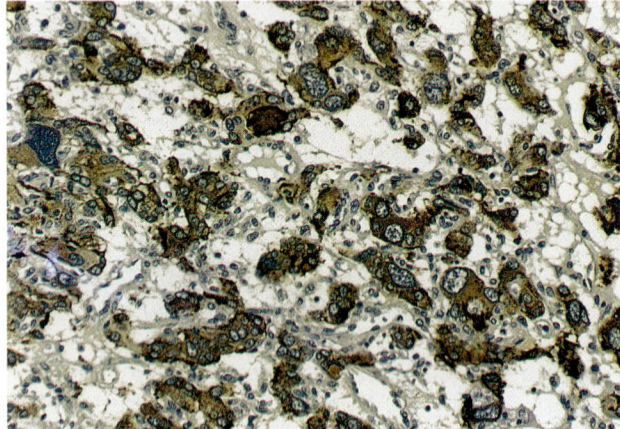

FIGURE 21-40
Pheochromocytoma. A. The cut surface of an adrenal tumor from a patient with episodic hypertension is reddish brown with a prominent area of fibrosis. Foci of hemorrhage and cystic degeneration are evident. **B.** A photomicrograph of the tumor shows polyhedral tumor cells with ample finely granular cytoplasm. Note the enlarged hyperchromatic nuclei. **C.** Many of the tumor cells show positive immunohistochemical staining for chromogranin A, a marker of neuroendocrine differentiation.

Pathology: In sporadic cases of pheochromocytoma, 80% of tumors are unilateral, 10% are bilateral, and 10% are in extraadrenal locations. By contrast, two thirds of those occurring in the context of MEN are bilateral. The tumors range in size from small lesions measuring 1 cm across to large masses of more than 2 kg. Most tumors are 5 to 6 cm in diameter and weigh 80 to 100 g.

Pheochromocytomas tend to be encapsulated, spongy, reddish masses, with prominent central scars, hemorrhage, and foci of cystic degeneration (Fig. 21-40A). The histological appearance is highly variable. Typically, circumscribed nests *(zellballen)* of neoplastic cells are present. The tumor cells range from polyhedral to fusiform and show a granular, amphophilic, or basophilic cytoplasm and vesicular nuclei. Eosinophilic globules are usually seen in the cytoplasm. Cellular pleomorphism is often prominent and may include multinucleated tumor giant cells (see Fig. 21-40B). The tumor is traversed by numerous capillaries. Less commonly, the architectural pattern features trabecular or solid formations, with only indistinct *zellballen.*

By electron microscopy, membrane-bound, dense core granules are seen, corresponding to stored catecholamines. Immunohistochemical stains attest to the neuroendocrine nature of the tumor and reveal the presence of neuron-specific enolase, chromogranin (Fig. 21-40C), and synaptophysin.

In 5 to 10% of cases, pheochromocytoma proves to be malignant, although this figure may be higher for extraadrenal tumors. There are no reliable histological criteria to distinguish malignant from benign pheochromocytoma, and malignancy is only determined by the biological behavior of the tumor (i.e., metastases). Both benign and malignant pheochromocytomas evidence mitoses, cellular pleomorphism, invasion of the capsule or blood vessels, and necrosis. Metastases are most common in the regional lymph nodes, bone, lung, and liver.

Clinical Features: With few exceptions, the clinical features associated with pheochromocytoma are caused by the release of catecholamines by the tumor. Patients with pheochromocytoma come to medical attention because of (1) asymptomatic hypertension discovered on a routine physical examination, (2) symptomatic hypertension that is resistant to antihypertensive therapy, (3) malignant hypertension (e.g., encephalopathy, papilledema, proteinuria), (4) myocardial infarction or aortic dissection, or (5) paroxysms of convulsions, anxiety, or hyperventilation.

In the typical case, episodic catecholamine release leads to a paroxysm or crisis, lasting up to several hours, with severe throbbing headache, sweating, palpitations, tachycardia, abdominal pain, and vomiting. An elevated blood pressure, often to an extreme degree, is characteristic. A paroxysm is often precipitated by activities that place pressure on the abdominal contents (including the tumor), such as exercise, lifting, bending, or vigorous abdominal palpation. Although anxiety may be a prominent feature of a paroxysm, emotional stress is not an initiating factor.

More than 90% of patients with pheochromocytoma exhibit hypertension, which is sustained in two thirds of patients and is similar to essential hypertension. In these patients, blood pressure rises to even higher levels during a paroxysm. In one third of patients, hypertension is only episodic. Frequently, episodic hypertension becomes sustained, and in many untreated patients, the condition evolves into malignant hypertension.

There are other consequences of excess catecholamine levels. Orthostatic hypotension results from decreased plasma volume and poor postural tone. An increased basal metabolic rate, sweating, heat intolerance, and weight loss may mimic hyperthyroidism. Angina and myocardial infarction occur in the absence of coronary artery disease. The cardiac complications are attributed to myocardial necrosis caused by elevated catecholamine levels (*catecholamine cardiomyopathy*).

Pheochromocytoma is diagnosed by finding increased urinary levels of catecholamine metabolites, particularly vanillylmandelic acid, metanephrine, and unconjugated catecholamines. The definitive treatment for pheochromocytoma is surgical extirpation of the tumor. α-Adrenergic blocking agents are used to control hypertensive crises, and β-adrenergic receptor antagonists are helpful adjuncts.

Paraganglioma Is a Pheochromocytoma in an Extraadrenal Site

Paragangliomas arise in paraganglia in any location, including the retroperitoneum, the posterior mediastinum, and the urinary bladder. Bladder paraganglioma may present as a peculiar syndrome of headaches and paroxysmal hypertension on urination. Paragangliomas may also arise in the base of the skull, in the neck, in vagal or aortic bodies, or in any organ that contains paraganglionic tissue, such as the larynx and small intestine. They arise in such paraganglia as the glomus jugulare, the carotid body, and other vasoreceptor bodies. Most (90%) paragangliomas of the head and neck are benign; those in the retroperitoneum are more often malignant.

Carotid body tumor is a prototypic paraganglioma that arises at the carotid bifurcation, forming a palpable mass in the neck. Interestingly, carotid body tumors are 10 times more frequent in persons living at high altitude than those at sea level, suggesting that these tumors actually represent a hyperplastic response to prolonged sensing of hypoxia by the carotid body.

Autosomal dominant transmission of paragangliomas has been described in some families, and hereditary paraganglioma was the first hereditary tumor syndrome that was reported to be caused by a germline mutation in a gene encoding a mitochondrial protein. Genetic linkage is traced to the *SDHD* gene (11q23), which encodes a subunit of cytochrome B that has been proposed to participate in oxygen sensing. Curiously, all affected persons, whether male or female, have inherited the disease from their father.

NEUROBLASTOMA

Neuroblastoma is a malignant tumor of neural crest origin that is composed of neoplastic neuroblasts and originates in the adrenal medulla or sympathetic ganglia. The neuroblast is derived from primitive sympathogonia and represents an intermediate stage in the development of the sympathetic ganglion neurons (see Fig. 21-38). **Neuroblastoma is one of the most important malignant tumors of childhood, accounting for up to 10% of all childhood cancers and 15% of cancer deaths among children.** The overall incidence is 1 in 7000. The peak incidence is in the first 3 years. The tumor is congenital in some cases and has even been found in premature stillborns. In fact, neuroblastoma accounts for half of all cancers diagnosed in the first month of life. Occasional cases are encountered in adolescents or adults. Although the occurrence of neuroblastoma is sporadic, a few instances of familial tumors are recorded.

Pathogenesis: Embryogenesis of the adrenal medulla and presumably of other parts of the sympathetic nervous system continues during the first year of life. Persistence and transformation of these embryonal structures may be related to the pathogenesis of neuroblastoma. Neuroblastoma is characterized by frequent deletions on chromosome 1 (1p35-36), with unbalanced translocation with 17q. Extrachromosomal double minutes and homogeneously staining regions (HSRs) are found on chromosome 2. The HSRs represent amplification of N-*myc*, an abnormality that plays a key role in determining the aggressiveness of neuroblastoma. It is thought that the locus on chromosome 1 encodes a gene that suppresses the amplification of N-*myc*.

Pathology: Neuroblastoma can originate in any location where cells derived from the neural crest are present (i.e., from the posterior cranial fossa to the coccyx). One third of tumors are in the adrenal gland, another third in other abdominal sites, and 20% in the posterior mediastinum.

Neuroblastomas range in size from minute, barely discernible nodules to tumors readily palpable through the abdominal wall. They are round, irregularly lobulated masses that weigh 50 to 150 g or more (Fig. 21-41A). The cut surface is soft and friable, with a variegated maroon color. Areas of necrosis, hemorrhage, calcification, and cystic change are frequently present.

Microscopically, the tumor is composed of dense sheets of small, round to fusiform cells with hyperchromatic nuclei and scanty cytoplasm, which are often compared with lymphocytes. Mitoses are frequent. Characteristic rosettes are defined by a rim of dark tumor cells in a circumferential arrangement around a central pale fibrillar core (see Fig. 21-41B). Pseudorosettes, featuring tumor cells clustered radially around small vessels, are also present. The electron microscopic appearance of neuroblastoma cells is distinctive. The malignant neuroblasts exhibit peripheral dendritic processes containing longitudinally oriented microtubules and neurosecretory granules and filaments in the cytoplasm.

Neuroblastomas readily infiltrate the surrounding structures and metastasize to regional lymph nodes, the liver, lungs, bones, and other sites. Metastasis to the orbit may result in proptosis. Occasionally, metastases may be found earlier than the primary tumor.

1168   The Endocrine System

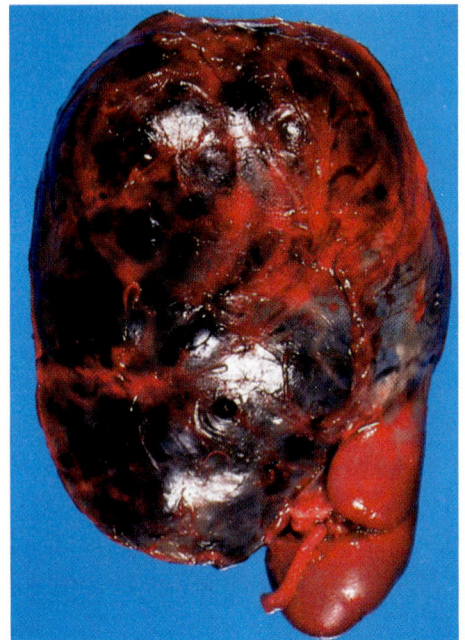
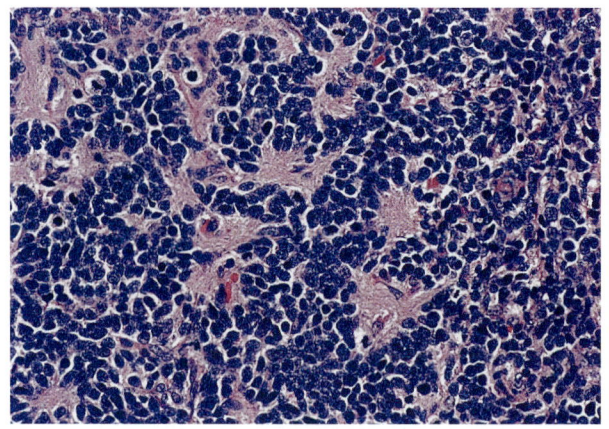

FIGURE 21-41
Neuroblastoma. **A.** A large, lobulated, hemorrhagic and cystic tumor, adherent to the upper pole of the kidney, was removed from a child who presented with an abdominal mass. **B.** A photomicrograph illustrates the characteristic rosettes, formed by small, regular, dark tumor cells arranged around a central, pale fibrillar core.

Clinical Features: The signs and symptoms of neuroblastoma are highly variable, owing to the numerous sites of the primary tumor and its metastases. The presenting sign is often an enlarging abdomen in a young child. Physical examination discloses a firm, irregular, nontender mass. Hepatic metastases enlarge the liver and occasionally produce ascites. Marked irritability may reflect pain from bony metastases. Respiratory distress accompanies large masses in the thorax, and tumors in the pelvis obstruct the bowel or ureters. Spinal cord compression may lead to gait disturbance and sphincter dysfunction. Severe diarrhea may be caused by secretion of vasoactive intestinal peptide by the neuroblastoma.

Urinary excretion of catecholamines and their metabolites is almost invariably elevated in patients with neuroblastoma. The urine contains increased amounts of norepinephrine, vanillylmandelic acid (VMA), homovanillic acid (HVA) and dopamine.

A number of prognostic factors have been identified:

- **Age:** The best prognosis is seen in children under the age of 2 years.
- **Site:** Extraadrenal tumors tend to be better differentiated and, accordingly, have a better prognosis.
- **Stage:** Survival is 90% in stage I (tumor confined to the organ of origin) and decreases to less than 3% in stage IV (widespread metastases). An exception is stage IVS (special), in which the characteristic chromosomal abnormalities of neuroblastoma are absent. Even with metastases to the liver and bone marrow, patients with stage IVS often undergo spontaneous remissions and have a 60 to 90% survival rate.
- **Grade:** Low-grade (better differentiated) tumors carry a better prognosis than do high-grade (undifferentiated) neuroblastomas.
- **VMA/HVA ratio:** A ratio of less than 1 indicates a deficiency of dopamine β-hydroxylase activity in aggressive tumors and suggests an unfavorable outcome.

- **Genomic alterations:** Amplification of N-*myc* occurs in 30% of cases and, as noted above, is negatively correlated with survival. Deletion of chromosome 1p and gain in 17q portend a bleak prognosis, whether they occur independently or together. Some neuroblastomas express the nerve growth factor receptor that is encoded by the *TRK* gene. A high level of *TRK* expression strongly predicts prolonged survival.

Localized neuroblastomas are treated by surgical resection alone. Patients with disseminated tumor are given chemotherapy and sometimes irradiation.

Ganglioneuroma Is a Mature Tumor Variant of Neuroblastic Tumors

Ganglioneuroma, like neuroblastoma, is a tumor of neural crest origin, which is found in older children and young adults. Ganglioneuroma is benign and arises in sympathetic ganglia, typically in the posterior mediastinum. Up to 30% of these tumors occur in the adrenal medulla. In keeping with its degree of differentiation, ganglioneuroma does not manifest the chromosomal abnormalities characteristic of neuroblastoma.

Pathology: Ganglioneuromas are well encapsulated and display a myxoid, glistening, cut surface. Microscopically, they show well-differentiated, mature ganglion cells, associated with spindle cells in a loose, abundant fibrillar stroma (Fig. 21-42). The fibrils represent neurites extending from the tumor cell bodies. The cytoplasmic processes of the ganglion cells contain neurosecre-

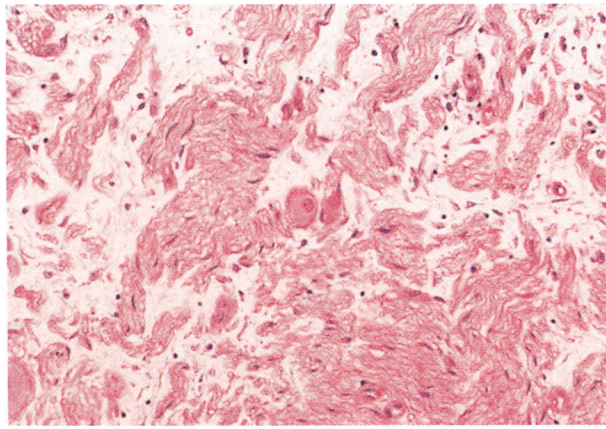

FIGURE 21-42
Ganglioneuroma. A photomicrograph shows mature ganglion cells interspersed among wavy spindle cells embedded in a myxoid matrix.

tory granules and may even form synaptic junctions. Typical neuroendocrine substances, such as neuron-specific enolase and certain peptide hormones, are readily demonstrated. As mentioned above, a neuroblastoma may differentiate into a ganglioneuroma.

Thymus

The theories underlying the historical categorization of the thymus as an endocrine organ have long been discredited. Nevertheless, we now know that the thymus elaborates a number of factors (thymic hormones) that play a key role in the maturation of the immune system and the development of immune tolerance. On this basis, inclusion of the thymus in a chapter on endocrine pathology is appropriate.

ANATOMY AND FUNCTION

Embryologically, the thymus derives from the third pair of pharyngeal pouches, with an inconstant contribution from the fourth pair. The organ is irregularly pyramidal, with its base located inferiorly and its two lobes fused in the midline. Its fibrous capsule extends into the parenchyma, forming septa that delimit lobules. The thymus is largest in relation to total body size and weight at birth, at which time it averages about 25 g. It continues to grow until puberty, and then may weigh 45 g.

Microscopically, the lobules display an outer cortex and an inner medulla. The cortex consists of densely packed lymphocytes, which in this location are termed *thymocytes*. *Hassall corpuscles* are medullary structures that are focally keratinized, concentric aggregates of epithelial cells characteristic of the thymus.

The thymus has now emerged as the key site for the differentiation of T lymphocytes (see Chapter 4). The thymus also has a small population of neuroendocrine cells, which may explain the occurrence of neuroendocrine tumors in this organ. The thymus also exhibits a complement of myoid cells, which have many structural and functional features of striated muscle cells but are nevertheless regarded as epithelial cells. Myoid cells may play a role in the autoimmune pathogenesis of myasthenia gravis.

Beginning at puberty, the thymus starts to involute and continues to diminish in size into adulthood. Initially, cortical thymocytes are decreased relative to the epithelial cells. Eventually, the thymus consists of islands of epithelial cells depleted of lymphocytes and contains aggregates of Hassall corpuscles separated by adipose tissue.

AGENESIS AND DYSPLASIA

Alterations in the thymus vary from complete absence (*agenesis*) or severe *hypoplasia* to a situation in which the thymus is small but exhibits a normal architecture. Some small glands exhibit *thymic dysplasia,* characterized by an absence of thymocytes, few if any Hassall corpuscles, and only epithelial components. A number of developmental abnormalities of the thymus are associated with immune deficiencies (see Chapter 4) and hematological disorders.

Severe combined immunodeficiency features defects of both T and B lymphocytes and is associated with severe thymic dysplasia.

DiGeorge syndrome is caused by a failure in the development of the third and fourth branchial pouches, resulting in agenesis or hypoplasia of the thymus and parathyroid glands, congenital heart defects, dysmorphic facies, and a variety of other congenital anomalies. As a result, the patients exhibit hypocalcemia and a deficiency of cellular immunity, with a particular susceptibility to *Candida* infections.

Nezelof syndrome is similar to DiGeorge syndrome except for the absence of parathyroid and cardiac involvement.

Wiskott-Aldrich syndrome is a sex-linked, recessive, hereditary disease in which severe immunodeficiency is associated with a hypoplastic thymus, eczema, and thrombocytopenia.

Reticular dysgenesis refers to a severe form of immune deficiency characterized by a vestigial thymus and developmental failure of bone marrow stem cells, resulting in lymphopenia, granulocytopenia, and death in utero or in the neonatal period.

Swiss-type hypogammaglobulinemia is an autosomal recessive disorder featuring severe thymic hypoplasia or dysplasia. Infants with this condition have no lymphocytes or Hassall corpuscles in the thymus and die within a few years from a variety of infections. The anomaly represents a failure of the thymic anlage in the neck to descend into the mediastinum.

Ataxia telangiectasia is an autosomal recessive trait featuring diffuse telangiectasia, cerebellar ataxia, and frequent occurrence of lymphoma. The involuted thymus shows no epithelial differentiation or Hassall corpuscles.

Pineal Gland

ANATOMY AND FUNCTION

The pineal gland is only 5 to 7 mm in maximal diameter and weighs barely 100 to 180 mg. Shaped like a minute pine cone, it is located below the posterior edge of the corpus callosum and between the superior colliculi.

Microscopically, the pineal gland is composed of cords and clusters of large epithelial-like cells, termed *pinealocytes*. A second cell type is similar to brain astrocytes.

The pineal gland produces a number of neurotransmitter substances, among which the most abundant and readily demonstrable is melatonin. Although in lower animals melatonin has a significant depigmenting effect, such an action has not been shown in mammals. Since melatonin levels are distinctly higher at night than during waking hours, it has been suggested that it may function as a sleep inducer.

Serotonin and several peptides are also produced by the pineal. Significant among the peptides is arginine vasotocin, a hormone that has important antigonadotropic activity in animals. Melatonin may act as a releasing factor for arginine vasotocin.

About the time of puberty, calcifications in the pineal gland can be shown in autopsy specimens or by various radiological techniques.

NEOPLASMS

Tumors of the pineal gland are curiosities, representing less than 1% of brain tumors.

 Pathology:

- **Germ cell tumors:** These are the most frequent pineal neoplasms and are apparently derived from misplaced germ cells. Germinomas, or dysgerminomas, account for about 60% of pineal tumors and are indistinguishable from their gonadal counterparts.
- **Pineocytoma:** This benign tumor is a solid, well-circumscribed mass that replaces the pineal body. Microscopically, small tumor cells with round nuclei and eosinophilic cytoplasm appear as nests separated by thin strands of connective tissue. The overall appearance is similar to that of a paraganglioma, but no neurosecretory granules are present.
- **Pineoblastoma:** This highly malignant tumor is extremely rare and occurs in young adults. Soft masses, often showing hemorrhagic and necrotic areas, invade and infiltrate the surrounding structures. Microscopically, pineoblastoma consists of small oval cells, with dark nuclei and scanty cytoplasm, resembling medulloblastoma or neuroblastoma. Mitoses are generally numerous.

Clinical Features: Regardless of histological type, tumors of the pineal gland manifest with signs and symptoms related to their impact on the surrounding structures, including headaches and visual and behavioral disturbances. In children, these tumors are frequently associated with precocious puberty, predominantly in boys. The prognosis of pineal tumors is poor in the case of pineoblastoma but is also guarded in cases of pineocytoma. Even nonneoplastic pineal cysts pose a great threat to life because of the difficulties involved in their removal.

SUGGESTED READING

Books

DeGroot LJ (ed): *Endocrinology.* 4th ed. Philadelphia: WB Saunders, 2001.

DeLellis RA: *Tumors of the parathyroid gland. Atlas to tumor pathology*, 3rd series. Fascicle 16. Washington, DC: Armed Forces Institute of Pathology, 1993.

Felig P, Baxter JD, Frohman, LA (eds): *Endocrinology and metabolism.* 4th ed. New York: McGraw-Hill, 2001.

Kornstein MJ: *Pathology of the thymus and mediastinum.* Philadelphia: WB Saunders, 1995.

Lack EE: *Tumors of adrenal glands and extra-adrenal paraganglia. Atlas of tumor pathology*, 3rd series. Fascicle. Washington, DC: Armed Forces Institute of Pathology, 1997.

Livolsi VA, Asa SL (eds): *Endocrine pathology.* Philadelphia: Churchill Livingstone, 2002.

Rosai J, Carcangina ML, DeLellis RA: *Tumors of the thyroid gland. Atlas of tumor pathology,* 3rd series. Fascicle. Washington, DC: Armed Forces Institute of Pathology, 1993.

Wenig BM, Heffnes CS, Adair CF: *Atlas of endocrine pathology.* Philadelphia: WB Saunders, 1997.

Wilson JD, Foster DW (eds): *Williams textbook of endocrinology,* 9th ed. Philadelphia: WB Saunders, 1998.

Review Articles

Alsanea O, Clark OH: Familial thyroid cancer. *Curr Opin Oncol* 13:44–51, 2001.

Baloch ZW, LiVolsi VA: Follicular patterned lesions of the thyroid. *Am J Clin Pathol* 117:143–150, 2002.

Boscaro M, Barzon L, Falio F, Sonino N: Cushing's syndrome. *Lancet* 357:783–791, 2001.

Dayan, CM, Daniels GH: Chronic autoimmune thyroiditis. *N Engl J Med* 335:99–107, 1996.

Eng C: The RET proto-oncogene in multiple endocrine neoplasia type 2 and Hirschsprung's disease. *N Engl J Med* 335:943–951, 1996.

Faglia G, Spada A: Genesis of pituitary adenomas: State of the art. *J Neurooncol* 54:95–110, 2001.

Ganguly A: Primary aldosteronism. *N Engl J Med*: 339(25): 1828, 1998.

Gimm O: Thyroid cancer. *Cancer Lett* 163:143–156, 2001.

Hoff AO, Cote GJ, Gagel RF: Multiple endocrine neoplasias. *Annu Rev Physiol* 62:377–411, 2000.

Hull KL, Harvey S: Growth hormone resistance: Clinical states and animal models. *J Endocrinol* 163:165–172, 1999.

Johnson SB, Eng TY, Giaccone G, Thomas CR: Thymoma: Update for the new millennium. *Oncologist* 6:239–246, 2001.

Lloyd RV: Molecular pathology of pituitary adenomas. *J Neurooncol* 54:111–119, 2001.

Marx, S: Hyperparathyroid and hypoparathyroid disorders. *N Engl J Med* 343(25):1863–1875, 2000.

Neumann PH, Hoegerle S, Manz T, et al.: How many pathways to pheochromocytoma. *Semin Nephrol* 22(2):89–99, 2002.

Parks JS, Brown MR, Hurley DL, et al.: Heritable disorders of pituitary development. *J Clin Endocrinol Metab* 84:4362–4370, 1999.

Peterson P, Uibo R, Krohn K: Adrenal autoimmunity: results and developments. *Trends Endocrinol Metab* 11(7):285–290, 2000.

Phay JE, Moley JF, Lairmore TC: Multiple endocrine neoplasias. *Semin Surg Oncol* 18:324–332, 2000.

Puxeddu E, Fagin J: Genetic markers in thyroid neoplasia. *Endocrinol Metab Clin North Am* 30(2):493–513, 2001.

Reincke M, Beuschlein F, Slawik M, Borm K: Molecular adrenocortical tumourigenesis. *Eur J Clin Invest* 30(suppl 3):63–68, 2000.

Savage MO, Burren CP, Blair JC, et al.: Growth hormone insensitivity: Pathophysiology, diagnosis, clinical variation and future perspectives. *Horm Res* 55(suppl 2):32–35, 2001.

Schusshem DH, Skarulis MC, Agarwal SK, et al.: Multiple endocrine neoplasia type 1: New clinical and basic findings. *Trends Endocr Metab* 12(4):173–178, 2001.

Shane, E: Clinical review 122, Parathyroid carcinoma. *J Clin Endocr Metab* 86(2):485–493, 2001.

Speiser, PW: Congenital adrenal hyperplasia owing to 21-hydroxylase deficiency. *Endocrinol Metab Clin* 30(1):31–59, 2001.

Stassi G, DeMaria R: Autoimmune thyroid disease: New models of cell death in autoimmunity. *Nat Rev/Immunol* 2:195–204, 2002.

Ten S, New M, Maclaren N: Addison's disease 2001. *J Clin Endocrinol Metab* 86: 2909–2922, 2001.

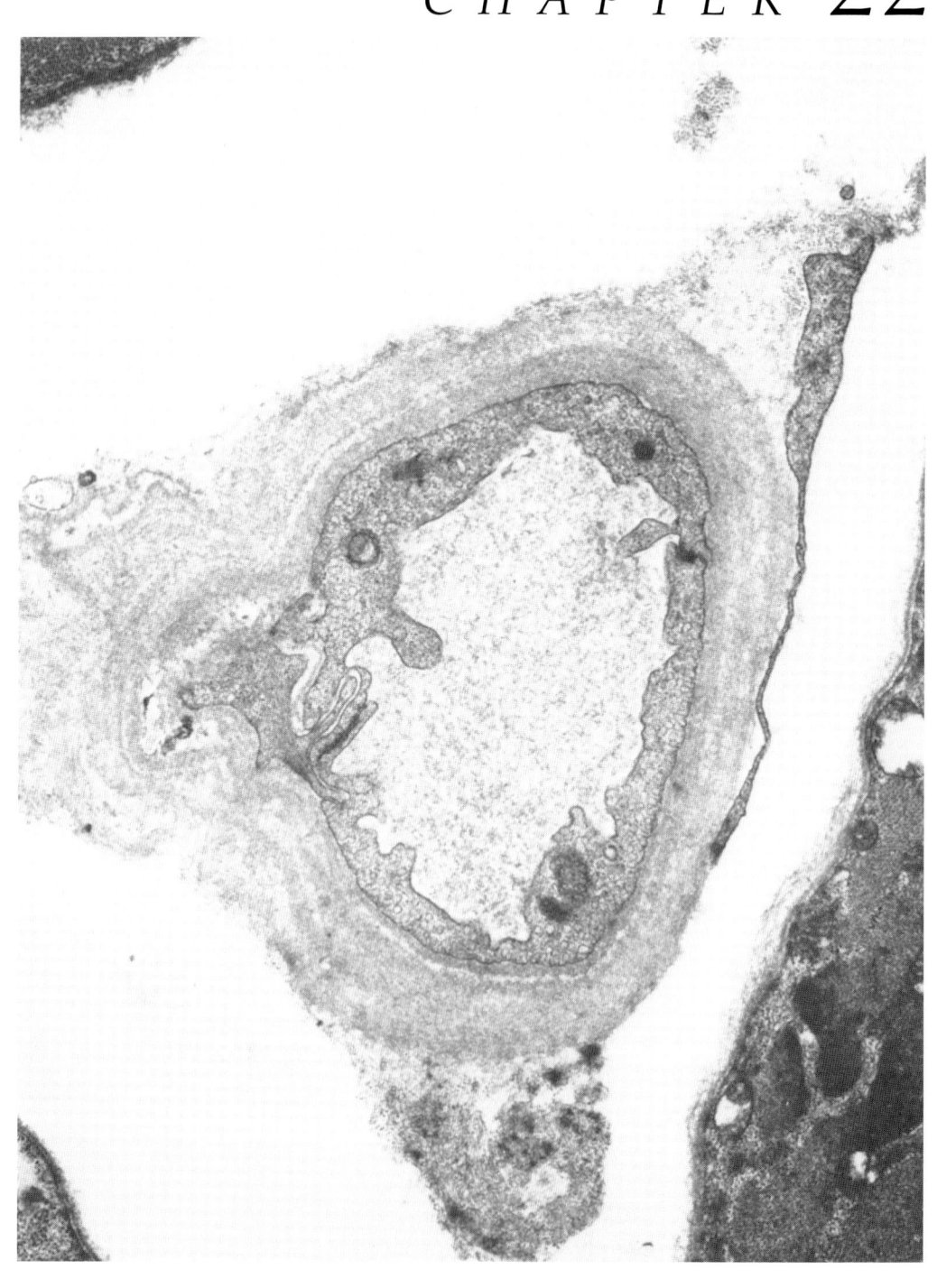

CHAPTER 22

Diabetes Mellitus

Barry J. Goldstein

Type 1 Diabetes Mellitus

Type 2 Diabetes Mellitus

Complications of Diabetes

Atherosclerosis

Diabetic Microvascular Disease

Diabetic Nephropathy

Diabetic Retinopathy

Diabetic Neuropathy

Infections

Pregnancy

FIGURE 22-1 (see opposite page)
Electron micrograph of a muscle capillary from a 56-year-old woman with T2DM. Note the thickened basement membrane, a characteristic late lesion in this disease.

Almost a century ago, the noted physician Sir William Osler defined diabetes mellitus as "a syndrome due to a disturbance in carbohydrate metabolism from various causes, in which sugar appears in the urine, associated with thirst, polyuria, wasting and imperfect oxidation of fats." Although he described the salient clinical features of the disease, Osler also emphasized the diverse causes of diabetes.

Today, diabetes is a major health problem that is affecting increasing numbers of persons in the developed world. Currently, two major forms of diabetes are recognized, categorized by their underlying pathophysiology. Type 1 diabetes mellitus, also called *insulin-dependent (IDDM) or juvenile-onset diabetes*, is caused by autoimmune destruction of the insulin-producing β cells in the pancreatic islets and affects less than 10% of all patients with diabetes. By contrast, type 2 diabetes mellitus, also termed *non-insulin-dependent (NIDDM) or maturity-onset diabetes*, is typically associated with obesity and results from a complex interrelationship between resistance to the metabolic action of insulin in its target tissues and inadequate secretion of insulin from the pancreas (Table 22-1).

Gestational diabetes also develops in a few percent of pregnant women, owing to the insulin resistance of pregnancy combined with a β-cell defect, but almost always abates following parturition. Diabetes can also occur secondary to other endocrine conditions or drug therapy, especially in patients with Cushing syndrome or during treatment with glucocorticoids. Other rare clinical syndromes are associated with either frank hyperglycemia or abnormal glucose metabolism. Because these conditions are uncommon and have a well-defined genetic etiology that differs from the more common forms of diabetes, they are not considered in detail.

The current criteria for the diagnosis of diabetes mellitus are based on determining the abnormal glucose threshold levels that are most closely associated with the chronic complications of this disorder. In particular, the hyperglycemia of diabetes causes the "microvascular" changes characteristic of diabetic retinopathy and renal glomerular damage. In a younger patient with hyperglycemia and elevated plasma ketones or frank ketoacidosis, the diagnosis of type 1 diabetes due to absolute insulin deficiency is obvious. Type 2 diabetes typically develops gradually over many years before it is recognized, most often in an overweight person with a genetic predisposition. Currently accepted criteria include a fasting plasma glucose level of at least 126 mg/dL or a glucose level above 200 mg/dL taken any time of day in a patient with overt symptoms of polyuria and polydipsia. The normal fasting plasma glucose level is less than 110 mg/dL; patients with fasting glucose levels of 110 up to 126 mg/dL have "impaired fasting glucose," and need to be followed closely because they are at high risk of developing diabetes over time.

TYPE 1 DIABETES MELLITUS

Type 1 diabetes mellitus (T1DM) is a life-long disorder of glucose homeostasis that results from the autoimmune destruction of the β cells in the islets of Langerhans. The disease is characterized by few if any functional β cells in the islets of Langerhans and extremely limited or nonexistent insulin secretion. As a result, body fat rather than glucose is preferentially metabolized as a source of energy. In turn, oxidation of fat overproduces ketone bodies (acetoacetic acid and β-hydroxybutyric acid), which are released into the blood from the liver and lead to metabolic ketoacidosis. Hyperglycemia results from unsuppressed hepatic glucose output and reduced glucose disposal in skeletal muscle and adipose tissue and leads to glucosuria and dehydration from loss of body water into the urine. If uncorrected, these effects ultimately lead to coma and death (Fig. 22-2)

Epidemiology: T1DM is most common among northern Europeans and their descendants and is not seen as frequently among Asians, blacks and Native Americans. For example, the incidence of T1DM in Finland is 20 to 40 times that in Japan. Although the disorder can develop at any age, the peak age of onset coincides with puberty. Some older patients may present with autoimmune β-cell destruction that has developed slowly over many years. An increased incidence in late fall and early winter has been documented in many geographical areas.

Pathogenesis: A variety of factors have been incriminated in the pathogenesis of T1DM.

Genetic Factors

Fewer than 20% of those with T1DM have a parent or sibling with the disease. In identical (monozygotic) twins in which one twin is diabetic, both members of the pair are affected in less than half of cases. This lack of complete concordance suggests that environmental factors contribute in a major way to the development of the disease. However, certain genetic factors are important, especially the antigens of the major histocompatibility complex (MHC). **Some 95% of patients with type T1DM express either HLA-DR3 or HLA-DR4, or both, compared with 20% of the general population.**

TABLE 22-1 Comparison of Type 1 and Type 2 Diabetes Mellitus

	Type 1 Diabetes	Type 2 Diabetes
Age at onset	Usually before 20	Usually after 30
Type of onset	Abrupt; often severe with ketoacidosis	Gradual; usually subtle; often asymptomatic
Usual body weight	Normal	Overweight
Genetics (parents or siblings with diabetes)	<20%	>60%
Monozygotic twins	50% concordant	90% concordant
HLA associations	+	No
Islet cell antibodies	+	No
Islet lesions	Early—inflammation Late—atrophy and fibrosis	Fibrosis, amyloid
β Cells	Markedly reduced	Normal or slightly reduced
Blood insulin	Markedly reduced	Elevated or normal
Clinical management	Insulin absolutely required	Diet, exercise, oral drugs, insulin

There is evidence that susceptibility to T1DM is associated with the *DQ* locus and a single amino acid substitution at a specific site (codon 57) in the DQ β-chain domain. Fully 96% of patients are homozygous for this polymorphism, compared with only 19% of healthy unrelated persons. It is postulated that this mutation might modulate an autoimmune T-cell response directed against the β cell. However, in addition to codon 57, some 20 independent chromosomal regions have thus far been associated with susceptibility to T1DM. Interestingly, the children of fathers with T1DM are three times more likely to develop the disease than are children of diabetic mothers, suggesting genetic imprinting of the paternal susceptibility gene.

Autoimmunity

The concept of an autoimmune pathogenesis for T1DM is supported by the observation that patients who die shortly after the onset of the disease often exhibit an infiltrate of mononuclear cells in and around the islets of Langerhans, termed *insulitis* (Fig. 22-3). Among the inflammatory cells, $CD8^+$ T lymphocytes predominate, although some $CD4^+$ cells are also present. The infiltrating inflammatory cells also elaborate cytokines, for example, IL-1, IL-6, interferon-α, and nitric oxide, which may further contribute to the pathogenesis of β cell injury.

An autoimmune origin for T1DM was initially suggested by the demonstration of circulating antibodies against components of the β cells of the islets (including insulin itself) in most newly diagnosed children with diabetes. Many of these patients develop islet cell antibodies months or years before the production of insulin by the islets decreases and clinical symptoms appear, a clinical state known as "prediabetes" (Fig. 22-4). However, these antibodies are regarded as a response to the β-cell antigens released during the destruction of β cells by cell-mediated immune mechanisms, rather than the initial cause of β-cell depletion. The

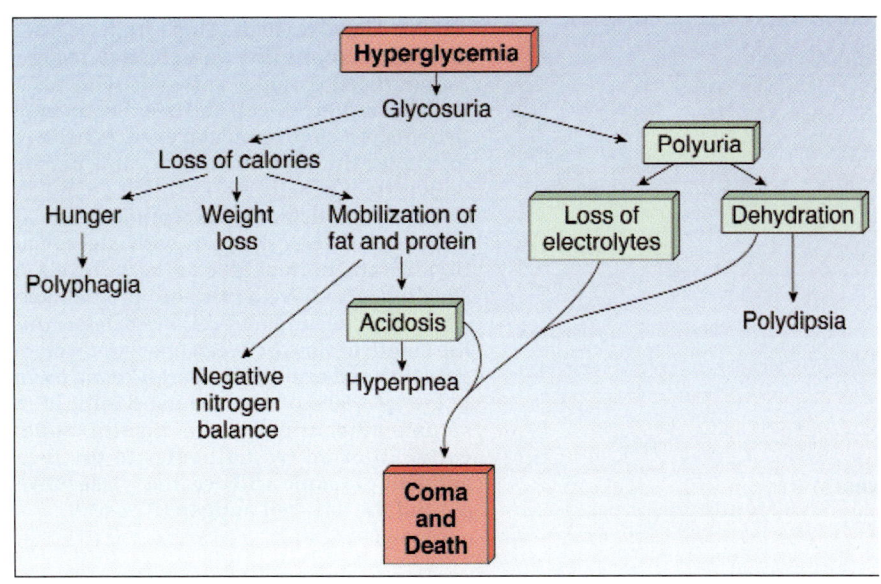

FIGURE 22-2
Symptoms and signs of uncontrolled hyperglycemia in diabetes mellitus.

1176   Diabetes Mellitus

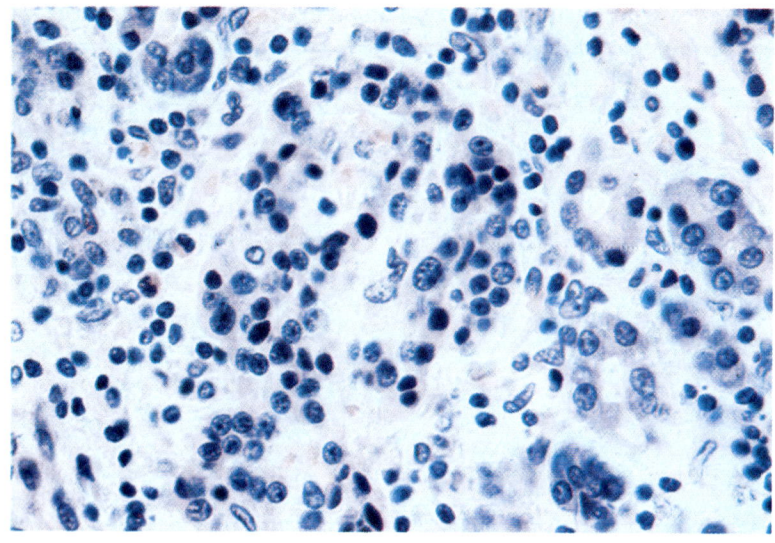

FIGURE 22-3
Insulitis in type 1 diabetes mellitus. A mononuclear inflammatory infiltrate is seen in and around the islet.

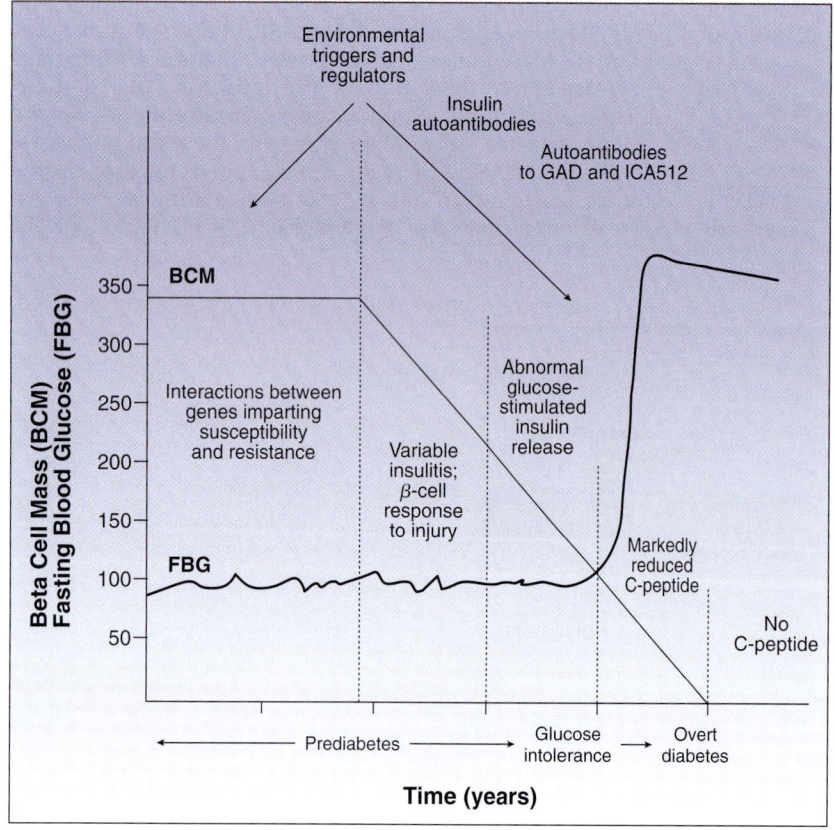

FIGURE 22-4
Pathogenetic stages in the development of T1DM. The disease develops from an initial genetic susceptibility to defective recognition of β-cell epitopes and ends with essentially complete β-cell destruction in most patients. An environmental event is believed to trigger the immune attack, and persons with certain genetic markers (HLA-DR3 and -DR4) are particularly susceptible to the autoimmune disease. Patients with islet cell antibodies and normal blood glucose levels are considered to have a state of "prediabetes." The rate of decline in β-cell mass determines the length of time between onset of β-cell destruction and eventual hyperglycemia owing to loss of >90% of functioning β cells. In the serum, autoantibodies to insulin appear early, followed by antibodies to the β-cell antigens glutamic acid decarboxylase (GAD-65) and the islet cell antigen (ICA-512).

detection of antibodies to islet cells and islet antigens (GAD-65, ICA-512, insulin, etc.) in a blood sample is a useful tool for establishing the diagnosis of type 1 diabetes.

Cell-mediated immune mechanisms are fundamental to the pathogenesis of T1DM, and cytotoxic T lymphocytes sensitized to β cells in T1DM persist indefinitely, possibly for a lifetime. Patients transplanted with a donor pancreas or a preparation of purified islets must be treated with immunosuppressive drugs. Ten percent of patients with T1DM manifest at least one other organ-specific autoimmune disease, including Hashimoto thyroiditis, Graves disease, myasthenia gravis, Addison disease, or pernicious anemia. Interestingly, most patients with polyendocrine immune syndromes (see Chapter 20) possess HLA DR3 and DR4 histocompatibility antigens.

The destruction of β-cells in T1DM generally develops slowly, and specific stages of the disease have been described (Fig. 22-4). Clinically apparent diabetes with hyperglycemia or ketoacidosis manifests only when 90% of the insulin-secreting cells have been eliminated and insulin deprivation becomes severe.

Environmental Factors

What triggers the immunological injury to the islets of Langerhans? Viruses and chemicals have been implicated as causative factors in at least some cases of T1DM. For example, the disease occasionally develops after infection with mumps or group B coxsackie viruses. Children and young adults who were infected in utero with rubella also occasionally develop diabetes, presumably after viral injury of the fetal pancreas.

Certain viral and dietary proteins may share antigenic epitopes with human cell-surface proteins and trigger the autoreactive disease process by "molecular mimicry." For example, bovine serum albumin contains subunits of MHC class II proteins, and a coxsackie B virus protein has homology to the human GAD-65 islet antigen protein. Geographical and seasonal differences in the incidence of T1DM further suggest that environmental factors are important in the pathogenesis of this disorder.

Pathology: The most characteristic early lesion in the pancreas of T1DM is a lymphocytic infiltrate in the islets *(insulitis),* sometimes accompanied by a few macrophages and neutrophils (see Fig. 22-3). **As the disease becomes chronic, the β cells of the islets are progressively depleted; eventually insulin-producing cells are no longer discernible.** The loss of β cells results in variably sized islets, many of which appear as ribbonlike cords that are difficult to distinguish from the surrounding acinar tissue. Fibrosis of the islets is uncommon. The deposition of amyloid in the islets of Langerhans in type 2 diabetes is absent. The exocrine pancreas in chronic T1DM often exhibits diffuse interlobular and interacinar fibrosis, accompanied by atrophy of the acinar cells.

Clinical Features: T1DM classically manifests with acute metabolic decompensation characterized by ketoacidosis and hyperglycemia. Severe ketoacidosis may be preceded by several weeks to months of increased urine output (polyuria) and increased thirst (polydipsia). Excessive diuresis results from glucosuria, and increased appetite (polyphagia) and weight loss are due to inefficient energy use from defective carbohydrate metabolism. Often the clinical onset of T1DM coincides with another acute illness, such as a febrile viral or bacterial infection.

TYPE 2 DIABETES MELLITUS

Type 2 diabetes mellitus (T2DM) is a heterogeneous disorder characterized by reduced tissue sensitivity to insulin and impaired insulin secretion. The disease usually develops in adults, with an increased prevalence in obese persons and in the elderly. Recently, T2DM has been appearing in increasing numbers in younger adults and adolescents, owing to worsening obesity and lack of exercise in this age group. **Hyperglycemia in T2DM is not caused by the destruction of β cells but is rather a failure of the β cells to meet an increased demand for insulin in the body.** T2DM affects more than 16 million Americans, almost half of whom are undiagnosed. Almost 10% of persons older than 65 years of age are affected, and 80% of patients with T2DM are overweight (Fig. 22-5). T2DM is most prevalent in ethnic minority groups in the United States, including blacks, Hispanics, Asians, and Native Americans.

Pathogenesis: T2DM results from a complex interplay between underlying resistance to the action of insulin in its metabolic target tissues (liver, skeletal muscle, and adipose tissue) and a reduction in glucose-stimulated insulin secretion, which fails to compensate for the increased demand for insulin. Progression to overt diabetes in susceptible populations occurs most commonly in patients exhibiting both of these defects (Fig. 22-6).

Genetic Factors

Multifactorial and multigenic inheritance is a key contributor to the development of T2DM. Sixty percent of patients have either a parent or a sibling with the disease. In some populations, notably Native Americans and some indigenous populations found in Pacific Island nations, adoption of a more affluent lifestyle has led to the occurrence of T2DM in 30 to 50% of the population. Both monozygotic twins are almost always affected with the disease. No association with genes of the MHC, as seen in T1DM, has been found. Despite the high familial prevalence of the disease, the inheritance pattern is complex and thought to be due to multiple interacting susceptibility genes. Constitutional factors such as obesity (which itself has strong genetic determinants), hypertension, and the amount of exercise influence the phenotypic expression of the disorder and have complicated the genetic analyses.

Glucose Metabolism

In a normal person, the extracellular concentration of glucose in fed and fasting states is maintained in a tightly limited range. This rigid control is mediated by the opposing ac-

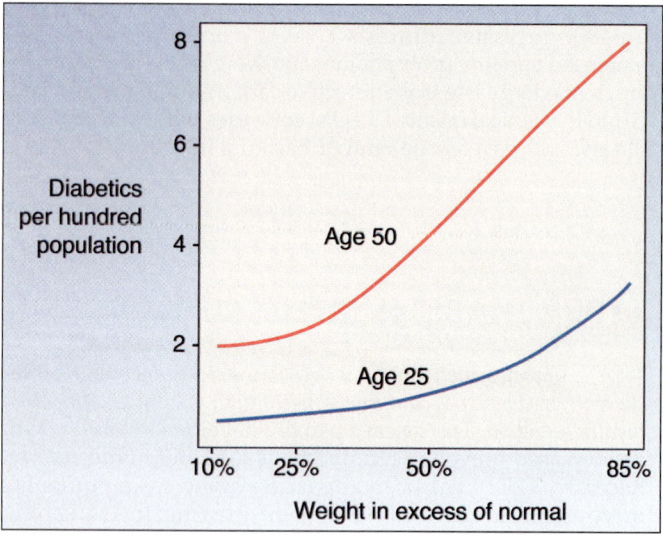

FIGURE 22-5
Occurrence of diabetes in relation to body weight in young and older adults. In persons over 50 years of age, the risk of diabetes increases linearly with body weight more than 25% above normal.

tions of insulin and glucagon. Following a carbohydrate-rich meal, absorption of glucose from the gut leads to an increase in blood glucose, which stimulates insulin secretion by the pancreatic β cells and the subsequent insulin-mediated increase in glucose uptake by skeletal muscle and adipose tissue. At the same time, insulin suppresses hepatic glucose production by (1) inhibiting gluconeogenesis, (2) enhancing glycogen synthesis, (3) blocking the effects of glucagon on the liver, and (4) antagonizing the release of glucagon from the pancreas.

β Cell Function

Persons with T2DM exhibit impaired β-cell insulin release in response to glucose stimulation, a defect that can appear early in the progression of the disease. Mild-to-moderate hyperglycemia can alter the coupling set-point between glucose levels and insulin secretion by a process known as *glucose toxicity*. This functional abnormality is specific for glucose, since the β cells retain the ability to respond to other secretagogues, such as amino acids. A rare autosomal dominant form of inherited diabetes, known as *maturity-onset diabetes of the young (MODY)*, features mutations in glucokinase, an important glucose sensor of the β cell. Other mutations affecting β-cell development and function have also been identified in MODY kindreds. However, mutations in these genes do not account for the typical prevalent forms of T2DM. β Cell function may also be affected by the chronically elevated plasma levels of free fatty acids that occur in obese persons.

Insulin Resistance

Peripheral insulin resistance is a fundamental component in the pathogenesis of T2DM. In obesity, several products released from adipose cells (including free fatty acids and cytokines such as tumor necrosis factor-α and adiponectin) affect peripheral insulin sensitivity. Plasma levels of these products are strongly influenced by body fat distribution, especially visceral–abdominal (upper body) versus subcutaneous (hips/buttocks; lower body) adiposity. There is a higher prevalence of insulin resistance and T2DM in persons with the former.

The insulin receptor is a heterotetrameric glycoprotein composed of two extracellular α subunits that bind insulin and two transmembrane β subunits that express insulin-stimulated tyrosine kinase activity. Activation of the receptor kinase leads to tyrosine phosphorylation of several insulin receptor substrate (IRS) proteins. Adaptor proteins bind to these sites, after which their latent signaling activity becomes activated. In turn, these signaling kinases phosphorylate lipid and protein substrates, effects that lead to the translocation of glucose transport proteins and activation of glucose and lipid metabolism, depending on the specific target cell type (liver, skeletal muscle, or adipose tissue). In obese persons, the release of inhibitory mediators from adipose tissue interferes with the insulin signaling cascade by disrupting the propagation of protein-tyrosine phosphorylation. Hyperinsulinemia, secondary to insulin resistance, also down-regulates the number of insulin receptors on the plasma membrane.

The "Insulin Resistance / Metabolic Syndrome"

Resistance to the action of insulin in target tissues and compensatory hyperinsulinemia are closely tied to a diverse set of cardiovascular risk factors that are prevalent in both obese, sedentary persons and in patients with T2DM. These risk factors, together termed the *metabolic syndrome*, include mild hypertension (perhaps related to a failure of endothelial-dependent vascular relaxation) and a dyslipidemia, characterized by reduced HDL cholesterol, increased circulating triglycerides, and small, dense, low-density lipoprotein (LDL) particles (Table 22-2).

 Pathology: A variety of microscopic lesions are found in the islets of Langerhans of many, but not all, patients with T2DM. Unlike T1DM, in T2DM

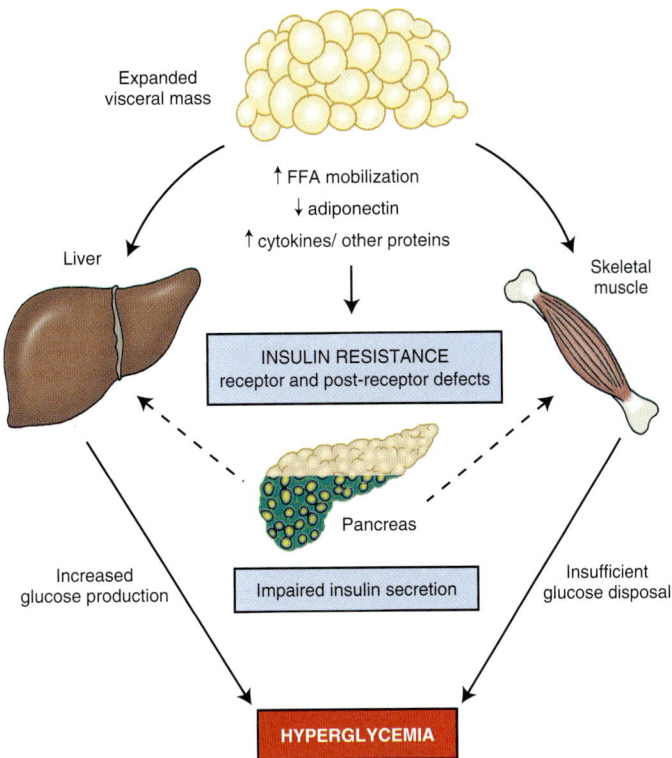

FIGURE 22-6
Pathogenesis of obesity-related T2DM. The expanded visceral fat mass in upper-body obesity elaborates several factors that contribute to tissue insulin resistance. These include an increase in circulating free (nonesterified) fatty acids and other cytokines and proteins that inhibit insulin action, as well as a decrease in factors that enhance insulin signaling, such as adiponectin. These changes result in a block to insulin action in liver and skeletal muscle at the level of the insulin receptor and at postreceptor signaling sites, resulting in a failure of insulin to suppress hepatic glucose production and to promote glucose uptake into muscle. The resulting hyperglycemia is normally countered by increased insulin secretion by pancreatic β cells. In persons with T2DM, the combination of resistance to insulin action and a genetically determined impairment of the β-cell response to hyperglycemia results in hyperglycemia, and T2DM ensues.

TABLE 22-2 Components of the Insulin Resistance/Metabolic Syndrome

Clinical Signs	Laboratory Abnormalities	Comorbid Illnesses
Central (upper body) obesity Acanthosis nigricans (hypertrophic, hyperpigmented skin changes)	Elevated fasting and/or postprandial glucose Insulin resistance with hyperinsulinemia Dyslipidemia Abnormal thrombolysis Hyperuricemia Endothelial and vascular smooth muscle dysfunction	Hypertension (usually mild) Atherosclerosis Hyperandrogenism with polycystic ovary syndrome

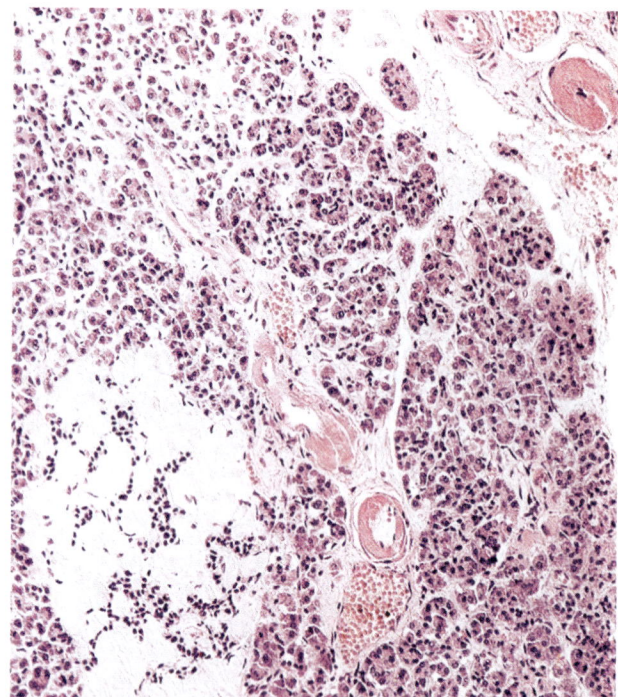

FIGURE 22-7
Amyloidosis (hyalinization) of an islet in the pancreas of a patient with T2DM. The blood vessel adjacent to the islet shows the advanced hyaline arteriolosclerosis characteristic of diabetes.

there is no consistent reduction in the number of β cells, and no morphological lesions of these cells have been found by light or electron microscopy.

In some islets, fibrous tissue accumulates, sometimes to such a degree that they are obliterated. Islet amyloid is often present (Fig. 22-7), particularly in patients over 60 years of age. This type of amyloid is composed of a polypeptide molecule known as *amylin*, which is secreted with insulin by the β cell. Importantly, as many as 20% of aged nondiabetic persons also have amyloid deposits in their pancreas, a finding that has been attributed to the aging process itself.

COMPLICATIONS OF DIABETES

The discovery of insulin in the early years of the 20th century promised to cure diabetes, but as diabetics lived longer, it became apparent that they were subject to numerous complications (see Fig. 22-1). **It is now clearly established that the severity and chronicity of hyperglycemia in both T1DM and T2DM are the major pathogenetic factors leading to the "microvascular" complications of diabetes including retinopathy, nephropathy, and neuropathy. Thus, control of blood glucose remains the major means by which the development of microvascular diabetic complications can be minimized.** It has been more difficult to demonstrate that glucose control can prevent atherosclerosis and its complications (coronary artery disease, peripheral vascular disease, and cerebrovascular disease). These "macrovascular" complications are especially common in insulin-resistant patients with T2DM, since they tend to be older and frequently harbor additional vascular risk factors.

 Pathogenesis: A variety of biochemical mechanisms have been proposed to account for the development of pathological changes in diabetes.

PROTEIN GLYCOSYLATION: Glucose binds nonenzymatically, by attaching to a wide variety of proteins. This process, termed *glycosylation*, occurs roughly in proportion to the severity of hyperglycemia. Numerous cellular proteins are modified in this manner, including hemoglobin, components of the crystalline lens, and proteins in cellular basement membranes. A specific fraction of the glycosylated hemoglobin in circulating red blood cells (hemoglobin A_{1c}) is measured routinely to monitor the overall degree of hyperglycemia that occurred during the preceding 6 to 8 weeks. Nonenzymatic glycosylation of hemoglobin is irreversible, and the level of hemoglobin A_{1c}, therefore, serves as a maker for glycemic control, as well as ongoing protein damage in the body due to excessive blood glucose.

The initial glycosylation products (known chemically as Schiff bases) are labile and can dissociate rapidly. With time, these labile products undergo complex chemical rearrangements to form stable *advanced glycosylation products*, consisting of a glucose derivative covalently bound to the protein amino group. As a result, the structure of the protein is permanently altered, and its function may be affected. For example, albumin and IgG do not normally bind to collagen, but they adhere to glycosylated collagen. Unstable chemical bonds in the proteins containing advanced glycosylation products can lead to physical cross-linking of nearby proteins, which may contribute to the characteristic thickening of the vascular basement membranes in diabetes. Importantly, unlike the initial labile glycosylation products, advanced glycosylation products can continue to cross-link proteins despite a return of blood glucose to a normal level. Thus, in a canine model of diabetic retinopathy (see below), this complication is prevented only if blood glucose is strictly controlled within 2 months of the initiation of hyperglycemia. Patients with diabetic retinopathy have higher levels of these products than do diabetics without this complication. Moreover, compounds that inhibit the formation of advanced glycosylation products provide some protection against diabetic complications in experimental animals.

THE ALDOSE REDUCTASE PATHWAY: By mass action, hyperglycemia also increases the uptake of glucose in tissues that do not depend on insulin. Some of the increased flux of glucose is metabolized by aldose reductase, leading to the accumulation of sorbitol This sugar alcohol has been suspected to play a role in diabetic complications in a variety of tissues, including peripheral nerves, retina, lens, and kidney. Although aldose reductase has a low affinity for glucose, it generates appreciable amounts of sorbitol in these tissues when blood glucose levels are elevated. The mechanism by which an accumulation of sorbitol causes tissue injury is not fully understood. In the lens, the accumulation of this alcohol may simply create an osmotic gradient that causes an influx of fluid and consequent swelling. Sorbitol may also be directly toxic to cells. Increased intracellular sorbitol has been linked to decreased myoinositol (a precursor of phosphoinositides), lowered activity of protein kinase C, and inhibition of the plasma membrane sodium pump.

PROTEIN KINASE C ACTIVATION: In patients with hyperglycemia, specific isoforms, mainly PKC-β and PKC-δ, are activated by diacylglycerol (DAG) synthesized from glycolytic intermediates. The activation of PKC may lead to (1) increased production of extracellular matrix and cytokines, (2) enhanced microvascular contractility, (3) increased microvascular permeability, and (4) proliferation of endothelial and smooth muscle cells. PKC also induces the activation of phospholipase A$_2$ and inhibits the activity of Na$^+$/K$^+$-ATPase. Inhibition of PKC-β by a selective inhibitor prevents or reverses a number of vascular abnormalities in vitro and in vivo.

EXCESSIVE REACTIVE OXYGEN SPECIES: In various cell types, hyperglycemia increases the production of reactive oxygen species by mitochondrial oxidative phosphorylation. Reactive oxygen species have been implicated in many types of cell injury (see Chapter 1).

Atherosclerosis is a Dangerous Complication of Diabetes

Cardiovascular disease, including atherosclerotic heart disease and ischemic stroke, is the major cause of death among adults with diabetes, accounting for more than half of all deaths in this population. The extent and severity of atherosclerotic lesions in medium-sized and large arteries are increased in patients with long-standing diabetes. The usual protective effect of female sex is eliminated by diabetes, and coronary artery disease develops at a younger age than in nondiabetic persons. Moreover, mortality from myocardial infarction is higher in diabetic than in nondiabetic patients. As indicated above, patients with T2DM frequently exhibit multiple risk factors of the metabolic syndrome that contribute to the development of atherosclerosis.

Atherosclerotic peripheral vascular disease, particularly of the lower extremities, is a common complication of diabetes. Vascular insufficiency leads to ulcers and gangrene of the toes and feet, complications that ultimately necessitate amputation. Indeed, diabetes accounts for 40% of nontraumatic limb amputations in the United States.

Diabetic microvascular disease is a cause of renal failure and blindness. The mechanism(s) whereby hyperglycemia promotes atherosclerosis is the subject of considerable study. A number of pathogenetic factors have been proposed, including glycosylated LDLs that are poorly cleared by the liver, glycosylation and cross-linking of cellular proteins (which can damage the vessel wall), a defect in lipoprotein lipase that impairs the clearance of chylomicrons and leads to postprandial hypertriglyceridemia and accumulation of atherogenic remnant lipoprotein particles. Enhanced platelet aggregation, increased plasma fibrinogen levels, and defective endothelial production of nitric oxide with impaired vasodilation of the arterial wall are also observed in patients with diabetes.

Hyaline arteriolosclerosis (see Fig. 22-7) **and capillary basement membrane thickening** (Figs. 22-1 and 22-8) **are characteristic vascular changes in those with diabetes.** The frequent occurrence of hypertension contributes to the development of the arteriolar lesions. In addition, deposition of basement membrane proteins, which may also become glycosylated, increases in diabetes. Aggregation of platelets in the smaller blood vessels and impaired fibrinolytic mechanisms have also been suggested to play a role in the pathogenesis of diabetic microvascular disease.

Whatever the pathogenetic processes, the effects of microvascular disease on tissue perfusion and wound healing are profound. For example, it is believed to reduce blood flow to the heart, which is already compromised by coronary atherosclerosis. Healing of chronic ulcers that develop from trauma and infection of the feet in diabetic patients is commonly defective, in part because of microvascular disease. The major complications of diabetic microvascular disease involve the kidney and the retina.

Diabetic Nephropathy

Of patients with T1DM, 30 to 40% ultimately develop renal failure. A somewhat smaller proportion (up to 20%) of patients with T2DM are similarly affected. Conversely, since diabetes is such a common condition, diabetic nephropathy accounts for one third of all new cases of renal failure. Although some patients with T1DM die from uremia, most who develop nephropathy succumb to cardiovascular disease, the risk of this complication being 40 times greater in diabetics with end-stage renal disease. The prevalence of diabetic nephropathy increases with the severity and duration of the hyperglycemia. **Kidney disease due to diabetes is the most common reason for renal transplantation in adults.**

Initially, hyperglycemia leads to glomerular hypertension and renal hyperperfusion (Fig. 22-9). Increased glomerular pressure favors the deposition of protein in the mesangium, resulting in glomerulosclerosis and eventually in renal failure. Advanced glycosylation products and lipoprotein abnormalities may contribute to changes in the chemical composition of the glomerular basement membrane. In addition, growth factors (e.g., transforming growth factor-β) have been implicated in some of the cellular abnormalities in . diabetic nephropathy. Regardless of the underlying mechanism, strict control of blood glucose levels retards the development of diabetic nephropathy. Treatment with angiotensin-converting enzyme (ACE) inhibitors, which reduce systemic blood pressure, glomerular hypertension, and renal perfusion, retards the progression of diabetic nephropathy.

Eventually, the glomeruli in the diabetic kidney exhibit a unique lesion termed *Kimmelstiel-Wilson disease or nodular glomerulosclerosis* (see Chapter 30). Two micro-

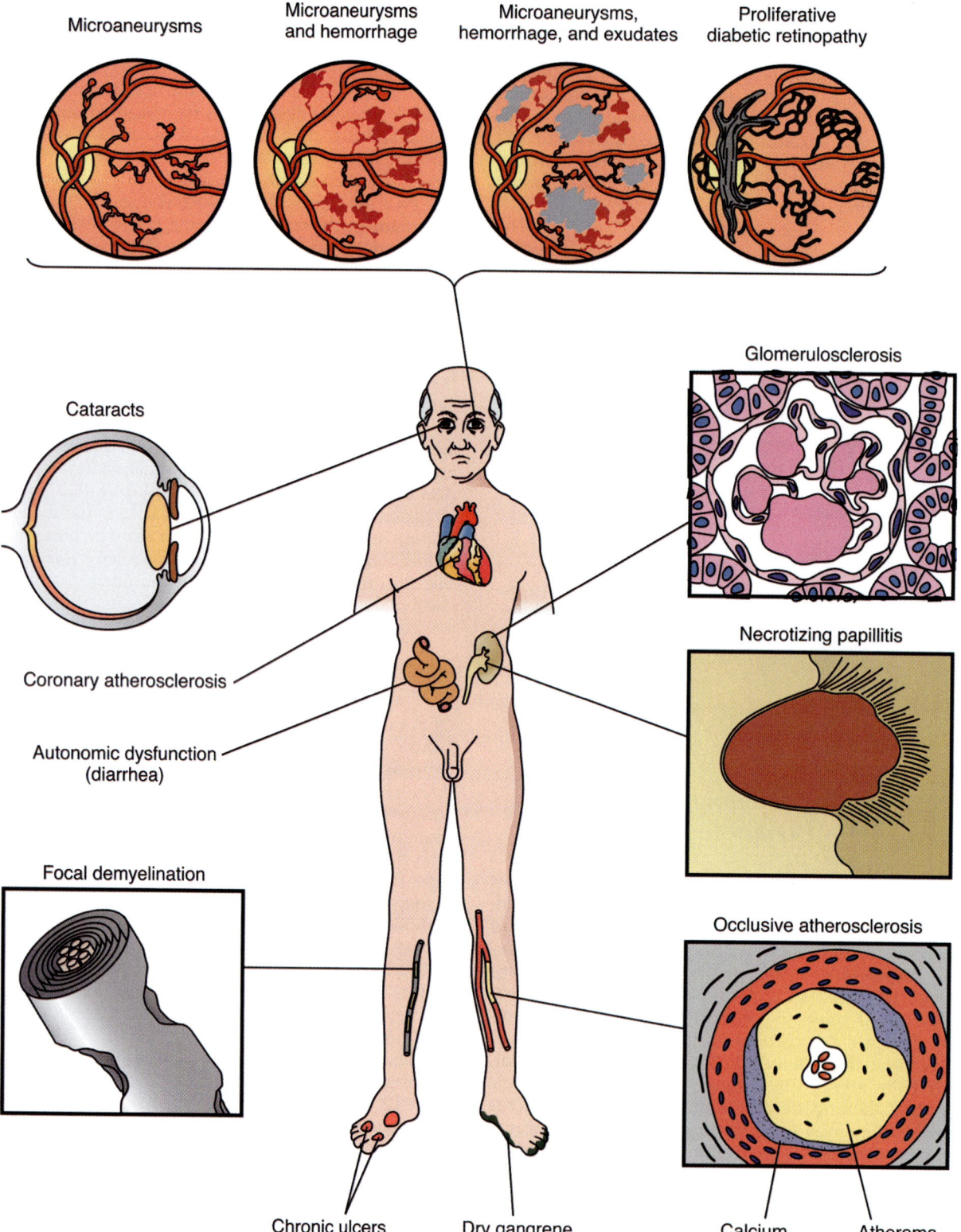

FIGURE 22-8
Secondary complications of diabetes. The effects of diabetes on a number of vital organs result in complications that may be incapacitating (cerebral and peripheral vascular disease), painful (neuropathy), or life threatening (coronary artery disease, pyelonephritis with necrotizing papillitis).

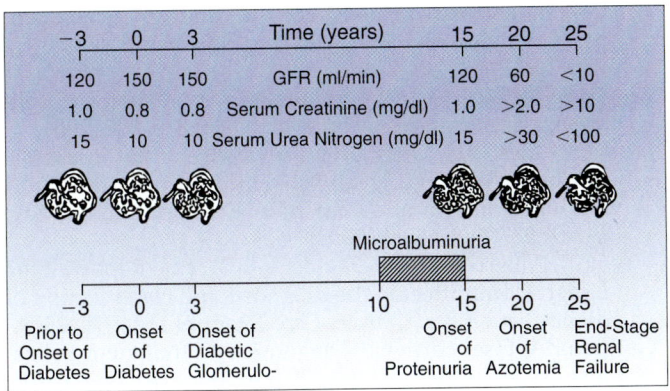

FIGURE 22-9
Natural history of diabetic nephropathy. Initially, renal hypertrophy and hyperfiltration lead to an increase in the glomerular filtration rate (GFR). Once the decline in renal function begins, on average at least 10 years after the onset of diabetes, leakage of a small amount of serum albumin into the urine (microalbuminuria) is the first abnormality that is easily and reliably measured. The elevation in serum creatinine and gross proteinuria occur much later.

scopic patterns are observed. In the more common one, spherical masses of basement membrane-like material accumulate in the lobules of the glomeruli (Fig. 22-10). The other form is characterized by more diffuse, although somewhat irregular, deposition of this material throughout the glomerulus. The latter change must be differentiated from membranous nephropathy. The onset of glomerular disease is heralded clinically by the appearance of small amounts of serum albumin in the urine. Proteinuria increases with the passage of time, and renal function progressively declines.

Diabetic Retinopathy

Diabetic retinopathy is the most important cause of blindness in the Unites States in persons under the age of 60 years, the risk being higher in T1DM than in T2DM. In fact, 10% of patients with T1DM of 30 years' duration become legally blind. Nevertheless, since there are many more patients with T2DM, this group contains most patients with diabetic retinopathy. Retinopathy is the most devastating ophthalmic complication of diabetes, although glaucoma, cataracts, and corneal disease also occur with increased frequency. Like nephropathy, the prevalence of retinopathy in diabetes is related to the duration and degree of glycemic control. Diabetic retinopathy is discussed in detail in Chapter 30.

Diabetic Neuropathy Affects Sensory and Autonomic Innervation

Peripheral sensory impairment and autonomic nerve dysfunction are among the most common and distressing complications of diabetes. Changes in the nerves are complex, and abnormalities in axons, the myelin sheath, and Schwann cells have all been found. In addition, disease of the small blood vessels of the nerves contributes to the disorder. Evidence suggests that hyperglycemia increases the perception of pain, independent of any structural lesions in the nerves.

Peripheral neuropathy is initially characterized by pain and abnormal sensations in the extremities. However, fine touch, pain detection, and proprioception are ultimately lost. As a result, the diabetic tends to ignore irritation and minor trauma to the feet, joints, and lower extremities. Thus, peripheral neuropathy can be a major factor in the development of ulcers of the feet, which so commonly plague patients with severe diabetes. It also plays a role in the painless destructive joint disease that occasionally occurs.

Although autonomic nerve dysfunction is subtle, abnormalities in the neurogenic regulation of cardiovascular and gastrointestinal functions frequently result in postural hypotension and problems of gut motility, such as diarrhea. Erectile dysfunction and retrograde ejaculation are common complications of autonomic dysfunction, although vascular disease is often a contributing factor. Occasionally, diabetics develop a hypotonic urinary bladder, which results in the retention of urine and predisposes to infection.

Infections Principally Involve the Kidney

Bacterial and fungal infections complicate the lives of diabetic patients in whom hyperglycemia is poorly controlled. Multiple abnormalities in the host response to microbial invasion have been described in such patients. Leukocyte function is compromised, and the immune response is blunted. Prior to the use of insulin, tuberculosis and purulent infections were life threatening. Fortunately, with good control, the diabetic patient today is much less susceptible to infections. However, urinary tract infections continue to pose a

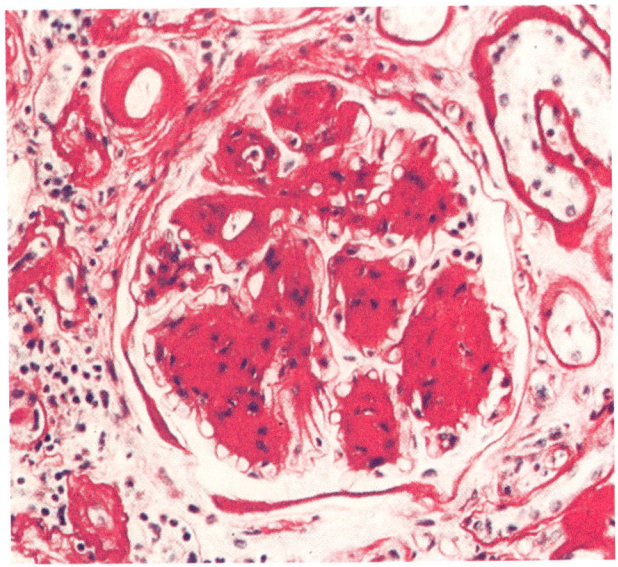

FIGURE 22-10
Diabetic glomerulosclerosis. A periodic acid–Schiff stain demonstrates nodular accumulations of basement membrane-like material in the glomerulus.

problem, because glucose in the urine provides an enriched culture medium. In addition, patients with autonomic neuropathy often have a dystonic bladder that retains urine. Pyelonephritis is a constant threat for patients with diabetes, and necrotizing papillitis may be a devastating complication of renal infection.

Pregnancy May Be Complicated by Diabetes

Although gestational diabetes develops in only a few percent of seemingly healthy women during pregnancy, it continues after parturition in a small proportion of these patients. Pregnancy is a state of insulin resistance, but only pregnant women with compromised β-cell insulin secretion become diabetic. These abnormalities in the amount and timing of pancreatic insulin secretion make these women highly susceptible to overt T2DM later in life.

Diabetic mothers with poor glycemic control may give birth to large infants, making labor and delivery difficult and necessitating a cesarean section. Tight glucose control in the diabetic mother is necessary to prevent overstimulation of the fetal pancreas during gestation. Fetuses exposed to hyperglycemia in utero may develop hyperplasia of the pancreatic β cells, which may secrete insulin autonomously and cause hypoglycemia at birth and in the early neonatal period.

Infants of diabetic mothers show a 5 to 10% incidence of major developmental abnormalities. These include anomalies of the heart and great vessels and neural tube defects, such as anencephaly and spina bifida. The frequency of these lesions relates to the control of maternal diabetes during early gestation.

SUGGESTED READING

Book

Goldstein BJ, Gorstein F (guest eds). *Diabetes mellitus, clinics in laboratory medicine,* vol. 21, no. 1. Philadelphia: WB Saunders, March 2001.

Review Articles

Atkinson MA, Eisenbarth GS: Type 1 diabetes: New perspectives on disease pathogenesis and treatment. *Lancet* 358(9277):221–229, 2001.

Bell GI, Polonsky KS: Diabetes mellitus and genetically programmed defects in beta-cell function. *Nature* 414(6865):788–791, 2001.

Brownlee M: Biochemistry and molecular cell biology of diabetic complications. *Nature* 414(6865):813–820, 2001.

Ford ES, Giles WH, Dietz WH: Prevalence of the metabolic syndrome among US adults—Findings from the Third National Health and Nutrition Examination Survey. *JAMA* 287(3):356–359, 2002.

Gavin JR, Alberti KGMM, Davidson MB, et al.: Report of the Expert Committee on the diagnosis and classification of diabetes mellitus. *Diabetes Care* 23(suppl:1):1–S19, 2000.

Gottlien PA, Eisenbarth GS: Diagnosis and treatment of pre-insulin dependent diabetes. *Annu Rev Med* 49:391–405, 1998.

Harris MI: Diabetes in America: Epidemiology and scope of the problem. *Diabetes Care* 21(suppl 3):C11–C14, 1998.

Kahn BB, Flier JS: Obesity and insulin resistance. *J Clin Invest* 106(4):473–481, 2000.

Kukreja A, MacLaren NK: Autoimmunity and diabetes. *J Clin Endocrinol Metab* 84:4371–4378, 1999.

Marker J, Maclaren N: Immunopathology of immune-mediated (type 1) diabetes. *Clin Lab Med* 21(1):15–30, 2001.

Martin S, Wolf-Eichbaum D, Duinkerken G, et al.: Development of type 1 diabetes despite severe hereditary B-cell deficiency. *N Engl J Med* 345:1036–1040, 2001.

McGowan T, McCue P, Sharma K: Diabetic nephropathy. *Clin Lab Med* 21(1):111–146, 2001.

Meier M, King GL: Protein kinase C activation and its pharmacological inhibition in vascular disease. *Vasc Med* 5(3):173–185, 2000.

Rosenbloom A, Arslanian S, Brink S, et al.: Type 2 diabetes in children and adolescents. *Pediatrics* 105(3):671–680, 2000.

Saltiel AR: New perspectives into the molecular pathogenesis and treatment of type 2 diabetes [Review]. *Cell* 104(4):517–529, 2001.

Saltiel AR, Kahn CR: Insulin signalling and the regulation of glucose and lipid metabolism. *Nature* 414(6865):799–806, 2001.

Stumvoll M, Gerich J: Clinical features of insulin resistance and beta cell dysfunction and the relationship to type 2 diabetes. *Clin Lab Med* 21(1):31–51, 2001.

Unger RH: Lipotoxic diseases. *Annu Rev Med* 53:319–336, 2002.

Zimmet P, Alberti KGMM, Shaw J: Global and societal implications of the diabetes epidemic. *Nature* 414(6865):782–787, 2001.

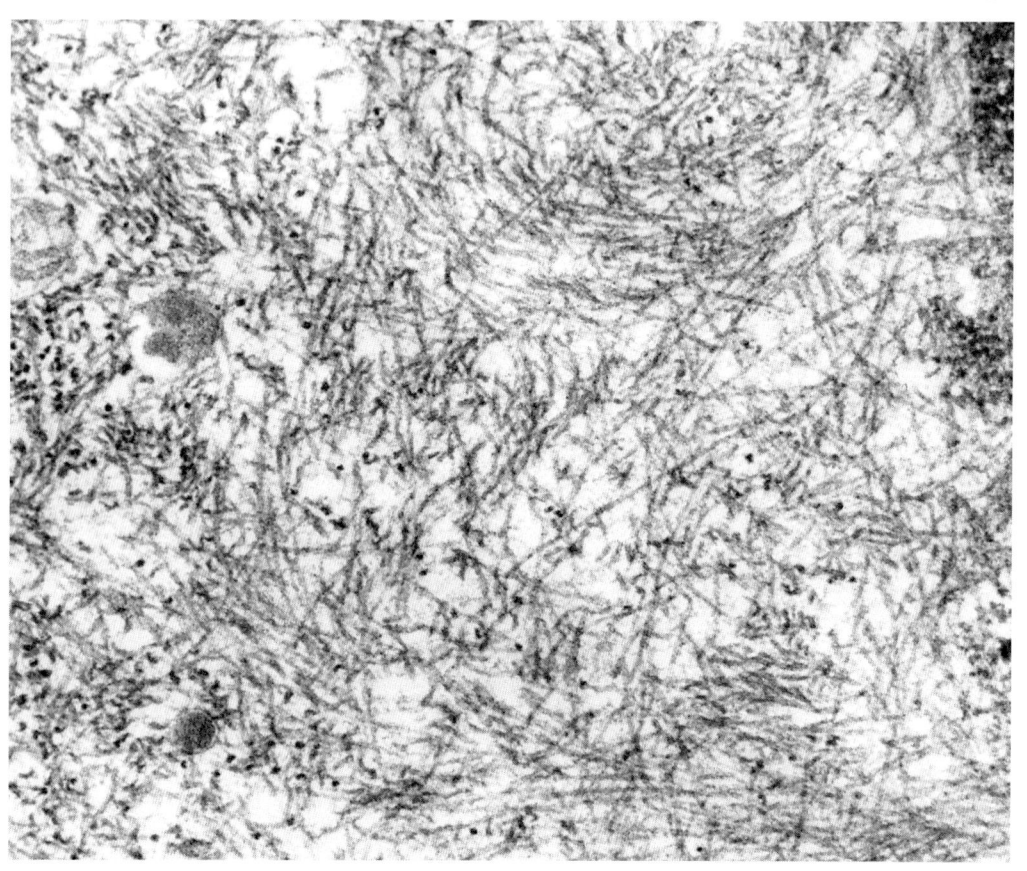

CHAPTER 23

The Amyloidoses

Robert Kisilevsky

Common Components of Amyloid

Staining Properties of Amyloid Deposits

Structure of Amyloid

Definition of Amyloid

Clinical Classification of the Amyloidoses
Primary Amyloidosis
Secondary Amyloidosis
Familial Amyloidosis
Isolated Amyloidosis

Classification of Amyloidoses by the Type of Protein
Aβ2M Amyloid
AL Amyloid
AA Amyloid
APrP Amyloid
ATTR Amyloid (Transthyretin Amyloid)
Other Amyloids

A General Scheme of Amyloidogenesis

Morphological Features of Amyloidoses

Clinical Features of Amyloidoses

Amyloid Treatment Strategies

FIGURE 23-1 *(see opposite page)*
Amyloid deposits in tissue. Parallel and interlacing arrays of fibrils are evident in this electron micrograph.

Amyloid refers to a group of diverse extracellular protein deposits that have (1) common morphological properties, (2) affinities for specific dyes, and (3) a characteristic appearance under polarized light. **Although they vary in amino acid sequence, all amyloid proteins are folded in such as way as to share common ultrastructural and physical properties.**

Disorders associated with amyloid deposition have been known for more than 300 years, but it was not until Virchow's time in the mid-19th century that attempts were made to define the nature of the tissue deposits by their staining properties. Amyloid stained blue with acidified iodine, which was then in use for demonstrating cellulose or starch. This staining not only led to coining of the term *amyloid* (starchlike), but also incorrectly suggested its fundamental nature. Neither starch nor cellulose is a constituent of amyloid, and a different complex carbohydrate is responsible for its iodine-staining properties. Amyloid deposits are composed of two classes of constituents:

A DISEASE-SPECIFIC FIBRILLOGENIC PROTEIN: The nature of this protein varies with the underlying disease. The tertiary structure of the protein and the manner in which it interacts with other molecules are responsible for the characteristics of amyloid. **The specific fibrillogenic protein in various types of amyloid is now the determining factor in the classification of amyloid.**

A SET OF COMMON COMPONENTS FOUND IN ALL AMYLOIDS

- The **amyloid P component (AP)** is a pentagonal, doughnut-shaped protein that is present in all types of amyloid. AP is identical with, and is derived from, a normal circulating serum protein, termed *serum amyloid P (SAP)*. SAP is also a structural component of normal basement membranes.
- **Other molecular building blocks of basement membranes** are present in amyloid and include laminin, collagen type IV, and perlecan (a heparan sulfate proteoglycan). The glycosaminoglycan side chain of perlecan is heparan sulfate. This carbohydrate side chain is probably responsible for the iodine-staining properties of amyloid. It also plays a crucial role in altering the conformation of the disease-specific fibrillogenic proteins.
- **Apolipoprotein E (apoE)** is a constituent of high-density lipoproteins and plays a role in cholesterol transport.

Not all amyloids are the same, and the protein responsible for the fibrillary characteristics varies significantly. For example, in amyloid associated with multiple myeloma, the fibrillogenic component is a product of immunoglobulin light chains produced by myeloma cells. In amyloid associated with inflammatory diseases, the fibrillogenic component is derived from an acute phase protein that is produced by the liver and is unrelated to immunoglobulins. In these two cases, amyloid is deposited systemically.

In other situations, amyloid is deposited only locally. Amyloid in medullary carcinoma of the thyroid is restricted to the tumor deposits, and its fibrillogenic component is derived from a polypeptide hormone related to calcitonin. In the pancreas, amyloid located either in an islet cell tumor or in the islets in type 2 diabetes is derived from a peptide hormone secreted with insulin (amylin, or islet amyloid polypeptide [IAPP]). In Alzheimer disease, the amyloid is restricted to the brain and its blood vessels; yet it is derived from a plasma membrane protein that is found not only in the central nervous system but distributed ubiquitously in the body.

Although the nature of amyloid deposits varies widely and the conditions under which they occur are disparate, a century of usage has entrenched the term *amyloidosis* as connoting a single disease. This notion has today been replaced by the concept that the term should be used generically to designate a group of diseases. **Thus, amyloidosis is characterized by proteinaceous tissue deposits with common morphological, structural, and staining properties but with variable protein composition.**

STAINING PROPERTIES OF AMYLOID DEPOSITS

The staining properties and general appearance of amyloid are governed primarily by the nature of its protein. Because of its compact structure, amyloid has few morphological features visible by light microscopy. When routine stains are used, amyloid is amorphous, glassy, and almost cartilage-like, properties that are responsible for its so-called hyaline appearance. On staining with hematoxylin and eosin, amyloid stains no differently from many other proteins. However, the specific nature and underlying organization of the amyloid proteins, as well as those of associated molecules (glycosaminoglycans and amyloid P component), allow amyloid to be stained in specific ways.

CONGO RED: All amyloids stain red with the Congo red dye (Fig. 23-2A). When the sections stained with Congo red are viewed under polarized light, the deposits exhibit a red-green birefringence (see Fig. 23-2B). The fibrillary deposits organized in one plane have one color, and those organized perpendicular to that plane have the other color. **Congo red is the stain most commonly used for the diagnosis of amyloidosis.**

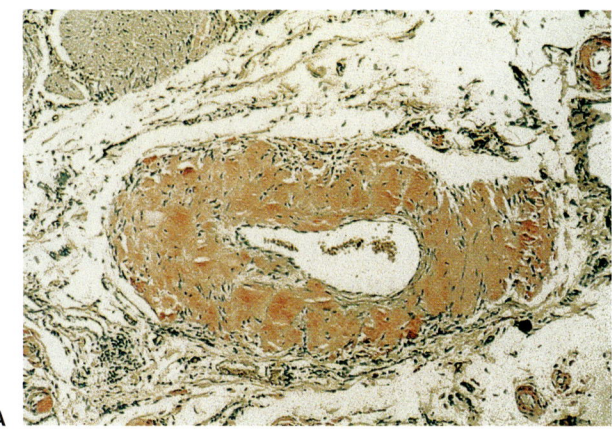 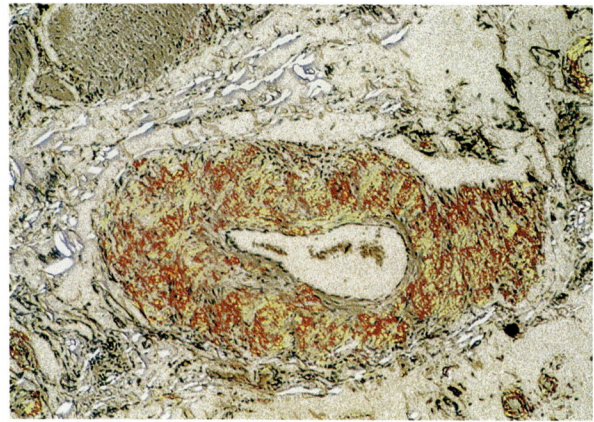

FIGURE 23-2
AL amyloid involving the wall of an artery stained with Congo red is shown under ordinary light (A) and polarized light (B). Note the red–green birefringence of the amyloid. Collagen has a silvery appearance.

THIOFLAVIN T: Although not entirely specific for amyloid, staining with thioflavin t allows the amyloid to fluoresce when viewed in ultraviolet light.

ALCIAN BLUE: The presence of glycosaminoglycans in all amyloid deposits is demonstrated with a variety of Alcian blue stains, which cause the glycosaminoglycans to appear blue.

SPECIFIC ANTIBODIES: The success in isolating various amyloid proteins has led to the preparation of both polyclonal and monoclonal antibodies directed against the different proteins. In turn, immunohistochemical techniques have been devised to demonstrate the presence of AP component, as well as the specific protein present in each type of amyloid.

STRUCTURE OF AMYLOID

All amyloids have a similar ultrastructural appearance, regardless of which protein is responsible for the fibrillary component. By electron microscopy, groups of fibers are arranged in parallel arrays, with each group having a different orientation (see Fig. 23-1). These parallel arrays orient the specific dyes, such as Congo red, and thus give amyloid the ability to rotate polarized light, a property that yields its classic birefringence. Although the individual fibrils vary considerably in length, all have a diameter of 7 to 13 nm. When isolated, individual fibrils usually consist of two or more intertwining strands, each 3.0 to 3.5 nm thick, which are twisted about each other as a shallow helix. However, the structure of the fibril and the composition of amyloid in situ seem to be similar to those of basement membrane microfibrils, on whose surface are the protein-specific filaments organized into 3- nm tight helical protofibrils.

The secondary and tertiary organization of the protein that constitutes the amyloid fibril has been explored by x-ray diffraction and infrared spectroscopy. The individual protein subunits appear to be organized primarily as a **β-pleated sheet**. However, in the case of the amyloid peptide found in inflammatory diseases, there is an abundant α-helical structure as well as one segment organized into a β-pleated sheet. Similar findings have now been made with the amyloid peptides responsible for amyloid in Alzheimer disease and in the pancreatic islets in adult-onset (type 2) diabetes. The individually folded polypeptide subunits are stacked into fibrils. The precise manner and mechanism by which this occurs may be different for each amyloid. The interactions between the polypeptide monomers are responsible for most of the crossed β-pleated sheet structure.

In all amyloids, highly charged glycosaminoglycans, SAP, the other basement membrane components (laminin and collagen IV), and apoE, are present in close association with the amyloid deposits. In at least six types of amyloid, the basement membrane form of heparan sulfate proteoglycan (perlecan) has been identified as the charged component. But, other heparan sulfate proteoglycans may play a similar role in other forms of amyloid (e.g., agrin in Alzheimer disease). The interaction of amyloid protein precursors with the common components probably changes the conformational stability of the disease-specific protein, shifting it in favor of amyloidogenic intermediates, which in turn interact as β-pleated sheets. Thus, the basic fibril seems not to be formed simply as a result of the primary structure of the precursor or the protein fragment. Fibril formation is most likely influenced by the manner in which the protein fragment interacts with additional components. The common secondary and tertiary organization of the proteins then results in uniform structural and staining properties.

DEFINITION OF AMYLOID

The staining and structural properties of amyloid allow a general definition, based primarily on its morphological characteristics.

- All forms of amyloid stain positively with Congo red and show red–green birefringence when viewed under polarized light.

- Ultrastructurally, all forms of amyloid consist of interlacing bundles of parallel arrays of fibrils, which have a diameter of 7 to 13 nm.
- The protein in the amyloid fibrils contains a large proportion of crossed β-pleated sheet structure.

CLINICAL CLASSIFICATION OF THE AMYLOIDOSES

The classification of amyloidosis has undergone a major change (Table 23-1), primarily because of the realization that the specific protein found in each type of amyloid overlaps previous groupings. For example, the amyloid protein of familial Mediterranean fever (an inherited disorder) and that deposited secondarily in a variety of inflammatory disease are one and the same. Similarly, the proteins found in "primary" amyloidosis and in amyloid associated with a variety of plasma cell dyscrasias are identical. The amyloid of isolated cardiac amyloidosis and that of senile systemic amyloidosis are also indistinguishable.

The older clinical classifications did not take protein structure into account. For example, familial Mediterranean fever and familial amyloidotic polyneuropathy were grouped together as "familial" forms of amyloid, a classification that implies a similar process in each disease. This concept is not supported by current information. The older classification is still used in clinical medicine, and the newer groupings, based on the protein type, are now coming into general use. For this reason, both classifications must be reviewed.

The older classification is based on the clinical presentation of the patient and categorizes amyloidosis as primary, secondary, familial, or isolated. Primary, secondary, and familial amyloidoses are usually, but not always, systemic diseases, in which patients frequently present with renal dysfunction or heart failure. The liver, spleen, gastrointestinal tract, tongue, and subcutaneous tissues are also frequent sites of amyloid deposition. Isolated amyloidosis is, by definition, restricted to a single organ.

Primary Amyloidosis Refers to the Presentation of Amyloid without Any Preceding Disease

In one third of these cases, primary amyloidosis is the harbinger of frank **plasma cell neoplasia**, such as multiple myeloma or other B-cell lymphomas. In this respect, primary amyloidosis forms part of the spectrum of amyloid disorders associated with B-cell dysfunction but differs from other types in that the amyloid appears before, rather than after, the overt malignancy. Regardless of whether amyloidosis or the B-cell neoplasm presents first, the type of amyloid protein is the same.

Secondary Amyloidosis Complicates Inflammatory Conditions

Secondary amyloidosis is associated with a previously existing, persistent inflammatory disorder, which may or may not have an immunological basis. Patients with rheumatoid arthritis, ankylosing spondylitis, and occasionally systemic lupus erythematosus may develop secondary amyloidosis. Most other patients with secondary amyloidosis have conditions that are complicated by long-standing inflammation (e.g., lung abscess, tuberculosis, or osteomyelitis). These disorders were the most common causes of systemic amyloidosis in the past, but the use of antibiotics and modern surgical

TABLE 23-1 Classification of Amyloids

Amyloid Protein	Protein Precursor	Clinical Setting
AA	apoSAA	Persistent acute inflammation
AL	κ or λ light chain	Multiple myeloma, plasma cell dyscrasias, and primary amyloid
AH	γ chain	Waldenström macroglobulinemia
ATTR	Transthyretin	Familial amyloidotic polyneuropathy (FAP), normal TTR in senile systemic amyloid
AApoAI	apoAI	FAP Iowa
AGel	Gelsolin	Familial amyloidosis, Finnish
ACys	Cystatin C	Hereditary cerebral hemorrhage with amyloid (HCHWA), Icelandic
ALys	Lysozyme	Hereditary systemic amyloidosis, Ostertag-type
AFib	Fibrinogen	Hereditary renal amyloidosis
Aβ	β-protein precursor	Alzheimer disease
		Down syndrome, HCHWA Dutch
APrP	Prion protein	CJD[a], scrapie, BSE[a], GSS[a], Kuru
ACal	(Pro)calcitonin	Medullary carcinoma of the thyroid
AANF	Atrial naturetic factor	Isolated atrial amyloid
AIAPP	Islet amyloid polypeptide	Type 2 diabetes, insulinomas
AIns	Insulin	Islet amyloid in the degu (a rodent)
AApoAII	ApoAII (murine)	Amyloid in senescence accelerated mice

[a] CJD, Creutzfeldt-Jakob disease; BSE, bovine spongiform encephalopathy; GSS, Gerstmann-Straussler-Sheinker syndrome.

techniques have drastically reduced the frequency of this complication.

Currently, secondary amyloidosis also occurs in persons who develop chronic skin abscesses as a result of subcutaneous self-administration of narcotics, and patients with cystic fibrosis who now live long enough with recurrent lung infections to develop amyloidosis as a complication. Secondary amyloidosis is also seen in patients with specific cancers, such as Hodgkin disease and renal cell carcinoma. The amyloid protein deposited secondary to these malignancies is identical to that seen in rheumatoid arthritis, chronic infections, and familial Mediterranean fever.

Familial Amyloidoses Show an Ethnic Distribution

Several geographical populations display genetically inherited forms of amyloidosis.

FAMILIAL MEDITERRANEAN FEVER (FMF): This autosomal recessive disease is found predominantly in the Mediterranean basin among Sephardic Jews and Turks, although Armenians and Arabs may also be affected. More than 90% of the Jewish patients in Israel are of Sephardic origin. FMF is characterized by polymorphonuclear leukocyte dysfunction and recurrent episodes of serositis, including peritonitis. Since there is recurrent inflammation, the type of amyloid protein deposited is the same as that in amyloidosis secondary to acquired inflammatory disorders. The gene for Mediterranean fever *(MEFV)* has been mapped to the short arm of chromosome 16, encoding a protein termed *pyrin* or more poetically, *mare nostrin*. It is expressed in neutrophils and is thought to be a transcription factor that regulates other genes involved in the suppression of inflammation.

FAMILIAL AMYLOIDOTIC POLYNEUROPATHY (FAP): This is usually an autosomal dominant genetic disorder, in which at least 60 mutations, scattered throughout the amyloidogenic protein, have been described. Each protein gives rise to a clinical variant of the disease. FAP exhibits a predilection for peripheral and autonomic nerves. The most common variant is due to a methionine for valine substitution at residue 30 in **transthyretin**, the protein responsible for this form of amyloidosis. This met30 variant has been described primarily in three nationalities, namely, Swedish, Portuguese, and Japanese. Interestingly, the demographic distribution of FAP in Japan occurs primarily in a region where the Portuguese had established a colony. Portugal, the area where this disorder is most frequent, was originally visited and settled by Viking seamen. Whether the mutation responsible for this form of familial amyloidosis originated in Scandinavia or whether identical mutations arose in different geographical populations remains to be determined.

HEREDITARY CONGOPHILIC ANGIOPATHY (ICELANDIC): Also termed hereditary cerebral hemorrhage with amyloid (HCHWA), this form of amyloidosis is the result of a mutation in cystatin-c, a protease inhibitor.

HEREDITARY CONGOPHILIC ANGIOPATHY (DUTCH): HCHWA (Dutch) is similar clinically and pathologically to the Icelandic variety but results from a mutation in the amyloid-forming segment of the Aβ protein precursor of Alzheimer disease (see below). These patients do not, however, manifest dementia.

Isolated Amyloidosis

Isolated amyloidosis has been described in the major arteries, lung, heart, and various joints and in association with endocrine tumors that secrete polypeptide hormones. In endocrine tumors, the amyloid is usually part of a hormone or a prohormone. By far, the most common organ-specific amyloids are those found in the aorta in atherosclerosis, in Alzheimer disease, and in type 2 diabetes.

Aortic Atherosclerosis and Arterial Inflammations

Amyloid has long been known to be present in the wall of the aorta at sites of atherosclerosis and in arteries with inflammation (e.g., giant cell arteritis) associated with elastic lamina. The amyloid peptide isolated in these conditions has been designated *medin*, classified as **Amed,** and shown to be a 50-residue proteolytic fragment derived from lactadherin. This precursor was previously described in milk fat-globule membranes and is also synthesized by smooth muscle cells of the arterial media. The function of this protein is unknown.

Alzheimer Disease

In the most common form of dementia, Alzheimer disease, Aβ amyloid is restricted to the brain and its vessels. The deposited protein, a 4-kilodalton peptide called the *Aβ protein*, is a fragment of a larger Aβ-protein precursor (AβPP), which is a normal cell membrane constituent. The longer part of AβPP is extracellular, with the remainder traversing the cell membrane and ending in a cytoplasmic portion of approximately 100 amino acids. The Aβ protein itself is a segment of 40 to 43 amino acids that lies immediately outside and partially within the cell membrane. AβPP is present not only in the cells of the central nervous system but also in most other tissues. There are at least five mRNA splicing products of the *AβPP* gene, several of which have been identified in the brain, but only one of which (AβPP-695) is brain specific. It is generally accepted, but has never been demonstrated, that the Aβ protein giving rise to Aβ amyloid is derived from a cell in the central nervous system. Since AβPP is present in so many cell types, it is still possible that the source of Aβ for the vascular amyloid or the brain parenchymal amyloid in Alzheimer disease is extracerebral.

Aβ Protein is derived from AβPP by a series of proteolytic steps, catalyzed by enzymes termed *secretases*. The α secretase cuts within the Aβ-protein segment and thus precludes its involvement in producing the Aβ-protein fragment. The β and γ secretases, respectively, cut at the amino- and carboxy-terminal ends of Aβ-protein, thereby generating the 40- to 43-residue amyloidogenic fragment. Mutations adjacent to these cleavage sites (but not within the Aβ-protein) are associated with several familial forms of Alzheimer disease, suggesting that amyloid is important in the pathogenesis of Alzheimer disease.

The gene for AβPP is located on chromosome 21, which likely explains the observation that patients with **Down syndrome** (trisomy 21) all develop the morphological lesions of Alzheimer disease by 35 years of age. Several other genes, in addition to AβPP, have been implicated in both the pathogenesis of Alzheimer disease and the deposition of Aβ. These include a locus on chromosome 19 that codes for apoE, one of the common constituents of all amyloids. The E_4 isoform of apoE is linked to Alzheimer disease. Loci on chromosomes 1 and 4, which code for two related proteins, called *presenilins*, have also been linked to Alzheimer disease. Mutations in these proteins influence γ secretase activity and thus the production and processing of Aβ protein. In tissue culture, the Aβ protein in a random conformation is innocuous to neurons. However, folding of the protein into a β sheet containing protofibrils and its organization into Aβ in vivo confers neuronal toxicity in vitro and in vivo. There is also evidence that TGF-β1 may contribute to amyloid deposition in Alzheimer disease through its capacity to induce amyloid-binding proteins.

Diabetes

The amyloid deposited in the islets of Langerhans in type 2 diabetes is also derived from a larger precursor, a peptide related to a variant of calcitonin, termed *islet amyloid polypeptide (IAPP)*, or *amylin*. Like insulin, this novel hormone is produced by the β cells of the islets and seems to have a profound effect on glucose uptake by the liver and striated muscle cells. In transgenic mice that synthesize human amylin, overproduction of this protein leads to islet amyloid. These observations imply that islet amyloid is involved in the pathogenesis of type 2 diabetes, although the subject requires further study.

Senile Cardiac Amyloidosis

Isolated amyloid deposition may occur in the heart, particularly in men, after the age of 70 years. This disorder is usually asymptomatic, but occasionally, extensive deposits in the myocardium may cause heart failure. The amyloid precursor responsible is **transthyretin**.

CLASSIFICATION OF AMYLOIDOSES BY THE TYPE OF PROTEIN

Isolation and characterization of many of the fibrillar proteins in the various forms of amyloid has prompted a reconsideration of the groupings into which each specific disorder should be placed. It is now apparent that (1) specific forms of secondary amyloidosis share a common protein with primary amyloidosis, (2) familial Mediterranean fever should be grouped with secondary forms occurring in association with inflammatory disorders and some cancers, and (3) there are isolated forms of amyloidosis that involve single-organ systems that have the same type of protein found in familial amyloidotic polyneuropathy. The presence of amyloid deposits with identical proteins in seemingly distinct clinical entities implies that common pathological processes occur. These various amyloid proteins are designated A (amyloid), followed by a letter or abbreviation that refers to the specific origin of the protein. Currently, 24 different amyloidogenic proteins have been isolated and identified from human or animal tissues.

The most common clinically related amyloids are (1) AMed and atherosclerosis (2) Aβ and Alzheimer disease, (3) AIAPP (islet amyloid polypeptide) and type 2 diabetes, and (4) Aβ2M and chronic dialysis. The first three are covered above.

Aβ2M Amyloid Is Associated with Renal Dialysis

The deposition of amyloid formed from $β_2$-microglobulin (β2M) is a relatively new disease, characterized by a **destructive arthropathy, owing to amyloid deposition in the major joints of patients undergoing chronic renal dialysis.** Because dialysis has been in common use for only 25 to 30 years and more than 8 to 10 years are required before the manifestations of Aβ2M become apparent, the disease did not appear as a clinical entity until the early 1980s. Today, most (50–75%) patients undergoing dialysis for more than 10 years manifest this disorder. Aβ2M amyloid is deposited in the subchondral bone and periarticular tissues as well as in the gastrointestinal tract. The circulating level of β2M, which serves as the precursor pool for amyloid deposition, is markedly increased in patients with renal failure. The intact normal protein is deposited, and neither proteolytic processing nor a mutation is involved in the pathogenesis of Aβ2M deposition.

AL Amyloid Derives from Immunoglobulin Light Chains

The first amyloid protein to be isolated and sequenced was AL amyloid, which was derived from patients who had primary amyloidosis or multiple myeloma. **AL amyloid usually consists of the variable region of immunoglobulin light chains (L, light) and can be derived from either the κ or λ moieties.** Occasionally, the AL amyloid subunit is larger than the variable end of light chains, in which case it may represent the complete immunoglobulin light chain. Within an individual patient, the sequence of AL amyloid protein is constant, regardless of the organ from which the amyloid is isolated. The amino acid sequence of the variable region of urinary Bence Jones protein corresponds to the patient's AL protein. Since the light chains produced by the neoplastic cells in plasma cell dyscrasias are unique to each patient, **AL amyloid isolated from different persons differs in its amino acid sequence.**

AL protein is common to primary amyloidosis and amyloidosis associated with either multiple myeloma, B-cell lymphomas, or other plasma cell dyscrasias. AL protein in isolated nodules of lung amyloid is a product of focal aggregates of plasma cells. Since one third of patients who first present with "primary" amyloidosis subsequently develop plasma cell abnormalities or frank myeloma, "primary" amyloidosis, multiple myeloma, and immunoblastic lymphomas apparently form a spectrum of a single disorder. In some cases, the malignant disease presents first as multiple myeloma or lymphoma; in other cases, it is announced by AL deposits in various tissues.

Only some patients with multiple myeloma develop AL amyloid, probably because some κ or λ chains are more fibrillogenic than others. The mechanism by which AL amyloid is deposited is summarized in Figure 23-3.

Classification of Amyloidoses by the Type of Protein 1193

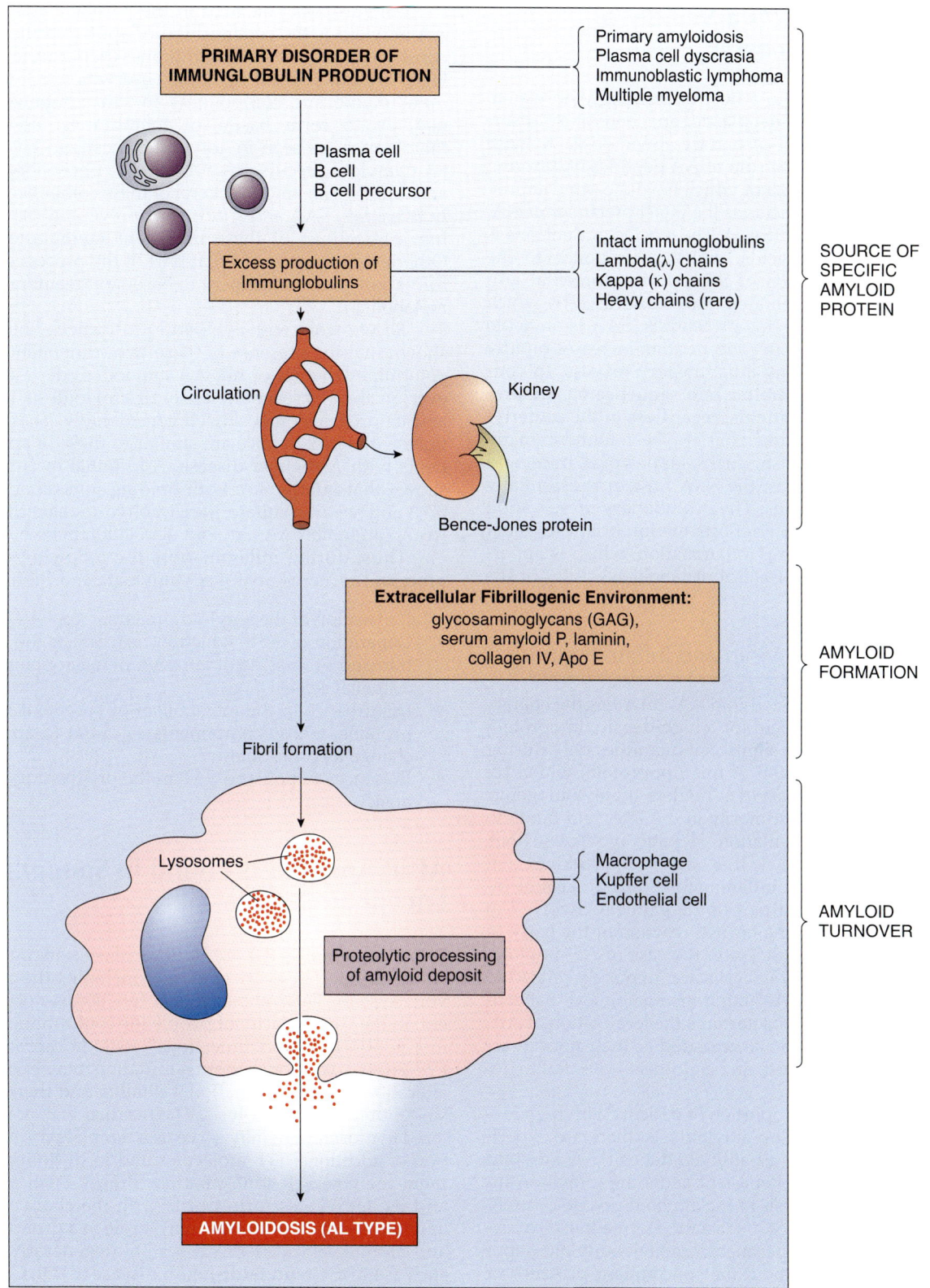

FIGURE 23-3
The mechanism of AL amyloid deposition.

AA Amyloid Reflects a Variety of Inflammatory Processes

AA amyloid is common to a host of seemingly unrelated, persistent inflammatory, neoplastic, and hereditary disorders that lead to so-called secondary amyloidosis. As with AL amyloid, there is a spectrum of AA peptides of differing size within AA deposits, all of which have the same amino-terminal sequence. This includes the intact precursor of AA, namely serum amyloid A (SAA). The most prevalent size is a peptide of 76 amino acids, which corresponds to the amino-terminal two thirds of SAA. In experimental animals, intact SAA is incorporated into AA fibrils, after which it undergoes postfibrillogenic proteolysis. SAA is an acute phase protein, whose serum concentration increases rapidly up to 1000-fold during any inflammatory process. **In contrast to AL protein, the amino acid sequence of AA proteins is identical in all patients, regardless of the underlying disorder.** The SAA protein has also been found in many other species, including fish, ducks, guinea pigs, mice, and monkeys. In these animals, the SAA protein is essentially the same as that in humans. The evolutionary preservation of the amino acid sequence reflects the important role that SAA probably plays during inflammation, which is apparently concerned with cholesterol metabolism at sites of tissue injury.

Deposition of AA Amyloid and Inflammation

Circulating SAA is converted into AA. SAA has the characteristics of an apolipoprotein for a high-density lipoprotein (HDL); yet it is present in significant quantities only during inflammation. Denaturation of this lipoprotein, which releases a subunit termed *apoSAA*, renders it amyloidogenic. ApoSAA is synthesized primarily in the liver and binds to HDL on entering the circulation. Hepatic apoSAA mRNA synthesis is induced by IL-1, IL-6, and TNF, cytokines that are released by activated inflammatory cells at sites of inflammation. Thus, at least part of the pathway involved in AA deposition involves the normal reaction of the body to acute inflammatory stimuli. As in the case of AL amyloid, macrophages and endothelial cells are intimately related to AA amyloid deposition. Although the anatomical distribution of these cells seems to determine the localization of AA, amyloid deposition cannot be regarded as their normal activity. Why do inflammatory and endothelial cells fail to degrade SAA completely?

While only a small proportion of patients with high levels of SAA actually develop amyloidosis, there are experimental models in which all animals deposit AA amyloid within a matter of days. Persistent acute inflammation induces not only the synthesis of the amyloid precursor SAA, but also the appearance of a substance termed *amyloid enhancing factor (AEF)*. In experimental models, amyloid deposition does not occur without the concomitant presence of AEF, which has characteristics analogous to those of a crystallization nidus, serving as a template for AA amyloid fibril formation. In this respect it has features analogous to those of the "infectious" particle that plays a role in transmissible spongiform encephalopathies, the prion protein (see below). When injected intravenously, AEF localizes to macrophages and endothelial cells, thereby altering their metabolic processing of SAA.

An additional element in the pathogenesis of murine AA amyloid is the codeposition of apoE and the structural constituents of basement membranes (perlecan, laminin, collagen IV, and SAP). Despite the observation that these basement membrane components in vitro organize spontaneously to form basement membranes, no basement membranes are seen in amyloid deposits in vivo. At least four amyloid precursors—SAA, IAPP, phosphorylated Tau, and AβPP—can bind to several of these components in vitro. In two cases, SAA and AβPP, they prevent the normal binding interactions of these basement membrane proteins. Other evidence suggests that part of the process of amyloid formation is a derangement in basement membrane protein metabolism.

Recent work with apoE and SAP "knock-out" mice has shown that the presence of these two components does not determine whether or not AA amyloid is deposited. However, in their absence the onset of amyloidosis is delayed, and its progression is slowed considerably. These observations with apoE in mice are similar to those of apoE4 in patients with Alzheimer disease. Additional recent work has shown that interference with binding interactions between SAA and heparan sulfate, the carbohydrate side chain of perlecan, can inhibit AA amyloid deposition in vivo.

Thus, during inflammation, the following coincident processes are necessary for AA amyloid deposition (Fig. 23-4):

- Generation of the amyloid precursor apoSAA
- Generation of AEF, which in turn affects the conformation and processing of apoSAA in macrophages and endothelial cells
- Disturbance in the metabolism of basement membrane proteins, whose components can bind to apoSAA and change its conformation
- Presence of apoE and SAP in the progression of amyloidosis

APrP Amyloid Is Found in Spongiform Encephalopathies

Prion proteins (PrPs) are natural plasma membrane constituents found in a variety of cells, including the central nervous system. Their physiological function is not yet apparent. In the vast majority of people the conformation of PrP is in a nonfibrillar, non-"infectious" state. In rare instances, a PrP protein, with or without a mutation, may experience an alteration in its conformational stability and then an altered susceptibility to proteolysis. The residual PrP, now in an altered conformation, may serve as a template for the association of additional PrP molecules and in so doing confer on them the new PrP conformation (PrPsc). Such altered PrP and its aggregates form fibrils with the characteristics of amyloid and are believed to play a role in a group of human and animal central nervous system degenerative diseases such as **kuru, Creutzfeldt-Jakob disease (CJD), Gerstmann-Straussler-Sheinker disease (GSS), scrapie, and bovine spongiform encephalopathy (BSE, mad cow disease) (see Chapter 28).** In the case of kuru and BSE, the evidence is clear that ingestion of tissue contaminated with PrPsc can induce the PrPsc conformation and the disease in recipients. Cases of CJD have been reported after surgical implantation of tissue transplants or the use of pituitary extracts from infected individuals. Such clinical experience highlights the human

Classification of Amyloidoses by the Type of Protein

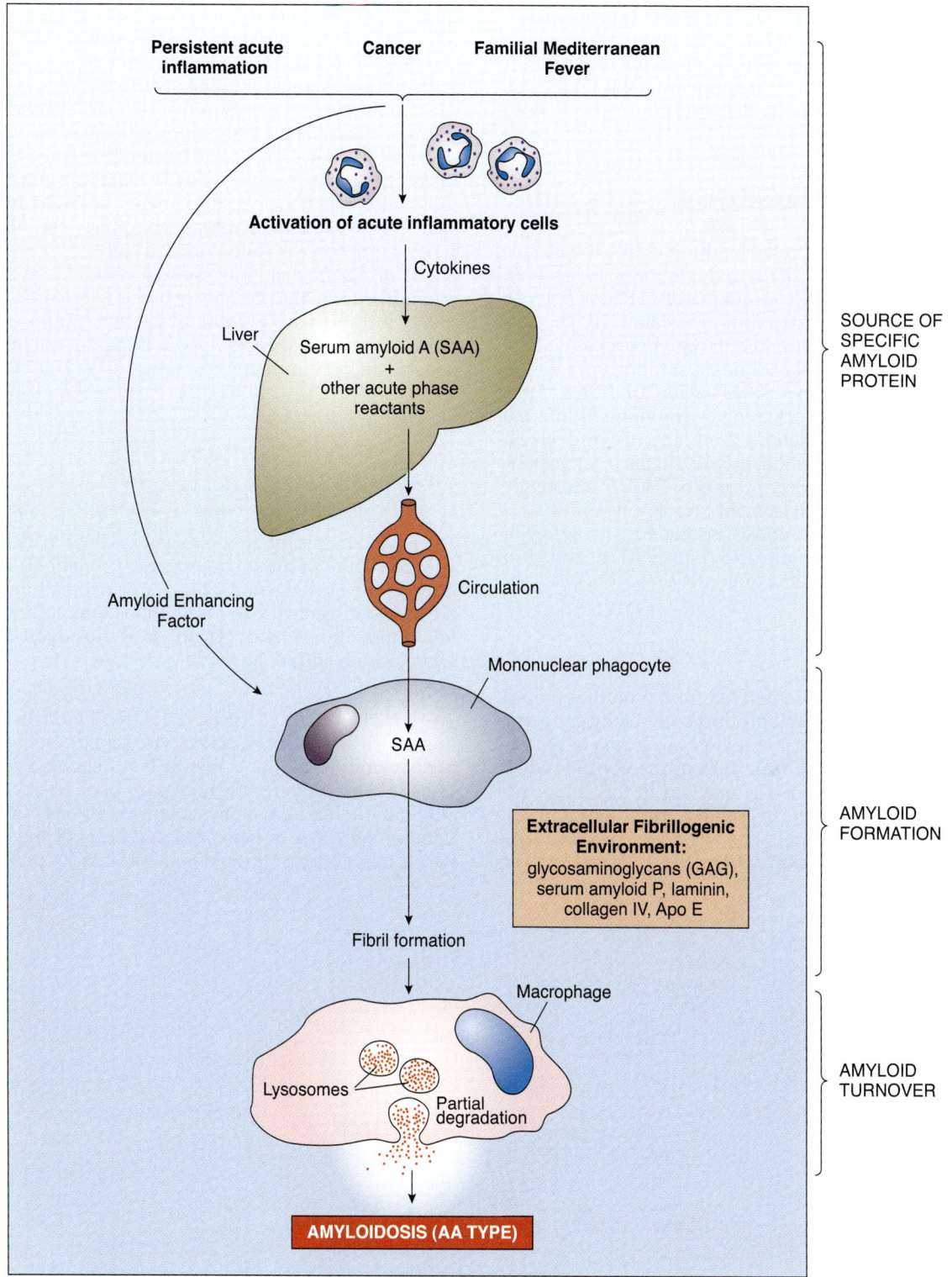

FIGURE 23-4
The mechanism of AA amyloid deposition. A variety of diseases is associated with the activation of polymorphonuclear leukocytes and macrophages, which in turn leads to the synthesis and release of acute phase reactants by the liver, including SAA. SAA in the presence of amyloid-enhancing factor (AEF) is likely released substantially intact by macrophages. In a fibrillogenic environment the released product complexes with glycosaminoglycans and SAP as AA amyloid. This deposit is then processed by macrophages.

and veterinary health issues related to the transmission of PrP conformational disorders. Nevertheless, the "infectious" nature of PrPsc is not one of replication of the exogenous transferred PrPsc, but rather the influence it has on the conformation of the endogenous PrP and the medical consequences that ensue.

ATTR Amyloid (Transthyretin Amyloid)

Transthyretin (TTR) is secreted by the liver into the plasma, where it serves as a carrier of thyroid hormones and as a retinal binding protein. At least 60 mutants of TTR have been described, each responsible for a clinical variant FAP. The most common form of familial amyloidotic polyneuropathy (FAP) is caused by a methionine for valine substitution in TTR at position 30. This mutation lowers the stability of the tetrameric native TTR, allowing the formation of a monomeric intermediate with altered conformation. There is a satisfying correlation between the mutations that give rise to the most unstable tetramers and the most severe forms of FAP. Interestingly, normal TTR is deposited in isolated cardiac amyloidosis and in a systemic form of amyloidosis associated with aging, indicating that an altered amino acid sequence is not an absolute requirement for the deposition of ATTR.

Other Amyloids

Other forms of amyloid are derived from a normal preprohormone or from a hormonal product secreted by endocrine tissue or endocrine tumors. Medullary carcinoma of the thyroid originates from the C-type cells of the thyroid, which normally secrete calcitonin. The amyloid in this tumor is a fragment of procalcitonin. In isolated atrial amyloid, the peptide is atrial natriuretic factor. Amyloid proteins have been characterized in the skin, where they are related to keratin. There are other examples of isolated forms of human amyloidosis for which there is little structural information. An example is amyloid in osteoarthritic joints associated with aging, a frequent finding at autopsy.

Conformational instability of several other proteins with amyloid-like fibril formation is believed to play a role in several other diseases (see Chapter 28). Thus, phosphorylated tau protein, complexed with heparan sulfate, has been identified as paired helical filaments in the neurons of patients with Alzheimer disease. Similarly the filaments in Lewy bodies in patients with Parkinson disease are composed of α synuclein. This protein rapidly forms such filaments in vitro in the presence of heparin/heparan sulfate. Finally, intranuclear protein filaments composed of long polyglutamine sequences appear to play a role in neurodegeneration in Huntington disease.

A GENERAL SCHEME OF AMYLOIDOGENESIS

The requirements for amyloidogenesis in vivo include (1) an adequate pool of an amyloidogenic protein, (2) a nidus or nucleus for fibrillogenesis, (3) conformational instability of the amyloidogenic protein (mutations, proteolysis, and protein interactions) and (4) amyloid turnover. These are schematically interrelated in Figure 23-5.

AN ADEQUATE PRECURSOR POOL: In some settings, such as ATTR associated with senile systemic or senile cardiac amyloid, the constitutive hepatic synthesis of transthyretin provides the necessary pool. In other forms of amyloid, such as AA, a physiological response as part of inflammation leads to increased synthesis of the precursor, which inadvertently provides the necessary pool. Alterna-

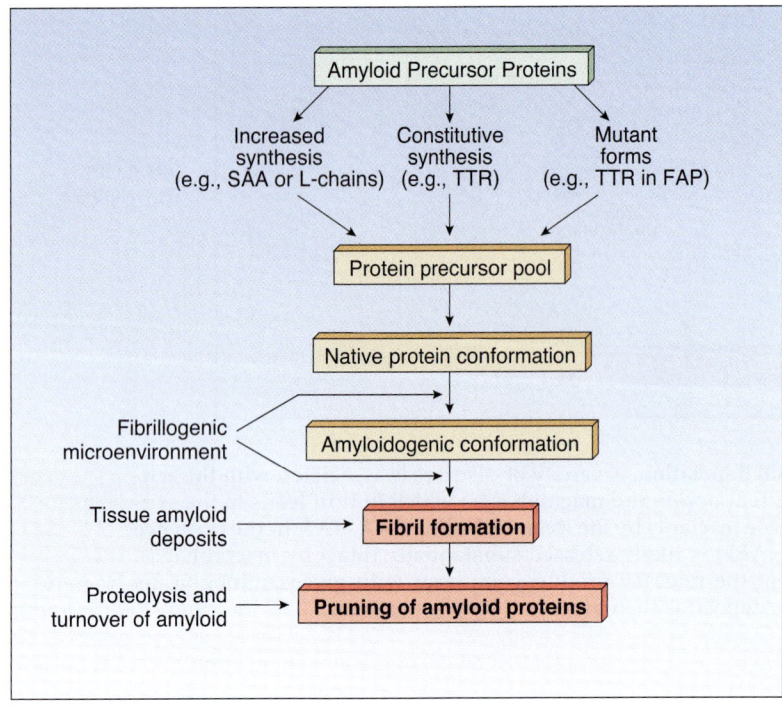

FIGURE 23-5
General scheme for amyloidogenesis.

tively, mutations may alter a nonamyloidogenic protein, providing it with an amyloidogenic sequence and generating the required pool.

ANATOMICAL LOCALIZATION OF AMYLOID: The physiological function of the amyloid precursor probably determines the location of the specific form of amyloid. For instance, SAA, the precursor of AA, may target high density lipoproteins (HDL) to macrophages and endothelial cells. Mishandling of SAA by such cells would set the stage for local AA deposition. Similarly, a mutation may not only provide an amyloidogenic sequence, but may also cause the protein to interact with different cells. Thus, the same protein in mutant and normal forms may be involved in amyloid at different anatomical sites. For example, normal TTR is found in the heart in senile cardiac amyloidosis. Yet in FAP, the same protein in its mutant form is deposited as ATTR in the peripheral nervous system.

ALTERED MICROENVIRONMENTS, FIBRILLIZATION NUCLEI AND CONFORMATIONAL INSTABILITY: An appropriate microenvironment is necessary for the precursor protein to present as amyloid. This environment likely involves changes in the metabolism of basement membrane proteins and direct molecular interactions of these proteins with the amyloidogenic protein. Examples include SAA, tau, α synuclein, IAPP, or Aβ and their interaction with heparan sulfate. In these cases, this interaction changes the conformation of the amyloidogenic protein, thereby increasing its β-sheet content. A fibrillization nucleus may aid and abet this process by driving the equilibrium away from the native conformation in favor of the amyloid one.

PROTEOLYSIS AND TURNOVER: In some forms of amyloid, proteolysis of the precursor may be part of its processing or posttranslational modification. These prefibrillogenic steps generate a normal peptide or protein, which under appropriate conditions may lead to amyloid deposition. The conversion of AβPP into Aβ in Alzheimer disease is an example. Proteolysis of amyloid precursors, which generates the varied sizes of peptides found in individual deposits, is inferred to occur at a step beyond the incorporation of the precursor into the amyloid fibrils. Proteases in various tissues process the fibrils until further degradation becomes difficult. Thus, the size of the residual amyloid peptides varies in any given deposit.

MORPHOLOGICAL FEATURES OF AMYLOIDOSES

When first deposited, amyloid fibrils are usually in close association with subendothelial basement membranes (Fig. 23-6). **Because amyloid accumulates along stromal networks, the deposits take on the architectural framework of the organs involved.** The morphological differences in amyloid deposition from one organ to the next simply reflect the differing stromal organization of each tissue. For example, in the medulla of the kidney, amyloid is laid down in a longitudinal fashion, parallel to the tubules and vasa recta. By contrast, in the glomerulus (Figs. 23-7 and 23-8), amyloid appears in a pattern determined by the lobular architecture of that structure. Splenic amyloid may be associated with either the stroma of the red pulp or that of the white pulp. On gross examination, amyloid in the red pulp imparts a diffusely pale and waxy appearance, the so-called lardaceous spleen.

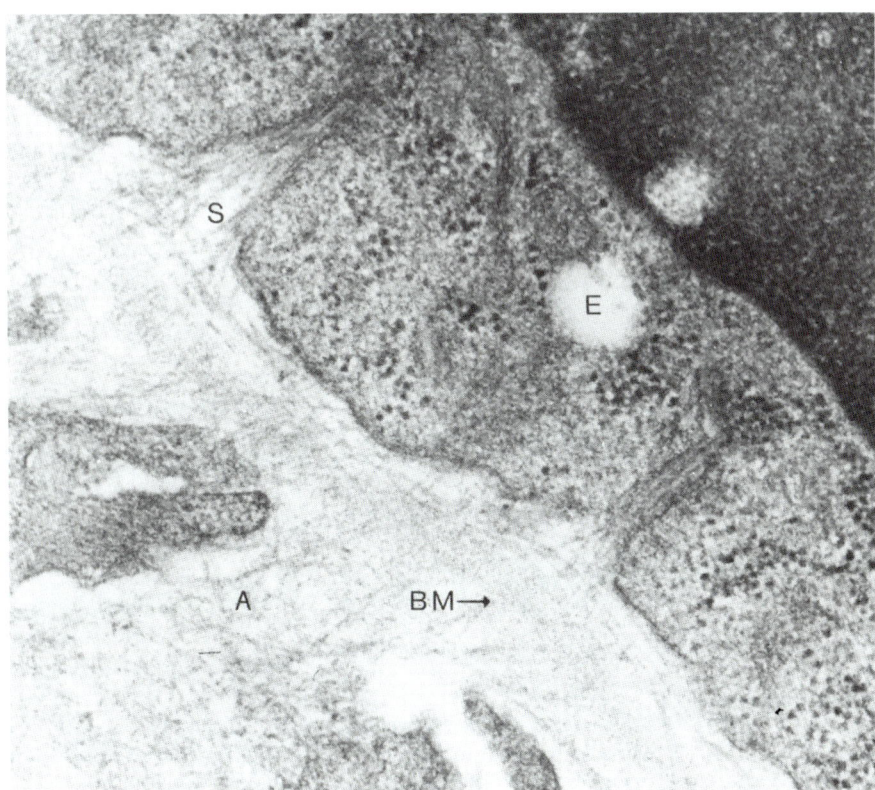

FIGURE 23-6
Electron micrograph of glomerular amyloid *(A)* illustrating its location relative to the basement membrane *(BM)*. Amyloid spicules *(S)* extend into the cytoplasm of the glomerular epithelial cells *(E)*.

The Amyloidoses

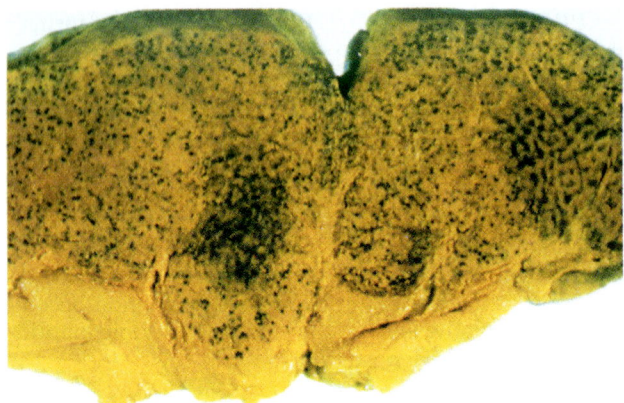

FIGURE 23-7
A kidney containing AA amyloid stained with the iodine reaction. Note the dotlike staining of the glomeruli in the cortex and the linear array in the medulla.

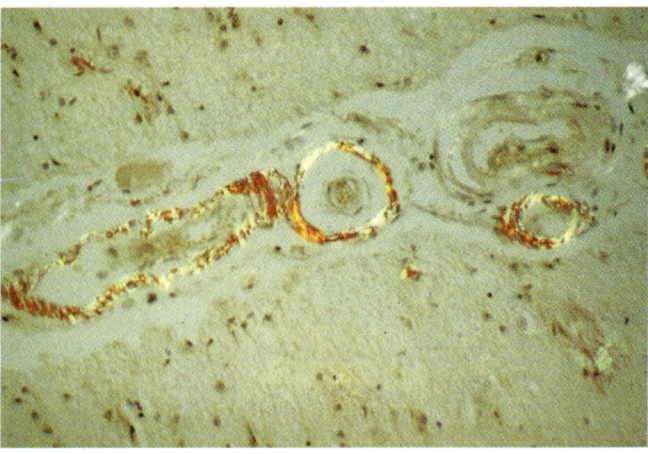

FIGURE 23-9
Cerebrovascular amyloid in a case of Alzheimer disease. The section was stained with Congo red and examined under polarized light.

The cut surface of the spleen containing white pulp amyloid is different and shows multiple pale foci scattered throughout the organ, an appearance labeled *sago spleen*. Deposits in the liver follow the arteries of the portal triads or are laid down along central veins and radiate into the parenchyma along the liver cell plates.

Amyloid adds interstitial material to sites of deposition, thereby increasing the size of affected organs. This increase may be counterbalanced by the deposition of amyloid in blood vessels (Fig. 23-9), an effect that impairs circulation and may lead to organ atrophy. Affected organs may, therefore, increase or decrease in size. Since compact amyloid deposits are essentially avascular, the involved organs are commonly pale and firm.

Regardless of whether amyloid is laid down in a systemic or local fashion, the deposits tend to occur between parenchymal cells and their blood supply. Amyloid may eventually entrap the parenchymal cells, may have a direct toxic effect on these cells through the interaction of protofibrils and cell membranes, or may interfere with their nutrition. **In any event, amyloidosis leads to cell strangulation, atrophy, and death** (Fig. 23-10).

CLINICAL FEATURES OF AMYLOIDOSES

No single set of symptoms points unequivocally to amyloidosis as a diagnosis. The symptomatology of amyloidosis is governed by both the underlying disease and the type of

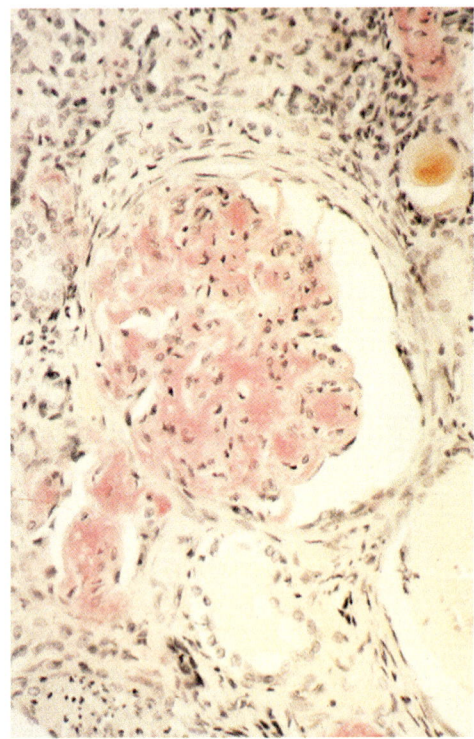

FIGURE 23-8
The microscopic appearance of AA amyloid from the glomeruli of the specimen in Figure 23-7. Note the lobular pattern of the amyloid deposit and the involvement of the afferent arteriole.

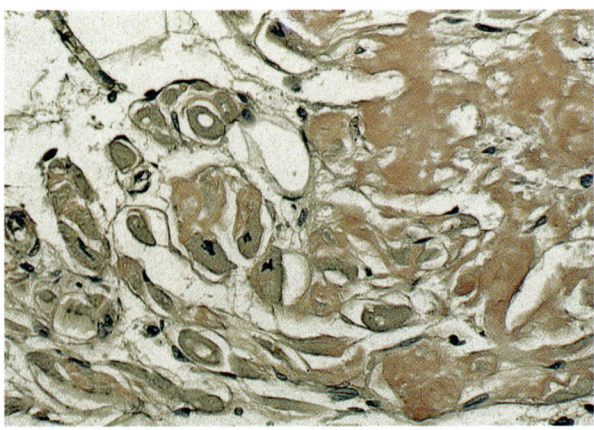

FIGURE 23-10
Myocardial amyloid (AL type), showing the encroachment upon, and strangulation of, individual myocardial fibers.

protein deposited. It is not uncommon for amyloidosis to be found as a completely unexpected disorder, with no clinical manifestations. In other cases, unexplained renal and cardiac complications may be the presenting conditions.

KIDNEY: Patients with multiple myeloma, chronic long-standing inflammatory disorders, or familial Mediterranean fever who develop the nephrotic syndrome should be suspected of having amyloidosis. Proteinuria, particularly in patients with plasma cell dyscrasias, may be overlooked if the patient is already excreting a Bence Jones protein. Progressive glomerular obliteration may ultimately lead to renal failure and uremia.

HEART: Amyloid involvement of the myocardium should be suspected in systemic forms of amyloidosis in which congestive failure or cardiomegaly is associated with low voltage on the electrocardiogram. Entrapment of the conduction system leads to arrhythmias, which in turn can result in sudden death. Not only does congestive failure secondary to cardiac amyloidosis respond poorly to digitalis therapy, but amyloid fibrils also sequester and concentrate digoxin, thereby precipitating digitalis toxicity and fatal arrhythmias. Amyloid deposition within the myocardium may also impair ventricular distensibility and filling, an effect that appears clinically as a **restrictive form of cardiomyopathy.** In some instances, cardiac amyloidosis has masqueraded as constrictive pericarditis.

GASTROINTESTINAL TRACT: The ganglia, smooth muscle vasculature, and submucosa of the gastrointestinal tract may all be affected by amyloid. Deposits in these locations alter gastrointestinal motility and absorption. Patients complain of either constipation or diarrhea, occasionally in association with malabsorption. Enlargement of the tongue is classic, and interference with its motor function may be severe enough to affect speech and swallowing.

PERIPHERAL NERVES: The familial polyneuropathic forms of amyloid usually manifest as paresthesias, with loss in temperature and pain sensation of the extremities.

In all systemic forms of amyloidosis, the patient's course is usually unremitting and ultimately fatal. Patients with multiple myeloma and AL amyloidosis generally die within 1 to 2 years, either from the malignancy itself or from cardiac or renal complications. Patients with AA amyloidosis secondary to long-standing inflammatory disease have a more protracted course, but death may be expected within 5 years of the diagnosis, usually from cardiac or renal failure. Persons who suffer deposition of ATTR of the familial type have an extended course of 15 to 25 years. Symptoms may begin at any age but are usually postpubertal, with death most common in the fifth and sixth decades. Successful treatment of the underlying condition, such as multiple myeloma or an inflammatory disorder, may on occasion lead to resorption and resolution of amyloid deposits. These clinical observations indicate that amyloid does turn over, albeit slowly.

Even when one suspects amyloidosis, the diagnosis ultimately rests on its histological demonstration in biopsy specimens. Amyloid is readily demonstrated in gingival and rectal biopsy specimens and in abdominal subcutaneous fat. It is commonly visualized in renal biopsies taken as part of a general investigation of impaired renal function. The availability of antisera specific for the various amyloid proteins now allows determination of the specific forms of amyloid.

AMYLOID TREATMENT STRATEGIES

Strategies for antiamyloid therapy flow from the processes of amyloidogenesis outlined above.

REDUCTION IN THE AMYLOID PRECURSOR CONCENTRATION: Since an adequate amyloid precursor pool is necessary for fibrillogenesis, attempts have been made to limit the availability of such precursors. A clinical example involves mutant ATTR in familial. Liver transplantation in patients with FAP replaces the abnormal TTR with its normal counterpart. In such patients, one can demonstrate a gradual reduction in amyloid load. In some patients such an approach leads to clinical improvement.

INHIBITION OF NIDUS (NUCLEUS) FORMATION: Colchicine is the drug of choice in preventing the development of amyloidosis in patients with familial mediterranean fever (FMF). Experimentally, this drug acts by preventing the generation of AEF (the nidus), thereby preventing the appearance of amyloid.

INCREASING THE STABILITY OF AMYLOIDOGENIC PROTEINS: Some amyloidogenic proteins (e.g., TTR) are natural carriers of other ligands. The presence of such ligands on the amyloid precursor stabilizes its conformation. In the case of TTR, analogues of the natural ligand may exert the same effect, opening an interesting therapeutic avenue.

INHIBITION OF MOLECULAR INTERACTIONS: The recent recognition that amyloid fibril formation may be the product of interactive processes between two or more molecular components suggests that interference with such interactions may inhibit amyloidogenesis. Experimentally, this approach has proved successful with several different forms of amyloid, but its effectiveness in human amyloidosis remains to be demonstrated.

ACCELERATION OF AMYLOID REMOVAL: Patients with AL amyloid who are treated with an iodinated analogue of doxorubicin resorb considerable amounts of their amyloid. The agent binds with high affinity to several amyloids, including AL. On theoretical grounds, displacement of some of the components from amyloid fibrils may make the remainder more susceptible to proteolytic digestion. Treatment of human amyloidosis has, however, not been attempted.

SUGGESTED READING

Bellotti V, Mangione P, Merlini G: Review: Immunoglobulin light chain amyloidosis: The archetype of structural and pathogenic variability. *J Struct Biol* 130:280–289, 2000.

Benson MD, Uemichi T: Transthyretin amyloidosis. *Amyloid* 3:44–56, 1996.

Buxbaum JN, Tagoe CE: The genetics of the amyloidoses. *Annu Rev Med* 51:543–569, 2000.

Caughey B: Interactions between prion protein isoforms: The kiss of death? *Trends Biochem Sci* 26:235–242, 2001.

Chen SM, Berthelier V, Yang W, Wetzel R: Polyglutamine aggregation behavior *in vitro* supports a recruitment mechanism of cytotoxicity. *J Mol Biol* 311:173–182, 2001.

Cohlberg JA, Li J, Uversky VN, Fink AL: Heparin and other glycosaminoglycans stimulate the formation of amyloid fibrils from α-synuclein *in vitro*. *Biochemistry* 41:1502–1511, 2002.

Damas AM, Saraiva MJ: Review: TTR amyloidosis—Structural features leading to protein aggregation and their implications on therapeutic strategies. *J Struct Biol* 130:290–299, 2000.

Glenner GG: Amyloid deposits and amyloidosis: The β-fibrilloses (Part I). *N Engl J Med* 302:1283–1292, 1980.

Glenner GG: Amyloid deposits and amyloidosis: The β-fibrilloses (Part II). *N Engl J Med* 302:1333–1341, 1980.

Goedert M, Jakes R, Spillantini MG, et al.: Assembly of microtubule associated protein tau into Alzheimer-like filaments induced by sulphated glycosaminoglycans. *Nature* 383:550–553, 1996.

Haass C: The molecular significance of amyloid beta-peptide for Alzheimer's disease. *Eur Arch Psychiatry Clin Neurosci* 246:118–123, 1996.

Hamilton JA, Benson MD: Transthyretin: A review from a structural perspective. *Cell Mol Life Sci* 58:1491–1521, 2001.

Kahn SE, Andrikopoulos S, Verchere CB: Islet amyloid: A long-recognized but underappreciated pathological feature of type 2 diabetes. *Diabetes* 48:241–253, 1999.

Kazatchkine MD, Husby G, Arak S, et al.: Nomenclature of amyloid and amyloidosis—WHO-IUIS Nomenclature Sub-Committee. *Bull WHO* 71:105–108, 1993.

Kisilevsky R: Review: Amyloidogenesis-unquestioned answers and unanswered questions. *J Struct Biol* 130:99–108, 2000.

Kisilevsky R, Fraser PE: Aβ amyloidogenesis: Unique or variation on a systemic theme? *Crit Rev Biochem Mol Biol* 32:361–404, 1997.

Kisilevsky R, Gruys E, Shirahama T: Does amyloid enhancing factor (AEF) exist? Is AEF a single biological entity? *Amyloid* 2:128–133, 1995.

Kisilevsky R, Lemieux LJ, Fraser PE, et al.: Arresting amyloidosis *in vivo* using small-molecule anionic sulphonates or sulphates: Implications for Alzheimer's disease. *Nat Med* 1:143–148, 1995.

Merlini G, Bellotti V, Andreola A, et al.: Protein aggregation. *Clin Chem Lab Med* 39:1065–1075, 2001.

Park K, Verchere CB: Identification of a heparin binding domain in the N-terminal cleavage site of pro-islet amyloid polypeptide—Implications for islet amyloid formation. *J Biol Chem* 276:16611–16616, 2001.

Peterson SA, Klabunde T, Lashuel HA, et al.: Inhibiting transthyretin conformational changes that lead to amyloid fibril formation. *Proc Natl Acad Sci USA* 95:12956–12960, 1998.

Porte D, Kahn SE: β-Cell dysfunction and failure in type 2 diabetes—Potential mechanisms. *Diabetes* 50:S160–S163, 2001.

Prusiner SB: Shattuck lecture—Neurodegenerative diseases and prions. *N Engl J Med* 344:1516–1526, 2001.

Skinner M: AL amyloidosis: The last 30 years. *Amyloid* 7:13–14, 2000.

Spillantini MG, Tolnay M, Love S, Goedert M: Microtubule-associated protein tau, heparan sulphate and α-synuclein in several neurodegenerative diseases with dementia. *Acta Neuropathol* 97:585–594, 1999.

Westermark P: Classification of amyloid fibril proteins and their precursors: An ongoing discussion. *Amyloid* 4:216–218, 1997.

Zoghbi HY, Orr HT: Glutamine repeats and neurodegeneration. *Annu Rev Neurosci* 23:217–247, 2000.

CHAPTER 24

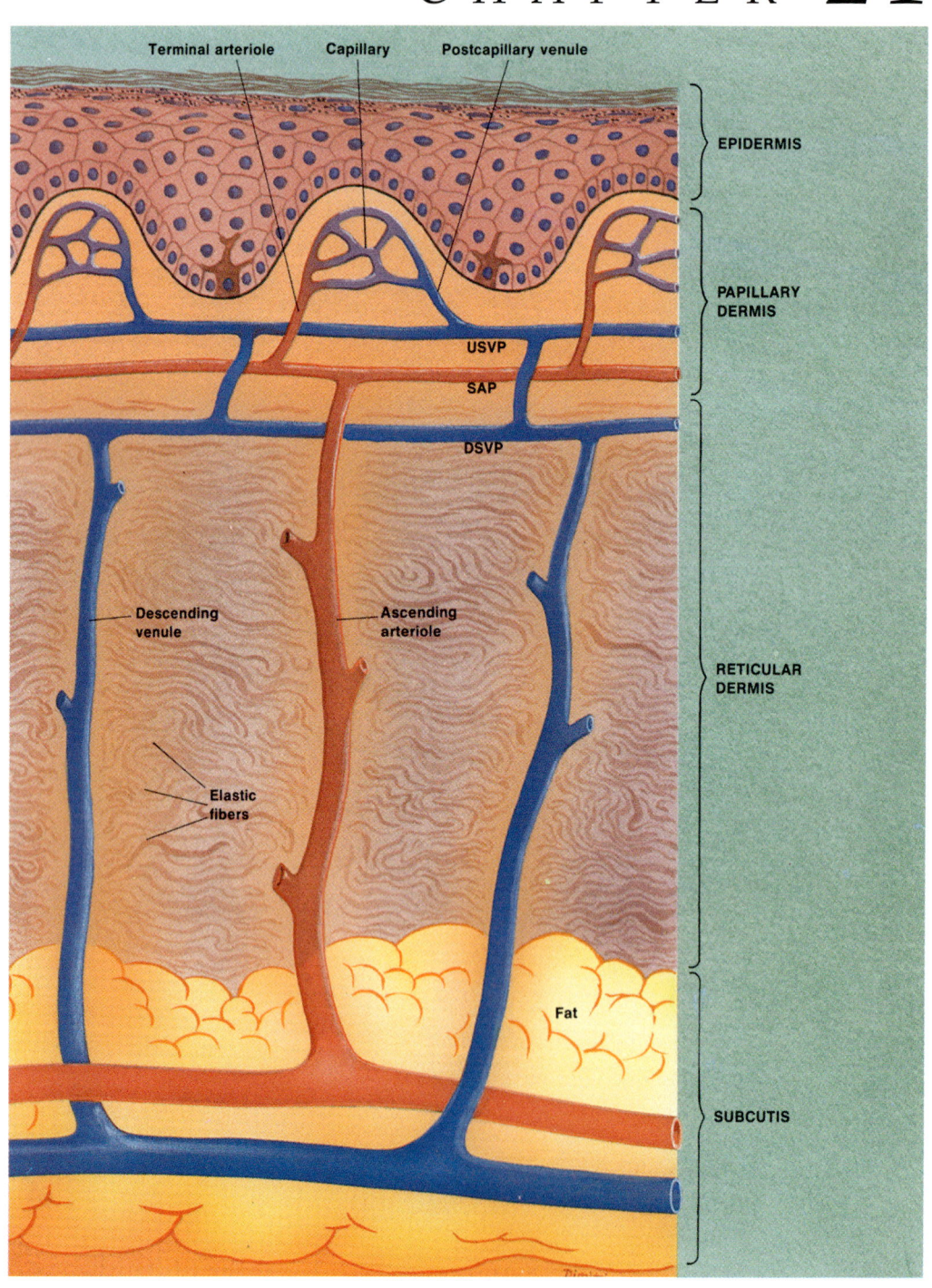

The Skin

Craig A. Storm
David E. Elder

Anatomy and Physiology of the Skin

Diseases of the Epidermis
Ichthyoses
Darier Disease
Psoriasis
Pemphigus Vulgaris

Diseases of the Basement Membrane Zone (Dermal–Epidermal Interface)
Epidermolysis Bullosa
Bullous Pemphigoid
Dermatitis Herpetiformis
Erythema Multiforme
Systemic Lupus Erythematosus
Lichen Planus

Inflammatory Diseases of the Superficial and Deep Vascular Bed
Urticaria and Angioedema
Cutaneous Necrotizing Vasculitis
Allergic Contact Dermatitis
Granulomatous Dermatitis
Sarcoidosis
Granuloma Annulare

Disorders of the Dermal Connective Tissue
Scleroderma

Inflammatory Disorders of the Panniculus
Erythema Nodosum
Erythema Induratum

Acne Vulgaris: A Disorder of the Pilosebaceous Unit

Infections and Infestations
Impetigo
Superficial Fungal Infections
Deep Fungal Infections
Viral Infections
Arthropod Infestations

Primary Neoplasms of the Skin
Common Acquired Melanocytic Nevus (Mole)
Dysplastic (Atypical) Nevus
Melanocytic Dysplasia
Malignant Melanoma
Benign Tumors of Melanocytes
Verrucae
Keratosis
Basal Cell Carcinoma
Squamous Cell Carcinoma
Merkel Cell Carcinoma
Adnexal Tumors
Fibrohistiocytic Tumors
Mycosis Fungoides
HIV Infection

FIGURE 24-1 (see opposite page)
The dermis and its vasculature. The dermis is divided into two distinct anatomical regions. The papillary dermis with its vascular plexus and the epidermis usually react together in diseases that are primarily limited to the skin. The reticular dermis and the subcutis are altered in association with systemic diseases that manifest in the skin. *DSVP*, deep superficial venular plexus; *SAP*, superficial arterial plexus; *USVP*, upper superficial venular plexus.

The skin is an optimal organ for studying fundamental principles of pathology because the lesions on its surface are readily apparent. Except for diseases of highly specialized tissues—for instance, those of the alveolus or glomerulus or the demyelinating diseases of the central nervous system—all classes of disease are seen in the skin. Some diseases, such as the blistering ones, are manifested only in the skin (except for some involvement of the mucous membranes).

Considering the imperatives of appearance in human interactions, an alteration in the appearance of the skin may, at times, be the most important feature of cutaneous disease. Many cutaneous diseases have only minor symptoms, and some have no symptoms at all. Few are life threatening, and many are self-limited. However, even the self-limited, asymptomatic cutaneous diseases are often of great concern to the patient. For example, the symptoms of acne are systemically minor, but the disease can change a life. Although scalp hair is unneeded, baldness may cause considerable distress. Vitiligo, a completely asymptomatic, progressive, depigmentary disorder, may turn an otherwise normal black person into a recluse or an outcast.

ANATOMY AND PHYSIOLOGY OF THE SKIN

The skin is a protective barrier; microorganisms find it almost impossible to penetrate the epidermis from the outside, and water loss is limited from the inside. The skin is vital in regulating temperature and in protecting against ultraviolet light. A wide variety of sensory receptors communicate details related to the immediate environment. The skin plays a prominent role in immunological regulation through the skin-associated lymphoid tissues (SALT), which consist of lymphocytes and antigen-presenting cells that travel between the skin and regional lymph nodes via the lymphatics and bloodstream. Keratinocytes, Langerhans cells, mast cells, lymphocytes, and macrophages all serve functions related to immunity. Epidermal keratinocytes produce a variety of cytokines, notably interleukin (IL)-1α and IL-1β as well as eicosanoids. This ability of keratinocytes to produce products that mediate immunity and inflammation is necessary in an organ relentlessly exposed to the external environment. Langerhans cells, the dendritic antigen-presenting cells of the skin, are bone marrow-derived, epidermal, immigrant cells. They play an important role in the development and regulation of contact hypersensitivity, allograft rejection, and graft-versus-host disease.

KERATINOCYTES: The epidermis is a multilayered sheet of keratin-producing cells. A progressive change in morphology occurs from the replicating columnar cells of the basal layer *(stratum basalis)* through the spinous layer *(stratum spinosum)* and the granular layer *(stratum granulosum)* to the nonviable flattened cells of the cornified layer *(stratum corneum)* (Fig. 24-2). The basal cells harbor most of

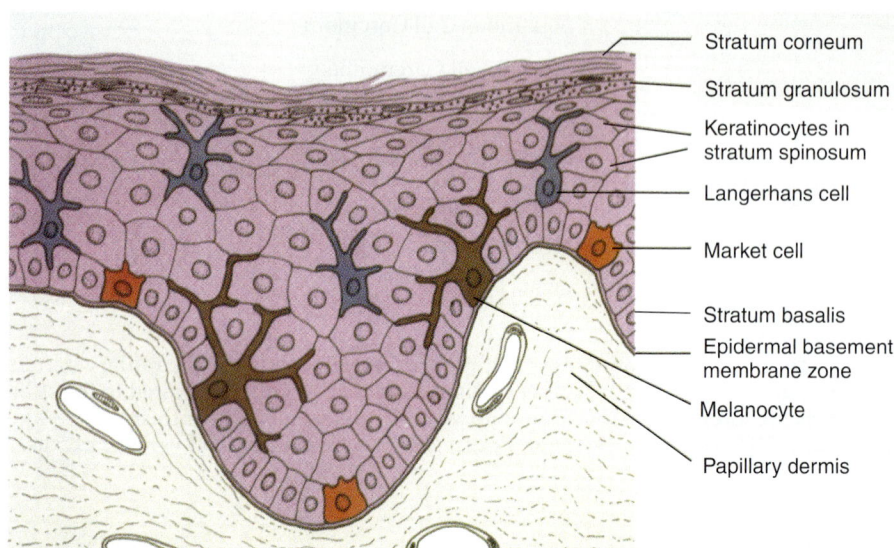

FIGURE 24-2
Normal epidermis and the epidermal immigrant cells. Keratinocytes form the multilayered epidermis, protecting against water loss and bacterial invasion. Melanocytes provide color as well as protection against ultraviolet radiation. Langerhans cells are among the cells responsible for the skin's function as an immunological organ. Merkel cells may represent one of the enablers of tactile function of the skin.

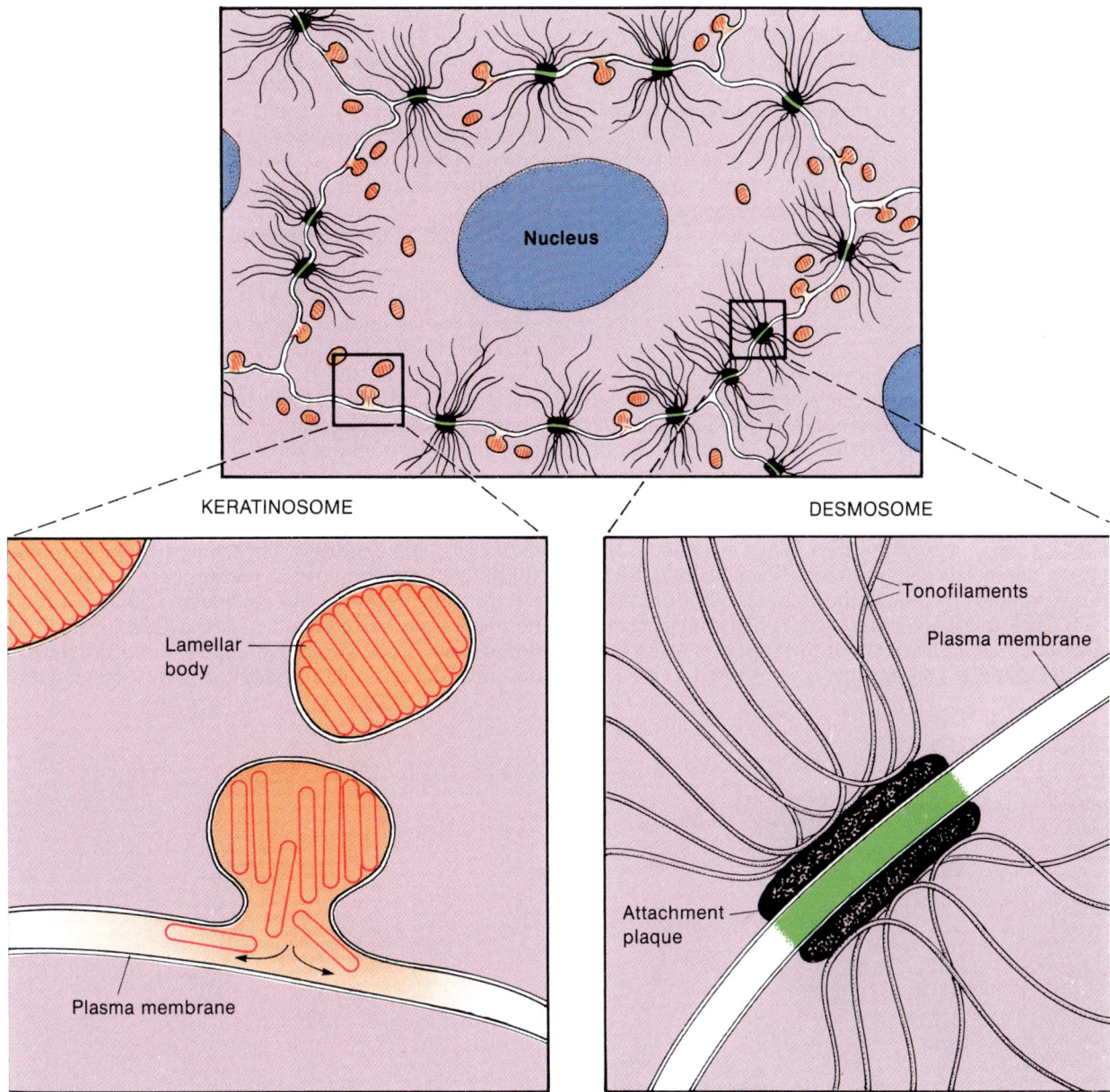

FIGURE 24-3
The keratinocyte, keratinosome, and desmosome. The keratinocyte cytoplasm is dominated by delicate keratin fibrils, the tonofilaments. These are part of the cytoskeleton of the cell and loop within the attachment plaque of the desmosome. The lamellar body of the keratinocyte extrudes its contents into the intercellular space. This material probably has a role in cellular cohesion.

the mitotic activity of the epidermis. As the keratinocytes approach the superficial aspects of the epidermis, they become anucleate and form what are essentially flattened plates of dead cells on the surface of the skin (the cornified layer). Keratinocytes synthesize a sulfur-poor, filamentous protein, the *tonofibril*, which is related to the keratin molecule of the stratum corneum. Tonofibrils are composed of varying blends of acidic and basic intermediate keratin filaments, resulting in over 30 different keratins that are responsible for structures such as the stratum corneum, hair, and nails. Bundles of tonofibrils converge on, and terminate at, the plasma membrane in attachment plates called *desmosomes* (Fig. 24-3).

Keratinocytes are also distinguished by two other structural products: *keratohyaline granules* and *Odland bodies*. Keratohyaline granules are the defining feature of the granular layer and are composed of a histidine-rich, electron-dense, basophilic protein, *profilaggrin*, which is associated with intermediate filaments. Odland bodies, also known as keratinosomes or membrane-coating granules, are the only structurally distinctive, secretory product of the epidermis (Fig. 24-3). They form in the outer spinous and granular layers and discharge their contents into the intercellular spaces, appearing there as lamellar masses parallel to the surface of the skin. Odland bodies and the discharged lamellated products are most clearly manifested in the outer granular layer and are related to the epidermal barrier function.

The epidermis harbors immigrant cells of neuroectodermal and mesenchymal origin that do not synthesize keratin but which have their own highly distinctive organelles. They appear in varying numbers and at varying levels of the epidermis. Two of these cells, melanocytes and Langerhans cells, are dendritic. The third, the Merkel cell, is associated with a terminal neuronal axon.

MELANOCYTES: Melanocytes are dendritic cells that are largely responsible for the color of the skin; they originate in the neural crest. The melanocytes lie in the basal layer of the epidermis and are separated from the dermis by the epidermal basement membrane zone. A single melanocyte supplies dendrites to over 30 keratinocytes (Fig. 24-4).

The *melanosome* is a cytoplasmic membrane-bound complex in which melanin is synthesized. When melanin synthesis is active, the melanosome contains filaments that are arranged in a parallel array along the long axis of the organelle (Fig. 24-4). The orderly internal structure of the melanosome is progressively obliterated, and it then appears as an electron-opaque granule. This granule is transferred to the keratinocyte, where it protects the nuclear material from ultraviolet light by forming a supranuclear cap.

Melanin is responsible for the diverse coloration of humans and other animals. Interestingly, the black cloud that obscures the retreat of a squid is secreted by a gland that synthesizes massive quantities of melanin. Skin color is largely based on the number, size, and packaging of melanosomes in keratinocytes. In hair and epidermal keratinocytes, melanins are packaged to absorb and reflect visible light, thereby forming the integumentary colors.

LANGERHANS CELLS: These cells arrive in embryonic skin in the last month of the first trimester, following the melanocytes by a month. With the arrival of these HLA-DR–positive cells, the skin acquires the ability to recognize and process antigens, at which time it becomes a part of the immune system. Uncommon in the dermis, these cells are distributed throughout the nucleated layers of the epidermis, where they constitute about 4% of the cells. They are difficult to see in routine light microscopic preparations because their cytoplasm is translucent and is formed of a perikaryon and dendrites. The Langerhans cells do not form specialized attachments to the apposed keratinocytes. In electron micrographs, the cytoplasm contains a moderate number of specialized organelles, the *Birbeck granules*. In two dimensions, these structures appear to be racquet-shaped, but three-dimensional reconstruction has shown them to be

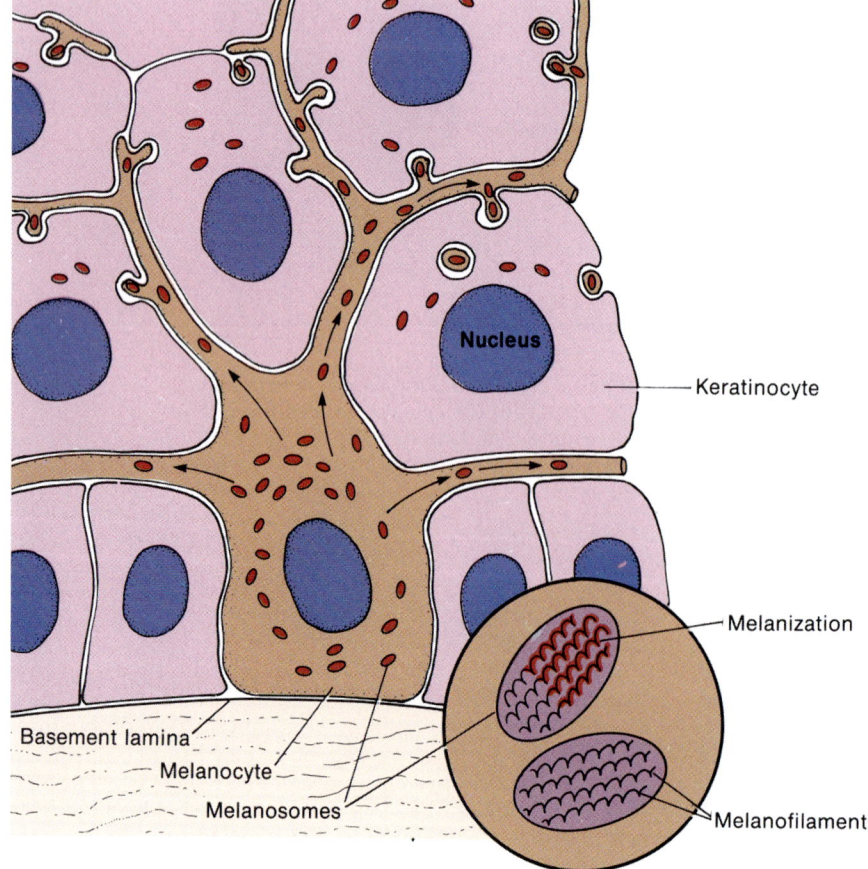

FIGURE 24-4
A melanocyte supplies over 30 keratinocytes with melanin granules by way of complex dendritic cytoplasmic extensions. Melanin granules are transferred to keratinocytes and come to lie in a supranuclear cap, a site indicating their protective function. Pigment granules are actually formed in the melanocytes within distinctive organelles—the melanosomes. Pigment is synthesized on small filaments within this organelle *(inset).*

Anatomy and Physiology of the Skin

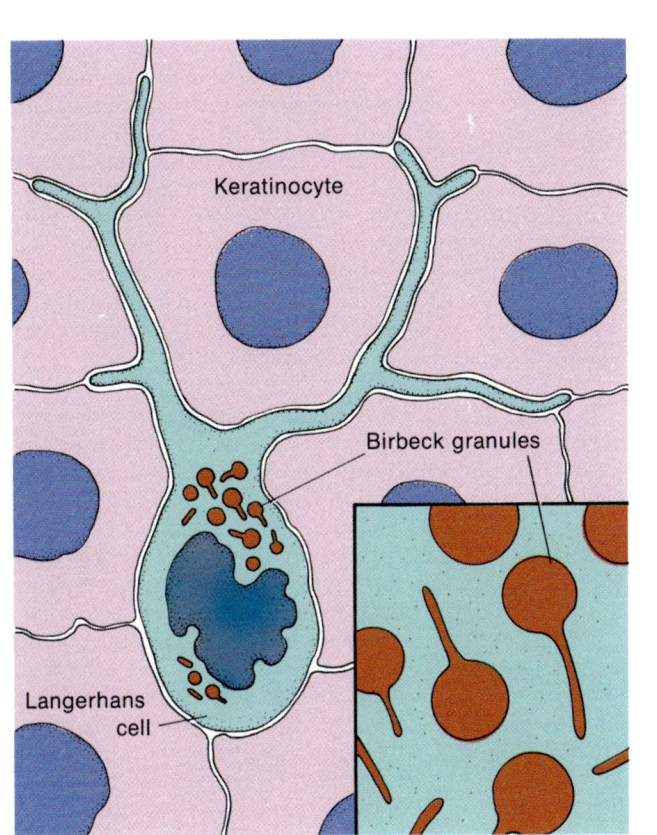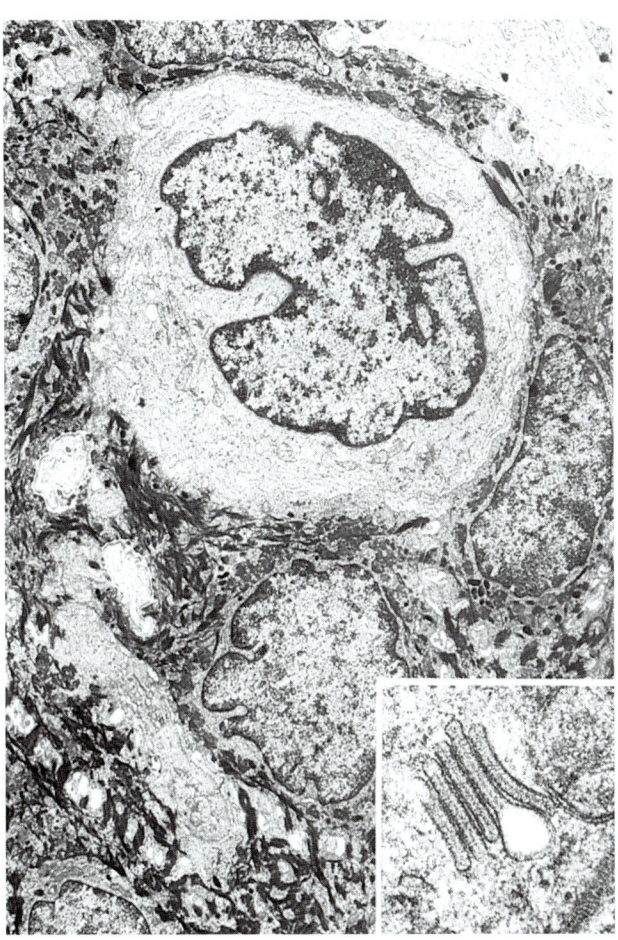

FIGURE 24-5
The dendritic Langerhans cell can recognize and process antigens. A. The unique racket-shaped organelles, called *Birbeck granules*, may be important in antigen presentation. B. An electron micrograph of a Langerhans cell shows a high-power view of the racket-shaped organelles (inset). The Langerhans cell body *(mid-lower portion)* is pale compared to the surrounding keratinocytes, whose cytoplasm contains electron-dense packets of tonofilaments. A dendrite is present *(upper right corner)*.

cup-shaped (Fig. 24-5). The function of these unique organelles that are derived from the plasma membrane is probably related to the role of Langerhans cells as antigen-presenting cells (antigenic material being internalized into Birbeck granules).

In Langerhans cell histiocytoses (see Chapter 20), Birbeck granules are attached to the plasma membrane of the proliferating cells and are in direct communication with the extracellular space. Furthermore, they have a fuzzy coat of clathrin, a feature of "coated pits," suggesting a relationship to receptor-mediated antigen processing and recognition. Langerhans cells express MHC I, MHC II, and receptors for Fc IgG and Fc IgE. They are identified by the immunohistochemical demonstration of CD1 or, less specifically, by S-100 protein.

MERKEL CELLS: Although still classified as "immigrant" cells, evidence is accumulating that Merkel cells may actually not be immigrants to the epidermis but, rather, specialized basal keratinocytes. They form desmosomes with keratinocytes and express keratins 8, 18, and 20 in a fashion similar to that of keratinocytes. The cells project short, blunt cytoplasmic fingers into adjacent keratinocytes. Merkel cells do not appear in all areas of the epidermis, but are seen in special regions such as the lips, oral cavity, external root sheath of the hair follicles, and the palmar skin of the digits. They have a distinctive organelle, a membrane-bound, dense-core granule, 100 nm or larger in width (Fig. 24-6). Immunohistochemical and ultrastructural studies suggest that the Merkel cell has a neurosecretory function. The basal aspect of the cell is apposed to a small nerve plate, which is connected to a myelinated axon by a short, nonmyelinated axon. This complex structure may function as a tactile mechanoreceptor.

BASEMENT MEMBRANE: The basement membrane zone (BMZ) serves as an interface between the dermis and the epidermis and is as diverse in function as it is complex in

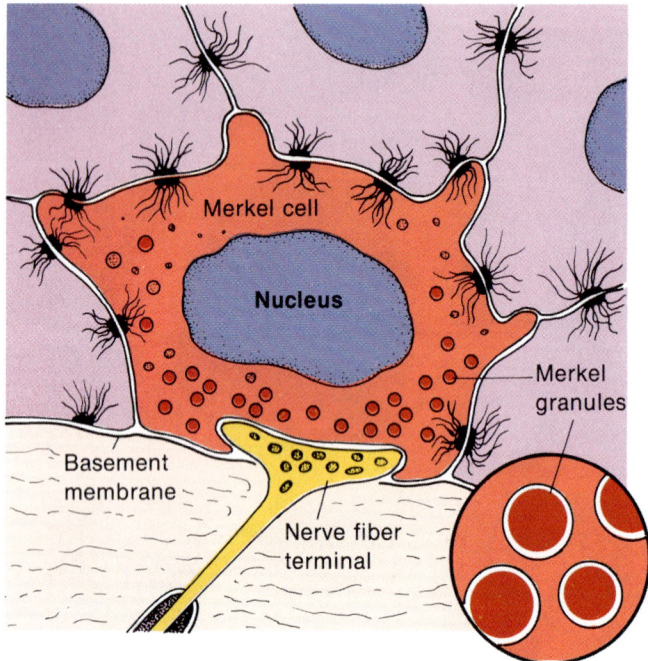

FIGURE 24-6
The Merkel cell, which differs from other immigrant cells, forms desmosomes with keratinocytes and is attached to a small nerve plate (nerve fiber terminal). The membrane-delimited, dense core granule is distinctive *(inset).*

structure (Fig. 24-7). It is responsible for dermal–epidermal adherence and probably functions as a selective macromolecular filter. It is also a site of immunoglobulin and complement deposition in certain cutaneous diseases. Most of the structures of the BMZ are elaborated by cells of the epidermis. The basal lamina is the primary organizational feature of the BMZ and is responsible for epithelial cell polarity as well as some keratin gene expression. Ultrastructurally, the basal lamina includes the following:

- **Deep aspects of the basal keratinocytes** including the plasma membrane and the tonofilaments that attach to the deep face of the hemidesmosome
- **Hemidesmosome,** with its subdesmosomal dense plate
- **Anchoring filaments** that extend from the subdesmosomal dense plates across the lamina lucida and insert into the lamina densa
- **Lamina lucida,** an electron-lucent layer containing adherence proteins
- **Lamina densa,** composed principally of type IV collagen
- **Anchoring fibrils,** which are arrays of type VII collagen extending from the inner face of the lamina densa for a short distance into the papillary dermis
- **Microfibrils,** which feature delicate, long, elastic fibrils that blend with the underlying elastic fibrillary system of the skin

Certain antigenic components have been identified in the BMZ, some of which play identified roles in cutaneous disease. Laminin is a glycoprotein present in the lamina lucida and lamina densa of all BMZs. It assists in the organization of macromolecules of the BMZ and promotes attachment of cells to the extracellular matrix. Laminin binds to type IV collagen. Bullous pemphigoid (BP) antigens were identified with antibodies from patients with the blistering disorder bullous pemphigoid. The antigens BPAG1 and BPAG2 (type XVII collagen) are normal constituents of the dermal–epidermal junction but are absent in BMZs around adnexal structures and blood vessels. These BP antigens are located in the hemidesmosomes and the cytoplasm of the basal keratinocytes. Type IV collagen is present in the lamina densa of all BMZs. It is the most superficial component of the complex collagen fiber network of the dermis and is important in dermal–epidermal attachment. Type VII collagen is present on the deep aspect of the basal lamina in anchoring fibrils. Anchoring fibril antigens (AF-1 and AF-2) reside within anchoring fibrils and possibly within the lower lamina densa.

The **dermis** is a complex organization of connective tissue deep to the BMZ and is composed predominantly of collagen, which is embedded in a ground substance rich in hyaluronic acid. The dermis consists of two zones:

PAPILLARY DERMIS: The papillary dermis is a narrow zone immediately deep to the BMZ of the epidermis. This region is pale pink with the hematoxylin and eosin stain and has little organization when viewed with the light microscope (Fig. 24-1). Delicate collagen fibrils are the most apparent structures. This delicate connective tissue extends as a sheath about blood vessels, nerves, and adnexal structures. This entire network of collagen is known as the *adventitial dermis.*

The papillary dermis is generally altered in conjunction with epidermal disease and with disorders affecting the superficial vascular bed. The epidermis, papillary dermis, and superficial vascular bed react jointly and influence each other in complex ways. Some primary skin diseases with few, if any, systemic manifestations, such as psoriasis and lichen planus, involve these superficial structures.

RETICULAR DERMIS: The reticular dermis is deep to the papillary dermis and contains most of the dermal collagen, which is organized into coarse bundles and associated with elastic fibers (Fig. 24-1). The reticular dermis and subcutis (also recognized as a cutaneous structure) are less common sites of pathological change and, when diseased, are often manifestations of systemic disease. Scleroderma (progressive systemic sclerosis) and erythema nodosum are examples.

CUTANEOUS VASCULATURE: The skin receives 10 times the amount of blood needed for its nutrition, and cutaneous circulating blood has a number of functions. For example, the skin, via its vascular network, is important in temperature regulation. Also, many aspects of cutaneous inflammation involve the superficial cutaneous vasculature.

An ascending arteriole arises from arteries in the subcutis and directly crosses much of the reticular dermis (Fig. 24-1). In the outer part of the reticular dermis, in conjunction with other similar ascending arteries, a superficial arteriolar plexus is formed. From this plexus a terminal arteriole extends into each dermal papilla, where an arterial capillary is formed. The arterial capillary makes a U-turn and on its descent becomes a venous capillary and a postcapillary venule. The venules then join to form a complex venular plexus in the reticular dermis, immediately deep to the papillary dermis. The venular end of this vascular structure is important in the mediation of the cutaneous inflammatory response.

The lymphatic vessels of the skin form a random network, beginning as lymphatic capillaries near the epidermis. A superficial lymphatic plexus is then formed, from which

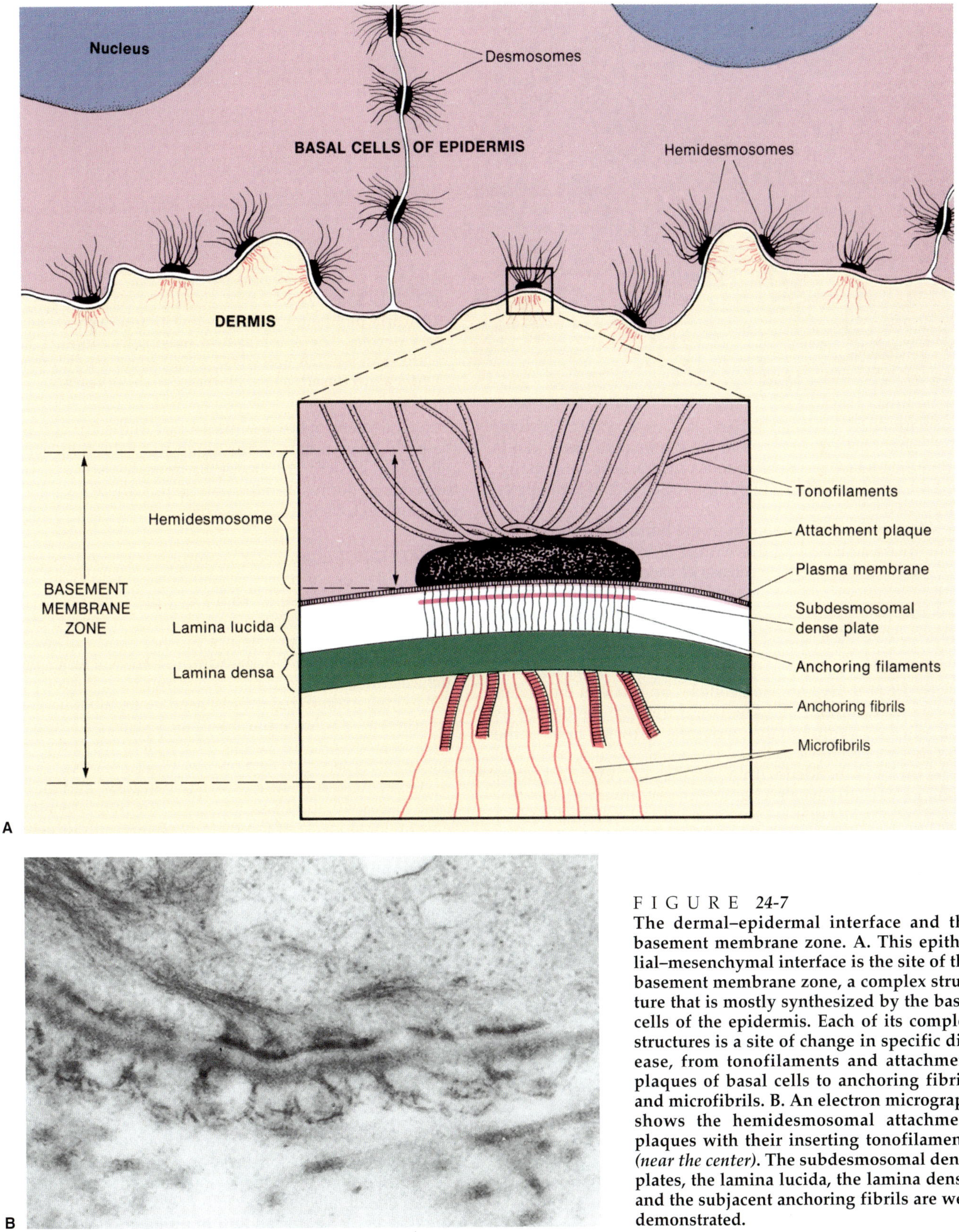

Anatomy and Physiology of the Skin 1209

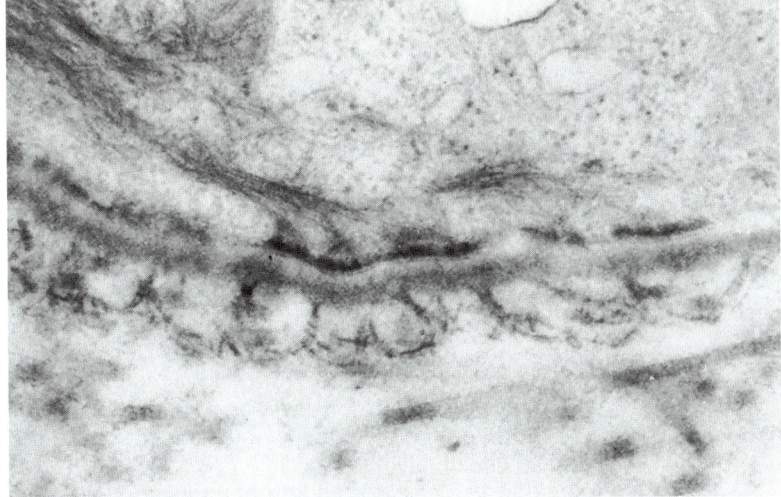

FIGURE 24-7
The dermal–epidermal interface and the basement membrane zone. A. This epithelial–mesenchymal interface is the site of the basement membrane zone, a complex structure that is mostly synthesized by the basal cells of the epidermis. Each of its complex structures is a site of change in specific disease, from tonofilaments and attachment plaques of basal cells to anchoring fibrils and microfibrils. B. An electron micrograph shows the hemidesmosomal attachment plaques with their inserting tonofilaments (*near the center*). The subdesmosomal dense plates, the lamina lucida, the lamina densa, and the subjacent anchoring fibrils are well demonstrated.

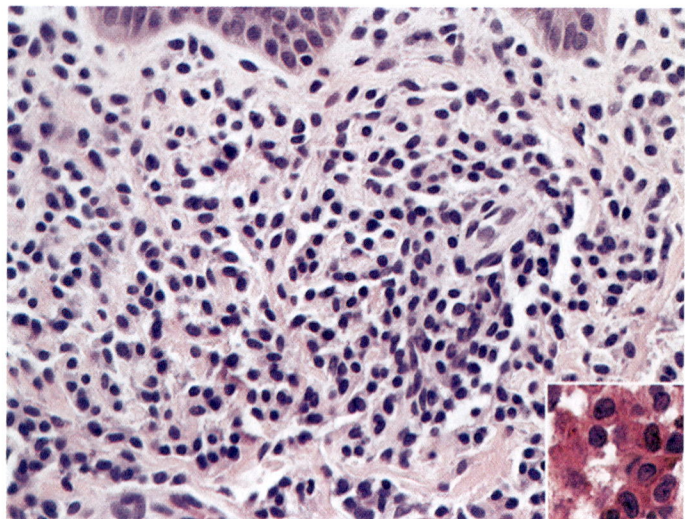

FIGURE 24-8
Urticaria pigmentosa. Mast cells fill and expand the papillary dermis. The cytoplasm of mast cells contains chloracetate esterase-rich granules, giving them a red hue in this Leder stain (*inset*), a useful distinguishing feature.

lymphatic channels drain to regional lymph nodes. The lymphatic channels are involved in the drainage of tissue fluids and in the metastasis of cutaneous cancers, especially malignant melanoma. Cutaneous lymphatics have, at best, an incomplete basal lamina.

Mast cells are derived from the bone marrow and are normally present around the venules of the skin, where they provide for the immediate release of vasoactive and chemotactic substances. Mast cells mediate all types of inflammation, and they proliferate in a spectrum of diseases termed *urticaria pigmentosa* (Fig. 24-8).

HAIR FOLLICLES: Hair follicles originate in the primitive epidermis and grow downward through the dermis as well as upward through the epidermis. Growing hairs of the scalp and beard have bulbs of epithelial and mesenchymal tissue firmly embedded within the subcutis. A vertical cross-section of a bulb reveals a cap of actively dividing, keratin-synthesizing cells that become arrayed in layers that join at the top of the bulb to form the cylindrical hair shaft. The differentiating hairs form the roof of the epithelial bulb and interact with an island of melanocytes that contribute melanin to the passing keratinocytes. This process results in hair color. The colored keratinocytes lose their nuclei as they form the final product, the cylindrical hair shaft. Curly hair is formed from angulated bulbs, and straight hair develops from round bulbs.

THE HAIR CYCLE: Hair grows in a cyclical fashion. At any given time, 90% of hairs are normally in the *anagen* phase, the actively growing phase. These growing hairs have a mosaic distribution and are interspersed with hairs that show no evidence of active growth, termed *telogen* hairs. Hairs in the process of ceasing growth, known as *catagen* hairs, still have hair shafts. Catagen hairs end in the lower reticular dermis as slightly widened clublike structures, each surrounded by a rim of nucleated keratinocytes. The hair bulbs are no longer evident, and the lamina densa surrounding the catagen hair is strikingly thickened.

As the telogen phase (resting follicle) is reached, the end of the hair retreats to the level of the arrector pili muscle. The hair shaft may be missing, since it is no longer tethered at the base, leaving only a remnant of the original follicle. However, a delicate vascularized mesenchymal tract, the *telogen*

tract, extends from the attenuated tip. At the top of this tract, the early anagen hair forms again from the follicular stem cells. With growth, it follows the delicate pathway through the reticular dermis into the panniculus, there forming a mature anagen follicle and a new hair.

ALOPECIA: Alopecia, commonly known as *baldness,* refers to the loss of hair. *Common alopecia,* which affects both men and women, results from a complex and poorly understood interaction of heritable and hormonal factors. Men castrated before puberty retain scalp hair and fail to grow a beard. On the other hand, the administration of testosterone to such castrated men results in the growth of a beard and may lead to male-pattern baldness. The loss of scalp hair results in replacement of a large terminal hair follicle by a diminutive *vellus* hair follicle, the source of the delicate "fuzz" on the cheeks of women and on the upper cheeks of men.

Growing hair is the site of active mitosis, and many systemic diseases cause cessation of mitosis in this location and subsequent alopecia. If the malady passes, mitotic activity is renewed and regrowth occurs. If a patient is subjected to a potent antimitotic regimen, such as chemotherapy for advanced cancer, hair follicles stop growth, hair is lost, and a telogen follicle follows. With cessation of therapy, hair cycling resumes. Almost any kind of follicular inflammation can induce the telogen phase. If fibrosis distorts the telogen tract (the regrowth pathway), permanent loss of that follicle and alopecia result.

Alopecia areata is a circumscribed area of hair loss, usually on the scalp, although other body areas may be involved. Less commonly, there may be loss of all scalp hair **(alopecia totalis)**, and rarely all hair **(alopecia universalis)**. A brisk lymphocytic infiltrate is found around the hair bulb and results in the formation of telogen hairs and hair loss. The findings of alopecia areata may actually result from a heterogeneous group of diseases. This histological pattern and the association of this phenomenon with the inheritance of HLA class II alleles (especially HLA-DQ3) has been interpreted as evidence for an autoimmune etiology. Generally, scarring does not occur, and hair may regrow normally after varying time periods. Occasionally, especially when hair loss is extensive, alopecia is permanent.

VELLUS HAIRS: These fine hairs may play a role in touch perception in many mammals, but in humans they have no function. Microscopically, vellus hairs are diminutive anagen hairs, with a small active bulb high in the reticular dermis, together with small sebaceous glands.

SEBACEOUS FOLLICLES: These structures develop with puberty and are clinically important because they are the site of acne. Sebaceous follicles have a minute vellus hair at the base. The central face exhibits large sebaceous glands that dwarf the vellus hairs and fill the follicular canal with sebum.

DISEASES OF THE EPIDERMIS

Ichthyoses Feature Epidermal Thickening and Scales

The ichthyosiform dermatoses, many of which are heritable, comprise a heterogeneous group of cutaneous diseases characterized by striking thickening of the stratum corneum. The term *ichthyosis* reflects the similarity of the diseased skin to coarse, fish-like scales (Fig. 24-9). There are four major ichthyoses: (1) ichthyosis vulgaris, (2) X-linked ichthyosis, (3) lamellar ichthyosis, and (4) epidermolytic hyperkeratosis. Several rare ichthyoses are associated with other abnormalities such as abnormal lipid metabolism, neurological disorders, bone diseases, and cancer.

Pathogenesis: Three general defects are involved in the excessive epidermal cornification of the ichthyoses:

- **Increased cohesiveness** of the cells of the stratum corneum, possibly related to altered lipid metabolism
- **Abnormal keratinization,** manifested as impaired tonofilament formation and keratohyaline synthesis, and as excessive cornification
- **Increased basal cell proliferation,** associated with a decrease in transit time of keratinocytes across the epidermis

Pathology: All ichthyoses (with the possible exception of lamellar ichthyosis) have a stratum corneum that is disproportionately thick in comparison with the nucleated epidermal layers. Virtually all diseases characterized by thickening of the nucleated epidermal layers also exhibit hyperkeratosis. For example, chronic scratching or rubbing of normal skin causes a thickened epidermis and dermal changes, a condition known as *lichen simplex chronicus.* In this entity, the nucleated epidermal layer and the compacted stratum corneum may each be three times normal thickness. By contrast, in ichthyosis, the stratum corneum may be five times thicker than normal, but it overlies a disproportionately thin nucleated epidermis.

Ichthyosis Vulgaris

Ichthyosis vulgaris is an autosomal dominant disorder of keratinization characterized by mild hyperkeratosis and reduced or absent keratohyaline granules in the epidermis. Scaly skin results from increased cohesiveness of the stratum corneum. The attenuated stratum granulosum consists of a single layer with small defective keratohyaline granules. Decreased or absent synthesis of *profilaggrin,* a keratin filament "glue," is responsible for these defects.

Ichthyosis vulgaris is the prototype of disproportionate corneal thickening. The stratum corneum is loose and has a basket-weave appearance, which differs little from the normal except in amount. The granular layer is greatly diminished and often appears absent (Fig. 24-9). Ultrastructurally, the keratohyaline granules are small and spongelike, a feature indicating defective synthesis. The basal and spinous layers appear entirely normal. **Thus, the primary defect in ichthyosis vulgaris is in the granular and cornified layers, the epidermal zones responsible for the final stage of keratinization and cornification.**

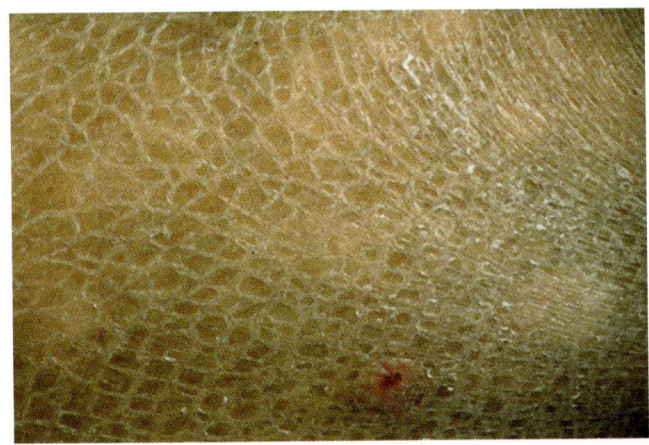
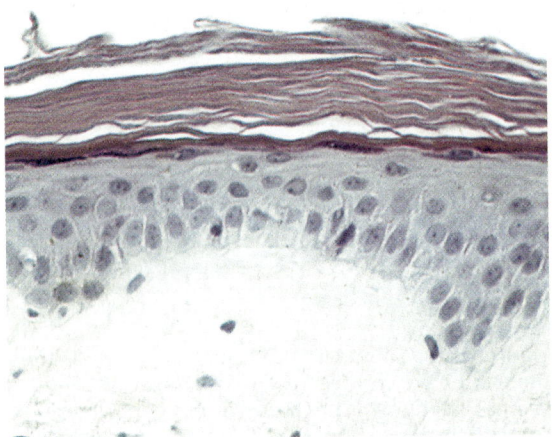

FIGURE 24-9
Ichthyosis vulgaris. A. Noninflammatory fishlike scales are evident on the thigh of a patient with a strong family history of ichthyosis vulgaris. B. There is disproportionate thickening of the stratum corneum relative to the normal thickness of the nucleated epidermal layer. The stratum granulosum is thin and focally absent.

Clinical Features: Ichthyosis vulgaris is the most common of the ichthyoses and begins in early childhood. A family history of this condition is often obtained. Small white scales occur on the extensor surfaces of the extremities and on the trunk and face. The disease is lifelong, but most patients can be maintained free of scales with topical treatment.

A clinical and histological state similar to ichthyosis vulgaris is occasionally associated with other diseases or may follow the use of drugs that affect cholesterol metabolism. Lymphomas, especially Hodgkin disease, may be associated with ichthyosis, and other neoplasms, systemic granulomatous disorders, and connective tissue disease are also occasionally complicated by the disorder. It is possible that drugs produce ichthyosis by interfering with pathways of cholesterol metabolism similar to those involved in the rare ichthyoses. In these uncommon keratotic diseases, cutaneous changes are apparently due to abnormalities in lipid metabolism, for instance, phytanic acid storage disease (*Refsum disease*).

X-linked ichthyosis

This condition is a heritable epidermal disorder characterized by delayed dissolution of the desmosomal disks in the stratum corneum, owing to a deficiency of steroid sulfatase. Steroid sulfatase normally degrades the Odland body product, cholesterol sulfate, which provides cellular adhesion in the lower stratum corneum. Failure of steroid sulfatase action on cholesterol sulfate leads to persistent cohesion of the stratum corneum, but in this disease the granular layer is preserved.

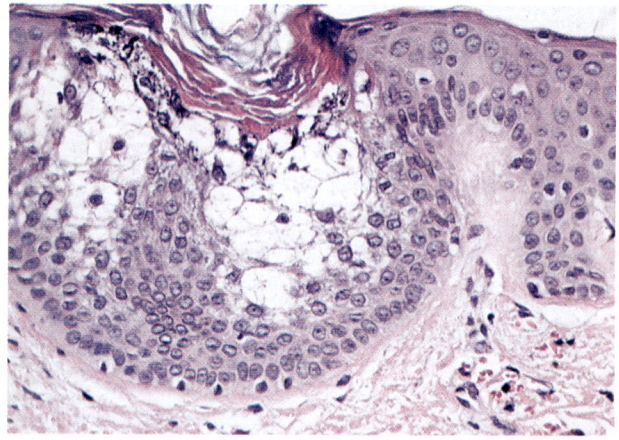

FIGURE 24-10
Epidermolytic hyperkeratosis. The keratinocytes of the stratum spinosum have clumped tonofilaments. As a result, their cytoplasm is relatively clear. In the outer stratum spinosum, the clumped fibrils are further compacted and whorl about the nuclei, resulting in dark cytoplasm condensed about the nuclei. These cells separate from each other to produce epidermolysis. A normal portion of epidermis is seen on the *right*.

Lamellar ichthyosis

This autosomal recessive congenital disorder of cornification is characterized by severe and generalized ichthyosis. It is typified by increased cohesiveness of the stratum corneum, accompanied by numerous keratinosomes and an abnormally large amount of intercellular substance. The disease is genetically heterogeneous, but mutations in the gene encoding the transglutaminase 1 enzyme (*TGM1*; chromosome 14q11), with a resulting defect in lamellar body secretion, often underlies the disorder.

Epidermolytic hyperkeratosis

This type of ichthyosis is a congenital, autosomal dominant disease that features generalized erythroderma, ichthyosiform skin, and blistering. The disease results from mutations in the *K1* and *K10* keratin genes, which encode the keratins in the suprabasal epidermis. These mutations cause faulty assembly of keratin tonofilaments and impair their insertion into desmosomes. These flaws prevent normal development of the cytoskeleton, resulting in epidermal "lysis" and a tendency to form vesicles.

In epidermolytic hyperkeratosis, the spinous keratinocytes contain thick, eosinophilic tonofilaments that whorl around the nucleus in a concentric fashion (Fig. 24-10). The cytoplasm has a clear zone peripheral to the perinuclear tonofilaments, but at the periphery of the cell, these filaments again become condensed. The stratum corneum is disproportionately thickened (Fig. 24-11).

 Clinical Features: Epidermolytic hyperkeratosis manifests with blistering at or shortly after birth. The disease may be generalized or localized to only several areas of the body. The lesions tend to appear dark and even verrucous. Other than the cosmetic disfigurement, the major problem is secondary bacterial infection.

The major ichthyoses are compared in Table 24-1.

Darier Disease Is a Genetic Disorder of Keratinization

Darier disease, also called *keratosis follicularis*, is an autosomal dominant disorder of keratinization characterized by multifocal keratoses.

 Pathogenesis: Darier disease is linked to a defect in the intercellular matrix, with the responsible gene located on chromosome 12q23-24.1. The specific gene, *ATP2A2*, encodes a calcium pump of the endoplasmic reticulum, and its mutation may exert a direct effect on the calcium-dependent assembly of desmosomes. The wide range of neuropsychiatric problems among patients with Darier disease may also be related to *ATP2A2* mutations.

Diseases of the Epidermis

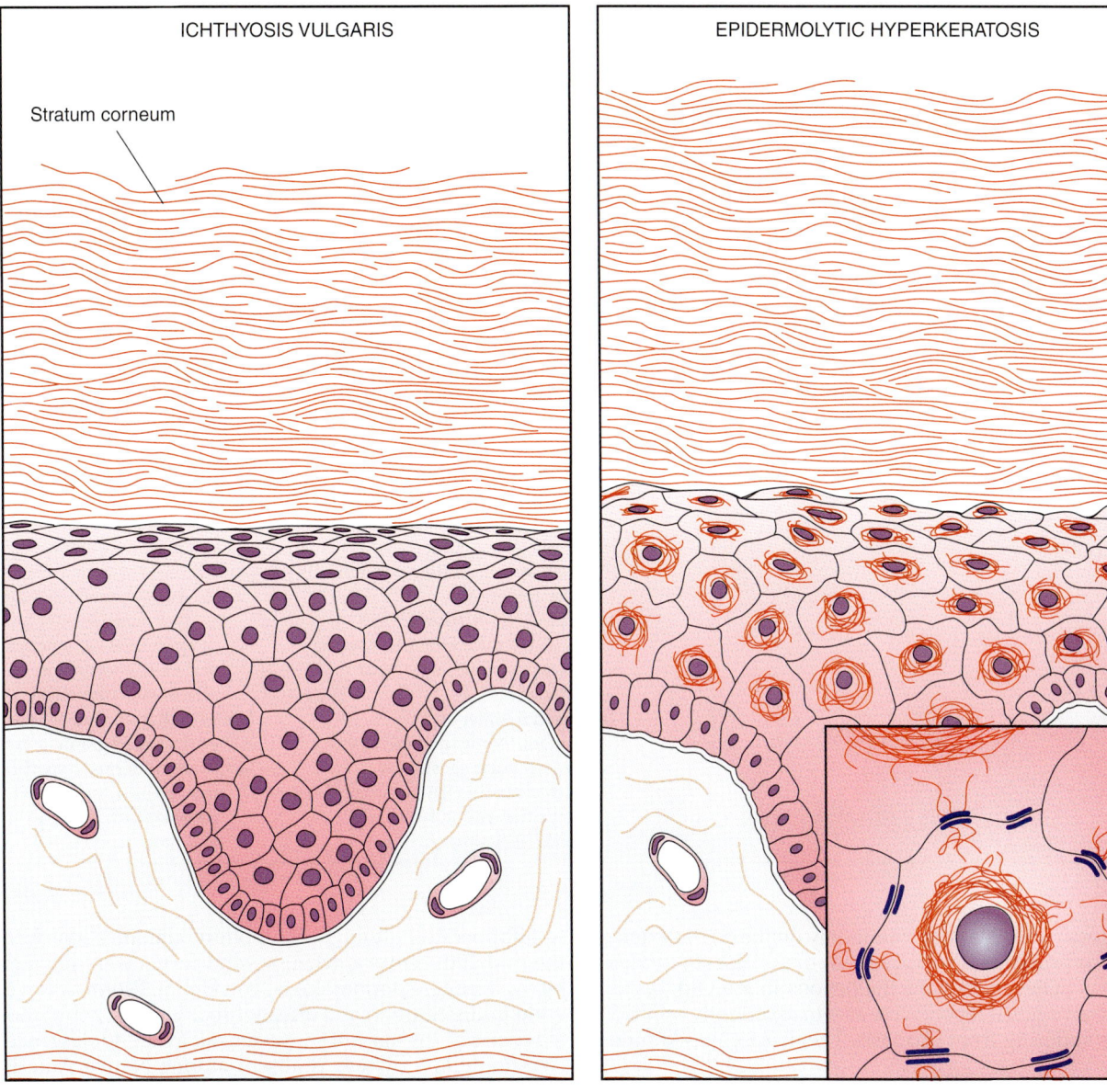

FIGURE 24-11
A. Ichthyosis vulgaris and (B) epidermolytic hyperkeratosis. Both diseases are characterized by thickening of the stratum corneum relative to the nucleated layers. Epidermolytic hyperkeratosis is characterized by abnormal keratin synthesis, manifested by whorled keratin filaments about the nucleus *(inset)*.

Pathology: Microscopically, the warty papule of Darier disease has a suprabasal cleft. Above and to the side of the cleft, dyskeratotic keratinocytes with eosinophilic cytoplasm contain keratin fibrils that whorl about the nucleus (Fig. 24-12). The roof of the cleft is formed by a column of compact keratotic material. In the stratum spinosum, some of these cells, called *corps ronds*, have pyknotic nuclei. The eosinophilic seedlike remnants of dyskeratotic cells in the stratum corneum are termed *corps grains*.

Clinical Features: Darier disease first appears late in childhood or in adolescence as skin-colored papules that later become crusted. The affected area displays numerous warty elevations, each 2 to 4 mm in diameter. The chest, nasolabial folds, back, scalp, forehead, ears, and groin are sites of predilection.

Psoriasis Is a Proliferative Skin Disease Characterized by Scaly Plaques

Psoriasis is a disease of the dermis and epidermis that is characterized by persistent epidermal hyperplasia. It is a chronic, frequently familial disorder that features large,

TABLE 24-1 A Comparisoin of the Major Ichthyoses

Type of Ichthyosis	Mode of Inheritance	Present at Birth	Pathogenetic Mechanism	Histology
Ichthyosis vulgaris	Autosomal dominant	No; onset in childhood	Normal epidermal turnover Retention keratosis due to defective dissolution of adhesive mechanisms in the stratum corneum	Hyperkeratosis, loosely woven, disproportionately thick in relationship to a relatively thin stratum spinosum Thin granular layer with abnormal keratohyaline granules
Sex-linked ichthyosis	X-linked recessive	Yes; onset may be in infancy	Normal epidermal turnover Constitutional absence of steroid sulfatase and arylsulfatase-C Retention keratosis due to a failure to break down cholesterol sulfate, an important substance in stratum corneum adhesion	Compact, disproportionately thick stratum corneum. Normal granular layer. Stratum spinosum only slightly thick
Epidermolytic hyperkeratosis	Autosomal recessive	Yes	Increased germinative cell replication and decreased cellular transit time through the epidermis Defect in keratin genes *K1* and *K10*, the differentiation-specific keratins of the suprabasal epidermis	Tonofilaments aggregate at the cell periphery and have a distorted association with desmosomes, which may lead to dyshesion (acantholysis) of epidermal keratinocytes and vesicle formation; entire skin is rarely involved
Lamellar ichthyosis	Autosomal recessive	Yes	Increased number of keratinosomes and increased intercellular substance; defects in transglutaminase acylation and in lamellar body secretion	Moderate hyperkeratosis; normal or thickened granular layer Moderate epidermal hyperplasia; may be psoriasiform with parakeratosis; entire skin and nails are involved

erythematous, scaly plaques, commonly on the dorsal extensor cutaneous surfaces. Psoriasis is one of the oldest diseases known. It is believed that the injunctions in the Old Testament directed against lepers were also inadvertently applied to persons suffering from psoriasis. The disease was known to Hippocrates, although its modern classification dates to the mid-19th century, when several forms were recognized by the Viennese dermatologist von Hebra. Psoriasis is worldwide in distribution and affects 1 to 2% of the population. It may arise at any age but shows a peak in late adolescence. Interestingly, the disease is absent among Native Americans and shows a low incidence among Asians.

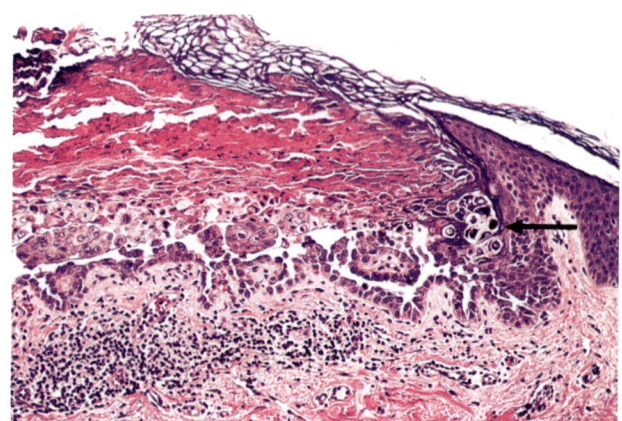

FIGURE 24-12
Darier disease. Virtually the entire epidermis exhibits focal acantholytic dyskeratosis. A small portion of normal epidermis is present *(right)*. In the lesion, there is a suprabasal cleft with a few dyshesive (acantholytic) keratinocytes surmounted by hyperkeratosis and parakeratosis. The cleft is not a vesicle because true vesicles contain inflammatory cells and tissue fluid. Dyskeratosis is present above the cleft.

 Pathogenesis: The pathogenesis of psoriasis remains poorly understood and is likely multifactorial.

GENETIC FACTORS: Psoriasis unquestionably has a genetic component, although only one third of patients with psoriasis have a positive family history of the disease. The more severe the illness, the greater the likelihood of a familial background. The genetic basis for psoriasis rests on a number of observations: (1) an increased incidence of the disease among relatives and offspring of patients with psoriasis, (2) 65% concordance for psoriasis in monozygotic twins, and (3) increased occurrence of certain HLA haplotypes in affected persons. The frequency of HLA-B13, HLA-B17. HLA-Bw57, and particularly HLA-Cw6, are all increased. In fact, persons with the HLA-Cw6 phenotype are 10 to 15 times more likely to develop psoriasis than is the general population.

ENVIRONMENTAL FACTORS: The entire epidermis of any person with the psoriatic phenotype can express clinical lesions. In this context, a variety of stimuli, such as physical injury *(Köbner's phenomenon),* infection, certain drugs, and photosensitivity, may produce psoriatic lesions in apparently normal skin. The pathogenesis of the psoriatic plaques may be appreciated by contrasting the effect of chronic cutaneous trauma in persons with and without psoriasis. Chronic irritation of the skin of a normal person—for instance, that caused by repeated rubbing—produces a tough, scaly, cutaneous plaque that is psoriasiform both clinically and histologically. However, with cessation of the trauma, the lesion disappears. In the psoriatic patient, even less trauma produces a psoriatic plaque that may persist for years after the initial injury.

ABNORMAL CELLULAR PROLIFERATION: There is evidence to suggest that deregulation of epidermal proliferation and an abnormality in the microcirculation of the dermis are responsible for the development of psoriatic lesions (Fig. 24-13). Abnormal proliferation of keratinocytes is possibly related to defective epidermal cell surface receptors. A decrease in the activity of adenylyl cyclase in the lower proliferative compartment of the epidermis has been attributed to faulty β-adrenergic receptors. The decrease in cAMP alters cutaneous responses to trauma in complex ways that are not fully understood.

An increase in cAMP-regulated proteinases and augmented polyamines of low molecular weight are postulated to be associated with a growth factor-like effect and induction of neutrophilic inflammation. Acute inflammation follows an increase in phospholipase A_2, which enhances the production of arachidonic acid. In turn, the lipooxygenase metabolites of arachidonic acid, notably leukotriene B_4, exert potent neutrophilic chemotactic effects.

MICROCIRCULATORY CHANGES: In psoriatic skin, the capillary loops of the dermal papillae become venular, showing multiple layers of basal lamina material, wide lumina, and "bridged" fenestrations between endothelial cells. The vascular change, which occurs in concert with a striking increase in neutrophilic chemotactic factors, leads to diapedesis of many neutrophils at the tips of dermal papillae and subsequent migration into the epidermis (the "squirting papillae") (Fig. 24-13). This unusual pattern of neutrophilic inflammation is responsible for the dense collections of neutrophils in the stratum corneum *(Munro microabscesses)* as well as for the scattering of neutrophils throughout the epidermis *(spongiform pustules).*

IMMUNOLOGICAL FACTORS: T lymphocytes have been proposed to contribute to the pathogenesis of psoriatic lesions. The eruption of such lesions coincides with the infiltration of T cells into the epidermis. By contrast, resolution of psoriatic plaques, whether spontaneous or induced by treatment, is preceded by the disappearance of, or reduction in the number of, epidermal T cells. Streptococcal superantigens reportedly induce the expression of cutaneous lymphocyte antigens, which enable T cells to migrate to the skin. Finally, T lymphocytes from psoriatic patients can produce lesional plaques in apparently normal skin when transferred to nude mice.

In summary, the keratinocytes of persons afflicted with psoriasis possess a genetically determined phenotype that exhibits a capacity for hyperproliferation and altered differentiation. A number of environmental stimuli may trigger the release of cytokines and growth factors by the keratinocytes and other cell types in the epidermis. The ensuing immune and inflammatory responses contribute to the full development of psoriatic lesions.

Pathology: The most distinctive pathological changes are seen at the periphery of a chronic psoriatic plaque. The epidermis is thickened and displays both hyperkeratosis and parakeratosis. Parakeratosis may manifest as circumscribed, ellipsoidal foci, or it may be diffuse, in which case the granular layer is diminished or absent. The nucleated layers of the epidermis are thickened several-fold in the rete pegs and are frequently thinner over the dermal papillae (Fig. 24-14). In turn, the papillae are elongated and appear as sections of cones, with their apices toward the dermis. In chronic lesions, the papillae tend to appear as bulbous clubs with short handles (Figs. 24-14 and 24-15). The rete ridges of the epidermis have a profile reciprocal to that of the dermal papillae, resulting in interlocked mesepnchymal and epithelial clubs, with alternatively reversed polarity (Fig. 24-15). The capillaries of the papillae are dilated and tortuous. In a very early lesion, the changes may be limited to dilation of capillaries and a few neutrophils "squirting" into the epidermis. Epidermal hyperplasia and hyperkeratosis are hallmarks of more-chronic lesions.

Ultrastructurally, the capillaries are venulelike; neutrophils may emerge at their tips and migrate into the epidermis above the apices of the papillae. Neutrophils may become localized in the epidermal spinous layer or in small Munro microabscesses in the stratum corneum and may be associated with circumscribed areas of parakeratosis (Fig. 24-16). The dermis below the papillae exhibits a varying number of mononuclear inflammatory cells, mostly lymphocytes, around the superficial vascular plexus. There is little extension of the inflammatory process into the subjacent reticular dermis.

The psoriasiform histological pattern is common in cutaneous pathology. Seborrheic dermatitis, reaction to chronic trauma (lichen simplex chronicus), and cutaneous T-cell lymphoma (mycosis fungoides) all exhibit psoriasiform epidermal change.

Clinical Features: The severity of psoriasis varies from annoying scaly lesions over the elbows to a serious debilitating disorder involving most of the skin and often associated with arthritis. A single lesion of psoriasis may be a small focus of scaly erythema or an enormous confluent plaque covering much of the trunk (Fig. 24-14). A typical plaque is 4 to 5 cm in diameter, is sharply demarcated at its margin, and is covered by a surface of silvery scales. When the scales are detached, pinpoint foci of bleeding, originating from the dilated capillaries in the dermal papillae, dot the underlying glossy erythematous surface *(Auspitz sign).*

Of all patients with psoriasis, 7% develop seronegative arthritis (see Chapter 26). The tendency to arthropathy has a genetic component and is linked to several HLA haplotypes, particularly HLA-B27. Psoriatic arthritis closely resembles its rheumatoid counterpart, but it is usually milder and causes little disability.

Psoriasis is a disease of intermittent activity and variable presentation, but familial psoriasis is unusually severe. In some variations of the disease, neutrophilic pustules

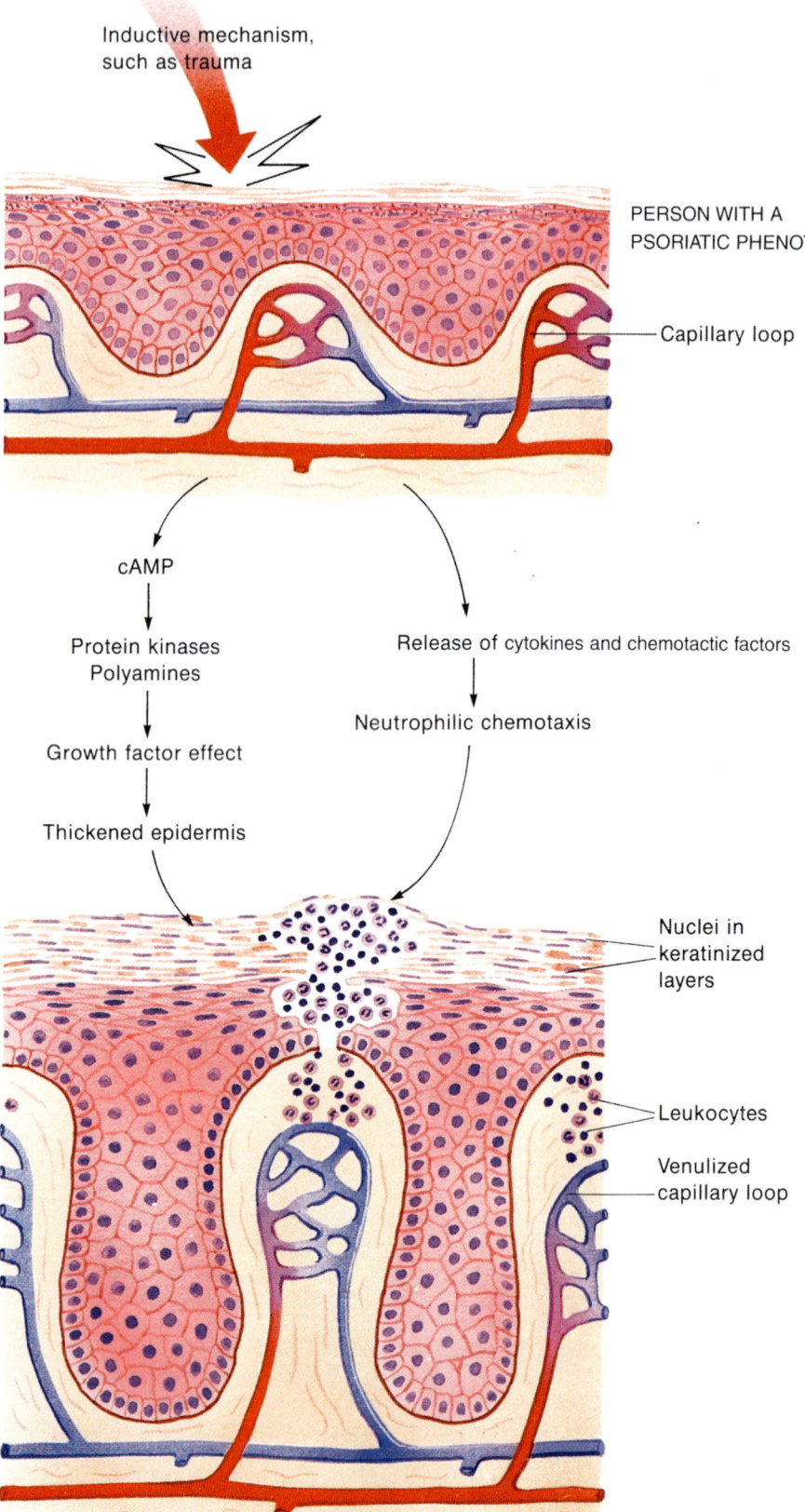

FIGURE 24-13
Pathogenetic mechanisms in psoriasis. The drawing depicts the deregulation of epidermal growth, venulization of the capillary loop, and a unique form of neutrophilic inflammation. The altered epidermal growth is thought to be caused by defective epidermal cell surface receptors. This results in a decrease in cAMP, together with the effects indicated. The decrease in cAMP is also likely to be related to the increased production of arachidonic acid, which in turn leads to activation of LTB-4. This potent neutrophilic chemotactic agent acts on a venulized capillary loop. Neutrophils then emerge from the tips of the capillary loop at the apex of the dermal papilla rather than from the postcapillary venule, as is the rule in most inflammatory skin diseases.

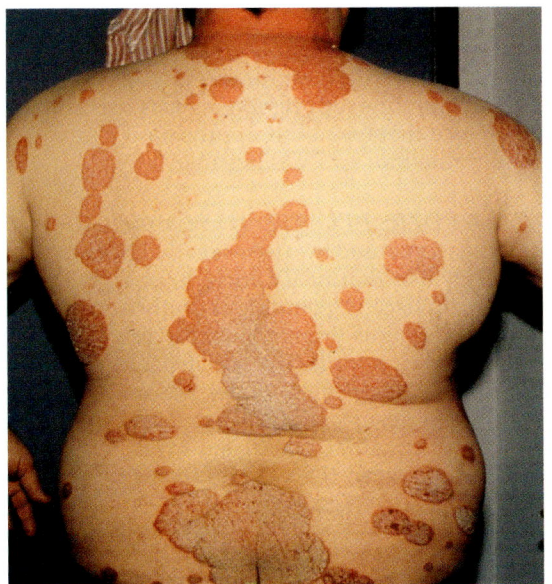
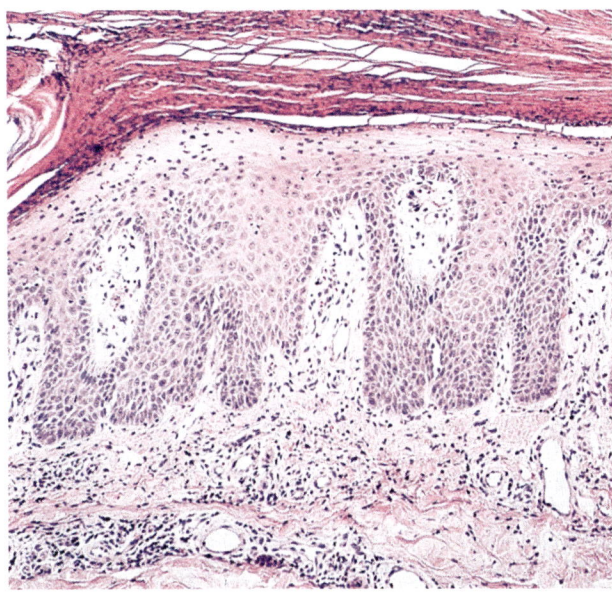

FIGURE 24-14
Psoriasis. This disorder is the prototype of psoriasiform epidermal hyperplasia. **A.** A patient with psoriasis shows large, confluent, sharply demarcated, erythematous plaques on the trunk. **B.** Microscopic examination of a lesion demonstrates that the rete ridges are uniformly elongated, as are the dermal papillae, giving an interlocking pattern of alternately reversed "club's." The dermal papillae are edematous and reside beneath a thinned epidermis (suprapapillary thinning). There is striking parakeratosis, which is the scale observed clinically.

dominate the pathological process *(pustular psoriasis)*. Severe intractable psoriasis has been observed in some patients with acquired AIDS, but the cause is not known.

Psoriasis has long been treated with coal tar or wood tar derivatives and anthralin, a strong reducing agent. Topical and systemic corticosteroids have also been used. Severe, generalized psoriasis justifies systemic treatment with methotrexate, although hepatic toxicity remains a threat (see Chapter 14). Phototherapy ("PUVA") after the administration of psoralens (ultraviolet-absorbing compounds that

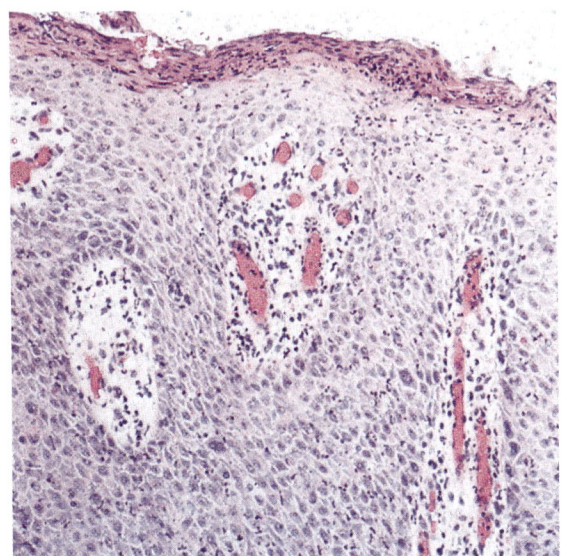

FIGURE 24-15
Psoriasis. The clubbed papillae contain tortuous dilated venules. The prominent venules are part of the venulization of capillaries, which may be of histogenetic importance in psoriasis. The papilla to the *right* has one cross-section of its superficial capillary venule loop, which is normal. The papilla in the *center* shows numerous cross-sections of its venule, indicating striking tortuosity.

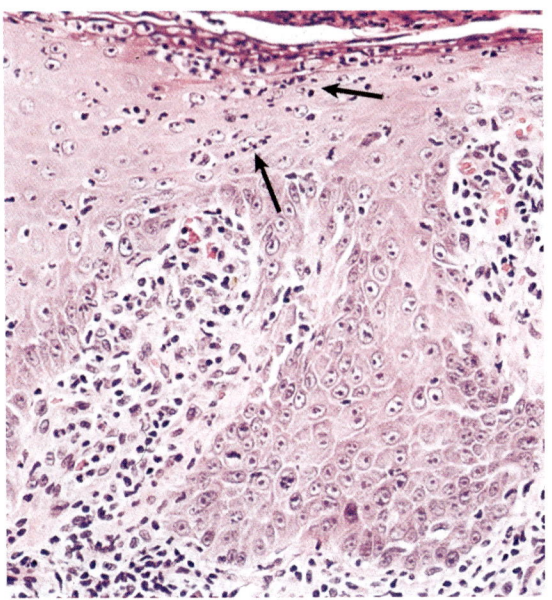

FIGURE 24-16
Psoriasis. Neutrophils migrate into the epidermis, emerging from the venulized capillaries at the tips of the dermal papillae. They migrate to the upper stratum spinosum and stratum corneum *(arrows).* In some forms of psoriasis, pustules are common clinical lesions.

bind to DNA) has proved effective in many severe cases. More recently, synthetic derivatives of vitamin A and vitamin D have been added to the list of pharmacological treatments.

Pemphigus Vulgaris Is a Blistering Skin Disorder Caused by Antibodies to Keratinocytes

Dyshesive disorders are cutaneous maladies in which blister formation is secondary to diminished cohesiveness of the epidermal keratinocytes. Pemphigus vulgaris (Greek, *pemphix*, "bubble"), the prototype of dyshesive diseases, is a chronic, blistering skin disorder caused by the action of antibodies to surface antigens on stratified squamous cells. The malady occurs most commonly between 40 and 60 years of age, but it is reported in all age groups, including children. All races are susceptible to pemphigus vulgaris (PV), but persons of Jewish or Mediterranean heritage are at greater risk.

Pathogenesis: PV is an autoimmune disease caused by antibodies to a keratinocyte antigen. Circulating IgG antibodies in patients with PV react with an epidermal surface antigen called *desmoglein 3*, a desmosomal protein. Antigen–antibody union results in dyshesion, which is augmented by the release of plasminogen activator and, hence, the activation of plasmin. This proteolytic enzyme acts on the intercellular substance and may be the dominant factor in dyshesion. Internalization of the pemphigus antigen–antibody complex, disappearance of attachment plaques, and retraction of perinuclear tonofilaments may all act in concert with proteinases to cause dyshesion and vesiculation (Fig. 24-17).

Pathology The blister in PV forms because of the separation of the stratum spinosum and outer epidermal layers from the basal layer. This suprabasal dyshesion results in a blister that has an intact basal layer as a floor and the remaining epidermis as a roof (Figs. 24-18 and 24-19). Desmoglein 3 is concentrated in the lower epidermis, explaining the location of the blister. The blister contains a moderate number of lymphocytes, macrophages, eosinophils, and neutrophils. Distinctive, rounded keratinocytes, termed acantholytic cells, are shed into the vesicle during the process of dyshesion. The basal cells remain adherent to the basal lamina and form a layer of "tombstone cells." The dyshesion may extend along the dermal adnexa and is not always strictly suprabasal. The subjacent dermis shows a moderate infiltrate of lymphocytes, macrophages, eosinophils, and neutrophils, predominantly around the capillary venular bed.

Clinical Features: The characteristic lesion of PV is a large, easily ruptured blister that leaves extensive denuded or crusted areas. The lesions are most common on the scalp and mucous membranes and in the periumbilical and intertriginous areas. Without corticosteroid treatment, the disease is progressive and usually fatal, and much of the cutaneous surface may become denuded. Immunosuppressive agents are also useful for maintenance therapy. With appropriate treatment, the 10-year mortality rate for PV is less than 10%.

DISORDERS RELATED TO PEMPHIGUS VULGARIS: Other diseases caused by dyshesion that have a pathogenetic mechanism like that of PV include pemphigus vegetans, pemphigus foliaceus, pemphigus erythematosus, and drug-induced pemphigus (most commonly associated with penicillamine and captopril). The specific antigen of pemphigus foliaceus is *desmoglein 1*, a desmosomal protein. Autoantibodies to desmoglein 1 cause dyshesion in the outer spinous and granular epidermal layers (Fig. 24-20). The differences between the various forms of pemphigus are

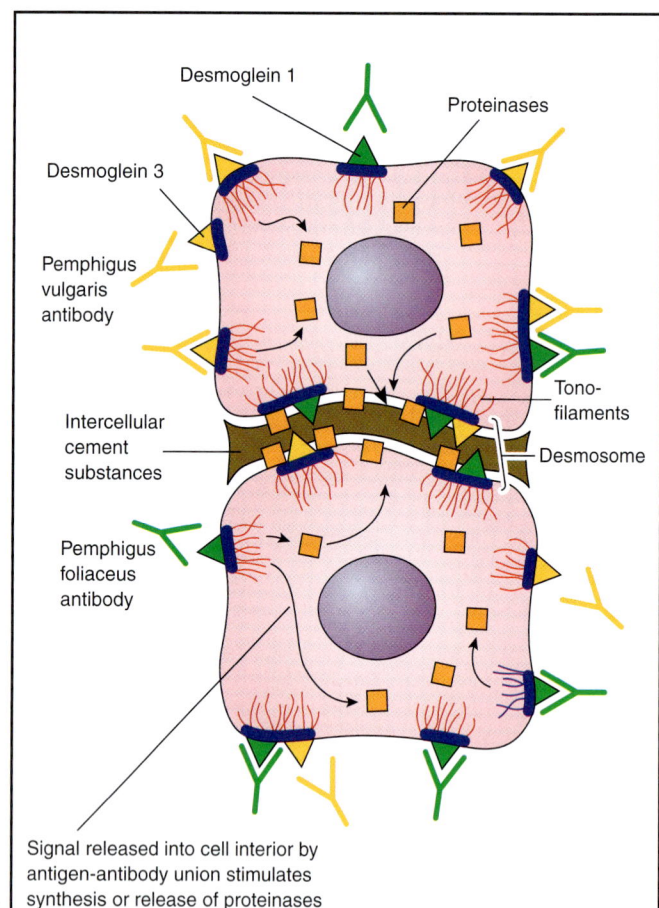

FIGURE 24-17
Pemphigus vulgaris. A pathogenetic mechanism of suprabasal dyshesion is shown. (1) A circulating autoantibody binds to an antigen on the outer leaflet of the plasma membrane (desmosome) of the keratinocyte, especially in the basal regions. (2) Antigen–antibody union results in release of a proteinase (plasmin). (3) The proteinase interacts with intercellular cement, initiating dyshesion. (4) Desmosomes deteriorate, tonofilaments clump about the nucleus, the cells round up, and separation is complete. (5) A vesicle, which is usually suprabasal, forms. Alternatively, acantholysis may occur by direct interference with desmosomal and adherence junction attachments.

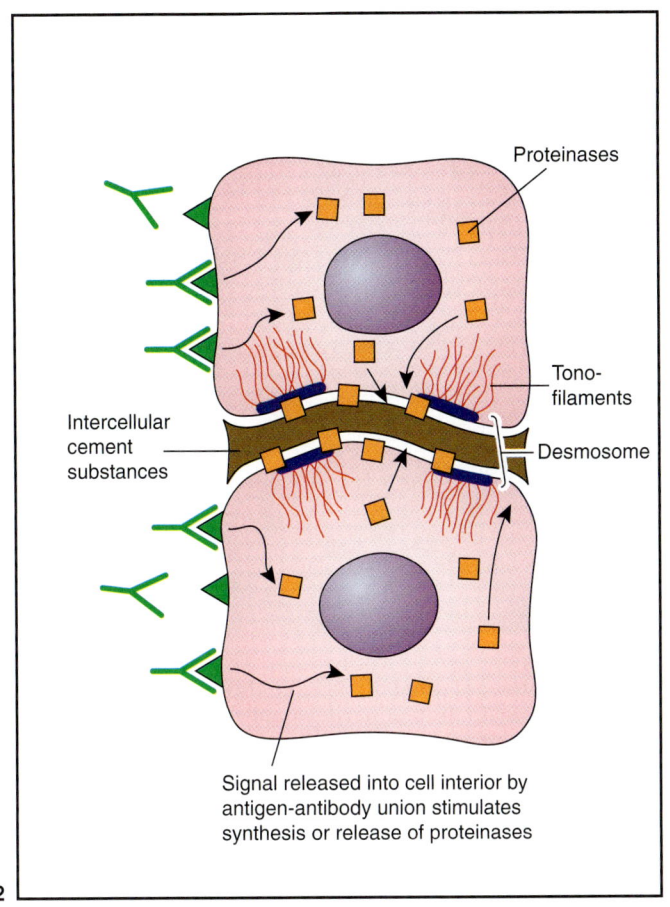
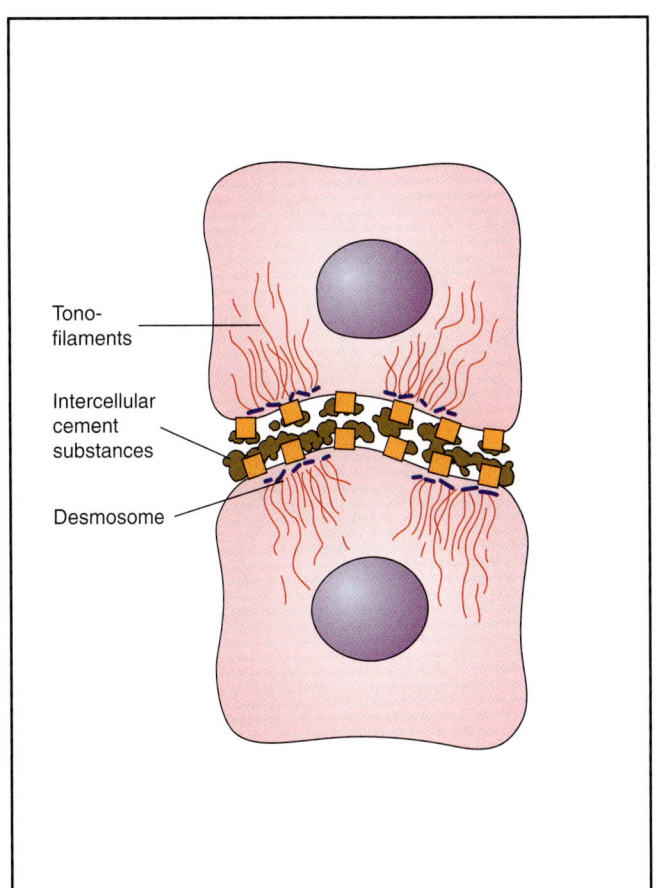
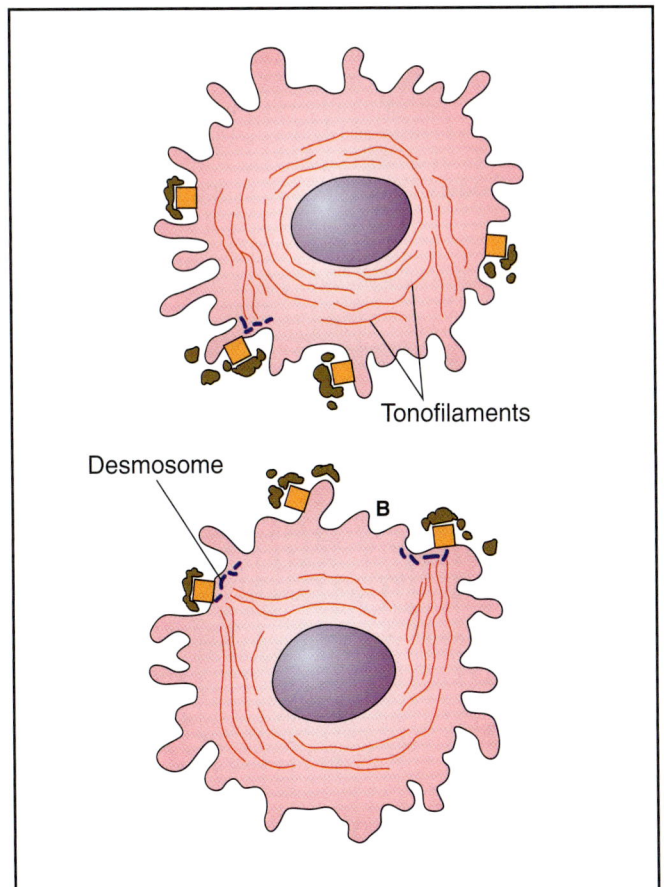
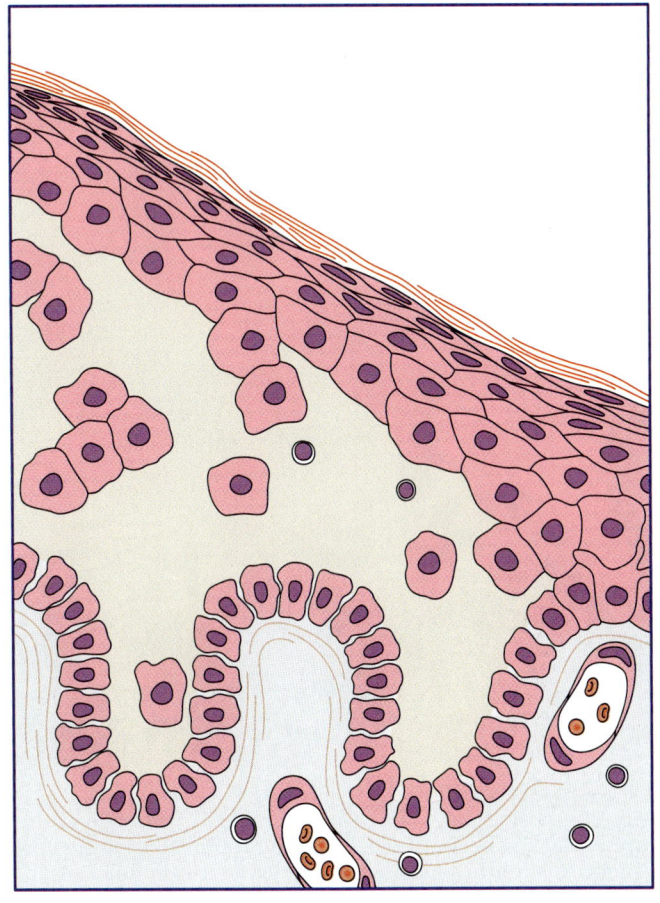

FIGURE 24-17 *(continued)*

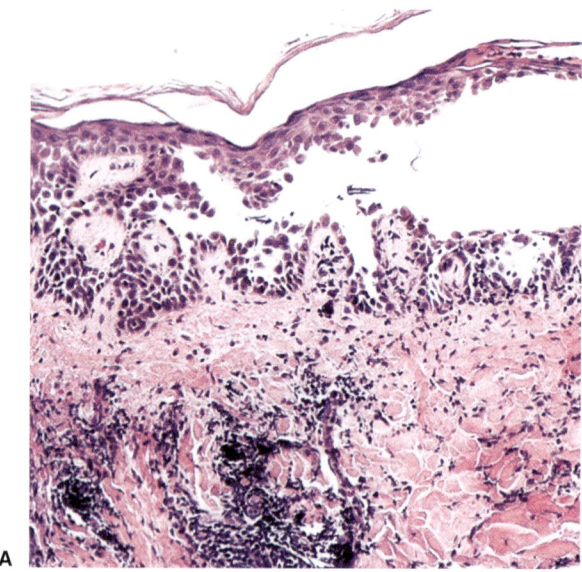
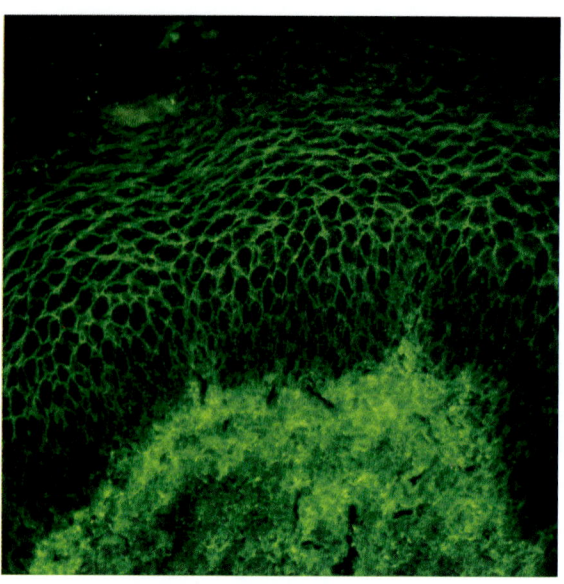

FIGURE 24-18
Pemphigus vulgaris. A. Suprabasal dyshesion leads to an intraepidermal blister containing acantholytic keratinocytes. B. Direct immunofluorescence examination of perilesional skin reveals antibodies, usually of the IgG type, deposited in the intercellular substance of the epidermis, yielding a lacelike pattern outlining the keratinocytes.

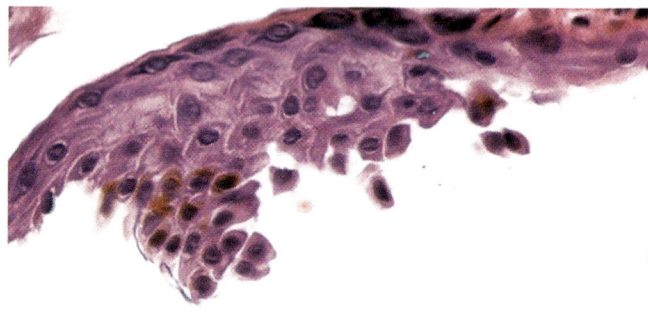

outlined in Table 24-2. Paraneoplastic pemphigus has been described in association with cancers, usually lymphoproliferative tumors.

Pemphigus may be associated with other autoimmune diseases, such as myasthenia gravis and lupus erythematosus, and may also be seen with benign thymomas. Other diseases may mimic the histological appearance of PV, namely, familial benign chronic pemphigus *(Hailey-Hailey disease)* and transient acantholytic dermatosis *(Grover disease)*. However, IgG antibodies do not react with epidermal antigens in these entities.

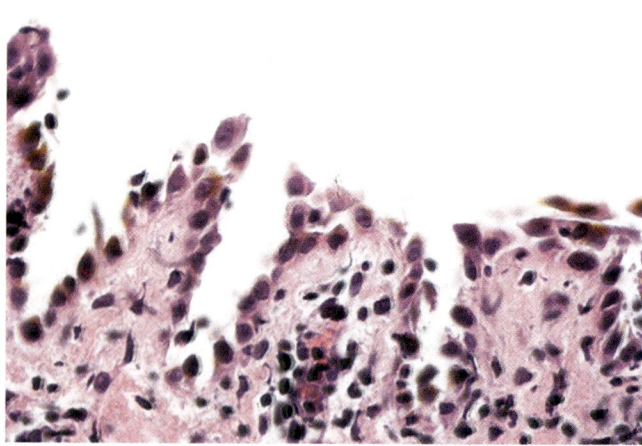

FIGURE 24-19
Pemphigus vulgaris. High-power magnification of the suprabasal dyshesion reveals crisply delineated basal keratinocytes slightly separated from each other and totally separated from the stratum spinosum. The basal keratinocytes are firmly attached to the epidermal basement membrane zone.

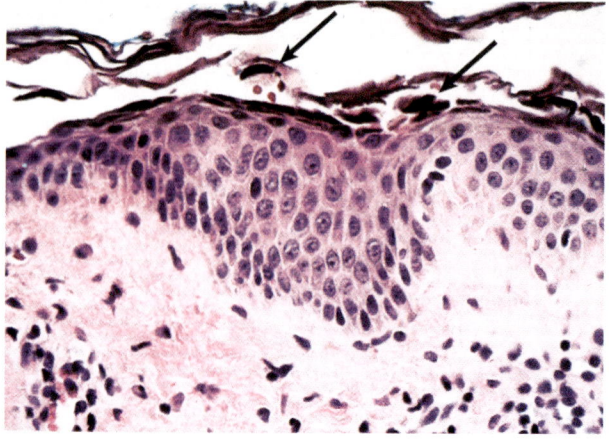

FIGURE 24-20
Pemphigus foliaceus. The dyshesion develops in the outer stratum spinosum and stratum granulosum. (Compare with that of pemphigus vulgaris; Fig. 24-19.) Dyshesive and dyskeratotic keratinocytes of the stratum granulosum *(arrows)* are important hallmarks.

TABLE 24-2 Diseases of the Pemphigus Group: Reactive Antibodies of the IgG Type to Antigen on the Plasma Membranes of Stratified Squamous Epithelia

Type of Pemphigus	Clinical Features	Pathology
Pemphigus vulgaris	Flaccid, easily ruptured bullae commonly involving the scalp, periumbilical region, intertriginous areas, and mucous membranes Commonly occurs during the fourth and fifth decades of life Occurs predominantly in persons of Jewish origin and other Mediterranean peoples	Suprabasal dyshesive vesicle with a sparse infiltrate of lymphocytes, macrophages, and eosinophils; antigen is desmoglein 3 (in desmosomes)
Pemphigus vegetans	A variant of pemphigus vulgaris, but healing in intertriginous areas is characterized by complex papillary epidermal hyperplasia, resulting in verrucous or vegetating lesions	The same as for pemphigus vulgaris with superimposed extensive epidermal hyperplasia Eosinophils may be numerous
Pemphigus foliaceus	Bullae occur early in the course of the disease but may not be present; the disease may be eczematoid, with shallow erosions, scales, and crusting; the scalp, face, throat, back, and abdomen are commonly involved, but mucous membrane involvement is uncommon; not fatal if untreated; question of slight predominance in Jews	Dyshesion is in the spinous layer; granular cells may peel apart; appearance is of shedding granular cells one by one Variable number of inflammatory cells Neutrophils may be numerous with formation of subcorneal pustules Antigen is desmoglein 1 (in desmosomes)
Pemphigus erythematosus	Similar to pemphigus foliaceus but dominated by lupuslike changes on the butterfly area of the face Immunologically, patients have pemphigus antibodies, antinuclear antibodies, and immune-complex deposits of lupus erythematosus	Same as for pemphigus foliaceus

DISEASES OF THE BASEMENT MEMBRANE ZONE (DERMAL–EPIDERMAL INTERFACE)

Epidermolysis Bullosa Features Blister Formation in the Basement Membrane Zone

Epidermolysis bullosa (EB) comprises a heterogeneous group of disorders loosely bound by their hereditary nature and by a tendency to form blisters at the sites of minor trauma. The clinical spectrum of the disease ranges from a minor annoyance to a widespread, life-threatening blistering disease. These blisters are almost always noted at birth or shortly thereafter. The classification of these disorders is based on the site of blister formation in the basement membrane zone (BMZ) (Table 24-3). The different mechanisms of blister formation that underlie each of the three major categories of EB are shown in Figure 24-21.

Epidermolytic EB

This disorder also known as *EB simplex*, is a group of autosomal dominant skin diseases that display blister formation as a result of disruption of basal keratinocytes. Epidermolytic EB has been attributed to mutations of genes encoding cytokeratin intermediate filaments, which likely provide mechanical stability to the epidermis. The blisters develop in response to minor trauma, such as merely rubbing the skin, but heal without scarring (thus, the term *simplex*). Although

TABLE 24-3 Classification of Epidermolysis Bullosa (Selected Variants)

Class	Site of Blister Formation	Name of Variant	Healing Residuum	Heredity	Molecular Defect	Chromosomal Defect
Epidermolytic	Within the basal keratinocytic layer	Localized epidermolysis bullosa simplex Generalized epidermolysis bullosa simplex	None None	Autosomal dominant Autosomal dominant	Keratins 5 and 14	12q11-13 and 17q21
Junctional	Lamina lucida	Epidermolysis bullosa letalis Generalized atrophic benign epidermolysis bullosa	None or atrophic skin Atrophic skin	Autosomal recessive Autosomal recessive	Laminin 5 Integrins α6β4 Collagen type XVII	1q25-31, 1q3, and 18q11.2 1q32 and 10q23.4
Dermolytic	Immediately deep to the lamina densa	Dystrophic epidermolysis bullosa Dystrophic epidermolysis bullosa	Scars, nails deformed Scars, teeth, and nails deformed	Autosomal dominant Autosomal recessive	Collagen type VII	3p21

EPIDERMOLYTIC EB

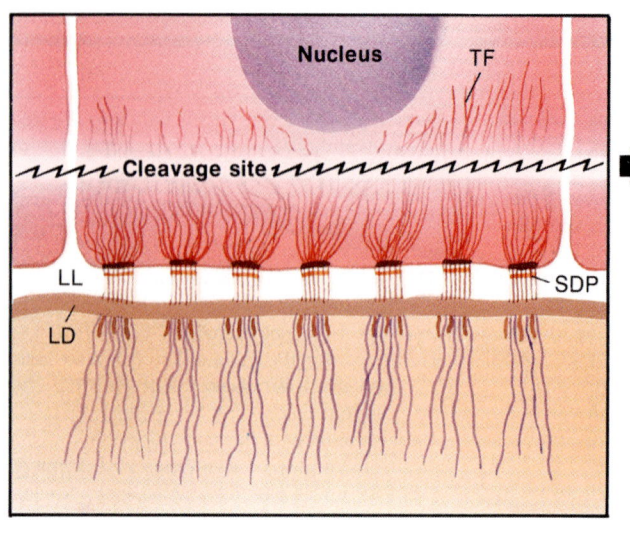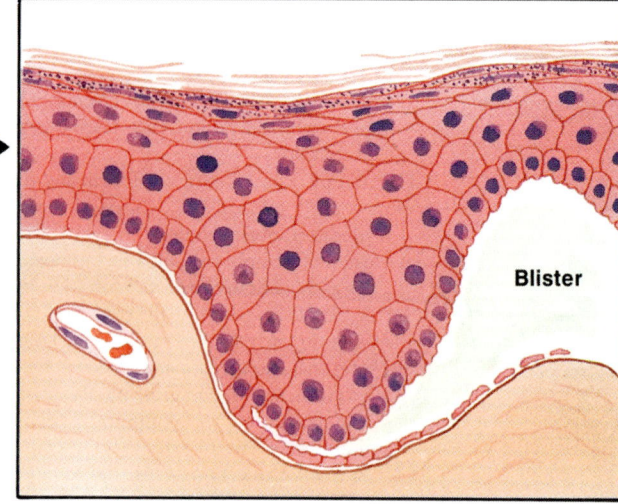

JUNCTIONAL EB

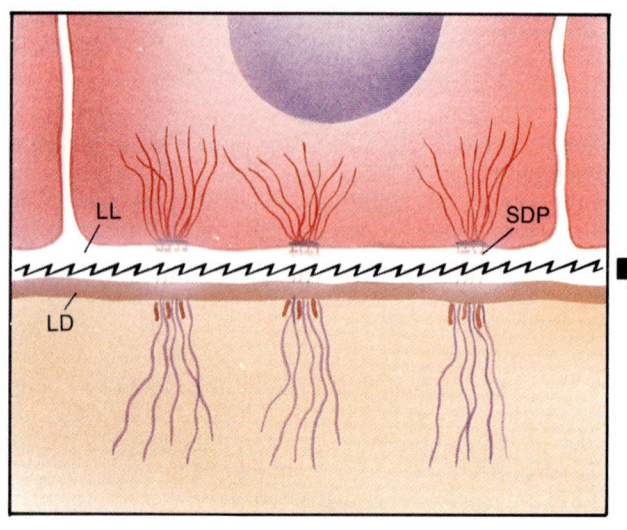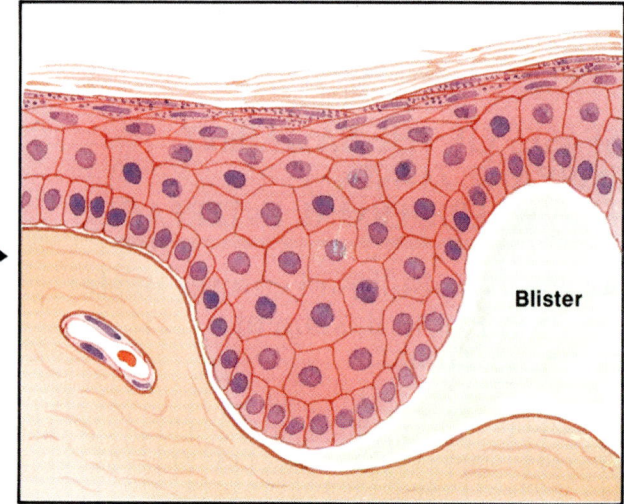

DERMOLYTIC EB

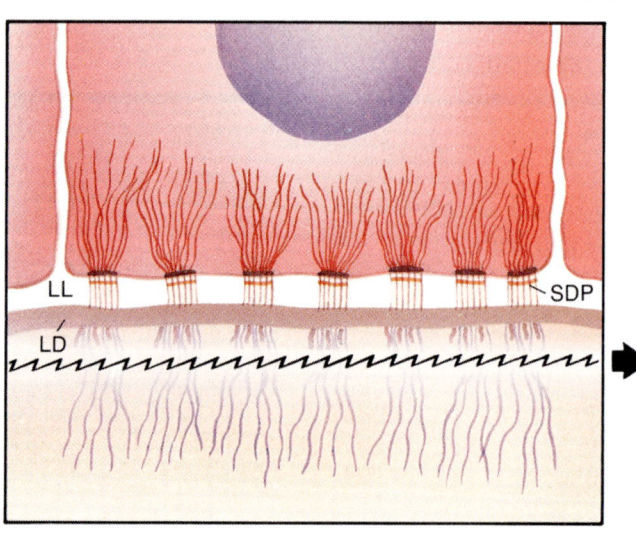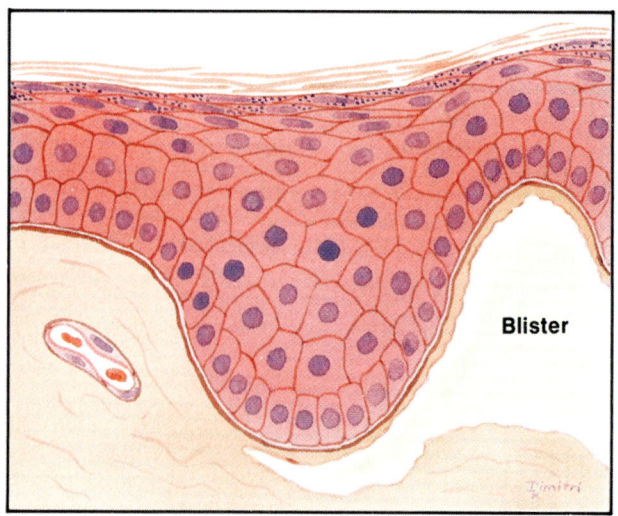

epidermolytic EB is cosmetically disturbing and sometimes debilitating, it is not life threatening.

Pathology: Cytolysis of the basal keratinocytes is the basis of blister formation in the epidermolytic variety of EB. Initially, small, subnuclear, cytoplasmic vacuoles develop, increase in size, and coalesce. The formation of these vacuoles reflects the presence of abnormal keratins 5 and 14, which aggregate about the keratinocyte nuclei. The plasma membrane ruptures when the large vacuole reaches it, after which the cell is lysed. An intraepidermal vesicle results from the lysis of several basal keratinocytes. The roof of the vesicle is an almost intact epidermis with a fragmented basal layer. The floor of the vesicle shows bits of basal cell cytoplasm attached to the lamina densa, which is seen as a well-preserved pink line at the base of the vesicle. Inflammatory cells are sparse.

Junctional EB

This type of EB is a heritable, autosomal recessive skin disease in which blisters form within the lamina lucida. The clinical expression ranges from a benign disease with no effect on the life span to a severe condition that may be fatal within the first 2 years of life.

Pathogenesis: In the severe form, mutations in the genes for certain isoforms of laminin and the integrins have been reported. The benign form has been attributed to mutations in the gene coding for type XVII collagen. Both varieties heal without scarring, but there may be residual atrophy of the skin. There may also be associated abnormalities of nails and teeth.

Pathology: An intact epidermis forms the roof of the vesicle in junctional EB. The plasma membranes of the basal keratinocytes are unchanged. The floor of the vesicle is an intact lamina densa, as in epidermolytic EB, but the attached fragments of basal cell cytoplasm are lacking. The blister, therefore, occurs within the lamina lucida. Both lesional and uninvolved skin shows fewer basal hemidesmosomes, which have poorly developed attachment plaques and subbasal dense plates.

Dermolytic EB

Also known as *dystrophic EB* dermolytic EB is a heritable skin condition in which blisters are located immediately deep to the lamina densa. Dermolytic disease may be either dominant or recessive, the latter being more severe. In both variants, healed blisters are characterized by atrophic ("dystrophic") scarring. There may be associated abnormalities of nails and teeth.

Pathogenesis: The development of dermolytic EB is attributed to a defect in anchoring fibrils. An abnormal architecture and a reduced number of these fibrils have been demonstrated in apparently normal skin of affected newborns. The basic defect is a mutation in the gene encoding collagen type VII on chromosome 3 (3p21). Anchoring fibrils comprise a net in the upper dermis through which fibers of collagen types I and III course. This structure serves to anchor the epidermis to the underlying dermis, and its disruption results in subepidermal bullae arising in the sublamina densa zone.

Pathology: The roof of the vesicle is normal epidermis with an attached, intact lamina lucida and lamina densa. The base of the vesicle is formed by the outer part of the papillary dermis. Ultrastructurally, there are fewer anchoring fibrils in the dominant variant and a virtual absence of fibrils in the recessive form. A corresponding decrease in the anchoring fibril proteins AF-1 and AF-2 occurs in the two variants.

Bullous Pemphigoid (BP) Is an Autoimmune Blistering Disease That Involves Basement Membrane Proteins

BP is a common, autoimmune, blistering disease with clinical similarities to pemphigus vulgaris (thus, the term *pem-*

FIGURE 24-21

Epidermolysis bullosa. Three distinct mechanisms of blister formation are shown. Electron microscopic images are diagrammed on the *left*; light microscopic images are on the *right*. Epidermolytic EB is caused by disintegration of the lowermost regions of the epidermal basal cells. The bottom portions of the basal cells cleave, and the remainder of the epidermis lifts away. Small fragments of basal cells remain attached to the basement membrane zone. Junctional EB is characterized by cleavage in the lamina lucida. Dermolytic EB is associated with rudimentary and fragmented anchoring fibrils. The entire basement membrane zone and epidermis split away from the dermis in relationship to these flawed anchoring fibrils. *LL*, lamina lucida; *LD*, lamina densa; *SDP*, subdesomosomal dense plate.

phigoid) but in which acantholysis is absent. The disease is most common in the later decades of life, but it shows no predilection regarding race or gender.

Pathogenesis: Like pemphigus vulgaris, BP is an autoimmune disease, but in this case complement-fixing IgG antibodies are directed against two basement membrane proteins, BPAG1 and BPAG2. BPAG1 is a 230-kd protein located in the intracellular portion of the basal cell hemidesmosome. BPAG2 is a 180-kd protein that traverses the plasma membrane and extends into the upper lamina lucida. The antigen–antibody complex may injure the basal cell plasma membrane through the formation of the C5b–C9 membrane attack complex (see Chapter 4). In turn, this damage may interfere with the elaboration of adherence factors by basal keratinocytes. Of greater importance is the production of the anaphylatoxins C3a and C5a following activation of the complement cascade. These molecules cause degranulation of mast cells and the release of factors chemotactic for eosinophils, neutrophils, and lymphocytes. Levels of IL-5 and eotaxin, known to play significant roles in the recruitment and function of eosinophils, are increased in the blister fluid of BP patients. The eosinophil granules contain tissue-damaging substances, including eosinophil peroxidase and major basic protein. These molecules, together with proteases of neutrophilic and mast cell origin, cause dermal–epidermal separation within the lamina lucida (Fig. 24-22).

Pathology: The blisters of BP are subepidermal, with the roof of the blister formed by intact epidermis and the base by the lamina densa of the BMZ (Fig. 24-23). The blisters contain numerous eosinophils, together with fibrin, lymphocytes, and neutrophils. In BP, apparently normal skin shows migration of mast cells from the venule toward the epidermis. With the onset of erythema, eosinophils appear in the upper dermis and are occasionally arranged along the epidermal BMZ. Ultrastructurally, the first site of dermal–epidermal separation is in the lamina lucida and is associated with the disruption of anchoring filaments. Immunofluorescent studies demonstrate linear deposition of C3 and IgG along the epidermal BMZ and antibodies directed against BPAG1 and BPAG2 in the serum (Fig. 24-24).

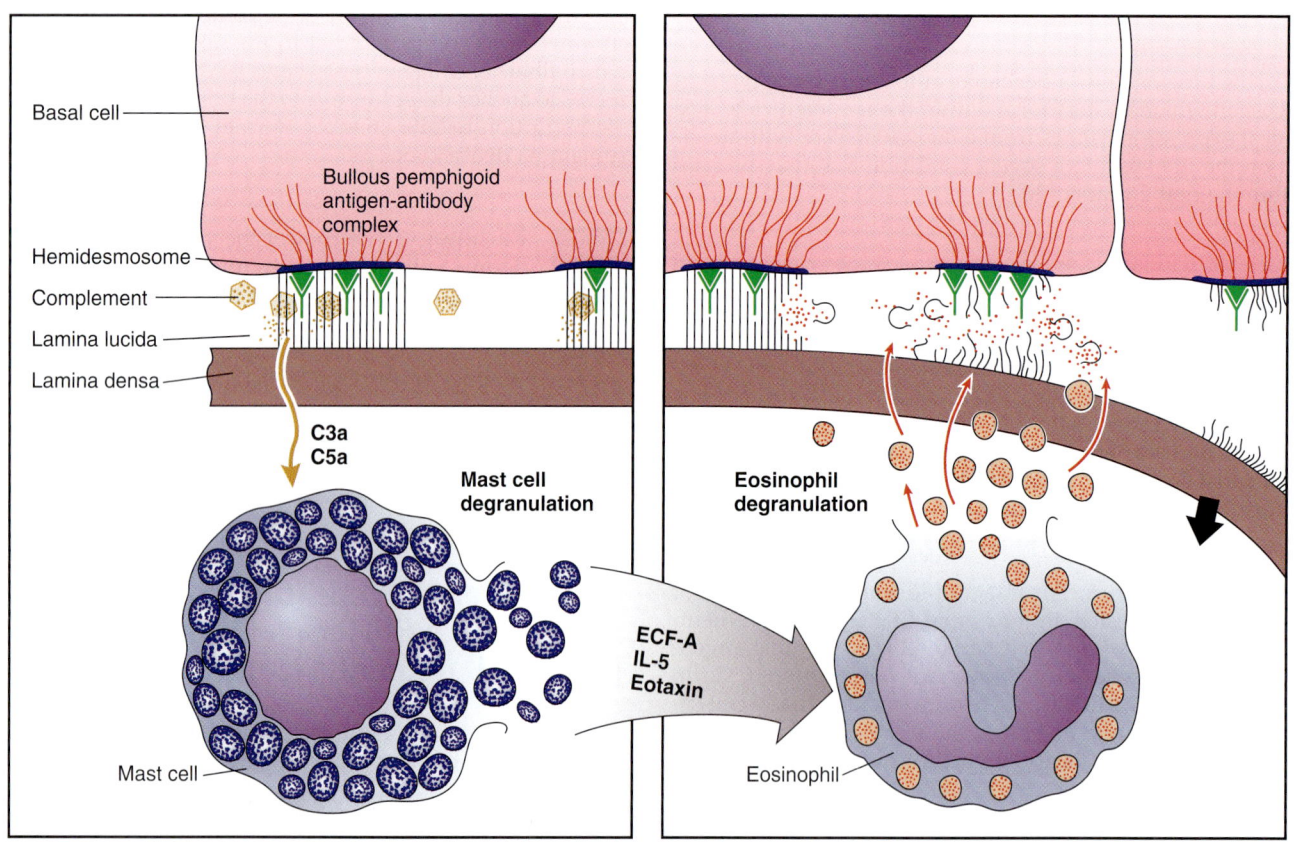

FIGURE 24-22

Bullous pemphigoid. Pathogenetic mechanisms of blister formation are outlined. A circulating antibody to an apparently normal glycoprotein—BP antigen—in the lamina lucida precipitates the pathogenetic events in bullous pemphigoid. **A.** Antigen–antibody union activates complement, and the anaphylatoxins C3a and C5a are produced. These degranulate mast cells, resulting in the release of eosinophilic chemotactic factors. **B** and **C.** The tissue-damaging substances of eosinophilic granules cause vesicle formation at the lamina lucida, with some breakdown of the lamina densa. *ECF-A*, eosinophil chemotactic factor-A.

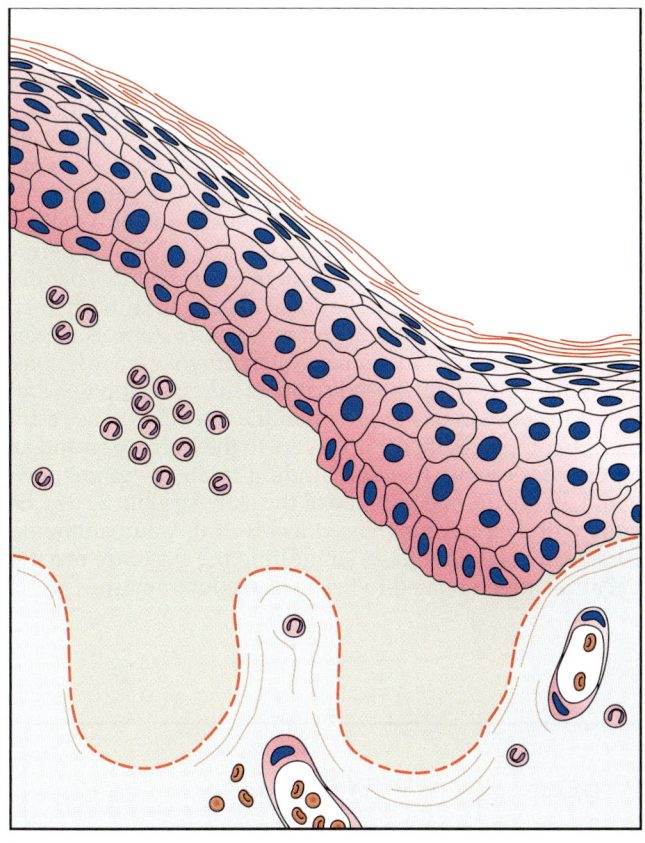

FIGURE 24-22 (continued)

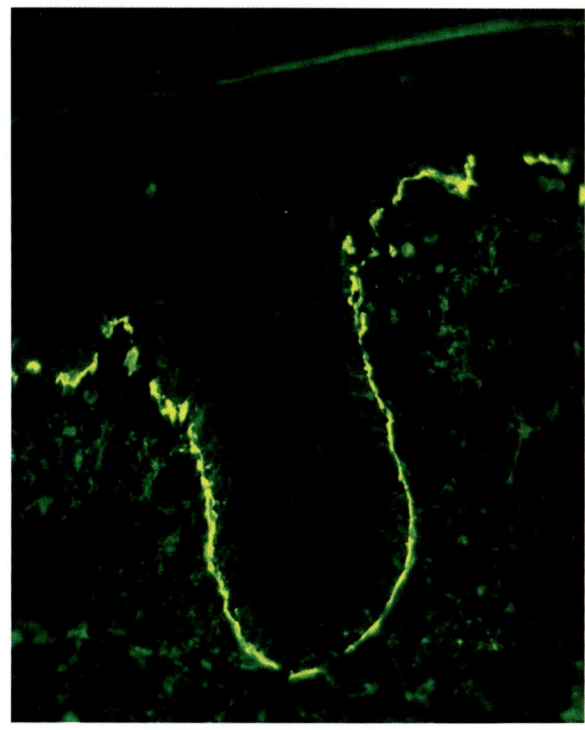

FIGURE 24-24
Bullous pemphigoid. Direct immunofluorescence study discloses linear deposition of IgG (and C3) along the dermal–epidermal junction. Ultrastructurally, these antibodies and complement are present in the lamina lucida.

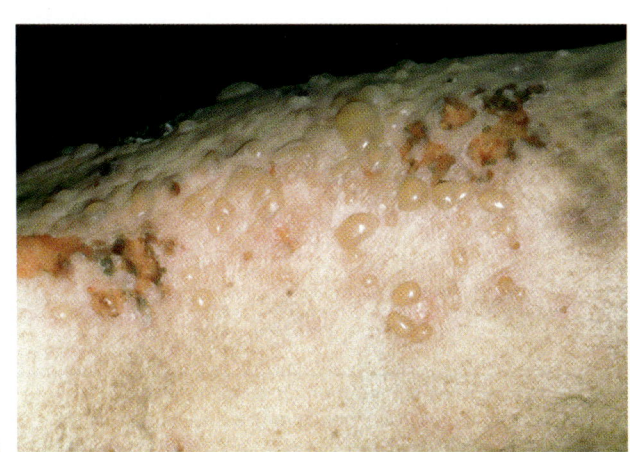

FIGURE 24-23
Bullous pemphigoid. A. The skin shows multiple tense bullae on an erythematous base and erosions, distributed primarily on the medial thighs and trunk. B. A subepidermal blister has an edematous papillary dermis as its base. The roof of the blister consists of the intact, entire epidermis, including the stratum basalis. Inflammatory cells, fibrin, and fluid fill the blister.

Clinical Features: The blisters of BP are large and tense and may appear on normal-appearing skin or on an erythematous base (Fig. 24-23). The medial thighs and flexor aspects of the forearms are commonly affected, but the groin, axillae, and other cutaneous sites may also develop blisters. The disease is self-limited but chronic, and the patient's general health is usually unaffected. The course of the disease is greatly shortened by systemic administration of corticosteroids.

Dermatitis Herpetiformis Reflects Gluten Sensitivity

Dermatitis herpetiformis (DH) is an intensely pruritic cutaneous eruption related to gluten sensitivity, which is characterized by urticaria-like plaques and small vesicles over the extensor surfaces of the body.

 Pathogenesis: DH is associated with gluten sensitivity in patients of the HLA-B8, HLA-DR3, and HLA-DQw2 haplotypes. The gluten-sensitive enteropathy is often subclinical (see Chapter 14). Gluten is a protein found in wheat, barley, rye, and oats. The cutaneous lesions are related to granular deposits of IgA at the dermal–epidermal interface, mainly at the tips of the dermal papillae. IgA immune complexes at the tips of dermal papillae are more prominent in perilesional skin than in normal-appearing skin. Importantly, a gluten-free diet controls the disease, whereas reintroduction of gluten provokes new lesions.

Genetically predisposed patients may develop IgA antibodies to components of gluten in the intestines. The resulting IgA complexes then gain access to the circulation and are deposited, possibly through binding to an as yet unknown ligand, in the dermal papillae of the skin (see Fig. 24-26). Patients with DH have increased levels of IgA autoantibodies to tissue transglutaminase, suggesting the existence of a dermal autoantigen related to tissue transglutaminase.

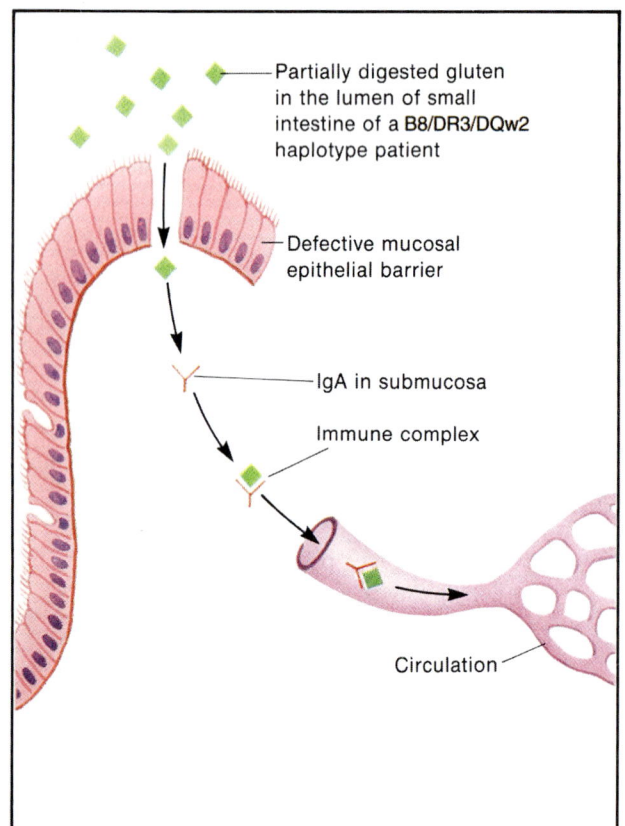

1. Formation of immune complexes in submucosa of small intestine. Passage of immune complexes into the circulation.

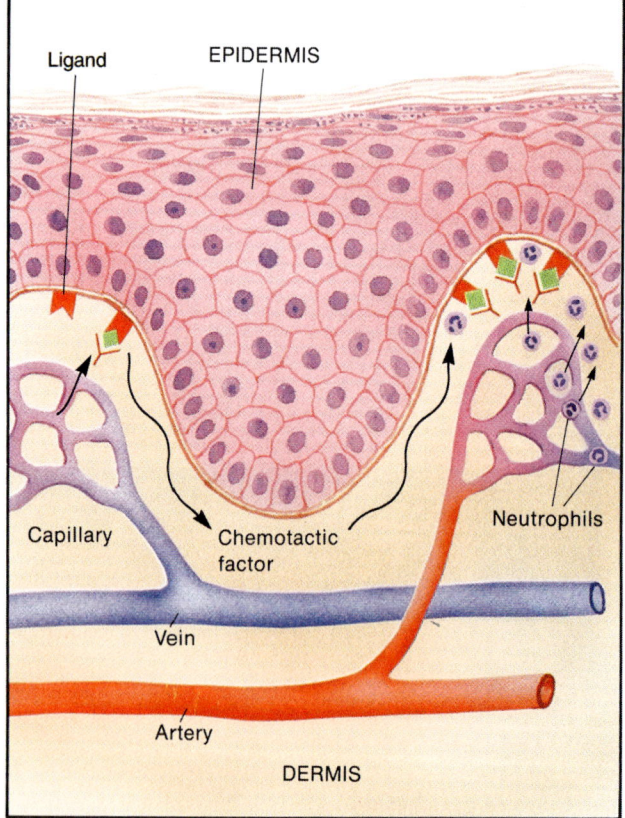

2. Ligand–immune complex union releases neutrophil chemotactic factor. Neutrophils migrate to the tips of the papillae.

FIGURE 24-25
Dermatitis herpetiformis. Proposed pathogenesis for cutaneous lesions. The disease is initiated in the small intestine and is likely expressed in the skin because of the presence of a ligand immediately deep to the lamina densa.

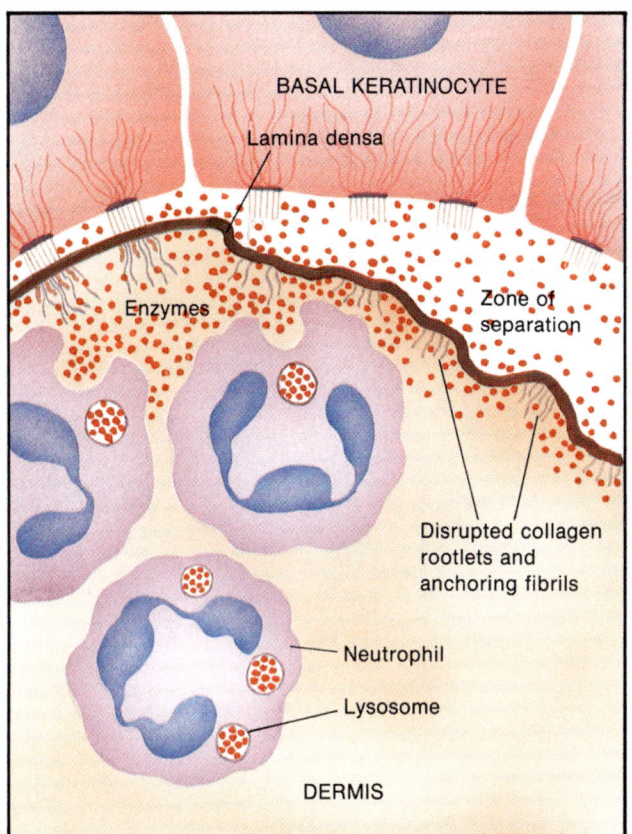
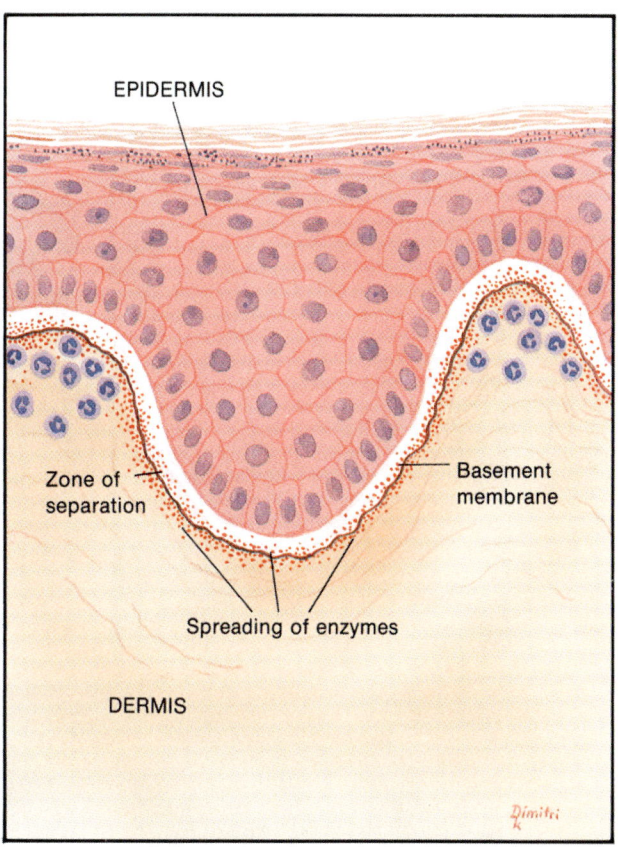

3. Dissolution of basal rootlets and anchoring fibrils by enzymes released by neutrophils. Early dermo-epidermal separation.

4. Concentration of neutrophils at the tips of the papillae. Spreading of enzymes along basement membrane. Lifting away of lamina densa.

FIGURE 24-25 *(continued)*

IgA immune complexes are inefficient in complement activation (alternate pathway), and few neutrophils are attracted to the site. However, the neutrophils that do accumulate elaborate leukotrienes, which attract more neutrophils. The release of lysosomal enzymes by the inflammatory cells cleaves the epidermis from the dermis. The immune complexes are deposited deep to the lamina densa in intimate relationship to the collagen rootlets (microfibrils) which, along with anchoring fibrils, are important in the attachment of the lamina densa to the subjacent papillary dermis (Fig. 24-25).

 Pathology: Within 24 hours after cessation of dapsone therapy, erythematous urticarial plaques develop about the elbows and knees. A delicate perivenular lymphocytic infiltrate appears, together with a row of neutrophils immediately deep to the lamina densa in the dermal papillae. During the next 12 hours, the neutrophils aggregate in clusters of 10 to 25 at the tips of the dermal papillae to create a diagnostic histological appearance.

There are two related mechanisms of dermal–epidermal separation. One is associated with the sheetlike spread of a layer or two of neutrophils at the dermal–epidermal interface. In this situation, the entire epidermis detaches from the papillary dermis (Fig. 24-26). The roof of such a vesicle contains the epidermis; the floor is composed of the lamina densa and the papillary dermis. In contrast to bullous pemphigoid, eosinophils are uncommon early in the course of DH.

In the second mechanism of vesicle formation, many neutrophils accumulate rapidly in the tips of the dermal papillae. The release of neutrophilic lysosomal enzymes in the superficial portion of the dermal papillae results in (1) uncoupling of the epidermis from the dermis at the tips of dermal papillae, (2) disruption of the BMZ in the lamina lucida and superficial part of the papillae, and (3) tearing of the epidermis across the adjacent rete ridges. In the resulting vesicle, the roof has alternating tears across its epidermal covering, and the floor shows residual epidermal pegs alternating with the basal half of dermal papillae.

Clinical Features: The lesions of DH are especially prominent over the elbows, knees, and buttocks (Fig. 24-26). The intensely pruritic vesicles may become grouped in a fashion similar to that in herpes simplex infections (therefore, the term *herpetiformis*) and are almost invariably rubbed until broken. Thus, patients may present with only crusted lesions and no intact vesicles. Although the disease is of varying severity and characterized by remissions, it is disturbingly chronic. The healing lesions

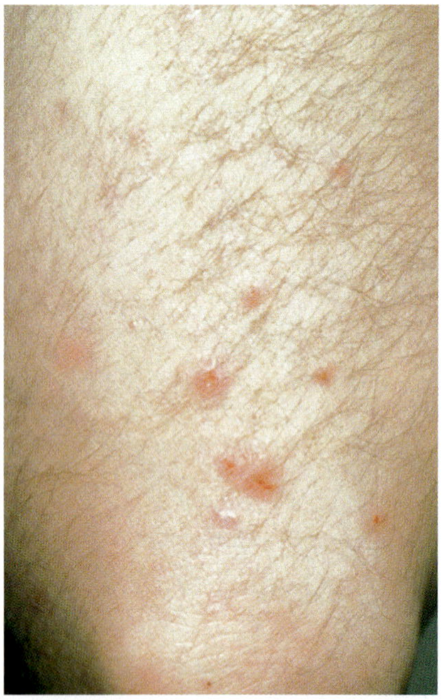

FIGURE 24-26

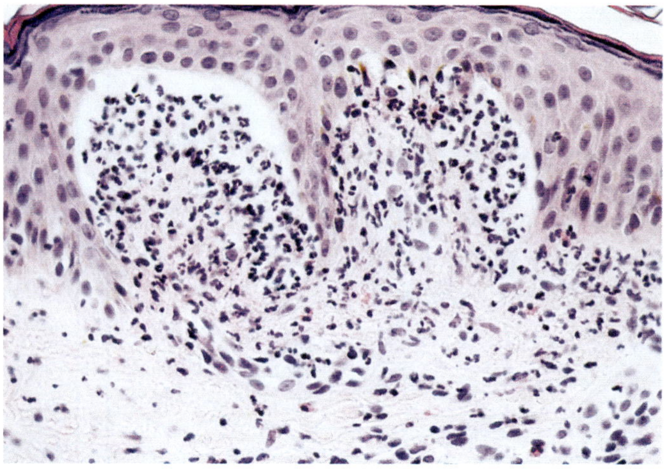

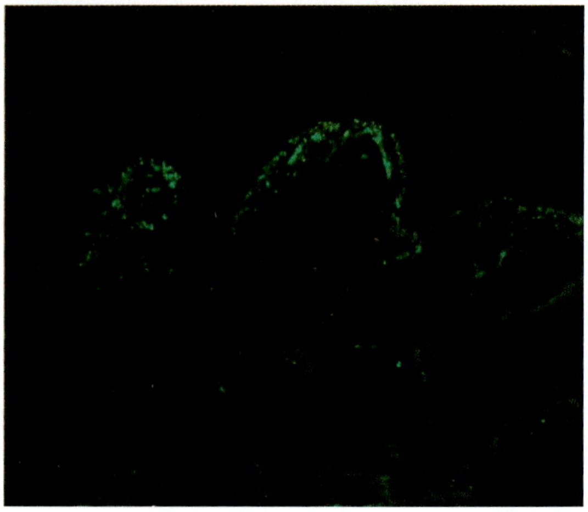

Dermatitis herpetiformis. A. Pruritic, symmetric, grouped vesicles on an erythematous base are seen on the elbows and knees. B. Dermal papillary abscesses of neutrophils with vesicle formation at the dermal–epidermal junction are characteristic. C. Direct immunofluorescence reveals IgA deposited in dermal papillae in association with (but not necessarily directly upon) anchoring fibrils and elastic tissue fibers. This is the site of neutrophil infiltration and subepidermal vesicle formation.

often leave scars. Other than a gluten-free diet, treatment with dapsone or sulfapyridine controls the signs and symptoms of DH by an unknown mechanism.

Erythema Multiforme Is Often a Reaction to a Drug or Infection

Erythema multiforme (EM) is an acute, self-limited disorder that varies from a few erythematous macules and blisters (EM minor) to a life-threatening, widespread ulceration of the skin and mucous membranes (EM major; Stevens-Johnson syndrome). This phenomenon is usually a reaction to a drug or an infectious agent, in particular, herpes simplex infection.

 Pathogenesis: The list of agents thought to provoke EM is long and includes herpesvirus, *Mycoplasma,* and sulfonamides. However, a precipitating factor can be demonstrated in only half of cases. In postherpetic EM, the deposition of viral antigens, IgM and C3 can be identified in a perivascular location and at the epidermal BMZ. The combination of infiltrating lymphocytes and the presence of antigen–antibody complexes within the lesions suggest that both humoral and delayed types of hypersensitivity mechanisms contribute to the pathogenesis of EM.

 Pathology: The dermis in EM shows a sparse infiltrate of lymphocytes about the superficial vascular bed and at the dermal–epidermal interface. The

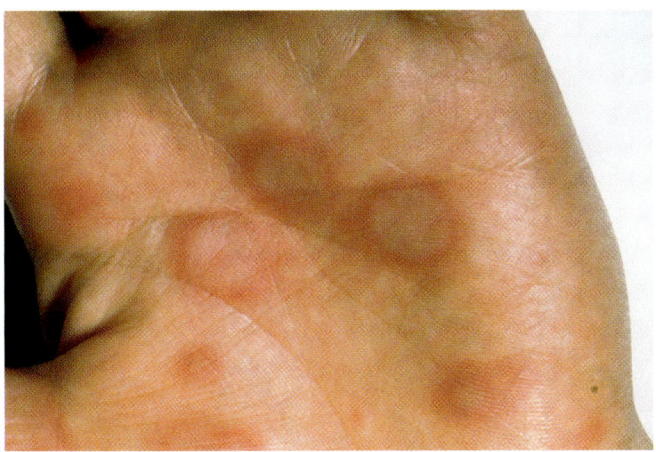

FIGURE 24-27
Erythema multiforme. Steroid-responsive "target" papules, characterized by central bullae with surrounding erythema, appeared after antibiotic therapy.

characteristic morphological feature in the epidermis is the presence of apoptotic keratinocytes, which have a pyknotic nucleus and an eosinophilic cytoplasm. Apoptosis may be extensive and associated with a subepidermal vesicle, whose roof is an almost completely necrotic epidermis. Because of the acute onset of the disease, in most cases there is little or no change in the stratum corneum.

Clinical Features: The characteristic "target" or "iris" lesions of EM have a central, dark red zone, occasionally with a blister, surrounded by a paler area (Fig. 24-27). In turn, the latter is encompassed by a peripheral red rim. Urticarial plaques are common. The presence of vesicles and bullae usually predicts a more severe course. EM is a common condition, with a peak incidence in the second and third decades of life. It is occasionally encountered in association with other presumably immunological cutaneous disorders, including erythema nodosum, toxic epidermal necrolysis, and necrotizing vasculitis. *Stevens-Johnson syndrome* refers to an unusually severe form of EM that involves several mucosal surfaces and internal organs and is frequently fatal.

Systemic Lupus Erythematosus Is an Immune Complex Disease

Systemic lupus erythematosus (SLE), the paradigm of immune complex disease, is characterized by a variety of autoantibodies and other immune abnormalities indicating B-cell hyperactivity (see Chapters 4 and 16). Although cutaneous involvement may be severe and cosmetically devastating, it is not life-threatening. However, the nature and pattern of immune reactants in the skin serve as an excellent guide to the likelihood of systemic disease.

Pathogenesis: Although an impressive case can be made for the pathogenetic significance of immune complexes in the renal disease of SLE, they are not likely to be solely responsible for the production of the cutaneous lesions. In this respect, immune complexes are present in both lesional and normal-appearing skin in SLE. The deposition of immune reactants along the epidermal BMZ (positive lupus band test) of "normal" skin is important in the diagnosis of SLE. The epidermal injury in the cutaneous lesions seems to be initiated by exogenous agents such as ultraviolet light and perpetuated by cell-mediated immune reactions similar to those in graft-versus-host disease. The manifestations of epidermal injury include (1) vacuolization of basal keratinocytes, hyperkeratosis, and diminished epidermal thickness; (2) release of DNA and other nuclear and cytoplasmic antigens to the circulation; and (3) deposition of DNA and other antigenic determinants in the epidermal BMZ (lamina densa and immediately subjacent dermis) (Fig. 24-28). Thus, epidermal injury, local immune-complex formation, deposition of circulating immune complexes, and lymphocyte-induced cellular injury all seem to act in concert.

The various forms of cutaneous lupus erythematosus have been classified according to their chronicity, but considerable overlap in features is possible. There is an inverse relationship between the prominence of skin lesions and the extent of systemic pathology.

CHRONIC CUTANEOUS (DISCOID) LUPUS ERYTHEMATOSUS: This form of lupus is usually a disease of the skin alone. The disease manifestations are generally above the neck and appear on the face (especially in the malar area), scalp, and ears. The lesions begin as slightly elevated violaceous papules with a rough scale of keratin. As they enlarge, they assume a disk shape, with a hyperkeratotic margin and a depigmented center. The cutaneous lesions may culminate in disfiguring scars. Elevation of circulating antinuclear antibodies (ANA) is seen in less than 10% of patients.

Pathology: In discoid lupus, the nucleated epidermal layers are modestly thickened or somewhat thin. Hyperkeratosis and plugging of hair follicles are prominent features. The rete–papillae pattern of the dermal–epidermal interface is partially effaced. The basal keratinocytes are vacuolated, and eosinophilic apoptotic bodies are noted. The lamina densa is greatly thickened and reduplicated. On PAS staining, multiple layers of lamina densa extend into the subjacent dermis. The excessive quantity of lamina densa, a product of the basal keratinocytes, reflects a response of basal cells to damage. These changes all suggest that injury to basal keratinocytes is an essential pathogenetic characteristic of skin disease associated with lupus (Figs. 24-29 through 24-31).

The basal keratinocytes and BMZ contain a diffuse lymphocytic infiltrate that penetrates the basal layer focally. Deeper in the dermis, dense patches of helper and cyto-

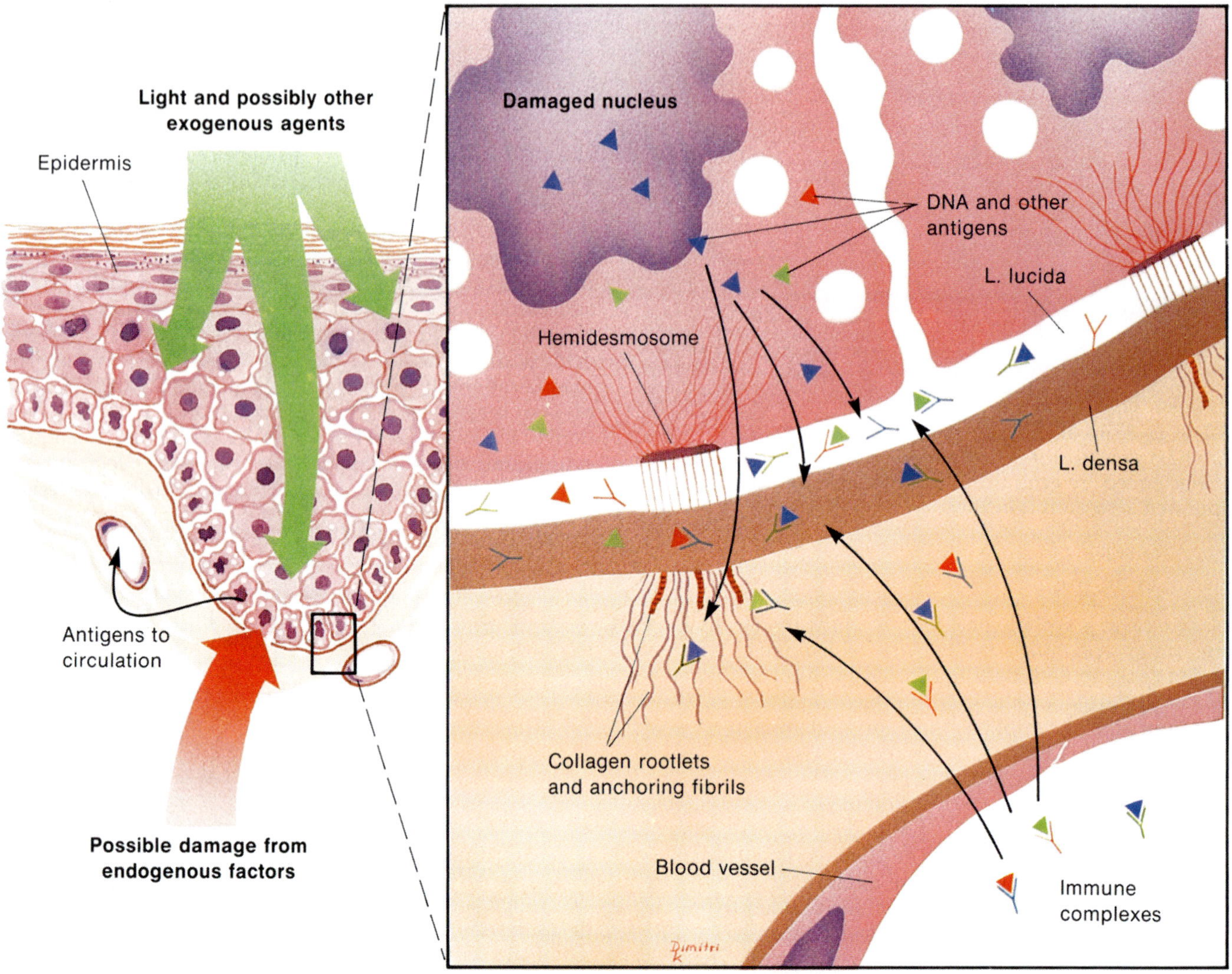

FIGURE 24-28

Lupus erythematosus. A cell-mediated immune reaction leads to epidermal cellular damage when initiated by light or other exogenous agents as well as endogenous ones. Such injury releases a large number of antigens, some of which may return to the skin in the form of immune complexes. Immune complexes are also formed in the skin by a reaction of local DNA with antibody that may also be deposited beneath the epidermal basement membrane zone.

toxic/suppressor T lymphocytes, often with plasma cells, are commonly found around skin appendages. Immune complexes are predominantly located deep to the lamina densa, but they are also seen on the lamina densa and within the lamina lucida. This pattern contrasts with that of BP, in which there are only two antigens, both precisely localized to the lamina lucida.

SUBACUTE CUTANEOUS LUPUS ERYTHEMATOSUS: This disorder primarily afflicts young and middle-aged white women. In contrast to discoid lupus, subacute cutaneous lupus may be accompanied by involvement of the musculoskeletal system and kidneys. Initially, scaly erythematous papules develop and then enlarge into psoriasiform or annular lesions, which may fuse. The skin changes are seen in the upper chest, upper back, and extensor surfaces of the arms, a distribution indicating that light exposure plays a role in the pathogenesis of the disorder. Significant scarring does not occur. About 70% of patients have circulating anti-Ro (ss-A) antibodies, and ANA levels are elevated in 70%.

 Pathology: Histologically, subacute cutaneous lupus features edema of the papillary dermis, thickening of the lamina densa, and prominent vacuolar degeneration of the basilar keratinocytes. There is some lymphocytic infiltration of the BMZ, but deeper patches of lymphocytes are not observed.

Diseases of the Basement Membrane Zone

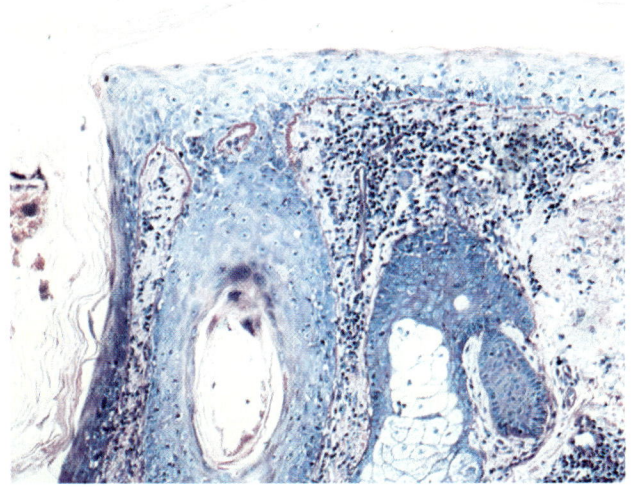

FIGURE 24-29
Lupus erythematosus. A variably cell-rich to cell-poor, bandlike, lymphocytic infiltrate is present in the papillary and adventitial dermis. There is epidermal atrophy arising from damage to the epidermis, which is mediated by infiltrating lymphocytes.

ACUTE SYSTEMIC LUPUS ERYTHEMATOSUS: Over 80% of patients with SLE have acute cutaneous manifestations during the course of their illness, in association with disease of the kidneys and joints. The rash is often the first manifestation of the disease and may precede the onset of systemic symptoms by a few months. The typical "butterfly" rash of SLE is a delicate erythema of the malar area of the face, which may pass in a few hours or a few days. Many patients exhibit a maculopapular eruption of the chest and ex-

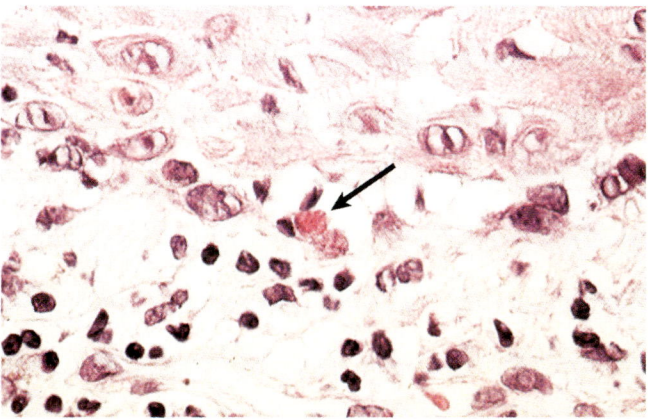

FIGURE 24-31
Lupus erythematosus. An active lesion shows striking basal vacuolization, with keratinocyte necrosis *(arrow)* forming a dense eosinophilic body (apoptotic/fibrillary/colloid body) that is surrounded by lymphocytes (satellitosis).

tremities, often developing after sun exposure. Both rashes heal without scarring. Lesions indistinguishable from discoid lupus may occur. ANA levels are elevated in more than 90% of patients.

 Pathology: Histologically, the earliest malar blush of acute cutaneous lupus may show only edema of the papillary dermis. More often, the changes are similar to those in the subacute form of lupus. In *bullous* SLE, blisters may occur subepidermally and beneath the lamina densa, where an autoantibody against type VII collagen, a component of anchoring fibrils, is deposited.

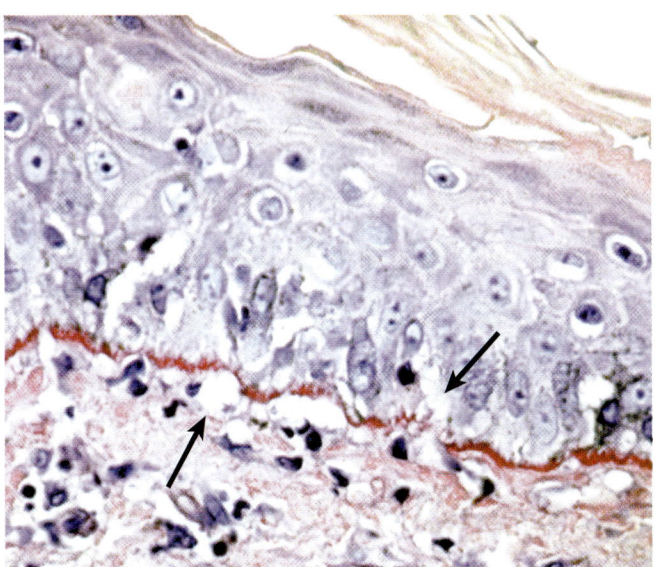

FIGURE 24-30
Lupus erythematosus. Basal cell necrosis with resultant basal keratinocytic migration and synthesis of new basement membrane zone leads to thickening of the epidermal basement membrane zone, as evident in this PAS stain. Notice the vacuoles *(arrows)* on either side of the basement membrane zone, an indicator of cellular injury.

Lichen Planus Is a Hypersensitivity Reaction with Lymphocytic Infiltrates at the Dermal–Epidermal Junction

"Lichenoid" tissue reactions are so named because the clinical lesions resemble certain lichens that form a scaly growth on rocks or tree trunks. Histologically, a lichenoid infiltrate is characterized by a bandlike infiltrate of lymphocytes that obscures the dermal–epidermal junction. The disease is characterized by reduced epidermal turnover and subsequent hyperkeratosis without parakeratosis. Lichen planus (LP) is the prototypic disorder of this group, which includes entities such as lichen nitidus and lichenoid drug eruptions.

 Pathogenesis: The etiology of LP is unknown. The disease is occasionally familial and may also accompany a variety of disorders thought to be au-

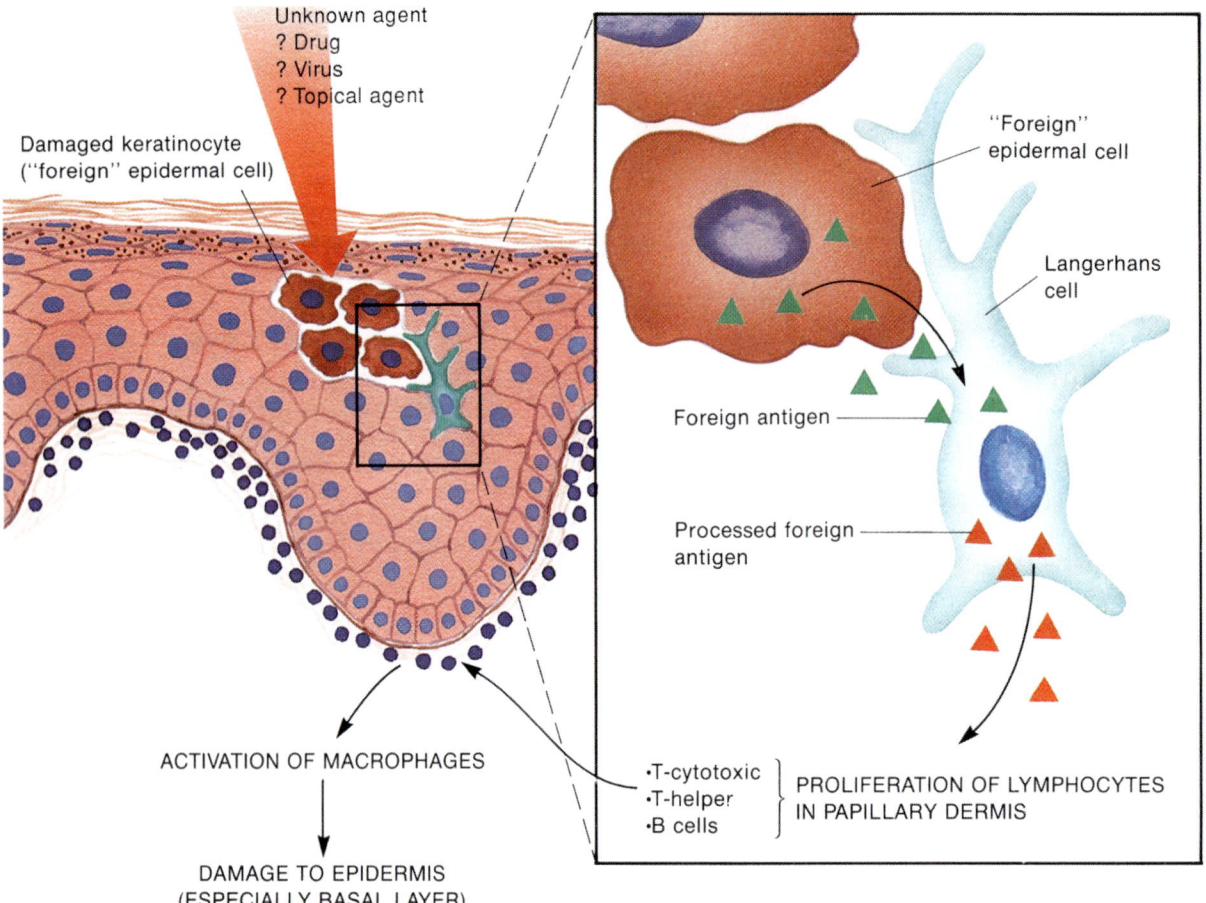

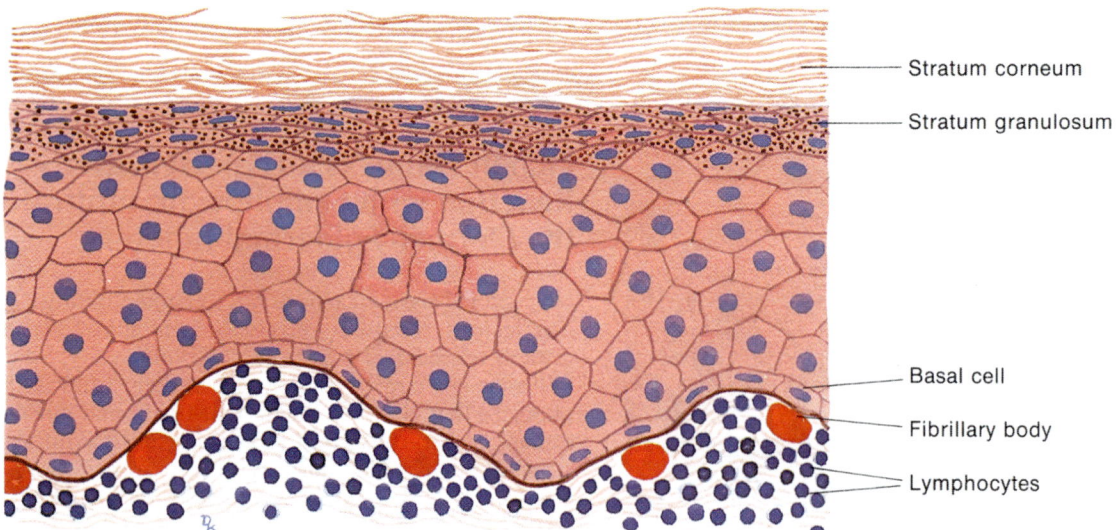

FIGURE 24-32
Lichen planus. Pathogenetic mechanisms are outlined. The disease is apparently initiated by epidermal injury. This injury causes some epidermal cells to be treated as "foreign." The antigens of such cells are processed by Langerhans cells. The processed antigen induces lymphocytic proliferation and macrophage activation. Macrophages, along with T lymphocytes, kill the epidermal basal cells, resulting in a reactive epidermal proliferation and the formation of fibrillary bodies.

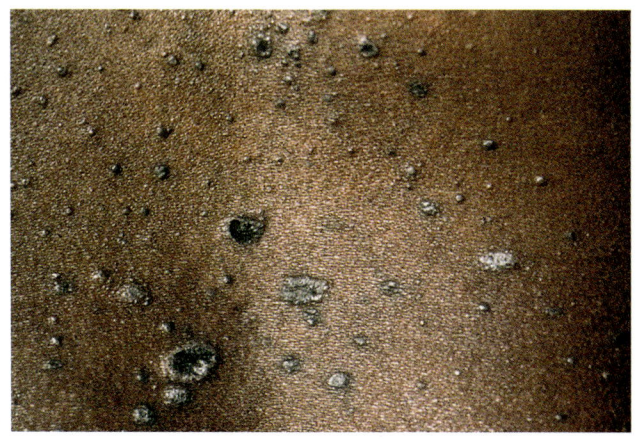
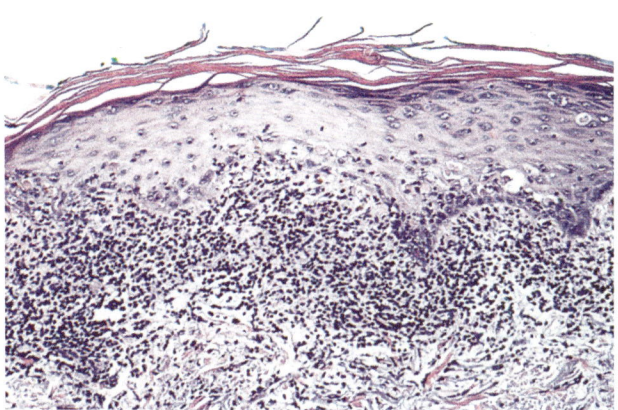

FIGURE 24-33
Lichen planus. **A.** The skin displays multiple flat-topped violaceous polygonal papules. **B.** A cell-rich, bandlike, lymphocytic infiltrate disrupts the stratum basalis. Unlike lupus erythematosus, there is usually epidermal hyperplasia, hyperkeratosis and wedgelike hypergranulosis.

toimmune, such as SLE and myasthenia gravis. LP is more frequent in patients with ulcerative colitis. Drugs such as gold, chlorothiazide, and chloroquine may induce lichenoid reactions. External agents such as photographic chemicals may evoke a lichenoid response. LP-like lesions are also often observed in the later stages of chronic graft-versus-host disease. Thus, it seems that immunological mechanisms play a role in the pathogenesis of LP (Fig. 24-32). The presence of apoptotic bodies and the demonstration of increased epidermal cell turnover provide evidence that the lesions of LP result from cell destruction and subsequent reactive epidermal proliferation. Evidence supports the notion that LP is a delayed type of hypersensitivity reaction, initiated and amplified by cytokines such as gamma interferon (IFN-γ) and IL-6, whose expression is due not only to infiltrating lymphocytes but also to stimulated keratinocytes.

Pathology: The epidermis in LP features compact hyperkeratosis with little or no parakeratosis. The stratum granulosum is thickened, frequently in a distinctive, focal, wedge-shaped pattern, with the base of the wedge abutting the stratum corneum. The stratum spinosum is variably thickened.

The distinctive pathological changes of LP are at the dermal–epidermal interface. The basal layer is no longer a distinctive row of cuboidal cells but is replaced by flattened or polygonal keratinocytes. The undulating interface between the dermal papillae and the rounded profiles of the rete ridges is obscured by a dense infiltrate of lymphocytes and macrophages, many of the latter containing melanin pigment (melanophages) (Fig. 24-33). The lymphocytes are principally of the helper/inducer phenotype. Sharply pointed ("saw-toothed") wedges of keratinocytes project into the inflammatory infiltrate.

Commonly admixed with the infiltrate (in the epidermis or dermis) are globular, fibrillary, eosinophilic bodies, 15 to 20 μm in diameter (Fig. 24-34), which represent apoptotic keratinocytes. These structures are variably termed *apoptotic, colloid, Civatte,* or *fibrillary bodies.* The fibrils within the apoptotic bodies are keratin filaments. An increased number of epidermal Langerhans cells is seen in early LP.

Clinical Features: LP is a chronic eruption characterized by violaceous, flat-topped papules, usually on the flexor surfaces of the wrists (Fig. 24-33).

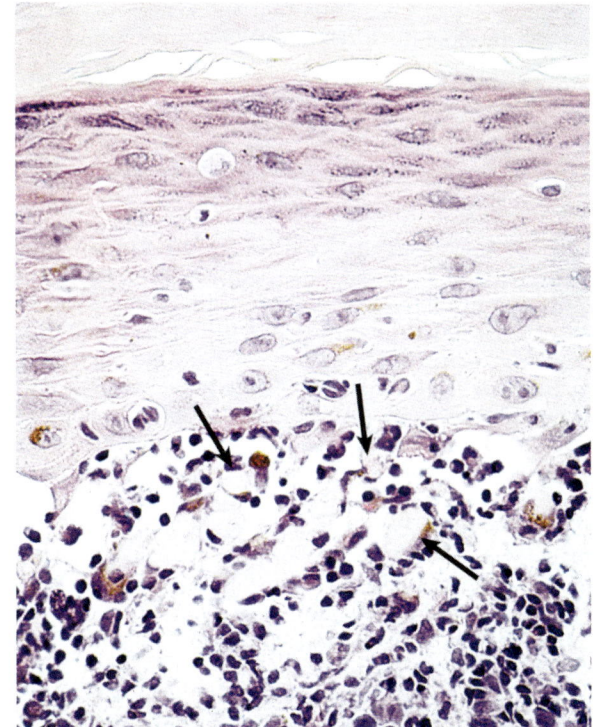

FIGURE 24-34
Lichen planus. Hypergranulosis and loss of rete ridges are noted. The site of pathological injury is at the dermal–epidermal junction where there is a striking infiltrate of lymphocytes, many of which surround apoptotic keratinocytes *(arrows).*

White patches or streaks may also be present on the oral mucous membranes. In most patients, the pruritic lesions resolve in less than a year, but they may occasionally persist for longer periods.

INFLAMMATORY DISEASES OF THE SUPERFICIAL AND DEEP VASCULAR BED

Urticaria and Angioedema Reflect Anaphylactic Reactions

Urticaria and angioedema are type I (IgE-dependent or anaphylactic) hypersensitivity reactions initiated by the degranulation of mast cells sensitized to a specific antigen. **Urticaria** or hives are raised, pale, well-demarcated pruritic papules and plaques that appear and disappear within a few hours. The lesions represent edema of the superficial portion of the dermis. **Angioedema** refers to a condition in which the edema involves the deeper dermis or subcutis, resulting in an egglike swelling. Both entities have a rapid onset and range in severity from simply annoying lesions to life-threatening anaphylactic reactions. The mainstays of treatment are avoidance of the offending agent and prompt administration of antihistamines.

Dermatographism is a linear hive with a rich pink flare produced by brisk stroking of the skin. It is found in approximately 4% of the population and represents an exaggerated IgE-dependent response. One may write on the skin of such persons and create a hive in the form of a legible word.

 Pathogenesis: Most cases of urticaria are IgE dependent, and the final pathway is an exaggerated permeability of venules secondary to the degranulation of mast cells. An almost endless list of materials may react with IgE antibodies on the surface of the mast cell. Urticaria occur in both atopic and nonatopic persons. Atopic persons have intensely pruritic skin eruptions, a family history of similar eruptions, and a personal or family history of allergies. They commonly exhibit an elevation of circulating IgE.

Initially, cutaneous venules react to the degranulation of mast cells and the release of their stored vasoactive mediators with increased permeability, resulting in rapidly forming edema. If the reaction persists, inflammatory cells are attracted to the area and a persistent urticarial plaque (lasting more than a day) results.

Hereditary angioedema is a serious autosomal dominant disorder caused by mutation of C1-esterase inhibitor.

 Pathology: In urticaria, the collagen fibers and fibrils are splayed apart by excess fluid. The lymphatic vessels are dilated, and the venules show margination of neutrophils and eosinophils. Vessels are cuffed by a few lymphocytes. A persistent urticarial reaction shows an increased number of lymphocytes and eosinophils, but neutrophils are sparse.

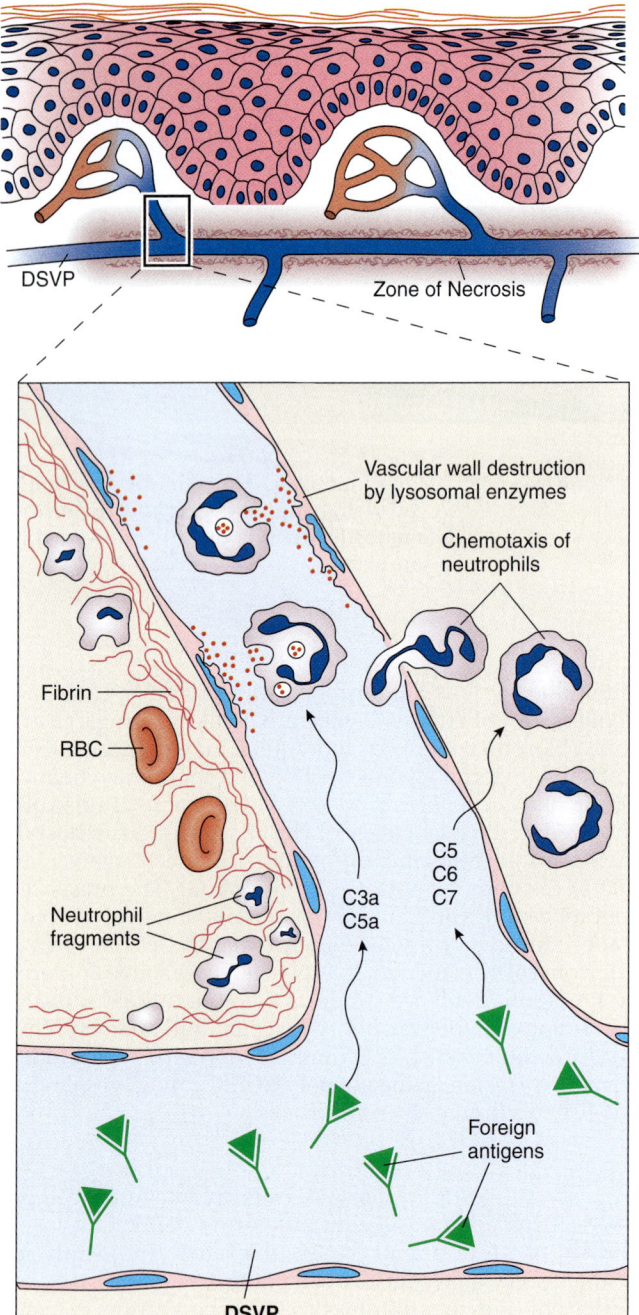

FIGURE 24-35
Cutaneous necrotizing vasculitis. The pathogenesis of vessel damage is depicted. The site of the vascular pathology is indicated in the *upper diagram*. Circulating immune complexes activate complement. There is neutrophilic chemotaxis *(C5a)* and neutrophilic destruction. Vascular damage occurs, with extravasation of erythrocytes, fibrin deposition, and leukocytoclasia. *RBC*, red blood cell; *DSVP*, deep superficial venular plexus.

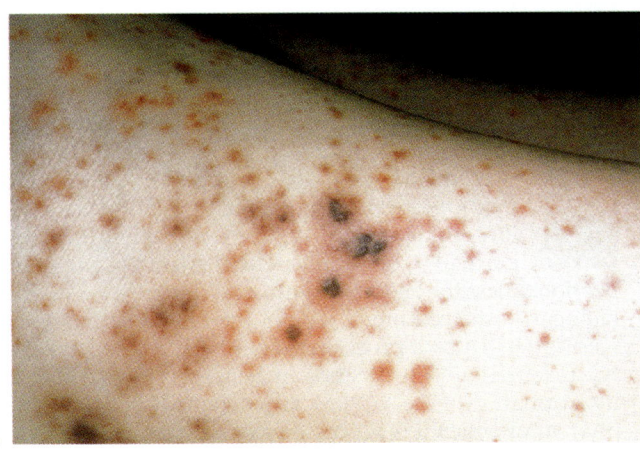
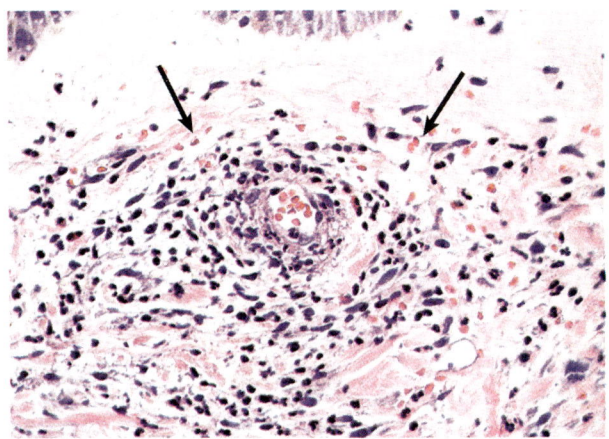

FIGURE 24-36
Cutaneous necrotizing vasculitis. A. Palpable purpuric tender papules on the legs of a 25-year-old woman. The condition resolved after therapy for streptococcal pharyngitis. B. The vessel is surrounded by pink fibrin and neutrophils, many of which have disintegrated (leukocytoclasis). Extravasated red blood cells *(arrows)* and inflammation give the classic clinical appearance of "palpable purpura."

Cutaneous Necrotizing Vasculitis Is an Immune Reaction That Features Neutrophilic Inflammation

Cutaneous necrotizing vasculitis (CNV) present as "palpable purpura," and has also been called *allergic cutaneous vasculitis, leukocytoclastic vasculitis,* and *hypersensitivity angiitis.*

Pathogenesis: In CNV, circulating immune complexes are deposited in the vascular walls, probably at sites of injuries, at branch points where turbulence is increased, or where the venous circulation is slowed, as in the lower extremities. The elaborated C5a complement component attracts neutrophils, which degranulate and release lysosomal enzymes, resulting in endothelial damage and fibrin deposition (Fig. 24-35).

CNV may be either primary, without a known precipitating event in about half of the cases, or associated with a specific infectious agent (e.g., hepatitis B virus or hepatitis C virus). It may also be a secondary process in a variety of chronic diseases, such as rheumatoid arthritis, SLE, and ulcerative colitis. CNV may also be associated with (1) underlying malignancies such as lymphoma, (2) a drug or some other allergy, or (3) an infectious process such as Henoch-Schönlein purpura.

Pathology: The lesions of CNV show vessel walls obliterated by a neutrophilic infiltrate. The endothelial cells are difficult to visualize, and the damage to the vessel is manifested by fibrin deposition and the extravasation of erythrocytes (Fig. 24-36). Many of the neutrophils are also damaged, resulting in dustlike nuclear remnants, a process known as *leukocytoclasia* (Fig. 24-37). The collagen fibers between affected vessels are separated by neutrophils, eosinophils, and leukocytoclastic cellular remnants, as well as the extravasated erythrocytes that account for the characteristic palpable purpura.

Clinical Features: CNV is distinguished by purpuric papules, which are red, palpable lesions, 2 to 4 mm in width, that do not blanch under pressure (palpable purpura) (Fig. 24-36). Multiple lesions characteristically appear in crops on the lower extremities or at sites of pressure. The lesions may be confined to the skin in an otherwise healthy person, or they may involve small blood vessels in the joints, gastrointestinal tract, or kidney. Individual lesions persist for up to a month and then resolve, leaving

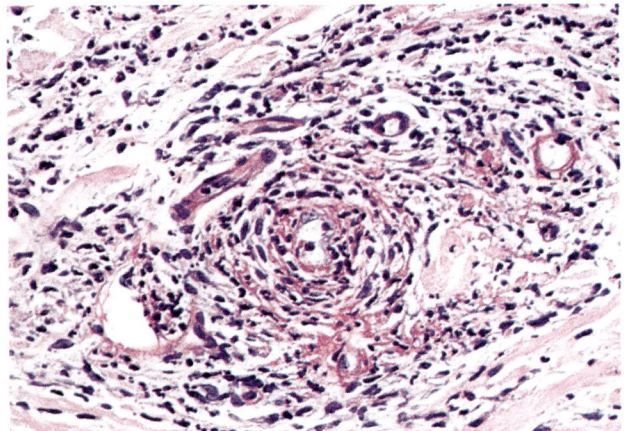

FIGURE 24-37
Cutaneous necrotizing vasculitis. The pink fibrillary-to-amorphous material about the vessels is called "fibrinoid" necrosis. The principal component is fibrin, but the material also contains degenerated cellular components, complement, and other serum constituents.

Allergic Contact Dermatitis Features Cell-Mediated Hypersensitivity to Exogenous Agents

Allergic contact dermatitis is a type IV hypersensitivity (cell-mediated) reaction in the skin following exposure to a sensitizing agent. Some of the most common sensitizing agents are members of the *Rhus* genus of plants. Some 90% of the population of the United States is sensitive to the common offenders: *R. radicans* (poison ivy), *R. diversiloba* (poison oak), and *R. vernix* (poison sumac). These plant dermatitides are so well known that the resultant disease is commonly labeled according to the offending plant. The patient definitively states "I have poison ivy" and comes to the physician for relief, not a diagnosis.

 Pathogenesis: The offending plant contains low-molecular-weight compounds called *haptens*, in particular, oleoresins. These are not active in sensitization unless they combine with a carrier protein. This likely happens at the cell membrane of the Langerhans cell in the *sensitization phase*, a process that has been studied as a prototype of antigenic sensitization in delayed-type hypersensitivity. Formation of the hapten-carrier complex requires about 1 hour, after which it is processed as an antigen by the Langerhans cells. These cells carry the antigen through the lymphatics to the regional lymph nodes and present the antigen to $CD4^+$ T lymphocytes (Fig. 24-38). After 5 to 7 days, some clones of these T lymphocytes become sensitized to the antigen, become activated, multiply, and circulate as memory

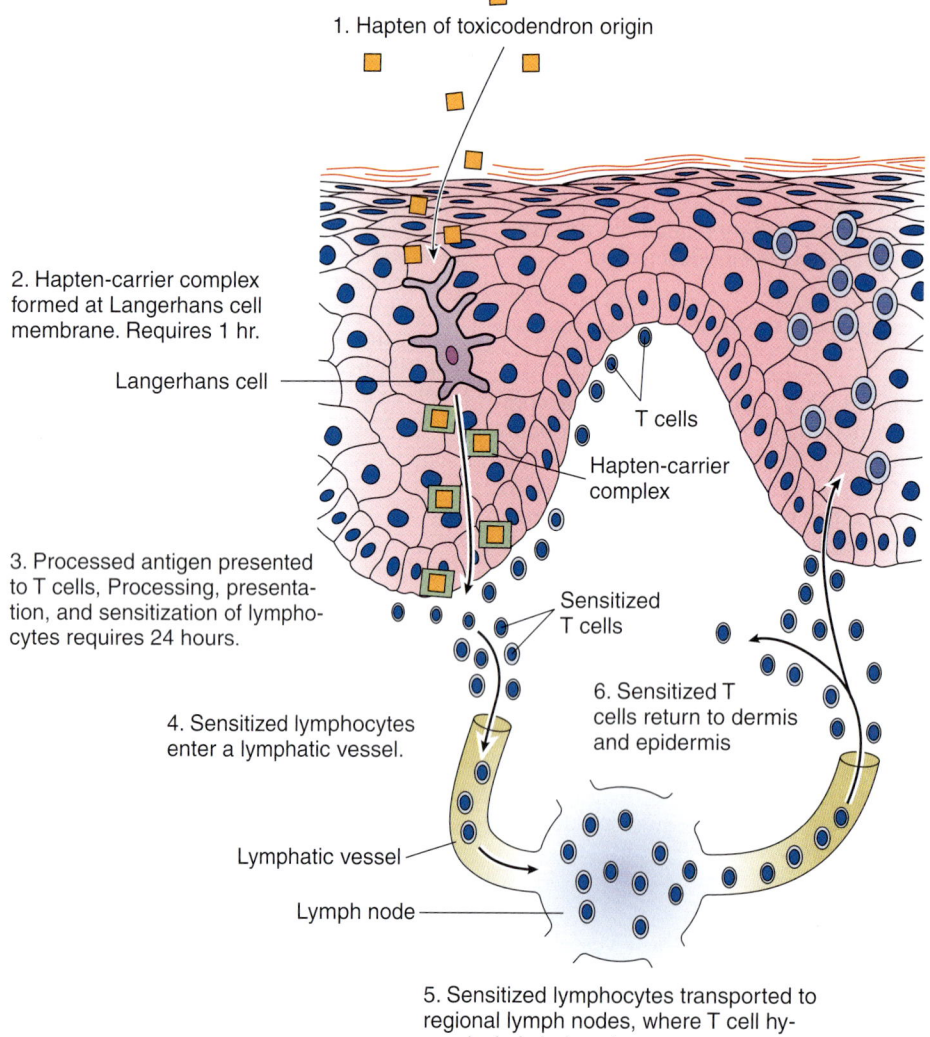

FIGURE 24-38
Allergic contact dermatitis. Pathogenetic mechanisms are shown.

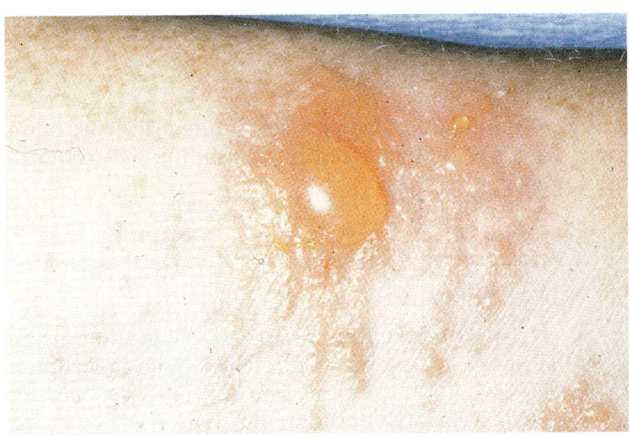 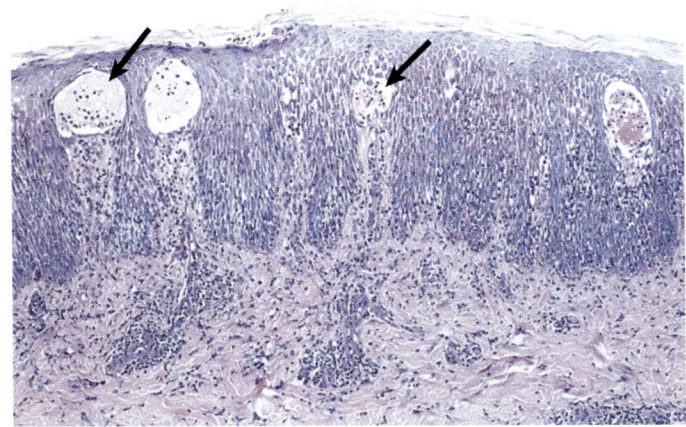

FIGURE 24-39
Allergic contact dermatitis. **A.** Vesicles and bullae developed on the volar forearm after application of perfume. **B.** Epidermal spongiosis and spongiotic vesicles *(arrows)* are present in this biopsy of "poison ivy." Infiltrating lymphocytes are apparent in the epidermis, where they effect the cell-mediated delayed hypersensitivity reaction.

cells in the bloodstream. Some migrate to the skin, ready to react with the antigen if they encounter it. IL-1, produced by Langerhans cells, supports the proliferation of $CD4^+$ Th1 lymphocytes, the effector cells of delayed hypersensitivity.

In the *elicitation phase*, the specifically sensitized T lymphocytes in the circulation enter the skin. At the site of antigen challenge, Langerhans cells, endothelial cells, perivascular dendritic cells, and monocytes process the antigen and present it to the specifically sensitized T cells, which then migrate into the epidermis. Cytokine production leads to the accumulation of more T cells and macrophages. This inflammatory infiltrate is responsible for epidermal cell injury. It is proposed that activated T cells in the skin, via IFN-α, induce apoptosis of keratinocytes by up-regulating the expression of Fas by the keratinocytes. Fas ligand enters the microenvironment after being expressed on the T-cell surface.

 Pathology: Allergic contact dermatitis is a model of *spongiotic dermatitis*, a reaction pattern in which there is edema in the epidermis. In the initial 24 hours following reexposure to the offending plant (elicitation phase), numerous lymphocytes and macrophages accumulate about the superficial venular bed and extend into the epidermis. The epidermal keratinocytes are partially separated by the edema fluid, creating a spongelike appearance *(spongiosis)* (Fig. 24-39). The stratum corneum contains coagulated eosinophilic fluid and plasma proteins. Later, numerous mononuclear inflammatory cells and eosinophils accumulate. Vesicles containing lymphocytes and macrophages are present, and large amounts of eosinophilic coagulated fluid accumulate in the stratum corneum.

 Clinical Features: When a person first comes into contact with poison ivy, no immediate reaction occurs. Five to 7 days after reexposure, the site of contact becomes intensely pruritic, after which erythema and small vesicles rapidly develop (Fig. 24-39). Over the next few days, the area enlarges, becomes fiery red, develops numerous vesicles, and exudes a large amount of clear proteinaceous fluid. During this evolution, pruritus is intense. The entire process lasts about 3 weeks. Exudation gradually subsides, and the whole area is covered by an irregular crust that eventually falls off. Pruritus diminishes, and healing occurs without scarring.

When a sensitized patient again comes into contact with poison ivy, the entire process is greatly accelerated. Within 24 to 48 hours, the lesions appear, spread rapidly, and produce the same clinical appearance. However, the reaction is usually more intense. Again, the lesions clear in about 3 weeks. Allergic contact dermatitis responds to topical or systemic administration of corticosteroids.

Granulomatous Dermatitis Is a Response to Indigestible Antigens

Granulomas, generally defined as localized collections of epithelioid macrophages, form in response to insoluble or slowly released antigens that produce either a focal nonallergic response or an allergic response in sensitized persons. Implicated antigens include foreign substances implanted accidentally into the skin (e.g., silicone in breast implants or endogenous antigens such as keratin). In many cases of granulomatous dermatitis, including sarcoidosis, the exact antigen is not known. Other common causes include mycobacterial and other infections (see Chapter 9) and granuloma annulare. Phagocytosis of the foreign particulate matter or processing of protein antigens is central to the activation of tissue macrophages as they are become the characteristic granulomatous epithelial cells (see Chapter 2).

Sarcoidosis May Lead to Skin Lesions

Sarcoidosis is a granulomatous disorder of unknown etiology that primarily affects the lungs but may also involve the skin, lymph nodes, spleen, eyes, and other organs (see Chapter 12). The granulomas of sarcoidosis are the classic epithelioid cell type, without caseation necrosis (Fig. 24-40). They

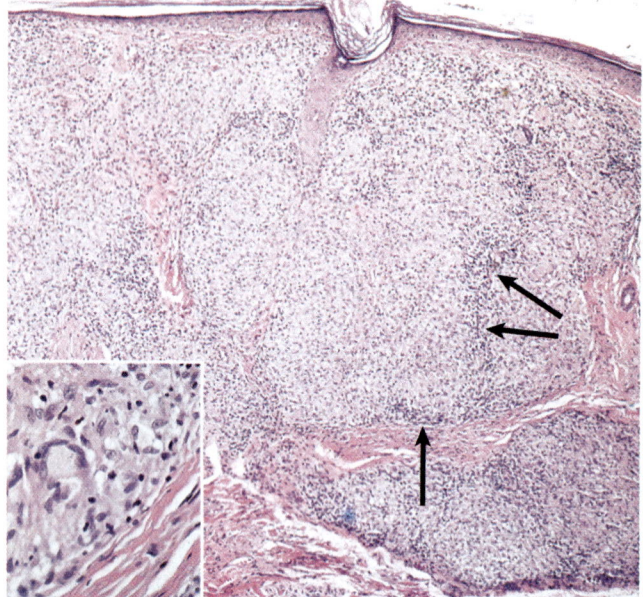

FIGURE 24-40
Sarcoidosis. Numerous large granulomas fill the reticular dermis. Around some of the granulomas are small cuffs of lymphocytes *(arrows)*. The granulomas are composed of epithelioid macrophages, some of which are multinucleated *(inset)*.

involve both the dermis and the subcutaneous tissue. The cutaneous manifestations of sarcoidosis are characterized by asymptomatic papules, plaques, and nodules of the dermis and subcutis. Some dermal plaques may be annular, and those that involve the subcutis appear as irregular nodules. In severe cases, the cutaneous lesions are so prominent that they simulate a diffuse infiltrative neoplasm.

Granuloma Annulare Is a Reaction to an Unknown Antigen

Granuloma annulare is a benign, self-limited disorder of unknown etiology, characterized by palisading "necrobiotic" granulomas in the skin.

 Pathogenesis: It is postulated that granuloma annulare is an immunologically mediated reaction to an unknown antigen. The disease has been reported to follow various conditions, such as insect bites, sun exposure, and viral infections. Antigenic stimuli are thought to include viral antigens, altered dermal collagen or elastic fibers, or proteins in the saliva of biting arthropods. The precise type of immune reaction is unclear, but both circulating immune complexes and cell-mediated immunity may be involved. The activated macrophages may themselves contribute to the disease process by releasing lysosomal enzymes and cytokines that in turn cause the focal collagen degeneration (so-called necrobiosis) characteristic of granuloma annulare.

 Pathology: Well-developed lesions contain a central area of acellular degenerated collagen and mucin deposition (necrobiosis) in the superficial to mid-reticular dermis (Fig. 24-41). This central area is surrounded by palisaded macrophages, each with the long axis of the nucleus radiating outward. Occasional multinucleated cells are found along with a superficial perivascular lymphocytic infiltrate.

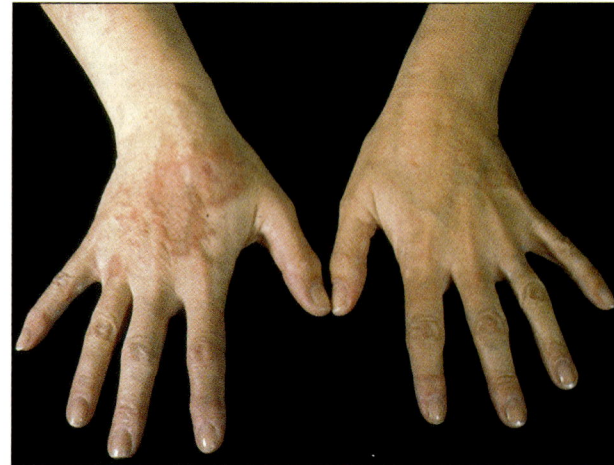
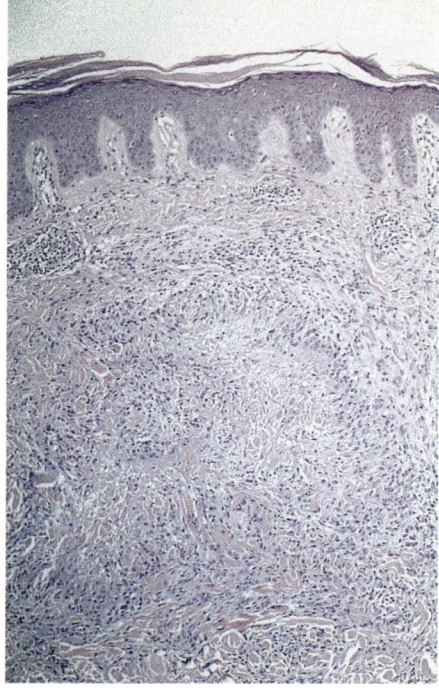

FIGURE 24-41
Granuloma annulare. **A.** The skin exhibits a typical annular plaque on the dorsal right hand. **B.** A central area of acellular degenerated collagen is surrounded by palisaded macrophages with the long axes of their nuclei radiating outward.

Clinical Features: The most common type of granuloma annulare occurs on the dorsum of the hands and feet, primarily in children and young adults (Fig. 24-41). The disease manifests as asymptomatic, skin-colored or erythematous annular plaques. About 15% of patients have disseminated granuloma annulare, with 10 or more lesions involving the trunk and neck. Granuloma annulare rarely requires treatment and usually has no medical consequences. In patients with significant cosmetic disfigurement, lesional injection of steroids is usually effective.

DISORDERS OF THE DERMAL CONNECTIVE TISSUE

Scleroderma Features Intense Fibrosis of the Skin

Scleroderma (Greek, *skleros*, hard), also known as *progressive systemic sclerosis*, is marked by fibrosis and tightening of the skin. The disease also displays variable structural and functional involvement of internal organs, including the kidneys, lungs, heart, esophagus, and small intestine. *Morphea* is similar to scleroderma, but it involves only patchy, circumscribed areas of the skin. The pathogenesis and systemic manifestations of scleroderma are discussed in Chapters 4 and 16.

Pathology: The initial cutaneous lesions of scleroderma are in the lower reticular dermis, but eventually the entire reticular dermis and even the papillary dermis are involved. There is diminished space among collagen bundles in the reticular dermis and a tendency for the collagen bundles to be enlarged, hypocellular, and parallel to each other. A patchy lymphocytic infiltrate containing a few plasma cells is common and may also be present in the underlying subcutaneous tissue. Sweat ducts are entrapped in the thickened fibrous tissue, and there is loss of the normal fat around eccrine structures. Hair follicles are completely obliterated (Fig. 24-42). In late stages of the disease, large areas of subcutaneous fat are replaced by newly formed collagen.

Clinical Features: Scleroderma shows a peak incidence in persons between 30 and 50 years of age, and women are afflicted four times as often as men. Patients with early scleroderma usually present with Raynaud phenomenon (see Chapter 10) or nonpitting edema of the hands or fingers. The affected areas become hard and tense. The skin of the face becomes masklike and expressionless, and the skin around the mouth exhibits radial furrows. In late stages of the disease, the skin over large parts of the body is thickened, densely fibrotic, and fixed to the underlying tissue. The prognosis is related to the extent of disease in visceral organs, particularly the lung and kidney.

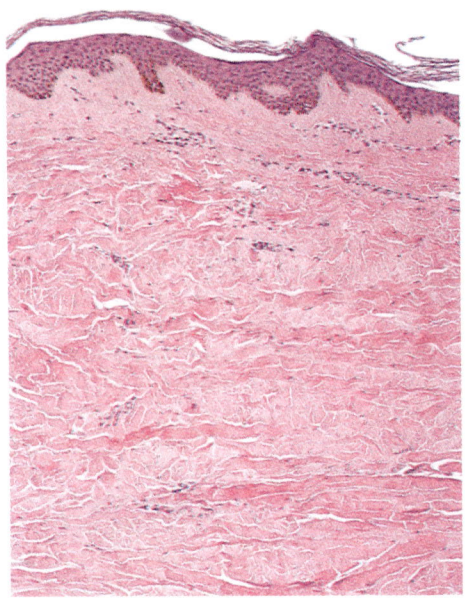

FIGURE 24-42
Scleroderma. The dermis is characterized by large, reticular collagen bundles that are oriented parallel to the epidermis. The large size and loss of basket-weave pattern of these collagen bundles are abnormal. No appendages are apparent because these structures have been destroyed.

INFLAMMATORY DISORDERS OF THE PANNICULUS

Panniculitis encompasses a heterogeneous group of diseases in which the principal focus of inflammation is in the subcutis (panniculus). The various disorders gathered under the umbrella of panniculitis are classified according to their location. *Septal panniculitis* refers to inflammation in the septa of the connective tissues, whereas *lobular panniculitis* denotes involvement of the fat lobules. These two entities may occur with or without accompanying vasculitis. For example, *polyarteritis nodosa* produces septal panniculitis (see Chapter 10).

Erythema Nodosum Is Related to Toxic and Infectious Agents

Erythema nodosum (EN) is a cutaneous disorder that manifests as self-limited, nonsuppurative, tender nodules over the extensor surfaces of the lower extremities. The disease has a peak incidence in the third decade of life and is three times more common in women than in men.

Pathogenesis: EN is triggered by exposure to a wide variety of agents, including drugs and microorganisms (bacteria, viruses, and fungi), and occurs in association with a number of benign and malignant systemic diseases. Common infections complicated by EN include streptococcal diseases (especially in children), tuberculosis, and *Yersinia* infection. In endemic areas, deep fungal infections (blastomycosis, histoplasmosis, coccidioidomycosis) are common causes. EN also frequently occurs after acute respiratory tract infections of unknown etiology, but which are likely viral. In drug-induced EN, the agents most commonly implicated are sulfonamides and oral contraceptives. Finally, Crohn disease and ulcerative colitis may be complicated by EN.

It is thought that EN represents an immunological response to foreign antigens, although the evidence is indirect. For example, patients with tuberculosis or coccidioidomycosis do not develop EN until the skin test becomes positive, and testing with Frei antigen for lymphogranuloma venereum may itself induce EN. The early neutrophilic inflammation suggests that EN may be a response to the activation of complement, with resulting neutrophilic chemotaxis. The subsequent chronic inflammation, foreign body giant cells, and fibrosis are secondary to necrosis of adipose tissue at the interface of the septa and lobules.

 Pathology: Early in the course of the disease, the lesions of EN are in the fibrous septa of the subcutaneous tissue, where neutrophilic inflammation is associated with the extravasation of erythrocytes. In chronic lesions, the septa are widened, with focal collections of giant cell macrophages around small areas of altered collagen, and an ill-defined lymphocytic infiltrate (Fig. 24-43). Giant cells and inflammatory cells extend into the lobule from the interface between the septum and the fat lobule. Secondary vascular involvement is occasionally noted.

 Clinical Features: EN typically manifests acutely on the anterior aspects of the lower limbs as dome-shaped, exquisitely tender, erythematous nodules.

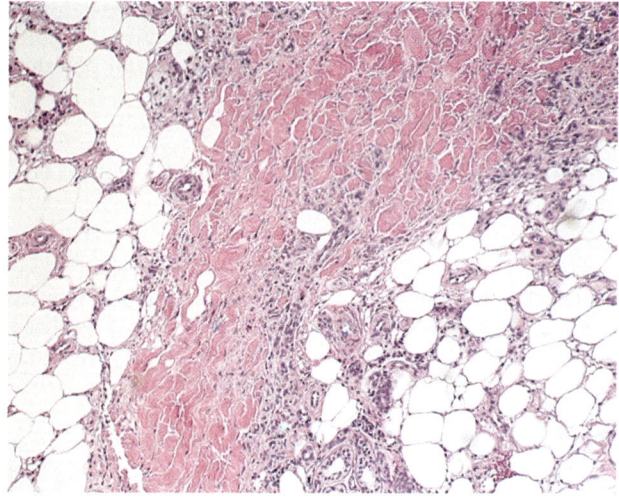

FIGURE 24-43
Erythema nodosum. The reticular dermis is present in *upper right*. Within the panniculus *(extending through the middle of the field)* is a widened septum. Lymphocytes and macrophages are present at its border with the adipose tissue lobules. The vessels palisading along the border of the septum are infiltrated by lymphocytes.

The nodules eventually become firm and less tender and disappear in 3 to 6 weeks. As some nodules heal, others arise, but all lesions resolve without residual scarring within 6 weeks.

Erythema Induratum Is Frequently Associated with *M. tuberculosis*

Erythema induratum (EI) refers to chronic, recurrent subcutaneous nodules or plaques on the legs, predominantly in women. EI was traditionally considered a "tuberculid" (i.e., a hypersensitivity reaction to mycobacteria or associated antigens at a distant site). The failure of lesional tissue to yield isolates of mycobacteria in culture or in laboratory animals eventually cast doubt on this historical concept. However, subsequent investigations using the polymerase chain reaction have detected a specific *M. tuberculosis* DNA sequence in over 75% of skin biopsy specimens with a histological diagnosis of EI.

 Pathology: In contrast to EN, EI manifests initially as a lobular panniculitis. This lesion is secondary to a vasculitis that produces ischemic necrosis of the fat lobule. The panniculus exhibits a dense, chronic inflammatory infiltrate within the lobules, which can form prominent tuberculoid granulomas or result in areas of coagulative necrosis. The lobular septa within the panniculus are relatively spared. The vascular changes are usually extensive and include (1) prominent infiltration of small and medium-sized arteries and veins by a dense lymphoid or granulomatous infiltrate, (2) endothelial swelling, which may progress to thrombosis, and (3) fibrous thickening of the intima. Extensive ischemic necrosis leads to subsequent ulceration of the overlying epidermis. Eventually, the lesions heal by fibrosis.

 Clinical Features: Patients with EI present with recurrent, tender, erythematous, subcutaneous nodules on the legs, particularly in the area of the calf. The lesions tend to ulcerate and heal with an atrophic scar. The course may last many years, and systemic steroids are usually necessary to control the disease.

ACNE VULGARIS: A DISORDER OF THE PILOSEBACEOUS UNIT

Acne vulgaris is a self-limited, inflammatory disorder of the sebaceous follicles that typically afflicts adolescents, results in the intermittent formation of discrete papular or pustular lesions, and may lead to scarring. In some cases, acne extends as long as the third decade. The condition is cosmetically disfiguring and often psychologically debilitating. Acne is so common that many regard it as a "rite of passage" through adolescence.

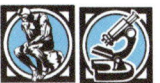

Pathogenesis and Pathology: The development of acne is related to (1) excessive hormonally induced production of sebum, (2) abnormal cornification of portions of the follicular epithelium, (3) a response to the anaerobic diphtheroid *Propionibacterium acnes,* and (4) rupture of the follicle and subsequent inflammation. The sebaceous follicle contains a vellus hair and prominent sebaceous glands. The change in hormonal status at puberty leads to the production of sebum in the follicle and to altered cornification in the neck of the sebaceous follicle (infundibulum), effects that produce dilation of the follicular canal. Another round of excessive sebum production is associated with the desquamation of squamous cells and the accretion of keratinous debris, a situation that provides a rich environment for the proliferation of *P. acnes*. These combined changes result in the formation of a distended, plugged follicle, termed a *comedone*. Neutrophils are attracted to the area by chemotactic factors released by *P. acnes*, where they release hydrolytic enzymes to form a follicular abscess *(pustule)*. They also attack the wall of the follicle, thereby permitting the escape of sebum, keratin, and bacteria into the perifollicular tissue, where they stimulate further acute inflammation and a perifollicular abscess (Fig. 24-44). The development of an allergy to *P. acnes* intensifies the inflammatory response. The fully evolved lesions show intense neutrophilic inflammation surrounding a ruptured sebaceous follicle. In addition, numerous macrophages, lymphocytes, and foreign body giant cells accumulate in response to the rupture of the sebaceous follicle.

Clinical Features: Acne vulgaris features a variety of skin lesions in different stages of development, including comedones, papules, pustules, nodules, cysts, and pitted scars. Comedones, the primary noninflammatory lesions of acne, are either open *(blackheads)* or closed *(whiteheads)*. The more advanced inflammatory lesions vary from small, erythematous papules to large, tender, purulent nodules and cysts.

Acne vulgaris is treated with topical cleansing and keratolytic and antibacterial agents. Severe cases are managed with topical vitamin A, systemic antibiotics, and synthetic oral retinoids (isotretinoin).

INFECTIONS AND INFESTATIONS

The skin is under constant assault from a countless variety of marauders and provides an effective but imperfect barrier against them. Bacteria, fungi, viruses, parasites, and insects sometimes succeed in penetrating our first line of defense.

Impetigo Is an Infection by Staphylococci or Streptococci

Superficial bacterial infections of the skin, known as *impetigo*, occur mostly in children, who are often infected through minor breaks in the skin. Adults tend to manifest impetigo as a sequel to an underlying disease process that somehow compromises the barrier function of the skin. Honey-colored crusted erosions or ulcers, often with central healing, are present most commonly on exposed areas such as the face, hands, and extremities (Fig. 24-45). A combination of topical and systemic antimicrobial agents directed against staphylococci or streptococci is the mainstay of therapy. **Ecthyma** occurs when the organism invade the superficial aspects of the skin to form a necrotizing ulcerated lesion in the dermis.

Pathology: Microscopically, an abundance of neutrophils is found beneath the stratum corneum. Bacterial organisms may be identified with special stains. Vesicles or bullae form and eventually rupture, allowing a thin, seropurulent discharge to appear. This discharge dries and forms the characteristic layers of exudate containing neutrophils and cellular debris. Reactive epidermal changes (spongiosis and elongation of the rete ridges) and superficial dermal inflammation are usually present.

Superficial Fungal Infections Are Caused by Dermatophytes

Dermatophytes are fungi that can infect nonviable keratinized epithelium, including stratum corneum, nails, and hair. They synthesize keratinases that digest keratin and provide sustenance for the organisms. Often, superficial fungal infections are caused by a change in the microenvironment of the skin, which allows overgrowth of transient or resident flora. For example, the use of immunosuppressive agents such as topical or systemic glucocorticoids may impair the cell-mediated immune response that normally eliminates dermatophytes from the skin. Excessive sweating or occlusion of a body part may provide an environment that "tips the balance" between fungal proliferation and elimination in favor of proliferation.

Of the 10 or so dermatophyte species that are common causes of human cutaneous infection, *Trichophyton rubrum* is the most common cause. A superficial infection caused by a dermatophyte is called a *dermatophytosis, tinea,* or *ringworm*. The tineas have distinctive clinical features depending on the site of infection. They are divided as follows: (1) *tinea capitis* (scalp; "ringworm"), (2) *tinea barbae* (beard), (3) *tinea faciei* (face), (4) *tinea corporis* (trunk, legs, arms, or neck, excluding the feet, hands, and groin), (5) *tinea manus* (hands), (6) *tinea pedis* (feet; "athlete's foot"; Fig. 24-46), (7) *tinea cruris* (groin, pubic area, and thigh; "jock itch"), and (8) *tinea unguium* (nails; "onychomycosis").

Other causes of superficial fungal infections are the *Candida* species and *Malassezia furfur*. *Candida* species require a warm, moist environment in which to flourish, such as that found on a baby's bottom encased in a wet diaper. *M. furfur* requires a moist, lipid-rich environment. *Tinea versicolor*, caused by *M. furfur*, is more common in young adults when sebum production is greatest. Variably sized, pigmented, sharply demarcated, round or oval macules with fine scales are present, predominantly on the upper trunk.

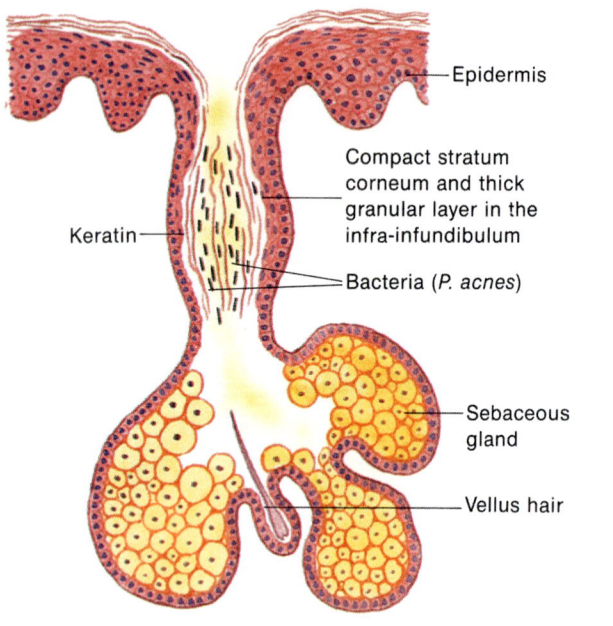
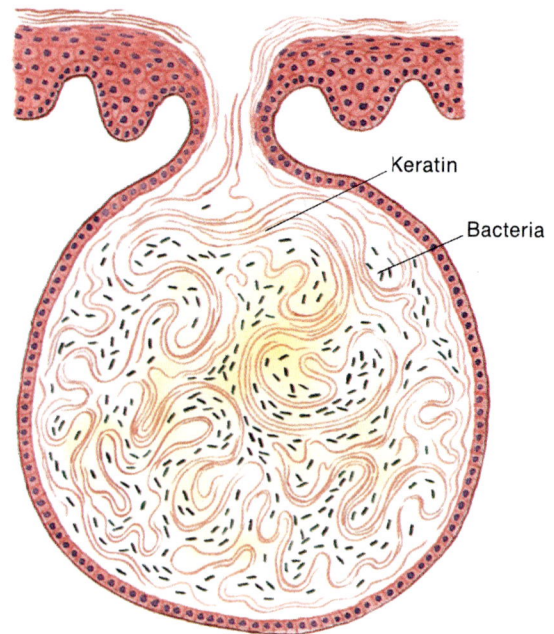
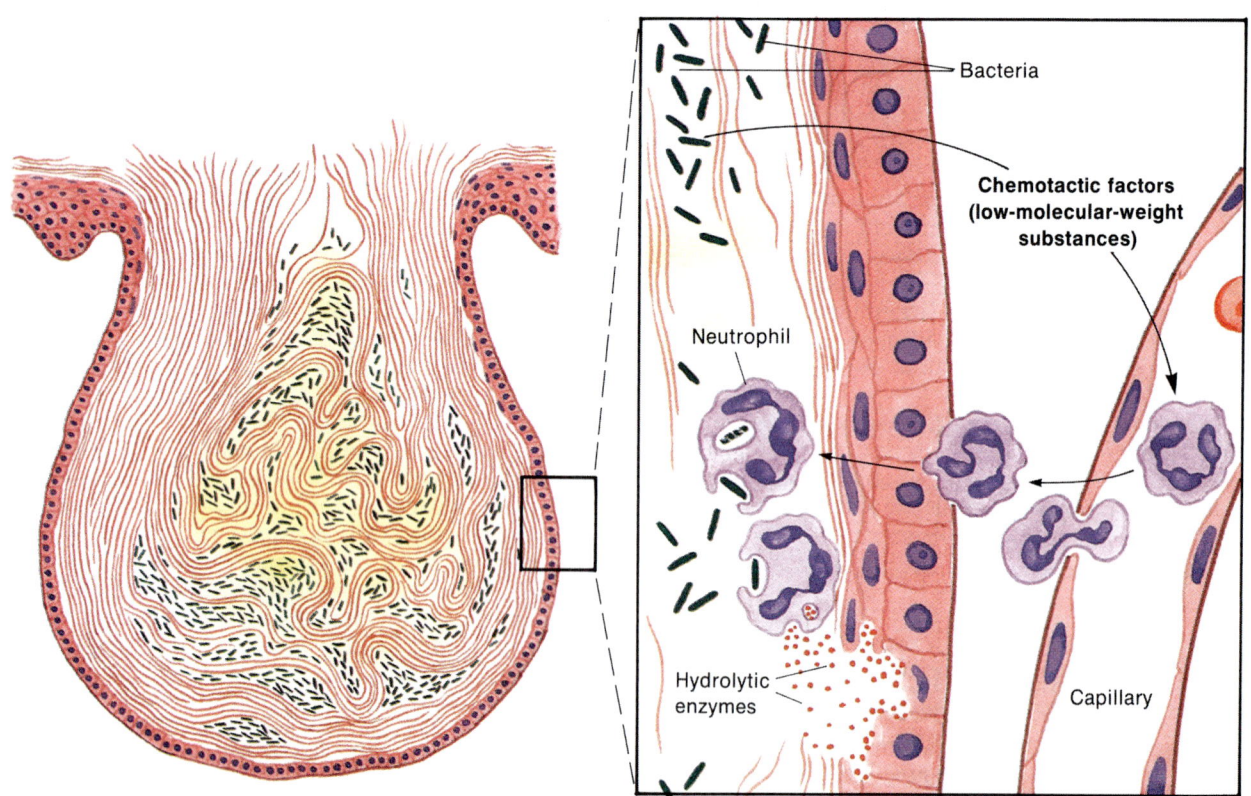

FIGURE 24-44
Acne vulgaris. The pathogenesis of follicular distention, rupture, and inflammation is depicted. Acne is a disease of the follicular canal of a sebaceous follicle. A compact stratum corneum and a thickened granular layer in the infrainfundibulum are the beginning of the formation of a comedone. Microcomedones (A), closed (B), and open (C) comedones form. Excessive sebum secretion occurs, and the bacterium *P. acnes* proliferates. The organism produces chemotactic factors, leading to neutrophil migration into the intact comedone. Neutrophilic enzymes are released, and the comedone ruptures, inducing a cycle of chemotaxis and intense neutrophilic inflammation (D and E).

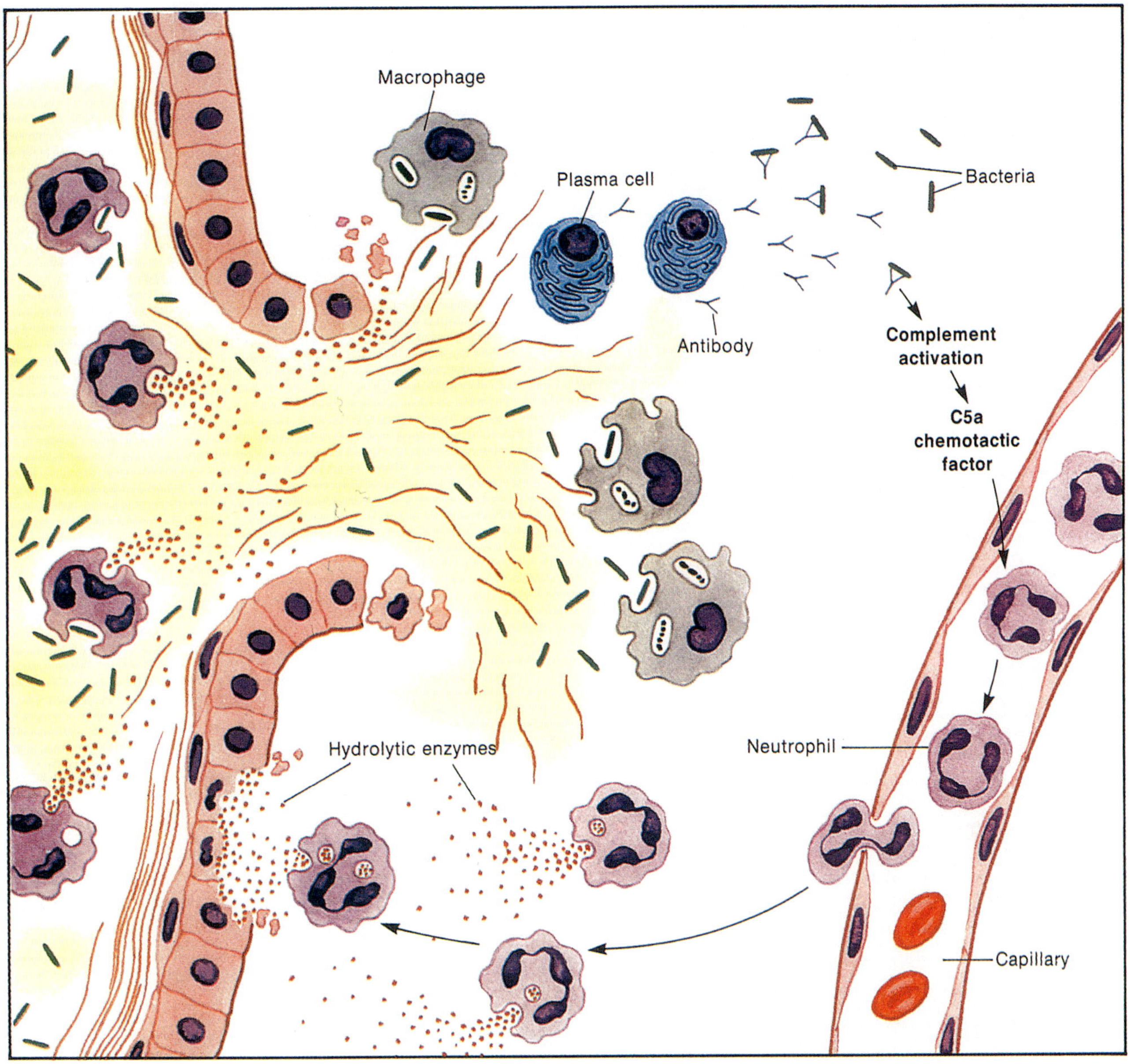

Infections and Infestations 1243

E. INFLAMMATION AND RUPTURE OF SEBACEOUS FOLLICLE

FIGURE 24-44 (continued)

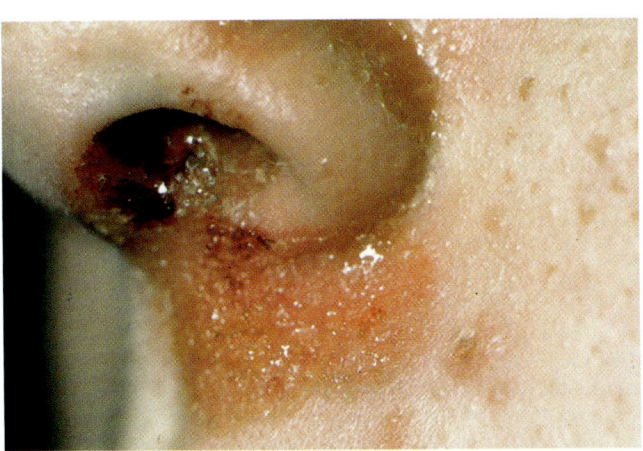

FIGURE 24-45
Impetigo contagiosa. Honey-colored crusts secondary to rupture of vesicopustules are seen in the nasal area of a child, an area commonly colonized by *Staphylococcus aureus*.

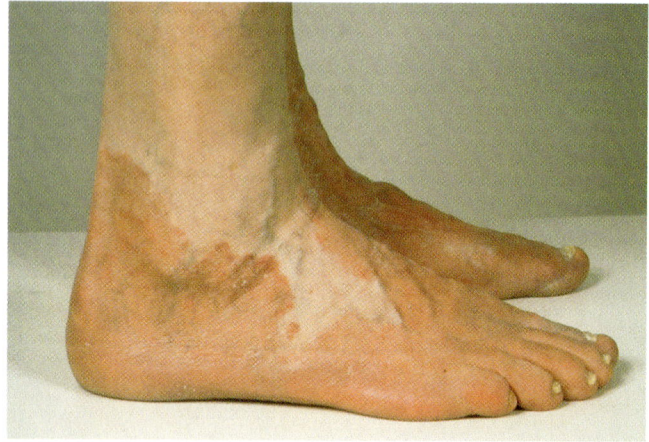
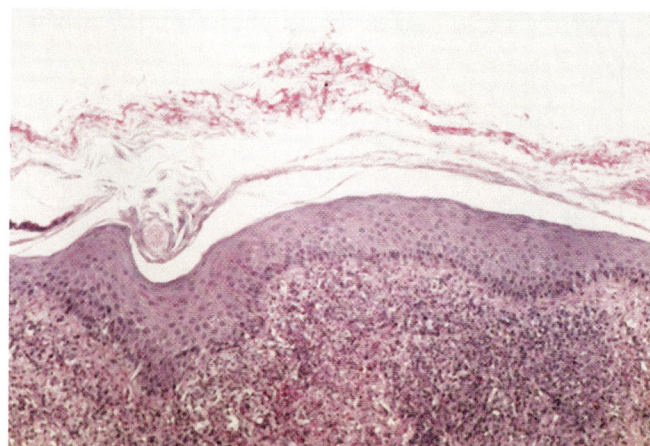
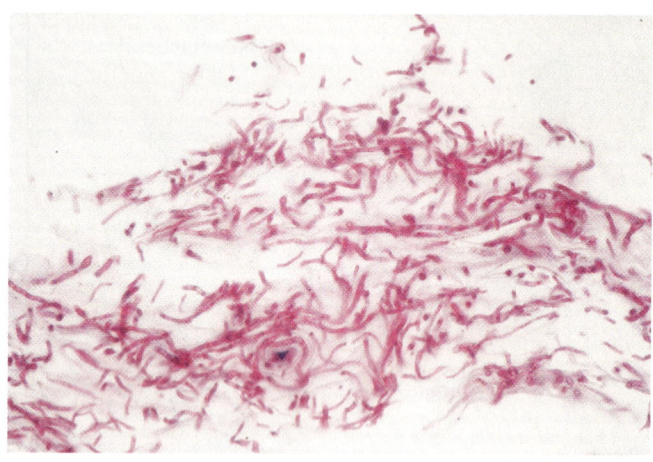

FIGURE 24-46
Dermatophytosis. A. Tinea pedis. A leading edge of scale and erythema in a moccasin distribution characterizes this infection, most commonly caused by *Trichophyton rubrum*. B. A dense inflammatory infiltrate is present in the epidermis and dermis and is associated with the presence of fungal hyphae in the stratum corneum. C. A higher power view of the fungal hyphae in the stratum corneum.

Special stains such as PAS show budding yeast and hyphal forms in the most superficial layers of the stratum corneum. Hyperkeratosis, epidermal hyperplasia, and chronic perivascular inflammation are noted in the dermis (Fig. 24-46).

Deep Fungal Infections Reflect Dissemination of Pulmonary Infections

Most invasive or systemic fungal infections arise from inhalation of aerosolized material contaminated with organisms such as *Histoplasma* or *Blastomyces*. A primary pulmonary infection may then spread to the skin or mucosa. Locally invasive fungal infections of the skin are rare and usually arise from traumatic implantation of organisms such as *Sporothrix* or *Fonsecaea*. An underlying immunocompromised state increases the likelihood of dissemination of fungal organisms.

Deep extension of a local cutaneous infection often results in a chancrelike lesion at the site of implantation. Intervening lymphatic vessels may become indurated and thickened. Nodules and ulcerations, especially those found bilaterally, suggest an internal source of infection.

The presence of certain morphological features or staining patterns may provide a clue to the identity of the organism. For example, the yeast form of *Blastomyces dermatitidis* displays notably refractile walls and a broad-based budding pattern, whereas the yeast form of *Histoplasma capsulatum* is much smaller, is often found within macrophages, and shows a narrow-based budding pattern. Staining a smear with India ink, or a tissue biopsy with mucicarmine, may show the thick capsule characteristic of the yeast *Cryptococcus neoformans*. Marked epidermal hyperplasia, intraepidermal microabscesses, and suppurative granulomatous inflammation in the dermis are some of the findings associated with these deep-seated fungal infections (Fig. 24-47).

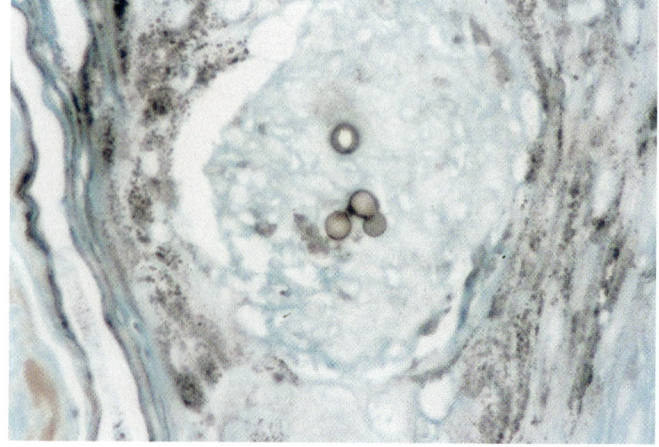

FIGURE 24-47
Blastomycosis. A period acid-Schiff stain highlights the organisms, which are thick-walled spores 8 to 15 microns in diameter. One of the organisms demonstrates broad-based budding.

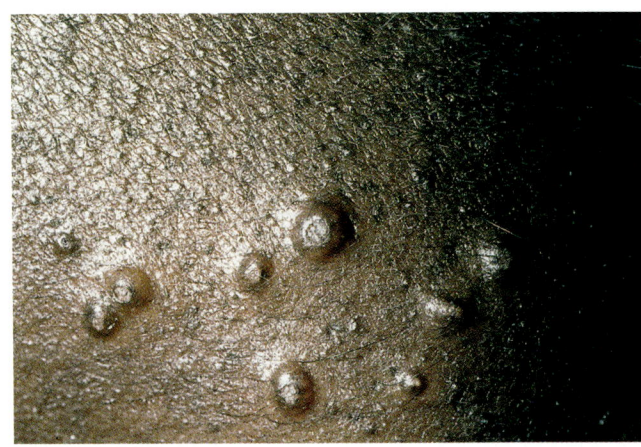 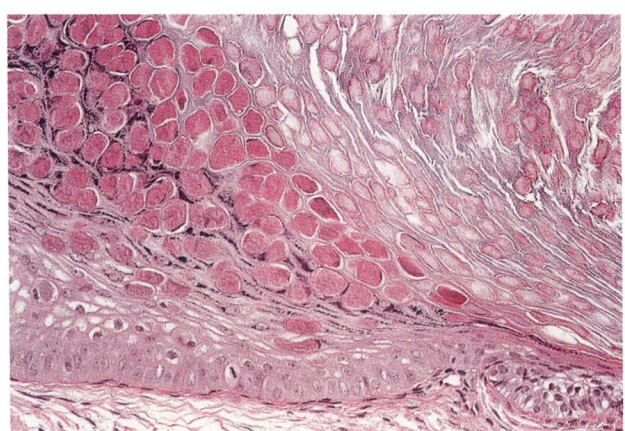

FIGURE 24-48
Molluscum contagiosum. A. Multiple umbilicated papules in an HIV-positive patient. B. The keratinocytes that are infected with this poxvirus show large eosinophilic cytoplasmic inclusions called "molluscum bodies."

Viral Infections Cause a Wide Variety of Skin Lesions

The dermatoses caused by viruses are numerous and include a wide spectrum of clinical manifestations (see Chapter 9). Some viruses, such as the poxvirus *molluscum contagiosum (MCV)* or the *human papillomaviruses (HPV)* (see below), manifest as benign epithelial proliferations that are transient and resolve spontaneously. Other viruses (e.g., measles or *parvovirus* [erythema infectiosum]) cause febrile illness with self-limited cutaneous eruptions (exanthems). Primary infection by most of the *human herpesviruses* is often asymptomatic but results in a state of latent infection. Upon reactivation, the virus causes a vesicular eruption.

Molluscum contagiosum is a common infection among children and sexually active adults. It is a self-limited infection that is easily spread by direct contact. Firm, dome-shaped, smooth-surfaced papules with a characteristic central umbilication are usually found on the face, trunk, and anogenital area. Microscopic examination shows epidermal cells containing large intracytoplasmic inclusion bodies ("*molluscum* bodies"), which are found within cup-shaped areas that also exhibit verrucous (papillomatous) epidermal hyperplasia. Numerous viral particles are present within these inclusion bodies (Fig. 24-48).

Arthropod Infestations Produce Pruritic Skin Lesions

Mites and lice, other insects, and spiders produce local lesions that may be intensely pruritic.

- *Scabies* is a severely pruritic, eczematous dermatitis caused by the mite *Sarcoptes scabei*. The female mite burrows beneath the stratum corneum on the fingers, wrists, trunk, and genital skin (Fig. 24-49). An intense lymphocytic and eosinophilic dermatitis is induced as a hypersensitivity reaction to the mite and its eggs and feces.

- *Pediculosis*, another pruritic dermatosis, may be caused by a variety of human lice. Eggs ("nits") of the lice may be found attached to hair shafts.

- **Biting insects** produce lesions that vary from small, pruritic papules to large, weeping nodules. The reaction depends on the particular arthropod species and the character of the host immune response. For example, tick bites tend to be large, with a striking lymphocytic and eosinophilic infiltrate. Lymphoid follicles may also form. Flea bites are usually urticarial, with a scant neu-

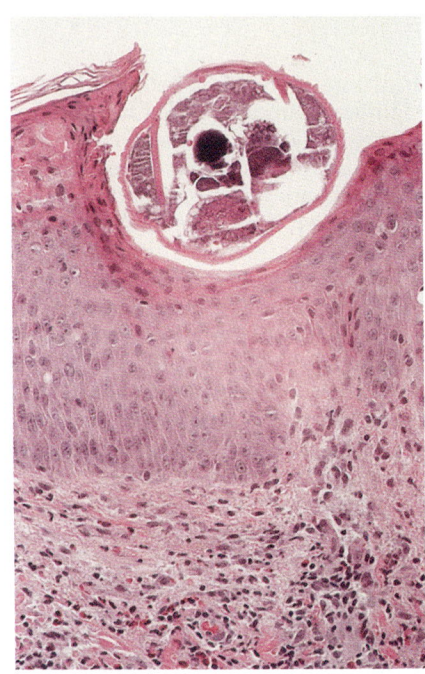

FIGURE 24-49
Scabetic nodule. A scabies mite is present in the stratum corneum.

PRIMARY NEOPLASMS OF THE SKIN

Cutaneous tumors constitute a paradigm for understanding neoplasia in general. These lesions are on the body surface, where their development and evolution may be readily observed. The availability of tumor tissue from the developmentally sequential lesions has permitted the correlation of studies of tumor cells in vitro with the observed behavior of clinical lesions.

The incidence of malignant melanoma, in particular, is increasing at an alarming rate. It is estimated that more than 1% of children born today will develop malignant melanoma. Although a diagnosis of malignant melanoma has traditionally carried with it an element of danger, the prognosis is actually excellent if the lesion is recognized and excised before it exhibits a vertical growth phase. If, however, the tumor extends beyond a critical depth in the dermis, many patients will die of metastatic disease.

Common Acquired Melanocytic Nevus (Mole) Is a Benign Pigmented Skin Lesion

Common acquired melanocytic nevus, is composed of a localized proliferation of melanocytes within the epidermis or dermis.

Pathogenesis: Most people who are exposed to a significant amount of light in the first 15 years of life, regardless of their skin color, develop 10 to 50 nevi on their skin. Black skin can develop nevi, but they are less common and are not associated with progression to melanoma. However, if they are located on the palms of the hands, the soles of the feet, or on the genital skin, the risk of melanoma is the same in all races. The nevi do not ordinarily develop in areas protected from light by at least two layers of clothing, such as the breasts of women. Red-haired, blue-eyed persons with milk-white skin are notable exceptions, in that they are exquisitely sensitive to light and form freckles, but they do not develop a significant number of nevi. There is an unequivocal causal relationship between ultraviolet light and melanocytic nevi (and malignant melanoma), but the relationship is complex; some people with fair skin form relatively few nevi, whereas some with dark skin develop numerous nevi. The ability to form nevi has been correlated with polymorphic variants of the melanocortin receptor and with subsequent variation in the ratio of red pheomelanin to brown eumelanin.

Epidemiological studies have shown melanocytic nevi to be precursor lesions to the development of melanoma. A person with 100 or more nevi that are 2 to 5 mm in greatest dimension has a threefold greater risk of developing melanoma than one with fewer than 25 similar nevi. Patients with clinically atypical-appearing nevi or histologically proven dysplastic nevi have an even greater risk of developing melanoma.

Melanocytic nevi begin to appear between the first and second years of life and continue to emerge for the first two decades of life. A nevus first appears as a small tan dot no bigger than 1 to 2 mm in diameter. During the next 3 to 4 years, the dot enlarges to become a uniform tan to brown area that is circular or oval. The peripheral outline usually remains regular. When the nevus is 4 to 5 mm in diameter, it is flat or slightly elevated, stops enlarging peripherally, and is sharply demarcated from the surrounding normal skin. Over the next 10 years, the lesion elevates, and its color pales to the point of becoming a tan taglike protrusion. For the next decade or two, it gradually flattens, and the skin may approximate a normal appearance. Most people show a gradual decrease in the number of nevi through the years. Notably, many melanoma patients tend to retain increased numbers of nevi, including atypical ones, in the later decades of life.

Pathology: At the inception of a melanocytic nevus, there is an increased number of melanocytes in the basal epidermis, with subsequent hyperpigmentation. The melanocytes eventually form nests, frequently at the tips of the rete ridges, and then migrate into the dermis where they form small clusters. As the lesion becomes elevated, the dermal nevus cells begin to differentiate in a manner reminiscent of Schwann cells, an evolution that gradually encompasses the entire dermal component, leaving a core of delicate neuromesenchyme. The nevus may eventually flatten and possibly even disappear. The histological classification of melanocytic nevi reflects the evolution of the lesions:

- **Junctional nevus:** The melanocytes form nests at the tips of the rete ridges in the epidermis.
- **Compound nevus:** Nests of melanocytes are seen in the epidermis, and some of the cells have migrated into the dermis (Fig. 24-50).
- **Dermal nevus:** Intraepidermal melanocytic growth has ceased (Fig. 24-51).

Dysplastic (Atypical) Nevus Shows Persistent Melanocytic Growth

Some common acquired nevi do not follow the expected pattern of growth, differentiation, and disappearance described above. Such lesions persist and are often more than 5 mm in greatest dimension. These nevi may show focal areas of aberrant melanocytic growth and become larger and more irregular peripherally. The irregular area is flat (macular) and extends asymmetrically from the parent nevus. Some clinically dysplastic nevi are entirely macular.

Germline mutations in the *CDKN2A* tumor-suppressor gene (also known as *p16* or *p16INK4a*), mapped to chromosome 9p21, have been found in some dysplastic nevus/melanoma patients and their family members. This gene encodes an inhibitor of cyclin-dependent kinase 4 (CDK4) that functions to suppress proliferation.

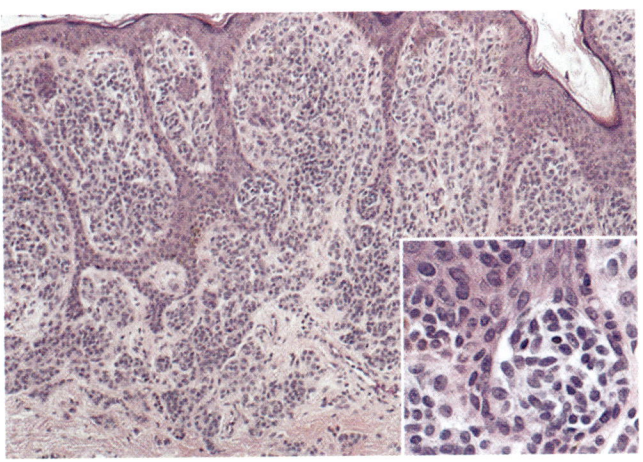

FIGURE 24-50
Compound melanocytic nevus. Melanocytes are present as nests within the epidermis and dermis. An intraepidermal nest of melanocytes is surrounded by keratinocytes (inset).

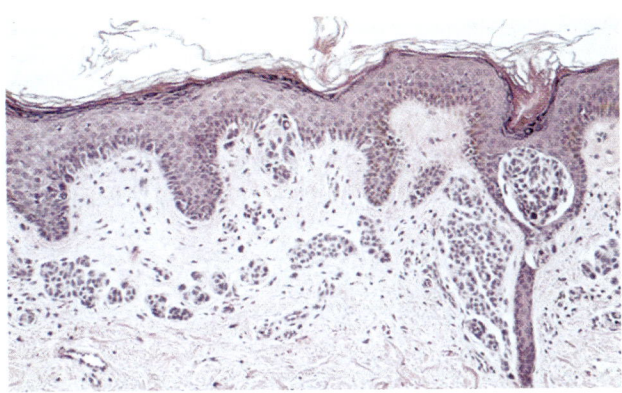

FIGURE 24-52
Compound nevus with melanocytic dysplasia. On the *right*, a compound nevus is apparent with both intraepidermal and dermal components. To the *left*, within the epidermis are single atypical melanocytes within the basal unit, as well as incipient lamellar fibroplasia. Dermal melanocytes are present *below*.

Melanocytic Dysplasia Features Architectural and Cytologic Atypia

Initially, the growth of melanocytes in the basal epidermis appears similar to that which occurs in the early stages of a common nevus. This area is abnormal in architectural pattern, not in cytological features. A band of eosinophilic connective tissue *(lamellar fibroplasia)* is seen around the rete ridges, which contain aberrantly growing melanocytes. These aberrant melanocytes may grow to become continuous streams of melanocytes extending from rete to rete ("bridging"). As these architectural features become more prominent, melanocytes with large atypical nuclei that are reminiscent of malignant cells may also appear in the areas of architectural disorder. This combination of architectural disorder and cytological atypia constitutes a dysplastic nevus (Figs. 24-52 and 24-53). Areas of dysplasia may also be associated with a subjacent lymphocytic infiltrate. More than one third of malignant melanomas have a precursor nevus, most of which show melanocytic dysplasia.

Malignant Melanoma Has Consequences Related to the Depth of Invasion

Radial Growth Phase Melanoma

The most frequently encountered form of melanoma is in the radial growth phase and is also termed *superficial spreading melanoma* (Fig. 24-54).

Pathology: Large epithelioid melanocytes are dispersed in nests and as individual cells throughout the entire thickness of the epidermis. These melanocytes may be only in the epidermis *(melanoma in situ)* or they may also extend into the papillary dermis. In the radial growth phase, no nest has growth preference (larger size) over the other nests (Fig. 24-55). Thus, the melanocytes of the radial growth phase grow in all directions: upward in the epidermis, peripherally in the epidermis, and downward from the epidermis into the dermis. Mitoses are not seen in dermal melanocytes. The enlargement of these lesions is at the periphery, hence the term *radial*. The melanocytes of the radial growth phase are typically associated with a brisk lymphocytic response. Melanomas in the radial growth phase have only rarely been observed to metastasize.

Clinical Features: Superficial spreading melanoma (SSM) tends to occur on skin that has been exposed intermittently to the sun. The tumor has been associated with a history of sunburn. Early melanomas in the radial growth phase have a slightly elevated and palpable border. The neoplasm is usually variably and haphazardly pigmented. Some parts are black or dark

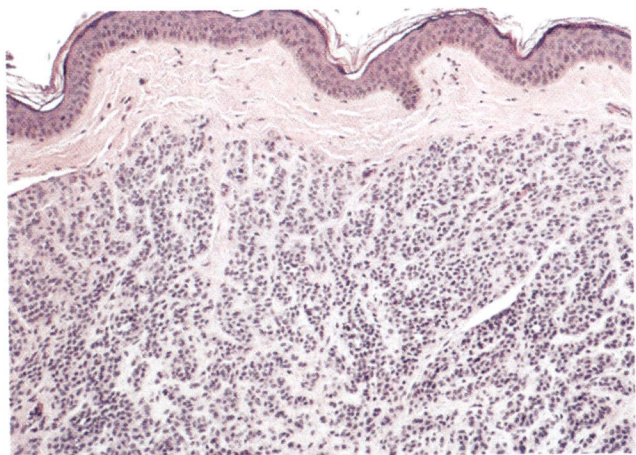

FIGURE 24-51
Dermal melanocytic nevus. The melanocytes are entirely confined to the dermis.

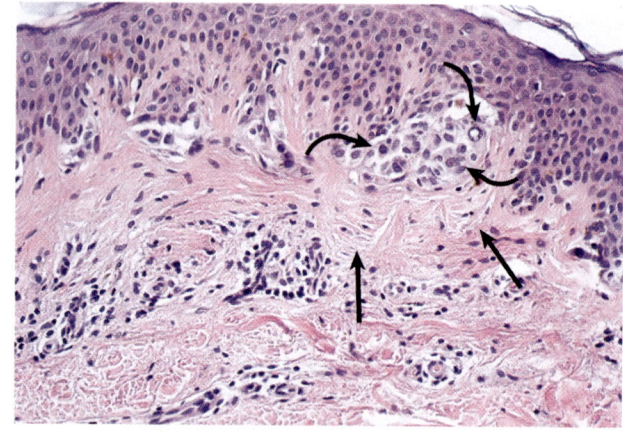
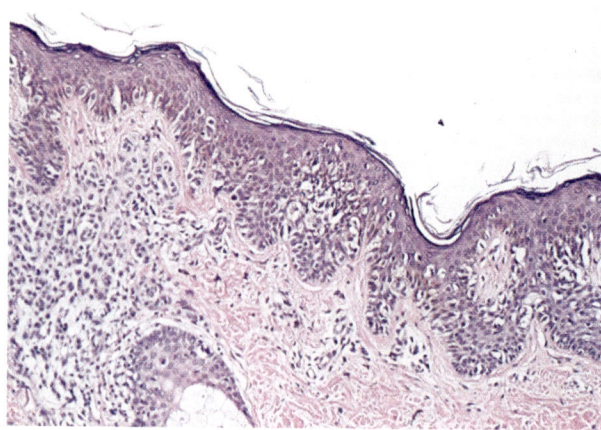
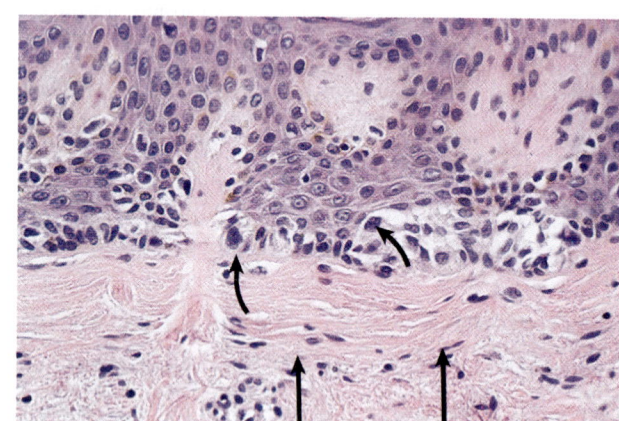

FIGURE 24-53
Dysplastic nevus. A. There is bridging of rete ridges by nests of melanocytes, melanocytes with cytological atypia *(curved arrows)*, lamellar fibroplasia *(straight arrows)*, and a scant perivascular lymphocytic infiltrate. B. To the *left* is a zone containing typical dermal nevic cells of a compound melanocytic nevus. In the epidermis on the *right* is a lentiginous proliferation of atypical melanocytes with lamellar fibroplasia. This photomicrograph is taken from the junction of the papular and macular components of this dysplastic nevus. Dysplasia usually develops in the macular portion, which takes up most of the field. C. These ellipsoid melanocytic nests resting above lamellar fibroplasia *(straight arrows)* exhibit large epithelioid melanocytes with atypia *(curved arrows)*.

brown, whereas other areas may be lighter brown, possibly mixed with pink or light blue tints. The entire lesion may be purely dark brown (see Fig. 24-54). With regard to lesions that are eventually documented to be melanoma, patients frequently state that a change in a nevus occurred. Such changes can include itching, increase in size, darkening, or bleeding and oozing, though the last signs tend to appear later. Even in the absence of such observations on the part of the patient, any lesion that prompts clinical suspicion of melanoma warrants an excisional biopsy. The "ABCD rule" is a convenient mnemonic that is commonly taught to patients to help them recognize changes in nevi that should prompt them to seek medical attention: **A**symmetry of shape, **B**order irregularity, **C**olor variation, and a **D**iameter more than 6 mm. However, not all early melanomas exhibit these attributes, and any changing lesion should be evaluated for excisional biopsy.

Vertical Growth Phase Melanoma

After a variable time (usually 1 to 2 years), the character of growth begins to change. Melanocytes exhibit mitotic activity and grow as spheroid nodules that expand more rapidly than the rest of the tumor in the surrounding papillary dermis (Fig. 24-56). The net direction of growth tends to be per-

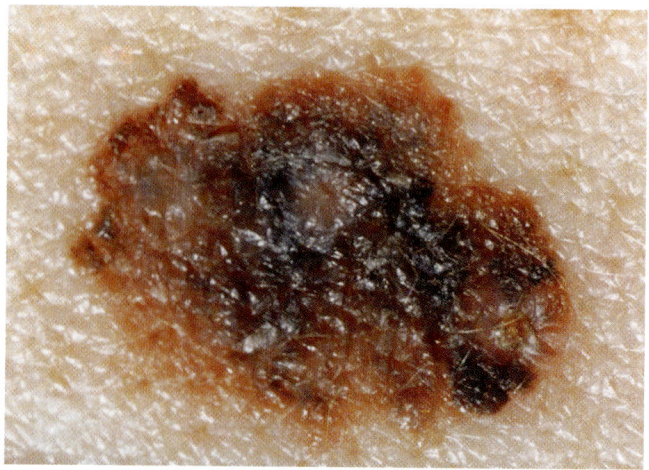

FIGURE 24-54
The clinical appearance of the radial growth phase in malignant melanoma of the superficial spreading type. The larger diameter is 1.8 cm.

Primary Neoplasms of the Skin

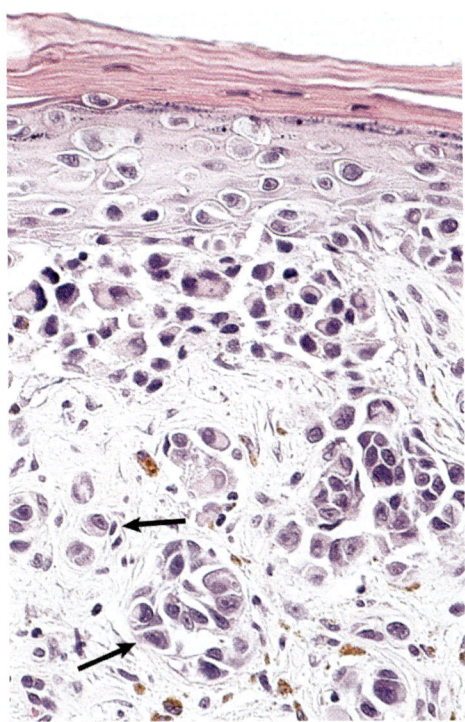

FIGURE 24-55
Malignant melanoma, superficial spreading type, radial growth phase. Melanocytes grow singly within the epidermis at all levels and as large, irregularly sized nests at the dermal–epidermal junction. Tumor cells are present in the papillary dermis *(arrows)*, but no nest shows preferential growth over the others.

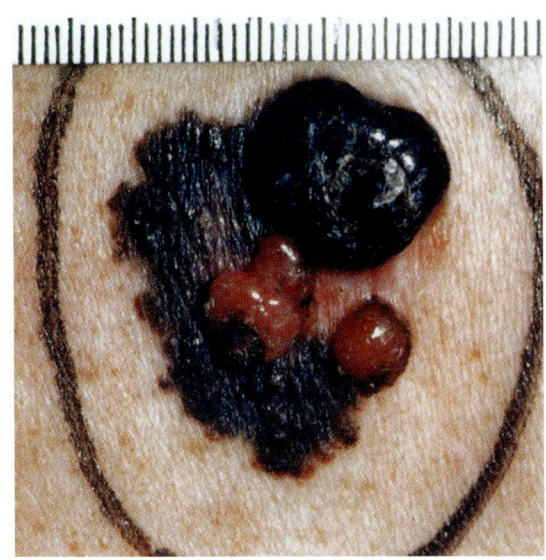

FIGURE 24-56
Malignant melanoma the superficial spreading type is represented by the relatively flat, dark, brown–black portion of the tumor. Three areas in this lesion are characteristic of the vertical growth phase. All are nodular in configuration; two have a pink coloration, and the largest is a rich, ebony black.

pendicular to that of the radial growth phase, hence the term *vertical* (Figs. 24-57 through 24-59).

thick, have no evident mitoses, and exhibit a brisk infiltrate of lymphocytes rarely metastasize. Vertical growth phase melanomas that are more than 3.6 mm thick, display more than 6 mitoses/mm^2, and do not contain tumor-infiltrating lymphocytes frequently metastasize. Lesions intermediate between these extremes can be recognized and their behavior predicted through the use of prognostic models, albeit imperfectly.

 Pathology: The more specific characteristics of vertical growth phase are as follows:

- The melanocytes tend to differ in appearance from those of the radial growth phase. For example, they may contain little or no pigment, whereas the cells of the radial growth phase are melanotic.
- The cellular aggregate that characterizes the vertical growth phase is larger than the clusters of melanocytes that form the intraepidermal and invasive components of the radial growth phase. The dominant site of tumor growth is shifted from the epidermis to the dermis.
- Tumors that extend into the lower half of the reticular dermis are considered to be in the vertical growth phase.
- The host immune response may be absent at the base of the vertical growth phase.
- Markers of cell cycle progression, such as Ki-67, increase in cells of the vertical growth phase.

Even when tumors enter the vertical growth phase, they may still lack the propensity to metastasize. For example, vertical growth phase melanomas that are less than 1.7 mm

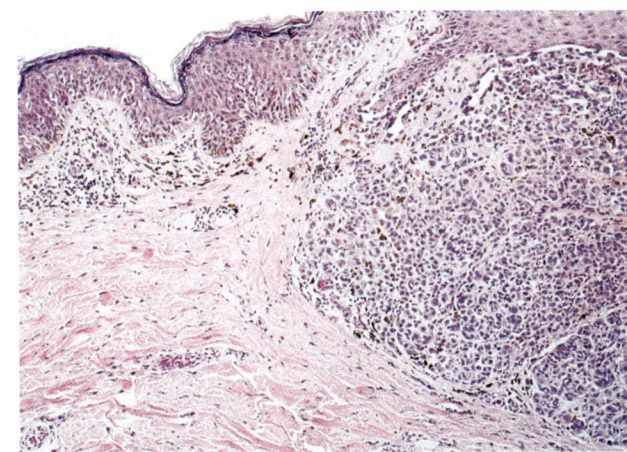

FIGURE 24-57
Malignant melanoma, superficial spreading type, vertical growth phase. Vertical growth is manifested by the distinct spheroid tumor nodule to the *right*. A focus of melanocytes clearly has a growth advantage (larger size) over other nests in the radial growth phase *(left)*. The nodule distorts the papillary dermal–reticular dermal junction and therefore is level III.

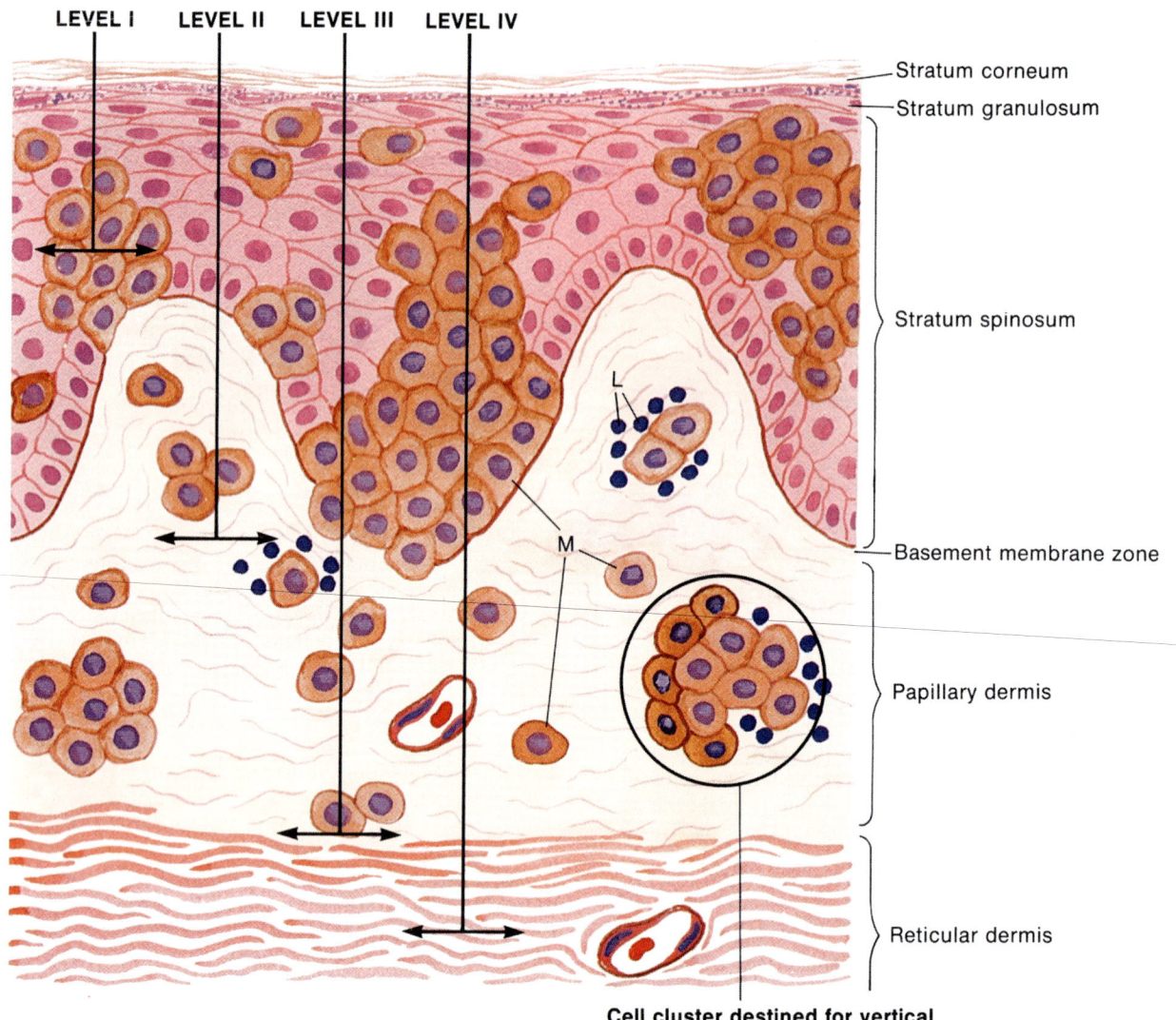

FIGURE 24-58
Malignant melanoma. In the radial growth phase, cells grow in the epidermis and are present in the dermis. They grow in all directions: outward, peripherally, and downward. The net direction of growth is peripheral—along the radii of an imperfect circle. Growth, as manifested by mitotic activity, is largely in the epidermis. No cells in the dermis seem to have a growth preference over others. The nest depicted here is shown as it evolves into the vertical growth phase in Figures 24-58 and 24-59. The anatomical landmarks of the levels of invasion are shown. Level III is not simply the occasional impingement of a tumor cell against the reticular dermis but indicates a collection of cells that fills and widens the papillary dermis and broadly abuts the reticular dermis. Level III invasion is usually a manifestation of the vertical growth phase. Level IV invasion should be designated only when tumor cells clearly permeate between otherwise unaltered collagen bundles of the reticular dermis.

Metastatic Melanoma

Metastatic melanoma arises from the melanocytes of the vertical growth phase. Initial metastases usually involve the regional lymph nodes, although hematogenous spread is also possible. When hematogenous spread occurs, metastases are unusually widespread in comparison with other neoplasms; virtually any organ may be involved. Many metastatic melanomas remain dormant for long periods, only to reappear years after excision of the primary tumor.

Nodular Melanoma

Occasionally, a melanoma "bypasses" the stepwise tumor progression described above and manifests all of its malignant characteristics in the initial lesion. Nodular melanoma is an uncommon form of the tumor (10%) and appears as a circumscribed, elevated, spheroidal nodule. It does not develop through a radial growth phase but is in the vertical growth phase when initially observed (Fig. 24-60). Histologically, nodular melanoma is composed of one or more nodules of

Primary Neoplasms of the Skin

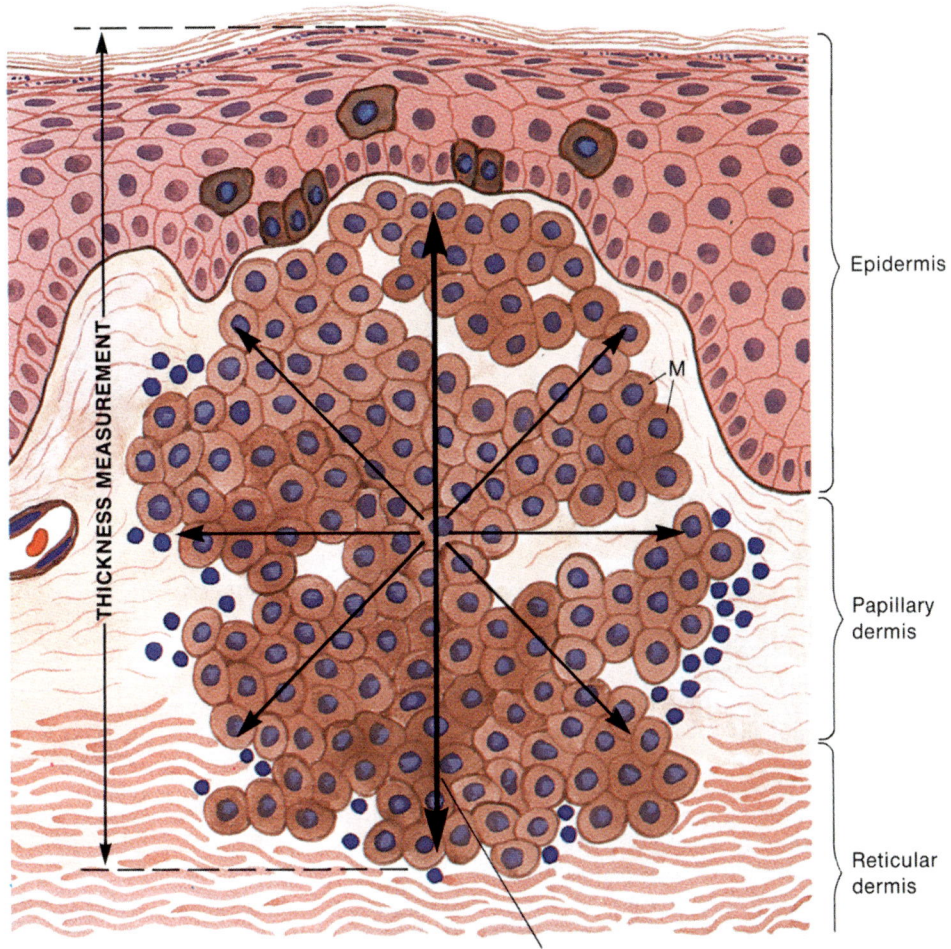

FIGURE 24-59
Malignant melanoma. The evolved vertical growth phase in malignant melanoma of the superficial spreading type is shown, with an indication of how thickness is measured. In this illustration, the vertical growth phase has extended into the reticular dermis. Small nodules of tumor cells that clearly have a growth preference over other tumor cells may be a manifestation of the vertical growth phase. Thickness measurements (arrows) are taken from the outermost granular layer across the tumor in its thickest part.

cells that grow in an expansile fashion in the dermis (Figs. 24-61 and 24-62).

Lentigo Maligna Melanoma

Lentigo maligna melanoma, also known as *Hutchinson's melanotic freckle*, is a large, pigmented macule that occurs on sun-damaged skin. It develops almost exclusively in fair-skinned, usually elderly, whites. Because it occurs on exposed body surfaces, it is probably related to chronic ultraviolet light exposure, without acute episodes of sunburn and often in outdoor workers.

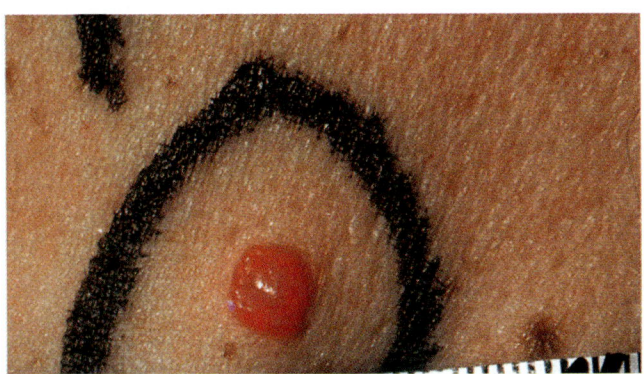

FIGURE 24-60
Malignant melanoma of the nodular type. The primary focus of growth of this 0.5-cm lesion is in the dermis.

 Pathology: In the radial growth phase, lentigo maligna melanoma (LMM) is a flat, irregular, brown- to-black patch that may cover a large part

1252   The Skin

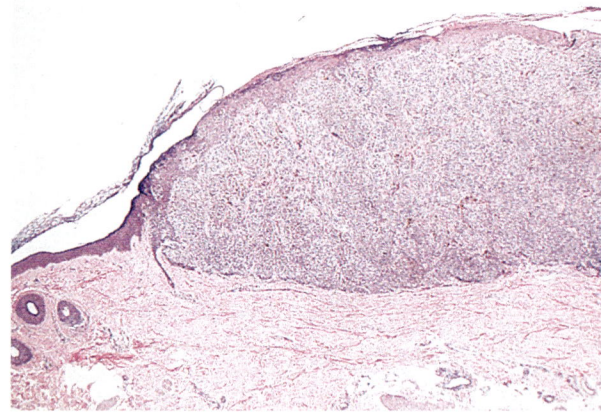

FIGURE 24-61
Malignant melanoma, nodular type. Intraepidermal growth is essentially absent. There is no radial growth lateral to the nodule. This tumor expands the papillary dermis and distorts the reticular dermal junction; it is therefore level III.

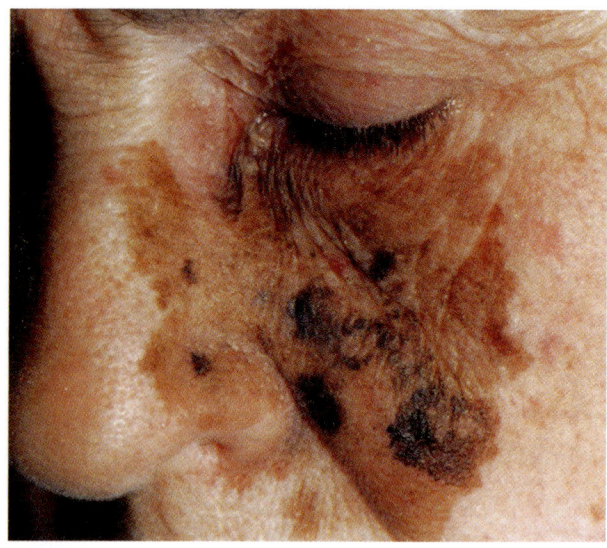

FIGURE 24-63
Malignant melanoma of the lentigo maligna type, radial growth phase.

of the face or dorsal hands (Fig. 24-63). The cells of the radial growth phase are predominantly in the basal layer, often forming contiguous or nearly contiguous rows of atypical single melanocytes but occasionally forming small nests that hang down into the papillary dermis (Fig. 24-64). In the radial growth phase of LMM, invasion is not as prominent or as extensive as in superficial spreading melanoma. Cells of the radial growth phase of LMM vary in size and are usually associated with effacement of the rete ridges and thinning of the epidermis. The subjacent dermis often shows a modest lymphocytic infiltrate and, with only rare exceptions, solar degeneration of the connective tissue.

In the vertical growth phase of LMM (Fig. 24-65), the cells tend to be spindle-shaped. These cells will occasionally provoke a connective tissue response to form a firm plaque (desmoplasia). Cells of the vertical growth phase may also grow along small nerves (neurotropism).

Acral Lentiginous Melanoma

Acral lentiginous melanoma is the most common form of melanoma in dark-skinned people and, as the name implies, is generally limited to the palms, soles, and subungual re-

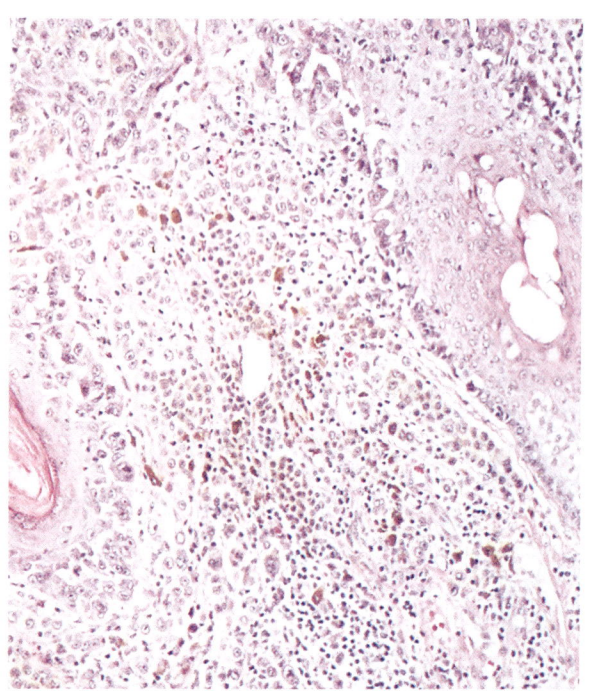

FIGURE 24-62
Malignant melanoma, vertical growth phase. The host response consists of lymphocytes infiltrating amid the melanocytes ("tumor-infiltrating lymphocytes").

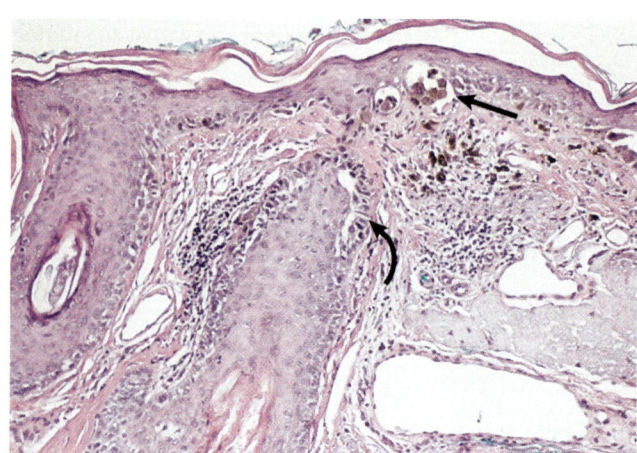

FIGURE 24-64
Lentigo maligna. Atypical melanocytes grow largely at the dermal–epidermal interface (straight arrow), with extension down the external root sheath of follicles (curved arrow). Upward growth of melanocytes is much less prominent than in intraepidermal malignant melanoma of the superficial spreading type.

Primary Neoplasms of the Skin

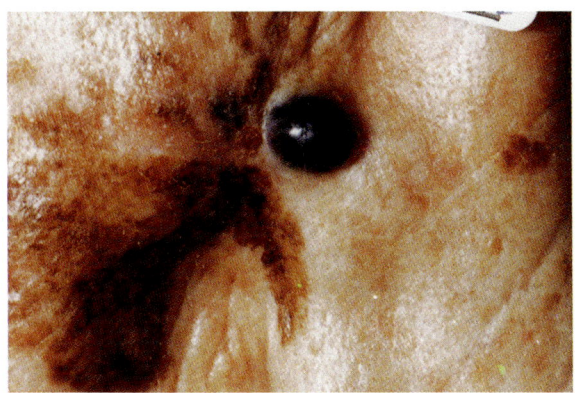

FIGURE 24-65
Lentigo maligna. The clinical appearance of the radial and vertical growth phase in malignant melanoma of the lentigo maligna type is shown. The lesion is 1 cm in diameter.

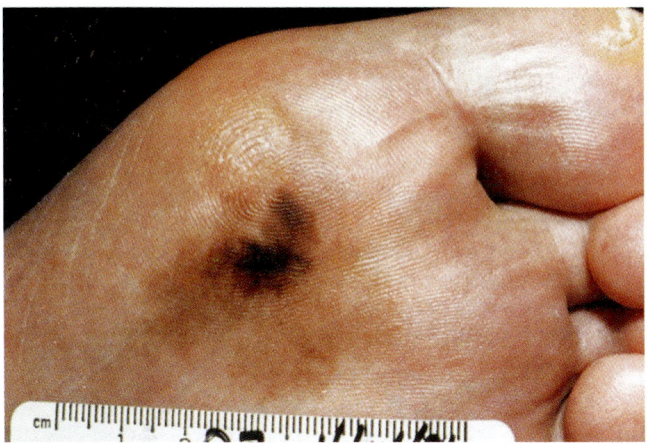

FIGURE 24-66
Malignant melanoma, acral lentiginous type (radial growth phase). The clinical appearance of the sole of the foot is depicted.

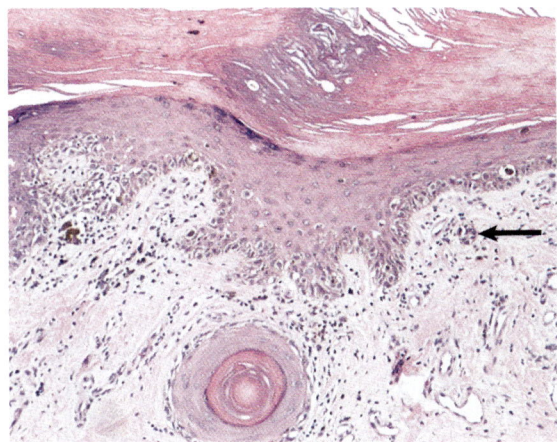

FIGURE 24-67
Malignant melanoma, acral lentiginous type, principally intraepidermal radial growth. Atypical melanocytes are present along the dermal–epidermal junction, with focal upward growth. A small dermal nest of atypical melanocytes is present (arrow).

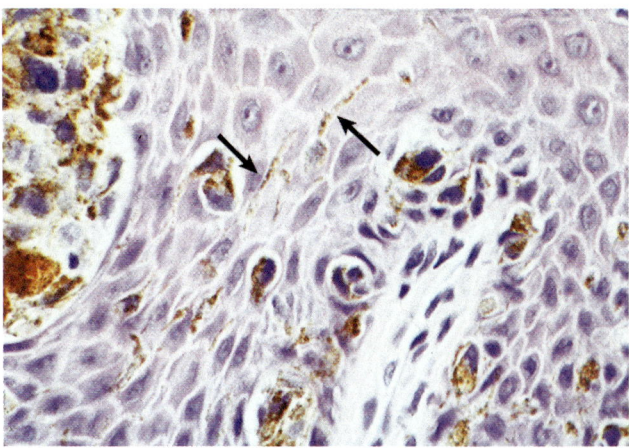

FIGURE 24-68
Malignant melanoma, acral lentiginous type. Large melanocytes with prominent dendrites (arrows) are present in the basilar region of the epidermis, with upward growth. The tumor cells contain numerous melanosomes, making the perinuclear and dendritic cytoplasms brown.

gions. A similar, though rare, tumor occurs on the mucous membranes and is called *mucosal lentiginous melanoma*.

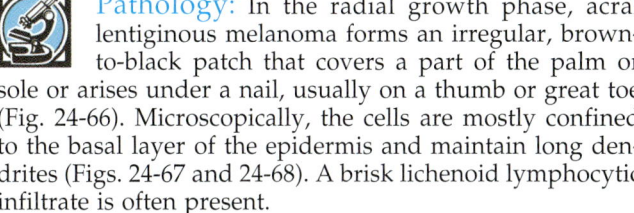

Pathology: In the radial growth phase, acral lentiginous melanoma forms an irregular, brown-to-black patch that covers a part of the palm or sole or arises under a nail, usually on a thumb or great toe (Fig. 24-66). Microscopically, the cells are mostly confined to the basal layer of the epidermis and maintain long dendrites (Figs. 24-67 and 24-68). A brisk lichenoid lymphocytic infiltrate is often present.

As the vertical growth phase develops, cells may grow upward in the epidermis and become more epithelioid. The vertical growth phase (Figs. 24-69 and 24-70) is similar to that

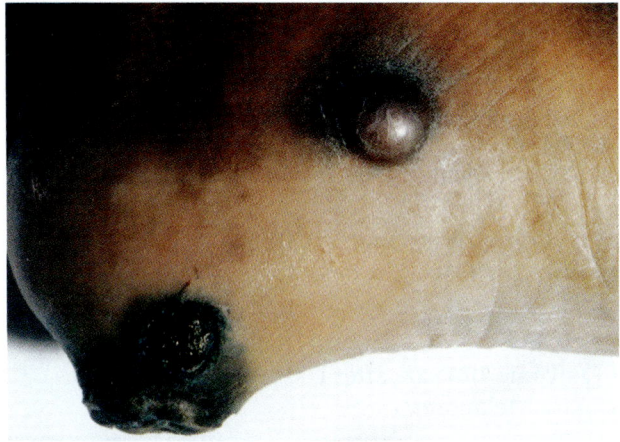

FIGURE 24-69
Malignant melanoma, the acral lentiginous type. The lesion on the heel is the primary tumor. The flat portion represents the radial growth phase, whereas the elevated portion indicates the vertical growth phase. The dark nodule on the instep is a metastasis.

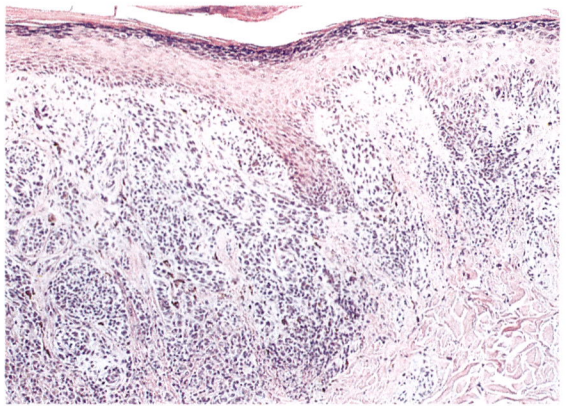

FIGURE 24-70
Malignant melanoma, acral lentiginous type, vertical growth phase. On the *left* is confluent growth of atypical dermal melanocytes filling and expanding the papillary dermis.

of lentigo maligna melanoma in that it commonly consists of spindle cells and occasionally includes neurotropism.

Staging and Prognosis of Melanoma

The prognosis of a patient whose tumor has entered the vertical growth phase is based on a number of attributes.

TUMOR THICKNESS: The evaluation of tumor thickness is recognized as the single strongest prognostic variable for melanoma that is apparently confined to the primary site. The thickness of a melanoma is measured from the most superficial aspect of the stratum granulosum to the point of deepest penetration of the tumor into the dermis (Fig. 24-59). The outcome may be predicted with some accuracy by dividing the tumors into four thickness groups without regard to the growth phase of the tumor. The prognosis up to 10 years after removal of the primary lesion may then be estimated from Table 24-4.

DERMAL MITOTIC RATE: In tumor cells of the vertical growth phase, the mitotic rate is highly predictive of survival. Survival becomes progressively worse as the mitotic rate increases. The 5-year survival is 99% for patients with a mitotic rate of zero, 85% with a mitotic rate of 0.1 to 6.0/mm^2, and 68% with a mitotic rate over 6 mitoses/mm^2.

LYMPHOCYTIC RESPONSE: The interaction of lymphocytes and tumor cells in the vertical growth phase is an important prognostic indicator. The cellular response is reported to be *infiltrative* when the lymphocytes actually infiltrate and disrupt the tumor, frequently forming rosettes about tumor cells (Fig. 24-71). If tumor-infiltrating lymphocytes (TILs) are present throughout the vertical growth phase or are seen across the entire base of the vertical growth phase, the infiltrate is said to be *brisk*. The higher the TIL grade, the better the prognosis.

LOCATION: Melanomas on the extremities have a better prognosis than those on the head, neck, or trunk (axial). However, melanomas on the sole of the foot or the subungual region have a prognosis similar to, or worse than, axial lesions.

SEX: For every site and thickness, women have a better prognosis than men. For example, women with axial melanomas that are 0.8 to 1.7 mm thick have a 10-year survival rate of almost 90% after excision of the lesion, whereas the comparable figure in men is only 60%.

REGRESSION: Many primary melanomas show some evidence of spontaneous regression in the radial growth phase component, indicated clinically by a change to a blue-white or white color. Microscopically, such regression is characterized by a widened papillary dermis, with melanophages and a lymphocytic infiltrate. Patients whose tumors show such changes have a somewhat poorer prognosis than those in whom regression is absent. It is thought that regression plays some sort of permissive role in the development of vertical growth phase.

TABLE 24-4 **Tumor Thickness as Sole Predictor of Outcome 10 Years after Definitive Therapy of Primary Melanoma**

Thickness (mm)	Survival (%)
<0.76	96
0.76–1.69	83
1.70–3.60	59
>3.60	29

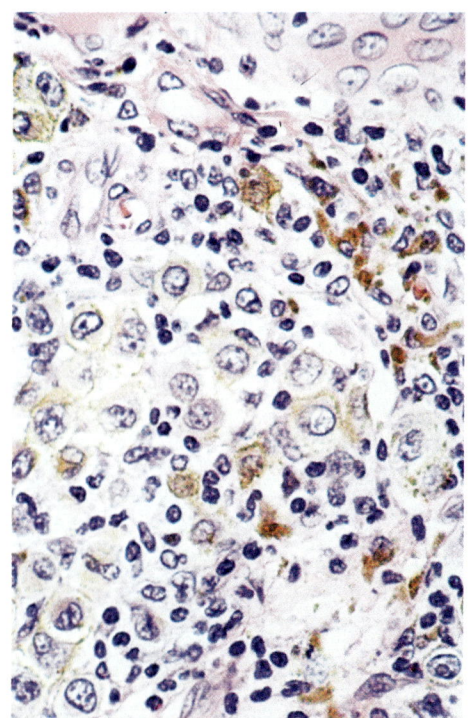

FIGURE 24-71
Malignant melanoma, vertical growth phase. Numerous tumor-infiltrating lymphocytes are arranged about individual tumor cells as satellites.

ULCERATION: The presence of ulceration in a primary melanoma has been associated with decreased survival. In one study, the survival rates were 92% and 66% for patients with and without ulceration, respectively.

LEVELS OF INVASION: The level of tumor invasion as outlined in the Clark system refers to the degree of tumor penetration within the anatomical layers of the skin (Fig. 24-58). It is a predictor of the likelihood of metastasis, although it is not as accurate as tumor thickness. Level IV invasion may predict lymph node metastases. The various levels are defined as follows. Level I: Tumor cells are situated entirely above the basement membrane (in situ). Level II: Invasive cells are present only in the papillary dermis without filling or expanding it (radial growth phase). Level III: The tumor has usually entered the vertical growth phase and impinges on the reticular dermis, forming small expansile nodules that widen the papillary dermis. Level IV: Tumor cells clearly invade between the collagen bundles of the reticular dermis. Level V: The tumor extends into the subcutaneous fat.

STAGE: The stage of the disease is perhaps the most important single factor influencing a patient's survival. Metastasis to regional lymph nodes has been associated with an estimated 40% decrease in 5-year survival, compared with patients with clinically localized tumors. The number of involved lymph nodes is also highly predictive of prognosis. Patients with one positive node have a 10-year survival of 40%, compared with 25% with 2 to 4 nodes and 15% with 5 or more nodes involved.

The tumor–node–metastasis (TNM) system of tumor staging incorporates features related to the primary tumor, to regional lymph nodes and soft tissues, and to distant metastases. The T (primary tumor) attributes of tumor thickness, presence or absence of ulceration, and level of invasion are classified after excision of the melanoma. The number of lymph nodes with metastatic tumor and the characterization of this tumor as micrometastasis or macrometastasis is a large part of the N (node) classification. *Micrometastasis* refers to nodal metastases that are diagnosed after sentinel or elective lymphadenectomy; *macrometastasis* refers to clinically detectable nodal metastases confirmed by therapeutic lymphadenectomy. The M (metastasis) properties incorporate the results of an evaluation for distant metastases at various anatomical sites. A TNM classification scheme is used to determine the pathological stage of disease, which in turn reflects the probability of survival (Table 24-5).

The current recommendations regarding excisional removal of confirmed melanomas state that a 5-mm margin of uninvolved tissue should be obtained with in situ melanoma, a 1-cm margin with a thickness of 1 mm or less, and a 2-cm margin should be taken with melanomas 1 to 4 mm thick or with Clark level IV with any thickness.

Benign Tumors of Melanocytes May Mimic Melanoma

Congenital Melanocytic Nevus

About 1% of white children are born with some form of pigmented lesion on their skin, sometimes as inconspicuous as

TABLE 24-5 Survival Rates by Staging Categories

Pathological Stage	Clinical Attributes[a]	10-Year Survival
I	Clinically localized tumor; 2.0 mm thick or less	79–88%
II	Clinically localized tumor; >2.0 mm thick	32–64%
III	Metastasis to regional lymph node(s)	18–63%
IV	Metastasis to distant sites	6–16%

[a] Adapted from TNM classification.

a small patch of pale tan hyperpigmentation. Rarely, the trunk or an extremity is covered by a large pigmented patch or plaque that is cosmetically deforming ("giant hairy" or "garment" nevus). Such areas display a striking increase in the number of intraepidermal and dermal melanocytes. These melanocytes may extend deep into the subcutaneous tissue. Malignant melanoma may develop in these large congenital melanocytic nevi. Some physicians attempt to remove these large lesions, but in many instances their size makes surgical removal problematic.

Spitz Tumor

Spitz tumors (also known as spindle and epithelioid cell nevi) occur in children or adolescents and, with less frequency, in adults. The Spitz tumor manifests as an elevated, spheroid, pink, smooth nodule, usually on the head or neck, and grows rapidly, increasing to a diameter of 3 to 5 mm within 6 months. The lesion is composed of large spindle or epithelioid melanocytes that extend into the epidermis and into the dermis (Fig. 24-72). The cells are so atypical that an incorrect diagnosis of melanoma may be made even though melanoma is exquisitely rare in childhood.

Blue Nevus

The blue nevus appears in childhood or late adolescence as a dark blue, gray, or black, firm, well-demarcated papule or nodule on the dorsum of the hands or feet or on the buttocks, scalp, or face. The clinical appearance may prompt an excisional biopsy to rule out nodular melanoma. Melanin-containing melanocytes with long, thin dendrites are present in the superficial to mid-dermis, where they are often admixed with numerous melanin-containing macrophages (Fig. 24-73).

Freckle and Lentigo

Freckles, or *ephelides,* are small, brown macules that occur on sun-exposed skin, especially in people with fair skin (Fig. 24-74). Freckles usually appear at about age 5. The pigmentation of a freckle deepens with exposure to sunlight and fades when light exposure ceases. A lentigo is a discrete, brown macule that appears at any age and on any part of the body (though a *solar lentigo,* or "liver spot," appears at an older age after long-term sun exposure) (Fig. 24-75). Unlike a freckle, the pigmentation of a lentigo does not depend on sun expo-

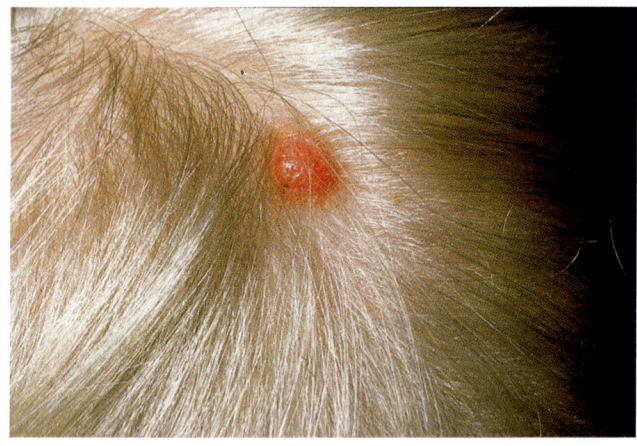
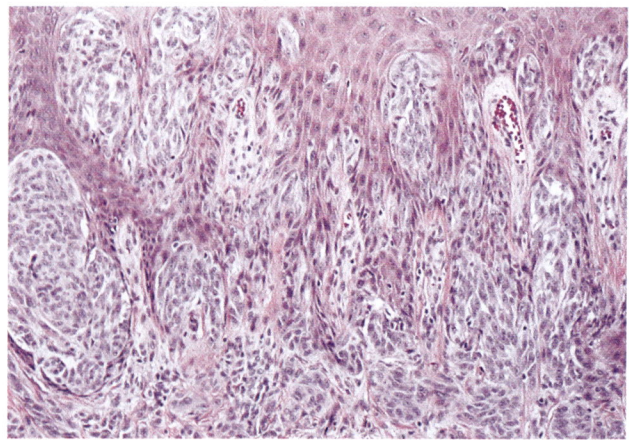
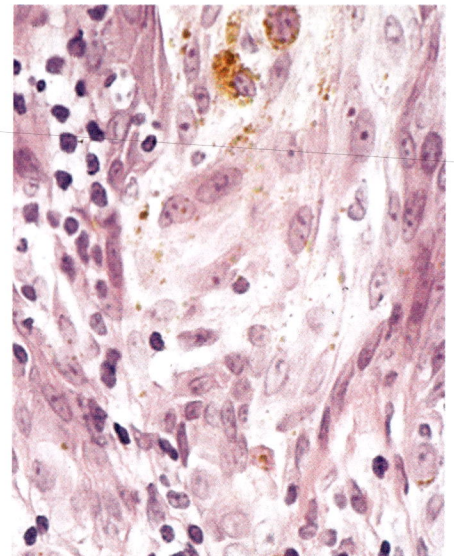
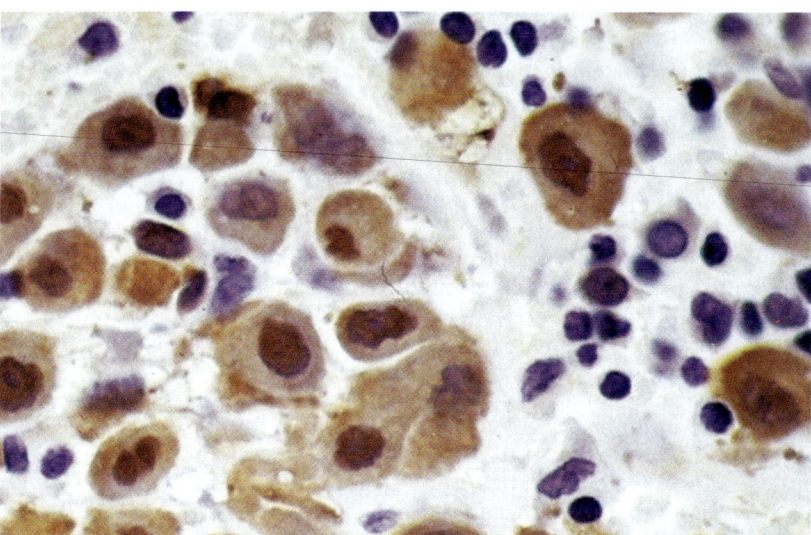

FIGURE 24-72
Spindle and epithelioid cell (Spitz) nevus. A. A symmetric pink nodule appeared suddenly in a child but then remained stable for several weeks until it was excised. B. Spitz tumors are composed of large melanocytes with prominent nuclei. Within a hyperplastic epidermis, the melanocytes are disposed in large nests. Even though the cells are large and, at first glance, suggest melanoma, they are much more uniform than the cells of most malignant melanomas. C. The melanocytes have amphophilic cytoplasm and prominent regular nuclei. D. Most melanocytic tumors, including Spitz tumors, are composed of cells that possess S-100 antigen, as shown by the brown reaction product found in them after immunohistochemical study. S-100 antigen is found in high concentration in most tumors of neural crest origin.

sure. Freckles show hyperpigmentation of the basal keratinocytes without a concomitant increase in the number of melanocytes. Lentigines, on the other hand, display elongated rete ridges, increased melanin pigment in both the basal keratinocytes and melanocytes, and an increased number of melanocytes. Larger lesions may need to be biopsied to rule out lentigo maligna melanoma.

Verrucae Are Warts Caused by Human Papillomavirus

Verrucae are cutaneous tumors. The lesions are circumscribed, symmetric, epidermal proliferations that are elevated above the skin and often appear papillary.

 Pathology:

- *Verruca vulgaris,* also known as the common wart, is an elevated papule with a verrucous (papillomatous) surface. They may be single or multiple and are most frequent on the dorsal surfaces of the hands or on the face. Histologically, verruca vulgaris displays hyperkeratosis and papillary epidermal hyperplasia (Fig. 24-76). *Koilocytes* (i.e., enlarged keratinocytes with a pyknotic nucleus surrounded by a halolike cleared area) are observed within the upper epidermis. Viral inclusions are

Primary Neoplasms of the Skin

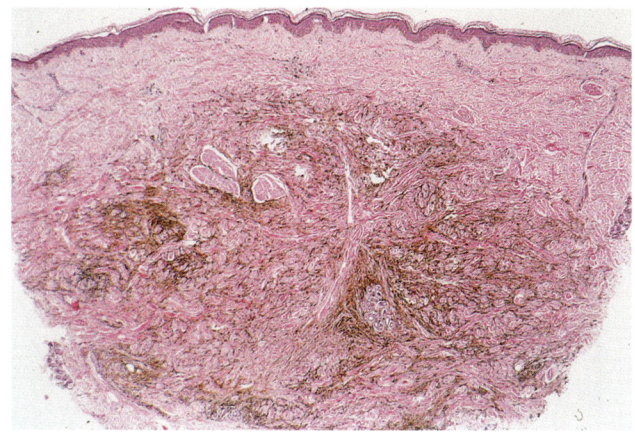 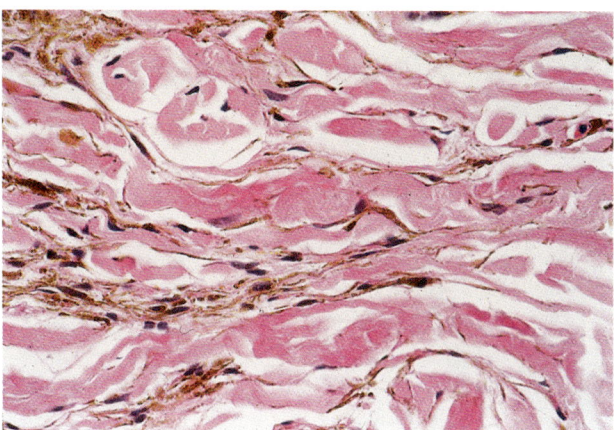

FIGURE 24-73
Blue nevus. **A.** Within the dermis there is a poorly defined but symmetric spindle cell proliferation that is dark brown. **B.** The lesion is composed of elongate cells with heavily pigmented dendrites and small bland nuclei.

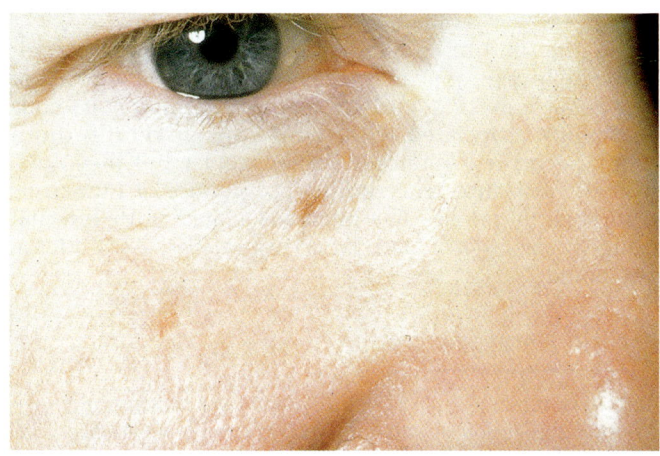

FIGURE 24-74
Freckle. A fair-complexioned man has a prominent brown macule that darkens in sunlight.

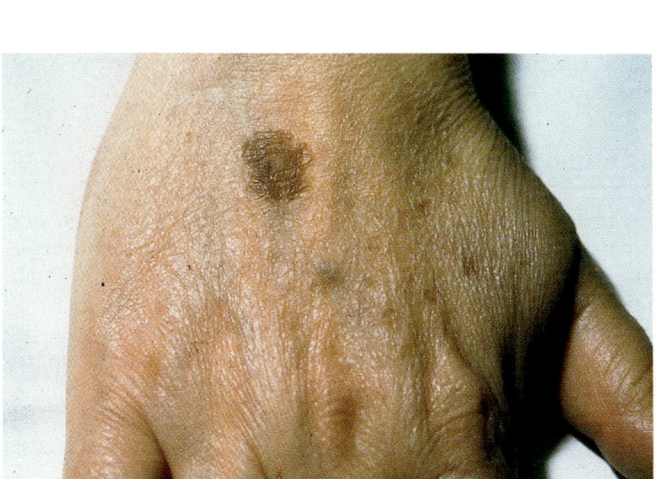

FIGURE 24-75
Lentigo. A 1-cm irregular patch of slightly variegated hyperpigmentation is present with a background of chronic solar damage.

difficult to identify (Fig. 24-77). Several HPV types, including types 2 and 4, have been demonstrated in verruca vulgaris. No malignant potential is recognized.

- **Plantar warts** are benign, frequently painful, hyperkeratotic nodules on the soles of the feet. Occasionally, similar lesions appear on the palms of the hands *(palmar warts)*. Histologically, plantar warts are endophytic or exophytic, papillary, squamous epithelial proliferations. The cells contain abundant cytoplasmic inclusions that are similar in appearance to the darker-staining keratohyaline granules. The nuclei of keratinocytes near the base of these warts also contain pink nuclear inclusions. HPV type 1 is the etiological agent.
- **Verruca plana** are small flat papules that appear on the face. Microscopically, they display slight elongation of the rete ridges (acanthosis), frequently striking hypergranulosis, and superficial koilocyte formation. HPV

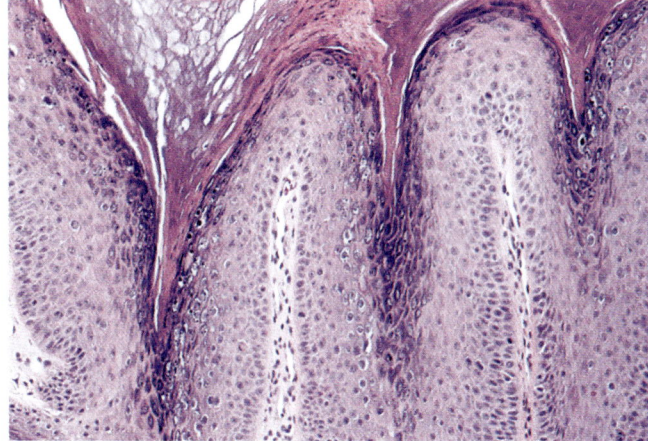

FIGURE 24-76
Verruca vulgaris. Verruca vulgaris is the prototype of papillary epidermal hyperplasia. Squamous epithelial-lined fronds have fibrovascular cores. The blood vessels within the cores extend close to the surface of verrucae, which makes them susceptible to traumatic hemorrhage and the resultant black "seeds" that patients observe.

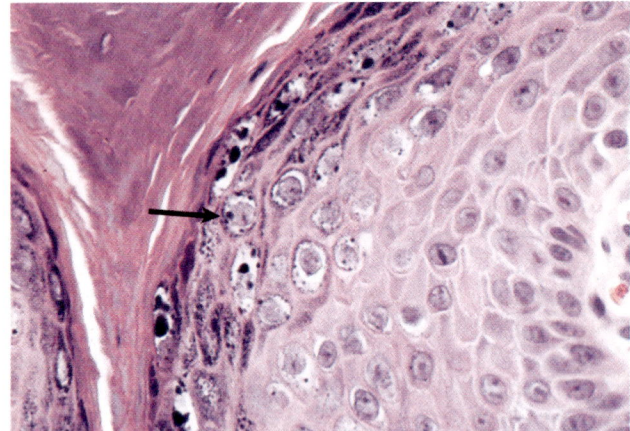
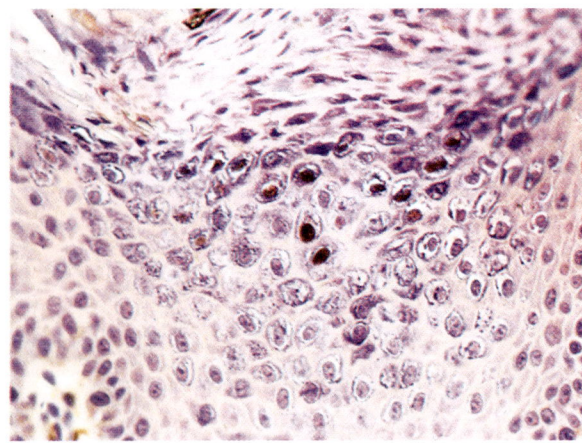

FIGURE 24-77
Verruca vulgaris. A. Characteristic cytopathic changes occur in the outer portion of the stratum spinosum and stratum granulosum, in which there is perinuclear vacuolization and prominent keratohyaline granules, with homogeneous blue inclusions *(arrow)*. B. Papilloma virus surface antigen is demonstrated in an immunohistochemical preparation as brown intranuclear reaction product.

types 3 and 10 are among the types that elicit these lesions. The lesions do not progress to cancer.
- *Condyloma acuminatum* represent warts occurring primarily around the genitalia, which are transmitted by sexual activity. Histologically, the lesion consists of a papillary squamous proliferation. Koilocytosis and an almost continuous cap of parakeratosis are usually present. HPV types 6 and 11 are the usual etiological agents. Squamous cell carcinoma may develop in the lesions, in which case HPV types 16 and 18 are usually identified.
- *Bowenoid papulosis,* also caused by HPV types 16 and 18, is characterized by multiple hyperpigmented papules on the genitalia. The lesions may be histologically identical to squamous cell carcinoma in situ in that they display disordered epithelial maturation and scattered keratinocyte atypia. The lesions also exhibit parakeratosis and irregular acanthosis. Bowenoid papulosis often regresses but, in some cases, may progress to dysplasia or malignancy.
- *Epidermodysplasia verruciformis* is a rare autosomal recessive disease characterized by impaired cell-mediated immunity and subsequently enhanced susceptibility to HPV infection. Warts similar to those of verruca plana, with confluence into patches, are widespread. The entity is first apparent in childhood, and squamous cell carcinoma develops in 30 to 60% of patients. HPV types 5, 8, 9, and 47 are the most commonly encountered viruses in lesions that display squamous cell carcinoma.

Keratosis Is a Benign Horny Growth Composed of Keratinocytes

Seborrheic Keratosis

Seborrheic keratoses are scaly, frequently pigmented, elevated papules or plaques whose scales are easily rubbed off. Although they are among the most common keratoses, the etiology is unknown. The lesions generally occur in the later years of life and tend to be familial. Clinically and microscopically, the lesions appear "pasted on" and are composed of broad anastomosing cords of mature stratified squamous epithelium associated with small cysts of keratin (horn cysts). Seborrheic keratoses are innocuous, but they are a cosmetic nuisance. The sudden appearance of numerous seborrheic keratoses has been associated with internal malignancies *(sign of Leser-Trélat),* especially gastric adenocarcinoma.

Actinic Keratosis

Actinic keratoses ("from the sun's rays") are keratinocytic neoplasms that develop in sun-damaged skin as circumscribed keratotic patches or plaques, commonly on the backs of the hands or the face. Microscopically, the stratum corneum is no longer loose and basket-weaved but is replaced by a dense parakeratotic scale. The underlying basal keratinocytes display significant atypia (Fig. 24-78). With time, actinic keratoses may unpredictably evolve into squamous cell carcinoma in situ and finally into invasive squamous cell carcinoma. However, most are stable, and many regress.

Keratoacanthoma

Keratoacanthomas are rapidly growing keratotic papules on sun-exposed skin that develop over a period of 3 to 6 weeks into crater-like nodules. They reach a maximum diameter of 2 to 3 cm. Spontaneous regression usually follows within 6 to 12 months, leaving an atrophic scar. Keratoacanthomas are best considered a variant of squamous cell carcinoma, although a plethora of opinions exists regarding this topic.

 Pathology: Histologically, keratoacanthomas are endophytic papillary proliferations of keratinocytes. The lesion is cup shaped, with a central, keratin-filled umbilication and overhanging ("buttressing")

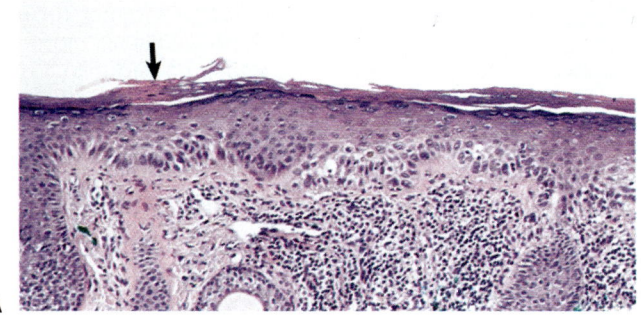
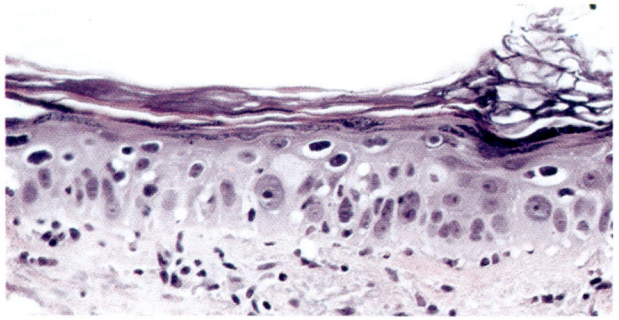

FIGURE 24-78
Actinic keratosis. **A.** A low-power view reveals cytological atypia within the stratum basalis and lower stratum spinosum with loss of polarity. A lichenoid, bandlike, lymphocytic infiltrate is frequently present. Parakeratosis is present here only in a small focus *(arrow).* **B.** High-power examination of an actinic keratosis reveals striking cytological atypia of the basal keratinocytes, the hallmark of actinic keratoses.

edges (Fig. 24-79). At the base of the keratin, the keratinocytes are large and contain an abundance of homogeneous, eosinophilic ("glassy") cytoplasm. At the lower aspect of the lesion, irregular tongues of squamous epithelium infiltrate the collagen of the reticular dermis. Older lesions show active fibroplasia in the dermis around the epithelial tongues. There may be focal lichenoid inflammation, and the dermis may be markedly infiltrated with neutrophils, lymphocytes, and eosinophils. Microabscesses of neutrophils and entrapped dermal elastic fibers may be present within the lesion.

Basal Cell Carcinoma Is a Locally Invasive Epidermal Neoplasm

Basal cell carcinoma (BCC) is the most common malignant tumor in persons with pale skin. Although it may be locally aggressive, metastases are exceedingly rare.

Pathogenesis: BCC usually develops on the sun-damaged skin of people with fair skin and freckles. However, unlike squamous cell carcinoma, BCC also arises on areas not exposed to intense sunlight. It is unusual to find BCC on the fingers and dorsal surfaces of the hands. The tumor is thought to derive from pluripotential cells in the basal layer of the epidermis, more specifically, in the bulge region of the hair follicle.

BCC is also a component of a number of heritable syndromes in which the tumor originates on skin that has had little light exposure. *Nevoid BCC syndrome* refers to the occurrence of multiple tumors in the context of a complex multisystem disease. The syndrome also includes pits (dyskeratoses) on the palms and soles, mandibular cysts, hypertelorism, and a predisposition to other neoplasms, including medulloblastoma. The BCCs of the syndrome appear at a young age and may number in the hundreds.

Germline mutations in the human tumor suppressor gene *PTCH,* mapped to chromosome 9q22, are responsible for the development of nevoid BCC syndrome. Somatic mutations in the *PTCH* gene have also been implicated in 20 to 30% of sporadic BCC.

Pathology: BCC is composed of nests of deeply basophilic epithelial cells with narrow rims of cytoplasm that are attached to the epidermis and protrude into the subjacent papillary dermis (Fig. 24-80). The central part of each nest contains closely packed keratinocytes that are slightly smaller than the normal epidermal basal keratinocytes and show occasional apoptosis. The pe-

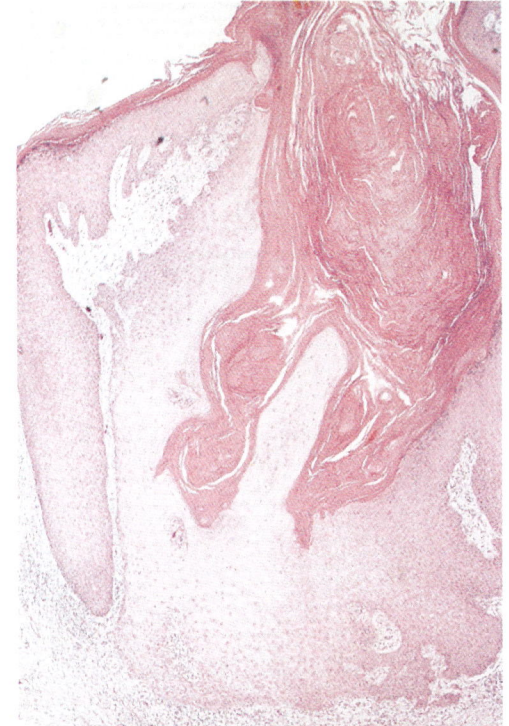

FIGURE 24-79
Keratoacanthoma. A keratin-filled crater *(right)* is lined by glassy proliferating keratinocytes that invade the dermis.

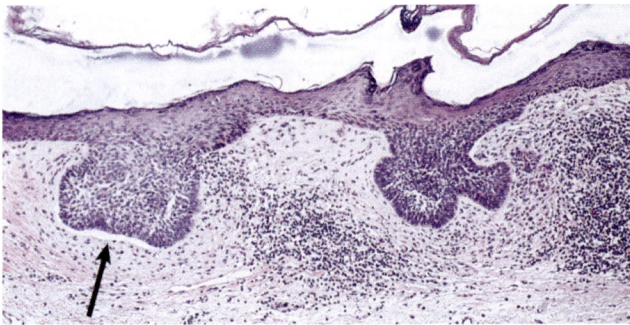

FIGURE 24-80
Basal cell carcinoma, superficial type. Buds of atypical basaloid keratinocytes extend from the overlying epidermis into the papillary dermis. The peripheral keratinocytes mimic the stratum basalis by palisading. The separation artifact *(arrow)* is present because of poorly formed basement membrane components and the hyaluronic acid-rich stroma that contains collagenase.

 Clinical Features: A number of common forms of BCC are recognized. Treatment usually involves various excision or eradication procedures.

- *Pearly papule* is the prototypic nodulocystic type of lesion and is so named because it resembles a 2- to 3-mm pearl (Fig. 24-81). It is covered by tightly stretched epidermis and is laced with small, delicate, branching vessels (telangiectasia).
- *Rodent ulcer* is a small crater in the center of the pearl.
- *Superficial* BCC appears as a scaly, red, sharply demarcated plaque (Fig. 24-80).
- *Morpheaform* BCC is a pale, firm, scarlike tumor that is ill-defined on and especially beneath the skin surface, making it particularly difficult to eradicate (Fig. 24-81).
- *Pigmented BCC* may grossly resemble malignant melanoma.

riphery of each nest shows an organized layer of polarized, columnar keratinocytes, with the long axis of each cell perpendicular to the surrounding BMZ ("peripheral palisading"). *Superficial, multicentric BCC* is composed of apparently isolated, but actually interconnected, nests that usually remain confined to the papillary dermis and manifest clinically as a spreading plaque. *Nodulocystic BCC* is also attached to the epidermis and exhibits the same cytological and architectural features as the superficial type of BCC but grows more deeply into the dermis. Usually, tumor cells of the dermal islands are associated with a mucinous ground substance and are surrounded by an array of fibroblasts and lymphocytes. The tumor nests are often separated from the adjacent stroma by thin clefts ("retraction artifact"), a feature that is sometimes helpful in distinguishing BCC from other adnexal neoplasms displaying basaloid cell proliferation. BCC with a particularly dense, sclerotic stroma is called *morpheaform BCC* because of a clinical resemblance to lesions of localized scleroderma, also known as *morphea*.

Squamous Cell Carcinoma Typically Resembles Differentiated Keratinocytes

Squamous cell carcinoma (SCC) is second only to BCC in incidence and may be caused by ultraviolet light, ionizing radiation, chemical carcinogens, and HPV. SCC is most common on the sun-damaged skin of fair persons with light hair and freckles and often originates in actinic keratoses. The tumor is exceedingly rare on normal black skin.

 Pathogenesis: Although SCC has multiple causes, ultraviolet light is the most common cause. SCC arising in sun-damaged skin has a low propensity to metastasize (<2%). It may also arise in association with chronic scarring processes such as osteomyelitis sinus tracts, burn scars, and areas of radiation dermatitis. In these settings, SCC has a greater propensity to metastasize.

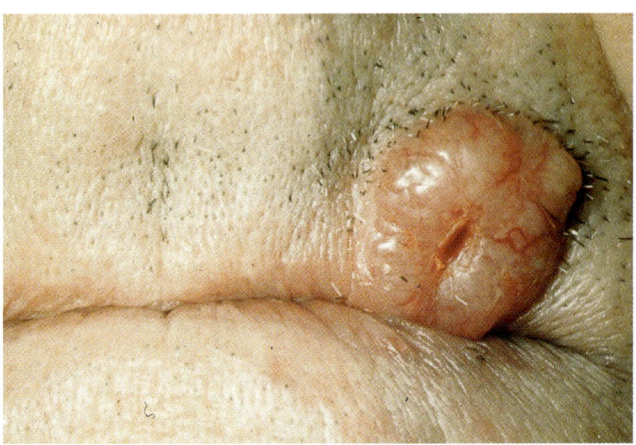
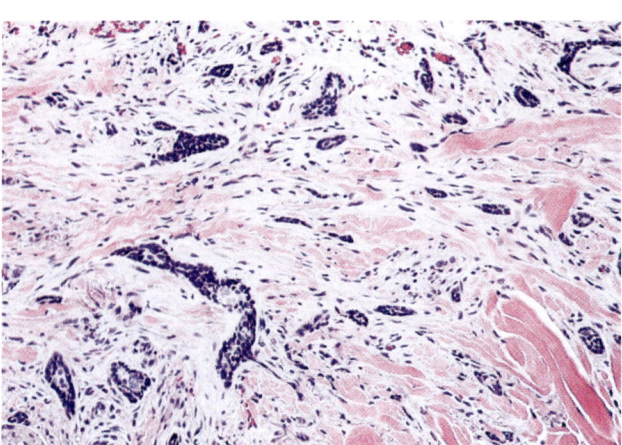

FIGURE 24-81
Basal cell carcinoma. A. The tumor exhibits typical rolled pearly borders with telangiectases and central ulceration. B. Microscopic examination shows a sclerosing and infiltrative lesion. Irregularly branching strands of tumor cells permeate the dermis, with induction of a cellular, fibroblastic, hyaluronic acid-rich stroma.

Mutations in *p53* are identified in over 90% of SCCs, as well as in many actinic keratoses.

 Pathology: SCC is composed of tumor cells that mimic in varying degrees the epidermal stratum spinosum and extend into the subjacent dermis (Fig. 24-82). The edges of many tumors show changes typical of actinic keratosis, namely, a variably thickened epidermis with parakeratosis and significant atypia of the basal keratinocytes.

Clinical Features: SCC characteristically arises in chronically sun-exposed areas such as the backs of the hands, the face, lips, and ears (Fig. 24-82). Early lesions are small, scaly or ulcerated, erythematous papules, which may be pruritic. SCCs are usually treated by electrosurgery, topical chemotherapy, excision, or radiation therapy.

Merkel Cell Carcinoma Is an Aggressive Tumor of Neurosecretory Cells That Displays Epithelial Differentiation

Merkel cell carcinoma (MCC) is typically a solitary, dome-shaped, red to violaceous nodule or indurated plaque that arises on the skin of the head and neck in elderly white patients. These are dangerous tumors that end in death of 30 to 65% of the patients within 5 years.

 Pathology: Most MCCs consist of large solid nests of undifferentiated cells that resemble small cell carcinoma of the lung. At its periphery, the tumor may show a trabecular pattern. Nuclear chromatin is dense and evenly distributed, and there is scant cytoplasm. Frequent mitotic figures and nuclear fragments are present. Immunohistochemical staining for cytokeratin 20 shows a characteristic "perinuclear dot" cytoplasmic focus of immunoreactivity. Tumor cells also stain positively with neuroendocrine markers such as chromogranin and synaptophysin.

Adnexal Tumors Differentiate toward Skin Appendages

Adnexal tumors generally appear as elevated small nodules on the skin. A familial history of similar tumors can often be elicited from patients. Frequently, the lesions appear at puberty. Although most of these tumors behave in a benign fashion, malignant counterparts are sometimes observed.

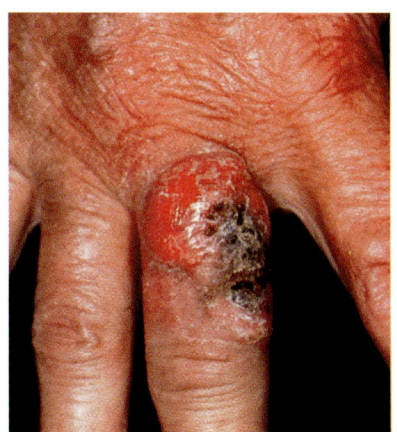
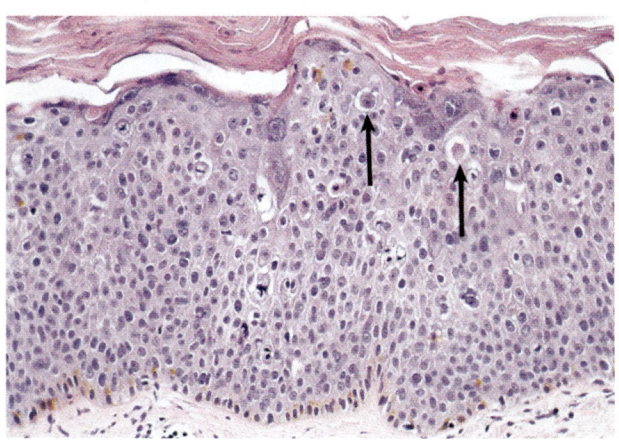
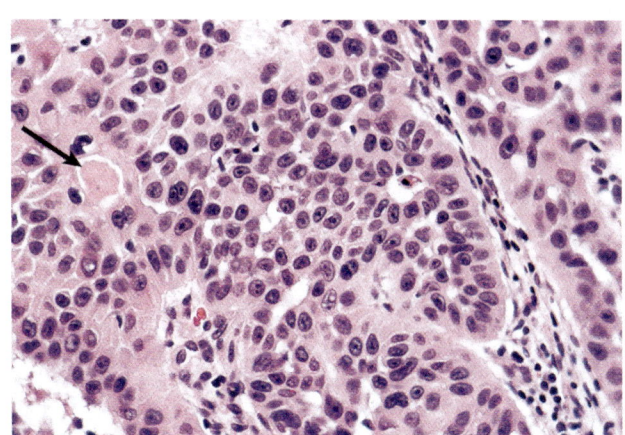

FIGURE 24-82
Squamous cell carcinoma. A. An ulcerated, encrusted, and infiltrating lesion is seen on the sun-exposed dorsal aspect of a finger. B) A microscopic view of the periphery of the lesion shows squamous cell carcinoma in situ. The entire epidermis is replaced by atypical keratinocytes. Mitoses and multinucleation of keratinocytes are apparent, as is apoptosis *(arrows)*. C. Squamous cell carcinoma, invasive component. High-power view reveals irregularly shaped lobules of strikingly atypical keratinocytes that have invaded to the level of the mid-reticular dermis. Apoptotic cells are present *(arrow)*. The pink, platelike cytoplasm, as well as intercellular bridges (desmosomes), are helpful diagnostic features in excluding other malignancies.

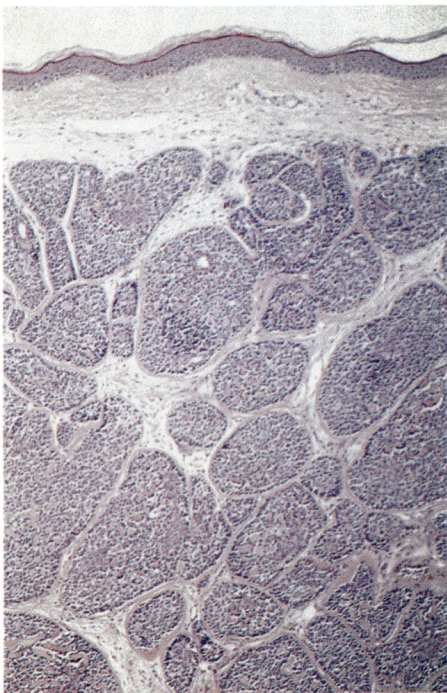

FIGURE 24-83
Cylindroma. Sharply circumscribed islands of basophilic epithelial cells reside in a jigsaw-puzzle-like array. Dense eosinophilic hyaline sheaths surround each island and form small circular cords within each island.

Cylindroma

Cylindroma is an adnexal neoplasm in which the cells show features of sweat gland differentiation. The lesions may be solitary or multiple elevated nodules around the scalp. An autosomal dominant, heritable variant features multiple tumors. Occasionally, cylindromas become large and cluster about the head, in which case they are termed *turban tumors*. Microscopic examination shows sharply circumscribed nests of deeply basophilic cells (Fig. 24-83). Each nest of cells is surrounded by a hyalinized, thickened BMZ.

Syringoma

Syringoma typically appears about the eyelid and upper cheek as a small, elevated, flesh-colored papule. Microscopically, small ducts resembling the intraepidermal portion of the eccrine sweat ducts are observed (Fig. 24-84).

Poroma

Poroma is a common, solitary neoplasm that histologically resembles a seborrheic keratosis but contains narrow ductal lumina and occasional cystic spaces. The pattern has been interpreted as eccrine sweat gland differentiation. The tumor is a firm, raised lesion, usually less than 2 cm in diameter, that develops on the sole or sides of the foot, the hands, or fingers. Microscopically, poromas extend from the lower portion of the epidermis into the dermis as broad, anastomosing bands of uniform, cuboidal cells. Occasional malignant lesions with ductal differentiation are termed *porocarcinomas*.

Trichoepithelioma

Trichoepithelioma is a neoplasm that differentiates toward hair structures. It usually occurs as a solitary lesion, but in the *multiple trichoepithelioma syndrome*, it is transmitted as an autosomal dominant trait. The lesions begin to appear at puberty, on the face, scalp, neck, and upper trunk. Microscopically, trichoepitheliomas resemble basal cell carcinomas but contain numerous "horn cysts" that are composed of keratinized centers surrounded by basophilic epithelial cells.

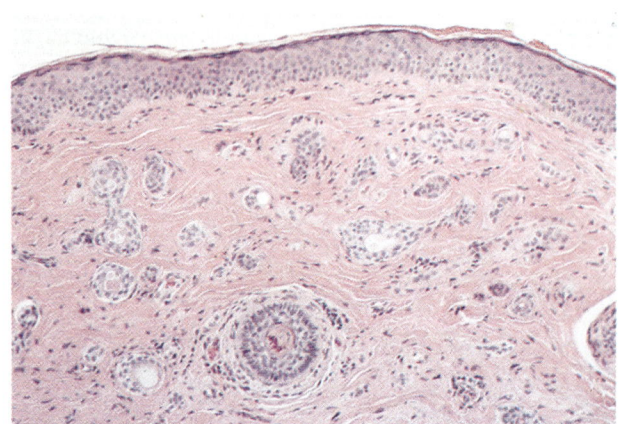
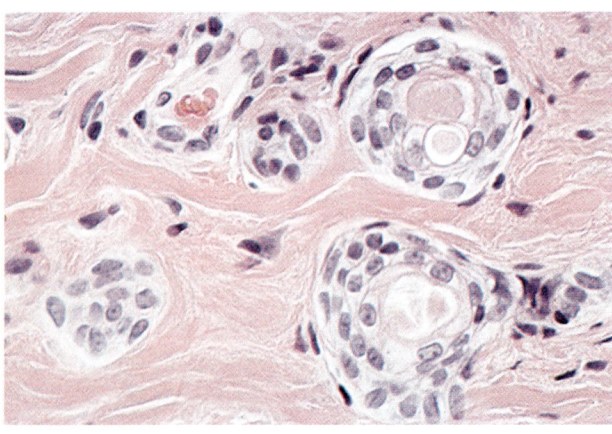

FIGURE 24-84
Syringoma. A. Within the upper dermis is a proliferation of epithelium-forming ducts, tubules, and solid islands amid a dense fibrous stroma. B. The ductal differentiation closely mimics that of the straight dermal eccrine duct, with a central lumen and cuticle formation. The enzyme complement of the cells and their immunophenotype support eccrine ductal derivation.

Fibrohistiocytic Tumors of the Skin Show a Varied Spectrum of Differentiation

Dermatofibroma

Dermatofibroma is a common, benign tumor composed of fibroblasts and macrophages, the former being the neoplastic cell. It occurs on the extremities as a dome-shaped, firm, rubbery nodule with ill-defined borders and variable pigmentation, ranging from pink to dark brown. The lesions are usually no more than 3 to 5 mm in diameter. Microscopically, the papillary and reticular dermis are replaced by fibrous tissue with a distinctive pattern. The fibroblasts tend to form ill-defined small cartwheels with a small vascular space at the center. The tumors are not well demarcated, and they blend with the surrounding dermis. The overlying epidermis is hyperplastic and frequently hyperpigmented.

Dermatofibrosarcoma Protuberans

Dermatofibrosarcoma protuberans, a tumor of intermediate malignant potential, is a slowly growing nodule or indurated plaque that appears most frequently on the trunk of young adults. Local recurrence after attempted complete excision is common, but metastases are rare. The most common histological pattern is a poorly circumscribed, monotonous population of spindle cells arranged in a dense "storiform" (pinwheel-like) array. The tumor extends into the subcutis along the fat septa and interstices, creating an infiltrative, honeycomb-like pattern. The tumor cells display CD34, an antigen found in endothelial cells and some neural tumor cells, as well as in dermal fibroblast-like dendritic cells, the probable cell of origin. Positive immunoreactivity to CD34 may be helpful in distinguishing this tumor from a dermatofibroma, which does not exhibit this antigen.

Atypical Fibroxanthoma

Atypical fibroxanthoma is a neoplasm of low-grade malignant potential that appears as a dome-shaped nodule on the sun-damaged skin of elderly persons. The tumor cells show bizarre cytological features. Microscopically, atypical spindle cells and epithelioid cells infiltrate and disrupt the dermis. Multinucleated cells, some with a finely vacuolated cytoplasm, may be prominent. Mitotic figures are numerous. This lesion must be distinguished from spindle-cell squamous-cell carcinoma and spindle-cell melanoma. Atypical fibroxanthoma stains negatively for cytokeratins and S-100 protein, thereby differentiating it from squamous cell carcinoma and melanoma, respectively. Treatment is by excision, but local recurrence is common.

Mycosis Fungoides Is a Variant of Cutaneous T-Cell Lymphoma

The etiology of mycosis fungoides (MF) is unknown, but it is thought that malignancy of helper T cells (CD4$^+$) may be caused by chronic exposure to an antigen.

Pathology: In the early stages of the disease, delicate, erythematous plaques appear, often in the area of the buttocks. Microscopically, these plaques tend to display psoriasiform changes in the epidermis. The early inflammatory cell infiltrates in the dermis are polymorphic and are often not diagnostic of MF.

Skin involvement becomes progressively more prominent and more infiltrative. The most important histological feature of MF is the presence of lymphocytes in the epidermis (*epidermotropism*). In late stages, the dermal infiltrate becomes dense to the point of forming tumor nodules. Increasing numbers of atypical lymphocytes that display hyperchromatic, convoluted (cerebriform) nuclei are seen in the papillary dermis and in the epidermis (Fig. 24-85). Circumscribed nests of these atypical lymphocytes eventually appear in the epidermis and are known as *Pautrier's microabscesses*. Polymerase chain reaction and Southern blotting techniques may reveal the presence of a T-cell receptor gene rearrangement and thus the presence of a clonal cell population.

Sézary syndrome refers to the systemic dissemination of MF. The characteristic feature is the presence of cerebriform lymphocytes in the peripheral circulation.

Clinical Features: MF affects older age groups, has a slight male predominance, and preferentially affects blacks over whites. The disorder is classically divided into three stages: patch, plaque, and tumor. In the patch stage, which may persist for months, eruptions consist of scaly, erythematous macules that may be slightly indurated. The lesions are usually found on the lower abdomen, buttocks, and upper thighs as well as the breasts of women and can mimic other dermatitides such as psoriasis or eczema (Fig. 24-85). The plaque stage displays lesions that are more infiltrated and circumscribed. As these plaques coalesce, the involvement becomes more widespread. Large, variably shaped nodules can form on existing indurated plaques or on apparently normal skin. Spread to lymph nodes or visceral involvement portends reduced survival. Therapeutic modalities include ultraviolet light, topical nitrogen mustard, and electron beam therapy.

HIV Infection Causes Various Skin Diseases

Kaposi Sarcoma

Kaposi sarcoma is a malignant tumor derived from endothelial cells. This vascular neoplasm is an important cutaneous sign observed in the AIDS pandemic and is discussed in Chapters 4 and 10. Human herpesvirus 8 (HHV-8) is thought to play a role in the pathogenesis of Kaposi sarcoma.

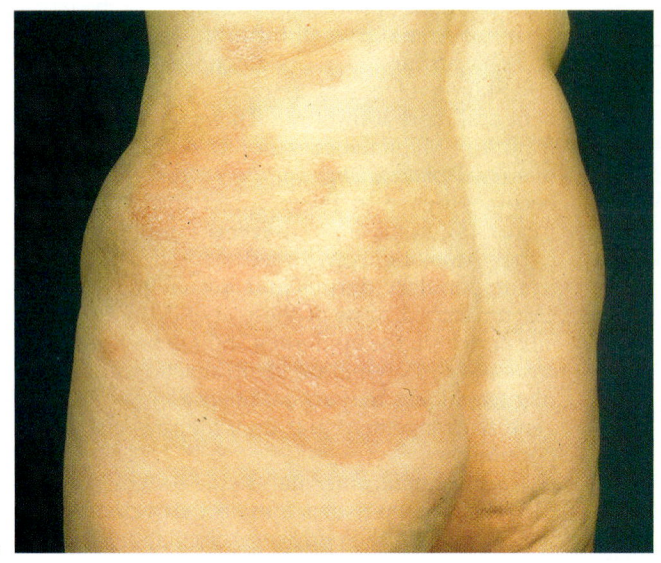
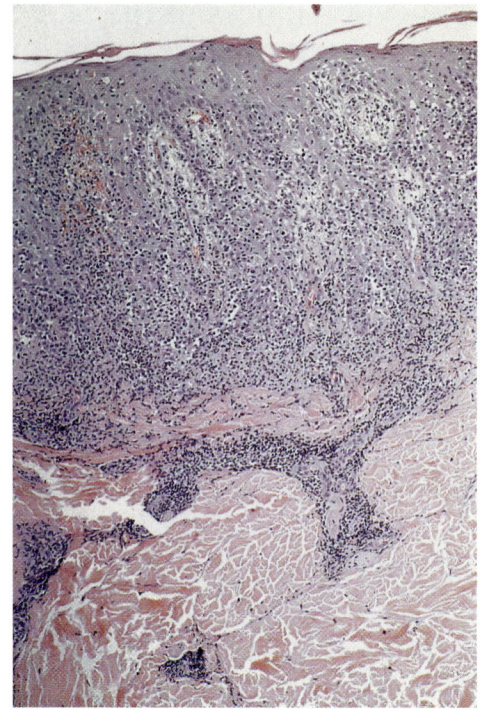
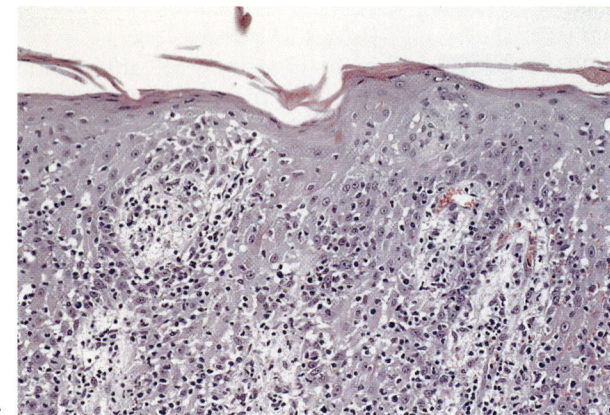

FIGURE 24-85
Mycosis fungoides. A. A 66-year-old woman presented with a 30-year history of erythematous scaly patches and plaques with telangiectases, atrophy, and pigmentation. B. The papillary dermis is expanded by an infiltrate of atypical lymphocytes. Lymphocytes with hyperchromatic nuclei infiltrate the thickened epidermis. C. A higher power view of (B).

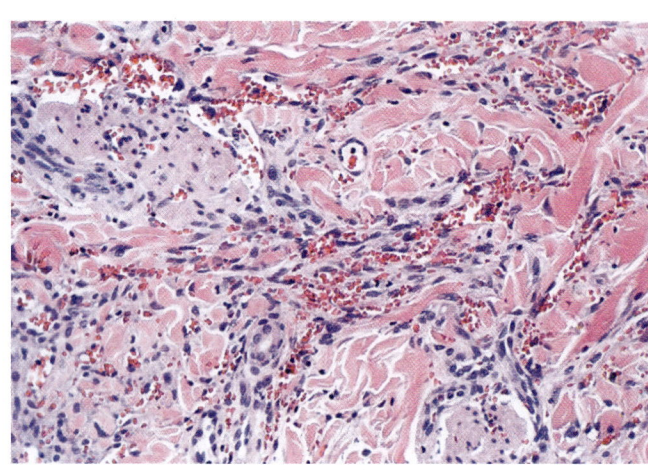

FIGURE 24-86
Kaposi sarcoma, plaque stage. Extending along the vascular arcades and amid reticular dermal collagen is a proliferation of endothelial cells. They form delicate vascular channels filled with red blood cells. Some endothelial cells are not canalized (have not formed lumina.)

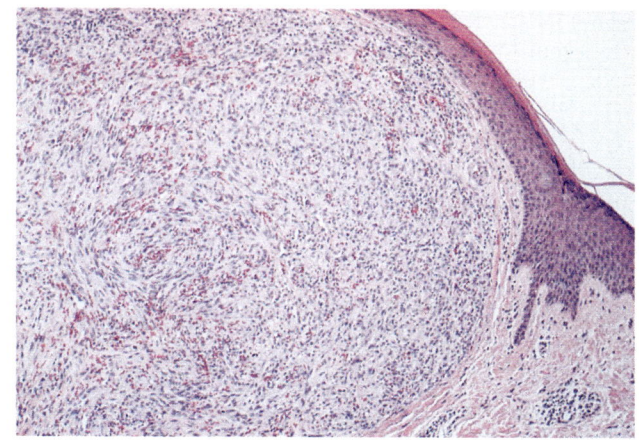
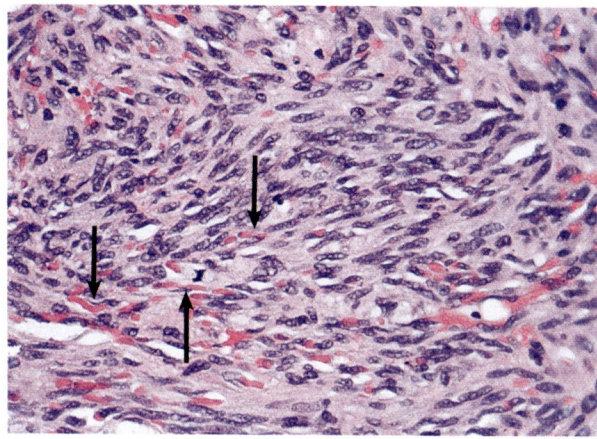

FIGURE 24-87
Kaposi sarcoma, nodule stage. A. A large nodule is composed of proliferating endothelial cells forming fascicles and vascular spaces. B. A higher-power view of (A) shows cytological atypia of the spindle cells. Red blood cells appear agglutinated (arrows). The endothelial cells, in which the agglutinated red blood cells are present, form slitlike spaces.

Pathology: All cases of Kaposi sarcoma, whether or not they are associated with HIV infection, evolve through three stages: patch, plaque, and nodule. In the patch stage, a subtle proliferation of irregular vascular channels, lined by a single layer of mildly atypical endothelial cells, radiates from preexisting blood vessels and extends almost imperceptibly into the surrounding reticular dermis. Extravasated red blood cells, hemosiderin deposition, and a sparse inflammatory infiltrate consisting of lymphocytes and plasma cells are commonly observed.

In the plaque stage (Fig. 24-86), the entire reticular dermis is involved, with frequent extension into the subcutis and formation of bundles of spindle cells. In the nodule stage (Fig. 24-87), well-circumscribed dermal nodules are composed of anastomosing fascicles of spindle cells surrounding numerous slitlike spaces.

Bacillary Angiomatosis

Bacillary angiomatosis is a pseudoneoplastic proliferation of capillaries that arises in response to infection with *Bartonella* species. Late-stage AIDS patients are at risk for infection with these organisms.

Pathology: The proliferative lesions appear as red-to-brown papules, often in large numbers, and may be confused with Kaposi sarcoma. Histologically, they appear as lobular proliferations of capillaries, with plump endothelial cells protruding into the lumina. These lesions are surrounded by an edematous stroma containing an inflammatory infiltrate composed of mononuclear cells, variable numbers of neutrophils and neutrophil fragments. Silver impregnation stains show dense masses of bacilli within the basophilic deposits. The lesions clear with antibiotic treatment.

Eosinophilic Folliculitis

Eosinophilic folliculitis is a chronic pruritic eruption of papules that are centered on hair follicles in AIDS patients. The lesions are most often found on the trunk and proximal extremities. An infiltrate composed of lymphocytes, macrophages, and numerous eosinophils is present in the perifollicular adventitial dermis and around the dermal blood vessels.

SUGGESTED READING

Books

Austen KF, Eisen AZ, Freedberg IM, et al.: *Dermatology in general medicine*, 5th ed. New York: McGraw-Hill, 1998.
Balch CM, Houghton AN, Sober AJ, et al (eds): *Cutaneous melanoma*, 3rd ed. St. Louis: Quality Medical, 1998.
Berger TG, James WD, Odom RB (eds.): *Diseases of the skin*, 9th ed. Philadelphia: WB Saunders, 2000.
Campbell JL, Habif TP, Quitadamo MJ, et al (eds.): *Skin disease*. St. Louis: Mosby, 2001.
Elder D, Elenitsas R, Jaworsky C, et al (eds): *Histopathology of the skin*, 8th ed. Philadelphia: Lippincott-Raven, 1997.
Farmer ER, Hood AF (eds): *Pathology of the skin*, 2nd ed. New York: McGraw-Hill, 2000.
Goldblum JR, Weiss SW (eds.): *Soft tissue tumors*, 4th ed. St. Louis: Mosby, 2001.
Smoller BR, Horn TD: *Dermatopathology in systemic disease*. New York: Oxford, 2001.
Sternberg SS: *Histology for pathologists*, 2nd ed. Philadelphia: Lippincott-Raven, 1997.

Reviews
Anatomy and Physiology of the Skin

Cotsarelis G, Paus R: The biology of hair follicles. *N Engl J Med* 341:491–497, 1999.

Fine JD: The skin basement membrane zone. *Adv Dermatol* 2:283–304, 1987.

Johnson KO: The roles and functions of cutaneous mechanoreceptors. *Curr Opin Neurobiol* 11:455–461, 2001.

McMillan JR, Shimizu H: Desmosomes: structure and function in normal and diseased epidermis. *J Dermatol* 28:291–298, 2001.

Rietschel RL: A simplified approach to the diagnosis of alopecia. *Dermatol Clin* 14:691–695, 1996.

Romani N, Ratzinger G, Pfaller K, et al.: Migration of dendritic cells into lymphatics—The Langerhans cell example: Routes, regulation, and relevance. *Int Rev Cytol* 207:237–270, 2001.

Smack DP, Korge BP, James WD: Keratin and keratinization. *J Am Acad Dermatol* 30:85–102, 1994.

Uchi H, Terao H, Koga T, et al.: Cytokines and chemokines in the epidermis. *J Dermatol Sci* 24:S29–38, 2000.

Diseases of the Epidermis

Elder JT, Nair RP, Henseler T, et al.: The genetics of psoriasis 2001. *Arch Dermatol* 137:1447–1454, 2001.

Hertl M: Humoral and cellular autoimmunity in autoimmune bullous skin disorders. *Int Arch Allergy Immunol* 122:91–100, 2000.

Nickoloff BJ: Skin innate immune system in psoriasis: Friend or foe? *J Clin Invest* 104:1161–1164, 1999.

Nousari HC, Anhalt GJ: Pemphigus and bullous pemphigoid. *Lancet* 354:667–672, 1999.

Prinz JC: Psoriasis vulgaris—A sterile antibacterial skin reaction mediated by cross-reactive T cells? An immunological view of the pathophysiology of psoriasis. *Clin Exp Dermatol* 26:326–332, 2001.

Ringpfeil F, Raus A, DiGiovanna JJ, et al.: Darier disease— Novel mutations in ATP2A2 and genotype-phenotype correlation. *Exp Dermatol* 10:19–27, 2001.

Travers JB, Hamid QA, Norris DA, et al.: Epidermal HLA-DR and the enhancement of cutaneous reactivity to superantigenic toxins in psoriasis. *J Clin Invest* 104:1181–1189, 1999.

Valdes-Flores M, Kofman-Alfaro SH, Jimenez-Vaca AL, et al.: Deletion of exons 1–5 of the STS gene causing X-linked ichthyosis. *J Invest Dermatol* 116:456–458, 2001.

Yang J, Ahn K, Cho M, et al.: Novel mutations of the transglutaminase 1 gene in lamellar ichthyosis. *J Invest Dermatol* 117:214–218, 2001.

Diseases of the Basement Membrane Zone

Bhattacharya M, Kaur I, Kumar B: Lichen planus: A clinical and epidemiological study. *J Dermatol* 27:576–582, 2000.

Callen JP: Collagen vascular diseases. *Med Clin North Am* 82:1217–1237, 1998.

Dieterich W, Laag E, Bruckner-Tuderman L: Antibodies to tissue transglutaminase as serologic markers in patients with dermatitis herpetiformis. *J Invest Dermatol* 113:133–136, 1999.

Engineer L, Bhol K, Kumari S, et al.: Bullous pemphigoid: interaction of interleukin 5, anti-basement membrane zone antibodies and eosinophils. A preliminary observation. *Cytokine* 13:32–38, 2001.

Fayyazi A, Schweyer S, Soruri A, et al.: T lymphocytes and altered keratinocytes express interferon-gamma and interleukin 6 in lichen planus. *Arch Dermatol Res* 291:485–490, 1999.

Fine J, Eady RAJ, Bauer, EA, et al.: Revised classification system for inherited epidermolysis bullosa: Report of the second international consensus meeting on diagnosis and classification of epidermolysis bullosa. *J Am Acad Dermatol* 42:1051–1066, 2000.

Leaute-Labreze C, Lamireau T, Chawki D, et al.: Diagnosis, classification, and management of erythema multiforme and Stevens-Johnson syndrome. *Arch Dis Child* 83:347–352, 2000.

Millard TP, McGregor JM: Molecular genetics of cutaneous lupus erythematosus. *Clin Exp Dermatol* 26:184–191, 2001.

Reunala TL: Dermatitis herpetiformis. *Clin Dermatol* 19:728–736, 2001.

Spirito F, Chavanas S, Prost-Squarcioni C, et al.: Reduced expression of the epithelial adhesion ligand laminin 5 in the skin causes intradermal tissue separation. *J Biol Chem* 276:18828–18835, 2001.

Yancey KB, Egan CA: Pemphigoid: Clinical, histologic, immunopathologic, and therapeutic considerations. *JAMA* 284:350–356, 2000.

Inflammatory Diseases of the Superficial and Deep Vascular Bed

Carugati A, Pappalardo E, Zingale C, et al.: C1-inhibitor deficiency and angioedema. *Mol Immunol* 38:161–173, 2001.

English JC, Patel PJ, Greer KE: Sarcoidosis. *J Am Acad Dermatol* 44:725–743, 2001.

Fang KS, Lawry M, Haas A: Papules on the hands. Granuloma annulare. *Arch Dermatol* 137:1647–1652, 2001.

Gibson LE: Cutaneous vasculitis update. *Dermatol Clin* 19:603–615, 2001.

Hsu S, Le EH, Khoshevis MR: Differential diagnosis of annular lesions. *Am Fam Physician* 64:289–296, 2001.

Thestrup-Pedersen K: Clinical aspects of atopic dermatitis. *Clin Exp Dermatol* 25:535–543, 2000.

Trautmann A, Akdis M, Brocker E, et al.: New insights into the role of T cells in atopic dermatitis and allergic contact dermatitis. *Trends Immunol* 22:530–532, 2001.

Wakelin SH: Contact urticaria. *Clin Exp Dermatol* 26:132–136, 2001

Disorders of the Dermal Connective Tissue

Hawk A, English JC: Localized and systemic scleroderma. *Semin Cutan Med Surg* 20:27–37, 2001.

Inflammatory Disorders of the Panniculus

Requena L, Sanchez Yus E: Panniculitis. Part I. Mostly septal panniculitis. *J Am Acad Dermatol* 45:163–183, 2001.

Requena L, Sanchez Yus E: Panniculitis. Part II. Mostly lobular panniculitis. *J Am Acad Dermatol* 45:325–361, 2001.

Acne Vulgaris

Federman DG, Kirsner RS: Acne vulgaris: pathogenesis and therapeutic approach. *Am J Manag Care* 6:78–87, 2000.

Infections and Infestations

Amagai M, Matsuyoshi N, Wang ZH, et al.: Toxin in bullous impetigo and staphylococcal scalded-skin syndrome targets desmoglein 1. *Nat Med* 6:1213–1214, 2000.

Rinaldi MG: Dermatophytosis: epidemiological and microbiological update. *J Am Acad Dermatol* 43:S120–124, 2000.

Sangueza OP, Fleet SL, Requena L: Update on the histologic findings of cutaneous infections. *Adv Dermatol* 16:361–423, 2000.

Primary Neoplasms of the Skin

Bale AE, Yu K: The hedgehog pathway and basal cell carcinomas. *Hum Mol Genet* 10:757–762, 2001.

Barnhill R: Malignant melanoma, dysplastic melanocytic nevi, and Spitz tumors. *Clin Plast Surg* 27:331–360, 2000.

Elder DE, Murphy GF: *Melanocytic tumors of the skin*. Washington, DC: Armed Forces Institute of Pathology (in press).

Goessling W, McKee PH, Mayer RJ: Merkel cell carcinoma. *J Clin Oncol* 20:588–598, 2002.

Goldstein BG, Goldstein AO: Diagnosis and management of malignant melanoma. *Am Fam Physician* 63:1359–1368, 2001.

Guillen DR, Cockerell CJ: Cutaneous and subcutaneous sarcomas. *Clin Dermatol* 19:262–268, 2001.

Kamino H, Salcedo E: Histopathologic and immunohistochemical diagnosis of benign and malignant fibrous and fibrohistiocytic tumors of the skin. *Dermatol Clin* 17:487–505, 1999.

Piepkorn, M: Melanoma genetics: an update with focus on the CDKN2A(p16)/ARF tumor suppressors. *J Am Acad Dermatol* 42:705–722, 2000.

Pollock PM, Trent JM: The genetics of cutaneous melanoma. *Clin Lab Med* 20:667–690, 2000.

Ratner D, Peacocke M, Zhang H, et al.: UV-specific p53 and PTCH mutations in sporadic basal cell carcinoma of sun-exposed skin. *J Am Acad Dermatol* 44:293–297, 2001.

Salasche S: Epidemiology of actinic keratosis and squamous cell carcinoma. *J Am Acad Dermatol* 42:S4–7, 2000.

Sanchez Yus E, Simon P, Requena L, et al.: Solitary keratoacanthoma. *Am J Dermatopathol* 22:305–310, 2000.

Schaffer JV, Bolognia JL: The clinical spectrum of pigmented lesions. *Clin Plast Surg* 27:391–408, 2000.

Schuchter LM: Review of the 2001 AJCC staging system for cutaneous malignant melanoma. *Curr Oncol Rep* 3:332–337, 2001.

Titus-Ernstoff L: An overview of the epidemiology of cutaneous melanoma. *Clin Plast Surg* 27:305–316, 2000.

White WL, Loggie BW: Sentinel lymphadenectomy in the management of primary cutaneous malignant melanoma: an update. *Dermatol Clin* 17:645–655, 1999.

Cutaneous Manifestations of HIV Infection

Aftergut K, Cockerell CJ: Update on the cutaneous manifestations of HIV infection: Clinical and pathologic features. *Dermatol Clin* 17:445–471, 1999.

Ensoli B, Sgadari C, Barillari G, et al.: Biology of Kaposi's sarcoma. *Eur J Cancer* 37:1251–1269, 2001.

Gasquet S, Maurin M, Brouqui P, et al.: Bacillary angiomatosis in immunocompromised patients. *AIDS* 12:1793–1803, 1998.

CHAPTER 25

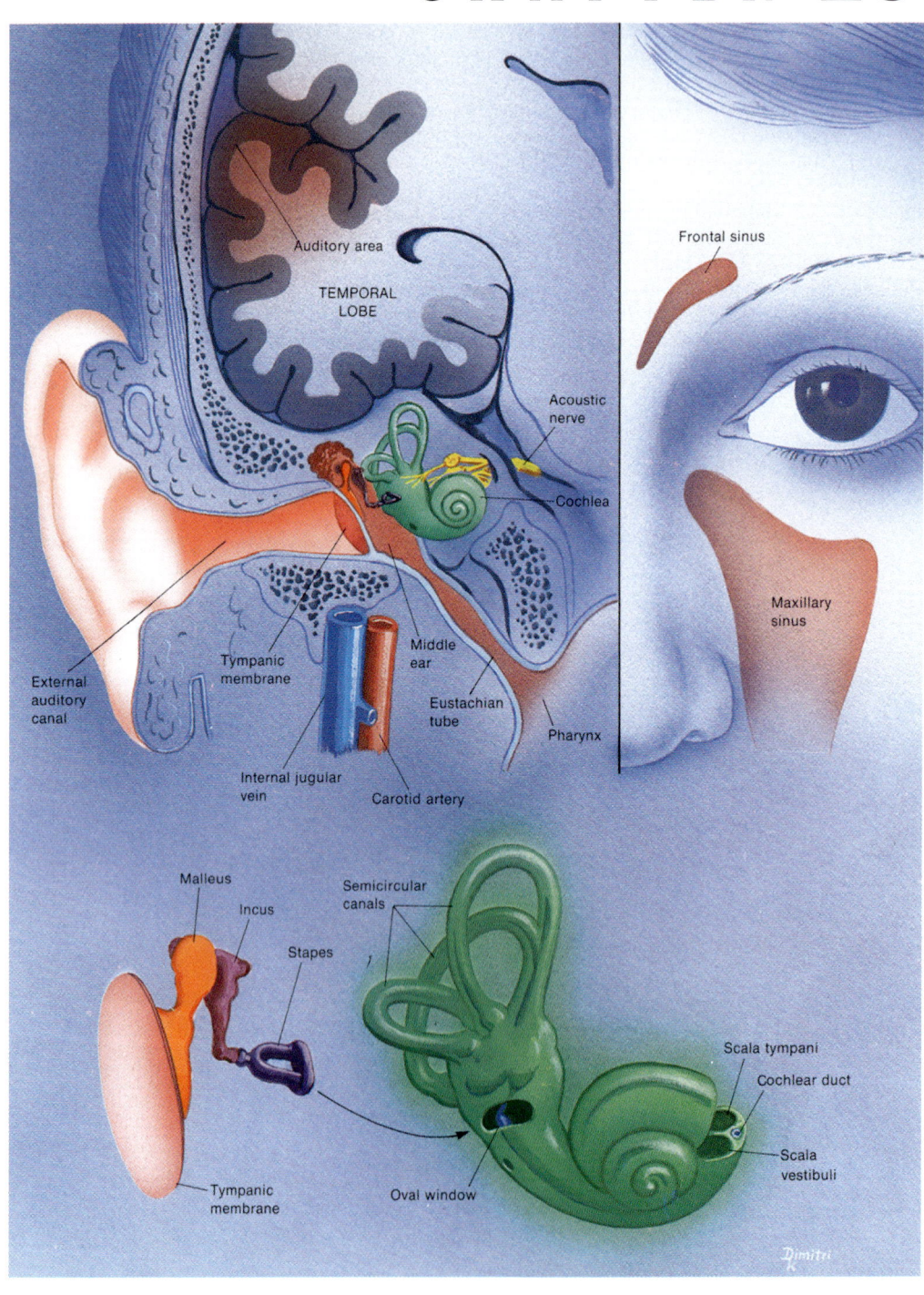

The Head and Neck

Bruce M. Wenig
Mary Cunnane
Károly Bálogh

Oral Cavity

Anatomy

Developmental Anomalies

Infections
Bacterial and Fungal Infections
Viral Infections

Benign Tumors
Leukoplakia and Erythroplakia

Squamous Cell Carcinoma

Diseases of the Lips

Diseases of the Tongue

Dental Caries (Tooth Decay)

Diseases of the Pulp and Periapical Tissues

Periodontal Disease

Odontogenic Cysts and Tumors
Ameloblastoma

Salivary Glands

Sjögren Syndrome

Pleomorphic Adenoma (Mixed Tumor)

Monomorphic Adenoma

Malignant Tumors
Mucoepidermoid Carcinoma
Adenoid Cystic Carcinoma
Acinic Cell Carcinoma

Nose and Paranasal Sinuses

Diseases of the Nasal Cavity and Paranasal Sinuses
Rhinitis
Nasal Polyps
Sinusitis
Syphilis
Leprosy
Rhinoscleroma
Fungal Infections
Leishmaniasis

(continued)

FIGURE 25-1 *(see opposite page)*
Anatomy of the ear. *(Top)* The relations of the external, middle, and inner ear. Note the tympanic membrane, the ossicles of the middle ear, the location of the eustachian tube, and the proximity of the meninges and the brain. *(Bottom)* Diagrammatic visualization of the tympanic membrane and the ossicles. The *arrow* indicates the normal position of the stapes in the oval window. A cross-section of the cochlea demonstrates the relation of the cochlear duct (carrying endolymph) to the scala tympani and scala vestibuli (filled with perilymph).

Wegener Granulomatosis

Nasal-Type Angiocentric T-Cell/Natural Killer (T/NK)-Cell Lymphoma

Benign Tumors

Malignant Tumors

Nasopharynx

Anatomy and Function

Hypoplasia and Hyperplasia of Pharyngeal Lymphoid Tissue

Inflammation

Tumors

Juvenile Nasopharyngeal Angiofibroma

Squamous Cell Carcinoma

Nasopharyngeal Carcinoma

Lymphomas of Waldeyer Ring

Plasmacytoma

Chordoma

Other Malignant Tumors

The Ear

External Ear

Middle Ear

Anatomy

Otitis Media

Internal Ear

Anatomy

Otosclerosis

Meniere Disease

Labyrinthine Toxicity

Viral Labyrinthitis

Acoustic Trauma

Tumors

Oral Cavity

The oral cavity is lined by nonkeratinized or only lightly keratinized squamous epithelium. The bacteria, spirochetes, viruses, fungi, and parasites normally found in the oral cavity are usually harmless. If the mucosa is injured or the defense mechanisms of the body are impaired, for instance by immunosuppression, the same organisms can cause disease, as in fusospirochetal gingivitis. Healthy persons may also carry pathogens such as *Corynebacterium diphtheriae* or meningococci in the oral cavity. Systemic diseases frequently affect the oral cavity, and although the oral mucosa is not necessarily a mirror to the body, it may reflect more than localized disease.

ANATOMY

The oral mucosa consists of the keratinized tissues of the attached gingiva and hard palatal mucosa and the nonkeratinized mucosa of the lower labial mucosa (inner lip mucosa) and buccal mucosa (inner cheek mucosa). It also included the nonattached gingiva, that is, the movable gingiva that continues into the maxillary and mandibular sulci, the ventral tongue, the floor of the mouth, the mucosa of the soft palate and tonsillar pillars, and the specialized keratinized gustatory mucosa of the dorsum of the tongue.

The keratinized tissues of the attached gingiva and hard palate may be orthokeratinized with a granular cell layer or it may be parakeratinized. The epithelium is three to four times the thickness of the epidermis of skin. Beneath the epithelium is the lamina propria, composed of fibrous tissue and blood vessels. Since there is no muscularis mucosa, a true "submucosa" is not present. The mucosa abuts the densely fibrous periosteum of the hard palate or the alveolus of the maxilla and mandible. Mucous glands are present in the lamina propria, particularly in the posterior hard palatal mucosa, with mature fatty tissue being prominent in the anterior hard palatal mucosa. Occasionally, rests of odontogenic epithelium with clear cells are found in the gingiva.

The crevicular epithelium is a continuation of the gingival epithelium as it turns inward toward the tooth surface and then toward the root of the tooth. This epithelium is nonkeratinized and often exhibits irregular hyperplasia, leukocyte exocytosis, and microulcerations because of the response of the epithelium to plaque in the gingival crevice. The nonkeratinized mucosa consists of the epithelium with a relatively thick spinous cell layer and the lamina propria. The term *submucosa* is sometimes loosely applied to the deep connective tissue just above the muscle layer, in which the minor salivary glands are often embedded.

The anterior two thirds of the dorsum of the tongue is covered by keratinized stratified squamous epithelium specialized to form filiform papillae (pointed projections of keratin), which are often associated with bacterial colonies.

Between these are the fungiform papillae that consist of mushroom-shaped elevations of the mucosa that contain taste buds. Separating the anterior two thirds from the posterior one third are the circumvallate papillae that contain taste buds at their base. The serous salivary glands of the posterior tongue empty into the crypts surrounding these papillae. The last group of papillae is the foliate papillae located in the posterior lateral tongue in a series of ridges. Each taste bud consists of a barrel-shaped collection of modified epithelial cells that extend vertically from the basal lamina to the epithelial surface, opening via a taste pore. They are innervated by terminal nerve twigs from the lamina propria.

DEVELOPMENTAL ANOMALIES

FACIAL CLEFTS: Failure of fusion of facial structures in the seventh week of embryonic life leads to the formation of facial clefts, the most common of which is cleft upper lip (harelip). It may be unilateral or bilateral and frequently occurs in association with cleft palate (see Chapter 6).

LINGUAL THYROID NODULE: During its normal development, the thyroid gland descends from the base of the tongue to its final position in the neck. Heterotopic functioning thyroid tissue or a developmental cyst *(thyroglossal duct*

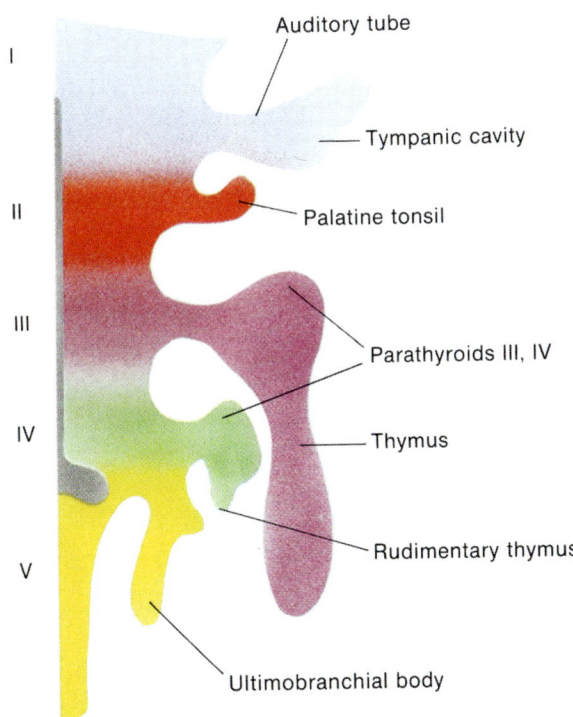

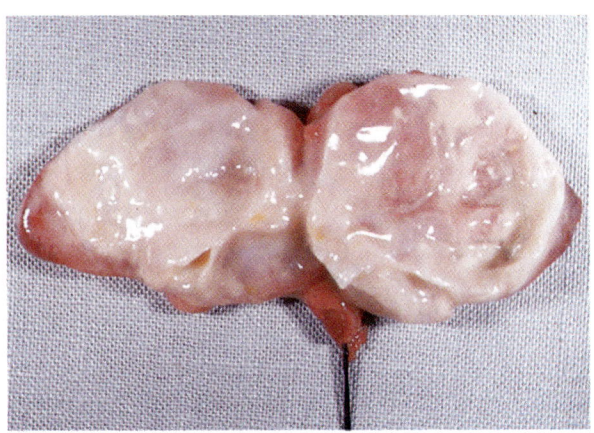

FIGURE 25-3
Branchial cleft cyst. Most of these cysts arise from the second branchial cleft and occur laterally in the neck. The cysts have a thin wall, contain turbid fluid, and are lined by stratified squamous or respiratory-type epithelium.

cyst) may occur anywhere along the path of descent. The most common location is at the foramen cecum of the tongue. There is a 4:1 female predilection, and symptoms such as dysphonia, sore throat, and awareness of a mass in the throat often become evident during adolescence and pregnancy. Radioisotope imaging typically shows radionuclide activity in the mouth but not the neck.

BRANCHIAL CLEFT CYST: Branchial cleft cysts originate from remnants of the branchial arches (Fig. 25-2). They occur on the lateral anterior aspect of the neck or in the parotid gland, mostly in young adults. The cyst contains thin, watery fluid and mucoid or gelatinous material. It is usually lined by squamous epithelium, although foci of ciliated respiratory or pseudostratified columnar epithelium also are seen (Fig. 25-3).

INFECTIONS

The following terms are used to describe localized inflammation of the oral cavity:

- *Cheilitis* (lips)
- *Gingivitis* (gum)
- *Glossitis* (tongue)
- *Stomatitis* (oral mucosa)

Bacterial and Fungal Infections Commonly Affect the Oral Cavity

SCARLET FEVER: Predominantly a disease of children, scarlet fever is caused by several strains of β-hemolytic streptococci (*Streptococcus pyogenes*). Damage to the vascular endothelium by the erythrogenic toxin results in a rash on the skin and in the oral mucosa. The tongue has a white coating, through which the hyperemic fungiform papillae project as small red knobs ("strawberry tongue").

APHTHOUS STOMATITIS (CANKER SORES): Aphthous stomatitis describes a common disease that is characterized

FIGURE 25-2
Branchial apparatus in humans. Schematic diagram of the pharyngeal pouches *(left half, ventral view)* in a human embryo of 6 weeks. Five pairs of pouches give rise to many important structures of the head, neck, and chest. A wide spectrum of congenital malformations results from abnormalities of the branchial apparatus.

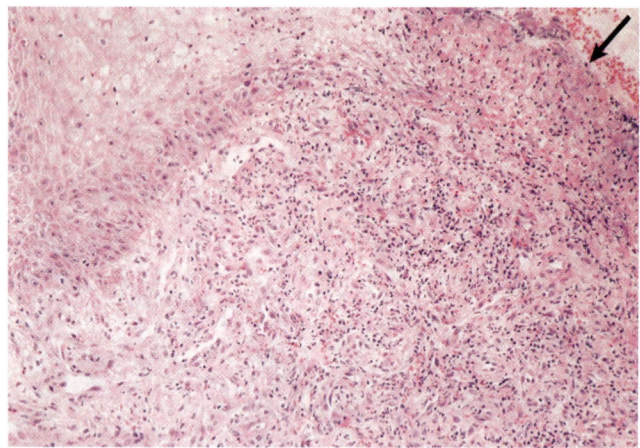

FIGURE 25-4
Pyogenic granuloma of the gingiva. The lesion displays vascular granulation tissue and inflammation. The epithelial surface is partly ulcerated (arrow).

by painful, recurrent, solitary or multiple, small ulcers of the oral mucosa. The causative agent is unknown. Bacteria, mycoplasma, viruses, autoimmune reactions, and hypersensitivity have been implicated but are unproved. Microscopically, the lesion consists of a shallow ulcer covered by a fibrinopurulent exudate. The underlying inflammatory infiltrate is composed of mononuclear and polymorphonuclear leukocytes. The lesions heal without scar formation.

PYOGENIC GRANULOMA: *Pyogenic granuloma is a reactive vascular lesion that commonly occurs in the oral cavity.* Usually some minor trauma to the tissues permits invasion of nonspecific microorganisms. In the oral cavity, pyogenic granulomas, ranging from a few millimeters to a centimeter, are most frequent on the gingiva. The lesion is seen as an elevated, red or purple, soft mass, with a smooth, lobulated, ulcerated surface. Microscopically, the nodule consists of highly vascular granulation tissue that shows varying degrees of acute and chronic inflammation (Fig. 25-4). With time, pyogenic granuloma becomes less vascular and comes to resemble a fibroma.

In pregnant women, particularly near the end of the first trimester, a gingival lesion may develop that grossly and microscopically is identical to pyogenic granuloma. Termed *pregnancy tumor,* it may or may not regress after delivery.

ACUTE NECROTIZING ULCERATIVE GINGIVITIS (VINCENT ANGINA): *Vincent angina represents an infection by two symbiotic organisms, one a fusiform bacillus and the other a spirochete (Borrelia vincentii).* The term *fusospirochetosis* is used to describe such an infection. The fact that these organisms are found in the mouths of many healthy persons suggests that predisposing factors are important in the development of acute necrotizing ulcerative gingivitis. The most important element appears to be decreased resistance to infection as a result of inadequate nutrition, immunodeficiency, or poor oral hygiene. Vincent infection is characterized by punched-out erosions of the interdental papillae. The ulceration tends to spread and eventually to involve all gingival margins, which become covered by a necrotic pseudomembrane.

Noma **(cancrum oris)** *is a severe fusospirochetal infection in persons who are malnourished, debilitated from infections, or weakened by blood dyscrasias, and features a rapidly spreading gangrene of the oral and facial tissues.* Large masses of tissue slough and leave the bones exposed (Figs. 9-39 and 25-5A), especially in children.

LUDWIG ANGINA: *Ludwig angina is a rapidly spreading cellulitis, or phlegmon, which originates in the submaxillary or sublingual space but extends locally to involve both.* The bacteria responsible for this infection originate from the oral flora, but this potentially life-threatening inflammatory process is uncommon in developed countries. A variety of aerobic or anaerobic microorganisms have been implicated in Ludwig angina. Patients often have chronic illnesses associated with immunosuppression.

Ludwig angina is most often related to dental extraction or trauma to the floor of the mouth. After extraction of a tooth, hairline fractures may occur in the lingual cortex of the mandible, providing microorganisms ready access to the submaxillary space. By following the fascial planes, the infection may dissect into the parapharyngeal space and from there into the carotid sheath. An infected (mycotic) aneurysm of the

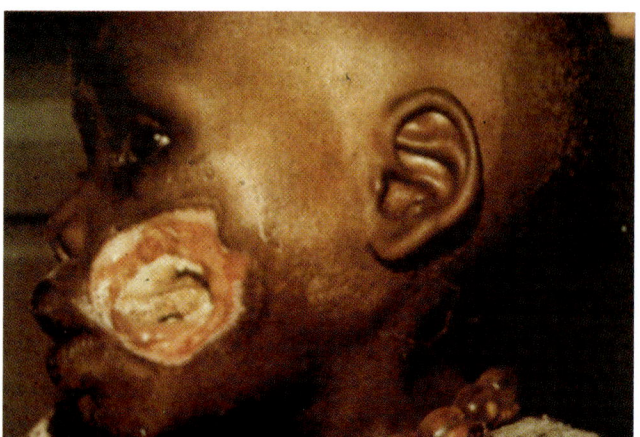
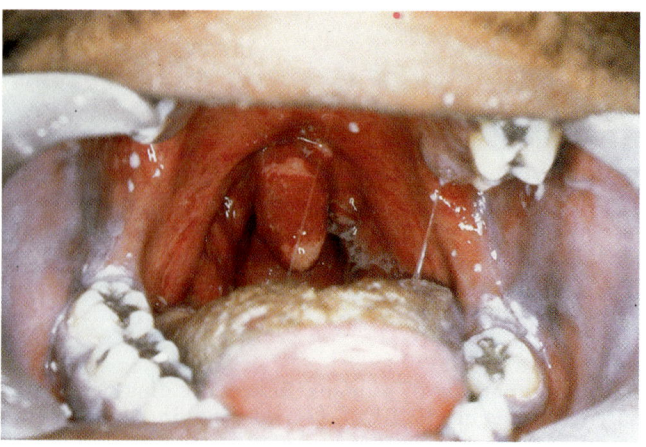

FIGURE 25-5
A. *Noma,* also referred to as *cancrum oris,* appears in this young boy as a large facial ulcerative lesion with exposure of subjacent soft tissues, including bone. B. Oral candidiasis.

internal carotid artery may result, and its erosion causes massive hemorrhage. The inflammation may also dissect into the superior mediastinum, involving the pleural space and pericardium.

DIPHTHERIA: Infection with *C. diphtheriae* is characterized by the formation of a patchy pseudomembrane, which often begins on the tonsils and pharynx but may also involve the soft palate, gingiva, or buccal mucosa.

TUBERCULOSIS: Primary tuberculous lesions of the oral mucosa are rare, and most lesions are the result of pulmonary disease. The bacilli are carried in the sputum and enter the mucosa through a small break, where they produce irregular, painful ulcers, most commonly on the tongue. A biopsy reveals caseating granulomatous inflammation that typifies the tuberculous granulomas.

SYPHILIS: The chancre of primary syphilis may form on the lips, tongue, or oropharyngeal mucosa after oral--genital contact with an infected person. It is accompanied by a regional lymphadenitis and heals spontaneously in a few weeks. If syphilis is not treated adequately, a diffuse mucocutaneous eruption of the secondary stage develops. The lesions in the oral mucosa appear as multiple gray–white patches overlying the ulcerated surface. They may undergo spontaneous remission but may also recur. After years of syphilitic infection, gummas may appear on the palate and tongue. They are firm nodular masses that eventually ulcerate and may lead to perforation of the palate.

ACTINOMYCOSIS: Branched, filamentous bacteria of the actinomyces group occasionally cause oral infections. The most common offender is *Actinomyces bovis*, but *A. israelii* is sometimes encountered. The organisms produce a chronic granulomatous inflammation and abscesses that drain by the formation of fistulas. Because actinomycetes are common inhabitants of the oral cavity of healthy persons, culture of the organism does not necessarily signify an infection. It is customary to distinguish cervicofacial (the most common form), pulmonary, and abdominal forms of actinomycosis, according to the site of the infection. In cervicofacial actinomycosis, the infection of the soft tissues may extend to adjacent bones, most commonly to the mandible.

CANDIDIASIS: Also termed *thrush* or *moniliasis*, candidiasis is caused by a yeastlike fungus, *Candida albicans*, which is a common surface inhabitant of the oral cavity, gastrointestinal tract, and vagina. To cause disease, the fungus must penetrate the tissues, albeit superficially. Oral candidiasis is most common in immunocompromised persons and diabetics, and the incidence in patients with AIDS is 40 to 90%. The oral lesions typically appear as white, slightly elevated, soft patches that consist mainly of fungal hyphae (Fig. 25-5B).

Viral Infections Present As Vesicular or Ulcerative Lesions

Herpes simplex virus (HSV) and cytomegalovirus (CMV) infections manifest as vesiculobullous and ulcerative lesions, respectively. Infection by Epstein-Barr virus (EBV) may occur as mucosal ulcerative lesions in the posterior oral cavity; alternatively, as seen in the EBV-related lesion termed *oral hairy leukoplakia*, EBV infection gives rise to shaggy white lesions on the lateral tongue and other mucosal surfaces. Oral hairy leukoplakia is most often, but not exclusively, associated with HIV infection.

Pathology: Herpetic and CMV infections are often accompanied by surface epithelial ulceration. At the edge of the mucosal HSV ulcer are large, multinucleated, epithelial cells with "ground glass" homogenized nuclei, often exhibiting nuclear molding. There may be an accompanying intraepithelial bulla. In CMV infections, the infected cells, usually of fibroblastic, monocytic, or endothelial cell origin, have large nuclei with prominent eosinophilic nucleoli.

HERPES SIMPLEX VIRUS TYPE 1: Herpes labialis (cold sores, fever blisters) and herpetic stomatitis are caused by HSV type 1 and are among the most common viral infections of the lips and oral mucosa in both children and young adults. Transmission occurs by droplet infection, and the virus can be recovered from the saliva of infected persons. The disease starts with painful inflammation of the affected mucosa, followed shortly by the formation of vesicles. These vesicles rupture and form shallow, painful ulcers, ranging from punctate size to a centimeter in diameter. Microscopically, the herpetic vesicle forms as a result of "ballooning degeneration" of the epithelial cells. Some epithelial cells show intranuclear inclusion bodies. The ulcers heal spontaneously without scar formation.

Once HSV has been introduced into the body, it survives in a dormant state in the trigeminal ganglion. It can be reactivated to cause recurrent herpetic lesions in diverse ways, including trauma, allergy, menstruation, pregnancy, exposure to ultraviolet light, and other viral infections. In the oral cavity, the recurrent vesicles almost invariably develop on a mucosa that is tightly bound to the periosteum, for example, the hard palate.

OTHER VIRAL INFECTIONS: Coxsackievirus causes herpangina, which is seen as an acute vesicular oropharyngitis. After a brief course, the infection confers immunity. Other viral infections that involve the oral mucosa are infectious mononucleosis (EBV), measles, rubella, chickenpox, and herpes zoster.

BENIGN TUMORS

Benign tumors that are common in other regions of the body are seen also in the oral cavity. These include pigmented nevi, fibromas, hemangiomas, lymphangiomas, and squamous papillomas. Trauma may lead to ulceration of these lesions, in which case, they may bleed or become infected.

A distinctive lesion limited to the oral cavity is peripheral giant cell granuloma. This is not a neoplasm but rather an unusual proliferative reaction to local injury that is seen as a mass on the gingiva or the alveolar process. This lesion has a variety of names, such as *epulis, giant cell reparative granuloma, giant cell tumor of gum,* and *osteoclastoma.* The adjective "peripheral" denotes the superficial, extraosseous location of the lesion, as opposed to the "central" giant cell granulomas that occur within the jawbones.

The prevailing view is that peripheral giant cell granuloma is not a neoplasm but rather an unusual proliferative reaction to local injury. In rare cases, it is caused by hyperparathyroidism, in which case, it can be regarded as a brown tumor of soft tissues. The lesion always occurs on the gingiva or the alveolar process and seems to originate from the deeper soft tissues. Most patients are young or middle-aged adults, but the lesion occurs in children and has been reported in edentulous elderly patients.

 Pathology: Peripheral giant cell granuloma is seen as a mass covered by mucous membrane, which can be ulcerated. The tumor varies from brown to black, depending on the amount of hemorrhage. Histological examination reveals a nonencapsulated lesion with numerous multinucleated giant cells embedded in a fibrous stroma that also contains ovoid or spindle-shaped mesenchymal cells (Fig. 25-6). The lesion is vascular and shows foci of old hemorrhage, with hemosiderin-laden macrophages and chronic inflammation. The origin of the multinucleated giant cells remains unclear, although immunohistochemical evidence suggests that they are derived from macrophages.

Leukoplakia and Erythroplakia Are Lesions of the Mucosa

The clinical appearance of premalignant or "incipient" lesions of the mucosal surfaces of the upper aerodigestive tract include leukoplakia, erythroplakia, or speckled leukoplakia,

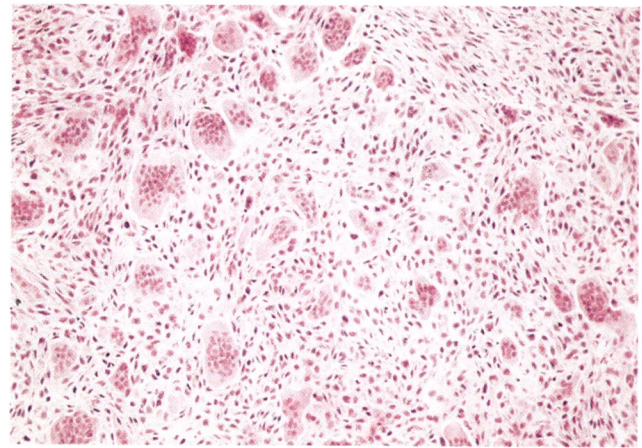

FIGURE 25-6
Peripheral giant cell granuloma. A protruding gingival mass contains multinucleated giant cells and spindle-shaped stromal cells.

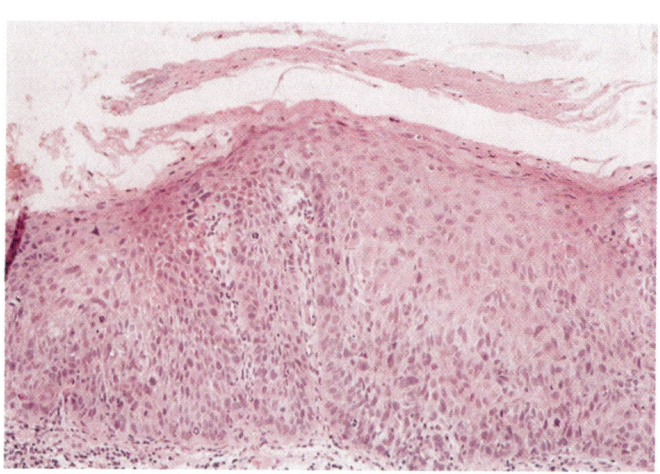

FIGURE 25-7
Leukoplakia. The lesion was seen as a white patch on the buccal mucosa of a heavy smoker. Histologically, epithelial hyperplasia, marked atypia, and parakeratosis are evident.

reflecting the presence of a white, red, or mixed white/red lesion, respectively. *Leukoplakia (Greek,* leukos, *"white" and* plax, *"plaque") refers to an asymptomatic white lesion on the surface of a mucous membrane.* Although not a tumor, oral leukoplakia and erythroplakia are discussed here because some lesions undergo transformation to squamous cell carcinoma. The disorders occur with equal frequency in both sexes, mostly after the third decade of life. A variety of diseases appear clinically as leukoplakia, including various keratoses, hyperkeratosis, and squamous carcinoma in situ. Thus, leukoplakia is not a histological diagnosis but rather a descriptive clinical term. Other clinical entities may also feature a white plaque on the oral mucosa, (e.g., candidiasis, lichen planus, psoriasis, and syphilis).

The causes of leukoplakia are diverse, the most common factors being use of tobacco products, alcoholism, and local irritation. The same factors also appear to be important in the etiology of oral carcinoma.

 Pathology: Leukoplakia occurs most often on the buccal mucosa, tongue, and floor of the mouth. The plaques may be solitary or multiple and vary in size from small lesions to large patches. Erythroplaia is commonly associated with ominous histopathological alterations, including severe dysplasia, carcinoma in situ, or invasive carcinoma. By contrast, leukoplakic lesions are not necessarily premalignant and may demonstrate a spectrum of histopathological changes, ranging from increased surface keratinization without dysplasia to invasive keratinizing squamous carcinoma (Fig. 25-7). Leukoplakic lesions, in contrast with erythroplakic lesions, tend to be well defined with demarcated margins. Although the probability of developing carcinoma in a leukoplakic lesion is low, there is still a risk (10–12%) of malignant transformation. The clinical appearance of a mixed white and red lesion, called *speckled leukoplakia,* carries an intermediate risk between "pure" leukoplakic and "pure" erythroplakic lesions for the development of a malignancy, but speckled leukoplakia should be viewed as a variant of erythroplakia.

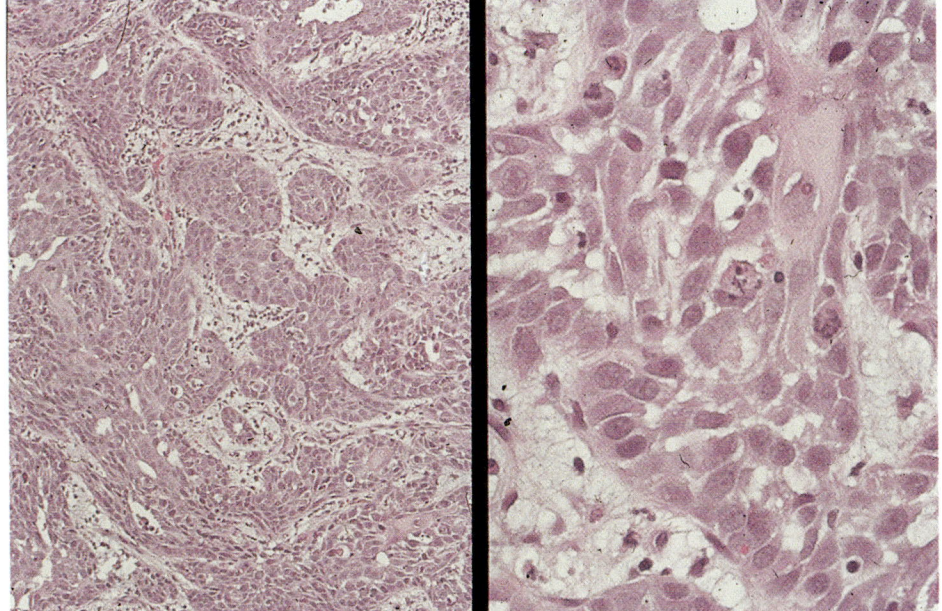

FIGURE 25-8
Squamous cell carcinoma. A. An infiltrative neoplasm is composed of cohesive nests of tumor. B. A less differentiated tumor displays cells with pleomorphic nuclei, prominent nucleoli, brightly eosinophilic cytoplasm indicating keratinization, and intercellular bridges connecting adjacent cells. B. A mitotic figure is seen to the *right of center.*

Oral hairy leukoplakia exhibits shaggy parakeratosis and edema. The EBV-infected epithelial cells have a vacuolated cytoplasm and are superficially located immediately beneath the keratin. The nuclei show dense central eosinophilic inclusions. Candidal hyphae are usually present, and HPV infection occurs concurrently in up to half of cases.

SQUAMOUS CELL CARCINOMA

Squamous cell carcinoma (SCC) is the most common malignant tumor of the oral mucosa and may occur at any site. It most frequently involves the tongue, followed in descending order by the floor of the mouth, alveolar mucosa, palate, and buccal mucosa. The male-to-female ratio is 2:1 for the gum but 10:1 for squamous carcinoma of the lip. There are substantial variations in the geographical distribution of oral cancer; for example, it is the single most common cancer of men in India.

Pathogenesis: Predisposing factors in the pathogenesis of oral cancer include the use of tobacco products, alcoholism, iron deficiency (Plummer-Vinson syndrome), physical and chemical irritants, chewing of betel nuts, ultraviolet light on the lips, and poor oral hygiene (craggy teeth and ill-fitting dentures). Not surprisingly, several of these factors also have been mentioned in connection with leukoplakia. Some SCCs of the head and neck have been associated with human papillomavirus (HPV) infection, but a direct cause and effect between the presence of HPV and the development of SCC has not been definitively established. Multiple separate epidermoid carcinomas may be found at the same time (synchronous) or at intervals (metachronous) in the oral mucosa, a situation termed *field cancerization*.

 Pathology: Invasive SCC of the oral cavity is similar to the same tumor in other sites and is generally preceded by carcinoma in situ. Variations in differentiation in SCC have led to a system of grading tumors. Accordingly, grade I carcinoma is well differentiated and frequently keratinizing (Fig. 25-8). At the other end of the spectrum, grade IV carcinomas are so poorly differentiated that their origin is difficult to determine on morphological grounds. Oral carcinoma metastasizes mainly to the submandibular, superficial, and deep cervical lymph nodes. More than half of patients who die of SCC of the head and neck have distant, blood-borne metastases, most commonly in the lungs, liver, and bones.

The histological grade of the carcinoma does not necessarily correlate with prognosis. However, SCCs that infiltrate in a pushing fashion, with large, cohesive cords and islands of cells, have a better prognosis than tumors that infiltrate in small irregular cords or single cells. These patterns of infiltration also correlate with the incidence of lymph node metastases.

BENIGN DISEASES OF THE LIPS

The lips are affected by a variety of degenerative, inflammatory, and proliferative processes. Some of these, particularly those expressed in the skin and mucous membranes, are systemic; others reflect localized disease (Figs. 25-9 and 25-10).

BENIGN DISEASES OF THE TONGUE

MACROGLOSSIA: All the components of the tongue may be involved by various localized or systemic diseases, some of which

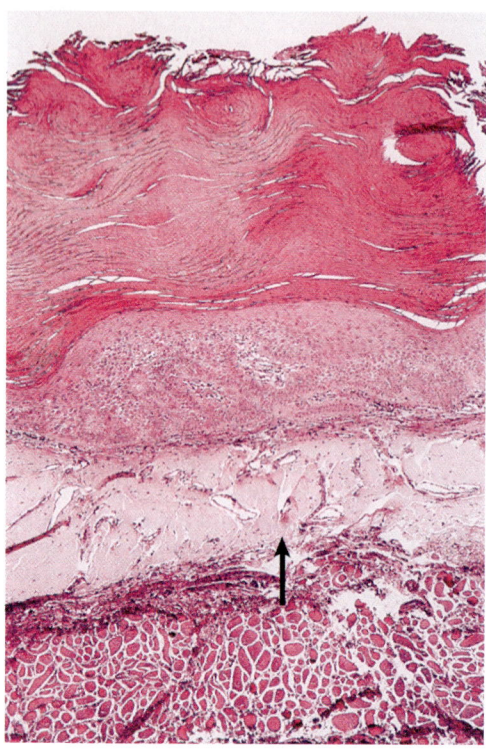

FIGURE 25-9
Solar cheilitis. A lesion analogous to a solar keratosis is present in the vermilion border of the lower lip. Hyperkeratosis and epithelial hyperplasia and dysplasia are evident. The light band under the epithelium *(arrow)* represents solar elastosis (damaged collagen) resulting from ultraviolet radiation.

can lead to enlargement of the tongue. If present at birth, macroglossia is usually due to diffuse lymphangioma or hemangioma, although rarely enlargement is caused by congenital neurofibromatosis or true muscle hypertrophy. An enlarged tongue that protrudes from the mouth occurs in congenital hypothyroidism, Hurler syndrome, glycogen-storage disease type II (Pompe disease), Beckwith-Wiedemann syndrome, and Down syndrome. Acquired macroglossia is due to amyloidosis, acromegaly, and infiltration or lymphatic obstruction by tumors.

GLOSSITIS: Inflammation of the tongue, termed *glossitis*, can be caused by various microorganisms, physical effects, chemical agents, or systemic diseases. Some forms of glossitis are associated with vitamin deficiencies, including pernicious anemia, riboflavin deficiency, pellagra, and pyridoxine deficiency.

DENTAL CARIES (TOOTH DECAY)

Caries is the most prevalent chronic disease of the calcified tissues of the teeth. It affects persons of both sexes and every age group throughout the world, and its incidence has markedly increased with modern civilization.

 Pathogenesis: Dental caries results from the interactions of several factors.

BACTERIA: Dental caries is a chronic infectious disease of the enamel, dentin, and cementum of teeth, the organisms being part of the indigenous oral flora. Tooth surfaces are normally colonized by numerous microorganisms, and unless the surface is cleaned thoroughly and frequently, colonies of bacteria coalesce into a soft mass known as *dental plaque.*

Carious lesions result primarily from leaching of mineral in dental tissues by acids that are produced from food residues by microorganisms on tooth surfaces. Numerous streptococci, lactobacilli, and actinomycetes in the oral flora have these characteristics. Indirect evidence points strongly to *Streptococcus mutans* as the primary etiological agent that initiates caries. Deeper in the enamel and dentin, organisms other than *S. mutans* may be more capable of maintaining the destructive process.

SALIVA: Saliva has a high buffering capacity that helps neutralize microbially produced acids in the mouth. In addition, it contains several bacteriostatic factors, such as lysozyme, lactoferrin, the lactoperoxidase system, and secretory immunoglobulins. Removal of the major salivary

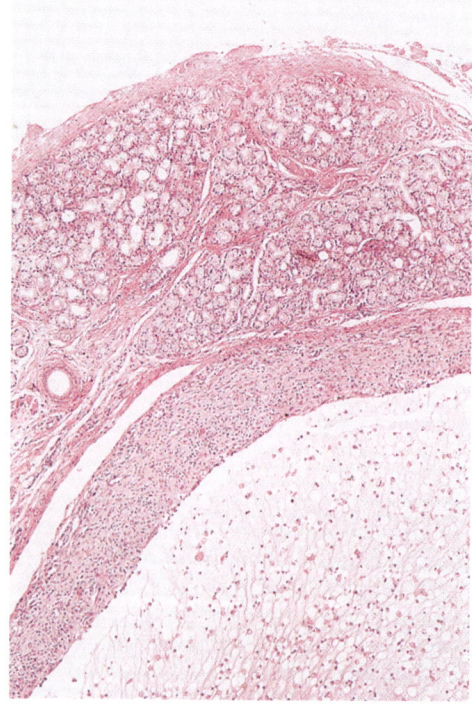

FIGURE 25-10
Mucocele of lower lip. This cystic lesion is associated with the minor salivary glands and is probably caused by trauma that permits escape of mucus. The cyst has a fibrous wall and is lined by granulation tissue. The lumen is filled with mucus that contains numerous macrophages.

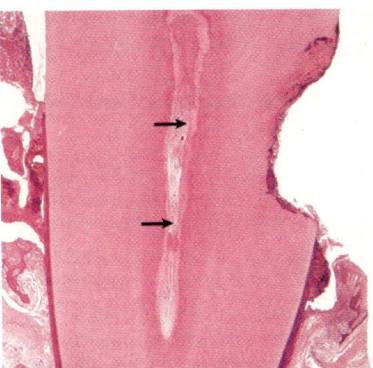

FIGURE 25-11
Dental caries. A large cavity close to the gingival margin is illustrated. *Arrows,* band of secondary dentin that lines the pulp chamber. This newly formed dentin is opposite the area of tooth destruction and was produced by the stimulated odontoblasts.

glands in rats results in a 10-fold increase in caries. In humans, *xerostomia* (chronic dryness of the mouth from lack of saliva) results in rampant caries.

DIETARY FACTORS: One of the most important factors in the development of caries is a high-carbohydrate diet. The roughage in raw and unrefined foods cleanses the teeth. Additionally, roughage necessitates more mastication, which further contributes to cleansing of the teeth. By contrast, soft and refined foods tend to stick to the teeth and also require less chewing.

FLUORIDE: The presence of fluoride in the drinking water protects against dental caries. Fluoride is incorporated into the crystal lattice structure of enamel, where it forms fluoroapatite, a less acid-soluble compound than the apatite of enamel. The fluoridation of drinking water in many communities has been followed by a dramatic reduction in the incidence of dental caries in children whose teeth were formed while they drank fluoride-containing water.

Pathology: Caries begins with the disintegration of the enamel prisms after decalcification of the interprismatic substance, events that lead to the accumulation of debris and microorganisms (Figs. 25-11 and 25-12). These changes produce a small pit or fissure in the enamel. When the process reaches the dentinoenamel junction, it spreads laterally and also penetrates the dentin along the dentinal tubules. A substantial cavity then forms in the dentin, producing to a flask-shaped lesion with a narrow orifice. Decalcification of dentin leads to focal coalescence of the destroyed dentinal tubules. Only when the vascular pulp of the tooth is invaded does an inflammatory reaction *(pulpitis)* appear, accompanied for the first time by pain.

DISEASES OF THE PULP AND PERIAPICAL TISSUES

The dental pulp consists of delicate connective tissue enclosed within the calcified walls of dentin. The pulp chamber is lined by odontoblasts and has a minute apical foramen through which blood vessels, lymphatics, and small nerves penetrate.

PULPITIS: Inflammation of the dental pulp, known as *pulpitis,* results from invasion by the oral bacteria involved in dental caries. Pain in acute pulpitis reflects increased pressure in the pulp chamber, caused by edema and exudate. This increased pressure also facilitates the spread of inflammation. Acute pulpitis may be accompanied by the formation of a small pulp abscess, and several small abscesses may lead to necrosis of the entire pulp. Chronic pulpitis may be the outcome of a subsiding acute inflammation or may be a chronic inflammation from its onset.

Acute or chronic pulpitis, if untreated, ultimately results in complete necrosis of the dental pulp. The infection may spread through a root canal into the periapical region, thereby leading to more serious lesions.

APICAL (OR PERIAPICAL) GRANULOMA: The most common sequel of pulpitis is the formation of chronically inflamed periapical granulation tissue (Fig. 25-13). The inflammatory tissue gradually becomes surrounded by a fibrous capsule, and when the tooth is extracted, the encapsulated granuloma is found attached to the root.

RADICULAR CYST (APICAL PERIODONTAL CYST): The squamous epithelium of an apical granuloma proliferates, forming a cavity, or cyst, lined by stratified squamous epithelium.

PERIAPICAL ABSCESS: As a result of pulpitis, an abscess may develop around the root of the tooth, either directly or after the formation of periapical granulomas and cysts.

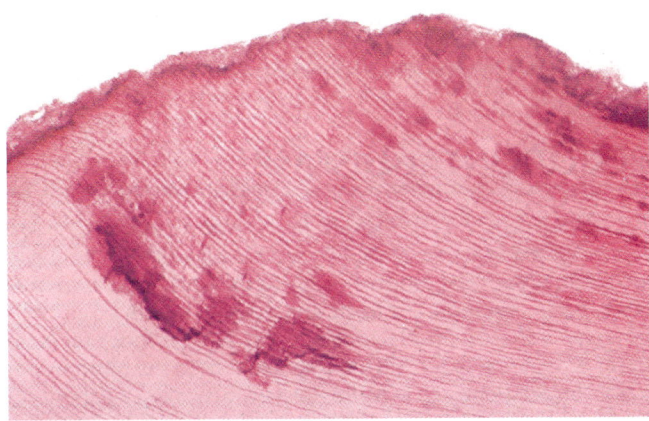

FIGURE 25-12
Dental caries. Deposits of debris cover the surface. Bacterial colonies *(dark purple)* have extended into dentinal canals.

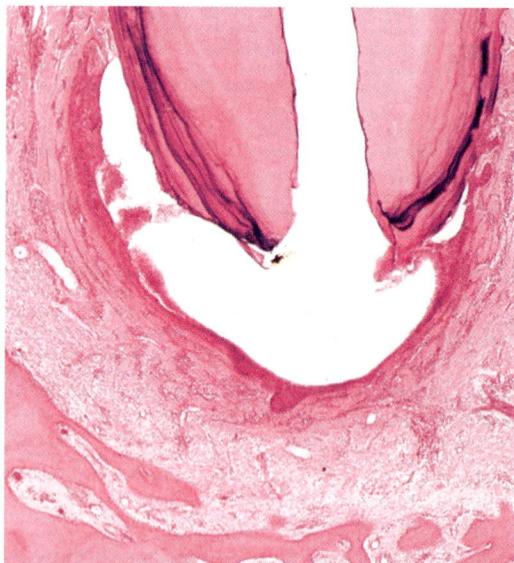

FIGURE 25-13
Advanced caries with periapical granuloma.

 OSTEOMYELITIS: A periapical abscess, if not contained, rapidly extends to the adjacent bone, where it produces osteomyelitis. Bacteriological cultures in all stages of pulpitis and periapical infections grow *Staphylococcus aureus, Staphylococcus epidermidis,* various streptococci, or mixed organisms.

Pathology: Osteomyelitis of the mandible or maxilla is an uncommon complication of odontogenic disease, usually of periapical infection. Like osteomyelitis of other bones, it may become localized or propagate within the jawbones. The infection may break through the cortical bone and spread in various tissue spaces of the head and neck, causing cellulitis *(phlegmon)* or abscesses. The purulent exudate may discharge into the surface of the mucous membranes or skin and create fistulas. In advanced cases, the infection follows the line of gravity in the tissue planes and ultimately reaches the mediastinum. These grave complications of osteomyelitis caused by dental infection were often lethal in the preantibiotic era but are rare today.

PERIODONTAL DISEASE

Periodontal disease refers to acute and chronic disorders of the soft tissues surrounding the teeth, which eventually lead to the loss of supporting bone. The gingiva (gum) is the part of the oral mucosa that surrounds the teeth and ends in a thin edge (free gingiva) adheres closely to the teeth. The periodontal ligament is composed of collagen fibers that hold the tooth in position by suspending it in the socket (alveolus) of the jawbone. These structures form the periodontium.

Chronic periodontal disease typically occurs in adults, particularly in persons with poor oral hygiene. However, many persons with apparently impeccable habits but a strong family history of periodontal disease, manifest the disorder. Chronic periodontitis causes loss of more teeth in adults than does any other disease, including caries.

  Pathogenesis and Pathology: Periodontal disease is caused by the accumulation of bacteria under the gingiva in the periodontal pocket. As the mass of bacteria adhering to the surface of tooth *(dental plaque)* ages and mineralizes, it forms *calculus* (tartar). Adult periodontitis is associated very strongly with *Bacteroides gingivalis.* In addition, *Bacteroides intermedius, Actinomyces* species, *Haemophilus* species, and a few other microorganisms may also participate.

The inflammation often starts as a marginal gingivitis, which, if untreated, progresses to chronic periodontitis. Once initiated, periodontitis continues to progress in the absence of treatment. Chronic inflammation (Fig. 25-14) weakens and destroys the periodontium, causing loosening and eventual loss of teeth.

Special Forms of Periodontal Disease

Hematological disorders may affect the oral tissues. Agranulocytosis causes necrotizing ulcers anywhere in the oral and pharyngeal mucosa, but involvement of the gingiva is particularly common. Infectious mononucleosis often results in gingivitis and stomatitis, with exudate and ulceration. Acute and chronic leukemias of all types cause oral lesions. The most common involvement of oral tissues is seen in acute monocytic leukemia, in which 80% of the patients exhibit gingivitis, gingival hyperplasia, petechiae, and hemorrhage. Necrosis and ulceration of the gingiva lead to severe superimposed infection, which may cause loss of teeth and alveolar bone. A hemorrhagic diathesis may be reflected in gingival hemorrhage.

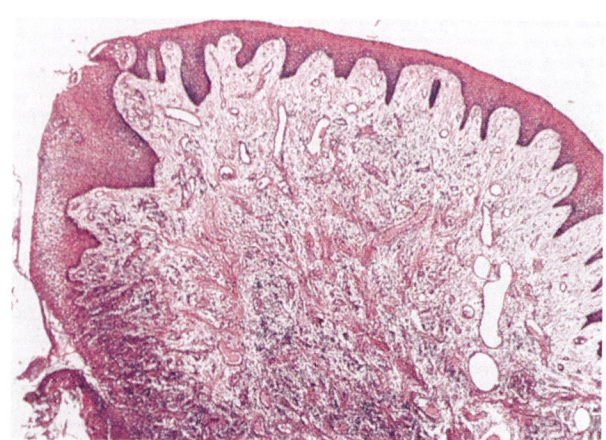

FIGURE 25-14
Hyperplastic chronic gingivitis. A section of gingiva in a case of periodontal disease shows a hyperplastic epithelium overlying chronically inflamed granulation tissue.

Scurvy (vitamin C deficiency) is of historical interest but in less dramatic forms is still encountered, particularly in poor, neglected, or ignorant persons. Scurvy tends to affect the marginal and interdental gingiva, which becomes swollen and bright red and readily bleeds and ulcerates. Hemorrhage into the periodontal membrane causes loosening and loss of teeth.

ODONTOGENIC CYSTS AND TUMORS

A variety of odontogenic cysts and tumors arise in the jawbones and the adjacent soft tissues. Their pathogenesis can be understood on the basis of dental histogenesis (Fig. 25-15).

ODONTOGENIC CYSTS: Odontogenic cysts include inflammatory cysts and developmental cysts. The most common is the radicular, or apical, periodontal cyst, which involves the apex of an erupted tooth, usually after an infection of the dental pulp. The cyst is lined by stratified squamous epithelium derived from the epithelial rests of Malassez.

DENTIGEROUS CYSTS: These cysts are associated with the crown of an impacted, embedded, or unerupted tooth, most often involving the mandibular and maxillary third molars. The cyst forms after the crown of the tooth has completely developed, and fluid accumulates between the crown and the overlying enamel epithelium. Dentigerous cysts tend to be unilocular and are lined by a thin layer of stratified squamous epithelium. Pressure by an enlarging cyst can cause marked resorption of bone and adjacent teeth. Among the potential complications of a dentigerous cyst are (1) recurrence after incomplete removal, (2) development of an ameloblastoma from the cyst lining or from epithelial rests of Malassez, and (3) progression to squamous cell carcinoma.

Ameloblastoma Originates in the Enamel Organ

Ameloblastomas are tumors of epithelial odontogenic origin and represent the most common clinically significant odontogenic tumor. They are slow-growing, locally invasive tumors that generally follow a benign clinical course.

 Pathology: Most ameloblastomas arise in the mandible, and most of these occur in the ramus or molar area. Ameloblastomas in the maxilla are

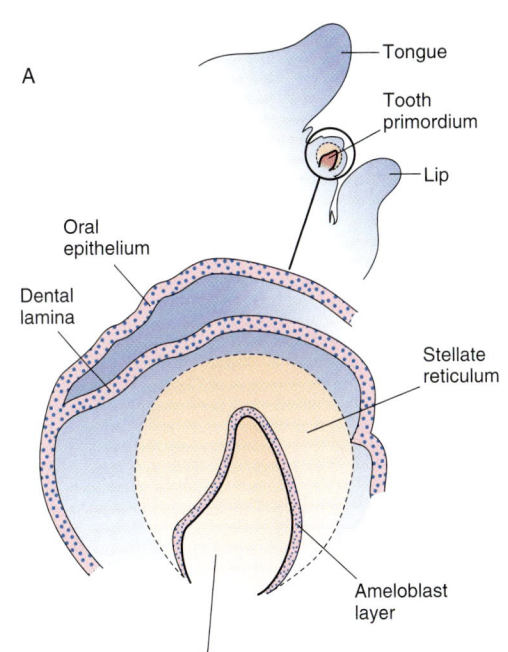
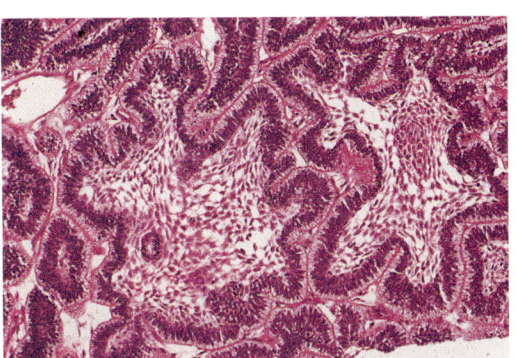

FIGURE 25-15

Development of teeth and odontogenic tumors. Diagrammatic representation of the normal development of a tooth and the mode of formation of a dentigerous cyst and ameloblastoma. A. Sagittal section of the lower jaw of a human embryo at 14 weeks, through the primordium of the lower central incisor. The enamel organ at this stage is a double-walled sac, composed of an outer convex wall and an inner concave wall. Between the two are looser ectodermal cells (stellate reticulum). The stellate reticulum gives rise to dentigerous cysts, whereas the ameloblasts may form an ameloblastoma. B. Ameloblastoma is characterized by cellular islands in which the nuclei at the periphery align in a perpendicular manner referred to as *palisading*; the central portion, referred to as *stellate reticulum*, has a looser (less cellular) appearance.

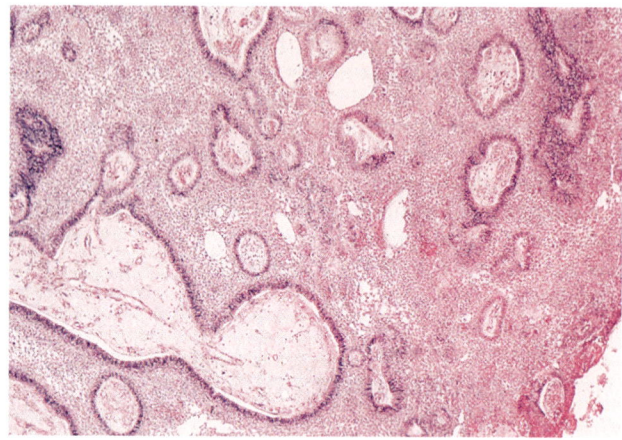

FIGURE 25-16
Ameloblastoma. A common histological pattern is characterized by confluent islands of epithelium. The peripheral cells form bands that separate the tumor from the stroma. Several microcysts are present.

most common in the molar area, but they can also involve the maxillary antrum or floor of the nasal cavity. The tumor tends to grow slowly as a central lesion of bone. Radiographs show a multilocular cystlike appearance, with a smooth periphery, expansion of the bone, and thinning of the cortex. Ameloblastomas are divided into three types: the conventional solid or multicystic type, representing 85% of cases; the unicystic type, accounting for 13% of cases; and the peripheral (extraosseous) type, constituting 1% of cases.

Microscopically, ameloblastoma resembles the enamel organ in its various stages of differentiation, and a single tumor may show various histological patterns. Accordingly, the tumor cells resemble ameloblasts at the periphery of the epithelial nests or cords, where columnar cells are oriented perpendicularly to the basement membrane (Fig. 25-15B and 25-16). The centers of these cell nests consist of loosely arranged, larger, polyhedral cells that resemble the stellate reticulum of the developing tooth. Frequently, the complete breakdown of these looser areas results in the formation of microcysts.

The prognosis of ameloblastoma is favorable. Incompletely excised tumors recur, but malignant transformation does not occur.

Salivary Glands

The salivary glands, which develop as buds of the oral ectoderm, are tubuloalveolar structures that secrete saliva. The major salivary glands are paired organs. The parotid glands secrete serous saliva, whereas the submandibular and sublingual glands produce mixed serous and mucous saliva. The minor salivary glands are widespread, being present under the mucosa of the lips, cheeks, palate, and tongue. Lymph nodes are normally embedded in the parotid gland. The intraparotid lymph nodes may be involved in a variety of inflammatory, reactive, or proliferative processes, including malignant lymphoma.

XEROSTOMIA: Xerostomia refers to chronic dryness of the mouth from the lack of saliva and has many causes. Diseases that involve the major salivary glands and produce xerostomia include mumps, Sjögren syndrome, sarcoidosis, radiation-induced atrophy (Fig. 25-17), and drug sensitivity (antihistamines, tricyclic antidepressants, hypotensive drugs, phenothiazines).

SIALORRHEA: Increased salivary flow is associated with many conditions, for example, acute inflammation of the oral cavity, as in aphthous stomatitis, Parkinson disease, rabies, mental retardation, nausea, and pregnancy.

ENLARGEMENT: Unilateral enlargement of the major salivary glands is due to inflammation, cysts, or neoplasms. Bilateral enlargement is caused by inflammation (mumps, Sjögren syndrome), granulomatous disease (sarcoidosis), or diffuse neoplastic involvement (leukemia or malignant lymphoma).

SIALOLITHIASIS: Calcific stones occur in the ducts of salivary glands, most commonly in the submandibular gland. The most important consequence of stone formation is obstruction of the duct, often followed by inflammation distal to the occlusion.

PAROTITIS: Acute suppurative parotitis is caused by the ascent of bacteria (usually *S. aureus*) from the oral cavity when the salivary flow is reduced. It is most frequently seen

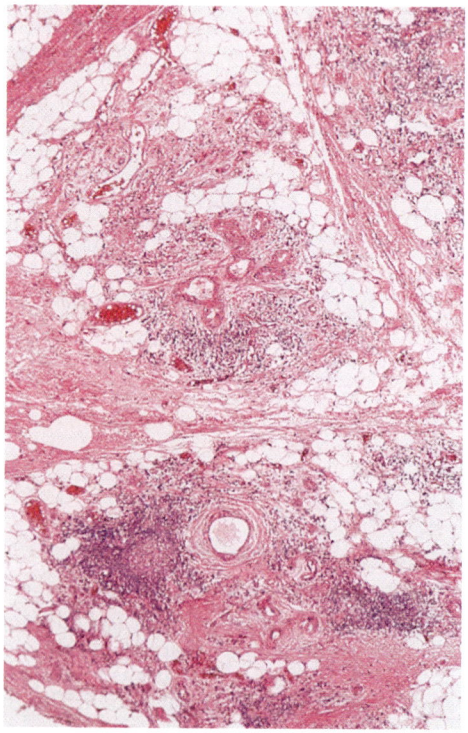

FIGURE 25-17
Chronic sialadenitis. Severe chronic inflammation and marked atrophy of the submandibular gland are present after irradiation of an adjacent oral cancer. The atrophic acini have been replaced by fat.

in debilitated or postoperative patients. Acute and chronic parotitis is often associated with stricture of the salivary ducts or obstruction by stones. The stagnant secretions serve as a medium for retrograde bacterial invasion.

Epidemic parotitis (mumps) is an acute viral disease of the parotid glands that spreads with infected saliva. The submandibular and sublingual salivary glands also may be involved. In addition to infection of the salivary glands in mumps, pancreatitis and orchitis are not uncommon. Microscopically, the salivary glands are densely infiltrated by lymphocytes and macrophages and exhibit degenerative changes and necrosis of the epithelial cells. Mumps is discussed in more detail in Chapter 9.

SJÖGREN SYNDROME

Sjögren syndrome is a chronic inflammatory disease of the salivary and lacrimal glands; it may be restricted to these sites or may be associated with a systemic collagen vascular disease. Involvement of the salivary glands leads to dry mouth *(xerostomia)*, and disease of the lacrimal glands results in dry eyes *(keratoconjunctivitis sicca)*. The pathogenesis and clinical features of Sjögren syndrome are discussed in Chapter 4.

Pathology: The parotid glands and sometimes the submandibular glands in Sjögren syndrome are unilaterally or bilaterally enlarged, but their lobular appearance is preserved. Histologically, an initial periductal round cell infiltrate gradually extends to the acini, until the glands are completely replaced by a sea of polyclonal lymphocytes, immunoblasts, germinal centers, and plasma cells. Proliferating myoepithelial cells surround remnants of the damaged ducts and form so-called epimyoepithelial islands (Fig. 25-18). The term *benign lymphoepithelial lesion* has been introduced to describe these characteristic microscopic changes. Similar changes can be seen in the

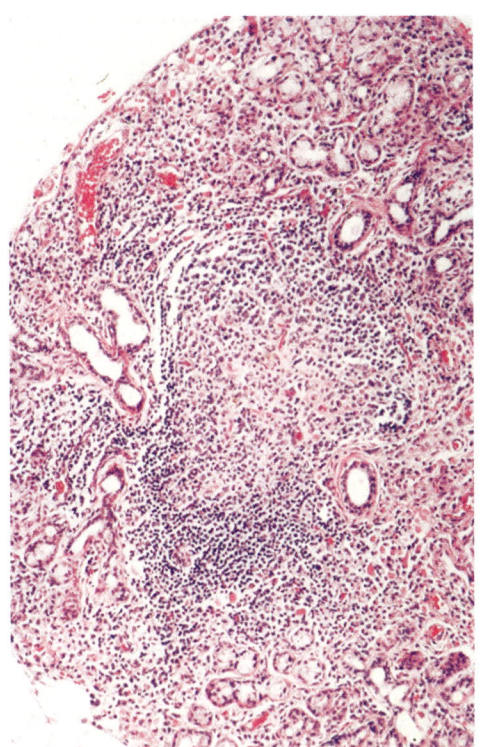

FIGURE 25-19
Sjögren syndrome. A lip biopsy shows lobules of mucous glands infiltrated by lymphocytes and plasma cells. Slightly dilated ducts without acini indicate glandular atrophy.

lacrimal glands and in the minor salivary glands. Focal lymphocytic sialadenitis can also be demonstrated in minor salivary glands obtained by labial biopsy in most patients with Sjögren syndrome (Fig. 25-19). Late in the course of the disease, the affected glands become atrophic, with fibrosis and fatty infiltration of the parenchyma. The lymphoid infiltrates in Sjögren syndrome may contain monotypic cells that have restricted immunoglobulin patterns, which may not be invasive and may remain localized.

Mikulicz syndrome refers to a symmetric enlargement of the salivary and lacrimal glands due to a specific disease, such as leukemic infiltrates, malignant lymphoma, amyloidosis, tuberculosis, or sarcoidosis. The use of this term in such situations is not warranted, because it is ambiguous.

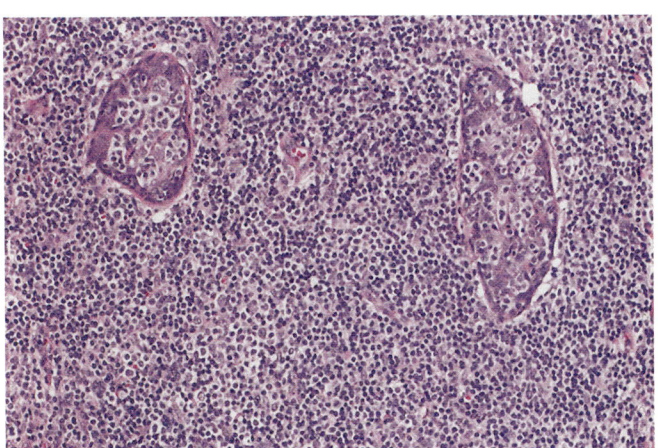

FIGURE 25-18
Sjögren syndrome. There is infiltration of the involved salivary gland by a mixed chronic inflammatory cell infiltrate. Extension of the infiltrate into epithelial (ductal) structures results in metaplasia and characteristic epimyoepithelial islands.

PLEOMORPHIC ADENOMA (MIXED TUMOR)

Pleomorphic adenoma, the most common tumor of the salivary glands, is a benign neoplasm characterized by a biphasic appearance, which represents an admixture of epithelial and stromal elements. Two thirds of all tumors of the major salivary glands, and about half of those in the minor ones, are pleomorphic adenomas. The tumor is nine times more frequent in the parotid than in the submandibular gland and usually arises in the superficial lobe of the parotid. It occurs most fre-

1282 | The Head and Neck

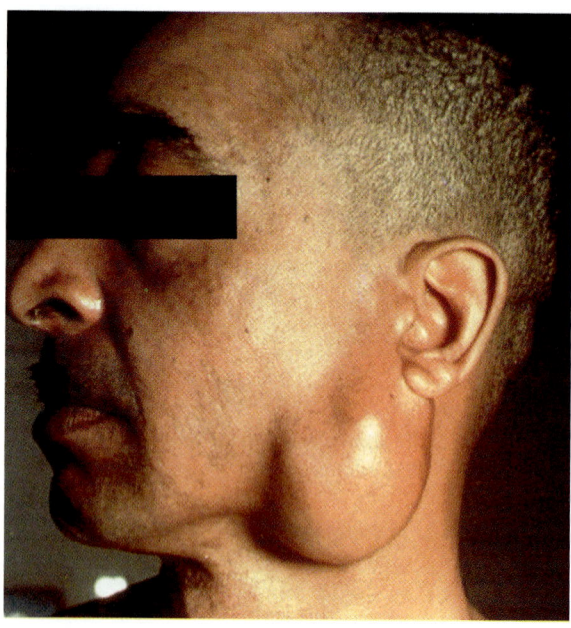

FIGURE 25-20
Pleomorphic adenoma of the parotid. A conspicuous tumor mass is seen at the angle of the jaw.

quently in middle-aged persons and shows a female preponderance.

Pathology: Pleomorphic adenoma is seen as a slowly growing, painless, movable, firm mass that has a smooth surface (Fig. 25-20). Tumors that arise deep in the parotid gland may grow between the ramus of the mandible and the styloid process and stylomandibular ligament into the parapharyngeal space, where they are seen as swellings of the lateral pharyngeal or tonsillar regions.

Microscopically, pleomorphic adenoma shows a mixture of epithelial tissue intermingled with myxoid, mucoid, or chondroid areas (Fig. 25-21 and 25-22) (Fig. 25-20). The older term *mixed tumor* referred to this peculiar mixture of epithelial cells and mesenchymal ground substance. However, the neoplasm is now considered to be of epithelial origin: hence the label "adenoma."

The epithelial component of pleomorphic adenoma consists of two cell types, ductal and myoepithelial cells. The cells lining the ducts form tubules or small cystic structures and contain clear fluid or eosinophilic, PAS-positive material. Around the epithelial cells of the ducts are smaller myoepithelial cells, which constitute the main cellular component. The myoepithelial cells form well-defined sheaths, cords, or nests (see Fig. 25-21) and are often separated by a cellular ground substance that resembles cartilaginous, myxoid, or mucoid material.

 Clinical Features: Pleomorphic adenomas have a fibrous capsule, and as they grow, the surrounding fibrous tissue condenses around them. The tumors become larger and tend to protrude focally into the adjacent tissues, thereby becoming nodular (see Fig. 25-22). At surgery, these tumor projections can be missed if the tumor is not carefully dissected to leave an intact capsule and an adequate margin of surrounding glandular parenchyma. Tumor implanted during surgery or tumor nodules left behind continue to grow as recurrences in the scar tissue of the previous operation. When the recurrent tumor is removed, the facial nerve may have to be sacrificed. Recurrence of pleomorphic adenoma represents local growth and does not reflect malignancy.

On rare occasions, carcinomas arise in pleomorphic adenomas and are referred to as *carcinoma ex pleomorphic adenoma*. In this situation a pleomorphic adenoma that has been present for many years may begin to grow rapidly or become painful. Histological examination reveals an unequivocal carcinoma in an otherwise benign pleomorphic adenoma. These tumors are usually high-grade malignancies such as poorly differentiated adenocarcinoma and undifferentiated adenocarcinoma, but virtually any type of salivary gland malignancy may occur in this setting, including mucoepidermoid or adenoid cystic carcinomas.

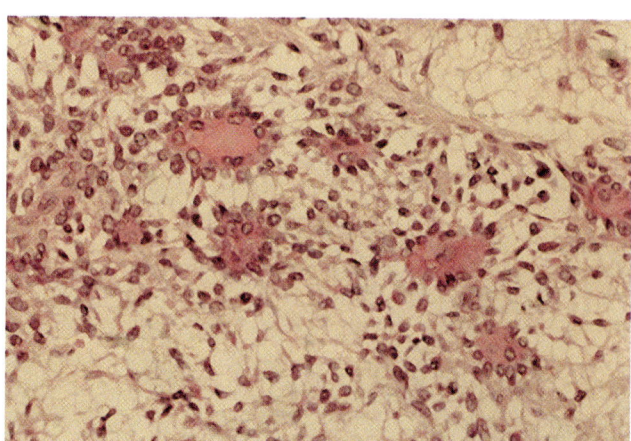
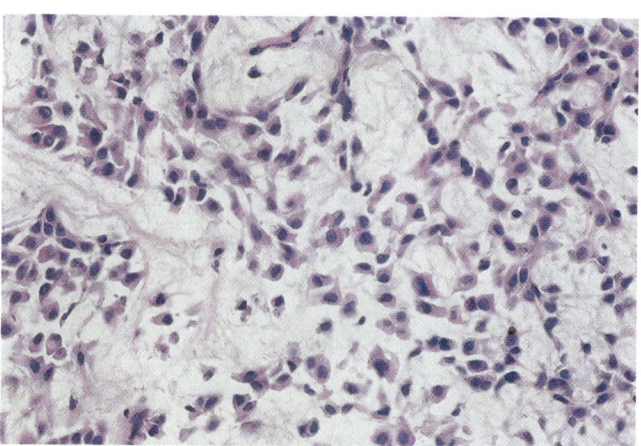

FIGURE 25-21
A. Cellular components of pleomorphic adenomas include an admixture of glands and myoepithelial cells within a chondromyxoid stroma. B. Myoepithelial cells may have a variety of appearances, including plasmacytoid and spindle-shaped cells.

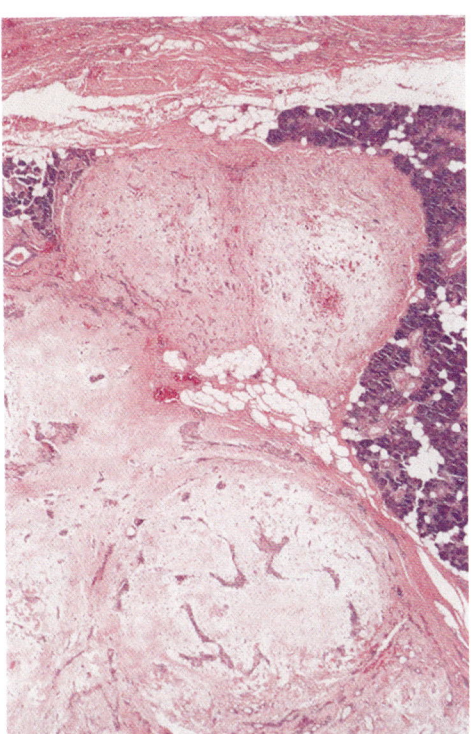

FIGURE 25-22
Pleomorphic adenoma of the parotid gland. The tumor contains characteristic myxoid and chondroid portions. The tumor is partly encapsulated, but a nodule protruding into the parotid gland lacks a capsule. If such nodules are not included in the resection, the tumor will recur.

MONOMORPHIC ADENOMA

A small proportion (5–10%) of benign epithelial tumors of the salivary glands consist of epithelium arranged in a regular, usually glandular, pattern without a mesenchyme-like component. Monomorphic adenomas include (1) Warthin tumor (papillary cystadenoma lymphomatosum), (2) basal cell adenoma, (3) oxyphilic adenoma or oncocytoma, (4) canalicular adenoma, (5) myoepithelioma, and (6) clear cell adenoma.

WARTHIN TUMOR: Warthin tumor is a benign neoplasm of the parotid gland, composed of cystic glandular spaces embedded in dense lymphoid tissue. This tumor is the most common monomorphic adenoma. Although the neoplasm is clearly benign, it can be bilateral (15% of cases) or multifocal within the same gland. Warthin tumor is the only tumor of the salivary glands that is more common in men than in women. These lesions generally occur after the age of 30 years, with most arising after age 50 years.

Pathology: The tumor is composed of glandular spaces that tend to become cystic and show papillary projections. The cysts are lined by characteristic eosinophilic epithelial cells *(oncocytes)* and are embedded in dense lymphoid tissue with germinal centers (Fig. 25-23).

The histogenesis of this peculiar tumor has been much debated. Lymph nodes, which are normally found in the parotid gland and in its immediate vicinity, usually contain a few ducts or small islands of salivary gland tissue. It has been suggested that Warthin tumors arise from the proliferation of these salivary gland inclusions.

ONCOCYTOMA (OXYPHIL ADENOMA): These rare benign tumors are composed of nests or cords of oncocytes, most of which occur in the parotid glands of elderly persons. Oncocytes are benign epithelial cells that are swollen with mitochondria, which impart a granular appearance to the cytoplasm. They can be found scattered or in small clusters among the epithelial cells of various normal organs (e.g., the thyroid and parathyroid glands). For unknown reasons, oncocytes begin to appear in early adulthood, and their number increases with age. Their function is unknown.

MALIGNANT SALIVARY GLAND TUMORS

Salivary gland tumors account for about 5% of all neoplasms of the head and neck. Most (75%) occur in the parotid glands, 10% arise in the submandibular glands, and 15% are located in minor salivary glands (mucoserous glands) of the upper aerodigestive tract. Less than 1% present in the sublingual glands.

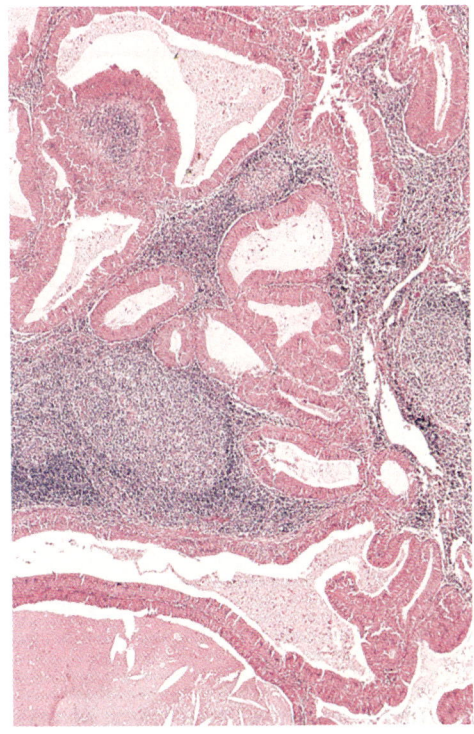

FIGURE 25-23
Warthin tumor. Cystic spaces and ductlike structures are lined by oncocytes. Follicular lymphoid tissue is present.

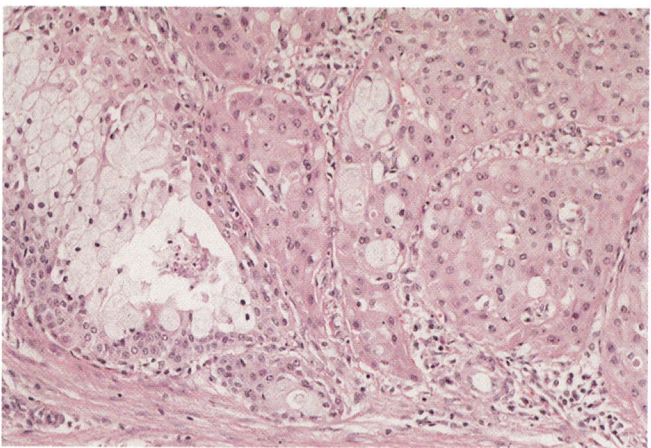

FIGURE 25-24
Mucoepidermoid carcinoma is characterized by an admixture of mucocytes, epidermoid cells, and intermediate cells. The mucocytes are clustered and have a clear cytoplasm with eccentrically situated nuclei. Epidermoid cells are squamouslike cells but lack keratinization and intercellular bridges. Intermediate cells (best seen at *lower left*) are smaller than epidermoid cells.

Mucoepidermoid Carcinoma Features Neoplastic Squamous and Mucus-Secreting Cells

Mucoepidermoid carcinoma is a malignant salivary gland tumor composed of a mixture of neoplastic squamous cells, mucus-secreting cells, and epithelial cells of an intermediate type. It originates from ductal epithelium, which has a considerable potential for metaplasia. This neoplasm accounts for 5 to 10% of major salivary gland tumors and 10% of those in the minor salivary glands. Within the major salivary glands, more than half of mucoepidermoid carcinomas arise in the parotid gland. In the minor salivary glands, they develop most frequently in the palate. Although the tumor may occur in adolescents, most tumors are seen in adults and are more common in women.

 Pathology: Mucoepidermoid carcinoma grows slowly and is seen as a firm painless mass. Microscopically, low-grade (well-differentiated) tumors form irregular solid, ductlike, and cystic spaces that include the presence of epidermoid cells, mucus-secreting cells and intermediate cells (Fig. 25-24). Intermediate-grade tumors tend to be (1) more solid in growth, (2) composed of a greater percentage of epidermoid and intermediate cells, and (3) possessed of fewer mucus-secreting cells. High-grade (poorly differentiated) carcinomas exhibit a markedly pleomorphic cell population lacking evidence of differentiation. However, scattered mucus-secreting cells are present.

Clinical Features: Even low-grade (well-differentiated) mucoepidermoid carcinomas can metastasize, but the 5-year survival is better than 90%, regardless of the primary site. High-grade (poorly differentiated) mucoepidermoid carcinomas have a much lower survival rate (20–40%).

Adenoid Cystic Carcinoma Invades Locally but Usually Recurs

Adenoid cystic carcinoma, previously termed cylindroma, *is a slowly growing malignant neoplasm of the salivary gland, which is notorious for its tendency to invade locally and to recur after surgical resection.* It constitutes 5% of all tumors of the major salivary glands and 20% of those of the minor salivary glands. One third of neck tumors arise in the major salivary glands and two thirds in the minor ones. They occur not only in the oral cavity but also in the lacrimal glands, nasopharynx, nasal cavity, paranasal sinuses, and lower respiratory tract. They are most common in persons between 40 and 60 years of age.

 Pathology: Histologically, adenoid cystic carcinomas present varying patterns. The tumor cells are small, have scant cytoplasm, and grow in solid sheets or as small groups, strands, or columns. Within these structures, the tumor cells interconnect to enclose cystic spaces, resulting in a solid, tubular or cribriform (sievelike) arrangement (Fig. 25-25). The tumor cells produce a homogeneous basement membrane material that gives them the characteristic *cylindromatous* appearance.

The tumors probably originate from cells that are differentiating toward intercalated ducts and toward myoepithelium. Adenoid cystic carcinoma tends to infiltrate the perineural spaces (Fig. 25-26) and is frequently painful. For these reasons, they are often diagnosed in an advanced stage. Although most adenoid cystic carcinomas do not metastasize for many years, they are difficult to eradicate completely, and their long-term prognosis is poor.

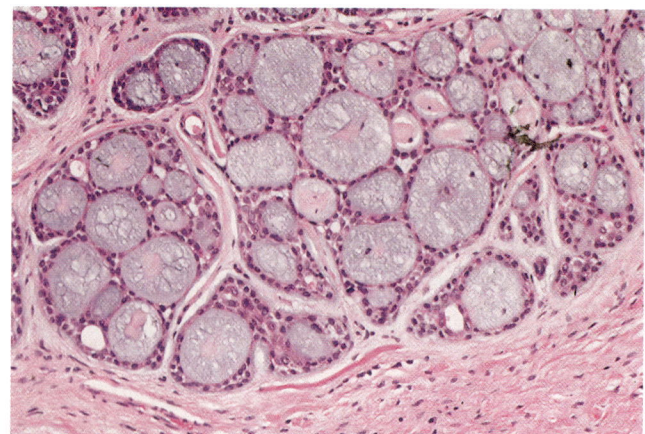

FIGURE 25-25
Adenoid cystic carcinoma showing cribriform growth in which cystlike spaces are filled with basophilic material. The cyst spaces are really pseudocysts surrounded by myoepithelial cells.

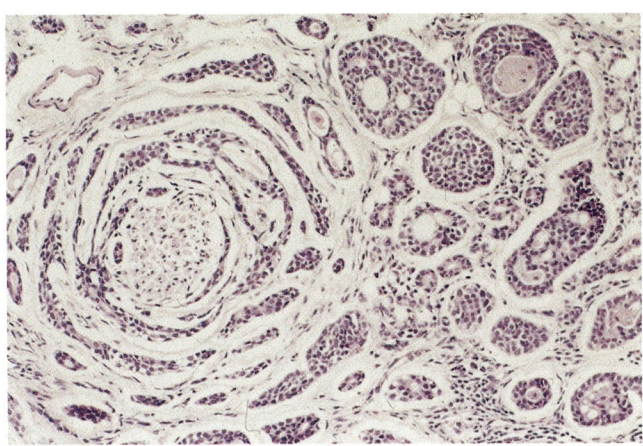

FIGURE 25-26
Adenoid cystic carcinomas are noted for their propensity to grow around (and into) nerves, as seen on the *left* of this illustration.

Acinic Cell Carcinoma Arises from Epithelial Secretory Cells

Acinic cell carcinoma is an uncommon tumor of the parotid gland (10% of all salivary gland tumors). It is occasionally encountered in the other salivary glands and occurs principally in young men between the ages of 20 and 30 years. It is seen as an encapsulated, round mass, usually less than 3 cm across, and is sometimes cystic. Microscopically, acinic cell carcinomas are composed of uniform cells with a small central nucleus and abundant basophilic cytoplasm, similar to the secretory (acinic) cells of the normal salivary glands. The tumor may metastasize to the regional lymph nodes.

After surgical resection of the tumor, most (90%) patients survive for 5 years, but local recurrence may be expected in one third of patients, and only half survive for 20 years.

Nose and Paranasal Sinuses

ANATOMY

The apertures of the nostrils (anterior nares) lead into the nasal vestibule, a space lined by skin that contains hairs and sebaceous glands. Beyond the nares, the nasal cavity is divided by the median septum into two symmetric chambers, termed the *nasal fossae.* Each nasal fossa has an olfactory region, consisting of the superior nasal concha and the opposed part of the septum, and a respiratory region, which constitutes the rest of the cavity. On the lateral wall are the inferior, middle, and superior nasal conchae (turbinates), overhanging the corresponding nasal passages or meatuses. The paranasal sinuses are paired air spaces that communicate with the nasal cavity.

The mucous membrane covering the respiratory portion of the nasal cavity has a ciliated, columnar epithelium with interspersed goblet cells. The anatomical interrelations favor certain routes of spread of disease and therefore play an important role in the development of complications (Table 25-1; Fig. 25-27).

DISEASES OF THE EXTERNAL NOSE AND NASAL VESTIBULE

Virtually all diseases of the skin can occur on the external nose, including lesions due to solar damage (e.g., actinic keratosis, basal cell carcinoma, squamous cell carcinoma, and malignant melanoma). The numerous sebaceous glands of the nose are a frequent site of acne vulgaris.

Rhinophyma refers to a protuberant bulbous mass on the nose caused by marked hyperplasia of the sebaceous glands and chronic inflammation of the skin in acne rosacea.

Pyogenic granuloma is an inflammatory lesion often seen on the anterior nasal septum. It consists of exuberant granulation tissue secondary to trauma.

NOSEBLEED (EPISTAXIS): Trauma to the nose or nasal mucosa is the most common cause of nosebleed. Hypertension, a variety of hematological abnormalities, inflammatory conditions, and neoplastic diseases of the nasal mucosa may cause bleeding from the nose. Epistaxis frequently originates in a triangular area of the anterior nasal septum called *Little area.* In this region, the epidermis is thin, and not infrequently, numerous dilated blood vessels, or telangiectasias, are apparent. Little area is also the location of ulcerations and perforations, which may be caused by various diseases or by trauma to the nasal septum (Table 25-2).

DISEASES OF THE NASAL CAVITY AND PARANASAL SINUSES

Rhinitis Is Usually Viral or Allergic

Rhinitis is defined as inflammation of the mucous membranes of the nasal cavity and sinuses. The causes range from the common cold to unusual infections such as diphtheria, anthrax, and glanders.

TABLE 25-1 Pathological Processes in the Nose and Paranasal Sinuses and Their Relation to Adjacent Structures

Nasopharynx ⇌ Nasal cavity	⇌ Maxillary sinus ⇌ Intraorbital, oral, and odontogenic disease
	⇌ Ethmoid sinuses ⇌ Intraorbital and intracranial disease
	⇌ Frontal sinus ⇌ Intraorbital and intracranial disease
	⇌ Sphenoid sinus ⇌ Cranial and intracranial disease

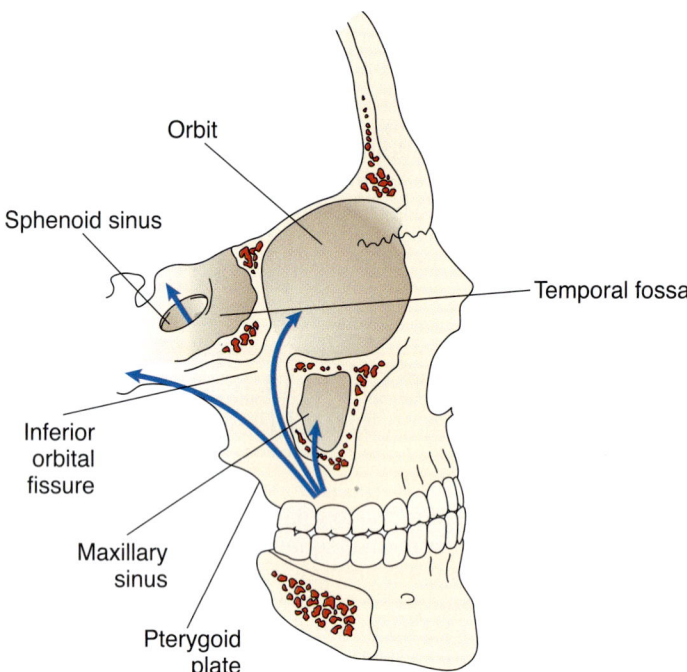

FIGURE 25-27
Pathways of infection to the intracranial cavity. Osseous pathways of infection from the jaws. *Arrows*, the direction of spread from the teeth to the maxillary sinus and through the inferior orbital fissure to the orbit. A deeper route is along the lateral pterygoid lamina up to the base of the skull, where, medial to the foramen ovale, a small aperture admits the vein of Vesalius. Through this small vein, the pterygoid plexus communicates with the cavernous sinus.

VIRAL RHINITIS: The most common cause of acute rhinitis is viral infection, especially the common cold *(acute coryza)*. In viral rhinitis, the agent replicates in the epithelial cells, after which the degenerating epithelial cells are shed. The mucosa is edematous and engorged and is infiltrated by neutrophils and mononuclear cells. Clinically, mucosal swelling is manifested as nasal stuffiness. Abundant mucus secretion and increased vascular permeability lead to *rhinorrhea* (the free discharge of a thin nasal mucus).

Viral rhinitis is usually followed within a few days by secondary infections caused by the normal denizens of the nasal and pharyngeal mucus. The abundant serous discharge then becomes mucopurulent, after which the surface epithelium is shed. The epithelial cells regenerate rapidly after the inflammation subsides.

ALLERGIC RHINITIS: Numerous allergens are constantly present in our environment, and sensitivity to any one of them can cause allergic rhinitis. In this condition, airborne allergenic particles (e.g., pollens, molds, animal allergens) are deposited on the nasal mucosa. Often called *hay fever*, allergic rhinitis may be acute and seasonal or chronic and perennial.

TABLE 25-2 **Causes of Perforation of the Nasal Septum**

Trauma
Specific infections (tuberculosis, syphilis, leprosy)
Wegener granulomatosis
Lupus erythematosus
Chronic exposure to dust (containing arsenic, chromium, copper, etc.)
Cocaine abuse
Malignant tumors

 Pathogenesis: The few plasma cells present in the nasal mucosa normally produce immunoglobulin E (IgE). Mast cells in the nasal mucosa or free in nasal secretions also bear specific IgE directed against allergens. On contact with an allergen, the mast cells release cytoplasmic granules containing a variety of chemical mediators and enzymes. Some mediators are preformed and thus act rapidly (e.g., histamine); others are slowly eluted from the granule matrix (e.g., heparin or trypsin); and still others are newly synthesized (e.g., leukotrienes). Thus, an immediate, rapidly apparent reaction may give way to a prolonged inflammatory reaction as the various mediators exert their specific effects. The released mediators cause the signs and symptoms of allergic rhinitis, and many of the responses are attributable to histamine acting through its H_1 receptor.

 Pathology: The increased capillary permeability mediated by vasodilator substances results in edema of the nasal mucosa, especially of the inferior turbinates. Microscopic examination of the nasal secretions or mucosa reveals numerous eosinophils. The late phase of mast cell–mediated reactions is associated with persistent edema of the nasal mucosa and is seen clinically as nasal obstruction.

CHRONIC RHINITIS: Repeated bouts of acute rhinitis may lead to the development of chronic rhinitis. Often a deviated nasal septum is a contributory factor. Chronic rhinitis is characterized by thickening of the nasal mucosa because of persistent hyperemia, hyperplasia of the mucous glands, and **infiltration by lymphocytes and plasma cells.**

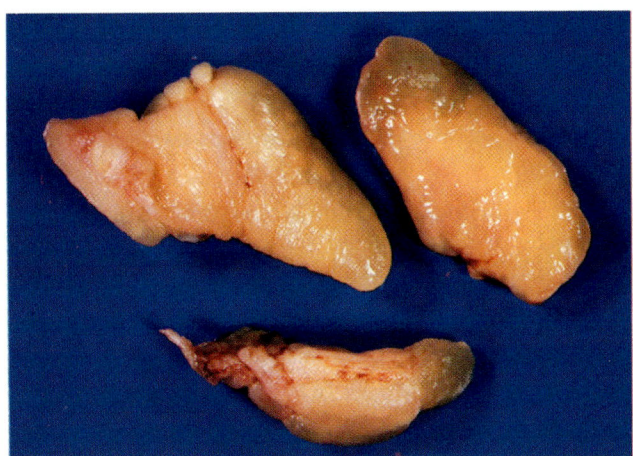

FIGURE 25-28
Nasal polyps. These smooth, pale, polypoid masses were removed from a patient with chronic rhinitis.

Nasal Polyps Are Focal Inflammatory Swellings

Sinonasal inflammatory polyps are nonneoplastic lesions of the mucosa. Most polyps arise from the lateral nasal wall or the ethmoid recess. They may be unilateral or bilateral, single or multiple. Symptoms include nasal obstruction, rhinorrhea, and headaches. The etiology involves multiple factors, including allergy, cystic fibrosis, infections, diabetes mellitus, and aspirin intolerance (Fig. 25-28).

Microscopically, sinonasal allergic polyps are lined externally by respiratory epithelium and contain mucous glands within a loose mucoid stroma, which is infiltrated by plasma cells, lymphocytes, and numerous eosinophils. Thickening of the basement membrane and goblet cell hyperplasia are usually prominent (Fig. 25-29).

Sinusitis Is a Bacterial Infection

Sinusitis refers to an inflammation of the mucous membranes of the paranasal sinuses.

 Pathogenesis: Any condition (inflammation, neoplasm, foreign body) that interferes with drainage or aeration of a sinus renders it liable to infection. If the ostium of a sinus is blocked, the secretion or exudate accumulates behind the obstruction.

Acute sinusitis is a disorder of less than 3 weeks' duration, caused predominantly by the extension of infection from the nasal mucosa. In most cases, a rich bacterial flora is found, with *Haemophilus influenzae* and *Branhamella catarrhalis* most frequently present. Maxillary sinusitis may also be due to odontogenic infections, in which case, bacteria from the roots of the first and second molar teeth penetrate the thin bony plate that separates them from the floor of the maxillary sinus.

Chronic sinusitis is a sequel of acute inflammation, either as a result of incomplete resolution of the infection or because of recurrent acute complications. In contrast to acute sinusitis, the purulent exudate in chronic sinusitis almost always includes anaerobic bacteria.

 Pathology: Acute or chronic sinusitis may be followed by a number of complications:

- **Mucocele:** *The term* mucocele *refers to the accumulation of mucous secretions in a nasal sinus.* Infection of a mucocele results in a sinus filled with mucopurulent exudate, termed *pyocele*. Purulent exudate in the sinus is termed *empyema* (Fig. 25-30). Mucoceles occur most often in the anterior compartments ("cells") of the ethmoid sinus and in the frontal sinus. The lesions develop slowly and by pressure cause resorption of bone (pressure atrophy). Mucoceles of the anterior ethmoid or frontal sinuses may be large enough to displace the contents of the orbit and occasionally may erode into the central nervous system.
- **Osteomyelitis:** Bone infection results from the extension of a suppurative infection in the frontal sinus to the bone. Infection of the walls of a nasal sinus may spread through Volkmann canals to the periosteum, producing periostitis and a subperiosteal abscess. If these occur on the orbital side of the bone, orbital cellulitis or an orbital abscess forms. The skin overlying the infection is often markedly edematous, and subcutaneous cellulitis or a subcutaneous abscess also may develop. Osteomyelitis also may spread rapidly between the outer and inner tables of the skull.

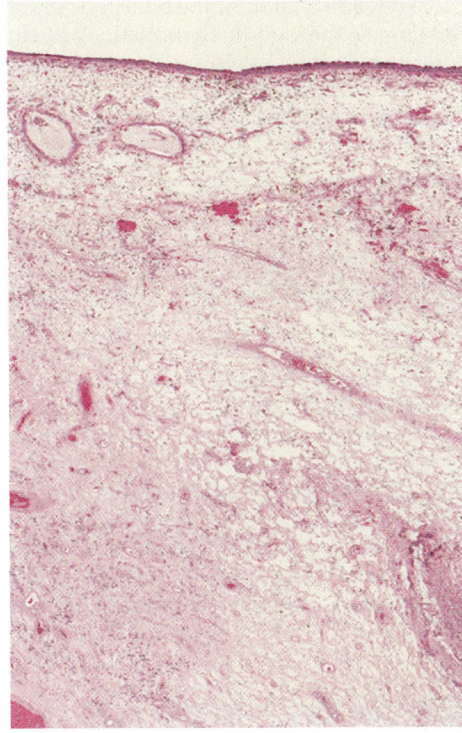

FIGURE 25-29
Nasal inflammatory polyp. An intranasal mass features an intact surface epithelium *(top)* and an edematous stroma, with a chronic inflammatory cell infiltrate.

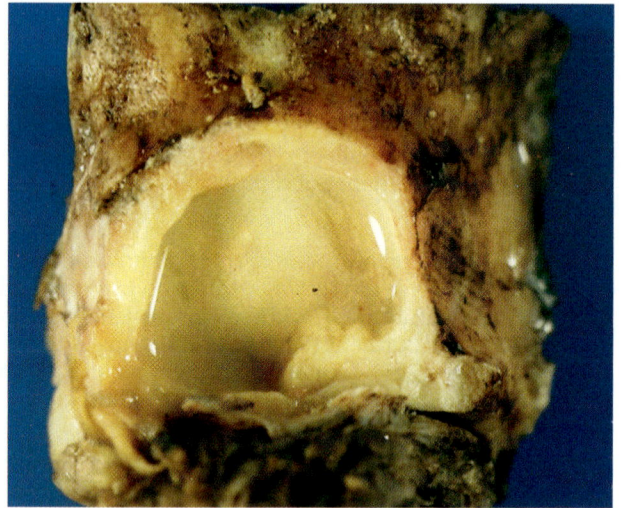

FIGURE 25-30
Empyema of the maxillary sinus (sagittal section). Infection followed chronic obstruction of the orifice caused by adenocarcinoma of the nasal mucosa.

- **Septic thrombophlebitis:** Infection in the sinuses may penetrate the bone and spread to the frontal and diploe venous systems. The spread of septic thrombophlebitis to the cavernous venous sinus through the superior ophthalmic veins is a life-threatening complication.
- **Intracranial infections:** Spread of infection to the cranial cavity also may complicate sinusitis. Lesions include epidural, subdural, and cerebral abscesses and purulent leptomeningitis. These consequences may develop without extensive destruction of the bone, because the infection can spread through the lymphatics or veins. Before the days of chemotherapy, these dreaded complications often led to death within a few days. With proper treatment, they are today uncommon.

Syphilis May Destroy the Nasal Bridge

Although a primary chancre in the nose is rare, the mucosal lesions of secondary syphilis are commonly observed in the nose and nasopharynx. In tertiary syphilis, the inflammatory process may involve large portions of the nasal mucosa, the underlying cartilage, and bone. Perichondrial or periosteal gummas may destroy nasal cartilage and bone. The ensuing collapse of the nasal bridge produces so-called saddle nose. Destruction of the bony walls of the nose may also lead to perforation of the nasal septum, hard palate, wall of the orbit, or maxillary sinus. For the full spectrum of syphilis, see Chapter 9.

Leprosy Is Spread through Nasal Secretions

Because *Mycobacterium leprae* multiplies more readily at a lower body temperature, it frequently infects cooler body sites, such as the nares and the anterior nasal mucosa. Indeed, nasal involvement is commonly the first manifestation of leprosy.

 Pathology: The skin around the nares and the anterior nasal mucosa shows nodules, ulceration, or perforations. Nasal involvement is important because leprosy is spread through nasal secretions that teem with bacilli. Tuberculoid and intermediate forms of leprosy, which account for most cases, are microscopically characterized by chronic granulomatous inflammation. Patients with deficient cellular immunity develop lepromatous leprosy, in which numerous foamy macrophages (so-called lepra cells) contain many phagocytosed mycobacteria. Leprosy is discussed in more detail in Chapter 9.

Rhinoscleroma Is a Chronic Bacterial Infection of the Nose

Rhinoscleroma (scleroma) is a chronic inflammatory process that usually begins in the nose and remains localized to that site, although it may extend slowly into the nasopharynx, larynx, and trachea. Rarely, rhinoscleroma is seen in other locations, including the paranasal sinuses, orbital tissues, skin, lips, oral mucosa, gastrointestinal tract, and cervical lymph nodes. Cases of intracranial invasion also have been described.

 Epidemiology: Rhinoscleroma is endemic in some Mediterranean countries and in parts of Asia, Africa, and Latin America. Indigenous cases also have been recognized in the United States. The disease occurs in both sexes and at any age. Poor domestic and personal hygiene are common to most patients. Epidemiological evidence suggests that household relationships are the decisive factor in the development of this disorder.

 Pathogenesis: Although the gram-negative diplobacillus, *Klebsiella rhinoscleromatis*, also known as *von Frisch bacillus*, was identified more than a century ago, Koch's postulates were fulfilled only in the 1970s. Experimental disease was produced by repeatedly injecting bacilli suspended in sterile mucin into the same site. The organisms are present in the throats of many healthy persons, but the mode of transmission is unknown.

 Pathology: The infected tissues appear firm, greatly thickened, irregularly nodular, and often ulcerated. Microscopically, the granulation tissue is strikingly rich in plasma cells, lymphocytes, and foamy macrophages (Fig. 25-31). The characteristic large macrophages, referred to as *Mikulicz cells*, contain masses of phagocytosed bacilli.

Diseases of the Nasal Cavity and Paranasal Sinuses

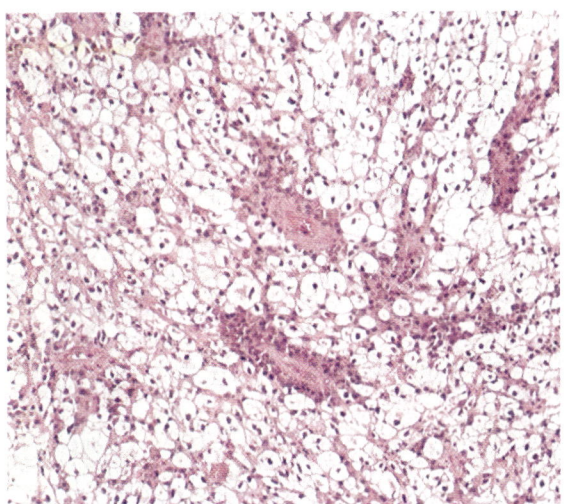

FIGURE 25-31
Scleroma. Granulation tissue contains numerous foamy macrophages (Mikulicz cells).

Serological tests are valuable in establishing the diagnosis of rhinoscleroma, because specific antibodies are present in many patients. The disease is successfully treated with various antibiotics.

Fungal Infections Are Usually Opportunistic

Pathogenic fungi occasionally involve the nose and paranasal sinuses as part of a cutaneous or mucocutaneous infection, particularly in immunodeficient persons.

Candidiasis is the most common fungal infection of the nasal mucosa, usually accompanying oral and pharyngeal candidiasis (*thrush*).

Aspergillosis is uncommon and generally occurs in a paranasal sinus. The fungi may disseminate to the venous sinuses, meninges, and brain. Aspergillosis of the sinonasal tract may be noninvasive or invasive. Noninvasive types of aspergillus sinusitis include allergic fungal sinusitis (AFS) and sinus mycetoma (so-called fungus balls).

AFS represents a hypersensitivity reaction to fungal antigens and occurs in patients who are atopic or immunologically "hypercompetent." The pathogenesis of AFS is similar to that of allergic bronchopulmonary aspergillosis. The disease occurs at all ages but is most commonly seen in children or young adults. It primarily involves the maxillary and ethmoid sinuses, although any sinus may be involved.

Fungus balls or aspergilloma occur in immunologically competent patients, usually with chronic sinus disease associated with poor drainage. In this setting, the fungus can proliferate and form a dense mass of hyphae that causes nasal obstruction (Fig. 25-32). Evidence of bone destruction and ocular symptoms may be present.

Invasive fungal sinusitis usually affects immunocompromised or immunosuppressed patients. In the rare *rhinocerebral aspergillosis,* the organisms disseminate to the venous sinuses, meninges, and brain, and few patients survive.

Rhinosporidiosis of the nose is produced by the enigmatic *Rhinosporidium seeberi,* an organism whose source remains unknown. The microbe is classified among the fungi, although it has not been grown in culture and has not been transmitted experimentally. The disease is endemic in Sri Lanka and in parts of India, Central America, and South America.

The nasal mucosa afflicted with rhinosporidiosis contains vascular polypoid masses. Occasionally, similar lesions occur in the mucosa of other parts of the upper respiratory tract, the conjunctiva, the ear, or the skin. Microscopically, the polyps show marked chronic inflammation and characteristic

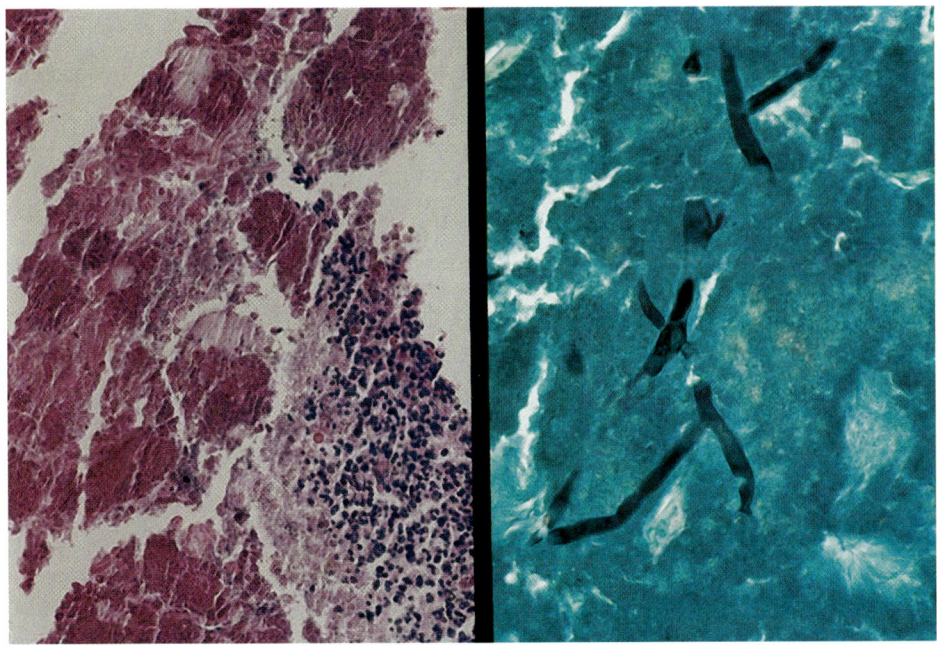

FIGURE 25-32
Allergic fungal sinusitis. (*Left panel*) Allergic mucin appears as amorphous, acellular eosinophilic material; adjacent mixed inflammatory cell infiltrate is present. (*Right panel*) *Aspergillus* species are branched septate fungi (Gomori methenamine silver stain).

spherical sporangia. The sporangia, 50 to 350 μm in diameter, have a thick, homogeneous wall and contain clear cytoplasm and innumerable small endospores. The rupture of the sporangia evokes a foreign-body giant cell reaction. The treatment of choice is surgical removal of the lesions.

Leishmaniasis

The nose is a frequent site of the mucocutaneous form of leishmaniasis, caused by *Leishmania braziliensis* (see Chapter 9). The nasal disease, known as *espundia*, occurs in Central and South America. The initial lesion is a cutaneous sore that heals within a few months. In some patients, mucocutaneous lesions develop in the nose or upper lip after an interval of months or years. The infection probably spreads by nasal contact with contaminated fingers.

 Pathology: The infected mucosa exhibits polypoid inflammatory lesions and superficial ulcers. In the earlier phases of the infection, many macrophages contain parasites. Later, a tuberculoid type of granulomatous response develops. Such lesions contain few recognizable parasites. Bacterial infection may supervene and lead to destruction of the soft tissues and collapse of the anterior cartilaginous nasal septum.

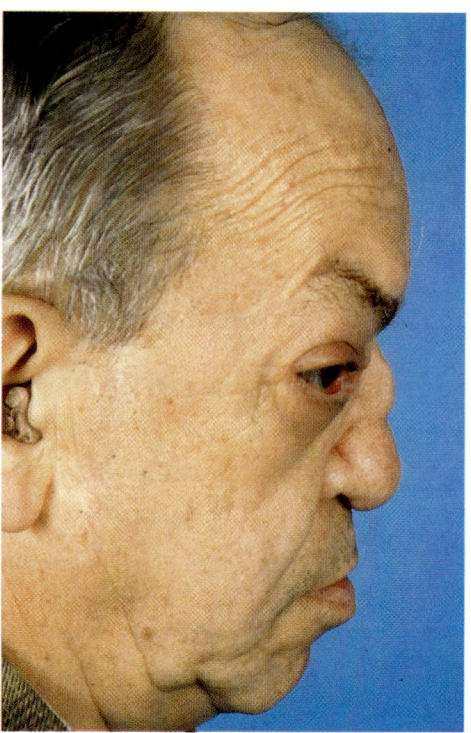

FIGURE 25-33
Saddle nose deformity of Wegener granulomatosis.

Wegener Granulomatosis May Manifest in the Nose

Wegener granulomatosis affects the lower airways (see Chapter 10).

 Pathology: In its fully developed form, this uncommon disease involves the lungs, kidneys, and small arteries throughout the body. The sinonasal tract may be affected as part of the systemic process or may have disease localized to this region. The disease often first manifests as septal perforation and mucosal ulceration. There is slowly progressive destruction of the nose and paranasal sinuses with development of saddle nose deformity (Fig. 25-33). The resulting "runny nose," sinusitis, and nosebleeds may be accompanied by constitutional symptoms, such as fever, malaise, and weight loss. Microscopically, the nasal lesions reveal ischemic-type necrosis, vasculitis, mixed chronic inflammatory cell infiltrate, scattered multinucleated giant cells, and microabscess formation. Well-formed granulomas are not seen in Wegener granulomatosis. Elevated serum levels of antineutrophil cytoplasmic antibodies (ANCA) are associated with active disease.

Nasal-Type Angiocentric T-Cell/Natural Killer (T/NK)-Cell Lymphoma Is an Aggressive, Highly Lethal Disease

Nasal-type angiocentric T/NK-cell lymphoma *has supplanted the previous designations of* lethal midline granuloma, midline malignant reticulosis, *and* polymorphic reticulosis. *Nasal-type angiocentric T/NK cell lymphoma manifests as necrotizing, ulcerating mucosal lesions of the upper respiratory tract* (Fig. 25-34A). If untreated, the lymphoma is invariably fatal.

 Pathology: The polymorphism of the atypical lymphocytic infiltrate is a characteristic feature that distinguishes the nasal-type T/NK-cell lymphoma from a conventional lymphoma. Similar necrotizing infiltrates can also occur in the upper airways, lungs, and alimentary tract, but any organ may be involved. Characteristically, the malignant cellular infiltrate surrounds small-to-medium-sized blood vessels (angiocentric) and infiltrates through the vascular wall (angioinvasive), often occluding the lumen in a thrombuslike manner and resulting in adjacent tissue necrosis (ischemic-type) (Fig. 25-34B). An association with EBV infection has been established with this type of lymphoma.

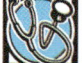 Clinical Features: The clinical course of nasal-type T/NK-cell lymphoma is characterized by an insidious onset, with symptoms of nonspecific rhinitis or sinusitis. Gradually, the nasal mucosa becomes

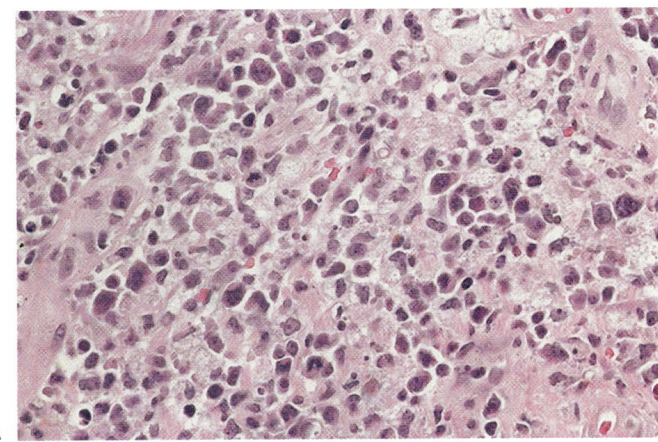
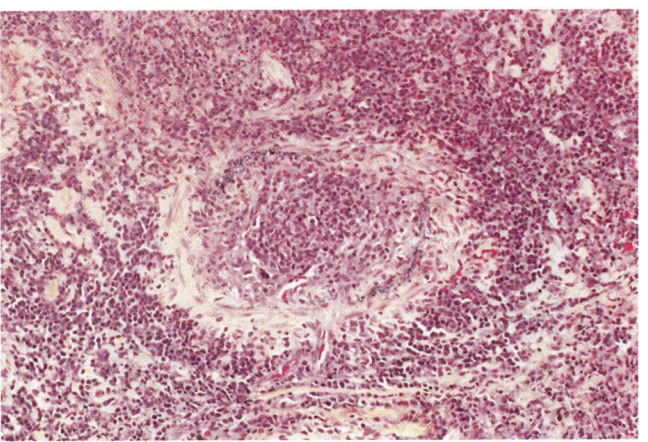

FIGURE 25-34
Angiocentric T/NK cell lymphoma. A. A malignant cellular infiltrate shows dyshesive cell growth; special stains confirmed this infiltrate as a lymphoma. B. Cellular infiltrate growing around and into a medium-sized blood vessel with disruption of the external elastic membrane and occlusion of the vessel lumen (elastic stain).

focally swollen and indurated and eventually ulcerated. The ulcers are covered by a black crust, under which the lesions progress to erode cartilage and bone. This destruction causes defects of the nasal septum, hard palate, and nasopharynx, with serious functional consequences. Frequently, the skin of the midface also becomes involved, hence the descriptive name *lethal midline granuloma*. In half of patients, the disease remains localized, but an equal proportion exhibit widespread dissemination of the lymphoma. Unlike Wegener granulomatosis, serum levels of ANCA are not elevated in nasal-type T/NK-cell lymphoma. Death is due to secondary bacterial infection, aspiration pneumonia, or hemorrhage from an eroded large blood vessel.

The infiltrates of nasal-type T/NK cell lymphoma are, at least initially, radiosensitive, and remission with cytotoxic agents has also been reported.

Benign Tumors of the Nose

SQUAMOUS PAPILLOMA: The most frequent benign tumor of the nasal cavity is squamous papilloma, which almost always occurs in the nasal vestibule. The lesion is often indistinguishable from a wart (verruca vulgaris).

INVERTED PAPILLOMA: This tumor involves the lateral nasal wall and may spread into the paranasal sinuses. Inverted papillomas occur mainly in middle-aged persons. As the name implies, they show characteristic inversions of the surface epithelium into the underlying stroma (Fig. 25-35). HPV types 6/11 and rarely other types (16/18, 33, 40, 57) have been found in inverted papillomas, but a cause-and-effect relationship remains to be proved. Although histologically benign, the tumors may erode bone by pressure. Unless surgical resection extends beyond the boundaries of the grossly visible lesion, they frequently recur. In 5% of cases, inverted papillomas give rise to squamous cell carcinoma.

Malignant Tumors of the Nose

Carcinomas of the Nasal Cavity and Paranasal Sinuses

More than half of carcinomas of the nasal cavity and paranasal sinuses originate in the antrum of the maxillary si-

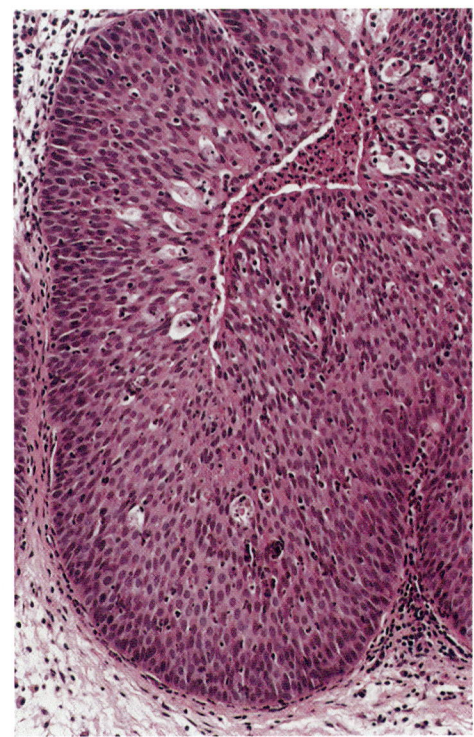

FIGURE 25-35
Sinonasal inverted papilloma. Epithelial nests are growing downward (inverted) into the submucosa. They are composed of a uniform cellular proliferation, which displays an inflammatory cell infiltrate and scattered microcysts.

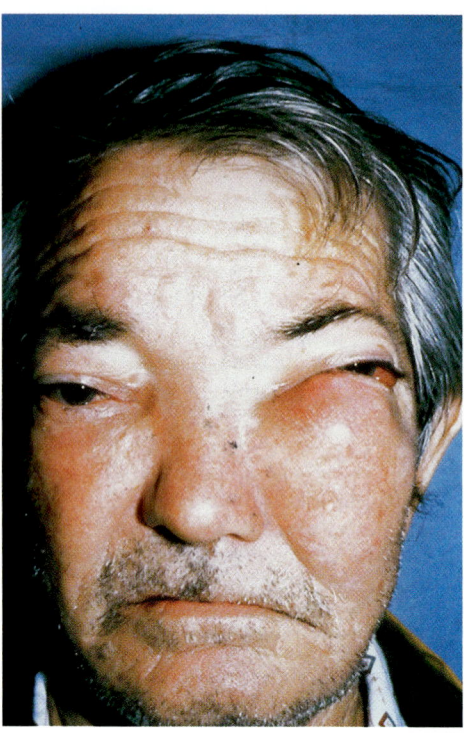

FIGURE 25-36
Squamous cell carcinoma of the maxillary sinus caused an obvious facial deformity, owing to invasion outside the confines of the sinus. Involvement of the orbit and facial nerve is evident. The latter is defined by drooping of the mouth to the side of the facial nerve paralysis.

nus, one third in the nasal cavity, 10% in the ethmoid sinus, and 1% in the sphenoid and frontal sinuses (Fig. 25-36). Most cancers of the nasal cavity and paranasal sinuses are squamous cell tumors. Some 15% are adenocarcinomas, transitional cell carcinomas, or undifferentiated carcinomas.

 Pathogenesis: Several industrial chemicals have been implicated in the causation of cancer of the nose and sinuses, including nickel, chromium, and aromatic hydrocarbons. Occupational settings that reportedly carry an increased risk for cancer of the nose and sinuses (but for which a specific chemical agent has not been identified) are woodworking in the furniture industry, the use of cutting oils, and employment in the leather textile industries.

Tumors in nickel workers are squamous cell cancers, which usually arise from the middle turbinate. The latency period varies from 2 to 32 years. The tumors related to other occupational exposures are predominantly adenocarcinomas and occur mostly in the maxillary and ethmoid sinuses. Because of the industrial setting in which many cancers of the nose and sinuses arise, they are much more common in men and occur after age 50 years.

Cancers of the nasal cavity and sinuses grow relentlessly and invade adjacent structures but typically do not give rise to distant metastases. The usual survival is only a few years.

Olfactory Neuroblastoma

Olfactory neuroblastoma (esthesioneuroblastoma) is an unusual malignant tumor of the nose of likely neural crest origin. The tumor has a slight male predominance and occurs over a wide age range from 3 years to the ninth decade.

Pathology: This cancer arises from the olfactory mucosa that covers the superior third of the nasal septum, the cribriform plate, and the superior turbinate. Olfactory neuroblastoma is usually polypoid and highly vascular and displays diverse histological patterns, depending on the amount of intercellular neurofibrillary material (Fig. 25-37). The tumor cells are slightly larger than lymphocytes, exhibit round nuclei with an even distribution of chromatin, and have an inconspicuous cytoplasm. In some cases, the tumor cells form pseudorosettes (Homer Wright rosettes) or true neural rosettes (Flexner-Wintersteiner rosettes). By electron microscopy, olfactory neuroblastoma reveals intracytoplasmic secretory granules and cytoplasmic

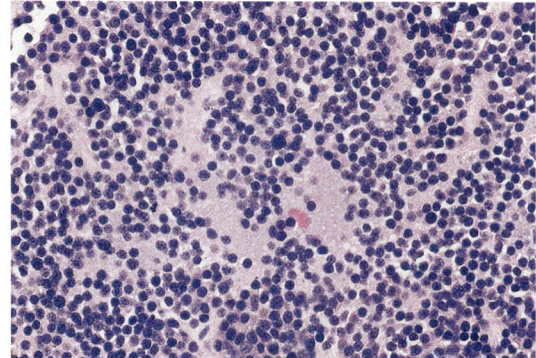
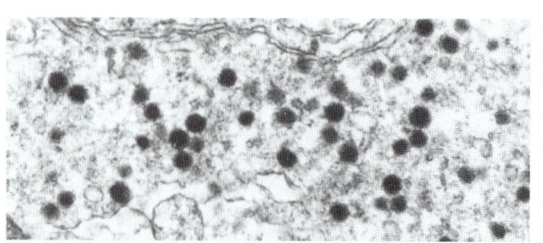

FIGURE 25-37
Olfactory neuroblastoma. **A.** This tumor is composed of small round cells with hyperchromatic nuclei and a background eosinophilic stroma representing neurofibrillary matrix. **B.** An electron micrograph shows intracytoplasmic, secretory-type, membrane-bound granules with dense cores.

fibrils and microtubules, similar to those of neuroblastomas at other sites (Fig.25-37B).

 Clinical Features: Olfactory neuroblastomas slowly invade and destroy bony structures and are readily spread through the lymphatics to involve regional and distant lymph nodes. Hematogenous metastases are less frequent. The 5-year survival rate is 50%, and death is usually due to invasion of the cranial cavity.

Nasopharynx

ANATOMY AND FUNCTION

The nasopharynx is continuous anteriorly with the nasal cavities; its roof is formed by the body of the sphenoid bone, and its posterior wall is formed by the cervical vertebrae. On the lateral walls of the nasopharynx are the openings of the eustachian tubes.

The nasopharynx of the newborn is covered by pseudostratified ciliated columnar epithelium. With advancing age, it is replaced by a stratified squamous epithelium over large areas (80%). The mucosa contains numerous mucous glands and abundant lymphoid tissue.

WALDEYER RING: The circular band of lymphoid tissue located at the opening of the oropharynx into the respiratory and digestive tracts is referred to as Waldeyer ring. The lymphoid tissue on the superior posterior wall forms the nasopharyngeal tonsils, which, when hyperplastic, are better known as adenoids. The palatine tonsils, situated laterally where the pharynx connects with the oral cavity, are covered by stratified squamous epithelium, which dips into the lymphoid tissue and lines the infoldings (crypts). The crypts normally contain desquamated epithelium, lymphocytes, some neutrophils, and saprophytic organisms, including bacteria, *Candida*, and actinomycetes. Virulent pathogens may also be present in the pharynx of healthy persons (e.g., *C. diphtheriae*, meningococcus).

Waldeyer ring is well developed in children and contains follicles with germinal centers. In fact, the largest collection of B lymphocytes in the normal child is found in the tonsils. The pharyngeal lymphoid tissue diminishes considerably on reaching adulthood, and with increasing age, it gradually involutes but does not totally disappear. Tonsillectomy and adenoidectomy, less widely practiced today than formerly, result in a major loss of pharyngeal lymphoid tissue. The removal of tonsils and adenoids is not followed by a decrease in serum immunoglobulins and does not alter the serological response to several human respiratory viruses. However, secretory IgA is decreased locally in the nasopharynx. Interestingly, tonsillectomy triples the risk of developing Hodgkin disease later in life.

HYPOPLASIA AND HYPERPLASIA OF PHARYNGEAL LYMPHOID TISSUE

Bruton sex-linked agammaglobulinemia represents a congenital absence of pharyngeal lymphoid tissue (see Chapter 4). This familial disease affects only male offspring, who have minimal or no lymphoid tissue in their tonsils, pharynx, and intestines (Peyer patches and appendix). On the other hand, they have a normally developed thymus.

Atrophy of pharyngeal lymphoid tissue is commonly seen in advanced states of AIDS and in chronically immunosuppressed patients. Local radiation therapy also results in marked loss of lymphoid tissue in Waldeyer ring.

Hyperplasia of nasopharyngeal lymphoid tissue follows infections or chronic irritation of the pharynx by dust, smoke, and fumes. In some primary immunodeficiency syndromes (dysgammaglobulinemia type I or nodular lymphoid hyperplasia), the tonsils may be enlarged, presumably reflecting an adaptive response by the immune system.

INFLAMMATION

Pharyngitis and tonsillitis are among the most common diseases of the head and neck. Inflammation of the nasopharynx occurs predominantly in children, although it is also frequent in adolescence and in early adulthood. Viral or bacterial infections may be limited to the palatine tonsils, but the nasopharyngeal tonsils or adjacent pharyngeal mucosa may also be involved, often as part of a general upper respiratory tract infection. In the latter case, the initial infecting agent is most often a virus spread by droplet or by direct contact. Viral pharyngitis is usually caused by influenza, parainfluenza, adenovirus, respiratory syncytial virus, and rhinovirus.

Infectious mononucleosis is often accompanied by a sore throat. Unlike most other viral diseases, infectious mononucleosis typically produces an exudative pharyngitis.

S. pyogenes is the most important cause of pharyngitis and tonsillitis, because of the possibility of serious suppurative and nonsuppurative sequelae. **Diphtheria** is still an important cause of pharyngitis in some countries. These infections are characterized by an exudate or, in the case of diphtheria, a pseudomembrane, on the tonsils and pharynx.

Acute tonsillitis is a bacterial infection, usually with *S. pyogenes* (group A β-hemolytic streptococci). Follicular tonsillitis is characterized by pinpoint exudates that can be extruded from the crypts.

Pseudomembranous tonsillitis refers to a necrotic mucosa covered by a coat of exudate, for instance in diphtheria or in *Vincent angina*. The latter is caused by fusiform bacilli and spirochetes that are present in the normal bacterial flora of the mouth. These organisms become pathogenic when the local or systemic resistance is low (e.g., after mucosal injury or in malnutrition).

Recurrent or chronic tonsillitis is not as common as once believed, and enlarged tonsils in children do not necessarily mean chronic tonsillitis. However, repeated infections can cause enlargement of the tonsils and adenoids to a degree that may obstruct the air passages. In children, repeated bouts of streptococcal tonsillitis may be associated with rheumatic fever or glomerulonephritis, and the patient may benefit from tonsillectomy.

Peritonsillar abscess (quinsy) is usually the sequel of inappropriately treated acute bacterial tonsillitis. If it is not recognized and managed appropriately, it may lead to several life-threatening situations: (1) aided by gravity, it may dissect inferiorly to the pyriform sinus, with obstruction of, or rupture into, the airway; (2) a peritonsillar abscess may extend laterally into the parapharyngeal space (parapharyngeal abscess) and weaken the wall of the carotid artery; or (3) the abscess may penetrate along the carotid sheath inferiorly into the mediastinum or, superiorly, to the base of the skull or into the cranial cavity, with disastrous consequences.

Adenoids is a term that stems from the time when lymph nodes were called lymph "glands" and lymphoid tissue was thought to be "glandlike." Adenoids represent chronic inflammatory hyperplasia of the pharyngeal lymphoid tissue. This condition is often accompanied by chronic tonsillitis or rhinitis, almost always in children. Enlarged adenoids may cause partial or complete block of the eustachian tube, leading to otitis media.

TUMORS OF THE NASOPHARYNX

Juvenile Nasopharyngeal Angiofibroma Is a Tumor of Adolescent Boys

Juvenile angiofibroma is an uncommon, highly vascular neoplasm of the nasopharynx, which is histologically benign but locally aggressive.

Pathology: The tumor is rounded or nodular and has a sessile or pedunculated attachment to the upper posterior or lateral nasopharyngeal wall. Angiofibroma may grow into the fissures and foramina of the skull or may destroy bone and spread into adjacent structures, such as the nasal cavity, paranasal sinuses, orbit, middle cranial fossa, or pterygomaxillary fossa.

Histologically, angiofibroma has vascular and stromal components (Fig. 25-38). The blood vessels vary in size and shape, and their walls are characterized by the absence of a smooth muscle layer or the presence of irregularly arranged smooth muscle. These defects in the vessel wall preclude vasoconstriction, thereby contributing to brisk bleeding after trauma. Biopsies are, therefore, dangerous and contraindicated. Although many surgeons still advocate a surgical approach, good results can be obtained with radiation therapy.

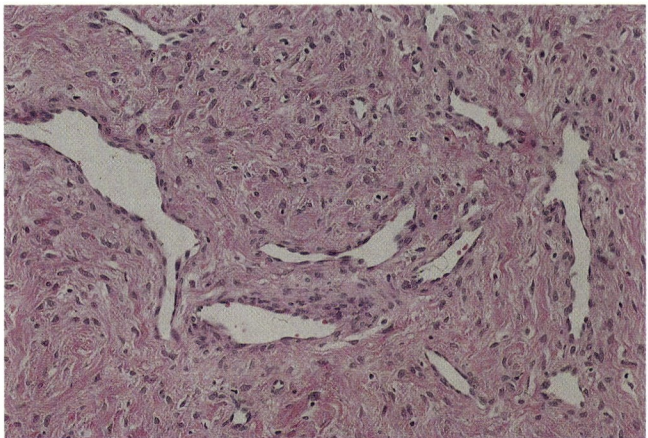

FIGURE 25-38
Nasopharyngeal angiofibroma is composed of slitlike vascular structures in a collagenous stroma.

Squamous Cell Carcinoma

The oropharynx, including the tonsillar bed and the anterior and posterior faucial pillars, is a common site for squamous carcinomas. These tumors tend to be less differentiated and biologically more aggressive than their counterparts in the anterior oral cavity. SCCs of the oropharynx often metastasize early because of the rich lymphatic network in this region. The primary lymphatics drain into the superior deep jugular and submandibular lymph nodes and, to a somewhat lesser degree, into the retropharyngeal lymph nodes.

Nasopharyngeal Carcinoma Is Related to EBV

Nasopharyngeal carcinoma (NPC) is an epithelial cancer of the nasopharynx that is classified into keratinizing and nonkeratinizing subtypes. Nonkeratinizing carcinoma is associated with EBV infection.

 Epidemiology: *The undifferentiated subtype of nonkeratinizing carcinoma is particularly common in southeast Asia and parts of Africa.* By far the most common cancer of the nasopharynx, nasopharyngeal carcinoma is the most frequent of all malignant tumors in the Chinese. In Hong Kong, nasopharyngeal undifferentiated carcinoma represents 18% of all cancers, compared with a worldwide prevalence of 0.25%. Chinese born in the United States have about a 20-fold greater mortality from carcinoma of the nasopharynx than do persons of other races. There is also a high incidence in Tunisia and East Africa.

 Pathogenesis: Various environmental risk factors for nasopharyngeal carcinoma (diet, inhalation of various substances, ethnic customs) have been sought, but no association has been positively demonstrated. Recent studies point to a possible combined role for environmental and genetic factors in the pathogenesis of nasopharyngeal carcinoma. There is an association with the A2/sin HLA profile in the Chinese, suggesting a genetic susceptibility.

EBV is present in the tumor cells and B lymphocytes of patients with NPC. Moreover, 85% of patients also have antibodies to EBV and contain anti-EBV IgA in the serum. EBV genomes are detected in 75 to 100% of nonkeratinizing and undifferentiated types of NPC. The detection of EBV genomes in the keratinizing subtype is variable and, if present, is generally limited to scattered dysplastic intraepithelial cells. For more details on EBV infection, see Chapters 5 and 9.

 Pathology: Nasopharyngeal carcinoma is seen as either keratinizing (squamous cell) tumors or nonkeratinizing ones. The keratinizing tumors occur in an older population and do not bear the same relation to EBV infection as do the nonkeratinizing types. The latter are classified as differentiated or undifferentiated. Differentiated nonkeratinizing nasopharyngeal carcinomas display a stratified appearance and distinct cell margins. By contrast,

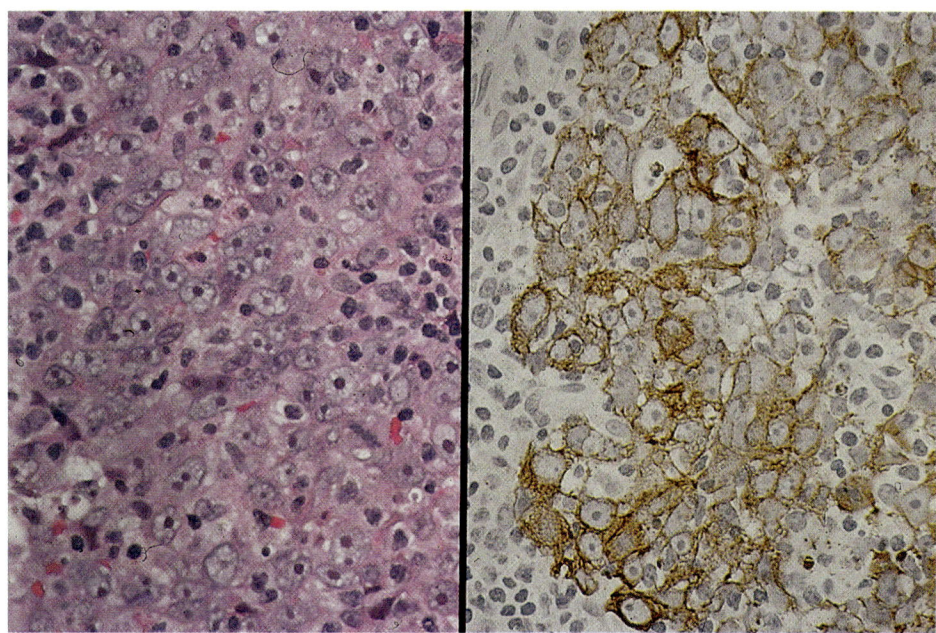

FIGURE 25-39
Nasopharyngeal nonkeratinizing carcinoma, undifferentiated type. The *left panel* shows the presence of cells with large nuclei and prominent eosinophilic nucleoli. The *right panel* shows that these cells are cytokeratin positive, indicating an epithelial cell proliferation.

undifferentiated tumors exhibit clusters of poorly delimited or syncytial cells bearing large oval nuclei and scant eosinophilic cytoplasm (Fig. 25-39). The undifferentiated variant often features a conspicuous lymphoid infiltrate, accounting for the obsolete (and misleading) term *lymphoepithelioma*. Both subtypes are immunoreactive with cytokeratin. The presence of cytokeratin and absence of hematological or lymphoid markers in the neoplastic cells distinguish nasopharyngeal undifferentiated carcinoma from malignant lymphoma.

Clinical Features: Because of their location, most nasopharyngeal carcinomas remain asymptomatic for a long time. Palpable cervical lymph node metastases are the first sign of disease in about half of cases, and even then, many patients have no complaints referable to the nasopharynx. The tumor infiltrates neighboring regions, such as the parapharyngeal space, orbit, and cranial cavity, resulting in neurological symptoms and disturbances of hearing. Invasion of the base of the skull leads to involvement of the cranial nerves. Neoplasms growing in the fossa of Rosenmüller and in the lateral wall of the nasopharynx produce symptoms referable to the middle ear. Obstruction of the eustachian tube is common. The rich lymphatic network draining the nasopharynx is the route of frequent and early metastases to the cervical lymph nodes.

Nasopharyngeal undifferentiated carcinoma is radiosensitive, and more than half of patients with tumor restricted to the nasopharynx survive 5 or more years. Metastasis to the cervical lymph nodes considerably reduces the survival rate, and cranial nerve involvement or distant metastasis carries a dismal prognosis.

Lymphomas of Waldeyer Ring Are Mostly Diffuse B-Cell Tumors

Lymphomas constitute 5% of head and neck cancers. In this region, Waldeyer ring is by far the most common site of origin of lymphoma. The palatine tonsils are the most common primary site of lymphoma, followed by the lymphoid tissue of the nasopharynx and the base of the tongue. Enlargement of a single tonsil in any age group, or bilateral painless tonsillar enlargement in adults, suggests the possibility of a lymphoma. In these cases, the cervical lymph nodes are most often involved by metastases.

Histologically, 90% of nasopharyngeal lymphomas are diffuse, and more than half have been classified as large cell lymphomas. In the United States and Asia, the vast majority of lymphomas of Waldeyer's ring are of B-cell origin.

Plasmacytoma

Three fourths of all extramedullary plasmacytomas occur in the head and neck, with a strong predilection for the nasopharynx, nasal cavity, and paranasal sinuses. Like extramedullary plasmacytomas in other body sites, these tumors are best considered as part of a spectrum of plasma cell disorders. The tumors may remain localized or may evolve into systemic plasma cell myeloma.

Chordoma Arises from the Remnants of the Embryonic Notochord

Chordoma, a malignant tumor derived from notochordal cellular remnants is uncommon in persons younger than the

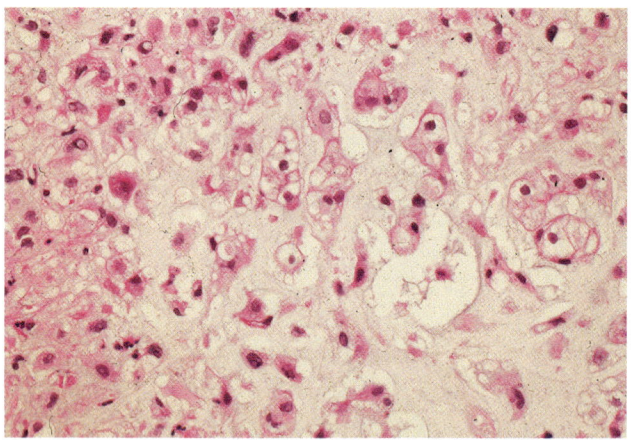

FIGURE 25-40
Chordoma. Large vacuolated (physaliferous) tumor cells are evident.

4th decade of life. In one third of cases, these tumors extend into the nasopharynx. In the cranial region, they originate from the area of the sphenooccipital synchondrosis. Histologically, they exhibit large vacuolated (*physaliferous*) cells surrounded by abundant intercellular matrix (Fig. 25-40). Chordomas usually grow slowly, but they infiltrate bone and are ordinarily not accessible to complete surgical removal. Few patients with chordomas of the cranial region survive longer than 5 years.

Other Malignant Tumors

Other malignant tumors of the nasopharynx are rare. They may arise from various components of the mucosa or adjacent supportive soft tissues and skeleton. *Embryonal rhabdomyosarcoma* (Fig. 25-41) arises in the pharyngeal tissues of young children. This highly malignant tumor invades contiguous structures and metastasizes by both the bloodstream and the lymphatics. *Kaposi sarcoma* has been reported in the nasopharyngeal mucosa of patients with AIDS.

The Ear

EXTERNAL EAR

The elastic cartilage of the auricle and that of the external ear canal are continuous and are covered by skin. The external auditory canal ends blindly at the tympanic membrane (eardrum), which separates the external ear from the middle ear. The outer surface of this airtight membrane is covered by squamous epithelium, which is continuous with the skin of the external ear canal. Its inner surface is lined by the cuboidal epithelium of the middle ear. Between these two epithelial covers of the tympanic membrane is a middle layer of dense fibrous tissue.

KELOIDS: Keloids are particularly common on the ear lobes after piercing for earrings or other trauma (see Chapter 3). They are much more frequent in blacks and Asians than in whites. The lesions can attain considerable size and tend to recur. Histologically, keloids are composed of thick, hyalinized bundles of collagen in the deep dermis (see Fig. 3-14).

CAULIFLOWER EARS: These deformities are particularly common in wrestlers and boxers and are the result of repeated mechanical trauma to the external ear. Blows to the ears cause subperichondrial hematomas, which organize and deform the ears.

RELAPSING POLYCHONDRITIS: This rare, chronic disorder of unknown origin is characterized by intermittent inflammation that destroys the cartilaginous structures in the ears, nose, larynx, tracheobronchial tree, ribs, and joints. It may involve hyaline cartilage, elastic cartilage, or fibrocartilage.

 Pathogenesis: The cause of the cell damage is obscure, although immune mechanisms are suspected. Antibodies to cartilage, type II collagen, and chondroitin sulfate have been demonstrated in the serum of patients during acute attacks. The presence of immune complexes has been demonstrated in the involved cartilage. Relapsing polychondritis occurs alone or in association with one of the connective tissue diseases. Noncartilaginous tissues, such as the sclera and cardiac valves, also may be affected. Aortitis can cause fatal rupture of the aorta.

 Pathology: Microscopically, the perichondrium is infiltrated with lymphocytes, plasma cells, and neutrophils, which also extend into the adjacent cartilage (Fig. 25-42). The chondrocytes die, and the cartilaginous matrix degenerates and fragments. Ultimately, the cartilage is destroyed and replaced by granulation tissue and fibrosis.

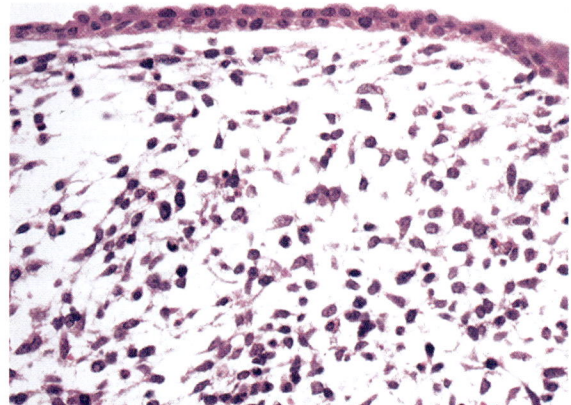

FIGURE 25-41
Embryonal rhabdomyosarcoma from a 3-year-old girl. This highly malignant tumor arose in the parapharyngeal space and invaded the adjacent structures. The oval or tadpole-shaped tumor cells under the epithelium have hyperchromatic, eccentric nuclei and immunohistochemical and ultrastructural features of rhabdomyoblasts.

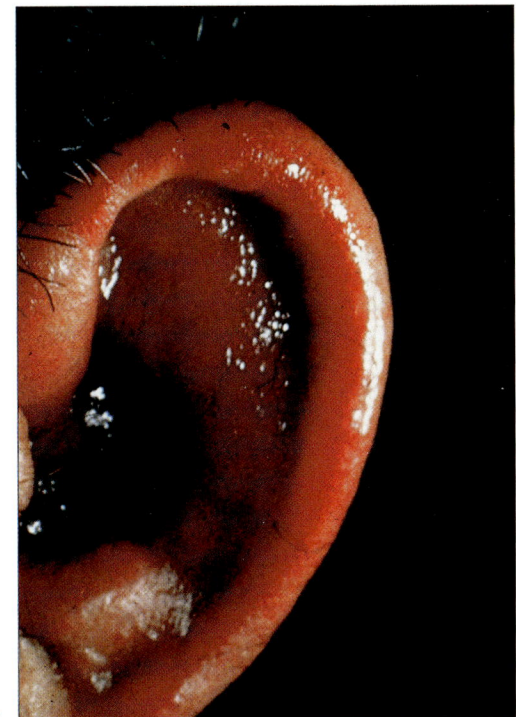
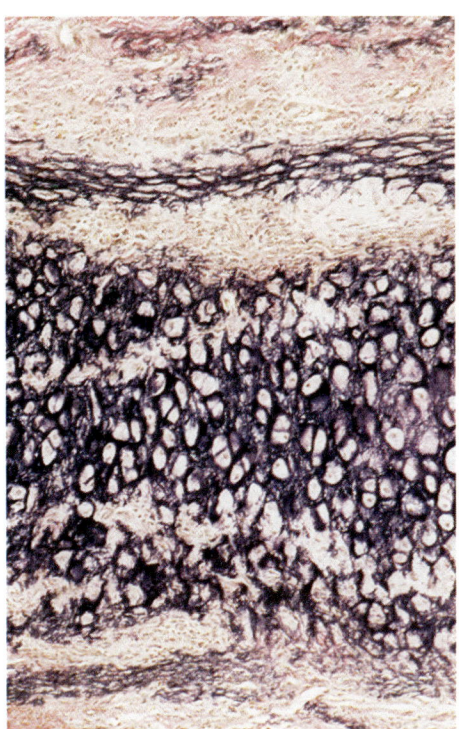

FIGURE 25-42
Relapsing polychondritis. **A.** The ear is beefy red. **B.** The perichondrium and elastic cartilage are infiltrated and partially destroyed by inflammatory cells and replaced by fibrosis.

MALIGNANT OTITIS EXTERNA: This infection of the external auditory canal is caused by *Pseudomonas aeruginosa*. The infection may spread through the skin and cartilage to cause mastoiditis or osteomyelitis of the skull, thrombosis of the venous sinuses, meningitis, and death. Malignant otitis externa occurs primarily in elderly diabetics but has also been reported in patients with blood dyscrasias (e.g., leukemia, granulocytopenia).

AURAL POLYPS: These benign inflammatory lesions arise from within the external ear canal or extrude into the canal from the middle ear. Aural polyps are composed of ulcerated and inflamed granulation tissue, which bleeds readily. Polyps arising in the middle ear are the result of chronic otitis media.

MIDDLE EAR

Anatomy

The middle ear, or tympanic cavity, is an oblong space in the temporal bone lined by a mucous membrane (see Fig. 25-1). Together with the mastoid, it forms a closed mucosal compartment, also referred to as the *middle ear cleft*. Most of the lateral wall consists of the tympanic membrane. Anteriorly, the eustachian tube connects the middle ear with the nasopharynx and provides an air passage to equalize air pressure on both sides of the tympanic membrane. The three auditory ossicles—the malleus, incus, and stapes—form a chain that connects the tympanic membrane with the oval window (on the medial wall of the tympanic cavity) and conducts sound across the middle ear space. The freedom of motion of the ossicles, particularly that of the stapes in the oval window, is more important for hearing than is an intact tympanic membrane. The middle ear opens posteriorly into the mastoid antrum, a honeycomb of small, aerated, bony compartments (air cells) lined by a thin mucous membrane, which is continuous with that of the middle ear.

Otitis Media Often Results from Obstruction of the Eustachian Tube

Otitis media refers to inflammation of the middle ear, which is usually the result of an upper respiratory tract infection that extends from the nasopharynx.

 Pathogenesis: The infection almost invariably penetrates through the mastoid antrum into the mastoid cells. In the presence of an infection in the nasopharynx, microorganisms may reach the middle ear by ascending through the eustachian tube. Acute otitis media may be due to viral or bacterial infections or to obstruction of the eustachian tube without microorganisms. In the case of viral otitis media, the process may resolve without suppuration, or the middle ear may be secondarily invaded by pus-forming bacteria.

Obstruction of the eustachian tube is important in the production of middle ear effusion. When the pharyngeal end of the eustachian tube is swollen, air cannot enter the tube. Air in the middle ear is then absorbed through the mucosa, and negative pressure causes transudation of plasma and occasionally bleeding. Antibiotics usually cure or suppress the condition.

ACUTE SEROUS OTITIS MEDIA: Obstruction of the eustachian tube may result from sudden changes in atmospheric pressure (e.g., during flying in an aircraft or deep-sea diving). This effect is particularly severe in the presence of an upper respiratory tract infection, an acute allergic reaction, or viral or bacterial infection at the orifice of the eustachian tube. Inflammation may also occur without bacterial invasion of the middle ear. More than half of children in the United States have had at least one episode of serous otitis media before their third birthday. It has become increasingly evident that repeated bouts of otitis media in early childhood often contribute to unsuspected hearing loss, which is due to residual (usually sterile) fluid in the middle ear.

CHRONIC SEROUS OTITIS MEDIA: Recurrent or chronic serous effusion of the middle ear is due to the same conditions that cause acute obstruction of the eustachian tube. Carcinoma of the nasopharynx may be the cause of chronic serous otitis media in an adult and should always be suspected when a unilateral effusion occurs in the middle ear of an adult.

Pathology: In chronic serous otitis media, mucus-producing (goblet) cell metaplasia may be seen in the mucosal lining of the middle ear. If the obstruction occurs acutely, there may be accompanying hemorrhage, for example, in the mastoid cells. Extravasation of blood and the degradation of erythrocytes liberate cholesterol. Cholesterol crystals stimulate a foreign-body reaction and the formation of granulation tissue, referred to as a *cholesterol granuloma*. Large cholesterol granulomas may destroy tissue in the mastoid or antrum. If the cholesterol granuloma is allowed to persist for many months, the granulation tissue may become fibrotic, a process that eventually results in complete obliteration of the middle ear and mastoid by fibrous tissue.

ACUTE SUPPURATIVE OTITIS MEDIA: One of the most common infections of childhood, acute suppurative otitis media, is caused by virulent pyogenic bacteria that invade the middle ear, usually through the eustachian tube. *S. pneumoniae* (pneumococcus) is the most common causative agent in all age groups (30–40%). *H. influenzae* causes about 20% of cases and is less frequent with increasing age. If the purulent exudate in the middle ear accumulates, the eardrum ruptures, and the pus is then discharged. In most cases, the infection is self-limited, and even without therapy tends to heal.

ACUTE MASTOIDITIS: Infection of the mastoid bone was a common complication of acute otitis media before the advent of antibiotics, and it is still seen, albeit rarely, in cases of inadequately treated otitis media. Characteristically, the mastoid air cells are filled with pus, and the thin osseous intercellular walls become destroyed. Extension of the infection from the mastoid to contiguous structures causes complications (Fig. 25-43).

CHRONIC SUPPURATIVE OTITIS MEDIA AND MASTOIDITIS: Neglected or recurrent infection of the middle ear and mastoid process may eventually produce a chronic inflammation of the mucosa or destruction of the periosteum covering the ossicles (Fig. 25-44). Chronic otitis media is much more common in persons who had ear disease in early childhood, which may have arrested normal development of the air cells in the mastoid.

Pathology: The inflammatory process tends to be insidious, persistent, and destructive. By definition, the eardrum is always perforated in chronic otitis media. Painless discharge *(otorrhea)* and varying degrees of hearing loss are constant symptoms. Exuberant granulation tissue may form polyps, which can extend through the perforated eardrum into the external ear canal.
Cholesteatoma is a mass of accumulated keratin and squamous mucosa that results from the growth of squamous epithelium from the external ear canal thorough the perforated eardrum into the middle ear. In that location, it continues to produce keratin. Microscopically, cholesteatomas are identical to epidermal inclusion cysts and are surrounded by granulation tissue and fibrosis. The keratin mass frequently becomes infected and shields the bacteria from antibiotics. The principal dangers of cholesteatoma arise from erosion of bone, a process that may lead to the destruction of important contiguous structures (e.g., auditory ossicles, facial nerve, labyrinth).

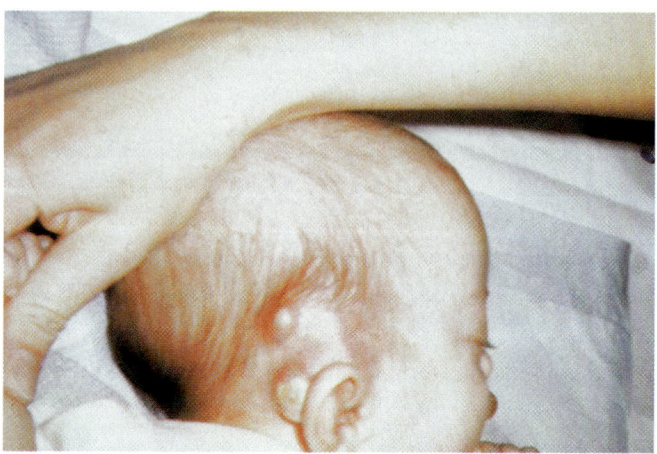

FIGURE 25-43
An unusual complication of otitis media, acute mastoiditis, appears as large bulging lesions above the child's ear.

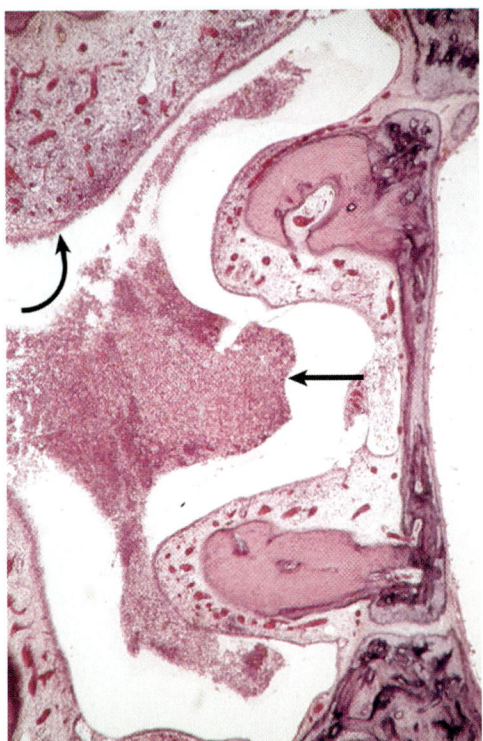

FIGURE 25-44
Chronic suppurative otitis media. A purulent exudate (*straight arrow*) is present in the middle ear cavity. The entire mucosa (*curved arrow*) is thickened by chronic inflammation and granulation tissue. The footplate and the crura of the stapes are at right.

COMPLICATIONS OF ACUTE AND CHRONIC OTITIS MEDIA: As a result of antibiotic treatment, complications of otitis media are now rare. However, a potential for serious, and even fatal, complications still exists with any suppurative inflammation of the middle ear. The following cranial and intracranial complications may develop:

- Destruction of the facial nerve
- Deep cervical or subperiosteal abscess, when the cortical bone of the mastoid process is eroded
- Petrositis, when the infection spreads to the petrous portion of the temporal bone through the chain of air cells
- Suppurative labyrinthitis, as a result of infection of the internal ear
- Epidural, subdural, or cerebral abscess, after extension of the infection through the inner table of the mastoid bone
- Meningitis, when the infection extends to the meninges
- Thrombophlebitis of the sigmoid sinus, which occurs when the infection spreads through the dura to the posterior cranial fossa

Jugulotympanic Paraganglioma Arises from Middle Ear Paraganglia

Jugulotympanic paraganglioma, is the most frequent benign tumor of the middle ear. The tumors grow slowly but, over the years, cause extensive destruction of the middle ear and may extend into the internal ear and cranial cavity. Metastases are rare.

Histologically, paragangliomas of the middle ear are identical to those arising in other locations and show characteristic lobules of cells embedded in a richly vascular connective tissue (Fig. 25-45). The paraganglial cells are of neural crest origin and contain varying amounts of catecholamines, mostly epinephrine and norepinephrine.

INTERNAL EAR

Anatomy

The petrous portion of the temporal bone contains the labyrinth, which shelters the end organs for hearing (the cochlea) and equilibrium (the vestibular labyrinth; see Fig. 25-1). The complex cavities of the osseous labyrinth contain the membranous labyrinth, which forms a series of communicating membranous sacs and ducts. The osseous labyrinth is filled with a clear fluid, the perilymph. The perilymphatic system is continuous with the subarachnoid space through the cochlear aqueduct, which provides direct exchange with the cerebrospinal fluid. The membranous labyrinth contains a different fluid, the endolymph, which circulates in a closed system. Because of the lack of barriers between the cochlear and vestibular labyrinths, injury or disease of the inner ear frequently affects both hearing and equilibrium.

The cochlea is coiled upon itself like a snail shell and makes two and one-half turns. There are three compartments in the cochlea; two of these contain perilymph and the third (the cochlear duct) contains endolymph. The cochlear duct encompasses the end organ for hearing, the organ of Corti, which rests on the basement membrane. The organ of Corti is arranged as a spiral, with three rows of outer hair cells and a row of inner hair cells. When the hairs of these neuroepithelial cells are bent or distorted by sonic vibration, the mechanical force is converted into electrochemical im-

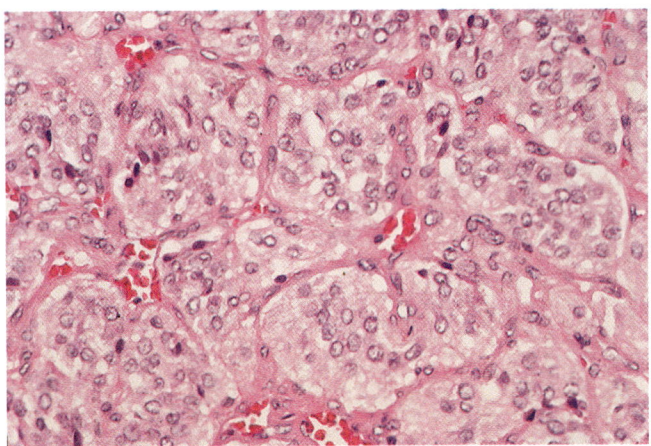

FIGURE 25-45
Jugulotympanic paraganglioma. Tumor cell nests are composed of cells with ill-defined cell borders and prominent eosinophilic cytoplasm (chief cells); difficult to identify by light microscopy are the peripherally situated sustentacular cells.

pulses and is interpreted in the temporal cortex as sound. The vestibular portion of the membranous labyrinth consists of the utricle, the saccule, and the semicircular canals. Each of these structures contains the specialized neuroepithelium that is the end organ for equilibrium.

Otosclerosis Results in Progressive Deafness

Otosclerosis refers to the formation of new spongy bone about the stapes and the oval window, which results in progressive deafness. The condition is an autosomal dominant hereditary defect and is the most common cause of conductive hearing loss in young and middle-aged adults in the United States. Ten percent of white and 1% of black adult Americans have some otosclerosis, although 90% of cases are asymptomatic. The female-to-male ratio is 2:1, and both ears are usually affected. The pathogenesis of otosclerosis is obscure.

 Pathology: Although any part of the petrous bone may be affected, otosclerotic bone tends to form at particular points. The most frequent site (80–90%) is immediately anterior to the oval window. The focus of sclerotic bone extends posteriorly and may infiltrate and replace the stapes. This process progressively immobilizes the footplate of the stapes, and the developing bony ankylosis (Fig. 25-46) is functionally manifested as a slowly progressive conductive hearing loss.

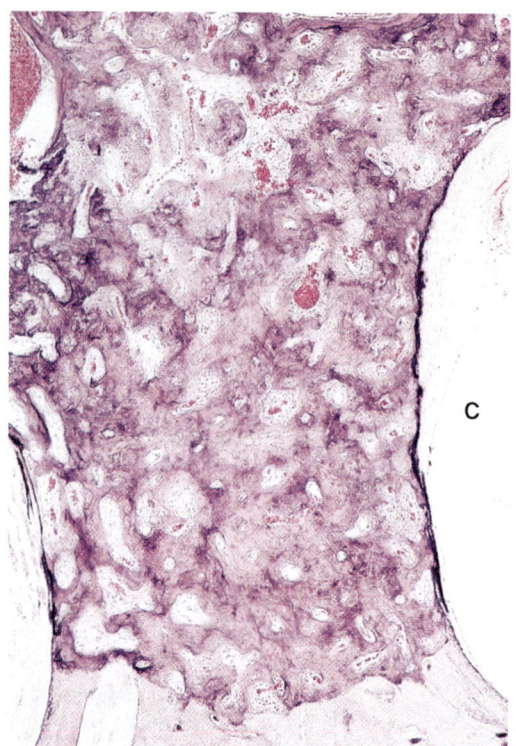

FIGURE 25-47
Otosclerosis. In the lateral wall of the cochlea, the basophilic and more vascular bone is well demarcated. C, organ of Corti.

Histologically, the initial lesion of otosclerosis is resorption of bone, with formation of highly cellular fibrous tissue, which contains wide vascular spaces and osteoclasts (Fig. 25-47). The focus of resorbed bone is later replaced by immature bone. By repeated remodeling, this bone develops into more mature bone.

Otosclerosis is successfully treated by surgical mobilization of the auditory ossicles.

Meniere Disease Refers to the Triad of Vertigo, Sensorineural Hearing Loss, and Tinnitus

A wide variety of etiologic factors have been suggested, but the cause of Meniere disease remains uncertain. Its pathological correlate is hydropic distention of the endolymphatic system of the cochlea. Meniere disease is most common in the fourth and fifth decades and is bilateral in 15% of patients.

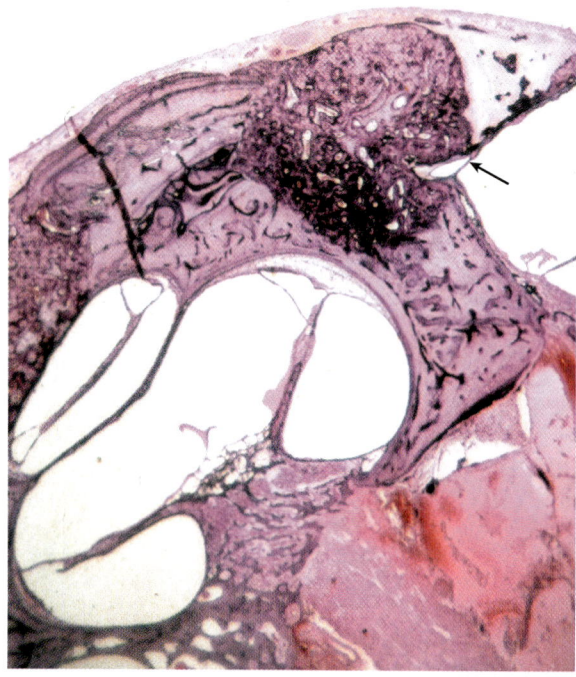

FIGURE 25-46
Otosclerosis. Otosclerotic foci appear as dark purple areas in the bony labyrinth. At the anterior margin of the oval window (*arrow*), otosclerosis has immobilized the footplate of the stapes by bony ankylosis.

 Pathology: Microscopically, the earliest change is dilatation of the cochlear duct and saccule. As the disease *(hydrops)* progresses, the entire endolymphatic system becomes dilated, and the membranous wall frequently tears (Fig. 25-48). Ruptures are sometimes followed by collapse of the membranous labyrinth, but atrophy of the sensory and neural structures is rare. It is thought that the symptoms of Meniere disease occur when endolym-

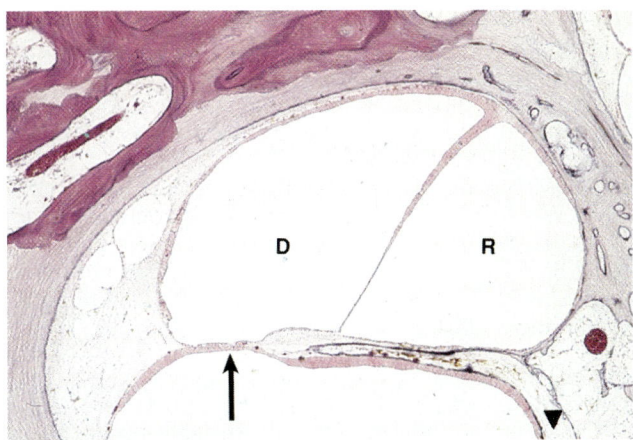

FIGURE 25-48
Meniere disease. The cochlear duct (D) is markedly distended, and the Reissner membrane (R) is pushed back by endolymphatic hydrops. Neither the organ of Corti (arrow) nor the spiral ganglion (arrowhead) is in its usual location.

phatic hydrops causes rupture, and the endolymph escapes into the perilymph.

 Clinical Features: The attacks of vertigo, which are accompanied by nausea and vomiting and are often incapacitating, last less than 24 hours. Weeks or months go by before another episode, and in time, the remissions become longer. The hearing loss recovers between attacks but later becomes permanent. Meniere disease seems to be improved by a low-salt diet and the administration of diuretics.

Labyrinthine Toxicity is a Drug-Induced Cause of Deafness

The best known drugs that produce ototoxic side effects are the aminoglycoside antibiotics, which cause irreversible damage to the vestibular or cochlear sensory cells. Other antibiotics, diuretics, antimalarial drugs, and salicylates may also cause transient or permanent sensorineural hearing loss. Among the antineoplastic agents, cisplatin frequently causes temporary or permanent hearing loss. The labyrinth of the embryo is especially sensitive to some drugs (congenital deafness due to thalidomide, quinine, and chloroquine).

Viral Labyrinthitis Can Result in Congenital Deafness

Viral infections are becoming increasingly recognized as the cause of several inner ear disorders, particularly deafness. Most cases represent invasion of the labyrinth by the virus. CMV and rubella are the best known prenatal viral infections that cause congenital deafness through maternal-to-fetal transmission. CMV antigen has been demonstrated in the cells of the organ of Corti and neurons of the spiral ganglia.

Mumps is the most common cause of deafness among the postnatal viral infections. The infection can cause rapid hearing loss, which is unilateral in 80% of cases. By contrast, prenatal infection of the labyrinth with rubella is usually bilateral, with permanent loss of cochlear and vestibular function. A number of other viruses are suspected to cause labyrinthitis, including influenza and parainfluenza viruses, EBV, herpesviruses, and adenoviruses. Temporal bone specimens of such cases reveal severe damage to the organ of Corti, with almost total loss of both inner and outer hair cells.

Acoustic Trauma

Noise-induced hearing loss is a significant health problem in industrialized countries. Occupational or recreational exposure to loud tones or noises may cause temporary or permanent loss of hearing. The earliest damage occurs in the external hair cells of the organ of Corti. The loss of sensory hairs is followed by deformation, swelling, and disintegration of the hair cells.

Tumors

SCHWANNOMA: Nearly all schwannomas in the internal auditory canal arise from the vestibular nerves. Vestibular schwannomas, which account for about 10% of all intracranial tumors, are slow growing and encapsulated. Larger tumors protrude from the internal auditory meatus into the cerebellopontine angle and may deform the brainstem and adjacent cerebellum (see Fig. 28-136). Schwannomas cause slowly progressive vestibular and auditory symptoms. Neurofibromatosis, type 2, is characterized by a high incidence of bilateral vestibular schwannomas. Histologically, these tumors are indistinguishable from other vestibular schwannomas (see Chapter 28). For a more detailed discussion of acoustic neurinomas, see Chapter 28.

MENINGIOMA: Meningiomas of the cerebellopontine angle take origin from the meningothelial cells in the arachnoid villi. The favored sites for these tumors are the sphenoid ridge and the petrous pyramid. Meningiomas may extend into the adjacent temporal bone or dural sinuses (Fig. 25-49).

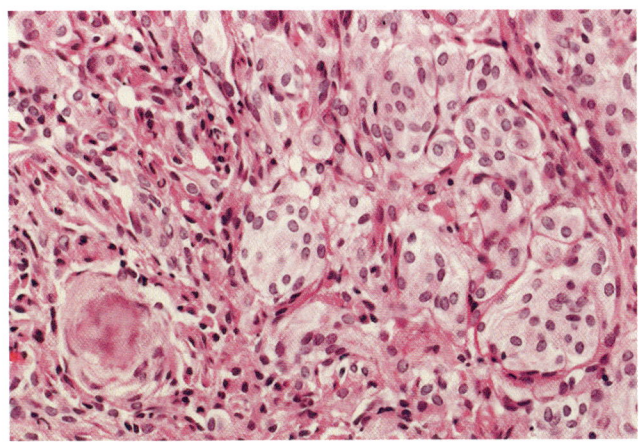

FIGURE 25-49
Meningioma. Small cell nests are composed of cells with uniform round nuclei; toward the left of the illustration a psammomatoid body appears as an acellular eosinophilic structure.

SUGGESTED READING

Books

Barnes I (ed): *Surgical pathology of the head and neck*, 2nd ed. rev. exp. New York: Marcel Dekker, 2001.

Ellis GL, Auclair PL, Gnepp DR: *Surgical pathology of the salivary glands.* Philadelphia: WB Saunders, 1991.

Friedmann I, Arnold W: *Pathology of the ear.* Edinburgh: Churchill Livingstone, 1992.

Fu Y-S, Wenig BM, Abemayor E, Wenig BL (eds): *Head and neck pathology with clinical correlations.* Philadelphia: Churchill Livingstone, 2001.

Gnepp DR (ed): *Diagnostic surgical pathology of the head and neck.* Philadelphia: WB Saunders, 2001.

Grundmann E, Krueger GRF, Ablashi DV (eds): *Nasopharyngeal carcinoma.* Stuttgart: Gustav Fischer Verlag, 1981.

Hawke M, Jahn AF (eds): *Disease of the ear: Clinical and pathological aspects.* Philadelphia: Lea & Febiger, 1986.

Hooks JJ, Jordan GH: *Viral infections in the oral cavity.* New York: Elsevier-North Holland, 1982.

Konigsmark BW, Gorlin RJ: *Genetic and metabolic deafness.* Philadelphia: WB Saunders, 1976.

McCarthy PL, Shklar G: *Diseases of the oral mucosa*, 2nd ed. Philadelphia: Lea & Febiger, 1980.

Michaels L (ed): *Ear, nose and throat histopathology.* New York: Springer-Verlag, 1987.

Nager GT: *Pathology of the ear and temporal bone.* Baltimore: Williams & Wilkins, 1993.

Neville BW, Damm DD, Allen CM, Bouquot JE (eds): *Oral and maxillofacial pathology*, 2nd ed. Philadelphia: WB Saunders, 2002.

Regezi JA, Sciubba J: *Oral pathology: Clinical-pathologic correlations*, 2nd ed. Philadelphia: WB Saunders, 1993.

Robertson PB, Greenspan JS: *Perspectives on oral manifestations of AIDS: Diagnosis and management of HIV-associated infections.* Littleton, MA: PSG Publishing, 1988.

Robinson HBG, Miller AS: *Colby, Kerr and Robinson's color atlas of oral pathology*, 5th ed. Philadelphia: JB Lippincott, 1990.

Schuknecht HF: *Pathology of the ear.* Cambridge, MA: Harvard University Press, 1974.

Tala H, Moutsopoulos HM, Kassan SG (eds): *Sjögren's syndrome: Clinical and immunological aspects.* New York: Springer-Verlag, 1987.

Wenig BM: *Atlas of head and neck pathology.* Philadelphia: WB Saunders, 1993.

Wenig BM: General principles of head and neck pathology. In: Harrison LB, Sessions RB, Hong WK (eds): *Head and neck cancer.* Philadelphia: Lippincott-Raven, 1999.

Review Articles

General

Batsakis JG, Luna MA: Midfacial necrotizing lesions. *Semin Diagn Pathol* 4:90–103, 1987.

Feinmesser R, Miyazaki I, Cheung R, et al.: Diagnosis of nasopharyngeal carcinoma by DNA amplification of tissue obtained by fine-needle aspiration. *N Engl J Med* 326: 17–21, 1992.

Saul SH, Kapadia SB: Primary lymphoma of Waldyer's ring. *Cancer* 56:157, 1985.

Swanson JA, Hoecker JL: Otitis media in young children. *Mayo Clin Proc* 71:179–183, 1996.

Wenig BM: Nose/sinuses. In: Fletcher CM (ed): *Diagnostic histopathology of tumors*, 2nd ed. London: Churchill Livingstone, 2000.

Wenig BM: Squamous cell carcinoma of the upper aerodigestive tract: Precursors and problematic variants. *Mod Pathol* 2002;15:229–254.

Wenig BM: Nasal cavity, paranasal sinuses, and nasopharynx. In: Weidner N, Cote RJ, Suster S, Weiss LM (eds): *Modern surgical pathology.* Philadelphia: WB Saunders, 2003.

Wenig BM: The ear. In: Weidner N, Cote RJ, Suster S, Weiss LM (eds): *Modern surgical pathology.* Philadelphia: WB Saunders, 2003.

Oral Cavity

Kramer IRH, Lucas RB, Pindborg JJ, Sobin LH: Definition of leukoplakia and related lesions: An aid to studies on oral precancer. *Oral Surg* 46:518, 1978.

Shaw JH: Causes and control of dental caries. *N Engl J Med* 316:996–1004, 1987.

Williams RC: Periodontal disease. *N Engl J Med* 322:373–382, 1990.

Nose and Paranasal Sinuses

Batsakis JG, Luna MA: Midfacial necrotizing lesions. *Semin Diagn Pathol* 4:90–103, 1987.

Fienberg R, et al: Correlation of antineutrophil cytoplasmic antibodies with the extrarenal histopathology of Wegener's (pathergic) granulomatosis and related forms of vasculitis. *Hum Pathol* 24:160–168, 1993.

Lee NK, et al: Head and neck squamous cell carcinomas associated with human papillomaviruses and an increased incidence of cervical pathology. *Otolaryngol Head Neck Surg* 99:296–301, 1988.

Naclerio RM: Allergic rhinitis. *N Engl J Med* 325:860–869, 1991.

Vokes EE, Weichselbaum RR, Lippman SM, Hong WK: Head and neck cancer. *N Engl J Med* 328:184–186, 1993.

Wald ER: Sinusitis in children. *N Engl J Med* 326:319–323, 1992.

Wu TC, et al: Association of human papillomavirus with nasal neoplasia. *Lancet* 341:522–524, 1993.

Nasopharynx

De The G, Ito Y (eds): *Nasopharyngeal carcinoma: Etiology and control.* Lyon: IARC Scientific Publications, no. 20, 1978.

Feinmesser R, Miyazaki I, Cheung R, et al.: Diagnosis of nasopharyngeal carcinoma by DNA amplification of tissue obtained by fine-needle aspiration. *N Engl J Med* 326: 17–21, 1992.

Saul SH, Kapadia SB: Primary lymphoma of Waldeyer's ring. *Cancer* 56:157, 1985.

Ear

Melamed Y, Shupak A, Bitterman H: Medical problems associated with underwater diving. *N Engl J Med* 326: 30–35, 1992.

Nadol JB: Hearing loss. *N Engl J Med* 329:1092–1102, 1993.

Swanson JA, Hoecker JL: Otitis media in young children. *Mayo Clin Proc* 71:179–183, 1996.

Original Articles

Bedi GC, Westra WH, Gabrielson E, et al.: Multiple head and neck tumors: evidence for common clonal origin. *Can Res* 26:251–261, 1995.

Califano J, van der Riet P, Westra W, et al.: Genetic progression model for head and neck cancer: implications for field cancerization. *Cancer Res* 56:2484–2487, 1996.

Decker J, Goldstein JC: Risk factors in head and neck cancer. *N Engl J Med* 306:1151–1155, 1982.

Dyson N, Howley PM, Münger K, Harlow E: The human papillomavirus-16 E7 oncoprotein is able to bind the retinoblastoma gene product. *Science* 243:934–937, 1989.

Gillison ML, Koch WM, Capone RB, et al.: Evidence for a causal association between human papillomavirus and a subset of head and neck cancers. *J Natl Cancer Inst* 92:709–720, 2000.

MacMillan C, Kapadia SB, Finkelstein SD, et al.: Lymphoepithelial carcinoma of the larynx and hypopharynx: study of eight cases with relationship to Epstein-Barr virus (EBV) and p53 gene alterations, and review of the literature. *Hum Pathol* 27:1172–1179, 1996.

McKaig RG, Baric RS, Olshan AF: Human papillomavirus and head and neck cancer: Epidemiology and molecular biology. *Head Neck* 20:250–265, 1998.

Mork J, Lie K, Glattre E, et al.: Human papillomavirus infection as a risk factor for squamous-cell carcinoma of the head and neck. *N Engl J Med* 344:1125–1131, 2001.

Pacchioni D, Negro F, Valente G, Bussolati G: Epstein-Barr virus by in situ hybridization in fine-needle aspiration biopsies. *Diagn Mol Pathol* 3:100–104, 1994.

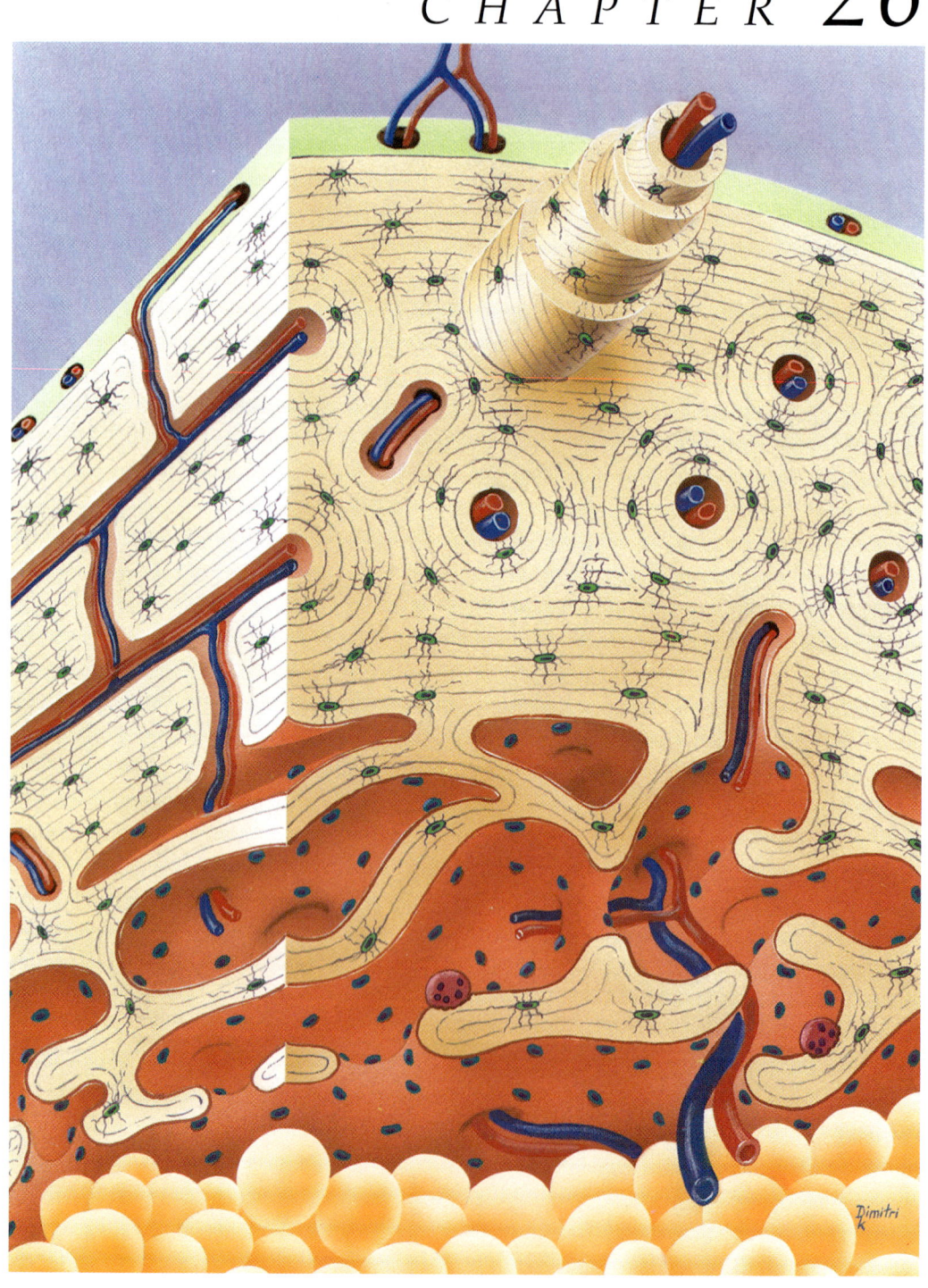

CHAPTER 26

Bones and Joints

Alan L. Schiller
Beverly Y. Wang
Michael J. Klein

Bones

Anatomy

Bone Marrow

Blood Supply

Periosteum

Bone Matrix

Cells of Bone

Microscopic Organization of Bone Tissue

Cartilage

Bone Formation and Growth

Primary Ossification

Secondary Ossification

Formation of the Metaphysis

Obliteration of the Growth Plate

Disorders of the Growth Plate

Cretinism

Morquio Syndrome

Achondroplasia

Scurvy

Asymmetric Cartilage Growth

Modeling Abnormalities

Osteopetrosis, Marble Bone Disease, or Albers–Schönberg Disease

Progressive Diaphyseal Dysplasia

Delayed Maturation of Bone

Osteogenesis Imperfecta

Enchondromatosis

Fracture

Fracture Healing

Stress Fracture

Osteonecrosis (Avascular Necrosis, Aseptic Necrosis)

Reactive Bone Formation

Heterotopic Calcification Tissue

Myositis Ossificans

FIGURE 26-1 (see opposite page)
Anatomy of bone. A schematic representation of cortical and trabecular bone. The longitudinal section (*left*) shows the vasculature entering the periosteum via the periosteal perforating arteries and coursing through the bone perpendicular to the long axis in Volkmann canals. The vessels that proceed longitudinally, or parallel to the long axis, are located in haversian canals. Each artery is accompanied by a vein. Within the cortex, osteocytes reside in lacunae, and their cell processes extend into the canaliculi. The cross-sectional view (*right*) illustrates the various types of lamellar bone in the cortex. Circumferential lamellar bone is located adjacent to the periosteum and borders the marrow space. Concentric lamellar bone surrounds the central haversian canals to form an osteon. Each layer of the concentric lamellar bone displays a change in the pitch of the collagen fibers, such that each layer has a different arrangement of collagen. The interstitial lamellar bone occupies the space between osteons. The marrow space is filled with fat, and its trabecular bone is contiguous with the cortex. Multinucleated osteoclasts are present, and palisaded osteoblasts surround the bone surfaces. The perforating arteries from the periosteum and the nutrient artery from the marrow space communicate within the cortex via haversian and Volkmann canals.

Infections

Osteomyelitis

Tuberculosis

Syphilis

Langerhans Cell Histiocytosis

Eosinophilic Granuloma

Hand-Schüller-Christian Disease

Letterer-Siwe Disease

Metabolic Bone Diseases

Osteoporosis

Secondary Osteoporosis

Osteomalacia and Rickets

Vitamin D Metabolism

Dietary Deficiency of Vitamin D

Intestinal Malabsorption

Disorders of Vitamin D Metabolism

Renal Disorders of Phosphate Metabolism

Defective Mineralization

Primary Hyperparathyroidism

Actions of Parathyroid Hormone

Renal Osteodystrophy

Paget Disease of Bone

Gaucher Disease

Fibrous Dysplasia

Benign Tumors of Bone

Nonossifying Fibroma

Solitary Cyst

Aneurysmal Bone Cyst

Osteoid Osteoma

Osteoblastoma

Solitary Chondroma

Chondroblastoma

Chondromyxoid Fibroma

Malignant Tumors of Bone

Osteosarcoma

Chondrosarcoma

Giant Cell Tumor

Ewing Sarcoma

Multiple Myeloma

Joints

Classification of Synovial Joints

Structures of the Synovial Joint

Osteoarthritis

Rheumatoid Arthritis

Spondyloarthropathy

Juvenile Arthritis

Gout

Primary Gout

Gout Due to Inborn Errors of Metabolism

Secondary Gout

Calcium Pyrophosphate Dihydrate-Deposition Disease (Chondrocalcinosis and Pseudogout)

Calcium Hydroxyapatite-Deposition Disease

Hemophilia, Hemochromatosis, and Ochronosis

Tumors and Tumorlike Lesions of Joints

Ganglion

Synovial Chondromatosis

Pigmented Villonodular Synovitis

Soft Tissue Tumors

Tumors and Tumorlike Conditions of Fibrous Origin

Nodular Fasciitis

Fibromatosis

Malignant Fibrous Histiocytoma

Tumors of Adipose Tissue

Lipoma

Liposarcoma

Rhabdomyosarcoma

Smooth Muscle Tumors

Smooth Muscle Tumors

Synovial Sarcoma

Bones

The functions of bone are classified as mechanical, mineral storage, and hematopoietic. The mechanical functions of bone include protection for the brain, spinal cord, and chest organs; rigid internal support for the limbs; and deployment as lever arms in the skeletal muscle. Bone is the principal reservoir for calcium and stores other ions such as phosphate, sodium, and magnesium. The bones also serve as hosts for the hematopoietic bone marrow.

The mechanical properties of bone are related to its construction and internal architecture. Although extremely light, bone has a high tensile strength. This combination of strength and light weight results from its hollow tubular shape, the layering of bone tissue, and the internal buttressing of the matrix.

The term *bone* can refer to both an organ and a tissue. The "organ" is composed of bone tissue, cartilage, fat, marrow elements, vessels, nerves, and fibrous tissue. Bone "tissue" is described in microscopic terms and is defined by the relation of its collagen and mineral structure to the bone cells.

ANATOMY

Macroscopically two types of bone are recognized.

- **Cortical bone** is dense, compact bone, whose outer shell defines the shape of the bone. Cortical bone composes 80% of the skeleton, and because of its density, its functions are principally biomechanical.
- **Coarse cancellous bone** (also termed *spongy, trabecular,* or *marrow bone*) is found at the ends of long bones within the medullary canal. Cancellous bone has a high surface-to-volume ratio and contains many more bone cells per unit volume than does cortical bone. Changes in the rate of bone turnover are manifested principally in cancellous bone.

All bones contain both cancellous and cortical elements (Fig. 26-1), but their proportions differ. The body, or shaft, of a long tubular bone, such as the femur, is composed of cortical bone, and its marrow is formed principally by fat. Toward the ends of the femur, the cortex becomes thin, and coarse cancellous bone becomes the predominant structure. By contrast, the skull is formed by outer and inner tables of compact bone, with only a small amount of cancellous bone within the marrow space, called the *diploë*.

The anatomical structures of bone are defined in relation to a transverse cartilage plate, which is present in the growing child. This structure is termed *the growth plate, the epiphyseal cartilage plate,* or *the physis* (Fig. 26-2). The terms *epiphysis, metaphysis,* and *diaphysis* are defined in relation to the growth plate.

- **The epiphysis** is the area of the bone that extends from the subarticular bone plate to the base of the growth plate.
- **The metaphysis** describes the region from the side of the growth plate facing away from the joint to the area where the bone develops its fluted or funnel shape. The metaphysis contains coarse cancellous bone.
- **The diaphysis** corresponds to the body or shaft of the bone and is the zone between the two metaphyses in a long tubular bone.

The metaphysis blends into the diaphysis and represents the area where the coarse cancellous bone dissipates. It is the area of bone that is particularly important in hematogenous infections, tumors, and malformations of the skeleton.

Two additional terms are essential to an understanding of the organization of bone:

- **Endochondral ossification** is the process by which bone tissue replaces cartilage.
- **Intramembranous ossification** refers to the mechanism by which bone tissue supplants membranous or fibrous tissue laid down by the periosteum.

All bones in the body are formed by at least some intramembranous ossification. Some bones (e.g., the calvaria of the skull) are forged purely by intramembranous ossification. Microscopically, it cannot be determined whether bone formation resulted from replacement of cartilage or of fibrous tissue. Because bone tumors tend to recapitulate their embryological origins, it is not surprising that cartilaginous tumors of the frontal bone have not been seen, because the calvaria of the skull do not originate from cartilage.

Bone Marrow

The bone marrow resides in the space enclosed by the cortical bone, called the *marrow space* or *medullary canal*. It is supported by a delicate connective tissue framework that enmeshes the marrow cells and the blood vessels. Three types of marrow are evident to the naked eye:

- **Red marrow** corresponds to hematopoietic tissue and is found in virtually all bones at the time of birth. At the time of adolescence, the red marrow is confined to the axial skeleton, which includes the skull, vertebrae, sternum, ribs, scapulae, clavicles, pelvis, and the proximal humerus and femur. Red marrow may also be pathological, depending on the age of the patient and the site of the marrow. For example, the presence of red marrow in the femoral diaphysis of a 55-year-old man is abnormal and may reflect underlying disease, such as leukemia.

1308 Bones and Joints

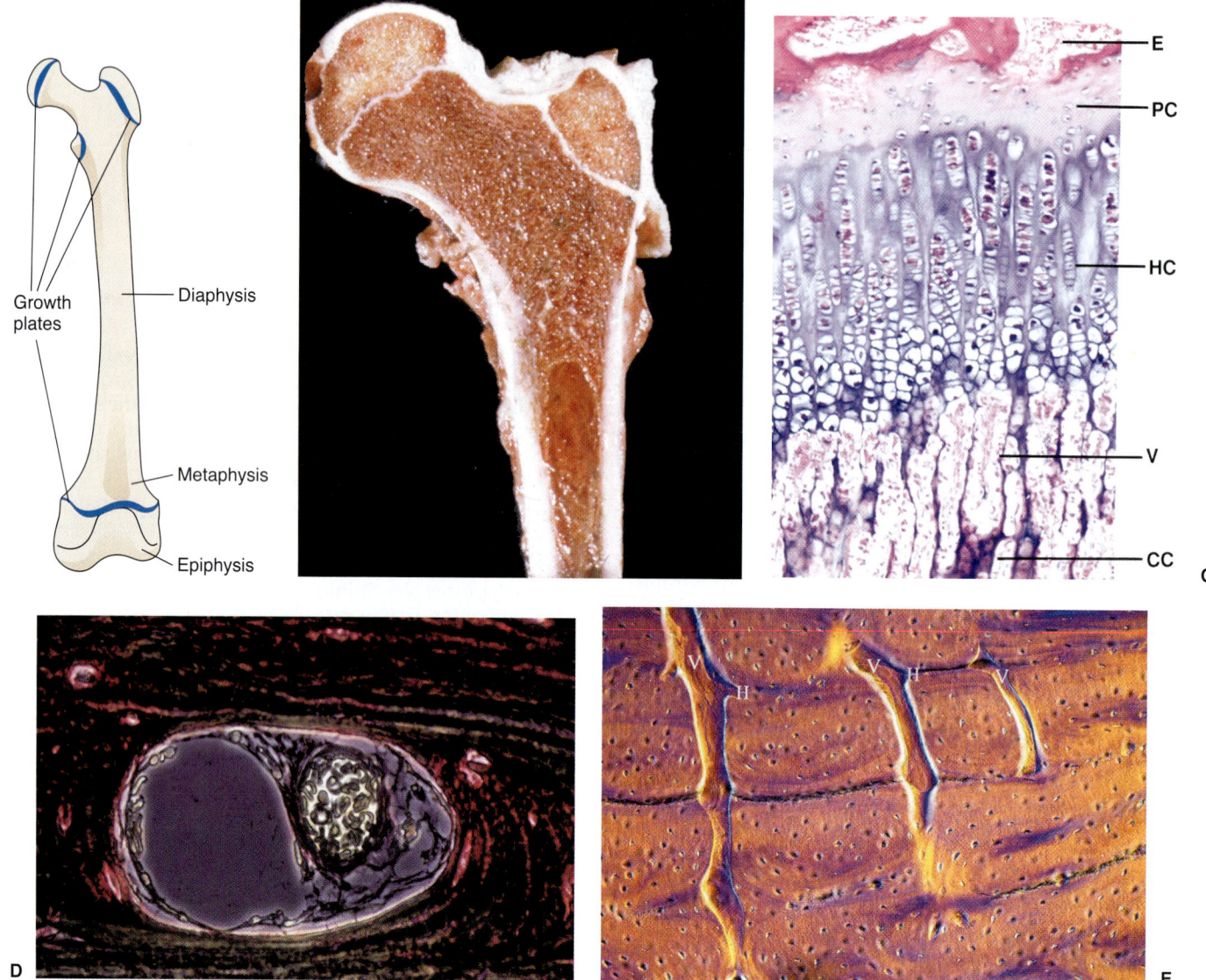

FIGURE 26-2
Anatomy of a long bone. A. Diagram of the femur illustrates the various compartments. B. Coronal section of the proximal femur illustrates the various anatomical parts of a long bone. The epiphysis of the femoral head and the apophysis of the greater trochanter are separated from the metaphysis by their respective growth plates. The cortex and the medullary cavity are well visualized. The medullary cavity contains cancellous bone until the metaphysis narrows into the diaphysis (shaft) of the bone, which is almost completely devoid of bone and filled with marrow. C. A section of the epiphysis with a zone of proliferating cartilage cells. Beneath this zone, the hypertrophic cartilage cells are arrayed in columns. At the *bottom*, the calcifying matrix is invaded by blood vessels. E, epiphysis; PC, proliferative cartilage; HC, hypertrophic cartilage; CC, calcified cartilage; V, vascular invasion. D. Haversian canal containing a venule (thin-walled wider vessel on *left*) and an arteriole (thicker-walled narrow vessel on the *right*.) E. Volkmann canals. In this photograph, three Volkmann canals are seen running parallel to each other *(v)* and perpendicular to the cortex. The openings of two haversian canals *(h)* are visible.

- **Yellow marrow** appears microscopically as fat tissue and is found in the bones of the limbs. Yellow marrow in a normally hematopoietic area, such as a vertebral body, is abnormal at any age.
- **Gray or white marrow** is deficient in hematopoietic elements and is often fibrotic. **It is always a pathological tissue in a nongrowing adult bone or in areas distant from the growth plate in a child.**

Blood Supply Enters Bone Through Specialized Canals

The long tubular bones are provided with blood from two sources and contain canals to supply the tissues.

- **Nutrient arteries** enter the bone through a nutrient foramen and supply the marrow space and the internal one third to one half of the cortex.
- **Perforating arteries** are small straight vessels that extend inward from the periosteal arteries on the external surface of the periosteum (the fibrous capsule of the bone). The perforating arteries anastomose in the cortex with branches from the nutrient arteries coming from the marrow space.
- **Haversian canals** are spaces in the bone of the cortex that course parallel to the long axis of the bone for a short distance and then branch and communicate with other similar canals. Each canal contains one or two blood vessels, lymphatics, and some nerve fibers.
- **Volkmann canals** are spaces within the cortex that run perpendicular to the long axis of the cortex to connect adjacent haversian canals. Volkmann canals also contain blood vessels.

Each artery has its paired vein and, perhaps, free nerve endings. Drainage of the veins proceeds either from the cortex outward to the periosteal veins or inward into the marrow space and out the nutrient veins.

Periosteum Covers All Bones

The periosteum is a specialized connective tissue that covers all bones of the body and can form bone. The internal layer of the periosteum, termed the *cambium layer*, is applied to the surface of the bone and consists of loosely arranged collagenous bundles, with spindle-shaped connective tissue cells and a network of thin elastic fibers. The outer *fibrous layer* is contiguous with soft tissue planes and fascia. It is composed of dense connective tissue containing blood vessels.

Bone Matrix Is Organic and Mineralized

Bone tissue is composed of cells (10% by weight), a mineralized phase (hydroxyapatite crystals, representing 60% of the total tissue), and an organic matrix (30%). Thus, with the exception of the cells, bone is a biphasic structure comprising an organic and an inorganic matrix.

The **mineralized matrix** consists of poorly crystalline hydroxyapatite, $Ca_{10}(PO_4)_6(OH)_2$. Because of its net negative charge, this material can neutralize substantial amounts of acid. Other important ions in bone are carbonate, citrate, fluoride, chloride, sodium, magnesium, potassium, and strontium.

The **organic matrix** consists of 88% type I collagen, 10% other proteins, and 1 to 2% lipids and glycosaminoglycans. **Thus, type I collagen essentially defines the organic matrix.** Other proteins include the following:

- **Osteocalcin** is a protein produced by osteoblasts, and blood levels of this protein serve as a useful marker of bone formation.
- **Osteopontin** and **sialoprotein** are bone matrix proteins containing the amino acid sequence *Arg-Gly-Asp,* which is recognized by the cell-attachment proteins termed *integrins*. Thus osteopontin and bone sialoprotein probably help anchor cells to the bone matrix.

Cells of Bone Maintain Its Structure

There are four types of cells in bone tissue, each of which has specific functions related to the formation, resorption, and remodeling of bone.

OSTEOPROGENITOR CELL: The osteoprogenitor cell, which ultimately differentiates into osteoblasts and osteocytes, is itself derived from a primitive stem cell. The stem cell can develop into adipocytes, myoblasts, fibroblasts, or osteoblasts. The osteoprogenitor cell is found in the marrow, periosteum, and all the supporting structures within the marrow cavity. This cell is not readily recognized by light microscopy because it appears as a small, nonspecific, stellate or spindle-shaped cell. In response to an appropriate signal, the osteoprogenitor gives rise to an osteoblast.

OSTEOBLAST: Osteoblasts are the protein-synthesizing cells that produce and mineralize bone tissue. Precursor cells are turned into osteoblasts under the influence of the transcription factor CBFA-1. These large mononuclear and polygonal cells are arrayed in a line along the bone surface (Fig. 26-3A). Underlying the layer of osteoblasts is a thin, eosinophilic zone of organic bone matrix that has not yet been mineralized, termed *osteoid*. The time from the deposition of osteoid to its mineralization is known as the *mineralization lag time*. Reflecting its protein synthetic capacity, the osteoblast has a complex cytoplasm containing abundant endoplasmic reticulum, a prominent Golgi apparatus, and mitochondria with calcium-containing granules. Cytoplasmic processes that extend into the osteoid are in contact with cells embedded within the matrix, called *osteocytes*. The syncytium of osteocytes and osteoblasts probably serves to prevent bone calcium (99% of the body's calcium) from equilibrating with the general extracellular space. When the osteoblast is inactive, it flattens on the surface of bone tissue. The osteoblast contains alkaline phosphatase, manufactures osteocalcin, and has parathyroid hormone receptors. Collagenase secreted by the osteoblasts may also facilitate osteoclastic activity. Finally, a number of growth factors, including transforming growth factor-β (TGF-β), insulin-like growth factor-1 (IGF-1), IGF-2, platelet-derived growth factor (PDGF), interleukin-1 (IL-1), fibroblast growth factor (FGF), and tumor necrosis factor-α TNF-α, are produced by osteoblasts and play an important role in regulating growth and differentiation of bone.

OSTEOCYTE: The osteocyte is an osteoblast that is completely embedded in bone matrix and is isolated in a lacuna

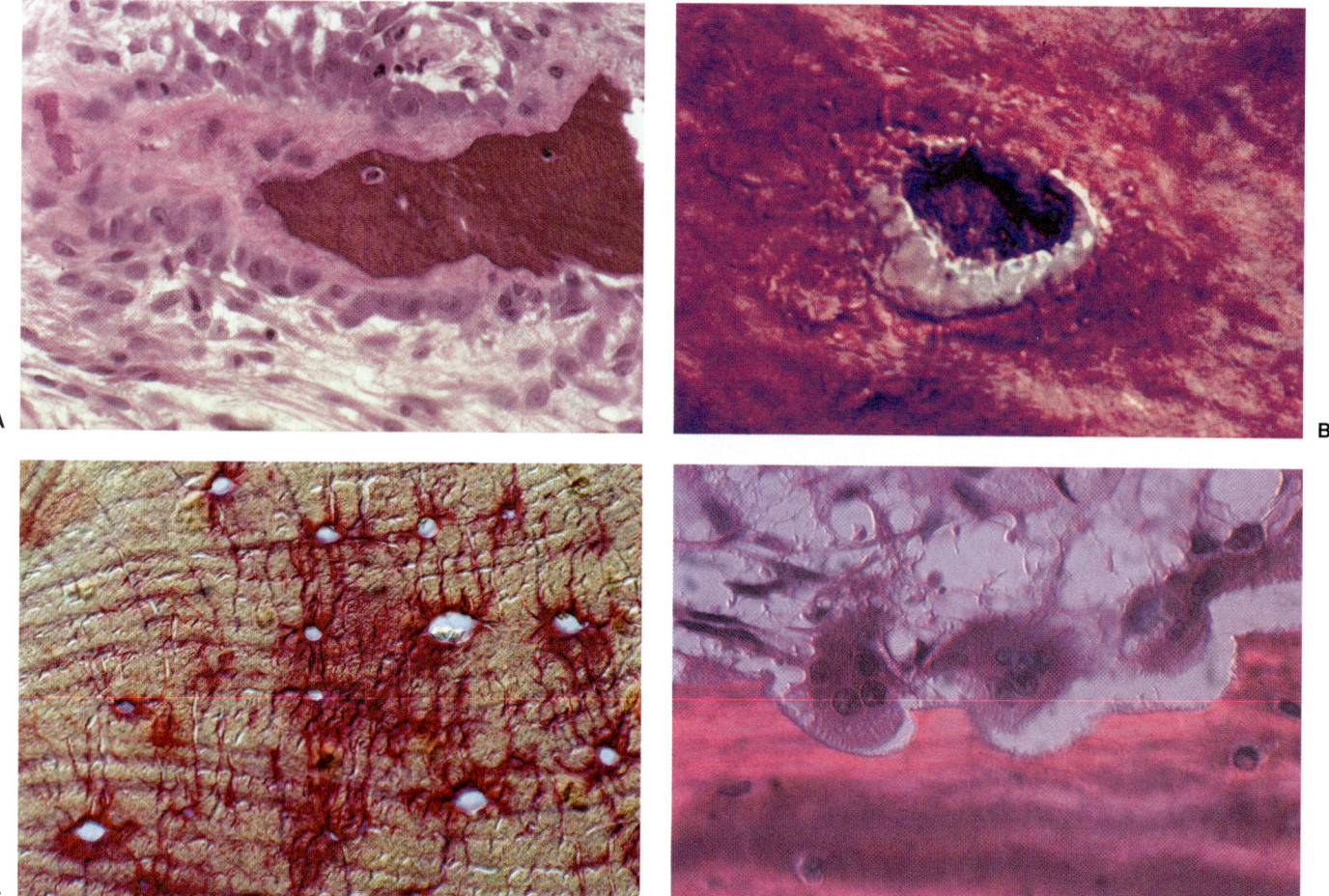

FIGURE 26-3
A. The cells of bones. A developing bone spicule demonstrates a prominent layer of plump osteoblasts lining the pink osteoid seam. The dark purple layer beneath the osteoid seam is mineralized bone. B. Osteocyte. Osteocytes represent trapped osteoblasts surrounded by bone matrix. The space surrounding the cell is called a *lacuna*. At this power, a few cytoplasmic extensions of the cell can be seen extending into narrow channels in the bone, called *canaliculi*. C. The extensive intercommunication of osteocyte processes via their canalicular network in cortical bone is visible in this section. D. Osteoclasts. These are multinucleated giant cells found on bone surfaces within small scalloped reabsorption pits, called *Howship lacunae*.

(see Fig. 26-3B). Although osteocytes are responsible for depositing small quantities of bone around lacunae, with time this cell loses its capacity for protein synthesis, and the Golgi apparatus and endoplasmic reticulum become inconspicuous. The osteocyte has numerous processes that extend through bony canals, called *canaliculi*, and communicate with those from other osteocytes (see Fig. 26-3C). The cytoplasmic processes contain actin filaments and are separated from processes of other osteocytes by tight gap junctions. Recent evidence suggests the osteocyte may be the bone cell that recognizes and responds to mechanical forces.

OSTEOCLAST: The osteoclast, which is the exclusive bone-resorptive cell, is of hematopoietic origin and is a member of the monocyte/macrophage family. It is a multinucleated cell that contains many lysosomes and is rich in hydrolytic enzymes. Osteoclasts are found on the surfaces of bones in small depressions, termed *Howship lacunae* (see Fig. 26-3D). Osteoclasts are highly polarized cells. The most strikingly polarized structure of the cell is its *ruffled membrane*, a complex infolding of plasmalemma, juxtaposed to the bone surface, which is visualized by electron microscopy (Fig. 26-4). The ruffled membrane is the osteoclast's resorptive organelle and forms only when the cell is in contact with, and is actively degrading, bone. Osteoclastic resorption is a multistep process that involves attachment of the cell to bone by integrins. A tight gasketlike seal isolates an extracellular compartment that forms between bone and the osteoclast ruffled membrane. A proton pump then acidifies this compartment to a pH of 4.5, in effect creating a giant extracellular lysosome. This proton-rich environment mobilizes bone mineral, thereby exposing the organic matrix of bone to degradation by lysosomal enzymes. Degraded fragments of bone are transported to the opposite side of the osteoclasts and then released to the extracellular space. Although the machinery of an osteoclast is superbly suited for bone resorption, it functions only if the matrix is mineralized. **In**

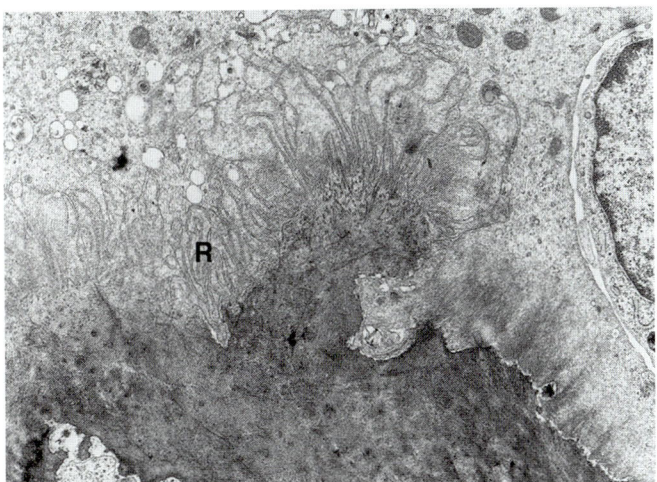

FIGURE 26-4
Osteoclast. An electron micrograph shows the ruffled membrane (R), which consists of a complex infolding of the plasma membrane juxtaposed to bone.

Microscopic Organization of Bone Tissue

Microscopic examination reveals two types of bone tissue: lamellar bone and woven bone (Fig. 26-6). Both varieties may be mineralized or unmineralized, the latter being termed *osteoid*.

Lamellar Bone

Lamellar bone is produced slowly and is highly organized. As the stronger bone tissue, it forms the adult skeleton. **Anything other than lamellar bone in the adult skeleton is abnormal.** Lamellar bone is defined by three characteristics: (1) a parallel arrangement of type I collagen fibers, (2) few osteocytes in the matrix, and (3) uniform osteocytes in lacunae parallel to the long axis of the collagen fibers. There are four types of lamellar bone. (Fig 26-7).

- **Circumferential bone** forms the outer periosteal and inner endosteal lamellar envelopes of the cortex.

fact, any bone that is lined by osteoid or unmineralized cartilage is protected from osteoclastic activity. In rickets, the growth plate does not calcify normally; it therefore grows without osteoclastic resorption and becomes very thick.

The resorptive action of osteoclasts initiates the constant remodeling of bone that is a normal part of skeletal maintenance (Fig. 26-5).

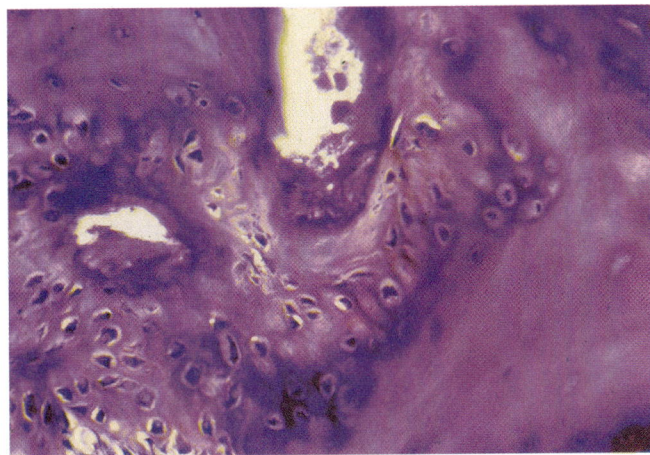

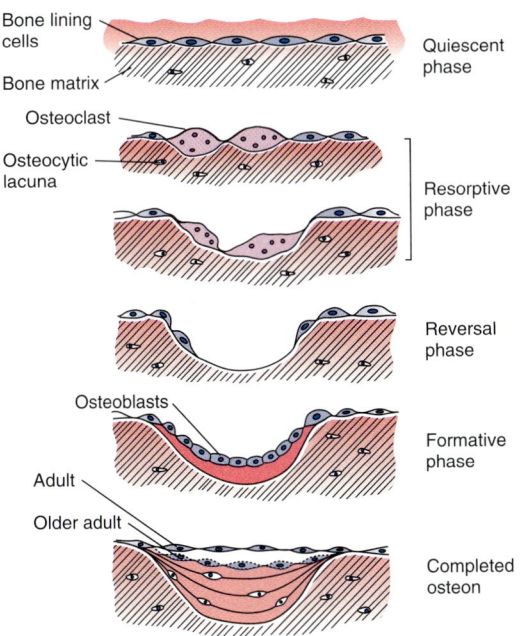

FIGURE 26-5
Bone-remodeling sequence. Bone remodeling is initiated by the appearance of osteoclasts on a bone surface previously lined by fusiform cells. After development of a resorption bay, osteoclasts are replaced by osteoblasts, which deposit new bone. The bone loss that attends aging (senile osteoporosis) is due to incomplete filling of resorption bays.

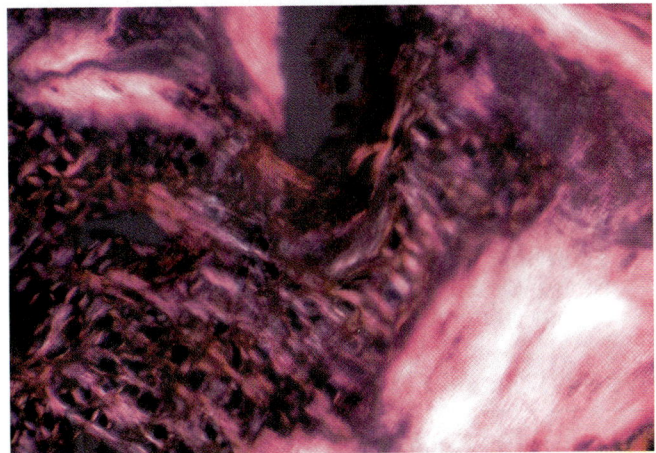

FIGURE 26-6
Woven bone. A. In this section, the woven bone constitutes early fracture repair. Note that in the area of new bone there are many osteocytes that vary in size but are mainly large with prominent lacunae (compare with area of mature bone at *lower right*). B. This is the same section viewed in polarized light. Note that the collagen fibers are disposed in a pattern resembling the loose fiber pattern of coarsely woven burlap.

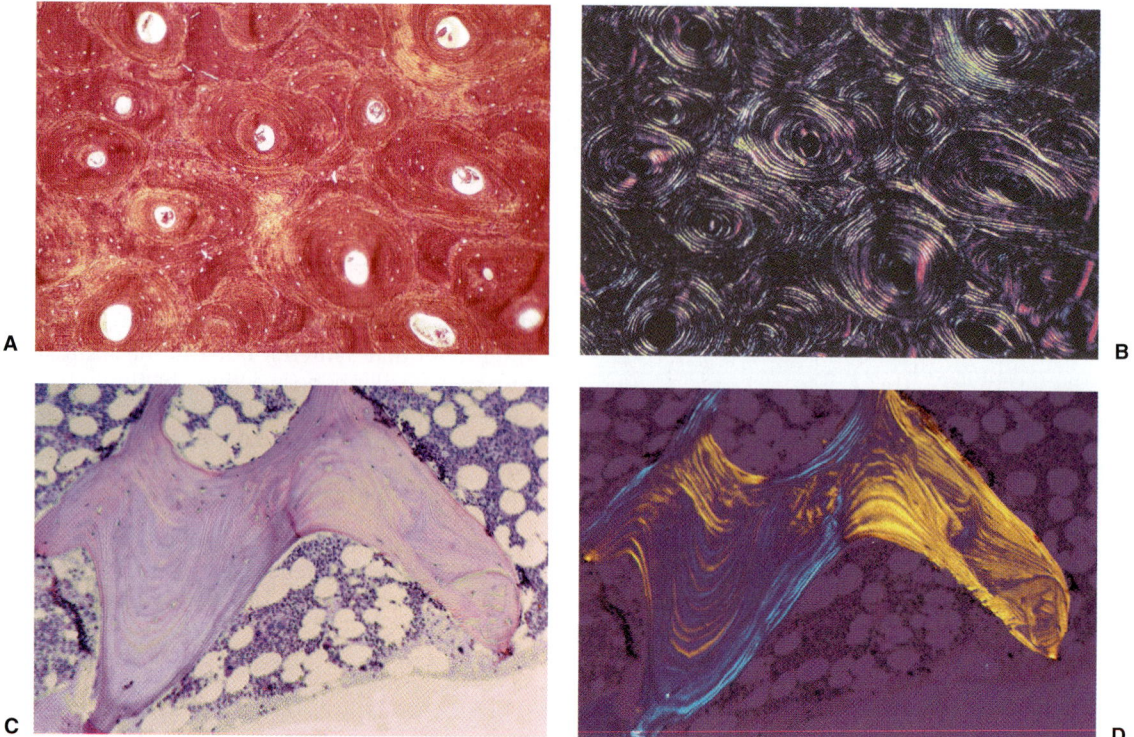

FIGURE 26-7
Cortical lamellar bone. A. Lamellae of the compacta (cortex) are arranged concentrically about haversian canals. B. The same field in polarized light shows the alternating light and dark layered arrangement of the collagen fibers. C. Lamellae of the spongiosa in a single mature trabecula are shown in a bright field view. D. Polarized light demonstrates that the lamellae are arranged in light and dark layers, but these layers are in long plates rather than in a concentric arrangement.

- **Concentric lamellar bone** is arranged around the haversian canals. In two dimensions, concentric lamellar bone and its haversian artery and vein constitute the *osteon* (see Fig. 26-1). In three dimensions, the osteons comprise the haversian system. These cylinders of bone around the haversian canals run parallel to the long axis of the cortex and are the strongest bone made. The osteons form only if there is appropriate stress. For example, a paralyzed limb in a child has a cortex composed exclusively of poorly formed haversian systems and circumferential lamellar bone.
- **Interstitial lamellar bone** represents remnants of either circumferential or concentric lamellar bone that have been remodeled and are wedged between the osteons.
- **Trabecular lamellar bone** forms the coarse cancellous bone of the medullary cavity. It exhibits plates of lamellar bone perforated by marrow spaces.

Woven Bone

Woven bone is identified by (1) an irregular arrangement of type I collagen fibers, hence the term *woven*; (2) numerous osteocytes in the matrix; and (3) variation in the size and shape of the osteocytes (see Fig. 26-6A and B).

Woven bone is deposited more rapidly than lamellar bone. It is haphazardly arranged and of low tensile strength, serving as a temporary scaffolding for support. It is not surprising that woven bone is found in the developing fetus, in areas surrounding tumors and infections, and as part of a healing fracture. **The presence of woven bone in the adult skeleton always represents a pathological condition and indicates that reactive tissue has been produced in response to some stress in the bone.**

Cartilage

In contrast to bone, cartilage does not contain blood vessels, nerves, or lymphatics. It may be focally calcified to provide some internal strength in the appropriate areas.

Cartilage Matrix

Like bone, cartilage may be viewed as an organic and inorganic biphasic material. The inorganic phase is composed of calcium hydroxyapatite crystals, equivalent to those found in bone matrix. However, the organic matrix is quite different from that of bone. Essentially, cartilage is a hyperhydrated structure, with water forming some 80% of its weight. The remaining 20% is composed principally of two macromolecular substances, namely type II collagen and proteoglycans. The water content is extremely important in the function of articular cartilage because it enhances the resilience and lubrication of the joint. The proteoglycans are complex macromolecules composed of a central linear protein core, to which are attached long side arms of polysaccharides called *glycosaminoglycans*. These molecules are polyanionic because of the regular presence of carboxyl groups and sulfates along the molecules. Cartilage glycosaminoglycans comprise three long-chain, unbranched, repeating, polydimeric saccharides: chondroitin-4-sulfate, chondroitin-6-sulfate, and keratan sulfate. The chondroitin sulfates are the most abundant, accounting for 55 to 90% of the cartilage matrix, depending on the age of the tissue.

Types of Cartilage

There are three types of cartilage:

- **Hyaline cartilage:** This is the prototypic cartilage, constituting the articular cartilage of the joints, the cartilaginous anlage of developing bones, the growth plates, the costochondral cartilages, the cartilages of the trachea, bronchi, and larynx, and the nasal cartilages. Hyaline cartilage is the most common cartilage in tumors, in fracture callus, and in areas of relative avascularity.
- **Fibrocartilage:** This tissue is essentially hyaline cartilage that contains numerous type I collagen fibers for tensile and structural strength. It is found in the annulus fibrosus of the intervertebral disk, tendinous and ligamentous insertions, menisci, the symphysis pubis, and insertions of joint capsules. Fibrocartilage may also occur in a fracture callus.
- **Elastic cartilage** is found in the epiglottis, in the arytenoid cartilages of the larynx, and in the external ear.

Chondrocytes

Chondrocytes are derived from primitive mesenchymal cells that are similar to the precursors of bone cells. The chondroblast gives rise to the chondrocyte. As in bone, the cell that destroys calcified cartilage is the osteoclast.

BONE FORMATION AND GROWTH

Bone tissue grows only by appositional growth, defined as the deposition of new matrix on the surface by adjacent surface cells. By contrast, virtually all other tissues, especially cartilage, increase by interstitial cell proliferation within the matrix as well as by appositional growth. The development of bone in the fetus follows a stereotyped sequence.

Most of the skeleton (except the bones of the calvaria and the clavicles) develops from cartilage anlagen that are present during fetal development. Thus, bone is first represented by tissue cartilage, which is eventually resorbed and replaced by bone, in a process termed *endochondral ossification*. The development of bone can be illustrated by using a limb as an example.

Primary Ossification

The process of primary ossification follows a temporal sequence:

1. **Cartilage anlage:** By 5 weeks of gestation, a thin layer of mesenchymal cells forms between the ectoderm and endoderm of the limb bud and condenses into a core of hyaline cartilage. This cartilaginous anlage becomes the precursor of the future long bone of that limb. The fibrous capsule of the cartilage anlage is called a *perichondrium*. The width of the cartilaginous anlage is increased by appositional growth of chondroblasts, which deposit cartilage matrix on the internal surface of the perichondrium. At the same time, the anlage increases in length by a combination of appositional and interstitial growth of the chondrocytes. At this stage, the long "bone" is actually composed of cartilage.
2. **The primary center of ossification:** The vascular bed increases, and the perichondrium deposits woven bone on the surface of the cartilage core. This circumferential sleeve of woven bone is the primary center of ossification, because it is the first bone tissue to be formed, and the perichondrium is thereafter termed *periosteum* (Fig. 26-8A).
3. **Cylinderization:** Within the cartilaginous anlage, chondrocytes form proliferating columns, which eventually undergo focal calcification. Calcification is the signal for osteoclastic resorption and invasion of vessels into the cartilaginous mass. Thus, the earliest endochondral ossification occurs after the cartilage is hollowed out from the

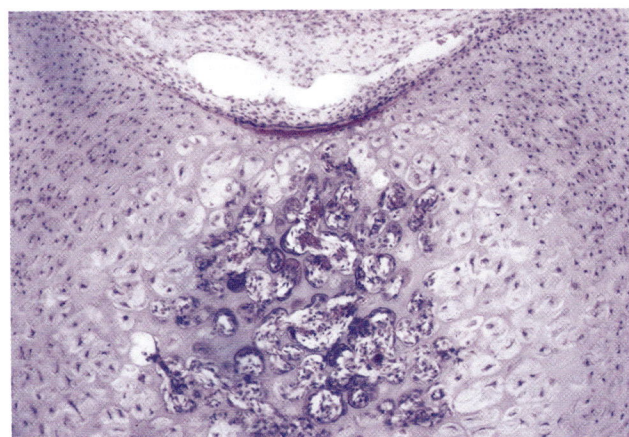 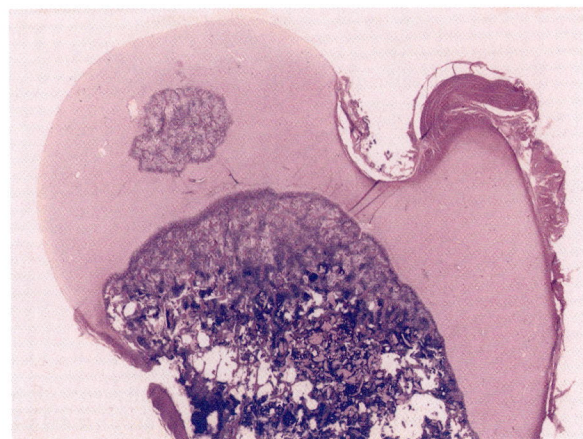

FIGURE 26-8
Primary ossification. **A.** This section of a short tubular bone demonstrates the first true bone tissue deposited on the outside of the midshaft of the cartilage model along with very early hollowing of the center of the cartilage model to form mixed spicules of cartilage and bone (primary spongiosa). **B.** The secondary ossification center is demonstrated in this femoral head.

center of the anlage. This "cavitation" of the cartilaginous core forms the future marrow space. The progressive hollowing of the diaphysis is termed *cylinderization*.

4. **Primary spongiosum:** The swollen, hypertrophied chondrocytes within the central cartilage begin to die, and capillary invasion becomes more extensive. The surfaces of the calcified cartilage cores become enveloped by woven bone laid down by osteoblasts, which arrive through the pluripotential mesenchymal tissue that enters with the capillaries. This cartilaginous core, surrounded by woven bone, is called *primary spongiosum*, or *primary trabecula*. It is the first bone formed after the replacement of cartilage in the process of endochondral ossification.

Cavitation continues along the future diaphysis toward each end of the bone. Meanwhile, the bone enlarges in width by appositional bone growth from the ever-increasing periosteal sleeve, which makes additional woven bone for the future cortex.

Secondary Ossification

Programmed events similar to those in the primary spongiosum take place in the cartilaginous ends of the future bone. Resting (reserve) cartilage is stimulated to become columns of proliferating cartilage, which then progress to hypertrophied chondrocytes and, eventually, calcified cartilage.

1. **The secondary center of ossification** (Fig. 26-8B): Also termed the *epiphyseal center of ossification*, this structure is formed at the ends of the bone when cartilage is resorbed. The centrifugal enlargement of the secondary ossification is called *hemispherization* and occurs simultaneously with the longitudinal development of the marrow cavity of the diaphysis.

2. **Formation of the growth plate:** Eventually, as the ends of the bone expand during hemispherization and cylinderization occurs in the future diaphysis, a zone of cartilage is trapped between the end of the bone and the diaphysis. This cartilage is destined to be the *growth plate* (Fig. 26-9A). The growth plate is a layer of modified cartilage between the diaphysis and the epiphysis, and its structure is essentially unchanged from early fetal life to skeletal maturity. **The growth plate controls the longitudinal growth of bones and ultimately determines adult height.**

3. **Structure of the growth plate:** The chondrocytes of the growth plate are arranged in vertical rows, which, in three dimensions, are really helices. When viewed longitudinally, the growth plate, proceeding from the epiphysis to the metaphysis, is divided into zones (Figs. 26-2B and 26-9).

The **reserve (resting) zone** is supplied by the epiphyseal arteries and has small chondrocytes and very little matrix. An additional peripheral zone, known as the *zone of Ranvier*, lies directly under the perichondrium.

The **proliferative zone** is the next deeper zone, in which active proliferation of chondrocytes occurs both longitudinally and transversely, although the main growth thrust is in the longitudinal direction. In a very active growth plate, the proliferative zones form more than half the thickness of the growth plate.

The **hypertrophic zone** is the next cartilaginous area and is characterized by a substantial increase in the size of the chondrocytes. The intercellular matrix is prominent, and

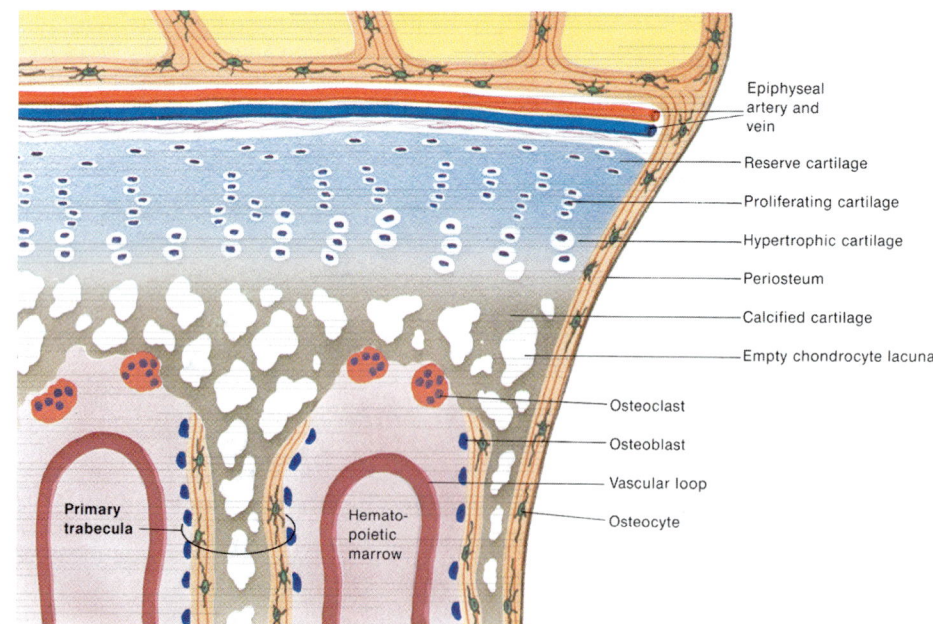

FIGURE 26-9
Anatomy of the growth (epiphyseal) plate. A. Normal growing epiphyseal plate. The epiphysis is separated from the epiphyseal plate by transverse plates of bone that seal the plate so that it grows only toward the metaphysis. The various zones of cartilage are illustrated. As the calcified cartilage migrates toward the metaphysis, the chondrocytes die, and the lacunae are empty. At the interface of the epiphyseal plate and the metaphysis, osteoclasts bore into the calcified cartilage, accompanied by a capillary loop from the metaphyseal vessels. Osteoblasts follow the osteoclasts and lay down osteoid on the cartilage core, thereby forming the bone primary spongiosum, or primary trabeculae.

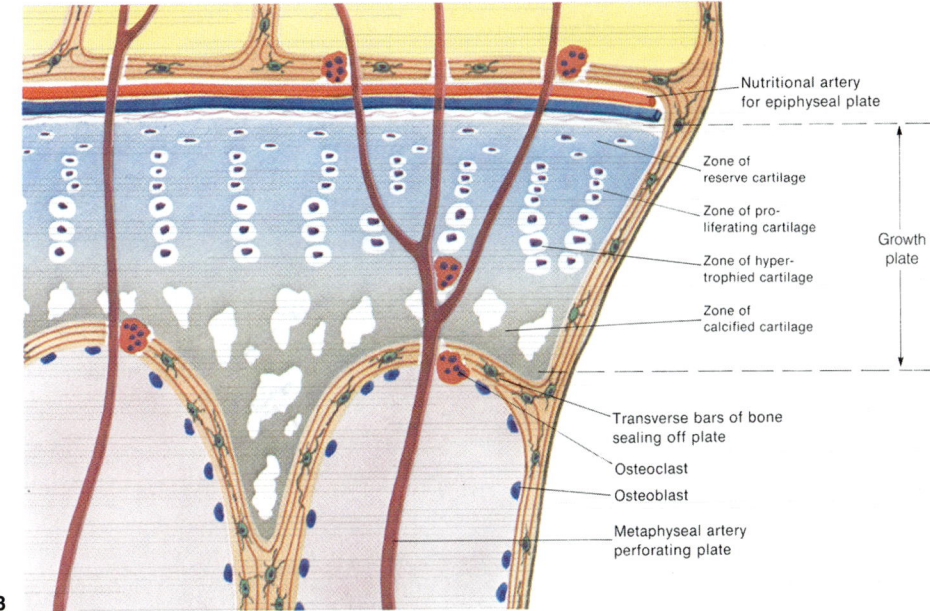

FIGURE 26-9 (continued)
B. Normal closure. The epiphyseal cartilage has ceased to grow, and metaphyseal vessels penetrate the cartilage plate. Transverse bars of bone separate the plate from the metaphysis.

a dense zone, called the *territorial matrix*, surrounds chondrocytes.

The **zone of calcification** is the cartilaginous zone closest to the metaphysis, where the matrix becomes mineralized.

The **zone of ossification** is the area where a coating of bone is laid down on the surface of the calcified cartilage. Capillaries grow into the calcified cartilage and give access to osteoclasts, which resorb much of the calcified matrix. Residual vertical walls of calcified cartilage act as scaffolding for the deposition of bone.

The molecular mechanisms governing endochondral growth are beginning to be understood. For example, mutations of the FGF-3 receptor lead to either growth arrest or acceleration. Similarly, development of a normal growth plate depends on the expression of parathyroid hormone-related protein. Failure to produce this protein leads to severe growth retardation and distorted growth plates.

Formation of the Metaphysis

The formation of the metaphysis, which is called *funnelization*, occurs at the ring of DeLaCroix, a periosteal cuff of bone surrounding the epiphyseal cartilage. Here a wave of periosteal osteoclasts resorbs the cortex, so that a fluted or funnel shape begins to appear. At the same time, endosteal osteoblastic bone is deposited to keep pace with, and to offset, some of the osteoclastic resorption. The net result is the funnel or fluted shape of the bone.

Obliteration of the Growth Plate

The growth plate is normally obliterated at a specific age for each bone (Fig. 26-9B). Closure of the growth plate is induced by sex hormones and occurs earlier in girls than in boys. The renewal of chondrocytes slows and ultimately ceases. The entire plate is eventually replaced by bone. In some persons, a transverse bony plate representing the site of closure can be seen radiologically.

DISORDERS OF THE GROWTH PLATE

Cretinism Leads to Defective Cartilage Maturation

Cretinism, the syndrome that results from maternal iodine deficiency (see Chapter 21), has profound effects on the skeleton. Linear growth is severely impaired, resulting in dwarfism, with the limbs disproportionately short in relation to the trunk. The delayed closure of the fontanelles of the skull causes an unusually large head. There is a delay in the closure of the epiphyses, as well as radiological stippling of these zones. Shedding of deciduous teeth and eruption of permanent teeth are retarded.

 Pathology: In cretinism, the chondrocytes do not follow the orderly progression of the endochondral sequence. Instead, the maturation of the hypertrophied zone is retarded, and the zone of proliferative cartilage is narrow. Endochondral ossification, therefore, does not proceed appropriately, and transverse bars of bone in the metaphysis seal off the growth plate. Although the growth plates may remain open, the failure of endochondral ossification produces severe dwarfism. The misshapen epiphyses seen on radiography reflect incomplete penetration of the secondary centers of ossification of the epiphysis.

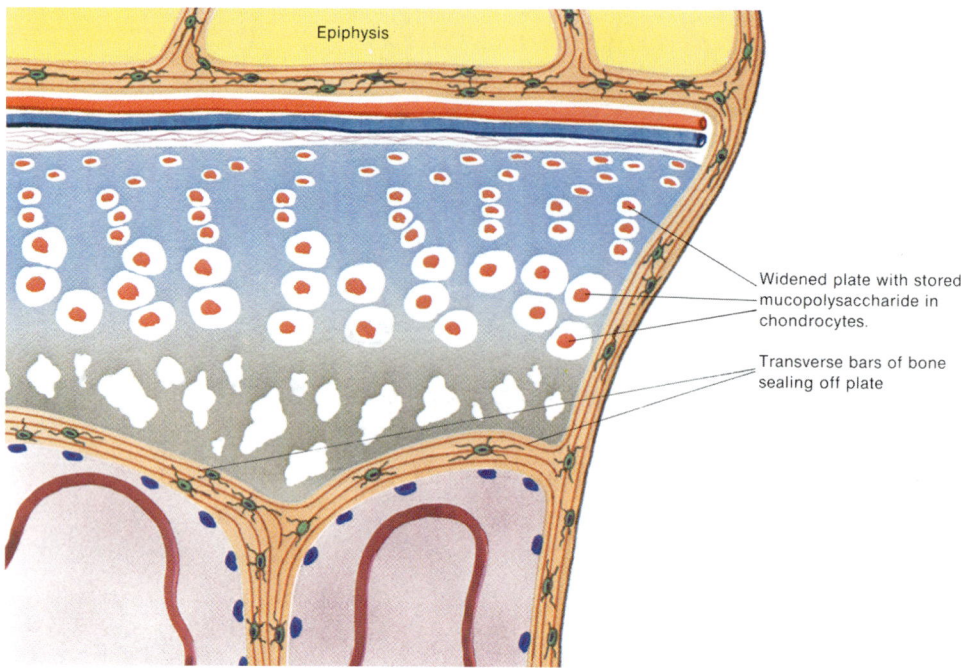

FIGURE 26-10
The growth (epiphyseal) plate in the mucopolysaccharidoses. These disorders are characterized by disorganized and abbreviated columns of swollen chondrocytes that are engorged with mucopolysaccharides. There is interference with the normal endochondral sequence, and the epiphyseal plate is sealed off by transverse bars of bone from the metaphysis. Dwarfism results from the lack of vascular penetration into the epiphyseal plate. Such penetration normally sustains new bone formation, thereby allowing continued lengthening of the bone.

Morquio Syndrome Features Mucopolysaccharide Deposition in Chondrocytes

Many of the mucopolysaccharidoses (see Chapter 6) involve skeletal deformities, which can be attributed to the deposition of mucopolysaccharides (glycosaminoglycans) in the developing bones (Fig. 26-10). An example is Morquio syndrome (mucopolysaccharidosis type IV), which leads to a particularly severe form of dwarfism, in addition to dental defects, mental retardation, corneal opacities, and increased urinary excretion of keratan sulfate.

Pathology: Mucopolysaccharides accumulate in the chondrocytes, a process that ultimately interferes with the normal endochondral sequence. The result is a disorganized growth plate, which is also sealed off by transverse bars of bone. This syndrome is an inherited deficiency with several phenotypes, caused by absence or reduction in the activity of lysosomal enzymes involved in the degradation of keratan sulfate in glycosaminoglycans, especially in the cartilage, cornea, and intervertebral disks.

Clinical Features: Symptoms are characterized by typical skeletal changes (e.g., femoral head dysplasia, vertebral deformities, and dwarfism). Corneal clouding, disturbances of heart valve function, hearing defects, and keratan sulfaturia are other systemic consequences.

Achondroplasia Is an Inherited Dwarfism Caused by Arrest of the Growth Plate

Achondroplasia refers to a syndrome of short-limbed dwarfism and macrocephaly and represents a failure of normal epiphyseal cartilage formation. It is the most common genetic form of dwarfism (1:15,000 live births) and is inherited as an autosomal dominant trait. Most cases represent new mutations. The mean adult height in achondroplasia is 131 cm (51 inches) in men and 125 cm (49 inches) in women. Achondroplastic dwarfs have normal mentation and an average life span. However, some patients develop severe kyphoscoliosis and its complications.

Pathogenesis: Achondroplasia is caused by an activating mutation in the FGF-3 receptor on chromosome 16 (4p16.3). The achondroplastic mutation negatively regulates chondrocyte proliferation and differentiation and arrests the development of the growth plate.

Consistent with this observation, an inactivating FGF-3 receptor mutation leads to accelerated longitudinal growth. The recently described *pseudoachondroplasia,* has the same phenotype but its associated mutations are in the cartilage oligomeric matrix protein *(COMP)* gene locus on chromosome 19.

Pathology: The growth plate in achondroplasia is greatly thinned, and the zone of proliferative cartilage is either absent or extensively attenuated (Fig. 26-11). The zone of provisional calcification, if present, undergoes endochondral ossification, but at a greatly reduced rate. A transverse bar of bone often seals off the growth plate, thereby preventing further bone formation and causing dwarfism. Interestingly, the secondary centers of ossification and the articular cartilage are normal. Because intramembranous ossification is undisturbed, the periosteum functions normally, and the bones become very short and thick. For the same reasons, the head of the dwarf appears unusually large, compared with the bones formed from the cartilage of the face. The spine is of normal length, but the limbs are abnormally short.

Scurvy Reflects Vitamin C Deficiency

Scurvy, the clinical expression of vitamin C deficiency, is today a rare disease (see Chapter 8).

Pathogenesis: Vitamin C is a cofactor in the hydroxylation of proline and lysine. Hydroxyproline and hydroxylysine are important in stabilizing the helical structure of collagen and in cross-linking the tropocollagen fibers into the proper molecular structure of collagen. Wound healing and bone growth are, therefore, impaired in patients with scurvy. Furthermore, the basement membrane of capillaries is damaged by this condition, and widespread capillary bleeding is common.

Pathology: The skeletal changes of scurvy reflect the lack of osteoblastic function. Woven bone is not formed because osteoblasts cannot produce and normally cross-link collagen. At the growth plate, the chondrocytes continue to grow. The zone of calcified cartilage may actually become more prominent, because it is more heavily calcified. Osteoclasts resorb this zone, but the primary spongiosum does not form properly, and there is irregular vascular perforation of the cartilage plate (Fig. 26-12). Fractures and capillary bleeding occur, leading to further disorganization in the metaphysis—hence the German term Trümmerfeld ("field of ruin") for this area of the sub-epiphyseal plate. The subperiosteal bleeding may be so severe that it leads to diminution of the cortex, reduced appositional growth, and osteoporosis. Dislocation of the growth plate also may occur.

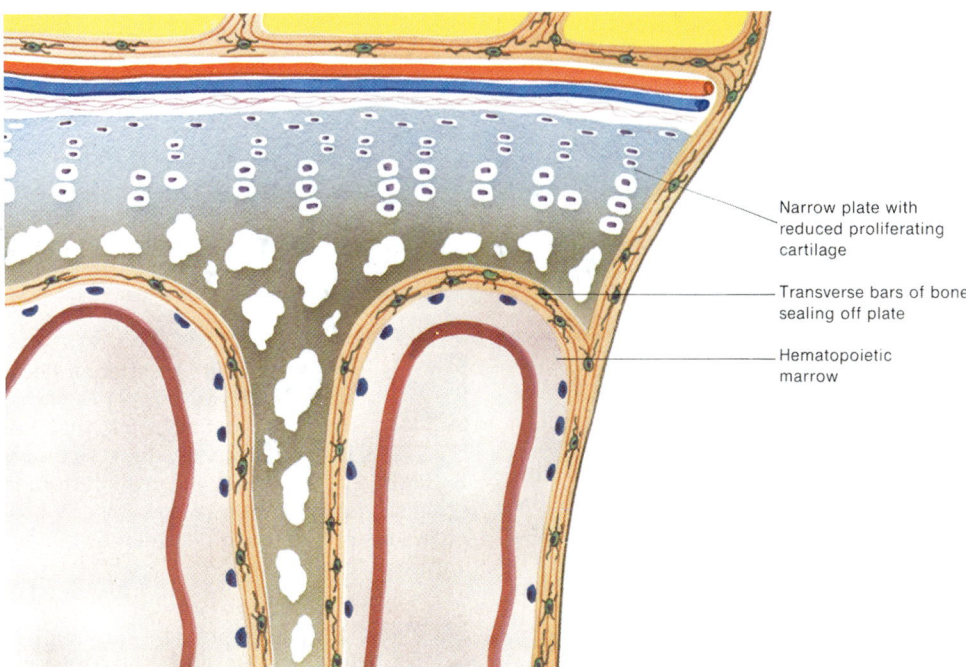

FIGURE 26-11

The growth (epiphyseal) plate of an achondroplastic dwarf. In achondroplasia, the epiphyseal plate is reduced in thickness, and the zones of proliferating cartilage are attenuated. Osteoclastic activity is inconspicuous, and the interface between the plate and the metaphysis is often sealed by transverse bars of bone that prevent further endochondral ossification. As a result, the bones are shortened.

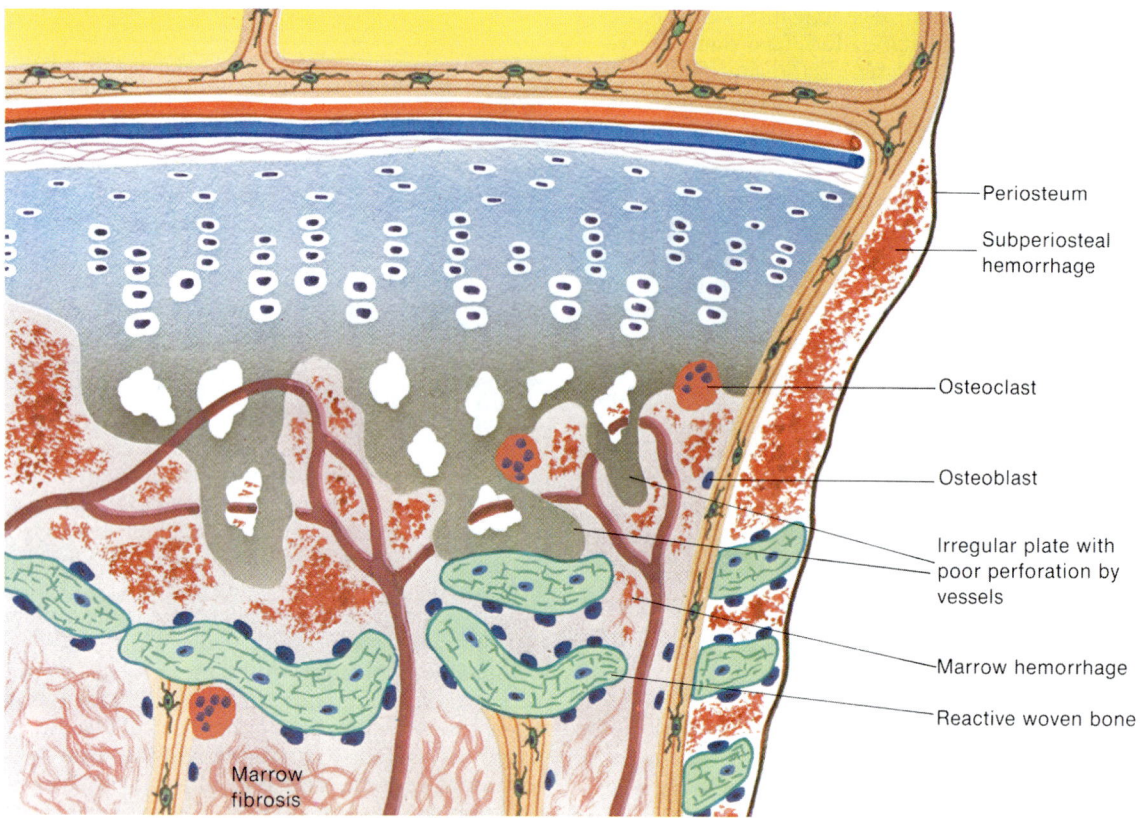

FIGURE 26-12
The growth (epiphyseal) plate in scurvy. Defective collagen formation leads to capillary fragility and periosteal hemorrhage. Osteoclasts do not perforate the plate in a regular fashion. There is often extensive hemorrhage in this region. Microfractures cause secondary microcalluses; reactive bone is, therefore, seen in this region.

Children with scurvy have visible bone deformities, similar to those associated with rickets. In adults, bone deformities are not seen, but subperiosteal bleeding may occur, leading to joint and muscle pain.

Asymmetric Cartilage Growth Causes Spinal Disorders and Tumors

Asymmetric cartilage growth, such as occurs in patients with knock-knees and bowed legs, develops when one part of the growth plate, either medial or lateral, grows faster than the other. Most cases are hereditary, but mechanical forces, such as trauma near the growth plate, may stimulate one side to grow faster or in an asymmetric fashion.

To correct a severe condition in a child, the growth of this portion of the plate is retarded by surgically implanting a staple or a brace, thereby allowing the opposite side of the plate to grow. In an adult, because the growth plates have already closed, surgical osteotomy (fracture) is used. Aside from the cosmetic appearance, these conditions may require correction to prevent future incongruity, eventual loss of articular cartilage, and joint destruction.

Scoliosis and Kyphosis

Scoliosis *is an abnormal lateral curvature of the spine, usually affecting adolescent girls.* **Kyphosis** *refers to an abnormal anteroposterior curvature.* When both conditions are present, the term **kyphoscoliosis** is used.

 Pathogenesis: A vertebral body grows in length (height) from the endplates of the vertebrae, which correspond to the growth plates of the long tubular bones. As in tubular bones, the vertebral bodies increase in width by appositional bone growth from the periosteum. In scoliosis, for unknown reasons, one portion of the endplate grows faster than the other, thereby producing a lateral curvature of the spine.

 Clinical Features: The treatment is appropriate stress on the vertebral body through the use of braces or internal fixation to straighten the spine. If kyphoscoliosis is severe, the patient may eventually develop chronic pulmonary disease, cor pulmonale, and joint problems, particularly involving the hip.

Osteochondroma

Osteochondroma is a developmental defect (hamartoma) of the skeleton, which arises from a defect at the ring of Ranvier of the growth plate. Solitary osteochondroma is the most common form of the lesion. The tumor may have to be removed if it is cosmetically displeasing or presses upon an artery or nerve.

Pathogenesis: The ring of Ranvier guides the growth of the growth cartilage toward the metaphysis. If the ring of Ranvier is absent or defective, growth cartilage grows laterally into the soft tissue. Vessels originating in the marrow cavity of the bone extend into this cartilage mass. Continuation of this process results in a cartilage-capped, bony, stalked osteochondroma (Fig. 26-13), which is in direct continuity with the marrow cavity of the parent bone. Loss of distal chromosome 8q is associated with osteochondroma.

Pathology: Osteochondromas tend to grow away from the joint. In radiographs, a cartilaginous mass is in direct continuity with the parent bone and lacks an underlying cortex. On histological examination, a cartilage-capped, bony mass is surrounded by a surface fibrous membrane, which actually represents the perichondrium. Active endochondral ossification deep to the cartilage cap allows the bony protuberance to lengthen.

HEREDITARY MULTIPLE OSTEOCHONDROMATOSIS: This inherited autosomal dominant disorder is characterized by numerous osteochondromas. Although not as common as solitary osteochondroma, the heritable variety is not rare. It occurs predominantly in men, but because of its variable expression, a seemingly unaffected woman from an afflicted family may transmit the disorder.

Pathology: In severe cases of hereditary osteochondromatosis, dwarfism may result because of lateral displacement of the longitudinal growth plate by the osteochondroma. Metacarpals may be shortened, and fixed pronation or supination may develop if the lesions occur in the forearm and interfere with the function of the wrist. Further orthopedic difficulties may be caused by unequal leg length and disturbed joint function because of encroaching osteochondromas. Each individual lesion in multiple osteochondromatosis is identical to a solitary osteochondroma. In multiple osteochondromatosis, however, there is a long-term increased risk of developing a chondrosarcoma in the cartilage cap, although this is a rare event.

Hereditary multiple exostoses (EXT) is one of the most common inherited musculoskeletal disorders with an incidence of about 1/50,000. EXT is genetically heterogeneous with at least 3 chromosomal loci: *EXT1* (8q24.1), *EXT2* (11p11-p13), and *EXT3* (19p). Loss of function of the *EXT1* or *EXT2* gene is the main cause of EXT.

Hemihypertrophy

Hemihypertrophy refers to a number of conditions that stimulate the growth plate in one limb to undergo rapid and prolonged endochondral ossification. As a consequence, the limb is much longer than the contralateral one. An infection in the metaphyseal area may stimulate the growth plate to grow rapidly. An arteriovenous malformation may also cause the growth plate to grow faster than its counterpart. Fractures and tumors near

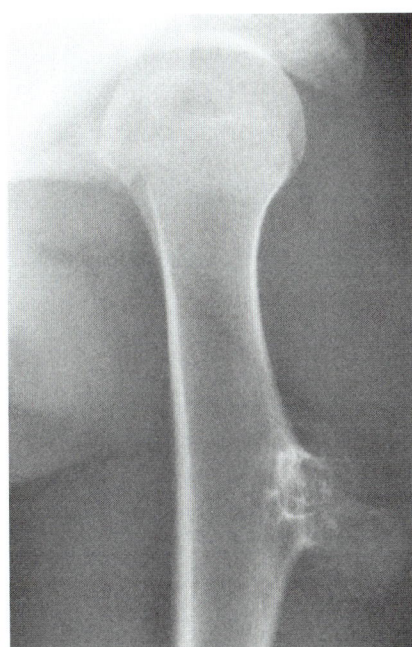
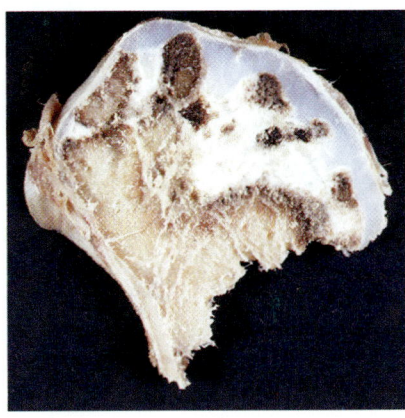

FIGURE 26-13
Osteochondroma. **A.** A radiograph of an osteochondroma of the humerus shows a lesion that is directly contiguous with the marrow space. **B.** The cross-section of an osteochondroma shows the cap of calcified cartilage overlying poorly organized cancellous bone.

the growth plate may produce the same result. In some cases, hemihypertrophy is part of an inherited syndrome. Children with isolated hemihypertrophy are at increased risk for neoplasms.

MODELING ABNORMALITIES

Osteopetrosis (Marble Bone Disease, Albers–Schönberg Disease) Features Abnormally Dense Bone

Osteopetrosis, also known as marble bone disease *or* Albers–Schönberg disease, *is a group of at least nine, rare, inherited disorders.* The most common autosomal recessive form is a severe, sometimes fatal disease affecting infants and children. Death of infants with this severe variant is attributable to marked anemia, cranial nerve entrapment, hydrocephalus, and infections. A more benign form, transmitted as an autosomal dominant trait and seen in adulthood or adolescence, is associated with mild anemia or no symptoms at all.

 Pathogenesis: **The sclerotic skeleton of osteopetrosis is the result of failed osteoclastic bone resorption.** The disease is caused by mutations in genes that govern osteoclast formation or function. For example, mutation of genes encoding proteins necessary for the generation of macrophages, which are osteoclast precursors, prompts one form of osteopetrosis distinguished by an absence of osteoclasts. Mutation of the oncogene *c-src,* which is necessary for osteoclast polarization, results in another type of osteopetrosis. In the latter form of the disease, abundant, yet ineffective, osteoclasts fail to polarize, as evidenced by the lack of a ruffled membrane.

Because osteoclast function is arrested, osteopetrosis is characterized by (1) the retention of the primary spongiosum with its cartilage cores, (2) lack of funnelization of the metaphysis, and (3) a thickened cortex. The result is short, blocklike, radiodense bones, hence the term *marble bone disease* (Fig. 26-14). These bones are extremely radiopaque and weigh two to three times more than normal bone. However, they are basically weak because the bone structure is intrinsically disorganized and cannot remodel along lines of

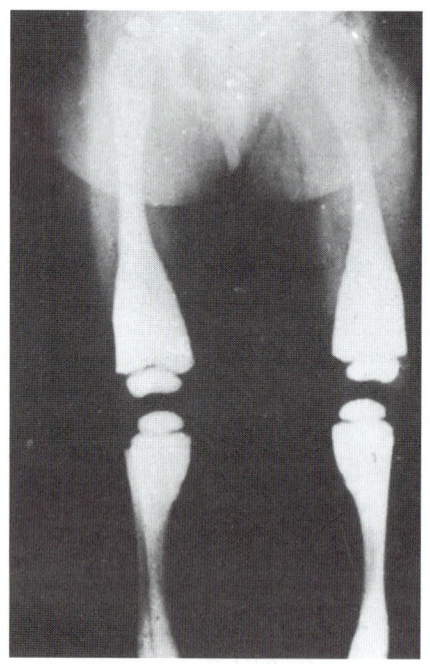
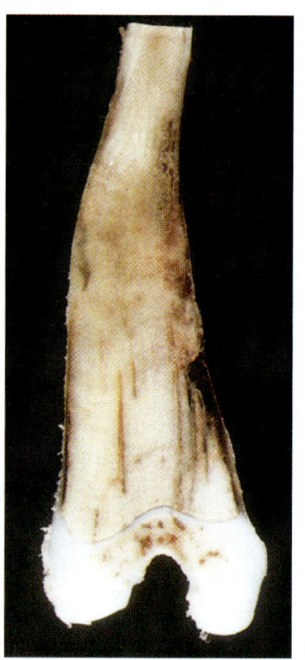
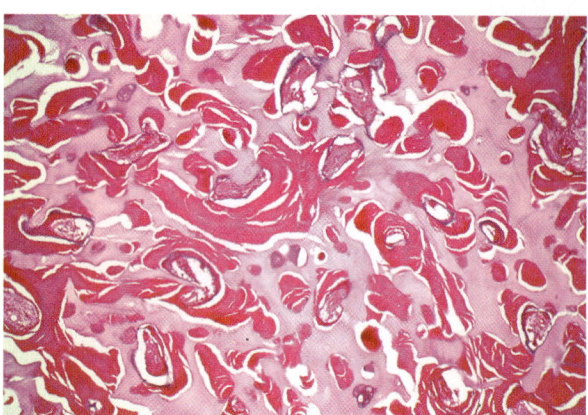

FIGURE 26-14
Osteopetrosis. **A.** A radiograph of a child shows markedly misshapen and dense bones of the lower extremities, characteristic of "marble bone disease." **B.** A gross specimen of the femur shows obliteration of the marrow space by dense bone. **C.** A photomicrograph of the bone of a child with autosomal recessive osteopetrosis demonstrates disorganization of bony trabeculae by retention of primary spongiosa (mixed spicules) and further obliteration of the marrow space by secondary spongiosa. The result is complete disorganization of the trabeculae and absence of marrow.

stress. The mineralized cartilage is also weak and friable. As a result, the bones in osteopetrosis fracture easily.

Autosomal dominant osteopetrosis (ADO) type II is the most frequent type of osteopetrosis, (incidence 5/100,000), and is associated with frequent fracture in 75% of patients. Its gene is located on chromosome 1p21. Deficiency of carbonic anhydrase II has been identified as the primary defect in the autosomal recessive syndrome of osteopetrosis with renal tubular acidosis and cerebral calcification. An abnormal chromosome 11q12-13 region is linked to ADO type I, osteoporosis–pseudoglioma syndrome, and malignant infantile osteopetrosis.

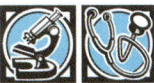 **Pathology and Clinical Features:** On gross examination the bones in osteopetrosis are widened in the metaphysis and diaphysis, resulting in the characteristic "Erlenmeyer flask" deformity. Histologically, the bone tissue is extremely irregular, and almost all areas contain a cartilage core. Depending on the mutation, osteoclasts may be absent, present in normal numbers, or even abundant. In the case of osteopetrosis characterized by normal or increased numbers of osteoclasts, the molecular defect lies in a gene involved in the function of osteoclasts, rather than their formation.

The suppression of hematopoiesis in osteopetrosis is not due to encroachment of mineralized tissue on the marrow, but rather to its replacement by sheets of abnormal osteoclasts or extensive fibrosis. Marrow suppression in patients with the malignant form of osteopetrosis is sufficient to cause severe anemia and even pancytopenia. To compensate for the encroachment on the marrow space, extramedullary hematopoiesis occurs in the liver, spleen, and lymph nodes, with resulting enlargement of these structures. The narrowing of neural foramina causes cranial nerve involvement, and subsequent strangulation of nerves leads to blindness and deafness. Osteopetrosis is treated by bone marrow transplantation, which gives rise to a new clone of functional osteoclasts.

Progressive Diaphyseal Dysplasia Features Thickened Long Bones

Progressive diaphyseal dysplasia (Camurati–Engelmann disease) is an autosomal dominant disorder of children in which cylinderization does not proceed appropriately, resulting in symmetric thickening in, and increased diameter of, the diaphyses of long bones. It is due to increased bone formation linked to a mutation in the propeptide of TGF-β. The disease particularly affects the femur, tibia, fibula, radius, and ulna. Patients have pain over the affected areas, fatigue, muscle wasting, atrophy, and gait abnormalities.

DELAYED MATURATION OF BONE

Osteogenesis Imperfecta Relates to Abnormal Type I Collagen

Osteogenesis imperfecta (OI) refers to a group of mainly autosomal dominant, heritable disorders of connective tissue, caused by mutations in the gene for type I collagen, affecting the skeleton, joints, *ears, ligaments, teeth, sclerae, and skin* (see Chapter 6). There are at least four types of OI, each with a different genetic structural abnormality and clinical features.

 Pathogenesis: The pathogenesis of OI involves mutations of *COL1A1* and *COL1A2* genes, which encode the α1 and α2 chains of type I procollagen, the major structural protein of bone. These two genes are located in chromosomes 17 (17q21.3-q22) and 7 (7q21.3-q22), respectively. While *COL1A1* mutations are seen in all types of OI, mutations of *COL1A2* are found in types II, III, and IV OI. Mutations of *COL1A1* affect three fourths of the type I collagen molecules, with half of the molecules containing one abnormal proα1 chain and one quarter containing two abnormal proα1 chains. By contrast, mutations in *COL1A2* affect only half of the synthesized collagen molecules.

Osteogenesis Imperfecta Type I

OI type I is the mildest phenotype and is inherited as an autosomal dominant trait. It is characterized by multiple fractures after birth, blue sclera, and hearing abnormalities. In some patients abnormalities of the teeth are also conspicuous.

 Pathology and Clinical Features: The initial fractures usually occur after the infant begins to sit and walk. There may be hundreds of fractures a year with minor movement or trauma. On radiological examination, the bones are extremely thin, delicate, and abnormally curved (Fig. 26-15). When a fracture occurs, the fracture callus may be extensive enough to resemble a tumor. As the child grows, the fractures tend to decrease in severity and frequency, and stature is generally unaffected.

The sclerae are very thin, with the blue color being attributable to the underlying choroid. The progressive hearing loss, which develops to total deafness in adulthood, results from fusion of the auditory ossicles. The joint laxity associated with the condition eventually leads to kyphoscoliosis and flat feet. Because of hypoplasia of the dentine and pulp, the teeth are misshapen and bluish yellow.

Osteogenesis Imperfecta Type II

OI type II is a lethal, perinatal disease with an autosomal dominant inheritance pattern. Affected infants are stillborn or die within a few days, in a sense being crushed to death. They exhibit markedly short stature and severe deformities of the limbs, and almost all of the bones sustain fractures during delivery or during uterine contractions in labor. As in OI type I, the sclerae are blue.

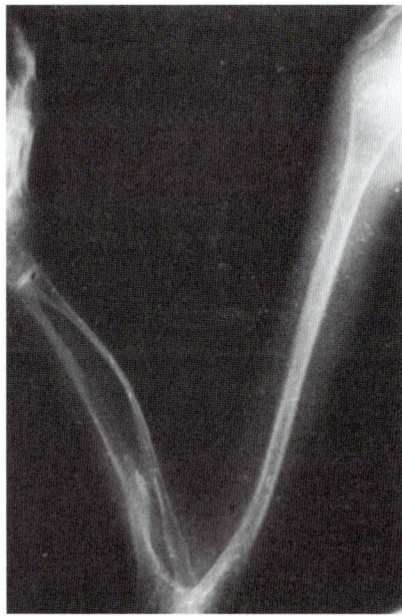

FIGURE 26-15
Osteogenesis imperfecta. A radiograph illustrates the markedly thin and attenuated humerus and bones of the forearm. There is a fracture callus in the proximal ulna.

Osteogenesis Imperfecta Type III

OI type III is the progressive, most severely deforming type of disease and is characterized by many bone fractures, growth retardation, and severe skeletal deformities. The inheritance pattern is autosomal dominant, although (rarely) autosomal recessive forms are reported. Fractures are present at birth, but the bones are less fragile than in the type II form. These patients eventually develop severe shortening of their stature because of progressive bone fractures and severe kyphoscoliosis. Although the sclerae may be blue at birth, they become white shortly thereafter. Abnormalities of the teeth are common.

Osteogenesis Imperfecta Type IV

OI type IV is similar to type I except that the sclerae are normal. The condition is heterogeneous in its presentation, and there may or may not be dental disease. In this disorder, abnormal cross-linkages of collagen result in thin, delicate, and weak collagen fibrils. This inappropriate collagen does not allow the bone cortex to mature, so that at birth the cortex of the bone resembles that of a fetus. The cortex is composed of woven bone and small areas of lamellar bone. Over a period of years, the cortex matures, but this may not occur until adolescence or even later. In any event, the frequency of fractures tends to decrease over a long period. These patients are vigorously treated with orthopedic devices, including rods inserted into the medullary cavities to prevent the dwarfing effect of multiple fractures.

There is no single treatment for OI. Recently, osteoprogenitor cells for bone marrow transplantation, growth factors, bisphosphonates, and gene therapy to improve collagen synthesis have been undergoing clinical trials in an attempt to modify the course and severity of the disease. Because exuberant fracture callus occurs, it is not surprising that rare cases of OI have been interpreted as osteosarcoma.

Enchondromatosis Is Marked by Multiple Cartilaginous Tumors

Enchondromatosis, also termed Ollier disease *is a bone disorder characterized by the development of numerous cartilaginous masses that lead to bony deformities.* The condition is not strictly a disease of delayed maturation of bone, but one in which residual hyaline cartilage, anlage cartilage, or cartilage from the growth plate does not undergo endochondral ossification and remains in the bones. As a consequence, the bones show multiple, tumorlike masses of abnormally arranged hyaline cartilage (enchondromas), with zones of proliferative and hypertrophied cartilage (Fig. 26-16). These tumors tend to be located in the metaphyses. As growth continues, the enchondromas settle in the diaphysis of adolescents and adults.

Enchondromatosis is asymmetric and may cause bone deformities. Whether enchondromas represent true neoplasms is debated, but they exhibit a strong tendency to undergo malignant change into chondrosarcomas in adult life. Therefore a patient with enchondromatosis who has increasing pain or an increasing abnormality at one site should be evaluated to rule out an underlying sarcoma.

Solitary enchondroma has histological features similar to Ollier disease and principally affects the tubular bones of the hands and feet. It undergoes malignant change only rarely.

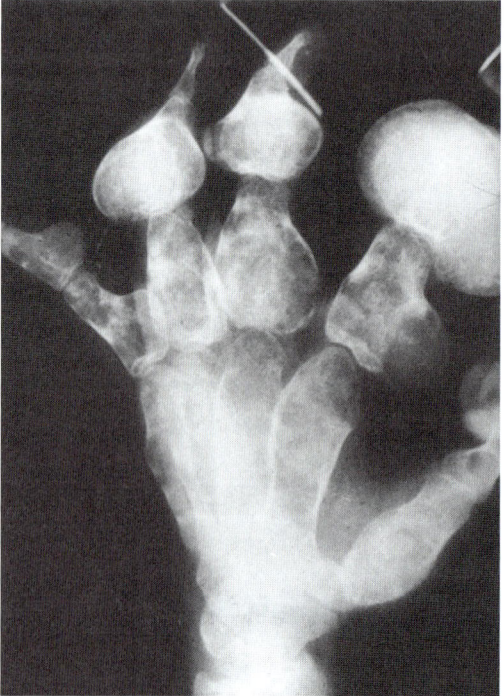

FIGURE 26-16
Multiple enchondromatosis (Ollier disease). A radiograph of the hand shows bulbous swellings that represent cartilage masses composed of hyaline cartilage, which is sometimes admixed with more primitive myxoid cartilage.

Maffucci syndrome is characterized by multiple enchondromas and cavernous hemangiomas. This condition usually manifests in early childhood and may lead to significant skeletal deformities. Chondrosarcoma develops in as many as half of all patients with Maffucci syndrome. The incidence of malignant tumors in other organs is also increased in patients with Mafucci syndrome.

FRACTURE

The most common bone lesion is a fracture, which is defined as a discontinuity of the bone. A force perpendicular to the long axis of the bone results in a transverse fracture. If the applied force is in the long axis of the bone, the resulting fracture is caused by compression. A torsional force results in a spiral fracture, and combined tension and compression shear forces cause angulation and displacement of the fractured ends.

A force powerful enough to fracture a bone also injures the adjacent soft tissues. In this situation, there is often (1) extensive muscle necrosis, (2) hemorrhage because of shearing of capillary beds and larger vessels of the soft tissues, (3) tearing of tendinous insertions and ligamentous attachments, and (4) even nerve damage, caused by stretching or direct tearing of the nerve.

Fracture Healing

In the repair of a bone fracture, anything other than the formation of bone tissue at the fracture site represents incomplete healing. The healing of a fracture is divided into three phases: the inflammatory phase, the reparative phase, and the remodeling phase (Fig. 26-17). The duration of each phase depends on the patient's age, the site of fracture, the patient's overall health and nutritional status, and the extent of soft tissue injury. Local factors, such as vascular supply and mechanical forces at the site, also play a role in healing.

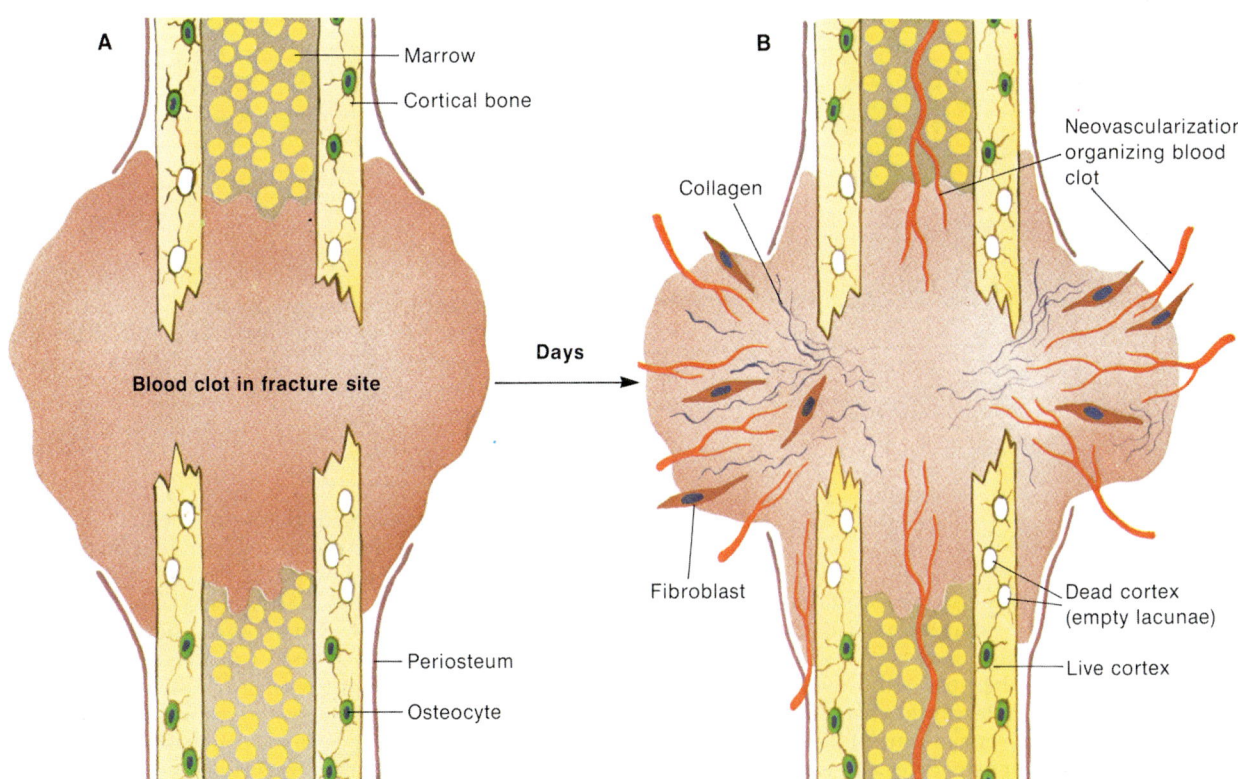

FIGURE 26-17
Healing of a fracture. **A.** Soon after a fracture is sustained, an extensive blood clot forms in the subperiosteal and soft tissue, as well as in the marrow cavity. The bone at the fracture site is jagged. **B.** The inflammatory phase of fracture healing is characterized by neovascularization and beginning organization of the blood clot. Because the osteocytes in the fracture site are dead, the lacunae are empty. The osteocytes of the cortex are necrotic well beyond the fracture site, owing to the traumatic interruption of the perforating arteries from the periosteum. **C.** The reparative phase of fracture healing is characterized by the formation of a callus of cartilage and woven bone near the fracture site. The jagged edges of the original cortex have been remodeled and eroded by osteoclasts. The marrow space has been revascularized and contains reactive woven bone, as does the periosteal area. **D.** In the remodeling phase, during which the cortex is revitalized, the reactive bone may be lamellar or woven. The new bone is organized along stress lines and mechanical forces. Extensive osteoclastic and osteoblastic cellular activity is maintained.

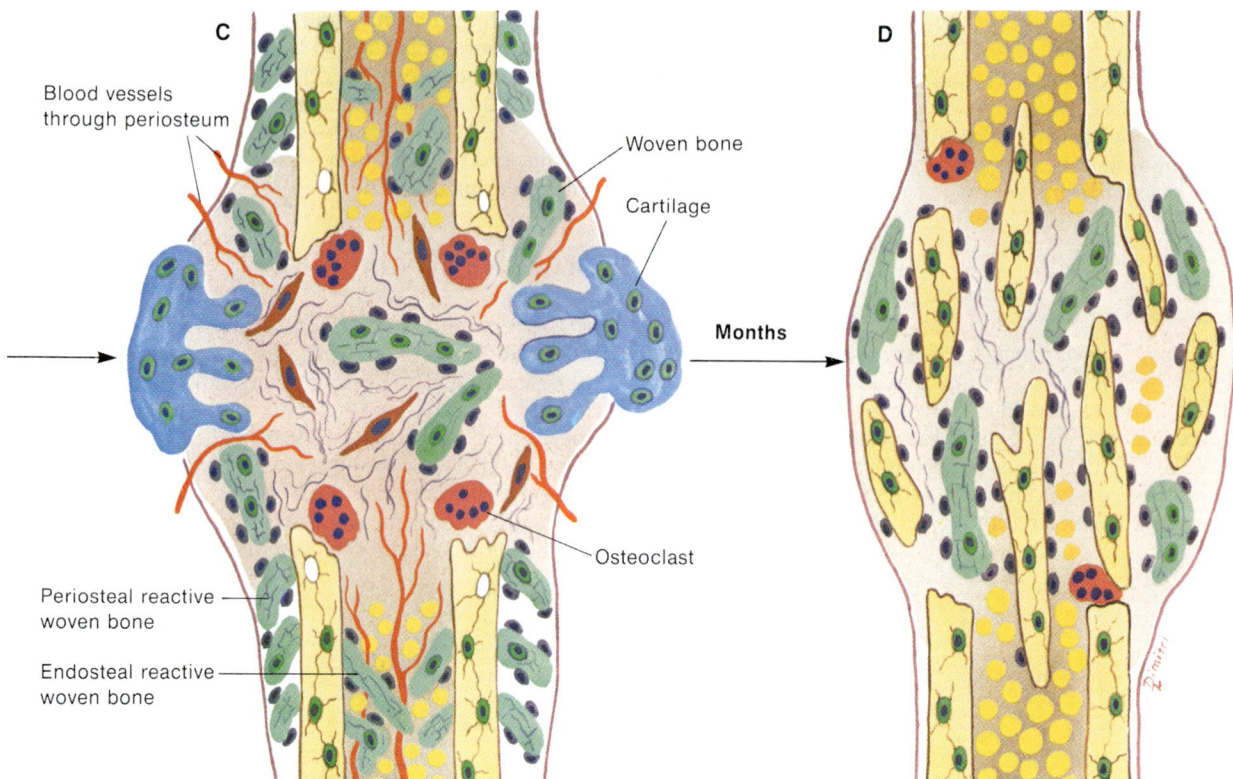

FIGURE 26-17 (continued)

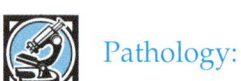 Pathology:

The Inflammatory Phase

In the first 1 to 2 days after a fracture, rupture of blood vessels in the periosteum and adjacent muscle and soft tissue leads to extensive hemorrhage. Extensive necrosis of bone at the fracture site also occurs because of the disruption of large vessels in the bone and the interruption of the cortical vessels (i.e., the Volkmann and haversian canals). **The hallmark of dead bone is the absence of osteocytes and empty osteocyte lacunae.**

In 2 to 5 days, the hemorrhage forms a large clot, which must be resorbed so that the fracture can heal. Neovascularization begins to occur peripheral to this blood clot By the end of the first week, most of the clot is organized by invasion of blood vessels and early fibrosis.

The earliest bone, which is invariably woven bone, has formed after 7 days. **This corresponds to the "scar" of bone.** Because bone formation requires a good blood supply, the woven bone spicules begin to appear at the periphery of the clot. Pluripotential mesenchymal cells from the soft tissue and within the bone marrow give rise to the osteoblasts that synthesize the woven bone. In most fractures, cartilage also is formed and is eventually resorbed by endochondral ossification. The granulation tissue containing bone or cartilage is termed a *callus*. Woven bone also forms inside the marrow cavity at the periphery of the blood clot because vascular tissue is also present in this location.

The Reparative Phase

The reparative phase begins following the first week after the fracture and extends for months, depending on the degree of movement and the fixation of the fracture. By this time, the acute inflammatory cells have dissipated. The reparative process involves the differentiation of pluripotential cells into fibroblasts and osteoblasts. Repair proceeds from the periphery toward the center of the fracture site and accomplishes two objectives: (1) it organizes and resorbs the blood clot and, (2) more importantly, it furnishes neovascularization for the construction of the callus, which will eventually bridge the fracture site. The events leading to repair are as follows:

1. Armies of osteoclasts within the haversian canals form cutting cones that bore into the cortex toward the fracture site. A new vessel accompanies the cutting cone, supplying nutrients to these cells and providing more pluripotential cells for cell renewal.
2. At the same time, the external callus, which is found on the surface of the bone and is formed from the periosteum and the soft tissue mesenchymal cells, continues to grow toward the fracture site.
3. Simultaneously, an endosteal, or internal, callus forms within the medullary cavity and grows outward toward the fracture site.

4. The cortical cutting cones reach the fracture site, and the ends of the fractured bone begin to appear beveled and smooth, as the site is remodeled by osteoclasts.
5. The same is true of the endosteal surface of the cortex, as the internal callus works its way to the fracture site.
6. Where there are large areas of cartilage, new blood vessels invade the calcified cartilage, after which the endochondral sequence duplicates the normal formation of bone at the growth plate.

The Remodeling Phase

Several weeks after the fracture, the ingrowth of callus has sealed the bone ends, and remodeling begins. In the remodeling phase, the bone is reorganized so that the original cortex is restored. Occasionally, the bone is strong enough to qualify as a clinically healed fracture, but biologically, the fracture may not be truly healed and may continue to undergo remodeling for years. For instance, the callus of rib fractures may remain throughout life because the continual respiratory movement of the ribs shears blood vessels and preserves extensive cartilage callus. In a child, in whom the growth plates are still open, the normal modeling process of growing bone overtakes the callus, so that a fracture may not be recognizable in later life. Similarly, normal modeling in a child may correct the angulation of a bone at the fracture site. If the fracture is near the growth plate, differential growth rates of the growth plate also correct the angulation. In an adult, however, because the plates are closed, angulation often requires correction with external or internal devices.

Special Considerations

There are unusual nuances to fracture healing that deserve mention.

PRIMARY HEALING: A fracture does not necessarily result in bone displacement and soft tissue injury. For example, a drill hole in the bone cortex or a controlled fracture, such as an osteotomy created with a fine saw during orthopedic surgery, does not displace bone. In this situation, there is almost no soft tissue reaction and callus formation because the bone is rigidly fixed. The fracture callus grows directly into the fracture site by a process called *primary healing*. This results in rapid reconstitution of the cortex, including restoration of the haversian systems. Similarly, if a fracture site is held in rigid alignment by metal screws and plates, there is also little external callus. The cortical cutting cones will then be prominent and will heal the fracture site quickly.

NONUNION: If a fracture site does not heal, the condition is termed *nonunion*. Causes of nonunion include interposition of soft tissues at the fracture site, excessive motion, infection, poor blood supply, and other factors mentioned above. Continued movement at the unhealed fracture site may also lead to *pseudoarthrosis*, a condition in which jointlike tissue is formed. Pluripotential tissue cells become histologically indistinguishable from synovial cells, secrete synovial fluid, and form a jointlike structure. In such cases, the fracture never heals, and the jointlike material must be removed surgically for the fracture to heal properly.

Stress Fracture Results from the Accumulation of Microfractures

Stress fracture, also known as fatigue or march fracture, *refers to the accumulation of stress-induced microfractures, which eventually results in a true fracture through the bone cortex.*

 Pathogenesis: A stress fracture occurs in bones in which the cortex has few osteons and forms only when stress is applied to the cortex. If the ill-prepared cortex (e.g., in the fifth metatarsal) undergoes repeated mechanical stress (e.g., from jogging, skiing, or ballet dancing), the bone produces cutting cones in an attempt to implant osteons. If the stress continues and microfractures accumulate, periosteal and endosteal calluses develop to strengthen the bone while active remodeling takes place. An actual fracture occurs as the last event if the stresses are continually applied during remodeling.

 Clinical Features: Stress fractures produce pain and swelling over the affected bone. **At the site of a future stress fracture, callus forms before the fracture occurs.** When the actual fracture takes place, the pain becomes more severe. In the early stages of this condition, before the actual fracture, the radiological appearance may resemble that of a tumor. A biopsy will show that the cortex is riddled with cutting cones for remodeling, which is also the case with the reactive bone at the periphery of an invasive tumor.

OSTEONECROSIS (AVASCULAR NECROSIS, ASEPTIC NECROSIS)

Osteonecrosis refers to the death of bone and marrow in the absence of infection (Fig. 26-18). Causes of osteonecrosis are listed in Table 26-1. Necrotic bone heals differently in the cortex and in the underlying coarse cancellous bone.

 Pathology: **Necrotic coarse cancellous bone** heals by a process called *creeping substitution*, in which the necrotic marrow is replaced by invading, or creeping, neovascular tissue, which provides the pluripotential cells needed for bone remodeling. Although the necrotic bony trabeculae may be resorbed directly by osteoclastic activity, they are more commonly surrounded by new woven or lamellar bone generated by the osteoblastic activity of the

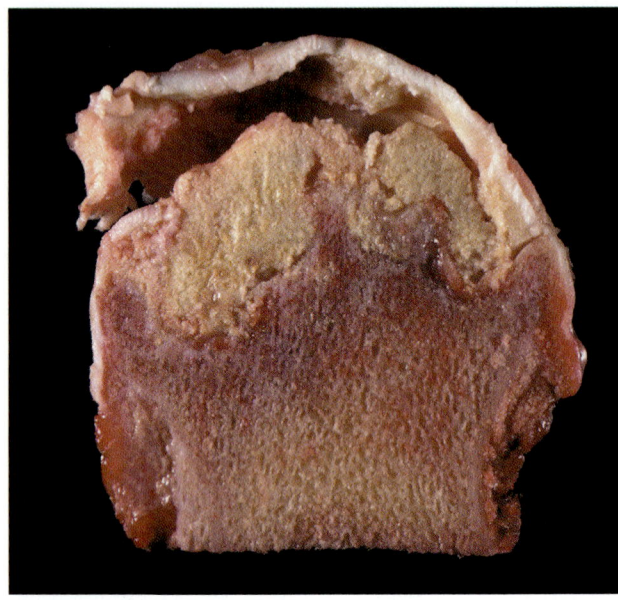

FIGURE 26-18
Osteonecrosis of the head of the femur. A coronal section shows a circumscribed area of subchondral infarction with partial detachment of the overlying articular cartilage and subarticular bone.

granulation tissue. Eventually, the sandwich composed of necrotic bone in the center and the surrounding viable bone is remodeled by osteoclastic activity, and new bone is laid down through intramembranous bone formation.

Necrotic cortical bone is healed by a cutting cone. The cutting cone, as discussed above, forms by way of the preexisting vascular channels in the cortex. The appropriate signals reach this vascular channel and stimulate neovascularization by the surrounding pluripotential mesenchymal tissue. Osteoclasts make their way into the necrotic compact cortical bone, with osteoblasts trailing behind. As a result, tunnels bore their way into the necrotic cortex, thereby leading to new bone formation. This is a slow process, and the bone is often laid down de novo as lamellar bone.

Legg-Calvé-Perthes disease refers to osteonecrosis in the femoral head in children, and *idiopathic osteonecrosis* occurs in a similar location in adults. In both conditions, collapse of the femoral head may lead to joint incongruity and eventual severe osteoarthritis. Collapse of the subchondral bone results from several mechanisms:

- Necrotic bone may sustain stress fractures and compaction over a long period.
- The portion peripheral to the necrotic bone may undergo neovascularization. On radiological examination, there is a lucent area surrounding the necrotic zone.
- The rigid articular cartilage and subchondral bone may actually crack as the subchondral necrotic zone collapses, producing a fracture.

A radiograph in avascular necrosis often shows the necrotic zone to be radiodense because of (1) relative osteoporosis in the surrounding viable bone compared with the unchanged necrotic bone; (2) the addition of new bone through creeping substitution; (3) the formation of calcium soaps, which arise as a result of the necrosis of marrow fat; and (4) actual compaction of the preexisting dead bone. It is possible that focal end-arterial vascular insufficiency may precede these events, because the necrotic zone tends to be wedge shaped.

TABLE 26-1 Causes of Osteonecrosis

Trauma, including fracture and surgery
Emboli, producing focal bone infarction
Systemic diseases, such as polycythemia, lupus erythematosus, Gaucher disease, sickle cell disease, and gout
Radiation, either internal or external
Corticosteroid administration
Specific focal bone necrosis at various sites—for instance, in the head of the femur (Legg–Calvé–Perthes disease) or in the navicular bone (Köhler disease)
Organ transplantation, particularly renal, in patients with persistent hyperparathyroidism
Osteochondritis dissecans, a condition of unknown etiology in which a piece of articular cartilage and subchondral bone breaks off into a joint. It is thought that a focal area of bone necrosis occurs and eventually detaches.
Autografts and allografts
Thrombosis of local vessels secondary to the pressure of adjacent tumors or other space-occupying lesions
Idiopathic factors, as in the high incidence of osteonecrosis of the head and the femur in alcoholics. Necrotic bone heals differently in the cortex and in the underlying coarse cancellous bone.

REACTIVE BONE FORMATION

Reactive bone is intramembranous bone that is formed in response to stress on bone or soft tissue. Conditions such as tumors, infections, trauma, or generalized or focal disease can stimulate bone formation.

 Pathology: The periosteum may respond with a so-called sunburst pattern (Fig. 26-19), as seen with certain tumors, or a progressive layering of the periosteum, which produces an *onionskin pattern* of the cortex. The endosteal or the marrow surface may produce new bone, so that on radiological studies, the cortex appears to be thickened, and the coarse cancellous bone appears to be denser.

The reactive bone may be either woven or lamellar, depending on the rates of deposition of the reactive bone. For example, reactive bone around an indolent infection, such as a chronic osteomyelitis, may be laid down de novo as lamellar bone from the periosteum. In this case, the bone has time to respond to the persistent stress. Similarly, a benign tumor may stimulate a lamellar bone reaction. By contrast, a rapidly growing tumor is more likely to promote woven bone formation as a response to the rapid growth of the tumor cells. Invariably, reactive bone is of the intramembranous type, because it is derived from the periosteum or the endosteal tissue of the marrow.

Heterotopic Calcification Affects Soft Tissues

Reactive bone formation must be distinguished from *heterotopic calcification*, which is the deposition of acellular minerals in soft tissue. Reactive bone formation, or heterotopic bone formation, involves the production of woven or lamellar bone, which may or may not be mineralized. Radiologically, these entities are usually distinctive. Reactive bone often has a spicular or trabeculated pattern, whereas heterotopic calcification has an irregular, splotchy, amorphous appearance. Heterotopic calcification tends to occur in necrotic soft tissue or in cartilage and is usually denser than bone on radiography. Heterotopic calcification appears in two forms:

- **Metastatic calcification** occurs in conditions in which there is an increase in the calcium–phosphorus product. Thus, hypercalcemic states or hyperphosphatemic conditions predispose normal soft tissues to calcification.
- **Dystrophic calcification** is seen in abnormal soft tissues such as tumors, degenerative diseases such as arteriosclerosis, and areas subjected to trauma. In addition, loss of neurological function, as seen in quadriplegia and hemiplegia, predisposes the affected parts to soft tissue calcification.

Myositis Ossificans Is Formation of Reactive Bone in Muscle after Injury

Myositis ossificans, also termed *heterotopic ossification,* affects young persons and, although it is entirely benign, often mimics a malignant neoplasm.

 Pathogenesis: The lesion typically results from blunt trauma to the muscle and soft tissues, usually of the lower limb. Peripheral neovascularization of the resulting hematoma leads in a short time to the formation of bone spicules in the soft tissue, because the local environment is similar to that of an initial hematoma in a healing fracture. Because myositis ossificans often occurs near a bone, such as the femur or tibia, on radiography it may be misdiagnosed as a malignant bone-forming tumor.

 Pathology: Histologically, woven bone is formed within the granulation tissue (Fig. 26-20). In an early lesion of myositis ossificans, the cells of the woven bone and surrounding soft tissue are pleomorphic and show abundant mitoses, a histological appearance that also resembles a malignant tumor. **The key feature that distinguishes myositis ossificans from a neoplasm is that the bone matures peripherally, whereas it is immature or not formed at all in the center of the lesion.** The phenomenon of peripheral maturity with central immaturity is called the *zonation effect* and clearly indicates a reactive process. A neoplasm has an opposite zonation effect, because the most mature tissue of the tumor is located centrally. In a well-developed lesion, this phenomenon may be seen radiographically (Fig. 26-20).

The growth pattern of myositis ossificans reflects the ingrowth of neovascular tissue from the peripheral portion into the center of the damaged area. In the late stages, the lesion may contain cartilage and even lamellar bone. Thus, in a well-developed lesion, it may mimic a sesamoid bone in the soft tissue.

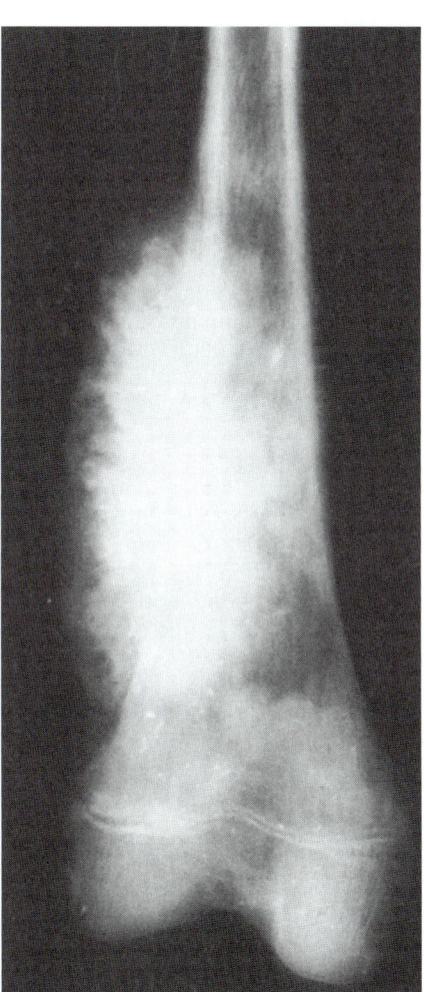

FIGURE 26-19
Reactive bone formation. A radiograph of a resected femur bearing an osteosarcoma shows a sunburst pattern of hyperdense new bone in the distal diaphysis and metaphysis. This radiodensity is due to woven bone produced by the sarcoma and the periosteal reaction of the host bone. The epiphyseal plate is represented as a transverse lucent line that separates the metaphysis from the epiphysis. The radiating radiodense bone extends beyond the periosteum into the soft tissues, obscuring the underlying bone architecture.

INFECTIONS

Osteomyelitis Is a Bacterial Infection of Bone

Osteomyelitis is defined as an inflammation of the bone and bone marrow. Although any infectious agent may cause it, the term is

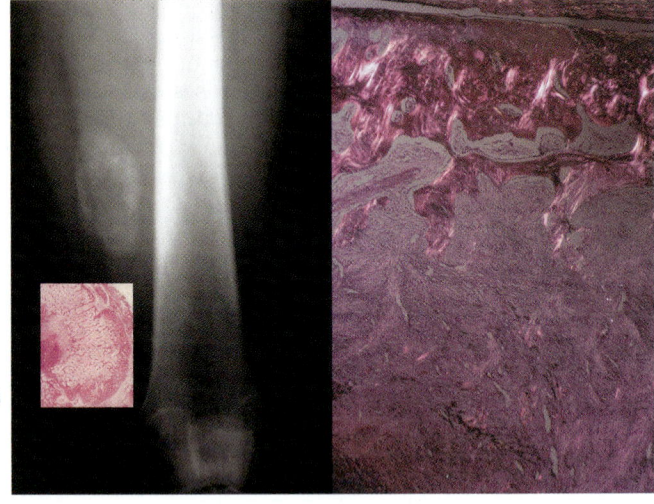

FIGURE 26-20
Myositis ossificans circumscripta. A. Radiograph of the thigh shows a soft tissue mass with a radiolucent center and ossification that becomes denser at the periphery. B. Inset demonstrates the mass at low power magnification. There is progression from a circumscribed, hemorrhagic center through fibrous tissue, discontinuous trabeculae, and finally, to compact bone, corresponding to the bony shell seen in the radiograph. C. Higher magnification in polarized light demonstrates progression of bone formation to compacta and even the presence of a small amount of lamellar bone.

most often used to mean inflammation caused by bacterial infection. The most common pathogens are *Staphylococcus* species, but other organisms, such as *Escherichia coli, Neisseria gonorrhoeae, Haemophilus influenzae,* and *Salmonella* species, are also seen. The organisms are introduced either through the hematogenous route or by direct introduction of the organisms into the bone.

Direct Penetration

Infection by direct penetration or extension of bacteria is now the most common cause of osteomyelitis in the United States. Bacterial organisms are introduced directly into the bone by penetrating wounds, fractures, or surgery. Staphylococci and streptococci are still commonly incriminated, but in 25% of postoperative infections, anaerobic organisms are detected. Rarely, a gram-negative organism may seed a hip after a urological or gastrointestinal surgical procedure.

Hematogenous Osteomyelitis

Infectious organisms may reach the bone from a focus elsewhere in the body through the bloodstream. Often the focus itself, (e.g., a skin pustule or infected teeth and gums) poses little threat. Some suggest that even the mere brushing of teeth creates a temporary bacteremia, which may allow organisms to reach the bone.

The most common sites affected by hematogenous osteomyelitis are the metaphyses of the long bones, such as in the knee, ankle, and hip. The infection principally affects boys aged 5 to 15 years, but it is occasionally seen in older age groups as well. Drug addicts may develop hematogenous osteomyelitis from infected needles.

  Pathogenesis and Pathology: Hematogenous osteomyelitis primarily affects the metaphyseal area because of the unique vascular supply in this region (Fig. 26-21). Normally, arterioles enter the calcified portion of the growth plate, form a loop, and then drain into the medullary cavity without establishing a capillary bed. This loop system permits slowing and sludging of blood flow, thereby allowing bacteria time to penetrate the walls of the blood vessels and to establish an infective focus within the marrow. If the organism is virulent and continues to proliferate, it creates increased pressure on the adjacent thin-walled vessels because they lie in a closed space, the marrow cavity. Such pressure further compromises the vascular supply in this region and produces bone necrosis. The necrotic areas coalesce into an avascular zone, thereby allowing further bacterial proliferation.

If the infection is not contained, pus and bacteria extend into the endosteal vascular channels that supply the cortex and spread throughout the Volkmann and haversian canals of the cortex. Eventually, pus forms underneath the periosteum, shearing off the perforating arteries of the periosteum and further devitalizing the cortex. The pus flows between the periosteum and the cortex, isolating more bone from its blood supply, and may even invade the joint. Eventually, the pus penetrates the periosteum and the skin to form a draining sinus (Fig. 26-22). A sinus tract that extends from the cloaca to the skin may become epithelialized by epidermis that grows into the sinus tract. When this occurs, the sinus tract invariably remains open, continually draining pus, necrotic bone, and bacteria.

Periosteal new bone formation and reactive bone formation in the marrow tend to wall off the infection. At the same time, osteoclastic activity resorbs bone. If the infection is virulent, this attempt to contain it is overwhelmed, and the infection races through the bone, with virtually no bone formation but extensive bone necrosis. More commonly, pluripotential cells modulate into osteoblasts in an attempt to wall off the infection. Several lesions may develop:

- **Cloaca** is the hole formed in the bone during the formation of a draining sinus.
- **Sequestrum** is a fragment of necrotic bone that is embedded in the pus.
- **Brodie abscess** consists of reactive bone from the periosteum and the endosteum, which surrounds and contains the infection.
- **Involucrum** refers to a lesion in which periosteal new bone formation forms a sheath around the necrotic sequestrum. An involucrum that involves an entire bone may exist for several years before a patient seeks medical attention.

In very young children (1 year old or younger) afflicted with osteomyelitis, the adjacent joint is often involved because the periosteum is loosely attached to the cortex. From the age of 1 year to puberty, subperiosteal abscesses are common. Spread to adjacent joints may also occur in adults.

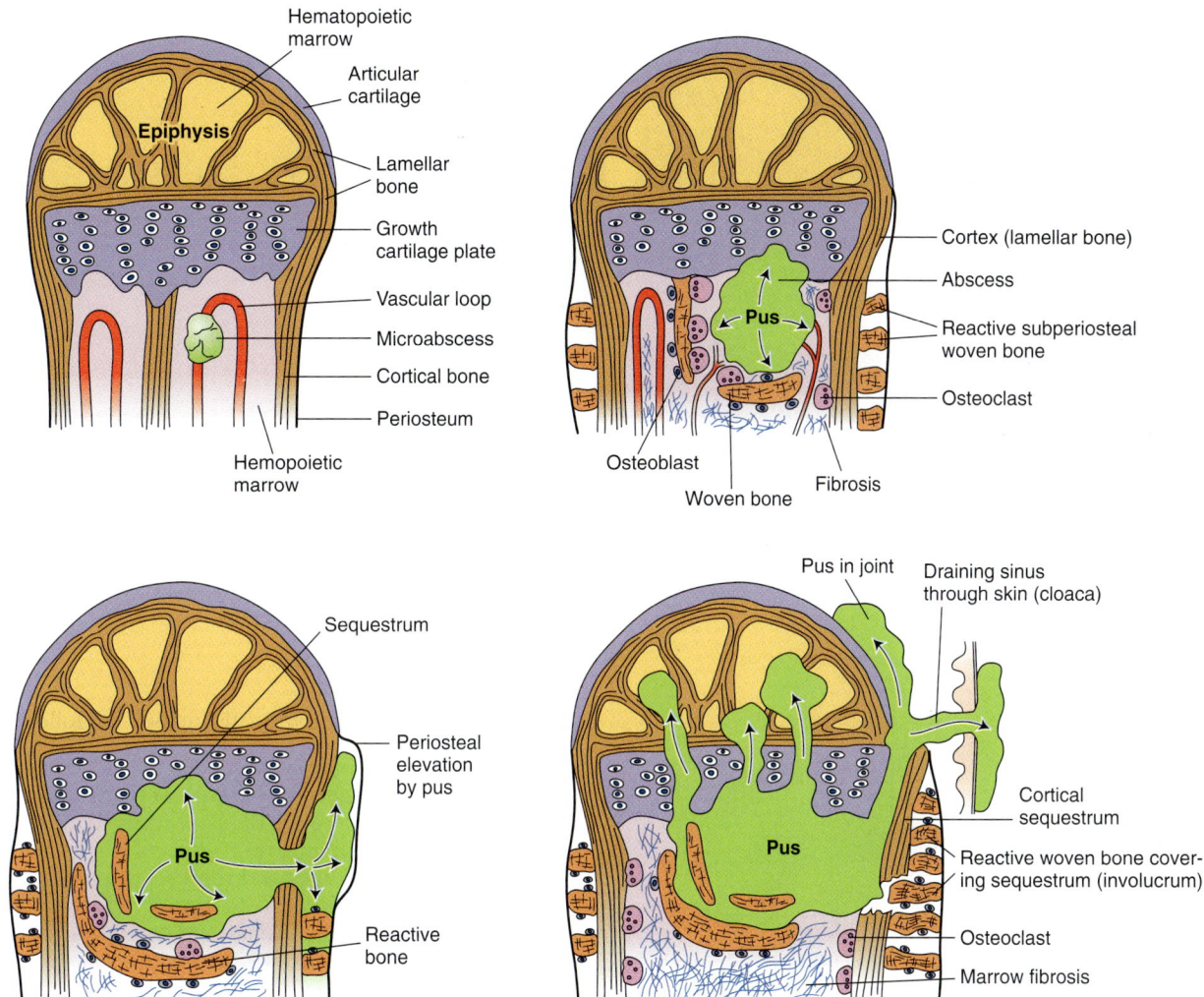

FIGURE 26-21
Pathogenesis of hematogenous osteomyelitis. A. The epiphysis, metaphysis, and growth plate are normal. A small, septic microabscess is forming at the capillary loop. B. Expansion of the septic focus stimulates resorption of adjacent bony trabeculae. Woven bone begins to surround this focus. The abscess expands into the cartilage and stimulates reactive bone formation by the periosteum. C. The abscess, which continues to expand through the cortex into the subperiosteal tissue, shears off the perforating arteries that supply the cortex with blood, thereby leading to necrosis of the cortex. D. The extension of this process into the joint space, the epiphysis, and the skin produces a draining sinus. The necrotic bone is called a *sequestrum*. The viable bone surrounding a sequestrum is termed the *involucrum*.

Vertebral Osteomyelitis

In adults, osteomyelitis frequently involves vertebral bodies (Fig. 26-23). The intervertebral disk is not a barrier to bacterial osteomyelitis, particularly staphylococcal infection. Infections travel from one vertebra to the next by directly traversing the intervertebral disk. Some investigators consider that the intervertebral disk is actually the primary source of infection, so-called diskitis. The disk expands with pus and is eventually destroyed as the pus bores into the adjacent vertebral bodies.

Half or more of the cases of vertebral osteomyelitis are caused by *Staphylococcus aureus*. Twenty percent represent infections with *E. coli* and other enteric organisms, many of which originate from the urinary tract. *Salmonella* species are also seen in the vertebral bodies, as are *Brucella* species. The predisposing factors are intravenous drug abuse, upper urinary tract infections, urological procedures and hematogenous spread of organisms from other sites. Back pain, with point tenderness over the area of infection, is associated with low-grade fever and an increased sedimentation rate.

Occasionally, a paravertebral abscess draining the bone may "point" and emerge in the groin or elsewhere. Vertebral osteomyelitis may lead to (1) vertebral collapse with paravertebral abscesses, (2) spinal epidural abscesses, with cord compression from the abscess or from displaced fragments of the infected bone, and (3) compression fractures of the vertebral body, leading to neurological deficits.

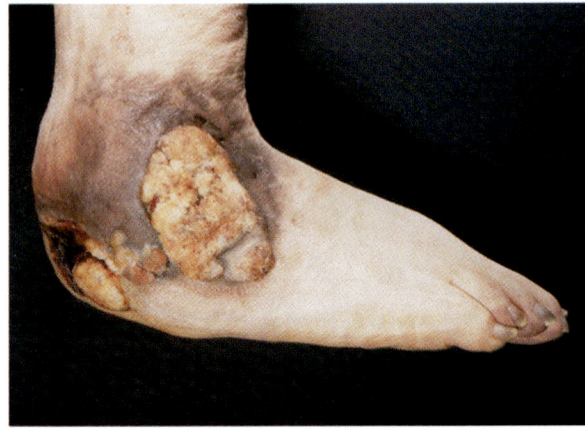
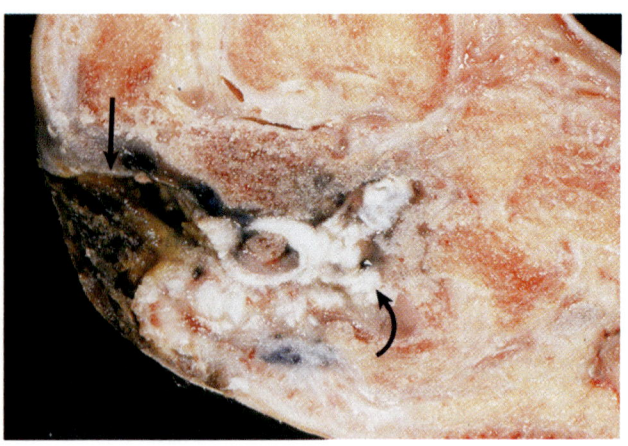

FIGURE 26-22
Chronic osteomyelitis. **A.** In this patient with chronic osteomyelitis, the skin overlying the infected bone is ulcerated and a draining sinus (*dark area*) is evident over the heel. **B.** After amputation of the foot, a sagittal section shows a draining sinus (*straight arrow*) that connects the infected bone with the surface of the ulcerated skin. The white tissue (*curved arrow*) is invasive squamous cell carcinoma, which arose in the skin.

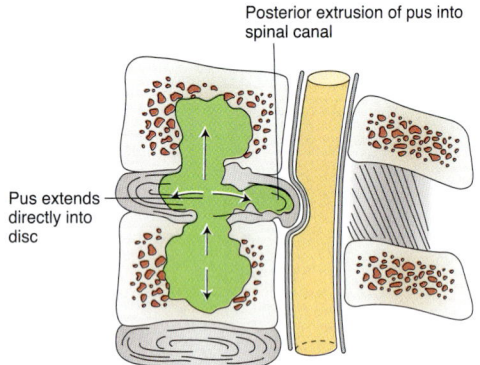
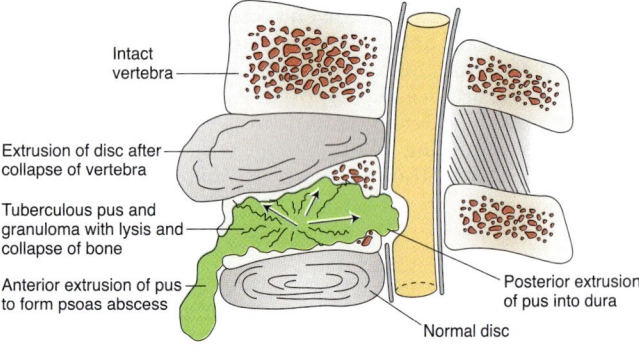

FIGURE 26-23
Osteomyelitis of the vertebral body. **A.** Bacterial osteomyelitis expands from one vertebral body to the next by direct invasion of the intervertebral disk and may actually push posteriorly into the spinal canal. The sequence of events in the marrow cavity is similar to that in a long bone. **B.** In tuberculous osteomyelitis, the bone is destroyed by resorption of bony trabeculae, which results in mechanical collapse of the vertebrae and extrusion of the intervertebral disk. Tuberculous organisms cannot penetrate the intervertebral disk directly; rather, they extend from one vertebra to the next after mechanical forces destroy and extrude the intervertebral disk.

Complications

The complications of osteomyelitis include the following:

- **Septicemia:** Dissemination of organisms through the bloodstream may occur as a result of bone infection. It is unusual for osteomyelitis to result from septicemia.
- **Acute bacterial arthritis:** Joint infection is secondary to osteomyelitis at all ages and represents a medical emergency. Direct digestion of cartilage by inflammatory cells destroys the articular cartilage and produces osteoarthritis. Rapid intervention to prevent this complication is mandatory.
- **Pathological fractures:** Osteomyelitis may lead to fractures, which heal poorly and may require surgical drainage.
- **Squamous cell carcinoma:** This cancer develops in the bone or in the sinus tract of long-standing chronic osteomyelitis, often years after the initial infection. In such cases, squamous tissue arises from the epithelialization of the sinus tract and eventually undergoes malignant transformation (see Fig. 26-22).
- **Amyloidosis:** This systemic disease was a common complication of chronic osteomyelitis in the preantibiotic era, and patients often would die of cardiac and renal disease. Currently, it is rare among inhabitants of industrialized countries.
- **Chronic osteomyelitis:** Chronic infection of bone may follow acute osteomyelitis. Chronic osteomyelitis, especially that involving the entire bone, is incurable because necrotic bone or sequestra function as foreign bodies in avascular areas, and antibiotics do not reach the bacteria. Chronic osteomyelitis is, therefore, treated symptomatically with surgery or antibiotics for the duration of the patient's life.

 Clinical Features: Hematogenous osteomyelitis in children occurs as a sudden illness, with fever and systemic toxicity, or as a subacute illness in which local manifestations predominate. Swelling, erythema, and tenderness over the involved bone are characteristic. The leukocyte count is often conspicuously increased, but it is normal in so many cases that absence of leukocytosis does not rule out the disease.

The treatment of osteomyelitis depends on the stage of the infection. Early osteomyelitis is treated with intravenous antibiotics for 6 or more weeks. Surgery is used to drain and decompress the infection within the bone or to drain abscesses that do not respond to antibiotic therapy. As mentioned above, in long-standing, chronic osteomyelitis, antibiotics alone are not curative, and extensive surgical debridement of necrotic bone is often required.

Tuberculosis of Bone Reflects a Primary Focus Elsewhere

Tuberculosis of bone invariably originates at other foci, usually the lungs or lymph nodes (see Chapter 9). When the bone infection is caused by the rare bovine type of tubercle bacillus, the initial focus is often in the gut or tonsils. The mycobacteria spread to the bone hematogenously, and only rarely is there direct spread from a lung or lymph node.

Tuberculous Spondylitis (Pott Disease)

Tuberculous spondylitis, that is, infection of the spine, is a feared complication of childhood tuberculosis. The disease affects the bodies of the vertebrae, sparing the lamina and spines and the adjacent vertebrae (see Figs. 26-23 and 26-24).

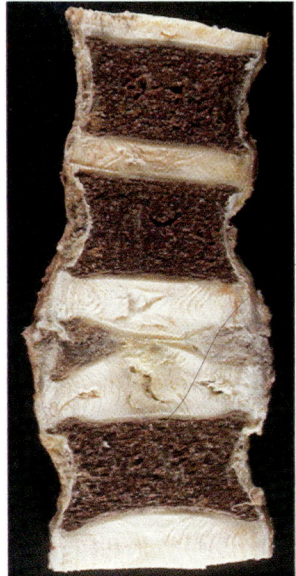

FIGURE 26-24
Tuberculous spondylitis (Pott disease). A vertebral body is almost completely replaced by tuberculous tissue. Note the preservation of the intervertebral disks.

With antibiotic treatment, Pott disease is rare. The thoracic vertebrae are usually affected, especially the eleventh thoracic vertebra; the lumbar and cervical vertebrae are less commonly involved.

 Pathology: The pathological process in tuberculous spondylitis is similar to that at other sites. The tuberculous granulomas first produce caseous necrosis of the bone marrow, an effect that leads to slow resorption of bony trabeculae and, occasionally, to cystic spaces in the bone. **Because there is little or no reactive bone formation, collapse of the affected vertebra is usual, after which kyphosis and scoliosis ensue.** The intervertebral disk is crushed and destroyed by the compression fracture, rather than by invasion of organisms. The typical hunchback of bygone days was often the victim of Pott disease.

If the infection ruptures into the soft tissue anteriorly, pus and necrotic debris drain along the spinal ligaments and form a *cold abscess*, a term that signifies the absence of acute inflammation. A *psoas abscess* forms near the lower lumbar vertebrae and dissects along the pelvis, to emerge through the skin of the inguinal region as a draining sinus. Such a process may occur without any prior symptoms and may be the first manifestation of tuberculous spondylitis. Paraplegia results from vascular insufficiency of the spinal nerves, rather than from direct pressure.

Tuberculous Arthritis

Hematogenous spread of tuberculosis may bring organisms to the joint capsule, synovium, or intracapsular portion of the bone. Tuberculosis induces granulomas in synovial tissue, which then becomes edematous and papillary and may fill the entire joint space. Massive destruction of the articular cartilage results from undermining granulation tissue in the bone. The destroyed joint is replaced by bone, an effect that leads to an immovable joint *(bony ankylosis)*.

Tuberculous Osteomyelitis of the Long Bones

Infection of the long bones is the least common bone manifestation of tuberculosis. Tuberculosis of a long bone occurs near the joint, where it also produces arthritis. For unknown reasons, the greater trochanter of the femur is a common site for this disease.

Syphilis of Bone is Today Rare

Syphilis causes a slowly progressive, chronic, inflammatory disease of bone, which is characterized by granulomas, necrosis, and marked reactive bone formation. It may be acquired through sexual contact, or it may be passed through the placenta from mother to fetus (see Chapter 9). The bone changes in syphilis depend on the age of the patient, the endosteal and periosteal changes, and the presence or absence of gummas.

Pathology:

Congenital Syphilis

Involvement of bone in congenital syphilis may appear as early as the fifth month of gestation and is fully developed at birth. The spirochetes are ubiquitous in the epiphysis and periosteum, where they produce osteochondritis (epiphysitis) and periostitis, respectively (Fig. 26-25). If the disease is severe, the epiphysis may become dislocated, leaving the child with a functionless limb *(pseudoparalysis of Parrot)*.

The knee is most often affected by congenital syphilis. The growth plate is irregularly widened and displays a yellow discoloration. The zone of calcified cartilage is destroyed, and a sea of lymphocytes, plasma cells, and spirochetes fills the marrow spaces. Because the periosteum is stimulated to produce reactive new bone, the thickness of the cortex may actually be doubled. The inflammatory infiltrate permeates the cortex through the Volkmann and haversian canals and settles in the elevated periosteum. Ultimately, as the affected bones grow they become short and deformed.

Acquired Syphilis

Acquired syphilis in adults produces lesions of the bone early in the tertiary stage, 2 to 5 years after inoculation of the organisms. Periostitis is predominant because the growth plates have already closed. The bones most commonly affected are the tibia, nose, palate, and skull. The tibial lesions are marked by periostitis, with deposition of new bone on the medial and anterior aspects of the shaft, a process that leads to the *saber shin* deformity. The skull thickness also increases because of periosteal stimulation.

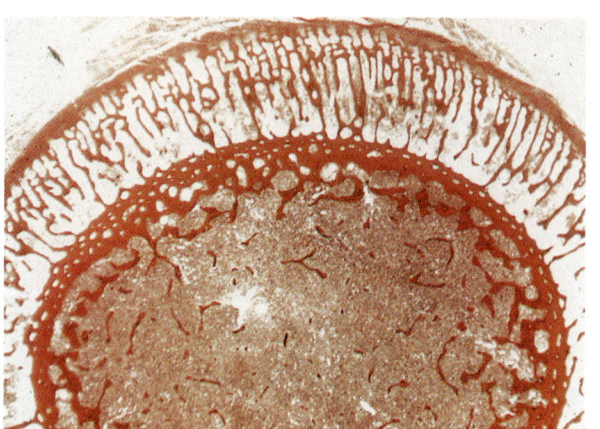

FIGURE 26-25
Congenital syphilis of bone. A cross-section of a tubular bone infected by syphilis shows marked periosteal new bone formation. The medullary cavity is filled with a lymphoplasmacytic infiltrate that replaces the normal marrow fat. The cortex is irregularly destroyed by osteoclastic resorption, a process that stimulates periosteal new bone formation.

The formation of gummas is most common during the tertiary stage of the disease. The bone adjacent to gummas is slowly replaced by fibrous marrow. Ultimately, perforations occur through the cortex. The markedly irregular, thickened periosteal surfaces, which are perforated by pits and serpiginous ulcerations, are characteristic of syphilis. Lysis and collapse of the nasal and palatal bones produce the classic *saddle nose*—perforation, destruction, and collapse of the nasal septum.

LANGERHANS CELL HISTIOCYTOSIS

Langerhans cell histiocytosis (LCH) is a generic term (previously referred to as histiocytosis X) *for three entities characterized by the proliferation of Langerhans cells in various tissues:* (1) eosinophilic granuloma, a localized form; (2) Hand-Schüller-Christian disease, a disseminated variant; and (3) Letterer–Siwe disease, a fulminant and often fatal generalized disease (see Chapter 20). The term *histiocyte* is synonymous with tissue macrophage, and the label *histiocytosis* was originally based on the presumption that the proliferated cells were histiocytes.

 Pathology: The histological appearance of the bones in all three variants of LCH is identical and is characterized by collections of large, phagocytic cells with pale, eosinophilic, foamy cytoplasm and convoluted nuclei (Fig. 26-26). By electron microscopy these cells have the typical racquet-shaped, tubular structures, *Birbeck granules,* seen in the Langerhans cells of the skin (Fig. 26-26C). Numerous scattered eosinophils are located throughout the lesions, occasionally forming collections called *eosinophilic abscesses.* Multinucleated giant cells of the foreign body (Touton) type are often seen in the lesion, as are chronic inflammatory cells.

The lesions of LCH may occur in any part of the body, including bones, skin, brain, lungs, lymph nodes, liver, and spleen. Although cholesterol deposition is prominent in the macrophages, there is no defined abnormality related to cholesterol metabolism, and these patients do not exhibit hypercholesterolemia.

The radiological findings in the bones in all three diseases are identical. The lesions may occur in the metaphysis or diaphysis of a long bone, or in a flat bone, especially in the skull. They are visualized as punched-out lytic defects, with virtually no reactive bone. Such lesions may lead to fractures and periosteal callus formation.

Eosinophilic Granuloma Is a Self-Limited Disease

Eosinophilic granuloma, in either its solitary or multiple varieties, accounts for 70% of all cases of LCH. It is usually encountered in the first two decades of life, but occasionally occurs in older persons. There are typically one or two lytic

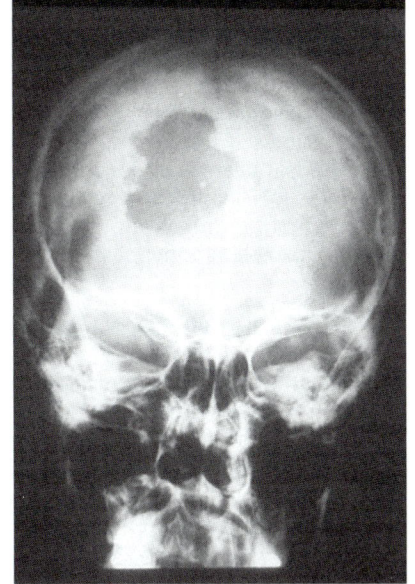
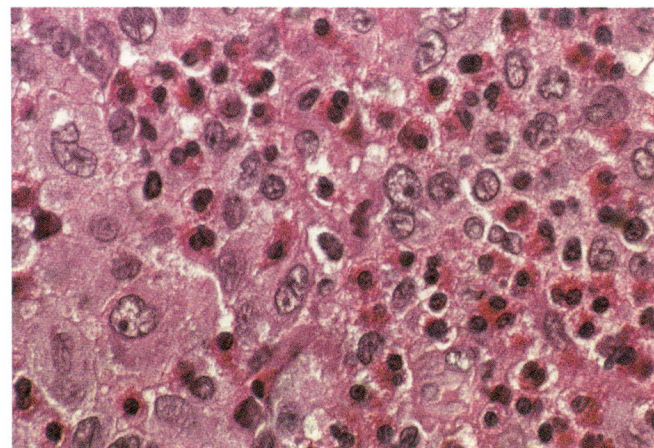
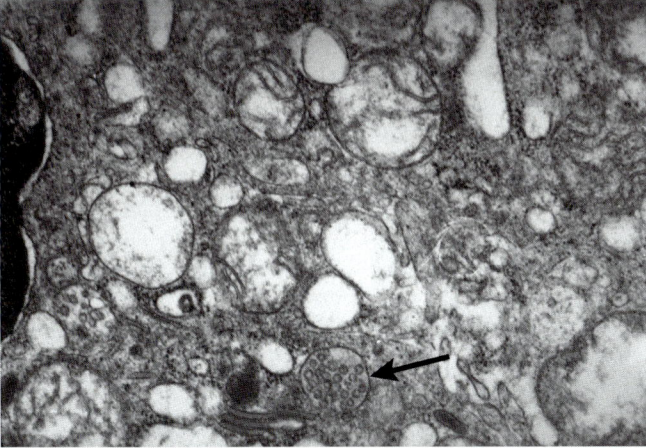

FIGURE 26-26
Eosinophilic granuloma. A. A radiograph of the skull shows a large, lytic lesion. B. A photomicrograph shows large, plump histiocytes (Langerhans cells) with vesicular, occasionally grooved nuclei and eosinophils. C. Electron micrograph of a Langerhans histiocyte demonstrates Birbeck granules (arrow).

areas in bones of the axial or appendicular skeleton (Fig. 26-26A) or the vertebrae. These lesions may cause mild pain or may be an incidental finding on a routine chest radiograph. Foci of disease in the lower thoracic or upper lumbar vertebrae may lead to collapse and pathological fractures. Eventual recovery is the rule.

Hand-Schüller-Christian Disease Is a Childhood Disease

Hand-Schüller-Christian disease occurs in younger children (aged 2 to 5 years) and is more widespread than eosinophilic granuloma. It represents some 20% of all cases of LCH. Radiolucent bony lesions characterize the disorder, most frequently in the calvaria, ribs, pelvis, and scapulae. Involvement of the jaw bone results in the loss of teeth, evident radiologically as "floating teeth." A lesion may infiltrate the retroorbital space, producing exophthalmos. Infiltration of the stalk of the hypothalamus by the proliferated Langerhans cells leads to diabetes insipidus. Twenty percent of patients have lymphadenopathy and lung infiltrates.

Crusty, red, weepy skin lesions occur at the hairline and on the extensor surfaces of the extremities, abdomen, and occasionally soles of the feet. Deafness results from involvement of the external auditory canal and mastoid air cells. One third of affected patients demonstrate disease in the liver and spleen, and 40% have bone lesions, half of which involve the skull. Thus, the classic triad of Hand-Schüller-Christian disease, **(1) radiolucent lesions of the skull, (2) diabetes insipidus, and (3) exophthalmos,** occurs in only one third of patients.

Letterer-Siwe Disease Is a Potentially Fatal Disease of Infants

Letterer–Siwe disease is an aggressive systemic malady that occurs in children younger than 2 years and accounts for 10% of cases of LCH. Affected children fail to thrive and become cachectic. Multiple organ involvement culminates in massive hepatosplenomegaly, lymphadenopathy, anemia, leukopenia, and thrombocytopenia. Widely scattered, seborrheic skin lesions, which are often hemorrhagic, are usual. The bone lesions are not prominent initially, but progressive marrow replacement and pulmonary infiltration occasionally cause death.

Clinical Features: Eosinophilic granuloma is a self-limited disease, and most of the lesions disappear if left alone. A bone lesion may have to be curetted and packed with bone chips. Sometimes the biopsy itself is enough to stimulate repair of the lytic lesion. A collapsed vertebra may actually reconstitute itself over time. Hand-Schüller-Christian disease may require radiation therapy for some bone and retroorbital lesions. Diabetes insipidus seems to be irreversible, despite irradiation of the pituitary region. Drugs such as corticosteroids, cyclophosphamide, and tumoricidal agents may also be used to treat Hand-Schüller-Christian disease. Similarly aggressive therapy for Letterer-Siwe disease may improve the prognosis.

Metabolic Bone Diseases

Metabolic bone diseases are defined as disorders of metabolism that result in secondary structural effects on the skeleton, including diminished bone mass due to decreased synthesis or increased destruction, reduced bone mineralization, or both. Because metabolic bone diseases are systemic, a biopsy of any bone should reveal the abnormality, even though its severity may differ in various parts of the skeleton (Fig. 26-27).

OSTEOPOROSIS

Osteoporosis is a metabolic bone disease characterized by diffuse skeletal lesions in which normally mineralized bone is decreased in mass to the point that it no longer provides adequate mechanical support. Although osteoporosis reflects a number of causes, it is always characterized by loss of skeletal mass. The remaining bone exhibits a normal ratio of mineralized to nonmineralized (i.e., osteoid) matrix. Bone loss and eventually fractures are the hallmarks of osteoporosis, regardless of the underlying causes (Fig 26-28). The etiology for bone loss is diverse but includes smoking, vitamin D deficiency, low body mass index, hypogonadism, a sedentary lifestyle, and glucocorticoid therapy.

 Epidemiology: In normal persons of both sexes, bone mass peaks between the ages of 25 and 35 years and begins to decline in the fifth or sixth decade. Bone loss with age occurs in all races, but because of higher peak bone mass, blacks are less prone to osteoporosis than are Asians and whites. The bone loss associated with normal aging in women has been divided into two phases: one due to menopause and one due to aging. The latter affects men as well as women. At a certain point, the loss of bone suffices to justify the label *osteoporosis* and renders weight-bearing bones susceptible to fractures. The most common fractures occur in the neck and intertrochanteric region of the femur (hip fracture, Fig 26-28), the vertebral bodies, and the distal radius *(Colles fracture)*. In whites in the United States, 15% of persons have had a hip fracture by the age of 80 years, and by age 90 years; this figure increases to 25%. Women are at twice the risk of hip fracture as men, although among blacks and some Asian populations, the incidence is equal among the sexes. Compared with other osteoporotic fractures, hip fractures incur the greatest morbidity, mortality, and direct medical costs. The female predominance is particularly striking for vertebral fractures, in which the female-to-male ratio is 8:1. A subset of women in the early postmenopausal years is at particular risk of vertebral fractures, which are rare in middle-aged men. The propensity of men to sustain hip fractures as opposed to vertebral ones also reflects factors other than bone mass, such as loss of proprioception.

Pathogenesis: *Regardless of the cause of osteoporosis, it always reflects enhanced bone resorption relative to formation.* Thus this family of diseases should be viewed in the context of the remodeling cycle. Bone resorption and bone formation exist simultaneously. All osteoblasts and osteoclasts belong to a unique temporary structure, known as the basic multicellular unit, or *BMU*. The BMU is responsible for bone remodeling throughout life. Persons younger than 35 or 40 years completely replace bone resorbed during the remodeling cycle. With age, less bone is replaced in resorption bays than is removed, leading to a small deficit at each remodeling site. Given the thousands of remodeling sites in the skeleton, the net bone loss, even in a short time, can be substantial.

Osteoporosis is classified as either primary or secondary. **Primary osteoporosis,** by far the more common variety, is of uncertain origin and occurs principally in postmenopausal women (type 1) and elderly persons of both sexes (type 2). **Secondary osteoporosis** is a disorder associated with a defined cause, including a variety of endocrine and genetic abnormalities.

Type 1 primary osteoporosis is due to an absolute increase in osteoclast activity. Given that osteoclasts initiate bone remodeling, the number of remodeling sites increases in this state of enhanced osteoclast formation, a phenomenon known as *increased activation frequency.*

The increased number of osteoclasts that appears in the early postmenopausal skeleton is the direct result of estrogen withdrawal. The effects of estrogen lack are not, however, targeted directly to the osteoclast, but rather to cells derived from marrow stroma, which secrete cytokines that recruit osteoclasts. These cytokines, which are believed to be estrogen sensitive, include IL-1 and IL-6, TNF, and macrophage colony-stimulating factor (MCSF).

Type 2 primary osteoporosis, also known as **senile osteoporosis**, has a more complex pathogenesis than does type 1. Type 2 osteoporosis generally appears after age 70 years and reflects attenuated osteoblast function. Thus, although osteoclast activity is no longer increased, the number of osteoblasts and the amount of bone produced per cell are insufficient to replace the bone removed during the resorptive phase of the remodeling cycle.

Primary osteoporosis has been linked to a number of factors that influence peak bone mass and the rate of bone loss:

- **Genetic factors:** The development of clinically significant osteoporosis is related, in largest part, to the maximal amount of bone in a given person, referred to as *the peak bone mass*. The determinants of peak bone mass are to a large extent genetic. In general, peak bone mass is greater in men than in women and in blacks than in whites or Asians. There is a higher concordance of peak bone mass in monozygotic than in dizygotic twins.

Osteoporosis   1335

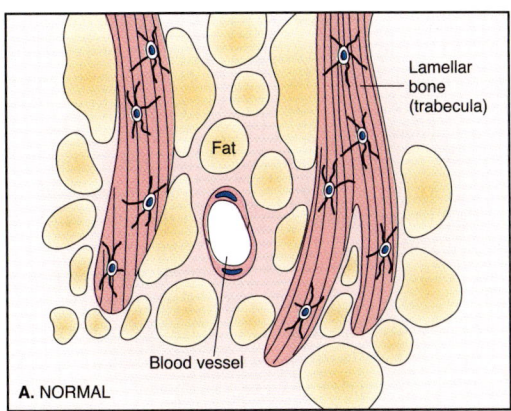

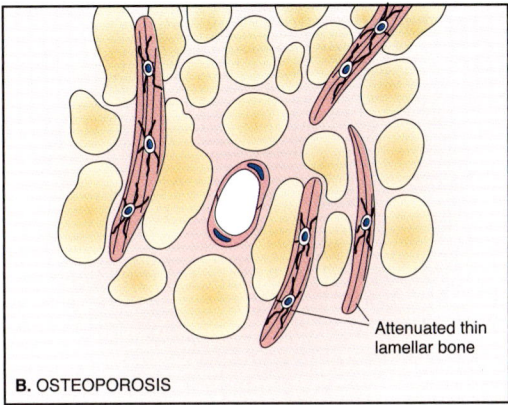
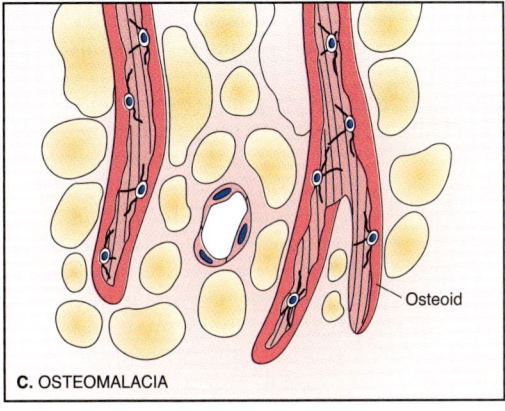

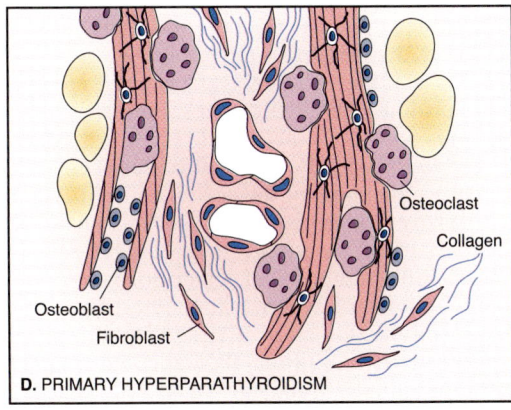
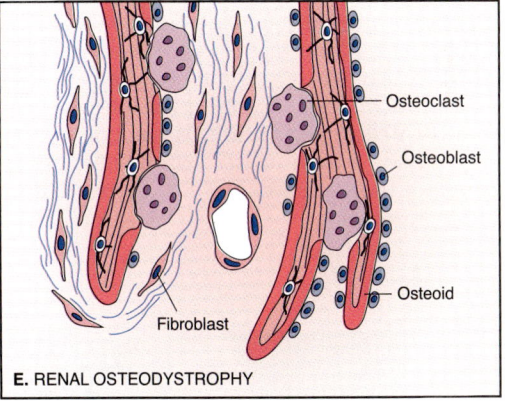

FIGURE 26-27

Metabolic bone diseases. **A.** Normal trabecular bone and fatty marrow. The trabecular bone is lamellar and contains evenly distributed osteocytes. **B.** Osteoporosis. The lamellar bone exhibits discontinuous, thin trabeculae. **C.** Osteomalacia. The trabeculae of the lamellar bone have abnormal amounts of nonmineralized bone (osteoid). These osteoid seams are thickened and cover a larger than normal area of the trabecular bone surface. **D.** Primary hyperparathyroidism. The lamellar bone trabeculae are actively resorbed by numerous osteoclasts that bore into each trabecula. The appearance of osteoclasts dissecting into the trabeculae, a process termed *dissecting osteitis,* is diagnostic of hyperparathyroidism. Osteoblastic activity also is pronounced. The marrow is replaced by fibrous tissue adjacent to the trabeculae. **E.** Renal osteodystrophy. The morphological appearance is similar to that of primary hyperparathyroidism, except that prominent osteoid covers the trabeculae. Osteoclasts do not resorb osteoid, and wherever an osteoid seam is lacking, osteoclasts bore into the trabeculae. Osteoblastic activity, in association with osteoclasts, is again prominent.

Women of reproductive age whose mothers have postmenopausal osteoporosis exhibit a lower bone mineral density than do women in the general population. The bone mineral density (BMD) has been the most commonly used index for the definition and study of osteoporosis. Genetic factors are thought to play an important role in regulating BMD. In men, there are different phenotypic variations of BMD alterations. Although these have been associated with various chromosomal loci, the actual causative genes are not as yet identified.

- **Calcium intake:** The average calcium intake of postmenopausal women in the United States is below the recommended value of 800 mg/day. However, whether this seeming dietary deficiency contributes to the development of osteoporosis is controversial, in view of a number of studies to the contrary. Nevertheless, it has been recommended that both premenopausal and postmenopausal women increase the intake of calcium and vitamin D.

- **Calcium absorption and vitamin D:** Absorption of calcium in the intestine decreases with age. Because calcium absorption is largely under the control of vitamin D, attention has been directed to the role of this steroid hormone in osteoporosis. Compared with controls, persons with osteoporosis demonstrate somewhat lower circulating levels of $1,25(OH)_2D$, the active form of vitamin D that promotes calcium absorption in the intestine. This decrease has been attributed to an age-related decrease in the activity of 1α-hydroxylase in the kidney, the enzyme that catalyzes the formation of $1,25(OH)_2D$. The decrease in 1α- hydroxylase activity has been attributed to decreased stimulation of the enzyme by parathyroid hormone (PTH), as well as an age-related decrease in the response of the renal tubule to PTH. Interestingly, the administration of estrogens to postmenopausal women with osteoporosis increases both the circulating level of $1,25(OH)_2D$ and calcium absorption. It has been suggested that decreased 1α-hydroxylase activity in the kidney may stimulate the secretion of PTH, thereby contributing to bone resorption.

- **Exercise:** Physical activity is necessary for the maintenance of bone mass, and athletes often have increased bone mass. By contrast, the immobilization of a bone (e.g., prolonged bed rest, application of a cast) leads to accelerated bone loss. As a matter of current interest, the weightlessness of space flight results in severe bone loss (33% of trabecular bone mass in 25 weeks). Despite earlier expectations, there is no evidence that vigorous exercise in this setting substantially increases bone mass or helps prevent osteoporosis.

- **Environmental factors:** Cigarette smoking in women has been correlated with an increased incidence of osteoporosis. It is possible that the decreased level of active estrogens produced by smoking (see Chapter 8) is responsible for this effect.

In summary, the two major determinants of primary osteoporosis are estrogen deficiency in postmenopausal women and the aging process in both sexes. The possible mechanisms for these effects are summarized in Figure 26-29.

Pathology: The ratio of osteoid to mineralized bone is normal in persons with osteoporosis. Newer densitometric and imaging techniques, such as computerized tomography, are sufficiently sensitive and precise to detect small deficiencies of bone.

Because of the abundance of cancellous bone in the spine, osteoporotic changes are generally most conspicuous in that location. In vertebral body fractures caused by osteoporosis, the vertebra is deformed, with anterior wedging and collapse. If the vertebral body is not fractured, there is a general outline of both endplates, with a virtual absence of cancellous bone.

Histologically, osteoporosis is characterized by decreased thickness of the cortex and reduction in the number and size of trabeculae of the coarse cancellous bone. Whereas senile osteoporosis tends to feature reduced trabecular thickness, postmenopausal osteoporosis exhibits disrupted connections between trabeculae. The loss of trabecular connectivity, which is attended by diminished biomechanical strength and ultimately leads to fracture, is due to perforation of the trabeculae by resorbing osteoclasts in remodeling sites. In histological sections, the loss of connectivity results in the appearance of "isolated" islands of bone (see Fig. 26-27).

Clinical Features: Postmenopausal osteoporosis usually becomes recognizable within 10 years after the onset of the menopause, whereas senile osteoporosis generally becomes symptomatic after age 70 years. Until recently, most patients were unaware of their disease until they had a fracture of a vertebra, hip, or other bone. However, the development of sensitive screening techniques now permits early diagnosis. Compression fractures of the vertebral bodies often occur after trivial trauma or may even follow lifting a heavy object. With each compression fracture, the patient becomes shorter and develops kyphosis (*dowager's hump*). Serum calcium and phosphorus levels remain normal.

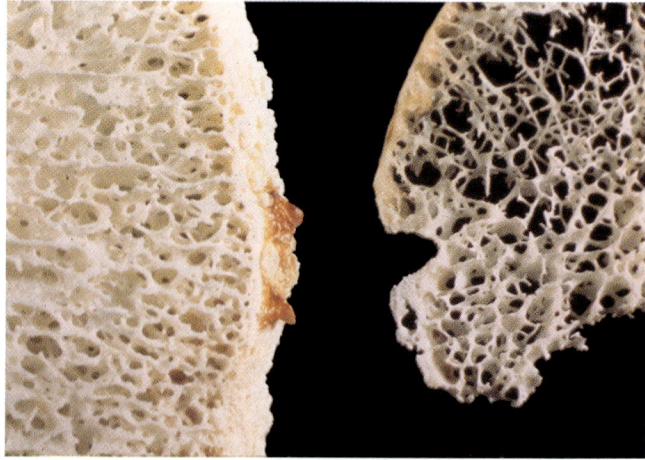

FIGURE 26-28
Osteoporosis. Femoral head of an 82-year-old female with osteoporosis and a femoral neck fracture *(right)* compared with a normal control cut to the same thickness *(left)*.

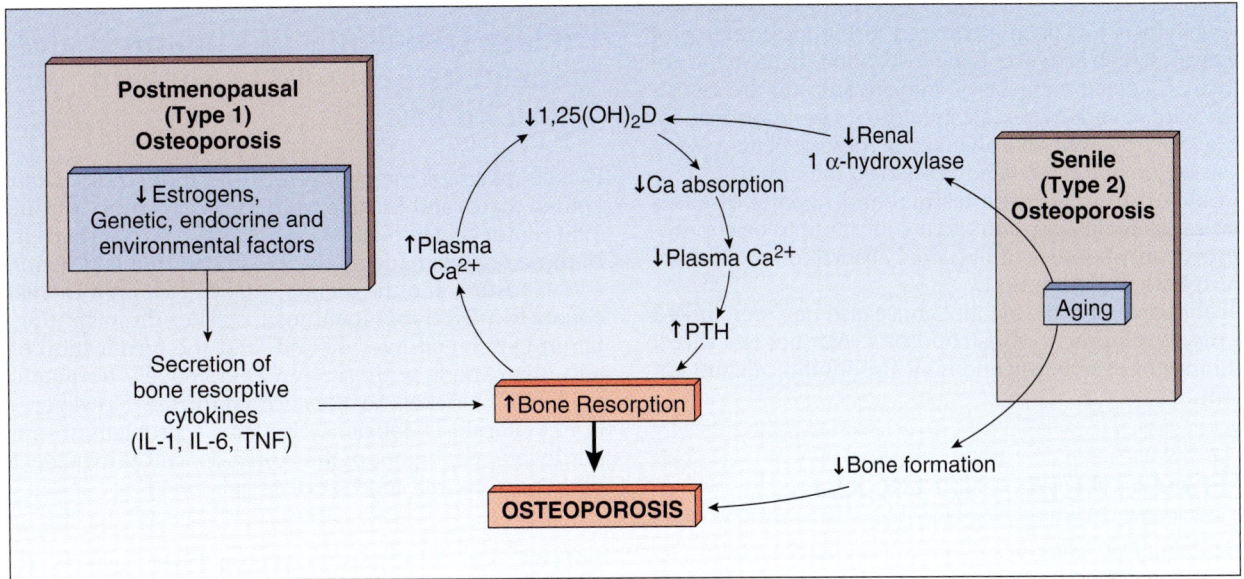

FIGURE 26-29
Pathogenesis of primary osteoporosis.

Estrogen therapy is an effective if controversial means of preventing postmenopausal osteoporosis. Because hormone treatment carries with it slightly increased risks of breast and endometrial cancers, other bone-specific antiosteoporotic drugs have been developed. A new class of inorganic compounds, known as *bisphosphonates*, appears particularly promising. All successful antiosteoporotic agents thus far developed block or slow the rate of bone resorption but do not stimulate bone formation. Thus, the drugs may prevent progression of the disease but cannot cure the patient who already has osteoporosis. Dietary supplementation with calcium in elderly patients has been shown to reduce the risk of osteoporotic fractures by half.

Secondary Osteoporosis Reflects Extraosseous Metabolic Disorders

Osteoporosis develops in association with a large number of other conditions. Causes of secondary osteoporosis include adverse effects of drug therapy, endocrine disorders, eating disorders, immobilization, marrow-related disorders, disorders of the gastrointestinal or biliary tract, renal disease, and cancer.

- **Endocrine conditions:** The most common form of secondary osteoporosis is iatrogenic and results from corticosteroid administration. Bone loss may also result from an excess of endogenous glucocorticoids, as in Cushing disease. Corticosteroids inhibit osteoblastic activity, thereby reducing bone formation. They also impair vitamin D-dependent intestinal calcium absorption, an effect that leads to increased secretion of PTH and increased bone resorption.

Estrogen is a key hormone for maintaining bone mass. Estrogen deficiency is the major cause of age-related bone loss in both sexes; estrogen deficiency or a low level of bioavailable estrogen decreases bone mass in elderly males. Its role in bone metabolism is focused on the role of proinflammatory cytokines: IL-1, IL-6, TNF-α, and RANK-L (receptor activator nuclear factor-kappa B ligand), GM-CSF, M-CSF, and PGE$_2$. It is thought that these cytokines act upon both osteoclasts and osteoblasts via mediation by estrogen receptors.

Hyperparathyroidism causes osteoclast recruitment and increased osteoclastic activity, resulting in secondary osteoporosis (see below). In both sexes, hyperparathyroidism secondary to calcium malabsorption increases remodeling, worsening the cortical thinning and porosity and predisposing to hip fractures.

Hyperthyroidism causes accelerated turnover of bone and increases osteoclastic activity. Although thyrotoxicosis is associated with some secondary osteoporosis, bone loss is limited.

Hypogonadism in both men and women is accompanied by osteoporosis. In women with primary gonadal failure (Turner syndrome) or with secondary amenorrhea as a result of pituitary disease, estrogen deficiency is likely the cause. Hypogonadal men (e.g., Klinefelter syndrome, hemochromatosis) are at risk of osteoporosis because of a deficiency of anabolic androgens. Similarly, hypogonadism contributes to bone loss in 25% of elderly males. In men, there is also evidence of decreased bone density in androgen-deprivation therapy for prostatic carcinoma.

- **Hematological malignancies:** A variety of hematological cancers, particularly multiple myeloma, are accompanied by significant bone loss. The malignant plasma cells of multiple myeloma secrete osteoclast-activating factor, which is presumably responsible for secondary osteoporosis. Some leukemias and lymphomas are also associated with osteoporosis. The bone loss found in systemic

- **Malabsorption:** Gastrointestinal and hepatic diseases that cause malabsorption often contribute to osteoporosis, probably because of impaired absorption of calcium, phosphate, and vitamin D.
- **Alcoholism:** Chronic alcohol abuse also has been linked to the development of osteoporosis. Alcohol is a direct inhibitor of osteoblasts and may also inhibit calcium absorption.

mastocytosis has been attributed to the local release of heparin, which activates bone resorption. Even in the absence of skeletal metastases, some neoplasms are associated with severe hypercalcemia due to bone resorption. Osteoclastic activity is enhanced in these patients, owing to secretion of PTH-related protein by the tumor.

OSTEOMALACIA AND RICKETS

Osteomalacia (soft bones) *is a disorder of adults characterized by inadequate mineralization of newly formed bone matrix.* **Rickets** *refers to a similar disorder in children, in whom the growth plates (physes) are open.* Thus children with rickets manifest defective mineralization not only of bone (osteomalacia) but also of the cartilaginous matrix of the growth plate. Diverse conditions associated with osteomalacia and rickets include abnormalities in vitamin D metabolism, phosphate deficiency states, and defects in the mineralization process itself.

Vitamin D Metabolism Influences Bone Mineralization

Vitamin D is ingested in food or synthesized in the skin from 7-dehydrocholesterol under the influence of the ultraviolet component of sunlight (Fig. 26-30). The vitamin is first hydroxylated in the liver at carbon 25 to form its major circulating metabolite, 25-hydroxyvitamin D. It is then again hydroxylated in the proximal renal tubule at carbon 1 to produce the active hormone 1,25-dihydroxyvitamin D, (1,25(OH)$_2$D). Exposure to sunlight provides sufficient vitamin D for bone growth and mineralization, even in the face of an inadequate dietary source.

Receptors for 1,25(OH)$_2$D are not only present in classic targets, such as intestine, bone, and kidney but are expressed in many cells. This steroid hormone is a general inducer of differentiation, for example, influencing the maturation of hematopoietic and dermal cells, as well as a number of cancers. In the intestine, 1,25(OH)$_2$D stimulates the absorption of calcium and phosphate. It is also essential for osteoclast maturation. Although 1,25(OH)$_2$D enhances bone resorption in vitro, this effect does not occur in vivo, probably because of suppressed secretion of PTH. Regardless of the mechanism, 1,25(OH)$_2$D, in concert with PTH, serves to maintain the concentrations of calcium and phosphate in the blood that are required for proper mineralization of bone. **The principal determinant of the formation of 1,25(OH)$_2$D is the serum calcium concentration.** A decrease in the level of blood calcium stimulates the release of PTH, which acts to augment synthesis of 1,25(OH)$_2$D by the kidney.

Hypovitaminosis D can result from (1) inadequate exposure to sunlight, (2) deficient dietary intake, or (3) defective intestinal absorption. In addition there are hereditary and acquired disorders of vitamin D metabolism.

Dietary Deficiency of Vitamin D and Inadequate Exposure to Sunlight Cause Rickets

Rickets plagued the children of the industrial cities of the United States and Europe from the 17th century through the 19th century. Less than 100 years ago, 85% of urban children in these regions had rickets. These children had insufficient sun exposure, and the dietary intake of vitamin D was inadequate to avert hypovitaminosis D. The administration of vitamin D-rich cod liver oil and later the fortification of milk and other foods with vitamin D effectively terminated the epidemic of rickets in Western countries. However, nutritional vitamin D deficiency remains a problem in some underdeveloped regions of the world, as well as in neglected elderly persons and food faddists.

Intestinal Malabsorption Decreases the Availability of Vitamin D

In industrialized countries, diseases that are associated with intestinal malabsorption cause osteomalacia more often than does poor nutrition. **Intrinsic diseases of the small intestine, cholestatic disorders of the liver, biliary obstruction, and chronic pancreatic insufficiency are the most frequent causes of osteomalacia in the United States.**

Malabsorption of vitamin D and calcium complicates a number of small intestinal diseases, including celiac disease, Crohn disease, scleroderma, and the postsurgical blind-loop syndrome. In obstructive jaundice, the lack of bile salts in the intestine impairs the absorption of lipids and lipid-soluble substances, among which is fat-soluble vitamin D. Furthermore, with sufficient liver damage, the hydroxylation of vitamin D is reduced. Interestingly, biliary cirrhosis, a disease characterized by intestinal malabsorption and vitamin D deficiency, leads to osteoporosis rather than osteomalacia. This surprising finding indicates that vitamin D is essential not only for mineralization but also for the synthesis of bone collagen.

Disorders of Vitamin D Metabolism Are Inherited or Acquired

Vitamin D metabolism can be disturbed either by defective 1α-hydroxylation of vitamin D in the kidney or by insensitivity of the target organ to 1,25(OH)$_2$D. Two autosomal recessive diseases associated with rickets are together known as *vitamin D-dependent rickets*.

Vitamin D-dependent rickets type I results from an inherited deficiency of renal 1α-hydroxylase activity. The clinical and biochemical changes of rickets appear during the first year of life, and these children exhibit hypocalcemia, hypophosphatemia, and high levels of serum PTH and alkaline phosphatase. The disease is controlled by the administration of 1,25(OH)$_2$D.

Vitamin D-dependent rickets type II represents inherited mutations of the vitamin D receptor, which render end organs insensitive to 1,25(OH)$_2$D. The manifestations of rickets usually become evident early in life but may ap-

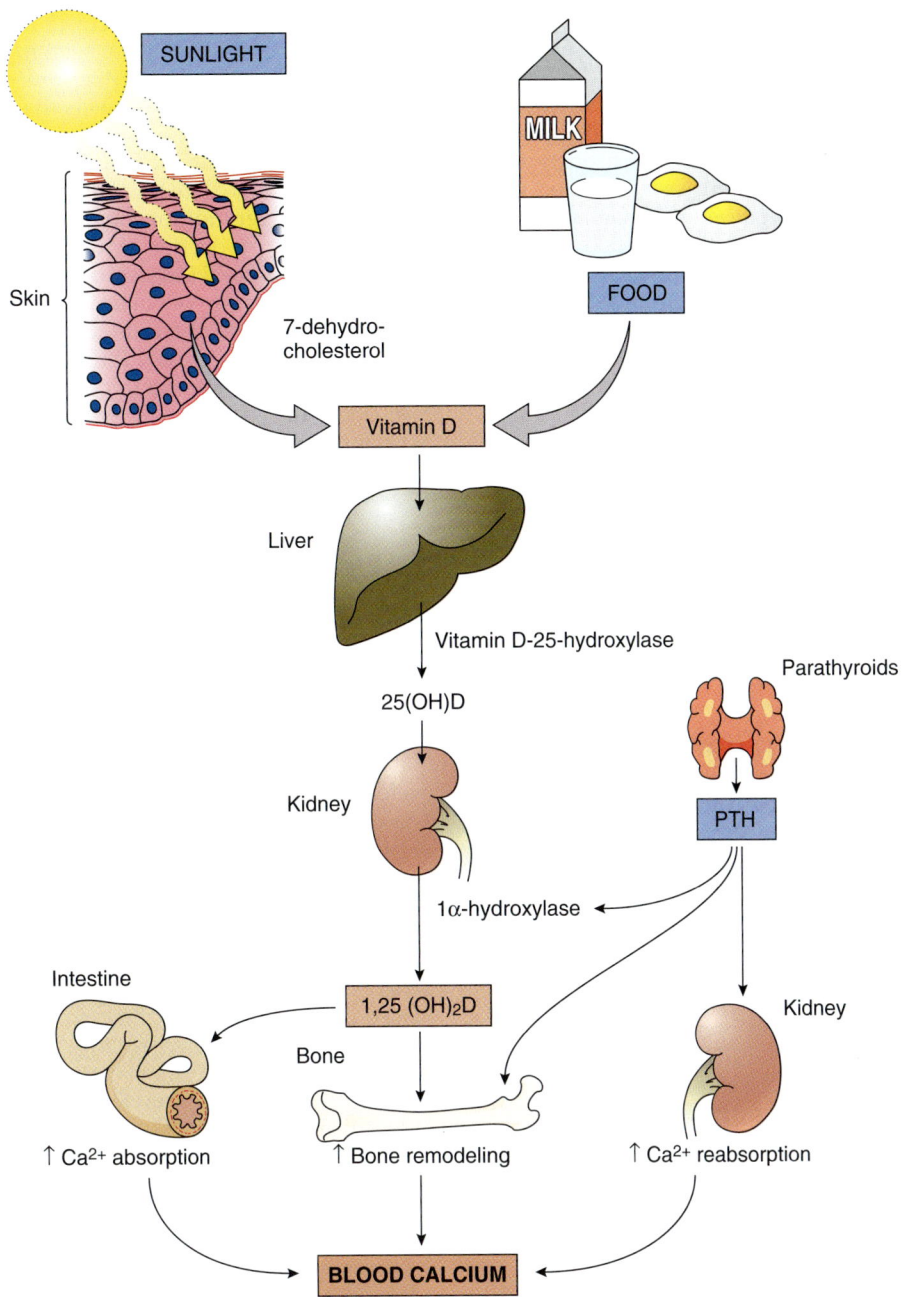

FIGURE 26-30
Metabolism of vitamin D and the regulation of blood calcium.

pear at any time up to adolescence. The serum concentration of $1,25(OH)_2D$ is very high. Patients do not respond to $1,25(OH)_2D$ but are helped by repeated intravenous administration of calcium.

Acquired alterations in vitamin D metabolism include defective renal 1α-hydroxylation and end-organ insensitivity. Some of the causes of impaired α-hydroxylation are hypoparathyroidism, tumor-induced osteomalacia, chronic renal diseases, and osteomalacia of old age. Osteomalacia occasionally complicates the treatment of epilepsy with anticonvulsant drugs, particularly phenobarbital and phenytoin. It is believed that these drugs block the action of $1,25(OH)_2D$ on target organs.

Renal Disorders of Phosphate Metabolism Interfere with Vitamin D Metabolism

Both rickets and osteomalacia may result from impaired reabsorption of phosphate by the proximal renal tubules, with resulting hypophosphatemia.

X-LINKED HYPOPHOSPHATEMIA: This condition, also termed *vitamin D-resistant rickets* or *phosphate diabetes*, is the most common type of hereditary rickets and is inherited as a dominant trait. Mutations in the *PHEX* (phosphate-regulating) gene on the X chromosome (Xp22) impair transport of phosphate across the luminal membrane of proximal renal tubular cells. Although renal phosphate wasting is central to the disease, osteoblast function is also impaired. In boys, florid rickets appears during childhood, whereas girls often suffer only hypophosphatemia. The disease is treated with life-long administration of phosphate and $1,25(OH)_2D$. Histologically, the bones of patients with X-linked hypophosphatemia show severe osteomalacia and contain wide osteoid seams. They also exhibit characteristic hypomineralized areas surrounding osteocytes, known as "halos." The presence of these structures indicates that osteocytes are responsible for the terminal mineralization of bone.

FANCONI SYNDROMES: These inborn errors of metabolism are characterized by renal wastage of phosphate, glucose, bicarbonate, and amino acids. They are all characterized by renal tubular acidosis and result in rickets and osteomalacia. Fanconi syndromes include Wilson disease, tyrosinemia, galactosemia, glycogen-storage disease, and cystinosis. Renal tubular damage that leads to phosphate wastage may also be acquired, as in lead or mercury intoxication, amyloidosis, and Bence-Jones proteinuria.

TUMOR-ASSOCIATED OSTEOMALACIA: This disorder is a phosphate-wasting syndrome that is associated with predominantly benign and occasionally malignant tumors of soft tissue and bone. The typical laboratory features are hypophosphatemia, hyperphosphaturia, low serum concentrations of $1,25(OH)_2D$, and elevated serum alkaline phosphatase. Oncogenic osteomalacia mimics the clinical phenotype of X-linked hypophosphatemia and autosomally dominant hypophosphatemia. The paraneoplastic phosphaturic factors secreted by the tumor, or *phosphatonins,* cause renal tubular phosphate wasting and prevent tubular conversion of 25-hydroxyvitamin D into $1,25(OH)_2D$. Phosphatonins thus appear to have the same effect as the inherited mutations of the *PHEX* gene seen in x-linked hypophosphatemia. Removal of the primary tumor is often curative.

Defective Mineralization

Hypophosphatasia is a rare autosomal recessive disease in which a low activity of alkaline phosphatase in the blood and bones is associated with inadequate bone mineralization, resulting in rickets and osteomalacia. No effective treatment is available.

Some bisphosphonates used in the treatment of Paget disease and high doses of fluoride impair mineralization of newly forming bone matrix and may lead to osteomalacia.

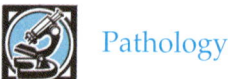 Pathology:

OSTEOMALACIA: Osteomalacia, like osteoporosis, causes an osteopenic radiological pattern. The only findings may be compression fractures of the vertebrae and de-creased bone thickness, as occur in osteoporosis. However, some specific findings may be seen in osteomalacia, including the pseudofractures of *Milkman-Looser syndrome*. These are radiolucent transverse defects that are most common on the concave side of a long bone, medial side of the neck of the femur, ischial and pubic rami, ribs, and scapula.

Histologically, defective mineralization in osteomalacia results in **exaggeration of the osteoid seams,** both in thickness and in the proportion of trabecular surface covered (see Figs. 26-27 and 26-31). Osteoid seams reflect a time lag between the deposition of collagen and the appearance of the calcium salt. Although adults add 1 μm of new matrix to the surfaces of bone every day, it requires 10 days to mineralize this new bone. The normal thickness of osteoid seams, therefore, does not exceed 12 μm. Areas of pseudofracture display abundant osteoid and may function as stress points for true fractures. These areas do not evoke formation of callus and do not extend through the entire diameter of the bone.

RICKETS: Rickets is a disease of children and, therefore, results in extensive changes at the physeal plate (Fig. 26-32), which does not become adequately mineralized. The calcified cartilage and the zones of hypertrophy and proliferative cartilage continue to grow because osteoclastic activity does not resorb the cartilage growth plate. As a consequence, the growth plate is conspicuously thickened, irregular, and lobulated. Endochondral ossification proceeds very slowly and preferentially at the peripheral portions of the metaphysis. The result is a flared, cup-shaped epiphysis. The largest part of the primary spongiosum is composed of lamellar or woven bone that, importantly, remains unmineralized.

On histological examination, the growth plate exhibits striking changes. The resting zone is normal, but the zones of proliferating cartilage are greatly distorted. The ordered progression of helix-forming chondrocytes is lost and is replaced by a disorderly profusion of cells separated by small amounts of matrix. The resulting lobulated masses of proliferating and hypertrophied cartilage are associated with increasing width of the growth plate, which may be 5 to 15 times the normal width. The zone of provisional calcification is poorly defined, and only a minimal amount of primary

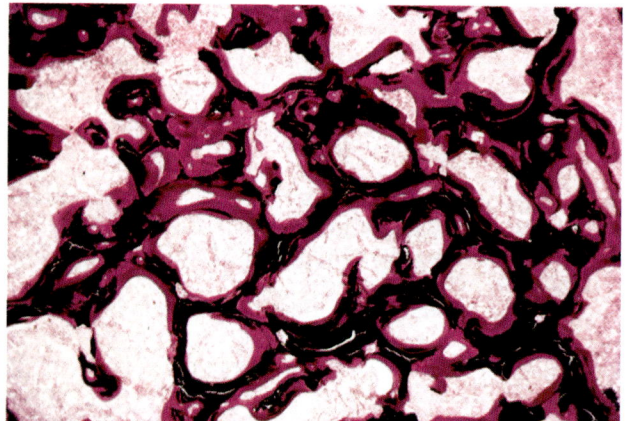

FIGURE 26-31
Osteomalacia. The surfaces of the bony trabeculae (*black*) **are covered by a thicker than normal layer of osteoid** (*red*) **with the von Kossa stain, which colors calcified tissue black.**

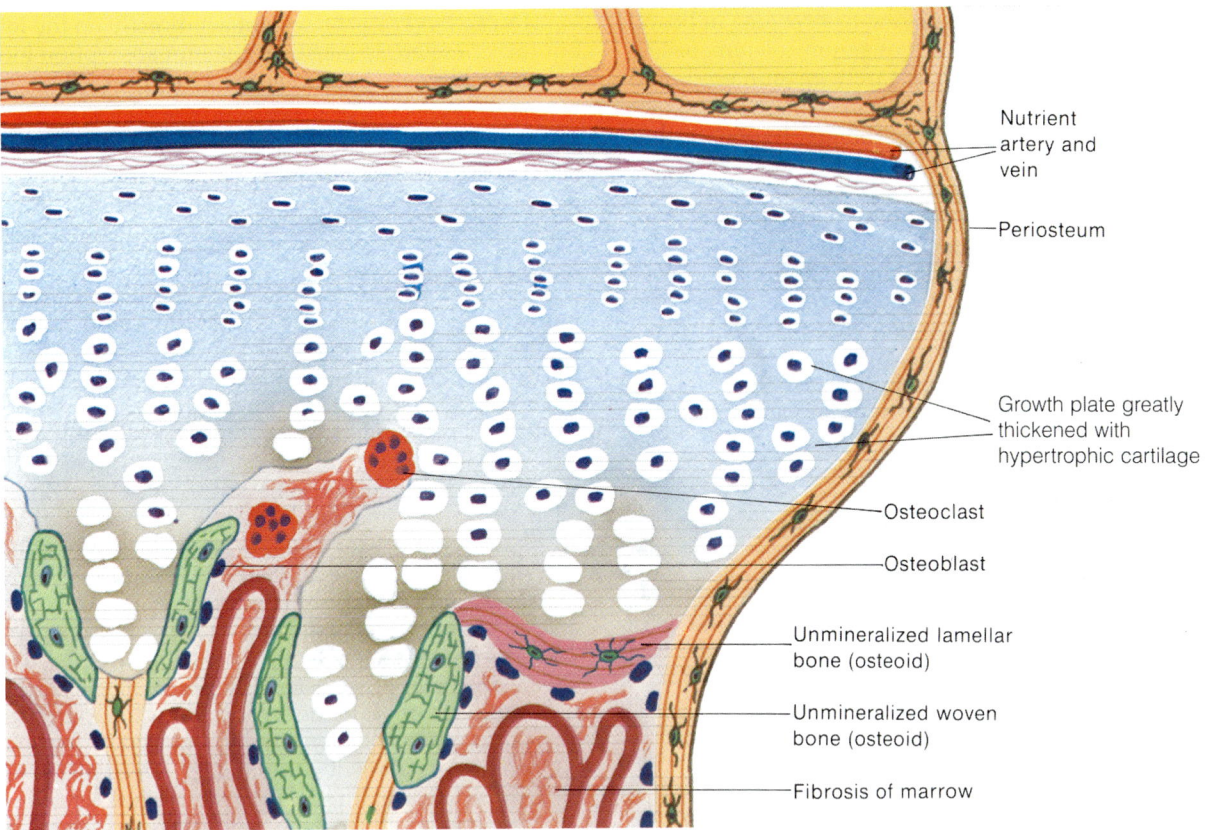

FIGURE 26-32
The growth plate in rickets. The growth plate is thickened and disorganized, with a large zone of hypertrophic cartilage cells. Irregular perforation of the cartilage plate by osteoclasts occurs because there is little calcified cartilage. The woven bone on the surface of some of the primary trabeculae is unmineralized and therefore easily fractured. Such microfractures often lead to hemorrhage at the interface between the plate and the metaphysis.

spongiosum is formed. Masses of proliferating cartilage extend into the metaphyseal region, without any apparent vascular invasion and with little osteoclastic activity.

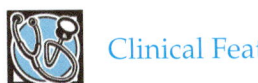 **Clinical Features:**

OSTEOMALACIA: The clinical diagnosis of osteomalacia is often difficult. Patients have nonspecific complaints, such as muscle weakness or diffuse aches and pains. In mild forms of the disease, only slowly progressive changes in bone are seen, and many patients are totally asymptomatic for years. In advanced cases, poorly localized bone pain and tenderness are common, especially in the spine, pelvis, and proximal parts of the extremities. In such cases, the diagnosis of osteomalacia may be made only after an acute fracture, the most common sites being the femoral neck, pubic ramus, spine, or ribs. Muscular weakness and hypotonia lead to a waddling gait in severe cases, and some patients are not able to walk at all.

RICKETS: Children with rickets are apathetic and irritable and have a short attention span. They are content to be sedentary, assuming a Buddha-like posture. Rachitic children are short and exhibit characteristic changes of bones and teeth. Flattening of the skull, prominent frontal bones *(frontal bossing),* and conspicuous suture lines are typical. There is delayed dentition, with severe dental caries and enamel defects. The chest has the classic *rachitic rosary* (a grossly beaded appearance of the costochondral junctions that is produced by enlargement of the costal cartilages) and indentations of the lower ribs at the insertion of the diaphragm. *Pectus carinatum* ("pigeon breast") reflects an outward curvature of the sternum.

The overall musculature is weak, and abdominal weakness leads to a "potbelly." The limbs are shortened and deformed, with severe bowing of the arms and forearm and frequent fractures. The femoral head may dislocate from the growth plate (slipped capital femoral epiphysis).

PRIMARY HYPERPARATHYROIDISM

Primary hyperparathyroidism refers to a metabolic bone disease characterized by generalized bone resorption caused by inappropriate secretion of PTH. Early in the 20th century, bone disease in patients diagnosed with primary hyperparathyroidism was often advanced and crippling. Owing to screening of hospitalized patients for abnormalities of serum calcium, severe primary hyperparathyroidism is rarely encountered, and clinically significant bone disease is unusual.

The histological changes of primary hyperparathyroidism are known as *osteitis fibrosa*. This term applies to all circumstances of markedly accelerated remodeling and may be seen in Paget disease and hyperthyroidism and even in some patients with postmenopausal osteoporosis. Almost all (90%) the cases of primary hyperparathyroidism are caused by one or more parathyroid adenomas, whereas hyperplasia of all four glands accounts for only 10%. Rarely, hyperparathyroidism complicates a parathyroid carcinoma. Because PTH promotes excretion of phosphate in the urine and stimulates osteoclastic bone resorption, low serum phosphate and high serum calcium levels are characteristic.

Parathyroid Hormone Regulates Extracellular Calcium

The effects of PTH are mediated by its effects on bone, kidney, and (indirectly) intestine.

BONE: PTH mobilizes calcium from bone, the major reservoir of calcium in the body. It increases the resorption of bone in the context of accelerated remodeling. Thus, enhanced bone formation is also a component of hyperparathyroidism. Depending on the relative increase in bone resorption and formation, respectively, the secretion of excess PTH may result in decreased, normal, or increased bone mass.

KIDNEY: PTH stimulates the reabsorption of calcium by the thick ascending and granular portions of the distal renal tubules. It also enhances phosphate excretion in the proximal and distal convoluted tubules by directly inhibiting sodium-dependent phosphate transport. In addition, the hormone augments the activity of 1α-hydroxylase in the proximal tubules, thereby stimulating the production of [1,25 (OH)$_2$D].

INTESTINE: PTH does not act directly on the intestine, but rather enhances intestinal calcium absorption indirectly by increasing renal synthesis of 1,25(OH)$_2$D.

Pathogenesis and Pathology: The histogenesis of osteitis fibrosa may be classified into three stages.

- **Early stage:** Initially, osteoclasts are stimulated by the increased PTH levels to resorb bone. From the subperiosteal and endosteal surfaces, osteoclasts bore their way into the cortex as cutting cones. This process is termed *dissecting osteitis* because each osteon is continually hollowed out by osteoclastic activity (see Figs. 26-27 and 26-33A). At the same time, collagen fibers are laid down in the endosteal marrow, and additional osteoclasts penetrate the bone. In contrast to myelofibrosis of hematological origin, in which fibrous tissue is randomly distributed in the marrow space, the collagen of osteitis fibrosa is deposited adjacent to trabeculae. This observation suggests that the stromal cells depositing matrix material are osteoblast precursors.
- **Osteitis fibrosa:** In the second stage, the trabecular bone is resorbed and the marrow is replaced by loose fibrosis, hemosiderin-laden macrophages, areas of hemorrhage from microfractures, and reactive woven bone. This combination of features constitutes the "osteitis fibrosa" portion of the complex.
- **Osteitis fibrosa cystica:** As primary hyperparathyroidism progresses and hemorrhage continues, cystic degeneration ultimately occurs, leading to the final stage of the disease. The areas of fibrosis that contain reactive woven bone and hemosiderin-laden macrophages often display many giant cells, which are actually osteoclasts. Because of its macroscopic appearance, this lesion has been termed a *brown tumor* (Fig. 26-33B). This is not a true tumor, but rather a repair reaction as an end stage of hyperparathyroidism.

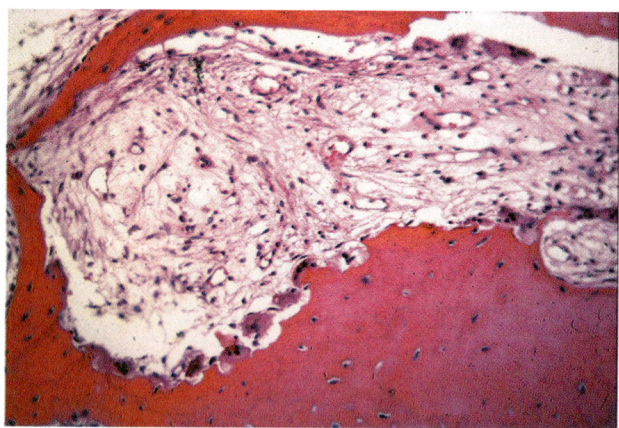
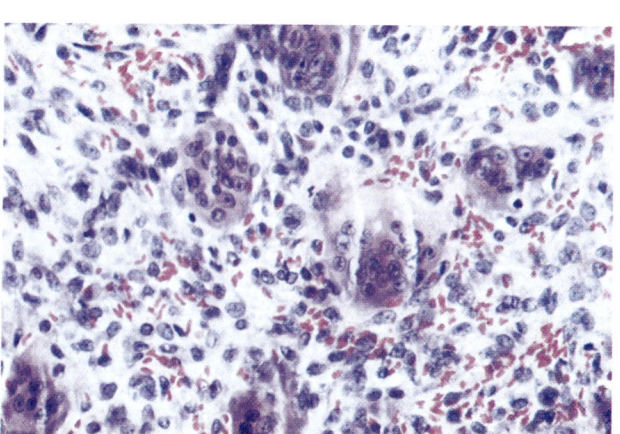

FIGURE 26-33

A. Primary hyperparathyroidism. Section through compact bone shows tunneling reabsorption of a haversian canal. Numerous osteoclasts and stromal fibrosis are evident. B. A section of tissue obtained from a "brown tumor" reveals numerous giant cells in a cellular, fibrous stroma. Scattered erythrocytes are present throughout the tissue.

The skeletal radiographs of most persons with primary hyperparathyroidism are normal. Some patients exhibit mottled bone cortices, with an irregular frayed surface in the outer table of the skull, tufts of the terminal digits, and shafts of the metacarpals (Fig. 26-34). A distinctive radiological peculiarity, referred to as *subperiosteal bone resorption*, is evident in the subperiosteal outer surface of the cortex and reflects dissecting osteitis. Resorption around the tooth sockets causes the lamina dura of the teeth to disappear, a well-known finding on x-ray.

A classic feature of osteitis fibrosa cystica is the presence of multiple, localized, lytic lesions, which represent hemorrhagic cysts or masses of fibrous tissue. These eccentric and well-demarcated lesions are separated from the soft tissue by a periosteal shell of bone. **The focal, tumorlike, lytic lesions always occur in the context of an abnormal skeleton produced by hyperparathyroidism.** If a single lesion is examined without considering the rest of the skeleton, it may be mistaken for a primary giant cell neoplasm of bone.

 Clinical Features: The symptoms of primary hyperparathyroidism are related to the abnormality of calcium homeostasis and have been summarized as *"stones, bones, moans, and groans."* The "stones" refer to kidney stones, and the "bones" to the skeletal changes. The "moans" describe psychiatric depression and other abnormalities associated with hypercalcemia, and the "groans" characterize the gastrointestinal irregularities associated with a high serum calcium level.

Primary hyperparathyroidism is treated with surgical removal of the parathyroid adenomas. When parathyroid hyperplasia is the cause of the disease, three and a half glands are usually removed. The remaining fragment suffices to ensure that the patient does not develop hypocalcemia. After surgery, the histological appearance of the affected skeleton gradually normalizes.

A familial type of primary hyperparathyroidism is associated with mutations in the calcium-sensing receptor (*CASR*) gene, located on chromosome 3 (3q13.3).

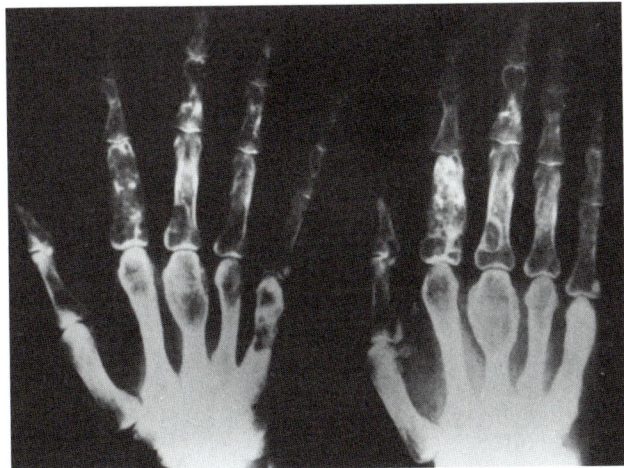

FIGURE 26-34
Primary hyperparathyroidism. A radiograph of the hands reveals bulbous swellings ("brown tumors") and numerous cavities, both representing bone resorption.

RENAL OSTEODYSTROPHY

Renal osteodystrophy is a complex metabolic bone disease that occurs in the context of chronic renal failure. Severe renal osteodystrophy is most common in patients maintained on long-term dialysis, because they live long enough to develop conspicuous bone disease.

 Pathogenesis: The pathogenesis of renal osteodystrophy is similar to that of osteomalacia, with secondary hyperparathyroidism exerting its influence by way of osteoclastic resorption of bone (see Fig. 26-27). The sequence of events that leads to renal osteodystrophy may be summarized as follows:

1. In chronic renal disease, a reduced glomerular filtration rate leads to retention of phosphate, thereby producing **hyperphosphatemia.** High serum phosphate levels drive down the serum calcium levels.
2. Tubular injury causes a reduction in 1α-hydroxylase activity, with a resulting deficiency of 1,25(OH)$_2$D.
3. Intestinal calcium absorption is, in turn, decreased, worsening the **hypocalcemia.**
4. Hypocalcemia stimulates the elaboration of parathyroid hormone. In fact, most patients with end-stage renal disease have substantial hyperparathyroidism. However, PTH does not effectively promote intestinal calcium absorption or renal tubular resorption of calcium because of failure to produce adequate 1,25(OH)$_2$D.
5. Perhaps because of hyperparathyroidism and hyperphosphatemia, a substantial proportion of patients with end-stage renal disease have increased bone mass. Renal osteosclerosis is particularly prominent in vertebrae where, owing to alternating bands of radiopaque and normally dense bone, the lesion is named *"rugger jersey spine."*

The adynamic variant of renal osteodystrophy (ARO) is characterized by arrested bone remodeling. More than 40% of adults who are treated with hemodialysis and more than 50% of those who are treated with peritoneal dialysis have bone biopsy evidence of ARO. Also, the development of adynamic bone during the treatment of secondary hyperparathyroidism with large intermittent doses of calcitriol can aggravate growth retardation in prepubertal children who undergo peritoneal dialysis. Adynamic bone is characterized histopathologically by an overall reduction in cellular activity in bone, with the numbers of both osteoblasts and osteoclasts diminished. These changes can be due to either direct inhibitory effects of systemic factors on osteoblastic function or indirect changes in osteoblastic activity mediated through PTH-dependent mechanisms. Old bone accumulates because it is not remodeled, thereby leading to structural compromise of the skeleton and increased tendency to fractures.

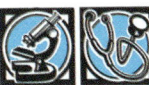 Pathology and Clinical Features: As a result of these effects of chronic renal failure, renal osteodystrophy is characterized by varying degrees of osteomalacia, osteitis fibrosa, osteomalacia, osteosclerosis, and adynamic bone disease (Fig. 26-35). Combinations of osteitis fibrosa and osteomalacia are

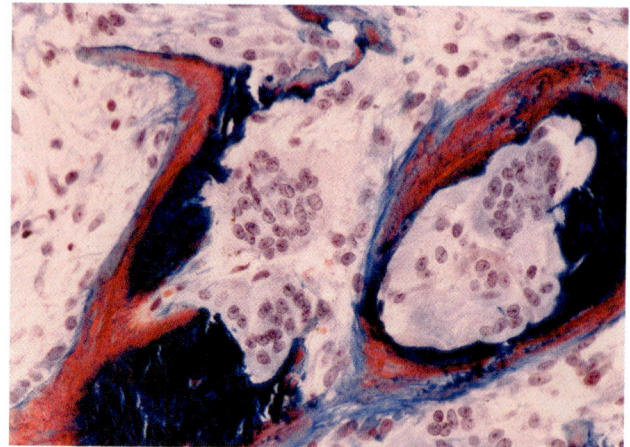
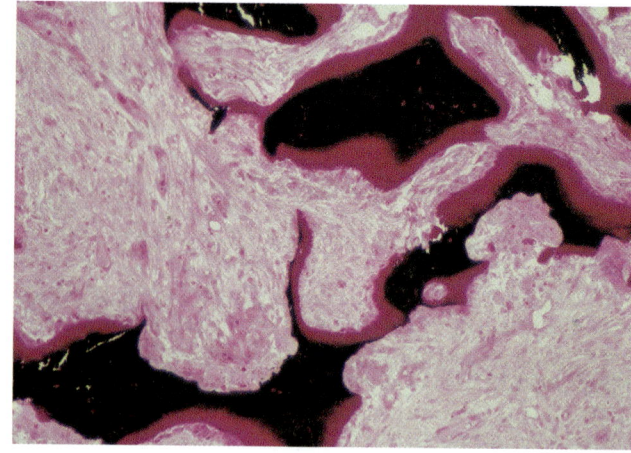
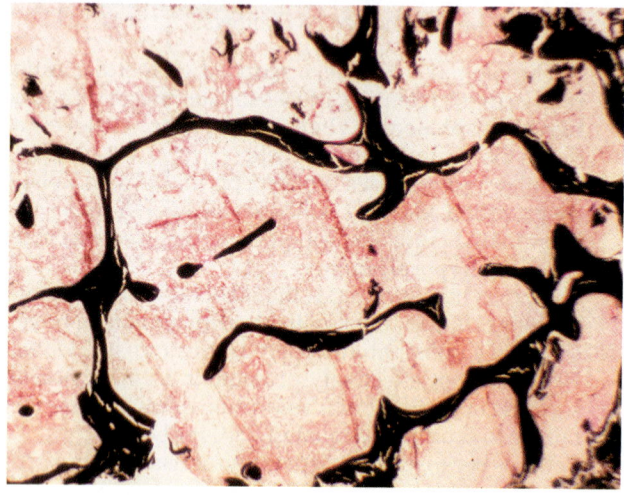

FIGURE 26-35

Renal osteodystrophy. **A.** Osteitis fibrosa. Several large multinucleated osteoclasts are reabsorbing these bone spicules, and the paraosseous tissue is fibrotic. Note that the osteoclastic reabsorption takes place only on the mineralized *(blue)* portions of the trabeculae. In this undercalcified section, the unmineralized bone (osteoid) appears *red*. **B.** Osteomalacia. This is a Von Kossa stain prepared on an undercalcified section. The mineralized bone is *black* and the abundant osteoid appears *magenta*. Osteoid is thick and lines a large proportion of the bone surfaces. Surfaces not covered by the osteoid demonstrate scalloped Howship lacunae and contain abundant osteoclasts. **C.** Adynamic bone disease in which remodeling is attenuated, with a paucity of osteoblasts, osteoclasts, and osteoid (Von Kossa stain).

particularly common. Hyperphosphatemic patients with terminal chronic renal disease may display metastatic calcification at various sites, including the eyes, skin, muscular coats of arteries and arterioles, and periarticular soft tissues.

The management of renal osteodystrophy involves not only the treatment of renal failure but also the control of phosphate levels by appropriate drug therapy and infusions. Occasionally, parathyroidectomy is required to control hyperparathyroidism, and the administration of vitamin D may also be necessary.

PAGET DISEASE OF BONE

Paget disease is a chronic condition characterized by lesions of bone resulting from disordered remodeling, in which excessive bone resorption initially results in lytic lesions, to be followed by disorganized and excessive bone formation

 Epidemiology: Paget disease is common and generally affects men and women older than 60 years. In predisposed populations, 3% of elderly persons manifest the disease at autopsy or on radiographic examination. The disorder has an unusual worldwide distribution, afflicting populations of the British Isles and following their migrations throughout the world. Persons of English descent living in the United States, Australia, New Zealand, and Canada have a high incidence of the disease. Northern Europeans also have more Paget disease than southern Europeans. The disorder is almost nonexistent in Asia and in the indigenous populations of Africa and South America. For unknown reasons the incidence of Paget disease appears to have decreased over the last several decades.

 Pathogenesis: Sir James Paget, who coined the term *osteitis deformans* for this disease more than a century ago, thought that the cause was likely an infection of bone. Since then, virtually every type of disease process, including neoplasia, has been proposed as the cause. Although Paget disease resembles a metabolic disease histologically, its clinical tendency to involve one bone or only a few bones does not fulfill the definition of a metabolic disorder. A hereditary predisposition has been suggested by reports of almost 100 families in which Paget disease seems to be transmitted as an autosomal dominant trait. The gene locus of familial Paget disease was recently identified in chromosome 18 (18q21-22).

An abundance of evidence indicates that Paget may indeed have been correct and that the disease named after him is of viral origin. Virtually all patients exhibit nuclear inclusions consistent with the structure of a virus in osteoclasts and osteoclast precursors, which are not found in any other skeletal disease other than giant cell tumors of bone. They consist of microfilaments in a paracrystalline array and have been compared with the inclusions in the brains of patients with subacute sclerosing encephalitis (see Chapter 29). This similarity has suggested the possibility that a slow virus may be involved (Fig. 26-36). Support for this hypothesis has come from the finding that the marrow of Paget disease patients contains paramyxovirus nucleocapsid transcripts.

Paget disease is characterized by a localized increase in osteoclast formation that leads to bone resorption. The increased osteoclastogenic nature of the bone microenvironment is mediated by common factors, including increases in IL-6 and RANK ligand. The latter, a recently described osteoclast stimulatory factor, appears to mediate the effects of most osteotropic factors on osteoclast formation. Osteoclasts and osteoclast precursors from Paget patients are abnormal and appear hyperresponsive to vitamin D and RANK-L.

 Pathology: The lesions of Paget disease may be solitary or may occur at multiple sites. They tend to localize to the bones of the axial skeleton, including the spine, skull, and pelvis. The proximal femur and tibia may also be involved in the polyostotic form of the disease. Solitary Paget disease rarely involves the humerus, but in polyostotic disease, lesions involving this bone are common.

Paget disease is an example of bone remodeling gone awry. The disease is triphasic, as follows:

1. **"Hot" or osteoclastic resorptive stage:** Radiologically, there is a characteristic, sharply defined, flame-shaped or wedge-shaped lysis of the cortex, which may mimic a tumor (Fig 26-37A). Histologically, there is widespread osteolysis, with marrow fibrosis and dilation of marrow sinusoids.
2. **Mixed stage of osteoblastic and osteoclastic activity:** By x-ray, the bones are larger than normal. In fact, Paget disease is one of only two diseases that produce **larger than normal bones** (the other is fibrous dysplasia, discussed below). The cortex in the mixed phase is thickened, and the accentuation of the coarse cancellous bone makes the bone look heavy and enlarged (Fig. 26-37B and C). Involvement of vertebral bodies leads to a "picture frame" appearance (see Fig. 26-37D), as the cortices and endplates become greatly exaggerated in comparison with the coarse cancellous bone of the vertebral body. Although the bone is abnormal, the distorted, coarse cancellous bone and cortex still tend to align along stress lines. The pelvis is often thickened in the area of the acetabulum. Histologically, there is evidence of both irregular osteoclast activity and osteoblast activity.
3. **"Cold" or burnt-out stage:** This period is characterized histologically by little cellular activity and radiologically by thickened and disordered bones.

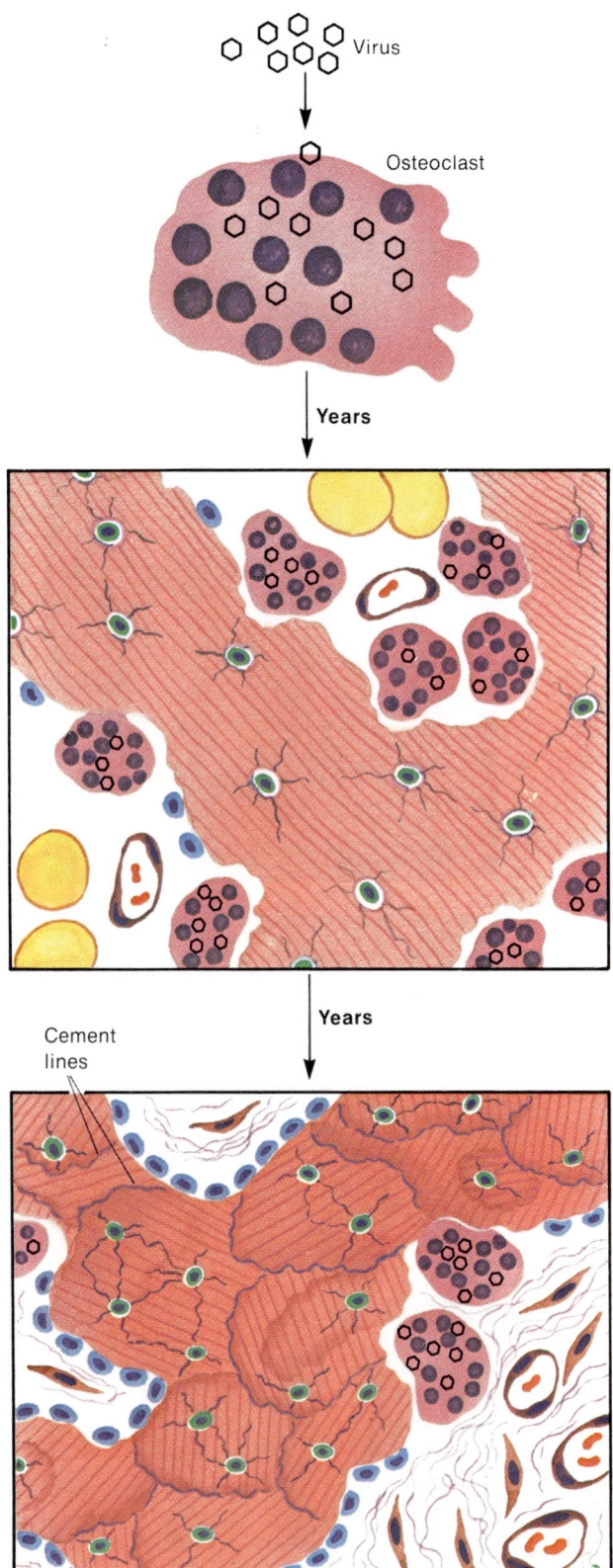

FIGURE 26-36

Hypothetical viral etiology of Paget disease of bone. A virus infects osteoclastic progenitors or osteoclasts and stimulates osteoclastic activity, thereby leading to excessive resorption of bone. Over a period of years, the bone develops a characteristic mosaic pattern, produced by chaotically juxtaposed units of lamellar bone that form irregular cement lines. The adjacent marrow is often fibrotic, and there is a mixture of osteoclasts and osteoblasts on the surface of the bone.

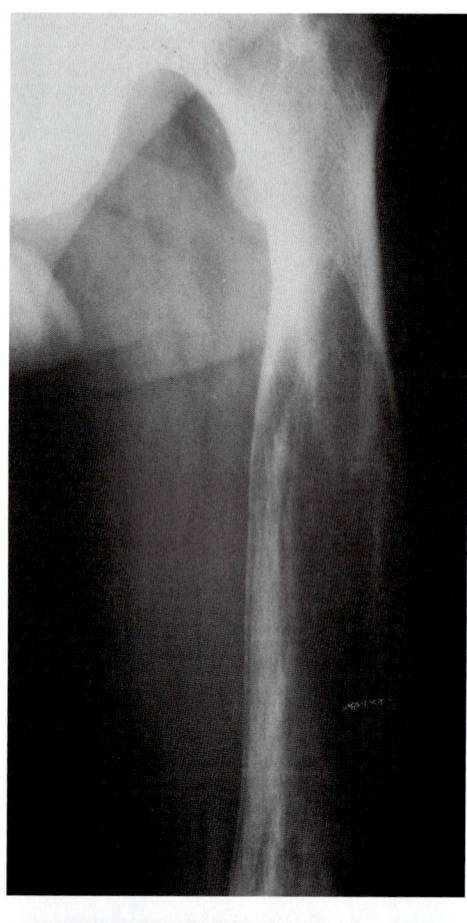
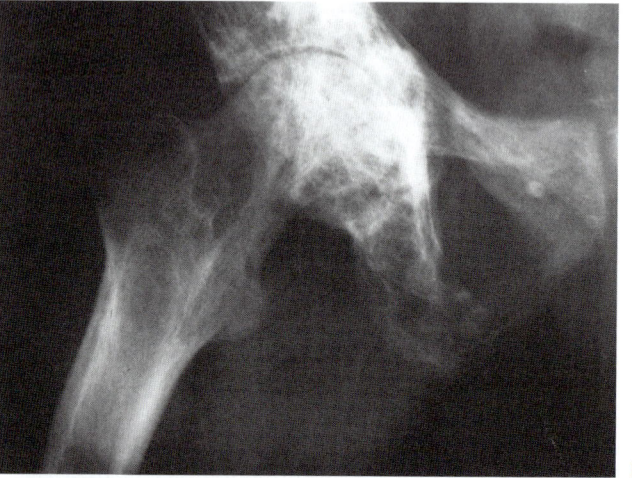
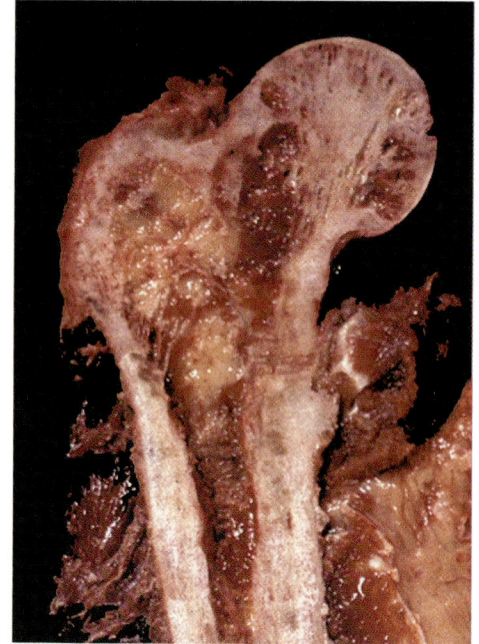
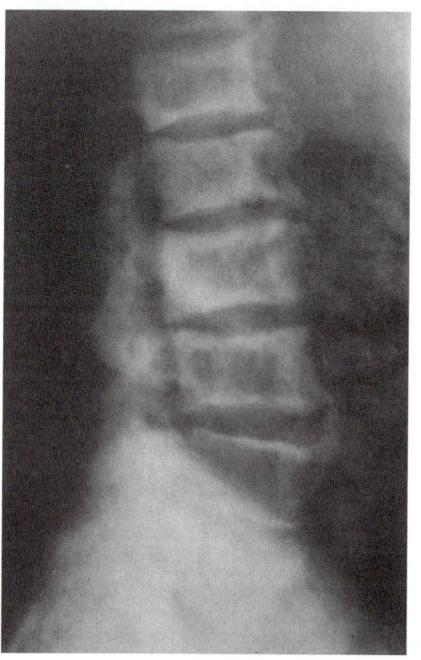

FIGURE 26-37
Paget disease. **A.** A radiograph of early Paget disease shows cortical dissolution, increased diameter of the diaphysis, and an advancing, wedge-shaped area of cortical reabsorption ("flame sign"). Proximal to the edge of this wedge, the femur appears entirely normal. **B.** Later Paget disease of the proximal femur and pelvis shows cortical disorganization and irregular coarse trabeculations. **C.** Gross specimen of proximal femur showing cortical thickening and coarse trabeculations of the femoral head and neck. **D.** Paget disease of the spine shows shortening and widening of the lumbar vertebral bodies. Their cortices and endplates are thickened and have a "picture-frame" appearance.

The disease need not progress through all three stages, and in polyostotic disease, various foci may appear in different stages.

The osteoclast is the pathological cell of Paget disease, and its appearance is characteristic. Whereas normal osteoclasts contain fewer than a dozen nuclei, those of Paget disease are huge and may encompass more than 100 (Fig. 26-38). The nuclei may contain intranuclear inclusions that demonstrate viruslike particles ultrastructurally.

Because active Paget disease is a disorder of accelerated remodeling, its histological features are those of severe osteitis fibrosa. Numerous osteoclasts, large active osteoblasts, and peritrabecular marrow fibrosis are encountered. The rapid remodeling leads to disruption of trabecular architecture. Trabeculae are characteristically distorted and irregular, with a high surface-to-volume ratio. Bone collagen is often arranged in a woven rather than lamellar pattern.

With time, the lesions of Paget disease burn out and become inactive. The diagnostic hallmark of this stage is the abnormal arrangement of lamellar bone, in which islands of irregular bone formation, resembling pieces of a jigsaw puzzle, are separated by prominent *cement lines*. The result is a *mosaic pattern* in the bone, which can be seen particularly well under polarized light. In the cortex of an affected bone, the osteons tend to be destroyed, and concentric lamellae are incomplete. Although the changes in lamellar bone are diagnostic, it is common to see woven bone as part of the pathological process. In this situation, the woven bone is a reactive phenomenon, as in a microcallus, and represents a temporary bridge between islands of the mosaic bone of Paget disease.

Clinical Features: The most common focal symptom of Paget disease is pain in the affected bone, although its cause is not clear. The pain may be related to microfractures, to the stimulation of free nerve endings by dilated blood vessels adjacent to the bones, or to weight bearing in weaker bones. The diagnosis is primarily made by x-ray findings.

SKULL: Involvement of the skull is particularly common in Paget disease. The skull exhibits localized lysis, generally in the frontal and parietal bones, which is termed *osteoporosis circumscripta*. Alternatively, there may be thickening of the outer and inner tables, which is most pronounced in the frontal and occipital bones. The skull becomes very heavy and may collapse over the C1 vertebra, thereby compressing the brain and spinal cord. Hearing loss is occasioned by involvement of the ossicles and bony impingement on the eighth cranial nerve at the foramen. *Platybasia* (flattening of the base of the skull) impinges on the foramen magnum, thereby compressing the medulla and upper spinal cord.

The jaws may be grossly misshapen, and the teeth may fall out. Often, the facial bones increase in size, especially the maxillary bones, producing so-called *leontiasis ossea* (lionlike face).

PAGETIC STEAL: Occasionally, patients feel lightheaded, a symptom due to so-called pagetic steal, in which blood is shunted from the internal carotid system to the bones rather than directed to the brain.

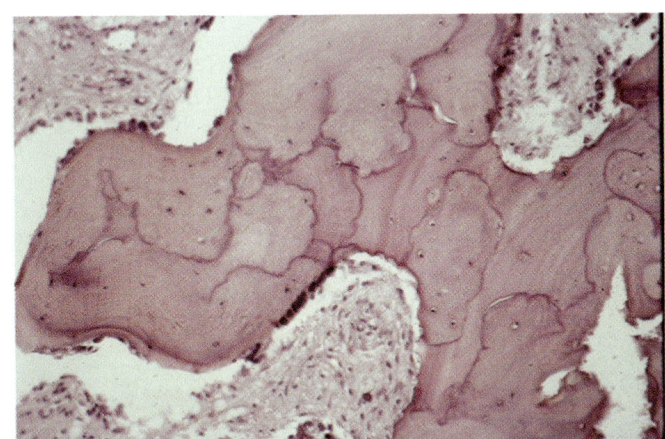
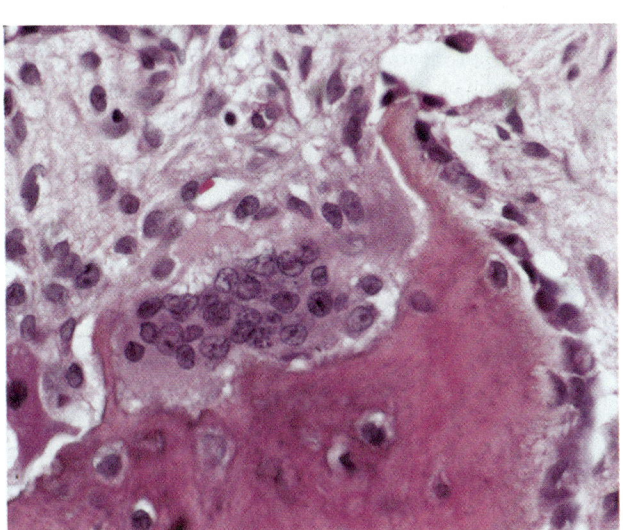
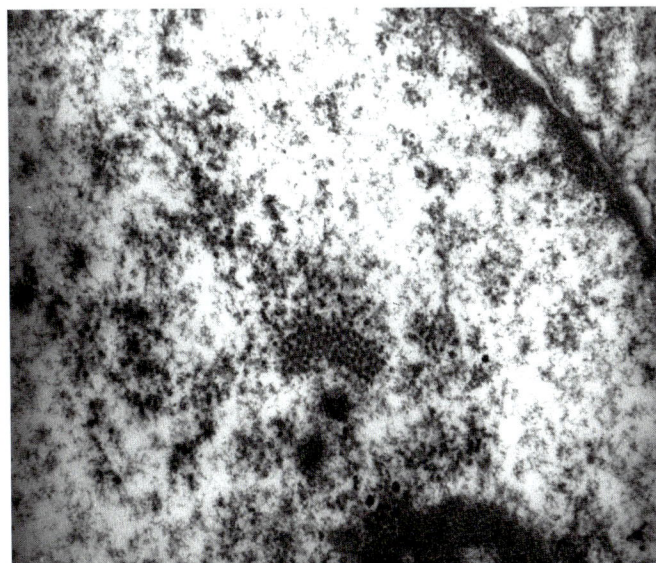

FIGURE 26-38
Paget disease. A. A section of bone shows prominent and irregular basophilic cement lines. B. An osteoclast in pagetic bone contains many more nuclei than a usual osteoclast. A few of the nuclei contain eosinophilic intranuclear inclusion-like particles. C. On electron microscopy, the nuclei of the osteoclasts contain particles that resemble paramyxovirus in their shape and orientation.

FRACTURES AND ARTHRITIS: Bone fractures are common in Paget disease, the bones snapping transversely like a piece of chalk. Incomplete fractures without displacement are called *infractions*. Involvement of the pelvis leads to hip problems. The loss of subchondral bone compliance causes secondary osteoarthritis and destruction of the articular cartilage.

HIGH-OUTPUT CARDIAC FAILURE: With extensive Paget disease, blood flow to the bones and subcutaneous tissue increases remarkably, requiring increased cardiac output. In the presence of underlying cardiac disease, it may be severe enough to result in cardiac failure.

SARCOMATOUS CHANGE: Neoplastic transformation may occur in a focus of Paget disease, usually in the femur, humerus, or pelvis. This complication occurs in less than 1% of all cases and usually arises in patients with severe Paget disease. However, the incidence of bone sarcoma is still 1000 times higher than that in the general population. Interestingly, the skull and vertebrae, the bones most commonly involved by Paget disease, rarely undergo sarcomatous change. The sarcoma is usually osteogenic but may be fibrosarcoma or chondrosarcoma.

GIANT CELL TUMOR: This lesion is not a neoplasm but rather a reactive phenomenon, similar to the "brown tumor" of hyperparathyroidism. Giant cell tumor represents an overshoot of osteoclastic activity and an associated fibroblastic response. Radiation therapy to the giant cell tumor is curative in many cases.

The serum calcium and phosphorus levels in Paget disease are normal, even though the turnover rate of bone increases more than 20-fold. Although hypercalcemia is rare, it does occur if the patient is immobilized. The collagen structure of bone in Paget disease is entirely normal, but because of the accelerated bone turnover, levels of collagen breakdown products (hydroxyproline and hydroxylysine) increase in the serum and urine. Hydroxyproline excretion may reach 1000 mg/day (normal, <40 mg). The serum alkaline phosphatase level is the most useful laboratory test in diagnosing Paget disease. It increases enormously and correlates with osteoblastic activity. The alkaline phosphatase levels are disproportionately high with skull involvement, but tend to be low when only the pelvis is affected. A sudden increase in the activity of serum alkaline phosphatase may reflect sarcomatous change within a lesion.

Fortunately, most patients with Paget disease are asymptomatic and require no treatment. Fractures, osteoarthritis, and other orthopedic complications are treated symptomatically. Drugs directed at abnormal osteoclast function, including calcitonin, bisphosphonates, and mithramycin, may be useful.

GAUCHER DISEASE

Gaucher disease is an autosomal recessive hereditary storage disease that affects the bones and other organs. It is the most common lysosomal storage disease, with an estimated birth frequency of 1/50,000 in the white population. The disease is panethnic and has its highest prevalence in the Ashkenazi Jewish population.

Pathogenesis: The faulty gene encodes for β-glucocerebrosidase and is located on chromosome 1q21, with more than 200 mutations thus far described. Gaucher disease reflects deficient activity of the lysosomal hydrolase, β-glucocerebrosidase (acid β-glucosidase) and causes monocytes and macrophages to store excessive amounts of glucocerebroside in lysosomes. The resulting distended cells are called Gaucher cells, and their presence in various tissues is the hallmark of the disease.

Pathology and Clinical Features: Histologically, Gaucher cells are enlarged macrophages, up to 100 μm in diameter, which exhibit cytoplasmic linear inclusions. Ultrastructurally, these inclusions are tubulelike lysosomes. Virtually all patients with Gaucher disease type I have some abnormality of the skeleton.

FAILURE OF REMODELING OF THE DISTAL FEMUR AND PROXIMAL TIBIA: This is the most common, although the least troublesome, skeletal abnormality in Gaucher disease. The defect is manifested as an absence of appropriate flaring, and therefore, funnelization and cylinderization are abnormal (Fig. 26-39). The resulting bone has an Erlenmeyer flask shape, similar to that seen in other modeling deformities (e.g., osteopetrosis).

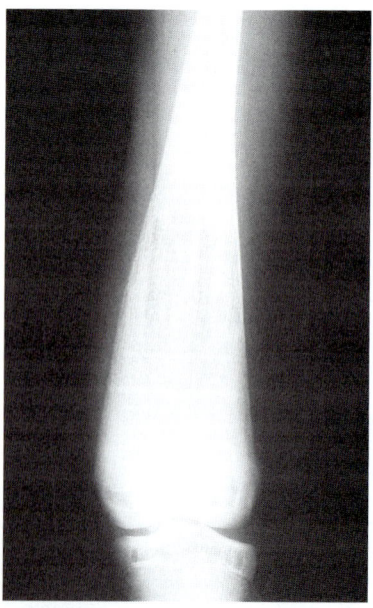

FIGURE 26-39

Gaucher disease. A radiograph of the distal femur shows the characteristic flaring of the metaphysis and distal diaphysis.

GAUCHER CRISIS: This event occurs in only a few patients with the disease, but it is intensely painful and disabling. The crisis results from acute infarction of a large segment of bone, usually the spine, pelvis, or femoral head. The lesion may even be multifocal in one or several bones. In many cases, Gaucher crisis occurs after an acute viral illness. The patients have sudden, severe, and progressive pain, which is localized to an anatomical focus. Fever, tenderness in the area of the bone, and soft tissue swelling are characteristic. Gaucher crisis lasts for 2 or more weeks and then gradually improves.

LOCALIZED AND DIFFUSE BONE LOSS: Localized lucent lesions, cortical thinning, and loss of coarse cancellous bone are seen radiologically. Bone loss is usually most severe in the axial skeleton and the proximal appendicular skeleton. On histological examination, areas of decreased bone mass contain marrow packed with Gaucher cells. These patients are generally asymptomatic until a fracture or osteonecrosis occurs.

OSTEOSCLEROTIC LESIONS: Increased bone formation occurs in the medullary cavity of the long bones and pelvis. Reactive new bone forms in areas that have undergone osteonecrosis, as evidenced by the presence in these zones of dead bone, fat necrosis, and calcification of fat. Occasionally, osteosclerotic lesions are present in the flat bones of the skull.

CORTICOMEDULLARY OSTEONECROSIS: This is the most disabling of the skeletal problems associated with Gaucher disease and occurs most commonly in young patients between the ages of 8 and 35 years. It affects the femoral head or proximal humerus or, less commonly, a femoral or tibial condyle, talus, or capitulum. Corticomedullary osteonecrosis may involve the shaft of long bones as well. It is bilateral in more than half of patients and is often multifocal. The pathogenesis of this lesion is not clear.

PATHOLOGICAL FRACTURES: The vertebrae, the long bones, and even the pelvis may have spontaneous fractures.

HEMATOGENOUS OSTEOMYELITIS AND SEPTIC ARTHRITIS: These infections are not uncommon in patients with Gaucher disease, and the incidence of postoperative wound infection is also high. The most common agents are coliform or anaerobic organisms. It may be that bacteria are deposited in areas of bone infarction, or perhaps the phagocytic cells filled with glucocerebroside are incompetent and cannot respond to the invading bacteria.

Enzyme replacement therapy for Gaucher disease is effective, and hematopoietic stem cell gene therapy is also promising.

FIBROUS DYSPLASIA

Fibrous dysplasia is a peculiar developmental abnormality of the skeleton characterized by a disorganized mixture of fibrous and osseous elements in the interior of affected bones. It occurs in children or adults and may involve a single bone (monostotic) or many bones (polyostotic). In 5% of cases of fibrous dysplasia, the skeletal lesions are associated with skin pigmentation and endocrine dysfunction, in which case the term *McCune-Albright syndrome* is applied.

Pathogenesis: Activating mutations in the α subunit of the stimulatory guanine nucleotide-binding protein (G$_S$α), which is linked to adenylyl cyclase, have been described in bone cells from patients with fibrous dysplasia and McCune-Albright syndrome. The result would be constitutive activation of adenylyl cyclase and increased levels of cyclic AMP, thereby enhancing certain functions of the affected cells (e.g., c-*fos* protooncogene, c-*jun*, IL-6, and IL-11).

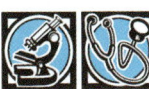

Pathology and Clinical Features:

MONOSTOTIC FIBROUS DYSPLASIA: Monostotic fibrous dysplasia is the most common form of the disease and is most often seen in the second and third decades, without any predilection for either sex. The bones commonly involved are the proximal femur, tibia, ribs, and facial bones, although any bone may be involved. The disease may be asymptomatic or it may lead to a pathological fracture.

POLYOSTOTIC FIBROUS DYSPLASIA: One fourth of patients with polyostotic fibrous dysplasia exhibit disease in more than half of the skeleton, including the facial bones. Symptoms usually are seen in childhood, and almost all patients have pathological fractures, limb deformities, or limb-length discrepancies. Polyostotic fibrous dysplasia is more common in females. Sometimes the disease becomes quiescent at puberty, whereas pregnancy may stimulate the growth of lesions.

MCCUNE-ALBRIGHT SYNDROME: This condition is characterized by endocrine dysfunction, including acromegaly, Cushing syndrome, hyperthyroidism, and vitamin D-resistant rickets. The most common endocrine abnormality is precocious puberty in girls (boys rarely have McCune-Albright syndrome). As a result, premature closure of the growth plates may lead to abnormally short stature. The most frequent extraskeletal manifestations of McCune-Albright syndrome are the characteristic skin lesions. These are pigmented macules ("café-au-lait" spots) with irregular ("coast of Maine") borders, which do not cross the midline of the body and are usually located over the buttocks, back, and sacrum. These macules have a tendency to overlie the skeletal lesions.

The radiographic features of fibrous dysplasia are distinctive. The bone lesion has a lucent ground-glass appearance with well-marginated borders and a thin cortex. The bone may be ballooned, deformed, or enlarged, and involvement may be focal or may encompass the entire bone (Fig. 26-40A).

All forms of fibrous dysplasia have an identical histological pattern (see Fig. 26-40B,C). Benign fibroblastic tissue is arranged in a loose, whorled pattern. Irregularly arranged, purposeless spicules of woven bone that lack osteoblastic

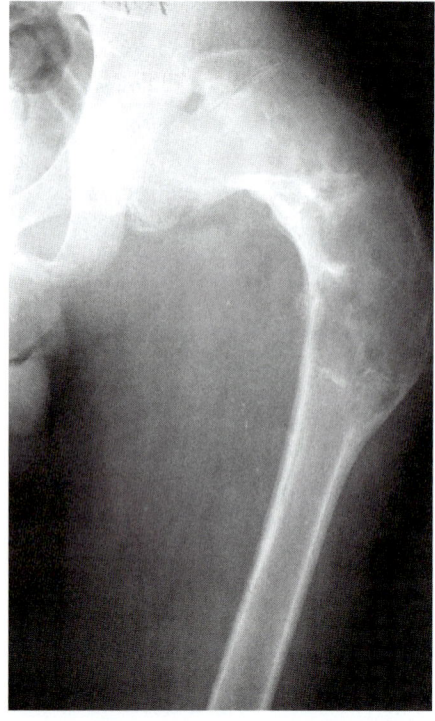
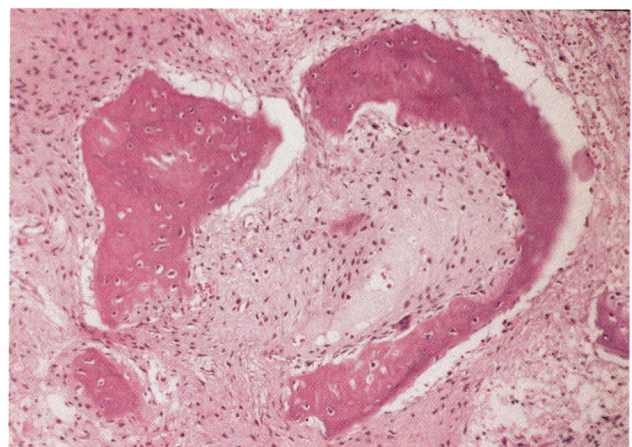
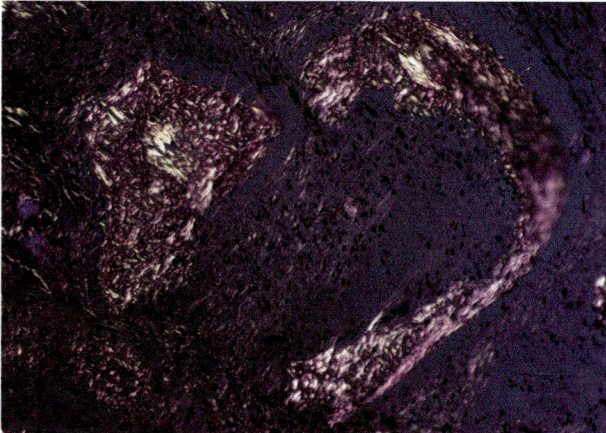

FIGURE 26-40
Fibrous dysplasia. A. A radiograph of the proximal femur shows a "shepherd's crook" deformity caused by fractures sustained over the years. Irregular, marginated, ground-glass lucencies are surrounded by reactive bone. The shaft has an appearance that has been likened to a soap bubble. **B.** Histologically, fibrous dysplasia consists of moderately cellular fibrous tissue in which irregular, curved spicules of woven bone develop without discernible appositional osteoblast activity. **C.** The same section in polarized light demonstrates not only that the spicules are woven, but also that their fiber pattern extends imperceptibly into the fiber pattern of the surrounding stroma.

rimming are embedded in the fibrous tissue. In 10% of cases, irregular islands of hyaline cartilage are also present. Occasionally, cystic degeneration occurs, with hemosiderin-laden macrophages, hemorrhage, and osteoclasts congregated about the cyst. Rarely (<1% of cases), malignant degeneration (osteosarcoma, chondrosarcoma, or fibrosarcoma) has been reported, but most of these cases involved prior radiation therapy. Treatment of fibrous dysplasia consists of curettage, repair of fractures, and prevention of deformities.

BENIGN TUMORS OF BONE

Bone tumors of all kinds are uncommon but are nevertheless important neoplasms, because many occur in children and young persons and are potentially lethal. A primary bone tumor may arise from any one of the cellular elements of bone. Most neoplasms of bone occur near the metaphyseal area, and more than 80% of primary tumors occur in either the distal femur or the proximal tibia (Fig. 26-41). In the growing child, these areas are characterized by conspicuous growth activity and are, therefore, more likely to develop a tumor.

Nonossifying Fibroma Is a Solitary Lesion of Childhood

Nonossifying fibroma, also termed fibrous cortical defect, *is a benign tumor that occurs in the metaphysis of a long bone, most commonly the tibia or femur.* The disorder is very common and may be present in as many as 25% of all children between ages 4 and 10 years, after which it characteristically regresses. Whether nonossifying fibroma is a neoplastic or developmental lesion remains controversial. Most cases are asymptomatic, although pain or fracture through the thin

Benign Tumors of Bone   1351

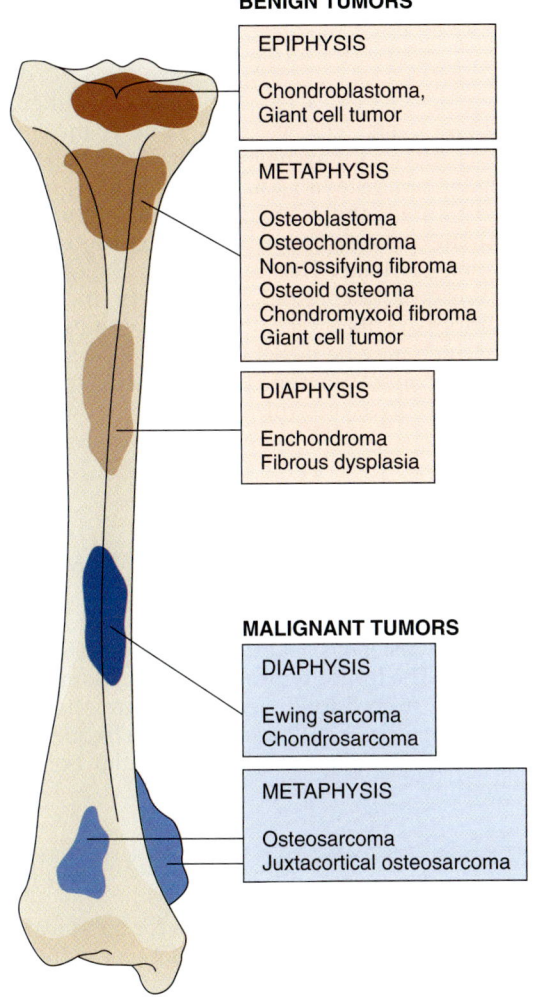

FIGURE 26-41
Location of primary bone tumors in long tubular bones.

thirds of all solitary bone cysts occur in the upper (proximal) humerus or femur, usually in the metaphysis adjacent to the growth plate.

Pathogenesis: Solitary bone cyst seems not to be a true neoplasm but rather a disturbance of bone growth with superimposed trauma. Secondary organization of a hematoma or some abnormality of the metaphyseal vessels causes accumulation of fluid. The "tumor" then grows by expansion of the fluid cavity, and the resulting pressure causes resorption of bone, mediated by the neighboring osteoclasts. The process is slow, so that as the endosteal surface of the cortex is resorbed, a thin periosteal shell of new bone is laid down. This sequence results in a thin, well-marginated, radiolucent bone lesion (Fig. 26-42), which is never greater in diameter than the growth plate and is particularly susceptible to pathological fracture.

Pathology: Solitary bone cyst is lined by fibrous tissue, a few giant cells, hemosiderin-laden macrophages, chronic inflammatory cells, and reactive bone. Osteoclasts are present in the advancing front of the cyst and allow expansion of the lesion. The cyst contains masses of amorphous proteinaceous material.

cortex overlying the lesion occasionally calls attention to the condition.

Pathology: Radiologically, nonossifying fibromas are identified by a cortical, eccentric position and by well-demarcated, central lucent zones surrounded by scalloped, sclerotic margins. On gross examination, the lesion is granular and dark red to brown. Microscopically, bland spindle cells are arranged in an interlacing, whorled pattern in which multinuclear giant cells and foamy macrophages may be seen. The rare, symptomatic or expanded lesions are treated with curettage and bone grafting.

Solitary Bone Cyst Occurs in Children and Adolescents

Solitary, or unicameral, bone cyst is a benign, fluid-filled, unilocular, lesion. There is a male predilection (3:1). More than two

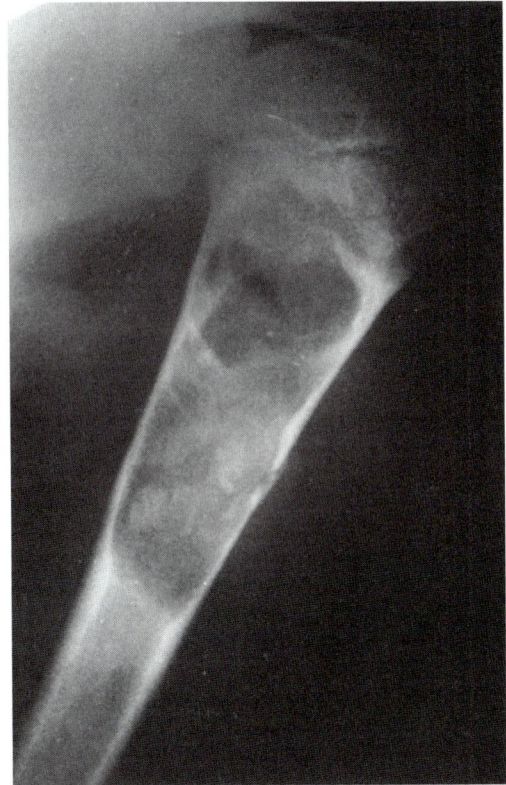

FIGURE 26-42
Solitary bone cyst. A radiograph of the proximal humerus of a child (note the epiphyseal plate) shows a large, well-demarcated, lytic epiphyseal and diaphyseal lesion. The cortex is thinned, but there is no cortical distortion or malformation of the shape of the bone.

Clinical Features: Most solitary bone cysts are entirely asymptomatic until a pathological fracture calls attention to the lesion. Once the diagnosis is confirmed by other imaging studies and by finding clear fluid by needle aspiration, intralesional corticosteroids are administered. Curettage and deposition of bone chips are performed only when the cyst is not controlled by injection.

Aneurysmal Bone Cyst Is Not a True Tumor

Aneurysmal bone cyst is an uncommon, expansive, hyperemic lesion arising within a bone or on its surface. It occurs in children and young adults, with a peak incidence in the second decade. The lesion has been observed at every skeletal site but is most frequent in the long bones and the vertebral column. Its pathogenesis is obscure, but it may represent cystic vascular transformation of an underlying lesion such as chondroblastoma, osteoblastoma, fibrous dysplasia, or giant cell tumor.

 Pathology: The periosteum around an aneurysmal bone cyst is ballooned but intact. In the spine, aneurysmal bone cyst may actually extend across more than one bone. By magnetic resonance imaging (MRI), fluid-fluid levels may be seen as blood cells separate from plasma. The cut surface of the lesion resembles a sponge permeated with blood and blood clots (Fig. 26-43). The walls and the septa of the aneurysmal cyst are composed of granulation tissue containing multinucleated giant cells, with occasional osteoid trabeculae.

 Clinical Features: Although some aneurysmal bone cysts tend to grow slowly, most expand rapidly and may reach an enormous size. The lesions usually manifest with pain and swelling, sometimes in relation to trauma, and often develop in a short period of time. The bone cyst may "blow out," that is, rupture and produce local hemorrhage. The treatment of choice is extraperiosteal excision and curettage. At surgery, incision of the cyst decompresses its internal pressure, resulting in brisk bleeding, which may be difficult to control. In sites such as the vertebral column or the pelvis, selective arterial embolization has been successful.

Osteoid Osteoma Is a Painful Lesion

Osteoid osteoma is a small, painful, benign lesion of bone composed of osseous tissue (the nidus) and surrounded by a halo of reactive bone formation. The tumor typically occurs in young persons, ranging in age from 5 to 25 years. Boys are affected more commonly than girls (3:1). Osteoid osteoma frequently arises in the cortex of the diaphysis of the tubular bones of the lower extremity.

 Pathology: Osteoid osteoma is a spherical, hyperemic tumor, about 1 cm in diameter, which is considerably softer than the surrounding bone (Fig. 26-44) and easily enucleated at surgery. Microscopically, the tumor is composed of thin, irregular, trabeculae within a cellular granulation tissue containing osteoblasts and osteoclasts. The trabeculae are more mature in the center, which is often partially calcified. Reactive, sclerotic bone surrounds the nidus.

 Clinical Features: Pain, typically nocturnal, is out of proportion to the size of the lesion. It is often exacerbated by the intake of alcoholic beverages and promptly relieved by aspirin, possibly because of the high prostaglandin content of the tumor. Surgical excision or electrocautery is curative and leaves the patient very grateful to the surgeon.

Osteoblastoma

Osteoblastoma is an uncommon, benign neoplasm that is histologically similar to osteoid osteoma but larger and not accompanied by nocturnal pain relieved by aspirin. It stimulates less bone reaction and appears as a purely radiolucent lesion, with only a thin shell of surrounding bone. Osteoblastoma occurs in persons between the ages of 10 and 35 years, with no sex predilection, and mainly affects the spine and long bones.

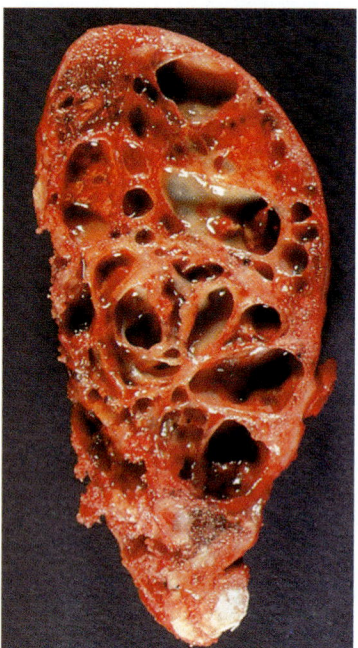

FIGURE 26-43
Aneurysmal bone cyst. In cross-section, the lesion consists of a spongy mass containing multiple blood-filled cysts. Some of the septa between the cysts contain bony tissue.

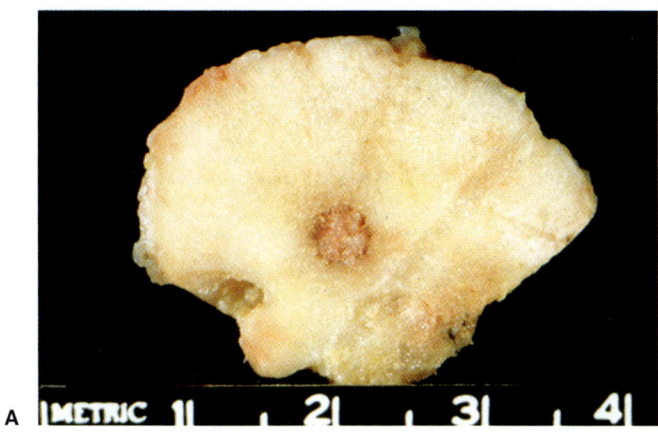
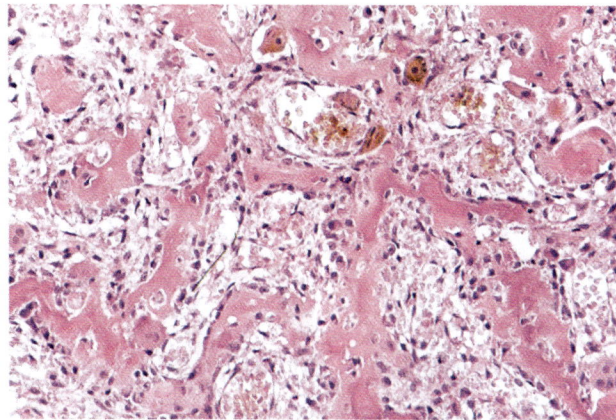

FIGURE 26-44
Osteoid osteoma. A. A gross specimen of an osteoid osteoma shows the central nidus, which is embedded in dense bone. B. A photomicrograph of the nidus reveals irregular trabeculae of woven bone surrounded by osteoblasts, osteoclasts, and fibrovascular marrow.

Curettage cures small osteoblastomas, but larger lesions may require wide resection.

Solitary Chondroma Features Hyaline Cartilage

Solitary chondroma (enchondroma) is a benign, intraosseous tumor composed of well-differentiated hyaline cartilage. Although it has been debated whether it represents a true neoplasm or a hamartoma, recent cytogenetic analyses indicate a clonal origin for these lesions, suggesting that they are in fact neoplasms. The diagnosis is made at any age, and many cases are entirely asymptomatic.

Pathology: Most cases of solitary chondroma occur in the metacarpals and phalanges of the hands, the remainder being in almost any other tubular bone. The tumor is small and grows slowly. Radiologically, it appears as a well-delimited radiolucent area, sometimes containing stippled calcifications. On gross examination, solitary chondroma has the semitranslucent appearance of hyaline cartilage, often with a few calcified areas. Microscopically, the cartilaginous tissue is well differentiated, with sparse chondrocytes.

Asymptomatic chondromas are best left untreated. When pain intervenes, curettage and bone grafting are the treatment of choice.

Chondroblastoma Occurs in the Epiphyses of Long Bones

Chondroblastoma is an uncommon, benign chondrogenic tumor that favors the upper femur, tibia, and humerus. It is more common in males than in females (2:1), and 90% of cases occur in young persons between the ages of 5 and 25 years.

Pathology: Chondroblastoma grows slowly, and on radiological examination, displays an eccentric, radiolucent appearance with sharply defined borders (Fig. 26-45). On gross examination, the tumor is soft and compact with scattered gray or hemorrhagic areas. Microscopically, primitive chondroblasts are arranged as sheets of round-to-polyhedral cells that have well-defined cytoplasmic borders and large, ovoid nuclei, often with prominent nuclear grooves. The cartilage matrix appears primitive and is variably calcified, which accounts for the mottled pattern often seen in computed tomography (CT) scans. Chondroblastoma causes bone destruction by stimulating osteoclastic resorption. In fact, these tumors may perforate the cortex, although they remain confined by the periosteum.

Clinical Features: Because of its paraarticular location, the symptoms of chondroblastoma tend to be related to a joint, with moderate pain, mild swelling, and functional limitation of joint movement. If neglected, the tumor may on rare occasions attain a large size, destroy the epiphyseal area, and invade the joint. Curettage is the treatment of choice, although in 10% of cases, the tumor recurs.

Chondromyxoid Fibroma

Chondromyxoid fibroma is a rare, benign cartilage-like tumor of bone that occurs in the femur or tibia of children and young adults. The tumor is also found occasionally in almost any bone.

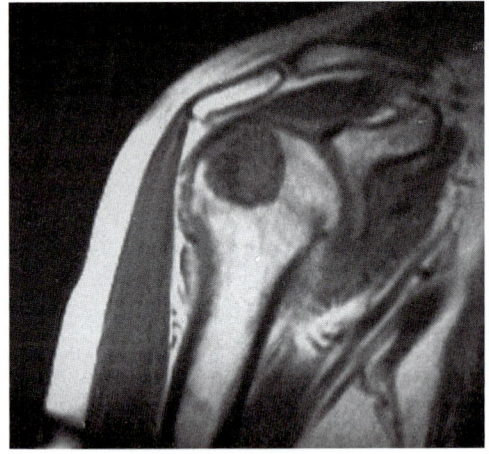 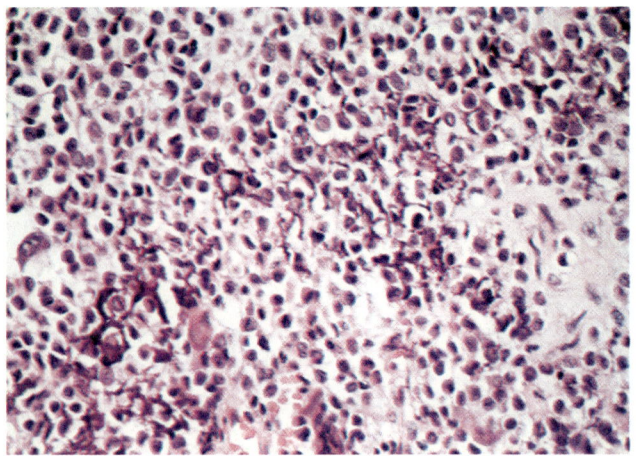

FIGURE 26-45
Chondroblastoma. A. A magnetic resonance image of the shoulder of a child shows a prominent lytic lesion of the head of the humerus that involves the epiphysis and extends across the epiphyseal plate. B. The histological appearance of a chondroblastoma is defined by plump, round cells (chondroblasts) surrounded by a mineralized matrix.

Pathology: Radiologically, chondromyxoid fibroma is identified as an eccentric, lucent defect with a thin scalloped border of sclerotic bone. On gross examination, the tumor is a firm, lobulated, grayish white or yellowish mass that replaces bone and thins the cortex. Microscopically, sparsely cellular lobules show spindle and stellate cells and multinucleated giant cells embedded within a chondroid or myxoid matrix. The lobules are usually separated by bands of highly cellular tissue composed of plump, round, mononuclear cells and multinucleated cells similar to those seen in chondrosarcoma. The distinct lobulation of the tumor and its characteristic sclerotic borders are important, since in some instances, the presence of large, pleomorphic cells in its chondroid matrix has led to an erroneous diagnosis of chondrosarcoma.

Chondromyxoid fibroma is best treated by surgical excision because the tumor tends to recur after simple curettage.

MALIGNANT TUMORS OF BONE

Osteosarcoma Is the Most Common Primary Malignant Bone Tumor

Osteosarcoma, also termed osteogenic sarcoma, is a highly malignant bone tumor characterized by formation of bone tissue by tumor cells. It represents one fifth of all bone cancers and is most frequent in adolescents between the ages of 10 and 20 years, affecting boys more often than girls (2:1).

Pathogenesis: Almost two thirds of cases of osteosarcoma exhibit mutations in the retinoblastoma *(Rb)* gene (see Chapter 5), and many tumors also contain mutations in the *p53* gene. Thus, osteosarcoma takes its place among cancers related to the inactivation of tumor-suppressor genes. The tumor is more common in tall persons. Interestingly, osteosarcomas in dogs are more frequent in large breeds. When it arises in older persons, osteosarcoma is almost always a complication of Paget disease or radiation exposure. For example, radium watch dial painters who wetted their brushes by licking them developed osteosarcoma many years later as a result of the deposition of radium in their bones. Moreover, osteosarcoma has also developed in adults and children previously subjected to external, therapeutic radiation. Several preexisting benign bone lesions are associated with an increased risk of later osteosarcoma, including fibrous dysplasia, osteomyelitis, and bone marrow infarcts. Although trauma may call attention to an existing osteosarcoma, there is no evidence that it ever causes the tumor.

Pathology: Osteosarcoma often arises in the vicinity of the knee, that is, the lower femur (Fig. 26-46A), upper tibia, or fibula, although any metaphyseal area of a long bone may be affected. The proximal humerus is second to the knee area as a site of osteosarcoma, and 75% of osteosarcomas arise adjacent to the knee or shoulder.

Radiological evidence of bone destruction and bone formation is characteristic, the latter representing neoplastic bone. Often, the periosteum produces an incomplete rim of reactive bone adjacent to the site where it is lifted from the cortical surface by the tumor. When this appears on an x-ray as a shell of bone intersecting the cortex at one end and open at the other end, it is referred to as *Codman triangle.* A "sunburst" periosteal reaction is also often superimposed (see Fig. 26-19).

The gross appearance of the tumor is highly variable, depending on the relative amounts of bone, cartilage, stroma, and blood vessels. The cut surface may show any combination of hemorrhagic, cystic, soft, and bony areas. The neoplastic tissue may invade and break through the cortex, spread into the marrow cavity, elevate or perforate the periosteum, or grow into the epiphysis and even reach the joint space.

Histological examination reveals malignant cells with osteoblastic differentiation producing woven bone (Fig. 26-46B). The malignant cells stain prominently for alkaline phosphatase and osteonectin. The tumorous bone is laid down haphazardly and not aligned along stress lines. Often, foci of malignant cartilage cells or pleomorphic giant cells are intermixed. In areas of osteolysis, nonneoplastic osteoclasts are found at the advancing front of the tumor.

Osteosarcoma spreads through the bloodstream to the lungs. In fact, almost all patients (98%) who die of this disease have lung metastases. Less commonly, the tumor metastasizes to other bones (35%), the pleura (33%), and the heart (20%).

 Clinical Features: Osteosarcoma presents with mild or intermittent pain around the knee or other involved areas. As the pain becomes more intense, the area becomes swollen and tender. The adjacent joint becomes functionally limited. The serum alkaline phosphatase activity is increased in half of patients and may decrease after amputation, only to increase again with recurrence or metastasis. Metastatic disease heralds rapid clinical deterioration and death.

Historically, osteosarcoma was treated exclusively by amputation or disarticulation of the involved limb, but the prognosis for 5-year survival did not exceed 20%. More-recent developments in chemotherapy and limb-sparing surgery have resulted in 5-year disease-free rates as high as 60%. Resection of isolated pulmonary metastases appears to prolong survival.

Juxtacortical Osteosarcoma

Juxtacortical osteosarcoma is a rare variant of osteosarcoma that occurs on the periosteal surface of the bone, especially the lower posterior metaphysis of the femur (72% of cases). Unlike classic osteosarcoma, most patients are older than 25 years, and the tumor is more common in women. Juxtacortical osteosarcoma spares the deep cortex and medulla of the bone and grows external to the shaft (Fig. 26-47). Usually, Codman triangle is not evident radiologically, because the periosteum is not elevated. Most cases of juxtacortical osteosarcoma are low-grade lesions, which do not require adjunctive chemotherapy. Surgical excision is the treatment of choice, and the prognosis is good, with a 5-year survival of more than 80%.

Chondrosarcoma Is a Cartilaginous Malignancy Whose Grade Determines Prognosis

Chondrosarcoma is a malignant tumor that originates from cartilage cells and maintains its cartilaginous nature throughout its evolution. Some patients have a history of enchondromas, solitary osteochondroma, or hereditary multiple osteochondromas. Most have no known preexisting lesion. Chondrosarcoma is the second most common primary malignant bone tumor, occurring more commonly in men than in women (2:1). It is most frequently seen in the fourth to sixth decades (average age, 45 years).

 Pathology: Chondrosarcoma occurs in three anatomical variants:

CENTRAL CHONDROSARCOMA: This form arises in the medullary cavity of pelvic bones, ribs, and long bones, although any site may be affected. Radiologically, poorly defined borders, a thickened shaft, and perforation of the cor-

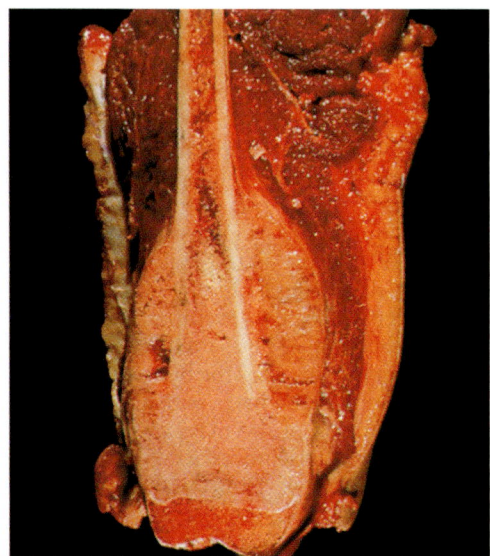
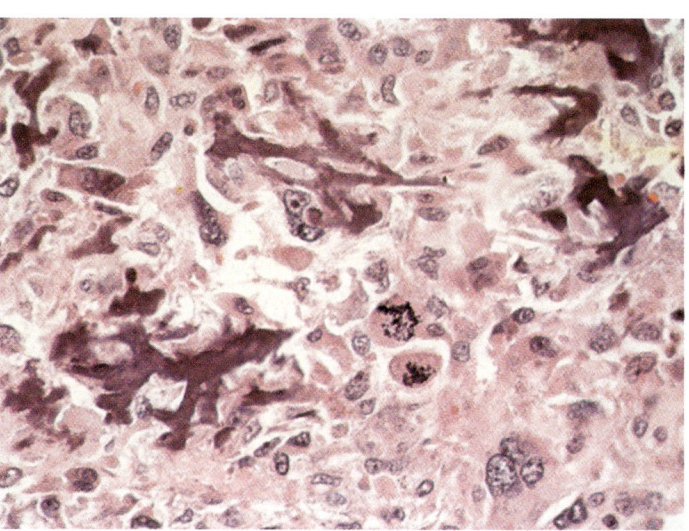

FIGURE 26-46
Osteosarcoma. A. The distal femur contains a dense osteoblastic malignant tumor that extends through the cortex into the soft tissue and the epiphysis. B. A photomicrograph reveals pleomorphic malignant cells, tumor giant cells, and mitoses. The tumor produces woven bone that is focally calcified.

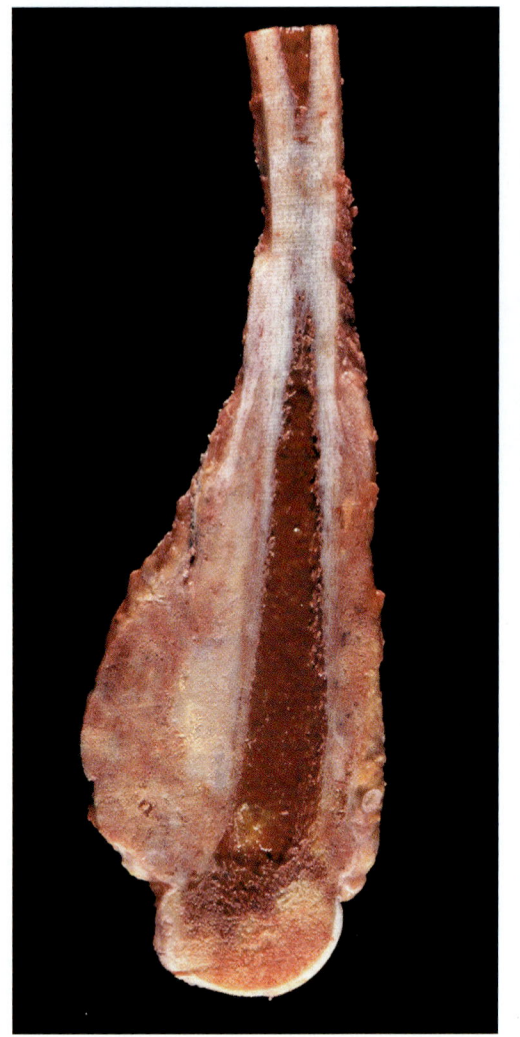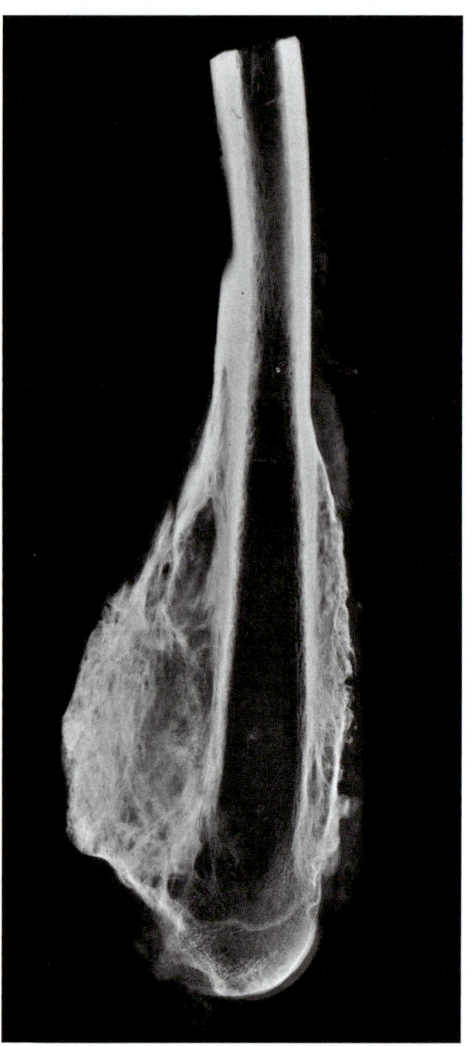

FIGURE 26-47
Juxtacortical osteosarcoma. A. The posterior surface of the femur has a tumor on its posterior surface. The medullary cavity is not involved. B. An x-ray of the specimen demonstrates that the tumor produces bone matrix (it is radiodense) and at the same time does not invade the medullary cavity.

tex characterize these tumors. There are usually stippled radiopacities or ringlike ossifications representing calcification or endochondral ossification in the tumor (Fig 26-48A). Although central chondrosarcoma may penetrate the cortex, extension beyond the periosteum is uncommon. On gross examination, the neoplastic cartilaginous tissue is compressed inside the bone and exhibits areas of necrosis, cystic change, and hemorrhage (Fig 26-48B). The cortex of the bone and the intertrabecular spaces of the marrow are infiltrated by the tumor.

Central chondrosarcoma begins with deep pain, which becomes more intense with time. In most cases, the tumor cannot be palpated, but in untreated cases, large masses may eventually form.

PERIPHERAL CHONDROSARCOMA: This variant is less common than the central variety of chondrosarcoma and arises outside the bone, almost always in the cartilaginous cap of an osteochondroma. It occurs after the age of 20 years and never before puberty. The most frequent location of peripheral chondrosarcoma is the pelvis, followed by the femur, vertebrae, sacrum, humerus and other long bones. It arises only rarely distal to the knee or elbow. Radiologically, characteristic radiopacities representing calcification or ossification of the neoplastic cartilage are virtually pathognomonic for the lesion. Macroscopically, peripheral chondrosarcoma tends to be a large bosselated mass that surrounds the base of an osteochondroma and invades the bone.

Peripheral chondrosarcoma is usually seen as a slowly growing mass. Expansion of the mass causes pain and local symptoms. In the pelvis, the lumbosacral plexus may be compressed, and tumors in the vertebrae may cause paraplegia.

JUXTACORTICAL CHONDROSARCOMA: This is the least common variety of chondrosarcoma and is similar to central chondrosarcoma in its predilection for middle-aged men. It tends to be situated in the metaphysis of long bones, lying on the outer surface of the cortex. Thus it is probably periosteal or parosteal in origin. Radiologically, it may be entirely translucent or focally calcified. The symptoms of juxtacortical chondrosarcoma are dominated by swelling, with little accompanying pain.

Histologically, chondrosarcomas are composed of malignant cartilage cells in various stages of maturity (Fig. 26-48C). Occasionally, a well-differentiated chondrosarcoma is difficult to distinguish from a benign tumor on cytological grounds alone. Zones of calcification are often conspicuous and are seen radiographically as splotches or bulky masses. Chondrosarcoma expands by stimulating osteoclastic resorption of bone and often breaks through the cortex. Most chondrosarcomas grow slowly, but hematogenous metastases to the lungs are common in poorly differentiated variants.

There is a positive correlation between histological grade, histomorphology, and the degree of karyotypic complexity. Trisomy 7 is associated with chondrosarcoma. Rearrangement of the short arm of chromosome 17 is associated with high-grade chondrosarcoma. Alterations of 12q13 are associated with tumors exhibiting myxoid features. Extraskeletal myxoid chondrosarcomas have a classical translocation (9;22)(q31;q12).

 Clinical Features: Chondrosarcoma is one of the few tumors in which microscopic grading has a significant prognostic value. The 5-year survival rate for low-grade chondrosarcomas is 80%, for moderate-grade tumors about 50%, and for high-grade tumors only 20%. Wide excision is the usual treatment.

Giant Cell Tumor of Bone Occasionally Metastasizes

Giant cell tumor of bone is a locally aggressive, potentially malignant neoplasm characterized by the presence of osteoclastic, multinucleated, giant cells randomly and uniformly distributed in a

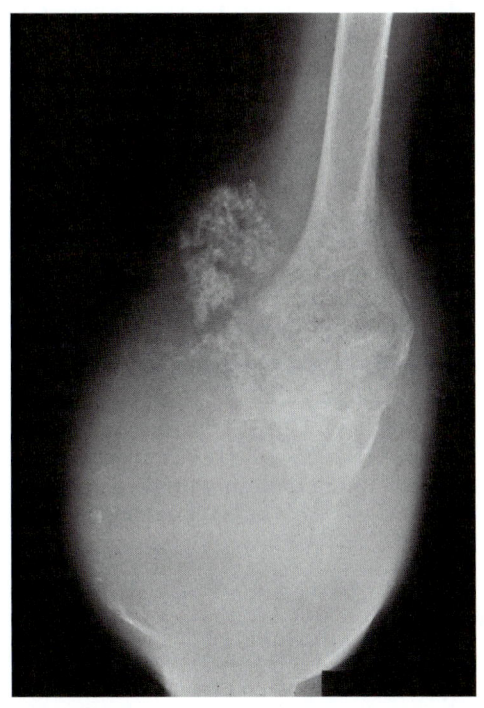

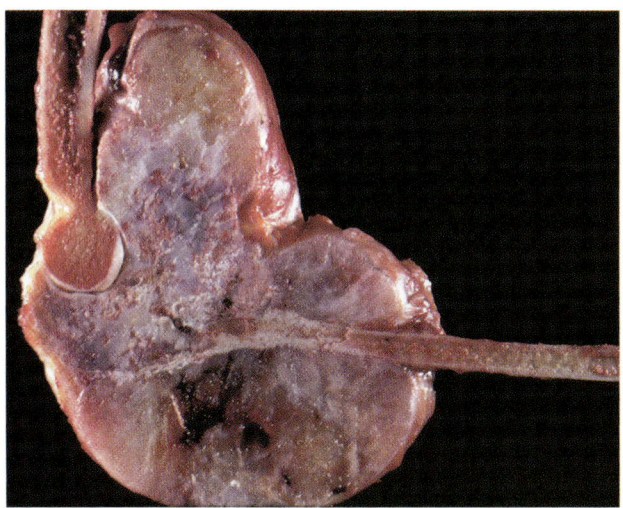

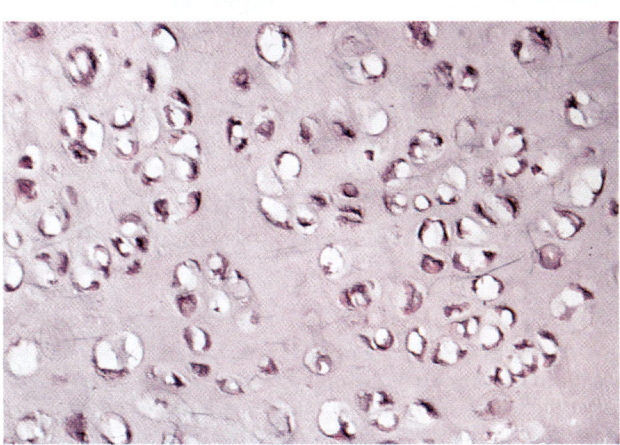

FIGURE 26-48
Chondrosarcoma. A. Radiograph demonstrates a large, destructive mass replacing the proximal ulna. There is a huge soft tissue mass containing aggregates of ring-shaped and popcornlike calcifications. **B.** Resected gross specimen demonstrates lobulated hyaline cartilage with calcifications, ossification, and focal liquefaction. **C.** A photomicrograph of a chondrosarcoma shows malignant chondrocytes with pronounced atypia.

background of proliferating mononuclear cells. It usually occurs in the third and fourth decades, has a slight predilection for women, and seems to be more common in Asia than in Western countries. Giant cell tumors in the elderly may be secondary to irradiation. Paget disease may produce a giant cell reactive lesion that closely resembles a true giant cell tumor. The neoplasms are thought to arise from primitive stromal cells that can modulate into osteoclasts.

Pathology: In most cases (90%), giant cell tumor of bone originates at the junction between the metaphysis and the epiphysis of a long bone, with more than half being situated in the knee area (distal femur and proximal tibia; Fig. 26-49A). The lower end of the radius, humerus, and fibula are also occasionally involved. The neoplasm is often a lytic lesion that grows slowly enough to allow a periosteal reaction. Thus, radiologically, the tumor tends to be surrounded by a thin, bony shell and expands the bone. Often, it has a multiloculated or "soap bubble" appearance, representing endosteal resorption of the bone.

On gross examination, giant cell tumor is clearly circumscribed, and its cut surface is soft and light brown, without bone or calcification. Numerous hemorrhagic areas result in the appearance of a sponge full of blood. In some cases, cystic cavities and necrotic areas are present. Giant cell tumor is often limited by the periosteum, although aggressive forms penetrate the cortex and the periosteum, even reaching the joint capsule and the synovial membrane.

Microscopically, giant cell tumor exhibits two types of cells (Fig. 26-49B). The mononuclear ("stromal") cells are plump and oval, with large nuclei and scanty cytoplasm. Large osteoclastic giant cells, some with more than 100 nuclei, are scattered throughout the richly vascularized stroma. Diffuse interstitial hemorrhage is common. On low power examination, the tumor often appears as a syncytium of nuclei with poor demarcation of cytoplasmic borders and random distribution of the giant cells. It is thought that the mononuclear cells are the neoplastic and proliferative components of giant cell tumor (mitotic activity is common in the mononuclear cells but is not observed in the giant cells). Indeed, the diagnosis of malignancy in a giant cell tumor depends upon the morphology of the mononuclear cells rather than that of the multinucleated cells.

Clinical Features: All giant cell tumors must be viewed as potentially malignant, because after simple curettage they may metastasize to distant sites, particularly the lungs. Virtually all metastases have occurred after an initial surgical intervention. Most of these patients may enjoy an essentially normal life span, especially if the metastatic deposits are few and can be surgically removed. Thus, some hold that local recurrence of the tumor reflects inadequate resection and that distant metastases result from dislodgment of tumor fragments during surgery.

True malignancy in giant cell tumor may be occasionally observed as either a sarcomatous lesion arising in a typical giant cell tumor or as a pure sarcoma after a giant cell tumor has been curetted. Recurrence as pure sarcoma may occur spontaneously or after local radiation therapy. About 6% of giant cell tumors demonstrate sarcomatous transformation.

Giant cell tumors manifest with pain, usually in the joint adjacent to the tumor. Microfractures and pathological fractures are frequent, owing to thinning of the cortex. The tumor is usually treated with thorough curettage and bone grafting, although more aggressive management, including en bloc resection or even amputation, may be necessary. Local recurrence after simple curettage has been reported in one third to one half of cases, and 5 to 10% metastasize.

Ewing Sarcoma Is a Primitive Neuroectodermal Tumor of Childhood

Ewing sarcoma (EWS) is an uncommon malignant bone tumor composed of small, uniform, round cells. It represents only 5% of all bone tumors and is found in children and adolescents, with two thirds of cases occurring in patients younger than

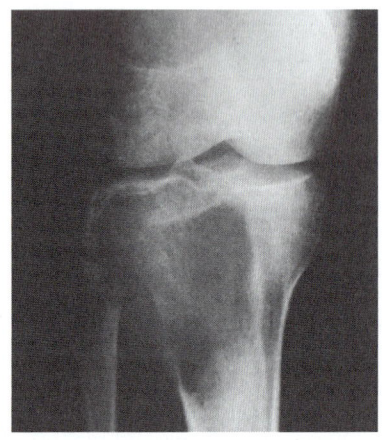
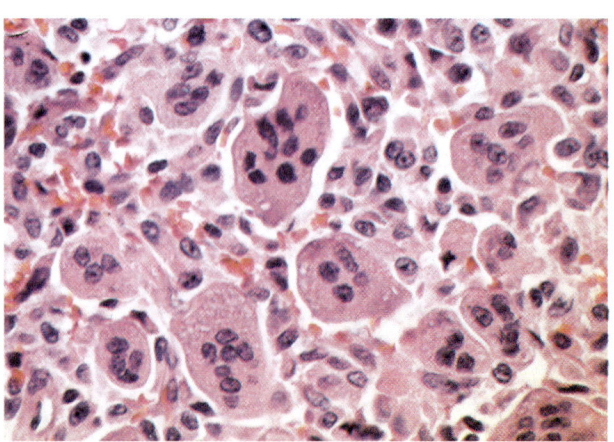

FIGURE 26-49
Giant cell tumor of bone. A. Radiograph of the proximal tibia shows an eccentric lytic lesion with virtually no new bone formation. The tumor extends to the subchondral bone plate and breaks through cortex into the soft tissue. B. Photomicrograph shows osteoclast-type giant cells and plump, oval, mononuclear cells. The nuclei of both types of cells are identical.

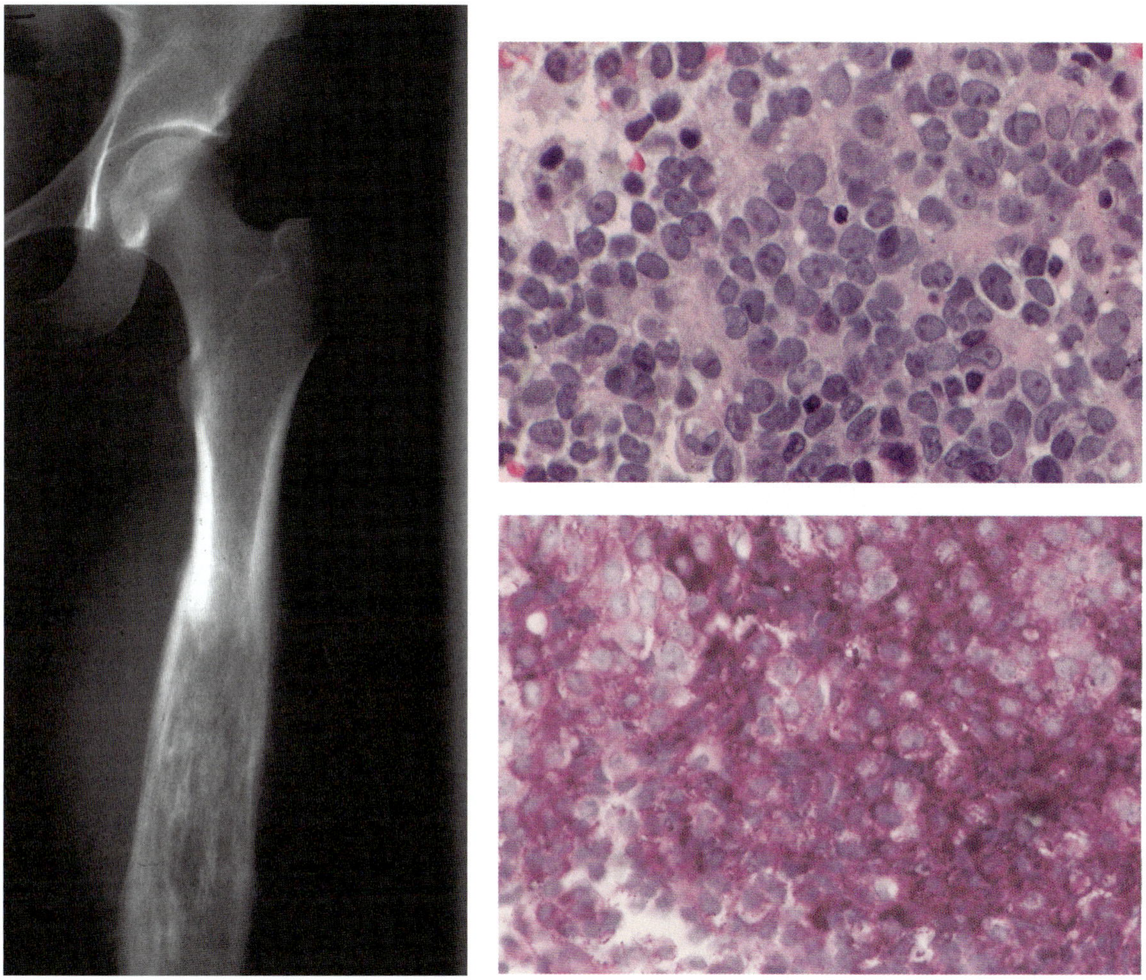

FIGURE 26-50

Ewing sarcoma. **A.** A clinical x-ray demonstrates expansile cortical destruction with poor circumscription and a delicate interrupted periosteal reaction. **B.** A biopsy specimen shows fairly uniform small cells with round, dark blue nuclei, paucity of mitotic activity, and poorly defined cytoplasm. **C.** A PAS stain demonstrates abundant intracellular glycogen.

20 years. Boys are affected more often than girls (2:1). EWS is very rare in blacks.

Pathogenesis: EWS is thought to arise from primitive marrow elements or immature mesenchymal cells. Virtually all (90%) of these tumors have a reciprocal translocation between chromosomes 11 and 22 [t(11;22)p(13;q12)], which results in the fusion of the amino terminus of the *EWS1* gene to the carboxy terminus of the *FLI-1* gene, which encodes a transcription factor. The resulting fusion protein, EWS/FLI-1, is an aberrant transcription factor whose target genes are not yet identified. A less common translocation t(21;22) leads to an *EWS/ERG* gene fusion and gives rise to a variant of EWS with a significantly worse prognosis.

Pathology: EWS is primarily a tumor of the long bones in childhood, especially the humerus, tibia, and femur, where it occurs as a midshaft or metaphyseal lesion. It tends to parallel the distribution of red marrow, so when it arises in the third decade or later, it affects the pelvis and spine. However, no bone is immune from involvement.

The radiographic findings are variable and depend upon the interaction of the tumor with the host bone. There is often a destructive process in which the border between normal bone and the lesion is indistinct (Fig. 26-50A). The onion-skin pattern of periosteal bone that is sometimes seen on radiological examination represents circumferential discontinuous layers of periosteal new bone associated with a lytic lesion involving the medulla and endosteal surface of the cortex. Since some patients present with fever and weakness as well as bone pain, it is not surprising that their condition may be mistaken for osteomyelitis.

On gross examination, EWS is typically soft and grayish white, often studded by hemorrhagic foci and areas of necrosis. The tumor may infiltrate the medullary spaces without destroying the bony trabeculae. It may also diffusely infiltrate the cortical bone or form nodules in which the bone is completely resorbed. In many cases, the tumor mass penetrates the periosteum and extends into the soft tissues.

Microscopically, EWS cells appear as sheets of closely packed, small, round cells with little cytoplasm, which are up to twice the size of a lymphocyte (Fig. 26-50B).). Fibrous strands separate the sheets of cells into irregular nests. There is little or no interstitial stroma, and mitoses are infrequent. In some areas, the neoplastic cells tend to form rosettes. An important diagnostic feature is the presence of substantial amounts of glycogen in the cytoplasm of the tumor cells, which is well visualized with the PAS stain (Fig 26-50C).

EWS metastasizes to many organs, including the lungs and brain. Other bones, especially the skull, are common sites for metastases (50–75% of cases).

 Clinical Features: Ewing sarcoma initially presents with mild pain, which becomes more intense and is followed by swelling of the affected area. Nonspecific symptoms, including fever and leukocytosis, commonly follow. In some cases, a soft tissue mass is encountered.

In the past, the prognosis of EWS was dismal, with 5-year survival rates of only 5% after surgery or radiation therapy. The use of chemotherapy, combined with irradiation and surgery, has now led to 5-year disease-free survivals of 60 to 75%.

Multiple Myeloma Produces Lytic Lesions

Malignant tumors of plasma cells may be either local (plasmacytoma) or diffuse (see Chapter 20). Multiple myeloma occurs most often in older persons (average age, 65 years) and affects men twice as often as women. Because myeloma cells secrete cytokines that recruit osteoclasts, the lesions are unique in that they are almost exclusively lytic. The bones most frequently involved are the skull (Fig. 26-51), spine, ribs, pelvis, and femur. Pathological fractures are common. On microscopic examination, sheets of plasma cells show varying degrees of maturity. Amyloid deposits, in both skeletal and extraskeletal sites, are seen in 10% of patients.

Despite irradiation and chemotherapy, the prognosis is poor (the median survival time is 32 months). The cause of death is usually infection or kidney failure. Solitary plasmacytoma has a better prognosis, with a 60% 5-year survival.

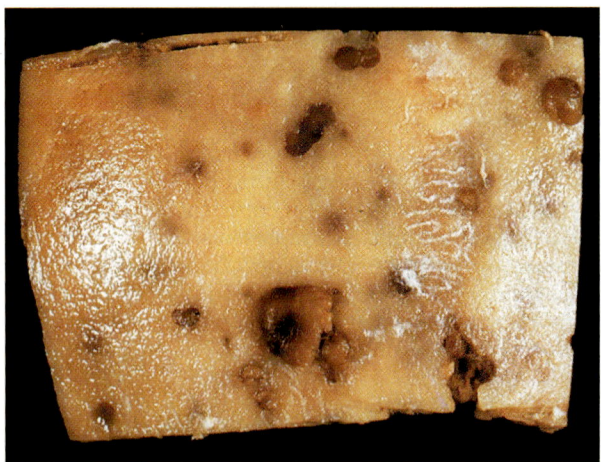

FIGURE 26-51
Multiple myeloma. A segment of the skull from a patient with multiple myeloma reveals numerous punched-out, lytic lesions.

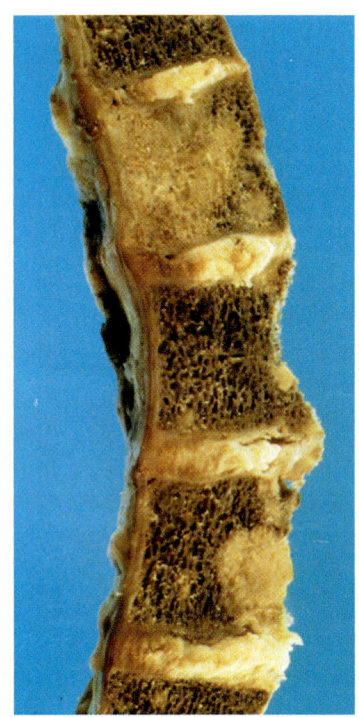

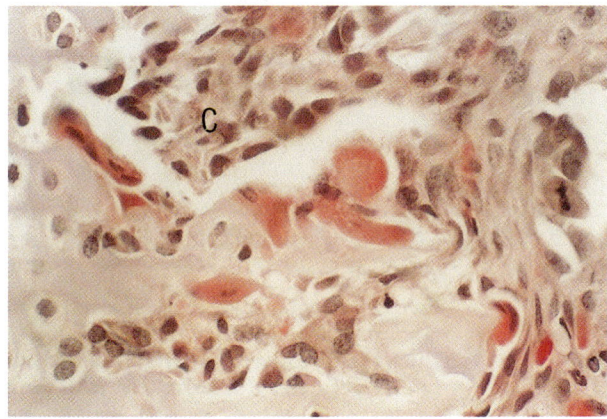

FIGURE 26-52
A. Metastatic carcinoma to bone. A section through the vertebral column reveals conspicuous nodules of metastatic tumor. B. Tumor-induce osteolysis. Breast cancer (C) metastatic to bone recruits numerous osteoclasts (*red-staining cells*), which resorb bone and lead to osteolytic lesions.

Metastatic Tumors Are the Most Common Malignant Tumors in Bone

Carcinomas compose most metastatic lesions to bone, specifically tumors of the breast, prostate, lung, thyroid, and kidney. It is estimated that skeletal metastases are found in at least 85% of cancer cases that have run their full clinical course. The vertebral column is, by far, the most commonly affected bony structure. Tumor cells usually arrive in the bone by way of the bloodstream; in the case of spinal metastases, the vertebral veins often transport them.

Some tumors (thyroid, gastrointestinal tract, kidney, neuroblastoma) produce mostly lytic lesions by stimulating osteoclasts. A few neoplasms (prostate, breast, lung, stomach) stimulate osteoblastic components to make bone, creating dense foci on radiographs (Fig. 26-52A). However, most deposits of metastatic cancer in the bones have mixtures of both lytic and blastic elements (Fig. 26-52B).

Joints

A joint (or articulation) is a union between two or more bones, whose construction varies with the function of that joint. There are two types of joints: (1) **a synovial or diarthrodial joint,** which is a movable joint, such as the knee or elbow, that is lined by a synovial membrane; and (2) **a synarthrosis,** which is a joint that has little movement.

Synarthroses are further divided into four subclassifications:

- **A symphysis** is an articulation joined by fibrocartilaginous tissue and firm ligaments that allows little movement. Examples are the symphysis pubis and the ends of vertebral joints.
- **A synchondrosis** is found at the ends of bones and has articular cartilage but is not associated with synovium or a significant joint cavity. An example of such a joint is the sternal manubrial joint.
- **A syndesmosis** connects bones by fibrous tissue without any cartilaginous elements. The distal tibiofibular articulation and the cranial sutures are syndesmoses.
- **A synostosis** is a pathological bony bridge between bones, as occurs with ankylosis of the spine.

Diseases of diarthrodial joints are among the oldest pathological conditions known, having been found in the fossil bones of dinosaurs. One third of the population of the United States older than 50 years develop some form of clinically significant joint disease.

CLASSIFICATION OF SYNOVIAL JOINTS

The synovial, or diarthrodial, joints are classified according to the type of movement they permit.

- **A uniaxial joint** allows movement around only one axis. Examples include a hinge joint such as the elbow and a pivot (rotational) joint, such as the radioulnar joint.
- **A biaxial joint** allows movement around two axes, as the condyloid joint of the wrist axis is oriented in the long diameter and the other along the short diameter of the articular surfaces. This joint permits four-way movement: flexion, extension, abduction, and adduction. In a saddle joint, such as the carpometacarpal joint of the thumb, the joint surfaces allow movement as in a condyloid joint.
- **Polyaxial joints** permit movement in virtually any axis. In a ball-and-socket joint, such as is found in the shoulder and hip, all movements, including rotation, are possible.
- **A plane joint,** represented by the patella, allows the articular surfaces to glide over one another.

UNIT LOAD: The concept of unit load is the most important principle in the understanding of joint function. The unit load is the compressive force, expressed as kilograms per cubic centimeter of articular cartilage. The unit load is fairly constant over the hip, knee, and ankle (20–26 kg/cm^3 along the articular surfaces). Because the articular cartilage is injured if the load exceeds these values, a number of mechanisms protect the joint from exceeding the unit load.

The adjacent muscles are the major shock-absorbing structures that protect the joint. In addition, deformation, even to the extent of microscopic fractures of the coarse cancellous bone, also helps to protect the joint. Moreover, deformation of the joint allows increasing the contact area with increasing load. Diarthrodial joints may have intraarticular structures such as ligaments and menisci. The menisci hold distributed force along the articular surface and allow two planes of motion, such as flexion and rotation. However, 90% or more of the absorption of energy across the knee joint is by active muscle contraction, and only 10% or less is by secondary mechanisms, such as absorption of force by the coarse cancellous bone of the knee joint. **Thus, virtually any structure is sacrificed, even to the point of a bone fracture, to protect the articular cartilage from forces that exceed the critical unit load.**

STRUCTURES OF THE SYNOVIAL JOINT

Movement plays a major role in the formation of a joint. A lack of movement retards joint development and may result in a rare but extremely crippling disease termed *arthrogryposis*, which is characterized by joint fusion.

Synovium

Synovial joints are partially lined on their internal aspects by the synovium. The synovial lining is not a true membrane because there is no basement membrane separating the synovial lining cells from the subsynovial tissue. The synovium is composed of one to three layers of synovial lining cells and is made up of two types of cells, distinguishable only by electron microscopy. **Type A cells** are macrophages that contain lysosomal enzymes and dense bodies. **Type B cells** secrete hyaluronic acid. The synovial cell membranes are disposed in villi and microvilli, an arrangement that creates an enormous surface area. It is estimated that the knee alone has 100 m^2 of synovial lining. The synovium controls a number of functions, including (1) diffusion in and out of the joint; (2) ingestion of debris; (3) secretion of hyaluronate, immunoglobulins, and lysosomal enzymes; and (4) lubrication of the joints by secretion of glycoproteins. The clear, sticky, viscid synovial fluid is present in small amounts, not exceeding 1 to 4 mL. It is the chief source of nourishment for chondrocytes of the articular cartilage, which lacks a blood supply. The synovial fluid is an ultrafiltrate that functions as a molecular sieve. It does not contain tissue thromboplastin and therefore has no clotting capacity. α_2-Macroglobulin is absent, although in disease states, this protein may accumulate. Hyaluronate is a very large molecule and has a great affinity for water because of its high number of negative charges.

Articular Cartilage

The hyaline cartilage that covers the articular ends of the bones does not participate in endochondral ossification and is well suited for its dual role of absorbing shocks and lubricating the surface of the movable joint. On gross examination, the articular cartilage is glistening, smooth, white, and semirigid and is generally not thicker than 6 mm.

Histological Characteristics

Although the articular surface appears smooth on gross examination, scanning electron microscopy reveals gentle waves and pits that correspond to the underlying lacunae of the surface chondrocytes. There are four histological zones in the articular cartilage (Fig 26-53).

- **Tangential or gliding zone:** This is the region closest to the articular surface, where the chondrocytes are elongated, flattened, and parallel to the long axis of the surface. Within this zone, a condensation of type II collagen fibers forms the so-called skin of the articular cartilage.
- **Transitional zone:** The chondrocytes in this slightly deeper zone are larger, ovoid, and more randomly distributed than those in the tangential zone. The standard hyaline cartilage matrix is present, and by electron microscopy, the collagen fibers are arranged transverse to the articular surface.
- **Radial zone:** The next deeper zone is the radial zone, where the chondrocytes are small and are arranged in short columns like those seen in the epiphyseal plate. In this area, the collagen fibers are large and are oriented perpendicular to the long axis of the articular surface.
- **Calcified zone:** Small chondrocytes and a heavily calcified matrix characterize the deepest region.

The calcified zone is separated from the radial zone by a transverse, undulating, heavily calcified "blue line" (evident on hematoxylin–eosin staining) called the *tidemark*. The tidemark is the interface between mineralized and unmineralized cartilage. Above the tidemark on the joint side, all of the cartilage receives its nutrition from the synovial fluid by diffusion. Deep to the tidemark, the calcified cartilage is nourished by epiphyseal blood vessels.

The tidemark is the area where the cartilage cells are renewed. As a result of cell division, true articular chondrocytes migrate upward toward the joint surface. Cell division below the tidemark occurs in the calcified cartilage, if there is appropriate stimulation. For example, in acromegaly, when the epiphyseal plates have already closed, the bones may grow in minute increments, because growth hormone stimulates the calcified cartilage remnant of the epiphyseal cartilage anlage. Because the joints in acromegaly do not keep pace, joint incongruity leads to severe osteoarthritis. Deep to the calcified cartilage, the transverse bony plate, termed the *subchondral bone plate,* supports the articular cartilage. It is directly contiguous with the coarse cancellous bone of the epiphysis.

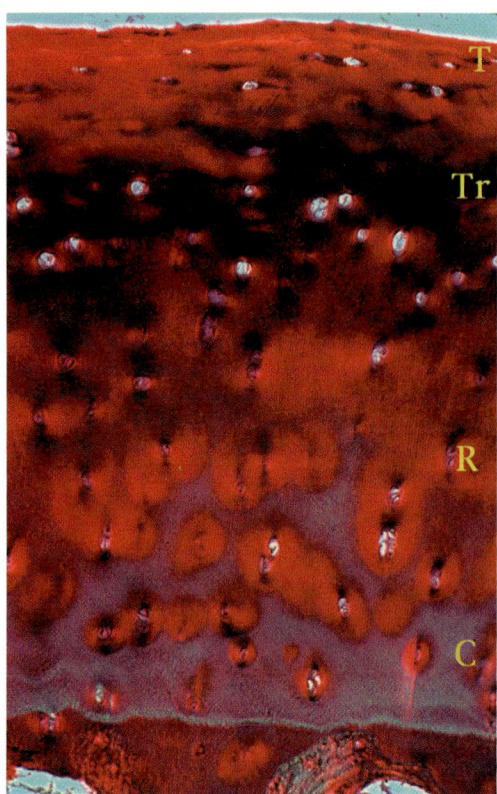

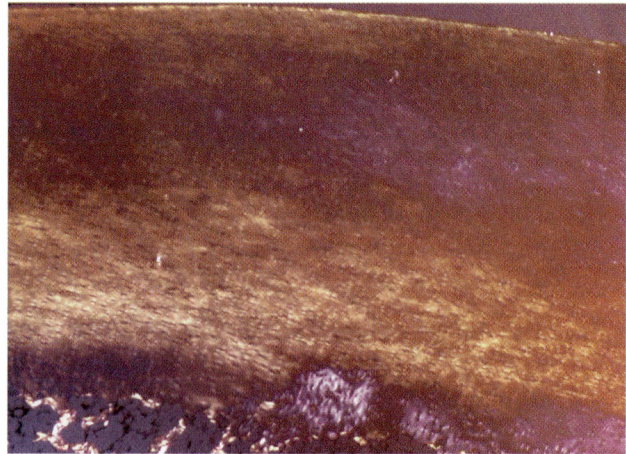

FIGURE 26-53

A. Articular hyaline cartilage demonstrating tangential zone *(T)*, transitional zone *(Tr)*, radial zone *(R)*, and calcified zone *(C)*. The chondrocyte lacunae change shape in conformation with the direction of the collagen arcades in the cartilage. B. Articular cartilage, polarized light. The tangential and radial zones have the highest concentration of collagen fibers and appear bright yellow.

OSTEOARTHRITIS

Osteoarthritis is a slowly progressive destruction of the articular cartilage that is manifested in the weight-bearing joints and fingers of older persons or the joints of younger persons subjected to trauma. Osteoarthritis is the single most common form of joint disease. The disorder is not a single nosological entity but rather a group of conditions that have in common the mechanical destruction of a joint.

Primary osteoarthritis is a disorder in which the destruction of the joints to results from an intrinsic defect of the joint cartilage. The prevalence and severity of primary osteoarthritis increases with age. Persons aged 18 to 24 years have a rate of 4%, whereas 85% of those who are aged 75 to 79 years are afflicted. Before the age of 45 years, the disease predominantly affects men. After age 55 years, however, osteoarthritis is more frequent in women. Many cases of primary osteoarthritis seem to exhibit a familial clustering, suggesting that hereditary factors predispose to the disease.

Primary osteoarthritis has variously been called *wear and tear arthritis* and *degenerative joint disease*. Progressive degradation of articular cartilage leads to joint narrowing, subchondral bone thickening, and eventually a nonfunctioning, painful joint. Although osteoarthritis is not primarily an inflammatory process, a mild inflammatory reaction may occur within the synovium.

Secondary osteoarthritis has a known underlying cause, including congenital or acquired incongruity of joints, trauma, crystal deposits, infection, metabolic diseases, endocrinopathies, inflammatory diseases, osteonecrosis, and hemarthrosis.

Chondromalacia is a term applied to a subcategory of osteoarthritis that affects the patellar surface of the femoral condyles of young persons and produces pain and stiffness of the knee.

Pathogenesis: Factors that play a major role in the etiology of osteoarthritis include the following.

INCREASED UNIT LOAD: Abnormal force on the cartilage may result from a number of factors, but it is often attributable to pathological incongruities of the joint. For example, in congenital hip dysplasia, a fairly common abnormality, the socket of the acetabulum is shallow, covering only 30 to 40% of the femoral head (normal, 50%). As a result, there is less surface area covered by cartilage and an increased load on the articular cartilage. When the critical unit load is exceeded, death of chondrocytes leads to degradation of the articular cartilage.

RESILIENCE OF THE ARTICULAR CARTILAGE: Because articular cartilage binds extensive amounts of water, it normally has a swelling pressure of at least 3 atm. A disruption in the water bonding resulting from the events discussed above leads to decreased resilience.

STIFFNESS OF THE SUBCHONDRAL COARSE CANCELLOUS BONE: The structure of the bone adjacent to a joint is also an important factor in the maintenance of articular cartilage. Mechanical forces are not transferred to articular cartilage by normal stress, but rather are dissipated by microfractures of the coarse cancellous bone. Damage to the coarse cancellous bone results in an increased unit load on the cartilage because of an increase in the stiffness of subchondral bone, for example, in Paget disease.

BIOCHEMICAL ABNORMALITIES: The biochemical changes of osteoarthritis primarily involve proteoglycans. Proteoglycan content and aggregation decrease, and the chain length of the glycosaminoglycans is reduced. The collagen fibers are thicker than normal, and the arcades of Benninghoff are disrupted. The water content of osteoarthritic cartilage increases. The reduction in proteoglycans allows more water to be bound to the collagen fibers. Thus, osteoarthritic cartilage, or any cartilage that is fibrillated, tends to swell more than normal cartilage.

Although the synthesis of matrix by chondrocytes is augmented in the early stages of osteoarthritis, protein synthesis eventually tends to decrease, suggesting that the cells reach a point at which they fail to respond to reparative stimuli. Similarly, whereas chondrocytes in early osteoarthritic cartilage replicate, cell replication diminishes with advanced disease. Acid cathepsin, which attacks the protein cores of the matrix macromolecules, increases in osteoarthritic cartilage. Although collagenase is not present in normal cartilage, it is found in osteoarthritic cartilage.

GENETIC FACTORS: Studies of identical twins have demonstrated genetic contributions to the prevalence of osteoarthritis. Genetic analysis of patients with a type of familial, early-onset osteoarthritis revealed a variety of mutations in the gene for type II collagen *(COL2A1)*, the major collagen species of articular cartilage.

Pathology: The joints commonly affected by osteoarthritis are the proximal and distal interphalangeal joints of the upper extremity, knees and hips, and the cervical and lumbar segments of the spine. Radiologically, osteoarthritis is characterized by (1) narrowing of the joint space, which represents the loss of articular cartilage; (2) increased thickness of the subchondral bone; (3) subchondral bone cysts; and (4) large peripheral growths of bone and cartilage, called *osteophytes*. The histological changes follow a well-described sequence.

1. The earliest histological changes of osteoarthritis involve the loss of proteoglycans from the surface of the articular cartilage, manifested as decreased metachromatic staining. At the same time, empty lacunae in the articular cartilage indicate the death of chondrocytes (Fig. 26-54). The viable chondrocytes enlarge, aggregate into groups or clones, and become surrounded by basophilic staining matrix called the *territorial matrix*.
2. Osteoarthritis may arrest at this stage for many years before it proceeds to the next stage, which is characterized by fibrillation (i.e., development of surface cracks parallel to the long axis of the articular surface). These fibrillations may persist for many years before further progression occurs.
3. As fibrillations propagate, synovial fluid begins to flow into the defects. The cracks are progressively oriented more vertically, tending to parallel the long axis of the collagen fibrils. Synovial fluid works its way deeper into the articular cartilage along the cracks. Eventually, pieces of articular cartilage break off and lodge in the synovium,

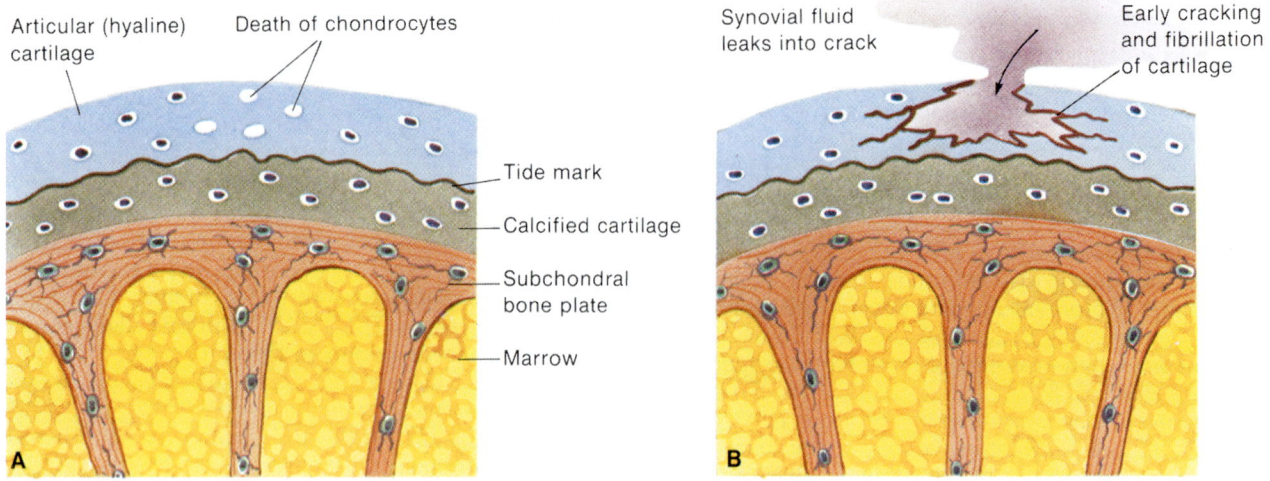
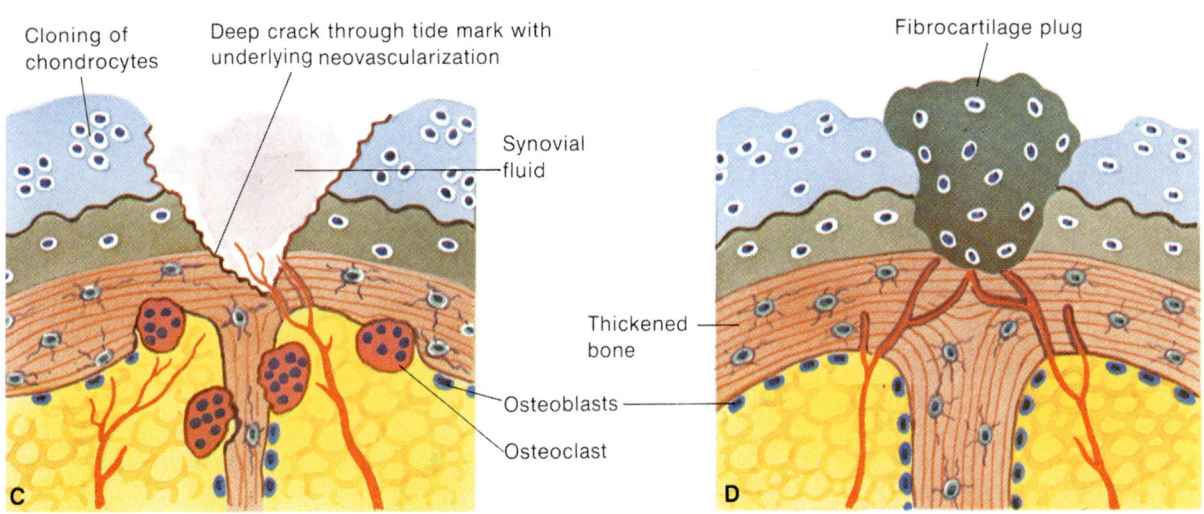
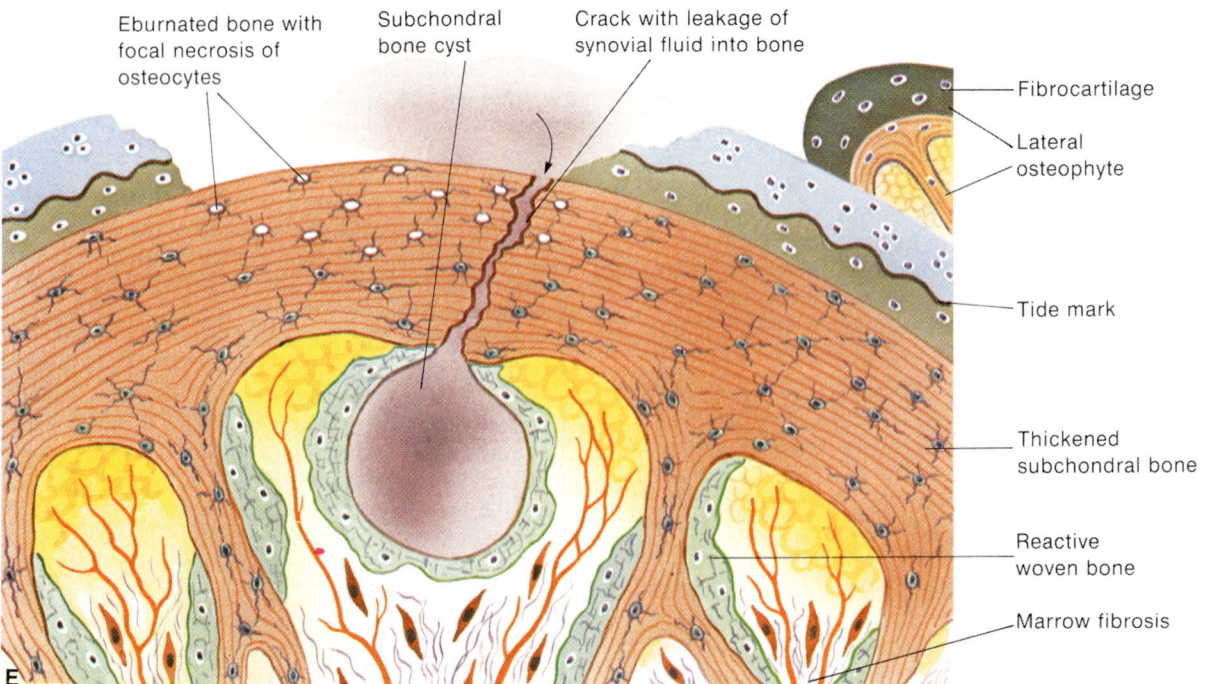

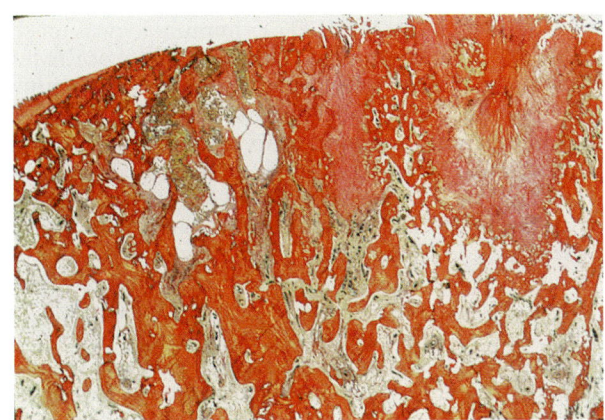 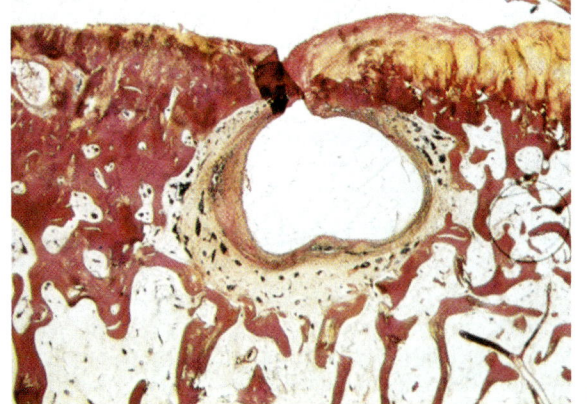

FIGURE 26-55
Osteoarthritis. A. A femoral head with osteoarthritis shows a fibrocartilaginous plug *(far right)* extending from the marrow onto the joint surface. Eburnated bone is present over the remaining surface. B. A section through the articular surface of an osteoarthritic joint demonstrates focal absence of the articular cartilage, thickening of subchondral bone *(left)*, and a subchondral bone cyst.

thereby inducing inflammation and a foreign-body giant cell reaction. The result is a hyperemic and hypertrophied synovium.

4. As the crack extends down toward the tidemark and eventually crosses it, neovascularization from the epiphysis and subchondral bone extends into the area of the crack, inducing subchondral osteoclastic bone resorption. Adjacent osteoblastic activity also occurs and results in a thickening of the subchondral bone plate in the area of the crack. As neovascularization progressively extends into the area of the crack, mesenchymal cells invade, and fibrocartilage forms as a poor substitute for the articular hyaline cartilage (Fig. 26-55A). These fibrocartilaginous plugs may persist, or they may be swept into the joint. The subchondral bone becomes exposed and burnished as it grinds against the opposite joint surface, which is undergoing the same process. These thick, shiny, smooth areas of subchondral bone are referred to as *eburnated* (ivory-like) bone (see Figs. 26-54 and 26-55B).

5. In some areas, the eburnated bone eventually cracks, allowing synovial fluid to extend from the joint surface into the subchondral bone marrow, where it eventually leads to a *subchondral bone cyst* (see Fig. 26-55B). These cysts increase in size as synovial fluid is forced into the space but cannot exit. Eventually, osteoclasts resorb bone and osteoblasts attempt to wall off the area. The result is a subchondral bone cyst filled with synovial fluid, with a well-marginated, reactive bone wall.

6. An osteophyte develops, usually in the lateral portions of the joint, when the mesenchymal tissue of the synovium modulates into osteoblasts and chondroblasts to form a mass of cartilage and bone. On gross examination, osteophytes are pearly grayish bone nodules appearing on the peripheral portion of the joint surface. These osteophytes, or bony spurs, also occur at the lateral portions of the intervertebral disks, extending from the adjacent vertebral bodies. They produce the "lipping" pattern seen on radiological studies as osteoarthritis of the spine. In the fingers, osteophytes at the distal interphalangeal joints are termed *Heberden nodes*.

 Clinical Features: The signs and symptoms of osteoarthritis are related to the location of the involved joints and the severity and duration of the joint deterioration. The physical findings vary. The involved joints may be enlarged, tender, and boggy and may demonstrate crepitus. Deep, achy joint pain that follows activity and is relieved by rest is the clinical hallmark of osteoarthritis. Pain is usually a manifestation of significant joint destruction and arises in the periarticular structures, because articular cartilage lacks a nerve supply. Discomfort also is caused by short periods of stiffness, which is frequently experienced in the morning or after periods of minimal activity. Restricted joint motion is a harbinger of severe disease and may result from joint or muscle contractures, intraarticular loose bodies, large osteophytes, and loss of congruity of the joint surfaces.

At present there is no specific treatment to prevent or arrest osteoarthritis. Therapy is directed at specific orthopedic

FIGURE 26-54
Histogenesis of osteoarthritis. A and B. The death of chondrocytes leads to a crack in the articular cartilage that is followed by an influx of synovial fluid and further loss and degeneration of cartilage. C. As a result of this process, cartilage is gradually worn away. Below the tidemark, new vessels grow in from the epiphysis, and fibrocartilage (D) is deposited. E. The fibrocartilage plug is not mechanically sufficient and may be worn away, thus exposing the subchondral bone plate, which becomes thickened and eburnated. If there is a crack in this region, synovial fluid leaks into the marrow space and produces a subchondral bone cyst. Focal regrowth of the articular surface leads to the formation of osteophytes.

conditions and includes exercise, weight loss, and other supportive measures. In disabling osteoarthritis, joint replacement may be necessary.

RHEUMATOID ARTHRITIS

Rheumatoid arthritis (RA) is a systemic, chronic inflammatory disease in which chronic polyarthritis involves diarthrodial joints symmetrically and bilaterally. The proximal interphalangeal and metacarpophalangeal joints, elbows, knees, ankles, and spine are commonly affected. The onset is usually in the third or fourth decade, but the prevalence increases with age until age 70 years. However, RA may occur at any age. The disease afflicts 1 to 2% of the adult population, and its incidence is greater in women than in men (3:1). The excess incidence of RA in women is firmly established before the menopause, after which the frequency for men and women increases uniformly. Commonly, the joints of the extremities are affected simultaneously and often in a symmetric pattern. The course of the disease varies and is often punctuated by remissions and exacerbations. The broad spectrum of clinical manifestations ranges from barely discernible to severe, destructive, mutilating disease.

It is now thought that classic RA comprises a heterogeneous group of disorders. Patients who are persistently seronegative for rheumatoid factor probably have disease of a different etiology than do those who are seropositive. There are also rheumatoid-like diseases that are associated with underlying maladies, such as inflammatory bowel disease and cirrhosis.

 Pathogenesis: A number of factors have been implicated in the development of RA.

GENETIC FACTORS: A contribution of hereditary factors to the susceptibility to RA is suggested by the increased frequency of the disease in first-degree relatives of affected persons and by the concordance for the illness in monozygotic twins (30%). In addition, it is generally agreed that certain major histocompatibility genes are expressed in a nonrandom manner in patients with RA. An important genetic locus that predisposes to RA is present in HLA II genes, and a specific set of HLA-DR alleles (DR4, DR1, DR10, DR14) is consistently increased in these patients. These alleles share a pentapeptide sequence motif (shared epitope) in a hypervariable segment of the **HLA-DRB1 gene**, which forms the rheumatoid pocket on the HLA molecule. It is likely that the binding properties of this pocket influence the type of peptides that can be bound by RA-associated HLA-DR molecules, thereby affecting the immune response to these peptides. Interestingly, seropositive RA (poor prognosis) is associated with a high frequency of an arginine in the shared epitope, whereas seronegative disease (good prognosis) commonly exhibits a lysine in the same position, further suggesting that the physical characteristics of the rheumatoid pocket influence the immune response in RA.

HUMORAL IMMUNITY: Immunological mechanisms play an important role in the pathogenesis of RA. Lymphocytes and plasma cells accumulate in the synovium, where they produce immunoglobulins, mainly of the IgG class. In addition, immune-complex deposits are present in the articular cartilage and the synovium. Increased serum levels of IgM, IgA, and IgG are also found in patients with RA.

Some 80% of patients with classic RA are positive for **rheumatoid factor** (RF). This factor actually represents multiple antibodies, principally IgM, but sometimes IgG or IgA, directed against the Fc fragment of IgG. Significant titers of RF are also found in patients with related collagen vascular diseases, such as systemic lupus erythematosus, progressive systemic sclerosis, and dermatomyositis. RF also occurs in a wide variety of nonrheumatic disorders, including pulmonary fibrosis, cirrhosis, sarcoidosis, Waldenström macroglobulinemia, tuberculosis, kala azar, lepromatous leprosy, and viral hepatitis. Even healthy elderly persons, particularly women, occasionally test positive for RF.

Although patients with classic RA may be seronegative, the presence of RF in high titer is frequently associated with severe and unremitting disease, many systemic complications, and a serious prognosis. The presence of IgG RF is sometimes associated with the development of systemic complications, such as necrotizing vasculitis.

Immune complexes (IgG RF + IgG) and complement components are found in the synovium, synovial fluid, and extraarticular lesions of patients with RA. Furthermore, patients with seropositive RA have lower levels of complement in their synovial fluid than do those who suffer the seronegative type.

CELLULAR IMMUNITY: It has also been postulated that cell-mediated immunity contributes to RA. Abundant T lymphocytes in the rheumatoid synovium are frequently Ia positive ("activated") and of the helper type. They are often in close contact with HLA-DR–positive cells, which are either macrophages or dendritic Ia-positive cells.

T cells may directly or indirectly interact with macrophages through the production of cytokines that inhibit the migration and proliferation of the latter. Such substances have been found in rheumatoid synovial fluid and in supernatants from rheumatoid tissue explants. These studies provide strong evidence that the joint destruction in RA reflects local production of cytokines, especially TNF and IL-1

INFECTIOUS AGENTS: Neither infectious bacteria nor viruses have been detected in the joints of patients with RA. Structures resembling viruses have been reported early in the course of the disease. Most patients with RA develop antibodies against a nuclear antigen in B cells infected with Epstein-Barr virus (EBV). This antigen is termed RA-associated nuclear antigen (RANA) and is closely related to the nuclear antigen encoded by EBV (EBNA). Moreover, EBV is a polyclonal B-cell activator that stimulates the production of RF. Interestingly, the peripheral blood of many patients with RA contains an increased number of EBV-infected B cells.

LOCAL FACTORS: Synovial cells cultured from rheumatic joints exhibit a decreased response to glucocorticoids and increased production of hyaluronate. These cells release a peptide (connective tissue-activating peptide) that may influence the function of other cells, producing increased amounts of prostaglandins, particularly prostaglandin E_2 (PGE_2).

A hypothetical scenario consistent with the evidence presented earlier might be constructed as follows:

1. In a genetically susceptible person, an unknown agent (possibly a virus, such as EBV) infects a joint or some other tissue and stimulates the formation of antibodies.
2. These immunoglobulins act as new antigens, that is, they trigger the production of antiidiotype antibodies (RF).
3. Immune complexes that contain RF are deposited in the synovium and activate the complement cascade. This effect increases vascular permeability and the uptake of immune complexes by leukocytes, which in turn release lysosomal enzymes, activated oxygen species, and other injurious products.
4. Activated macrophages in the synovium present unknown antigens to T cells, thereby stimulating the production of cytokines, which amplify inflammation, tissue injury, and the proliferation of synovial cells.

 Pathology: The early synovial changes of RA are edema and the accumulation of plasma cells, lymphocytes, and macrophages (Fig. 26-56). There is a concomitant increase in vascularity and exudation of fibrin in the joint space, which may result in small fibrin nodules that float in the joint *(rice bodies)*.

PANNUS FORMATION: The synovial lining cells, which are normally only 1 to 3 layers thick, undergo hyperplasia and form layers 8 to 10 cells deep. Multinucleated giant cells are often found among the synovial cells. **The result is a synovial lining thrown into numerous villi and frondlike folds that fill the peripheral recesses of the joint** (Fig. 26-57A). As the synovium undergoes hyperplasia and hypertrophy, it creeps over the surface of the articular cartilage and adjacent structures. This inflammatory synovium, now containing mast cells, is termed a *pannus* (cloak). The pannus covers the articular cartilage and isolates it from the synovial fluid. Lymphocytes aggregate into masses and eventually develop follicular centers (*Allison–Ghormley Bodies*; Fig. 26-57B). **The pannus erodes the articular cartilage and the adjacent bone, probably through the action of collagenase produced by the pannus** (Fig. 26-57C). Since PGE_2 and IL-1 stimulate osteoclasts and are actively produced in the rheumatoid synovium, they may mediate bone erosion.

The characteristic bone loss of RA is juxtaarticular, that is, it is immediately adjacent to both sides of the joint. The pannus penetrates the subchondral bone; it may involve tendons and ligaments, leading to deformities and instabilities. (Fig 26-58). Eventually, the joint is destroyed and undergoes fibrous fusion, termed ankylosis (Fig. 26-58). Long-standing cases may lead to bony bridging of the joint *(bony ankylosis)*. The pannus may destroy cartilage by depriving it of its nourishment; alternately, it may stimulate T lymphocytes to secrete a factor causing the release of lysosomal enzymes. In turn, this process may lead to secondary osteoarthritis.

Changes in the synovial fluid include a massive increase in volume, increased turbidity, and decreased viscosity. The protein content and the number of inflammatory cells in the fluid increase, correlating with the activity of the rheumatoid process. In some cases, the leukocyte count exceeds $50,000/\mu L$, with 95% polymorphonuclear leukocytes.

Rheumatoid Nodules

RA is a systemic disease that also involves tissues other than the joints and tendons. A characteristic lesion, termed the *rheumatoid nodule,* is found in extraarticular locations. This structure has a centrally located core of fibrinoid necrosis, which is a mixture of fibrin and other proteins, such as degraded collagen (Fig. 26-59). A surrounding rim of macrophages is arranged in a radial, or palisading, fashion. Peripheral to the macrophages is an outer circle of lymphocytes, plasma cells, and other mononuclear cells. The overall appearance resembles a peculiar granuloma surrounding a core of fibrinoid necrosis. Rheumatoid nodules, which are usually found in areas of pressure (e.g., the skin of the elbows and legs), are movable, firm, rubbery, and occasionally tender. A large nodule may ulcerate. Recurrence after surgical removal is common.

Rheumatoid nodules may also be seen in lupus erythematous and rheumatic fever. They are sometimes found in visceral organs, such as the heart, lungs, and intestinal tract, and even the dura. Nodules in the bundle of His may cause cardiac arrhythmias; in the lungs, they produce fibrosis and even respiratory failure (see Chapter 12).

RA also may be accompanied by acute necrotizing vasculitis, which can affect virtually any organ.

 Clinical Features: The clinical diagnosis of RA is imprecise and is based on a number of criteria, such as the number and types of joints involved, the presence of rheumatoid nodules and RF, and radiographic features characteristic of the disease.

The onset of RA may be acute, slowly progressing, or insidious. Most patients give a history of slowly developing fatigue, weight loss, weakness, and vague musculoskeletal discomfort, which eventually localizes to the involved joints. Diseased joints tend to be warm, swollen, and painful. The pain is heightened by motion and is most severe after periods of disuse. Unabated disease causes progressive destruction of the joint surfaces and periarticular structures. Eventually, patients manifest severe flexion and extension deformities, associated with joint subluxation, which may terminate in joint ankylosis.

The natural history of RA is variable, and in most patients, the activity of the disease waxes and wanes. One fourth of patients seem to recover completely. Another fourth remain for many years with only slight functional impairment, whereas half have serious progressive and disabling joint disease. There is an increased mortality from a variety of infections, gastrointestinal hemorrhage and perforation, vasculitis, heart and lung involvement, amyloidosis, and subluxation of the cervical spine. In fact, the survival of patients with active RA is comparable to that observed in Hodgkin disease and diabetes.

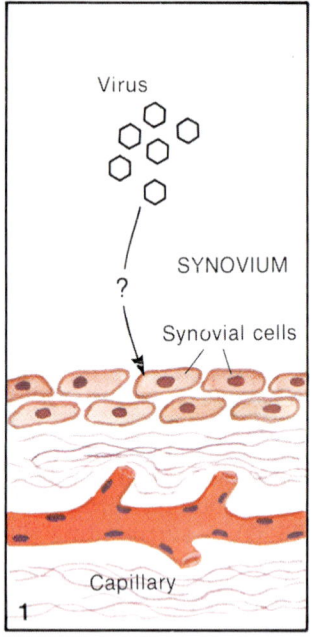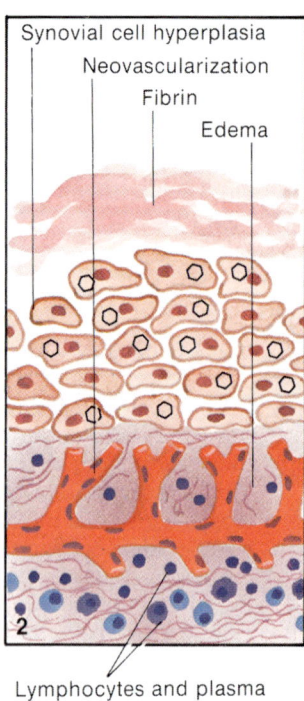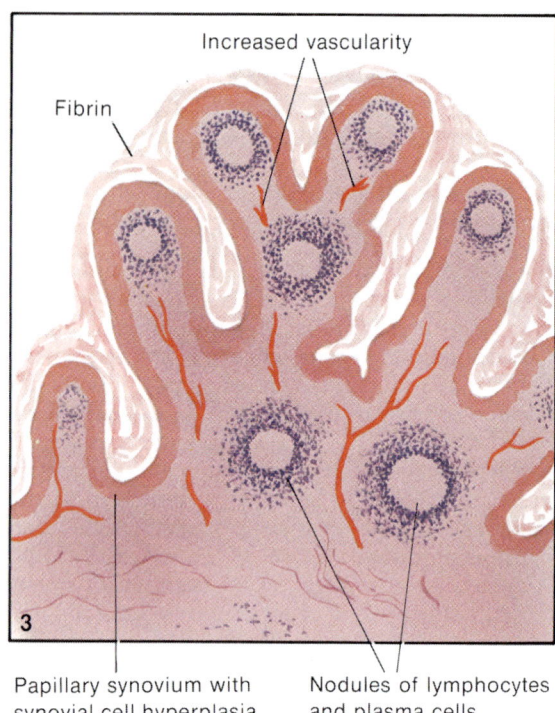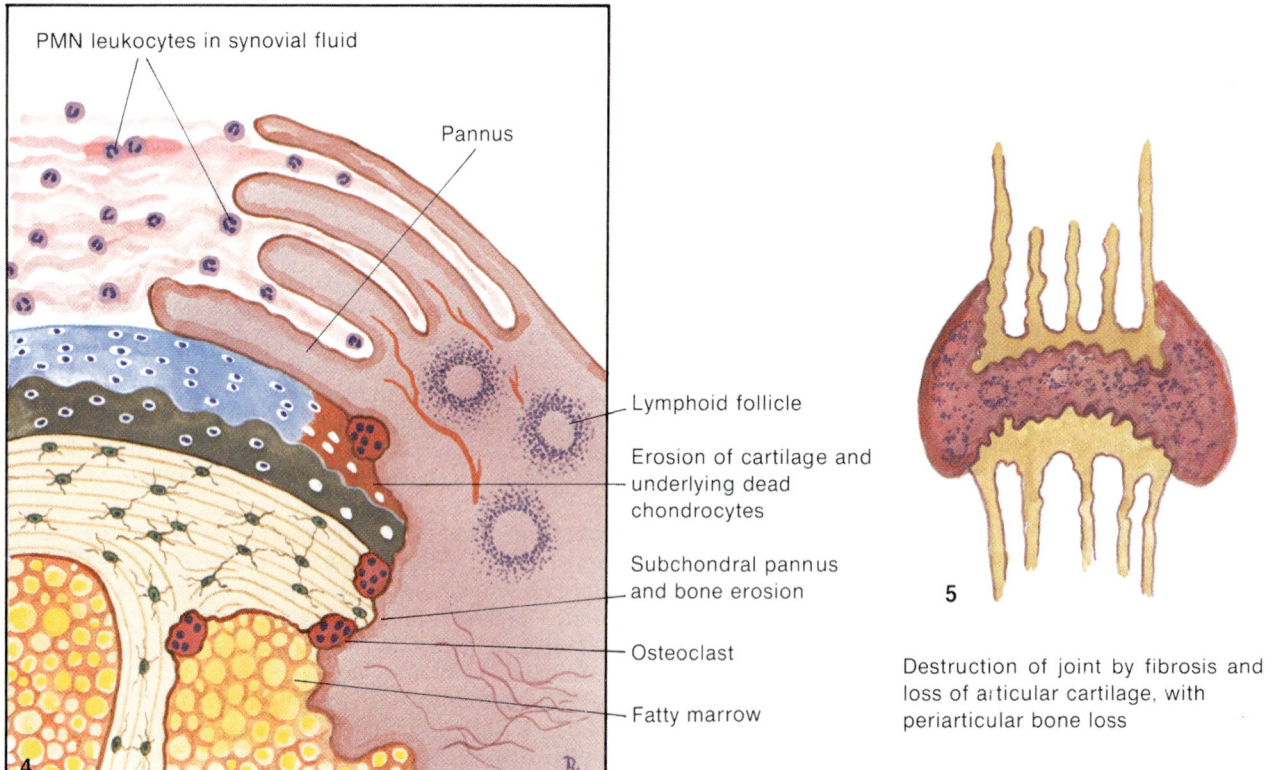

FIGURE 26-56

Histogenesis of rheumatoid arthritis. 1. A virus or an unknown stress may stimulate the synovial cells to proliferate. 2. The influx of lymphocytes, plasma cells, and mast cells, together with neovascularization and edema, leads to hypertrophy and hyperplasia of the synovium. 3. Lymphoid nodules are prominent. 4. Proliferating synovium extends into the joint space, burrows into the bone beneath the articular cartilage, and covers the cartilage as a pannus. The articular cartilage is eventually destroyed by direct resorption or deprivation of its nutrient synovial fluid. The synovial tissue continues to proliferate in the subchondral region, as well as in the joint. 5. Eventually, the joint is destroyed and becomes fused, a condition termed *ankylosis*.

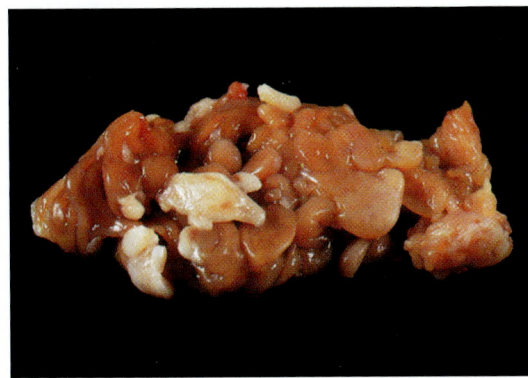
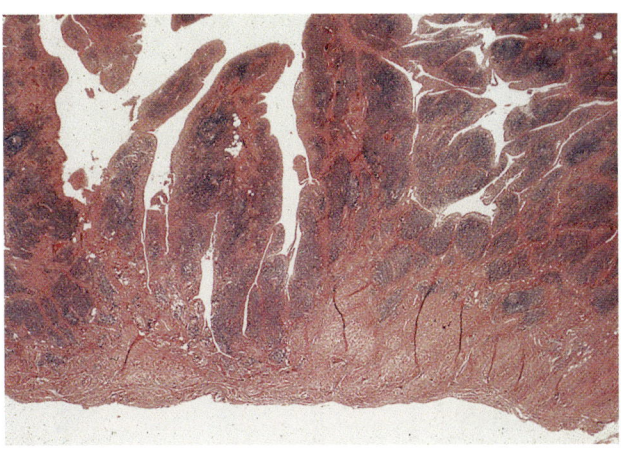
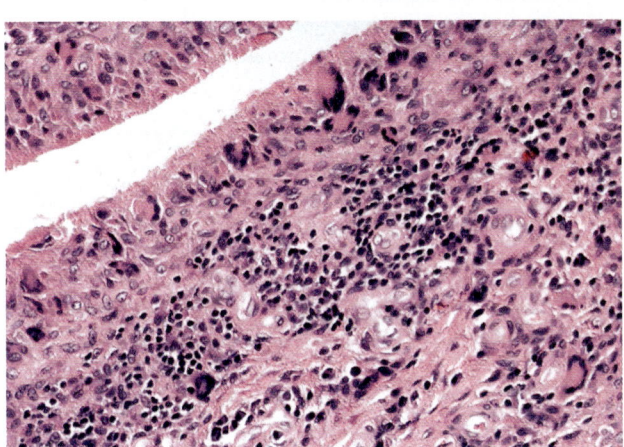

FIGURE 26-57
Rheumatoid arthritis. A. Hyperplastic synovium from a patient with rheumatoid arthritis shows numerous fingerlike projections, with focal pale areas of fibrin deposition. The brownish color of the synovium reflects hemosiderin accumulation derived from old hemorrhage. B. A microscopic view reveals prominent lymphoid follicles (Allison-Ghormley bodies), synovial hyperplasia and hypertrophy, villous folds, and thickening of the synovial membrane by fibrosis and inflammation. C. A higher-power view of the inflamed synovium demonstrates hyperplasia and hypertrophy of the lining cells. Numerous giant cells are on and below the surface. The stroma is chronically inflamed.

The drugs used to suppress the inflammatory process of the synovium and to induce a remission are essentially of three classes:

- **Antiinflammatory agents** include aspirin, nonsteroidal antiinflammatory drugs, phenylbutazone, glucocorticoids, and even intraarticular corticosteroid injections.
- **Remission-inducing drugs** are gold salts, penicillamine, and antimalarial drugs, such as chloroquine.
- **Immunosuppressive drugs** are used in patients with severe progressive disease who do not respond to other medications.

Spondyloarthropathy Refers to Seronegative Arthritis Mostly Linked to HLA-B27

A number of clinical entities were formerly classified as variants of RA but are now recognized to be distinct disorders. These forms of arthritis are now termed *spondyloarthropathies* and include ankylosing spondylitis, Reiter syndrome, psoriatic arthritis, and arthritis associated with inflammatory bowel disease. These conditions share the following features:

- Seronegativity for RF and other serological markers of RA
- Association with class I histocompatibility antigens, particularly HLA-B27
- Sacroiliac and vertebral involvement
- Asymmetric involvement of only few peripheral joints
- A tendency to inflammation of periarticular tendons and fascia
- Systemic involvement of other organs, especially uveitis, carditis, and aortitis
- Preferential onset in young men

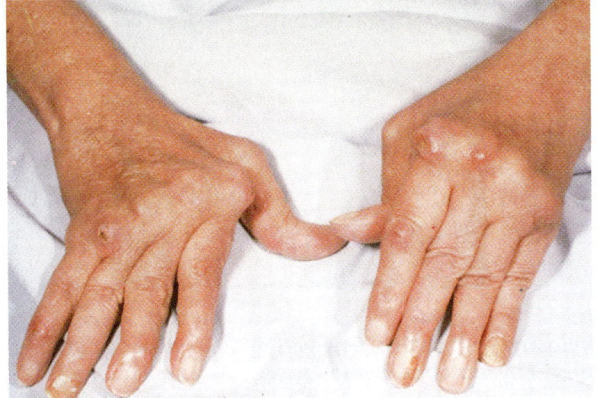

FIGURE 26-58
Rheumatoid arthritis. The hands of a patient with advanced arthritis show swelling of the metacarpal phalangeal joints and the classic ulnar deviation of the fingers.

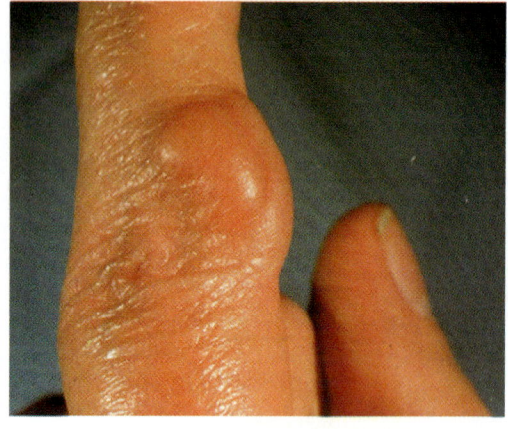
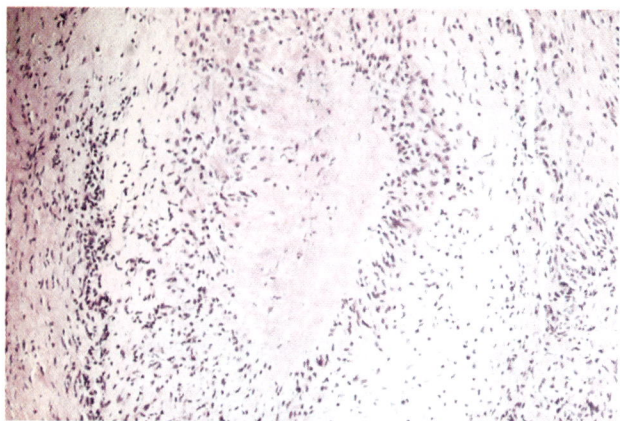

FIGURE 26-59
Rheumatoid nodule. A. A patient with rheumatoid arthritis has a mass on a digit. B. Microscopic view of a rheumatoid nodule shows a central area of necrosis surrounded by palisaded macrophages and a chronic inflammatory infiltrate.

Ankylosing Spondylitis

Ankylosing spondylitis is an inflammatory arthropathy of the vertebral column and sacroiliac joints. It may be accompanied by asymmetric, peripheral arthritis (30% of patients) and systemic manifestations. Ankylosing spondylitis is most common in young men, and the peak incidence is at about age 20 years. **More than 90% of patients are positive for HLA-B27 (normal, 4 to 8%), although the disorder affects only 1% of persons with this haplotype.**

Pathology: Ankylosing spondylitis begins at the sacroiliac joints bilaterally and then ascends the spinal column by involving the small joints of the posterior elements of the spine. The result is ultimate destruction of these joints, after which the spine becomes fused posteriorly. The unburdened vertebral bodies become square and osteoporotic, because the main force of gravity is borne by the fused posterior elements. In such cases, the intervertebral disk undergoes ossification and may disappear. Eventually, bony fusion of the vertebral bodies ensues (Fig. 26-60).

Although a few patients with ankylosing spondylitis rapidly develop crippling spinal disease, most are able to maintain their employment and live a normal life span. However, up to 5% of patients develop AA amyloidosis and uremia, and a few manifest severe cardiac involvement.

Reiter Syndrome

Reiter syndrome is a triad that includes (1) seronegative polyarthritis, (2) conjunctivitis, and (3) nonspecific urethritis. The disorder is almost exclusively encountered in men and usually follows venereal exposure or an episode of bacillary dysentery. As in ankylosing spondylitis, Reiter syndrome is associated with HLA-B27 antigen in up to 90% of patients. In fact, after an attack of dysentery, 20% of HLA-B27–positive men develop Reiter syndrome.

The pathological features of Reiter arthritis are comparable to those of RA. More than half of patients develop mucocutaneous lesions similar to those of pustular psoriasis (*keratoblennorrhagicum*) over the palms, soles, and trunk. In most patients, the disease remits within a year, but in 20%, progressive arthritis develops, including ankylosing spondylitis.

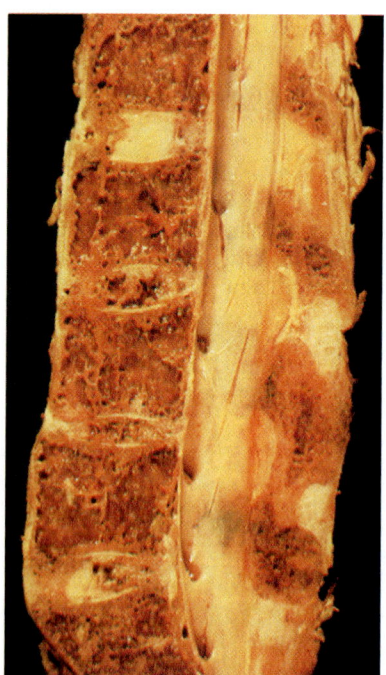

FIGURE 26-60
Ankylosing spondylitis. The vertebrae have been cut longitudinally. The vertebral bodies are square and have lost most of their trabecular bone, owing to osteoporosis from disuse. Bone bridges fuse one vertebral body to the next across the intervertebral disks. Portions of the intervertebral disk are replaced by bone marrow. Bony bridges also fuse the posterior elements, a condition termed *ankylosis*.

Psoriatic Arthritis

Of all patients with psoriasis, particularly in those with severe disease, 7% develop an inflammatory seronegative arthritis. HLA-B27 has been linked to psoriatic spondylitis and inflammation of the distal interphalangeal joints, and HLA-DR4 has been associated with a rheumatoid pattern of involvement. The joint disease is usually mild and only slowly progressive, although a mutilating form is occasionally encountered.

Enteropathic Arthritis

Ulcerative colitis and Crohn disease are accompanied by seronegative peripheral arthritis in 20% of cases and spondylitis in 10%. This form of arthritis also is seen in patients with Whipple disease and after certain bacterial infections of the gut. No particular tissue type is associated with peripheral arthritis, but most patients with ankylosing spondylitis are HLA-B27 positive. It has been proposed that HLA-B27 and proteins from enteric bacteria are structurally related in a manner that potentially affects antigen presentation to the T-cell receptor. Resection of the affected bowel in ulcerative colitis relieves the arthritis, but in Crohn disease, this complication often does not resolve.

Juvenile Arthritis Applies to Any Inflammatory Arthritis in Children

Juvenile arthritis, or Still disease, refers to a number of different chronic arthritic conditions in children. At one time, this term signified a variant of RA that was characterized by chronic synovitis and extraarticular symptoms. However, it is now recognized that in addition to RA, many children with juvenile arthritis eventually develop ankylosing spondylitis, psoriatic arthritis, and other connective tissue diseases.

- **Seropositive arthritis:** Fewer than 10% of children with arthritis are positive for RF and have a polyarticular presentation. Females predominate (80%) among children with seropositive Still disease, and in most cases (75%), antinuclear antibodies are present. There is an association with HLA-D4, and more than half of the children eventually develop severe arthritis.
- **Polyarticular disease without systemic symptoms:** One fourth of juvenile arthritis patients (90% girls) have disease of several joints, are seronegative, and do not manifest systemic symptoms. Fewer than 15% of these patients eventually develop severe arthritis.
- **Polyarticular disease with systemic symptoms:** Twenty percent of children with polyarticular juvenile arthritis have prominent systemic symptoms that include high fever, rash, hepatosplenomegaly, lymphadenopathy, pleuritis, pericarditis, anemia, and leukocytosis. Most (60%) of these patients are boys who are negative for RF, and one fourth of all of these children are left with severe arthritis.
- **Pauciarticular arthritis:** Children with involvement of only a few large joints, such as the knee, ankle, elbow, or hip girdle, account for half of all cases of juvenile arthritis and fall into two general groups. The larger group (80%) is mainly girls who are negative for RF but exhibit antinuclear antibodies and are positive for HLA-DR5, HLA-DRw6, or HLA-DRw8. Of these patients, one third have ocular disease characterized by chronic iridocyclitis (inflammation of the iris and ciliary body). Only a small minority of these children have residual polyarthritis or ocular damage. The smaller group of children with a pauciarticular presentation is composed almost exclusively of boys, is negative for both RF and antinuclear bodies, and is positive for HLA-B27 (75%). A few have acute iridocyclitis, which resolves spontaneously. Some of these boys subsequently develop ankylosing spondylitis.

GOUT

Gout is a heterogeneous group of diseases in which the common denominator is an increased serum uric acid level and the deposition of urate crystals in the joints and kidneys. Although all patients with gout display hyperuricemia, fewer than 15% of all persons with hyperuricemia have gout.

Gout is characterized by acute and chronic arthritis. The varieties of gout are classified according to the etiology of the hyperuricemia into primary and secondary forms. **Primary gout** refers to hyperuricemia in the absence of any other disease, whereas **secondary gout** occurs in association with another illness that results in hyperuricemia. Of all cases of hyperuricemia, one third are primary and the remainder secondary.

 Pathogenesis: Uric acid results from the catabolism of purines derived either from the diet or synthesized de novo. In most mammals, relatively insoluble uric acid is converted to highly soluble allantoin by urate oxidase. The loss of this enzyme during the course of human evolution has imposed a narrow balance between uric acid production and tissue deposition of urates. In humans, uric acid is eliminated from the body only in the urine. Thus, the level of uric acid in the blood (normal, <7.0 mg/dL in men, <6.0 in women) reflects the difference between the amount of purines ingested and synthesized and the extent of renal excretion. Gout can result from (1) overproduction of purines, (2) augmented catabolism of nucleic acids as a result of increased cell turnover, (3) decreased salvage of free purine bases, or (4) decreased urinary excretion of uric acid (Fig. 26-61). A high dietary intake of purine-rich foods, particularly meat, by an otherwise normal person does not lead to hyperuricemia and gout.

Primary Gout Reflects Idiopathic Hyperuricemia

Most cases (85%) of idiopathic gout result from an as-yet-unexplained impairment of uric acid excretion by the kidneys. In the remainder, there is a primary overproduction of uric acid, but only in a minority of cases has the underlying abnormality been identified.

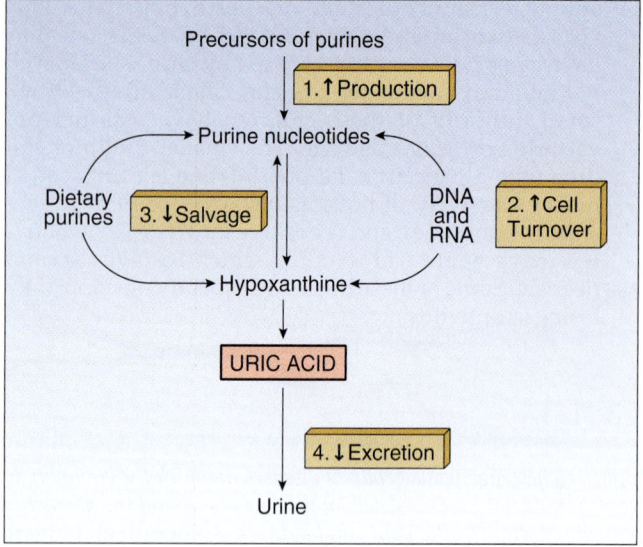

FIGURE 26-61
Pathogenesis of hyperuricemia and gout. Purine nucleotides are synthesized de novo from nonpurine precursors or derived from preformed purines in the diet. Purine nucleotides are catabolized to hypoxanthine or incorporated into nucleic acids. The degradation of nucleic acids and dietary purines also produces hypoxanthine. Hypoxanthine is converted to uric acid, which in turn is excreted into the urine. Hyperuricemia and gout result from *(1)* increased de novo purine synthesis, *(2)* increased cell turnover, *(3)* decreased salvage of dietary purines and hypoxanthine, and *(4)* decreased uric acid excretion by the kidneys.

GENETIC FACTORS: A familial tendency to gout has been recognized since the time of Galen. Hyperuricemia is common among the relatives of persons with gout. It has been proposed that primary hyperuricemia in some persons is inherited as an autosomal dominant trait with variable expression, in some as an X-linked abnormality, and in others as instances of multifactorial inheritance. Precocious gout exhibits a strong familial tendency, a feature that is consistent with the fact that the early onset of many diseases with multifactorial inheritance (e.g., atherosclerosis, diabetes) is likely to be associated with a clearly visible genetic component. The consensus today is that multiple genes control the level of serum uric acid.

Gout Can Be Due to Inborn Errors of Metabolism

Although the specific cause of an abnormally high rate of urate production is not identifiable in most cases of primary gout, two inborn errors of metabolism that result in an elevated level of phosphoribosyl pyrophosphate (PP-ribose-P) are known. In this respect, the rate-limiting step in purine synthesis is the condensation of glutamine with PP-ribose-P to form phosphoribosylamine. An increased intracellular concentration of PP-ribose-P accelerates the biosynthesis of purines. PP-ribose-P, through the activity of hypoxanthine phosphoribosyl transferase (HPRT), also condenses with, and thereby salvages, purine bases (hypoxanthine and guanine) derived from the catabolism of nucleic acids.

LESCH-NYHAN SYNDROME: This condition represents an inherited, X-linked (Xq26-q27) deficiency of HPRT, a defect that leads to accumulation of PP-ribose-P and in turn to enhanced purine synthesis. Children with this syndrome are clinically normal at birth but exhibit delays in development and neurological dysfunction within the first year. Most are mentally retarded and exhibit self-mutilation. They are hyperuricemic and eventually develop gouty arthritis. In addition, obstructive nephropathy and hematological abnormalities are often present.

Secondary Gout Often Results from DNA Turnover

A number of conditions result in hyperuricemia and secondary gout. As in primary gout, secondary hyperuricemia may reflect urate overproduction or decreased urinary excretion of uric acid. Increased production of uric acid is most commonly associated with increased turnover of nucleic acids, as seen in leukemias and lymphomas and after chemotherapy for cancer. Accelerated ATP degradation may also lead to overproduction of uric acid and occurs in glycogen-storage diseases and tissue hypoxia. Ethanol intake is a cause of secondary hyperuricemia, in part owing to accelerated ATP catabolism and (to a lesser degree) decreased renal excretion of uric acid. Reduced urate excretion may result from primary renal disease. Dehydration and diuretics increase tubular reabsorption of uric acid and lead to hyperuricemia. In fact, various drugs are implicated in 20% of patients with hyperuricemia.

Saturnine gout was described in 18th century England, where this disease was prevalent among the upper classes with lead plumbing in their houses (Saturn is the symbol for lead). It is now recognized that these patients were afflicted with lead nephropathy. The Romans had a similar problem, because they drank from vessels containing lead.

 Epidemiology: Primary gout is a disease of adult men, and only 5% of cases occur in women. It is rare in children before the age of puberty and in women during the reproductive period. The peak incidence is in the fifth decade. This sex distribution can be traced to the fact that at all ages, the mean serum urate concentration in women is lower than that in men, although it increases after menopause. A family history is elicited in many patients with gout, but environmental factors also play an important role. Positive correlations exist between the prevalence of hyperuricemia in a population and the mean values for weight, protein intake, alcohol consumption, social class, and intelligence. Thus, gout is a disease that exemplifies the interplay between genetic predisposition and environmental influences.

 Pathology: When sodium urate crystals precipitate from supersaturated body fluids, they absorb fibronectin, complement and a number of other proteins on their surfaces. Neutrophils that have ingested urate crystals release activated oxygen species and lysosomal enzymes, which mediate tissue injury and promote an inflammatory response.

The presence of long, needle-shaped crystals that are negatively birefringent under polarized light is diagnostic of gout (Fig. 26-62). Monosodium urate monohydrate crystals may be found intracellularly in leukocytes of the synovial fluid. A *tophus* is an extracellular soft-tissue deposit of urate crystals surrounded by foreign-body giant cells and an associated inflammatory response of mononuclear cells. These granuloma-like areas are found in cartilage, in any of the soft tissues around joints, and even in the subchondral bone marrow adjacent to joints.

Macroscopically, any chalky white deposit on the surfaces of intraarticular structures, including articular cartilage, suggests gout. Radiologically, gouty arthritis exhibits characteristic, punched-out, juxtaarticular, lytic ("rat bite") lesions that are associated with only minimal reactive new bone (Fig. 26-63). In contrast to RA, there is no juxta-articular osteopenia in gout.

Urate deposits in the kidney occur in the interstitium between renal tubules, especially at the apices of the medulla. These deposits are grossly visible as small, shiny, golden-yellow, linear streaks in the medulla.

Clinical Features: The clinical course of gout may be divided into four stages: (1) asymptomatic hyperuricemia, (2) acute gouty arthritis, (3) intercritical gout, and (4) chronic tophaceous gout. Renal stones occur in any stage except the first. In most cases, symptomatic gout appears before the renal stones, which usually require 20 to 30 years of sustained hyperuricemia.

- **Asymptomatic hyperuricemia** often precedes clinically evident gout by many years.
- **Acute gouty arthritis** was well characterized by Thomas Sydenham, who described his own disease in the 1600s. It is a painful condition that usually involves one joint and is unaccompanied by constitutional symptoms. Later in the course of the disease, polyarticular involvement with fever is common. At least half of patients are first seen with a painful and red first metatarsophalangeal joint (great toe), designated *podagra*. Eventually, 90% of all patients have such an attack. Commonly, a gouty attack begins at night and is exquisitely painful, simulating an acute bacterial infection of the affected joint. A large meal or drinking alcoholic beverages may trigger an attack, but other specific events such as trauma, certain drugs, and surgery may also be responsible. Even when untreated, an acute attack of gout is self-limited.
- **The intercritical period** is the asymptomatic interval between the initial acute attack and subsequent episodes. These periods may last up to 10 years, but later attacks tend to be increasingly severe and prolonged and polyarticular.
- **Tophaceous gout** eventually appears in the untreated patient in the form of tophi in the cartilage, synovial membranes, tendons, and soft tissues.

Renal failure is responsible for 10% of deaths in persons with gout. One third of gout patients have mild albuminuria, a reduced glomerular filtration rate, and decreased renal concentrating ability. However, the contribution of urate nephropathy to chronic renal dysfunction is unclear, and hypertension, preexisting kidney disease, and the intake of analgesic drugs may be more important. In patients with severe gout caused by inherited enzyme deficiencies, and in those with a precocious presentation, urate nephropathy remains a prominent feature of the clinical course. **Urate stones** constitute 10% of all renal calculi in patients in the United States and up to 40% in Israel and Australia. The prevalence of urate stones correlates with the serum concentration of uric acid and affects up to 25% of gout patients. They also have an increased frequency of calcium-containing stones, in which case the uric acid may serve as a nidus for a calcium stone.

TREATMENT: The treatment of gout is designed to (1) decrease the severity of acute attacks, (2) reduce serum urate levels, (3) prevent future attacks, (4) promote the dissolution of urate deposits, and (5) alkalinize the urine to prevent stone formation. The principal drugs used to interrupt the inflammatory process, thereby preventing or controlling the acute attack, are nonsteroidal antiinflammatory agents. Colchicine has been employed for hundreds of years and has been administered prophylactically during the intervals between gouty attacks to prevent recurrent episodes. Uricosuric drugs that interfere with urate reabsorption by the renal tubule are often useful.

A drug worthy of special attention is **allopurinol**, a competitive inhibitor of xanthine oxidase, the enzyme that converts xanthine and hypoxanthine to uric acid. This drug causes a prompt decrease in uricosemia and uricosuria. It is used in patients who have renal insufficiency and those who are resistant to other uricosuric drugs. It also may be administered to patients undergoing chemotherapy for hematopoietic proliferative disorders, which increases the rate of urate production.

CALCIUM PYROPHOSPHATE DIHYDRATE-DEPOSITION DISEASE (CHONDROCALCINOSIS AND PSEUDOGOUT)

Calcium pyrophosphate dihydrate (CPPD)-deposition disease refers to the accumulation of this compound in synovial membranes (pseudogout), joint cartilage (chondrocalcinosis), ligaments, and tendons. The disease can be idiopathic, associated with trauma, linked to a number of metabolic disorders, or, in rare cases, hereditary.

CPPD-deposition disease is principally a condition of old age, with half of the population older than 85 years being afflicted. Most cases in the elderly are without symptoms. Because fully two thirds of these patients manifest preexisting joint damage, it is believed that trauma and the aging process in cartilage promote nucleation of CPPD crystals. In asymptomatic cases, punctate or linear calcifications may be present in any fibrocartilage or hyaline cartilage surface. For example, radiography of the knee may disclose linear streaks that outline the menisci.

1374   Bones and Joints

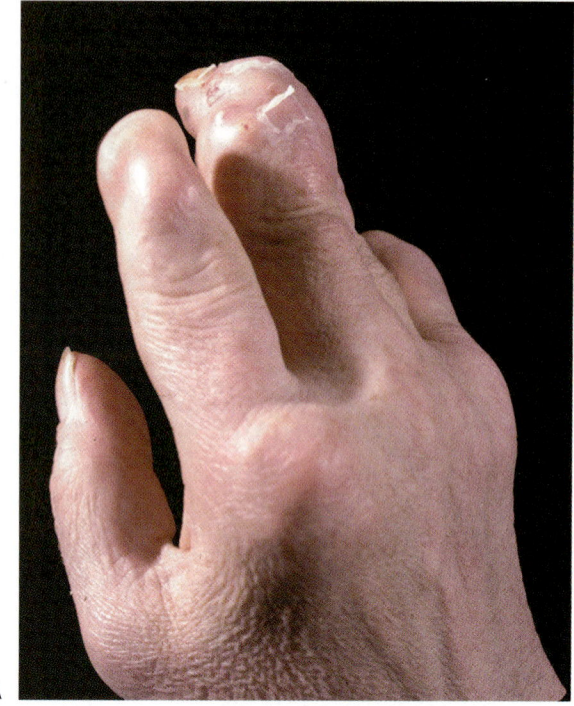
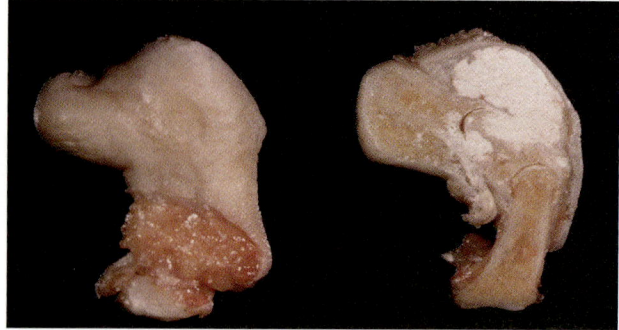
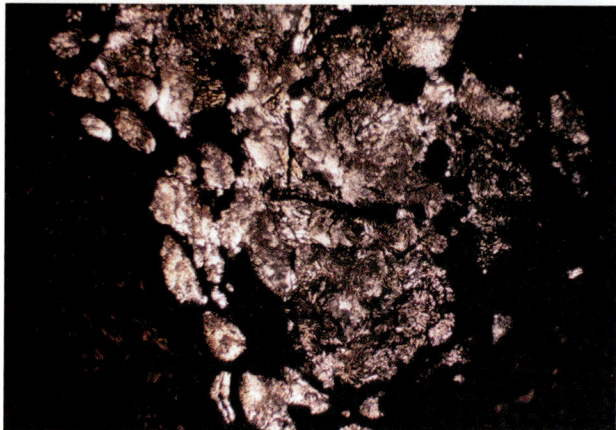
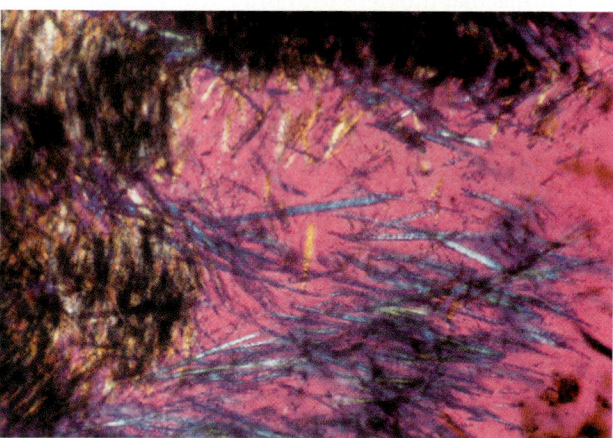
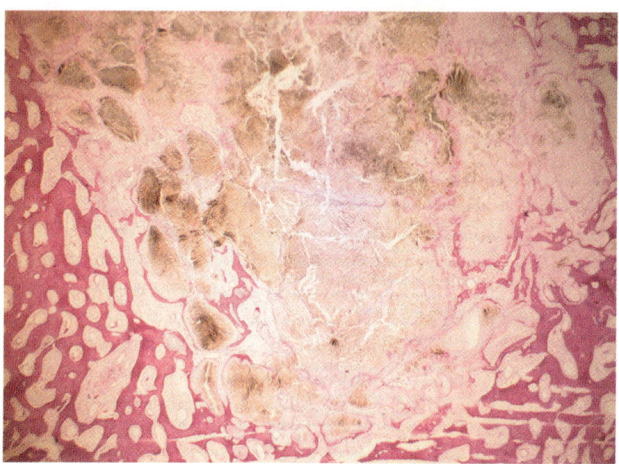

FIGURE 26-62
Gout. A. Gouty tophi of the hands appear as multiple rubbery nodules, one of which is ulcerated. B. A cross-section of a digit demonstrates a tophaceous collection of toothpaste-like urate crystals. C. Histologic section in bright field demonstrates brownish monosodium urate crystals within the bone. D. High-power micrograph in polarized light with a quartz compensator plate demonstrates negative birefringence of the crystals (those having their long axes parallel to the slow compensator axis are yellow). E. A section through the tophus (if usual aqueous processing is used) demonstrates a foreign body reaction around a pink, amorphous lesion from which the urate crystals have been dissolved in processing.

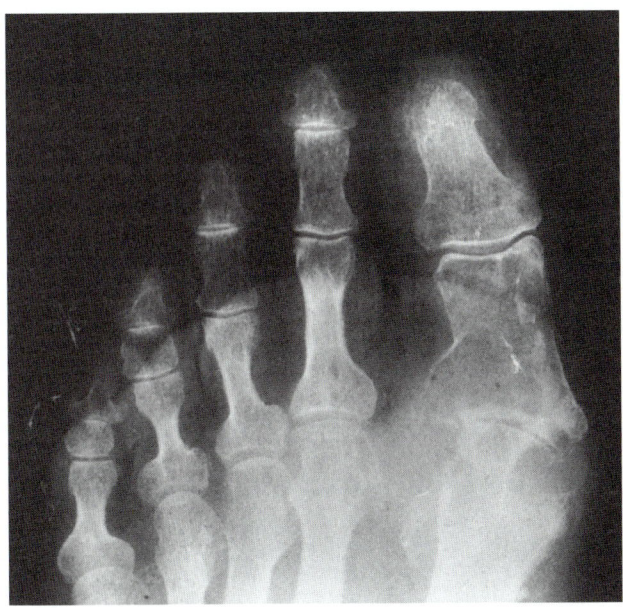

FIGURE 26-63
Gout. A radiograph of the first metatarsophalangeal joint shows a lytic lesion that destroys the joint space. There is an adjacent soft tissue tophus, as well as surrounding edema.

two joints. Some 25% of patients with CPPD-deposition disease have an acute onset of goutlike symptoms manifesting as inflammation and swelling of the knees, ankles, wrists, elbows, hips or shoulders. Metatarsophalangeal joints, which are frequently affected in gout, are usually spared. The synovial fluid exhibits abundant leukocytes containing CPPD crystals.
- **Pseudorheumatoid arthritis** is a variant of CPPD-deposition disease in which multiple joints are chronically involved. The symptoms are mild and resemble those of RA.
- **Pseudoosteoarthritis** has symptoms similar to those of osteoarthritis.
- **Pseudoneurotrophic disease** is characterized by joint destruction severe enough to resemble a neurotrophic joint.

On gross examination, CPPD deposits appear as chalky white areas on the cartilaginous surfaces (Fig. 26-64A). Unlike needle-shaped urate crystals, they are stubby, short, and rhomboid ("coffin shaped") and have weak positive birefringence under polarized light (Figs 26-64B and C). In contrast to urate crystals, CPPD crystals do not dissolve in water and are easily found in tissue sections. Only few mononuclear cells and macrophages surround foci of crystal deposition.

 Pathogenesis: The major predisposing abnormality in patients with CPPD-deposition disease is an excessive level of inorganic pyrophosphate in the synovial fluid. This material derives from the hydrolysis of nucleoside triphosphates in the chondrocytes of the joint. Increased pyrophosphate levels in the synovial fluid can result from either increased production or decreased catabolism.

CPPD deposition is commonly found in the knees after trauma and after surgical removal of the meniscus. It is possible that released nucleotides after injury to the articular cartilage serve as a substrate for nucleotide triphosphate pyrophosphohydrolase (NTP), thereby increasing the production of pyrophosphate. A number of other disorders are associated with the deposition of CPPD crystals, including hyperparathyroidism, hypothyroidism, hemochromatosis, Wilson disease, and ochronosis. Iron and copper are presumed to inhibit pyrophosphatase, accounting for decreased degradation of pyrophosphate.

Hypophosphatasia is a heritable condition in which the activity of alkaline phosphatase (the enzyme that hydrolyzes pyrophosphate) in serum and tissue is deficient. As a result, pyrophosphate is not adequately metabolized and accumulates in the synovial fluid.

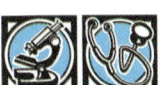 **Pathology and Clinical Features:** A minority of patients with CPPD-deposition disease who are symptomatic are classified according to the nature of joint involvement.

- **Pseudogout** refers to self-limited attacks of acute arthritis lasting from 1 day to 4 weeks and involving one or

CALCIUM HYDROXYAPATITE-DEPOSITION DISEASE

Calcium hydroxyapatite-deposition disease is an acute or chronic arthritis characterized by hydroxyapatite crystals within leukocytes and mononuclear cells in joint tissue and synovial fluid. Calcium hydroxyapatite (HA) is the major mineral of bone and teeth and is the compound deposited in dystrophic and metastatic calcification. HA crystals are frequently encountered in the synovial fluid of joints involved by osteoarthritis, but there is reason to believe that severe HA deposition is a distinct entity. The joints most frequently involved are the knee, shoulder, hip, and fingers. Attacks may last several days.

HEMOPHILIA, HEMOCHROMATOSIS, AND OCHRONOSIS

Hemophilia, hemochromatosis, and ochronosis (see Chapter 6) all produce joint disease with degradation of the matrix and destruction of the articular cartilage.

Hemophilia gives rise to severe forms of arthritis because of extensive bleeding into joints (hemarthrosis), particularly the knees, elbows, ankles, shoulders, and hips. In addition to the effects within the articular cartilage matrix, synovial proliferation also simulates RA.

Hemochromatosis is complicated by arthritis in half of affected patients. The hands, hips, and knees may be involved in recurrent attacks.

Ochronosis is a rare, autosomal recessive disease caused by a defect in homogentisic acid oxidase. The deposi-

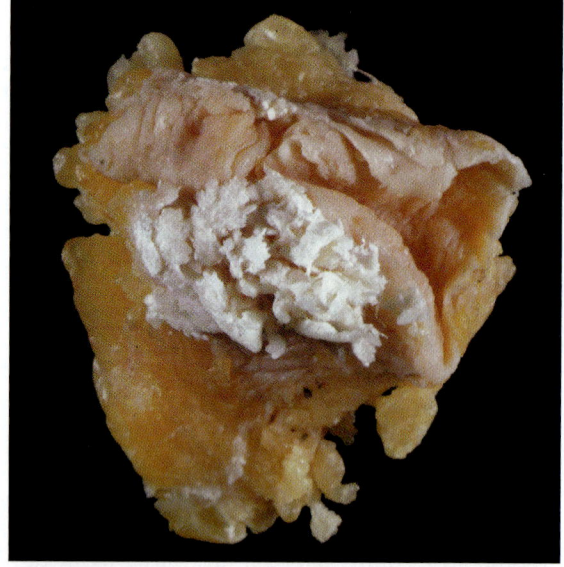
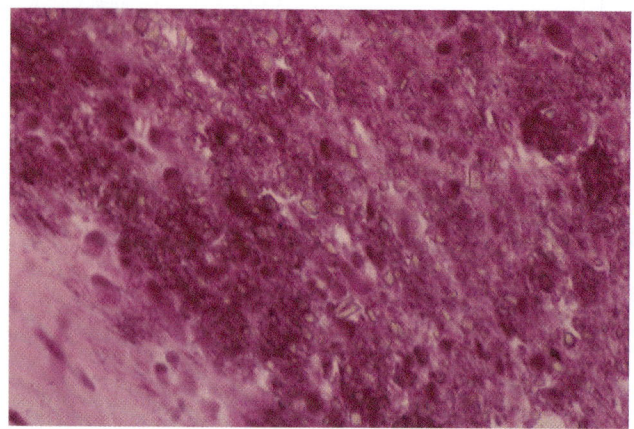
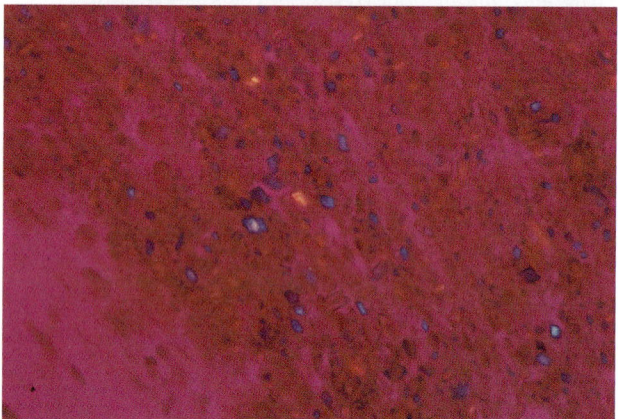

FIGURE 26-64
Calcium pyrophosphate-deposition disease (CPPD). A. Gross specimen demonstrates chalky-white calcific material. B. A histological section shows purplish crystals coated with hematoxylin. The crystals that are not coated are clearly rhomboid. C. Polarized microscopy with a quartz compensator reveals that the crystals show weak positive birefringence.

tion of ochronotic pigment in the cartilage of the joints, including the intravertebral disks, eventually causes them to become brittle and degenerate.

TUMORS AND TUMORLIKE LESIONS OF JOINTS

True neoplasms of the joints are rare. The most common malignant lesions of the synovium are metastatic carcinomas, particularly adenocarcinoma of the colon, breast, and lung. Lymphoproliferative diseases (e.g., leukemia) may also involve the synovium, mimicking other conditions, such as RA. It is unusual for primary malignant bone tumors to extend into the joint, although they may invade the joint capsule from the soft tissues.

Ganglion is a Small Fluid-Filled Cyst

A ganglion is a thin-walled, simple cyst containing clear mucinous fluid, which occurs most commonly on the extensor surfaces of the hands and feet, especially the wrist. The cyst arises either from the synovium or from areas of myxoid change in the connective tissue, possibly after trauma. If the lesion is painful, it can be readily removed surgically, although a blow with the family Bible was the traditional treatment for a ganglion on the dorsum of the wrist.

Baker's cyst refers to a herniation of the synovium of the knee joint into the popliteal space. It is most often seen in association with various forms of arthritis, in which the intraarticular pressure is increased.

Synovial Chondromatosis Features Cartilage Nodules in a Joint

Synovial chondromatosis is a benign, self-limited disease in which hyaline cartilage nodules, which form in the synovium, detach from that structure and float in the synovial fluid in a manner similar to grains of sand between gears. The chronic irritation produced by these foreign bodies stimulates the synovium to secrete large amounts of synovial fluid and also causes bleeding in the synovial membrane. Synovial chondromatosis involves the large diarthrodial joints of young and middle-aged men, affecting the knee in most cases, but also the hip, elbow, shoulder, and ankle. Patients have pain, stiffness, and locking of the joint, with associated bloody effusions.

Unlike the cartilage that detaches from the articular surface in osteoarthritis, in synovial chondromatosis fragments of hyaline cartilage are formed de novo in the synovium.

Therefore, they do not have a tidemark and thus differ from true articular cartilage. Occasionally, the cartilage nodules, while still residing in the synovium, undergo endochondral ossification, in which case, the disease is called *synovial osteochondromatosis*. If these nodules detach, the bony portions die, but the cartilage fragments remain viable and enlarge because they are nourished by synovial fluid. Evacuating the joint and performing a partial synovectomy treat the condition.

Pigmented Villonodular Synovitis Is a Benign Neoplasm of the Synovial Lining

Pigmented villonodular synovitis is characterized by an exuberant proliferation of synovial lining cells with extension into the subsynovial tissue. It involves a single joint, usually occurs in young adults, and is equally distributed between male and female subjects. The most common site (80%) is the knee, although pigmented villonodular synovitis also occurs in the hip, ankles, calcaneocuboid joint, elbow, and tendon sheaths of the fingers and toes.

Pathology: The tumors arise on the synovium of tendon sheaths, bursae, and diarthrodial joints. The lesions of pigmented villonodular synovitis invade the joint and erode the bone (Fig 26-65A). They may insinuate through joint capsules into soft tissue and encompass nerves and arteries, sometimes necessitating radical surgical excision. The synovium develops enlarged folds and nodular excrescences (Fig. 26-65B). Microscopically, the tumor is composed of bland mononuclear cells with scattered multinucleated giant cells in which the nuclei are arrayed peripherally. Hemosiderin-laden macrophages reflect previous hemorrhage (see Fig. 26-65C and D).

Localized nodular synovitis is a similar condition of the knee that involves only one portion of the synovium rather than the entire membrane. The symptoms are limited to pain, joint locking, and joint effusions.

Localized nodular tenosynovitis, also called **giant cell tumor of the tendon sheath**, involves the tendon sheaths of the hands and feet. **It is the most common soft tissue tumor of the hand.** The lesion occurs mostly in young and middle-aged women and involves the flexor surface of the middle or index finger.

The treatment for all forms of pigmented villonodular synovitis is surgical. Radiation therapy produces fibrosis of the proliferating synovial tissue, but amputation is occasionally necessary.

Soft Tissue Tumors

The term *soft tissue tumor* refers to neoplastic conditions that arise in certain extraskeletal mesodermal tissues of the body, including skeletal muscle, fat, fibrous tissue, blood vessels, and lymphatics. Tumors of peripheral nerves are included in the category of soft tissue tumors, despite their derivation from the neuroectoderm.

In the context of soft tissue tumors, the term *benign* is relative, because so-called benign tumors may have a limited capacity for invasive growth and may recur locally. Soft tissue tumors are rare, accounting for less than 1% of all cancers in the United States. Benign soft tissue neoplasms are 100 times more common than malignant ones.

A group of genetic disorders that are associated with soft tissue tumors includes neurofibromatosis type 1, tuberous sclerosis, Osler-Weber-Rendu disease, and mesenteric fibromatosis in Gardner syndrome. Burns in childhood produce scars, which in rare instances lead to soft tissue fibroblastic tumors many years later. Radiation injury has been reported to be associated with the development of sarcomas years after exposure. Claims that trauma is the cause of a soft tissue tumor are usually made in cases in which possible compensation is involved. There is no scientific evidence to support this association, and injury merely draws attention to a preexisting tumor.

A few important general principles relate to soft tissue tumors:

- Superficial tumors tend to be benign.
- Deep lesions are often malignant.
- Large tumors are more often malignant than small ones.
- Rapidly growing tumors are more likely to be malignant than tumors that develop slowly.
- Calcification may exist in both benign and malignant tumors.
- Benign tumors are relatively avascular, whereas most malignant ones are hypervascular.
- Some soft tissue tumors are classified on the basis of genetic or molecular findings.

TUMORS AND TUMORLIKE CONDITIONS OF FIBROUS ORIGIN

Nodular Fasciitis May Be Mistaken for Sarcoma

Nodular fasciitis is a benign but rapidly growing reactive lesion that probably results from trauma and commonly affects the superficial tissues of the forearm, trunk, and back (Fig. 26-66). Most cases occur in adults, and the rapid growth of this lesion usually prompts the patient to seek medical attention. Histologically, nodular fasciitis may be mistaken for a sarcoma, because it is hypercellular and has abundant mitoses and numerous, pleomorphic, spindle-shaped cells. Its true nature is revealed when it is recognized that the entire "mass" is the counterpart of granulation tissue in response to trauma. The lesion is self-limited and is cured by surgical excision.

Fibromatosis Is Locally Aggressive

Fibromatosis, also known as desmoid tumor, *is a locally invasive, slowly growing, collagenous mass that may occur virtually anywhere in the body.* Although they do not metastasize, the lesions of fibromatosis are locally invasive, and surgical resection is often followed by a local recurrence. An increased

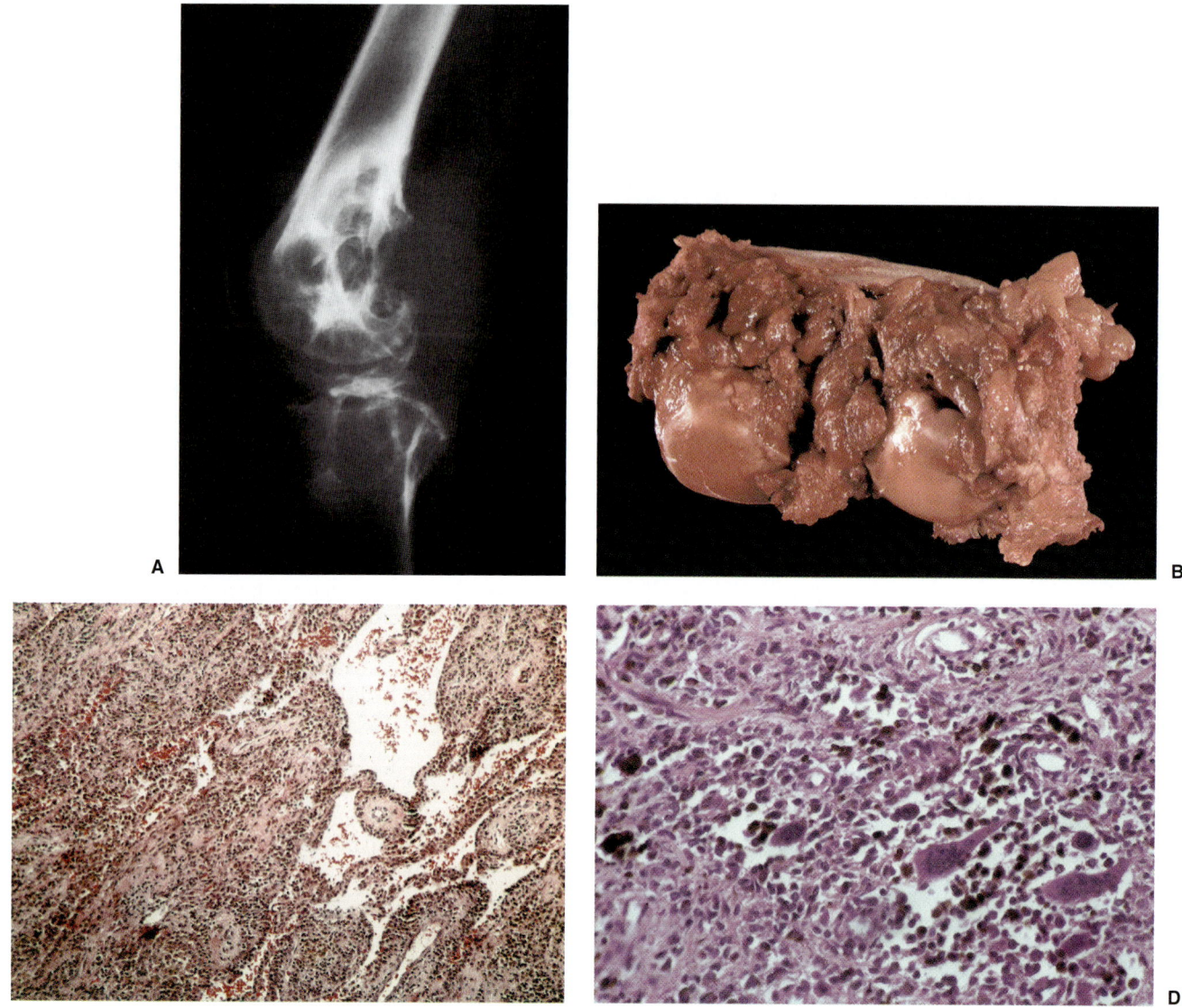

FIGURE 26-65
Pigmented villonodular synovitis. A. Radiograph of the knee demonstrates confluent erosions of the distal femur and proximal tibia and a soft tissue mass within the joint. B. Gross specimen shows massive destruction of the femoral condyles. Note brown color and nodular thickenings. C. Low-power microscopy demonstrates thickened villous synovium. D. At higher power, the cellular infiltrate mainly consists of mononuclear macrophages, many of which contain brown hemosiderin pigment, and multinucleated giant cells.

incidence of fibromatosis has been reported in diabetics, alcoholics, and epileptics. Thus, this "tumor" may represent a reaction to repeated trauma at a specific site.

Pathology: On gross examination, the lesions of fibromatosis tend to be large, firm, and whitish, with poorly demarcated borders and a whorled cut surface. They frequently originate in a muscular fascia. Microscopic examination reveals sheets and interdigitating fascicles of benign-appearing spindle cells (fibroblasts) with little mitotic activity. Because microscopic tongues of tumor extend between preexisting structures, surgical "shelling out" of the lesion is followed by recurrences in half of cases. Complete surgical excision is curative.

Specific forms of fibromatosis are identified by their characteristic locations:

- **Palmar fibromatosis** (Dupuytren contracture) is the single most common form of fibromatosis, occurring in 1 to 2% of the general population but in as many as 20% of persons older than 65 years. In half of cases, the lesion is bilateral, and in 10% of cases, it is associated with fibromatosis in other locations. Fibrous nodules and cordlike bands in the palmar fascia eventually lead to flexion contractures of the fingers, particularly the fourth and fifth digits.
- **Plantar fibromatosis** is similar to palmar fibromatosis, except that it is less frequent and involves the plantar aponeurosis.

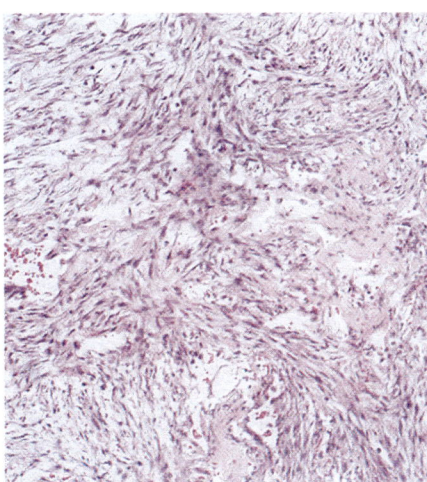

FIGURE 26-66
Nodular fasciitis. Swirls of tightly woven spindle cells and collagen are admixed with a few lymphoid cells and vascular channels.

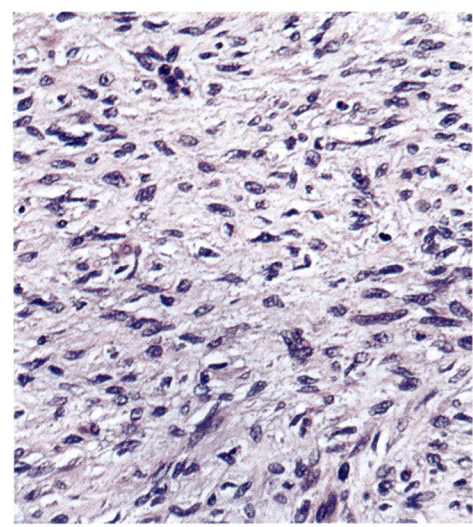

FIGURE 26-67
Fibrosarcoma. A photomicrograph demonstrates irregularly arranged neoplastic fibroblasts.

- **Penile fibromatosis** (Peyronie disease) is the least common of the localized fibromatoses and is characterized by an induration of, or mass in, the shaft of the penis, causing it to curve toward the affected side *(penile strabismus).* The lesion leads to urethral obstruction and pain on erection.

Fibrosarcoma Has a Guarded Prognosis

Fibrosarcoma is a malignant tumor of fibroblasts, which is most commonly found in the thigh, particularly around the knee. This neoplasm typically occurs in adults, although it may be encountered in any age group and may even be congenital. Congenital (infantile) fibrosarcoma (CFS) has a chromosomal translocation, t(12;15)(p13;q26) that contains an *ETV6-NTRK3* fusion gene and has a poor prognosis. Fibrosarcomas arise from connective tissue, such as fascia, scar tissue, periosteum, and tendons. Macroscopically, the tumors are sharply demarcated and frequently exhibit necrosis and hemorrhage. They are characterized histologically by pleomorphic fibroblasts (Fig. 26-67), which often form densely interlacing bundles and fascicles, producing a "herringbone" pattern. The prognosis for fibrosarcoma is at best guarded; the survival at 5 years is only 40% and that at 10 years, 30%. Poorly differentiated fibrosarcomas have a worse prognosis than well-differentiated ones.

Malignant Fibrous Histiocytoma Is the Most Common Soft Tissue Sarcoma

Malignant fibrous histiocytoma (MFH) is a soft tissue tumor that contains foci of histiocytic (macrophage) differentiation and is the most frequent sarcoma encountered after radiation therapy. MFH typically occurs in older adults, but cases have been recorded at all ages. In half of cases, MFH arises in the deep fascia or within a skeletal muscle, and the tumor has been reported in association with surgical scars and foreign bodies.

Pathology: Histologically, MFH displays a highly variable morphological pattern, with areas of spindle-shaped tumor cells arrayed in an irregularly whorled (storiform) pattern adjacent to pleomorphic fields (Fig. 26-68). The spindle cells tend to be well differentiated and resemble fibroblasts. There are occasional plump cells (histiocytes), abundant mitoses, a few xanthomatous cells, and a moderate chronic inflammatory reaction. Some tumors contain numerous tumor giant cells, which exhibit an intense eosinophilia. The extent of collagen deposition varies and sometimes dominates the microscopic pattern. A few tumors reveal a conspicuous myxoid stroma. MFH possesses neither the ultrastructural nor the immunophenotypic profile of histiocytes (macrophages) but instead is more closely related to primitive mesenchymal cells or fibroblasts; its karyotype demonstrates numerous complex chromosomal aberrations.

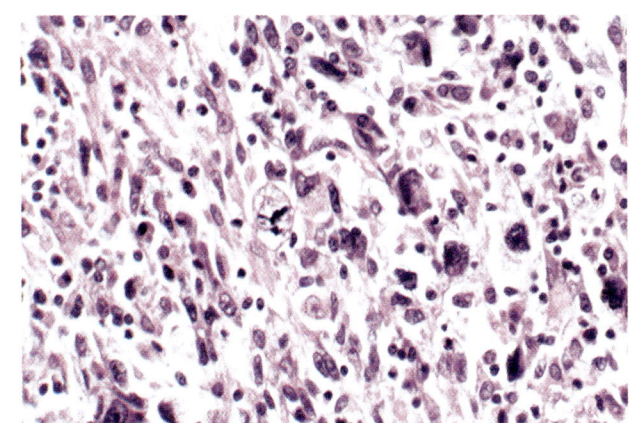

FIGURE 26-68
Malignant fibrous histiocytoma. An anaplastic tumor exhibits spindle cells, plump lipid-laden histiocytes, tumor giant cells, an abnormal mitosis *(center),* and a mild chronic inflammatory infiltrate.

TUMORS OF ADIPOSE TISSUE

Lipoma Closely Resembles Normal Fat

Lipoma is composed of well-differentiated adipocytes and is the most common soft tissue mass. This benign, circumscribed tumor can originate at any site in the body that contains adipose tissue, but most appear in the subcutaneous tissues of the upper half of the body, especially on the trunk and neck. Lipomas are encountered mainly in adults, and patients with multiple tumors often have relatives with a similar history.

Pathology: On gross examination, lipomas are encapsulated, soft, yellow lesions that vary in size and may become very large. Deeper tumors are often poorly circumscribed. Histologically, a lipoma is often indistinguishable from normal adipose tissue. Lipomas are adequately treated by simple local excision.

ANGIOLIPOMA: This is a small, well-circumscribed, subcutaneous lipoma that exhibits extensive vascular proliferation and usually appears shortly after puberty. Angiolipoma is often multiple and painful.

Liposarcoma May Attain a Huge Size

The second most common sarcoma in adults, liposarcoma composes 20% of all malignant soft tissue tumors. The neoplasm arises after age 50 years and is most frequent in the deep thigh and retroperitoneum. Liposarcomas tend to grow slowly but may become extremely large.

Pathogenesis: The myxoid variant of liposarcoma is another example of the growing list of human cancers that are associated with specific chromosomal translocations that result in the synthesis of an abnormal fusion protein. In the case of liposarcoma, most tumors exhibit a translocation between chromosomes 12 and 16, [t(12;16)(q13;p11)], in which the *TLS/FUS* gene on chromosome 16 is fused with the *CHOP* gene on chromosome 12. The *TLS/FUS* gene product is a novel RNA-binding protein with substantial homology to the EWS protein of Ewing sarcoma, whereas the CHOP protein is a transcriptional repressor.

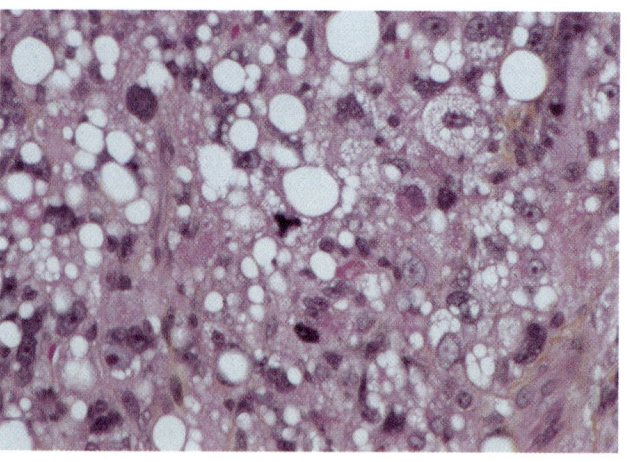

FIGURE 26-69
Liposarcoma. Pleomorphic cells are present, many containing lipid vacuoles that indent the nuclei or completely displace them to one side (signet ring cells).

Pathology: On gross examination the typical liposarcoma measures 5 to 10 cm in diameter, although some measuring 40 cm in diameter and weighing in excess of 20 kg have been encountered. On cut section the appearance of the tumor varies, depending on the proportions of adipose, mucinous, and fibrous tissue. Poorly differentiated liposarcomas grossly appear similar to brain tissue and display necrosis, hemorrhage, and cysts. Microscopically, the most common pattern is one of variably differentiated, "signet ring" lipoblasts embedded in a vascularized myxoid stroma (Fig. 26-69). Poorly differentiated liposarcomas show uniform round cells with vesicular nuclei, which may be difficult to distinguish from other small cell sarcomas. Well-differentiated liposarcomas can be confused with lipomas.

Local recurrence rates and metastases after surgery are high for round cell and pleomorphic liposarcomas, and the 5-year survival for these tumors is less than 20%. By contrast, the 5-year survival for patients with well-differentiated and myxoid tumors exceeds 70%.

RHABDOMYOSARCOMA

Rhabdomyosarcoma is a malignant tumor that displays features of striated muscle differentiation. It is uncommon in mature adults but is the most frequent soft tissue sarcoma of children and young adults. The histogenesis of rhabdomyosarcoma is controversial, but probably most of these tumors derive from primitive mesenchyme that has retained the capacity for skeletal muscle differentiation. Alternatively, rhabdomyosarcoma may arise from embryonal muscle tissue that is displaced into the soft tissues during embryogenesis.

Pathology: Most cases of rhabdomyosarcoma can be classified according to four histological categories.

EMBRYONAL RHABDOMYOSARCOMA: This form is most common in children between the ages of 3 and 12 years and frequently involves the head and neck, genitourinary tract, and retroperitoneum. The morphological appearance varies from that of a highly differentiated tumor containing rhabdomyoblasts, with large eosinophilic cytoplasm and cross-striations (Fig. 26-70A), to that of a poorly differentiated neoplasm.

BOTRYOID EMBRYONAL RHABDOMYOSARCOMA: This tumor, also known as *sarcoma botryoides,* is distinguished by the formation of polypoid, grapelike tumor masses. Microscopically, the malignant cells are scattered in an abundant myxoid stroma. Botryoid foci may occur in any type of embryonal rhabdomyosarcoma, but they are most common in tumors of hollow visceral organs, including the vagina (see Chapter 18) and bladder.

ALVEOLAR RHABDOMYOSARCOMA: This neoplasm occurs less frequently than the embryonal type and principally affects young persons between ages 10 and 25 years; rarely, it may be seen in elderly patients. It is most common in the upper and lower extremities, but it can also be distributed in the same sites as the embryonal type. Typically, club-shaped tumor cells are arranged in clumps that are outlined by fibrous septa. The loose arrangement of the cells in the center of the clusters leads to the "alveolar" pattern (see Fig. 26-70B). The tumor cells exhibit intense eosinophilia, and occasional multinucleated giant cells are identified. Malignant rhabdomyoblasts, recognizable by their cross-striations, occur less commonly in the alveolar variant than in embryonal rhabdomyosarcoma, being present in only 25% of cases. Most alveolar rhabdomyosarcomas express *PAX3-FKHR* or *PAX7-FKHR* gene fusions, resulting from t(2;13)(q35;q14) or t(1;13)(p36;q14) translocations, respectively. In patients with localized tumors, the type of fusion does not correlate with the clinical outcome. However, in the presence of metastatic disease, *PAX3-FKHR*–positive tumors have a worse prognosis than do *PAX7-FKHR*–positive ones

PLEOMORPHIC RHABDOMYOSARCOMA: The least common form of rhabdomyosarcoma is found in the skeletal muscles of older persons, often in the thigh. This tumor differs from the other types of rhabdomyosarcoma in the pleomorphism of its irregularly arranged cells. Large, granular, eosinophilic rhabdomyoblasts, together with multinucleated giant cells, are common. Cross-striations are virtually nonexistent.

The historically dismal prognosis associated with most rhabdomyosarcomas has improved in the past two decades as a result of the introduction of combined therapeutic modalities, including surgery, radiation therapy, and chemotherapy. Today, more than 80% of patients with localized or regional disease are cured. Factors indicating a worse prognosis include patient age above 10, a tumor size greater than 5 cm, alveolar and pleomorphic histological subtypes, and advanced stage of disease.

SMOOTH MUSCLE TUMORS

LEIOMYOMA: This benign soft tissue tumor usually arises in the subcutaneous tissues or from the walls of blood vessels. Leiomyomas are painful lesions that appear as firm, yellow, circumscribed nodules. Microscopically, intersecting fascicles of regular smooth cells are evident. Simple excision is curative.

LEIOMYOSARCOMA: This malignant soft tissue neoplasm is an uncommon tumor of adults that typically arises from the wall of blood vessels in the extremities. Macroscopically, leiomyosarcomas tend to be well circumscribed, but they are larger and softer than leiomyomas and often exhibit necrosis, hemorrhage, and cystic degeneration. Histologically, the tumor cells are arranged in fascicles, often with palisaded nuclei. Well-differentiated tumor cells have elongated nuclei and eosinophilic cytoplasm; poorly differentiated ones show severe nuclear atypism. Leiomyosarcoma is differentiated from leiomyoma mainly by a high mitotic activity, which

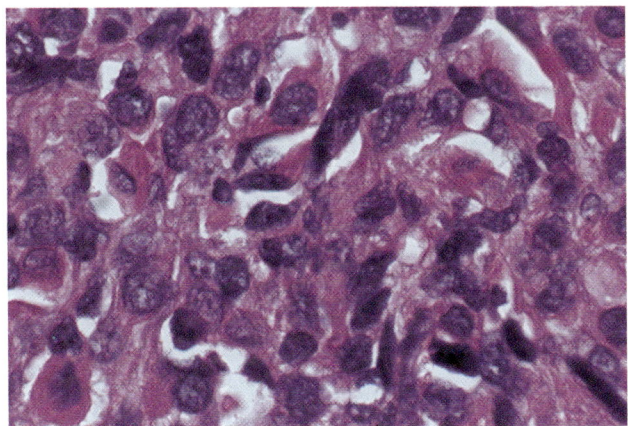
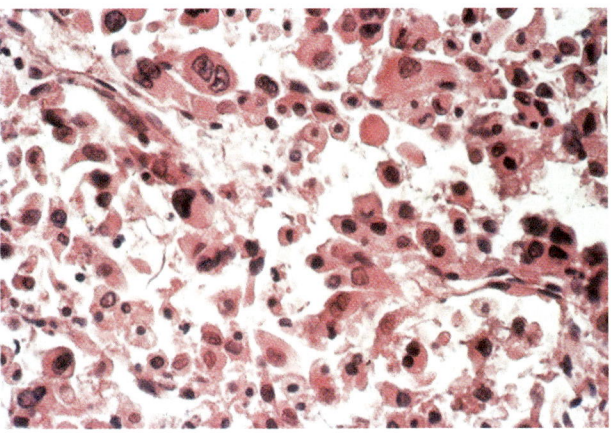

FIGURE 26-70
Rhabdomyosarcoma. A. The tumor contains polyhedral and spindle-shaped tumor cells with enlarged, hyperchromatic nuclei and deeply eosinophilic cytoplasm. A few cells have clearly visible cross striations. B. Alveolar rhabdomyosarcoma. The neoplastic cells are arranged in clusters that display an alveolar pattern.

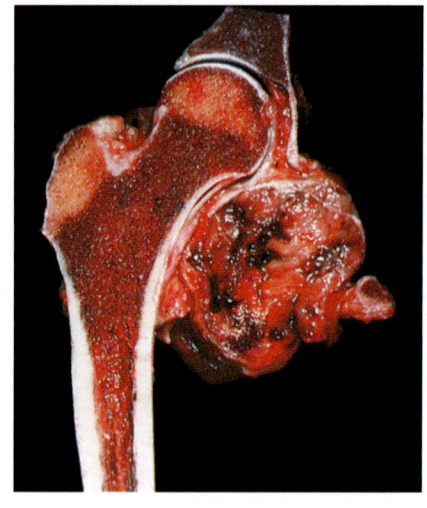
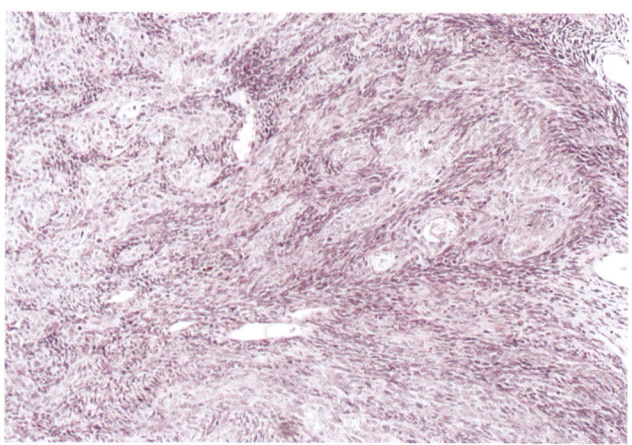

FIGURE 26-71

Synovial sarcoma. A. Section of the upper femur and acetabulum reveals a tumor adjacent to the hip joint and the neck of the femur. **B.** A microscopic view demonstrates the biphasic appearance of a synovial sarcoma. Irregular spaces are lined by plump, synovial-like neoplastic cells. The intervening tissue contains cells with similar nuclei.

also indicates the prognosis. Most leiomyosarcomas eventually metastasize, although dissemination may be seen as late as 15 or more years after resection of the primary tumor.

VASCULAR TUMORS

Benign vascular tumors (hemangiomas) are among the most common soft tissue tumors and are the most frequent neoplasms of infancy and childhood. By contrast, angiosarcomas are among the rarest of soft tissue tumors, accounting for less than 1% of all sarcomas. Vascular tumors are discussed in detail in Chapter 10.

SYNOVIAL SARCOMA

Synovial sarcoma is a highly malignant soft tissue tumor that arises in the region of a joint, usually in association with tendon sheaths, bursae, and joint capsules. Fewer than 10% of synovial sarcomas are intraarticular. Although the tumor bears a microscopic resemblance to the synovium, its origin from this tissue has not been established. Synovial sarcoma occurs principally in adolescents and young adults as a painful or tender mass, usually in the vicinity of a large joint, particularly the knee.

 Pathogenesis: Synovial sarcomas display a specific, balanced chromosomal translocation involving chromosomes X and 18 [t(x;18)(p11.2;q11.2)]. This translocation results in the fusion of the *SYT* (synteny) gene on chromosome 18 to the *SSX* gene (a transcriptional repressor) on the X chromosome, leading to the production of a hybrid protein, SYT-SSX1 or SYT-SSX2. The **SYT-SSX2** protein is associated with a better prognosis if the disease is localized.

 Pathology: On gross examination, synovial sarcomas are usually circumscribed, round or multilobular masses attached to tendons, tendon sheaths, or the exterior wall of the joint capsule (Fig. 26-71A). The tumors tend to be surrounded by a glistening pseudocapsule and in many instances are cystic. They range from small nodules to masses of 15 cm or more in diameter, the average being 3 to 5 cm.

Microscopically, synovial sarcoma is classically described as having a **biphasic pattern** (see Fig. 26-71B). Fluid-filled glandular spaces lined by epithelium-like tumor cells are embedded in a sarcomatous, spindle cell background. These elements vary in proportion, distribution, and cellular differentiation, with the spindle cells usually considerably more numerous than the glandular elements. If the "epithelial" component is lacking, the tumor is referred to as *monophasic synovial sarcoma*. Although monophasic synovial sarcoma resembles fibrosarcoma, its atypical spindle cells are plumper and swirled rather than being arranged in a herringbone pattern. Synovial sarcoma usually expresses cytokeratin or epithelial membrane antigen.

The recurrence rate of synovial sarcoma is high, and metastases occur in more than 60% of cases. The 5-year survival rate is about 50%, and those who die usually have extensive lung metastases.

SUGGESTED READING

Books

Avioli LV, Krane SM (eds): *Metabolic diseases and clinically related disorders*, 3rd ed. Philadelphia: WB Saunders, 1997.

Collins DH: *Pathology of bone.* London: Butterworth, 1966.

Dahlin DC, Unni KK: *Bone tumors: General aspects and data on 8,542 cases.* 4th ed. Springfield, IL: Charles C Thomas, 1986.

Farvus M (ed): *Primer on the metabolic bone diseases and disorders of mineral metabolism.*: American Society for Bone and Mineral Research, 1990.

Fechner RE, Mills SE: *Tumors of bones and joints. Atlas of tumor pathology.* Fascicle 8, 3rd series. Washington, DC: Armed Forces Institute of Pathology, 1993.

Glimcher MJ: On the form and function of bone: From molecules to organs: Wolff's law revisited. In: Kelley WN, Harris ED Jr, Ruddy S, Sledge CB: *Textbook of rheumatology,* 5th ed. Philadelphia: WB Saunders, 1997.

Kempson RL, Fletcher CM, Evans HL, et al.: *Tumors of the soft tissues. Atlas of tumor pathology.* Fascicle 30. 3rd series. Washington, DC: Armed Forces Institute of Pathology, 2001.

Marcus R, Feldman D, Kelsey J (eds): *Osteoporosis.* San Diego: Academic Press, 1996.

Rodman GP, Shumacher HR (eds): *Primer on the rheumatic diseases,* 8th ed. Atlanta: Arthritis Foundation, 1983.

Scriver CR, Beaudet AL, Sly SW, Valle D (eds): *The metabolic basis of inherited disease,* 6th ed. New York: McGraw-Hill, 1989.

Unni KK: Dahlin's bone tumors. General aspects and data on 11,087 cases. 5th ed. Philadelphia: Lippincott-Raven, 1996:263–283.

Veis A (ed): *Chemistry and biology of mineralized connective tissue.* New York: Elsevier-North Holland, 1981.

Vogelstein B, Kinzler KW: *The Genetic Basis of Human Cancer,* 2nd ed. New York: McGraw-Hill Medical Publishing, 2002.

Weiss SW, Goldblum JR: *Enzinger and Weiss's soft tissue tumors,* 4th ed. St. Louis: CV Mosby, 2001.

Review Articles

The ADHR Consortium: Autosomal dominant hypophosphatemic rickets is associated with mutations in FGF23. *Nat Genet* 26:345-348, 2000.

Barton NW, Brady RO, Dambrosia JM, et al.: Replacement therapy for inherited enzyme deficiency—macrophage-targeted glucocerebrosidase for Gaucher's disease. *N Engl J Med* 324:1464–1470, 1991.

Biermann JS: Common benign lesions of bone in children and adolescents. *J Pediatr Orthop* 22:268–273, 2002.

Byers PH: Osteogenesis imperfecta: perspectives and opportunities. *Curr Opin Pediatr* 12:603–609, 2000.

Dagher R, Pham TA, Sorbara L, et al.: Molecular confirmation of Ewing sarcoma. *J Pediatr Hematol/Oncol* 23: 221–223, 2001.

de Vernejoul MC, Benichou O: Human osteopetrosis and other sclerosing disorders: Recent genetic developments. *Calcif Tissue Int* 69:1–6, 2001.

Forlino A., Marini JC: Osteogenesis imperfecta: Prospects for molecular therapeutics. *Mol Genet Metab* 71:225–232, 2000.

Fuchs B, Pritchard DJ: Etiology of osteosarcoma. *Clin Orthop* 397:40–52, 2002.

Gallacher SJ: Paget disease of bone. *Curr Opin Rheumatol* 5:351=N356, 1993.

Gigante M, Matera MG, Seripa D, et al.: Ext-mutation analysis in Italian sporadic and hereditary osteochondromas. *Int J Cancer* 95:378–383, 2001.

Haynes MK, Smith JA: Rheumatoid arthritis—A molecular understanding. *Ann Intern Med* 136:908–922, 2002.

Hendy GN, D'Souza-Li L, Yang B, et al.: Mutations of the calcium-sensing receptor (CASR) in familial hypocalciuric hypercalcemia, neonatal severe hyperparathyroidism, and autosomal dominant hypocalcemia. *Hum Mutat* 16:281–296, 2000.

Hruska KA, Teitelbaum SL: Renal osteodystrophy. *N Engl J Med* 333:166–174, 1995.

Huvos AG. Malignant surface lesions of bone. *Curr Diagn Pathol* 7:247–250, 2001.

Inman RD, Scofield RH: Etiopathogenesis of ankylosing spondylitis and reactive arthritis. *Curr Opin Rheumatol* 6:360–370, 1994.

Klein MJ, Kenan S, Lewis MM: Osteosarcoma: Clinical and pathological considerations. *Orthop Clin North Am* 20: 327–345, 1989.

Kuivaniemi H, Tromp G, Prockop D: Mutations in fibrillar collagens (types I, II, III, and XI), fibril-associated collagen (type IX), and network-forming collagen (type X) cause a spectrum of diseases of bone, cartilage, and blood vessels. *Hum Mutat* 9:300–315, 1997.

Maiya S, Grimer RJ, Ramaswamy R, Deshmukh NS: Osteosarcoma occurring in osteogenesis imperfecta tarda. *Int Orthop* 26:126–128, 2002.

Marcus R: Normal and abnormal bone remodeling in man. *Annu Rev Med* 38:129–143, 1987.

Manolagas AC, Jilka RL: Bone marrow, cytokines, and bone remodeling: Emerging insights into the pathophysiology of osteoporosis. *N Engl J Med* 332:305–311, 1995.

Manolagas SD. Birth and death of bone cells: Basic regulatory mechanisms and implications for the pathogenesis and treatment of osteoporosis. *Endocr Rev* 21:115–137, 2000.

Nuovo MA, Dorfman HD, Sun CC, Chalew SA: Tumor-induced osteomalacia and rickets. *Am J Surg Pathol* 13:588–599, 1989.

Ollier W, Barton A: Genetic approaches to the investigation of rheumatoid arthritis. *Curr Opin Rheumatol* 13:260–269, 2002.

Qualman SJ, Morotti RA: Risk assignment in pediatric soft-tissue sarcomas: An evolving molecular classification. *Oncol Rep* 4:123–130, 2002.

McCormick G, Duncan G, Tufaro F: New perspectives in the molecular basis of hereditary bone tumors. *Mol Med Today* 5:481–486, 1999.

Ragland BD, Bell WC, Lopez RR, Siegal GP: Cytogenetics and molecular biology of osteosarcoma. *Lab Invest* 82:365–373, 2002.

Ralston SH: Genetic control of susceptibility to osteoporosis. *J Clin Endocrinol Metab* 87:2460–2466, 2002.

Raney RB: Soft-tissue sarcoma in childhood and adolescence. *Curr Oncol Rep* 4:291–298, 2002.

Reddy SV, Kurihara N, Menaa C, Roodman GD: Paget's disease of bone: A disease of the osteoclast. *Rev Endocr Metab Disord* 2:195–201, 2001.

Riggs BL: The mechanisms of estrogen regulation of bone resorption. *J Clin Invest* 106:1203–1204, 2000.

Roodman GD: Studies in Paget's disease and their relevance to oncology. *Semin Oncol* 28(4 suppl 11):15–21, 2001.

Salusky IB, Goodman WG: Adynamic renal osteodystrophy: Is there a problem? *J Am Soc Nephrol* 12:1978–1985, 2001.

Sandberg AA, Bridge JA: Updates on the cytogenetics and molecular genetics of bone and soft tissue tumors: Congenital (infantile) fibrosarcoma and mesoblastoma nephroma. *Can Gene Cytogene* 132:1–13, 2002.

Schiller AL: Diagnosis of borderline cartilage lesions of bone. *Semin Diagn Pathol* 2:42–61, 1985.

Scully RE, Mark EJ, McNeely WF, et al.: Case 29-2001 Oncogenic osteomalacia. *N Engl J Med* 345:903–908, 2001.

Seufert J, Ebert K, Muller J, et al.: Octreotide therapy for tumor-induced osteomalacia. *N Engl J Med* 345:1883–1888, 2001.

Sledge CB: Structure, development, and function of joints. *Orthop Clin North Am* 6:619–629, 1975.

Sorensen PHB, Lynch JC, Qualman SJ, et al.: PAX3-FKHR and PAX7-FKHR gene fusions are prognostic indicators in alveolar rhabdomyosarcoma: A report from the children's oncology group. *J Clin Oncol* 20:2672–2679, 2002.

Tallini G, Dorfman H, Brys P, et al.: Correlation between clinicopathological features and karyotype in 100 cartilaginous and chordoid tumors. A report from the Chromosomes and Morphology (CHAMP) Collaborative Study Group. *J Pathol* 196:194–203, 2002.

Unger S, Hecht JT: Pseudoachondroplasia and multiple epiphyseal dysplasia: New etiologic developments. *Am J Med Genet* 106:244–250, 2001.

Weiss SW: Soft tissue sarcomas: Lessons from the past, challenges for the future. Mod Pathol 15:77–86, 2002.

CHAPTER 27

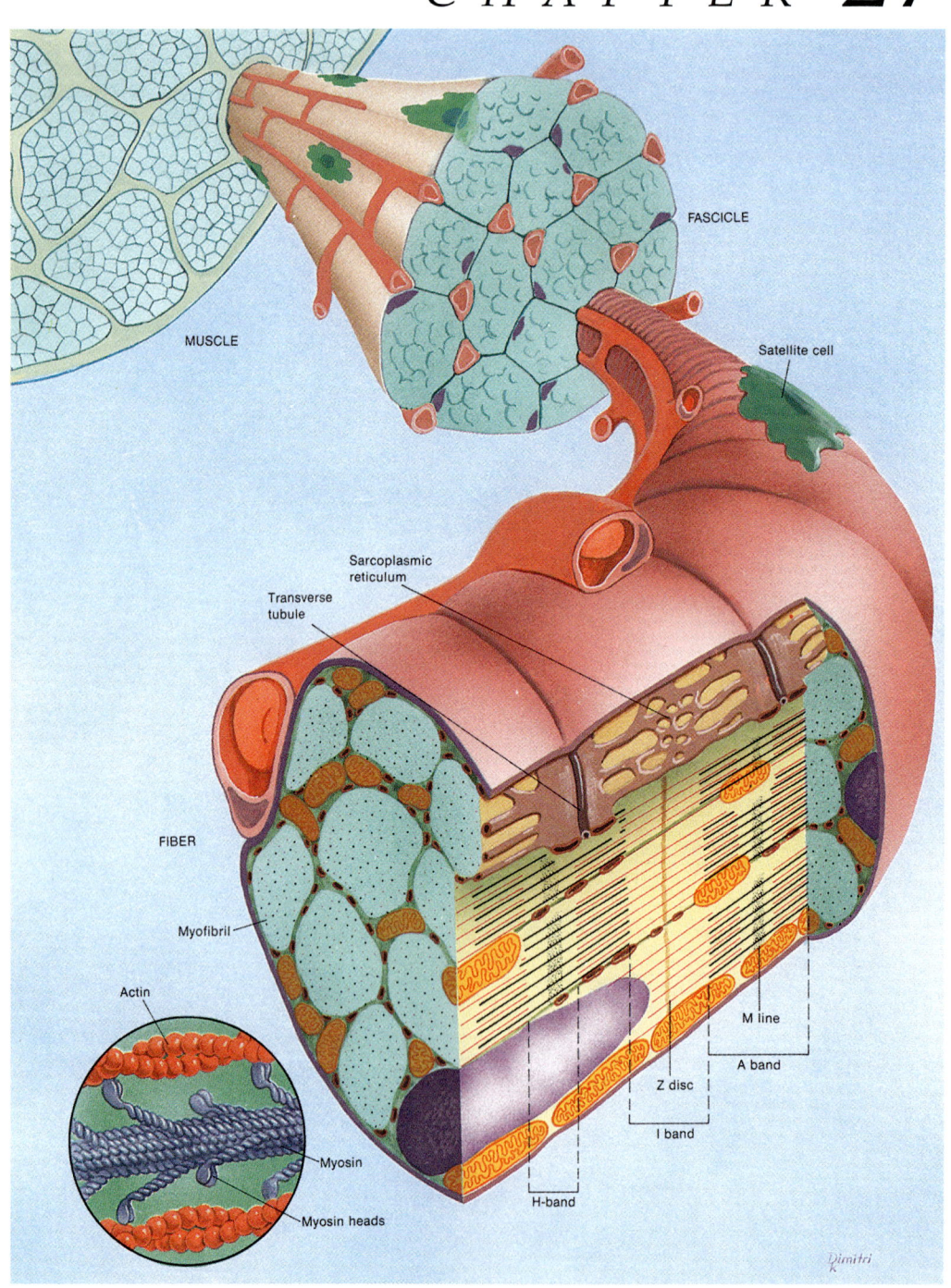

Skeletal Muscle

Lawrence C. Kenyon
Mark T. Curtis

Embryology and Anatomy
Structure of the Myofiber

Histochemistry

Histochemistry

Muscle Biopsy

General Pathological Reactions

Muscular Dystrophy
Duchenne and Becker Muscular Dystrophies
Myotonic Dystrophy

Central Core Disease
Rod (Nemaline) Myopathy
Central Nuclear Myopathy (Myotubular Myopathy)

Inflammatory Myopathies
Polymyositis
Inclusion Body Myositis
Granulomatous Myositis
Vasculitis

Myasthenia Gravis

Lambert-Eaton Syndrome

(continued)

FIGURE 27-1 *(see opposite page)*
Anatomy of skeletal muscle. The composite drawing demonstrates the morphological features of striated muscle from grossly visible to macromolecular levels. In the *upper left*, a portion of a muscle is contained by a distinct outer connective tissue layer called the *epimysium* or *fascia*. Fascicles are groups of muscle fibers separated by connective tissue septa called *perimysium*. Within the fascicle, individual muscle fibers (myofibers) are closely packed and are surrounded by an intricate array of microvasculature and a barely perceptible network of connective tissue called the *endomysium*. The enlarged fascicle also shows scattered, flattened cells (*green*), called *satellite cells*, lying on the surface of the fiber. Each muscle fiber is covered by a basement membrane (*orange*) and packed with bundles of myofilaments called *myofibrils*. The endoplasmic reticulum (sarcoplasmic reticulum) forms an extensive, complex tubular network with periodic dilations (cisternae) around each myofibril. The cisternae are closely apposed to the transverse tubules, which are derived from the cell membrane (sarcolemma) and form a transverse network, which resembles chicken wire, around each myofibril, giving extensive communication between the internal and external environments. The cross-striations of striated muscle are created by the arrangement of the myofilaments of the myofibril. The dark A band results from the thick myosin filaments and the thinner, partially overlapping actin filaments. In the middle portion of the myosin filaments where the actin does not overlap, there is a lighter band called the H zone or H band. In the middle of the H band, the center of each myosin filament thickens, forming intermolecular bridging with the adjacent myosin filament and giving rise to the M line. The finer actin filaments are anchored on the dark Z disk of the lighter I band. With contraction, the myosin filaments pull the actin filaments, causing the H zone to disappear, the A band to widen, and the I band to shrink. The mitochondria are scattered throughout the sarcoplasm among the myofibrils. In the final enlargement, the myosin filament is covered with myosin heads that attach to receptor sites on the surrounding actin filaments. The movement of these heads, with attachment and detachment, pulls the actin filaments, ratchet fashion, past the myosin filament.

Inherited Metabolic Diseases

Glycogen-Storage Diseases (Glycogenoses)

Lipid Myopathies

Mitochondrial Diseases

Myoadenylate Deaminase Deficiency

Familial Periodic Paralysis

Rhabdomyolysis

Denervation

Spinal Muscular Atrophy

Type II Fiber Atrophy

Critical Illness Myopathy

EMBRYOLOGY AND ANATOMY

The myoblast is a primitive cell that fuses with other myoblasts to form a cylindrical multinucleated myotube. The periphery of the myotube rapidly accumulates myofibrils, containing myosin and actin, which become arrayed in the cross-banded pattern characteristic of striated muscle (Fig. 27-1).

The myotube matures completely when it is innervated by the terminal axon of a lower motor neuron. Before innervation, the sarcolemma of the myotube contains diffusely distributed nicotinic receptors for acetylcholine on its surface membrane. When innervation occurs, these receptors become highly concentrated at the motor endplate. Although an individual muscle fiber is innervated by only a single nerve ending, a given motor neuron innervates numerous muscle fibers.

The muscle fibers responsible for movement are referred to as *extrafusal* fibers, whereas those contained within stretch receptors (muscle spindle organs) are known as *intrafusal* fibers. Most primary myopathies feature damage to the extrafusal fibers but not the intrafusal fibers. The result is that the muscle spindle organs, which are usually inconspicuous in routine histologic preparations, become more prominent as the extrafusal fibers disappear.

The Myofiber Comprises Distinct Functional Units

After innervation the nuclei of each fiber move from the center to arrange themselves in a regular pattern beneath the sarcolemma (see Fig. 27-3A). The myofiber has a distinctive architecture that is visualized by electron microscopy. Muscle contraction is produced by the actin filaments sliding past the myosin filaments (see Figs. 27-1 and 27-2). A few definitions are in order.

- **Sarcomere:** Functional unit of the myofibril that extends from one Z band to the next
- **Z band:** A distinct electron-dense band that anchors the thin actin filaments
- **I band:** Zone of the actin filaments as they extend from the Z band into the A band.
- **A band:** Structure composed of the thick myosin filaments. Actin filaments overlap the myosin filaments to a variable extent, depending on the degree of muscle contraction. The thin filaments form a hexagonal array around each thick filament.
- **H zone:** Pale region in the midportion of the A band where the actin filaments end
- **M line:** Zone of intermolecular bridging and thickening of the myosin filaments at the midline of the A band, which forms a thin, slightly darker electron-dense band.

During contraction, the sliding actin filaments advance farther into the A band, producing a shorter sarcomere length. As a result, the lengths of the I band and H zone decrease, whereas that of the A band remains nearly constant.

The *sarcoplasmic reticulum* surrounds each myofibril and forms an elaborate membranous network that has irregular dilations (cisternae) juxtaposed to a transverse tubular network derived from the sarcolemma. The *transverse tubular system* (T tubule system) is arranged across the fiber like chicken wire, each ring wrapping around an individual myofibril (see Fig. 27-1). This arrangement allows an electrical stimulus to proceed along the surface of the muscle fiber and to become diffusely and rapidly internalized by way of the transverse tubular system. The electrical signal is translated into a chemical signal between the transverse tubule and the cisternae of the sarcoplasmic reticulum. This process releases calcium from the sarcoplasmic reticulum into the vicinity of myofibrils, where the chemical signal triggers muscle contraction.

The lower motor neuron and the fibers that it innervates are referred to as the **motor unit**. The size of a motor unit varies. In limb muscles, a single motor unit can comprise as many as several hundred myofibers. By contrast, each motor unit of the extraocular muscles may have as few as 20 myofibers. The muscles of the eye are also exceptional because a single fiber may have more than one motor endplate.

Myofiber Types Are Slow or Fast Twitch

After innervation, a characteristic metabolic profile develops for different muscle fibers. In lower mammals, some muscles have a deep red color (type I), whereas others are pale (type II).

TYPE I FIBERS (RED, SLOW TWITCH): If a nerve stimulates a dark (red) muscle, the resulting contraction is slower and more prolonged than when a nerve excites a pale (white) muscle. For this reason, red muscles have been classified as "slow twitch." Type I fibers tend to have more oxygen-storing red pigment (myoglobin) and more mitochondria. The corresponding mitochondrial enzymes of the Krebs cycle and the carrier proteins of the electron-transport chain are all present in greater amounts in the red, slow-twitch muscle than in the white, fast-twitch muscle. The alkaline histo-

Embryology and Anatomy

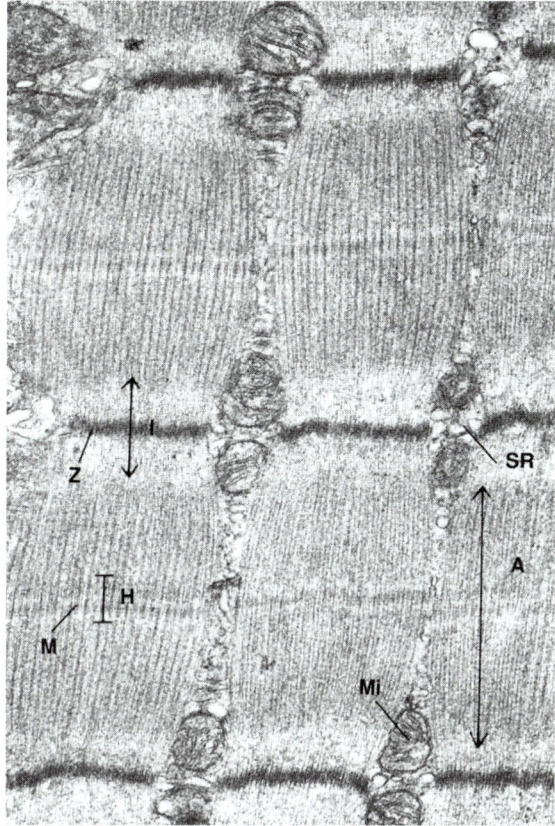

FIGURE 27-2
Normal muscle. This electron micrograph of the biceps muscle demonstrates the ultrastructure of the sarcomere. The thin dark band, the Z disk (Z), bisects the broad, pale I band (I), a zone composed of the thin actin filaments. The broad, dark band, made up of the thick myosin filaments and overlapping actin filaments, is the A band (A). The middle of the A band consists of the pale H zone (H), which in turn is bisected by a slightly darker M line (M), representing a zone of intermolecular bridging of myosin. Small membrane-bound vesicles compose the sarcoplasmic reticulum (SR) and the transverse tubules. Pairs of mitochondria (Mi) tend to be located between myofibrils at the level of the I bands.

chemical reaction for myosin ATPase gives a crisp distinction between the two fiber types. Type I fibers remain almost unstained at high (alkaline) pH, whereas type II fibers stain darkly (Fig. 27-3).

Functionally, type I muscles have a greater capacity for long, sustained contractions, and they resist fatigue. A training program to increase endurance produces little change in size of type I fibers, but conditioning of these fibers results in a proliferation of mitochondria and an expanded capacity for generating energy.

TYPE II FIBERS (WHITE, FAST TWITCH): Stimulation of type II fibers elicits a faster, shorter, and more powerful contraction than occurs in type I fibers. Glycogen, phosphorylase, and other enzymes in the Embden-Meyerhof pathway, which produce energy by anaerobic glycolysis, are present in higher concentrations in white muscle. Type II muscle fibers are suitable for rapid contractions of brief duration and react to strength training with hypertrophy. Androgenic steroids induce hypertrophy of type II fibers, and disuse of the muscle results in their selective atrophy.

The lower motor neuron influences fiber type. During embryonic development of mammals, the early muscle cells begin to express type-specific contractile proteins before muscle is innervated. Thus, the phenotype of a myofiber seems to be a genetically determined property of the cell, rather than one that is determined by the nerve supply. However, the innervation of muscle can alter the types of myofibers. For example, after denervation injury, reinnervation of a slow-twitch muscle by the nerve from a fast-twitch muscle causes the newly innervated type I fibers to assume the staining characteristic of type II fibers. It is thought that the pattern or rate of discharge of the lower motor neuron plays an important role in this process. Because the lower motor neuron can determine the fiber type, it follows that all the muscle fibers in a given motor unit are of the same type. A cross-section of muscle that has been stained with the alkaline ATPase reaction demonstrates a random mixture of fiber types (see Fig. 27-3B), because the motor units interdigitate extensively with each other.

In humans, no muscles are composed exclusively of one fiber type. However, the proportion of fiber types does vary from muscle to muscle. For example, the soleus muscle is composed of predominantly type I fibers (≥80%). The pattern of fiber types in a given muscle varies between persons, a difference that is apparently genetically determined. Some evidence indicates that changing the use of a muscle over a long period through intensive training may alter the pattern of muscle fiber types.

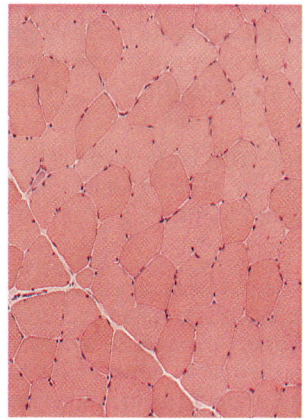 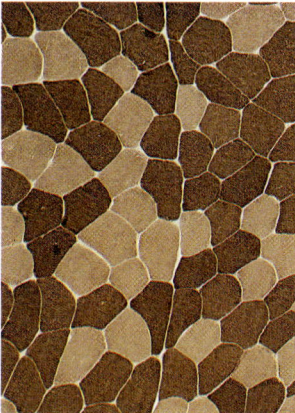

FIGURE 27-3
Normal muscle. A. Hematoxylin and eosin stain. In this transverse frozen section of the vastus lateralis, the polygonal myofibers are separated from each other by an indistinct, thin layer of connective tissue, the endomysium. The thicker band of connective tissue, the perimysium, demarcates a bundle or fascicle of fibers. All of the nuclei in this field are located at the periphery of the cells. Occasional nuclei are contained within satellite cells but cannot be distinguished from those of the myofibers by light microscopy. B. Myofibrillar (myosin) ATPase. Type I fibers are pale, at high (alkaline) pH; type II fibers are dark. Note the intermixture of fiber types.

HISTOCHEMISTRY

Application of enzyme histochemical reactions to frozen tissue is helpful in the interpretation of pathological changes in muscle biopsy specimens.

NONSPECIFIC ESTERASE: With this stain, type I fibers are slightly darker than type II fibers. The nonspecific esterase reaction is important in identifying denervation atrophy, because many of the atrophic denervated fibers are selectively stained, whether they are type I or type II (see Fig. 27-23). Macrophages are also intensively stained by this reaction, as are motor endplates, owing to their acetylcholine esterase activity.

NADH-TETRAZOLIUM REDUCTASE: The reaction product in the NADH–tetrazolium reductase (NADH-TR) reaction is reduced tetrazolium (formazan), which appears as a dark precipitate. Myofibrils are outlined as unstained areas. Because type I fibers have many mitochondria, they appear dark with this stain. The NADH-TR stain does not distinguish the two fiber types as clearly as does the ATPase reaction. In addition, the identity of the fiber type is often not maintained in pathological states. Abnormal collections of mitochondria are darkly stained in primary mitochondrial disorders. Also, excessive staining occurs in atrophic fibers as a result of denervation, whether they were originally type I or type II. Target fibers characteristic of denervation are best recognized with this stain (see Fig. 27-24).

SUCCINATE DEHYDROGENASE (SDH): SDH reduces tetrazolium in the presence of the substrate, succinate, and the staining pattern closely resembles that of NADH-TR. This stain is the most sensitive histochemical index of mitochondrial proliferation caused by mutations of mtDNA, presumably because the genetic defect does not interfere with the electron carrier function (see Fig. 27-21B).

CYTOCHROME C OXIDASE: This histochemical reaction reduces diaminobenzidine in the presence of cytochrome c, producing a brownish color (see Fig. 27-21C).

ALKALINE PHOSPHATASE: Muscle fibers are normally unstained with the alkaline phosphatase reaction, but regenerating ones are selectively stained. Small blood vessels (probably arterioles) appear black. Cases of dermatomyositis often exhibit abnormal staining of the blood vessels in perifascicular and endomysial connective tissue, which can be a helpful sign of the inflammatory nature of the disease.

PERIODIC ACID–SCHIFF (PAS): The PAS reaction demonstrates the basement membrane of muscle fibers and capillaries. Within the fiber, most of the PAS-positive material is glycogen, a finely granular material distributed around the myofibrils throughout the fiber. The PAS stain is helpful in the diagnosis of glycogen-storage diseases.

OIL RED ORCEIN: This stain (in frozen tissue) marks neutral lipid and is particularly useful in the evaluation of lipid storage myopathies such as carnitine deficiency (see Fig. 27-20).

MODIFIED GOMORI TRICHROME STAIN: This stain is performed on frozen tissue and is the most versatile stain in evaluation of myopathies. Various inclusions and abnormalities are easily seen with this stain, including nemaline rods (see Fig. 27-11A), ragged red fibers in mitochondrial disorders (see Fig. 27-21A), and rimmed vacuoles in inclusion body myositis (see Fig. 27-14B).

MUSCLE BIOPSY

Since the normal muscle pattern is more constant within a specific muscle, it is advantageous to limit the biopsy to the same muscle from case to case. Samples from either the quadriceps femoris or the biceps brachii are suitable for biopsy in most primary muscle diseases (myopathies). Biopsy of the gastrocnemius muscle and the sural nerve is often performed in patients with a suspected peripheral neuropathy. However, some neuromuscular conditions are more focal, and judgment must be exercised accordingly.

Biopsy sampling from a moderately involved muscle is the most informative. Unaffected muscles may have little or no pathological changes, whereas a severely weak muscle may be largely replaced by adipose and fibrous connective tissue (see end-stage muscle, Fig. 27-5).

GENERAL PATHOLOGICAL REACTIONS

Necrosis is a common response of myofibers to injury in primary muscle diseases (myopathies). Widespread acute necrosis of skeletal muscle fibers *(rhabdomyolysis)* releases cytosolic proteins, including myoglobin, into the circulation, an event that may result in myoglobinuria and acute renal failure. In many human myopathies, necrosis occurs in a segment along the length of the fiber, leaving two intact portions that flank the site of damage (Fig. 27-4). The injury quickly elicits two responses: an influx of blood-borne macrophages into the necrotic cytoplasm and activation of the satellite cells, a population of dormant myoblasts located in close proximity to each fiber. As the monocytes gradually phagocytose the necrotic debris and remove it, the satellite cells become active myoblasts and proliferate. Within 2 days, they begin to fuse, both to each other and to the ends of the intact fiber remnants, to form a joining multinucleated segment. This regenerating fiber is smaller in diameter than the parent fiber, and it has basophilic cytoplasm and large, vesicular nuclei with prominent nucleoli.

Regeneration can restore normal structure and function of muscle fibers within a few weeks after a single episode of injury, as in the inherited disorder myophosphorylase deficiency (see below). With subacute or chronic disorders, fiber necrosis proceeds concurrently with fiber regeneration, gradually leading to atrophy of muscle fibers and fibrosis.

MUSCULAR DYSTROPHY

In the middle of the 19th century, physicians discovered that progressive weakness of the voluntary muscles could

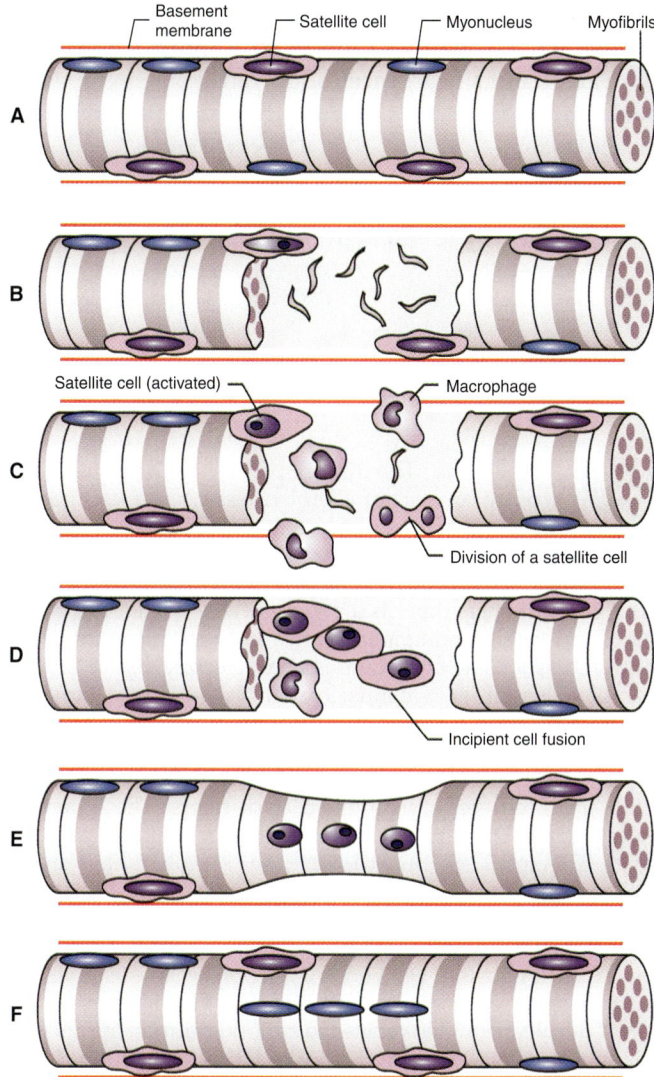

FIGURE 27-4
Segmental necrosis and regeneration of a muscle fiber. A. A normal muscle fiber contains myofibrils and subsarcolemmal nuclei and is covered by a basement membrane. Scattered satellite cells are situated on the surface of the sarcolemma, inside the basement membrane. These cells are dormant myoblasts, capable of proliferating and fusing to form differentiated fibers. They constitute 3 to 5% of the nuclei, as observed in a cross-section of skeletal muscle. B. In many muscle diseases (e.g., Duchenne muscular dystrophy or polymyositis), injury to the muscle fiber causes segmental necrosis with disintegration of the sarcoplasm, leaving a preserved basement membrane and nerve supply (not shown). C. The damaged segment attracts circulating macrophages that penetrate the basement membrane and begin to digest and engulf the sarcoplasmic contents (myophagocytosis). Regenerative processes begin with the activation and proliferation of the satellite cells, forming myoblasts within the basement membrane. Macrophages gradually leave the site of injury with their load of debris. D. At a later stage, the myoblasts are aligned in close proximity to each other in the center of the fiber and begin to fuse. E. Regeneration of the fiber segment is prominent, as indicated by the large, pale, vesicular, centrally located nuclei. F. The fiber is nearly normal except for a few persistent central nuclei. Eventually, the normal state (A) is restored.

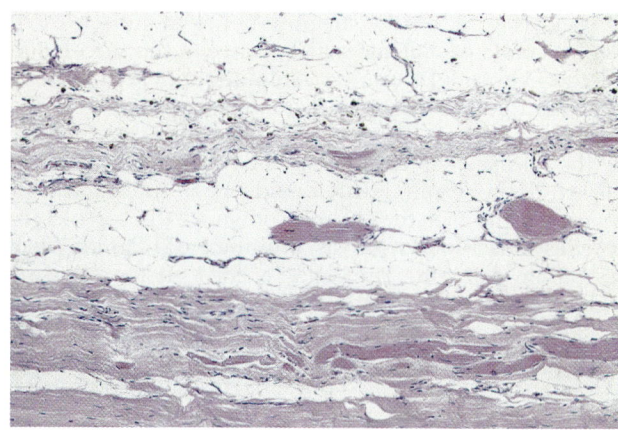

FIGURE 27-5
End-stage neuromuscular disease. In this section of the deltoid muscle stained by hematoxylin and eosin, skeletal muscle has been largely replaced by fibrofatty connective tissue. The few surviving muscle fibers have a deeper eosinophilia than does the abundant collagenous component.

be caused by either a disorder of the nervous system or primary degeneration of muscles. *Muscular dystrophy* was the name applied to primary muscular degeneration. It was frequently found to be hereditary (or at least familial) and relentlessly progressive. Morphological study of muscle tissue from these patients showed necrosis of muscle fibers, with regenerative activity, progressive fibrosis, and infiltration of the muscle with fatty tissue (Fig. 27-5). Little or no inflammation was recognized. In subsequent years, numerous variants of this type of muscle disease were described, and a classification of hereditary, progressive, noninflammatory degenerative conditions of muscle has evolved.

Duchenne and Becker Muscular Dystrophies Are Inherited Noninflammatory Myopathies

Duchenne muscular dystrophy is a severe, progressive, X-linked, inherited condition characterized by progressive degeneration of muscles, particularly those of the pelvic and shoulder girdles. It is the most common noninflammatory myopathy in children. A milder form of the disease is known as *Becker muscular dystrophy* (see Chapter 6 for the molecular genetics of both diseases). The serum creatine kinase activity is greatly increased in both conditions.

 Pathogenesis: Duchenne muscular dystrophy is caused by mutations of a large gene on the short arm of the X chromosome (Xp21). This gene codes for *dystrophin*, a 427-kd protein localized on the inner surface of the sarcolemma. Dystrophin links the subsarcolemmal cytoskeleton to the exterior of the cell through a transmembrane complex of proteins and glycoproteins that binds to laminin. Dystrophin is absent or greatly reduced in amount, often as a result of deletions of the gene (Fig. 27-6). Dystrophin-deficient muscle fibers thus lack the normal interaction between the sarcolemma and the extracellular matrix. This disruption may be responsible for the observed increased osmotic fragility of dystrophic muscle, the excessive influx of calcium ions, and the release of soluble muscle enzymes such as creatine kinase into the serum. Further evidence to support this hypothesis is the fact that a breakdown of the sarcolemma precedes muscle cell necrosis, and the basal lamina seems to separate from the sarcolemma early in the course of Duchenne muscular dystrophy.

Becker muscular dystrophy is allelic to Duchenne dystrophy, and mutations of the genes produce an altered dystrophin, usually a truncated protein. This mutated protein is localized to the surface membrane of muscle fibers, but the immunocytochemical staining is often less intense or focally absent (see Fig. 27-6). The abnormal protein apparently retains sufficient function to yield a less severe phenotype. Other muscle diseases closely resemble Duchenne and Becker dystrophies but are inherited in a recessive autosomal fashion. Some of these patients have mutations that affect the expression of transmembrane proteins or glycoproteins and interrupt the link between the cytoskeleton and extracellular matrix (Table 27-1)

TABLE 27-1 **Muscular Dystrophies and Congenital Myopathies Caused by Abnormalities in the Sarcolemma or Extracellular Matrix**

Muscle Disease	Defective Proteins
Sarcoglycanopathies	Sarcoglycans α–ε (muscle fiber plasma membrane proteins)
Dysferlinopathies (Limb girdle and Miyoshi myopathy)	Dysferlin (muscle fiber plasma membrane protein)
Caveolinopathies (hereditary rippling muscle disorder, RMD)	Caveolin-3 (muscle fiber plasma membrane protein)

 Pathology: The disease process in Duchenne dystrophy consists of (1) relentless necrosis of muscle fibers, (2) a continuous effort at repair and regeneration, and (3) progressive fibrosis. The degenerative process eventually outstrips the regenerative capacity of the muscle. As a consequence, there is a progressively decreasing number of muscle fibers and increasing amounts of fibrofatty connective tissue. The end stage is characterized by an almost complete loss of skeletal muscle fibers, but relative sparing of the muscle spindle fibers (intrafusal fibers) (see Fig. 27-5).

In the early stage of the disease, necrotic fibers and regenerating fibers tend to occur in small groups, together with scattered, large, hyalinized dark fibers. The latter are overly contracted and are thought to precede fiber necrosis (Figs. 27-7 and 27-8). Breakdown of the sarcolemma is one of the earliest ultrastructural changes. Macrophages invade necrotic fibers and reflect a scavenging function rather than an inflammatory process.

The diagnosis of Duchenne dystrophy can be established by polymerase chain reaction (PCR) analysis of genomic DNA derived from leukocytes in a blood sample. In practice, diagnosis using this method is limited to large deletions of the gene. About 30% of the patients have small rearrangements or point mutations of the gene, and they can be evaluated by muscle biopsy, which shows little or no detectable dystrophin by immunoblot or immunocytochemical staining.

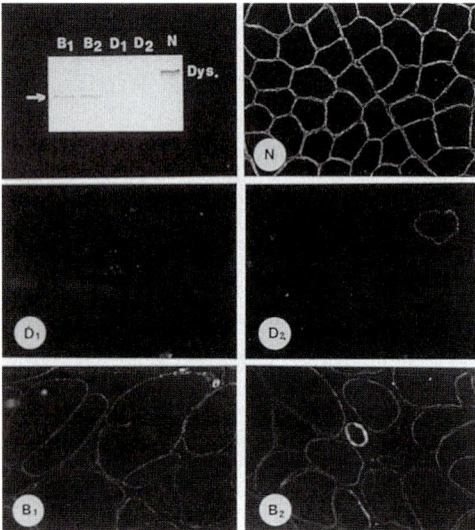

FIGURE 27-6
Dystrophin analysis in Duchenne and Becker muscular dystrophies. Immunofluorescence stain for dystrophin. The sections illustrate a normal subject *(N)*, two patients with Duchenne dystrophy *(D)*, and two with Becker dystrophy *(B)*. Dystrophin is normally concentrated at the surface membrane of every muscle fiber, but in Duchenne dystrophy, the protein is absent or is only barely detected in a small proportion of muscle fibers. Becker dystrophy exhibits hypertrophic muscle fibers with reduced expression of dystrophin. The immunoblot *(upper left)* of normal muscle shows a band near the top of the gel corresponding to the 427-kd protein dystrophin. Dystrophin is undetectable in Duchenne dystrophy. In Becker dystrophy, a weaker band has migrated farther down the gel relative to the normal protein, and it corresponds to a smaller, truncated protein. The combined analysis (immunolocalization and immunoblot) of the dystrophin protein is diagnostic of this group of dystrophies (dystrophinopathies).

 Clinical Features: Boys with Duchenne muscular dystrophy have markedly increased serum creatine kinase levels from birth and morphologically abnormal muscle even in utero. Clinical weakness is not detectable during the first year, but usually becomes so by the age of 3 or 4 years. The weakness is noted mainly around the pelvic and shoulder girdles (proximal muscle weakness) and is relentlessly progressive. "Pseudohypertrophy" (enlargement of a muscle due to abundant replacement of muscle fibers by fibroadipose tissue) of the calf muscles eventually develops. Patients are usually wheelchair bound by the age of 10 years and bedridden by 15 years. The most common causes of death are complications of respiratory insufficiency caused by muscular weakness or cardiac arrhythmia owing to myocardial involvement. Other extraskeletal manifestations include gastrointestinal dysfunction (due to degeneration of smooth muscle) and intellectual impairment. Many boys affected with Duchenne dystrophy exhibit variable degrees of mental retardation, apparently due to the lack of dystrophin in the central nervous system.

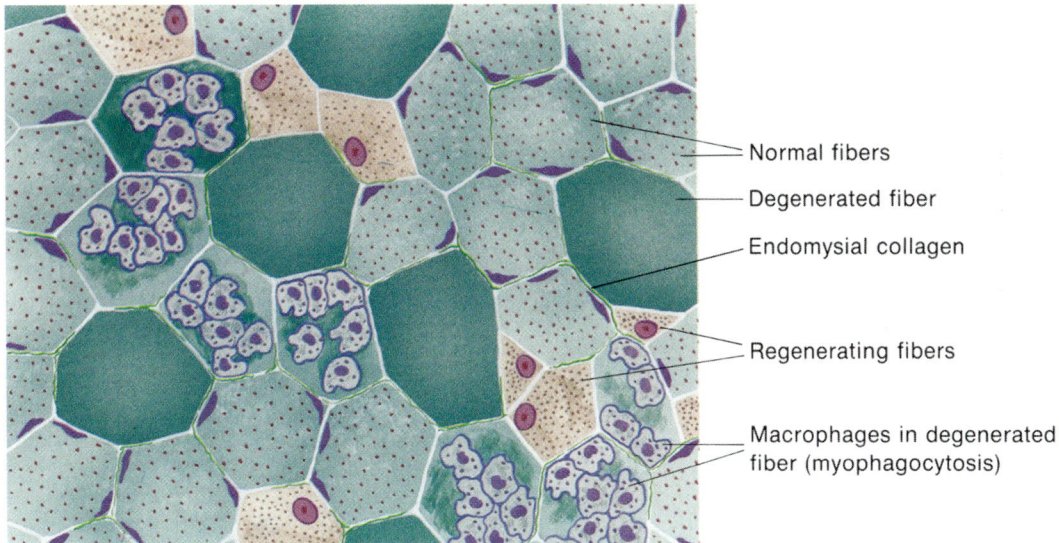

FIGURE 27-7
Duchenne muscular dystrophy. The pathological changes in skeletal muscle are illustrated by staining with the modified Gomori trichrome stain. Some fibers are slightly larger and darker than normal. These represent overcontracted segments of sarcoplasm situated between degenerated segments. Other fibers are packed with macrophages (myophagocytosis), which remove degenerated sarcoplasm. Other fibers are smaller than normal and have granular sarcoplasm. These fibers have enlarged, vesicular nuclei with prominent nucleoli and represent regenerating fibers. Developing endomysial fibrosis is represented by the deposition of collagen around individual muscle fibers. The changes are those of a chronic, active noninflammatory myopathy.

Occasional cases that are indistinguishable from Duchenne muscular dystrophy occur in girls. These patients represent a genetically different disease or nonrandom inactivation of the X chromosome.

CARRIER DETECTION: Because Duchenne muscular dystrophy is inherited as an X-linked recessive disease, the condition is passed from a mother who is a heterozygous carrier of the abnormal gene. Alternatively, the disease can stem from a spontaneous somatic mutation of the gene, which occurs at a high rate and accounts for 30% of cases. Until recently, the best method of detecting carriers was multiple determinations of serum creatine kinase levels, which are moderately increased in 75% of heterozygotes. There is

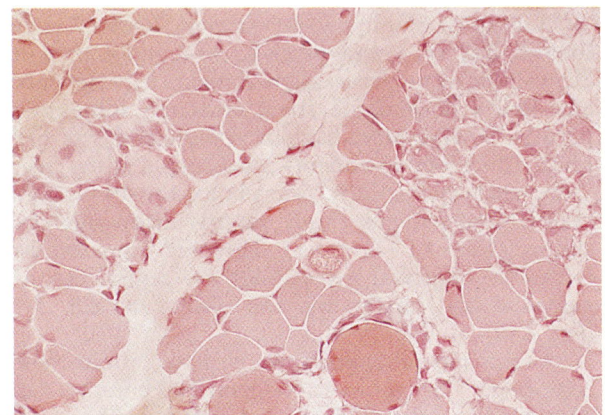 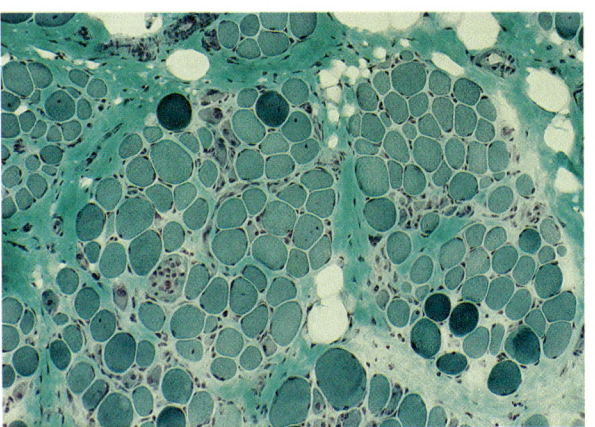

FIGURE 27-8
Duchenne muscular dystrophy. A. Hematoxylin and eosin stain. A section of vastus lateralis muscle shows necrotic muscle fibers, some of them invaded by macrophages. The endomysial septa are thickened, indicating fibrosis. B. Modified Gomori trichrome stain. A similar section demonstrates dark-staining enlarged fibers, which represent overly contracted fibers. Calcium influx across the defective surface membrane overwhelms mechanisms that maintain a low resting Ca^{2+} concentration and triggers excessive contraction. There is conspicuous perimysial and endomysial fibrosis.

considerable variability in the expression of the carrier state, probably because of variations in the random inactivation of the X chromosome. Some carriers can now be detected by dystrophin immunolocalization performed on a muscle biopsy specimen. This procedure shows a characteristic mosaic pattern of deficient and normal myofibers. Molecular probes detect more than two thirds of persons who carry large deletions.

Myotonic Dystrophy Is Characterized by Impaired Muscle Relaxation

Myotonic dystrophy, the most common form of adult muscular dystrophy, is an autosomal dominant disorder characterized by slowing muscle relaxation (myotonia) and progressive muscle weakness and wasting. The prevalence has been estimated to be as high as 14 per 100,000, although it may be higher because of the difficulty in detecting minimally affected persons. The age at onset and severity of symptoms show extreme variations. Myotonic dystrophy can be separated into two clinical groups: adult onset and congenital.

Pathogenesis: The gene for myotonic dystrophy has been localized to the long arm of chromosome 19 (19q13.3), and most cases seem to be descended from one original mutation. This mutation is the expansion of a CTG repeat near the 3′ end of the gene. Normal persons have fewer than 30 copies of this trinucleotide repeat, whereas it is present in 50 copies or more in minimally affected patients with myotonic dystrophy. An interesting genetic characteristic of this disease is the phenomenon of *anticipation* (i.e., an earlier age at onset and increasing severity of symptoms in successive generations). The number of trinucleotide repeats increases with successive generations, and the size of the repeat sequence correlates with the severity of symptoms. The gene for myotonic dystrophy encodes a novel serine–threonine protein kinase. The mechanism of injury brought about by the expansion of CTG repeats in myotonic dystrophy, as in other trinucleotide repeat disorders, is not clearly understood at present (see Chapter 1).

Pathology: The pathological changes of adult myotonic dystrophy are highly variable, even in muscles from the same patient. Most patients display atrophy of type I fibers and hypertrophy of type II fibers. Internally situated nuclei are a constant feature. The ATPase reaction shows many ring fibers, in which there is a circumferential concentration of heavily stained sarcoplasm. Necrosis and regeneration, although occasionally present, are not prominent (as they are in Duchenne muscular dystrophy).

The muscle of congenital myotonic dystrophy shows myofiber atrophy, frequent central nuclei, and failure of fiber differentiation. These pathological features closely resemble those of the X-linked recessive type of myotubular myopathy (see below).

Clinical Features: In addition to skeletal muscle, myotonic dystrophy affects many systems, including the heart, smooth muscle, central nervous system, endocrine glands, and eye. The diagnosis is based on clinical features, the family history, and the characteristic electromyography, which exhibits myotonic discharges. The demonstration of an expanded trinucleotide repeat is predictive in utero and can be diagnostic in patients.

Adult myotonic dystrophy features slowly progressive muscle weakness and stiffness, principally in the distal limbs. The facial and jaw muscles are virtually always affected, and ptosis can be severe. Extramuscular features of myotonic dystrophy are sometimes present and include cataracts, testicular atrophy with diminished fertility, and variable degrees of personality deterioration. A few patients exhibit involvement of smooth muscle, with disorders of the gastrointestinal tract, gallbladder, and uterus. Cardiac arrhythmias and, less commonly, cardiomyopathy have been reported.

Congenital myotonic dystrophy is seen only in the offspring of women who themselves exhibit symptoms of myotonic dystrophy. The infants are born with severe muscle weakness, but myotonia is inconspicuous or absent, although it appears in later childhood. A significant number of these patients suffer mental retardation.

CONGENITAL MYOPATHIES

Occasionally, a newborn manifests generalized hypotonia, with decreased deep tendon reflexes and muscle bulk. Many of these children have a difficult perinatal period because of weak respiration and consequent pulmonary complications. Some have "malignant" hypotonia, which is progressive and results in death within the first 12 months of life. *Werdnig-Hoffman disease* and *infantile acid maltase deficiency* (*Pompe disease*) are examples.

Other hypotonic patients have a "benign" course. Although the hypotonia persists throughout their lives, it shows little or no progression. Patients become ambulatory and live a normal life span, although sometimes complicated by secondary skeletal complications of the hypotonia. This group of patients is subsumed in the category of "congenital myopathies." Morphological study of the muscle of these patients rarely reveals distinctive structural abnormalities of myofibers. Three of the most common forms of congenital myopathies are central core disease, nemaline (rod) myopathy, and central nuclear myopathy (Fig. 27-9).

Some generalizations can be made about these three conditions. They all have congenital hypotonia, decreased deep tendon reflexes, decreased muscle bulk, and delayed motor milestones. In addition, the morphological abnormality expressed in the muscle biopsy specimen in all three conditions is usually limited to type I (red) fibers. Furthermore, these patients often have an abnormal predominance of type I fibers or possibly, a failure to develop type II (white) fibers. The skeletal muscle does not show signs of active myofiber necrosis or fibrosis, and patients do not have increased serum creatine kinase activity.

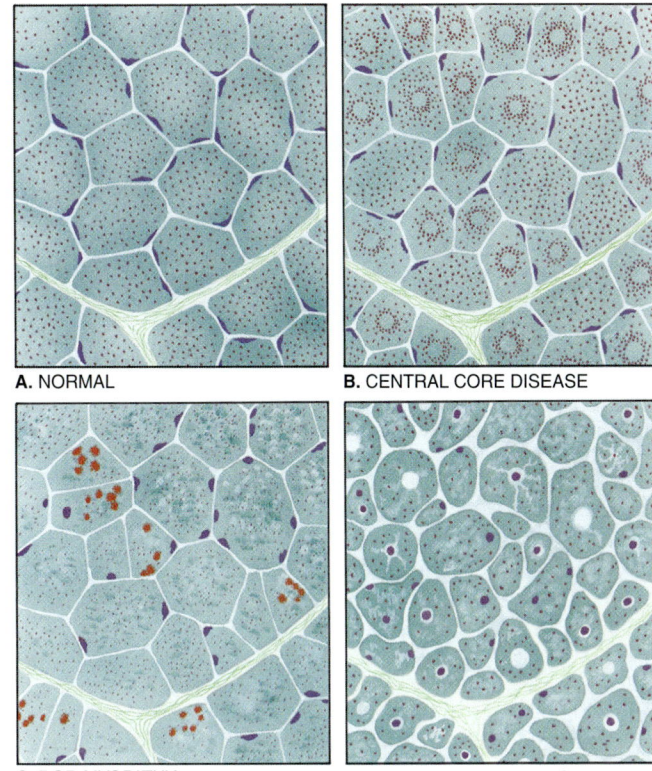

FIGURE 27-9

Congenital myopathies. **A. Normal.** A frozen section of normal skeletal muscle stained with modified Gomori trichrome is depicted. The nuclei are *purple*, the membranous organelles (mitochondria and sarcoplasmic reticulum) are *red*, myofibrils are *light green*, and perifascicular collagen is *light green*. The fibers are of uniform size and somewhat polygonal. **B. Central core myopathy.** Many type I fibers are slightly smaller than normal and contain a round central core that runs the length of the muscle fiber. The core is devoid of membranous organelles and is surrounded by a condensed ring. "Core fibers" resemble target fibers (see Fig. 27-24), although no neuropathic process has yet been demonstrated in central core disease. **C. Rod (nemaline) myopathy.** Many type I fibers are slightly smaller than normal and contain reddish aggregates of rods. In transverse section, many of the rods appear as granules because they are oriented in parallel to the longitudinal axis of the fiber. **D. Central nuclear myopathy (myotubular myopathy).** Many type I fibers are smaller and rounder than normal. Some contain a single, central nucleus, whereas others contain a round central pale zone, representing the zone between adjacent longitudinally arranged nuclei. These fibers resemble the myotube stage during embryonic development of skeletal muscle.

Central Core Disease Exhibits Congenital Muscle Weakness

Central core disease is an autosomal dominant condition characterized by congenital hypotonia, with proximal muscle weakness, decreased deep tendon reflexes, and delayed motor development. The disease has been traced to a mutation on the long arm of chromosome 19 (19q13.1) that codes for the ryanodine receptor, the calcium-release channel of the sarcoplasmic reticulum. Occasional cases are sporadic or show autosomal recessive inheritance. The typical patient becomes ambulatory, although muscle strength never develops to a normal level.

 Pathology: Muscle biopsy reveals a striking predominance of type I fibers. Many or all of these fibers display a central zone of degeneration that exhibits a loss of staining in the NADH-TR reaction (Fig. 27-10B). This central core abnormality extends throughout the entire length of the fiber. The central core is difficult to see with the hematoxylin and eosin stain (see Fig. 27-10A) but can often be demonstrated with the PAS reaction. By electron microscopy, the central core is characterized by a loss of mitochondria and other membranous organelles, with or without disorganization of the myofibrils. Membranous organelles tend to condense around the margin of the central core. The structure of the periphery of the fiber is otherwise unremarkable.

The central core anomaly bears a striking resemblance to the target fibers seen in active denervating conditions (see Fig. 27-24), although there is no evidence of denervation. The motor endplates are architecturally unremarkable, and no extrajunctional nicotinic acetylcholine receptors are present in the muscle membrane.

Mutations of the ryanodine receptor gene also cause one form of *malignant hyperthermia,* a potentially fatal disorder triggered by the use of anesthesia for surgery. Both central core disease and this adverse response to anesthesia coexist in some patients.

Rod (Nemaline) Myopathy Displays Inclusions That Derive from the Z Band

Rod myopathy includes a heterogeneous group of diseases that have in common the accumulation of rodlike inclusions within the sarcoplasm of skeletal muscle. The disease was initially named "nemaline" myopathy because the inclusions within the muscle fiber were interpreted as a tangled, threadlike mass. In reality, they are clusters of rod-shaped structures.

The classic congenital form of rod myopathy is characterized by congenital hypotonia and delayed motor milestones of variable clinical severity, with associated secondary skeletal changes such as kyphoscoliosis. Some patients exhibit severe involvement of muscles of the face, pharynx, and neck. Later-onset (childhood and adult) forms tend to be associated with some muscle degeneration, increased serum creatine kinase levels, and a slowly progressive course. A few patients originally designated as having limb girdle muscular dystrophy have eventually been found to have rod myopathy. The cause of the condition is unknown, and inheritance seems to be either autosomal dominant or autoso-

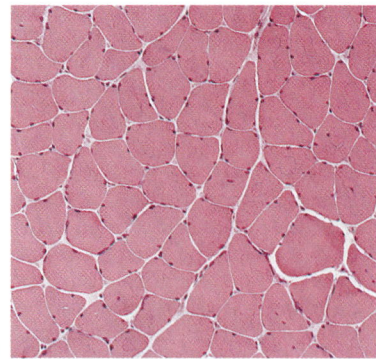
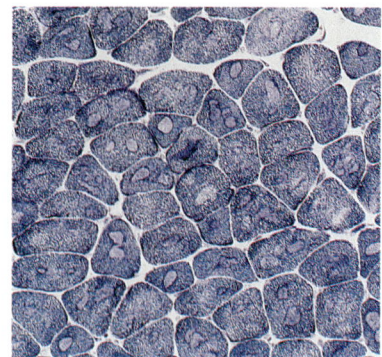

FIGURE 27-10
Central core disease. A. Hematoxylin and eosin stain. A section of vastus lateralis muscle appears nearly normal. B. Stained for NADH-tetrazolium reductase, the same muscle shows a distinct circular zone of pallor in the center of most muscle fibers. A thin zone of excessive staining surrounds the core lesion. All of the myofibers in this case were type I, as demonstrated by the myofibrillar ATPase stain (not shown). Note the close resemblance of the core lesions to the target formations found in the muscle fibers of neurogenic disorders (see Fig. 27-24).

mal recessive. The genes responsible for rod myopathy so far identified include slow α-tropomyosin, nebulin, skeletal muscle α-actin, β-tropomyosin, and slow troponin T. Mutations in the ryanodine receptor gene have also been associated with nemaline rod formation.

Pathology: The findings on muscle biopsy consist of a variable predominance of type I fibers and the accumulation of rod-shaped structures within their sarcoplasm. The aggregates of these inclusions are often located in subsarcolemmal regions near nuclei. They are brilliant red to dark red when stained with the modified Gomori trichrome stain (see Figs. 27-9 and 27-11A) and may or may not be visible with hematoxylin and eosin. The rods are almost always positive with the phosphotungstic acid hematoxylin (PTAH) stain and are negative with the ATPase and NADH-TR reactions. Ultrastructural studies demonstrate that the inclusions are indeed rod shaped and arise from the Z band, which they resemble ultrastructurally (Fig. 27-11B).

Rods have been described in a variety of neuromuscular diseases, including denervation atrophy, muscular dystrophy, and inflammatory myopathies. Experimental tenotomy (cutting a tendon) induces formation of rods in the muscle when the nerve supply remains intact. In rod myopathy, however, the inclusions constitute the predominant pathological change.

Central Nuclear Myopathy (Myotubular Myopathy) Resembles the Myotubular Stage of Embryogenesis

Central nuclear myopathy (myotubular myopathy) refers to a group of clinically and genetically heterogeneous inherited conditions that have in common the presence of a centrally located nucleus in skeletal muscle cells. Autosomal recessive, autosomal dominant, and X-linked recessive (Xq28) varieties have been recognized. In X-linked inheritance, the newborn is strikingly weak and hypotonic and may die of respiratory insufficiency during the neonatal period. The autosomal dominant form tends to be of later onset and is associated with modestly increased serum creatine kinase levels. It has a slowly progressive course and, like rod myopathy, resembles the so-called limb girdle muscular dystrophy syndrome. Some patients exhibit a striking involvement of the facial and extraocular musculature.

Pathology: Biopsy specimens from patients with central nuclear myopathy are variable, but are characterized by type I fiber predominance (Fig. 27-12). Many of these fibers are small and round, with a single central nucleus, accounting for the name of the disease. In this respect, they resemble the myotubular stage in the embryogenesis of skeletal muscle. This apparent immature state suggests a possible defect in the nerve supply to the muscle fiber, because the lower motor neuron requires subsequent maturation of the fiber. However, studies of the lower motor neuron, including the motor endplate, have failed to demonstrate any abnormality in these patients. Mutations of a gene for a tyrosine phosphatase cause the X-linked form of myotubular myopathy.

The later-onset forms of myotubular myopathy are characterized morphologically by more-mature muscle fibers, in which the fibers are larger, have more numerous myofibrils, and display single central nuclei that appear more mature.

INFLAMMATORY MYOPATHIES

The inflammatory myopathies represent a heterogeneous group of acquired disorders, all of which feature symmetric proximal muscle

Inflammatory Myopathies

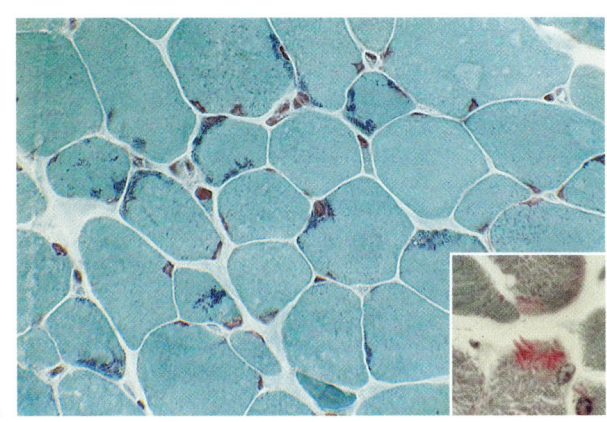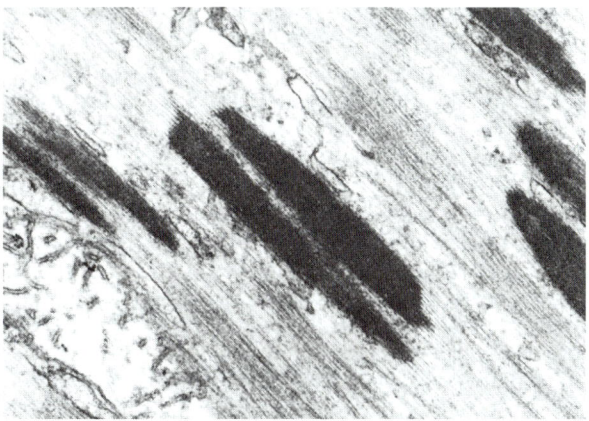

FIGURE 27-11
Rod (nemaline) myopathy. (*A*) Muscle fibers contain dark aggregates of rods and granules (modified Gomori trichrome stain). As shown in the inset, these rods tend to be located at the fiber periphery near nuclei. (*B*) An electron micrograph of the same biopsy shows that the structures are rod-shaped and are derived from the Z-disc.

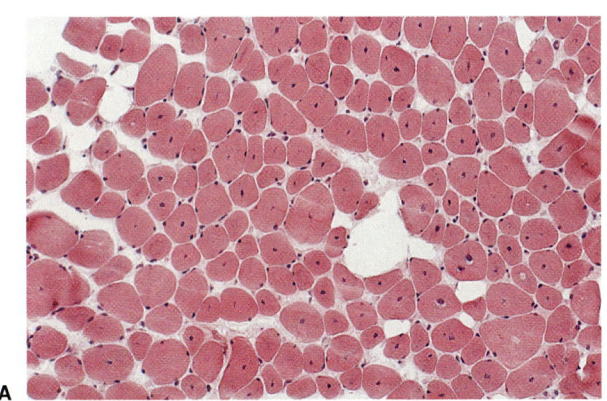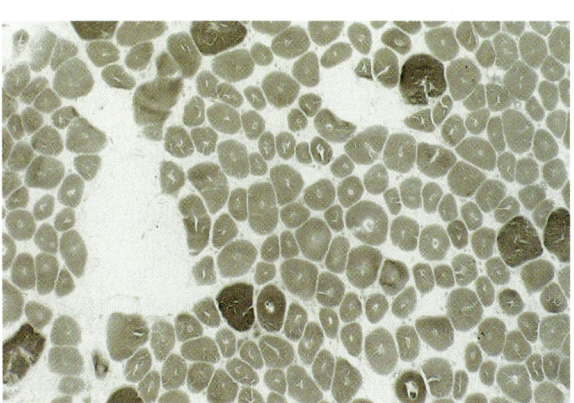

FIGURE 27-12
Central nuclear (myotubular) myopathy. A. Hematoxylin and eosin stain. Many muscle fibers contain a single central nucleus, and most of the affected muscle fibers are abnormally small. These fibers resemble the late myotube stage of fetal development of skeletal muscle. B. Myofibrillar (myosin) ATPase stain. The section demonstrates a type I phenotype in the fibers with central nuclei. It also illustrates type I fiber predominance, which is a general feature of congenital myopathies. C. Electron micrograph. Normal-appearing nuclei occupy the centers of muscle fibers in myotubular myopathy.

weakness, increased serum levels of muscle-derived enzymes, and nonsuppurative inflammation of skeletal muscle.

Inflammatory myopathies are uncommon, the annual incidence being 1 in 100,000. Dermatomyositis afflicts children and adults, whereas polymyositis almost always occurs after the age of 20 years. Both disorders occur more commonly in females than in males. By contrast the incidence of inclusion body myositis is three times greater in men than in women, and the disorder usually occurs after age 50 years.

The inflammatory myopathies are thought to have an autoimmune origin because of (1) their association with other autoimmune and connective tissues diseases, (2) pathological evidence of autoimmune mechanisms of muscle cell injury, (3) detection of autoantibodies in serum, and (4) a beneficial response to immunosuppressive agents in polymyositis and dermatomyositis (but not inclusion body myositis). No specific target autoantigens in muscle or blood vessels have been identified. The most common morphological characteristics in the inflammatory myopathies are (1) the presence of inflammatory cells, (2) necrosis and phagocytosis of muscle fibers, (3) a mixture of regenerating and atrophic fibers, and (4) fibrosis.

Clinical Features: All the inflammatory myopathies manifest as insidious proximal and symmetric muscle weakness, gradually increasing over a period of weeks to months. Patients have problems with simple activities that require the use of proximal muscles, including lifting objects, climbing steps, or combing hair. Dysphagia and difficulty in holding up the head reflect involvement of the pharyngeal and neck-flexor muscles. Some patients with inclusion body myositis have distal muscle weakness of the limbs that equals or exceeds that of proximal muscles. In advanced cases, the respiratory muscles may be affected. The weakness progresses over weeks or months and leads to severe muscular wasting.

Dermatomyositis is distinguished from the other myopathies by the presence of a characteristic rash on the upper eyelids, face, trunk, and occasionally other body surfaces. It may occur alone or in association with scleroderma, mixed connective tissue disease, or other autoimmune conditions. When dermatomyositis occurs in a middle-aged man, it is associated with an increased risk of epithelial cancer, most commonly carcinoma of the lung. By contrast, polymyositis and inclusion body myositis have only a chance association with malignancy.

Patients with inflammatory myopathies have increased serum creatine kinase and other muscle enzyme levels. Antinuclear and anticytoplasmic antibodies exist in all of these diseases, with specificity to several different antigens. Treatment of polymyositis and dermatomyositis with corticosteroids is usually successful, but inclusion body myositis is generally resistant to all therapy.

Polymyositis Features Muscle Damage Mediated by Cytotoxic T Cells

Pathogenesis: Polymyositis is thought to be related to direct muscle cell damage produced by cytotoxic T cells, and there is no evidence of a microangiopathy, such as that found in dermatomyositis (see below). In these disorders, healthy muscle fibers are initially surrounded by CD8+ T lymphocytes (Fig. 27-13) and macrophages, after which the muscle fibers degenerate. In contrast to normal muscle tissue, the affected muscles in polymyositis express MHC-I antigen on the sarcolemma. Because cytotoxic T cells attack antigenic targets in association with MHC-I molecules, these findings support an immunopathological basis for this disorder.

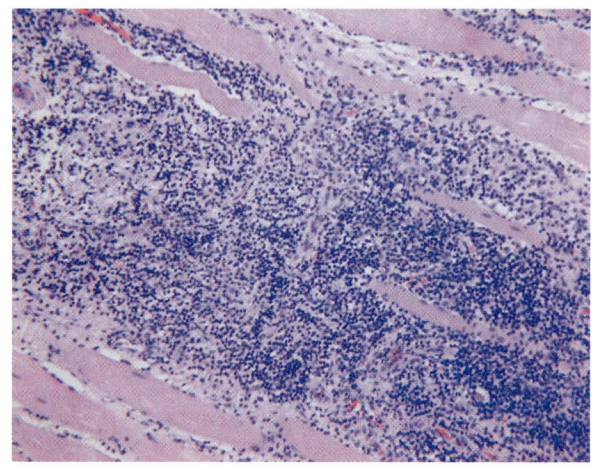 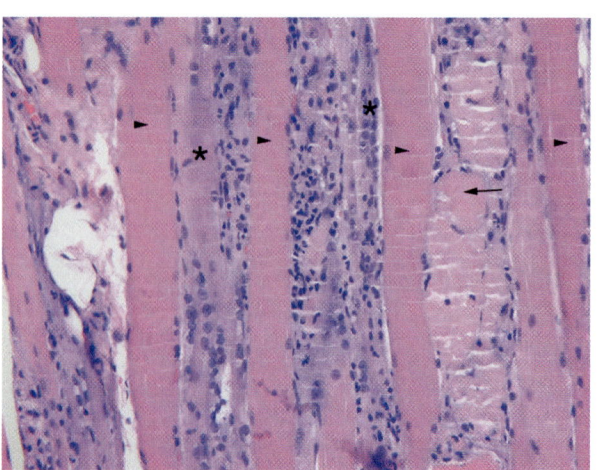

FIGURE 27-13

Polymyositis. A. Hematoxylin and eosin stain. A section of affected muscle shows an inflammatory myopathy. Mononuclear inflammatory cells infiltrate chiefly the endomysium. The field includes single-fiber necrosis. **B.** Region of healing inflammatory myopathy demonstrates intact fibers *(arrowheads)*, necrotic fibers *(arrow)*, and regenerating fibers characterized by enlarged nuclei and basophilic cytoplasm *(asterisk)*.

Inflammatory Myopathies

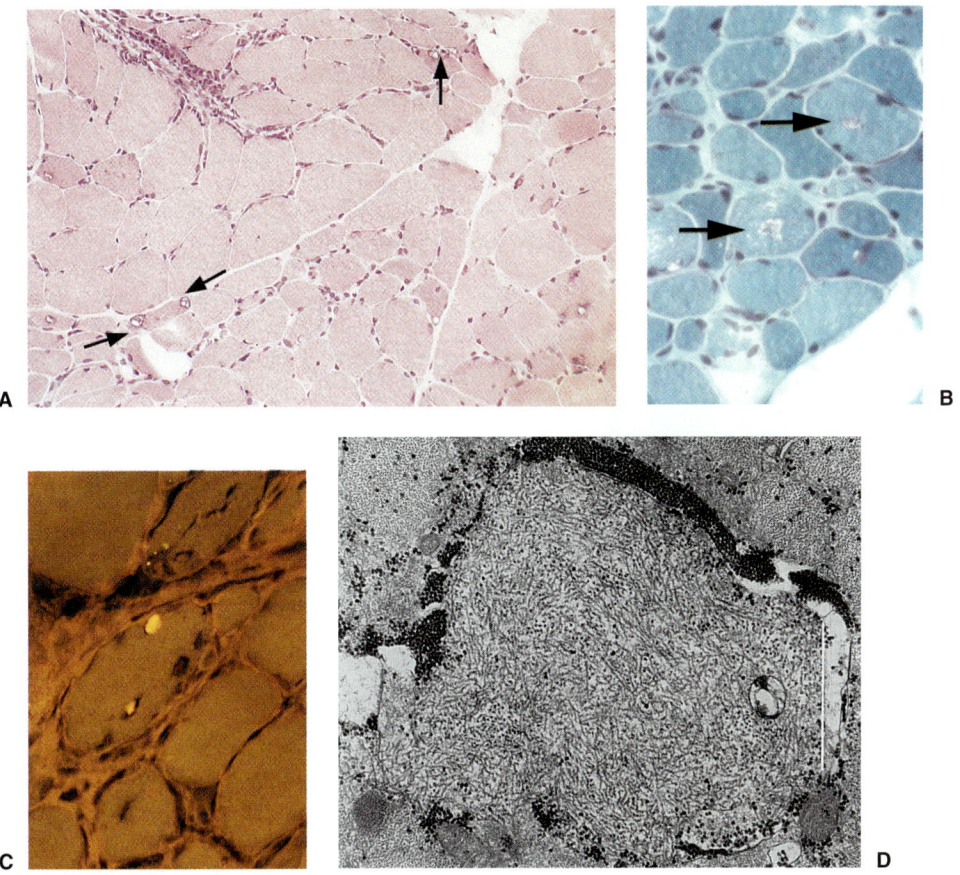

FIGURE 27-14
Inclusion body myositis (IBM). A. Hematoxylin and eosin stain. The features in IBM resemble those of polymyositis, but the muscle fibers also exhibit rimmed vacuoles *(arrows)* corresponding to enlarged lysosomes. The hyaline inclusions are sparse and difficult to visualize with this stain. B. Modified Gomori trichrome stain shows granular basophilic rimming of vacuoles. C. Congo red stain. The inclusion has weak congophilia, but the color signal is strong because it has been enhanced by fluorescence excitation. D. An electron micrograph shows the characteristic filaments of the amyloid inclusions.

The role of autoantibodies against nuclear antigens and cytoplasmic ribonucleoproteins in the pathogenesis of muscle injury is unknown. There is a frequent association between polymyositis and anti-Jo-1, an antibody against histidyl-tRNA synthetase, with the concomitant presence of interstitial lung disease, Raynaud phenomenon, and nonerosive arthritis.

Although viral infections may trigger polymyositis, muscle tissue has not yielded a virus on culture. An inflammatory myopathy indistinguishable from polymyositis occurs in many cases of human HIV-1 infection, but the role of the retrovirus is unclear.

 Pathology: Inflammatory cells infiltrate connective tissue mostly within the fascicles (i.e., endomysial inflammation) and invade apparently healthy muscle fibers (see Fig. 27-13). Angiopathy is absent. Isolated degenerating or regenerating fibers are scattered throughout fascicles. Perifascicular atrophy is not present in polymyositis (see below).

Inclusion Body Myositis Manifests Amyloid Deposits

The pathological features of inclusion body myositis resemble those of polymyositis and consist of single-fiber necrosis and regeneration with predominantly endomysial cytotoxic T cells. In addition, basophilic granular material is seen at the edge of slitlike vacuoles (rimmed vacuoles) within the muscle fibers. The fibers also contain small eosinophilic cytoplasmic inclusions, often located near the rimmed vacuoles (Fig. 27-14A and B). The inclusions are stained by Congo red and represent a form of intracellular amyloid (see Fig. 27-14C). The substance is immunoreactive for β-amyloid protein, the same type of amyloid present in the senile plaques of Alzheimer disease. The pathogenic significance of these inclusions is not understood. Small groups of angulated fibers are present. By electron microscopy, the granules of rimmed vacuoles contain membranous whorls. Distinctive filaments are found in the vicinity of the rimmed vacuoles (see Fig. 27-14D). The pathognomonic features of inclusion body myositis include the Congo red-positive inclusions and the characteristic filaments in the cytoplasm (or rarely in nuclei) of muscle fibers.

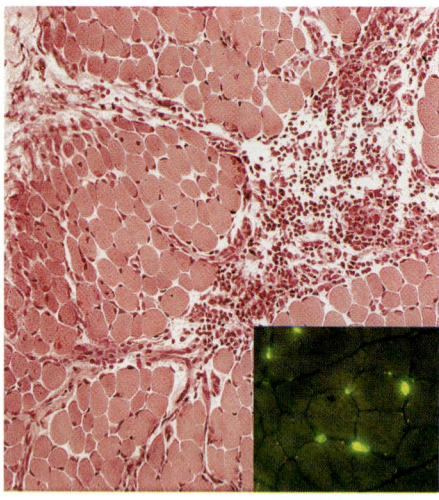

FIGURE 27-15
Dermatomyositis. Hematoxylin and eosin stain. The inflammatory cells infiltrate predominantly the perimysium rather than the endomysium. The periphery of muscle fascicles shows most of the muscle fiber atrophy and damage, resulting in a pattern of injury characteristic of dermatomyositis, termed *perifascicular atrophy*. Immunofluorescence *(inset)* reveals that the walls of many capillaries display C5b-9 (membrane attack complex), reflecting the altered microvasculature typical of dermatomyositis. A few small regenerating fibers are also stained by this method.

Dermatomyositis Is Caused by an Immune-Mediated Microangiopathy

 Pathogenesis: This myopathy is characterized by (1) immune complexes of IgG, IgM, and complement components, including membrane attack complement C5b-9 in the walls of capillaries and other blood vessels; (2) microangiopathy with loss of capillaries; (3) signs of injury and atrophy of myofibers; and (4) perivascular infiltrates of B cells and T cells with a predominantly CD4-helper phenotype (Fig. 27-15). These features suggest that muscle injury in dermatomyositis is produced primarily by complement-mediated cytotoxic antibodies directed against the microvasculature of skeletal muscle tissues. In fact, the presence of complement on the capillaries precedes inflammation or damage to the muscle fibers and is the most specific lesion of dermatomyositis. This microangiopathy is thought to lead to ischemic injury of individual muscle fibers and eventually to fiber atrophy. True infarcts may result from the involvement of larger intramuscular arteries. The rash, which clinically distinguishes dermatomyositis from the other types of inflammatory myopathies, is presumably related to the same microangiopathy.

 Pathology: Dermatomyositis features lymphoid infiltrates around blood vessels and in connective tissue of the perimysium (see Fig. 27-15). The infiltrates are composed of B cells and T cells, with a high ratio of helper cells (CD4$^+$) to cytotoxic/suppressor (CD8$^+$) T cells.

Immune complexes in the walls of blood vessels (see Fig. 27-15, inset) are associated with microangiopathy. The intramuscular blood vessels exhibit endothelial hyperplasia, fibrin thrombi, and obliteration of capillaries. Perifascicular atrophy consists of one or more layers of atrophic fibers located at the periphery of the fascicles. The combination of perifascicular atrophy and immune complexes in capillary walls is virtually diagnostic of dermatomyositis, even in the absence of inflammation. The abnormal staining of the endomysial connective tissue with the alkaline phosphatase reaction reflects damage to the blood vessels.

Granulomatous Myositis

Inflammatory myopathy can also occur in the setting of sarcoidosis. Whereas 60% of patients with sarcoidosis may have granulomas in their muscle tissue (Fig. 27-16), only a few patients display evidence of chronic myopathy with weakness and muscle wasting.

Vasculitis

Vasculitis can be present in skeletal muscle in the setting of periarteritis nodosa (PAN) (Fig. 27-17), Wegener granulomatosis, collagen vascular disease, and immune-mediated hypersensitivity states. In such instances, skeletal muscle may show neurogenic changes secondary to nerve damage.

MYASTHENIA GRAVIS

Myasthenia gravis is an acquired autoimmune disease characterized by abnormal muscular fatigability and caused by circulating antibodies to the acetylcholine (Ach) receptor at the myoneural junction. It occurs in all races and is twice as common in women as in

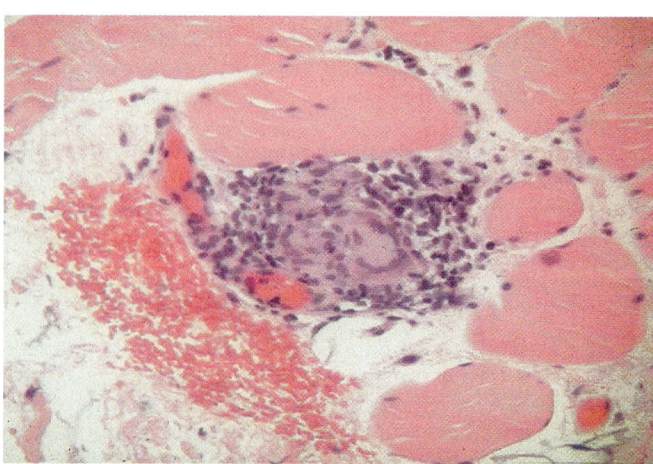

FIGURE 27-16
Sarcoid myopathy. Hematoxylin and eosin stain. Intramuscular granuloma with Langhans giant cell from a patient with sarcoidosis.

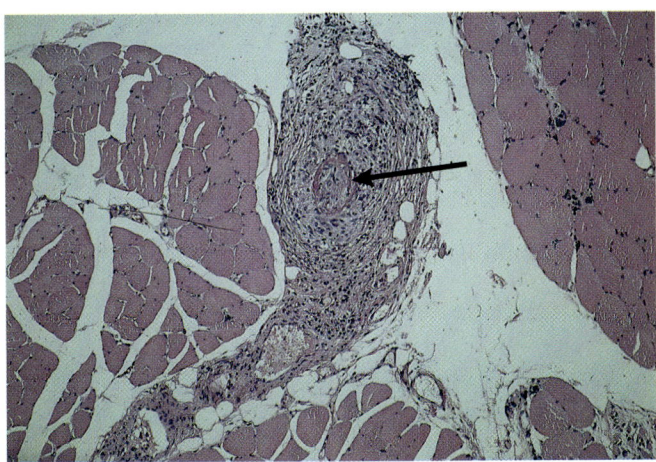

FIGURE 27-17
Periarteritis nodosa (PAN). Hematoxylin and eosin stain. PAN is one of the forms of necrotizing vasculitis that can affect skeletal muscle. Fibrinoid necrosis is present in a blood vessel wall *(arrow).*

men. The disease typically begins in young adults, but cases in children and the very old have also been described.

 Pathogenesis: Myasthenia gravis is mediated by an immunological attack on the Ach receptor of the motor endplate. Polyclonal antibodies attach to various epitopes of the receptor protein, thereby reducing the number of receptors.

In myasthenia gravis, the antigen–antibody complex binds complement components and produces shedding of the terminal portions of the folds of the neuromuscular junction, which are rich in Ach receptors. The IgG antibodies are bivalent and cross-link the receptor proteins remaining in the postsynaptic membrane. This effect increases the rate of endocytosis of the receptors, exceeding the muscle fiber's ability to replace them. The combination of a reduced area of the postsynaptic membrane, a decreased number of Ach receptors per unit area, and a widened synaptic space results in muscle weakness and abnormal fatigability. The antireceptor antibodies do not act by directly blocking binding of Ach to prevent neuromuscular transmission.

The thymus clearly plays an important role in the pathogenesis of myasthenia gravis. Up to 40% of patients have an associated thymoma, and surgical removal of the tumor is often curative. As many as 75% of the remaining patients have thymic hyperplasia, and in such cases, thymectomy is often an effective treatment. Ach receptors have been demonstrated on the surface of some thymic cells in both thymoma and thymic hyperplasia. Thus, there is evidence to suggest that in myasthenia gravis, thymic T lymphocytes activate B lymphocytes to produce antireceptor antibodies.

 Pathology: By light microscopy, the pathological changes in myasthenia gravis are not impressive. At best, a muscle biopsy may reveal atrophy of type II muscle fibers. Focal collections of lymphocytes may be present within the fascicles, particularly in autopsy tissue. By electron microscopy, most muscle endplates are abnormal, even in muscles that are not weakened. There is simplification of the sarcolemmal secondary folds, breakdown and loss of the crests of the folds, and widening of the clefts.

 Clinical Features: Patients with myasthenia gravis show considerable variation in the severity of the condition, and as in other autoimmune diseases, the symptoms tend to wax and wane. Weakness of the extraocular muscles is typically severe and causes ptosis and diplopia. In fact, myasthenia gravis may remain confined to these muscles. More frequently, the disease progresses to other muscles, such as those associated with swallowing, the trunk, and extremities. Patients with myasthenia gravis also have a high incidence of other autoimmune diseases.

The overall mortality of myasthenia gravis is about 10%, often owing to respiratory insufficiency because of muscle weakness. In addition to thymectomy, corticosteroid therapy, methotrexate, and anticholinesterase drugs are used alone or in combination. Plasmapheresis acts to reduce the titers of anti-Ach receptor antibodies and can ameliorate symptoms, but the clinical improvement is short-lived.

LAMBERT-EATON SYNDROME

Lambert-Eaton syndrome is a paraneoplastic disorder that manifests as muscular weakness, wasting, and fatigability of the proximal limbs and trunk. Also termed *myasthenic–myopathic syndrome,* the disease is usually associated with small cell carcinoma of the lung, although it may also occur in patients with other malignant diseases and rarely in the absence of an underlying malignancy. There is neurophysiological evidence for a defect in the release of acetylcholine at the nerve terminals. Like myasthenia gravis, the disease seems to have an autoimmune basis, because it can be transferred to mice by IgG from patients and it responds to treatment with corticosteroids. The pathogenic IgG autoantibodies recognize voltage-sensitive calcium channels that are expressed both in motor nerve terminals and in the cells of the lung cancer. The calcium channels, which are necessary for release of Ach, are greatly reduced in the presynaptic membrane in these patients, thereby interfering with neuromuscular transmission.

INHERITED METABOLIC DISEASES

Skeletal muscle is dramatically affected by a variety of endocrine and metabolic diseases, such as Cushing syndrome, Addison disease, hypothyroidism, hyperthyroidism, and conditions associated with hepatic or renal failure. In the following discussion, however, primary hereditary abnormalities in the metabolism of skeletal muscle result in abnormal muscular function.

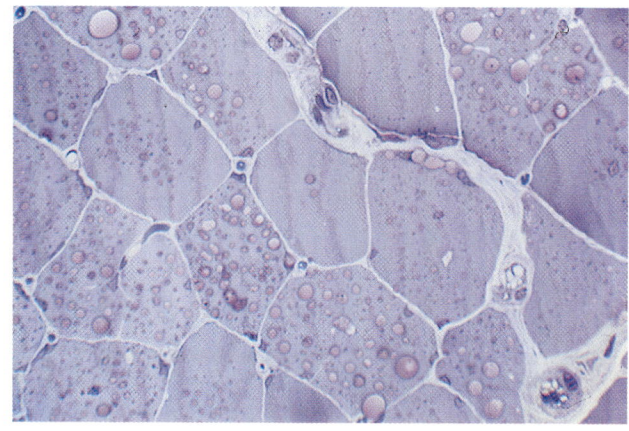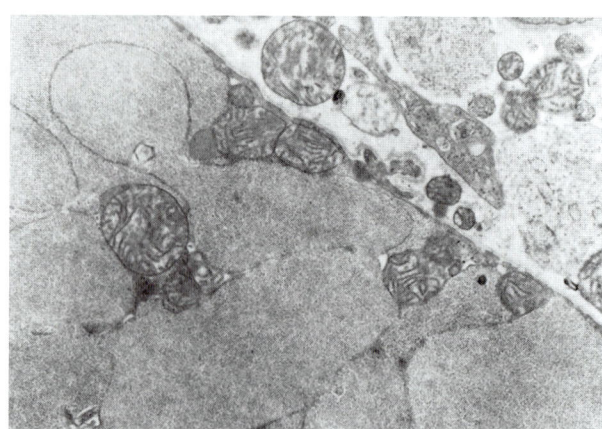

FIGURE 27-18
Acid maltase deficiency—adult onset. A. Semithin plastic section of muscle stained with toluidine blue. Vacuoles in muscle fibers contain metachromatic (slightly reddish) glycogen, which contrasts with the orthochromatic (bluish) staining of other structures. B. An electron micrograph shows an accumulation of glycogen particles within lysosomes.

Glycogen-storage diseases (Glycogenoses) Are Genetic Disorders That Produce Variable Effects on Muscle

Glycogen-storage diseases are autosomal recessive, inherited, metabolic disorders characterized by an inability to degrade glycogen (see Chapter 6).

Type II Glycogenosis (Acid Maltase Deficiency, α-1,4-Glucosidase Deficiency, Pompe Disease)

Various genetic mutations affect the acid maltase activity of muscle and lead to distinctly different clinical syndromes. Acid maltase is a lysosomal enzyme that is expressed in all cells and participates in the degradation of glycogen. When the enzyme is deficient, glycogen is not broken down, accumulates within lysosomes, and remains membrane bound (Fig. 27-18).

 Pathology: In all forms of glycogenosis due to acid maltase deficiency, the morphological changes are distinctive and almost pathognomonic (Fig. 27-18). The muscle in Pompe disease displays massive accumulation of membrane-bound glycogen and disappearance of the myofilaments and other sarcoplasmic organelles. Surprisingly, there is very little regeneration, and apparently inactive satellite cells are present on the surface of muscle fibers that have been almost completely destroyed by the disease process.

The pathological features of late infantile, juvenile, and adult-onset forms of type II glycogenosis are milder. The morphological changes range from an overt vacuolar myopathy demonstrated by routine histology to very subtle accumulation of membrane-bound glycogen particles detectable only by electron microscopy. Vacuoles observed by light microscopy are empty or they contain PAS-positive granular material that is removed by diastase, indicating that it is composed of glycogen.

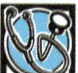 **Clinical Features:** The first acid maltase deficiency to be recognized, described by Pompe, is the most severe form and occurs in the neonatal or early infantile stage. These patients have severe hypotonia and areflexia and clinically resemble patients with Werdnig-Hoffmann disease (see below under Denervation). Sometimes the patients have an enlarged tongue and cardiomegaly and die of cardiac failure, usually within the first 2 years of life. Many tissues are affected, but the most significant involvement is in skeletal and cardiac muscle, the central nervous system (CNS), and the liver. The serum creatine kinase level is only slightly to moderately increased. Patients with later-onset forms of the disease have a mild, but relentlessly progressive, myopathy. Glycogen accumulates in other organs, but clinical expression of the disorder is usually limited to muscle.

Type III Glycogenosis (Debranching Enzyme Deficiency, Cori Disease, Limit Dextrinosis, Amylo-1,6-Glucosidase Deficiency)

Type III glycogenosis is a rare, autosomal recessive disease that affects children or adults. In these patients, phosphorylase hydrolyzes 1,4-glycosidic linkages of the terminal glucose chains of glycogen, but not beyond the site of a branch point, owing to the absence of the debranching enzyme. Glycogen without surface glucose chains is referred to as "limit dextrin." Hepatomegaly and growth retardation are usual. The muscle symptoms vary, and the most severe and consistent involvement is related to liver dysfunction in children. Rarely, these patients appear in adulthood with a slowly progressive myopathy. Electron microscopy reveals large masses of glycogen granules free in the sarcoplasm.

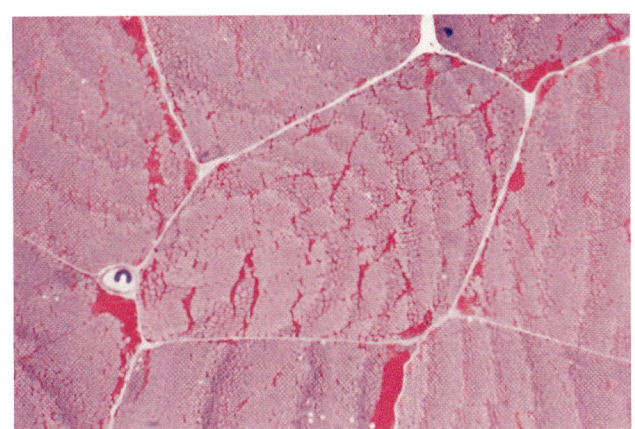
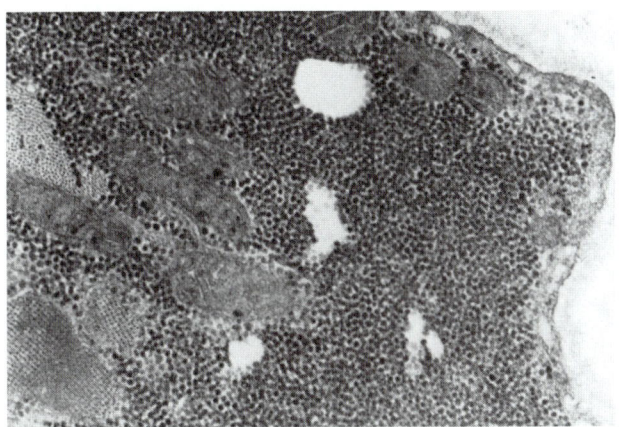

FIGURE 27-19
McArdle disease (myophosphorylase deficiency). **A.** Transverse semithin plastic section of muscle stained by periodic acid–Schiff (PAS) and toluidine blue. PAS-positive glycogen accumulates predominantly in the subsarcolemmal region. **B.** An electron micrograph demonstrates an abnormal mass of glycogen particles just beneath the sarcolemma. The glycogen is not surrounded by a membrane, in contrast to the lysosomal glycogen storage of acid maltase deficiency.

Type V Glycogenosis (McArdle Disease, Myophosphorylase Deficiency)

Type V glycogenosis is a more common metabolic myopathy that is usually not progressive or severely debilitating. The enzyme, myophosphorylase, is a tissue-specific protein of normal skeletal muscle. In the absence of enzyme activity, skeletal muscle glycogen cannot be cleaved at 1,4-glycosidic chains to produce glucose for energy production during periods of physical exertion. As a result, muscle cramps occur with exercise. The patient also cannot produce lactate during ischemic exercise, a defect that is the basis for a metabolic test for the condition.

Pathology: The tissue may appear completely normal, except for the absence of phosphorylase activity. However, there is usually evidence of subtle abnormal accumulation of glycogen granules within the sarcoplasm, predominantly within the subsarcolemmal area (Fig. 27-19). The specific diagnosis can be made by the histochemical reaction for myophosphorylase, but it must be confirmed by biochemical assay of the muscle enzyme activity or by analysis of genomic DNA.

Clinical Features: If patients avoid strenuous exercise, the abnormality does not seriously interfere with their lives. However, prolonged, vigorous exercise can lead to widespread necrosis of myofibers and release of soluble muscle proteins such as creatine kinase and myoglobin into the circulation. This event, in turn, can produce myoglobinuria and renal failure.

Muscle biopsy should be performed several weeks after an episode of symptoms to allow regeneration of the muscle.

Type VII Glycogenosis (Phosphofructokinase Deficiency)

Phosphofructokinase (PFK) deficiency is less common than McArdle disease but causes an identical syndrome. PFK is a key enzyme in the Embden-Meyerhof pathway, which catalyzes the conversion of fructose-6-phosphate to fructose-1,6-diphosphate. In muscle, this enzyme is composed of four identical subunits (M_4), whereas in erythrocytes, the tetramer contains two different subunits (the M and L subunits), each under separate genetic control. As a result, a genetic lack of the muscle subunit results in a complete absence of PFK activity in muscle, but only a 50% decrease in activity in erythrocytes. In the latter cells, the remaining active enzyme is made up of four normal L subunits.

Patients with type VII glycogenosis often have slight anemia or low-grade hemolysis. The morphological findings are similar to those in McArdle disease, except that patients exhibit phosphorylase activity in the muscle. By contrast, a histochemical reaction for PFK shows little or no staining for the enzyme. The diagnosis is substantiated by biochemical analysis of the enzyme activity in muscle.

Lipid Myopathies Are Caused by Defective Fat Metabolism

Occasionally, a muscle biopsy specimen from a patient with exercise intolerance or muscle weakness contains an excess amount of neutral lipids. Such conditions are caused by a variety of metabolic disorders affecting lipid metabolism, of which more than a dozen have been identified. In brief, lipid myopathies may involve (1) deficient transport of fatty acids into the mitochondria (carnitine-deficiency syndromes and carnitine palmityl transferase deficiency), (2) defects in a variety of enzymes that mediate β-oxidation of fatty acids, (3) abnormalities in respiratory chain enzymes, and (4) defects in triglyceride use. Only disorders involving carnitine metabolism are discussed here.

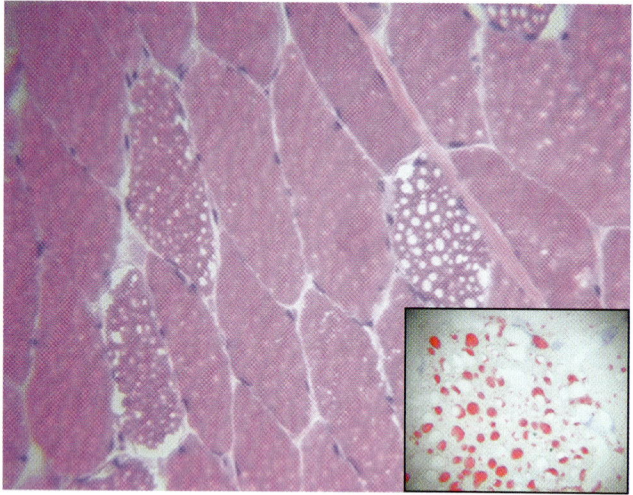

FIGURE 27-20
Lipid storage myopathy. Hematoxylin and eosin-stained frozen section. Numerous cytoplasmic vacuoles are present in the muscle fibers. Oil red-orcein stain *(inset)* demonstrates that the cytoplasmic vacuoles contain neutral lipid.

Carnitine Deficiency

Carnitine, which is synthesized in the liver and is present in large quantities in skeletal muscle, is necessary for the transport of long-chain fatty acids into the mitochondria. Patients with muscle carnitine deficiency, an autosomal recessive condition, have progressive proximal muscle weakness and atrophy and often show signs of denervation and peripheral neuropathy. The absence of carnitine leads to massive accumulation of lipid droplets in the sarcoplasm outside the mitochondria, a change readily evident in a muscle biopsy specimen (Fig. 27-20). Sometimes oral carnitine therapy alleviates the symptoms. Carnitine deficiency in skeletal muscle also occurs as part of a systemic disorder that can affect the CNS, heart, and liver.

Carnitine Palmityl Transferase Deficiency

As in carnitine deficiency, persons with carnitine palmityl transferase deficiency cannot metabolize long-chain fatty acids because of an inability to transport these lipids into the mitochondria, where they undergo β-oxidation. After prolonged exercise, these patients have muscular pain, which may progress to myoglobinuria. Prolonged fasting can produce the same symptoms. After such an episode, fibers regenerate and restore muscle structure. Biopsy specimens show no excess sarcoplasmic lipid or other microscopic abnormalities, and the diagnosis depends on the biochemical assay for carnitine palmityl transferase activity.

Mitochondrial Diseases Reflect Mutant nDNA or mtDNA

Inherited defects of mitochondrial metabolism are an uncommon but conceptually important group of disorders. Historically, diseases of muscle were recognized first and designated mitochondrial myopathies, but others affect both the CNS and muscle and are known as the *mitochondrial encephalomyopathies*. The nervous system, skeletal muscle, heart, kidney, and other organs can be affected in different combinations as part of a multisystem disease.

The inherited diseases of mitochondria are classified genetically into two broad groups, defects of either nuclear DNA (nDNA) or mitochondrial DNA (mtDNA). Point mutations, deletions, and duplications of mtDNA have been identified and linked to several syndromes of the mitochondrial encephalomyopathies. This group of syndromes is discussed here.

 Pathogenesis: Most mitochondrial proteins are encoded by nDNA, but 13 of the approximately 80 polypeptide subunits of the respiratory chain complexes are specified by mtDNA. Defects in these proteins constitute the mitochondrial encephalomyopathies.

The diseases of mtDNA have a maternal form of inheritance, contrasting with the mendelian pattern of nDNA mutations. mtDNA of the zygote is derived exclusively from the oocyte. The zygote and its daughter cells have many mitochondria, each of which contains several copies of the maternally derived mitochondrial genome. Mutations in copies of mtDNA are passed on randomly to subsequent generations of cells. During growth of the fetus or later, it is likely that some cells contain only mutant genomes (mutant homoplasmy), whereas others have only normal genomes (wild-type homoplasmy). Still others receive a mixed population of mutant and normal mtDNA (heteroplasmy). In turn, clinical expression of a disease produced by a given mutation of mtDNA depends on the total content of mitochondrial genomes and the proportion that is mutant. **The fraction of mutant mtDNA must exceed a critical value for a mitochondrial disease to become symptomatic.** This threshold varies in different organs and is presumably related to the energy requirements of the cells.

 Pathology: In skeletal muscle, the pathological signature of a defect of mtDNA is the accumulation of mitochondria. The excessive number of organelles is expressed as aggregates of reddish granular material in the sarcoplasm, as demonstrated by the modified Gomori trichrome stain (Fig. 27-21A). The abnormality has been termed a *ragged red fiber* because of the irregular contour of the reddish deposits at the fiber periphery. Pathogenic mutations of mtDNA in these diseases often impair the activity of complex IV (cytochrome oxidase). Three of the subunits are encoded by mtDNA, and they are required for function of the assembled electron transport carrier. Hence, histochemical stains for ragged red fibers often demonstrate deficient cytochrome oxidase activity (see Fig. 27-21C). By contrast, the ragged red fibers stain intensely for succinate dehydrogenase (SDH, complex II), a complex that is exclusively encoded by nDNA (see Fig. 27-21B). SDH is one of the many proteins synthesized in the cytoplasm and imported into the mitochondria and presumably reflects the proliferation of mitochondria. The defects of mitochondria (see Fig. 27-21D) result in atrophy of myofibers and accumulation of sarcoplasmic lipid and glycogen. Death of nerve cells and reactive astrocytosis occurs in the CNS.

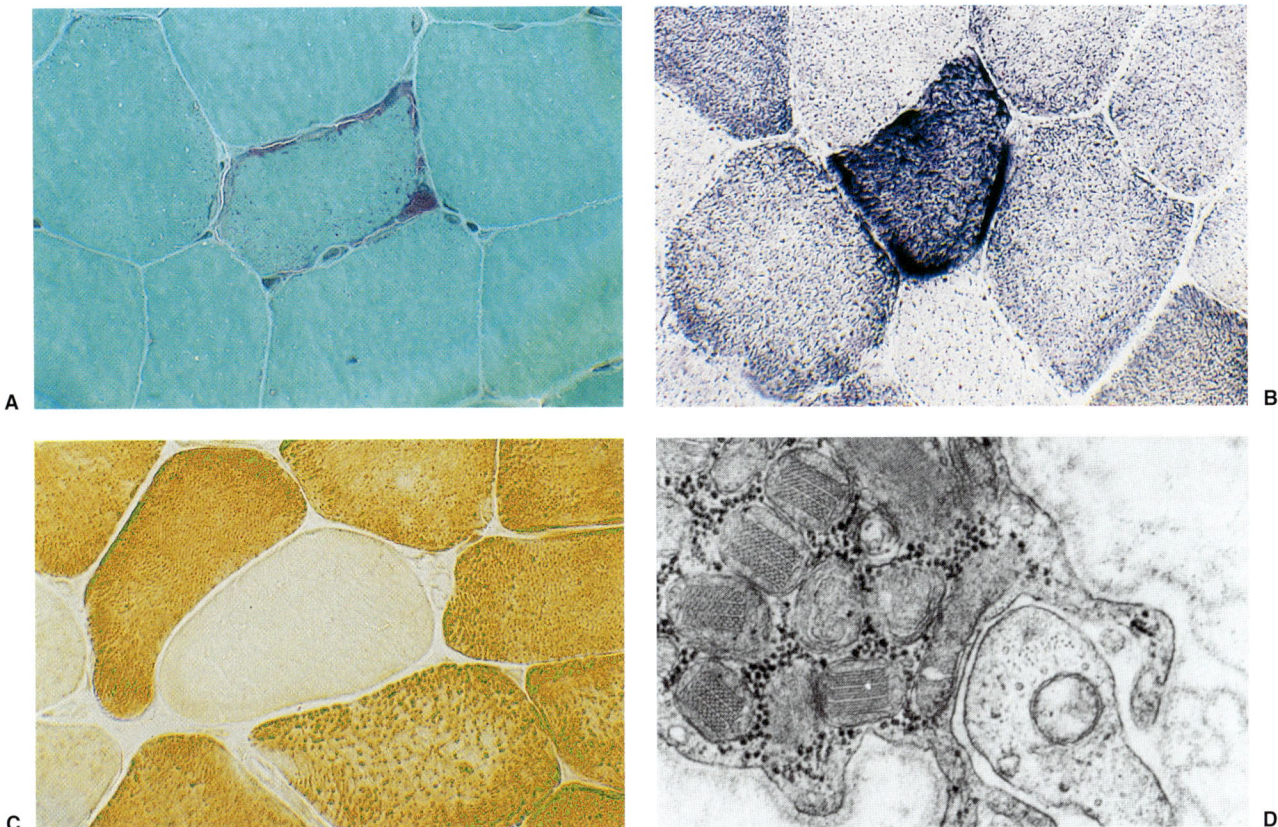

FIGURE 27-21
Mitochondrial myopathy caused by deletions of mitochondrial DNA (mtDNA). A. Modified Gomori trichrome. A ragged red fiber shows prominent proliferation of reddish, granular mitochondria, located chiefly in a subsarcolemmal region. B. Succinate dehydrogenase (SDH) stain. A ragged red fiber shows overexpression of SDH, an electron-transport carrier that is entirely encoded by nuclear DNA (nDNA). C. Another ragged red fiber displays lack of histochemical staining for cytochrome oxidase. Three subunits of this electron-transport carrier are coded by mtDNA, and the mutations have interfered with function in this fiber. D. An electron micrograph reveals mitochondria with ultrastructural abnormalities, including paracrystalline inclusions.

Clinical Features: The clinical manifestations of the encephalomyopathies vary, but usually begin in childhood. Some patients begin with muscle weakness and later develop a brain disorder. Others present with a neurological disease of the brain and may or may not have overt muscle weakness, even though muscle biopsy indicates a mitochondrial disorder. Other organs, such as the heart, are often affected as part of a multisystem disorder.

Three neurological syndromes have been designated (1) *Kearns-Sayre syndrome* (progressive ophthalmoplegia, retinal pigmentary degeneration, cardiac arrhythmias, and other features), (2) *MELAS* (mitochondrial myopathy, encephalopathy, lactic acidosis, and strokelike episodes), and (3) *MERRF* (myoclonic epilepsy and ragged red fibers). Most patients with Kearns-Sayre syndrome have large deletions of mtDNA that are not familial. MELAS and MERRF usually display point mutations of mitochondrial genes for certain transfer RNAs and show a maternal pattern of inheritance.

Myoadenylate Deaminase Deficiency Is a Frequent Cause of Mild Weakness

Adenosine monophosphate deaminase (AMP-DA) is present in large quantities in skeletal muscle, particularly in type II fibers. AMP-DA is an important enzyme in the regulation of the purine nucleotide cycle and helps to maintain the ATP/ADP ratio during exercise. A group of patients with mild proximal muscle weakness and exercise intolerance exhibit complete absence of AMP-DA activity. It is a common, autosomal recessive condition, occurring in 1 to 2% of all muscle biopsy specimens. There is a question as to whether AMP-DA deficiency represents a separate disease entity or a malady that is unmasked by other neuromuscular diseases.

Familial Periodic Paralysis Reflects Impaired Electrolyte Flux

Familial periodic paralysis refers to a group of autosomal dominant disorders characterized by episodes of muscular weakness or even

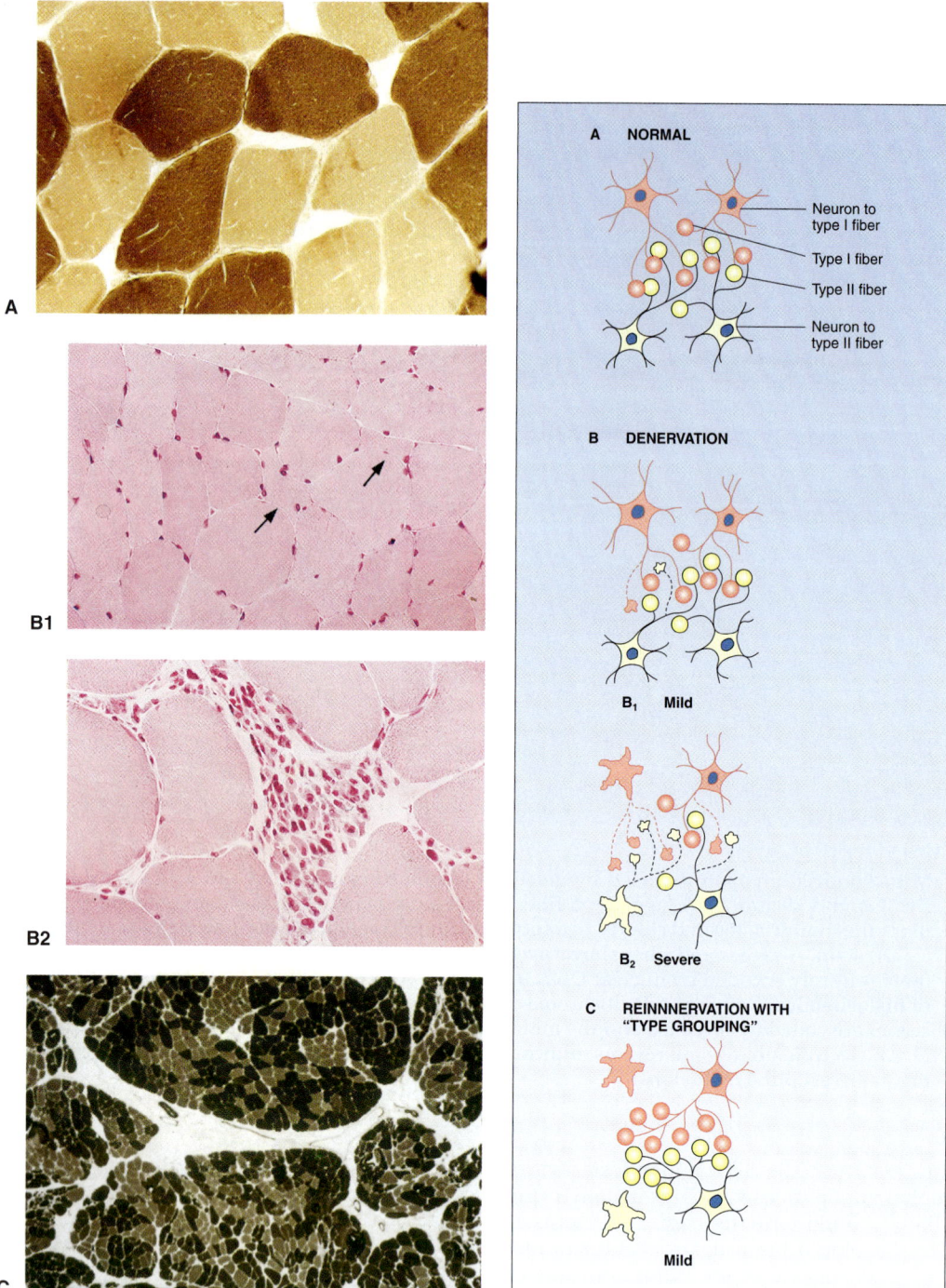

FIGURE 27-22

Denervation/reinnervation. (A) As shown in the photomicrograph, the normal intermixed distribution of type I (*pale*) and type II (*dark*) muscle fibers is shown by staining for ATPase. In the drawing, two neurons (*red*) innervate type I muscle fibers, and two neurons (*yellow*) supply type II fibers. (B) Denervation; hematoxylin and eosin stain. With early (mild) denervation (B1), portions of the axonal tree degenerate, resulting in angular atrophy of scattered type I and II muscle fibers. With more advanced (severe) denervation (B2), entire lower motor neurons or numerous axonal processes degenerate, causing small groups of angular atrophic fibers to appear as illustrated in the photomicrograph. (C) Reinnervation; myofibrillar ATPase. As neurons degenerate, surviving neurons sprout more nerve endings and reinnervate some of the denervated fibers. These reinnervated fibers become either type I or type II, according to the type of neuron that reinnervates them. This process results in fewer, but larger, motor units and the appearance of clusters of fibers of one type adjacent to clusters of the other type, a pattern called "type grouping." The photomicrograph demonstrates type grouping. (Compare with the normal pattern illustrated in Fig. 27-3B or 27-19A.) This field would appear normal except for a few atrophic fibers if it were stained with hematoxylin and eosin.

complete paralysis, followed by a rapid recovery. The disorders are related to abnormalities in sodium and potassium fluxes into and out of muscle cells. During an attack, the surface of the muscle fibers does not propagate an action potential, although the delivery of calcium inside the muscle fiber results in contraction. Muscle biopsy specimens taken during the attack exhibit no detectable abnormalities of recent onset. Later, permanent mild myopathic features and sarcoplasmic vacuoles appear. The vacuoles correspond to dilated or remodeled sarcoplasmic reticulum and transverse tubules. In some cases, a distinct subpopulation of fibers (type IIB) contains large numbers of tubular aggregates that are derived from the tubular network of the sarcoplasmic reticulum.

There are three clinically and genetically distinct syndromes—hypokalemic, hyperkalemic, and normokalemic periodic paralysis. The hypokalemic type has been linked to mutations of the gene that encodes a voltage-gated calcium channel of skeletal muscle; the hyperkalemic and normokalemic forms reflect mutations in the *SCN4A* gene on chromosome 17q, which specifies the sodium channel.

RHABDOMYOLYSIS

Rhabdomyolysis refers to the dissolution of skeletal muscle fibers and the release of myoglobin into the circulation, an event that may result in myoglobinuria and acute renal failure. The disorder may be acute, subacute, or chronic. During acute rhabdomyolysis, the muscles are swollen, tender, and profoundly weak.

Occasionally, an episode of rhabdomyolysis may complicate or follow influenza. Some patients develop rhabdomyolysis with apparently mild exercise and probably have some form of metabolic myopathy. After recovery, a subsequent biopsy may reveal muscle that is morphologically normal. Rhabdomyolysis also may complicate heat stroke or malignant hyperthermia after administration of an anesthetic such as halothane. Alcoholism is occasionally associated with either acute or chronic rhabdomyolysis.

The pathological changes in rhabdomyolysis correspond to an active, noninflammatory myopathy, with scattered necrosis of muscle fibers and varying degrees of degeneration and regeneration. Clusters of macrophages are seen in and around muscle fibers, but these are not accompanied by lymphocytes or inflammatory cells.

DENERVATION

The pathology of denervation reflects lesions of the lower motor neuron. Lesions of the upper motor neuron, as occur in multiple sclerosis or stroke, result in paralysis and atrophy. However, the lower motor neuron in these conditions remains intact, and the pathological changes reflect a nonspecific diffuse atrophy rather than denervation atrophy.

A muscle biopsy is a highly sensitive test for detecting a lesion of the lower motor neuron, but the pattern of denervation does not identify the cause of the lesion. For example, it does not distinguish between a disease such as amyotrophic lateral sclerosis, a disorder of motor neurons, and a peripheral neuropathy due to diabetes mellitus. The morphological changes indicate whether the denervation is recent or chronic.

When a skeletal muscle fiber becomes separated from contact with its lower motor neuron, it invariably atrophies, owing to the progressive loss of myofibrils. On cross-section, the atrophic fiber has a characteristic angular configuration, seemingly compressed by surrounding normal muscle fibers (Fig. 27-22). If the fiber is not reinnervated, the atrophy proceeds to complete loss of myofibrils, and the nuclei condense into aggregates. In the end stage, the muscle fibers disappear and are replaced chiefly by adipose tissue.

The early phase of denervating disease is characterized by irregularly scattered, angular, atrophic fibers. As the disease progresses, these fibers are seen in groups, at first in small clusters of several fibers, and later in progressively larger groups (see Fig. 27-22B). These fibers are excessively dark when stained for nonspecific esterase (Fig. 27-23) and NADH-TR reactions, in contrast to atrophy caused by disuse or wasting. With the ATPase reaction, the groups of denervated fibers are a mixture of type I and type II fibers. **Virtually all of the known denervating conditions exhibit no selective denervation of one type of motor neuron.**

Another abnormality occasionally present in a denervating condition is the "target fiber" (Fig. 27-24), seen in 20% of cases. This change is apparently transient, occurring during or shortly after the process of denervation or reinnervation and indicating that the process is active. The lesion consists of central pallor of the muscle fiber, which is surrounded by a condensed zone that in turn is surrounded by a normal zone of sarcoplasm. Target fibers are difficult to see with the hematoxylin and eosin stain but are clearly demonstrated by the NADH-TR stain, which shows greatly reduced staining in the central zone, reflecting a reduced number or absence of mitochondria.

With every episode of denervation, there is an effort at reinnervation. In a slowly progressive denervating process, reinnervation may actually keep pace with denervation. New sprouting nerve endings make synaptic contact with the muscle fiber at the site of the previous motor endplate. Shortly after denervation, the muscle fiber becomes covered with nicotinic Ach receptors (extrajunctional receptor), a situation similar to that in the myotubular phase of embryogenesis. This denervated state induces the sprouting of new nerve endings from adjacent surviving nerve. With reinnervation, the extrajunctional receptor again disappears from the sarcolemma, except at the point of synaptic contact.

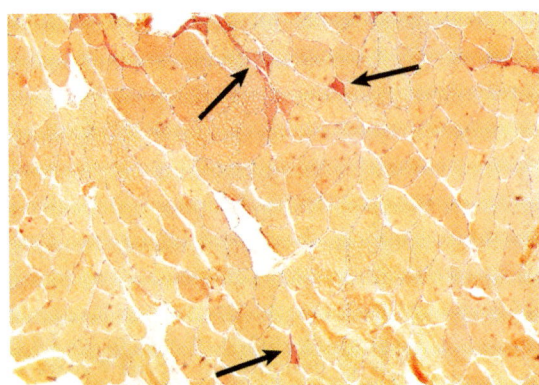

FIGURE 27-23

Denervation. In this frozen section of the biceps muscle subjected to the nonspecific esterase reaction, a few irregularly scattered, angular, atrophic fibers *(arrows)* are excessively dark stained. This pattern is highly characteristic of atrophy due to denervation.

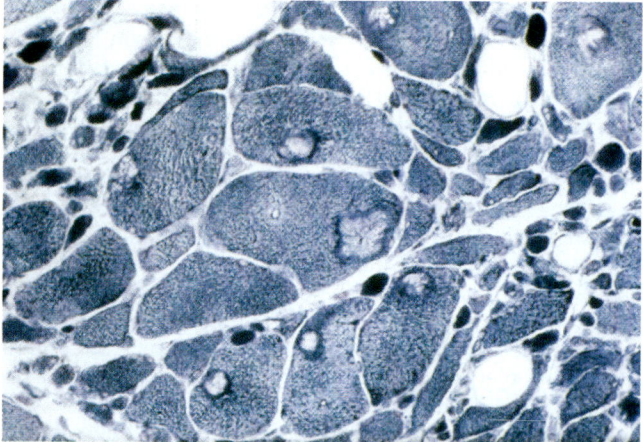

FIGURE 27-24
Target fiber. A cross-section of striated muscle treated with the NADH-TR stain demonstrates several "target fibers," a characteristic feature of some cases of denervation. Because the enzyme reaction creates a product (formazan) that selectively fixes to membranous organelles, the centers of the target areas appear devoid of mitochondria and sarcoplasmic reticulum. The myofibrils may or may not be intact.

In a chronic denervating condition, reinnervation of each surviving motor unit gradually becomes larger. As a lower motor neuron of a specific type takes over the innervation of a given field of fibers, fiber groups of one type are seen adjacent to groups of another type. This pattern is designated *type grouping* and is pathognomonic of denervation followed by reinnervation (see Figs. 27-22C and 27-25).

Patients with striking type grouping often have symptoms of muscle cramping in addition to progressive muscular weakness. After a single episode of denervation, such as occurs with poliomyelitis, reinnervation often leads to a remarkable recovery of strength. Years later, a biopsy shows a conspicuous pattern of type grouping, with scattered pyknotic nuclear clumps (see Fig. 27-25A). In such cases, there are neither angular atrophic fibers nor target fibers.

Occasionally, a biopsy specimen reveals an abnormal prominence of one fiber type over the other. This situation is designated *type predominance* and may involve either type I or type II fibers. The reason for this effect is often not clear, but there is frequently evidence of denervation. It could be that in type predominance, reinnervation favors one type of lower motor neuron over another.

It is not uncommon to see occasional muscle fibers undergoing necrosis or regeneration in neuropathic conditions. In these patients, a modest increase in serum creatine kinase levels reflects muscle degeneration. This finding is common in patients with slowly progressive forms of spinal muscular atrophy, as in Kugelberg-Welander disease and Kennedy disease.

Spinal Muscular Atrophy Reflects Progressive Degeneration of Anterior Horn Cells

Spinal muscular atrophy (SMA) is characterized by degeneration of anterior horn cells of the spinal cord and represents the second most common, lethal, autosomal recessive disorder after cystic fibrosis. Childhood SMA is classified into type I (*Werdnig-Hoffmann disease*), type II (intermediate), and type III (*Kugelberg-Welander disease*). The survival motor neuron gene (5q11.2-13.3) is absent in virtually all (99%) cases of SMA.

WERDNIG-HOFFMANN DISEASE (INFANTILE SMA): *Werdnig-Hoffmann disease results in progressive and se-*

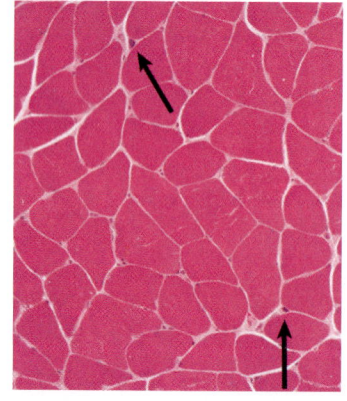 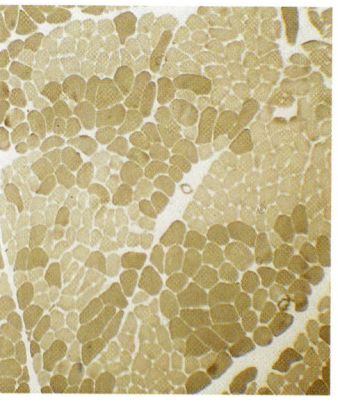

FIGURE 27-25
Type grouping. A. Biopsy of the biceps obtained from a 27-year-old woman who had contracted poliomyelitis at age 7 years. A section of the biceps stained with hematoxylin and eosin shows muscle fibers that vary slightly in size and shape. The scattered black "dots" (*arrows*) among some of the fibers are pyknotic nuclear clumps in extremely atrophic fibers that were not reinnervated. The fiber types cannot be distinguished with this stain. B. A similar case stained for ATPase. Striking type grouping reflects reinnervation. Groups of type II fibers (*dark*) are adjacent to groups of type I fibers. As a result, there are fewer but larger motor units. The absence of angular atrophic fibers or target fibers suggests that there is no active denervation.

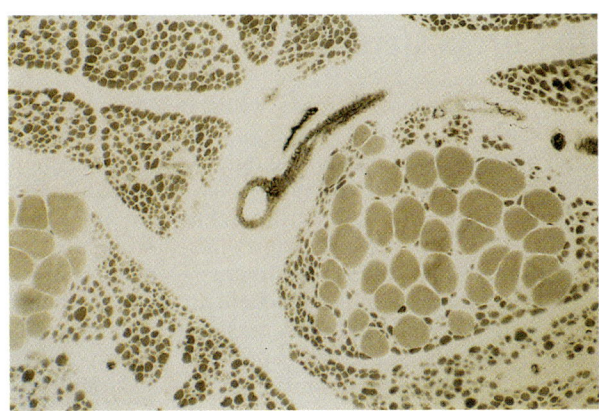

FIGURE 27-26
Werdnig-Hoffman disease (infantile spinal muscular atrophy). This cross-section of skeletal muscle stained for myofibrillar ATPase is derived from an infant with severe hypotonia. It shows groups of extremely atrophic, rounded type I and type II fibers and clusters of markedly hypertrophied type I fibers.

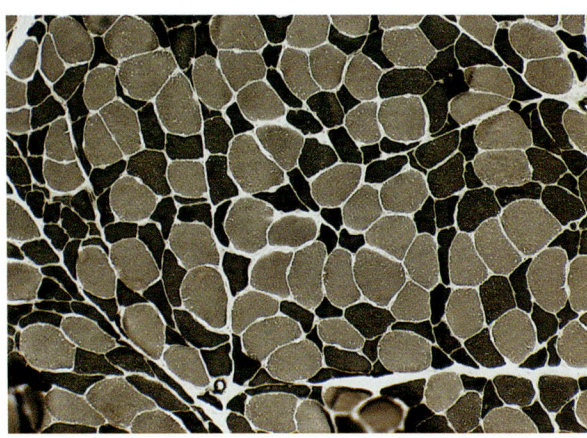

FIGURE 27-27
Type II fiber atrophy. This biopsy of the vastus lateralis muscle was taken from a 48-year-old man with proximal muscle weakness because of endogenous corticosteroid toxicity (Cushing syndrome). Virtually all of the angular atrophic fibers are type II. This form of atrophy closely mimics denervation atrophy when visualized with the hematoxylin and eosin stain.

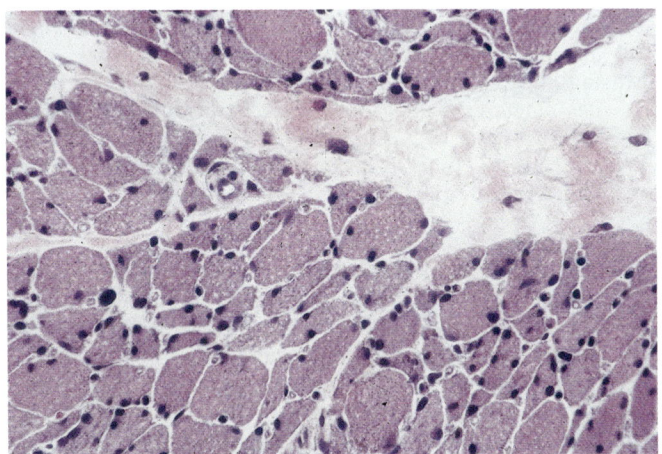

FIGURE 27-28
(A) Critical illness myopathy frequently shows atrophic muscle with angular muscle fibers (Hematoxylin and eosin) (B) Normal skeletal muscle shows both thin and thick myofilaments (electron micrograph) (C) Critical illness myopathy shows a marked loss of thick myosin filaments, whereas α actin(thin) filaments are intact (electron micrograph).

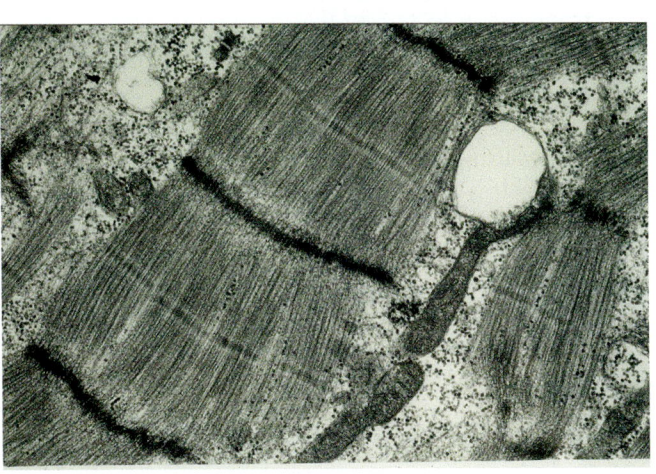

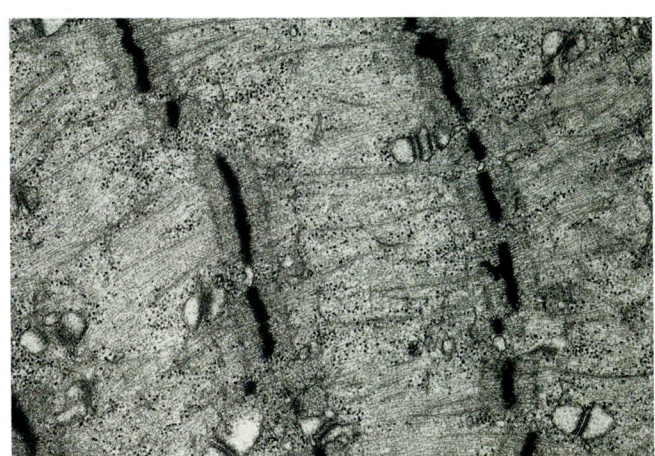

vere weakness in early infancy, the infants seldom living beyond the first year of life. The denervation seems to begin in utero after the establishment of motor units. The histological pattern is virtually pathognomonic (Fig. 27-26). Groups of minute, rounded, atrophic fibers are still identifiable with the ATPase reaction as being either type I or type II. In addition, there are fascicles of normal muscle fibers and almost invariably clusters of hypertrophied type I fibers. In addition to the absent survival motor neuron gene, a second gene (neuronal apoptosis inhibitory protein gene) has also been implicated in the pathogenesis of Werdnig-Hoffmann disease.

KUGELBERG–WELANDER DISEASE (JUVENILE SMA): *This variant is a later-onset form of SMA and is not necessarily progressive.* Previously, these patients were often designated as having limb-girdle muscular dystrophy. The electromyographic pattern of denervation helps to identify these patients. The muscle biopsy specimen shows type grouping and other evidence of a neurogenic disorder but can resemble a myopathy in a small sample because of coexisting necrotic fibers and regenerating fibers.

Type II Fiber Atrophy Resembles Denervation Myopathy

A commonly misinterpreted pathological pattern in muscle biopsy specimens is atrophy resulting from disuse, wasting, upper motor neuron disease, and corticosteroid toxicity. This diffuse, nonspecific atrophy is manifested histologically by selective angular atrophy of type II fibers. With the hematoxylin and eosin stain, it is sometimes impossible to distinguish this pattern of atrophy from that of denervation. However, with the ATPase reaction, all of the angular atrophic fibers are type II (Fig. 27-27). Furthermore, these abnormal fibers do not stain heavily with the nonspecific esterase reaction or the NADH-TR reaction. Type II atrophy is a common condition that is often related to a more chronic problem.

STEROID MYOPATHY: Corticosteroid therapy can produce muscle weakness, and the muscle biopsy is characterized histologically by type II atrophy. This pathological feature raises an important point clinically, because patients with polymyositis are often treated with large doses of corticosteroids. If the patient develops worsening weakness, the physician must decide whether the symptom represents a relapse of the polymyositis and requires an increase in the dosage of corticosteroids. Alternatively, the weakness may represent steroid myopathy, in which case a decreased dosage is indicated.

In weakness caused by corticosteroid toxicity, patients do not demonstrate an increased serum creatine kinase level and histologically manifest selective atrophy of type II fibers, in the absence of muscle fiber degeneration and inflammation. By contrast, fiber degeneration and inflammation would be expected in recurrent polymyositis, a process that is reflected in increased serum creatine kinase activity.

Critical Illness Myopathy Is Associated with Corticosteroid Therapy

Patients on high-dose steroids while being given neuromuscular blocking agents may experience severe weakness in spite of removal of paralyzing agents. Such patients may have "critical illness myopathy," also known as myosin heavy chain depletion syndrome. Electron microscopic analysis of skeletal muscle from these patients demonstrates loss of thick myosin filaments from muscle fibers (Fig. 27-28). The underlying mechanism of the myosin depletion is not understood, but cessation of corticosteroid therapy frequently results in reappearance of myosin thick filaments and resultant restoration of muscle strength.

SUGGESTED READING

Books

Carpenter S, Karpati G: *Pathology of skeletal muscle*, 2nd ed. New York, Oxford University Press, 2001.

DiMauro S: Mitochondrial encephalomyopathies. In: Rosenberg RN (ed): *Molecular and genetic basis of neurological disease.* Stoneham: Butterworth, 1993: 665–694.

Emery AEH: *Duchenne muscular dystrophy,* rev. ed. Oxford Monographs on Medical Genetics, vol 15. New York: Oxford University Press, 1988.

Engel AG, Franzini-Armstrong C (eds): *Myology,* 2nd ed. New York: McGraw-Hill, 1994.

Karpati G (ed): *Structural and molecular basis of skeletal muscle diseases.* Basal, ISN Neuropath Press, 2002.

Mastaglia FL, Walton OF, Detchant L (eds): *Skeletal muscle pathology,* 2nd ed. Edinburgh: Churchill Livingstone, 1992.

Walton JA (ed): *Disorders of voluntary muscle,* 5th ed. London: Churchill Livingstone, 1988.

Review Articles

Ahn AH, Kunkel LM: The structural and functional diversity of dystrophin. *Nat Genet* 3:283–291, 1993.

Asbury AK, McKhann GM, McDonald WI (eds): Diseases of the central nervous system. *Clin Neurol* 1:11–15, 1992.

Beggs AH, Kunkel LM: Improved diagnosis of Duchenne/Becker muscular dystrophy. *J Clin Invest* 85:613–619, 1990.

Cullen MJ, Mastaglia FL: Morphological changes in dystrophic muscle. *Br Med Bull* 36:145–152, 1980.

DiMauro S, Bresolin E, Hays AP: Disorders of glycogen metabolism of muscle. *Crit Rev Clin Neurobiol* 1:83–116, 1984.

DiMauro S, Trevisan C, Hays A: Disorders of lipid metabolism in muscle. *Muscle Nerve* 3:369–388, 1980.

Mastaglia FL, Ojeda VJ: Inflammatory myopathies: Part 1. *Ann Neurol* 17:215–227, 1985.

Mastaglia FL, Ojeda VJ: Inflammatory myopathies: Part 2. *Ann Neurol* 17:317–323, 1985.

Plotz PH, Dalakas M, Leff RL, et al: Current concepts in the idiopathic inflammatory myopathies: Polymyositis, dermatomyositis and related disorders. *Ann Intern Med* 111:143–157, 1989.

Worton RG, Thompson MW: Genetics of Duchenne muscular dystrophy. *Annu Rev Genet* 22:601–629, 1988.

CHAPTER 28

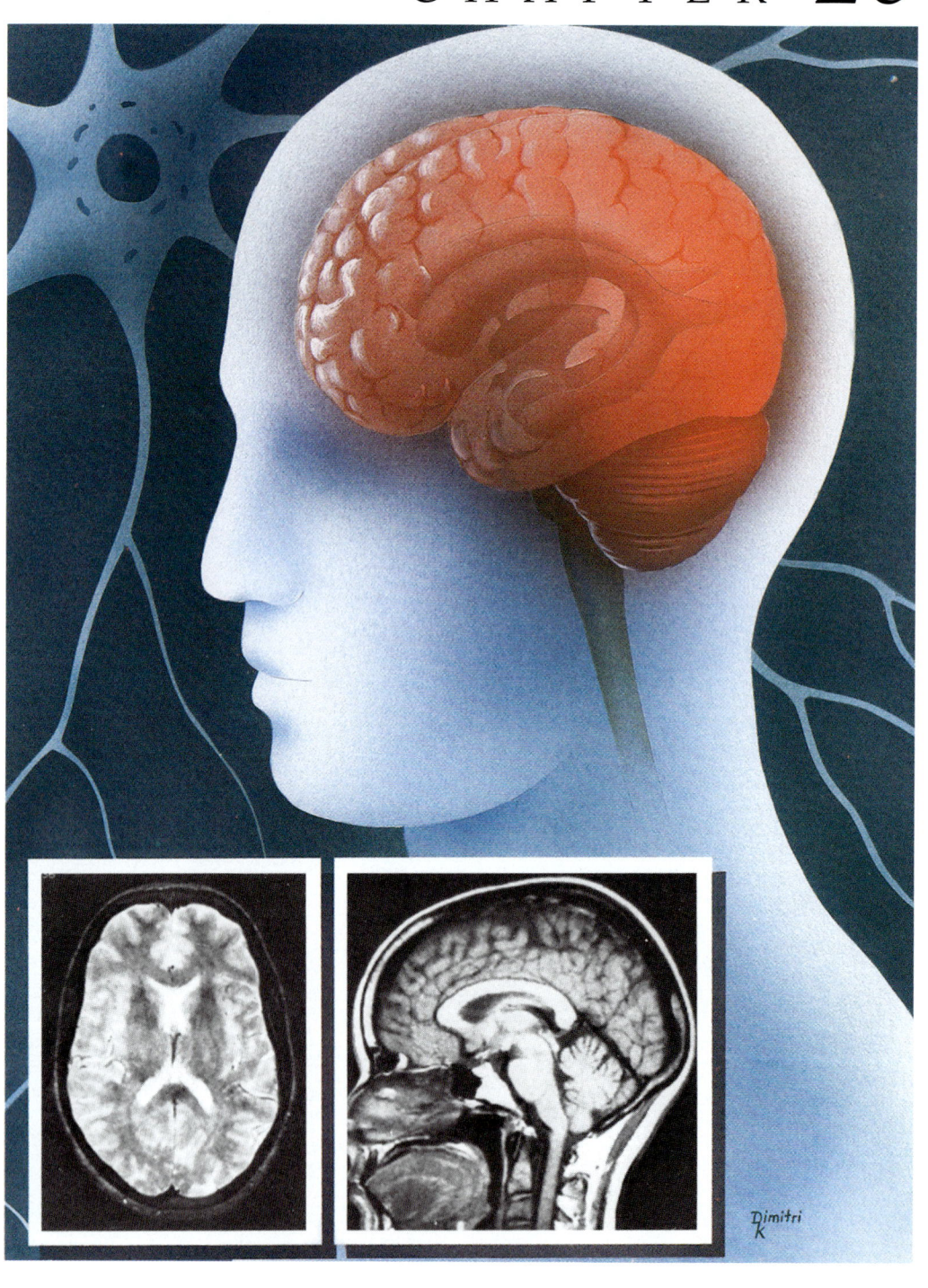

The Nervous System

John Q. Trojanowski: The Central Nervous System
Thomas W. Bouldin: The Peripheral Nervous System

The Central Nervous System

Cells of the Nervous System

Neurons
Astrocytes
Oligodendroglia
Ependyma
Microglia

Congenital Malformations

Neural Tube Defects (Dysraphic States)
Malformations of the Spinal Cord
Arnold-Chiari Malformation
Congenital Hydrocephalus
Disorders of Cerebral Gyri
Congenital Defects
Epilepsy

Trauma

Epidural Hematoma
Subdural Hematoma
Subarachnoid Hemorrhage
Cerebral Contusion

Penetrating Wounds
Spinal Cord Injuries

Circulatory Disorders

Vascular Malformations
Cerebral Aneurysms
Cerebral Hemorrhage
Cerebral Ischemia and Infarction

Cerebrospinal Fluid

Hydrocephalus

Infectious Diseases

Meningitis
Cerebral Abscess
Viral Encephalomyelitis
Prion Diseases (Spongiform Encephalopathies)

Demyelinating Diseases

Leukodystrophies
Multiple Sclerosis
Postinfectious and Postvaccinal Encephalomyelitis
Central Pontine Myelinolysis

(continued)

FIGURE 28-1 *(see opposite page)*
The brain. The anatomical structures of the brain are well visualized by magnetic resonance imaging.

Neuronal Storage Diseases

Tay-Sachs Disease

Hurler Syndrome

Gaucher Disease

Niemann-Pick Disease

Metabolic Neuronal Diseases

Phenylketonuria

Cretinism

Wilson Disease

Metabolic Disorders

Alcoholism

Hepatic Encephalopathy

Subacute Combined Degeneration of the Spinal Cord

Neurodegenerative Diseases

Parkinson Disease

Amyotrophic Lateral Sclerosis

Trinucleotide Repeat Expansion Syndromes

Alzheimer Disease

Tumors of the CNS

Tumors Derived from Astrocytes

Ependymoma

Medulloblastoma

Ganglioglioma

Neoplasms of Mesenchymal Origin

Neoplasms Derived from Ectopic Tissues

Tumors of Germ Cell Origin

Hemangioblastoma

Lymphoma

Metastatic Tumors

Colloid Cyst

Hereditary Intracranial Neoplasms

The Peripheral Nervous System

Anatomy

Reactions to Injury

Axonal Degeneration

Segmental Demyelination

Peripheral Neuropathies

Diabetic Neuropathy

Uremic Neuropathy

Critical Illness Polyneuropathy

Alcoholic Neuropathy

Acute Inflammatory Demyelinating Polyneuropathy (Guillain-Barré Syndrome)

Dorsal Root Ganglionitis (Sensory Neuronopathy)

Vasculitic Neuropathy

Neuropathies Associated with Monoclonal Gammopathy

Amyloid Neuropathy

Paraneoplastic Neuropathies

Toxic Neuropathy

Hereditary Neuropathies

Neuropathies as a Complication of AIDS

Chronic Idiopathic Axonal Neuropathy

Nerve Trauma

Traumatic Neuroma

Plantar Interdigital Neuroma (Morton Neuroma)

Tumors

Schwannoma

Neurofibroma

Malignant Peripheral Nerve Sheath Tumor (Malignant Schwannoma, Neurofibrosarcoma)

The Central Nervous System

The nervous system is the most complex organ system in the body (Fig. 28-1), and its major components (brain, spinal cord, peripheral nerves, and ganglia) are intimately interconnected to enable rapid communications. The sensory, motor, cognitive, memory, and autonomic functions of the nervous system have distinct anatomical correlates, although defects in one area may have significant effects on the functionality of other regions. Despite this intricate organization and the fact that neurons are the most asymmetric cells in the body, with extensions (e.g., axons) that extend up to meters away from the parent cell body, the nervous system is governed largely by the same principles that control the function of cells in the rest of the body.

TOPOGRAPHY: The functional properties of the nervous system are topographically localized, and neurological diseases are also regionally distributed. The selective vulnerability of different nervous system cells and regions to disease processes is one of the most profound unresolved enigmas of neuropsychiatric illnesses. For example, Huntington disease is primarily characterized by selective degeneration of neurons in the caudate nuclei, whereas Parkinson disease targets the nigrostriatal system, and amyotrophic lateral sclerosis singles out upper and lower motor neurons of cerebrum, brainstem, and spinal cord. Similarly, infectious diseases have distinct topographic predilections; poliomyelitis involves the anterior horn cells of the spinal cord and the motor nuclei of the brainstem, herpes simplex preferentially affects the temporal lobes, and rabies seeks out the medulla. Vascular diseases and demyelinating conditions also display regional preferences within the nervous system, and a degree of topographic predictability characterizes most brain tumors.

AGE: The nervous system is affected by neuropsychiatric disorders throughout the life span, but individual diseases commonly manifest a predilection for selected age groups. For example, inborn errors of metabolism, such as Tay-Sachs disease, the leukodystrophies, and several tumors, are encountered largely in childhood. Multiple sclerosis shows a strong preference for young adults, rarely having its onset before puberty or after the age of 40 years. Huntington disease typically strikes youthful and middle-aged adults. Parkinson disease is rarely evidenced before the later decades of life, and Alzheimer disease tends to be a malady of the aged brain.

CELLS OF THE NERVOUS SYSTEM

Neurons Are the Effector Cells of the Nervous System

Although mature neurons do not divide, the dogma that neurons are never generated after birth has been overturned in the past decade. However, the functional significance of the production of small numbers of new neurons in the adult brain is unknown. The nervous system indeed loses neurons with progressive aging, but these losses may not be as profound as suggested earlier.

The need for structural stability in the nervous system is counterbalanced by the need for plasticity in neuronal net-

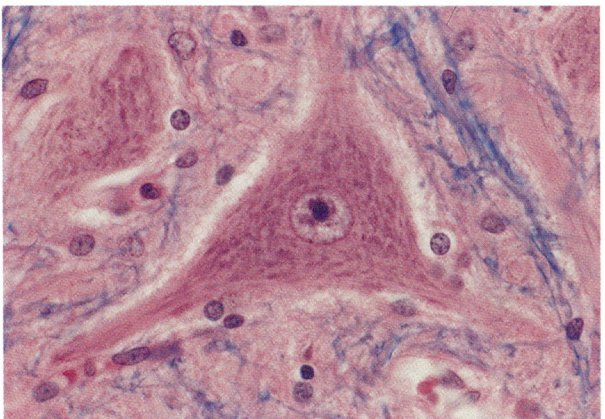

FIGURE 28-2
Neuron. Nerve cells are typically pyramidal with a round nucleus and prominent nucleolus. The granularity of the cytoplasm is imparted by rough endoplasmic reticulum (Nissl substance), but over 95% of the volume of large neurons is invested in its processes (axons and dendrites) that extend for very long distances (~1 m for some motor neurons), making neurons the most highly asymmetric cells in humans and other mammals.

works. The fact that neurons of the central nervous system (CNS) cannot effectively regenerate axons over long distances limits the ability of the CNS to respond to many different types of injuries. Thus, an infarct that transects the internal capsule creates a permanent motor deficit because transected axons do not regenerate to reestablish lost connections. Since CNS neurons do not remyelinate efficiently after injury, a demyelinating disease like multiple sclerosis causes permanent functional deficits.

ANATOMY: Neurons have a variety of shapes and sizes, but certain features are common to all of them. Microscopically, the centrally located, round nucleus contains a prominent nucleolus. The cytoplasm is abundant, and the ribosome-studded endoplasmic reticulum forms prominent basophilic granules known as Nissl bodies (Fig. 28-2). Some neurons, such as those in substantia nigra or locus ceruleus, contain cytoplasmic pigment termed *neuromelanin* (Fig. 28-3).

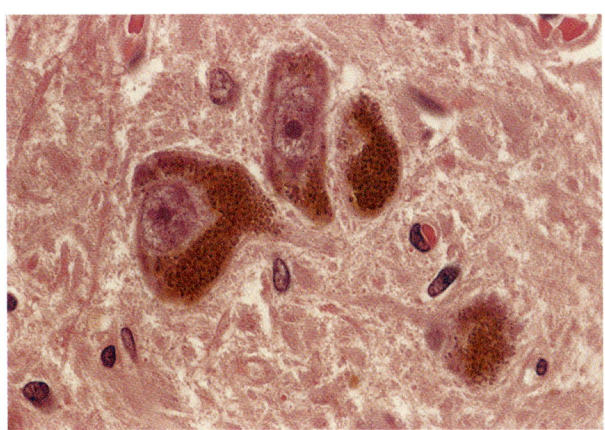

FIGURE 28-3
Pigmented neurons. Neurons of the substantia nigra and locus ceruleus are heavily pigmented with neuromelanin.

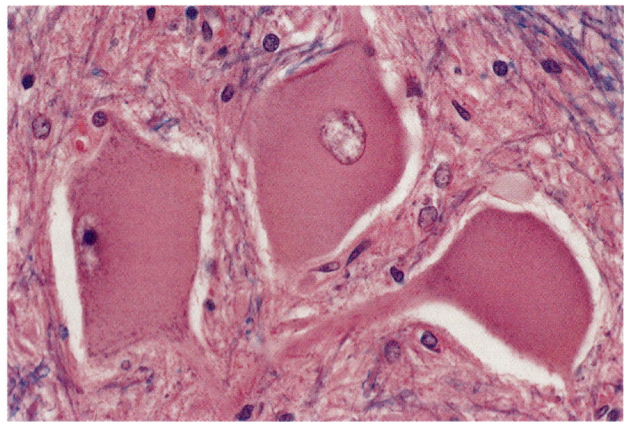

FIGURE 28-4
Chromatolysis. An injured neuron appears swollen with pale cytoplasm and marginated Nissl substance near the plasma membrane.

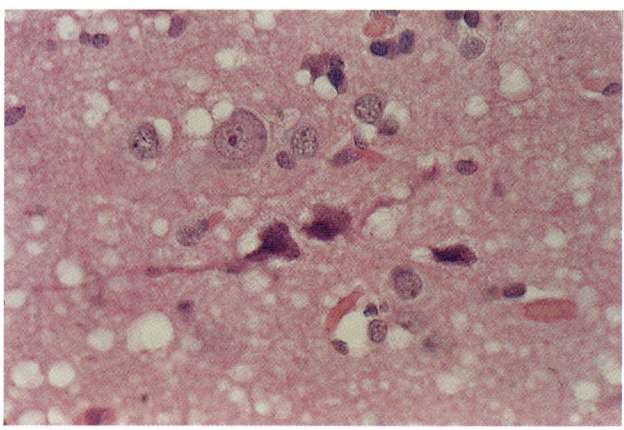

FIGURE 28-6
Atrophy. In this case of Creutzfeldt-Jakob disease, a prion disease, injured neurons are shriveled and hyperchromatic, and there is the classic spongiform change (large white vacuoles) that is a hallmark of most prion diseases.

Neurons are also highly asymmetric, with numerous branching projections (axons and dendrites) that serve to connect neurons into extended networks or functional multicellular units. Dendrites are best demonstrated by silver impregnation or antibodies to dendritic markers such as MAP2. Each neuron usually gives rise to a single axon, which may extend for more than a meter to arborize in terminal synapses with the processes of other neurons. Some axons are surrounded by a myelin sheath; others are unmyelinated.

Neurons react to injury in several ways that may be reversible or culminate in cell death.

CHROMATOLYSIS: Injured neurons swell, the cytoplasm expands, and the Nissl substance disperses near the plasma membrane (Fig. 28-4). The nucleus assumes an eccentric position. This process is known as chromatolysis and is a common response to injury (e.g., axonal transaction). It may be reversible, but it also may be a harbinger of cell death (Fig. 28-5).

ATROPHY: The loss of neurons in the brain may be appreciated on gross examination as a global or regional reduction (atrophy) in brain volume or weight. Single neurons may also atrophy or shrivel and become hyperchromatic (Fig. 28-6).

NEURONOPHAGIA: Injuries that kill neurons create cellular debris and elicit phagocytosis by immune cells (i.e., brain macrophages or brain microglia). This phagocytic response is termed *neuronophagia* (Fig. 28-7).

INTRANEURONAL INCLUSIONS: Diverse nuclear and cytoplasmic inclusions affect neurons, particularly in viral encephalitides (Figs. 28-8 and 28-9) and in neurodegenerative diseases characterized by intracytoplasmic amyloid deposits (see below).

Astrocytes Support Neurons and Promote Repair

Astrocytes are star-shaped glial cells that far outnumber neurons throughout the CNS. Although they have long

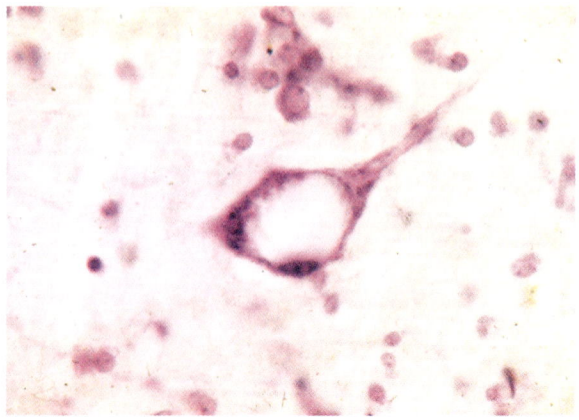

FIGURE 28-5
Hydropic degeneration. Fluid-filled vacuoles distend the cytoplasmic compartment and displace the nucleus.

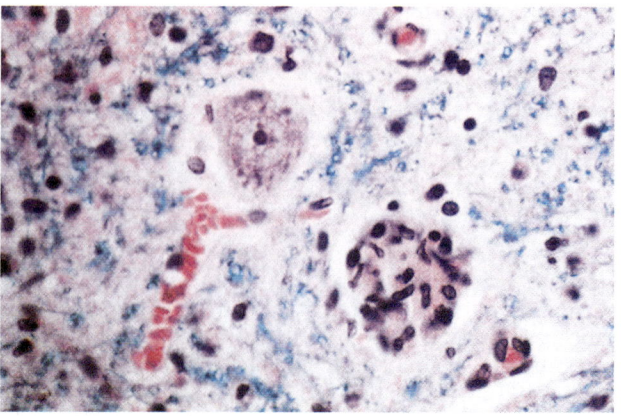

FIGURE 28-7
Neuronophagia. Leukocytes may accumulate at sites of neuronal necrosis and engulf these cells, as shown here in poliomyelitis.

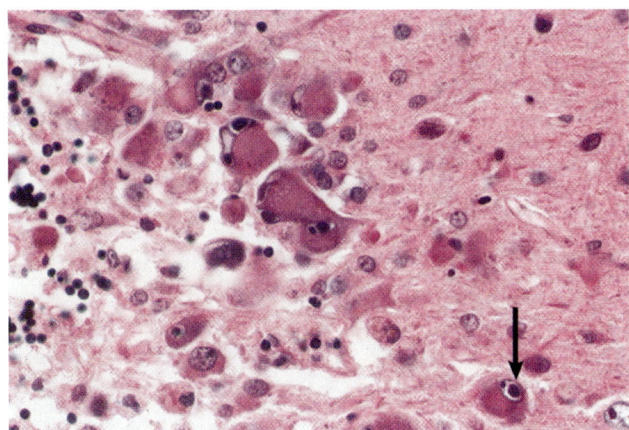

FIGURE 28-8
Intranuclear inclusions. Cytomegalovirus induces intranuclear inclusions with prominent clear halos *(arrow)*. These inclusions are demonstrated in the Purkinje cells of a patient with acquired immunodeficiency syndrome (AIDS).

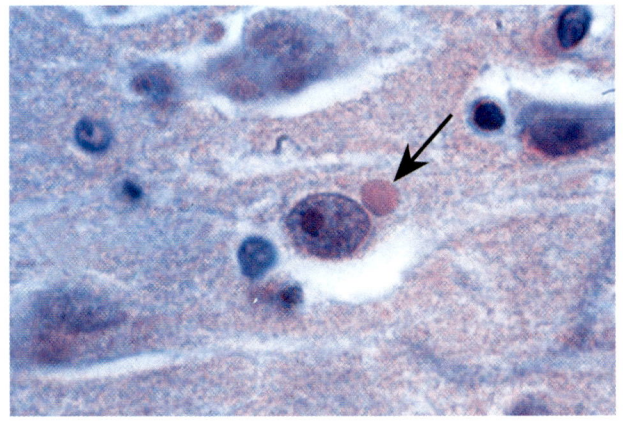

FIGURE 28-9
Negri body. Rabies encephalitis is characterized by round, eosinophilic cytoplasmic inclusions that resemble an erythrocyte *(arrow)*.

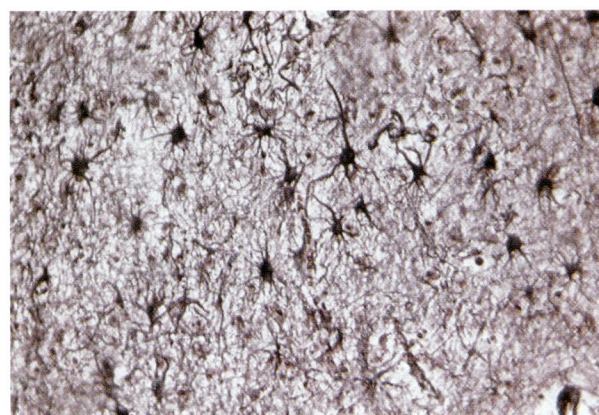

FIGURE 28-10
Astrocytes. Astrocyte proliferation in the brain of a patient with tertiary syphilis demonstrated with silver carbonate staining.

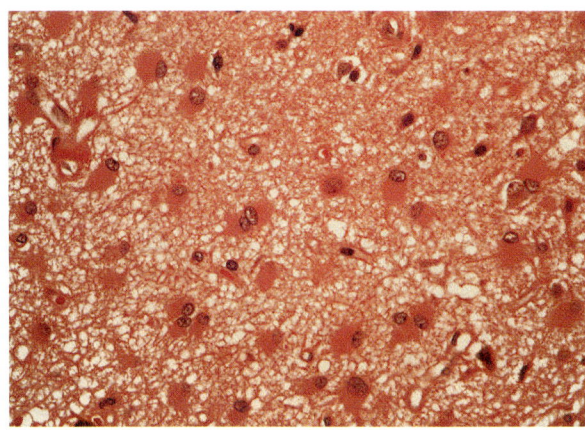

FIGURE 28-11
Astrocytes. Hematoxylin and eosin (H&E)-stained reactive astrocytes are plump with pink cytoplasm (gemistocytic astrocytes).

been thought to serve a supportive purpose, more-recent studies also implicate them in signaling functions (e.g., as components of the tripartite synapse) previously considered the sole domain of neurons. Astrocytes also play a prominent role in the CNS response to injury.

ANATOMY: Multiple species of CNS astrocytes have been identified, but the two best-known subtypes are *fibrillary astrocytes* in white matter, and *protoplasmic astrocytes* in gray matter. By light microscopy, both types of astrocytes display a round nucleus, 7 to 10 μm in diameter, with homogeneous chromatin and scant cytoplasm. However, immunostains for glial fibrillary acidic protein (GFAP) or silver impregnation reveal processes extending in all directions from the astrocyte cell body (Fig. 28-10), some of which terminate as foot processes on blood vessels. By electron microscopy, both types of astrocytes contain a meshwork of fine glial filaments formed by polymers of GFAP.

REACTIONS: Astrocytes proliferate locally in response to injuries (e.g., trauma, abscess, tumors, infarcts, and hemorrhages). This process, referred to as *astrocytosis* or *gliosis*, is readily demonstrated by GFAP immunostaining (Figs. 28-10 through 28-12). Astrocytosis evolves in hours to days and

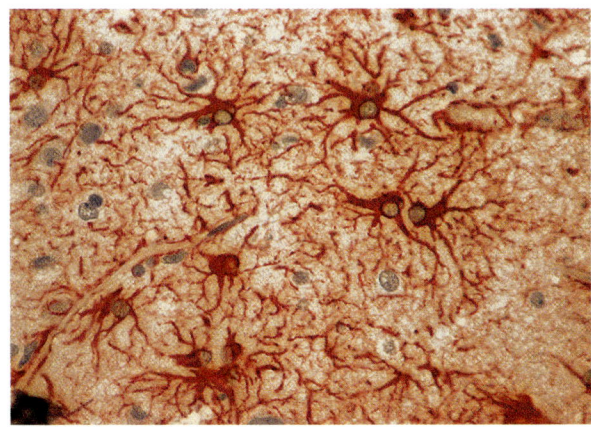

FIGURE 28-12
Reactive astrocytes. The glial processes of astrocytes stain intensely for glial fibrillary acidic protein (GFAP).

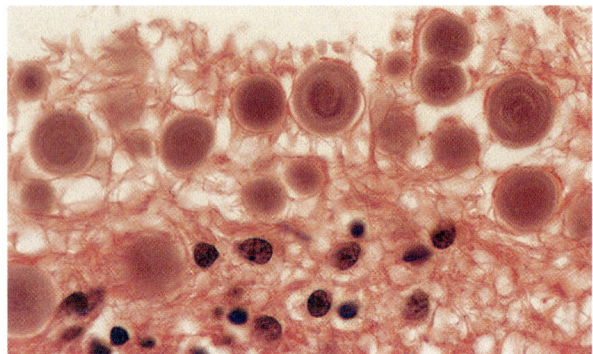

FIGURE 28-13
Corpora amylacea. These are amorphous, basophilic bodies that accumulate in the subependymal areas of elderly persons.

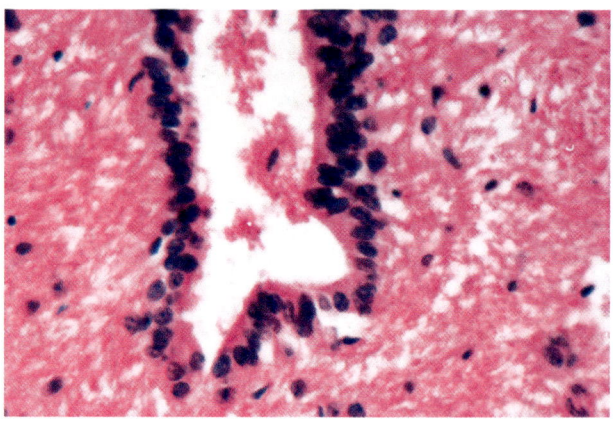

FIGURE 28-15
Ependyma. The central canal of the spinal cord is lined by a single layer of closely aligned, cuboidal-to-columnar ependymal cells.

persists to an extent that is usually commensurate with the severity of the initiating injury. The consequence is a "glial scar" composed of reactive astrocytes and their processes. Astrocytes may also undergo neoplastic transformation to result in the most common primary brain tumors, namely, gliomas or astrocytomas.

Corpora amylacea are 5- to 20-nm basophilic and amorphous structures formed by aggregates of carbohydrates and proteins. These bodies accumulate with normal aging with a predilection for subpial and subependymal regions (Fig. 28-13). Although they appear extracellular by light microscopy, they evolve within processes of astrocytes.

Oligodendroglia Are the Myelin-Producing Cells of the CNS

Oligodendroglia are related to astrocytes insofar as they are both of neurectodermal origin. In sections stained with hematoxylin and eosin or Luxol fast blue, oligodendroglia have dark, round nuclei with a thin rim of cytoplasm. In the gray matter, many oligodendroglia are disposed as "satellites" around neurons, whereas oligodendrocytes in the white matter are arrayed longitudinally between myelinated fibers (Fig. 28-14). Oligodendroglia synthesize myelin during the late gestational period and through early postnatal life subsequently maintaining these lipid membranes to insulate axons. In diseases that affect oligodendrocytes (e.g., in multiple sclerosis and progressive multifocal leukoencephalopathy), demyelination impairs axonal function. Oligodendrogliomas are a less common type of glioma than astrocytic neoplasms.

Ependyma Regulates Fluid Transport

A single layer of ependymal cells lines the four ventricular chambers, the aqueduct of Sylvius, the central canal of the spinal cord, and the filum terminale. These cells vary from cuboidal to flat (Fig. 28-15) and modulate fluid transfer between the cerebrospinal fluid (CSF) and the CNS. During gestation, some viral infections target the ependymal cells, an event responsible in part for aqueductal stenosis and congenital hydrocephalus. Ependymomas, which result from the neoplastic transformation of ependymal cells, generally arise within a ventricle, but they also present as intramedullary tumors of the spinal cord and filum terminale.

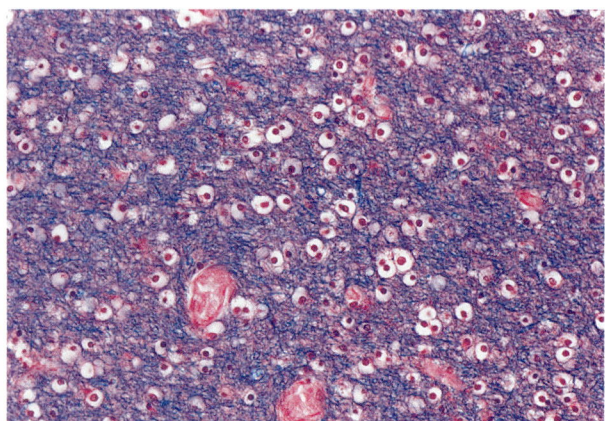

FIGURE 28-14
Normal white matter. In this section stained with H&E plus Luxol fast blue for myelin, the white matter contains oligodendroglia, with small nuclei and clear cytoplasm. They are often aligned along the myelinated axons.

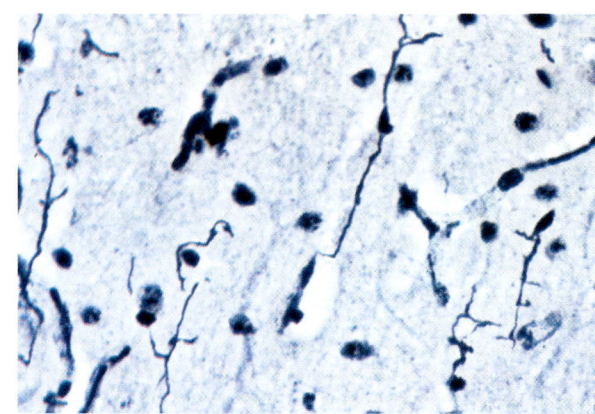

FIGURE 28-16
Microglia. CNS macrophages, termed *microglia*, show a few elongated processes in silver carbonate stains.

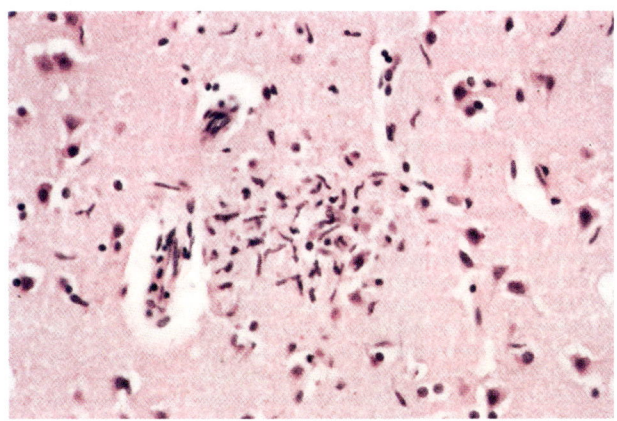

FIGURE 28-17
Glial nodule. Microglia and astrocytes create cellular nodules in response to viral, protozoan, or rickettsial infections.

Microglia Are Macrophages of the CNS

Microglia are phagocytic macrophage-derived cells of the CNS, accounting for 5% of all glial cells.

ANATOMY: Resting microglia are identified in tissues stained with hematoxylin and eosin by their hyperchromatic, elongated nuclei surrounded by a thin rim of cytoplasm. When stained with silver for microglial markers, they appear filiform and display fine processes (Fig. 28-16). Microglia may be scattered in the neuropil or disposed around neurons or blood vessels.

REACTIONS: Microglia proliferate and show reactive changes in areas of injury. Two patterns are recognized, namely, focal microglial nodules and diffuse microgliosis. *Microglial nodules* are formed of microglia and astrocytes (Fig. 28-17), and are typical responses to viral or other infections. Some reactive microglia exhibit a prominent elongated nucleus, in which case they are referred to as *rod cells*. In response to necrosis, microglia become phagocytic, accumulate lipids and other cellular debris, and are designated *gitter cells* (Fig. 28-18). Although the embryonic derivation of microglia continues to be debated, it appears that phagocytic microglia in CNS inflammations are blood-derived monocytes.

CONGENITAL MALFORMATIONS

The development of the CNS proceeds according to a precise schedule, and each morphological event is the cornerstone for those that follow. For example, myelination is initiated late in embryonic development only after the neurons and oligodendroglia have differentiated and migrated to their appropriate destinations; interruption of these processes results in flawed myelination. **Thus, congenital anomalies reflect interruptions in the completion of critical developmental processes.**

Accordingly, the characteristics of a congenital malformation are defined more by the time of the insult than by the nature of the injury itself. Although specific congenital malformations may have many causes, they tend to share a common time-related target. For instance, anoxia and radiation induce anencephaly (see below) when administered to rats early in the eighth day of pregnancy but only a little later cause cleft palate.

Neural Tube Defects (Dysraphic States) Reflect Impaired Closure of the Dorsal Aspect of the Vertebral Column

Spina Bifida

Spina bifida is a neural tube defect most common in the lumbosacral region (Fig. 28-19). It is further classified according to the extent of the defect.

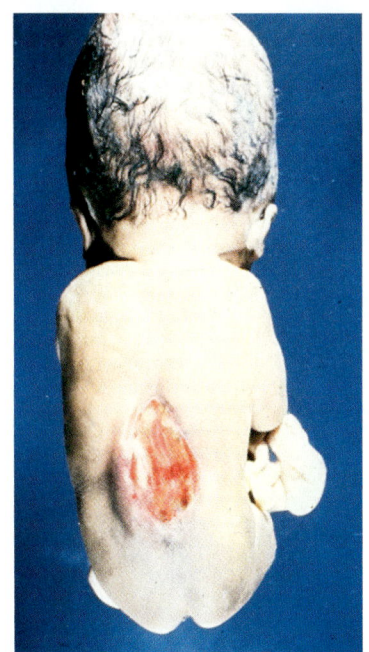

FIGURE 28-19
Spina bifida with meningomyelocele. The deformity is evident at birth as an elliptical, cutaneous defect over the lumbar spine.

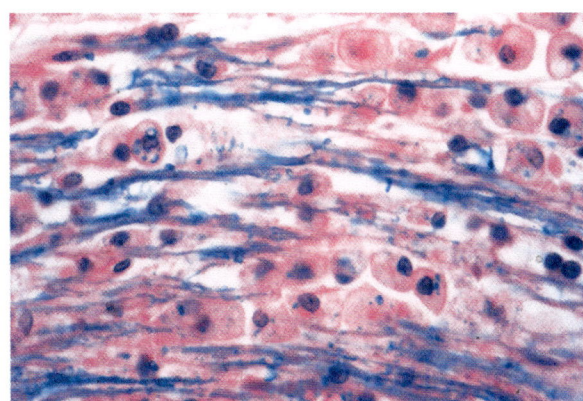

FIGURE 28-18
Macrophages. Section from a patient with central pontine myelinolysis. Macrophages, activated microglia, and other cells accumulate at sites of tissue destruction.

1420   The Nervous System

- **Spina bifida occulta:** This defect is restricted to the vertebral arches and is usually asymptomatic. It is frequently manifested externally only by a dimple or small tuft of hair.
- **Meningocele:** This condition features a more extensive bony and soft tissue defect that permits protrusion of the meninges as a fluid-filled sac. The lateral aspects of the sac are characteristically covered by skin, whereas the apex is usually ulcerated.
- **Meningomyelocele:** This term refers to a still more extensive defect that exposes the spinal canal and causes the nerve roots (particularly those of the cauda equina) to be entrapped in subcutaneous scar tissue (Fig. 28-20). Characteristically, the spinal cord appears as a flattened, ribbonlike structure.
- **Rachischisis:** In this extreme defect, the spinal column is converted into a gaping canal, often without a recognizable spinal cord (Fig. 28-21).

Neural tube defects are also discussed in Chapter 6.

Pathogenesis: Spina bifida is induced readily in rats and chicks at the eighth to ninth gestational day by chemicals such as trypan blue or by hypervitaminosis A. It probably results from a failure of neural tube closure, but the validity of this concept is uncertain. Maternal folic acid deficiency has been associated with an increased incidence of neural tube defects, and folic acid has therefore, been approved for inclusion as a food supplement in commercial flour.

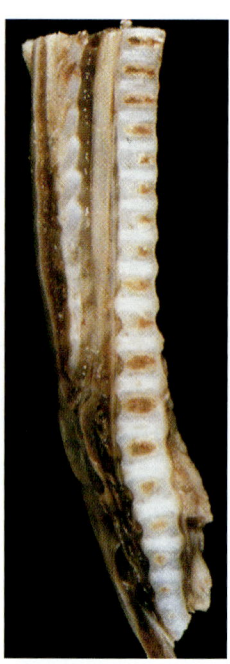

FIGURE 28-21
Rachischisis. A view of the vertebral column shows a bony, cutaneous defect with segmental absence of the spinal cord.

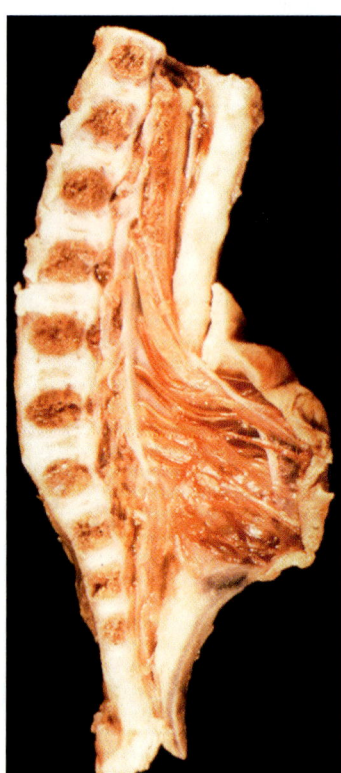

FIGURE 28-20
Meningomyelocele. A sagittal section of the vertebral column discloses nerve roots arching through the saccular defect.

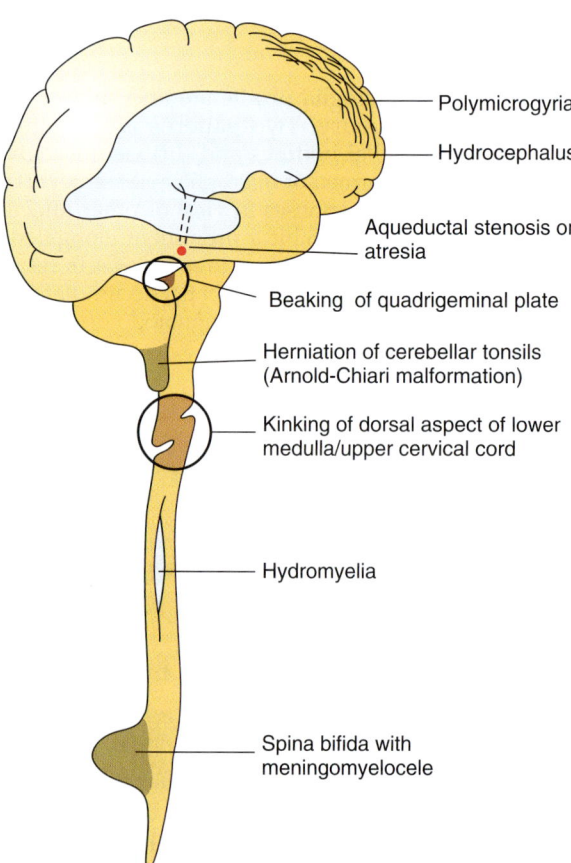

FIGURE 28-22
Arnold-Chiari malformation and associated lesions.

Congenital Malformations

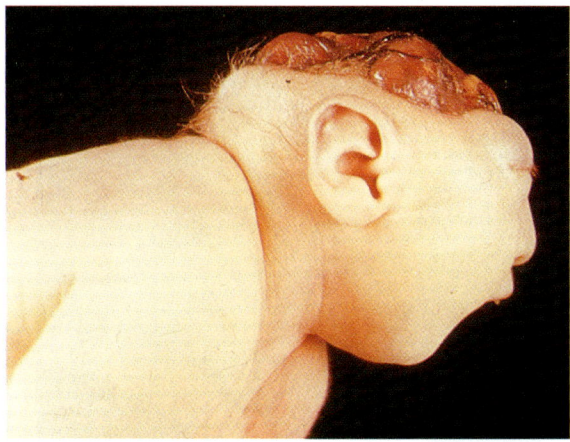

FIGURE 28-23
Anencephaly. Absence of a calvarium exposes a mass of vascularized tissue (cerebrovasculosa), in which there are rudimentary neuroectodermal structures. The lesion is bounded anteriorly by normally formed eyes and posteriorly by the brainstem.

Clinical Features: The spectrum of neurological deficits in neural tube defects ranges from no symptoms in spina bifida occulta to lower limb paralysis, sensory loss, and incontinence with meningomyelocele. One must be aware of potential associated malformations such as Arnold-Chiari malformation, hydrocephalus, polymicrogyria, and hydromyelia of the spinal central canal (Fig. 28-22).

Anencephaly

Anencephaly refers to the congenital absence of all or part of the brain (Fig. 28-23). Among CNS malformations, anencephaly is second in incidence to spina bifida (0.5–2.0 per 1000 births, with a modest female predominance). Anencephalic fetuses are either stillborn or die within the first few days of life.

Pathogenesis: The pathogenesis of anencephaly is unclear, but it may be due to failed closure of the anterior neuropore or disturbed angiogenesis. The concurrence of anencephaly with other neural tube defects, such as spina bifida, suggests they all may result from shared pathogenic mechanisms.

Pathology: The cranial vault in anencephaly is absent, and the cerebral hemispheres are a discoid mass of highly vascularized, poorly differentiated neural tissue, the so-called *cerebrovasculosa*. This structure lies on the flattened base of the skull, behind two well-formed eyes, which mark the anterior margin of disturbed organogenesis. A well-differentiated retina attests to the preservation of the eyes, and short segments of the optic nerve extend posteriorly. The posterior aspect of the malformation forms a variable transitional zone with a recognizable midbrain, but most often the entire brainstem and cerebellum are rudimentary. The upper spinal cord is hypoplastic, and a dysraphic bony defect of the posterior spinal column (rachischisis) may involve the cervical area. Vertebral and basilar arteries usually are identifiable in a tangle of meningeal vessels (Fig. 28-24A).

The cerebrovasculosa corresponds to the residual underdeveloped cerebral hemispheres typically containing islands of immature neural tissue (see Fig. 28-24B). It also encloses cavities partially lined by ependyma with or without choroid plexus. However, the mass is composed predominantly of abnormal vascular channels that vary considerably in size.

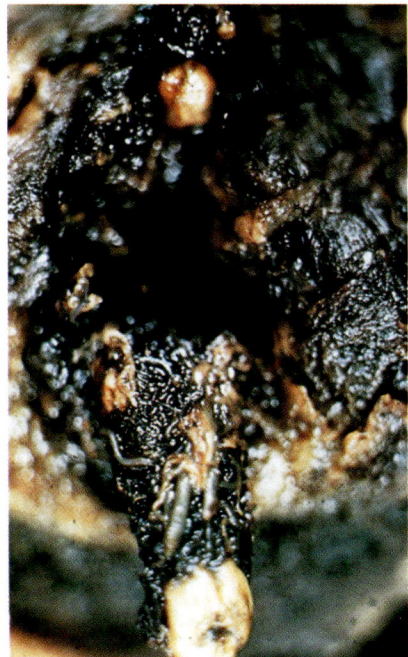
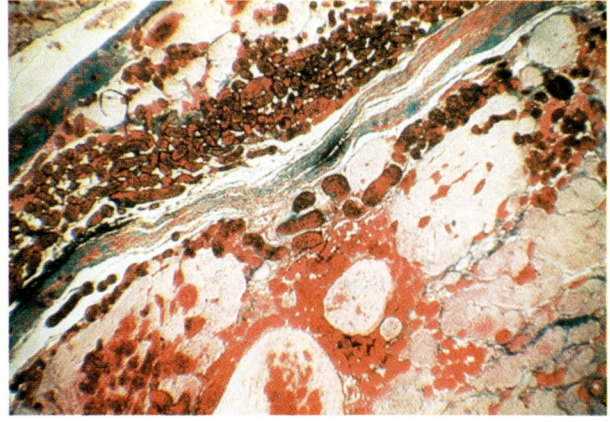

FIGURE 28-24
Anencephaly. A. Inferior view of the discoid mass (cerebrovasculosa) that replaces the brain in anencephaly shows a well-formed medulla encircled by a plexus of abnormal blood vessels. B. A microscopic section shows that the cerebrovasculosa contains islands of neural tissue and an abundance of thin-walled blood vessels.

Malformations of the Spinal Cord are Uncommon Congenital Disorders

The spinal cord may harbor congenital malformations that are less apparent at birth than neural tube defects. They include rare duplications, ranging from complete (*dimyelia*) to partial duplications of spinal cord into two separate structures (*diastematomyelia*).

Hydromyelia refers to dilation of the central canal of the spinal cord (see Fig. 28-22).

SYRINGOMYELIA: In this congenital malformation, a tubular cavitation (syrinx) extends for variable distances along the entire length of the spinal cord, which may or may not communicate with the central canal. The condition is usually encountered in adults, although many cases are thought to represent a congenital malformation. Clearly, some cases are caused by trauma, ischemia, or tumors. The syrinx is filled with a clear fluid closely resembling CSF. The symptoms of syringomyelia are related to the extent of the syrinx and its concomitant destruction of cells and fibers. Motor and sensory deficits occur at various levels, reflecting the anatomical location of the lesions in the spinal cord.

Syringobulbia is a variant of syringomyelia in which slitlike cavities are located in the medulla.

Arnold-Chiari Malformation Involves the Medulla and Cerebellum

Arnold-Chiari malformation is a condition in which the brainstem and cerebellum are compacted into a shallow, bowl-shaped posterior fossa with a low-positioned tentorium. It is often associated with syringomyelia or a lumbosacral meningomyelocele (see Fig. 28-22), and the symptomatology depends on the severity of the defect.

Pathogenesis: Arnold-Chiari malformation may result when a meningomyelocele anchors the lower end of the spinal cord and causes downward growth of the vertebral column, thereby creating traction on the medulla (see Fig. 28-22). However, other features of this malformation (curvature of the medulla, beaking of the quadrigeminal plate) are not explained by this mechanism. Other proposed mechanisms include increased intracranial pressure associated with hydrocephalus or limited size of the posterior fossa.

Pathology: In Arnold-Chiari malformation, the caudal aspect of the cerebellar vermis is herniated through an enlarged foramen magnum (Fig. 28-25) and protrudes onto the dorsal aspect of the cervical cord, often reaching the level of C3 to C5. The herniated tissue is bound in position by thickened meninges and shows pres-

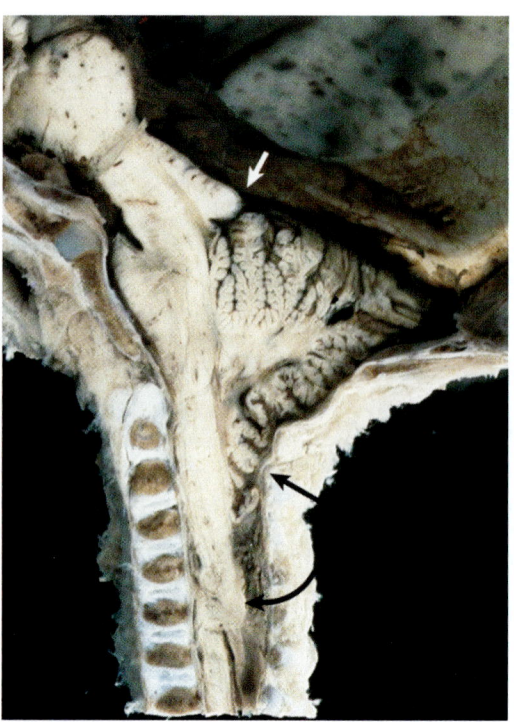

FIGURE 28-25
Arnold-Chiari malformation. The cerebellar vermis is herniated below the level of the foramen magnum (*straight arrow*). **The downward displacement of the dorsal portion of the cord causes the obex of the fourth ventricle to occupy a position below the foramen magnum. The beaking of the inferior colliculus of the quadrigeminal plate** (*white arrow*) **and the S-shaped angulation of the upper cervical cord are seen** (*curved arrow*).

sure atrophy (i.e., depletion of Purkinje and granular cells). The brainstem also is displaced caudally. Typically, the displacement is more exaggerated dorsally than ventrally, and landmarks such as the obex of the fourth ventricle are more caudal than ventral structures such as the inferior olive. From a lateral perspective, the lower medulla is angulated in its midsegment, thereby creating a dorsal protrusion (Fig. 28-26). The foramina of Magendie and Luschka are compressed by the bony ridge of the foramen magnum. The cerebellum is flattened to a discoid contour, and the quadrigeminal plate is often deformed by a "beak-shaped" dorsal protrusion of the inferior colliculi. Hydrocephalus results from obstruction of the foramina of Magendie and Luschka.

Congenital Hydrocephalus Refers to an Excessive Amount of CSF and Ventricular Enlargement

The fluid accumulations are in varied locations and have many causes, as discussed below in the section on cerebrospinal fluid.

Congenital atresia of the aqueduct of Sylvius is the most common cause of congenital hydrocephalus (Fig. 28-27). It occurs with an incidence of 1 in 1000 live births. Histo-

Congenital Malformations

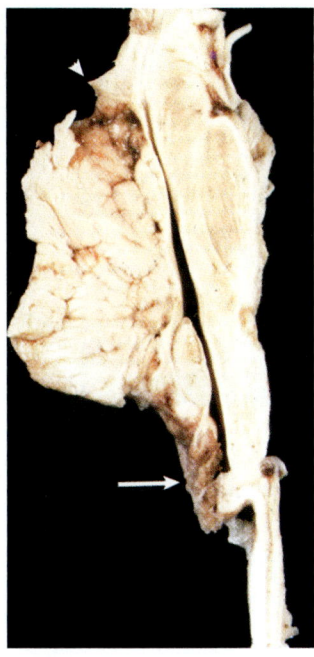

FIGURE 28-26
Arnold-Chiari malformation. A sagittal section of the brainstem illustrates the features enumerated in Figure 28-22. A tongue of cerebellar vermis extends downward over the dorsum of the cervical cord *(arrow)*. Note the sharp beak of the inferior colliculus *(arrowhead)*.

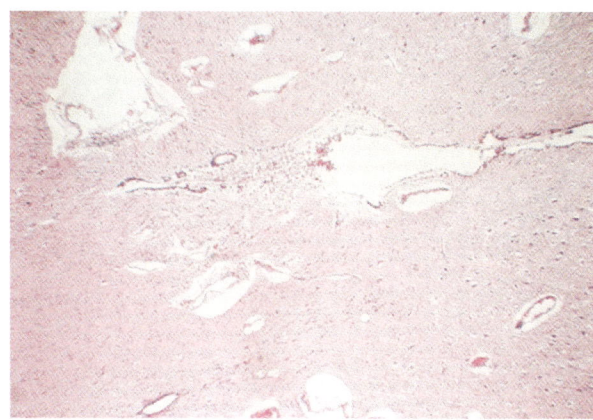

FIGURE 28-28
Neonatal hydrocephalus. Multiple atretic canals replace the normal single aqueduct of Sylvius.

logical examination of the midbrain may disclose multiple atretic channels (Fig. 28-28) or an aqueduct narrowed by gliosis (Fig. 28-29), which may result from transplacental transmission of viruses that induce ependymitis.

Disorders of Cerebral Gyri Are Frequently Associated with Mental Retardation

Abnormalities of the cerebral gyri, which are frequently associated with mental retardation, include a spectrum of entities exemplified by the following:

- **Polymicrogyria** refers to the presence of small and excessive gyri (Fig. 28-30).

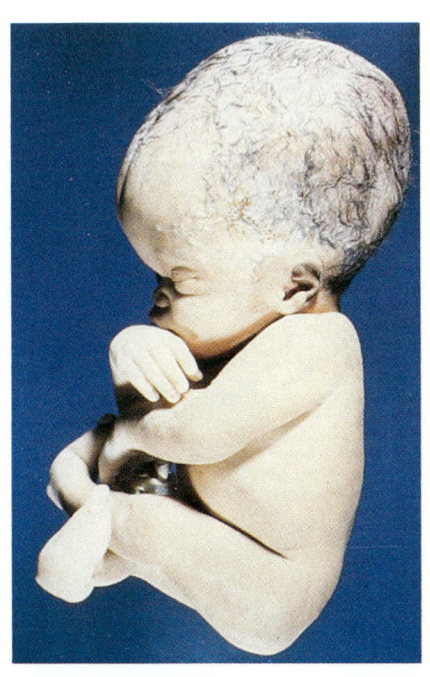
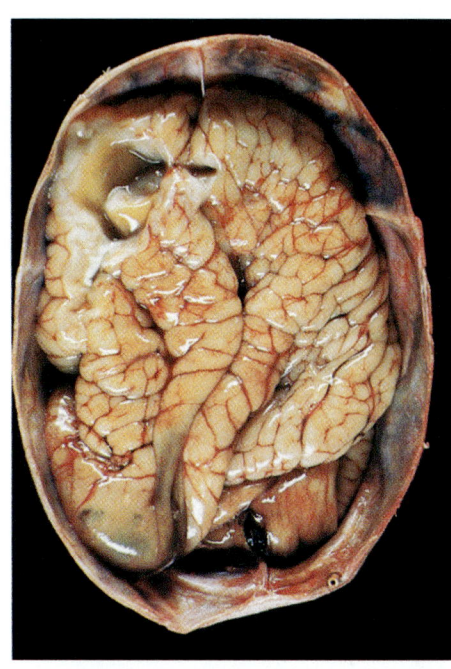

FIGURE 28-27
Congenital hydrocephalus. A. Hydrocephalus occurring before the fusion of the cranial sutures causes pronounced enlargement of the head. B. Removal of the calvaria demonstrates an atrophic and collapsed cerebral cortex.

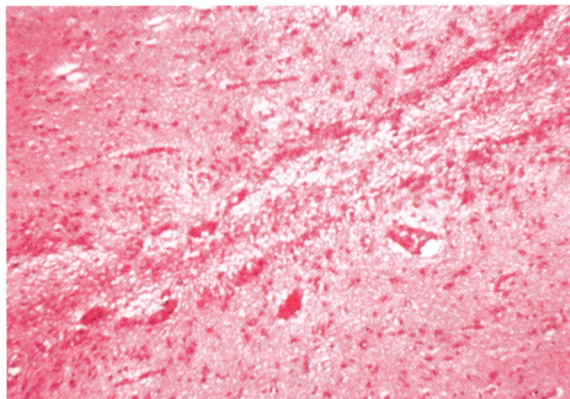

FIGURE 28-29
Neonatal hydrocephalus. The aqueduct of Sylvius is occluded by astrogliosis, a possible response to an intrauterine viral infection.

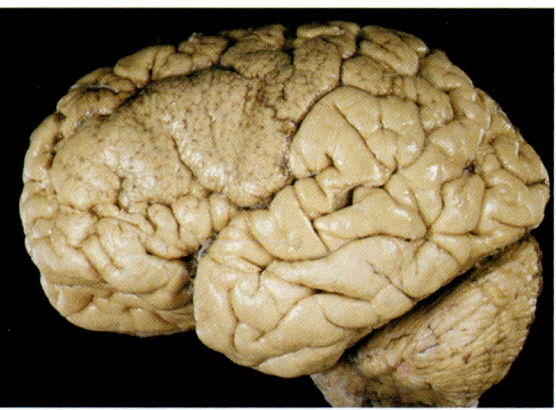

FIGURE 28-31
Pachygyria. The occurrence of broad gyri marks a deformity of embryonic development.

- **Pachygyria** is a condition in which the gyri are reduced in number and unusually broad (Fig. 28-31).
- **Lissencephaly** is a congenital disorder in which the cortical surface of the cerebral hemispheres is smooth or has imperfectly formed gyri. Some 60% of patients with lissencephaly show deletions in the region of the *LIS1* gene on chromosome 17p13.3, which encodes a protein involved in cytoskeletal dynamics that plays a role in cell proliferation and motility.

    Gyral malformations arise from disturbances in neuronal migration, a highly patterned event of the first trimester of embryonic development. The primitive neurons move centrifugally from the germinal epithelia to populate the cortex. The number of neurons and their positions in the cortex are determining factors in the cortical infolding that creates sulci and gyri.

- **Heterotopias** are focal disturbances in neuronal migration that lead to nodules of ectopic neurons and glia, usually in white matter. They are often are associated with mental retardation and seizures and may be caused by maternal alcoholism.

Congenital Defects Are Often Associated with Chromosomal Abnormalities

Derangements of the larger autosomes, 1 through 12, are incompatible with sustained intrauterine life, and affected fetuses are spontaneously aborted. Structural and functional abnormalities attributable to gross chromosomal derangements are best exemplified by trisomies of chromosomes 13 to 15 and chromosome 21 (Down syndrome).

Down Syndrome

Down syndrome (trisomy 21) is characterized by mental retardation, distinctive facial features, and other anomalies. Although most cases reflect trisomy of chromosome 21, they rarely result from translocations or mosaicism. Down syndrome is discussed in detail in Chapter 6. The brain is moderately reduced in weight and is shortened in its anteroposterior dimension. There is a simple gyral pattern, with disproportionately slender superior temporal gyri (Fig. 28-32). The

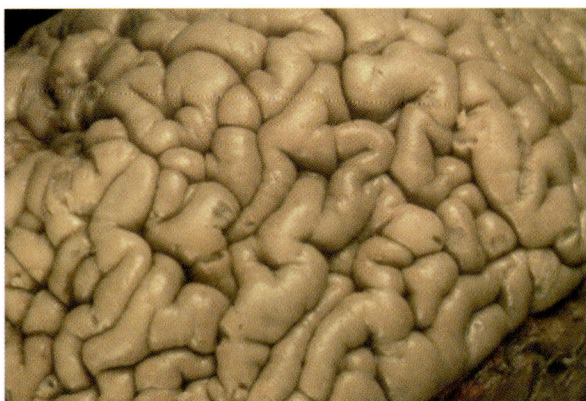

FIGURE 28-30
Polymicrogyria. The surface of the brain exhibits an excessive number of small, irregularly sized, randomly distributed gyral folds.

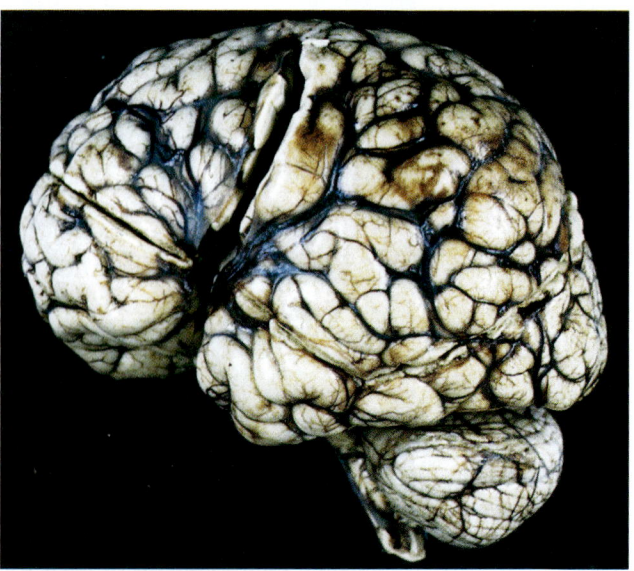

FIGURE 28-32
Down syndrome. Mild microcephaly and underdevelopment of the superior temporal gyri are noted.

cytoarchitecture of the Down syndrome cortex closely approximates normal patterns, although patients typically develop changes of Alzheimer disease pathology (see below) by the fourth decade of life.

Trisomy 13–15

Trisomy 13-15 has an incidence of 1 per 5000 births, with a modest female predominance. The congenital deformities involve the brain, facial features, and extremities. The complex is dominated by holoprosencephaly, arrhinencephaly, microphthalmia, cyclopia, low-set ears, harelip, and cleft palate. The extremities exhibit polydactyly and "rocker bottom" feet.

HOLOPROSENCEPHALY: This term refers to a microcephalic brain in which the interhemispheric fissure is absent. The horseshoe-shaped cerebral hemispheres have fused frontal poles, across which the gyri show an irregular horizontal orientation (Fig. 28-33). A common ventricular chamber is created by lateral displacement of the posterior portions of the cerebral hemispheres. Bilobed caudate nuclei and thalami are prominent. Holoprosencephaly is rarely compatible with life beyond a few weeks or months.

ARRHINENCEPHALY: The absence of the olfactory tracts and bulbs (rhinencephalon) is associated with holoprosencephaly or occurs as a solitary malformation (Fig. 28-34).

ABSENCE OF THE CORPUS CALLOSUM: This anomaly is a regular feature of holoprosencephaly, but it can also be a solitary lesion. Absence of the corpus callosum may occur without significant impairment of interhemispheric functional coordination, but it is occasionally associated with seizures. The corpus callosum physically tethers and functionally interconnects the hemispheres, and its absence permits the lateral ventricles to drift outward and upward (Fig. 28-35), a position that is radiographically diagnostic.

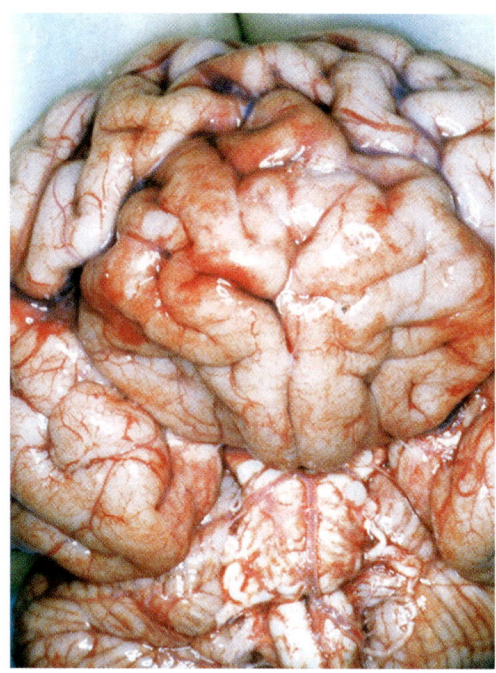

FIGURE 28-34
Arrhinencephaly. Absence of the olfactory system frequently accompanies holoprosencephaly.

Epilepsy Features Paroxysmal, Transient Disturbances (Seizures) in Brain Function

Seizures impair consciousness and cause abnormal motor activity or sensory or mental disturbances. Epilepsy has a prevalence of 6 per 1000, and newborns and infants are particularly vulnerable. Most seizures (75%) occur without a

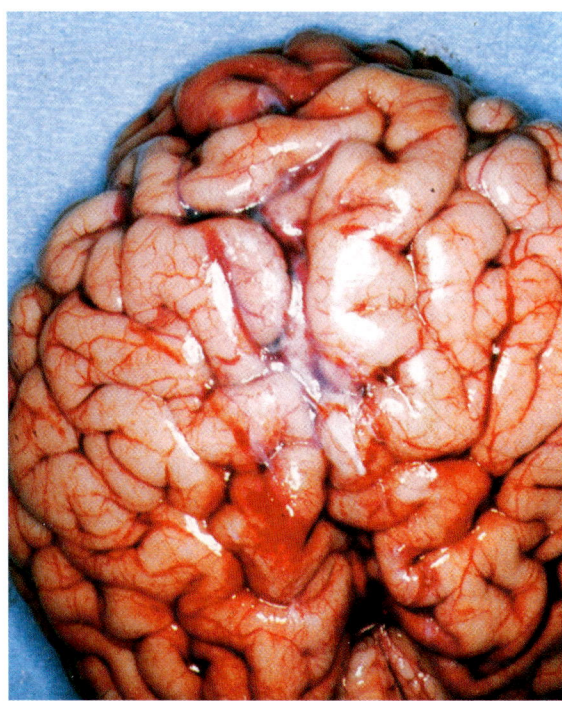

FIGURE 28-33
Holoprosencephaly. A view from the superior aspect of the brain shows the absence of the anterior interhemispheric fissure.

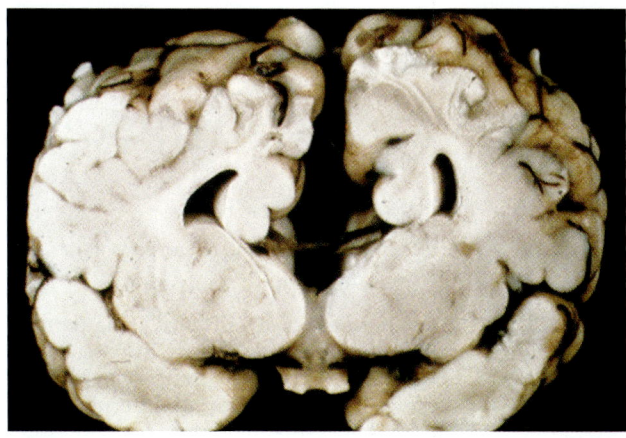

FIGURE 28-35
Congenital absence of the corpus callosum. The lateral ventricles are laterally displaced and the cingulate gyri occupy the position of the absent corpus callosum.

1426 The Nervous System

demonstrable organic lesion and are classed as idiopathic epilepsy. Most of these cases are sporadic, although hereditary forms are recognized.

 Pathology: Careful studies of the brains of patients who had idiopathic epilepsy often reveal neuronal loss and reactive gliosis. The affected areas include the hippocampus, cerebellum, thalamus, and cerebral neocortex. Whether these changes are the cause of idiopathic epilepsy or result from the anoxia that occurs with generalized seizures is still debated. Heterotopias are occasionally found, and less commonly, epilepsy may be initiated by an intracranial tumor, arteriovenous malformation, or brain scar from a penetrating wound. Such lesions are more likely to cause seizures the closer they are to the motor cortex or surface of the brain.

TRAUMA

Epidural Hematoma Is Accumulation of Blood between the Calvaria and the Dura

Epidural hematoma usually results from a blow to the head, and unless treated promptly, it generally fatal.

 Pathogenesis: The intracranial dura is securely bound to the inner aspect of the calvaria and is thus analogous to the periosteum. The middle meningeal arteries occupy the space between the dura and the calvaria. They are grooved into the inner table of the bone, and their branches splay across the temporal–parietal area, generally as three major vessels. The temporal bone is one of the thinnest bones of the skull and is particularly vulnerable to fracture, so that seemingly minor trauma may fracture it and transect branches of the middle meningeal artery. The result is life-threatening epidural hemorrhage (Fig. 28-36).

  Pathology and Clinical Course: Transection of the middle meningeal artery permits the escape of arterial blood into the epidural space, thereby separating the dura from the calvaria. The hematoma enlarges relentlessly (Fig. 28-37). During the initial 4 to 8 hours, the intracranial events are largely asymptomatic. When the hematoma attains a volume of 30 to 50 mL, symptoms that reflect a space-occupying lesion appear. Because the supratentorial compartment has a fixed volume, the introduction of a space-occupying mass displaces an equal volume from this region. The earliest volumetric adjustments before symptoms appear are accomplished by the downward displacement of CSF through the aperture in the tentorium. If the hematoma continues to enlarge, intracranial pressure eventually exceeds the venous pressure. The large venous sinuses are then compressed, resulting in circulatory stagnation and cerebral ischemia. During this interval of global cerebral hypoxia, diffuse cortical impairment is manifested by confusion and disorientation.

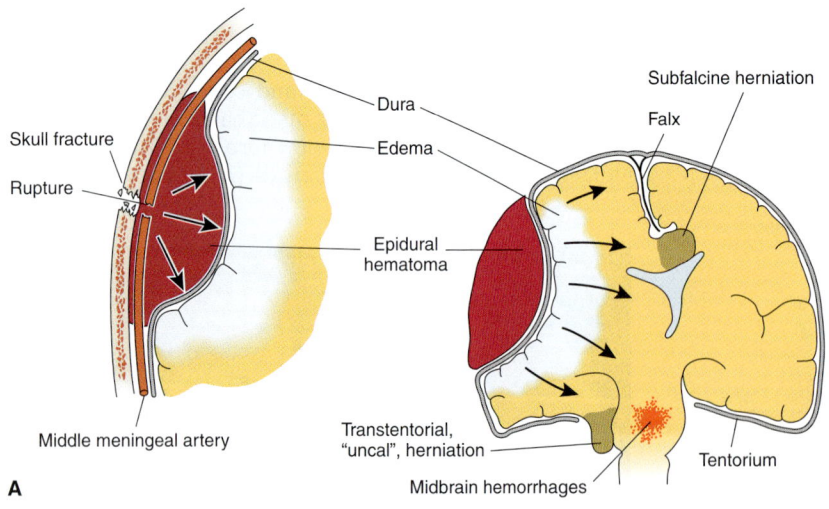
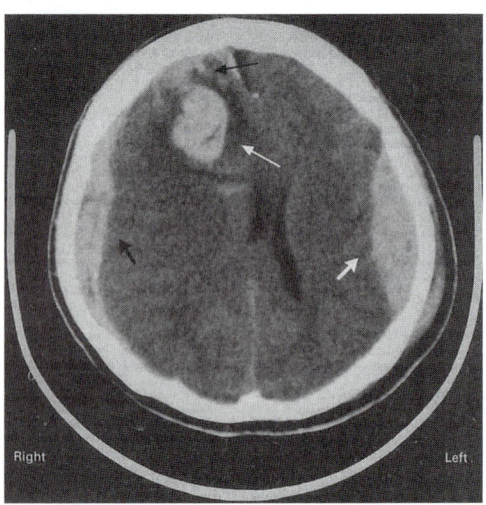

FIGURE 28-36
Development of an epidural hematoma. A. Transection of a branch of the middle meningeal artery by the sharp fracture initiates bleeding under arterial pressure that dissects the dura from the calvaria and produces an expanding hematoma. After an asymptomatic interval of several hours, transtentorial herniation becomes life-threatening. **B.** CT scan of post-traumatic intracranial hemorrhages. The film shows an epidural hematoma (thick white arrow, left side): a laminated subdural hematoma (thick black arrow, right side); an intraparenchymal hematoma (thin white arrow, right side); and a subarachnoid hemorrhage (thin black arrow, right frontal region).

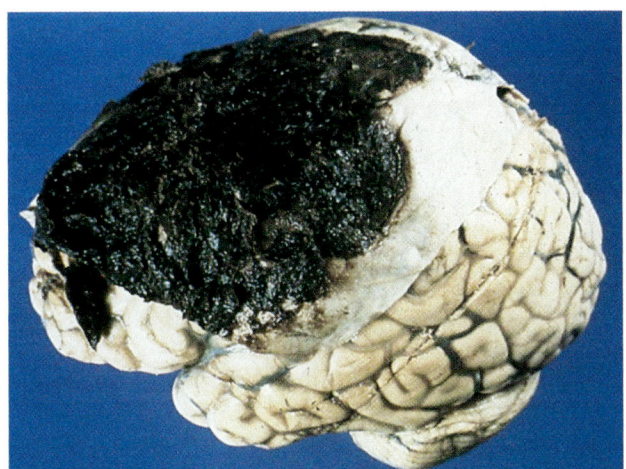

FIGURE 28-37
Epidural hematoma. A discoid mass of fresh hemorrhage overlies the frontal–parietal cortex.

The *Cushing reflex* is a protective response that augments cerebral circulation and increases cerebral oxygenation. The heart rate slows to increase ventricular filling, and myocardial contraction becomes more forceful. The blood pressure, particularly systolic pressure, increases. If bleeding continues, the hematoma can attain a size of about 60 mL within 6 to 10 hours. After compensatory mechanisms have been exhausted, the brain is shifted laterally away from the side of the lesion. The medial temporal lobe on the side of the hematoma is compressed against the midbrain to displace it downward through the opening created by the tentorium, a fatal event known as *transtentorial herniation* (Fig. 28-38). This herniation compresses the tissues of the uncus of the hippocampus against the midbrain and also against contiguous structures, such as the third nerve. Thus, the oculomotor nerve is compressed against the edge of the tentorium, causing third-nerve palsy. The pupil, generally on the side of the lesion, becomes fixed and dilated.

The herniated uncus also compresses the vasculature of the midbrain, especially the paired mesencephalic veins (great veins of Rosenthal). Venous stagnation in the midbrain causes further hypoxia and impairs neuronal function. Damage to the reticular formation is expressed clinically as a decline in the level of consciousness. Shortly thereafter, hemorrhage (Figs. 28-38 through 28-40) and necrosis of the brainstem occur, after which injury to the reticular formation becomes irreversible (Fig. 28-41). Death is imminent or, if the supratentorial pressure is relieved, unconsciousness is permanent. **Epidural hematomas are invariably progressive and, when not recognized and evacuated, are fatal in 24 to 48 hours.**

Concussion is defined as the transient loss of consciousness due to trauma. The blow to the head that causes an epidural hematoma does not necessarily have to produce a concussion. Consciousness is a positive neurological activity that depends on the function of specific neurons, especially in the brainstem reticular formation. Concussion is exemplified in the boxing ring, as the consequence of a blow that deflects the head upward and posteriorly, often with a rotatory component. These motions impart a quick torque on the brainstem and cause functional paralysis of the neurons of the reticular formation. By contrast, a blow to the temporal–parietal area may lead to a skull fracture but does not gener-

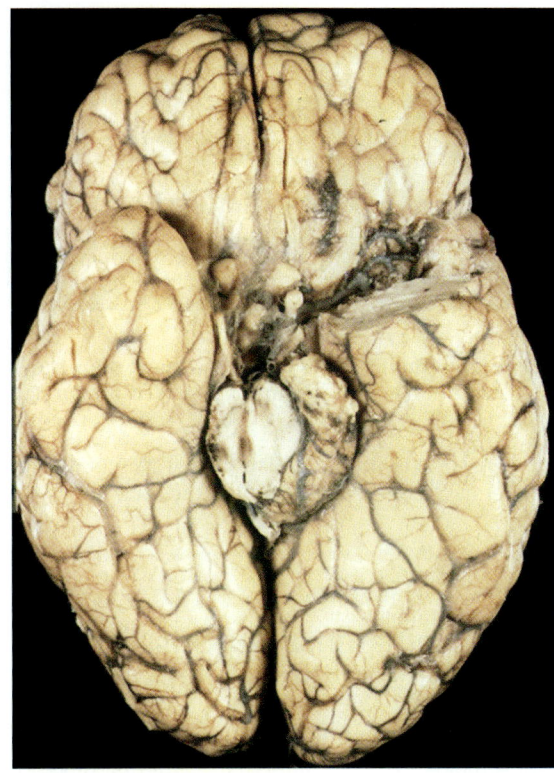

FIGURE 28-38
Transtentorial herniation. The uncus of the hippocampus is herniated downward to displace the midbrain, which is the site of secondary ("Duret") hemorrhages.

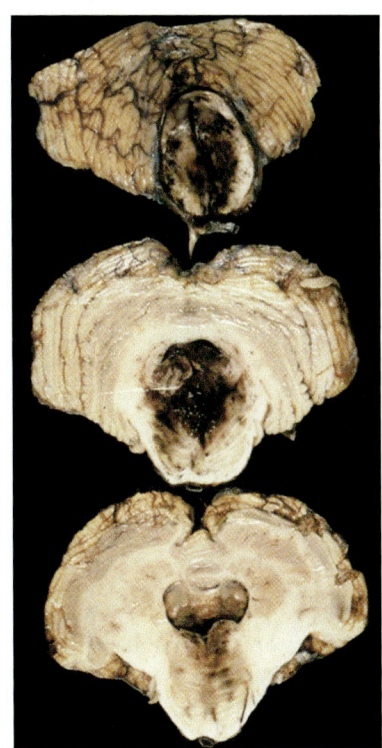

FIGURE 28-39
Transtentorial herniation. Duret hemorrhages in a case of transtentorial herniation tend to be midline and to occupy the brainstem from the upper midbrain to midpons.

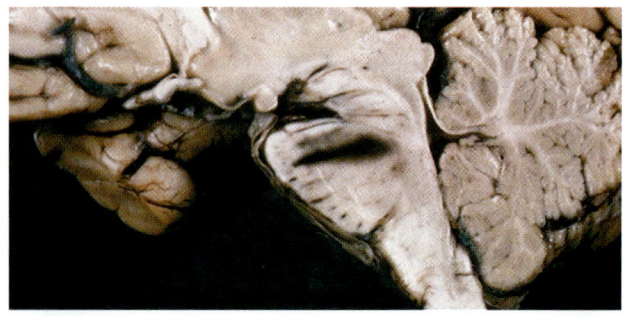

FIGURE 28-40
Transtentorial herniation. A sagittal section reveals the longitudinal distribution of Duret hemorrhages *(red-brown streaks).*

ally cause a concussion, because lateral movement of the cerebral hemispheres is prevented by the falx.

Subdural Hematoma Reflects Torn Bridging Veins in the Subdural Space

Subdural hematoma is a significant cause of death after head injuries from falls, assaults, vehicular accidents, and sporting mishaps.

 Pathogenesis: The cerebral hemispheres are tethered loosely by blood vessels and cranial nerves and float in the CSF. Drainage from the cerebral hemispheres flows upward through veins that cross the subarachnoid space and arachnoid and traverse the subdural space to breach the dura and enter the dural sinus.

When the frontal or occipital portion of the moving head strikes a fixed object or when the stationary head is struck by a blunt object, the cerebral hemispheres are displaced in an anteroposterior direction and hit forcefully against the inner aspect of the occipital or frontal bone. The soft cerebral tissues become compact and then recoil, producing a rippling effect through brain parenchyma. Because the dura adheres to the skull and the arachnoid is attached to the cerebrum, the disparate movement of these membranes produces a shearing effect in the subdural space, which tears the veins that pass through this compartment (Fig. 28-42). Unlike the epidural space, the subdural space can expand. Since bleeding in this situation is from veins, it usually stops spontaneously after an accumulation of 25 to 50mL, from a local tamponade effect. However, this also can compress severed bridging veins and cause thrombosis. Because the brain is symmetric and a force applied in the sagittal plane similarly affects both cerebral hemispheres, it is not surprising that subdural hematomas are frequently bilateral.

Pathology: A subdural hematoma, even when it is limited and too small to cause symptoms, can induce important tissue responses. Contact between the hematoma and the dura causes irritation and leads to the formation of granulation tissue over the subsequent several weeks. This process creates a membrane above the hematoma, termed the *outer membrane* (Fig. 28-43). Fibroblasts migrate from this membrane to invade the subjacent hematoma and form a fibrous membrane subjacent to the blood clot. Two weeks are required for this *inner membrane* to become visible (Fig. 28-44).

A subdural hematoma, static in size and generally asymptomatic, has the potential for three routes of evolution:

- The hematoma may be reabsorbed and leave only a small amount of telltale hemosiderin.
- The hematoma may remain static, with the potential for calcification.
- The hematoma may enlarge.

Expansion of the hematoma, together with the onset of symptoms, commonly results from rebleeding, usually within 6 months. Since granulation tissue is vulnerable to minor trauma, even that caused by shaking the head, it can rebleed and create a new hematoma subjacent to the outer membrane. A series of events similar to those described above ensues, including formation of a second inner membrane. Such episodes of sporadic rebleeding expand the lesion periodically and at unpredictable intervals. Alternatively, it has been postulated that lysis of the original hematoma may create a hyperosmotic state that attracts fluid across the inner membrane and enlarges the lesion. If true, this process is of less consequence than rebleeding as a cause of symptoms. Remarkably, during the genesis of a subdural hematoma, the severance of the cortical bridging veins is so precisely localized to the subdural space that it compartmentalizes blood away from the CSF. **Thus, the absence of blood in the CSF does not negate the presence of a subdural hematoma.**

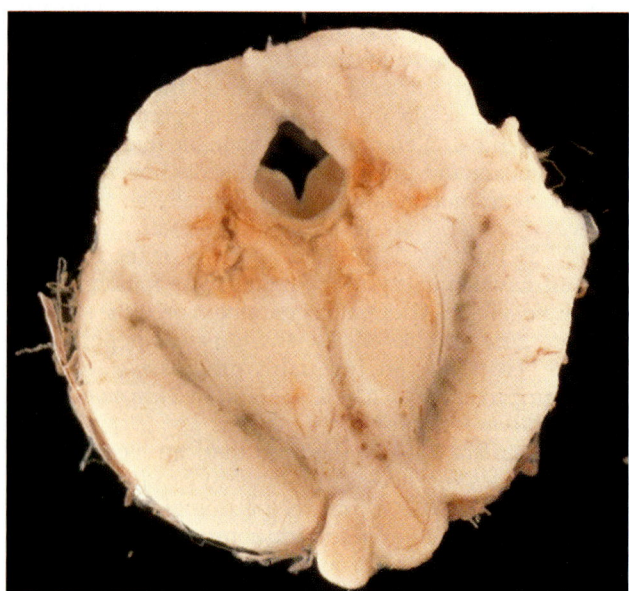

FIGURE 28-41
Transtentorial herniation in a cross-section of the midbrain of a patient who survived but remained unconscious for several months. Hemosiderin-stained areas *(orange-brown)* **mark the sites of previous Duret hemorrhages.**

Trauma 1429

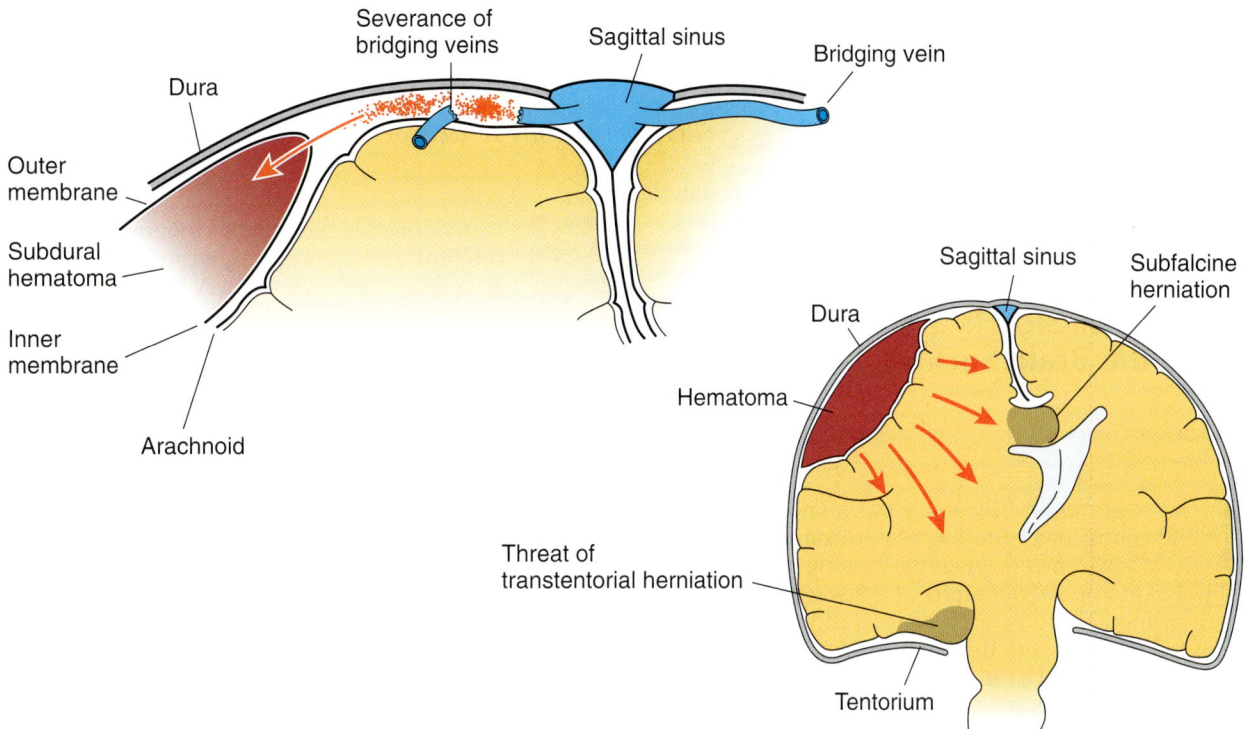

FIGURE 28-42
Development of a subdural hematoma. With head trauma, the dura moves with the skull, and the arachnoid moves with the cerebrum. As a result, the bridging veins are sheared as they cross between the dura and the arachnoid. Venous bleeding creates a hematoma in the expansile subdural space. Subsequent transtentorial herniation is life threatening.

Clinical Features: Subdural hematomas cause diverse clinical manifestations. Stretching of the meninges induces headaches, pressure on the motor cortex produces contralateral weakness, and focal cortical irritation can initiate seizures. Bilateral subdural hematomas may impair cognitive function and lead to a mistaken diagnosis of dementia, or rebleeding may cause a lethal transtentorial herniation.

Subarachnoid Hemorrhage Refers to Any Bleeding into the Subarachnoid Space

Subarachnoid hemorrhage may be seen in association with traumatic head injuries (e.g., cerebral contusion or laceration). However, it is rarely an isolated finding in the case of

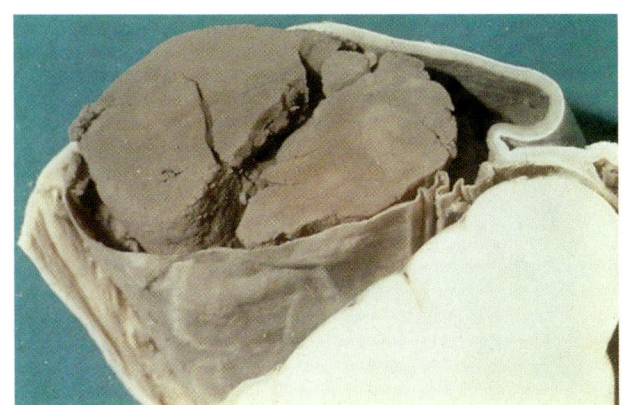

FIGURE 28-43
Subdural hematoma. A chronic subdural hematoma is encapsulated by an outer membrane (*thin brown layer beneath the thicker white dura*).

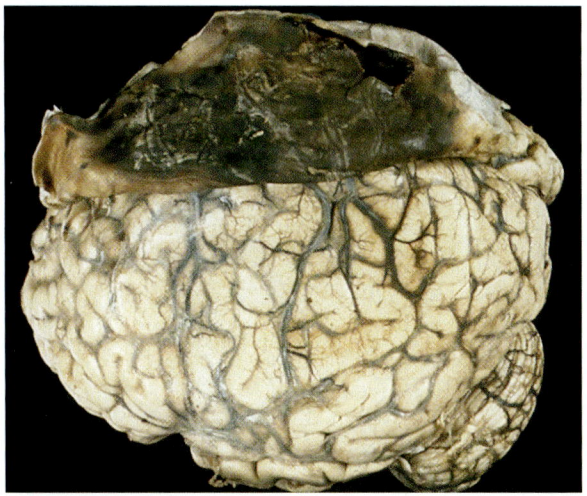

FIGURE 28-44
Subdural hematoma. The left leaf of the dura has been deflected upward to disclose a subdural hematoma that is thinly encapsulated by an inner membrane.

trauma and usually complicates hemorrhage in other parts of the brain. **Two thirds of cases of subarachnoid hemorrhages reflect the rupture of a preexisting arterial aneurysm** (see below). In 10% of cases, an arteriovenous malformation is demonstrated. The remaining instances result from a variety of conditions, including blood dyscrasias, infections, vasculitis, and tumors. Subarachnoid hemorrhage and cerebral aneurysms are discussed more fully below.

Cerebral Contusion Is a Traumatic Bruise of the Brain Surface

 Pathogenesis: Like subdural hematomas, cerebral contusions generally result from anteroposterior displacements when the moving head strikes a fixed object. Anteroposterior shifts of the soft tofulike brain renders it vulnerable to bruises or lacerations as a consequence of forces applied to the head, especially in the midsagittal plane. The severity of the contusion corresponds to the velocity of the acceleration and the abruptness of the deceleration of the head. When the contusion occurs at the point of impact, the lesion is referred to as a *coup* (Fr., "blow") injury (Fig. 28-45). If the side of the brain opposite the impact site strikes the skull, the resulting abrasions are contralateral to the point of initial contact and are termed a *contrecoup* injury (see Fig. 28-45).

The distant location of contrecoup lesions underscores the anatomical features that determine the nature of the injury, as illustrated by Fig. 28-45, in which the occipital bone is the site of impact. There is no injury to the subjacent cortex, but the impact causes disparate motion of the cerebrum and the skull, so that the frontal and temporal poles strike the bony surfaces of the frontal and middle fossae.

 Pathology: If the force of the impact is mild, the cerebral contusion is limited to the cortex and the apex of gyri (Fig. 28-46A). A greater force destroys larger expanses of cortex, creates deep cavitary lesions that extend into the white matter, or lacerates the cortex and causes hemorrhage (see Fig. 28-46B). Together with edema, hemorrhage can create a mass lesion, which threatens life by transtentorial herniation.

Contusions are permanent. The bruised, necrotic tissue is promptly phagocytosed by macrophages and eliminated in large part via the bloodstream. Astrocytosis then leads to local scar formation, which persists as telltale evidence of a prior contusion (Fig. 28-47).

The consequences of traumatic brain injury may be internal and subtle to demonstrate. The parasagittal cortex is anchored to arachnoid villi *(pacchionian granulations)*, whereas the lateral aspects of the cerebrum move more freely. This anatomical feature, together with the differential density of gray and white matter, permits generation of shearing forces between different brain regions, leading to diffuse axonal shearing injuries, particularly in vehicular accidents. Shearing injuries can distort or disrupt axons, causing them to retract into "spheroids" as well as lose their myelin. This type of injury typically occurs in parasagittal white matter and may be accompanied by multiple small hemorrhages. If the injury is severe, the patient becomes

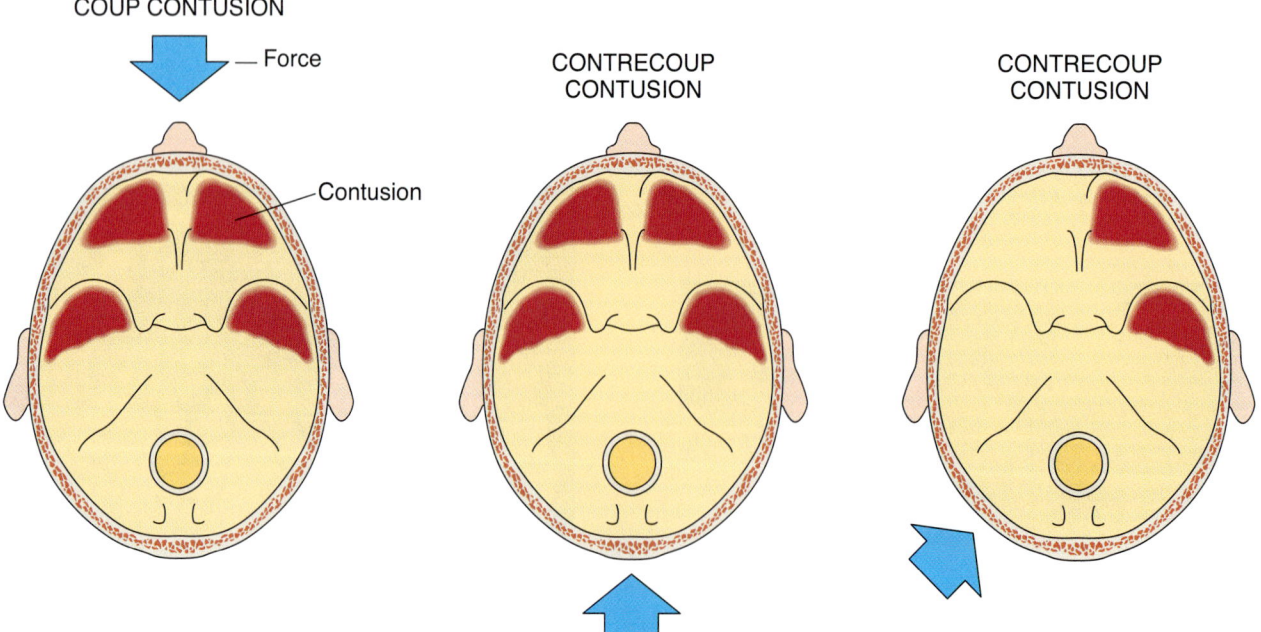

FIGURE 28-45

Mechanisms of cerebral contusion. The cerebral hemispheres float in the CSF. Rapid deceleration or acceleration of the skull causes the cortex to impact forcefully into the anterior and middle fossae. The position of a contusion is determined by the direction of the force and the intracranial anatomy.

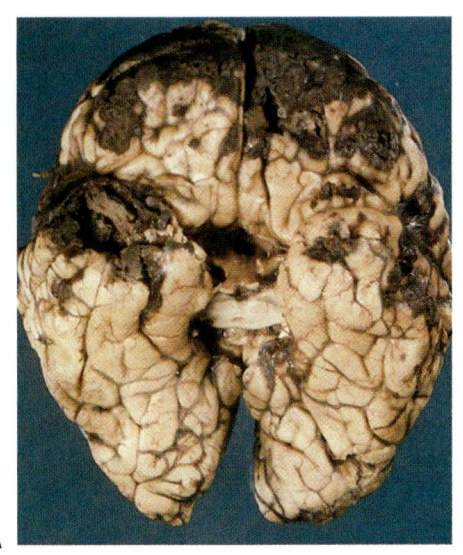
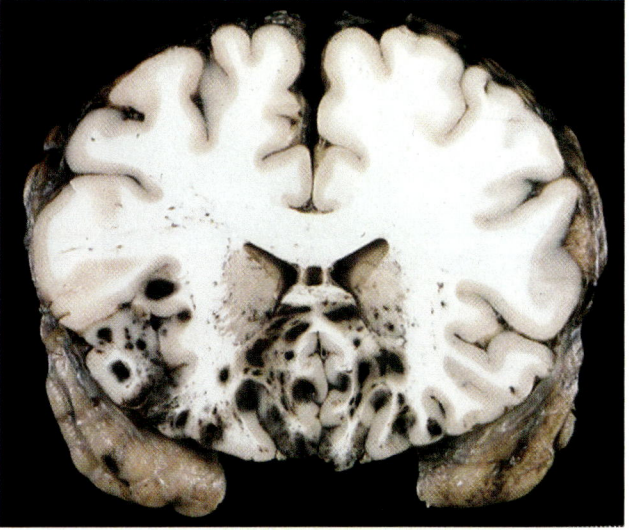

FIGURE 28-46
Recent cerebral contusions. A. Multiple areas of hemorrhage mark the poles of the frontal and temporal lobes. B. A coronal section of *A* shows underlying parenchymal hemorrhages.

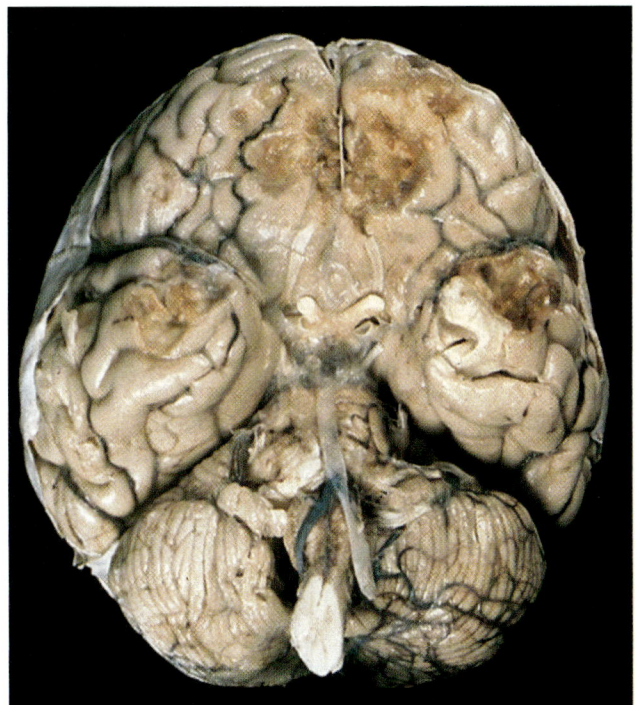
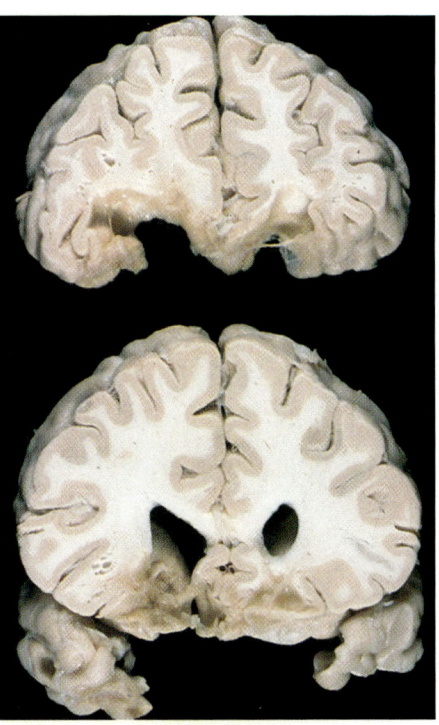

FIGURE 28-47
Remote cerebral contusion. A. Previous cerebral contusions are evidenced by a ragged appearance and focal excavation of blood. B. Coronal section through the old cerebral contusions discloses cystic areas that mark previous hemorrhages (*brown areas*).

1432   The Nervous System

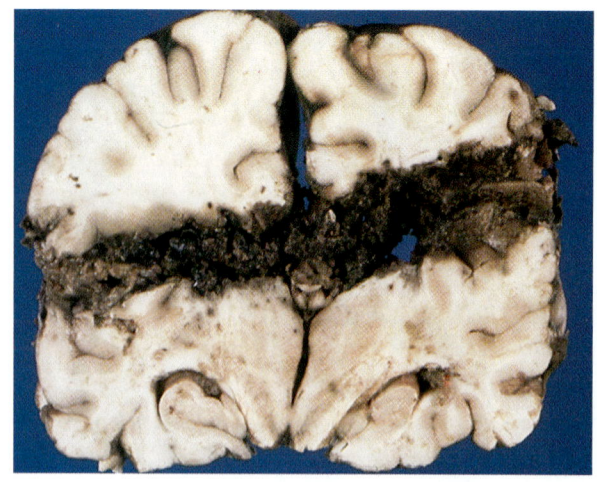
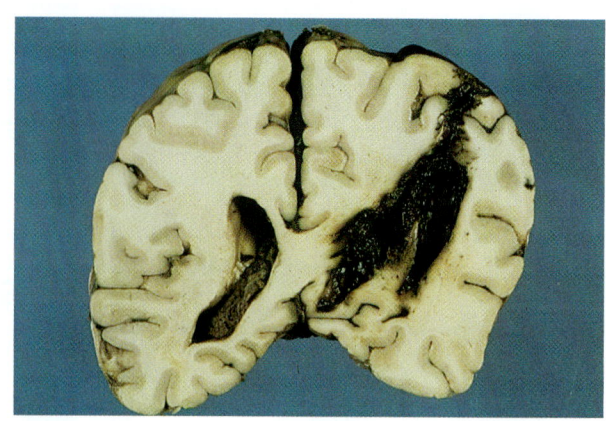

FIGURE 28-48
Penetrating wound. A. A .32-caliber bullet created a hemorrhagic tract through the cerebrum. B. A butcher knife was plunged deep into the brain, causing lethal hemorrhage.

comatose, although magnetic resonance imaging may show only small hemorrhages and focal edema.

Penetrating Wounds Produce Hemorrhage and Blast Effects

Penetrating objects such as bullets and knives enter the cranium and traverse the brain with variable velocities. In the absence of direct injury to the vital brain centers, the immediate threat to life is hemorrhage (Fig. 28-48). As noted above, bleeding creates a space-occupying mass, which may culminate in lethal transtentorial herniation. In the case of the cerebellum, herniation of the cerebellar tonsils into the foramen magnum is followed by compression of the medulla, thereby disabling vital cardiac and respiratory centers.

Velocity contributes a blast effect to a projectile (Fig. 28-49). As a high-velocity bullet traverses the brain, it disrupts tissues by its own mass as well as by a centrifugal blast that enlarges the diameter of the cylinder of disruption. Thus, a high-velocity bullet can cause immediate death through an explosive increase in intracranial pressure. This pressure forcefully herniates the cerebellar tonsils into the foramen magnum, causing immediate death.

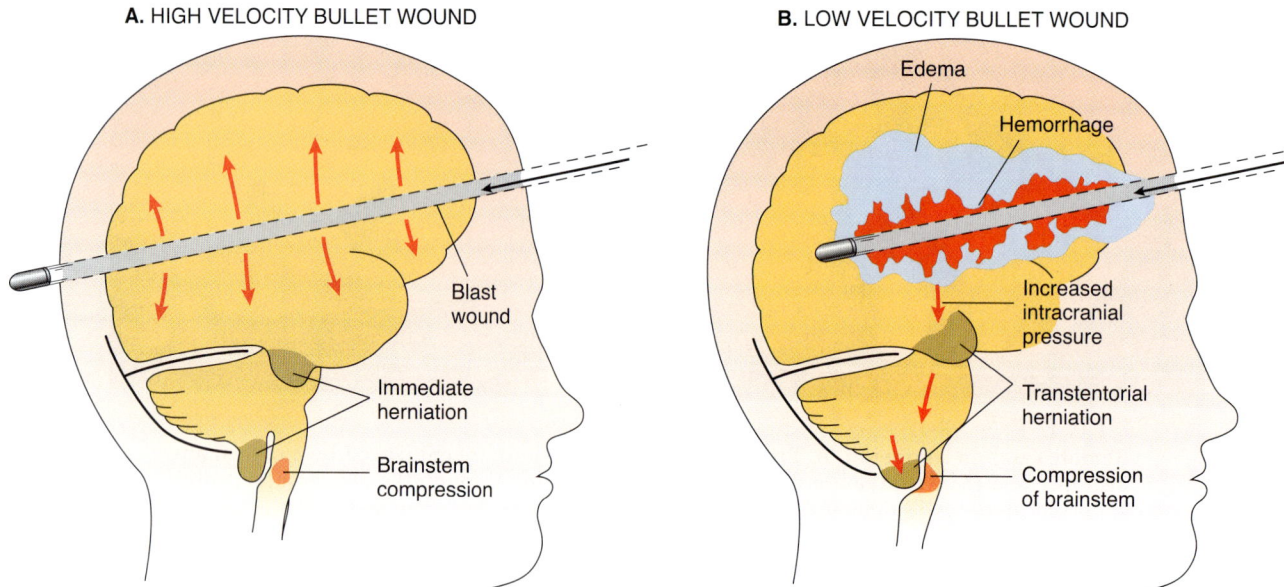

FIGURE 28-49
Consequences of high- and low-velocity bullet wounds. A. The "blast effect" of a high-velocity projectile causes an immediate increase in supratentorial pressure and results in death because of impaction of the cerebellum and medulla into the foramen magnum. B. A low-velocity projectile increases the pressure at a more gradual rate through hemorrhage and edema.

Seizures are a threat in healed penetrating wounds, usually occurring 6 to 12 months after the trauma. Collagenous tissue is displaced into the brain from the scalp or dura, and fibroblasts subsequently proliferate to form a dense scar. The precise mechanism by which a scar activates neurons and leads to seizures remains obscure.

Spinal Cord Injuries Often Lead to Paraplegia or Quadriplegia

Traumatic lesions of the spinal cord may result from direct injury to the cord by penetrating wounds (e.g., stab wounds, bullets) or indirect injury as a consequence of fractures or displacement of vertebrae. The spinal cord may be contused not only at the site of injury but also above and below the point of trauma. Traumatic injury may be complicated by compromise of the arterial supply to the cord, with resulting infarction.

The bodies of the vertebrae are separated by intervertebral disks and are stabilized in normal alignment by two longitudinal ligaments, as well as by the posterior bony processes. The anterior spinal ligament adheres to the ventral surface of the vertebral bodies, whereas the posterior spinal ligament is affixed to the dorsal vertebral column. As a result of extreme flexion or extension (Fig. 28-50), the angulation of the bony vertebral column brings the spinal cord forcefully

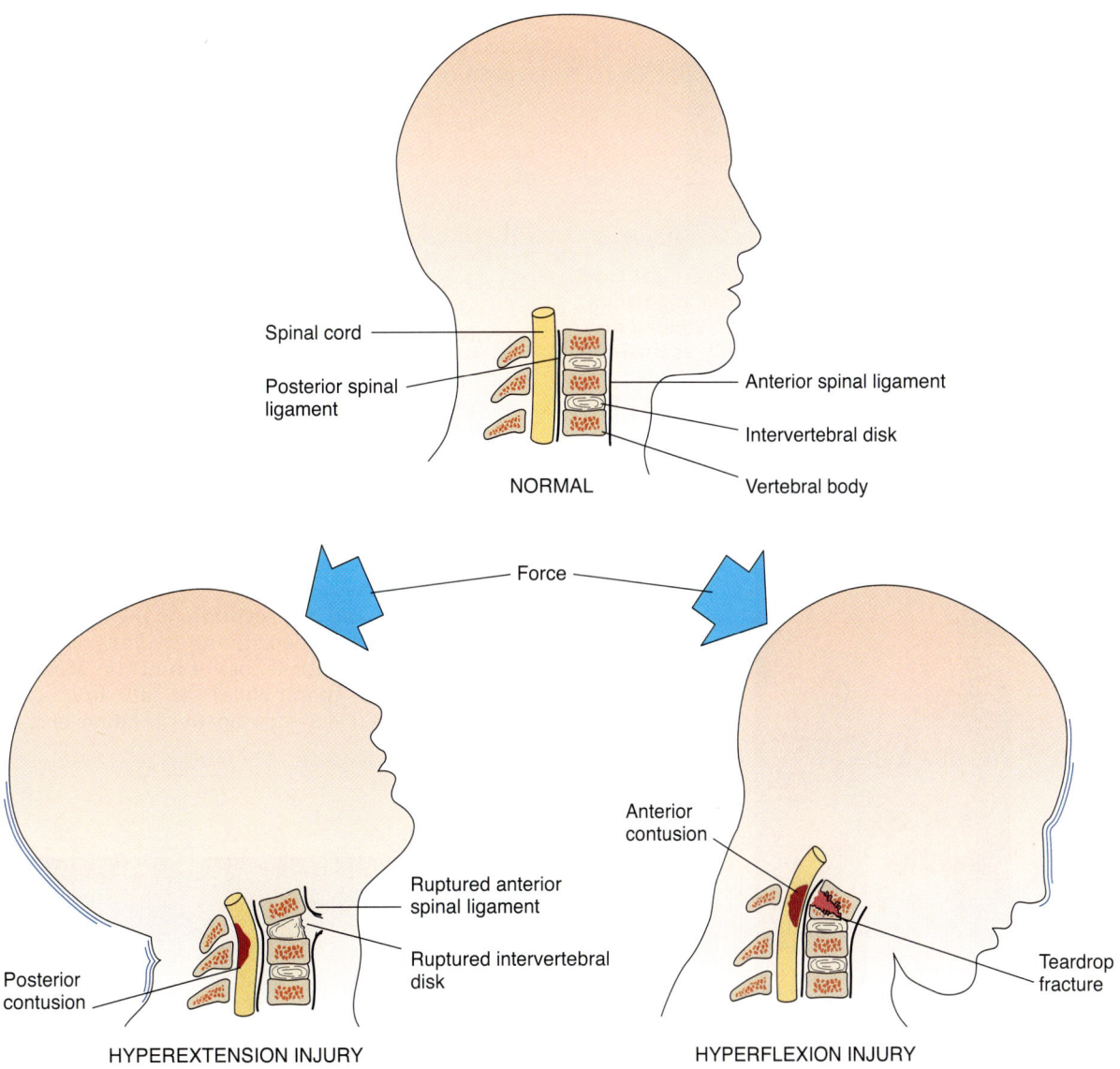

FIGURE 28-50

Spinal injury. Numerous different angles of force can be applied to the highly vulnerable cervical spine. Posterior (hyperextension) and anterior (hyperflexion) injuries are the most common. Hyperextension injury causes rupture of the anterior spinal ligament and excessive posterior angulation. Hyperflexion injury causes compression associated with a "teardrop" fracture of a vertebral body and produces excessive forward angulation of the cord.

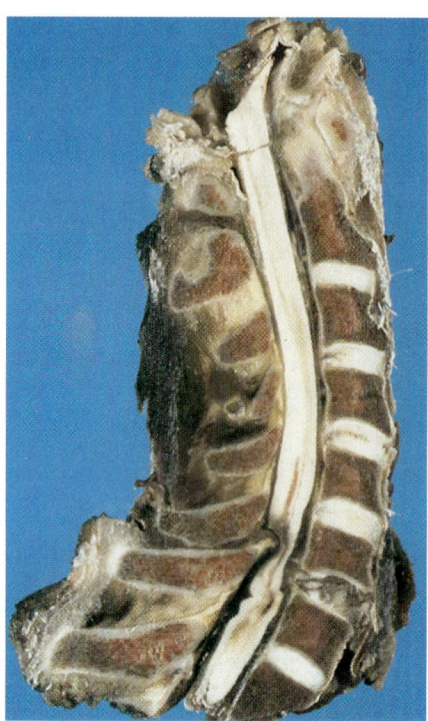

FIGURE 28-51
Cervical contusion. Hyperextension injury of cervical cord from a blow to the forehead resulted in posterior angulation. The anterior spinal ligament ruptured, the intervertebral disk fragmented, and the cord was brought forcibly against the posterior process of the underlying fixed vertebral body.

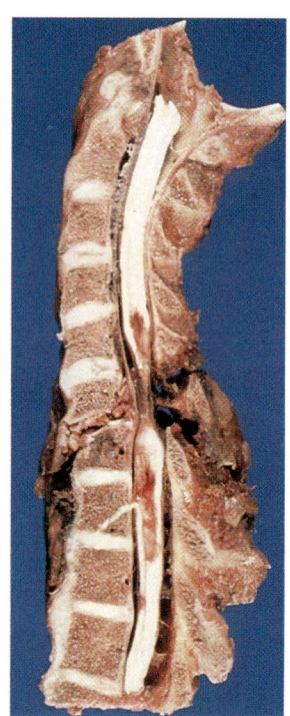

FIGURE 28-52
Cervical contusion. Hyperflexion injury caused forward angulation of the cervical cord, with fracture of the anterior lip of the underlying vertebral body. The cord is angulated over the superior–posterior ridge of the fixed underlying cervical body.

into contact with bone or, alternatively, interferes with the regional circulation.

HYPEREXTENSION INJURY: When the forehead is struck from the front and driven posteriorly (e.g., as a result of diving head first into shallow water), the posterior displacement of the head (hyperextension) tears the anterior spinal ligament, thereby permitting sharp posterior angulation of the spinal canal. At the point of angulation, the posterior aspect of the spinal cord is brought into forceful and damaging contact with the posterior process of the stationary vertebral body, which lies immediately caudal to the angulation (Fig. 28-51).

HYPERFLEXION INJURY: When the head or shoulders are struck from behind by an object of considerable weight or when this region of a falling human body (generally in a flexed position) strikes a stationary object, the head is driven forcefully forward and downward (hyperflexion). The impact forces one vertebral body down upon the underlying one. The anterior lip of the underlying vertebral body is fractured, with forward slippage and downward displacement of the overlying vertebra. This distortion of the spinal canal results in sharp forward angulation of the spinal cord. The anterior surface of the angulated cord is driven forcefully into the posterior superior edge of the stable underlying vertebral body (Fig. 28-52).

The consequences of a spinal cord injury vary with the severity of the trauma.

- **Concussion of the spinal cord** is the mildest injury and represents a transient and reversible disturbance of spinal cord function.
- **Contusion of the spinal cord** is the result of more severe trauma, ranging from a minor transient bruise to hemorrhagic spinal cord necrosis. The spinal cord necrosis and edema caused by a severe contusion are referred to as *myelomalacia*, and a hematoma within the spinal cord is termed *hematomyelia* (Fig. 28-53).
- **Lacerations and transections of the spinal cord**, usually produced by penetrating wounds, are irreversible and result in complete loss of function. Paralysis of the lower limbs (paraplegia) or all four extremities (quadriplegia) depends on the location and extent of the injury.

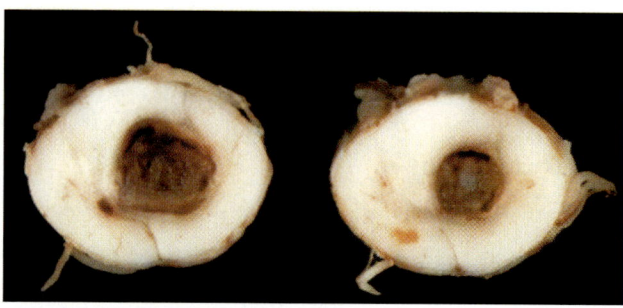

FIGURE 28-53
Cervical contusion. A cross-section of a contused spinal cord shows central hemorrhage ("hematomyelia with myelomalacia").

CIRCULATORY DISORDERS

Vascular Malformations May Lead to Hemorrhage

- **Arteriovenous malformation** (Fig. 28-54): This is the most common congenital vascular malformation and has the greatest clinical significance. Seizure disorders and intracranial hemorrhages, usually subarachnoid or intracerebral, commonly arise in the second or third decades. The abnormal blood vessels are thought to form during embryogenesis as a result of a focal communication between cerebral arteries and veins. The resulting congeries of abnormal vessels are typically located in the cerebral cortex and the contiguous underlying white matter. The malformation enlarges with time and tends to involve a larger area.
- **Cavernous angioma:** This congenital anomaly is far less common than arteriovenous malformations. It is similar to cavernous angiomas elsewhere (e.g., liver) in being formed by large, irregular, thin-walled vascular channels. Although most cavernous angiomas are asymptomatic, they may cause intracranial bleeding, epilepsy, or focal neurological disturbances.
- **Telangiectasia:** This focal aggregate of uniformly small vessels with intervening neural parenchyma may initiate seizures but rarely ruptures.
- **Venous angioma:** This structure consists of a focus of a few enlarged veins and is distributed randomly in the spinal cord or brain. The lesion is generally asymptomatic, and overlaps in part with cavernous angiomas.

Cerebral Aneurysms Rupture and Lead to Fatal Hemorrhage

Intravascular pressure and weakness in arterial walls lead to the formation of cerebral aneurysms. Some of the causes are as follows:

- **Developmental defects** give rise to berry (saccular, medial defect) aneurysms (Fig. 28-55).
- **Atherosclerosis** (Fig. 28-56) results in aneurysms that produce a mass effect.
- **Hypertension** is associated with arteriolar lipohyalinosis and induces Charcot-Bouchard aneurysms (Fig. 28-57)
- **Bacterial infection** leads to mycotic aneurysms.
- **Trauma** on rare occasions causes dissecting aneurysms.

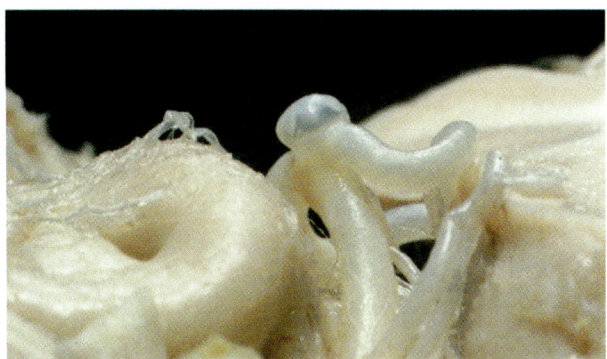

FIGURE 28-55
Berry aneurysm. A thin-walled aneurysm protrudes from an arterial bifurcation in the circle of Willis.

Berry Aneurysms

 **Pathogenesis and Pathology:** Berry (saccular) aneurysms are the consequence of arterial defects that are presumed to arise

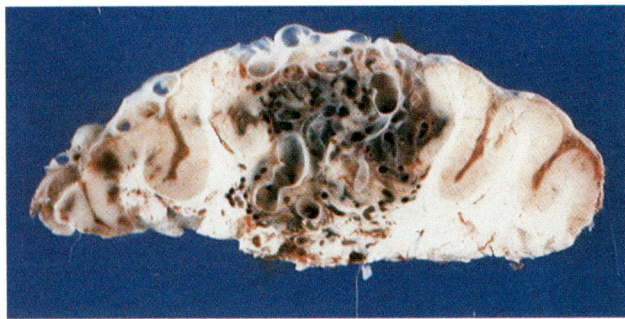

FIGURE 28-54
Arteriovenous malformation. Abnormal blood vessels replace the cortical gray matter and extend deeply into the white matter.

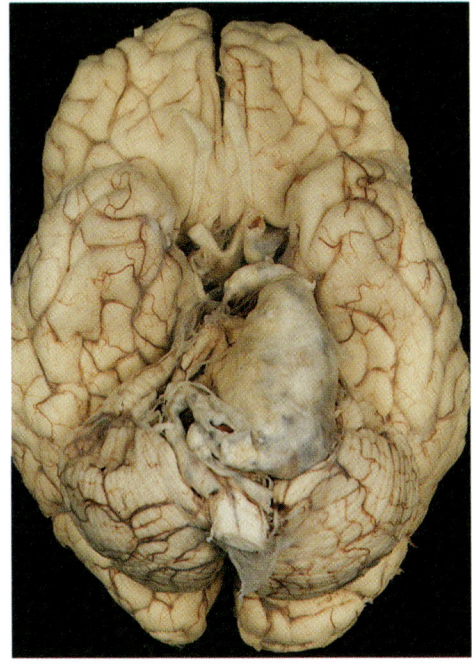

FIGURE 28-56
Atherosclerotic aneurysm. Fusiform dilation of the basilar and internal carotid arteries has resulted from severe atherosclerosis.

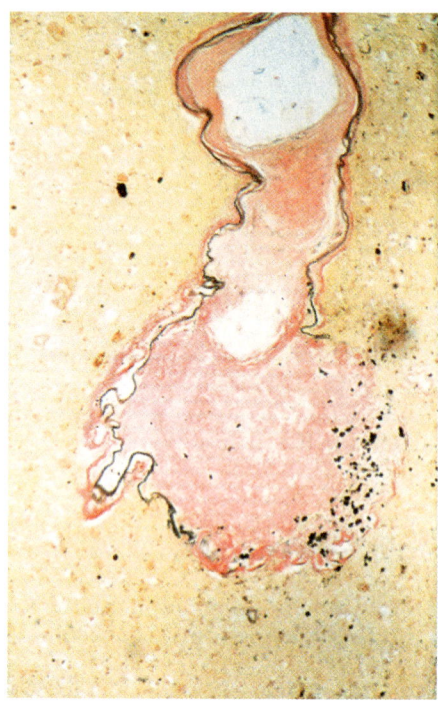

FIGURE 28-57
Charcot-Bouchard aneurysm. Chronic hypertension caused deposition of lipid in, and hyalinization of, the arterial wall. A microaneurysm arises from the damaged wall of the arteriole. The hemosiderin-laden macrophages attest to previous hemorrhage.

during embryogenesis when arteries bifurcate (Fig. 28-58). The muscular layer of a blood vessel that bifurcates into two branches may fail to interdigitate adequately across the branch point, thereby creating a point of congenital muscular weakness that is bridged only by endothelium, the internal elastic membrane, and a thin adventitia. Over time, the blood flow from the parent vessel exerts pressure at the point of bifurcation that expands the congenital defect. The internal elastic membrane may degenerate or fragment, after which a saccular aneurysm evolves that is precariously covered only by a layer of adventitia.

More than 90% of saccular aneurysms occur at branch points in the carotid system. They are about equally distributed at the junction of (1) the anterior cerebral and anterior communicating arteries, (2) the internal carotid–posterior communicating–anterior cerebral–anterior choroidal arteries, and (3) the trifurcation of the middle cerebral artery. In 20% of cases, multiple berry aneurysms are present. Clinically silent berry aneurysms occur in as many as 25% of persons older than 55 years.

 Clinical Features: **Rupture of a berry aneurysm results in life-threatening subarachnoid hemorrhage, with a 35% mortality during the initial hemorrhage.** Rupture produces intracerebral or intraventricular hemorrhage in up to one third of patients. A sudden severe headache characteristically heralds the onset of subarachnoid hemorrhage and may be followed by coma. Patients who survive for 3 to 4 days often manifest a progres-

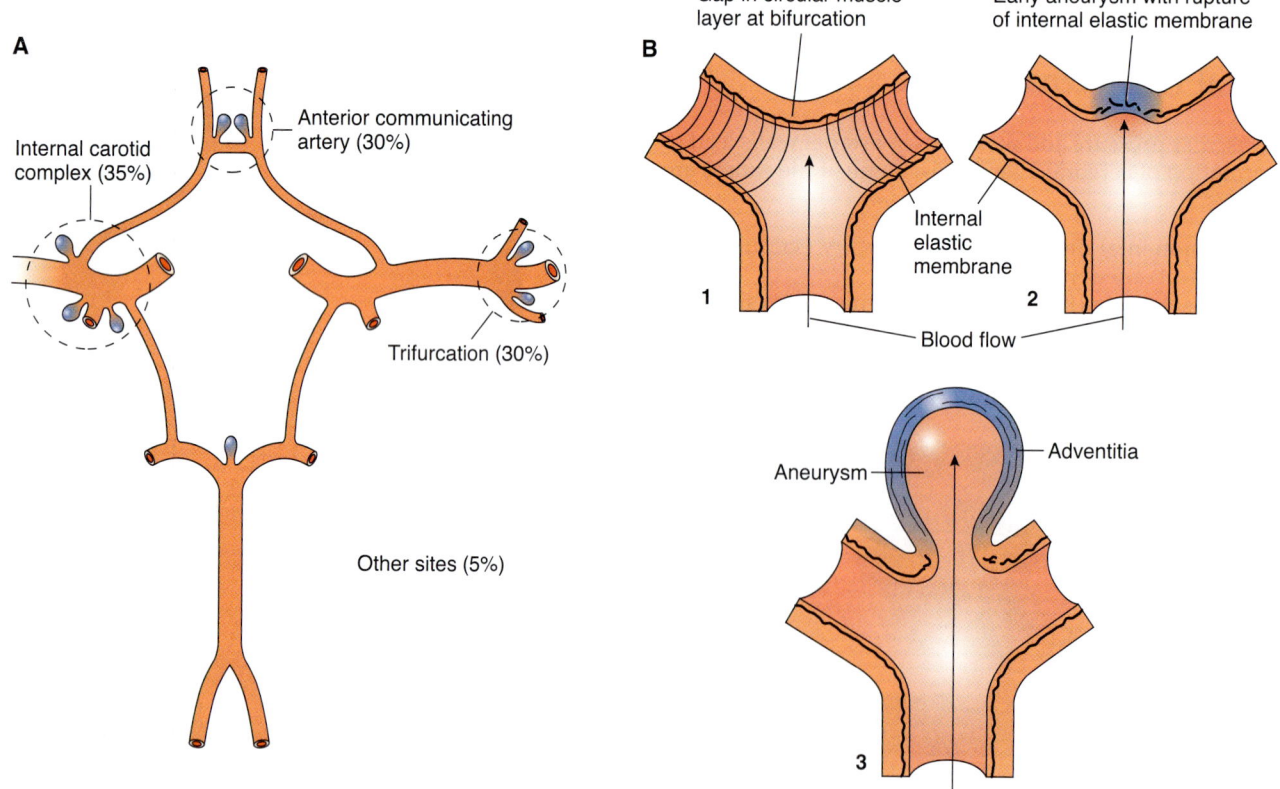

FIGURE 28-58
Saccular aneurysm. A. The incidence of saccular aneurysms (berry aneurysms), which preferentially involve the carotid tributaries, is shown. B. The lesion evolves as a result of blood acting on an early embryonic defect.

sive decline in consciousness, which may be caused by arterial spasms that lead to cerebral ischemia and infarction. Survivors of the initial episode often rebleed, in which case the prognosis is worse. Enlargement of a saccular aneurysm forms a mass that may compress cranial nerves and produce palsies or impinge on parenchymal structures and induce neurological symptoms.

Atherosclerotic Aneurysms

Aneurysms caused by atherosclerosis are localized mainly in major cerebral arteries (vertebral, basilar, and internal carotid) that are favored sites of atherosclerosis. Fibrous replacement of the media and destruction of the internal elastic membrane weaken the arterial wall and cause aneurysmal dilation (Fig. 28-59). As they enlarge, atherosclerotic aneurysms tend to be fusiform and elongate. Thus, an enlarging atherosclerotic aneurysm of the basilar artery will encroach upon the cerebellopontine angle, compress cranial nerves, and produce neurological deficits (see Fig. 28-56). Atherosclerotic aneurysms rarely rupture, and the major complication is thrombosis.

Mycotic Aneurysms

Infections of arterial walls result from septic emboli that usually originate in an infected cardiac valve. The embolus flows through the carotid circulation and typically lodges in a distal branch of the middle cerebral artery, where bacteria proliferate, induce inflammation, destroy the affected arterial wall, and lead to the formation of an aneurysm. Rupture of the aneurysm can cause intracerebral or subarachnoid hemorrhage. Alternatively, microorganisms may be released and produce a cerebral abscess or meningitis.

Cerebral Hemorrhage Causes Stroke (Apoplexy)

Cerebral hemorrhages that occur without trauma are referred to as "spontaneous," although most are caused by a

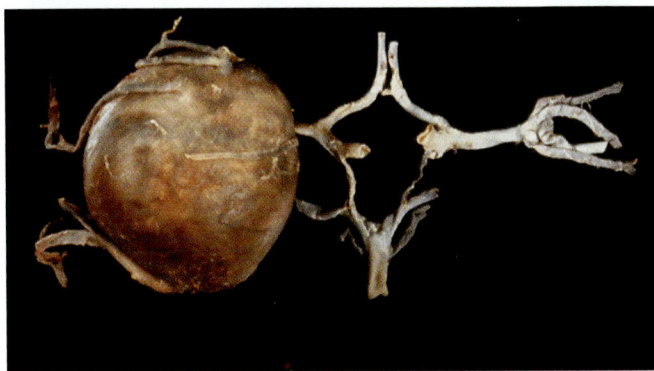

FIGURE 28-59
Giant saccular aneurysm. A large aneurysm of the middle cerebral artery created a mass lesion *(on the left)*, which produces symptoms that may be mistaken clinically for those of a tumor.

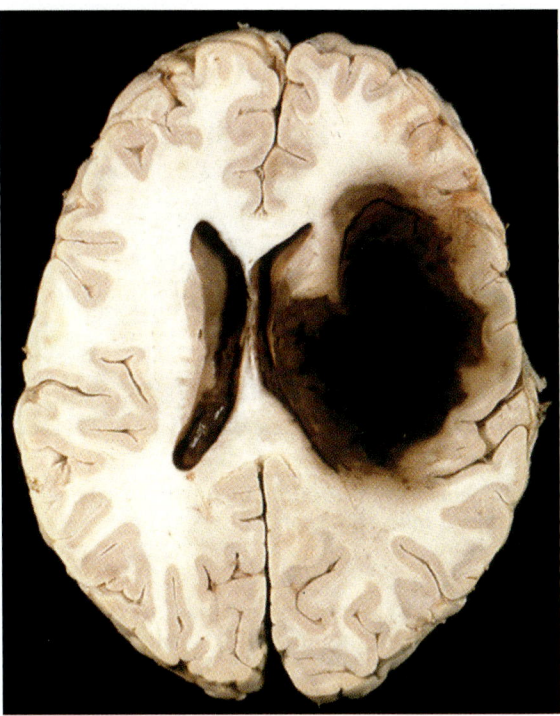

FIGURE 28-60
Cerebral hemorrhage. A spontaneous cerebral hemorrhage near the external capsule produced a hematoma that threatened to rupture into a lateral ventricle.

vascular anomaly (see above) or are the consequence of longstanding hypertension. **Hypertensive intracerebral hemorrhage** occurs at preferential sites, which in order of frequency are (1) the basal ganglia–thalamus (65%), (2) pons (15%), and (3) cerebellum (8%) (Figs. 28-60 through 28-62).

Hypertension compromises the integrity of cerebral arterioles by causing the deposition of lipid and hyaline material in their walls, an alteration referred to as *lipohyalinosis* (see Fig. 28-57). Weakening of the wall leads to the formation of *Charcot-Bouchard* aneurysms, which are located mainly along the trunk of a vessel rather than at its bifurcation.

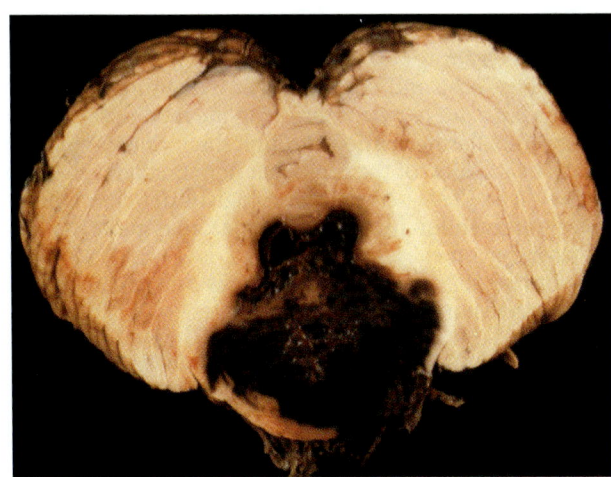

FIGURE 28-61
Pontine hemorrhage. A spontaneous hemorrhage in the midpons nearly occupies it completely.

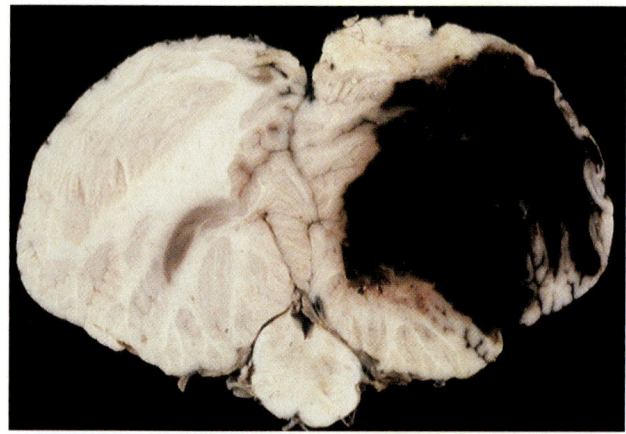

FIGURE 28-62
Cerebellar hemorrhage. A spontaneous hemorrhage has destroyed a lateral lobe of the cerebellum.

The onset of symptoms in the case of a hypertensive cerebral hemorrhage (hemorrhagic stroke) is abrupt, and weakness usually dominates. When hemorrhage is progressive, as is common, death occurs within hours to days. As the hematoma enlarges, it may cause death by transtentorial herniation or it may rupture into a lateral ventricle and lead to massive intraventricular hemorrhage (Fig. 28-63).

INTRAVENTRICULAR HEMORRHAGE: Rupture of a cerebral blood vessel into a ventricle rapidly distends the entire ventricular system, including the fourth ventricle, with blood. The blood rarely emerges from the foramina of Magendie and Luschka, but death rapidly ensues from distention of the fourth ventricle and compression of vital centers in the medulla.

PONTINE HEMORRHAGE: In this catastrophic event, the loss of consciousness reflects damage to the reticular formation, an injury that overshadows all other specific cranial nerve deficits. The initial hemorrhage is generally in the midpons. With minimal enlargement, it encroaches upon vital medullary centers, commonly resulting in death before the patient arrives at the hospital.

CEREBELLAR HEMORRHAGE: Bleeding into the cerebellum causes abrupt ataxia and is accompanied by a severe occipital headache and vomiting. The expanding hematoma threatens life acutely by compressing the medulla or by producing cerebellar herniation through the foramen magnum. Surgical evacuation of the cerebellar hematoma is life saving and may leave few serious neurological deficits, whereas surgical intervention for cerebral hematomas generally has a very poor outcome.

Spontaneous cerebral hemorrhages due to causes other than hypertension include

- Leakage from an arteriovenous malformation
- Erosion of a blood vessel by a primary or secondary neoplasm
- A bleeding diathesis, as exemplified by thrombocytopenic purpura
- Endothelial injury by microorganisms, notably rickettsiae
- Embolic infarction, with consequent hemorrhage into the area of necrosis

Cerebral Ischemia and Infarction Represent the Major Causes of Stroke

Inadequate perfusion of the brain results from generalized low blood flow due to extracranial events that lead to global ischemia (cardiac arrest, external hemorrhage) or from occlusive cerebrovascular disease (cerebral artery thrombosis), which produces regional ischemia and often a localized infarct. Global ischemia also results from hypoxia (near-drowning, carbon monoxide poisoning, suffocation).

Global Ischemia

The pattern of injury produced by global ischemia (or hypoxia) reflects the anatomy of the cerebral vasculature and the selective vulnerability of individual neurons to oxygen deprivation (Fig. 28-64).

WATERSHED INFARCTS: The anterior, middle, and posterior cerebral arteries perfuse partially overlapping territories, but there are no anastomoses between their terminal branches (Fig. 28-65). For example, the anterior cerebral arteries mainly perfuse the medial aspects of both cerebral hemispheres. However, they also perfuse the parasagittal cortex by variably overlapping with the distribution of the middle cerebral arteries. Since this overlap zone is not as richly perfused as the primary territories of the anterior and middle cerebral arteries, reduced blood flow in these arteries will diminish perfusion more severely in the partial overlap zone (watershed area), thereby causing a parasagittal watershed infarct.

LAMINAR NECROSIS: This lesion also reflects the topography of the cerebral vasculature (Figs. 28-66 and 28-67). The cerebral cortex is perfused by short "penetrators," which originate at right angles from pial blood vessels and then penetrate gray matter, where they form a plexus of capillar-

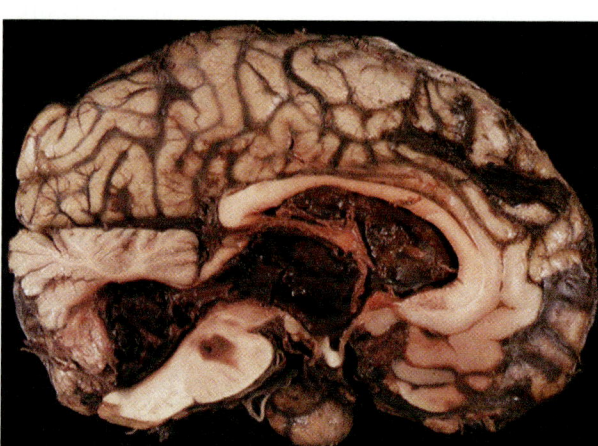

FIGURE 28-63
Intraventricular hemorrhage. A sagittal section of the brain shows ventricular chambers filled with blood. The patient died rapidly from compression of the brainstem by blood in the fourth ventricle.

Circulatory Disorders 1439

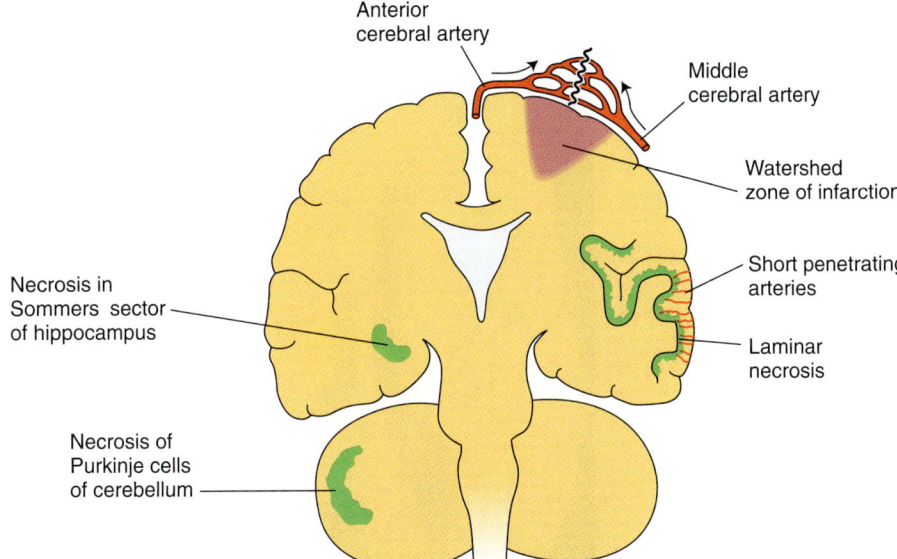

FIGURE 28-64
Consequences of global ischemia. A global insult induces lesions that reflect the vascular architecture (watershed infarcts, laminar necrosis) and the sensitivity of individual neuronal systems (pyramidal cells of Sommer sector, Purkinje cells).

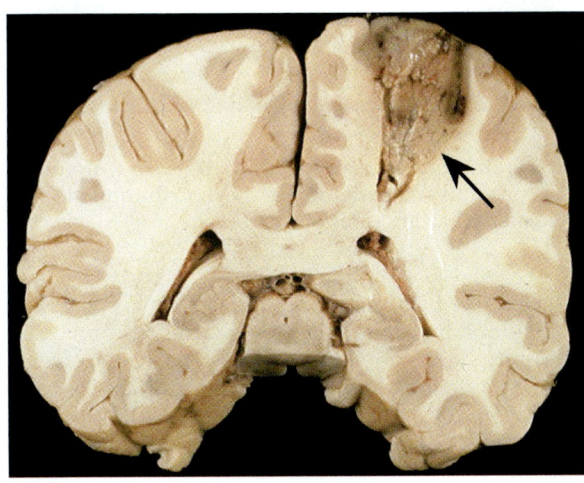

FIGURE 28-65
Watershed infarct. A coronal section through the brain shows a recent infarct (arrow) between the distributions of the anterior and middle cerebral arteries.

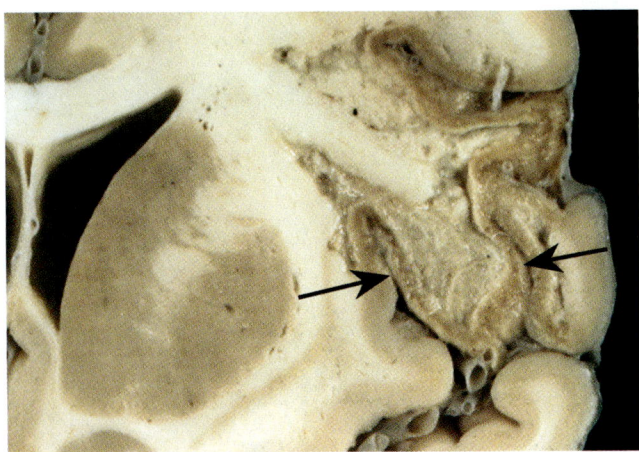

FIGURE 28-66
Laminar necrosis. A more restricted zone of infarction (relative to that shown in Fig. 28-65) (arrows) is seen within the cerebral cortex.

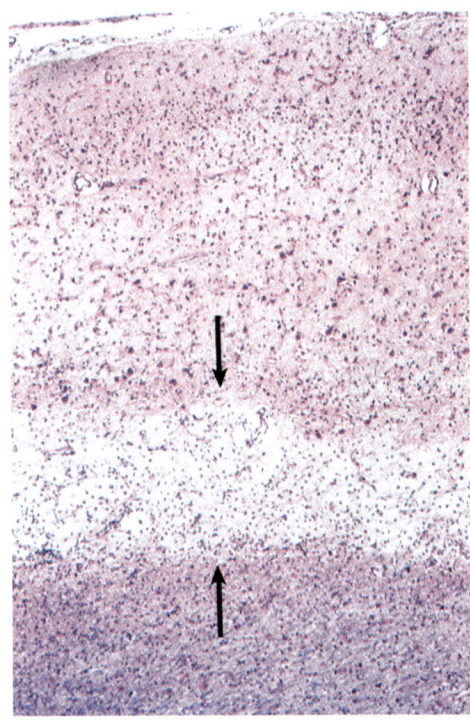

FIGURE 28-67
Laminar necrosis. Microscopic view of Fig. 28-66 shows that the zone of infarction (arrows) selectively involves layers IV–VI of cortex.

ies in cortical layers V and VI. A loss of circulatory pressure will selectively diminish perfusion of this terminal capillary plexus and cause laminar necrosis in the deeper layers of neocortex. However, the selective vulnerability of neurons to ischemia/hypoxia also contributes to this laminar pattern of involvement.

Selective neuronal sensitivity to a lack of oxygen is expressed most dramatically in the Purkinje cells of the cerebellum and the pyramidal neurons of Sommer sector in the hippocampus. Because of their exquisite vulnerability to hypoxia/ischemia, these neurons succumb more readily than do their neighbors to similar degrees of oxygen deprivation, thereby resulting in localized necrosis.

Regional Ischemia and Cerebral Infarction

The prevalence and progressive nature of atherosclerosis are reflected in the fact that cerebrovascular occlusive disease remains a major cause of morbidity and mortality. Atherosclerosis predisposes to vascular thrombosis and embolic events, both of which result in localized ischemia and subsequent cerebral infarction (Fig. 28-68).

Pathology: Although cerebral infarcts are traditionally designated either "hemorrhagic" or "bland," these descriptors are somewhat simplistic. In general, infarcts caused by embolization are hemorrhagic, whereas those initiated by local thrombosis are ischemic (or bland). Emboli occlude vascular flow abruptly, after which

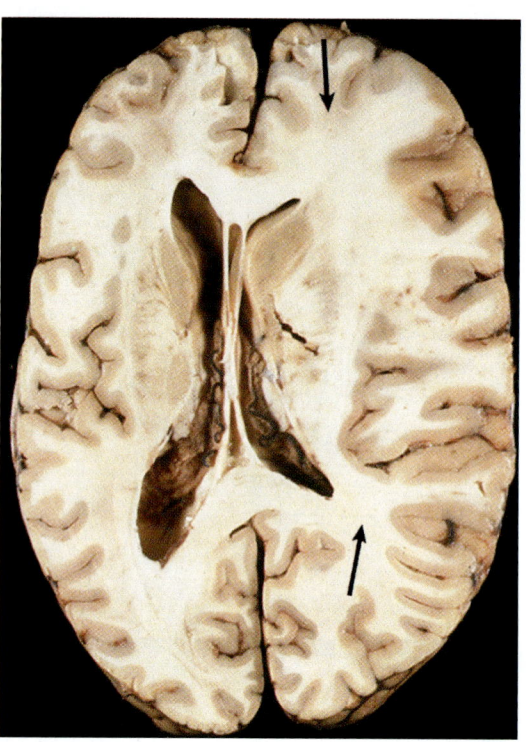

FIGURE 28-69
Recent cerebral infarct. A horizontal section of the brain shows expansion and softening in the distribution of the right middle cerebral artery *(between arrows).*

the distal segments of affected blood vessels become necrotic and leak blood into the region. By contrast thrombosis progresses more slowly and gradually deprives downstream arteries of blood flow, thereby guarding against secondary hemorrhage.

An infarct of the brain acutely transforms the affected tissue into necrotic, friable debris (Fig. 28-69), which is ultimately phagocytosed and eliminated by macrophages (Fig. 28-70). Initially capillaries proliferate at the margin of the infarct, become numerous by the fifth day, and improve perfusion of the infarct penumbra. Subsequently, the necrotic area is slowly eliminated by phagocytosis to form

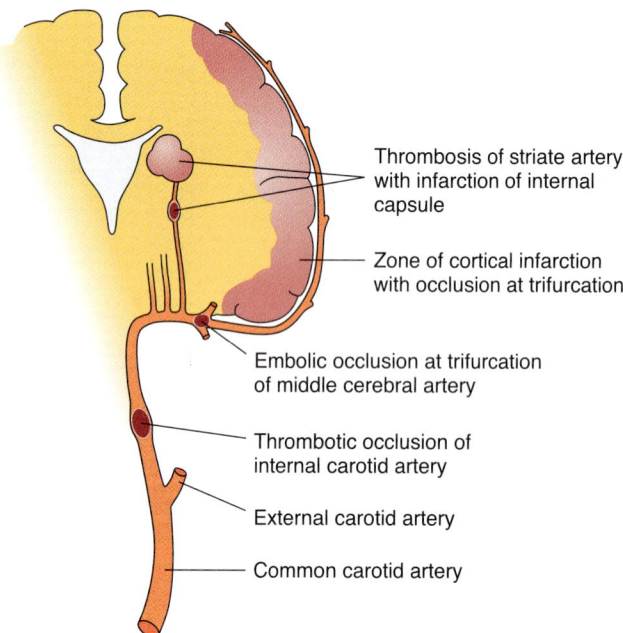

FIGURE 28-68
Distribution of cerebral infarcts. The normal distribution of the cerebral vasculature defines the pattern and size of infarcts and, consequently, their symptoms. Occlusion at the trifurcation causes cortical infarcts with motor and sensory loss and often aphasia. Occlusion of a striate branch transects the internal capsule and causes a motor deficit.

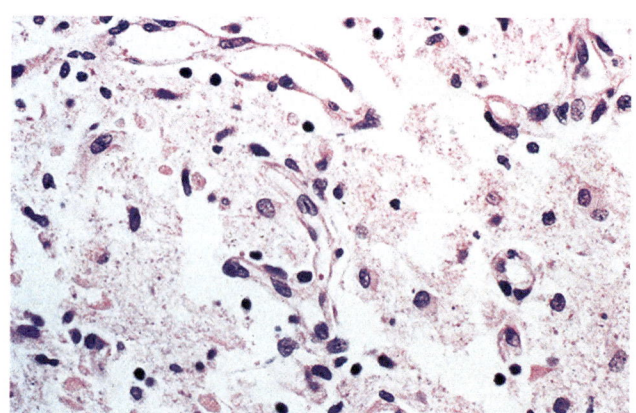

FIGURE 28-70
Recent cerebral infarct. A microscopic view of material in Fig. 28-69 shows destruction of the parenchyma with debris-laden macrophages and proliferated capillaries.

Circulatory Disorders

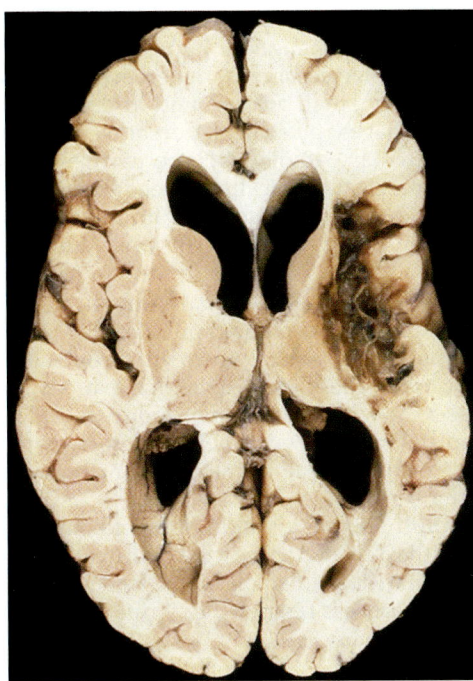

FIGURE 28-71
Remote cerebral infarct. A horizontal section of the brain demonstrates an end-stage infarct with a cyst traversed by atretic vessels.

a gliosis-lined cystic cavity. If the area of the infarction is large, the residual cyst is bridged by a cobweb of atretic blood vessels (Fig. 28-71). Although cerebral infarcts are examples of coagulative necrosis, large brain infarcts eventually fragment and liquefy (liquefactive necrosis).

Clinical Features: The diversity of the neurological deficits caused by stroke directly reflect the consequences of occluding different cerebral vessels. For example, the lengthy and slender striate arteries, which take origin from the proximal middle cerebral artery, are commonly occluded by atherosclerosis and thrombosis. The resultant infarct often transects the internal capsule and produces hemiparesis or hemiplegia (Fig. 28-72). Similarly, the trifurcation of the middle cerebral artery is a favored site for lodgment of emboli and for thrombosis secondary to atherosclerotic damage. Occlusion of the middle cerebral artery at this site deprives the parietal cortex of circulation and produces motor and sensory deficits. When the dominant hemisphere is involved, these lesions are commonly accompanied by aphasia.

Localized ischemia is associated with three distinct clinical syndromes:

- **Transient ischemic attack (TIA)** refers to focal cerebral dysfunction that lasts less than 24 hours and is often of only a few minutes' duration. Although it is followed by complete neurological recovery, a TIA signifies an increased risk of a cerebral infarct.
- **Stroke in evolution** describes the progression of neurological symptoms while the patient is under observation. This syndrome is uncommon and usually reflects propagation of a thrombus in the carotid or basilar arteries.
- **Completed stroke** is the term for a stable neurological deficit resulting from a cerebral infarct.

Regional Occlusive Cerebrovascular Disease

The various occlusive cerebrovascular diseases that lead to cerebral infarcts may be classified into five categories, in accord with the caliber and nature of the involved vessel:

- Large extracranial and intracranial vessels, such as the carotid, vertebral, and basilar arteries
- Arteries of the circle of Willis and their immediate branches
- Parenchymal arteries and arterioles
- Capillaries
- Large veins and dural sinuses

THE LARGE EXTRACRANIAL AND INTRACRANIAL ARTERIES: These arteries are frequent sites of atherosclerosis (Fig. 28-73). The most notable example is the common carotid artery, in which atherosclerotic plaques are particularly prominent at the site of its bifurcation into external and internal branches. Occlusion or stenosis of an internal carotid artery affects the ipsilateral hemisphere, but this can be offset by the variable collateral circulation through the anterior and posterior communicating arteries. Most often, occlusion of a carotid artery produces infarcts restricted to all or some portion of the distribution of the middle cerebral artery (see Fig. 28-68).

THE CIRCLE OF WILLIS: The various branches of this major vascular network of the brain may be occluded, but the consequences depend on the configuration of the circle. Thus, a large anterior communicating artery can provide collateral circulation to a frontal lobe whose arterial supply has been compromised by occlusion of the internal carotid artery. The middle cerebral artery is most often occluded by thrombosis complicating atherosclerosis in the circle of Willis. Because the trifurcation of the middle cerebral artery is a site of a major stepdown in vascular caliber, it is the pre-

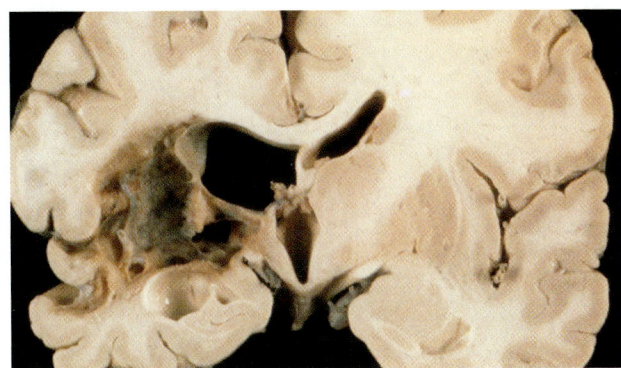

FIGURE 28-72
Remote cerebral infarction. Occlusion of the striate vessels resulted in an infarct in the region of the internal capsule and basal ganglia. Resorption of destroyed brain tissue led to cyst formation, with dilation of the adjacent ventricle.

1442   The Nervous System

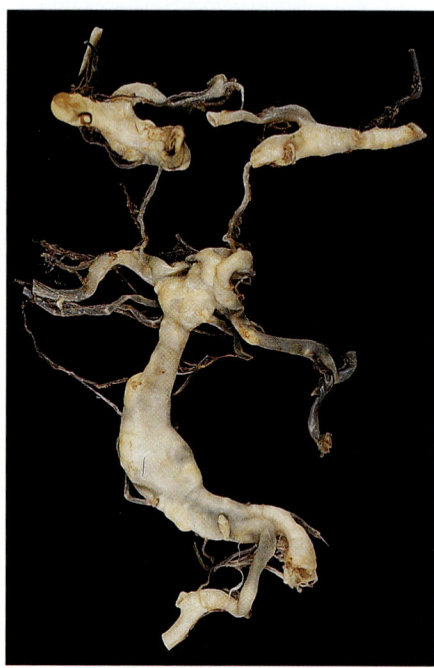

FIGURE 28-73
Atherosclerosis of the cerebral vasculature. The large vessels (the vertebral, basilar, internal carotid, and middle cerebral arteries) in this dissected specimen show significant atherosclerosis. The smaller vessels are less involved.

dominant site occluded by emboli, most of which emanate from the heart (Fig. 28-74).

THE PARENCHYMAL ARTERIES AND ARTERIOLES: These vessels rarely become atherosclerotic, but they are damaged by hypertension and become stenotic because of atherosclerosis, thereby causing small so-called lacunar infarcts. When multiple, these minute infarcts can impair cognition and create the entity termed *multiple infarct dementia.*

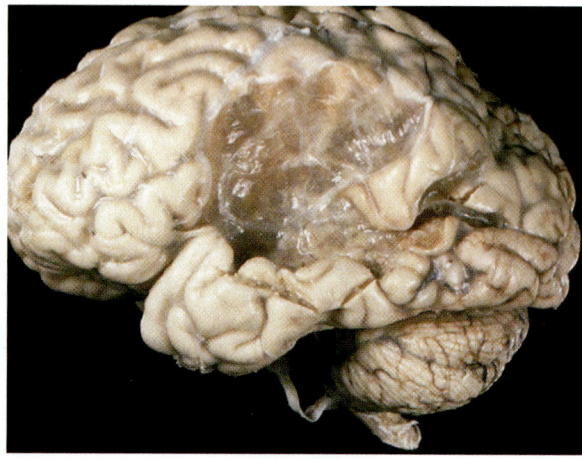

FIGURE 28-74
Remote cerebral infarction. Occlusion of the middle cerebral artery at its trifurcation resulted in an infarct that has become cystic.

Hypertensive encephalopathy refers to the neurological complications of malignant hypertension (see Chapter 10). As in other affected organs, hypertension can cause fibrinoid necrosis of small arteries and arterioles, as well as minute hemorrhages (petechiae). Cerebral edema may complicate the vascular pathology. Hypertensive encephalopathy usually manifests clinically as headache and vomiting that progress to coma and death. With modern antihypertensive therapy, malignant hypertension is uncommon.

THE CAPILLARY BED: Small emboli, notably those composed of fat or air, occlude capillaries (Fig. 28-75).

Fat emboli are carried downstream through the cerebral vessels until the caliber of the embolus exceeds that of the blood vessel, at which point they lodge and block blood flow. The distal capillary endothelium becomes hypoxic and permeable, and petechiae develop, most commonly in the white matter.

Air emboli liberate a multitude of bubbles that further fragment as they encounter vascular bifurcations until they impede vascular flow in small blood vessels. In this situation, petechiae are less restricted to white matter than those caused by fat emboli.

THE CEREBRAL VEINS: The cerebral veins empty into large venous sinuses, the most prominent of which is the sagittal sinus because it accommodates the venous drainage from the superior portions of the cerebral hemispheres (Fig. 28-76). Venous sinus thrombosis in the brain is a potentially lethal complication of the following:

- Systemic dehydration, as occurs in an infant with gastrointestinal fluid loss
- Phlebitis, caused for example by mastoiditis or bacteremia

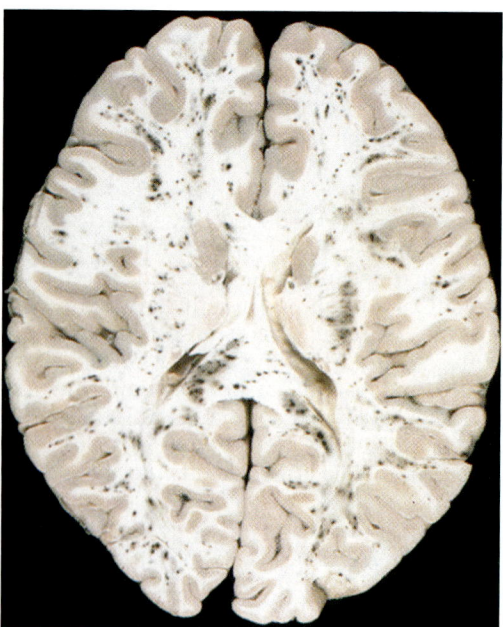

FIGURE 28-75
Fat embolization. Horizontal section of the brain from a patient who had massive trauma exhibits numerous petechiae throughout the white matter.

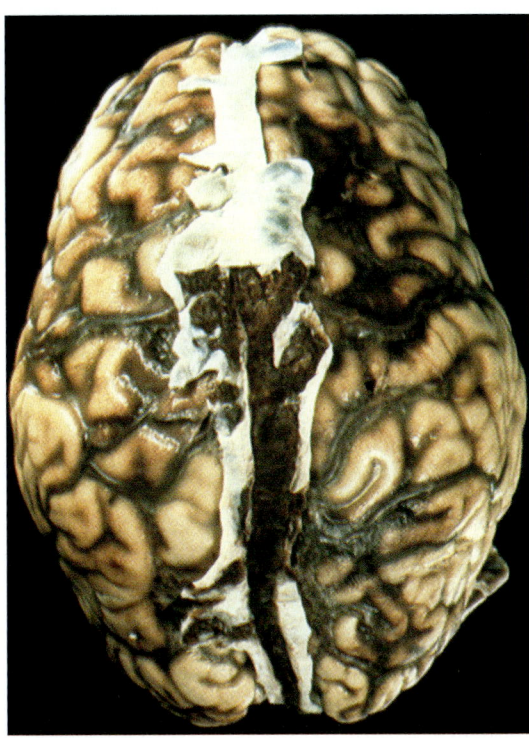

FIGURE 28-76
Sagittal sinus thrombosis. Removal of the dura reveals that the sagittal sinus is filled with clotted blood. Secondary thrombosis of the veins in the cerebral cortex has led to bilateral hemorrhagic infarcts.

- Obstruction by a neoplasm, notably a meningioma
- Sickle cell disease

Because venous obstruction causes stagnation upstream, abrupt thrombosis of the sagittal sinus results in bilateral hemorrhagic infarctions of the frontal lobe regions. A more indolent occlusion of the sinus (due to invasion by a meningioma) permits the recruitment of collateral circulation through the inferior sagittal sinus, which lies at the lower edge of the falx and empties into the straight sinus.

CEREBROSPINAL FLUID (CSF)

The CSF constitutes an "accessory circulatory system" adapted to the needs of the CNS. CSF flows from its intraventricular origin to its sites of reabsorption, principally through the arachnoid villi and into the dural sinuses. The fluid transports metabolites to CNS cells, serves as a medium for clearing metabolic waste, and protects or "cushions" structures contained within it.

The volume of CSF in the adult CNS is about 150 mL. It is formed principally by the choroid plexus at a rate of approximately 500 mL/day and is reabsorbed by the arachnoid villi. A small volume of CSF also flows in the subarachnoid compartment through the Virchow-Robin spaces. With advancing age, the choroid plexus becomes fibrotic and contains cholesterol and calcium deposits, although CSF is produced throughout life.

The choroid plexus stretches along the roof of the third ventricle, passes through the foramina of Monro, and then angles posteriorly to span the lateral ventricles. The choroid plexus does not enter the aqueduct of Sylvius. However, the posterior aspect of the fourth ventricle is covered by choroid plexus, which extends laterally through the foramen of Luschka into the immediate subarachnoid space of the cerebellopontine angle.

Hydrocephalus Refers to Dilation of the Ventricles by Accumulated CSF

When obstruction to the flow of CSF in the brain is within the ventricles, hydrocephalus is designated *noncommunicating* (Fig. 28-77). *Communicating* hydrocephalus occurs when there is no obstruction in the ventricular system, but reabsorption of CSF by the arachnoid villi is impaired.

NONCOMMUNICATING HYDROCEPHALUS: The flow of CSF through the ventricular system may be obstructed by (1) congenital malformations, (2) neoplasms, (3) inflammation, or (4) hemorrhage. The aqueduct of Sylvius is the most common location of obstructive congenital malformations. Choroid plexus tumors and ependymomas that arise in the ventricles can obstruct CSF flow and produce hydrocephalus. Parenchymal tumors, such as gliomas, may compress the aqueduct or ventricles and thereby cause hydrocephalus. Viral ependymitis during embryogenesis may result in congenital aqueductal stenosis (see Fig. 28-29).

COMMUNICATING HYDROCEPHALUS: An impairment of reabsorption of CSF with resultant communicating hydrocephalus can complicate subarachnoid hemorrhage, meningitis, and the spread of tumor within the subarachnoid space.

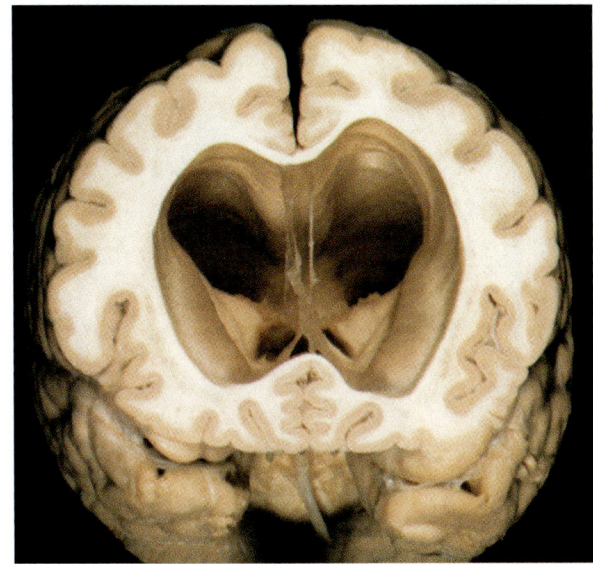

FIGURE 28-77
Hydrocephalus. Coronal section of the brain from a patient who died of a brain tumor that obstructed the aqueduct of Sylvius shows marked dilation of the lateral ventricles.

Pathology: In hydrocephalus of all etiologies, the cerebral hemispheres are enlarged, and the ventricular system is dilated behind the point of obstruction. The external pattern of the gyri tends to be less prominent as sulci are compressed. The white matter is reduced in volume, and the basal ganglia and thalamus are attenuated (see Figs. 28-77 and 28-78).

When hydrocephalus develops *in utero* or in early life, usually because of obstruction at the aqueduct of Sylvius, the ventricles expand behind the point of obstruction, the cranial sutures separate, the head enlarges, and the cortex becomes thin. Histological examination of the obstructed aqueduct reveals multiple small, irregular, ependyma-lined canals (see Fig. 28-28). In some cases, a single aqueduct or a cluster of aborted canals are surrounded by gliosis, suggesting that an intrauterine viral infection caused inflammatory ependymitis (see Fig. 28-29). Without surgical CSF drainage or shunting, hydrocephalus is slowly progressive and lethal.

 Clinical Features: Because the infantile cranium expands easily, symptoms of increased intracranial pressure are generally absent. Convulsions are common, and optic atrophy with blindness can occur. Weakness and spasticity are frequent, but cognition may be spared, although severe ventricular dilation results in dementia. Surgical shunting of CSF controls hydrocephalus in some children.

In adults, the onset of hydrocephalus and increased intracranial pressure is heralded by headache, vomiting, and papilledema. If the obstruction is not relieved, mental deterioration ensues. Curiously, for reasons that are not known, CSF pressure is not increased in a rare dementing syndrome known as *normal pressure hydrocephalus*.

Hydrocephalus ex vacuo refers to enlargement of the ventricular system as a compensatory response to severe brain atrophy and is unrelated to obstructive lesions (Fig. 28-79).

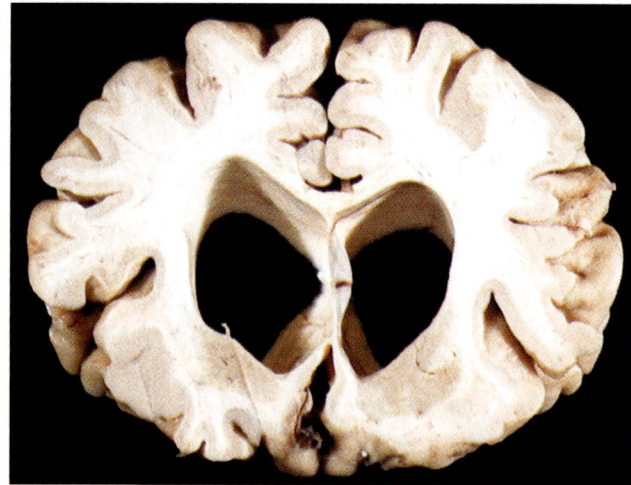

FIGURE 28-79
Hydrocephalus ex vacuo. Atrophy of the cerebral cortex in an aged, demented person is associated with enlargement of the ventricles.

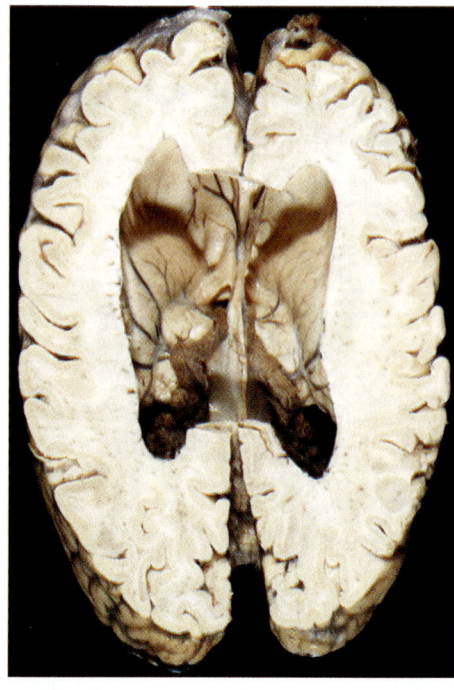

FIGURE 28-78
Hydrocephalus. A horizontal section of the brain from a patient with obstructive hydrocephalus caused by a neoplasm emphasizes the enlargement of the lateral ventricles.

INFECTIOUS DISEASES

Many organisms infect the CNS, but most localize at preferred CNS sites. For example, poliovirus targets spinal and brainstem motor neurons, herpes simplex virus localizes to the temporal lobes, progressive multifocal leukoencephalopathy (JC virus) preferentially involves cerebral white matter, and bacteria generally cause meningitis. Bacteria can also invade brain and result in cerebritis or brain abscess or enter the subdural space to induce subdural empyema.

Fungi such as *Cryptococcus neoformans* infect the leptomeninges, whereas *Aspergillus fumigatus* produces cerebral abscesses or leptomeningitis. *Treponema pallidum* causes syphilis by entering the CNS through the bloodstream. It can reside in the CNS for prolonged periods, where it propagates to induce distinct clinical syndromes such as dementia paralytica and tabes dorsalis. It can also invade the meninges, where it initiates fibrosis and an obliterative endarteritis, a condition termed *meningovascular syphilis*.

Rickettsial infections, such as Rocky Mountain spotted fever, target endothelial cells to produce petechiae, cerebral edema, and encephalopathy. *Toxoplasma gondii* has low virulence in healthy adults, but transplacental transmission enables infection of the fetal brain, resulting in paraventricular necrosis and calcification of the basal ganglia and thalamus. Immunocompromised adults (e.g., AIDS) may also be infected with this organism. Thus, anatomical localization, specific tissue responses, and the age and immunological status of the patient are critical for understanding intracranial infections.

Meningitis Is a Dangerous Infection Caused by a Variety of Microorganisms

Leptomeningitis denotes an inflammatory process localized to the pia/arachnoid (Fig. 28-80A). This compartment houses the CSF, an excellent culture medium for most microorganisms. The response of CSF to infections varies with the organism and extent of infection, including changes in its cellular, protein, sugar, and electrolyte composition and in its serological reactivity (see Fig. 28-80B).

Pachymeningitis refers to inflammation of the dura and is usually a consequence of contiguous extracranial infection such as chronic sinusitis or mastoiditis. The dura is a substantial barrier to infection, and inflammation is usually restricted to its outer surface.

Bacterial Meningitis

With few exceptions, all forms of meningitis are initiated by microorganisms, suppurative bacteria being the principal offenders.

Suppurative Meningitis

- *Escherichia coli:* In the newborn, whose resistance to gram-negative bacteria has not yet fully developed, *E. coli* is the prime cause of meningitis. The transplacental transfer of maternal IgG imparts protection to the newborn against many bacteria. However, *E. coli* and similar gram-negative organisms require IgM for neutralization, an immunoglobulin that does not cross the placenta.

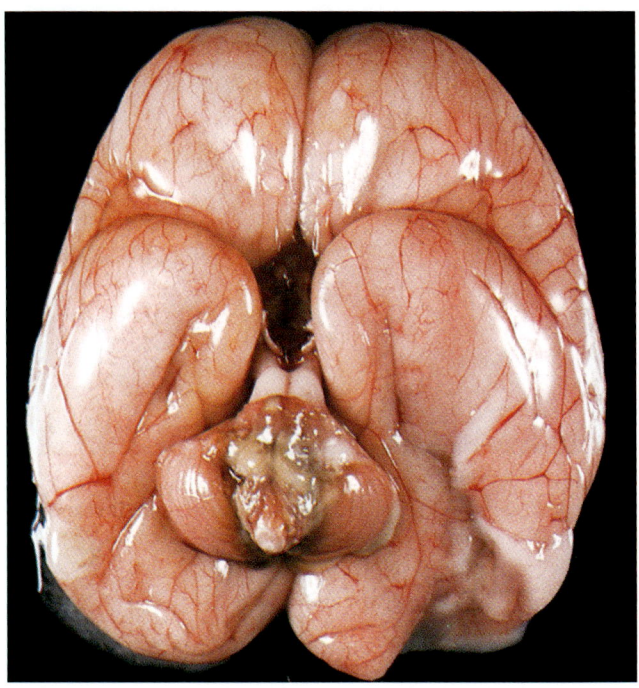

FIGURE 28-81
Escherichia coli **meningitis.** The brain of an infant who died of *E. coli* meningitis shows a purulent exudate *(creamy white areas)* in the leptomeninges at the base of the brain.

Consequently, in infancy gram-negative organisms quickly produce a purulent meningitis with a high mortality (Fig. 28-81).

- *Haemophilus influenzae:* Environmental exposure to *H. influenzae*, a gram-negative organism, is somewhat de-

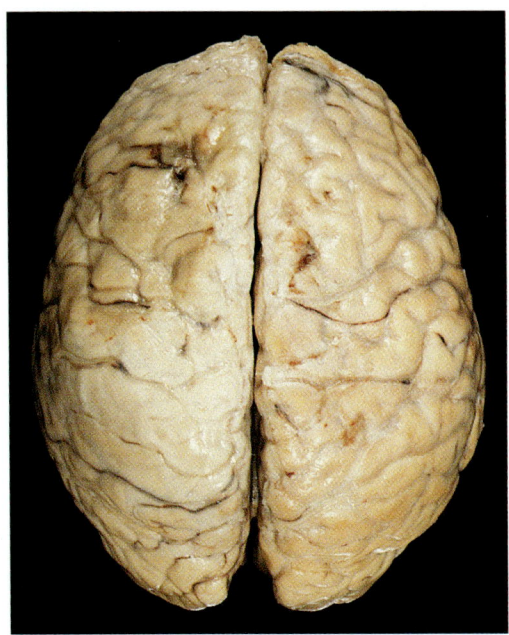
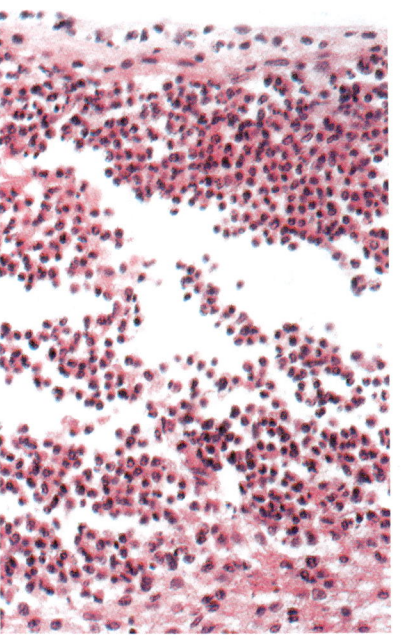

FIGURE 28-80
Purulent meningitis. A. A creamy exudate opacifies the leptomeninges. **B.** A microscopic section shows the accumulation of numerous neutrophils in the subarachnoid space.

1446　The Nervous System

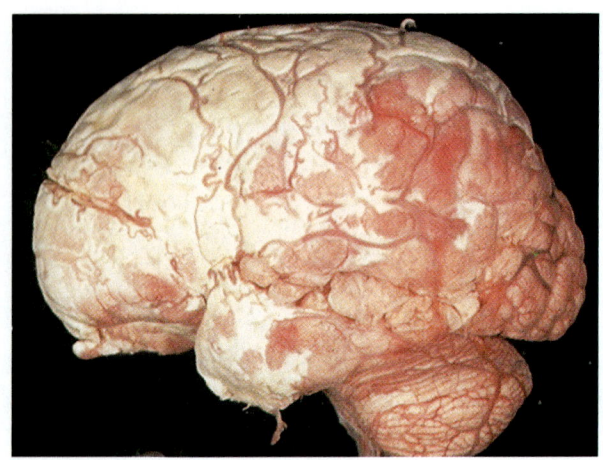

FIGURE 28-82
Haemophilus influenzae meningitis. A loculated fibrinous exudate involves the meninges.

layed, and the incidence of meningitis is maximal between 3 months and 3 years (Fig. 28-82).
- **Streptococcus pneumoniae:** The pneumococcus predominates as a cause of meningitis later in life. Patients with a history of basilar skull fracture have an unusually high incidence of pneumococcal meningitis, which often recurs after treatment.
- **Neisseria meningitidis:** The meningococcus resides in the nasopharynx, and airborne transmission in crowded places (e.g., schools or barracks) causes "epidemic meningitis." Initially, bacteremia causes fever, malaise, and petechial rash, but intravascular coagulopathy may cause lethal adrenal hemorrhages *(Waterhouse-Friderichsen syndrome)*. Untreated meningococcal bacteremia is prone to initiate an acute fulminant meningitis.

Although organisms reach the intracranial compartment by way of the bloodstream, it is not clear how they exit (Fig. 28-83).

Because most organisms initiate a purulent or suppurative response, the presence of polymorphonuclear leukocytes in the CSF is the most definitive index of meningitis (see Fig. 28-80B). Yet lymphocytes are the hallmark of tuberculosis and the viral meningitides, as well as of some chronic infections, such as those due to *C. neoformans*.

 Pathology: Macroscopic examination reveals an exudate (leukocytes, fibrin) opacifying the arachnoid. The exudate may be mild and equivocal to the naked eye or prominent enough to obscure blood vessels. Purulent exudates are conspicuous over the cerebral hemispheres (see Fig. 28-80A) but may extend to the base of the brain and from intracranial to intraspinal and subarachnoid spaces, which are in continuity. Although the pia is an effective barrier against the spread of infection, and cerebral abscesses rarely complicate meningitis, the pia forms sleeves

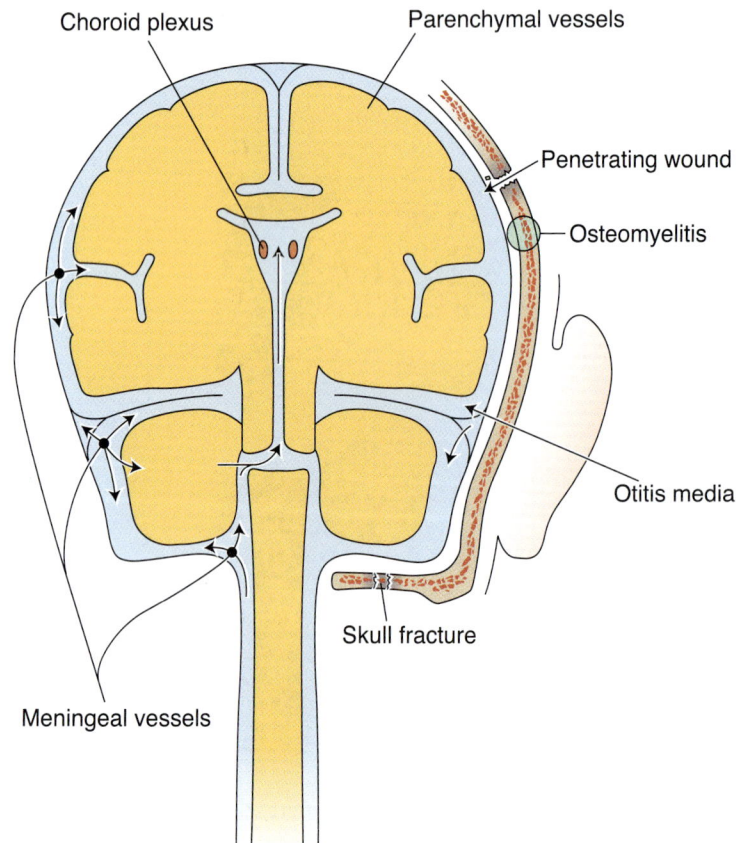

FIGURE 28-83
Routes of entry of infectious organisms into the cranial cavity.

around blood vessels that penetrate the brain *(Virchow-Robin spaces)* in continuity with the subarachnoid space.

H. influenzae elicits a dense exudate, rich in leukocytes and fibrin, that creates a barrier to antibiotics (see Fig. 28-82).

Clinical Features: Suppurative meningitides share similar symptoms (albeit with a rapid or insidious onset) including headache, vomiting, fever, and convulsions (especially in children). Classic signs of meningitis include cervical rigidity, knee pain with hip flexion (Kernig sign), and knee/hip flexion when the neck is flexed (Brudzinski sign). In untreated cases, delirium gives way to coma and death.

Tuberculous Meningitis and Tuberculomas

Tuberculous granulomas in the meninges are analogous to those elsewhere (Fig. 28-84). Epithelioid cells, Langhans giant cells, and lymphocytes surround areas of caseous necrosis. Inadequately treated tuberculous meningitis results in meningeal fibrosis, communicating hydrocephalus, and arteritis, the last leading to infarcts. Since tuberculous meningitis has a predilection for the base of the brain, such infarcts are often in the distribution of the striate arteries. Untreated tuberculous meningitis is fatal in 4 to 6 weeks. Parenchymal tuberculosis produces *tuberculomas* (i.e., solitary masses with central caseous necrosis surrounded by granulomatous tissue [Fig. 28-85]).

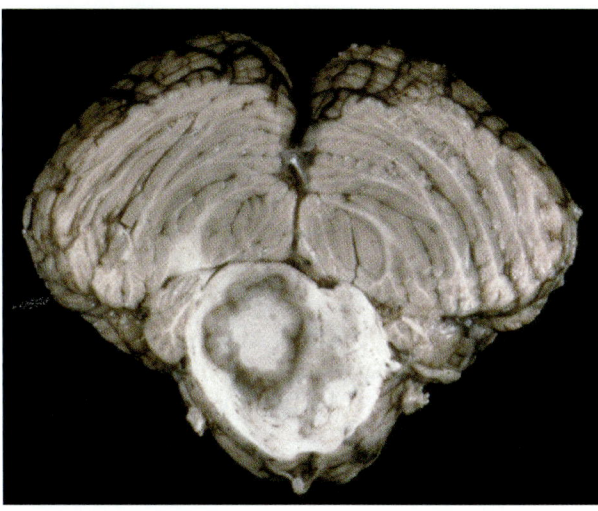

FIGURE 28-85
Tuberculoma. A spherical mass is present in the tegmentum of the pons. The caseous center is encapsulated by a rim of darker granulomatous tissue.

Most cases of tuberculous meningitis follow hematogenous dissemination, although multiple portals of CNS entry are available for tubercle bacilli.

Pott disease refers to tuberculosis of the spine, in which an epidural granulomatous mass destroys the spine and causes spinal cord compression (Fig. 28-86). Pott disease was

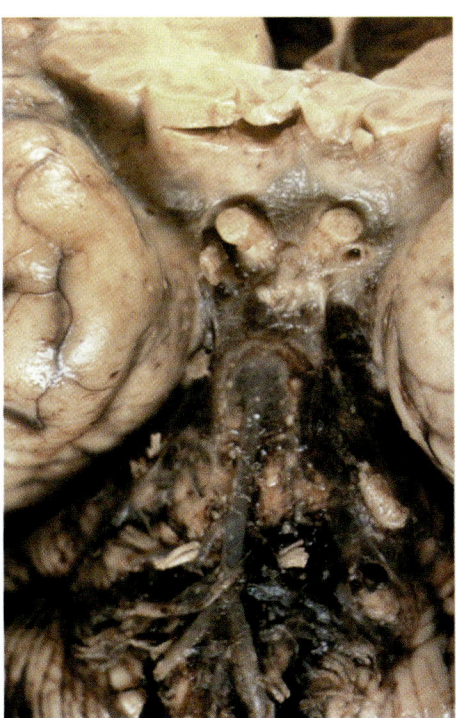

FIGURE 28-84
Tuberculous meningitis. The meninges covering the base of the brain (especially over the optic chiasm and interpeduncular fossa) are opacified by the meningeal exudate.

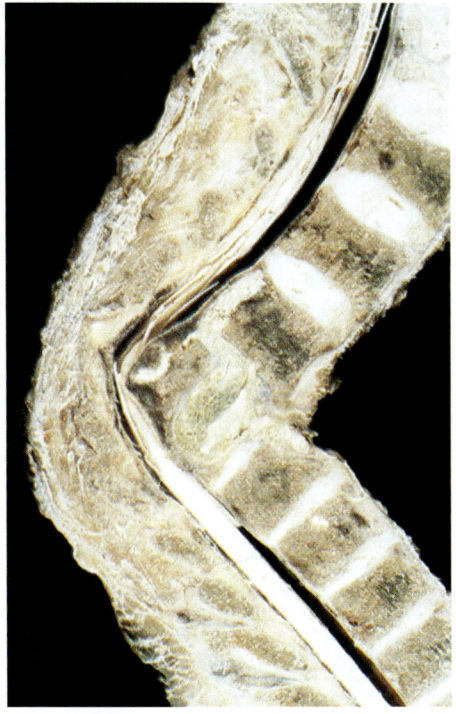

FIGURE 28-86
Pott disease. Tuberculosis of the spine caused a destructive spondylitis, with resulting kyphosis and compression of the spinal cord.

formerly responsible for many so-called hunchbacks, a condition that is rare today.

Viral Meningitis

Infection of the meninges may be the most common viral disease of the CNS, but unlike bacterial meningitis, it is usually benign and leaves no sequelae. The most common causative agents are enteroviruses (e.g., coxsackievirus B, echovirus), but mumps, lymphocytic choriomeningitis, Epstein-Barr, and herpes simplex viruses are responsible for many sporadic cases.

Viral meningitis (predominantly a disease of children and young adults) is heralded by a sudden febrile illness with a severe headache. The CSF contains excess lymphocytes and a slight increase in protein but, unlike bacterial meningitis, no decrease in CSF glucose.

Cryptococcal Meningitis

Cryptococcal meningitis is an indolent infection in which the virulence of the causative agent marginally exceeds the resistance of the host. In most instances, it acts opportunistically in immunocompromised persons, but the organism on rare occasion can establish meningitis in an immunologically competent host. *C. neoformans* customarily enters the human host by the inhalation of contaminated particulates. Birds are a major reservoir, and their inhaled excreta initiate a pneumonitis, after which the fungi enter the bloodstream and attain the intracranial compartment.

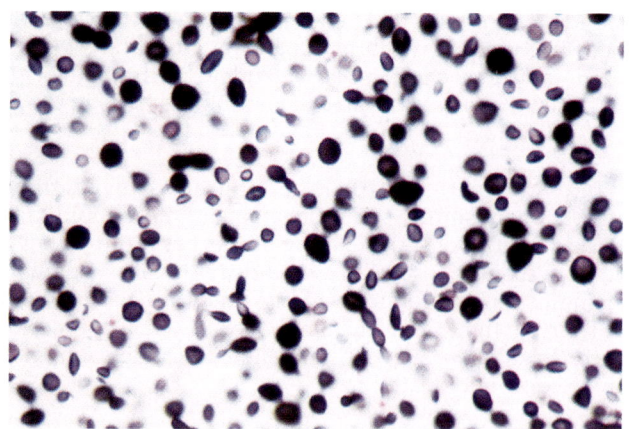

FIGURE 28-87
Cryptococcal meningitis. The cryptococcal organisms vary in size (between 5 and 15 μm in diameter. They reproduce by budding.

Pathology: The tissue response to *C. neoformans* in the meninges is typically sparse. The lesions are widely disseminated in the meninges, ependyma, and choroid plexus. To the naked eye, they appear as discrete white nodules, a millimeter or so in diameter. Microscopically, organisms may abound, particularly in the Virchow–Robin spaces. An occasional multinucleated giant cell, sometimes with phagocytosed organisms, is accompanied by scant epithelioid cells and a scattering of lymphocytes.

Cryptococcal organisms are encapsulated spheres, 5 to 15 μm in diameter. They have an external gelatinous capsule and reproduce by budding (Fig. 28-87). When a drop of contaminated CSF is mixed with India ink, microscopic examination shows a clear halo about the encapsulated organism. This capsule sheds specific antigens that can be detected in the CSF by the latex cryptococcal antigen test.

C. neoformans usually causes only meningitis, but rare cases of infection show collections of organisms within the brain parenchyma, forming gelatinous pseudocysts (Fig. 28-88).

Amebic Meningoencephalitis

Two genera of amebae, *Naegleria* and *Acanthamoeba*, penetrate the intracranial compartment by way of the cribriform plate, via the olfactory nerves. Persons exposed to brackish water while swimming may be infected by *Naegleria*, which produces a fulminant, usually fatal, leptomeningitis. By light microscopy, the trophozoites of *Naegleria* appear similar to macrophages. Infection by *Acanthamoeba*, whose trophozoites resemble *Naegleria* (Fig. 28-89), is also fatal, but with a more protracted course. In addition to meningitis, *Acanthamoeba* produces parenchymal abscesses and a granulomatous tissue reaction. The organism has a distinctive double serrated cell wall.

Syphilitic (Luetic) Meningitis and Related Lesions

The spirochete of syphilis, *T. pallidum*, enters the bloodstream from the primary lesion, the chancre. The onset of secondary syphilis is marked by a maculopapular rash on the skin and mucous membranes. A few lymphocytes and plasma cells and increased protein in the CSF reflect entry of blood-borne spirochetes into the meninges. The organisms do not survive for long and the CSF reverts to normal. On oc-

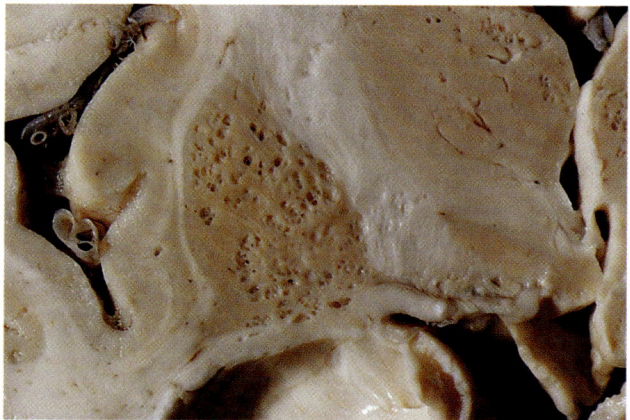

FIGURE 28-88
Cryptococcal infection. The historic term for cryptococcus, *Torula histolytica*, referred to the propensity of this organism to create a lytic, spongy lesion in the parenchyma, which is shown here in the basal ganglia from a patient who died of acquired immunodeficiency syndrome (AIDS).

Infectious Diseases 1449

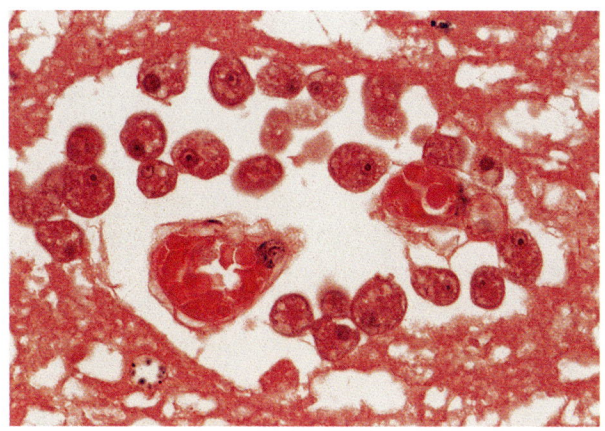

FIGURE 28-89
Acanthamoeba infection. The protozoa bear a close resemblance to macrophages *(arrows)*.

TABES DORSALIS: The initial lesion in this disorder is a variant of chronic meningitis. The dorsal nerve roots proximal to the dorsal root ganglia are met by a conical sleeve of arachnoid filled with CSF, which can be the site of syphilitic inflammation. Fibrous tissue generated by the inflammation constricts nerve roots to cause axonal (wallerian) degeneration. The axons that course cephalad in the posterior fasciculus do not synapse with intramedullary neurons as do all other ascending pathways in the cord. They are, rather, direct extensions of posterior root axons, so that wallerian degeneration initiated in the dorsal spinal nerves extends into the posterior fasciculi. This is the most readily visualized morphological lesion of tabes dorsalis and accounts for the loss of position sense in the lower extremities. The serological reaction of the CSF generally reverts to negative before the onset of tabetic symptoms.

LUETIC DEMENTIA: *T. pallidum* may also lodge latently in the brain for decades. The spirochetes replicate sluggishly and escape eradication, only to cause *dementia paralytica* years after the initial infection. The morphological features of luetic dementia include the following:

- Focal loss of cortical neurons (Figs. 28-90 and 28-91)
- Disfigurement of the topography of the residual nerve cells ("wind-blown appearance")

casion, however, the transient spirochete initiates a fibroblastic response in the meninges, accompanied by an obliterative endarteritis (Fig. 28-90) that induces multiple small infarcts in the cerebral cortex. Plasma cells, the hallmark of syphilis, surround the arterioles of the cerebral cortex in luetic meningovascular syphilis.

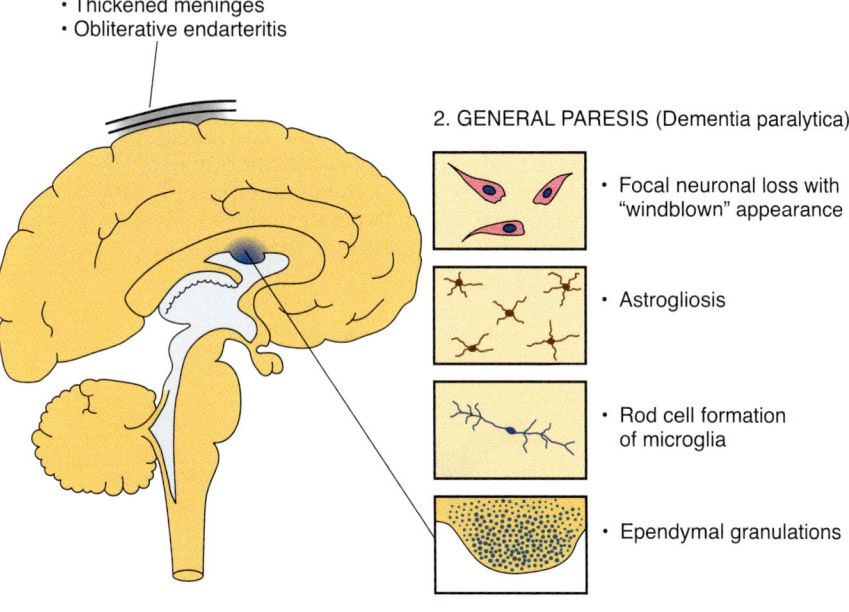

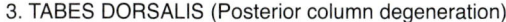

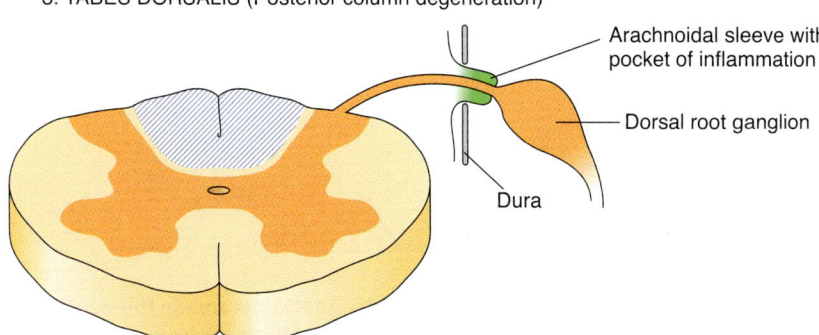

FIGURE 28-90
Involvement of the central nervous system in syphilis.

1450 The Nervous System

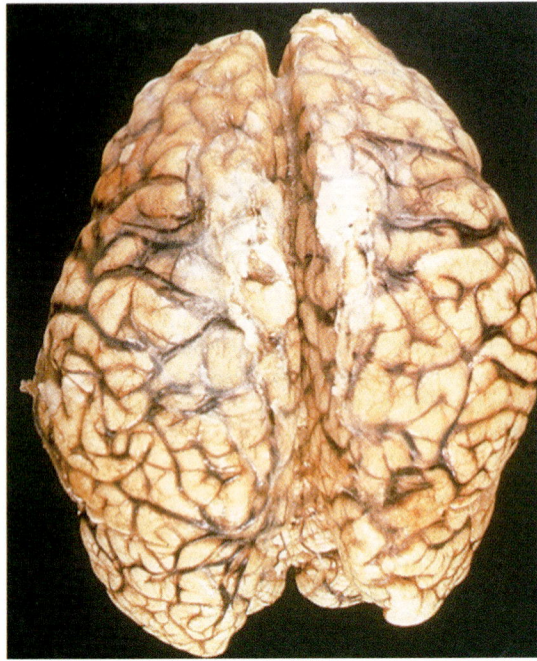

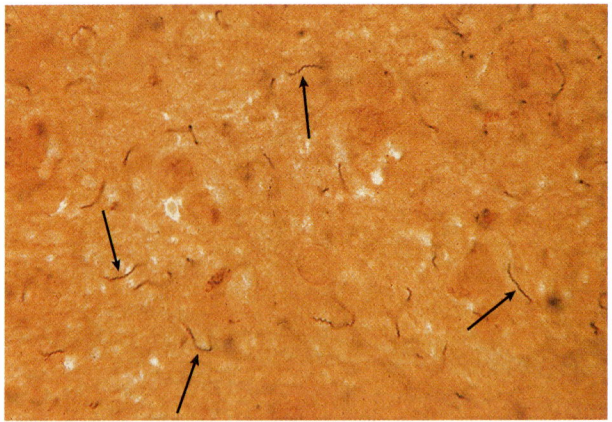

FIGURE 28-91
Tertiary syphilis (general paresis). A. The brain shows cortical atrophy, most marked in the frontal lobes. B. Spirochetes are evident with a silver stain (arrows).

- Marked gliosis
- Conversion of microglia into elongated forms encrusted with iron ("rod cells")
- Nodular ependymitis

Cerebral Abscess Is a Potentially Fatal Space-Occupying Lesion

The cortex and subjacent white matter contain a rich capillary bed. It is, therefore, not surprising that blood-borne microorganisms lodge in this location, where they replicate and elicit an acute inflammatory and edematous reaction termed *cerebritis* (Fig. 28-92). Within days, liquefactive necrosis causes an expanding abscess (Figs. 28-93 and 28-94) and threatens life by transtentorial herniation or rupture into a ventricle.

Astrocytes predominate in cerebral repair, but fibroblasts also contribute to the formation of a capsule around abscesses. If the abscess is not drained or treated with antibiotics, pressure builds within it. Both the abscess and surrounding edema compress blood vessels, thereby disposing the affected region to ischemia. The region below an abscess also is susceptible to the growth of microorganisms that escape from the "mother" abscess, and frequently "daughter" abscesses form beneath the primary lesion. They can carry the inflammatory process to the ventricles, from which the infection can pass across the ependyma through the foramina of Magendie and Luschka and onto the meninges, with a fatal outcome.

Viral Encephalomyelitis Reflects Localization in Specific CNS Areas

The manifestations of viral infections of CNS parenchyma are heterogeneous, both clinically and pathologically (Fig.

28-95). Thus, poliomyelitis affects spinal and brainstem motor neurons, rabies localizes to the brainstem, and herpes simplex targets the temporal lobes. Subacute sclerosing panencephalitis and progressive multifocal leukoencephalopathy afflict the cerebral hemispheres, the former generally in childhood and the latter in immunocompromised persons. The mechanisms of viral tropism may reflect specific binding of viruses to sites on the plasma membranes of CNS cells, the ability of viruses to remain latent, or selective replication in distinct intracellular microenvironments. Since axons project over long distances, viruses that enter a neuron may be

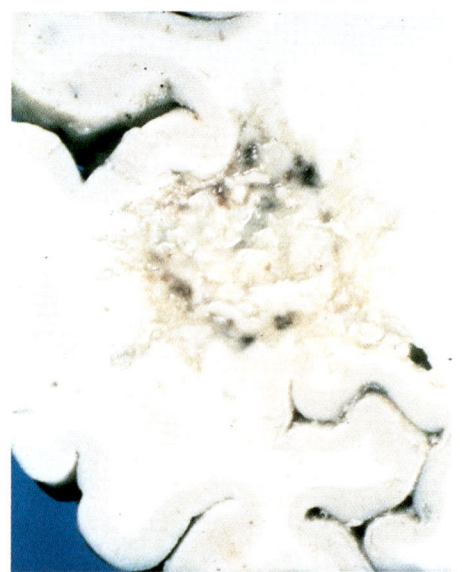

FIGURE 28-92
Cerebritis. An irregular, soft, gelatinous area in the white matter is the prodromal phase of a cerebral abscess.

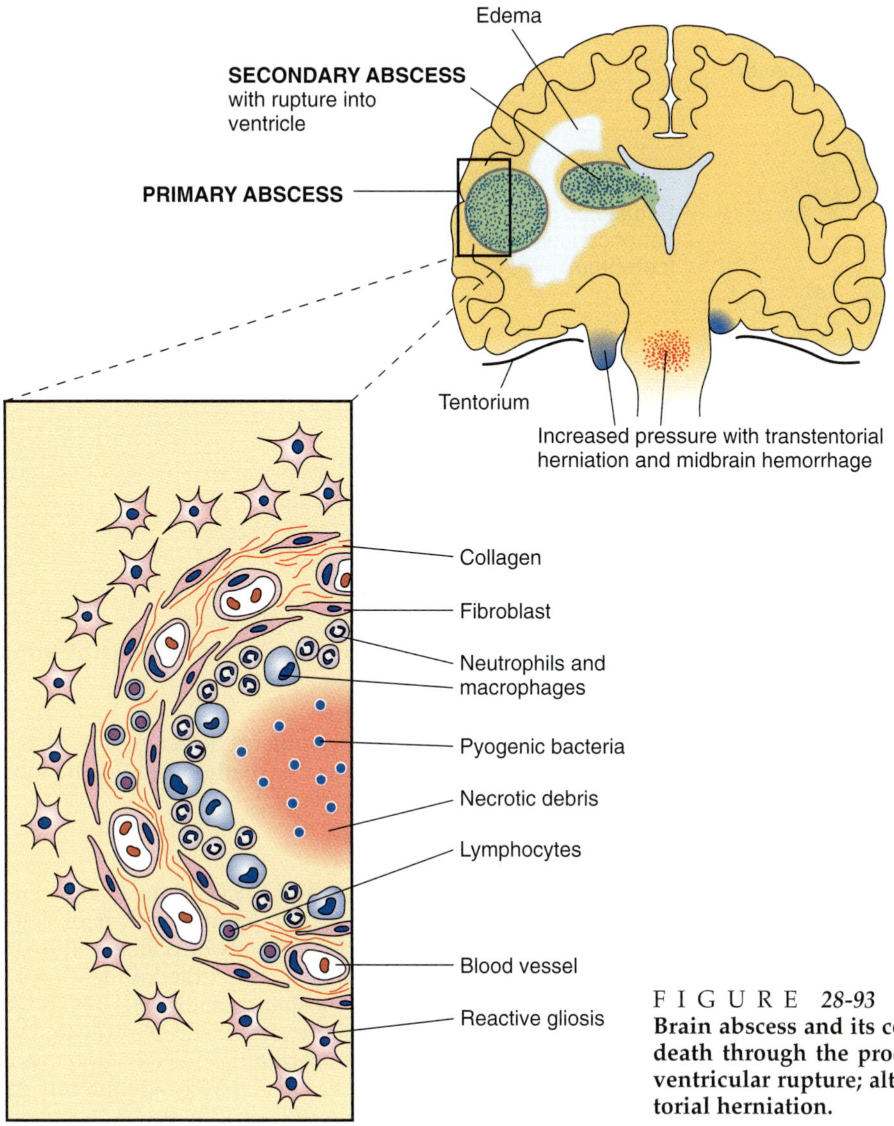

Infectious Diseases

FIGURE 28-93
Brain abscess and its complications. A cerebral abscess may cause death through the production of secondary abscesses with intraventricular rupture; alternatively, death may result from transtentorial herniation.

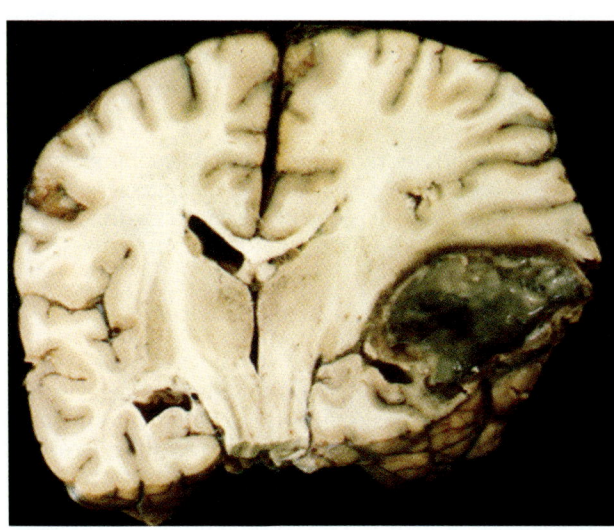

FIGURE 28-94
Cerebral abscess. A young man with chronic otitis media developed an abscess in the temporal lobe, which then ruptured into the temporal horn of the lateral ventricle.

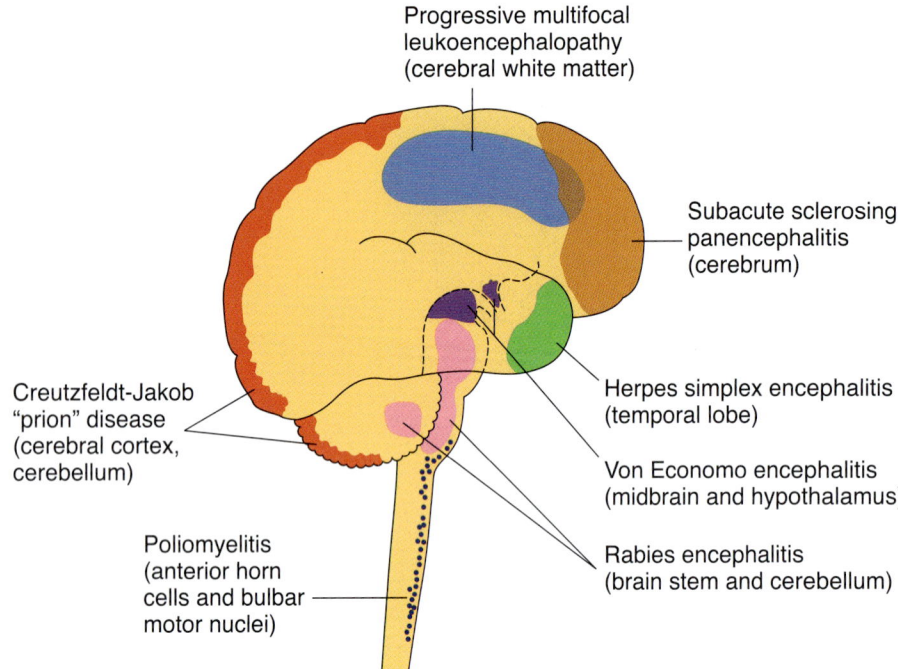

FIGURE 28-95
Distribution of the lesions of viral encephalitides.

transported by orthograde and retrograde axonal and dendritic transport mechanism to sites distant from their point of entry, as exemplified by rabies and herpesviruses.

 Pathology: The classic hallmark of most CNS viral infections is the presence of **perivascular lymphocytes** around arteries and arterioles (Fig. 28-96), but a more diagnostic feature is the formation of viral inclusion bodies (Fig. 28-97). However, inclusion bodies are not seen in all viral infections (e.g., poliomyelitis).

The characteristics of the most common inclusions are as follows:

- **Herpes simplex and herpes zoster infection:** The inclusions are small, intranuclear, and eosinophilic and cannot be distinguished from each other by their morphological appearance (see Fig. 28-101).
- **Rabies:** The eosinophilic Negri body in the cytoplasm is unequivocal evidence of rabies encephalitis (see Fig. 28-9).
- **Progressive multifocal leukoencephalopathy:** The intranuclear inclusions that characterize this disease reflect the presence of papovavirus (JC virus) in oligodendroglia. They are associated with mild enlargement of the nucleus and exhibit a "ground glass" appearance (see Fig. 28-104).
- **Subacute sclerosing panencephalitis:** The intranuclear inclusions are basophilic and are rimmed by a prominent halo.
- **Cytomegalovirus infection:** Eosinophilic inclusions are present in both the nucleus and cytoplasm of astrocytes and neurons. They are most conspicuous in the enlarged nucleus, where they are sharply defined and surrounded by a halo (see Fig. 28-8 and Fig. 28-103).

Viral particles also may be visualized by electron microscopy, but in situ hybridization, polymerase chain reaction (PCR), and immunohistochemistry detect viral particles most reliably and are more effective methods for the diagnosis of viral infections (see Fig. 28-103).

 Clinical Features: The onset of most viral encephalitides is abrupt. The more specific neurological deficits (e.g., the paralysis of poliomyelitis or difficulty in swallowing in rabies) reflect the localization of the viral infection. Although most encephalitides run a brief course, the tempo can vary. For example, the clinical course of subacute sclerosing panencephalitis may extend over years, whereas herpes simplex virus may reside latently in the gasserian ganglion for decades and may do the same in the brain. Thus, viral infections also may be implicated in chronic cerebral disorders.

Poliomyelitis

The term poliomyelitis *refers to any inflammation of the gray matter of the spinal cord, but in common usage, it implies an infection by poliovirus.* The organism is one of the enteroviruses, which are small, nonenveloped, single-stranded, RNA viruses.

 Epidemiology: Historical evidence suggests that poliomyelitis has occurred in epidemic form since antiquity. The medical triumph over this disease in the 20th century depended on many years of prior research that culminated in the development of effective vaccines to prevent the disease. Persons infected with poliovirus shed large amounts of virus in their stools, and infection spreads

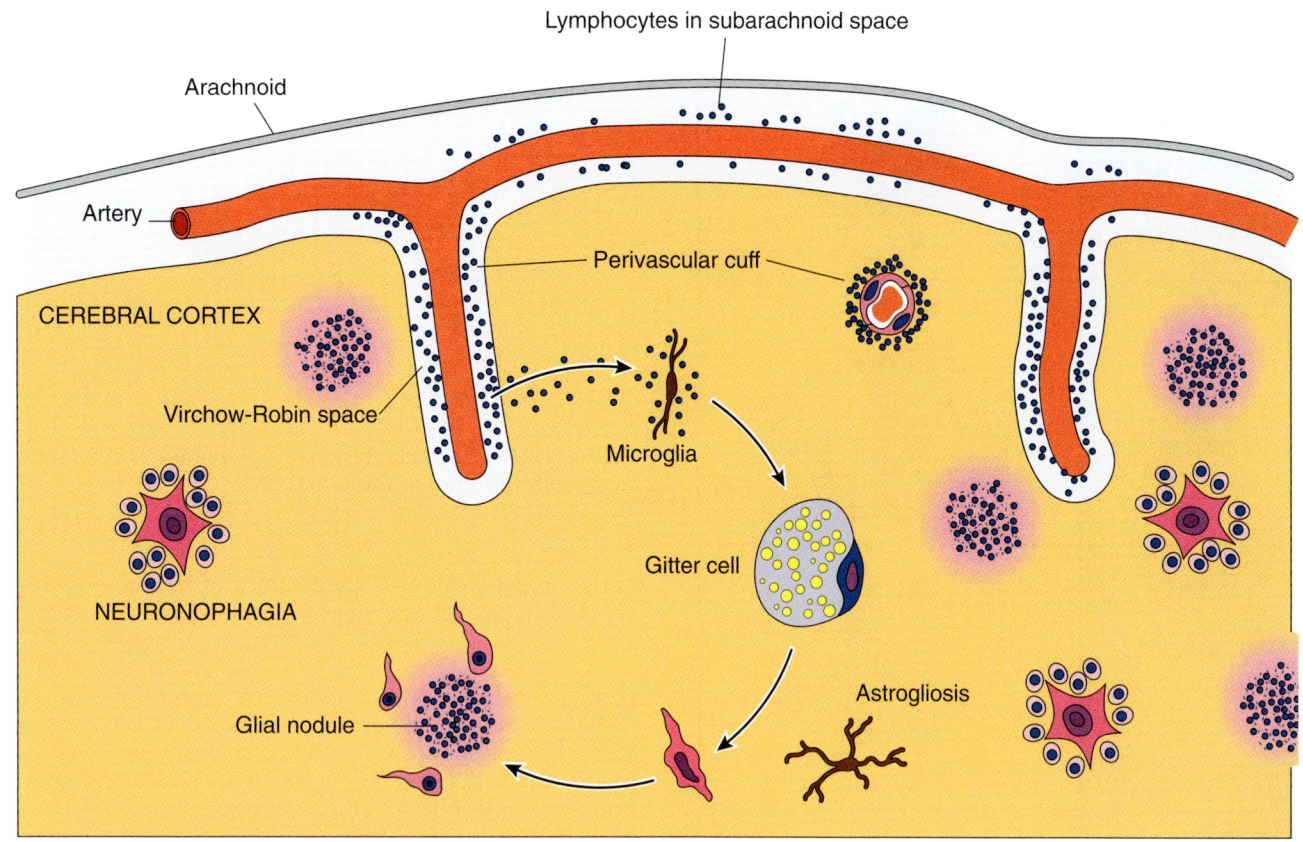

FIGURE 28-96
The lesions of viral encephalitis.

by the fecal–oral route. The agent spreads rapidly among children in close quarters where there are opportunities for fecal–oral contact.

 Pathology: Binding sites on motor neurons and the favorable intracellular conditions for viral replication permit the virus to enter these cells and replicate. The infected cells undergo chromatolysis (see Fig. 28-4 and Fig. 28-98), after which they are phagocytosed by macrophages (neuronophagia; see Fig. 28-7). The initial inflammatory response transiently includes polymorphonuclear leukocytes, which are followed by lymphocytes that surround blood vessels in the spinal cord and brainstem. The inflammation may also extend into the meninges. The motor cortex usually shows no inflammation but may contain "glial nodules," (i.e., focal collections of microglia and lymphocytes) (see Fig. 28-17). Although the immunological response of the host to poliovirus is limited, it may halt progression of clinical disease. Sections of spinal cord in cases of healed poliomyelitis show a paucity of neurons, with secondary degeneration of the corresponding ventral roots and peripheral nerves.

 Clinical Features: After infection with poliovirus, nonspecific symptoms such as fever, malaise, and headache are followed in several days by signs of meningitis and shortly thereafter by paralysis. In severe cases, the muscles of the neck, trunk, and all four limbs may be rendered powerless, and paralysis of the respiratory muscles may become life threatening. Patients with milder cases exhibit an asymmetric and patchy paralysis, most prominently in the lower limbs.

Improvement begins in about a week, and only some of the muscles affected at the outset remain permanently paralyzed. The mortality varies from 5 to 25%, with death usually resulting from respiratory failure. The development in the 1950s of effective vaccines against poliovirus has largely eliminated the disease.

Rabies

Rabies is an encephalitis caused by rabies virus, an enveloped, single-stranded RNA virus of the rhabdovirus group. Rabies has been recognized throughout recorded history. Lower animals harbor a reservoir of this zoonosis and transmit the lethal encephalitis to humans. Dogs, wolves, foxes, and skunks are the principal reservoirs, but the infection also extends to bats and domestic animals, including cattle, goats, and swine. The infectious agent is transmitted to humans through contaminated saliva introduced by a bite. In the United States, where dogs are routinely vaccinated against rabies, the few human rabies infections (one to five per year) usually result from exposure to rabid wild an-

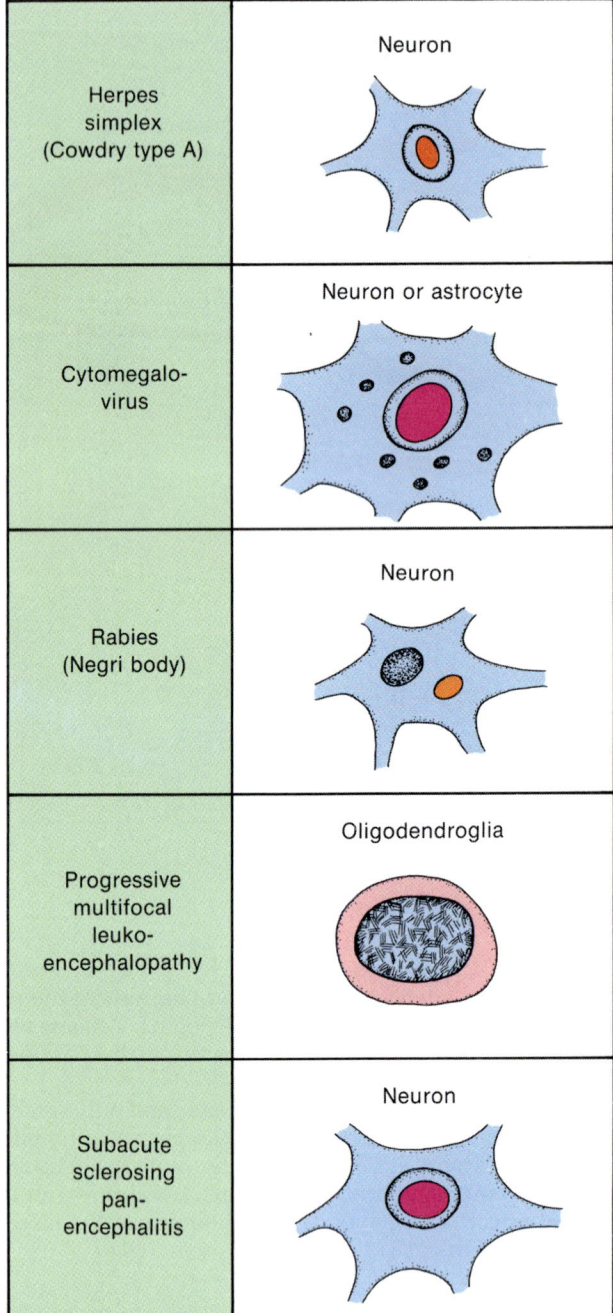

FIGURE 28-97
Inclusion bodies in viral encephalitides.

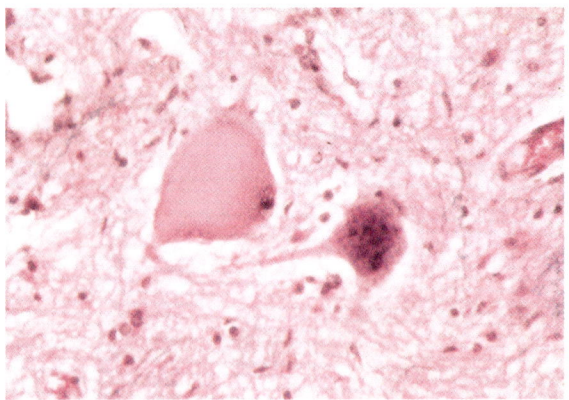

FIGURE 28-98
Poliomyelitis. Chromatolysis and neuronal necrosis are seen in the anterior horn of the spinal cord.

varies in proportion to the distance of transport, being as short as 10 days or as long as 3 months.

 Pathology: Lymphocytes aggregate about small arteries and veins in the brainstem. Scattered neurons show chromatolysis and neuronophagia, and glial nodules develop. The inflammation is centered in the brainstem and spills into the cerebellum and hypothalamus. Negri bodies (see Fig. 28-9) in the hippocampus, brainstem, and cerebellar Purkinje cells confirm the diagnosis of rabies.

 Clinical Features: Destruction of brainstem neurons by rabies virus initiates painful spasms of the throat, difficulty swallowing, and a tendency to aspirate fluids. These symptoms prompted the original designation "hydrophobia." The clinical symptoms also reflect a general encephalopathy, characterized by irritability, agitation, seizures, and delirium. The CSF displays a typical viral response, including (1) a modest increase in the number of lymphocytes, (2) a moderate increase in protein content, and (3) unaltered glucose levels and CSF pressure. The illness progresses to death within one to several weeks, unless postexposure vaccination is administered in a timely manner.

Herpes Simplex Encephalitis and Related Infections

Herpesviruses include herpes simplex (types 1 and 2), varicella-zoster virus, cytomegalovirus, Epstein-Barr virus, and simian B virus.

HERPES SIMPLEX VIRUS TYPE 1 (HSV-1): Herpes simplex virus type 1 is largely responsible for the "cold sore." The region of the vesicular lesion on the lip is innervated from the gasserian ganglion through its mandibular nerve trunk. HSV-1 may reside latently within the gasserian ganglion, where it proliferates during periods of stress and is transmitted centrifugally through the nerve trunk to the lip.

imals. In areas of Asia, Africa, and South America, however where rabies is endemic, most human infections result from dog bites. In those areas of the world, rabies kills more than 50,000 persons annually.

 Pathogenesis: The virus enters a peripheral nerve and is transported by retrograde axoplasmic flow to the spinal cord and brain. The latent interval

Infectious Diseases 1455

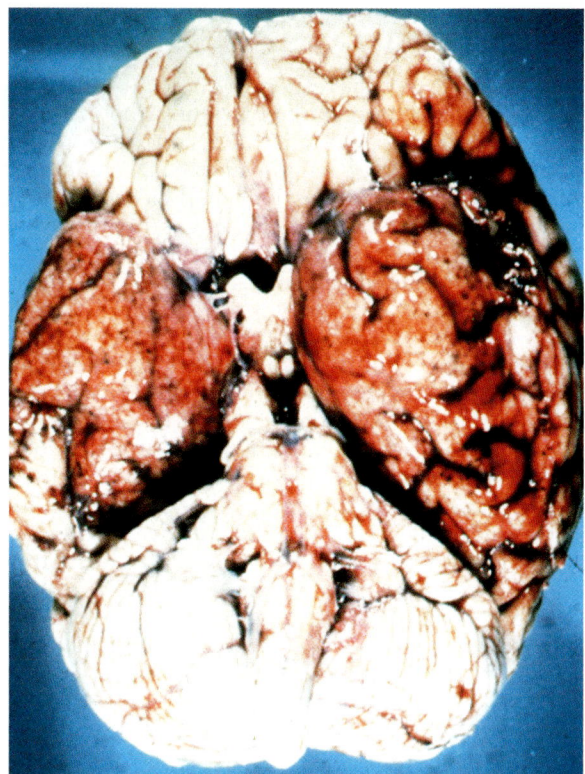

FIGURE 28-99
Herpes simplex encephalitis. The temporal lobes are preferentially involved by a hemorrhagic, necrotizing inflammation.

Herpes encephalitis is a major viral infection of the human nervous system. In adults, the encephalitis is caused principally by HSV-1 and localizes predominantly in one or both temporal lobes.

 Pathology: Herpes encephalitis is a fulminant infection. The temporal lobes become swollen, hemorrhagic, and necrotic (Fig. 28-99). The in-

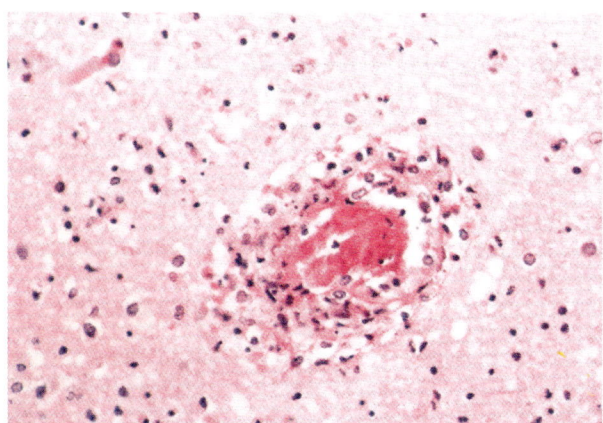

FIGURE 28-100
Herpes simplex encephalitis. A microscopic view of material shown in Fig. 28-99 shows a necrotizing arteritis in a temporal lobe.

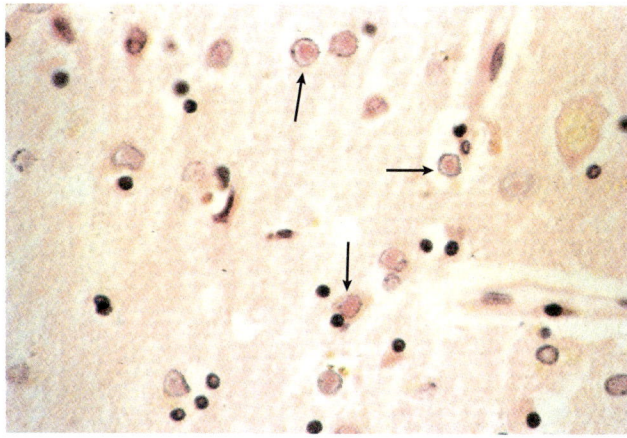

FIGURE 28-101
Herpes simplex encephalitis. The infected neurons display small, intranuclear, eosinophilic inclusions that lack halos (arrows).

flammatory exudate is predominantly lymphocytic and perivascular. The small arteries and arterioles become hemorrhagic and edematous (Fig. 28-100). Intranuclear inclusions occur in both neurons and in glial cells. The inclusions are eosinophilic and usually surrounded by a halo (Fig. 28-101). The detection of viral proteins by immunohistochemical techniques is diagnostically reliable.

HERPES SIMPLEX VIRUS TYPE 2 (HSV-2): In women, HSV-2 initiates a vesicular lesion on the vulva, coupled with a latent infection in the pelvic ganglia. Newborns acquire HSV-2 from the birth canal and thereafter have an encephalitis. At this age, the neural tissues are extremely vulnerable, and the infection promptly causes extensive liquefactive necrosis in the cerebrum and cerebellum (Fig. 28-102).

VARICELLA-ZOSTER VIRUS: Herpes zoster causes a disease that is anatomically analogous to the gasserian gan-

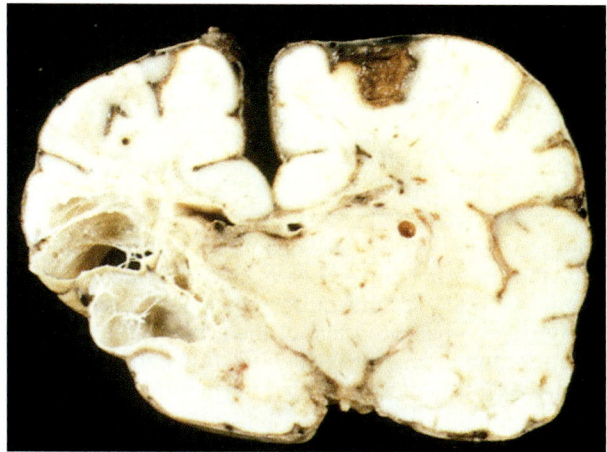

FIGURE 28-102
Herpes simplex type 2 encephalitis. The brain of an infant born to a mother with genital herpes shows conspicuous cavitary lesions.

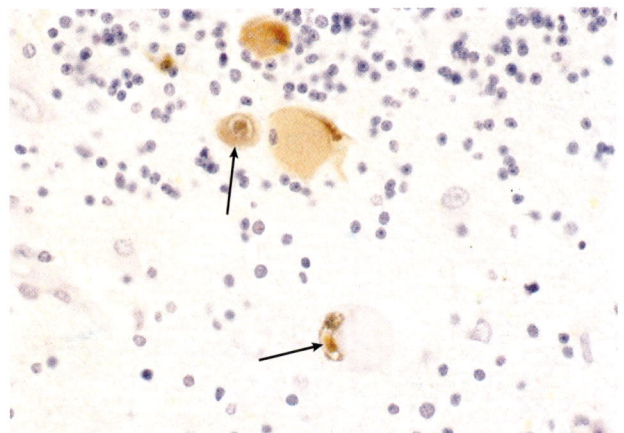

FIGURE 28-103
Cytomegalovirus (CMV) encephalitis. Immunohistochemical localization of CMV antigens demonstrates intranuclear and intracytoplasmic inclusions within Purkinje cells of the cerebellum (arrow).

glion–cold sore complex of herpes simplex. The cutaneous vesicular eruption of "shingles" occurs in the distribution of a dermatome whose dorsal root ganglion harbors the varicella-zoster virus. The infection elicits only mild inflammation and rarely spreads to the CNS.

CYTOMEGALOVIRUS: This agent crosses the placenta to induce encephalitis in utero. The lesions in the embryonic CNS predominate in the periventricular areas and are characterized by necrosis and calcification. Because of the proximity of these lesions to the third ventricle and the aqueduct, they are prone to induce hydrocephalus. Cytomegalovirus is one of the agents of the so-called TORCH (toxoplasmosis, other [congenital syphilis and viruses], rubella, cytomegalovirus, and herpes simplex virus) complex of newborns. In adults, cytomegalovirus initiates encephalitis in immunocompromised hosts (see Fig. 28-8 and Fig. 28-103).

SIMIAN B VIRUS: This virus contaminates the saliva of lower primates and is transmitted to humans through a bite, causing fulminant encephalitis and myelitis.

Arthropod-Borne Viral Encephalitis

Arthropod-borne viruses, termed *arboviruses*, are heterogeneous and are transmitted between vertebrates by blood-sucking vectors (e.g., mosquitoes, ticks). Togaviridae and Bunyaviridae constitute most of the arboviruses that cause human encephalitis. Arbovirus infections are zoonoses of animals, and humans are infected when bitten by virus-harboring arthropods. Humans do not continue viral propagation. The various encephalitides caused by arboviruses are named principally for the location where they were first noted (Table 28-1), for example, Eastern, Western, and Venezuelan equine encephalitis, St. Louis encephalitis, Japanese B encephalitis, and California encephalitis.

 Pathology: The response of the brain does not differentiate among the various arboviruses that cause encephalitis, and the lesions vary from mild meningitis with scattered lymphocytes to severe inflammation of gray matter, thrombosis of small blood vessels, and prominent necrosis. No inclusions are present in the infected neurons. In necrotic foci, neuronophagia is evident, and if the patient survives, demyelination and gliosis may develop.

 Clinical Features: The arthropod-borne encephalitides share many features, but each type has a different course. For example, Eastern equine encephalitis is commonly a fulminant disease that kills in a few days, whereas Venezuelan equine encephalitis tends to be benign. Mild cases of arbovirus encephalitis may be manifested only by a mild flulike syndrome and are not diagnosed as encephalitis. In severe cases, the onset is abrupt, with high fever, headache, vomiting, and meningeal signs, followed by lethargy and coma. Most victims die within 5 days. Young children often survive but may be left with mental retardation, epilepsy, and other neurological sequelae.

Encephalitis Lethargica (von Economo Encephalitis)

Beginning in 1916 and lasting for 5 years, the agent of encephalitis lethargica induced a severe encephalitis pandemic. Although the identity of the infectious agent is disputed, the characteristic perivascular cuffs of lymphocytes in the midbrain and hypothalamus argued for a viral cause. The dominant symptom was somnolence, which persisted for weeks. An occasional patient was left with parkinsonism (see below), but other victims developed Parkinson disease ("postencephalitis parkinsonism") a decade or so later, suggesting that subclinical injury to neurons of the substantia nigra compromised their longevity.

TABLE 28-1 Insect-Borne Viral Encephalitis

Virus	Insect Vector	Distribution
St. Louis encephalitis	Mosquito	North and South America
Western equine encephalitis	Mosquito	North and South America
Venezuelan equine encephalitis	Mosquito	North and South America
Eastern equine encephalitis	Mosquito	North America
California encephalitis	Mosquito	North America
Murray Valley encephalitis	Mosquito	Australia, Papua New Guinea
Japanese B encephalitis	Mosquito	Eastern and southeastern Asia
Tick-borne encephalitis	Tick	Eastern Europe, Scandinavia

Subacute Sclerosing Panencephalitis

Subacute sclerosing panencephalitis (SSPE) is a chronic, lethal, viral infection of the brain caused by the measles virus. First recognized in 1933 and named "subacute inclusion-body encephalitis," its features were defined later as an encephalitis of insidious onset, predominantly in childhood. The course is protracted, and inflammation occurs primarily in cerebral gray matter. However, in adults, SSPE may follow a more rapid course.

Pathogenesis: SSPE is a consequence of infection with the measles virus, and most patients give a history of measles in childhood. The underlying mechanisms for the persistence of the virus within infected cells is uncertain, but its presence for years in the brain leads to a chronic neurodegenerative process.

Pathology and Clinical Features: The infection is highlighted by prominent intranuclear inclusions in neurons and oligodendroglia, marked gliosis in affected gray and white matter (hence *sclerosing*), patchy loss of myelin, and ubiquitous perivascular lymphocytes and macrophages. In some cases, affected neurons contain neurofibrillary tangles (see below). Over a period of years, the classic disease leads insidiously to cognitive deficits, behavioral changes, motor and sensory impairments, and ultimately death. The CSF typically contains an increased titer against the measles virus.

Progressive Multifocal Leukoencephalopathy

Progressive multifocal leukoencephalopathy (PML) is a relentlessly destructive focal disease caused by JC virus, which principally affects the white matter in brain. PML manifests dementia, weakness, visual loss, and ataxia, leading to death in most patients within 6 months. The infection exemplifies the fundamental characteristics of neurotropic viruses, such as selectivity for specific cell types, notably oligodendroglia (Fig. 28-104), with demyelination caused by damage to oligodendrocytes (Fig. 28-105). In contrast to many viruses, JC virus is oncogenic (Fig. 28-106).

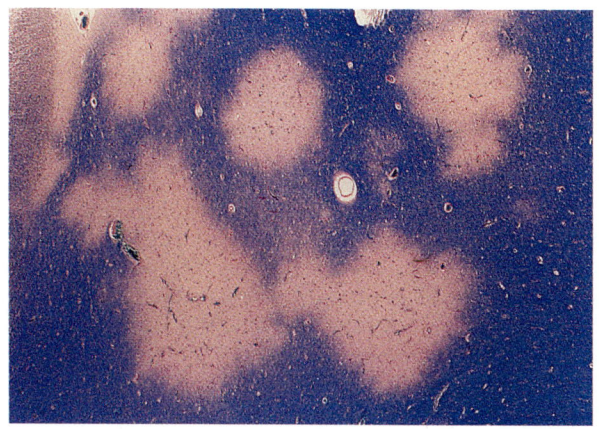

FIGURE 28-105
Progressive multifocal leukoencephalopathy. A luxol fast blue stain for myelin in the brain demonstrates conspicuous demyelination *(pale pink–brown areas).*

JC virus is a papovavirus closely analogous to simian virus 40 (SV40 virus). Most commonly, PML is a terminal complication in immunosuppressed patients, such as those treated for cancer or lupus erythematosus, organ transplant patients, and persons with AIDS. In fact, PML now occurs in 3% or more of AIDS patients in the United States and Europe.

Pathology: The typical lesions of PML appear as widely disseminated discrete foci of demyelination near the gray–white junction in the cerebral hemispheres and the brainstem (see Fig. 28-105). The characteristic lesion of PML exhibits the following morphological features:

- It is spherical, measuring several millimeters in diameter.
- A central area is largely devoid of myelin.

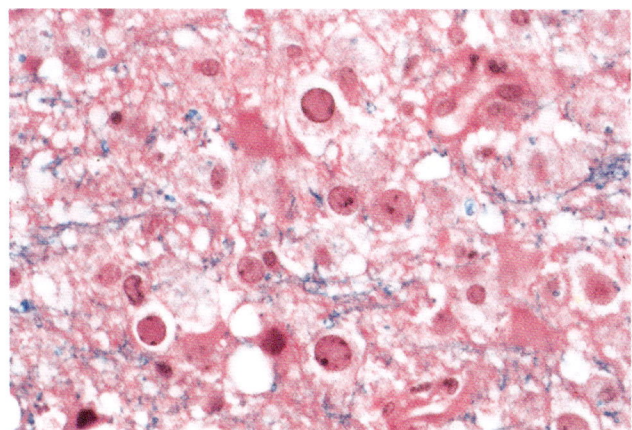

FIGURE 28-104
Progressive multifocal leukoencephalopathy. The oligodendroglia are enlarged and exhibit intranuclear inclusions.

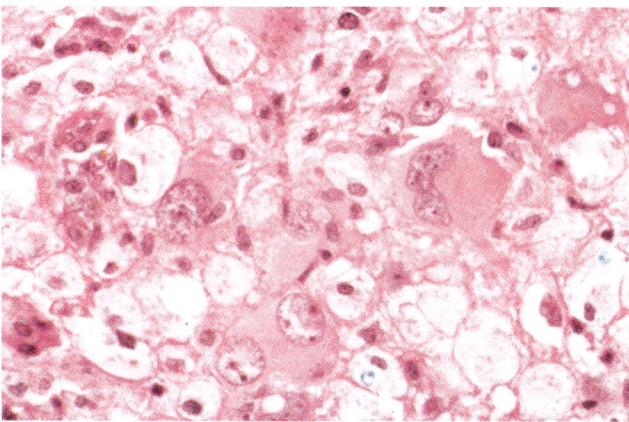

FIGURE 28-106
Progressive multifocal leukoencephalopathy. The astroglia display marked nuclear pleomorphism.

- Axons are retained.
- Few oligodendrocytes are seen.
- The lesion is infiltrated by macrophages, without necrosis.
- Pleomorphic astrocytes are present (see Fig. 28-106).

A pathognomonic feature of PML is a peripheral area of demyelination that contains enlarged oligodendrocytes, with homogeneously dense, hyperchromatic, intranuclear inclusions, which lack a halo and have a ground-glass appearance (see Fig. 28-104). Electron microscopy discloses intranuclear, crystalline arrays of spherical virions, 35 to 40 nm in diameter. The pleomorphic astrocytes appear anaplastic and contain multiple irregular nuclei, which display dense chromatin. Astrocytomas have developed in some patients with PML.

AIDS Encephalopathy

Many AIDS patients manifest a clinical encephalopathy and harbor brain lesions at autopsy. Some have an opportunistic infection in the brain (e.g., toxoplasmosis, cytomegalovirus [see Fig. 28-8], herpes simplex, progressive multifocal leukoencephalopathy, or a primary lymphoma). However, in most AIDS patients with encephalopathy, the disease is attributable to an active infection of the CNS by the retrovirus itself. **Dementia is the most common clinical manifestation of AIDS encephalopathy** *(AIDS dementia complex),* which ranges from mild to severe cognitive impairment, with paralysis and loss of sensory functions.

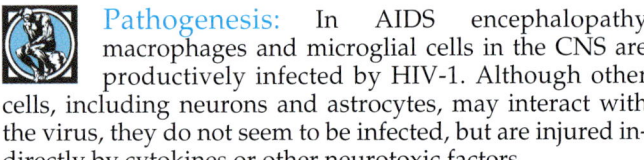

Pathogenesis: In AIDS encephalopathy macrophages and microglial cells in the CNS are productively infected by HIV-1. Although other cells, including neurons and astrocytes, may interact with the virus, they do not seem to be infected, but are injured indirectly by cytokines or other neurotoxic factors.

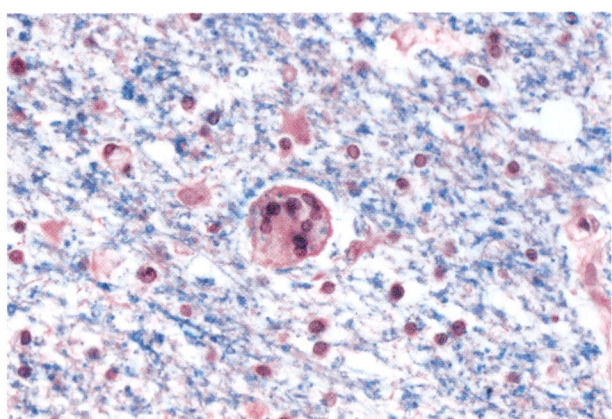

FIGURE 28-107
Acquired immunodeficiency syndrome (AIDS) encephalopathy. This higher-power view of material shown in Fig. 28-108 shows a multinucleated macrophage and diffuse astrogliosis.

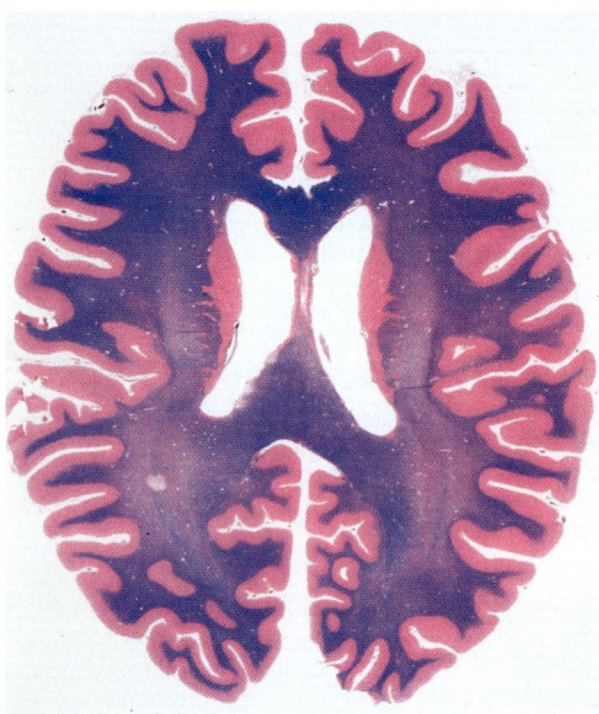

FIGURE 28-108
Acquired immunodeficiency syndrome (AIDS) encephalopathy. A horizontal section of the brain stained for myelin demonstrates a symmetric pallor, predominantly in the corona radiata, indicating demyelination.

Pathology: On gross examination, AIDS encephalopathy is characterized by mild cerebral atrophy, with dilation of the lateral ventricles and slight prominence of the gyri and sulci. The histological changes are usually in the subcortical gray and white matter. **The hallmark of AIDS encephalopathy is the presence of multinucleated giant cells of the monocyte/macrophage lineage associated with microglial nodules** (Fig. 28-107). In addition, myelin pallor (Fig. 28-108), reflecting diffuse demyelination, intense astrogliosis, and loss of neurons are commonly found.

Vacuolar myopathy is another disorder attributed to HIV infection, although it is less frequent than encephalopathy. It is characterized by marked vacuolation of the posterior and lateral columns, principally at the thoracic level of the spinal cord. Ataxia and spastic paraparesis dominate the clinical presentation.

Congenital HIV encephalopathy and myelopathy differ from the adult disease more in their intensity than in their specific attributes. Calcification of the basal ganglia and thalamus are more common in childhood infections and can be visualized radiographically.

Prion Diseases (Spongiform Encephalopathies) Are Transmissible Neurodegenerative Diseases

Prion diseases comprise a group of neurodegenerative conditions characterized clinically by slowly progressive ataxia and demen-

TABLE 28-2 Prion Diseases

I. Human
   A. Creutzfeldt-Jakob disease (CJD)
      1. Sporadic (85% of all CJD cases; incidence 1 per million worldwide)
      2. Inherited mutation of the prion gene, autosomal dominant transmission (15% of all CJD cases)
      3. Iatrogenic
         a. Hormone injection
            Human growth hormone (55 cases)
            Human pituitary gonadotropin (5 cases)
         b. Tissue grafts
            Dura mater (11 cases)
            Cornea (1 case)
            Pericardium (1 case)
         c. Medical devices (inadequate sterilization)
            Depth electrodes (2 cases)
            Surgical instruments (not definitely proven)
      4. New variant CJD (vCJD)
   B. Gerstmann-Staussler-Scheinker disease (GSS; inherited prion gene mutation, autosomal dominant transmission)
   C. Fatal familial insomnia (FFI; inherited prion gene mutation, autosomal dominant transmission)
   D. Kuru (confined to the Fore people of Papua New Guinea, formerly transmitted by cannibalistic ritual)
II. Animal
   A. Scrapie (sheep and goats)
   B. Bovine spongiform encephalopathy (BSE; "mad cow disease")
   C. Transmissible mink encephalopathy
   D. Feline spongiform encephalopathy
   E. Captive exotic ungulate spongiform encephalopathy (nyala, gemsbok, eland, arabian oryx, greater kudu)
   F. Chronic wasting disease of deer and elk
   G. Experimental transmission to many species, including primates and transgenic mice

---

tia and pathologically by accumulations of fibrillar or insoluble prion proteins, degeneration of neurons, and vacuolization termed **spongiform degeneration** (Fig. 28-109). The classic spongiform encephalopathies include several syndromes including kuru, Creutzfeldt-Jakob disease (CJD), Gerstmann-Straussler-Scheinker syndrome, and fatal familial insomnia (Table 28-2). In addition, similar diseases occur in animals, including scrapie in sheep and goats, bovine spongiform encephalopathy (BSE; mad cow disease), transmissible mink encephalopathy, and chronic wasting disease in mule deer and elk.

Prion diseases encompass infectious and autosomal dominant (due to prion gene mutations) forms, but in most cases, the mode of acquisition is uncertain. In addition to their many singular clinical and molecular pathological features, prion diseases are currently under intense scrutiny because of recent data that indicate a link between BSE ("mad cow disease") and a new variant of human CJD, namely vCJD.

Pathogenesis: All spongiform encephalopathies are transmissible, and inadvertent human transmission of CJD has followed the administration of contaminated human pituitary growth hormone, corneal transplantation from a diseased donor, insufficiently sterilized neurosurgical instruments, and surgical implantation of contaminated dura. The infectious agent is not a conventional virus, as implied by the earlier term "slow virus" sheep scrapie, but an unprecedented protein termed the *prion (proteinaceous infectious particles).*

The human prion gene *(PRNP)* is located on the short arm of chromosome 20 and consists of a single exon encoding 254 amino acid residues. The normal prion gene product, prion protein (PrP), is a constitutively expressed cell-surface glycoprotein that is bound to the plasmalemma by a glycolipid anchor. The highest levels of PrP messenger RNA (mRNA) are found in CNS neurons, but the function of the protein is unknown. Remarkably, the normal cellular prion protein, termed *cellular PrP* or PrP^C, and the pathogenic (infectious) prion protein, known as scrapie PrP or PrP^{SC}, do not differ in amino acid sequence. However, they have different three-dimensional conformations and patterns of glycosylation. Specifically, PrP^C is rich in α-helix configuration, whereas the β-pleated sheet content of PrP^{SC} is predominant. This conformational change is presumed to underlie the conspicuous resistance of PrP^{SC} to proteinase digestion as well as the prion-propagation mechanism, whereby normal host PrP^C is converted to PrP^{SC}. The newly converted proteins then change other PrP^C proteins into pathogenic PrP^{SC}. The result is an autocatalytic, exponentially expanding accrual of abnormal PrP^{SC}. Accumulation of PrP^{SC} compromises cell function and results in neurodegeneration by mechanisms that remain to be elucidated but may be similar to those of other neurodegenerative diseases characterized by brain amyloidosis (see below).

Pathology: The cardinal morphological features of prion diseases are neuronal degeneration and loss, gliosis, spongiform degeneration (small microcysts), and accumulations of insoluble prions with properties of amyloid (see Fig. 28-109). These lesions are most prevalent in the cortical gray matter, but they also involve the deeper nuclei of the basal ganglia, hypothalamus, and cerebellum.

The various human prion diseases have distinctive features.

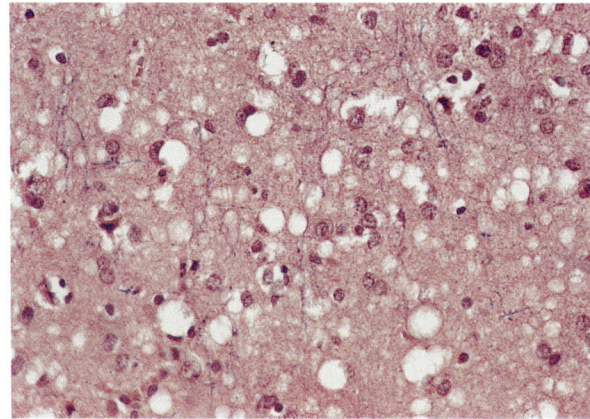

FIGURE 28-109
Creutzfeldt-Jakob disease. A. Spongiform degeneration of the gray matter is characterized by individual and clustered vacuoles, with no evidence of inflammation.

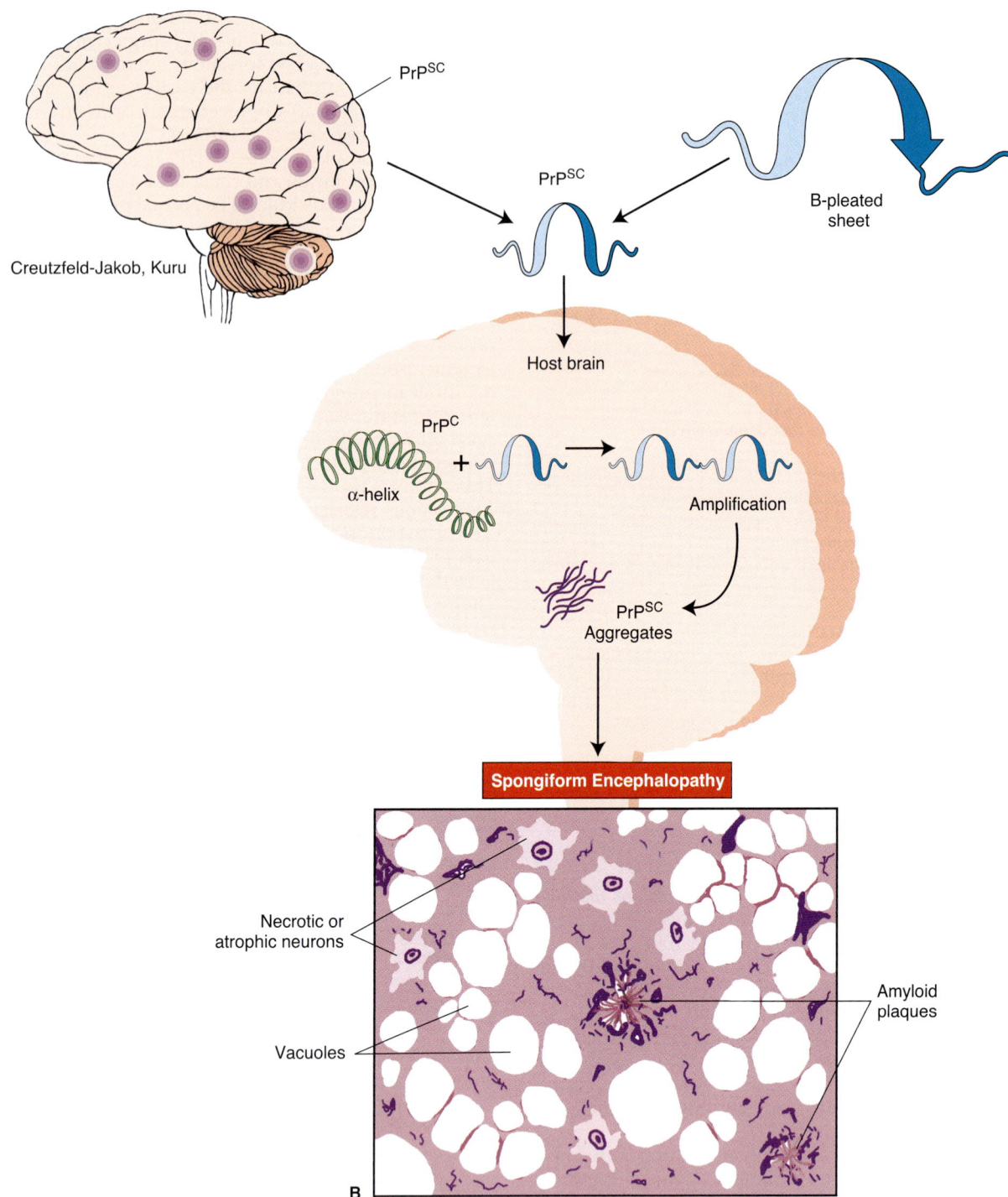

FIGURE 28-109 B. Pathogenesis of prion diseases.

KURU: In 1956, a medical officer in New Guinea provided an account of kuru, a progressive, fatal neurological disorder, in members of an isolated tribe. The disease takes its name from the word "trembling" in the language of the Fore people. The transmission of kuru was linked to ritualistic cannibalism in which women and children ate human brain.

Kuru was the first human prion disease shown to be transmissible. The disease formerly reached epidemic proportions in the Fore people but was eliminated after the cessation of cannibalism. The initial and most prominent clinical feature of kuru is ataxia of the limbs and trunk, owing to severe involvement of the cerebellum. In 70% of kuru cases, insoluble, fibrillar prion proteins accumulate extracellularly as amyloid or "kuru" plaques, and spongiform change is present in both the cerebral hemispheres and cerebellum. Late in the clinical course, some patients manifest dementia. Like all prion diseases, kuru is lethal.

CREUTZFELDT-JAKOB DISEASE (CJD): This rare, subacute encephalopathy was first fully described by Jakob in 1921. Symptoms begin insidiously, but within 6 months, the patient exhibits severe dementia and within a year is usually dead. The involvement of the cerebellum adds ataxia to the predominant symptom of dementia and distinguishes CJD clinically from Alzheimer disease.

CJD is by far the most common form of human prion disease and can be classified into four types based on etiology:

- **Sporadic CJD:** The sporadic form occurs worldwide, with an incidence of 1 per million, and accounts for 75% of all cases of CJD. The mode of acquisition is unknown; patients do not exhibit the mutations associated with the inherited forms of CJD or other prion diseases, and there is no history of iatrogenic exposure. A normal polymorphism, which codes either for methionine (M) or valine (V), occurs at codon 129 of the prion gene. Susceptibility to all forms of CJD is influenced by this polymorphism, with a disproportionate number of patents homozygous at this locus. The frequencies for the white population are 51% M/V, 37% M/M, and 12% V/V.

    Sporadic CJD exhibits prototypical histological features of the spongiform encephalopathies: microcystic neuropil vacuolation (see Fig. 28-109), astrogliosis, and neuronal loss. No host inflammatory response is seen. Clinically, sporadic CJD is characterized by the classic triad of dementia, myoclonus, and periodic spike–wave complexes in the electroencephalogram (EEG). The dementia is rapidly progressive, with death occurring within 4 to 12 months. However, longer courses of 2 to 5 years are well documented. Some 15% of cases are first seen with ataxia similar to that of kuru, with dementia following later.
- **Inherited CJD:** *Familial CJD* constitutes 15% of prion diseases, with an incidence of 1 per 10 million. Several different mutations of the prion gene have been documented in various kindreds. The mutated PrP causes familial CJD, fatal familial insomnia, and Gerstmann-Straussler-Scheinker disease.

GERSTMANN-STRAUSSLER-SCHEINKER SYNDROME (GSS): This disorder was described in 1936 as a spinocerebellar ataxia with dementia. Patients exhibit progressive limb and truncal ataxia over 2 to 10 years. At autopsy, prominent prion protein amyloid or kurulike plaques, neuron loss, and spongiform change are found in the cerebellum, cerebrum, and brainstem. Dementia is a late feature of the disease.

FATAL FAMILIAL INSOMNIA (FFI): This human prion disease is characterized by a profound disturbance of sleep–wake cycles and intractable insomnia. Dysautonomia, abnormal endocrine function, and signs of pyramidal and cerebellar dysfunction are common. Although cognitive function usually remains intact, dementia may supervene. The most conspicuous neuropathological finding is neurodegeneration of specific thalamic nuclei. The disease has been described in several Italian families and is caused by a point mutation in codon 178 of the *PRNP* gene, leading to a substitution of aspartic acid by asparagine. Sporadic forms of FFI also occur. Interestingly, the same mutation is found in another prion disease, a subtype of inherited CJD termed *CJD^{178}*. The two disorders differ in that fatal insomnia contains a codon for methionine at the polymorphic locus 178, whereas the CJD^{178} allele at this locus codes for valine.

- **Iatrogenic CJD:** As listed in Table 28-2, a number of iatrogenic cases of CJD have been documented, but most of the causes have been eliminated. For example, recombinant human growth hormone has supplanted human pituitary-derived preparations for therapy.
- **New variant CJD:** New variant CJD (vCJD) was identified by a surveillance program in the United Kingdom following the BSE epidemic that devastated the cattle industry. A group of patients was identified that differed from other patients with sporadic CJD in several important characteristics, the most striking of which is age. The mean age at onset of symptoms for sporadic CJD is 65 years; it is 26 years for vCJD patients. Other differences include a longer duration of illness for vCJD (median, 12 months vs. 4 months) and an atypical clinical presentation, with vCJD patients showing various behavioral changes or sensory disturbances (dysesthesias) and none of the characteristic EEG findings of sporadic CJD. At autopsy, vCJD is characterized by prominent spongiform change in the basal ganglia and thalamus and extensive PrP plaques in the cerebrum and cerebellum. The plaques are distinctive in that they are surrounded by a zone of spongiform change, a feature that is not found in sporadic CJD but is seen in scrapie. Finally, brains from vCJD patients contain much more PrP than brains from sporadic CJD patients. Since physicochemical analysis revealed that the vCJD PrP^{SC} exhibits characteristics distinct from CJD PrP^{SC} but similar to the prions in BSE that were transmitted to mice and primates, BSE is likely the source of the new CJD variant.

DEMYELINATING DISEASES

Demyelinating diseases are disorders in which the etiology relates to a selective loss of myelin. Thus, multiple sclerosis is viewed as a demyelinating disease, whereas necrosis due to infarcts or abscesses, traumatic contusions, and secondary demyelination caused by wallerian degeneration, are not so classified.

Leukodystrophies Reflect Inherited Disturbances in the Formation and Preservation of Myelin

Metachromatic Leukodystrophy

Metachromatic leukodystrophy (MLD), the most common leukodystrophy, is an autosomal recessive disorder of myelin metabolism that is characterized by the accumulation of a cerebroside (galactosyl sulfatide) in the white matter of the brain and peripheral nerves. MLD predominates in infancy, but rare "juvenile" or "adult" cases have been described. The disorder is lethal within several years.

 Pathogenesis: MLD is caused by a deficiency in the activity of arylsulfatase A, a lysosomal enzyme involved in the degradation of myelin sulfatides. Accordingly, there is progressive accumulation of sulfatides within the lysosomes of myelin-forming Schwann cells and oligodendrocytes.

 Pathology: In MLD, the accumulated sulfatides form cytoplasmic spherical granules, 15 to 20 μm in diameter, which stain metachromatically with cresyl violet and toluidine blue. The brain shows diffuse myelin loss, accumulation of metachromatic material in white matter, and prominent astrogliosis. Demyelination of peripheral nerves is less severe.

Krabbe Disease

Krabbe disease is a rapidly progressive, invariably fatal, autosomal recessive neurological disorder caused by a deficiency of galactocerebroside β-galactosidase. The condition appears in young infants and is defined by the presence of perivascular aggregates of mononuclear and multinucleated "globoid cells" in the white matter, hence the alternative name *globoid cell leukodystrophy*. The globoid cells are macrophages that contain undigested galactocerebroside (galactosylceramide).

Krabbe disease appears in the early months of life and progresses to death within 1 to 2 years. Severe motor, sensory, and cognitive impairments reflect the diffuse involvement of the nervous system.

 Pathogenesis: The brains of patients with Krabbe disease show almost complete loss of oligodendroglia and myelin. It has been hypothesized that the enzyme deficiency results in toxic, alternative metabolites that destroy oligodendroglia, thereby producing demyelination.

 Pathology: At autopsy, the brain is small, and the loss of myelin is diffuse, but the cerebral cortex is normal. Marbled areas of partial and total demyelination are present. Astrogliosis is typically severe. As demyelination proceeds, clusters of globoid cells are found around blood vessels. These cells measure up to 50 μm in diameter and contain as many as 20 peripherally located nuclei. In end-stage disease, the number of globoid cells decreases, and in areas of severe myelin loss, only scattered globoid cells remain. By electron microscopy, the globoid cells contain crystalloid-like inclusions with straight or tubular profiles.

Adrenoleukodystrophy

Adrenoleukodystrophy (ALD) refers to an X-linked (Xq28), inherited disorder in which dysfunction of the adrenal cortex and demyelination of the nervous system are associated with high levels of saturated very-long-chain fatty acids (VLCFAs) in tissue and body fluids. ALD occurs in children between the ages of 3 and 10 years, and neurological symptoms precede the signs of adrenal insufficiency. The disease progresses rapidly, and the body is quickly reduced to a vegetative state, which may persist for several years before death supervenes.

 Pathogenesis: The cause of ALD involves an enzyme mutation that impairs the capacity to degrade VLCFAs. A defect in the peroxisomal membrane prevents the normal activation of free VLCFAs by the addition of coenzyme A (CoA). As a result of the inability to degrade VLCFAs, these fatty acids accumulate in gangliosides and myelin. Pathological changes in the brain and adrenal are considered to reflect the accumulation of abnormal cholesterol esters and the toxic effects of VLCFAs.

 Pathology: ALD is characterized in brain by confluent, bilaterally symmetric demyelination. The most severe lesions are in the subcortical white matter of the parietooccipital region, which then extend rostrally (while sparing cortex) to result in a severe loss of myelinated axons and oligodendrocytes. Gliosis and perivascular infiltrates of mononuclear cells (mostly lymphocytes) are prominent in affected areas. Scattered macrophages contain PAS-positive and sudanophilic material. Peripheral nerves are affected, but less so than the brain. The adrenals are atrophic, and electron microscopy of cortical cells reveals pathognomonic cytoplasmic, membrane-bound, curvilinear inclusions or clefts (lamellae) containing VLCFAs. Similar inclusions occur in Schwann cells and CNS macrophages.

Alexander Disease

Alexander disease is a rare neurological disorder of infants and children that is characterized by a loss of myelin in the brain and a striking accumulation of irregular, extracellular fibers (Rosenthal fibers; Fig. 28-110). Clinically, these children have psychomotor retardation, progressive dementia, and paralysis, and eventually die.

 Pathogenesis: The disease is caused by mutations in the gene encoding GFAP (glial fibrillary acidic protein), which leads to aggregates of fibrous structures, known as Rosenthal fibers, formed by GFAP in astrocytes. It is not yet clear how this process impairs myelin formation and induces degeneration of oligodendrocyte and myelin degeneration.

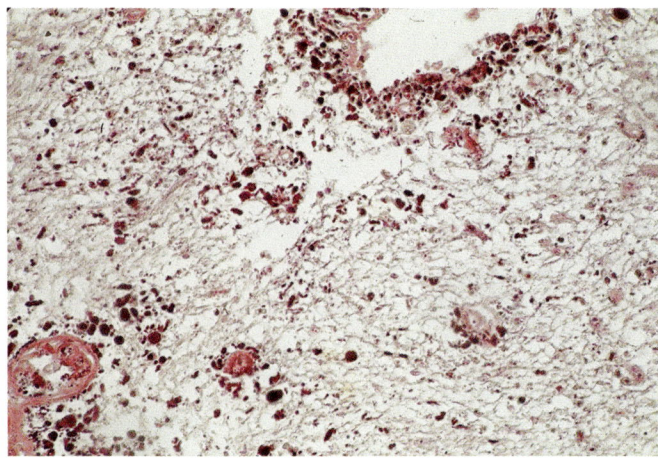

FIGURE 28-110
Alexander disease. Rosenthal fibers are aggregated beneath the pia and about blood vessels.

Pathology: Alexander disease features the presence of abundant Rosenthal fibers (GFAP filaments with associated protein chaperones, e.g., α-B-crystallin). These irregular, beaded and fibrous lesions are deposited in the subpial regions of brain and spinal cord as well as the white matter, especially around blood vessels, where astrocyte end feet terminate (see Fig. 28-110). Small Rosenthal fibers are present in glial processes. Larger Rosenthal fibers appear as irregular elongated or spiral extracellular accumulations. The content of myelin in the white matter is strikingly deficient. Interestingly, myelin is well preserved in the peripheral nerves, where Schwann cells express little or no GFAP.

Multiple Sclerosis Features Patches of Demyelination throughout the White Matter

Multiple sclerosis (MS) is a chronic demyelinating disease that is the most common chronic CNS disease of young adults in the United States, with a prevalence of 1 per 1000. The disorder affects sensory and motor functions and is characterized by exacerbations and remissions over many years. MS is acquired at a mean age of 30 years, with women afflicted almost twice as often as men.

Pathogenesis: The etiology of MS remains obscure, but experimental and clinical studies point to a genetic predisposition to MS and an immune pathogenesis. MS is principally a disease of temperate climates. Persons who emigrate before the age of 15 years from areas with a low prevalence of MS to more temperate endemic areas acquire an increased risk of developing disease, suggesting that environmental factors generate susceptibility to the disease.

GENETIC FACTORS: A genetic predisposition to MS is suggested by familial aggregation of the disease, an increased risk in second- and third-degree relatives of MS patients, and a 25% concordance for MS in monozygotic twins. Susceptibility is also linked to a number of major histocompatibility complex (MHC) alleles (e.g., HLA-DR2), thereby implying that immune mechanisms are involved in the pathogenesis. Indeed, siblings with MS may share the same T-cell receptor haplotype.

IMMUNE FACTORS: The evidence supporting a role for immune mechanisms in MS also comes from the microscopic appearance of the lesions. For example, chronic MS lesions demonstrate perivascular lymphocytes, macrophages, and numerous CD4$^+$ (helper-inducer subset), as well as CD8$^+$ T cells. Moreover, the CD4$^+$ T cells isolated from the CSF of MS patients appear to be oligoclonal. Although the target antigen has not been identified, the data suggest an immune response to a specific protein of the CNS. Further support for immune mechanisms comes from the experimental production of an antigen-specific, T cell-mediated, autoimmune disease, termed *experimental allergic encephalitis* (*EAE*). Injection of myelin basic protein into experimental animals, including nonhuman primates, elicits a demyelinating disorder that is similar to MS.

INFECTIOUS AGENTS: A wide variety of viruses have been implicated in the etiology of MS, including vaccinia, mumps, rubella, herpes simplex, and measles. However, to date no direct evidence exists for the involvement of any infectious agent.

 Pathology: **The demyelinated plaque is the hallmark of MS** (Fig. 28-111A). Plaques, rarely more than 2 cm in diameter, accumulate in great numbers in the brain and spinal cord. They are discrete, with smoothly rounded contours, and are usually in white matter, although they occasionally breach the gray–white junction. The lesions exhibit a preference for the optic nerves, chiasm, and paraventricular white matter (see Fig. 28-111B), although the CNS distribution of MS plaques is highly random. Plaques are also frequent in the spinal cord.

The evolving plaque is marked by the following morphological hallmarks:

- Selective loss of myelin in a region of axonal preservation (see Fig. 28-111C)
- A few lymphocytes that cluster about small veins and arteries (Fig. 28-112)
- An influx of macrophages
- Considerable edema

When neurons are within the boundaries of a plaque, the neuronal cell bodies are remarkably spared, but the same is not true of axons, which may degenerate. The number of oligodendrocytes is moderately diminished, and as the plaque ages, it becomes more discrete and less edematous. This sequence serves to emphasize the focal nature of the injury, its selectivity, and its severity, because demyelination is total within the area of the plaque. Characteristically, axons in the plaques lose their myelin abruptly (see Fig. 28-111C). Old MS plaques are dense and exhibit gliosis. This "scar" impairs the structural integrity of the axons.

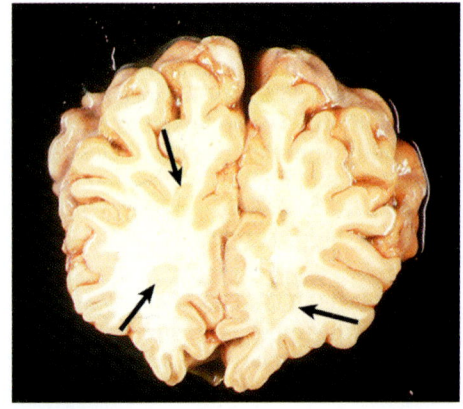
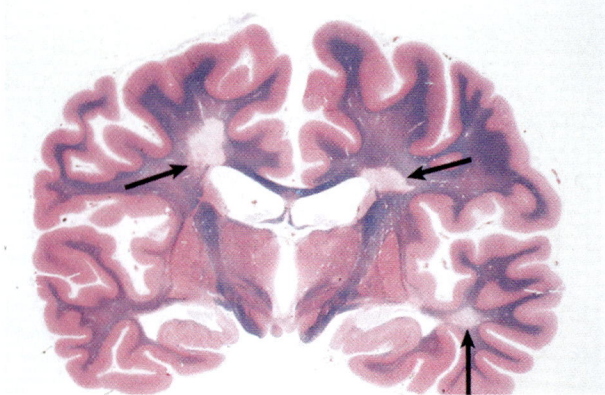
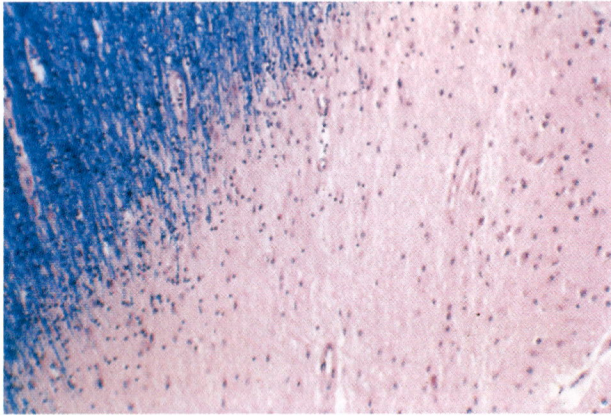

FIGURE 28-111
Multiple sclerosis. A. In this unfixed brain, the plaques of multiple sclerosis in the white matter *(arrows)* assume the darker color of the cerebral cortex. B. Coronal section of the brain from a patient with long-standing multiple sclerosis, stained for myelin, shows discrete areas of demyelination *(arrows)* with characteristic involvement of the superior angles of the lateral ventricles. C. Higher magnification of *B* shows the edge of a plaque and emphasizes the regional character of the lesion. Both motor and sensory fibers lose their myelin but retain axonal continuity as they traverse the lesion.

Clinical Features: MS usually has its onset during the third or fourth decades and is punctuated thereafter by abrupt and brief episodes of clinical progression, interspersed with periods of relative stability. However, some patients with MS suffer a relentless course without any remissions. Each exacerbation reflects the formation of additional demyelinated MS plaques. The visual system and the paraventricular areas are particularly vulnerable to the disease, whereas the peripheral nerves are uniformly spared. MS typically begins with symptoms relating to lesions in the optic nerves, brainstem, or spinal cord. Blurred vision or the loss of vision in one eye is often the presenting complaint. When the initial lesion is in the brainstem, the early symptoms are double vision and vertigo. Plaques within the spinal cord produce weakness of one or both legs and sensory symptoms in the form of numbness in the lower extremities. Many of the initial symptoms are partially reversible within a few months.

Unfortunately, in most patients with MS, the disease follows a chronic relapsing and remitting course, with development of permanent lesions. In established cases, the degree of functional impairment is highly variable, ranging from minor disability to severe incapacity, with widespread paralysis, dysarthria, severe visual defects, incontinence, and dementia. The patients usually die of respiratory paralysis or urinary tract infections while they are in terminal coma. Most patients with MS survive 20 to 30 years after the onset of symptoms. In some patients, treatment with interferon-β has been reported to be helpful.

Postinfectious and Postvaccinal Encephalomyelitis Are Immune Responses to Viral Antigens

Some viral exanthems (e.g., measles, varicella, rubella) are in rare instances followed about 3 to 21 days after the rash by an encephalomyelitis. The disease is characterized by focal perivascular demyelination and conspicuous mononuclear cell infiltrates around small to medium-sized venules in the

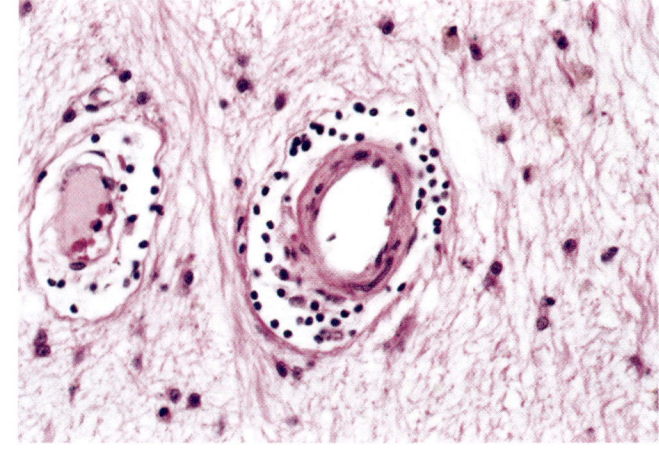

FIGURE 28-112
Multiple sclerosis. An end-stage lesion features astrogliosis, thick-walled blood vessels, moderate perivascular inflammation, and a secondary loss of axons.

white matter of the brain and spinal cord. This disorder is suspected to be immune mediated, but the precise pathogenesis remains unclear.

In children, postinfectious encephalomyelitis is heralded by the sudden onset of headache, vomiting, fever, and meningeal signs. In severe cases, these symptoms may be followed by paraplegia, incontinence, and stupor, and 15 to 20% of patients die. A similar syndrome termed *postvaccinal encephalomyelitis,* may follow immunization against infectious agents (e.g., smallpox, rabies). The use of more-purified vaccines that are free of cross-reacting antigenic contaminants has nearly eliminated this complication.

Central Pontine Myelinolysis Occurs in Alcoholics

Central pontine myelinolysis is a rare demyelinating disorder that affects the pons. Discrete areas of selective demyelination occur in the pons (Fig. 28-113), although the lesions often are too small to have clinical manifestations and are discovered only at autopsy. In a few patients, quadriparesis, pseudobulbar palsy, or severe depression of consciousness ("pseudocoma") may occur. Central pontine myelinolysis is thought to arise from overly rapid correction of hyponatremia in alcoholics or malnourished persons.

NEURONAL STORAGE DISEASES

Neuronal storage diseases are inherited enzyme deficiencies that result in the accumulation of normal metabolic products within lysosomes. These disorders are discussed in detail in Chapter 6, and only the highlights of the neurological manifestations are presented here.

Tay-Sachs Disease Reflects the Neuronal Accumulation of a Ganglioside

Tay-Sachs disease (amaurotic familial idiocy) is a lethal, autosomal recessive disorder caused by an inborn deficiency of hexosaminidase A, which permits the accumulation of ganglioside in CNS neurons. The disease is fatal in infancy and early childhood. Retinal involvement increases macular transparency and is responsible for a *cherry-red spot* in the macula.

The brain is the major site of storage of gangliosides, and progressively enlarges during infancy. On histological examination, lipid droplets are seen in the cytoplasm of distended nerve cells of the CNS and peripheral nervous system. Electron microscopy reveals the lipid within lysosomes in the form of whorled "myelin figures." The neural tissues respond with a diffuse astrogliosis. An affected infant appears normal at birth but shows a delay in motor development by age 6 months. Thereafter, progressive deterioration leads to flaccid weakness, blindness, and severe mental impairment. Death usually supervenes before the end of the second year.

Hurler Syndrome Represents Storage of Mucopolysaccharides

Hurler syndrome is an autosomal recessive disturbance in glycosaminoglycan metabolism that results in the intraneuronal accumulation of mucopolysaccharides. The clinical variants of this syndrome are distinguished by variable involvement of visceral organs and the nervous system. The disease is typically expressed in infancy or early childhood as dwarfism, corneal opacities, skeletal deformities, and hepatosplenomegaly. The intraneuronal storage distends the cytoplasmic compartment and is accompanied by astrogliosis and progressive mental deterioration.

Gaucher Disease Features the Deposition of Glucocerebrosides

Gaucher disease is an autosomal recessive genetic disorder characterized by a deficiency of glucocerebrosidase and the accumulation of glucocerebroside, principally in macrophages. The CNS is most severely involved in the infantile type (type II) of Gaucher disease. Although intraneuronal accumulation of glucocerebroside is not conspicuous, neuronal loss is severe and is accompanied by diffuse astrogliosis. These infants fail to thrive and die at an early age.

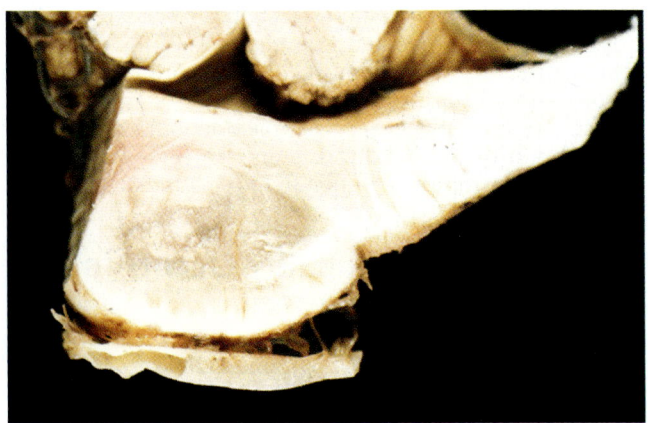
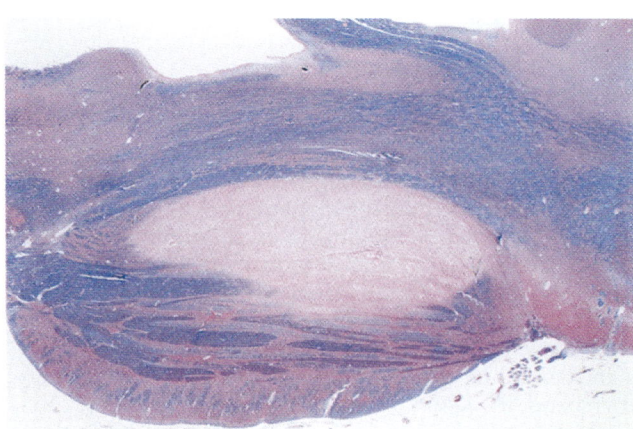

FIGURE 28-113
Central pontine myelinolysis. A. Sagittal section of the brainstem shows a soft lesion in the tegmentum of the pons. B. A section of A stained for myelin reveals a sharply demarcated loss of myelin *(pale pink area).*

Niemann-Pick Disease Displays the Accumulation of Sphingomyelin

Niemann-Pick disease is an autosomal recessive disorder in which intraneuronal storage of sphingomyelin results from a deficiency of sphingomyelinase. The clinical symptoms occur early, and the disease is marked by failure of the infant to develop and thrive. The mononuclear phagocyte system is targeted for storage, but the nervous system may predominate symptomatically during infancy. The brain becomes atrophic and shows marked astrogliosis. Retinal degeneration may produce a cherry-red spot, similar to that in Tay-Sachs disease.

METABOLIC NEURONAL DISEASES

Phenylketonuria Leads to Retention of Phenylalanine

Phenylketonuria (PKU) is an autosomal recessive disorder caused by a deficiency in phenylalanine hydroxylase (see Chapter 6). Phenylalanine accumulates in the blood and tissues because conversion of phenylalanine to tyrosine is blocked. The condition becomes apparent in the early months of life and leads to mental retardation, seizures, and impaired physical development. Untreated patients rarely obtain an IQ above 50. Although there are no consistent alterations, the brain may be underweight and deficient in myelination.

Cretinism Reflects Infantile Hypothyroidism

Severe hypothyroidism in infancy, termed *cretinism*, alters the functional capacity of the CNS. The disorder is reversible by the early administration of thyroxine, but when untreated, clinical disease emerges. The brain acquires a near-normal weight, has appropriate neuronal cytoarchitecture, and is well myelinated. However, stunted growth and cognitive impairments become evident.

Wilson Disease Exhibits Excess Copper in the Brain

Wilson disease, an autosomal recessive disease, is an inherited disorder of copper metabolism caused by mutations of the *WD* gene that affects brain and the liver; thus the synonym "hepatolenticular degeneration" (see Chapter 14). Defective biliary excretion of copper favors the deposition of copper in the brain. Symptoms of cerebral intoxication appear clinically in the second decade, evidenced in athetoid movements. Before, during, or after the appearance of neurological symptoms, an insidiously developing cirrhosis of the liver may result in hepatic failure. The deposition of copper in the limbus of the cornea produces a visible golden-brown band, the *Kayser-Fleischer ring* (see Chapter 29).

Macroscopically, the lenticular nuclei of the brain show a light golden discoloration, and in 25% of cases, small cysts or clefts are evident in the putamen or in deep layers of the neocortex. Histologically, mild neuron loss and gliosis characterize the disease.

METABOLIC DISORDERS

Alcoholism Is Associated with Several CNS Manifestations

The problems caused by alcoholism reflect poor nutrition and intoxication. Four cerebral lesions warrant consideration (Fig. 28-114):

- Wernicke syndrome (see Fig. 28-115)
- Central pontine myelinolysis (see Fig. 28-113)
- Cortical atrophy
- Atrophy of the superior aspect of the vermis of the cerebellum (Fig. 28-116)

Wernicke Syndrome

Wernicke syndrome is secondary to thiamine (vitamin B_1) deficiency and is characterized clinically by the rapid onset of a disturbance in thermal regulation, altered consciousness, ophthalmoplegia, and nystagmus, and pathologically by lesions in the hypothalamus and mamillary bodies, the periaqueductal regions of the midbrain, and the tegmentum of the pons (Fig. 28-114). The syndrome arises most commonly in association with chronic alcoholism, although it may appear in patients whose nutrition is sustained by infusions that lack thiamine.

Wernicke syndrome may progress rapidly to death, but it is reversed by the administration of thiamine. In fatal cases, petechiae occur around capillaries in the mamillary bodies, hypothalamus, periaqueductal region, and the floor of the fourth ventricle. Over time, hemosiderin deposition identifies regions where petechiae occurred. Neurons and myelin are spared, but the mamillary bodies atrophy.

Wernicke-Korsakoff syndrome refers to a state of disordered recent memory often compensated for by confabulation. The histological changes are distinguished from those of Wernicke syndrome by degeneration of neurons in the medial–dorsal nucleus of the thalamus. Thus, Wernicke syndrome and Korsakoff psychosis occur concurrently in chronic alcoholism, but their causes may be different.

Many chronic alcoholics display cerebral atrophy, but the cause of this is not entirely clear, and the relative roles of alcohol toxicity, malnutrition, and other factors remain to be defined. Similar uncertainties prevail with regard to the atrophy of the Purkinje and granular cells of the cerebellum. These alterations are the most common corollary of chronic alcoholism and are ostensibly the cause of truncal ataxia, which persists during periods of sobriety. As noted above, central pontine myelinolysis is an iatrogenic complication caused by the rapid correction of hyponatremia.

Hepatic Encephalopathy Occurs in End-Stage Liver Disease

Hepatic encephalopathy is a common clinical expression of liver failure, manifested as delirium, seizures, and coma (see Chapter 14). In general, the clinical symptoms greatly exceed their morphological correlates, which are restricted to the appearance of altered astroglia (termed *Alzheimer type II astrocytes*), which show enlarged nuclei and marginated chromatin, especially in the thalamus.

Metabolic Disorders 1467

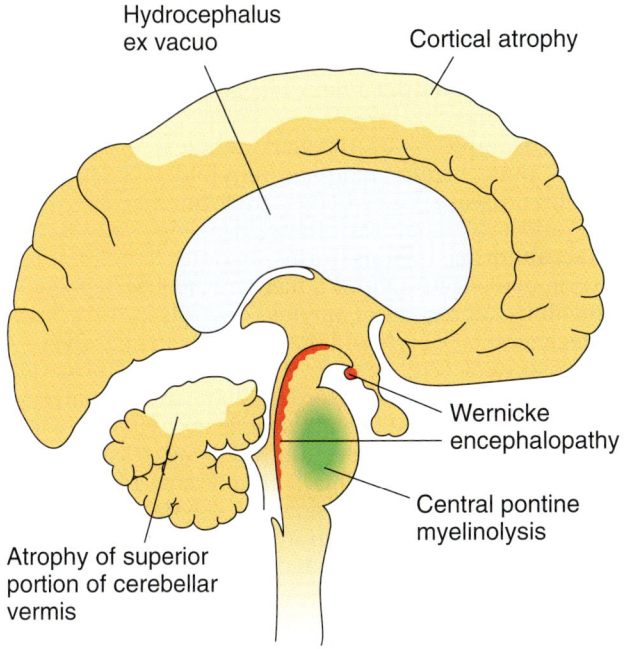

FIGURE 28-114
Regions of the brain with lesions associated with chronic alcoholism.

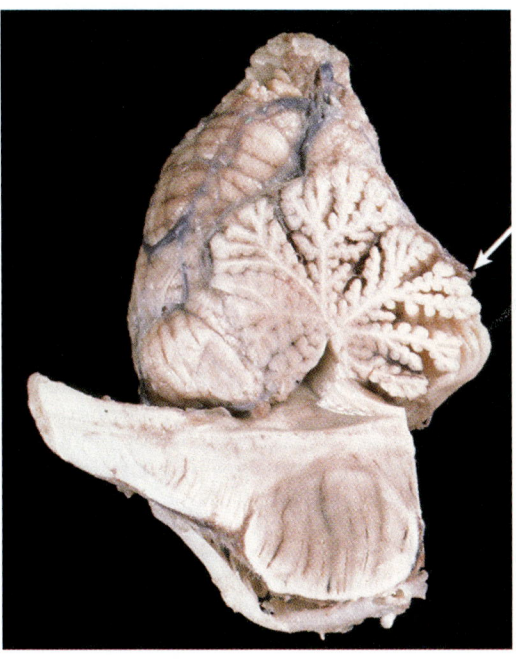

FIGURE 28-116
Chronic alcoholism. The superior and anterior portions of the cerebellar vermis (arrow) are atrophic.

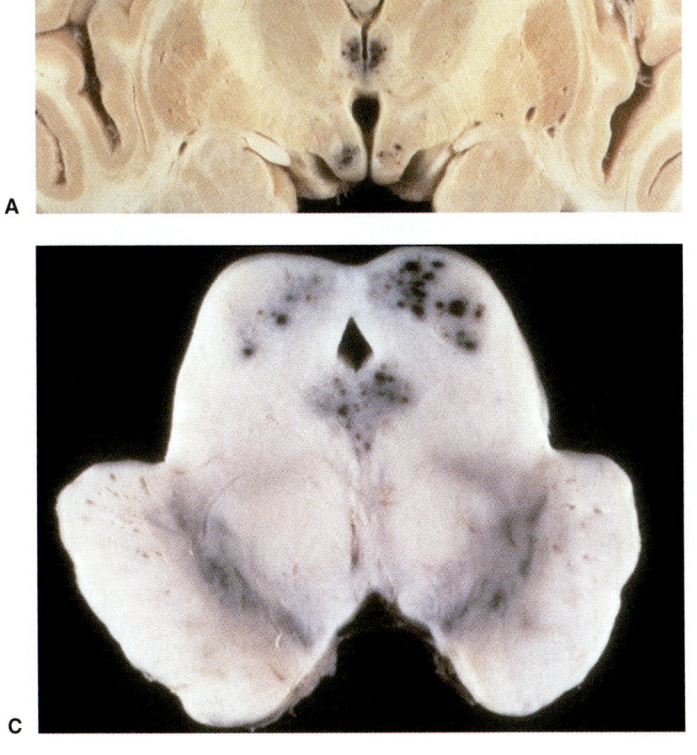

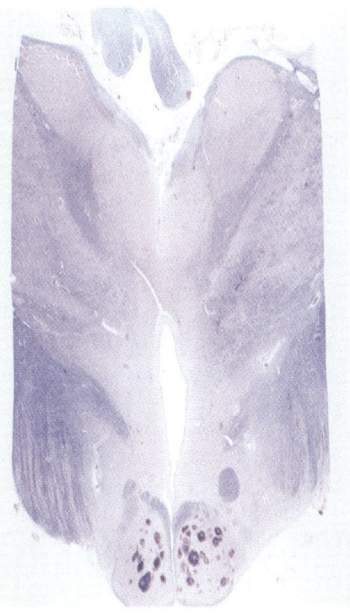

FIGURE 28-115
Wernicke encephalopathy. A. The mamillary bodies and the paraventricular regions exhibit petechiae. B. A histological section of A, stained with Luxol fast blue shows selective involvement of the mamillary bodies. C. The quadrigeminal plate and periaqueductal regions display conspicuous petechiae.

Subacute Combined Degeneration of the Spinal Cord Is a Complication of Pernicious Anemia

Subacute combined degeneration of the spinal cord results from a lack of vitamin B_{12} (pernicious anemia) and leads to lesions in the posterolateral portions of the spinal cord (see Chapters 14 and 20). Initially, there is symmetric myelin and axonal loss at the thoracic level of the spinal cord (see Fig. 28-121). Astrogliosis is mild in the acute lesions, but with time, the affected spinal cord exhibit gliosis and atrophy, especially in the posterolateral areas of the cord. A burning sensation in the soles of the feet and other paresthesias herald the onset of this rapidly progressive and poorly reversible neurological disorder. Weakness emerges in all four limbs, followed by defective postural sensibility, incoordination, and ataxia. In addition to pernicious anemia, subacute combined degeneration may complicate a rare case of extensive gastric resection and other malabsorption syndromes. Because vitamin B_{12} is not found in plants, some extreme vegetarians who eschew all animal products, even milk and eggs, have developed subacute combined degeneration after many years on the restricted diet.

NEURODEGENERATIVE DISEASES

The heterogeneous group of neurodegenerative diseases includes Parkinson disease, amyotrophic lateral sclerosis, Huntington disease, the spinocerebellar ataxias, Alzheimer disease, and several other less common disorders. Some of these conditions primarily involve specific neuroanatomical systems (Parkinson and Huntington disease, amyotrophic lateral sclerosis) or wider regions of the nervous system (Alzheimer disease). However, emerging data now implicate a number of different abnormal proteins that form aggregates with the properties of amyloid (congophilic and fibrillar, with a β-pleated sheet structure). The deposition of amyloid is a common factor in the onset and progression of many sporadic and hereditary neurodegenerative disorders, as summarized in Table 28-3.

For example, neurofibrillary tangles containing tau (NFTs) plus senile plaques amyloid-β (Aβ) define Alzheimer disease. Lewy bodies are formed by α-synuclein fibrils and are signatures of Parkinson disease. As noted above, abnormal prions form amyloid deposits. Thus, growing evidence provides a mechanistic link between the filamentous aggregates of amyloid deposits in the CNS and the degeneration of affected brain regions in neurodegenerative disorders (Fig. 28-117). Inexplicably, almost all of these neurodegenerative disorders share an enigmatic symmetry. Missense mutations in the gene encoding the disease protein cause an early onset and highly aggressive familial disorder as well as the hallmark brain lesions of the disease. However, the same brain lesions also characterize the corresponding wild-type protein in sporadic variants of these conditions. Notably, many of the familial forms of these diseases are autosomal dominant, which means that the bearer of a mutation will develop the disease if he lives to the age of disease onset, and that there are few, if any, "escapees." It is not clear how filamentous protein aggregates cause disease. It could result from sequestration of the disease protein or other macromolecules and organelles into the aggregates, thereby rendering them unavailable to perform their normal functions. Although aggregation of the disease protein could be a protective response initially, as the aggregates enlarge, they might physically occlude axons and dendrites or block the movement of material within the cytoplasm of affected cells. In view of parallels between the brain amyloidoses in many of these neurodegenerative disorders, clarification of this mysterious symmetry in one disease could have a significant impact on understanding mechanisms underlying all of these disorders (Fig. 28-117).

TABLE 28-3 Representative Neurodegenerative Diseases with Filamentous Amyloid Lesions

Disease	Lesion	Components	Location
Alzheimer disease	Senile plaques	Amyloid-β	Extracellular
	Neurofibrillary tangles	tau	Intracytoplasmic
Amyotrophic lateral sclerosis	Spheroids	Neurofilament subunits/ superoxide dismutase (SOD-1)	Intracytoplasmic
Dementia with Lewy bodies	Lewy bodies	α-Synuclein	Intracytoplasmic
Frontotemporal dementias	Neurofibrillary tangles	tau	Intracytoplasmic
Multiple system atrophy	Glial inclusions	tau	Intracytoplasmic
Parkinson disease	Lewy bodies	α-Synuclein	Intracytoplasmic
Prion diseases	Prion deposits	Prions	Extracellular
Trinucleotide repeat diseases	Inclusions	Polyglutamine tracts	Intracellular

Sporadic and hereditary neurodegenerative diseases characterized by prominent filamentous brain lesions. Frontotemporal dementias (as exemplified by Pick disease and corticobasal degeneration) form a group of disorders known as taupathies because filamentous tau inclusions are the hallmarks of these disorders. Dementia with Lewy bodies, multiple system atrophy, and Parkinson disease (together with several other rare disorders) form a group of disorders known as α-synucleinopathies because filamentous α-synuclein inclusions are neuropathological signatures of these diseases.

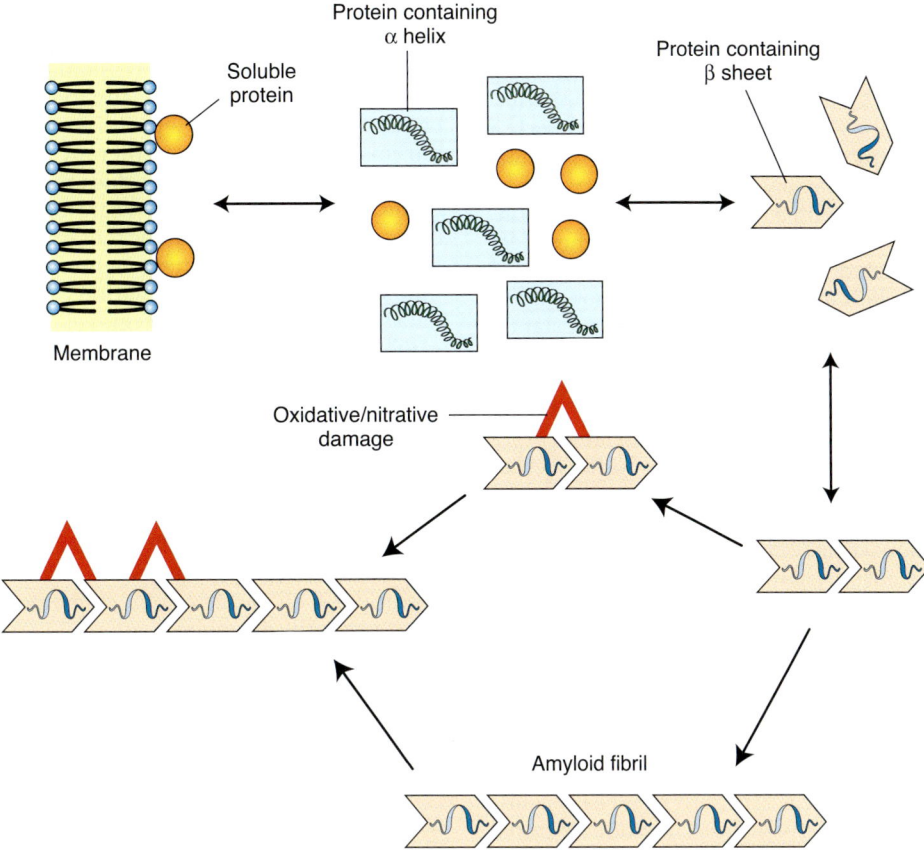

FIGURE 28-117
Filamentous protein aggregates: Targets of novel therapies for CNS neurodegenerative diseases. The schematic depicts the stepwise conversion of normal soluble proteins that either lack secondary structure *(orange balls)* or have an α-helical secondary structure *(blue boxes)*. They may interact normally with other structures such as organelle membranes *(box at the upper left)*. Spontaneously or due to mutations, the proteins can adopt a β-sheet structure *(unconnected arrowheads)*, which is reversible. However, if the proteins go on to form dimers, trimers, tetramers, and so forth, then they assemble into amyloid fibrils *(connected arrowheads)*. This process also may be driven by posttranslational modifications such as oxidative/nitrative damage *(red carats)*. These changes may act in several ways to promote fibrillogenesis, including cross-linking proteins or inducing conformational changes that stabilize the protein polymers into fibrils, thereby promoting formation of amyloid deposits, senile plaques, neurofibrillary tangles, Lewy bodies glial cytoplasmic inclusions, and prion amyloid lesions.

Parkinson Disease Is a Common Movement Disorder

First described in 1817, Parkinson disease (PD) is a neurological disorder characterized pathologically by the loss of neurons, primarily in the substantia nigra, and the accumulation of Lewy bodies, formed by filamentous α-synuclein aggregates. Clinically, PD features tremors at rest, muscular rigidity, expressionless countenance, emotional lability, and, less commonly, cognitive impairments, including dementia late in the disease course.

Epidemiology: PD typically appears in the sixth to eighth decades of life. The disease is frequent, and more than 2% of the population in North America eventually develop PD. The prevalence has remained unchanged for at least the past 40 years, and no racial differences are apparent, but men are more affected than women. Although most cases are sporadic, missense mutations in the α-synuclein gene are responsible for rare cases of autosomal dominant, early-onset, familial PD. Moreover, the demonstration that wild-type α-synuclein (a synaptic protein of unknown function) is the major building block of the aggregated filaments in Lewy bodies has led to a paradigm shift in thinking about the mechanisms underlying familial and sporadic PD. It has also led to the recognition of a number of other diseases (e.g., multiple system atrophy, dementia with Lewy bodies, progressive autonomic failure, REM sleep behavior disorder) that are also characterized by the accumulation of filamentous α-synuclein inclusions. These disorders are now designated *α-synucleinopathies* and are considered brain-specific amyloidoses. Lewy bodies and other α-synuclein inclusions share properties common to amyloid deposits within and outside the brain.

Pathogenesis: The vast majority of cases of PD are idiopathic, but the disease has been recorded after viral encephalitis (von Economo encephalitis) and after intake of the toxic chemical 1-methyl-4-phenyl-1,2,3,6-tetrahydropyridine (MPTP). The substantia nigra is a component of the extrapyramidal system that relays information to the basal ganglia through dopaminergic synapses. Normal aging is associated with a loss of neurons in the substantia nigra and reduced levels of dopamine, but these features are more exaggerated in PD. Lewy bodies, composed of filamentous α-synuclein aggregates, are seen not only in neurons and their processes (Lewy neuritis) in the substantia nigra, but also in other brain regions.

Accumulating evidence suggests that oxidative stress produced by the autooxidation of catecholamines during melanin formation injures the neurons in the substantia nigra by promoting the misfolding of α-synuclein and the formation of filamentous inclusions. A byproduct of the illicit synthesis of a meperidine analogue, MPTP, induced a PD-like syndrome in intravenous drug users. Since MPTP inhibits mitochondrial electron transport, it may produce parkinsonism by mechanisms similar to those of naturally occurring PD.

 Pathology: Gross examination of the brain in PD reveals a loss of pigmentation in the substantia nigra and locus ceruleus (Fig. 28-118A). Other brain regions are affected to a lesser extent. On microscopic examination, pigmented neurons are scarce, and small extracellular deposits of melanin are derived from necrotic neurons. Some residual nerve cells are atrophic, and a few contain Lewy bodies, which are visualized as spherical, eosinophilic cytoplasmic inclusions. (Fig. 28-118B) By electron microscopy, Lewy bodies exhibit amyloid-like filaments formed by insoluble α-synuclein.

 Clinical Features: PD is characterized by slowness of all voluntary movements and muscular rigidity throughout the entire range of movement. Most patients have a coarse tremor of the distal extremities, which is present at rest and disappears with voluntary movement. The face is expressionless (masklike), and a reduced rate of swallowing leads to drooling. There is an increased incidence of depression and dementia. In early parkinsonism, substitution therapy with levodopa is beneficial. However, this therapy does not rectify the underlying disorder and after several years becomes ineffective. Another emerging symptomatic therapy that shows promise for the treatment of PD patients who no longer respond to levodopa is deep brain stimulation. Preliminary clinical trial data suggest that dopaminergic cell transplants may become viable therapies for PD in the future.

Striatonigral degeneration is a rare disorder that mimics PD so closely that it is rarely diagnosed during life. At autopsy, the corpus striatum (caudate and putamen) is visibly atrophied, and microscopic examination shows severe loss of neurons in this region. Less severe changes occur in the substantia nigra and locus ceruleus This condition is also recognized with Shy-Drager disease and olivopontocerebellar atrophy as part of a syndrome complex known as *multiple system atrophy*. This syndrome is characterized by filamentous α-synuclein inclusions primarily in white matter oligodendroglia, known as glial cytoplasmic inclusions. They also occur to a lesser extent in neurons, where they exhibit the morphological features of Lewy bodies that are similar to those in PD.

Progressive supranuclear palsy is another unusual neurological disorder that is clinically similar to PD but adds a progressive paralysis of vertical eye movements. The course of the disease is relentless, with death within 5 to 10 years. The pathological changes in the brain are more widespread than in PD, with loss of neurons in the globus pallidus, subthalamic nucleus, red nucleus, tectum, periaqueductal gray matter, and dentate nuclei. Neurofibrillary tangles (NFTs) formed by filamentous tau aggregates are noted. Thus, this disease combines clinical features of PD with dementia and is a prototypical form of *neurodegenerative taupathy*, since the sole inclusions are tau-rich NFTs.

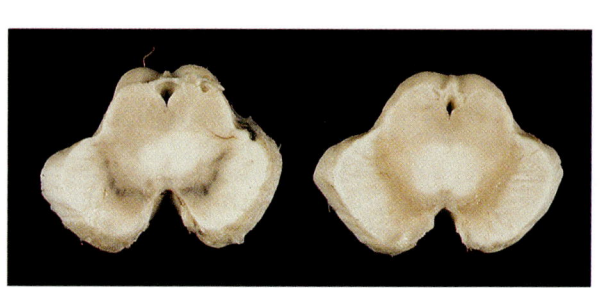
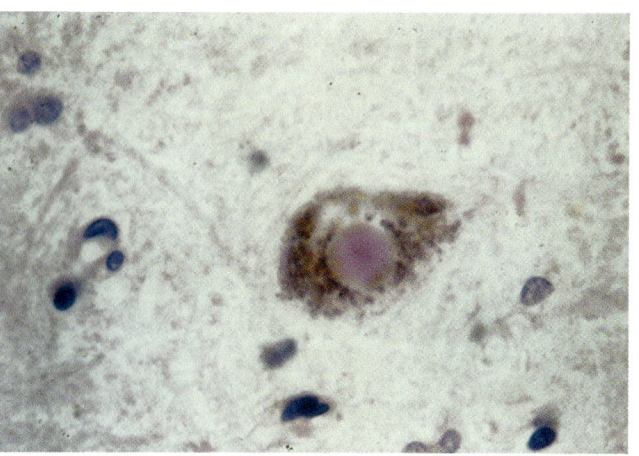

FIGURE 28-118
Parkinson Disease. A. The normal substantia nigra of the midbrain *(left)* is heavily pigmented, whereas the same region from a patient with PD *(right)* has lost neurons and neuromelanin. **B.** A microscopic section of the substantia nigra from a patient with PD shows a Lewy body (a spherical eosinophilic inclusion surrounded by a halo within the cytoplasm of a pigmented dopaminergic neuron.)

Amyotrophic Lateral Sclerosis Leads to Profound Weakness and Death

Amyotrophic lateral sclerosis (ALS) is a degenerative disease of motor neurons of the brain and spinal cord that results in progressive weakness and wasting of the extremities and eventually impairment of the respiratory muscles.

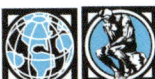 Epidemiology and Pathogenesis: ALS is a worldwide disease with an incidence of 1 in 100,000. The frequency of the disease peaks in the fifth decade of life, and it is rare in persons younger than 35 years. There is a 1.5- to 2.0-fold excess of ALS in men. Restricted geographical areas with a particularly high incidence of ALS exist in Guam and parts of Japan and Papua New Guinea, but these cases differ from ALS in the rest of the world. Cases in the Chamorro people indigenous to Guam are characterized by abundant accumulations of tau-rich NFTs and are now classified as *neurodegenerative taupathies*. Moreover, ALS on Guam is part of a spectrum of disorders that includes dementia and parkinsonism.

Familial ALS cases, with an autosomal dominant pattern, account for 5% of all cases of ALS. The gene for familial ALS is located on chromosome 21q and has been associated with missense mutations in the gene that codes for superoxide dismutase 1 *(SOD1)*. Interestingly familial ALS caused by *SOD1* mutations is not due to deficient SOD activity. Transgenic mice that have two normal copies of the murine SOD gene but also express the human mutant SOD1 protein develop a syndrome that closely resembles ALS. This finding indicates that the mutant *SOD1* gene in ALS results in a gain of toxic function. Aggregation of SOD1 and other proteins, such as neurofilament subunits, presumably impairs the survival of motor neurons.

 Pathology: ALS affects motor neurons in three locations: (1) the anterior horn cells of the spinal cord; (2) the motor nuclei of the brainstem, particularly the hypoglossal nuclei; and (2) the upper motor neurons of the cerebral cortex. The injury to the motor neurons leads to degeneration of their axons, visualized in striking alterations of the lateral pyramidal pathways in the spinal cord.

The defining histological change in ALS is a loss of large motor neurons accompanied by mild gliosis (Fig. 28-119A). This change is most evident in the anterior horns of the lumbar cord, the cervical enlargements of the spinal cord, and the hypoglossal nuclei, where neurofilaments may also aggregate in axons to form inclusions termed *spheroids*. There is also a loss of the giant pyramidal Betz cells in the motor cortex of the cerebrum. The most striking secondary change in the spinal cord is a loss of myelinated fibers in the lateral corticospinal tracts (see Fig. 28-121), which imparts a pallor to these areas when they are viewed with myelin stains. The anterior nerve roots are atrophic (Fig. 28-119B), and the affected muscles are pale and shrunken.

 Clinical Features: ALS begins as weakness and wasting of the muscles of a hand, often accompanied by painful cramps of the muscles of the arm. Irregular rapid contractions of the muscles that do not move the limb (fasciculations) are characteristic. The disease is inexorably progressive, with increasing weakness of the limbs leading to total disability. Speech may become unintelligible, and respiratory weakness supervenes. Despite the dramatic wasting of the body, intellectual capacity tends to be preserved to the end, although a few ALS patients also suffer dementia. The clinical course does not usually extend beyond a decade.

Trinucleotide Repeat Expansion Syndromes Comprise a Heterogeneous Group of Hereditary Neurodegenerative Diseases

A large group of neurological diseases can now be classified on a genetic basis as trinucleotide repeat expansion

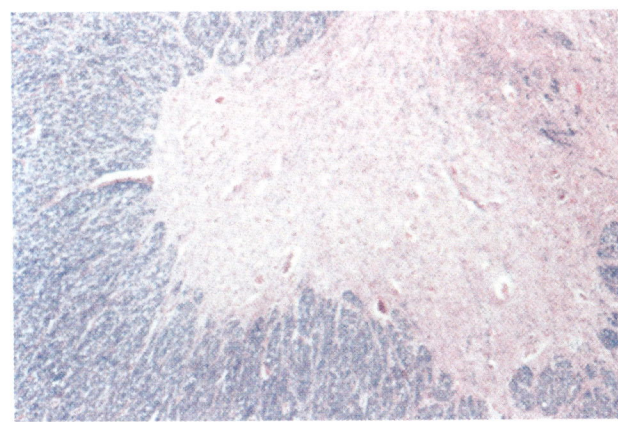
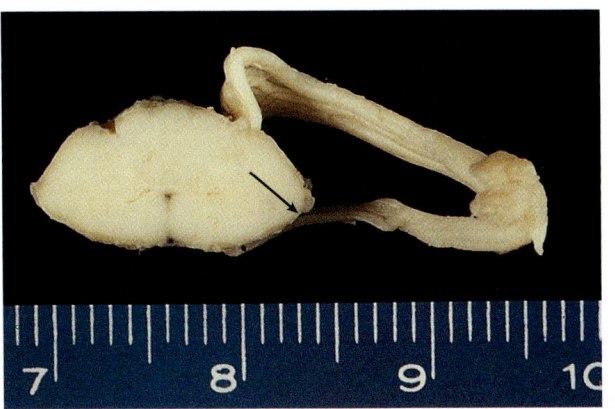

FIGURE 28-119
Amyotrophic lateral sclerosis. A. Photomicrograph of severe loss of spinal cord anterior horn motor neurons without evidence of inflammation. B. The ventral root *(arrow)* is grossly atrophic as a result of anterior horn neuron loss.

syndromes (Table 28-4). The first such disorder to be identified was fragile X syndrome in 1991, followed by spinal and bulbar muscular atrophy and myotonic dystrophy. The triplet repeat mutation disorders now include Huntington disease and Friedreich ataxia, but the number of disorders included in this category continues to expand as new mutations lead to the identification of additional variants of these diseases.

Trinucleotide repeats are a normal feature of many genes, and expansion of the number of triplet repeats confers pathogenicity. Some triplet repeat diseases show only a small expansion compared with the normal counterpart (e.g., Huntington disease), whereas in others, the expansion is quite large (e.g., fragile X syndrome and Friedreich ataxia). This class of diseases includes examples of all forms of inheritance, including X-linked, autosomal dominant, and autosomal recessive. In some of these disorders, the expansion mutation lies within the coding region of a gene segment and results in the production of an abnormal ("toxic") protein, as appears to be the case for most of the autosomal dominant CAG expansion disorders. In others, the expansion occurs in a noncoding region of the gene and presumably interferes with transcription or message processing. The resulting decreased level of protein production constitutes a loss-of-function mutation (as appears to be the case with the GAA expansion of Friedreich ataxia). Our knowledge is still embryonic, but discovery of the mutations sets the stage for characterizing the normal protein function and elucidating the sequential steps in the pathogenesis of disease, which then could lead to better therapies.

Huntington Disease

Huntington disease (HD) is an autosomal dominant genetic disorder characterized by involuntary movements of all parts of the body, deterioration of cognitive function, and often severe emotional disturbance. First described by a medical student in 1872, the disorder principally affects whites of northwestern European ancestry, with an incidence of 1 in 20,000. Genealogical studies indicate that all cases of HD derive from the spread of an original focus in northern Europe; the disease is notably rare in Asia and Africa.

 Pathogenesis: The *HD* gene is located on chromosome 4 (4p16.3) and codes for a novel protein, *huntingtin*. In 1993, it was discovered that the genetic alteration at this locus consists of expansion of a trinucleotide (CAG) repeat. The repeat is located within the coding region of the gene and results in production of an altered protein, which contains a polyglutamine tract near the N terminus. In agreement with the dominant mode of inheritance, the triplet expansion likely results in a toxic gain of function. HD is an example of a true autosomal dominant disorder, since one abnormal allele suffices to cause disease.

The huntingtin gene product is widely expressed in tissues throughout the body and in all regions of the CNS by neurons and glia. However, its function is unknown. It is thought that critical proteins may interact specifically with the expanded polyglutamine tract and become dysfunctional in affected cells. Alternatively, amyloid-like aggregates of mutant huntingtin may impede intracellular trafficking.

As with other CAG repeat expansion diseases, a strong inverse correlation is seen between the magnitude of the expansion and the age of clinical onset, and the most numerous repeats are seen in juvenile-onset cases. Interestingly, CAG length is more unstable and tends to be longer when inherited from the father than in maternal transmission. As a result, transmission of the *HD* mutation from the father results in clinical disease some 3 years earlier than when it is passed from the mother. Moreover, the ratio of children with juvenile-onset HD who inherit the expanded CAG allele from their father to those who inherit it from their mother is 10:1.

Sporadic (new mutation) cases of HD were thought to be rare, but genetic testing now reveals increasing numbers of these patients. Most new mutations arise from unstable transmission of triplet repeats from an asymptomatic parent whose alleles exhibit repeat lengths in the zone between the normal (<30) and HD (>36) ranges (referred to as "intermediate alleles").

 Pathology: On gross examination of brains from patients who died of HD, the frontal cortex is symmetrically and moderately atrophic, whereas the

TABLE 28-4 Charcot-Marie-Tooth Disease (CMT) and Related Hereditary Neuropathies

Type of CMT	Inheritance	Gene	Mutation	Pathology
Demyelinating neuropathies				
1A	Dominant	Peripheral myelin protein 22 *(PMP22)*	Duplication or point mutation	Demyelinating neuropathy; axonal loss also present
1B	Dominant	Myelin protein zero *(P0)*	Point mutation	Demyelinating neuropathy; axonal loss also present
X	X-linked	Connexin 32 (Gap junction protein β1)	Point mutation	Demyelinating neuropathy; axonal loss also present
DSS	Dominant	*PMP22* or *P0*	Point mutations	Demyelinating neuropathy; axonal loss also present
HNPP	Dominant	*PMP22*	Deletion or point mutation	Demyelinating neuropathy with tomacula
Axonal neuropathies				
2A	Dominant	Kinesin 1B *(KIF1B)*	Point mutation	Axonal neuropathy
2E	Dominant	Neurofilament light chain *(NEFL)*	Point mutation	Axonal neuropathy

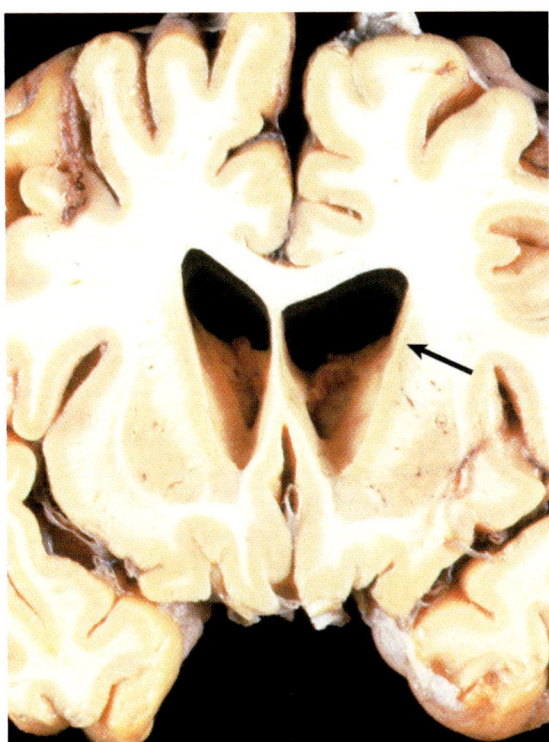

FIGURE 28-120
Huntington disease. The caudate nuclei (arrow) are markedly atrophic bilaterally, leading to enlarged lateral ventricles.

lateral ventricles appear disproportionately enlarged, owing to the loss of the normal convex curvature of the caudate nuclei (Fig. 28-120). There is symmetric atrophy of the caudate nuclei, with lesser involvement of the putamen. Microscopically, the neuronal population of the caudate and putamen, particularly the small neurons, is greatly depleted, and there is an accompanying moderate astrogliosis. The cortical neurons are similarly, but less severely, depleted. Amyloid-like aggregates of huntingtin have been detected in neurons, especially in nuclei. Accumulations of the mutant protein also occur in neuronal processes, which could impair communication between neurons through their axons and dendrites. Biochemical assays at the termination of the disease show a marked decrease in γ-aminobutyric acid (GABA) and glutamic acid decarboxylase.

Clinical Features: The symptoms of HD are usually first seen at about age 40 years, but 5% of persons with the disorder develop neurological signs before 20 years of age, and a comparable proportion develop manifestations after age 60 years. Cognitive and emotional disturbances precede the onset of abnormal movements by several years in more than half of patients. Because of the prominent involvement of the extrapyramidal system, choreoathetoid movements progress to total incapacitation. Subsequent involvement of the cortex leads to a severe loss of cognitive function and intellectual deterioration, often accompanied by paranoia and delusions. The interval from the onset of symptoms to death averages 15 years.

The Inherited Spinocerebellar Ataxias

The spinocerebellar ataxias represent a heterogeneous category of disease that features (1) a broad but system-based topography, (2) a genetic contribution, and (3) a precocious loss of neurons and neural tracts in the cerebellum, brainstem, and spinal cord. The symptoms reflect the topography of the lesions. Thus, ataxia and intention tremor suggest involvement of the cerebellum; rigidity and tremor reflect degeneration of the brainstem; and losses of deep tendon reflexes, vibration sense, and pain sensation are caused by disease of the spinal cord.

Because there is greater anatomical and clinical uniformity among cases from a particular family than among random cases from different families, case reports have generally focused on specific families, and the original authors' names have been appended to the different syndromes. For example, an inherited form of cerebelloolivary degeneration is designated "cerebelloolivary degeneration of Holmes," which is distinguished from the sporadic "cerebelloolivary degeneration of Marie." These cases also share many features with "olivopontocerebellar degeneration of Menzel." A similar complexity pertains to the nosology of spinal cord degeneration. This complex nosology is now being clarified by the identification of the genetic defects that cause these disorders, and many inherited ataxias, including Machado-Joseph disease and Friedreich ataxia, have been shown to be triplet repeat expansion disorders.

Friedreich Ataxia

Friedreich ataxia is the most common inherited ataxia, with a prevalence in European populations of 1 in 50,000. Although the inheritance pattern is autosomal recessive, many cases arise sporadically as new mutations without a family history. The onset of symptoms is usually before age 25 years, followed by an unremitting and progressive course of about 30 years before death. The hallmark of Friedreich ataxia is a combined ataxia of both the upper and lower limbs. Dysarthria, lower-limb areflexia, extensor plantar reflexes, and sensory loss also occur in most patients. Frequently associated systemic abnormalities are deformities of the skeletal system, (e.g., scoliosis, pes cavus), hypertrophic cardiomyopathy (which commonly causes death), and diabetes mellitus.

 Pathogenesis: The genetic defect in Friedreich ataxia was mapped to chromosome 9 in 1988. The candidate gene *(X25)* encodes a mitochondrial protein *(frataxin)* of 210 amino acid residues, which is involved in iron transport into mitochondria. In 1996, a mutation consisting of an unstable expansion of a trinucleotide (GAA) repeat was found in the first intron of the frataxin gene (9q13.3-21.1). The recessive pattern of inheritance suggests that this expansion results in a loss of function, which is consistent with an absence of frataxin mRNA transcripts in patients with Friedreich ataxia. The expansion mutation probably interferes with transcription or RNA processing. In normal persons, the highest levels of frataxin gene expression are found in the heart and spinal cord. It is, therefore, likely that a lack of frataxin is responsible for both the neuropathological manifestations of

1474   The Nervous System

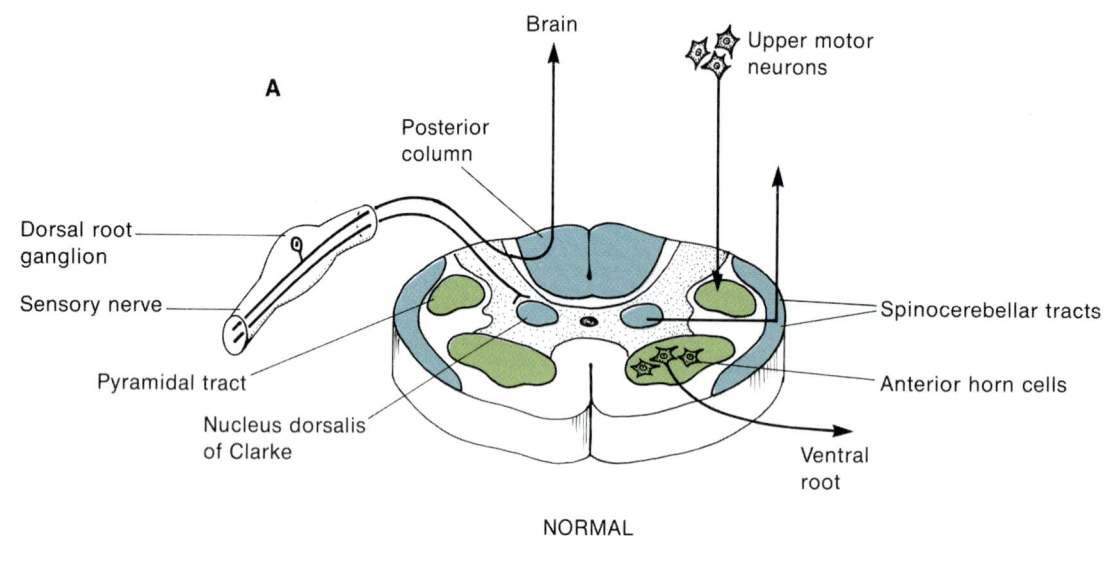
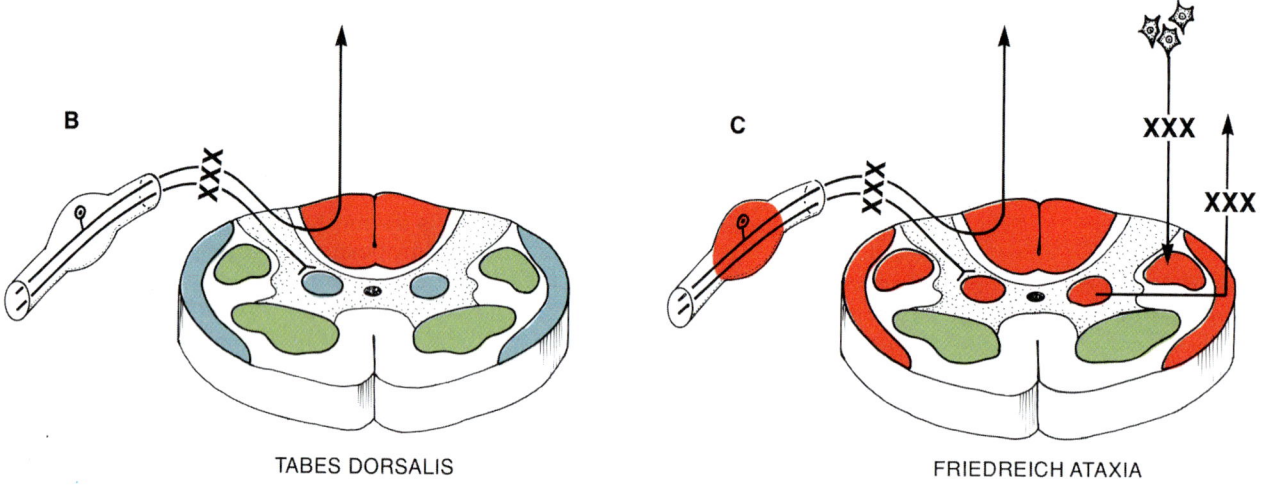
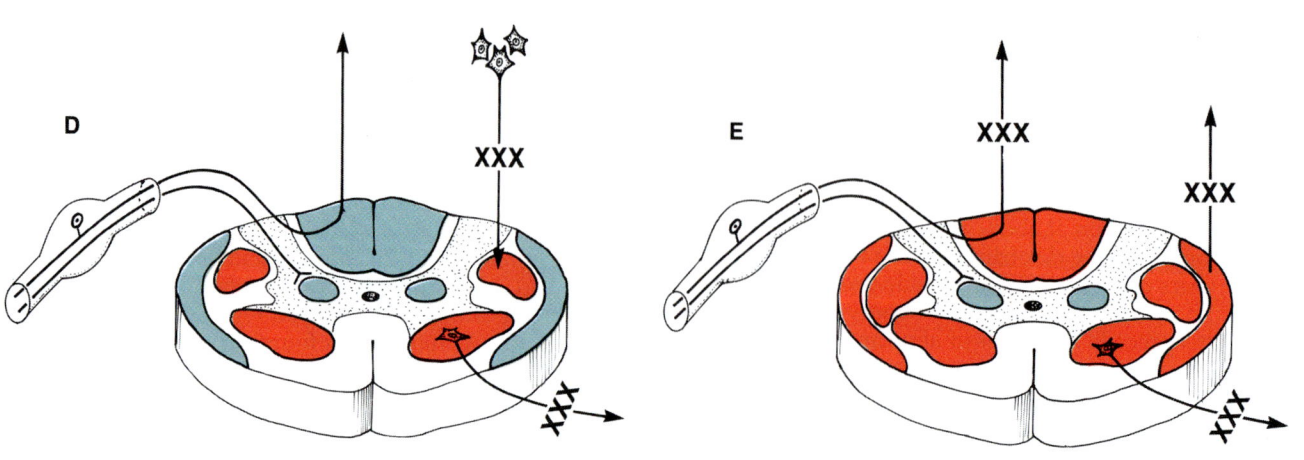

FIGURE 28-121
Degenerative disorders of the spinal cord. Many ascending (blue) and descending (green) pathways traverse the spinal cord. The four diseases illustrated differentially disrupt these pathways (red), depending on the location of the primary pathological process.

Friedreich ataxia and the cardiomyopathy. There is a strong inverse correlation between the size of the triplet expansion and the age of disease onset, and a direct relationship with the rate of clinical progression and the frequency of hypertrophic cardiomyopathy.

The clinical spectrum of Friedreich ataxia is broader than previously thought. Many patients have sporadic ataxia, in which the typical clinical features of Friedreich ataxia are not fully expressed or in which atypical signs or symptoms are present. In such cases, identification of a GAA repeat expansion in the frataxin gene confirms the diagnosis of Friedreich ataxia. In one study, a significant proportion of patients (14%) with proven GAA expansion of the frataxin gene have an onset after 25 years of age (26 to 51), and 12% have retained lower-limb reflexes.

Pathology: The most prominent postmortem findings in Friedreich ataxia are seen in the spinal cord. The classic lesion consists of degeneration of three major pathways: the posterior columns, corticospinal pathways, and the spinocerebellar tracts (Fig. 28-121). Posterior column degeneration accounts for the sensory loss experienced by patients with Friedreich ataxia and results from loss of the parent neuronal cell bodies, which are located in the dorsal root ganglia. In advanced cases, this degeneration can be appreciated grossly as shrinkage of the dorsal spinal roots and posterior funiculi. Similarly, atrophy of the spinocerebellar tracts, with attendant ataxia, follows neuronal degeneration in the dorsal nucleus of Clarke. The corticospinal tracts show the most pronounced degeneration more distally in the cord, with gradually less pronounced atrophy as the cord is followed proximally toward the brainstem. This process is referred to as a "dying back" phenomenon.

Alzheimer Disease Is the Principal Cause of So-Called Senility

Alzheimer disease (AD) is an insidious and progressive neurological disorder characterized clinically by loss of memory, cognitive impairment, and eventual dementia and pathologically by Aβ-containing senile plaques and neurofibrillary tangles formed by tau filaments. Although Alzheimer's original patients were restricted to patients younger than 65 of age and were said to suffer "presenile dementia," the term *Alzheimer disease* now refers to dementias that display characteristic pathological changes.

Epidemiology: Although AD is a worldwide disease, its distribution has been best studied in Western countries. **It is the most common cause of dementia in the elderly, accounting for more than half of all cases.** The prevalence of the condition is closely related to age. Before age 65 years, the prevalence of AD is at most 1 to 2%, whereas it is 10% or more after age 85 years. Women are affected twice as often as men. Most cases of AD are sporadic, but a familial variant is recognized.

Pathogenesis: Although the cause of AD has not been fully elucidated, there have been significant advances in our understanding of the origin of both AD-associated amyloid and NFTs.

AMYLOID β-PROTEIN (Aβ): Increasing evidence points to the importance of the deposition of Aβ protein in the neuritic plaques of AD. These plaques are located in areas of the cerebral cortex that are linked to intellectual function and are a constant feature of AD. However, there are examples of cognitively intact elderly persons whose brains displayed the same burden of senile plaques as is seen in AD, thereby raising questions about whether or not it is the extracellular senile plaques or some intracellular process involving Aβ metabolism that compromises neuronal function in AD. The core of these plaques contains a distinct form of Aβ peptide, which is predominantly 42 amino acids in length. Aβ is derived by proteolysis from a much larger (695 amino acids) membrane-spanning amyloid precursor protein (APP). Full-length APP has an extracellular region, a transmembrane sequence, and a cytoplasmic domain. The region comprising Aβ serves to anchor the amino-terminal portion of APP to the membrane. The physiological functions of APP and Aβ remain obscure.

The normal degradation of APP involves a proteolytic cleavage in the middle of the Aβ domain, with the release of a fragment extending from the middle of the Aβ domain to the amino terminus of APP. This fragment is not amyloidogenic. Proteolysis at either end of the Aβ domain then releases intact and highly amyloidogenic Aβ that accumulates in senile plaques as amyloid fibrils.

The deposition of Aβ appears to be necessary but not sufficient for the pathogenesis of AD because of the following considerations:

- Patients with **Down syndrome** (trisomy 21) develop the clinical and histopathological features of AD, including deposition of Aβ in neuritic plaques, generally by age 40 years. The gene for APP is located on chromosome 21, and the additional dose of the gene product in trisomy 21 may predispose to precocious accumulation of Aβ.
- Some patients with the familial form of AD carry mutant APP genes or mutant presenilin genes. These mutations lead to increased production of Aβ, the amyloidogenic fragment of APP.
- Transgenic mice expressing mutant human APP genes develop senile plaques in the brain that are very similar to those of AD. However, these mice lack other critical features of AD such as NFTs and evidence of neurodegeneration, such as significant loss of neurons.

Neurons and glial cells are sites of APP synthesis in the brain, but Aβ also accumulates in the walls of cerebral blood vessels (Fig. 28-122).

NEUROFIBRILLARY TANGLES: NFTs are composed of paired helical filaments that consist of an abnormal form of a microtubule-associated protein (MAP) termed *tau*. In AD, the phosphorylation of tau at aberrant sites results in a protein that does not associate with microtubules but instead aggregates in the form of paired helical filaments. The release of tau from microtubules deprives cells of its microtubule stabilizing effects, thereby impairing axonal transport

1476 The Nervous System

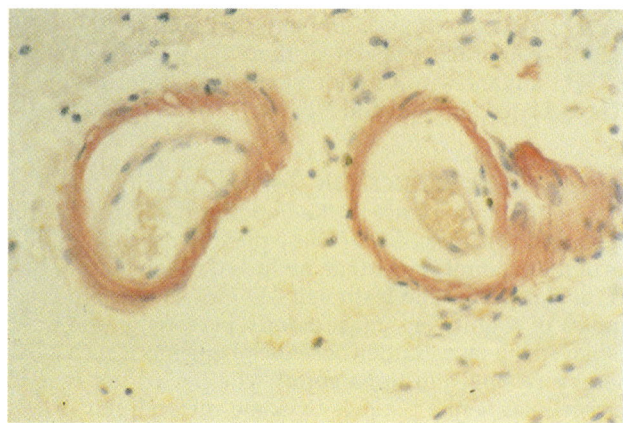

FIGURE 28-122
Congophilic angiopathy. The cerebral blood vessels stain with Congo red, indicating the presence of amyloid.

and compromising neuronal function. Indeed, mutations in the *tau* gene on chromosome 17 cause familial frontotemporal dementia with parkinsonism. Interestingly, transgenic mouse models that overexpress mutant or wild-type tau develop a neurodegenerative phenotype, with neuron loss and defective axonal transport.

Remarkably, most cases of AD are also associated with abundant Lewy bodies. Thus AD features a "triple" brain amyloidosis, owing to accumulations of filamentous tau, Aβ, and α-synuclein.

GENETIC FACTORS: As mentioned above, mutations of the *APP* gene have been associated with certain early-onset familial variants of AD. Additional genetic associations (Table 28-5) involve the apolipoprotein E (apoE) genotype and the genes for PS-1 and PS-2.

TABLE 28-5 Genetic Factors in Alzheimer Disease (AD)

Gene	Chromosome	Disease Association
Amyloid precursor protein (*APP*)	21	Mutations of the *APP* gene are associated with early-onset familial AD
Presenilin 1 (*PS1*)	14	Mutations of the *PS1* gene are associated with early-onset familial AD
Presenilin 2 (*PS2*)	1	Mutations of the *PS2* gene are associated with Volga German familial AD
Apolipoprotein E (*apoE*)	19	Presence of the ϵ4 allele is associated with increased risk and younger age of onset of both inherited and sporadic forms of late-onset AD

APOLIPOPROTEIN E: ApoE has long been known for its role in cholesterol metabolism. Its relevance to dementia was uncovered in 1993, when it was reported that specific apoE alleles are susceptibility factors for sporadic and late-onset familial subtypes of AD. The human apoE gene is found on chromosome 19 (19q13.2). The three common alleles, ε2, ε3, and ε4, all occur in North American apoE genotypes. An increased risk of late-onset familial and sporadic AD is associated with inheritance of the ε4 allele, particularly the homozygous ε4/ε4 genotype, which occurs in 2% of the population. Conversely, the ε2 allele may confer some protection. The age at which symptoms appear in late-onset AD also correlates with the ε4 allele; ε4/ε4 homozygotes exhibit

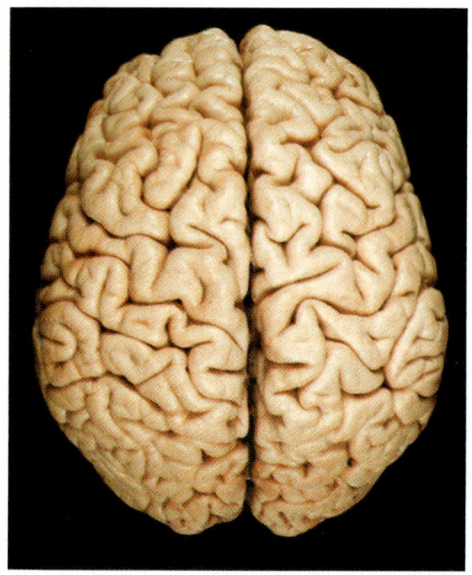
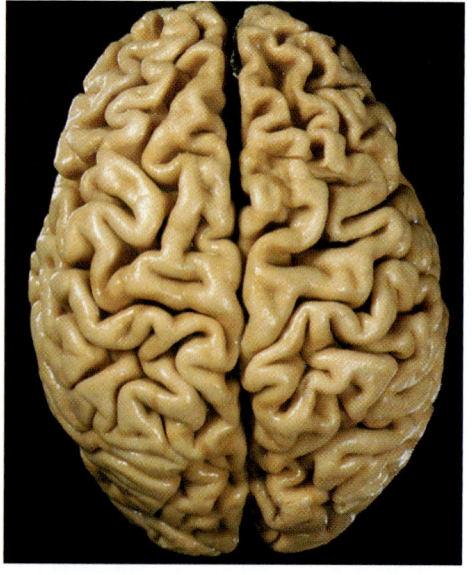

FIGURE 28-123
Alzheimer disease. A. Normal brain. B. The brain of an AD patient shows cortical atrophy with thin gyri and prominent sulci.

Neurodegenerative Diseases

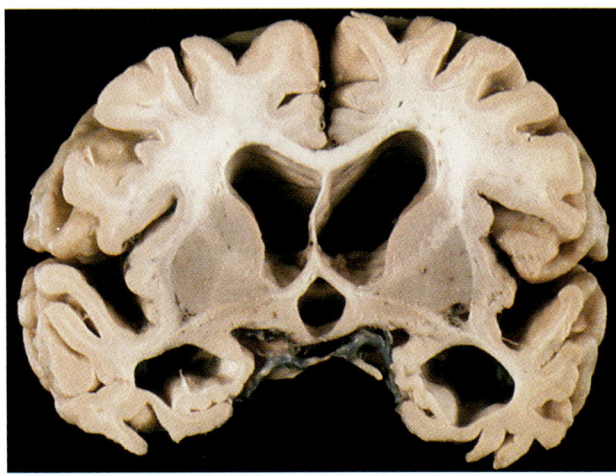

FIGURE 28-124
Alzheimer disease. Severe atrophy of hippocampus and cortex causes ventricular enlargement (hydrocephalus ex vacuo).

the earliest age at onset (<70 years), whereas patients with the ε2 allele experience the latest onset (>90 years). The presence of the ε4 allele has also been correlated with an increased number of senile plaques in AD patients, but the apoE genotype is not an absolute determinant of AD and cannot be used to predict who will develop AD. The mechanisms whereby these different apoE alleles influence the risk of AD remain poorly understood.

PRESENILIN: Two genes with significant homology are associated with different kindreds of familial AD. Mutations of the *PS1* gene located on chromosome 14, are associated with the most common form of autosomal dominant early-onset AD. The *PS2* gene resides on chromosome 1 and is associated with AD in Volga German pedigrees. Importantly, presenilin mutations occur in half of all inherited AD, compared with only a few percent for mutant *APP* genes. Both presenilin genes code for proteins characterized by multiple transmembrane domains. There is some evidence to suggest that PS1 and PS2 mutant proteins alter the processing of β-APP, thereby favoring increased production and deposition of Aβ. Cellular processing of APP releases Aβ fragments of varying lengths, but the Aβ42 variant (see above) appears to be particularly amyloidogenic. It is the Aβ molecule whose production is enhanced by mutant *PS1*.

Pathology: During the course of AD, neurons are lost and gliosis occurs. The gyri narrow, the sulci widen, and cortical atrophy becomes apparent. The brain loses approximately 200 g in an interval of 3 to 8 years (Fig. 28-123). The atrophy is bilateral and symmetric and targets the frontal and hippocampal cortex (Fig. 28-124).

The microscopic changes in AD (Fig. 28-125) are dominated by the presence of (1) senile plaques, (2) NFTs, and (3) neuron loss. Other lesions such as Lewy bodies and granulovacuolar degeneration are also present. Identical morphological alterations occur in lesser intensity in the cerebrum of

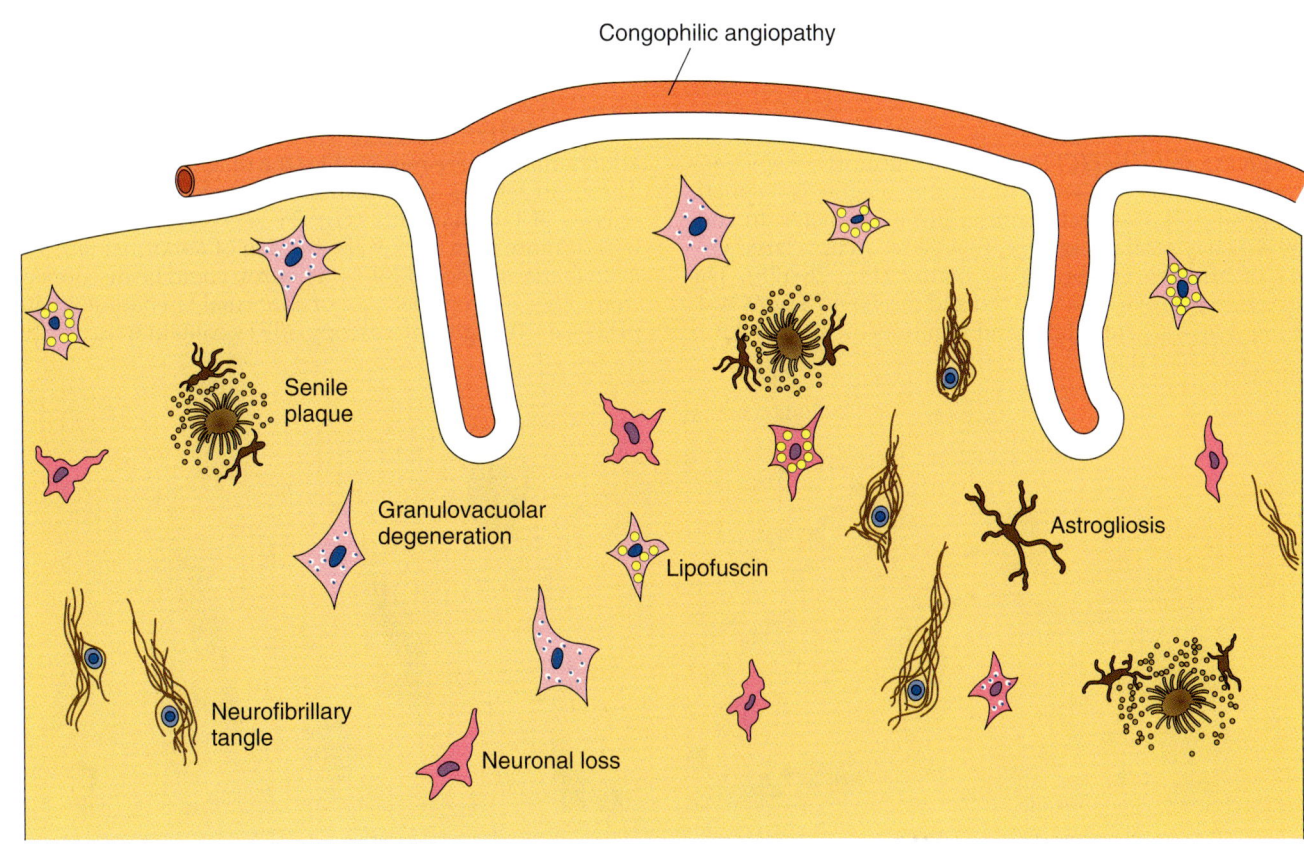

FIGURE 28-125
Microscopic lesions of Alzheimer disease.

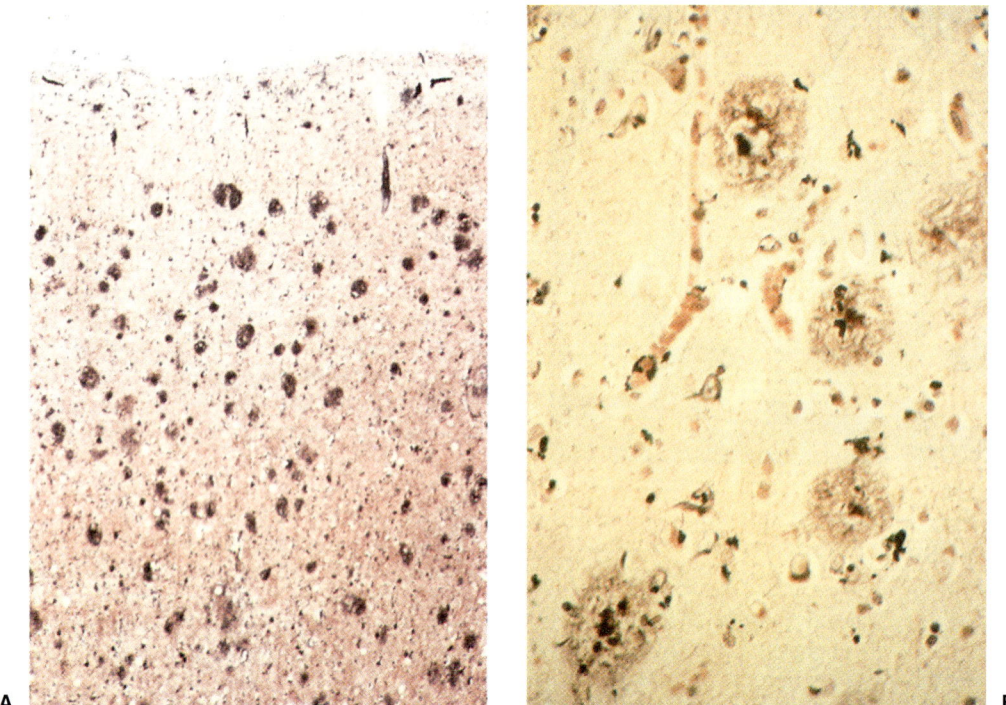

FIGURE 28-126
Alzheimer disease. A. Section of AD cerebral cortex stained with silver reveals abundant senile plaques (SPs). B. A higher-magnification view of A shows the irregular size and spherical shape of SPs formed by fibrillar Aβ deposits.

a large proportion of elderly persons with symptoms as minor as forgetfulness, and a prodromal phase of AD known as mild cognitive impairment (MCI) shows lesser changes than those in full blown AD.

SENILE (NEURITIC) PLAQUES: The most conspicuous histological lesion, the senile or neuritic plaque, is a spherical deposit of Aβ several hundred μm in diameter. In end-stage disease, senile plaques converge to occupy large volumes of affected cerebral gray matter (Fig. 28-126). The plaques are positive for congo red and thioflavin S (amyloid-binding dyes), argentophilic, and immunoreactive for Aβ at the core and periphery. They are surrounded by reactive astrocytes, microglia and tau, and display α-synuclein immunoreactive neuronal processes (dystrophic neuritis).

NEUROFIBRILLARY TANGLES: Like senile plaques, abundant NFTs are required for the diagnosis of definite AD. These structures are formed by large intracytoplasmic masses of tau filaments (Fig. 28-127). Neuronal processes harbor more than 90% of the burden of abnormal tau. Thus, even in the absence of NFTs, a neuron could be disconnected from other neurons because of abnormal tau pathology in its processes. By light microscopy, NFTs contain irregular bun-

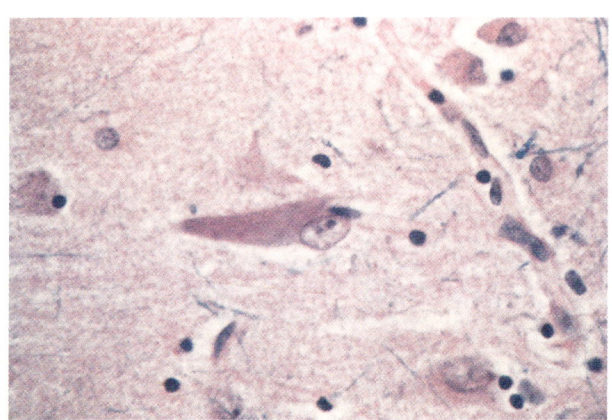 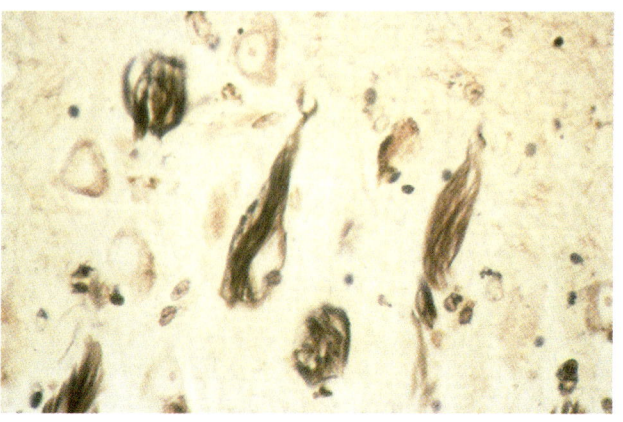

FIGURE 28-127
Alzheimer disease. A. The cytoplasm of a neuron in an AD brain is distended by a NFT. B. A silver stain of A demonstrates the fibrillary character of NFTs.

dles of fibrils that are positive for congo red and thioflavin S, argentophilic, and immunoreactive for tau. Electron microscopy reveals the tangles to be composed of paired, 10-nm thick, helical filaments. Western blots demonstrate abundant insoluble tau proteins.

NFTs also occur in neurodegenerative diseases other than AD, including *dementia pugilistica,* postencephalitic parkinsonism, Guam ALS/parkinsonism dementia complex, Pick disease, corticobasal degeneration, sporadic frontotemporal dementias, hereditary FTDP-17, etc. Indeed, hereditary and sporadic neurodegenerative diseases characterized by abnormal forms of tau are now classified as *taupathies,* since they may share common mechanisms of brain degeneration.

GRANULOVACUOLAR DEGENERATION: This morphological change is not diagnostic of AD and is largely restricted to the cytoplasm of hippocampal pyramidal cells, where it is evident as circular clear zones containing basophilic and argentophilic granules (Fig. 28-128).

HIRANO BODIES: Like granulovacuolar degeneration, these structures are found almost exclusively in hippocampal pyramidal neurons, especially in their processes. Hirano bodies are eosinophilic rods, 10 to 15 μm thick. They are not unique to AD but are seen in the brains of normal elderly persons and in patients with other neurological conditions.

Proposed mechanisms underlying the development of AD are illustrated in Figure 28-129.

 Clinical Features: Patients with AD come to medical attention because of a gradual loss of memory and cognitive function, difficulty with language, and changes in behavior. Persons with mild cognitive impairment (MCI) are increasingly being recognized, since they progress to full blown dementia at a rate of about 15% per year. AD progresses inexorably, so that previously intelligent and productive persons eventually become demented, mute, incontinent, and bedridden. Bronchopneumonia is the usual lethal outcome of AD.

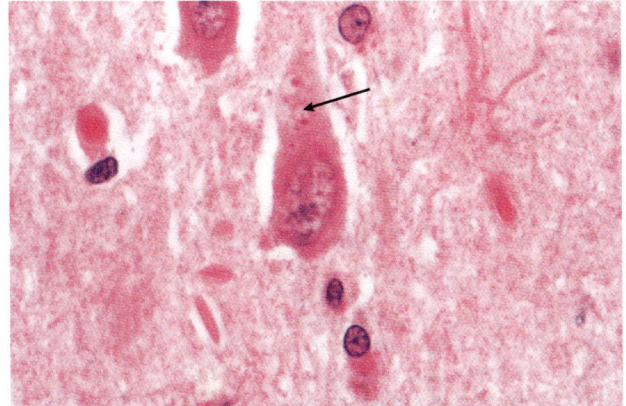

FIGURE 28-128
Alzheimer disease. A section of the AD hippocampus shows granulovacuolar degeneration *(arrow)* in a pyramidal neuron.

Pick Disease

Pick disease *(lobar sclerosis)* is manifested clinically as loss of executive function followed by a dementia that can be indistinguishable from AD. This disorder is prototypical of frontotemporal dementias, and most cases are sporadic, although Pick disease kindreds have been described. Sporadic Pick disease becomes symptomatic in midadult life and progresses relentlessly to death over a period of 3 to 10 years.

The cortical atrophy in Pick disease is initially unilateral and localized to the frontotemporal regions, but it becomes bilateral with disease progression. The atrophy may attain extreme proportions, so that the affected gyri are reduced to a thin edge *(knife-blade atrophy).* Histologically, the involved cortex is markedly depleted of neurons and displays conspicuous astrogliosis. Many residual neurons contain intensely argentophilic and tau immunoreactive cytoplasmic inclusions termed *Pick bodies.* By electron microscopy, these structures are formed by densely aggregated straight tau filaments.

TUMORS OF THE CNS

Tumors within the intracranial compartment can be classified according to five origins:

- **Neuroectoderm,** principally gliomas
- **Mesenchymal structures,** notably meningiomas and schwannomas
- **Ectopic tissues,** such as craniopharyngiomas, dermoid and epidermoid cysts, lipomas, and dysgerminomas
- **Retained embryonal structures** (e.g., paraphyseal cysts)
- **Metastases**

Intracranial tumors constitute only 2% of all "aggressive" neoplasms, and most affect older persons. However the frequency of several types of brain tumors in childhood imparts clinical significance to their appearance in the young. Gliomas account for 60% of primary intracranial neoplasms, meningiomas for 20%, and all others for 20% (Fig. 28-130). Tumors of neuroectodermal origin are predominantly glial, and they are presumed to be derived from astrocytes (astrocytomas), oligodendroglia (oligodendrogliomas), or ependyma (ependymomas). Each of these tumors exhibits varying degrees of anaplasia, from well-differentiated tumors that are difficult to distinguish from normal tissue to anaplastic tumors that do not resemble CNS tissue at all.

BENIGN VERSUS MALIGNANT: The descriptive terms *benign* and *malignant* require qualification when used in reference to brain tumors, especially gliomas. For example, even a very well differentiated astrocytoma infiltrates freely through the surrounding brain tissue and has a poorly defined margin. The term *benign* may be applied to this lesion, because its growth is indolent and permits survival for 5 to 10 years. However, unlike "benign" neoplasms elsewhere, many astrocytomas are eventually fatal, owing in part to their transformation over time into more "malignant" anaplastic astrocytomas or glioblastomas and in part to encroachment upon vital centers. Unlike malignant tumors elsewhere, high-grade gliomas rarely metastasize outside the CNS.

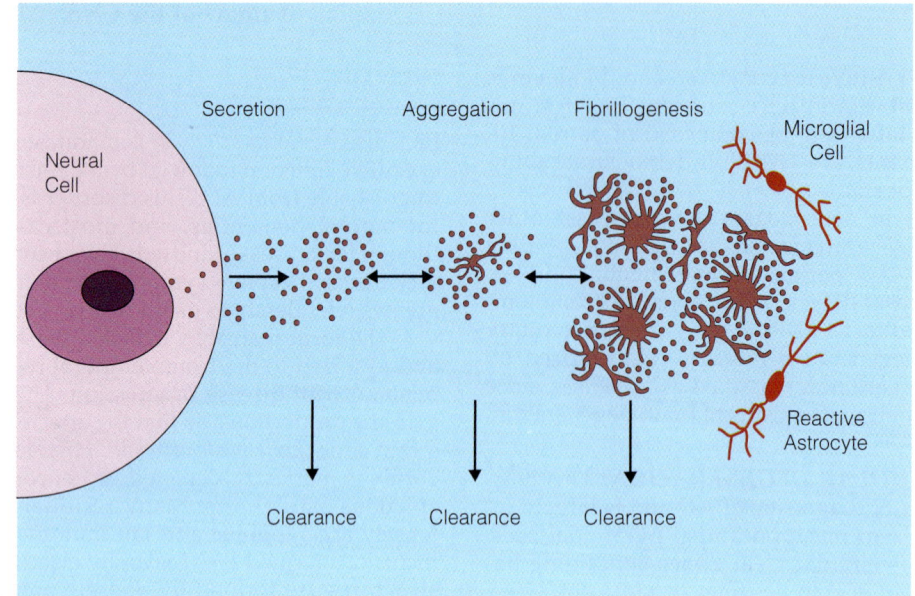

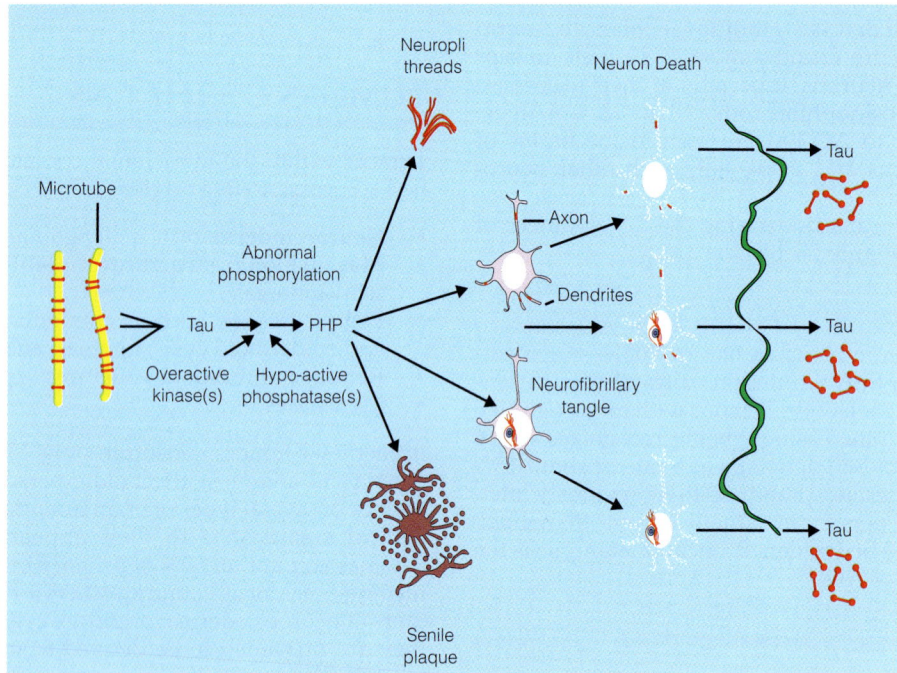

FIGURE 28-129
Mechanisms of amyloidosis and brain degeneration in Alzheimer disease. A. This schematic illustrates a hypothetical mechanism for the formation of senile plaques (SPs) from soluble Aβ peptides (red balls) produced inside cells (orange sphere, left) and secreted into the extracellular space. Amyloidogenic Aβ may encounter fibril-inducing cofactors (green curvilinear profiles) and go on to form A fibrils (yellow linear profiles) to deposit in SPs (far right). SPs are surrounded by reactive astrocytes and microglial cells, which secrete cytokines that may contribute to the toxicity of the SPs. These steps may be reversible. Increasing Aβ clearance or reducing its production, as well as modulating the inflammatory response, may be effective therapeutic interventions for AD, in combination with therapies that target brain degeneration caused by NFTs. B. This schematic illustrates a hypothetical mechanism leading to the conversion of normal human CNS tau (solid rectangles) overlying 2 microtubules (curvilinear profiles, left) into paired helical filaments (PHFs). PHFs are generated in neuronal perikarya and their processes. Overactive kinase(s) or hypoactive phosphatase(s) may contribute to this effect. Abnormally phosphorylated tau forms PHFs in neuronal processes (neuropil threads) and neuronal perikarya (NFTs). Tau in PHFs loses the ability to bind microtubules, thus causing their depolymerization, disruption of axonal transport, and degeneration of neurons. Accumulation of PHFs in neurons could exacerbate this process by physically blocking transport in neurons. The death of affected neurons (neurons drawn with interrupted lines on the right) would release tau and increase the levels of tau in the CSF of AD patients. NFT formation may be reversible, and drugs that block NFT formation, reverse it, or stabilize MTs may be effective therapeutic interventions for AD.

AGE OF THE PATIENT AND LOCATION OF THE TUMOR: Most tumors in the intracranial or intraspinal compartment have predictable geographical localizations. Thus, astrocytic neoplasms occur predominantly in the cerebral hemispheres in middle life and old age, in the cerebellum and pons in childhood, and in the spinal cord in young adults. Oligodendrogliomas predominantly involve the cerebrum in adults, whereas ependymomas have their highest incidence in fourth ventricle during the first 3 decades of life, followed in frequency by intramedullary lesions that arise from the ependymal lining of the spinal canal and from the filum terminale. Inexplicably, ependymomas are least common in the lateral ventricles, which have the largest ependymal surface.

Some tumors, such as the craniopharyngiomas, medulloblastomas, and germinomas, have highly specific sites of origin. A few tumors, notably the third ventricular cyst, are rigidly restricted to a single position in the septum pellucidum, where the lesion regularly abuts against the foramen of Monro, lifts the fornix, and compresses the medial aspects of the internal capsules. Thus, the symptoms of intracranial pressure (hydrocephalus), personality changes, bilateral leg weakness, and urinary incontinence relate to the position of this expansible mass, which is cytologically benign but may kill by virtue of its location and surgical inaccessibility. Meningiomas arise from widely distributed arachnoid villi but display preferred sites of origin (see below).

Within the rigidly defined volume of the intracranial compartment, a new growth compromises space. In the case of meningiomas, the mass displaces the brain, rather than infiltrating it. Glioblastoma multiforme infiltrates and destroys neural tissue. Most tumors are also associated with regional edema, which is disproportionately abundant in the immediate environs of a metastatic tumor and adds to the mass effect of the metastasis. Tumors positioned adjacent to the ventricles, particularly the fourth ventricle or the aqueduct of Sylvius, are prone to obstruct these conduits and cause hydrocephalus.

NEURONAL TUMORS: Infrequently, the neuroectoderm gives rise to a neoplasm of neuronal heritage. These tumors occur most often in childhood, and their cellular composition is usually primitive. An important example is the medulloblastoma, which arises in the cerebellum, generally in the first decade of life. This entity is usually situated in the vermis; its growth is rapid, and regional infiltration is extensive.

Although even highly anaplastic tumors rarely metastasize outside the cranial cavity, certain tumors, notably medulloblastoma and less commonly ependymoma and pineal parenchymal tumor, have a marked propensity to disseminate or "seed" by way of the CSF throughout the CNS. The implants generally involve the subarachnoid compartment over the spinal cord and cauda equina. In conformity with the principle that a cell must be capable of replication to undergo neoplastic transformation, medulloblastomas and the better-differentiated ganglionic tumors typically occur during infancy or childhood. In fact, many tumors probably have their origin during embryonic development. It is intriguing to consider that residual embryonic neural progenitor cells or stem cells of the adult brain undergo neoplastic transformation, which then culminates in the emergence of gliomas and neuronal tumors. Interestingly, although esthesioneuroblastomas of the olfactory mucosa occurs in adults, the olfactory epithelium is a neural structure that re-

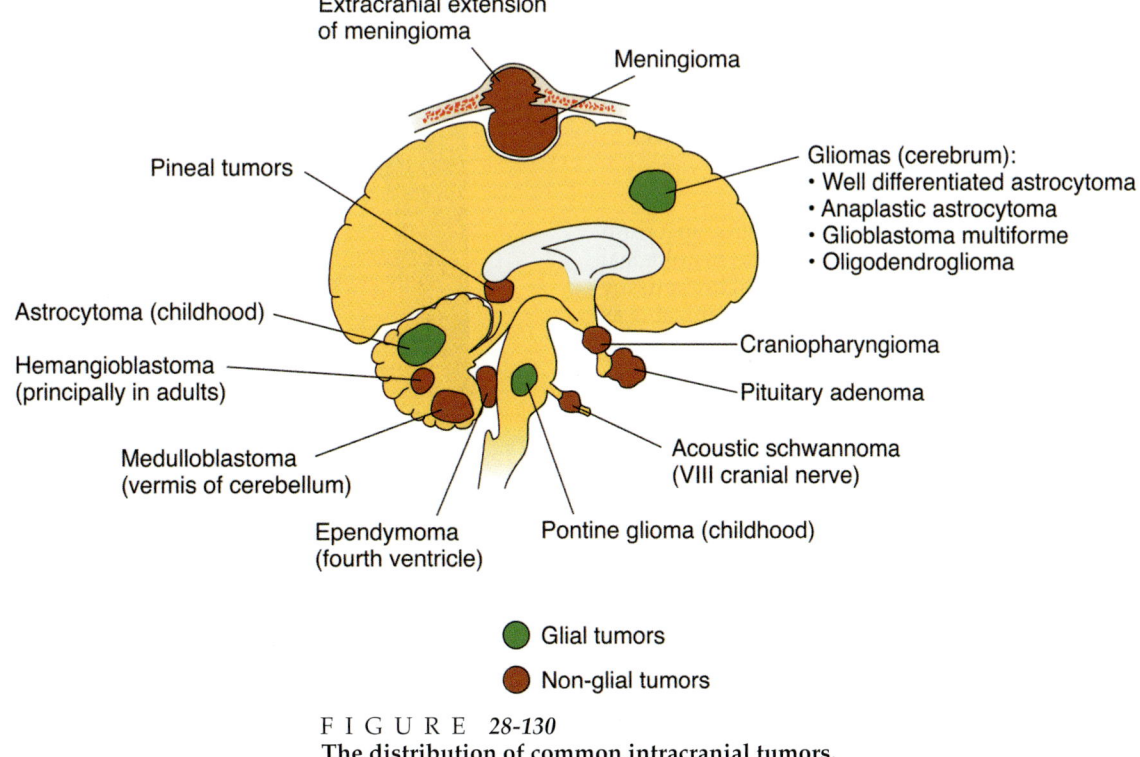

FIGURE 28-130
The distribution of common intracranial tumors.

tains its proliferative potential throughout adult life to replace the olfactory neurons that turn over continuously.

SYMPTOMS OF INTRACRANIAL TUMORS: An infiltrative neoplasm that destroys functional neural tissue creates a neurological deficit, which may be sensory or motor or both, depending on the function of the affected brain region. Cognitive functions are not infrequently impaired. Alternatively, a neoplasm that "irritates" a functional area may initiate an involuntary release of neuronal activity that manifests as seizures. These include (1) motor seizures, (2) subtle visual and olfactory seizures ("uncinate fits"), and (3) seizure disorders that stem from vegetative centers of the brain. Meningiomas and the well-differentiated gliomas, such as astrocytomas, oligodendrogliomas, and gangliomas, are most likely to be associated with seizures.

The mass of a neoplasm, combined with edema or hydrocephalus, causes increased intracranial pressure, which leads to headaches and vomiting. A mass effect, if progressive, ultimately causes various herniations of neural tissue:

- **Transtentorial herniation:** The medial aspect of the hippocampus (uncus) herniates through the tentorium (see Fig. 28-38), where it interferes with the circulatory dynamics of the midbrain. This effect causes a decline in the level of consciousness as a result of impaired function of the reticular formation. This herniation can compress the third nerve against the tentorium and cause a third nerve palsy, resulting in a fixed dilated pupil. Shortly thereafter, midbrain necrosis and hemorrhage lead to permanent loss of consciousness and death (see Fig. 28-39).
- **Foramen magnum herniation:** As a result of increased pressure in the posterior fossa, cerebellar tonsils herniate into the foramen magnum. Compression of the cardiac and respiratory centers is lethal.
- **Subfalcine herniation:** The cingulate gyrus herniates beneath the falx, which on rare occasions may result in infarction in the territories supplied by the pericallosal vessels, with weakness of, or sensory loss in, the legs.

Tumors Derived from Astrocytes Show Varying Histologic Grades

Neoplasms derived from astrocytes display a wide spectrum of differentiation, ranging from tumors whose histological structure is remarkably similar to that of normal brain tissue to highly aggressive growths that are hardly recognizable as of glial origin. These tumors can be divided according to their increasing anaplasia into three broad categories: astrocytoma, anaplastic astrocytoma, and glioblastoma multiforme. Recognition of these glial neoplasms is facilitated by their immunopositivity for GFAP, but the abundance of GFAP diminishes with increasing malignancy.

Astrocytoma

Astrocytoma is a glioma composed of well-differentiated astrocytes. It comprises 20% of primary intracranial neoplasms. It frequents (1) the cerebral hemispheres in adults (Fig. 28-131); (2) the optic nerve, walls of the third ventricle, midbrain, pons, and cerebellum in the first two decades of life (Fig. 28-132); and (3) the spinal cord, predominantly in the thoracic and cervical segments, in young adults.

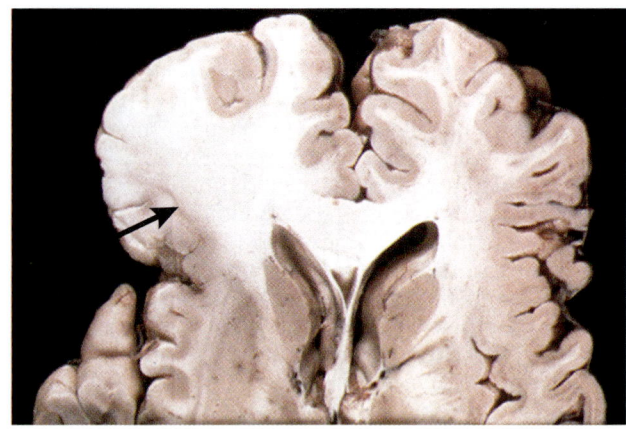

FIGURE 28-131
Astrocytoma. A poorly demarcated, expansile mass occupies the left frontal lobe *(arrow).*

 Pathology: On macroscopic examination, astrocytomas are poorly demarcated and insidiously infiltrate surrounding brain. Childhood astrocytomas of the cerebellar hemispheres are frequently cystic. Astrocytomas of the cerebrum often contain microcysts, and some contain enough calcospherites to be visible radiographically. Microscopically, astrocytomas feature small glial cells with unremarkable nuclei and cytoplasmic processes (Fig. 28-133). The astrocytoma variants are:

- **Fibrillary astrocytoma:** This tumor, particularly in the cerebral hemispheres of adults, has prominent glial processes.
- **Gemistocytic astrocytoma:** Abundant eosinophilic cytoplasm encases the tumor cell nuclei.

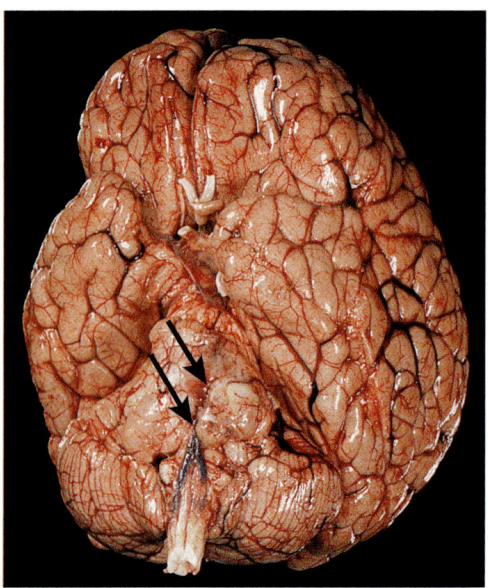

FIGURE 28-132
Astrocytoma. During childhood, the brainstem is a common site of astrocytomas. Note entrapment of the basilar artery *(arrows).*

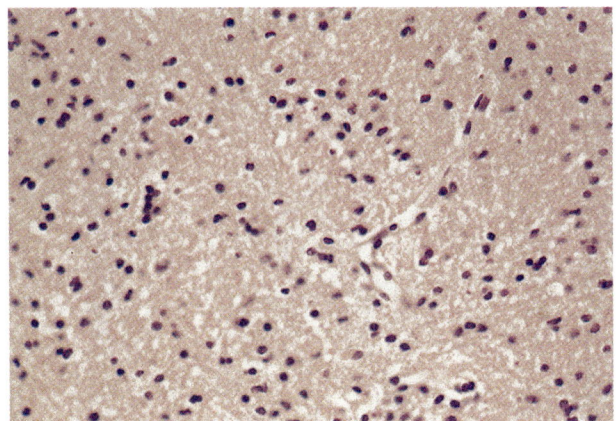

FIGURE 28-133
Astrocytoma. A microscopic section shows a moderately cellular, well-differentiated astrocytoma with minimal pleomorphism.

- **Juvenile pilocytic astrocytoma:** This neoplasm occurs in children and is characterized by abundant, hairlike glial processes. The cells typically contain Rosenthal fibers, similar to those seen in Alexander disease, albeit less abundant.

The life expectancy of patients with astrocytoma varies widely, but approximates 5 years. Transformation to a higher degree of anaplasia, often to glioblastoma multiforme, occurs in 10% of cases or more, in which case life expectancy is considerably shortened.

Anaplastic Astrocytoma

Anaplastic astrocytoma is distinguished from the other astrocytomas by (1) greater cellularity, (2) cellular pleomorphism, and (3) anaplasia (Fig. 28-134). The topographic distribution parallels that of astrocytoma. The growth of the tumor is rapid, and life expectancy averages 3 years.

Glioblastoma Multiforme

Glioblastoma multiforme is the extreme expression of anaplasia among the glial neoplasms and accounts for 40% of all primary intracranial tumors.

 Pathology: Most glioblastomas have constituent cells with recognizable astrocytic properties, including GFAP positivity, but they display (1) marked pleomorphism, (2) frequent mitoses, (3) regional zones of necrosis, and (4) endothelial proliferation. The last feature probably reflects the release of angiogenic growth factors by these high-grade tumors. Hyperplasia of fibroblasts is also produced by glioblastomas located in or near the meninges and may actually attain malignant proportions. In such cases, the sarcomatous growth intermingles fibrosarcoma with the glioma, resulting in a *gliosarcoma*.

Glioblastomas typically infiltrate extensively, and frequently cross the corpus callosum to result in a bilateral lesion likened to a butterfly because of its gross configuration and mottled red/yellow color (Fig. 28-135). The colors represent multiple areas of recent (red) and remote (yellow) hemorrhage. The cardinal histological features of glioblastoma multiforme are as follows:

- **Marked cellularity,** with variable degrees of cellular pleomorphism and multinucleated cells (Fig. 28-136)
- **Serpentine areas of necrosis** surrounded by zones of crowded tumor cells ("palisading necrosis"); Fig. 28-137)
- **Endothelial cell proliferation** formed by clusters of small vessels, referred to as "glomeruloid" formations (Fig. 28-138)

Glioblastomas predominate in the later decades of life, with twice the frequency of astrocytomas. The clinical course rarely exceeds 18 months from the time of diagnosis, regardless of therapeutic intervention.

Oligodendroglioma Arises in the White Matter and Grows Slowly

Oligodendrogliomas occur predominantly in the white matter of the cerebral hemispheres of adults.

Pathology: Histologically, the tumors have small rounded nuclei like normal oligodendrocytes (Figure 28-139), but they also exhibit increased cell density and cellular pleomorphism. Calcospherites, which on occasion are visualized radiographically, are scattered randomly throughout the lesion. The slow growth is reflected in few mitotic figures and necrosis, although markers of cell proliferation demonstrate that dividing cells are not uncommon in oligodendrogliomas. Loss of heterozygosity (LOH) for chromosomes 1p or 19q may emerge as a useful molecular signatures for these tumors.

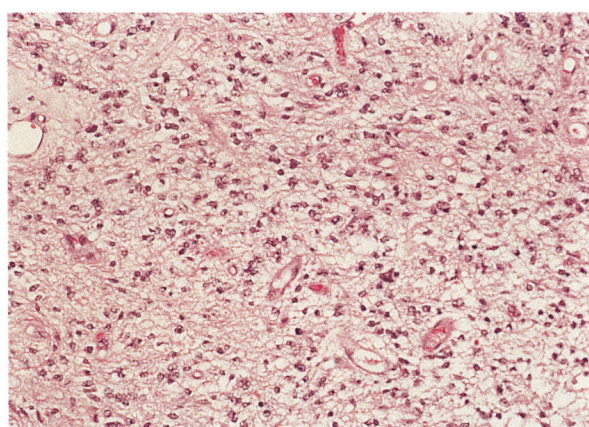

FIGURE 28-134
Anaplastic astrocytoma. Anaplasia introduces hypercellularity of astrocytes with nuclear pleomorphism and increased vascularity.

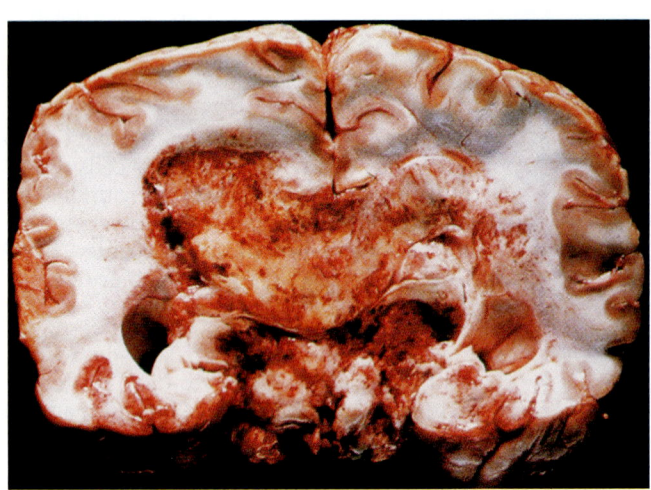
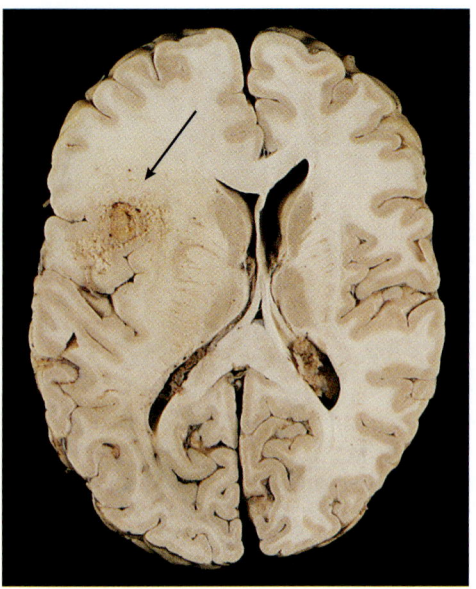

FIGURE 28-135
Glioblastoma multiforme. A. The tumor occupies the splenium of the corpus callosum with bilateral extension into white matter, where it has a variegated red and yellow appearance ("butterfly tumor"). B. Horizontal section of the brain from another patient with a glioblastoma multiforme reveals a partially necrotic and edematous mass in the left insula (*arrow*).

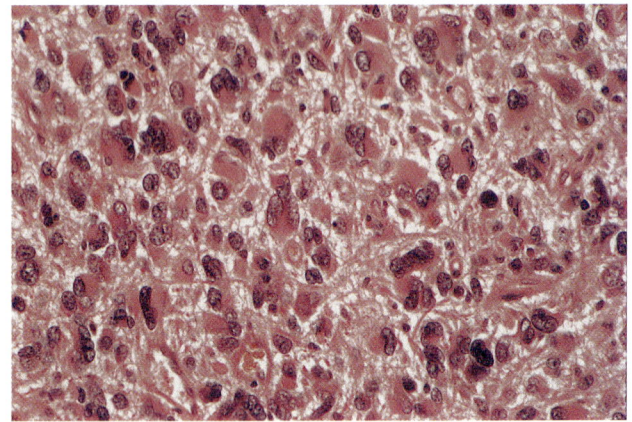

FIGURE 28-136
Glioblastoma multiforme. Malignant gliomas show marked nuclear pleomorphism with bizarre multinucleated glial cells.

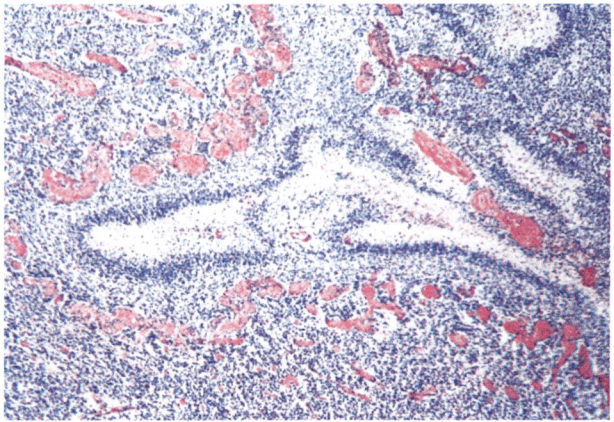

FIGURE 28-137
Glioblastoma multiforme. Photomicrograph shows a highly vascularized tumor with serpentine areas of necrosis, bordered by hypercellular zones (palisading).

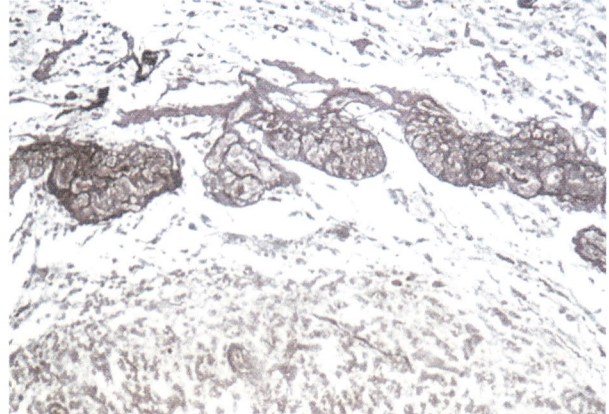

FIGURE 28-138
Glioblastoma multiforme. Silver staining shows proliferated endothelial cells in glomeruloid structures near the tumor.

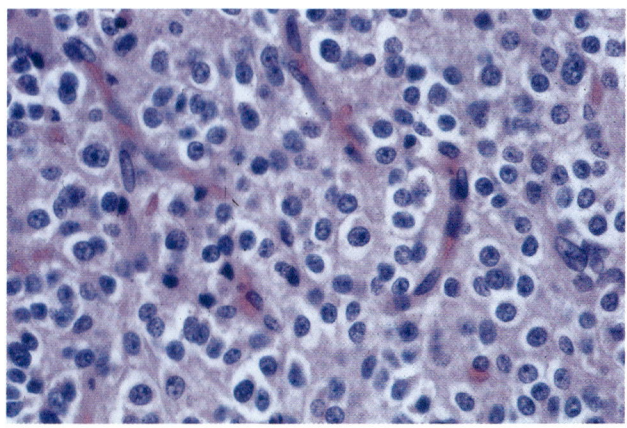

FIGURE 28-139
Oligodendroglioma. The tumor is composed of cells that resemble normal oligodendrocytes.

The symptoms of oligodendroglioma are frequently ushered in by seizures. Although the lesion is infiltrative, its slow growth permits survival for 5 to 10 years.

Ependymoma Originates in the Lining of the Cavities That Contain Cerebrospinal Fluid

Ependymoma is most common in the fourth ventricle (Fig. 28-140A), *producing obstruction and resulting in hydrocephalus.* This neoplasm is second only to astrocytoma as an intramedullary tumor of the spinal cord, where it arises from the ependymal lining of the central canal or the filum terminale. Spinal astrocytomas are most often seen at the lumbosacral level, whereas intramedullary astrocytoma, is usually located in the cervical–thoracic region. There are no specific ependymal cell markers, but LOH for chromosome 22q may provide a molecular signature.

The cells of an ependymoma characteristically have an "epithelial" appearance, similar to that of normal ependymal cells. They possess ovoid nuclei, with coarse chromatin material and well-defined plasma membranes. The cells of an ependymoma form clefts or may arrange around blood vessels, creating an anuclear mantle of glial processes about the adventitia (see Fig. 28-140B). The tumor generally grows slowly, but it can seed the subarachnoid space.

CHOROID PLEXUS PAPILLOMA: This benign variant of ependymoma, is distinctive enough to warrant separate classification. Choroid papilloma occurs most commonly in young boys and usually arises in a lateral ventricle. Hydrocephalus is the major complication. On gross examination, choroid papilloma appears as an intraventricular papillary mass. Microscopically, it duplicates the structure of the normal choroid plexus. Transthyretin immunoreactivity is a reliable marker for these tumors. Choroid plexus papillomas can also transform into carcinomas if they are not excised.

Medulloblastoma Is a Childhood Cerebellar Tumor

Medulloblastoma, the most common intracranial neuroblastic lesion, derives from the transient, cerebellar, external granular cell layer of neuronal progenitor cells, or from their derivatives, that have migrated aberrantly into deeper regions of the cerebellar cortex. It arises exclusively in the cerebellum and has its highest frequency toward the end of the first decade. The tumor infiltrates aggressively and frequently disseminates through the CSF.

Medulloblastomas are characterized by cells with hyperchromatic, round-to-oval nuclei and scant cytoplasm, which often crowd together with no structural pattern. The neuroblastic character of the cells is occasionally expressed in rosette formation, a distinctive feature of embryonic and neoplastic neuroblasts. The detection of neuronal and progenitor cell markers (neurofilament proteins, synaptophysin, nestin) may be diagnostically informative in distinguishing these tumors from metastatic epithelial tumors (frequently positive for epithelial keratins), lymphomas (usually positive for leukocyte markers) or other neuroectodermal malignancies. A number of genetic abnormalities have been detected in medulloblastomas (e.g., c-*myc* and N-*myc* amplification, LOH for chromosome 17q, etc.), but none are specific.

Children with medulloblastoma are first seen with cerebellar dysfunction or hydrocephalus. Similar to embryonic neuroblasts, the tumor is highly sensitive to ionizing radiation, but unfortunately, subarachnoid dissemination is frequent. The 10-year survival rate is only 50%.

Ganglioglioma Is Composed of Mature and Immature Neurons in a Stroma of Glia

Ganglioglioma is a rare brain tumor that commonly expresses its presence in seizures during the first two decades of life. The neuronal constituents are represented by (1) small

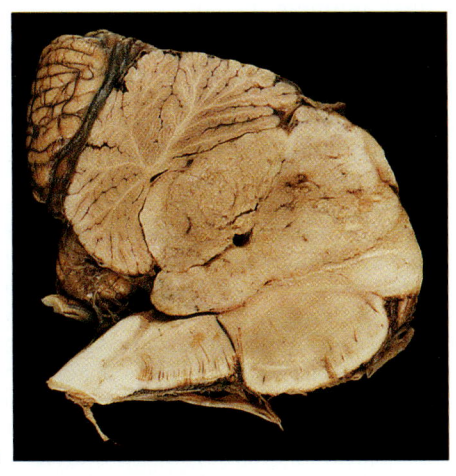
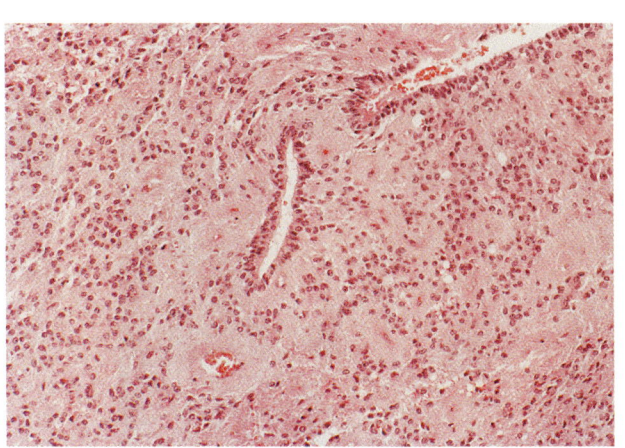

FIGURE 28-140
Ependymoma. A. The fourth ventricle is distended by a well-demarcated mass that flattens the pons and elevates the cerebellum. B. A microscopic section of the tumor in A shows randomly arranged cells in a fibrillary matrix with clefts lined by tumor cells.

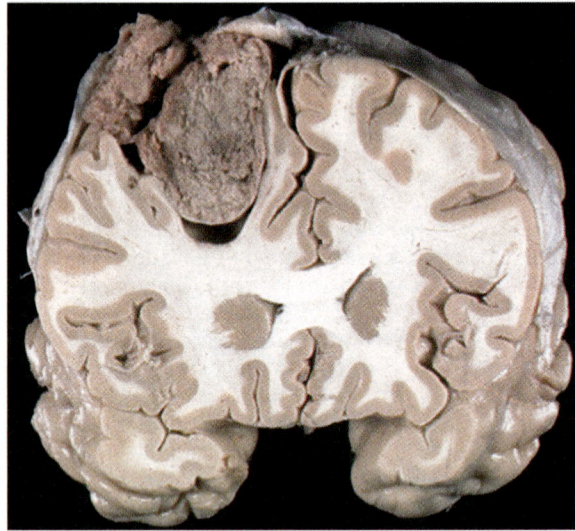

FIGURE 28-141
Meningioma. A tumor that arises from the arachnoid indents the underlying cortex.

rounded nuclei of neuroblasts, (2) intermediate forms, (3) large nuclei with prominent nucleoli and the well-defined cytoplasm of neurons, and (4) the expression of multiple neuronal marker proteins. The matrix of ganglioglioma is formed by astrocytes. This tumor grows indolently and is often cured by surgical removal.

Neoplasms of Mesenchymal Origin Are External to the Brain

Meningioma

Meningiomas are intracranial tumors that arise from the arachnoid villi and produce symptoms by compressing adjacent brain tissue. They account for almost 20% of all primary intracranial neoplasms. Meningiomas occur at almost any intracranial site but are most common in parasagittal regions of the cerebral hemispheres, the olfactory groove, and the lateral sphenoid wing. They occur with a 60:40 female-to-male incidence, but in the spinal canal, this ratio approaches 10:1. The peak frequency is in the fourth to fifth decades, but there is a significant incidence in young adults. In some cases the tumor forms a discoid mass (meningioma en plaque) (Fig. 28-141). Meningiomas have a propensity to erode contiguous bone (Fig. 28-142). The superficial position of meningiomas, coupled with neural displacement rather than infiltration, invites total surgical excision. However, tumors at the base of the brain often invade the skull, thereby limiting complete resection and making recurrence common.

 Pathogenesis: Meningiomas typically arise in one of three settings:

- Sporadic cases (most common)
- Iatrogenic cases caused by prior radiation therapy to the cranium
- In association with a genetic disorder, especially neurofibromatosis type 2 (NF2)

Most meningiomas arise sporadically. Many such tumors exhibit loss, partial deletion, or mutation of the *NF2* locus (22q12), suggesting that perturbations of the this tumor-suppressor gene are involved not only in NF2 (see below), but also in the origin of many sporadic meningiomas (and schwannomas).

The induction of meningiomas by radiation therapy involves a latent period of a decade or more and is directly related to the radiation dosage. Low-dose scalp irradiation for tinea capitis was widely used until 1960. For these patients, the average interval between the treatment and the detection of a meningioma was 35 years. With higher radiation doses, such as those used for head and neck cancers, the interval may be as short as 5 years. Meningiomas also occur in conjunction with several genetic syndromes, most importantly NF2. An association has also been reported with basal cell nevus syndrome (Gorlin syndrome), and rare, familial, multiple meningioma syndromes have been documented.

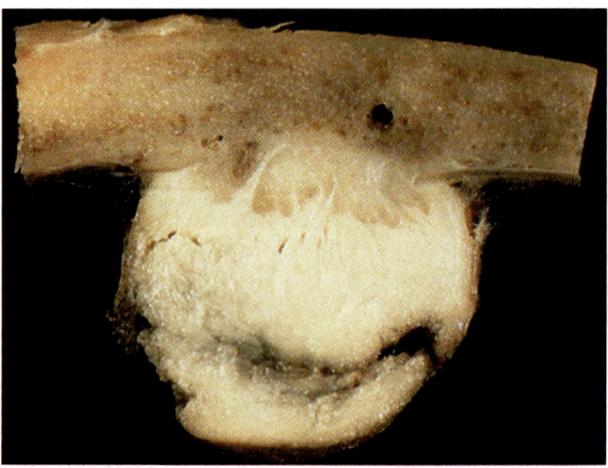

FIGURE 28-142
Meningioma. The bone in the overlying calvaria is infiltrated by a locally aggressive meningioma.

 Pathology: On gross examination, most meningiomas appear as well-circumscribed, firm, bosselated masses of variable size. The cut surface presents a gray appearance similar to that of uterine leiomyomas. The histological hallmark of meningiomas is a whorled pattern of "meningothelial" cells (Fig. 28-143), in association with psammoma bodies (laminated, spherical calcospherites). Although this morphological appearance is distinctive, in many meningiomas it is obscured by a predominantly fibroblast-like proliferation. Some meningiomas are dominated by blood vessels *(angiomatous meningioma)*; others have a papillary appearance *(papillary meningiomas)*; a rare lesion features microcystic formations *(microcystic meningioma)*. The different subtypes of meningioma do not differ significantly in their biological behavior. Meningiomas are negative for GFAP and keratins, but positive for epithelial membrane antigen.

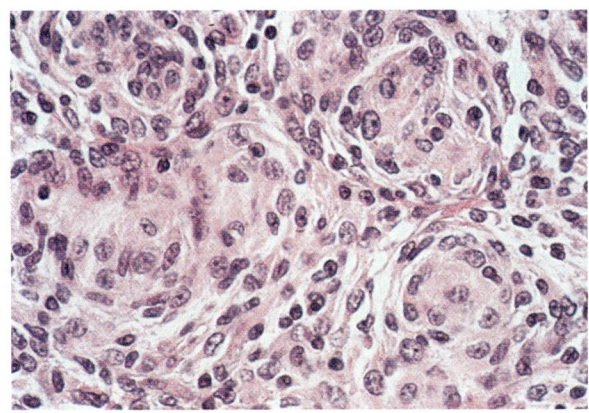

FIGURE 28-143
Meningioma. A microscopic section shows whorled meningothelial cells.

Clinical Features: The indolent growth of meningiomas enables them to enlarge slowly for years before becoming symptomatic, during which time they displace the brain but do not infiltrate it. Thus, seizures rather than neurological deficits frequently characterize their clinical presentation, particularly with tumors at parasagittal sites situated over the convexity of the hemispheres. In other locations, meningiomas compress a variety of functional structures. Thus, tumors of the olfactory groove produce anosmia; those in the suprasellar region lead to visual deficits; meningiomas in the cerebellopontine angle cause cranial nerve palsies; and those in the spinal column result in dysfunction of the spinal nerve roots and spinal cord.

Because the meninges, are innervated by pain fibers, headaches are common. Penetration of the calvaria may create a tumor mass on the external surface of the skull. Meningiomas that are not completely excised tend to recur, and some may transform into malignant and invasive meningiomas, although these more aggressive variants rarely arise de novo.

Schwannoma

Schwannoma is a tumor derived from Schwann cells, which produce both collagen and myelin. This tumor is also known as neurilemmoma, perineural fibroblastoma, and neurinoma. Histologically, schwannomas appear as interwoven fascicles of spindle cells. Occasionally, parallel arrays of tumor cells are noted at the ends of a fibrillar bundle and are referred to as a *Verocay body*. Fortunately, Schwannomas are rarely malignant, and nuclear pleomorphism, when limited to occasional cells, does not predict accelerated growth.

Acoustic neuromas are intracranial schwannomas that are restricted to the eighth nerve (Fig. 28-144). Interestingly, the tumor invariably begins at the transition from oligodendroglia to Schwann cells along CNS axons that form peripheral nerves. This junction corresponds anatomically to the position of the internal auditory meatus. Thus, acoustic neuromas may cause tinnitus and deafness as they expand the bony meatus. These neurinomas can also protrude into the cerebellopontine angle and compress other nerves.

Schwannomas also arise on spinal nerve roots. On occasion, they are entirely within the spinal canal, although at other times, they span a bony foramen, with a "dumb-bell" configuration. Together with meningiomas, schwannomas compose most intradural–extramedullary neoplasms. Tumors of Schwann cells also occur on peripheral nerves as schwannomas and neurofibromas. As mentioned above, some schwannomas exhibit deletions or mutations of the *NF2* gene.

Neoplasms Derived from Ectopic Tissues Compress Adjacent Structures

Craniopharyngioma

Craniopharyngiomas are solid and cystic lesions located above the sella turcica that arise from the epithelium of Rathke's pouch. This structure is a part of the embryonic nasopharynx that migrates cephalad and gives origin to the anterior lobe of the hypophysis (Fig. 28-145A). Some cystic lesions are lined by squamous epithelium, whereas others, referred to as *adamantinomas*, are solid and resemble tumors of dentigerous origin (see Fig. 28-145B). Craniopharyngiomas generally become symptomatic in the first two decades of life, creating visual deficits and headaches. They may cause pituitary failure, including diabetes insipidus.

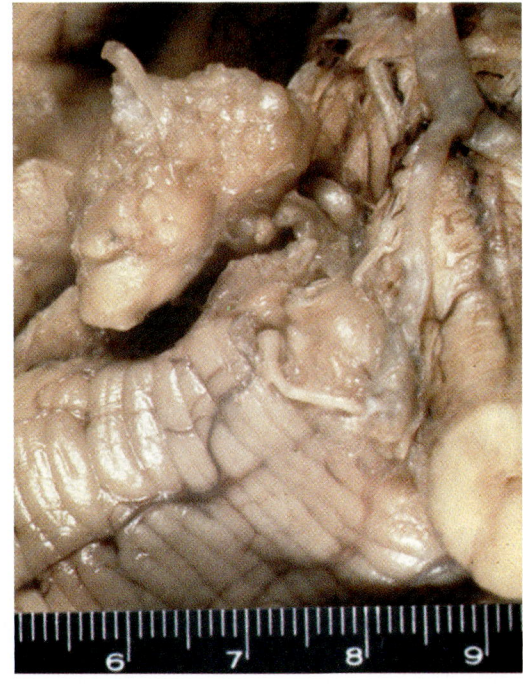

FIGURE 28-144
Acoustic neuroma. A tumor in the cerebellar pontine angle arises from the eighth cranial nerve.

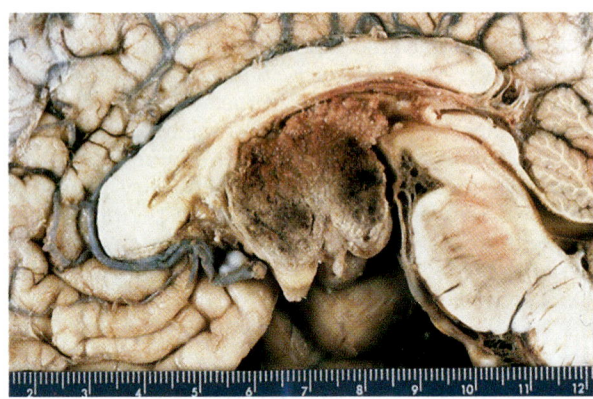
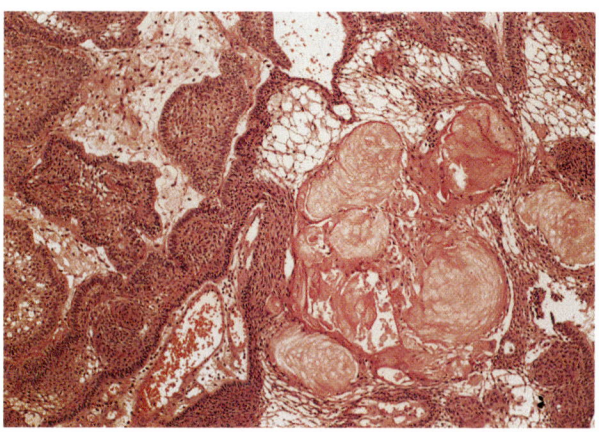

FIGURE 28-145
Craniopharyngioma. A. The tumor arises above the sella turcica as a spherical mass that impinges on the optic chiasm, hypothalamus, and third ventricle. B. Microscopic section shows cords of epithelial cells interspersed with keratin debris.

Dermoid and Epidermoid Cysts

Dermoid and epidermoid cysts result from misdirected embryonic development. The term *dermoid* refers to cysts lined by squamous epithelium, skin appendages, and hair. These cysts extend into bones of the skull and occasionally into the intracranial compartment. The displaced squamous cells proliferate and develop into a cyst, which fills with desquamated keratotic debris that resembles "mother of pearl." The intracranial lesions tend to occur in the posterior fossa or about the sella turcica. Although these cysts are not true neoplasms, accumulating debris causes expansion of the intracranial mass, thereby leading to symptoms.

Lipoma

Lipomas arise from rudiments of adipose tissue carried inward as the brain forms during embryogenesis. They are positioned (1) along the superior aspect of the corpus callosum (Fig. 28-146), (2) the dorsum of the quadrigeminal plate, and (3) the dorsal sagittal plane of the spinal cord near the cauda equina. Lipomas enlarge slowly, if at all, but may enmesh cranial or spinal nerves and interfere with nerve conduction. Most lipomas of the CNS are encountered incidentally at postmortem examination and histologically mimic normal adipocytes.

Tumors of Germ Cell Origin Are Similar to Gonadal Neoplasms

Neoplasms that originate from misplaced germ cells occur within the cranial cavity and, less commonly, in the spinal cord. Such tumors are almost invariably located in midline structures, especially in the area of the pineal gland, but also at sites immediately adjacent to this gland, in the cerebellopontine angle, and around the sella turcica. Intracranial germ cell tumors display a number of phenotypes that parallel gonadal neoplasms, including seminoma, choriocarcinoma, embryonal carcinoma, endodermal sinus tumor, and teratoma.

Intracranial germ cell tumors are seen primarily in young adult men, and the symptoms depend on the location of the expanding mass. Destruction of the pineal gland by a germ cell tumor may produce precocious puberty, particularly in boys. In that location it may compress the superior colliculus and restrict ocular motion. Compression of the aqueduct of Sylvius leads to hydrocephalus.

Hemangioblastoma Is a Cerebellar Tumor That Is Often Syndromic

Hemangioblastoma is a highly vascularized tumor that originates predominantly in the cerebellum. Although its name suggests that it arises from endothelial cells, the true cell of origin is still debated. Hemangioblastoma features endothelium-lined canals interspersed with plump cells (Fig. 28-147). **In 20% of cases, these cells secrete erythropoietin and induce polycythemia.** A rare hemangioblastoma arises in the spinal cord, and on occasion they originate above the tentorium. Hemangioblastoma usually becomes clinically apparent as an expanding mass between the ages of 20 and 40 years.

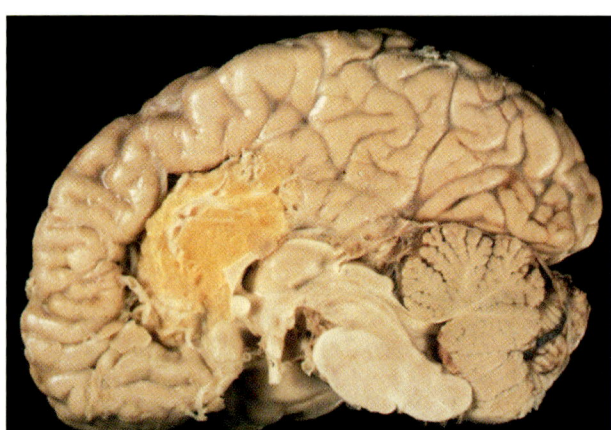

FIGURE 28-146
Lipoma. A soft yellow mass is seen in the dorsal, midsagittal axis of the brain.

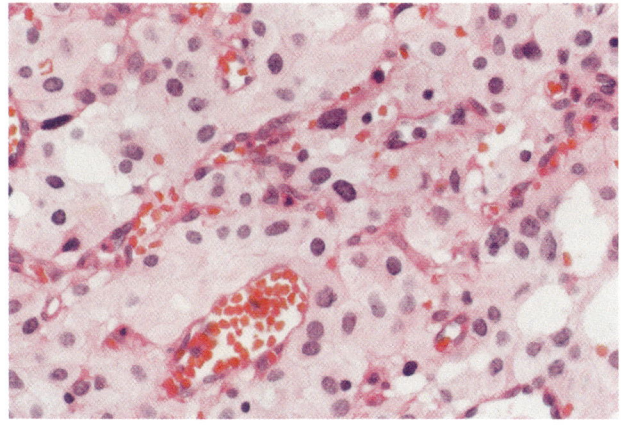

FIGURE 28-147
Hemangioblastoma. The tumor is composed of cells with abundant pink cytoplasm and is traversed by thin-walled vascular channels.

Lindau syndrome refers to the hereditary occurrence of a cerebellar hemangioblastoma that is not associated with other lesions.

Von Hippel-Lindau syndrome is a hereditary variant in which cerebellar hemangioblastoma is associated with retinal hemangiomas and other tumors, owing to mutations in the tumor suppressor *VHL* gene (see Chapter 5).

Lymphoma Can Originate in the CNS

Lymphoma arises as a primary B-cell lesion in the brain in a manner analogous to its occurrence in the stomach, small bowel, or testis, but the overwhelming majority of lymphomas are metastatic to the brain from other sites. In the brain, primary lymphoma often arises deep in the cerebral hemispheres, commonly in bilateral periventricular positions (Fig. 28-148A,B). A mixture of small and large lymphocytes is angiocentric (see Fig. 28-148C). Lymphomas often arise in the context of immunosuppression as well as in AIDS. In some instances they have been linked etiologically to infection with Epstein-Barr virus.

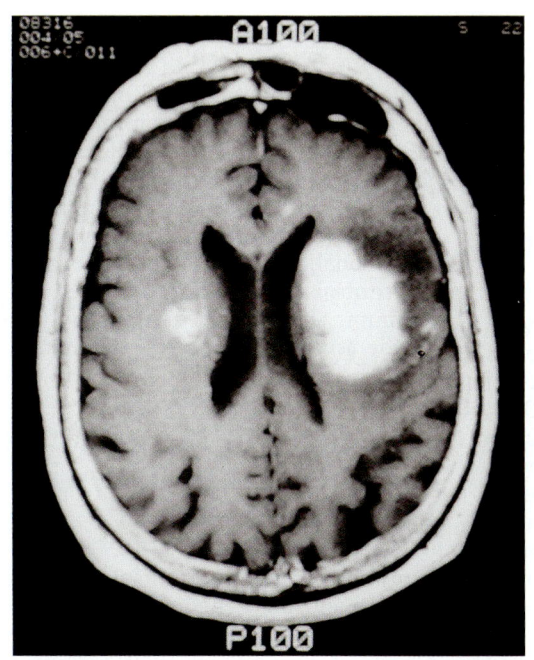
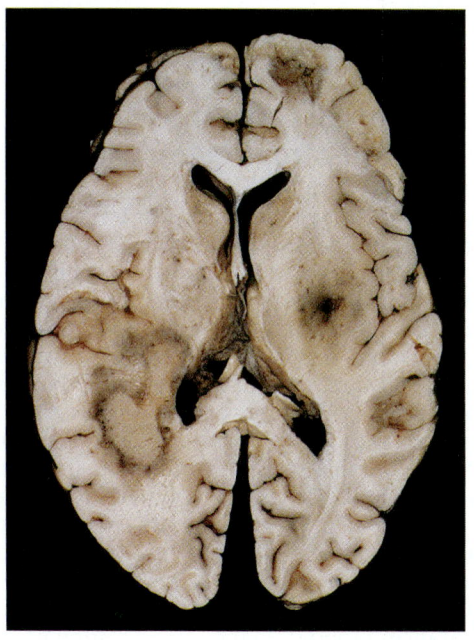

FIGURE 28-148
Primary lymphoma of the brain. A. Magnetic resonance imaging shows a multicentric lymphoma localized near the ventricles. B. A multiplicity of variegated grey–black lesions is distributed through both hemispheres of a patient with AIDS. C. Microscopic section of the tumor reveals an angiocentric focus of neoplastic lymphocytes stained for a B-cell antigen.

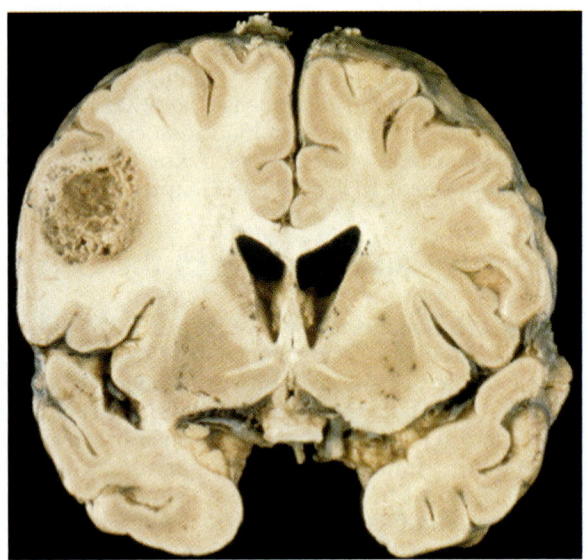

FIGURE 28-149
Metastatic carcinoma. A discrete, spherical lesion in the cerebral cortex *(left)* is surrounded by edematous parenchyma.

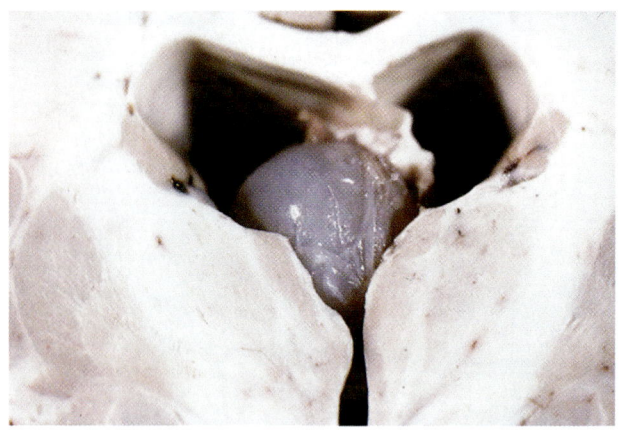

FIGURE 28-150
Colloid cyst. The lesion arises in the roof of the third ventricle and impinges on the foramen of Monro to produce hydrocephalus.

Extracranial lymphomas may secondarily involve the CNS, usually late in the course of the disease. The meninges, epidural space, and nerve roots are most commonly affected.

Metastatic Tumors Are the Most Common Intracranial Neoplasms

Metastatic tumors reach the intracranial compartment through the bloodstream, generally in patients with advanced cancer. Tumors of different organs vary in their incidence of intracranial metastases. For example, a patient with disseminated melanoma has a greater than 50% likelihood of acquiring intracranial metastases, whereas the incidence of such metastases in carcinoma of the breast and lung is 35%, and that for cancer of the kidney or colon is only 5%. Certain carcinomas, such as those of the prostate, liver, and adrenals, and sarcomas of all types rarely establish intracranial metastases. Most metastatic lesions seed to the gray–white junction, reflecting the rich capillary bed in this area. Carcinomas may spread to the calvaria and extend into the intracranial compartment.

A metastasis contrasts with a primary glioma in its discrete appearance, globoid shape, and prominent halo of edema (Fig. 28-149). Metastases to the leptomeninges permit tumor cells to grow in the CSF, suspended as if they were in tissue culture.

Colloid Cyst Exerts Pressure Effects

Colloid cysts (paraphyseal cyst, third ventricular cyst) are distinctive for their anterior, midline location in the tegmental portion of the third ventricle (Fig. 28-150). In this location, they (1) occlude the foramina of Monro, (2) elevate and compress the fornix, and (3) press on the lateral wall of the third ventricle. These effects result in hydrocephalus, alterations in personality, weakness of the lower legs, and loss of bladder control. Colloid cysts are lined by ciliated cuboidal epithelium. The lesions enlarge slowly, usually over decades, by the accumulation of desquamated and secretory products. The origin of colloid cysts remains uncertain.

Hereditary Intracranial Neoplasms Are Often Associated with Extracranial Tumors

A number of hereditary disorders are associated with CNS tumors, and the genetic bases of the major syndromes are listed in Table 28-6. Other inherited diseases in which neoplasms of systemic organs figure prominently include the

TABLE 28-6 Hereditary Syndromes Associated with Intracranial Tumors

Disease	Chromosome Locus	Gene (Protein)	Nervous System Tumor(s)
Neurofibromatosis 1	17q11	*NF1* (neurofibromin)	Neurofibroma
			Neurofibrosarcoma
			Juvenile pilocytic astrocytoma of the optic nerves ("optic glioma")
Neurofibromatosis 2	22q12	*NF2* (schwannomin/merlin)	Schwannoma
			Meningioma
			Ependymoma (spinal cord)
Tuberous sclerosis	9q34	*TSC1* (hamartin)	Subependymal giant cell
	16p13.3	*TSC2* (tuberin)	Astrocytoma
von Hippel-Lindau syndrome	3p25	*VHL*	Hemangioblastoma

expression of nervous system tumors. For example, malignant gliomas arise in patients with Li-Fraumeni syndrome, and medulloblastomas are associated with the gastrointestinal tumors of Turcot syndrome.

Neurofibromatosis (von Recklinghausen Disease)

NF occurs in two distinct forms, both of which are inherited as autosomal dominant traits (see Chapter 6). NF2 is usually characterized by bilateral acoustic neuromas. However, the disease can be diagnosed in patients with a unilateral eighth nerve tumor if two of the following are present: neurofibroma, meningioma, glioma, or schwannoma.

Tuberous Sclerosis (Bourneville Disease)

Tuberous sclerosis is an autosomal dominant disease characterized by hamartomas (tubers) of the brain, retina, and viscera. This disease reflects disordered migration and arrested maturation of the neuroectoderm, resulting in formation of "tubers" of the cerebral cortex and of subependymal astrocytic nodules (Fig. 28-151A). The tubers are discrete cortical areas composed of bizarre cells with neuronal and glial features. The subependymal nodules have been likened to "candle drippings" and provide the substrate for gemistocytic astrocytomas (see Fig. 28-151B). In addition to the intracranial lesions, the syndrome includes (1) facial angiofibromas (adenoma sebaceum), (2) cardiac rhabdomyomas, and (3) mesenchymal tumors of the kidney (angiomyolipomas). Most tuberous sclerosis patients have seizures and are mentally retarded. Mutations in two genes have been linked to tuberous sclerosis. *TSC1* (9q34) codes for a protein termed *hamartin*. *TSC2* (16p13) encodes *tuberin*, a protein with homology to a GTPase-activating protein. Both genes seem to act as tumor suppressors.

Lindau Syndrome

As mentioned above, some hemangioblastomas of the cerebellum assume a hereditary pattern (Lindau syndrome). An identical tumor may occur in the retina (von Hippel-Lindau syndrome). In the latter syndrome, cysts also occur in the kidneys and pancreas.

Sturge-Weber Syndrome (Encephalofacial Angiomatosis)

Sturge-Weber syndrome is a rare, nonfamilial congenital disorder characterized by angiomas of the brain and face. The facial lesion is usually unilateral and is termed a *port wine stain (nevus flammeus)*. The leptomeninges exhibit large angiomas, which in severe cases may occupy an entire hemisphere. Cerebral calcification and atrophy often underlie the intracranial angiomas. The link between angiomas of the face and the brain has been attributed to the continuity of the embryological vascular supply of the telencephalon, the eye, and the overlying skin. In most instances, Sturge-Weber syndrome is associated with mental deficiency.

The Peripheral Nervous System

ANATOMY

The peripheral nervous system is external to the brain and spinal cord and includes (1) cranial nerves, (2) dorsal and

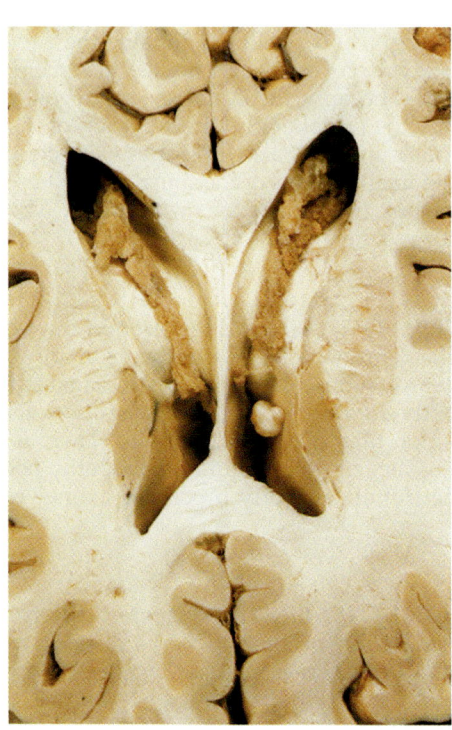
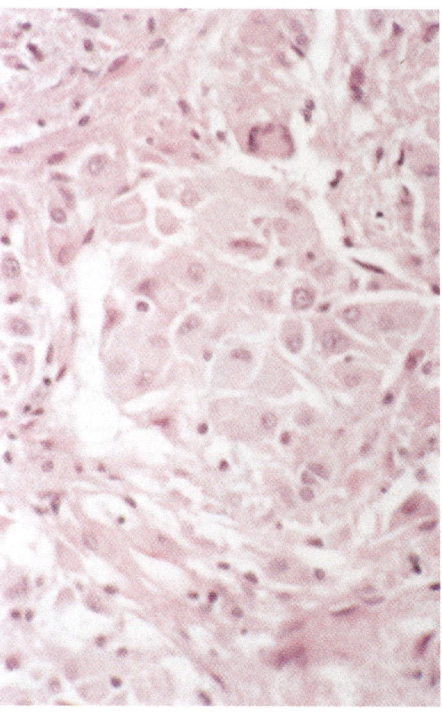

FIGURE 28-151
Tuberous sclerosis. A. Horizontal section of the brain shows subependymal astrocytic nodules in the lateral ventricles ("candle drippings"). B. A giant cell astrocytoma has developed from one of the subependymal hamartomas.

ventral spinal roots, (3) spinal nerves and their continuations, and (4) ganglia. Peripheral nerves carry somatic motor, somatic sensory, visceral sensory and autonomic fibers.

The somatic motor and preganglionic autonomic fibers arise from neuronal cell bodies within the CNS. The sensory and postganglionic autonomic fibers originate from neuronal cell bodies within ganglia located on cranial nerves, dorsal roots, and autonomic nerves. The neurons and satellite cells of the ganglia and all of the Schwann cells are derived from the neural crest.

The peripheral nerves, but not their ganglia, have a blood–nerve barrier analogous to the blood–brain barrier. Endoneurial connective tissue surrounds the individual nerve fibers, which are bundled into fascicles by the perineurial connective tissue. Epineurial connective tissue binds the fascicles together and contains the nutrient arteries.

Peripheral nerve fibers are either myelinated or unmyelinated (Fig. 28-152). Myelinated fibers range from 1 to 20 μm in diameter, whereas unmyelinated ones are considerably smaller, measuring 0.4 to 2.4 μm. Myelin is an elaboration of the Schwann cell plasmalemma and is necessary for saltatory nerve conduction. Schwann cells ensheathe both the myelinated and the unmyelinated fibers. The axon determines whether the ensheathing Schwann cell differentiates into a myelin-forming cell. Myelin-sheath thickness, internodal length (i.e., the distance between two nodes of Ranvier), and conduction velocity are proportional to the axonal diameter.

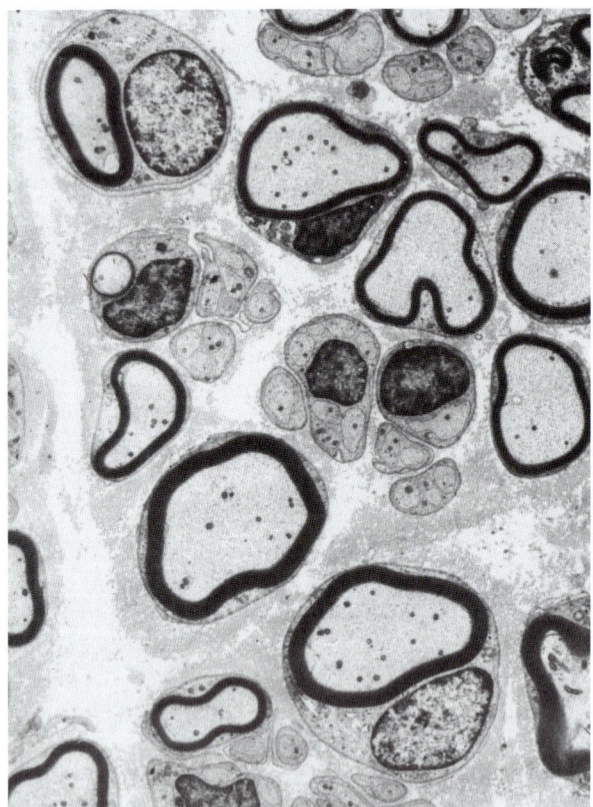

FIGURE 28-152
Structure of peripheral nerve. Electron micrograph of a peripheral nerve shows myelinated fibers interspersed with groups of unmyelinated fibers. Note that unlike myelinated axons, several unmyelinated axons may share a Schwann cell.

REACTIONS TO INJURY

Peripheral nerve fibers display only a limited number of reactions to injury. The major types of nerve fiber damage are axonal degeneration and segmental demyelination. The peripheral nervous system differs from the CNS in having the capacity for functionally significant axonal regeneration and remyelination.

Axonal Degeneration May Be Followed by Regeneration

Degeneration (necrosis) of the axon occurs in many neuropathies and reflects significant injury of the neuronal cell body or its axon. Axonal degeneration is quickly followed by breakdown of the myelin sheath and Schwann cell proliferation. Myelin degradation is initiated by Schwann cells and completed by macrophages, which infiltrate the nerve within 3 days after axonal degeneration. If the degeneration is restricted to the distal axon, regenerating axons may sprout within 1 week from the intact, proximal axonal stump. There are several types of axonal degeneration.

DISTAL AXONAL DEGENERATION: In many neuropathies, axonal degeneration is initially restricted to the distal ends of the larger, longer fibers (Fig. 28-153). Peripheral neuropathies characterized by the selective degeneration of distal axons are known as *dying-back neuropathies* (distal axonopathies) and are typically seen as distal ("glove-and-stocking") neuropathies.

In distal axonal degeneration, the neuronal cell body and proximal axon remain intact. Therefore, axonal regeneration and return of nerve function may be possible if the cause of the distal axonal degeneration can be identified and removed. This must occur before the dying-back degeneration extends enough centripetally to involve the proximal axon and cell body. Recovery is also limited in some dying-back neuropathies, because the distal axonal degeneration involves not only the peripherally directed axon of the dorsal root-ganglion neuron, but also its centrally directed axon traveling in the dorsal columns of the spinal cord. These centrally directed axons, like other axons within the CNS, have little capacity for regeneration.

NEURONOPATHY: Axonal degeneration may result from death of the neuronal cell body, as occurs in dorsal root ganglionitis. Neuropathies showing selective damage to the neuronal cell body are referred to as *neuronopathies* and are much less common than distal axonopathies. There is little potential for recovery of function in neuronopathy because death of the neuronal cell body precludes axonal regeneration.

WALLERIAN DEGENERATION: This term refers to the axonal degeneration that occurs in a nerve distal to a transection or crush of the nerve. In some instances the distal nerve regenerates.

Segmental Demyelination Is Common in Many Neuropathies

The loss of myelin from one or more internodes (segments) along a myelinated fiber reflects Schwann cell dysfunction (Fig. 28-153). This condition may be caused by direct injury to the Schwann cell or myelin sheath *(primary demyelination)*, or it may result from underlying axonal abnormalities *(secondary demyelination)*.

The loss of the myelin sheath is not accompanied by degeneration of the underlying axon. Macrophages infiltrate the nerve and clear the myelin debris. Degeneration of the internodal myelin sheath is followed sequentially by (1) Schwann cell proliferation, (2) remyelination of the demyelinated segments, and (3) recovery of function. The remyelinated internodes have shortened internodal lengths. Repeated episodes of segmental demyelination and remyelination of peripheral nerves, as occurs in chronic demyelinating neuropathies, lead to the accumulation of supernumerary Schwann cells around axons *(onion-bulbs)* and clinically apparent nerve enlargement *(hypertrophic neuropathy;* Fig. 28-154).

A. INTACT MYELINATED FIBER

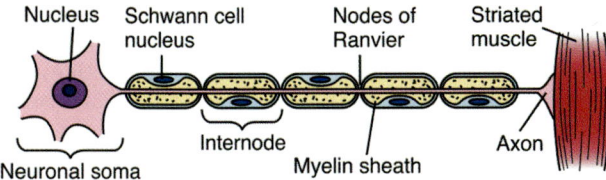

B. DISTAL AXONAL DEGENERATION

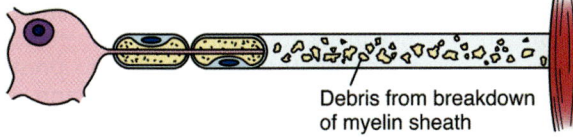

C. DEGENERATION OF CELL BODY AND AXON

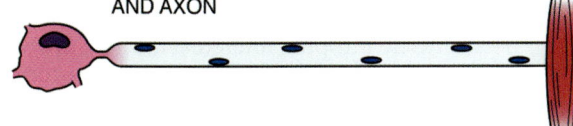

D. SEGMENTAL DEMYELINATION

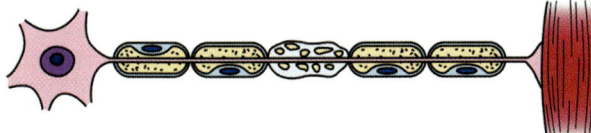

E. REMYELINATION

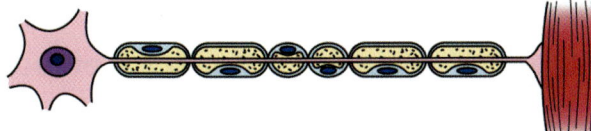

F. REGENERATING AXON

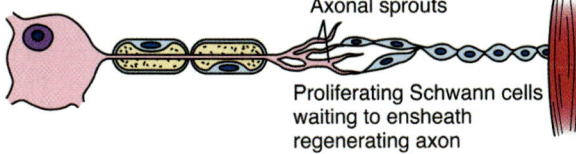

G. REGENERATED NERVE FIBER

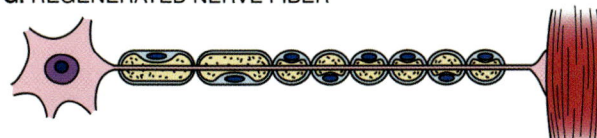

FIGURE 28-153
Basic responses of peripheral nerve fibers to injury.

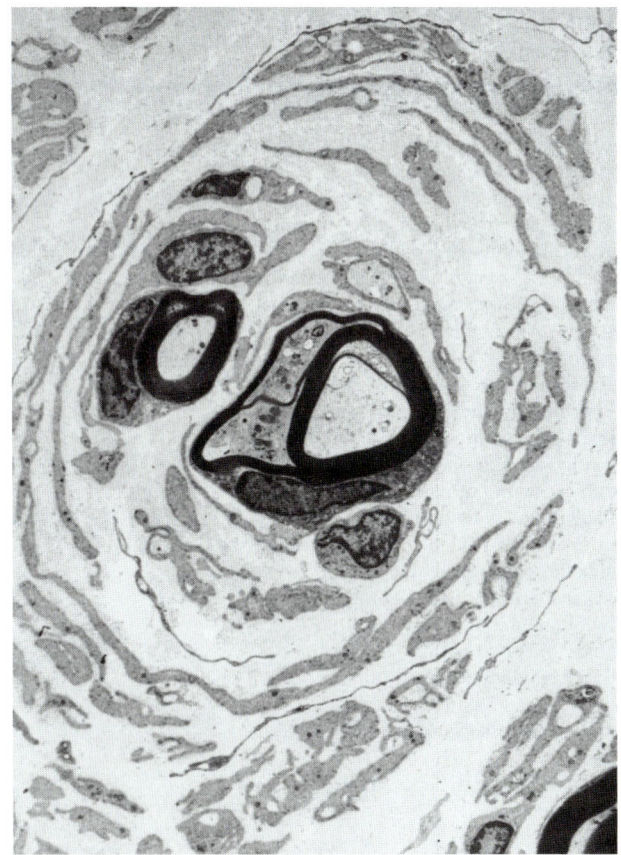

FIGURE 28-154
Onion-bulb formation in peripheral nerve. Electron micrograph shows multiple layers of flattened Schwann cell processes encircling two myelinated axons. Onion-bulb formations are common in the demyelinating form of Charcot-Marie-Tooth disease.

PERIPHERAL NEUROPATHIES

Peripheral neuropathy is a process that affects the function of one or more peripheral nerves. The disease may be restricted to the peripheral nervous system, involve both the peripheral and central nervous systems, or affect multiple organ systems. Peripheral neuropathies are encountered in all age groups and may be hereditary or acquired.

The causes of peripheral neuropathy are diverse (Table 28-7). Diabetic neuropathy is the most common neuropathy in the United States. Other common causes of neuropathy include alcoholism, renal failure, neurotoxic drugs, autoimmune diseases, monoclonal gammopathy, Charcot-Marie-Tooth disease, and HIV infection.

Pathology: The pathological findings in most neuropathies are limited to mainly axonal degeneration, mainly segmental demyelination, or a combination of both. When axonal degeneration predominates, the neuropathy is classified as an *axonal neuropathy;* when segmental demyelination predominates, the neuropathy is classified as *demyelinating neuropathy*. Most (80–90%) neuropathies are axonal. Electrophysiological studies often help to differentiate between axonal and demyelinating neuropathies. Nerve-conduction velocity is typically near normal in axonal neuropathies but conspicuously decreased in demyelinating neuropathies.

Many neuropathies do not show additional disease-specific histological features beyond axonal loss or demyelination, so that clinicopathological correlation is necessary to establish causation. A small number of neuropathies have disease-specific histological features, such as necrotizing arteritis (vasculitic neuropathy), granulomatous inflammation (leprosy, sarcoid), amyloid deposits (amyloid neuropathy), abnormalities of the myelin sheath (IgM paraproteinemic neuropathy, hereditary neuropathy with liability to pressure palsies), or abnormal accumulations in Schwann cells (leukodystrophy) or axons (giant axonal neuropathy).

Clinical Features: The major clinical manifestations of peripheral neuropathy are muscle weakness, muscle atrophy, altered sensation, and autonomic dysfunction. Motor, sensory, and autonomic functions may be equally or preferentially affected. Sensory abnormalities may reflect predominant involvement of large-diameter fibers (position and vibration sense) or small-diameter fibers (pain and temperature). The tempo of the neuropathy may be acute (days to weeks), subacute (weeks to months), or chronic (months to years). The disease may be localized to one nerve (*mononeuropathy*) or several nerves (*mononeuropathy multiplex*), or it may be diffuse and symmetric (*polyneuropathy*).

TABLE 28-7 Etiological Classification of Neuropathies

Immune mediated
Acute inflammatory demyelinating polyneuropathy
Acute motor axonal neuropathy
Acute motor sensory axonal neuropathy
Chronic inflammatory demyelinating polyneuropathy
Multifocal motor neuropathy
Dorsal root ganglionitis (sensory neuronopathy)
Neuropathies associated with monoclonal gammopathy
Vasculitic neuropathy
Metabolic
Diabetic polyneuropathy and mononeuropathies
Uremic neuropathy
Hepatic neuropathy
Hypothyroid neuropathy
Porphyric neuropathy
Critical illness polyneuropathy
Neuropathy associated with deficiency of vitamin B_1, B_6, B_{12}, or E
Alcoholic neuropathy
Toxic and drug-induced neuropathies
Amyloid neuropathy
AL amyloid neuropathy
Familial amyloid neuropathy
Hereditary neuropathies
Neuropathies associated with infections
Leprosy
Human immunodeficiency virus
Cytomegalovirus
Herpes zoster
Lyme disease
Diphtheria (toxin)
Paraneoplastic neuropathies
Sarcoid neuropathy
Radiation neuropathy
Traumatic neuropathy
Chronic idiopathic axonal neuropathy

Diabetic Neuropathies Reflect Metabolic or Ischemic Damage

Peripheral neuropathy is a common complication of diabetes mellitus. The neuropathy may manifest as a distal sensory or sensorimotor polyneuropathy, autonomic neuropathy, mononeuropathy, or mononeuropathy multiplex. The mononeuropathies may involve cranial nerves (cranial neuropathy), nerve roots (radiculopathy), or proximal peripheral nerves. **Distal, predominantly sensory, polyneuropathy is the most common form of diabetic neuropathy.**

Pathogenesis: The pathogenesis of the nerve fiber injury in diabetes is unknown. It has long been held that the metabolic alterations of diabetes are responsible for the distal symmetric polyneuropathy, and that nerve ischemia caused by the small-vessel disease causes mononeuropathies. There is some evidence, however, to suggest that local nerve ischemia may also play a role in the pathogenesis of symmetric polyneuropathy.

Pathology: The distal symmetric polyneuropathy of diabetes is characterized pathologically by a mixture of axonal degeneration and segmental demyelination, with axonal degeneration predominating. The axonal loss involves fibers of all sizes, but occasionally preferentially affects the large myelinated fibers *(large-fiber neuropathy)* or the small myelinated fibers and unmyelinated fibers *(small-fiber neuropathy)*. There may also be loss of neurons in the dorsal root ganglia and anterior horns, but this appears to be a consequence of centripetal progression of dying-back axonal degeneration rather than a neuronopathy.

Uremic Neuropathy May Complicate Chronic Renal Failure

Uremic neuropathy is a distal sensorimotor axonal polyneuropathy. The pathogenesis of the nerve fiber damage is not known, but the disease usually stabilizes or improves with long-term dialysis. Uremic neuropathy is characterized pathologically by both distal axonal degeneration and segmental demyelination, with axonal degeneration predominating and preferentially involving large-diameter fibers. The neuropathy resolves after renal transplantation.

Critical Illness Polyneuropathy Is Associated with Sepsis and Multiorgan Failure

Critical illness polyneuropathy is a distal axonal neuropathy that develops in severely ill patients. The pathogenesis of the condition is obscure. The acute, predominantly motor, neuropathy may first become apparent when the patient cannot be weaned from ventilatory support. A *critical illness myopathy* may also occur in these patients.

Alcoholic Neuropathy Usually Results from Nutritional Deficiencies

Alcoholic neuropathy is a distal sensorimotor axonal polyneuropathy that is generally attributed to nutritional deficiencies and possibly to a direct toxic effect of ethanol on the peripheral nervous system. Peripheral nerves show loss of nerve fibers from axonal degeneration of the dying-back type. Axonal neuropathy is also associated with a lack of vitamins B_1, B_6, B_{12}, or E but is much less common in the United States than is alcoholic neuropathy. The toxic axonal neuropathy associated with isoniazid therapy for tuberculosis is due to the drug's interference with the metabolism of vitamin B_6.

Acute Inflammatory Demyelinating Polyneuropathy (Guillain-Barré Syndrome) Is Immune-Mediated

Acute inflammatory demyelinating polyneuropathy (AIDP) is an acquired, immune-mediated neuropathy that often follows immunization or viral, bacterial and mycoplasmal infections. It may also be sporadic or complicate surgery, cancer, or HIV infection. AIDP is the most common cause of acute polyneuropathy in children and adults. Motor dysfunction usually predominates over sensory or autonomic disturbances. Some 5% of cases are seen with ophthalmoplegia, ataxia, and areflexia *(Fisher syndrome)*. The muscular paralysis may cause respiratory embarrassment, and the autonomic involvement may result in cardiac arrhythmias, hypotension, or hypertension. Resolution of the neuropathy begins 2 to 4 weeks after onset, and most patients make a good recovery. Lumbar puncture characteristically reveals an increased protein level in the CSF and no pleocytosis. The increased protein level is attributable to the inflammation of the spinal roots. Current evidence suggests that the demyelination is immunologically mediated, and plasmapheresis and intravenously administered gamma globulin have proven beneficial.

AIDP may involve all levels of the peripheral nervous system, including spinal roots (polyradiculoneuropathy), ganglia, craniospinal nerves, and autonomic nerves. The distribution of the lesions varies from case to case. Involved regions show endoneurial infiltrates of lymphocytes and macrophages, segmental demyelination, and relative sparing of axons. The lymphoid infiltrates are often perivascular, but there is no true vasculitis. Macrophages are frequently found adjacent to degenerating myelin sheaths and have been observed to strip off and phagocytose the superficial myelin lamellae. Such macrophage-mediated demyelination is rarely observed in other neuropathies.

Acute motor axonal neuropathy and *acute motor sensory axonal neuropathy* manifest clinically as the Guillain-Barré syndrome and are often associated with prior *Campylobacter jejuni* infection.

Chronic inflammatory demyelinating polyneuropathy (CIDP) is similar to Guillain-Barré syndrome but has a chronic course characterized by multiple relapses or a slow continuous progression. The nerves in CIDP may show numerous onion bulbs, owing to recurring episodes of demyelination, Schwann cell proliferation, and remyelination. Corticosteroid therapy is effective in CIDP but not in Guillain-Barré syndrome, suggesting that the two neuropathies may have a different immune-mediated pathogenesis.

Multifocal motor neuropathy is a rare, slowly progressive, multiple mononeuropathy that may be mistaken clinically for motor neuron disease. The neuropathy is characterized pathologically by demyelination, suggesting that it is related to CIDP. There is often an associated increased titer of anti-GM_1 antibodies, but no role for these antibodies in the pathogenesis of the disorder has been demonstrated. The neuropathy responds to intravenously administered gamma globulin.

Dorsal Root Ganglionitis (Sensory Neuronopathy) Is Idiopathic or Paraneoplastic

This neuronopathy typically manifests as a subacute or chronic sensory polyneuropathy with sensory ataxia. Although the pathogenesis of neuronal degeneration is unknown, an immune mechanism is likely, and the disorder has occurred in association with Sjögren syndrome. Paraneoplastic sensory neuronopathy is frequently associated with anti-Hu antibodies (antineuronal autoantibodies). The dorsal root ganglia show infiltration by lymphocytes and loss of sensory neurons.

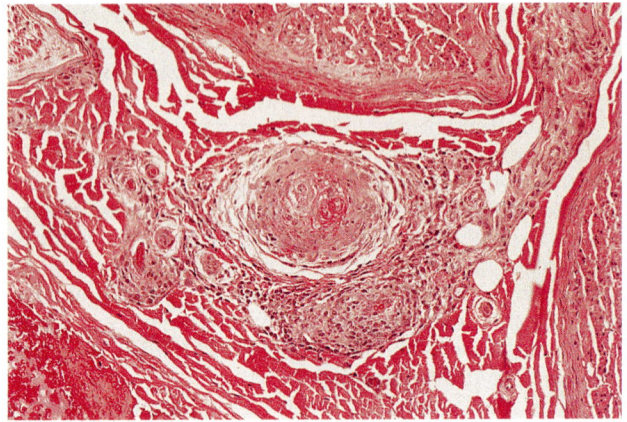

FIGURE 28-155
Vasculitic neuropathy in a patient with polyarteritis nodosa. Photomicrograph of a cross-section of a sural nerve reveals an inflamed epineurial artery with a disorganized wall and thrombosis in its lumen.

Vasculitic Neuropathy Is Ischemic

Vasculitis may involve the nutrient arteries of nerves as a manifestation of a more widespread, multiorgan disease, such as polyarteritis nodosa, rheumatoid arthritis, cryoglobulinemia, HIV infection, or cancer. In about a third of cases, the necrotizing arteritis appears limited to the peripheral nervous system *(nonsystemic vasculitic neuropathy)*. Vasculitic neuropathy is characterized pathologically by axonal degeneration and occurs as a mononeuropathy or mononeuropathy multiplex (Fig. 28-155).

Neuropathies May Be Associated with Monoclonal Gammopathy

Monoclonal gammopathy may cause an amyloid neuropathy, a cryoglobulinemia-associated vasculitic neuropathy, a chronic axonal polyneuropathy, or a chronic demyelinating polyneuropathy. The monoclonal gammopathy may be of undetermined significance (MGUS) or due to a plasma cell neoplasm. The pathogenesis of the paraproteinemia-associated axonal polyneuropathy is unknown. Chronic demyelinating polyneuropathy often occurs with an IgM MGUS or Waldenström macroglobulinemia, in which the paraprotein binds to myelin-associated glycoprotein (MAG), suggesting that anti-MAG antibodies are involved in the pathogenesis of demyelination. Anti-MAG antibody neuropathy is characterized pathologically by extensive segmental demyelination, a variable number of onion bulbs, axonal loss, and a distinctive widening of the myelin lamellae (Fig. 28-156). Paraproteinemic neuropathy may rarely present as the POEMS syndrome (polyneuropathy, organomegaly, endocrinopathy, monoclonal gammopathy, and skin changes).

Amyloid Neuropathy Features a Distal Sensorimotor Axonal Polyneuropathy

In addition to its effects on sensory and motor nerves, amyloid infiltration of the peripheral nervous system often leads to prominent autonomic dysfunction. Although the disorder may be hereditary, it more commonly complicates light-chain (AL) amyloidosis associated with primary systemic amyloidosis or multiple myeloma. A point mutation in the transthyretin (prealbumin) gene is responsible for most cases of dominantly inherited, familial amyloid polyneuropathy. Pathologically, amyloid neuropathy is characterized by the deposition of amyloid in peripheral nerves, dorsal root ganglia, and autonomic ganglia. The interstitial amyloid deposits are both endoneurial and epineurial and frequently involve the walls of blood vessels. The deposition of amyloid is accompanied by loss of myelinated and unmyelinated fibers. Postulated mechanisms for the nerve-fiber damage include direct mechanical injury of nerve fibers and ganglion cells by amyloid deposits and nerve ischemia caused by amyloid infiltration of the vasa nervorum.

Carpal tunnel syndrome is a chronic entrapment neuropathy of the median nerve at the wrist and represents another complication of systemic amyloidosis. The nerve entrapment results from amyloid infiltration of the flexor retinaculum. Many other conditions, including occupational injuries, are also associated with carpal tunnel syndrome.

Paraneoplastic Neuropathies Often Precede Recognition of Cancer

In addition to neuropathies, other paraneoplastic diseases of the nervous system include chronic encephalomyelitis,

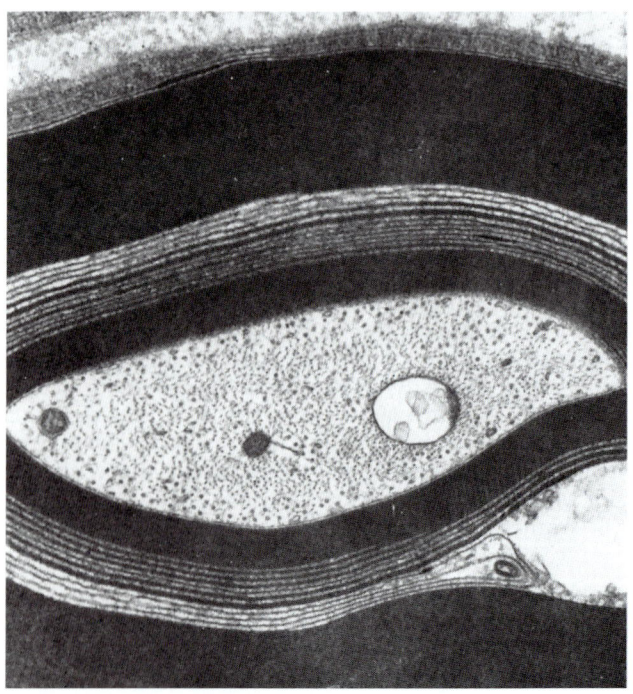

FIGURE 28-156
Paraproteinemic neuropathy. An electron micrograph shows a myelinated fiber with multiple, abnormally widely spaced, myelin lamellae from a patient with an IgM monoclonal gammopathy of unknown significance and a chronic demyelinating neuropathy.

necrotizing myelopathy, cerebellar degeneration, and the Eaton-Lambert syndrome. Several different clinicopathological types of paraneoplastic neuropathy have been defined.

- **Paraneoplastic sensorimotor polyneuropathy:** This distal polyneuropathy is characterized by axonal degeneration and demyelination, with axonal loss predominating.
- **Paraneoplastic sensory neuronopathy:** Less commonly, paraneoplastic neuropathy may manifest as a subacute sensory neuronopathy due to a dorsal root ganglionitis. Similar histological changes may also occur in the CNS (*paraneoplastic encephalomyelitis*). Anti-Hu antibodies are often present in these patients, and small cell carcinoma of the lung is the usual cause.
- **Inflammatory demyelinating polyneuropathy:** Guillain-Barré and chronic inflammatory demyelinating polyneuropathy may be associated with cancer.
- **Paraneoplastic vasculitic neuropathy:** Vasculitic neuropathy may rarely complicate cancer.

Not all neuropathies associated with cancer result from remote effects of the neoplasm on the nervous system. Cancer may cause neuropathy by direct compression or infiltration of nerves or nerve roots. Cancer patients may also develop chemotherapy-induced toxic neuropathy or radiation-induced neuropathy (brachial or lumbosacral plexopathy).

Toxic Neuropathy Is Mostly Iatrogenic

A wide variety of environmental agents and industrial compounds cause peripheral neuropathy (Table 28-8), but most cases of toxic neuropathy are caused by drugs. Most toxic neuropathies are characterized by axonal degeneration, usually of the dying-back type. Amiodarone, buckthorn toxin, and diphtheria toxin are notable for producing demyelinating neuropathies. Persons with hereditary neuropathy may be especially vulnerable to drug-induced peripheral neuropathy.

TABLE 28-8 **Agents Associated with Toxic Neuropathy**

Drugs	Environmental and Industrial Agents
Amiodarone	Acrylamide
Chloramphenicol	Allyl chloride
Colchicine	Arsenic
Dapsone	Buckthorn toxin
Disulfiram	Carbon disulfide
Ethambutol	Chlordecone
Gold	Dimethylaminopropionitrile
Isoniazid	Diphtheria toxin
Metronidazole	Ethylene oxide
Misonidazole	*n*-Hexane (glue sniffing)
Nitrofurantoin	Methyl *n*-butyl ketone
Nucleoside analogues (antiretrovirals)	Lead
Paclitaxel (taxanes)	Mercury
Phenytoin	Methyl bromide
Platinum	Organophosphates
Pyridoxine (vitamin B_6)	Polychlorinated biphenyls
Suramin	Thallium
Thalidomide	Trichloroethylene
Vincristine	Vacor

TABLE 28-9 **Inherited Diseases Associated with Neuropathy**

Abetalipoproteinemia
Fabry disease (α-galactosidase A deficiency)
Familial amyloid polyneuropathies
Apolipoprotein A_1 amyloidosis
Gelsolin amyloidosis
Transthyretin amyloidosis
Friedreich ataxia
Giant axonal neuropathy
Hereditary motor and sensory neuropathies (Charcot-Marie-Tooth disease)
Hereditary motor neuropathies (spinal muscular atrophies)
Hereditary sensory and autonomic neuropathies
Leukodystrophies
Adrenoleukodystrophy
Globoid cell leukodystrophy
Metachromatic leukodystrophy
Porphyrias
Refsum disease (phytanic acid storage disease)
Tangier disease

Hereditary Neuropathies Are the Most Common Form of Chronic Neuropathy in Children

Peripheral neuropathy is a manifestation of a variety of inherited diseases (Table 28-9) and is often of unrecognized cause in adults.

CHARCOT-MARIE-TOOTH DISEASE (CMT): CMT is a genetically and pathologically heterogeneous group of slowly progressive distal sensorimotor polyneuropathies that manifest in childhood or early adult life. It is the most common inherited neuropathy and among the most common inherited neurological disorders. CMT may be broadly divided into demyelinating and axonal forms. *CMT1*, the most common type, has autosomal dominant inheritance and a chronic demyelinating polyneuropathy with onion bulbs and axonal loss. The less common *CMT2* shows autosomal dominant inheritance and dying-back axonal neuropathy. X-linked (*CMTX*) and autosomal recessive (*CMT4*) types have also been described. Mutations in a growing number of genes have been associated with the CMT phenotype. The subtypes of CMT are defined by their specific genetic defects (Table 28-10).

Dejerine-Sottas syndrome resembles CMT1, but is much more severe, with onset in early infancy. Peripheral nerves show a severe demyelinating neuropathy with onion bulbs and axonal loss.

Hereditary neuropathy with liability to pressure palsies typically manifests with recurrent mononeuropathies. The nerves show demyelination, distinctive sausage-shaped thickenings (tomacula) of the myelin sheaths, and axonal loss.

TABLE 28-10 Charcot-Marie-Tooth Disease (CMT) and Related Hereditary Motor and Sensory Neuropathies (HMSN)

Disease	Inheritance	Linkage	Candidate Gene	Pathology
CMT1A (HMSN IA)	Dominant	Chromosome 17	Peripheral myelin protein-22 (PMP22)	Chronic demyelinating polyneuropathy with numerous onions bulbs and nerve hypertrophy; distal axonal degeneration also is present
CMT1B (HMSN IB)	Dominant	Chromosome 1	Myelin protein zero (P_0) (a protein of PNS myelin)	
CMTX1	Dominant	Chromosome X	Connexin-32 (a gap junction protein)	
CMT2 (HMSN II)	Dominant	Chromosome 1	Unknown	Distal axonal degeneration
Dejerine-Sottas syndrome (HMSN III)	Recessive or dominant	Chromosome 17 or 1	PMP22 or P_0	Chronic demyelinating neuropathy with onion bulbs and nerve hypertrophy; distal axonal degeneration also is present
Hereditary liability to pressure palsies	Dominant	Chromosome 17	PMP22	Chronic demyelinating neuropathy with focally thickened myelin sheaths (tomacula) and axonal degeneration

Neuropathies Are a Complication of AIDS

Peripheral neuropathy is a common complaint in persons infected with HIV. The neuropathy may manifest clinically as a distal symmetric polyneuropathy, a mononeuropathy, or a lumbosacral polyradiculopathy.

- **Distal sensory polyneuropathy** is the most common type of neuropathy associated with HIV infection. The disorder is characterized by distal axonal degeneration and usually occurs during the later stages of AIDS. The pathogenesis of the axonal degeneration is obscure, and there is no effective therapy.
- **Inflammatory demyelinating polyneuropathy** associated with AIDS may be acute or chronic. The disorder is thought to be immunologically mediated. It typically occurs early in the course of HIV infection, before the full onset of AIDS. The neuropathy often responds to plasmapheresis, intravenous gamma globulin, or corticosteroids.
- **Cytomegalovirus infection** of the peripheral nervous system is responsible for some of the mononeuropathies and lumbosacral polyradiculopathies associated with AIDS.
- **Vasculitic neuropathy** may cause mononeuropathy and mononeuropathy multiplex in some AIDS patients.
- **Toxic neuropathy** is caused by several drugs used in the therapy of AIDS. These drug-induced axonal neuropathies are clinically similar to AIDS-associated distal sensory polyneuropathy.

Chronic Idiopathic Axonal Neuropathy

In 10 to 20% of patients who have peripheral neuropathy, no cause is apparent despite careful and extensive investigation. These cryptogenic neuropathies typically occur in older patients as chronic, distal, sensorimotor axonal polyneuropathy and have an indolent course.

NERVE TRAUMA

Traumatic Neuroma Is a Mass of Regenerating Axons and Scar Tissue

Traumatic neuroma forms at the end of the proximal stump of a nerve that has been disrupted physically. After transection of a peripheral nerve, regenerating axonal sprouts arise within 1 week from the distal ends of the intact axons in the proximal nerve stump. If the severed ends of the proximal and distal nerve stumps are closely approximated, the regenerating axonal sprouts may find and reinnervate the distal stump. The regenerating axons advance in the distal stump at a rate of about 1 mm/day. However, in many instances, the severed ends of the nerve are not closely approximated, and there is considerable scar tissue between the proximal and distal stumps. The wide gap between the proximal and distal stumps prevents the regenerating sprouts from successfully reinnervating the distal stump. In this situation, the regenerating axons grow haphazardly into the scar tissue at the end of the proximal stump to form a painful swelling known as a traumatic or *amputation neuroma.*

Plantar Interdigital Neuroma (Morton Neuroma) Is a Painful Lesion of the Foot

Plantar interdigital neuroma is a painful, sausage-shaped swelling of the plantar digital nerve between the second and third or third and fourth metatarsal bones. It is probably caused by repeated nerve compression. The swelling is not a true neuroma, because it results from endoneurial, perineurial, and epineurial fibrosis rather than a mass of regenerating axons. The fibrotic nerve also shows nerve fiber loss and areas of myxoid degeneration. Morton neuroma is particularly common in women who wear high heels.

TUMORS

Primary tumors of the peripheral nervous system are of neuronal or nerve sheath origin. The neuronal tumors (e.g., neuroblastoma and ganglioneuroma) usually arise from the adrenal medulla or sympathetic ganglia. The common nerve sheath tumors are schwannoma and neurofibroma.

Schwannoma May Arise in Any Nerve

Schwannoma is a benign, slowly growing, typically encapsulated neoplasm of Schwann cells that originates in cranial nerves, spinal roots, or peripheral nerves. These tumors usually are seen in adults and only very rarely undergo malignant degeneration.

VESTIBULAR SCHWANNOMA (ACOUSTIC SCHWANNOMA): Intracranial schwannomas account for 8% of all intracranial tumors. They arise from the eighth cranial nerve within the internal auditory canal or at the meatus and cause unilateral, sensorineural hearing loss and tinnitus. The slowly growing tumor enlarges the meatus, extends medially into the subarachnoid space of the cerebellopontine angle *(cerebellopontine angle tumor)*, and compresses the fifth and seventh cranial nerves, brainstem, and cerebellum. The posterior fossa mass may also lead to increased intracranial pressure, hydrocephalus, and tonsillar herniation. Most vestibular schwannomas are unilateral and are not associated with NF. Bilateral vestibular schwannomas are a defining feature of NF2.

INTRASPINAL AND PERIPHERAL SCHWANNOMAS: Intraspinal schwannomas are intradural or extramedullary tumors that arise most often from the dorsal (sensory) spinal roots. They produce radicular (root) pain and spinal cord compression. More-peripheral schwannomas usually arise on nerves of the head, neck, and extremities.

 Pathology: Schwannomas tend to be oval and well demarcated and vary in diameter from a few millimeters to several centimeters. The nerve of origin, if large enough, may be identifiable. The cut surface is firm and tan to gray, and often shows focal hemorrhage, necrosis, xanthomatous change, and cystic degeneration. Microscopically, the proliferating Schwann cells form two distinctive histological patterns (Fig. 28-157).
Antoni A pattern is characterized by interwoven fascicles of spindle cells with elongated nuclei, eosinophilic cytoplasm, and indistinct cytoplasmic borders. The nuclei may palisade in areas to form structures known as *Verocay bodies*.
Antoni B pattern features spindle or oval cells with indistinct cytoplasm in a loose vacuolated background.

Degenerative changes in schwannomas are common and include collections of foam cells, recent or old hemorrhage, foci of fibrosis, and hyalinized blood vessels. Scattered atypical nuclei are frequently encountered in schwannomas, but mitotic figures are uncommon.

Neurofibroma Features Several Cell Types

Neurofibroma is a benign, slowly growing tumor of peripheral nerve composed of Schwann cells, perineurial-like cells, and fibroblasts. A distinction between neurofibroma and schwannoma is warranted because of the close association of neurofibroma with neurofibromatosis 1 (NF1) and its potential for sarcomatous degeneration to malignant peripheral nerve sheath tumor.

Neurofibromas may be solitary or multiple and may arise on any nerve. They are found in both children and adults. Most commonly, neurofibromas involve skin, major nerve plexuses, large deep nerve trunks, retroperitoneum, and gastrointestinal tract. Most *solitary cutaneous neurofibromas* occur outside the context of NF and do not have the potential for sarcomatous degeneration. The presence of multiple neurofibromas or one large plexiform neurofibroma is virtually diagnostic of NF1 and should prompt a careful search for other stigmata of the disease.

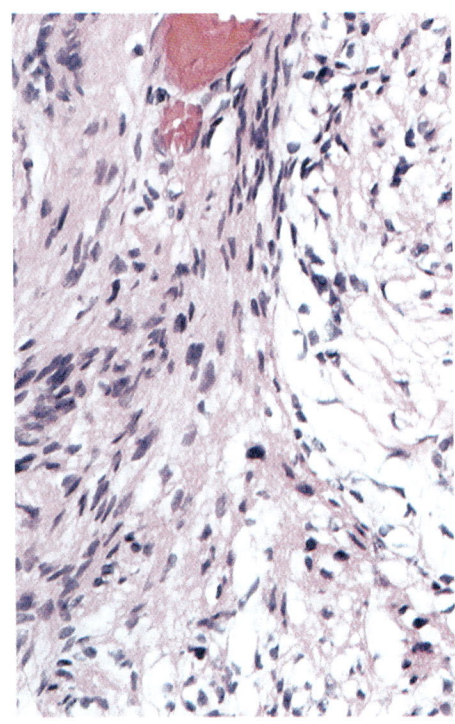

FIGURE 28-157
Schwannoma. A photomicrograph shows the characteristically abrupt transition between the compact Antoni type A histological pattern *(left)* and the spongy Antoni type B histological pattern *(right)*.

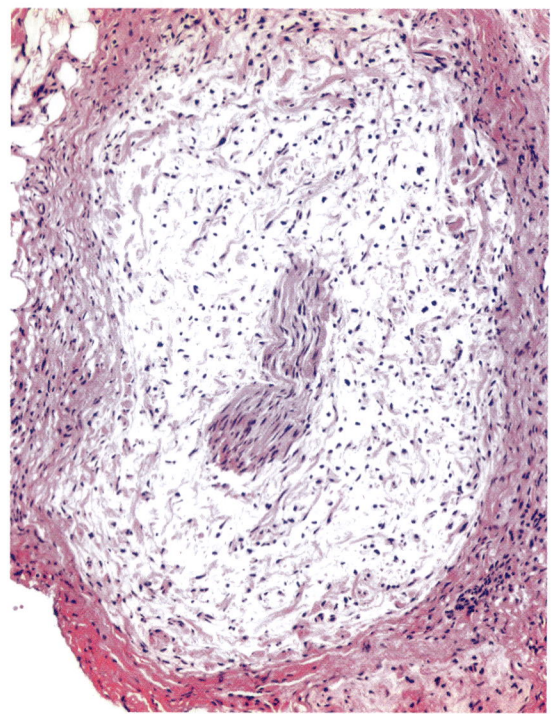

FIGURE 28-158
Neurofibroma. Photomicrograph shows that the proliferating spindle-shaped Schwann cells form small strands that course haphazardly through a myxoid matrix.

Pathology: On gross examination, a neurofibroma arising in a large nerve appears as a poorly circumscribed, fusiform enlargement. The diffuse, intrafascicular growth of the tumor within multiple nerve fascicles may so enlarge the nerve's fascicles that they appear grossly to be the cords of a nerve plexus (*plexiform neurofibroma*). Neurofibroma may involve long segments of the nerve, making complete surgical excision impossible. When they arise from small nerves, the nerve of origin may not be apparent. Cutaneous neurofibromas originate from dermal nerves and are seen as soft nodular or pedunculated skin tumors.

The cut surface of a neurofibroma is soft and light gray, and the enlarged nerve fascicles of the plexiform neurofibroma may be prominent. Microscopically, a tumor arising in a large nerve is characterized by an endoneurial proliferation of spindle cells with elongated nuclei, eosinophilic cytoplasm and indistinct cell borders (Fig. 28-158). Interspersed among the spindle cells are an extracellular myxoid matrix, wavy bands of collagen and residual nerve fibers. The coursing of nerve fibers through the neurofibroma contrasts with the pattern in schwannoma, in which nerve fibers are pushed peripherally into the tumor capsule. The neurofibromatous proliferation often extends beyond the nerve fascicle into the adjacent tissue.

Some 2 to 5% of NF1-associated neurofibromas exhibit sarcomatous transformation to malignant peripheral nerve sheath tumor. The presence of increased cellularity and mitotic figures heralds malignant transformation.

Malignant Peripheral Nerve Sheath Tumor (Malignant Schwannoma, Neurofibrosarcoma)

Malignant peripheral nerve sheath tumor (MPNST) is a poorly differentiated, spindle cell sarcoma of peripheral nerve of uncertain histogenesis. The tumor may arise de novo or from malignant transformation of a neurofibroma. MPNST is most common in adults and typically arises in larger nerves of the trunk or proximal limbs. **About half of these sarcomas occur in patients with neurofibromatosis.** There is an increased incidence of MPNST at sites of previous irradiation.

MPNST manifests grossly as an unencapsulated, fusiform enlargement of a nerve. Microscopically, the neoplasm resembles fibrosarcoma. The tumor is prone to local recurrence and blood-borne metastases.

SUGGESTED READING

The Central Nervous System

Alison MR (ed): *Cancer handbook.* London: Nature Publishing Group, 2001.

Clark CM, Trojanowski JQ (eds): *Neurodegenerative dementias: Clinical features and pathological mechanisms.* New York: McGraw-Hill, 2000.

Esiri M, Lee VM-Y, Trojanowski JQ (eds): *The neuropathology of dementia.* Cambridge: Cambridge University Press, In press, 2002.

Geschwind D, Gregg J (eds): *Microarrays for the neuroscience: an essential guide,* Boston: MIT Press, 2002.

Graham DI, Lantos PL (eds): *Greenfield's neuropathology,* 7th ed. London: Hodder Arnold Press, 2002.

Kleihues P, Cavenee WK (eds): *Pathology and genetics of tumors of the nervous system,* 2nd ed. Lyon: International Agency for Cancer Research, 2000.

Rosenberg RN, Prusiner SB, Di Mauro S, et al. (eds): *The molecular and genetic basis of neurological and psychiatric disease,* 3rd ed, Woburn: Butterworth Heineman Press, In press, 2002.

The Peripheral Nervous System

Asbury AK, Thomas PK (eds): *Peripheral nerve disorders 2.* Oxford: Butterworth-Heinemann, 1995.

Dyck PJ, Thomas PK, Griffin JW, et al. (eds): *Peripheral neuropathy,* 3rd ed. Philadelphia: WB Saunders, 1993.

Enzinger FM, Weiss SW: *Soft tissue tumors,* 3rd ed. St. Louis: Mosby-Year Book, 1995.

Midroni G, Bilbao JM: *Biopsy diagnosis of peripheral neuropathies.* Boston: Butterworth-Heinemann, 1995.

Ouvrier RA: Peripheral neuropathies. In: Berg BO (ed): *Principles of child neurology.* New York: McGraw-Hill, 1996: 1607–1655.

Schaumburg HH, Berger AR, Thomas PK: *Disorders of peripheral nerves,* 2nd ed. Philadelphia: FA Davis, 1992.

CHAPTER 29

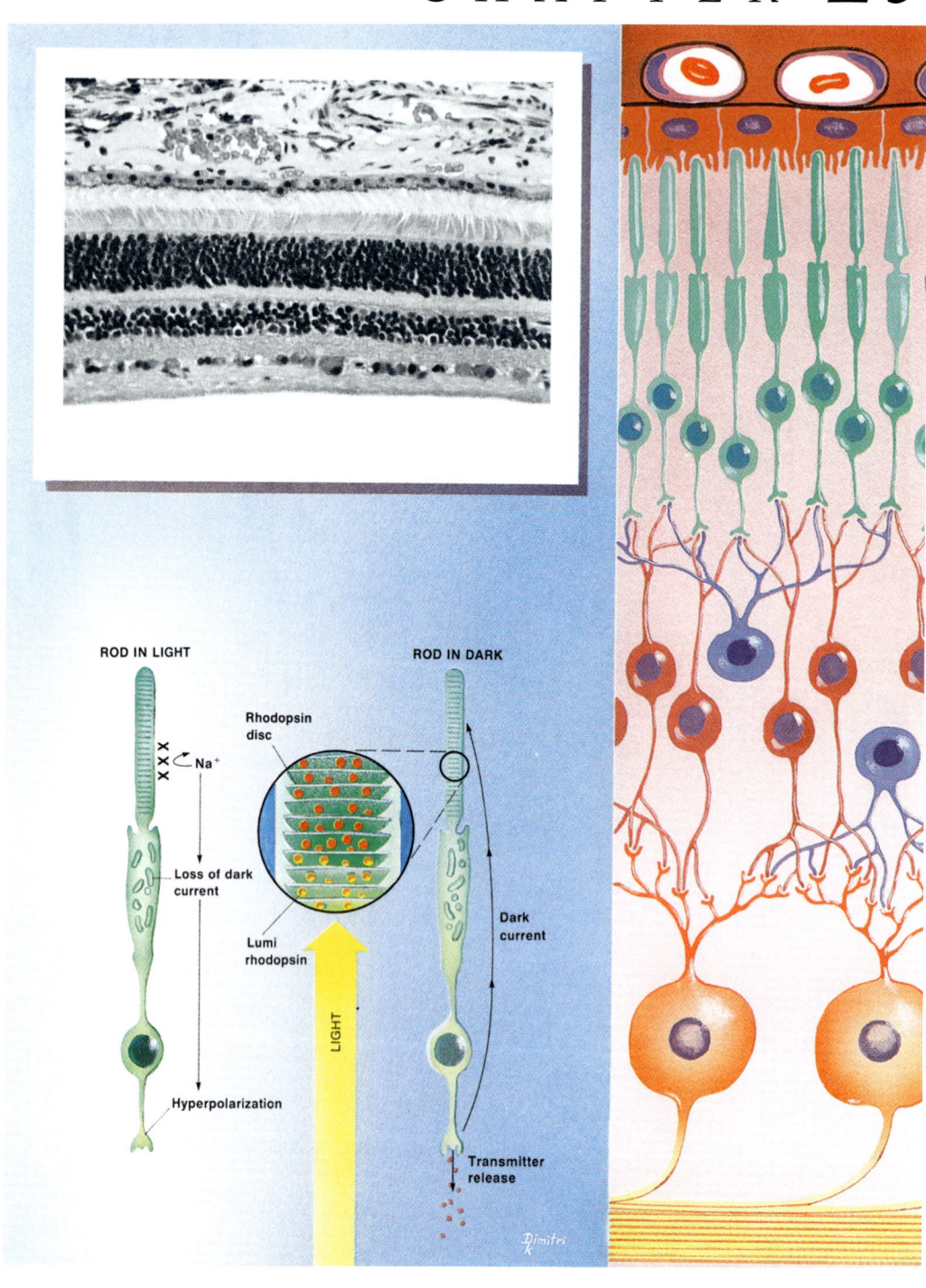

The Eye

Gordon K. Klintworth

Physical and Chemical Injuries

The Eyelids

The Orbit
Exophthalmos of Hyperthyroidism

The Conjunctiva
Hemorrhage
Conjunctivitis
Pinguecula and Pterygium

The Cornea
Herpes Simplex
Onchocerciasis
Arcus Lipoides (Arcus Senilis)
Band Keratopathy
Corneal Dystrophies
Cataracts
Presbyopia

The Uvea
Sympathetic Ophthalmitis
Sarcoidosis

The Retina
Retinal Hemorrhage
Retinal Occlusive Vascular Disease
Diabetic Retinopathy
Retinitis Pigmentosa
Macular Degeneration
Cherry-red Spot at the Macula
Angioid Streaks
Retinopathy of Prematurity

The Optic Nerve
Optic Nerve Head Edema
Optic Atrophy

Glaucoma
Types of Glaucoma
Effects of Increased Intraocular Pressure

Myopia

Phthisis Bulbi

Neoplasms
Malignant Melanoma
Retinoblastoma
Metastatic Intraocular and Orbital Neoplasms

FIGURE 29-1 *(see opposite page)*
The retinal basis of vision. The retina, the specialized tissue that responds to light, contains neurons arranged in distinct layers. In the vertebrate retina, light passes through the entire eye before reaching the photoreceptors (rods and cones). The outer segment of each photoreceptor is its light-sensitive region. The rod outer segment contains a dense stack of disc membranes in which the photoprotein, rhodopsin, is embedded. The biochemical transduction of light into neural impulses depends on ion fluxes.

The unprotected position of the eye makes it vulnerable to a host of injuries from physical trauma, toxic chemicals, solar radiation, adverse climatic conditions, and the harmful effects of light. Countless antigens and a myriad of microorganisms cause ocular disease in susceptible persons. The eye is also affected in numerous systemic diseases, and the recognition of ocular manifestations in these disorders aids in the clinical diagnosis of many conditions. Although life-threatening neoplasms are uncommon, many ocular afflictions cause severe visual impairment and frequently blindness.

PHYSICAL AND CHEMICAL INJURIES

Physical trauma to the eye commonly causes ecchymosis of the highly vascular eyelids (black eye); when this occurs, other parts of the eye also may be injured. Superficial disruptions of the corneal epithelium follow traumatic abrasions, prolonged wearing of a contact lens, foreign bodies on the eye, exposure to ultraviolet light, and exposure to caustic chemicals. Blunt trauma increases the intraorbital pressure momentarily, causing the bones in the floor of the orbit to fracture into the maxillary sinus *(blowout fracture)*. The inferior rectus muscle may become entrapped in the fracture, thereby causing the eye to sink into the orbit *(enophthalmos)*.

An almost infinite variety of foreign materials can injure the eye. Whereas small particles often lodge in the superficial ocular tissues, some penetrate into or through the eye. A foreign particle may damage the eye during entry or because of secondary infection after the introduction of microorganisms. Some foreign bodies provoke a prominent acute inflammatory or granulomatous reaction. Others, such as those containing iron, cause retinal degeneration and even discoloration of the ocular tissues *(siderosis bulbi)*, effects that may not be evident for several years. Other complications of ocular injuries include cataracts, retinal detachment, and glaucoma.

The eye is commonly injured by a variety of household and industrial chemicals that enter it accidentally or as a result of a malicious act. The damage created depends on the nature of the chemical.

THE EYELIDS

The more important conditions that affect the eyelids include the following:

Blepharitis is inflammation of the eyelids. It is common and sometimes produces an acute, red, tender, inflammatory mass.

Hordeolum (or sty) refers to an acute, inflammatory, focal lesion of the eyelid. Acute inflammation involving the meibomian glands is termed an *internal hordeolum,* whereas acute folliculitis of the glands of Zeis is an *external hordeolum.*

Chalazion is a granulomatous inflammation centered around the meibomian glands or the glands of Zeis. It is thought to represent a reaction to extruded lipid secretions. A chalazion usually produces a painless swelling in the eyelid.

Inflammatory pseudotumor of the orbit describes an idiopathic chronic inflammatory reaction associated with a variable degree of fibrosis. It is a common cause of proptosis and partial immobility of the eyeball.

Xanthelasma refers to a yellow plaque of lipid-containing macrophages, usually involving the nasal aspect of the eyelids. It is often seen in older persons and patients with disorders of lipid metabolism (e.g., familial hypercholesterolemia, primary biliary cirrhosis).

THE ORBIT

Exophthalmos *or* **proptosis** *is an abnormal forward protrusion of the eyeball.* The term *exophthalmos* is used mainly when the condition is bilateral; *proptosis* refers to a unilateral protrusion of the eye. Numerous conditions cause forward protrusion of the eye. The most common cause is thyroid disease, followed by orbital dermoid cysts, and hemangiomas. Other orbital conditions can cause proptosis: various inflammatory lesions, lymphomas, developmental anomalies, vascular problems, and neoplasms all contribute cases. Proptosis also results from lesions of the paranasal sinuses and intracranial cavity.

Exophthalmos of Hyperthyroidism Continues Despite Treatment

Exophthalmos due to Graves disease may precede or follow other manifestations of thyroid dysfunction. Exophthalmos resulting from thyroid disease usually occurs in early adult life, especially in women (female-to-male ratio, 4:1). It may be severe and progressive, particularly in middle life, when exophthalmos no longer correlates well with the state of thyroid function. Dysthyroid exophthalmos may be associated with edema of the eyelids, chemosis (edema of the conjunctiva), and limited ocular motion. The pathogenesis of exophthalmos is discussed in Chapter 21.

Clinical Features: Although it is usually bilateral, one eye may be involved earlier or more extensively than the other. Other ocular manifestations of hyperthyroidism include retraction of the upper eyelid (owing to increased sympathetic tone) and a characteristic stare or apparent proptosis resulting from exposure of the conjunctiva above the corneoscleral limbus.

Complications of severe exophthalmos include several potentially blinding complications: corneal exposure with subsequent ulceration, and optic nerve compression. Paradoxically, thyroidectomy may increase the incidence and severity of exophthalmos associated with hyperthyroidism.

THE CONJUNCTIVA

Hemorrhage

Conjunctival hemorrhage follows blunt trauma, anoxia, or severe bouts of coughing. It also occurs spontaneously, often first noted on arising after sleep. Conjunctival hemorrhages do not extend into the cornea because of the barrier imposed by the close apposition of the corneal epithelium to the underlying substantia propria.

Conjunctivitis Is Infectious or Allergic

Microorganisms lodging on the surface of the eye frequently cause conjunctivitis, keratitis (corneal inflammation), or a corneal ulcer. The eye may also become infected by hematogenous spread from a focus of infection elsewhere. Iatrogenic infections of the eye are always a distinct possibility in ophthalmic surgical procedures, such as corneal grafts and intraocular instillation of prosthetic lenses. Adenoviruses and other pathogens may be introduced into the eye by a physician using infected eyedrops or a contaminated tonometer (an instrument used to measure intraocular pressure).

At some stage in life, virtually everyone has viral or bacterial conjunctivitis. This most common of eye diseases is characterized by hyperemic conjunctival blood vessels (pink eye). The inflammatory exudate that accumulates in the conjunctival sac commonly crusts, causing the eyelids to stick together in the morning. The conjunctival discharge may be purulent, fibrinous, serous, or hemorrhagic and contains inflammatory cells that vary with the etiological agent. In keeping with the seasonal nature of many allergens, allergic conjunctivitis sometimes occurs only during a particular time of the year.

Trachoma

Trachoma is a chronic, contagious conjunctivitis caused by Chlamydia trachomatis. Different serotypes of *C. trachomatis* cause ocular, genital, and systemic infections (trachoma, inclusion conjunctivitis, and lymphogranuloma venereum) in millions of people (see Chapter 9).

 Epidemiology: About 500 million people are afflicted by trachoma, an acute, infectious, cicatrizing keratoconjunctivitis caused by *C. trachomatis*

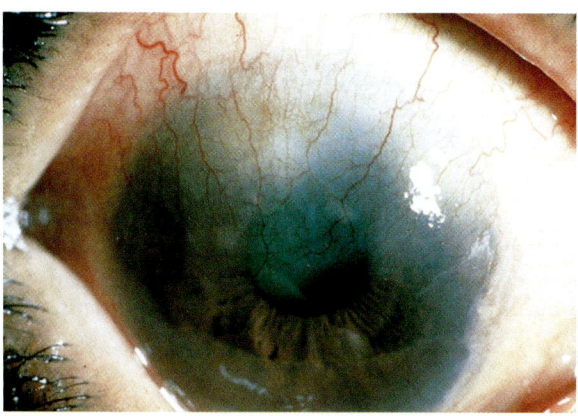

FIGURE 29-2
Trachoma. A clinical photograph of the cornea of a patient with severe trachoma shows extensive fibrovascular opacity (pannus) in the superior cornea.

(serotypes A, B, and C). **This infection is the most common cause of blindness in the world and is especially prevalent in Asia, the Middle East, and parts of Africa.** Trachoma is not very contagious, but overcrowding and poor hygienic conditions favor its transmission by fingers, fomites, and flies. Spontaneous healing is common in children, but in adults, the disease progresses more rapidly and rarely heals in the absence of treatment.

 Pathology: Trachoma is virtually always bilateral and involves the upper half of the conjunctiva more extensively than the lower (Fig. 29-2). The cellular infiltrate is predominantly lymphocytic, and conjunctival lymph follicles with necrotic germinal centers are characteristic. Eventually lymphocytes and blood vessels invade the superior portion of the cornea between the epithelium and Bowman's zone *(trachomatous pannus)*. Scarring of the conjunctiva and eyelids distorts the eyelids. On microscopic examination, the desquamated conjunctival epithelium exhibits glycogen-rich intracytoplasmic inclusion bodies and large macrophages containing nuclear fragments *(Leber cells)*. Secondary bacterial infection is a common complication.

Other Chlamydial Infections

Chlamydia is responsible for a purulent conjunctivitis *(inclusion blennorrhea)* that develops in newborns, who become infected during passage through the birth canal. The infection is also acquired by swimming in nonchlorinated pools (swimming pool conjunctivitis) or from discharges of lesions of the conjunctiva, urethra, or cervix uteri.

In adults and older children, *Chlamydia* causes a chronic follicular conjunctivitis with focal lymphoid hyperplasia *(inclusion conjunctivitis)* and intracytoplasmic inclusion bodies indistinguishable from those of trachoma. In contrast to trachoma, however, the lower tarsal conjunctiva is involved. Scarring and necrosis do not develop, and keratitis is rare and mild.

Ophthalmia Neonatorum

Ophthalmia neonatorum is a severe, acute conjunctivitis with a copious purulent discharge, especially in the newborn, caused by Neisseria gonorrhoeae. The infection, a common cause of blindness in some parts of the world, is complicated by corneal ulceration, perforation, and scarring and panophthalmitis. The infant usually becomes infected while passing through the birth canal of an infected mother. Aside from gonorrhea, ophthalmia neonatorum has other causes, including other pyogenic bacteria and *C. trachomatis*. Today, newborns are routinely treated with penicillin eye drops.

Pinguecula and Pterygium

Pinguecula is a yellowish conjunctival lump usually located nasal to the corneoscleral limbus. It is the most common conjunctival lump. Despite its yellowish appearance, the lesion does not contain fat; rather, it consists of sun-damaged connective tissue identical to that in similarly injured skin (actinic elastosis).

Pterygium is a fold of vascularized conjunctiva that grows horizontally onto the cornea in the shape of an insect wing (hence the name). It is often associated with a pinguecula and frequently recurs after excision.

THE CORNEA

Herpes Simplex Causes Corneal Ulcerations

Herpesvirus (HSV) has a predilection for the corneal epithelium, where it causes keratitis, but it can invade the corneal stroma and occasionally other ocular tissues.

PRIMARY INFECTION BY HSV TYPE 1: Subclinical or undiagnosed localized ocular lesions are caused by HSV type 1 in childhood. These infections are accompanied by regional lymphadenopathy, systemic infection, and fever. HSV type 2 rarely causes ocular infection, but when it does, it can produce widespread lesions of the cornea and retina. An exception occurs in the newborn, who becomes infected during passage through the birth canal of a mother who harbors genital herpes. Most corneal lesions due to HSV are asymptomatic plaques of diseased epithelial cells that contain replicating virus. These usually heal without ulceration, but an acute unilateral follicular conjunctivitis may occur. Corneal ulcers appear after the serum antibody levels increase.

REACTIVATION OF HSV INFECTION: Latent in the trigeminal ganglion, HSV may pass down the nerves and reactivate the infection. In contrast to primary infection by the virus, reactivation disease is characterized by ulceration of the cornea and a more severe inflammatory reaction.

Recurrence of corneal ulcers due to HSV may be precipitated by ultraviolet light, trauma, menstruation, emotional and physical stress, exposure to light or sunlight, vaccination, and other factors.

 Pathology: HSV causes multiple, minute, discrete, intraepithelial corneal ulcers *(superficial punctate keratopathy)*. Although some of these lesions heal, others enlarge and eventually coalesce to form linear or branching fissures (dendritic ulcers, from Gk., *dendron*, "tree"). The epithelium between the fissures desquamates, causing sharply demarcated, irregular geographical ulcers. The corneal ulcers are readily seen in the patient after the cornea has been stained with fluorescein. The affected epithelial cells, which may become multinucleated, contain eosinophilic, intranuclear inclusion bodies *(Lipschütz bodies)*.

The lesions of the corneal stroma vary in reactivated HSV infection. Typically, a central disc-shaped corneal opacity develops beneath the epithelium, owing to edema and a minimal inflammatory cell infiltrate *(disciform keratitis)*. The corneal stroma may become markedly thinned, and Descemet's membrane may bulge into it *(descemetocele)*. Corneal perforation can also occur.

Onchocerciasis Leads to Blindness in Tropical Regions

The nematode *Onchocerca volvulus*, which is transmitted by bites of infected blackflies, is by far the most important helminthic infection of the eye (see Chapter 9). **This parasite accounts for blindness in at least half a million people in regions of Africa and Latin America in which it is endemic.** Microfilaria released from fertilized adult female worms migrate into the superficial cornea, bulbar conjunctiva, aqueous humor, and other ocular tissues. After the demise of the intracorneal microfilaria, an inflammatory response causes corneal opacification and visual impairment *(river blindness)*. Less frequently, endophthalmitis, retinal lesions, and optic atrophy occur. Treatment with ivermectin is highly effective.

Arcus Lipoides (Arcus Senilis)

Arcus lipoides (formerly called arcus senilis *because of its frequency in the elderly) is a white arc due to lipid deposition in the peripheral cornea.* It may also form an entire ring, in which case the term *annulus lipoides* is more appropriate. Although not necessarily associated with increased serum lipid levels, arcus lipoides accompanies certain disorders of lipid metabolism, and its presence alerts the perceptive clinician to the systemic disorder.

Band Keratopathy Is a Horizontal Band across the Cornea

Band keratopathy refers to an opaque horizontal band across the superficial central cornea. The opacification in band keratopathy may contain calcium phosphate (calcific band keratopathy) or noncalcified protein (chronic actinic keratopathy).

In **calcific band keratopathy,** calcium phosphate deposits in a horizontal band across the superficial central cornea in conditions associated with hypercalcemia. However, the disorder most often occurs in the absence of an increased serum calcium concentration, as in chronic uveitis and other ocular disorders.

Chronic actinic keratopathy occurs worldwide but is most severe in regions in which people spend a considerable amount of time outdoors. Their unprotected eyes are exposed to excessive ultraviolet light, such as that reflected from desert, water, or snow.

Corneal Dystrophies Comprise Varied Genetic Disorders

The corneal dystrophies encompass a heterogeneous group of hereditary, noninflammatory diseases of the cornea. Most corneal dystrophies are autosomal dominant or recessive, but rare cases are X-linked recessive. The corneal dystrophies have traditionally been classified according to the primary layer that is involved: (1) the outer layer composed of epithelium, basement membrane, and Bowman's layer; (2) the stroma; and (3) the endothelium and Descemet's membrane. A shortcoming of such a classification is its artificiality, because many of the conditions involve more than one layer.

EPITHELIAL DYSTROPHIES: The different epithelial dystrophies are characterized by a variety of distinct abnormalities, which include (1) microcysts or accumulations of anomalous material within the cytoplasm of the corneal epithelium, (2) defects in the epithelial basement membrane, and (3) deposition of a finely fibrillar substance in Bowman's layer. In some epithelial dystrophies, faulty desmosomes may permit the separation of adjacent epithelial cells, leading to the accumulation of fluid-filled microcysts. A loss of hemidesmosomes between the epithelium and Bowman's layer leads to painful, recurrent erosions that begin in early childhood. Although there may be a slow decrease in visual acuity, epithelial dystrophies do not ordinarily cause blindness. Patients with one corneal dystrophy of the corneal epithelium *(Meesmann dystrophy)* have dominant mutations in the *KRT3* or *KRT12* genes, which encode keratin 3 and keratin 12, respectively. The mutations result in aggregations of abnormal cytokeratin filaments and severely impair cytoskeletal function in the affected cells.

STROMAL DYSTROPHIES: The stromal dystrophies are clear-cut entities in which different substances (e.g., amyloid, glycosaminoglycans, unidentified proteins, and a variety of lipids) accumulate within the corneal stroma because of inherited metabolic disorders. Each stromal dystrophy causes a characteristic form of corneal opacification. The age of onset and the rate of progression vary with the particular disorder. Although the clinical manifestations may be limited to the cornea, other tissues are involved in some of these dystrophies. Several inherited corneal disorders, including granular corneal dystrophy and lattice corneal dystrophy, are distinctly different mutations in the same gene, namely, the *TFGBI (BIGH3)* gene on chromosome 5 (5q). Another predominantly stromal corneal dystrophy *(macular corneal dystrophy)* results from a defect in the CHST6 gene on chromosome 16 (16q), which encodes a sulfotransferase that catalyzes the transfer of sulfate groups to the *N*-acetyl glucosamine and galactose moieties in keratan sulfate.

ENDOTHELIAL DYSTROPHIES: Several different endothelial dystrophies are recognized, usually accompanied by abnormalities in Descemet's membrane, the basement membrane of the corneal endothelium. In one dystrophy of the corneal endothelium *(Fuchs dystrophy)*, wartlike excrescences form on Descemet's membrane, and progressive visual loss follows corneal edema and the degeneration of the endothelial cells. Missense mutations in the *COL8A2* gene encoding the α_2 chain of type VIII collagen have been identified in some patients with early-onset Fuchs dystrophy and posterior polymorphous corneal dystrophy, both of which affect the corneal endothelium and its basement membrane (Descemet's membrane).

THE LENS

Cataracts Are Opacifications in the Crystalline Lens

Cataracts are a major cause of visual impairment and blindness throughout the world and are the outcome of numerous conditions.

Pathogenesis: Cataracts can be caused by diabetes or by deficiencies in riboflavin or tryptophan. A variety of cataracts result from genetic disorders. Others are related to the actions of toxins, drugs, or physical agents. Substances that may cause cataracts include dinitrophenol, naphthalene, ergot, phospholine iodide (topical), corticosteroids, and phenothiazines. Physical agents that cause cataracts are heat, ultraviolet light, trauma, intraocular surgery, and ultrasound.

Ocular diseases that may be complicated by cataracts include uveitis, intraocular neoplasms, glaucoma, retinitis pigmentosa, and retinal detachment. Cataracts also are associated with congenital rubella virus infection, aging, some skin diseases (atopic dermatitis, scleroderma), and various systemic diseases. A wide variety of cataracts are inherited and some of them are associated with other ocular or systemic abnormalities. Cataracts can result from mutations in the heat shock transcription factor-4 *(HSF4)* gene, as well as in genes that encode many specific lens proteins.

Pathology: The most common cataract in the United States is associated with aging (age-related cataract). Clefts appear between the lens fibers, and degenerated lens material accumulates in these spaces (morgagnian corpuscles, incipient cataract). The degenerated lens material exerts osmotic pressure, causing the damaged lens to increase in volume by imbibing water. Such a swollen lens may obstruct the pupil and cause glaucoma *(phacomorphic glaucoma)*.

In a mature cataract (Fig. 29-3), the entire lens degenerates, and its volume diminishes because lenticular debris escapes into the aqueous humor through a degenerated lens capsule (hypermature cataract). After becoming engulfed by macrophages, the extruded lenticular material may obstruct the aqueous outflow and produce glaucoma (phacolytic

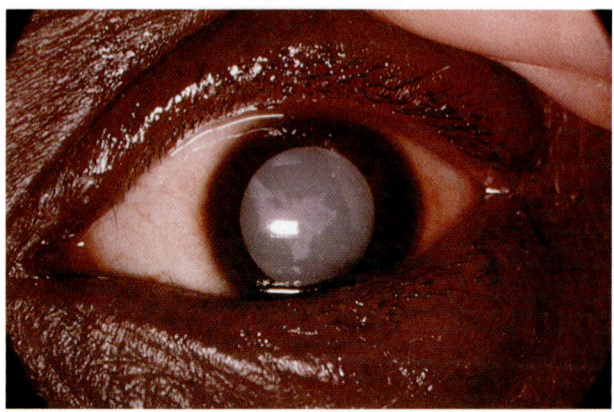

FIGURE 29-3
Cataract. The white appearance of the pupil in this eye is due to complete opacification of the lens ("mature cataract").

glaucoma). The compressed lens fibers in the center of the lens normally harden with aging (simple nuclear sclerotic cataract) and may become brown or black. If the peripheral portion of the lens, or lens cortex, becomes liquefied *(morgagnian cataract)*, the sclerotic nucleus may sink within the lens by gravity.

Fortunately, cataractous lenses can be surgically removed, and optical devices can be provided to permit focusing of light on the retina (spectacles, contact lenses, implantation of prosthetic lenses).

Presbyopia Is a Failure of Accommodation

Presbyopia is an impairment of vision associated with aging, in which the near point of distinct vision becomes located farther from the eye. At the equator of the crystalline lens, the cuboidal subcapsular cells differentiate into elongated lens fibers throughout life. Once formed, these lens fibers persist indefinitely. Older fibers become displaced into the center of the lens, causing it to enlarge with age. After this process has occurred for many years, the lens loses its elasticity, an effect that interferes with its normal tendency to become spherical, thereby diminishing the power of accommodation. As a result, most persons after age 40 years begin to have difficulty reading and require spectacles for near vision.

Phacoanaphylactic Endophthalmitis Is an Autoimmune Disorder

Phacoanaphylactic endophthalmitis is an immunologically evoked, granulomatous response to lens proteins. The inflammatory lesion occurs around or within the lens (or its remains) in an eye with a traumatized or cataractous lens or after surgical removal of a cataractous lens. A similar reaction may occur spontaneously in the contralateral eye months or years later. This autoimmune reaction to unique lens proteins, which are normally sequestered from the immune system, can be provoked experimentally by immunization with autologous lens material.

THE UVEA

A variety of inflammatory conditions affect the uveal tract. Inflammation of the uvea *(uveitis)* also encompasses inflammation of the iris (iritis), the ciliary body *(cyclitis)*, and the iris plus the ciliary body *(iridocyclitis)*. Inflammation of the iris and ciliary body typically causes a red eye, photophobia, moderate pain, blurred vision, a pericorneal halo, ciliary flush, and slight miosis. A flare is common in the anterior chamber on slit-lamp biomicroscopy, and keratic precipitates or a *hypopyon* also develop.

Posterior synechiae are adhesions that develop between the iris and the lens.

Peripheral anterior synechiae are adhesions between the peripheral iris and the anterior chamber angle. Both types of synechiae are complications of iritis and can cause glaucoma.

Sympathetic Ophthalmitis Is an Autoimmune Uveitis

In sympathetic ophthalmitis, the entire uvea develops granulomatous inflammation after a latent period, in response to an injury in the other eye. Perforating ocular injury and prolapse of uveal tissue often lead to a progressive, bilateral, diffuse, granulomatous inflammation of the uvea. This uveitis develops in the originally injured eye (exciting eye) after a latent period of 4 to 8 weeks. The latent period may, however, be as short as 10 days or as long as many years. The uninjured eye (sympathizing eye) becomes affected at the same time as the injured eye or shortly thereafter. Vitiligo and graying of the eyelashes sometimes accompanies the uveitis. Nodules containing reactive retinal pigment epithelium, macrophages, and epithelioid cells commonly appear between Bruch's membrane and the retinal pigment epithelium *(Dalen-Fuchs nodules)*. Experimental studies suggest that the antigen responsible for sympathetic ophthalmitis resides in the photoreceptors of the retina (arrestin).

Sarcoidosis Often Affects the Eye

Ocular involvement occurs in one fourth to one third of patients with sarcoidosis and is frequently the initial clinical manifestation. Although any of the ocular and orbital tissues may be involved, this granulomatous disease has a predilection for the anterior segment of the eye. Ocular involvement is usually bilateral and most often takes the form of a granulomatous uveitis. Other ocular manifestations of sarcoidosis include calcific band keratopathy, cataracts, retinal vascularization, vitreous hemorrhage, and bilateral enlargement of the lacrimal and salivary glands *(Mikulicz syndrome)*.

THE RETINA

Retinal Hemorrhage Is of Varied Etiology

Retinal hemorrhages are a feature of many disorders, including hypertension, diabetes mellitus, and central retinal vein occlusion. The appearance varies with the location. Hemorrhage in the nerve fiber layer spreads between axons and causes a flame-shaped appearance on funduscopy, whereas deep retinal hemorrhages tend to be round. When located between the retinal pigment epithelium and Bruch's membrane, blood appears as a dark mass and clinically may resemble a melanoma.

After accidental or surgical perforation of the globe, choroidal hemorrhages may detach the choroid and displace the retina, vitreous body, and lens through the wound.

Retinal Occlusive Vascular Disease Is an Important Cause of Blindness

Vascular occlusion results from thrombosis, embolism, stenosis (as in atherosclerosis), vascular compression, intravascular sludging or coagulation, or vasoconstriction (e.g., in hypertensive retinopathy or migraine). Thrombosis of the ocular vessels may accompany primary disease of these vessels, as in giant cell arteritis.

Certain disorders of the heart and of major vessels, such as the carotid arteries, predispose to emboli that lodge in the retina and are evident on funduscopic examination at points of vascular bifurcation. Within the optic nerve, emboli in the central retinal artery frequently lodge in the vessel where it passes though the scleral perforations (lamina cribrosa).

Pathology: The effect of vascular occlusion depends on the size of the vessel involved, the degree of resultant ischemia, and the nature of the embolus. Small emboli often do not interfere with retinal function, whereas septic emboli may cause foci of ocular infection. Retinal ischemia of any cause frequently results in the appearance of white fluffy patches that resemble cotton on ophthalmoscopic examination *(cotton-wool patches)*. These round spots, which are seldom wider than the optic disc, consist of aggregates of swollen axons in the nerve-fiber layer of the retina. The affected axons contain numerous degenerated mitochondria and dense bodies related to the lysosomal system, which accumulate because of impaired axoplasmic flow. Histologically, in cross-section, the individual swollen axons resemble cells *(cytoid bodies)*. Cotton-wool spots are reversible if the circulation is restored in time.

Central Retinal Artery Occlusion

Like the neurons in the rest of the nervous system, those in the retina (Fig. 29-4) are extremely susceptible to hypoxia. Central retinal artery occlusion (Figs. 29-5 and 29-6) may follow thrombosis of the retinal artery, as in atherosclerosis or giant cell arteritis, or embolization to that vessel. Intracellular edema, manifested by retinal pallor, is prominent, especially in the macula, where the ganglion cells are most numerous. The foveola (i.e., the vascularized choroid beneath the center of the macula) stands out in sharp contrast as a prominent *cherry-red spot*. The lack of retinal circulation reduces the retinal arterioles to delicate threads (see Fig. 29-6).

Permanent blindness follows central retinal artery obstruction, unless the ischemia is of short duration. Unilateral blurred vision, lasting a few minutes *(amaurosis fugax)*, occurs with small retinal emboli.

Central Retinal Vein Occlusion

Central retinal vein occlusion results in flame-shaped hemorrhages in the nerve-fiber layer of the retina, especially around the optic disc. The hemorrhages reflect the high intravascular pressure that dilates and ruptures the veins and collateral vessels (Fig. 29-7). Edema of the optic disc and retina occurs because of an impaired absorption of interstitial fluid.

Vision is disturbed but may recover surprisingly well, considering the severity of the funduscopic changes. An intractable closed-angle glaucoma, with severe pain and repeated hemorrhages, commonly ensues 2 to 3 months after central retinal vein occlusion (100-day glaucoma, thrombotic glaucoma, neovascular glaucoma). This distressing complication is caused by neovascularization of the iris and adhesions between the iris and the anterior chamber angle *(peripheral anterior synechiae)*.

Hypertensive Retinopathy Relates to the Severity of Hypertension

Increased blood pressure commonly affects the retina, causing changes that can readily be seen with the ophthalmoscope (Figs. 29-8 and 29-9).

Pathology: Features of hypertensive retinopathy include the following:

- Arteriolar narrowing
- Hemorrhages in the retinal nerve fiber layer (flame-shaped hemorrhages)
- Exudates, including some that radiate from the center of the macula (macular star)
- Fluffy white bodies in the superficial retina (cotton-wool spots)
- Microaneurysms

In the eye, arteriolosclerosis accompanies long-standing hypertension and commonly affects the retinal and choroidal vessels. The lumina of the thickened retinal arterioles become narrowed, increasingly tortuous, and of irregular caliber. At sites where the arterioles cross veins, the latter appear kinked *(arteriovenous nicking)*. However, the venous diameter before the site of compression is not wider than that after it. Thus, the kinked appearance of the vein is not due to compression by a taut sclerotic artery. Rather, it reflects sclerosis within the venous walls, because the retinal arteries and veins share a common adventitia at sites of arteriovenous crossings.

By funduscopy, abnormal retinal arterioles appear as parallel white lines at sites of vascular crossings *(arterial sheathing)*. Initially, the narrowed lumen of the retinal vessels

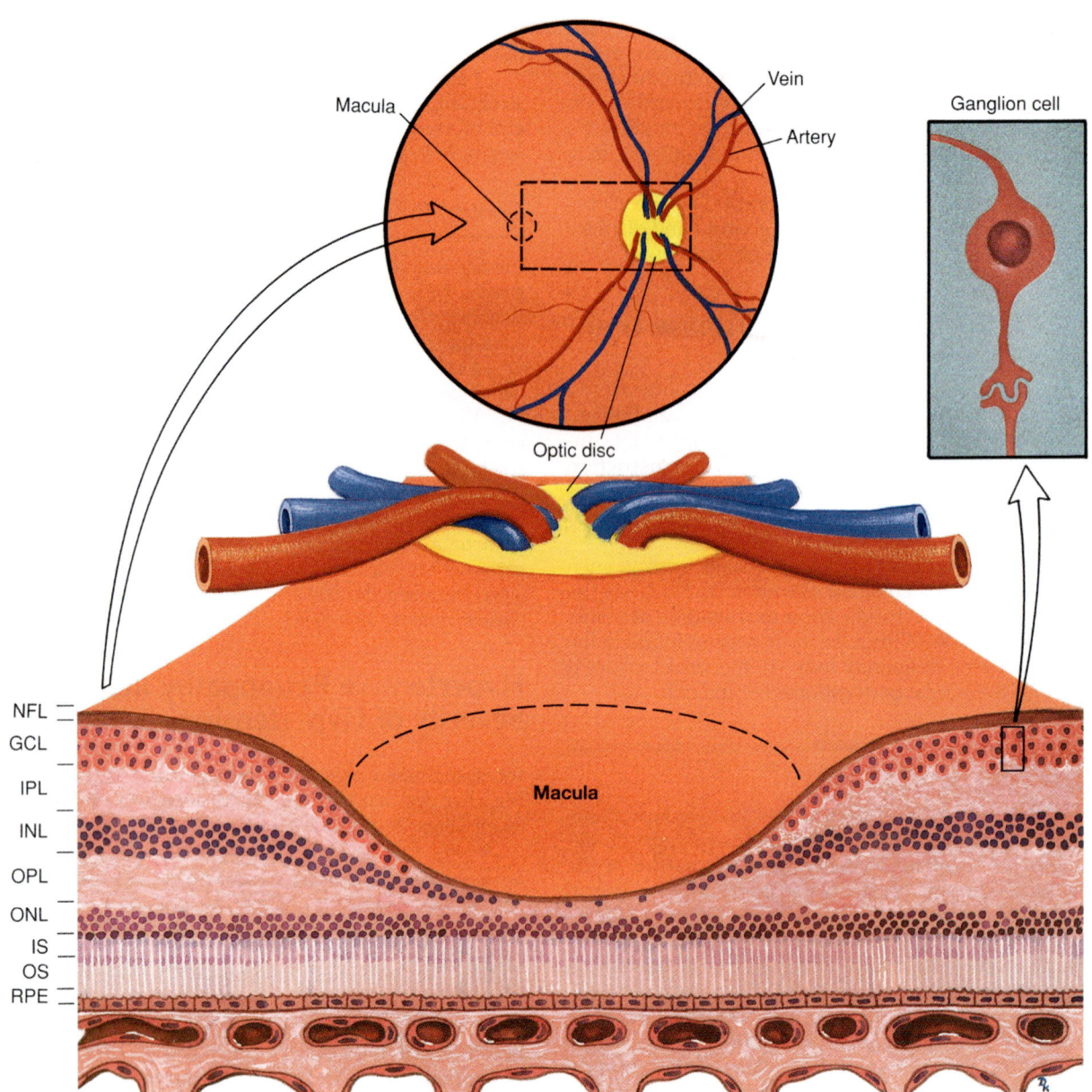

FIGURE 29-4
The normal retina. Constituents of the normal retina are arranged in distinct layers. These include the nerve fiber layer *(NFL)*, ganglion cell layer *(GCL)*, inner plexiform layer *(IPL)*, inner nuclear layer *(INL)*, outer plexiform layer *(OPL)*, outer nuclear layer *(ONL)*, inner segments *(IS)* and outer segments *(OS)* of the photoreceptors, and the retinal pigment epithelium *(RPE)*. The axons from the ganglion cells enter the nerve fiber layer and converge toward the optic disc. The inner retina contains arteries and veins. The retina is thinnest at the center of the macula, where bare photoreceptors rest on the retinal pigment epithelium. Only one cell thick in most of the retina, the ganglion cell layer is multilayered at the macula.

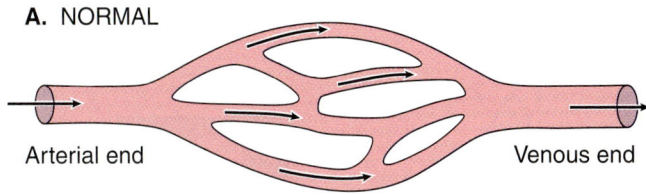

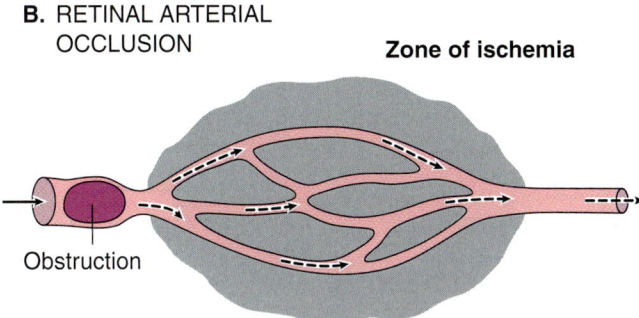

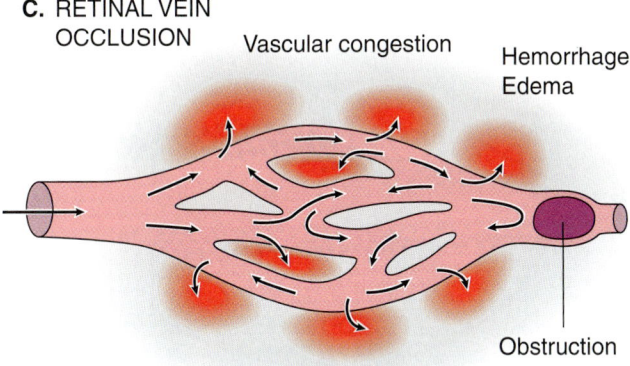

FIGURE 29-5

Occlusion of the retinal artery and vein. A. In the retina, as in other parts of the body, blood normally flows through a capillary network. B. When the retinal arteries become occluded (e.g., with an embolus) a zone of retinal ischemia ensues. This is accompanied by impaired neuronal function and visual loss, and the ischemic retina becomes pale. Because the intravascular pressure within the ischemic tissue is low, hemorrhage is inconspicuous. C. With retinal vein occlusion, vascular congestion, hemorrhage, and edema are prominent, whereas ischemia is mild and neuronal function remains intact.

decreases the visibility of the blood column and makes it appear orange on ophthalmoscopic examination *(copper wiring)*. However, as the blood column eventually becomes completely obscured, light reflected from the sclerotic vessels appears as threads of silver wire *(silver wiring)*.

Small superficial or deep retinal hemorrhages often accompany retinal arteriolosclerosis. **Malignant hypertension** is characterized by a necrotizing arteriolitis, with fibrinoid necrosis and thrombosis of the precapillary retinal arterioles.

The Retina

Diabetic Retinopathy Is Primarily a Vascular Disease

The eye is frequently involved in diabetes mellitus, and ocular symptoms occur in 20 to 40% of diabetics even at the clinical onset of the disease. Virtually all patients with type 1 (insulin-dependent) diabetes and many of those with type 2 (non–insulin-dependent) diabetes develop some background retinopathy (see below) within 5 to 15 years of the onset of diabetes (Figs. 29-10 to 29-12). The more dangerous proliferative retinopathy does not appear until at least 10 years of diabetes, after which the incidence increases rapidly and remains high for many years. **The frequency of proliferative retinopathy correlates with the degree of glycemic control; the better the control, the lower the rate of retinopathy.**

Retinal ischemia can account for most features of diabetic retinopathy, including the cotton-wool spots, capillary closure, microaneurysms, and retinal neovascularization. Ischemia results from narrowing or occlusion of retinal arterioles (as from arteriolosclerosis or platelet and lipid thrombi) or from atherosclerosis of the central retinal or ophthalmic arteries.

 Pathology: The retinopathy of diabetes is characterized by background and proliferative stages.

BACKGROUND (NONPROLIFERATIVE) DIABETIC RETINOPATHY: This stage exhibits venous engorgement, small hemorrhages *(dot and blot hemorrhages),* capillary microaneurysms, and exudates. These lesions usually do not impair vision unless associated with macular edema. The retinopathy begins at the posterior pole but eventually may involve the entire retina.

On funduscopy, the first discernible clinical abnormality in background diabetic retinopathy is engorged retinal veins, with localized sausage-shaped distentions, coils, and loops. This is followed by small hemorrhages in the same areas, mostly in the inner nuclear and outer plexiform layers. With time, "waxy" exudates accumulate, chiefly in the vicinity of the microaneurysms. The retinopathy of elderly diabetic persons frequently displays numerous exudates *(exudative diabetic retinopathy),* whereas this is not a feature in diabetic patients with type 1 disease. Because of the hyperlipoproteinemia of diabetics, the exudates are rich in lipid and thus appear yellowish *(waxy exudates).*

PROLIFERATIVE RETINOPATHY: After many years, diabetic retinopathy becomes proliferative. Delicate new blood vessels grow along with fibrous and glial tissue toward the vitreous body. Neovascularization of the retina is a prominent feature of diabetic retinopathy and of other conditions caused by retinal ischemia. Tortuous new vessels first appear on the surface of the retina and optic nerve head and then grow into the vitreous cavity. The newly formed friable vessels bleed easily, and the resultant vitreal hemorrhages obscure vision. Neovascularization is associated with the proliferation and migration of astrocytes, which grow around the new vessels to form delicate white veils (gliosis).

1512   The Eye

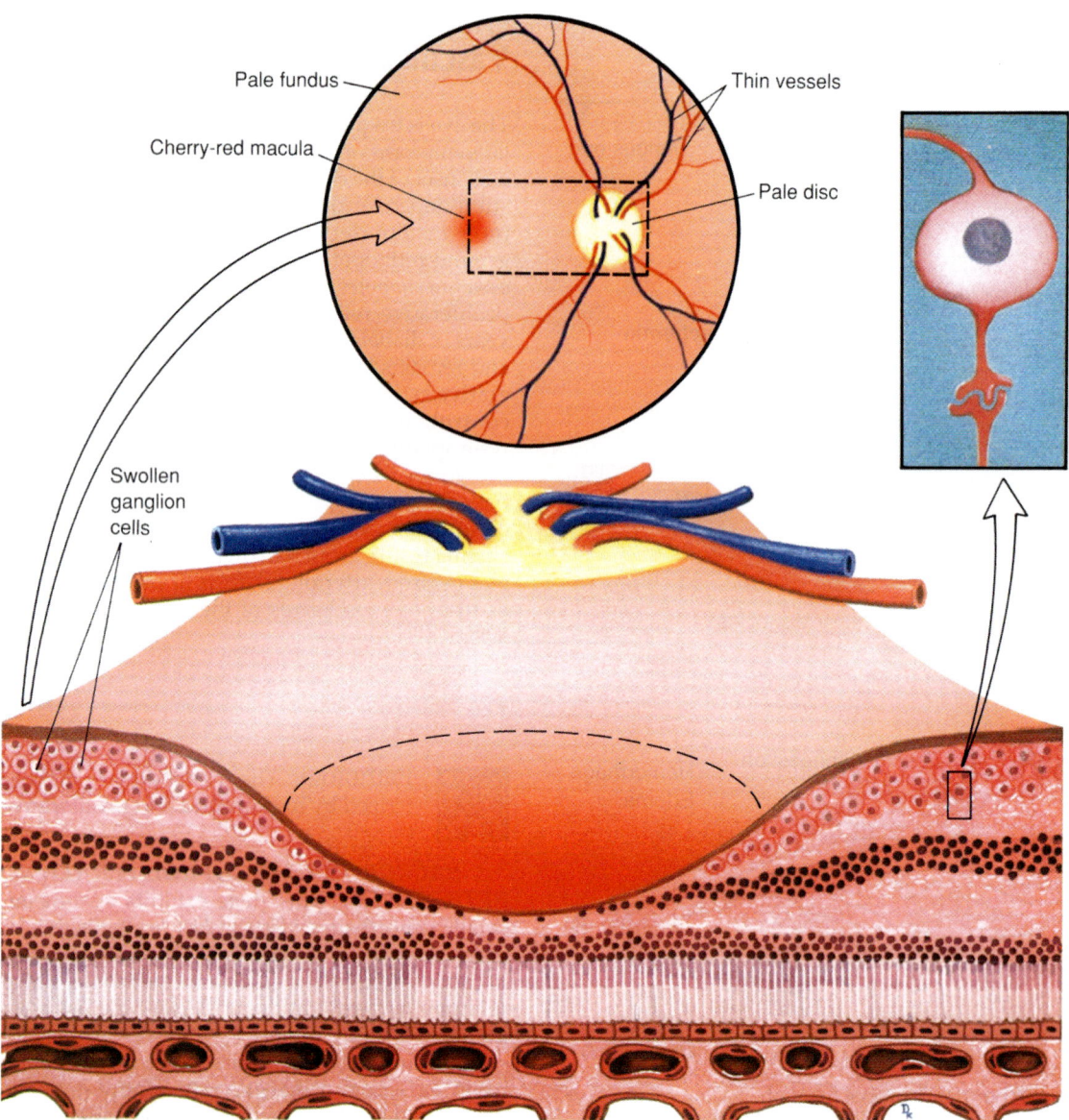

FIGURE 29-6
Central retinal artery occlusion. When the central retinal artery becomes occluded (e.g., with an embolus), the entire retina becomes edematous and pale. Decreased blood flow makes the retinal vessels less visible on funduscopic examination. The macula becomes cherry-red, owing to the prominent, but normal, underlying vasculature of the choroid.

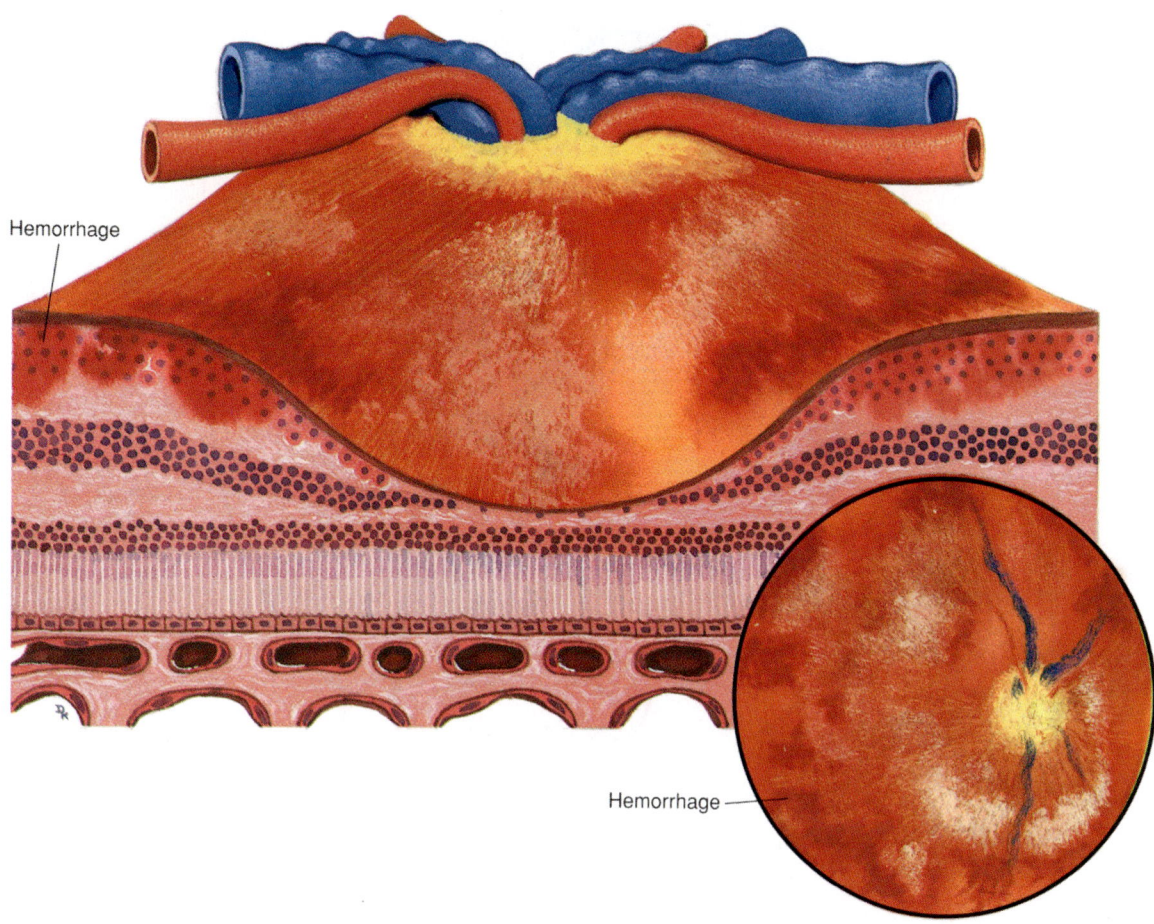

FIGURE 29-7
Central retinal vein occlusion. In contrast to central retinal artery occlusion, central retinal vein occlusion produces considerable vascular engorgement and retinal hemorrhage as a consequence of increased intravascular pressure.

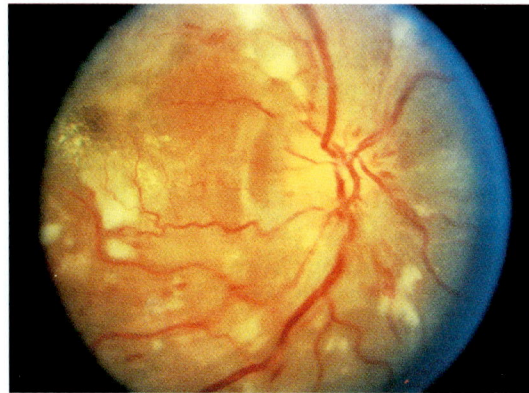

FIGURE 29-8
Hypertensive retinopathy. A photograph of the ocular fundus in a patient with extensive retinopathy. The optic nerve head is edematous; the retina contains numerous exudates and "cotton-wool" spots.

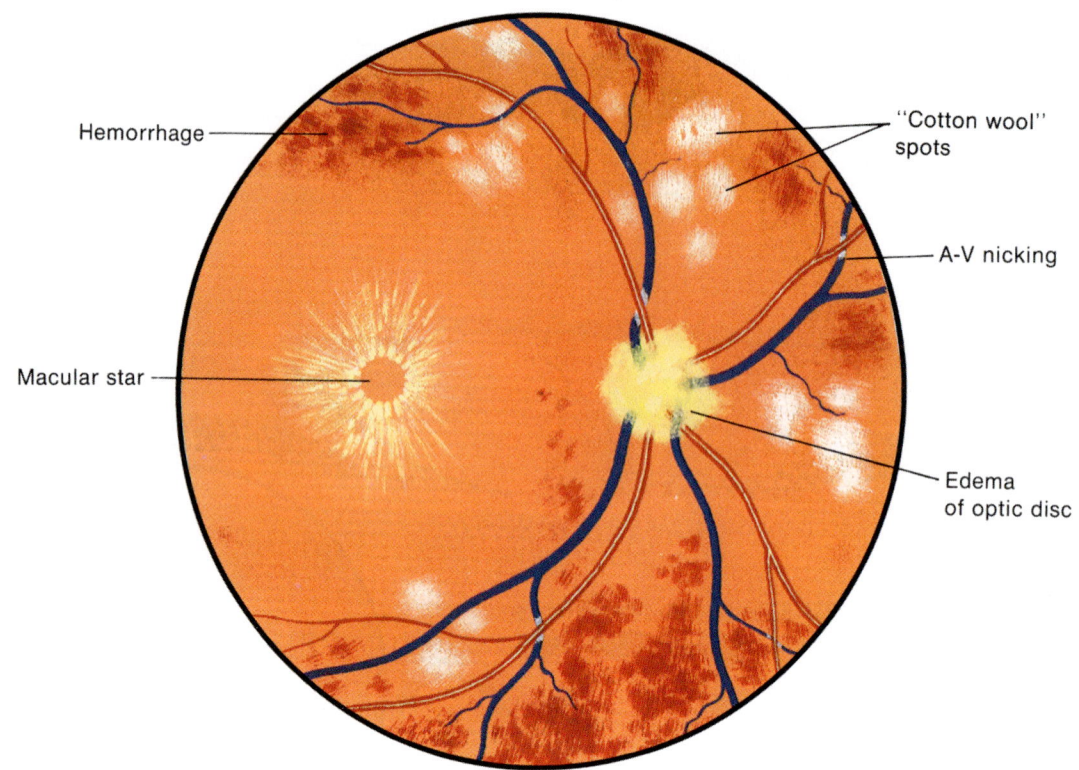
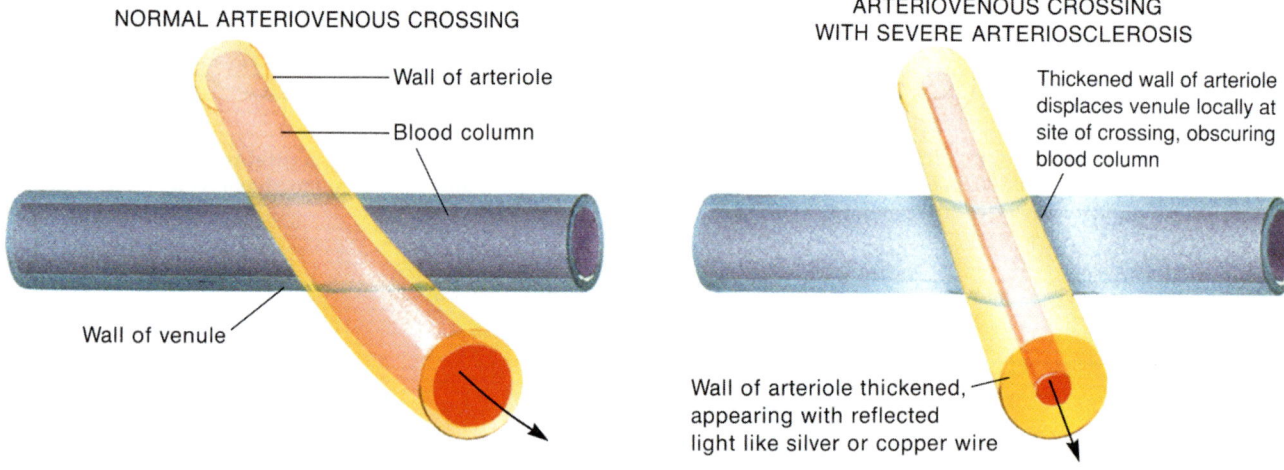
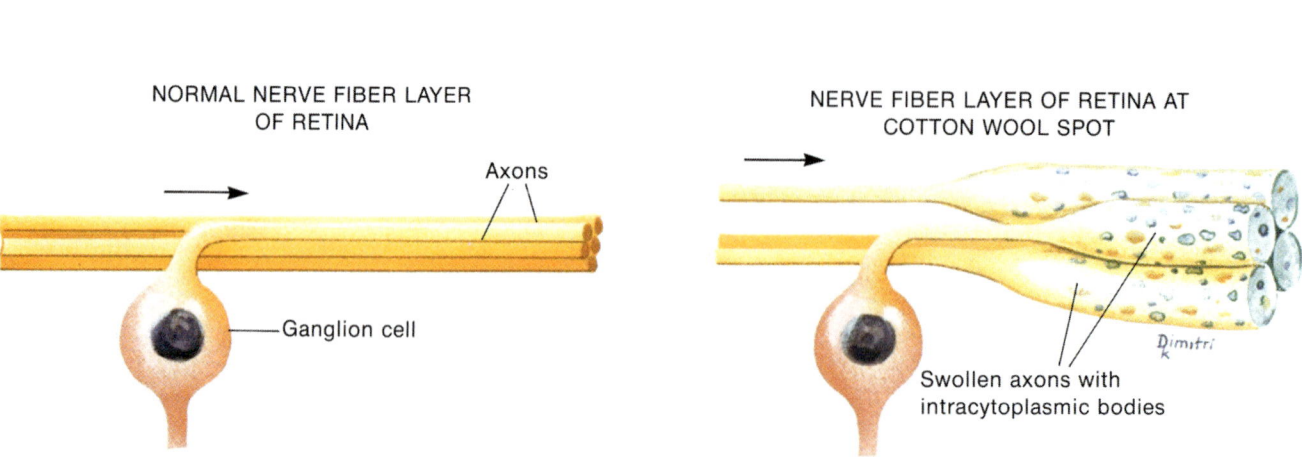

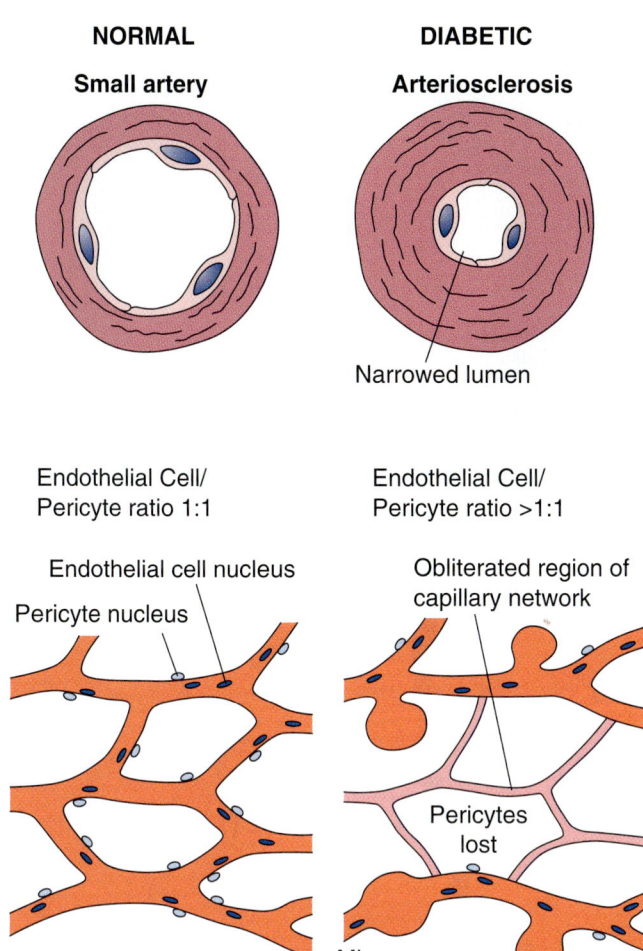

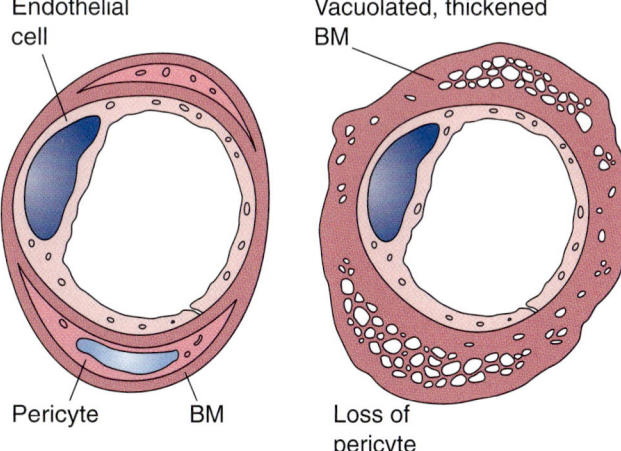

FIGURE 29-10
Diabetic retinopathy. In diabetic retinopathy, the microvasculature is abnormal. Arteriosclerosis narrows the lumen of the small arteries. Pericytes are lost, and the endothelial cell-to-pericyte ratio is greater than 1. Capillary microaneurysms are prominent, and portions of the capillary network become acellular and show no blood flow. The basement membrane of the retinal capillaries is thickened and vacuolated.

FIGURE 29-9
Hypertensive retinopathy. Various abnormalities develop within the retina in hypertension. The commonly associated arteriolosclerosis affects the appearance of the retinal microvasculature. Light reflected from the thickened arteriolar walls mimics silver or copper wire. Blood flow through the retinal venules is not well visualized at the sites of arteriolar–venular crossings. This effect is due to a thickening of the venular wall rather than to an impediment to blood flow caused by compression; the column of blood proximal to the compression is not wider than the part distal to the crossing. Impaired axoplasmic flow within the nerve fiber layer, caused by ischemia, results in swollen axons with cytoplasmic bodies. Such structures resemble cotton on funduscopy ("cotton-wool spots"). Hemorrhages are common in the retina, and exudates frequently form a star around the macula.

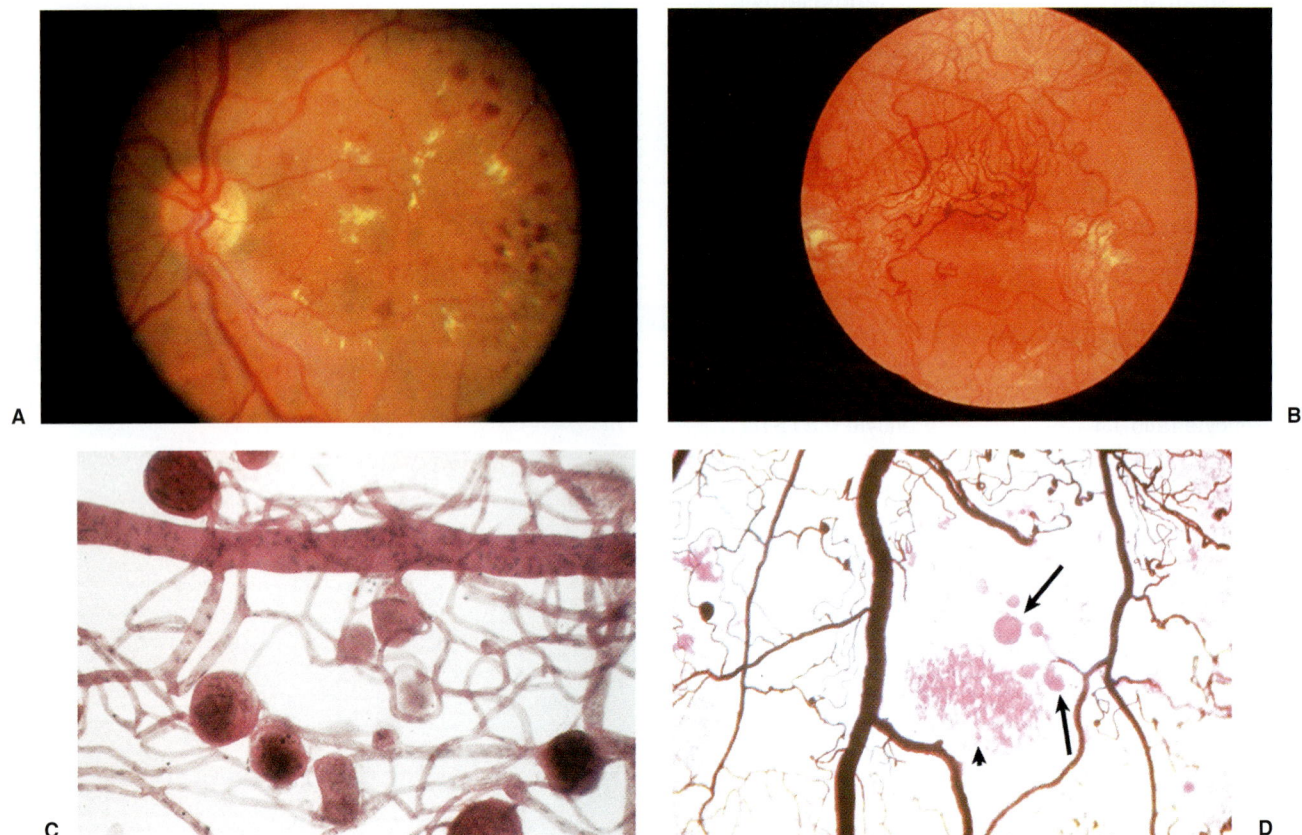

FIGURE 29-11
Diabetic retinopathy. **A.** The ocular fundus in a patient with background diabetic retinopathy. Several yellowish "hard" exudates, which are rich in lipids, are evident, together with several relatively small retinal hemorrhages. **B.** A vascular frond has extended anterior to the retina in the eye with proliferative diabetic retinopathy. **C.** Numerous microaneurysms are present in this flat preparation of a diabetic retina. **D.** This flat preparation from a diabetic was stained with periodic acid–Schiff (PAS) after the retinal vessels had been perfused with India ink. Microaneurysms *(arrows)* and an exudate *(arrowhead)* are evident in a region of retinal nonperfusion.

The proliferating fibrovascular and glial tissue contracts, often causing retinal detachment and blindness. Frequently, features of hypertensive and arteriolosclerotic retinopathy are associated with diabetic retinopathy.

Diabetic retinopathy, glaucoma, and age-related maculopathy are the leading causes of irreversible blindness in the United States. Blindness in diabetic retinopathy results when the macula is involved, but it also follows vitreous hemorrhage, retinal detachment, and glaucoma. Once blindness ensues, it heralds an ominous future for the patient, because death from ischemic heart disease or renal failure often follows. In fact, the mean life expectancy in such cases is less than 6 years, and only one fifth of blind diabetics survive 10 years. Laser phototherapy and strict glycemic control early in the course of proliferative retinopathy have proved effective in controlling this complication.

Diabetic Iridopathy

In diabetics with severe retinopathy, a fibrovascular layer frequently grows along the anterior surface of the iris and in the anterior chamber angle. Because such iris neovascularization *(rubeosis iridis)* is a feature of several conditions associated with retinal ischemia, it is believed to be due to an angiogenic factor produced by the ischemic retina.

 Pathology: A fibrovascular membrane leads to adhesions between the iris and the cornea *(peripheral anterior synechiae)* and between the iris and lens *(posterior synechiae),* while traction by the fibrovascular membrane pulls the iris pigment epithelium around the pupillary margin *(ectropion uveae).* The friable new vessels on the iris bleed easily and cause *hyphema* (hemorrhage within the anterior chamber of the eye). Neovascularization of the iris is clinically important because it frequently culminates in a blind, painful eye, owing to secondary glaucoma *(neovascular glaucoma).*

Hyperglycemia leads to glycogen storage in the pigmented epithelium of the iris, a phenomenon analogous to that produced in the renal tubules by glycosuria *(Armanni-Ebstein phenomenon).* When tissue sections of diabetic eyes are processed in the usual manner, the pigment epithelium of the iris sometimes contains numerous vacuoles, which imparts a lacy appearance. The vacuoles result from the loss of glycogen in the preparation of tissue sections. Glycogen stor-

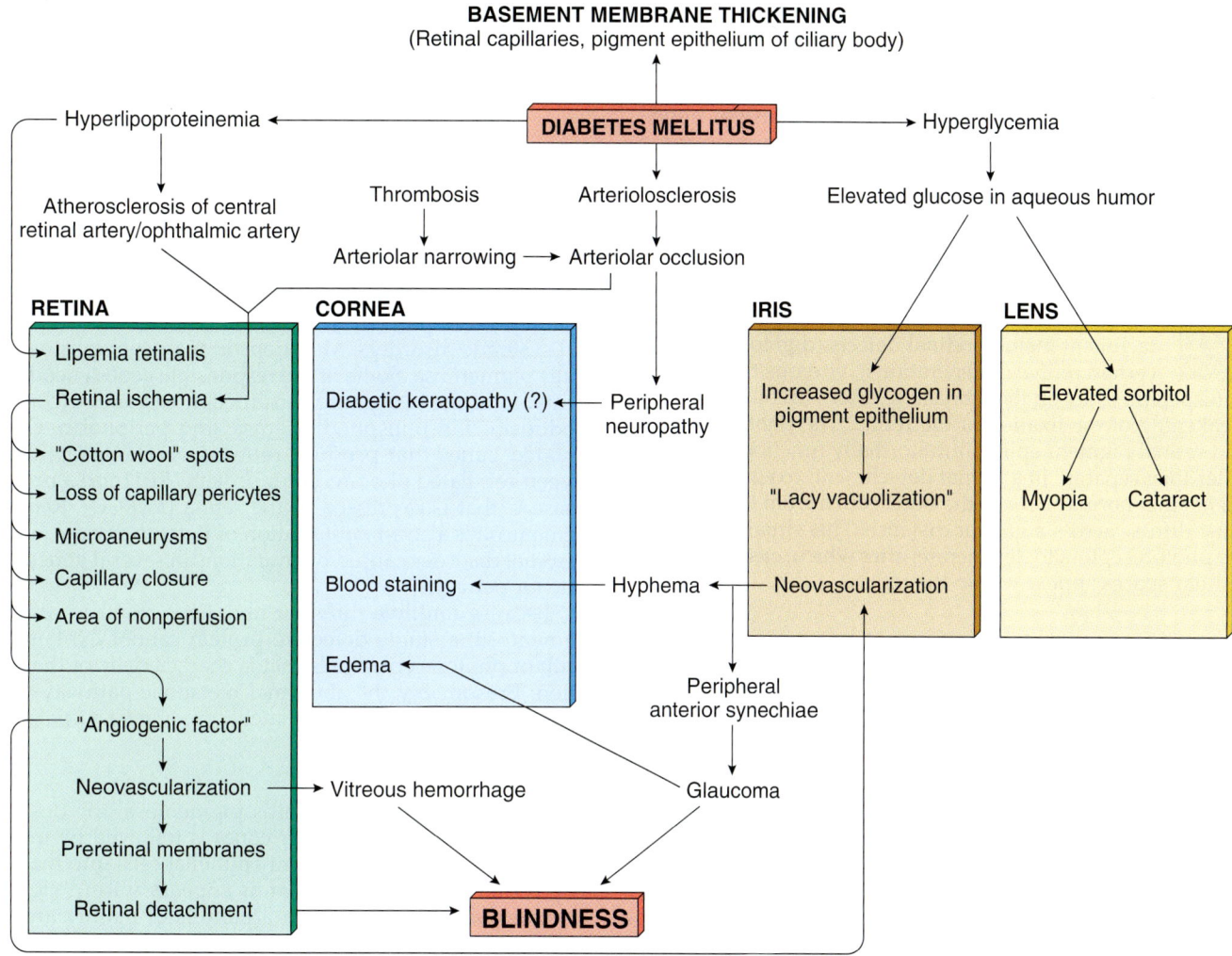

FIGURE 29-12
Effect of diabetes on the eye.

age within the pigment epithelium of the iris is thought to account for the scattering of the iris pigment observed clinically in diabetic patients.

Diabetic Cataracts

Patients with type 1 diabetes often develop bilateral "snowflake" cataracts. These consist of a blanket of white needle-shaped opacities in the lens immediately beneath the anterior and posterior lens capsule. The opacities coalesce within a few weeks in adolescents, and within days in children, until the whole lens becomes opaque. Snowflake cataracts can be produced experimentally in young animals and result from an osmotic effect caused by the accumulation of sorbitol, the alcohol derived from glucose (see Chapter 22). The increased sorbitol content of the lens causes imbibition of water and enlargement of the lens.

Age-related cataracts occur in diabetics at an earlier age than in the general population and progress more rapidly to maturity. A sudden temporary myopia, caused by increased refractive power in the lens, may be the presenting manifestation of diabetes.

Other Ophthalmic Manifestations of Diabetes

Diabetic persons are at increased risk for inflammation of the anterior segment of the eye, phycomycosis (mucormycosis) of the orbit, and primary open-angle glaucoma. They are also prone to the *Argyll Robertson pupil* (unequal and irregularly shaped pupils that react to accommodation but not to light). Cranial nerve palsies occur, especially of the oculomotor nerve. Some patients with long-standing diabetes develop recurrent corneal erosions, which are thought to be due to impaired innervation of the cornea.

Retinal Detachment Separates the Sensory Retina from the Pigment Epithelium

During fetal development, the space between the sensory retina and the retinal pigment epithelium is obliterated when these two layers become apposed. However, the sensory retina readily separates from the retinal pigment epithelium when fluid (liquid vitreous, hemorrhage, or exudate) accumulates within the potential space between these structures. Such a separation is a common cause of blindness. Laser treatment has greatly improved the prognosis for patients with detached retina.

Pathogenesis: Factors predisposing to retinal detachment include retinal defects (due to trauma or certain retinal degenerations), vitreous traction, diminished pressure on the retina (e.g., after vitreous loss), and weakening of the fixation of the retina. The photoreceptors and retinal pigment epithelium normally function as a unit. After they separate in a retinal detachment, oxygen and nutrients that normally reach the outer retina from the choroid must diffuse across a greater distance. This situation causes the photoreceptors to degenerate, after which, cystlike extracellular spaces appear within the retina.

Pathology: Three varieties of retinal detachment are recognized—rhegmatogenous, tractional, and exudative.

RHEGMATOGENOUS RETINAL DETACHMENT: This condition is associated with a retinal tear and often with degenerative changes in the vitreous body or peripheral retina. Full-thickness holes in the retina are not complicated by retinal detachment unless liquid vitreous gains access to the potential space between the retina and the retinal pigment epithelium. Even then, some vitreoretinal traction seems to be necessary for retinal detachment to occur. Retinal detachment follows intraocular hemorrhage (e.g., after trauma) and is a potential complication of cataract extractions and several other ocular operations.

TRACTIONAL RETINAL DETACHMENT: In some instances, the retina is detached by being pulled toward the center of the eye by adherent vitreoretinal adhesions, as occurs in proliferative diabetic retinopathy, in retinopathy of prematurity, and after intraocular infection.

EXUDATIVE RETINAL DETACHMENT: Accumulation of fluid in the potential space between the sensory retina and the retinal pigment epithelium causes a detached retina in disorders such as choroiditis, choroidal hemangioma, and choroidal melanoma.

Retinitis Pigmentosa Is a Heritable Cause of Blindness

Retinitis pigmentosa *(pigmentary retinopathy) is a generic term that refers to a variety of bilateral, progressive, degenerative retinopathies characterized clinically by night blindness and constriction of peripheral visual fields and pathologically by the loss of retinal photoreceptors (rods and cones) and pigment accumulation within the retina.*

Pathogenesis: Multiple genetic disorders result in retinitis pigmentosa. Some are isolated ocular disorders, with autosomal dominant, autosomal recessive, or X-linked recessive inheritance; in others, the pigmentary retinopathies are associated with neurological and systemic disorders. Mutations in many genes cause retinitis pigmentosa. Some of the responsible genes encode for members of the rod phototransduction cascade, including rhodopsin, rod phosphodiesterase, and peripherin. Other mutated genes that produce retinitis pigmentosa encode oxygen-regulated photoreceptor protein *(RP1)* and a protein kinase C that is expressed in the retina *(PRKCG)*. Retinitis pigmentosa is also a manifestation of Refsum disease, a peroxisomal disorder caused by mutations in several genes that code for peroxins.

Because multiple different mutations result in retinitis pigmentosa, a single defective protein cannot explain the death of photoreceptor cells that is characteristic of the condition. Presumably the abnormal metabolic pathways that result from all mutations ultimately converge at a final common point.

Pathology: In retinitis pigmentosa, the destruction of rods and later cones is followed by migration of retinal pigment epithelial cells into the sensory retina (Fig. 29-13). Melanin appears within slender processes of spidery cells and accumulates mainly around small branching retinal blood vessels (especially in the equatorial portion of the retina), like spicules of bone. The retinal blood vessels then gradually attenuate, and the optic nerve head acquires a characteristic waxy pallor.

Clinical Features: The clinical manifestations of retinitis pigmentosa, as well as the appearance and distribution of the retinal pigmentation, vary with the causes of the retinopathy. Half of all patients with retinitis pigmentosa have a family history of the disease. Patients with autosomal recessive and X-linked disease are more severely affected and usually are seen in childhood with night blindness and peripheral field defects. Autosomal dominant forms of retinitis pigmentosa tend to be less severe, and symptoms begin later in life. As the condition progresses, contraction of the visual fields eventually leads to tunnel vision. Central vision is usually preserved until late in the course of the disease. In a few cases, the macula becomes involved, and blindness ensues.

Macular Degeneration Is Principally Age-Related

The center of the macula, the foveola, is the point of greatest visual acuity. In this area, a high concentration of cones rests

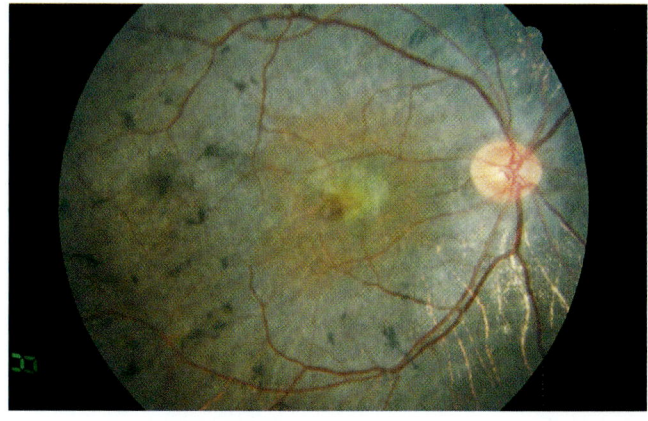
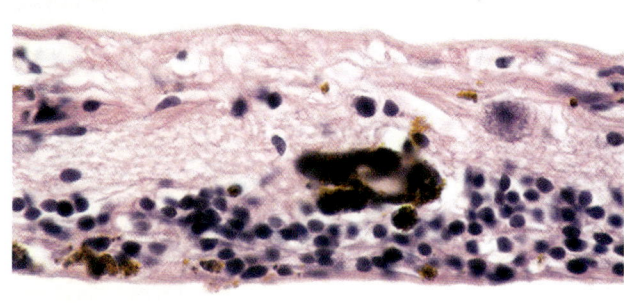

FIGURE 29-13
A. Fundus photograph of the retina of a patient with pigmentary retinopathy (retinitis pigmentosa) shows attenuated retinal vessels and foci of retinal pigmentation. **B.** Microscopic appearance of a severely degenerated retina in pigmentary retinopathy. Note the focal accumulations of pigmented cells (derived from retinal pigmented epithelium) within the retina.

on the retinal pigment epithelium. Surrounding the macula, the retina has a multilayered concentration of ganglion cells. With aging, in certain drug toxicities (e.g., chloroquine), and in several inherited disorders, the macula degenerates, and central vision is impaired.

The most common cause of reduced vision in the United States is age-related maculopathy. This condition is sometimes associated with a subretinal fibrovascular tissue and sometimes bleeding into the subretinal space (hemorrhagic macular degeneration). Laser photocoagulation has proved beneficial. Interestingly, in one series of patients with age-related macular degeneration, mutations in the *ABCR* gene (ATP–binding cassette transporter–retina) were found. *ABCR* codes for a rod cell protein (rim protein) that is thought to be a transporter involved in molecular recycling. Mutations in this gene may allow degraded material *(drusen)* to accumulate and interfere with retinal function.

Cherry-Red Spot at the Macula Describes a Bright Central Foveola

In lysosomal storage diseases, including the gangliosidoses, myriad intracytoplasmic lysosomal inclusions within the multilayered ganglion cell layer of the macula impart a striking pallor to the affected retina. As a result, the central foveola appears bright red because of the underlying choroidal vasculature (Fig. 29-14). A cherry-red spot also occurs at the macula after central retinal artery occlusion but for a different reason. Edema causes the entire retina to appear pale, which highlights the subfoveolar vascular choroid.

Angioid Streaks

Angioid streaks refer to the vessellike appearance of fractures in Bruch's membrane when the posterior segment of the eye is examined clinically. In a variety of systemic conditions, Bruch's membrane fractures spontaneously, thereby causing characteristic irregular lines that radiate beneath the retina from the optic nerve head (angioid streaks).

Retinopathy of Prematurity Results from Oxygen Toxicity

Retinopathy of prematurity, also termed retrolental fibroplasia, *is a bilateral, iatrogenic, retinal disorder that occurs predominantly in premature infants who have been treated after birth with oxygen.* The entity was originally called *retrolental fibroplasia* because of a mass of scarred tissue behind the lens in advanced cases. In the United States and in some other countries more than a half-century ago, retinopathy of prematurity (Fig. 29-15) was the leading cause of blindness in infants. This bilateral, iatrogenic ocular disorder is almost restricted to premature infants administered high concentrations of oxygen. When a premature infant is exposed to excessive amounts of oxygen (e.g., in an incubator), the developing retinal blood vessels become obliterated, and the peripheral retina, which is normally avascular until the end of fetal life, does not vascularize. The more mature the retina, the less the vasoobliterative effect of hyperoxia. When the infant eventually returns to ambient air, an intense proliferation of vascular endothelium and glial cells begins at the junction of the avascular and vascularized portions of the retina. This becomes apparent 5 to 10 weeks after removal of the infant from the incubator and, as in diabetic retinopathy, it is thought to result from the liberation of an angiogenic factor produced by the avascular and ischemic peripheral retina. This angiogenic factor is also believed to account for the neovascularization of the iris that sometimes accompanies the retinopathy of prematurity. In 25% of cases, retinopathy progresses to a cicatricial phase, characterized by retinal detachment, a fibrovascular mass behind the lens (retrolental), and blindness.

THE OPTIC NERVE

Optic Nerve Head Edema Often Reflects Increased Intracranial Pressure

Optic nerve head (optic disc) edema refers to a swelling of the optic nerve head where it enters the globe. The condition is also

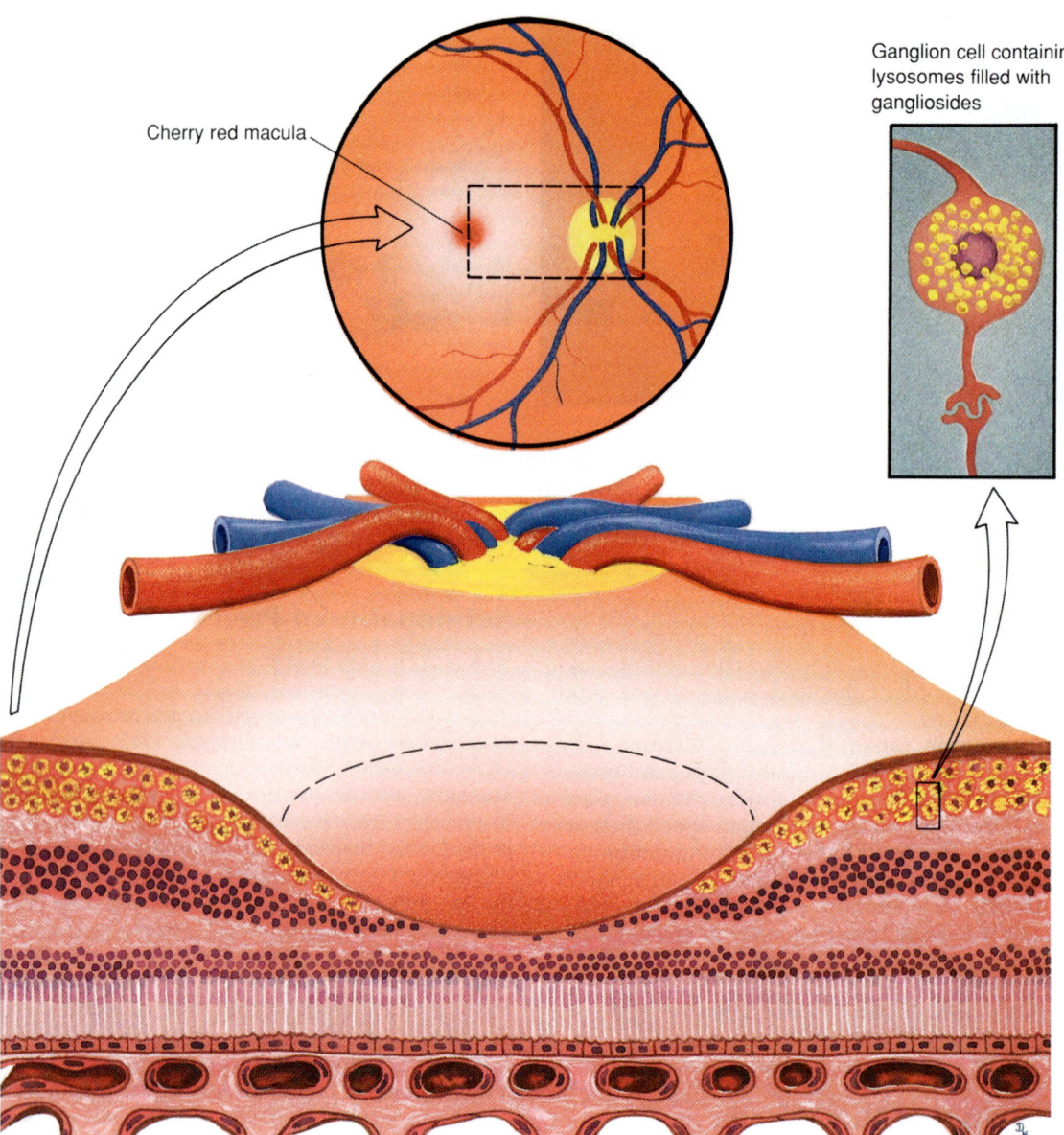

FIGURE 29-14
Cherry-red macula. A cherry-red spot appears at the macula in several lysosomal storage diseases that are characterized by intracytoplasmic accumulations within the retinal ganglion cells, such as granulocyte–macrophage-2 (GM_2) gangliosidosis type II (Tay-Sachs disease). The macula develops this appearance because the pallor created by the deposits within the multilayered ganglion cells enhances the visibility of the underlying normal choroidal vasculature.

known by the misnomer *papilledema,* which is imprecise because no optic papilla exists. Optic nerve head edema can result from various causes, the most important of which is **increased intracranial pressure.** The term *papilledema* is still widely used in that context. Other important causes of optic nerve head edema are (1) obstruction to the venous drainage of the eye (as may occur with compressive lesions of the orbit), (2) an infarct of the optic nerve (ischemic optic neuropathy), (3) inflammation of the optic nerve close to the eyeball (optic neuritis, papillitis), and (4) multiple sclerosis.

Edema of the optic nerve head is characterized clinically by a swollen optic disc that displays blurred margins and dilated vessels (Fig. 29-16). Frequently, hemorrhages (Fig. 29-17), exudates, and cotton-wool spots are seen, and concentric folds of the choroid and retina may surround the nerve head. Acutely, optic nerve head edema results in few if any visual symptoms. As the condition becomes established, swelling of the optic nerve head enlarges the normal blind spot. After many months, atrophic changes lead to a loss of visual acuity.

Optic Atrophy Results From a Loss of Axons in the Nerve

Optic atrophy is a thinning of the optic nerve caused by a loss of axons within its substance. The nerve axons within the optic nerve are lost in many conditions. Possible causes include (1)

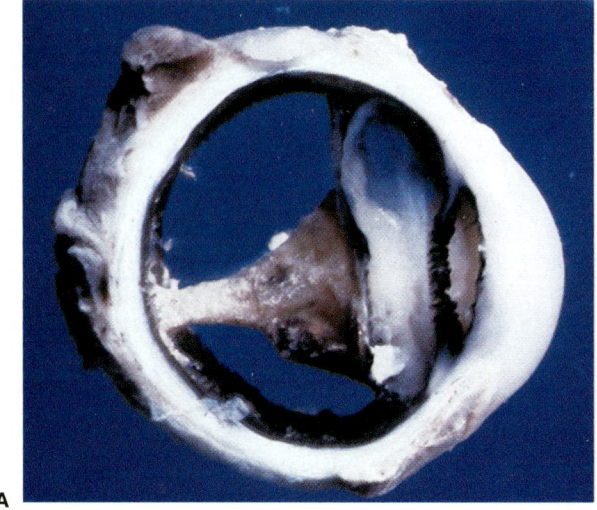
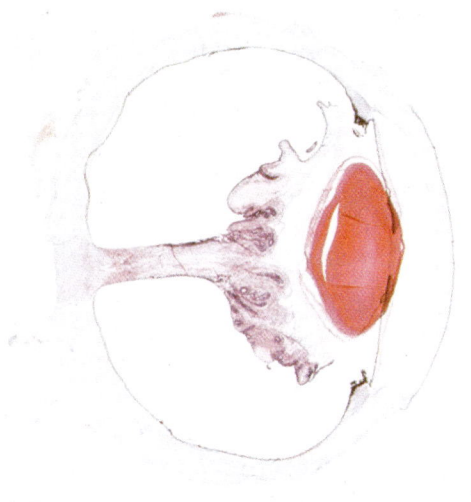
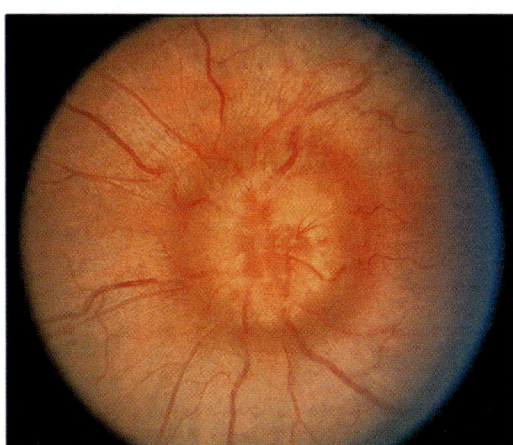

FIGURE 29-15
Retinopathy of prematurity. A. Horizontal section through an eye with advanced retinopathy of prematurity (retrolental fibroplasia) shows a totally detached retina adherent to a fibrovascular mass behind the lens. B. Whole mount of an eye with advanced retinopathy of prematurity provides a view corresponding to the macroscopic eye illustrated in *A*. C. Light-microscopic view of an early angiogenic focus in the retina with retinopathy of prematurity.

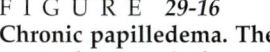
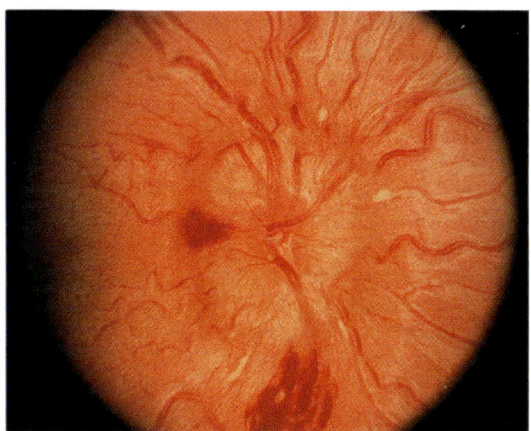

FIGURE 29-16
Chronic papilledema. The optic nerve head is congested and protrudes anteriorly toward the interior of the eye. It has blurred margins, and the vessels within it are poorly seen. In contrast to acute papilledema, the veins are not so congested, and hemorrhage is not a feature.

FIGURE 29-17
The optic nerve head is markedly congested, with dilated veins and a blurred margin. A small hemorrhage is evident within the optic nerve head at its junction with the retina. Several small "cotton-wool" spots are present within the adjacent retina.

1522   The Eye

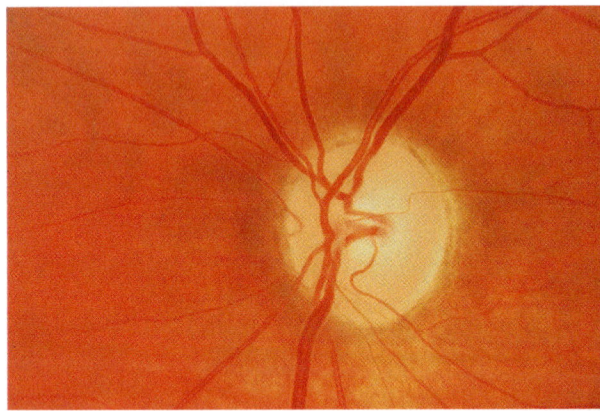

FIGURE 29-18
Optic atrophy. The margin of the optic nerve head is sharply demarcated from the adjacent retina. Because the myelinated axons in the optic nerve are markedly diminished, the optic nerve head appears much whiter than normal.

long-standing edema of the optic nerve head, (2) optic neuritis, (3) optic nerve compression, (4) glaucoma, and (5) retinal degeneration. Optic atrophy also can be caused by some drugs, such as ethambutol and isoniazid. The optic nerve head is usually flat and pale in optic atrophy (Fig. 29-18), but when this disorder follows glaucoma, the disc is excavated (*glaucomatous cupping*). Optic atrophy can follow mutations in the *OPA1*, *OPA3*, and *WFS1* genes. Multiple mutations in the mitochondrial genome are associated with *Leber hereditary optic neuropathy*.

GLAUCOMA

Glaucoma refers to a collection of disorders that feature an optic neuropathy accompanied by a characteristic excavation of the optic nerve head and a progressive loss of visual field sensitivity. In most cases, glaucoma is produced by increased intraocular pressure *(ocular hypertension)*; however, increased intraocular pressure does not necessarily cause glaucoma.

After being produced by the ciliary body, the aqueous humor enters the posterior chamber (the space between the iris and the zonules) before passing through the pupil to the anterior chamber (between the iris and the cornea). From that site, it drains into veins by way of the trabecular meshwork and Schlemm canal (Fig. 29-19). A delicate balance between the production and drainage of the aqueous humor maintains intraocular pressure within its physiological range (10–20 mm Hg). In certain pathological states, aqueous humor accumulates within the eye, and the intraocular pressure increases. Temporary or permanent impairment of vision results from pressure-induced degenerative changes in the retina and optic nerve head (Fig. 29-20) and from corneal edema and opacification.

Glaucoma almost always follows a congenital or acquired lesion of the anterior segment of the eye that mechanically obstructs the aqueous drainage. The obstruction may be located between the iris and lens, in the angle of the anterior chamber, in the trabecular meshwork, in Schlemm's canal, or in the venous drainage of the eye.

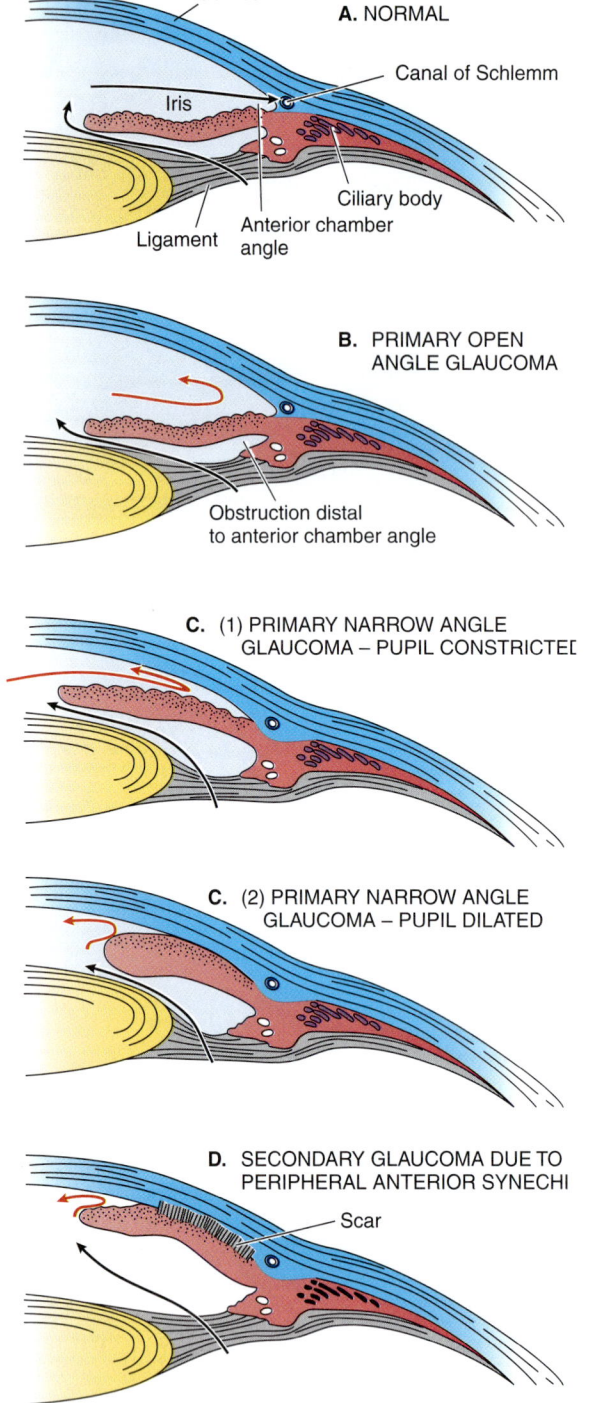

FIGURE 29-19
Pathogenesis of glaucoma. The anterior segment of the eye is affected differently in various forms of glaucoma. A. Structure of the normal eye. B. In primary open-angle glaucoma, the obstruction to the aqueous outflow is distal to the anterior chamber angle, and the anterior segment resembles that of the normal eye. C. In primary narrow-angle glaucoma, the anterior chamber angle is open, but narrower than normal when the pupil is constricted (C1). When the pupil becomes dilated in such an eye, the thickened iris obstructs the anterior chamber angle (C2), causing increased intraocular pressure. D. The anterior chamber angle can become obstructed by a variety of pathological processes, including an adhesion between the iris and the posterior surface of the cornea (peripheral anterior synechia).

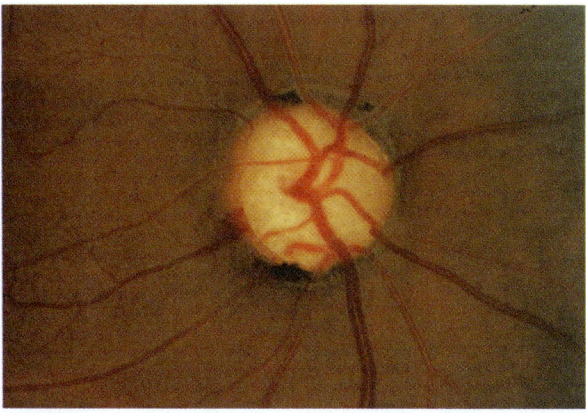

FIGURE 29-20
Optic nerve head in glaucoma. The anterior part of the optic nerve is depressed ("optic cupping"), and the blood vessels crossing the margin of the optic nerve head are displaced nasally. The fundus appears dark because this eye from a black patient contains numerous pigmented melanocytes in the choroid.

Types of Glaucoma

Congenital Glaucoma (Infantile Glaucoma, Buphthalmos)

Congenital glaucoma refers to glaucoma caused by obstruction to the aqueous drainage by developmental anomalies. The disorder develops even though the intraocular pressure may not increase until early infancy or childhood. Most cases of congenital glaucoma occur in boys (65%), and an X-linked recessive mode of inheritance is common. The developmental anomaly usually involves both eyes and, although often limited to the angle of the anterior chamber, may be accompanied by a variety of other ocular malformations. Congenital glaucoma is associated with a deep anterior chamber, corneal cloudiness, sensitivity to bright lights *(photophobia),* excessive tearing, and buphthalmos. The term *buphthalmos* (Gk. *bous,* "ox"; *ophthalmos,* "eye") designates the enlarged eyes of congenital glaucoma that result from expansion caused by increased intraocular pressure beneath a pliable sclera. Several genes for congenital glaucoma have been identified. Homozygous mutations in the cytochrome P4501B1 gene *(CYP1B1)* account for some cases of autosomal recessive primary infantile glaucoma. Congenital glaucoma associated with developmental anomalies of the eye (secondary congenital glaucoma) results from mutations in the forkhead transcription factor gene *(FKHL7),* pituitary homeobox 2 gene *(PTX2),* or paired box 6 gene *(PAX6).*

Primary Open-Angle Glaucoma

Primary glaucoma develops in a person with no apparent underlying eye disease. The disorder is subdivided into *open-angle glaucoma,* in which the anterior chamber angle is open and appears normal, and *closed-angle glaucoma,* in which the anterior chamber is shallower than normal, and the angle is abnormally narrow.

Primary open-angle glaucoma is the most frequent type of glaucoma and a major cause of blindness in the United States. It affects 1 to 3% of the population older than 40 years and occurs principally in the sixth decade. The intraocular pressure increases insidiously and asymptomatically, and although almost always bilateral, one eye may be affected more severely than the other. With time, damage to the retina and optic nerve causes an irreversible loss of peripheral vision.

 Pathogenesis: The angle of the anterior chamber is open and appears normal, but increased resistance to the outflow of the aqueous humor is present within the vicinity of Schlemm's canal. Persons with diabetes mellitus and myopia have an increased risk of primary open-angle glaucoma.

Primary open-angle glaucoma has been mapped to several loci on chromosomes 1, 2, 3, 7, and 8. Some cases of primary open-angle glaucoma are due to more than a dozen different mutations in the *MYOC (TGRR)* gene on chromosome 1 (1q21-q31). When primary open-angle glaucoma occurs in association with the nail–patella syndrome, mutations involve the Lim homeobox transcription factor *1(LMX1B)* gene. A susceptibility to normal tension glaucoma is associated with an intronic polymorphism of the *OPA1* gene, as well as with a mutation in the *OPTN* gene.

Primary Closed Angle Glaucoma

Primary closed-angle glaucoma occurs after age 40 years.

 Pathogenesis: The disorder afflicts persons whose peripheral iris is displaced anteriorly toward the trabecular meshwork, thereby creating an abnormally narrow angle. When the pupil is constricted *(miotic),* the iris remains stretched so that the chamber angle is not occluded. However, when the pupil dilates *(mydriasis),* the iris obstructs the anterior chamber angle, thereby impairing aqueous drainage and resulting in sudden episodes of intraocular hypertension. This is accompanied by ocular pain, and halos or rings are seen around lights. In such persons, the intraocular pressure may also increase if the pupil becomes blocked (e.g., by a swollen lens) and aqueous humor accumulates in the posterior chamber.

 Clinical Features: **Acute closed-angle glaucoma is an ocular emergency, and it is essential to start ocular hypotensive treatment within the first 24 to 48 hours if vision is to be maintained.** Primary closed-angle glaucoma affects both eyes, but it may become apparent in one eye 2 to 5 years before it is noted in the other. The intraocular pressure is normal between attacks, but after many episodes, adhesions form between the iris and the trabecular meshwork and cornea *(peripheral anterior synechiae)* and accentuate the block to the outflow of the aqueous humor.

Secondary Glaucoma

The causes of secondary glaucoma are many and include inflammation, hemorrhage, neovascularization of the iris, and adhesions. In secondary glaucoma, the anterior chamber angles may be open or closed. Because the underlying disorder is usually limited to one eye, secondary glaucoma tends to be unilateral.

Low-Tension Glaucoma

Low-tension glaucoma refers to an entity in which the characteristic visual-field defect and all of the ophthalmoscopic features of chronic open-angle glaucoma occur without an increase in intraocular pressure. The characteristic visual-field defect and all of the ophthalmoscopic features of chronic simple (open-angle) glaucoma often occur in the elderly without an increase in intraocular pressure. Although some eyes may be hypersensitive to normal intraocular pressure, many cases of low-tension glaucoma probably represent an infarction of the optic nerve head.

Effects of Increased Intraocular Pressure

Prolonged ocular hypertension has several effects on the eye:

- In adults, increased intraocular pressure leads to a characteristic cupped excavation of the optic nerve head (glaucomatous cupping), accompanied by a nasal displacement of the retinal blood vessels. In infants, cupping of the optic disc tends to be less prominent.
- The cornea or sclera bulges at weak points, such as sites of scars in the outer coat of the eye.
- Optic atrophy, with loss of axons, gliosis, and thickening of the pial septa, follows the retinal degeneration and damage to the nerve fibers at the optic disc.
- The ganglion cell layer of the retina degenerates, thereby impairing vision. The outer retina, which derives its nutrition from the underlying choroid, remains intact.
- When the intraocular pressure is increased before age 3 years, the pliable eye sometimes enlarges extensively *(buphthalmos)*. After the first few years of life, a rigid sclera prevents glaucomatous eyes from enlarging under the increased pressure.

MYOPIA

Myopia is a refractive ocular abnormality in which light from the visualized object focuses at a point in front of the retina because of a longer than usual anteroposterior diameter of the eye. Myopia affects more than 70 million persons in the United States, requiring correction with glasses or contact lenses. Popular controversial procedures for correcting myopia include forms of refractive surgery by use of an excimer laser such as laser-assisted in situ keratomileusis (LASIK). Myopia usually begins in young persons and varies in severity. A mild form *(stationary or simple myopia)* is generally nonprogressive after the cessation of body growth, whereas a genetically determined "progressive myopia" is more severe. The causes of myopia are complex, but some inherited types have been mapped to different chromosomes (Xq28, 12q21-q23, and 18p11.31). Myopia is a feature of *Stickler syndrome,* an autosomal dominant disorder characterized by progressive myopia beginning during childhood and leading to retinal detachment and blindness. Separate genetic variants of this condition result from mutations in three collagen genes (*COL11A2, COL11A1,* and *COL11A2*).

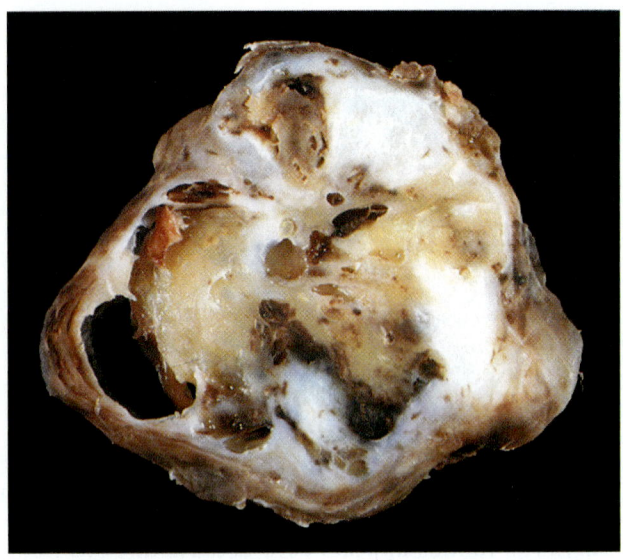

FIGURE 29-21
Section through an eye with phthisis bulbi, exemplifying the markedly disorganized nature of the intraocular contents of such atrophic disordered globes.

PHTHISIS BULBI

Phthisis bulbi refers to a nonspecific, end-stage eye that is disorganized and atrophic. This condition (Fig. 29-21) is most common after trauma to, or inflammation of, the eye. The eye is small and soft, and the choroid and ciliary body are separated from the sclera. The sclera is thickened, wrinkled, and indented owing to the loss of intraocular pressure. The cornea is flattened, shrunken, and opaque. The intraocular contents are disorganized by diffuse scarring, and detachment of the sensory retina is invariably encountered. The lens is displaced and often calcified. A typical finding in phthisis bulbi is intraocular bone formation, which seems to be derived from the hyperplastic pigment epithelium. Eyes afflicted with phthisis bulbi are often enucleated.

NEOPLASMS

The eye and adjacent structures contain a wide variety of cell types, and as one might expect, benign and malignant neoplasms arise from them. **Intraocular neoplasms arise mostly**

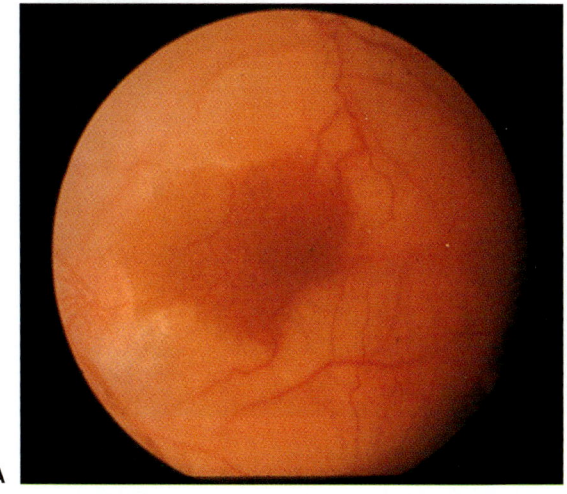 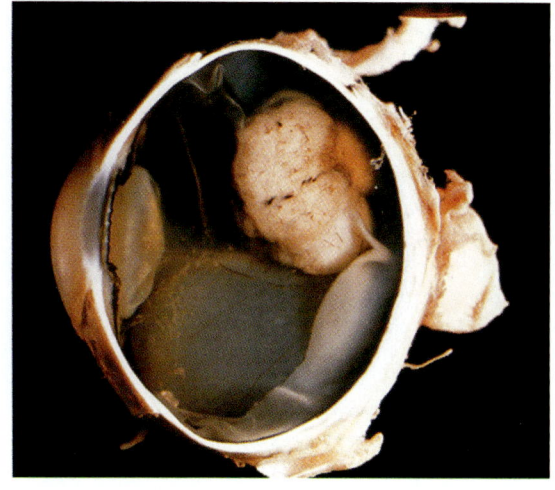

FIGURE 29-22
Malignant melanoma. **A.** Malignant melanoma of the choroid is apparent as a dark mass visible beneath the retinal blood vessels. **B.** A mushroom-shaped melanoma of the choroid is present in this eye. Choroidal melanomas commonly invade through Bruch's membrane and result in this appearance.

from immature retinal neurons (retinoblastoma) and uveal melanocytes (melanoma). Although the retinal pigment epithelium often undergoes reactive proliferation, it seldom becomes neoplastic.

Malignant Melanoma Arises from Melanocytes in the Uvea

Uveal melanoma is a malignant neoplasm that originates from melanocytes or nevi in the uvea. Malignant melanoma is the most common primary intraocular malignancy. It may arise from melanocytes in any part of the eye, the choroid being the most common site.

 Pathology: Choroidal melanomas are mostly circumscribed and invade Bruch's membrane, causing a mushroom-shaped mass (Fig. 29-22). By contrast, some tumors are flat (diffuse melanoma) and cause a gradual deterioration of vision over many years. Some do not become apparent until extraocular dissemination has occurred. Orange lipofuscin pigment is evident over the surface of some choroidal melanomas.

Microscopically, uveal melanomas may be composed mainly of variable numbers of spindle-shaped cells without nucleoli (spindle A cells), spindle-shaped cells with prominent nucleoli (spindle B cells), and polygonal cells with distinct cell borders and prominent nucleoli (epithelioid cells). The cells vary in their amount of pigmentation, and some cells may contain abundant cytoplasmic lipid ("balloon cell degeneration"). Variable amounts of necrosis are common in uveal melanomas.

Melanomas of the ciliary body and iris may extend circumferentially around the globe (ring melanoma). Melanomas in the iris are seen clinically 1 to 2 decades earlier than those in the choroid and ciliary body, perhaps because they are more easily seen.

Aside from hematogenous spread, uveal melanomas disseminate by traversing the sclera to enter the orbital tissues, usually at sites where blood vessels and nerves pass through the sclera. Unlike melanomas of the skin, those of the uvea do not spread by lymphatics because the eye lacks these structures. Intraocular melanomas sometimes cause cataract, glaucoma, retinal detachment, inflammation, and even hemorrhage.

The usual treatment for most uveal melanomas is enucleation of the eye, but some are treated with other methods, such as radiotherapy or local excision. More than half of patients with uveal melanomas survive for 15 years after enucleation. Deaths have been reported within 5 years from spindle A melanomas, but tumors composed purely of epithelioid cells have the worst prognosis. Anecdotally, the diagnosis of metastatic ocular melanoma has been made intuitively by astute clinicians who discovered an enlarged liver in a patient with a "glass eye."

Retinoblastoma Originates from Immature Neurons

Retinoblastoma the most common intraocular malignant neoplasm of childhood (Fig. 29-23) affecting 1:20,000 to 1:34,000 children. The tumor most frequently is seen within the first 2 years of life and sometimes even at birth. The presenting signs include a white pupil (leukocoria), squint (strabismus), poor vision, spontaneous hyphema, or a red, painful eye. Secondary glaucoma is a frequent complication. Light entering the eye commonly reflects a yellowish color similar to that from the tapetum of a cat (cat's eye reflex). Most retinoblastomas occur sporadically and are unilateral. Some 6 to 8% of retinoblastomas are inherited. Up to 25% of sporadic retinoblastomas and most inherited retinoblastomas are bilateral.

Retinoblastomas are related to inherited or acquired deletions of, or mutations in, the retinoblastoma *(Rb)* tumor-

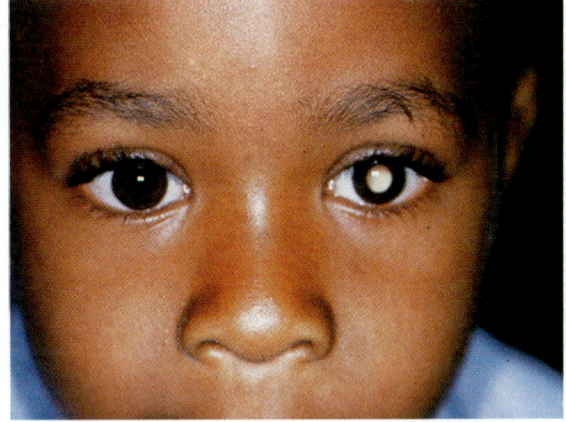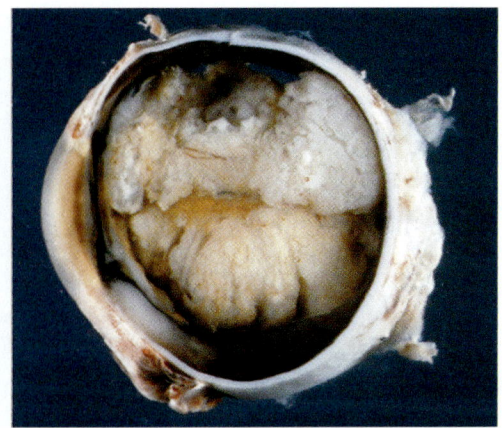

FIGURE 29-23
Retinoblastoma. **A.** The white pupil (leukocoria) in the left eye is the result of an intraocular retinoblastoma. **B.** This surgically excised eye is almost filled by a cream-colored intraocular retinoblastoma with calcified flecks.

suppressor gene, located on the long arm of chromosome 13 (13q14) (see Chapter 5).

 Pathology: Some retinoblastomas grow toward the vitreous body and can be seen with an ophthalmoscope (endophytic retinoblastoma). Others extend between the sensory retina and the retinal pigment epithelium, thereby detaching the retina (exophytic retinoblastoma). A few retinoblastomas are both endophytic and exophytic. The retina often contains several distinct foci of tumor in the same eye, some of which represent multifocal origin, whereas others reflect tumor implantations from dissemination through the vitreous body.

Retinoblastoma is a cream-colored tumor that contains scattered, chalky white, calcified flecks within yellow necrotic zones, which may be detected radiologically. The tumors are intensely cellular and display several morphological patterns. In some instances, densely packed, round neoplastic cells with hyperchromatic nuclei, scant cytoplasm, and abundant mitoses are randomly distributed. In other retinoblastomas, the cells are arranged radially around a central cavity *(Flexner-Wintersteiner rosettes),* as they differentiate toward photoreceptors. In some cases, the cellular arrangement resembles the *fleur-de-lis (fleurette).* Viable tumor cells align themselves around blood vessels, and necrotic areas with calcification are seen a short distance from the vascularized regions.

Retinoblastomas disseminate by several routes. They commonly extend into the optic nerve, from where they spread intracranially. They also invade blood vessels, especially in the highly vascular choroid, before metastasizing hematogenously throughout the body. Bone marrow is a common site of blood-borne metastases, but surprisingly, the lung is rarely involved.

Retinoblastomas are almost always fatal if left untreated. However, with early diagnosis and modern therapy, survival is high (about 90%). Rarely, spontaneous regression occurs for reasons that remain unknown. Patients with inherited retinoblastomas, presumably as a consequence of the loss of *Rb* gene function, have an increased susceptibility to other malignant tumors, including osteogenic sarcoma, Ewing sarcoma, and pinealoblastoma.

Metastatic Intraocular and Orbital Neoplasms

Metastatic neoplasms in the eye are more common than those that arise within the ocular tissues. Sometimes an ocular metastasis is the initial clinical manifestation of the cancer, but most cases are diagnosed only after death. Leukemias and cancers of the breast and lung account for most cases of intraocular metastases, usually to the posterior choroid. Neuroblastoma frequently metastasizes to the orbit in infancy and childhood. The orbit may be invaded by malignant neoplasms of the eyelid, conjunctiva, paranasal sinuses, nose, nasopharynx, and intracranial cavity.

SUGGESTED READING

Eagle RC Jr: Eye pathology: An atlas and basic Text. Philadelphia: WB Saunders, 1999.

Garner A, Klintworth GK (eds): *Pathobiology of ocular disease: A dynamic approach,* 2nd ed. New York: Marcel Dekker, 1994.

Klintworth GK: The eye pathologist, an eye pathology tutor and disease database. http://emsweb.mc.duke.edu/eyepath.nsf

Klintworth GK, Eagle RC Jr: Eye and ocular adnexa. In: Damjanov I, Linder J (eds). *Anderson's pathology,* 10th ed. St. Louis: Mosby, 1996: 2832–2875.

Scroggs MW, Klintworth GK: The eye and ocular adnexa. In: Sternberg SS (ed): *Diagnostic surgical pathology,* 2nd ed. New York: Raven Press, 1994:949–980.

Spencer WH (ed): *Ophthalmic pathology: An atlas and textbook,* 4th ed, 3 vols. Philadelphia: WB Saunders, 1996.

Yanoff M, Fine BS: *Ocular pathology,* 5th ed. St. Louis: Mosby-Year Book, 2002.

CHAPTER 30

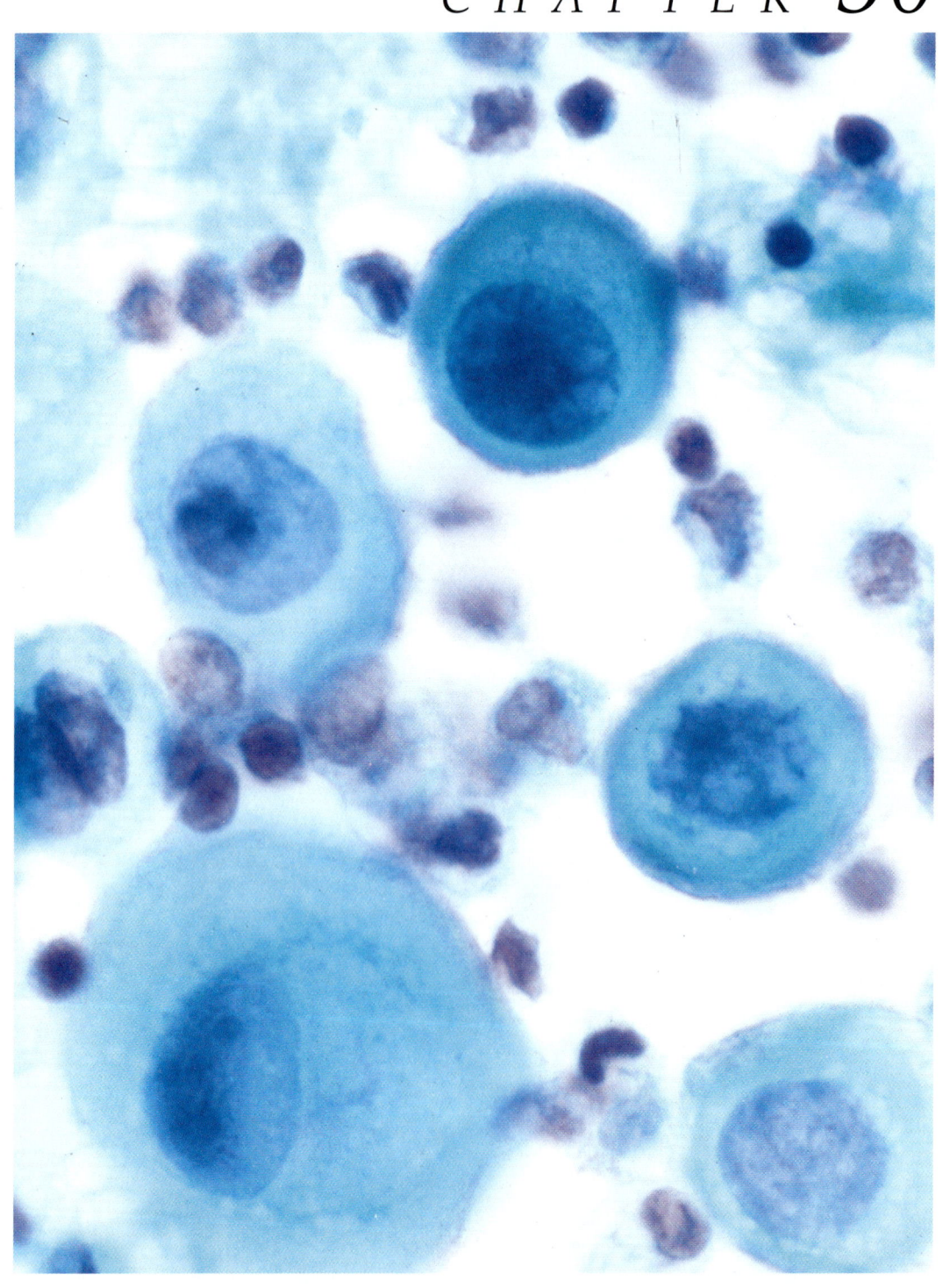

Cytopathology

Marluce Bibbo

Applications of Cytopathology

Early Detection of Asymptomatic Cancer

Symptomatic Cancers

Tumor Recurrence

Cytological Methods

Cells in Body Fluids

Abrasive Cytology

Fine-Needle Aspiration Cytology

Advantages of Cytopathology

Limitations of Cytopathology

Accuracy of Cytological Methods

Causes of Error in Cytology

Morphological Parameters in Cytological Evaluation

Morphological Parameters in Cytological Evaluation

Specimen Cellularity

Cell Arrangement

Variations in Cell Size and Shape

Cytoplasmic Features

Features of Malignancy in the Nucleus

Extracellular Material and Background

Reporting Systems

FIGURE 30-1 *(see opposite page)*
Cytological preparation of pleural fluid from a patient with mesothelioma.

Abrasive Cytology Dislodges Cells from Body Surfaces

Cervical smears are obtained by means of a spatula or small brush. Other abrasive methods include endoscopic brushing of the mucosal surfaces of the gastrointestinal, respiratory, and urinary tracts; the balloon technique for obtaining cells from the esophagus; and scraping of cutaneous, oral, vaginal, or conjunctival lesions to detect herpesvirus inclusions. Washing (or lavage) of mucosal or serosal surfaces during endoscopy or open surgery may be considered a combined exfoliative and abrasive method, because it samples both cells that are shed spontaneously and those that are dislodged mechanically.

Triage of Lumps and Bumps Is Accomplished by Fine-Needle Aspiration Cytology

Virtually any organ or tissue can be sampled by fine-needle aspiration, which uses aspiration under negative pressure through a thin-gauge needle. Superficial organs (e.g., thyroid, breast, lymph nodes, prostate, skin, and soft tissues) are easily targeted. Deep organs (e.g., lung, mediastinum, liver, pancreas, kidney, adrenal gland, and retroperitoneum) are aspirated with guidance by fluoroscopy, computed tomography, or ultrasound.

A combination of air-dried, Romanowsky-stained smears and alcohol-fixed smears stained by the Papanicolaou method are preferred by most American cytopathologists. A separate pass can be made for cell block preparation, which allows characterization of the tumor architectural features in the tissue fragments. Immunocytochemical stains are readily performed in sections from the paraffin embedded block.

Examples of cytological preparations from various organs are shown in Figs. 30-1 through 30-14.

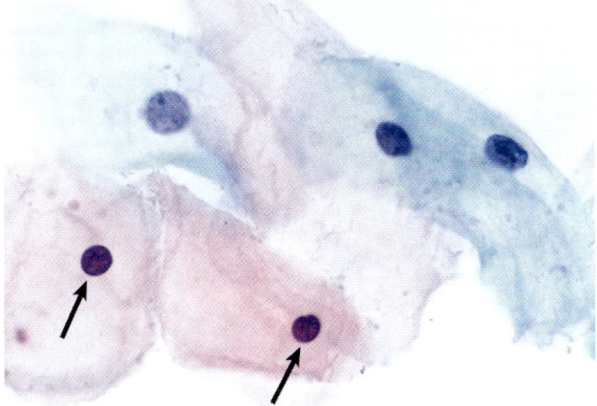

FIGURE 30-2
Normal cervical Papanicolaou (Pap) smear. Large squamous cells from the superficial and intermediate layers of the epithelium are illustrated. The cells have abundant cytoplasm that varies in staining from pink to blue. The nuclei are small, and the nuclear–cytoplasmic ratio is low. The most superficial cells have pyknotic nuclei *(arrows)*.

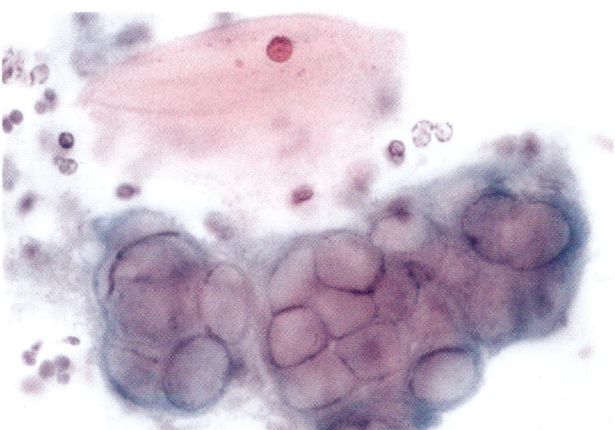

FIGURE 30-3
Herpes simplex virus infection in a cervical smear. Note multinucleation of squamous cells, nuclear molding, margination of the chromatin, and "ground glass" appearance of the nuclei. A normal superficial squamous cell serves for comparison.

ADVANTAGES OF CYTOPATHOLOGY

Cytology has both advantages and limitations compared with the examination of histological samples (biopsy).

Less trauma is produced by cytological techniques than by biopsy. Thus, there are fewer complications such as hemorrhage or perforation. For example, aspirating pleural fluid with a thin needle is much less traumatic than obtaining a piece of the pleura by open biopsy or with a large needle. Similarly, brushing the surface of an endobronchial tumor or a colonic lesion is less likely to cause hemorrhage than is removing a piece of the tissue. Because of the small diameter of the needle used for fine-needle aspiration, the risk of hemorrhage, infection, or tumor spread is negligible compared with that associated with large-core needle biopsy or punch biopsy. For example, acute pancreatitis, a serious complication of large-core needle biopsy or open biopsy of the pancreas, is vanishingly rare with fine-needle aspiration.

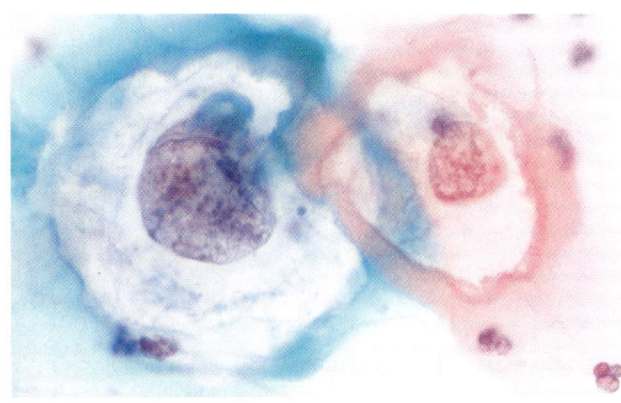

FIGURE 30-4
Papillomavirus infection in a cervical smear. Two superficial squamous cells exhibit *koilocytotic atypia,* a term that denotes the presence of sharply demarcated, large perinuclear vacuoles, combined with alterations in the chromatin pattern.

1532 Cytopathology

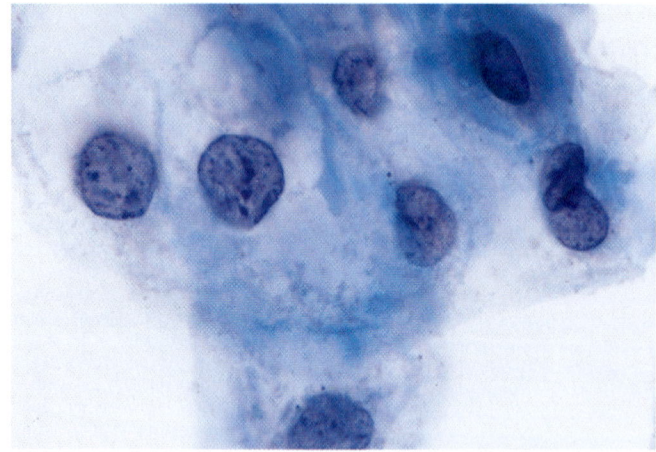

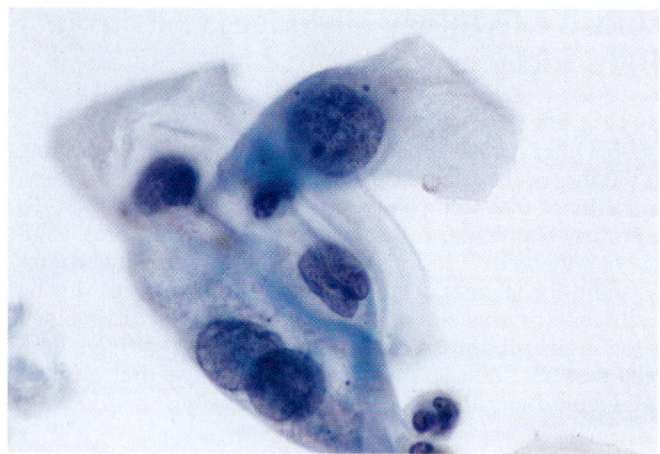

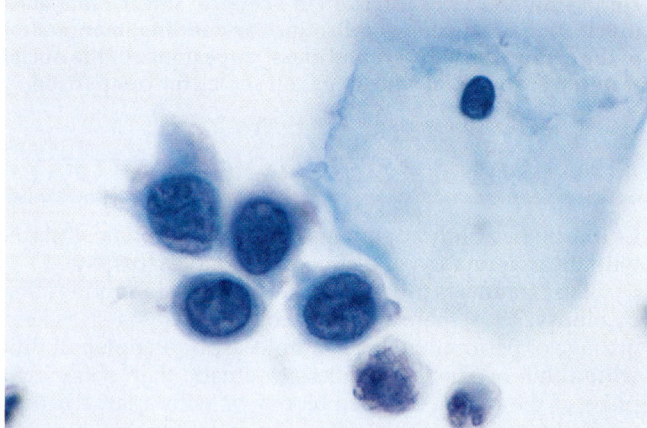

FIGURE 30-5
Spectrum of squamous intraepithelial lesions (SILs) in cervical smears. A. Low-grade SIL (mild dysplasia, CIN1). The dysplastic cells have abundant cytoplasm. The nucleus is enlarged and hyperchromatic. B. High-grade SIL (moderate dysplasia, CIN2). The dysplastic cells have a higher nuclear–cytoplasmic ratio than do mildly dysplastic cells. C. High-grade SIL (severe dysplasia, CIN3/carcinoma in situ). Multiple dysplastic squamous cells with scant cytoplasm and very high nuclear–cytoplasmic ratios are seen. Note the normal superficial squamous cell.

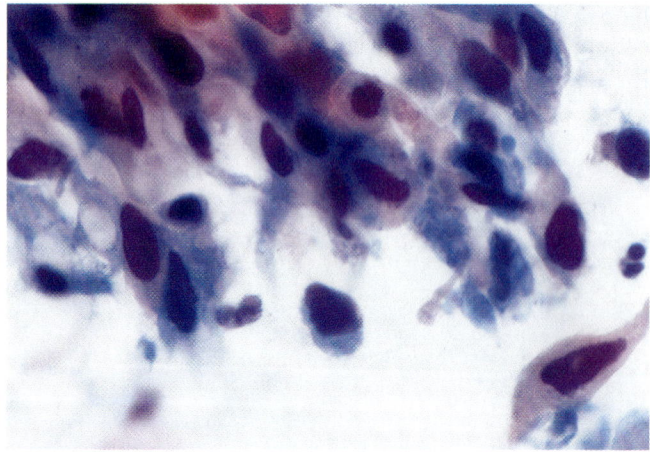

FIGURE 30-6
Invasive squamous cell carcinoma of the cervix. Pleomorphic elongate squamous cells, with enlarged, irregular and hyperchromatic nuclei.

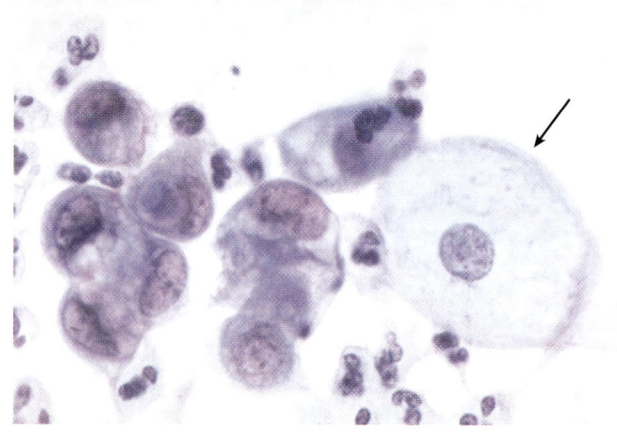

FIGURE 30-7
Endometrial adenocarcinoma in a cervical smear. A cluster of medium-sized malignant cells displays cytoplasmic vacuoles. The nuclei are eccentric and have irregular nuclear membranes and abnormally distributed chromatin. Note the benign squamous cell (arrow).

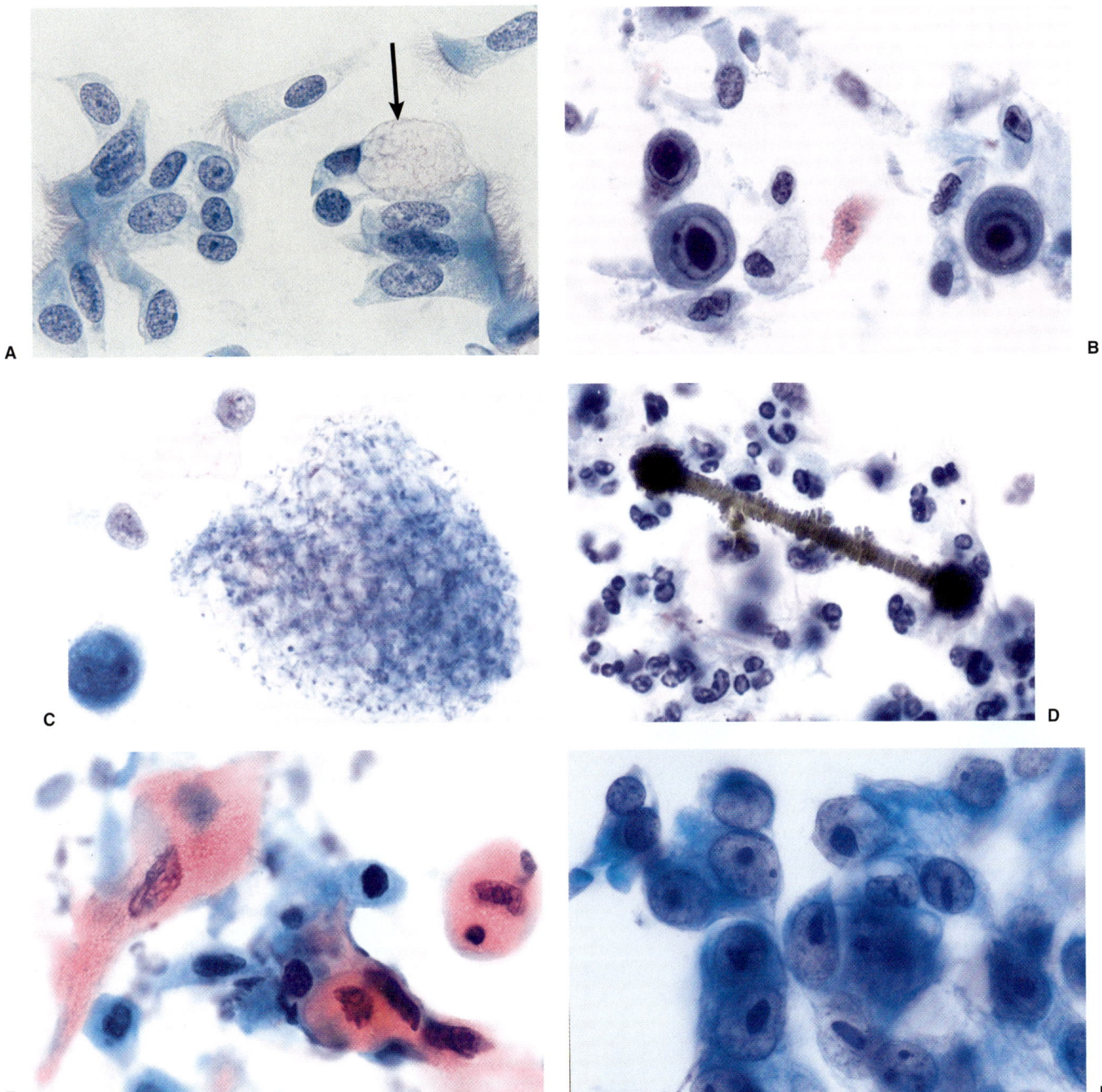

FIGURE 30-8
Cytology of the respiratory tract. A. Normal bronchial epithelial cells in a bronchial brush specimen. Note the ciliated columnar cells with uniform and basally located nuclei. The chromatin is finely granular and evenly dispersed; the nuclear membrane is smooth and regular. Note the goblet cell *(arrow)*. B. Cytomegalovirus (CMV) infection in a bronchial washing. Note the large basophilic nuclear inclusions surrounded by a halo and marginated chromatin, forming the typical target-shaped appearance. C. *Pneumocystis carinii* in a bronchoalveolar lavage specimen. This foamy alveolar cast composed of small cysts, each with an eccentric dot, is characteristic of *P. carinii*. Bronchial cells and an alveolar macrophage are evident. D. Ferruginous body in the sputum. This long, yellow, beaded structure with clubbed ends is formed by the precipitation of iron and protein complexes on asbestos fibers. E. Squamous cell carcinoma in a bronchial brush specimen. Highly atypical squamous cells show marked variation in size and shape. The nuclei are hyperchromatic and irregular. The orange color in some of the cells denotes the presence of keratin. F. Adenocarcinoma cells in bronchial brush specimen. A cluster of epithelial cells with highly atypical nuclei, prominent nucleoli, and cytoplasmic vacuoles is seen.

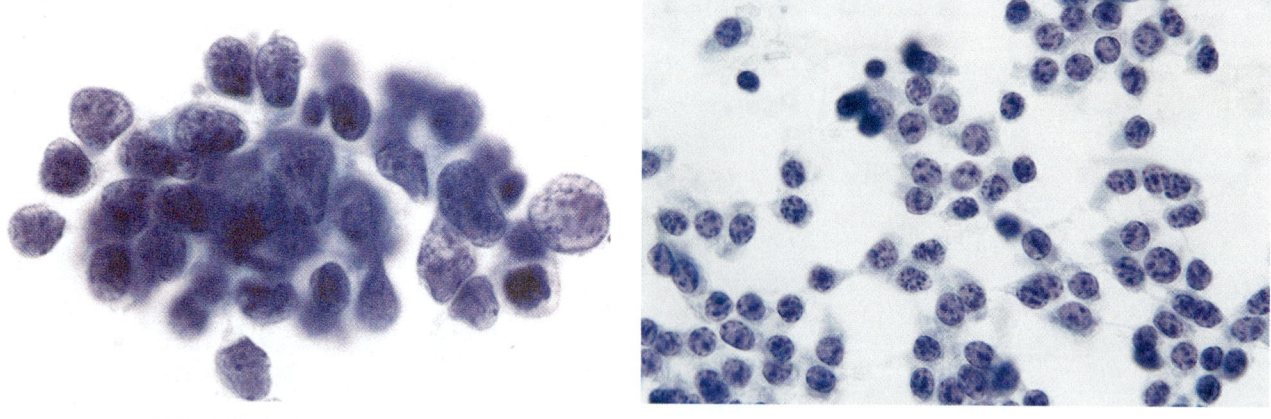

FIGURE 30-8 (continued)
G. Small cell carcinoma in a bronchial brush specimen. The cells are small, the cytoplasm is scanty, and the nuclei are molded where they abut adjacent ones. H. Carcinoid tumor in a fine-needle aspirate of the lung. These small cells are arranged in loosely cohesive sheets. They have scant cytoplasm and uniform round nuclei. The chromatin is evenly dispersed.

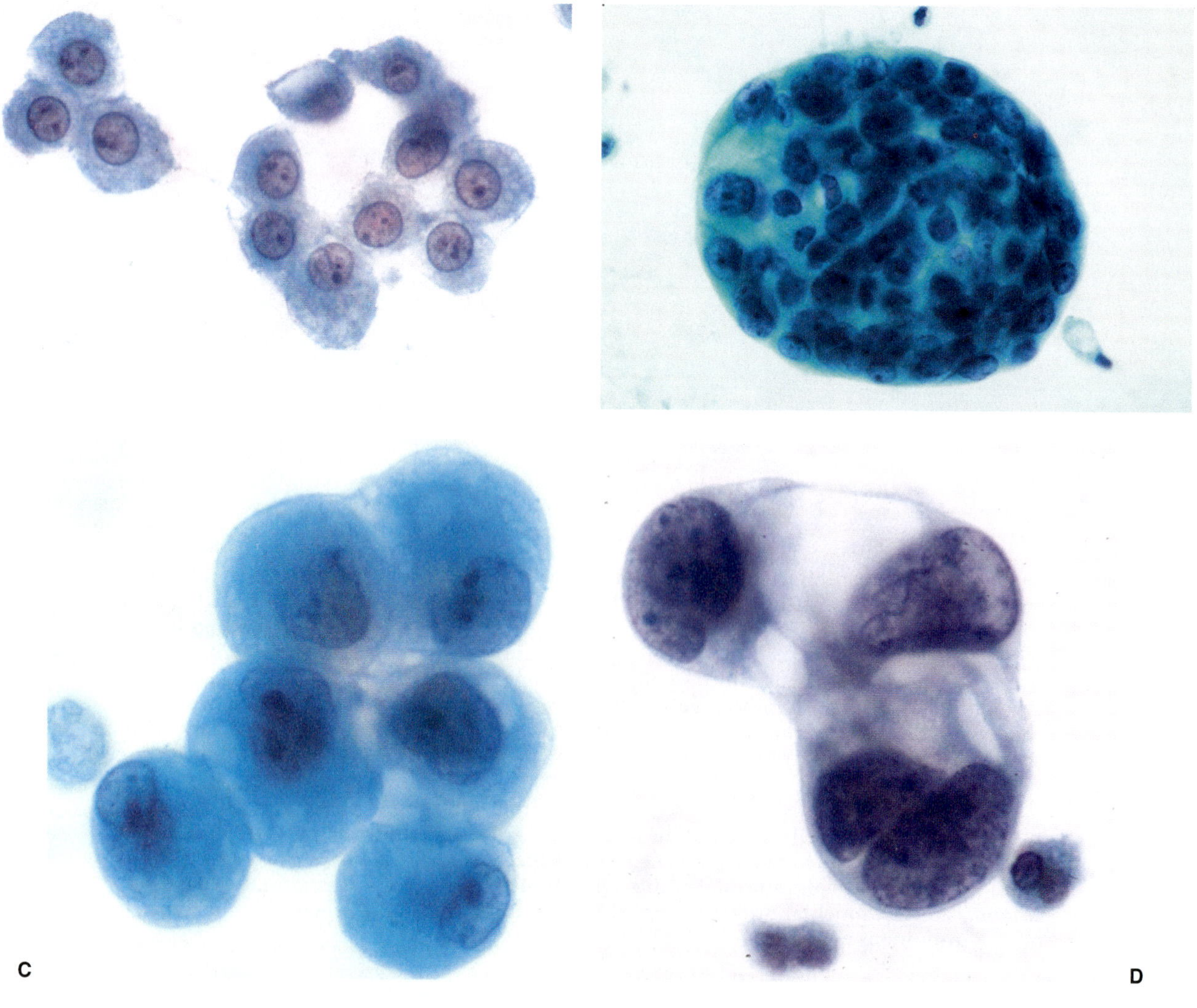

Advantages of Cytopathology   1535

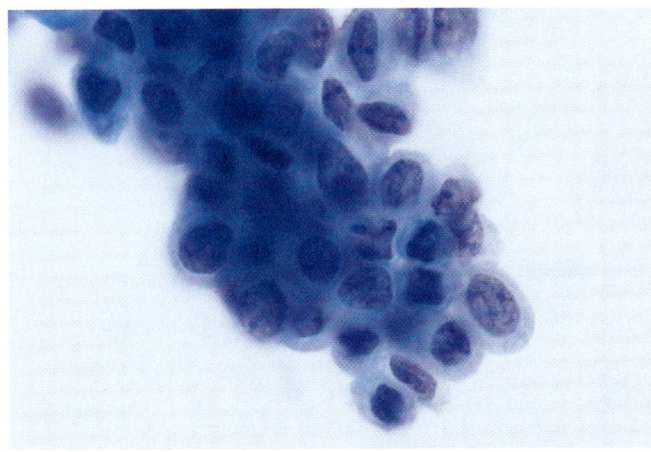
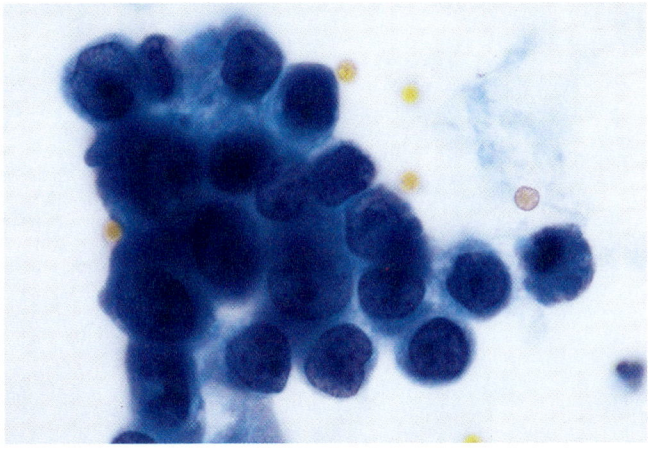

FIGURE 30-10
Cytology of the urinary tract. A. Low-grade papillary transitional cell carcinoma from the renal pelvis. Architecturally, the cells form a papillary structure, and the nuclei are crowded and hyperchromatic. B. High-grade transitional cell carcinoma in urine. Highly pleomorphic cells with varying sized, hyperchromatic, irregular nuclei are evident.

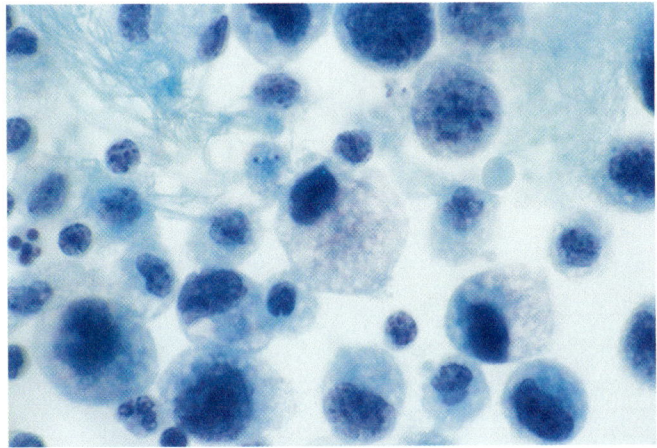
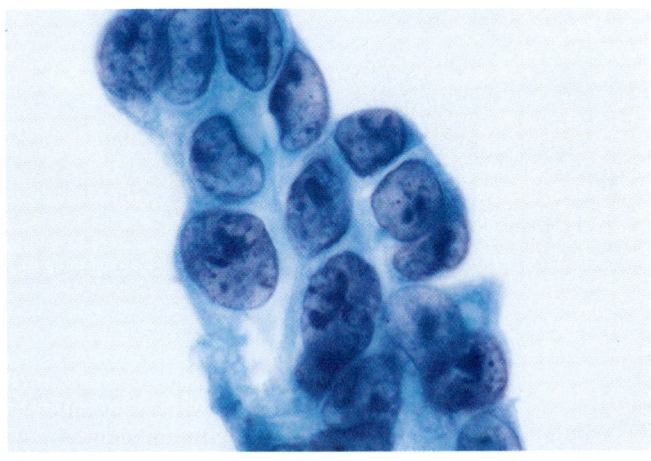

FIGURE 30-11
Cytology of the alimentary tract. A. Gastric carcinoma in brushing specimen. Note cytoplasmic vacuoles in tumor cells. B. Adenocarcinoma of the colon. The malignant nuclei display variation in size and shape and prominent nucleoli.

←

FIGURE 30-9
Cytology of effusions. A. Benign mesothelial cells in pleural fluid. The nuclei are small, round, and uniform. The nuclear membrane is smooth, and the nucleoli are small. B. Metastatic breast carcinoma. Note "cannon ball" appearance of the tumor cells. C. Cells of a malignant mesothelioma in pleural fluid. The cytoplasm resembles that of normal mesothelial cells, but the nuclei are large, hyperchromatic, and irregular. The chromatin is abnormally distributed, the nucleoli are prominent, and the nuclear membrane has irregular indentations. D. Metastatic ovarian adenocarcinoma in ascitic fluid. The nuclei exhibit malignant criteria, and the cytoplasm contains secretory vacuoles.

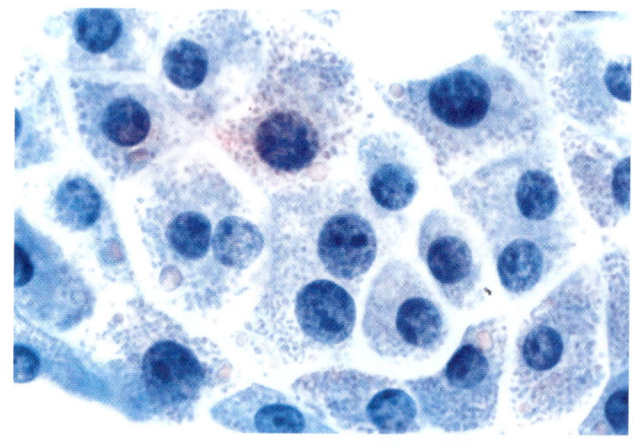 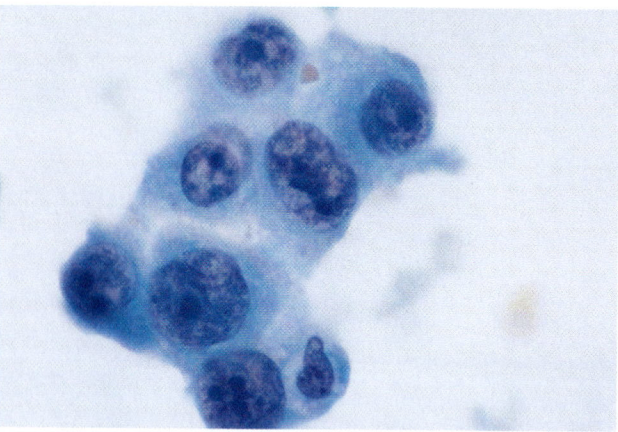

FIGURE 30-12
Fine-needle aspiration (FNA) cytology of the breast. A. Apocrine metaplasia. These benign cells have abundant and granular cytoplasm. B. Mammary duct carcinoma. The cells vary in size and shape and are poorly cohesive. The nuclei are hyperchromatic, with irregular membranes and clumping of the chromatin. The nucleoli are prominent.

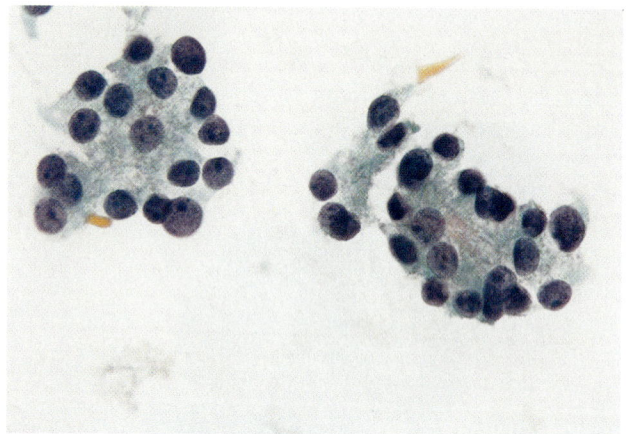 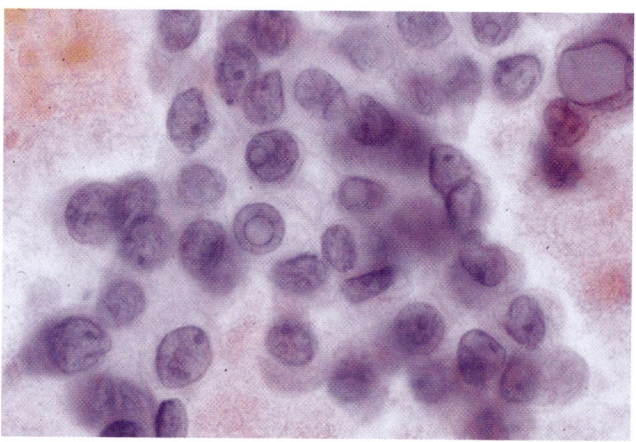

FIGURE 30-13
Fine-needle aspiration (FNA) cytology of the thyroid. A. Follicular neoplasm. The tumor cells form small follicles with scant colloid and mild nuclear atypia. B. Papillary carcinoma. A papillary frond of the tumor shows nuclei with nuclear grooves and intranuclear inclusions.

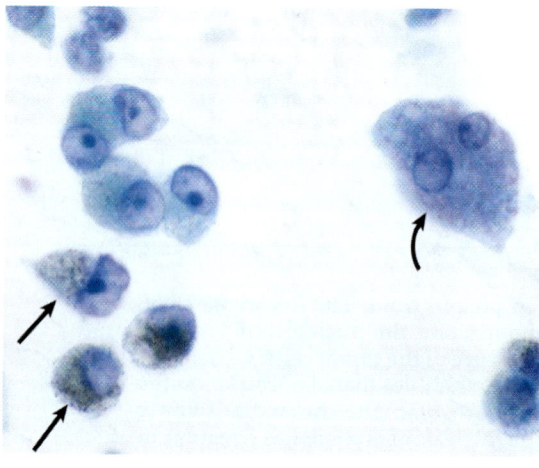

FIGURE 30-14
Metastatic malignant melanoma in a fine-needle aspirate of the liver. Poorly cohesive tumor cells exhibit eccentric nuclei and prominent nucleoli. The cytoplasm contains fine melanin granules *(straight arrows)*. A benign binucleated hepatocyte is evident *(curved arrow)*.

The complications of anesthesia are of no concern, because collection of cytological samples usually does not require general or local anesthesia.

A larger sampling surface is available for cytological methods. This is particularly important in endoscopic procedures and assessment of the intraperitoneal spread of cancer cells during laparotomy. In peritoneal washings, a very large area of the peritoneum is sampled, whereas biopsy samples are limited to a few, small, grossly visible foci. A focus of flat in situ carcinoma of the bladder that is not evident on cystoscopy is more likely to be discovered by cytological examination of urine or bladder washings than by random biopsy samples.

Tumors that are difficult to access by biopsy may be sampled by cytological methods. Examples include cerebrospinal fluid cytology to diagnose meningeal carcinomatosis, brushing or washing a gastrointestinal tract stricture that does not permit passage of the biopsy instrument, and fine-needle aspiration of a peripheral carcinoma of the lung that is beyond the reach of a bronchoscope.

A rapid diagnosis is one of the major advantages of cytological methods. Direct smears and fine-needle aspirates can be read within a few minutes of the collection. Fluids that need laboratory preparation can be processed, if necessary, in less than an hour.

Greater convenience is afforded by the collection of cytological specimens than with biopsy. In most instances, no prior preparation of the patient is necessary, and the sampling is done as an office procedure. For endoscopically collected specimens, no preparations are needed beyond those required routinely for visualization.

An increased detection rate of malignancy in endoscopic procedures is achieved by combining cytological sampling (washing or brushing) with biopsy. In turn, this reduces the possibility that a repeated diagnostic procedure will be required.

Greater cost-effectiveness of use of cytology for cancer detection has been amply demonstrated. Often, it eliminates needless tests, procedures, and surgical operations.

LIMITATIONS OF CYTOPATHOLOGY

Classification of the type of tumor is generally more difficult with cytological samples than with biopsy specimens because of the small size of cytological samples and the loss of tissue pattern. Cytological interpretation relies heavily on morphological alterations of individual cells and to a lesser degree on the relation between the cells (e.g., formation of acini or squamous pearls, molding of cells, papillary arrangement). The patterns of tumor infiltration and invasion of the adjacent structures and vascular channels are important histological parameters in the determination of malignancy but cannot be evaluated by cytology. For example, the differential diagnosis between follicular adenoma and well-differentiated follicular carcinoma of the thyroid depends on the absence or presence of capsular and vascular invasion, rather than the appearance of the tumor cells. Because such invasion cannot be determined by aspiration of the lesion, a diagnosis of "follicular neoplasm" is rendered by the cytopathologist; further classification of the tumor requires histological examination of the excised tumor.

The small size of the specimen may preclude accurate classification of some neoplasms with mixed elements, such as adenosquamous carcinoma, carcinosarcoma, or synovial sarcoma, if only one component of the tumor is sampled. In exfoliative cytology, carcinomas are more readily diagnosed than sarcomas, because epithelial neoplasms have a higher tendency to shed tumor cells. For the same reason, malignant mixed mesodermal tumor of the female genital tract is frequently diagnosed as adenocarcinoma on examination of the peritoneal fluid or cervicovaginal smears.

The extent and depth of invasion cannot be assessed by cytological examination. For example, it is not possible to distinguish with certainty between in situ and invasive transitional cell carcinoma of the bladder by cytological examination of the urine, between microinvasive and deeply invasive squamous carcinoma of the cervix with cervical smears, or between intraductal carcinoma and invasive duct carcinoma of the breast by needle aspiration.

ACCURACY OF CYTOLOGICAL METHODS

The accuracy of cytological diagnosis depends on several factors, including the experience of the specimen collector, the sampling method, the sample adequacy, the target organ, and the expertise of the examiner. False-positive diagnoses are rarely made by experienced cytopathologists; thus, the specificity of a malignant diagnosis approaches 100%. The sensitivity of the test, however, is in the range of 80 to 90% for most specimen types. The existence of false-negative results indicates that the absence of malignant cells in cytological samples does not completely rule out the possibility of malignancy. Unless a benign cause for a lesion can be established by cytological examination (e.g., fibroadenoma of the breast, benign cyst of the thyroid, liver abscess, granuloma of the lung), further investigation, including histological biopsy, is warranted to exclude a malignant etiology.

Higher sensitivity has been achieved by some endoscopic brushing methods, particularly for alimentary tract cancers, whereas for some specimen types, the sensitivity is lower. For example, cytological examination of cerebrospinal fluid detects only one third of primary neoplasms of the central nervous system and only one half of metastatic cancers, because only tumors that communicate with the ventricles or meninges can shed cells. For urinary tract cancers, the sensitivity of cytology depends on the type and grade of the tumor. Low-grade transitional cell carcinomas, which by definition have little or no nuclear atypia, are difficult to detect, whereas high-grade neoplasms are usually diagnosed correctly.

CAUSES OF ERROR IN CYTOLOGY

Several factors contribute to erroneous cytological interpretations:

- **Inadequate sampling** is one of the major causes of false-negative diagnoses in cytology. For example, in obtaining a smear of the uterine cervix, it is critical to sample the transformation zone, because most precancerous lesions of the cervix arise in this area. Thus, an adequate cervical smear should contain squamous cells as well as endocervical material (columnar cells, mucus, and metaplastic squamous cells). The adequacy of a sputum specimen is assessed by the presence of pulmonary macrophages, which indicates a deep cough sample. Examples of inadequate cytological samples include (1) a peritoneal washing specimen that lacks mesothelial cells, (2) a smear of a cutaneous vesicle that is obtained to search for viral changes but lacks squamous cells, and (3) a gastric brushing specimen that contains blood and inflammatory cells but no epithelial cells.

- **Poor fixation of the smears or inadequate preservation of a fluid** is another preventable cause of error in cytology. For the Papanicolaou staining method, cells must be fixed in 95% ethanol or by a spray fixative immediately after smearing on the slide. A few seconds of delay in fixation can cause air-drying artifacts that create substantial difficulties in interpretation. To circumvent problems of poor fixation, liquid-based Paps have been introduced recently and are becoming popular. Cervical scrapings are rinsed in special fixative solutions, which improves cell preservation and the sensitivity of the test.

Cells in body fluids undergo degeneration at a rate that varies according to the type of fluid. Generally, cells are better protected in fluids with a high protein concentration, such as effusions, than in those that contain little protein (e.g., urine or cerebrospinal fluid). To prevent cell degeneration, fluids must be transported to the laboratory and processed rapidly. Refrigeration slows cell degeneration and bacterial growth for a few hours or a day, but if delay is inevitable, a preservative should be used. Addition of an equal volume of 50% ethanol is a good method for preservation of fluids. Formaldehyde, a commonly used fixative for histological samples, is not appropriate for cytological preparations.

Suboptimal laboratory preparation and staining can cause considerable difficulty in the interpretation of cytological smears. Examples include (1) inadequate cell concentration or poor adhesion to the glass slide, (2) thick smears containing multiple layers of cells, (3) poor fixation, and (4) inadequate or excessive exposure of the cells to various staining reagents.

MORPHOLOGICAL PARAMETERS IN CYTOLOGICAL EVALUATION

Specimen Cellularity Is Influenced by Various Factors

In general, abrasive methods produce more cells than spontaneously exfoliated samples. For example, samples of a lung neoplasm obtained by bronchial washing or brushing are likely to have a larger number of tumor cells than a sputum specimen.

In fine-needle aspiration, larger needles produce more cellular samples than very thin ones. Important factors for obtaining adequately cellular samples include (1) placement of the needle or brush in the proper position, (2) application of optimal pressure or suction, (3) adequate movement of the device within the target tissue, and (4) avoidance of dilution of cells with excessive blood.

The type of tissue sampled greatly influences the cellularity of the specimen. Epithelial cells are generally detached with greater ease than stromal cells or fibrous tissue. Malignant cells have lower cohesiveness than their benign counterparts; thus they are more likely to exfoliate spontaneously or mechanically. Malignant neoplasms that have little connective tissue support (e.g., small cell carcinoma of the lung, lymphoma, malignant melanoma) produce more cellular samples than those with a generous fibrous stroma (e.g., scirrhous carcinoma of the breast). Carcinomas tend to exfoliate cells more readily than do sarcomas.

Cell Arrangement Is an Important Cytological Parameter

Although the tissue pattern is usually lost in cytological preparations, the relation between cells is a helpful criterion for cytological diagnosis. Cells may appear singly, in small groups, in monolayer sheets, or in three-dimensional clusters. Several cells may fuse, forming a large formation termed a *syncytium*. Cell clusters may form (1) papillary configurations with fibrovascular cores (papillary transitional cell carcinoma, papillary adenocarcinoma, malignant mesothelioma), (2) glandular or tubular structures (adenocarcinoma), (3) follicles (follicular adenoma of the thyroid), (4) rosettes (neuroblastoma), or (5) pearls (squamous cell carcinoma) (Table 30-1).

Variations in Cell Size and Shape Occur in Neoplasms

Depending on the type of neoplasm, the size of tumor cells varies greatly. Small cell carcinoma of the lung, some types of lymphoma, and many childhood tumors are composed of small regular cells. By contrast, squamous cell carcinoma, giant cell carcinoma, pleomorphic sarcomas, some endocrine carcinomas, and choriocarcinoma display very large cells. Malignant neoplasms tend to vary more in cell size than benign tumors, a feature termed *anisocytosis*. However, this rule does not apply to all neoplasms. Well-differentiated adenocarcinomas and low-grade transitional cell carcinomas, for example, have little anisocytosis. Conversely, marked anisocytosis may be seen in some benign conditions, such as lymph node hyperplasia or radiation effects.

Cell shape may vary widely from one tissue to another, but cells of the same type in normal tissues and in benign

TABLE 30-1 **Cell Arrangement**

Single	Glandular structures
Small groups	Follicles
Sheets	Rosettes
3D[a] clusters	Pearls
Papillary configuration	

[a] 3D, three-dimensional.

TABLE 30-2 Cytoplasm

Color	Vacuoles
Texture	Pigments
Halos	Other cell products
Inclusions	

neoplasms are generally uniform (monomorphic). By contrast, most malignant tumors exhibit marked variation in cell shape (pleomorphic).

Cytoplasmic Features May Reveal the Tissue Origin or Etiology

The cytoplasm is evaluated for color, texture, presence of inclusions, vacuoles, pigments, and other cell products (Table 30-2). With the Papanicolaou method, the cytoplasm assumes various shades of pink to blue; keratin is characterized by an orange color. The cytoplasm may vary in texture from homogeneous to granular or foamy. The presence of pigments, including melanin, hemosiderin, bile, lipofuscin, and carbon particles, is helpful in identifying the cell type. Single or multiple vacuoles in the cytoplasm indicate degenerative changes, secretory activity, or phagocytosis. Viral and chlamydial infections may form inclusions in the cytoplasm. Squamous cells infected by human papillomavirus show characteristic changes called *koilocytotic atypia*, which consists of a large perinuclear halo and nuclear abnormalities. The accumulation of immunoglobulin in the cytoplasm of reactive or neoplastic plasma cells forms an eosinophilic globule termed the *Russell body*. Small cytoplasmic concretions *(Michaelis-Gutmann bodies)* are seen in malakoplakia.

The Most Important Features of Malignancy Reside in the Nucleus

The size and shape of the nucleus, alterations of nuclear membrane and chromatin, prominence of the nucleolus, and mitotic activity are important parameters in cytological evaluation (Table 30-3). The nuclei of normal cells show little variation in size and shape. Modest nuclear enlargement occurs in normal cells during the S phase of the cell cycle and in reactive or regenerating cells. Malignant cells usually exhibit significant nuclear enlargement, which is frequently disproportionate to the enlargement of the cell and results in an increased nuclear-to-cytoplasmic ratio. In addition, significant variations in nuclear size *(anisokaryosis)* and nuclear shape are common in malignant neoplasms. The nuclei of most cancer cells, with the exception of some well-differentiated tumors, are abnormally shaped and have an irregular contour, with protrusions, indentations, and grooves. Molding of the nuclei against one another is seen in some tumors (classically in small cell carcinomas), probably owing to a rapid growth rate and scanty cytoplasm.

The nuclei of cancer cells are usually darker (*hyperchromatic*) than those of normal cells, and the chromatin tends to be coarser and unevenly distributed. Multinucleation per se is not helpful in the diagnosis of malignancy, because this feature may be seen in (1) normal cells (e.g., superficial urothelial cells, osteoclasts, syncytiotrophoblasts), (2) inflammatory conditions (e.g., multinucleated giant cells in granulomas), (3) benign neoplasms (e.g., giant cell tumor of the tendon sheath), or (4) malignant neoplasms (e.g., giant cell carcinoma, malignant fibrous histiocytoma, choriocarcinoma).

The nucleoli of cancer cells, particularly in poorly differentiated tumors, are often larger and more numerous than those in their benign counterparts. However, prominent nucleoli also can be seen in metabolically active benign cells. Furthermore, in some types of cancer (e.g., small cell carcinoma of the lung), tumor cells lack conspicuous nucleoli. Cytoplasmic invagination into the nucleus, which is seen in cross-section as a pale intranuclear inclusion, may occur in some benign and malignant neoplasms and may be helpful in their classification. For example, the presence of such cytoplasmic "inclusions" in a thyroid aspirate is a strong indication of papillary carcinoma.

Although increased mitotic activity can occur in both benign and malignant tumors, cancer cells in general have a higher rate of mitosis. Additionally, the presence of abnormal mitoses (abnormal distribution of chromosomes or presence of more than two mitotic poles) is a reliable criterion for the diagnosis of malignancy.

Extracellular Material and Background Surround the Cells

The background of the smear is evaluated for the presence of inflammation, blood, various extracellular substances, cell products, necrotic debris, and microorganisms. The

TABLE 30-4 Smear Background in Cytological Specimens

Inflammation (acute, chronic, granulomatous)
  Microorganisms
  Bacteria
  Fungi
  Helminths
  Protozoa (*Trichomonas vaginalis, Pneumocystis carinii,* amebae)
Necrotic debris
Blood, hemosiderin
Mucin
Amyloid
Colloid
Psammoma bodies
Ferruginous bodies
Curschmann spirals
Charcot-Leyden crystals
Renal casts
Urinary crystals

TABLE 30-3 Nucleus

Size	Intranuclear inclusion
Shape	Nucleolus
Altered chromatin	Mitotic activity

type of inflammation (acute, chronic, granulomatous) and some varieties of microorganisms, including bacteria, fungi, protozoa, and helminths, can be identified. Cell necrosis may occur in a variety of benign conditions (e.g., infections, trauma, ischemia, and irradiation) but may also be a prominent feature of many malignant neoplasms. Thus, in the absence of recognizable intact cells, a definitive diagnosis cannot be made on a sample composed entirely of necrotic debris. However, when present in association with malignant cells, necrosis generally indicates an invasive cancer. In this way, necrosis may help to distinguish an invasive squamous cell carcinoma of the uterine cervix from carcinoma in situ. This criterion, however, cannot be generalized to all types of cancers. For instance, carcinoma in situ of the breast may also contain foci of necrosis (comedocarcinoma). Common entities found in the smear background are listed in Table 30-4.

REPORTING SYSTEMS

Various methods have been used for reporting the results of cytological tests. Papanicolaou devised a numerical classification system that ranged from class I for the absence of abnormal cells to class V for conclusive evidence of cancer. In the early years of cytopathology, this classification was widely adopted, but it proved inadequate as the field expanded. Most laboratories have replaced the Papanicolaou classification with **narrative reports for nongynecological cytology** similar to the terminology used in histopathological reporting.

In 1988, a group of pathologists and gynecologists met in Bethesda, Maryland, in an attempt to standardize **gynecological cytology reports**. The group concluded that the Papanicolaou classification was unacceptable in the modern practice of cytopathology and proposed a new reporting classification that has since become known as the **Bethesda system**. This reporting system, with revisions, has been adopted by most laboratories in the United States (Table 30-5).

Each cytology report should include the following elements:

- A statement regarding the adequacy of the specimen for evaluation
- A general categorization (optional) (e.g., "Negative for intraepithelial lesion or malignancy" or "Epithelial cell abnormality"
- An interpretation/result

SUGGESTED READING

Books

Atkinson BF (ed): *Atlas of diagnostic cytopathology.* Philadelphia: WB Saunders, 1992.
Bibbo M (ed): *Comprehensive cytopathology,* 2nd ed. Philadelphia: WB Saunders, 1997.
DeMay RM: *The art and science of cytopathology.* Chicago: ASCP Press, 1996.
Koss LG: *Diagnostic cytology and its histopathologic bases,* 4th ed. Philadelphia: JB Lippincott, 1997.
Koss LG, Woyke S, Olszewski W: *Aspiration biopsy: Cytologic interpretation and histologic bases,* 2nd ed. Tokyo: Igaku-Shoin, 1992.
Kurman RJ, Solomon D: *The Bethesda System for reporting cervical/vaginal cytologic diagnoses: Definitions, criteria, and explanatory notes for terminology and specimen adequacy.* New York: Springer-Verlag, 1994.
Silverberg SG, DeLellis RA, Frable WJ (eds): *Principles and practice of surgical pathology and cytopathology,* 3rd ed. New York: Churchill Livingstone, 1997.

Review Articles

Bigner SH, Johnston WW: The cytopathology of cerebrospinal fluid: II. Metastatic cancer, meningeal carcinomatosis and primary central nervous system neoplasms. *Acta Cytol* 25:461–479, 1981.
Christopherson WM: Cytologic detection and diagnosis of cancer: Its contributions and limitations. *Cancer* 51:1201–1208, 1983.
Ehya H: Effusion cytology: The value and limitations of cytologic examination. *Clin Lab Med* 11:443–467, 1991.
Frable WJ: Needle aspiration biopsy: Past, present, and future. *Hum Pathol* 20:504–517, 1989.
Gharib H, Goellner JR. Fine needle aspiration biopsy of the thyroid: An appraisal. *Ann Intern Med* 118:282–289, 1993.
Hajdu SI: Cytology from antiquity to Papanicolaou. *Acta Cytol* 21:668–676, 1977.
Hajdu SI, Ehya H, Frable WJ, et al.: The value and limitations of aspiration cytology in the diagnosis of primary tumors: A symposium. *Acta Cytol* 33:741–790, 1989.

TABLE 30-5 Bethesda System 2001

Specimen adequacy
  Satisfactory for evaluation
  Unsatisfactory for evaluation . . . (specify reason)
Interpretation/result:
Negative for intraepithelial lesion or malignancy
Other
  Endometrial cells (in a woman ≥40 years of age)
Epithelial cell abnormalities
  Atypical squamous cells
    of undetermined significance (ASC-US)
    cannot exclude HSIL (ASC-H)
  Low-grade squamous intraepithelial lesion (LSIL)
    encompassing: HPV/mild dysplasia/CIN1
  High-grade squamous intraepithelial lesion (HSIL)
    encompassing: moderate and severe dysplasia, CIS/CIN2 and CIN 3
    with features suspicious for invasion (if invasion is suspected)
  Squamous cell carcinoma
  Atypical
    endocervical cells (NOS or specify in comments)
    endometrial cells (NOS or specify in comments)
    glandular cells (NOS or specify in comments)
  Atypical
    endocervical cells, favor neoplastic
    glandular cells, favor neoplastic
  Endocervical adenocarcinoma in situ
  Adenocarcinoma
    endocervical
    endometrial
    extrauterine
    not otherwise specified (NOS)
Other malignant neoplasms (specify)

Hajdu SI, Melamed MR: Limitations of aspiration cytology in the diagnosis of primary neoplasms. *Acta Cytol* 28:337–345, 1984.

Kline TS: Survey of aspiration biopsy cytology of the breast. *Diagn Cytopathol* 7:98–105, 1991.

Koss LG: Cytology: Accuracy of diagnosis. *Cancer* 64(suppl):249–252, 1989.

Solomon D: Bethesda System 2001. *Acta Cytol* 45:1077-1078, 2001.

Wakely PE, Kneisl JS: Soft tissue aspiration cytopathology. *Cancer Cytopathol* 90:292-298, 2000.

Zakowski MF: Fine needle aspiration cytology of tumors: Diagnostic accuracy and potential pitfalls. *Cancer Invest* 12:505–515, 1994.

Figure Acknowledgments

Specific acknowledgment is made for permission to use the following material:

Chapter 1, Figure 2. Okazaki H, Scheithauer BW: Atlas of Neuropathology. New York, Gower Medical Publishing, 1988. By permission of the author.

Chapter 3, Figure 19. Okazaki H, Scheithauer BW: Atlas of Neuropathology. New York, Gower Medical Publishing, 1988. By permission of the author.

Chapter 5, Figure 6. Reprinted from Bullough PG, Vigorita VJ: Atlas of Orthopaedic Pathology. New York, Gower Medical Publishing, 1984 with permission from Elsevier.

Chapter 5, Figure 18. Reprinted from Bullough PG, Boachie-Adjei O: Atlas of Spinal Diseases. New York, Gower Medical Publishing, 1988 with permission from Elsevier.

Chapter 6, Figure 33. Reprinted from Bullough PG, Vigorita VJ: Atlas of Orthopedic Pathology. New York, Gower Medical Publishing, 1988 with permission from Elsevier.

Chapter 7, Figure 1. Courtesy of Dr. David C. Walker, The iCAPTURE Centre/UBC Pulmonary Research, St. Paul's Hospital.

Chapter 7, Figures 4, 19, 31. Courtesy of UBC Pulmonary Registry, St. Paul's Hospital.

Chapter 7, Figures 6, 7, 13. Courtesy of Dr. Greg J. Davis, Dept. of Pathology, University of Kentucky College of Medicine.

Chapter 7, Figure 23. Courtesy of Dr. Ken Berry, Dept. of Pathology, St. Paul's Hospital.

Chapter 7, Figure 27. Courtesy of Dr. Kevin C. Kain, Centre for Travel and Tropical Medicine, Toronto General Hospital.

Chapter 7, Figure 36: Courtesy of Dr. Alex Magil, Dept. of Pathology, St. Paul's Hospital.

Chapter 8, Figure 14. Okazaki H, Scheithauer BW: Atlas of Neuropathology. New York, Gower Medical Publishing, 1988. By permission of the author.

Chapter 8, Figure 16. Reprinted from McKee PH: Pathology of the Skin. Copyright Gower Medical Publishing, 1989, with permission from Elsevier.

Chapter 9, Figures 21A, 21B, 28, 54A, 71, 83, 89, 90, 98A, and 98B. Reprinted from Farrar WE, Wood MJ, Innes JA, Tubbs H: Infectious Diseases Text and Color Atlas, 2nd ed. Copyright Gower Medical Publishing, 1992, with permission from Elsevier.

Chapter 12, Figure 40. Travis WB, Colby TV, Koss MN, Muller NL, Rosado-de-Christenson ML, and King, TE: Nonneoplastic Disorders of the Lower Respiratory Tract, Washington DC: American Registry of Pathology, 2002.

Chapter 12, Figure 55. Courtesy of the Armed Forces Institute of Pathology.

Chapter 12. The authors would like to gratefully acknowledge Dr. Bruce Wenig for the contribution of Figure 5 and Dr. Anthony Gal for the contribution of Figure 70.

Chapter 13, Figures 6A, 10A, 12, 15, 16, 24, 26, 28, 45, 47, 54A, 63, 64. Reprinted from Mitros FA: Atlas of Gastrointestinal Pathology. New York, Gower Medical Publishing, 1988 with permission from Elsevier.

Chapter 13, Figure 12. Courtesy of Dr. Cecilia M. Fenoglio-Preiser.

Chapter 14, Figure 47. Yanoff M: Ocular Pathology: A Color Atlas. New York, Gower Medical Publishing, 1988.

Chapter 14, Figure 63. Thung SN, Gerber MA: Histopathology of liver transplantation. In Fabry TL, Klion FM (eds): Guide to Liver Transplantation. New York, Igaku-Shoin Medical Publishers, 1992.

Chapter 17, Figure 4 and 10. Weiss MA, Mills SE: Atlas of Genitourinary Tract Diseases. New York, Gower Medical Publishers, 1988.

Chapter 17, Figure 46. Blackwell KL, Bostwick DG, Zincke H, et al: J. Urol 1994; 151(6):1565-1570. Reproduced with permission.

Chapter 18, Figures 5, 6, 17, 18, 23, 30, 32, 35, 37, 38, 43, 51, 65, 71, 72, and 78. Reprinted with permission of Stanley J. Robboy, MD, and Gynecologic Pathology Associates, Durham and Chapel Hill, North Carolina.

Chapter 18, Figures 14, 18, 19, 23, 25, 28, 33, 36. Robboy SJ, Anderson MC, and Russell P (eds): Pathology of the Female Reproductive Tract. London, Churchill-Livingstone, 2002, pp. 111-112, 147, 167, 140, 203, 248, 322, 354.

Chapter 18, Figures 66A and 66B. Reprinted from Woodruff JD, Parmley TH: Atlas of Gynecologic Pathology. New York, Gower Medical Publishing, 1988 with permission from Elsevier.

Chapter 20, Figure 41. Courtesy of Becton-Dickinson.

Chapter 21, Figure 13. Sandoz Pharmaceutical Corporation.

Figure Acknowledgments

Chapter 22, Figure 3. Reprinted from Atkinson and Eisenbarth: Lancet 2001; 358:221, with permission from Elsevier.

Chapter 22, Figure 9. Courtesy of the American Diabetes Association.

Chapter 24, Figures 9A, 23A, 26A (Courtesy W. Witmer), 27, 33A, 36A, 39A, 41A, 45, 46A, 47, 48, 49, 72A, 73, 74, 75, 81A, 85A. Elder AD, Elenitsas R, Johnson BL, et al: Synopsis and Atlas of Lever's Histopathology of the Skin. Lippincott Williams & Wilkins, Philadelphia, 1999, p 2, clin. fig. IA1; p 163, clin. fig. IVE3; p 167, clin. fig. IVE4.b; p 124, clin. fig. IIIH1.a; p 105, clin. fig. IIIF1.a; p 115, clin. fig. IIIG1.a; p 85, clin. fig. IIIB1a.a; p 219, clin. fig. VE3.a; clin. fig. IVA2.b; p 7, clin. fig. IC1; p 212, fig. VD1.d; p 51, clin. fig. IIE1.f and IIE1.1; p 226, clin. fig. VE5.f; p 283, clin. fig. VIB3.g; p 280, clin. fig. VIB3.q and VIB3.s; p 10, clin. fig. ID1.b; p 31, clin. fig. IIC1.a; clin. fig. IIF2.a; p 96, clin. fig. IIID1.d.

Chapter 26, Figures 22A, 22B, 43, 55B, 60, and 71A. Reprinted from Bullough PG: Atlas of Orthopaedic Pathology, 2nd ed. New York, Gower Medical Publishing, 1992 with permission from Elsevier.

Chapter 28, Figures 57 and 135A. Okazaki H, Scheithauer BW: Atlas of Neuropathology. New York, Gower Medical Publishing, 1988, By permission of the author.

Index

Page numbers in *italic* designate figures; page numbers followed by the letter *t* designate tables.

A

AA amyloidosis, 1194, *1195*
α₁-Antiproteinases, 73
α₁-Antitrypsin deficiency, 16, 682, 787, 798
A bands, 1388
ABCD rule, for malignant melanoma, 1248
ABCR gene, 1519
Abdominal aortic aneurysm, 510–512, *511*
Aberrant (ectopic) pancreas, 812
Abetalipoproteinemia, 703
ABO antigens, in peptic ulcer, 679–680
Abortion, spontaneous, 990
Abrasion (injury), 338
Abrasion cytology, 1531, *1535*
Abruptio placentae, in smokers, 318, *319*
Abscess, 25, *26*, 75
   appendiceal/periappendiceal, 732
   Brodie, 1329
   cerebral, 323, *324*, 1450, *1450, 1451*
   cold, 1331
   eosinophilic, 1066, *1066*, 1332, *1332*
   liver, 792–793
      amebic, 449–450, *450*
      cholangitic, 792
      pyogenic, 792
   periapical, 1277
   peritonsillar (quinsy), 1293–1294
   psoas, 1331
Absence of corpus callosum, 1425, *1425*
Absorption, nutrient, 697, *698*
Acantholytic dermatosis, transient, 1220
Acanthosis, 1040, *1040*
Acanthosis nigricans, 209
Acetaldehyde, in alcoholic organ injury, 322
Acetaminophen toxicity, 22–24, *24*, 873–874
Achalasia, 665, *666*, 672
Achondroplasia, 1316–1317, *1317*
Acid(s)
   arachidonic, 52–53, 52t, *53*
   ascorbic, 352–353, *353*
   bile, *698*, 699
   folic, 352
   gastric, hypersecretion, 674
   hydrochloric, 680
   hypochlorous, 73–74
Acid maltase deficiency (Pompe disease), 1401–1402, *1402*
Acinar cell carcinoma, 820
Acinic cell carcinoma, salivary gland, 1285
Acinus, hepatic, 743
Acne vulgaris, 1241–1242, *1243*
Acoustic neuroma, 1487, *1487*

Acoustic (vestibular) schwannoma, 1498–1499
Acoustic trauma, 1301
Acral lentiginous melanoma, *1252*, 1252–1254, *1253, 1254*
Acrodermatitis enteropathica, 354–355
ACTH
   excess, 1132, 1158–1163
   insufficiency, 5, 1158
ACTH-dependent adrenal hyperfunction, 1158–1161, *1159*
ACTH-independent adrenal hyperfunction, 1160–1162
Actinic keratopathy, 1507
Actinic keratosis, 1258, *1259*
Actinomycosis, 406, *406*
   genital tract, 934
   oral, 1273
Activated protein C resistance, 1061
Active hyperemia, 284
Acute cholecystitis, *806*, 806–807
Acute decompression sickness (bends), 293
Acute hemorrhagic erosive gastritis, 674–675, *675*
Acute hemorrhagic pancreatitis, 813, 815, *815*
Acute inflammation, 42, *44*
   leukocyte recruitment in, *65*, 65–70, *66, 67*
   leukocyte transmigration in, 68–70, *69*
   outcomes of, 75
Acute intermittent porphyria, 791
Acute monoblastic leukemia, 1081, *1081*
Acute mountain sickness, 337
Acute myeloid leukemia, 1079–1082, *1080*, 1081t
   therapy-induced, 1081
Acute necrotizing ulcerative gingivitis (Vincent angina), 1272, *1272*
Acute pancreatitis, 812–816
Acute phase proteins, 81, 81t
Acute phase response, to inflammation, 81, 81t
Acute postinfectious glomerulonephritis, 849–851, *850, 851*
Acute promyelocytic leukemia, 1080
Acute rejection, 140–141, *141*
Acute renal failure, urinalysis in, 870t
Acute suppurative lymphadenitis, 1086
Acute tubular necrosis, 308, *309*, 867–869, *868*, 868t, *869*
ADA (adenosine deaminase) deficiency, 146t, 147

Addison disease (primary adrenocortical insufficiency), 1156–1157, *1157*
Addressins, 57–58, 120
Adenocarcinoma
   bladder, 900
   cervical, 952–953
   colorectal, 729, *729*, *1527, 1535*
   endometrial, 958–961, 959t, *960, 961*, 961t
      clear cell, 960, *961*
      endometrioid, 959
      with squamous differentiation, 959, *960*
   gallbladder, 808, *808*
   gastric, 168, *168*, 686–688
      diffuse or infiltrating, 686, *687*, 688
      polypoid (fungating), 686, *688*
      ulcerating, 686, *686*, 688
   ovarian
      clear cell, 975
      endometrioid, 974–975
      mucinous, 974, *975*
      serous, 973–974, *974*
   pancreatic, 817, *818, 819*, 820
   papillary, 169, *169*
   prostate
      histological features, *922*
      intraepithelial neoplasia, 922, *922*
      metastasis to spine, 924, *924*
      prostate-specific antigen (PSA) test, 924, *924*
      TNM staging, *924*, 924–925, 925t
   renal, 316
   scirrhous, 169, *169*
   serous peritoneal, 985
   small-intestinal, 705–706
   vaginal clear cell, 940, *940*
Adenoid cystic carcinoma, 1284, *1284*
Adenoids, 1294
Adenoma, 168, *168*
   adrenal, *1160*, 1160–1161
   colorectal, 721–727
      tubulovillous, *723*, 723–724
      villous, 722–723, *723*
   corticotrope, 1132
   gastric tubular, 684
   gonadotrope, 1132
   hepatic, 326, 796, *797*
   lactotrope (prolactinoma), 1131
   null cell, 1133
   parathyroid, 1151, *1151*
   pituitary, 1130–1133, 1130t, *1131*
   renal, 880
   salivary gland, 1282, *1282, 1283*

1545

Adenoma (contd.)
    oxyphil (oncocytoma), 1283
    pleomorphic, *1282, 1283*
        Warthin tumor, 1283, *1283*
    silent, 1133
    small-bowel, 705
    somatotrope, 1131–1132, *1132*
    thyroid, 1141, 1144, *1145*
        Hürthle cell, 1144, *1145*
        toxic, 1141
    thyrotrope, 1132–1133
Adenomatoid tumor, 984
    testicular, 918
Adenomatous polyposis, familial, 193
Adenomatous polyps
    colorectal, 721–727
    gastric, 684
Adenomyosis, 954, *955*
Adenosarcoma, uterine, 962
Adenosine deaminase (ADA) deficiency, 146t, 147
Adenosis
    sclerosing, 1002, *1004*
    vaginal, 939, *939*
Adenosquamous carcinoma, 169
Adenovirus, 364
Adhesion molecules, *66,* 66–68, *67*
    in metastasis, 177–180
    of vessel wall, 474
Adhesions
    focal (focal contacts), 88
    intrauterine (Asherman syndrome), 954
    small-bowel, 705
Adipocyte complement–related protein, 346
Adipose tissue, tumors of, *1379,* 1380
Adrenal adenoma, *1160,* 1160–1161
Adrenal cancer, metastatic, 1163
Adrenal cortical carcinoma, 1161, *1161*
Adrenal cortical insufficiency, 1156–1158
    acute, 1158
    primary (Addison disease), 1156–1157, *1157*
Adrenal disorders
    cortex, 1153–1170
        adrenal cysts, 1163
        adrenal hyperfunction, 1158–1163, *1159*
        adrenal insufficiency, 1156–1158
        congenital adrenal hyperplasia, 1154–1156, *1155, 1156*
        primary aldosteronism (Conn syndrome), 1163
    medulla and paraganglia, 1163–1168, *1164*
        ganglioneuroma, 1168–1169, *1169*
        neuroblastoma, 1167–1168, *1168*
        paraganglioma, 1167–1168
        pheochromocytoma, 1164–1167, *1165, 1166*
    metastatic cancer, 1163
Adrenal gland anatomy
    cortex, 1153
    medulla and paraganglia, *1163,* 1163–1164
Adrenal hyperfunction, 1158–1163, *1159*
    ACTH-dependent, 1158–1161, *1159*
    ACTH-independent, 1160–1162
        adrenal adenoma, *1160,* 1160–1161

adrenal cortical carcinoma, 1161, *1161*
corticosteroid-induced, 1161–1162
Adrenal hyperplasia
    bilateral micronodular (Carney complex), 1161
    clinical features, 1161–1162, *1162, 1163*
    diffuse, 1160
    nodular, 1160
Adrenal insufficiency, 1156–1158
Adrenalitis, autoimmune, 1157, *1157*
Adrenal myolipoma, 1163
Adrenoleukodystrophy, 1462–1463
Adult T-cell leukemia/lymphoma, 1109
Adventitial dermis, *1204,* 1208
Adynamic renal osteodystrophy (ARO), 1343
Aflatoxins, 201, *202*
    in liver cancer, 798
African trypanosomiasis (sleeping sickness), 454–456, *455*
Agammaglobulinemia, Bruton X-linked, 143–145, 145t, 1293
Age
    infection risk and, 361
    peptic ulcer and, 679
    stomach cancer and, 686
Agenesis, 219
    anorectal, 711
    renal, 831
    renal pelvis and ureter, 889–890
    uterine, 953
Aggressive NK cell leukemia, 1108–1109
Aging, 34–38
    cardiac atrophy in, 6
    cellular basis, 35–36, *36*
    diseases of premature, 37, *37*
    functional/structural changes, 35
    genetic factors, 36–37
    in vitro studies, 36–37
    maximal life span, *34,* 34–35
    oxidative damage and, 37–38
    summary hypothesis, 38
Agranulocytosis, 1062, 1278
Agricultural chemicals, toxicity, 328–329
AIDS-associated Castleman's disease, 152–153
AIDS/HIV, 147–153
    cancer risk in, 206–207
    epidemiology, 147–148
    fungal infections in, *1245*
    gastrointestinal disorders in, 731–732, 732t
    HIV-associated nephropathy in, 841–842, *842*
    immunology, 151
    Kaposi sarcoma, 1263–1264, *1264, 1265*
    M. avium-intracellulare complex and, 427–428
    neoplasia in
        bacillary angiomatosis, 1263–1264
        Kaposi sarcnoma, *1263,* 1263–1273, *1264*
        skin, 1262–1264
    pathology and clinical features, 151–153, *152*
    Pneumocystis carinii pneumonia, 446–447, *447*

transmission and pathogenesis, 148–151, *149, 150*
AIDS lymphadeonopathy, 1088
Air embolism, 292–293
    cerebral, 1442
Air pollutants, 329–330
Airway inflammation, neurokinins in, 58
AJCC staging, of melanoma, 1254t
Alagille syndrome, 796
AL amyloid, 1192, *1193*
Albers-Schönberg disease, *1320,* 1320–1321
Albinism, 261
    oculocutaneous, 261, 1064
Albumin synthesis, 746
Alcoholic cardiomyopathy, 320
Alcoholic cerebellar degeneration, 322
Alcoholic hyaline, 14
Alcoholic liver disease, 773–778
    cirrhosis, 777–779, *780,* 798
    dose-response relationship in, 773, *774*
    epidemiology, 773–774, *774*
    ethanol metabolism and, 774, *775*
    fatty liver and associated lesions, 774–777, *775, 776, 777*
    hepatitis, 777, *778, 779*
Alcoholic neuropathy, 1495
Alcoholism, 320–322
    B vitamin deficiency in, 349–350
    central pontine myelinolysis in, 1465, *1465*
    fetal alcohol syndrome, 322
    Mallory-Weiss syndrome in, 670
    osteoporosis in, 1337
    pancreatitis in, 813, 816
    systemic effects, *320,* 320–322
    Wernicke-Korsakoff syndrome, 1468
    Wernicke syndrome, 1466–1468, *1467*
Aldose reductase pathway, in diabetes mellitus, 1181
Aldosteronism
    glucocorticoid-remediable, 501
    primary (Conn syndrome), 1162–1163
Alexander disease, *1462,* 1462–1463
Alkaptonuria (ochronosis), *260,* 260–261
Alkylating agents, as carcinogens, 201
Allergic contact dermatitis, *1236,* 1236–1237, *1237*
Allergic cutaneous vasculitis, *1234, 1235,* 1235–1236
Allergic granulomatosis and angiitis (Churg-Strauss syndrome), 506, *506*
Allergic (Henoch-Schönlein) purpura, 859–860, 1052
Allergic rhinitis, 1286
Allergy
    basophilia in, 1064, 1065t
    eosinophilia in, 1054t, 1064
Allison-Ghormley bodies, 1366, 1367, *1367, 1369*
Alopecia, 1210
Alopecia areata, 1210
Alopecia totalis, 1210
Alpha cell tumors (glucagonoma), 823, *823*
Alpha storage pool disease (grey platelet syndrome), 1056
Alport syndrome (hereditary nephritis), 848–849, *849*

Index

Altitude-related illnesses, 337–338
Aluminum toxicity, 333
Alveolar edema, 302, *303*
Alveolar fibrosis, 114
Alveolar injury, 112, *113*
Alveolar rhabdomyosarcoma, 1381
Alzheimer disease, 1191–1192
Alzheimer type II astrocytes, 1468
Amblyopia, in alcoholism, 322
Amebiasis, 447–450, *448, 449, 450*
  hepatic abscess in, 449–450, *450*
  intestinal, 449, *449*
Amebic meningitis, 1448, *1449*
Amebic meningoencephalitis, primary, 456
Amelia, 223
Ameloblastoma, 1279–1280, *1280*
Amenorrhea, obesity and, 347
Ames test, 199
Ammonia, in hepatic encephalopathy, 755
Amniotic fluid embolism, 293, *293*
Amniotic membrane rupture, smoking and, *319*
Amphetamines, 324
Ampulla of Vater, carcinoma of, 706, 809
Amylin, 821
Amylo-1,6-glucosidase deficiency (Cori disease), 1402
Amyloid
  definition, 1189–1190
  staining properties, 1188–1189, *1189*
  structure, *1186*, 1199
Amyloid neuropathy, 1496
Amyloidosis, 1186–1200
  Alzheimer disease, 1191–1192, 1195–1196, 1475–1479, *1476, 1476t, 1477, 1478, 1479, 1480*
  in cancer, 209
  classification by protein type, 1192–1196, *1195*
  clinical classification, 1190–1192
  clinical features, 1198–1199
  common components, 1188
  familial, 1191
    familial amyloidotic polyneuropathy, 1191
    familial Mediterranean fever, 1191
    hereditary congophilic angiopathy (Icelandic), 1191
  general scheme of pathogenesis, *1196*, 1196–1197
  in inclusion body myositis, 1399, *1399*
  isolated, 1191
  morphological features, *1197*, 1197–1198, *1198*
  neurodegenerative diseases of, 1456t
  osteomyelitis in, 1330
  primary, 1190
  with renal dialysis, 1192
  secondary, 1190–1191
  senile cardiac, 1192
  treatment strategies, 1199
  in type 2 diabetes, *1178*
Amyloid P component, 1188
Amyotrophic lateral sclerosis, 208, 1471, *1471*
Anaerobic glycolysis, 27–28
Anal canal, epidermoid cancers of, 731

Analgesic nephropathy, 873–874
Anaphase lag, 230
Anaphylactic shock, 305
Anaphylactic skin reactions, 1234–1235
Anaphylatoxins, 50, *51*
Anaplasia, 170, *171*
Anaplastic astrocytoma, 1483, *1483*
Anaplastic large-cell lymphoma, 1110, *1111*
Anaplastic (undifferentiated) thyroid carcinoma, 1149, *1149*
ANCA (idiopathic crescentic) glomerulonephritis, 859
ANCA necrotizing vasculitis, 860, *860*
ANCAs
  in glomerulonephritis, 837
  in renal disease, 858–859
Anchoring fibrils, 107
Androblastoma, 980–981, *981*
Anemia, 1028–1048
  aplastic, 1031, *1031*, 1031t
  autoimmune hemolytic, 209
  in cancer, 209
  of chronic disease, 1033
  of chronic renal disease, 1033
  classification, 1028t, *1029–1030*, 1030t
  Fanconi, 1054
  hemoglobinopathies, 1041–1044
    double heterozygosities, 1043
    hemoglobin C disease, 1043–1044
    hemoglobin E disease, 1044
    sickle cell disease, *1041*, 1041–1043, *1042*
    sickle cell trait, 1043
  hemolytic, 1038–1040
    acanthosis, 1040, *1040*
    in burn injury, 1048
    G6PD deficiency, 1040–1041
    hereditary elliptocytosis, 1039–1040
    hereditary spherocytosis, 1039, *1039*
    hypersplenism, 1047–1048
    immune, 1044–1046
    mechanical red cell fragmentation sydromes, 1046–1047, *1047*
    paroxysmal nocturnal hemoglobinurua, 1047
    of prematurity, vitamin E in, 354
  iron deficiency, *1032*, 1032–1033
  in lead poisoning, 331, 1033–1034
  megaloblastic, 114–1037, *1035, 1036, 1037*
  microangiopathic, 209
  myeloplastic, 1033
  normocytic normochromic, 1048
  pernicious, *1034, 1035*, 1036, 1468, 1478
  pure red cell aplasia, 1031–1032
    acute self-limited, 1032
    chronic relapsing, 1032
    Diamond-Blackfan syndrome, 1032
  pyridoxine-responsive, 352
  refractory, 1078
  thalassemia, 1037–1038
    alpha, 1038
    beta, 1037–1038
    heterozygous β, 1038
    homozygous β (Cooley anemia), 1037–1038, *1038*
Anencephaly, 221–223, *222, 1421*, 1421–1422
Aneuploidy, 230

Aneurysm, 492
  abdominal aortic (dissecting), 510–512, *510–514, 511*
  berry, 286
  cerebral, 1430, *1435*, 1435–1437, *1436, 1437*
    atherosclerotic, *1435*, 1437
    berry, *1435*, 1435–1437
    Charcot-Bouchard, *1436*, 1437
    mycotic, 1437
    saccular, *1436.1427*, 1437
  of cerebral arteries, 512
  dissecting, *512*, 512–513
  mycotic, 513–514
  syphilitic, 513, *513*
Aneurysmal bone cyst, *1351*, 1351–1352
Angelman syndrome, 266–267
Angiitis
  allergic granulomatosis and (Churg-Strauss syndrome), 506, *506*
  hypersensitivity, 505–506
Angina
  intestinal abdominal, 697
  Ludwig, 1272–1273
  Vincent (acute necrotizing ulcerative gingivitis), 1272, *1272*, 1293
Angiocentric T cell/NK cell lymphoma, 1290–1291, *1291*
Angiodysplasia (vascular ectasia), intestinal, 720–721
Angioedema, 1234–1235
  hereditary, 52, 1235
Angiofibroma, juvenile nasopharyngeal, 1294, *1294*
Angiofollicular lymph node hyperplasia (Castleman disease), 1088
Angiogenesis, 80
  tumor, 179, 183
  in wound healing, *102*, 104–106
Angioid retinal streaks, 1519
Angiolipoma, 1380
Angioma
  cavernous, 1435
  spider, 757
  venous, 1435
Angiomatosis
  bacillary, 1265
  encephalofacial (Sturge-Weber syndrome), 1491
Angiomyolipoma, 880
Angioplasty, restenosis after, 492–493
Angiosarcoma, 517
Ankylosing spondylitis, 1370, *1370*
Ann Arbor staging system, for Hodgkin lymphoma, 1114t
Annular pancreas, 812
Anogenital warts, 370
ANO incompatibility, 275
Anorectal agenesis, 711
Anorectal fistula, 711
Anorectal malformations, 710–711
Anorectal stenosis, 711
Anorexia, in cancer, 207
Anovulatory bleeding, 955–956, 956t
Anoxia, necrosis in, 27
Anthracosis, 12, *13*
Anthrax, 403–404
  septicemic, 404

Cytopathology refers to diagnostic techniques that are used to examine cells from various body sites to determine the cause or nature of disease. Cytological methods date to the mid-19th century, when investigators detected abnormal cells in body fluids such as urine, sputum, effusions, and gastric secretions. In 1928, George Papanicolaou, while studying the hormonal effects of the menstrual cycle on squamous cells exfoliated from human uterine cervix, initiated the modern era of diagnostic cytology by discovering cellular abnormalities that were associated with uterine cancer. Despite initial skepticism, cytological examination, popularly termed the **"Pap" test**, has been widely accepted as the most reliable screening test for the early detection of cancer and precancerous conditions of the uterine cervix. Sporadic attempts to collect diagnostic samples from tumors by means of a needle were documented as early as the mid-19th century, but it was not until the 1920s that this method was used systematically. Despite remarkable success with this technique, needle aspiration did not become popular until the 1970s. The past 30 years have witnessed a tremendous surge in the application of cytology to numerous human organs. It is now considered a routine modality in the diagnosis and surveillance of cancer.

APPLICATIONS OF CYTOPATHOLOGY

Screening Is Important for Early Detection of Asymptomatic Cancer

The most important application of cytopathology in the area of cancer prevention is the examination of scrapings and brushings from the cervix. Widespread screening of the female population by Pap smears has conspicuously reduced the incidence of cervical cancer in the United States and many other countries. For example, in Iceland, an 80% decline in mortality from cervical cancer has been achieved. Similarly, in Canada, the incidence of cervical cancer was reported to be 4.5 cases per 100,000 in screened populations, compared with 29 cases in unscreened ones.

The bladder, lung, esophagus, and endometrium are other organs in which cytopathology is useful in the detection of early cancers. Although economic considerations preclude mass screening for such tumors, it is feasible to screen specific populations at high risk for the development of certain cancers. Examples of such surveys include sputum cytology in uranium mine workers, who have a high incidence of lung cancer, and urine cytology in industrial workers exposed to chemical carcinogens, who have a high frequency of bladder cancer. In China, where esophageal cancer is very common, cytological screening by the balloon technique has achieved 90% accuracy in detecting this tumor.

Many Symptomatic Cancers Are Diagnosed by Cytology

Cytological sampling by needle aspiration is less complicated than an open biopsy, and most organs are now accessible to such studies. Diagnosis by cytological tests is particularly important in the case of advanced malignant tumors that are not amenable to surgical treatment. Examples of such neoplasms include pancreatic carcinoma with metastases, hepatocellular carcinoma, and small cell carcinoma of the lung. A definitive diagnosis in such instances precludes the necessity of surgical intervention.

Cytological Methods Detect Tumor Recurrence

For some types of cancers, cytology is the most feasible surveillance method to detect recurrence. The best example is periodic urine cytology, usually at 3-month intervals, to monitor the recurrence of cancer of the urinary tract. In patients with ovarian carcinoma, after the initial surgery and completion of chemotherapy, an exploratory laparotomy is performed to assess the response of the tumor to treatment ("second-look" operation). Even in the absence of grossly visible residual or recurrent tumor, peritoneal washings are examined to assess the presence of malignant cells. Cytological methods are also used in evaluation of cancer patients who develop an effusion, neurological symptoms, lymphadenopathy, or nodules in the skin, lung, or liver.

CYTOLOGICAL METHODS

Spontaneously Shed Cells in Body Fluids Can Be Detected

Examples include sputum, cerebrospinal fluid, urine, effusions in body cavities (pleura, pericardium, peritoneum), nipple discharge, and vitreous and aqueous humors of the eye. The number of cells in such specimens usually does not suffice to allow adequate assessment by direct smearing of the fluid on a glass slide. Thus, cytology laboratories use various cell-concentration techniques, such as centrifugation or membrane filtration, to prepare the specimens.

Antibiotics, pseudomembranous colitis and, 711, *711*
Antibodies
 antinuclear, in lupus erythematosus, 158
 antiphospholipid, 157
 cytotoxic, 675–676
 intrinsic factor, 676
Antibody-dependent cell-mediated cytotoxicity, 206
Anticoagulants
 circulating, 1058
 lupus, 1058, 1061
Antidiuresis, inappropriate in cancer, 207–208
Antigen-antibody (immune) complexes, 51
Antigen-presenting cells (APCs), *125*, 125–126
Antigens, tumor, 204–206, *205*
Anti-glomerular basement membrane glomerulonephritis, 857–858, *859*
Antineutrophil cytoplasmic antibodies (ANCA), 504
Antiphospholipid antibody syndrome, 1061
Antithrombin deficiency, 1061
Antral membrane, congenital, 674
Anus, imperforate, 711
Aorta, 292
 Takayasu arteritis, 598
Aortic stenosis, calcific, 14
Aortic wall, dissecting aneurysm of, *512*, 512–513
Aortitis, syphilitic, 409–410, *410*, 513, *513*
APC gene, 193, 727
APCs (antigen-presenting cells), *125*, 125–126
Apgar score, 270, 271t
Aphthous stomatitis (canker sores), 1271–1272
Apical/periapical granuloma, 1277, *1277*
AP kinase pathway, 99
Aplasia, 220
 germ cell, *910*
 pure red cell, 1031–1032
 red cell, 209
Aplastic anemia, 1031, *1031*, 1031t
Aplastic renal dysplasia, 832
Apocrine metaplasia, *1536*
Apolipoprotein E, 487, 1188
 Alzheimer disease and, 1476–1477
Apolipoproteins, 493t
Apoptosis, 29–34
 DNA damage and, 30
 in equilibrium, 33
 in fetal development, 29
 in infection, 30
 inhibition in cancer, 81
 initiation, 30–31, *31*
 mediation, 31–33, *32*
 mitochondrial mediation, 31–33, *32*
 morphology, 29, *29*, *30*
 oncogene action and, 191
 physiological function, 29–30
 p53 in, 33
 quantitative assays, *33*, 33–34
 viral cytoxicity and, 22
Appendiceal anatomy, 732

Appendiceal disorders
 mucocele, 733, *733*
 neoplasms, 733, *735*
Appendicitis, *732*, 732–733
 tuberculous, 733
Appropriate for gestational age (AGA) classification, 269
APrP amyloidosis, 1194–1196
Aqueduct of Sylvius, congenital atresia, 1422, *1423*, *1424*
Arachidonic acid, 52–53, 52t, *53*
Arachidonic acid-derived contracting factors, 60
Arachidonic acid-derived relaxing factors, 60
Arachidonic acid metabolites, 53–56
Arachnodactyly, 244, *244*
Arcus lipioides (archus senilis), 1506
Argentaffin cells, 673
Argyll-Robertson pupil, 1517
Argyrophil cells, 673
Arias-Stella reaction, 953, *953*
Armanni-Ebstein phenomena, 1516–1517
Arnold-Chiari malformation, *1420*, 1422, *1422*, *1423*
Aromatic amines, as carcinogens, 201
Arrhenoblastoma, 980–981, *981*
Arrhinencephaly, 1425, *1425*
Arsenic toxicity, 332–333
Arteries, *472*, 475–479
 cerebral, occlusion of, *1441*, 1441–1443
 coronary, *280*
 elastic, 476–477
 muscular, 477–479
Arteriolar vasoconstriction, 45
Arteriolar vasodilation, 45
Arterioles, 282–283, *283*, 478
Arteriolosclerosis, 502–503
 benign, 502, *502*
 malignant (accelerated) hypertension, 502–503
Arteriosclerosis, hyaline, in diabetes mellitus, *1180*, 1181, *1183*
Arteriovenous malformation, 1435, *1435*
Arteritis (*see also* Vasculitis)
 giant cell, 506–507, *507*
 Takayasu, 508, 861, 861t
Arthritis
 acute gouty, 1373
 bacterial, 378
 enteropathic, 1371
 in Gaucher disease, 1349
 juvenile (Still disease), 1371
 neurokinins in, 58
 osteoarthritis, 1363–1366, *1364*, *1365*
 psoriatic, 1371
 rheumatoid, 1088, 1366–1371
 septic, 383, 1349
 seronegative (spondyloarthropathy), 1369–1371
 tuberculous, 1331
 in ulcerative colitis, 718, *718*
Arthropathy, in hemochromatosis, 785
Arthropod-borne viral encephalomyelitis, 1456–1457, 1456t
Arthropod infestations, *1245*, 1245–1246
Arthus reaction, 135–136, *137*

Articular cartilage, 1362, *1362*
Asbestosis, 203–204
Ascariasis, 459–460, 459t, *460*
Ascites, 285, 297, 304
 chylous, 304
 in portal hypertension, 761, *761*
Aseptic necrosis
 of bone, 1325–1327, *1326*, 1326t
 of femoral head, 321
Asherman syndrome, 954
Aspartic proteinases, 73
Aspergilloma, 431
Aspergillosis, 430–432, 1289, *1289*
 allergic bronchopulmonary, 431
 aspergilloma, 431
 invasive, 430–431, *431*
Aspiration, amniotic fluid, 270, *270*
Aspiration pneumonia, in tracheoesophageal fistula, 663–664
Aspirin
 gastritis and, 674
 mechanism of action, 55
 in peptic ulcer disease, 679
 renal toxicity, 873–874
 Reye syndrome, 790
Aspirin-triggered lipoxin, 55
Astrocytes, 1416–1418, *1417*, *1418*, *1419*
 Alzheimer type II, 1468
Astrocytoma, *1482*, 1482–1483, *1483*
 anaplastic, 1483, *1483*
Astrocytosis, *1417*, 1417–1418
Asymmetric cartilage growth, 1317–1320
Asynchrony, nuclear to cytoplasmic, 1034
Ataxia
 Friedreich, 240, 1473–1475
 inherited spinocerebellar, 1473–1475
Ataxia telangiectasia, 194, 1169
Atheroembolism, renal, 863, *864*
Atherogenesis, 484t
Atheroma, components, 484t
Atherosclerosis, 287–288, 483–498 (*see also* Hypertension)
 abdominal aortic aneurysm and, 510–512, *511*
 abdominal pain in, 697
 amyloid in, 1191
 atherogenesis, 484t
 atheroma components, 484t
 complications, *491*, 491–492, *492*
 in diabetes mellitus, 1181
 epidemiology, 484
 hereditary disorders and, 497–499, 497t
 apolipoprotein E, 487
 familial hypercholesterolemia, 496, 497, 497t, *498*, 499
 high-density lipoprotein, 487497
 lipoprotein (a) (Lp[a]), 487497
 hypercoagulability in, 1062
 obesity and, 346
 pathogenesis, 484–488, 484t, *486*, *487*
 encrustation hypothesis, 484
 hemodynamic hypothesis, 485
 insudation hypothesis, 484
 intima cell mass/neointima formation hypothesis, 485
 monoclonal hypothesis, 485
 reaction to injury hypothesis, 484–485

unifying hypothesis, 485–489, *486, 487, 488*
pathology, *487, 488,* 488–492, *489, 490*
  fatty streak, *486,* 489
  fibrinofatty plaque, *487,* 488–490
  intimal cell mass, 489
restenosis after angioplasty, 492–493
risk factors and predictors, 493–494, 494t
smoking and, 315, *315*
thrombosis and, 287–288
Atherosclerotic cerebral aneurysm, *1435,* 1437
Atresia, 220
  anorectal, 711
  biliary, 795–796
  congenital of aqueduct of Sylvius, 1422, *1423, 1424*
  gastric partial, 674
  of small intestine, 691
  vaginal, 939
Atrial fibrillation, 288
Atrial natriueretic factor, 499
Atrophic endometrium, 953
Atrophic gastritis, 676, *676*
Atrophy, 4–6, *6, 9*
  acute yellow (massive hepatic necrosis), 770, *770*
  of brain, *5*
  chronic inflammation and, 5–6
  endocrine insufficiency and, 5
  functional demand and, 5
  ischemia and, 5
  of neurons, 1416, *1416*
  nutritional inadequacy and, 5
  optic, 1520–1521, *1521*
  spinal muscular, *1409,* 1409–1411, *1410*
Atypical fibroxanthoma, 1263
Aural polyps, 1297
Autocrine stimulation, of oncogenes, 185
Autoimmune adrenalitis, 1157, *1157*
Autoimmune atrophic gastritis, 675–676
Autoimmune chronic pancreatitis, 816
Autoimmune disease, 153–162
  bullous pemphigoid, 1223–1226, *1224, 1225*
  chronic inflammation and, 76
  dermatomyositis, 161–162
  diabetes mellitus type 1, 1175–1177, *1176*
  Hashimoto thyroiditis, *1139, 1142,* 1142–1143
  mechanisms of, 153–154
  mixed connective tissue disease (MCTD), 162
  polyglandular autoimmune syndromes, 1156–1157
  polymyositis, 161–162
  primary adrenocortical insufficiency (Addison disease), 1156–1157
  rheumatoid arthritis, 1366–1371
  scleroderma, 159–161, *160*
  Sjögren syndrome, 158–159, *159,* 1281, *1281*
    lymphoma in, 1094
  systemic lupus erythematosus, 155, 155–158, *157, 158,* 853–856, *855,* 855t, 1229–1231, *1230, 1231*
  theories of

molecular mimicry, 154
polyclonal B-cell activation, 154
self-antigen theory, 154
T-cell abnormality theory, 154
tissue injury in, 154–155
Autoimmune hemolytic anemia, 209, 1044–1045
Autoimmune hepatitis, 773
Autosomal dominant polycystic kidney disease (ADPKD), *833,* 833–834
Autosomal recessive polycystic kidney disease (ARPKD), *833,* 834, *834*
Avascular necrosis of bone, 1325–1327, *1326,* 1326t
Azo dyes, as carcinogens, 201
Azurophilic granules, 70, *71*

B

Babesiosis, 444
Bacillary angiomatosis, 1265
Bacillus anthracis, 403–404
Bacterial arthritis, 378
Bacterial endocarditis, 287, 289, 378
  in drug abuse, 323, *324*
Bacterial infections, 376–406 (*see also specific infections*)
  actinomycosis, 406, *406*
  bejel, 411
  by branching filamentous organisms, *406,* 406–407
  Campylobacter jejuni, 393–394
  childhood, 381–384
  chlamydial, 414–417
  cholera, 391–393, *394*
  clostridial, 397–401, *398–399*
  diphtheria, 381–382, *382*
  Echerichia coli, 387–389, *388*
  endotoxins, 376–377
  enteropathogenic, 387–395 (*see also* Diarrhea)
  exotoxins, 376
  fusospirochetal, 413–414, *414*
  Haemophilus influenzae, 382–383
  leprosy (Hansen disease), 425–427
  leptosporosis, 412–413, *413*
  Lyme disease, 411–412
  mycoplasmal, 420–429, 420t (*see also* Mycoplasmal infections)
  Neisseria meningitides, 383, 383–384
  nocardiosis, 407, *407*
  pertussis (whooping cough), 382
  pinta, 411
  psittacosis (ornithosis), 416–417
  pulmonary, 395–397
  Q fever, 420
  relapsing fever, 413
  rickettsial, 417, 417–420, 417t
  Rocky Mountain spotted fever, 417–418, *418*
  spirochetal, 407–411, 407t (*see also* Syphilis)
  typhus, 418–420, *419*
  yaws, 411
Bacterial killing
  nonoxidative, 74
  oxidative, 73–74
Bacterial meningitis, 47, 1445–1448

Bacterial opsonization, 50
Bactericidal/permeability-increasing protein (BPI), 74
B acute lymphoblastic leukemia/lymphoma, 1091–1093, *1092*
Baker's cyst, 1376
Balanitis, 903–904
Band keratophathy, 1506–1507
Barr body, 236
Barrett epithelium, 9
Barrett esophagus, 667, *668*
Bartholin gland cyst, 934
Bartonellosis, 405–406
Basal cell carcinoma, skin, 1259–1260, *1260*
Basement membrane zone, 1207–1208, *1209*
  diseases of, 1221–1223, 1221t, *1222*
    bullous pemphigoid, 1223–1226, *1224, 1225*
    dermatitis herpetiformis, 700–701, *701, 1226–1227,* 1226–1228, *1228, 1230–1231,* 1230–1232, *1232*
    epidermolysis bullosa, 1221–1223, 1221t, *1222*
    erythema multiforme, 1228–1229, *1229*
    lichen planus, 1231–1234, *1232, 1233*
    systemic lupus erythematosus, 1229–1231, *1230, 1231*
  glomerular, *829,* 829–830, *830*
  in wound repair, 88–95, *89,* 89t, *91,* 91t
Basophilia, 1064, 1065t
Basophils, 62, *63,* 1026
B-cell lymphoproliferative diseases, in AIDS, 153
bcl-2 protein, 191
Becker muscular dystrophy, 262–264, *263,* 1391–1394, *1392,* 1392t, *1393*
Beckwith-Wiedemann syndrome, 881
Behçet disease, 509–510
Bejel, 411
Benign arteriolosclerosis, 502, *502*
Benign essential gammopathy, 1101, *1102*
Benign prostatic hypertrophy (nodular prostatic hyperplasia), 918–920, *919, 920, 921*
Benign recurrent intrahepatic cholestasis, 750
Beri-beri (thiamine deficiency), 349, *350*
Bernard-Soulier syndrome, 1055–1056, *1056*
Berry aneurysm, 286, *1435*
Bethesda reporting system, 946
Bethesda reporting system 2001, 1540, 1540t
Bezoars, 689, *690*
Bicornuate uterus, 953
Bilateral micronodular adrenal hyperplasia (Carney complex), 1161
Bile acids, *698,* 699
Bile duct carcinoma (cholangiocarcinoma), 800, *800,* 809
Bile duct microhamartoma (von Meyenburg complexes), 797
Bile infarct (bile lake), 753
Bilharziasis (schistosomiasis) (*see under* Helminthic infections)
Biliary atresia, 795–796
Biliary cirrhosis, primary, 779–780, *780*

Biliary obstruction, 751–753, *752, 753*
  extrahepatic, 781–782, *782*
Bilirubin disorders, 747–753
  hyperbilirubinemia, 747–749
  jaundice, 747, *747*
Bilirubin encephalopathy, 273
Bilirubin metabolism, 747
Biological aging, 34–38
Biopsy
  bone marrow, 1023, *1025,* 1025t
  muscle, 1390
Birbeck granules, 1066, *1066,* 1206–1207, *1207,* 1332, *1332*
Birth injury, 275–276
  cranial, 275
  fractures, 275, 276
  peripheral nerve, 276
Bladder
  anatomy, 888
  congenital disorders, 891–892
    diverticula, 892
    extrophy, *891,* 891–892
    urachal remnants, 892
    vesicoureteral valve incompetence, 892
  cystitis, 892–894
  neoplasia
    benign, *895,* 895–896, *896*
    benign transitional cell papilloma, 897, *899*
    malignant, 896–900, *897,* 897t
Bladder cancer, 896–900, *897,* 897t
  adenocarcinoma, 900
  epidemiology, 212, 896
Bladder papilloma, 897, *898*
Blastomycosis, 437, *438,* 1244, *1244*
  South American, 438, *438*
Bleeding (*see also* Hemorrhage)
  dysfunctional uterine, 955–956, 956t
  gastrointestinal, major causes, 734
Blepharitis, 1504
Blood, components of, *43*
Blood flow, velocity, *478*
Blood supply
  of bone, 1309
  wound healing and, 109
Blood vessels (*see also* Vessel wall)
  aneurysms, 510–514, *511* (*see also* Aneurysms)
  atherosclerosis, 483–498 (*see also* Atherosclerosis; Thrombosis)
  coagulation, *480,* 480–483, *481, 482* (*see also* Coagulation)
  embryonic development, 474–479, *475*
  fibromuscular dysplasia, 503–504
  hypertension, 498–503 (*see also* Hypertension)
  lymphatic diseases, 515
  lymphatic system tumors, 518–519
  Mönckberg medial sclerosis, 503
  Raynaud phenomenon, 503, *504*
  tumors
    benign, 515–517, *516*
    malignant, 517–518
  vasculitis, 504–510, 504t (*see also* Vasculitis)
  veins, *514,* 514–515 (*see also* Varicose veins)
  vessel wall, 474–475, *476,* 476t, *477*

Bloom syndrome, 194–195
Blue nevus, 1255, *1257*
B lymphocytes, 124
  immune-response interactions, 129
Bodies
  Allison-Ghormley, 1366, 1367, *1367, 1369*
  Barr, 236
  Döhle, *1063*
  Hirano, 1479, *1480*
  Howell-Jolly, *1029*
  inclusion, in viral encephalomyelitis, 1453, *1454*
  Lewy, 11, 1468
  Mallory, 11, *779*
  Negri, *1417, 1454*
  Odland, 1205–1206, *1206*
  reticulate, 414
  rice, 1366, 1367, *1367, 1368*
  Sciller-Duval, 978, *978*
Boils (furuncles), 377
Bone
  anatomy, *1304,* 1307–1313, *1308*
  delayed maturation, *1321,* 1321–1322
    echondromatosis (Ollier disease), *1322,* 1322–1323
  fibrous dysplasia, 1348–1349
  formation and growth, *1313,* 1313–1315, *1314, 1315*
  fracture, 1323–1326
    fracture healing, *1323–1324,* 1323–1326
  growth plate disorders, 1315–1320
    achondroplasia, 1316–1317, *1317*
    asymmetric cartilage growth, 1317–1320
    cretinism, 1138, 1145–1146, 1313, 1321
    Morquio syndrome, 1315–1316, *1316*
    in scurvy, 1317–1318, *1318*
  infections
    osteomyelitis, 1327–1331, *1330*
    syphilitic, 1331
    tuberculosis, *1330,* 1330–1331
  lamellar, 1311–1312, *1312*
    concentric, *1304,* 1312
  Langerhans cell histiocytosis, 1332–1334
    eosinophilic granuloma, 1332–1333, *1333*
    Hand-Schüller-Christian disease, 1333
    Letter-Siwe disease, 1333–1334
  metabolic diseases of, 1333–1348, *1335*
  metastases to, *1360,* 1360–1361
  microscopic organization, *1311,* 1311–1313, *1312*
  modeling abnormalities
    osteopetrosis (Albers-Schönberg disease, marble bone disease), *1320,* 1320–1321
    progressive disphyseal dysplasia, 1321
  osteonecrosis, 1325–1327, *1326,* 1326t
  Paget disease of, 1344–1348, *1345, 1346, 1347*
  reactive bone formation, 1326–1327, *1327*
    heterotrophic calcification, 1327
    myositis ossificans, 1327, *1328*
  tumors
    benign, 1350–1354, *1351*
    malignant, 1354–1360
  woven, *1311,* 1312

Bone cyst, aneurysmal, *1351,* 1351–1352
Bone destruction, in multiple myeloma, 1103
Bone marrow
  anatomy, 1020–1025, *1021,* 1307–1308, *1308*
  embryology, *1020*
  in multiple myeloma, 1099t, *1100,* 1100–1101
  reactive lymphoid hyperplasia, 1085
Bone marrow biopsy, 1023, *1025*
Bone matrix, 1309
Borrelia burgdorferi, 411–412
Borrelia recurrenti, 413
Botryoid embryonal rhabdomyosarcoma, 1381
Botulism, 400–401
Bourneville disease (tuberous sclerosis), 1491, *1491*
Bovine spongiform encephalopathy (mad cow disease), 1194–1196
Bowen disease, 937
Bowenoid papulosis, 905–906, 1256
Brachial palsy, 276
Brain, in prematurity, 270
Brain abscess, 323, *324*
Brain lesions, in TORCH complex, 224
BRCA1/BRCA2 genes, 193, 1006–1007
Breast
  anatomy and development, *996,* 998
  benign tumors, 1004–1006
    fibroadenoma, 1004, *1005*
    intraductal papilloma, 1006, *1006*
  carcinoma, 1006–1014
    colloid (mucinous), 1010, *1011*
    frequency by type, 1008t
    in situ, 1007–1009, *1008, 1009*
    intraductal, *1536*
    invasive, 1009–1011, *1010*
    male, 1014
    medullary, 1011, *1012*
    metaplastic, 1011
    metastatic patterns, 1012
    oncogene expression, 1013, *1013*
    pathogenesis, 1006–1007
    prognostic factors, 1012–1014, *1014*
    staging, 1012
    treatment, 1014
    tubular, 1010
  congenital anomalies, 1000
  duct ectasia, 1001
  fat necrosis, 1001
  fibrocystic change, 1001–1004, *1002, 1003*
    nonproliferative, 1001–1002, *1003–1004*
    proliferative, 1002–1004
  gynecomastia, 1000, *1999*
  hormonal control, 998–1000, *999*
  juvenile (pubertal) hypertrophy, 1000
  male, 1000, *1000,* 1014
  mastitis
    acute, 1001
    granulomatous, 1001
  Paget disease of nipple, 1009–1010, *1010*
  phyllodes tumor, 1014–1015, *1015*
Breast cancer
  BRCA1/BRCA2 genes in, 193
  epidemiology, 212, 213

Breast tissue, ectopic, 934
Brenner tumor, 971, *973*
Brodie abscess, 1329
Bronchi, nornal epithelium, *1533*
Bronchial carcinoma, small cell, *1534*
Bronchiectasis, in cystic fibrosis, 250
Bronchitis
 in cystic fibrosis, 250
 smoking and, 316, *318*
Bronchoconstriction, neurokinins in, 58
Bronchopulmonary dysplasia, 272–273
Bronchopulmonary foregut malformation, 664
Bronze diabetes, 784, *784*
Brown tumors, 1342, *1342*
Brucellosis, 401–402
Brunn buds, 894
Brunn nests, 894
Bruton X-linked agammaglobulinemia, 143–145, 145t, 1293
Buboes, 402
Budd-Chiari syndrome, 304, 790
Buerger disease (thromboangiitis obliterans), 508–509, *510*
Bullous pemphigoid, 1223–1224, *1224*, *1225*
Buphthalmos, 1523–1524
Burkitt lymphoma, 185, 197–198, 1106–1108, *1108*
 epidemiology, 212, 213
Burns, 335–337
 cutaneous, 335–336, *336*
 electrical, 336–337, *337*
 infections in, 378
 inhalation, 336
Buscke and Lowenstein tumor, 906, *906*
Byler syndrome, 751

C

Cachexia, 207
Cadherins, in metastasis, 178–179
Cadmium toxicity, 333
Caenorhabdis elegans, aging studies, 36
Café au lait spots, 246
Caisson disease, 293
Calcific aortic stenosis, 14
Calcification, 14, *14*
 arterial, 488, *489*
 dystrophic, 14, *14*, 1327
 ectopic, 354
 heterotropic, 1327
 metastatic, 14, 1327
Calcific cystitis, 892
Calcific keratopathy, 1506–1507
Calcifying pancreatitis, chronic, 816–817, *817*
Calcium hydroxyapatite deposition disease, 1375, *1376*
Calcium metabolism, in hyperparathyroidism, 1341–1343, *1342*
Calcium pyrophosphate dihydrate deposition disease, 1373–1375, *1376*
Calculi, renal
 calcium stones, 876
 cystine stones, 877
 infection stones, 876
 staghorn, 876, *877*
 uric acid, 876
Caliectasis, 872, *873*
Caloric restriction, aging and, 38
Campylobacter jejuni, 393–394, 694
Canalization, in thrombi, 287, *288*
Cancer (*see also specific types*)
 adrenal metastatic, 1163
 adrenocortical, 1160, *1161*
 as altered differentiation, 182
 bile duct, 800, *800*
 bladder, 316
 chemical carcinogenesis, 199–203, *200*
 chronic inflammation and, 76, 80–81
 clonal origin of, *181*, 181–182
 common types, 210t, 211
 epidemiology, *210*, 210–213
 esophageal, 316, *671*, 671–672
 grading of, 180, *180*
 growth of, 182–183
  dormancy period, 183
  doubling times, 183
  tumor angiogenesis, 183
 histological diagnosis, 170–180
  electron microscopy, 171, *172*
  of metastasis, 171
  tumor markers, 171–172, *173*, 174–175t
  vs. benign tumors, 170, *170*
  vs. parent tissue, 170–171
 immunology, 204–207, *205*
 invasive properties, 173–175, *175*, *177*
 laryngeal, 316
 liver, 798–800, *799*, *800*
 lung, 315–36, *316*
 metastasis, 175–180
  hematogenous, 176, *176*
  lymphatic, 176–177, *177*
  by seeding, 177
  skip, 177
  steps in, 177–180, *178*
  target organs in, 179–180
 molecular genetics, 193–195
  DNA methylation, 194
  DNA repair genes, 194–195
  hereditary cancer syndromes, 195, 196t, *197*
  oncogenes, 184–191
  telomerase and, 195
  tumor suppressor genes, 191–194
 mortality, *210*, 210–211
 pancreatic, 316, *317*, 817–820, *818*, *819*
 parathyroid, 1152
 penile, 905–906
 physical carcinogenesis, 203–204
  asbestos, 203–204
  UV radiation, 203
 radiation-related, 342–344, *343*
 staging of, 180–181
 stomach, 677, 685–689
 systemic effects, 207–208
 thyroid, 1144–1149
 viruses and, 195–198
Cancer chemotherapy, impaired phagocytosis in, 74–75
Cancer risk, of oral contraceptives, 326
Cancrum oris (noma), 414, *414*
Candida esophagitis, 667
Candidiasis, 429–430, 429t, *430*
 in AIDS, 152
 chronic mucocutaneous, 146
 disseminated, 430
 endocardial, 430
 female genital, 934
 intestinal, 695
 nasal, 1289
 oral (thrush), 430, *1272*, *1273*
 vulvovaginitis, 430
Capillaries, 282–283, *283*, 478
Capillary filtration, 297
Capillary hemangioma, 516
Capillary lymphangioma, 518
Caput succedaneum, 275
Carbon monoxide, 330
Carbon tetrachloride, 22
Carbuncles, 377
Carcinoembryonic antigen (CEA), 172
Carcinogens
 chemical, 201
 occupational, 326–333, 327t
Carcinoid tumors, *1534*
 colorectal, 731
 gastric, 689
 islet cell, 823, *824*
 of small intestine, 706–708, *707*
 thymic, 1122
Carcinoma
 acinar cell, 820
 adenoid cystic, 1284, *1284*
 adenosquamous, 169
 adrenal cortical, 1160, *1161*
 ampullary, 706
 basal cell, skin, 1259–1260, *1260*
 bile duct, 809
 breast, 1006–1014 (*see also* Breast *and specific lesions*)
  medullary, 1011, *1012*
  metaplastic, 1011
  tubular, 1010
 cervical
  endometrial, *1532*
  in situ, *175*
  squamous cell, *1532*
 colloid, 169
 endometrial (*see also* Adenocarcinoma)
  secretory, 960
 esophageal, 211, *671*, 671–672
 gastric, *1535*
 hepatocellular, 798–800, *799*
 histological diagnosis, 172
 intraductal, *1536*
 medullary, 169
 Merkel cell, skin, 1261
 mucoepidermoid, salivary gland, 1284, *1284*
 nasal cavity and paranasal sinuses, 1292, *1292*
 nasopharyngeal, 198
  Epstein-Barr virus and, 1294–1295, *1295*
  squamous cell, 1294
 oral cavity, squamous cell, 1275, *1275*
 parathyroid, 1152
 renal cell, 882–884, *883*, 883t
 renal transitional cell, 884
 salivary gland

Carcinoma *(contd.)*
  acinic cell, 1285
  adenoid cystic carcinoma, 1284, *1284*
  mucoepidermoid, 1284, *1284*
  skin
    basal cell, 1259–1260, *1260*
    Merkel cell, 1261
    squamous cell, 1260–1261, *1261*
  small cell
    bronchial, *1534*
    thymic, 1122
  squamous cell, 182
    of bone, 1329
    cervical, *949*, 949–951, *950, 1532*
    nasopharyngeal, 1293
    oral cavity, 1275, *1275*
    skin, 1260–1261, *1261*
    vaginal, 940, 940t
    verrucous, 937–938
    vulvar, *937*, 937–938, 938t
  terminology, 168–169
  thymic, 1122
  thyroid
    anaplastic (undifferentiated), 1148–1149, *1149*
    familial medullary, 1164, *1165*
    follicular, 1147, *1147*
    medullary, 1147–1149, *1148*
    papillary, 1145–1147, *1146*
  transitional cell, 168–169, *169*
    bladder, 898–900
  grades 1 through 3, 898–900, *899*
  in situ, *898*
    renal, *1535*
Carcinosarcoma, 169
  uterine, 962
Cardiac anomalies, in TORCH complex, 225
Cardiac glands, 673
Cardiac involvement, in lupus erythematosus, 157
Cardiac output, 292
Cardiac scarring, 114
Cardiogenic shock, 305
Cardiomyopathy, 288
Cardiovascular defects, in Marfan syndrome, 244
Cardiovascular disease, smoking and, *314*, 315
Caretaker genes, 194–195
Carney complex (bilateral micronodular adrenal hyperplasia), 1161
Carpal tunnel syndrome, 1496
CARS (compensated antiinflammatory response system), 308
Cartilage, 1312
  articular, 1362, *1362*
  elastic, 1313
  fibrocartilage, 1313
  hyaline, 1313
  types, 1313
Cartilage anlage, 1313
Cartilage growth, asymmetric, 1318–1319
Cartilage matrix, 1312–1313
Caruncles, urethral, 905
Caseous necrosis, 26, *27*
Caspase, 31
Castleman disease, 1088
  AIDS-associated, 152–153

Casts, renal, 869
Catalase, 20
Cataracts, 1507–1508, *1508*
  diabetic, 1517
  radiation-related, 341
Catenins, in metastasis, 178–179
Cat-scratch disease, 405, *405*, 1089
Cauliflower ear, 1296
Cavernous angioma, 1435
Cavernous hemangioma, 516, *516*
Cavernous lymphangioma, 518–519
Cavernous transformation, 758
CD4/CD8 cells, *122, 123*, 128–129
CD (cluster of differentiation) numbers, 120
Cecal volvulus, 704–705
Celiac disease (gluten-sensitive enteropathy), 672, 700–702, *701, 702*
Cell arrangement, 1538, 1538t
Cell–cell adhesion molecules, 474
Cell cycle, 107–108, *108*
  of malignant cells, 170–171
  in oncogene action, *190*, 190–191
Cell death, 24–34
  apoptosis, 22
    in developmental processes, 29
    in DNA damage, 30
    Fas receptor in, 30–31, *31*
    in infection, 30
    initiation signals, 30
    morphology, 29, *29, 30*
    p53 activation, 33
    physiological function, 29–30
    quantitative assays, 33–34, *35*
  necrosis, 24–29
    mechanisms, 24–25
    types, 25–26
Cell injury, 1–38
  cell death, 24–34
  mechanisms and morphology, 15–24
    chemotoxicity, 22–24
    hydropic swelling, 15–16, *16*
    ionizing radiation, 21, 22
    ischemia/reperfusion injury, 20–21
    ischemic injury, 16
    oxidative stress, 16–20, *18, 19*, 19t, *20*
    subcellular changes, 16, *16, 17*
    viral cytoxicity, 21–22, *23*
  reactions, 1–15
    atrophy, 4–6, *6, 9*
    calcification, 14, *14*
    dysplasia, 9, *9*
    hyalinization, 14
    hyperplasia, 7–8, *8*
    hypertrophy, 6–7, *7*
    intracellular storage, 10–14
    metaplasia, 8–9, *9*
Cell membrane-associated molecules, 51
Cell migration, in wound repair, 86–88, *87*
Cells *(see also specific types)*
  antigen-presenting (APCs), *125*, 125–126
  argentaffin, 673
  argyrophil, 673
  Askanazy, 1143, 1144, *1145*
  of bone, 1309–1311, *1310, 1311*
  chromaffin, 1164
  dendritic, 77, 126
  detection in body fluids, 1530

  endothelial, 86
  enterochromaffin, 673, 823, *824*
  epidermal, 106–107
  epithelial, 88
  foam, 255
  Gaucher, 253, *253*
  goblet, 691
  heart failure, *284*, 285
  HeLa, 197
  hepatocytes, 743–745
  of immune system, 120–127
  inflammatory, 59–65
  Kupffer, 745–746
  labile, 108
  Langerhans, *1204*, 1206–1207, *1207*
  Langhans giant, 79, *80*
  Leydig, 889
  mast, 62, *63*, 1210, *1210*
  Merkel, *1204*, 1207, *1208*
  mucous neck, 673
  myeloid-to-erythroid ratio, 1023, *1025*, 1025t
  natural killer (NK), 55, 124, 138, *140*
  of nervous system, 1415–1419
  Paneth, 691
  parietal (oxynic), 673
  permanent, 108
  plasma, 77
  precursor, 1023, *1023, 1024*
  progenitor, *1022*, 1022–1023
  Reed-Sternberg, *1012*, 1111, *1111, 1115*
  Sertoli, 889
  Sézary, *1110*
  smooth muscle, 86
  stable, 108, 109
  stem, 108–109, 120–121, *121*, 1022, *1022*
  Warthin-Finkeldey, 1089
  zymogen (chief), 673
Cellular adhesion molecules *(see Adhesion molecules)*
Cellular atypia, 170, *171*
Cellular bases of disease, 4
Cellular migration, in wound healing, 107
Cellulitis
  facial, 383
  Ludwig angina, 1272–1273
  streptococcal, 380, *380*
Celomic metaplasia, 982
Central chondrosarcoma, 1355–1356, *1357*
Central core disease, *1395*, 1395–1396
Central diabetes insipidus, 1133, *1133*
Central nervous system (CNS)
  cerebrospinal fluid (CSF), 1443–1444
  chromosomal abnormalities, 1424–1425
  circulatory disorders, 1435–1443
    cerebral aneurysm, *1345, 1435*, 1435–1437, *1436, 1437*, 1443–1445.1425, *1444*
    cerebral hemorrhage/stroke, *1437*, 1437–1438, *1438*
    cerebral ischemia/infarction, 1438–1443, *1439, 1440, 1441*
    regional ischemia and cerebral infarction, *1440*, 1440–1441, *1441*
    vascular malformations, 1435, *1435*
  congenital disorders, epilepsy, 1425–1426
  congenital malformations, 1419–1426

in chromosomal abnormalities, *1424,* 1424–1425, *1425*
neural tube defects, 1419–1422
degenerative diseases, Pick disease, 1479, *1480*
demyelinating diseases, 1461–1465
in alcoholism (central pontine myelinolysis), 1465, *1465*
leukodystrophies, 1461–1462
multiple sclerosis, 1463–1464, *1464*
postinfectious/postvaccinal encephalomyelitis, 1464–1465
healing in, 112–114
infectious diseases, 1444
cerebral abscess, 1450, *1450, 1451*
meningitis, 1445–1458
prion diseases (spongiform encephalopathies), 1458–1462, 1459t, *1460*
viral encephalomyelitis, 1450–1458, *1452*
metabolic disorders
alcoholism, 1466–1468, *1467*
hepatic encephalopathy, 1468
subacute combined spinal degeneration, 1468
metabolic neuronal diseases
cretinism, 1466
phenylketonuria (PKU), 1466
Wilson disease (hepatolenticular degeneration), 1466
neurodegenerative diseases, 1468–1479, 1468t
Alzheimer disease, 1475–1479, 1476t, *1477, 1478, 1479, 1480*
amyotrophic lateral sclerosis, 1471, *1471*
Parkinson disease, 1469–1470, *1470*
progressive supranuclear palsy, 1471
striatonigral degeneration, 1471
trinucleotide repeat expansion syndromes, 1472–1475, *1474*
neuronal storage diseases, 1465–1466
Gaucher disease, 1466
Hurler syndrome, 1466
Niemann-Pick disease, 1466
Tay-Sachs disease, 1465–1466
regional occlusive cerebrovascular disease, *1441,* 1441–1443
trauma, 1426–1435
cerebral contusion, *1430,* 1430–1432, *1431*
epidural hematoma, *1426,* 1426–1428, *1427, 1428*
penetrating wounds, *1432,* 1432–1433
spinal cord injuries, *1433,* 1433–1434
subarachnoid hemorrhage, 1429–1430
subdural hematoma, 1428–1429, *1429*
tumors, 1479–1491, *1481*
acoustic neuroma, 1487, *1487*
anaplastic astrocytoma, 1483, *1483*
astrocytoma, *1482,* 1482–1483, *1483*
benign vs. malignant, 1479
choroid plexus papilloma, 1485
colloid cysts, 1490, *1490*
craniopharyngioma, 1487, *1488*
dermoid/epidermoid cysts, 1488–1489
ependymoma, 1485, *1485*
ganglioglioma, 1485–1486
germ cell, 1488
glioblastoma multiforme, 1483, *1484*
hemangioblastoma, *1488,* 1488–1489
hereditary intracranial/extracranial, 1490–1491, 1490t
in Lindau syndrome, 1489, 1491
lipoma, 1488, *1488*
medulloblastoma, 1485
meningioma, 1312, *1494,* 1494–1495, *1495.1294*
metastatic, 1489–1490, *1490*
in neurofibromatosis, 1491
neuronal, 1481–1482
oligodendroglioma, 1483–1485, *1484*
primary lymphoma, 1489, *1489*
schwannoma, 1487, *1487*
in Sturge-Weber syndrome (encephalofacial angiomatosis), 1491
symptoms of intracranial, 1482
in tuberous sclerosis (Bourneville disease), 1491, *1491*
Central nuclear (myotubular) myopathy, 1396, *1397*
Central pontine myelinolysis, 322
Cephalohematoma, 275
Cerebal edema, 303
Cerebral abscess, 1450, *1450, 1451*
Cerebral aneurysm, 512, 1430, *1435,* 1435–1437, *1436, 1437*
Cerebral contusion, *1430,* 1430–1432, *1431*
Cerebral edema
altitude-related, 337
in hepatic failure, 756
Cerebral hemorrhage, *1437,* 1437–1438, *1438*
Cerebral ischemia/infarction, 297, 1438–1443, *1439, 1440, 1441*
global, 1438–1440, *1439, 1440*
regional, *1440,* 1440–1441, *1441*
Cerebral venous thrombosis, 1442–1443, *1443*
Cerebritis, 1450, *1450*
Cerebrospinal fluid (CSF), 1443–1444
transport, 1418
Cerebrovascular amyloid, *1198*
Cervical carcinoma
endometrial, *1532*
epidemiology, 212
in situ, *175*
squamous cell, *1532*
Cervical dysplasia, *9*
Cervical glandular intraepithelial neoplasia (CGIN), 951
Cervical intraepithelial neoplasia (CIN), *945,* 945–949, *946, 947*
Cervical metaplasia, 8–9, *9*
Cervicitis, 942, *944*
Cervix, 941–952
adenocarcinoma, 952–953
anatomy, 941–942, *942, 943, 944*
benign neoplasia, 942–945
endocervical polyp, 942–943, *945*
leiomyoma, 943–945
microglandular hyperplasia, 943
cervicitis, 942, *944*
squamous cell neoplasia, 945–952

cervical intraepithelial neoplasia (CIN), *945,* 945–949, *946, 947*
human papillomavirus and, 947, *947*
incidence, 951t
invasive squamous cell carcinoma, 949–951, *950*
microinvasive squamous cell carcinoma, 949, *949*
staging, 951t
Cestodes intestinal tapeworms, 469–471, 469t
c-*fos* oncogene, 189
C granules, 70, *71*
Chagas disease, 454, *454,* 665
Chalazion, 1504
Chancre, 408–409, *409* (*see also* Syphilis)
Chancroid, 386, 903, 931
Charcot-Bouchard aneurysm, *1436,* 1437
Charcot-Marie-Tooth disease, 243, 1497, 1498t
Chédiak-Higashi syndrome, 1063–1064
Cheilosis
in riboflavin deficiency, 351, *351*
solar, *1276*
CHEK2 gene, 1006–1007
Chemical carcinogenesis, 199–203, *200*
agents of, 199–201
endogenous and environmental factors in, 201–203
mutagenicity and, 199
in pancreatic cancer, 817
progression of, 199
Chemical esophagitis, 668–669
Chemical gastropathy, 677–678
Chemical peritonitis, 736
Chemicals, environmental, 326–333
Chemokines, 56, 56–57
CXC (CC), 57
functional classes, 57
Chemotaxis, 68, *69*
Chemotoxicity, 22–24
acetaminophen, 22–24, *24*
carbon tetrachloride, 22
unmetabolized chemicals, 24
Cherry-red macula, 1519, *1520*
Cherry-red spot sign, 1465
in Tay-Sachs disease, 254
Chickenpox, 370, *370, 371*
Chief cells, 1149
Childhood bacterial infections, 381–384
Chlamydial infections, 414–417, 931–932
C. pneumoniae, 417
C. psittaci, 416–417
C. trachomatis, 414, 415–416
lymphogranuloma venereum, *415,* 415–416
sexually transmitted, 415
trachoma, 416
penile lesions, 903
Chloroform, 328
Cholangiocarcinoma, 800, *800*
Cholangitic liver abscess, 792
Cholangitis, primary sclerosing, 780–781, *781*
Cholecystitis
acute, *806,* 806–807
chronic, 807, *807*

1554   **Index**

Cholelithiasis (gallstones), 802–806
  cholesterol stones, *803*, 803–804
  oral contraceptives and, 326
  pancreatitis in, 813, 816
  pigment stones, 804, *804*
Cholera, 391–393, *394*
Cholestasis, 751–753, *752*, *753*
  benign recurrent intrahepatic, 750
  cellular mechanisms, 751–752, *752*
  in drug-induced hepatotoxicity, 790
  familial intrahepatic cholestasis (Byler syndrome), 751
  intrahepatic of pregnancy, 750
  morphological features, *752*, 752
Cholestatic hepatitis, 768–769
Cholesteatoma, 1298
Cholesterol, *494*, 494–496, *495*
  atherosclerosis and, 493
  familial hypercholesterolemia, 496, *497*, *498*, *499*
Cholesterol clefts, renal, 863, *864*
Cholesterol granuloma, 1298
Cholesterolosis, 807–808
Cholesterol transport pathway, *495*
Chondroblastoma, 1353, *1354*
Chondrocalcinosis, 1373–1375, *1376*
Chondrocytes, 1313
Chondroma, 167, *167*
  solitary (enchodroma), 1352–1353
Chondromatosis, synovial, 1376–1377
Chondromyxoid fibroma, 1353–1354
Chondrosarcoma, 167, 169, *169*, 1355–1357
  central, 1355–1356, *1357*
  juxtacortical, 1356–1357
  peripheral, 1356
Chordoma, 1295–1296, *1296*
Chorioamnionitis, 986
Choriocarcinoma, 978, 993, *993*, 993t
  epidemiology, 212
Choristoma, 168, 278
Choroid plexus papilloma, 1485
Chromaffin cells, 1164
Chromatolysis, in neuronal injury, 1416, *1416*
Chromomycosis, *438*, 439
Chromosomal abnormalities
  autosomal dominant, *242*, 242–243, 243t
    biochemical basis, 243
    connective tissue, 243–247
    new vs. inherited mutations, 243
  autosomal recessive, 247–252, *248*, 248t
    cystic fibrosis, 249, 249–251, *250*
    lysosomal storage disorders, 251–258
  autosomal syndromes, 231–236, 232t
    chromosomal breakdown, 236
    deletion syndromes, 234t, 235–236
    translocation syndromes, 235–236
    trisomy 13, 235
    trisomy 13–15, 1425
    trisomy 18, 235
    trisomy 21 (Down syndrome), 231–235, 232t, *233*, *234*, *1424*, 1424–1425
    trisomy 22, 235
    X-linked, 261–266, 261t
      Fabry disease, 266
      fragile X syndrome, 264–266, *265*, *266*

hemophilia A (factor VIII deficiency), 264
muscular dystrophies, *260*, 262–264
X-linked dominance, 261–262, *262*
  congenital CNS malformations in, *1424*, 1424–1425, *1425*
  connective tissue diseases, 243–247
    achondroplastic dwarfism, 247
    Ehlers-Danlos syndromes, 244–245, 245t
    familial hypercholesterolemia, 257
    Marfan syndrome, 243–244, *244*
    neurofibromatosis, 246, *246*
  inborn errors of amino acid metabolism, 258–260, 258t, *259*
    albinism, 261
    alkaptonuria (ochronosis), *260*, 260–261
    phenylketonuria (PKU), 258–260, *259*
    tyrosinemia, 260
  of number, 230–236
    efects of, 231
    gestational stage and, 231
    nomenclature, 231, 231t
    nondisjunction, 230–231
    sex chromosomes, 236–242, *239*
  of sex chromosomes, 236–242, *239*
    female multiple-X, 239
    Klinefelter syndrome (47,XXY), 237–238, *238*
    Turner syndrome (45X),*239*, 238–239
    X chromosome, 236–237
    Y chromosome, 236
    YYY male, 238
  single gene, 239–242
    mutations, 241–243, *242*, *243*
  structural, 227–230, *228*, *229*
    deletions, 228
    inversions, 228–230
    isochromosomes, 230
    reciprocal translocations, 227–228, *228*, *229*
    ring chromosomes, 230
    Robertsonian translocation, 228
Chromosomal banding, 226–227
Chromosomal breakdown syndromes, 236
Chromosomal deletions, 228
Chromosomal inversions, 228–230
Chromosomal translocation, 185, *186*
Chromosomes
  fluorescence in situ hybridization (FISH), 226, *227*
  normal complement, *226*, 226–227
  ring, 230
  structure, 226, *226*
Chronic autoimmune (Hashimoto) thyroiditis, *1139*, *1142*, 1142–1143
Chronic calcifying pancreatitis, 816–817, *817*
Chronic cholecystitis, 807, *807*
Chronic discoid lupus erythematosus, 158
Chronic eosinophilic leukemia, 1075–1076
Chronic granulomatous disease, 1063–1064
Chronic idiopathic myelofibrosis, 1070t, 1071t, 1074, *1074*
Chronic inflammation, 5–6, 7–8
  cancer and, 80–81
  cells involved in, 76, 76–78

acute inflammatory cells, 78
dendritic cells, 77
fibroblasts, 77–78, *78*
lymphocytes, 77, *77*
monocyte/macrophages, *76*, 76–77
plasma cells, 77
cellular components, 76–78
definition, 42, 44
granulomatous, 79, 79–80, *80*
inflammatory cells, 76–78
injury and repair in, 78–79
Chronic inflammatory demyelinating polyneuropathy, 1495
Chronic interstitial cystitis (Hunner ulcer), *893*, 893–894
Chronic lymphocytic leukemia/small lymphocytic lymphoma, 1095–1098, *1097*, *1098*
Chronic mucocutaneous candidiasis, 146
Chronic myelogenous leukemia, 1067–1071, 1070t, *1071*, 1071t, *1072*
Chronic osteomyelitis, *1329*, 1329–1330
Chronic pancreatitis, 816–817, *817*
Chronic rejection, 141, *141*
Churg-Strauss syndrome, 506, *506*, 860
Chylous ascites, 304
Circulating anticoagulants, 1058
Circulation, normal, 282–283, *283*
Cirrhosis, 111, *111*, 303, 753–754, *754*, 754t
  alcoholic, 320, *321*, 777–779, *780*, 798
  causes, 754t
  cryptogenic, 754–755
  endocrine complications in, 756–757
  heritable disorders associated with, 785–788
    α₁-antitrypsin deficiency, 787
    cystic fibrosis, 787
    inborn errors of metabolism, 787–788
    Wilson disease (hepatolenticular degeneration), 785–787, *786*
  Indian childhood, 788
  macronodular, *754*, 754–755
  micronodular (Laennec), 754
  portal hypertension in, 758
  primary biliary, 779–780, *780*
  pulmonary complications in, 756
  vs. focal nodular hyperplasia, *797*, 797
c-jun oncogene, 189
Clear cell adenocarcinoma
  endometrial, 960
  ovarian, 975
  vaginal, 940, *940*
Cleft lip/left palate, 268, *268*
Clefts, facial, 1271
Clonal thrombocytosis, 1057
Clonorchiasis, 467–468, *468*
Clonorchis sinensis, 793–794, *794*
Clostridial infections
  botulism, 400–401
  C. difficile colitis, 401
  food poisoning *(C. perfringens)*, 397
  gas gangrene, 399–400
  necrotizing enteritis, 397–399
  tetanus, 400, *400*
Clostridium difficile colitis, 711, *711*
Clostridium perfringens, 694
Clot lysis, 483

Index

Clotting factors, 746
c-*myc* protooncogene, 185, 190
Coagulation, *480*, 480–483, 480t, *481, 482,* 482t
  endothelial regulation, 481–483, *482,* 482t
  fibrinolysis, 483, *493*
  mechanisms, *480,* 480–481
  platelet adhesion, 481
  versus thrombosis, 479
Coagulation abnormalities, 1056–1062
  in cancer, 209
  circulating anticoagulants, 1058
  disseminated intravascular coagulation (DIC), 82, 1058–1059, *1059, 1060*
  fibrinolysis, 1059
  hemophilia B, 1056–1057
  in hepatic failure, 756
  hypercoagulability, 1059–1060, 1061t
    acquired, 1061
    inherited, 1060–1061
  in liver disease, 1057
  in multiple myeloma, 1103
  in vitamin K deficiency, 1058
  von Willebrand disease, 1057
Coagulation cascade, *480*
Coagulative necrosis, 25, *25*
Cobalt toxicity, 333
"Cobblestone" colon, *713*
Cocaine, 324
Coccidiodomycosis, *433, 436,* 436–437, *437*
  disseminated, *436, 437*
$^{14}CO_2$-cholyl-glycine breath test, 700
Codominance, 240
Cold abscess, 1331
Cold agglutinin disease, 7–45, *1045*
Cold hemolysin disease (paroxysmal cold hemoglobinemia), 1045–1046
Colic, renal, 876
Colitis
  collagenous, *719,* 719–720, *720*
  ischemic, *720, 720*
  lymphocytic, 719–720
  pseudomembranous, 711, *711*
Collagen abnormalities
  Alport syndrome (hereditary nephritis), 848–849, *849*
  osteogenesis imperfecta, *1321,* 1321–1322
Collagenous colitis, *719,* 719–720, *720*
Collagens, *103*
  fibrillar, 92
  in wound repair, 91t, 92–95
Collagen synthesis, *84,* 86
Collectins, 50
Colloid adenoma, of thyroid, 1144, *1145*
Colloid carcinoma, 169
  breast, 1010, *1011*
Colloid cysts, 1490, *1490*
Colony-forming units (CFUs), *1022,* 1022–1023, *1023*
Colony-stimulating factors, 81
Colorectal cancer, 727–731, *1535*
  adenocarcinoma, *727,* 727–730, *728*
  carcinoid tumors, 731
  Dukes classification, 161
  epidemiology, 212, 213
  epidermoid of anal canal, 731
  hereditary nonpolyposis colorectal cancer (HNPCC) syndrome, 194, 729–730, *730,* 730t
  lymphoma, 731
  molecular genetics, 727–728, *728*
  pathogenesis, 727
  pathology, 728–729, *729*
  risk factors, 728
  staging, 728–729, 730t
  ulcerative colitis and, 719
Colorectal polyps
  adenomatous (premalignant), 721–727
    cancer and, 724
    familial adenomatous polyposis (FAP), *724,* 724–725, *725*
    serrated adenoma, 724
    tubular adenoma, *722, 722*
    tubulovillous adenomas, *723,* 723–724
    villous adenomas, 722–723, *723*
  nonneoplastic, 725–727
    hyperplastic (metaplastic) polyps, 725, *726*
    inflammatory polyps, 726, *726*
    juvenile (retention) polyps, 726, *726*
    lymphoid polyps, 726–727
Comedocarcinoma, of breast, 1007–1008, *1009*
Common acquired melanocytic nevus (mole), 1246, *1247*
Common cold (coryza), 363, 1286
Common variable immunodeficiency (CVID), 145, 145t
Compensated antiinflammatory response system (CARS), 308
Competence genes, 189
Complement activation, *49,* 49–50
  alternative pathway, 50
  classical pathway, *49,* 49–50
  mannose-binding pathway, 50
Complementary adhesion molecules, *66,* 66–68, *67*
Complement deficiencies, 51t, 52
Complement-mediated cytotoxicity, 206
Complement system, 49–52, *50*
  biological components, 50, *51*
  deficiency diseases, 51–53, 51t
  regulation, 50–52, *51,* 51t
Complete blood count (CBC), normal adult values, 1028t
Compound nevus, 1246, *1247*
Concentric lamellar bone, *1304,* 1312
Concussion, 1427–1428
  spinal cord, 1434
Condylomata acuminatum (genital warts), 370, 903, 932, *933,* 1258
Condylomata lata, 226, 409, *410,* 931
Confluent hepatic necrosis, 769–770, *770*
Congenital adrenal hyperplasia, 1154–1156, *1155, 1156*
  21-hydroxylase deficiency (CAH), 1154
  11β-hydroxylase deficiency, 1154–1156
Congenital anomalies
  arteriovenous malformation, 1435, *1435*
  of breast, 1000
  central nervous system (CNS), 1419–1426
  of cerebral vasculature, 1435, *1435*
  congenital lymphangiectasia (Milroy disease), 704
  esophagus, 663–665
  gallbladder, 802, *803*
  hepatic fibrosis, 798
  intestinal
    large bowel, 709–711
    small intestine, 691–692
  of kidney, 831–835
  oral cavity
    branchial cleft cyst, 1271.*1265*
    facial clefts, 1271
    lingual thyroid nodule, 1271
  of pancreas, 812
  renal pelvis and ureter, 889–890, *890*
  rubella and, 365–366
  thyroid, 1135
  of urinary bladder, *891,* 891–892
  uterus, 953
Congenital atresia of aqueduct of Sylvius, 1422, *1423, 1424*
Congenital Chagas disease, 454
Congenital esophageal stenosis, 664
Congenital hepatic fibrosis, 798
Congenital hydrocele, 901, *901*
Congenital hydrocephalus, 1422–1423, *1423, 1424*
Congenital hypothyroidism (cretinism), 1138, 1145–1146, 1313, 1321
Congenital lymphangiectasia (Milroy disease), 704
Congenital megacolon (Hirschsprung disease), 709–710, *710*
Congenital megaureter, 890
Congenital melanocytic nevus, 1255
Congenital muscular dystrophy, 1394
Congenital myopathies, 1394–1396, *1395*
Congenital syphilis, 225–226, 410–411
Congenital toxoplasmosis, 446, *446*
Congestion, *284,* 284–285, *285*
Congestive heart failure, 299–301, *300, 301, 302*
  hepatic congestion in, 791, *792*
Conjunctival diseases, 1505–1506 (*see also* under Eye)
Connective tissue tumors, vulvar, 936
Conn syndrome (primary aldosteronism), 1163
Contracture, wound, *105,* 107, 115–116
Contusion, 3378
  cerebral, *1430,* 1430–1432, *1431*
  spinal cord, 1434, *1434*
Cooley anemia (homozygous β thalassemia), 1037–1038, *1038*
Copper deficiency, 355
Cori disease, 1402
Cornea, *93*
Corneal diseases, 1506–1507 (*see also* under Eye)
  arcus lipioides (archus senilis), 1506
  band keratopathy, 1506–1507
  herpes simplex ulcerations, 1506–1507
  onchocerciasis, 1506
Corneal dystrophies, 1507
Coronary artery, *280*
Coronavirus, in SARS, 364
Corpora amyllacea, 1418, *1418*
Corpus callosum, absence of, 1425, *1425*
Corpus luteum cyst, 967

Index

Cortical necrosis, in shock, 866–867, *867*
Corticomedullary osteonecrosis, 1349
Corticosteroid-induced Cushing syndrome, 1161–1162
Corticosteroids
 gastritis and, 674
 in inflammatory disease, 52–53
Corticosteroid synthesis, *1155*
Corticotrope adenoma, 1132
Coryza (common cold), 363, 1286
Cotton embolism, 294
Coup/contrecoup lesions, 1430, *1430*
COX-1, as inflammatory mediator, 53–54, *54*
COX-2, as inflammatory mediator, 54, *54*
Coxiella burnetti, 420
Cranial birth injury, 275
Cranial hemorrhage
 subarachnoid, 275
 subdural, 275
Craniopharyngioma, 1133, *1133,* 1487, *1488*
Cranioschischisis, 222
C-reactive protein, atherosclerosis and, 494
Crescentic glomerulonephritis, 858–859, *859,* 859t
CREST variant, of scleroderma, 161
Cretinism, 1138, 1313, 1315, 1466
Creutzfeld-Jacob disease, 1194–1196
Creutzfeld-Jakob disease, 1194–1200, 1198–1200, *1459,* 1461
 iatrogenic, 1461
 new variant, 1461
Crib death (SIDS), 276–277
Cri du chat syndrome, 228, 236
Crigler-Najjar syndrome, 747
Critical illness myopathy, *1410,* 1411
Critical illness polyneuropathy, 1495
Crohn disease, 697, 713–716, *714, 715, 716*
 appendicitis in, 733
 cancer risk and, 706
 vs. ulcerative colitis, 719t
Croup, 363
Cryoglobulinemic vasculitis, 860, *860*
Cryptococcal meningitis, 1448, *1448*
Cryptococcosis, 432–434, *433, 434*
Cryptorchidism, 906–907, *907*
Cryptosporidiosis, 450
Crypts of Lieberkuhn, 709
Curling (stress) ulcers, 674
Cushing disease, 1132, 1158–1161, *1159*
Cushing reflex, 1427
Cushing syndrome, 1161–1163, *1162*
 in cancer, 207
Cushing (stress) ulcers, 674
Cutaneous diphtheria, 382
Cutaneous necrotizing vasculitis, *1234, 1235,* 1235–1236
Cutaneous vasculature, *1202,* 1208–1210, *1209*
Cyanide, 329
Cyanocobalamin (vitamin B$_{12}$), 352
Cyclooxygenation, 52
Cyclosporine, nephrotoxicity, 880
Cylinderization, of cartilage, 1313–1314
Cylindroma, 1262, *1262*
Cyst(s)
 adrenal, 1163

 aneurysmal bone, *1351,* 1351–1352
 Baker's, 1376
 Bartholin gland, 934
 bladder, 894–896, *895*
 bone
  aneurysmal, 1350–1351, *1351*
  solitary, *1350,* 1351–1352
 colloid, 1490, *1490*
 congenital gastric, 674
 dentigerous, 1279
 dermoid, 976–977, *977*
 dermoid/epidermoid, 1488–1489
 echinococcal, *471*
 follicular, 934
 liver, 797
 mesenteric, 736
 mucinous, 934
 odontogenic, 1279
 omental, 736
 ovarian, 966–969, *967, 968*
 pancreatic, 812
 radicular (apical periodontal), 1277
 thyroglossal duct, 1135
Cystadenoma, 970, *972*
 mucinous pancreatic, 817
 pancreatic, 817
 serous pancreatic, 817
Cysteine proteinases, 73
Cystic disease
 of kidney
  acquired, 835
  congenital, 832–835
 of liver, 797–798
Cysticercosis, 469, 469–470
Cystic fibrosis, 12, 249, 249–251, *250,* 692
 pancreatitis in, 816
Cystic fibrosis transmembrane conductance regulator (CFTCR), 249, 249–250
Cystic hygroma, 518–519
Cystic infarcts, 296, *296*
Cystic lymphagioma (cystic hygroma, cavernous lymphangioma), 518–519
Cystic medial necrosis of Erdheim, 513
Cystine stones, 877
Cystinosis, 258
Cystitis, 892–894
 calcific, 892
 chronic, 893, 893–894
  chronic interstitial cystitis (Hunner ulcer), *893,* 893–894
  malakoplakia, 894, *894*
 hemorrhagic, 892, *893*
 pseudomembranous, 892
 suppurative, 892
 ulcerative, 892
Cystitis glandularis, 9, 895
Cytochrome P450, 6
Cytogenetics, 226–266
 in cancer diagnosis, 1068, *1070*
Cytokines, 60
 in inflammation, 75
 in ischemia/reperfusion injury, 21
 in metastasis, 179
 in septicemia, *306,* 306–307
 in wound regeneration, 97
Cytology
 abrasion, 1531, *1535*

 causes of error, 1537–1538
 fine-needle aspiration, 1531, *1536*
 morphological parameters, 1538–1540, 1538t, 1539t
Cytomegalovirus, 373–375, *375,* 932, *1533*
 intranuclear inclusions, *1417*
 in TORCH complex, 224
Cytomegalovirus encephalitis, 1456, *1456*
Cytomegalovirus esophagitis, 667–668, *668*
Cytopathology, 1528–1541
 advantages, 1531, 1536
 applications, 1530
 limitations, 1537
 methods, *1528,* 1530–1531, *1531, 1532, 1533, 1534, 1535, 1536*
 morphological parameters, 1538–1540, 1538t, 1539t
 reporting systems, 1540, 1540t
Cytotoxic antibodies, 675–676
Cytotoxic edema, 303
Cytotoxicity, immunological, 206, *206*

D

Darier disease (keratosis follicularis), 1212, *1214*
DCC gene, 727
Death domains, 31
Debranching enzyme deficiency (Cori disease), 1402
Decompression sickness, 293
Decorin, 94t
Deep venous thrombosis (DVT), 515
 in pancreatic cancer, 820
Defensins, 74
Degeneration, granulovacuolar, 1479, *1479*
Dehiscence, 115
Dehydration, 304
Dejerrine-Sottas syndrome, 1497
Delacroix, ring of, 1315
Deletion syndromes, 234t, 235–236
Delta cell tumors (somatostatinoma), 823
Delta storage pool disease, 1056
Dementia, luetic, 1449–1450, *1450*
Demyelinated plaque, 1464, *1464*
Demyelinating diseases, 1461–1465
Dendritic cells, 126
 in chronic inflammation, 77
Dental caries (tooth decay), 1276–1277, *1277*
Dental defects, in congenital syphilis, 226
Dentigerous cysts, 1279
Denys-Drash syndrome, 881
De Quervain thyroiditis, 1143, *1143*
Dermal nevus, 1246, *1247*
Dermatitis
 allergic contact, *1236,* 1236–1237, *1237*
 exfoliative, 209
 granulomatous, 1237
 radiation, 341, *342*
 spongiotic, 1237
 stasis, 514, *514*
 vulvar acute, 934–935, *935*
 vulvar chronic, 935–936, *936*
Dermatitis herpetiformis, *1226–1227,* 1226–1228, *1228*
 celiac disease and, 700–701, *701*
Dermatofibroma, 1263
Dermatofibrosarcoma protuberans, 1263

Index

Enterocolitis
  neonatal necrotizing, 272, 711
  radiation, 721
  Yersinia, 694
Enteropathic arthritis, 1371
Enteropathy-associated T-cell lymphoma, 1109
Environmental chemicals, 326–333
Environmental factors, in peptic ulcer disease, 679
Environmental metaplastic (multifocal atrophic) gastritis, *676*, 676–677
Enzymes, proteolytic, 179
Eosinophilia, 1064, 1064t
  in cancer, 209
Eosinophilic abscess, 1332, *1332*
Eosinophilic granuloma, 1065, *1065*
Eosinophilic microabcesses, 1066, *1066*
Eosinophils, 62, *63*, 1026
  bactericidal proteins of, 74
Ependyma, 1418, *1418*
Ependymoma, 1485, *1485*
Epidermal cells, 106–107
Epidermodysplasia, 197
Epidermodysplasia verruciformis, 1258
Epidermolysis bullosa, 669, 1221–1223, 1221t, *1222*
Epidermolytic hyperkeratosis, 1212, *1212*, *1213*, 1214t
Epidermylosis bullosa, 95
Epidural hematoma, *1426*, 1426–1428, *1427*, *1428*
Epiglottitis, 383
Epilepsy, 1425–1426
Epiphrenic diverticula, 665
Epiphyseal plate, 1314, *1314*
Epispadias, 900
Epistaxis (nosebleed), 1285, 1286t
Epithelial cells, in wound repair, 88
Epithelial dysplasia, in ulcerative colitis, 719, *719*
Epithelioma, 167–168, *168*
Epstein-Barr virus, 197–198, 372–373, *374*, *375*
  nasopharyngeal carcinoma and, 1294–1295, *1295*
  in posttransplant lymphoproliferative disorder, 1116–1117, *1117*
Erdheim, cystic medial necrosis of, 513
Erectile dysfunction, 902, 902t
Erysipelas, 380, *380*
Erythema gangrenosum, 396
Erythema induratum, 1240
Erythema multiforme, 1228–1229, *1229*
Erythema nodosum, *1239*, 1239–1240
Erythma gyratum repens, 209
Erythroblastosis fetalis, 273–275, *274*, *275*
Erythrocytosis, in cancer, 208
Erythroplakia, 1274, *1274*
Erythropoietin, 1025
Escherichia coli, 694
  diarrhea, 387–388, *388*
  neonatal infections, 389
  pneumonia, 389
  sepsis, 389
  urinary tract infections, 388–389
E-selectin, 67

Esophageal cancer, 316, *671*, 671–672
  epidemiology, 211
  smoking and, 316
Esophageal disorders, 663–672
  congenital, 663–665
    bronchopulmonary foregut malformation, 664
    congenital esophageal stenosis, 664
    rings and webs, 664, *664*
    Plummer-Vinson (Paterson-Kelly) syndrome, 664, 672
    Schatzki ring, 664, *664*
    tracheoesophageal fistula, 663–664, *664*
  esophageal varices, 669, *669*, 759–760
  esophagitis, 666–669
    Barrett esophagus, 667, *668*
    chemical, 668–669
    infective, 667–668, *668*
    mechanical, 669
    reflux, 666–667
    in systemic illness, 669
  hiatal hernia, 666, *666*
    paraesophageal, 666
    sliding, 666
  lacerations and perforations, 669–670, *670*
  motor disorders, 665–666
    achalasia, 665, *665*, 672
    in scleroderma, 666
  neoplasms, 670–672
    benign, 670, *670*
    carcinoma, *671*, 671–672
Esophageal varices, 759–760
Esophagitis, reflux, in alcoholics, 321
Esophagus, anatomy, 663
Essential thrombocythemia, 1070t, 1071t, 1074–1075, *1075*
Estrogen therapy, osteoporosis and, 1336
Ethylene glycol, 328
Euploidy, 230
Ewing sarcoma, 1358–1360, *1359*
Exercise-induced hypertrophy, 6–7, *7*
Exfoliative dermatitis, 209
Exogenous pigments, 12, *13*
Exopthalmos, of hyperthyroidism, 1504–1505
Exotoxins
  bacterial, 376
  streptococcal, 378–379
Exstrophy, of urinary bladder, *891*, 891–892
Extracellular matrix
  in chronic inflammation, 78
  in wound repair, 88–95, 89t, 90, 91t
Extrahepatic biliary obstruction, 781–782, *782*
Extramedullary plasmacytoma, 1099, 1103
Extranodal marginal-zone B-cell lymphoma of mucosa-associated lymphoid tissue (MALT), 1104, *1104*
Extranodal NK/T-cell lymphoma, nasal type, 1109
Exudate, 46
  fibrinous, 46
  purulent, 46, *47*
  serous, 46
Eye, *1502*, 1502–1526
  conjunctival diseases, 1505–1506
    chlamydial conjunctivitis, 1505

    hemorrhage, 1505
    infectious vs. allergic, 1505
    ophthalmia neonatorum, 1506
    pinguecula, 1506
    pterygium, 1506
    trachoma, 1505, *1505*
  corneal diseases, 1506–1507
  lens disorders, 1507–1508
    cataracts, 1507–1508, *1508*
    phacoanaphylactic endophthalmitis, 1508
    presbyopia, 1508
  myopia, 1320
  neoplasms, 1524–1526
    malignant melanoma, 1525, *1525*
    metastatic, 1526
    retinoblastoma, 1525–1526, *1526*
  optic nerve, 1519–1522
    glaucoma, 1522–1524, *1523*, *1531*
    in increased intracranial pressure, 1519–1520, *1521*
    optic atrophy, 1520–1521, *1521*
  orbital disorders, 1504–1505
    exophthalmos of hyperthyroidism, 1504–1505
  phthisis bulbi, 1524, *1524*
  physical and chemical injuries, 1504
  retinal disorders, 1508–1509
    angioid streaks, 1519
    cataracts, 1517
    cherry-red macula, 1519, *1520*
    diabetic cataracts, 1517
    diabetic iridopathy, 1516–1517
    diabetic retinopathy, 1511, *1516*, 1516–1517, *1517*
    hemorrhage, 1508–1509
    hypertensive retinopathy, 1509–1511, *1513*, *1514*
    macular degeneration, 1518–1519
    retinal detachment, 1518
    retinitis pigmentosa, 1518, *1519*
    retinopathy of prematurity, 1519, *1521*
    vascular occlusion, 1509, *1510*, *1511*, *1512*, *1513*
  uveal disorders, 1508
    in sarcoidosis, 1508
    sympathetic ophthalmitis, 1508
    synechiae, 1508

F

Fabry disease, 266
Facial cellulitis, 383
Facial clefts, 1271
Facial nerve palsy, 276
Factor V Leiden hypercoagulability, 1061
Fallopian tube, 965–966
  anatomy, 965
  ectopic pregnancy, 965–966, *966*
  salpingitis, 965
  tumors, 966
Familial adenomatous polyposis (FAP), 193, *724*, 724–725, *725*
  attenuated, 725
  Gardner syndrome, 725
  Turcot syndrome, 725
Familial amyloidoses, 1191
Familial benign chronic pemphigus (Hailey-Hailey disease), 1220

Index

Familial hereditary pancreatitis, 816
Familial hypercholesterolemia, 496, 497, *498, 499*
Familial hypoparathyroidism, 1150
  isolated, 1150
Familial intrahepatic cholestasis (Byler syndrome), 751
Familial Mediterranean fever, 1191
Familial medullary thyroid carcinoma, *1165*, 1165–1167
Familial paroxysmal polyserositis (familial Meditarranean fever), 735–736, 1191
Familial periodic paralysis, 1405
Fanconi anemia, 1054
Fanconi syndrome, 1340
Fasciitis, nodular, 170, *170*, 1377, *1379*
Fasciola hepatica, 793–794, *794*
Fascioliasis, 468
Fasciolopsiasis, 469
Fas receptor, in apoptosis, 30–31, *31*
Fatal familial insomnia, 1461–1462
Fat embolism, 294, *294*
  cerebral, 1442, *1442*
Fat necrosis, 26, *26*
Fatty liver
  alcoholic, 774–777, *775, 776, 777*
  nonalcoholic, 778
  toxicity-related, 789–790
Female multiple-X syndromes, 239
Female reproductive system (*see also* Subtopics)
  cervix, 941–952
  embryology, 929
  fallopian tube, 965–966
  genital infections, 929–934, 930t
  menstrual cycle, *952*, 952–953
  ovary, 966–981
  peritoneum, 981–984 (*see also* Endometriosis)
  placenta and gestational disease, 985–994
  uterus, 952–965
  vagina, 939–941
  vulva, 934–939
Feminization, in alcoholics, 321
Femoral head, aseptic necrosis of, 321
Fenestrae, 69
  hepatic, 745
Ferritin, 12
Fetal alcohol syndrome, 223–224, 322
Fetal hydantoin syndrome, 223
Fetal radiation injury, 340
Fetal thyroid adenoma, 1144, *1145*
Fetal tobacco syndrome, 316–219, *318*
Fetal wound repair, 114
Fever, 81–82
  in cancer, 207
FHIT gene, 193
Fibers, microfibrillar, 244
Fibrillar collagens, 92
Fibrillation, atrial, 288
Fibrillin, 93, 94t
Fibrillin-1, 244
Fibrils, anchoring, 107
Fibrinoid necrosis, 26, *27*
Fibrinolysis, 483, *493*, 1059
Fibrinolytic factors, 61
Fibrinous exudate, 46

Fibrinous pericarditis, 46, *47*
Fibrinous pleuritis, 46, *47*
Fibroadenoma, 169
  of breast, 1004, *1005*
Fibroblast proliferation, *103*, 103–104
Fibroblasts, 86, *103*
  in chronic inflammation, 77–78, *78*
Fibrocartilage, 1313
Fibrocystic breast change, 1001–1004, *1002, 1003, 1004*
Fibrohistiocytic skin tumors, 1263
Fibrolamellar hepatocellular carcinoma, 799, *799*
Fibroma
  chondromyxoid, 1353–1354
  medullary, 880
  nonossifying, 1350–1351
  ovarian, 979, *979*
Fibromatosis
  palmar (Dupuytren contracture), 1378
  penile (Peyronie disease), 1378
  plantar, 1378
Fibromuscular dysplasia, 503–504, 863
Fibronectins, 94t, 95
Fibrosarcoma, 1379, *1379*
Fibrosis
  congenital hepatic, 798
  idiopathic retroperitoneal, 890, *891*
  periportal, 771
  peritubular/tubular, 909, *910*
  pulmonary, 285
  retroperitoneal, 737
  thyroid, 1144, *1144*
Fibrous dysplasia, 1349–1350
  McCune-Albright syndrome, 1349–1350, *1350*
  monostotic, 1349
  polyostotic, 1349
Fibrous histiocytoma, malignant, *1379*, 1379–1380
Fibroxanthoma, atypical, 1263
Filariasis, lymphatic (elephantiasis), *457*, 457–458
Filopodia, 88
Fine-needle aspiration
  technique, 1531, *1536*
  of thyroid, *1536*
Finkeldey giant cells, *365*
Fistula
  anorectal, 711
  in Crohn disease, 715–716
  tracheoesophageal, 663–664, *664*
  umbilical, 692
FK506 (tacrolimus), nephrotoxicity, 880
Flatus, high altitude–related, 337
Flow cytometry, 1068, *1068, 1069*
Fluid, interstitial, 283
Flukes, liver, 793–794, *794*
Fluorescence in situ hybridization (FISH), *226, 227*, 1068, *1070*
Fluoride, in tooth decay prevention, 1276
Foam cells, 255
Focal contacts (focal adhesions), 88
Focal nodular hepatic hyperplasia, 797, *797*
Focal proliferative lupus nephritis, 156, *157*
Focal segmental glomerulosclerosis, 840–841, 840t, *841*

Folic acid deficiency, 352, 704, *1034*, 1034–1037, *1035, 1037*
  neural tube defects and, 223
  tropical sprue and, 704
Follicle cysts, 955–967, *967*
Follicles
  hair, 1210
  sebaceous, 1211
Follicle-stimulating hormone (FSH), 1132–1133
  insufficiency, 5
Follicular cysts, 934
Follicular hyperplasia, of lymph nodes, 1086–1088, *1088*
Follicular lymphoma, 1103–1104, *1104*
Follicular thyroid adenoma, 1144, *1145*
Follicular thyroid carcinoma, 1147, *1147*
Folliculitis, eosinophilic, 1265
Food poisoning, 378, 397, 694
Foramen magnum, herniation, 1482
Foreign body giant cells, 79, *80*
Foreign-body sarcoma, 204
Fractures, 1323–1327
  birth injury, 275, *276*
  healing of, *1323–1324*, 1323–1326
  in Paget disease of bone, 1348
  stress, 1325
Fragile X syndrome, 264–266, *265, 266*
Frameshift mutations, 240
Freckles, 1255–1256, *1257*
Friedreich ataxia, 240–241, 1473–1475
Fructose intolerance, hereditary, 788
Fundic gland polyps, 685
Fungal infections, 429–440
  aspergillosis, 430–432, *431*
  blastomycosis, 437–438, *438*
  candidal, 429–430, 429t, *430*
  chlamydial conjunctivitis, 1505–1506
  chromomycosis, *438*, 439
  coccidiodomycosis, *433, 436*, 436–437, *437*
  cryptococcosis, 432–434, *433, 434*
  dermatophyte, 439–440
  histoplasmosis, 434–436, *435, 436*
  intestinal, 695
  mycetoma, 440, *440*
  mycotic aneurysm, 513–514
  nasal cavity, 1289–1290
  paracoccidiodomycosis (South American blastomycosis), *438*, 438
  Pneumocystis carinii pneumonia, 446–447, *447*
  skin, 1241–1244, *1243*
  sporotrichosis, *438*, 438
Furuncles (boils), 377
Fusospirochetal infections, 413–414, *414*

G

GABA, in hepatic encephalopathy, 755
Galactosemia, 788
Gallbladder, 802–808
  anatomy, 801–802
  cholecystitis
    acute, *806*, 806–807
    chronic, 807, *807*
  cholelithiasis (gallstones), 802–806, *803*
  cholesterolosis, 807–808
  congenital anomalies, 802, *803*

Index

hydrops of (mucocele), 806, *806*
neoplasia
  benign, 808
  malignant, *808*, 808–809
strawberry, 807–808
Gallstones, 802–806, *803*
Ganglioglioma, 1485–1486
Ganglion, 1376
Ganglioneuroma, 1168–1169, *1169*
Ganglionitis, dorsal root, 1495
Gangliosidoses, 1465–1466
Gangrenous stomatitis (noma), 414, *414*
Gardnerella, 931
Gardner syndrome, 725
Gas gangrene, 399–400
Gasoline, 328
Gastric adenocarcinoma, 168, *168*
Gastric cancer, epidemiology, 211, 213
Gastric lymphoma, 689
Gastric outlet obstruction, Pyloric obstruction, 684
Gastrinoma (Zollinger-Ellison syndrome), 822–823
Gastritis
  acute hemorrhagic erosive, 674–675, *675*
  atrophic, 676, *676*
  chronic, 675–678
    autoimmune atropic, 675–676
    Helicobacter pylori, 677
    multifocal atrophic (environmental metaplastic), *676*, 676–677
    reactive (chemical) gastropathy, 677–678
    Menetrier disease (hyperplastic hypersecretive gastropathy), *678*, 678–679
Gastroesophageal reflux disease (GERD), in alcoholics, 321
Gastrointestinal bleeding, major causes, *734*
Gastrointestinal disorders
  appendix, 733–745, 737–749
  in cystic fibrosis, 250
  esophagus, 663–672
  large intestine, 708–732
  peritoneum, 733–736
  small intestine, 690–708
  stomach, 672–690
Gastrointestinal obstruction, major causes, *735*
Gastrointestinal stromal tumors (GIST), 670–671, 684, *685*, 705
  malignant, 689, 708
Gastropathy, hyperplastic hypersecretive (Menetrier disease), *678*, 678–679
Gaucher cells, 253, *253*
Gaucher disease, 251–254, *253*, *1348*, 1348–1349, 1465
  sphingolipidases and, 251, *252*
  type 1 (chronic nonneuropathic), 253
  type 2 (neuropathic), 253–254
  type 3 (subacute neuropathic), 254
Gell and Coombs hypersensitivity classification, 130t
Gene amplification, 185
Genes
  competence, 189
  DNA repair, 194–195

mutator (caretaker), 194–195
mutator (DNA mismatch repair), 184
retinoblastoma *(Rb)*, 191–193, *192*
tumor suppressor, 184, 191–194
types, 240
Genetic disorders
  chromosomal abnormalities, 226–266
  epidemiology, *217*, 217–218
  of genetic imprinting, 266–267
    Angelman syndrome, 266–267
    Prader-Willi syndrome, 266–267
  mitochondrial diseases, 266
  of morphogenesis, 219–221
  multifactorial inheritance, 267–268, 267t, *268*
    cleft lip/left palate, 268, *268*
  prenatal diagnosis, 268–269
  principles of teratology, 218–219
  screening for, 268
  terminology, 216–217
Genetic factors
  in aging, 36–37, 38
  in Alzheimer disease, 1476, 1476t
  in breast cancer, 1006–1007
  in celiac disease, 700
  in diabetes mellitus, type 1, 1174–1175
  in osteoarthritis, 1366–1368, *1367*
  in peptic ulcer disease, 679–680
  in rheumatoid arthritis, 1366
  in stomach cancer, 686
Genetic imprinting, 266–267
Genital infections, female, 929–934, 930t
Genital ulcers, 386
Genital warts (condyloma acuminatum), 370, 903, 932, *933*, 1258
Germ cell aplasia, *910*
Germ cell tumors
  of CNS, 1488
  ovarian, *976*, 976–979
  of pineal gland, 1169
  thymic, 1122
Gerstmann-Straussler-Scheinker syndrome, 1194–1196, 1459, 1461
Gestational disease, 985–994 (*see also* Placenta; Pregnancy)
  choriocarcinoma, 993, *993*, 993t
  gestational trophoblastic disease, *990*, 990–994, 992t
  placental site trophoblastic tumor, 993–994
Ghon complex, 423
Ghrelin, 345
Giant cell arteritis, 506–507, *507*, 861, 861t
Giant cell granuloma, oral, *1274*, *1274*
Giant cells, 130
  Finkeldey, 365
  foreign body, 79, *80*
  Langhans, 79, *80*
Giant cell thyroiditis, 1143, *1143*
Giant cell tumor
  of bone, 1357–1358, *1358*
  vs. Paget disease of bone, 1348
Giardiasis, 450–451
Gigantism, 1131
Gilbert syndrome, 747
Gingivitis, 1278, *1278*
  acute necrotizing ulcerative (Vincent angina), *1272*, *1272*

Glanders, 405
Glands
  cardiac, 673
  pyloric, 673
Glanzmann thrombasthenia, 1056
Glaucoma, 1522–1524, *1523*, *1531*
Gleason grading, of prostate cancer, *922*, 923, *923*
Glioblastoma multiforme, 1483, *1484*
Gliosis, *1417*, 1417–1418
Glomerular basement membrane, *829*, 829–830, *830*, 849
Glomerular disease, 835–859
  acute postinfectious glomerulonephritis, 849–851, *850*, *851*
  Alport syndrome (hereditary nephritis), 848–849, *849*
  in amyloidosis, 846–848, *847*, *848*
  anti-glomerular basement membrane glomerulonephritis, 857–858, *859*
  crescentic glomerulonephritis, 858–859, *859*, 859t
  diabetic glomerulosclerosis, 843–846, *845*, *846*
  focal segmental glomerulosclerosis, 840–841, 840t, *841*
  HIV-associated nephropathy, 841–842, *842*
  IgA nephropathy, *856*, 856–857, *857*
  light-chain/heavy chain deposition, 848
  lupus glomerulonephritis, 853–856, *855*, 855t
  membranoproliferative glomerulonephritis
    type I, 851–852, *852*, *853*, 951t
    type II, 852–853, *853*, *854*
  membranous glomerulopathy, *842*, 842–843, *843*, *844*, *845*
  minimal-change glomerulonephropathy, 837–840, *839*, *840*
  nephritic (glomerulonephritic) syndrome, 836, 836t
  nephrotic syndrome, 835–836, 835t, 836t
  pathogenesis, 837, *838*
  pathology, 837–839, 839t
  thin basement membrane nephropathy, 849
Glomerulonephritis
  acute postinfectious, 849–851, *850*, *851*
  anti-glomerular basement membrane, 857–858, *859*
  crescentic, 858–859, *859*, 859t
  lupus
    diffuse proliferative, 156, *158*
    focal proliferative, 156, *157*
    membranous, 156
  membranoproliferative
    type I, 851–852, *852*, *853*, 951t
    type II, 852–853, *853*, *854*
  membranous, 52
Glomerulopathy
  membranous, *842*, 842–843, *843*, *844*, *845*
  in multiple myeloma, 1101
Glomerulosclerosis, focal segmental, 840–841, 840t, *841*
Glomerulus (glomeruli), *825*, *828*, *829*, *830*
  renal, 111–112, *112*

Glomus tumor (glomangioma), 516–517, *517*
Glossitis, 1276
Glucagon-like peptide, 346
Glucagonoma (alpha cell tumor), 823, *823*
Glucocorticoid-remediable aldosteronism, 501
Glucocorticoids, in inflammation, 75
Gluconeogenesis, 746
Glucose homeostasis, 746
Glucose-6-phosphate dehydrogenase (G6PD) deficiency, 1040–1041
Glutathione peroxidase, 20
Gluten sensitivity, dermatitis herpetiformis in, 700–701, *701*, *1226–1227*, 1226–1228, *1228*, *1230–1231*, 1230–1232, *1232*
Glycogenoses, *257*, 257–258
Glycogenosis, 787–788
Glycogen storage diseases (glycogenoses), 1401–1403
  liver disease in, 787–788
  type II (acid maltase deficiency, Pompe disease), 1401–1402, *1402*
  type III (debranching enzyme deficiency, Cori disease), 1402
  type V (McArdle disease), 1402–1403, *1403*
  type VII (phosphofructokinase deficiency), 1403
Glycolysis, anaerobic, 27–28
Glycoproteins, matrix, 93–95, 94t
Glycosaminoglycans (GAG), 95, 255–256
Goblet cells, 691
Goiter
  drug-induced, 1137
  endemic, 1137
  iodide-induced, 1137
  nontoxic, 1135, *1136*
  toxic multinodular, 1141
Goitrous hypothyroidism, 1137
Gonadal radiation injury, 341, *341*
Gonadoblastoma, 979
Gonadotrope adenoma, 1132
Gonadotropic syndromes, in cancer, 208
Gonorrhea, 384–386, *385*, *386*, *929*, *930*
Goodpasture syndrome, 134, *134*
Gout, 1371–1373, *1372*, *1374*, *1375*, *1380*, 1380–1382, *1382*, *1401*
  pseudo-, 1373–1375, *1376*
  tophaceous, 1373
G phases, of cell cycle, 108
G-protein abnormalities, in cell death, 24
G-protein-coupled receptors, 99
G-protein-mediated pathways, 64, *64*
Graft-versus-host disease, 669
Granulaomatous disease, chronic, 1063–1064
Granulations
  pacchionian, 1430
  toxic, 1063
Granulation tissue, 102, *102*, 103
Granules
  Birbeck, 1066, *1066*, 1206–1207, *1207*, *1332*, *1332*
  keratohyaline, 1205–1206, *1206*
  neutrophil, 70, *71*

Granulocytes, 1025–1026
Granulocytosis, paraneoplastic, 209
Granuloma annulare, *1238*, 1238–1239
Granuloma inguinale, 386–387, *387*, 903, 931
Granulomas, 79, *79*, 80
  apical/periapical, 1277, *1277*
  cholesteol, 1298
  in Crohn disease, 714–715, *715*
  eosinophilic, 1065, *1065*
  granuloma inguinale, 903
  peripheral giant cell oral, 1274, *1274*
  pyogenic, 116, 936, 1285
  pyogenous, *1272*, *1272*
  in schistosomiasis, 467
  talc, 324, *324*
Granulomatosis
  allergic and angiitis (Churg-Strauss syndrome), 506, *506*
  Wegener, *507*, 507–508, 860, *1290*, *1290*
Granulomatous (giant cell) arteritis, 506–507, *507*
Granulomatous dermatitis, 1237
Granulomatous inflammation, 79, *79*, 80
Granulomatous (sarcoid) myositis, 1400, *1400*
Granulomatous thyroiditis, 1143, *1143*
Granulosa cell tumor, 979–980, *981*
Granulovacuolar degeneration, 1479, *1479*
Graves disease, 134, 1138–1141, *1139*, *1140*
Gray (radiation measure), 339
Grey platelet syndrome (alpha storage pool disease), 1056
Ground-glass hepatocytes, 771, *772*
Growth factor receptors, in oncogene activation, 186–188, *187*
Growth factors
  in bone marrow kinetics, 1023, 1025
  in metastasis, 179
  in oncogene activation, 185–186
  in tumor angiogenesis, 183
  in wound healing, 104, *105*, 105t6
Growth plate disorders, 1315–1320
GTPases, 99
Guillain-Barré syndrome, 1495
Gunshot wounds, 338, *339*
Gynecomastia, 7, 1000, *1999*
Gyral malformations, 1423–1424, *1424*

H

HAART (highly active antiretroviral therapy), 153
Haemophilus influenzae, 382–383
Hageman factor, 48, *48*
Hailey-Hailey disease, 1220
Hairball (trichobezoar), 689, *690*
Hair cycle, 1210, 12104
Hair follicles, 1210
Hairs, vellus, 1211
Hairy cell leukemia, 1099, *1099*
Hairy leukoplakia, 1273
Hallocinogens, 323
Hamartoma, 168, *168*
  in pediatric patients, 278
Hand-Schüller-Christian disease, 1065, 1333
Hansen disease (leprosy), 1288
Haploidy, 230
Haplosufficiency, 243

Haptotaxis, 57
Hashimoto thyroiditis, *1139*, *1142*, 1142–1143
  lymphoma in, 1094
HBV genome, 762–763
Head and neck
  ear, *1268*, 1296–1301, *1297–1302*
    external, *1268*, 1296–1299
    internal, 1299–1301, *1968*
    middle, *1268*, 1297–1299
  nasopharynx, 1293–1296
  nose and nasal vestibule, 1285, 1285t, 1286t
  oral cavity, 1270–1279
  salivary glands, 1280–1281, *1281*
Heart
  circulatory function, 292
  healing of, 112, *113*, 114
  senile atrophy, 6
Heart failure
  congestive, 299–301, *300*, *301*, *302*
    hepatic congestion in, 791, *792*
  in hemochromatosis, 784
Heart failure cells, *284*, 285
Heat shock proteins, 58
HeLa cells, 197
Helicobacter heilmannii, 677
Helicobacter pylori, 677, 678, 681–682.677, *682*
  in stomach cancer, 686
Helminthic infections, 457–471
  ascariasis, 793
  cestodes intestinal tapeworms, 469–471, 469t
    cysticercosis, *469*, 469–470
    echinococcosis, *470*, 470–471, *471*
  filiarial nematodes, 457–459
    loiasis, 458–459, *459*
    lymphatic filariasis (elephantiasis), *457*, 457–458
    onchocerciasis (river blindness), 458, 1306
  intestinal nematodes, 459–462, 459t
    ascariasis, 459–460, 459t, *460*
    hookworms, 460–461, *461*
    pinworms (enterobiasis), 462
    strongyloidiasis, *461*, 461–462
    trichuiasis, 459t, 460, *460*
  tissue nematodes, 462–464
    cutaneous larva migrans, 464, *464*
    dracunculiasis, 464, *465*
    trichinosis, 462–463, *463*
    visceral larva migrans (toxocariasis), 464
  trematodes (flukes), 464–469, 793–794, *794*
    clonorchiasis, 467–468, *468*
    fascioliasis, 468
    fasciolopsiasis, 469
    paragonimiasis, 468
    schistosomiasis (bilharziasis), 464–467, *465*, *466*, *467*
Hemangioblastoma, *1488*, 1488–1489
Hemangioma, 515–516, *516*
  capillary, 516
  cavernous, 516, *516*
  hepatic, 797
  infantile, 797

juvenile (strawberry), 516
multiple hemangiomatous syndrome, 516
in pediatric patients, 278
Hemangionendothelioma, 517
Hemangiopericytoma, 517–518
Hemangiosarcoma, 800–801
  hepatic, 791
Hemarthrosis, 287
Hematocele, 902
Hematogenous osteomyelitis, 1328, *1329*, 1349
Hematological malignancy, osteoporosis in, 1337
Hematological syndromes, in cancer, 208–209
Hematoma, 286–287
  aortic wall (dissecting aneurysm), *512*, 512–513
  epidural, *1426*, 1426–1428, *1427, 1428*
  retroplacental, 988
  subdural, 1428–1429, *1429*
Hematomyelia, 1434, *1434*
Hematopoiesis, *121*, 121–123, *122*, 1021, *1021*
Hematopoietic disorders, polycythemia, 1048
Hematopoietic system, embryology, 1020, *1021*
Hemihypertrophy, of epiphyseal plate, 1319–1320
Hemochromatosis
  hereditary, *13, 14*, 782–785, *783, 784*
  joint disease in, 1375–1376
  liver cancer and, 798
Hemodynamic disorders, 280–310
  edema, 297–299
    cerebral, 303
    congestive heart failure, *300*, 300–301, *301, 302*
    effusion in, 303–304
    in hepatic cirrhosis, 303
    in nephrotic syndrome, 303
    pulmonary, *301*, 301–303, *302, 303*
  embolism, 290–294
    pulmonary, *290*, 290–292
    systemic arterial and infarcts, 292–294, *293*
  fluid loss and overload, 304
  infarction, 295–297, *296*
  normal circulation, 282–283, *283*
  of perfusion, 293–287
    hemorrhage, 285–297
    hyperemia, 283–285
  shock, 304–310
    classification, 305, *305*
    multiple organ dysfunction syndrome (MODS), 307–308
    septic, 305–307
  thrombosis, 287–290
Hemoglobin C disease, 1043–1044
Hemoglobin E disease, 1044
Hemoglobinemia, paroxysmal cold, 1045–1046
Hemoglobinopathies, 1041–1044
  double heterozygosities, 1043
  hemoglobin C disease, 1043–1044
  hemoglobin E disease, 1044

hemoglobin H disease, 1038
sickle cell disease, *1041*, 1041–1043, *1042*
sickle cell trait, 1043
Hemoglobin oxygen affinity, 1044
Hemoglobinuria, paroxysmal nocturnal, 1047
Hemolytic anemia, of prematurity, vitamin E in, 354
Hemolytic disease of newborn, 1046, *1046*
Hemolytic-uremic syndrome, *864*, 865, 1055
Hemopericardium, 304
Hemoperitoneum, 287
Hemophilia, joint disease in, 1375–1376
Hemophilia A (factor VIII deficiency), 264
Hemophilia B, 1056–1057
Hemorrhage, 285–297 (*see also* Bleeding)
  cerebral, *1437*, 1437–1438, *1438*
    in aneurysmal rupture, 1435–1437
  conjunctival, 1505
  Duret, *1427*, 1427, *1428*
  intracranial, in newborn, 275
  intraventricular, in newborn, 272, *272*
  in Meckel diverticulum, 692
  in peptic ulcer disease, 684
  retinal, 1508–1509
    high altitude related, 337
  subarachnoid, 512, 1429–1430
Hemorrhagic cystitis, 892, *893*
Hemorrhagic fevers, viral, 368–369, 368t
Hemorrhagic gastritis, acute, 674–675, *675*
Hemorrhagic pancreatitis, 813
  acute, 815, *815*
Hemorrhagic stroke, *1437*, 1437–1438, *1438*
Hemorrhoids, 721
Hemosiderin, 12
Hemosiderosis, 12–14, *13*
Hemostasis, 479–483 (*see also* Thrombosis)
  coagulation, *480*, 480–483, 480t, *481, 482*, 482t
  normal
    coagulation cascade in, 1051–1052
    platelets in, 1048–1051, *1049, 1050*
  thrombolysis and plasminogen activation, 1051
Hemostatic disorders, 1051–1062
  of blood vessels, 1051–1052
    allergic (Henoch-Schönlein purpura), 859–860, 1052
    extravascular dysfunction, 1052
    hereditary hemorrhagic telangiectasia (Rendu-Osler-Weber syndrome), 758, 1052
  coagulation abnormalities, 1056–1062
  of platelets, 1052–1057
  principal causes of bleeding, 1051t
Hemothorax, 287
Henle, loop of, 830
Henoch-Schönlein purpura, 859–860, 1052
Heparin-like molecules, 60
Hepatic adenoma, 796, *797*
Hepatic encephalopathy, 755, 1466
Hepatic failure, 754–755
  coagulation defects in, 756
  complications, 755
  hypoalbuminemia in, 756
Hepatic fibrosis, congenital, 798
Hepatic hemangioma, 797

Hepatic necrosis
  confluent, 769–770, *770*
  massive (acute yellow atrophy), *770*, 770
  piecemeal, 770, *771*
  submissive confluent, 770
Hepatic schistosomiasis, 467, *467*
Hepatic sinusoids, *745*, 745–746
Hepatic vein thrombosis, 759
Hepatitis, 761–773
  alcoholic, 777, *778, 779*
  autoimmune, 773
  cholestatic, 768–769
  drug-induced, 790, *791*
  herpes, 372
  neonatal, 794–796, *795*, 795t
  viral
    acute, 768–770
    causes, 761t
    chronic, 770–773
    comparative features, 773
    pathology, 768–773
Hepatitis A, 762, *762, 763*
Hepatitis B, 762–767–758, *765, 766*
  chronic, *766*, 766–767
  clinical features, 764–767, *765, 766*
  complications, 770–772, *771*
  epidemiology, 763–764
  fulminant, 766
  pathogenesis, 764, *764*
Hepatitis B virus (HBV), 198
Hepatitis C, 767, *768, 769*
  complications, 770–772, *771*
  liver cancer and, 798
Hepatitis D, 767
Hepatitis E, 767–768
Hepatoblastoma, 800
Hepatocellular carcinoma, 798–800, *799*
  fibrolamellar, 799, *799*
Hepatocellular necrosis, zonal, 789, *789*
Hepatocytes, 743–745
  ground-glass, 771, *772*
Hepatolenticular degeneration (Wilson disease), 785–787, *786*, 1466
Hepatorenal failure, 756
Hereditary angioedema, 52, 1234
Hereditary cancer syndromes, 195, 196t, *197*
Hereditary congophilic angiopathy (Dutch), 1191
Hereditary congophilic angiopathy (Icelandic), 1191
Hereditary disorders, atherosclerosis in, 497–499, 497t
Hereditary elliptocytosis, 1039–1040
Hereditary hemochromatosis, *783*, 783–785, *784*
Hereditary hemorrhagic telangiectasia (Osler-Weber-Rendu syndrome), 758, 1052
Hereditary multiple osteochondromatatosis, 1319
Hereditary neuropathies, 1497–1498, 1497t, 1498t
Hereditary nonpolyposis colorectal cancer (HNPCC) syndrome, 194, 729–730, *730*, 730t
Hereditary platelet disorders, 1055–1056
Hereditary spherocytosis, 1039, *1039*

Index

Hermaphroditism, 907–908, 908t
HER2/neu oncogene, 1013, *1013*
Hernia, 705
  congenital diaphragmatic, 674
  hiatal, 666, *666*
  scrotal inguinal, 902
Herniation
  forman magnum, 1482
  subfalcine, 1482
  transtentorial, 1427, *1427*, 1428, 1482
Heroin, 322–323
Herpes encephalitis, 372
Herpes hepatitis, 372
Herpes labialis (cold sores, fever blisters), 1273
Herpesviruses, 369–375, 932
  cytomegalovirus, 373–375, *375*
  encephelomyelitis in, 1454–1456, *1455*
  Epstein-Barr virus, 197–198, 372–373, *374, 375*, 1116–1117, 1294–1295
  genital herpes, 903
  herpes simplex, *371*, 371–372, 371t, 1454–1456, *1455, 1531*
    corneal ulcerations in, 1506–1507
  herpes zoster (shingles), 370, *370*, 371
  human herpesvirus 8 (HHV8), 198
  oral manifestations, 1273
  skin infections, 1245
  varicella-zoster, 369–371, *370, 371*
Herpetic esophagitis, 667–668, *668*
Herpetic stomatitis, 1273
Heterotopia, 220, 1424
Heterotropic calcification tissue, 1327
Hiatal hernia, 666, *666*
  paraesophageal, 666
  sliding, 666
Hidradenoma, 936
High-density lipoproteins (HDLs), 496, 487497
High endothelial venules (HEVs), *126*, 127
Highly active antiretroviral therapy (HAART), 153
Hilus cell tumor, 981
Hirano bodies, 1479, *1480*
Hirschsprung disease (congenital megacolon), 709–710, *710*
Histiocytic necrotizing lymphadenitis (Kikuchi disease), 1089
Histiocytoma, malignant fibrous, *1379*, 1379–1380
Histiocytosis
  Langerhans cell, *1065*, 1065–1066, *1066*, 1332–1334
  sinus, 1090, *1090*
Histoplasmosis, 434–436, *435, 436*, 1244
  disseminated, 435, *435*
HIV, therapy for, 153 (*see also* AIDS/HIV)
HIV-1, life cycle, 148–151, *149, 150, 152*
HIV-2, 153
HIV-associated nephropathy, 841–842, *842*
HIV-associated skin neoplasms, 1263–1264, *1264, 1265*
Hodgkin lymphoma, *1111*, 1111–1117, *1112, 1115*
  Ann Arbor staging system, 1114t
  classical, *1115*, 1115–1116
  clinical features, *1113*, 1113–1114
  epidemiology, 213, 1111–1113
  histological classification, 1114–1116, 1114t, *1115*
  lymphocyte-depleted, 1116
  lymphocyte-rich, 1116
  mixed-cellularity, 1116, *1116*
  nodular lymphocyte predominant, 1114–1115
  nodular sclerosis, 1114, 1114t, 1116, *1116*
  Reed-Sternberg cells, *1012*, 1111, *1111, 1115*
Holoprosencephaly, 1425, *1425*
Homocysteine, atherosclerosis and, 493
Homogeneous staining regions (HSRs), *186, 187*
Homozygous β thalassemia (Cooley anemia), 1037–1038, *1038*
Hookworms, 460–461, *461*
Hordeolum (sty), 1504
Hormone(s)
  follicle-stimulating (FSH), 1132–1133
  inflammatory (cytokines), 55, 55–57, *56*
  luteinizing (LH), 1132
  melanocyte-stimulating, 345
Hormone replacement therapy
  complications, 326
  hepatotoxicity, 790–791, *791*
Howell-Jolly bodies, *1029*
Human papillomavirus (HPV), 197, 375–376, 932, *933*, 1245, *1256*, 1256–1258, *1257*
  cervical neoplasia and, 947, *947*
Human parvovirus B19, 366
Human T-cell leukemia virus (HTLV-1), 195
Hunner ulcer, *893*, 893–894
Huntingdon disease, 240, 250, 1472–1475, *1473*
Hurler syndrome, 1465
Hürthle cell adenoma, 1143, *1144, 1145*
Hutchinson-Guilford progeria, 37, *37*
Hutchinson teeth, 226
Hutchinson triad, 226
Hyaline, 14
Hyaline arteriosclerosis, in diabetes mellitus, *1180*, 1181, *1183*
Hyaline cartilage, 1313
Hyaline membrane, 272, *272*
Hyaline-vascular angiofollicular lymph node hyperplasia, 1088
Hyaluronan, 95
Hydatidiform mole
  complete, 990–992, *991*, 992t
  invasive, 992
  partial, 992, 992t
Hydrocarbons, aromatic halogenated, 329
Hydrocele, 901, *901*
Hydrocephalus, 1443–1444
  communicating, 1443
  congenital, 1422–1423, *1423, 1424*
  ex vacuo, 1444, *1444*
  noncommunicating, 1443, *1443, 1444*
Hydrogen peroxide, bactericidal activity, 73
Hydromyelia, 1420, 1422
Hydronephrosis, 877, *877*
Hydropericardium, 297
Hydropic swelling, 15, 15–16, *16*
Hydrops, of gallbladder, 806, *806*

Hydrops fetalis, 273, *274*, 1038
Hydrostatic pressure, 45
Hydrothorax, 297
Hydroureter, 890
21-Hydroxylase deficiency, 1154
Hydroxyl radicals, bactericidal activity, 74
Hygroma, cystic, 518–519
Hyperacute rejection, 140, *141*
Hyperbilirubinemia, unconjugated, 747–749
  benign recurrent intrahepatic cholestasis, 750
  Crigler-Najjar syndrome, 747
  Dubin-Johnson syndrome, 749–750, *750*
  familial intrahepatic cholestasis (Byler syndrome), 751
  Gilbert syndrome, 747
  intrahepatic cholestasis of pregnancy, 750
  MRP proteins in, 749–751
  neonatal, 751
  obstructive mechanisms in, 751–753, *752, 753*
  Rotor syndrome, 750
  in sepsis, 751
Hypercalcemia
  in cancer, 208
  in hypervitaminosis D, 354
  nephrocalcinosis in, 876, 876t
  pancreatitis and, 814
Hypercholesterolemia, familial, 496, 497, *498, 499*
Hypercoagulable states, in cancer, 209
Hyperemia, 283–285
  active, 284
  passive (congestive), *284*, 284–285, *285*
Hypereosinophilic syndrome, 1075–1076
Hyper-IgM syndrome, 145, 146t
Hyperkeratosis, epidermolytic, 1212, *1212, 1213*, 1214t
Hyperlipidemia, pancreatitis and, 813–814
Hypermethylation, 194
Hyperparathyroidism, primary, 1341–1343, *1342*
Hyperphenylalaninemia
  malignant, 259
  as term, 258
Hyperphosphatemia, 1343
Hyperplasia, 7–8, *8*
  adrenal, 1160
    congenital, *1155*, 1155–1156, *1156*
  atypical of breast, 1004
  cervical, microglandular, 943
  in chronic inflammation, 8, *8*
  demand-induced, 7–8
  endometrial, *957*, 957–958, *958*
  hepatic
    focal nodular, 797, *797*
    nodular regenerative, 797
  hormone-induced, 7
  immune system in, 7–8
  lymph node
    angiofollicular (Castleman disease), 1088
    follicular, 1086–1088, *1088*
    interfollicular, 1088
    reactive, *1086–1087*, 1086–1088
  mast cell (reactive mastocytosis), 1067
  nodular lymphoid, 726–727

nodular prostatic (benign prostatic hypertrophy), 918–920, *919, 920, 921*
parathyroid, 1151–1152, *1152*
primary parathyroid, 1151, *1151*
reactive lymphoid, of bone marrow, 1085
thymic, 1120, *1120*
Hyperplastic hypersecretive gastropathy (Menetrier disease), *678*, 678–679
Hyperplastic (metaplastic) polyps, 725, *726*
Hypersensitivity, 130–140
  classification, 130t
  delayed-type, 138, *139*
  type I (immediate-type), 130–132, 130t, *131*
  type II (non-IgE), 130t, 132–134, *133, 134, 135*
  type III (immune complex/vasculitis), 134–136, *136, 137*
  type IV (cell-mediated), 136–140, *138, 139, 140*
  vs. toxicity, 327
Hypersensitivity angiitis, 505–506, *1234, 1235*, 1235–1236
Hypersensitivity (drug-induced) tubulointerstitial nephritis, 874, *874*
Hypersplenism, 1047–1048
  in alcoholism, 321
Hypertension, 498–503
  acquired, 502
  arteriolosclerosis and, 502–503, *504*
  atherosclerosis and, 493
  epidemiology, 498–499
  malignant (accelerated), 502–503
  molecular genetics of, 501–502
  pathogenesis, 499, *500, 501*
  in pheochromocytoma, 1164
  portal, *757*, 757–761, *759*, 797
  preeclampsia/eclampsia, 865, *865, 866*, 986–988, *987*
  in primary aldosteronism (Conn syndrome), 1163
  pulmonary, 285
  renal disease in, *861*, 861–863, *862*
Hypertensive encephalopathy, 1442
Hypertensive intracerebral hemorrhage, 1437, *1438*
Hypertensive nephropathy, malignant, 862–863, *863*
Hypertensive nephrosclerosis, *861*, 861–863, *862*
Hypertensive retinopathy, 1509–1511, *1513, 1514*
Hyperthecosis, stromal, *969*, 969
Hyperthermia, 335–337
  malignant, 335
  systemic, 335
Hyperthyroidism, 1138–1141
  exopthalmos of, 1504–1505
  Graves disease, 1138–1141, *1139, 1140*
  immune mechanisms, 1138–1139, *1139*
  osteoporosis in, 1337
  toxic adenoma, 1141
  toxic multinodular goiter, 1141
Hypertrophic intestinal tuberculosis, 695
Hypertrophy, 6–7, *7*
  cellular mechanisms, 7
  exercise-induced, 6–7, *7*
  functional demand and, 6–7, *7*
  juvenile (pubertal) of breast, 1000
  physiological (hormonal), 6
Hyperuicemia, *1380*, 1380–1382, *1382, 1401*
Hyperuricemia, 1371–1373, *1372, 1374, 1375*
Hyperviscosity syndrome, 1103
Hypervitaminosis D, 354
Hypoalbuminemia, 756
  in cancer, 209
Hypocalcemia, 1343
  in cancer, 208
Hypochlorous acid, 73–74
Hypoethylation, 194
Hypogammaglobinemic sprue, 704
Hypogammaglobulinemia, 703–704
  Swiss-type, 1169
  transient of infancy, 145, 145t
Hypoglycemia, in cancer, 208
Hypogonadism, osteoporosis in, 1337
Hypokalemia, in primary aldosteronism (Conn syndrome), 1163
Hypoparathyroidism
  familial, 1150
  familial isolated, 1150
  idiopathic, 1150
  pseudohypoparathyroidism, 1150, *1150*
  pseudopseudohypoparathyroidism, 1150
Hypophosphatasia, 1340
Hypophosphatemia, 1376
  X-linked, 1339
Hypopituitarism, *1129*, 1129–1130
  empty sella syndrome, 1130, *1130*
  isolated gonadotropin deficiency (Kallman syndrome), 1130
Hypoplasia, 220
  renal, 831
  thymic, 1169
Hypospadias, 900
Hypospermatogenesis, 909
Hypothalamic-pituitary axis
  disorders of, 1134, 1134t
  in inflammation, 81
Hypothermia, 334
Hypothyroidism, 1135–1138, *1136, 1137*
  congenital (cretinism), 1137–1138, 1145–1146, 1313, 1321, 1466
  goitrous, 1137
  primary (idiopathic), 1137
Hypotonia, malignant, 1394
Hypovolemia, in portal hypertension, 761, *761*
Hypovolemic shock, 305
Hypoxia, hemoglobinopathy and, 1044
H zone, 1388

I

Iatrogenic drug injury, 325, *325*
Iatrogenic neutropenia, 74–75
I bands, 1388
Ichthyoses, 1211–1212
  epidermolytic hyperkeratosis, 1212, *1212, 1213*, 1214t
  ichthyosis vulgaris, *1211*, 1211–1212, *1213*
  lamellar ichthyosis, 1212, 1214t
  lichen simplex chronicus, 1211
  X-linked ichthyosis, 1212, 1214t
Idiopathic crescentic glomerulonephritis, 858–859, *859*, 859t
Idiopathic hypereosinophilic syndrome, 1064
Idiopathic(primary) hypoparathyroidism, 1150
Idiopathic (primary) hypothyroidism, 1137
Idiopathic inflammatory bowel disease
  collagenous colitis, *719*, 719–720, *720*
  Crohn disease, 713–716, *714, 715, 716*
  lymphocytic colitis, *719*, 719–720, *720*
  ulcerative colitis, *716*, 716–719, *717, 718*, 719t
Idiopathic myelofibrosis, chronic, 1070t, 1071t, 1074, *1074*
Idiopathic pancreatitis, 814
Idiopathic portal hypertension, 758
Idiopathic (immune cytopenic) purpura, 1053, *1053*
Idiopathic retroperitoneal fibrosis, 890, *891*
IgA deficiency, selective, 145, 145t
IgA myeloma, 1101
IgA nephropathy, *856*, 856–857, *857*
IgD myeloma, 1101
IgE hypersensitivity, 130–132, 130t, *131*
IgE myeloma, 1101
IgG myeloma, 1101
Ileus, meconium, 692
Immune (antigen-antibody) cmplexes, 51
Immune cytopenic (idiopathic) purpura, 1053, *1053*
Immune hemolytic anemias, 1044–1046
  autoimmune, 1044–1045
    alloimmune hemolytic anemia, 1046
    cold agglutinin disease, 7–45, *1045*
    cold hemolysin disease (paroxysmal cold hemoglobinemia), 1045–1046
    hemolytic disease of newborn, 1046, *1046*
    hemolytic transfusion reactions, 1046
Immune system
  autoimmune disease, 153–162
  biology of, 120–130
    cellular components, 120–127
    cellular/humoral responses, 128–130
  cancer and, 204–207, *205*
  evaluation, 141–143, *142*
  immunodeficiency diseases, 143–153
    adenosine deaminase (ADA) deficiency, 146t, 147
    AIDS, 147–153 (*see also* AIDS/HIV)
    Bruton X-linked agammaglobulinemia, 143–145, 145t, 1293
    chronic mucocutaneous candidiasis, 146
    combined, 146–147, 146t
    common variable immunodeficiency (CVID), 145, 145t
    DiGeorge syndrome, 145–146
    hyper-IgM syndrome, 145, 146t
    primary antibody, 143–145, 145t
    primary T cell, 145–146
    purine nucleoside phophorylase deficiency, 146t, 147
    selective IgA, 145, 145t
    severe combined immunodeficiency (SCID), 146–147, 146t, 1169
    transient hypogammaglobulinemia of infancy, 145, 145t
    Wiskott-Aldrich syndrome, 147

Immunocompromise
    in alcoholism, 321
    infection risk and, 362
    infective esophagitis in, 667–668, 668
    M. avium-intracellulare complex and, 427
    in multiple myeloma, 1103
    polyclonal lymphoproliferation in, 198
    Toxoplasma encephalitis in, 446
    Toxoplasma lymphadenopathy syndrome, 445, 445–446
Immunoglobulins (Igs), 68
    in metastasis, 177
Immunohistochemical tumor markers, 171–172, 173
Immunological cytotoxicity, 206, 206
Immunological factors, in celiac disease, 700
Immunoproliferative small intestinal disease (alpha chain disease, Mediterranean lymphoma), 1104
Imperforate anus, 711
Imperforate hymen, 939
Impetigo, 380, 380
Inborn errors of, amino acid metabolism, 258–260, 258t, 259
Inclusion bodies, in viral encephalomyelitis, 1453, 1454
Inclusion body myositis, 1399, 1399
Inclusions, intranuclear, 1416, 1417
Indian childhood cirrhosis, 788
Indian filing, 1010, 1011
Infancy
    diseases of, 267–278
        biliary atresia, 795–796
        birth injury, 275–276
        erythroblastosis fetalis, 273–275, 274, 275
        infantile hepatic hemangioma, 797
        neonatal hepatitis, 794–796, 795, 795t
        neonatal (physiological) jaundice, 751
        neoplasms, 277, 277–278
        organ inmmaturity, 269–270, 270
        prematurity and growth retardation, 269–277, 270
        respiratory distress syndrome (RDS), 270–273, 271, 272, 606
        sudden infant death syndrome (SIDS), 276–277
        transient hypogammaglobulinemia, 145, 145t
    hemolytic disease of newborn, 1046, 1046
Infantile hepatic hemangioma, 797
Infarct(s)
    bile (bile lake), 753
    cerebral
        laminar necrosis, 1438–1439, 1439
        watershed, 1438, 1439
    cystic, 296, 296
    pale, 295, 295–296
    red, 295, 295–296
    renal, 866, 866
    septic, 296, 296
    of small intestine, 695–697, 696, 697
    watershed, 297
Infarction
    cerebral, 297, 1440, 1440–1441, 1441
    fatal, 296–297
    hepatic, 792

    intestinal, 297
    mechanisms of, 295–297, 296
    myocardial, 288, 295, 296.297
    pulmonary, 291, 296
Infections
    atherosclerosis and, 494
    bacterial, 376–406, 380–381, 692–685 (*see also* Bacterial infections *and specific diseases*)
    bone, 1327–1332
        syphilitic, 1331–1332, 1332
        tuberculous, 1331, 1331
    central nervous system, 1444
    complement system and, 52–53
    epidemiology, 361t
    female genital, 929–934, 930t
    female peritoneal, 981–984 (*see also* Endometriosis)
    fungal, 429–440 (*see also* Fungal infections *and specific diseases*)
    helminthic, 457–471 (*see also* Helminthic infections)
    host factors in, 361–362, 361t
    intestinal, large bowel, 711, 711
    of oral cavity, 1271–1273
    placental, 986
    of prosthetic devices, 378
    protozoal, 441–456 (*see also* Protozoal infections *and specific diseases*)
    respiratory, 378
    skin, 1241–1246
        deep fungal, 1244, 1244
        dermatophyte (superficial fungal), 1241–1244, 1243
        impetigo, 1241, 1243
    small intestine, 693–695
    terminology, 361
    viral, 362–377 (*see also* Vital infections *and specific diseases*)
Infectious mononucleosis, 372–373, 374, 375, 1085, 1088–1089, 1120, 1293–1294
Infective esophagitis, 667–668, 668
Infectivity, 361
Infertility
    in endometriosis, 983, 983–984
    male, 908–909, 908t, 909, 910
    radiation-related, 341
Inflammation, 41–82
    acute, 44, 44
        leukocyte functions in, 70–73, 73
        leukocyte recruitment in, 65, 65–70, 66, 67
        leukocyte transmigration, 68–70, 69
        outcomes of, 75
    cell-derived mediators, 52–58
        arachidonic acid, 52–53, 52t, 53
        arachidonic acid metabolites, 53–56
        cytokines, 55, 55–57, 56
        neurokinins, 58
        platelet-activating factor (PAF), 53, 53–54
        reactive oxygen species (ROS), 57–58
        stress proteins, 58
    cells of, 59–65
    chronic, 5–6, 7–8, 42, 44, 75–79
        cells involved in, 76, 76–78
        cellular components, 76–78
        injury and repair in, 78–79

    definition, 42
    extracellular matrix mediators, 58–59, 59
    general considerations, 42–45
    granulomatous, 79, 79, 80
    mediators of, 44
    plasma-derived mediators, 48–52
        complement, 49, 49–50
        Hageman factor, 48, 48
        kinins, 49
    regulation of, 75
    suppurative, 48
    systemic manifestations of, 81–82, 81t
    in wound healing, 100–102
Inflammatory cells, 59–65
    activation pathways, 64–65
        G-protein-mediated, 64, 64
        JAK-STAT, 65, 65
        TNFR, 64–65, 65
    acute in chronic inflammation, 78
    bactericidal activity, 73–75, 73t
    basophils, 62, 63
    dendritic cells, 77
    endothelial cells, 59–61, 60, 61
    eosinophils, 62, 63
    fibroblasts, 77–78, 78
    lymphocytes, 77, 77
    mast cells, 62, 63
    monocyte/macrophages, 61, 62
    neutrophils, 59, 60
    plasma cells, 77
    platelets, 62–63, 63
    polymorphonuclear nucleocytes (PMNs), 59–61, 60, 61
Inflammatory myopathies, 1396–1400
    dermatomyositis, 1399–1400, 1400
    granulomatous (sarcoid) myositis, 1400, 1400
    inclusion body myositis, 1399, 11399
    polymyositis, 1398, 1398–1399
    vasculitis in periarteritis nodosa, 1400, 1400
Inflammatory polyps, colorectal, 726, 726
Inflammatory pseudotumor of orbit, 1504
Inflammatory skin diseases, 1233–1238
    allergic contact dermatitis, 1235–1236, 1236, 1237
    cutaneous necrotizing vasculitis, 1234, 1235, 1235–1236
    granuloma annulare, 1238, 1238–1239
    granulomatous dermatitis, 1237
    pannicular, 1239–1240
        erythema induratum, 1240
        erythema nodosum, 1239–1240, 1240
    sarcoidosis, 1237–1238, 1238
Influenza, 363
Inguinal hernia, 902
Inhalational (pulmonary) anthrax, 404
Inhalation burns, 336
Inherited Creutzfeld-Jakob disease, 1461
Inherited metabolic diseases
    lipid myopathies, 1403, 1404
    mitochondrial diseases, 1404, 11405
    myoadenylate deaminase deficiency, 1404–1405
Inositol trisphosphate (IP$_3$), 64
Insomnia, fatal familial, 1461–1462
Insulinoma, 821–822, 822

Insulin resistance, 1178
Insulin resistance/metabolic syndrome, 1178, *1180*, 1180t
Insulitis, 1175, *1176*
Integrin receptors, 99
Integrins, 68, 88, 88t
   in metastasis, 179
Interferon-γ, in macrophage activation, 55
Interfollicular lymph node hyperplasia, 1088
Interleukins, 55
   in bone marrow kinetics, 1025
   in inflammation, 75
Interstitial edema, 303
Interstitial fluid, 283
Interstitial lung disease, 650–6261
Interstitial (edematous) pancreatitis, 813
Interstitium, vascular, 283
Intestinal abdominal angina, 697
Intestinal amebiasis, 449, *449*
Intestinal infarction, 297
Intestinal metaplasia, *676*, 676–677
Intestinal tuberculosis, 694–695
   hypertrophic, 695
   ulcerative, 694
   ulcerohypertrophic, 695
Intracellular storage, 10–14
   cholesterol, 10
   fat, 10
   glycogen, 10
   inherited lysosomal diseases, 10
Intracranial hemorrhage
   cerebellar, 1438
   intraventricular, 1438
   in newborn, 275
   pontine, 1438
Intracranial pressure increase, 1519–1520, *1521*
Intraductal carcinoma in situ, 1007–1009, *1008, 1009, 1536*
Intraductal papilloma, 1006, *1006*
Intrahepatic cholestasis of pregnancy, 750
Intramural pseudodiverticulosis, 665
Intranuclear inclusions, 1416, *1417*
Intrauterine adhesions (Asherman syndrome), 954
Intrauterine devices (IUDs), trauma related to, 954
Intravenous leiomyomatosis, 964
Intraventricular hemorrhage, in newborn, 272, *272*
Intrecellular storage, abnormal proteins, 10–14, *11, 13*
Intrinsic factor antibodies, 676
Intussusception, 704
Invasive aspergillosis, 430–431, *431*
Invasive (infiltrating) ductal carcinoma, *1008, 1009, 1009*
Involucrum, 1329
Involution failures, 220
Iodide-induced goiter, 1137
Ionizing radiation, 21, *22*
Iron metabolism, 782–783
Iron-overload syndromes, 12–14, *13*
   hereditary hemochromatosis, *783*, 783–785, *784*
   secondary,779t, 785

Iron storage disorders, 12–14
Ischemia, 16
   definition, 5
Ischemia/reperfusion injury, 20–21
Ischemic colitis, 720, *720*
Ischemic injury, 16
Ischemic renal tubular necrosis, 868, 868t, *869*
Ischemic stroke, 1438–1443, *1439, 1440, 1441*
Islet cell tumors, 821–825
   alpha cell tumors (glucagonoma), 823, *823*
   beta cell tumors (insulinomas), 821–822, *822*
   delta cell tumors (somatostatinoma), 823
   D$_1$ tumors (VIPomas, Verner-Morrison syndrome), 823
   in ectopic hormone syndromes, 825
   enterochromaffin cell (carcinoid) tumors, 823, *824*
   gastrinoma (Zollinger-Ellison syndrome), 822–823
   in multiple endocrine neoplasia (MEN), 823
Islets of Langerhans, 820–821, *821,* 821t
Isochromosomes, 230
Isolated amyloidosis, 1191–1192
Isolated gonadotropin deficiency (Kallman syndrome), 1130

J
JAK-STAT pathway, 65, *65*
Jaundice, 747, *747*
   in bile duct carcinoma, 809
   cholestatic, 747
   in liver failure, 755
   neonatal (physiological), 751
   in sepsis, 751
Jock itch, 1241
Joint disorders, 1360–1377
   arthritis
     enteropathic, 1371
     juvenile (Still disease), 1371
     psoriatic, 1371
     rheumatoid, 1366–1371
   calcium hydroxyapatite deposition disease, 1374, *1374*
   calcium pyrophosphate dihydrate deposition, 1373–1375, *1376*
   gout, 1371–1373, *1372, 1374, 1375, 1380,* 1380–1382, *1382, 1401*
   in hemachromatosis, 1374–1375
   in hemophilia, 1374–1375
   osteoarthritis, 1363–1366, *1364, 1365*
   tumors and tumorlike lesions, 1376–1377
Joints, synovial
   classification, 1361
   structures, 1361–1362, *1362*
Jugulotympanic paraganglioma, 1299, *1299*
Junctional nevus, 1246
Juvenile arthritis (Still disease), 1371
Juvenile (strawberry) hemangioma, 516
Juvenile (pubertal) hypertrophy, of breast, 1000
Juvenile nasopharyngeal angiofibroma, 1294, *1294*
Juvenile (retention) polyps, 726, *726*

Juxtacortical chondrosarcoma, 1356–1357
Juxtacortical osteosarcoma, 1355
Juxtacrine functions, of PAF, 53
Juxtaglomerular apparatus, 830–831

K
Kala azar (visceral leishmaniasis), 793
Kallikrein, 48, *48*
Kallman syndrome, 1130
Kaposi sarcoma, 152, 198, 518, *1263,* 1263–1264, *1264, 1265*
Karyolysis, 25
Karyorrhexis, 25
Kasabach-Merritt syndrome, 1056
Kawasaki disease, 508, *509,* 860, *860*
Kayser-Fleischer rings, 786, *786,* 1466
Keloids, 115, *115*
   aurual, 1296
Keratinocytes, 106–107, *1204,* 1204–1205, *1205*
Keratinosomes, 1204, *1205*
Keratitis, in riboflavin deficiency, 351, *351*
Keratocanthoma, 1258–1259, *1259*
Keratohyaline granules, 1205–1206, *1206*
Keratomalacia, in vitamin A deficiency, 348–349
Keratopathy, band, 1506–1507
Keratosis
   actinic, 1258, *1259*
   seborrheic, 1258
Keratosis follicularis (Darier disease), 1212, *1214*
Kernicterus, 273, 747
Kerosene, 328
Kidney(s) (*see also* Renal *entries*)
   anatomy, *825,* 828–831
     blood vessels, 828
     glomerular basement membrane, *829,* 829–830, *830*
     glomerulus (glomeruli), *825,* 828, *829, 830*
     interstitium, 831
     juxtaglomerular apparatus, 830–831
     tubules, 830
   calculi (stones), 876–877, *877*
   congenital anomalies, 831–835
     autosomal dominant polycystic kidney disease (ADPKD), *833,* 833–834
     autosomal recessive polycystic kidney disease (ARPKD), *833,* 834, *834*
     ectopic kidney, 831
     glomerulocystic disease, 834
     horseshoe kidney, 831, *831*
     medullary sponge kidney, 835
     nephronophthisis-medullary cystic disease complex, 834–835
     Potter sequence (oligohydramnios sequence), 831
     renal agenesis, 831
     renal dysplasia, 831–835, *832*
     renal hypoplasia, 831
   glomerular diseases, 835–859, 836t
   healing of, 111–112, *112*
   lead poisoning and, 331
   mercury poisoning and, 332
   neoplasia
     benign, 880–881
     malignant, 881–884

Kidney(s) *(contd.)*
  obstructive uropathy/hydronephrosis, 877, *877*
  in plasma cell neoplasia, 1101
  in shock, 308, *309*
  transplant rejection, 877–880, *878*, 878t, *879*
  tubulointerstitial disease, 867–876
    acute tubular necrosis, 306, *309*, 867–869, *868*, 868t, *869*
    analgesic nephropathy, 873–874
    drug-induced (hypersensitivity), 874, *874*
    light-chain cast nephropathy, in multiple myeloma, 874–875, *875*
    nephrocalcinosis, 876, 876t
    pyelonephritis, 869–872, *870*, *871*
    urate nephropathy, *875*, 875–876
  vascular disease, 859–867
    cortical necrosis in shock, 866–867, *867*
    hypertensive, 861–863
    preeclampsia, 865, *865*, *866*
    renal artery stenosis, 863
    renal atheroembolism, 863, *864*
    renal infarcts, 866, *866*
    renal vasculitis, 859–861, 860t
    sickle cell nephropathy, 865–866
    thrombotic microangiopathy, 863–865, *864*, *865*
Kikuchi disease (histiocytic necrotizing lymphadenitis), 1089
Kimmelsteil-Wilson nodules, 845, *845*
Kininases, 75
Klebsiella pneumonia, 395
Klinefelter syndrome (47,XXY), 237–238, *238*
Knudson's two-hit hypothesis, of retinoblastoma, 191, *192*
Köbner's phenomenon, 1215
Korsakoff psychosis, 321–322
Korsakoff syndrome, 350
Krabbe disease, 1462
Krukenberg tumor, 688, *688*, 981, *981*
Kugelberg-Welander disease, 1409
Kupffer cells, 745–746
Kuru, 1194–1196, 1461
Kwashiorkor, *347*, 347–348
Kyphoscoliosis, 1318
Kyphosis, 1318

L

Labile cells, 108
Labyrinthine toxicity, 1301
Laceration, 3378
Lactoferrin, 74
Lactose-intolerance test, 700
Lactotrope adenoma (prolactinoma), 1131
Laennec (micronodular) cirrhosis, 754
Lambert-Eaton syndrome, 1401
Lamellar bone, 1311–1312, *1312*
  concentric, *1304*, 1312
Lamellar ichthyosis, 1212, 1214t
Lamellipodia, 88
Laminar necrosis, cerebral, 1438–1439, *1439*
Laminins, 89t, 91t, 93–95
Langerhans cell histiocytosis, *1065*, 1065–1066, *1066*, 1332–1334

  Hand-Schüller-Christian disease, 1333
  Letter-Siwe disease, 1333–1334
Langerhans cells, *1204*, 1206–1207, *1207*
Langhans giant cells, 79, *80*
Large-bowel anatomy, 708
Large-bowel disorders, 708–732
  in AIDS, 731–732, 732t
  colorectal polyps, 721–727
    adenomatous (premalignant), 721–727, *722*, *723*, *724*
    familial adenomatous polyposis (FAP), 724–725, *725*, *733*
    nonneoplastic, 725–727, *726*
    serrated adenoma, 724
  congenital, 709–711
    anorectal malformations, 710–711
    congenital megacolon (Hirschsprung disease), 709–710, *710*
  diverticular disease, 712–713
    diverticulitis, 713
    diverticulosis, *712*, 712–713
  endometriosis and obstruction, 730–731
  idiopathic inflammatory bowel disease, 713–720
    collagenous colitis, *719*, 719–720, *720*
    Crohn disease, 713–716, *714*, *715*, *716*, 719t
    lymphocytic colitis, *719*, 719–720, *720*
    ulcerative colitis, *716*, 716–719, *717*, *718*, 719t
  infections, 711
    neonatal necrotizing enterocolitis, 711
    pseudomembranous colitis, 711, *711*
  malignant tumors, 727–731
  melanosis coli, 731
  radiation enterocolitis, 721
  solitary rectal ulcer syndrome, 721
  stercoral ulcers, 731
  vascular, 720–721
    angiodysplasia (vascular ectasia), 720–721
    hemorrhoids, 721
    ischemic colitis, 720, *720*
Larva migrans
  cutaneous, 464, *464*
  visceral, 464
Laryngeal cancer, smoking and, 316
Lateral aberrant thyroid gland, 1135
Laxatives, in acquired megacolon, 709–710
Lead poisoning, 330–332, *331*, 1033–1034
Legg-Calvé-Perthes disease, 1326
Legionnaires disease, 395–396, *396*
Leiomyoma, 1381
  cervical, 943–945
  uterine, *963*, 963–964
Leiomyomatosis, intravenous, 964
Leiomyosarcoma, 1381–1382
  uterine, *964*, 964–965, *965*
Leishmaniasis, 451–452, *452*, *453*, 1290
  diffuse cutaneous, 451
  localized, 451
  mucocutaneous, 451–452
  visceral (kala azar), 452, *453*, 793
Lens disorders, 1507–1508 *(see also under Eye)*
Lentigo, solar, 1255–1256, *1257*
Lentigo maligna melanoma, 1250–1251, *1252*

Leprosy (Hansen disease), 425–427, 1288
  lepromatous, *426*, 427, *427*
  tuberculoid, 425, *426*
Leptin, 345
Leptospirosis (Weil syndrome), 794
Leptosporosis (Weil syndrome), 412–413, *413*
Lesch-Nyhan syndrome, 1372
Letterer-Siwe disease, 1065, *1065*, 1333–1334
Leukemia
  acute monoblastic, 1081, *1081*
  acute myeloid, 1079–1082, *1080*, 1081t
  acute promyelocytic, 1080
  aggressive NK cell, 1108–1109
  chronic eosinophilic, 1075–1076
  chronic lymphocytic, 212
  chronic lymphocytic leukemia/small lymphocytic lymphoma, 1095–1098, *1097*, *1098*
  chronic myelogenous, 1067–1071, 1070t, *1071*, 1071t, *1072*
  developmental biology, 182
  hairy cell, 1099, *1099*
  mast cell, 1067
  in neurofibromatosis, 246
  neutrophilic, 1075
  precursor T-acute lymphoblastic, 1093, *1093*
  T-cell
    large granular lymphocyte, 1108
    lymphocytic, 1107
    prolymphocytic, 1108
Leukemia/lymphoma, adult T-cell, 1109
Leukemoid reaction, 81, 1063
Leukocyte adhesion molecules, 474
Leukocyte positioning, 68, *69*
Leukocytes *(see also White cell disorders and specific disorders)*
  in phagocytosis, 70, *71*
  polymorphonuclear (PMNs), 44, *45*
  transmigration of, 68–70, *69*
  in wound repair, 86, *87*
Leukocytoclastic vasculitis, *1234*, *1235*, 1235–1236
Leukocytosis, 81
Leukodystrophies, 1462–1463
  adrenoleukodystrophy, 1462–1463
  Alexander disease, *1462*, 1462–1463
  Krabbe disease, 1462
  metachromatic leukodystrophy, 1462
Leukoencephalopathy, progressive multifocal, *1457*, 1457–1458
Leukopenia, 81
Leukoplakia, *1274*, *1274*
  hairy, 1273
Leukotrienes, in inflammation, 54
Lewy bodies, 1468
Leydig cells, 889
Leydig cell tumors, 917, *917*
Libman-Sacks endocarditis, 157, 289
Lichen planus, 1231–1234, *1232*, *1233*
Lichen sclerosus, 935–936, *936*
Lichen simplex chronicus, 935, *935*, 1211
Liddle syndrome, 501
Lieberkuhn, crypts of, 709
Life span, maximal, *34*, 34–35
Li-Fraumeni syndrome, 193

Index

Ligand–receptor binding, 64
Light chain amyloidosis, 1192, *1193*
Light-chain cast nephropathy, 1101
   in multiple myeloma, 874–875, *875*
Light-chain disease, 1100, 1102
Light-chain/heavy chain deposition, glomerular, 848
Limit dextrinosis, 1402
Lindau syndrome, 1489, 1491
Lingual thyroid nodule, 1271
Lip disorders, 1275
   mucocele, *1276*
   solar cheilitis, *1276*
Lipid metabolism, *494*, 494–496, *495*
Lipid myopathies, 1403, *1404*
   carnitine deficiency, 1403, *1404*
   carnitoyl palmityl transferase deficiency, 1403
Lipid peroxidation, 19, *20*
Lipofuscin, 12
Lipoma, 170, *170*, 1380
   cerebral, 1488, *1488*
   intestinal, 705
Lipooxygenation, 52
Lipopolysaccharide (LPS), 55
Lipoprotein (a) (Lp[a]), 487497
Liposarcoma, 1380–1381
Lipoxins, 75
   in inflammation, 54–55
Lips
   benign diseases of, 1275, *1276*
   mucocele, *1276*
   solar cheilitis, *1276*
Liquefactive necrosis, 25–26, *26*
Lisch nodules, 246
Listeriosis, 404
Liver
   anatomy, *742*, 743–746, *744*, *745*
   bilirubin metabolism, 747–753
   functions, 746–747
   healing of, 111
   in prematurity, 270
   regenerative capacity, 746–747
Liver disease
   abscess
     amebic, 449–450, *450*
     bacterial, 792–793
   alcoholic, 773–778
   cancer
     cholangiocarcinoma (bile duct carcinoma), 800, *800*
     epidemiology, 212, 213
     hemangiosarcoma, 800–801
     hepatoblastoma, 800
     hepatocellular carcinoma, 798–800, *799*
     fibrolamellar, *800*
     metastatic, 801, *801*
   cirrhosis, 753–754, *754*, 754t
     heritable disorders associated with, 785–788
     Indian childhood, 788
     primary biliary, 779–780, *780*
     vs. focal nodular hyperplasia, 797, *797*
   coagulation abnormalities in, 1058
   congestion in, 285, *286*
   extrahepatic biliary obstruction, 781–782, *782*
   hepatic failure, 754–756
   hepatitis
     autoimmune, 773
     viral, 761–773, 761t
   infantile
     biliary atresia, 795–796
     neonatal hepatitis, 794–796, *795*, 795t
   infantile cholestasis syndromes, 794–796, *795*, 795t
   iron-overload syndromes, 782–785
     hereditary hemochromatosis, 783–785, *784*, *785*
     secondary, 779t, 785
   neoplasia
     benign, *796*, 796–798, *797*
     malignant, 798–800, *799*
   parasitic infestations, *793*, 793–794, *794*
   porphyrias, 791
   portal hypertension, *757*, 757–761, *759*, 797
   primary sclerosing cholangitis, 780–781, *781*
   schistosomiasis, 467, *467*
   toxic liver injury, 788–791
     drug-induced disease, 790–791, *791*
   transplantation in, 801, *802*
   in ulcerative colitis, 718
   vascular, 791–792, *792*
     congestive heart failure, 791, *792*
     infarction, 792
     in shock, 792
Liver lobules, *742*, *743*, *744*
Lobular carcinoma, invasive, 1010, *1011*
Lobular carcinoma in situ, 1008–1009, *1011*
Lobular disarray, 768, *769*
Lobules, liver, *742*, *743*–746, *744*, *745*
Loiasis, 458–459, *459*
Loop of Henle, 830
Low birth weight
   classification, 269
   smoking and, 319
Low-density lipoproteins (LDLs), *494*, 494, 496
LSD, 324
L-selectin, 67
Ludwig angina, 1272–1273
Luetic dementia, 1449–1450, *1450*
Lung cancer, smoking and, 315–36, *316*
Lungs (see also Pulmonary entries; Respiratory entries)
   bacterial infections, 395–397 (see also Pneumonia)
   healing of, 112, *113*, 114
   hyperemia in, 285, *285*
   in prematurity, 269–270, *270*
Lupus anticoagulant, 1061
Lupus erythematosus, 1229–1231
   chronic discoid, 158
   drug-induced, 158
   subacute cutaneous, 158
   systemic (SLE), 52, 155–158, 1229–1231, *1230*, *1231*
     acute systemic, 1231
     chronic cutaneous, 1229–1230, *1231*
     lupus glomerulonephritis, 853–856, *855*, 855t
     lymphadenopathy in, 1089
     pathogenesis, *155*, 155–156
     pathology and clinical features, 156–159, *158*, *159*
     splenomegaly in, 1120
     subacute cutaneous, 1230
Lupus-like diseases, 158
   chronic discoid lupus, 158
   drug-induced lupus, 158
Lupus nephritis
   focal proliferative, 156, *157*
   membranous, 156
   mesangial, 156, *157*
   proliferative, diffuse, 156, *158*
Luteal phase defect, 956
Luteinizing hormone (LH), 1132
Lyme disease, 411–412
Lymphadenitis, 75
   acute suppurative, 1086
   histiocytic necrotizing (Kikuchi disease), 1089
Lymphadenopathy, 1088
   AIDS, 153, 1087
   phenytoin-induced, 1089
Lymphadenopathy syndrome, *Toxoplasma*, *445*, 445–446
Lymphangiectasia, congenital (Milroy disease), 704
Lymphangiitis, 75, 515
Lymphangioma
   capillary, 518
   cystic (cystic hygroma, cavernous lymphangioma), 518–519
   in pediatric patients, 278
Lymphangiosarcoma, 519
Lymphatic filariasis (elephantiasis), *457*, 457–458
Lymphatic system, 283, 479
   malignant lymphomas, 1091–1117, 1091t, 1092t
   posttransplant lymphoproliferative disorder, 1116–1117, *1117*
   spleen, *1118*, 1118–1120, 1119t
   thymus, 1120–1122
   tumors, 518–519
Lymphedema, 298, *299*, 515
   radiation, 519
Lymph flow, 45
Lymph nodes
   anatomy, 1084–1085, *1086*–*1087*
   hyperplasia
     angiofollicular (Castleman disease), 1087
     follicular, 1086–1088, *1088*
     interfollicular, 1088
     mixed-pattern, 1088–1089
     reactive, 1085–1089
Lymphocytes, 123–124, *124*
   in chronic inflammation, 77, *77*
   perivascular, in viral encephalomyelitis, 1452, *1453*
   quantitation by flow cytometry, 143
Lymphocytic colitis, *719*, 719–720, *720*
Lymphocytopenia, 1086
Lymphocytosis, 1085, *1085*
   acute infectious, 1085
Lymphogranuloma venereum, *415*, 415–416, 903, 932, 1089

Lymphoid hyperplasia
    nodular, 726–727
    reactive of bone marrow, 1084–1085
Lymphoid polyps, 726–727
Lymphoma, 1091–1117 (see also Leukemia)
    anaplastic large-cell, 1110, *1111*
    angiocentric T cell/NK cell, 1290–1291, *1291*
    B acute lymphoblastic leukemia/lymphoma, 1091–1093, *1092*
    Burkitt, 185, 197–198, 212, 213, *1008*, 1106–1108
    chronic lymphocytic leukemia/small lymphocytic lymphoma, 1095–1098, *1097, 1098*
    colorectal, 730
    developmental biology, 182
    diffuse large B-cell, 1106, *1106*
    enteropathy-associated T-cell, 1109
    extranodal marginal-zone B-cell of mucosa-associated lymphoid tissue (MALT), 1104, *1104*
    follicular, 1103–1104, *1104*
    gastric, 689
    hepatosplenic T-cell, 1109
    histological diagnosis, 172
    Hodgkin, 213, *1111*, 1111–1117, *1112, 1115*
    lymphoplasmacytic/Waldenström microglobinemia, 1098
    malignant, 1091–1117
        testicular metastasis, 918
    mantle cell, *1105*, 1105–1106
    mature (peripheral) B-cell, 1094–1098, 1094t, 1095t, *1096, 1097*
    mature T-cell and NK-cell, 1108–1110
    mediastinal (thymic) diffuse large B-cell, 1105, 1106
    Mediterranean, 706, *707*
    mycosis fungoides and Sézary syndrome, 1109–1110, *1110*
    mycosis fungoides variant, 1263, *1265*
    plasmacytoid, 1063
    primary CNS, 1489, *1489*
    primary effusion, 152, 1106
    primary of small bowel, 706–707
    Richter syndrome, 1097
    subcutaneous panniculitis-like T-cell, 1109
    thyroid, 1149
    T-lymphoblastic, 1092, *1092*
    of Waldeyer's ring, 1295–1296
    western-type intestinal, 706
    WHO classifications, 1190t, 1191t
Lymphoplasmacytic lymphoma/Waldenström microglobinemia, 1098
Lymphopoiesis, *121*, 121–123, *122*
Lymphopoietic system
    benign disorders, 1085–1090
    intestinal and bronchial lymphoid tissue, 1085
Lynch syndrome (hereditary nonpolyposis colon cancer), 194
Lysergic acid diethylamide (LSD), 324
Lysis, of thrombi, 289
Lysosomal hydrolases, 74
Lysosomal storage diseases, 251–258
    cystinosis, 258
    Gaucher disease, 251–254, *253*
    glycogenoses, *257*, 257–258
    mucopolysaccharidoses, 255–257, 255t
    Niemann-Pick disease, 255
    sphingolipidases and, 251, *252*
    Tay-Sachs disease (GM$_2$ gangliosidosis type 1), *254*, 254–255
Lysozymes, 74

M

α_2-Macroglobulin, 73
Macroglossia, 1275–1276
Macrophage-mediated cytotoxicity, 206, *206*
Macrophages, 129–130
    microglia as, 1419, *1419*
    in wound repair, 86, *87*
Macrovesicular steatosis, 789
Macula, cherry-red, 1519, *1520*
Macular degeneration, 1518–1519
Mad cow disease (bovine spongiform encephalopathy), 1459
Maffucci syndrome, 1323
Major histocompatibility complex (MHC), 61–62, 127–128, *128*
    class II molecules, 127
    class I molecules, 127
    clinical tissue typing, 127–128
Malabsorption
    abetalipoproteinemia, 703
    in cancer, 209
    celiac disease (gluten-sensitive enteropathy), 700–702, *701, 702*
    congenital lymphangiectasia, 704
    hypogammaglobulinemia, 703–704
    intestinal, 697–700, *698*
    laboratory evaluation, 700
    lactase deficiency, 700
    radiation enteritis, 704
    tropical sprue, folate deficiency and, 704
    Whipple disease, 702, *703*
Malakoplakia, 894, *894*
Malaria, *441*, 441–444, *442–443, 444*
Malassezia furfur, *1241, 1244*
Male reproductive system
    anatomy, 889
    circulatory disturbances
        erectile dysfunction, 902, 902t
        priapism, 902, 902t
        scrotal edema, 902
    cryptorchidism, 906–907, *907*
    disorders of sexual differentiation, 907–908, 908t
    embryology, 889
    infertility, 908–909, 908t, *909, 910*
    inflammatory disorders, 902–904, 902t
        balanitis, 903–904
        sexually transmitted, 903, *903*
    neoplasia, 905–906
    penile disorders
        congenital, 900
        inflammation, 903–904
    prostate disorders, 918–925
    prostatic disorders, 918–925
        cancer, 921–925, *922*
        nodular hyperplasia (benign prostatic hypertrophy), 918–920, *919, 920, 921*
        prostatitis, 918
    scrotal masses, 900–902, *901*
    testis, epididymis, and vas deferens
        epididymitis, 910, *910*
        orchitis, 910–911, *911*
        testicular neoplasms, 911–918, 911t
    urethritis, 904–905
Malformation, definition, 218–219
Malignancy (see also Cancer; Neoplasia; *specific diseases*)
    cell nuclear indications, 1539, 1539t
    eosinophilia in, 1064
    hematological, osteoporosis in, 1337
Malignant fibrous histiocytoma, *1379*, 1379–1380
Malignant (accelerated) hypertension, 502–503
Malignant hypertensive nephropathy, 862–863, *863*
Malignant hyperthermia, 335
Malignant melanoma, 1210, 1247–1258
    ABCD rule, 1248
    acral lentiginous melanoma, *1252*, 1252–1254, *1253, 1254*
    fine-needle aspiration, *1536*
    histological diagnosis, 172, *172*
    lentigo maligna melanoma, 1251–1252, *1253*
    metastatic melanoma, 1250
    nodular melanoma, 1250–1251, *1251, 1252*
    ocular, 1525, *1525*
    radial growth phase melanoma, 1247–1248, *1249, 1250*
    staging and prognosis, *1254*, 1254–1255, 1254t
    vertical growth phase melanoma, 1248–1249, *1249, 1250, 1251*
    vs. benign melanocytic tumors, 1255–1256
        blue nevus, 1255, *1257*
        congenital melanocytic nevus, 1255
        freckle and lentigo, 1255–1256, *1257*
        Spitz tumor, 1255, *1256*
    vs. pigmented basal cell carcinoma, 1259
    vulvar, 938
Mallory bodies, 11, *779*
Mallory-Weiss syndrome, 321, 670
MALT (mucosa-associated lymphoid tissue), 1104, *1104*
Manganese deficiency, 355
Mannose-binding lectin, 50
Mantle cell lymphoma, *1105*, 1105–1106
Marantic endocarditis, 289
Marasmus, 347
Marble bone disease, *1320*, 1320–1321
Marfan syndrome, 243–244, *244*
MARS (mixed inflammatory response syndrome), 308
Mast cell leukemia, 1067
Mast cell proliferation, 1066–1067, *1067*
Mast cells, 62, *63*, 1210, *1210*
Mast cell sarcoma, 1067
Mastitis
    acute, 1001
    granulomatous, 1001

Index

Mastocytoma, 1067
Mastocytosis
  localized, 1067
  reactive, 1067
  systemic, 1067
Matrix
  bone, 1309
  cartilage, 1312–1313
  provisional, 90, 101–102
  stromal (connective tissue), 90–92
Matrix glycoproteins, 93–95, 94t
Mature (peripheral) B-cell lymphoma, 1094–1098, 1094t, 1095t, *1096*, *1097*
Maximal life span, *34*, 34–35
May-Heggin anomaly, 1052
McArdle disease, 259, 1402–1403, *1403*
McCune-Albright syndrome, 1349–1350, *1350*
Measles (rubeola), 364–365, *365*
Meckel diverticulum, 692, *692*
Meconium ileus, 692
Mediastinal (thymic) diffuse large B-cell lymphoma, 1106
Medin, 1191
Meditarranean fever, familial, 1191
Mediterranean fever, familial (familial paroxysmal polyserositis), 735–736, 1191
Mediterranean lymphoma, 706, *707*
Medullary carcinoma, 169
  breast, 1011, *1012*
  thyroid, 1147–1149, *1148*
Medullary fibroma, 880
Medulloblastoma, 1485
Megacolon
  acquired, 709–710
  in Chagas disease, 454
  congenital (Hirschsprung disease), 709–710, *710*
Megaesophagus, in Chagas disease, 454
Megaloblastic anemia, 114–1037, *1035*, *1036*, *1037*
Megaureter, congenital, 890
Meiotic segregation, *228*
Melanins, 12, *13*
Melanocortins, in obesity, 345
Melanocytes, *1204*, 1206, *1206*
Melanocyte-stimulating hormone, 345
Melanoma, malignant (*see* Malignant melanoma)
Melanosis coli, 731
Melioidosis, 397, *397*
Membrane, hyaline, 272, *272*
Membrane attack complex (MAC), 49, 52, 132
Membranes, congenital pyloric and antral, 674
Membranoproliferative glomerulonephritis
  type I, 851–852, *852*, *853*, 951t
  type II, 852–853, *853*, *854*
Membranous glomerulonephritis, 52
Membranous glomerulopathy, *842*, 842–843, *843*, *844*, *845*
Membranous lupus nephritis, 156
Mendelian trait, 229
Menetrier disease (hyperplastic hypersecretive gastropathy), *678*, 678–679

Meniere disease, 1300–1301, *1301*
Meningioma, 1301, *1301*, 1302, *1302*, *1486*, 1486–1487
Meningitis, 1445–1458
  amebic, 1448, *1449*
  bacterial, 47, 1445–1448
  Escherichia coli, 1445, *1445*, 1447
  Haemophilus influenzae, 1445–1446, *1446*
  Neisseria meningitidis, 1446
  purulent, 1445, *1445*
  routes of entry, *1446*
  Streptococcus pneumoniae, 1446
  tubercular in Pott disease, 1447–1448, *1448*
  tuberculous meningitis and tuberculoma, *1447*, 1447–1448
  in congenital syphilis, 226
  cryptococcal, 1448, *1448*
  neonatal *E. coli*, 389
  syphilitic (luetic), 1448–1450, *1449*, *1450*
  viral, 1448
Meningocele, 222, *223*, 1420
Meningococcemia, *383*, 383–384
Meningoencephalitis, primary amebic, 456
Meningomyelocele, 1420, *1420*
Meningovascular syphilis, 226, 410
Menopause, 5, *6*
  hormone replacement therapy, 326
  smoking and early, 316
Menstrual cycle, *952*, 952–953, 998–1000, *999*
Menstrual disorders, obesity and, 347
Mental retardation
  in Down syndrome, 234
  in fetal alcohol syndrome, 224
  in neurofibromatosis, 246
Mercury poisoning, 332–333, *869*
Merkel cell carcinoma, 1261
Merkel cells, *1204*, 1207, *1208*
Mesangial lupus nephritis, 156, *157*
Mesenteric cysts, 736
Mesenteric vein thrombosis, 697
Mesothelial tumors, 984
Mesothelioma, 203–204, 737
  diffuse malignant, 984
  papillary, 984, *984*
Metabolic bone disease, 1333–1348, *1335*
  Gaucher disease, 1338–1349, *1348*
  osteomalacia/rickets, 1338–1341
  osteoporosis, 1334–1337, *1335*
    primary, 1333–1335, *1335*, *1336*
    secondary, 1337–1338
  Paget disease of bone, 1344–1348, *1345*, *1346*, *1347*
  primary hyperparathyroidism, *1335*, 1341–1343
  renal osteodystrophy, *1335*, 1342–1343, *1343*
Metabolic disorders, of skeletal muscle, 1401–1405
Metachromatic leukodystrophy, 1462
Metalloproteinases, 73
  in wound regeneration, 95–97, 96t, 97t
Metals, as carcinogens, 201
Metal toxicity, 330–333, 1033–1034
Metaplasia, 8–9, *9*
  bladder, 895

  celomic, 982
  in chronic inflammation, 78
  intestinal, *676*, 676–677
  nephrogenic, 895–896
  pseudopyloric, 677
  squamous, 8–9, *9*
Metaplastic carcinoma, of breast, 1011
Metastasis, 175–180
Metastatic calcification, 14, 1327
Methanol, 328
Microangiopathic anemia, 209
Microangiopathy, thrombotic, 863–865, *864*, *865*, 865t
Microcirculation, 282–283, *283*
Microfibrillar fibers, 244
Microglandular hyperplasia, cervical, 943
Microglia, 1419, *1419*
Microhamartoma, bile duct (von Meyenburg complexes), 797
Micronodular (Laennec) cirrhosis, 754
Microvascular disease, in diabetes mellitus, *1170*, 1181, *1182*
Microvesicular steatosis, 789, *790*
Microvilli, 698
Microwave radiation, 344
Midgut volvulus, 704–705
Miliary tuberculosis, 423–424, *424*
Milroy disease (congenital lymphangiectasia), 515, 704
Minamata disease, 332–333
Minimal-change glomerulonephropathy, 837–840, *839*, *840*
Missense mutations, 240
Mitochondrial mediation, of apoptosis, 31–33, *32*
Mitochondrial myopathies, 1404, 11405
Mitochondrial oxidative damage, in aging, 37
Mitochondrial pathway, of oncogene action, 191
Mitochondrial permeability transition pore (MPTP), 29
Mitosis, 107–108, *108*
  of malignant cells, 170–171
Mixed connective tissue disease (MCTD), 162
Mixed inflammatory response syndrome (MARS), 308
Molds, 429 (*see also* Fungal infections)
Molluscum contagiosum, 932, *1245*, *1245*
Mönckberg medial sclerosis, 503
Monoclonal gammopathy, 1496–1497
  of unknown significance (MGUS), 1101, 1102
Monocyte/macrophages, 1026
  in acute inflammation, 61, *62*
  in chronic inflammation, 76, 76–77
  in wound healing, 101–102
Monocytosis, 1064–1065
Mononuclear-phagoctye and immunoregulatory effect (M-PIRE system), 1026
Mononuclear phagocytes, 124–125
Mononucleosis, infectious, *1085*, 1088–1089, 1293–1294
Monosomy, 230
Monostotic fibrous dysplasia, 1349

Monotopic effect, 221
Morphea, 1239, 1260
Morpheaform bsal cell carcinoma syndrome, 1259
Morphogenetic disorders, 219–221 (*see also* Congenital anomalies)
　congenital syphilis, 225–226
　fetal alcohol syndrome, 223–224
　fetal hydantoin syndrome, 223
　neural tube defects, 221–223, *222*
　　anencephaly, 221–223, *222*
　thalidomide-induced malformations, 223, *223*
　TORCH complex, *224*, 224–225, 225t
　types, 219–221, *220*
Morquio syndrome, 1315–1316, *1316*
Morton neuroma (plantar interdigital neuroma), 1498–1499
Mosaicism, 231
Motor neuropathy, subacute, 208
M phase, of cell cycle, 108
M-PIRE system, 1026
MRP proteins, 749–751
Mucinous (colloid) adenocarcinoma, ovarian, 974, *975*
Mucinous (colloid) carcinoma, breast, 1010, *1011*
Mucinous cysts, 934
Mucocele, 733, *733*, 1287, *1288*
　of gallbladder (hydrops), 806, *806*
　of lip, *1276*
Mucocutaneous candidiasis, chronic, 146
Mucocutaneous leishmaniasis, 451–452
Mucocutaneous lymph node syndrome (Kawasaki disease), 508, *509*
Mucopolysaccharidoses, 255–257, 255t
　Gaucher disease, 1466
　Hurler syndrome, 256–257, 1465
　Morquio syndrome, 1315–1316, *1316*
Mucosa-associated lymphoid tissue (MALT), 1104, *1104*
Mucous neck cells, 673
Mulberry molars, 226
Multicystic renal dysplasia, 832, *832*
Multidrug-resistance proteins (MRPs), 749–751
Multifactorial inheritance, 267–268, 267t, *268*
Multifocal atrophic (environmental metaplastic) gastritis, 676, 676–677
Multifocal motor neuropathy, 1495
Multinodular nontoxic goiter, 1135, *1136*
Multiple endocrine neoplasia (MEN), 682, 1164–1165
　familial medullary thyroid carcinoma, *1165*, 1165–1167
　type 1 (Werner syndrome), 823, 1164–1165
　type 2A (Sipple syndrome), 1165
　type 2B, 1165
Multiple hemangiomatous syndromes, 516
Multiple melanoma, in bone, 1360, *1360*
Multiple myeloma, 212, 1099–1103, 1099t, *1100, 1102, 1103*
　biclonal, 1100
　plasmocytosis in, 1085–1086
　renal complications, 874–875, *875*

Multiple sclerosis (MS), 1463–1464, *1464*
Multisystem organ dysfunction syndrome (MODS), 82, 307–308
Mumps, 366–367, *367*
Muscle, skeletal, 1386–1411
Muscular arteries, 477–479
Muscular dystrophy, *260*, 262–264, *1391*, 1391–1394
　Becker, 262–264, *263*, 1391–1394, *1392*, 1392t, *1393*
　congenital, 1394
　Duchenne, 262–264, *263*, 1391–1394, *1392*, 1392t, *1393*
　myotonic dystrophy, 1394
Mutagens, chemical, 199
Mutations, 240–243, 241t, *242, 243*
　fragile X syndrome, 240
　frameshift, 240
　Friedreich ataxia, 240–241
　functional consequences, 241–242, *242*
　Huntingdon disease, 240, 250, 1472–1475, *1473*
　missense, 240
　mutation hotspots, 242, *242*
　myotonic dystrophy, 240
　nonsense, 240
　oncogenes and, 185
　point, *241*
　synonymous, 240
Mutator genes, 194–195
Myasthenia gravis, 1401
　thymona in, 1121
Mycetoma, 440, *440*
Mycobacterial infections, 420–429, 420t
　atypical, 428–429, 428t
　leprosy (Hansen disease), 425–427, *426, 427*
　M. avium-intracellulare complex, 427–428, *428*, 428t
　M. pneumoniae, 420–421
　tuberculosis, 421–425
Mycobacterium bovis, 694
Mycobacterium chelonae, 429
Mycobacterium fortuitum, 429
Mycobacterium kansasii, 429
Mycobacterium marinum, 429
Mycobacterium scrofulaceum, 429
Mycobacterium tuberculosis, in erythema induratum, 1239–1240, *1240*
Mycobacterium ulcerans, 429
Mycoplasma, 931
Mycosis fungoides (lymphoma variant), 1263, *1265*
Mycosis fungoides and Sézary syndrome, 1109–1110, *1110*
Mycotic aneurysms, 513–514
Mycotic cerebral aneurysm, 1437
Myelinolysis, central pontine, 322
Myelodysplastic diseases
　acute myeloid leukemia, 1079–1082, *1080*, 1081t
　chronic eosinophilic leukemia and hypereosinophilic syndrome, 1075–1076
　chronic idiopathic myelofibrosis, 1070t, 1071t, 1074, *1074*
　chronic myelogenous leukemia, 1067–1072, 1070t, *1071*, 1071t, *1072*

　essential thrombocythemia, 1070t, 1071t, 1074–1075, *1075*
　hematopoietic manifestations, 1076–1079, 1076t, *1077*
　myeloid sarcoma, 1082–1083, *1083*
　neutrophilic leukemia, 1075
　polycythemia vera, 1070t, 1071t, 1072–1074
　5q-syndrome, 1078
　refractory anemia, 1078
　　with excess blasts, 1078–1079
　　with ringed sideroblasts, 1078
　refractory cytopenia with multilineage dysplasia, 1078
　WHO classifications, 1070t, 1071t, 1076t
Myelofibrosis, chronic idiopathic, 1070t, 1071t, 1074, *1074*
Myelogenous leukemia, chronic, 1067–1071, 1070t, *1071*, 1071t, *1072*
Myeloid sarcoma, 1082–1083, *1083*
Myeloid-to-erythroid ratio, 1023, *1025*, 1025t
Myeloma
　multiple, 212, 874–875, *875*
　nonsecretory, 1100
　solitary osseous, 1099, 1103
Myelomalacia, 1434, *1434*
Myelomeningocele, 222, *223*
Myeloperoxidase deficiency, 1064
Myeloplastic anemia, 1033
Myelopoietic cells
　of bone marrow, 1020–1025
　peripheral, 1025–1026
Myeloproliferative disease, basophilia in, 1064
Myoadenylate deaminase deficiency, 1404–1405
Myocardial amyloid, *1198*
Myocardial infarction, *114*, 288, *295, 296, 297*
Myocarditis, in Chagas disease, 454, *454*
Myofiber, 1388–1389, *1389*
　type I (slow twitch, red), 1388–1389, *1389*
　type II (fast twitch, white), 1389, *1389*
Myofibroblasts, 86, *105*
Myolipoma, adrenal, 1163
Myopathy
　congenital, 1394–1396, *1395*
　　central core disease, *1395*, 1395–1396
　　central nuclear (myotubular), 1396, *1397*
　　rod (nemaline), 1396, *1397*
　critical illness, 1410, 1411
　lipid, 1403, *1404*
　steroid, 1411
Myophosphorylase deficiency (McArdle disease), 1402–1403, *1403*
Myopia, 1320
Myositis
　dermatomyositis, 1399–1400, *1400*
　inclusion body, 1399, *1399*
　polymyositis, *1398*, 1398–1399
　sarcoid (granulomatous), 1400, *1400*
Myositis ossificans, 1327, *1328*
Myotonic dystrophy, 240, 1394
Myxedema, 1136
Myxedema madness, 1136

Index

N

Naegleria fowleri, 456
Nasal cavity
   angiocentric T cell/NK cell lymphoma, 1290–1291, *1291*
   benign tumors, 1291, *1291, 1292*
   leishmaniasis, 1290
   leprosy (Hansen disease), 1288
   malignant tumors, 1291, *1291, 1292*
   rhinoscleroma, 1288–1289, *1289*
   Wegener granulomatosis, 1290, *1290*
Nasal inverted papilloma, 1291, *1291, 1292*
Nasal polyps, 1287, *1287*
Nasogastric intubation, 669
Nasopharyngeal angiofibroma, juvenile, 1294, *1294*
Nasopharyngeal cancer, 198, 211
Nasopharynx, 1293–1296
   anatomy and function, 1293
   inflammation, 1293–1294
   lymphoid hypoplasia and hyperplasia, 1293
   tumors, 1294–1296
   Waldeyer's ring, 1293
Natural killer cell-mediated cytotoxicity, 206, *206*
Natural killer (NK) cells, 55, 124
Necrosis, 24–29
   acute tubular, 308, *309*, 867–869, *868*, 868t, *869*
   aseptic of femoral head, 321
   caseous, 26, *27*
   causes, 26–29, *28*
   cerebral laminar, 1438–1439, *1439*
   coagulative, 25, *25*
   confluent hepatic, 769–770, *770*
   fat, 26, *26*
   fibrinoid, 26, *27*
   hepatic
      massive (acute yellow atrophy), 770, *770*
      piecemeal, 770, *771*
      submissive confluent, 770
   inflammation and, 52
   liquefactive, 25–26, *26*
   mechanisms, 24–25, 26–29, *28*
   of muscle, 1390–1391, *1391*
   papillary, 871, *871*, 873
   proximal tubular, 332
   renal tubular, 867–869, *868*, 868t, *869*
   types, 25–26
   zonal hepatocellular, 789, *789*
Necrotizing enteritis, 397–399
Necrotizing enterocolitis, in newborn, 272
Negative thymic selection, 123
Negri bodies, *1417*
Neisseria gonorrhoeae, 384–386, *385, 386*
Neisseria gonorrhoeae (see also Gonorrhea; Syphilis)
Neisseria meningitides, 383, *383*–384
Nematodes (see under Helminthic infections and specific diseases)
Neonatal hepatitis, 794–796, *795*, 795t
Neonatal herpes, 372
Neonatal hydrocephalus, 1422–1423, *1423, 1424*
Neonatal (physiological) jaundice, 751

Neonatal necrotizing enterocolitis, 711
Neonatal pneumonia, 381
Neonatal sepsis, 381
Neonatal thrombocytopenia, 1054
   Fanconi anemia, 1054
   neonatal alloimmune chrombocytopenia, 1054
   nonimmune, 1054
   Wiscott-Aldrich syndrome, 1054
Neoplasia, 165–213
   benign versus malignant, 167
   bladder, benign metaplasia and proliferation, *895*, 895–896, *896*
   classification and terminology, 167–169
      benign, 167–168
      malignant, 168–169
   definition, 166
   dysplasia as stage in, 9
   esophageal, 670–672
      benign, *670*, 670–671
      carcinoma, *671*, 671–672
   gallbladder, *808*, 808–809
   gastric
      benign, 684–685
      malignant, 685–689
   hepatic, 790–791
   histological diagnosis, 170–180
   HIV-associated, 1263–1264, *1264, 1265*
   of infancy, 277, *277*–278
   liver, benign, *796*, 796–798, *797*
   ocular, 1524–1526
   oral cavity, benign, 1273–1274
   pancreatic
      endocrine pancreas, 820–825
      exocrine pancreas, 816–820
   peritoneal, 736–737
   renal, 848
      benign, 880–881
      malignant, 881–884
   renal pelvis and ureters, 891
   skin, 1246–1265
   small-bowel, 705–708
   testicular, 911–918, 911t
Nephritic (glomerulonephritic) syndrome, 836, 836t
Nephroblastoma (Wilms tumor), 881–882, *882*
Nephrocalcinosis, 876, 876t
Nephrogenic diabetes insipidus, 1133
Nephrogenic metaplasia, 895–896
Nephrogenic rests, 881
Nephrolithiasis, 876–877, *877*
Nephroma, mesoblastic, 881
Nephronophthisis–medullary cystic disease complex, 834–835
Nephropathy
   diabetic, 1181–1183, *1183*
   lead, 331, *332*
Nephrosclerosis, hypertensive, *861*, 861–863, *862*
Nephrotic syndrome, 303, 835–836, 835t, 836t
   in cancer, 209
Nerve trauma, 1498–1499
Nervous system
   age and, 1415
   alcoholism and, 321–322

   cells of, 1415–1419
      astrocytes, 1416–1418, *1417, 1418, 1419*
      ependyma, 1418, *1418*
      microglia, 1419, *1419*
      neurons, *1415*, 1415–1416, *1416*
      oligodendroglia, 1418, *1418*
   healing in, 112–114
   topography, 1415
Nescator americanus, 460–461
Nescator duodenale, 460–461, *461*
Nests, thyroid, 1135
Neural tube defects
   anencephaly, *1421*, 1421–1422
   Arnold-Chiari malformation, *1420*, 1422, *1422, 1423*
   congenital hydrocephalus, 1422–1423, *1423, 1424*
   gyral malformations, 1423–1424, *1424*
   spinal cord malformations, *1420*, 1422
      hydromyelia, *1420*, 1422
      syringobulbia, 1422
      syringomyelia, 1422
Neural tube defects (dysraphic states), 1419–1422
   spina bifida, *1419*, 1419–1421, *1420*
Neuroblastoma, 1167–1168, *1168*
   olfactory, *1292*, 1292–1293
Neurodegenerative diseases, 1468–1479, 1468t
Neuroendocrine tumors, histological diagnosis, 172
Neurofibrillary tangles, 11, 1475, *1477, 1478*, 1478–1479
Neurofibroma, 246, *246*, 1499–1500, *1500*
   plexiform, 246
Neurofibromatosis, 193
   type I (von Recklinghausen's disease), 245, *245*, 1491
   type II (central), 246–247
Neurokinins, in inflammation, 58
Neurological syndromes, in cancer, 208
Neuroma
   plantar interdigital (Morton neuroma), 1498–1499
   traumatic, 114, 1498
Neuronal storage diseases, 1465–1466
Neurons, *1415*, 1415–1416, *1416*
Neuropathic ulcers, 115
Neuropathy, diabetic, 1183
Neuropeptide Y, 346
Neurophagia, 1416, *1416*
Neurotoxicity
   of lead, 331
   mercury, 332–333
Neutropenia, 1062, 1062t
   iatrogenic, 74–75
Neutrophil granules, 70, *71*
Neutrophilia, 1062–1063, 1062t, *1063t*
Neutrophilic leukemia, 1075
Neutrophils, 1025–1027
   in ischemia/reperfusion injury, 21
Nevoid basal cell carcinoma syndrome, 1259
Nevus
   blue, 1255, *1257*
   common acquired melanocytic nevus (mole), 1246, *1247*

1574   Index

(contd.)
   compound, 1246, *1247*
   dermal, 1246, *1247*
   dysplastic (atypical), 1246
   junctional, 1246
Newborn, hemolytic disease of, 1046, *1046*
New variant Creutzfeld-Jakob disease, 1461
Nezelof syndrome, 1169
NF-1 gene, 193
Niacin deficiency (pellagra), *350,* 350–351
Nickel toxicity, 333
Nidogen/entactin, 91t
Niemann-Pick disease, 255, 1466
Nitric oxide, 60
   bactericidal activity, 74
   as inflammatory mediator, 58
   in ischemia/reperfusion injury, 21
Nitric oxide synthase, 475
Nitrosamines
   as carcinogens, 201
   in stomach cancer, 685–686
NK cell leukemia, 1107–1109
Nocardiosis, 407, *407*
Nodular adrenal hyperplasia, 1160
Nodular fasciitis, 170, *170,* 1377, *1379*
Nodular lymphoid hyperplasia, 726–727
Nodular melanoma, 1250–1251, *1251, 1252*
Nodular prostatic hyperplasia (benign prostatic hypertrophy), 918–920, *919, 920, 921*
Nodular sclerosis Hodgkin lymphoma, 1114, 1114t, 1116, *1116*
Nodular synovitis, 1375, 1377
Nodular tenosynovitis, 1377
Nodules
   cartilage, 1375
   Kimmelsteil-Wilson, 845, *845*
   lingual thyroid, 1271
   Lisch, 246
   rheumatoid, 1367–1369, *1369*
   typhoid, 390
Noma, 414, *414,* 1272, *1272*
Nonalcoholic steatohepatitis, 346–347
Nonbacterial thrombotic endocarditis, 209
Nonfibrillar collagens, 92
Nonossifying fibroma, 1350–1351
Nonreceptor protein kinases, 188, *188*
Nonsecretory myeloma, 1100
Nonsense mutations, 240
Nonvenereal treponematoses, 411
Normocytic normochromic anemia, 1048
Norwalk virus, 367–368, 694
Nose and paranasal sinuses, 1286–1292
   fungal infections, 1288–1289, *1289*
   Hansen disease (leprosy), 1288
   leishmaniasis, 1289
   malignant tumors, 1291, *1291*
   nasal polyps, 1286, 1287, *1287*
   nosebleed, 1285, 1286t
   rhinitis, 1286
   rhinoscleroma, 1288, *1288*
   sinusitis, 1286–1287, *1287*
   syphilis, 1287
   Wegener granulomatosis, 1289, *1289*
Nosebleed (epistaxis), 1285, 1286t
NSAIDs, 873–874
   mechanism of action, 54
   in peptic ulcer disease, 679

Nuclear to cytoplasmic asynchrony, 1034
Null cell adenoma, 1133
Nutritional disorders, 344–354
   obesity, 344–347, *345, 346, 347* (see also Obesity)
   protein-calorie malnutrition, *347,* 347–348
   trace mineral deficiencies, 354–355
   vitamin deficiencies, 348–354

O

Obesity, 344–347, *345, 346*
   in Cushing sydrome, 1162
   in diabetes mellitus type 2, 1177, *1178, 1179*
   pancreatitis and, 814
Obstruction
   gastrointestinal, major causes, *735*
   ureteral, 890, *891*
Obstructive renal dysplasia, 832
Obstructive uropathy, 877, *877*
Occupational carcinogens, 326–333, 327t
Ochronosis, 1375–1376
Ocular defects
   in congenital syphilis, 226
   in Marfan syndrome, 244
   in TORCH complex, 224–225
Ocular diseases
   diabetic retinopathy, 1183
   oculocutaneous albinism, 1064
   smoking and, 316
   Wilson disease (hepatolenticular degeneration), 786, *786*
Oculocutaneous albinism (OCA), 261, 1064
Oculoglandular tularemia, 403
Odland bodies, 1205–1206, *1206*
Odontogenic cysts and tumors, *1279,* 1279–1280
Olfactory neuroblastoma, *1292,* 1292–1293
Oligodendroglia, 1418, *1418*
Oligodendroglioma, 1483–1485, *1484*
Oligohydramnios (Potter) sequence, 831
Oligomeorrhea, obesity and, 347
Oliguria, 304
Ollier disease (echondromatosis), *1322,* 1322–1323
Omental cysts, 736
Onchocerciasis (river blindness), 458, 1506
Oncocytma, 1133
Oncocytoma, renal, 880
Oncogenes
   activation mechanisms, 184–185, *186, 187*
      chromosomal translocation, 185, *186*
      gene amplification, 186
      mutation, 185
   HER2/neu, 1013, *1013*
   mechanisms of action, 185–191, *187, 188, 189, 190*
      bcl-2 protein and apoptosis, 191
      cell cycle control, *190,* 190–191
      DNA viruses, 193
      growth factor receptors, 186–188, *187*
      growth factors, 185–186
      nonreceptor protein kinases, 188, *188*
      nuclear regulatory proteins, 189–190
      Ras oncogenes, 188–189, *189*
   mechanisms of activation
      chromoasomal translocation, 185, *186*

      gene amplification, 186
      growth factors, 186–187
      mutation, 185
   in pancreatic cancer, 819
Oncotic pressure, 45
Ophthalmia neonatorum, 1506
Opsonins, 50, *51,* 70
Opsonization, 50
Optic atrophy, 1520–1521, *1521*
Optic nerve
   glaucoma, 1522–1524, *1523,* 1531
   in increased intracranial pressure, 1519–1520, *1521*
   optic atrophy, 1520–1521, *1521*
Oral candidiasis (thrush), *1272,* 1273
Oral cavity, 1270–1276
   anatomy, 1270–1271
   congenital anomalies
      branchial cleft cyst, 1271.*1265*
      facial clefts, 1271
      lingual thyroid nodule, 1271
   dental caries (tooth decay), 1276–1277, *1277*
   infections, 1271–1273
      bacterial and fungal, 1271–1273
      viral, 1273
   leukoplakia and erythroplakia, 1274, *1274*
   lip disorders, 1275, *1276*
   neoplasms
      benign tumors, 1273–1274
      squamous cell carcinoma, 1275, *1275*
      odontogenic cysts and tumors, *1279,* 1279–1280
      pulp and periapical tissues, 1277–1278
      squamous cell carcinoma, 1275, *1275*
      tongue disorders, 1275–1276
Oral contraceptives, 955
   side effects, *325,* 325–326
Orbit, inflammatory pseudotumor of, 1504
Orchitis, 910
Organelles, changes due to injury, 16, *17*
Organ inmmaturity, in prematurity, 269–270, *270*
Organization, of inflammatory response, 99
Orthopnea, 301
Osler-Weber-Rendu syndrome (hereditary hemorrhagic telangiectasia), 758, 1052
Osmotic pressure, 45
Ossification
   funnelization (mesophysis formation), 1315
   growth-plate obliteration, 1315, *1315*
   primary, *1313,* 1313–1314
   secondary, *1313, 1314,* 1314–1315
   zone of, 1315
Osteitis, dissolving, *1335,* 1342, *1342*
Osteitis deformans, 1344
Osteitis fibrosa cystica, 1342
Osteoarthritis, 1363–1366, *1364, 1365*
Osteoblastoma, 1352–1353
Osteoblasts, 1309, *1310*
Osteochondroma, 1319, *1319*
   hereditary multiple osteochondromatosis, 1319
Osteoclasts, *1310,* 1310–1311
   in Paget disease of bone, 1347, *1347*

Osteocytes, 1309–1310, *1310*
Osteodystrophy, renal, *1335*, 1343–1344, *1344*
Osteogenesis imperfecta, 1321–1322
  type I, 1321, *1321*
  type II, 1321
  type III, 1321
  type IV, 1321–1322
Osteoid osteoma, 1352–1353, *1353*
Osteomalacia, 1338–1341
Osteomyelitis, 377, 1327–1330, *1330*
  chronic, *1329*, 1329–1330
  complications, 1329–1330
  of dental origin, 1278
  hematogenous, 1328–1329, *1329*, 1349
  sinusitis in, 1287
  tuberculous of long bones, 1331
  vertebral, 1329, *1330*
Osteonecrosis, 1325–1327, *1326*, 1326t
  corticomedullary, 1349
Osteopetrosis, *1320*, 1320–1321
Osteopontin, 59
Osteoporosis, 1334–1337, *1335*
  primary, 1334–1337, *1335*, *1336*
  secondary, 1337–1338
  smoking and, 316
Osteoprogenitor cells, 1309
Osteosarcoma, 1354–1355, *1355*
  juxtacortical, 1355
Oteitis fibrosa, 1342
Oteitis fibrosa cystica, *1335*, 1342
Otitis externa, malignant, 1297
Otitis media, 1297–1299
  acute mastoiditis, 1298, *1298*
  acute serous, 1298
  acute suppurative, 1298
  chronic serous, 1298
  chronic suppurative, 1298–1299, *1299*
Otosclerosis, 1300, *1300*
Ovary, 966–981
  anatomy and embryology, 966
  cystic lesions, 966–967
    corpus luteum cyst, 967
    follicle cysts, 955–967, *967*
    theca lutein cysts, 967
  polycystic ovary (Stein-Levanthal) syndrome, *960*, 967–969
  stromal hyperthecosis, 969, *969*
  tumors, 969–981 (*see also specific lesions*)
    adenocarcinoma
      endometrioid, 974–975
      mucinous, 974, *975*
      serous, 973–974, *974*
        benign, 970–971
        borderline, 971–973, *973*
        choriocarcinoma, 978
        classification, 970t
        clear cell adenocarcinoma, 975
        cystadenoma, 970, *972*
        dysgerminoma, 976, *977*
        epidemiology, 213
        epithelial, 969–976, *970*, *971*, *972*
        fibroma, 979, *979*
        germ cell, *976*, 976–979
        gonadoblastoma, 979
        granulosa cell tumor, 979–980, *981*
        hilus cell, 981

    Krukenberg, 981, *981*
    malignant, 973–976
    metastatic, 981, *981*
    Sertoli-Leydig cell, 980–981, *981*
    sex cord/stromal, 979–981
    staging, 975t
    steroid cell, 981
    teratoma, 976–978, *977*, *978*
    thecoma, 979
    transitional cell tumor (Brenner tumor), 971, *973*
    yolk sac tumor, 978, *979*
Overhydration, 304
Oxidative stress, 16–20, *18*, *19*, 19t, *20*
  in aging, 37–38
  ionizing radiation in, 21, 22
Oxygen delivery, hemoglobinopathy and, 1044
Oxyphil adenoma (oncocytoma), 1283

P
p53
  in apoptosis, 33
  in carcinogenesis, 192–193
  in colorectal adenocarcinoma, 728
  function, 33
  homeostasis, 33
  inactivation, 33
Pacchionian granulations, 1430
Pachygyria, 1424, *1424*
Paget disease
  of bone, 1344–1348, *1345*, *1346*, *1347*
    vs. giant cell tumor, 1348
  of nipple, 1009–1010, *1010*
  vulvar, *938*, 938–939
Pagetic steal, 1348
Pain, in inflammation, 82
Pale infarcts, *295*, 295–296
Palmar fibromatosis (Dupuytren contracture), 1378
Palsy
  brachial, 276
  facial nerve, 276
  progressive supranuclear, 1471
Pancreas
  aberrant (ectopic), 812
  anatomy and physiology, 812, 820–821, *821*, 821t
  annular, 812
  divisum, 812
Pancreatic diseases
  congenital anomalies, 812
  neoplasms, 817–820
    cancer, 316, *317*, 812, 817–820, *818*, *819*
    cystadenoma, 817
    islet cell, 820–825
    pancreatic pseudocyst, 815, *815*
    pancreatitis (*see also* Pancreatitis)
      acute, 812–816
      chronic, 816–817
Pancreatic islets, 820–821, *821*, 821t
Pancreatic pseudocyst, 815, *815*
Pancreatic tissue, ectopic, 674
Pancreatitis
  acute, 812–816
    hemorrhagic, 813, 815, *815*
    pathogenesis, 813–814, *814*

  alcoholism and, 320
  chronic
    calcifying, 816–817, *817*
    cancer risk and, 819
    complications, 817, *818*
    idiopathic, 816
    pathogenesis, 816
    pathology, 816–817, *817*
  in cystic fibrosis, 250, *250*
  familial hereditary, 816
  interstitial (edematous), 813
Panencephalitis, subacute sclerosing, 1457
Paneth cells, 691
Pannus formation, 1367, *1369*
Papanicolaou (Pap) smear, 1531, 1539, 1540
Papillary adenocarcinoma, 169, *169*
Papillary carcinoma in situ, 1009
Papillary dermis, *1204*, 1208
Papillary mesothelioma, 984, *984*
Papillary necrosis, 871, *871*, 873
Papillary thyroid carcinoma, 1145–1147, *1146*
Papilloma, 168
  bladder, 897, *898*, *899*
    transitional cell, 897, *899*
  exophytic, 897
  inverted, 897
    choroid plexus, 1485
    condylomata acuminata, 370, 903, 932, *933*, 1258
    intraductal, 1006, *1006*
    nasal inverted, 1291, *1291*, *1292*
    sinonasal, 1291, *1291*
Papule, pearly, 1260, *1260*
Papulosis, bowenoid, 905–906, 1256
Paracellular diapedesis, 69
Paracoccidiodomycosis (South American blastomycosis), 438, *438*
Paracrine functions, of PAF, 53
Paradoxical pulmonary embolism, 293
Paraesophageal hernia, 666
Paraganglioma, jugulotympanic, 1299, *1299*
Paragonimiasis, 468
Paralysis
  familial periodic, 1405
  phrenic nerve, 276
Paraneoplastic granulocytosis, 209
Paraneoplastic neuropathies, *1496*, 1496–1497, *1497*
Parasitic infections
  rickettsial vasculitis, 510
  schistosomiasis, 294
Parathyroid disorders, 1150–1153, *1152*, *1153*
  hypoparathyroidism, 1150, *1150*
  parathyroid adenoma, 1151, *1151*
  parathyroid carcinoma, 1152
  primary hyperparathyroidism, 1150–1152
  primary parathyroid hyperplasia, 1151–1152, *1152*
Parietal (oxynic) cells, 673
Parkinson disease, 1468–1471, *1470*
Parotitis, 1280–1281
Paroxysmal cold hemoglobinemia, 1045–1046
Paroxysmal nocturnal dyspnea, 301
Paroxysmal nocturnal hemoglobinuria, 1047

Index

Passive (congestive) hyperemia, *284*, 284–285, *285*
Patent ductus arteriosus, 272
Pathology, definition, 4
Pearly papule, 1260, *1260*
Pediculosis, 1245
Pelger-Huet anomaly, 1063
Peliosis hepatitis, 790, *791*
Pellagra (niacin deficiency), *350*, 350–351
Pelvic inflammatory disease (PID), *930*, 933
Pemphigoid, 669
    bullous, 1223–1224, *1224*, *1225*
Pemphigus, familial benign chronic (Hailey-Hailey disease), 1220
Pemphigus erythematosus, 1221t
Pemphigus foliaceus, 1221t
Pemphigus vegetans, 1221t
Pemphigus vulgaris, *1218*, 1218–1221, *1219*, *1220*, 1221t
Penetrating wounds, of head, *1432*, 1432–1433
Penile fibromatosis (Peyronie disease), 1378
Penis
    cancer, 905–906
        bowenoid papulosis, 905–906
        invasive squamous cell carcinoma, 906
        squamous cell carcinoma in situ, 905–906
        verrucous carcinoma, 906, *906*
    circulatory disturbances, 902
    congenital disorders, 900
    inflammatory disorders, 902–904, 902t
        balanitis, 903–904
        Peyronie disease, 904, 1378
        sexually transmitted diseases, 903, *903*
Pepsinogen I, 680
Peptic ulcer disease, 679–684
    diseases associated with, *682*, 682–684
    duodenal, *683*
    environmental factors, 679
    gastric, *683*
    genetic factors, 679–680
    Helicobacter pylori in, 681–682.*677*, *682*
    hydrochloric acid and, 680
    malignant transformation, 684
    in Meckel diverticulum, 692
    pathogenesis, 681–682.*677*, *682*
    pathology, *683*, 683–684
    physiological factors
        in duodenal ulcers, 680
        in gastric ulcers, 680–681
Peptide, glucagon-like, 345–346
Perforation
    esophageal, 670
    gastric, 689
    of peptic ulcer, 684, 692
Perfusion (driving) pressure, 292
Periapical abscess, 1277
Pericardial effusion, 304
Pericarditis
    constrictive, *100*
    fibrinous, *46*, *47*
Pericytes, 86, 478
Periodontal disease, 1278, *1278*
    in agranulocytosis, 1278
Periosteum, 1309
Peripheral chondrosarcoma, 1356

Peripheral giant cell oral grauloma, 1274, *1274*
Peripheral nervous system
    healing in, 114
    tumors, 1499–1500
Peripheral neuropathies, 1494–1498, 1494t (*see also* Neuropathy)
    in cancer, 208
    in lead poisoning, 331
Peripheral vascular resistance, 292
Periportal fibrosis, 771
Peritoneal dialysis, peritonitis caused by, 736
Peritoneal effusion, 304
Peritoneum, female reproductive, 981–984 (*see also* Endometriosis)
    mesothelial tumors, 984
    pseudomyxoma peritonei, *985*, *985*
    serous tumors, 984–985, *985*
Peritonitis
    chemical, 736
    peritoneal dialysis and, 736
    spontaneous bacterial, 736, 761
    tuberculous, 736
Peritonsillar abscess (quinsy), 1293–1294
Peritubular/tubular fibrosis, 909, *910*
Perlecan, 91t
Permanent cells, 108
Pernicious anemia, 675–676, *1034*, *1035*, *1036*, 1468, 1478
Peroxisome proliferator–related receptors, 346
Peroxynitrite, 21
Pertussis (whooping cough), 382
Petechiae, *287*, *287*
Peutz-Jeghers syndrome, *705*, *705*, *706*
Peyer patches, 690, 693
Peyronie disease (penile fibromatosis), 904, 1378
p16 gene, 896
Phacoanaphylactic endophthalmitis, 1508
Phacomatoses, 195
Phagocytes, mononuclear, 124–125, 129–130
Phagocytosis, 70, *71*
    congenital defects in, 74–75, 74t
Phagolysosomes, 70
Pharyngitis, 1293
    streptococcal, 379–380
Phencyclidine (PCP), 323
Phenylketonuria (PKU), 258–260, *259*, 1466
Phenytoin-induced lymphadenopathy, 1089
Pheochromocytoma, 1164–1167, *1165*, *1166*
Philadelphia chromosome, 185
Phimosis, 900
Phlebothrombosis, 515
Phocomelia, 223
Phosphatases, 75
Phosphatidylinositol biphosphate (PIP$_2$), 64
Phosphatidylinositol-3 kinase (PI3K), 33, 99
Phosphofructokinase deficiency, 1403
Phospholipase C, 99
Phospholipid metabolism, of cell membranes, 64
Phospholipidosis, 790
Phthisis bulbi, 1524, *1524*
Phyllodes tumor, 1014–1015, *1015*
Physical injuries, 338–344

Phytobezoar, 689
Pick disease, 1479, *1480*
Pickwickian syndrome, 347
Piecemeal hepatic necrosis, 770, *771*
Pigmented villonodular synovitis, 1377, *1378*
Pigments, exogenous, 12, *13*
PI3K, 33
Pineal gland, 1169
Pineoblastoma, 1169
Pineocytoma, 1169
Pinguecula, 1506
Pinta, 411
Pinworms (enterobiasis), 462
Pituitary disorders, 1129–1134
    hypopituitarism, *1129*, 1129–1130
    of hypothalamic-pituitary axis, 1133–1134.1128t
    pituitary adenomas, 1130–1133, 1130t, *1131*
    of posterior pituitary, 1133, *1133*
Placenta
    anatomy, 986
    embryonal development, 985
    infections, 986
        chorioamnionitis, 986
        villitis, 986
    placenta accreta, *988*, 988–989
    retroplacental hematoma, 988
Placental site trophoblastic tumor, 993–994
Placenta previa, smoking and, 318, *319*
Plague, 402
Plantar fibromatosis, 1378
Plantar interdigital neuroma (Morton neuroma), 1498–1499
Plantar warts, 1256
Planter warts, 370
Plaque
    atherosclerotic, *487*, *488*, 488–490, *489*
        rupture, 491
    demyelinated, 1464, *1464*
    senile (neuritic), 1478, *1478*
Plasma cell angiofollicular lymph node hyperplasia, 1088
Plasma cells, in chronic inflammation, 77
Plasmacytoid lymphoma, 1063
Plasmacytoma, 1295
    extramedullary, 1099, 1103
Plasmacytosis, 1085–1086
Plasminogen, 48, *48*, 1051
Plasminogen activator inhibitors, 73
Platelet-activating factor (PAF), *53*, 53–54, 132
Platelet adhesion, 481
Platelet-derived growth factor (PDGF), 186
Platelet-derived growth factor (PDGF) receptor, 188
Platelet disorders, 1048–1057
    acquired qualitative, 1056
    hemolytic-uremic syndrome, 1055
    hereditary
        alpha storage pool disease (grey platelet syndrome), 1056
        Bernard-Soulier syndrome, 1055–1056
        delta storage pool disease, 1056
        Glanzmann thrombasthenia, 1056
        Kasabach-Merritt syndrome, 1056

purpura
- idiopathic (immune cytopenic), 1053, *1053*
- posttransfusion, 1054
- thrombotic thrombocytopenic, 1054–1055
- splenic sequestration, 1055
- thrombocytopenia, 1052–1053, 1053t
  - May-Heggin anomaly, 1052
  - neonatal, 1054
  - pregnancy-associated, 1054
- thrombocytosis, 1056
  - clonal, 1056
  - reactive, 1056

Platelets, inflammatory response, 62–63, *63*
Pleomorphic rhabdomyosarcoma, 1381
Pleomorphism, 170, *171*
Pleural effusion, 303–304
Pleuritis, fibrinous, 46, *47*
Plexiform neurofibroma, 246
Plummer-Vinson (Paterson-Kelly) syndrome, 664, 672
PMNs, 59–61, *60, 61, 65,* 65–70, *66, 67,* 1025–1026
- in phagocytosis, 70–73, *71*
- in wound repair, 86, *87*

Pneumatosis cystoides intestinalis, 708
Pneumonia
- aspiration, in tracheoesophageal fistula, 663–664
- chlamydial, 417
- *E. coli,* 389
- mycoplasmal, 420–421
- neonatal, 381
- *Pneumocystis carinii,* 151, 446–447, *447, 1533*
- streptococcal, 381

Pneumonic tularemia, 403
Point mutations, 240, *241*
Polyarteritis nodosa, 505, *505,* 860, *860*
Polychondritis, relapsing, 1296, *1297*
Polycyclic aromatic hydrocarbons, as carcinogens, 201
Polycystic kidney disease
- autosomal dominant, *833,* 833–834
- autosomal recessive, *833,* 834, *834*

Polycystic ovary (Stein-Leventhal) syndrome, *960,* 967–969
Polycythemia
- absolute, 1048
- relative, 1048
- secondary, 1048

Polycythemia vera, 1070t, 1071t, 1072–1074
Polyglandular autoimmune syndromes, 1157
Polymicrogyria, 1423, *1424*
Polymyositis, 161–162, *1398,* 1398–1399
Polyneuropathy, in alcoholism, 322
Polyostotic fibrous dysplasia, 1349
Polyps
- aural, 1296
- colorectal, 721–727
- endocervical, 942–943, *945*
- endometrial, *956,* 956–957
- fibroepithelial vaginal, 939
- gastric, 684–685
  - fundic gland, 685
- hyperplastic, 684
- tubular adenoma (adenomatous polyps), 684
- nasal, 1287, *1287*
- in ulcerative colitis, *717*

Polytopic effect, 221
Pompe disease, 259, 1401–1402, *1402*
Poroma, 1262
Porphyria, acute intermittent, 791
Porphyria cutanea tarda, 791
Portal hypertension, *757,* 757–761, *759,* 797
- intrahepatic, 758
- posthepatic, *757,* 758–759, *759*
- prehepatic, 758
- systemic complications, 759–760

Positive thymic selection, 123
Postinfectious/postvaccinal encephalomyelitis, 1464–1465
Postpericardiotomy syndrome, 304
Posttransfusion purpura, 1054
Posttransplant lymphoproliferative disorder, 1116–1117, *1117*
Pott disease, *1330,* 1330–1331, 1447–1448, *1448*
Potter complex, *220,* 221
Potter sequence (oligohydramnios sequence), 831
Potter syndrome, 890
PPC4 gene, 193
p15/p16 genes, 193
Prader-Willi syndrome, 266–267
Precursor T-acute lymphoblastic leukemia, 1093, *1093*
Preeclampsia/eclampsia, 865, *865, 866,* 986–988, *987*
Pregnancy
- amniotic fluid changes in, *270*
- drug abuse in, 324
- ectopic, 965–966, *966*
- endometrium of, 953, *953*
- gestational trophoblastic disease, *990,* 990–994, 992t
- hypertensive disease in
  - preeclampsia, 865, *865, 866*
  - preeclampsia/eclampsia, 986–988, *987*
- intrahepatic cholestasis of, 750
- multiple gestations, 989, *989*
- spontaneous abortion, 990

Pregnancy-associated thrombocytopenia, 1054
Prekallikrein, 48, *48*
Premature aging, diseases of, 37
Prematurity, 269–277, *270*
- Apgar score, 270, 271t
- hemolytic anemia, vitamin E in, 354
- neonatal necrotizing enterocolitis in, 711
- organ immaturity, 269–270, *270*
- respiratory distress syndrome (RDS), 270–273, *271, 272,* 606
- retinopathy of, 1519, *1521*

Presbyopia, 1508
Presenilin, 1478
Pressure, perfusion, 292
Priapism, 902
Primary adrenocortical insufficiency (Addison disease), 1156–1157, *1157*
Primary aldosteronism (Conn syndrome), 1163

Primary amebic meningoencephalitis, 456
Primary biliary cirrhosis, 779–780, *780*
Primary effusion lymphoma, 152, 1106
Primary healing, 109–111, *110*
Primary hyperparathyroidism, 1150–1152, *1335,* 1337, *1341,* 1341–1342
Primary (idiopathic) hypothyroidism, 1137
Primary parathyroid hyperplasia, 1151–1152, *1152*
Primary pigmented nodular adrenocortical disease (Carney complex), 1161
Primary sclerosing cholangitis, 780–781, *781*
Prion diseases (spongiform encephalopathies), 10, 1458–1462, *1459,* 1459t
- Creutzfeld-Jakob disease, 1198–1200, 1459, *1459,* 1461
- fatal familial insomnia, 1461–1462
- Gerstmann-Straussler-Scheinker syndrome, 1459, 1461
- kuru, 1461

Prion proteins, 1194–1195
Progenitor cells, *1022,* 1022–1023
Progeria, 37, *37*
Progesterone deficiency, 956
Programmed cell death, 29–34
Progression factors, 189
Progressive disphyseal dysplasia, 1321
Progressive multifocal leukoencephalopathy, *1457,* 1457–1458
Progressive supranuclear palsy, 1471
Progressive systemic sclerosis (scleroderma), *1238,* 1239, *1239*
Proinflammatory molecules, 50, *51*
Prolactinoma, 1131
Prolapse, rectal, 721
Proliferating cell nuclear antigen (PCNA), 172
Prostaglandin deficiency, 674
Prostanoids, as inflammatory mediators, 53–54
Prostate
- benign prostatic hypertrophy (nodular prostatic hyperplasia), 918–920, *919, 920, 921*
- cancer, 921–925
  - adenocarcinoma, 921–925, *922*
  - epidemiology, 212, *213*

Prostate-specific acid phosphatase (PSAP), 172
Prostate-specific antigen (PSA) test, 924, *924*
Protease inhibitors, 75
- in pancreatitis, 813

Protein(s)
- abnormal stored, 10–14, *11, 13*
- acute phase, 81, 81t
- adipocyte complement-related, 346
- bactericidal/permeability-increasing (BPI), 74
- C-reactive, atherosclerosis and, 494
- eosinophilic bactericical, 74
- heat shock, 58
- hydroxyl radicals and, 19
- prion, 1194–1195
- SPARC (secreted protein acidic and rich in cysteine), 59
- stress, 58

Proteinase inhibitors, 73
Proteinases, 71–73, *72*, 72t
Protein C deficiencies, 1061
Protein folding, *11*, 11–12
Protein kinase C, 64
  in diabetes mellitus, 1181
Protein S deficiencies, 1061
Protein tyrosine kinase receptors, *98*, 98–99
Proteolytic enzymes, in metastasis, 179
Proteolytic inactivation, of complement system, 51
Prothombotic agents, 61
Prothrombinase complex, 480–481
Protooncogenes, 184 (*see also* Oncogenes)
Protozoal diseases, 441–456
  African trypanosomiasis (sleeping sickness), 454–456, *455*
  amebiasis, 447–450, *448*, *449*, *450*, 793, *793*
  babesiosis, 444
  Chagas disease, 454, *454*
  cryptosporidiosis, 450
  giardiasis, 450–451
  intestinal, 695, *696*
  leishmaniasis, 451–452, *452*, *453*
    visceral (kala azar), 793
  of liver, 793, *793*
  malaria, *441*, 441–444, *442–443*, *444*
  primary amebic meningoencephalitis, 456
  schistosomiasis, 758
  toxoplasmosis, *445*, 445–446
Provisional matrix, 90, 101–102
Proximal tubular necrosis, 332
P-selectin, 67
Pseudocyst, pancreatic, 815, *815*
Pseudodiverticulosis, intramural, 665
Pseudogout, 1373–1374, *1374*
Pseudohermaphroditism
  female, 908, 908t
  male, 908, 908t
Pseudohypoparathyroidism, 1150, *1150*
Pseudomembranous colitis, 711, *711*
Pseudomembranous cystitis, 892
Pseudomembranous tonsillitis, 1293
Pseudomonas aeruginosa, 396
Pseudomonas infection, in cystic fibrosis, 251
Pseudomyxoma peritonei, 985, *985*
Pseudopseudohypoparathyroidism, 1150
Pseudopyloric metaplasia, 677
Psittacosis (ornithosis), 416–417
Psoas abscess, 1331
Psoriasis, 1213–1218, *1216*, *1217*
Psoriatic arthritis, 1371
Psychosis, Korsakoff, 321–322
11p-syndrome, 236
PTEN gene, 193
Pterygium, 1506
Pubertal hypertrophy, of breast, 1000
Puerperal sepsis, 380–381
Pulmonary (inhalational) anthrax, 404
Pulmonary disease, in cystic fibrosis, 250
Pulmonary edema, 285, *285*, 301, 301–303, *302*, *303*
  altitude-related, 337
Pulmonary embolism, *290*, 290–292
  fate of, 292
  with infarction, 291
  without infarction, 291

massive, 291, *291*
paradoxical, 293
saddle, 291, *291*
Pulmonary hypertension, 285
Pulmonary infarction, 291, 296
Pulmonary infections
  Enterobacter, 395
  Klebsiella, 395
  Legionnaires disease, 395–396, *396*
  melioidosis, 397, *397*
  Pseudomonas aeruginosa, 396
Pulmonary surfactant, 270–273, *271*, *272*
Pulpitis, 1277
Pure red cell aplasia, 1031–1032
  acute self-limited, 1032
  chronic relapsing, 1032
  Diamond-Blackfan syndrome, 1032
Purine nucleoside phophorylase deficiency, 146t, 147
Purpura, 287
  Henoch-Schönlein, 859–860, 1052
  idiopathic (immune cytopenic), 1053, *1053*
  posttransfusion, 1054
  purpura simplex, 1052
  senile, 1052
  thrombotic thrombocytopenic, 865, 1054–1055
Purse-string closure, 106
Purulent effusion, 46, *47*
Purulent exudate, 46, *47*
Pyelonephritis
  acute, 870–872, *871*
  chronic, *872*, 872–873, *873*
  papillary necrosis in, 871, *871*, 973
  xanthogranulomatous, 872–873
Pyelophlebitis
  portal vein, 732
  suppurative, 758
Pyknosis, 25
Pylephlebitic liver abscess, 792, *792*
Pyloric glands, 673
Pyloric membrane, congenital, 674
Pyloric obstruction, in peptic ulcer disease, 684
Pyogenic gram-positive cocci, 377–381
Pyogenic granuloma, 116, 936, 1285
Pyogenic liver abscess, 792
Pyogenous granuloma, 1272, *1272*
Pyometra, 954
Pyridoxine (vitamin B₆), 351–352

Q
Q fever, 420
13q-syndrome, 236
Quinsy (peritonsillar abscess), 1293–1294

R
Rachischisis, 1420, *1420*
Rad, 339
Radial growth phase melanoma, 1247–1248, *1249*, *1250*
Radiation (*see also* Radiation injury)
  breast cancer and, 1006
  electromagnetic, 344
  microwave, 344
  in multiple myeloma, 1100
  thyroid cancer and, 1145

Radiation dermatitis, 341, *342*
Radiation enteritis, 703
Radiation enterocolitis, 721
Radiation esophagitis, 669
Radiation injury, 338–344, *341*, 341–342
  carcinogenic, 342–344, *343*
  linear no-threshold hypothesis, 343
  localized, *341*, 341–342
  whole-body, 339–341, *340*
Radiation lymphedema, 519
Radiation vasculitis, 510
Radicular (apical periodontal) cyst, 1277
Radon, 344
Rales, 301
ras oncogene, 188–189, *189*, 727
Raynaud phenomenon, 503, *504*, 1239
Rb gene, 191–193, *192*
Reactive bone formation, 1326–1327, *1327*
  myositis ossificans, 1327, *1328*
Reactive oxygen species (ROS), 16–18, *18*, *19*, 19t
  in apoptosis, 31–33, *32*
  bactericidal activity, 73–74, 73t
  in diabetes mellitus, 1181
  cellular defenses, 20
  hydrogen peroxide, 18–19, 19t
  hydroxyl radicals, *19*, 19–20, *20*
  as inflammatory mediators, 57–58
  in necrosis, 28–29
  peroxynitrite, 20
  superoxide, 18, *19*, 19t
Reactive thrombocytosis, 1056
Receptors, peroxisome proliferator–related, 346
Reciprocal translocations, 227–228, *228*, *229*
Rectal atresia, 711
Rectal prolapse, 721
Rectal ulcer, 721
Red blood cells
  disorders of, 1028–1048, 1028t (*see also* Anemia)
  normal structure and function, *1026*, 1026–1028, *1027*, 1028t
Red infarcts, *295*, 295–296
Reed-Sternberg cells, *1012*, 1111, *1111*, 1115
Reepithelialization, 106–107
Reflux, vesicoureteral, 892
Reflux esophagitis, 666–667
Reflux gastropathy, 677–678
Refractory anemia, 1078–1079
Regeneration, 107–109
Regional occlusive cerebrovascular disease, *1441*, 1441–1443
Reiter syndrome, 903, 905, 1370
Rejection, transplant (*see* Transplant rejection)
Relapsing fever, 413
Relapsing polychondritis, 1296, *1297*
Remodeling, 95–97
  of vessel wall, 477
Renal agenesis, 831
Renal artery stenosis, 863
Renal atheroembolism, 863, *864*
Renal calculi (stones), 876–877, *877*
Renal cancer
  renal cell carcinoma, 882–884, *883*, 883t
  transitional cell carcinoma, 884

Wilms tumor (nephroblastoma), 881–882, *882*
Renal colic, 876
Renal disease
　anemia of chronic, 1033
　in systemic lupus erythematosus, 156–157, *157*
　Wegener granulomatosis, *507*, 507–508
Renal dysplasia, 831–835, *832*
　types, 832, *832*
Renal failure
　acute, urinalysis in, 869t
　in gout, 1373
　hepatorenal, 756
Renal glomerulus (glomeruli), 111–112, *112*
Renal hypoplasia, 831
Renal infarcts, 866, *866*
Renal oncocytoma, 880
Renal osteodystrophy, *1335*, 1343–1344, *1344*
　adynamic (ARD), 1343
Renal papillary necrosis, 871, *871*, 873
Renal pelvis and ureter
　congenital disorders, 889–890
　tumors, 891
　ureteritis and obstruction, 890, *891*
Renal transitional cell carcinoma, *1535*
Renal tubular necrosis, acute, 306, *309*, 867–869, *868*, 868t, *869*
Renal tubules, 830
　cortical, 111
　medullary, 111
Rendu-Osler-Weber syndrome (hereditary hemorrhagic telangiectasia), 758, 1052
Renin–angiotensin–aldosterone system, 499
　in shock, 308
Reproductive disease, in cystic fibrosis, 250
Reproductive system (*see* Female reproductive system; Male reproductive system)
Respiratory disease
　in lupus erythematosus, 157
　Wegener granulomatosis, *507*, 507–508
Respiratory distress syndrome, of newborn, 270–273, *271*, *272*, 606
Respiratory infections, 378
Respiratory syncytial virus, 364
Respiratory tract, normal epithelium, *1533*
Respiratory tract cytology, *1533*
Respiratory viruses, 363–364
　adenovirus, 364
　common cold, 363
　croup, 363
　influenza, 363
　respiratory syncytial virus, 364
　severe acute respiratory syndrome (SARS), 364
Restenosis after angioplasty, 492–493
Rests, nephrogenic, 881
Retention (juvenile) polyps, 726, *726*
Reticular dermis, *1202*, 1208
Reticular dysgenesis, 1169
Reticulate bodies, 414
Retina, normal, *1510*
Retinal detachment, 1518
Retinal disorders, 1508–1509 (*see also under* Eye)

Retinal hemorrhage, high altitude related, 337
Retinitis pigmentosa, 1518, *1519*
Retinoblastoma, 191–193, *192*, 228, 1525–1526, *1526*
Retinoids, 20
　in cancer development, 182
Retinopathy
　diabetic, 1183
　of prematurity, 1519, *1521*
RET protooncogene, 1146, 1165, *1165*
Retroperitoneal fibrosis, 737
Retroplacental hematoma, 988
Reye syndrome, 790
Rhabdomyolysis, 1405–1406
Rhabdomyosarcoma, 1380–1381, *1381*
　alveolar, 1381
　embryonal (sarcoma botryoides), 940–941, *941*, 1296, *1296*, 1381
　pleomorphic, 1381
Rhagades, 226
Rheumatoid arthritis, 1088, 1366–1371
　genetic factors, 1366
　immune factors, 1365
　pannus formation, 1365–1367, *1366*, *1367*, *1369*
Rheumatoid factor, 1366
Rheumatoid nodules, 1367, *1368*
Rh incompatibility, 273–275, *274*
Rhinitis, 1286
　in congenital syphilis, 226
Rhinoscleroma, 1288–1289, *1289*
Rhinosporidiosis, 1289–1290
RhoGAM, 275
Rhus sp. (poison ivy), 1236
Riboflavin deficiency, 351, *351*
Rice bodies, 1366, 1367, *1367*, *1368*
Richter syndrome, 1098
Rickets, 1341, *1341*
Rickettsial infections, *417*, 417–420, 417t
　Q fever, 420
　Rocky Mountain spotted fever, 417–418, *418*
　typhus
　　louse-borne (epidemic), 418–419, *419*
　　murine (endemic), 419
　　scrub, 419–420
Rickettsial vasculitis, 510
Riedel thyroiditis, 1144, *1144*
Ring chromosomes, 230
Ring of Delacroix, 1315
Rings, esophageal, 664, *664*
River blindness (onchocerciasis), 458, 1506
Robertsonian translocation, 228
Rocky Mountain spotted fever, 417–418, *418*
Rodent ulcer, 1260
Rod (nemaline) myopathy, 1396, *1397*
Roentgen, 339
Rolling, 66, *66*, 68, *69*
Rotaviruses, 367, 694
Rotor syndrome, 750
Rubella, 365–366
　in TORCH complex, 224
Rupture
　amniotic membranes, *319*
　atherosclerotic plaues, 491
　gastric, 689
　splenic, 1120

S

Saber shin, 226
Saccular cerebral aneurysm, *1436*, 1437, *1437*
Sacrococcygeal teratoma, 278
Sagittal sinus thrombosis, *1443*
Saliva, 1276
Salivary glands, 1280–1281, *1281*
　malignant tumors
　　adenoid cystic carcinoma, 1284, *1284*
　　mucoepidermoid carcinoma, 1284, *1284*
　　monomorphic adenoma, 1283, *1283*
　　oncocytoma (oxyphil) adenoma, 1283
　　Warthin tumor, 1283, *1283*
　parotitis, 1280–1281
　pleomorphic adenoma, 1282, *1282*, *1283*
　sialolithiasis, 1280
　sialorrhea, 1280
　Sjögren syndrome, 1280, 1281, *1281*
　xerostomia, 1280, *1280*
Salmonella enterocolitis, 389–390
Salmonellosis
　nontyphoidal, 693–694
　typhoid fever, 693
Salpingitis, 965
　tuberculous, 933
Salt-wasting congenital adrenal hyperplasia, 1154
Sandhoff disease, 254
Sarcoid (granulomatous) myositis, 1400, *1400*
Sarcoidosis, 1237–1238, *1238*
　uveitis in, 1508
Sarcoma, 168–169, *169*
　endometrial stromal, 961–962, *962*
　Ewing, 1358–1360, *1359*
　foreign-body, 204
　Kaposi, 152, 198, 518, 1263–1264, *1264*, *1265*
　mast cell, 1067
　myeloid, 1082–1083, *1083*
　synovial, 1382, *1382*, *1383*
Sarcoma botryoides (embryonal rhabdomyocsarcoma), 940–941, *941*
Sarcomatous change, in Paget disease of bone, 1348
Sarcomere, 1388
SARS (severe acute respiratory syndrome), 364
Scabies, 1245, *1245*
Scalded skin syndrome, 377
Scarlet fever, 80, 380, 1271
Scarring, 75, 114
　excessive (keloid formation), 115, *115*
Schatzki ring, 664, *664*
Schilling test, 700, 1036
Schistosomiasis (bilharziasis), 294, 464–467, *465*, *466*, *467*, 758
　hepatic, 467, *467*
　urogenital, 467
Schmidt syndrome (polyglandular autoimmune syndrome type 2), 1157
Schwannoma, 1300, 1301, 1302, 1487, *1487*, 1498–1499, *1499*
SCID (severe combined immunodeficiency), 146–147, 146t
Scirrhous adenocarcinoma, 169, *169*

Scleroderma, 159–161, *160*, 1239, *1239*
  CREST variant, 161
  esophageal stenosis in, 666
Scleroproteins, 92, *93*
Sclerosing adenosis, 1002, *1004*
Sclerosing cholangitis, primary, 780–781, *781*
Sclerosis, Mönckberg medial, 503
Scoliosis, 1318
Scrapie, 1194–1196, 1459
Scrotal cancer, 906
Scrotal edema, 902
Scrotal inguinal hernia, 902
Scrotal masses, 900–902, *901*
Scrub typhus (Tsutsugamushi fever), 419–420
Scurvy, 352–353, *353*, 1052, 1317–1318, *1318*
Sebaceous follicles, 1211
Seborrheic keratosis, 1258
Secondary hyperparathyroidism, 1153, *1153*
Secretory leukocyte proteinase inhibitor (SLPI), 73
Seizure disorders, 1425–1426
Selectins, 67, 120
Selective IgA defiency, 145, 145t
Senile atrophy, 6
Senile cardiac amyloidosis, 1192
Senile (neuritic) plaque, 1478, *1478*
Senile purpura, 1052
Sensorimotor peripheral neuropathy, in cancer, 208
Sepsis
  Escherichia coli, 389
  jaundice in, 751
  neonatal, 381
  puerperal, 380–381
Septate vagina, 939
Septic arthritis, 383, 1349
Septicemia, 306–307, 378
Septicemic anthrax, 404
Septic infarcts, 296, *296*
Septic shock, 305–307
Septic thrombophlebitis, 1288
Sequestration crisis, in sickle cell disease, 1043
Sequestrum, 1329
Serine proteinases, 73
Serosanguineous exudate, 46
Serous adenocarcinoma
  endometrial, 960
  ovarian, 973–974, *974*
  peritoneal, 985
Serous borderline tumors, peritoneal, 984–985, *985*
Serous exudate, 46
Serpins, 73
Serrated adenoma, 724
Sertoli cells, 889
Sertoli-Leydig cell tumors
  ovarian, 980–981, *981*
  testicular, 917–918, *918*
Serum protein electrophoresis (SPEP), *142*, 142–143
Serum sickness, 135, 504
Severe acute respiratory syndrome (SARS), 364
Severe combined immunodeficiency (SCID), 146–147, 146t, 1169

Sex cord/stromal tumors, ovarian, 979–981
Sex distribution
  chemical carcinogenicity, 203
  in life span, 35
  peptic ulcer disease, 679
  stomach cancer, 686
  tumor type, 210t, 211, *211*
Sex hormones, oral contraceptives, side effects, 325, 325–326
Sexually transmitted diseases (STDs), 384–387
  AIDS/HIV, 518
  chancroid, 386, 931
  chlamydial, *414, 415*, 415–417, 931–932
  condyloma acuminatum, 370, 903, 932, *933*, 1258
  cytomegalovirus, 932
  Gardnerella, 931
  gonorrhea, 384–386, *385, 386*, 929, *930*
  granuloma inguinale, 386–387, *387*, 931
  herpesvirus, 932
  human papillomavirus (HPV), 932
  lymphogranuloma venereum, *415*, 415–416, 932
  Molluscum contagiosum, 932
  Mycoplasma, 931
  pelvic inflammatory disease (PID), *930*, 933
  penile lesions, 903, *903*
  syphilis, 225–226, *408*, 408–411, *409*, 794, 929–931, 1273, 1288, 1331–1332, *1332*, 1448–1450, *1449, 1450*
  trichomoniasis, 933
  urethritis in, 904
Sézary syndrome, 1109–1110, *1110*
Shigellosis, 391, 693
Shingles (herpes zoster), 370, *370, 371*
Shock
  anaphylactic, 305
  cardiogenic, 305
  classification, 305, *305*
  complications, *307*
  endotoxic, 305–307, *306*
  hepatic congestion in, 792
  hypovolemic, 305
  in inflammatory conditions, 82
  meningococcal, *383*, 383–384
  multiple organ dysfunction syndrome (MODS), 307–308
  neurogenic, 305, *307*
  renal cortical necrosis in, 866–867, *867*
  renal tubular necrosis in, 867–869, *868*, 868t, *869*
  septic, 305–307
  toxic shock syndrome, 378, 934
  vascular compensatory mechanisms, 308
Sialolithiasis, 1280
Sialorrhea, 1280
Sickle cell disease, *1041*, 1041–1043, *1042*
Sickle cell nephropathy, 865–866
Sickle cell trait, 1043
Sievert (radiation measure), 339
Sigmoid volvulus, 705
Silent adenoma, 1133
Simian B virus, 1456
Simian immunodeficiency virus (SIV), 153
Sinonasal papilloma, 1291

Sinus histiocytosis, 75, 1090, *1090*
Sinusitis, 1287–1288
  mucocele in, 1287, *1288*
  in osteomyelitis, 1287
  septic thrombophlebitis in, 1288
Sinusoids, hepatic, 745, 745–746
Sipple syndrome (MEN type 2A), 1165
Situs inversus, 674
Sjögren syndrome, 158–159, *159*, 1281, *1281*
  lymphoma in, 1094
Skeletal deformities, in Marfan syndrome, 244
Skeletal disorders, in alcoholism, 321
Skeletal muscle, 1386–1411
  biopsy, 1390
  in cancer, 208
  congenital myopathies, 1394–1396, *1395*
    central core disease, *1395*, 1395–1396
    central nuclear (myotubular) myopathy, 1396, *1397*
    rod (nemaline) myopathy, 1396, *1397*
  denervation/reinervation, 1406–1407, 1406–1411
    critical illness myopathy, *1410*, 1411
    Kugelberg-Weilander disease, 1409
    spinal muscular atrophy, 1409–1411
    steroid myopathy, 1411
    type grouping, 1409, *1409*
    type II fiber atrophy, 1409–1411, *1410*
    type predominance, 1409
    Werdig-Hoffman disease, 1409, *1410*
  embryology and anatomy, 1388–1389
    myofiber, 1388–1389, *1389*
  enzyme histochemistry, 1390
  general pathological reactions, 1390–1391, *1391*
  histochemistry, 1390
  inflammatory myopathies, 1396–1400
    dermatomyositis, 1399–1400, *1400*
    granulomatous (sarcoid) myositis, 1400, *1400*
    inclusion body myositis, *1399*, 11399
    polymyositis, *1398*, 1398–1399
    vasculitis in periarteritis nodosa, 1400, *1400*
  inherited metabolic diseases, 1401–1405
    familial periodic paralysis, 1405
    glycogen-storage diseases (glycogenoses), 1401–1403
    lipid myopathies, 1403, *1404*
    mitochondrial diseases, 1404, 11405
    myoadenylate deaminase deficiency, 1404–1405
  Lambert-Eaton syndrome, 1401
  muscular dystrophy, *1391*, 1391–1394
    congenital, 1394
    Duchenne and Becker, 1391–1394, *1392*, 1392t, *1393*
    myotonic dystrophy, 1394
  myasthenia gravis, 1401
  rhabdomyolysis, 1405–1406
Skin, 1202–1265
  acne vulgaris, 1241, *1242–1243*
  anatomy and function, *1204*, 1204–1211, *1205, 1206, 1207, 1208, 1209, 1210*
  basement membrane zone diseases, 1221–1231, 1221t, *1222*

epidermolysis bullosa, 1221–1223, 1221t, *1222*
connective-tissue disorders, 1239, *1239*
epidermal diseases, 1211–1221, 1221t
infections and infestations, 1241–1246
  arthropod, 1245, *1245*
inflammatory diseases of vascular bed, 1234–1239
inflammatory pannicular disorders, 1239–1240
  erythema induratum, 1240
  erythema nodosum, 1239–1240, *1240*
neoplasms, 1246–1265
  dermatofibroma, 12556
  malignant melanoma, 1246–1257
stages of healing, 100t
in systemic lupus erythematosus, 156
wound healing in, 109–111, *110*
Skin cancer, 209
  basal cell carcinoma, 1258–1259, *1259*
  epidemiology, 212
  malignant melanoma, 1246–1257
  UV radiation in, 203
Skin sensitivity testing, 143
Skull fractures, in newborn, 275
Sleep apnea, in crib death, 276
Sleeping sickness (African trypanosomiasis), 454–456, *455*
Sliding hernia, 666
Slow-reacting substance of anaplylaxis (SRS-A), 54
Small-bowel disease, 690–708
  congenital, 691–692
    atresia and stenosis, 691
    duplications, 691–692
    malrotation, 692
    Meckel diverticulum, 692, *692*
    meconium ileus in cystic fibrosis, 692
  Crohn disease, 697
  infections, 693–695
    bacterial diarrhea, 693–694
    fungal, 695
    parasitic, 695, *696*
    tuberculosis, 694–695
    viral gastroenteritis, 694
  ischemic
    acute, 695–697, *697*
    arterial occlusion, 695–697, *696*, *697*
    mesenteric vein thrombosis, 696–697, *697*
    nonocclusive, 695–696
    sorbitol-induced, 697
  malabsorption, 697–700
    abetalipoproteinemia, 703
    congenital lymphangiectasia, 704
    hypogammaglobulinemia, 703–704
    radiation enteritis, 704
    tropical sprue, 704
    Whipple disease, 702, *703*
  mechanical obstruction, 704–705
  neoplasms, 705–708
    benign, 705
    malignant, 705–708
  pneumatosis cystoides intestinalis, 708
  vascular diseases, 695–697
Small cell carcinoma
  bronchial, *1534*
  thymic, 1122

Small for gestational age (SGA) classification, 269
Small intestine, anatomy, 690–691
Smallpox (variola), 366, *367*
Small storage granules, 70, *71*
Smoking, 314–319
  asbestos exposure and, 204
  atherosclerosis and, 493
  cardiovascular complications, 314, *315*
  diseases related to, *314*
  fetal tobacco syndrome, 316–219, *318*
  lung cancer and, 315–36, *316*
  mortality from, 314, *315*
  nonneoplastic diseases and, 316, *318*
  pancreatic cancer and, 817
  passive, 319
  in peptic ulcer disease, 679
  thromboangiitis obliterans and, 508–509, *510*
Smooth muscle, of vessel wall, 475
Smooth muscle cells, in wound repair, 86
Smooth muscle tumors, 1381–1382
Sodium retention, 299, *300*
Soft tissue tumors, 1365–1381
  of adipose tissue, 1378–1379
  angiolipoma, 1380
  fibromatosis, 1377
  fibrosarcoma, 1379, *1379*
  liposarcoma, 1380, *1380*
  malignant fibrous histiocytoma, *1379*, 1379–1380
  nodular fasciitis, 1377, *1379*
  rhabdomyosarcoma, *1380*, 1380–1381
  smooth muscle, 1381–1382
    leiomyoma, 1381
    leiomyosarcoma, 1381–1382
Solar cheilitis, *1276*
Solar cheilosis, *1276*
Solar lentigo, 1255–1256, *1257*
Solitary bone cyst, *1350*, 1351–1352
Solitary echondroma, 1322
Solitary osseous myeloma, 1099, 1103
Solitary rectal ulcer syndrome, 721
Solvents and vapors, toxicity, 328
Somatostatinoma (delta cell tumor), 823
Somatotrope adenoma, 1131–1132, 1131–1132.*1125*, *1132*
South American blastomycosis, 438, *438*
Space of Disse, 745, *745*
SPARC (secreted protein acidic and rich in cysteine), 59
Specific granules, 70, *71*
Spermatocele, *901*, 902
S phase, of cell cycle, 108
Spherocytosis, hereditary, 1039, *1039*
Sphingomyelin, 255
Sphingomyelinase, 255
Spider angiomas, 757
Spina bifida, 222, 222–223, *223*, *1419*, 1419–1421, *1420*
Spina bifida occulta, 1420
Spinal cord, subacute combined degeneration, 1468
  in pernicious anemia, 1478
Spinal cord disorders, in cancer, 208
Spinal cord injuries, *1433*, 1433–1434
  concussion, 1434

contusion, 1434, *1434*
hyperextension injury, 1434, *1434*
hyperflexion injury, 1434, *1434*
Spinal cord malformations, *1420*, 1422
Spinal muscular atrophy, 1409–1411
Spine, tuberculosis of (Pott disease), 1447–1448, *1448*
Spirochetal infections, 407–411, 407t, 792 (*see also* Syphilis)
Spitz tumor, 1255, *1256*
Spleen, *1118*, 1118–1120, 1119t
  congestion in, 285, *286*
  red pulp, 1118–1119
  white pulp, 1118, *1118*
Splenic disorders
  accessory spleens, 1119
  congenital absence (asplenia), 1119
  hypersplenism, 1047–1048, 1119
  rupture, 1120
  splenomegaly, 1119–1120, 1119t
    congestive, 1120
    cyst- and tumor-related, 1120
    infiltrative, 1120
    reactive, 1119
Splenomegaly, 1119–1120, 1119t
  in portal hypertension, 760–761
Spondylitis, tuberculous (Pott disease), *1330*, 1330–1331
Spondyloarthropathy, 1369–1371
  ankylosing spondylitis, 1370, *1370*
  enteropathic arthritis, 1371
  psoriatic arthritis, 1371
  Reiter syndrome, 1371
Spongiform encephalopathies, 10, 1194–1196
Spongiotic dermatitis, 1237
Spontaneous abortion, 990
Spontaneous bacterial peritonitis, 761
Spontaneous decay, 50–51
Sporadic Creutzfeld-Jakob disease, 1461
Sporotrichosis, 438, *438*
Sprue
  hypogammaglobinemic, 704
  nontropical (celiac disease), 672, 700–702
  tropical, folate deficiency and, 704
Squamous cell carcinoma, 900
  bladder, 900
  cervical, *1532*
    invasive, 949–951, *950*
    microinvasive, 949, *949*
  developmental biology, 182
  nasopharyngeal, 1294
  oral cavity, 1275, *1275*
  penile
    in situ, 905–906
    invasive, 906
    verrucous, 906, *906*
  skin, 1259–1260, *1260*
  vaginal, 940, 940t
  vulvar, *937*, 937–938, 938t
  verrucous, 937–938
Squamous cell neoplasia, cervical, cervical intraepithelial neoplasia (CIN), 945, 945–949, *946*, *947*
Squamous epithelial lesions, *1532*
Squamous metaplasia, 8–9, *9*
Stable cells, 108, *109*

Staghorn calculi, 876, *877*
Staphylococcus aureus, 377–378, 694
Starling principle, 45
Starvation, atrophy and, *5*
Stasis dermatitis, 514, *514*
Steatohepatitis, nonalcoholic, 346–347
Steatosis
    macrovesicular, 789
    microvesicular, 789, *790*
Stein-Leventhal (polycystic ovary) syndrome, 960, 967–969
Stem cells, 108–109, 120–121, *121*, 1022, *1022*
Stenosis
    anorectal, 711
    calcific aortic, *14*
    congenital esophageal, 664
    congenital pyloric, 673–674
    renal artery, 863
    small intestine, 691
Stercoral ulcers, 731
Steroid cell tumor, ovarian, 981
Steroid myopathy, 1411
Stevens-Johnson syndrome, 1229
Still disease (juvenile arthritis), 1371
Stomach, anatomy, *672*, 672–673
Stomach cancer, 677, 685–689
    carcinoid tumors, 689
    environmental factors, 685–686
    gastric lymphoma, 689
    malignant gastrointestinal stromal tumor, 689
    pathogenesis, 685–686
    pathology, 686–689
        advanced disease, *686*, 686–687, *687*
        early disease, *687*, 687–688, *688*
    peptic ulcer and, 684
Stomach disorders
    bezoars, 689, *690*
    congenital, 673–674
        diaphragmatic hernia, 674
        pyloric stenosis, 673–674
        rare, 674
    gastritis, 674–679
        acute hemorrhagic erosive, 674–675, *675*
        atrophic, *676*, 676
        chronic, 675–678
    mechanical, 689
        diverticula, 689
        rupture, 689
        volvulus, 689
    neoplasia
        benign, 684–685, *685*
        malignant, 685–689 (*see also* Stomach cancer)
    peptic ulcer disease, 679–684
Stomatitis, herpetic, 1273
Storage disorders, liver disease in, 787–788
Strawberry gallbladder, 807–808
Strength, wound, 107
Streptococcal cellulitis, 380, *380*
Streptococcal glomerulonephritis, 849–851, *850, 851*
Streptococcus pneumoniae, 381
Streptococcus pyogenes, 378–380, *379, 380*
Stress fracture, 1325
Stress proteins, 58
Stress (Curling, Cushing) ulcers, 674
Striatonigral degeneration, 1471
Stroke
    completed, 1441
    in evolution, 1441
    hemorrhagic, *1437*, 1437–1438, *1438*
    ischemic, 1438–1443, *1439, 1440, 1441*
    transient ischemic attacks (TIAs), 1441
Stromal hyperthecosis, 969, *969*
Stromal (connective tissue) matrix, 90–92
Stromal tumors, endometrial, 961–962, *962, 963*
Stroma ovarii, 977
Strongyloidiasis, *461*, 461–462
Sturge-Weber syndrome (encephalofacial angiomatosis), 1491
Subacute combined degeneration, of spinal cord, 1468
Subacute motor neuropathy, 208
Subacute sclerosing panencephalitis, 1457
Subacute thyroiditis, 1143, *1143*
Subarachnoid hemorrhage, 512, 1429–1430
Subcutaneous panniculitis-like T-cell lymphoma, 1109
Subdural hematoma, 1428–1429, *1429*
Subfalcine herniation, 1482
Sudden infant death syndrome (SIDS), 276–277
Sulfur dioxide pollution, 329–330
Superoxide
    bactericidal activity, 73
    as inflammatory mediator, 57–58
Superoxide dismutase (SOD), 20
Suppurative cystitis, 892
Suppurative inflammation, 48
Suppurative lymphadenitis, acute, 1086
Suppurative pyelophlebitis, 758
Surfactant, pulmonary, 270–273, *271, 272*
Sweat test, for cystic fibrosis, 250, *251*
Swiss-type hypogammaglobulinemia, 1169
Sympathetic ophthalmitis, 1508
Syndecans, 59
Syndrome of apparent mineralocorticoid excess (AME), 501
Synechiae, 1508
Synonymous mutations, 240
Synovial chondromatosis, 1376–1377
Synovial joints
    classification, 1361
    structures, 1361–1362, *1362*
Synovial sarcoma, 1382, *1382, 1383*
Synovitis
    nodular, 1377
    pigmented villonodular, 1377, *1378*
Synovium, 1361–1362
Syphilis, *408*, 408–411, *409*, 794, 929–931, 1288
    congenital, 225–226, 410–411
    meningovascular, 226, 410
    oral lesions, 1273
    primary, 408–409, *409*
    secondary, 409, *409*
    tertiary, 409–410, *410*
Syphilitic aneurysm, 513, *513*
Syphilitic aortitis, 409–410, *410*
Syphilitic (luetic) meningitis, 1440–1450, *1449, 1450*

Syringobulbia, 1422
Syringoma, 936, 1262, *1262*
Systemic inflammatory response (SIRS), 305–307, *306*
Systemic lupus erythematosus (SLE) (*see under* Lupus erythematosus)
Systemic mastocytosis, 1067

T

Tabes dorsalis, 1449
Tacrolimus (FK506), nephrotoxicity, 880
Takayasu arteritis, 508, 861, 861t
Talc embolism, 294, *295*
Talc granuloma, 324, *324*
Tangles, neurofibrillary, 11, 1475, *1477, 1478*, 1478–1479
Tapeworms, 469–471, 469t, 794 (*see also* Helminthic infections)
Tattoos, 12
Tay-Sachs disease (GM_2 gangliosidosis type 1), *254*, 254–255, 1465
TCDD, 329
T-cell lymphocytic leukemia, 1108
T cell–mediated cytotoxicity, 206, *206*
T-cell receptors, 124, *124*
Telangiectasia, 1435
    hereditary hemorrhagic (Rendu-Osler-Weber syndrome), 758, 1052
Telomerase, 195
Telomeres, 36, 195
Temporal (giant cell) arteritis, 506–507, *507*
Tenascins, 59
Tenosynovitis, nodular, 1377
Teratocarcinoma, 182
    testicular, 915, *916*
Teratogenesis, definition, 219
Teratogens, 218
Teratoma, 976–978, *977, 978*
    sacrococcygeal, 278
    testicular, 915, *916*
Tertiary granules, 70, *71*
Tertiary hyperparathyroidism, 1153
Testicular cancer, 911–918, 911t
    carcinoma in situ, 913
    epidemiology, 212
    histogenesis, 912, *912*
    Leydig cell tumors, 917, *917*
    metastases, 918
    nomenclature, 913
    nonseminatous germ cell tumors, 914–918.*909, 916*
    seminoma, 913–914, *914*
    Sertoli cell tumors, 917–918, *918*
    teratocarcinoma, 915, *916*
    teratoma, 915, *916*
    yolk sac carcinoma, 915, *916*, 917, *917*
Testicular dysgenesis (Klinefelter syndrome), 237–238, *238*
Testis, undescended (cryptorchidism), 906–907, *907*
Tetanus, 400, *400*
Tethering, *65, 66, 68, 69*
Thalassemia, 1037–1038
    alpha, 1037–1038
    beta, 1037–1038
Thalassemia trait, 1038
Theca lutein cysts, 967

Index

Thecoma, 979
Thermal disorders
  focal alterations, 334–335
  hyperthermia, 335–337
  hypothermia, 334
Thermal injury, neurokinins in, 58
Thermal regulation, 334
Thiamine deficiency (beri-beri), 349, *350*
Thin basement membrane nephropathy, 849
13q-syndrome, 236
Thoroughfare channels, of microciruclation, 282
Thrombasthenia, Glanzmann, 1056
Thromboangiitis obliterans (Buerger disease), 508–509, *510*
Thrombocythemia, essential, 1070t, 1071t, 1074–1075, *1075*
Thrombocytopenia, 286
  in alcoholism, 321
  drug-induced, 1054
  neonatal, 1054
  pregnancy-associated, 1054
Thrombocytosis, 1056
  in cancer, 209
  clonal, 1056
  primary, 1061
  reactive, 1056
  secondary, 1061
Thromboembolism, 292, *293*
Thrombolysis, plasminogen activation in, 1051
Thrombomodulin, 60
Thrombophlebitis, 515
  septic, 1288
Thrombosis, 479
  arterial and atherosclerosis, 287–288
  cardiac, 288–289, *289*
  cerebral venous, 1442–1443, *1443*
  coronary, 287–288, 542–543, *543*
  deep venous (DVT), 515
  hepatic vein, 759
  mesenteric vein, 696–697, *697*
  mural, 489–491
  sagittal sinus, *1443*
  venous, 209, *289*, 289–290
  versus coagulation, 479
  in wound healing, 100
Thrombospondins, 59
Thrombotic microangiopathy, 863–865, *864, 865*, 865t
Thrombotic thrombocytopenic purpura, 865, 1054–1055
Thrombus, 287
Thrush, 430
Thymic disorders, 1120–1122
  carcinoid tumor, 1122
  dysplasia, 1169
  germ cell tumors, 1122
  hyperplasia, 1120, *1120*
  hypoplasia, 1169
  small cell carcinoma, 1122
  thymoma, *1121*, 1121–1122
Thymic selection, 123
Thymoma, *1121*, 1121–1122
  malignant, 1121–1122
  in myasthenia gravis, 1121

Thymus
  agenesis and dysplasia, 1169
  anatomy and function, 1168–1169
  in myasthenia gravis, 1401
Thyroglossal duct cyst, 1135
Thyroid, fine-needle aspiration, *1536*
Thyroid cancer, 1144–1149
  anaplastic (undifferentiated) thyroid carcinoma, 1149, *1149*
  familial medullary carcinoma, *1165*, 1165–1167
  follicular thyroid carcinoma, 1147, *1147*
  lymphoma, 1149
  medullary thyroid carcinoma, 1147–1149, *1148*
  papillary thyroid carcinoma, 1145–1147, *1146*
Thyroid disorders, 1134–1149 (*see also* Hyperthyroidism; Hypothyroidism; Thyroid cancer)
  cancer, 1144–1149
  congenital anomalies, 1135
  familial medullary thyroid carcinoma, *1165*, 1165–1167
  follicular adenoma, 1144, *1145*
  hyperthyroidism, 1138–1141
  hypothyroidism, 1135–1138, *1136, 1137*
  nontoxic goiter, 1135, *1136*
  smoking and, 316
  thyroiditis, 1141–1144
Thyroid gland
  anatomy and function, 1134
  lingual, 1134
Thyroid hormone, in obesity, 345
Thyroiditis
  chronic autoimmune (Hashimoto), 1093, *1139, 1142*, 1142–1143
  Riedel, 1144, *1144*
  silent, 1143
  subacute, 1143, *1143*
Thyroid nodule, lingual, 1271
Thyroid-stimulating hormone (TSH), 1132
Thyrotrope adenoma, 1132
Tinea (ringworm), 1241
Tissue, granulation, 102, *102*, 103
Tissue factor, 480
Tissue inhibitors of metalloproteinases (TMPs), 73
Tissue plasminogen activator (tPA), 1051
Tissue typing, 127–128
T-lymphoblastic lymphoma, 1093, *1093*
T lymphocytes, *123*, 124 (*see also* T-cell entries)
  immune-response interactions, 128–129
TNF-α
  in apoptosis, 30–31, *31*
  in ischemia/reperfusion injury, 21
TNFR pathway, 64–65, *65*
TNM staging, prostate cancer, *924*, 924–925, 925t
Tongue disorders, 1275–1276
  glossitis, 1276
  macroglossia, 1275–1276
Tonsillitis, 1293
Tooth disorders
  dental caries, 1276–1277, *1277*
  periodontal disease, 1278, *1278*

  pulp and periapical tissues, 1277–1278, *1278*
Tophaceous gout, 1373, *1374*
TORCH complex, *224*, 224–225, 225t
Toxic acute tubular necrosis, 867–868
Toxic adenoma, 1141
Toxic granulation, 1063
Toxicity-related fatty liver, 789–790
Toxic liver injury, 788–790
Toxic multinodular goiter, 1141
Toxic neuropathy, 1496
Toxic shock syndrome, 378, 934
Toxocariasis, 464
Toxoplasma lymphadenopathy syndrome, *445*, 445–446
Toxoplasmosis, *445*, 445–446, 1089, *1089*
  congenital, 446, *446*
  in TORCH complex, 224
Tracheoesophageal fistula, 663–664, *664*
Trachoma, 416, 1505, *1505*
Transcellular diapedesis, 69
Transformation zone, cervical, 941–942, *942, 943, 944*
Transient acantholytic dermatosis (Grover disease), 1220
Transient hypogammaglobulinemia of infancy, 145, 145t
Transient ischemic attacks (TIAs), 1441
Transitional cell carcinoma, 168–169, *169*, 898–900
  grades 1 through 3, 898–900, *899*
  in situ, *897*, 897–898
  papilloma, 899
  renal, 884, *1535*
  staging, 898–899, 898t
Transitional cell papilloma, bladder, 897, *899*
Transitional cell tumor, ovarian (Brenner tumor), 971, *973*
Translocation syndromes, 235–236
Transplant rejection, 140–141, *141*
  graft-versus-host disease, 141
  of implanted tumors, 204, *205*
  liver, 801, *802*
  renal, 877–880, *878*, 878t, *879*
Transtentorial herniation, 1427, *1427*, 1428, 1482
Transthyretin amyloidosis, 1196
Transudate, 46
Trauma
  acoustic, 1301
  central nervous system, 1426–1435
  uterine, 954
Traumatic neuroma, *114*, 1498
Trematodes (flukes), 464–469 (*see also under* Helminthic infections)
Treponema pallidum, 408, *409*, 929 (*see also* Syphilis)
Treponematoses, nonvenereal, 411
Triad, Hutchinson, 226
Trichinosis, 462–463, *463*
Trichloroethylene, 328
Trichobezoar, 689, *690*
Trichoepithelioma, 1262
Trichomoniasis, 933
Trichuiasis, 459t, 460, *460*
Trigone, 888

Trinucleotide repeat expansion syndromes, 1472–1475, *1474*
Triorthocresyl phosphate (TOCP), 329
Trisomy, 230
Trisomy 13, 235
Trisomy 13–15, 1425
Trisomy 18, 235
Trisomy 21 (Down syndrome), 231–235, 232t, *233, 234, 1424,* 1424–1425, 1475
Trisomy 22, 235
Trophic ulcers, 115
Tropical phagedenic ulcers, 413–414, *414*
Trousseau syndrome, 820
Trypanosoma brucei, 454–456, *455*
Trypanosoma cruzi, 454
Trypanosomiasis (sleeping sickness), 454–456, *455*
TSH
  deficiency, 5
  in hypertrophy, 6
Tsutsugamushi fever (scrub typhus), 419–420
Tubercular skin disorder, erythema induratum, 1240
Tuberculoid leprosy, 425, *426*
Tuberculoma, *1447,* 1447–1448
Tuberculosis, 26, 27, *421,* 421–425
  genital tract, 933–934
  intestinal, 694–695
  miliary, 423–424, *424*
  oral, 1273
  primary, *422, 423,* 423–424
  secondary (cavitary), *424,* 424–425
Tuberculous appendicitis, 733
Tuberculous arthritis, 1331
Tuberculous endometritis, 933–934
Tuberculous meningitis, *1447,* 1447–1448
Tuberculous peritonitis, 736
Tuberculous salpingitis, 933
Tuberculous spondylitis (Pott disease), *1330,* 1330–1331
Tuberous sclerosis (Bourneville disease), 1491, *1491*
Tubular adenoma, 684
  colorectal, 722, *722*
Tubular carcinoma, breast, 1010
Tubules
  renal, 830
  renal cortical, 111
  renal medullary, 111
Tubulorrhexis, 111
Tubulovillous adenomas, 723–724
Tularemia, *402,* 402–403, 1089
  oculoglandular, 403
  pneumonic, 403
  typhoidal, 403
  ulceroglandular, 403
Tumor(s) *(see also* Neoplasia *and specific lesions)*
  blood vessels
    benign, 515–517, *516*
    malignant, 517–518
  bone
    benign, 1350–1354, *1351*
    malignant, 1351–1361
  breast *(see also under* Breast)
    benign, 1004–1006
    phyllodes tumor, 1014–1015, *1015*
    brown, 1342, *1342*
    Buscke and Lowenstein, 906, *906*
    central nervous system (CNS), 1479–1491, *1481*
    fallopian tube, 966
    giant cell of bone, 1357–1358, *1358*
    giant cell vs. Paget disease of bone, 1348
    of infancy and childhood, 278
    Krukenburg, 688, *688*
    ovarian, 969–981, 970t
    renal pelvis and ureters, 891
    smooth muscle, 1381–1382
    soft tissue, 1377–1381
    uterine, 956–965, 962t
    vascular, 1382
Tumor antigens, 204–206, *205*
Tumor embolism, 294
Tumor markers, 171–172, *173,* 174–175t
Tumor suppressor genes, 184, 191–194
TUNEL assay, 34
Tunica adventitia, 477
Tunica albuginea, 889
Tunica intima, 476
Tunica media, 476–477
Turcot syndrome, 725
Turner syndrome (45X), 230, 238–239, *239*
Twinning, 989, *989*
Two-hit hypothesis, of retinoblastoma, 191, *192*
Type grouping, 1409, *1409*
Type predominance, 1409
Typhoidal tularemia, 403
Typhoid fever, *390,* 390–391, *392–393,* 693
Typhoid nodules, 390
Typhus
  louse-borne (epidemic), 418–419, *419*
  murine (endemic), 419
  scrub (Tsutsugamushi fever), 419–420
Tyrosinase-positive/negative oculocutaneous albinism, 261
Tyrosine kinases, 64
Tyrosinemia, 260, 788

U
Ulcer(s)
  genital, 386
  Hunner, *893,* 893–894
  neuropathic, 115
  peptic, 679–684
  rodent, 1260
  solitary rectal ulcer syndrome, 721
  stercoral, 731
  stress (Curling, Cushing), 674
  trophic, 115
  tropical phagedenic, 413–414, *414*
Ulcerating gastric adenocarcinoma, 686, *686, 688*
Ulceration, 115
Ulcerations, corneal, 1506–1507
Ulcerative colitis, *716,* 716–719, *717, 718,* 719t
  colorectal cancer and, 719
  differential diagnosis, 718–719, 719t
  extraintestinal manifestations, 718, *718*
Ulcerative cystitis, 892
Ulcerative intestinal tuberculosis, 694

Ulceroglandular tularemia, 403
Ulcerohypertrophic intestinal tuberculosis, 695
Undescended testes (cryptorchidism), 906–907, *907*
Unilateral multicystic renal dysplasia, 832, *832*
Uniparental disomy, 266
Urachal remnants, 892
Urate nephropathy, *875,* 875–876
Uremic neuropathy, 1495
Ureteral obstruction, 890, *891*
Ureteritis, 890, *891*
Ureteritis cystica, 895, *895*
Ureteropelvic junction obstruction, 890
Ureters
  anatomy, 888
  congenital disorders, 889–890, *890*
  dilation, 890
  ectopic, 890
Urethra
  female, 888
  male, 888
Urethral cancer, 905
Urethral caruncles, 905
Urethritis, 904–905
  nonspecific infectious, 904
  in Reiter syndrome, 905
  sexually transmitted, 904
  urethral caruncles, 905
Urethritis cystica, 894, *895*
Uric acid alculi, 876
Urinalysis, in acute renal failure, 869t
Urinary tract *(see also* Urinary tract infections *and individual organs)*
  anatomy, 888–889
  embryology, 889
  inflammatory disorders, 902–904, 902t
  penis, urethra, and scrotum, 900–902, *901*
  renal pelvis and ureter, 889–890, *890*
Urinary tract cytology, 1535
Urinary tract infections, *Escherichia coli,* 388–389
Urogenital schistosomiasis, 467
Urolithiasis, 876–877, *877*
Urothelium, 888–889, *999*
Urticaria, 1234–1235
Urticaria pigmentosa, 1067
Uterine adenosarcoma, 962
Uterine agenesis, 953
Uterus, 952–965
  adenomyosis, 954, *955*
  anatomy, 952
  bicornuate, 953
  congenital anomalies, 953
  endometritis, 954, *954*
  endometrium of pregnancy (Arias-Stella reaction), 953, *953*
  hormonal effects, 955–956, 956t
  traumatic lesions, 954
    adhesions (Asherman syndrome), 954
    from IUDs, 954
  tumors, 956–965, 962t
    endometrial adenocarcinoma, 958–961, 959t, *960, 961,* 961t
    endometrial hyperplasia and, *957,* 957–958, *958*

endometrial polyp, *956*, 956–957
endometrial stromal, 961–962, *962*, *963*
intravenous leiomyomatosis, 964
leiomyoma, *963*, 963–964
leiomyosarcoma, *964*, 964–965, *965*
Uterus didelphys, 953
Uterus duplex bicornis, 953
Uterus septus, 953
Uveal disorders, 1508
Uveal melanoma, 1525, *1525*

V

Vagina, 939–941
  anatomy, 939
  malignant tumors, 940–941
    clear cell adenocarcinoma, 940, *940*
    embryonal rhabdomyosarcoma (sarcoma botryoides), 940–941, *941*
    squamous cell carcinoma, 940, 940t
  nonneoplastic conditions, 939–940
    atrophic vaginitis, 939
    benign tumors, 940
    congenital anomalies, 939
    fibroepithelial polyp, 939
    vaginal adenosis, 939, *939*
    septate, 939
Vaginal adenosis, 939, *939*
Vaginal atresia, 939
Vaginitis, atrophic, 939
Vanishing bile duct syndrome, 801, *802*
Varicella zoster, 369–371, *370*, *371*, 1455–1456
Varices, esophageal, 515, 669, *669*, 759–760
Varicocele, *901*, 902
Varicose veins
  esophageal varices, 515, 669, *669*
  hemorrhoids, 515
  of legs, 514, *514*
  varicocele, 515
Variola (smallpox), 366, *367*
Vascular cell adhesion molecules (VCAMs), 474
Vascular disease
  in diabetes mellitus, *1170*, 1181, *1182*
  in drug-related hepatotoxicity, 790, *791*
  of large bowel, 720–721
  of liver, 791–792, *792*
  renal, 859–867
  vasculitis (*see* Vasculitis)
Vascular occlusion, retinal, 1509, *1510*, *1511*, *1512*, *1513*
Vascular tumors, 1382
Vasculature, cutaneous, *1202*, 1208–1210, *1209*
Vasculitic neuropathy, 1496, *1496*
Vasculitis, 134–136, *136*, *137*, 504–510, 504t
  allergic granulomatosis and angiitis (Churg-Strauss syndrome), 506, *506*
  Behçet disease, 509–510
  cryoglobulinemic, 860, *860*
  cutaneous necrotizing, *1234*, *1235*, 1235–1236
  giant cell arteritis (temporal arteritis, granulomatous arteritis), 506–507, *507*
  hypersensitivity angiitis, 505–506
  Kawasaki disease (mucocutaneous lymph node syndrome), 508, *509*
  pathogenesis, 504
  polyarteritis nodosa, 505, *505*
  radiation, 510
  renal, 859–861, 860t
    large-vessel, 861
    medium-sized vessel, 860
    small vessel, 859–860
  rickettsial, 510
  skeletal muscle in periarteritis nodosa, 1400, *1400*
  Takayasu arteritis, 508
  thromboangiitis obliterans (Buerger disease), 508–509, *510*
  Wegener granulomatosis, *507*, 507–508
Vasculogenesis, 104
Vasoactive inflammatory mediators, 45
Vasoactive intestinal peptide (VIP), 823
Vasoconstriction, in shock, 308
Vasodilation, in portal hypertension, 761, *761*
Vasogenic edema, 303
Vector-borne diseases
  anthrax, 403–404
  bacterial, 400–405
  bartonellosis, 405–406
  brucellosis, 401–402
  cat-scratch disease, 405, *405*, 1089
  fascioliasis, 468
  glanders, 405
  larva migrans, 464, *464*
  leptosporosis, 412–413, *413*
  listeriosis, 404
  of liver, 793–794
  Lyme disease, 411–412
  malaria, 441, 441–444, *442–443*, *444*
  plague, 402
  psittacosis (ornithosis), 416–417
  rabies, 1453–1454
  rickettsial, 417, 417–420, 417t
  tularemia, *402*, 402–403, 1089
  typhus
    louse-borne (epidemic), 418–419, *419*
    murine (endemic), 419
    scrub, 419–420
Vegetations, endocardial, 288
Veins, 283, 478
Vellus hairs, 1211
Velocity, of blood flow, *478*
Venocclusive disease, hepatic, 758–759
Venous angioma, 1435
Venous diseases
  deep venous thrombosis (DVT), 515
  varicosities, *514*, 514–515
Venous thrombosis, *289*, 289–290
  in cancer, 209
  cerebral, 1442–1443, *1443*
  hepatic vein, 759
Venules, 283
  high endothelial (HEVs), *126*, 127
Verner-Morrison syndrome (VIPoma), 823
Verrucae (warts), 370, *1256*, 1256–1258, *1257*
  syphilitic, 931
Verruca plana, 1256
Verruca vulgaris (common wart), 370, 1256, *1257*
Verrucous penile squamous cell carcinoma, 906, *906*

Versican, 94t
Vertebral osteomyelitis, 1329, *1330*
Vertical growth phase melanoma, 1248–1249, *1249*, *1250*, *1251*
Vesicoureteral reflux, 892
Vesicoureteral valve, congenital incompetence, 892
Vessel wall, 474, *475*, *476*, *477*, 477t
  endothelial cells, 474–475
  smooth muscle cells, 475
VHL gene, 193
Vibrio cholerae, 391–393, *394*
Vibrio parahaemolyticus, 393
Villitis, 986
Villous adenomas, 722–723, *723*
Vincent angina (acute necrotizing ulcerative gingivitis), *1272*, 1272, 1293
VIPoma (Verner-Morrison syndrome), 823
Viral cytotoxicity, 21–22, *22*, *23*
  apoptosis and, 22
  direct, 21–22
  immunologically mediated, 22
Viral encephalomyelitis, 1450–1458, *1452*
  AIDS encephalopathy, 1458, *1458*
  arthropod-borne, 1456–1457, 1456t
  cytomegalovirus, 1456, *1456*
  demyelination in, 1465
  encephalitis lethargica (von Economo encephalitis), 1457
  herpesvirus, 1454–1456, *1455*
  inclusion bodies in, *1454*
  poliomyelitis, 1452–1453, *1454*
  postinfectious/postvaccinal, 1464–1465
  progressive multifocal leukoencephalopathy, *1457*, 1457–1458
  rabies, 1453–1454
  subacute sclerosing panencephalitis, 1457
Viral gastroenteritis, 694
Viral hepatitis, 761–773, 761t
Viral infections (*see also* specific organisms and diseases)
  female reproductive tract, 932, *933*
  hemorrhagic fevers, 368–369, 368t
    ebola, 368–369
    West Nile virus, 369
    yellow fever, 368
  herpesvirus, 369–375
    cytomegalovirus, 373–375, *375*
    Epstein-Barr virus, 197–198, 372–373, *374*, *375*, 1116–1117, 1294–1295
    herpes simplex, *371*, 371–372, 371t
    varicella-zoster, 369–371, *370*, *371*
  human papillomavirus (HPV), 375–376
  intestinal, 367–368 (*see also* Diarrhea)
    Norwalk virus, 367–368
    rotavirus, 367
  oral cavity, 1273
  respiratory, 363–364
  viral exanthems, 364–365, *365*
    human parvovirus B19, 366
    measles (rubeola), 364–365, *365*
    mumps, 366–367, *367*
    rubella, 365–366
    smallpox (variola), 366, *367*
Viral labyrinthitis, 1301, *1302*
Viral meningitis, 1448

Viral pancreatitis, 813
Viral rhinitis, 1286
Virulence, 361
Viruses
 DNA, 193, 197–198
  Epstein-Barr virus (EBV), 197–198, 372–373, *374*, *375*, 1116–1117, 1294–1295
  hepatitis B (HBV), 198
  herpesviruses, 198, 369–375
  human herpesvirus 8 (HHV8), 198
  human papillomavirus (HPV), 197
  human T-cell leukemia virus (HTLV-1), 195
 Norwalk, 694
 rotavirus, 694
 simian B, 1456
Visceral larva migrans (toxocariasis), 464
Visceral leishmaniasis (kala azar), 452, *453*, 793
Vitamin A, 20
 deficiency, 322, *348*, 348–349
 toxicity, 349
Vitamin B$_6$ (pyridoxine), 351–352
Vitamin B$_{12}$ (cyanocobalamin), 352
Vitamin B complex, 349–352
Vitamin B$_{12}$ deficiency, *1034*, 1034–1037, *1035*, *1037*, 1478
Vitamin C (ascorbate), 20
 deficiency (scurvy), 352, *353*, 1052, 1317–1318, *1318*
  hemorrhage in, 286
Vitamin D, 353–354
 bone disorders and, 1338–1339, *1339*
 deficiency, 353–354
 toxicity, 354
Vitamin deficiencies, in alcoholism, 322
Vitamin E (α-tocopherol), 20, 354
Vitamin K, 354
Vitamin K deficiency, 1058
Volvulus, 704–705
 gastric, 689
 midgut, 704
 sigmoid, 704
von Economo encephalitis, 1457
von Gierke disease, 257–258
von Hippel-Lindau disease, 882
von Hippel-Lindau syndrome, 193, 886, 1489
von Meyenburg complexes (bile duct microhamartomas), 797
von Recklinghausen disease (neurofibromatosis type I), 245, *245*, 1491
von Willebrand disease, 1057
Vulva, 934–939
 anatomy, 934–939
 benign tumors, 936
 dermatoses, 934–936
  acute dermatitis, 934–935, *935*
  chronic dermatitis, 935–936, *936*
 developmental anomalies and cysts, 934–939
 malignancy/premalignancy, 936–939
  malignant melanoma, 938
  Paget disease, *938*, 938–939
  squamous cell carcinoma, *937*, 937–938, 938t
  verrucous carcinoma, 937–938
  vulvar intraepithelial neoplasia (VIN), 936–937
Vulvovaginitis, candidal, 430

W

WAGR complex, 277, 881
Waldenström microglobulinemia, 1098
Waldeyer's ring, 1293
 lymphoma of, 1295–1296
Warthin-Finkeldey cells, 1089
Warthin tumor, 1283, *1283*
Warts, *1256*, 1256–1257, *1257*
 anogenital, 370
 bowenoid papulosis, 1258
 common (verruca vulgaris), 370, 1256, *1257*
 epidermodysplasia verruciformis, 1258
 genital (condyloma acuminatum), 370, 903, 932, *933*, 1258
 plantar, 370, 1257
 syphilitic, 931
 verruca plana, 1257
Warty (basaloid) vulvar dysplasia, 936–937
Waterhouse-Friderichsen syndrome, 309, *310*, 384, 1158
Watershed infarct, 297
 cerebral, 1438, *1439*
Webs, esophageal, 664, *664*
Wegener granulomatosis, *507*, 507–508, 860, 1290, *1290*
Weil syndrome (leptospirosis), 794
Werdig-Hoffman disease, 1409, *1410*
Werner syndrome (MEN type 1), 37, 1164
Wernicke encephalopathy, 320, 321, *321*
Wernicke-Korsakoff syndrome, 1468
Wernicke syndrome, 1466–1468, *1467*
West Nile virus, 369
Whipple disease, 702, *703*
White cell disorders
 diagnostic techniques, 1067–1070, *1068*, *1069*, *1070*
 myeloproliferative diseases, 1070, 1070t, 1071t (*see also* Leukemia; Lymphoma)
 nonmalignant, 1062–1070
  mast cell proliferation, 1066–1067, *1067*
  neutropenia, 1062, 1062t
  neutrophilia, 1062–1063, *1063*, 1063t
  qualitative, 1063–1066
WHO classification
 acute myeloid leukemia, 1081t
 mature B-cell neoplasms, 1190t
 mature T-cell and NK-cell neoplasms, 1092t
 myelodysplastic diseases, 1070t, 1071t, 1076t
 plasma cell myeloma, 1099t
Whooping cough (pertussis), 382
Wilms tumor (nephroblastoma), 193, 277, 881–884, *882*
Wilms tumor aniridia syndrome, 228
Wilson disease (hepatolenticular degeneration), 785–787, *786*, 1466
Wiskott-Aldrich syndrome, 147, 1054, 1169
Wound contracture, *105*, 107, 115–116

Wound healing, 84–116
 basic processes, 86–99
  cell migration, 86–88, *87*
  cell proliferation, 97
  extracellular matrix, 88–90, 89t, 90, 91t
  mediation pathways, 97–99, *98*
  remodeling, 95–97, 96t, 97t
 conditions modifying, 109–116
  local factors, 109
  site-specific factors, 109–114
 excessive, 116
 fetal, 114
 heart, 112, *114*, 115
 kidney, 111–112, *112*
 liver, 111, *111*
 lung, 111
 nervous system, 111–114, *114*
 regeneration, 107–109
  cellular proliferation, 108–109
  mitosis, 107–108, *109*
  stem vs. stable cells in, 109
 repair, 99–107
  organization, 99
  sequence of, 100–107, 100t, *101–102*, *103*, 103t, *104*, *105*, 106t
 skin, 109–111, *110*
 suboptimal, 114–116, *115*
Wounds
 deep penetrating, 338, *339*
 gunshot, 338, *339*
Wound strength, 107
Woven bone, *1311*, 1312
WT-1 gene, 193

X

Xanthelasma, 1504
Xanthine oxidase, 20–21
Xanthogranulomatous pyelonephritis, 872–873
Xanthoma, 10, 499, 873
X chromosome abnormalities, 236–237
Xeroderma pigmentosum, 194, 203
Xerophthalmia, in vitamin A deficiency, 348–349
Xerostomia, 1280, *1280*
X-linked agammaglobulinemia, Bruton, 143–145, 145t, 1293
X-linked dominance, 261–262, *262*
X-linked genetic diseases, 261–266, 261t
X-linked hypophosphatemia, 1339
X-linked ichthyosis, 1212, 1214t
X-linked lymphoproliferative syndrome, 198, 206–207
Xylose absorption, 700

Y

Yaws, 411
Y chromosome abnormalities, 236
Yeasts, 429 (*see also* Fungal infections)
Yellow atrophy, hepatic acute, 770, *770*
Yellow fever, 368
Yersinia enterocolitica, 395, 694
Yersinia pseudotuberculosis, 395, 694
Yolk sac carcinoma
 ovarian, 978, *979*
 testicular, 915, *916*, *917*, 917
YYY male syndrome, 238

Z

Zahn, lines of, 287, *288*
Z bands, 1388, 1396, *1397*
Zelballen, *1166*, 1166–1167
Zenker diverticulum, 665
Zinc deficiency, 354–355
Zollinger-Ellison syndrome (gastrinoma), 822–823
Zonal hepatocellular necrosis, 789, *789*
Zones
   of articular cartilage, 1362, *1362*
   basement membrane, 1207–1208, *1209*
   of calcification, 1315
   myofiber H, 1388
   of ossification, 1315
   transformation (*see* Transformation zone)
Zoon balanitis, 903–904
Zoonotic infections (*see* Vector-borne infections *and specific diseases*)
Zymogen (chief) cells, 673